CRITICAL CARE MEDICINE

PRINCIPLES OF DIAGNOSIS
AND MANAGEMENT
IN THE ADULT

Fourth Edition

CRITICAL CARE MEDICINE

PRINCIPLES OF DIAGNOSIS AND MANAGEMENT IN THE ADULT

Joseph E. Parrillo, MD
Chairman, Heart and Vascular Hospital
Hackensack University Medical Center
Professor of Medicine
Rutgers New Jersey Medical School
Hackensack, New Jersey

R. Phillip Dellinger, MD, MS
Professor of Medicine
Cooper Medical School of Rowan University
Director, Critical Care
Cooper University Hospital
Camden, New Jersey

ELSEVIER
SAUNDERS

ELSEVIER
SAUNDERS

1600 John F. Kennedy Blvd.
Ste 1800
Philadelphia, PA 19103-2899

CRITICAL CARE MEDICINE: PRINCIPLES OF DIAGNOSIS AND MANAGEMENT IN THE ADULT
ISBN: 978-0-323-08929-6

Library of Congress Cataloging-in-Publication Data

Critical care medicine : principles of diagnosis and management in the adult / [edited by] Joseph E. Parrillo, R. Phillip Dellinger.—4th ed.
p. ; cm.
Includes bibliographical references and index.
ISBN 978-0-323-08929-6 (hardcover : alk. paper) I. Parrillo, Joseph E. II. Dellinger, R. Phillip.
[DNLM: 1. Critical Care. 2. Intensive Care Units. WX 218]
RC86.7
616'.028—dc23

2013014389

Executive Content Strategist: William R. Schmitt
Senior Content Development Specialist: Janice M. Gaillard
Publishing Services Manager: Patricia Tannian
Senior Project Manager: Sharon Corell
Senior Book Designer: Louis Forgione

Printed in China.

Last digit is the print number: 9 8 7 6 5 4 3 2

To our families
Gale, Nicholas, and Jenny Parrillo
and
Kate, Walker, Lauren, Reid, and Meg Dellinger

To our families

Cody, Nicholas, and Jenny Peterson

and

Kate, Walter, Thomas, Sara, and Abby Mellinger

Contributors

Wissam Abouzgheib, MD, FCPP
Section Head, Interventional Pulmonary and Assistant Professor of Medicine, Pulmonary and Critical Care, Cooper University Hospital, Camden, New Jersey

David Anthony, MD
Staff Anesthesiologist and Intensivist, Cardiothoracic Anesthesiology, Anesthesiology Institute, Cleveland, Ohio

Shariff Attaya, MD
Fellow, Cardiovascular Disease, Rush University Medical Center, Chicago, Illinois

Robert A. Balk, MD
Director of Pulmonary and Critical Care Medicine, Internal Medicine, Rush University Medical Center, Professor of Medicine, Rush Medical College, Chicago, Illinois

Richard G. Barton, MD
University of Utah Medical Center, Department of Surgery, Salt Lake City, Utah

Thaddeus Bartter, MD
Interventional Pulmonologist, University of Arkansas for Medical Sciences, Little Rock, Arkansas

C. Allen Bashour, MD
Associate Professor of Anesthesiology, Staff, Department of Cardiothoracic Anesthesia, Anesthesia Institute, Cleveland Clinic, Lerner College of Medicine of Case Western Reserve University, Cleveland, Ohio

Carolyn Bekes, MD
Professor of Medicine, Cooper Medical School of Rowan University, Chief Medical Officer, Cooper University Hospital, Camden, New Jersey

Emily Bellavance, MD
Assistant Professor of Surgery, Division of Surgical Oncology, Department of Surgery, University of Maryland School of Medicine, Baltimore, Maryland

Karen Berger, PharmD
Neurocritical Care Clinical Pharmacist, New York Presbyterian/Weill Cornell Medical Center, New York, New York

Julian Bion
Professor of Intensive Care Medicine, University of Birmingham, Birmingham, United Kingdom

Thomas P. Bleck, MD, FCCM
Professor, Neurological Sciences, Neurosurgery, Internal Medicine, and Anesthesiology, Rush Medical College, Associate Chief Medical Officer, Critical Care, Rush University Medical Center, Chicago, Illinois

Frank Bowen, MD
Department of Cardiothoracic Surgery, Cooper University Hospital, Camden, New Jersey

Susan S. Braithwaite, MD
Visiting Clinical Professor, Medicine, University of Illinois-Chicago, Chicago, Illinois, Staff Physician, Saint Francis Hospital, Evanston, Illinois

Pietro Carioni, MD
Dipartimento di Fisiopatologia Medico-Chirurgica e dei Trapianti, Università degli Studi di Milano, Dipartimento di Anestesia, Rianimazione ed Emergenza Urgenza, Fondazione IRCCS Ca' Granda–Ospedale Maggiore Policlinico, Milan, Italy

Eleonora Carlesso, MD
Dipartimento di Fisiopatologia Medico-Chirurgica e dei Trapianti, Università degli Studi di Milano, Milan, Italy

Rodrigo Cartin-Ceba, MD
Consultant, Pulmonary and Critical Care Medicine, Mayo Clinic, Rochester, Minnesota

Maurizio Cecconi, MD, MD (UK), FRCA
Consultant in Anaesthesia and Intensive Care Medicine, St. George's Healthcare NHS Trust, Honorary Senior Lecturer, St. George's University of London, London, United Kingdom

Louis Chaptini, MD
Assistant Professor of Medicine, Section of Digestive Diseases, Yale University School of Medicine, New Haven, Connecticut

Lakhmir S. Chawla, MD
Associate Professor, Department of Medicine, George Washington University Medical Center, Washington, District of Columbia

Ismail Cinel, MD, PhD
Professor of Anesthesiology, Marmara University School of Medicine, Director, Intensive Care Unit, Chief Medical Officer, Marmara University Education and Research Hospital, Istanbul, Turkey

T. R. Craig, PhD, MRCP, MB, BCh, BAO
Specialist Registrar, Critical Care Medicine, Regional Intensive Care Unit, Royal Hospitals, Belfast HSC Trust, Belfast, Northern Ireland, United Kingdom

Brendan D. Curti, MD
Director, Biotherapy and Genitourinary Oncology Research, Earle A. Chiles Research Institute, Portland, Oregon

Quinn A. Czosnowski, PharmD
Assistant Professor of Clinical Pharmacy, Department of Pharmacy Practice and Pharmacy Administration, University of the Sciences, Philadelphia, Pennsylvania

Marion Danis, MD
Chief, Bioethics Consultation Service, Department of Bioethics, National Institutes of Health, Bethesda, Maryland

R. Phillip Dellinger, MD, MS
Professor of Medicine, Cooper Medical School of Rowan University, Director, Critical Care, Cooper University Hospital, Camden, New Jersey

Fedele J. DePalma, MD
Gastroenterology Associates, Newark, Delaware

Jose Diaz-Gomez, MD
Staff Anesthesiologist/Intensivist, Cardiothoracic Anesthesiology, Cleveland Clinic, Assistant Professor of Anesthesiology, Cleveland Clinic Lerner College of Medicine at Case Western Reserve University, Cleveland, Ohio

Hisham Dokainish, MD, FRCPC, FASE, FACC
Associate Professor of Medicine, McMaster University, Director of Echocardiography, Hamilton Health Sciences, Hamilton, Ontario, Canada

Guillermo Domínguez-Cherit, MD, FCCM
Director, División of Pulmonary, Anesthesia, and Critical Care, Instituto Nacional de Ciencias Medicas y Nutrición "Salvador Zubiran," Mexico City, Distrito Federal, Mexico

David J. Dries, MSE, MD
Assistant Medical Director, Department of Surgery, HealthPartners Medical Group/Regions Hospital, St. Paul, Minnesota, Professor of Surgery and Anesthesiology, Department of Surgery, University of Minnesota, Minneapolis, Minnesota

Lakshmi Durairaj, MD
Associate Professor, Division of Pulmonary Critical Care and Occupational Medicine, University of Iowa Hospitals and Clinics, Iowa City, Iowa

Adam B. Elfant, MD
Associate Professor of Medicine, Associate Head Division of Gastroenterology, Cooper University Hospital, Camden, New Jersey

E. Wesley Ely, MD, MPH
Professor of Medicine, Department of Allergy, Pulmonary and Critical Care Medicine, Vanderbilt University Medical Center, Nashville, Tennessee

Henry S. Fraimow, MD
Associate Professor of Medicine, Division of Infectious Diseases, Cooper Medical School of Rowan University, Camden, New Jersey

John F. Fraser, MB ChB, PhD, MRCP, FFARCSI, FRCA, FCICM
Professor in Intensive Care Medicine, Director of Critical Care Research Group, University of Queensland School of Medicine, The Prince Charles Hospital, Brisbane, Australia

Yaakov Friedman, BA, MD
Associate Professor of Medicine, Rosalind Franklin University of Medicine, Chicago, Illinois

Brian M. Fuller, MD
Assistant Professor, Anesthesiology and Emergency Medicine, Division of Critical Care, Washington University School of Medicine, St. Louis, Missouri

Ognjen Gajic, MD, MSc
Professor of Medicine, Pulmonary and Critical Care Medicine, Mayo Clinic, Rochester, Minnesota

Luciano Gattinoni, MD, FRCP
Dipartimento di Fisiopatologia Medico-Chirurgica e dei Trapianti, Università degli Studi di Milano, Dipartimento di Anestesia, Rianimazione ed Emergenza Urgenza, Fondazione IRCCS Ca' Granda–Ospedale Maggiore Policlinico, Milan, Italy

Nandan Gautam, MRCP, DICM, FRCP, FFICM
Consultant, Medicine and Critical Care, University Hospital, Birmingham, United Kingdom

Martin Geisen, MD
Clinical and Research Fellow, Department of Intensive Care Medicine, St. George's Healthcare NHS Trust, London, United Kingdom

Fredric Ginsberg, MD
Associate Professor of Medicine, Division of Cardiovascular Disease, Cooper Medical School of Rowan University, Camden, New Jersey

H. Warren Goldman, MD, PhD
Professor and Chairman of Neurosurgery, Cooper Medical School of Rowan University, Chief of Neurosurgery, Cooper University Hospital, Medical Director, Cooper Neurological Institute, Cooper University Hospital, Camden, New Jersey, Professor of Surgery, Rutgers Robert Wood Johnson Medical School, New Brunswick, New Jersey

Bala K. Grandhi, MD, MPH
Assistant Director, Internal Medicine Residency Program, Central Michigan University, Saginaw, Michigan

A. B. J. Groeneveld, Prof. Dr., FCCP, FCCM
Professor Doctor, Intensive Care, Erasmus MC, Rotterdam, Netherlands

David P. Gurka, PhD, MD, FACP, FCCP
Associate Professor of Medicine, Department of Medicine, Rush Medical College, Director, Section of Critical Care Medicine, Division of Pulmonary and Critical Care Medicine, Department of Medicine, Director, Surgical Intensive Care Unit, Assistant Chief Medical Officer for Critical Care and Safety Quality, Rush University Medical Center, Chicago, Illinois

Marilyn T. Haupt, MD
Chair and Interim Program Director, Internal Medicine, Central Michigan University College of Medicine, Saginaw, Michigan

Dustin M. Hipp, MD, MBA
Resident Physician, Department of Pediatrics, Baylor College of Medicine, Texas Children's Hospital, Houston, Texas

Michael J. Hockstein, MD
Medical Director, 4G SICU, Department of Surgery, Medstar Washington Hospital Center, Washington, District of Columbia

Steven M. Hollenberg, MD
Professor of Medicine, Cooper Medical School of Rowan University, Director, Coronary Care Unit, Cooper University Hospital, Camden, New Jersey

Robert C. Hyzy, MD
Associate Professor, Division of Pulmonary and Critical Care Medicine, Department of Internal Medicine, University of Michigan, Ann Arbor, Michigan

Hani Jneid, MD, FACC, FAHA, FSCAI
Assistant Professor of Medicine, Director of Interventional Cardiology Research, Baylor College of Medicine, The Michael E. DeBakey VA Medical Center, Houston, Texas

Laura S. Johnson, MD
Trauma Surgery, Washington Hospital Center, Washington, District of Columbia

Robert Johnson, MD
General Surgery, Thoracic Surgery, Saint Louis University Hospital, St. Louis, Missouri

Amal Jubran, MD
Professor of Medicine, Pulmonary and Critical Care Medicine, Loyola University Medical Center, Loyola University Medical Center, Maywood, Illinois, Section Chief, Pulmonary and Critical Care Medicine, Edward Hines Jr. Veterans Affairs Hospital, Hines, Illinois

George Karam, MD
Professor of Medicine, Department of Medicine, Louisiana State University Health Sciences Center, Baton Rouge, Louisiana

Steven T. Kaufman, MD
Assistant Professor of Medicine, Endocrinology, Diabetes, and Metabolism, Cooper University Hospital, Camden, New Jersey

Jason A. Kline, MD
Assistant Professor of Medicine, Nephrology, Cooper Medical School of Rowan University, Camden, New Jersey

Zoulficar Kobeissi, MD
Assistant Professor of Clinical Medicine, Department of Medicine, Weill Cornell Medical College/The Methodist Hospital, Houston, Texas

Anand Kumar, MD
Associate Professor, Section of Critical Care Medicine, Section of Infectious Diseases, University of Manitoba, Winnipeg, Canada, Rutgers Robert Wood Johnson Medical School, Camden, New Jersey

Neil A. Lachant, MD
Chief, Section of Hematology, Cooper Cancer Institute, Cooper University Hospital, Professor of Medicine, Cooper Medical School of Rowan University, Camden, New Jersey

Franco Laghi, MD
Professor of Medicine, Division of Pulmonary and Critical Care Medicine, Loyola University of Chicago, Stritch School of Medicine, Chicago, Illinois, Edward Hines Jr. Veterans Administration Hospital, Hines, Illinois

Rekha Lakshmanan, MD
Intensivist, Critical Care, Mercy Hospital St. Louis, St. Louis, Missouri

Stephen E. Lapinsky, MB, BCh, MSc, FRCPC
Professor, Department of Medicine, University of Toronto, Site Director, Intensive Care Unit, Mount Sinai Hospital, Toronto, Ontario, Canada

Marc Laufgraben, MD, MBA
Associate Professor of Medicine, Division of Endocrinology, Diabetes, and Metabolism, Cooper Medical School of Rowan University, Camden, New Jersey

G. G. Lavery, MD, FJFICMI, FFARCSI
Clinical Director, HSC Safety Forum, Public Health Agency, Consultant, Critical Care, Royal Hospital, Belfast HSC Trust, Belfast, Northern Ireland, United Kingdom

Kenneth V. Leeper, Jr., MD
Professor of Medicine, Division of Medicine/Pulmonary and Critical Care, Emory University School of Medicine, Atlanta, Georgia

Dan L. Longo, MD
Deputy Editor, New England Journal of Medicine, Professor of Medicine, Harvard Medical School, Boston, Massachusetts

Ramya Lotano, MD, FCCP
Assistant Professor of Medicine, Department of Medicine, Cooper University Hospital, Camden, New Jersey

Vincent E. Lotano, MD
Hospital of the University of Pennsylvania Division of Thoracic Surgery, Director of Thoracic Surgery, Pennsylvania Hospital, Philadelphia, Pennsylvania

Dennis G. Maki, MD
Ovid O. Meyer Professor of Medicine, Divisions of Infectious Diseases and Pulmonary/Critical Care Medicine, Attending Physician, Center for Trauma and Life Support, University of Wisconsin Hospital and Clinics, Madision, Wisconsin

Andrew O. Maree, MD, MSc
Consultant Cardiologist, Waterford Regional Hospital, Waterford, Ireland

Paul E. Marik, MD, FCCM, FCCP
Chief, Division of Pulmonary and Critical Care Medicine, Department of Internal Medicine, Eastern Virginia Medical School, Norfolk, Virginia

John Marini, MD
Professor of Medicine, Pulmonary and Critical Care Medicine, University of Minnesota, Director of Pysiologic and Translational Research, Regions Hospital, St. Paul, Minnesota

John C. Marshall, MD, FRCSC
Professor of Surgery, Department of Surgery and the Interdepartmental Division of Critical Care Medicine, University of Toronto, St. Michael's Hospital, Toronto, Ontario, Canada

Henry Masur, MD
Chief, Critical Care Medicine Department, Clinical Center, National Institutes of Health, Bethesda, Maryland

Dirk M. Maybauer, MD, PhD
Professor in Anaesthesia and Critical Care Medicine, Philipps University of Marburg, Marburg, Germany, Assistant Professor in Anesthesiology and Critical Care Medicine, The University of Texas Medical Branch, Galveston, Texas

Marc O. Maybauer, MD, PhD, EDIC, FCCP
Professor in Anaesthesia and Critical Care Medicine, Philipps University of Marburg, Marburg, Germany, Assistant Professor in Anesthesiology and Critical Care Medicine, The University of Texas Medical Branch, Galveston, Texas

Christopher B. McFadden, MD
Assistant Professor, Medicine, Cooper Medical School of Rowan University, Camden, New Jersey

Todd A. Miano, PharmD
Pharmacy Clinical Specialist, Surgical Critical Care, Hospital of the University of Pennsylvania, Philadelphia, Pennsylvania

Thomas R. Mirsen, MD
Associate Professor, Neurology, Cooper Medical School of Rowan University, Camden, New Jersey

Manoj K. Mittal, MBBS
Neurocritical Care Fellow, Neurology, Mayo Clinic, Rochester, Minnesota

Rui Moreno, MD, PhD
Professor, Unidade de Cuidados Intensivos Neurocríticos, Hospital de São José, Centro Hospitalar de Lisboa Central, E.P.E., Lisboa, Portugal

Nick Murphy, MB BS, FRCA, DipICM
Honorary Senior Lecturer, Clinical Medicine, University of Birmingham, Consultant Intensivist, Critical Care, Queen Elizabeth Hospital, Birmingham, Edgbaston, Birmingham, United Kingdom

Katie M. Muzevich, PharmD, BCPS
Department of Pharmacy, Virginia Commonwealth University Health System, Richmond, Virginia

Girish B. Nair, MD
Fellow, Pulmonary and Critical Care Medicine, Winthrop University Hospital, Rock Hill, South Carolina

Michael S. Neiderman, MD
Chairman, Department of Medicine, Winthrop University Hospital, Mineola, New York, Professor of Medicine, Department of Medicine, SUNY at Stony Brook, Stony Brook, New York

Hollis O'Neal, MD, MSc
Assistant Professor of Clinical Medicine, Pulmonary and Critical Care Medicine, Louisiana State University Health Sciences Center, Baton Rouge, Louisiana

Matthew Ortman, MD
Assistant Professor of Medicine, Rutgers Robert Wood Johnson Medical School, University of Medicine and Dentistry of New Jersey, Cooper Medical School of Rowan University, Division of Cardiology, Department of Medicine, Cooper University Hospital, Camden, New Jersey

Luis Ostrosky-Zeichner, MD, FACP, FIDSA
Associate Professor of Medicine and Epidemiology, Division of Infectious Diseases, University of Texas Medical School at Houston, Houston, Texas

Igor Ougorets, MD
Overlook Hospital, Summit, New Jersey

Igor F. Palacios, MD
Director of Interventional Cardiology, Division of Cardiology, Massachusetts General Hospital—Harvard Medical School, Boston, Massachusetts

Paul M. Palevsky, MD
Chief, Renal Section, VA Pittsburgh Healthcare System, Professor of Medicine and Clinical and Translational Science, University of Pittsburgh, Pittsburgh, Pennsylvania

Amay Parikh, MD, MBA, MS
Instructor of Clinical Medicine, Department of Medicine, Columbia University Medical Center, New York, New York

Sea Mi Park, MD, PhD
Clinical Research Fellow, Weill Cornell Medical Center, New York, New York

Joseph E. Parrillo, MD
Chairman, Heart and Vascular Hospital, Hackensack University Medical Center, Professor of Medicine, Rutgers New Jersey Medical School, Hackensack, New Jersey

Steven Peikin, MD, FACG, AGAF
Professor of Medicine and Head, Division of Gastroenterology and Liver Diseases, Cooper Medical School of Rowan University and Cooper University Hospital, Camden, New Jersey

Priscilla Peters, BA, RDCS, FASE
Echocardiographic Clinical Specialist, Cooper University Hospital, Assistant Professor of Medicine, Robert Wood Johnson School of Medicine, Camden, New Jersey

Juan Gabriel Posadas-Calleja, MD, MsC, FCCP
Department of Critical Care Medicine, University of Calgary, Alberta Health Services, Alberta, Canada

Melvin R. Pratter, MD
Head, Division of Pulmonary and Critical Care Medicine, Pulmonary and Critical Care, Cooper University Hospital, Professor of Medicine, Cooper Medical School of Rowan University, Camden, New Jersey

S. Sujanthy Rajaram, MD, MPH
Assistant Professor of Medicine, Department of Medicine, Cooper University Hospital, Cooper Medical School of Rowan University/Rutgers Robert Wood Johnson Medical School, Camden, New Jersey

Annette C. Reboli, MD
Founding Vice Dean, Professor of Medicine, Infectious Diseases Division, Cooper Medical School of Rowan University and Cooper University Hospital, Camden, New Jersey

John H. Rex, MD, FACP
Vice President and Head of Infection, Global Medicines Development, AstraZeneca Pharmaceuticals, Boston, Massachusetts, Adjunct Professor, Department of Medicine, Section of Infectious Diseases, University of Texas Medical School–Houston, Houston, Texas

Andrew Rhodes, FRCA, FRCP, FFICM
Clinical Director, Critical Care, St. George's Hospital, London, United Kingdom

Fred Rincon, MD, MSc, MBE
Assistant Professor, Neurology and Neurosurgery, Thomas Jefferson University, Philadelphia, Pennsylvania

Axel Rosengart, MD, PhD, MPH
Director, Critical Care and Emergency Neurology and Neurosurgery, Professor of Neurology and Neuroscience, and Neurosurgery, Weill Cornell Medical Center, New York, New York

Andrea M. Russo, MD
Professor of Medicine, Rutgers Robert Wood Johnson Medical School, Cooper Medical School of Rowan University, Director, Cardiac Electrophysiology, Cooper University Hospital, Camden, New Jersey

Rebecca L. Ryszkiewicz, MD, RDMS
Fellow in Emergency Medicine Ultrasound, Department of Emergency Medicine, Eastern Virginia Medical School, Norfolk, Virginia

Sajjad A. Sabir, MD
Assistant Professor of Medicine, Cooper Medical School of Rowan University, Cooper Structural Heart Disease Program Director, Interventional Echocardiography, Division of Cardiology, Cooper University Hospital, Camden, New Jersey

Jeffrey R. Saffle, MD, FACS
Professor, Surgery, University of Utah Health Center, Salt Lake City, Utah

Rommel Sagana, MD
Assistant Professor, Pulmonary/Critical Care, University of Michigan, Ann Arbor, Michigan

Raul Sanchez, MD
Department of Medicine, The Methodist Hospital, Houston, Texas

Gregory A. Schmidt, MD
Professor of Medicine, Pulmonary Diseases, Critical Care, and Occupational Medicine, University of Iowa, Iowa City, Iowa

Christa Schorr, RN, MSN
Director of Databases for Quality Improvement and Research Program Director of Critical Care Research Trials, Medicine–Critical Care, Cooper University Hospital, Camden, New Jersey

Curtis N. Sessler, MD
Orhan Muren Professor of Medicine, Internal Medicine, Virginia Commonwealth University Health System, Director, Center for Adult Critical Care, Medical College of Virginia Hospitals & Physicians, Richmond, Virginia

Michael C. Shen, MD
Department of Medicine, The Methodist Hospital, Houston, Texas

Henry Silverman, MD, MA
Professor of Medicine, University of Maryland School of Medicine, Baltimore, Maryland

Sabine Sobek, MD
Instructor, Department of Medicine, Northwestern University Feinberg School of Medicine, Perioperative Hospital, Internal Medicine, Northwestern Memorial Hospital, Chicago, Illinois

Michael Sterling, MD, FACP, FCCM
Assistant Director, Emory Center for Critical Care, Emory Midtown Hospital, Medical Director Surgical Intensive Care Unit and Assistant Professor of Medicine, Division of Pulmonary, Allergy, and Critical Care Medicine, Emory University School of Medicine, Atlanta, Georgia

Robert W. Taylor, MD
Mercy Medical Center, Department of Critical Care, St. Louis, Missouri

Christopher B. Thomas, MD
Assistant Professor of Clinical Medicine, Pulmonary and Critical Care Medicine, Louisiana State University Health Sciences Center, Baton Rouge, Louisiana, Co-Director, Division of Critical Care, Anesthesia Medical Group, Nashville, Tennessee

Martin J. Tobin, MD
Division of Pulmonary and Critical Care, Medicine, Edward Hines Jr. Veterans Affairs Hospital and Loyola University of Chicago, Stritch School of Medicine, Hines, Illinois

Simon K. Topalian, MD
Assistant Professor of Medicine, Cooper Medical School of Rowan University, Interventional Echocardiography, Division of Cardiology, Cooper University Hospital, Camden, New Jersey

Sean Townsend, MD
Vice President of Quality and Safety, California Pacific Medical Center, Clinical Assistant Professor of Medicine, University of California, San Francisco, San Francisco, California

Richard Trohman, MD
Co-Director of Section, Cardiology, Rush University Medical Center, Chicago, Illinois

Stephen Trzeciak, MD, MPH
Associate Professor of Medicine and Emergency Medicine, Cooper Medical School of Rowan University, Cooper University Hospital, Camden, New Jersey

Mykola V. Tsapenko, MD, PhD
Critical Care Medicine, Charleston Area Medical Center, Charleston, West Virginia

Constantine Tsigrelis, MD
Assistant Professor of Medicine, Cooper Medical School of Rowan University, Attending Physician and Director, Infectious Diseases–ICU Clinical Service, Division of Infectious Diseases, Cooper University Hospital, Camden, New Jersey

Zoltan G. Turi, MD
Professor of Medicine, Cooper Medical School of Rowan University, Director, Cooper Vascular Center, Director, Cooper Structural Heart Disease Program, Camden, New Jersey

Alan R. Turtz, MD
Associate Professor, Surgery, Rutgers Robert Wood Johnson Medical School, Attending Neurosurgeon, Cooper University Hospital, Camden, New Jersey

Ulug Unligil, MD
Critical Care Fellow, Section of Critical Care Medicine, University of Manitoba, Winnipeg, Canada

Jean-Louis Vincent, MD, PhD
Director, Department of Intensive Care, Erasme Hospital, Université Libre de Bruxelles, Brussels, Belgium

Lawrence S. Weisberg, MD
Professor of Medicine, Cooper Medical School of Rowan University, Head of Nephrology, Cooper University Hospital, Camden, New Jersey

Steven Werns, MD
Professor of Medicine, Cooper Medical School of Rowan University, Adjunct Professor of Medicine, Robert Wood Johnson Medical School, Director, Invasive Cardiovascular Services, Cooper University Hospital, Camden, New Jersey

Eelco F. M. Wijdicks, MD, PhD
Professor of Neurology, College of Medicine, Mayo Clinic, Rochester, Minnesota

Sergio L. Zanotti-Cavazzoni, MD, FCCM
Assistant Professor of Medicine, Division of Critical Care Medicine, Cooper Medical School of Rowan University, Director, Critical Care Medicine Fellowship Program, Division of Critical Care Medicine, Cooper University Hospital, Camden, New Jersey

Janice L. Zimmerman, MD
Professor, Clinical Medicine, Department of Medicine, Weill Cornell Medical College, New York, New York, Adjunct Professor of Medicine, Baylor College of Medicine, Head, Critical Care Division, Department of Medicine, Director, Medical Intensive Care Unit, The Methodist Hospital, Houston, Texas

Preface

Few fields in medicine have grown, evolved, and changed as rapidly as critical care medicine has during the past 40 years. From its origins in the postoperative recovery room and the coronary care unit, the modern intensive care unit (ICU) now represents the ultimate example of medicine's ability to supply the specialized personnel and technology necessary to sustain and restore seriously ill persons to productive lives. While the field continues to evolve rapidly, sufficient principles, knowledge, and experience have accumulated in the past few decades to warrant the production of a textbook dedicated to adult critical care medicine. We chose to limit the subject matter of our book to the critical care of *adult* patients to allow the production of a comprehensive textbook in a single volume.

This book was envisioned to be multidisciplinary and multiauthored by acknowledged leaders in the field but aimed primarily at practicing critical care physicians who spend the better part of their time caring for patients in an ICU. Thus, the book would be appropriate for critical care internists as well as for surgical or anesthesia critical care specialists. The goal was to produce the acknowledged "best practice" standard in critical care medicine.

The first edition of the textbook was published in 1995, co-edited by Joe Parrillo and Roger Bone. The book sold exceedingly well for a first edition text. After the untimely death of Roger Bone in 1997, Phil Dellinger joined Joe Parrillo as the co-editor for the second, third, and now this fourth edition. As co-editors, we have labored to produce a highly readable text that can serve equally well for comprehensive review and as a reference source. We felt that it was important for usability and accessibility to keep the book to a single volume. This was a challenge, because critical care knowledge and technology have expanded significantly during the past decade. By placing emphasis on clear, concise writing and keeping the focus on critical care medicine for the adult, this goal was achieved.

Our view of critical care medicine is mirrored in the organization of the textbook. Modern critical care is a multidisciplinary specialty that includes much of the knowledge and technology contained in many disciplines represented by the classic organ-based subspecialties of medicine, as well as the specialties of surgery and anesthesiology. The book begins with a section consisting of chapters on the technology, procedures, and pharmacology that are essential to the practicing critical care physician. This section is followed by sections devoted to the critical care aspects of cardiovascular, pulmonary, infectious, renal, metabolic, neurologic, gastrointestinal, and hematologic-oncologic diseases. Subsequent chapters are devoted to important social, ethical, and other issues such as psychiatric disorders, severity of illness scoring systems, and administrative issues in the ICU. This fourth edition has significant content additions and revisions, including a new chapter devoted to bedside ICU ultrasound. Online videos are also available featuring a variety of content areas, including echocardiograms and bedside ultrasounds of a variety of exam sites.

Each chapter is designed to provide a comprehensive review of pertinent clinical, diagnostic, and management issues. This is primarily a clinical text, so the emphasis is on considerations important to the practicing critical care physician; also presented, however, are the scientific (physiologic, biochemical, and molecular biologic) data pertinent to the pathophysiology and management issues. We have aimed for a textbook length that is comprehensive but manageable. Substantial references (most now online) are provided for readers wishing to explore subjects in greater detail. We have identified key points and key references to highlight the most important issues within each chapter. Continued popular features of this fourth edition include a color-enhanced design and clinically useful management algorithms.

We have been fortunate to attract a truly exceptional group of authors to write the chapters for *Critical Care Medicine: Principles of Diagnosis and Management in the Adult.* For each chapter, we have chosen a seasoned clinician-scientist actively involved in critical care who is one of a handful of recognized experts on his or her chapter topic. We have continued the international flavor of our authorship. To provide uniformity in content and style, one or both of us have edited and revised each chapter.

We wish to thank the highly dedicated people who provided us with the assistance needed to complete a venture of this magnitude. Our thanks go to Linda Rizzuto, who provided valuable organizational and editorial input; to Ellen Lawlor, for her administrative assistance; and to the excellent editorial staff at Elsevier, including William Schmitt, Janice Gaillard, and Sharon Corell.

Joseph E. Parrillo
Hackensack, New Jersey

R. Phillip Dellinger
Camden, New Jersey

Contents

Video Contents

CRITICAL CARE MEDICINE

PRINCIPLES OF DIAGNOSIS AND MANAGEMENT IN THE ADULT

PART 1

CRITICAL CARE PROCEDURES, MONITORING, AND PHARMACOLOGY

1

Cardiac Arrest and Cardiopulmonary Resuscitation

Stephen Trzeciak

CHAPTER OUTLINE

EPIDEMIOLOGY AND GENERAL PRINCIPLES

Sudden cardiac arrest is defined as the cessation of effective cardiac mechanical activity as confirmed by the absence of signs of circulation. Sudden cardiac arrest is the most common fatal manifestation of cardiovascular disease and a leading cause of death worldwide. In North America alone, approximately 350,000 persons annually undergo resuscitation for sudden cardiac arrest. Approximately 25% of sudden cardiac arrest events are due to pulseless ventricular arrhythmias (i.e., ventricular fibrillation [VF] or pulseless ventricular tachycardia [VT]), whereas the rest can be attributed to other cardiac rhythms (i.e., asystole or pulseless electrical activity [PEA]).[1] Patients who suffer cardiac arrest due to VF or VT have a much higher chance of surviving the event compared with patients who present with PEA/asystole.[2] Patients with ventricular arrhythmias have a better prognosis because (1) ventricular arrhythmias are potentially treatable with defibrillation (i.e., "shockable" initial rhythm) to restore circulation, whereas the other initial rhythms are not, and (2) ventricular arrhythmias are typically a manifestation of a cardiac cause of cardiac arrest (e.g., acute myocardial infarction), whereas the other initial rhythms are more likely to be related to a noncardiac cause and perhaps an underlying condition that is less treatable. The success with cardiopulmonary resuscitation (CPR) for VF as compared to other rhythms across varying levels of rescuer intervention is displayed in Table 1.1. The basic principles of resuscitation are an integral part of training for many health care providers (HCPs). Because timely interventions for cardiac arrest victims have the potential to be truly lifesaving, it is especially important for critical care practitioners to have a sound understanding of the evaluation and management of cardiac arrest.

A number of critical actions (chain of survival) must occur in response to a cardiac arrest event. The *chain of survival* paradigm (Fig. 1.1) for the treatment of cardiac arrest has five separate and distinct elements: (1) immediate recognition that cardiac arrest has occurred and activation of the emergency response system; (2) application of effective CPR; (3) early defibrillation (if applicable); (4) advanced cardiac life support; and (5) initiation of postresuscitation care (e.g., therapeutic hypothermia).[3]

CARDIOPULMONARY RESUSCITATION AND ADVANCED CARDIAC LIFE SUPPORT

For CPR to be effective in restoring spontaneous circulation, it must be applied immediately at the time of cardiac arrest. Therefore, immediate recognition that a cardiac arrest has occurred and activation of the emergency response system is essential. Patients become unresponsive at the time of cardiac arrest. Agonal gasps may be observed in the early moments after a cardiac arrest event, although normal breathing ceases. Pulse checks (i.e., palpation of femoral or carotid arteries for detection of a pulse) are often unreliable, even when performed by experienced HCPs.[4] Because delays in initiating CPR are associated with worse outcome, and prolonged attempts to detect a pulse may result in a delay in initiating CPR, prolonged pulse checks are to be avoided. CPR should be started immediately if the patient is unresponsive and either has agonal gasps or is not breathing.[3]

Table 1.1 Estimates of Success of Cardiopulmonary Resuscitation Based on 31 Published Reports

	Hospital Discharge Rate (%)	
Intervention Category	All Rhythms	Ventricular Fibrillation
BLS	5	12
BLS + defibrillation	10	16
ACLS	10	17
BLS + ACLS	17	26
BLS + defibrillation + ACLS	17	29

ACLS, advanced cardiac life support; BLS, basic life support.
Adapted from Cummins RO, Ornato JP, Thies WH, et al: Improving survival from sudden cardiac arrest: The "chain of survival" concept. Circulation 1991;83:1832-1847.

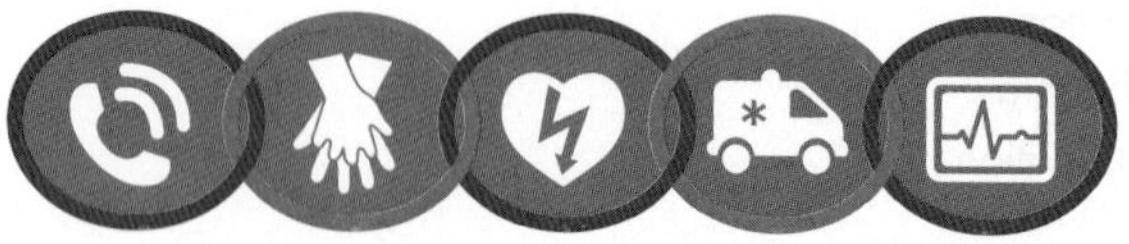

Figure 1.1 The American Heart Association chain of survival paradigm. This figure represents the critical actions needed to optimize the chances of survival from cardiac arrest. The links (from left to right) include (1) immediate recognition of cardiac arrest and activation of the emergency response system; (2) early and effective cardiopulmonary resuscitation; (3) defibrillation (if applicable); (4) advanced cardiac life support; and (5) post–cardiac arrest care (including therapeutic hypothermia if appropriate). (Reprinted with permission from Travers AH, Rea TD, Bobrow BJ, et al: Part 4: CPR overview: 2010 American Heart Association Guidelines for Cardiopulmonary Resuscitation and Emergency Cardiovascular Care. Circulation 2010;122(18 Suppl 3):S676-684.)

CHEST COMPRESSIONS

In CPR, chest compressions are used to circulate blood to the heart and brain until a pulse can be restored. The mechanism by which chest compressions generate cardiac output is through an increase in intrathoracic pressure plus direct compression of the heart. With the patient lying in the supine position, the rescuer applies compressions to the patient's sternum. The heel of one hand is placed over the lower half of the sternum and the heel of the other hand on top in an overlapping and parallel fashion. The recommended compression depth in adults is 2 inches. The recommended rate of compression is 100 or more per minute. "*Push hard, push fast*" is now the American Heart Association (AHA) mantra for CPR instruction. This underscores the importance of vigorous chest compressions in achieving return of spontaneous circulation (ROSC).[5] In addition, incomplete recoil of the chest impairs the cardiac output that is generated, and thus the chest wall should be allowed to recoil completely between compressions. Owing to rescuer fatigue, the quality of chest compressions predictably decreases as the time providing chest compressions increases, and the persons providing chest compressions (even experienced HCPs) may not perceive fatigue or a decrease in the quality of their compressions.[6] Therefore, it is recommended that rescuers performing chest compressions rotate every 2 minutes.

The quality of CPR is a critical determinant of surviving a cardiac arrest event.[7] Minimization of interruptions in chest compressions is imperative. Interruptions in chest compressions during CPR have been quite common historically, and the "hands off" time has been shown to take up a substantial amount of the total resuscitation time.[7] Potential reasons for "hands off" time include pulse checks, rhythm analysis, switching compressors, procedures (e.g., airway placement), and pauses before defibrillation ("preshock pause"). All of these potential reasons for interruptions must be minimized. Pauses related to rotating compressors or pulse checks should take no longer than a few seconds.[5] Eliminating (or minimizing) preshock pauses has been associated with higher likelihood of ROSC and improved clinical outcome.[8]

DEFIBRILLATION

The next critically important action in the resuscitation of patients with cardiac arrest due to pulseless ventricular arrhythmias (i.e., VF or pulseless VT) is rapid defibrillation. Delays in defibrillation are clearly deleterious, with a sharp decrease in survival as the time to defibrillation increases.[9] With the advent of automatic external defibrillators (AEDs) and their dissemination into public places, both elements of effective CPR (both effective chest compressions and rapid defibrillation) can be performed by lay rescuers in the field for patients with out-of-hospital cardiac arrest. Figure 1.2 shows the importance of rapid defibrillation, with decreasing success of resuscitation with increasing time to defibrillation.

RESCUE BREATHING

The most recent AHA recommendations regarding ventilation during CPR depends on who the rescuer is (i.e., trained HCPs versus lay person).[5] For trained HCPs, the recommended ventilation strategy is a cycle of 30 chest compressions to two breaths until an endotracheal tube is placed, and then continuous chest compressions with one breath every 6 to 8 seconds after the endotracheal tube is placed. Excessive ventilations can be deleterious from a hemodynamic perspective due to increased intrathoracic pressure and reduction in the cardiac output generated by CPR and thus should be avoided during resuscitation. Excessive ventilation could also potentially result in alkalemia.

For lay persons who are attempting CPR in the field for a victim of out-of-hospital cardiac arrest, rescue breathing is no longer recommended. Rather, the recommended strategy is compression-only (or "hands-only") CPR.[5] The rationale is that compression-only CPR can increase the number of effective chest compressions that are delivered to the patient (i.e., minimizes interruptions for rescue breaths), and does not require mouth-to-mouth contact. Mouth-to-mouth contact is one of the perceived barriers to CPR in the field. By removing this element, the hope is that an increase in attempts at bystander CPR will result. Hands-only CPR has been found to be not inferior to conventional

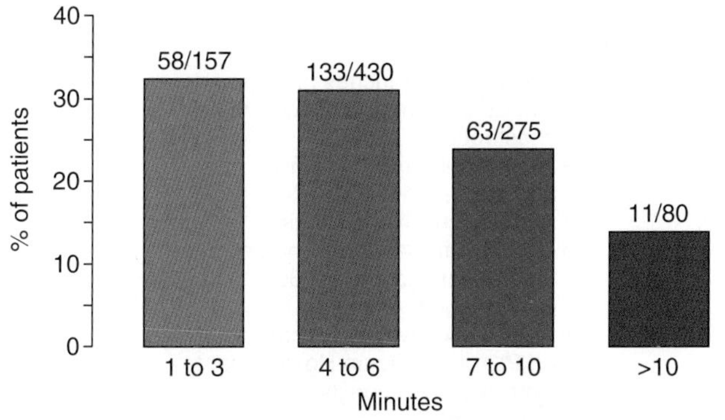

Figure 1.2 Relationship between the time interval before attempted defibrillation and the proportion of patients discharged from the hospital alive after out-of-hospital cardiac arrest. (Adapted from Weaver WD, Cobb LA, Hallstrom AP, et al: Factors influencing survival after out-of-hospital cardiac arrest. J Am Coll Cardiol 1986; 7:752-757.)

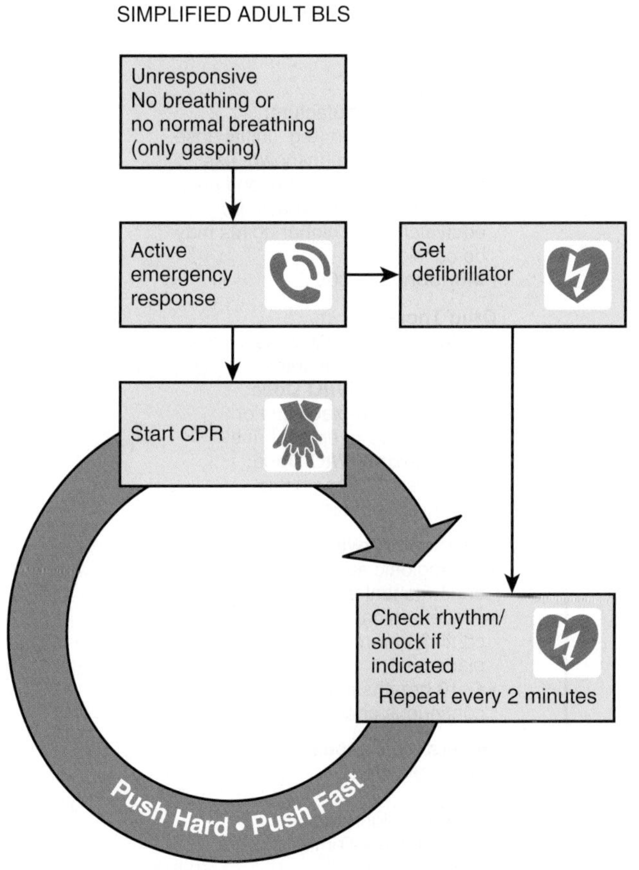

Figure 1.3 American Heart Association simplified basic life support algorithm. BLS, basic life support; CPR, cardiopulmonary resuscitation (Reprinted with permission from Berg RA, Hemphill R, Abella BS, et al: Part 5: Adult basic life support: 2010 American Heart Association Guidelines for Cardiopulmonary Resuscitation and Emergency Cardiovascular Care. Circulation 2010;122(18 Suppl 3):S685-705.)

CPR including rescue breaths for victims of out-of-hospital cardiac arrest,[10-12] and thus hands-only CPR has become the preferred technique to teach lay rescuers.

Figure 1.3 displays the AHA algorithm for adult basic life support.

ADVANCED CARDIAC LIFE SUPPORT

There are several additional elements of resuscitation that are intended specifically for trained HCPs (e.g., advanced cardiac life support [ACLS]), and these elements include pharmacologic therapy. Figure 1.4 displays the AHA algorithm for ACLS.[13]

The primary goal of pharmacologic interventions is to assist the achievement and maintenance of spontaneous circulation. The mainstay of pharmacologic interventions is vasopressor drugs. Epinephrine (1 mg) is administered by intravenous (IV) or intraosseous (IO) route every 3 to 5 minutes during CPR until ROSC is achieved.[13] If IV/IO access cannot be established, epinephrine could be administered via endotracheal tube, but at a higher dose (2-2.5 mg). Vasopressin (40 mg IV/IO) can be substituted for the first or second dose of epinephrine. Amiodarone is the preferred antiarrhythmic agent. In patients with VF/VT not responding to CPR, defibrillation, and vasopressor therapy, amiodarone is recommended (300 mg IV/IO for the first dose, 150 mg IV/IO for the second dose).[13] Recently, the use of atropine for PEA/asystole was removed from the ACLS algorithm. Along these lines, there is also insufficient evidence to recommend routine administration of sodium bicarbonate during CPR.

It is notable that the impact of recommended ACLS therapies on outcome from cardiac arrest remains a matter of debate. Some studies have shown that ACLS interventions did not improve clinical outcomes when compared to basic life support alone.[14]

POSTRESUSCITATION CARE

Even if ROSC is achieved with CPR and defibrillation, cardiac arrest victims are at extremely high risk of dying in the hospital, and many who survive sustain permanent crippling neurologic sequelae. Approximately 50% to 60% of patients successfully resuscitated from out-of-hospital cardiac arrest do not survive. After ROSC, global ischemia/reperfusion (I/R) injury results in potentially devastating neurologic disability. The primary cause of death among postresuscitation patients is brain injury. However, clinical trials have shown that mild therapeutic hypothermia after ROSC can improve outcomes. These landmark clinical trials have dramatically transformed the classical thinking about anoxic brain injury after cardiac arrest; this condition is in fact *treatable*. Early therapeutic interventions such as hypothermia initiated in the post-ROSC period can improve the trajectory of the long-term disease course. Accordingly, the postresuscitation care is now considered to be a crucial fifth link in the chain of survival paradigm (see Fig. 1.1).[15]

GENERAL APPROACH

Patients resuscitated from cardiac arrest should be admitted to a critical care unit with the following capabilities:[16]

- Critical care support to optimize cardiovascular indices and vital organ perfusion, and prevent repeat cardiac arrest (or provide rapid treatment of rearrest if it occurs)

ADULT CARDIAC ARREST

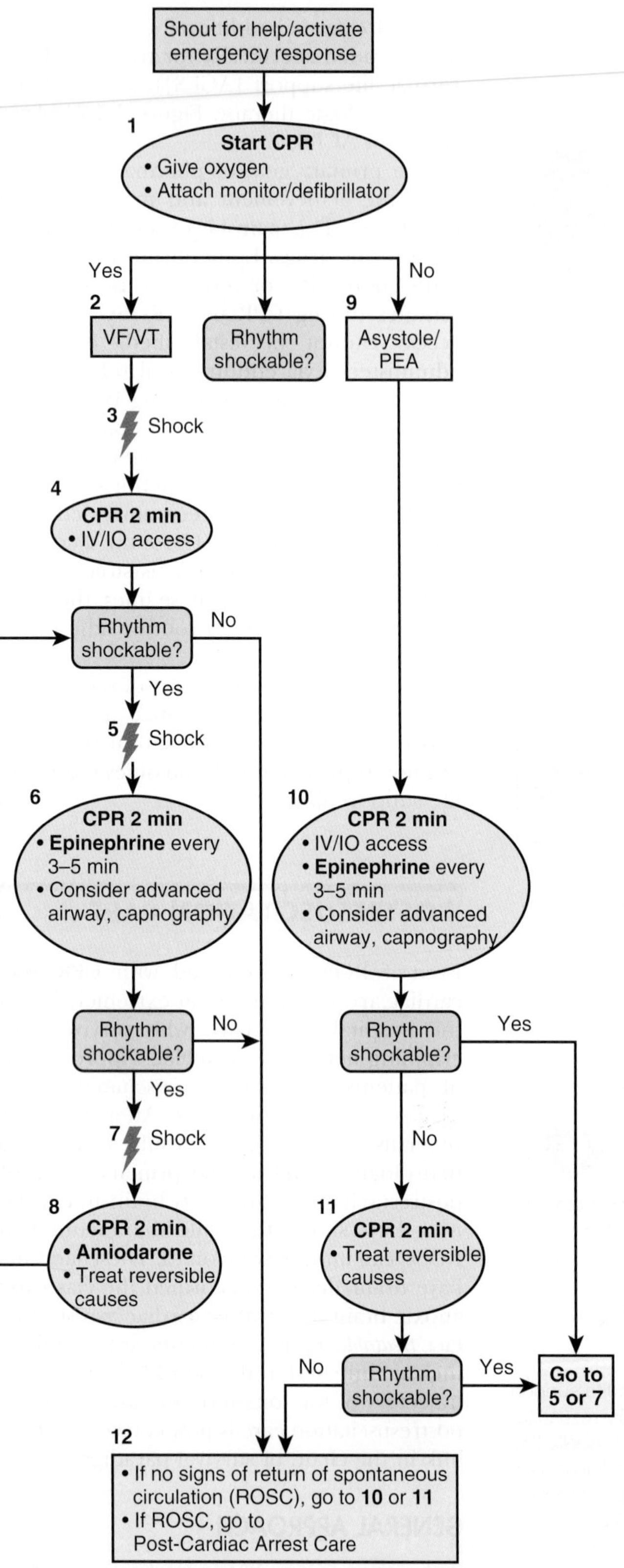

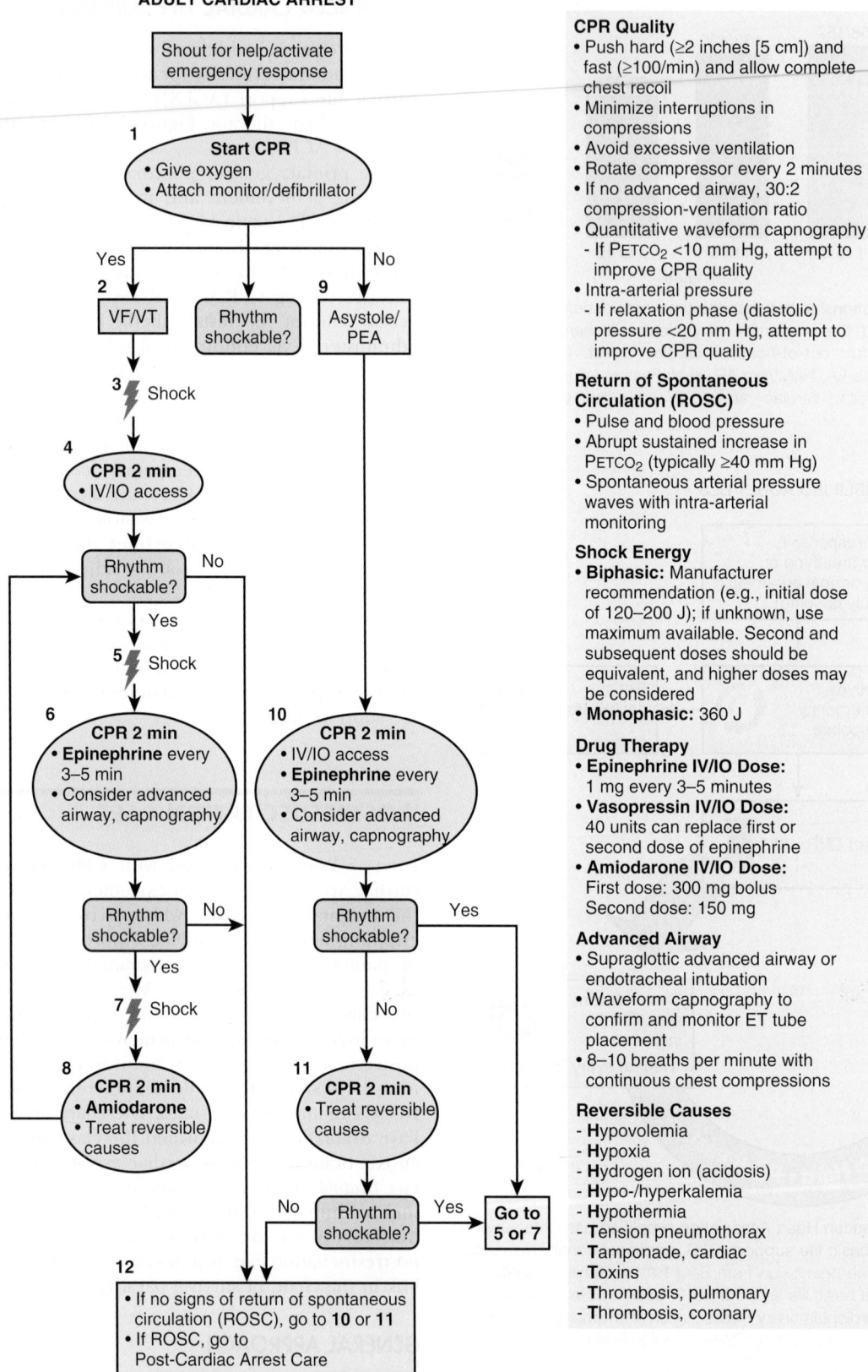

CPR Quality
- Push hard (≥2 inches [5 cm]) and fast (≥100/min) and allow complete chest recoil
- Minimize interruptions in compressions
- Avoid excessive ventilation
- Rotate compressor every 2 minutes
- If no advanced airway, 30:2 compression-ventilation ratio
- Quantitative waveform capnography
  - If P_{ETCO_2} <10 mm Hg, attempt to improve CPR quality
- Intra-arterial pressure
  - If relaxation phase (diastolic) pressure <20 mm Hg, attempt to improve CPR quality

Return of Spontaneous Circulation (ROSC)
- Pulse and blood pressure
- Abrupt sustained increase in P_{ETCO_2} (typically ≥40 mm Hg)
- Spontaneous arterial pressure waves with intra-arterial monitoring

Shock Energy
- **Biphasic:** Manufacturer recommendation (e.g., initial dose of 120–200 J); if unknown, use maximum available. Second and subsequent doses should be equivalent, and higher doses may be considered
- **Monophasic:** 360 J

Drug Therapy
- **Epinephrine IV/IO Dose:** 1 mg every 3–5 minutes
- **Vasopressin IV/IO Dose:** 40 units can replace first or second dose of epinephrine
- **Amiodarone IV/IO Dose:** First dose: 300 mg bolus Second dose: 150 mg

Advanced Airway
- Supraglottic advanced airway or endotracheal intubation
- Waveform capnography to confirm and monitor ET tube placement
- 8–10 breaths per minute with continuous chest compressions

Reversible Causes
- **H**ypovolemia
- **H**ypoxia
- **H**ydrogen ion (acidosis)
- **H**ypo-/hyperkalemia
- **H**ypothermia
- **T**ension pneumothorax
- **T**amponade, cardiac
- **T**oxins
- **T**hrombosis, pulmonary
- **T**hrombosis, coronary

Figure 1.4 American Heart Association advanced cardiac life support (ACLS) algorithm. CPR, cardiopulmonary resuscitation; IO, intraosseous; IV, intravenous; PEA, pulseless electrical activity; ROSC, return of spontaneous circulation; VF, ventricular fibrillation; VT, ventricular tachycardia. (Reprinted with permission from Neumar RW, Otto CW, Link MS, et al: Part 8: Adult advanced cardiovascular life support: 2010 American Heart Association Guidelines for Cardiopulmonary Resuscitation and Emergency Cardiovascular Care. Circulation 2010;122(18 Suppl 3):S729-767.)

- Interventional cardiac catheterization for possible percutaneous coronary intervention (PCI) if needed
- Mild therapeutic hypothermia (33°-34° C) for 12 to 24 hours in attempts to prevent permanent neurologic injury
- Systematic application of an evidence-based approach to neurologic prognostication to refrain from inappropriately early final determinations of poor neurologic prognosis (i.e., prevent inappropriately early withdrawal of life support before the neurologic outcome can be known with certainty)

CRITICAL CARE SUPPORT

I/R triggers profound systemic inflammation. In clinical studies, ROSC has been associated with sharp increases in circulating cytokines and other markers of the inflammatory response. Accordingly, some investigators have referred to the post–cardiac arrest syndrome as a "sepsis-like" state. The clinical manifestations of the systemic inflammatory response may include marked hemodynamic derangements such as sustained arterial hypotension similar to septic shock. Hemodynamic instability occurs in approximately 50% of patients who survive to intensive care unit admission after ROSC, and thus the need for aggressive hemodynamic support (e.g., continuous infusion of vasoactive agents and perhaps advanced hemodynamic monitoring) should be anticipated.[17]

In addition to a systemic inflammatory response, an equally important contributor to post-ROSC hemodynamic instability is myocardial stunning. Severe, but potentially reversible, global myocardial dysfunction is common following ROSC. The cause is thought to be I/R injury, but treatment with defibrillation (if applied) could also contribute. Although the myocardial dysfunction occurs in the absence of an acute coronary event, myocardial ischemia may be an ongoing component of myocardial depression if an acute coronary syndrome caused the cardiac arrest. Severe myocardial stunning may last for hours but often improves by the 24-hour mark after ROSC. An echocardiogram may be helpful in hemodynamic assessment after ROSC to determine if global myocardial depression is present, as this may impact decisions on vasoactive drug support (e.g., dobutamine) or mechanical augmentation (e.g., intra-aortic balloon counterpulsation) until the myocardial function recovers. However, when needed, clinicians should be aware that β-adrenergic agents may increase the likelihood of dysrrhythmia.

Although there are no data on whether specific blood pressure or other hemodynamic goals are beneficial,[18] expert opinion (and clinical intuition) suggests that hemodynamics and organ perfusion should be optimized.[15] Rapidly raising the blood pressure in patients who remain markedly hypotensive after ROSC is prudent, because postresuscitation arterial hypotension has been associated with sharply lower survival rate.[17] Whether or not postresuscitation hypotension has a cause-and-effect relationship with worse neurologic injury or is simply a marker of the severity of the I/R injury that has occurred remains unclear.

Regarding respiratory system support, exposure to hyperoxia (excessively high partial pressure of arterial oxygen [Pa_{O_2}]) has been associated with poor clinical outcome among adult patients resuscitated from cardiac arrest and admitted to an intensive care unit.[19] These data corroborate the findings of numerous laboratory studies in animal models in which hyperoxia exposure after ROSC worsens brain histopathologic changes and neurologic function.[20-24] A paradox may exist regarding oxygen delivery to the injured brain, where inadequate oxygen delivery can exacerbate cerebral I/R injury, but excessive oxygen delivery can accelerate formation of oxygen free radical and subsequent reperfusion injury. Although clinical data on this topic are few at the present time (and specifically no interventional studies have been performed), expert opinion advocates limiting unnecessary exposure to an excessively high postresuscitation Pa_{O_2} by titrating the fraction of inspired oxygen down after ROSC as much as possible to maintain an arterial oxygen saturation of 94% or more.[15]

Seizures are not uncommon after anoxic brain injury, and it is important to be vigilant in clinical assessment for any motor responses that could represent seizure activity so that they can be treated promptly with anticonvulsant medications. Continuous electroencephalography monitoring (if available) can be useful, especially if continuous administration of neuromuscular blocking agents becomes necessary for any reason.

CARDIAC CATHETERIZATION

Acute coronary syndrome is the most common cause of sudden cardiac arrest. Clinicians should have a high clinical suspicion of acute myocardial ischemia as the inciting event for the cardiac arrest when no other obvious cause of cardiac arrest is apparent. Although ST-segment myocardial infarction is an obvious indication for PCI, other more subtle electrocardiogram abnormalities may indicate that an acute ischemic event caused the cardiac arrest. In patients with no obvious noncardiac cause of cardiac arrest, a clinical suspicion of coronary ischemia, an abnormal electrocardiogram after ROSC, and consultation with an interventional cardiologist is warranted and coronary angiography should be considered. Recent studies and experience indicate that inducing hypothermia simultaneously with emergent PCI is feasible.

THERAPEUTIC HYPOTHERMIA

Therapeutic hypothermia (TH), also called mild therapeutic hypothermia or targeted temperature management, is a treatment strategy of rapidly reducing the patient's body temperature after ROSC for the purposes of protection from neurologic injury. The body temperature is typically reduced to 33° to 34° C for 12 to 24 hours. After ROSC the severity of the reperfusion injury can be mitigated, despite the fact that the initial ischemic injury has already occurred. Reperfusion injury refers to tissue and organ system injury that occurs when circulation is restored to tissues after a period of ischemia, and is characterized by inflammatory changes and oxidative damage that are in large part a consequence of oxidative stress. Neuronal cell death after I/R injury is not instantaneous, but rather a dynamic process. In animal models of cardiac arrest, brain histopathologic changes may not be found until 24 to 72 hours after cardiac arrest.[15] This indicates that a distinct therapeutic window of

Table 1.2 Therapeutic Hypothermia Versus Normothermia for Management of Comatose Survivors of Cardiac Arrest*

	Patient Response: No. Affected/Total			
Outcome Measure	Normothermia	Hypothermia	**Risk Ratio (95% CI)**†	***P* Value**‡
Favorable neurologic outcome§	54/137 (39%)	75/136 (55%)	1.40 (1.08-1.81)	0.009
Death	76/138 (55%)	56/137 (41%)	0.74 (0.58-0.95)	0.02

*Neurologic outcome and mortality rate at 6 months in a randomized trial of therapeutic hypothermia versus normothermia in comatose survivors of out-of-hospital cardiac arrest due to ventricular fibrillation or pulseless ventricular tachycardia.

†The risk ratio was calculated as the rate of a favorable neurologic outcome or the rate of death in the hypothermia group divided by the rate in the normothermia group. CI, confidence interval.

‡Two-sided *P* values are based on Pearson's chi square tests.

§A favorable neurologic outcome was defined as a cerebral performance category of 1 (good recovery) or 2 (moderate disability). One patient in the normothermia group and one in the hypothermia group were lost to neurologic follow-up.

Reprinted with permission from Hypothermia After Cardiac Arrest Study Group: Mild therapeutic hypothermia to improve the neurologic outcome after cardiac arrest. N Engl J Med 2002;346(8):549-556.

opportunity exists. In theory, TH may protect the brain by attenuating or reversing all of the following pathophysiologic processes: disruption of cerebral energy metabolism, mitochondrial dysfunction, loss of calcium ion homeostasis, cellular excitotoxicity, oxygen free radical generation, and apoptosis. Two clinical trials of TH were published in 2002.[25,26] These trials showed improved outcomes with TH for comatose survivors of witnessed out-of-hospital cardiac arrest with VF as the initial rhythm. The survival data for the largest of these clinical trials (i.e., the Hypothermia After Cardiac Arrest Study Group) appear in Table 1.2 and Figure 1.5.

The current AHA guidelines for CPR and emergency cardiovascular care recommend 12 to 24 hours of TH for comatose survivors of out-of-hospital cardiac arrest due to VF or pulseless VT.[16] TH may also be considered for victims of in-hospital cardiac arrest and other arrest rhythms. Figure 1.6 displays the AHA algorithm for post–cardiac arrest care including TH.[16]

Appropriate selection of candidates for TH is clearly important. If a patient does not follow verbal commands after ROSC is achieved, this indicates that the patient is at risk for brain injury and TH should be strongly considered. If a patient is clearly following commands immediately after ROSC, then significant brain injury is less likely and it is probably reasonable to withhold TH. There are multiple potential methods for inducing TH including specialized external or intravascular cooling devices for targeted temperature management, or a combination of conventional cooling methods such as ice packs, cooling blankets, and cold (4° C) IV saline infusion. Compared to the use of specialized cooling devices, overshoot (body temperature < 31° C) is a not uncommon occurrence with use of ice packs, cooling blankets, and cold saline.[27] Regardless of what method is used, effective achievement of target temperature may be aided by the use of a uniform physician order set for TH induction.[28] The current recommendation is to maintain TH for 12 to 24 hours.[16] Whether or not a longer duration of therapy could be beneficial is currently unknown.

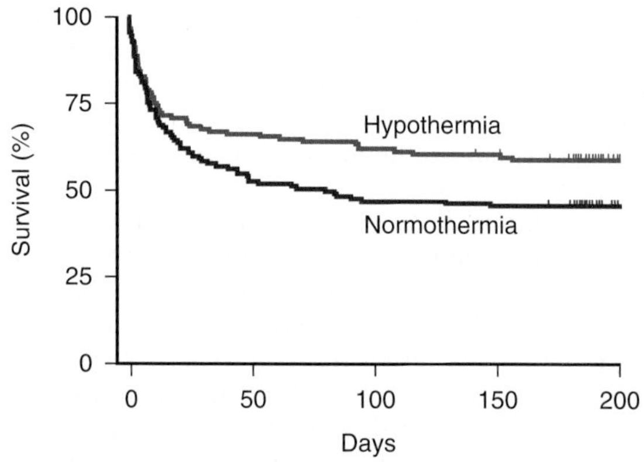

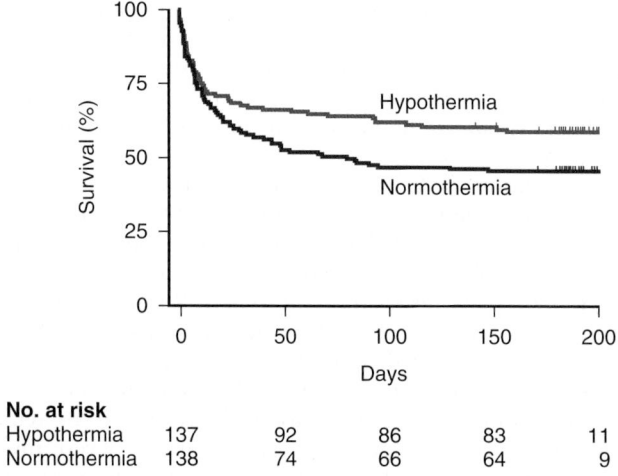

No. at risk					
Hypothermia	137	92	86	83	11
Normothermia	138	74	66	64	9

Figure 1.5 Cumulative survival in the normothermia and hypothermia groups from a randomized trial of therapeutic hypothermia in comatose survivors of out-of-hospital cardiac arrest due to ventricular fibrillation or pulseless ventricular tachycardia. Censored data are indicated by tick marks. (Reprinted with permission from Hypothermia After Cardiac Arrest Study Group: Mild therapeutic hypothermia to improve the neurologic outcome after cardiac arrest. N Engl J Med 2002;346(8):549-556.)

Shivering with TH induction is very common and should be anticipated. Shivering can be detrimental to the patient by making goal temperature more difficult (or impossible) to achieve. Therefore, immediate recognition and treatment of shivering is imperative. Adequate sedation and analgesics are an essential component of TH, especially the induction phase, and often the administration of additional sedative and opioid agents will be sufficient to ameliorate shivering. If shivering persists despite sedatives or opioid agents, neuromuscular blocking agents may be required. If neuromuscular blocking agents are used, they are often only necessary in the induction phase of TH when the temperature is dropping at a fast rate. Once target temperature is achieved, patients often stop shivering. It is prudent to try

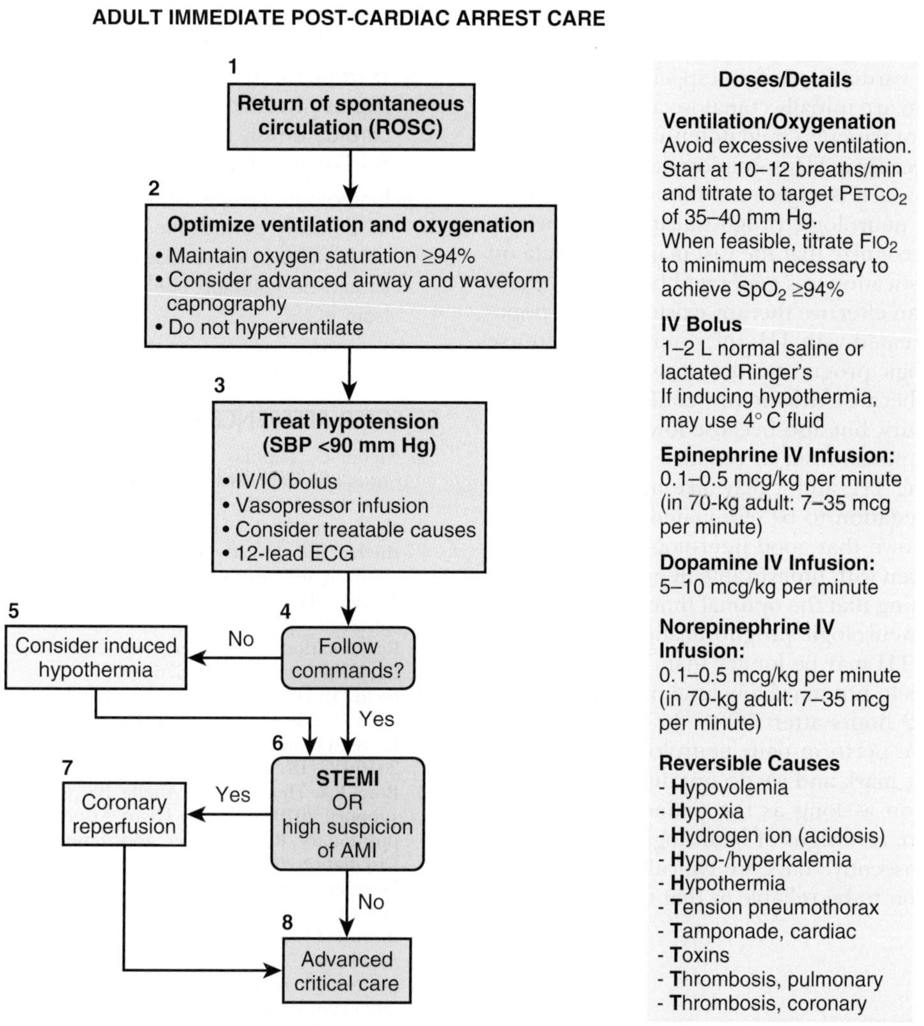

Figure 1.6 American Heart Association post–cardiac arrest care algorithm. AMI, acute myocardial infarction; ECG, electrocardiogram; IO, intraosseous; IV, intravenous; ROSC, return of spontaneous circulation; SBP, systolic blood pressure; STEMI, ST-segment elevation myocardial infarction. (Reprinted with permission from Peberdy MA, Callaway CW, Neumar RW, et al: Part 9: Post-cardiac arrest care: 2010 American Heart Association Guidelines for Cardiopulmonary Resuscitation and Emergency Cardiovascular Care. Circulation 2010;122(18 Suppl 3):S768-786.)

to limit neuromuscular blocking agents to the induction phase of TH, and they likely can be withheld thereafter. Unnecessarily prolonged neuromuscular blockade should be avoided because prolonged neuromuscular weakness may persist after discontinuation and could potentially make the patient's neurologic assessment at a later time point more challenging. When using neuromuscular blocking agents for the induction of TH, their administration may be titrated to the resolution of shivering rather than complete paralysis, which may result in the administration of a much lower dose of neuromuscular blocker.

A number of potential complications are possible with TH including bradycardia, a "cold diuresis" resulting in hypovolemia and electrolyte derangements, hyperglycemia, coagulopathy, and perhaps increased risk of secondary infection. However, these potential complications are often not severe when they do occur, and in terms of risk-benefit determinations, the risk of anoxic brain injury usually greatly outweighs the risks of complications.

If TH is not initiated, fever must be avoided. Fever is not uncommon in the post–cardiac arrest population because of the intense proinflammatory response to I/R and must be treated aggressively with antipyretic therapies and other techniques (e.g., cooling blankets). Fever is clearly detrimental in brain-injured patients because it increases cerebral metabolic rate.

NEUROLOGIC PROGNOSTICATION

Neurologic prognostication is often extremely difficult in the first few days after resuscitation from cardiac arrest.[29] Although some neurologic examination findings may suggest poor prognosis, few of these signs on examination are sufficiently reliable upon which to base treatment decisions (e.g., support withdrawal). These critically important decisions should hinge on neurologic examination findings in which the false-positive rate (FPR) (i.e., the rate of predicting a poor outcome that ultimately proves not to be poor) approaches zero. An abundance of clinical data exists on neurologic assessment after cardiac arrest, and few examination findings have a sufficiently low false-positive rate in the first 72 hours after ROSC to form the basis of a limitation of support decision.[15,30] In particular, neurologic prognostication immediately (e.g., first 24 hours) after resuscitation from cardiac arrest is especially unreliable. Among patients who are initially comatose after ROSC, one quarter to one half of patients could potentially have a favorable outcome, especially if TH is employed. In general, the recommended approach is to wait a minimum of 72 hours after ROSC before neurologic prognostication.[30] However, it is important to recognize that the vast majority of data on neurologic prognostication was generated before the era of TH, that is, before an effective therapy existed. In the population of patients treated with TH, the optimal time course for making neurologic prognostication may be significantly different, not only because the therapy could modulate the degree of brain injury, but also because low body temperature decreases the metabolism of sedative agents that are typically used during TH, and it may take much longer for the effects of the sedation to be eliminated. Recently published data have shown that good neurologic outcome can potentially occur even with unfavorable neurologic findings at 72 hours, suggesting that the optimal time interval to wait before attempting neurologic prognostication in the population treated with TH may be longer than 72 hours.[31] Our general approach is to not make any final neurologic prognostication until 72 hours after ROSC. In the population treated with TH, we perform daily neurologic assessments beyond the 72-hour mark and we do not make final neurologic prognostication as long as the patient continues to improve. If there are zero signs of neurologic improvement over 2 or more consecutive days, we typically deem neurologic prognostication to be reliable at that time.

KEY POINTS

- The quality of CPR (especially in quality of and minimization of interruptions in chest compressions) is probably the single most important treatment-related determinant of outcome from cardiac arrest. Therefore, *"push hard, push fast."*
- Cellular damage from ischemia/reperfusion injury is a dynamic process, and a therapeutic window exists after resuscitation from cardiac arrest in which the effects can be attenuated.

KEY POINTS (Continued)

- Therapeutic hypothermia is the first proven therapy to improve neurologic outcome after resuscitation from cardiac arrest, indicating that brain injury related to cardiac arrest is in fact a treatable condition.
- Neurologic prognostication is notoriously challenging in the early period after resuscitation from cardiac arrest, and in most cases attempts at prognostication should be withheld until at least the 72-hour mark from ROSC.

SELECTED REFERENCES

1. Nichol G, Thomas E, Callaway CW, et al: Regional variation in out-of-hospital cardiac arrest incidence and outcome. JAMA 2008;300(12):1423-1431.
2. Nadkarni VM, Larkin GL, Peberdy MA, et al: First documented rhythm and clinical outcome from in-hospital cardiac arrest among children and adults. JAMA 2006;295(1):50-57.
3. Travers AH, Rea TD, Bobrow BJ, et al: Part 4: CPR overview: 2010 American Heart Association Guidelines for Cardiopulmonary Resuscitation and Emergency Cardiovascular Care. Circulation 2010;122(18 Suppl 3):S676-S684.
4. Field JM, Hazinski MF, Sayre MR, et al: Part 1: Executive summary: 2010 American Heart Association Guidelines for Cardiopulmonary Resuscitation and Emergency Cardiovascular Care. Circulation 2010;122(18 Suppl 3):S640-S656.
5. Berg RA, Hemphill R, Abella BS, et al: Part 5: Adult basic life support: 2010 American Heart Association Guidelines for Cardiopulmonary Resuscitation and Emergency Cardiovascular Care. Circulation 2010;122(18 Suppl 3):S685-S705.
6. Manders S, Geijsel FE: Alternating providers during continuous chest compressions for cardiac arrest: Every minute or every two minutes? Resuscitation 2009;80(9):1015-1018.
7. Abella BS, Alvarado JP, Myklebust H, et al: Quality of cardiopulmonary resuscitation during in-hospital cardiac arrest. JAMA 2005;293(3):305-310.
8. Edelson DP, Abella BS, Kramer-Johansen J, et al: Effects of compression depth and pre-shock pauses predict defibrillation failure during cardiac arrest. Resuscitation 2006;71(2):137-145.
9. Kitamura T, Iwami T, Kawamura T, et al: Conventional and chest-compression-only cardiopulmonary resuscitation by bystanders for children who have out-of-hospital cardiac arrests: A prospective, nationwide, population-based cohort study. Lancet 2010;375(9723):1347-1354.
10. Hupfl M, Selig HF, Nagele P: Chest-compression-only versus standard cardiopulmonary resuscitation: A meta-analysis. Lancet 2010;376(9752):1552-1557.

The complete list of references can be found at www.expertconsult.com.

2

Airway Management in the Critically Ill Adult

G. G. Lavery | T. R. Craig

CHAPTER OUTLINE

Appropriate management of the airway is the cornerstone of good resuscitation. It requires judgment (airway assessment), skill (airway maneuvers), and constant reassessment of the patient's condition. Although complex procedures sometimes are lifesaving and always carry the potential to impress, the timely use of simple airway maneuvers often is very effective and may avoid the need for further intervention.

STRUCTURE AND FUNCTION OF THE NORMAL AIRWAY

Critical care staff members require an understanding of structure and function in order to successfully manage the airway and the conditions that may affect it. The relevant information can be gained from a variety of sources.[1-5] The airway begins at the nose and oral cavity and continues as the pharynx and larynx, which lead to the trachea (beginning at the lower edge of the cricoid cartilage) and then the bronchial tree. The airway[1] provides a pathway for airflow between the atmosphere and the lungs;[2] facilitates filtering, humidification, and heating of ambient air before it reaches the lower airway;[3] prevents nongaseous material from entering the lower airway;[6] and allows phonation by controlling the flow of air through the larynx and oropharynx.[4]

THE NOSE

The nose has a midline septum separating two cavities that communicate externally via the external nares (nostrils). Each cavity has a roof formed by the nasal cartilages, frontal bones, cribriform plate, ethmoid, and body of sphenoid. Portions of the maxilla and palatine bones make up the nasal floor (which also forms part of the roof of the oral cavity). The medial wall of each nasal cavity is formed by the nasal septum, the vomer, and ethmoid bones. The lateral wall lies medial to the orbit, the ethmoid, and maxillary sinuses and has three horizontal bony projections—the superior, middle, and inferior nasal conchae. These structures greatly increase the surface area, and the overlying mucosa is highly vascular, supplied by the maxillary arterial branch of the external carotid artery and the ethmoidal branch of the ophthalmic artery. The (nonolfactory) sensory innervation of the nasal mucosa is supplied by two divisions of the trigeminal nerve.

THE ORAL CAVITY

The teeth form the lateral wall of the oral cavity, while the floor is the tongue—a mass of horizontal, vertical, and transverse muscle bundles attached to the mandible and the hyoid bone. The sulcus terminalis, a V-shaped groove, divides the anterior two thirds of the tongue (sensory innervation from the lingual nerve and taste from the chordae tympani) from the posterior one third (sensory supply from the glossopharyngeal nerve). All intrinsic and extrinsic muscles of the tongue are supplied by the hypoglossal nerve, except the palatoglossus, which is supplied by the vagus nerve.

THE PHARYNX

The adult pharynx is a midline structure, running anterior to the cervical prevertebral fascia, from the base of the skull to the level of the sixth cervical vertebra (approximately 14 cm), and continuing as the esophagus. It is a muscular tube with three portions: the nasopharynx, oropharynx, and laryngopharynx (or hypopharynx). It contains three groups of lymphoid tissue: the adenoids, the pharyngeal tonsil (on the posterior wall), and the palatine (lingual) tonsils and has the inner opening of the eustachian tube on each lateral wall. The vagus nerve supplies all but one of the pharyngeal muscles. Sensory supply is via branches of the glossopharyngeal and vagus nerves. The pharynx provides a common pathway for the upper alimentary and respiratory tracts and is concerned with swallowing and phonation.

THE LARYNX

The larynx sits anterior to the laryngopharynx and the fourth to the sixth cervical vertebrae and is posterior to the infrahyoid muscles, the deep cervical fascia, and the subcutaneous fat and skin that cover the front of the neck. Laterally lie the lobes of the thyroid gland and carotid sheath. The larynx acts as a sphincter at the upper end of the respiratory tract and is the organ of phonation. The epiglottis and the thyroid, cricoid, and paired arytenoid, cuneiform, and corniculate cartilages, together with the interconnecting ligaments, make up the skeleton of the larynx, which has a volume of 4 mL. Two pairs of parallel horizontal folds project into the lumen of the larynx—the false vocal cords (lying superiorly) and the true vocal cords (inferiorly). The opening between the true cords is called the glottis. The larynx communicates above with the laryngopharynx and below with the trachea, which begins at the lower edge of the cricoid ring.

The superior aspect of the epiglottis is innervated by the glossopharyngeal nerve, whereas the vagus, via its superior laryngeal nerve (SLN) and recurrent laryngeal nerve (RLN) branches, innervates the larynx, including the inferior surface of the epiglottis. The external (motor) branch of the SLN supplies the cricothyroid muscle, and the internal branch is the sensory supply to the larynx down to the vocal cords. The RLN supplies all of the intrinsic laryngeal muscles and is the sensory supply to the larynx below the cords. Injury to the SLN causes hoarseness secondary to a loss of tension in the ipsilateral vocal cord. Complete unilateral RLN palsy inactivates both ipsilateral adductor and abductor muscles. Vocal cord adduction, however, is maintained by the unopposed SLN-innervated cricothyroid muscle. With bilateral RLN palsy, both cords are in adduction as a result of the unopposed action of the cricothyroid muscle. On inspiration, the adducted vocal cords then act like a Venturi device, generating a negative pressure that pulls the cords together, producing inspiratory stridor—the characteristic sign of upper airway obstruction. Laryngospasm, a severe form of airway obstruction, may be triggered by mechanical stimulation of the larynx or by cord irritation due to aspiration of oral secretions, blood, or vomitus.

In health, the laryngeal abductor muscles contract early in inspiration, separating the vocal cords and facilitating airflow into the tracheobronchial tree. Movements of the thyroid and arytenoid cartilages alter the length and tension of the vocal cords, and sliding and rotational movements of the arytenoid cartilages can alter the shape of the glottic opening between the vocal cords. Fine control of the muscles producing these movements allows vocalization as air passes between the vocal cords in expiration. The sound volume is increased by resonance in the sinuses of the face and skull.

THE TRACHEOBRONCHIAL TREE

The trachea is a fibrous tube, 2 cm in diameter, running in the midline for 10 to 15 cm from the level of the sixth cervical vertebra to its bifurcation (carina) at the level of the fourth thoracic vertebra. The walls include 15 to 20 incomplete cartilaginous rings limited posteriorly by fibroelastic tissue and smooth muscle.

The cervical trachea lies anterior to the esophagus, with the RLN in the groove between the two. Anteriorly lie the cervical fascia, infrahyoid muscles, isthmus of the thyroid, and the jugular venous arch. Laterally lie the lobes of the thyroid gland and the carotid sheath. In the thorax, the trachea is traversed anteriorly by the brachiocephalic artery and vein (which may be damaged or eroded by the tracheostomy tube). To the left are the common carotid and subclavian arteries and the aortic arch. To the right are the vagus nerve, the azygos vein, and the pleurae. The carina lies anterior to the esophagus behind the bifurcation of the pulmonary trunk.

The bronchial tree is similar in structure to the trachea. Two main bronchi diverge from the carina. The right main bronchus is shorter, wider, and more vertical and runs close to the pulmonary artery and the azygos vein. The left main bronchus passes under the arch of the aorta, anterior to the esophagus, thoracic duct, and descending aorta.[7]

OVERVIEW OF AIRWAY FUNCTION

In the nose, inspired gas is filtered, humidified, and warmed before entering the lungs. Resistance to gas flow through the nose is twice that of the mouth, explaining the need to mouth-breathe during exercise when gas flows are high. Warming and humidification continue in the pharynx and tracheobronchial tree. Between the trachea and the alveolar sacs, airways divide 23 times. This network increases the cross-sectional area for the gas exchange process but also reduces the velocity of gas flow. Hairs on the nasal mucosa filter inspired air, trapping particles greater than 10 μm in diameter. Many particles settle on the nasal epithelium. Particles 2 to 10 μm in diameter fall on the mucus-covered bronchial walls (as airflow slows), initiating reflex bronchoconstriction and coughing. Ciliated columnar epithelium lines the respiratory tract from the nose to the respiratory bronchioles (except at the vocal cords). The cilia beat at a frequency of 1000 to 1500 cycles per minute, enabling them to move particles away from the lungs at a rate of 16 mm per minute. Particles less than 2 μm in diameter may reach the alveoli, where they are ingested by macrophages. If ciliary motility is defective as a result of smoking or an inherited disorder (e.g., Kartagener's syndrome or another ciliary dysmotility syndrome), the "mucus escalator" does not work, so more particles are allowed to reach the alveoli, thereby predisposing the patient to chronic pulmonary inflammation.[8]

The larynx prevents food and other foreign bodies from entering the trachea. Reflex closure of the glottic inlet occurs during swallowing[6] and periods of increased intrathoracic (e.g., coughing, sneezing) or intra-abdominal (e.g., vomiting, micturition) pressure. In unconscious patients, these reflexes are lost, so glottic closure may not occur, increasing the risk of pulmonary aspiration.

ASSESSING ADEQUACY OF THE AIRWAY

Adequacy of the airway should be considered in four aspects:

- *Patency.* Partial or complete obstruction will compromise ventilation of the lungs and likewise gas exchange.
- *Protective reflexes.* These reflexes help maintain patency and prevent aspiration of material into the lower airways.
- *Inspired oxygen concentration.* Gas entering the pulmonary alveoli must have an appropriate oxygen concentration.
- *Respiratory drive.* A patent, secure airway is of little benefit without the movement of gas between the atmosphere and the pulmonary alveoli effected through the processes of inspiration and expiration.

PATENCY

Airway obstruction most frequently is due to reduced muscle tone, allowing the tongue to fall backward against the postpharyngeal wall, thereby blocking the airway. Loss of patency by this mechanism often occurs in an obtunded or anesthetized patient lying supine. Other causes include the presence of blood, mucus, vomitus, or a foreign body in the lumen of the airway or edema, inflammation, swelling, or enlargement of the tissues lining or adjacent to the airway.

Upper airway obstruction has a characteristic presentation in the spontaneously breathing patient: noisy inspiration (stridor), poor expired airflow, intercostal retraction, increased respiratory distress, and paradoxical rocking movements of the thorax and abdomen.[9] These resolve quickly if the obstruction is removed. In total airway obstruction, sounds of breathing are absent entirely, owing to complete lack of airflow through the larynx. Airway obstruction may occur in patients with an endotracheal tube (ET) or tracheostomy tube in situ due to mucous plugging or kinking of the tube or the patient's biting down on a tube placed orally. If such patients are spontaneously breathing, they will have the same symptoms and signs just described. Patients on assisted (positive-pressure) breathing modes will have high inflation pressures, decreased tidal and minute volumes, increased end-tidal carbon dioxide levels, and decreased arterial oxygen saturation.

PROTECTIVE REFLEXES

The upper airway shares a common pathway with the upper gastrointestinal tract.[6] Protective reflexes, which exist to safeguard airway patency and to prevent foreign material from entering the lower respiratory tract, involve the epiglottis, the vocal cords, and the sensory supply to the pharynx and larynx.[10] Patients who can swallow normally have intact airway reflexes, and normal speech makes absence of such reflexes unlikely. Patients with a decreased level of consciousness (LOC) should be assumed to have inadequate protective reflexes.

INSPIRED OXYGEN CONCENTRATION

Oxygen demand is elevated by the increased work of breathing associated with respiratory distress[11] and by the increased metabolic demands in critically ill or injured patients. Often, higher inspired oxygen concentrations are required to satisfy tissue oxygen demand and to prevent critical desaturations during maneuvers for managing the airway. A cuffed ET, connected to a supply of oxygen, is a sealed system in which the delivered oxygen concentration also is the inspired concentration. A patient wearing a facemask, however, inspires gas from the mask and surrounding ambient air. Because the patient will generate an initial inspiratory flow in the region of 30 to 60 L per minute, and the fresh gas flow to a mask is on the order of 5 to 15 L per minute, much of the tidal inspiration will be "room air" entrained from around the mask. The entrained room air is likely to dilute the concentration of oxygen inspired to less than 50%, even when 100% oxygen is delivered to the mask.[12] This unwelcome reduction in inspired oxygen concentration can be mitigated by (1) using a mask with a reservoir bag, (2) ensuring that the mask is fitted firmly to the patient's face, (3) using a high rate of oxygen flow to the mask (15 L per minute), and (4) supplying a higher oxygen concentration if not already using 100%.

RESPIRATORY DRIVE

A patent, protected airway will not produce adequate oxygenation or excretion of carbon dioxide without adequate respiratory drive. Changing arterial carbon dioxide tension (PCO_2), by changing H^+ concentration in cerebrospinal fluid (CSF), stimulates the respiratory center, which in turn controls minute volume and therefore arterial PCO_2 (negative feedback).[11,13] This assumes that increased respiratory drive can produce an increase in minute ventilation (increased respiratory rate or tidal volume, or both, per breath), which may not occur if respiratory mechanics are disturbed. Brain injury and drugs such as opioids, sedatives, and alcohol are direct-acting respiratory center depressants.

Ventilation can be assessed qualitatively by looking, listening, and feeling. In a spontaneously breathing patient, listening to (and feeling) air movement while looking at the extent, nature, and frequency of thoracic movement will give an impression of ventilation. These parameters may be misleading, however. Objective assessment of minute ventilation requires PCO_2 measurement in arterial blood or monitoring of end-tidal carbon dioxide, which can be used as a real-time measure of the adequacy of minute ventilation.[13] If respiratory drive or minute ventilation is inadequate, positive-pressure respiratory support may be required, and any underlying factors should be addressed if possible (e.g., depressant effect of sedatives or analgesics).

MANAGEMENT OF THE AIRWAY

The aims of airway management are to provide an adequate inspired oxygen concentration; to establish a patent, secure airway; and to support ventilation if required.

PROVIDING AN ADEQUATE INSPIRED OXYGEN CONCENTRATION

Although oxygen can be administered via nasal cannula, this method does not ensure delivery of more than 30% to 40% oxygen (at most). Other disadvantages include lack of humidification of gases, patient discomfort with use of flow rates greater than 4 to 6 L per minute, and predisposition to nasal mucosal irritation and potential bleeding.[14] Therefore, despite being more intrusive for patients, facemasks are superior for oxygen administration. The three main types of facemasks are shown in Figure 2.1:

- The anesthesia-type facemask (mask A in Fig. 2.1) is a solid mask (with no vents) with a cushioned collar to provide a good seal. It is suitable for providing very high oxygen concentrations (approaching 100%) because entrainment is minimized and the anesthetic circuit normally includes a reservoir of gas. These masks become unacceptable for many *awake* patients within a few minutes because of the association with heat, moisture, and claustrophobia.
- The simple facemask has vents that allow heat or humidity out but that also entrain room air. These masks have no seal and are relatively loose-fitting. Such masks may have a reservoir bag (approximately 500 mL) sitting inferior to the mask (B2 in Fig. 2.1), or may have no reservoir (B1 in Fig. 2.1). Using a simple facemask, without a reservoir bag, it is difficult to deliver an inspired oxygen concentration in excess of 50% even with tight application and 100% oxygen flow to the mask. Under the same conditions, a simple mask with a reservoir bag can produce an inspired oxygen concentration of about 80%.
- The Venturi mask (C in Fig. 2.1) has vents that entrain a known proportion of ambient air when a set flow of 100% oxygen passes through a Venturi device.[14] Thus, the inspired oxygen concentration (usually 24% to 35%) is known.

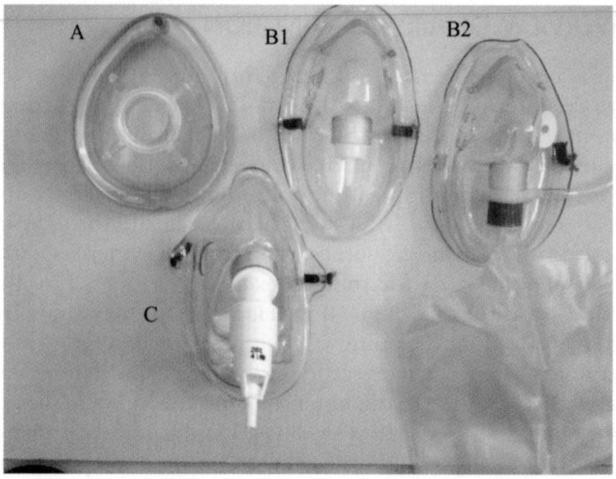

Figure 2.1 Facemasks: anesthesia mask (**A**); simple facemask (**B1**); simple facemask with reservoir bag (**B2**); Venturi mask (**C**).

ESTABLISHING A PATENT AND SECURE AIRWAY

Establishing a patent and secure airway can be achieved using simple airway maneuvers, further airway adjuncts, tracheal intubation, or a surgical airway.

AIRWAY MANEUVERS

Simple airway maneuvers involve appropriate positioning, opening the airway, and keeping it open using artificial airways if needed.

Positioning for Airway Management

In the absence of any concerns about cervical spine stability (e.g., with trauma, rheumatoid arthritis, or severe osteoporosis), raising the patient's head slightly (5 to 10 cm) by means of a small pillow under the occiput can help in airway management. This adjustment extends the atlanto-occipital joint and moves the oral, pharyngeal, and laryngeal axes into better alignment, providing the best straight line to the glottis ("sniffing" position).[15,16]

Clearing the Airway

Acute airway obstruction in the obtunded patient often due to the tongue or extraneous material—liquid (saliva, blood, gastric contents) or solid (teeth, broken dentures, food)—in the pharynx. In the supine position, secretions usually are cleared under direct vision using a laryngoscope and a rigid suction catheter.[17] In some cases, a flexible suction catheter, introduced through the nose and nasopharynx, may be the best means of clearing the airway. A finger sweep

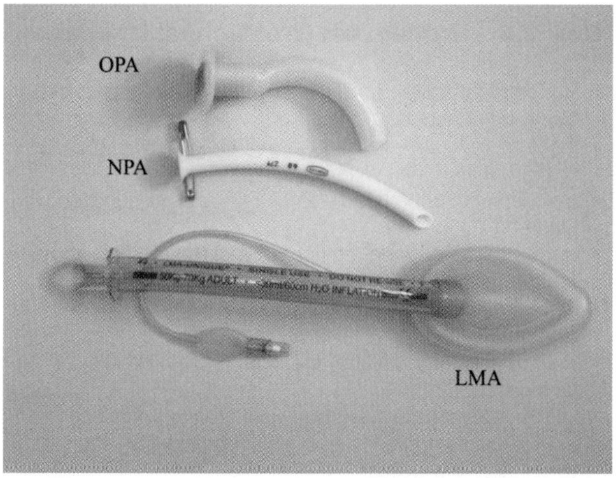

Figure 2.2 Artificial airways: oropharyngeal airway (OPA); nasopharyngeal airway (NPA); laryngeal mask airway (LMA).

Box 2.1 Contraindications to Insertion of Oropharyngeal and Nasopharyngeal Airways

Contraindications to Oropharyngeal Airways

Inability to tolerate (gagging, vomiting)
Airway swelling (burns, toxic gases, infection)
Bleeding into the upper airway
Absence of pharyngeal or laryngeal reflexes
Impaired mouth opening (e.g., with trismus or temporomandibular joint dysfunction)

Contraindications to Nasopharyngeal Airways

Narrow nasal airway in young children
Blocked or narrow nasal passages in adults
Airway swelling (burns, toxic gases, infection)
Bleeding into the upper airway
Absence of pharyngeal or laryngeal reflexes
Fractures of the midface or base of skull
Clinical scenarios in which nasal hemorrhage would be disastrous

of the pharynx may be used to detect and remove larger solid material in unconscious patients without an intact gag reflex. During all airway interventions, if cervical spine instability cannot be ruled out, relative movement of the cervical vertebrae must be prevented—most often by manual inline immobilization.[17,18]

Triple Airway Maneuver

The triple airway maneuver often is beneficial in obtunded patients if it is not contraindicated by concerns about cervical spine instability. As indicated by its name, this maneuver has three components: head tilt (neck extension), jaw thrust (pulling the mandible forward), and mouth opening.[19] The operator stands behind and above the patient's head. Then the maneuver is performed as follows:

- Extend the patient's neck with the operator's hands on both sides of the mandible.
- Elevate the mandible with the fingers of both hands, thereby lifting the base of the tongue away from the posterior pharyngeal wall.
- Open the mouth by pressing caudally on the anterior mandible with the thumbs or forefingers.

Artificial Airways

If the triple airway maneuver or any of its elements reduces airway obstruction, the benefit can be maintained for a prolonged period by introducing an artificial airway into the pharynx between the tongue and the posterior pharyngeal wall (Fig. 2.2).

The oropharyngeal airway (OPA) is the most commonly used artificial airway. Simple to insert, it is used temporarily to help facilitate oxygenation or ventilation before tracheal intubation. The OPA should be inserted with the convex side toward the tongue and then rotated through 180 degrees. Care must be taken to avoid pushing the tongue posteriorly, thereby worsening the obstruction. The nasopharyngeal airway (NPA) has the same indications as for the OPA but significantly more contraindications[20] (Box 2.1). It is better tolerated than the OPA, making it useful in semiconscious patients in whom the gag reflex is partially preserved. These artificial airways should be considered to be a temporary adjunct—to be replaced with a more secure airway if the patient fails to improve rapidly to the point at which an artificial airway no longer is needed. Such airways should not be used in association with *prolonged* positive-pressure ventilation.

ADVANCED AIRWAY ADJUNCTS

Advanced airway adjuncts fill the gap between simple airway maneuvers and the insertion of a tracheal tube or surgical airway. These devices can be used to facilitate safe reliable airway management and manual ventilation in the prehospital or emergency resuscitation setting, often without expert medical presence.

The laryngeal mask airway (LMA) is a small latex mask mounted on a hollow plastic tube.[21-26] It is placed "blindly" in the lower pharynx overlying the glottis. The inflatable cuff helps wedge the mask in the hypopharynx, sitting obliquely over the laryngeal inlet. Although the LMA produces a seal that will allow ventilation with gentle positive pressure, it does not definitively protect the airway from aspiration. Indications for use of the LMA in critical care are (1) as an alternative to other artificial airways, (2) the difficult airway, particularly the "can't intubate–can't ventilate" scenario, and (3) as a conduit for bronchoscopy. It is possible to pass a 6.0-mm ET through a standard LMA into the trachea, but the LMA must be left in situ. The intubating LMA (ILMA), which was developed specifically to aid intubation with a tracheal tube, has a shorter steel tube with a wider bore, a tighter curve, and a distal silicone laryngeal cuff.[27-30] A bar present near the laryngeal opening is designed to lift the epiglottis anteriorly. The ILMA allows the passage of a specially designed size 8.0 ET.

In recent years, many modified LMAs have reached clinical practice. They have been designed with the intention of promoting easier insertion, improving reliability of the laryngeal seal, and allowing safe gastric drainage of gastric fluid.

Box 2.2 Orotracheal Intubation: Indications and Relative Contraindications

Indications

Long-term correction or prevention of airway obstruction
Securing the airway and protecting against pulmonary aspiration
Facilitating positive-pressure ventilation
Enabling bronchopulmonary toilet
Optimizing access to pharynx, face, or neck at surgery

Contraindications (Relative)

Possibility of cervical spine instability
Impaired mouth opening (e.g., trismus, temporomandibular joint dysfunction)
Potential difficult airway
Need for surgical immobilization of maxilla or mandible (wires, box frame)

Box 2.3 Procedure: Orotracheal Intubation

- Position patient and induce anesthesia ± neuromuscular blockade (if needed).
- Perform manual ventilation using triple airway maneuver and oropharyngeal airway
- Hold laryngoscope handle (left hand) near the junction with blade.
- Insert the blade along the right side of the tongue—moving tongue to the left.
- Advance tip of the blade in the midline between tongue and epiglottis.
- Pull upward and along the line of the handle of the laryngoscope.
- Lift the epiglottis upward and visualize the vocal cords.
- Do *not* use the patient's teeth as a fulcrum when attempting to visualize the glottis.
- Stop advancing tube when cuff is 2 to 3 cm beyond the cords.
- Connect to a bag-valve system and pressurize it by squeezing bag.
- Inflate cuff until audible leak around tube stops.
- Check correct tube position (auscultation) and assess cuff pressure.
- Check end-tidal CO_2 trace.

The Combitube (esophageal-tracheal double-lumen airway) is a combined esophageal obturator and tracheal tube, usually inserted blindly.[31-35] Whether the "tracheal" lumen is placed in the trachea or esophagus, the Combitube will allow ventilation of the lungs and give partial protection against aspiration. The Combitube also is a potential adjunct in the "cannot intubate–cannot ventilate" situation. Disadvantages include the inability to suction the trachea when the device is sitting in its most common position (in the esophagus). Insertion also may cause trauma, and the Combitube is contraindicated in patients with known esophageal disease or injury or intact laryngeal reflexes and in persons who have ingested caustic substances.

TRACHEAL INTUBATION

If the foregoing interventions are not effective or are contraindicated, tracheal intubation is required. This modality will provide (1) a secure, potentially long-term airway; (2) a safe route to deliver positive-pressure ventilation if required; and (3) significant protection against pulmonary aspiration. *Orotracheal intubation* is the most widely used technique for clinicians practiced in direct laryngoscopy (indications and contraindications in Box 2.2). Normally, anesthesia with or without neuromuscular blockade is necessary for this procedure, which is summarized in Box 2.3.

Tracheal intubation requires lack of patient awareness (as in the unconscious state or with general anesthesia) and the abolition of protective laryngeal and pharyngeal reflexes. The drugs commonly used to achieve these states are shown in Table 2.1. Anesthesia is achieved using an intravenous induction agent, although intravenous sedatives (e.g., midazolam) theoretically may be used. Opioids often are used in conjunction with induction agents because they may reduce the cardiovascular sequelae of laryngoscopy and intubation (tachycardia and hypertension) and may contribute to the patient's unconsciousness.

Abolition of protective laryngeal and pharyngeal reflexes sometimes is achieved by inducing a deep level of unconsciousness using one or more of the aforementioned agents, followed by inhalation of high concentrations of a volatile anesthetic agent (e.g., sevoflurane, isoflurane). This technique sometimes is used in the difficult airway scenario to obtain conditions suitable for tracheal intubation in a patient who is still breathing spontaneously.

Table 2.1 Drugs Used to Facilitate Tracheal Intubation

Drug	Dose (Intravenous)
Induction Agent	
Propofol	1-2.5 mg/kg
Opioids	
Fentanyl	1.0-1.5 μg/kg
Morphine	0.15 mg/kg
Nondepolarizing Agents	
Atracurium	0.4-0.5 mg/kg
Vecuronium	0.1 mg/kg
Rocuronium	0.45-0.6 mg/kg
Depolarizing Agent	
Succinylcholine (suxamethonium)	1.0-1.5 mg/kg

More often, a muscle relaxant is used to abolish the protective reflexes, abduct the vocal cords, and facilitate tracheal intubation. In the elective situation, nondepolarizing neuromuscular blocking agents are used. These drugs have the disadvantage of requiring several minutes to exert their effect, during which the patient must receive ventilation via a mask, thus allowing the possibility of gastric dilation and pulmonary aspiration. In patients at high risk of the latter (e.g., nonfasting patients), a depolarizing muscle relaxant (succinylcholine) is used because it produces suitable

Box 2.4 Procedure: Nasotracheal Intubation (Blind and Under Direct Vision)

Preparation and Assessment of the Patient

1. Use a nasal decongestant such as phenylephrine to reduce bleeding.
2. Provide local anesthesia to the nasal mucosa.
3. Examine each nostril for patency and deformity.
4. Choose the most patent nostril, and use an appropriate-size ET.
5. After induction of anesthesia, position the head and neck as for oral intubation.

Blind Nasotracheal Intubation	*Nasotracheal Intubation (Direct Vision)*
• Keep patient breathing spontaneously.	• Patient may be apneic with or without relaxants.
• Insert well-lubricated ET into the nostril (concavity forward, bevel lateral).	• Gently advance ET through the nose.
• While passing ET along nasal floor, listen for audible breathing through the tube.	• When ET tip is in oropharynx, perform laryngoscopy.
• Advance ET, rotating as needed to maintain clear breath sounds.	• Visualize ET in pharynx and advance toward glottis.
• ET will pass through cords, and patient may cough.	• Advance ET through cords into trachea, under direct vision if possible.
• Technique takes time, so it is not suitable for a patient experiencing desaturation.	• Use Magill forceps if required to guide tip while advancing ET.
• Do not force passage of ET, because this could cause bleeding.	• Try to avoid damaging cuff if using forceps to help passage through cords.

ET, endotracheal tube.

conditions for intubation within 15 to 20 seconds, and mask ventilation is not required. Succinylcholine has several side effects—among them hyperkalemia, muscle pains, and (rarely) malignant hyperpyrexia.

Nasotracheal intubation shares the problems and contraindications associated with the NPA.[20] The technique usually is employed when there are relative contraindications to the oral route (e.g., anatomic abnormalities, cervical spine instability). Nasotracheal intubation may be achieved under direct vision or with use of a blind technique, either with the patient under general anesthesia or in the awake or lightly sedated patient with appropriate local anesthesia (Box 2.4). If orotracheal or nasotracheal intubation is required but cannot be achieved, then a surgical airway is required (see later).

With a need for isolation of one lung from another, a double-lumen tube (having one cuffed tracheal lumen and one cuffed bronchial lumen fused longitudinally) can be used.[36] The main indications are (1) to facilitate some pulmonary or thoracic surgical procedures; (2) to isolate a lung containing contaminated fluid (e.g., in lung abscess) or blood, thereby preventing contralateral spread; and (3) to enable differential or independent lung ventilation (ILV). ILV allows each lung to be treated separately—for example, to deliver positive-pressure ventilation with high positive end-expiratory pressure (PEEP) to one lung while applying low levels of continuous positive airway pressure (CPAP) only to the other. Such a strategy may be advantageous in cases of pulmonary air leak (bronchopleural fistula, bronchial tear, or severe lung trauma) or in severe unilateral lung disease requiring ventilatory support.[37,38]

PROVIDING VENTILATORY SUPPORT

If a patient has no (or inadequate) spontaneous ventilation, then a means of generating gas flow to the lower respiratory tract must be provided. Negative pressure, mimicking the actions of the respiratory muscles, occasionally is used in some patients who require long-term ventilation. In acute care, however, ventilation is achieved using positive pressure, which requires an unobstructed airway; in the nonintubated patient, this is best achieved by proper positioning, the triple airway maneuver, and use of an OPA or NPA. In a patient without an ET in place, particularly if some degree of airway obstruction exists, positive-pressure ventilation often will cause gastric distention and (potentially) regurgitation and pulmonary aspiration.

BAG-VALVE-MASK VENTILATION

Ventilation with a mask requires an (almost) airtight fit between mask and face. This is best achieved by firmly pressing the mask against the patient's face using the thumb and index finger (C-grip) while pulling the mandible upward toward the mask with the other three fingers. The other hand is used to squeeze the reservoir bag, generating positive pressure. Excessive pressure from the C-grip on the mask may lead to backward movement of the mandible with subsequent airway obstruction, or a tilt of the mask with leakage of gas. If a proper seal is difficult to attain, placing a hand on each side of the mask and mandible is advised, with a second person manually compressing the reservoir bag (four-handed ventilation). Bag-valve-mask systems have a self-reinflating bag, which springs back after compression, thereby drawing gas in through a port with a one-way valve. It is important to have a large reservoir bag with a continuous flow of oxygen attached to this port in order to ensure a high inspired oxygen concentration.[39,40] Bag-valve-mask ventilation usually is a short-term measure in urgent situations or is used in preparation for tracheal intubation.

PROLONGED VENTILATION USING A SEALED TUBE IN THE TRACHEA

Ventilation of the lungs with a bag-valve-mask arrangement is difficult if required for more than a few minutes or if the patient needs to be transported. In these instances, ventilation through a sealed tube in the trachea is indicated. Orotracheal or nasotracheal intubation, surgical cricothyrotomy, and tracheostomy all achieve the same result: a cuffed tube in the trachea, allowing the use of positive-pressure ventilation and protecting the lungs from aspiration. Mechanical ventilation is discussed in Chapter 9.

APNEIC OXYGENATION

Apneic oxygenation is achieved using a narrow catheter that sits in the trachea and carries a flow of 100% oxygen. The catheter may be passed into the trachea via an ET or under direct vision through the larynx. This apparatus can be set up as a low-flow open system (gas flow rate of 5 to 8 L per minute) or as a high-pressure (jet ventilation) system[41] and can be used to maintain oxygenation with a difficult airway either at intubation or at extubation (see later).

PHYSIOLOGIC SEQUELAE AND COMPLICATIONS OF TRACHEAL INTUBATION

Laryngoscopy is a noxious stimulus that, in an awake or lightly sedated patient, would provoke coughing, retching, or vomiting and laryngospasm. In clinical practice, however, laryngoscopy and tracheal intubation usually are performed after induction of anesthesia, and in emergency situations, the patient often is hypoxic and hypercarbic, with increased sympathetic nervous system activity. Thus, the physiologic effects of laryngoscopy and tracheal intubation tend to be masked.

Laryngoscopy and intubation cause an increase in circulating catecholamines and increased sympathetic nervous system activity, leading to hypertension and tachycardia. This represents an increase in myocardial work and myocardial oxygen demand, which may provoke cardiac dysrhythmias and myocardial hypoxia or ischemia. Laryngoscopy increases cerebral blood flow and intracranial pressure—particularly in patients who are hypoxic or hypercarbic at the time of intubation.[42] This rise in intracranial pressure will be exaggerated if cerebral venous drainage is impeded by violent coughing, bucking, or breath-holding.

Coughing and laryngospasm occur frequently in patients undergoing laryngoscopy and intubation when muscle relaxation and anesthesia are inadequate. Increased bronchial smooth muscle tone, which increases airway resistance, may occur as a reflex response to laryngoscopy or may be due to the physical presence of the ET in the trachea; in its most severe form, termed bronchospasm, this increased tone causes audible wheeze and ventilatory difficulty. Increased resistance to gas flow will occur because the cross-sectional area of the ET is less than that of the airway. This difference usually is unimportant with positive-pressure ventilation but causes a significant increase in work of breathing in spontaneously breathing patients. Resistance is directly related to $1/r^4$ (where r is the radius of the ET) and will be minimized by use of a large-bore ET. Gas passing through an ET, bypassing the nasal cavity, also loses the beneficial effects of warming, humidification, and the addition of traces of nitric oxide (NO).[43]

The effects of intubation on functional residual capacity (FRC) are complex. In patients under anesthesia, a fall in FRC is well documented. This decrease may be due to the loss of respiratory muscle tone following induction of anesthesia and the relatively unopposed effect of the elastic recoil in the lungs.[43] The increased resistance to gas flow due to the presence of the ET may slow expiration, producing intrinsic PEEP (and therefore an increase in FRC) if the next inspiration begins before expiration is complete.

Laryngoscopy and intubation may cause bruising, abrasion, laceration, bleeding, or displacement or dislocation of the structures in and near the airway (e.g., lips, teeth or dental prostheses, tongue, epiglottis, vocal cords, laryngeal cartilages). Dislodged structures such as teeth or dentures may be aspirated, blocking the airway more distally. Less common complications include perforation of the airway with the potential for the development of a retropharyngeal abscess or mediastinitis. Over time, erosions due to pressure and ischemia may develop on the lips or tongue (or external nares and anterior nose in patients with a nasotracheal tube) and in the larynx or upper trachea.[44] These lesions result in a breach of the mucosa with the potential for secondary infection. In the case of the lips and tongue, such lesions are (temporarily) disfiguring and painful and may inhibit attempts to talk or swallow.

The mucosa of the upper trachea (subglottic area) is subjected to the pressure of the cuff of the ET. This pressure reduces perfusion of the tracheal mucosa and, combined with the mechanical movement of the tube (from patient head movements, nursing procedures, or rhythmic flexion with action of the ventilator), tends to cause mucosal damage and increase the risk of superficial infection. These processes may lead to ulceration of the tracheal mucosa, fibrous scarring, contraction, and ultimately stenosis, which can be a life-limiting or life-threatening problem. Although irrefutable evidence is lacking, most clinicians believe that limiting the period of orotracheal or nasotracheal intubation and reducing cuff pressures may reduce the frequency of this complication.[44]

Any tube in the trachea has a significant effect on the mechanisms protecting the airway from aspiration and infection. The mucus escalator may be inhibited by mucosal injury and by the lack of warm humidified airflow over the respiratory epithelium.[45] The disruption of normal swallowing results in the pooling of saliva and other debris in the pharynx and larynx above the upper surface of the tube's inflatable cuff, which may become the source of respiratory infection if the secretions become colonized with microorganisms, or may pass beyond the cuff into the lower airways—that is, pulmonary aspiration (silent or overt).[46,47] The former may occur as a result of (1) colonization of the gastric secretions and the regurgitation of this material up the esophagus to the pharynx or (2) transmission of microorganisms from the health care environment to the pharynx via medical equipment or the hands of hospital staff or visitors (cross-infection).[45,47-50]

The presence of a tube traversing the larynx and sealing the trachea makes phonation impossible. The implications of this limitation for patients and their families often are ignored. If patients cannot tell caregivers about pain, nausea, or other concerns, they may become frustrated, agitated, or violent. This may result in the excessive use of sedative or psychoactive drugs, which prolong time on ventilation and stay in the intensive care unit (ICU), with the risk of infection increased accordingly.[51] The inability to communicate may therefore be a real threat to patient survival. Potential solutions involve the use of letter and picture boards, "speaking valves" (with tracheostomy), laryngeal microphones, or computer-based communication packages. The involvement and innovations of disciplines such as the speech and language center may be advantageous.

THE DIFFICULT AIRWAY

The difficult airway has been defined as "the clinical situation in which a conventionally trained anesthetist experiences difficulty with mask ventilation of the upper airway, tracheal intubation, or both."[52] It has been a commonly documented cause of adverse events including airway injury, hypoxic brain injury, and death under anesthesia.[53-59] The frequency of difficulty with mask ventilation has been estimated to be between 1.4% and 7.8%,[60-62] while tracheal intubation using direct laryngoscopy is difficult in 1.5% to 8.5% and impossible in up to 0.5% of general anesthetics.[58,63] The incidence of failed intubation is approximately 1:2000 in the nonobstetric population and 1:300 in the obstetric population.[64] In the critical care unit, up to 20% of all critical incidents are airway related,[65-67] and such incidents may occur at intubation, at extubation, or during the course of treatment (as with the acutely displaced or obstructed ET or tracheostomy tube).

RECOGNIZING THE POTENTIALLY DIFFICULT AIRWAY

Many conditions are associated with airway difficulty (Table 2.2), including anatomic abnormalities, which may result in

Table 2.2 Conditions Associated with Difficult Airway

Causative Factors	Associated Conditions/Disorders
Abnormal facial anatomy/development	Small mouth or large tongue Dental abnormality Prognathia Obesity Advanced pregnancy Acromegaly Congenital syndromes*
Inability to open mouth	Masseter muscle spasm (dental abscess) Temporomandibular joint dysfunction Facial burns Postradiotherapy fibrosis Scleroderma
Cervical immobility/abnormality	Short neck/obesity Poor cervical mobility (e.g., ankylosing spondylitis) Previous cervical spine surgery Presence of cervical collar Postradiotherapy fibrosis
Pharyngeal or laryngeal abnormality	High or anterior larynx Deep vallecula: inability to reach base of epiglottis with blade of scope Anatomic abnormality of epiglottis or hypopharynx (e.g., tumor) Subglottic stenosis
Injury	Traumatic debris Obstructing foreign bodies Basilar skull fracture Bleeding into airway or adjacent swelling/hematoma Fractured maxilla/mandible Cervical spine instability (confirmed or potential) Laryngeal fracture or disruption
Infections	Epiglottitis Abscess Croup, bronchiolitis Laryngeal papillomatosis Tetanus/trismus
Connective tissue/inflammatory disorders	Rheumatoid arthritis: temporomandibular joint or cervical spine involvement, cricoarytenoid arthritis Ankylosing spondylitis Scleroderma Sarcoidosis
Endocrine disorders	Goiter: airway compression or deviation Hypothyroidism, acromegaly: large tongue

*Visit http://www.erlanger.org/craniofacial and http://www.faces-cranio.org for specific details.

Data from Criswell JC, Parr MJA, Nolan JP: Emergency airway management in patients with cervical spine injuries. Anaesthesia 1994;49:900-903; and Morikawa S, Safar P, DeCarlo J: Influence of head position upon upper airway patency. Anaesthesiology 1961;22:265.

an unusual appearance, thereby alerting the examiner. The goal is to identify the potentially difficult airway and develop a plan to secure it. Factors including age older than 55 years, body mass index greater than 26 kg/m^2, presence of a beard, lack of teeth, and a history of snoring have been identified as independent variables predicting difficulty with mask ventilation—in turn associated with difficult tracheal intubation.[61,68]

Mallampati[69] developed a grading system (subsequently modified[64]) that predicted ease of tracheal intubation at direct laryngoscopy. The predictive value of the Mallampati system has been shown to be limited[70,71] because many factors that have no influence on the Mallampati classification—mobility of head and neck, mandibular or maxillary development, dentition, compliance of neck structures, and body shape—can influence laryngeal view.[53,66,72,73] A study of a complex system including some of these factors found the rate of difficult intubation to be 1.5%, but with a false-positive rate of 12%.[74] A risk index based on the Mallampati classification, a history of difficult intubation, and five other variables lacked sufficient sensitivity and specificity.[75] Airway management should be based on the fact that the difficult airway cannot be reliably predicted.[76,77] This is a particularly important consideration in the critical care environment.

THE OBSTRUCTED AIRWAY

Although the most common reason for an obstructed airway in the unintubated patient is posterior displacement of the tongue in association with a depressed level of consciousness, it is the less common causes that provide the greatest challenges. It is important to elucidate the level at which the obstruction occurs and the nature of the obstructing lesion. Obstruction may be due to infection or edema (epiglottitis, pharyngeal or tonsillar abscess, mediastinal abscess), neoplasm (primary malignant or benign tumor, metastastic spread, direct extension from nearby structures), thyroid enlargement, vascular lesions, trauma, or foreign body or impacted food.[14,78]

Airway lesions above the level of the vocal cords are considered to lie in the upper airway and commonly manifest with stridor.[79] If breathing is labored and associated with difficulty breathing at night, rather than just noisy breathing, then the narrowing probably is more than 50%. Patients with these lesions usually fall into one of two groups: (1) those who can be intubated, usually under inhalational induction, with the ENT (ear-nose-throat) surgeon immediately available to perform rigid bronchoscopy or tracheostomy if required, or (2) those who require a tracheostomy performed while under local anesthesia. In patients with midtracheal obstruction, computed tomography (CT) imaging usually is necessary to discover the exact level and nature of the obstruction and to allow planning of airway management for nonemergency clinical presentations.[79] Tracheostomy often is not beneficial because the tube may not be long enough to bypass the obstruction. In such instances, fiberoptic intubation often may be useful.[79] Lower tracheal obstruction often is due to space-occupying lesions in the mediastinum and necessitates multidisciplinary planning involving ENT, cardiothoracic surgery, anesthesia, and critical care team members.

TRAUMA AND THE AIRWAY

Airway management in the trauma victim provides additional challenges because the victim often has other life-threatening conditions and preparation time for management of the difficult airway is limited. Approximately 15% of severely injured patients have maxillofacial involvement, and 5% to 10% of patients with blunt trauma have an associated cervical spine injury (often associated with head injury).[80]

Problems encountered in trauma patients include presence in the airway of debris or foreign bodies (e.g., teeth), vomitus, or regurgitated gastric contents; airway edema; tongue swelling; blood and bleeding; and fractures (maxilla and mandible). Patients must be assumed to have a full stomach (requiring bimanual cricoid pressure and a rapid-sequence induction for intubation), and many will have pulmonary aspiration before the airway is secured. An important consideration in most cases is the need to avoid movement of the cervical spine at laryngoscopy or intubation.[17,18] Direct injury to the larynx is rare but may result in laryngeal disruption, producing progressive hoarseness and subcutaneous emphysema. Tracheal intubation, if attempted, requires great care and skill because it may cause further laryngeal disruption. With Le Fort fractures, airway obstruction or compromised respiration requiring immediate airway control is present in 25% of cases.[81] Postoperative bleeding after operations to the neck (thyroid gland, carotid, larynx) may compress or displace the airway, leading to difficulty in intubation.

THE AIRWAY PRACTITIONER AND THE CLINICAL SETTING

Although airway difficulties often are due to anatomic factors as discussed, it is important to recognize that the inability to perform an airway maneuver also may be due to a practitioner's inexperience or lack of skill.[82-87] Expert opinion and clinical evidence also identify lack of skilled assistance as a factor in airway-related adverse events.[88-91] As might be expected, inexperience and lack of suitable help may contribute to failure in optimizing the conditions for laryngoscopy (Box 2.5). Airway and ventilatory management performed in the prehospital setting or in the hospital but outside an operating room (OR) carries a higher frequency of adverse events and a higher mortality rate when compared with those performed using anesthesia in an OR.[92-96] In the critical care unit, all invasive airway maneuvers are potentially difficult.[97] Positioning is more difficult

Box 2.5 Common Errors Compromising Successful Intubation

- Poor patient positioning
- Failure to ensure appropriate assistance
- Faulty light source in laryngoscope or no alternative scope
- Failure to use a longer blade in appropriate patients
- Use of inappropriate tracheal tube (size or shape)
- Lack of immediate availability of airway adjuncts

on an ICU bed than on an OR table. The airway structures may be edematous after previous laryngoscopy or presence of an ET. Neck immobility, or the need to avoid movement in a potentially unstable cervical spine, may be other contributing factors.[98-100] Poor gas exchange in ICU patients reduces the effectiveness of preoxygenation and increases the risk of significant hypoxia before the airway is secured.[101] Cardiovascular instability may produce hypotension or hypoperfusion, or may lead to misleading oximetry readings (including failure to record any value at all), a further confounding factor for the attending staff.[102,103]

MANAGING THE DIFFICULT AIRWAY

Management of the difficult airway can be considered in the framework of three possible clinical scenarios with progressively increasing risks for the patient: (1) the anticipated difficult airway; (2) the unanticipated difficult airway; and (3) the difficult airway resulting in a "cannot intubate/cannot ventilate" situation.

Requirements for clinicians involved in airway management include the following:

- Expertise in recognition and assessment of the potentially difficult airway. This involves the use of the assessment techniques noted previously and a "sixth sense."[76]
- The ability to formulate a plan (with alternatives).[52,53,104-106]
- Familiarity with algorithm(s) that outline a sequence of actions designed to maintain oxygenation, ventilation, and patient safety. The American Society of Anesthesiologists (ASA) guidelines[52] and the composite plan from the Difficult Airway Society (DAS)[104] are shown in Figures 2.3 and 2.4. The latter summarizes four airway plans (A to D), available from the DAS website (www.das.uk.com).
- The skills and experience to use a number of airway adjuncts, particularly those relevant to the unanticipated difficult airway.

THE ANTICIPATED DIFFICULT AIRWAY

The anticipated difficult airway is the "least lethal" of the three scenarios—with time to consider strategy, optimize patient status, and obtain appropriate adjuncts and personnel. The key questions are as follows:

1. Should the patient be kept awake or be anesthetized for intubation?
2. Which technique should be used for intubation?

Awake Intubation

Awake intubation is more time-consuming, requires experienced personnel, is less pleasant for the patient (compared with intubation under anesthesia), and may have to be abandoned as a result of the patient's inability or unwillingness to cooperate. Because spontaneous breathing and pharyngeal or laryngeal muscle tone is maintained, however, it is significantly safer. The techniques available are fiberoptic and retrograde intubation. It also may be used in patients judged to be at risk for a difficult airway, whereupon an initial direct laryngoscopic view allows intubation.

Fiberoptic Intubation. Fiberoptic intubation is a technique in which a flexible endoscope with a tracheal tube loaded along its length is passed through the glottis. The tracheal tube is then pushed off the endoscope and into the trachea, and the endoscope is withdrawn. An informed patient, trained assistance, and adequate preparation time make fiberoptic intubation less stressful. The nasotracheal route is used most often and requires the use of nasal vasoconstrictors. Nebulized local anesthetic is delivered to the airway via facemask. Sedation may be given, but ideally the patient should remain breathing spontaneously and responsive to verbal commands. The procedure often is time-consuming and tends to be used in elective situations[107] (Box 2.6).

Box 2.6 Indications for Fiberoptic Intubation

Anticipated difficult intubation
Avoidance of dental damage in high-risk patient
Direct laryngeal trauma
Other need for awake intubation

Retrograde Intubation. For retrograde intubation,[108,109] local anesthesia is provided and the cricothyroid membrane is punctured by a needle through which a wire or catheter is passed upward through the vocal cords. When it reaches the pharynx, the wire is visualized, brought out through the mouth, and then used to guide the ET through the vocal cords before it is withdrawn. This technique also can be used to guide a fiberoptic scope through the vocal cords. Owing to time constraints, it is not suitable for emergency airway access and is contraindicated in any patient with an expanding neck hematoma or coagulopathy.

Intubation Under Anesthesia

It may be decided, in spite of the safety advantage of awake intubation, to anesthetize the patient before attempted intubation. Preparation of the patient, equipment, and staff is paramount (Box 2.7). Adjuncts such as those described later should be available, either to improve the chances of intubation or to provide a safe alternative airway if intubation cannot be achieved.

UNANTICIPATED AIRWAY DIFFICULTY

The unanticipated difficult airway allows only a short period to solve the problem if significant hypoxemia, hypercarbia, and hemodynamic instability are to be avoided. The patient usually is anesthetized, may be apneic, and may have received muscle relaxants, and previous initial attempt(s) at intubation may have been unsuccessful. If appropriate equipment, assistance, and experience are not immediately at hand, little time is available to obtain them. Nevertheless, it is essential to maintain oxygenation and avoid hypercarbia if possible—commonly by mask ventilation with 100% oxygen. The four-handed technique often is used.

If the practitioner is inexperienced, if the patient has had no (or a relatively short-acting) muscle relaxant, and if ventilation is not a problem, it may be appropriate to let the patient recover consciousness. An awake intubation can then be planned either after a short period of recovery or on another occasion. With an experienced practitioner, it may be appropriate to continue, using techniques to

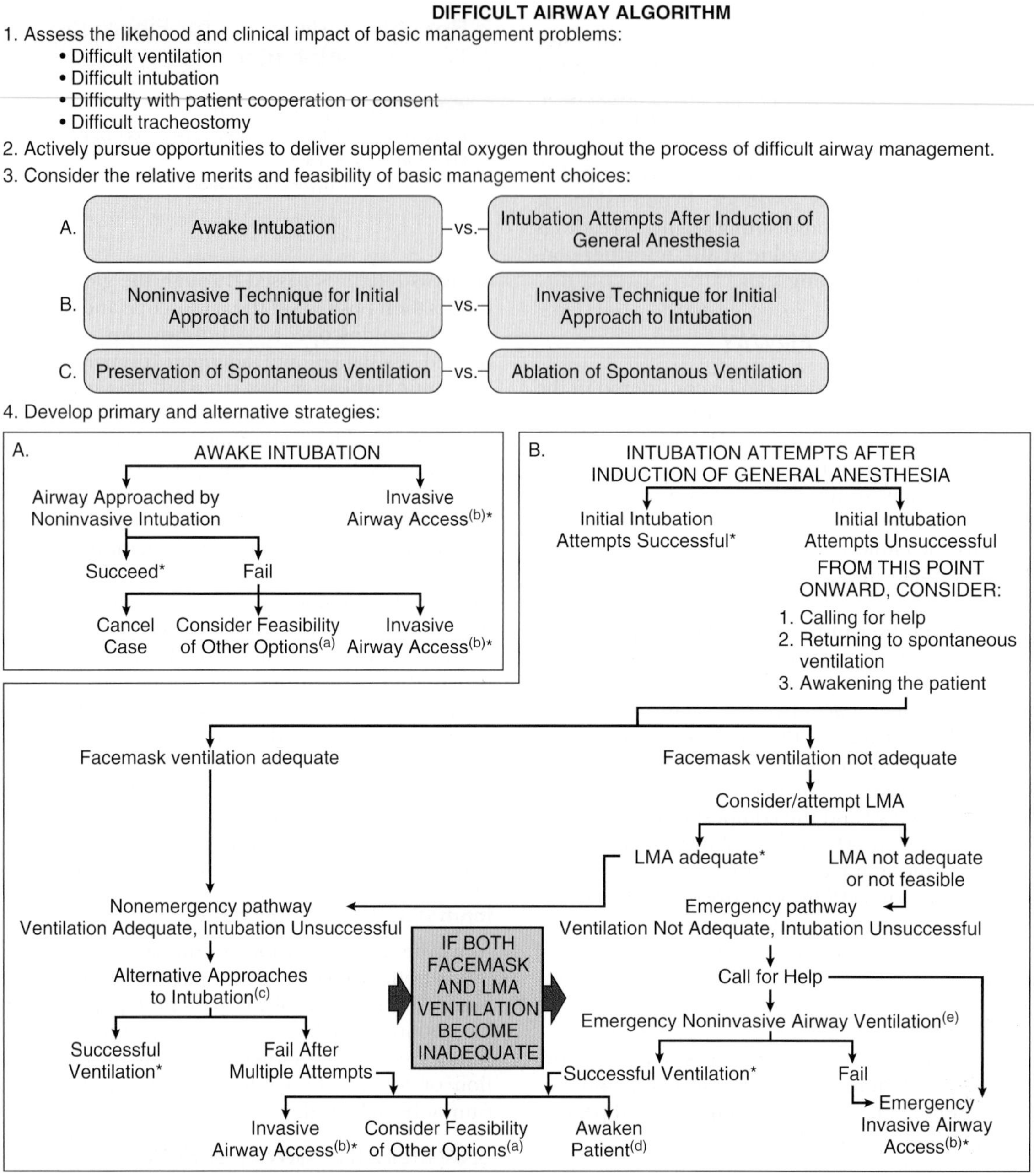

* Confirm ventilation, tracheal intubation, or LMA placement with exhaled CO_2.

a. Other options include (but are not limited to) surgery utilizing facemask or LMA anesthesia, local anesthesia infiltration, and regional nerve blockade. Pursuit of these options usually implies that mask ventilation will not be problematic. Therefore, these options may be of limited value if this step in the algorithm has been reached via the Emergency Pathway.

b. Invasive airway access includes surgical or percutaneous tracheostomy and cricothyrotomy.

c. Alternative noninvasive approaches to difficult intubation include (but are not limited to) use of different laryngoscope blades, LMA as an intubation conduit (with or without fiberoptic guidance), fiberoptic intubation, intubating stylet or tube changer, light wand, retrograde intubation, and blind oral or nasal intubation.

d. Consider re-preparation of the patient for awake intubation or canceling surgery.

e. Options for emergency noninvasive airway ventilation include (but are not limited to) rigid bronchoscope, esophageal-tracheal Combitube ventilation, and transtracheal jet ventilation.

Figure 2.3 Algorithm for managing the difficult airway. (Adapted from Practice guidelines for management of the difficult airway: An updated report by the American Society of Anesthesiologists Task Force on Management of the Difficult Airway. Anaesthesia 2003;98:1269.)

improve the chances of visualizing and intubating the larynx. As discussed next, various adjuncts may be useful in this situation and also in the anticipated difficult airway when it has been decided to intubate with the patient under anesthesia.

Bimanual Laryngoscopy

Application of pressure on the cricoid area or the upper anterior tracheal wall, or both, by the laryngoscopist (a technique sometimes termed bimanual laryngoscopy) may improve laryngeal view.[110,111] When the view is optimized, an

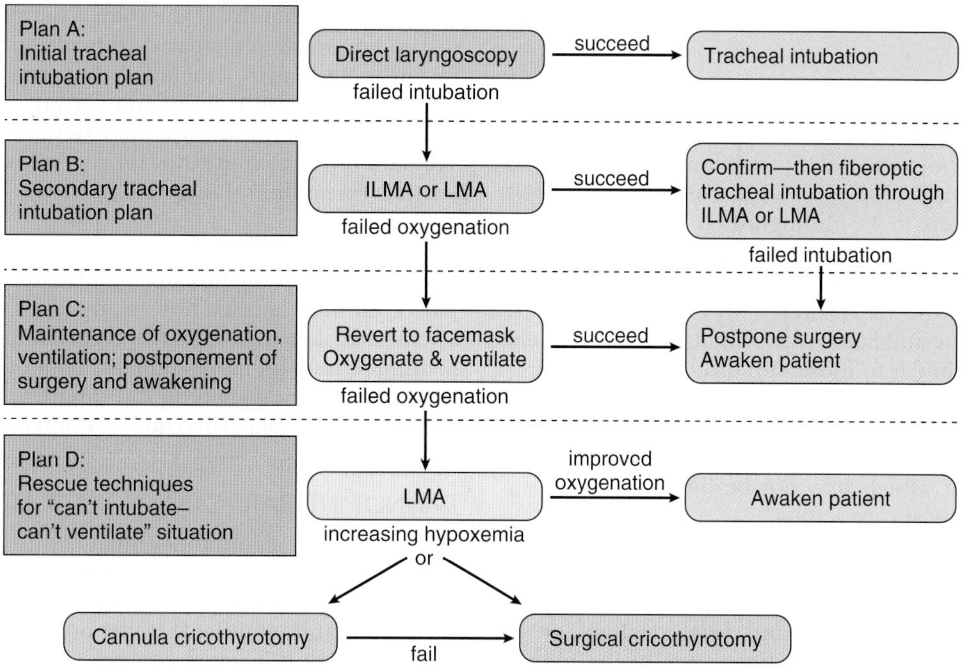

Figure 2.4 A four-component algorithm for managing the difficult airway. (From Difficult Airway Society: Difficult Airway Society Composite Plan. Anaesthesia 2004;59:675-694.)

Box 2.7 Checklist for Anticipated Difficult Intubation of Patient Under General Anesthesia

- Prepare and assess the patient.
- Prepare and test the equipment.
- Ensure skilled assistance with knowledge of BURP/bimanual laryngoscopy.
- Have available:
  - A range of tracheal tubes lubricated and cuffs tested for patency (*women:* 7.0 to 7.5 mm in internal diameter; *men:* 7.5 to 9.0 mm in internal diameter).
  - Endotracheal tube stylets
  - Laryngeal mask airway (LMA)
  - A range of laryngoscopes including specialized blades and handles
- Check battery and bulb function.
- Check functioning of suction devices.
- Use optimal patient position.
- Preoxygenation with 100% oxygen for 3 to 5 minutes if possible
- Provide other equipment as desired:
  - Gum elastic bougie*
  - Lighted stylet*
  - Combitube*
  - Intubating LMA*
  - Fiberoptic scope*

*Depending on choice of individual practitioner.
BURP, *b*ackward, *u*pward, and *r*ightward *p*ressure.

assistant maintains the pressure and thus the position of the larynx, freeing the hand of the laryngoscopist to perform the intubation. The use of "blind" cricoid pressure, or BURP (backward, upward, and rightward pressure), by an assistant may impair laryngeal visualization.[112-114]

Stylet ("Introducer") and Gum Elastic Bougie

The *stylet* is a smooth, malleable metal or plastic rod that is placed inside an ET to adjust the curvature—typically into a J or hockey-stick shape to allow the tip of the ET to be directed through a poorly visualized or unseen glottis.[115] The stylet must not project beyond the end of the ET, to avoid potential laceration or perforation of the airway.

The *gum elastic bougie* is a blunt-ended, malleable rod which at direct laryngoscopy may be passed through the poorly or nonvisualized larynx by putting a J-shaped bend at the tip and passing it blind in the midline upward beyond the base of the epiglottis. Then, keeping the laryngoscope in the same position in the pharynx, the ET can be "railroaded" over the bougie, which is then withdrawn. For many critical care practitioners, it is the first-choice adjunct in the difficult intubation situation.[111,116]

Different Laryngoscope or Blade

Greater than 50 types of curved and straight laryngoscope blades are available, the most commonly used being the curved Macintosh blade.[20] Using specific blades in certain circumstances has been both encouraged[117-119] and discouraged.[120] In patients with a large lower jaw or "deep pharynx," the view at laryngoscopy is often improved significantly, by using a size 4 Macintosh blade (rather than the more common adult size 3). This ensures the tip of the blade can reach the base of the vallecula to lift the epiglottis. Other blades, such as the McCoy, may be advantageous in specific situations.[121,122]

Lighted Stylet

A lighted stylet (light wand) is a malleable fiberoptic light source that can be passed along the lumen of an ET to facilitate blind intubation by transillumination. It allows the tracheal lumen to be distinguished from the (more posterior) esophagus on the basis of the greater intensity of light visible through anterior soft tissues of the neck as the ET passes beyond the vocal cords.[123] In elective anesthesia, the intubation time and failure rate with light wand–assisted intubation were similar to those with direct laryngoscopy,[124] and in a large North American survey, the light wand was the preferred alternative airway device in the difficult intubation scenario.[125] A potential disadvantage is the need for low ambient light, which may not be desirable (or easily achieved) in a critical care setting.

Video Laryngoscopy

Video laryngoscopes are intubation devices that combine modified laryngoscope blades and video technology to provide the operator with an indirect view of the glottis. Examples of video laryngoscopes include the Storz, Glidescope, McGrath, and Pentax airway scope. They are potentially useful teaching tools as they provide the operator and student with identical views.

Depending upon the manufacturer, the devices vary in design; the blades can be standard Macintosh or angulated. Video laryngoscopes with a standard Macintosh blade such as the Storz device are inserted into the oral cavity using the standard direct laryngoscope technique. After insertion, an image of the airway appears on screen. In comparison, insertion of a video laryngoscope with an angulated blade such as the Glidescope, requires insertion into the middle of the oral cavity without a tongue sweep. Once the blade tip is at the base of the tongue the device is rotated so the tip of the blade is directed at the epiglottis. A precurved stylette endotracheal tube is pushed through the glottis. The stylet is withdrawn as the ET reaches the vocal cords and the ET is advanced downward.[126] The Pentax airway scope has a video display incorporated into the handle. The transparent blade has two channels, one for the ET and the second to facilitate suctioning.[127] The McGrath laryngoscope also had a camera mounted on a blade allowing the operator to focus on the patients face and the screen simultaneously.[128]

In contrast, optical laryngoscopes do not have a video attachment but instead uses a lens to provide a view of the glottis not obtained with direct laryngoscopy. The Airtraq optical laryngoscope has a blade with an optical channel and a guiding channel for the ET. It permits glottic visualization in a neutral head position.[129]

Multiple controlled and observational studies suggest that video laryngoscopy can provide superior views of the glottis compared to direct laryngoscopy.[130,131] They may be particularly useful in patients with cervical instability, either by providing a better glottic view or by a reduction in upper cervical movement during intubation.[132,133] However, an improved laryngeal view does not always equate to a successful intubation. Intubation time can also be prolonged with the video laryngoscope, especially in inexperienced hands.[134] The role of the video laryngoscope in the known or anticipated difficult airway is unclear. A recent meta-analysis concluded that data on these devices in the patient with a difficult airway are inadequate.[131] Current data do not suggest these devices should supersede standard direct laryngoscopy for routine or difficult airways. Further research in this area is needed.

Fiberoptic Intubation

The fiberoptic bronchoscope can be used in the unanticipated difficult airway if it is readily available and the operator is skilled.[58,135,136] With an anesthetized patient, the technique may be more difficult. Loss of muscle tone will tend to allow the epiglottis and tongue to fall back against the pharyngeal wall. This can be counteracted by lifting the mandible.

CANNOT INTUBATE–CANNOT VENTILATE

"Cannot intubate–cannot ventilate" is an uncommon but life-threatening situation best managed by adherence to an appropriate algorithm.[52,53,104] All personnel involved will be pressured (and motivated) by the potential for severe injury to the patient. Efficient teamwork will be more likely in an environment that is relatively calm. Although it may be difficult, shouting, impatience, anger, and panic should be avoided in such situations. Figure 2.5 presents a simple flow sheet summarizing the appropriate actions.[137]

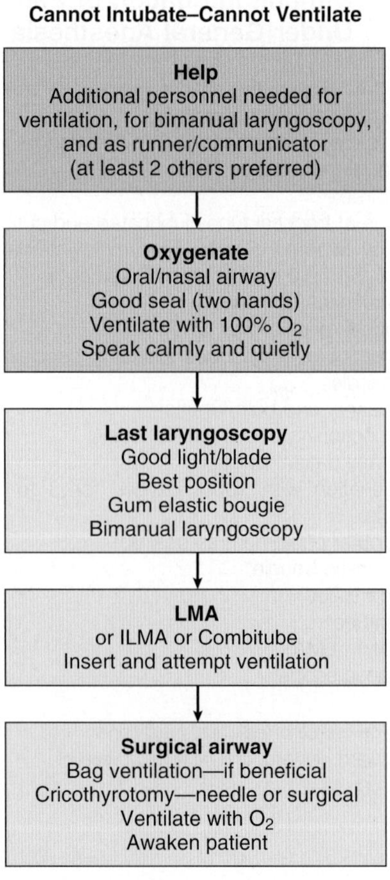

Cannot Intubate–Cannot Ventilate
Help
Additional personnel needed for ventilation, for bimanual laryngoscopy, and as runner/communicator (at least 2 others preferred)
Oxygenate
Oral/nasal airway
Good seal (two hands)
Ventilate with 100% O_2
Speak calmly and quietly
Last laryngoscopy
Good light/blade
Best position
Gum elastic bougie
Bimanual laryngoscopy
LMA
or ILMA or Combitube
Insert and attempt ventilation
Surgical airway
Bag ventilation—if beneficial
Cricothyrotomy—needle or surgical
Ventilate with O_2
Awaken patient

Figure 2.5 Flow chart for the "cannot intubate–cannot ventilate" scenario.

CONFIRMING TUBE POSITION IN THE TRACHEA

A critical factor in the difficult airway scenario, potentially leading to death or brain injury, is failure to recognize misplacement of the ET. Attempted intubation of the trachea may result in esophageal intubation. This alone is not life-threatening unless it goes unrecognized.[138] Thus, confirmation of ET placement in the trachea is essential.

Visualizing the ET as it passes between the vocal cords into the trachea is the definitive means of assessing correct tube positioning. This may not always be possible, however, owing to poor visualization. In addition, the laryngoscopist may be reluctant to accept that the ET is not in the trachea. Several clinical observations support the presence of the ET in the trachea.

Chest wall movement with positive-pressure ventilation (manual or mechanical) is usual but may be absent in patients with chronic obstructive pulmonary disease (COPD), obesity, or decreased compliance (e.g., in severe bronchospasm). Although condensation of water vapor in the ET suggests that the expired gas is from the lungs, this also may occur with esophageal intubation. The *absence of water vapor* usually is indicative of esophageal intubation. *Auscultation of breath sounds* (in both axillae) supports correct tube positioning but is not absolute confirmation.[139] Apparent inequality of breath sounds heard in the axillae may suggest intubation of a bronchus by an ET that has passed beyond the carina. Of note, after emergency intubation and clinical confirmation of the ET in the trachea, 15% of ETs may still be inappropriately close to the carina.[140]

The use of capnography to detect *end-tidal carbon dioxide* is the most reliable objective method of confirming tube position and is increasingly available in critical care.[141] False-positive results may be obtained initially when exhaled gases enter the esophagus during mask ventilation[142] or when the patient is generating carbon dioxide in the gastrointestinal tract (as with recent ingestion of carbonated beverages or bicarbonate based antacids).[143] A false negative result (ET in trachea but no carbon dioxide gas detected) may be obtained when pulmonary blood flow is minimal, as in cardiac arrest.[144] Visualizing the trachea or carina through a *fiberoptic bronchoscope*, which may be readily available in critical care, also will confirm correct placement of the ET.

SURGICAL AIRWAY

The indication for a surgical airway is inability to intubate the trachea in a patient who requires it, and the techniques available are cricothyrotomy and tracheostomy.

CRICOTHYROTOMY

Cricothryotomy may be performed as a percutaneous (needle) or open surgical procedure (Box 2.8). The indication for both these techniques is the "cannot intubate–cannot ventilate" situation. Although needle cricothyrotomy is an emergency airway procedure, the technique is similar to that for "mini-tracheostomy," which is performed electively. Unlike the other surgical airway techniques, a needle cricothyrotomy does *not* create a definitive airway. It will not allow excretion of carbon dioxide but will produce satisfactory oxygenation for 30 to 40 minutes. It can be viewed as a form of apneic ventilation (see later discussion). There are several methods of connecting the intravenous cannula to a gas delivery circuit with the facility to ventilate, using equipment and connections readily available in the hospital. The appropriate method thus should be thought out in advance and available on the difficult airway trolley or bag. New commercial kits that come preassembled also are available.

Box 2.8 Procedure: Needle and Surgical Cricothyrotomy

The cricothyroid membrane is diamond-shaped and lies between the thyroid and the cricoid cartilages. Inject subdermal lidocaine and epinephrine (adrenaline) for local anesthesia.

Needle Cricothyrotomy	***Surgical Cricothyrotomy***
• Identify the cricothyroid membrane and the midline. • Insert a 14-gauge intravenous cannula and syringe through the skin and membrane. • Continuously apply negative pressure until air enters the syringe. • Stop at this point and push the cannula off the needle into the trachea. • The insertion of the cannula into the trachea allows apneic (low-pressure) ventilation or jet (high-pressure) ventilation.	• Make a 1.5-cm skin incision over the cricothyroid membrane. • Incise the superficial fascia and subcutaneous fat. • Divide the cricothyroid membrane (short blade, blunt forceps, or the handle of a scapel often is used). • Insert (6.0) cuffed tracheostomy tube through membrane between the thyroid and cricoid cartilages.

A surgical cricothyrotomy allows a cuffed tube to be inserted through the cricothyroid membrane into the lower larynx or upper trachea. This allows positive-pressure ventilation for considerable periods and also protects against pulmonary aspiration.

TRACHEOSTOMY

A tracheostomy is an opening in the trachea—usually between the second and third tracheal rings or one space higher—that may be created surgically or made percutaneously.[145-149] The indications for and contraindications to tracheostomy are summarized in Box 2.9. In comparison with long-term orotracheal or nasotracheal intubation, tracheostomy often contributes to a patient who is less agitated, requires less sedation, and who may wean from ventilation more easily.[51,150] This increased ability to wean is sometimes attributed to reduced anatomic dead space. The potential reduction in sedation after tracheostomy, however, is a much greater advantage to weaning

Box 2.9 Tracheostomy: Indications and Contraindications

Indications for Tracheostomy

Inability to maintain a patent airway
Suspected cervical spine instability (percutaneous technique only)
Prevention of damage to vocal cords and (possibly) subglottic stenosis
Abnormal anatomy (percutaneous only)
Upper airway obstruction
High inotrope or ventilatory requirement (relative)
Requirement for tracheobronchial toilet with suctioning
Part of larger surgical procedure (e.g., laryngectomy)

Contraindications to Tracheostomy

Prolonged orotracheal or nasotracheal intubation
Local inflammation
Failure to wean from ventilation
Bleeding disorder (relative)
Absence of protective airway reflexes
Arterial bleeding in neck/upper thorax

Box 2.10 Tracheostomy: Benefits and Complications

Benefits

Comfort
Reduced need for sedation
Improved weaning from ventilation
Improved ability to suction trachea
Prevention of ulceration of lips and tongue or healing of such ulcers
Reduced upper airway injury
Potential for speech and oral nutrition

Complications

Misplacement of tube
Primary hemorrhage
Pneumothorax or tension pneumothorax; hemothorax
Surgical emphysema
Infection
Late hemorrhage—erosion of innominate (or other) vessels
Tracheoesophageal fistula

than the small reduction in dead space. The benefits and complications of tracheostomy are listed in Box 2.10. Percutaneous tracheostomy is becoming increasingly common and typically is carried out by medical staff in the ICU (Box 2.11).

Another technique involving retrograde (inside-out) intubation of the trachea has been developed: A specially designed tracheal tube is used to keep the neck tissues under tension until tube placement has been accomplished.[147] It is a more time-consuming technique that at present is not widely practiced.

Box 2.11 Procedure: Bronchoscopy-Assisted Percutaneous Tracheostomy

- Withdraw endotracheal tube (ET) until the cuff lies at or just below the cords.
- Pass a flexible bronchoscope down ET to distal end.
- Make a 1.5- to 2-cm transverse incision at midpoint between cricoid cartilage and suprasternal notch.
- Strip away tissue down to pretracheal fascia using blunt dissection (forceps).
- Under direct vision, use a 14-gauge cannula to puncture anterior tracheal wall (in midline).
- Advance cannula into trachea, aspirate air, and insert Seldinger guidewire.
- Dilate around guidewire using dilator(s) or special forceps.
- Pass tracheostomy tube over guidewire into trachea.
- Pass bronchoscope through tracheostomy to check position.

Although no consensus exists on what defines prolonged tracheal intubation, or when tracheostomy should be performed,[151] most ICUs convert the intubated airway to a tracheostomy after 1 to 3 weeks, with earlier tracheostomy becoming increasingly favored.[150,151]

Conventional wisdom states that the tracheostomy procedure is more complex and time-consuming than a surgical cricothyrotomy and should be performed only by a surgeon.[152] Studies in the elective ICU situation suggest that cricothyrotomy is simpler and (at worst) has a similar complication rate.[153,154] Although needle cricothyrotomy has long been advocated as a life-saving emergency intervention,[155] recent work suggests that surgical cricothyrotomy is the more advantageous procedure.[156] In patients with unfavorable anatomy, surgical cricothyrotomy is a viable alternative to elective tracheostomy.[153] Surgical cricothyrotomy has been viewed as a temporary airway that should be converted to tracheostomy within a few days, but it may be used successfully as a definitive (medium-term) airway,[157,158] thereby avoiding conversion from cricothyrotomy to tracheostomy, which can cause significant morbidity.[159,160]

EXTUBATION IN THE DIFFICULT AIRWAY PATIENT (DECANNULATION)

The patient with a difficult airway still poses a problem at extubation, because reintubation (if required) may be even more difficult than the original procedure. Between 4% and 12% of surgical ICU patients require reintubation[161] and may be hypoxic, distressed, and uncooperative at the time of reintubation. The presence of multiple risk factors for difficult intubation,[100] as well as acute factors such as airway edema and pharyngeal blood and secretions, makes reestablishing the airway in such patients challenging. Before extubation of any critical care patient, the critical care team should have formulated a strategy that includes a plan for reintubation.

Stylets (airway exchange catheters) that allow gas exchange either by jet ventilation or by insufflation of oxygen may be useful in extubating the difficult airway patient.[53,162,163] The stylet is placed through the ET, with care taken to ensure that the distal end has not reached as far as the carina. The ET can then be removed after a successful leak test. The stylet may remain in situ until the situation is judged to be stable.[100]

TUBE DISPLACEMENT IN THE CRITICAL CARE UNIT

ENDOTRACHEAL TUBE

ET displacement in the ICU is a life-threatening emergency that may result in significant morbidity.[164] Although tube dislodgement sometimes is viewed as unavoidable, often preventable factors are involved.[165-167] Changes in patient posture or head position cause significant movement of the tube within the trachea.[168,169] The frequency of tube displacement can be reduced by good medical and nursing practice,[170] attention to the arrangements and ergonomics around the bed, achieving appropriate sedation levels, and ensuring adequate ICU nurse staffing.[171,172] Experience and the ability to anticipate possible glitches constitute an important part of prevention. The management of ET displacement starts with an assessment of whether the patient can manage without the ET.[167] If replacement is required, preparations for a potentially difficult reintubation are indicated.

TRACHEOSTOMY TUBE

Adverse events with tracheostomy tubes are quite common.[167,173] Displacement may be a life-threatening event,[174] especially if the tube has been in place less than 5 to 7 days[151] (before a well-defined tract between skin and trachea is formed) or if the procedure has been performed percutaneously (so that the external opening of the tract may not easily admit a new tube of the same size). The option to leave the patient without a tube should be considered, and if this option is pursued, the tracheostomy opening should be dressed to make it (to some degree) "airtight"—thus facilitating effective coughing. If the patient needs a tube but replacing the tracheostomy is not possible, then oral reintubation should be performed, after which the tracheostomy should be dressed. With a more mature tracheostomy (more than 7 days old), it usually is possible to insert a new tube through the mature tract between skin and trachea.[151]

Tracheostomy tubes may be displaced from the lumen of the trachea but appear to be normal when viewed externally. Difficulty with breathing, ventilation, or tracheal suctioning or the presence of a pneumothorax, pneumomediastinum, or surgical emphysema may be due to tracheostomy tube displacement. Fiberoptic assessment of the tube position and patency may be very useful. Assessing tracheostomy tube position on the chest x-ray film is of no value.

Box 2.12 Predictors for Poor Airway Outcomes

- Use of a supraglottic airway (only) in patients with a recognized airway difficulty
- Cases in which awake fiberoptic intubation was indicated, but not used
- Failure to use capnography or failure to interpret capnography trace correctly
- Airway maneuvers in obese patients, in the emergency department or the intensive care unit
- Use of emergency cannula cricothyrotomy (60% failure rate)
- Displacement of a tracheostomy tube
- Events related to emergence, recovery, and extubation

From Cook TM, Woodall N, Frerk C (eds): The NAP4 report: Major complications of airway management in the UK: Results of the Fourth National Audit Project of the Royal College of Anaesthetists and the Difficult Airway Society. Br J Anaesth 2011;106:617-631. Available at http://www.rcoa.ac.uk/index.asp?PageID=1089. Accessed 30 March 2011.

THE NAP4 PROJECT

The Royal College of Anaesthetists (UK) national audit project (NAP4) provided significant insight into contemporary airway management.[175] The project, using a 2-week national sample, estimated that approximately 2.9 million general anesthetics are administered in the United Kingdom's National Health Service (NHS) each year. Airway management involved a supraglottic airway device (SAD) in 56% of cases, a tracheal tube in 38%, and a facemask in 5%.

The study looked at airway complications during anesthesia and also in airway management in emergency departments and ICUs across the NHS hospital system. There were 16 deaths associated with the 2.9 million anesthetics and an additional 108 patients who suffered severe or moderate harm. Airway management in the ICU and emergency department was judged to be responsible for 22 deaths with an additional 28 patients suffering severe or moderate harm.

Failure to plan (ahead) appeared to be a common causative factor in a large number of poor airway outcomes. This was sometimes due to (1) poor assessment (no recognition that there was a potential problem needing a plan), (2) failure to plan even when potential problems were recognized, and (3) failure to have alternative plan(s) (in the event that "Plan A" was not successful). Many poor outcomes are the result of repeated use of an approach that has already (sometimes repeatedly) failed.[176,177]

NAP4 revealed a number of scenarios or patient-related factors that seemed to predispose to poor airway outcomes. These predictors are summarized in Box 2.12.

COMMON PROBLEMS IN AIRWAY MANAGEMENT

PROBLEM 2.1 Ineffective (Spontaneous) Breathing Despite Artificial Airway

UNDERLYING CAUSES

1. Obstructed airway
2. Depressed respiratory drive (influence of drugs)
3. Inefficient respiratory effort (e.g., from fractured ribs or diaphragmatic injury)
4. Pulmonary pathologic process (pneumonitis, contusion, collapse, consolidation)

ACTION

Attempt to deliver 100% oxygen. Check airway. When airway obstruction has been corrected or ruled out, the patient's respiratory status should improve unless another underlying pathologic process is present. If no improvement is obtained, manually ventilate the patient. If respiratory status still fails to improve, proceed to tracheal intubation with manual or mechanical ventilation. Investigate and treat any underlying condition.

PROBLEM 2.2 Ineffective Manual Ventilation Despite Artificial Airway

POTENTIAL CAUSES

1. Obstructed airway
2. Poor seal or poor technique with mask or manual ventilation
3. Pulmonary pathologic process (pneumonitis, contusion, collapse, consolidation)

ACTION

Attempt to deliver 100% oxygen at 15 to 20 L per minute. Check and readjust airway and patient head position. When airway obstruction has been corrected or ruled out, use a two-handed approach for mask and airway, with an assistant squeezing the bag. If no improvement is obtained, check for availability of someone with more airway experience. If no such person is available, proceed to tracheal intubation with manual or mechanical ventilation. Investigate and treat any underlying condition.

PROBLEM 2.3 Unilateral Chest Movements in the Intubated Ventilated Patient

POTENTIAL CAUSES

1. Bronchial intubation
2. Bronchial obstruction
3. Lung collapse, pneumothorax
4. Hemothorax, pleural effusion
5. Consolidation, absent lung (pneumonectomy)

ACTION

If bronchial intubation is suspected, deflate the tracheal tube cuff and slowly withdraw the tube 1 to 2 cm. Reinflate the cuff, and manually ventilate the patient while auscultating both sides of the chest. Is air entry present and equal on both sides? Be suspicious if the tube has to be withdrawn more than 3 to 4 cm or if the tube length at the teeth is much less than the expected correct length; another underlying cause may be involved. In an adult, the average distance from the vocal cords to the carina is 12 cm. The tip of an 8.0 (adult) tracheal tube typically is 6.5 cm below the upper surface of the balloon, which must sit below the vocal cords. Therefore, if the upper surface of a cuff is only 3 cm below the vocal cords, the tip will be within 2 to 3 cm of the carina. It is easy to inadvertently intubate a bronchus or leave the tip of the tube close enough to enter the bronchus with head movement or when moving the patient. In adults with normal bronchial anatomy, the tube tip usually will pass into the right main bronchus.

PROBLEM 2.4 Sudden Airway or Ventilatory Compromise in Ventilated Patient with Orotracheal Tube

A ventilated patient with an orotracheal tube in place may suddenly develop dyspnea, hypoxemia, hypercarbia, and a seesaw respiratory pattern. The mechanical ventilator alarm will sound.

POTENTIAL CAUSES

1. Failure of oxygen or air supply to the ventilator
2. Ventilator disconnection or obstruction in ventilator circuit
3. Obstructed tracheal tube
   - Plugged by mucus or clot
   - Kink in tracheal tube
   - Biting on tube (previous biting may have narrowed the tube)
   - Obstruction of tube tip by side wall of lower airways or carina
4. Patient's fighting against ventilator
5. Respiratory fatigue (e.g., with weaning from mechanical support or new infection)
6. Pneumothorax or tension pneumothorax
7. Rapid development of large hemothorax or pleural effusion

ACTION

Disconnect the patient from the ventilator, and ventilate through the tracheal tube manually. Have the ventilator and circuit checked by another appropriate staff member. High resistance or inability to inflate the lungs suggests tube obstruction or an intrathoracic problem. The (recent) inability to pass a suction catheter down the lumen is suggestive of tube obstruction. If the patient's condition is stable or improving, a small fiberoptic bronchoscope or laryngoscope (if readily available) may be passed down the tube. An obstruction may be removed by suction catheter, or removal of the tube and use of mask ventilation (to reverse hypoxemia and hypercarbia), followed by reintubation, may be required. If no answer to the problem is found, consider whether the patient's condition could be due to a tension pneumothorax. If appropriate, use needle decompression. Otherwise, order emergency chest film and continue either manual or mechanical ventilation as appropriate.

PROBLEM 2.5 Sudden Airway or Ventilatory Compromise in Ventilated Patient with Tracheostomy

A ventilated patient with a tracheostomy may suddenly develop dyspnea, hypoxemia, hypercarbia, and a seesaw respiratory pattern. The mechanical ventilator alarm will sound.

POTENTIAL CAUSES

Causes may include all those listed for Problem 2.4.

ACTION

Appropriate interventions are the same as for Problem 2.4, with an appreciation of the fact that tracheostomy tubes are shorter, more curved, and more rigid than tracheal tubes. They rarely kink but may become blocked with secretions or blood.[31,178] Suctioning the tube may resolve this. Double-skinned tracheostomy tubes may be unblocked by removing the inner tube (containing the obstruction) for washing, leaving the outer tube in place to maintain a clear airway. Such double-skinned tubes are safer for patients discharged to general wards. Tracheostomy tubes also may become obstructed when the distal opening is blocked by a mucosal flap, the side wall of the trachea, or (rarely) the carina.

KEY POINTS

- The difficult airway may be unanticipated despite expert preassessment. Airway practitioners must have plans to deal with this scenario.
- Use of the appropriate size and type of laryngoscope blade in conjunction with other adjuncts and techniques is an important element of successful tracheal intubation—particularly with the unanticipated difficult airway.
- Airway difficulty in critical care is common and may be precipitated long after intubation by acute events such as tube dislodgement or obstruction.
- Tube dislodgement in critical care is potentially avoidable and may be influenced by staffing levels, sedation policy, and other bedside factors.
- Surgical cricothyrotomy is a relatively simple procedure and may be used to establish a medium-term airway, avoiding the need for tracheostomy.
- In critical care, removal of a tracheal tube may precipitate an acute difficult airway scenario. A protocol for handling a difficult reintubation should always be in place.
- All critical care physicians should be familiar with one or more difficult airway algorithms and the practical skills they require.

SELECTED REFERENCES

52. Practice guidelines for management of the difficult airway: An updated report by the American Society of Anesthesiologists Task Force on Management of the Difficult Airway. Anesthesiology 2003;98:1269-1277.
60. Kheterpal S, Han R, Tremper KK, et al: Incidence and predictors of difficult and impossible mask ventilation. Anesthesiology 2006;105:885-891.
63. Crosby ET, Cooper RM, Douglas MJ, et al: The unanticipated difficult airway with recommendations for management. Can J Anaesth 1998;45:757-776.
66. Beckmann U, Baldwin I, Hart GK, et al: The Australian Incident Monitoring Study in Intensive Care: AIMS-ICU. An analysis of the first year of reporting. Anaesth Intensive Care 1996;24:320-329.
104. Henderson JJ, Popat MT, Latto IP, et al: Difficult Airway Society guidelines for management of the unanticipated difficult intubation. Anaesthesia 2004;59:675-694.
105. Benumof JL: Laryngeal mask airway and the ASA difficult airway algorithm. Anaesthesiology 1996;84:686-699.
114. Levitan RM, Kinkle WC, Levin WJ, et al: Laryngeal view during laryngoscopy: A randomized trial comparing cricoid pressure, backward-upward-rightward pressure, and bimanual laryngoscopy. Ann Emerg Med 2005;47:548-555. Epub 2006 Mar 14.
130. Niforopoulou P, Pantazopoulos I, Demestiha T, et al: Video-laryngoscopes in the adult airway management: A topical review of the literature. Acta Anaesthesiol Scand 2010;54:1050-1061.
137. Lavery GG, McCloskey BV: The difficult airway in adult critical care. Crit Care Med 2008;36(7):2163-2173.
149. Groves DS, Durbin CG, Jr: Tracheostomy in the critically ill: Indications, timing and techniques. Curr Opin Crit Care 2007;13:90-97.

The complete list of references can be found at www.expertconsult.com.

3

Assessment of Cardiac Filling and Blood Flow

Martin Geisen | Maurizio Cecconi | Andrew Rhodes

CHAPTER OUTLINE

The accurate assessment and manipulation of the circulation are important parts of the management of critically ill patients. The principal objective of cardiorespiratory manipulation is to ensure optimal oxygen delivery. Adequate cellular respiration, adequate delivery of substrates and pharmaceuticals, and eventual recovery of organs and tissues are possible only when this has been achieved. This chapter deals with the physiologic principles governing the cardiovascular system and discusses interpretation of hemodynamic data in a clinical context. With the increasing number of medical devices available to monitor the circulation, this chapter also outlines the principles underlying the design and function of these devices, as well as their uses and limitations (Tables 3.1 to 3.4).

CARDIAC FILLING

One of the fundamental concepts of hemodynamic optimization of the critically ill patient is the manipulation of cardiac output as a main determinant of blood flow and oxygen delivery. Cardiac output is defined as the product of stroke volume (SV) and heart rate (HR). Although options to control heart rate are limited, clinical studies investigating hemodynamic optimization protocols have been largely focused on interventions to increase stroke volume. The stroke volume of the heart is determined by the complex interaction of three components: preload, contractility, and afterload. A thorough understanding of the physiology and pathophysiologic principles that define these components is essential for the clinician to successfully control and improve cardiovascular dynamics.

Our current understanding of the relationship between preload and contractility and their effect on stroke volume is based on the experiments of Dario Maestrini, Otto Frank, and Ernest Starling. Culminating in Starling's "law of the heart," which states that the force of myocardial contraction is directly proportional to the end-diastolic myocardial fiber length (or "preload"), as determined by the ventricular end-diastolic volume (EDV).[1,2] It is this relationship, commonly known as the Frank-Starling mechanism that matches venous return to cardiac output (Fig. 3.1).

The most common intervention used by clinicians to improve stroke volume—the administration of fluids—is aimed at increasing venous return as a main determinant of EDV. In this regard two factors are important to consider: the position of an individual heart on the Frank-Starling curve and the expected response to fluid administration, as well as giving the right amount of fluid in order to achieve a hemodynamic response. The dynamics of venous return have been extensively described by Arthur Guyton, whose theories contribute to our current understanding of the circulation and may help to optimize venous return.[3,4]

PRELOAD

Based on Ernest Starling's observations, preload is defined as the tension developed by the stretch of the myocardial fibers: An increase in venous return leads to an increase in EDV which in turn increases myocardial sarcomere length, resulting in an increase of contractility and a rise in stroke volume and cardiac output. Conversely, a decrease in venous return will reduce EDV, resulting in a decreased stroke volume and cardiac output. This mechanism matches the mechanical activity of both ventricles under changing

Table 3.1 Primary Measured Hemodynamic Data

Parameter/Formula	Normal Range
Arterial blood pressure (BP)	
Systolic (SBP)	90-140 mm Hg
Diastolic (DBP)	60-90 mm Hg
Mean arterial pressure (MAP): [SBP + (2 × DBP)]/3	70-105 mm Hg
Right atrial pressure (RAP)	2-6 mm Hg
Right ventricular pressure (RVP)	
Systolic (RVSP)	15-25 mm Hg
Diastolic (RVDP)	0-8 mm Hg
Pulmonary artery pressure (PAP)	
Systolic (PASP)	15-25 mm Hg
Diastolic (PADP)	8-15 mm Hg
Mean pulmonary artery pressure (MPAP): [PASP + (2 × PADP)]/3	10-20 mm Hg
Pulmonary artery occlusion pressure (PAOP)	6-12 mm Hg
Left atrial pressure (LAP)	6-12 mm Hg
Cardiac output (CO): HR × SV/1000	4.0-8.0 L/min

HR, heart rate; SV, stroke volume.

Table 3.2 Derived Hemodynamic Data

Derived Parameter/Formula	Normal Range
Cardiac index (CI): CO/BSA	2.5-4.0 L/min/m^2
Stroke volume (SV): CO/HR × 1000	60-100 mL/beat
Stroke volume index (SVI): CI/HR × 1000	33-47 mL/m^2/beat
Systemic vascular resistance (SVR): 80 × (MAP − RAP)/CO	1000-1500 dyn·s/cm^5
Systemic vascular resistance index (SVRI): 80 × (MAP − RAP)/CI	1970-2390 dyn·s/cm^5/m^2
Pulmonary vascular resistance (PVR): 80 × (MPAP − PAOP)/CO	<250 dyn·s/cm^5
Pulmonary vascular resistance index (PVRI): 80 × (MPAP − PAOP)/CI	255-285 dyn·s/cm^5/m^2

BSA, body surface area; CO, cardiac output; HR, heart rate; MAP, mean arterial pressure; MPAP, mean pulmonary artery pressure; RAP, right atrial pressure; PAOP, pulmonary artery occlusion pressure.

Table 3.3 Hemodynamic Parameters—Adult

Parameter/Formula	Normal Range
Left ventricular stroke work (LVSW): SV × (MAP − PAOP) × 0.0136	58-104 g-m/beat
Left ventricular stroke work index (LVSWI): SVI × (AP − PAOP) × 0.0136	50-62 g-m/m^2/beat
Right ventricular stroke work (RVSW): SV × (MPAP − RAP) × 0.0136	8-16 g-m/beat
Right ventricular stroke work index (RVSWI): SVI × (MPAP − RAP) × 0.0136	5-10 g-m/m^2/beat
Coronary artery perfusion pressure (CPP): Diastolic BP − PAOP	60-80 mm Hg
Right ventricular end diastolic volume (RVEDV): SV/EF	100-160 mL
Right ventricular end systolic volume (RVESV): EDV − SV	50-100 mL
Right ventricular ejection fraction (RVEF): SV/EDV	40-60%

BP, blood pressure; CO, cardiac output; EF, ejection fraction; HR, heart rate; MAP, mean arterial pressure; MPAP, mean pulmonary artery pressure; PAOP, pulmonary artery occlusion pressure; RAP, right atrial pressure; SV, stroke volume; SVI, stroke volume index.

Table 3.4 Oxygenation Parameters—Adult

Parameter/Formula	Normal Range
Partial pressure of arterial oxygen (Pao_2)	80-100 mm Hg
Partial pressure of arterial carbon dioxide ($Paco_2$)	35-45 mm Hg
Bicarbonate (HCO_3^-)	22-28 mEq/L
pH	7.38-7.42
Arterial oxygen saturation (Sao_2)	95-100%
Mixed venous oxygen saturation ($S\dot{v}o_2$)	60-80%
Arterial oxygen content (Cao_2): (0.0138 × Hb × Sao_2) + (0.0031 × Pao_2)	17-20 mL/dL
Venous oxygen content (Cvo_2): (0.0138 × Hb × $S\dot{v}o_2$) + (0.0031 × Pvo_2)	12-15 mL/dL
Arteriovenous oxygen content difference [$C(a-v)O_2$]: $Cao_2 - Cvo_2$	4-6 mL/dL
Oxygen delivery (Do_2): Cao_2 × CO × 10	950-1150 mL/min
Oxygen delivery index (Do_2I): Cao_2 × CI × 10	500-600 mL/min/m^2
Oxygen consumption (Vo_2): $C(a-v)O_2$ × CO × 10	200-250 mL/min/m^2
Oxygen consumption index (Vo_2I): $C(a-v)O_2$ × CI × 10	120-160 mL/min/m^2
Oxygen extraction ratio (O_2ER): [($Cao_2 - C\dot{v}o_2$)/Cao_2] × 100	22-30%
Oxygen extraction index (O_2EI): [($Sao_2 - S\dot{v}o_2$)/Sao_2] × 100	20-25%

CI, cardiac index; CO, cardiac output; Hb, hemoglobin.

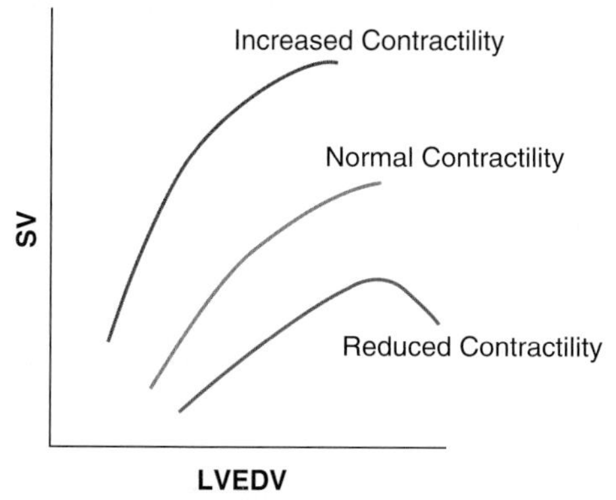

Figure 3.1 Graph demonstrating the Frank-Starling principle: The effect of preload on stroke volume in three different myocardial contractility states. LVEDV, left ventricular end diastolic volume; SV, stroke volume.

physiologic conditions and functions independent of nervous supply.

Preload is determined by the following factors:

- Circulating blood volume
- Venous capacitance (i.e., sympathetic stimulation resulting in venoconstriction, mechanical compression)
- Posture: The Trendelenburg position (supine, head down) increases venous return. Clinically, a passive leg raise test may be performed to assess volume responsiveness by autotransfusion of approximately 300 mL of blood from the splanchnic and lower limb compartments to the central circulation, increasing preload.
- Intracavitary pressures: Abdominal hypertension and increased intrathoracic pressures (i.e., during positive-pressure ventilation and application of positive end-expiratory pressure [PEEP]) can oppose venous return.
- Ventricular compliance: Ventricular compliance determines the relationship between EDV and end-diastolic pressure (i.e., diastolic dysfunction or impaired relaxation as in ventricular hypertrophy).
- Heart rate: The filling time influences EDV.
- Atrial contraction: Atrial contraction contributes to EDV and may be impaired (i.e., in atrial fibrillation).

INDICATORS OF PRELOAD

In vivo measurement of sarcomere length is not possible. To assess this variable in the clinical setting, ventricular end-diastolic pressures have been traditionally used as surrogate parameters to estimate EDV. Although EDV can be assessed by echocardiography, continuous monitoring of this parameter is currently not possible. Static indices of preload include traditional parameters assessing filling pressures or volumes as well as parameters derived from recently introduced techniques based on thermodilution (see later), which have been classified as volumetric indices of preload. Recently, parameters based on the cyclic changes in intrathoracic pressure during mechanical ventilation have been introduced as estimates of preload responsiveness under certain circumstances, although they do not measure preload per se. These dynamic indices of preload can play a role in predicting an increase of stroke volume after an increase of preload, or in other words, the "fluid responsiveness" of the ventricle.

STATIC INDICATORS OF PRELOAD

These parameters give an estimate of preload, but their ability to predict a response to fluid administration is limited. Static preload indices have been defined for both sides of the heart:

Static indices of the left side of the heart:

- Left ventricular end-diastolic volume (LVEDV)
- Left ventricular end-diastolic pressure (LVEDP)
- Left atrial pressure (LAP)
- Pulmonary artery occlusion or "wedge" pressure (PAOP or PAWP)

Static indices of the right side of the heart:

- Right ventricular end-diastolic volume (RVEDV)
- Right ventricular end-diastolic pressure (RVEDP)
- Right atrial pressure (RAP)
- Central venous pressure (CVP)

It is generally postulated that EDVs correspond to myocardial sarcomere length just prior to ventricular contraction and that end-diastolic pressures correspond with EDVs.

For the left side of the heart these relationships are as follows:

$$PAOP = LAP = LVEDP \approx LVEDV$$

For the right side of the heart these relationships are as follows:

$$CVP = RAP = RVEDP \approx RVEDV$$

It is important to note that these assumptions do not hold true in most clinical conditions and all parameters are influenced by physiologic and technologic factors. Ventricular pressures and volumes both are influenced by ventricular compliance, so there is only a poor relationship between the two, and the traditional assumption that CVP, RAP, PAOP, and LAP estimate LVEDP as an indicator of LVEDV has to be questioned. PAOP reflects left ventricular function only if the vascular system between the catheter tip and the left ventricle is free from any pathologic condition that could influence the pressures detected by the catheter.

PAOP *overestimates* LVEDP in the following conditions:

- Chronic mitral stenosis
- PEEP
- Left atrial myxoma
- Pulmonary hypertension

PAOP *underestimates* LVEDP in the following conditions:

- Poorly compliant left ventricle
- LVEDP greater than 25 mm Hg

PAOP readings are accurate only if the tip of the pulmonary artery catheter (PAC) is appropriately wedged in West lung zone 3, corresponding to the lower third of the lung where continuous blood flow can be assumed.

The PAOP does not predict preload and bears little or no relationship to the subsequent response to a volume challenge. It is important to realize, however, that pressure is one of the driving forces responsible for edema formation in the lungs. In this regard, the PAOP may function as more of a safety limit rather than as a guide to therapy.[5-7]

The CVP reflects RAP and has been traditionally used as a marker of right ventricular preload and, assuming a relationship between CVP, RVEDP, and RVEDV, of left ventricular preload. However, CVP does not accurately reflect left ventricular preload and has been shown to correlate poorly with blood volume.[5-7] The main clinical value of measuring CVP is to provide information about the right side of the heart, as in cases of right ventricular failure or in assessing the right ventricular response to pulmonary hypertension. A low CVP in the setting of clinical signs of tissue hypoperfusion may be predictive of a benefit from fluid administration, and a rapid significant rise of CVP during a fluid challenge may indicate that the heart is not fluid responsive.[8-12]

VOLUMETRIC INDICATORS OF PRELOAD

Based on cardiac output measurements using thermodilution and incorporating indicator passage times, volumetric preload parameters have been introduced as an alternative to conventional "static" parameters and have become available with thermodilution-based monitoring techniques such as the PAC, pulse contour continuous cardiac output (PiCCO), and EV1000 systems. The continuous end-diastolic volume index (CEDVI), derived from a modified PAC is a surrogate of RVEDV. Global end-diastolic volume index (GEDVI), intrathoracic blood volume index (ITBVI), and extravascular lung water index (EVLWI) are parameters provided by devices that require transpulmonary thermodilution for the measurement of cardiac output based on pulse pressure analysis (i.e., PiCCO and EV1000 systems, see later). GEDVI represents the total intracardiac volume, and the volume of the descending aorta has been shown to be a better indicator of preload than CVP.[13,14]

DYNAMIC INDICATORS OF PRELOAD (OR PRELOAD RESPONSIVENESS)

Based on the study of heart-lung-interactions a number of so-called dynamic preload indicators have been introduced. Although these parameters are not measures of preload per se, they play an important role in the prediction of the hemodynamic response (i.e., by an increased cardiac output) to an increase in preload (preload or "volume" responsiveness). Generally, these parameters are based on the observation that transient changes in preload occur during mechanical ventilation.[15,16]

Stroke Volume Variation

During mechanical ventilation each positive-pressure breath induces a decrease in venous return. In conditions of decreased volume status, when the right ventricle is responsive to an increase in preload, a reduction in right ventricular outflow will occur and result in a decrease of left ventricular preload after the number of cardiac cycles it takes to pump blood through the lung (pulmonary transit time). If the left ventricle is preload responsive as well, a transient decrease in stroke volume will occur. This cyclic variation in stroke volume (stroke volume variation, SVV) can indicate volume responsiveness if it reaches a certain degree and may describe the response to a volume challenge in relation to changes in cardiac output.[17-21]

Pulse Pressure Variation

Similar to SSV, a marked respiratory variation of the arterial pulse pressure (pulse pressure variation, PPV) has been found to accurately predict volume responsiveness.[22-24]

SVV, PPV, and systolic pressure variation (SPV) are automatically calculated by an array of cardiac output monitors.

Plethysmographic Variability Index

The pulse oximeter plethysmographic waveform has been shown to display respiratory variations during mechanical ventilation, which can be predictive of volume responsiveness. Calculation of the plethysmographic variability index (PVI) is performed by measuring changes of the perfusion index (PI = pulsatile infrared signal/nonpulsatile infrared signal × 100) over at least one respiratory cycle.[25-27]

Indices Derived by Echocardiography

Finally, respiratory variations of the inferior vena cava diameter as measured by transthoracic echocardiography (TTE) or the superior vena cava (SVC) diameter as measured by transesophageal echocardiography (TEE) have been shown to accurately predict volume responsiveness.[28,29]

It is important to note that these variables are reliable only during controlled mechanical ventilation. Other conditions in which the use of these parameters cannot be advised are as follows:

- Cardiac arrhythmias
- Application of low tidal volumes (i.e., <8 mL/kg)
- Open chest conditions
- Right ventricular failure

CONTRACTILITY

Ventricular contractility, or inotropy, describes the strength of ventricular contraction. It is defined as the tension developed by myocardial fibers at a given preload and afterload and the velocity of the shortening of the myocardial sarcomeres. It represents the intrinsic ability of the myocardium to generate a force independent of filamental stretch or ventricular loading conditions. Contractility is influenced by the following factors:

Factors that *increase* myocardial contractility:

- Circulating catecholamines
- Drugs (inotropes, digoxin, calcium solutions)
- Metabolic state (i.e., hyperthermia)
- Sympathetic nervous system activity
- Increased heart rate

The following factors *reduce* myocardial contractility:

- Hypoxia or hypercapnia
- Metabolic state (acidosis, hypothermia, hyperkalemia, hypocalcemia)
- Drugs (e.g., β-adrenergic receptor antagonists, digoxin)

- Acute and chronic cardiomyopathies
- Parasympathetic nervous system activation

Contractility is difficult to assess in the clinical setting. The temporal rate of change of ventricular pressure (dP/dt) and its maximum value (peak dP/dt) can be derived invasively (i.e., in the cardiac catheterization laboratory) or estimated less invasively with varying accuracy by echocardiography and some cardiac output monitoring devices. This parameter has been shown to be related to ventricular function in clinical studies. Echocardiography provides additional functional assessment of ventricular wall motion and blood velocity kinetics. Parameters such as the fractional area change (FAC) and ejection fraction (EF) are no accurate measures of contractility but are related to the contractile state of the myocardium and can be used to guide therapy.

AFTERLOAD

The afterload of the heart may be considered as the ventricular wall tension required to eject the stroke volume during systole. According to the law of LaPlace, afterload relates to the stress within the wall of the ventricle developing during systolic ejection:

$$T = (P \times r)/2$$

where T = tension, P = intraventricular pressure, and r = intraventricular radius. In this equation afterload is mainly dependent on wall thickness and ventricular radius. At a given pressure, an increase in ventricular radius (i.e., dilatation of the ventricle) will increase afterload. An increase in wall thickness (i.e., ventricular hypertrophy) will reduce afterload.

Afterload for the left ventricle is increased by the following factors:

- Anatomic obstruction (e.g., aortic valve stenosis, subvalvular obstruction)
- Raised systemic vascular resistance (SVR)
- Decreased elasticity of the aorta and great vessels
- Increased ventricular volume

Afterload for the right ventricle is increased by the following factors:

- Anatomic obstruction (e.g., pulmonary valve stenosis)
- Raised pulmonary vascular resistance (PVR) (e.g., pulmonary hypertension, pulmonary embolism, hypoxia, and hypercarbia)
- Increased ventricular volume

The *Anrep effect* describes an intrinsic regulatory mechanism of the heart in response to an acute increase in afterload, which results in an initial reduction in stroke volume followed by an increase in EDV, which restores the stroke volume toward near-normal values.

INDICATORS OF AFTERLOAD

SVR and PVR are the most commonly used indicators of afterload in the clinical setting for the left and right ventricle, respectively. Vascular resistance can be described as the mechanical property of the vascular system opposing flow of blood into a vascular bed. There are two main components of vascular resistance:

- *Flow component*—frictional opposition to blood flow through the vessels, with blood viscosity being the major determinant: Vascular resistance increases with an increase in viscosity.
- *Frequency-dependent or "reactive" component*—related to the compliance of the vessel walls and the inertia of the ejected blood. A low vascular compliance increases vascular resistance.

SVR and PVR cannot be measured directly and thus are calculated from Ohm's law:

$$V = I \times R$$

where V = voltage, I = current, and R = resistance. Applied to cardiovascular physiology this principle looks as follows:

$$\Delta P = \text{CO} \times R$$

in which ΔP is the pressure gradient, CO (cardiac output) is "flow," and R is the resistance.

SVR is calculated as follows:

$$\text{SVR (dyn} \cdot \text{s/cm}^5) = 80 \times (\text{MAP} - \text{RAP})/\text{CO}$$

where MAP = mean arterial pressure (mm Hg), RAP = right atrial pressure (mm Hg), and CO = cardiac output. To convert from mm Hg to dyne × second/cm^5 the multiplication by 80 is necessary. Normal values for SVR range from 800 to 1200 dyne × second/cm^5. If standardized to body surface area, SVR is quoted as SVRI (SVR index) with normal values for SVRI ranging from 1900 to 2400 dyne × second/cm^5/m^2.

The following factors affect SVR:

- *Vessel diameter:* According to the law of Hagen-Poiseuille resistance is inversely related to the fourth power of the radius. This means that a decrease in vessel diameter during vasoconstriction will result in a significant increase in SVR. Vasodilation decreases SVR.
- *Compliance* of the systemic circulation
- *Blood viscosity and hematocrit*

In the same way as SVR, PVR may be calculated using the pressure differential across the pulmonary vasculature, between the mean pulmonary artery pressure (MPAP) and PAOP:

$$\text{PVR (dyne} \times \text{second/cm}^5) = 80 \times (\text{MPAP} - \text{PAOP})/\text{CO}$$

Values for PVR are normally below 250 dyne × second/cm^5. Again, PVR is often quoted as the PVR index or PVRI with a normal range between 255 to 285 dyne × second/cm^5/m^2.

The following factors affect PVR:

- *Vessel diameter:* Pulmonary vasoconstriction increases PVR (i.e., during hypoxia), and vasodilation reduces PVR.
- *Positive-pressure ventilation* increases PVR.
- *Established pulmonary hypertension* increases PVR.
- *Compliance* of the pulmonary circulation affects PVR.
- *Blood viscosity and hematocrit* affect PVR.

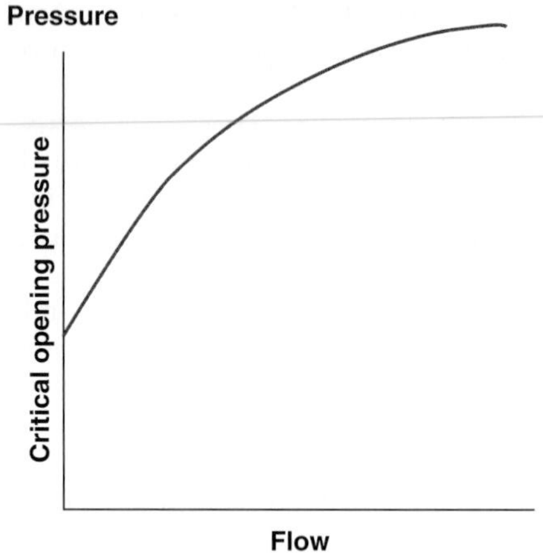

Figure 3.2 Relationship among pressure, flow, and resistance. The critical opening pressure reflects the pressure in the vasculature at zero flow. The important point to recognize is that this is not at the origin of the graph. This means that even when the flow is zero, a baseline pressure exists. Estimating systemic vascular resistance by calculating the gradient of pressure and flow for any given point will therefore be inaccurate, because the "line" is actually nonlinear and does not go through the zero origin.

CLINICAL LIMITATIONS OF SYSTEMIC VASCULAR RESISTANCE AND PULMONARY VASCULAR RESISTANCE

Although the concept of vascular resistance permits an intuitive understanding of the circulation, a number of limitations make it unreasonable to use SVR and PVR to guide therapy. First, because SVR and PVR are derived variables, errors inherent in the measurement of their components (i.e., filling pressures) are multiplied, making the derived number less accurate. Further, these calculations assume a linear relation between pressure and flow, which does not exist in vivo (Fig. 3.2). It is therefore wise to use these parameters with caution and consider their limitations in clinical practice.

CLINICAL INTERPRETATION OF INDICATORS OF PRELOAD

It has already been stressed that accurate assessment of the preload status of the heart is important because it may allow for the application of interventions resulting in an improvement of cardiovascular dynamics. However, without knowing whether the heart will actually respond to an increase of a certain status of volume or preload, this information is only of limited value. This concept—the individual response of cardiac output to a volume challenge—has become known as *volume responsiveness*.[30] Intravascular volume expansion is often the initial intervention in patients with circulatory failure. However, only approximately 50% of patients given a fluid challenge will respond by increasing cardiac output. The ability to distinguish fluid-responsive patients from nonresponders is important to avoid inappropriate and potentially harmful fluid challenges in situations in which other interventions (i.e., inotropes or vasopressors) should be preferentially used. Consequences of inappropriate fluid therapy include pulmonary edema, deterioration in gas exchange, and cardiac failure.

There are currently a number of parameters available with different monitoring modalities that can be used as estimates of preload and may predict volume responsiveness under defined conditions.

STATIC INDICATORS OF PRELOAD

Conventional static markers of cardiac preload, such as CVP and PAOP, are poor predictors of fluid responsiveness. CVP and PAOP reflect intracavitary pressures that frequently show poor correlation with transmural pressures, which are actually related to EDV through chamber compliance. Therefore, EDV is overestimated (i.e., under the application of PEEP) or underestimated (i.e., in concentric left ventricular hypertrophy) in many clinical situations. Furthermore, static parameters do not determine the position of the heart on the "individual" Frank-Starling curve as contractile function is not taken into the account. A patient may fail to respond to a fluid challenge because of ventricular dysfunction or poor ventricular compliance (see Fig. 3.1). It is important to realize, however, that pressure is one of the driving forces responsible for edema formation in the lungs. So although the PAOP is considered to have limited utility for predicting and guiding fluid challenges, it does have a role to play in determining how much volume should be administered to patients and may be regarded as more of a safety limit, rather than as a guide to therapy.[5,6]

VOLUMETRIC INDICATORS OF PRELOAD

The continuous end-diastolic volume (CEDV), global end-diastolic volume (GEDV), and intrathoracic blood volume (ITBV) are computed by some monitoring systems. Although CEDV and GEDV seem to be better indicators of preload than static parameters, they are still poor predictors of a response to a fluid challenge in most situations. Extravascular lung water (EVLW) has been shown to help in the identification of noncardiogenic pulmonary edema and has the potential to increase the safety of fluid therapy in patients with structural lung disease or acute lung injury (ALI) and acute respiratory distress syndrome (ARDS).[31,32]

DYNAMIC INDICATORS OF PRELOAD

A number of dynamic parameters have been described that allow the clinician at the bedside to predict with some accuracy which patients will or will not respond to a fluid challenge. These parameters include the SVV, PPV, SPV, and the PVI and changes of vena cava diameters as derived by echocardiography. Generally, an SPV, PPV, SVV, or PVI variation greater than approximately 10% suggests that the patient will be volume responsive (Fig. 3.3). As stressed earlier in this chapter, these parameters require controlled mechanical ventilation and a tidal volume of at least 8 mL/kg of body weight to be maintained in order to remain reliable. Further, the presence of arrhythmias and severe tricuspid regurgitation precludes the safe use of these variables.[16]

The Passive Leg-Raising Test

Patients who are critically ill seldom fulfill criteria to allow for dynamic preload indices to be accurate predictors of volume responsiveness. The passive leg-raising test has been suggested to overcome these limitations: Traditionally performed by lifting the legs up at a 45-degree angle in a supine position, approximately 150 mL of blood can be recruited

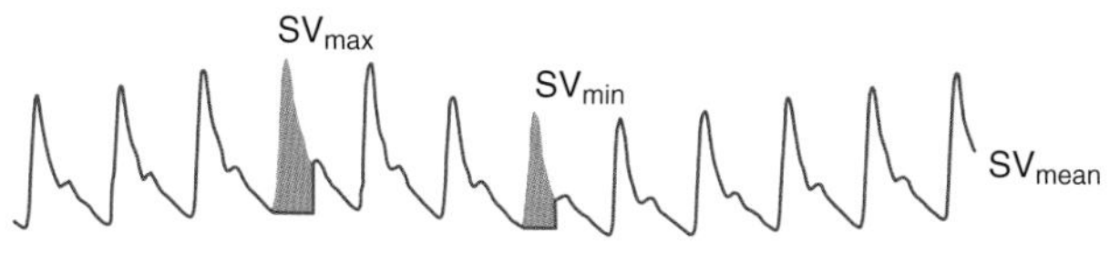

Figure 3.3 Stroke volume variation (SVV). The arterial pressure trace can be used to generate stroke volume (SV) on a beat-to-beat basis. The variation in SV—SVV—with mechanical ventilation is a useful marker for identifying patients who are likely to respond to an increase in intravascular volume. This tracing demonstrates the fluctuations in SV in a patient with an increased SVV.

to increase venous return in order to predict a response of cardiac output to a noninvasive, endogenous fluid challenge. However, by starting the passive leg raising from a 45-degree semirecumbent position, a substantial increase of mobilized venous blood can be achieved by adding venous blood from the splanchnic compartment to that from the lower extremities, increasing the sensitivity of the maneuver for the prediction of fluid responsiveness. It is important to note that when performing the passive leg raising, the monitoring modality used must be able to track changes in cardiac output within a time frame of approximately 60 to 90 seconds.[33-35]

The Diagnostic Fluid Challenge

In the care of critically ill patients situations do exist in which the preceding parameters are not reliable and a passive leg-raising test may be contraindicated owing to technical constraints or based on the patient's underlying illness, such as in brain injury with elevated intracranial pressure. In this scenario the clinician may rely on the administration of fluids as a diagnostic intervention to indicate a potential benefit from further fluid therapy by assessing the response of various hemodynamic parameters, with stroke volume being the parameter most widely used in studies investigating fluid responsiveness, with an increase of 10% to 20% indicating a positive response. Although the optimal volume to function as a fluid challenge has yet to be determined, it can be recommended in this situation to use the CVP as an indicator of a sufficient challenge of the right ventricle to ensure that an adequate preload has been achieved.[36,37]

It is important to recognize, however, that identification of a patient who is fluid responsive is not the same as saying that the patient should be given fluid without an appreciation of the clinical context. Most healthy patients will be volume responsive; however, few will benefit from volume challenges. In critically ill patients, other clinical factors need to be taken into account. Does the patient actually need a higher cardiac output? Or is cardiac output adequate, so that further increase may actually cause harm?

HEMODYNAMIC STATUS AND BLOOD FLOW

Cardiac output (or blood flow) is an important variable to be considered in a critically ill patient. Although arterial pressure has been used as the target for therapy, this focus is perhaps related more to convenience in measurement than to a sound physiologic rationale. When patients become critically ill, it is extremely difficult to predict cardiac output from routine clinical assessment, so sensible and logical use of vasoactive therapy requires monitoring of both pressure and flow. Arterial blood pressure often is mistakenly used as a surrogate marker for blood flow; however, no direct relationship between pressure and flow exists. Moreover, clinical estimation of cardiac output can be difficult and inaccurate, although clinical assessment must not be ignored. Often these signs constitute the only tool that a clinician may have to estimate a patient's hemodynamic status before admission to a critical care unit. At this stage the response of clinical assessment to simple therapeutic maneuvers can give important information. If, however, the patient fails to respond in a suitable fashion, monitoring of these variables becomes necessary in order to direct therapy.

Cardiac output is the volume of blood ejected by the left ventricle per minute. It is the product of heart rate and stroke volume. It should be borne in mind that excessive heart rates will reduce diastolic ventricular filling time, with a negative impact on stroke volume. Heart rhythm also is essential in determining cardiac output, and in general any rhythm other than sinus rhythm will result in a reduction in stroke volume. For example, the loss of atrial contribution to diastolic ventricular filling in atrial fibrillation results in a subsequent reduction in stroke volume and hence cardiac output.

Cardiac output should not be considered in isolation from other relevant variables. The concept of oxygen delivery describes the relationship between cardiac output and arterial oxygen content:

$$\text{Oxygen delivery} = \text{Arterial } O_2 \text{ content} \times \text{Cardiac output}$$

This variable (oxygen delivery) has been used in many studies, especially in the high-risk surgical population, as a target for resuscitation.

MEASUREMENT OF CARDIAC OUTPUT

The ideal method of measuring cardiac output would be noninvasive, accurate, continuous, safe, easy to use, and operator independent; would provide rapid data acquisition; and would be cost effective. None of the cardiac output monitoring devices currently available possesses all of these properties. Conventional thermodilution remains the clinical gold standard for accuracy in cardiac output measurement; however, newer, less invasive monitoring methods that provide continuous cardiac output data are establishing a role in patients' hemodynamic management.[38]

THE FICK PRINCIPLE

Fick described the following relationship in the nineteenth century: $Q = M/(A - V)$. That is, the uptake or release of a substance (M) by an organ is the product of the blood flow (Q) through that organ and the arteriovenous concentration difference (A − V) of the substance in question.

Applying the Fick principle to cardiac output measurement of the pulmonary blood flow over 1 minute may be achieved by measuring the arteriovenous oxygen content difference across the lungs and the rate of oxygen uptake. Oxygen uptake may be determined using spirometry by measuring the expired gas volume over a known time and calculating the difference in oxygen concentration between the expired gas and that of inspired gas. Accurate collection of the gas is difficult, unless the patient has an endotracheal tube, because of the leaks that occur around a facemask or mouthpiece. Analysis of the gas is straightforward if the inspired gas is air, but if it is oxygen-enriched air, two possible problems need to be taken into consideration: (1) the addition of oxygen may fluctuate, producing an error due to the nonconstancy of the inspired oxygen concentration, and (2) measurement of small changes in oxygen concentration at the top end of the scale is difficult. Blood oxygen content is measured via blood gas analysis. In the absence of intrapulmonary or intracardiac shunts, the pulmonary blood flow is equal to the systemic blood flow and thus cardiac output.

The technique just described based on the Fick principle may thus be used as an accurate and reliable static measure of cardiac output, but it remains a time-consuming and largely laboratory-based tool. Several variants of the basic method have been devised, but usually their accuracy is less reliable.

THERMODILUTION

As mentioned earlier, thermodilution from the PAC is considered to be the gold standard of cardiac output measurement for accuracy and acceptability in the clinical setting. Newer methods are routinely validated against the PAC thermodilution technique. A bolus of 5 to 10 mL of cold 0.9% NaCl or 5% dextrose is injected through the proximal port of a PAC into the right atrium. Temperature changes are measured by a distal thermistor in the pulmonary artery. A plot of temperature change against time gives a thermodilution curve from which cardiac output can be calculated from the Stewart-Hamilton equation (Fig. 3.4). Application of this equation assumes three major conditions: complete mixing of blood and indicator, no loss of indicator between place of injection and place of detection, and constant blood flow. For accurate results with this technique, it is important to ensure adherence to these conditions.

The degree of change in the temperature is inversely proportional to the cardiac output.

- Increased blood flow (and cardiac output) = minimal temperature change
- Decreased blood flow (and cardiac output) = pronounced temperature change

Modern PACs are able to provide a continuous reading of cardiac output. They contain an electrical heating coil that sits in the right atrium, which heats up the blood in a semirandom binary fashion. The pulsed heating bursts can be detected by the thermistor in the pulmonary artery, which after autocorrelation with the inputting signal can provide continuous cardiac output. It has to be noted, however, that this technique has a latency of 7 to 10 minutes.

DYE/INDICATOR DILUTION

A number of techniques are available to measure cardiac output with the use of either a dye (indocyanine green) or an indicator (lithium). The concept is exactly the same as that for thermodilution: injection of a substance into the right side of the heart and detection of the same substance distally, either in the pulmonary artery or in the aorta. A curve is generated, which is replotted semilogarithmically to correct for recirculation of the dye. Cardiac output is calculated from the injected dose, the area under the curve (AUC), and the duration of effect (short duration indicates high cardiac output) from the Stewart-Hamilton equation:

$$\dot{Q} = \frac{V(T_B - T_I)K_1K_2}{T_B(t)dt}$$

$\dot{Q}$ = cardiac output
V = volume of injectate
T_B = blood temperature
T_I = injectate temperature
K_1K_2 = computer constants
$T_B(t)dt$ = change in blood temperature over time

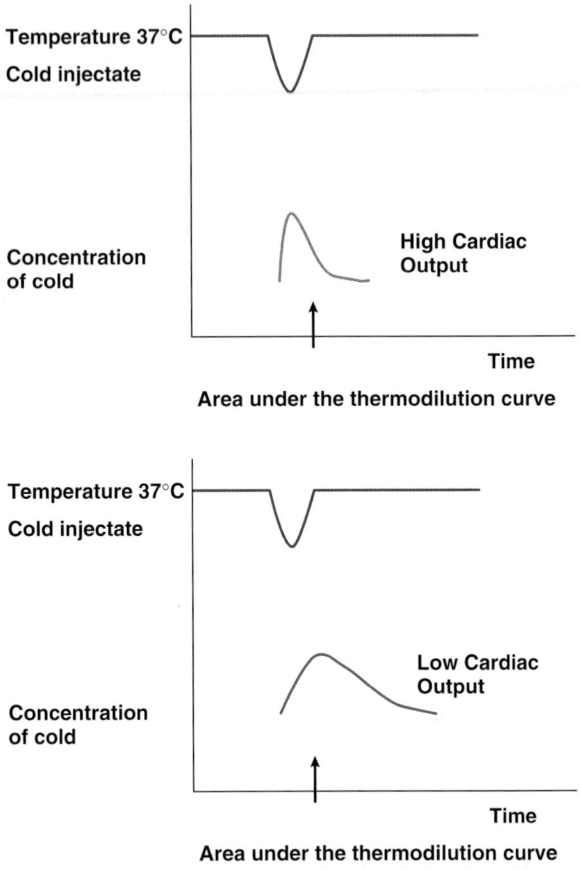

Figure 3.4 Thermodilution curves: A plot of temperature change versus time following a bolus of cold injectate. Cardiac output is inversely proportional to the area under the thermodilution curve. With a large cardiac output, the bolus is pumped rapidly past the thermistor, so the area is small.

ARTERIAL PULSE PRESSURE ANALYSIS

Arterial pulse pressure analysis is a technique of measuring and monitoring stroke volume on a beat-to-beat basis from the arterial pulse pressure waveform. This technique has several advantages over technologies such as the PAC, including its less invasive nature, as arterial access is available in most patients. Changes in both stroke volume and cardiac output are then shown on an almost continuous basis. A fair amount of less invasive cardiac output monitoring devices based on pulse pressure analysis are now commercially available and have resulted in a decreased use of the pulmonary catheter in most institutions (Table 3.5).

The fluctuations of blood pressure around its mean value occur as a specific volume of blood—the stroke volume—is forced into the aorta by each cardiac contraction. The magnitude of this pressure change, the pulse pressure, is a function of the magnitude of the stroke volume. On a beat-to-beat basis, the only factor that determines changes in pulse pressure is change in stroke volume, owing to the relatively slow nature of reactive vascular changes. In order to translate the pressure waveform into an accurate stroke volume, however, an estimate of the arterial compliance and resistance must be made. The greater the compliance, the less will be the vascular resistance to the pulsatile increase in the arterial pressure, and the less will be the pressure

Table 3.5 Less Invasive Hemodynamic Monitoring Devices

Modality	Device	Features	Requirements	CCO Response	Additional Variables		
Pulse Pressure Analysis							
Calibrated	PiCCOplus/ PiCCO$_2$	Thermistor-tipped arterial catheter	Central venous line	3 seconds	CVP GEDV EVLW	SVV PPV	Scvo$_2$
	LiDCOplus	Lithium dilution set	Arterial catheter	Beat-by-beat	—	SVV PPV	—
	EV1000/ VolumeView	Thermistor-tipped arterial catheter	Central venous line		CVP GEDV EVLW	SVV	Scvo^2
Uncalibrated	PulsioFlex	Specific arterial pressure transducer	Arterial catheter		—	SVV PPV	Scvo$_2$
	LiDCOrapid	—	Arterial catheter	Beat-by-beat	—	SVV PPV	—
	FloTrac/Vigileo	Specific arterial pressure transducer	Arterial catheter	20 seconds	—	SVV	Scvo$_2$
	PRAM MostCare	Specific arterial kit	Arterial catheter	Beat-by-beat	—	SVV PPV	—
Noninvasive	Nexfin	Finger pressure cuff	—	Beat-by-beat	—	SVV PPV	—
Doppler							
Transesophageal	CardioQ/ CardioQ-ODM	Esophageal probe	—	Beat-by-beat	—	—	—
Transthoracic	USCOM	Transthoracic probe	—	Intermittent	—	—	—
Applied Fick Principle							
Partial CO$_2$ rebreathing	NICO	Rebreathing loop	—	Every 3 minutes	—	—	—
Bioimpedance/Bioreactance							
Endotracheal bioimpedance	ECOM	Specific endotracheal tube	Arterial catheter	Continuous	—	—	—
Thoracic/whole body impedance	BioZ	Specific electrodes	—	Continuous	—	—	—
Thoracic bioreactance	NICOM	Specific electrodes	—	Continuous	—	SVV	
Plethysmographic Analysis							
Plethysmogram—variability	MASIMO	Specific transcutaneous probe	—	—	—	PVI	—

CCO, continuous cardiac output; CVP, central venous pressure; EVLW, extravascular lung water index; GEDV, global end-diastolic volume index; PPV, pulse pressure variation; PVI, plethysmographic variability index; SVV, stroke volume variation.

required to distend the vessel to accommodate a given stroke volume.

The need to incorporate arterial compliance and resistance into the measurement system has hindered this technology for many years. The origins of the pulse contour method for estimation of beat-to-beat stroke volume are based on the Windkessel model described by Otto Frank in 1899. Only recently have methods been described that can compensate or correct for these compliance or resistance changes to provide an accurate determination of stroke volume. Different technologies address this by different methods. Both lithium dilution and thermodilution techniques have been validated to calibrate pulse pressure tracking systems. Other devices are being marketed with the ability to self-calibrate after identifying vascular compliance and resistance directly from the pressure waveform.[39]

PROPRIETARY SYSTEMS REQUIRING CALIBRATION

PiCCO System

The PiCCO system[40] (Pulsion Medical Systems, Munich, Germany) utilizes a pulse contour method of tracking arterial pressure to derive changes in stroke volume. This system consists of a thermistor-tipped catheter, which is placed in the femoral or brachial artery. The device identifies the systolic area by recognizing the dicrotic notch on the arterial waveform. The systolic area is divided by the aortic impedance to calculate stroke volume. Transpulmonary thermodilution, requiring a central venous line, is used to calibrate the system in order to account for individual aortic compliance. In addition to tracking cardiac output and stroke volume, this technology also can provide dynamic indicators of volume responsiveness (SVV, SPV, and PPV), as well as a number of volumetric markers of preload (GEDV, ITBV, and EVLW). This system has been shown to be interchangeable with the pulmonary catheter in terms of the accuracy of measuring cardiac output and has been validated in a broad spectrum of clinical settings.[40]

LiDCOplus System

The LiDCOplus[41-44] (LiDCO, Cambridge, UK) tracks the power of the arterial waveform, rather than the contour, in order to track changes in stroke volume. A theoretical advantage is that the effect of reflected waves is reduced because the device does not need to identify specific parts of the arterial waveform. Because the morphologic pattern is not assessed, this technology also decreases (but does not negate) the effects of damping on the pressure system. This system can be calibrated by any independent form of cardiac output monitoring device but is sold with the proprietary lithium dilution cardiac output modality. The LiDCOplus technology also tracks the dynamic parameters of preload: SVV, SPV, and PPV.

EV1000 System

The EV1000 system has been recently introduced as a monitoring device based on pulse pressure analysis. Its components include a proprietory thermistor-tipped femoral arterial catheter and a separate sensor connected to the EV1000 monitor. Calibration by transpulmonary thermodilution is required and the system offers additional hemodynamic variables (GEDV, EVLW, SVV). Initial evaluation studies have shown a good agreement with the PiCCO system in the measurement of cardiac output and volumetric indices.[45,46]

Uncalibrated Systems

PulsioFlex System. This system (Pulsion Medical Systems, Munich, Germany), based on the PiCCO pulse contour algorithm, uses a proprietary transducer (ProAQT) integrated into the PulsioFlex system and does not require calibration. The device has recently been introduced by Pulsion Medical Systems, and initial clinical validation studies have shown good agreement with cardiac output measurements using transpulmonary thermodilution.[47]

LiDCOrapid System. This uncalibrated device uses the same algorithm as the LiDCOplus system, which has been well validated. Nomograms are used for the estimation of cardiac output instead of indicator dilution.

Flotrac. The Flotrac system (Edwards Lifesciences, Irvine, CA) consists of a proprietary transducer and a separate monitor (Vigileo). The technology assesses the variance of the arterial waveform in comparison with specific demographic characteristics of the patient to identify changes in stroke volume and analyzes statistical properties of the arterial pressure waveform to account for individual vascular resistance and compliance. Recent software updates have considerably improved the response time to changes in vascular dynamics (approx. 20 seconds), although concerns remain regarding the accuracy of cardiac output measurements in acute hemodynamic changes. Nonetheless, the Flotrac/Vigileo system has been integrated into protocols of hemodynamic optimization showing an improvement in clinical outcomes.[48-51]

Nexfin. The Nexfin system has been introduced recently as a totally noninvasive monitor of cardiac output. This system operates by applying a stepwise approach: An arterial pressure signal generated by combining photoelectric plethysmography with an intermittently inflated pressure cuff to maintain a constant arterial diameter. This finger arterial pressure signal is converted to a brachial arterial pressure waveform, which is used to calculate cardiac output. The current algorithm uses individualized components of a three-element Windkessel model, with age, gender, height, and weight as input parameters, incorporating the nonlinear effect of mean pressure and the influence of individual characteristics on aortic mechanical properties. Clinical studies have shown adequate correlation with cardiac output derived by thermodilution. The device offers the possibility of monitoring cardiac output at a very early clinical stage and may be instrumental in early treatment initiation.[52]

Masimo System. Although this is not a pulse pressure analysis-based monitor by definition, the Masimo system has the potential for use as an uncalibrated system for hemodynamic optimization. This device provides automated measurement of the PVI from a disposable finger sensor by measuring changes in perfusion index (PI = pulsatile infrared signal/nonpulsatile infrared signal × 100) over a time interval including at least one complete respiratory cycle.[25-27]

TRANSESOPHAGEAL DOPPLER[53-56]

The esophageal Doppler cardiac output monitor, described in the early 1970s, provides a safe and minimally invasive means of continuously monitoring the circulation. In comparison to suprasternal probes, esophageal probes have the advantage of less positional variety due to the smooth muscle tone of the esophagus and less signal interference from bone, soft tissue, and lung due to the close proximity of the aorta to the esophagus. The esophageal Doppler monitor measures blood flow velocity in the descending thoracic aorta using a flexible ultrasound probe. When these data are combined with the aortic cross-sectional area, other hemodynamic variables including stroke volume and cardiac output can be calculated. With the currently marketed device (CardioQ, Deltex, Chichester, UK) aortic cross-sectional area is assumed, providing minimally invasive, continuous cardiac output assessment. Abrupt changes in cardiac output are much better followed with Doppler systems than with the PAC-based continuous cardiac output systems.

Despite several potential sources of error, good correlation has been observed between measures of cardiac output made simultaneously with the esophageal Doppler monitor and with conventional thermodilution. Esophageal Doppler ultrasonography has been used for intravascular volume optimization both in the perioperative period and in the critical care setting.[29,32-35] One of the main advantages of the technique is the capability of rapid data acquisition after esophageal probe insertion.

Identification of the descending aortic waveform is essential for the correct use of the esophageal Doppler cardiac output monitor. Waveforms from other structures, such as the pulmonary artery, azygos vein, or celiac axis, may be encountered, leading to misinterpretation. After the characteristic descending aortic waveform is acquired, the signal is optimized before data acquisition by movement of the probe a centimeter up or down until the waveform indicates the best possible velocity and color intensities, followed by rotation of the probe to optimize the signal further if possible. The "peak velocity" display is used as a reference to the highest identified wave.

Esophageal Doppler waveform analysis has been increasingly evaluated as a method for determining optimal cardiac preload. The key preload parameter of interest is the flow time (FT)—the time required from the start of the waveform upstroke to return to baseline. FT represents the duration of left ventricular systole and makes up one third of the cardiac cycle (cycle time). Because the FT is heart rate dependent, it typically is corrected (FTc) to a rate of 60 beats per minute to compensate for the change in duration of systole. The FTc reflects the afterload status of the circulation. Decreased levels commonly are seen in hypovolemic patients, but caution in interpretation is advised because this pattern also can be seen with profound vasoconstriction. A more sensible use of this device is in following the effects of a fluid challenge. Because stroke volume can be determined on a beat-to-beat basis, it is easy to see the effects on the circulation of a small fluid bolus. Diagrammatic representations of characteristic Doppler waveform patterns are shown in Figure 3.5.

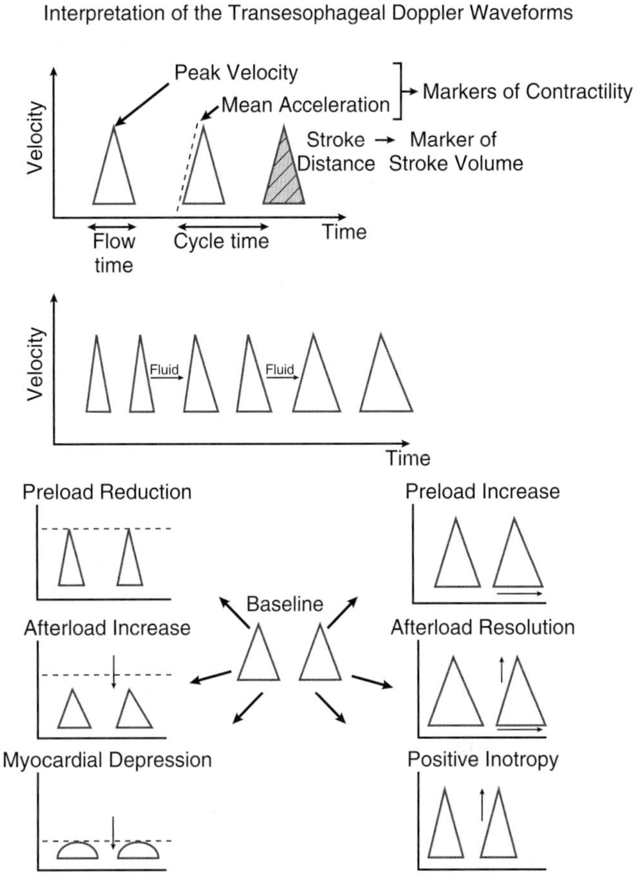

Figure 3.5 Diagrammatic representation of characteristic Doppler waveform patterns. The characteristic flow "triangles" generated in an esophageal Doppler study can be used to monitor cardiac output and stroke volume. The width of the base of the triangle (flow time) when corrected for heart rate provides an estimate of afterload. This diagram demonstrates the changes that are seen after a volume challenge in a variety of clinical conditions.

ECHOCARDIOGRAPHY[57,58]

TTE and TEE both are evolving tools in the critical care setting, and particularly TEE has become a standard of care for intraoperative monitoring in patients undergoing cardiac valvular replacement or repair. TEE has been used for a number of years for acute hemodynamic monitoring and diagnostic purposes in the cardiothoracic critical care setting and its use in the general critical care setting is now becoming commonplace.

Echocardiography provides a dynamic assessment of cardiac function, allowing visualization of cardiac chamber dimensions, functional assessments such as estimation of ventricular ejection fractions, detection of regional and global wall motion abnormalities, detection of valvular abnormalities, and exclusion of pericardial effusion. It also can be used to derive cardiac output from measurement of blood flow velocity by recording the Doppler shift of ultrasound signals reflected from the red blood cells. The time-velocity integral, which is the integral of instantaneous blood flow velocities during one cardiac cycle, is obtained for the blood flow in the left ventricular outflow tract (other sites can be used). This is multiplied by the cross-sectional area and the heart rate to give cardiac output. The results for cardiac output measured by this device in skilled hands are comparable to those obtained with use of the PAC.

The main disadvantages of the method are that a skilled operator is needed, the probe is large and therefore heavy sedation or anesthesia is needed, the equipment is very expensive, and an expert user is needed to adjust the probe to give continuous cardiac output readings. Nonetheless, echocardiography has an important and established clinical role. The modality is covered in detail in Chapter 8.

BIOIMPEDANCE AND BIOREACTANCE

Transthoracic bioimpedance is a technique initially developed as a noninvasive method of studying cardiovascular function during space flight. The underlying principle is the occurrence of changes in electrical impedance of the thoracic cavity with ejection of blood during systole.[37] In this model, the thorax is assumed to be a cylinder having electrical length between neck and xiphoid and has a basic impedance. A constant small current is passed between two outer electrodes attached to the skin (BioZ system) or an endotracheal tube (ECOM system), voltage change is sensed by two inner electrodes, and impedance is derived according to the equations described by Sramek and Bernstein.[59] Impedance is recognized to change with the cardiac cycle (related to changes in blood volume). The rate of change of impedance is a reflection of cardiac output. It is thought to be useful in estimating trends in cardiac output but not for absolute measurements. Contraction of the heart produces a cyclic change in transthoracic impedance of approximately 0.5%, unfortunately giving a rather low signal-to-noise ratio. Stroke volume and cardiac output can be measured continuously and at fixed intervals using this technique. Studies suggest that transthoracic bioimpedance is accurate in healthy volunteers, but its reliability decreases in critically ill patients, including those with sepsis or increased lung water, and in persons with pacemakers. Clinical evaluation studies have so far shown conflicting results and the technique has not gained wide clinical acceptance to date.[60-62]

BIOREACTANCE

As opposed to bioimpedance, this technique is based on the delivery of an oscillating electrical current and its modification by changes in stroke volume. The currently available NICOM system (Cheetah Medical, Inc., Vancouver, WA, USA) provides estimation of cardiac output by analyzing the variations in the frequency spectra of the electrical oscillations. Initial clinical validation studies have shown promising results.[63,64]

APPLICATION OF THE FICK PRINCIPLE

The NICO (Novametrix) system is a noninvasive device that applies Fick's principle on CO_2 and relies solely on airway gas measurement. The method actually calculates effective lung perfusion—that part of the pulmonary capillary blood flow that has passed through the ventilated parts of the lung. The effects of unrecognized ventilation-perfusion inequality in patients may explain why the results with this method show a lack of agreement between thermodilution and CO_2-rebreathing cardiac output.[65-68]

ASSESSMENT OF ADEQUACY OF THE CIRCULATION

Resuscitation of critically ill patients is a complex process. The rationale for most resuscitation maneuvers is that the delivery of oxygen to the tissues is inadequate, resulting in tissue hypoxia. Resuscitation is therefore aimed at increasing the oxygen delivery to a level at which enough oxygen is brought to the tissues to ensure efficient metabolism, so that normal cellular processes can occur. Part of this process entails measuring cardiac output and then increasing this variable to an "adequate" level. Unfortunately, this strategy is complicated as a result of the fact that all patients' cardiac output requirements differ—no "normal" level of flow can be specified for any patient in any given situation. In order to assess adequacy of perfusion, therefore, a number of surrogate markers need to be assessed that give an estimate of the underlying metabolic status. The cardiac output then needs to be assessed in combination with these surrogate markers of metabolism in order to ensure that resuscitation is improving the clinical situation.

CLINICAL ASSESSMENT

The first step in the hemodynamic assessment must be a thorough clinical assessment. Pulse rate and quality, respiratory rate, skin temperature, capillary refill time, core-peripheral temperature gradient, level of consciousness, and urine output are strongly related to cardiovascular dynamics, and a change in these clinical parameters may indicate deterioration as well as a positive response to a hemodynamic intervention. Skin mottling, pallor, and diaphoresis are alarming signs that need immediate and appropriate intervention. Recent studies have shown a strong relationship between clinical and microcirculatory parameters and underline their importance in hemodynamic assessment.[69-71]

Mixed Venous Oxygenation[72-75]

$S\bar{v}O_2$ is the oxygen saturation of mixed venous blood in the pulmonary artery. It reflects the overall venous saturation after the blood has been fully mixed in the right side of the heart. $S\bar{v}O_2$ is related to the balance between oxygen delivery (DO_2I) and the ability to extract oxygen, or the oxygen extraction ratio (O_2ER). Under normal circumstances, oxygen consumption is independent of supply until oxygen delivery falls below the anaerobic threshold. The normal O_2ER is approximately 25%, giving an $S\bar{v}O_2$ of 75%. In the face of a reduction in oxygen delivery, the tissues maintain oxygen consumption by increasing oxygen extraction, so $S\bar{v}O_2$ decreases. However, $S\bar{v}O_2$ does not necessarily vary with cardiac output. Not all patients can increase their O_2ER if DO_2I falls. Clinically, the response of $S\bar{v}O_2$ to an increase in cardiac output or oxygen delivery can aid hemodynamic manipulation. $S\bar{v}O_2$ can be measured by sampling blood from the distal lumen of a PAC and then measuring oxyhemoglobin saturation by means of co-oximetry, or by using an oximetric PAC that is able to continuously display $S\bar{v}O_2$. A flow diagram of a published protocol using PAC-derived parameters is shown in Figure 3.6.

It has been suggested that $S\bar{v}O_2$ should be monitored and the key variables manipulated to keep it within the normal range (65% to 75%). In practice, this means ensuring that

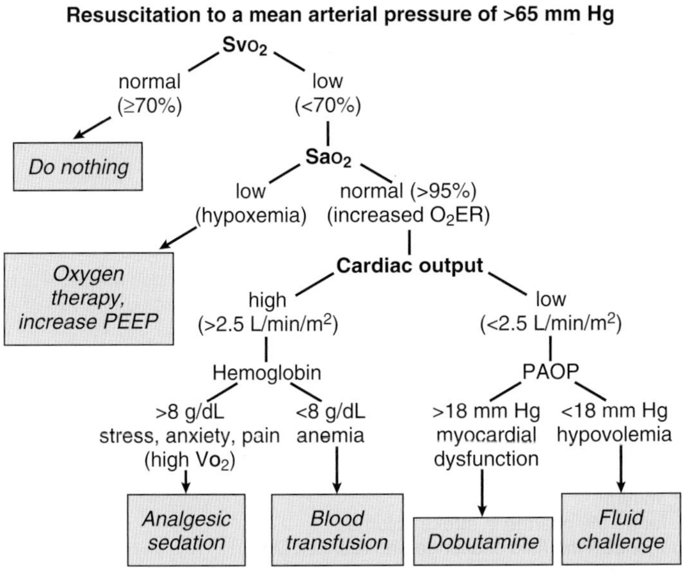

Figure 3.6 Flow chart for Pinsky-Vincent protocol. A diagnostic and treatment algorithm for the use of pulmonary artery catheter–derived variables. O_2ER, oxygen extraction ratio; PAOP, pulmonary artery occlusion pressure; PEEP, positive end-expiratory pressure; Sao_2, arterial oxygen saturation; Vo_2, oxygen consumption. (Adapted from Pinsky MR, Vincent JL: Let us use the PAC correctly and only when we need it. Crit Care Med 2005;33:1119-1122.)

the hemoglobin concentration and arterial oxygen saturation are normal and then either increasing cardiac output or decreasing oxygen utilization (such as by sedation or cooling). Thus, $S\bar{v}o_2$ monitoring provides a means of assessing the adequacy of cardiac output for a given patient. This strategy has been used with success in post–cardiac surgery patients and has been suggested for use in critically ill patients.

Central Venous Oxygen Saturation

In patients without PACs in place, central venous oxygen saturation ($Scvo_2$) may be measured by sampling from the distal lumen of a central venous line in the SVC. This variable bears some relationship to the mixed venous oxygen saturation, although because the venous blood is not totally mixed in the SVC, the relationship should be considered as representing a guide rather than reflecting reality. In practice, the central venous oxygen saturation should be used as a screening tool, rather than as an accurate marker of adequacy. If the level is very low, then the inference can be made that the circulation is inadequate; however, near-normal levels do not preclude underlying problems. The use of this variable in this fashion has proved successful in reducing mortality rates for early severe sepsis and is recommended as a target for therapy by the Surviving Sepsis Campaign.[74-76]

Blood Lactate

Blood lactate levels represent the balance between lactate production and lactate metabolism. The liver is responsible for the major part of lactate metabolism. Inadequate oxygen delivery and tissue hypoxia, irrespective of the underlying cause, results in increased lactate generation. In critically ill patients, high blood lactate levels develop from a combination of inadequate oxygen delivery secondary to poor perfusion (in terms of both perfusion pressure and flow), impaired cellular oxygen utilization from mitochondrial damage, and reduced hepatic clearance of lactate. A resolving lactic acidosis along with clinical signs of improved perfusion is an important indicator of improving perfusion after resuscitation. Lactate levels and lactate clearance have been shown to predict mortality risk and morbidity, and studies investigating protocols aimed at decreasing lactate levels have shown the potential role of lactate as a treatment goal.[77-80]

Venous-to-Arterial CO_2 Difference (Pco_2 Gap)

Oxygen-derived parameters, namely $S\bar{v}o_2$ and $Scvo_2$, may falsely indicate adequate tissue perfusion in the presence of anaerobic metabolism due to microcirculatory compromise. In this situation, a decrease in oxygen consumption (Vo_2) may occur, either because of impaired oxygen delivery or reduced oxygen demand resulting in normal levels of $S\bar{v}o_2$ or $Scvo_2$. In hypoxic conditions due to impaired tissue perfusion a rise in the partial pressure of CO_2 (Pco_2) is usually seen, widening the gap between arterial and venous Pco_2. Recent clinical studies have suggested that the venous-to-arterial CO_2 difference using a central venous and an arterial blood sample ($P(cv - a)CO_2$ or Pco_2 gap) may be used as a complementary tool to unmask inadequate tissue perfusion in patients who are apparently resuscitated to target goals, namely, an $Scvo_2$ of 70%. Further prospective clinical studies will show if this parameter has the potential to function as a treatment goal in the resuscitation of critically ill patients with hemodynamic compromise.[81-83]

GOAL-DIRECTED THERAPY

The concept of goal-directed therapy refers to the protocolized assessment and manipulation of hemodynamic variables in the resuscitation of critically ill patients. This approach became fashionable in the late 1980s and early 1990s, with a resurgence of interest in the early 2000s. Initially these protocols were relatively simple and consisted of measures to increase oxygen delivery and consumption to predefined targets. It was soon recognized that the same targets could not be used for every single group of patients undergoing different conditions and procedures, so protocols have now been refined for different patient populations.

HEMODYNAMIC OPTIMIZATION OF THE HIGH-RISK SURGICAL PATIENT

Many different protocols have been used for the management of the high-risk surgical patient.[84-92] Initially all such protocols targeted an oxygen delivery index of 600 mL/minute/m^2 with the use of fluids and positive inotropic agents. Measurement of cardiac output was performed through a PAC. Currently, many different protocols have been devised, some targeting oxygen delivery, some the mixed venous oxygen saturation, and some ensuring adequate volume loading by targeting a maximal stroke volume. The newer protocols reflect the more modern technologies, so they typically involve less invasive strategies and

Hemodynamic optimization of the high-risk surgical patient

Identify high-risk patients [severe cardiac/respiratory disease; age >70 years with limited physiologic reserve in 1 or more organs; extensive planned surgery; acute massive blood loss (>2.5 L); acute abdominal catastrophe (e.g., perforated viscus); acute renal failure; late-stage vascular disease involving the aorta]

↓

Maintain $Sa{O_2}$ >94%; Hb 8-10 g/dL; Temp 37°C; MAP 60-100 mm Hg

↓

Ensure central venous and arterial lines in situ

↓

Take arterial blood gas and central venous oxygen sample ($Scv{O_2}$)

↓

Commence hemodynamic flow monitoring (e.g., LiDCO/PiCCO/transesophageal Doppler/PAFC)

↓

Record $D{O_2}I$

↓

Every 15 minutes check $D{O_2}I$

↓

If $D{O_2}I$ <600 mL/min/m²

- Give a 250-mL fluid challenge and check for a 10% change in stroke volume
- if the patient is stroke volume responsive—give a further 250-mL fluid challenge and recheck $D{O_2}I$

↓

- if the patient is not stroke volume responsive—start dopexamine at 0.25 μg/kg/min (to a maximum of 1.0 μg/kg/min) if the $D{O_2}I$ <600 mL/min/m²
- Decrease dopexamine if HR >20% above baseline

If $D{O_2}I$ >600 mL/min/m²

- Continue to observe $D{O_2}I$ every 15 minutes for 8 hours postoperatively

Figure 3.7 Pearse protocol for management of the high-risk surgical patient. $D{O_2}I$, oxygen delivery index; Hb, hemoglobin concentration; HR, heart rate; LiDCO, lithium dilution cardiac output; MAP, mean arterial pressure; PAFC, pulmonary artery flotation catheter; PiCCO, pulse contour continuous cardiac output; $Sa{O_2}$, arterial oxygen saturation; $Scv{O_2}$, saturation of central venous oxygen. (Adapted from Pearse RM, Dawson D, Fawcett J, et al: Early goal-directed therapy after major surgery reduces complications and duration of hospital stay. Crit Care 2005;9:687-693.)

techniques. Data suggesting one protocol over another are essentially lacking, so it is best to choose appropriate monitoring technologies and therapeutic end points in accordance with the particular characteristics of the patient group being treated and depending on availability of appropriate devices and trained practitioners. Two protocols for optimization are shown in Figures 3.6 and 3.7.

EARLY GOAL-DIRECTED THERAPY OF SEVERE SEPSIS

Resuscitation of patients with severe sepsis and septic shock has been studied with an early goal-directed approach[74] (Fig. 3.8). In this approach, cardiac output has not actually been measured; however, a number of surrogate markers of adequacy of the circulation have been targeted. Volume loading is instigated early in this protocol and then targeted against markers of lactate metabolism and central venous oxygen saturation. If these markers fail to fall, then oxygen utilization is decreased by sedation and mechanical ventilation, and oxygen delivery is increased with the use of red blood cell transfusion and a positive inotrope. It should be noticed that although different parameters are being used, this strategy is very similar in principle to that used in the high-risk surgical group of patients.

CONCLUSIONS

Resuscitation of critically ill patients is a complex process. Several simple steps need to be taken to ensure delivery of an appropriate level of resuscitation. First, the patient should attain an optimal level of preload. This is best achieved by identifying the group of patients who are likely to benefit from volume loading and then providing this intervention, while at the same time not giving excess intravascular volume to patients who are unlikely to benefit from it. If it is impossible to predict which patients will benefit, then the fluid should be given under tightly controlled circumstances in the form of a fluid challenge with close monitoring of the circulation. After appropriate volume resuscitation, the circulation of some patients will still be inadequate for their metabolic demands. These patients may then benefit from either a reduction in oxygen requirements or an increase in oxygen delivery. This approach necessitates the monitoring of the circulation and the metabolic status.

KEY POINTS

- Isolated measurements of either right atrial pressure or pulmonary artery pressure are not good markers for identifying patients who will respond to a fluid challenge.
- Dynamic measurements of pulse or stroke volume variation can predict volume responsiveness with a high degree of sensitivity and specificity.
- No "normal" cardiac output can be specified for any patient, so cardiac output must be compared with other markers of metabolic status.
- Cardiac output can be measured by a number of techniques. Less important than how it is measured is how this knowledge is applied.

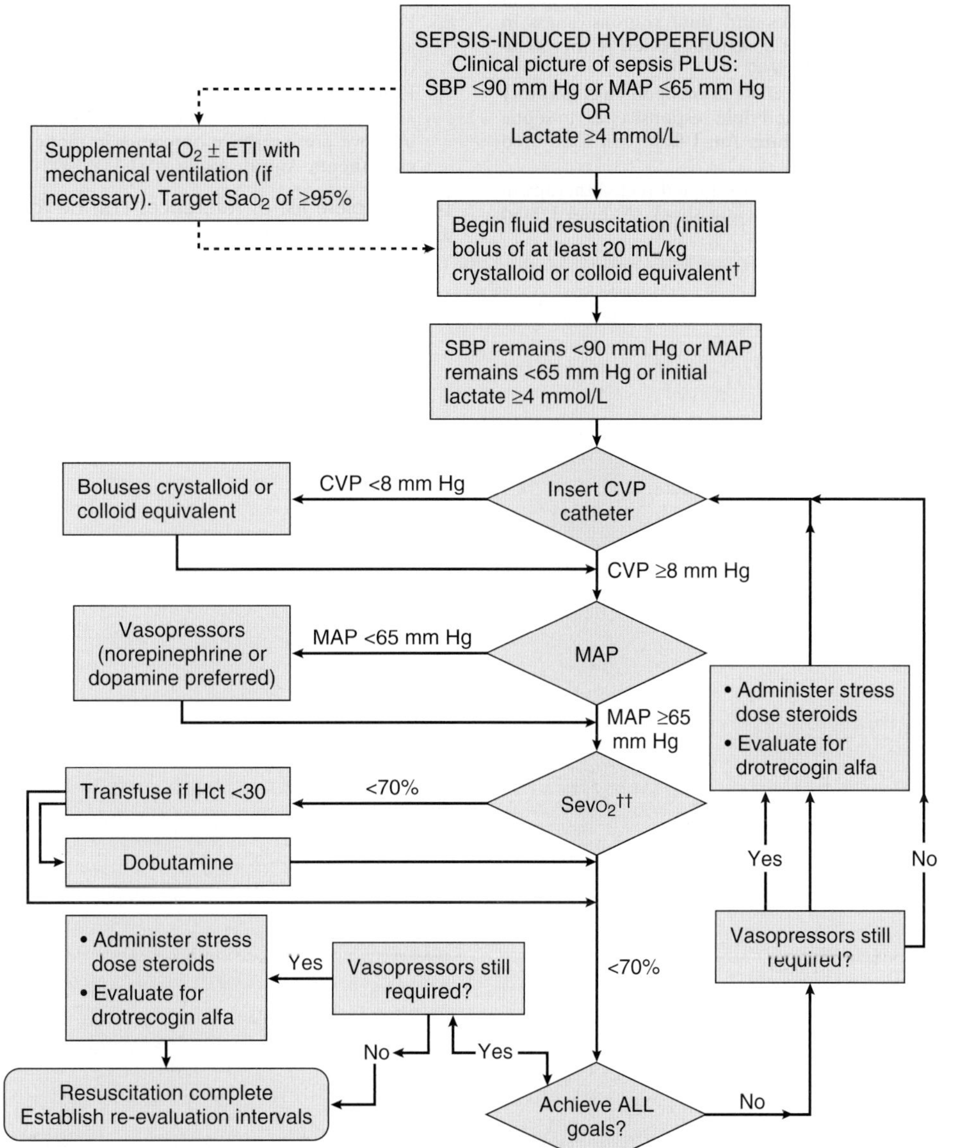

† In circumstances where MAP is judged to be critically low, vasopressors may be started at any point in this algorithm.
†† If pulmonary artery catheter is used, a mixed venous O_2 saturation is an acceptable surrogate and 65% would be the target.

Figure 3.8 Rivers protocol for hemodynamic management in severe sepsis or septic shock. This treatment algorithm provides a framework for the management of the hemodynamic disturbances associated with severe sepsis and septic shock. CVP, central venous pressure; ETI, endotracheal intubation; Hct, hematocrit; MAP, mean arterial pressure; SaO_2, arterial oxygen saturation; SBP, systolic blood pressure; $ScvO_2$, saturation of central venous oxygen.

SELECTED REFERENCES

9. Kumar A, Anel R, Bunnell E, et al: Pulmonary artery occlusion pressure and central venous pressure fail to predict ventricular filling volume, cardiac performance, or the response to volume infusion in normal subjects. Crit Care Med 2004;32:691-699.
12. Marik PE, Baram M, Vahid B: Does central venous pressure predict fluid responsiveness? A systematic review of the literature and the tale of seven mares. Chest 2008;134:172-178.
16. Marik PE, Cavallazzi R, Vasu T, Hirani A: Dynamic changes in arterial waveform derived variables and fluid responsiveness in mechanically ventilated patients: A systematic review of the literature. Crit Care Med 2009;37:2642-2647.
23. Michard F, Boussat S, Chemla D, et al: Relation between respiratory changes in arterial pulse pressure and fluid responsiveness in septic patients with acute circulatory failure. Am J Resp Crit Care Med 2000;162:134-138.
74. Rivers E, Nguyen B, Havstad S, et al: Early goal directed therapy in the treatment of severe sepsis and septic shock. N Engl J Med 2001;345:1368-1377.
77. Jansen TC, van Bommel J, Bakker J: Blood lactate monitoring in critically ill patients: A systematic health technology assessment. Crit Care Med 2009;37:2827-2839.
79. Jansen TC, van Bommel J, Schoonderbeek FJ, et al: Early lactate-guided therapy in intensive care unit patients: A multicenter, open-label, randomized controlled trial. Am J Respir Crit Care Med 2010;182:752-761.
82. Vallée F, Vallet B, Mathe O, et al: Central venous-to-arterial carbon dioxide difference: An additional target for goal-directed therapy in septic shock? Intensive Care Med 2008;34:2218-2225.
85. Pearse RM, Dawson D, Fawcett J, et al: Early goal-directed therapy after major surgery reduces complications and duration of hospital stay. Crit Care 2005;9:687-693.
92. Hamilton MA, Cecconi M, Rhodes A: A systematic review and meta-analysis on the use of preemptive hemodynamic intervention to improve postoperative outcomes in moderate and high-risk surgical patients. Anesth Analg 2011;112:1392-1402.

The complete list of references can be found at www.expertconsult.com.

4

Arterial, Central Venous, and Pulmonary Artery Catheters

Jean-Louis Vincent

CHAPTER OUTLINE

ARTERIAL CATHETERS

WHAT DO THEY OFFER?

The placement of an arterial catheter permits (1) reliable and continuous monitoring of arterial pressure and (2) repeated blood sampling. Analysis of the arterial pulse pressure curve may also have other applications, including assessment of fluid responsiveness and estimation of cardiac output. The appearance of arterial pressure waves will vary according to the site at which the artery is sampled. As the arterial pressure wave is conducted away from the heart, three effects are observed: The wave appears narrower; the dicrotic notch becomes smaller; and the perceived systolic and pulse pressures rise and the perceived diastolic pressure falls.

ARTERIAL PRESSURE MEASUREMENT

The optimal range of arterial pressure depends on individual patient characteristics, on underlying diseases, and also on treatment. Hence, it is impossible to give an optimal range of arterial pressure that is applicable in all patients. When arterial pressure needs to be evaluated accurately, oscillometric measurements become unreliable,[1] and insertion of an arterial catheter is indicated.

Four potential indications for insertion of an arterial catheter for measurement of arterial pressure are recognized:

1. *Hypotensive states associated with (a risk of) altered tissue perfusion.* Hypotension that is resistant to fluid administration requires the administration of vasopressor agents, and invasive measurement of arterial pressure is then necessary to titrate this form of therapy. Norepinephrine is the vasopressor agent most commonly used in this setting. A mean arterial pressure (MAP) of 65 to 70 mm Hg is usually targeted, but this level must be adapted to the individual patient and the clinical scenario; in particular, elderly patients with atherosclerotic disease may require higher levels than younger individuals with normal arteries.
2. *Intravenous vasodilator therapy.* Vasodilating therapy (e.g., nitrates and hydralazine) is a mainstay in the management of heart failure, because it can increase cardiac output. Close monitoring of arterial pressure is essential to avoid excessive hypotension.
3. *Severely hypertensive states.* Extreme hypertension may result in organ impairment, especially of the brain and the heart. Sodium nitroprusside or calcium entry blockers usually are used to lower arterial pressure, and careful, accurate monitoring is essential to titrate the antihypertensive therapy.
4. *Induction of hypertension.* Hypertension is sometimes induced in patients with neurologic diseases. Severe cerebral edema with intracranial hypertension, in particular, requires vasopressor support to maintain cerebral perfusion pressure (the gradient between the MAP and the

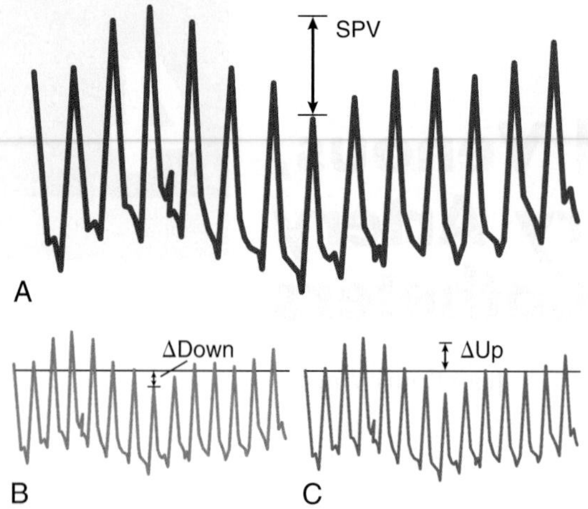

Figure 4.1 The systolic pressure variation (SPV) is the difference between the maximum and the minimum systolic blood pressures during one ventilatory cycle (**A**). The SPV is the sum of the ΔDown (**B**) and the ΔUp (**C**). (From Perel A, Pizov R, Cotev S: Systolic blood pressure variation is a sensitive indicator of hypovolemia in ventilated dogs subjected to graded hemorrhage. Anesthesiology 1987;67:498.)

intracranial pressure); likewise, hypertension may be used to treat or prevent the development of vasospasm secondary to subarachnoid hemorrhage, as part of the so-called triple-H therapy (hypertension, hypervolemia, hemodilution). Norepinephrine usually is used for this purpose.

FLUID RESPONSIVENESS

Variations in arterial pressure during positive-pressure ventilation have been used as a measure of fluid responsiveness. The transient increases in intrathoracic pressure influence venous return in patients who are likely to respond to fluid administration. This fluctuation in ventricular filling will translate into fluctuations in arterial pressure a few beats later. Accordingly, the greater the degree of systolic arterial pressure, or pulse pressure, variation during the respiratory cycle, the greater will be the increase in cardiac output in response to fluid administration (Fig. 4.1). However, this observation is valid primarily in patients without spontaneous respiratory movements and without significant arrhythmias, and only when a sufficient tidal volume is applied.[2,3]

CARDIAC OUTPUT ASSESSMENT

The pulse contour analysis also can serve to estimate cardiac output less invasively than with the pulmonary artery catheter (PAC). Because the only determinants of arterial pressure are the stroke volume and the resistance and compliance factors of the blood and arteries, analysis of the pulse contour trace can help to monitor cardiac output over time. This can be done with regular calibrations whenever changes in vascular tone or blood volume occur, or even in the absence of calibration. These measurements are still approximations, so further technological developments can be expected to improve accuracy.

BLOOD SAMPLING

The presence of an arterial catheter can greatly facilitate blood sampling, especially in terms of enabling easy access to the circulation for regular monitoring of blood gases, such as may be required in severe respiratory failure or with acute metabolic alterations. Sensors can measure blood gases continuously, but widespread use of such sensors is limited by their cost.

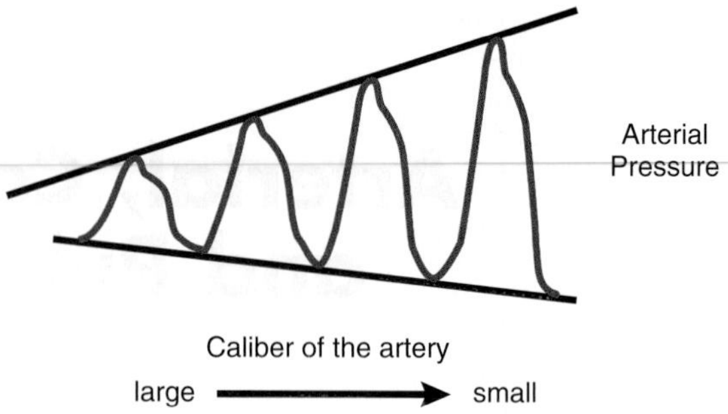

Figure 4.2 Schematic representation of an arterial pressure tracing showing that the pulse pressure increases as arterial size decreases.

ACCESS

For placement of arterial catheters, usually the radial artery is used. The femoral artery can be easily cannulated and gives a better signal, but presence of a femoral catheter interferes more with patient mobility and warrants concern about infection.[4] Use of other sites, such as the brachial or the axillary artery or even the dorsalis pedis artery,[5] can be considered. An important point to keep in mind is that the pulse pressure increases from the core to the periphery. In other words, the systolic pressure is overestimated in smaller arteries (Fig. 4.2). Hence, it may be better to rely more on mean values than on systolic or diastolic pressures.

COMPLICATIONS

The most feared complication with use of arterial catheters is ischemia. With any suspicion of ischemia, the catheter must be removed immediately. Allen's test, to determine occlusive arterial lesions distal to the wrist, is unreliable and is no longer widely used. The accidental disconnection of arterial lines can be associated with severe hemorrhage and even exsanguination. Infectious complications are rare.

CENTRAL VENOUS CATHETERS

WHAT DO THEY OFFER?

The central venous catheter can facilitate fluid administration. It also allows measurement of the central venous pressure (CVP) and enables access to central venous blood for sampling.

FLUID ADMINISTRATION

The large-bore central venous catheter allows fluids to be administered fast and reliably in the presence of acute hemorrhage. Placement of a central catheter is therefore essential in patients with hemorrhage due to polytrauma or with other forms of acute bleeding. It also allows irritant or hypertonic fluids to be administered, such as parenteral solutions, potassium-enriched solutions, and some therapeutic agents. Central venous lines also can be convenient in patients who need prolonged intravenous therapy when peripheral venous access becomes problematic.

MEASUREMENT OF CENTRAL VENOUS PRESSURE

CVP is identical to right atrial pressure (RAP) (in the absence of vena cava obstruction) and to right ventricular (RV) end-diastolic pressure (in the absence of tricuspid regurgitation). It is thus equivalent to the right-sided filling pressure. CVP is determined by the interaction of cardiac function and venous return, which is itself determined by the blood volume and the compliance characteristics of the venous system. Hence, an elevated CVP can reflect an increase in blood volume as well as an impairment in cardiac function. Because the CVP evaluates the right-sided filling pressures, CVP can be increased in the presence of pulmonary hypertension, even if left ventricular (LV) function is normal. The normal value in healthy persons is very low, not exceeding 5 mm Hg. Thus, the CVP value may not be much lower than normal in the presence of hypovolemia. In general, a CVP below 10 mm Hg can be considered to indicate that the patient is more likely to respond to fluid resuscitation, but exceptions to this rule exist. A high CVP suggests a certain blood volume but does not guarantee sufficient LV filling.

Clinically, CVP can be assessed by evaluation of the degree of jugular distention[6] or liver enlargement. A single CVP measurement is not very useful and is not a good indicator of a positive response to fluids; an increase in CVP without a concurrent increase in cardiac output is not only useless but also harmful, because it will lead to increased edema formation.

ACCESS TO BLOOD IN SUPERIOR VENA CAVA

Measuring the central venous oxygen saturation ($ScvO_2$) is a surrogate for measurement of the true mixed venous oxygen saturation ($S\bar{v}O_2$). Although absolute values of $ScvO_2$ are not identical to single $S\bar{v}O_2$ values, trends in $ScvO_2$ over time follow the same pattern as trends in $S\bar{v}O_2$, making $ScvO_2$ a useful measure in patients who do not require an arterial catheter.[7] $ScvO_2$ can be obtained either intermittently (by withdrawal of blood samples) or continuously (with the use of a catheter equipped with fiberoptic fibers).

TRACE ANALYSIS

Analysis of the CVP waveform can provide some interesting information. In particular, a large y descent indicates a restrictive cardiac state, but not all restrictive patterns are associated with this finding.

ACCESS

The central venous catheter generally is introduced via the internal jugular vein; the subclavian vein also can be used, although the risk of pneumothorax may be somewhat higher with this route. Peripherally inserted central catheters can also be placed, via the cephalic vein, basilic vein, or brachial vein. Introduction of a femoral catheter through the abdominal inferior vena cava to the right atrium can also yield reliable CVP measurements.[8] The use of femoral catheters, however, is associated with a greater risk of infections and thrombophlebitis.[9]

COMPLICATIONS

Complications of central venous catheterization are related primarily to puncture of the central vein: Hemothorax can be life-threatening, especially in the presence of severe respiratory failure. In the presence of unilateral pathology, the catheter must be introduced on the affected side. Arterial puncture resulting in a local hematoma is not uncommon, but hematoma formation usually is without major consequences. Bedside ultrasonography can help guide the introduction of the catheter into the vein. Excessive advancement of a long catheter in a small patient can result in arrhythmias; such arrhythmias have been described with advancement of the catheter tip into the right ventricle, but this problem can be identified by the presence of an RV trace on the monitor display.

Catheter-related infections constitute the major long-term complication. Adherence to basic hygiene guidelines can decrease the incidence of catheter-related sepsis. Triple-lumen catheters may be associated with a higher incidence of catheter-related infection,[10] primarily as a result of increased catheter manipulation. The use of antimicrobial-coated catheters may decrease the risk of infections,[11] but fears remain about the risks of development of resistant organisms.[12] Routine replacement of catheters after 3 to 7 days is not recommended.[13]

PULMONARY ARTERY CATHETERS

WHAT DO THEY OFFER?

PACs allow collection of data on right atrial, pulmonary artery, and pulmonary artery occlusive pressures (Fig. 4.3); flow (cardiac output); and oxygenation ($S\bar{v}O_2$).

PRESSURES

Right Atrial Pressure

As indicated earlier, the RAP is identical to the CVP in the vast majority of cases.

Pulmonary Artery Occlusion Pressure

When the balloon on the catheter is inflated, it causes an obstruction (becomes wedged) in a small branch of the pulmonary artery, interrupting the flow of blood locally (but blood flow continues normally in the rest of the pulmonary circulation), so that (assuming the absence of an abnormal obstacle) a continuous column of blood is present between the tip of the PAC and the left atrium. This pulmonary artery occlusion pressure (PAOP), or pulmonary artery wedge pressure (PAWP), generally reflects the left atrial pressure well. Nevertheless, a number of steps must be taken to ensure the adequacy of the measurement.

A first question is whether the PAOP reflects the pressure in the pulmonary veins and not the alveolar pressure. The tip of the catheter should be in a West zone III position, where a continuous column of blood exists between the

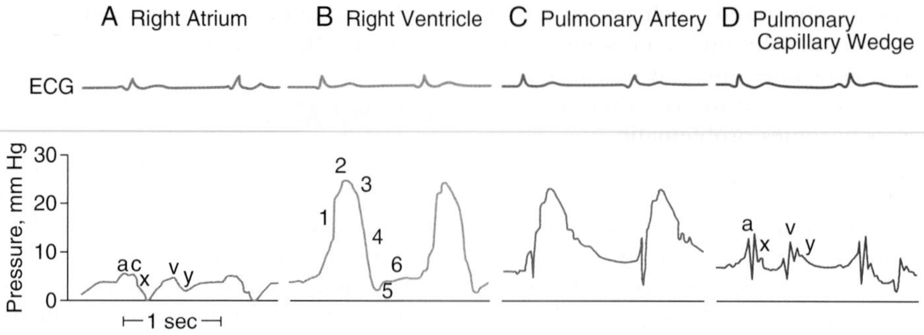

Figure 4.3 Pressure waveforms. **A,** The normal right atrial (RA) tracing. The a wave is the RA pressure rise resulting from atrial contraction and follows the P wave of the electrocardiogram (ECG). On simultaneous ECG and RA tracings it usually occurs at the beginning of the QRS complex. The c wave, caused by closure of the tricuspid valve, follows the a wave and is coincident with the beginning of ventricular systole. Atrial relaxation (x descent) is followed by a passive rise in RA pressure resulting from atrial filling during ventricular systole and occurs during the T wave of the simultaneously recorded ECG. The y descent reflects the opening of the tricuspid valve and passive atrial emptying. **B,** The normal right ventricular (RV) tracing. The sharp rise in RV pressure (1) is due to isometric contraction and is followed by a rapid pressure decrease (2) as blood is ejected through the pulmonary valve. This rapid ejection is followed by a phase of more reduced pressure decrease, which is often reflected in a small step in the downslope of the RV pressure waveform (3). The subsequent sharp decline in RV pressure (4) occurs as a result of isometric relaxation and is noted once the RV pressure falls below the pulmonary artery (PA) pressure (with consequent closure of the pulmonary valve). As RV pressure falls below RA pressure, the tricuspid valve opens, and passive refilling (5) of the right ventricle occurs, followed by atrial contraction, causing a biphasic wave of ventricular filling to appear on the RV tracing (6). **C,** The normal pulmonary arterial waveform. A pulmonary artery systolic elevation is caused by ejection of blood from the right ventricle, followed by a decline in pressure as RV pressure falls. As RV pressure falls below pulmonary artery pressure, the pulmonary valve closes, which causes a momentary rise in the declining pulmonary artery pressure. This is the dicrotic notch characteristic of the pulmonary arterial (and also the systemic arterial) waveform. The pulmonary artery systolic wave usually occurs in synchrony with the T wave of the ECG. Pulmonary artery diastolic pressure (PADP) does not fall below RA pressure and therefore is higher than right ventricular end-diastolic pressure (RVEDP): it is an approximation to left ventricular end-diastolic pressure (LVEDP). **D,** The normal pulmonary artery occlusion pressure (PAOP) waveform. The waveform of the pulmonary capillary wedge pressure (PCWP) is subject to the same mechanical variables as the RA waveform, but because of the damping that occurs through the pulmonary circulation, the waves and descents often are less distinct. Similarly, the mechanical events are recorded later in the cardiac cycle, as seen on the ECG. Thus, the a wave is not seen until after the QRS complex, and the v wave occurs after the T wave of the ECG. The PCWP is a closer approximation to LVEDP than is PADP. (From Grossman W: Cardiac catheterization. In Braunwald E (ed): Heart Disease: A Textbook of Cardiovascular Medicine, 3rd ed. Philadelphia, WB Saunders, 1992.)

catheter tip and the left atrium (Fig. 4.4). These considerations are less important with fluid optimization and with today's lower positive end-expiratory pressures (PEEPs).

To exclude a possible influence of airway pressure on PAOP readings, the changes in PAOP can simply be compared with the changes in pulmonary artery pressure (PAP) during the respiratory cycle. If PAOP reflects the pressure within the pulmonary veins, these changes should be identical, because the pulmonary artery and vein should be subjected to identical changes in intrathoracic pressures. If, on the other hand, the catheter tip is not in a West zone III, the changes in PAOP will be more significant than the changes in PAP. In these latter conditions, either fluid administration or some reduction in the PEEP level may abolish the differences.

The next question is whether the measured pressure is truly a transmural pressure—that is, the pressure difference between the vascular structures and the environmental structures. In other words, will changes in surrounding intrathoracic pressures influence the pressures measured? In the case of intrathoracic pressures, the changes in pleural pressure are particularly relevant. Hence, all measurements should be performed at end-expiration, when the pleural pressure is closest to zero. A marked fall in intrapleural pressure, as with a Mueller maneuver (forced inspiration against resistance), may dramatically increase the transmural pressures. A more common problem in the intensive care unit (ICU) is the increase in pleural pressure due to positive-pressure ventilation, sometimes with high PEEP levels.

One method of combating this problem could be to subtract the esophageal pressure from the measured PAOP, but this approach has a number of technological limitations. Simple disconnection of the respirator to measure PAOP after obtaining an equilibration state is not recommended, because the measured PAOP will not represent the real value when PEEP is applied. A better method consists of measuring the lowest (nadir) PAOP, within seconds after a very transient disconnection from the ventilator, to identify the true transmural pressure before a new equilibrium is reached.[14] Such a maneuver suppresses the high intrathoracic pressure and eliminates the influence of the extramural pressure, but the values obtained may not be valid in the presence of intrinsic PEEP. Other methods have been suggested, some relatively sophisticated[15] and others more simple, involving subtraction of approximately one third of the PEEP level from the measured PAOP, for example. The question is whether this is really so important, because absolute PAOP values are not very helpful.

In respiratory failure, PAOP does not represent true capillary pressure, which may be somewhat higher. The true capillary pressure may be estimated from the measurement of the intersection point of the rapid and slow pressure decay curves recorded after a rapid interruption of the blood flow; such measurements of capillary pressure are possible from the pressure trace. This pressure is

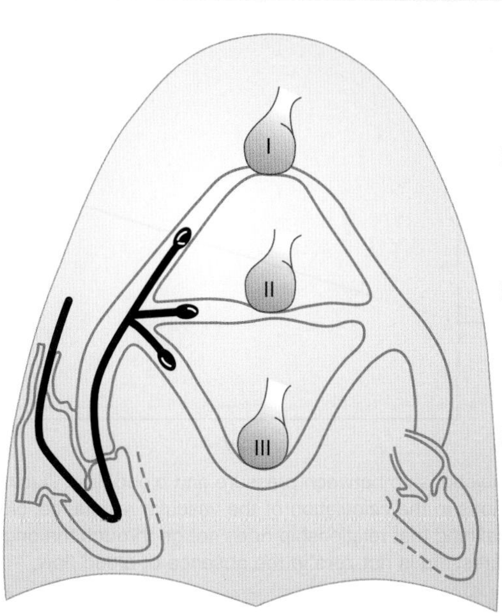

Figure 4.4 The position of the pulmonary artery catheter tip in relation to the zones of the theoretical lung model described by West. For pulmonary artery occlusion pressure (PAOP) to be a valid estimate of "left heart" filling pressure, a continuous column of blood must exist between the catheter tip and the left atrium. In zones I and II, pulmonary vasculature is either totally or partially compressed by the intra-alveolar pressure, and measurements of PAOP will be misleading. PA, alveolar pressure; Pa, pulmonary artery pressure; Pv, pulmonary venous pressure. (From Marini JJ: Respiratory Medicine and Intensive Care for the House Officer. Baltimore, Williams & Wilkins, 1991.)

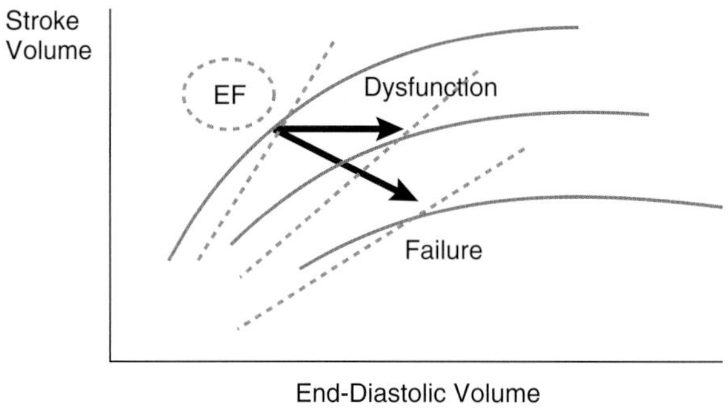

Figure 4.5 Ventricular function curve depicting the difference between ventricular dysfunction (decrease in the ventricular ejection fraction [EF] but preservation of stroke volume) and ventricular failure (defined as the inability of the heart to pump enough flow). The EF, the ratio between stroke volume and end-diastolic volume, is represented by the *dashed lines;* it is decreased in all cases.

well correlated with extravascular lung water in animal experiments. The need to know these values is questionable, however, because the primary goal remains to keep these hydrostatic pressures as low as possible while maintaining adequate cardiac output.

PAOP may not adequately reflect LV end-diastolic pressure. It may be lower in patients with aortic regurgitation or higher in the presence of significant tachycardia or mitral valve disease. LV end-diastolic pressure may not even accurately predict LV end-diastolic volume. This was already demonstrated many years ago with radionuclide techniques.[16] Preload is more directly defined as the end-diastolic volume. A stiff, noncompliant ventricle can result in a relatively high end-diastolic pressure for a given end-diastolic volume. An evaluation of end-diastolic volumes can be obtained less invasively with echocardiographic techniques. Likewise, the use of transthoracic thermodilution techniques allows the estimation of intrathoracic blood volume and global end-diastolic volumes. However, these assessments of end-diastolic volumes do not give additional information about the likelihood of fluid responsiveness.

In sum, then, a given level of cardiac filling pressures does not provide much information about fluid responsiveness, but monitoring can be very helpful to guide a fluid challenge.[17] During fluid administration, the goal is to obtain a significant increase in cardiac output (by the Frank-Starling mechanism), with the least increment in cardiac filling pressures, in order to minimize the risk of edema formation. The goal is not to keep the cardiac filling pressures within predefined arbitrary limits; rather, PAOP is a direct determinant of edema formation in the lungs. The key principle is to keep the PAOP as low as possible, provided that all of the other organs are happy.

Pulmonary Artery Pressures

Normally the pulmonary vasculature is a low-resistance circuit, so that the diastolic PAP should be equal to or only slightly higher than the PAOP. An increased pressure gradient between the diastolic PAP and the PAOP indicates active primary pulmonary hypertension related to pulmonary vascular changes (hypoxia) or diseases (primary pulmonary artery hypertension). Pulmonary hypertension may result in RV dilation with septal shifts that may compromise LV function.

CARDIAC OUTPUT

The reference method for measurement of cardiac output is use of the Fick equation; however, this equation is difficult to apply in practice. The indicator dilution technique has been used instead. Indocyanine green clearance has been used for many years, but this method is time-consuming and quite difficult to perform. The thermodilution technique developed by Ganz is a convenient technique which today allows the almost continuous measurement of cardiac output. The presence of tricuspid insufficiency is the major limitation to this technique. Other techniques, including transpulmonary and lithium dilution techniques, have been developed but are somewhat less precise.

The thermodilution technique estimates cardiac output over several cardiac cycles, whereas other techniques, including those based on pulse contour analysis, may assess beat-to-beat variations. These techniques may be useful for estimating the influence of changes in intrathoracic pressures on the stroke volume variation, an estimate of fluid responsiveness.

RIGHT VENTRICULAR VOLUMES

The use of a modified PAC equipped with a fast response thermistor also allows evaluation of the right ventricular ejection fraction (RVEF) (Fig. 4.5). With knowledge of the stroke volume, it becomes easy to calculate the end-systolic and end-diastolic volumes. This measurement can be particularly useful in the presence of RV failure, but this also is a situation in which the measurement is least reliable: tricuspid regurgitation secondary to pulmonary hypertension.

MIXED VENOUS OXYGEN SATURATION

$S\bar{v}O_2$ represents the balance between oxygen consumption and oxygen supply. According to the Fick equation:

$$VO_2 = \text{cardiac output} \times (CaO_2 - CvO_2)$$

where VO_2 is oxygen uptake and CaO_2 and CvO_2 are the arterial and mixed venous oxygen content, respectively. If the dissolved oxygen in the blood is neglected for the purposes of calculation, then

$$VO_2 = \text{cardiac output} \times Hb(SaO_2 - S\bar{v}O_2) \times C$$

and

$$S\bar{v}O_2 = SaO_2 - (VO_2/\text{cardiac output} \times Hb \times C)$$

where Hb is hemoglobin.

Accordingly, a decrease in $S\bar{v}O_2$ can reflect either a decrease in SaO_2 (hypoxemia), anemia, or a relative inadequacy of cardiac output in relation to the oxygen demand of the tissues.

$S\bar{v}O_2$ can be measured continuously using catheters equipped with fiberoptic fibers, and measurements are helpful to guide therapy. $ScvO_2$ has been proposed as a surrogate for $S\bar{v}O_2$, but the relationship between $ScvO_2$ and $S\bar{v}O_2$ is rather vague. Indeed, the $ScvO_2$ is lower than $S\bar{v}O_2$ in healthy conditions (as a result of the low O_2 extraction by the kidneys) but is higher than $S\bar{v}O_2$ in critically ill patients (because of relative increase in O_2 extraction in the kidneys and in the gut).[18] Moreover, O_2 extraction is high in the coronary circulation, and this is missed in the measurement of $ScvO_2$.

DERIVED VARIABLES

Hemodynamic assessment can include a number of derived variables, including resistance, ventricular stroke work, oxygen transport, oxygen consumption, and venous admixture, as described next.

Resistance. In steady-flow conditions, Ohm's law indicates that resistance is the ratio between the pressure drop and the flow in the system. In the pulmonary circulation, the inflow pressure would be the mean PAP and the outflow pressure would be PAOP; for the systemic circulation, these would be the MAP and the CVP, respectively. In either case, flow would be cardiac output. This approach is limited, however, by the fact that the extrapolated intercept of the PAP–cardiac output relationship represents the average closing pressure of the small pulmonary arterioles, and the slope represents the upstream arterial resistance. Accordingly, the increased PAP in pulmonary hypertension can be explained by both an increase in pulmonary vascular closing pressure and an increase in vascular tone, and pulmonary vascular resistance (PVR) is not a good reflection of vasomotor tone in the pulmonary vasculature. Pulmonary hemodynamics are therefore best assessed by altering blood flow to better evaluate this relationship (Fig. 4.6).

Calculation of systemic vascular resistance (SVR) is not very helpful either. It is better to base clinical decisions on primary variables. Simply stated, a relatively high cardiac output in relation to arterial pressure reflects a low SVR state, whereas a relatively low cardiac output reflects a high SVR state.

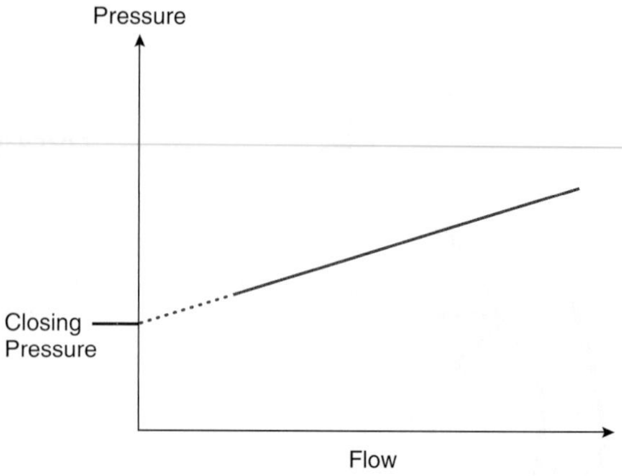

Figure 4.6 Relationship between pressure and blood flow, illustrating the limitations in the calculation of the vascular resistance. Note that the line defining that relationship does not go through the origin, because the pressure is not zero in the absence of blood flow.

Ventricular Stroke Work. The work developed by the ventricles is determined by the ventricular work as derived from the product of flow and the pressure generated. The relationship between stroke work and the respective filling pressure represents a better assessment of contractility than does the stroke volume. LV stroke work index (LVSWI) can be calculated using the equation

$$LVSWI = SVI(MAP - PAOP) \times 0.0136$$

where SI represents the stroke volume index.

Oxygen-Derived Variables. Oxygen transport can be assessed as the product of cardiac output and the arterial oxygen content, according to the equation

$$DO_2 = \text{cardiac output} \times CaO_2$$
$$= \text{cardiac output} \times ([Hb] \times SaO_2 \times 1.39) + 0.0031 \times PaO_2$$

Calculations of this variable benefit from combining measurements of cardiac output, Hb, and SaO_2 but have the limitation that the corresponding oxygen demand is unknown. Some studies suggested that maintaining supranormal DO_2 in the perioperative period or early after trauma may result in better outcomes.

Oxygen consumption also can be calculated from the product of cardiac output and the arteriovenous oxygen difference, according to the formula

$$VO_2 = \text{cardiac output} \times (CaO_2 - C\bar{v}O_2)$$

where $C\bar{v}O_2$ is calculated in the same way as for CaO_2, using the SvO_2 instead of the SaO_2.

The difficulty is in evaluating the oxygen requirements (or the oxygen demand) of the body. VO_2 assessment may perhaps be useful to evaluate the caloric need of the critically ill patient.

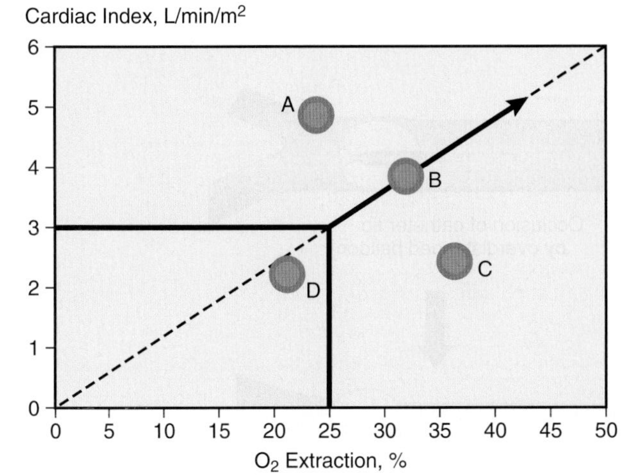

Figure 4.7 Diagram illustrating the relationship between cardiac index and O_2 extraction. Four typical examples are given: hyperkinetic state (**A**), anemia (**B**), low cardiac output state (**C**), and profound anesthesia (**D**).

The calculation of oxygen extraction (oxygen extraction ratio, or O_2ER) is accomplished by determining the ratio of $\dot{V}O_2$ to DO_2, or in a simplified way:

$$\begin{aligned} O_2ER = VO_2/DO_2 &= (CaO_2 - CvO_2)/CaO_2 \\ &= (SaO_2 - SvO_2)Hb/SaO_2 \times Hb \\ &= (SaO_2 - SvO_2)/SaO_2 \end{aligned}$$

Accordingly, when SaO_2 is close to 100%, in the absence of hypoxemia, O_2ER mirrors SvO_2. Its calculation can be useful in the presence of hypoxemia, when SaO_2 is decreased. Also, the relationship between cardiac output and O_2ER can be helpful to compare the central and the peripheral components of oxygen delivery (Fig. 4.7). This relationship is independent of Hb, so it can be helpful in evaluating the cardiovascular status in the presence of anemia.[19]

Venous Admixture. Venous admixture can be calculated by the Berggren equation:

$$Qs/Qt = \frac{Cc'O_2 - CaO_2}{Cc'O_2 - CvO_2}$$

in which Qs is shunt flow, Qt is total pulmonary blood flow, and $Cc'O_2$ represents the capillary oxygen content (assuming an oxygen saturation of 100%). This may help to assess the effects of various interventions (PEEP or other respiratory conditions, administration of vasoactive agents) on pulmonary hemodynamics.

COMPLICATIONS

Complications of pulmonary artery catheterization can be divided into seven categories as listed in Box 4.1. Many of these can be prevented, and most are relatively uncommon.

Complications of venous access are the same as for the insertion of a central venous catheter. Arrhythmias are common but usually are without major consequence, except in moribund patients. It has been suggested that lidocaine should be given prophylactically in predisposed patients, but this usually is not necessary. Likewise, complete atrioventricular block may develop in patients with left bundle branch block, but this is exceptional. Knot formation will be rare if the catheter is advanced carefully and if its presence in the pulmonary artery is confirmed before further advancement into the right ventricle. In particular, care should be taken not to advance the catheter by more than 30 to 35 cm into the right ventricle. Thrombotic complications have become rare with the development of heparin-coated catheters. The appearance of an infiltrate beyond the tip of the PAC on the chest film should suggest an evolving thrombotic event, which should lead to consideration of the withdrawal of the catheter. Endothelial lesions have been found at autopsy, but their clinical relevance is doubtful. Endocarditis is very rare. Valvular damage may occur as a result of improper handling of the catheter (in particular, its withdrawal with the balloon still inflated). Catheter-related infections remain a risk, but they do not seem to be any more common than with central venous catheters.

Box 4.1 Complications of Pulmonary Artery Catheter Insertion

- Complicated vascular access (pneumothorax, hematoma)
- Arrhythmias (e.g., heart block, ventricular tachycardia/fibrillation)
- Catheter knotting
- Pulmonary thrombosis and infarction
- Endothelial or valvular damage
- Colonization and bacteremia
- Pulmonary artery rupture

Pulmonary artery rupture is the most feared complication: Although it is exceptionally rare, it is associated with a high mortality rate. The usual cause is overinflating the balloon in the presence of resistance to inflation, particularly in the presence of preexisting PAH; other, less common causes are shown in Figure 4.8. The cardinal sign of rupture is the development of hemoptysis. The reaction to this event should not be to pull out the catheter entirely, but rather to withdraw it slightly and then inflate the balloon. If the hemorrhage does not stop, a thoracotomy may be necessary to repair the pulmonary artery.

TECHNICAL LIMITATIONS

Invasive measurements of pressures are based on fluid-filled systems with disposable transducers. The transducer includes a deformable membrane with a Wheatstone bridge modifying the electrical resistance and, correspondingly, the intensity of a current. Reliability is ensured by the excellent linearity between the pressure signal and the electrical signal generated by the transducer, in a range of frequency values largely exceeding the range of frequencies found in the human body.

Reliability is less secure in the intermediary system made of tubes and stopcocks along the extent of the pressure

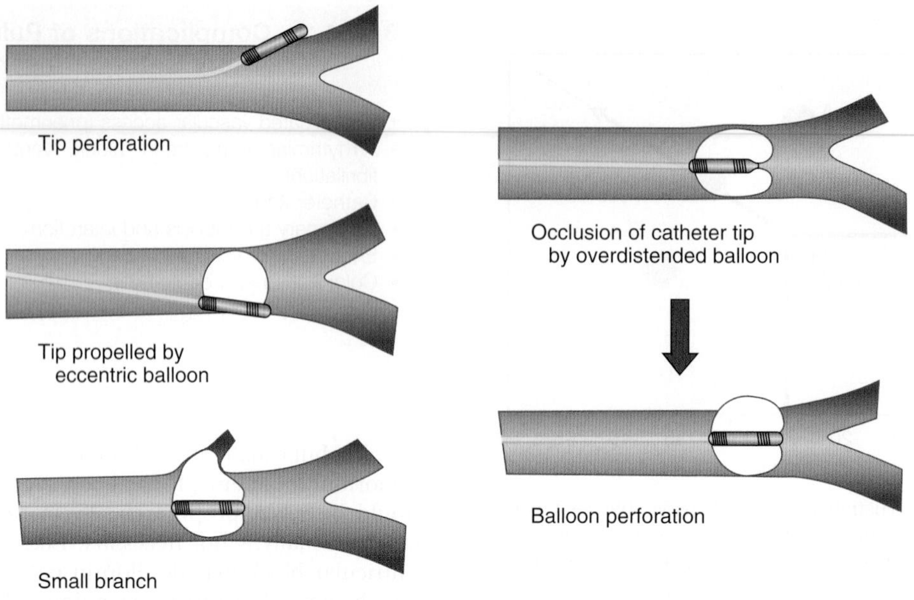

Figure 4.8 Possible mechanisms of pulmonary artery rupture (other than the most common cause, overinflating the balloon in the presence of resistance to inflation). (From Barash PG, Nardi D, Hammond G, et al: Catheter-induced pulmonary artery perforation. Mechanisms, management, and modifications. J Thorac Cardiovasc Surg 1981;82:5.)

system. These can modify the morphology of the trace, resulting in damping. Motion artifacts can further complicate the tracings. The presence of air bubbles also may alter the signal. Use of fluid-filled catheters to measure pressures provides reliable estimates of mean vascular pressures.

Three steps must be followed to guarantee reliable measurements:

1. The first step is appropriate zeroing, which is accomplished by opening the transducer to atmospheric pressure (taken as the zero value). All pressures must be measured with reference to an arbitrary reference point. This zero reference pressure level should ideally be where it is least influenced by location on the body. In humans, it is thought to be at the level of the right atrium, so the reference level usually is placed in the midchest (midaxillary) position at the level of the fourth intercostal space. In healthy persons, the CVP referred to that region does not change with supine versus upright position. An alternative reference is 5 cm vertically below the sternal angle. Obviously, errors in zeroing are relatively more important for measurements of cardiac filling pressures than for arterial pressure measurements, because the errors are quantitatively identical but proportionally greater.
2. The second step is calibration, which is now done automatically by today's electronic systems.
3. The third step is ensuring the good quality of the trace. Shaking the catheter should result in large pressure variations on the screen. A damped system will underestimate systolic pressures. The liquid column should be continuous, without air bubbles in the system. Excessive tubing length, or multiple stopcocks and connectors, may decrease the resonant frequency, resulting in "whipped" traces. Likewise, the presence of bubbles must be carefully avoided. Transient flushing should be followed by an abrupt return of the pressure trace to its actual value.

APPLICATIONS: DIAGNOSIS VERSUS MONITORING

Today the PAC is more useful in guiding therapy rather than in identifying abnormalities, this latter role having largely been taken over by noninvasive, mainly echocardiographic techniques (Table 4.1). In the past, analysis of waveforms was used—for example, the abnormal v waves of mitral regurgitation. Likewise, an increase of all pressures to identical levels should suggest pericardial tamponade. These findings should still alert the clinician to possible abnormalities, but echocardiographic techniques have largely replaced the use of the PAC for identifying valvular disease. The use of echocardiographic techniques for monitoring, however, is hampered by the difficulty of keeping the probe in the esophagus for prolonged periods of time, and results are very operator dependent.

To illustrate the need to integrate different variables, rather than focusing on just one variable, some suggested applications follow:

- *Interpretation of a cardiac output value:* It is important to consider the four determinants of cardiac output (Fig. 4.9).[20] Interpretation should start by considering the stroke volume (cardiac output divided by heart rate) and relating this to an index of ventricular filling (PAOP) and an index of ventricular afterload (arterial and pulmonary artery pressures); an inotropic agent should be added only when preload and afterload have been optimized.
- *Fluid status:* Low cardiac filling pressures may be normal or reflect hypovolemia. The measurement of cardiac output and $S\bar{v}O_2$ will help determine fluid needs. Indeed, hypovolemia typically is associated with a low

Table 4.1 Pulmonary Artery (PA) Catheterization Versus Echocardiographic Techniques for Management of Selected Disorders: Relative Value

	PA Catheterization		Echocardiography	
Disorder	Diagnosis	Monitoring	Diagnosis	Monitoring
Tamponade	+	++	+++	+
Hypovolemia	++	+++	++	+
Valvular disease	+	++	+++	+
Heart failure	++	+++	++	+
Right ventricular failure	++	+++	+++	++
Septic shock	+	+++	+	+

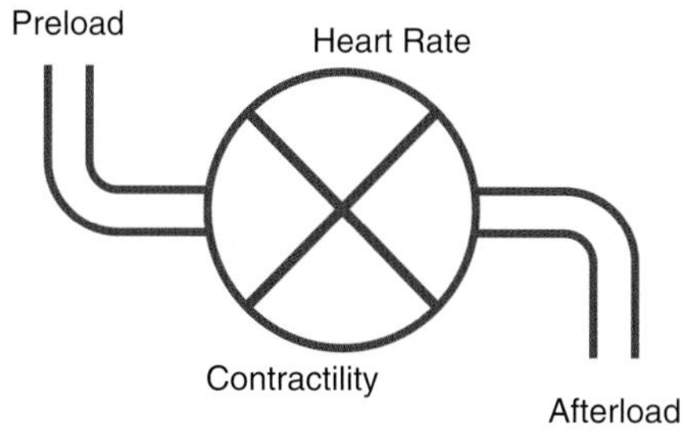

Figure 4.9 The four determinants of cardiac output.

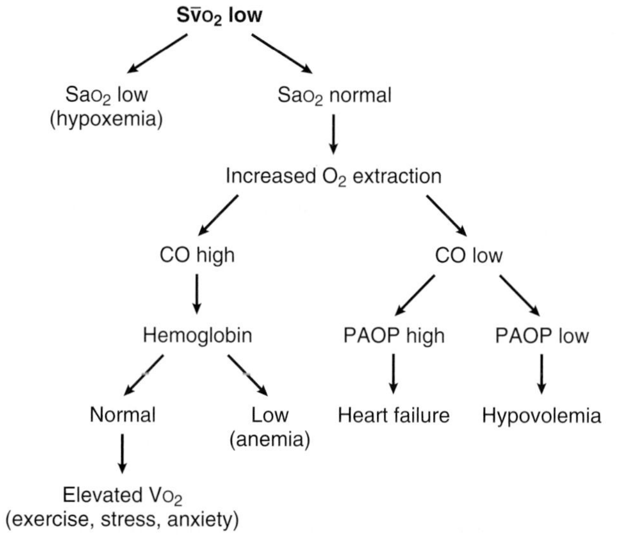

Figure 4.10 Interpretation of a low $S\bar{v}O_2$ (mixed venous oxygen saturation). CO, cardiac output; PAOP, pulmonary artery occlusion pressure; SaO_2, arterial oxygen saturation; VO_2, oxygen uptake.

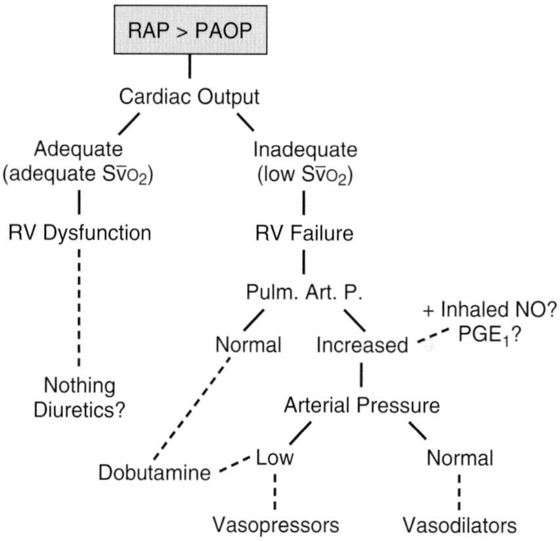

Figure 4.11 Interpretation of a reversed gradient between the right atrial pressure (RAP) and the pulmonary artery occlusion pressure (PAOP). NO, nitric oxide; PGE_1, prostaglandin E_1; RV, right ventricular; $S\bar{v}O_2$, mixed venous oxygen saturation.

cardiac output and a low $S\bar{v}O_2$ (Fig. 4.10). By contrast, hypervolemia in the presence of normal cardiac function will be manifested by high cardiac filling pressures associated with a relatively high cardiac output and normal or high $S\bar{v}O_2$.

- *Hemodynamic versus nonhemodynamic pulmonary edema:* The distinction between hemodynamic and nonhemodynamic types of lung edema no longer requires pulmonary artery catheterization; the clinical history and less invasive (e.g., echocardiographic) measurements usually are sufficient to separate the two. Nevertheless, invasive hemodynamic monitoring can reveal that patients thought to meet only the acute lung injury/acute respiratory distress syndrome (ALI/ARDS) criteria sometimes have unexpectedly high PAOP.[21]
- *RV dysfunction versus failure:* A reverse gradient between RAP and PAOP (i.e., a higher RAP than PAOP) indicates RV dysfunction or failure and usually is secondary to pulmonary hypertension, as will be immediately apparent from the measurements of pulmonary artery pressures. RV dysfunction is manifested by RV dilation (and thus a decrease in RVEF) with no limitation on cardiac output. This is the most common situation in patients with ARDS, who usually maintain a hyperkinetic state. Rather, RV failure refers to a state in which cardiac output is no longer sustained at adequate levels.[22] These different entities are illustrated in Figure 4.11.
- *LV dysfunction versus failure:* Here the gradient between PAOP and RAP will be higher than the typical 3 to 5 mm Hg. As with the right ventricle, in LV dysfunction the ventricular volumes may increase (so the ejection fraction will decrease), but the cardiac output may be simultaneously preserved; such a situation may exist in septic shock.

LV failure is more common and is manifested by a decrease in cardiac output and $S\bar{v}O_2$.

ASSESSING EFFECTS OF INTERVENTIONS

The PAC can be used to monitor the effectiveness of various interventions:

- *Fluid challenge:* A fluid challenge technique is indicated whenever the benefit of fluid administration is in doubt.[17] Ideally, fluid administration will result in increases in cardiac output and tissue perfusion without major increases in cardiac filling. An increase in PAOP in the absence of a significant change in cardiac output and $S\bar{v}O_2$ indicates that fluid administration will only result in an increased risk of edema and should be discontinued.
- *Inotropic agents:* The use of inotropes aims to increase cardiac output and possibly decrease PAOP. Lack of an increase in cardiac output after administration of a β_1-adrenergic inotropic agent indicates a desensitization of the β-adrenergic receptors and is associated with a worse prognosis.[23]
- *Vasopressors:* The use of pure vasoconstrictors is expected to increase arterial pressure but also cardiac filling pressures. An excessive increase in cardiac filling pressures with use of such an agent suggests the need for addition of an inotropic agent (e.g., dobutamine).
- *Vasodilators:* The administration of vasodilators may rapidly reduce arterial pressure so that continuous arterial pressure monitoring is usually indicated. Moreover, a reduction in vascular tone in the presence of hypovolemia may reduce venous return and thus cardiac output.

CLINICAL INDICATIONS FOR PULMONARY ARTERY CATHETER INSERTION

The improvement in noninvasive diagnostic techniques means that today the PAC is used primarily for monitoring. Potential indications include the following:

- *Severe circulatory shock:* The PAC can be used to help guide fluid challenges and titrate inotropic agents. Shock due to hypovolemia (as in polytrauma or with other forms of massive bleeding) does not require insertion of a PAC, because management of such patients generally is quite straightforward.
- *RV failure:* The PAC can be used to monitor pulmonary artery pressures, the gradient between RAP and PAOP, cardiac output, and $S\bar{v}O_2$.
- *Acute respiratory failure due to pulmonary edema:* Whether lung edema is hemodynamic or nonhemodynamic, the strategy should be to keep the hydrostatic pressures as low as possible, but this requires measurements of cardiac output and $S\bar{v}O_2$ to make sure the systemic circulation is not compromised.
- *Complex fluid management in the presence of impending renal failure:* Sometimes it is difficult to evaluate the fluid status in oliguric patients, in whom hypovolemia may compromise renal function but hypervolemia obviously must be avoided.
- *Dynamic assessment of cardiac function in specific conditions:* The best example is that of the patient who is difficult to wean from mechanical ventilation, possibly owing in part to cardiac dysfunction.

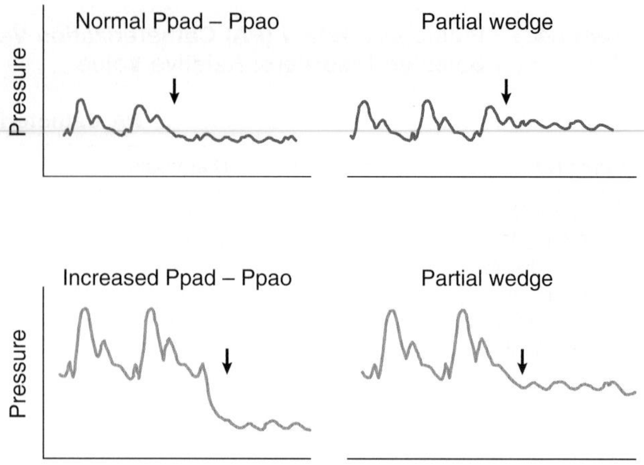

Figure 4.12 Schematic depiction of partial occlusion when the gradient between the pulmonary artery diastolic pressure (Ppad) and the pulmonary artery occlusion pressure (Ppao) is normal (*top*) or is increased (*bottom*). *Arrow* denotes balloon inflation. (From Leatherman JW, Shapiro RS: Overestimation of pulmonary artery occlusion pressure in pulmonary hypertension due to partial occlusion. Crit Care Med 2003;31:93-97.)

PULMONARY ARTERY OCCLUSION PRESSURE AND PARTIAL OCCLUSION

Partial occlusion of the pulmonary artery in the presence of pulmonary hypertension may be difficult to recognize and can lead to significant overestimation of the PAOP, denoted Ppao on Figure 4.12. A useful clue to partial occlusion is occurrence of a substantial increase in the PAOP without a concomitant change in the pulmonary artery diastolic pressure, denoted Ppad on the figure. If the Ppad – PAOP gradient is normal and the underlying disease process would predict increased PVR, partial occlusion should be suspected. Partial occlusion may occur if a catheter is either too proximal or too distal in the pulmonary artery, and appropriate repositioning may be corrective. The best PAOP may be obtained in some circumstances by further advancing the catheter with the balloon fully inflated and at other times by retracting the catheter to the original pulmonary artery position and attempting to occlude with 1.0 to 1.2 mL of air, instead of full inflation. It is imperative never to inflate against resistance. Figures 4.12 and 4.13 offer further information on diagnosis and management of partial occlusion.

DOES THE USE OF A PULMONARY ARTERY CATHETER IMPROVE OUTCOME?

The use of the PAC has been challenged on the basis that it has not been shown to improve outcomes.[21,24-26] An improvement in outcome, however, has not been demonstrated with other monitoring techniques either. Moreover, a number of studies have indicated that the use of the PAC can influence therapy.[27] If use of a PAC does not result in better outcomes, important and challenging questions arise about the beneficial effects of many therapeutic

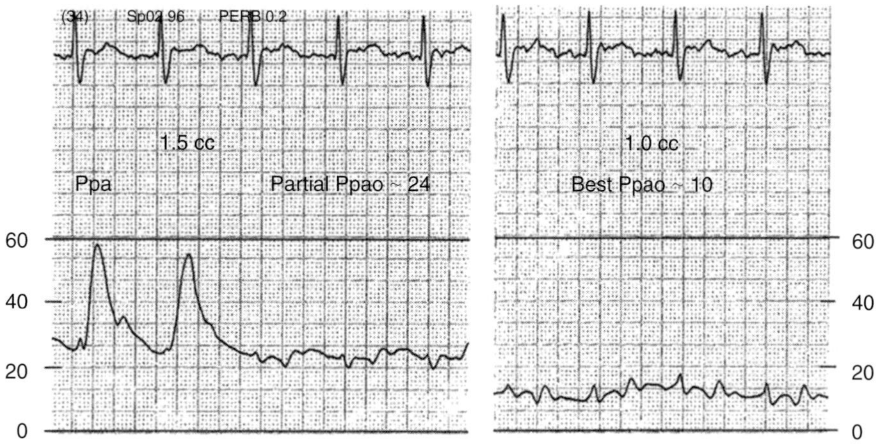

Figure 4.13 Partial pulmonary artery occlusion pressure (Ppao) measured when 1.5 cc of air was used to inflate the catheter balloon (*left graph*); a much lower Ppao was obtained with a 1.0-cc inflation (*right graph*). Review of the chest roentgenogram revealed that the catheter tip was too peripheral, so it was withdrawn to a more proximal location. Ppa, pulmonary artery pressure. See text for definition of partial and best Ppao values. Scale in mm Hg. (From Leatherman JW, Shapiro RS: Overestimation of pulmonary artery occlusion pressure in pulmonary hypertension due to partial occlusion. Crit Care Med 2003;31:93-97.)

Table 4.2 Components and Common Errors in Hemodynamic Monitoring

Component	Common Errors
1. Measure	Catheter misplacement Errors in pressure measurements No consideration of $S\bar{v}O_2$
2. Interpret	Interpretation of cardiac output without consideration of $S\bar{v}O_2$ Neglect of PAP/PAOP gradient Neglect of inversed RAP/PAOP gradient
3. Apply	Treating as if the data were not available Giving diuretics for a high PAOP without other consideration

PAP, pulmonary artery pressure; PAOP, pulmonary artery occlusion pressure; RAP, right atrial pressure; $S\bar{v}O_2$, mixed venous oxygen saturation.

interventions in the ICU. Some evidence suggests that the use of the PAC may improve outcomes in the most severely ill subsets of critically ill patients.[28,29] Errors in measurements from the PAC were identified many years ago,[30] and another consideration is the considerable interobserver variability in interpretation of PAC tracings.[31] Clearly, not all ICU patients need a PAC and insertion should be reserved for complex cases.[32] If a PAC is considered necessary, it is important to respect the three successive steps (Table 4.2): to take adequate and full measurements; to interpret the results correctly; and to apply the gathered information for the patient's benefit. Unfortunately, potential errors are associated with each step. Some of these issues can be addressed with better teaching and improved basic knowledge of hemodynamics and basic physiology.

KEY POINTS

- No simple guidelines for monitoring are available or applicable in all cases; monitoring should be tailored to each patient's needs.
- Each variable, taken individually, has limitations and is subject to error and difficulty in interpretation. Variables should be combined and integrated to provide a global picture of the clinical situation.
- A monitoring technique cannot improve outcome by itself; each of the three components of monitoring is important with any monitoring technique:
  - Accurate collection of data
  - Interpretation of the data
  - Application of the information obtained
- Cardiac output is an adaptive value that must constantly adjust to the oxygen requirements of the organs.
- Separation of the four determinants of cardiac output—heart rate, contractility, preload, and afterload—is useful to consider the various interventions that can be used to increase it.
- Measurements of mixed venous oxygen saturation are essential to interpret cardiac output measurements.
- The relationship between cardiac filling pressures and volumes is relatively weak. Pressure measurements are important, however, because pressures (rather than volumes) are the primary determinant of edema formation.
- The calculation of derived variables, such as vascular resistances, ventricular work, and oxygen-derived variables, is of limited usefulness.

SELECTED REFERENCES

2. Magder S: Hemodynamic monitoring in the mechanically ventilated patient. Curr Opin Crit Care 2011;17:36-42.
4. Lorente L, Santacreu R, Martin MM, et al: Arterial catheter-related infection of 2,949 catheters. Crit Care 2006;10:R83.
7. Rivers E, Anders DS, Powell D, et al: Central venous oxygen saturation monitoring in the critically ill patient. Curr Opin Crit Care 2001;7:204-211.
13. O'Grady NP, Alexander M, Burns NA, et al: Guidelines for the prevention of intravascular catheter–related infections. Clin Infect Dis 2011;52:e162-e193.
17. Vincent JL, Weil MH: Fluid challenge revisited. Crit Care Med 2006;34:1333-1337.
18. Varpula M, Karlsson S, Ruokonen E, et al: Mixed venous oxygen saturation cannot be estimated by central venous oxygen saturation in septic shock. Intensive Care Med 2006;32:1336-1343.
20. Vincent JL: Understanding cardiac output. Crit Care 2008;12:174.
21. Wheeler AP, Bernard GR, Thompson BT, et al: Pulmonary-artery versus central venous catheter to guide treatment of acute lung injury. N Engl J Med 2006;354:2213-2224.
27. Mimoz O, Rauss A, Rekik N, et al: Pulmonary artery catheterization in critically ill patients: A prospective analysis of outcome changes associated with catheter-prompted changes in therapy. Crit Care Med 1994;22:573-579.
32. Vincent JL, Rhodes A, Perel A, et al: Update on hemodynamic monitoring: A consensus of 16. Crit Care 2011;15:229.

The complete list of references can be found at www.expertconsult.com.

5 Cardiac Pacing

Matthew Ortman | Andrea M. Russo

CHAPTER OUTLINE

Cardiac pacing and arrhythmia management are of paramount importance in the critical care setting. Whether or not arrhythmia is the primary concern, the critical care physician needs to be proficient in arrhythmia recognition, temporary pacing, and basic device troubleshooting of previously implanted cardiac devices. This chapter is meant to be a practical review of an admittedly broad and expansive topic, focusing on issues that are most likely to arise on a day-to-day basis in the intensive care unit.

The following topics will be discussed: (a) indications for permanent pacing, (b) indications for temporary pacing, (c) conditions that are generally reversible or transient, where pacing is not typically required, (d) techniques for temporary pacing, including esophageal, transcutaneous, epicardial, and transvenous modalities, (e) complications related to pacing, and (f) additional considerations related to permanent pacing.

INDICATIONS FOR PERMANENT PACEMAKER IMPLANTATION

Bradycardia is the most common indication for pacing and is a common finding during the clinical evaluation of healthy individuals, as well as patients who are ill. Bradyarrhythmias may be caused by either intrinsic dysfunction of the sinus node (SN) or atrioventricular (AV) conduction system, or may be due to a response of normal tissues to extrinsic factors. In some cases, even profound bradycardia may be asymptomatic and have no immediate or long-term consequences. When deciding if a permanent pacemaker is in the best interests of the patient, the physician must analyze the clinical status of the patient, as well as the specific cardiac rhythm disorder, while considering the risks and benefits of permanent pacing.

The American College of Cardiology Foundation (ACCF), the American Heart Association (AHA), and the Heart Rhythm Society (HRS) have jointly engaged in the production of guidelines for cardiac implantable electronic device (CIED) implantation, with publication of updated Guidelines for Device-Based Therapy of Cardiac Rhythm Abnormalities in 2008.[1] These recommendations are primarily evidence-based, and this publication includes an extensive review of the literature on the topic. As with other guideline documents, recommendations are classified as class I, II, or III as follows:

- Class I: Benefit >>> Risk; the procedure/treatment *should* be performed/administered.
- Class II: Conditions for which there is conflicting evidence or divergence of opinion about the usefulness/efficacy of the procedure.
  - Class IIa: Benefit >> Risk; *it is reasonable* to perform the procedure/administer treatment, although additional studies with focused objectives are still needed.
  - Class IIb: Benefit ≥ Risk; the procedure/treatment *may be considered*, although additional studies with broad objectives are needed or additional registry data would be helpful.
- Class III: Risk ≥ Benefit; the procedure/treatment should *not* be performed/administered because it is not helpful and may be harmful.

The level of evidence or weight of evidence to support these recommendations is ranked as follows:

- Level of evidence A: Data derived from multiple randomized clinical trials or meta-analyses.
- Level of evidence B: Data derived from a single randomized trial or nonrandomized studies.
- Level of evidence C: Consensus opinion of experts, case studies, or standard of care.

Indications for permanent pacemaker implantation can be divided into the following categories: (1) pacing for bradycardia due to SN and AV node dysfunction; (2) pacing for special conditions, such as carotid sinus hypersensitivity, neurocardiogenic syncope, and cardiac transplantation; (3) pacing for prevention and treatment of arrhythmias; and (4) pacing for hemodynamic indications, including cardiac resynchronization therapy (CRT) and hypertrophic cardiomyopathy (HCM). As SN and AV node dysfunction are the most common indications for permanent pacemaker implantation, and are the most commonly encountered problems that require pacing in the intensive care setting, these indications will be the main focus of this chapter.

PACING INDICATIONS FOR SINUS NODE DYSFUNCTION

"Sinus node dysfunction" (SND) may be due to a problem of SN impulse formation or propagation, and may present with sinus bradycardia, chronotropic incompetence, or sinus arrest. SND may also be associated with "tachy-brady syndrome," in which rapidly conducted, paroxysmal atrial arrhythmias alternate with periods of sinus bradycardia or prolonged postconversion pauses.

SND is the most common cause of bradyarrhythmias in clinical practice. The typical age at the time of diagnosis of SND appears to be in the seventh or eighth decade of life, with a mean or median age of 71 to 74 years in randomized clinical trials evaluating pacemaker therapy.[2-4] However, clinical manifestations of SND may occur at any age and may be secondary to any one of several potential causes, including destruction of the SN, ischemia, infarction, infiltrative disease, surgical trauma, autonomic dysfunction, or endocrinologic abnormalities.[1,5]

Clinical manifestations of SND are diverse, and symptoms may include fatigue, reduced exercise tolerance, dyspnea on exertion, presyncope, lightheadedness, dizziness, or syncope. In the absence of any clearly reversible cause of bradycardia, the only effective treatment for symptomatic bradycardia in patients with SND is permanent pacing. Box 5.1 outlines recommendations for permanent pacing in patients with SND.[1]

PACING INDICATIONS FOR ACQUIRED ATRIOVENTRICULAR BLOCK

AV block refers to impairment of conduction of electrical impulses from the atria to the ventricles, and can occur at the level of the AV node, within the His-Purkinje system, or below the His-Purkinje system. In general, block at the level of the His-Purkinje system has a high risk of progression to complete heart block and carries a poor prognosis without pacemaker implantation.

Electrocardiographic classification of AV block includes first-degree, second-degree, and third-degree (complete) block. First-degree AV block (or first-degree AV delay) refers to a prolonged PR interval (>200 ms) without failure of conduction to the ventricle, and is usually due to delay of impulse conduction through the AV node or through atrial tissue. Second-degree AV block refers to failure of an atrial impulse to conduct to the ventricle, and this may be preceded by fixed or gradually lengthening PR intervals. Mobitz type I second-degree AV block (or Wenckebach block) is characterized by progressive PR interval prolongation prior

Box 5.1 Recommendations for Permanent Pacing in Sinus Node Dysfunction (SND)

Class I

1. Permanent pacemaker implantation is indicated for SND with documented symptomatic bradycardia, including frequent sinus pauses that produce symptoms. (Level of evidence: C)
2. Permanent pacemaker implantation is indicated for symptomatic chronotropic incompetence. (Level of evidence: C)
3. Permanent pacemaker implantation is indicated for symptomatic sinus bradycardia that results from required drug therapy for medical conditions. (Level of evidence: C)

Class IIa

1. Permanent pacemaker implantation is reasonable for SND with heart rate less than 40 beats/min when a clear association between significant symptoms consistent with bradycardia and the actual presence of bradycardia has not been documented. (Level of evidence: C)
2. Permanent pacemaker implantation is reasonable for syncope of unexplained origin when clinically significant abnormalities of sinus node function are discovered or provoked in electrophysiologic studies. (Level of evidence: C)

Class IIb

1. Permanent pacemaker implantation may be considered in minimally symptomatic patients with chronic heart rate less than 40 beats/min while awake. (Level of evidence: C)

Class III

1. Permanent pacemaker implantation is not indicated for SND in asymptomatic patients. (Level of evidence: C)
2. Permanent pacemaker implantation is not indicated for SND in patients for whom the symptoms suggestive of bradycardia have been clearly documented to occur in the absence of bradycardia. (Level of evidence: C)
3. Permanent pacemaker implantation is not indicated for SND with symptomatic bradycardia due to nonessential drug therapy. (Level of evidence: C)

From Epstein AE, DiMarco JP, Ellenbogen KA, et al. American College of Cardiology/American Heart Association Task Force on Practice Guidelines (Writing Committee to Revise the ACC/AHA/NASPE 2002 Guideline Update for Implantation of Cardiac Pacemakers and Antiarrhythmia Devices); American Association for Thoracic Surgery; Society of Thoracic Surgeons. ACC/AHA/HRS 2008 Guidelines for Device-Based Therapy of Cardiac Rhythm Abnormalities: A report of the American College of Cardiology/American Heart Association Task Force on Practice Guidelines. Circulation 2008;117:e350-e408.

to a nonconducted P wave, with a shorter PR interval on the conducted beat occurring after the blocked beat. Mobitz II second-degree AV block is characterized by a fixed PR interval prior to the dropped P wave, often associated with a wide QRS complex.

Mobitz I second-degree AV block is frequently benign and is most often localized to block within the AV node, although there are rare exceptions. Although Mobitz I second-degree AV block has a low risk of progression to complete heart block, Mobitz II second-degree AV block is a more severe conduction disturbance with a higher risk of progression to complete heart block. Although the anatomic level of block for individuals with 2:1 AV block may be at the level of the AV node or below the AV node, the level of block is more likely to be below the His-Purkinje system if the QRS complex is wide. However, if a preexisting bundle branch block is present, the block may be either at the level of the AV node or below the AV node.

Third-degree AV block refers to absence of impulse conduction from the atria to the ventricles, and this may be congenital or acquired. Permanent pacing is often indicated for acquired complete block without reversible causes. AV block may also occur in patients with SND, and 20% of patients with SND will have some degree of AV block.[4] In addition, following permanent pacemaker implantation for SND, the risk of developing AV block within 5 years of follow-up is 3% to 35%.[6-9]

Acquired AV block is most often due to aging or related to calcification of the conduction system. Ischemic heart disease, myocardial infarction, and traumatic surgical causes (such as cardiac valve surgery) are other common causes. Less common causes of AV block include infection (syphilis, Lyme disease, endocarditis), infiltrative disease (sarcoidosis, malignancy), neuromuscular disease, or drugs (beta blockers, calcium channel blockers, digoxin, or membrane-active antiarrhythmic agents).

Patients with AV block may be asymptomatic, or may have symptoms that vary from mild lightheadedness, dizziness, shortness of breath, or fatigue to presyncope and loss of consciousness. The decision regarding permanent pacemaker implantation should take into account whether or not symptoms are attributable to bradycardia, as well as the cause and "level" of AV block. Completely reversible causes of AV block, such as electrolyte disturbances or Lyme disease, should be excluded. Permanent pacing indications for acquired AV block are summarized in Box 5.2. Pacing indications for chronic bifascicular block and pacing for AV block associated with acute myocardial infarction are outlined in Boxes 5.3 and 5.4.

OTHER PERMANENT PACING INDICATIONS

In specific situations, permanent pacing may also be clinically indicated in some patients with carotid sinus hypersensitivity, neurocardiogenic syncope, or obstructive hypertrophic cardiomyopathy, and following cardiac transplantation.[1] Historically, antitachycardia pacemakers were occasionally utilized to treat recurrent supraventricular arrhythmias, but they are rarely used in contemporary practice with the availability of catheter ablation therapy. Pace termination of ventricular tachycardia is frequently utilized for the treatment of monomorphic ventricular tachycardia as part of implantable cardioverter-defibrillator (ICD) therapy, and can also be used to terminate frequent arrhythmia episodes using a temporary transvenous pacing system in the intensive care setting (Fig. 5.1).

Pacing may be useful in the prevention of pause-dependent, polymorphic ventricular tachycardia as well (Fig. 5.2). Permanent pacing is indicated for pause-dependent ventricular tachycardia, with or without QT prolongation (class I indication, level of evidence C), and is reasonable for high-risk patients with congenital long

Box 5.2 Recommendations for Permanent Pacing for Acquired Atrioventricular (AV) Block in Adults

Class I

1. Permanent pacemaker implantation is indicated for third-degree and advanced second-degree AV block at any anatomic level associated with bradycardia with symptoms (including heart failure) or ventricular arrhythmias presumed to be due to AV block. (Level of evidence: C)
2. Permanent pacemaker implantation is indicated for third-degree and advanced second-degree AV block at any anatomic level associated with arrhythmias and other medical conditions that require drug therapy that results in symptomatic bradycardia. (Level of evidence: C)
3. Permanent pacemaker implantation is indicated for third-degree and advanced second-degree AV block at any anatomic level in awake, symptom-free patients in sinus rhythm, with documented periods of asystole 3.0 seconds or longer or any escape rate less than 40 beats/min, or with an escape rhythm that is below the AV node. (Level of evidence: C)
4. Permanent pacemaker implantation is indicated for third-degree and advanced second-degree AV block at any anatomic level in awake, symptom-free patients with atrial fibrillation and bradycardia with 1 or more pauses of at least 5 seconds or longer. (Level of evidence: C)
5. Permanent pacemaker implantation is indicated for third-degree and advanced second-degree AV block at any anatomic level after catheter ablation of the AV junction. (Level of evidence: C)
6. Permanent pacemaker implantation is indicated for third-degree and advanced second-degree AV block at any anatomic level associated with postoperative AV block that is not expected to resolve after cardiac surgery. (Level of evidence: C)
7. Permanent pacemaker implantation is indicated for third-degree and advanced second-degree AV block at any anatomic level associated with neuromuscular diseases with AV block, such as myotonic muscular dystrophy, Kearns-Sayre syndrome, Erb dystrophy (limb-girdle muscular dystrophy), and peroneal muscular atrophy, with or without symptoms. (Level of evidence: B)
8. Permanent pacemaker implantation is indicated for second-degree AV block with associated symptomatic bradycardia regardless of type or site of block. (Level of evidence: B)
9. Permanent pacemaker implantation is indicated for asymptomatic persistent third-degree AV block at any anatomic site with average awake ventricular rates of 40 beats/min or faster if cardiomegaly or LV dysfunction is present or if the site of block is below the AV node. (Level of evidence: B)
10. Permanent pacemaker implantation is indicated for second- or third-degree AV block during exercise in the absence of myocardial ischemia. (Level of evidence: C)

Class IIa

1. Permanent pacemaker implantation is reasonable for persistent third-degree AV block with an escape rate greater than 40 beats/min in asymptomatic adult patients without cardiomegaly. (Level of evidence: C)
2. Permanent pacemaker implantation is reasonable for asymptomatic second-degree AV block at intra- or infra-His levels found at electrophysiologic study. (Level of evidence: B)
3. Permanent pacemaker implantation is reasonable for first- or second-degree AV block with symptoms similar to those of pacemaker syndrome or hemodynamic compromise. (Level of evidence: B)
4. Permanent pacemaker implantation is reasonable for asymptomatic type II second-degree AV block with a narrow QRS complex. When type II second-degree AV block occurs with a wide QRS, including isolated right bundle branch block, pacing becomes a class I recommendation. (Level of evidence: B)

Class IIb

1. Permanent pacemaker implantation may be considered for neuromuscular diseases such as myotonic muscular dystrophy, Erb dystrophy (limb-girdle muscular dystrophy), and peroneal muscular atrophy with any degree of AV block (including first-degree AV block), with or without symptoms, because there may be unpredictable progression of AV conduction disease. (Level of evidence: B)
2. Permanent pacemaker implantation may be considered for AV block in the setting of drug use or drug toxicity when the block is expected to recur even after the drug is withdrawn. (Level of evidence: B)

Class III

1. Permanent pacemaker implantation is not indicated for asymptomatic first-degree AV block. (Level of evidence: B)
2. Permanent pacemaker implantation is not indicated for asymptomatic type I second-degree AV block at the supra-His (AV node) level or that not known to be intra- or infra-His. (Level of evidence: C)
3. Permanent pacemaker implantation is not indicated for AV block that is expected to resolve and is unlikely to recur (e.g., drug toxicity, Lyme disease, or transient increases in vagal tone or during hypoxia in sleep apnea syndrome in the absence of symptoms). (Level of evidence: B)

From Epstein AE, DiMarco JP, Ellenbogen KA, et al: American College of Cardiology/American Heart Association Task Force on Practice Guidelines (Writing Committee to Revise the ACC/AHA/NASPE 2002 Guideline Update for Implantation of Cardiac Pacemakers and Antiarrhythmia Devices); American Association for Thoracic Surgery; Society of Thoracic Surgeons. ACC/AHA/HRS 2008 Guidelines for Device-Based Therapy of Cardiac Rhythm Abnormalities: A report of the American College of Cardiology/American Heart Association Task Force on Practice Guidelines. Circulation 2008;117:e350-408.

Box 5.3 Recommendations for Permanent Pacing in Chronic Bifascicular Block

Class I

1. Permanent pacemaker implantation is indicated for advanced second-degree AV block or intermittent third-degree AV block. (Level of evidence: B)
2. Permanent pacemaker implantation is indicated for type II second-degree AV block. (Level of evidence: B)
3. Permanent pacemaker implantation is indicated for alternating bundle branch block. (Level of evidence: C)

Class IIa

1. Permanent pacemaker implantation is reasonable for syncope not demonstrated to be due to AV block when other likely causes have been excluded, specifically ventricular tachycardia (VT). (Level of evidence: B)
2. Permanent pacemaker implantation is reasonable for an incidental finding at electrophysiologic study of a markedly prolonged HV (from the bundle of His to the ventricles) interval (100 ms or greater) in asymptomatic patients. (Level of evidence: B)
3. Permanent pacemaker implantation is reasonable for an incidental finding at electrophysiologic study of pacing-induced infra-His block that is not physiologic. (Level of evidence: B)

Class IIb

1. Permanent pacemaker implantation may be considered in the setting of neuromuscular diseases such as myotonic muscular dystrophy, Erb dystrophy (limb-girdle muscular dystrophy), and peroneal muscular atrophy with bifascicular block or any fascicular block, with or without symptoms. (Level of evidence: C)

Class III

1. Permanent pacemaker implantation is not indicated for fascicular block without AV block or symptoms. (Level of evidence: B)
2. Permanent pacemaker implantation is not indicated for fascicular block with first-degree AV block without symptoms. (Level of evidence: B)

AV, atrioventricular.
From Antman EM, Anbe DT, Armstrong PW, et al: ACC/AHA guidelines for the management of patients with ST-elevation myocardial infarction—Executive summary: A report of the American College of Cardiology/American Heart Association task force on practice guidelines (writing committee to revise the 1999 guidelines for the management of patients with acute myocardial infarction). Circulation 2004;110:588-636.

Box 5.4 Recommendations for Permanent Pacing for Atrioventricular (AV) Block Associated with Acute Myocardial Infarction

Class I

1. Permanent ventricular pacing is indicated for persistent second degree AV block in the His-Purkinje system with alternating bundle branch block or third-degree AV block within or below the His-Purkinje system after ST-segment elevation myocardial infarction. (Level of evidence: B)
2. Permanent ventricular pacing is indicated for transient advanced second- or third-degree infranodal AV block and associated bundle branch block. If the site of block is uncertain, an electrophysiologic study may be necessary. (Level of evidence: B)
3. Permanent ventricular pacing is indicated for persistent and symptomatic second- or third-degree AV block. (Level of evidence: C)

Class IIb

1. Permanent ventricular pacing may be considered for persistent second- or third-degree AV block at the AV node level, even in the absence of symptoms. (Level of evidence: B)

Class III

1. Permanent ventricular pacing is not indicated for transient AV block in the absence of intraventricular conduction defects. (Level of evidence: B)
2. Permanent ventricular pacing is not indicated for transient AV block in the presence of isolated left anterior fascicular block. (Level of evidence: B)
3. Permanent ventricular pacing is not indicated for new bundle branch block or fascicular block in the absence of AV block. (Level of evidence: B)
4. Permanent ventricular pacing is not indicated for persistent asymptomatic first-degree AV block in the presence of bundle branch or fascicular block. (Level of evidence: B)

From Epstein AE, DiMarco JP, Ellenbogen KA, et al: American College of Cardiology/American Heart Association Task Force on Practice Guidelines (Writing Committee to Revise the ACC/AHA/NASPE 2002 Guideline Update for Implantation of Cardiac Pacemakers and Antiarrhythmia Devices); American Association for Thoracic Surgery; Society of Thoracic Surgeons. ACC/AHA/HRS 2008 Guidelines for Device-Based Therapy of Cardiac Rhythm Abnormalities: A report of the American College of Cardiology/American Heart Association Task Force on Practice Guidelines. Circulation 2008;117:e350-408.

QT syndrome (class IIb indication, level of evidence B).[1] Atrial-based pacing ("AAI" or "DDD" mode) is considered the preferred pacing mode for prevention of polymorphic ventricular tachycardia associated with the congenital long QT syndrome. Pacing the left ventricle can improve hemodynamics in patients with dilated cardiomyopathy and bundle branch block by altering the activation sequence and influencing regional contractility, and is particularly effective in patients with left bundle branch block. This is referred to as "biventricular pacing" or "cardiac resynchronization therapy" and is beyond the scope of this chapter.

INDICATIONS FOR TEMPORARY PACING

Temporary pacing is typically reserved for situations in which an electrical disturbance is transient or reversible—for example, Lyme carditis, drug overdose, or inferior wall infarction—or when there is an ongoing contraindication

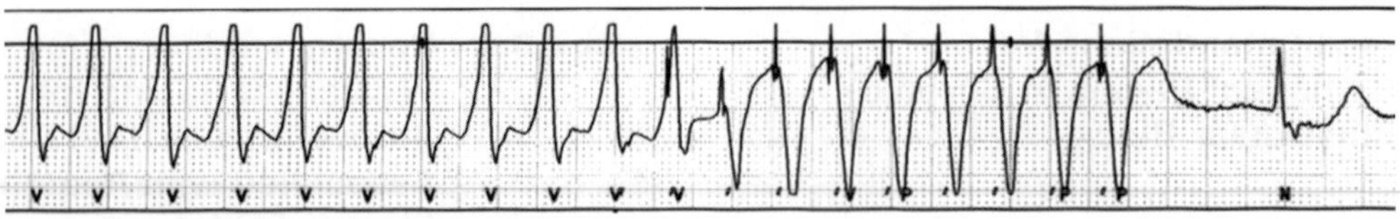

Figure 5.1 Telemetry strip demonstrating antitachycardia pacing. Pacing is delivered at a rate that is slightly faster than the underlying ventricular tachycardia, ultimately terminating the arrhythmia.

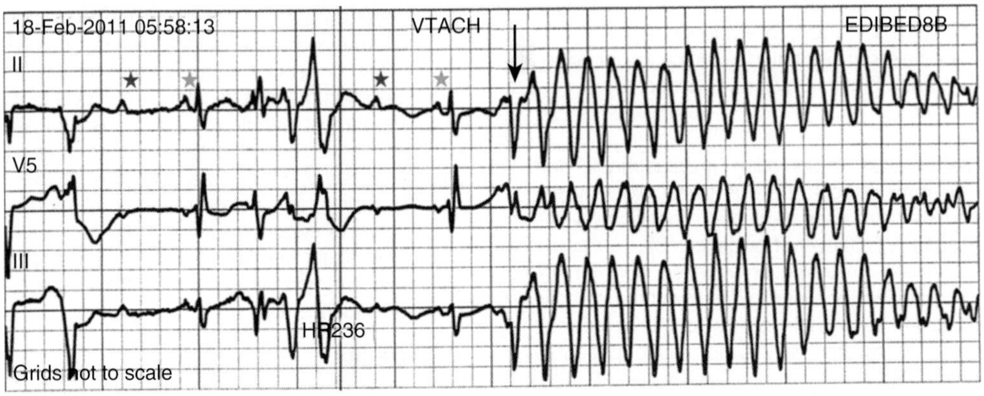

Figure 5.2 Telemetry strip demonstrating torsades de pointes. The rhythm is sinus with both conducted (*green stars*) and nonconducted (*red stars*) P waves. Premature ventricular complexes emerge from a dramatically prolonged QT-U complex (*black arrow*), eventually initiating polymorphic ventricular tachycardia.

to the implantation of a permanent device, most often because of infection.

ATRIOVENTRICULAR NODAL DYSFUNCTION

The "level" of AV block—whether at the level of the AV node or below the AV node in the His-Purkinje conduction system—is critical in determining the need for temporary pacing. AV nodal block improves with measures that accelerate AV nodal conduction, like atropine, dopamine, and isoproterenol. Infranodal block—that is, block below the level of the AV node at the bundle of His or bundle branches—may paradoxically worsen with these agents owing to downstream block in an already diseased His-Purkinje system. The origin of the escape rhythm—whether "proximal" or "distal" in the cardiac conduction system—predicts both its rate and stability. Complete heart block at the level of the AV node is associated with an escape rhythm arising from the AV junction, His bundle, or proximal fascicles; a narrow QRS morphologic pattern; and a heart rate in excess of 60 beats per minute. Infranodal block is associated with an escape rhythm arising from the bundle branches or even ventricular myocardium, a wide and often bizarre QRS morphologic pattern, and a heart rate in the range of 40 beats per minute.[10] Complete heart block with a junctional escape rhythm does not typically require temporary pacing, unless accompanied by hypotension. In contrast, complete heart block with a ventricular escape rhythm is inherently unstable and usually requires temporary pacing, even if hemodynamically stable. History can be quite helpful in risk stratification. A history of syncope in a patient who presents with advanced second-degree AV block may portend a higher degree of AV block or pause-dependent torsades de pointes, and there should be a very low threshold for temporary pacing.[11]

HIGH-GRADE AND PAROXYSMAL ATRIOVENTRICULAR BLOCK

In the critical care setting, it is crucial to distinguish between paroxysmal and vagally mediated AV block. Vagally mediated AV block due to *extrinsic*, parasympathetic input is characterized by progressive sinus slowing, progressive PR prolongation, Mobitz type I second-degree AV block immediately before the onset of complete heart block, and sinus slowing during the episode (Fig. 5.3). In contrast, high-grade AV block due to an *intrinsic* failure of a diseased His-Purkinje system—also termed "paroxysmal" AV block—is characterized by a constant sinus rate, or even sinus acceleration during the episode (Fig. 5.4). Patients with paroxysmal AV block *usually* have some sort of baseline conduction abnormality on their surface 12-lead electrocardiogram—most commonly, right bundle branch block—but this finding is not absolute. The hallmark of paroxysmal AV block is *immediate* transition from apparently normal conduction to complete AV block and ventricular asystole. This is usually triggered by a pause after a premature atrial or ventricular depolarization, but vagally mediated sinus slowing can have the same effect, complicating the interpretation of these events. Vagally mediated heart block is typically benign, is atropine responsive, and does *not* require temporary pacing. Paroxysmal AV block can be fatal and requires temporary transvenous pacing until a permanent pacemaker can be placed.[12]

ELECTROLYTE AND METABOLIC DERANGEMENT

Hyperkalemia can precipitate complete AV block and can also elevate pacing thresholds in permanent pacemaker systems.[13-15] A progressive increase in extracellular potassium raises the resting membrane potential, inactivating

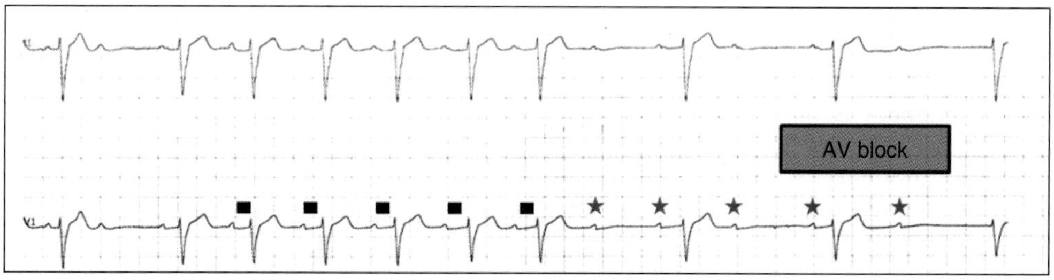

Figure 5.3 Telemetry strip demonstrating vagally mediated complete heart block. There is progressive PR prolongation (*black boxes*) and sinus *slowing* (*red stars*) just before the development of complete heart block, reflecting parasympathetic innervation of both the sinus and atrioventricular nodes.

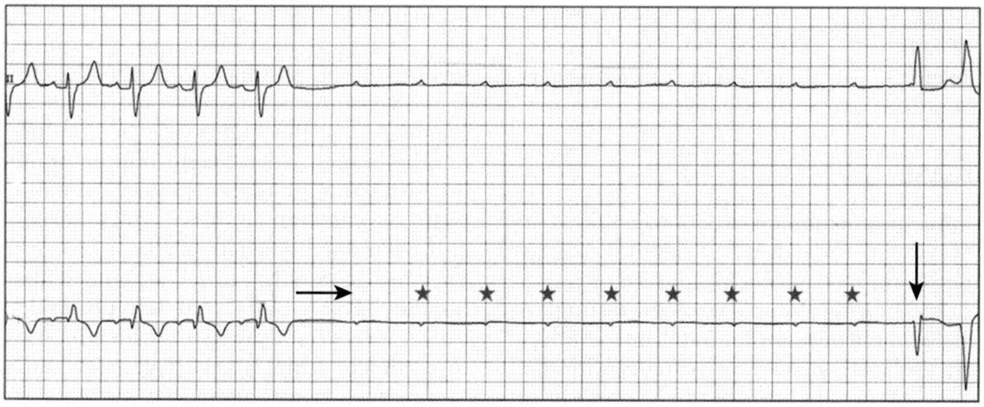

Figure 5.4 Telemetry strip demonstrating paroxysmal atrioventricular (AV) block. There is a brief sinus pause (*horizontal black arrow*) followed by multiple, nonconducted P waves (*red stars*) with associated sinus acceleration, reflecting an intrinsic failure of AV nodal conduction. The nearly 7-second pause is eventually interrupted by a junctional escape complex (*vertical black arrow*).

voltage-gated sodium channels that depend upon a sufficiently negative resting membrane potential for normal function. The effect is more pronounced in the atrium and ventricle than the cells of the specialized conduction system, explaining why the characteristic changes in the P wave and QRS complex typically precede sinoatrial (SA) and AV nodal dysfunction: "peaked" T waves and QT shortening (potassium level 5.5 mEq/L); PR prolongation and QRS widening (potassium level 6.5 mEq/L); a "sinoventricular" rhythm, due to the apparent absence of atrial activity (potassium level 8-9 mEq/L); and lastly, a "sine wave" pattern due to merging of the QRS and T wave that predicts impending cardiac arrest (potassium level 10 mEq/L).[16] Nevertheless, the 12-lead electrocardiogram may be entirely normal in cases of pronounced hyperkalemia, and AV block may occur in isolation.[17-20] Therefore, a routine metabolic evaluation is indicated in all patients with new conduction deficits.

The initial management of hyperkalemia-induced heart block is medical. If 12-lead electrocardiographic findings are pathognomonic for hyperkalemia, empiric treatment is appropriate while laboratory studies are pending. The administration of calcium chloride or calcium gluconate acutely antagonizes the electrical effects of potassium, partially restoring normal SA automaticity and conduction velocity. The effect is short-lived, however, and does nothing to correct extracellular potassium levels. Insulin, albuterol, and other catecholamines reduce extracellular potassium through activation of the Na^+/K^+-ATPase pump, and sodium polystyrene sulfonate (Kayexalate) facilitates its gastrointestinal excretion. Dialysis is the most definitive treatment but requires peritoneal or vascular access. Temporary pacing may be helpful, but prohibitively high capture thresholds may be problematic. In patients with a preexisting cardiac device, pacing outputs can be increased if there is intermittent "failure to capture," but the underlying metabolic disturbance takes precedence.

Case reports and animal studies suggest a link between metabolic acidosis and heart block, and metabolic acidosis frequently accompanies hyperkalemia in the setting of chronic kidney disease.[21] The administration of sodium bicarbonate acutely raises extracellular pH and indirectly lowers extracellular potassium, and may improve responsiveness to vasopressors in emergent situations.[22]

Hyponatremia, hypokalemia, hypomagnesemia, and hypocalcemia have not been implicated in heart block.

DRUG SIDE EFFECTS

A number of drugs can cause severe sinus bradycardia, AV block, or both. β-Adrenergic blockers and calcium channel blockers are both negatively chronotropic and inotropic, and their administration can result in significant bradycardia and hypotension, particularly in overdose. Digoxin toxicity may present with high-grade or complete AV block, further compounded by atrial or ventricular tachycardia due to increased automaticity. Amiodarone, dronedarone, and sotalol—class III antiarrhythmic drugs with mixed antiarrhythmic effects—frequently cause bradycardia due to SA or AV conduction defects. Some studies suggest that drug-induced AV block—particularly at therapeutic levels—is a predictor of future conduction disorders.[23]

Clearly, the initial treatment is discontinuation of the offending drug(s). Directed therapy may occasionally be useful as well, but the evidence is largely anecdotal. β-Adrenergic blocker toxicity may respond to glucagon, and calcium channel blocker toxicity may respond to calcium or glucagon in refractory cases.[24-28] Vasopressors are occasionally necessary because of the vasodilatory and negative inotropic effects of these drugs. Digoxin toxicity can be treated with digoxin antibody fragments (Digibind).[29] If hemodynamic instability persists in the setting of severe bradycardia, temporary pacing is indicated. β-Adrenergic blockers and calcium channel blockers increase pacing thresholds in permanent devices; if failure to capture is noted in a patient with suspected overdose of these agents, a temporary increase in pacing output may solve the problem.[30]

INFECTIOUS DISEASE

Lyme disease is the most common tick-borne illness in North America.[31] Erythema migrans is sufficient for diagnosis, but most patients cannot recall a tick exposure or rash.[32] The diagnosis of Lyme carditis requires serologic testing for confirmation, and *Borrelia burgdorferi* IgM and IgG antibodies are positive in the vast majority of patients with the disease.[33] Regardless of patient history, the diagnosis of Lyme carditis should always be entertained in a patient presenting with heart block in an endemic area. Typically, Lyme carditis affects the AV node and is associated with a stable, junctional escape rhythm, but more diffuse involvement of the His-Purkinje system with a slower, more unstable escape is also possible.[34] Although conduction deficits regress rapidly and completely with appropriate antibiotic therapy, temporary pacing is occasionally necessary.

Infective endocarditis can be complicated by a broad spectrum of conduction disturbances, including first-degree AV delay, bundle branch block, and complete heart block. Any new conduction deficit suggests perivalvular abscess, due to the proximity of the compact AV node and bundle branches to the membranous septum.[35,36] Conduction disturbances most commonly complicate aortic valve endocarditis, but the tricuspid valve and mitral valve are also susceptible.[37-39] Perivalvular abscess and heart block are indications for surgical repair.[40] Serial 12-lead electrocardiography should be performed in all patients with endocarditis, and temporary pacing should be strongly considered for any progressive conduction disturbance.

Lymphocytic and giant cell myocarditis are typically associated with acute systolic dysfunction, but they can also be complicated by severe electrical abnormalities, including complete heart block. Lymphocytic myocarditis carries a more favorable prognosis than giant cell myocarditis, but permanent pacemaker dependency is possible with either condition.[41]

AFTER MYOCARDIAL INFARCTION

Official guidelines for temporary and permanent pacing after ST-segment elevation myocardial infarction were last updated in 2004, and permanent pacemaker indications following myocardial infarction were updated in 2008 as previously discussed.[1,42] Recommendations for temporary pacing are largely based on expert opinion, in addition to case reports, case series, and published summaries from before the reperfusion era.

The need for temporary pacing is frequently made at the time of percutaneous intervention by the interventional cardiologist, but familiarity with official guidelines and an understanding of the risk of progression is critical in the appropriate management of the patient after myocardial infarction. Clearly, myocardial infarction complicated by asystolic arrest and symptomatic bradycardia justifies temporary transvenous pacing. Temporary transvenous pacing is recommended when an ST-segment elevation myocardial infarction is complicated by new bifascicular block or complete bundle branch block *and* concomitant Mobitz type II second-degree AV block, regardless of the culprit artery. It is also recommended for alternating bundle branch block, regardless of the status of AV conduction. Alternating bundle branch block—right bundle branch block alternating with left bundle branch block, or bifascicular block with right bundle branch block and alternating left anterior and posterior fascicular block—is a marker of severe His-Purkinje disease. In particular, bifascicular block with right bundle branch block and left posterior fascicular block carries a very poor prognosis with a high risk of progression to complete heart block (Fig. 5.5A and B).[43] In cases of Mobitz type II second-degree AV block with normal intraventricular conduction, fascicular block, and old bundle branch block, transvenous pacing is given a less stringent recommendation. Temporary transcutaneous pacing is recommended in every other scenario, with the exception of normal AV nodal and intraventricular conduction, isolated first-degree AV block, isolated left anterior or posterior fascicular block, and isolated old bundle branch block (Table 5.1).

The culprit artery has prognostic implications. Complete heart block complicating anterior wall myocardial infarction—usually involving the proximal left anterior descending artery—is due to necrosis of the interventricular septum and irreversible damage to the His-Purkinje conduction system. In contrast, complete heart block in inferior wall infarction—usually involving the proximal right coronary artery (RCA)—is vagally mediated and atropine sensitive in the first hours of infarction.[44] Local accumulation of adenosine in the days after infarction may lead to persistent, atropine-insensitive AV block, but permanent pacing is rarely indicated.[45] Because the RCA supplies the SA nodal artery in 90% of cases, a proximal RCA infarction may also be complicated by sinus bradycardia, SA exit block, and sinus arrest; these, too, are typically transient in nature and atropine responsive.

TORSADES DE POINTES

Torsades de pointes is a polymorphic (or "twisting" around the baseline) ventricular arrhythmia associated with QT prolongation. Because the QT interval is directly proportional to heart rate—that is, the QT interval lengthens at slow heart rates and shortens at fast heart rates—torsades de pointes is usually a self-terminating and recurrent arrhythmia. It can rarely degenerate into ventricular fibrillation

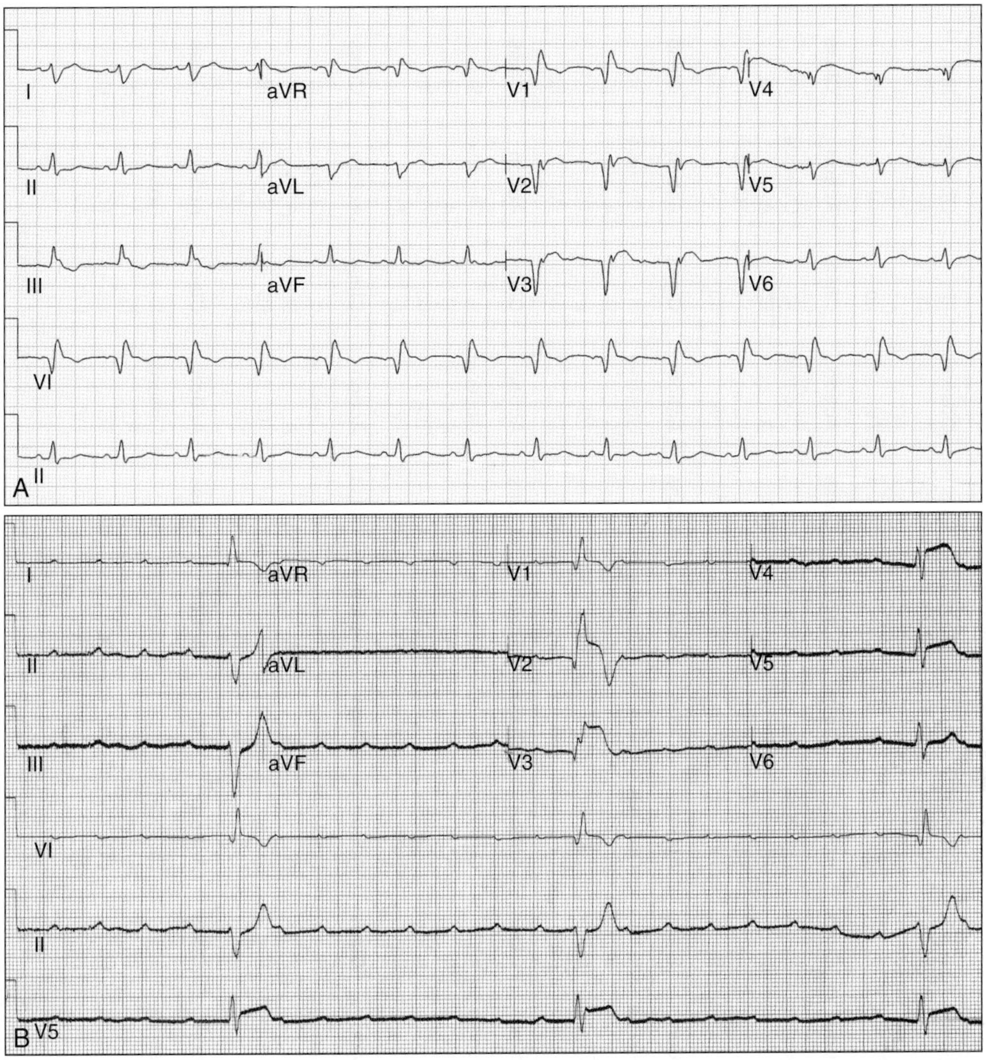

Figure 5.5 Bifascicular block following acute, left anterior descending coronary artery infarction. **A,** A 12-lead electrocardiogram demonstrating sinus rhythm with normal atrioventricular (AV) nodal conduction, but right bundle branch block and left posterior fascicular block. There are also pathologic Q waves in leads V_1 to V_4, consistent with an anterior wall infarction due to occlusion of a proximal left anterior descending artery. **B,** A 12-lead electrocardiogram of the same patient, 1 week later. There is now high-grade AV block with a right bundle branch block and left anterior fascicular block, due to necrosis of the His-Purkinje system that has left only the left posterior fascicle capable of conduction.

and require external defibrillation, but this development is uncommon. The underlying QT prolongation can be either congenital or acquired, the latter of which is by far more common in the critical care setting and most often is due to administration of a culprit drug or severe electrolyte disturbance.

The most important considerations in the management of torsades de pointes are appropriate recognition of the problem, correction of the underlying cause(s), and avoidance of QT-prolonging drugs that can further exacerbate the problem. Although this arrhythmia is polymorphic by definition, not all polymorphic ventricular arrhythmias are due to torsades de pointes. Polymorphic ventricular tachycardia may complicate acute coronary syndrome, but it is typically associated with a suggestive clinical history and ST-segment deviation. Temporary or permanent pacemaker malfunction with ventricular undersensing can lead to "R on T" pacing, and certain pacemaker settings that minimize ventricular pacing can predispose to "long-short" sequences and polymorphic ventricular arrhythmias as well.[46-49] If ventricular tachycardia is reliably initiated with pacing, pacemaker reprogramming may resolve the problem; electrophysiology consultation should be sought immediately.

The administration of magnesium sulfate (1-2 g over 5-10 minutes) is acutely effective in most patients.[50] If ineffective, isoproterenol (1-4 μg/minute) can accelerate the heart rate and thereby shorten the QT, but this should be avoided in long QT syndrome—particularly long QT type 1—because of the potential for proarrhythmia.

Temporary pacing is indicated in patients who fail electrolyte supplementation and pharmacologic augmentation of the heart rate, or patients with severe AV conduction disturbances. Temporary pacing shortens the action potential and QT interval but also truncates the progressive, post-PVC (premature ventricular contraction) pauses that typically trigger an episode (see Fig. 5.2).[51] Typically, pacing at a rate of 90 to 100 beats per minute is sufficient to

Table 5.1 Recommendations for Treatment of Atrioventricular and Intraventricular Conduction Disturbances During STEMI

Intraventricular Conduction	Normal		First-Degree AV block				Mobitz I Second-Degree AV Block				Mobitz II Second-Degree AV Block			
			Anterior MI		Nonanterior MI		Anterior MI		Nonanterior MI		Anterior MI		Nonanterior MI	
Normal	Action	Class	Action	Class	Action	Class	Action	Class	Action	Class	Action	Class	Action	Class
	Observe	I	Observe	I	Observe	I	Observe	IIb	Observe	IIa	Observe	III	Observe	III
	A	III	A	III	A	III	A*	III	A	III	A	III	A	III
	TC	III	TC	IIb	TC	IIb	TC	I	TC	I	TC	I	TC	I
	TV	III	TV	III	TV	III	TV	III	TV	III	TV	IIa	TV	IIa
Old or new fascicular block (LAFB or LPFB)	Action	Class	Action	Class	Action	Class	Action	Class	Action	Class	Action	Class	Action	Class
	Observe	I	Observe	IIb	Observe	IIb	Observe	IIb	Observe	IIb	Observe	III	Observe	III
	A	III	A	III	A	III	A*	III	A	III	A	III	A	III
	TC	IIb	TC	I	TC	IIa	TC	I	TC	I	TC	I	TC	I
	TV	III	TV	III	TV	III	TV	III	TV	III	TV	IIa	TV	IIb
Old bundle branch block	Action	Class	Action	Class	Action	Class	Action	Class	Action	Class	Action	Class	Action	Class
	Observe	I	Observe	III	Observe	III	Observe	III	Observe	III	Observe	III	Observe	III
	A	III	A	III	A	III	A*	III	A	III	A	III	A	III
	TC	IIb	TC	I	TC	I	TC	I	TC	I	TC	I	TC	I
	TV	III	TV	IIb	TV	IIb	TV	IIb	TV	IIb	TV	IIa	TV	IIa
New bundle branch block	Action	Class	Action	Class	Action	Class	Action	Class	Action	Class	Action	Class	Action	Class
	Observe	III	Observe	III	Observe	III	Observe	III	Observe	III	Observe	III	Observe	III
	A	III	A	III	A	III	A*	III	A	III	A	III	A	III
	TC	I	TC	I	TC	I	TC	I	TC	I	TC	IIb	TC	IIb
	TV	IIb	TV	IIa	TV	IIa	TV	IIa	TV	IIa	TV	I	TV	I
Fascicular block and RBBB	Action	Class	Action	Class	Action	Class	Action	Class	Action	Class	Action	Class	Action	Class
	Observe	III	Observe	III	Observe	III	Observe	III	Observe	III	Observe	III	Observe	III
	A	III	A	III	A	III	A*	III	A	III	A	III	A	III
	TC	I	TC	I	TC	I	TC	I	TC	I	TC	IIb	TC	IIb
	TV	IIb	TV	IIa	TV	IIa	TV	IIa	TV	IIa	TV	I	TV	I
Alternating left and right bundle branch block	Action	Class	Action	Class	Action	Class	Action	Class	Action	Class	Action	Class	Action	Class
	Observe	III	Observe	III	Observe	III	Observe	III	Observe	III	Observe	III	Observe	III
	A	III	A	III	A	III	A*	III	A	III	A	III	A	III
	TC	IIb	TC	IIb	TC	IIb	TC	IIb	TC	IIb	TC	IIb	TC	IIb
	TV	I	TV	I	TV	I	TV	I	TV	I	TV	I	TV	I

LAFB indicates left anterior fascicular block; LPFB, left posterior fascicular block; RBBB, right bundle-branch block; A, atropine; TC, transcutaneous pacing; TV, temporary transvenous pacing; STEMI, ST elevation myocardial infarction; AV, atrioventricular; and MI, myocardial infarction.

Four possible actions, or therapeutic options, are listed and classified for each bradyarrhythmia or conduction problem:

1. Observe: continued ECG monitoring, no further action planned.
2. A, and A*: atropine administered at 0.6 to 1.0 mg IV every 5 minutes to up to 0.04 mg/kg. In general, because the increase in sinus rate with atropine is unpredictable, this is to be avoided unless there is symptomatic bradycardia that will likely respond to a vagolytic agent, such as sinus bradycardia or Mobitz I, as denoted by the asterisk above.
3. TC: application of transcutaneous pads and standby transcutaneous pacing with no further progression to transvenous pacing imminently planned.
4. TV: temporary transvenous pacing. It is assumed, but not specified in the table, that at the discretion of the clinician, transcutaneous pads will be applied and standby transcutaneous pacing will be in effect as the patient is transferred to the fluoroscopy unit for temporary transvenous pacing.

From Epstein et al: Circulation 2008;117:e350-408.

suppress ventricular ectopy, but rates as fast as 140 beats per minute may be necessary.[52] Patients with preexisting cardiac devices can be adjusted at the bedside to achieve the same effect. In patients with normal AV nodal conduction, atrial pacing is preferred.

CONDITIONS THAT DO NOT NORMALLY REQUIRE PACING

HYPOTHERMIA

Hypothermia can produce dramatic electrocardiographic abnormalities—PR prolongation, QRS widening, and QT prolongation, in addition to both atrial and ventricular arrhythmias—and familiarity with this condition is increasingly important in the critical care setting owing to the widespread adoption of therapeutic hypothermia in survivors of cardiac arrest.[53,54] Moderate (32° C to 33.9° C) hypothermia causes a reduction in cardiac output that is mediated by sinus bradycardia, but this is accompanied by an increase in myocardial contractility and proportional decrease in basal metabolism. No specific treatment is needed, and attempts to increase the heart rate with drug or temporary pacing are counterproductive.[55] Deep hypothermia (<30° C) is associated with increased risk of atrial and ventricular arrhythmias, reduced responsiveness to electrical and pharmacologic cardioversion, and increased sensitivity to mechanical manipulation.[56] One case report describes the successful resuscitation of two severely hypothermic patients with transcutaneous pacing,[57] and another describes the near immediate initiation of ventricular fibrillation with transvenous pacing.[58] The role of temporary pacing—whether transcutaneous or transvenous—is limited, and should be reserved for extreme situations of hemodynamic and electrical instability. The primary treatment is rewarming.

HYPOTHYROIDISM

Severe hypothyroidism is most commonly seen in the elderly and is most often precipitated by infections. Case reports have established that severe hypothyroidism and myxedema coma can cause a range of AV conduction abnormalities, including complete heart block. The symptoms of hypothyroidism can be vague, and the electrocardiographic manifestations—P wave flattening, low QRS voltage and intraventricular conduction delays, QT prolongation, and T wave flattening or inversion—are nonspecific. Thyroid hormone replacement can quickly normalize conduction but may take up to several weeks in some patients.[59-61] Patients who present with new conduction abnormalities—particularly the elderly and infirm—should be routinely screened for hypothyroidism. Temporary pacing may be needed in cases of advanced AV block, but thyroid hormone supplementation is usually curative.

OBSTRUCTIVE SLEEP APNEA

Obstructive sleep apnea has been associated with cyclic patterns of SA and AV nodal conduction disturbances, occasionally resulting in prolonged periods of asystole during sleep.[62] In general, nocturnal arrhythmias are less clinically relevant than those during the day, and the need for intervention should be taken in the context of the clinical situation. Atropine has been shown to abolish cyclic variation and nocturnal bradycardia, suggesting that autonomic influences play a role.[63] One study suggested that atrial overdrive pacing reduces the number of central and obstructive apneic episodes,[64] but subsequent studies have shown no benefit and pacing does *not* have a role in the chronic management of this disorder.[65-67] Continuous positive airway pressure abolishes conduction disturbances in the majority of patients, suggesting that hypoxia plays a role in the pathophysiology of the condition. It is the therapy of choice.[68]

PREOPERATIVE ANESTHESIA

Preexisting His-Purkinje disease—complete right or left bundle branch block, or bifascicular block, for example—does *not* routinely require temporary pacing before surgery. Patients with complete heart block with junctional, and particularly ventricular escape complexes, should be considered for temporary pacing due to the potentially suppressive effects of general anesthesia. Patients with underlying left bundle branch block who require Swan-Ganz catheterization have a small risk of procedurally related complete heart block due to catheter-induced right bundle branch block.[69] In these situations, right-sided heart catheterization should be performed under fluoroscopy, and transcutaneous pacing should be immediately available. The presence of an "rS" complex in lead V_1 may reflect left-to-right septal activation and left bundle branch *delay*, rather than complete left bundle branch block; the risk of catheter-induced heart block may be lower in these circumstances.[70]

SEIZURE

Severe sinus bradycardia and prolonged periods of asystole complicate less than 0.4% of seizures.[71] "Ictal bradycardia" is felt to be vagally mediated, but there is disagreement in the epilepsy community about its potential contribution to sudden death.[72,73] Although the majority of episodes terminate spontaneously, some patients are ultimately referred for pacemaker implantation. In the critical care setting, continuous electrocardiographic and encephalographic monitoring can be quite helpful if clinical features suggest prodromal seizure activity. The most appropriate management—including the potential need for temporary pacing—is unclear.

SPINAL CORD INJURY AND TRACHEAL SUCTIONING

Severe cervical injury is nearly universally associated with sinus bradycardia, sinus pauses, and hypotension in the days after injury, but these changes typically resolve within 2 to 6 weeks.[74] Endotracheal intubation, tracheal suctioning, and repositioning can precipitate prolonged, vagally mediated pauses in these patients, presumably due to impairment of the sympathetic nervous system input during periods of increased parasympathetic tone. There have been case reports of asystolic cardiac arrest during tracheal suctioning, but supplemental oxygen therapy was at least partially effective in preventing further episodes, suggesting that hypoxia played a role.[75] The administration of atropine, theophylline, aminophylline, and isoproterenol—individually, or in combination—may attenuate these pauses, but their administration may be ineffective in the short-term and cumbersome in the long-term. There is no consensus on the issue, but some authors advocate placement of a permanent pacemaker in patients with a prolonged requirement of mechanical ventilation, due to the unpredictable nature of these events.[76] Temporary pacing can be considered on a case-by-case basis, but it is important to recognize that the primary underlying problem is autonomic in nature.

ESOPHAGEAL AND TRANSTHORACIC PACING

For reasons of efficacy and patient comfort, esophageal pacing has fallen out of favor in the last 2 decades in favor of transcutaneous and transvenous pacing techniques. Transthoracic pacing with direct, percutaneous placement of a needle into the heart is obsolete.

The esophagus lies immediately posterior to the left atrium, and an esophageal pill electrode was historically used to record atrial activity. Esophageal recording makes it very easy to identify atrial activity, which can be useful in the differentiation of ventricular tachycardia and supraventricular tachycardia with aberrant conduction.[77] The presence of AV dissociation is virtually pathognomonic for ventricular tachycardia, but atrial activity is often difficult to recognize on the 12-lead electrocardiogram, particularly with fast, wide complex arrhythmias. Nevertheless, there are easy-to-use algorithms that allow for the rapid and relatively accurate diagnosis of wide complex rhythms, often regardless of whether atrial activity is apparent on the 12-lead electrocardiogram.[78,79]

TRANSCUTANEOUS PACING

BACKGROUND

First described by Zoll in 1952 in the management of Stokes-Adams attacks, transcutaneous pacing involves the delivery of pacing stimuli though cutaneous patch electrodes.[80] It is the fastest and technically least challenging means of temporary pacing, and it does not introduce the risks associated with vascular access and transvenous pacing. The initial system required the subcutaneous insertion of 21-gauge needles and was limited by high pacing thresholds and significant pain. The technology has evolved over time, but these issues remain to some degree. Capture is still unsuccessful in a significant minority of patients, and it can be difficult to assess capture because of saturation artifact from pacing stimuli—particularly if pacing outputs are high (Fig. 5.6).[81] Transcutaneous pacing is still painful and generally requires the administration of sedation or analgesics. It is best tolerated in deeply anesthetized or unconscious patients, and most appropriate in situations in which pacing is required only briefly or intermittently, or as a bridging measure for placement of a transvenous system.

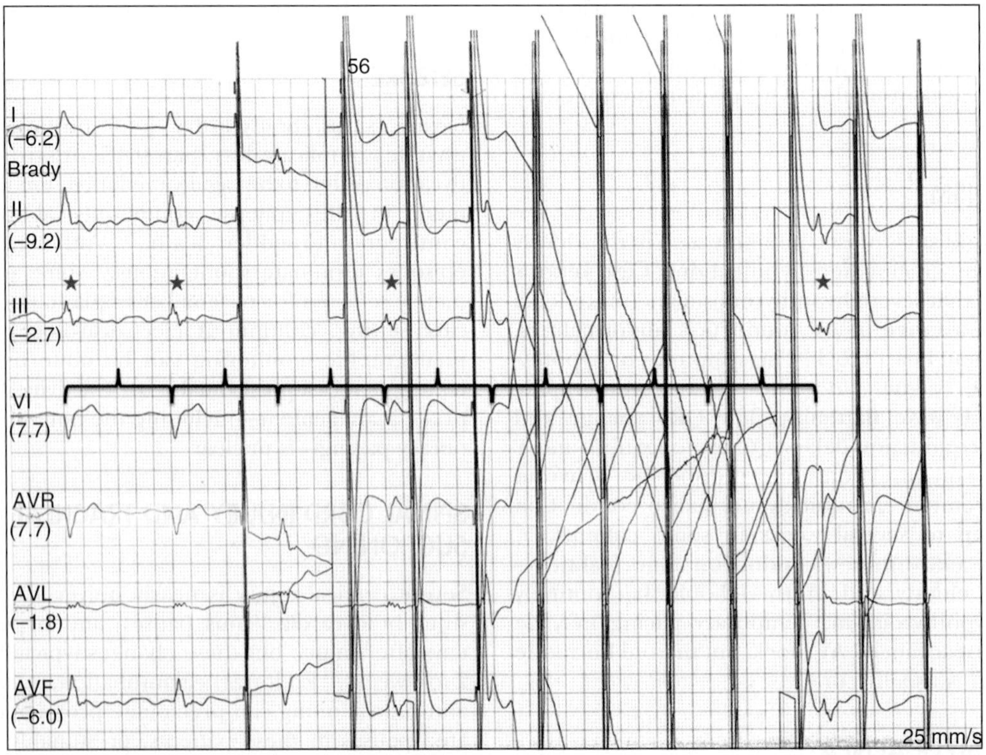

Figure 5.6 Telemetry strip demonstrating ineffective transcutaneous pacing. There is an underlying junctional rhythm (*red stars*) that "marches through" the pacing artifact without any change in rate or rhythm, proving that transcutaneous pacing fails to capture the myocardium. The pacing artifact saturates the tracing and makes interpretation quite difficult.

METHODS

Commercially available external defibrillators have both pacing *and* defibrillating capability. The skin should be cleaned thoroughly with alcohol, but preferably not shaved, because the pain associated with pacing is typically localized to small abrasions and local salt deposits on the skin.[82] The patch electrodes should be arranged in an anteroposterior position with one patch over the mid-dorsal spine at the left paravertebral position, and the other over the point of maximal impulse. If abrasions are present, the patches can be positioned in an adjacent area with intact skin. The external generator should be turned on at the lowest pacing output, and then increased in a step-wise fashion until reliable capture is observed on telemetry. It can be difficult to distinguish pacing artifact from capture, but the presence of a QRS complex and T wave—which represents cardiac depolarization and repolarization—is confirmatory. Capture should also be confirmed by the presence of a palpable or measurable pulse that matches the paced rate. The pacing outputs should be set *just above* capture threshold to minimize pacing artifact, pain, and risk of proarrhythmia.

Capture thresholds are predictably higher than with endocardial pacing, but most patients will capture at a pacing output of 40 to 70 mA. The capture threshold is proportional to the size of the patch electrode because of a reduction in current density—that is, larger electrodes require higher output for capture.[83] Higher impedance electrodes are preferred for pacing, but standard patch electrodes are more practical in daily practice. Hypoxia, acidosis, and prolonged periods of asystole may increase the pacing threshold.[84]

The pacing rate is dictated by the underlying rhythm and clinical indication. A patient with complete heart block and hemodynamic instability should be paced at 60 to 90 beats per minute, until transvenous pacing can be established. A patient with prolonged postconversion pauses or only intermittent heart block should be paced at 40 beats per minute to minimize pacing.

EPICARDIAL PACING

BACKGROUND

Permanent pacing is required in roughly 2% of coronary artery bypass grafting and up to 7.7% of valve surgery cases,[85-87] but transient SND, fascicular block, bundle branch block, and AV block are common within the first few days following surgery.[88] Epicardial pacing offers a safe and well-tolerated "bridge" to recovery, avoiding the need for transcutaneous and transvenous pacing. It also allows for prevention, diagnosis, and management of postoperative atrial arrhythmias, and the optimization of hemodynamics in the critical care setting.

METHODS

Epicardial wires are typically placed on the anterior right atrium and right ventricle at the conclusion of open heart surgery, then threaded through the right and left subcostal areas for attachment to an external pulse generator. Most surgeons will routinely implant both atrial and ventricular leads because AV synchrony and native conduction is preferred whenever possible, particularly in patients with preexisting systolic dysfunction.[89,90]

Pacing and sensing thresholds typically deteriorate rapidly over 3 to 5 days owing to local inflammation, and should be checked on a daily basis to ensure adequate safety margins, particularly in patients with ongoing pacemaker dependency. External pulse generators can deliver impulses up to 20 mA, but high outputs may only further exacerbate the local inflammation that produces high pacing thresholds.[91] Alternate locations—including the basal and lateral left ventricle—may be associated with more favorable pacing thresholds and cardiac performance.[92]

PREVENTION OF ATRIAL ARRHYTHMIAS

Atrial fibrillation complicates 20% to 50% of cardiac surgery cases, resulting in longer times in the hospital, increased hospital costs, and higher morbidity and mortality rates.[93] The administration of β-adrenergic blockers and amiodarone constitutes first-line therapy, but there is some data to support the use of atrial pacing in the postoperative setting.[94,95] One small, prospective study demonstrated a 17% absolute risk reduction of postoperative atrial fibrillation through the use of "overdrive" atrial pacing (AAI mode at a minimum of 80 beats per minute) for 24 hours on the second postoperative day, but longer-term follow-up was not reported in the study.[96] The trials have been small and heterogeneous in design, but meta-analysis suggests an absolute reduction of 10% of postoperative atrial fibrillation with overdrive atrial pacing.[97]

TREATMENT OF ATRIAL ARRHYTHMIAS

Rapid, "burst" atrial pacing can be easily performed at the bedside using a standard, external pulse generator. Typical atrial flutter and other macro-reentrant arrhythmias that involve the right atrium are often susceptible to pace termination, due to depolarization of the "excitable gap" of the circuit. Pace termination is simply performed by pacing the atrium at a sufficiently high pacing output to guarantee atrial capture at a rate that is slightly faster than the arrhythmia. One can start pacing at 10 mA and 10 to 20 beats per minute faster than the atrial rate for 5 to 10 seconds, but any of these parameters can be adjusted if initial attempts are unsuccessful. Because rapid ventricular pacing can easily precipitate ventricular fibrillation, it is essential to confirm the epicardial system is connected appropriately before any pacing attempt. Burst pacing may cause atrial flutter to degenerate into atrial fibrillation, which is often associated with a slower, better-tolerated heart rate.

DIAGNOSIS OF WIDE COMPLEX ARRHYTHMIAS

Atrial activity can be directly recorded by connecting the pin of the atrial wire to precordial lead V_1 of the 12-lead electrocardiogram, elucidating the mechanism of a tachycardia (Fig. 5.7).

RISKS

Some centers argue against the routine placement of epicardial wires because of their cost and potential risk, but their use remains nearly ubiquitous. The frequency of complications is far less than 1%, but case reports have described the inadvertent laceration of saphenous vein grafts,[98,99] right atrium,[100] and right ventricular outflow tract[101] with development of either pericardial tamponade or hemothorax following their removal, and infection attributed to abandonment and bacterial colonization of the wires.[102,103] Epicardial wires are almost always removed with gentle traction, and the prevailing thought is that their occasional abandonment does not constitute a risk to the patient. To minimize risk, they should be pulled after discontinuation of anticoagulation therapy in a monitored setting.

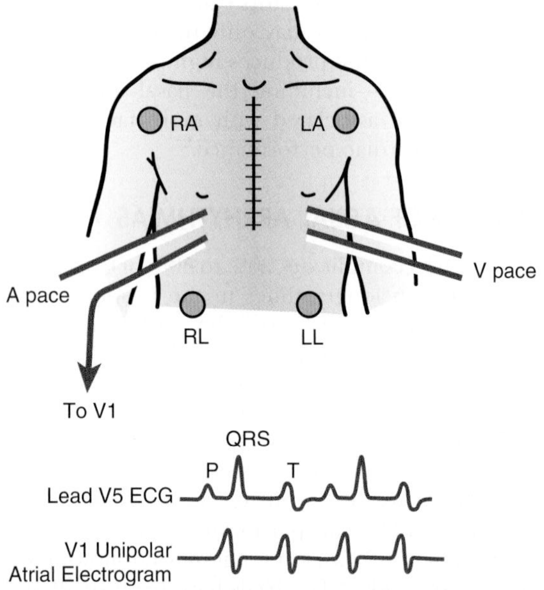

Figure 5.7 Temporary atrial pacing wires utilized for arrhythmia diagnosis. Epicardial pacing wires can be utilized for arrhythmia diagnosis in postoperative coronary artery bypass graft patients when P waves cannot be clearly visualized on surface electrocardiography. One of the epicardial atrial wires is clipped to lead V_1 on the standard electrocardiogram machine. The unipolar atrial electrogram now appears on lead V_1 referenced to surface lead V_5 in this figure, demonstrating two P waves for every QRS complex, making the diagnosis of atrial flutter.

TRANSVENOUS PACING

BACKGROUND

Cardiac pacing with an endocardial electrode was first introduced in 1959 and quickly supplanted transcutaneous pacing as the method of choice for temporary pacing.[104] Transvenous pacing is more reliable and more comfortable than transcutaneous pacing, but it also takes longer to initiate and introduces some degree of procedural risk.

METHODS

The internal jugular, subclavian, or femoral vein can be used, but the internal jugular is generally the preferred approach. The subclavian vein should be preserved for a permanent device, and the femoral vein carries a higher risk of infection, impedes patient movement, and requires fluoroscopic guidance. A variety of catheters are commercially available, the selection of which depends on operator preference, patient characteristics, and the availability of fluoroscopy (Fig. 5.8). Fluoroscopic imaging should be used routinely in patients with significant tricuspid regurgitation owing to the potential difficulty of catheter advancement across the tricuspid annulus in this setting. Fluoroscopic guidance should also be considered in patients with preexisting left bundle branch block and intermittent heart

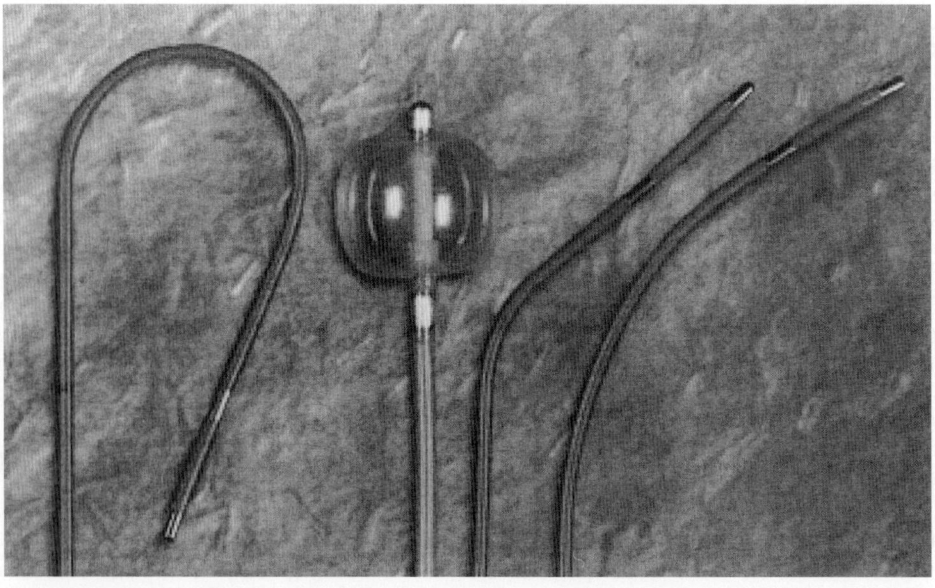

Figure 5.8 Temporary bipolar pacing catheters. *From left to right,* atrial J, semifloating balloon-tipped, and two ventricular catheters with different curves. (Courtesy of Daig Corporation/St. Jude Medical, Minneapolis, MN.)

block due to the potential for catheter-induced complete heart block.

Fluoroscopy simplifies catheter placement, but it may be unavailable, or a patient may simply be too unstable to transport to the catheterization laboratory in the critical care setting. If portable fluoroscopy is unavailable, the procedure is best performed "blindly" at the bedside using a "floppy," balloon-tipped catheter. Placement can be facilitated by electrocardiographic guidance, with or without pacing. If positioning is performed *with* pacing, the pacing catheter should be attached to an external pulse generator and set to pace at a rate slighter faster than the patient's intrinsic rate and at an intermediate pacing output (5 mA) to ensure capture. Catheter contact and position can be assessed by examination of the paced QRS morphologic appearance: an "LBBB" morphologic pattern with positive QRS complexes in leads II, III, and aVF (inferior frontal axis) suggests catheter position in the right ventricular outflow tract (Fig. 5.9) whereas an "LBBB" morphologic pattern with negative QRS complex in leads II, III, and aVF (superior frontal axis) suggests catheter position in the right ventricular apex (Fig. 5.10). If in the outflow tract, gentle withdrawal of the catheter will allow it to fall to a more inferior position and further advancement will guide it toward the apex. Deflating the balloon, then very gently advancing the catheter an additional 1 to 2 mm to wedge it in between the trabeculae of the right ventricle, can improve catheter stability. If positioning is performed *without* pacing, a pattern of ST-segment elevation on the local electrocardiogram indicates endocardial contact (Fig. 5.11).[105] The latter technique may be preferable in patients with complete heart block because even a brief period of overdrive pacing can extinguish a ventricular escape rhythm, resulting in immediate pacemaker dependency; therefore, transcutaneous pacing patches should be in place and available for use. If the pacing catheter has been advanced more than 40 cm without evidence of capture, it may have looped within the right atrium, or passed through the right atrium into the inferior vena cava. Either way, the catheter should be withdrawn with the balloon deflated, and then advanced again.

Once good contact has been established, the pacing threshold can be tested by reducing pacing output until loss of capture is noted on the monitor. Ideally, the pacing threshold should be less than 2 mA and sensing should be greater than 5 mV. To prevent inadvertent dislodgement during manipulation of the external pulse generator, the pacemaker should be sutured to the patient's skin with a redundant loop in two locations. A chest radiograph should be performed immediately to rule out pneumothorax and document catheter position.

SPECIAL CONSIDERATIONS IN TEMPORARY PACING

CONTRAINDICATIONS

Transvenous pacing should not be attempted in patients with a known superior vena cava (SVC) stenosis, and any resistance encountered during advancement of an intracardiac catheter should prompt the use of fluoroscopy (Fig. 5.12). Similarly, the presence of a mechanical tricuspid valve is an absolute contraindication, due to the potential for irreversible catheter entrapment.[106] Patients with any significant coagulopathy or ongoing need for anticoagulation may be better served with transcutaneous pacing, if at all possible. If transvenous pacing is necessary, it should be performed under fluoroscopic guidance to minimize the risk of lead perforation. Femoral access may be preferable in these circumstances, particularly if the need for transvenous pacing is felt to be short-lived.

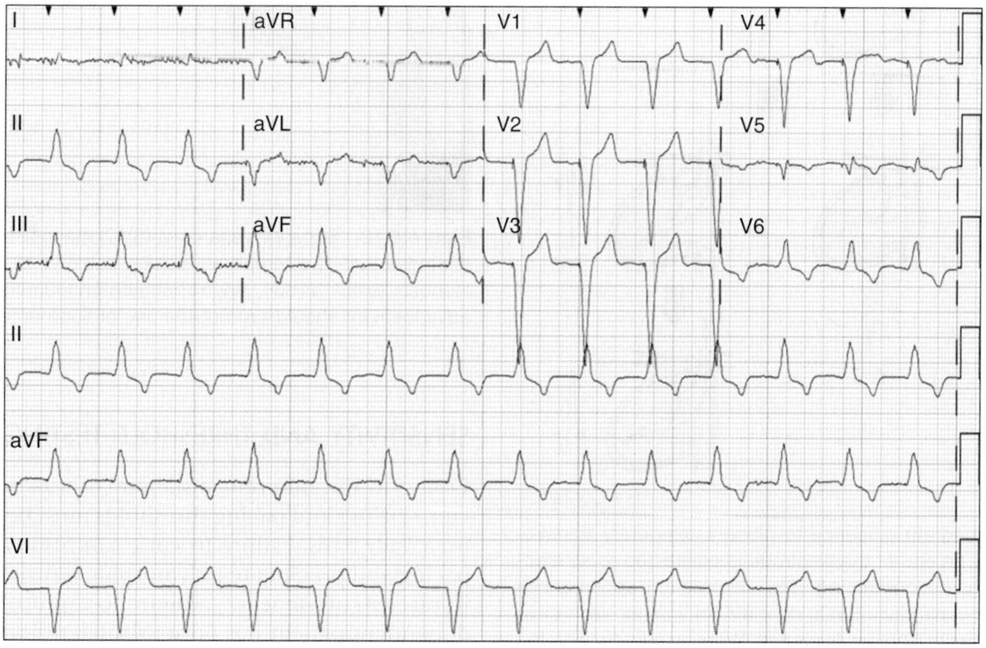

Figure 5.9 Paced morphologic pattern from right ventricular outflow tract. A paced QRS with a "left bundle branch block" morphologic pattern and "inferior" axis (positive QRS complexes in II, III, and aVF) suggests a pacing catheter position in the right ventricular outflow tract.

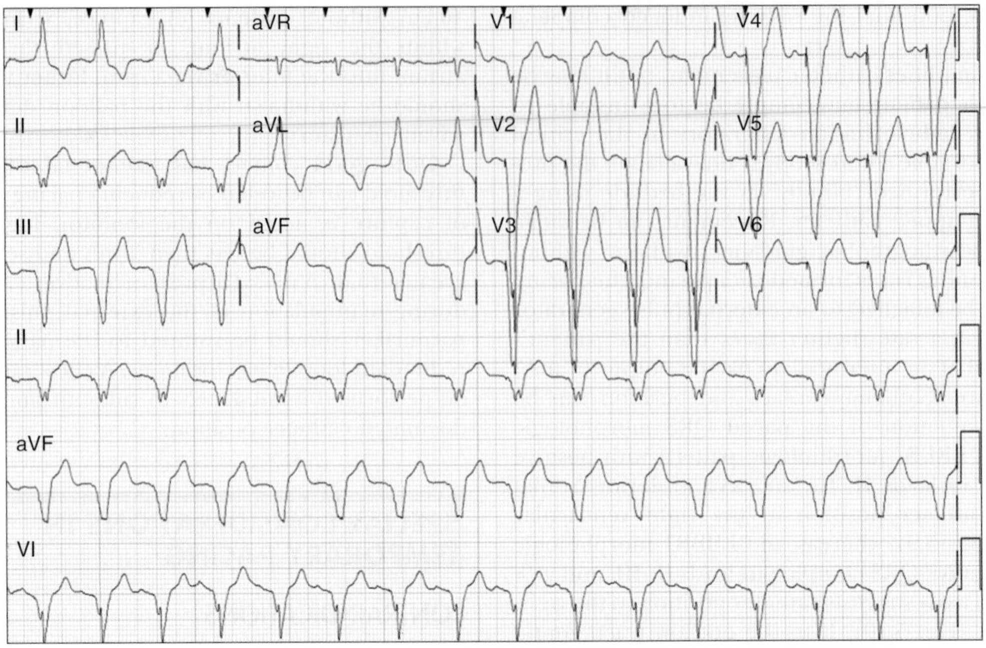

Figure 5.10 Paced morphologic pattern from right ventricular apex. A paced QRS complex with a "left bundle branch block" morphologic pattern and "superior" axis (negative QRS complexes in II, III, and aVF) suggests a pacing catheter position at the right ventricular apex.

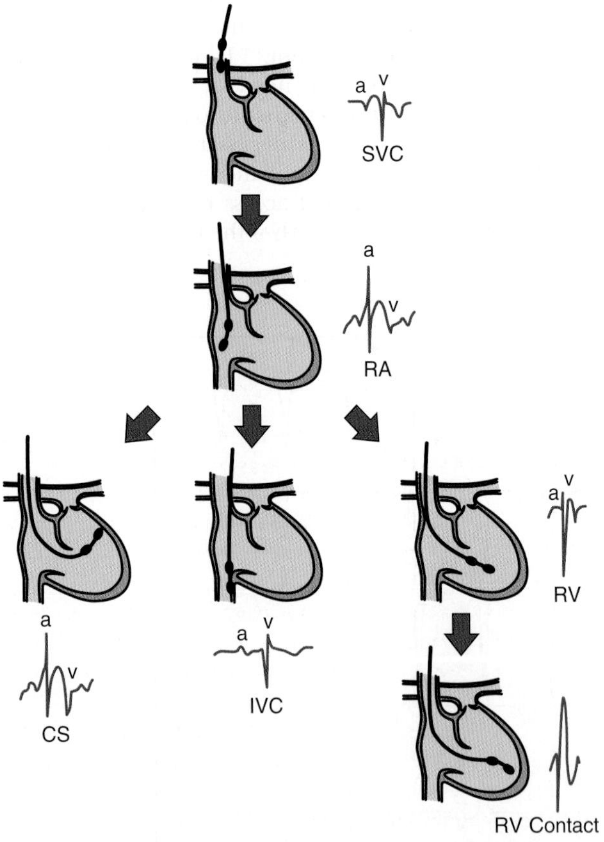

Figure 5.11 Electrogram guidance to place a temporary transvenous pacing lead. The end of the electrode is connected to an electrocardiogram to guide positioning. The electrogram appearances within the superior vena cava (SVC), right atrium, inferior vena cava (IVC), and right ventricle (RV) are illustrated. When in contact with the RV, the electrogram demonstrates an injury current with ST-segment elevation.

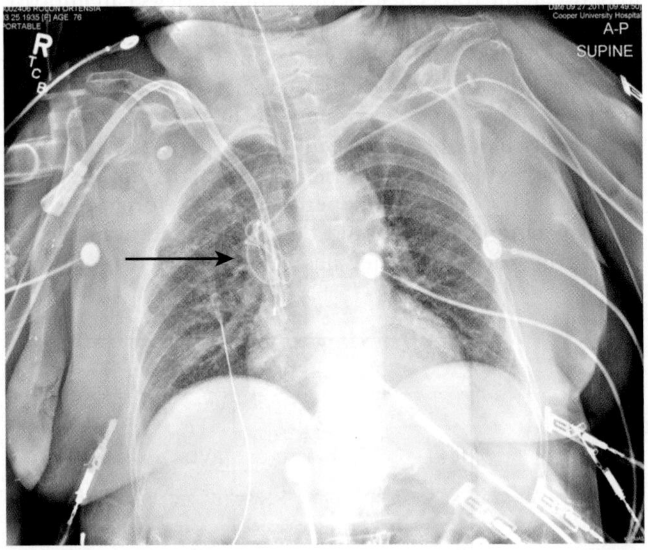

Figure 5.12 Superior vena cava (SVC) stenosis. There is extensive entanglement of a temporary pacing catheter at the site of an SVC stenosis (*black arrow*). Any resistance encountered during catheter advancement should prompt the use of fluoroscopy.

SENSITIVITY AND THRESHOLD TESTING

Owing to the inherent instability of a balloon-tipped catheter, sensing and pacing thresholds must be checked at least on a daily basis. Failure to sense can result in inappropriate pacing and precipitate polymorphic ventricular arrhythmias in rare circumstances.[107] Failure to capture in a pacemaker-dependent patient has obviously deleterious consequences, and it is imperative that the device be programmed with an adequate safety margin, typically two times the measured

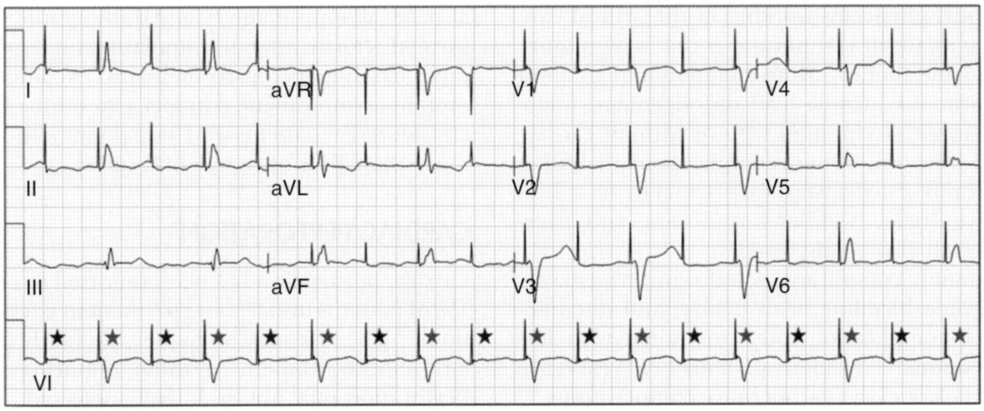

Figure 5.13 A 12-lead electrocardiogram demonstrating both capture (*red stars*) and failure to capture (*black stars*). Failure to capture can be easily recognized by the presence of pacing artifact without a subsequent QRS complex or T wave.

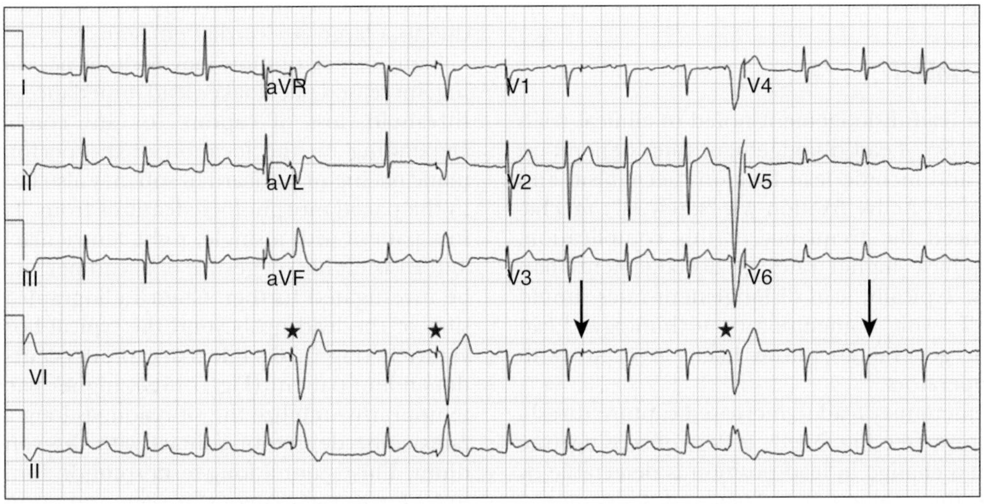

Figure 5.14 A 12-lead electrocardiogram demonstrating failure to sense. There is indiscriminate delivery of pacing artifact, independent of the underlying heart rate and rhythm (*black stars*). Pacing intermittently fails to capture when falling within the refractory period of the ventricular myocardium (*black arrows*).

threshold. Failure to capture can be easily recognized on the 12-lead electrocardiogram or telemetry monitor by the presence of pacing artifact without a subsequent QRS complex or T wave (Fig. 5.13). Failure to sense can be easily recognized by the indiscriminate delivery of pacing artifact, regardless of the underlying rhythm (Fig. 5.14).

INFECTION

Prevention of catheter-based infections is always important, but even more so in a patient who may ultimately require a permanent device. If a temporary pacemaker has been placed in emergent conditions, empiric coverage with a first- or second-generation cephalosporin is reasonable to minimize the likelihood of infection, particularly if femoral access has been chosen.

TIMING OF REIMPLANTATION

The timing depends on a number of factors, including (1) the stability of the temporary pacing system; (2) the pacing indication; and (3) ongoing contraindications to permanent implantation. In some circumstances—for example, in the setting of fungemia or endocarditis—a prolonged period of transvenous pacing is required. Permanent, "active fixation" pacing leads with retractable screws can be inserted through a peel-away venous sheath, and then attached to a permanent pulse generator on the patient's skin. In patients with recurrent ventricular tachyarrhythmias, a permanent defibrillator lead can be attached to an externalized defibrillator in the same fashion.[108] Permanent leads are more maneuverable than temporary leads, and the use of preformed stylets can facilitate delivery of the lead into the right atrium, if atrial pacing is desired. If AV synchrony is desired and SN function is normal, a VDD lead with atrial sensing and ventricular pacing capability can be placed.[109] In day-to-day clinical practice, dual-chamber and biventricular pacing with temporary pacing catheters is rarely, if ever, performed.

COMPLICATIONS OF PERMANENT PACEMAKER IMPLANTATION

Although pacemaker implantation is a well-established procedure with a low risk of major complications in experienced hands, physicians working in the critical care setting should be aware of complications that may require rapid recognition and therapy. More common implantation and lead complications include lead dislodgement, pneumothorax, hematoma, perforation with or without cardiac tamponade, and infection. Other complications including arrhythmias, thrombosis, inadvertent placement of a lead within the left ventricle, twiddler's syndrome, and pacemaker syndrome will also be discussed.

The most common complications following pacemaker implantation include bleeding, lead failure, and pneumothorax.[110] Higher complication rates are noted with less experienced operators.[110,111] Elderly patients (≥75 years) are also at increased risk of early postoperative complications.[112] Body mass index, congestive heart failure, use of anticoagulants, and passive atrial fixation leads are also independent predictors for development of short-term (within 2 months) pacemaker complications.[113]

LEAD DISLODGEMENT

The incidence of lead dislodgement noted in clinical trials is 1.8% to 2.6%.[4,114,115] Lead dislodgement rates depend on multiple factors and include lead fixation mechanism and operator experience. Active fixation (or "screw in") mechanisms have reduced the frequency of this complication. Atrial leads may have higher rates of dislodgement than ventricular leads. Typically, lead dislodgement rates should be less than 3% with contemporary technology. Lead complications in general are more likely to occur with inexperienced operators.[111]

Lead dislodgement may lead to increased capture thresholds, loss of capture (see Fig. 5.13), or loss of sensing (see Fig. 5.14). When a change in lead position is detectable by chest radiograph, this is referred to as "macro-dislodgement." However, loss of capture or undersensing can also be seen with "micro-dislodgement" of leads, where there is no detectable change in lead position on chest radiograph. In some cases of micro-dislodgement, intermittent undersensing of intrinsic complexes or a change in pacing threshold may be corrected by reprogramming the pacemaker sensitivity or output. However, large changes in lead position typically require lead revision. Intermittent motion of the cardiac lead may also result in increased ventricular ectopy, with a premature ventricular contraction morphologic pattern that is similar to the morphologic pattern of the paced complex.

PNEUMOTHORAX

Venous access may be obtained through subclavian or axillary puncture, as well as cephalic vein cut-down. Complications related to venous entry include bleeding, arterial injury due to inadvertent arterial puncture, pneumothorax, hemothorax, thrombosis, air embolism, arteriovenous fistula, and brachial plexus injury. The risk of pneumothorax related to subclavian venous puncture is 1% to 2%;[4,114] this risk may be reduced with contrast venography.

Pneumothorax typically presents early after the procedure, usually within 24 hours. Symptoms include chest pain, shortness of breath, or respiratory distress, which may be associated with hypotension or hypoxemia. Patients may also be asymptomatic. Chest radiography is typically performed shortly after the implantation procedure to document baseline lead placement and exclude pneumothorax, even in asymptomatic patients. Chest tube insertion may be considered in patients who have pneumothorax that involves more than 10% of the pleural space.

CARDIAC PERFORATION

Cardiac perforation has been reported to occur in less than 1% of patients undergoing permanent pacemaker implantation.[114] The risk may be higher in elderly patients, particularly elderly women, or those requiring anticoagulation. Perforation may not be initially detected, as some patients are asymptomatic. Alternatively, patients may report chest pain or shortness of breath. Lightheadedness or syncope may also occur, and can be associated with hemodynamic compromise in patients who develop cardiac tamponade due to a large pericardial effusion.

Signs of perforation may include pacemaker undersensing, increased pacemaker lead impedance, increased pacing threshold, loss of capture, or any combination thereof. Depending on the location of the perforation, diaphragmatic pacing or pericardial rub may also be noted. A change in the paced morphologic features from "LBBB" to "RBBB" in a patient with a single, right ventricular lead (Fig. 5.15A and B) is highly suggestive of a lead perforation and should be investigated further. Chest radiograph may show extension of the lead tip beyond the typical border of the right ventricle (Fig. 5.16). If loss of capture occurs in a pacemaker-dependent patient (Fig. 5.15C), higher pacing outputs may temporarily stabilize the situation, as long as the lead maintains some degree of contact with the ventricular myocardium. This is not a long-term solution but may obviate the need for transcutaneous or temporary transvenous pacing.

BLEEDING AND HEMATOMA

Hematoma is a common complication of pacemaker implantation, with increased risk in patients on anticoagulation. Although not life-threatening, a large hematoma can be quite painful, result in significant blood loss, and increase the risk of infection.[116] In most cases, hematomas can be managed conservatively with observation and analgesia alone. Placing a pressure dressing over the site, immobilizing the ipsilateral arm in a sling, and temporarily withholding anticoagulation are often effective. However, in some cases, hematomas may become large and very painful, with oozing or drainage from the site (Fig. 5.17). When concomitant infection cannot be excluded, open wound exploration in a sterile setting should be considered. Needle aspiration of the hematoma should *never* be attempted at the bedside as this increases the risk of infection.

Precautions should be taken to reduce the risk of bleeding pre- and postoperatively. As with any surgical procedure, the risk of bleeding associated with device implantation must be weighed against the risk of interruption of anticoagulation. Official guidelines recommend "bridging" anticoagulation with heparin products in patients with mechanical valves, atrial fibrillation, and venous thromboembolic disease at "high" risk for thromboembolism.[117] Nevertheless, there is a growing body of evidence in the

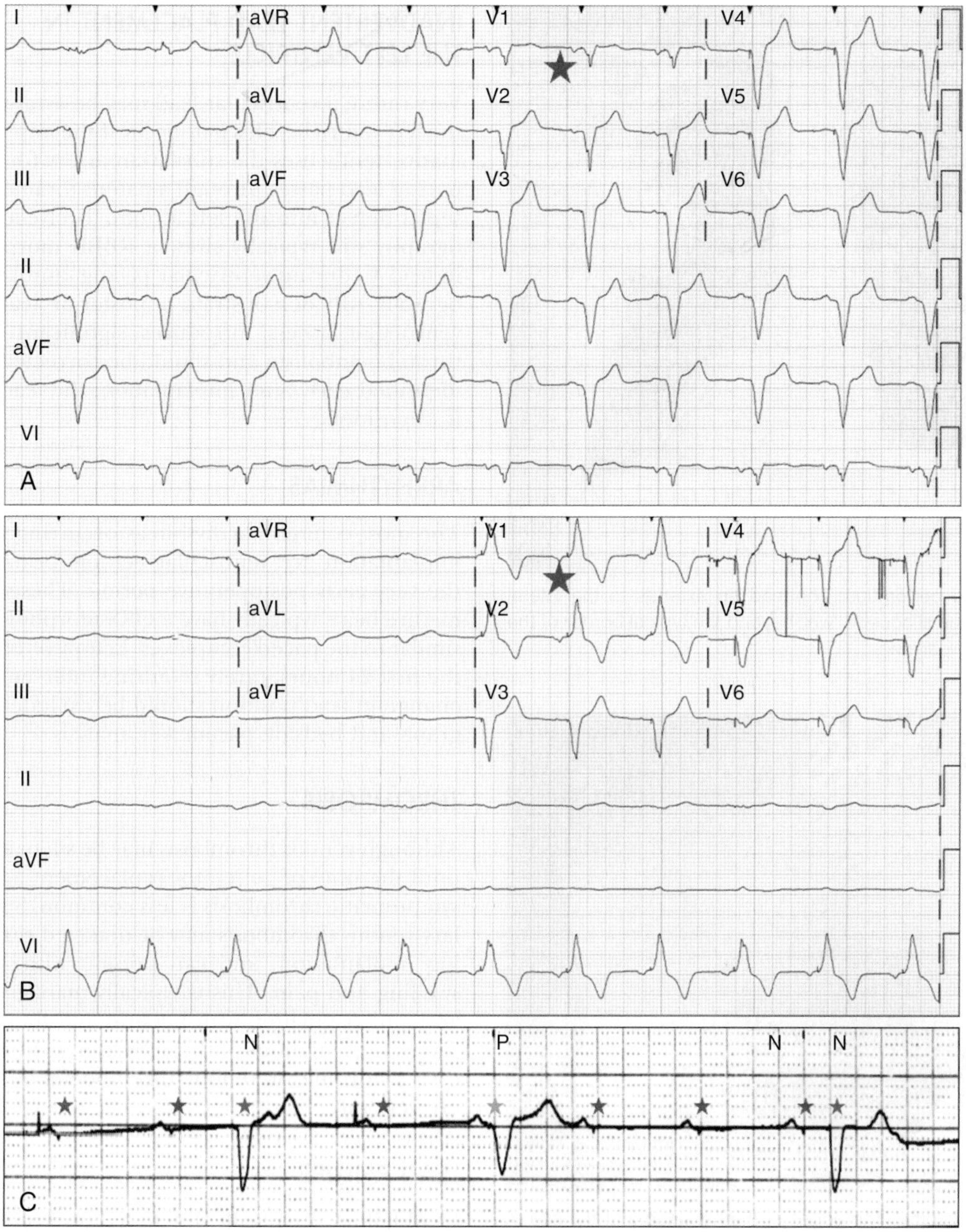

Figure 5.15 Lead perforation. **A,** A 12-lead electrocardiogram demonstrating sinus rhythm with synchronous ventricular pacing in a patient who had just undergone dual-chamber pacemaker placement. The paced morphologic pattern demonstrates a "left bundle branch block" appearance in lead V_1 (*red star*) with a leftward axis, consistent with normal lead position. **B,** A 12-lead electrocardiogram in the same patient demonstrating a "right bundle branch block" morphologic pattern in lead V_1 (*red star*) with a rightward axis, suggestive of lead perforation through the interventricular septum. **C,** Telemetry strip showing intermittent loss of ventricular capture shortly thereafter, due to progressive migration of the lead tip. There are sinus P waves with ventricular capture (*green stars*) and failure to capture (*red stars*) with pauses truncated by ventricular escape complexes (*blue stars*). The patient required emergent lead revision.

electrophysiology literature that continuation of warfarin may be safer than "bridging" with unfractionated and low–molecular-weight heparin.[118-120] There is no physician consensus about the optimal management of anticoagulation in this setting, but many physicians will implant pacemakers and defibrillators in fully anticoagulated patients.[121] A patient with a compelling indication for anticoagulation may be better served by early initiation of warfarin, rather than a prolonged interruption of anticoagulation in the perioperative period. That being said, most operators will not implant if the international normalized ratio is in excess of 3.0. In addition, most physicians will not implant devices while patients are actively taking dabigatran (Pradaxa), rivaroxaban (Xarelto) or apixaban (Eliquis); this may change with accumulated experience, but these agents should be withheld for five half-lives (roughly 48 hours) to minimize the risk of bleeding. Because there is significant variability in practice patterns, communication with the implanting physician about anticoagulation management is strongly recommended.

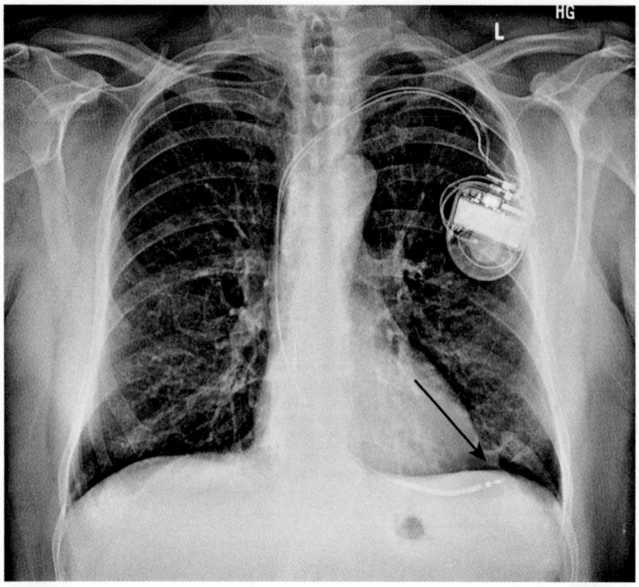

Figure 5.16 Lead perforation. The lead tip extends to the lateral border of the cardiac silhouette, well beyond the typical border of the right ventricle (*black arrow*).

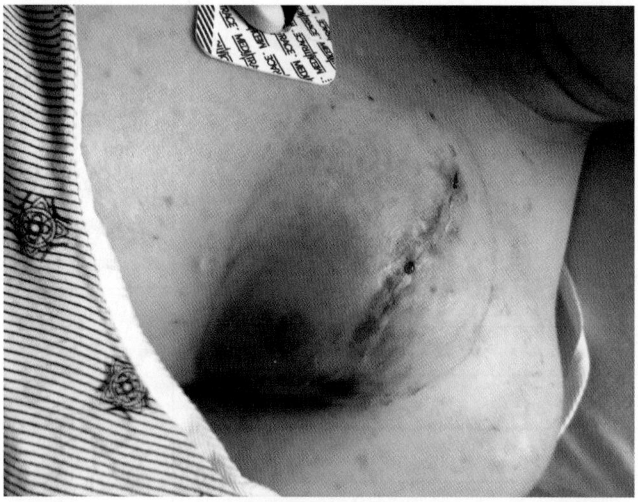

Figure 5.17 Hematoma. The edges of the hematoma at the site of pacemaker implantation are marked to follow the size and exclude continued expansion. A more erythematous area is noted on the medial lower edge of the hematoma. This may require drainage when large, tense, and painful, particularly if there is a need for early anticoagulation or if infection cannot be excluded.

Patients who have undergone device implant should not receive unfractionated or low-molecular-weight heparin for *at least* 6 hours after completion of the procedure, and low-molecular-weight heparin should be avoided in patients with significant renal insufficiency.[122] Dual antiplatelet therapy also increases the risk of pocket hematoma,[123,124] but these agents are not commonly held.

Thrombocytopenia and anemia are relative contraindications to device implantation, but a platelet count less than 50,000/μL and hemoglobin less than 7.0 g/dL are absolute contraindications for many implanters. Hematologic evaluation is recommended and transfusions may be necessary when pacemaker therapy is urgently required.

INADVERTENT LEAD PLACEMENT IN THE LEFT VENTRICLE

Very rarely, a ventricular lead may be errantly placed within the left ventricle. This may occur if the implanting physician inadvertently uses the subclavian artery for access, or if the pacing lead passes through a patent foramen ovale or atrial septal defect into the left atrium. Twelve-lead electrocardiography will typically show a RBBB morphologic pattern in lead V_1 during ventricular pacing, and lateral chest radiography will demonstrate a posterior lead position. Left ventricular access introduces significant risk of arterial thromboembolism and should be corrected immediately. If identified early after implantation, the lead should be easy to reposition.

ARRHYTHMIAS

The most common arrhythmias occurring after pacemaker implantation are ventricular ectopic beats, particularly in the very early postoperative period. These ventricular premature beats typically have a QRS morphologic appearance similar to the paced complexes. Ectopy often subsides within the first 24 hours, rarely requiring intervention. However, a change in lead position should be excluded by chest radiograph and bedside pacemaker analysis.

THROMBOSIS

Although venous thrombosis may be silent and not detected until the time of generator replacement and lead revision, symptomatic thrombosis is less common. Subclavian or axillary venous thrombosis may be detected early or late following implantation, and can present with upper extremity swelling and pain. This is typically managed with elevation and anticoagulation with heparin and then warfarin. More severe presentations of thrombosis, including superior vena cava syndrome or venous thromboembolic complications, are very rare.

LEAD FAILURE

Lead failure is typically due to fracture or insulation break, and this typically occurs long after initial implantation. Lead damage most often occurs close to the puncture site in the infraclavicular region (Fig. 5.18). Damage to the insulation may also occur at a site beneath the pulse generator due to abrasion, or may be the result of a suture being placed directly on the lead itself, in lieu of a suture sleeve. External trauma may also lead to lead damage and fracture.

Signs of insulation breaks include undersensing and reduced pacing lead impedance. Lead fractures may lead to high pacing lead impedance and loss of capture. Lead revision is indicated for lead fractures or insulation failure. Lead fracture typically requires replacement, but a localized insulation breach can often be repaired using a silicone repair kit.

TWIDDLER'S SYNDROME

Some patients may manipulate the pacemaker pulse generator, leading to dislodgement or fracture of the lead. This is called "twiddler's syndrome." Telemetry or electrocardiographic findings may include loss of capture and loss of sensing. In addition to demonstrating lead dislodgement, the twisted leads within the pacemaker pocket may also be visualized on chest radiograph (Fig. 5.19A). Suturing the pulse generator to the chest wall may help reduce motion of the pulse generator, although patients should always be instructed to avoid manipulation of the pocket. The operative appearance of the leads at the time of pacemaker lead revision is illustrated in Figure 5.19B.

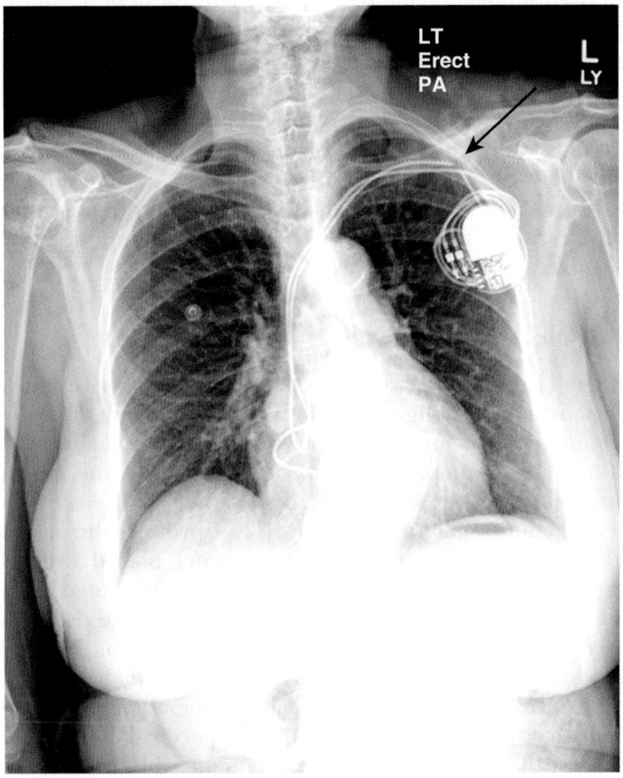

Figure 5.18 Lead fracture. Chest radiograph demonstrating unequivocal fracture of an atrial pacing lead (*black arrow*).

PACEMAKER SYNDROME

"Pacemaker syndrome" refers to a constellation of symptoms, such as fatigue, chest discomfort, dyspnea, cough, confusion, presyncope, or syncope, which are related to adverse hemodynamic effects resulting from loss of AV synchrony in patients with an implanted pacemaker. A significant drop in blood pressure may occur, and the diagnosis may be elusive in some cases unless specifically considered and confirmed by bedside evaluation. This can be corrected by reprogramming from the "VVI" mode to the "DDD" mode or "AAI" mode (in patients with intact AV conduction) or upgrading to a dual-chamber pacemaker, if a single-chamber ventricular device was implanted in a patient with sinus rhythm.

INFECTION

Care should be taken to avoid implantation of a permanent pacemaker in a patient with active infection, as this will increase the risk for device infection. Any active infection is a relative contraindication to permanent pacemaker implantation, although active bacteremia or fungemia are absolute contraindications. A fever or rising leukocytosis within 24 hours of implant should delay device implantation until a thorough investigation can be performed. Temporary pacing is appropriate in this setting, although that, too, has been associated with an increased risk of infection.[125] Patient characteristics also contribute to the risk of infection, and all modifiable risks should be optimized prior to device implantation.

Preoperative antibiotic administration has been shown to reduce the risk of device-related infection.[116] There is no standard regimen, but most administer a penicillin or first- or second-generation cephalosporin for coverage of staphylococcus.[126] Patients with a history of methicillin-resistant *Staphylococcus aureus* (MRSA) colonization or infection, recurrent or prolonged hospitalizations, or either a penicillin or cephalosporin allergy should be given vancomycin.

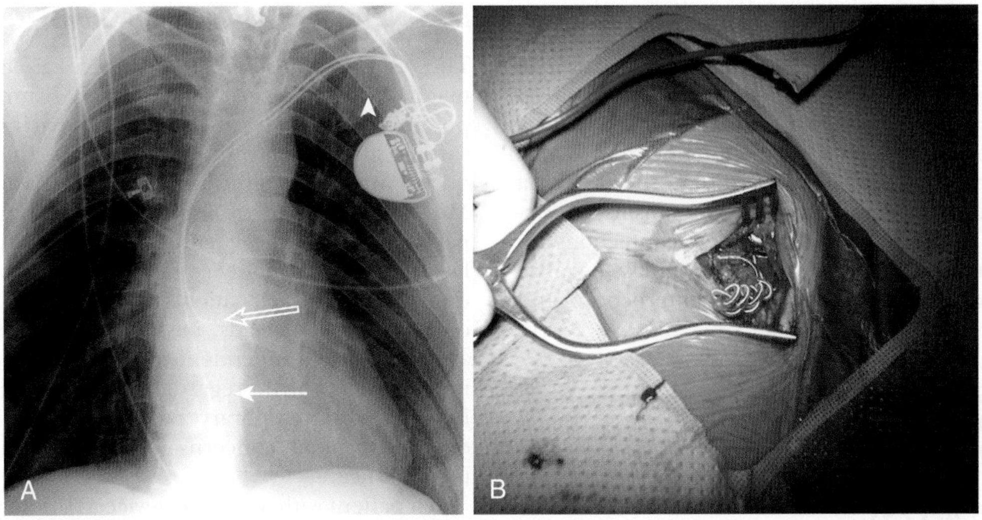

Figure 5.19 Pacemaker lead dislodgement due to twiddler's syndrome. **A,** Chest radiograph illustrating dislodgement of the atrial (*open arrow*) and ventricular leads (*solid arrow*) as well as significant lead entanglement in the vicinity of the pulse generator (*arrowhead*) in a patient with "twiddler's syndrome." **B,** Photograph taken at the time of lead revision, demonstrating significant entanglement of the leads.

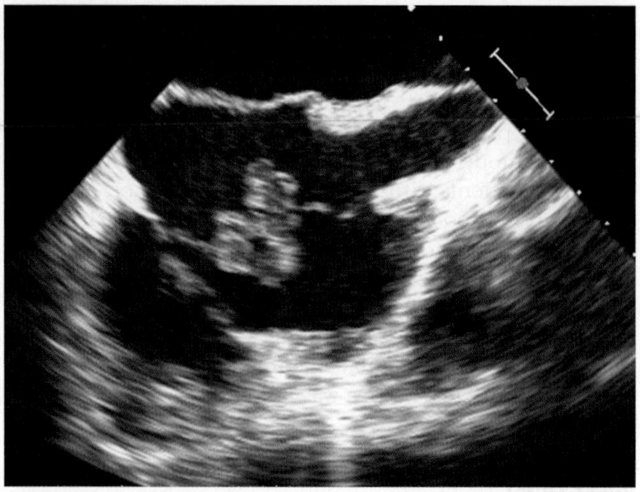

Figure 5.20 Endocarditis. The echocardiographic appearance of a large vegetation attached to an atrial lead.

Patients with a history of vancomycin-resistant enterococcus (VRE) should be given either linezolid or daptomycin. There are limited data on the efficacy of postoperative antibiotic administration, but most implanting physicians empirically continue antibiotics for 24 hours after the procedure.

Careful attention to surgical technique and sterile procedures are important in preventing infection of the implanted pacemaker system. Pacemaker infection may be superficial or deep, with an incidence of less than 2% following initial implantation procedures, although it may be higher following generator replacement or lead revisions.[4,127-129] Infections vary in severity from a superficial infection at the suture site with a local stitch abscess to a pocket infection or systemic infection with bacteremia. Erosion of the pacemaker pulse generator or leads may also be associated with infection.

Superficial skin infections or stitch abscesses may be treated and cured with antibiotic therapy. However, lead-associated endocarditis is a more serious complication and is associated with a high mortality rate. Systemic infections with bacteremia and endocarditis require device and lead extraction. Vegetations may develop on the pacemaker lead itself and become large, requiring extraction and removal of the pacing system for cure (Fig. 5.20). Infections may occur many months after device implantation, and hematogenous spread of organisms from a distant site may be a contributing factor. The most common organisms responsible for cardiac implantable electronic device infections are *S. aureus* (often methicillin-resistant) and coagulase-negative staphylococci followed by streptococci, enterococci, and gram-negative rods.[130,131]

SPECIAL CONSIDERATIONS IN PERMANENT PACING

INTRAVENOUS ACCESS

The vast majority of permanent device implants utilize the cephalic, axillary, or subclavian vein. Implants using the internal jugular and femoral vein are exceedingly rare. Devices are generally implanted on the nondominant side for reasons of patient convenience, but implants are usually less technically challenging on the left side. Devices should not be placed ipsilateral to the site of an arteriovenous fistula or graft, due to the short-term risk of vein thrombosis and long-term risk of vein stenosis.

If at all possible, subclavian access should be preserved in the critical care patient who may require permanent device implantation. If temporary venous access is required, the internal jugular or femoral vein should be used whenever possible. Peripherally inserted central catheter lines should not be placed ipsilateral to the side of the future permanent implant because of risk for venous thrombosis. Peripheral venography is not mandatory but can be helpful in very thin patients with a higher risk of pneumothorax and patients with signs of venous occlusion. It is therefore preferable to have an 18- or 20-gauge peripheral IV catheter in the upper extremity on the site of the planned implant, if at all possible.

MAGNET APPLICATION

Magnet application over a permanent pacemaker results in asynchronous pacing, such that pacing stimuli are delivered *regardless* of the underlying rhythm.[132] Prolonged periods of asynchronous pacing should be avoided in the critical care setting, when concomitant metabolic and electrolyte derangement may increase the risk of proarrhythmia with "R on T" pacing. In contrast, a magnet placed over an implantable cardioverter-defibrillator suspends detection of ventricular arrhythmias, but it does *not* cause the device to pace asynchronously. In the critical care setting, magnet application over a permanent pacemaker can be used to confirm capture, evaluate the morphologic appearance of the paced complex, and terminate pacemaker-mediated tachycardia. In the defibrillator patient who experiences inappropriate shocks for rapidly conducted atrial fibrillation, lead fracture, or oversensing of physiologic signals, magnet application may be lifesaving.

MAGNETIC RESONANCE IMAGING

The vast majority of implanted devices are not approved for magnetic resonance imaging (MRI) scanning due to the potential for lead heating, changes in pacing threshold, and cardiac stimulation with proarrhythmia. Current guidelines do not impose absolute contraindications against the use of MRI, but they do strongly recommend against its use in pacemaker-dependent patients and in patients with defibrillators, except in highly compelling circumstances.[133] Based on expert opinion, patients with new implants (<6 weeks old), abandoned leads, passive leads, or epicardial leads, and pacemaker-dependent patients with defibrillators are ineligible for MRI, regardless of the clinical indication. Patients with temporary pacemakers are also ineligible, owing to similar concerns for lead heating and external interference.

If a patient with a cardiac device absolutely needs an MRI, close coordination with the electrophysiologist and radiologist is mandatory to minimize risk. The device should be programmed in an asynchronous mode with rate responsiveness and other special pacing features deactivated to minimize the likelihood of unwarranted pacing. Cardiac resuscitation equipment should be immediately available, and device interrogation should be repeated immediately after the scan.[134] Since 2011, an "MRI-compatible" pacemaker has been available for commercial use in the United States (Advisa, MRI SureScan, Medtronic, Minneapolis, MN). In selected patients with no alternative, lead and pulse generator extraction may be an option.[135]

CONCLUSIONS

Multiple clinical trials have demonstrated the benefit of pacing therapy for the treatment of SND and AV conduction disturbances, as well as a variety of other conditions. Temporary pacing is particularly useful in the critical care setting and can be performed using a variety of techniques, including transcutaneous, transvenous, or epicardial approaches. Both temporary and permanent pacing can be associated with risks, but precautions can be taken to minimize risk whenever possible. Pacing may relieve symptoms, improve quality of life, or provide lifesaving therapy.

Many patients in the intensive care unit may develop bradyarrhythmias or have previously implanted permanent pacemakers already in place. Therefore, it is essential that critical care physicians are adept at arrhythmia recognition, recognize techniques for temporary pacing, and develop skills related to basic device troubleshooting to provide optimal care to patients in the intensive care setting.

KEY POINTS

- Bradyarrhythmias may be caused by either intrinsic dysfunction of the SN or AV conduction system, or may be due to a response of normal tissues to extrinsic factors.
- Temporary pacing is typically reserved for transient or reversible bradyarrhythmias, or when there is an ongoing contraindication to the implantation of a permanent device.
- Transcutaneous pacing is most appropriate in situations in which pacing is required only briefly or intermittently, or as a bridging measure for placement of a transvenous system.
- Complete heart block with a "junctional" escape rhythm does not typically require temporary pacing, unless accompanied by hypotension.
- Complete heart block with a "ventricular" escape rhythm usually requires temporary pacing, even if hemodynamically stable.
- There should be a very low threshold for temporary pacing in a patient with advanced second-degree AV block and history of syncope.
- Temporary pacing should be avoided in severely hypothermic patients due to the potential risk of catheter-induced ventricular fibrillation.

KEY POINTS (Continued)

- If there is an anticipated need for permanent pacing, the subclavian vein should be preserved for device placement.
- Heparin products, direct thrombin inhibitors, and factor Xa inhibitors should be withheld for at least 24 hours after pacemaker or defibrillator placement to minimize the risk of bleeding.
- It is imperative that the critical care physician recognize the electrocardiographic and radiographic signs of lead dislodgement and perforation.

SELECTED REFERENCES

1. Epstein AE, DiMarco JP, Ellenbogen KA, et al: American College of Cardiology/American Heart Association Task Force on Practice Guidelines (Writing Committee to Revise the ACC/AHA/NASPE 2002 Guideline Update for Implantation of Cardiac Pacemakers and Antiarrhythmia Devices); American Association for Thoracic Surgery; Society of Thoracic Surgeons. ACC/AHA/HRS 2008 Guidelines for Device-Based Therapy of Cardiac Rhythm Abnormalities: A report of the American College of Cardiology/American Heart Association Task Force on Practice Guidelines. Circulation 2008;117:e350-408.

12. Lee S, Wellens HJJ, Josephson ME: Paroxysmal atrioventricular block. Heart Rhythm 2009;6:1229-1234.

33. Wormser GP, Dattwyler RJ, Shapiro ED, et al: The clinical assessment, treatment, and prevention of Lyme disease, human granulocytic anaplasmosis, and babesiosis: Clinical practice guidelines by the Infectious Diseases Society of America. Clin Infect Dis 2006;43:1089-1134.

40. Bonow RO, Carabello BA, Chatterjee K, et al: ACC/AHA 2006 guidelines for the management of patients with valvular heart disease. Circulation 2006;114:e84-e231.

42. Antman EM, Anbe DT, Armstrong PW, et al: ACC/AHA guidelines for the management of patients with ST-elevation myocardial infarction—Executive summary: A report of the American College of Cardiology/American Heart Association task force on practice guidelines (writing committee to revise the 1999 guidelines for the management of patients with acute myocardial infarction). Circulation 2004;110:588-636.

45. Zimetbaum PJ, Josephson ME: Use of the electrocardiogram in acute myocardial infarction. N Engl J Med 2003;348:933-940.

93. Echahidi N, Pibarot P, O'Hara G, et al: Mechanisms, prevention, and treatment of atrial fibrillation after cardiac surgery. J Am Coll Cardiol 2008;51:793-801.

117. Douketis JD, Spyropoulos AC, Spencer FA, et al: Perioperative management of antithrombotic therapy: Antithrombotic therapy and prevention of thrombosis. Chest 2012;141:326S-350S.

118. Ahmed I, Gertner E, Nelson WB, et al: Continuing warfarin therapy is superior to interrupting warfarin with or without bridging anticoagulation therapy in patients undergoing pacemaker and defibrillator implantation. Heart Rhythm 2010;7:745-749.

133. Levine GN, Gomes AS, Arai AE, et al: Safety of magnetic resonance imaging in patients with cardiovascular devices: An American Heart Association scientific statement from the Committee on Diagnostic and Interventional Cardiac Catheterization, Council on Clinical Cardiology, and the Council on Cardiovascular Radiology and Intervention: Endorsed by the American College of Cardiology Foundation, the North American Society for Cardiac Imaging, and the Society for Cardiovascular Magnetic Resonance. Circulation 2007;116:2878-2891.

The complete list of references can be found at www.expertconsult.com.

6 Pericardial Tamponade: Clinical Presentation, Diagnosis, and Catheter-Based Therapies

Hani Jneid | Andrew O. Maree | Igor F. Palacios

CHAPTER OUTLINE

Pericardial diseases have variable clinical presentations, including acute pericarditis, asymptomatic pericardial effusion, and pericardial tamponade. Although pericarditis is often a self-limiting disorder responsive to nonsteroidal anti-inflammatory drugs or steroid therapy, pericardial tamponade is a life-threatening condition and requires immediate therapy. Echocardiography and cardiac catheterization are important diagnostic tools and help in guiding therapies. Percutaneous catheter-based therapies, including pericardiocentesis and percutaneous balloon pericardiotomy, are safe and effective therapeutic modalities. Percutaneous balloon pericardiotomy is a relatively novel catheter-based technique that is gradually replacing the more invasive surgical pericardial window procedures. Pericardiectomy remains the definitive therapy for certain conditions, such as constrictive pericardial disease.

ETIOLOGY OF PERICARDIAL EFFUSION AND TAMPONADE

Pericarditis or pericardial effusion or both may result from an infectious, metabolic, inflammatory, autoimmune, or neoplastic process (Box 6.1).[1-3] The frequency of specific causes depends on the geographic location, time period, and characteristics of the populations studied. In one European series of patients presenting with moderate and severe pericardial effusions, acute idiopathic pericarditis and iatrogenic causes accounted for most cases.[1] In a smaller series in the United States comprising patients presenting to a tertiary medical center with large pericardial effusions, malignancy was the most common cause.[4] Pericardial effusions occurring after radiation therapy, myocardial infarction, and surgical and interventional cardiac procedures are increasing in incidence. Uremia and hypothyroidism remain important causes but are seen less frequently given the prompt diagnosis and treatment of these disorders.

Pericardial fluid can be either a transudate or an exudate. Although transudative effusions typically occur in patients with congestive heart failure, exudative effusions may occur with most types of pericarditis and are characterized by a high concentration of proteins and fibrin. Pericardial effusions may be serous (or serosanguineous), suppurative, or hemorrhagic. Although the presence of suppurative effusion is pathognomonic for an acute infectious cause, usually bacterial, hemorrhagic pericardial effusion is commonly related to chronic infections, with tuberculosis a classic example, particularly in developing countries. In developed countries, hemorrhagic pericardial effusions are likely to be iatrogenic or malignant in origin. In a retrospective analysis of 150 patients in the United States who underwent pericardiocentesis for relieving cardiac tamponade, 64% of patients

Box 6.1 Etiology of Pericardial Effusion and Tamponade

- Idiopathic
- Infectious
  - Viral
  - Bacterial
  - Fungal
  - Others
- Metabolic
  - Uremia
  - Myxedema
- Collagen and other autoimmune disorders
  - Systemic lupus erythematosus
  - Rheumatoid arthritis
  - Rheumatic fever
  - Dressler's syndrome
  - Others
- Neoplastic
  - Primary
  - Pericardial metastasis
  - Local invasion
- Volume overload
  - Chronic heart failure
- Miscellaneous
  - Chest wall irradiation
  - Cardiotomy or thoracic surgery
  - Adverse drug reaction
  - Aortic dissection
  - Following myocardial infarction
  - Traumatic

had a hemorrhagic pericardial effusion (with iatrogenic causes and malignancy accounting for most cases).[5]

CLINICAL PRESENTATION

The clinical presentation of patients with pericardial effusion varies. Some patients are completely asymptomatic, whereas others develop pericardial tamponade and cardiovascular collapse.

The normal pericardium is a fibroelastic sac composed of visceral and parietal layers separated by the pericardial cavity and containing a thin layer (20 to 50 mL) of straw-colored fluid surrounding the heart.[3] The normal pericardium has a steep pressure-volume curve: It is distensible when the intrapericardial volume is small, but becomes gradually inextensible when the volume increases. In the presence of pericardial effusion, the intrapericardial pressure depends on the relationship between the absolute volume of the effusion, the speed of fluid accumulation, and pericardial elasticity. Although the rapid accumulation of small amounts of fluid (150 to 200 mL) can result in cardiac tamponade, the slow accumulation of larger effusions (>1 L, as in uremic pericardial effusions) is usually well tolerated.[6,7] The clinical presentation is not only related to the size of the effusion, but also, and more importantly, to the rapidity of fluid accumulation.

Pericardial tamponade is a clinical syndrome with defined hemodynamic and echocardiographic abnormalities, which result from the accumulation of intrapericardial fluid and impairment of ventricular diastolic filling.[7,8] The ultimate mechanism of hemodynamic compromise is the compression of cardiac chambers secondary to increased intrapericardial pressure.[8] Pericardial tamponade is usually a clinical diagnosis, with patients showing elevated systemic venous pressure, tachycardia, dyspnea, arterial pulsus paradoxus, muffled heart sounds, and evidence of electrical alternans on electrocardiogram (ECG).[3] Pulsus paradoxus, which describes the exaggerated inspiratory decline in arterial blood pressure (>10 mm Hg), is largely attributed to interventricular dependence within the confined pericardial space. Although its diagnostic utility was recognized many decades earlier,[9] various conditions may lead to its absence in patients with cardiac tamponade (e.g., in patients with concomitant aortic regurgitation, atrial septal defects, severe left ventricular dysfunction, aortic regurgitation, severe hypotension, pericardial adhesions, pulmonary artery obstruction, or positive-pressure ventilation).[8]

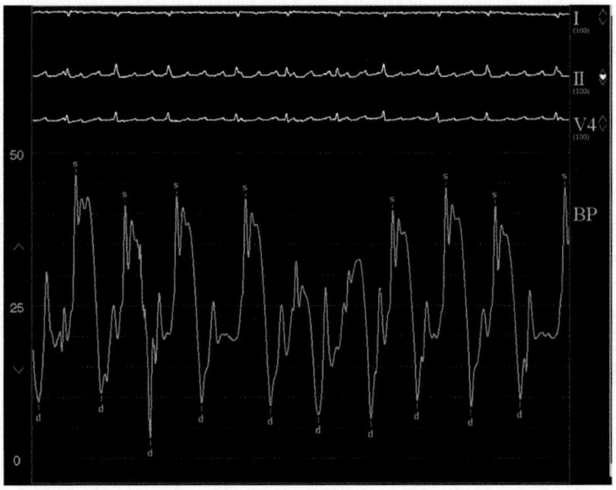

Figure 6.1 The patient is a 61-year-old woman with recent tricuspid valve repair presenting with increased dyspnea, orthopnea, and presyncope. She was hypotensive and had distended jugular veins and distant heart sounds on physical examination. The hemodynamic trace depicts elevated right ventricular pressure with exaggerated respiratory variation consistent with pericardial tamponade.

The ECG shows sinus tachycardia and low voltage. Electrical alternans, which describes the beat-to-beat alterations in the QRS complex reflecting cardiac swinging in the pericardial fluid, is a relatively specific sign for tamponade and is rarely seen with very large pericardial effusions alone.[10] Patients with pericardial effusions have an enlarged cardiac silhouette with clear lung fields on chest radiograph. The pericardial effusion has to reach 200 mL in volume to appear on the chest radiograph, and this volume occurs usually in slowly accumulating pericardial effusions (which are less likely to cause tamponade).[11] Rapidly accumulating small pericardial effusions may cause tamponade and have a normal chest radiograph.

The diagnosis of pericardial tamponade is best confirmed by a two-dimensional echocardiogram that shows a pericardial effusion, right atrial compression, and abnormal respiratory variations in the right and left ventricular dimensions and in the tricuspid and mitral valve flow velocities (Fig. 6.1).[12] The classic hemodynamic findings of pericardial tamponade include arterial pulsus paradoxus, elevation and diastolic equalization of right and left ventricular diastolic pressures with pericardial pressure, and depression of cardiac output.[8] Because patients with critical tamponade operate on the steep portion of the pericardial pressure-volume curve, drainage of even a small pericardial volume causes a dramatic reduction in intrapericardial pressure and rapid clinical and hemodynamic improvement (by shifting the stretched pericardium back to the flat portion of the pericardium pressure-volume curve).[8]

DIAGNOSTIC ROLE OF ECHOCARDIOGRAPHY

Echocardiography is recognized as a particularly useful imaging modality for pericardial disease.[13,14] Currently, two-dimensional echocardiography has become the gold standard diagnostic modality because it provides a highly sensitive and specific noninvasive imaging technique for pericardial disease.[12,15] It is also an important tool for the longitudinal follow-up of pericardial effusions over time (given a class IIa recommendation in the American Heart Association/American College of Cardiology guidelines for the clinical application of echocardiography).[12] Classically, a persistent echo-free space throughout the cardiac cycle between the parietal pericardium and the epicardium is pathognomonic for pericardial effusion by M-mode echocardiography.[13]

Two-dimensional echocardiography allows delineation of the size and distribution of the effusion, including loculated effusions, and helps assess the success of pericardiocentesis. The echocardiogram also can provide a reasonable estimate of the total volume of the effusion.[15] Circumferential effusion greater than 1 cm in width is considered large (>500 mL). Moderate effusions (100 to 500 mL) are usually circumferential but less than 1 cm, whereas small effusions (<100 mL) are usually localized posterior to the left ventricle and measure less than 1 cm. Classification criteria differ significantly among various echocardiographers and institutions. The typical echocardiographic signs of pericardial tamponade are listed in Box 6.2.

The nature of the pericardial fluid is difficult to identify by echocardiography. Increased echogenicity is suspicious, however, for the presence of proteins or cells or both in the pericardial fluid. Fibrin deposits localized in the epicardial surface can be identified as echogenic masses. In one study of 42 patients with tuberculous and viral or idiopathic pericardial effusions, intrapericardial echocardiogram abnormalities, such as a greater degree of pericardial thickening, frequency and thickness of exudative coating or deposits, and strands crossing the pericardial space, were useful criteria in the diagnosis of tuberculous pericardial effusion and in differentiating it from chronic idiopathic pericardial effusion.[16]

The classic echocardiographic signs of cardiac tamponade are right atrial and right ventricular diastolic collapse. The right atrium and right ventricle are compliant structures. As a result, increased intrapericardial pressure leads to their collapse when intracavitary pressures are only slightly exceeded by those in the pericardium. At end diastole (i.e., during atrial relaxation), right atrial volume is minimal, but pericardial pressure is maximal, causing the right atrium to buckle. Right atrial collapse, especially when it persists for more than one third of the cardiac cycle, is a highly sensitive but less specific sign for tamponade. Early diastolic collapse of the right ventricle (usually occurs in early diastole when the ventricular volume is still low) is present when the intrapericardial pressure exceeds the right ventricular pressure and is a highly specific sign for tamponade. Right ventricular collapse may not occur when the right ventricle is hypertrophied, or its diastolic pressure is greatly elevated. Left atrial collapse is seen in nearly 25% of patients and is specific for tamponade. Left ventricular collapse is less common because the wall of the left ventricle is more muscular. Dilation of the inferior vena cava with lack of inspiratory collapse (usually <50% reduction in its diameter) and swinging of the heart also are seen in patients with pericardial tamponade. Doppler echocardiography provides direct assessment of the ventricular filling patterns in pericardial tamponade.[11,12,17,18] Patients with pericardial tamponade have a marked increase in tricuspid and pulmonary valve flow velocities and a marked decrease in mitral and aortic valve flow velocities during inspiration compared with normal subjects and patients with effusions but not tamponade. Changes in left atrial inflow pattern and exaggerated respiratory variations in pulmonary venous flow velocity also are observed. In one study aiming to correlate clinical and echocardiographic findings prospectively, the highest specificity (98%) was seen in patients with right atrial and right ventricular collapse plus abnormal venous flow.[19] The sensitivity and specificity of any chamber collapse were 90% and 65%.[19]

In addition to echocardiography, computed tomography and magnetic resonance imaging are useful techniques in the evaluation of patients with pericardial disease. Their high resolution is useful in the assessment of pericardial thickness (particularly important in constrictive-effusive pericarditis) and in the detection of pericardial effusion, masses, and cysts.

Box 6.2 Echocardiographic Findings of Pericardial Tamponade

1. Abnormal inspiratory increase of right ventricular dimensions and abnormal inspiratory decrease of left ventricular dimensions
2. Right atrium collapse (>30% of cardiac cycle)
3. Right ventricular early diastolic collapse
4. Abnormal inspiratory increase in blood flow velocity through tricuspid and pulmonary valves and abnormal inspiratory decrease of mitral and aortic valve flow velocity
5. Respiratory variations of pulmonary and hepatic venous flow
6. Dilated inferior vena cava with lack of inspiratory collapse
7. Swinging heart

CATHETER-BASED DIAGNOSTIC AND THERAPEUTIC STRATEGIES

Cardiac catheterization historically has been the standard diagnostic modality for cardiac tamponade. Right-sided

Box 6.3 Cardiac Catheterization Findings of Cardiac Tamponade

1. Elevated filling pressures
2. Diastolic equalization of pressures
3. Absence or blunted y descent in the right atrium pressure tracing
4. Absence or blunted early diastolic dip in the right ventricular pressure tracing
5. Arterial pulsus paradoxus

heart catheterization can confirm the significance of a pericardial effusion and allows evaluation of hemodynamic changes occurring after pericardiocentesis. It usually shows two major findings in patients with pericardial tamponade: (1) elevation and equilibration of intracardiac diastolic pressures (usually 10 to 30 mm Hg) and (2) inspiratory increase in right-sided pressures and reduction in left-sided pressures (ventricular disconcordance), which are responsible for the presence of a pulsus paradoxus (Box 6.3).[8] With equalization of intrapericardial pressures, the mean right atrial, left atrial, diastolic pulmonary artery, and right and left ventricular end-diastolic pressures all are within 5 mm Hg of each other. In addition to producing elevation in the central venous pressure, cardiac tamponade produces characteristic changes in the waveforms of the hemodynamic tracings. With increasing severity of cardiac tamponade, the "y descent" and the early diastolic dip in the ventricular pressure tracings are gradually obliterated and eventually disappear. The absence of the y descent in the right atrial tracing is an important finding in pericardial tamponade. As pericardial fluid is removed, the intrapericardial pressure usually returns to the intrapleural pressure level, and the right atrial waveform normalizes with the reappearance of the diastolic y descent. If the right atrial pressure remains elevated after the pericardiocentesis, however, and a prominent y descent appears, the diagnosis of effusive-constrictive disease must be considered.[20] Although the latter condition is infrequent, it may be missed in some patients presenting with tamponade in whom it usually causes significant morbidity until they undergo surgical epicardiectomy. Pulsus paradoxus is another hallmark of pericardial tamponade; however, it may be absent in many conditions, or alternatively may be present in patients without cardiac tamponade, as previously stated.

PERICARDIOCENTESIS

INDICATIONS

Pericardiocentesis is the technique of catheter-based aspiration of pericardial fluid. It is a diagnostic and therapeutic modality in patients with pericarditis with pericardial effusion, pericardial effusion with pericardial tamponade, and effusive-constrictive pericarditis.

When the diagnosis of pericardial effusion has been made, it is important to determine whether the effusion is creating significant hemodynamic compromise. Many asymptomatic patients with large effusions do not require pericardiocentesis if they have no hemodynamic compromise, unless there is a need for fluid analysis for diagnostic purposes. In a prospective long-term follow-up of large idiopathic chronic pericardial effusion (up to 20 years), Sagrista-Sauleda and colleagues[21] concluded that large idiopathic chronic pericardial effusions were usually well tolerated for long periods in most patients with severe tamponade; however, they may develop unexpectedly at any time. Although pericardiocentesis was effective in resolving these effusions, recurrences were common, prompting the authors to recommend referral of these patients for pericardiectomy when recurrence occurs.[21] When cardiac tamponade occurs, the emergency drainage of pericardial fluid by pericardiocentesis is a lifesaving therapy in a patient who would otherwise develop pulseless electrical activity and cardiac arrest.

When performed, pericardiocentesis should achieve several objectives, as follows: (1) relief of tamponade, when present; (2) obtaining fluid for appropriate analyses; and (3) assessment of hemodynamics after pericardial fluid evacuation to exclude effusive-constrictive pericardial effusion. Elective pericardiocentesis is contraindicated in patients receiving anticoagulation and in patients with bleeding disorders or thrombocytopenia (platelet count <50,000/μL). Pericardiocentesis also is ill advised when the presence of pericardial fluid is not confirmed, and when the effusion is very small or loculated. When pericardial tamponade occurs, complicating acute aortic dissection, pericardiocentesis is contraindicated because of the risk of increased dP/dt and further hemorrhage and extension of the dissection. The patient instead should undergo direct aortic repair together with pericardial drainage in the operating room.

TECHNIQUE

Pericardiocentesis is most commonly performed via a subxiphoid approach under ECG and fluoroscopy guidance (Fig. 6.2A). Traditionally, pericardiocentesis has been performed in the cardiac catheterization laboratory with arterial and right-sided heart pressure monitoring. Today the procedure also is performed in the noninvasive laboratory, intensive care units, or even at the bedside under echocardiographic guidance.[22,23] Whichever modality is used, it is a safe procedure when performed by appropriately trained personnel.

Pericardiocentesis is a procedure based on the Seldinger technique of percutaneous catheter insertion. After the administration of local anesthesia (1% to 2% lidocaine) to the skin and deeper tissues of the left xiphocostal area, the pericardial needle is connected to an ECG lead. The needle is advanced from the left of the subxiphoid area while aiming toward the left shoulder (usually under fluoroscopic or echocardiographic guidance; however, blinded procedures are undertaken in cases of extreme emergencies). Often, a discrete pop is felt as the needle enters the pericardial space. ST-segment elevation is seen on the ECG lead tracing when the needle touches the epicardium and helps confirm the needle position (see Fig. 6.2B). The needle should be withdrawn slightly until the ST-segment elevation

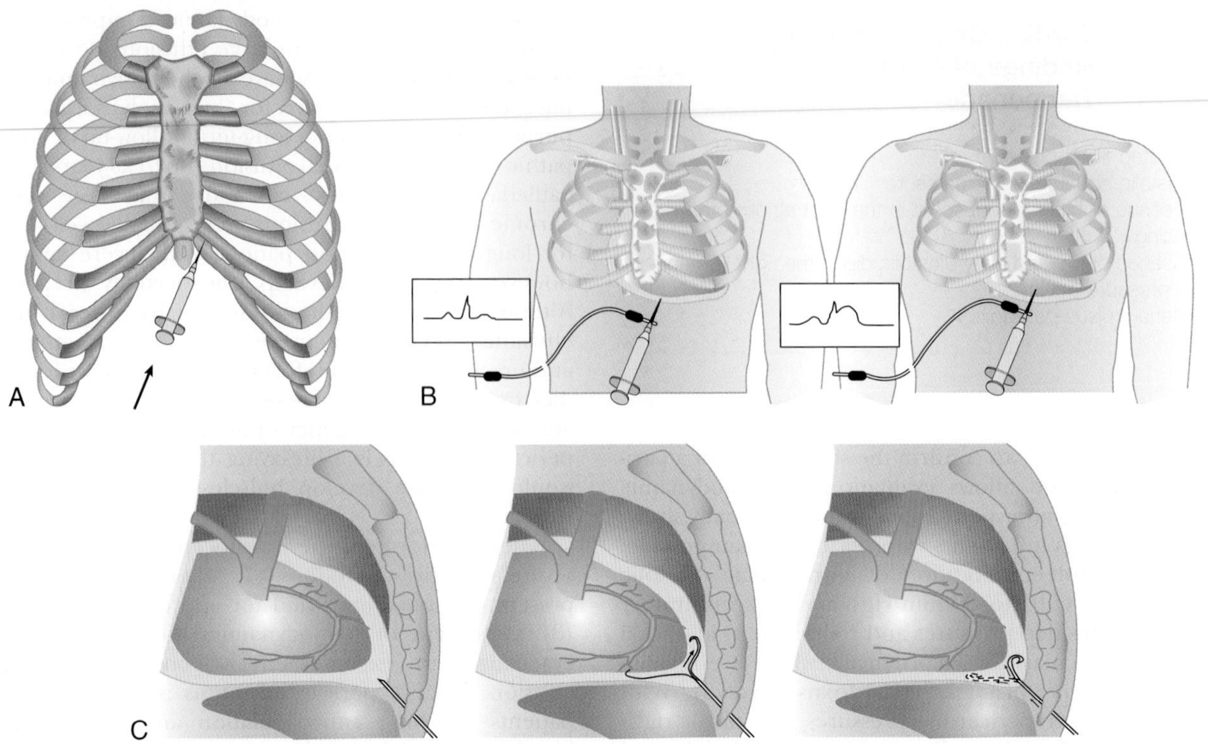

Figure 6.2 **A,** Diagrammatic representation of a pericardiocentesis procedure using the subxiphoid approach. **B,** The pericardial needle is connected to an electrocardiogram (ECG) lead. The needle is advanced from the left of the subxiphoid area aiming toward the left shoulder. ST-segment elevation is seen on the ECG lead tracing when the needle touches the epicardium. The needle should be retracted slightly until the ST-segment elevation disappears. **C,** After the pericardial space is entered with the pericardial needle, a guidewire is introduced in the pericardial space through the needle. The needle is removed, and a catheter is inserted in the pericardial sac over the guidewire (either anteriorly or inferiorly in the pericardial sac).

disappears. When the pericardial space is entered, a stiff guidewire is introduced into the pericardial space through the needle, which is thereafter removed, and a catheter is inserted into the pericardial sac over the guidewire (see Fig. 6.2C). The drainage catheter used (often a pigtail catheter, denoting its shape) has an end hole and multiple side holes. Intrapericardial pressure is measured by connecting a pressure transducer system to the intrapericardial catheter. Pericardial fluid is then removed. Samples of pericardial fluid should be sent for appropriate biochemical, cytologic, bacteriologic, and immunologic analyses to assist in the diagnosis of the cause of the effusion (the first sample is usually reserved for microbiologic studies).

In the presence of pericardial tamponade, aspiration of fluid should be continued until clinical and hemodynamic improvement occurs. The catheter is frequently left in place for continuous drainage and as a route to instill sclerosing or chemotherapeutic agents if needed. The catheter is secured to the skin with sterile sutures and covered with a sterile dressing. The success rate of pericardiocentesis increases and the incidence of complications decreases with the increasing size of the effusion.

COMPLICATIONS

The potential complications of pericardiocentesis include the laceration of the heart or a coronary vessel, sometimes causing fatal consequences. Puncture of the right atrium or the right ventricle with hemopericardial fluid accumulation, arrhythmias, air embolism, pneumothorax, and puncture of the peritoneal cavity or abdominal viscera all have been reported. Acute pulmonary edema may infrequently occur when the pericardial tamponade is decompressed too rapidly.

Other approaches of pericardiocentesis include the right xiphocostal, apical, right-sided, and parasternal approaches. Although these approaches may be useful under certain circumstances, they are associated with greater incidence of complications. The right xiphocostal approach is associated with higher incidence of right atrium and inferior vena cava injury. Puncture of the left pleura and the lingula is more frequent with the apical approach, and puncture of the left anterior descending and the internal mammary artery is more frequent with the parasternal approach.

Echocardiographically guided pericardiocentesis is a safe and effective technique.[23,24] In a series of 1127 therapeutic echocardiographically guided pericardiocenteses performed in 977 patients at the Mayo Clinic between 1979 and 1998, the procedural success rate was 97% overall, with a total complication rate of 4.7%.[24] Echocardiography allows identification of the ideal site of needle entry and trajectory and is especially useful in patients with loculated effusions. In contrast to pericardiocenteses performed in the cardiac catheterization laboratory, the left chest wall, rather than the subcostal, approach is often used with echocardiographically guided pericardiocenteses.

MANAGEMENT AFTER PERICARDIOCENTESIS

Pericardiocentesis does not completely evacuate the effusion in most cases, given particularly that active secretion and bleeding into the pericardial space may continue. It is best to leave the pericardial catheter in place for 24 to 72 hours after the initial fluid evacuation. The patient is admitted for continuous ECG monitoring and for assessment of the rate of pericardial drainage. The pericardial space should be drained every 8 hours and the catheter flushed with heparinized solution, and systemic antibiotics (usually a first-generation cephalosporin for empiric coverage of gram-positive bacteria) are administered for the duration of the catheter stay. Based on the cause of the effusion, the patient's clinical and hemodynamic condition, and the amount drained, the pericardial catheter is removed usually within 72 hours, and decisions for additional therapy are contemplated.

No special care is required after an uncomplicated pericardiocentesis. If pericardiocentesis is performed for cardiac tamponade, the patient is watched for signs of recurrent tamponade, and a follow-up echocardiogram is useful to monitor the resolution of the pericardial effusion and to detect signs of cardiac compression.

PREVENTION OF RECURRENT TAMPONADE

For many patients with pericardial effusion and tamponade, standard percutaneous pericardial drainage with an indwelling pericardial catheter is sufficient to avoid recurrence of pericardial effusion and tamponade. Patients who continue to drain more than 100 mL/24 hours 3 days after standard catheter drainage should be considered for more aggressive therapy. Reaccumulation of the pericardial fluid is particularly common in patients with malignant pericardial effusions. Additional therapeutic approaches are available to prevent pericardial fluid reaccumulation, including intrapericardial instillation of sclerosing agents, use of chemotherapy, radiotherapy, percutaneous balloon pericardial window, and surgical intervention.[25-28] Reaccumulation of fluid with recurrence of cardiac tamponade has been considered a definitive indication for an open surgical pericardial window or for percutaneous balloon pericardiotomy.[29]

OPEN SURGICAL PERICARDIAL WINDOW

Surgical procedures for creating a pericardial window range from a simple subxiphoid pericardial incision (pericardiotomy) to the removal of a variable portion of the pericardium (pericardiectomy). Although recurrence is higher with the pericardiotomy procedure, pericardiectomy often requires an anterior thoracotomy or sternotomy rather than a subxiphoid approach and is associated with a higher postoperative complication rate. Many physicians advocate the performance of subxiphoid pericardiotomy in critically ill patients with limited life expectancy, reserving pericardiectomy for patients with a relatively better prognosis.

Subxiphoid pericardiotomy allows for an adequate evacuation of the pericardial contents, direct inspection of the pericardial space to break down loculations, and the performance of pericardial biopsies and fluid sampling for diagnostic purposes. The procedure can be done safely and quickly under local anesthesia and provides prompt and long-term relief. Subxiphoid pericardiotomy alleviates the need for repeated pericardiocentesis and more invasive and difficult open drainage methods. Overall, the symptomatic recurrence of pericardial effusion after a surgical window is reported in the literature to be 5%.

PERCUTANEOUS BALLOON PERICARDIOTOMY

Patients with a malignant pericardial effusion and tamponade are likely to be suboptimal surgical candidates because of their overall poor health conditions and limited life expectancies. Palacios and colleagues[29,30] pioneered at Massachusetts General Hospital in Boston the technique of percutaneous balloon pericardial window (also called percutaneous balloon pericardiotomy) as an alternative and less invasive technique to surgical pericardial window. With this modality, adequate drainage of pericardial effusion is performed, and a pericardial window is created percutaneously under fluoroscopic guidance using a balloon-dilation catheter. The technique of percutaneous pericardial window is relatively simple and safe and is performed in the catheterization laboratory under local anesthesia with minimal discomfort. Conscious sedation with intravenous narcotics and a short-acting benzodiazepine is generally used.

PERCUTANEOUS BALLOON PERICARDIOTOMY TECHNIQUE

Percutaneous balloon pericardial window is offered as an alternative technique to the surgical pericardial window procedure for patients with persistent drainage from their indwelling intrapericardial catheter (≥3 days of >100 mL/24 hours drainage) or as primary therapy at the time of initial pericardiocentesis. The subxiphoid area around the indwelling pigtail pericardial catheter is infiltrated with local anesthesia (1% to 2% lidocaine). A small amount (5 to 10 mL) of iodinated contrast agent is injected in the pericardial space to help outline the parietal pericardium (Fig. 6.3A). A 0.038-inch stiff guidewire with a preshaped curve at the tip is advanced through the pigtail catheter into the pericardial space. The catheter is removed, leaving the guidewire in the pericardial space. After predilation of the skin and subcutaneous tissue along the track of the wire using a 10F dilator, a 20-mm-diameter × 3-cm-long balloon-dilation catheter (Boston Scientific, Watertown, MA) is advanced over the guidewire and positioned to straddle the parietal pericardium. Care should be taken to advance the proximal end of the balloon beyond the skin and the subcutaneous tissue to avoid dilation of the skin and subcutaneous tissue (and the resultant formation of a pericardial-cutaneous fistula) (see Fig. 6.3B). The balloon is inflated manually until the waist produced by the parietal pericardium disappears (see Fig. 6.3C). Biplane fluoroscopy is helpful to ascertain the correct position of the balloon straddling the parietal pericardium with the left lateral projection being particularly useful (see Fig. 6.3B and C). Two to three inflations are usually performed to have adequate opening of the parietal pericardium. The balloon-dilation catheter is

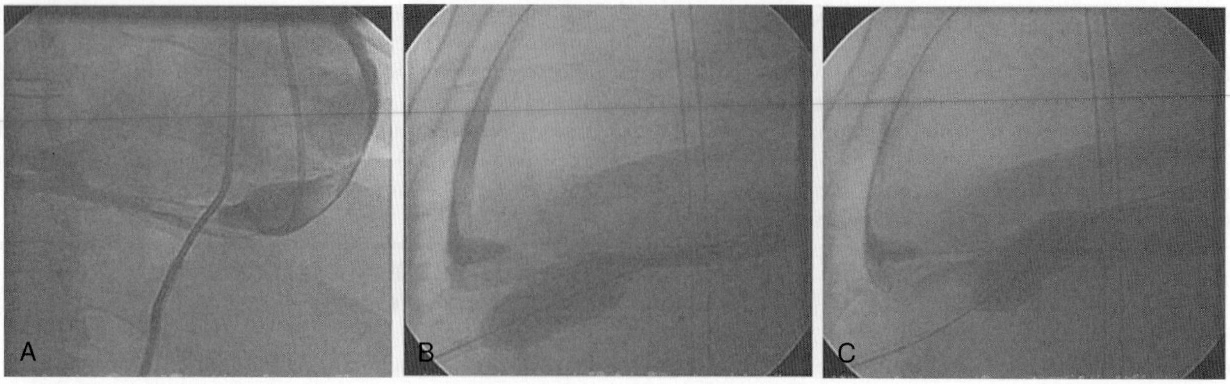

Figure 6.3 Computed tomography image of a percutaneous balloon pericardiotomy procedure. **A,** Injection of a small amount of iodinated contrast material confirms the intrapericardial location of the catheter. **B,** A left lateral projection shows an inflated dilating balloon catheter without a waist, indicating the need to reposition the balloon catheter to straddle the parietal pericardium. **C,** The balloon catheter is in the correct position and appears straddling the parietal pericardium in the left lateral projection.

removed, leaving the stiff guidewire in the pericardial space, where a new pigtail catheter is advanced over it and left indwelling in the pericardial space.

Patients are admitted to a regular medical ward unit after a percutaneous balloon pericardiotomy procedure and do not require a coronary unit admission. The pericardial catheter is aspirated every 6 to 8 hours and flushed with heparinized solution (5 mL, 100 U/mL). Pericardial drainage volumes are recorded, and the catheter is removed when there is less than 50 to 75 mL of pericardial drainage in 24 hours. Chest radiographs are obtained to check for the development of pleural effusion resulting from drainage of the pericardial fluid.

OUTCOME DATA AFTER PERCUTANEOUS BALLOON PERICARDIOTOMY

Palacios and colleagues[29] reported the first human experience with the technique of percutaneous balloon pericardiotomy in eight patients with malignant pericardial effusion and tamponade. The technique was successful in all patients with no immediate or late procedure-related complications. The mean time to radiologic development of a new or a significantly increased pleural effusion was 2.9 ± 0.4 days (range 2 to 5 days). No patient developed recurrence of the pericardial effusion or tamponade at a mean follow-up of 6 ± 2 months (range 1 to 11 months). Five patients died from their primary malignancy at 1, 4, 9, 10, and 11 months. A success rate of 87% was reported in the multicenter percutaneous balloon pericardial window registry, which enrolled 130 patients between 1987 and 1994 in 16 centers.[31,32] In this registry, three patients sustained pericardial bleeding and were considered to have a failed procedure and ended up undergoing surgical window procedures. Eight patients had recurrence of pericardial effusion (mean time to recurrence 54 ± 65 days), of whom seven ended up having surgical window procedures (with recurrence occurring in four of those patients).

COMPLICATIONS

Minor complications occurred in 13% of the patients.[31,32] The development of a large pleural effusion remains the major concern after percutaneous balloon pericardial window. Most patients develop a left pleural effusion within 24 to 48 hours of the procedure, which in most cases resolves spontaneously (presumably owing to the greater resorption capacity of the pleural surface). Thoracocentesis or chest tube placement was required in 15% of patients with preexisting pleural effusions compared with 9% of patients without preexisting pleural effusions.[31,32] It is desirable to aspirate most of the pericardial fluid before creating the window to limit the potential volume of fluid that can immediately leak to the pleural space. When the preprocedure chest radiograph reveals a large pleural effusion, the chance of requiring thoracentesis subsequent to the percutaneous pericardial window is higher, and the procedure should be performed only when its benefits outweigh the risks of thoracentesis or chest tube placement or both. It is not advised to perform the procedure in patients with marginal pulmonary reserve, as in postpneumonectomy patients, because the development of a pleural effusion may significantly compromise their respiratory function. Finally, an increased risk of bleeding from the pericardiotomy site occurs in patients with platelet or coagulation abnormalities. In these patients, a surgical procedure under direct visualization may be safer. Thoracoscopic techniques were developed to create a larger pericardial window and carry lower morbidity rates compared with open surgical techniques.[33] This technique allows adequate long-term drainage and the ability to obtain specimens for pathologic analysis.[33]

OTHER PERICARDIAL INTERVENTIONS

Percutaneous pericardial biopsy (PPB) is a relatively safe and feasible technique in the cardiac catheterization laboratory, and it can increase the diagnostic yield of pericardiocentesis and pericardial fluid analysis. One clinical scenario in which PPB may prove to be of particular importance is in the setting of tuberculous pericardial effusion because *Mycobacterium tuberculosis* is rarely cultured and a positive acid-fast stain is infrequently obtained from the pericardial fluid (which makes tuberculosis, unlike malignant pericarditis, a commonly missed diagnosis without the technique of PPB). PPB is also less invasive than surgical biopsy, and can be easily modified to obtain tissue samples from pericardial masses. PPB was initially described in 1988 by Endrys and colleagues,[34] who reported a series of 18 patients undergoing pericardial biopsy using an endomyocardial bioptome, and showed that PPB can be safely performed using conventional invasive cardiology techniques. Margey and colleagues[35] reported a case series of seven patients undergoing PPB for pericardial effusion, in whom they obtained a total of five biopsy specimens per patient with no complications. They demonstrated that pericardial biopsy adds incremental diagnostic value to the analysis of pericardial fluid alone, as it confirmed the absence of malignant invasion in four patients with neoplastic disease and the presence of lymphocytic and organizing effusive pericarditis in one and two patients, respectively.[35] Catheter-based intervention techniques in the pericardial space gained further momentum after a number of patients undergoing arrhythmia catheter ablation were found to have epicardial foci for the arrhythmia that could only be approached from the pericardial surface. Cardiologists also recognized that the pericardial space could be safely approach percutaneously even without a large collection of pericardial fluid present. Epicardial ablation has therefore become a therapeutic strategy for epicardial scar-related reentry, which is recognized as an important cause of ventricular tachycardia (especially in patients with nonischemic cardiomyopathy). Sosa and colleagues[36] were the first to show that the pericardial space can be safely entered with a blunt-tipped needle via a subxiphoid approach under fluoroscopic guidance. One should be aware that pericardial effusion and tamponade can occur as a result of these novel pericardial interventions.

KEY POINTS

- Patients with pericardial effusion have a variable clinical presentation; some are completely asymptomatic, whereas others develop tamponade and cardiovascular collapse.
- Pericardial tamponade is a clinical syndrome with defined hemodynamic and echocardiographic abnormalities, which result from the accumulation of intrapericardial fluid and impairment of ventricular diastolic filling.
- Two-dimensional echocardiography allows delineation of the size and distribution of the pericardial effusion, provides a reasonable estimate of its total volume, and helps assess the success of pericardiocentesis.

KEY POINTS (Continued)

- Pericardiocentesis is the technique of catheter-based aspiration of pericardial fluid and is a diagnostic and therapeutic modality.
- Pericardiocentesis is most commonly performed via the subxiphoid approach under ECG and fluoroscopy guidance in the cardiac catheterization laboratory with arterial and right-sided heart pressure monitoring. It also can be performed in the noninvasive laboratory or at the bedside using echocardiographic guidance.
- Percutaneous balloon pericardiotomy is an effective therapy for recurrent malignant pericardial effusion and is a less invasive alternative to surgical pericardial window.
- Surgical pericardiectomy is the definitive therapy for patients with constrictive pericardial disease.

SELECTED REFERENCES

1. Sagrista-Sauleda J, Merce J, Permanyer-Miralda G, et al: Clinical clues to the causes of large pericardial effusions. Am J Med 2000;109:95-101.
2. Troughton RW, Asher CR, Klein AL: Pericarditis. Lancet 2004;363: 717-727.
3. Lange RA, Hillis LD: Clinical practice: Acute pericarditis. N Engl J Med 2004;351:2195-2202.
8. Spodick DH: Acute cardiac tamponade. N Engl J Med 2003;349: 684-690.
10. Bruch C, Schmermund A, Dagres N, et al: Changes in QRS voltage in cardiac tamponade and pericardial effusion: Reversibility after pericardiocentesis and after anti-inflammatory drug treatment. J Am Coll Cardiol 2001;38:219-226.
11. Maisch B, Seferovic PM, Ristic AD, et al: Guidelines on the diagnosis and management of pericardial diseases: Executive summary. The Task Force on the Diagnosis and Management of Pericardial Diseases of the European Society of Cardiology. Eur Heart J 2004;25:587-610.
13. Feigenbaum H, Waldhausen JA, Hyde LP: Ultrasound diagnosis of pericardial effusion. JAMA 1965;191:711-714.
16. George S, Salama AL, Uthaman B, et al: Echocardiography in differentiating tuberculous from chronic idiopathic pericardial effusion. Heart 2004;90:1338-1339.
20. Sagrista-Sauleda J, Angel J, Sanchez A, et al: Effusive-constrictive pericarditis. N Engl J Med 2004;350:469-475.
30. Ziskind AA, Pearce AC, Lemmon CC, et al: Percutaneous balloon pericardiotomy for the treatment of cardiac tamponade and large pericardial effusions: Description of technique and report of the first 50 cases. J Am Coll Cardiol 1993;21:1-5.

The complete list of references can be found at www.expertconsult.com.

7 Intra-aortic Balloon Counterpulsation

Zoltan G. Turi | Simon K. Topalian

CHAPTER OUTLINE

The first and most widely utilized of the percutaneously placed cardiac assist devices, the intra-aortic balloon pump (IABP) displaces blood from the descending aorta during diastole, resulting in altered myocardial mechanics during systole. By raising diastolic perfusion pressure, the IABP has the potential to augment coronary flow. Unlike the majority of more recently developed and generally mechanically more complex devices, the IABP provides auxiliary rather than independent support of cardiac output. Although it uses complex software algorithms, it is the simplest of the invasive devices mechanically, is the lowest in profile, and is associated with relatively low failure rates. Its advantages include the feasibility of allowing insertion in the cardiac catheterization laboratory or operating room or at the bedside, as well as a relatively small footprint allowing placement in the vasculature with less morbidity than other devices in its class. The indications, complications, and relative effectiveness of the IABP have been studied extensively for nearly 4 decades. National Center for Health Statistics data show that at least 37,000 intra-aortic balloons were placed in the United States in 2004,[1] whereas some estimates range to more than 130,000 by 2010. There were close to 20,000 used in high-risk percutaneous coronary intervention (PCI) among U.S. centers contributing to the National Cardiovascular Data Registry (NCDR) during a recent 3-year period.[2] The primary hospital location where IABPs are placed is highly variable depending on patient acuity and types of procedures performed in individual institutions, but the cardiac catheterization laboratory has become the primary site,[3,4] and bedside placement in critical care units has declined to the low single-digit percentages.

HISTORY

Initial experiments aimed at altering the timing of phases of the cardiac cycle originated with animal experiments conducted by Adrian Kantrowitz in the early 1950s in the laboratory of Carl Wiggers at Western Reserve Medical School.[5] The focus was initially oriented toward improving coronary blood flow rather than augmentation of cardiac output. Appreciating that coronary flow (particularly in the left coronary circulation) occurs primarily in diastole, the concept was to delay the peak systolic pressure pulse to the diastolic phase of the cardiac cycle.[6] During the subsequent decade, this was followed by animal experiments attempting to use the diaphragm to provide the power for diastolic augmentation by wrapping it around the distal thoracic aorta.[7] Clauss and colleagues effectuated counterpulsation by withdrawing blood from the circulation during systole and restoring it during diastole,[8] but it was the work of Moulopoulos and associates[9] that introduced counterpulsation with a carbon dioxide–filled tube synchronized to the electrocardiogram (ECG) in canines. Kantrowitz subsequently changed the gas to helium, used in modern IABPs because it has only 5% of the density of CO_2 and allows faster inflation-deflation cycles and greater precision in timing. In addition, helium is inert, although it is less soluble and potentially more toxic in case of gas leak in the circulation. The IABP was introduced in humans in 1967 (Fig. 7.1). Initial favorable experience with intra-aortic counterpulsation in critically ill patients in cardiogenic shock (CS)[10,11] led to the first major multicenter trial. This trial demonstrated significant hemodynamic benefit but only a 17% survival to discharge rate.[12] A number of incremental improvements over the next 4 decades resulted in introduction of a percutaneous approach,[13] a second lumen for guidewire support of balloon advancement through the circulation,[14] increasing automation of the control consoles, and prefolded and progressively lower-profile balloons.[15]

PHYSIOLOGY

The classic concept of intra-aortic balloon counterpulsation involves inflation in synchrony with aortic valve closure, at the onset of isovolumic diastole and the appearance of the dicrotic notch, displacing blood comparable to the balloon's volume into the peripheral circulation during diastole. To accomplish further unloading, and to prevent interference with left ventricular (LV) ejection, balloon deflation has traditionally begun before opening of the aortic valve and the beginning of LV ejection, although as discussed subsequently, this may not be the optimal algorithm. An example of the effects of balloon counterpulsation on systolic and diastolic pressure is seen in Figure 7.2.

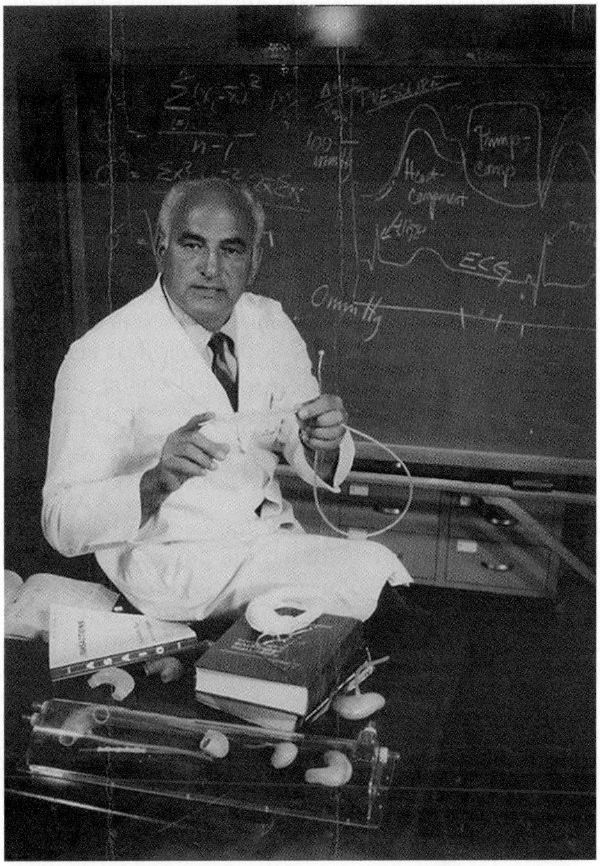

Figure 7.1 Adrian Kantrowitz with an early model of a working intra-aortic balloon pump used in patients circa 1967, the year of the initial human experience with the device.

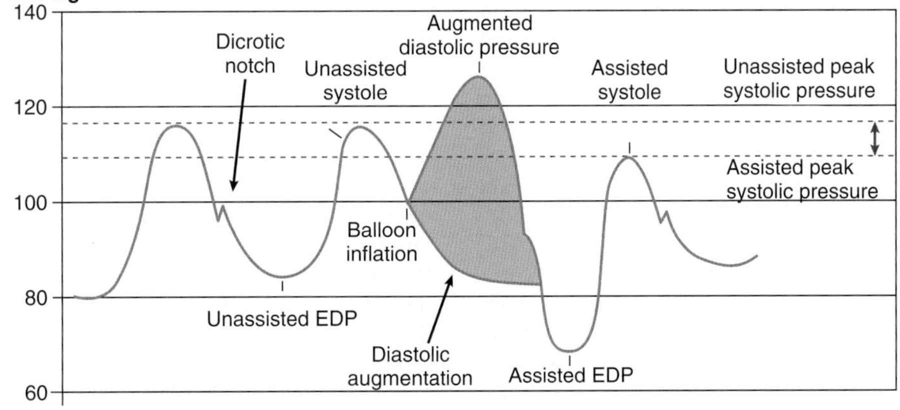

Figure 7.2 Systemic pressure response to an intra-aortic balloon pump. The console is set to trigger at 1:2, hence both unassisted and assisted systole and diastole are seen. Note decrease in systolic pressure with balloon counterpulsation (*double arrow*) and augmentation of diastolic pressure (area under curve in *blue*), thus decreasing afterload and increasing inflow pressure to the coronary and other vascular beds during diastole. EDP, end-diastolic pressure.

The hemodynamic response to institution of IABP is quite variable, and depends on a complex array consisting of the patient's intrinsic blood pressure, heart rate, heart rhythm, aortic compliance, overall peripheral vascular resistance, intravascular volume status, cardiac function, adjunctive pharmacotherapy, disease state of the coronary vasculature, and degree of preservation of coronary flow autoregulation. In addition, the exact location of the IABP in the vasculature, the volume of the balloon, the frequency of inflation (frequencies from 1:1 to 1:8 are available depending on manufacturer), and timing of inflation and deflation all play important roles. Thus, the "classic" response consisting of lowering the systolic blood pressure and augmentation of diastolic pressure may not be seen; this classic response is based on the initial experience in CS, which led to a 20% drop in systolic pressure and a 30% rise in diastolic pressure.[12] In fact, systolic pressure can increase secondary to improved cardiac output, can decrease, or can be unchanged, as can coronary blood flow. An important characteristic of the IABP in contrast to most mechanical assist devices is that it contributes to pulsatile flow, with theoretical benefits to end-organ perfusion beyond any actual change in mean flow or pressures.

DIASTOLE AND CORONARY BLOOD FLOW

Because the majority of coronary flow occurs in diastole, an increase in diastolic pressure has the potential to augment coronary flow as well as flow to other end organs. Diastolic pressure may in fact be augmented substantially, in part because balloon inflation is rapid, yielding an abrupt increase in volume and effecting a rapid rise on the pressure-volume curve. A variety of physical and biologic parameters, including compliance characteristics of the aorta and vascular bed, affect the degree of augmentation.[16] The extent of peak pressure rise has been reported in a range from minimal to near doubling of diastolic pressure.[17,18] However, increase in diastolic pressure and hence coronary perfusion pressure may not result in an increase in coronary flow because autoregulation modulates this potential and because in normal patients, end organs capable of autoregulation maintain flow without significant change.

Despite both several decades of experimentation in animal models and attempts to assess coronary flow in a variety of clinical settings in humans, the effect of IABP on coronary flow remains incompletely defined. Experimental and clinical data fail to show change in flow in native coronary arteries[19,20] or in bypass grafts[21] regardless of the severity of coronary stenosis.[22] Although total coronary blood flow may not increase, coronary blood flow velocity has consistently been demonstrated to rise.[17,23,24] In turn, data from a thrombolysis in myocardial infarction (MI) model suggest that the pulsatile waveform generated by IABP during diastole may contribute to improved time to coronary reperfusion without concomitant increase in coronary blood flow;[25] in all likelihood this improvement reflects the enhancement in peak flow velocity that may also help prevent reocclusion.[23] However, pulsatile flow may have additional benefit: in a randomized study comparing cardiopulmonary bypass with or without concomitant IABP, multiple parameters of whole-body perfusion were superior in the pulsatile flow setting.[26] In general, augmentation of blood flow appears most likely to occur in patients in profound shock.[17,24,27] Thus, most of the benefits of IABP are related to improvement in hemodynamics with secondary relief of ischemia. Amelioration of ischemia may in turn result in improved LV function and additional improvement in hemodynamics.

SYSTOLE AND MYOCARDIAL MECHANICS

Although the IABP is generally described as both improving myocardial oxygen supply and lowering myocardial oxygen demand, the predominant effect is the latter. This is based on decreased afterload and wall stress with increased stroke volume and cardiac output, in particular in patients with low-output states. In general, the magnitude of hemodynamic response is proportional to the extent of depression of cardiac function.[16] Because stroke volume improves, heart rate stays the same or tends to decrease even as cardiac output rises. Reduction in LV end-diastolic pressure and improved cardiac output is associated with lower left ventricular heart filling and pulmonary arterial pressures, whereas systolic pressure typically decreases and mean blood pressure stays the same in hemodynamically stable patients. In patients in shock, mean blood pressure rises and systolic pressure may increase as well. When IABP placement results in improved end-organ perfusion, as evidenced by signs such as better urine output, the overall prognosis is generally improved.[12] Reduction in left-sided heart filling and pulmonary artery pressures also leads to reduced right ventricular (RV) afterload; thus, IABP insertion may be helpful in some patients with right-sided heart failure.[28] Although ejection phase indices tend to improve with unloading, the extent of augmentation of cardiac output is limited by the overall reserve in LV systolic function. Thus, at the extremes of ventricular dysfunction, even with excellent positioning of the balloon and timing as well as large IABP volumes, the IABP may not provide sufficient augmentation of cardiac output in some patients. A variety of other parameters have been used to assess the effect of IABP in shock, most prominently the cardiac power index (mean systemic pressure times cardiac index), which is the strongest hemodynamic correlate of outcomes.[29]

EFFECTS ON ORGANS OTHER THAN THE HEART

The effect of IABP on flow to end organs other than the heart is also incompletely characterized. In the cranial circulation, as in the heart, net flow does not appear to increase in patients with a stable hemodynamic state. Further, with balloon deflation, there is some evidence for transient reversal of blood flow as well,[30] although this may be a consequence of early deflation (see discussion under "Timing"). Similarly, overall carotid flow is not changed in this setting.[31] During hypothermia while patients are under cardiopulmonary bypass, pulsatile augmentation as obtained by the IABP does appear to improve cerebral oxygenation.[32] Indirect evidence again suggests additional benefit in the setting of shock, with better cerebral blood flow, a setting in which there is modest clinical experience with using IABP in patients with refractory cerebral vasospasm.[33] Despite improvement in cardiac output with IABP, gastric tonometry has not shown improvement in the splanchnic circulation in CS patients,[34] and renal vein thermodilution has failed to show improvement in overall renal blood flow.[35] In cardiac surgery patients who subsequently developed low-output syndrome, however, IABP did have a positive effect on gastric tonometery.[36]

THE INTRA-AORTIC BALLOON PUMP APPARATUS

With the introduction of a separate guidewire lumen in the early 1980s,[14] the safety of IABP placement improved significantly. Previously, bulky 12 F or larger devices were placed via a surgical approach through an end-to-side graft to the femoral artery, with substantial associated morbidity. The device was then advanced through the femoral and iliac systems without a guidewire, frequently at the bedside with no fluoroscopic guidance. This led to a high rate of major vascular complications, in particular, iliac artery dissection but also aortic perforation and IABP malposition. The introduction of the percutaneous approach did not alleviate these problems until a guidewire lumen was added.[14]

There were conflicting demands on balloon design: first, to minimize the central lumen size as part of reducing overall profile, and second, at the same time to maintain a large enough lumen both for guidewires that could provide safe passage through the circulation as well as sufficient diameter for high-fidelity hemodynamic recordings. One solution to the latter has been the introduction of a line of catheters with a fiber-optic pressure measurement sensor.[37] In general, the guidewire lumens are designed to accommodate guidewires in the 0.018-inch to 0.030-inch range. The gas exchange lumen is concentrically placed around the guidewire lumen. Improvements in technology allowed for the introduction of tightly folded balloons prewrapped around the central lumen (Fig. 7.3); previously, a cumbersome process that sometimes led to device failure required the operator to wrap the balloon just before insertion.

BALLOON DIMENSIONS

The available IABP catheters range in gas volume from 25 to 50 mL and in shaft lengths from approximately 60 to 72 cm. The actual length of the balloon segment varies by manufacturer and balloon volume: Commercial balloon lengths are in the range of 16.5 to 26 cm. Although balloon volume does affect the degree of diastolic augmentation[38] and cardiac output[39] and may be particularly important in patients with severe, refractory CS, little difference was found in IABP effectiveness between 32-mL and 40-mL balloons in one study,[40] and risk to the patient is significantly higher if inflated balloon diameter approximates or exceeds aortic diameter (see "Complications"). Thus the decision for IABP size is typically based on patient size and severity of hemodynamic compromise, with the 40-mL balloon used in approximately three fourths of patients.[41] A special consideration for balloon volumes is patient air transport; rapid changes in altitude will lead to increased (during ascent) or decreased (with descent) volume, requiring monitoring to ensure that appropriate balloon volume is maintained.[42]

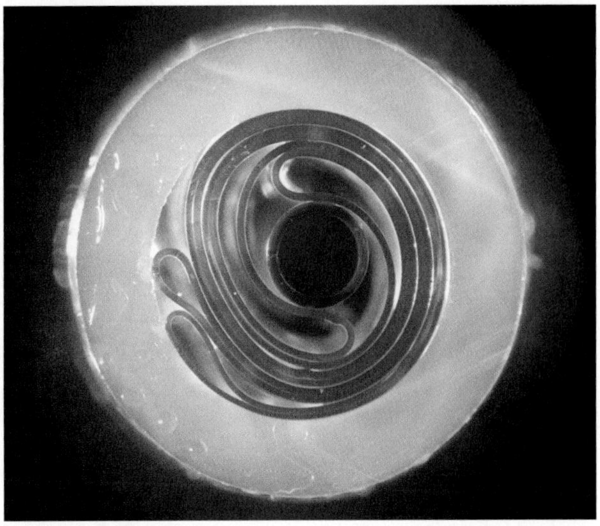

Figure 7.3 Magnified cross-sectional view of prefolded intra-aortic balloon (a 7.5 French wrap). The prefolding was a significant advance in technology in the early 1980s because it eliminated folding at the bedside, a process that occasionally led to tearing of the balloon membrane, and substantially reduced the overall profile of the device at insertion. (Courtesy of Datascope, Montvale, NJ.)

Because it is essential to locate the balloon below the origin of the left subclavian artery at the upper margin and above the renal arteries at the lower (a "safe zone"; Fig. 7.4), the tolerances are relatively low. Studies looking at the length of this segment in Japanese patients found a range of 21 to 25 cm, with good correlation between patient height and length of this segment (although in the relatively short Japanese population, the balloon lengths frequently exceeded the "safe zone" length for individual patients).[43] Recommendations vary by manufacturer: A 50-mL size I is generally recommended for patients taller than 6 feet (183 cm), and the 25-mL is used for patients shorter than 5 feet (152 cm). Recent changes in technology have allowed for larger diameter balloons to be available for shorter patients (e.g., a 50-mL IABP on an 8 F shaft is now available for patients 5′4″ [162 cm] and taller). In general, larger balloon sizes lead to improved unloading and augmentation with greater blood volume displacement. Early balloon models were designed to be occlusive during inflation, and experimental data have demonstrated optimal augmentation with 100% occlusion of the aorta.[38,39] Such full occlusion is generally avoided because of potential trauma to the aorta, ischemia to the spinal circulation, or abrasion of the balloon, which might contribute to a risk of rupture. The generally accepted value for ratio of balloon to aorta size is 80% to 90%; in the study by Igari[43] in Japanese patients, the range of commercially available balloon diameters was noted to be 14 to 15 mm, whereas aortic diameter mean at the level of the renal arteries was 17.5 ± 3.2 mm, within the accepted 80% to 90% range, although at least one 50-mL balloon has an expanded diameter of 18 mm (Arrow International, Inc., Reading, PA). In an earlier study in Americans, 90% of midthoracic aortas were larger than 19 mm.[44] Balloons are typically made of polyurethane or polyethylene, with materials chosen to allow rapid inflation-deflation cycles and tolerate an average of 100,000 to

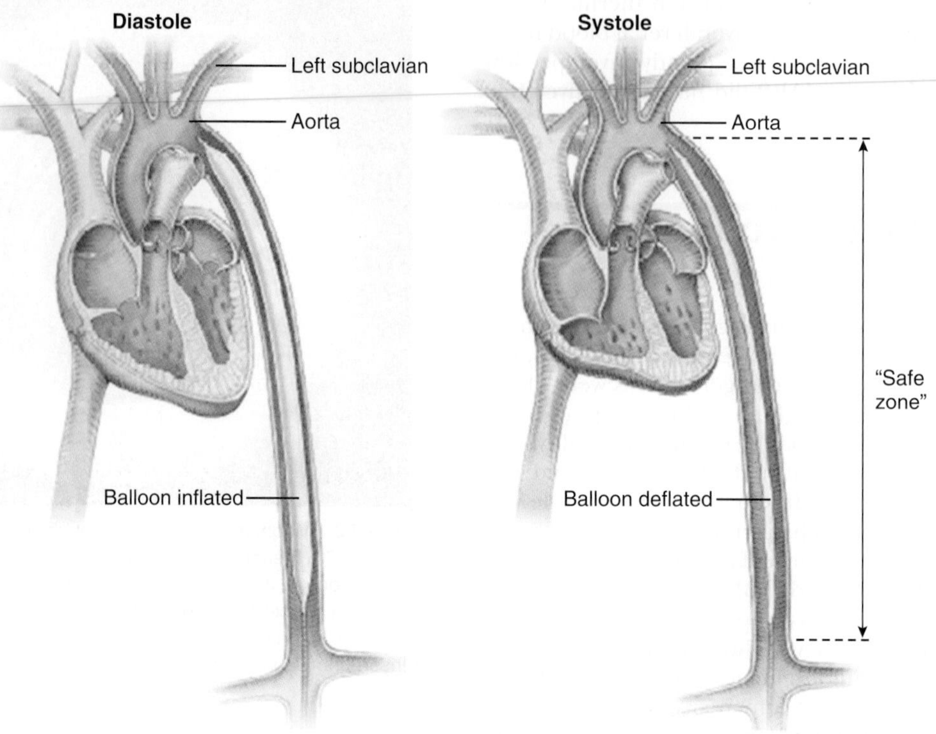

Figure 7.4 Location of intra-aortic balloon during inflation and deflation. Ideally the tip should be a few centimeters distal to the origin of the left subclavian artery and the proximal portion above the origins of the renal arteries, the "safe zone." (Adapted from figure provided by Teleflex Medical, Limerick, PA.)

150,000 cycles per day. Experimental materials with heparin and hydrophilic coatings have been developed to address thrombosis risk and trauma to the vasculature during device passage[45,46] but are not generally available.

BALLOON CONSOLE

IABPs are driven by complexly engineered consoles with extensive artificial intelligence designed to recognize electrocardiographic rhythms and hemodynamics, with the ability to trigger balloon inflation either from the ECG (including paced rhythms) or from pressure waveforms, although in some settings, such as during cardiopulmonary bypass, an automatic trigger at a preset rate can be used. Tachyarrhythmias and irregular rhythms have substantial influence on the effectiveness of the IABP, the former in part because of the disproportionately shorter diastolic filling periods, and the latter because of difficulties predicting the timing of occurrence of the dicrotic notch, although improved algorithms have been incorporated.[47] The central lumen of the balloon is typically connected to a transducer and separate ECG leads are connected to the console. A series of alarms identify leaks in the IABP circuit, high or low pressure, loss of trigger signals, blood in the gas line, low battery, and other anomalies that foreshadow or indicate impending or existing system failures. (Figure 7.5 demonstrates the control panel of a modern IABP console.) Modern IABPs using fiber-optic technology permit automatic calibration in patients after insertion and automatic recalibration on a periodic basis or whenever the algorithms detect a change in patient condition.

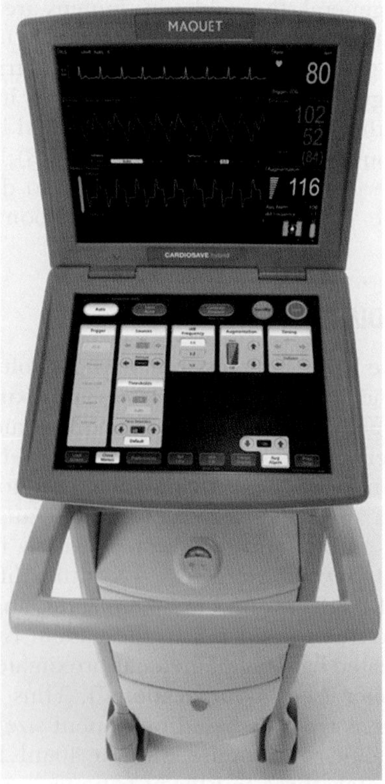

Figure 7.5 Intra-aortic balloon console showing continuous display of electrocardiogram, systemic pressure (note diastolic augmentation), and balloon pressure. (Courtesy of Datascope, Montvale, NJ.)

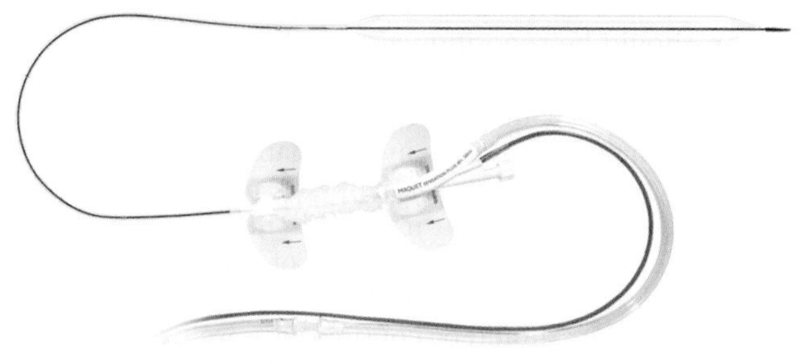

Figure 7.6 A modern intra-aortic balloon. A minimal size central lumen allows advancement over a guidewire. Low-profile balloons such as this one use fiber-optic cable for pressure monitoring. (Courtesy of Datascope, Montvale, NJ.)

PREPARATION

Balloon preparation requires establishing a vacuum in the gas lumen by drawing back on a large-volume syringe, and also flushing the central guidewire lumen (Fig. 7.6). If the procedure is to be done at the bedside without fluoroscopy, measuring the approximate distance along the course of the femoral and iliac arteries and then up the descending aorta is essential prior to IABP placement. The approximate depth to which it needs to be inserted should be noted on the shaft prior to beginning insertion. The ECG leads should be connected to the IABP console prior to introducing the catheter if ECG triggering is to be performed.

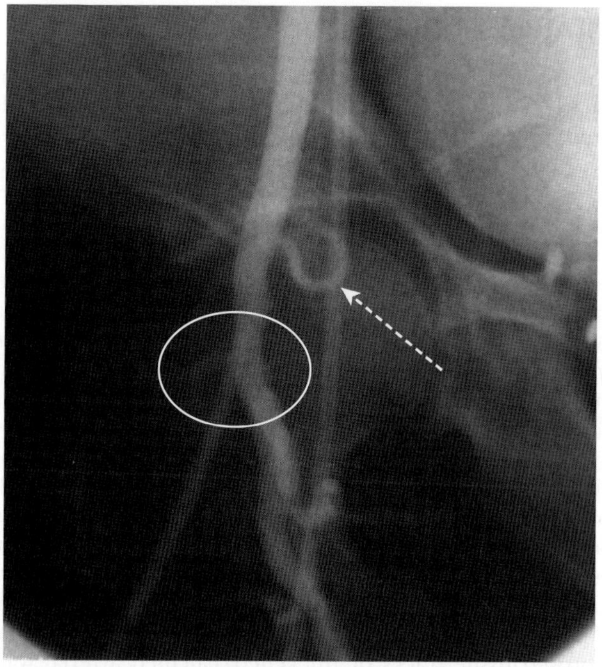

Figure 7.7 Optimal access for placement of an intra-aortic balloon pump, right femoral artery, left anterior oblique view. The sheath entry is above the femoral bifurcation near the center line of the femoral head (*circle*). Note the location of the inferior epigastric artery (IEA; *arrow*). The lowest inflection of the IEA lies just above the inguinal ligament; punctures below this point have a lower likelihood of subsequent retroperitoneal hemorrhage.

BALLOON INSERTION

Based on data from the Benchmark Registry, nearly two thirds of IABP insertions in the United States occur in the cardiac catheterization laboratory, one fourth in the operating room, and the remainder at the bedside in a variety of hospital locations. In contrast, outside the United States, the operating room and the catheterization laboratory each account for approximately 40% of placements, with the remaining 20% inserted at the bedside.[4]

The modern IABP is designed to be introduced percutaneously through the common femoral artery, which is the method used in 95% to 98% of cases, two thirds via the right common femoral artery.[41,48] A variety of disease states affect the ability to freely pass the device to the central aorta, in particular atherosclerosis, but also spasm and congenitally small vessels. Preprocedure assessment of the vascular tree is important: Diabetics, women, and patients with small body surface area in particular have small femoral arteries,[49] and there is a corresponding higher rate of vascular complications in these patients.[50] Pulses at the common femoral artery and below must be carefully documented before catheter insertion, and if there is suspected or confirmed peripheral vascular disease, angiography of the abdominal aorta, iliac artery, and lower extremities should be considered. This step is frequently not practical in the emergency setting or in patients with renal failure; in elective situations noninvasive evaluation should be performed, including ankle-brachial indices with pulse volume recordings, computed tomography, angiography, or magnetic resonance angiography.

FEMORAL ACCESS

Every effort should be made to ensure that femoral puncture is above the femoral bifurcation and below the inguinal ligament (Fig. 7.7). An excellent practice is to place a short 5 F or 6 F pilot sheath in the femoral artery and to perform angiography of the common femoral artery to confirm sheath entry below the inferior excursion of the inferior epigastric artery; punctures above this landmark correlate strongly with retroperitoneal hemorrhage.[51] Puncture below the femoral head drastically increases the likelihood of puncture into the femoral bifurcation vessels (77% of femoral bifurcations are at or below the inferior margin of the femoral head[49]), which in turn is associated with acute leg ischemia due to vascular obstruction, and pseudoaneurysm formation upon balloon removal is more likely because of lack of the anvil of the femoral head against which to perform manual compression. If the pilot sheath is found to have entered outside the common femoral artery on femoral angiography, consideration should be given to switching to the contralateral side. Using fluoroscopy to aid in puncturing the common femoral artery at a point over the lower half of the femoral head is a recommended technique to ensure proper sheath placement.

SHEATHLESS INSERTION

The use of a sheathless insertion technique has been recommended to reduce complications.[52] Sheaths typically add between 0.6 and 0.8 mm to the overall diameter required to place a device, so the sheath for an 8 F balloon approximates 10 F in outer diameter. "Going sheathless" therefore has the advantage of having the device occupy less space in the common femoral artery and has been described as reducing vascular complications with an odds ratio greater than 2:1.[53,54] Although retrospective analysis of large patient subsets presents compelling data that the sheathless approach is superior for reducing complications,[55] this finding has not been universally confirmed.[50,56] The latest data suggest that about 80% of IABPs are inserted with a sheath.[41] The sheathless approach is most compelling in diabetic patients, women, and patients with known peripheral vascular disease or small body surface area. Sheathless insertion of an IABP requires careful preparation of the tissue track to allow atraumatic entry of the balloon tip into the artery directly through the skin over a wire. Spreading of tissue and predilatation with a dilator are essential. Fibrosed tissue tracks or thickened/calcified arterial walls frequently resist sheathless entry. In some cases, a stiff guidewire provides an adequate rail along which to slide the naked balloon catheter into the vessel.

BALLOON ADVANCEMENT AND POSITIONING

Once suitable access is gained, guidewire passage to the aortic arch is ideally performed under fluoroscopic guidance. Without fluoroscopy at the bedside, approximating the distance from the femoral puncture to a point near the top of the descending aorta is imprecise and adds to the risk of trauma/ischemia to head and neck vessels, the aorta, or the renal arteries. In the critical care setting, transesophageal echocardiography is a suitable alternative to fluoroscopy for enabling precise balloon placement.[57] If fluoroscopy is not used, prompt postprocedure radiography to confirm location is imperative.

If guidewire passage meets resistance, alternative approaches include use of guidewires that are hydrophilic, steerable, or both.[58] If significant iliac stenosis is noted, balloon dilatation or stenting of the iliac artery is an accepted practice with high success rate both for achieving passage of the IABP and as an adjunct to preventing distal ischemia.[59,60] As more cardiologists become skilled in endovascular intervention, the ability to perform combined iliac stenting and IABP placement is expanding.[61]

Once the balloon has been advanced to a point 1 to 2 cm inferior to the left subclavian artery origin (see Fig. 7.4)—typically near the top of the descending aorta—the guidewire is withdrawn and the central lumen flushed. The vacuum port (minus its one-way valve) is connected to gas line tubing that in turn is connected to the console, and the dead space is purged and then filled with helium. The central catheter lumen is connected to a transducer on the console. After triggering is initiated, typically on every other beat, fluoroscopy should be used to confirm balloon location and filling, and pressure contours should be evaluated for appropriateness of timing (see later discussion under "Timing"). Once the timing is considered satisfactory, continuous pumping can be initiated. If necessary, the balloon should be repositioned with the console turned to standby to avoid trauma to the aorta.

The distal circulation should be assessed carefully after IABP placement. Distal ischemia is relatively common. The most likely cause of acute ischemia is obstruction of the artery by the catheter shaft itself. If ischemia occurs hours or days after insertion, the possibility of thrombus, typically secondary to stagnant blood in the confined space of a small or diseased vessel, should be considered as well. A technique for addressing distal limb ischemia—placement of a small sheath retrograde in the contralateral femoral artery and antegrade in the ipsilateral common femoral or superficial femoral artery—if performed by expert hands, can occasionally salvage an ischemic limb without forcing removal of the IABP[62] (Fig. 7.8). There is some evidence that IABP inflation properties and hemodynamic effects may be superior in the patient positioned horizontally than with the

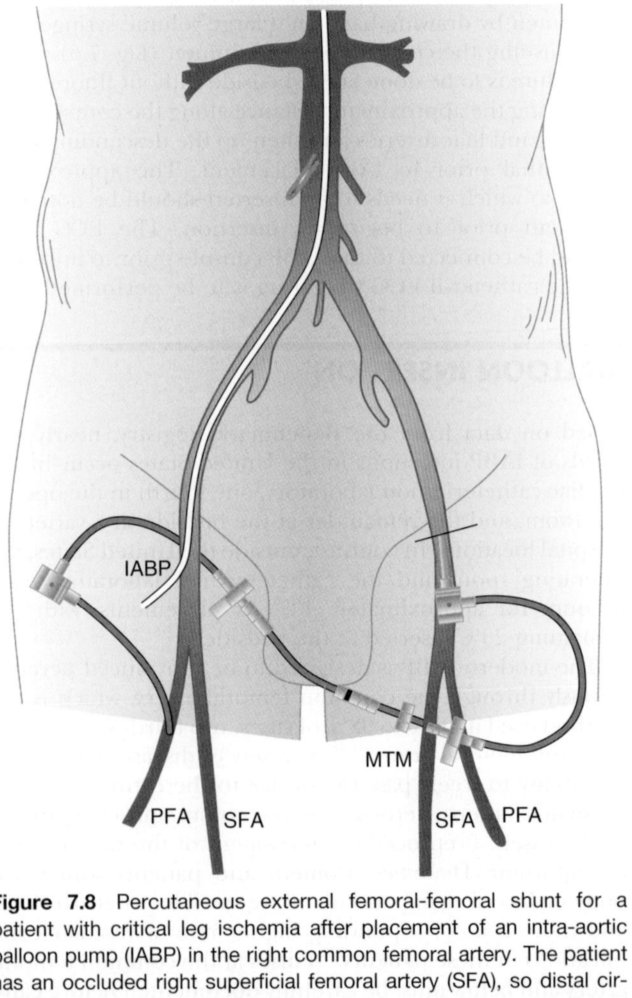

Figure 7.8 Percutaneous external femoral-femoral shunt for a patient with critical leg ischemia after placement of an intra-aortic balloon pump (IABP) in the right common femoral artery. The patient has an occluded right superficial femoral artery (SFA), so distal circulation depends on profunda femoris to superficial femoral collateral vessels. The antegrade sheath is placed directly into the profunda femoris. MTM, male-to-male adapter; PFA, profunda femoris artery. (From Merhi WM, Turi ZG, Dixon S, et al: Percutaneous ex-vivo femoral arterial bypass: A novel approach for treatment of acute limb ischemia as a complication of femoral arterial catheterization. Catheter Cardiovasc Intervent 2006;68:435-440.)

patient tilted at a 30-degree angle.[63] Postprocedure and subsequent monitoring of left arm pressures can lead to early diagnosis of inadvertent balloon advancement obstructing left subclavian artery inflow, a phenomenon to which the restless patient who flexes the thigh is predisposed.

ALTERNATE ACCESS ROUTES

Multiple alternatives to percutaneous femoral access have been described, all associated with higher complication rates. In part, this difference in rates is selection related: Patients with severe peripheral vascular disease have multiple comorbid conditions that affect IABP complications. In addition, introduction of a balloon into a peripheral vessel smaller than the common femoral artery or into a large central vessel through a surgical approach of necessity creates hazards associated with the introduction, maintenance, and withdrawal of the IABP.

Approaches described to date include the brachial, subclavian, axillary, iliac, transthoracic, and translumbar arteries. Although the brachial approach has been successful in isolated cases,[64,65] and sheathless entry reduces the overall diameter of lumen encroachment to less than 3 mm, the potential for complications is substantial. They include not only vascular injury and ischemia of the hand but also potential neurologic consequences from formation of thrombus on an indwelling catheter underneath the origin of the right common carotid artery (as the shaft traverses from the right subclavian artery to the innominate artery) as well as under the left common carotid artery and subclavian artery origin.[66]

Iliac insertion through a conduit has been used for patients in whom femoral access is not adequate or who are not candidates for ventricular assist devices: With retroperitoneal placement, patients can be at least partially ambulatory during prolonged counterpulsation.[67] Other routes of access that have been described are via the subclavian[68] and axillary arteries,[69,70] with or without conduits, and generally with an eye toward allowing modest ambulation during prolonged IABP use. A transthoracic approach has been described, with placement via the ascending aorta into the standard descending aortic location.[71,72] The morbidity rate associated with these surgical placements is significantly higher,[73] in part because they typically involve longer IABP indwelling times as well as the comorbidity issues already mentioned.

TIMING

The importance of IABP timing was understood from the time of the original Moulopolous study in 1962.[9] The timing of balloon inflation and deflation is designed to optimize afterload reduction and enhancement of diastolic pressure without interfering with ventricular ejection. Classically, it was considered optimal to inflate at the dicrotic notch, as soon as aortic valve closure occurred, and to deflate near the onset of ventricular depolarization, anticipating the beginning of mechanical systole (Fig. 7.9). In fact, significant enhancements to IABP efficiency can be obtained with refinements to these concepts.

LATE INFLATION AND EARLY DEFLATION

Gross errors in inflation and deflation lead to failure to obtain benefit from IABP and occasionally to significant hemodynamic compromise. Early in the history of IABP deployment, it was appreciated that inflation throughout the period from closure of the aortic valve to its subsequent opening was necessary for optimal hemodynamic effect.[16] Both late inflation and early deflation reduce augmented LV stroke volume and result in decreased peak diastolic coronary velocity;[23] the latter is demonstrated with transthoracic Doppler ultrasound, a tool that can potentially be used to optimize timing. An additional concern exists with early deflation: The abrupt decrease in IABP volume during diastole can lead to reversal of both coronary and other end organ (e.g., cerebral) flow back into the aorta, shunting blood from vital end organs.[30]

EARLY INFLATION

Early inflation results in increased afterload late in LV ejection with consequent impairment of LV systolic function. The ejection phase is shortened, LV end-systolic pressure rises, and stroke volume decreases; inflation, in the range of 130 to 190 ms before the dicrotic notch, results in a 20% decrease in stroke volume.[74] This effect may not be seen if early balloon inflation is less pronounced; no hemodynamic effect was noted when IABP inflation occurred 50 ms before the dicrotic notch. Regardless, although early inflation theoretically lengthens diastole and allows for a longer period of diastolic augmentation, the net effect does not appear to be salutary. In addition, early inflation carries theoretical risks associated with the increased afterload and wall stress, including aneurysm formation and rupture in the peri-MI period.

LATE DEFLATION

Similarly, late balloon deflation could be expected to interfere with ventricular ejection and decrease stroke volume. In fact, somewhat counterintuitively, a similar 110- to 180-ms delay in IABP deflation appears to have salutary effects and is associated with a stroke volume increase of 18%,[74] which apparently results from both an increase in diastolic filling period and an augmented decrease in afterload later in the cycle. This finding confirms a prior observation by Kern and associates[75] and suggests that, in general, most operators have timed deflation too early. The beneficial effect occurs with timing deflation to be simultaneous with LV ejection; delaying deflation beyond the range described, however, raises concerns similar to those described for early inflation.

ELECTROCARDIOGRAM TRIGGERING

When the ECG is used as the trigger, the descending slope of the T wave correlates best with the onset of diastole[38] and is the usual timing for balloon inflation. Deflation is typically timed to the R wave, which denotes a short time delay after the onset of electrical systole. Algorithms were developed early to effect prompt deflation and prevent inflation in the setting of ectopy, and IABP software recognizes

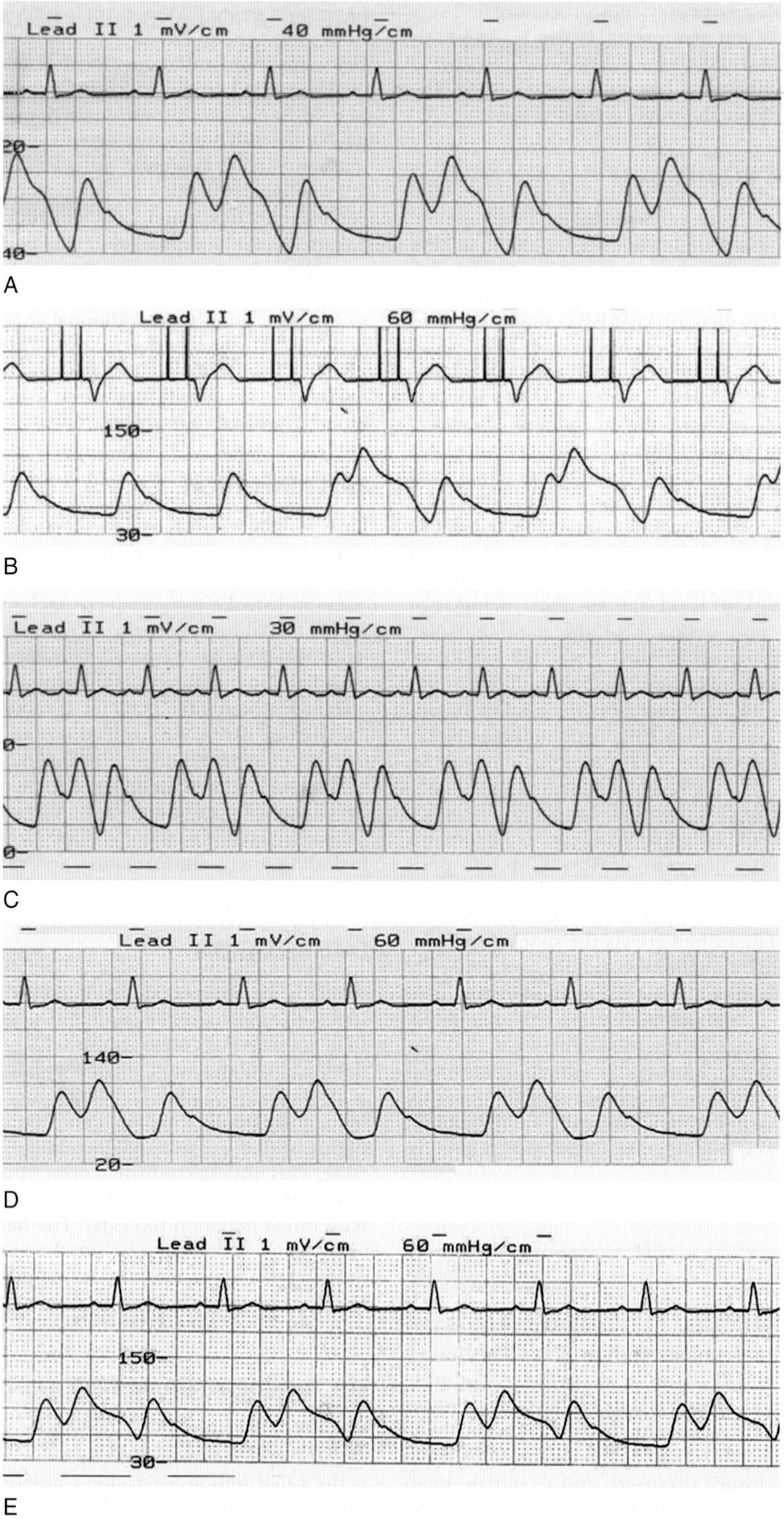

Figure 7.9 Examples of timing of intra-aortic balloon pump inflation and deflation with 1:2 balloon pumping. **A**, Optimal timing results in mild lowering of systolic pressure with diastolic augmentation. Also shown are examples of early inflation before the dicrotic notch (**B**), late inflation (**C**), early deflation (**D**), and late deflation (**E**).

pacemaker spikes in contrast to QRS complexes as well. As in the findings described previously,[74,75] deflation timed to the J point, with adjustment for the delay between onset of isovolumic systole and aortic valve opening, and perhaps slightly later, was shown early in the IABP literature to improve stroke volume.[38]

OTHER CONSIDERATIONS

A common problem has been proper timing in patients with underlying arrhythmias. Atrial fibrillation has been particularly vexing, with unpredictable beat-to-beat intervals. An algorithm to predict the occurrence of the distance between the QRS and the dicrotic notch was developed in the mid-1990s.[76] Newer dicrotic notch prediction algorithms using high-fidelity micromanometer pressure sensors have been described.[47] However, atrial fibrillation poses difficulties beyond timing alone; rapid ventricular rates result in a disproportionate decrease in the diastolic interval and limit the effectiveness of IABP because of the inherently short period of counterpulsation,[77] including subtraction of the fixed time interval required for shuttling helium into and out of the balloon. Operating at 1:2 rates may be required in this setting.

Lack of augmentation despite proper timing should result in troubleshooting the IABP console, checking with fluoroscopy to visualize inflation of the balloon and confirm the level of balloon placement, and excluding kinking of the gas line or other mechanical failures. Apparently normal IABP function with absence of hemodynamic improvement should raise a suspicion that the patient has a baseline hemodynamic state that will not benefit from LV unloading, in particular hypovolemia, sepsis, or profound hemodynamic collapse, as well as a number of conditions described subsequently (see "Contraindications").

Overall, timing of IABP should result in diastolic pressure augmentation and lowering of assisted peak systolic pressure when possible, with the former a generally used end point for patients with shock and the latter the primary goal in patients with more stable hemodynamics at the time of IABP insertion.

ADJUNCTIVE PHARMACOTHERAPY

Adjunctive pharmacotherapy typically includes heparinization. There are two theoretical reasons for anticoagulation: First, in patients receiving less than 1:1 counterpulsation, there is concern regarding clot formation on the balloon apparatus, and second, stagnant blood around the catheter shaft, especially in the common femoral artery, has been thought to raise the risk of thrombosis. The general consensus has been that anticoagulation should be administered if not contraindicated. The balloons themselves have a thrombogenic surface,[45] and occlusion of vessels requiring thromboembolectomy has been reported to be one of the most common complications, reaching nearly 3% in one series of 911 patients undergoing coronary artery bypass grafting (CABG).[53] Nevertheless, the thinking on this is in flux, with a growing evidence base that routine anticoagulation does not prevent thrombosis or thromboembolism but does increase bleeding risk. Thus, a recent study[78] compared routine heparin use versus selective anticoagulation only in those patients with an indication for heparin use other than IABP insertion. There was no difference in the rates of IABP-related complications including major limb ischemia, but anticoagulated patients had a higher incidence of non-access-site bleeding, predominantly gastrointestinal. A randomized trial had similar conclusions, although the course of counterpulsation was relatively brief.[79] Review of the best evidence to date leads to the somewhat controversial conclusion that anticoagulation may be best targeted to selected patients who are at risk of thrombosis or thromboembolism for reasons other than IABP use alone.[80]

A second adjunctive pharmacotherapy issue is the use of prophylactic antibiotics. Although fever, bacteremia, and sepsis were reported to be common (occurring at rates of 47%, 15%, and 12%, respectively) in one small study,[81] the infection rate in larger series has been less than 1%,[53] and the consensus is that the evidence base is too thin and the public health implications too unfavorable to recommend routine antibiotic use unless otherwise clinically warranted.[82] A third medication issue relates to sedation. Continuous bed rest in a critical care setting is frequently associated with disorientation or agitation. Balloon migration from leg bending and patient movement risks significant trauma to the aorta, renal arteries, and head and neck vessels. Careful sedation is essential. Finally, antiarrhythmic agents to slow and regularize the heart rate can have important benefits for lengthening diastole and optimizing balloon timing, both of which in turn enhance IABP augmentation.

BALLOON REMOVAL

Removal of the IABP poses several challenges. First, the ability to maintain hemodynamic stability without counterpulsation must be confirmed as part of the weaning process. Although cardiac output is disproportionately decreased with lowering of pumping ratios, such lowering appears superior to decreasing volumes as a weaning method, an approach confirmed by one small retrospective evaluation.[83] The balloon should not be turned off completely until the activated clotting time value confirms that anticoagulation has been effectively discontinued and the patient is ready for balloon removal, because thrombosis on the balloon surface occurs rapidly.[45] Most operators run the IABP at a low cycle rate, 1:3 to as low as 1:8 (depending on manufacturer), until anticoagulation has worn off sufficiently and the balloon can be removed. Nonfunctioning or stopped IABPs must be removed promptly, preferably within 20 minutes or less. A second challenge relates to the size of the deflated balloon. Because the balloon is delivered prefolded by the manufacturer (see Fig. 7.3), it passes readily through its delivery sheath during insertion. Once inflated, it will not refold when vacuum is applied, and the profile is too large for retrieval without bringing both the sheath and the balloon out of the body together.

Removing the balloon, especially after long indwelling times (mean indwelling time is 53 to 77 hours[41,48]), requires meticulous attention to several details. First, the balloon gas line should be aspirated to reduce the balloon profile. Second, it is essential to allow some bleeding after catheter removal and prior to compression to avoid stripping any clot off the balloon inside the common femoral artery. Because these are relatively large catheters, frequently deployed in patients with vascular disease who have a tenuous hemodynamic status even at the time of IABP removal, patients may not tolerate prolonged and aggressive compression of the groin. Recent discontinuation of heparin combined with a large arteriotomy size can result in significant difficulty in controlling hemorrhage and achieving hemostasis.

Surgical closure is sometimes preferable, particularly with severely obese patients, after very long indwelling times, with uncorrectable anticoagulation status, or with low or high punctures.[84] Vascular closure devices have been used successfully in small series[85,86] but require extreme caution; significant mortality risk is associated with infections related to vascular closure devices,[87] and assuring sterility at the time of IABP removal is difficult. When use of a closure device is required, the authors typically place a 0.018-inch stiff guidewire inside the lumen after extensive efforts to achieve sterility of both the field and the device, withdraw the IABP, and place the closure device over the wire; we cannot recommend this off-label approach, however, until a better evidence base is available. Finally, it is important to continue to monitor patients for adverse events because nearly 25% of IABP-related complications have been reported to occur *after* IABP removal.[88]

INDICATIONS

As with the original patients in 1968,[10] CS remained the most common indication for several decades, although later data suggest that circulatory support for percutaneous intervention has replaced hemodynamic instability in the acute MI setting as the primary indication for IABP insertion.[41] Other common indications are perioperative support for patients undergoing cardiac surgery, weaning from cardiopulmonary bypass, management of unstable angina, severe congestive heart failure, and with less evidence base, refractory ventricular arrhythmias or angina after MI as well as a host of miscellaneous settings largely defined by case reports (Box 7.1).

In general, indications can be divided into several categories: prophylactic versus therapeutic; hemodynamic support versus improved end-organ flow; and preoperative, intraoperative, or postoperative management. The rate of prophylactic use, defined as IABP insertion prior to percutaneous or surgical intervention, rose from 17.3% in 1992 to 31.3% in 2001 as a proportion of IABP use in the United States according to the Benchmark Registry.[4] The management and particularly the complications associated with these subcategories are substantially different. Box 7.1 lists indications for IABP use. The class I indications include CS if not quickly reversible with pharmacologic therapy, acute mitral insufficiency or ventricular septal rupture, recurrent ischemia or infarction, hypotension that does not respond to other interventions, and a low output state.

In general, use of an IABP identifies a high-risk population, with in-hospital mortality rate exceeding 20% among more than 22,000 patients (Fig. 7.10).[4,48,89] The Benchmark Registry examined the use of IABP in more than 5000 patients with acute MI; this represented 24% of all IABP placements at the 250 participating medical centers. Twenty-seven percent of the patients were in CS, an additional 12% needed support because of acute ventricular septal rupture or severe mitral insufficiency, and 5% underwent IABP placement for refractory LV failure. Thus, nearly half the patients with IABP placements and MI had hemodynamic settings in which balloon support was considered potentially life sustaining.[48] Recent data confirm extensive IABP use in high-risk patients undergoing PCI: 44.4% of CS patients, 10.3% of patients presenting with ST-segment elevation myocardial infarction (STEMI), 28.1% of those undergoing left main PCI, and 13.9% of patients with LV function less than 30%.[2]

Despite general acceptance of its utility in salvaging myocardium and decreasing mortality risk (even without a strong evidence base), and despite a significant associated complication rate, there are no separate American College of Cardiology/American Heart Association guidelines for placing an IABP.[90] However, indications for IABP use are included in the Guidelines for ST-Segment Elevation Myocardial Infaction[91] and in the more recent Guidelines for Percutaneous Coronary Intervention[92]; hemodynamic support devices are currently considered a class I indication in the setting of CS, although as described subsequently, the evidence base is in flux. It is important to note that severe hemodynamic deterioration, including CS, is not limited to acute MI patients with ST-segment elevation.[93]

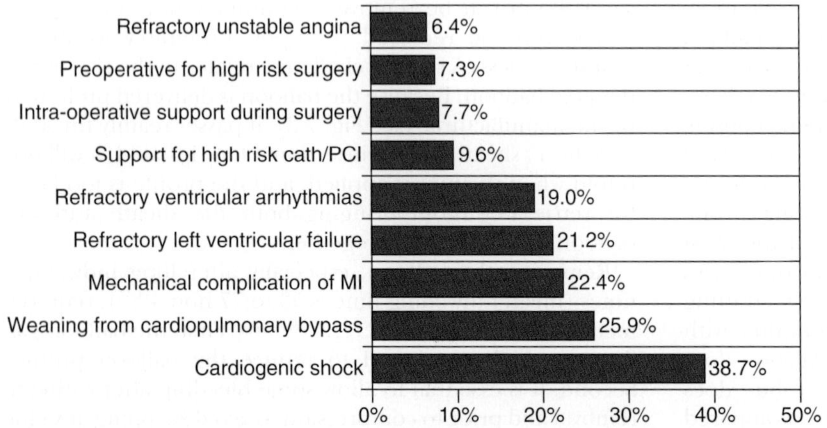

Figure 7.10 In-hospital mortality rate in 5495 patients with acute myocardial infarction (MI) enrolled in the Benchmark Registry. Note the threefold higher mortality rate among patients with rescue placement of intra-aortic balloon pumps (IABPs) compared with those in whom IABPs were inserted preoperatively for high-risk surgery, and the continuing high mortality rate for patients with cardiogenic shock. Cath, cardiac catheterization; PCI, percutaneous coronary intervention. (Adapted from Stone GW, Ohman EM, Miller MF, et al: Contemporary utilization and outcomes of intra-aortic balloon counterpulsation in acute myocardial infarction: The Benchmark Registry. J Am Coll Cardiol 2003;41:1940-1945.)

Box 7.1 Indications for Use of an Intra-aortic Balloon Pump

Acute ST-Segment Elevation Myocardial Infarction (STEMI)*

Class I Indications

Cardiogenic shock not promptly reversed with pharmacologic therapy
Acute mitral regurgitation
Ventricular septal rupture
Recurrent ischemia and infarction
Hypotension not responding to other interventions
Low-output state

Class II Indications

IIa: Refractory polymorphic ventricular tachycardia
IIb: Refractory pulmonary congestion

Additional Recommendations

In patients with cardiogenic shock after STEMI who are not candidates for revascularization
As a short- or long-term mechanical support as bridge to recovery or heart transplant

Other Settings†

Percutaneous Intervention

High-risk coronary angioplasty
- Acute coronary syndrome with hemodynamic instability
- Severe left ventricular (LV) dysfunction
- Unprotected left main vessel or single remaining vessel intervention

Hemodynamic support for decompensated patients undergoing structural heart disease interventions

Cardiac Surgery

Preoperative use
- Severe LV dysfunction
- Left main vessel disease
- Acute coronary syndrome
- Repeat thoracotomy

Perioperative or postoperative use
- Hemodynamic deterioration
- Inability to wean from bypass

Unstable Angina

Uncomplicated Myocardial Infarction (MI)‡

Congestive Heart Failure

Fulminant myocarditis
Decompensated aortic stenosis‡
Drug toxicity‡
Thyrotoxicosis‡
Multiple sclerosis‡
Lightning strike‡
Right ventricular (RV) failure‡
- RV infarction
- After heart transplantation
- Bridge to transplantation

Miscellaneous

Cardiopulmonary resuscitation‡
Noncardiac surgery
- Recent MI
- Left ventricular failure
- Unrevascularized myocardium
- Emergency surgery

*Based on Antman EM, Anbe DT, Armstrong PW, et al: ACC/AHA guidelines for the management of patients with ST-elevation myocardial infarction: A report of the American College of Cardiology/American Heart Association Task Force on Practice Guidelines (Committee to Revise the 1999 Guidelines for the management of patients with acute myocardial infarction). J Am Coll Cardiol 2004;44:E1-E211; and Levine GN, Bates ER, Blankenship JC, et al: 2011 ACCF/AHA/SCAI Guidelines for percutaneous coronary intervention: A report of the American College of Cardiology Foundation/American Heart Association Task Force on Practice Guidelines and the Society for Cardiovascular Angiography and Interventions. J Am Coll Cardiol 2011:58:2550-2583.
†Based on available literature (cited in text) without formal guidelines.
‡Minimal or inconsistent evidence base for indication.
Class I, conditions for which there is evidence for or general agreement that the procedure is benefical, useful, and effective; Class II, conditions for which there is conflicting evidence or a divergence of opinion about the usefulness or efficacy of a procedure.
Distribution of Indications from the Benchmark Registry[37]

Cardiogenic shock	18.8%
Acute mitral regurgitation or ventricular septal defect	5.5%
Refractory arrhythmia	1.7%
High-risk percutaneous intervention	20.6%
Preoperative cardiac surgery	13.0%
Perioperative and postoperative cardiac surgery	16.1%
Unstable angina (including post-MI)	12.3%
Refractory congestive heart failure	6.5%
Miscellaneous or information missing	5.5%

CARDIOGENIC SHOCK

The classic understanding of CS has been stunning or irreversible loss of a large amount of myocardium (≥40%) with resultant low output and compensatory elevated systemic vascular resistance to maintain central organ perfusion pressure. The definition of CS has varied, but the essential elements are persistent tissue hypoperfusion secondary to cardiac dysfunction in the presence of adequate filling pressure (and elevated left-sided heart filling pressure). The most common current definition is hypotension (blood pressure < 90 mm Hg systolic) for more than 30 minutes, with low cardiac index (less than 1.8 L/minute/m^2 without support or less than 2.2 L/minute/m^2 with support), and finally, elevated filling pressure (pulmonary artery wedge pressure > 15 mm Hg or LV end-diastolic pressure > 18 mm Hg or RV end-diastolic pressure > 10-15 mm Hg).[94] Data from the SHOCK (SHould we emergently revascularize Occluded Coronaries in cardiogenic shocK) trial have called several classic assumptions into question,[95] in part because some of the patients in this trial with CS had relatively preserved ejection fractions, whereas other patients with apparently much larger amounts of dysfunctional or nonfunctional heart muscle were hemodynamically compensated.

Although the incidence of CS has declined,[96] it remains significant; the most recent estimates are that it is seen in approximately 6% of acute MIs. Mortality rate, once described as high as 80% (though variable in the literature, primarily because of the multiple definitions used), has declined in part because of better interventional tools,[97] because patients with coronary artery disease are receiving better long-term medical therapy, which in turn helps limit infarct size, and because the pharmacotherapy for CS itself has improved. Mortality rate remains high, however, with a nearly 40% in-hospital death rate reported in the Benchmark Registry.[48]

IABP use in CS dates to the beginning of the IABP experience, and it results in predictable hemodynamic improvement in the majority of patients. IABPs have been shown to be beneficial in the setting of acute MI and CS when patients are *not* treated with PCI. The National Registry of Myocardial Infarction (NRMI) 2 compared results in patients with CS who received adjunct IABPs and those who did not.[98] Although mortality rate was not affected in patients undergoing primary angioplasty, those receiving only thrombolytic therapy had a significantly higher mortality rate (67% without IABP vs. 49% with IABP). Similar findings were shown in the SHOCK trial[99] as well as a meta-analysis of more than 10,000 STEMI patients with CS.[100] A small and underpowered randomized trial also suggested that patients with Killip class III or IV heart failure after MI have lower mortality rates when treated with fibrinolysis combined with IABP than when treated with fibrinolysis alone.[101] There is some basis for these findings from animal data, which suggest improved reperfusion when thrombolysis without other intervention is combined with IABP use.[25]

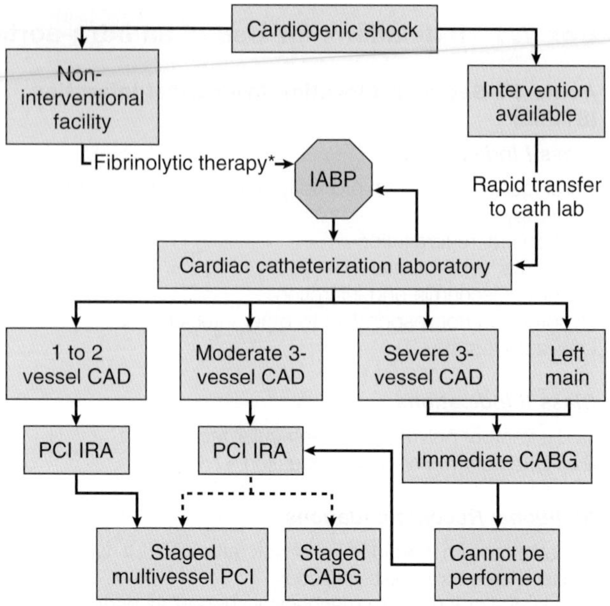

Figure 7.11 Algorithm for management of cardiogenic shock based on the SHOCK trial. Central to the treatment algorithm is rapid institution of intra-aortic balloon pump (IABP) treatment. For patients admitted to a hospital without interventional capacity, fibrinolytic therapy and IABP placement (if available) should be followed by rapid transfer to an interventional facility; if IABP treatment is unavailable, it can be started on the patient's arrival in the catheterization laboratory (cath lab) at an intervention-capable institution. *Fibrinolytic therapy should be given if there is more than a 90-minute delay until percutaneous coronary intervention (PCI) is available, less than 3 hours have passed since onset of infarction, and fibrinolysis is not contraindicated. CABG, coronary artery bypass grafting; CAD, coronary artery disease; IRA, infarct-related artery. (Adapted and modified from Hochman JS: Cardiogenic shock complicating acute myocardial infarction: Expanding the paradigm. Circulation 2003;107:2998-3002, used by permission of the American Heart Association.)

INTRA-AORTIC BALLOON PUMP USE AS AN ADJUNCT TO REVASCULARIZATION IN CARDIOGENIC SHOCK

Figure 7.11 provides an algorithm for CS management; it is notable that IABP is at the center of the algorithm, and part of early management in all patients except those with rapid response to initial pharmacologic interventions. Based largely on indirect evidence, it has been assumed that use of IABP as an adjunct to coronary intervention in CS improves outcomes.[102] Findings have included a nearly 60% reduction in the rate of major adverse events (ventricular fibrillation, cardiopulmonary resuscitation, prolonged hypotension) in the cardiac catheterization laboratory (odds ratio 2:1) after IABP insertion.[103] A trend toward lower 30-day and 1-year all-cause mortality rate has been demonstrated in patients in whom IABPs have been inserted within 1 day of presentation with CS,[104] albeit with a higher associated complication rate. Stabilization of patients with IABP and thrombolytic therapy and subsequent transfer for coronary intervention also appeared to have favorable effects on survival,[105] mimicking animal data showing that reperfusion combined with IABP is superior to reperfusion alone in salvaging heart muscle.[106] IABP plus mechanical ventilation may also have incremental benefit in CS management.[107]

However, a growing body of evidence suggests that IABP use may have at best modest benefits in CS when combined with acute intervention for revascularization. Most notably, the IABP SHOCK-II trial randomized IABP use in CS patients undergoing PCI.[108] No benefit of IABP was shown on 30-day mortality rate; a number of study design concerns exist (in particular between group crossovers and selection of a relatively low risk CS population) as well as the possibility that IABP placement before rather than after PCI (most patients had IABP placement after revascularization) would have shown additional benefit.[109] A smaller study, IABP SHOCK,[110] demonstrated no significant improvement in serial APACHE (Acute Physiology and Chronic Health Evaluation) II scores with IABP use. Several meta-analyses have come to similar conclusions,[100,111] albeit with evidence that IABP does have more readily demonstrable hemodynamic benefit; a more detailed examination of a small subset of patients did not confirm these hemodynamic benefits when compared to medical therapy alone.[112] The bottom line, that the routine use of IABP in CS patients undergoing PCI should remain a class I indication, is thus under considerable scrutiny.[113]

An important consideration for the use of IABP in shock is that the cause should not be hypovolemia. Similarly, patients with shock and preserved systolic function are unlikely to benefit; settings such as vigorous ejection fraction in patients who have volume-depleted hypertrophic left ventricles may lead to deterioration with IABP placement, even without outflow obstruction, whereas use of the device with dynamic outflow obstruction can lead to hemodynamic collapse.

Finally, consideration has been given to the use of IABP in RV infarction; isolated RV failure occurs in approximately 3% of patients with CS.[114] In this setting, patients commonly have severe hemodynamic decompensation and their overall prognosis is poor;[115] within the cohort of patients with CS, however, RV dysfunction is associated with inferior MI and a relatively better prognosis than CS based on LV dysfunction alone.[116] IABP use does not reliably result in hemodynamic improvement with RV infarction, and a variety of RV assist devices have been investigated, including pulmonary artery counterpulsation[117] and a right atrium–pulmonary artery bypass pump.[117,118] An occasional consideration in RV infarction is right-to-left shunting across a patent foramen ovale because of acute elevation in right-sided heart filling pressures, which result in a gradient that drives right-to-left atrial flow. Unloading of the left ventricle with an IABP can potentially exacerbate such shunting.[119]

MECHANICAL COMPLICATIONS OF ACUTE MYOCARDIAL INFARCTION

Afterload reduction has significant hemodynamic benefits in patients with abnormal unloading of the left ventricle into the right ventricle (ventricular septal rupture) or left atrium (severe mitral regurgitation).[120] The theoretical effect of counterpulsation in lowering afterload is in improving the ratio of forward flow through the aortic valve. The physiologic benefit in acute mitral insufficiency (mitral regurgitation) is widely accepted, resulting in a higher percentage of patients with severe mitral regurgitation and CS receiving IABP support than patients with CS alone.[121] The mechanism of benefit appears to be lowered aortic impedance with consequent improvement in cardiac output, and modest decrease in regurgitant fraction.[122] The IABP is in use in nearly all (98%) patients in this setting undergoing mitral valve repair, compared with less than half (43%) of those treated without surgery, a difference also influenced by selection issues. As with acute mitral regurgitation, 75% of ventricular septal rupture patients in the SHOCK registry underwent IABP placement.[123] Although systolic pressure did rise (from a median 81 mm Hg to 102 mm Hg) with institution of IABP in patients with ventricular septal rupture, mortality rate was dismal in both groups. In-hospital survival rate was only 13% with ventricular septal rupture, compared with 45% with severe mitral regurgitation. Nevertheless, IABP use is an essential element of intervention in acute ventricular septal rupture, and one goal of therapy has been stabilization before closure of the defect is undertaken.[124]

ACUTE MYOCARDIAL INFARCTION WITHOUT SHOCK

IABP use for uncomplicated acute MI is controversial. As with many modalities that lower myocardial oxygen demand, IABP theoretically helps decrease infarct size, even when reperfusion does not take place.[106] However, a number of older trials and two randomized trials from the past decade did not demonstrate compelling risk-to-benefit ratios with routine IABP use in acute MI patients undergoing PCI,[125,126] nor did a more recent study assessing myocardial infarct size using cardiac MRI.[127] The findings conform to a meta-analysis that showed no benefit along with a small increase in stroke and bleeding.[100] Economic analysis did not demonstrate significant increase in hospital costs in patients randomly assigned to undergo routine IABP insertion in this setting.[128] The potential benefit of the IABP in maintaining higher infarct artery patency has been demonstrated in two randomized studies showing that an open artery is more likely at 5 days[129] and at 3 weeks[130] in patients randomly assigned to IABP placement.

IABP has been used to manage recurrent ischemia and malignant ventricular arrhythmias in the peri-infarction setting, although the evidence base for these indications is less compelling, and both are class II indications (see Box 7.1) in patients with STEMI.[91]

UNSTABLE ANGINA

IABP use in unstable angina dates from an era in which the available alternatives were medical therapy and coronary bypass surgery, and IABP was utilized to stabilize patients before they were taken to the operating room. In certain settings, such as severe left main coronary artery disease discovered in the cardiac catheterization laboratory or in unstable angina with attendant hemodynamic instability, this approach is still appropriate.[131] Reducing myocardial oxygen demand frequently stabilizes these patients, and the IABP may have additional benefits during subsequent revascularization in the cardiac catheterization laboratory or operating room, as discussed later.

PROPHYLACTIC USE FOR CORONARY INTERVENTION

Prophylactic use of an IABP prior to PCI has generally been considered to be a sound strategy for high-risk patients, typically defined as having acute coronary syndrome with hemodynamic instability, severe LV dysfunction and extensive coronary disease, or left main/last remaining vessel intervention. Prophylactic IABP insertion in this setting had substantially better outcomes than rescue IABP placement according to retrospective multivariate analysis,[132] including evaluation of high-risk patients with severely depressed LV ejection fraction[133] undergoing angioplasty and patients undergoing unprotected left main PCI,[134] though the level of evidence base was generally weak. BCIS-1 (Balloon Pump-Assisted Coronary Intervention Study) randomly assigned patients to elective use of IABP prior to PCI in high-risk patients. Whereas it failed to demonstrate a significant benefit, a nonsignificant trend to decreased morality rate was seen (4.6% vs. 7.4%) and may reflect the underpowered nature of the trial. There was significant crossover in this study as well; crossover tends to dilute the power of studies that examine the use of already available technology, particularly when there is a perception on the part of clinicians that the device is efficacious, even if the efficacy is unproven.[135] IABP use in this setting is currently class IIb,[92] and is discussed further in this chapter under "Newer Technologies."

A partial explanation for the less-than-compelling evidence for the use of prophylactic IABP in this setting is the misconception that IABP provides adequate protection to allow prolonged ischemia in a critical vascular bed during coronary intervention. With total occlusion of flow to a large amount of myocardium, such as with unprotected left main angioplasty or angioplasty of a sole remaining vessel, hemodynamics may be preserved during the procedure, and ischemia and necrosis may be limited by lowering of myocardial oxygen demand effectuated by IABP. However, because cardiac output remains dependent on LV ejection, myocardial oxygen demand is substantially higher than when temporary cardiac or cardiopulmonary bypass is used, and significant stunning or necrosis or both of heart muscle can occur despite IABP use during high-risk angioplasty.

CARDIAC SURGERY

IABP is utilized in approximately 10% to 15% of patients undergoing cardiac surgery, with substantial rise in the rate in the past decade.[136] About half of this use is for coronary bypass patients; two-thirds of the CS patients in the Society of Thoracic Surgeons database had insertion of IABPs.[137] A number of studies have demonstrated a favorable influence on outcomes, including mortality rate.[138-140] Nevertheless, there is considerable variability in use among centers, reflecting a lack of consensus regarding indications for perioperative IABP use.[136,141] The vast majority of IABP insertions occur preoperatively.[136,137] The effectiveness of this approach has been controversial. One small randomized trial of high-risk patients demonstrated lower mortality rate, higher postoperative cardiac index, and shorter intubation time, intensive care unit (ICU) stay, and hospitalization in patients with preoperative IABP placement.[131] Mortality rate benefit was also observed in a retrospective single center experience[142] as well as a meta-analysis.[143] In contrast, a propensity analysis suggested excess mortality rate in nearly 2,000 patients receiving preoperative IABP insertion compared with 28,000 who did not.[144] Because of the limitations of propensity analysis, it is possible that selection bias determined the unfavorable outcomes associated with preoperative IABP use. Patients most likely to benefit from preoperative IABP insertion are those with depressed LV function, unstable angina or recent MI, or left main coronary artery disease or those who are undergoing repeat thoracotomy.

Several mechanisms can be postulated for superior outcomes with preoperative IABP insertion. Counterpulsation can provide hemodynamic support during anesthesia induction and during the stress of surgery before cardiopulmonary bypass is begun.[140,145] As already described, IABP with pulsatile flow during cardiopulmonary bypass also appears to have favorable effects on end-organ perfusion[26,146,147] with protection of both coronary and cerebral blood flow.[148] IABP insertion can also be used to assess prognosis; requirement for catecholamine support and overall hemodynamics 1 hour after institution of perioperative balloon pump insertion is highly predictive of overall outcome.[149]

Although studies have reported the mortality rate in high-risk patients treated with IABP as high as 53%, preoperative placement of an IABP was associated with substantially lower morbidity and mortality rates (24%), while postoperative insertion, in this case creating bias toward late insertion in situations with bad outcomes, was associated with a 63% mortality rate.[150] In the STS database, operative mortality rate in CS patients, the majority of whom received IABP, was high, ranging from 20% with isolated CABG to 33% for CABG and valve surgery and 58% for CABG and ventricular septal repair.[137] Similarly, a nonrandomized study of patients with an ejection fraction of 25% or less compared patients who were treated with preoperative IABP with those who were not. Mortality rate was 2.7% in the former group compared with 11.9% in the latter group, despite the presence of New York Heart Association (NYHA) class III or IV heart failure in 92% of the former and only 55% of the latter.[138] Several other post hoc analyses have found results consistent with advantages of preoperative IABP.[151,152]

Outcomes in addition to mortality rate that were superior in patients undergoing preoperative IABP insertion were duration of IABP support, length of hospital stay, and postoperative LV ejection fraction in a randomized study of high-risk patients with ejection fraction of 30% or less.[153] Similarly, preoperative use of an IABP in high-risk off-pump CABG patients appears to be favorable.[154,155] Thus, although the evidence base is incomplete, the overall preoperative use of IABP is growing.[136] Cost analysis appears to be favorable; combining high-risk cohorts randomly assigned to receive preoperative IABP placement or not,[131,145] costs were 36% less in patients with preoperative IABP insertion because of shorter IABP treatment time, shorter hospitalizations, and lower use of critical care facilities.[156]

CONGESTIVE HEART FAILURE

IABP has been used successfully in a variety of settings that results in congestive heart failure, including fulminant myocarditis[157] and severe decompensated aortic stenosis.[158] On the basis of case reports, the device has also been helpful as adjunctive therapy for myocardial depression secondary to drug toxicity,[159,160] myocardial contusion,[161] anaphylaxis,[162] thyrotoxicosis,[163] multiple sclerosis,[164] and even lightning strike.[165] Animal data suggest some benefit in the setting of RV failure;[166] the mechanism appears to be lowered pulmonary vascular resistance with consequent improvement in RV ejection.[28] IABP insertion has also improved outcomes in patients with acute RV failure after heart transplantation.[167]

Finally, IABP has been used as a bridge to transplantation, typically with placement in the axillary or external iliac arteries to allow ambulation during prolonged counterpulsation.[168] With development of a range of LV assist devices designed for long-term implantation, the use of IABP for this indication has waned.[169]

MISCELLANEOUS INDICATIONS

Limited data suggest that IABP placement during cardiopulmonary resuscitation has favorable effects.[170,171] The device has been used in pregnancy in patients undergoing heart surgery with an eye toward preserving uterine and fetal flow during cardiopulmonary bypass.[172] In patients at high risk for cardiac events during noncardiac surgery (e.g., recent MI, LV failure, unrevascularized ischemic myocardium),[173,174] IABP has been shown to have significant benefits for outcome,[175] although the evidence base consists largely of case reports;[176,177] a randomized trial has not been performed. Prophylactic IABP insertion seems particularly appropriate in high-risk patients undergoing emergency noncardiac surgery.[177]

USE OF THE INTRA-AORTIC BALLOON PUMP

Overall, the existing data suggest that IABP is underutilized. In more than 23,000 patients in CS reported by NRMI 2, only 31% were treated with IABP. As is the case for a number of other interventions, women were less likely to undergo IABP placement; there was an age and race difference as well, with lower rates in nonwhites and older patients.[178] A number of studies from the 1990s demonstrated less than 25% use of IABP in CS;[104,179] this figure contrasts with 86% utilization in the SHOCK trial.[102] Although some exclusion criteria in the latter may have improved suitability for IABP in the cohort enrolled in the study, the threefold higher use of the device in the SHOCK trial is consistent with wide underuse in clinical practice, similar to findings for a variety of pharmacologic and invasive interventions in acute MI.[90]

CONTRAINDICATIONS

The classic absolute contraindication to IABP use is aortic insufficiency (Box 7.2). Because the acute hemodynamic effects are so deleterious, animal and clinical investigations all date to the 1970s.[180] Increased retrograde volume displacement into the left ventricle during diastole greatly exacerbates wall stress, with greater potential for hemodynamic decompensation as well as LV pseudoaneurysm formation and LV rupture in the post-MI setting. The amount of aortic insufficiency that constitutes an absolute contraindication has no objective basis, but most operators use a threshold of trivial to mild. Similarly, the presence of aortic dissection or aortic aneurysm is considered an absolute contraindication because of the risk of extending dissection or causing aneurysmal rupture. Patent ductus arteriosus, like aortic insufficiency, theoretically has deleterious results from shunting of blood flow from the aorta with IABP induction, in this case increasing left-to-right shunting into the pulmonary artery. Generally, patients who have severe comorbid conditions at end of life or who exhibit brain death are considered to have contraindications to IABP placement.

Relative contraindications include placement of an indwelling foreign body into a patient with active infection including sepsis, severe peripheral vascular disease likely to result in limb ischemia, bleeding diathesis (although in practice, many patients who have low fibrinogen levels or are receiving aggressive anticoagulant or antiplatelet treatment undergo IABP placement), and contraindications to afterload reduction, such as dynamic LV outflow obstruction,[181] a condition that has on occasion been unmasked by institution of counterpulsation.[182] Patients with shock due to severe hypovolemia will not benefit from insertion and may deteriorate with IABP-induced afterload reduction.

Box 7.2 Contraindications to Use of Intra-aortic Balloon Pump

Absolute Contraindications

Aortic insufficiency*
Aortic dissection
Aortic aneurysm
Patent ductus arteriosus
Comorbidity with minimal survival expectancy
Brain death

Relative Contraindications

Hypovolemia
Severe peripheral vascular disease
Hypertrophic obstructive cardiomyopathy
Sepsis
Bilateral femoral-popliteal bypass grafts

*No evidence base exists for a minimal level of aortic insufficiency constituting an absolute contraindication.

COMPLICATIONS

From the initial experiences with IABPs in the 1960s, the significant complication rate has been the single largest drawback to its use (Table 7.1). The predominant complications have related to the access site, with bleeding and limb ischemia being the most common, but they also include infection, thrombocytopenia, stroke, device failure, and a variety of vascular misadventures. Table 7.1 describes complications of IABP from multiple registries, trials, and case reports. The complication rate associated with IABP is affected by the insertion of indwelling, typically 7 to 10 F devices into the femoral artery of patients with a high prevalence of diabetes, peripheral vascular disease, and other major comorbid conditions. As would be expected, duration of IABP use correlates with risk of complications overall,[183,184] including sepsis.[185,186] Thus, frequent reevaluation of the patient to confirm ongoing need for IABP is prudent. Death due to IABP has been relatively uncommon, with the rate typically less than 0.3% to as low as 0.05%,[41] and should be weighed against its considerable survival benefits.

The influence of procedure volume on outcomes has been demonstrated in a wide variety of cardiac procedures. Data from NRMI 2 found a significant correlation after multivariate analysis between number of IABP implants per year and CS mortality rate.[90] The study did not address complications related directly to IABP as a function of procedure volume for individual hospitals or operators. A higher rate of vascular complications was seen in the

Table 7.1 Complications with Use of Intra-aortic Balloon Pump (IABP) from the Benchmark Registry

Study Feature	All Benchmark Patients†	Patients with Myocardial Infarction Only‡
Year published	2001	2003
Total patients	16,909	5495
Reported Complication Rates		
All complications	7.0%	8.1%
Major*	2.8%	2.7%
Minor*	4.2%	5.4%
Vascular complications		
Limb ischemia	2.9%	2.3%
Major*	0.9%	0.5%
Vascular surgery	—	0.7%
Amputation	0.1%	0.1%
Hematologic complications		
Bleeding	2.4%	4.3%
Severe*	0.8%	1.4%
Infection	—	0.1%
Neurologic complications		
Stroke	—	0.1%
Death		
Due to IABP	0.05%	0.05%
Due to underlying morbidity	21.2%	20.0%
Others		
Deep vein thrombosis	—	0.1%
Bowel, renal, or spinal cord infarction	—	0.1%
Equipment malfunction	2.6%	2.3%
Balloon leak	1.0%	0.8%

**Major complications* are major limb ischemia, severe bleeding, balloon leak, and death attributable to IABP insertion or failure; *major limb ischemia* consists of loss of pulse, loss of sensation, or abnormal limb temperature or pallor requiring intervention, arterial repair, or amputation; *severe bleeding* is defined as bleeding that requires transfusion or surgical intervention or results in hemodynamic compromise. Independent risk factors for major complications were female gender, peripheral vascular disease, body surface area < 1.65 m^2, and age ≥ 75 years.

†Based on data from Ferguson JJ III, Cohen M, Freedman RJ Jr, et al: The current practice of intra-aortic balloon counterpulsation: Results from the Benchmark Registry. J Am Coll Cardiol 2001;38:1456-1462.

‡Based on data from Stone GW, Ohman EM, Miller MF, et al: Contemporary utilization and outcomes of intra-aortic balloon counterpulsation in acute myocardial infarction: The Benchmark Registry. J Am Coll Cardiol 2003;41:1940-1945.

quartile of hospitals performing the most IABP insertions in high-risk PCI in the NCDR database,[2] but after multivariate adjustment this difference was no longer present, likely reflecting substantially higher morbidity in that patient population.

Comparing overall complication rates among different series is hindered by lack of uniform definitions, variable demographics, comorbid conditions, duration of data collection, years when the data were collected (during which significant changes in technology may have occurred), and indications for IABP insertion. The rate of major complications has been reported to range from 2% to nearly 50%. However, the early data, which included surgical insertion, lack of a guidewire lumen for safer passage through the iliac arteries and aorta, and larger catheter and sheath sizes, were much worse than those in more recent series, with same center analyses describing as much as a fivefold decrease in major complications.[187] Thus, Kantrowitz and coworkers[188] reported a 47% complication rate over the first 15 years of IABP experience, and Alderman and colleagues[189] described a 42% rate of limb ischemia alone in their mid-1980s study. With improvements in technology, periprocedure pharmacology, patient selection, and management, the overall complication rates have declined to 15% in a large single hospital review published in 2000[50] and 6.5% in the Benchmark Registry, which incorporates the largest experience to date.[190] Although the series use variable definitions, the trend is unequivocal.

In general, diabetic patients and women have a higher complication rate,[188] coincident with the finding that these two populations also have significantly smaller femoral arteries.[49] A review of the existing literature on IABP complications shows peripheral vascular disease and female gender as nearly uniform markers of higher complication risk, with age, diabetes, size of catheter inserted, and smaller body surface area common but somewhat less consistent markers on multivariate analyses.[41,50]

VASCULAR COMPLICATIONS

Vascular complications including limb ischemia are the most common serious adverse events related to IABP insertion. Amputation is rare (0.1%),[41] but major limb ischemia, defined in the Benchmark Registry as "loss of pulse or sensation, or abnormal limb temperature or pallor requiring surgical intervention," occurred in 1.3% of cases.[190] Minor limb ischemia, defined as not requiring surgery and improving with balloon removal, occurred in another 1.2% in the same series. These numbers are consistent with steady improvement over the past decade: A smaller but still substantial earlier series from India involving 911 patients (with a much higher proportion of diabetic patients and likely significantly smaller body surface area) reported a 5.9% incidence of major vascular complications, and 5.8% rate of minor vascular complications.[53] This series used a 9.5 F shaft IABP, which has been shown to have higher vascular complication rates than the 8 F shaft balloons that have been available for the past decade.[191] Vascular complications, likely in part because of comorbid conditions, are associated with a much higher overall mortality rate—as much as a twofold increase.[88]

Trauma to the aorta has been reported, with paraplegia caused by spinal necrosis due to subadventitial hematoma,[192] cholesterol embolization to spinal and mesenteric arteries,[193] and aortic dissection[194] as well as no obvious cause in some patients. The presence of friable atheroma in the descending aorta has been associated with embolization.[195] IABP use has been identified as an independent predictor for neurologic complications of percutaneous intervention, although whether this is due to embolic phenomena or confounding variables has not been established.[196]

A complication particular to IABP is thrombocytopenia, occurring presumably because of destruction of platelets that adhere to the IABP surface, although the mechanism remains unclear. Critical care patients who have IABPs in place and are heparinized have a 7:1 odds ratio of a 50% drop in platelet count compared with patients without IABPs who are placed on heparin therapy at similar doses,[197] lowering the likelihood that heparin-induced thrombocytopenia is the etiologic factor.

MECHANICAL FAILURE

Several complications of mechanical failure of the balloon or console have serious consequences. Rupture of the balloon was more common early in the IABP era, with an incidence reported to range from 1.7%[198] to 5.2%.[199] Typically the diagnosis was made by the appearance of blood in the gas lumen, with triggering of alarms. The usual site of rupture has been at a point when the aorta is at its nadir in diameter along the course of the IABP. Small vessel size is associated with abrasion of the IABP (thus the observation that is it more common in women[200] likely correlates with their smaller body surface area); similar concerns arise for larger balloon sizes. Rupture of the balloon with a major gas leak, a rare event, has been reported to cause stroke secondary to gas embolization.[201] Hydrophilically coated balloons hold some promise for further reducing the risk of rupture through potentially decreasing abrasion of the balloon surface.[46] Fracturing of the IABP can occur with entrapment, including separation and migration of part of the device.[202] Clot may also form in the gas lumen after loss of balloon integrity and has been reported to interfere with balloon deflation, requiring use of a thrombolytic agent in the gas line to allow balloon deflation and removal of the balloon.[203]

TREATING COMPLICATIONS RELATED TO THE INTRA-AORTIC BALLOON PUMP

Several approaches to managing IABP-related complications have been proposed. Limb ischemia has traditionally been most successfully treated by removal of the IABP,[53,204] even in patients wholly dependent on the balloon, in order to avoid loss of limb. This situation has occasionally forced physicians and families to choose between loss of limb and patient survival. Surgical femoral-femoral shunting performed at the bedside with exteriorization of the graft has been described as one potential approach.[205] As previously mentioned, we have performed percutaneous nonsurgical external femoral-femoral shunting to effectively address limb ischemia by placing one sheath retrograde into the femoral artery contralateral to the IABP and another antegrade in the ipsilateral vessel, connecting the two sheaths with tubing and a flow regulator (see Fig. 7.5).[62] Infusion of prostaglandin E_1 through the balloon central lumen has been shown to relieve lower limb ischemia in a small series, presumably through increase in caliber of collateral vessels or relief of spasm in the common femoral or iliac system.[206]

NEWER TECHNOLOGIES

Kantrowitz, who began this work more than a half century ago, attempted to develop a permanent implantable IABP. Initial results of a pilot trial demonstrated substantial improvement in hemodynamics. The ability to use the device intermittently rather than continuously, theoretically without thromboembolic risk once fully endothelialized, and its location downstream from the head and neck vessels differentiate it from other ventricular assist devices.[207]

A number of other percutaneous extracorporeal assist devices have been developed, although they lack the flexibility of bedside insertion and the low profile of the IABP (Fig. 7.12). The TandemHeart device (CardiacAssist, Inc., Pittsburgh, PA) is a left atrial to femoroiliac bypass, powered by an external centrifugal pump that provides up to 4 L/minute of forward flow. It requires transseptal puncture, institution of cardiac bypass with much larger arterial cannulas than the IABP (21 F in the left atrium, 15 F to 17 F in the iliac artery), and in general is more complex with greater risk of complications, as shown in a randomized study comparing the two approaches in patients presenting with CS being considered for PCI.[208] It also cannot be shut off temporarily and requires more aggressive monitoring than balloon counterpulsation. Small randomized trials have been performed comparing the TandemHeart with IABP in patients with CS, demonstrating superior hemodynamics[208,209] with the TandemHeart device.

The Impella device (Abiomed, Danvers, MA) uses a miniaturized axial flow rotary pump fitted onto a pigtail catheter. It is placed retrogradely across the aortic valve. It pumps blood into the aorta and directly unloads the left ventricle.[210] The Impella 2.5 and 5.0 provide maximal flow of rates of 2.5 L/minute and 5.0 L/minute, respectively. Unlike the TandemHeart, it does not require transseptal puncture or extracorporeal circulation with the attendant complexity and risks but does require insertion of substantially larger hardware into the femoral artery than the IABP: A 13 F sheath is required for the Impella 2.5, whereas the shaft of the 5.0 device is 21 F. Both devices appear promising for circulatory support in a variety of settings but, unlike IABP, do not provide pulsatile flow.[211] Registry data utilizing Impella for high-risk PCI and for acute MI and CS showed consistent improvement in hemodynamics.[212,213] There are minimal data comparing IABP to Impella in patients with CS, with one small trial showing superior cardiac output during Impella use but an identical mortality rate.[214] In the setting of high-risk PCI, the PROTECT II trial compared prophylactic IABP to Impella: Hemodynamics were superior with Impella, but overall outcomes including 30-day major adverse events were similar, with some later trends that appeared to favor Impella use, albeit with study design and enrollment issues that may have confounded results. A caveat to Impella use in this setting relates to a higher adverse event rate in the setting of rotational atherectomy.[215] In a meta-analysis of three of the randomized clinical trials described previously,[208,209,214] hemodynamics consistently superior to IABP use were shown with TandemHeart and Impella, but these findings did not translate into a survival benefit;[216] it should be kept in mind that the TandemHeart and Impella devices are substantially more costly, complex

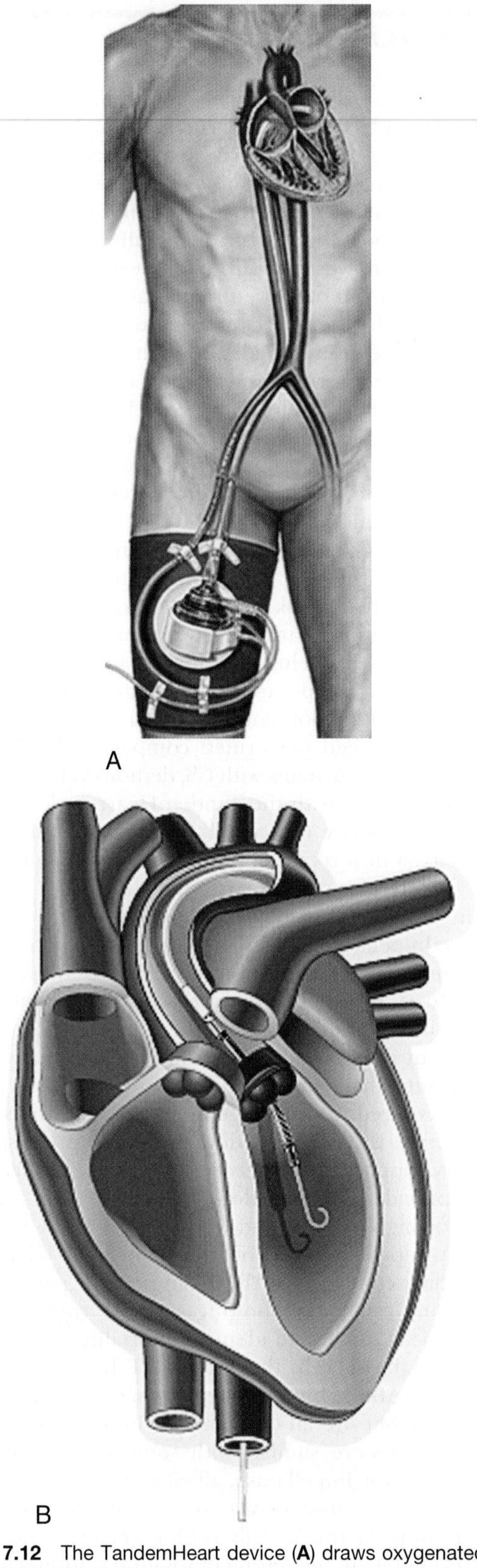

Figure 7.12 The TandemHeart device (**A**) draws oxygenated blood from a left atrial catheter placed across the interatrial septum and provides arterial return via a cannula placed into the femoral artery. The Impella catheter (**B**) draws blood from the left ventricle via a pigtail catheter placed retrograde across the aortic valve and pumps blood into the aorta. Although both devices actively provide systemic flow independent of left ventricular ejection, with superior hemodynamic results, neither delivers pulsatile flow and both require significantly larger arterial punctures than an intra-aortic balloon pump.

to institute and manage, and in the case of TandemHeart, appears to be associated with a higher complication rate.

Potential contraindications for both TandemHeart and Impella include aortic insufficiency and peripheral vascular disease. Aortic stenosis and presence of LV thrombus are contraindications for Impella use. Although post-MI ventricular septal rupture is uncommon, TandemHeart and Impella should be used with caution in that setting, because use of the devices could theoretically trigger right-to-left shunting because the substantial volume extraction from the left-sided heart circulation preferentially lowers LV pressure; however, despite the theoretical concern, a small series has documented benefit in this setting as well.[217] A number of other off-label uses of these devices have been described, including temporary support of the right ventricle[218] in RV infarction and as a bridge to ventricular assist devices and transplantation.

A vast array of other technologies is under development. The use of IABP in conjunction with assist devices that do not provide pulsatile flow may provide symbiotic preservation of end-organ circulation.[219,220]

KEY POINTS

- The IABP is the most widely utilized cardiac assist device, featuring modest though significant risk, straightforward percutaneous insertion, and excellent hemodynamic support.
- There is a wide range of indications for IABP use, from prophylactic support prior to percutaneous or surgical intervention to stabilization in the setting of CS.
- Unlike more complex ventricular assist devices, the IABP does not independently generate systemic output; thus, it provides auxiliary support of cardiac function.
- The primary benefit of IABP is decrease in afterload and secondary improvement in hemodynamics; diastolic perfusion pressure is augmented but end-organ total flow is usually not increased directly.
- Timing of IABP inflation and deflation, absence of arrhythmia, and length of diastole all contribute to the effectiveness of IABP.
- There is a growing evidence base for limiting anticoagulation use to clinical settings when there are indications other than IABP placement.
- A small but significant complication rate remains associated with IABP use, in particular, vascular compromise and bleeding.
- The routine use of IABP for high-risk PCI and acute MI with CS is under extensive review based on recent randomized trials; methodologic considerations in these studies make their impact on future guidelines uncertain.

SELECTED REFERENCES

36. Heinze H, Heringlake M, Schmucker P, et al: Effects of intra-aortic balloon counterpulsation on parameters of tissue oxygenation. Eur J Anaesthesiol 2006;23:555-562.

41. Ferguson JJ III, Cohen M, Freedman RJ Jr, et al: The current practice of intra-aortic balloon counterpulsation: Results from the Benchmark Registry. J Am Coll Cardiol 2001;38:1456-1462.
48. Stone GW, Ohman EM, Miller MF, et al: Contemporary utilization and outcomes of intra-aortic balloon counterpulsation in acute myocardial infarction: The benchmark registry. J Am Coll Cardiol 2003;41:1940-1945.
55. Erdogan HB, Goksedef D, Erentug V, et al: In which patients should sheathless IABP be used? An analysis of vascular complications in 1211 cases. J Card Surg 2006;21:342-346.
91. Antman EM, Anbe DT, Armstrong PW, et al: ACC/AHA guidelines for the management of patients with ST-elevation myocardial infarction: A report of the American College of Cardiology/American Heart Association Task Force on Practice Guidelines (Committee to Revise the 1999 Guidelines for the Management of patients with acute myocardial infarction). J Am Coll Cardiol 2004;44:E1-E211.
94. Reynolds HR, Hochman JS: Cardiogenic shock: Current concepts and improving outcomes. Circulation 2008;117:686-697.
108. Thiele H, Zeymer U, Neumann FJ, et al: Intraaortic balloon support for myocardial infarction with cardiogenic shock. N Engl J Med 2012;367(14):1287-1296.
110. Prondzinsky R, Lemm H, Swyter M, et al: Intra-aortic balloon counterpulsation in patients with acute myocardial infarction complicated by cardiogenic shock: The prospective, randomized IABP SHOCK Trial for attenuation of multiorgan dysfunction syndrome. Crit Care Med 2010;38:152-160.
127. Patel MR, Smalling RW, Thiele H, et al: Intra-aortic balloon counterpulsation and infarct size in patients with acute anterior myocardial infarction without shock: The CRISP AMI randomized trial. JAMA 2011;306:1329-1337.
215. O'Neill WW, Kleiman NS, Moses J, et al: A prospective randomized clinical trial of hemodynamic support with impella 2.5TM versus intra-aortic balloon pump in patients undergoing high-risk percutaneous coronary intervention: The PROTECT II Study. Circulation 2012;126(14):1717-1727.

The complete list of references can be found at www.expertconsult.com.

8 Echocardiography

Priscilla Peters | Hisham Dokainish

CHAPTER OUTLINE

Echocardiography has evolved to become a crucial noninvasive imaging modality in the critically ill patient. Its portability, safety, and widespread availability allow for the rapid diagnosis of life-threatening cardiac problems and rapid exclusion of cardiac disease in critically ill patients who present in an undifferentiated fashion. This chapter takes a systematic approach to the use of echocardiography in the critically ill, from the assessment of left ventricular (LV) and right ventricular (RV) function to valve disease, as well as pericardial disease, aortic disease, cardiac trauma, stroke, and rapid hemodynamic assessment.

APPROACH TO ECHOCARDIOGRAPHY

CARDIAC ANATOMY

Transthoracic echocardiography provides an excellent noninvasive means of assessing cardiac anatomy. Briefly, there are parasternal views, taken from approximately 2 cm leftward from the sternum and the fourth to fifth rib interspace, apical views, taken from the LV apex; subcostal views, taken from the epigastrium, and suprasternal views, taken from the sternal notch. Multiple images from different projections are needed to provide a complete view of the heart, manipulating the probe to provide long- and short-axis images of each structure interrogated.[1-3] The position of the echocardiographic transducer and the subsequent views produced are summarized in Figure 8.1.

BASIC ECHOCARDIOGRAPHIC PRINCIPLES

Echocardiography uses ultrasound (i.e., sound above the audible range) to evaluate the heart and proximal great vessels and typically combines two modalities: tissue imaging (M-mode and two-dimensional [2D]) and blood flow detection with velocity determination (Doppler). Cardiac tissue imaging is based on the transmission of ultrasound into the chest and its reflection by intrathoracic structures, which is determined by their acoustic properties. The two imaging modalities in general clinical use are M-mode and 2D imaging.

M-mode uses a single scan line or beam to produce what is known as the "ice-pick" or one-dimensional view through intracardiac structures along the path of the ultrasound beam. It has the advantage of an extremely high sampling rate (1000-3000 Hz compared to 20-60 Hz for traditional 2D imaging) because only a single beam path is interrogated. M-mode is useful for measuring linear dimensions (such as chamber dimensions) and for appreciating high-frequency motion (i.e., the vibration of a torn leaflet), as well as for timing of events, especially valve opening and closing. However, M-mode provides a very limited field of view and is now primarily used as an adjunct to 2D imaging.

Two-dimensional images are obtained from multiple sequential scan lines generated electronically (phased array) and processed to create a tomographic imaging plane with an expanded field of view. The time required to obtain all necessary scan lines reduces the frame rate to the range

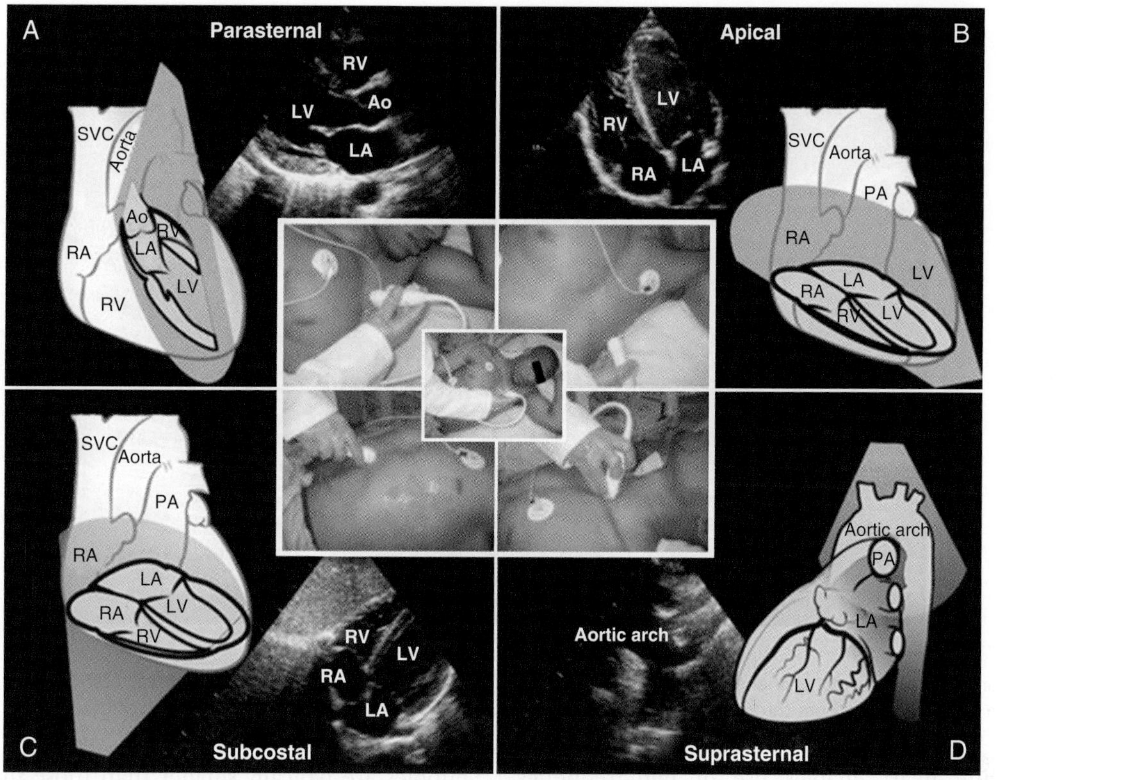

Figure 8.1 Line graphic demonstrating the four basic probe positions for transthoracic echocardiography. **A,** Parasternal long-axis (PLAX) imaging plane. **B,** Apical four-chamber (Ap4Ch) view. **C,** Subcostal view (Subx). **D,** Suprasternal notch view (SSN). Ao, aorta; LA, left atrium; LV, left ventricle; PA, pulmonary artery; RA, right atrium; RV, right ventricle; SVC, superior vena cava. (With kind permission of Springer Science+Business Media, Essential Echocardiography: A Practical handbook with DVD, Scott Solomon, Humana Press, May 2007.)

of 30 to 80 frames per second. Current ultrasound systems utilize both fundamental and harmonic imaging. Harmonic imaging transmits sound at a particular frequency (the *fundamental frequency*) but creates the image from sound reflected at twice the fundamental frequency, called the *second harmonic*, which improves image quality because the stronger harmonic signal undergoes considerably less distortion. This is particularly useful for endocardial border definition.

Doppler echocardiography uses ultrasound to determine blood flow velocity and direction within the heart. Two principal types of spectral Doppler techniques are used, termed *continuous wave* (CW) and *pulsed wave* (PW). CW uses two separate transducer crystals, one continuously transmitting and one continuously receiving the ultrasound signal. The high sampling rate of CW allows it to measure high velocities, but the source of any specific velocity measurement along the interrogated path cannot be differentiated (*range ambiguity*). On the other hand, PW uses one crystal, which alternates between sending and receiving an ultrasound pulse. The principal advantage of PW is that signals arise only from the area of interrogation, called the *sample volume* (*range resolution*); however, because the same crystal is used for sending and receiving the signal, a new pulse of ultrasound cannot be transmitted until the previous returning signal has been detected. This "pulsed" process results in too low a sampling rate to quantitate high velocities. PW and CW are thus complementary, with PW localizing the source of a signal and CW allowing for the unambiguous measurement of high velocities.[4] Color flow imaging is a form of PW in which information is coded with colors and superimposed on a 2D ultrasound image. Black and white identifies anatomic structures and color identifies blood flow velocities. Color Doppler has great utility in the evaluation of valvular regurgitant lesions and intracardiac shunts. An example of color Doppler identification of an atrial septal defect (ASD) with left-to-right shunting is shown in Figure 8.2. Pulsed Doppler can also evaluate the velocity of moving myocardium, which produces a signal of low velocity but high amplitude, named tissue Doppler imaging (TDI). Systolic and diastolic velocities within the myocardium and at the corners of mitral annulus can be recorded. Mitral annular velocities as measured by TDI are commonly used to evaluate diastolic function.[5]

ADDITIONAL ECHOCARDIOGRAPHIC MODALITIES

TRANSESOPHAGEAL ECHOCARDIOGRAPHY

When transthoracic echocardiography (TTE) image quality is suboptimal in certain patients in critical care—obesity, lung disease, uncooperative patient, ventilated patient, or when bandages or drainage tubes obscure the standard echo windows—transesophageal echocardiography (TEE) can be of great use.[6,7] TEE involves insertion into the esophagus of an endoscope-like probe with an ultrasound transducer on its tip. Image resolution is improved with TEE because the ultrasound beam is unimpeded by bone and air, and because

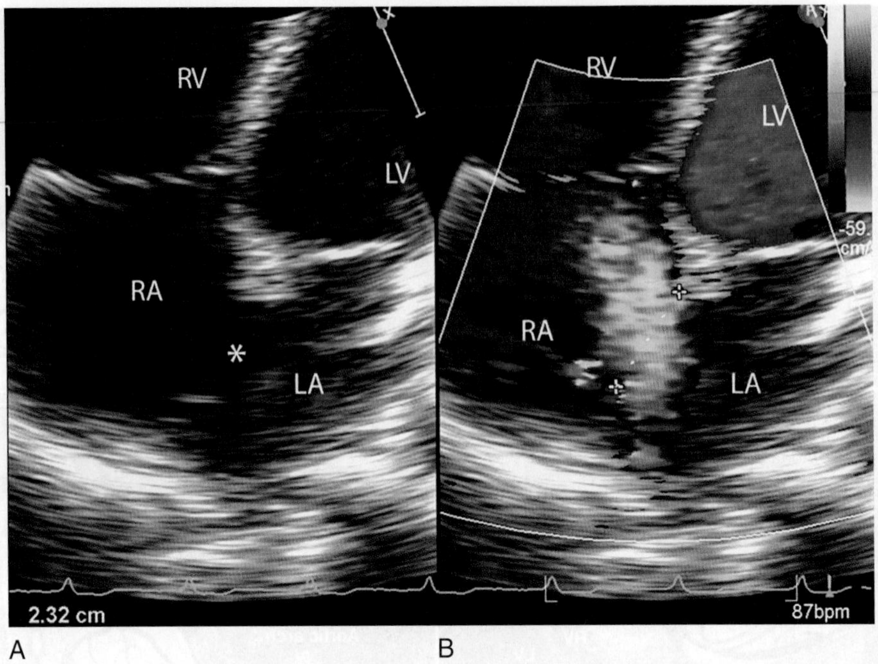

Figure 8.2 Color flow of secundum atrial septal defect (ASD). **A,** Apical image of dilated right-sided structures. Asterisk (*) indicates ASD. **B,** Color flow (*orange*) from left atrium through defect. LA, left atrium; LV, left ventricle; RA, right atrium; RV, right ventricle.

proximity to the heart enables use of high-frequency (7 MHz) probes. TEE can easily be performed at the bedside. Active esophageal disease is the major contraindication. A topical oral anesthetic spray is administered as well as an agent for conscious sedation. The TEE can be done with a nasogastric tube in place, but the nasogastric tube should be removed if there are any difficulties with passing the probe or in acquiring the images. Patients require blood pressure, respiratory, O_2 saturation, and heart rate monitoring during the procedure. A comprehensive transesophageal examination typically takes about 20 minutes for imaging, and then requires a period of recovery time.

CONTRAST ECHOCARDIOGRAPHY

SALINE CONTRAST

Echocardiographic contrast agents are substances that enhance the reflected ultrasound signal. Simple agitated saline contrast can be used to detect intracardiac shunts, commonly at the atrial level. To detect an intracardiac shunt, a contrast study can be done with agitated saline. In this technique, a 10-mL syringe containing 8 mL of normal saline is connected to a second 10-mL syringe containing 1 cm^3 of air via a three-way stopcock. Brisk exchange of the saline between the syringes creates microbubbles, which are then rapidly injected as an intravenous bolus, resulting in opacification of the right chambers of the heart. Saline contrast bubbles are too large to pass through the pulmonary capillaries but may appear in the left atrium and left ventricle as a result of passage across an intracardiac (ASD or patent foramen ovale [PFO]) or intrapulmonary communication; occasionally, a cough or Valsalva maneuver may transiently increase right-sided heart pressures and facilitate right-to-left crossover of bubbles.[8] Pulmonary arteriovenous malformations (AVMs) will demonstrate appearance of very small saline contrast in the left atrium; however, these bubbles are typically smaller than those that transit across an intracardiac shunt, and usually appear late after injection (after >7-10 beats) and persist after the right side of heart empties of contrast saline, representing the typical transit time of the contrast saline through the pulmonary bed and the AVM into the pulmonary veins. An example of saline contrast echocardiography with a right-to-left interatrial shunt is shown in Figure 8.3.

CONTRAST FOR LEFT VENTRICULAR OPACIFICATION

Commercially available contrast agents, specifically formulated to pass through the pulmonary capillary bed, can be used to opacify intracardiac chambers in order to enhance endocardial border definition. When activated, contrast agents yield perfluorocarbon microbubbles encapsulated in either a lipid or albumin shell, which exhibit lower acoustic impedance than blood and enhance the intrinsic backscatter of blood.[9] The most important clinical use of contrast agents in critical care is for left ventricular opacification (LVO), to be used when standard TTE images are suboptimal, which occurs in 25% or more of cases in the critical care setting.[10] These agents are useful in improving image quality in technically difficult echocardiograms and can provide significant additional diagnostic information, especially on LV function, the presence of LV apical thrombus, and detection of LV wall motion abnormalities.[11] Importantly, contrast for LVO has also been shown to reduce the need for other, more involved imaging modalities in the critical care population, such as TEE.[12-14] An example of contrast used for LVO in a patient with technically difficult echo windows is shown in Figure 8.4. In patients in whom contrast for LVO is used, the enhanced Doppler signals with the use of contrast can also be utilized for detection and measurement of faint tricuspid regurgitation (TR) signals for the estimation of pulmonary artery (PA) pressure, especially important in the critical care scenario.[10]

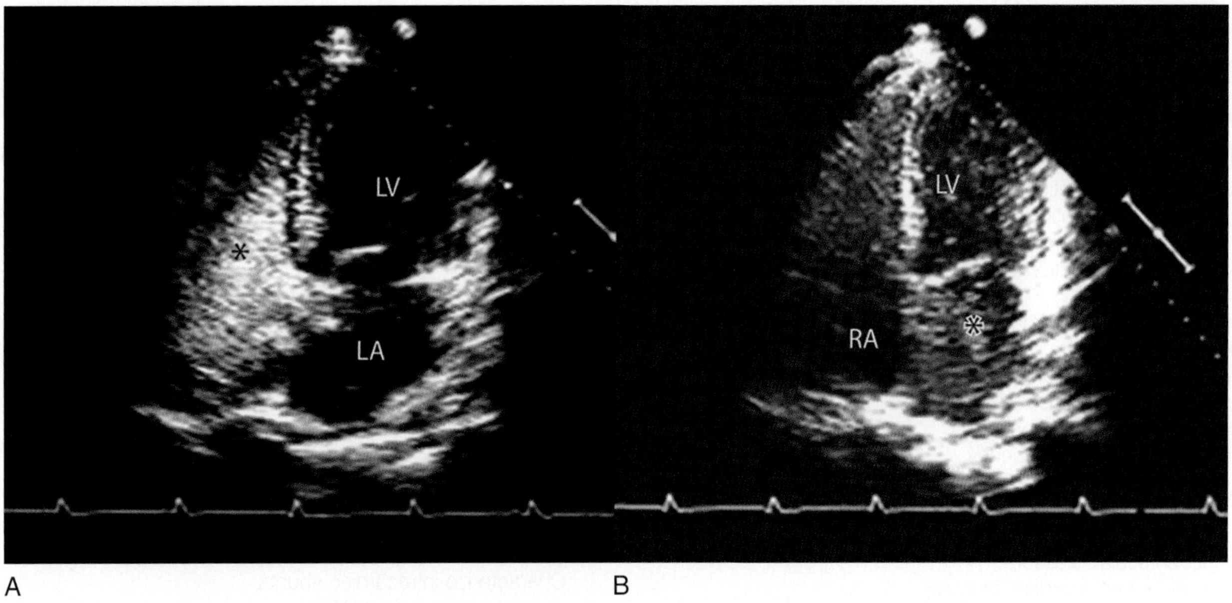

Figure 8.3 Young patient with hypoxia who had a saline contrast injection to rule out patent foramen ovale. **A,** Saline (*) enters right side of heart. **B,** Left side of heart opacifies with saline. LA, left atrium; LV, left ventricle; RA, right atrium.

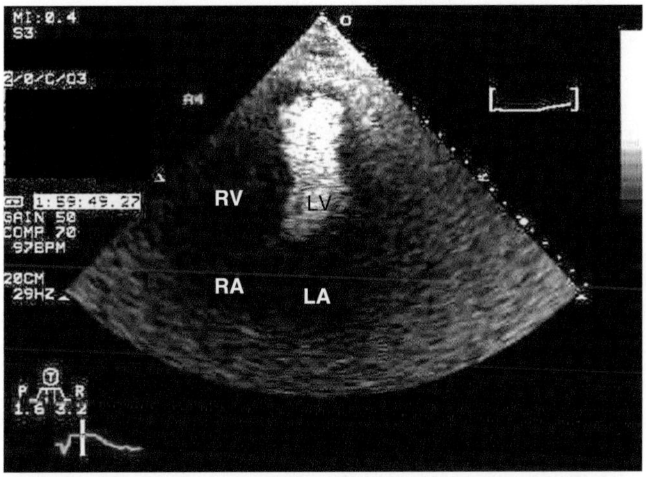

Figure 8.4 Apical four-chamber view with contrast enhancement demonstrating akinetic left ventricular apex during systole. LA, left atrium; LV, left ventricle; RA, right atrium; RV, right ventricle.

HANDHELD ECHOCARDIOGRAPHY

Handheld ultrasound devices are small, highly portable devices that can now be held in the palm of a hand. They can provide reasonable 2D and color Doppler images, have been shown to correlate reasonably well with full echocardiographic platforms, and detect clinically relevant findings.[15] Early concerns that unskilled users would obtain and subsequently misinterpret poor quality data have largely been ameliorated, and several reasonable studies suggest that noncardiology trained intensivists can successfully perform and correctly interpret a goal-directed transthoracic echocardiogram with a handheld device.[16,17] "Goal-directed" 2D imaging is typically limited to the assessment of biventricular size and function, and presence or absence of pericardial effusion. As handheld devices are technically adequate to evaluate major cardiac disease or trauma, a focused 2D study done by a trained individual with only a handheld device has great potential for rapid triage of patients in the emergency room or the intensive care area.[18-23] It is important to emphasize that unclear or ambiguous findings on handheld examination should be followed by a full study on a full echocardiographic platform to obtain accurate diagnosis; in addition, full Doppler interrogation for accurate detection of valve stenosis/regurgitation and accurate hemodynamic evaluation in suspected tamponade warrant comprehensive echocardiography on full-platform machines.

INDICATIONS FOR ECHOCARDIOGRAPHY

Although a broad range of critically ill patients are candidates for TTE to assess cardiac pathology and function, specific indications are summarized in Box 8.1. In general, any critical care patient with unexplained hypotension, pulmonary congestion, hemodynamic instability, known cardiac disease, a significant unexplained cardiac murmur, thoracic trauma, or suspected endocarditis are candidates for echocardiography. The most common use of TEE in critical care is inadequate or nondiagnostic TTE. Box 8.2 lists the major indications for use of TEE in critical care.

ASSESSMENT OF LEFT VENTRICULAR FUNCTION

SYSTOLIC FUNCTION

Although there are a variety of methods to assess LV systolic function by echocardiography (Doppler calculation of stroke volume, dP/dt using mitral regurgitation [MR] signal, tissue Doppler systolic velocity, and systolic strain and strain rate), the most commonly used and clinically relevant is the calculation or estimation of LV ejection fraction (EF).[24,25] As recommended in current guidelines,[24]

Box 8.1 Indications for Transthoracic Echocardiography in Critical Care

Hemodynamics

Left ventricular function
- Regional wall motion abnormalities
- Global dysfunction
- Transient dysfunction (sepsis, ischemic/catecholamine stunning)

Right ventricular function
Hypotension
Pericardial effusion/tamponade
Assess volume status
Outflow tract obstruction
Valvular stenosis/insufficiency

Hypoxia

Right ventricular function
Right ventricular pressure
Intracardiac/extracardiac shunting
Pulmonary embolus

Infections

Bacterial endocarditis

Trauma

Blunt thoracic trauma
Penetrating thoracic trauma

General

Assess proximal ascending aorta—dissection, hematoma
Source of murmur
Source of embolus
Procedural guidance (especially pericardiocentesis)

Table 8.1 Grading Left Ventricular Systolic Function by Left Ventricular Ejection Fraction

Systolic Function	Ejection Fraction
Hyperdynamic	>70%
Normal	55-70%
Mildly depressed	45-54%
Moderately depressed	30-44%
Severely depressed	<30%

calculation of left ventricular ejection fraction (LVEF) by method of discs (Fig. 8.5) is recommended, although visual estimation of LVEF is reliable when technically adequate images are evaluated by experienced echocardiographers.[26] EF (end-diastolic volume – end-systolic volume/end-diastolic volume) is dependent not only on intrinsic contractility but also on LV preload and afterload. Therefore, both factors should be considered when assessing LV systolic function. In general, LV systolic function is hyperdynamic when LVEF is greater than 70%, normal at 55% to 70%, mildly depressed at 45% to 54%, moderately depressed at 30% to 44%, and severely depressed at less than 30% (Table 8.1).[24] In the presence of regional dysfunction, EF

Box 8.2 Indications for Transesophageal Echocardiography in Critical Care

Inadequate or nondiagnostic transthoracic echocardiographic images
Evaluate suspected aortic dissection or trauma
Evaluate prosthetic valves, especially mitral
Investigate persistent hypoxemia
Detect presence of valvular vegetations
Identify complications of infective endocarditis:
- Abscesses
- Leaflet perforation
- Pseudoaneurysm formation
- Fistulas

Identify cardiac source of systemic embolus:
- Thrombus in left atrium and left atrial appendage
- Patent foramen ovale/atrial septal aneurysm
- Atheromatous debris of the aorta

Identify pulmonary embolus in transit
Characterize intracardiac shunts:
- Atrial septal defect (ASD)
- Ventricular septal defect (VSD)
- Anomalous pulmonary venous connections

Guide invasive procedures:
- Shunt closure
- Percutaneous balloon valvuloplasty

from multiple views should be integrated to accurately assess LV systolic function. To improve the accuracy of EF calculation by echocardiography, it is essential to avoid foreshortened apical views and to use intravenous contrast material when needed to enhance endocardial border definition (see Fig. 8.4). Aside from measurements of systolic function, 2D echocardiography is of great use in reliably assessing LV dimensions, wall thickness, volumes, and mass.[24] Reliable assessments of LV dimensions and EF, particularly when combined with knowledge of filling pressures, can be used to guide and assess the response to therapeutic measures of volume infusion or intravenous administration of inotropic/vasodilator or vasopressor drugs.

TDI-derived myocardial velocities (Fig. 8.6) have been utilized to assess global LV systolic properties.[27] This approach is dependent on TD technology to record mitral annulus and myocardial signals, which can be acquired from any area of the heart. However, because of their dependence on Doppler principles, they are of limited value when proper alignment cannot be achieved between the ultrasound beam and the plane of cardiac motion. TDI measurements of systolic annular velocity have been shown to reflect systolic dysfunction, even in the presence of normal LVEF (such as in hypertrophic cardiomyopathy [HCM] or infiltrative cardiomyopathy [ICM]).[27-29] Using speckle tracking imaging, a 2D echocardiographic technique that measures myocardial motion over time, myocardial deformation (strain) and rate of deformation (strain rate) can also be used to assess LV systolic function.[30,31] As in TDI, strain and strain rate can detect significant myocardial systolic abnormalities, even in the presence of preserved LVEF.[32,33] As with TDI, this is of particular importance in patients with diastolic heart failure, hypertensive heart disease, HCM, and

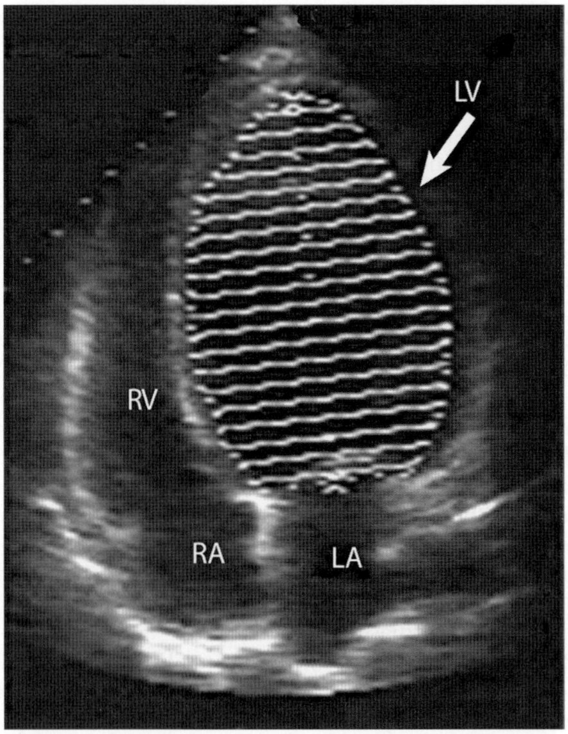

A

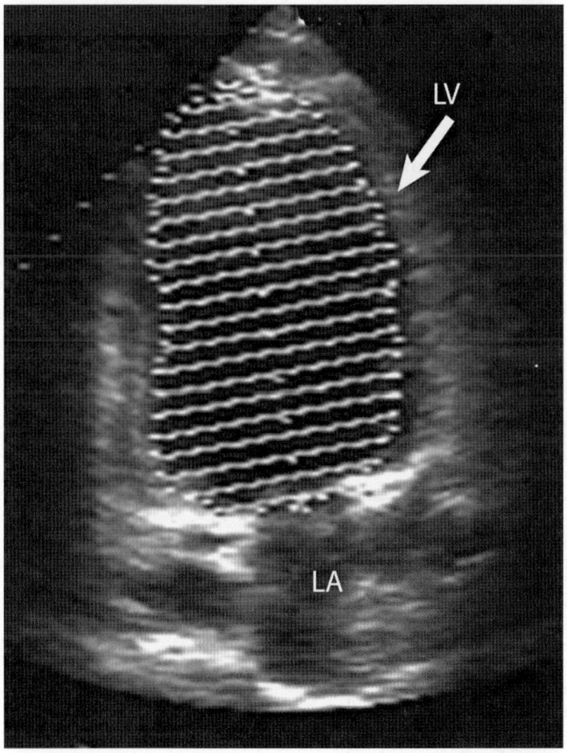

B

Figure 8.5 Left ventricular volumes and ejection fraction calculated using method of discs (*arrow*). **A,** Diastole; **B,** systole. LA, left atrium; LV, left ventricle; RA, right atrium; RV, right ventricle.

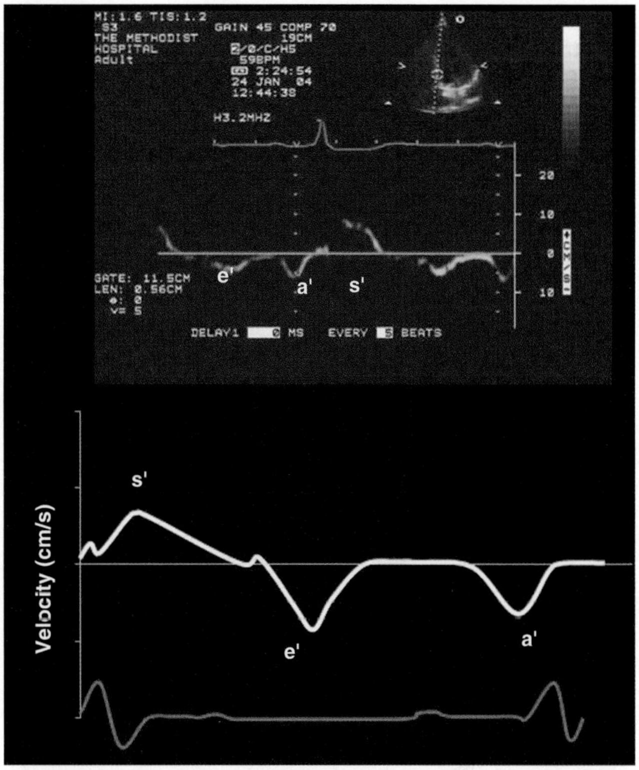

Figure 8.6 Example of tissue Doppler recording of the lateral mitral annulus from the apex. a′, late diastolic velocity; e′, early diastolic velocity; s′, systolic velocity.

infiltrative disease, when normal EF can coexist with significant and clinically important abnormalities of systolic function.

DIASTOLIC DYSFUNCTION

LV diastolic dysfunction in the intensive care unit (ICU) may be present as a result of cardiac as well as systemic disorders that can affect cardiac function: coronary and hypertensive heart disease, diabetes mellitus, amyloidosis, and HCM. A careful assessment of LV diastolic function by echocardiography can contribute essential information for the management of these patients.[34-36] In general, LV diastolic function refers to LV relaxation (measured as the rate of decay of LV systolic pressure during the isovolumic relaxation period) and LV chamber stiffness. In turn, chamber stiffness is calculated using measurements of LV volume and pressure during the diastolic filling period. However, prediction of LV filling pressures integrates the effects of the preceding hemodynamic variables as well as other factors such as RV filling, pericardial constraint, and LA function on LV diastolic function.

The recommended clinical approach for the assessment of LV diastolic function (European Association of Echocardiography [ASE] guideline algorithms) begins with the 2D examination to determine LV dimensions and volumes and the presence and extent of LV hypertrophy, using standard ASE criteria (Figs. 8.7 and 8.8).[37] Patients with a depressed EF or LV hypertrophy have impaired LV relaxation. Therefore, even in the absence of any corroborating Doppler information, one can still conclude that LV relaxation is impaired in these patients. Furthermore, this information can be combined with the mitral inflow pattern to predict filling pressures. It is also important to measure left atrial (LA) volume using apical four- and two-chamber views because LA volume is related to the extent of diastolic dysfunction when increase in LA volume parallels deterioration of LV diastolic function.[38] Mitral inflow is obtained using pulse Doppler, with a 1- to 2-mm sample volume placed at the level of mitral valve tips.[39] Early diastolic flow and velocity (E) occur in response to a positive pressure gradient between the LA and the LV, resulting from a rapidly decreasing LV pressure due to LV relaxation and early diastolic suction. In late diastole, LA contraction leads to another positive pressure gradient and late diastolic flow or the A velocity. With normal LV relaxation, early diastolic flow predominates and the E/A ratio is greater than 1. However, when LV relaxation is impaired, LV diastolic pressure is elevated and a reduced E velocity is observed. This leads to a higher LA preload and contraction velocity. Therefore, the E/A ratio decreases in the presence of impaired LV relaxation. Because LA pressure usually increases to maintain forward stroke volume, early diastolic transmitral pressure gradient increases, leading to a higher E velocity and E/A ratio. Because of the simulation to normal mitral inflow, this pattern is referred to as a pseudonormal mitral inflow pattern. In more advanced disease with markedly elevated LA pressure, the E velocity increases even further, resulting in a "restrictive" inflow pattern, in which E/A ratio is 2 or greater. It is possible to unmask the presence of impaired LV relaxation in these cases by performing a Valsalva maneuver. The decrease in venous return during the strain phase of Valsalva results in a decrease in LA pressure and E/A ratio.[40-42] TD-derived early diastolic mitral annular velocity (e′) can be recorded by pulsed Doppler at mitral annulus. When combined with E, E/e′ ratio is obtained, which has been shown to be a reasonable correlate of LV filling pressure,[41] although multiple diastolic echo-Doppler variables need to be synthesized to result in an accurate assessment of LV diastolic function.[43-45]

Pulmonary venous (PV) flow can also be analyzed to predict LV filling pressures. PV flow signals are readily recorded in the majority of patients seen in the outpatient laboratory but can be challenging in the critical care setting. Antegrade forward flow from the pulmonary vein into the left atrium occurs during systole (S) and early and mid-diastole (D). After atrial contraction, retrograde flow (Ar) from the left atrium into the pulmonary vein occurs. At the earlier stages of diastolic dysfunction where LV end-diastolic pressure is increased, the peak velocity and duration of Ar (velocity > 30 cm/second and Ar-A duration ≥ 35 ms) become more prominent.[42,46] Subsequently, with the rise in mean LA pressure, antegrade systolic flow decreases, whereas the D velocity increases with a shortening of its deceleration time. Assessment of PA systolic and diastolic pressures (see later) can provide helpful corroborating

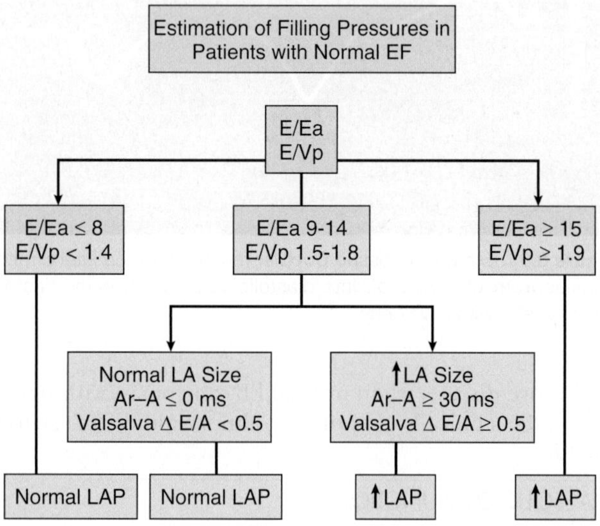

Figure 8.7 Algorithm for estimation of left ventricular filling pressures with normal ejection fraction.

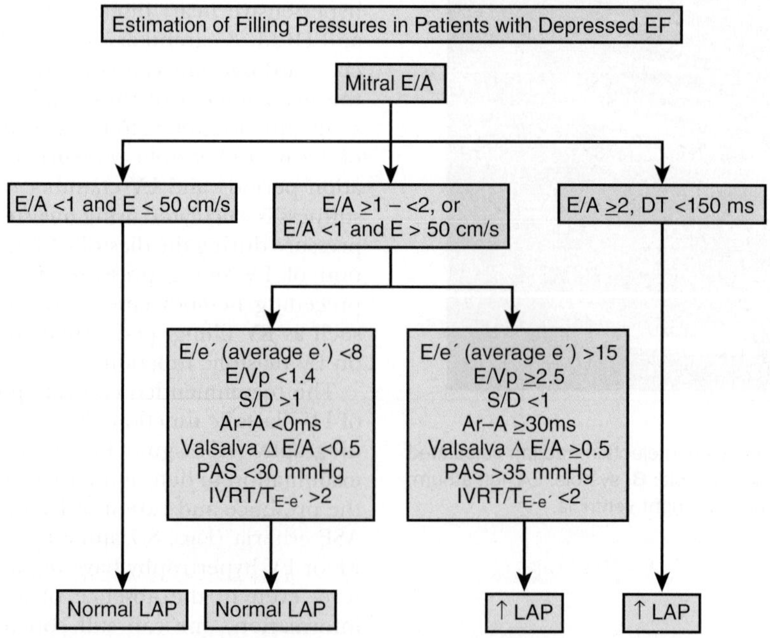

Figure 8.8 Algorithm for estimation of left ventricular filling pressures with depressed ejection fraction.

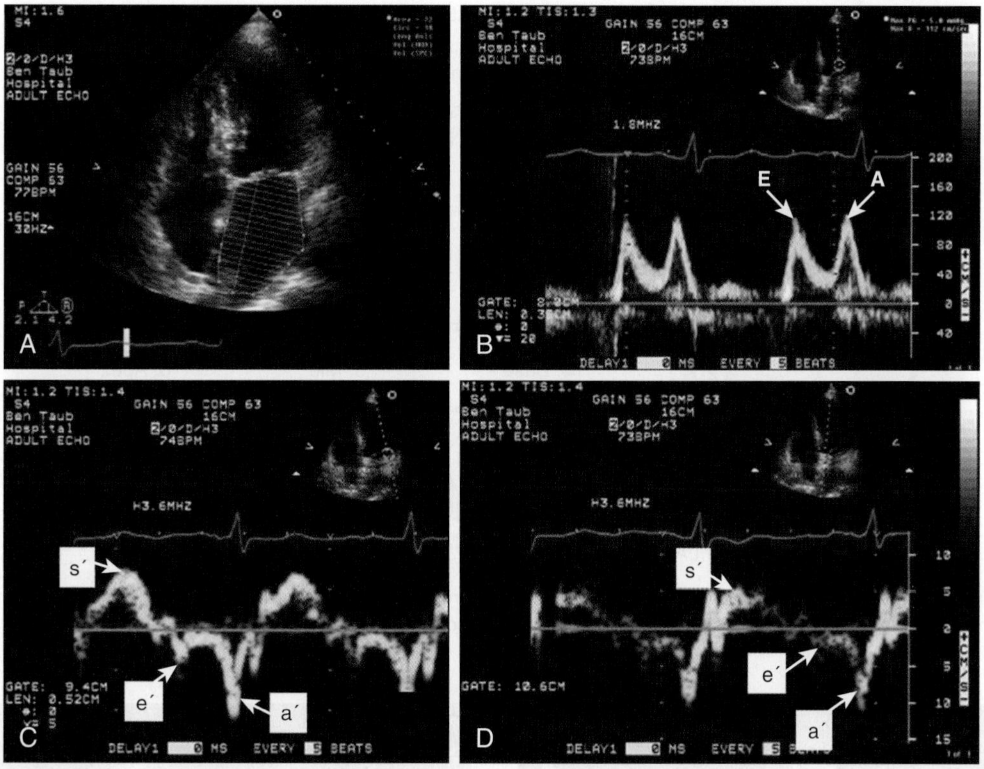

Figure 8.9 Integration of Doppler-derived data for assessment of left ventricular diastolic function. **A,** Measurement of left atrial volumes. **B,** Mitral inflow velocity. **C,** Doppler tissue imaging (DTI) of lateral mitral annulus. **D,** DTI of septal/medial mitral annulus.

evidence of the status of LV filling pressures. In the absence of pulmonary parenchymal and vascular disease, and in the presence of significant cardiac valvular disease or cardiomyopathy, one can reasonably infer that PA pressures are increased due to an elevated LA pressure. Figure 8.9 shows an example of a patient with preserved LVEF with elevated LV filling pressures as assessed by integrated diastolic assessment with multiple echo-Doppler variables.

ISCHEMIA/INFARCTION INCLUDING COMPLICATIONS

Echocardiography is essential for the assessment of LV regional function in the critical care setting when the diagnosis of ischemia/infarction is entertained. Adequate images, particularly when combined with harmonics and intravenous contrast, can provide comparable information to that obtained by TEE.[12,13] Furthermore, serial assessment of regional function is possible after the administration of thrombolytic drugs or percutaneous revascularization. In addition to technically good images, interpretation by an experienced echocardiographer is essential for achieving high accuracy. Regional function is determined by examining endocardial motion as well as local thickening. Abnormal LV regional function is usually determined when the dysfunction is observed in more than one plane, with particular LV segments corresponding to specific coronary artery distributions. An echocardiographic regional map for the identification of wall motion abnormalities and their correlation to coronary anatomy is shown in Figure 8.10. In general, thin (<5 mm in diameter), bright myocardial walls with abnormal motion are indicative of scars [?] (Fig. 8.11). When there is a wall with thin walls that moves opposite to adjacent, normal walls ("bulging"), aneurysm is often the cause (Fig. 8.12); in this case, thrombus in the aneurysm must be excluded to prevent systemic embolism. In addition to epicardial coronary artery disease, myocarditis, dilated cardiomyopathy (DCM), and abnormal conduction patterns (particularly RV pacing and left bundle branch block) can result in regional dysfunction. Therefore, final conclusions regarding cause of wall motion abnormalities should be made only after integration of clinical findings including electrocardiogram (ECG). In the setting of acute myocardial infarction, a number of studies have substantiated the prognostic power of echocardiography, particularly LVEF, LV diastolic function, RV function, and significant valve dysfunction.[47] Regional function is most reflective of long-term outcome when imaging is performed after recovery of myocardial stunning (usually a week to 10 days after presentation). However, in the acute setting, echocardiography may be obtained to help establish the diagnosis of an acute ischemic syndrome, determine the extent of myocardium at risk, identify apical clots (Fig. 8.13), and detect the presence of mechanical complications such as ventricular septal defect (VSD) (Fig. 8.14), contained cardiac rupture called pseudoaneurysms (Figs. 8.15 and 8.16), MR, pericardial effusion, and RV infarction, all of which may require urgent intervention.[48]

CARDIOMYOPATHY

HYPERTROPHIC CARDIOMYOPATHY

HCM is an inherited disorder that is characterized by unexplained LV hypertrophy in the absence of longstanding

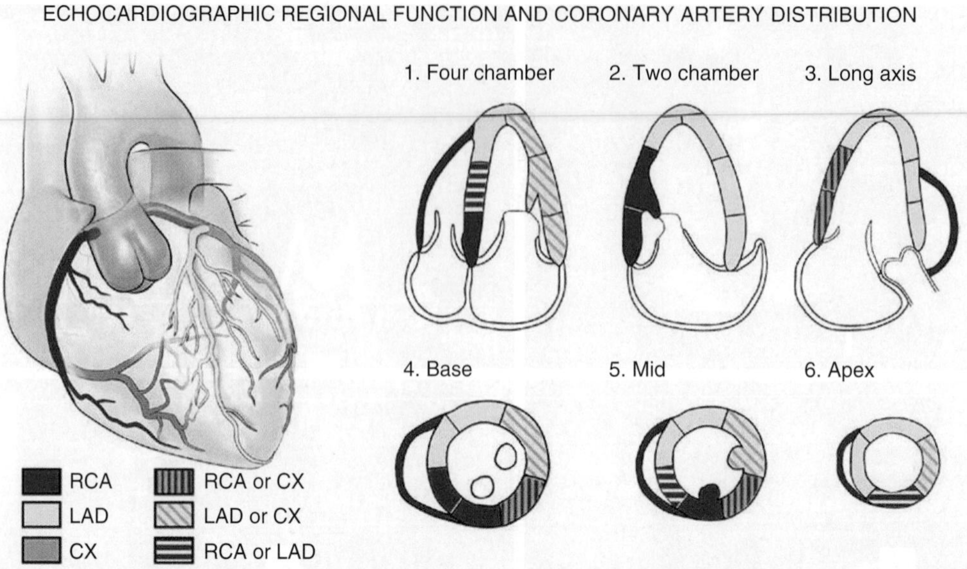

Figure 8.10 Graphic for relating coronary artery distribution to echocardiographic wall segments. Lang RM, et al. American Society of Echocardiography Recommendations for chamber quantification. J AM Soc Echocardiog 2005; 18 (12): 1440-63

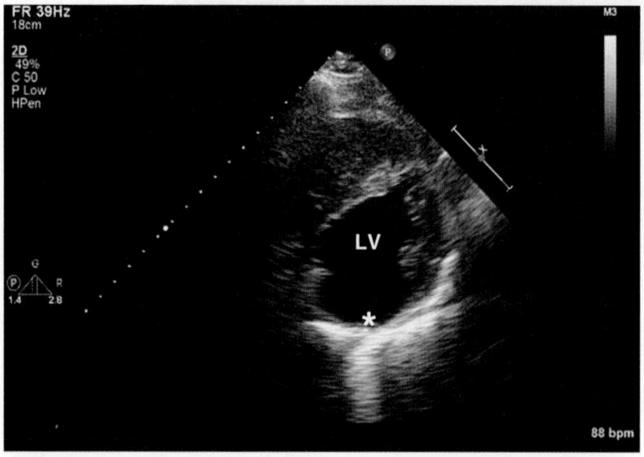

Figure 8.11 Short-axis view of the left ventricle demonstrating inferior infarction (*). Wall segment is thinned and bright. LV, left ventricle.

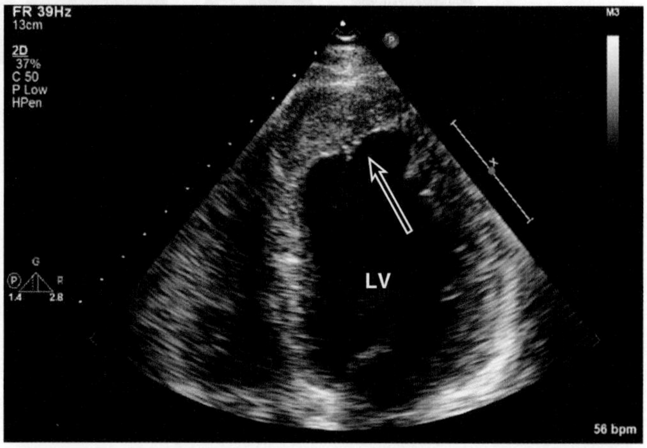

Figure 8.13 Apical four-chamber zoom view of the left ventricle (LV) demonstrating layered apical thrombus (*arrow*).

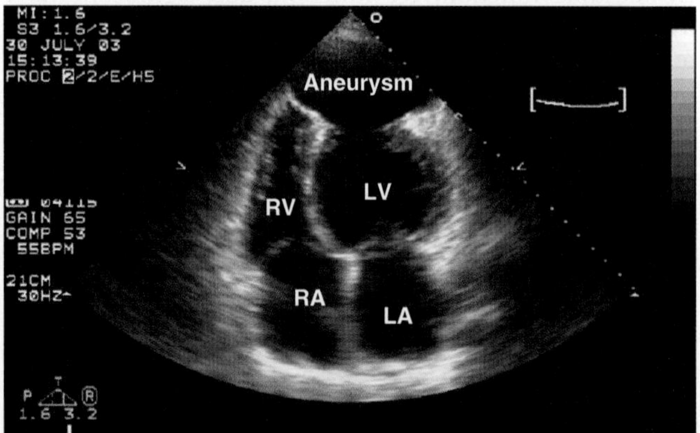

Figure 8.12 Apical four-chamber view demonstrating true left ventricular apical aneurysm. LA, left atrium; LV, left ventricle; RA, right atrium; RV, right ventricle.

hypertension or infiltrative disease.[49] At the pathologic level, there is myocyte disarray, with replacement of healthy myocytes with fibrosis. Therefore, on echocardiography, thick LV walls with elevated LV mass are seen. Early in the disease, LV function is usually hyperdynamic, although late in the disease, LVEF can become depressed ("burned-out HCM"). There are various morphologic types of HCM, including septal hypertrophy (Fig. 8.17), concentric (uniform) hypertrophy, apical hypertrophy, and hypertrophy concentrated in LV walls other than the septum. It is important to understand that LV obstruction with resultant dynamic gradients can occur in any of these morphologic types, thus the differentiation between obstructive and nonobstructive HCM. Echocardiography is uniquely positioned to differentiate these morphologic types, determine LV systolic function, assess for left ventricular outflow tract (LVOT) obstruction, identify associated MR, and determine LV filling pressures and PA pressure.[50] Obstruction in HCM is most often caused

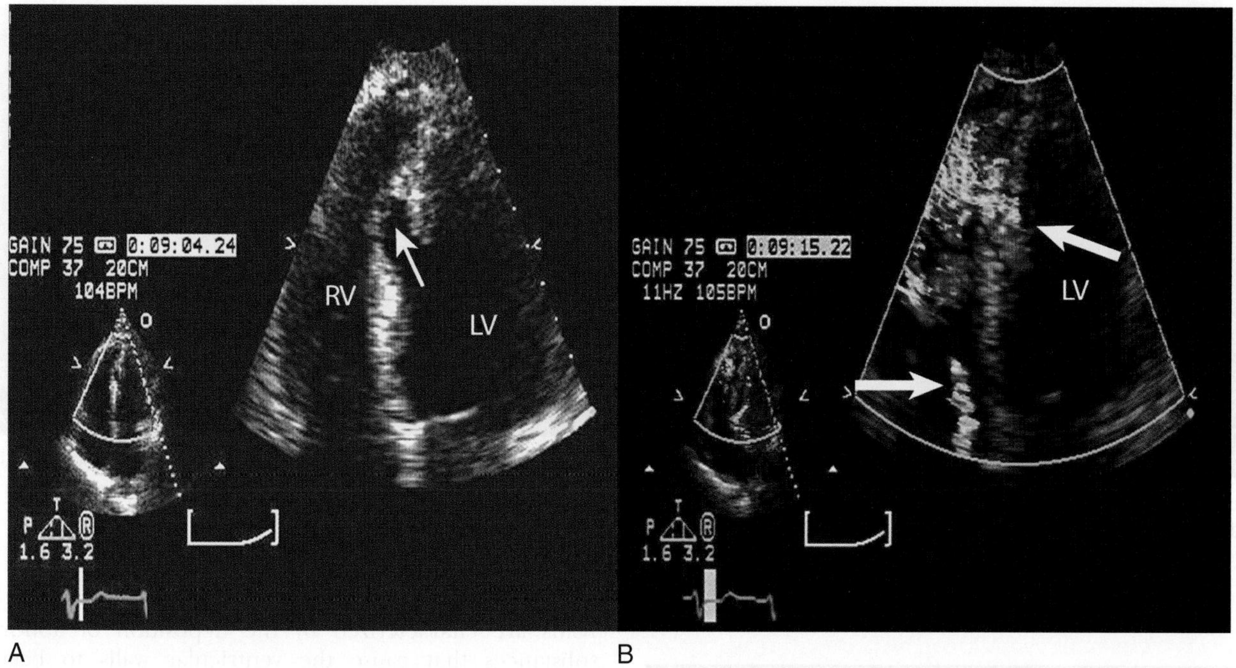

Figure 8.14 **A,** Four-chamber view demonstrating postinfarct ventricular septal defect (VSD) (*arrow*). **B,** Color flow demonstrating left-to-right shunting across ventricular septal defect (*upper arrow*) and tricuspid regurgitation (*lower arrow*). LV, left ventricle; RV, right ventricle.

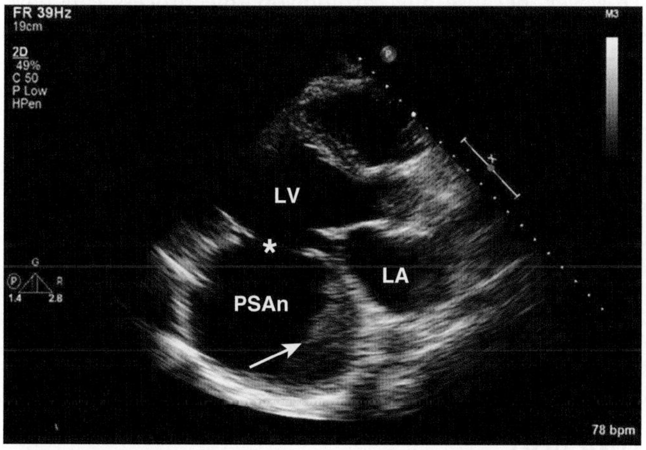

Figure 8.15 Long-axis view of inferobasal pseudoaneurysm. *Arrow* points to layered thrombus. LA, left atrium; LV, left ventricle; *, neck of pseudoaneurysm (PSAn).

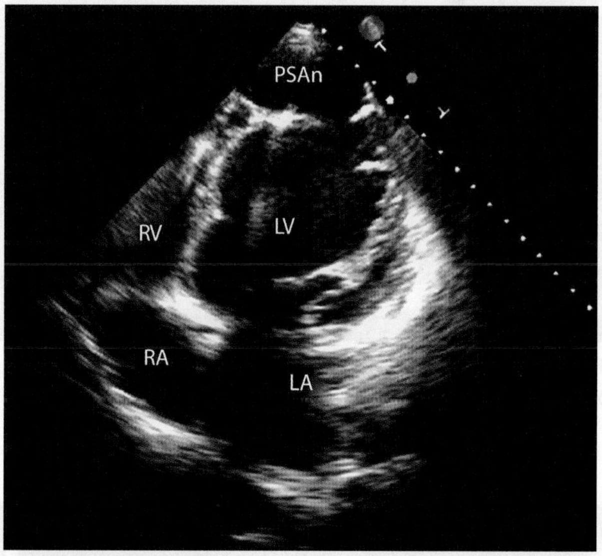

Figure 8.16 Pseudoaneurysm (PSAn) of the left ventricular apex. LA, left atrium; LV, left ventricle; RA, right atrium; RV, right ventricle.

by systolic anterior motion (SAM) of the mitral valve (Fig. 8.18), which physically obstructs the LVOT, resulting in a significant gradient. From the clinical point of view, HCM patients can present to critical care with hypotension, congestive heart failure, arrhythmias, stroke, and cardiac arrest; echocardiography is crucial in differentiating the underlying disease state and functional/morphologic associations with these presentations.

DILATED CARDIOMYOPATHY

DCM refers to nonischemic global LV systolic dysfunction often associated with RV dysfunction. Although viral myocarditis can cause this same picture, in general, DCM refers to familial inherited cardiomyopathy but can be caused by a variety of conditions including alcohol abuse, chemotherapeutic agents, and endocrine disorders. As genetic methods for diagnosing inherited DCM become more refined, an increasing proportion of idiopathic nonischemic cardiomyopathy is found to be inherited.[51] From the echocardiographic standpoint, DCM is readily diagnosed by dilated LV with depressed EF and often RV dysfunction; for final diagnosis, exclusion of a sufficient degree of coronary artery disease to explain degree of LV dysfunction is necessary.[52] Secondary MR and TR can be seen by color and spectral Doppler interrogation, and LV filling pressure and PA pressure assessments are important in clinical management. An example of a patient with DCM is seen in Figure 8.19.

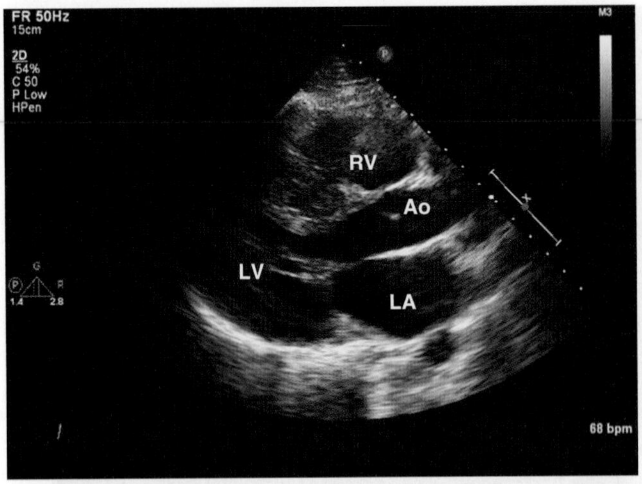

Figure 8.17 Long-axis view of patient with hypertrophic cardiomyopathy. Note marked septal thickness. Ao, aorta; LA, left atrium; LV, left ventricle; RV, right ventricle.

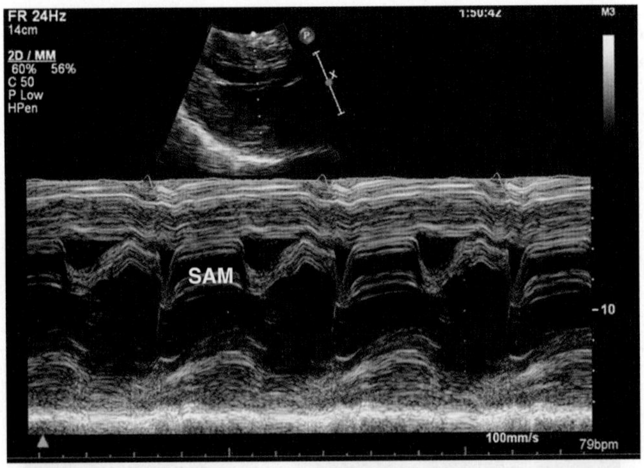

Figure 8.18 M-mode of classic systolic anterior motion (SAM) in hypertrophic cardiomyopathy.

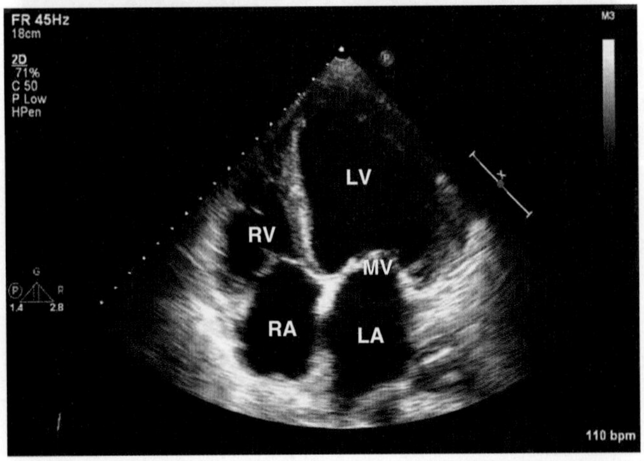

Figure 8.19 Apical four-chamber view of dilated cardiomyopathy. LA, left atrium; LV, left ventricle; MV, mitral valve; RA, right atrium; RV, right ventricle.

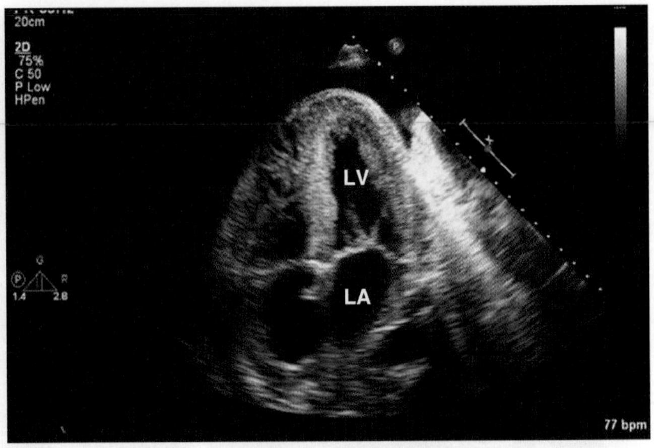

Figure 8.20 Apical four-chamber view of cardiac amyloidosis. Note bright thick walls. LA, left atrium; LV, left ventricle.

INFILTRATIVE/RESTRICTIVE CARDIOMYOPATHY

ICMs are characterized by the deposition of abnormal substances that cause the ventricular walls to become progressively rigid, thereby impeding ventricular filling.[53] This impedance to normal LV filling is termed "restrictive filling;" hence the other name, "restrictive cardiomyopathy." However, because any cardiomyopathic process can have restrictive filling (ischemic, dilated, hypertrophic), the preferred term is ICM. Some ICMs can cause LV and RV thickening, such as the archetypal ICM cardiac amyloidosis (Fig. 8.20), although others can cause ventricular thinning, such as sarcoidosis. From the echocardiographic point of view, thickened ventricular walls with restrictive LV filling and at time depressed LVEF are seen in amyloidosis;[54] the differentiation from HCM and hypertensive heart disease is made by the presence of low ECG voltages in ICM, as normal myocytes are replaced by amyloid. For sarcoidosis, many LV patterns can be seen, but focal LV aneurysms are typical; heart block on ECG is also often seen.

ASSESSMENT OF RIGHT VENTRICULAR FUNCTION

Echocardiographic assessment of RV function is challenging because of its complex shape. However, it is possible to integrate information from multiple views to reach reasonably accurate conclusions on RV size and function. In the parasternal short-axis view, the RV appears crescent-shaped, whereas in the apical four-chamber view it is triangular with its base along the tricuspid valve. Visually, assessment of RV size is usually done by comparing RV and LV transverse dimensions in the parasternal short-axis (Fig. 8.21) and apical views (Fig. 8.22). In general, the RV dimensions are one third of the LV dimensions. As the right ventricle dilates, its free wall bulges and in patients with moderate enlargement, RV dimensions are almost equal to those of the left ventricle. RV size is larger than LV size in patients with severe enlargement, with the right ventricle forming the cardiac apex. It is possible to measure RV end-diastolic and end-systolic dimensions and area in the apical four-chamber view; however, caution should be exercised to avoid tangential and foreshortened views. Normal RV

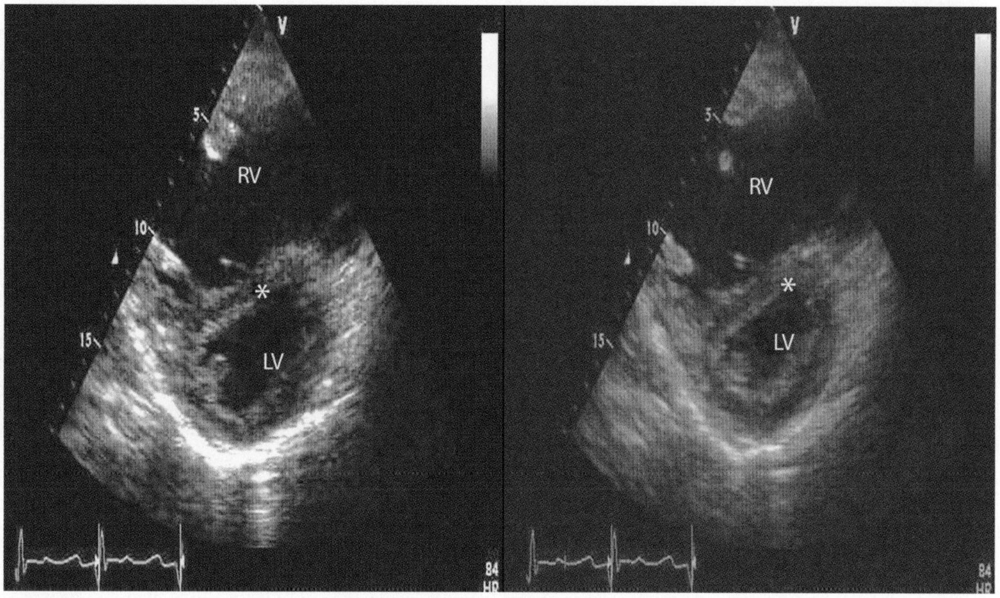

A B

Figure 8.21 Short-axis view of "D-shaped" left ventricle in systole **(A)** and diastole **(B)** with marked right ventricular enlargement. LV, left ventricle; RV, right ventricle.

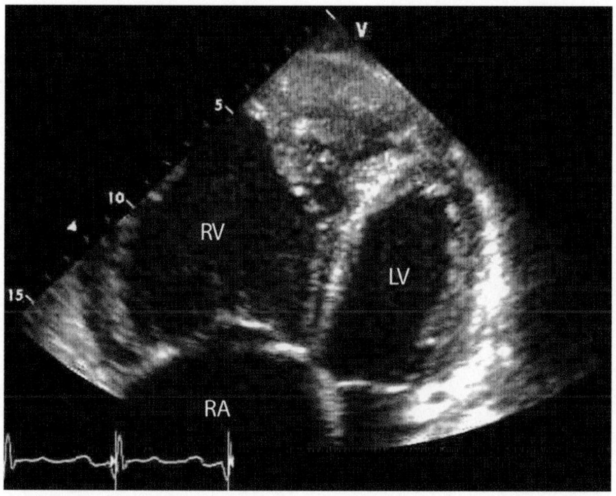

Figure 8.22 Apical four-chamber view of marked right ventricular dilatation. LV, left ventricle; RA, right atrium; RV, right venetricle.

dimension at the tricuspid annular level in the apical four-chamber view is less than 4.1 cm.[55] RV wall thickness is normally less than 0.5 cm and is most reliably measured by 2D echocardiography in subcostal views at the level of the tricuspid valve chordae tendinae.[55] If needed, contrast enhancement may be used. During TEE, RV size can be assessed in the midesophageal four-chamber view.

RV systolic function is estimated qualitatively in clinical practice as normal or mildly, moderately, or severely depressed function. It is also possible to obtain a quantitative measurement of RV systolic function by measuring RV fractional area change (FAC = end-diastolic area − end-systolic area/end-diastolic area) in the apical four-chamber view. This is a simple method with reasonable reproducibility and accuracy, and its normal value ranges to greater than 35%.[55] RV Tei index (TR duration − duration of systolic flow through the RV outflow tract/duration of systolic flow through the RV outflow tract) can be calculated as well, but it provides a combined assessment of RV systolic and diastolic function and is prone to various measurement errors.[56] The tricuspid annulus motion can provide useful information in patients with suboptimal visualization of RV free wall; normal tricuspid annular plane systolic excursion (TAPSE) is greater than 1.6 cm.[55] Additional information may be obtained by TD-derived tricuspid annulus systolic velocity.[57,58] Strain and strain rate[59] measurements have been applied in a number of diseases that affect the right ventricle, such as congenital heart disease, pulmonary embolism, and idiopathic pulmonary hypertension, and can indicate RV systolic abnormalities even in the presence of normal visual RV function, TAPSE, or FAC. Their routine clinical application, however, awaits additional improvements in the technique to enhance its reproducibility and to show the incremental information provided over 2D imaging and myocardial velocities.

Conditions of RV volume overload (e.g., ASD, severe TR or pulmonary regurgitation) result in diastolic flattening of the interventricular septum, which becomes rounded in systole, but RV pressure overload (primary pulmonary hypertension, acute or chronic thromboembolic disease, cor pulmonale) results in systolic and diastolic flattening of the interventricular septum ("D-shaped ventricle" in systole and diastole; see Fig. 8.21).[60] Acute RV dilatation can reduce LV filling through an increase in intrapericardial pressure, which in turn reduces LV transmural filling pressure.[61] An acute decline in RV function is usually accompanied by RV dilatation and decrease in RV systolic function in the presence of normal wall thickness. In the setting of an acute coronary syndrome, this may happen as a result of RV ischemia or infarction. The presence of normal/reduced PA pressures along with regional dysfunction can help identify these patients. Patients with chronic RV pressure overload (for example, idiopathic pulmonary hypertension) often

Table 8.2 Echocardiographic Assessment of Aortic Regurgitation Severity

Finding	Mild	Moderate	Severe
Central jets: color jet width/LVOT diameter	<25%	25-64%	≥65%
Vena contracta	<0.3 cm	0.3-0.6 cm	>0.6 cm
Pressure half-time	>500 ms	200-500 ms	<200 ms
LV end-diastolic dimension	Normal	5-6 cm	>6 cm
Regurgitant volume	<30 mL	30-59 mL	≥60 mL
Regurgitant fraction	<30%	30-49%	≥50%
Regurgitant orifice area	$<0.1\ cm^2$	$0.1\text{-}0.29\ cm^2$	$\geq 0.3\ cm^2$

LV, left ventricle; LVOT, left ventricular outflow tract.

Table 8.3 Echocardiographic Assessment of Mitral Regurgitation Severity

Finding	Mild	Moderate	Severe
Central jets: jet area by color Doppler/LA area	<20%	20-39%	>40%
Vena contracta	<0.3 cm	0.3-0.69 cm	≥0.7 cm
Pulmonary veins	Predominant systolic	Blunted systolic	Systolic reversal
LA size	Normal	Normal or dilated	Dilated
LV size	Normal	Normal or dilated	Dilated
Regurgitant volume	<30 mL	30-59 mL	≥60 mL
Regurgitant fraction	<30%	30-49%	≥50%
Regurgitant orifice area	$<0.2\ cm^2$	$0.2\text{-}0.39\ cm^2$	$\geq 0.4\ cm^2$

LA, left atrium; LV, left ventricle.

exhibit a dilated right ventricle with reduced contractility and increased wall thickness (see Fig. 8.22) in the presence of increased PA pressures and vascular resistance.[62]

DETERMINING VALVULAR FUNCTION AND DYSFUNCTION

Echocardiography provides important anatomic and physiologic information on cardiac valves. Valve morphologic features can be reliably assessed using 2D imaging. For example, the presence of thickening and calcification of aortic valves and the presence of prolapse/flail or rheumatic deformity of the mitral valve can be readily identified. Importantly, secondary changes such as chamber enlargement and LV/RV function can be followed serially, thus enabling timely decisions with respect to surgery or percutaneous interventions. Using 2D images and Doppler, it is possible to assess the severity of valvular stenosis or regurgitation and to calculate PA pressures.

EVALUATION OF MITRAL, TRICUSPID, AND AORTIC REGURGITATION

Similar principles apply to the assessment of mitral (MR), tricuspid (TR), and aortic (AR) regurgitation. Pulsed, CW, and color Doppler are useful, when combined, in identifying and accurately grading AR (Table 8.2), MR (Table 8.3), and TR (Table 8.4).[63] Echocardiographic assessment of regurgitant valves includes the 2D and comprehensive Doppler imaging in multiple views to identify the direction and size of regurgitant jets. Color Doppler has reasonable accuracy in assessing the severity of MR, TR, or AR when jets are central, although the severity of eccentric jets can be underestimated. In addition, several technical and physiologic factors can affect the size of the jet, irrespective of regurgitant volume, including color gain, pulse repetition frequency, filter settings, and atrial (or aortic)/ventricular pressures. Therefore, it is important to record blood pressures at the time of echocardiography. For MR and TR, the ratio of the jet area to LA or RA area has been used in clinical and research studies to assess these lesions; it is important that the Nyquist limit for color Doppler be greater than 55 cm/second for accurate assessment. For AR, the width of the jet at its origin is related to that of the LVOT to arrive at the ratio that expresses the severity of AR. It is also possible to measure the cross-sectional area of the regurgitant jet by planimetry and relate that to the corresponding area of the LVOT in the short-axis views. Figure 8.23 shows an image of severe MR, Figure 8.24 demonstrates significant posteriorly directed AR, and Figure 8.25 shows severe TR.

Table 8.4 Echocardiographic Assessment of Tricuspid Regurgitation Severity

Finding	Mild	Moderate	Severe
Central jets: jet area by color Doppler	$<5\ cm^2$	$5\text{-}10\ cm^2$	$>10\ cm^2$
Vena contracta	Not defined	Not defined, but <0.7 cm	>0.7 cm
PISA radius	≤0.5 cm	0.6-0.9 cm	>0.9 cm
RA size	Normal	Normal or dilated	Dilated
RV size	Normal	Normal or dilated	Dilated
Jet density	Soft	Dense	Dense
Jet contour	Parabolic	Variable	Triangular with early peak
Hepatic veins	Predominant systolic	Blunted systolic	Systolic reversal

PISA, proximal isovelocity surface area; RA, right atrium; RV, right ventricle.

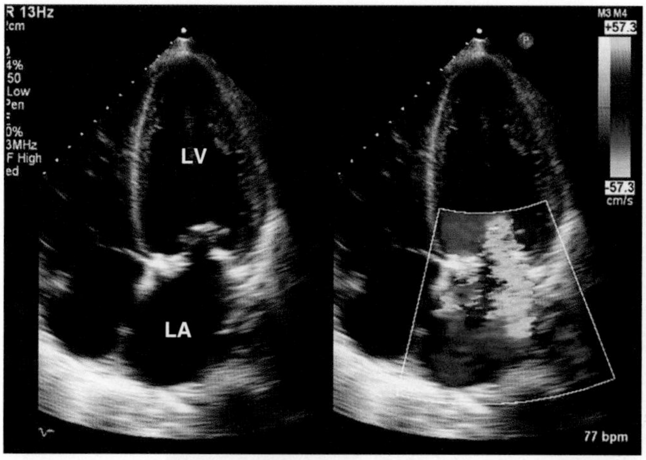

Figure 8.23 Apical four-chamber view demonstrating severe mitral regurgitation (*right panel*). LA, left atrium; LV, left ventricle.

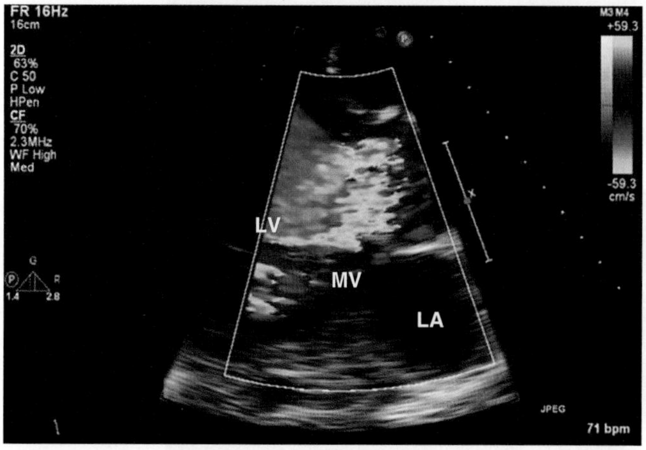

Figure 8.24 Long-axis view demonstrating severe posteriorly directed aortic regurgitation. LA, left atrium; LV, left ventricle; MV, mitral valve.

The "vena contracta" of the regurgitant jet, defined as the narrowest area of the jet that occurs at the orifice,[64] can be readily imaged and measured. As the regurgitant volume increases, vena contracta width increases (Fig. 8.26). The flow convergence method (proximal isovelocity surface area, or PISA, method) is a quantitative approach that can measure the regurgitant volume and the effective regurgitant orifice (ERO) area. Color flow mapping enables the visualization of the concentric hemispheres of flow as they approach the ERO (Fig. 8.27). The ERO area is calculated as:

$$6.28 \times r^2 \times V_a / V_{peak}$$

where V_a is the aliasing velocity, r is the maximal radius of the PISA, and V_{peak} is the peak velocity of the regurgitant signal by CW Doppler[65] (Fig. 8.27). This method is most reliable when jets are centrally located and the regurgitant orifice is adequately visualized.

The CW signal can provide useful information, as the brightness of these signals—in comparison with antegrade flow—increases with increasing severity of regurgitation. For patients with MR or TR who have severe lesions and a rapid rise in LA or RA pressure resulting in a large regurgitant "V" wave, early systolic peaking is seen (see Fig. 8.25,

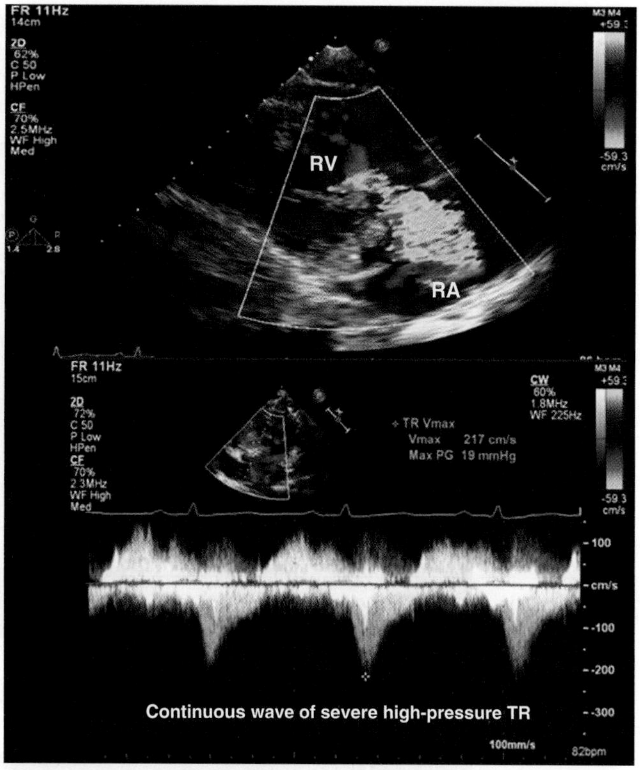

Figure 8.25 Severe tricuspid regurgitation (TR) (*upper panel*). Continuous wave Doppler demonstrating early peaking, low-velocity signal consistent with high right atrial pressure and severe TR (*lower panel*). RA, right atrium; RV, right ventricle.

lower panel). For AR, the deceleration time (pressure half-time = 0.29 × deceleration time) of the AR spectral Doppler signal is related to the rate at which aortic and LV pressures equilibrate in diastole, such that patients with hemodynamically significant lesions exhibit a rapid rise in LV diastolic pressure, leading to steep deceleration of AR velocity signal. In general, severe AR correlates with pressure half-time less than 250 ms, and mild AR with pressure half-time greater than 500 ms.[63] The pressure half-time is most reliable in cases with acute AR and may be prolonged in patients with chronic severe AR due to a concomitant increase in LV compliance (Fig. 8.28). For MR and TR, peak early diastolic filling velocity by PW (peak E-velocity) is increased in the setting of significant regurgitation because of the increased transvalvular flow generated by the regurgitant volume; in severe MR, a peak E velocity greater than 1.2 m/second is usually present. In addition, pulmonary and hepatic venous flow will show systolic reversal of flow in severe MR or TR, respectively, corresponding to the large regurgitant "V" wave in atrial pressure. In hemodynamically significant AR, diastolic flow reversal is noticed in the descending aorta. Normally, no (or only a minimal amount) flow reversal is seen in the descending aorta in early diastole. In patients with severe AR, holodiastolic flow reversal is observed.

In arriving at final conclusions, it is important to integrate all the findings obtained by 2D and Doppler.[63] For example, patients with chronic severe regurgitant lesions usually have dilatation of their cardiac chambers (for MR, LA and LV; for TR, right atrial [RA] and RV; for AR: LV) along with a large regurgitant volume. If the quality of the transthoracic

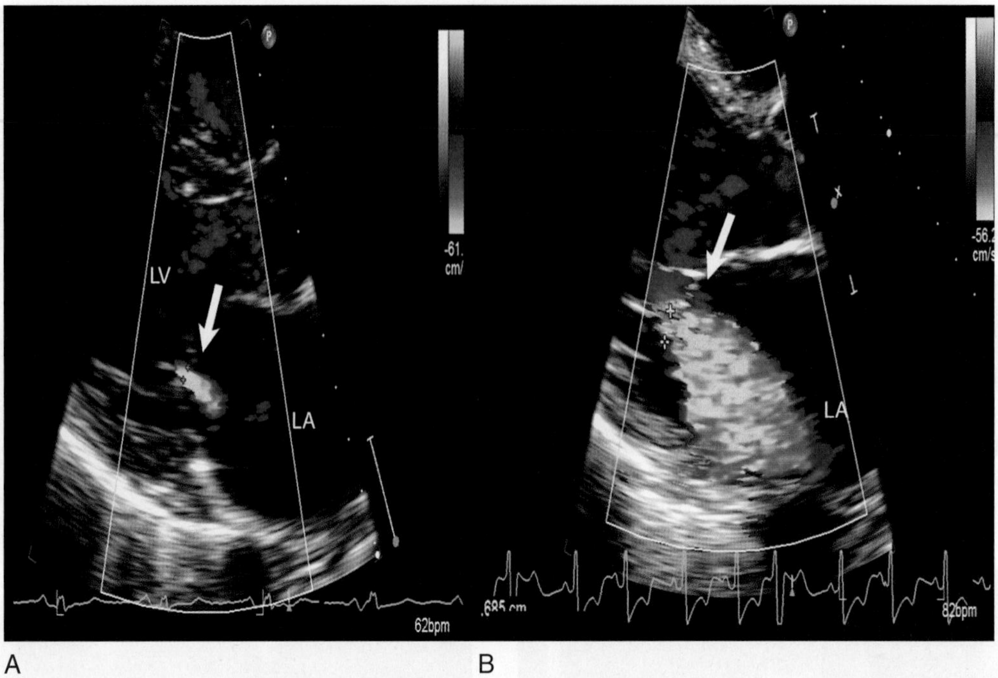

Figure 8.26 Vena contracta measurements (*arrows*) of mild **(A)** and severe **(B)** mitral regurgitation. LA, left atrium; LV, left ventricle.

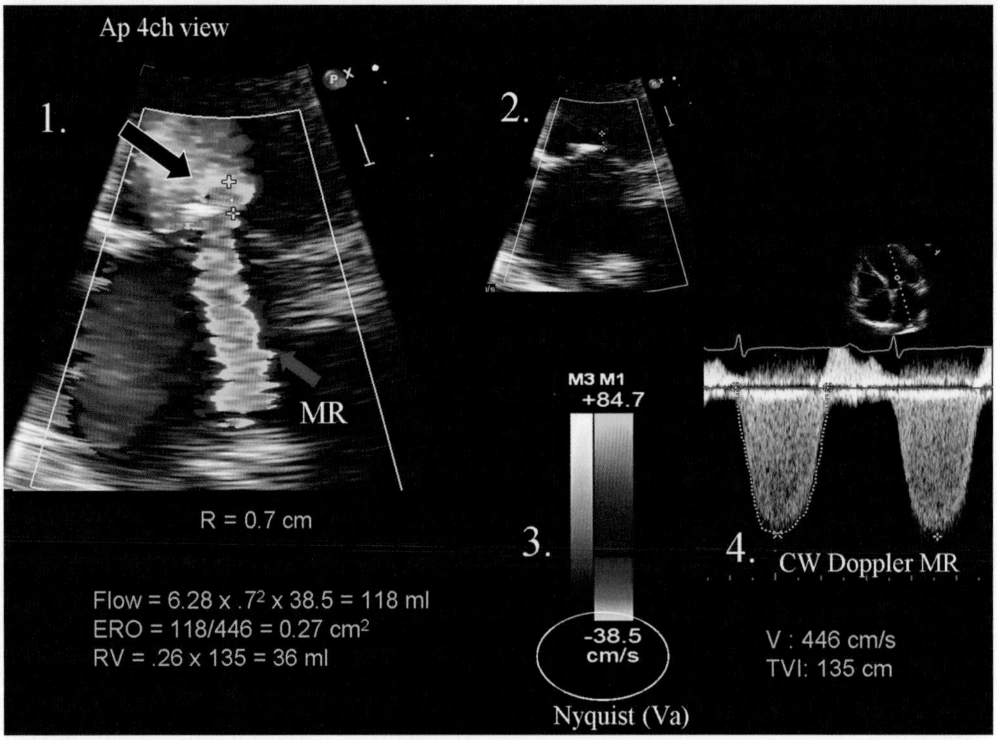

Figure 8.27 Moderate mitral regurgitation (MR) as calculated by the proximal isovelocity surface area method. *1*, Isolation and measurement of proximal color radius (*black arrow*). *2*, Confirmation of caliper placement without color. *3*, Nyquist (Va) velocity. *4*, Continuous wave (CW) Doppler of MR velocity and time velocity integral (TVI). *Red arrow*, MR jet.

images precludes the assessment of valvular disease, or the severity of MR or AR, it is reasonable to proceed to TEE. All of the preceding methods can be applied for the quantification of regurgitant lesions imaged by TEE. However, with respect to MR assessment by TEE, given the proximity of the TEE probe to the left atrium, MR jet area can be larger than that acquired by transthoracic imaging. In addition, TEE can provide unique information that is essential for successful mitral valve repair.

EVALUATION OF AORTIC STENOSIS

Patients with aortic stenosis (AS) have abnormally thickened or calcified valve leaflets along with reduced leaflet excursion, as seen by 2D echocardiography (Fig. 8.29).[66] In

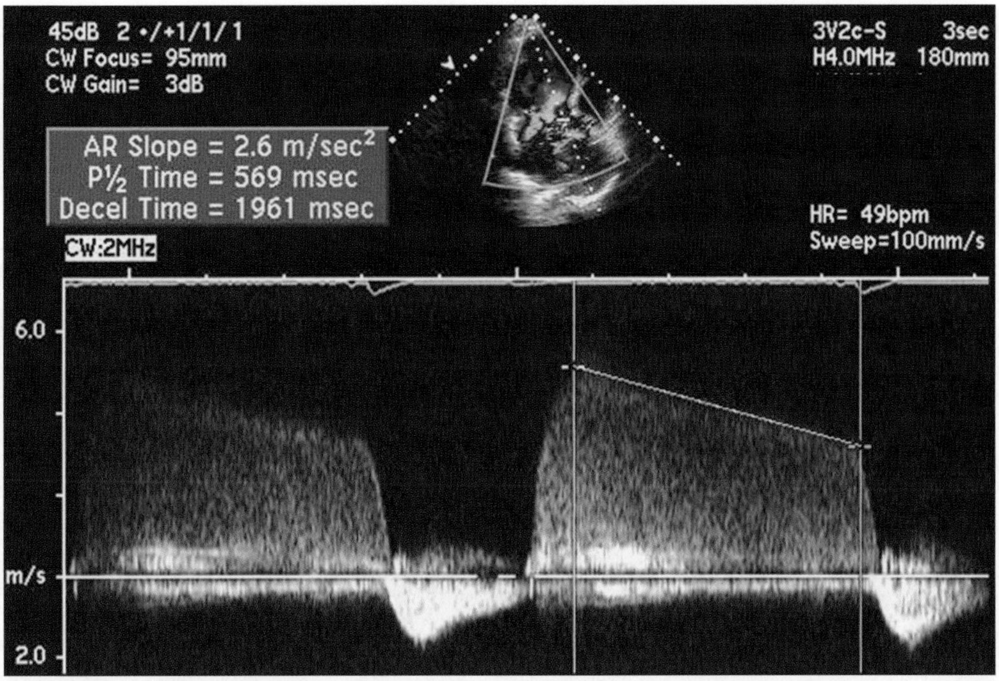

Figure 8.28 Example of online measurement of pressure half-time (P½ time) of the continuous wave spectral Doppler of aortic regurgitation.

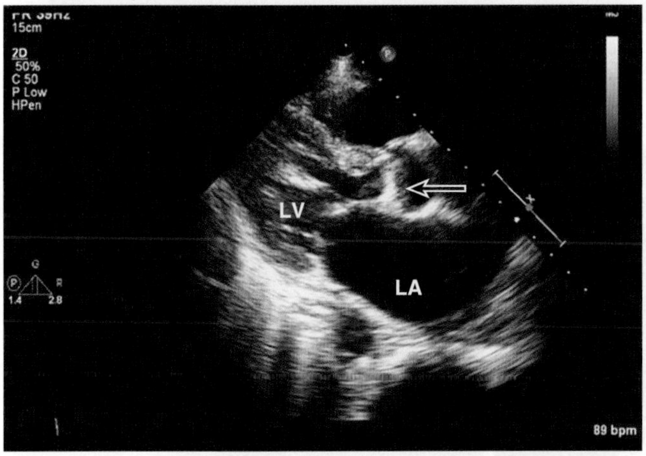

Figure 8.29 Two-dimensional image of calcific aortic stenosis (*arrow*). LA, left atrium; LV, left ventricle.

patients older than 70 years of age, the most common cause is degeneration of a trileaflet valve, although in patients younger than 70 years old, the most common cause is bicuspid aortic valve. In addition to morphologic changes of the aortic valve, 2D imaging is needed to determine LV dimensions, wall thickness, and EF. Such data are essential to assess the impact of AS on LV function, which is needed as part of the routine evaluation of patients with this disease. AS severity is assessed most reliably by the mean transvalvular systolic pressure gradient across the aortic valve and by the valve area, both of which are measured by Doppler echocardiography. Using the modified Bernoulli equation ($\Delta P = 4v^2$), the peak and mean gradients across the aortic valve can be calculated from the CW Doppler signal. An excellent correlation was observed between invasive and Doppler measurements of mean gradient when both measurements were simultaneously obtained.[67] However, several technical requirements are needed, including parallel alignment of the ultrasound beam with aortic flow and the use of multiple imaging windows (apical, right parasternal, subcostal, and suprasternal). Patients with a mild degree of AS may develop increased velocity and gradient when the transvalvular flow rate is increased, whether because of AR or the development of a hyperdynamic state; however, in this case the valve area will reflect the mild severity. Likewise, patients with severe AS may have lower than expected gradients with significantly depressed EF (Fig. 8.30), severe MR, severe RV dysfunction, severe TR, or intravascular volume depletion; again, in such cases, AV area is very useful to put the gradients in context of the stroke volume.

Aortic valve area is calculated using the continuity equation. The underlying principle is that the amount of blood flow through the LVOT and aortic valve will be the same because they are in continuity.[68] Aortic valve area (in cm^2) is given by systolic flow through LVOT/time velocity integral (TVI) of AS signal by CW (LVOT diameter^2 × 0.785 × LVOT TVI/aortic TVI) (see Fig. 8.30). The main source of error in this calculation is in the measurement of the LVOT diameter. However, when there is doubt, and in the absence of other significant valvular lesions, it is possible to use systolic flow through the RV outflow tract or diastolic mitral inflow in the numerator. Alternatively, LV stroke volume measured by 2D echocardiography (difference between end-diastolic and end-systolic volumes) may be used, provided adequate 2D images are present.

Some patients with severely depressed EF have only mildly or modestly elevated transvalvular gradients across the aortic valve, yet significant AS when the valve area is calculated (typically $<1\ cm^2$, see Fig. 8.30). It is reasonable to proceed to low dose (up to 20 µg/kg/minute) dobutamine echocardiography in these patients to assess not only LV

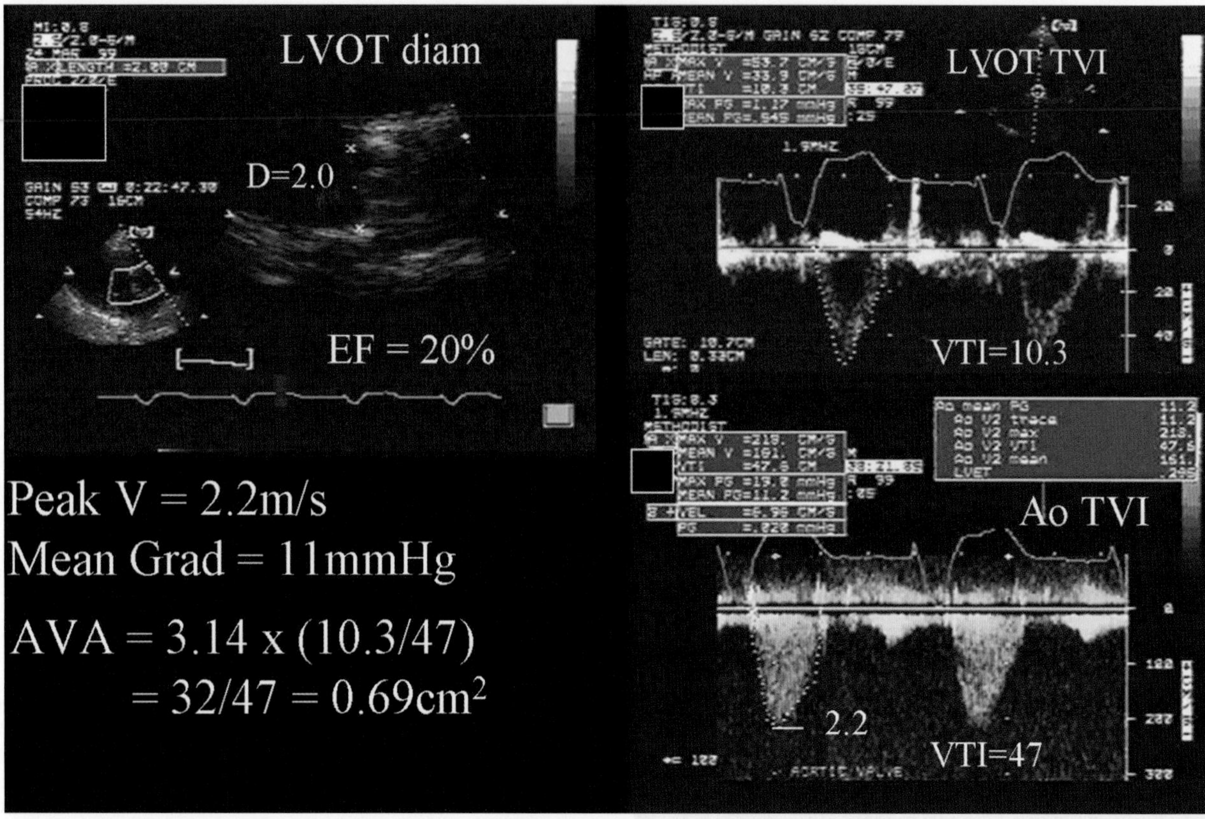

Figure 8.30 Assessment of aortic stenosis in a patient in Class III heart failure. Although the mean gradient is only 11 mm Hg, the calculated valve area is 0.69 cm^2. In this setting, the use of dobutamine may be efficacious. Ao, aorta; EF, ejection fraction; LVOT, left ventricular outflow tract; TVI, time velocity integral.

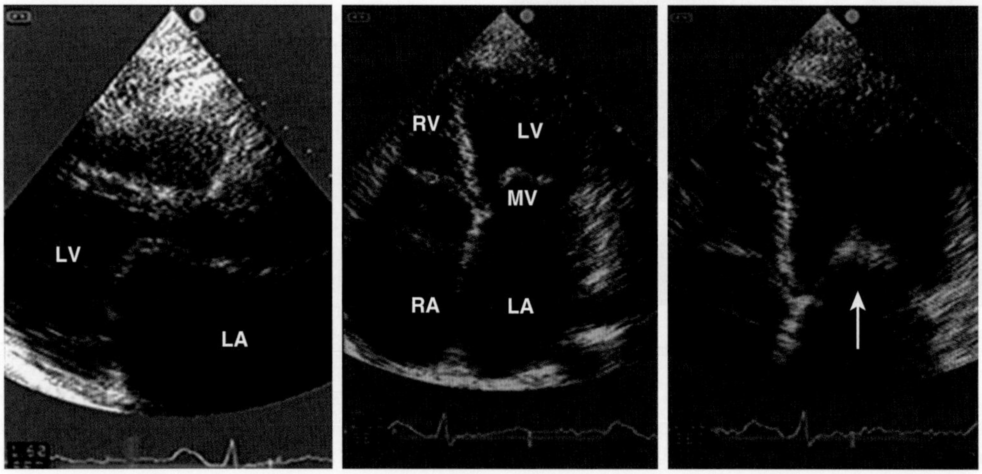

Figure 8.31 Long-axis view (*left*) of mitral stenosis demonstrating typical "hockey-stick" appearance of mitral valve. Four-chamber view (*right*) demonstrating doming of anterior leaflet, and marked dilatation of both atria and normal left ventricular and right ventricular size. This patient had rheumatic deformity of both the mitral and tricuspid valves. LA, left atrium; LV, left ventricle; MV, mitrial valve; RA, right atrium; RV, right ventricle.

contractile reserve but also the effect of increased transvalvular flow on the calculated aortic valve area.[69] Patients with dobutamine-induced increase in aortic valve area (>1 cm^2) are unlikely to have real AS, but their reduced valve area is largely the result of reduced flow rate. On the other hand, when there is an increase in gradient but still a severely reduced aortic valve area, valvular surgery should be considered because LV function and clinical status are likely to improve after valve replacement.

EVALUATION OF MITRAL STENOSIS

In patients with rheumatic mitral stenosis, 2D imaging shows the presence of valvular thickening and calcification along with abnormal leaflet mobility, such that there is doming of the anterior mitral leaflet along with reduced mobility of the posterior leaflet.[66] The anterior leaflet has a classic "hockey-stick" deformity when viewed in the parasternal long-axis and apical views (Figs. 8.31), and variable degrees of calcification, thickening, and subvalvular disease may be present. Direct planimetry of the mitral valve area is feasible in cases in which the mitral valve orifice is well visualized in the parasternal short-axis view. However, this measurement can be inaccurate when there is extensive calcification of valve leaflets, and when the short-axis plane is not positioned correctly at the level of valve tips. Color Doppler shows the PISA hemispheres on the LA side of the mitral valve during diastole (Fig. 8.32). Spectral Doppler can provide reliable transmitral pressure gradients and mitral valve area in most patients with mitral stenosis, as well as the hemodynamic impact on the right side of the heart with development of pulmonary hypertension (see Fig 8.33).

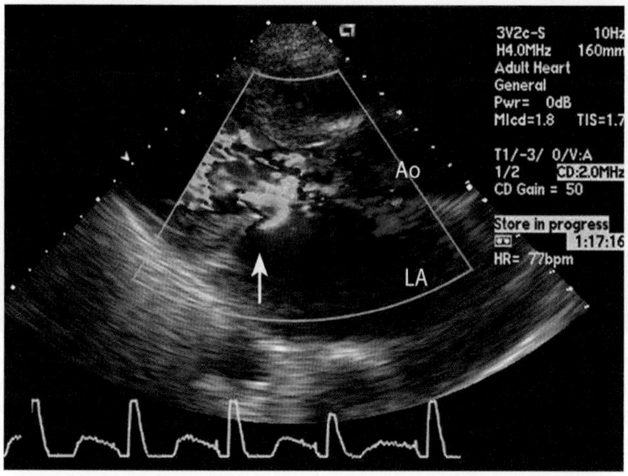

Figure 8.32 Parasternal long-axis view of a stenotic mitral valve demonstrating flow acceleration by color (proximal isovelocity surface area [PISA]) on the atrial side of the valve (*arrow*). Ao, aorta; LA, left atrium.

The current ultrasound systems have the capability to measure online peak and mean transvalvular gradients, using the modified Bernoulli equation (see earlier). Doppler-derived gradients have been shown to have excellent reproducibility and accuracy when compared to the simultaneously obtained LA-LV pressure gradient by cardiac catheterization. However, the transmitral pressure gradient is dependent on many variables other than the valve area. Therefore, the mean gradient can be increased with high transvalvular flow rate (whether because of a hyperdynamic flow state or MR), or short RR interval, even though mitral stenosis is only of a mild degree.

Mitral valve area is most easily calculated by Doppler, using the pressure half-time method. This method was originally conceived in the cardiac catheterization laboratory.[70] The severity of the stenosis is judged based on the time needed for the transmitral pressure gradient to decrease by 50% from its initial value in early diastole. This time increases with the severity of the stenosis, and mitral valve area (in cm^2) can be derived as 220/pressure half-time (in ms). Although simple and highly reproducible, its accuracy is limited in patients with abnormal LA or LV compliance, and those with significant AR.[71] The continuity equation is an additional method that is applicable in cases without significant AR and MR. In this method, the mitral valve area is calculated by systolic flow through the LVOT/TVI of mitral stenosis jet by CW.

EVALUATION OF PROSTHETIC VALVES

Echocardiography is the test of choice to assess prosthetic valve function.[72-74] From transthoracic windows, it is possible to identify the type of prosthetic valve, whether tissue or mechanical, the latter producing significant prosthetic

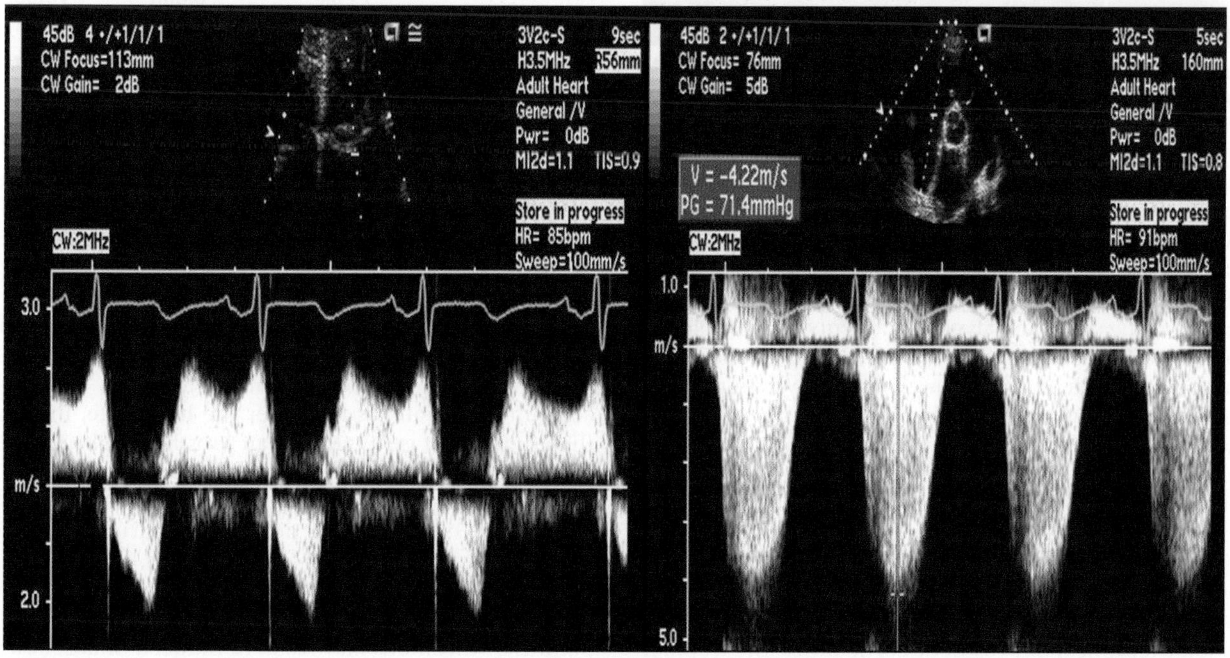

A B

Figure 8.33 **A,** Continuous wave (CW) Doppler display of mitral stenosis. Peak velocity is 2.2 m/second; time velocity integral, 67 cm; mean gradient, 11 mm Hg; mitral valve area, 1.3 cm^2, at a heart rate of 85 beats per minute. **B,** Tricuspid regurgitant signal from same patient demonstrating secondary pulmonary hypertension and a calculated right ventricular systolic pressure of at least 81 mm Hg, assuming a right atrial pressure of at least 10 mm Hg.

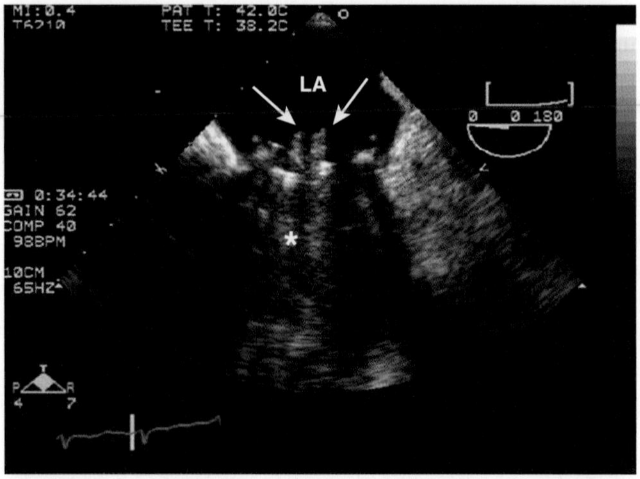

Figure 8.34 Transesophageal echocardiography of mechanical mitral valve open (*arrows*), demonstrating prosthetic artifact (*). LA, left atrium.

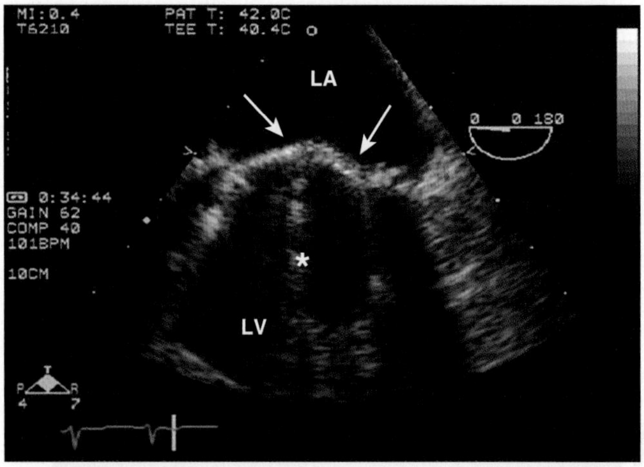

Figure 8.35 Transesophageal echocardiography of mechanical mitral valve when closed demonstrating artifact (*). LA, left atrium; LV, left ventricle.

echo artifact (Figs. 8.34 and 8.35). In some cases, large vegetations (Fig. 8.36) or thrombi may be visualized. However, in many situations of suspected prosthetic valve disease, TEE is needed because TTE images, especially with mechanical valves, can be obscured by echo artifact. Reliable recording of transvalvular gradients is possible by Doppler in almost all cases, provided the ultrasound beam is parallel to the direction of flow. Prosthetic valve gradients should be interpreted with the knowledge of the valve type, size, and position, as values vary depending on these variables (Table 8.5). Furthermore, consideration should be given to stroke volume/ventricular function/heart rate when conclusions are drawn about prosthetic valve function. It is very useful to compare Doppler-derived gradients to previous results (taking into consideration both flow and heart rates) in detecting possible changes in prosthetic valve function over time. For prosthetic aortic valves, the Doppler velocity index is calculated as peak velocity in LVOT/peak velocity across the valve by CW Doppler. Patients with normal function have a ratio that is 0.25 or greater. This ratio is particularly helpful in patients with increased transvalvular flow rate leading to increased mean gradient, as they will

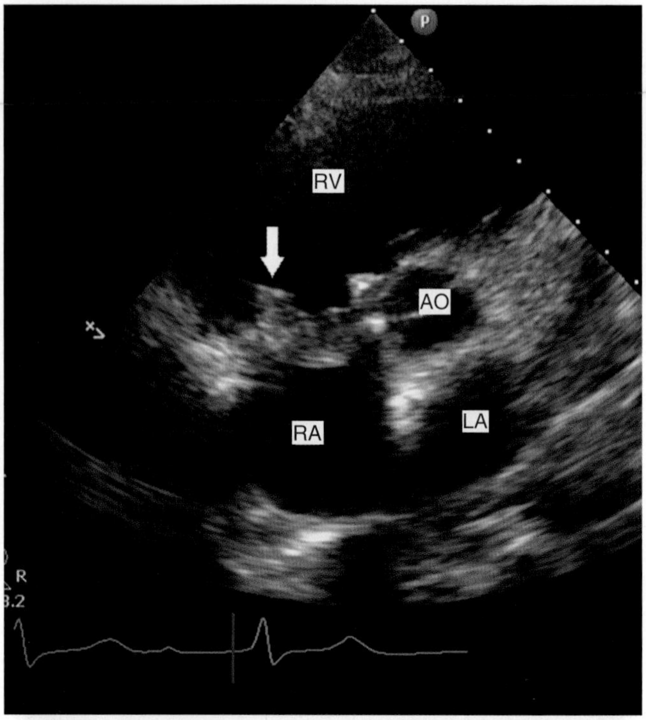

Figure 8.36 Basal short-axis TTE image of a bioprosthetic tricuspid valve with a large vegetation (*arrow*). The lesion caused both significant obstruction and regurgitation. AO, aorta; RA, right atrium; RV, right ventricle.

Table 8.5 Normal Doppler Values in Patients with Prosthetic Valves

Valve Type	Peak Velocity	Mean Gradient	Doppler Velocity Index
Aortic	≤3 m/sec*	≤25 mm Hg*	≥0.30
Mitral	<1.9 m/sec†	≤5 mm Hg†	
Tricuspid	<1.5 m/sec†	≤3 mm Hg†	
Pulmonary	≤3 m/sec*	≤25 mm Hg*	≥0.30

*Assuming normal stroke volume/ventricular function.
†Assuming normal heart rate (50-70 beats/min).

also have an increased flow velocity in the LVOT and therefore a normal Doppler velocity index.[75] Prosthetic mitral valves are best assessed by mean gradient, taking into account heart rate, as the faster the heart rate, the higher the gradient. In general, a mean prosthetic mitral gradient at a heart rate of 60 to 70 beats per minute should be less than 5 mm Hg in a normally functioning mitral prosthesis (Fig. 8.37). When there is doubt about structural or functional abnormalities of prosthetic valves, TEE should be considered. Complications of prosthetic valve endocarditis such as abscess are readily assessed by TEE (Fig. 8.38). A pannus or thrombus may result in reduced or absent leaflet motion and prosthetic valve stenosis. Depending on the thrombus burden and the clinical status of a given patient, TTE and TEE may be used to guide and follow the response to intravenous thrombolytic therapy. Although the severity and cause of prosthetic valve regurgitation may not be easily

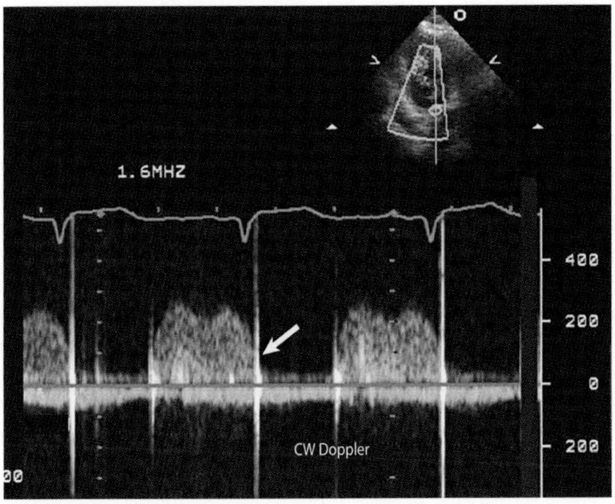

Figure 8.37 Continuous wave Doppler of an obstructed mechanical mitral valve prosthesis. Peak velocity 2.5 m/second; time velocity integral, 80 cm; mean gradient, 18 mm Hg; heart rate, 93 beats per minute. *Arrow* indicates mitral closing click.

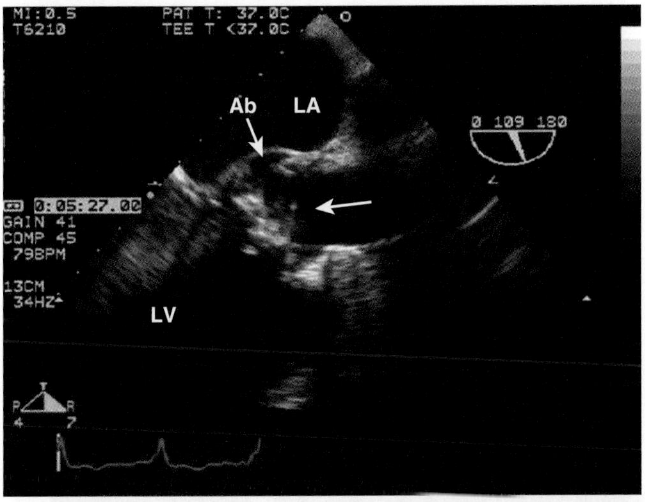

Figure 8.38 Transesophageal echocardiography of prosthetic aortic vegetation (*arrows*) and abscess/pseudoaneurysm formation (Ab). Pseudoaneurysm demonstrates systolic expansion and occurs in endocarditis when an abscess ruptures and allows communication with the systemic circulation. LA, left atrium; LV, left ventricle.

determined by TTE because of acoustic shadowing, TEE is extremely useful in evaluating the degree of regurgitation and in identifying the site of origin and direction of perivalvular leaks. Unlike prosthetic mitral valves, adequate visualization and Doppler interrogation of prosthetic aortic valves can be challenging by TEE. Therefore, if doubt remains, one should consider biplane fluoroscopy to assess the mobility of aortic valve discs. Normal Doppler values for prosthetic valves in the aortic, mitral, tricuspid, and pulmonary positions are shown in Table 8.5.

PERICARDIAL DISEASE

The detection of pericardial effusion generated much of the early interest in ultrasound as a useful cardiac diagnostic tool.[76] Today, echocardiography is routinely used to diagnose and manage pericardial disease. Pericardial effusion,

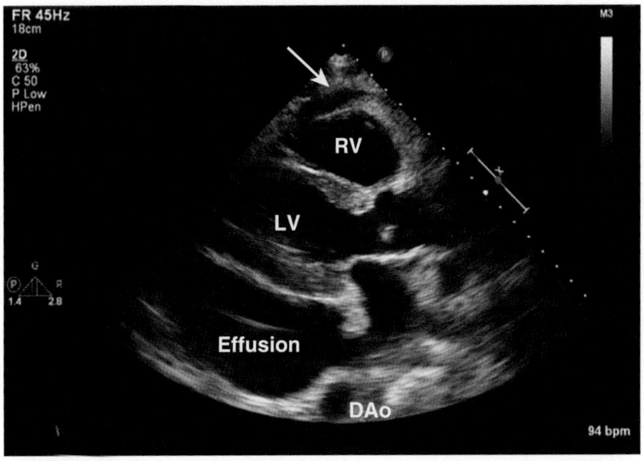

Figure 8.39 Long-axis view of large postoperative loculated posterior effusion. DAo, descending aorta; LV, left ventricle; RV, right ventricle.

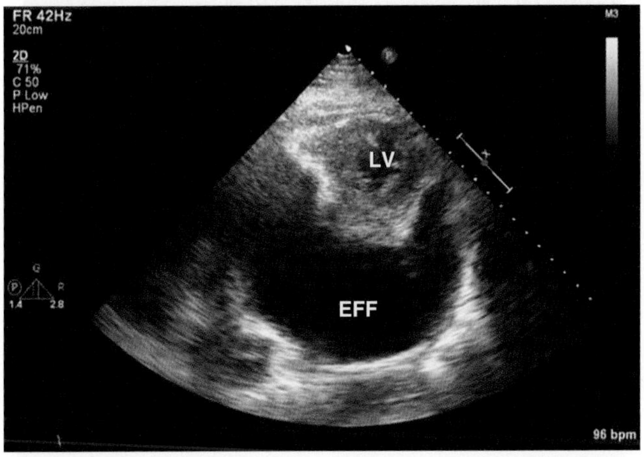

Figure 8.40 Short-axis view of the left ventricle demonstrating large posterior postoperative loculated collection of pericardial fluid (EFF). LV, left ventricle.

tamponade, and, to a lesser extent, pericardial constriction, can be readily and reliably assessed with echocardiography.

On 2D echocardiography, findings of pericardial effusion include an echo-free space adjacent to the heart as well as absence of pericardial motion (Fig. 8.39). Effusions are termed small, moderate, and large (Fig. 8.40) based on the visually estimated volume of fluid, its location (posterior only or circumferential), and the size of the heart relative to the size of the fluid space. The subcostal view is particularly useful for identifying pericardial effusions (Fig. 8.41). Large effusions may occasionally result in "swinging" of the heart within the pericardial space, a phenomenon that correlates with the electrical alternans noted on the ECG.[77] Loculated pericardial effusions can be identified in patients after cardiac surgery and in patients who sustain chest trauma. In these circumstances, the effusion is localized to a single area of the pericardial space. It is important to note that rapid development of a relatively small volume of fluid in a critical location may quickly result in hemodynamic compromise. Relatively small, localized hematoma in patients after cardiac surgery, percutaneous intervention, electrophysiology study, or trauma can create a compressive effect that compromises cardiac hemodynamics (Fig. 8.42).

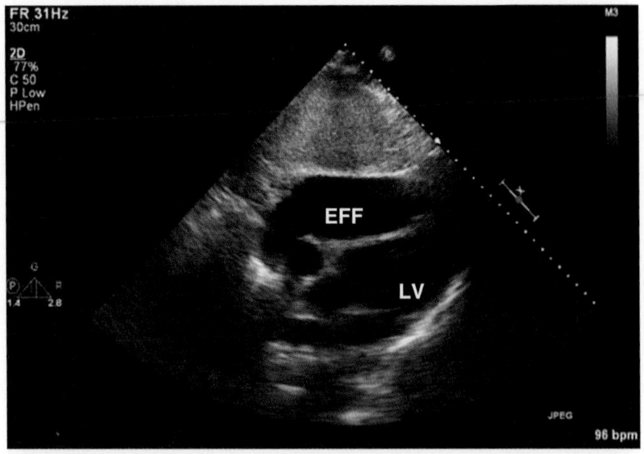

Figure 8.41 Subcostal view of inferoposterior pericardial effusion. The right ventricle is slit-like. LV, left ventricle.

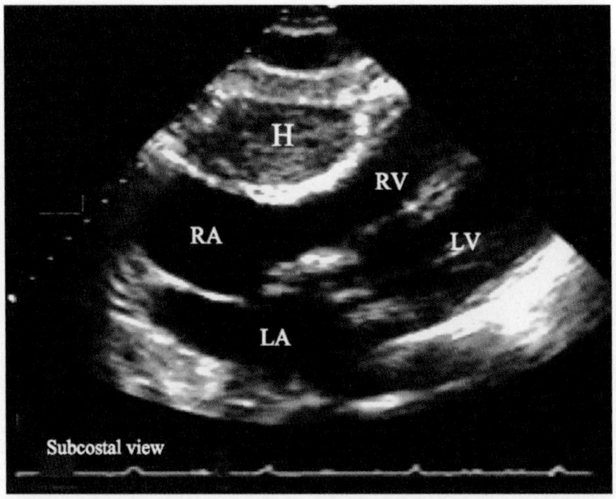

Figure 8.42 Subcostal view of intrapericardial hematoma (H). LA, left atrium; LV, left ventricle; RA, right atrium; RV, right ventricle.

Pericardial tamponade occurs when, in the presence of fluid accumulating in the pericardial space, the pressure in the pericardium exceeds the pressure in the cardiac chambers, resulting in impaired filling and reduction of stroke volume and cardiac output, eventuating tachycardia, hypotension, and jugular venous distention.[78] The physiologic consequences depend on the amount of fluid, the rate of accumulation, the distensibility of the pericardium, and the compliance of cardiac chambers.[79] Tamponade may result from accumulation of fluid, pus, blood, clots, or gas within the pericardium. There are several echocardiographic features of pericardial tamponade. Pericardial effusion, usually at least moderate in volume, must be present (unless acute as described earlier). As the pressure within the pericardium increases, cardiac chamber collapse will ensue.[80] Impairment of filling is sequential: The atria will collapse before the higher pressure ventricles.[81] The compressive effect of fluid is seen when the pressure is lowest in the chamber; RA collapse begins in late ventricular diastole (before or at the P wave) and should persist through at least one third of ventricular systole (Fig. 8.43). RA collapse occurs early in the course of tamponade but is a less specific marker than collapse of the right ventricle because the thin-walled right atrium can invert in the absence of tamponade when there is intravascular volume depletion. RV collapse occurs in early diastole.[82] This finding will manifest later in the continuum but is more specific for significant hemodynamic compromise.[83] RV collapse is best appreciated when the ultrasound beam is perpendicular to the RV outflow tract from subcostal or parasternal views (Fig. 8.44). Timing of the onset and duration of RV collapse can be appreciated with M-mode (Fig. 8.45). Right-sided chamber collapse may be absent when tamponade occurs in the setting of severely elevated right-sided filling pressures (pulmonary hypertension).[84] When the effusion is loculated behind the left ventricle in the setting of reduced LV volumes, as might be seen in postoperative patients, diastolic collapse of the LV may

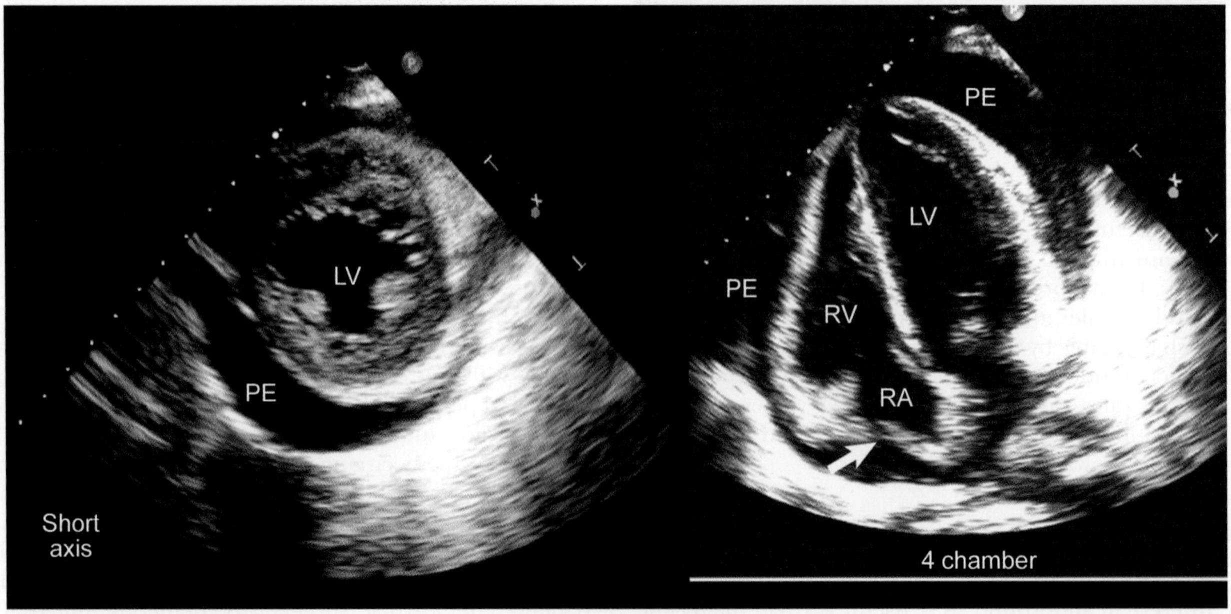

A B

Figure 8.43 Left ventricle short-axis view **(A)** of large circumferential pericardial effusion (*PE*). Apical four-chamber view **(B)** demonstrating right atrial collapse (*arrow*) and circumferential effusion. LA, left atrium; LV, left ventricle; RA, right atrium; RV, right ventricle.

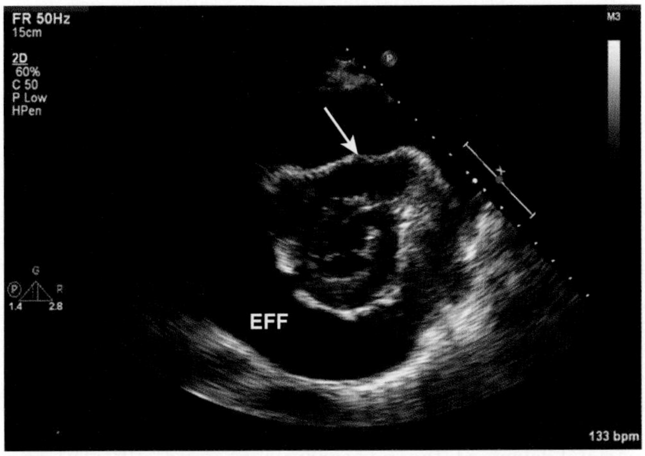

Figure 8.44 Short-axis view of the left ventricle demonstrating large circumferential effusion with right ventricular collapse (*arrow*). EFF, effusion.

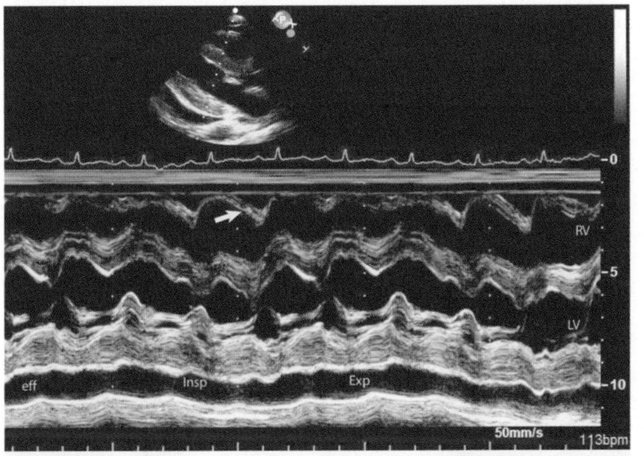

Figure 8.45 M-mode through the left/right ventricles in pericardial tamponade demonstrating right ventricular diastolic collapse (*arrow*). Note that the right ventricle fills at the expense of the left ventricle. eff, effusion; Exp, expiration; Insp, inspiration; LV, left ventricle; RV, right ventricle.

be the only indicator of hemodynamic compromise. A dilated inferior vena cava (IVC) that does not change dimension with respiration is also consistent with elevated intrapericardial pressures (Fig. 8.46), although this finding is nonspecific in intubated patients owing to positive intrathoracic pressures.

Reciprocal respiratory changes in RV and LV volumes become evident in tamponade, and increased right heart filling occurs at the expense of left heart filling in a process mediated by the pericardium. RV volume increases with inspiration, shifting the septum toward the left ventricle in diastole and toward the right ventricle in systole. RV volume decreases with expiration, normalizing septal motion as LV filling increases (Figs. 8.47 to 8.49). These findings correspond to the clinical finding of pulsus paradoxus. Transvalvular Doppler flow velocities demonstrate respirophasic changes in tamponade as well.[85] Initial transmitral velocities are enhanced with expiration and diminished (>25%) with inspiration in tamponade; transtricuspid flow augments with inspiration and diminishes with expiration (Figs. 8.50 and 8.51). Correspondingly, the RV outflow TVI increases with inspiration while the LV outflow TVI decreases. These

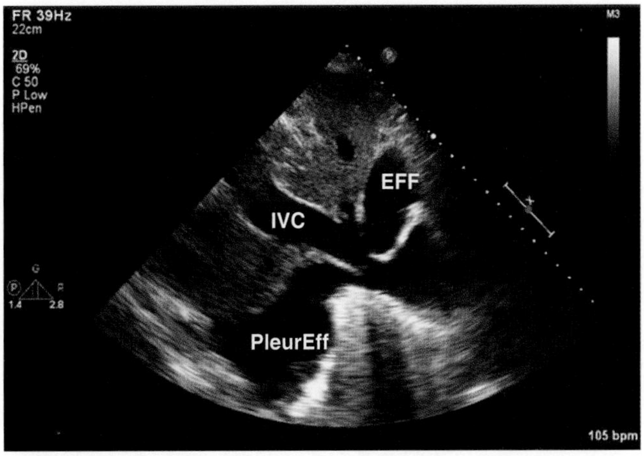

Figure 8.46 Subcostal view of inferior vena cava (IVC) plethora in tamponade. EFF, pericardial effusion; PleurEff, pleural effusion.

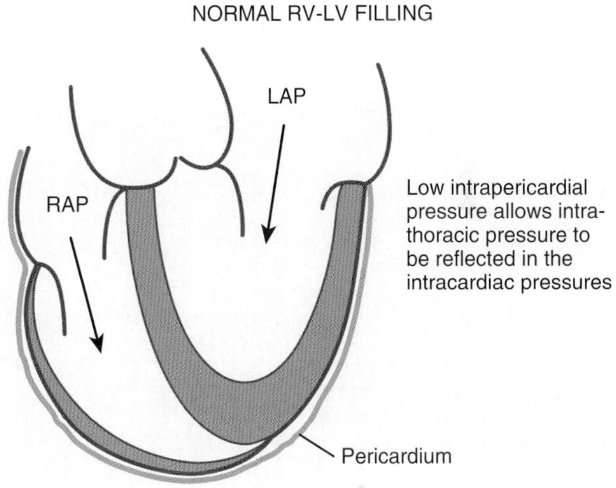

Figure 8.47 Diagram of normal ventricular filling. LAP, left atrial pressure; RAP, right atrial pressure. (Courtesy of Miguel Quinones, MD, Methodist DeBakey Heart Center, Houston, TX.)

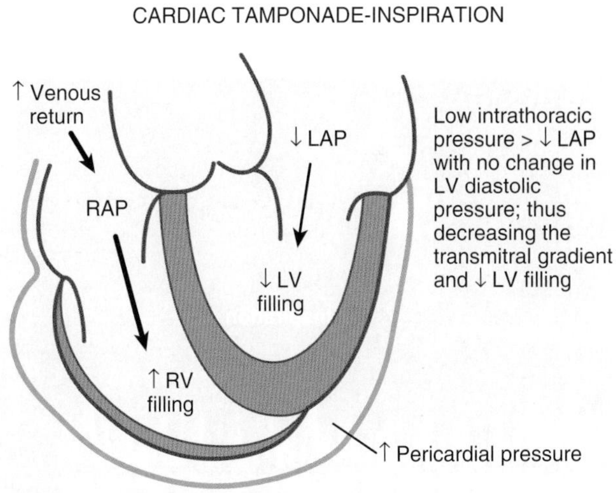

Figure 8.48 Alterations in left ventricular and right ventricular filling with inspiration in pericardial tamponade. LAP, left atrial pressure; LV, left ventricle; RAP, right atrial pressure; RV, right ventricle. (Courtesy of Miguel Quinones, MD, Methodist DeBakey Heart Center, Houston, TX.)

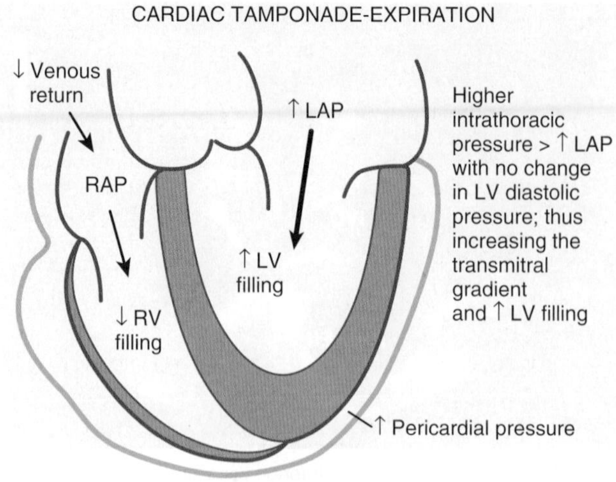

Figure 8.49 Ventricular filling pattern in cardiac tamponade during expiration. LAP, left atrial pressure; LV, left ventricle; RAP, right atrial pressure; RV, right ventricle. (Courtesy of Miguel Quinones, MD, Methodist DeBakey Heart Center, Houston, TX.)

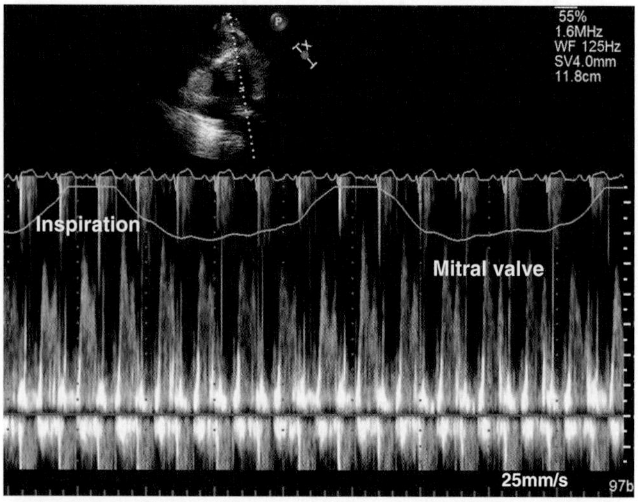

Figure 8.50 Doppler inflow of mitral valve in tamponade. Note respirometer.

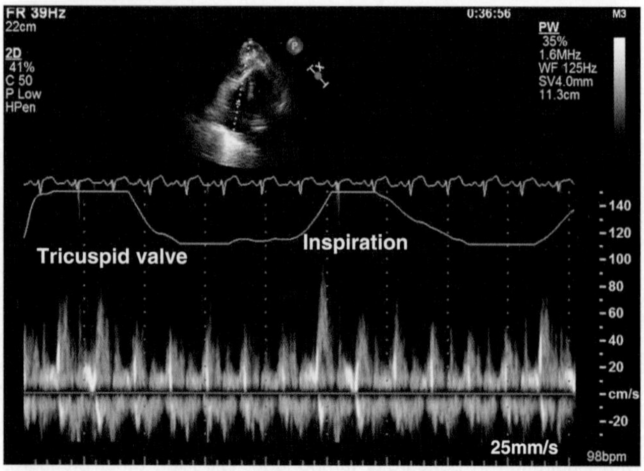

Figure 8.51 Doppler inflow of tricuspid valve in tamponade. Note respirometer.

are useful findings but can be difficult to demonstrate with precision in the acutely ill patient.

Echocardiography has been used to guide the percutaneous drainage of pericardial fluid.[86] Subcostal imaging is valuable in demonstrating the amount of inferior fluid in the typical location accessed by the subxiphoid needle approach, as well as determining the optimal site of puncture. Imaging from the cardiac apex in patients with large circumferential effusions can aid in determining needle position and guide advancement, although identifying the needle tip can occasionally be problematic. Once needle position is deemed appropriate and initial aspirate is obtained, an injection of a small amount of agitated saline confirms correct needle position within the pericardium[87] (Fig. 8.52).

Constrictive physiology is present when the visceral and parietal layers of the pericardium become adherent and fibrotic, resulting in marked impairment of LV filling. Chronic constrictive pericarditis is usually not associated with free pericardial fluid. The echocardiographic findings in constriction include a thickened pericardium (pericardial thickening may not be uniform); normal LV size with LA dilatation; abrupt termination of ventricular filling in

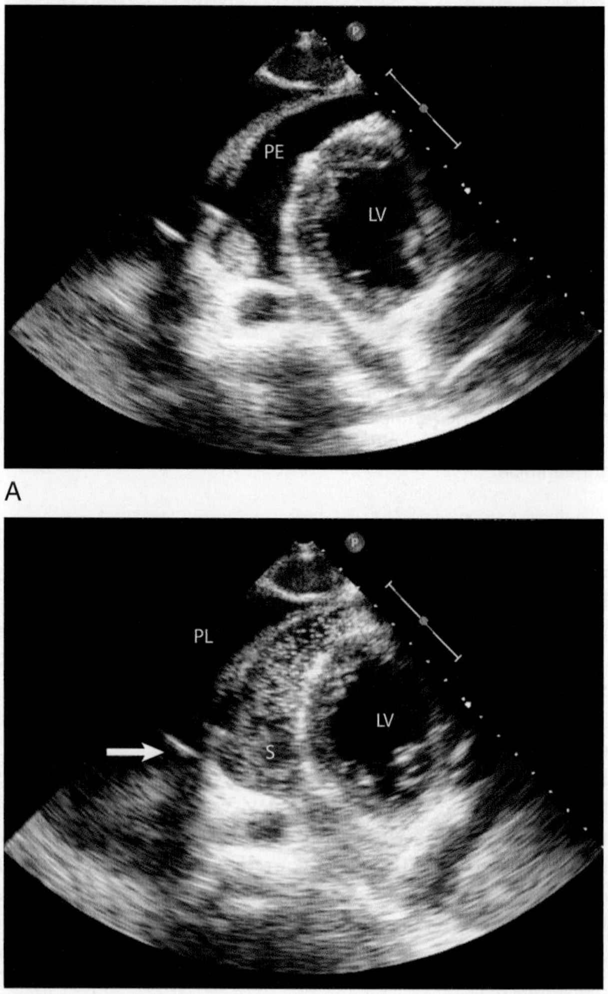

Figure 8.52 **A,** Pericardial effusion seen during pericardiocentesis before injection of saline, and, **B,** after injection of saline to confirm correct needle location *(arrow)* within the pericardial space. LV, left ventricle; PE, pericardial effusion; PL, pleural space; S, saline.

early diastole (best seen on M-mode); interventricular septal motion demonstrating a diastolic inward "bounce" in early diastole; and dilatation of the IVC. In addition, there is Doppler flow evidence of ventricular interaction with exaggerated respirophasic changes in transvalvular velocities, and dilated and plethoric IVC, like those seen in tamponade (Figs. 8.47 to 8.49, 8.53). Tissue Doppler imaging (TDI) evaluation of diastolic filling is useful in distinguishing between pericardial constriction and restrictive cardiomyopathy, as there is commonly substantial overlap of spectral Doppler findings in these entities because both share features of limited or restrictive ventricular diastolic filling. Data suggest that the mitral annulus early diastolic velocity (Ea) by TDI is usually higher in patients with constrictive pericarditis (Fig. 8.54) than in those with primary restrictive cardiomyopathy, as the rate of LV relaxation is impaired in patients with restrictive cardiomyopathy.[88,89]

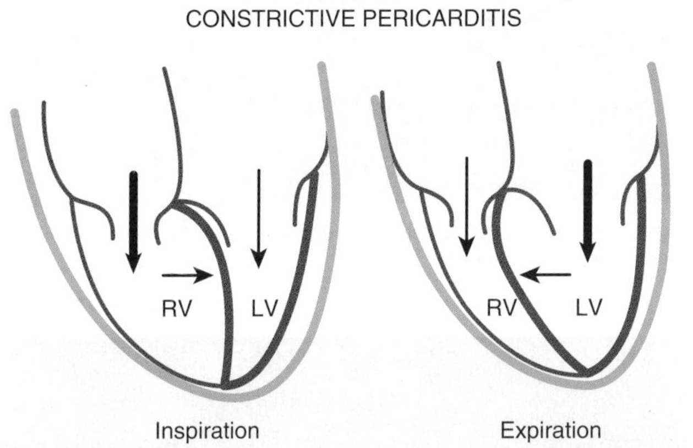

Figure 8.53 Ventricular interdependence in constrictive pericarditis. LV, left ventricle; RV, right ventricle. (Courtesy of Miguel Quinones, Methodist DeBakey Heart Center, Houston, TX.)

AORTIC DISEASE

Although TEE is the preferred method for evaluating the aorta, transthoracic imaging can visualize the proximal ascending aorta and can occasionally identify an intimal flap from aortic dissection (Fig. 8.55), either from the parasternal views or from the suprasternal notch. In addition, TTE can evaluate the integrity of the aortic valve and quantify the degree of AR; can recognize any LV wall motion abnormalities (but in this setting TTE cannot distinguish between primary ischemia and ischemia secondary to coronary extension of the dissecting flap); and can identify any associated pericardial effusion. It is important to note that, as seen in aortic aneurysms, patients with dissection very often have significant aortic dilation; thus, lack of aortic dilation may argue against dissection. However, overall, the sensitivity of

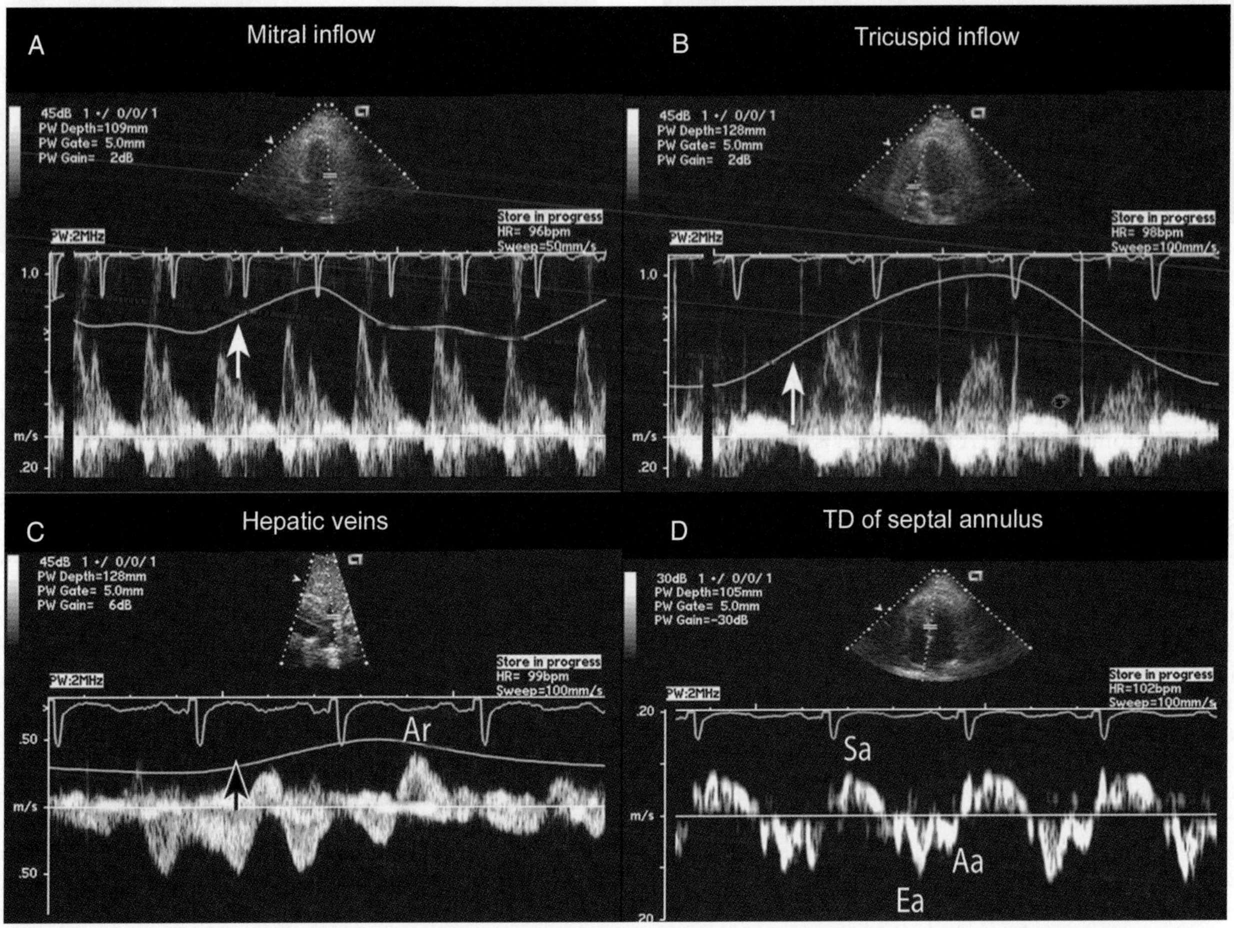

Figure 8.54 Doppler patterns in constrictive pericarditis. **A,** Respiratory variation *(arrow: inspiration)* in mitral inflow. **B,** Tricuspid inflow variability *(arrow: inspiration)*. **C,** Increase in diastolic hepatic flow reversal after expiration (Ar). **D,** Tissue Doppler of septal annulus; Ea velocity 10 cm/sec, consistent with pericardial constriction. Aa, late diastolic tissue velocity; Ea, early diastolic tissue velocity; Sa, systolic velocity.

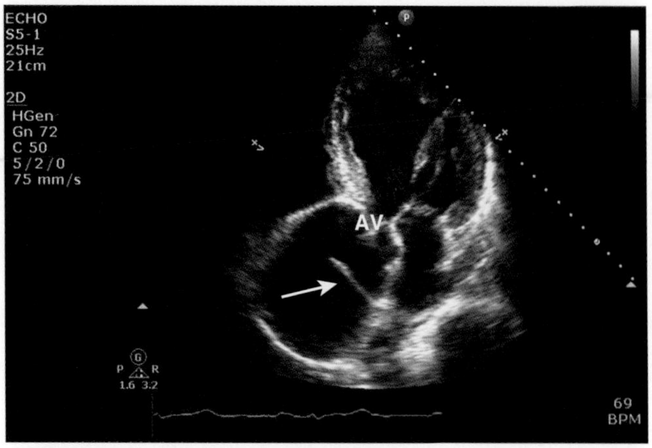

Figure 8.55 Transthoracic two-dimensional image from the apex demonstrating proximal aortic dissection flap (*arrow*). AV, aortic valve.

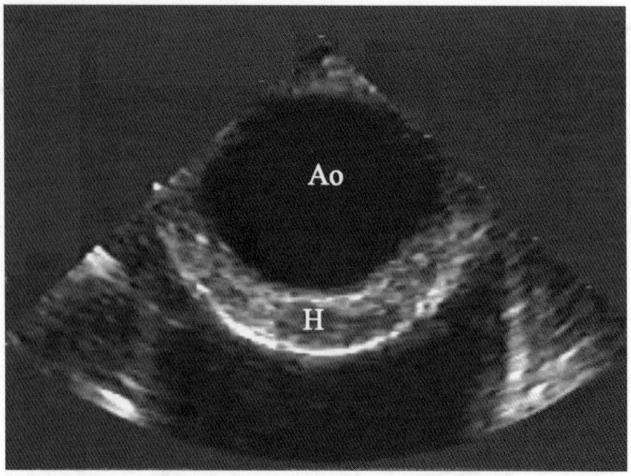

Figure 8.57 Transesophageal echocardiography of intramural hematoma (H). Ao, aorta.

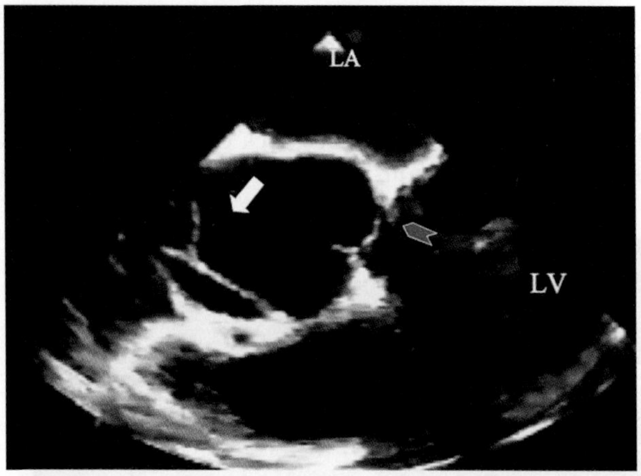

Figure 8.56 Transesophageal echocardiography image of proximal intimal dissection flap (*white arrow*). *Red arrow* indicates aortic valve. LA, left atrium; LV, left ventricle.

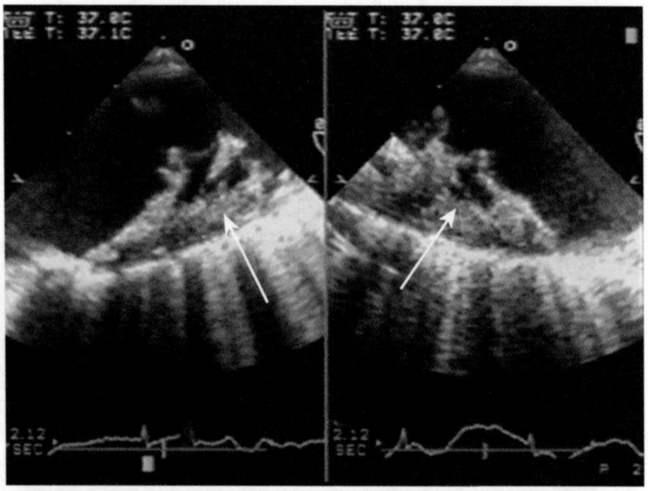

Figure 8.58 Transesophageal echocardiography of grade 5 atheromatous debris (*arrows*). This was an incidental finding.

TTE for the diagnosis of dissection in the aortic arch and descending aorta is low, and TEE (or other modalities such as computed tomography [CT] scanning) is often indicated. The close proximity of the esophagus to the aorta makes TEE the superior modality for the evaluation of aortic dissection, with both sensitivity and specificity of 98%.[90-94] The ascending aorta, aortic arch, and descending thoracic aorta can be visualized with excellent resolution. TEE can be performed rapidly and safely at the bedside. Particular attention must be given to ensuring adequate sedation to avoid hypertension, tachycardia, or gagging in patients with suspected dissection. Common features of dissection on TEE imaging include:

- An intimal flap that moves toward the false lumen in systole (Fig. 8.56)
- Color Doppler flow in both the true and the false lumens
- Color flow identification of entry/exit sites
- Stasis or thrombosis within the false lumen
- Intramural hematoma (IMH)

IMH, originally described as bleeding into the outer layers of the aortic media due to rupture of the vaso vasorum without a primary tear, appears as crescentic thickening of the aortic wall greater than 0.7 cm in the absence of a frank dissection flap (Fig. 8.57).[95] Considered a variant of overt aortic dissection, IMH is an important diagnosis to make, as data suggest IMH is a lethal condition when it involves the ascending aorta, and 16% of patients with IMH have evidence of evolution to classic aortic dissection on serial imaging.[96,97]

TEE is also very useful for identifying aortic atherosclerotic plaque (Fig. 8.58) in patients with systemic embolism (particularly stroke), as described in more detail subsequently.

CARDIAC TRAUMA

Blunt cardiac trauma occurs in the presence of evidence of external thoracic impact, such as chest wall contusions, hematomas, and fractured ribs/sternum, which is distinguished from great vessel trauma that can occur in rapid deceleration injuries. Virtually any cardiac structure can be impacted by blunt thoracic trauma and can result in significant risk of morbidity and death. Cardiac contusion is a common result of blunt thoracic trauma and is echocardiographically characterized by mainly RV—but also LV—global or regional dysfunction. Valve disruption with severe valvular regurgitation can occur; the most common valves to be disrupted are the tricuspid and mitral valves, respectively.[98] For cases of cardiac contusion, troponin levels can be helpful as negative serial troponins can argue against significant cardiac contusions.[99] Penetrating cardiac trauma is most often the result of bullet or knife penetration to the thorax but can occur from a variety of accidents. Echocardiographically, the most common manifestations of penetrating cardiac injuries are pericardial effusion/tamponade, although projectiles can at times be seen on echocardiography of the cardiac chambers. Although echocardiography has a vital role in the diagnosis and management of cardiac trauma, other imaging modalities such as radiography, CT, and magnetic resonance imaging (MRI) play important roles.

TEE is quite useful in the evaluation of the aorta following blunt injury, usually a result of high-speed deceleration accidents.[100,101] Traumatic disruption of the aorta usually involves the region of the aortic isthmus, the aortic segment between the left subclavian and the first intercostal arteries. Blunt injuries that can be identified by TEE include the more minor localized hematoma, limited intimal flaps, and mural thrombus (injuries not requiring surgical intervention), and the significant subadventitial rupture or complete transsection (injuries that require urgent surgical intervention). Subadventitial disruption commonly demonstrates a localized "thick medial flap" on TEE in association with significant change in the contour of the isthmus, or complete rupture with pseudoaneurysm formation can be seen.

INTRACARDIAC SHUNTS

Intracardiac shunts are either congenital (for example, ASD, VSD, PFO) or can be acquired, often in the setting of acute myocardial infarction (infarct-related VSD) or at times in the presence of penetrating cardiac trauma. From the critical care perspective, the important manifestations of cardiac shunts are heart failure and pulmonary hypertension from longstanding congenital lesions (for example, large ASD), stroke from right-to-left shunting in the presence of deep venous thrombosis, and persistent hypoxia resistant to oxygen therapy in the setting of right-to-left shunting. Although the discussion of congenital cardiac shunts is beyond the scope of this chapter,[102] any patient with history of cardiac surgery/intervention as a child or young adult should undergo echocardiography in the critical care setting to assess for congenital lesions, as should cyanotic or hypoxic individuals without such a history who are in critical care. Because paradoxic embolism—from the deep venous system into the vena cava, then right atrium and across into the left side of the heart—can cause embolic stroke, patients with stroke in critical care should, in the right clinical setting, be assessed for intracardiac shunt.[103] This is performed using color Doppler imaging of the interatrial septum, and if negative, followed by agitated saline contrast injection into the systemic veins, as described earlier. For patients in critical care with persistent hypoxia without obvious cause, right-to-left intracardiac shunting of deoxygenated blood can at times be the cause. In such scenarios, color Doppler interrogation including saline contrast injection under echocardiographic guidance as described previously can be of great utility (see Fig. 8.3).

HEMODYNAMIC ASSESSMENT

It is possible to calculate blood flow at several levels in the heart and aorta using Doppler echocardiography.[104] Such measurements of flow can be very useful in the ICU setting to derive LV stroke volume, cardiac output, regurgitant volumes of MR and AR, flow across an ASD or VSD, valve areas (by continuity principle), and the response to therapeutic measures such as intravenous administration of inotropic drugs or the effect of an intra-aortic balloon pump on systemic output. Stroke volume in mL (or cm^3) is calculated as the product of the cross-sectional area (cm^2) of the LVOT and the TVI (cm) by PW Doppler (Fig. 8.59) at this

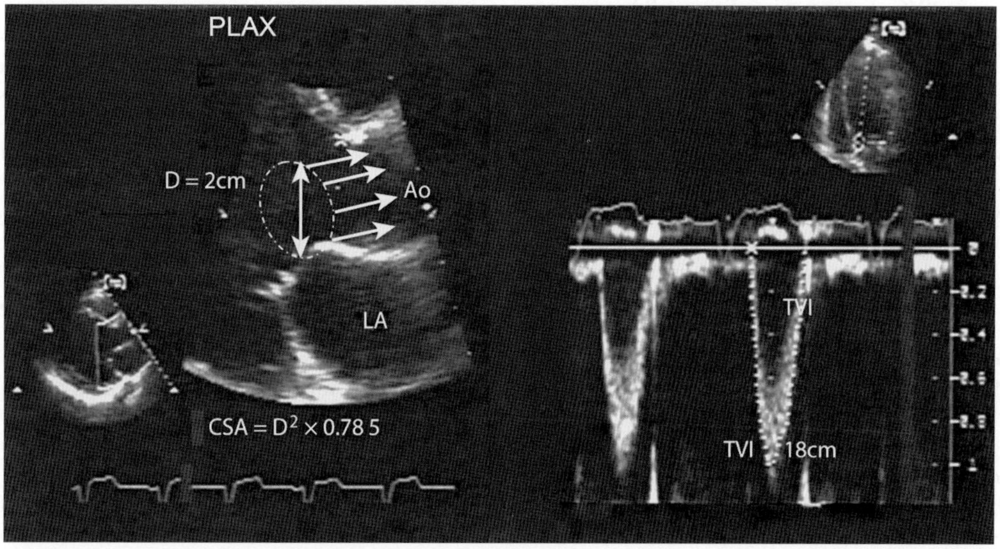

Figure 8.59 Method for stroke volume (SV) calculation using aortic annulus and aortic time velocity integral (TVI). SV = CSA × TVI. Ao, aorta; CSA, cross-sectional area; LA, left atrium; PLAX, parasternal long-axis view.

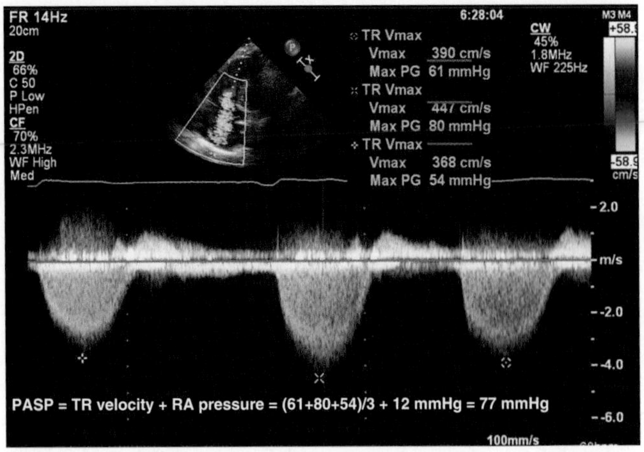

Figure 8.60 Method for calculation of right ventricular systolic pressure (see text). PASP, pulmonary artery systolic pressure; RA, right atrial; TR, tricuspid regurgitant velocity.

site.[105,106] Cardiac output can then be calculated as the product of stroke volume and heart rate. A number of studies have shown good accuracy of Doppler echocardiography when compared against measurements derived by thermodilution, including data obtained from patients in the ICU. Doppler-derived stroke volume can provide important clues in situations of reduced output (be it due to volume depletion or LV systolic dysfunction) as well as cases of high-output states such as sepsis and liver failure.

Peak PA systolic pressure is calculated from the peak Doppler velocity (v) of TR by CW (Fig. 8.60). Using the modified Bernoulli equation, the peak systolic gradient (ΔP) in mm Hg between the right ventricle and the right atrium is given by $4v^2$ (where v is in m/second). An estimate of RA pressure is then added to ΔP to estimate peak RV systolic pressure, and in the absence of pulmonary stenosis, peak PA systolic pressure.[107] RA pressure can be estimated from the change in IVC diameter with spontaneous breathing, as recorded from subcostal views. Normal variation or collapse of the IVC with breathing (>50%) implies normal RA pressure (0-5 mm Hg). Partial collapse (<50%) is generally estimated at 5 to 10 mm Hg, whereas no (or only minimal) change in IVC diameter implies an RA pressure of 15 mm Hg or more. When available, RA pressure can be obtained directly from a central venous pressure tracing, which is more accurate. In addition, hepatic venous flow may be used, particularly in patients on mechanical ventilation. Similar to pulmonary venous flow, a high RA pressure is associated with decreased RA filling from the hepatic veins during systole and increased filling during diastole (small S wave, large D wave). This measurement has been shown to have a good correlation with invasively measured RA pressure.[108]

STROKE AND OTHER SYSTEMIC EMBOLI

From 17% to 25% of all strokes are cardioembolic in origin.[109] Echocardiography, particularly TEE, is commonly used to search for potential cardiac sources of arterial emboli, the most common of which are atrial fibrillation (AF) with LA appendage thrombus, primary or metastatic LA tumor (see Fig. 8.61), atheromatous disease of the aorta (see Fig. 8.58), LV apical thrombus (see Fig. 8.13), and PFO with/without atrial septal aneurysm (ASA).[110,111] Although color Doppler may occasionally demonstrate a right-to-left shunt at the atrial level, injection of agitated saline in this setting is particularly useful in determining right-to-left bubble crossover (see Fig. 8.3). AF predisposes to thrombus formation in the body of the left atrium and in the LA appendage. Although transthoracic imaging can identify abnormalities that predispose to AF, such as mitral stenosis, TEE is necessary for a thorough assessment of the body of the left atrium and of the LA appendage, which is the most common site of thrombus formation in AF.[112,113] A significant association exists between aortic atheroma and stroke.[114] TEE reliably identifies aortic debris and can determine location, morphologic characteristics, and mobility of identified lesions (see Fig. 8.58).[113-115] The most common disorders associated with stroke identified by echocardiography are listed in Box 8.3.

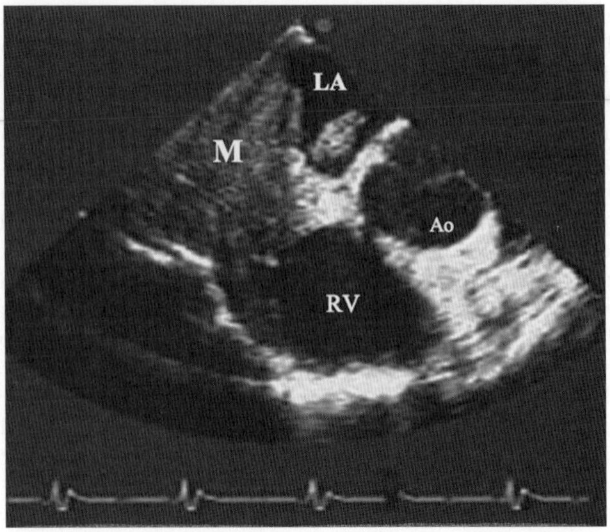

Figure 8.61 Transesophageal echocardiography of large mass (*M*) invading both atria with associated mobile thrombus in a patient who presented with bilateral upper extremity emboli and was found to have metastatic lung cancer. Ao, aorta; LA, left atrium; RV, right ventricle.

Box 8.3 Echocardiographic Evaluation of Cardiac Source of Embolus

- Intracardiac thrombus
  - Ventricular (apex)
  - Atrial (body of left atrium, left atrial appendage)
  - Prosthetic material (valves, monitoring lines, pacer wires)
  - Spontaneous contrast
- Valvular vegetations
- Patent foramen ovale/atrial septal defect
- Atrial septal aneurysm
- Intracardiac tumors
  - Primary (myxoma, fibroelastoma)
  - Metastatic (lung, breast)
- Mitral valve prolapse
- Mitral annular calcification
- Aortic annular calcium
- Atheromatous debris of the aorta

SUMMARY

Echocardiography with Doppler is a vital tool in the assessment of patients in critical care. Ventricular function and complications of myocardial infarction can be determined; the presence and significance of pericardial effusion can be assessed; hemodynamically significant valve disease can be quantified; presence and extent of infective endocarditis can be assessed; fundamental intracardiac hemodynamics can be calculated; cardiac complications of trauma can be noted; potential cardiac causes of stroke can be determined; and the assessment of aortic disease can reliably be accomplished. When TTE does not produce diagnostic images or when pertinent clinical questions remain unanswered, TEE can readily provide additional morphologic and hemodynamic information that can impact patient management and outcome in the critical care setting.

KEY POINTS

- Echocardiography is an invaluable noninvasive tool for the detection of cardiovascular abnormalities in the critical care setting.
- TEE should be used to provide more detailed or more comprehensive information when transthoracic images are inadequate. TEE may be considered for the evaluation of the aorta, for the assessment of native and prosthetic valves, and for the evaluation of intracardiac shunting.
- Commercially available contrast agents for LVO can now salvage many otherwise uninterpretable transthoracic studies.
- Echocardiography offers a number of reasonably accurate methods to assess global LV systolic properties, including EF using 2D imaging and tissue Doppler imaging. Stroke volume and cardiac output can also be reliably determined in most patients by echo-Doppler.
- Echocardiography now offers numerous methods to determine LV filling pressures with reasonable accuracy. A reliable assessment of LV dimensions and EF, when combined with knowledge of filling pressures, can be used to guide and assess the response to therapeutic measures.
- PA systolic and diastolic pressures can be calculated with confidence in many patients in the critical care setting.
- Mechanical complications of myocardial infarction, including acute MR, VSD, pseudoaneurysm formation, and LV thrombus, are readily evaluated with echocardiography.
- Although the echocardiographic assessment of the right ventricle is still challenging because of its complex shape, it is possible to integrate information from multiple views to reach reasonably accurate

KEY POINTS (Continued)

conclusions regarding RV size and function, particularly in the setting of RV pressure or volume overload.

- Echocardiography is particularly well suited to the evaluation of cardiac valve anatomy, morphologic features, and motion. The integration of 2D anatomy with spectral and color Doppler methods of quantifying obstructive and regurgitant lesions provides a comprehensive assessment of valvular disease. TEE may be needed to evaluate prosthetic valves and approaches to surgical repair.
- Pericardial effusion can be localized and quantified, and its hemodynamic impact can be assessed, with thoughtful application of imaging and Doppler techniques. In the setting of trauma and the cardiac surgical postoperative state, opportunistic loculated effusions must be identified.

SELECTED REFERENCES

6. Guarracino F, Baldassarri R: Transoesophageal echocardiography in the OR and ICU. Minerva Anestesiol 2009;75(9):518-529.

13. Yong Y, Fernandes V, Wu D, et al: Diagnostic accuracy and cost-effectiveness of contrast echocardiography on evaluation of cardiac function in technically very difficult patients in the intensive care unit. Am J Cardiol 2002;89:711-718.

16. Melamed R, Sprenkle MD, Ulstad VK, et al: Assessment of left ventricular function by intensivists using hand-held echocardiography. Chest 2009;135(6):1416-1420.

25. St John Sutton MG, Plappert T, Rahmouni H: Assessment of left ventricular systolic function by echocardiography. Heart Fail Clin 2009;5(2):177-190.

37. Nagueh SF, Appleton CP, Gillebert TC, et al: Recommendations for the evaluation of left ventricular diastolic function by echocardiography. J Am Soc Echocardiogr 2009;22:107-133.

43. Dokainish H, Nguyen JS, Sengupta R, et al: Do additional echocardiographic variables increase the accuracy of E/e′ for predicting left ventricular filling pressure in normal ejection fraction? An echocardiographic and invasive hemodynamic study. J Am Soc Echocardiogr 2010;23(2):156-161.

47. Mollema SA, Nucifora C, Bax JJ: Prognostic value of echocardiography after acute myocardial infarction. Heart 2009;95(21):1732-1745.

63. Zoghbi WA, Enriquez-Sarano M, Foster E, et al: Recommendations for evaluation of the severity of native valvular regurgitation with two dimensional and Doppler echocardiography. A report from the American Society of Echocardiography Nomenclature and Standards Committee and the Task Force on valvular regurgitation, developed in conjunction with the ACC Echocardiography Committee, the Cardiac Imaging Committee Council on Clinical Cardiology, the American Heart Association, and the European Society of Cardiology. J Am Soc Echocardiogr 2003;16:777-802.

66. Baumgartner H, Hung J, Bermejo J, et al: American Society of Echocardiography; European Association of Echocardiography. Echocardiographic assessment of valve stenosis: EAE/ASE recommendations for clinical practice. J Am Soc Echocardiogr 2009;22(1):1-23. (Erratum in J Am Soc Echocardiogr 2009;22(5):442.)

79. Little WC, Freeman G: Pericardial disease. Circulation 2006;113:1622-1632.

The complete list of references can be found at www.expertconsult.com.

9 General Principles of Mechanical Ventilation

Brian M. Fuller | Ismail Cinel | R. Phillip Dellinger

CHAPTER OUTLINE

Management of the mechanically ventilated patient is a cornerstone of critical care training and practice. The institution of mechanical ventilation can be a lifesaving measure. However, the mechanical ventilator also has potential for great harm and, in and of itself, does not reverse underlying disease. Limiting iatrogenic injury from ventilator-induced lung injury (VILI) should take high priority, along with acceptable levels of oxygenation and ventilation. The clinician should be aware of basic and advanced principles involving mechanical ventilation, allowing flexibility when applying evidence-based practices to the individual patient. Knowledge of guidelines and large clinical trials is vitally important, and the consideration of patient trajectory, individual physiology, timing of therapy, and severity of illness will make tailoring the ventilator prescription most effective.[1]

HISTORY

Hippocrates (460-370 BC) likely gave the first description of endotracheal intubation in his "Treatise on Air," in which he states that "One should introduce a cannula into the trachea along the jawbone so that air can be drawn into the lungs."[2] In 1530, Paracelsus (1493-1541) used a fire bellows connected to a tube inserted into a patient's mouth as a ventilator device.[3] The first known mechanical device designed specifically to provide ventilation for the patient was the foot pump developed by Fell and O'Dwyer in the 1880s.[4]

The first generation of mechanical ventilators focused primarily on the intermittent delivery of a bulk volume of gas to the patient with limited monitoring.[5]

Negative-pressure ventilators were invented and applied a negative pressure around the body or chest cavity. Two classic devices that provided negative-pressure ventilation were the iron lung and the chest cuirass or chest shell.[6] Iron lungs were widely used during the poliomyelitis epidemics of the 1930s and 1940s. These devices encased the patient from the neck down and applied negative pressure around the patient to expand the lungs. The chest cuirass was intended to alleviate the problems of patient access and "tank shock" that occurred secondary to venous pooling during the application of negative pressure associated with iron lungs.[7] Although the chest cuirass improved patient access and decreased the potential for tank shock, ventilation with this device was limited by the difficulties in maintaining an airtight seal between the shell and the patient's chest wall.

After the polio epidemic of the 1960s, the era of respiratory intensive care emerged, as positive-pressure ventilation via an artificial airway became commonplace.[6] Controlled mechanical ventilation eventually led to assisted modes of support, and positive end-expiratory pressure (PEEP) was introduced in the late 1960s. The improvements in mechanical ventilators came about as understanding was gained in manipulating variables of flow and pressure for patient benefit. Further technical evolution of ventilators included advances such as intermittent mandatory ventilation, and synchronous intermittent mandatory ventilation. Modern ventilators now boast microprocessors that serve both in the operating mechanism of the device and in the monitoring systems, enabling automatic adjustment of most aspects of the mechanical breath being delivered.

MECHANICAL VENTILATION

BASIC CONCEPTS

For a breath to be generated, a pressure gradient must exist. During normal spontaneous breathing, the diaphragm and other respiratory muscles create gas flow by lowering pleural, alveolar, and airway pressures relative to atmospheric pressure. Alveolar pressure is normally atmospheric at end-inspiration and end-expiration. Diaphragmatic and intercostal muscle activation during normal inspiration expands the chest and decreases intrapleural pressure from −5 cm H_2O to −8 cm H_2O. Alveolar pressure fluctuates from +1 cm H_2O during exhalation to −1 cm H_2O during inspiration.

A ventilation/perfusion ($\dot{V}/\dot{Q}$) mismatch occurs when areas of the lung are perfused but either poorly ventilated (low $\dot{V}/\dot{Q}$) or not ventilated at all (shunt). The latter is an intrapulmonary (IP) (capillary) shunt. Shunt may also be intracardiac (anatomic). Venous admixture, as a measure of less than fully oxygenated blood after passing through the lung, includes both low $\dot{V}/\dot{Q}$ areas of lung and IP shunt. Normal venous admixture is about 2% to 5%. Mechanical ventilation may increase the venous admixture to approximately 10% in the normal individual. Mechanical ventilation usually decreases venous admixture in alveolar lung disease, such as acute lung injury (ALI), improving the distribution of ventilation especially in previously underventilated lung areas. Pressures greater than alveolar opening and closing pressures expand the collapsed alveolus and prevent its collapse, respectively. However, if positive-pressure ventilation produces overdistention, redistribution of pulmonary blood flow to unventilated regions may occur, resulting in hypoxemia. *Dead space* refers to areas of the lung with a higher $\dot{V}/\dot{Q}$ ratio. *Anatomic dead space* is the volume of the conducting airways of the lungs, about 150 mL. *Alveolar dead space* refers to alveoli that are overventilated relative to perfusion; it is increased by any condition that reduces pulmonary blood flow, such as pulmonary embolism (PE) or with overdistention of the lung. *Mechanical dead space* refers to the rebreathed volume of the ventilator circuit; this volume behaves like an extension of the anatomic dead space. Mechanical ventilation can also increase dead space if it leads to overdistention.

An increased dead space fraction requires a greater minute ventilation to maintain alveolar ventilation and $Paco_2$ (partial pressure of carbon dioxide in arterial blood). Hyperventilation lowers $Paco_2$. Hypoventilation raises $Paco_2$; a modest elevation (50-70 mm Hg) reduces pH and is usually not by itself injurious in the mechanically ventilated patient. It has become increasingly recognized that hypercapnia during mechanical ventilation is well tolerated and may not be harmful. An exception occurs in the presence of increased intracranial pressure (ICP).

Although modern ventilators have evolved into complex machines, the basic premise remains: a ventilator is designed to replace or augment a patient's muscles in performing the work of breathing.[8] Ventilators use input power (electricity or compressed gas) to ventilate the lungs. To generate a breath (whether it be spontaneous or positive pressure), a pressure gradient must be generated from the airway opening to the alveoli. The volumes delivered and pressures generated largely depend on the mechanical properties of the respiratory system: the lungs and chest wall as well as the abdomen.[8] Each of these components has mechanical properties that determine the overall behavior of the respiratory system. Although the respiratory system can be quite complex, the main *variables* of interest are pressure, flow, and volume. The ventilator must generate a *pressure* to cause *flow* through an open circuit and therefore increase lung *volume*.[9] The pressure required to do this reflects a combination of the pressures to inflate the lung and chest wall. This can be illustrated by the equation of motion:[9,10]

$$\text{Muscle pressure} + \text{Ventilator pressure} = (\text{Elastance} \times \text{Volume}) + (\text{Resistance} \times \text{Flow})$$

Compliance describes the ease or difficulty of the respiratory system to expand in response to a delivered pressure and volume. Simplistically, compliance is defined by the change in volume (ΔV) divided by the change in pressure (ΔP), and the compliance of the respiratory system (C_{RS}) is $\Delta V/\Delta P_{alveolar}$. *Elastance* is the inverse of compliance, or the ratio of pressure change to volume change, and describes the tendency to recoil. *Resistance* describes the impedance to airflow through the respiratory system, or the ratio of pressure change to flow change. The *elastic load* is the pressure required to overcome the elastance of the respiratory system, and the *resistive load* is the pressure required to overcome flow resistance of the ventilator circuit, endotracheal tube, and airways.[8]

The equation of motion illustrates several basic principles. To drive gas into the patient, a ventilator can directly control either the pressure or the flow and volume applied at the airway. Despite its complexity a ventilator is simply a machine controlling one of these two variables (*control* variables). For example, in pressure control and pressure support ventilation (PSV), pressure is the control variable and is held constant, although flow and lung inflation will vary based on the patient's respiratory mechanics and inspiratory time (I time) (the latter set directly in pressure control and patient influence with pressure support). In volume ventilation, flow is the control variable and pressure and lung inflation vary with the patient's respiratory mechanics. Flow and volume are intimately linked: volume (L) = flow (L/second) × I time (second).

THE VENTILATOR CIRCUIT

The ventilator circuit consists of plastic tubing connecting the artificial airway or mask with the mechanical ventilator. Within the circuit may reside humidifiers, devices for the delivery of aerosolized medications, filters, suction catheters for secretion clearance, and heated wires.[11] The length and compliance (2-3 cm^3/cm H_2O) of the ventilator circuit are responsible for a volume of gas contained within the circuit, termed the *compressible volume.* This is partly responsible for the discrepancy between the set tidal volume delivered and the expiratory volume measured and displayed by the ventilator. The ventilator circuit also adds resistance to the system, but is minimal when compared to either the patient's inherent mechanics or the endotracheal tube. Although frequently colonized with bacterial pathogens, the routine change of the ventilator circuit for infection prevention (e.g., ventilator-associated pneumonia) is not recommended.

In the body, inspired gases are conditioned in the airway just before the carina so that they are fully saturated with water at body temperature by the time they reach the alveoli (37° C, 100% relative humidity, 44 mg/L absolute humidity, 47 mm Hg water vapor pressure). This portion of the airway acts as a heat and moisture exchanger (HME). Under normal conditions, about 250 mL of water is lost from the lungs each day to humidify the inspired gases.

Gases delivered from mechanical ventilators are typically dry, and the upper airways of patients being ventilated are functionally bypassed by artificial airways, necessitating the use of an external humidifying apparatus in the breathing circuit. Because the upper airway is bypassed during mechanical ventilation, the inspired gas temperature should be kept close to the body temperature. Inspired gases that bypass the upper respiratory tract through endotracheal tubes or tracheostomy tubes should be heated to at least 32° to 34° C at 95% to 100% relative humidity. The temperature probe for the heated humidifier should be placed inside the inspiratory limb of the ventilator circuit as close to the patient as possible. Moisture loss and subsequent dehydration of the respiratory tract result in epithelial damage.

An HME, which is placed between the artificial airway and the ventilator circuit, may be used to replace the traditional heated humidifier. During exhalation, moisture and heat from the patient are absorbed into the honeycomb structure of the exchanger and are transferred back to the patient during the next inhalation. Ventilator circuits with bacterial-viral filtering HMEs cost less to maintain and are less likely to colonize bacteria than those with heated humidifiers.[12,13] Contraindications for use of an HME are thick or large amounts of secretions, minute volume exceeding 10 L/minute, body temperature less than 32° C, and need for aerosolized medications.[14]

ALARMS AND SAFETY

Current ventilators are equipped with monitors that constantly or periodically assess the ventilator's operation and the patient's status (Fig. 9.1). These monitors are usually associated with alarms that visually or audibly notify the operator of any variation from the preset norm. Ventilator alarms can warn of potentially life-threatening events, must have an appropriate level of sensitivity and specificity, and must be evaluated clinically and in a clinical context.[15] There are some alarms related to *power input* (e.g., low battery, loss of power, loss of air supply) and *control circuit* (e.g., nonfunctioning ventilator, incompatible settings), but most alarms are related to measured *output,* such as pressure, volume, and flow.[8]

High-pressure alarms are triggered by patient factors (such as decreased compliance and increased resistance of the respiratory system) or by ventilator circuit malfunction (obstruction or kinking of the endotracheal tube). Low-pressure alarms are generally secondary to a leak in the system (ventilator circuit, endotracheal tube or cuff) or patient (large pressure loss from a bronchopleural fistula). A high expired volume alarm could be seen with improved pulmonary mechanics during pressure-control ventilation. Low expired volume could be secondary to patient-ventilator disconnect or a leak in the system or patient. A high-frequency alarm is secondary to either autotriggering or hyperventilation, and a low-frequency alarm indicates bradypnea or apnea.[8,15]

AUTOMATIC TUBE COMPENSATION

Traditionally, most clinicians apply some amount of pressure support during inspiration to compensate for the increased work of breathing related to artificial airway resistance. The amount of pressure support needed to counterbalance this resistance is highly variable, depending not only on the internal diameter of the endotracheal tube but also on flow, bend of the tube, and changing demands of the patient. This variability makes one level of pressure insufficient to meet these changing demands.[16]

Automatic tube compensation (ATC) compensates for endotracheal tube resistance via closed-loop control of calculated tracheal pressure. A ventilator with ATC compensates for the pressure drop across the endotracheal tube during inspiration by increasing the airway pressure and during expiration by decreasing airway pressure according to actual gas flow.[17-19] This technique uses a continuous calculation of the flow-dependent drop in pressure across the endotracheal tube. ATC is similar to PSV, but the pressure applied by the ventilator varies as a function of endotracheal tube resistance and flow demand. Most of the interest in ATC revolves around eliminating the imposed work of breathing during inspiration. During expiration, however, ATC may also compensate for that flow resistance by lowering the pressure in the expiratory limb transiently from its

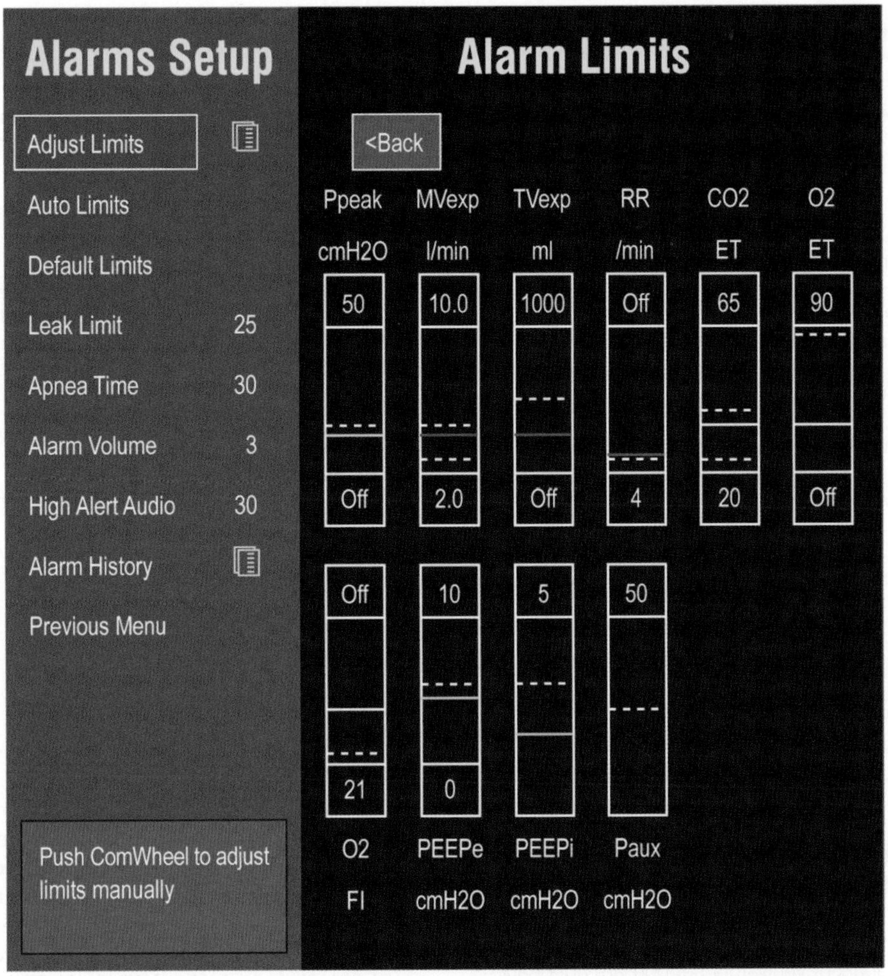

Figure 9.1 The alarm panel of a Draeger Evita 4 ventilator showing the alarms typically used on current ventilators. (Reproduced with permission from Draeger Medical, Inc., Lübeck, Germany.)

PEEP setting, helping reduce effective expiratory resistance and auto-PEEP.[17,20] In addition to overcoming the work of breathing imposed by the artificial airway, ATC may improve patient-ventilator synchrony by varying the flow commensurate with demand and may reduce air trapping by compensating for imposed expiratory resistance. During weaning trials, this technique may allow a more reliable prediction of patient performance when the tube is removed.

INDICATIONS FOR MECHANICAL VENTILATION

Mechanical ventilation is instituted for a number of reasons (Table 9.1).[21] Most commonly, these indications are a combination of a failure to adequately oxygenate, ventilate, or meet the metabolic demands of a physiologically stressed patient. Clinical indicators such as tachycardia, arrhythmias, hypertension, and tachypnea, use of accessory respiratory muscles, diaphoresis, and cyanosis are used to diagnose respiratory distress. Type I respiratory failure is hypoxemic respiratory failure, defined as a partial pressure of oxygen in arterial blood (Pa_{O_2}) less than 60 mm Hg. Type II respiratory failure is hypercarbic respiratory failure, defined as Pa_{CO_2} greater than 50 mm Hg, if elevated from patient baseline and associated with acidosis.[22] Blood pH is generally a better indicator than Pa_{CO_2} for adjusting minute ventilation. Hypercapnia should not prompt aggressive intervention if pH remains acceptable and the patient remains alert. Hypercapnia is generally well tolerated, but this clearly depends on the underlying pathophysiology and comorbid conditions of the patient (e.g., right ventricular dysfunction). However, a sustained pH of 7.65 or greater or 7.10 or less is often considered sufficiently dangerous in itself to require control of minute ventilation by mechanical ventilation. Mechanical ventilation may also be instituted to maintain normal blood pH, decrease work of breathing, assist left ventricular function in the setting of acute decompensated heart failure, or for airway protection in the setting of toxic overdose, traumatic brain injury, or any other significant acute central nervous system illnesses. Box 9.1 suggests guidelines for setting basic operating parameters in a mechanical ventilator.

MECHANICAL BREATH GENERATION

The breath generated by a mechanical ventilator can be separated into four *phases*: triggering, inspiration, cycling, expiration.

Table 9.1 Potential Indications for Mechanical Ventilation

Physiologic Mechanism	Clinical Assessment	Normal Range	Value(s)/Finding(s) Supporting Need for Mechanical Ventilation
Hypoxemia	P(A – a)O_2 gradient (mm Hg)	25-65	>350
	PaO_2/FIO_2 ratio	425-475	<300
	SaO_2	98%	<90% despite supplemental oxygen
Hypercarbia/inadequate alveolar ventilation	$PaCO_2$	35-45 mm Hg	Acute increase from patient's baseline pH <7.20 Mental status decline
Oxygen delivery/oxygen consumption imbalance	Elevated lactate	≤2.2 mg/dL	≥4 mg/dL despite adequate resuscitation
	Decreased mixed venous oxygen saturation	70%	<70% despite adequate acute resuscitation
Increased work of breathing	Minute ventilation	5-10 L/min	>15-20 L/min
	Dead space	0.15-0.30	≥0.5 (acute)
Inspiratory muscle weakness	NIP	80-100 cm H_2O	<20-30
	VC	60-75 mL/kg	<15-20
Acute decompensated heart failure	Jugular venous distention Pulmonary edema Decreased EF		Clinical judgment combined with the listed factors
Inadequate lung expansion	V_T (mL/kg)	5-8	<4-5
	VC (mL/kg)	60-75	<10-15
	Respiratory rate (breaths/min)	12-20	≥35

A – a, alveolar-arterial; EF, ejection fraction; NIP, negative inspiratory pressure; VC, vital capacity; V_T, tidal volume.

Box 9.1 Guidelines for the Initiation of Mechanical Ventilation

1. Choose the ventilator mode with which you are most familiar. The primary goals of ventilatory support are adequate oxygenation/ventilation, reduced work of breathing, synchrony between the patient and ventilator, and avoidance of high end-inspiratory alveolar pressures.
2. The initial FIO_2 (fraction of inspired oxygen) value should be 1.0. The FIO_2 thereafter can be titrated downward to maintain the SpO_2 (oxyhemoglobin saturation) at 92% to 94%. In severe acute respiratory distress syndrome (ARDS), >88% SpO_2 may be acceptable to minimize complications of mechanical ventilation.
3. Initial tidal volume (V_T) should be 8-10 mL/kg. Patients with acute respiratory failure (ARF) from neuromuscular disease often require V_T of 10-12 mL/kg to satisfy air hunger. In patients with ARDS, it is recommended to use a V_T of 6 mL/kg and to keep inspiratory plateau pressure (IPP) 30 cm H_2O or less.
4. Choose a respiratory rate and minute ventilation appropriate for the particular clinical requirements. Target pH, not $PaCO_2$. Initial respiratory rate is typically 10-12 breaths/min.
5. Use positive end-expiratory pressure (PEEP) in diffuse lung injury to support oxygenation and reduce the FIO_2.
6. In patients with COPD, avoid choosing settings that limit expiratory time and cause or worsen auto-PEEP.
7. When poor oxygenation, inadequate ventilation, or excessively high peak inspiration pressures are thought to be related to patient intolerance of ventilator settings and are not corrected by ventilator adjustment, consider initiating or increasing sedation or analgesia.

Adapted from Fundamental Critical Care Support, Des Plaines, IL, 2007, Society of Critical Care Medicine.

Triggering represents the change from expiration to inspiration and occurs either because of a drop in circuit pressure or diversion of flow (when patient triggered), or because of elapsed time. Sensitivity refers to a preset threshold of pressure or flow. When this threshold is reached, a mechanical breath is delivered. This threshold can be adjusted, and is usually set at −1 to −2 cm H_2O. If sensitivity is set too low, the ventilator will be triggered by any process that causes the airway pressure to drop below the set threshold. Such processes include patient motion, external compression, gastric suctioning, and air leaks in the circuit. Conversely, if the threshold is set too high, the work of breathing increases, as the patient must make a significant effort to overcome the threshold limit for inspiratory flow to occur. In the setting of pressure triggering, airway pressure is reduced (by patient effort) in the proximal circuit, the expiratory valve closes, pressurization of the inspiratory limb of the circuit occurs, and the patient receives a breath. Flow sensing was developed as an alternative to pressure triggering to reduce the delay in response time between neural input from the patient and delivery of gas volume by the ventilator.[23,24] In the setting of flow triggering, the patient's inspiratory effort induces a disruption of the constant flow in the ventilator inspiratory circuit. This change in flow signals the expiratory valve to close and for the ventilator to deliver the next breath. Flow triggering was initially demonstrated to decrease the work of breathing when compared to pressure triggering. However, with improvement in response time, monitoring, and feedback, pressure and flow triggering are similar in this regard.[25,26] Figure 9.2 is a representation of patient effort and ventilator response time.

During *inspiration*, pressurized gas is channeled from the ventilator to the patient after the exhalation valve closes.

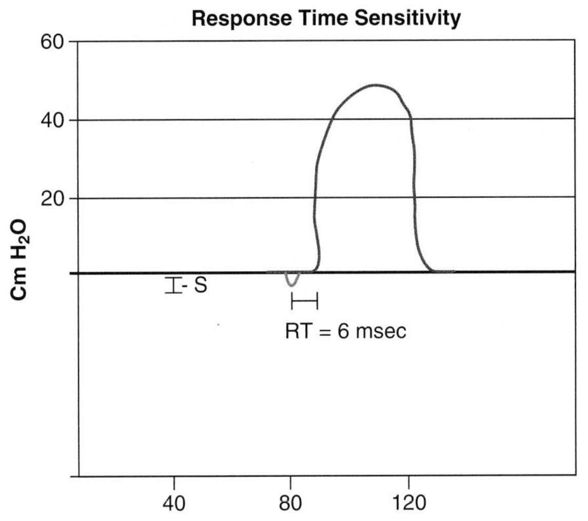

Figure 9.2 Pressure wave showing time relationship between patient inspiratory effort and ventilator response time (RT).

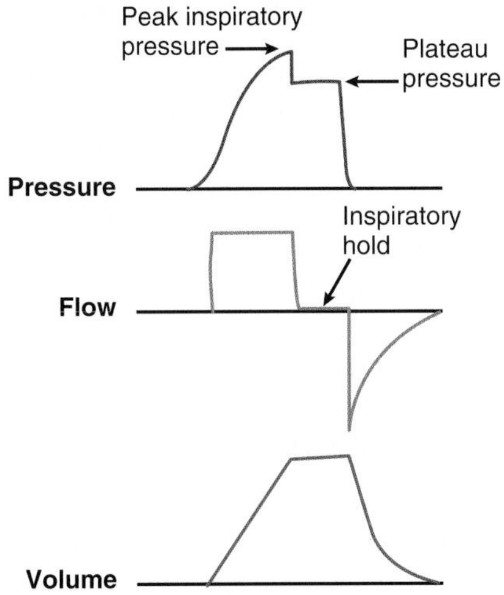

Figure 9.3 A plateau pressure measurement can be obtained in assist volume control mode by the performance of an inspiratory hold to better estimate the pressure in the lungs.

This phase can be controlled by how one sets flow or pressure in the ventilator proximal to the open inspiratory valve. For example, volume-assist control is flow controlled and pressure-assist control is pressure controlled. Choice of control variable is largely the discretion of the clinician, as either can be manipulated to achieve set goals. It should be noted, though, that in volume-targeted ventilation, excessive airway pressures can arise secondary to worsening pulmonary mechanics. In this situation, the pressure alarm will cause a pressure limit to cycle to expiration. At the end of inspiration in volume-targeted ventilation, an inspiratory hold maneuver can be performed (Fig. 9.3), which can distinguish the peak airway pressure from the plateau pressure (because flow is stopped, resistance is negligible). In pressure-targeted ventilation, minute ventilation is not guaranteed. It is a function of the compliance and resistance of the respiratory system. The clinician therefore should monitor these physiologic changes closely to avoid untoward changes in either airway pressure or Pa_{CO_2} levels.

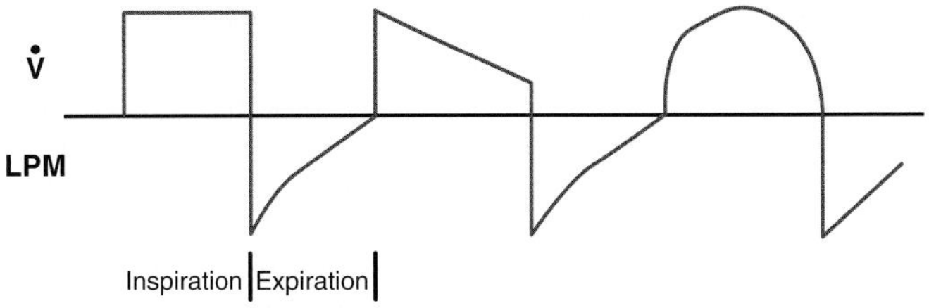

Figure 9.4 Depicted left to right are square, decelerating, and sine inspiratory flow waveforms as options for delivery of volume ventilation. Note that the square waveform produces the shortest inspiratory time and that the decelerating waveform does not return to zero flow at end inspiration. LPM, liters per minute; $\dot{V}$, flow.

With pressure control and pressure support (PS) breaths, the pattern of inspiratory flow is a natural decelerating pattern as the pressure gradient for flow decreases as pressure rises in the patient's lungs. The pattern of inspiratory flow with a flow-controlled breath is naturally square but can be computer altered to be *decelerating* or *sinusoidal* (Fig. 9.4). A square inspiratory flow pattern results in a rapid rise to a preset level (set by the clinician) followed by constant flow until cycling occurs. Decelerating flow results in a rapid rise to a maximum level followed by a gradual decrease until cycling. Sinusoidal flow pattern most closely represents normal physiologic breathing. It results in flow that gradually increases and then decreases during inspiration. The choice of inspiratory flow pattern should be based on patient characteristics, and a few common clinical scenarios should be familiar to the clinician. Square flow over time results in a shorter inspiratory time (I time), and therefore longer expiratory time (E time). For this reason it may be preferred in patients with obstructive physiology (chronic obstructive pulmonary disease [COPD] or asthma).[27,28] It is also usually tolerated better in patients with demand for high minute ventilation, such as severe metabolic acidosis or elevated ICP. In this situation, there is a potential for dyssynchrony to occur during the progression of the inspiratory phase if decelerating flow is chosen. The tradeoff is higher peak airway pressures with a square waveform, which may be ameliorated if it leads to a reduction in hyperinflation and iPEEP. Decelerating flow results in a longer I time and likely a better distribution of flow. With pulmonary pathophysiology involving heterogeneous distribution of injury (ALI as the prototype example), decelerating flow is likely the best choice, as the longer I time can lead to more homogeneous distribution of ventilation. The distribution of ventilation can be quite different when the flow pattern changes. A decelerating flow pattern yields the most even distribution under most abnormal airway conditions.[29] Studies have also demonstrated that a decelerating flow pattern improves the geographic distribution of lung vibration as a presumed surrogate of airflow.[30] The length of inspiration depends on several factors. In the pressure control mode of ventilation, the clinician directly controls the I time and I:E ratio. With pressure support the patient primarily controls I time. In flow-controlled (volume-targeted) ventilation, the I time is a function of set tidal volume (V_T) and flow rate (V_T/inspiratory flow rate) as well as flow wave characteristics (shape). The end-inspiratory alveolar pressure, as measured by an end-inspiratory hold, is the same for a given tidal volume regardless of the type of ventilator breath.

Cycling is the transition from inspiration to expiration (closing inspiratory valve and opening expiratory valve). It can occur due to a threshold of decrease in flow, elapsed time, or delivered volume. *Flow-cycled breaths* are PS breaths. Because flow rate decreases dramatically as patient inspiratory effort decreases and then ceases, the patient exerts control not only of initiation of breath but also of its termination. When a predetermined decrement in flow occurs, inspiration is terminated and the patient cycles to expiration. This is typically set at 25% of initial flow, but can be manipulated based on different clinical conditions. For example, if a large leak occurs (bronchopleural fistula or ventilator circuit leak) it may be wise to set the cycle at a higher percentage of initial flow to terminate inspiration at the appropriate time. Strength and duration of patient inspiratory effort influence tidal volume. For safety reasons, PS breaths can be cycled due to excessive pressures (e.g., coughing during inspiration) or elapsed time (e.g., secondary to a leak in the system which would prolong inspiration). In *time-cycled breaths* (pressure control), inspiration is terminated after a preset interval, regardless of whether preset pressure has been achieved or a desired tidal volume has been delivered. Pressure is maintained at a preset level throughout inspiration, yielding a square pressure waveform. Pressure-targeted ventilation is time cycled, and the time can be adjusted to yield a precise inspiration/expiration (I:E) ratio. In *volume-cycled breaths* (flow controlled), the clinician has selected the targeted tidal volume. Volume is delivered until that volume is reached. Airway pressure is directly dependent on the tidal volume and the mechanical characteristics of the patient's respiratory system. For safety reasons, volume-cycled breaths will be pressure cycled if airway pressures exceed the pressure alarm limit. In this situation, the delivered tidal volume will not reach the set volume target unless the pressure alarm limit is increased.

During expiration, flow from the ventilator is stopped, the exhalation valve opens, and gas is allowed out from the lungs. This release occurs passively. Inspiratory flow should cease prior to expiration. If this does not occur, the patient will develop auto-PEEP or intrinsic PEEP (iPEEP). This is most commonly seen in patients with expiratory flow limitation (COPD or asthma) or higher I:E ratios (see later).

VENTILATOR MODES

A ventilator mode describes ventilation over time and a set of specific combinations of breath characteristics delivered to a patient, including types of breaths, phase variables, and mandatory versus spontaneous breaths.[16] Clinician familiarity, unit, and institutional practice patterns determine to a large extent the mode that is employed. Also, data showing definitive improvement in clinically relevant outcomes when comparing one mode to another are lacking. Patient need and response to therapy should guide mode selection. Table 9.2 summarizes the features of some of the modes of mechanical ventilation, and Table 9.3 lists some of their advantages and disadvantages. Figure 9.5 also shows some characteristic waveforms of various modes of mechanical ventilation.

CONTINUOUS MANDATORY VENTILATION

With continuous mandatory ventilation (CMV), the patient has no influence on mechanical ventilation, and all breaths are mandatory. Patient-ventilator interaction is solely from the ventilator to the patient; it is time triggered and limited and cycled by the ventilator. Current ventilators do not have a CMV setting; this mode is essentially what is achieved when a patient on assist control (AC) ventilation has no interaction with the ventilator secondary to heavy sedation or neuromuscular blockade.

ASSIST CONTROL VENTILATION

In AC ventilation, a mandatory number of breaths are set and delivered with a set pressure or flow (assisted or unassisted), and if the patient's respiratory rate is higher than this backup setting (rate) additional assisted breaths to the preset pressure or flow are delivered. The target variable can be pressure (PC/AC) or volume (VC/AC).

Table 9.2 Overview of Features of Selected Modes of Mechanical Ventilation

Ventilator Mode	Trigger	Control	Cycling	Inspiratory Flow
Continuous mandatory ventilation (CMV)	Time	Flow or pressure	Volume or time	Selected or decelerating
Volume control/assist control (VC/AC)	Patient or time	Flow	Volume	Square, decelerating, or sinusoidal
Pressure control/assist control (PC/AC)	Patient or time	Pressure	Time	Decelerating
Synchronized intermittent mandatory ventilation (SIMV)	Patient or time	Pressure for patient breaths	Flow for spontaneous breaths	Decelerating for spontaneous breath
		Flow (VC) or pressure (PC) for ventilator breaths	Volume or time for ventilator breaths	Square (VC), decelerating (VC or PC), sinusoidal for spontaneous breaths
Stand-alone pressure-support ventilation (PSV)	Patient	None	Flow	Decelerating

Table 9.3 Potential Advantages and Disadvantages of Selected Modes of Mechanical Ventilation

Mode	Advantage(s)	Disadvantage(s)
Controlled mechanical ventilation (CMV)	Rests muscles of respiration	Requires use of heavy sedation/neuromuscular blockade
Assist volume control (AVC)	Reduced work of breathing Guarantees delivery of set tidal volume (unless peak pressure limit alarm is exceeded)	Potential adverse hemodynamic effects May lead to inappropriate hyperventilation and excessive inspiration pressures
Assist pressure control (APC)	Allows limitation of peak inspiratory pressures	Same as for AVC Potential hyperventilation or hypoventilation with lung resistance/compliance changes
Synchronized intermittent mandatory ventilation (SIMV)	Less interference with normal cardiovascular function	Increased work of breathing compared with assist control Patient may find it difficult to adjust to two different types of ventilator breaths
Stand-alone pressure-support ventilation (PSV)	Patient comfort Improved patient-ventilator interaction Decreased work of breathing	Apnea alarm is only backup Variable patient tolerance

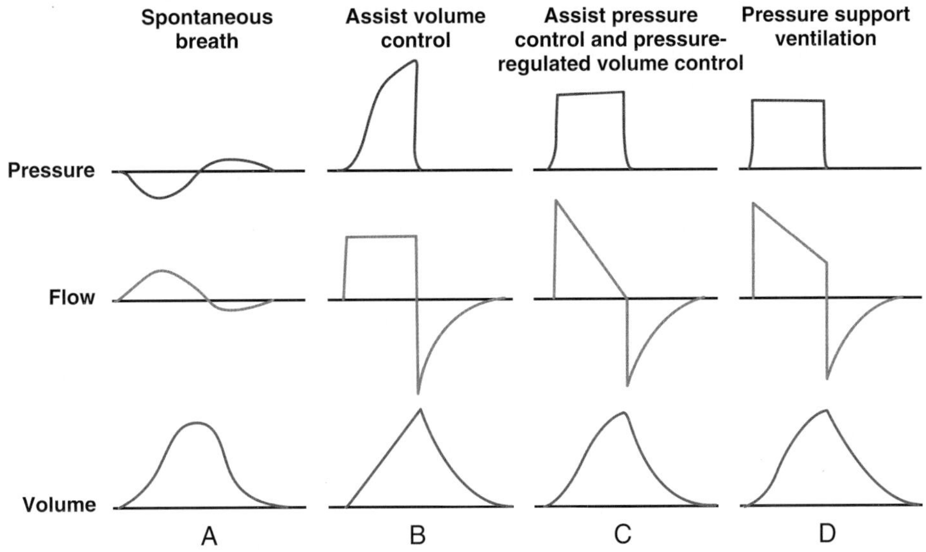

Figure 9.5 Characteristic pressure-flow waveforms with breathing spontaneously and various types of ventilation. **A,** Spontaneous breath. Such breaths are spontaneous, and inspiratory flow is achieved by the negative pressure generated by the respiratory muscles. Expiration occurs as these muscles relax. The combination of mandatory ventilator breaths (B or C) with spontaneous breaths (with or without pressure support) is called synchronized intermittent mandatory ventilation (SIMV). **B,** Assist volume control (AVC) ventilation. The flow is constant and pressure increases throughout inspiration. **C,** Assist pressure control (APC) ventilation or pressure-regulated volume control (PRVC). The pressure is constant and flow decreases throughout inspiration. In PRVC, the level of applied pressure may vary from one breath to the next. **D,** Pressure support ventilation. The pressure is constant and flow decreases throughout inspiration. When the flow reaches one fourth of its initial value, inspiration ends (flow-cycled). The flow and respiratory time are determined by patient effort and level of pressure support applied. The tidal volume varies from one breath to the next.

SYNCHRONIZED INTERMITTENT MANDATORY VENTILATION

With synchronized intermittent mandatory ventilation (SIMV), the ventilator delivers a mandatory number of breaths with a set pressure or flow (assisted or unassisted), similar to AC. However, spontaneous breaths are delivered upon patient triggering during a timing window created around the delivery of mandatory breaths. These spontaneous breaths can be totally driven by patient effort or pressure-enhanced as pressure-controlled/flow-cycled (PS) breaths. The ventilator will attempt to synchronize the delivery of this mandatory breath with the spontaneous effort of the patient (if effort is present). If the patient does not trigger a breath, then the ventilator will deliver a regularly scheduled mandatory breath (time triggered).

STAND-ALONE PRESSURE SUPPORT VENTILATION

This mode of ventilation is patient triggered, pressure controlled, flow cycled, with a decelerating flow inspiratory waveform. Cycling to expiration typically occurs when flow rate decreases to a set percentage of inspiratory flow (typically 25% of initial inspiratory flow). However, if there is a leak in the system, inspiratory flow may never decrease to the cycle threshold. In this situation, for safety purposes, flow can be time cycled as well. During inspiration, the ventilator will adjust flow to maintain the preset pressure, and tidal volume is dependent on patient effort, as well as the mechanics of the respiratory system. Pressurization rate to the goal pressure is determined by the rise time, which can be adjusted on many ventilators. If the rise time is set too low, increased work of breathing can occur; if set too high, preset pressure may be exceeded (overshoot), causing early cycling to expiration. PSV is effective at decreasing patient effort and work of breathing.[31-33] Data suggest that most clinicians view PSV as a weaning mode of mechanical ventilation, despite its being fully capable of appropriate full support in patients with respiratory failure intact respiratory drive.[34]

DUAL CONTROL MODES

The preceding modes of mechanical ventilation are classically referred to as "conventional" ventilator modes, which is purely arbitrary. Dual control modes of ventilation manipulate pressure or volume on either a breath-to-breath basis or within the same breath. Breath-to-breath modes include volume support (VS) and pressure-regulated volume control (PRVC), also called "pressure control volume guarantee." VS is PSV (pressure limited, flow cycled) that uses tidal volume as a feedback to adjust the pressure support level.[16] PRVC is pressure control ventilation (pressure limited, time cycled), but uses tidal volume as a conditional variable to adjust pressure to achieve desired tidal volume.

OTHER MODES OF MECHANICAL VENTILATION

AIRWAY PRESSURE RELEASE VENTILATION

Airway pressure release ventilation (APRV) has been described in the literature since 1987.[35] It is a time-triggered, pressure-controlled, time-cycled mode of mechanical ventilation that exactly resembles AC/PC with very extended I:E ratios if the patient is not spontaneously breathing.[36,37] It has been described as continuous positive airway pressure (CPAP) with an intermittent time-cycled release phase to a set lower pressure. Whereas conventional modes of mechanical ventilation elevate airway pressure up from a set baseline to accomplish tidal ventilation, APRV employs very high I:E ratios to maintain mean airway pressure, and brief deflations to accomplish ventilation. When APRV is used in acute respiratory distress syndrome (ARDS) (primary use) short T_{low} is used whereas this mode can be used in patients without ARDS with longer T_{low} and is often called "bilevel positive airway pressure" (BiPAP) in that circumstance (Fig. 9.6). The expiratory valve in APRV also facilitates spontaneous breathing throughout the ventilatory cycle, facilitating ventilation. Because this mode is primarily used with ARDS with long T_{high} and very short T_{low}, breathing occurs primarily during T_{high}. Pressure high (P_{high}) is the baseline airway pressure that occupies most of the ventilatory cycle. Pressure low (P_{low}) is the release pressure and is set at 0 cm H_2O. Time high (T_{high}) is the length of time for which P_{high} is maintained and T_{low} is the length of time for which P_{low} is maintained. This is primarily semantics, but the term *APRV* implies longer I:E ratios than BiPAP, and a P_{low} setting of 0 at all times.

Although outcome data are lacking compared to conventional ventilation using protective lung strategies, the

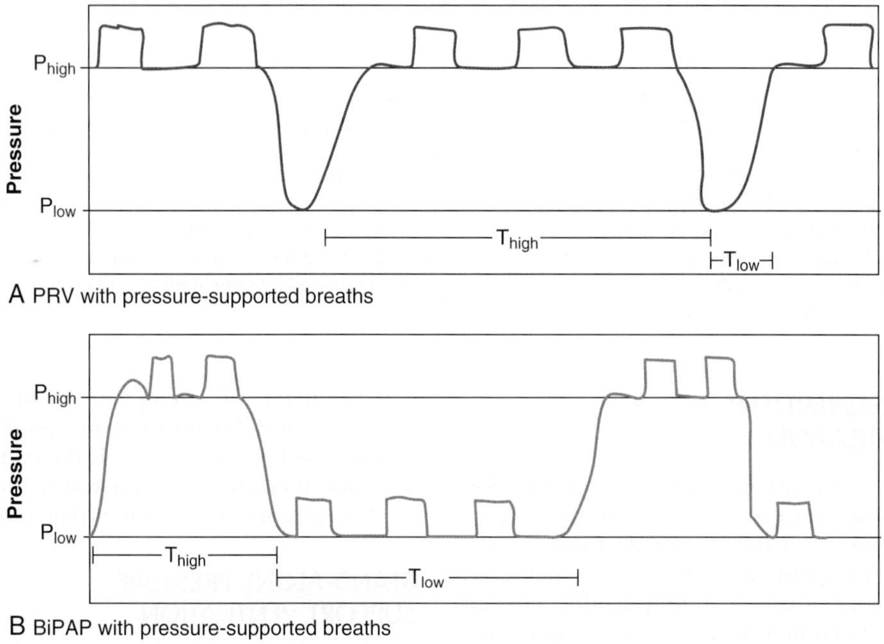

Figure 9.6 Pressure-time waveforms showing the use of airway pressure release ventilation (APRV). **A,** APRV with pressure-supported breaths. **B,** Bilevel positive airway pressure (BiPAP) with pressure-supported breaths.

reported advantages of APRV include sustained alveolar recruitment with improved oxygenation, higher mean airway pressures accomplished with lower Ppeak and Ppl, spontaneous breathing throughout the ventilatory cycle, and decreased use of sedation and neuromuscular blockade in severe ARDS.[37] The maintenance of spontaneous breathing may improve $\dot{V}/\dot{Q}$ matching by preferential ventilation of dependent lung regions, and the higher mean airway pressure, relative to Ppeak and Ppl, may limit VILI.

Alveolar recruitment is a pan-inspiratory phenomenon and alveoli that are recruited are more compliant than recruiting or nonrecruited alveoli. With prolonged elevated pressures, APRV likely recruits alveoli, which require a longer inflation with higher threshold opening pressures.[36,37] Sustained inflation maintains recruitment, decreases shunt and dead space, and employs the more compliant expiratory limb of the pressure-volume (PV) curve. Ventilation is determined by the stored kinetic energy at the high pressure, the intermittent release phase, and is augmented by spontaneous breathing. Although minute ventilation is decreased with this mode of ventilation, ventilation is also improved by a decrease in dead space.

Clinical data are limited but have shown improved oxygenation, less shunt and dead space, as well as decreased need for sedation and neuromuscular blockade.[37-41] Data on clinically relevant outcomes, such as mortality rates, mechanical ventilation days, and ICU days, are limited. This mode remains physiologically attractive for its effects on oxygenation and potential to limit VILI, but no specific recommendations can be made, given the lack of good outcome data.

HIGH-FREQUENCY OSCILLATORY VENTILATION

High-frequency oscillatory ventilation (HFOV) is very different from conventional bulk flow ventilation and uses respiratory frequencies much higher and tidal volumes much lower than conventional modes. It is similar to APRV in that it aims to elevate mean airway pressure to maximize recruitment and oxygenation, while limiting Ppeak.[42] Oxygenated, humidified gas (bias flow) passes in front of an oscillating membrane and generates very small tidal volumes at very high respiratory rates. This is actively driven by a piston pump that oscillates the diaphragm. This produces sinusoidal or somewhat erratic pressure waves that are actively driven in both inspiration and expiration (unique in that expiration is not passively driven by elastic recoil). This component is created by the backward movement of the diaphragm or piston of the oscillator. Resistance valves are used to apply a constant distending airway pressure, over which small tidal volumes are superimposed at a high respiratory frequency; in this fashion, it uncouples, for the most part, oxygenation and ventilation.

Given the fact the tidal volume is often less than anatomic dead space, HFOV relies on gas transport mechanisms much different from those employed by bulk flow ventilation. These mechanisms include some convective gas transport, but also molecular diffusion, pendelluft, coaxial flow, and Taylor dispersion.[43]

When initiating HFOV, the patient's endotracheal tube should be verified to be patent, as heavy secretions or kinks in the endotracheal tube will significantly harm ventilation. The mean airway pressure should be set at about 5 cm H_2O higher than that achieved with conventional settings. The bias flow delivers fresh gas into the ventilator circuit at 40 to 60 L/minute and helps maintain mean airway pressure.[43] The power control allows adjustment of amplitude (Δ pressure), which is set high enough to elicit vibrations of the patient to the lower abdomen or midthigh. Frequency helps determine ventilation and is set typically at 3 to 5 Hz. It should be noted, however, that at low frequencies, higher tidal volumes and bulk flow can be achieved, which assists in ventilation (and may contribute to VILI). Percentage of I time is set at 33% or 50%, depending on ventilation goals.

This effect would be predicted to be most beneficial when applied early in the course of severe ALI.[42,44] Recently completed clinical trials of the comparison of HFOV with ARDS net setting standard ventilation in patients at the onset of moderate or severe ARDS showed no benefit of HFOV, and one of the two trials showed increased mortality rate in the HFOV arm.[44,45] This would imply consideration of HFOV use only as salvage therapy in ARDS. The clinician should note that patients ventilated with HFOV will require heavy sedation or neuromuscular blockade.

EFFORT-ADAPTED MODES OF MECHANICAL VENTILATION

Early mechanical ventilators, such as the CMV mode setting, performed work on the patient and adapted the patient to the ventilator, with complete ventilator and physician control over breath characteristics and delivery. Although this can achieve adequate oxygenation and ventilation, it can come at a great expense to the patient, with side effects to include dyssynchrony, increased work of breathing, respiratory muscle weakness, and increased use of sedative infusions. Advances in ventilator technology, and increased recognition of the side effects of mechanical ventilation, have led to an increased awareness to adapt the ventilator to the patient, using the patient's physiology and demand to assist the respiratory muscles in proportion to effort and need. These effort-adapted modes of mechanical ventilation include proportional assist ventilation (PAV), neurally adjusted ventilatory assist (NAVA), and adaptive support ventilation (ASV).

PAV is a mode of partial support in which ventilator assist is delivered in proportion to patient effort. A defined level of assist, or unloading, relieves the resistive and elastic burden of the respiratory system.[46,47] The ventilator responds to the *mechanical output* of the patient and will amplify patient effort with a preset proportional amount of pressure support. The theory behind PAV is based on the equation of motion; based on changes in flow and volume, flow-proportional and volume-proportional pressure support is given. A percentage of effort is set by the clinician, and applied airway pressure develops as a function of volume to overcome elastance or a function of flow to overcome resistance.[46] Reported benefits of PAV include improved synchrony, better physiologic breathing pattern, and improved sleep quality.[48-54] A limitation of PAV is that it relies on the mechanical output from the patient, and therefore, continuous knowledge of the elastic and restrictive properties of the patient is a necessity. If PAV incorrectly estimates the mechanical properties, the ventilator may overassist, causing delayed inspiratory ending ("runaway phenomenon"). This problem has been improved by the development of PAV+ (PAV with load adjustable gain).

NAVA is similar to PAV in that it is also an effort-adapted mode of partial assist. Unlike PAV, which responds to the mechanical output from the patient, NAVA responds to the *neural input* from the electrical activity of the diaphragm (Edi). Pressure is applied in a linear proportion to Edi, and this requires the placement of an esophageal electrode (similar to nasogastric tube placement). The ventilator is triggered based on Edi or conventional signals (whichever comes first), therefore improving synchrony, as the time delay from patient effort to breathe is very brief. In addition, the amount of ventilator assistance varies based on Edi. As such, to achieve greater assistance, the patient must increase Edi. Reported benefits include improved synchrony[55-59] and preserved variability in breathing pattern.[46,60,61] High NAVA levels and high Edi may result in high inspiratory pressures and tidal volume delivery, especially in patients with unstable respiratory patterns or high respiratory drive.[62,63]

ASV ensures a set target minute ventilation based on measurements of the patient's E time constant and dynamic compliance, along with preset information of predicted body weight, minimum minute volume limit, and a pressure limit.[46] The ventilator attempts to minimize the work of breathing by combining the most effective combination of rate and tidal volume, while limiting pressure support. ASV potential benefits include decreased work of breathing and improved patient-ventilator interaction.

Effort-adapted modes of ventilator assist are physiologically attractive, especially considering that most conventional modes of mechanical ventilation are decades old. The decision to use these modes should be tailored to the individual patient. Patients with a high amount of dyssynchronous breaths and iPEEP secondary to obstructive physiology may benefit from a switch to these modes. They do not, however, ameliorate iPEEP, and extrinsic PEEP should be delivered appropriately. In patients who are severely hypoxemic or hemodynamically unstable, these modes should likely be avoided. All require an intact ventilator drive, and ongoing assessments of pulmonary mechanics is a necessity. Finally, the clinician must give up a significant amount of control with these modes of ventilation (which may be unappealing to some practitioners), and outcome data are currently lacking.

POSITIVE END-EXPIRATORY PRESSURE

CPAP maintains airway pressure above atmospheric pressure throughout the respiratory cycle by pressurization of the ventilator circuit. In mechanically ventilated patients, the purpose of CPAP is to achieve therapeutic PEEP in the presence of ALI or pulmonary edema (Fig. 9.7). In these patients PEEP serves to restore functional residual capacity (FRC), reduce IP shunt, shift ventilation to a more compliant portion of the PV curve, and prevent end-expiratory volume loss (derecruitment).[64] PEEP recruits previously nonaerated lung tissue and homogenizes regional distribution of tidal ventilation. The net effect on gas exchange reflects the balance between

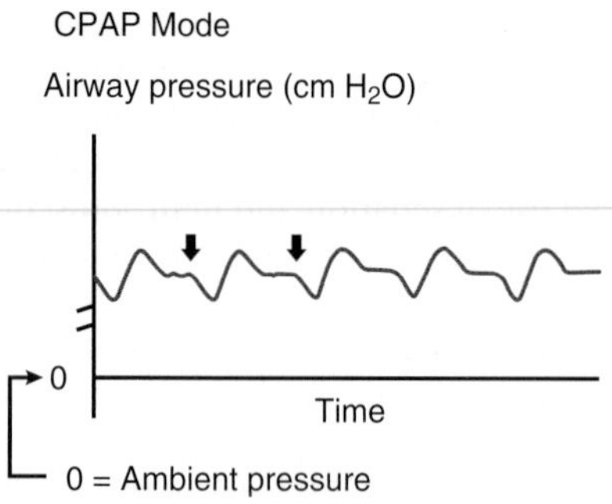

Figure 9.7 A pressure-time waveform in a patient with continuous positive airway pressure (CPAP) without application of pressure support ventilation is demonstrated. The patient is breathing spontaneously at an elevated baseline system pressure. With initiation of inspiration (*arrows*), pressure becomes more negative (but remains positive), and with expiration, pressure becomes more positive.

recruitment and overdistention. In the setting of obstructive physiology or expiratory flow limitation, PEEP serves less to improve oxygenation, but more to improve patient-ventilator synchrony and triggering.[27,28,65]

PEEP is not without side effects. Given the heterogeneous distribution of lung injury in ALI/ARDS, PEEP can overdistend more compliant lung units, contributing to VILI.[66] If PEEP leads to overdistention, it can augment dead space, increase pulmonary vascular resistance, and cause right-sided heart dysfunction. It can also decrease venous return and, in the setting of volume depletion, decrease cardiac output.

The optimal way to set PEEP is debated and controversial, as is the optimal level of PEEP to use.[67-82]

See Chapter 11 for a detailed discussion of PEEP application in ARDS.

MONITORING THE VENTILATED PATIENT

HEMODYNAMICS

Positive-pressure ventilation causes predictable physiologic changes and cardiopulmonary function is intimately linked—respiratory function alters cardiovascular function and vice versa.[83,84] The venous system is a low-pressure reservoir that contains about three fourths of our total blood volume.[83,85] This can be divided into the stressed and unstressed volume. The stressed volume contributes to the return of blood to the heart. The right ventricle's main function is to accept venous return and eject the optimal amount of blood into a (usually) highly compliant pulmonary vascular system.[84-87] This maintains a low right atrial pressure, thereby maximizing venous return and overall myocardial performance. A positive-pressure breath increases lung volume and increases intrathoracic pressure, which increases juxtacardiac pressure and therefore right atrial pressure. This can decrease venous return and therefore left ventricular preload several cardiac cycles later. At the same time, positive-pressure ventilation decreases left ventricular afterload by increasing the juxtacardiac pressure, therefore assisting ventricular contraction.

With respect to the mechanical ventilator, arterial blood pressure monitoring is commonplace in all intensive care units (ICUs). Though noninvasive cuff measurements can be adequate, invasive, continuous monitoring is much more informative when ventilator settings are dynamically changing. A fall in blood pressure temporally related to a ventilator change is a fairly specific indicator of a drop in cardiac output.[85] A narrow pulse pressure may indicate relative hypovolemia, although a widened pulse pressure may point to vasodilation or regurgitant cardiac valve disease. Pulse pressure variation (secondary to previously described heart-lung interactions) in mechanically ventilated patients is also the most accurate predictor of determining preload responsiveness.[88] Central venous pressure (CVP) is a reflection of right atrial pressure, and normally is low to maximize venous return. Despite the commonality of its use in determining volume status and preload responsiveness, data and physiology have shown that to be inaccurate.[89] This does not indicate the measurement of CVP is not of value. The absolute value and morphologic appearance (e.g., large v wave) of the CVP tracing can serve as valuable surrogates for right ventricular function, and an inspiratory fall in CVP can indicate preload responsiveness.[90] There are multiple other hemodynamic variables that could be measured in the mechanically ventilated patient, such as pulmonary artery occlusion pressure and mixed venous oxygenation, and these should be based on individual patient characteristics.

PULSE OXIMETRY

Pulse oximeters determine oxygen saturation by determining arterial blood light absorption at 660 nm and 940 nm wavelengths. The ratio of absorption of these two wavelengths is then calibrated against computer-stored algorithms to determine the oxygen saturation. Pulse oximeters are quite accurate at their upper range, but lose accuracy at lower oxygen saturations, require a good pulsatile signal, and have other limitations. These limitations include hypoperfusion, motion artifact, dyshemoglobinemias, ambient light, certain intravenous dyes, and deeply pigmented skin. Pulse oximetry is virtually ubiquitous in the ICU. Its use includes detection of hypoxemia, monitoring response to ventilator changes (such as PEEP setting), weaning F_{IO_2}, and as a surrogate for pulmonary gas exchange.[91]

END-TIDAL CAPNOGRAPHY

End-tidal capnography ($EtCO_2$) is a useful way to monitor the concentration of exhaled carbon dioxide (CO_2), plotting it against time. A normal capnogram consists of a low value at baseline during inspiration and while emptying CO_2-free dead space. This is followed by a steep increase as alveolar units empty CO_2, and this increases progressively until a plateau is reached. A normal value (e.g., when ventilation and perfusion are matched) is about 5 mm Hg less than the Pa_{CO_2}, and a normal shape consists of a low baseline, steep ascending portion, plateau, and steep decline. The $EtCO_2/Pa_{CO_2}$ gap can widen in patients with altered $\dot{V}/\dot{Q}$ relationships or changes in cardiac output; the morphologic pattern of the waveform can be altered in patients with endobronchial intubation, expiratory flow limitation, and ventilator dyssynchrony.

VENTILATOR WAVEFORMS

Modern ventilators allow continuous monitoring of pressure, volume, and flow waveforms, all of which are plotted against time. They are useful in readily identifying the mode of mechanical ventilation being used, as well as identifying physiologic abnormalities. Examination of the flow waveform can allow detection of iPEEP. A ripple-like waveform can indicate water or secretion buildup in the ventilator circuit. A prolonged expiratory flow pattern can indicate expiratory flow limitation. The pressure waveform allows calculation of compliance of the respiratory system, and an estimation of transalveolar pressure with an end-inspiratory hold maneuver to calculate plateau pressure. An initial overshoot in the pressure waveform may signal high patient effort or an overshoot on ramp speed. An upward inflection at the end of the pressure waveform could signal overdistention, and a dip in an otherwise square pressure waveform can signal patient effort and dyssynchrony.

MAINTAINING SUPPORT OF THE VENTILATED PATIENT

SEDATION AND ANALGESIA

Critically ill patients who are mechanically ventilated often require sedative and analgesic drugs, and pain is common among ICU patients.[92] The ideal sedative and analgesic regimen would provide adequate sedation and pain control, rapid onset of action, rapid recovery after discontinuation, minimal systemic accumulation, and minimal adverse effects—without raising health care costs.[93] The primary aim of these medications is to reduce the physiologic stress of respiratory failure and to improve the tolerance of mechanical ventilation. As more patients survive acute illness, the importance of goal-oriented sedation and analgesia has emerged, and the deleterious side effects of these medications is evident.[94]

Historically, mechanically ventilated patients have been treated with continuous infusions of benzodiazepines, opiates, and propofol.[95-97] Unfortunately, emerging data point to increased side effects associated with these medications, such as delirium, increased mechanical ventilation days, increased lengths of hospital stay, and higher mortality rate.[94,98,99] This has prompted interest in novel regimens with agents such as dexmedetomidine, an α_2-agonist with sedative and analgesic properties. Data have shown that dexmedetomidine use is associated with a reduction in delirium, improved cognitive function, and decrease in mechanical ventilation days.[100-104]

Regardless of the sedation regimen chosen, the mechanically ventilated patient should have sedation and analgesia titrated to a validated scale, such as the Richmond Agitation Sedation Scale, and delirium should be monitored at least daily, also with a validated scale (Confusion Assessment Method for the ICU [CAM-ICU]). All patients should be assessed daily for readiness to be liberated from the ventilator (spontaneous awakening trial [SAT]), and this should be paired with a spontaneous breathing trial (SBT).

POSITIONING

There is no optimal position for an individual patient and certainly no evidence-based gold standard. Predictable physiologic changes occur in patients when placed in the supine position, including reduced FRC, alteration in pleural pressure, reduced lung compliance, and change in $\dot{V}/\dot{Q}$ matching. The supine position should be avoided, as it is a risk factor for ventilator-associated pneumonia (VAP).[105,106] In patients with unilateral lung injury, the "good side" should be placed in the dependent position to optimize $\dot{V}/\dot{Q}$ match. Patients with severe hypoxemia (Pao_2:Fio_2 ratio < 100) should be considered for prone positioning early in the course of ALI, as this will likely improve oxygenation and may offer survival benefit in this patient cohort.[107]

SECRETION CLEARANCE

Secretion clearance is impaired in the mechanically ventilated patient owing to decreased mucociliary activity and inability to cough effectively. Removal of oral and tracheobronchial secretions is commonplace and standard care of the mechanically ventilated patient. Because of insufficient data and complications, scheduled and routine suctioning should be avoided, but the decision is based on patient assessment. The use of closed-circuit catheters is now commonplace, but data are conflicting with regard to patient benefit when compared to open-circuit catheters. Prior to the suctioning procedure, the caregiver should be aware of the potential for complications, such as hypoxia, airway trauma, and cardiac arrhythmias.

WEANING FROM MECHANICAL VENTILATION

Shortly after a patient is endotracheally intubated to initiate mechanical ventilation, thoughts should turn toward liberation from the ventilator. The withdrawal of mechanical support is a continuum from intubation until hospital discharge.[108,109] Depending on severity of illness, patient comorbid conditions, and critical care treatments needed, the timing of this may range from hours to weeks or months. There are several evidence-based guiding principles that shorten mechanical ventilation days across a broad cohort of critically ill patients.

The first step (and perhaps most important) in liberation from the ventilator is the targeted use of sedation, limitation of sedative and opioid infusions, and the monitoring for and aggressive treatment of delirium.[94] Patients should also undergo daily interruption of sedative medications (SAT), which has been shown to decrease ventilator days and ICU length of stay.[110] After awakening, the patient should be assessed for readiness to wean. The literature abounds with weaning predictors, all of which have modest sensitivity and specificity, including the frequency/tidal volume ratio.[109] Given this, as opposed to weaning predictors, the patient should undergo an SBT based on common sense, overall clinical trajectory, lack of hypoxia, and hemodynamic stability. The SAT should be paired with an SBT, as the SAT-SBT pairing decreases ventilator days, shortens ICU and hospital length of stay, and improves mortality rate.[111] An SBT can be conducted unassisted through a T-piece, on low-level PSV, or on CPAP, once or multiple times a day, and from 30 to 120 minutes; SIMV weaning is not recommended.[112-117] If a patient fails an SBT, a reason for that failure should be sought and corrected. This could include sedation, weakness, delirium, respiratory muscle fatigue, or left ventricular dysfunction. Also, after failing an SBT the patient should be placed immediately on comfortable full mechanical support, as delaying this and prolonging the SBT to the point of respiratory muscle exhaustion can delay extubation. After passing an SBT, the patient should be extubated unless a reason exists to leave the endotracheal tube in place (e.g., no cough reflex and heavy pulmonary secretions). The ability to predict successful extubation is challenging, and if the clinician never experiences a reintubation, he or she is likely not extubating patients based on the best available evidence.

COMPLICATIONS OF MECHANICAL VENTILATION

HEMODYNAMICS

Blood pressure is simply the product of cardiac output and systemic vascular resistance (BP = CO × SVR). Although the transition of positive-pressure ventilation is associated with a predictable set of physiologic responses, the overall hemodynamic response is largely a consequence of underlying patient comorbid conditions (such as left ventricular dysfunction) and preload status. Immediately after endotracheal intubation, worsening hemodynamics are usually secondary to a decrease in preload, as right atrial pressure will increase, or a drop in arteriolar tone from sedation and analgesia. Any change in hemodynamics in the mechanically ventilated patient should prompt a thorough and almost algorithmic evaluation for potential causes.

VENTILATOR-INDUCED LUNG INJURY

Mechanical ventilation can be a lifesaving intervention. However, it has great potential for harm, and the clinician's focus should extend beyond normalization of gas exchange to providing safe and physiologically sound mechanical ventilation. Perhaps nowhere is this demonstrated more significantly than with the concept of VILI. Most patients with ALI do not die of hypoxia, but rather multiple organ dysfunction syndrome (MODS).[118-121] Applied airway pressures in patients with ALI distribute in a heterogeneous fashion, leaving more compliant lung units overdistended, and others collapsed and nonrecruited. Respiratory system compliance is related to the amount of normally aerated lung tissue that remains, the so-called baby lung.[122] This heterogeneity leads to a maldistribution of ventilation, with some alveoli overdistended, others collapsed throughout the respiratory cycle, and others cyclically opening and closing. VILI is a spectrum, classically defined as barotrauma, atelectrauma, and volutrauma (stretch injury).[123] All of these can lead to biotrauma, or the decompartmentalization of the inflammatory response secondary to increased alveolar epithelial-capillary endothelial permeability. This results in the release of biologic inflammatory mediators and the spread of injury to distant organs, causing MODS and death. VILI is much more complex than the preceding definitions and involves tissue stress and strain modifiers, complex molecular mechanisms, as well as gene activation and up-regulation.[124,125]

Human studies support the concept of VILI and the importance of a protective ventilation strategy with low tidal volumes and the use of PEEP. Low tidal volume ventilation is the only intervention shown to consistently improve outcome in ALI, and support for protective lung ventilation to decrease VILI from several well-conducted clinical trials exists.[71,72,126] This includes data showing a decrease in inflammatory mediators in patients ventilated with a protective lung strategy. In the absence of a patient-specific factor to suggest otherwise, a protective ventilation strategy, consisting of low tidal volume ventilation, PEEP setting, and limitation of plateau pressure, should be attempted at all times. Emerging data suggest that these strategies should be employed not only in patients with ALI, but in all patients receiving mechanical ventilation, especially those with known risk factors for the development of ALI.[127]

VENTILATOR-ASSOCIATED PNEUMONIA

One of the most frequent complications of mechanical ventilation is the development of VAP.[128-139] VAP is discussed in Chapter 42.

GASTROINTESTINAL BLEEDING

Mechanical ventilation is a risk factor for gastrointestinal bleeding secondary to stress ulceration, trauma (especially traumatic brain injury), and major burns. Mechanical ventilation for longer than 48 hours is regarded as the most frequent risk factor.[140] The most effective treatment of stress ulceration is prevention. H_2-receptor antagonists and proton pump inhibitors have been shown to reduce the incidence of clinically important bleeding when compared to sucralfate and are considered the first-line therapy among many clinicians.[141-145]

VENOUS THROMBOEMBOLISM

Venous thromboembolism (VTE) refers to the development of deep venous thrombosis (DVT) or pulmonary embolism (PE) in the critically ill patient. Patients in whom DVT develops have worse clinical outcomes, including prolonged mechanical ventilation.[146] Furthermore, VTE is common and frequently asymptomatic in mechanically ventilated patients. Given the adverse clinical outcomes associated with VTE, thromboprophylaxis with low-molecular-weight heparin or unfractionated heparin, both administered subcutaneously, should be given unless contraindicated.[147-149]

NONINVASIVE POSITIVE-PRESSURE VENTILATION

Noninvasive positive-pressure ventilation (NIPPV) offers the potential to provide ventilatory assistance without an invasive artificial airway. NIPPV may be accomplished using a facemask or nasal mask fitted to the face and connected through standard ventilator tubing to either a standard mechanical ventilator or smaller ventilators made specifically to deliver noninvasive mechanical ventilation.

In patients with COPD and type II respiratory failure, NIPPV reduces dyspnea, decreases intubation rates, and improves mortality rates.[150-152] Similarly, in patients with cardiogenic pulmonary edema, NIPPV decreases intubation rates and improves survival.[152,153] NIPPV may also serve a critical role in decreasing mechanical ventilation days and improving weaning success, especially in patients with COPD recovering from type II respiratory failure.[154,155] Finally, immunocompromised patients, especially those with hematologic malignancies, should be considered for NIPPV.[156] Prior to initiation of NIPPV, the patient should be assessed for an adequate mental status for airway protection, hemodynamic stability, and lack of excessive secretions.

KEY POINTS

- High-pressure alarms are triggered by patient factors (such as decreased compliance and increased resistance of the respiratory system) or by ventilator circuit malfunction (obstruction or kinking of the endotracheal tube).
- Low-pressure alarms are generally secondary to a leak in the system (ventilator circuit, endotracheal tube or cuff) or patient (large pressure loss from a bronchopleural fistula).
- Automatic tube compensation (ATC) compensates for endotracheal tube resistance via closed-loop control of calculated tracheal pressure.
- The breath generated by a mechanical ventilator can be separated into four phases: triggering, inspiration, cycling, expiration.
- With pressure control and pressure support breaths the pattern of inspiratory flow is a natural decelerating pattern as the pressure gradient for flow decreases as pressure rises in the patient's lungs.
- In AC ventilation, a mandatory number of breaths are set and delivered with a set pressure or flow (assisted or unassisted), and if the patient's respiratory rate is higher than this backup setting (rate) additional assisted breaths to the preset pressure or flow are delivered. The target variable can be pressure (PC/AC) or volume (VC/AC).
- With SIMV, the ventilator delivers a mandatory number of breaths with a set pressure or flow (assisted or unassisted), similar to AC ventilation. However, spontaneous breaths are delivered upon patient triggering during a timing window created around the delivery of mandatory breaths. These spontaneous breaths can be totally driven by patient effort or pressure enhanced as pressure-controlled/flow-cycled (PS) breaths.
- Although outcome data are lacking compared to conventional ventilation using protective lung

Continued on following page

KEY POINTS (Continued)

strategies, the reported advantages of APRV include sustained alveolar recruitment with improved oxygenation, higher mean airway pressures accomplished with lower Ppeak and Ppl, spontaneous breathing throughout the ventilatory cycle, and decreased use of sedation and neuromuscular blockade in severe ARDS.[37]

- PAV is a mode of partial support in which ventilator assist is delivered in proportion to patient effort.
- NAVA is similar to PAV in that it is also an effort-adapted mode of partial assist. Unlike PAV, which responds to the mechanical output from the patient, NAVA responds to the neural input from the Edi. Pressure is applied in a linear proportion to Edi, and this requires the placement of an esophageal electrode (similar to nasogastric tube placement).

SELECTED REFERENCES

1. Marini JJ: Unproven clinical evidence in mechanical ventilation. Curr Opin Crit Care 2012;18(1):1.
32. Tokioka H, Saito S, Kosaka F: Effect of pressure support ventilation on breathing patterns and respiratory work. Intensive Care Med 1989;15(8):491-494.
34. Esteban A, Anzueto A, Frutos F, et al: Characteristics and outcomes in adult patients receiving mechanical ventilation. JAMA 2002;287(3):345-355.
39. Putensen C, Mutz NJ, Putensen-Himmer G, Zinserling J: Spontaneous breathing during ventilatory support improves ventilation-perfusion distributions in patients with acute respiratory distress syndrome. Am J Respir Crit Care Med 1999;159(4):1241.
63. Patroniti N, Bellani G, Saccavino E, et al: Respiratory pattern during neurally adjusted ventilatory assist compared with pressure support ventilation in acute respiratory failure patients. Intensive Care Med 2012;38(2):230-239.
84. Pinsky MR: Heart-lung interactions. Curr Opin Crit Care 2007; 13(5):528.
85. Magder S: Hemodynamic monitoring in the mechanically ventilated patient. Curr Opin Crit Care 2011;17(1):36.
103. Mirski MA, Lewin JJ, LeDroux S, et al: Cognitive improvement during continuous sedation in critically ill, awake and responsive patients: The Acute Neurological ICU Sedation Trial (ANIST). Intensive Care Med 2010;36(9):1505-1513.
107. Sud S, Friedrich JO, Taccone P, et al: Prone ventilation reduces mortality in patients with acute respiratory failure and severe hypoxemia: Systematic review and meta-analysis. Intensive Care Med 2010;36(4):585-599.
150. Nava S, Hill N: Non-invasive ventilation in acute respiratory failure. Lancet 2009;374(9685):250-259.

The complete list of references can be found at www.expertconsult.com.

10

Ventilatory Management of Obstructive Airway Disease

John Marini

CHAPTER OUTLINE

Positive-pressure ventilators have been in widespread clinical use for more than 4 decades. Our understanding of respiratory muscle function and ventilatory failure has undergone major revision over that period, helping to gear equipment and treatment strategies more effectively to patient requirements. Some of the more important advances in this area concern the interactions of patients having obstructive pulmonary disease (airflow obstruction [AO]) with the mechanical ventilator. Others concern physiologic principles important in withdrawing machine support from ventilator-dependent patients, many of whom have chronic obstructive pulmonary disease (COPD) or asthma. With these advances in mind, the purpose of this chapter is to provide an updated physiologic background for understanding mechanical ventilation in patients with AO, as well as to review selected aspects of this problem that are frequently overlooked and, though noteworthy, may be unfamiliar to many practitioners. Noninvasive ventilation, a modality of immense value in the treatment of alert patients with moderately severe obstructive illnesses, will not be extensively addressed here, as it is covered in other chapters of this text.

SPECIAL CHALLENGES OF PATIENTS WITH SEVERE AIRFLOW OBSTRUCTION

By assuming a major portion of the ventilatory workload, mechanical ventilation affords the opportunity to rest the respiratory muscles while maintaining pH homeostasis and oxygenation, thereby averting progressive ventilatory failure, respiratory arrest, or both. Unfortunately, these benefits are not cost-free—mechanical ventilation is expensive, uncomfortable, and inherently hazardous; few would dispute the desirability of avoiding the need for its implementation or of accelerating the process of its withdrawal. Although deceptively simple in concept, the management of patients with AO who require mechanical support often proves to be a rather complex clinical undertaking. To manage respiratory failure effectively in patients with severe AO, it is important to understand their distinctive problems. Patients with severe AO may be characterized by a number of salient clinical features. Paramount among these are increased work of breathing and mechanical compromise of the ventilatory pump that must contend with it. Such patients are also distinguished by their susceptibility to the hazards of machine support.

INCREASED WORK OF BREATHING

The mechanical breathing workload during passive ventilation can be quantified as the product of mean inflation pressure and minute ventilation. The mean inflation pressure (Pm) is approximated in a modification of the equation of motion of the respiratory system:

$$Pm = R(\text{flow}) + V_T/2C + PEEPi$$

In this equation R = resistance; V_T is tidal volume; C is respiratory system compliance (the inverse of elastance); and PEEPi is auto-PEEP, the positive end-expiratory alveolar pressure in excess of set PEEP because of dynamic hyperinflation (Fig. 10.1).

Increased resistance to airflow is responsible (directly or indirectly) for many of the physiologic disturbances that typify this disease. Flow resistance, an important determinant of Pm, is increased by structural and functional narrowing of the airway. Structural changes include a reduced number of airway channels, as well as narrowed cross-sectional airway caliber. In this already narrowed tapering network of tubes, the additional reduction of airway caliber caused by mucosal edema, functional compression, increased bronchomotor tone, or secretion accumulation noticeably increases the work of breathing because resistance relates linearly to the airway length but inversely to the fourth power of airway radius. For similar reasons, resistance within these critically narrowed airways is highly volume dependent, so that loss of lung volume is accompanied by loss of elastic recoil tension, reduction of cross-sectional area, tendency for expiratory airway collapse, and major increases in the frictional workload.[1,2]

Although each factor just enumerated contributes to AO, functional compression of the airway during exhalation is of overriding importance in many patients with components of emphysema or vigorous expiratory effort. Loss of elastic recoil encourages collapse of these narrowed bronchi as their transluminal distending pressure gradients decline (or reverse) during the course of exhalation. In most patients who require mechanical ventilatory support, dynamic airway collapse occurs even during tidal breathing, so the average airway resistance is often several times higher during exhalation than during the inspiratory phase of ventilation. This compressive mechanism underlies the phenomenon of air trapping and such hyperinflation-related consequences as loss of inspiratory power and reduced compliance of the respiratory system.

DYNAMIC HYPERINFLATION (AIR TRAPPING)

Expiration is normally a passive process that uses elastic energy stored during inflation to drive expiratory airflow. If the energy potential stored during inflation is insufficient to return the system to a relaxed equilibrium before the next inspiration begins, flow continues throughout expiration and alveolar pressure remains positive at end expiration, exceeding the clinician-selected PEEP value (Fig. 10.2).[3-9] This positive distending pressure within the alveoli increases the driving pressure for expiratory airflow and increases lung volume, thereby helping to overcome airflow resistance. Unfortunately, such hyperinflation also places the expiratory musculature at a mechanical disadvantage. Furthermore, because the hyperinflating end-expiratory alveolar pressure encourages deflation, it must first be counterbalanced by positive pressure applied to the central airway or by negative pleural pressure before inspiration can begin.[10,11] Thus PEEPi adds to the other components of the equation of motion to elevate the mean inflation pressure and inspiratory work of breathing. The process of air trapping contributes to an increase in the respiratory work of breathing in at least two other ways. Hyperinflation drives the respiratory system upward toward the least compliant portion of the pressure-volume relationship, incurring increased elastic work per liter of ventilation (see Fig. 10.1). At these higher volumes the lung approaches its elastic limit as the recoil tension of the distended rib cage becomes *expiratory* rather than inspiratory in nature. Finally,

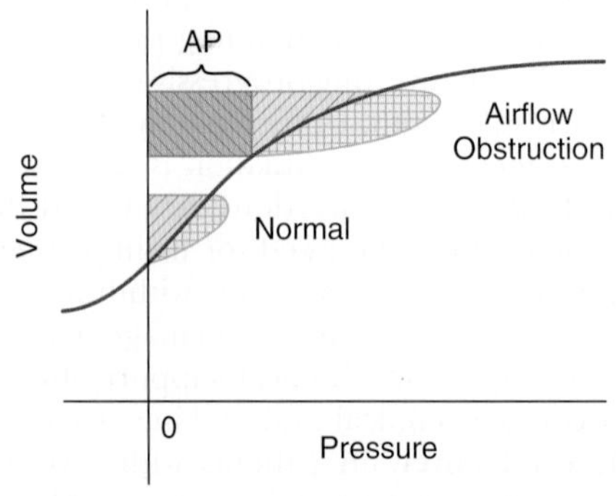

Figure 10.1 Depiction of the elements of the inspiratory equation of motion and their associated work of breathing. Stippled area is resistive work, and striped areas represent the elastic work associated with tidal volume and auto–positive end-expiratory pressure, respectively.

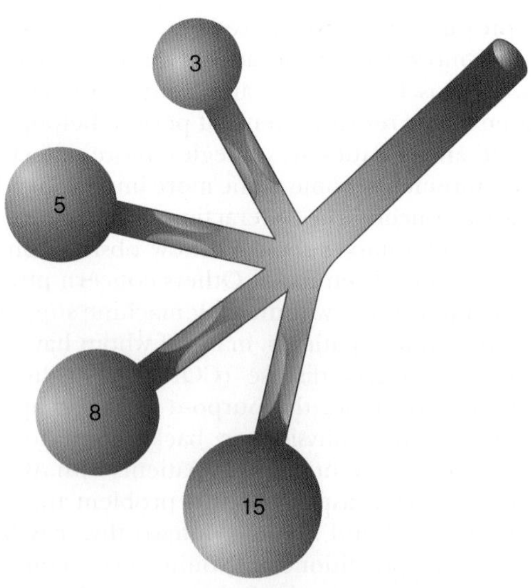

Figure 10.2 The auto–positive end-expiratory pressure (PEEP) effect. Auto-PEEP is the positive flow driving the difference between alveolar and airway opening pressures at end expiration. As depicted here, it can vary widely from site to site within the lung.

hyperinflation tends to convert more of the well-perfused ("zone 3") lung into less-well-perfused tissue, thereby increasing ventilatory deadspace and the minute ventilation requirement.

Generally, the resistance increase in patients with chronic AO and many of those with severe asthma concentrates within small airways.[1] Yet for certain asthmatic patients, the central airways and larynx contribute impressively to total resistance, accounting for the helpfulness of helium-oxygen (heliox) mixtures in some (but not all) patients during exacerbated asthma.[12] According to some reports, heliox helps to reduce air trapping in patients with COPD as well. Although there is some concern regarding the generalizability and accuracy of such observations, several mechanisms can be invoked, even if the *primary* site of expiratory obstruction is too peripheral for helium to reduce resistance there. These mechanisms include reduced inspiratory turbulence, faster expiratory flow in non–flow-limited channels with increased wave speed, modestly decreased CO_2 production, and perhaps reduced associated gas trapping.

Of note, dynamically positive end-expiratory alveolar pressure can also exist without hyperinflation, provided that airway collapse does not occur. In these instances expiratory muscle contraction increases pleural pressure, alveolar pressure, and the speed of expiratory airflow, obviating the need for hyperinflation to complete exhalation in the allotted time. Such mechanisms are employed by normal subjects during heavy exercise or when faced with major respiratory workloads. Indeed, many untrained normal subjects expire to positions below the equilibrium point of the respiratory system when exposed to PEEP. In this way the respiratory muscles can begin contraction from a mechanically advantageous position, and the expiratory muscles can share in the ventilatory work. Using this strategy, PEEP actually provides a boost to *inspiration,* experienced early in the cycle when the *expiratory* muscles relax. This "work-sharing" strategy, although effective for a normal individual, cannot be implemented by patients who experience dynamic airway collapse during tidal breathing. Because forceful expiratory efforts succeed not only in raising alveolar pressure but also in intensifying dynamic airway collapse, flow rate is determined strictly by lung volume and is not accelerated by expiratory muscle activity after the first third of expiration has been completed.

When dynamic collapse occurs during tidal respiration and breathing requirements are high, there is little alternative to hyperinflation, CO_2 retention, or both. At the chosen level of minute ventilation, maintaining the lower lung volume may be either too energy costly or physically impossible. For this reason, many patients with severe obstruction do not or cannot decrease their lung volumes when recumbent. Such considerations may help to explain the dyspnea experienced by most patients with severe AO on assuming horizontal positions. For the same recumbent angle, the lateral position allows slightly more decompression than does the supine position because lung volume influences airway caliber, airway resistance, and tendency for collapse as the lung deflates.[13] Patients with obesity have a lower resting lung volume and therefore exhibit higher airway resistance and tendency for dependent atelectasis and symptoms when airways are narrowed by bronchoconstriction or disease. Likewise, patients with acute respiratory distress syndrome have higher than normal airway resistance in dependent zones.

In fact, the distribution of gas trapping varies regionally throughout any diseased lung, depending on the local mechanical properties of the airways. Therefore, at the end of the expiratory cycle some zones remain patent, and some have sealed much earlier in the deflation cycle (see Fig. 10.2). Consequently, the end-expiratory value of auto-PEEP detected at the airway opening may not reflect the magnitude of gas trapping.[14] Clues to the presence of regional closure are often seen when the airway is occluded at end expiration; the auto-PEEP value shows an atypically slow rise to its final value as quasi-occluded small airways decompress into the common airway. In such cases, PEEP often eliminates this characteristic. During volume-controlled ventilation, plateau pressure tracks hyperinflation more reliably than direct measurements of PEEPi.

In some patients, especially those who passively receive ventilatory support, the problems presented by air trapping and dynamic hyperinflation are as much cardiovascular as pulmonary in nature. A relatively high fraction of the resulting positive alveolar pressure is transmitted to the pleural space, where it impedes venous return and confuses interpretation of hemodynamic pressure measurements made with pulmonary artery catheters (Fig. 10.3). Lung distention also adds to pulmonary vascular resistance, exacerbating the tendencies of patients with *cor pulmonale* toward low cardiac output and hypotension. Marked respiratory variation of systolic and pulse pressures during passive inflation indicates phasically adverse cardiac loading and strongly implies the possibility of dynamic hyperinflation (Fig. 10.4).

INCREASED MINUTE VENTILATION REQUIREMENT

Ventilation-perfusion ($\dot{V}/\dot{Q}$) mismatching is widespread in patients with severe AO, reducing the efficiency of carbon dioxide elimination.[1] It is not uncommon for the resting minute ventilation requirement to exceed 12 L per minute (twice the normal value) in patients with exacerbated

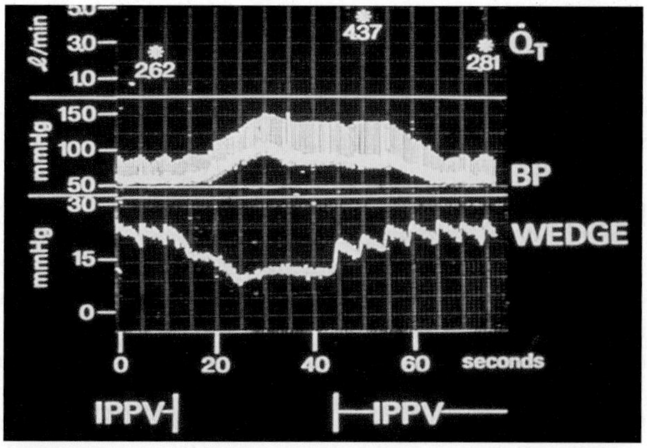

Figure 10.3 The hemodynamic impact of auto-PEEP (positive end-expiratory pressure) in a passively ventilated patient with severe airflow obstruction. A 40-second disconnection of the ventilator was associated with rising blood pressure and cardiac output despite a falling pulmonary artery wedge pressure.

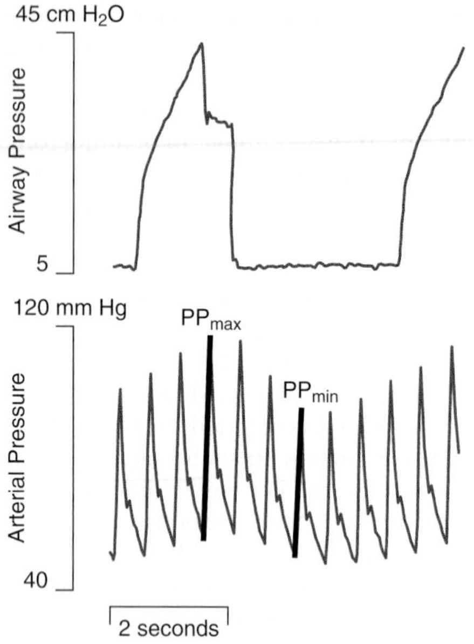

Figure 10.4 Marked respiratory variation of systemic arterial blood pressure, indicative of the relative variation in cardiac loading conditions associated with dynamic hyperinflation. PP, pulse pressure. (From Michard F, Teboul J-L: Using heart-lung interactions to assess fluid responsiveness during mechanical ventilation. Crit Care 2000;4:282-289.)

asthma or extensive emphysema and strong chemical drives to breathe. Not only do such increases in ventilation requirement act as a linear cofactor in the work of the breathing equation already discussed, but the high minute ventilation requirement itself increases most components of inspiratory pressure: flow, elastance (the reciprocal of compliance), tidal volume, and auto-PEEP. It is not surprising, therefore, that enormous increases in the oxygen consumption rate of the ventilatory muscles have been observed in patients with obstructive lung disease. During exacerbations, the oxygen consumed by ventilation and the metabolic demands associated with heightened vigilance, agitation, or anxiety may double the total body oxygen consumption observed during fully supported breathing. The prevalent combination of impaired $\dot{V}/\dot{Q}$ matching, hypoventilation, and diffusion impairment result in arterial oxygen desaturation that generally responds well to modest supplementation of inspired oxygen.

REDUCED MECHANICAL EFFICIENCY

In patients with exacerbated COPD or decompensated asthma, the oxygen consumed in the ventilatory task is disproportionate to the amount of mechanical work actually performed. The muscles of the hyperinflated ventilatory system are inefficiently aligned, force-length relationships of the shortened end-inspiratory fibers are suboptimal, and normally efficient coordination among the various muscles of the ventilatory group is often disrupted.[14-16] The energy cost of breathing, therefore, is greatly increased for the pressure and mechanical work actually generated by the breathing effort.

PROBLEMS AND HAZARDS OF VENTILATION WITH POSITIVE PRESSURE

Patients with AO who require mechanical ventilation present special challenges to the clinician for yet another reason: an unusual predisposition to its adverse consequences that are only loosely related to the airflow resistance. For reasons that are not entirely clear, patients with COPD have been reported to have an increased incidence of gastrointestinal ulceration and bleeding, especially during stress periods. This tendency is accentuated to an important degree by poor nutrition, stress, and the therapeutic use of high-dose corticosteroids. In modern intensive care unit practice, the incidence of ulceration has been greatly attenuated by the use of proton pump inhibitors and other means of acid suppression.

Even when able to cough with maximal force, patients with severe AO have difficulty in clearing contaminated secretions from the central and peripheral airways, predisposing to bronchial and lung infections. This tendency is accentuated when the airway is intubated or when noninvasive ventilation is provided with poorly humidified gas mixtures. These interventions accentuate the impediment to coughing efficiency, may encourage secretion thickening, and promote entry of contaminated secretions from the upper airway. In conjunction with mucus plugging, air trapping, and the tendency toward parenchymal infections, markedly inhomogeneous ventilation predisposes the ventilated patient with severe AO to the varied forms of barotrauma—pneumomediastinum, subcutaneous emphysema, and tension pneumothorax. Because the lungs cannot collapse, even a small pneumothorax in a ventilated patient with severe AO can rapidly develop a tension component, leading to ventilatory and circulatory compromise.

The hemodynamic sensitivity to positive-pressure ventilation of patients with AO arises for several reasons. The overexpanded lungs press outward on the chest wall, raising intrapleural pressure. When breathing efforts are silenced, as they are immediately after sedation and intubation, mean intrathoracic pressure abruptly changes from modestly negative to markedly positive. Increased pleural pressure raises the right atrial back-pressure to venous return. Simultaneously, increased peripheral vascular capacitance (caused in part by drug effects) and reduced peripheral vascular tone limit the rise in mean systemic pressure, the upstream driver of venous return. Blood pressure routinely falls, and cardiac output falls disproportionately to oxygen demand. Absolute values of measured central vascular pressures (central venous and wedge pressures) may therefore be misleadingly high and do not reflect intravascular filling and preload adequacy.[7] Marked respiratory variation of systolic and pulse pressures with the ventilatory cycle ("paradox") is a hemodynamic marker of relative hypovolemia caused by such mechanisms (see Fig. 10.4). Depending on choice of tidal volume, backup frequency, and set (and auto) PEEP, the afterload to right ventricular ejection may rise with any further lung expansion, whereas the tendency for alveolar deadspace creation is accentuated. Consequently, great care must be taken not to ventilate excessively and to provide adequate intravenous fluid support during this period. This advice pertains especially to patients with AO who require cardiac resuscitation.[17]

INTERACTIONS OF PRESSURE-TARGETED MODES WITH AUTO-PEEP

Pressure-targeted modes of ventilation, exemplified by pressure control, airway pressure release ventilation (APRV), and pressure support, have become increasingly popular to employ in the care of intubated patients, as well as in those receiving noninvasive ventilation by facemask. Because the development of auto-PEEP reduces the pressure difference between airway opening and alveolus that drives inspiration, it has a powerful influence on ventilation efficacy (Fig. 10.5). As already described, auto-PEEP varies not only with airway mechanics but also with the pattern of breathing and minute ventilation. For a fixed value of applied airway pressure, inspiratory tidal volume in patients with AO will be more sensitive to the frequency and the inspiratory time fraction (an expression of the inspiratory-to-expiratory [I:E] ratio) than are normal subjects or those with restrictive disease[18] (Fig. 10.6). Faster breathing frequencies, for example, allow auto-PEEP to build, and this auto-PEEP must first be counterbalanced for inspiratory airflow to begin. If the patient is passive or the amount of inspiratory muscle force remains constant, delivered tidal volume falls as the auto-PEEP builds.

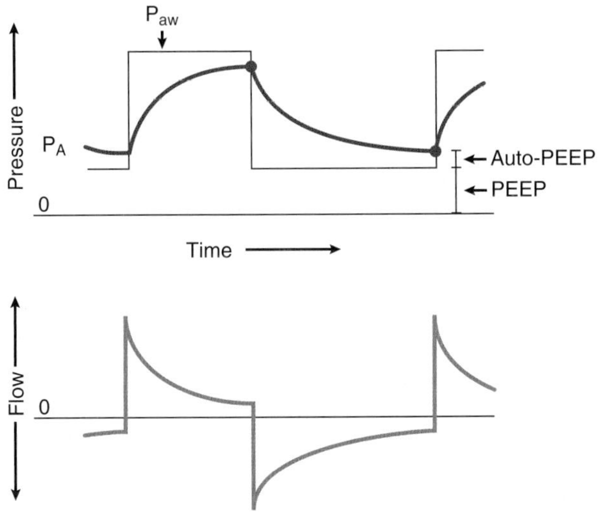

Figure 10.5 Interaction of alveolar (*red line*) and applied airway (*fine line*) pressures in a patient ventilated with pressure-targeted ventilation. Auto-PEEP diminishes the driving pressure of the subsequent ventilatory cycle.

This auto-PEEP/driving pressure interaction may result in an intriguing phenomenon resembling chaotic respiration during noninvasive ventilation with a leaky mask interface.[19] The coupled PEEPi and tidal volume form a "feed-forward" system in which a building auto-PEEP of one cycle adversely influences the tidal volume of the next one. But this smaller tidal volume also reduces the auto-PEEP that follows that restricted cycle, which in turn allows the subsequent breath—the third in the cycle—to have a larger effective driving pressure and tidal volume, and the cycling variation continues. This may account for some of the wide variability in breathing rhythm often observed in these patients.[20] If the mask leak volume is a function of the I:E ratio, it can be shown mathematically and experimentally that fractal and chaotic tidal volume delivery may occur, even when the patient's effort and mechanics remain unchanged (Fig. 10.7).[19] The consequences for comfort and sleep efficiency are likely to be significant, but clinical data are lacking on these issues at this time.

PRINCIPLES OF MANAGING THE VENTILATED PATIENT WITH SEVERE AIRFLOW OBSTRUCTION

Most patients hospitalized with exacerbations of asthma or COPD can be managed effectively by regimens that incorporate aggressive secretion clearance techniques,

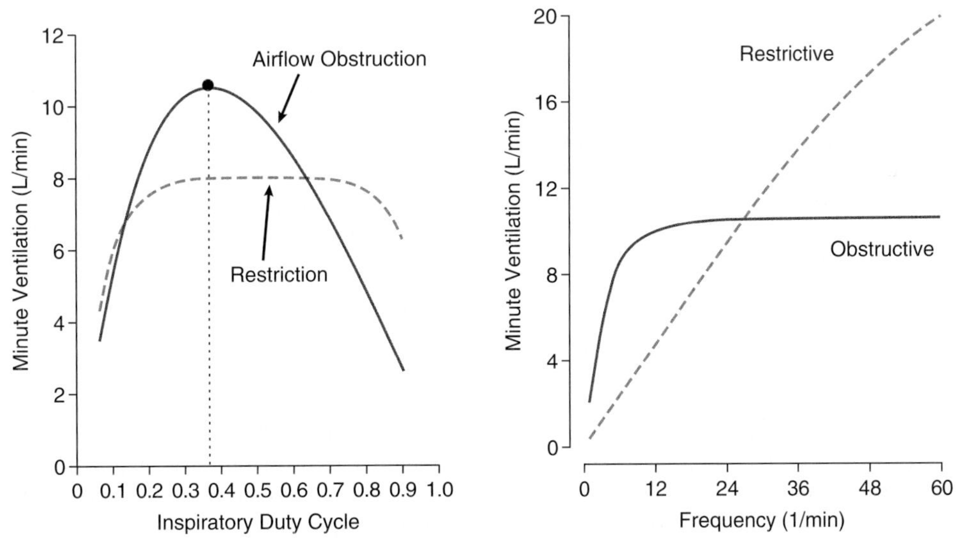

Figure 10.6 Relative sensitivity of patients with airflow obstruction to the settings of frequency and inspiratory time fraction for a fixed pressure target in pressure-controlled ventilation. This sensitivity is induced primarily by the impact of these settings on auto-PEEP (positive end-expiratory pressure).

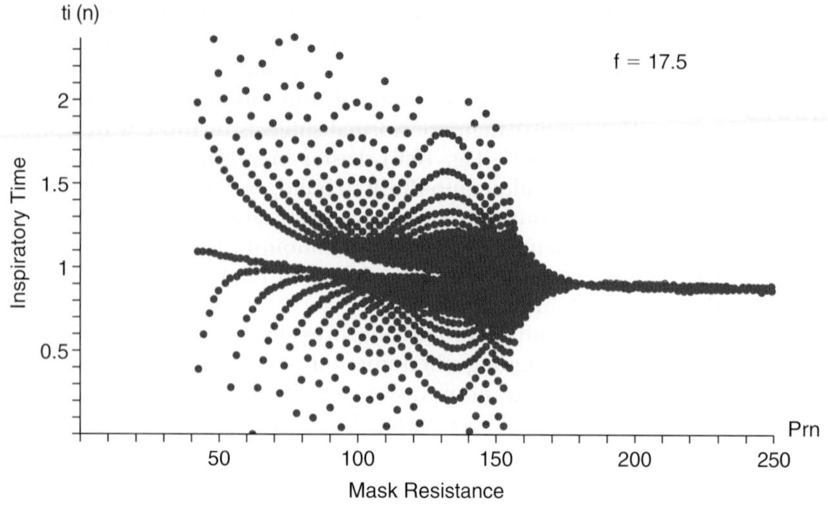

Figure 10.7 Theoretical behavior of tidal volume in response to pressure support by mask ventilation in a patient experiencing auto-PEEP (positive end-expiratory pressure). At a certain critical value of mask leak, there is wide cycle-to-cycle variation in tidal volume despite unchanging levels of pressure support and patient effort. Near "chaotic" behavior is a consequence of auto-PEEP. (Data from Hotchkiss JR, Adams AB, Dries DJ, et al: Dynamic behavior during noninvasive ventilation. Chaotic support? Am J Resp Crit Care Med 2001;163: 374-378.)

antibiotics, corticosteroids, intensified bronchodilators, hydration, cardiovascular support, secretion lubricants (e.g., guaifenesin), and supplemental oxygen. Noninvasive ventilation often helps as a temporizing measure for those with disease of *mild-moderate* severity, especially when cough is adequate to clear airway secretions and the patient is fully alert and accepting of a full facemask.[21-26] Only a minority of such patients treated in this way need translaryngeal intubation and institution of mechanical ventilatory support unless the problem is complicated by coexisting cardiovascular, infectious, or neuromuscular problems. When mechanical ventilation is required, however, the rationale underlying certain key management principles can easily be understood against a background of the physiologic derangements already described. These principles are as follows: (1) provide adequate support for muscle rest at adequate Pao_2 and pH; (2) do not overventilate; (3) minimize the minute ventilation requirement; (4) minimize risk of barotrauma; (5) maintain adequate bronchial hygiene; (6) prevent panic reactions; (7) establish appropriate nutrition. Each principle will be discussed in more detail:

Principle 1: Provide adequate support to rest the ventilatory muscles, while avoiding hypoxemia and profound acidemia.

Poised on the edge of decompensation, the ventilatory muscles must be rested adequately before withdrawal of machine support can be considered. Rest may allow recovery of energy reserves and restore the balance between ventilatory capability and demand. Indeed, benefits may accrue to muscle rest, even when it occurs intermittently on a chronic basis. Sufficient oxygen and mechanical support must be provided to achieve this goal, to permit restorative sleep, and to avoid significant hypoxemia (arterial oxygen saturation < 85%) and acidemia (pH < 7.2)—derangements that increase pulmonary vascular resistance; stimulate vigorous breathing; and inhibit mental, cardiac, and skeletal muscle functions.

Principle 2: Do not overventilate.

Profound respiratory acidosis and hypoxemia accentuate pulmonary hypertension, impair the right ventricle, and should be reversed. Nevertheless, although it is important to provide adequate ventilation and to reverse hypoxemia, overventilation is detrimental on several counts. Rapid reduction in the alveolar CO_2 tension tends to cause bronchoconstriction and impair neuromuscular and cardiovascular function. Furthermore, excess ventilation exacerbates dynamic hyperinflation and auto-PEEP, whereas moderate $Paco_2$ elevations are generally well tolerated.[27] Generally, it is a mistake to depress the $Paco_2$ below the level that the patient chronically maintains. Such a strategy may temporarily reset chemical drives, effectively increasing respiratory workload intensity once spontaneous breathing resumes. If $Paco_2$ falls sufficiently, the patient will not maintain unassisted breathing without intolerable effort, potentially delaying discontinuation of mechanical breathing assistance.

Principle 3: Minimize minute ventilation requirement.

Because hyperinflation, mean inflation pressure, and the adverse cardiovascular consequences of mechanical ventilation are intimately linked to the minute ventilation requirement, ventilatory deadspace and CO_2 output must be minimized and both metabolic acidosis and iatrogenic hyperventilation avoided or addressed.

Principle 4: Minimize the risk of barotrauma.

The predisposition of patients with severe AO to barotrauma must be combated by intelligent choices for tidal volume, ventilation frequency, PEEP, and machine settings of trigger sensitivity and flow. Reduction of the minute ventilation requirement decreases the mean or peak alveolar pressures, or both, reducing the incidence of barotrauma. The relative contributions of mean alveolar pressure, PEEP, dynamic cycling pressure, and peak static (plateau) ventilatory pressure to the risk of barotrauma are not clear. Based on epidemiologic evidence, however, peak airway inflation pressures in a passively inflated lung should be kept below 40 cm H_2O whenever possible. Selecting a tidal volume at the low end of the recommended range (6 to 8 mL/kg of ideal body weight) is probably best. The question of optimal flow setting is of no small importance: auto-PEEP and mean alveolar pressure are reduced by selection of relatively rapid flow settings when minute ventilation is high. Overall ventilation-perfusion matching may improve as well. Higher peak *dynamic* airway pressures engendered by these rapid flows are not entirely without risk, however; units served by low resistance pathways are in jeopardy from associated overdistention. For the same tidal inspiratory time, a constant ("square") flow waveform often serves better than a decelerating one. The risk of barotrauma can also be minimized by maintaining the lungs free of infection and the airways clear of secretions.

Principle 5: Maintain effective bronchial hygiene.

Secretion retention may dramatically increase airflow resistance and effectively seal off entire banks of functional alveoli, preventing their participation in ventilation. Thickened central airway secretions are a particular risk during mechanical ventilation, whether invasive or noninvasive (Fig. 10.8).[28] Apart from raising the end-inspiratory pressure, the resulting dynamic hyperinflation can detrimentally affect cardiovascular function, work of breathing, and ventilatory capability. In addition to effective suctioning, bronchodilators, adequate hydration, corticosteroids, mucolytics, mucolubricants, and infection control, frequent repositioning, mobilization, and physiotherapy are fundamental to secretion management. Percussive ventilation or vibro-percussive vest treatments often complement mobilization effectively when tolerated. Tracheotomies not only reduce resistance and provide improved access to the lower airway but also eliminate the direct connection between the pharynx and trachea established by tracheal intubation.

Principle 6: Prevent panic reactions.

In patients susceptible to dynamic airway collapse, an abrupt need to augment ventilation often precipitates a downward spiral in which the capability of the patient is overwhelmed by the imposed workload. Not only is minute ventilation increased during such episodes, but the resulting augmentation of dynamic hyperinflation impairs muscle strength and endurance. Respiratory acidosis, dyspnea, and anxiety result in an imbalance in the demand/capability relationship that creates a need for aggressive intervention. Anxiolytics, although hazardous to employ, may be extremely helpful in carefully selected circumstances.

Principle 7: Maintain appropriate nutrition, assure adequate hemoglobin concentration, and prevent obstipation.

In stressed and often malnourished patients, the nature and quantity of nutritional support can make the difference between eventual compensation and continued ventilatory insufficiency. Although reasonable caution is advisable, anemia should be reversed and an adequate number of calories should be provided, via the enteral route whenever possible. Care must be taken to ensure that bowel motility is normal; patients with AO frequently develop breathing discomfort because of abdominal distention within a compartment bounded by a hyperinflation-depressed diaphragm.

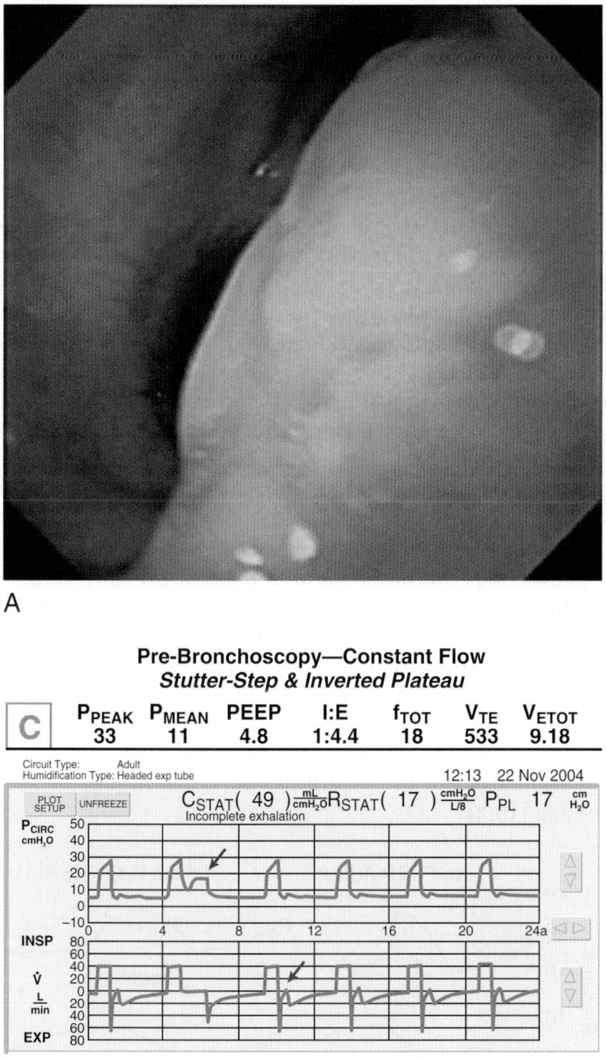

Figure 10.8 A, Central airway mucus retained in a ventilated patient with severe airflow obstruction. **B,** The resulting inverted plateau and stutter step deformations of the airway pressure and flow tracings during controlled, volume-cycled ventilation. (From Zamanian M, Marini JJ: Pressure-flow signatures of central-airway mucus plugging. Crit Care Med 2006;34:223-226.)

PRACTICAL MANAGEMENT OF THE VENTILATED PATIENT

INTUBATION

An understandable reluctance to initiate mechanical ventilation in patients with COPD or perennial asthma exists because ventilatory assistance may be needed for prolonged periods and because many such individuals are so chronically disabled as to be miserable or despondent at home—even when everything is going as well as possible from a physiologic viewpoint. The development of comfortable noninvasive systems, coupled with supportive trials and clinical experience, has given rise to the initial use of mask ventilation in those who are alert and can tolerate it. However, the most severely affected patients, especially those with copious, thick, and retained secretions, claustrophobia, anxiety, cardiovascular decompensation, or irreversible somnolence, continue to require intubation to stabilize their deteriorating conditions.[29]

A mounting load of secretions audibly retained within the central airways generally indicates that the patient is too weak or breathless to expectorate and often portends an imminent crisis. Hence, when this sign arises and cannot be easily reversed, most physicians consider it to be strong evidence favoring intubation for secretion management and ventilation support. Overt disorganization of the breathing rhythm and gasping or ataxic respirations strongly suggest approaching exhaustion.

INITIAL SUPPORT

POSTINTUBATION PROBLEMS

The first 24-hour period following tracheal intubation and initiation of positive-pressure ventilation may be highly dynamic for the patient with AO. Many of these individuals have depleted intravascular volume and impaired cardiovascular reflexes—features that prepare them poorly to compensate for the suddenly increased pleural pressure and impediment to venous return that usually accompany initiation of mechanical support. In this postintubation phase there is an understandable but unfortunate tendency for the physician to intentionally overventilate the patient, and many patients cough vigorously or fight against the rhythm imposed by the machine.

One reason for the agitation that some patients experience is a sudden buildup of positive intrathoracic pressure through the process of dynamic hyperinflation. When these intubated patients are deeply sedated and paralyzed, respiratory efforts cease and vasodilation occurs related to hypercapnia and sedation. The consequent rise of intrathoracic pressure, coupled with a fall in mean systemic vascular pressure, almost routinely depresses venous return and cardiac output (see Fig. 10.3). Therefore, the physician is well advised to remain alert to the predictable development of cardiovascular depression and hypotension following intubation or sedation and be prepared to intervene to reduce ventilation or to support the circulation at the initially selected level, or both. A catastrophic error is to misinterpret the development of sudden hypotension as the uncloaking of tension pneumothorax and then to undertake needle puncture of the chest wall. In such individuals it is also wise to remember the potential contribution of auto-PEEP to hypotension during cardiopulmonary resuscitation attempts.

Shortly after intubation there may be agitation, coughing, and retching related to tube insertion. When this interferes with comfort or ventilation, many lightly sedated patients benefit from 3 to 5 mL of 1% to 2% lidocaine instilled through the endotracheal tube. Instillation may be repeated one or two times, but care should be exercised, as lidocaine is easily absorbed via the lung. Fortunately, intolerance of tube placement gradually abates with sedation and the passage of time.

MACHINE SETTINGS

As a general rule, ventilation should be adequately supported during this initial phase, but it is better to underventilate cautiously than to overventilate the patient. One reasonable approach is to use assisted flow-regulated volume-controlled mechanical ventilation, delivered with a square wave profile, with the backup rate set to provide about two thirds of the estimated minute ventilation requirement. Although the flow setting is adjusted empirically to coordinate the cycle lengths of the patient and the ventilator, an initial peak flow setting of approximately four to six times the minute ventilation requirement (depending on whether the flow profile is square or decelerating, respectively) usually suffices to meet expiratory time requirements and minimize auto-PEEP without imposing undue risks that attend extraordinarily high peak cycling pressures. Assuming a minute ventilation of 12 L per minute, a constant flow setting of about 60 L per minute is usually appropriate. This yields an I:E ratio of approximately 1:4, which is considerably shorter than customary in a patient with normal mechanics who breathes at this level of minute ventilation. Reducing the I:E ratio still further may not improve gas trapping noticeably, as terminal rates of airflow are predictably very low. On the other hand, increasing airflow carries a high pressure and work cost in patients with such severe AO. For similar reasons, a constant inspiratory flow is preferable to a decelerating one when flow-controlled, volume-cycled ventilation is in use. Pressure-targeted ventilation is a sensible choice only if it is monitored closely or adjusted automatically by the ventilator to maintain tidal volume in response to changing airflow impedance.

The triggering threshold of the ventilator is set to be as sensitive as possible, and the auto-PEEP level is estimated when feasible to do so. (Measurement typically requires passive inflation to allow predictable occlusion of the circuit at end-expiration.) If auto-PEEP exceeds 5 cm of water and expiratory flow is limited during tidal breathing (which is almost invariably the case during the initial phase), an uncomfortable patient who makes spontaneous breathing efforts may benefit from the addition of a low level of end-expiratory pressure to counterbalance auto-PEEP and reduce the breathing workload (Fig. 10.9). PEEP levels in excess of 15 cm H_2O may be necessary in some instances to reestablish patency of some air channels.

The plateau pressure is a better guide to the degree of hyperinflation than is the measured level of auto-PEEP, for reasons already given. First, most machines do not allow estimation of auto-PEEP in a patient who is spontaneously triggering the ventilator and varies the length of the respiratory cycle. On the other hand, a plateau pressure estimate is usually recordable during triggered, as well as during controlled, volume-cycled breathing. Just as importantly, the auto-PEEP estimated by central airway occlusion is simply the volume-weighted average of those airways that remain open at end expiration, which generally have shorter time constants and better mechanical properties than those that seal earlier in the expiratory period at higher pressure (see Fig. 10.2).

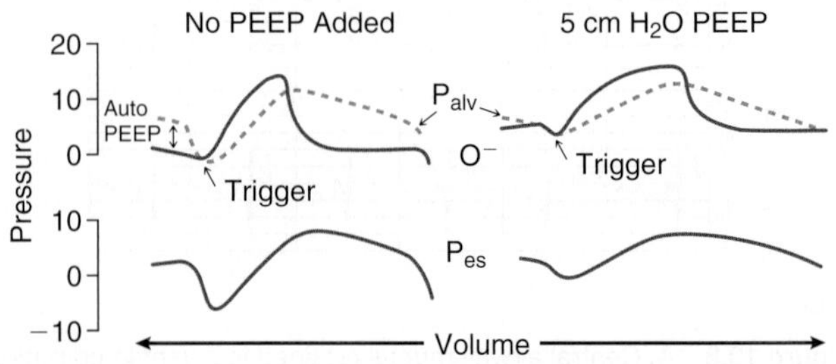

Figure 10.9 Work of breathing and ventilatory effort are improved in patients with tidal flow limitation by the addition of PEEP (positive end-expiratory pressure) marginally less than the original value of auto-PEEP. Airway pressure (*top*) and intrapleural pressure (*bottom*). P_{alv}, alveolar pressure; P_{es}, esophageal pressure.

The flow tracing gives some indication of the underlying presence of gas trapping but does not indicate its severity. For example, a severely obstructed airway may be totally occluded and therefore unable to transmit its high pressure to the pressure sensor located within the machine circuitry. Similarly, a narrow airway may give rise to an almost imperceptible flow at end expiration. Several features of the flow tracing are of value: High-frequency variations of the flow tracing suggest the presence of retained airway secretions or water in the external tubing. An abrupt transition between the earliest part of expiration and what follows ("hockey sticking") indicates a flow limitation during tidal breathing and the potential value of added PEEP if flow persists to the onset of the next breathing cycle (Fig. 10.10). Several signs appearing in the monitored airway pressure and flow signals have been reported that appear to be signatures of partial central airway occlusion, as by mucus plugging (see Fig. 10.8).[28]

SUPPORT PHASE MANAGEMENT

After the first hours of ventilatory support, rational management focuses not only on reversal of the underlying problems of infection, bronchospasm, secretion retention, and cardiac insufficiency but also on replenishing spent nutritional reserves and building endurance. It makes sense to support ventilation fully in patients intubated for ventilatory failure while fundamental pathologic processes and

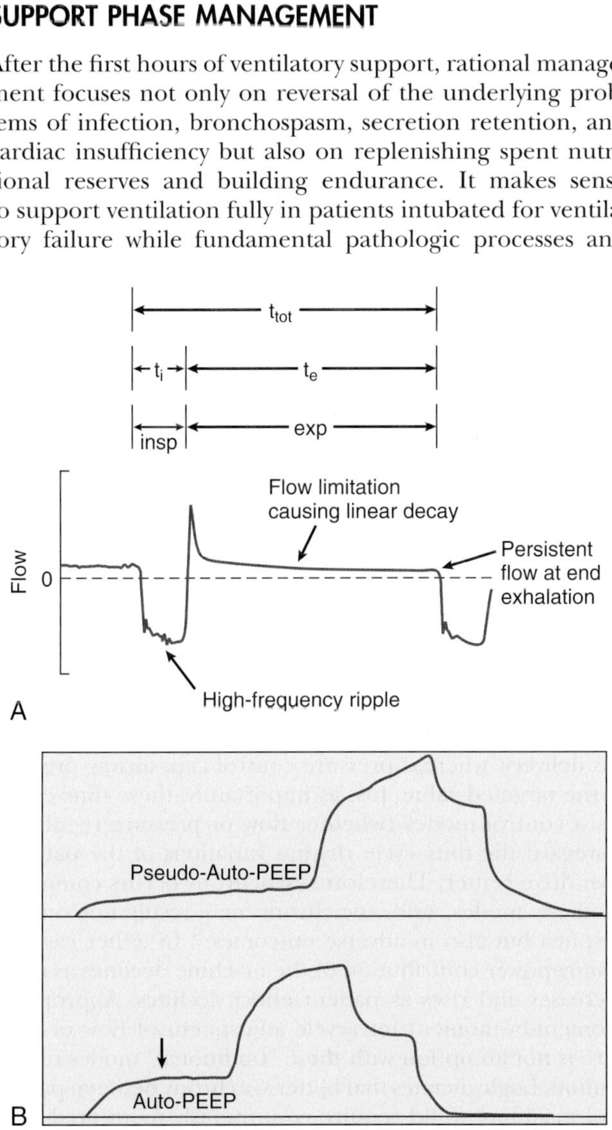

Figure 10.10 **A,** Typical flow tracing of a patient demonstrating flow limitation during tidal breathing. **B,** High-frequency ripple suggests secretions or circuit fluid, whereas "hockey sticking" and linear flow decay during expiration characterize flow limitation.

precipitating causes are being addressed—at least for the initial 24 to 48 hours. Because it is not known what intensity of ventilatory effort is best for patients with AO to undertake during the support phase of the illness, controversy exists as to the optimal mode of ventilation. During the support phase, the major ventilation objective as the acute problems causing deterioration are being addressed should be to provide sufficient breathing assistance to alleviate discomfort while not risking deconditioning of the ventilatory muscles. To this end, it is reasonable to use volume- or pressure-targeted assist-control (assisted mechanical ventilation) or synchronized intermittent mandatory ventilation (SIMV). In patients who are not deeply sedated and who breathe chaotically, the latter mode applied with pressure support sufficient to replicate the tidal volume of the mandated breaths may reduce the number of dyssynchronous "collisions" between the rhythms of patient and machine. Adequate sedation must be provided so as to assure comfort and reduce the minute ventilation requirement as other fundamental elements of ventilatory therapeutics are addressed (e.g., antibiotics, corticosteroids, regulation of intravascular volume, secretion expulsion or extraction, cardiovascular support). Assuring adequate oxygenation, ventilatory muscle rest, and restorative sleep deserve emphasis. Deep sedation and muscle relaxants, although occasionally necessary in achieving therapeutic objectives early in the ventilatory process, may prove detrimental when their use is prolonged unnecessarily. Not only does sedation present risks of muscle deconditioning and even neuromyopathy, but secretions tend to pool in dependent areas when breathing efforts and coughs are suppressed. As a general rule, deep sedation and paralysis should not be continued for longer than 40 to 72 hours after intubation.

Apart from improving expiratory resistance and reducing the minute ventilation requirement, another intervention aimed at reducing mean alveolar pressure and auto-PEEP is to modestly lengthen the available expiratory time (e.g., by increasing inspiratory flow rate). The flow rate should initially be set at approximately four times the minute ventilation requirement when using a constant inspiratory flow profile. Extending the expiratory time further is usually fruitless, unless minute ventilation is simultaneously reduced. Decelerating flow profiles are often poorly tolerated by the patient with severe AO who makes spontaneous efforts because the latter half of the inspiratory period may require higher flows than imposed by the tightly regulated and stereotyped flow waveform of the ventilator. Adjustments to the flow criterion off-switch that triggers expiration can help manage this problem during pressure-supported ventilation (Fig. 10.11).

PEEP AND CPAP IN SEVERE AIRFLOW OBSTRUCTION

The deliberate use of PEEP in patients with AO has historically been considered undesirable, but there is now ample reason to believe that most of these patients benefit from the application of low levels of PEEP or continuous positive airway pressure (CPAP).[5,10,11] When applied downstream of airways that collapse dynamically during the exhalation phase of tidal breathing, PEEP helps to improve the effective triggering responsiveness of the machine without

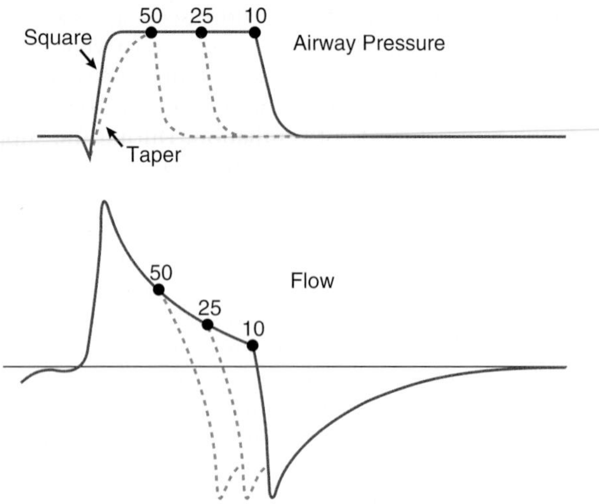

Figure 10.11 Adjustment of the expiratory flow trigger during pressure support can help to compensate for a slowly decelerating inspiratory flow profile that typifies patients with severe airflow obstruction. The appropriate adjustment in this schematic drawing might be from 25% to 50%.

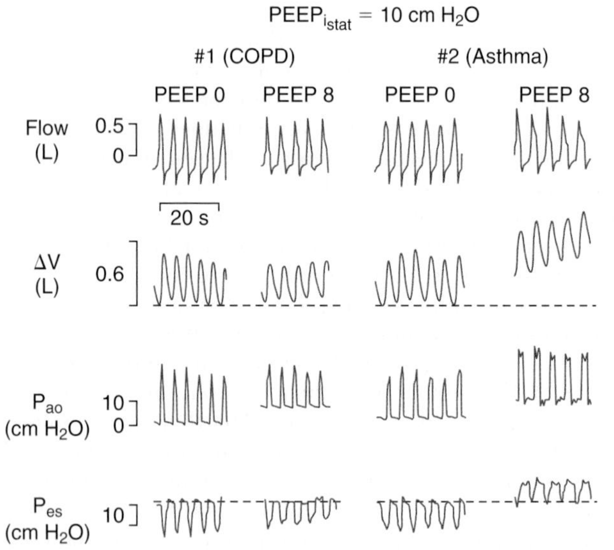

Figure 10.12 Differing responses of a flow-limited patient with chronic obstructive pulmonary disease (COPD) and a non–flow-limited patient with asthma to the application of PEEP (positive end-expiratory pressure). The rises of lung volume (V) and airway opening pressure (P_{ao}) in asthma and the absence of these features in the patient with COPD are demonstrated. (From Ranieri VM, Giuliani R, Cinnella G, et al: Physiologic effects of positive end-expiratory pressure in patients with chronic obstructive pulmonary disease during acute ventilatory failure and controlled mechanical ventilation. Am Rev Respir Dis 1993;147:5-13.)

significantly increasing the alveolar pressure or hyperinflation (Fig. 10.12). Most benefit is provided to patients receiving volume-controlled ventilation who do not experience proportionate increases of peak static or peak dynamic cycling pressures after PEEP application.[10,11,30] When using a fixed level of targeted pressure (pressure control or pressure support), tidal volume may increase after PEEP is applied. This occurs because the added PEEP counterbalances auto-PEEP to allow the applied inspiratory pressure

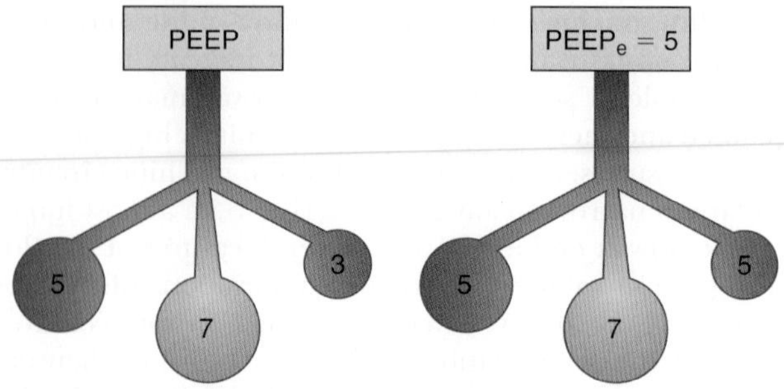

Figure 10.13 PEEP (positive end-expiratory pressure) evens the flow distribution by counterbalancing auto-PEEP in flow-limited channels with differing levels of gas trapping.

to more effectively drive inspiratory flow. In effect, PEEP improves the pressure gradient that drives *inspiratory* flow and delivers tidal volume. (Should minute ventilation increase with PEEP application, total PEEP may also rise.) Applied PEEP may also help to keep airways more widely patent, and thereby improve secretion clearance. Finally, the application of the external PEEP may help to even the distribution of ventilation among multiple units with heterogeneous time constants (Fig. 10.13).

NEWER MODES OF VENTILATION IN AIRFLOW OBSTRUCTION

Currently, the majority of ventilatory support of AO is still provided with modes of ventilation that are now decades old—flow-controlled, volume-cycled ventilation ("assist-control"); pressure assist control (pressure control, PCV); pressure support (PSV); and SIMV. When combined with PEEP/CPAP and an attentive provider, these time-tested options suffice for the majority of patients. Increasingly, however, practitioners have recognized the need to offload responsibility for minute-by-minute and even intrabreath adjustment of settings for flow and pressure delivery in response to changing conditions of mechanics or ventilatory demand. Patients with dyspnea generally need faster rise of pressure and flows to their target values, unimpeded inspiratory flow, and precise termination of the ventilator's inspiratory phase so as to avoid collisions between the patient's and the ventilator's cycling rhythms. Once set, however, a specified flow pattern regulates the ventilator's gas delivery, whereas pressure control caps airway pressure at the targeted value. Just as importantly, these time-cycled assist control modes (whether flow or pressure regulated) disregard the duty cycle rhythm variations of the patient's own drive center; Therefore, asynchrony occurs commonly in these modes, and asynchrony may result not only in dyspnea but also in adverse outcomes.[31] In either case the *relative* power contribution of the machine declines as effort increases and rises as patient effort declines. Appropriate moment-by-moment intracycle adjustment of flow or pressure is not an option with these "traditional" modes of ventilation. Logic dictates that better synchrony between patient and machine would require continuously monitored feedback and flexibility to adjust to the vagaries of patient need.

Of the newer modes of ventilation, four that have implications for AO have garnered considerable attention and have been incorporated into some of the latest equipment.

AIRWAY PRESSURE RELEASE VENTILATION AND BILEVEL VENTILATION

These modes were neither designed nor intended for patients with lengthy expiratory time constants. Airway pressure release ventilation does not take full advantage of its release phase in patients with lengthy expiratory time constants and therefore ineffectively ventilates unless the release frequency is high. The machine's inspiratory phase pressure is generally higher than that encountered during conventional ventilation, introducing the problems associated with sustained hyperinflation in patients with relatively flexible lungs. Wide variations of auto-PEEP and of release cycle volumes are to be expected. The addition of PEEP may not prove effective in mitigating this variation unless the release phase had been prolonged sufficiently to encounter flow limitation during tidal breathing.

PROPORTIONAL ASSIST VENTILATION

Proportional assist ventilation (PAV), a mode based on the equation of motion of the respiratory system that regulates delivered pressure in proportion to externally sensed inspiratory flow and volume, effectively mimics the actions of an auxiliary muscle in patients without gas trapping.[32-34] Quite unlike pressure support, which targets the same pressure for every breath, PAV takes resistance and compliance into account and is meant to provide help in proportion to effort (Fig. 10.14). Unfortunately, ventilatory impedance varies considerably in patients with AO, and a considerable fraction of inspiratory muscle effort is spent in counterbalancing variable auto-PEEP, an event that precedes the onset of inspiratory flow. Given the strong dependence of dynamic hyperinflation on minute volume ($\dot{V}_E$) and the expiratory time constant, PAV cannot easily fulfill its intended function in patients with severe OA and changing mechanics or minute ventilation needs. Despite these theoretical disadvantages, modern adaptations of PAV—which monitor respiratory mechanics on an ongoing basis—have shown at least equivalent comfort in patient trials, as well as no greater incidence of missed triggering events and greater tidal volume variability than pressure support, both in invasive and noninvasive settings.[35] Although reassuring, no outcome advantage over PSV has yet been convincingly demonstrated in any setting.

NEURALLY ADJUSTED VENTILATORY ASSIST

Neurally adjusted ventilatory assist (NAVA) is similar in concept to PAV in that it attempts to regulate the machine's power support moment by moment by sensing inspiratory effort from the patient.[34,36] The difference is that the diaphragmatic electromyogram (EMG) provides the signal, so the electrical timing and intensity of phrenic nerve traffic regulate the amplitude of the pressure delivered. NAVA depends on drive to breathe, not the lung's mechanical response. A thin, multielectrode esophageal catheter is used to pick up the strength and contour of the EMG signal, and failure to detect it has not been a major problem. The dynamic hyperinflation drawbacks of PAV in patients with AO are theoretically nullified by placing the "effort detector" closer to the respiratory drive controller—inspiratory efforts related to auto-PEEP are tracked and supported well before inspiratory flow actually begins. Inherent protective reflexes are believed to help the patient avoid overdistention, even if the machine's power boost factor is set inappropriately high. Despite its intuitive appeal, NAVA is still too new to the clinical arena to confirm its theoretical advantage.

ADAPTIVE SUPPORT VENTILATION

Adaptive support ventilation (ASV) is a mode that regulates machine output with pressure-targeted breaths delivered at a variable frequency and with variable pressure in accordance with breathing pattern feedback from the patient (Fig. 10.15). Its intent is to minimize the work of breathing and auto-PEEP, and it does this by optimizing the tidal volume and frequency combination that make up minute ventilation. As such, ASV is one step closer to closed-loop ventilation, in which clinical goals are set, monitored, and accomplished automatically. Once the clinician has determined the PEEP, F_{IO_2}, and cycling triggers for pressure

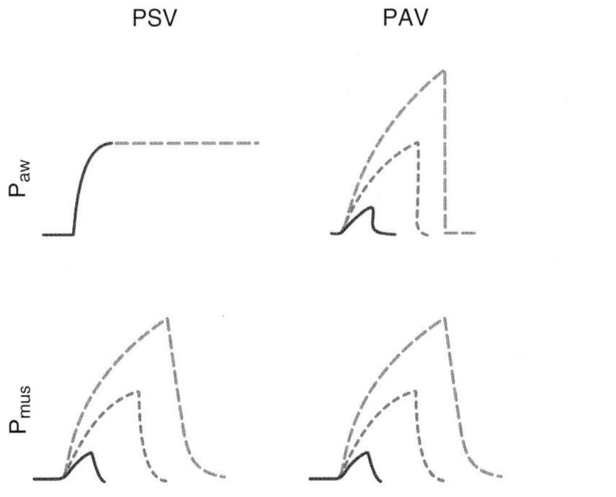

Figure 10.14 Comparison of pressure support (PSV) and proportional assist (PAV) in response to muscular efforts of varying intensity. The machine pressure mirrors the patient's muscular effort during PAV but not during PSV. (From Younes M: Proportional assist ventilation, a new approach to ventilatory support. Theory. Am Rev Respir Dis 1992;145:114-120.)

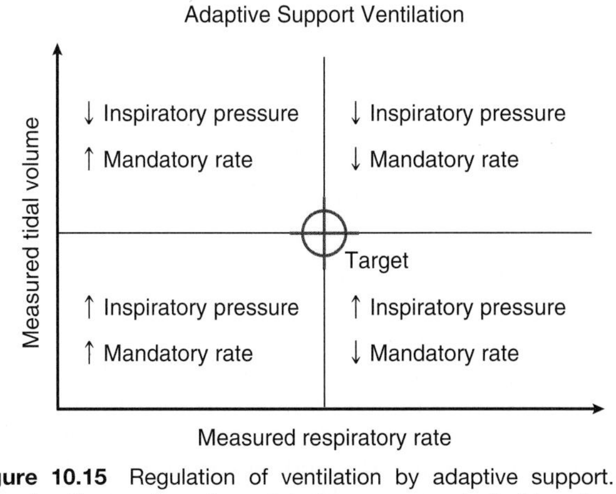

Figure 10.15 Regulation of ventilation by adaptive support. By changing the number of mandated pressure-controlled breaths and by regulating the pressure support rendered to each triggered cycle, adaptive support aims to keep breathing frequency and tidal volume within acceptable physiologic ranges (see text).

support, he or she must input the patient's ideal body weight (from which the series deadspace is estimated) and the fraction of estimated "normal" minute ventilation the machine should provide. It then varies the mandatory breath number and the pressure targets of a pressure-regulated SIMV algorithm. All the while, the machine tries to nudge the patient toward the ventilatory pattern optimum that *should* minimize deadspace, work of breathing, and auto-PEEP.

In observational studies ASV appears to regulate tidal volume and total breathing frequency effectively, without the need for clinician intervention. As with all advanced modes, however, its performance in severely stressful settings has not been validated and no convincing outcome benefit has yet been reported. As currently implemented, ASV lacks gas exchange feedback, does not calculate total physiologic deadspace, does not account for adjustment to the ideal optimum breathing pattern incurred by disease or deformity, and requires the clinician to specify what percentage of the ideal minute ventilation to shoot for. Nonetheless, it is a promising approach that modifies machine output in response to changing need and may prove to reduce the gas trapping that dysfunctional patterns of AO engender.

WEANING ("LIBERATION") PHASE

Protracted ventilator dependence is perhaps the most feared consequence of intubating patients with exacerbated COPD and perennial asthma. Not only are breathing workloads high, but the ability of the patient to sustain them is compromised by muscle weakness, hyperinflation, disadvantageous thoracic geometry, blunted ventilatory drive, and abnormal cardiovascular function. Rational management of the weaning patient with AO includes provision of adequate rest and nutritional support, enhancement of neuromuscular and cardiovascular function, and minimization of the breathing workload. Maintenance of positive mental attitude can greatly speed the weaning process.

Patients may fail to wean from mechanical ventilation for a wide variety of reasons. Among these are hypoxemia, cardiac arrhythmias, cardiovascular instability, and psychological dependence. However, imbalance between ventilatory capability and demand is perhaps the most common reason for failure to wean in patients with ventilatory failure either of itself or because it provokes one or more of the other factors just mentioned.[37,38]

PREDICTING READINESS FOR SPONTANEOUS BREATHING

In clinical practice a panel of indices has long been used to predict the outcome of the weaning trial. Most individual elements of these demand or capability panels can be classified as indicators of either one or the other, but not both. Some capability indicators depend on patient effort as well. Thus, a maximal inspiratory pressure measurement exceeding 30 cm H_2O and a minute ventilation requirement of less than 10 L per minute are standard components of the traditional predictive battery. Although minute ventilation has been criticized as unreliable when used alone, it is still a highly useful observation, particularly when referenced to blood gas measurements and integrated into an evaluation of other panel elements. When the patient is calm, a high degree of variation of minute ventilation suggests some degree of ventilatory reserve.[39] Because the product of minute ventilation and the average inspiratory pressure per breath are the main components of the breathing workload, minute ventilation must not be disregarded, even when more integrative indices are in use, such as the frequency-to–tidal volume ratio (rapid shallow breathing index, RSBI).[40] For example, a rising RSBI does not necessarily portend failure if minute ventilation rises as well. Published criteria for RSBI lose reliability in the presence of neuromuscular weakness, severe restriction, or chronic illness requiring ventilator support.[38]

Numerous other weaning outcome indices have been suggested over the years, but none stands alone as infallible, including the RSBI. The most successful of these indicators reliably relate power requirement to the ability of the patient to sustain it. Certain physiologic measurements such as the $P_{0.1}$ (a measurable indicator of ventilatory drive now offered on some of the newest ventilators) have predictive appeal. These are not universally available, however, and cannot be relied on for definitive judgment in every case. Because many factors may limit the patient's ability to be removed from the ventilator, more than one single indicator is usually necessary to observe. Alertness, degree of cardiovascular compensation, clinical trajectory over the preceding days, oxygenation status, secretion load, upper airway patency, coughing efficiency, and psychological well-being are as important as any single predictive measure based on mechanics and muscle strength. Successful weaning protocols take all such factors into account.[37,38,40]

Repeated failure to wean is often explained by cardiovascular factors such as ischemia and diastolic dysfunction. This is especially true when parameters based on ventilation appear favorable. Clues may appear in the form of cardiac dysrhythmias and an unfavorable excess of fluid intake over output. In part for such reasons, weaning protocols must be constructed carefully; failure to meet weaning criteria must be considered a cue to undertake a careful review of all potential factors that prevent success, not necessarily an indication to allow a bit more time with unchanging therapy.

WEANING APPROACHES

PREPARATIONS

Preparations for ventilator withdrawal should include ensuring adequate nocturnal rest with fully supported breathing, adequate nutrition, good circulatory reserve, avoidance of excessive intravascular volume and edema, treatment of infection, appropriate body positioning, and judicious sedation.[37,40] Obstipation, urinary retention, pleural effusions, gastric distention, musculoskeletal pain, severe anemia, and chemical imbalances must be avoided or reversed. During the full support phase of ventilation, care must be taken not to allow sedatives to accumulate or secretions to collect within the airways. Heat-moisture exchangers do not hydrate the airway secretions reliably, especially in low humidity environments or when high inspired concentrations of oxygen have been in use. Active humidification often proves the better choice when secretion load or clearance is problematic. Inspection of the central airway prior to attempted extubation may be rational when the patient has been ventilated for lengthy periods, as inspissated secretions may not have been adequately suctioned. Withdrawal of sedatives should be attempted on a daily basis in an effort to prevent oversedation, especially when the sedating drug is infused continuously. The patient must not depend on high levels of PEEP for either oxygenation or ventilatory comfort. It must be remembered that PEEP and CPAP aid ventilation in patients with flow limitation and auto-PEEP.

The use of frequent wakeups, intermittent dosing, and short-acting sedatives (especially in the hours prior to spontaneous breathing trials and weaning attempts) has helped to avoid the common problem of benzodiazepine metabolite hangover. When benzodiazepines are given for lengthy periods, lingering sedative effects may persist for up to a week after the last dose is given. Dexmedetomidine (Precedex), a sedative agent with relatively little hypnotic action, has proved helpful in some cases in which calm alertness is desired but difficult to otherwise achieve.[41] In well-selected cases, alertness-enhancing drugs such as modafinil (Provigil) have been helpful. Delirium that interferes with weaning occurs commonly and may benefit from such agents as quetiapine and olanzepine.[42]

SPECIFIC MODES

Considerable effort has gone into the delineation of the optimal weaning technique. It is generally true that the majority of patients do not need a lengthy period of gradual machine withdrawal once the primary problems that brought the patient to medical attention have been treated and the adverse effects of fluids and drugs given during their acute problems have been addressed.[43] It is also true, however, that a distinct subset of these patients with underlying AO or other chronic impairments not amenable to therapy cannot tolerate abrupt transitions to spontaneous breathing. More graded reloading is sometimes necessary because of fragile cardiovascular status, neuromuscular weakness, or psychological factors. Pressure support ventilation is generally to be preferred to SIMV, as the muscle and cardiovascular reloading process tends to be less sudden and more predictable. Intermittent T-piece weaning makes little sense to employ in these patients; each transition to fully spontaneous breathing abruptly imposes a full stress workload. All patients, however, should be *tested* with low-level pressure support or T-piece breathing before any gradual withdrawal of support is undertaken, as the latter may not be necessary.[44] Once the patient is breathing on low-level pressure support or from an oxygenated T-piece, observation should be continued at least 30 minutes, but generally less than 2 hours before decannulation of the airway is attempted. During the attempt at spontaneous breathing, the patient must be watched carefully and not allowed to fatigue because recovery from that condition may require more than a day to restore energy reserve.[45]

PERIEXTUBATION PHASE

In intubated patients suspected of upper airway obstruction, a cuff deflation test should be conducted before decannulating the airway. This is performed by elevating PEEP to 10 to 20 cm H_2O immediately in advance of deflation. An audible leak should be heard if the glottic space is not prohibitively tight. The sitting position, manipulation of head position and a temporary increase of PEEP may help break a “mucus seal” that otherwise prevents gas leakage. In questionable cases, advance preparations should be made for urgent intervention, should that prove necessary after tube extraction.

The immediate postextubation phase should be as carefully managed as the ventilated one. The first 24 hours off the ventilator are often difficult and tenuous, but in successful cases there should be progressive improvement. Coughing, deep breathing, adequate oxygenation, avoidance of arrhythmias, adequate bronchodilation and airstream hydration, maintenance of a clear central airway, and a mechanically efficient posture are crucial. Oral refeeding must be undertaken with extreme caution because swallowing difficulty in chronic dysfunction can persist days to weeks after extubation in patients who have been ventilated for lengthy periods. CPAP and intermittent noninvasive ventilation may be especially helpful in selected patients,[46] especially in the nighttime hours. Noninvasive ventilation maintains patency of an edematous upper airway and provides ventilation support during sleep. This is often important in patients who have received sedating medications or are sleep deprived. It must be used judiciously, however, and carefully applied. Ventilation by pressurized mask impedes secretion clearance, and if a humidifier is not used, mouth breathing during bilevel positive airway pressure (BiPAP) dries secretions and encourages displacement of oral material into the central airway. Therefore, it is common for patients who receive mask ventilation after extubation to require reintubation for clearance of thickened airway mucus.

KEY POINTS

- By assuming a major portion of the ventilator workload, mechanical ventilation affords the opportunity to rest the respiratory muscles while maintaining pH homeostasis and oxygenation, thereby averting progressive ventilatory failure or respiratory arrest, or both.
- Increased resistance to airflow and gas trapping is responsible (directly or indirectly) for many of the physiologic disturbances that typify AO.
- When dynamic collapse occurs during tidal respiration, and breathing requirements are high, there is little alternative to hyperinflation, CO_2 retention, or both.
- Ventilation-perfusion mismatching is widespread in patients with severe AO, reducing the efficiency of carbon dioxide elimination.
- Pressure-targeted modes of ventilation, exemplified by pressure control and pressure support, have become increasingly popular in the care of intubated patients, as well as those receiving noninvasive ventilation by facemask.
- Most patients hospitalized with exacerbations of asthma or COPD can be managed effectively by

Continued on following page

KEY POINTS (Continued)

regimens that incorporate aggressive secretion clearance techniques, antibiotics, corticosteroids, intensified bronchodilators, hydration, cardiovascular support, and supplemental oxygen.

- The first 24-hour period following tracheal intubation and initiation of positive-pressure ventilation is a highly dynamic one for the patient with AO.
- In the majority of cases, ventilatory support of AO is still currently provided with modes of ventilation that are now decades old—flow-controlled, volume-cycled ventilation ("assist-control"); PCV; PSV; and SIMV.
- Careful attention to the nature and quantity of sedation, coupled with daily attempts to awaken and test spontaneous breathing, accelerates liberation from mechanical ventilation.
- The postextubation phase should be as carefully managed as the ventilated one. The first 24 hours off the ventilator are often difficult and tenuous. During this phase, close attention to secretion clearance, sleep, upper airway patency, and fluid management will help to avert reintubation.

SELECTED REFERENCES

4. Laghi F, Goyal A: Auto-PEEP in respiratory failure. Minerva Anestesiol 2012;78(2):201-221.
5. Marini JJ: Dynamic hyperinflation and auto-positive end-expiratory pressure: Lessons learned over 30 years. Am J Respir Crit Care Med 2011;184(7):756-762.
11. Smith TC, Marini JJ: Impact of PEEP on lung mechanics and work of breathing in severe airflow obstruction. J Appl Physiol 1988;65:1488-1499.
14. Leatherman JW: Mechanical ventilation in obstructive lung disease. Clin Chest Med 1996;17:577-590.
20. Jubran A, Van de Graaff WB, Tobin MJ: Variability of patient-ventilator interaction with pressure support ventilation in patients with chronic obstructive pulmonary disease. Am J Respir Crit Care Med 1995;152:129-136.
23. Lightowler JV, Wedzicha JA, Elliott MW, Ram FS: Non-invasive positive pressure ventilation to treat respiratory failure resulting from exacerbations of chronic obstructive pulmonary disease: Cochrane Systematic Review and Meta-analysis. BMJ 2003;326:185.
31. Thille AW, Rodriguez P, Cabello B, et al: Patient-ventilator asynchrony during assisted mechanical ventilation. Intensive Care Med 2006;32(10):1515-1522.
34. Kacmarek RM: Proportional assist ventilation and neurally adjusted ventilatory assist. Respir Care 2011;56(2):140-152.
38. Epstein SK: Weaning from ventilatory support. Curr Opin Crit Care 2009;15(1):36-43.
42. Girard TD, Kress JP, Fuchs BD, et al: Efficacy and safety of a paired sedation and ventilator weaning protocol for mechanically ventilated patients in intensive care (Awakening and Breathing Controlled Trial): A randomised controlled trial. Lancet 2008;12; 371(9607):126-134.

The complete list of references can be found at www.expertconsult.com.

11

Mechanical Ventilation in Acute Respiratory Distress Syndrome

Luciano Gattinoni | Eleonora Carlesso | Pietro Caironi

CHAPTER OUTLINE

Since the first description of acute respiratory distress syndrome (ARDS) in 1967,[1] mechanical ventilation has been the primary "buying time" treatment for acute lung injury (ALI). Mechanical ventilation is not a "gas exchanger," but instead replaces, totally or partially, the force normally generated by the respiratory muscles to promote ventilation, providing muscle rest. The effects of mechanical ventilation on gas exchange are indirect and include (1) better clearance of carbon dioxide (CO_2) by the power of the mechanical ventilator to expand the diseased and collapsed lung; (2) improvement in oxygenation by preventing alveolar hypoxia caused by hypoventilation; (3) improvement in oxygenation by increasing inspiratory oxygen fraction, which affects alveolar partial pressure of oxygen (P_{AO_2}); (4) improvement in oxygenation by opening lung regions otherwise collapsed (alveolar recruitment); and (5) improving oxygenation by maintaining positive end-expiratory pressure (PEEP), preventing the collapse of the lung regions previously recruited during the inspiratory phase.

The negative effects of mechanical ventilation are interwoven with its positive effects. First, the driving force applied by the ventilator, if excessive, may alter, in different ways, the lung parenchyma and produce ventilator-induced lung injury (VILI). Second, the positive-pressure ventilation unavoidably turns the physiologically negative intrathoracic pressures into positive pressures. In consideration of this, the guiding principle of mechanical ventilation of ARDS patients should be that, whenever one manipulates the ventilator settings, one should refer to one polar star: The new setting is less harmful to the lung structure than the previous one.

HISTORY

Extensive reviews on the history of mechanical ventilation of ARDS can be found elsewhere.[2,3] In the 1970s, mechanical ventilation was recommended and performed with low PEEP and high tidal volume: ". . . larger tidal volumes (10 to 15 per kilogram) are preferable, having been used in several thousand ventilated patients with no evidence of development of pulmonary damage."[4] Today, this advice seems inconceivable. At that time, the main concerns were the putative harm of high inspiratory oxygen fraction and the hemodynamic impairment. It was later recognized in experimental and clinical settings[5-7] that high-volume/high-pressure mechanical ventilation could severely damage the lung parenchyma. Such lesions, primarily attributed to the excessive airway pressure, were collectively classified as *barotrauma*. In the same period, Suter and colleagues[8] published a report that, for the first time, systematically described the interaction between PEEP, lung mechanics, gas exchange, and hemodynamics.

In the 1980s, based on the work of Dreyfuss,[9,10] the focus progressively shifted from the potential harm of pressure to the harm of volume (overdistention), a concept that was popularized as *volutrauma*.[11] In the mid-1980s, the application of computed tomography (CT)[12,13] and the quantitative approach to CT analysis[14] led to the concept of *baby lung*,[15,16] which accounted for most of the previous observations on respiratory mechanics, gas exchange functionality, and potential harm of mechanical ventilation. The premise of this line of thought is that high pressure or excessive distention applied to a small fraction of the lung parenchyma (with a size similar to the lung of a baby) unavoidably leads to structural lesions of the lung regions open to ventilation. Total *lung rest* was achievable with the use of extracorporeal CO_2 removal, targeted to prevent the damages of high-pressure/high-volume ventilation.[17-19] The target of mechanical ventilation shifted toward lung protection, rather than normal gas exchange functionality. Hickling and associates[20] proposed the "permissive hypercapnia" strategy for ARDS, providing "gentle treatment" of the portion of the lung that remains open to ventilation (the baby lung) through less aggressive mechanical ventilation, at the acceptable price of an abnormally higher arterial partial pressure of carbon dioxide ($Paco_2$).

A large amount of experimental and clinical data over the years has supported the approach of a *lung protective strategy*.[21-25] Low tidal volume prevents the excessive global stress and strain of the baby lung, whereas higher PEEP prevents the regional excessive stress and strain by avoiding alveolar collapse and reopening during mechanical ventilation.[26] These mechanical events are associated with an inflammatory reaction of the epithelial and endothelial lung cells (*biotrauma/atelectrauma*) as shown by the seminal study of Tremblay and colleagues[27] (see also work of Dreyfuss and Saumon[11] and Tremblay and Slutsky[28]). The literature to date supports the thought that the harm of mechanical ventilation is due to excessive global or regional stress and strain.[29] This situation leads to two results—a physical rupture of the lung and a mechanically induced inflammation of the lung parenchyma, constituting VILI. The best "mechanical ventilation" would provide adequate gas exchange with the lowest amount of VILI.

PHYSIOLOGIC BASIS OF MECHANICAL VENTILATION

DRIVING FORCE

To ventilate the respiratory system, force is required. The driving force for ventilation under normal circumstances is provided by the respiratory muscles. During spontaneous breathing, the thoracic cage expands. This causes a decrease in intrathoracic pressure (pleural pressure, Ppl) relative to the atmosphere (in normal conditions approximately 2 mm Hg of ΔPpl is sufficient to expand the thoracic cage by 0.5 L). Because the lungs are connected in series with the thoracic cage, their volume is expanded to a near equal extent (not considering the blood shift[30]). The force that distends the lung is the pressure difference between the alveoli and the pleural cavity (the transpulmonary pressure, PL). As the lung expands, the alveolar pressure becomes subatmospheric, and gas flow is generated (*inspiration*). When the respiratory muscles relax, the potential energy accumulated in the respiratory system (lung and chest wall) returns the chest wall and the lung parenchyma to the resting position (*expiration*). In spontaneously breathing subjects, the driving force (muscular pressure, ΔPmusc) is spent partly to expand the chest wall (ΔPpl), partly to expand the lung (ΔPL), and partly to overcome the resistances to the gas flow. In *quasi-static* conditions, in which the resistances to gas flow are negligible:

$$\Delta Pmusc = \Delta Ppl + \Delta P_L$$

During positive-pressure mechanical ventilation, the rules are exactly the same, with the exception that ΔPmusc is substituted by the force provided by the ventilator, and the force is applied to the lung parenchyma and not to the chest wall. The driving pressure, which coincides with the airway pressure at plateau during an end-inspiratory pause (in quasi-static conditions), is spent first to expand the lung and second to expand the chest wall:

$$\Delta Paw = \Delta P_L + \Delta Ppl$$

In spontaneous breathing and during positive-pressure mechanical ventilation, the distending force of the lung is the transpulmonary pressure. During spontaneous breathing, pleural pressure is negative (facilitating venous return), whereas during mechanical ventilation it is positive (impairing venous return). What matters from the pulmonary perspective is the distending force (i.e., the transpulmonary pressure [ΔPL]), whereas what matters from the hemodynamic perspective is the pleural pressure (ΔPpl).

TRANSPULMONARY PRESSURE

At the same driving force applied to the whole respiratory system (lung and chest wall), the resulting transpulmonary pressure, ΔPL, may be extremely variable. If the lung is relatively "stiff," and the chest wall is relatively "soft" (e.g., during pulmonary fibrosis or ARDS of pulmonary origin), a greater fraction of the driving pressure is spent to distend the lung (high transpulmonary pressure). In contrast, if the lung is relatively soft, but the chest wall is relatively stiff (e.g., in the presence of an abdominal disease or severe obesity), most of the driving force is spent to move the chest wall (high pleural pressure).

To express this phenomenon quantitatively, it is convenient to consider the concept of *elastance*. The elastance of the whole respiratory system is the driving force (ΔPaw) required to increase the lung and the chest wall 1 L above their resting position (Etot = ΔPaw/1 L). Part of this driving force is spent to increase the lung volume of 1 L (EL = ΔPL/1L), and part is spent to increase the chest wall by the same amount (Ecw = ΔPpl/1 L). Transpulmonary pressure (ΔPL) can be expressed as the driving force times the ratio between lung elastance and total elastance of the respiratory system:

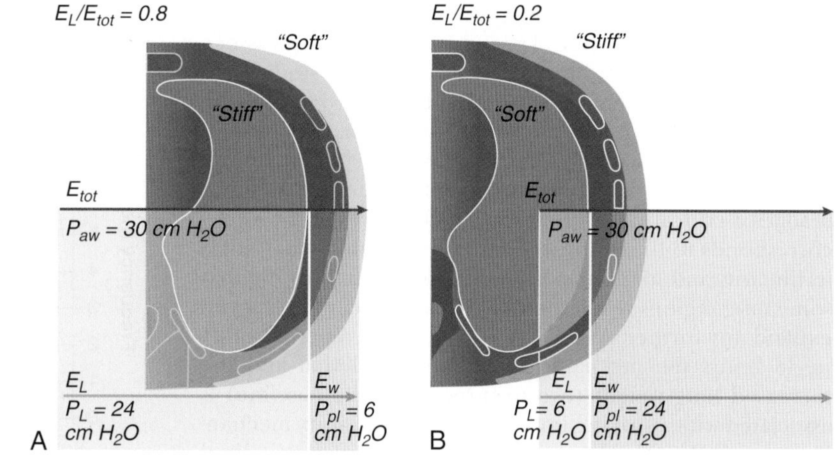

Figure 11.1 Two examples of EL/Etot variability in patients with acute lung injury/acute respiratory distress syndrome. **A,** EL/Etot = 0.2. **B,** EL/Etot = 0.8. This variability implies that for the same airway pressure applied (e.g., 30 cm H_2O), the resulting transpulmonary pressure (PL) may range from 6 to 24 cm H_2O.

$$\Delta P_L = \Delta Paw \times E_L/Etot$$

The transpulmonary pressure for a given driving pressure uniquely depends on the ratio of lung elastance to respiratory system elastance. In normal subjects EL/Etot is approximately 0.5, whereas in patients with ARDS it may range from 0.2 (e.g., in obese patients or in patients with high intra-abdominal pressure) to 0.8 (e.g., in patients with a very small baby lung and a normal chest wall elastance). This variability implies that for the same driving force applied and read on the ventilator display (e.g., 30 cm H_2O), the resulting transpulmonary pressure may range from 6 to 24 cm H_2O (Fig. 11.1).

FORCE-BEARING STRUCTURE OF LUNG PARENCHYMA

The transpulmonary pressure is applied to the force-bearing structure of lung parenchyma, the extracellular matrix, which constitutes the *lung skeleton*.[31] The lung skeleton is a complex and metabolically active structure that includes a network of several components—elastin, collagen, and proteoglycans. All these molecules are involved in determining the mechanical characteristics of the respiratory system. The elastin may be considered as an elastic spring, whereas the unextensible collagen, which is folded at end expiration and completely unfolded at a lung volume equal to total lung capacity, acts as a stop-length fiber.[32,33] The proteoglycans stabilize the collagen-elastin network, contributing to lung elasticity and alveolar stability at low and medium lung volumes.[34]

The matrix of elastin, collagen, and proteoglycans is arranged in two main fiber systems: (1) the *axial* system, which originates from the pulmonary hilum and runs deeply into the lung parenchyma down to the alveolar level, where it joins (2) the *peripheral* system, which originates from the visceral pleura and runs centripetally within the lung parenchyma.[31] The lung skeleton may be considered as a continuous elastic structure that reaches its extension limits at total lung capacity, a lung volume equal to about threefold the lung resting volume. At this level of alveolar distention, the collagen is completely unfolded, and further expansion is prevented. The epithelial and endothelial cells do not directly bear the applied forces because they are anchored to the extracellular matrix by a series of structural proteins (integrins), which are connected to the cytoskeleton. During lung expansion, the epithelial and the endothelial cells modify their shape.

It is well documented that mechanically induced cellular deformation activates a series of mechanosensors with the production of several inflammatory mediators, such as cytokines (interleukin 6, tumor necrosis factor-α, and interferon-γ),[27,35] metalloproteinases (enzymes involved in the remodeling of the matrix),[36] leukotrienes,[37] and interleukin 8,[38-40] the most powerful attractor of neutrophils.[41] Gross barotrauma (e.g., pneumothorax) is due to the stress at rupture of the lung skeleton, whereas intrapulmonary inflammation is primarily due to the excessive strain of the epithelial and endothelial cells.

CONCEPT OF STRESS AND STRAIN

Stress is the applied force, and strain is the linear deformation of material. In the whole lung, the rough approximation of stress is the transpulmonary pressure, whereas the approximation of the average strain is the change in volume relative to the lung resting volume. The ratio between alveolar stress and strain is defined as *lung-specific elastance* (Espec), which is mathematically defined as:

$$\Delta P_L = Espec \times \Delta V/V_0$$

where ΔV is the volume variation applied to the lung (i.e., the tidal volume), and V_0 is the lung resting volume (i.e., the functional residual capacity at atmospheric pressure [without any application of PEEP]). The lung-specific elastance is the transpulmonary pressure required to double the lung resting volume (i.e., the ΔPL when $\Delta V/V_0$ is equal to 1). In ARDS, lung-specific elastance is similar to normal,[16,42] reinforcing the concept of the baby lung (lung is small and not stiff), and questions the use of normalizing the tidal volume to the ideal body weight. The same tidal volume per kilogram may result in completely different strain according to the size of the baby lung (the V_0 of the previous equation). For example, a 70-kg man with ARDS may have, according to the severity of the lung injury, a residual baby lung equal to 60%, 40%, or 20% of his normal lung size. If the ventilator is set to deliver 10 mL/kg, the actual delivered tidal volume would generate an alveolar strain, which would result from the application, in normal lung, of a tidal volume equal to 17 mL/kg, 25 mL/kg, and 50 mL/kg, values associated with a significant lung injury in laboratory studies.[11,29]

Recently we attempted to quantify the relationship between stress-strain and VILI in healthy animals. We found that edema formation was a threshold phenomenon, induced by mechanical ventilation when the global strain reaches a critical value of about 2.[43] This threshold roughly corresponds to the point where the stress-strain curve loses its linearity and starts an exponential growth, indicating that some lung regions reach their own total capacity and cannot expand any further. At this level of strain, in a period of 24 to 48 hours the mechanical ventilation is lethal and the increased lung weight (two to three times the baseline) is associated with a striking impairment of respiratory mechanics, gas exchange, hemodynamics, inflammation, distal organs damage, and 100% mortality rate. This lethal strain, and associated stress, however, is rarely applied in clinical practice. To explain VILI in a diseased lung, therefore, alternative phenomena must be taken into account as the lung dishomogeneity and the presence of stress rise, which will be discussed later.

PATIENT CHARACTERIZATION

Using the least harmful mechanical ventilation setting requires a preliminary knowledge of the main pathophysiologic characteristics of the patient. The most relevant characteristics are the kind and amount of the lung injury, the chest wall elastance, and the lung recruitability.

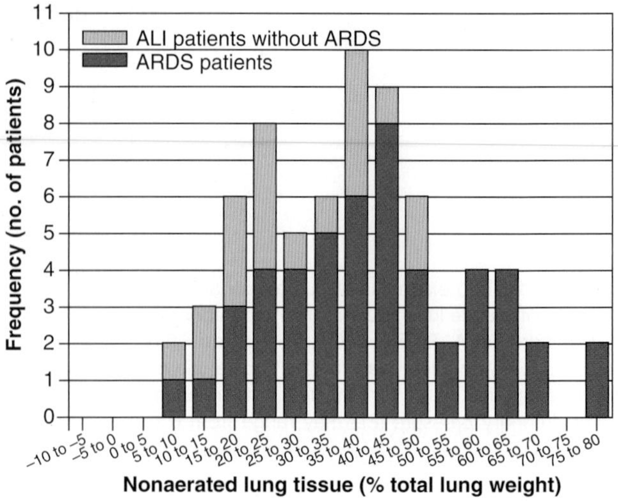

Figure 11.2 Frequency distribution of nonaerated lung tissue, expressed as a proportion of the total lung weight, recorded at 5 cm H_2O positive end-expiratory pressure in 68 patients with acute lung injury/acute respiratory distress syndrome (ALI/ARDS). *Green columns* represent patients with PaO_2/FIO_2 less than 300 (ALI without ARDS), whereas *purple columns* represent patients with PaO_2/FIO_2 less than 200 (ARDS). The nonaerated lung tissue was defined as the lung tissue having a physical density at computed tomography scan image analysis between +100 Hounsfield units (HU) and −100 HU, representing the portion of lung parenchyma that is consolidated or collapsed or both (i.e., the lung injury severity). (With permission from Gattinoni L, Caironi P, Cressoni M, et al: Lung recruitment in patients with the acute respiratory distress syndrome. N Engl J Med 2006;354:1775-1786.)

GAS EXCHANGE

OXYGEN

PaO_2, PaO_2-to-fraction of inspired oxygen ratio (PaO_2/FIO_2), and Riley's shunt fraction[44] are the most commonly used variables to assess the severity of lung injury. In particular, the PaO_2/FIO_2 thresholds of 300 and 200 were used to define ALI (300) and ARDS (200) according to the American-European Consensus Conference on ARDS.[45] Consequently, the PaO_2/FIO_2 ratio is perceived as a key variable by most intensive care unit (ICU) physicians: The lower the PaO_2/FIO_2 ratio, the greater the lung injury. This equivalence is highly questionable. First, in most large studies on ARDS, no association was found between hypoxemia and outcome.[46] In the large study showing a better outcome with low tidal volume compared with higher tidal volume, the PaO_2/FIO_2 ratio was significantly lower in the low tidal volume group despite ending with better outcome.[25] Finally, the PaO_2/FIO_2 ratio was not different in patients with early, intermediate, and late ARDS, suggesting that oxygenation was not dependent on the structural changes of lung parenchyma occurring with time.[47] In a study[48] in which the lung severity was assessed by CT scan (and defined as a fraction of the gasless tissue), we did not find significant changes of PaO_2/FIO_2 ratio over a wide range of nonaerated tissue (Fig. 11.2), and PaO_2/FIO_2 ratio was not associated with outcome.

Most data suggest that PaO_2/FIO_2 ratio is a weak indicator of the overall lung severity, with compensatory rearrangement of perfusion during ARDS limiting the deterioration of oxygenation. The same limits apply when PaO_2/FIO_2 ratio changes are used to assess lung recruitment. Because this maneuver is unavoidably associated with changes of perfusion (global or regional), the increase of PaO_2/FIO_2 ratio may be partly due to decrease of perfusion, as shown in the 1980s.[49-51] Most data suggest that the use of oxygenation variables alone to assess lung severity is misleading.

CARBON DIOXIDE

Although less considered, the variables derived from CO_2, as the total or alveolar deadspace, seem to be of greater value in assessing lung severity. It has been shown in ALI/ARDS patients that deadspace at entry is a strong predictor of outcome,[52] and that $PaCO_2$ for the same total ventilation steadily increases from early to intermediate and to late ARDS, reflecting the lung structural changes.[47] The PCO_2 response to prone position (in contrast to PO_2 response) is a strong prognostic index of mortality.[53] Most data suggest that CO_2-related variables (deadspace), more than PaO_2/FIO_2 ratio, reflect the severity of lung injury (and associated mortality rate) at the time of presentation and the structural changes of lung parenchyma occurring with time (fibrosis, *Pneumocystis*, and possibly perfusion defects).

RESPIRATORY MECHANICS, CHEST WALL ELASTANCE, AND LUNG VOLUME

In the original description of ARDS,[1] the low compliance (i.e., high elastance) of the respiratory system was a landmark of the syndrome. The respiratory system compliance is not considered in the current definition of ARDS, however.[45] For years, the low compliance was attributed uniquely to the lung component (lung stiffness and lack of surfactant). Quantitative CT shows, however, that the respiratory system compliance primarily reflects the size of lung open to gases (the baby lung[14,16]), suggesting that the intrinsic functioning lung elasticity in ARDS is close to normal (the lung is "small" rather than "stiff"). More than gas exchange, the respiratory system compliance indirectly assesses the lung injury severity (the smaller baby lung, the greater lung injury),[54] as confirmed in animal experiments.[55] Another variable also must be taken into account—the elastance of the chest wall. It has been shown in a significant portion of ALI/ARDS patients that the chest wall elastance is greater than normal because of increased intra-abdominal pressure, obesity, or severe edema.[56] In patients with extrapulmonary ARDS[57] and in obese patients,[58] the high elastance of the respiratory system may be due to the chest wall and to the lung derangement. Measurement of intra-abdominal pressure should be considered when selecting mechanical ventilator settings.

SEVERITY OF LUNG INJURY AND LUNG RECRUITABILITY

CT can be used to assess the severity of lung injury by measuring the fraction of nonaerated lung tissue at end expiration (end expiration pause at 5 cm H_2O). This fraction includes the lung tissue that is "consolidated" (i.e., not openable at 45 cm H_2O airway pressure) and the tissue that is collapsed but openable at 45 cm H_2O. These values were chosen to produce a minimal risk during the maneuver and because this is the most frequently used in the literature for recruitment maneuver.[59] In patients with elevated chest wall elastance, the resulting transpulmonary pressure could be insufficient, however, to overcome the opening pressure of some pulmonary units.

The total fractions of nonaerated lung tissue (consolidated plus recruitable) and the recruitable tissue alone (tissue that regains aeration at 45 cm H_2O airway pressure) are strongly associated with mortality rate. The data of Figure 11.2 show the inadequacy of the term ALI/ARDS, as currently defined, to describe the lung injury.[48] The data refer to a population of ALI/ARDS patients, classified according to the American-European Consensus Conference on ARDS,[45] in which a CT-based quantitative analysis of the whole lung parenchyma at 5 cm H_2O PEEP was performed. As shown in Figure 11.3, the fraction of the nonaerated lung tissue (consolidated or collapsed or both) may range from 5% to 70% of the entire lung parenchyma. Patients meeting ALI/ARDS criteria may have a baby lung size very close to that of normal subjects, or a baby lung that is just a small fraction of the expected normal lung. When the distending force is applied to the lungs by the mechanical ventilator, previously collapsed lung regions may open. Lung recruitability may be expressed as the amount of lung tissue regaining aeration when increasing the applied driving force from 5 to 45 cm H_2O. As shown in Figure 11.3, in some patients, lung recruitability was almost negligible, whereas in others it was equal to 25% to 35% of the entire lung parenchyma. Lung recruitability was strongly associated with the fraction of nonaerated tissue, suggesting that the greater the inflammatory edema, the greater the lung

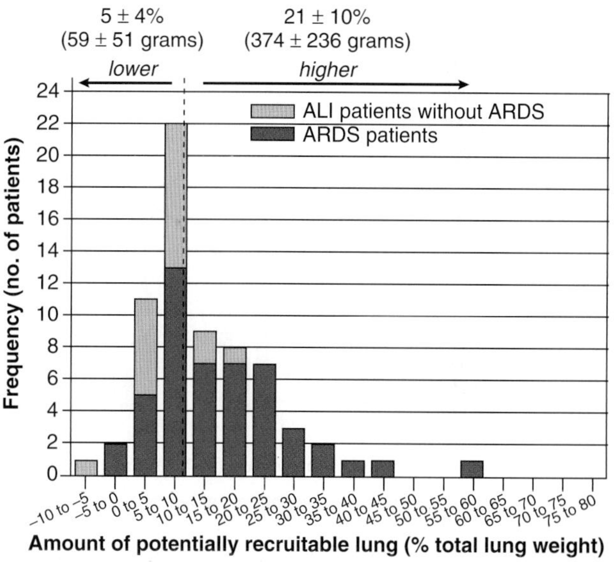

Figure 11.3 Frequency distribution of 68 patients with acute lung injury/acute respiratory distress syndrome (ALI/ARDS) according to the percentage of potentially recruitable lung, expressed as the percentage of total lung weight. ALI without ARDS was defined by a Pa_{O_2}/F_{IO_2} ratio less than 300, but not less than 200; ARDS was defined by a Pa_{O_2}/F_{IO_2} ratio less than 200. The percentage of potentially recruitable lung was defined as the proportion of lung tissue in which aeration was restored at airway pressures between 5 and 45 cm H_2O. (With permission from Gattinoni L, Caironi P, Cressoni M, et al: Lung recruitment in patients with the acute respiratory distress syndrome. N Engl J Med 2006;354:1775-1786.)

collapse. It seems that the best way to assess the overall lung severity and the related lung recruitability, both strongly associated with mortality rate, is the CT scan analysis. Physiologic variables are poor indicators of the severity of the lung injury. This relationship is shown in Figure 11.4—for a large variation of lung injury, ranging from 20% to 60% of the lung parenchyma, the values of Pa_{O_2}/F_{IO_2} ratio, lung compliance, and Pa_{CO_2} greatly overlap.

ARDS CLASSIFICATION

Although, in our opinion, the definition of ARDS should include a quantitative estimate of the lung edema, because this is not feasible in most of the ICU, alternative ways for defining ARDS have been sought. ARDS was first defined by Ashbaugh and coworkers in 1967.[1] Several other definitions have been introduced afterward, up to the American-European Consensus Conference (AECC) in 1994.[45] This conference defined ARDS as the acute onset of hypoxemia ($Pa_{O_2}/F_{IO_2} \leq 200$) with bilateral infiltrates seen at x-ray study and no evidence of left atrial hypertension, and these parameters were largely used for the enrollment of patients in clinical trials. In 2011, a panel of experts, under the initiative of the European Society of Intensive Care Medicine endorsed from the American Thoracic Society and Society of Critical Care Medicine, convened to develop what has been called the "Berlin definition."[60] The final Berlin definition is reported in Table 11.1. Stages of mild, moderate, and severe ARDS were related to increased mortality rates and increased median duration of mechanical ventilation in survivors.

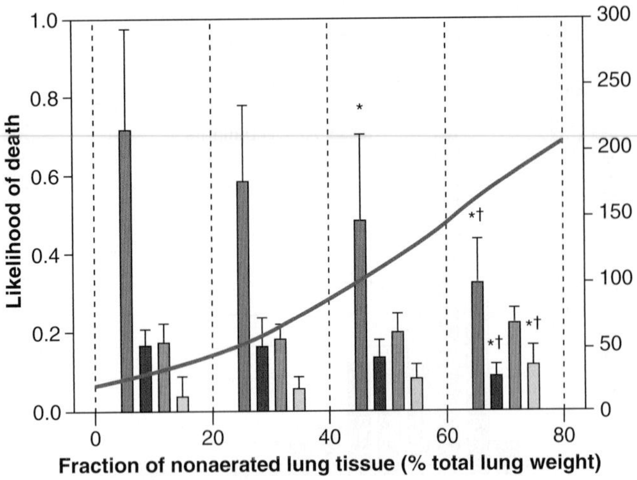

Figure 11.4 Mean ± standard deviation values of respiratory variables of a population of 68 patients with acute lung injury/acute respiratory distress syndrome. *Blue columns* represent PaO_2/FIO_2 ratio at positive end-expiratory pressure (PEEP) 5 cm H_2O (mm Hg), *red columns* represent respiratory system compliance at PEEP 5 cm H_2O (mL/cm H_2O), *green columns* represent deadspace fraction (%), and *gold columns* represent alveolar deadspace fraction (%). *$P < 0.05$ versus patients with a fraction of nonaerated tissue recorded at 5 cm H_2O PEEP less than 0.2. †$P < 0.05$ versus patients with a fraction of nonaerated tissue recorded at 5 cm H_2O PEEP ranging from 0.2 to 0.4. The *continuous purple line* represents the likelihood of death predicted by the fraction of nonaerated lung tissue recorded at 5 cm H_2O PEEP ($P = 0.015$). Weight is a poor surrogate of strain because ARDS patients with similar body weights may have completely different lung sizes and consequently different levels of strain at equal tidal volumes. This is confirmed by the plateau pressures measured in these different studies (see Fig. 11.5). As shown for the same tidal volume per ideal body weight, the plateau pressures are widely distributed with huge overlap between the studies. This reflects a wide distribution of the respiratory system compliance and consequently of the lung size.

Table 11.1 The Berlin Definition of ARDS

Defining Features	Criteria
Timing	Within 1 week of a known clinical insult or new/worsening respiratory symptoms
Chest imaging*	Bilateral opacities, not fully explained by effusions, lobar/lung collapse, or nodules
Origin of edema	Respiratory failure not fully explained by cardiac failure or fluid overload Need for objective assessment (e.g., echocardiography) to exclude hydrostatic edema if no risk factor is present
Oxygenation†	
Mild	$200 < PaO_2/FIO_2 \leq 300$ with PEEP or CPAP ≥ 5 cm H_2O‡
Moderate	$100 < PaO_2/FIO_2 \leq 200$ with PEEP ≥ 5 cm H_2O
Severe	$PaO_2/FIO_2 \leq 100$ with PEEP ≥ 5 cm H_2O

ARDS, acute respiratory distress syndrome; PaO_2, partial pressure of arterial oxygen; FIO_2, fraction of inspired oxygen; PEEP, positive end-expiratory pressure; CPAP, continuous positive airway pressure.
*Chest x-ray study or computed tomography scan.
†If altitude is higher than 1000 m, the following correction factor should be used: $PaO_2/FIO_2 \times$ (barometric pressure/760).
‡This may be delivered noninvasively in the "Mild" group.
From The ARDS Definition Task Force. Acute Respiratory Distress Syndrome—The Berlin definition. JAMA 2012;307(23):2526-2533.

MECHANICAL VENTILATION IN ACUTE RESPIRATORY DISTRESS SYNDROME: AVAILABLE EVIDENCE

SETTING TIDAL VOLUME

The main results of several outcome studies specifically designed to compare different tidal volumes are summarized in Table 11.2. A survival benefit was found in the study comparing 6 mL/kg tidal volume versus 12 mL/kg, the highest tidal volume range tested,[25] whereas no survival differences were found in the other studies, which compared intermediate values of tidal volumes.[21,23,24] As previously discussed, the tidal volume per ideal body weight is a poor surrogate of strain because ARDS patients with similar body weight may have completely different lung sizes and consequently different strain at equal tidal volume. This is confirmed by the plateau pressures measured in these different studies (Fig. 11.5). As shown for the same tidal volume per ideal body weight, the plateau pressures are widely distributed with huge overlap between the studies. This reflects a wide distribution of the respiratory system compliance and consequently of the lung size.

Despite the lack of information about stress and strain in each individual patient, most available data strongly suggest that a gentle ventilation is safer than the application of high volumes and pressures. This evidence does not mean that 6 mL/kg ideal body weight represents the ideal tidal volume. In a patient with a very small baby lung, it still may be harmful, inducing excessive strain, whereas if applied to a lung characterized by a large ventilatable area, it may be low. There is little doubt, however, that 12 mL/kg ideal body weight is excessively high and unnecessary. It is evident that low tidal volume ventilation, decreasing the global alveolar stress and strain, is advantageous compared with high tidal volume ventilation in different patients.

It has been suggested that a plateau pressure of 30 cm H_2O represents the safe limit for plateau pressure.[61] In a retrospective analysis, such a safe limit has been challenged, however.[62] This is understandable if we consider that the airway plateau pressure is a poor surrogate of stress owing to the high variability of the chest wall compliance. The same plateau pressure, 30 cm H_2O, may result in completely different stress values in different patients.

SETTING POSITIVE END-EXPIRATORY PRESSURE

The available evidence on the effects of higher versus lower levels of PEEP in ALI/ARDS patients is summarized in Table 11.3. As shown, despite the fact that the experimental data

Table 11.2 Different Tidal Volumes per Ideal Weight and Airway Plateau Pressures Investigated in Other Studies

Study	Group	No. of Patients	Tidal Volume (mL/kg)	Plateau Pressure (cm H_2O)	Mortality Rate (%)	*P* (Outcome)
Acute Respiratory Distress Syndrome Network[25]	Control	429	11.8 ± 0.8	33 ± 9	39.8	.007
	Treatment	432	6.2 ± 0.9	25 ± 7	31	
Brochard et al[23]	Control	58	10.3 ± 1.7	31.7 ± 6.6	37.9	NS
	Treatment	58	7.1 ± 1.3	25.7 ± 5	46.6	
Stewart et al[21]	Control	60	10.7 ± 1.4	26.8 ± 6.7	47	NS
	Treatment	60	7 ± 0.7	22.3 ± 5.4	50	
Brower et al[24]	Control	26	10.2 ± 0.1	30.6 ± 0.8	46	NS
	Treatment	26	7.3 ± 0.1	24.9 ± 0.8	50	
Amato et al[22]	Control	24	12 (768 ± 13)*	36.8 ± 0.9	71	<.001
	Treatment	29	<6 (348 ± 6)*	30.1 ± 0.7	38	

*Mean ± standard error values of tidal volume (mL/kg) were not provided in the report by Amato and colleagues. The value set by the physician and the mean ± standard error values of tidal volume in mL (over the first 36 hours) have been provided.
Studies cited in this table can be found in the complete list of references for the chapter, available online at www.expertconsult.com.

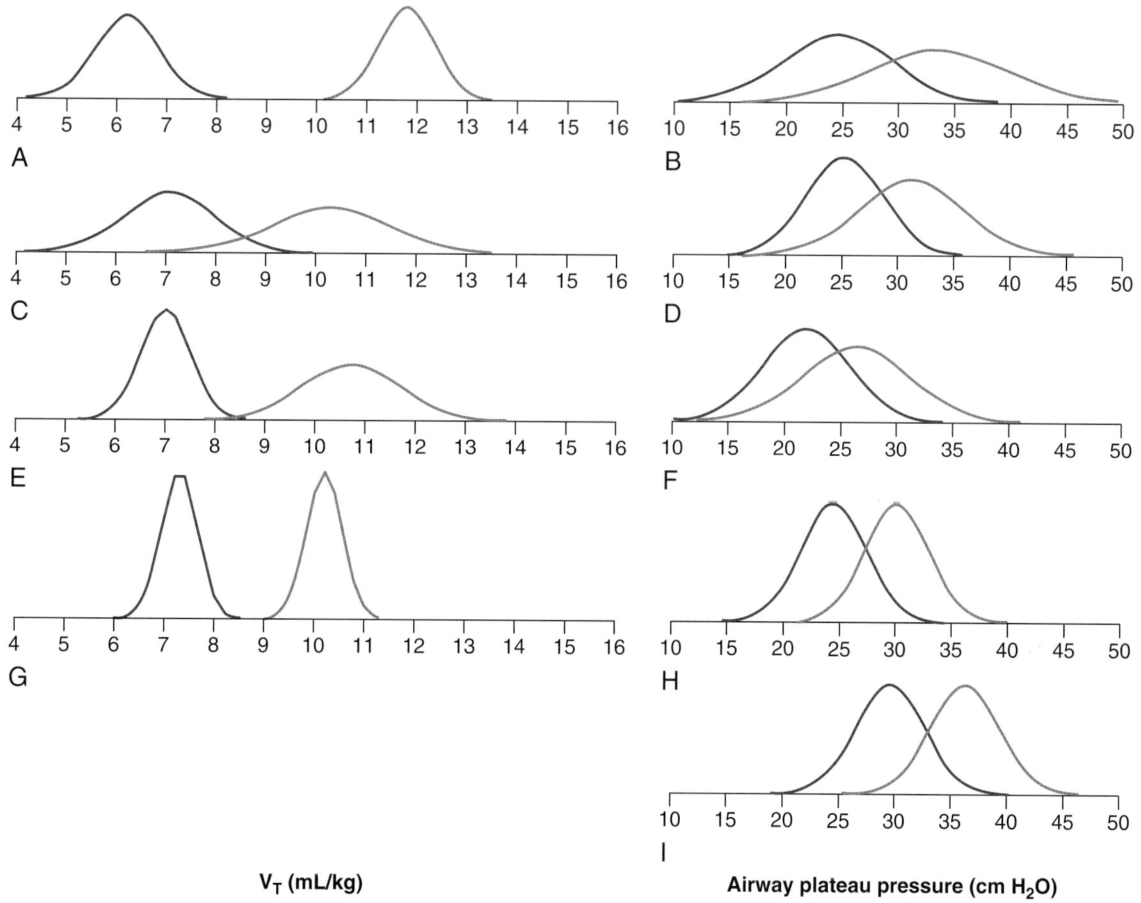

Figure 11.5 Distribution of tidal volume (VT) per ideal body weight (mL/kg) (*left column*) and of plateau pressure (*right column*) (*red line* = treated group; *blue line* = control group) in five randomized trials (computed from the reported mean ± standard deviation assuming a Gaussian distribution). Data taken from the following studies: **A** and **B,** Acute Respiratory Distress Syndrome Network;[25] **C** and **D,** The Multicenter Trial Group on Tidal Volume Reduction in ARDS;[23] **E** and **F,** Pressure- and Volume-Limited Ventilation Strategy Group;[21] **G** and **H,** Brower and associates;[24] **I,** Amato and associates.[22] (With permission from Gattinoni L, Carlesso E, Cadringher P, et al: Physical and biological triggers of ventilator-induced lung injury and its prevention. Eur Respir J Suppl 2003;47:15s-25s.)

Table 11.3 Summary of Available Evidence on the Effects of Higher PEEP in Patients with ALI/ARDS

Study	Population	Group	No. of Patients	PEEP (cm H_2O)	Tidal Volume (mL/kg)	Plateau Pressure (cm H_2O)	Mortality Rate (%)	*P* (Outcome)
Brower et al[63]	Unselected	Lower PEEP	273	8.9 ± 3.5 (first day)	6.1 ± 0.8 (first day)	24 ± 7 (first day)	27.5 (hospital discharge)	0.48
		Higher PEEP	276	14.7 ± 3.5 (first day)	6 ± 0.9 (first day)	27 ± 6 (first day)	24.9 (hospital discharge)	
Meade et al[64]	Unselected	Control	983	9.8 ± 2.7	6	<30	40.4 (hospital discharge)	0.19
		LOVS Group	983	14.6 ± 3.4	6	<40	36.4 (hospital discharge)	
Mercat et al[65]	Unselected	Minimal distention strategy	382	7.1 ± 1.8	6.1 ± 0.4	21.1 ± 4.7	31.2 (28 day)	0.31
		Increased recruitment strategy	385	14.6 ± 3.2	6.1 ± 0.3	27.5 ± 2.4	27.8 (28 day)	
Villar et al[126]	Selected	Control	45	9 ± 2.7 (first day)	10.2 ± 1.2 (first day)	32.6 ± 6.2 (first day)	55.5 (hospital discharge)	.41
		P flex	50	14.1 ± 2.8 (first day)	7.3 ± 0.9 (first day)	30.6 ± 6 (first day)	34 (hospital discharge)	
Ranieri et al[66]	Unselected	Control	19	6.5 ± 1.7	11.1 ± 1.9 (first day)	31.0 ± 4.5 (first day)	58 (28 day)	.19
		Lung Protective Strategy	18	14.8 ± 2.7	7.6 ± 1.1	24.6 ± 2.4	38 (28 day)	

ALI/ARDS, acute lung injury/acute respiratory distress syndrome; NS, not significant; PEEP, positive end-expiratory pressure; P flex, lower inflection point of the pressure-volume curve of the respiratory system.

Studies cited in this table can be found in the complete list of references for the chapter, available online at www.expertconsult.com.

provide striking evidence that PEEP may reduce the damages of mechanical ventilation, the largest studies comparing higher versus lower PEEP levels in unselected ALI/ARDS patients were unable to find any difference in outcome.[63-66] It has been suggested that PEEP should be of benefit in patients with higher lung recruitability and useless or harmful in patients with low lung recruitability.[67] Actually two meta-analyses seem to confirm this hypothesis. The meta-analysis by Phoenix and associates[68] showed a trend toward improved survival in the high PEEP group with no evidence of increase in barotrauma. The other meta-analysis by Briel and colleagues[69] on the largest three trials reported no treatment effect on hospital survival between higher and lower PEEP groups while a significant improved survival rate was found in patients in presence of ARDS defined as PaO_2/FIO_2 ratio equal or less than 200. In contrast, in patients with mild and moderate ARDS, higher PEEP seemed harmful. These results roughly account for what we know about the ARDS pathophysiology. In fact, the putative beneficial effect of PEEP on survival should be related to the prevention of excessive regional stress and strain by keeping open lung regions that would otherwise collapse.[26,70] When we studied lung recruitability in an unselected ALI/ARDS population, we found that it varied from 0% to more than 50% of the whole lung.[59] We found that severity of lung injury was associated with higher lung recruitability and more severe hypoxemia, greater deadspace, and lower compliance of the respiratory system. By arbitrarily dividing the study population into patients with higher or lower lung recruitability, we first observed that in the latter, the amount of recruitable lung was almost negligible, amounting to about 50 g of tissue weight. The response to the application of higher levels of PEEP was minimal and much lower than that observed in patients with higher lung recruitability.

SETTING RESPIRATORY RATE

Although extensive work has been devoted to understanding better how to set tidal volume and PEEP in ARDS, the potential importance of respiratory rate in the development of VILI has been scarcely investigated. Technology allows the use of respiratory rate from near zero breaths per minute using extracorporeal techniques to remove CO_2 to 2000 to 3000 breaths per minute, by employing high-frequency oscillation. Each tidal volume delivered may be considered as a stress cycle. Increasing the number of stress cycles may increase the lung damage. In experimental ARDS models, it has been observed that decreasing the respiratory rate decreases edema formation in isolated rabbit lung,[71] whereas an increase in respiratory rate, during spontaneous breathing, leads to an increase in edema formation.[72] It is conceivable that the respiratory rate may play a role in the pathogenesis of VILI when associated with a harmful tidal volume or inadequate PEEP. A different issue is the use of high-frequency oscillatory ventilation (HFOV), a technique that uses very high respiratory frequencies in association with very low tidal volumes and very high mean airway pressure, minimizing inspiratory overdistention and end-expiratory lung collapse.[73] Most patients treated with HFOV improved PaO_2/FIO_2 ratio and reduced oxygenation index over time. Clinical trials were not able to prove a survival benefit, however, a recent meta-analysis on six randomized controlled trials comparing HFOV to conventional ventilation suggested a survival benefit at 30 days.[74] Two clinical trials are currently ongoing with the aim of comparing HFOV with lung protective mechanical ventilation (OSCAR trial in the United Kingdom [ISRCTN10416500] and OSCILLATE trial in Canada [ISRCTN87124254]). In the absence of definitive evidence HFOV remains investigational for routine management of ARDS and should be reserved for patients unresponsive to conventional ventilator strategies.

SETTING INSPIRATORY-TO-EXPIRATORY RATIO

Mechanical ventilators provide a wide range of inspiratory-to-expiratory (I:E) ratios. Setting an adequate I:E ratio may be of great importance when ventilating patients with structural alterations of lung parenchyma, such as chronic obstructive pulmonary disease and emphysema, and during asthmatic exacerbation. In these conditions characterized by a time constant of the respiratory system greater than normal, a longer expiratory time must be provided to allow deflation of gas from the lungs before the next respiratory cycle, avoiding dynamic hyperinflation and intrinsic PEEP.[75] During ALI/ARDS, no convincing evidence has been provided for the advantages of setting an I:E ratio different from 1:1.

In the past, inverse ratio ventilation[76] was advocated as a tool to improve the effects of mechanical ventilation in ARDS.[77-79] Studies primarily showed an improvement of arterial oxygenation. Increased mean airway pressure, intrinsic PEEP, and a decrease in cardiac output were problematic.[80] Extreme forms of manipulating I:E ratio are not recommended; an I:E ratio in ALI/ARDS of 0.5 to 1.5 is appropriate.

INDIVIDUALIZING MECHANICAL VENTILATION IN PATIENTS WITH ACUTE RESPIRATORY DISTRESS SYNDROME

General principles underlying the application of mechanical ventilation in ALI/ARDS patients have been discussed. We now present the sequence of interventions that we believe are most appropriate for tailoring mechanical ventilation in an individual patient.[81]

The first intervention after admission to the ICU is to determine whether the patient has the criteria for ARDS diagnosis, keeping in mind that this syndrome consists of diffuse inflammatory lung edema. Patient history (research for possible etiologic factors leading to ARDS) and clinical observation (cyanosis, higher respiratory rate, use of accessory respiratory muscles, inspiratory crackles at lung auscultation mainly in the dependent lung regions) may suggest a possible lung inflammatory edema. Blood gas analysis and chest x-ray studies may confirm the initial diagnosis of the syndrome. The choice between an attempt of noninvasive respiratory support (facemask continuous positive airway pressure or noninvasive ventilation) or endotracheal intubation should be made on a clinical basis, according to the severity of illness, and whether the patient is stable or deteriorating. We pay particular attention to the improvement of Pa_{O_2} after oxygen administration and to Pa_{CO_2}. The lack of remarkable response in oxygenation to increased F_{IO_2} indicates a remarkable fraction of right-to-left intrapulmonary shunt, which is typical of ARDS. Low Pa_{CO_2} suggests that the respiratory muscles of the patient are still able to deal with the decreased compliance of the respiratory system (i.e., sustaining the increased respiratory effort), whereas normal or high levels of Pa_{CO_2} suggest a near exhaustion of the respiratory muscles and need of immediate ventilatory support.

Clinicians should be aware of the immediate possible consequences of intubation and initiation of mechanical ventilation. Sedation, either by itself or in association with muscle paralysis, produces a loss of respiratory muscle tone and a cranial shift of the diaphragm, promoting further lung collapse with immediate consequences in gas exchange. Mechanical ventilation produces an increase in intrathoracic pressure and decreased venous return. The intravascular volume status of the patient should be assessed before intubation, and hypovolemia should be corrected. The rate and the amount of fluid replacement should be decided for each individual patient. Inadequate fluid replacement may lead to a severe hemodynamic impairment immediately after beginning positive-pressure ventilation. An excessive fluid replacement in an inflamed lung with leaking capillaries may result in a dramatic increase of pulmonary edema with devastating consequences on gas exchange. Wiedemann and coworkers,[82] in a study published in the New England Journal of Medicine, compared a conservative and a liberal strategy of fluid management in 1000 patients with ALI. Although the primary end point (60-day mortality) was not significantly different, patients treated with the conservative strategy had better lung function and shorter duration of mechanical ventilation and intensive care without increasing nonpulmonary organ failures. For these reasons, we prefer to tailor fluid replacement according to the results of a fluid challenge test. Echocardiography also may be helpful in assessing the volumetric status.[83] After endotracheal intubation, the initial ventilatory setting employed is blind because the pathophysiologic characteristics of the patient have not yet been assessed. We usually set the ventilator (volume controlled) with a tidal volume equal to 6 to 8 mL/kg ideal body weight, F_{IO_2} equal to 0.7, and a respiratory rate of 15 breaths per minute, with an I:E ratio of 1:1. As soon as hemodynamic stability is obtained, a PEEP trial (preceded by a recruitment maneuver) is performed by applying in a random sequence of 5 to 15 cm H_2O PEEP with the patient under sedation and, sometimes, muscle paralysis. At each level of PEEP, we maintain tidal volume, respiratory rate, F_{IO_2}, and I:E ratio constant for about 20 minutes, after which we measure (1) arterial oxygenation, (2) respiratory system compliance, and (3) alveolar deadspace. Patients who, after the application of higher PEEP, improve at least two of these three parameters have a greater likelihood of having a higher lung recruitability. Alternatively, it is possible to target a specific saturation on the basis of pulse oximetry, if available, aiming at a hemoglobin oxygen saturation of 90%.

The improvement in arterial oxygenation alone, although commonly employed, may be misleading for the assessment of lung recruitment because it may be the result of a slight decrease in cardiac output or a modification of regional distribution of pulmonary blood flow or both. It has been shown that improvement in respiratory physiologic variables from a PEEP trial has low sensitivity (71%) and specificity

(59%) in assessing lung recruitability;[59] we prefer to obtain whole-lung CT scanning. In the CT scan facility, while maintaining the baseline ventilator setting, whole-lung CT scanning is performed at 5 cm H_2O PEEP at end expiration and 45 cm H_2O at end inspiration. The subsequent quantitative analysis of the CT scans allows us to obtain a precise assessment of lung recruitability. In patients with higher recruitability we apply PEEP greater than 15 cm H_2O, up to 20 cm H_2O and exceptionally greater than 20 but not exceeding 25 cm H_2O, whereas in patients with lower lung recruitability we apply a PEEP level not greater than 10 cm H_2O.

If CT scan is unavailable, and only the PEEP trial has been performed, we assign to the high-recruitment group patients with either a baseline PaO_2/FIO_2 ratio less than 150 when measured at 5 cm H_2O PEEP or patients who respond to 15 cm H_2O PEEP compared with 5 cm H_2O with a positive response of two of the following three variables: increased PaO_2, decreased alveolar deadspace, or increased compliance of the respiratory system.

We attempt to keep the plateau pressure less than 30 cm H_2O by modifying tidal volume and respiratory rate. As discussed earlier, however, tidal volume and plateau pressure are inadequate surrogates for alveolar stress and strain. We now measure, in each severe ARDS patient, the transpulmonary pressure by helium dilution technique, by employing an esophageal balloon (lung resting volume of 0 cm H_2O or 5 cm H_2O PEEP). With mechanical ventilation, a global pulmonary strain greater than about 1.5 (strain is dimensionless because it is the ratio of two volumes), or an end-inspiratory transpulmonary pressure greater than 20 cm H_2O, may cause VILI, with irreversible respiratory failure to follow.[11,29] These values of alveolar stress and strain are the ones at which the residual ventilatable lung reaches its near total lung capacity, with a full extension of the collagen fibers of the lung skeleton.

In some patients, we have observed that a tidal volume of 8 to 10 mL/kg ideal body weight determines a lung strain value less than 1 and a transpulmonary pressure value less than 14 cm H_2O. In these patients, we employ a tidal volume greater than 6 mL/kg ideal body weight, avoiding excessive hypercapnia or need for sedation. In contrast, in the most severe patients, in which the baby lung is extremely small, even a ventilation with 6 mL/kg ideal body weight may result in values of alveolar stress and strain higher than those required to reach total lung capacity. Evidence from the literature and physiologic reasoning strongly indicate that for these patients a safe form of mechanical ventilation does not exist.[84,85] We reserve to them the use of extracorporeal support. We acknowledge that measuring alveolar stress and strain may seem to be a physiologic curiosity or a research tool. Nonetheless, we have introduced them in our clinical practice as the most logical approach for VILI prevention.

Some authors advocate the use of other forms of mechanical ventilation in patients with ARDS.[86,87] The rationale of pressure support ventilation in ARDS relies on the possibility of decreasing the need for sedation, while preserving the contribution of spontaneous breathing, and with possible advantages on gas and flow pulmonary distribution.[88] During the full-blown phase of the illness, we prefer to keep the patient well sedated. This approach may help to reduce energy requirement and oxygen consumption and CO_2 production.

The onset of recovery is characterized by the control or reversal, or both, of the cause of ARDS. An increase of systemic oxygenation and respiratory system compliance follows. When a PaO_2 value greater than 80 mm Hg is obtained at FIO_2 of 0.4, we start the weaning from PEEP application, decreasing the PEEP level no more than 1 cm H_2O every 4 to 6 hours, and suspending the process if the oxygenation consistently deteriorates. Subsequently, after an appropriate adjustment of sedation, we shift from pressure-controlled or volume-controlled to pressure-support ventilation, initially setting the support at the same inspiratory pressure used during controlled ventilation. According to the patient's response, pressure-support level is progressively decreased, and the final phase of weaning is initiated at pressure support of 5 to 10 cm H_2O, FIO_2 lower than 0.4, and PEEP level equal to 5 cm H_2O.

POSSIBLE ADJUNCTS TO MECHANICAL VENTILATION

PRONE POSITION

Prone positioning, first proposed in 1974[89] and first applied in ARDS patients in 1976,[90] results in improved arterial oxygenation in most patients. After the introduction of CT scanning, showing lung consolidation located in the dependent lung regions and the aerated baby lung in the nondependent lung regions,[12,16] we integrated prone positioning as standard practice in clinical treatment of ARDS patients to improve systemic oxygenation.[91] The initial hypothesis was that better perfusion of the baby lung, located in the dependent lung regions after prone positioning, would provide advantages in gas exchange. The picture observed was quite different, however. We did observe an improvement in arterial oxygenation, but the mechanism was likely different because CT scans taken in the prone position showed a density redistribution toward the dependent lung areas.[92]

This observation led to our introduction of the "sponge model" as our pathophysiologic understanding of ARDS.[93] Whatever the position of the patient, the increased weight of the nondependent lung tissue squeezes the gas out of the dependent regions of the lung.[42] The mechanisms of improved gas exchange were different from that first hypothesized. It is not the aim of this chapter to discuss the possible physiologic mechanisms of prone positioning, which may be found elsewhere.[94-98] Taken together, all of the studies, including small and large series of patients, consistently showed that in 70% of the patients systemic oxygenation improves in prone compared with supine positioning,[98,99] without any change in the applied airway pressure. There is no doubt that in life-threatening severe hypoxemia a trial in the prone position is indicated.

A different issue is the effectiveness of the prone position in improving ARDS outcome. Is mechanical ventilation in ARDS less harmful in the prone compared with the supine position? Does mechanical ventilation induce less alveolar stress and strain in the prone position? There is a consistent physiologic rationale to believe that this is the case. In experimental settings[100-103] and in normal subjects and patients affected by ARDS, CT scan shows a more homogeneous distribution of gas throughout the lung parenchyma in the prone compared with the supine position.[98] This observation strongly suggests that the distribution of alveolar stress and strain is more homogeneous in the prone position. In experimental models of ARDS, there is evidence that prone positioning prevents or significantly delays the development of VILI.[103,104] Two large randomized studies on prone positioning were unable to show a significant benefit on outcome;[97,105] however, prone positioning was applied for only about a quarter of the day, and mechanical ventilation was not controlled. In a more recent trial,[106] in which prone positioning was applied for 20 hours per day and mechanical ventilation was strictly controlled, a positive benefit was found for the patients treated with prone positioning. On these bases the Prone-Supine II study[107] was organized to detect potential survival benefit of prone positioning avoiding the limitations of previous trials. Although, the study was not able to show a significant survival benefit in the general population, a favorable trend was detected in the subgroup of patients with severe ARDS. In a meta-analysis including 10 clinical trials on adults and children Sud and associates[108] found that prone ventilation reduced mortality rate in severely hypoxemic patients ($PaO_2/FIO_2 \leq 100$, $p = 0.01$) but not in patients with PaO_2/FIO_2 greater than 100 ($p = 0.36$). The authors' suggestion was that prone position may provide benefits in severely hypoxemic patients, but it should not be routinely used in all patients affected by acute hypoxemic respiratory failure. In a pooled analysis[107] of the four largest databases[99,105-107] of trials on prone position, the absolute mortality rate reduction in severe ARDS patients treated in prone position was approximately 10% (log-rank = 0.03). On the contrary, in patients with moderate ARDS prolonged prone position may be useless or possibly harmful.

EXTRACORPOREAL SUPPORT

Extracorporeal support of ARDS was first applied in 1972.[109] The first randomized trial ever performed in ALI/ARDS showed that patients treated with extracorporeal support or with conventional ventilation had similar mortality rates, equal to about 90%.[110] In the 1980s, our center introduced extracorporeal CO_2 removal in ARDS, aiming at lung rest with a suggestion of benefit.[111,112] A randomized study performed in 1994 did not show any survival benefit with extracorporeal CO_2 removal support.[113] The results of this trial may have been significantly influenced by bleeding complications in patients undergoing extracorporeal CO_2 removal. Despite the discouraging results, in Europe few centers continued to use veno-venous extracorporeal support as a last resource in selected series of patients.[114] In the United States, Bartlett and colleagues[115,116] continued to provide extracorporeal support associated with mechanical ventilation with less strict entry criteria and with encouraging results. The interest on extracorporeal membrane oxygenation (ECMO) renewed after the publication of CESAR trial in 2009,[117] which showed clear benefits on outcome when severely hypoxemic patients were treated with extracorporeal support in an expert high case volume center when compared to nonspecialized hospitals. The rebirth of the technique, however, occurred with its use as a rescue therapy during H1N1 flu epidemics in Australia and New Zealand in severely hypoxemic patients untreatable with conventional methods.[118] The approach was veno-venous with high blood flows. This report showed a survival rate higher than 70%, and an impressive number of centers in Europe, United States, South America, Canada, and Asia started to use ECMO in severely hypoxemic patients who do not receive benefits from maximal mechanical ventilation.[119-124] Survival rate ranged between 56% and 79%.

The impressive diffusion of ECMO led to the great improvement of this technology, and there are increasing numbers of reports describing simple forms of extracorporeal support, primarily aiming at CO_2 removal.[125] The actual indications for ECMO depend on the patient's need and the physician's request. The choice of the technique may vary from low-flow bypass with CO_2 removal to high-flow ECMO with total oxygenation support. If the aim is the treatment of life-threatening hypoxemia, the clear-cut indication is high-flow veno-venous ECMO. If the patient, however, presents with severe cardiac failure, veno-arterial ECMO must be used.

A simplified schema of the possible intervention is reported in Figure 11.6, which underlines the recent ARDS Berlin definition, which may be helpful in dictating the sequence of possible intervention when ARDS severity is increasing.

Therapeutic Options According to the Berlin Definition

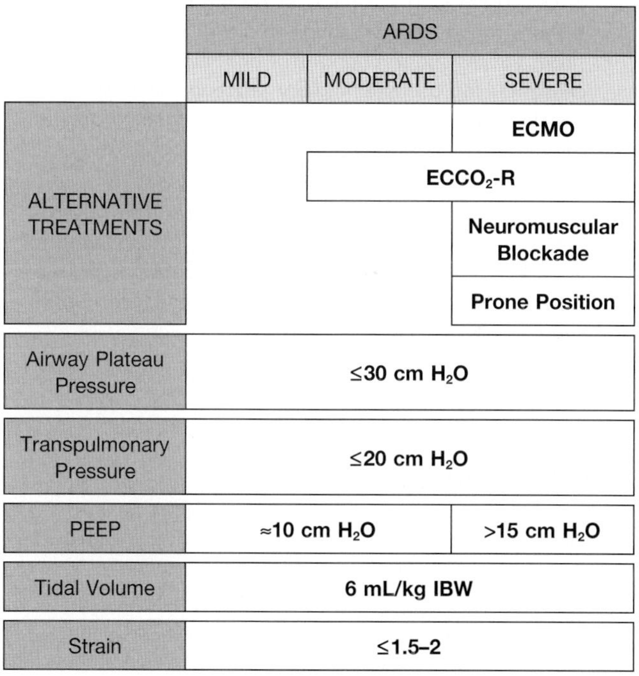
ARDS
MILD
MODERATE
SEVERE
ALTERNATIVE TREATMENTS
ECMO
ECCO2-R
Neuromuscular Blockade
Prone Position
Airway Plateau Pressure
≤30 cm H2O
Transpulmonary Pressure
≤20 cm H2O
PEEP
≈10 cm H2O
>15 cm H2O
Tidal Volume
6 mL/kg IBW
Strain
≤1.5–2

ARDS, acute respiratory distress syndrome; ECMO, extracorporeal membrane oxygenation; $ECCO_2$-R, extracorporeal CO_2 removal; PEEP, positive end-expiratory pressure; IBW, ideal body weight.

Modified from the Berlin definition of ARDS: an expanded rationale, justification, and supplementary material. Ferguson ND, Fan E, Camporota L, Antonelli M, Anzueto A, Beale R, Brochard L, Brower R, Esteban A, Gattinoni L, Rhodes A, Slutsky AS, Vincent JL, Rubenfeld GD, Thompson BT, Ranieri VM. Intensive Care Med. 2012 Oct;38(10):1573-82. Epub 2012 Aug 25. Erratum in: Intensive Care Med. 2012 Oct;38(10):1731-1732.

Figure 11.6 Simplified schema of possible ARDS intervention. ARDS, acute respiratory distress syndrome; ECMO, extracorporeal membrane oxygenation; $ECCO_2$-R, extracorporeal CO_2 removal; PEEP, positive end-expiratory pressure; IBW, ideal body weight.

KEY POINTS

- The targets of mechanical ventilation in ARDS have shifted from providing normal gas exchange to protecting the lung from VILI.
- Mechanical ventilation replaces the action of the respiratory muscles. The driving force of mechanical ventilation (airway pressure displayed on the ventilator) is spent partly to overcome the resistances to flow, partly to inflate the lung, and partly to inflate the chest wall.
- The distending force of the lung (the trigger of VILI) is the transpulmonary pressure (P_L)—the difference between the airway pressure (Paw) and the pleural pressure (Ppl). For the same driving force, in normal conditions, the transpulmonary pressure equals the driving force multiplied by the ratio between the lung elastance and the respiratory system elastance (lung elastance + chest wall elastance): $P_L = Paw \times E_L/Etot$. In normal subjects, this ratio is approximately 0.5; in ARDS patients, it may be 0.2 to 0.8. Consequently, the airway pressure alone may be misleading to assess the transpulmonary pressure imposed on the lung by mechanical ventilation (i.e., to assess the stress). We used airway pressure to indicate end-inspiratory pressure.
- The delivered tidal volume increases the lung volume and in the process produces strain on the lung. The ratio of change in lung volume over resting lung volume ($\Delta V/V_0$) is a rough approximation of the strain. Excessive strain causes shape changes of endothelial and epithelial cells inducing an inflammatory reaction. Because the resting volume (V_0, the baby lung) may vary largely in ARDS, the same tidal volume per ideal body weight may induce largely different strain values.
- Stress and strain, the triggers of VILI, are linked by a constant, specific lung elastance (Espec), accounting for the following relationship: P_L (stress) = Espec × $\Delta V/V_0$ (strain). The specific lung elastance is similar in normal subjects and in ARDS patients.
- Physiologic variables are generally poor indicators of the severity of lung injury, with the alveolar deadspace being the only variable associated with outcome. The severity of lung injury may be assessed by CT scan. The fraction of nonaerated lung tissue is strongly associated with mortality risk. The greater the lung injury, the smaller the baby lung, and the greater the stress-strain induced by mechanical ventilation.
- Among outcome studies testing different tidal volumes, only the study comparing the two extreme values tested (6 mL/kg versus 12 mL/kg) showed a significant benefit of lower tidal volume. Data from clinical studies and rationale from physiologic studies are strongly in favor of using the lowest tidal volume possible, likely associated with lower stress and strain, accepting hypercapnia as a side effect.
- All studies comparing lower versus higher PEEP randomly applied to *unselected* ARDS populations failed to show benefits on survival. In contrast, benefits of higher PEEP were found in more severe *selected* ARDS patients.
- The lung recruitability may vary greatly within the ARDS population (5% to 50% of the lung parenchyma) and is correlated with the overall lung injury severity. Higher PEEP possibly should be reserved only for patients with higher recruitability.
- When treating patients with ARDS, individual characteristics (lung injury severity, gas exchange, lung mechanics, abdominal pressure) should be assessed to tailor the least harmful mechanical ventilation setting according to the available evidence and physiologic rationale, providing the lowest stress and strain possible.
- In the severe ARDS, in which mechanical ventilation is more harmful, associated therapy such as prone positioning and extracorporeal support must be sought.

SELECTED REFERENCES

11. Dreyfuss D, Saumon G: Ventilator-induced lung injury: Lessons from experimental studies. Am J Respir Crit Care Med 1998; 157(1):294-323.
16. Gattinoni L, Pesenti A: The concept of "baby lung." Intensive Care Med 2005;31(6):776-784.
29. Gattinoni L, Carlesso E, Cadringher P, et al: Physical and biological triggers of ventilator-induced lung injury and its prevention. Eur Respir J Suppl 2003;47:15s-25s.
32. Maksym GN, Bates JH: A distributed nonlinear model of lung tissue elasticity. J Appl Physiol 1997;82(1):32-41.
43. Protti A, Cressoni M, Santini A, et al: Lung stress and strain during mechanical ventilation: Any safe threshold? Am J Respir Crit Care Med 2011;183(10):1354 (erratum, Am J Respir Crit Care Med 2012;185(1):115).
48. Gattinoni L, Caironi P, Cressoni M, et al: Lung recruitment in patients with the acute respiratory distress syndrome. N Engl J Med 2006;354(17):1775-1786.
58. Pelosi P, Croci M, Ravagnan I, et al: Total respiratory system, lung, and chest wall mechanics in sedated-paralyzed postoperative morbidly obese patients. Chest 1996;109(1):144-151.
70. Mead J, Takishima T, Leith D: Stress distribution in lungs: A model of pulmonary elasticity. J Appl Physiol 1970;28(5):596-608.
81. Marini JJ, Gattinoni L: Ventilatory management of acute respiratory distress syndrome: A consensus of two. Crit Care Med 2004; 32(1):250-255.
96. Pelosi P, Tubiolo D, Mascheroni D, et al: Effects of the prone position on respiratory mechanics and gas exchange during acute lung injury. Am J Respir Crit Care Med 1998;157(2):387-393.

The complete list of references can be found at www.expertconsult.com.

12

Bronchoscopy and Lung Biopsy in Critically Ill Patients

Thaddeus Bartter | Melvin R. Pratter | Wissam Abouzgheib

CHAPTER OUTLINE

Bronchoscopy plays an important role in the care of critically ill patients. Since the introduction of the flexible fiberoptic bronchoscope in 1968, flexible bronchoscopy has slowly gained importance as a diagnostic and a therapeutic tool. It has largely replaced rigid bronchoscopy in the intensive care unit (ICU) because of the lack of need for complete anesthesia, the ease of use, and the fact that with a flexible bronchoscope one can perform procedures on a critically ill ventilated patient through an endotracheal tube or tracheostomy tube.

Lung biopsy is often a procedure of last resort in a critically ill patient with lung disease who is not responding to therapy. Whereas many of these patients are on mechanical ventilation, the potential benefits of biopsy need to be carefully weighed against the potential risks.

This chapter will review bronchoscopy and lung biopsy in critically ill patients. By definition, a critically ill patient has one or more organs that are under stress and have limited functional reserve. Stresses that are usually well tolerated by healthy individuals may have serious or even fatal consequences for a patient in the ICU. This chapter will first review the physiologic stresses induced by bronchoscopy. It will then review diagnostic and therapeutic indications for bronchoscopy in the ICU. Finally, we will review the potential role of bronchoscopic and nonbronchoscopic approaches to lung biopsy.

FIBEROPTIC BRONCHOSCOPY–INDUCED PHYSIOLOGIC CHANGES

GENERAL CONSIDERATIONS

The act of cannulation of the airway is not a physiologically neutral event.[1-5] It stimulates both cardiovascular and respiratory responses. In the ICU, there are three common stimuli that provoke these reflexes: intubation, bronchoscopy, and suctioning. Even after the use of sedation and application of topical anesthesia, the passage of a bronchoscope through the larynx typically results in a 30% increase in mean arterial blood pressure and cardiac index, a 40% increase in heart rate, and an 86% increase in pulmonary arterial occlusion pressure.[1] The response seems to represent a reflex to mechanical stimulation of the larynx. A significant hemodynamic response occurs even when patients are anesthetized and paralyzed before the passage of a bronchoscope through the larynx and into the trachea, with conflicting data as to whether there is a difference in hemodynamic response between the nasal and the oral routes.[3,4] Topical anesthesia of the upper airway with lidocaine attenuates (but does not ablate) the cardiovascular responses.[3,5]

The significance of the cardiovascular changes associated with bronchoscopy is related primarily to their potential impact upon the heart and the brain. The increase in rate-pressure product has the potential to cause cardiac ischemia in patients with limited cardiac perfusion. In one small study, 3 of 10 monitored patients undergoing bronchoscopy, all of whom were 55 years old or older, developed electrocardiographic changes of ischemia.[2] In another study designed specifically to look at older patients, the incidence of ischemia was 17%.[6] Despite these findings, bronchoscopy has a low mortality rate from ischemia. In studies that have described complications from bronchoscopy (ranging from as few as 10 to as many as 48,000 procedures), the rate of death from ischemic events ranged from 0% to approximately 0.01%.[6-11]

A second potential cardiac complication of bronchoscopy is the triggering of arrhythmias. One study looking specifically for arrhythmias during bronchoscopy found an 11% incidence of "major arrhythmias."[12] As with ischemia, however, the reported mortality rate from arrhythmias has been very low; in two large studies of complications of bronchoscopy the mortality rate from arrhythmias ranged from 0% to 0.04%.[10,11]

With respect to the brain, both bronchoscopy and endotracheal suctioning cause significant increases in intracranial pressure.[2,13] Because mean arterial pressure and intracerebral pressure increase roughly in parallel, there is little overall change in cerebral perfusion pressure.[2,13] This may explain why no adverse intracerebral sequelae have been reported despite the observed increase in intracerebral pressure.[13] Nevertheless, we believe that close attention to intracerebral pressure is warranted whenever possible in brain-injured individuals undergoing bronchoscopy.

Bronchoscopy also affects the work of breathing, respiratory pressures, and lung volumes. Transnasal cannulation of the trachea leads to a decrease in inspiratory and expiratory flow, a decrease in vital capacity, and an increase in functional residual capacity.[14] Bronchoscopy through an endotracheal tube in a sedated but not ventilated patient leads to significant further decreases in flows and vital capacity and a marked increase in the work of breathing.[14,15]

BRONCHOSCOPY IN MECHANICALLY VENTILATED PATIENTS

Mechanical ventilation adds additional complexity to the physiologic effects of bronchoscopy. The details were elegantly delineated in a study by Lindholm and colleagues.[15] The first notable change is a dramatic increase in upper airway resistance. Airway narrowing related to endotracheal tube insertion by itself increases airway resistance. The subsequent introduction of a bronchoscope through the endotracheal tube greatly increases that resistance. The actual degree of increased airway resistance observed is related to the cross-sectional areas of both the endotracheal tube and the bronchoscope being inserted.[15] The increased resistance has implications for ventilator gas delivery. The first is a potential decrease in delivered volume. With a volume-cycled mode, pressure increases as needed to deliver the specified volume, but the set volume may not be delivered owing to a pressure pop-off set in the alarm/safety parameters of the ventilator. (Although peak pressures of 60 to 80 cm H_2O can be reached at the airway opening, note that the pressure gradient from the proximal obstruction limits the pressure delivered to the lung parenchyma.[15]) With a pressure-cycled mode of mechanical ventilation, the increase in upper airway resistance caused by bronchoscopic cannulation leads to an immediate decrease in delivered volume, the severity of which again depends upon the cross-sectional diameters of both the endotracheal tube and the bronchoscope. This effect can be countered by raising the applied pressure and the associated inspiratory airway pressure.

Whereas the driving pressure for inspiratory volumes depends upon external force (generated by the ventilator), exhalation is largely dependent upon the passive recoil of the lungs. The increase in airway resistance caused by introduction of the bronchoscope into the endotracheal tube thus has a disparate and more potentially dramatic effect upon expiratory volumes than upon inspiratory volumes. Sequential delivered volumes may be incompletely exhaled, causing a gradual buildup of intrathoracic volume and intrinsic positive end-expiratory pressure (auto-PEEP). Lindholm and colleagues[15] documented several cases of auto-PEEP greater than 18 cm H_2O. In one patient being bronchoscoped through an endotracheal tube with an internal diameter of 7 mm, auto-PEEP was recorded at 35 cm H_2O.

Suctioning adds another layer of complexity. In addition to the cardiovascular changes stimulated by suctioning mentioned earlier, suctioning can cause profound changes in intrathoracic pressures and lung volumes. Not only can the auto-PEEP induced during bronchoscopy be eliminated, but with prolonged suctioning negative intrathoracic pressure can be created.[15] This can lead to clinically relevant decreases in functional residual capacity, tidal volume, and minute ventilation, with potential for alveolar collapse, hypercarbia, and hypoxemia.

HYPOXEMIA

That bronchoscopy can cause hypoxemia is clear. The degree of hypoxemia ranges from mild to severe, and a variety of potential mechanisms are involved. The administration of benzodiazepines and narcotics can cause hypoxemia and respiratory depression in normal volunteers,[16] and one study showed a 35% incidence of desaturation after sedation even before bronchoscopy was performed.[17] The desaturation may not be completely due to central nervous system depression; Chhajed and coworkers[18] showed that hypoxemia during bronchoscopy could be corrected in most of their lung transplant patients by the insertion of a nasopharyngeal tube, indicating that in their population upper airway collapse was a major cause of hypoxemia. Apart from the effects of sedation upon oxygenation, bronchoscopy itself can cause hypoxemia. Changes in airway resistance and the impact of suctioning upon functional residual capacity are probably major factors.[19-22] Higher incidences of hypoxemia have been shown to correlate with the degree of prebronchoscopy pulmonary impairment, extent of suctioning, and performing a bronchoalveolar lavage (BAL).[20-25] Furthermore, the hypoxemia induced by bronchoscopy often does not resolve immediately upon removal of the bronchoscope; it can persist for more than 2 hours.[17,24,25] Hypoxemia represents another stress on top of the cardiovascular reflex changes cited earlier and may negatively impact organs at risk. Hypoxemia may play a significant role in cardiac ischemia and arrhythmias associated with bronchoscopy.[1]

Bronchoscopy through the endotracheal tube of a patient on a ventilator has been reported to cause an increase in Po_2 with an increase in Pco_2 and a decrease in Po_2 with no change in Pco_2.[14,15] The seemingly contradictory differences in findings probably reflect individual differences in how much patients are suctioned and the degree to which suctioning impacts functional residual capacity.

SUMMARY

In summary, bronchoscopy and other airway cannulations almost always trigger a reflex response that includes tachycardia and an increase in blood pressure. Bronchoscopy frequently causes hypoxemia, which may be of prolonged duration. For patients on ventilators, disparate physiologic changes can be created based on the mode of ventilation, the size of the endotracheal tube, the size of the bronchoscope, the duration of suctioning, and the flow rate that the suction channel of the bronchoscope is able to attain. Bronchoscopy can cause significant physiologic stress, and the critically ill patient may be less able to tolerate that stress than an otherwise healthy individual.

AIRWAY EVALUATION AND MANAGEMENT

INTUBATION AND ENDOTRACHEAL TUBE MANAGEMENT

Bronchoscopy can be an asset in the insertion and subsequent management of endotracheal tubes.[26,27] For patients with difficult airways, an endotracheal tube can be placed over a bronchoscope and slid into the trachea after direct visual intubation with the bronchoscope. A similar technique can be used for changing the endotracheal tube in a tenuous patient, especially if switching from nasal to oral or oral to nasal.[27] Bronchoscopy is valuable in the placement of tubes for single-lung ventilation or placement of double-lumen tubes.[27] Bronchoscopy also allows the bronchoscopist to position the tip of an endotracheal tube at a point approximately 2.5 cm above the carina under direct visualization or, when there is a process such as tumor compression of the trachea, to place the tube wherever needed for optimal ventilation.[26]

PERCUTANEOUS DILATIONAL TRACHEOSTOMY

Percutaneous dilational tracheostomy (PDT) has emerged as a primary method of tracheostomy for ICU patients. It has a lower incidence of overall complications than does open surgical tracheostomy, and it can be performed at the bedside, avoiding the risks of transporting a critically ill patient.[28-31] It also is more cost-effective.[29] PDT can be performed not only by surgeons, but also by trained intensivists and pulmonologists;[30] it has become a standard intensivist procedure in many institutions.[32,33] Although its overall safety profile is better than for open surgical tracheostomy, PDT does have a higher risk of posterior tracheal wall injury and false passage.[34] Bronchoscopy can be combined with PDT to allow direct endobronchial guidance for the procedure. Bronchoscopy has been suggested by several authors to be an important safety factor in PDT,[31,34-40] although its use is not universally practiced.[32,41] Direct visualization is a protection against inadvertent tracheal injury and a means of assessing an injury for intervention should it occur.[34,36,38] The most logical approach to PDT is a team approach[42] with at least two principal operators—one managing the bronchoscope and endotracheal tube and the second working at the neck to insert the tracheostomy tube.[31,34,39] The risk of using bronchoscopy for PDT is that of increased hypoventilation because the patient is being ventilated through the endotracheal tube during the procedure.[37] This can be obviated with the use of a pediatric bronchoscope for guidance; a large working channel is not needed for this application.

AIRWAY OBSTRUCTION AND ATELECTASIS

The upper airway can become obstructed via several mechanisms. Bronchoscopy is valuable in diagnosing all of them. When an endotracheal tube is inserted, it becomes part of the airway. Kinking of the endotracheal tube or luminal blockage by hardened, inspissated secretions causes the same physiologic problems as a primary tracheal process. Granulation tissue at the proximal end of a tracheostomy tube or at the distal end of a tracheostomy tube or endotracheal tube can cause obstruction and difficulty with inflation or deflation of the lungs. (This is much less common with endotracheal tubes than with tracheostomy tubes because of Murphy's eye, the distal side port, on endotracheal tubes.) Benign or malignant processes can cause strictures or compression of the trachea. Finally, edema of the vocal cords and periglottic structures can lead to upper airway obstruction that is not evident with an endotracheal tube in place but that can cause recurrent respiratory failure after extubation; performing extubation over a bronchoscope allows immediate evaluation of the upper airway as the endotracheal tube is withdrawn with immediate diagnosis of this problem.[27]

Foreign bodies can cause obstruction at various points in the airways. Traditionally, rigid bronchoscopy was used for management of foreign bodies given its capacity for airway control and the availability of tools larger than those that can be passed through a flexible bronchoscope.[43] Flexible bronchoscopes are the only choice, however, in an intubated patient, and the combination of larger channel scopes (2.8 mm and larger) for the passage of instruments and of different baskets and grasping tools makes flexible fiberoptic bronchoscopy a viable option in many cases.[26,43,44] For nonintubated patients, a flexible bronchoscope through a rigid bronchoscope is sometimes an optimal approach.[43]

Atelectasis is a common ICU problem and has been one of the most common indications for bronchoscopy in ICUs.[45,46] The argument is obvious: If standard "blind" suctioning is effective and useful, why not use suctioning under direct visualization for local airway obstruction due to secretions? One key study done by Marini and coworkers[47] challenged the assumption that bronchoscopy is an optimal approach to atelectasis. In their study of patients with radiologically evident atelectasis, one group underwent a regimen of initial bronchoscopy followed by regular chest physiotherapy and a second group received regular chest physiotherapy alone followed by delayed bronchoscopy at 48 hours only if atelectasis persisted. The authors showed early bronchoscopy to be the inferior approach; there was no difference in rate or degree of improvement between the two groups, and bronchoscopy led to more significant decreases in oxygenation.[47] The authors also looked at the presence or absence of air bronchograms, postulating that patients with air bronchograms had more distal consolidation (as opposed to proximal obstruction causing atelectasis) and would be more refractory to any attempts to re-expand consolidated lung. Their results strongly supported their postulate.[47]

These data are valuable and should lead to initial trials of chest physiotherapy in most cases of atelectasis, but they do not apply universally in clinical medicine. Some patients with chest trauma or spinal cord injury are not candidates for chest physiotherapy.[48] Patients with chest trauma or spinal cord injury are usually not candidates for chest physiotherapy. Some patients have atelectasis and a severe refractory hypoxemia as a result of shunting of blood through the atelectatic lung. In these patients, a 24-hour wait may be inappropriate, and bronchoscopy sometimes leads to marked improvement. Judicious use of bronchoscopy for atelectasis is thus a clinical decision involving the art of medicine.[48] Some patients with atelectasis have severe refractory hypoxemia as a result of shunting of blood through the atelectatic lung. In these patients, trying chest physiotherapy may be inappropriate because bronchoscopy often can lead to marked improvement almost immediately. Judicious use of bronchoscopy for atelectasis thus depends on the clinical situation. For patients who have a bronchoscope inserted for atelectasis, one technique that has been moderately successful is that of isolated segmental inflation; the bronchoscope or a ballooned catheter is wedged into the atelectatic segment, and pressure of at least 30 mm H_2O is applied through the bronchoscope or catheter.[45,48] This focal approach is more rational for focal atelectasis than are recruitment maneuvers applied to the whole chest because recruitment maneuvers are more likely to overdistend compliant alveoli than to open atelectatic alveoli.[45]

TRAUMA

The value of bronchoscopy for the evaluation of chest trauma was defined in a landmark paper by Hara and Prakash.[49] The authors looked at 53 cases of blunt trauma to the chest, neck, or both in which bronchoscopy was performed within 3 days of injury. Bronchoscopy was believed to be of clinical value in 53% of the 53 cases. They documented injury and tears of the upper and lower airways, contusion or hemorrhage, aspirated material, and plugging or secretions. Only one of eight major tracheal injuries was not completely diagnosed. These data give compelling evidence for visual bronchoscopic evaluation of the bronchial tree in all cases of significant blunt chest trauma.

SMOKE INHALATION

Inhalation injury is a unique form of trauma to the bronchial tree. Most inhalation injuries are due not to heat alone, but to the deposition in the bronchial tree of soot and gases, the products of combustion.[50] Early ventilatory support and aggressive pulmonary toilet probably improve outcomes for inhalation injury,[51,52] but the severity of inhalation injury may not become fully manifest for up to 5 days (usually 3 days).[52] Bronchoscopy has been advocated in the evaluation of patients with possible inhalation injury.[51-53] Some patients have mucosal injuries that are obvious to even an inexperienced bronchoscopist, but sometimes even when there is significant injury, the bronchoscopic appearance of the airways may be minimally abnormal. For patients who have relatively normal-appearing mucosae, biopsy specimens from segmental or subsegmental carinae can yield pathologic information that is predictive of the degree of inhalation injury (or lack thereof) and can be used to guide aggressiveness of management.[51,52] Another tool for evaluation of inhalation injury is the ventilation-perfusion scan,[50,53] but the objectivity and reproducibility of bronchoscopic endobronchial biopsy could lead one to argue that it should be the current standard of care for the diagnosis of possible inhalation injury.

HEMOPTYSIS

Hemoptysis can run the gamut from scant to massive. There are several definitions of massive hemoptysis, with varying quantities of blood specified over different intervals. The best definition of massive hemoptysis is functional: Massive hemoptysis is bleeding in quantities that threaten to cause death by asphyxiation from filling of the bronchial tree with blood or by exsanguination.[54,55] Patients with massive hemoptysis should always be admitted to the ICU.

Bronchoscopy plays two roles in massive hemoptysis—diagnostic and therapeutic. Most authors recommend bronchoscopy as soon as possible to localize the site of bleeding.[54-56] Rigid bronchoscopy and flexible bronchoscopy each have their advocates. The argument for rigid bronchoscopy is that it allows better visualization of the major airways, more aggressive suctioning, removal of clots, and local tamponade with packing materials.[56,57] The argument for flexible bronchoscopy is that it does not require the operating room or general anesthesia, it allows more thorough evaluation of the bronchial tree, and it allows directed intubation.[54,56] Intubation may be with a regular endotracheal tube in the trachea or in the left lung or with a double-lumen tube. (The right upper lobe takeoff is too proximal in the right bronchial tree to allow selective right main bronchus intubation.) If bleeding is too great, flexible bronchoscopy is of limited value; small amounts of blood can obscure the relatively small lens of a bronchoscope.[54] For massive hemoptysis, the goals of bronchoscopy are to identify the bleeding site and to stabilize the patient enough to allow arterial embolization, surgery, or a sequence of the two; embolization and surgery are usually the two most effective therapies. Several temporizing endobronchial therapies have been advocated: iced saline lavage, topical 1:20,000 epinephrine, endobronchial tamponade with packing or a Fogarty catheter, and endobronchial laser therapy.[54-56]

DIAGNOSIS OF INFECTION

Bronchoscopy is a valuable tool for the diagnosis of pulmonary infection in a critically ill patient. A variety of organisms, including *Mycobacterium tuberculosis, Pneumocystis jiroveci* (formerly *P. carinii*), fungi, viruses, and bacteria, are capable of causing severe pneumonia in critically ill patients. Given the broad differential diagnosis, it is important to try to determine the specific cause. Bronchoscopy offers access to lower airway secretions, which can lead to accurate diagnosis, focused therapy, and sometimes the withdrawing of unnecessary therapy. BAL is the most useful diagnostic modality. BAL can be performed in a patient who cannot or will not produce expectorated sputum or who is intubated. BAL samples alveoli more reliably than induced sputum. BAL fluid also is helpful for a broader range of diagnoses than induced sputum. In some cases, BAL recovery of organisms is not adequate alone, and biopsy is needed to confirm tissue invasion.

For BAL, the bronchoscope is wedged into a peripheral airway, and aliquots of sterile saline totaling at least 120 mL are instilled to ensure that alveolar spaces are reached. Box 12.1 summarizes the recommended method for BAL. Fluid retrieved via suctioning is sent for diagnostic studies. The BAL technique samples about 1 million alveoli, or 1% of the lung.[58] For some infections, the presence of an organism in the lung is pathognomonic for active infection, whereas for others quantitative cultures are needed to distinguish lower respiratory tract infection from upper airway contamination.

M. tuberculosis is a cause of pneumonia that should not be forgotten in critical care medicine. BAL is a sensitive tool for the diagnosis of *M. tuberculosis*, one of the organisms whose presence always means active infection.[59,60] BAL is more sensitive than gastric washings for the diagnosis of tuberculosis.[61] BAL or protected specimen brushings are often positive in patients who have pulmonary tuberculosis but negative sputum smears,[59,62,63] and BAL is also more sensitive than transbronchial biopsies for diagnosis of tuberculous pneumonia.[64] (For miliary tuberculosis, biopsy is of great value.[65]) The addition of molecular techniques such as polymerase chain reaction (PCR) can further increase the sensitivity of BAL for *M. tuberculosis*.[66]

P. jiroveci is a pathogen in immunocompromised individuals. Its incidence increased dramatically in the 1980s with the emergence of the acquired immunodeficiency syndrome (AIDS). In the 1960s and 1970s, only about 100 cases were diagnosed per year in the United States.[67] In the 1980s, thousands of cases were diagnosed.[67] Because the organism cannot be cultured, its detection depends on identification in respiratory secretions. BAL greatly increases the yield for *Pneumocystis* pneumonia over bronchial washings and brushings and is the diagnostic procedure of choice.[64,68,69] As with *M. tuberculosis, P. jiroveci* is an organism that can sometimes be difficult to see on smears, especially in patients with *Pneumocystis* pneumonia who do not have AIDS or who have AIDS but have received inhaled pentamidine.[70,71] PCR can increase the sensitivity of fluid examination with the caveat that some patients can have *Pneumocystis* colonization without infection, and the PCR method is sensitive enough to detect those cases.[72,73] In patients without AIDS or patients with AIDS receiving inhaled pentamidine, transbronchial biopsy increases the diagnostic yield.[70,74]

The diagnosis of fungal pulmonary infection is more problematic; some fungi can colonize the bronchial tree without being a cause of active infection. Fungal infection is a major issue in the immunocompromised host, but can occur in immunocompetent individuals and can be community-acquired.[75] *Candida* species often colonize the respiratory tract in critically ill patients; their isolation from BAL fluid alone is not diagnostic of tissue invasion.[75,76] *Aspergillus* runs the gamut of possibilities; it can colonize the upper airways without infection, and it can be difficult to detect sometimes when it is the cause of deep tissue infection. In the appropriate clinical and radiologic setting, a positive BAL for *Aspergillus* would be a reasonable criterion for starting therapy, but a negative BAL for *Aspergillus* is inadequate to rule out infection.[77] PCR would seem promising to increase sensitivity for *Aspergillus*, but published results have been variable, and it is not a standard tool.[78-80] Because of the possibility of colonization with *Aspergillus* and *Candida* species, lung biopsy showing tissue invasion is needed to confirm active infection by these fungi.[76,80] In contrast, *Cryptococcus neoformans*, although ubiquitous, does not routinely colonize the respiratory tract; its detection in samples of lung fluid is strong presumptive evidence for an active role in pulmonary infection.[81,82]

The endemic fungi, *Histoplasma capsulatum, Blastomyces dermatitidis*, and *Coccidioides immitis*, are capable of causing fulminant infection and cannot be ignored as diagnostic possibilities for pneumonia in patients who live in or travel through endemic areas.[81-86] Diagnosis is sometimes difficult, although the organism may be more plentiful and easier to identify in pulmonary secretions of patients who have

Box 12.1 Bronchoalveolar Lavage

- Wedge the bronchoscope into a peripheral area of whatever segment is most suspect radiologically. If there is no such segment, wedge into an upper lobe segment if *Pneumocystis* pneumonia is suspected or into a posterior lower lobe segment otherwise.
- Instill 30- to 60-mL aliquots of sterile nonbacteriostatic saline through the wedged bronchoscope until some fluid can be retrieved using suction. Discard approximately the first 20 mL of fluid.
- Attach a sterile specimen cup in line with the suction tubing, and instill further aliquots until at least 120 mL have been instilled and at least several milliliters of fluid have been obtained.
- Bilateral lavage has a higher yield than unilateral lavage.
- Have the fluid divided into two aliquots. One is plated using quantitative techniques; the second is centrifuged, stained, and examined for intracellular organisms and other diagnostic findings.
- Time from obtaining bronchoalveolar lavage fluid to plating of quantitative specimen should be <4 hours.

Data from references for this chapter (complete list available online).[58,99,148-150] fulminant disease. BAL fluid has a much higher yield than sputum.[87] If organisms are not seen on smear, fungal cultures can take weeks, an unacceptable interval for seriously ill patients. For *H. capsulatum*, an antigen can be detected in bodily fluids (including BAL) and is of clinical value.[86] The other two endemic fungi are more problematic when not demonstrable on staining of fluids or biopsy material, but promising techniques with antigen detection, DNA probes, and PCR are evolving and should become clinically available soon.[83,85,88,89]

Similar to fungi, viral pneumonias occur more frequently in immunocompromised hosts, but viruses play a role in community-acquired pneumonias as well.[90-92] In a multinational study, viruses alone were identified in 9% of community-acquired pneumonias, and viruses as copathogens were identified in an additional 9% of community-acquired pneumonias.[92] Viral pneumonia is relevant to the critical care setting; in the multinational study, 8% of patients with pure viral pneumonia were admitted to the ICU owing to severity of disease.[92] In another study using the most sensitive available virus detection technique, reverse transcriptase PCR, viruses were present as pathogens or co-pathogens in 23% of patients hospitalized for community-acquired pneumonia.[90] Analogous to the atypical pneumonias, no clinical characteristics reliably differentiate viral from bacterial pneumonia.[90,92,93]

The virology of viral pneumonia is different for pneumonia in immunocompetent and immunocompromised hosts. In immunocompetent individuals, the most common viruses are influenza A and B, parainfluenza, respiratory syncytial virus, and adenovirus.[93] In immunocompromised patients, the herpesviruses—herpes simplex, varicella zoster, and cytomegalovirus—are most common, with adenovirus, respiratory syncytial virus, and measles also occurring.[93,94] BAL is useful in the diagnosis of viral pneumonia; BAL fluid is an ideal substrate for most studies done to detect viral infection.[95,96] For all but herpes simplex virus and cytomegalovirus, the presence of the virus is diagnostic of infection.[95,97] Cytomegalovirus and herpes simplex virus can be present in BAL fluid in the absence of pneumonia; proof of tissue invasion is more specific for active infection.[95,97] Viral pneumonias are often difficult to diagnose, and cultures can take days to weeks. Newer diagnostic techniques such as reverse transcriptase PCR offer a more sensitive diagnostic tool.[98]

BAL is of major utility in the diagnosis of bacterial pneumonias. It has long been recognized that patients in the ICU often have colonization of the upper airways by several potentially pathogenic organisms, and that culture of upper airway secretions cannot be used to diagnose infections of the lower airways and lung parenchyma. Quantitative culture of BAL specimens has been proved to best obviate the issue of upper airway colonization, and BAL has thus emerged as the best currently available diagnostic test for bacterial pneumonia.[58,99] An alternative to BAL is the protected specimen brush (PSB). BAL allows the sampling of a much larger area of lung than does the PSB and logically would be a better diagnostic modality. Although the two modalities are equally accurate in some studies, for several reasons BAL has become the diagnostic procedure of choice for bacterial pneumonia (Box 12.2).[58,99] A third technique, the blind passage of a protected brush into the airways without bronchoscopic guidance, has been described.[100] This technique has a relatively lower sensitivity than BAL, which probably depends on which lobe is most involved with infection. For example the catheter cannot be passed into the upper lobes.[58,100] For this reason and the reasons cited in Box 12.2, BAL has evolved as the procedure of choice.[99]

Box 12.2 Reasons to Use Bronchoalveolar Lavage (BAL) Over Protected Specimen Brush for the Diagnosis of Lung Infiltrates

- BAL has a higher sensitivity.
- BAL is less expensive.
- BAL has a lower complication rate (pneumothorax or bleeding with protected specimen brush).
- BAL allows Gram stain of concentrated smear to look for extracellular organisms.
- BAL offers the opportunity to evaluate cells for intracellular organisms, additional proof of active infection.
- BAL is a tool for the diagnosis of infections other than bacterial infections.
- BAL yields specimens that can be used for probe techniques such as polymerase chain reaction.
- BAL is a tool for the diagnosis of other infiltrative processes (e.g., alveolar bleeding) that can mimic infection radiologically.

Data from references for this chapter (complete list available online).[58,99,101]

Two quantitative methods for bacterial growth of samples obtained by BAL have been described. The first is a simple log count; any bacteria present in greater than or equal to 10^4 colonies by quantitative methods is a pathogen unless proved otherwise.[58] (If PSB is used, a smaller area of lung is sampled and a concentration of $>10^3$ colonies is considered diagnostic of infection.[58]) The second, called the bacterial index, was described by Johanson and colleagues.[101] This method recognizes the fact that in careful studies numerous patients with pneumonia have more than one infecting organism.[23,92,101,102] For the bacterial index, the log numbers of each cultured organism are summed (10^4 *Staphylococcus aureus* + 10^3 *Pseudomonas aeruginosa* = bacterial index of 7). With this system, a bacterial index greater than 6 is a sign of moderate to severe pneumonia.[101] Although the bacterial index system seems more rational, single-organism quantification has become the de facto standard in current clinical practice.

Reinforcing the value of BAL for clinical management of bacterial infection is a study by Rodriguez and Fishman.[74] The authors performed quantitative cultures on BAL fluid and PSB from 32 ventilated patients not suspected to have pneumonia. There were six "false-positives," with quantitative cultures in the pneumonia range. Four of the six patients subsequently developed clinical pneumonia.

If a patient with suspected bacterial pneumonia has already been given antibiotics, the quantitative culture of distal airway secretions loses sensitivity.[103,104] A decrease in recovered organisms becomes significant within 12 hours of initiation of antimicrobial therapy and reaches 50%

between 24 and 48 hours.[105] This is not surprising because even quantitative cultures of lung tissue have a dramatic loss of sensitivity and specificity for patients who have received prior antibiotic therapy.[106] Despite this loss in sensitivity, BAL may make sense in the evaluation of critically ill patients with lung infiltrates who are receiving antibiotics as long as these limitations are recognized. BAL can detect organisms not being covered by the current antibiotic regimen, and BAL could help to define nonbacterial infectious agents or other noninfectious processes responsible for the clinical presentation.

When discussing the diagnostic utility of bronchoscopy for the diagnosis of severe lung infection, it is important to mention diagnoses that may be missed by the techniques discussed previously. The "atypical pneumonias"—principally *Legionella pneumophila*, *Mycoplasma pneumoniae*, and *Chlamydia pneumoniae* and *C. psittaci*—can be community-acquired. The myth that "atypical" and "typical" pneumonias can be distinguished clinically has been refuted. *Legionella* is particularly capable of causing severe disease, and the other organisms can be present as coinfectants in severe disease.[107-109] *Legionella* is not typically visible on Gram stain, does not grow on standard bacterial culture, and requires about 1 week to grow on special media when it is present. BAL material in a patient being evaluated for severe community-acquired pneumonia should be sent for direct fluorescent antibody staining for *Legionella* and for culture.[110] The direct fluorescent antibody staining is reasonably sensitive and very specific for *Legionella*,[107] and direct fluorescent antibody staining of pulmonary secretions and of urine are the most rapid diagnostic tools available. The direct fluorescent antibody of pulmonary secretions remains positive for at least 48 hours after institution of appropriate therapy.[110]

There is an importance to negative BAL for quantitative bacterial culture. A prospective study comparing management based upon quantitative cultures from invasive diagnostic techniques (BAL or PSB) with management based upon clinical data without quantitative cultures showed that the patients whose therapy was started or withheld based on quantitative bacterial studies had less antibiotic use, lower mortality rate, and less sepsis-related organ failure.[111] The importance of negative bacterial studies lies not only in the capacity to withhold or discontinue treatment for bacterial pneumonia, but also in the implication that other types of pulmonary infection or injury should be sought and that, in some cases, extrapulmonary sources of bacterial infection may be present.[58,111] The implications of BAL for a critically ill patient thus extend beyond the lungs.

In summary, bronchoscopic techniques for the diagnosis of pulmonary infection are valuable tools in intensive care medicine. BAL is the most valuable single tool, with diagnostic implications dependent on the organism being evaluated. It is important to remember that a wide spectrum of organisms can cause pneumonia in critically ill patients; the intensivist needs to consider tuberculosis, *Pneumocystis*, viruses, fungi, and atypical organisms in addition to typical bacteria.[112] When BAL fluid has been obtained, the diagnostic techniques of greatest value vary with the infecting organism. For some infecting organisms, detection of a causative organism can be difficult even in the presence of severe infection, and sensitive assays such as PCR can help in the rapid detection of the causative agent. In other cases, such as bacterial infection, organisms abound and it can be difficult to separate colonization from infection; in these cases, quantitative cultures are of greatest value. For other organisms, tissue samples are needed for definitive diagnosis. Table 12.1 summarizes diagnostic methods relevant to different lung infections. BAL fluid is the optimal substrate for almost every listed study with the exception of titers and biopsy material.

LUNG BIOPSY—SURGICAL AND TRANSBRONCHIAL

The decision of whether or when to perform an open lung biopsy is difficult and a matter of debate. Open lung biopsy is the gold standard for the diagnosis of severe cryptogenic lung disease.[113,114] When performed, it has a high diagnostic accuracy, although it is not 100% accurate; in one study with 25 patients who had biopsies and subsequent autopsies, the autopsy confirmed the open lung biopsy diagnosis in 76% of cases.[115] Open lung biopsy is useful not only in the diagnosis of infection (particularly infections for which tissue invasion is essential to prove clinical relevance), but also in the diagnosis of primary lung involvement by diseases such as malignancy, nonspecific inflammatory lung disease, and lung-related toxicities of therapeutic interventions. Box 12.3 demonstrates the breadth of possible diagnoses that can be made with open lung biopsy after other diagnostic studies are negative.

Box 12.3 Diagnoses with Open Lung Biopsy After Other Studies Are Negative

- Infection
  - Fungal infection
  - Mycobacterial infection
  - Pyogenic bacteria
  - Cytomegalovirus pneumonia
- Malignancy
  - Leukemia
  - Lymphoma
  - Angiosarcoma
  - Adenocarcinoma
  - Histiocytosis
  - Choriocarcinoma
- Cryptogenic organizing pneumonia
- Vasculitis
- Drug toxicity
- Interstitial fibrosis
- Diffuse alveolar damage
- Pulmonary embolism
- Wegener's granulomatosis
- Pulmonary alveolar proteinosis
- Idiopathic pulmonary fibrosis
- Interstitial pneumonitis
- Sarcoidosis
- Diffuse panbronchiolitis

Data from references for this chapter (complete list available online).[113,116-118]

Table 12.1 Diagnostic Techniques for Important Potentially Severe Pulmonary Infections

Important Organism	Presence in BAL Diagnostic?	Culture	Serology	Detection with Antibodies	Gene Amplification	Cytology/ Pathology/Other
M. tuberculosis	Yes	Usually positive—slow			PCR	Necrotizing granulomas
Legionella	Yes	Special media—slow	≥1:256 or 4-fold increase	IF of sputum or BAL	PCR±	DFA of urine or pleural fluid
"Typical" bacteria	No	BAL >10^4 PSB >10^3 BI >6				DFA—urinary pneumococcal antigen
Influenza virus (A, B, and C)	Yes	Positive—slow	4-fold increase	IF, ELISA (A and B)	PCR	Hemadsorption testing
Herpes simplex virus	No	Cell culture—cytopathic effects		IF, ELISA		Nuclear inclusions (Cowdry A bodies)
Cytomegalovirus	No	Cell culture—cytopathic effects		ELISA		Nuclear inclusions ("owl's eye")
Varicella-zoster virus	Yes	Cell culture—cytopathic effects				Nuclear inclusions (Cowdry A bodies) Typical rash helpful Tzanck preparation
Respiratory syncytial virus (rare)	Yes	Cell culture—cytopathic effects		IF	PCR	Eosinophilic cytoplasmic inclusions
Parainfluenza viruses (1-4)	Yes	Cell culture—cytopathic effects		IF	PCR	Hemadsorption testing Small eosinophilic cytoplasmic inclusions
Adenovirus	Yes	Cell culture—cytopathic effects		IF	PCR	Variable inclusion pattern
Cryptococcus	Yes	Slow				Antigen-serum Tissue invasion
Aspergillus	No					Tissue invasion
Candida	No					Tissue invasion
Coccidioides	Yes		High or increasing			
Histoplasma	Yes		≥1:64 or 4-fold increase	ELISA (cross-reacts with *Blastomyces*)		Can be hard to find even with culture Antigen-urine or serum Tissue invasion
Blastomyces	Yes			ELISA (cross-reacts with *Histoplasma*)		

BAL, bronchoalveolar lavage [fluid]; BI, bacterial index; DFA, direct fluorescent antibody; ELISA, enzyme-linked immunosorbent assay; IF, immunofluorescence testing (direct or indirect); PCR, polymerase chain reaction; PSB, protected specimen brush.

Data from references 84, 89, 90, 93, 96, 110, 112 for this chapter (complete list available online).

Open lung biopsy leads to a change in therapy in 57% to 75% of cases in which it is performed.[113,114,116-118] Open lung biopsy can be performed in patients with respiratory distress and patients on ventilators with a reasonable rate of perioperative complications; death attributed to the biopsy procedure itself is rare, and complications such as persistent air leak usually resolve over time.[114,116,117] Complication rates have been reported to be the same with video-assisted thoracic surgery as with thoracotomy.[118] Several recent studies have reported the frequent use of bedside open lung biopsy, which avoids transport of a critically ill patient and appears to have a morbidity rate similar to that of doing the biopsy in the operating room.[118-122]

Although open lung biopsy sounds promising, it has several drawbacks. First, authors who separated open lung biopsy results into "specific" (allowing focused therapy thought or known to have some efficacy) and "nonspecific" (a pattern of injury such as diffuse lung damage with no clear cause and no documented effective therapy) found that 38% to 46% of patients had nonspecific injury and no specific therapeutic benefit from the procedure.[114,118] Second, mortality rate is extremely high in this group despite specific diagnoses and the previously mentioned changes in therapy, particularly if the patients have respiratory compromise; for those patients, the short-term mortality rate ranges from 52% to 70%.[116-118] (Note that short-term mortality rate is believed by most authors to be related far more to the underlying disease than to the open lung biopsy procedure.[116-118]) Third, most patients already have received appropriate therapy; in most cases, the change in therapy would be discontinuation of unnecessary drugs or increased dosing of a drug already being given (usually steroids). In some, the benefit of open lung biopsy would be acknowledgment of end-stage disease and withdrawal of all therapy. The most important outcome of open lung biopsy would be a change in therapy that altered outcome from death to survival. Institution of a new potentially lifesaving therapeutic intervention as a result of open lung biopsy is uncommon.[114,116,117] In 1988, Warner and colleagues[117] discussed open lung biopsy in patients with respiratory compromise and said, "any complications of a procedure of unknown benefit is of concern." Some authors hold this opinion to this day. Most patients have received anti-infective drugs or steroids or both before open lung biopsy is considered, and one could argue that most patients who could respond would have responded before open lung biopsy. Nevertheless, that the controversy is "alive and well" is illustrated by a quote from Chuang and associates:[113] "It is not ethical to avoid open lung biopsy in patients with unclear diagnoses, as open lung biopsy is known to be the most sensitive and specific test available at this time."

Another controversy with respect to open lung biopsy concerns when to perform it. Two groups have reported open lung biopsy relatively early in the course of respiratory failure with diffuse infiltrates and have withheld therapies until and unless biopsy results demonstrated a specific indication.[121,122] Not unexpectedly, this approach led to a high number of new therapies, usually steroids or antiviral agents. Papazian and coworkers argued that their approach improved survival.[122] The data provide valuable support for a counterargument—that all patients with idiopathic diffuse lung disease should be treated with both steroids and antiviral agents. If this had been done in these two series, the added benefit of open lung biopsy would have been very small.

Given the controversies and the available data, a few principles would seem appropriate in considering whether or not open lung biopsy should be performed. First, in most cases, BAL (and perhaps transbronchial biopsy; see later) should be performed before open lung biopsy is considered. Second, patients who have three or more organs failing (lung plus two more) probably should not undergo biopsy; the prognosis is too poor.[114] Third, decisions about open lung biopsy should be based more upon the prior condition of the patient and the potential utility of the study than upon the degree of ventilatory distress or compromise of the patient; post-operative death related to the biopsy itself is rare. Open lung biopsy in a critically ill patient with undiagnosed pulmonary infiltrates remains a valuable tool that is uncommonly indicated but that will occasionally provide a diagnosis that results in lifesaving therapy.

Bronchoscopic transbronchial lung biopsy may fill the gap between "nontissue" procedures such as BAL and open lung biopsy with its large amount of tissue for pathologic examination and culture. Open lung biopsy by definition requires anesthesia and by definition causes a breach in pleural integrity and requires chest tube placement, with many patients having air leaks after the procedure.[116-118] Transbronchial lung biopsy requires only conscious sedation and would require chest tube placement only if a complication occurred, not as a matter of routine. As noted earlier in the discussion of infection, some diagnoses, such as invasive aspergillosis, *Candida* pneumonia, and cytomegalovirus pneumonia require tissue samples showing tissue invasion. Tissue samples can increase the diagnostic yield for other organisms such as *M. tuberculosis* and *P. jiroveci.*[123] Diagnoses such as cryptogenic organizing pneumonia and several others listed in Box 12.3 cannot be made without tissue. Transbronchial lung biopsy is reasonable with BAL or after a negative BAL in compromised patients with infiltrates of unknown cause.[123-125] It was formerly thought that to perform transbronchial lung biopsy in a patient on a ventilator carried too high a risk of complications to be warranted.[126] The available data challenge this concept. Two early studies[127,128] and several more recent studies[69,125,129,130] have evaluated the yield and complications of transbronchial lung biopsy in ventilated patients. All of these studies showed high yields similar to the yields for open lung biopsy. The pneumothorax rates varied from 0% to 24%. Bleeding was considered to be significant in 6% to 20%, with all cases self-limited. No fatalities occurred. When transbronchial lung biopsy in ventilated patients is compared with open lung biopsy, for which general anesthesia, incisions, violation of the visceral pleura, and a chest tube are requisites, it is apparent that transbronchial lung biopsy is underused in this population; it has a favorable risk-to-benefit ratio.

SPECIAL SITUATIONS

IMMUNOCOMPROMISED HOST

Immunocompromise is a recognized risk factor for respiratory infection. Years of elegant work have helped to define classic types of immunocompromise and patterns of infection that are more typical for the different types.[131-133] Long-recognized diseases causing immunocompromise include solid tumors on chemotherapy, hematologic malignancies, organ transplantation, chronic diseases for which cytotoxic or steroid therapy is given, human immunodeficiency virus (HIV) infection, and other less common acquired or congenital diseases.[126,133] Although immunocompromise definitely includes the preceding diseases, it has no clear boundaries. Patients with chronic insulin-dependent diabetes, alcoholics, patients with severe malnutrition, and patients on drugs such as infliximab, a tumor necrosis factor antagonist, almost certainly have degrees of immunocompromise that affect their susceptibility to infection.[134-138] The stresses of critical illness and organ dysfunction coupled with the broaching of natural defense systems (skin by central lines, lungs by intubation, urinary tract by catheters) put critically ill patients at increased risk for infection.

Many chronic illnesses probably also carry an increased risk for infection. Shelhamer and colleagues[133] recognized the difficulty with this issue and defined immunocompromise as "any condition, congenital or acquired, temporary or chronic, in which the response of the host to a foreign antigen is subnormal." For patients with classic known forms of immunocompromise, special diagnostic attention has to be paid to the possibility of *Pneumocystis* pneumonia, invasive fungal infection, infection with the herpesviruses, and tuberculosis. Three factors make this area gray rather than black-and-white: (1) Lack of knowledge that a patient is immunocompromised does not rule out immunocompromise, (2) degrees of immunocompromise exist, and (3) most of the pathogens discussed are capable of causing disease in "normal" hosts. For these reasons, some specific issues related to immunocompromise have been mentioned throughout this chapter, but in the clinical approach to a patient with severe respiratory disease, it makes sense to assume that any patient might be immunocompromised; the diagnostic workup should, as mentioned, cast a wide net.

THROMBOCYTOPENIA

Thrombocytopenia is an obvious risk factor for bleeding from invasive procedures. BAL has been shown to be safe and clinically useful in thrombocytopenic patients.[139] Bronchoscopic procedures and open lung biopsies have been performed safely in patients with thrombocytopenia.[118,140] Historically, procedures have been limited to BAL, or platelets have been given before bronchoscopic or surgical procedures.[118,140]

COMPLICATIONS AND DEATH

The true incidence of complications of bronchoscopy in the ICU is poorly defined. Most reviews of the topic[27,40,141-144] cite several older studies of bronchoscopy in general,[7-9,11,145] not specifically in critically ill patients. The two largest and most-cited reports are by Credle and colleagues[7] and Suratt and coworkers[11] and reviewed 24,521 (Credle) and "approximately 48,000" (Suratt) procedures. These were retrospective reports based on mailed questionnaires. Death rates were 0.01% and 0.03%.[7,11]

The next largest study was a retrospective single-institution study of 4273 bronchoscopies, which reported 0% mortality rate and a 0.5% frequency of major complications (pneumothorax, bleeding, respiratory failure requiring intubation).[9] Three prospective studies reported on 205 to 1146 flexible bronchoscopies and reported mortality rates of 0%,[9] 0.1%,[145] and 0.5%.[8] The highest reported mortality rate came out of a study from a consortium of expert bronchoscopists studying autofluorescence.[146] The study included the requisite of at least two endobronchial biopsies, and in a series of 300 cases the immediate postbronchoscopic mortality rate was 0.7%. Two retrospective studies[46,147] and one prospective study[69] reviewed bronchoscopies performed specifically on patients in the ICU. No procedure-related deaths were reported. Throughout these studies, only death rates are consistently noted; major and minor complications are variably defined.

Several principles emerge from the previously cited studies. The complication rates depend on the invasiveness of the procedure. The highest incidence of complications occurs with lung biopsy and then, in descending order, with brushings, BAL, and simple observation. For the patients expected to have the highest complication rate—patients on ventilators undergoing transbronchial biopsies—there is a pneumothorax rate of 24%, but no fatalities have been reported.[69,125,127-130] None of those studies involved large numbers of patients; it is inevitable that fatalities would occur in this subset of high-risk cases. Nevertheless, many years of experience with flexible fiberoptic bronchoscopy have led to the conclusion that its benefits outweigh its risks. No bronchoscopy should be done on a critically ill patient without a reason, but when a reason is present, bronchoscopy is often the unique or the safest method known of obtaining data that may affect care.

SUMMARY

Since its inception in 1968, flexible fiberoptic bronchoscopy has evolved into a major tool in the evaluation and management of critically ill patients. The bronchoscope allows evaluation of and sometimes management of airway problems. The bronchoscope follows the most natural pathway into the lung—the airway—and allows sampling of secretions and tissues from the alveolar level. The basic techniques have been defined for many years. What has been refined is our understanding of their utility and testing methodologies; increasing sensitivities and specificities over the years have greatly enhanced our capacities, particularly in the diagnosis of lung infections. Some lung infections require lung tissue for definitive diagnosis, as do several diagnoses that can cause diffuse lung disease and can sometimes mimic infection. Open lung biopsy is a time-honored approach with high diagnostic accuracy that may sometimes be an optimal approach. Transbronchial lung biopsy, even in a ventilated patient, has a clinical impact similar to that of open lung biopsy and is probably underused in critically ill patients with diffuse infiltrates who are failing empiric therapies. It is clear that the more ill the patient, the higher the risk of any invasive procedure, but the literature points the risk-to-benefit ratio of bronchoscopy in favor of performing bronchoscopy for the indications outlined in this chapter.

KEY POINTS

- Bronchoscopy has become a major tool in the evaluation of the airways and lung parenchyma of critically ill patients.
- Bronchoscopy stimulates a series of reflexes affecting blood pressure, heart rate, and intracerebral pressure, but this is true for any cannulation of the upper airway (e.g., suctioning), and bronchoscopy for the evaluation

KEY POINTS (Continued)

of lung problems in critically ill patients has a favorable risk-to-benefit ratio.

- Inserting a bronchoscope through an endotracheal tube causes upper airway obstruction and can cause hypoventilation or hyperinflation or both; the physiologic changes caused by the bronchoscope need to be understood and possibly compensated for.
- Bronchoscopy is a valuable tool for the diagnosis and management (especially intubation and percutaneous tracheostomy) of upper airway problems.
- Bronchoscopy with BAL is the most effective and accurate clinical tool currently available for the diagnosis of pulmonary infection in critically ill patients.
- The potential of bronchoscopy for the diagnosis of infection is being advanced at present not by bronchoscopic techniques but by the development and clinical application of extremely sensitive tools such as PCR assays.
- Critically ill patients with undiagnosed infiltrates occasionally benefit from lung biopsy; the results often affect management, but rarely affect outcome. Available data suggest that bronchoscopic transbronchial lung biopsy has yields similar to those for open lung biopsy with a more favorable risk-to-benefit ratio.

SELECTED REFERENCES

1. Lundgren R, Haggmark S, Reiz S: Hemodynamic effects of flexible fiberoptic bronchoscopy performed under topical anesthesia. Chest 1982;82:295-299.

15. Lindholm CE, Ollman B, Snyder JV, et al: Cardiorespiratory effects of flexible fiberoptic bronchoscopy in critically ill patients. Chest 1978;74:362-368.

30. Yarmus L, Pandian V, Gilbert C, et al: Safety and efficiency of interventional pulmonologists performing percutanoeus tracheostomy. Respiration 2012;84(2):123-127. Epub 2012 June 13.

47. Marini JJ, Pierson DJ, Hudson LD: Acute lobar atelectasis: A prospective comparison of fiberoptic bronchoscopy and respiratory therapy. Am Rev Respir Dis 1979;119:971-978.

49. Hara KS, Prakash UB: Fiberoptic bronchoscopy in the evaluation of acute chest and upper airway trauma. Chest 1989;96:627-630.

58. Chastre J, Combes A, Luyt CE: The invasive (quantitative) diagnosis of ventilator-associated pneumonia. Respir Care 2005;50:797-807; discussion 807-712.

120. Charbonney E, Robert J, Pache JC, et al: Impact of bedside open lung biopsies on the management of mechanically ventilated immunocompromised patients with acute respiratory distress syndrome of unknown etiology. J Crit Care 2009;24:122-128.

130. O'Brien JD, Ettinger NA, Shevlin D, et al: Safety and yield of transbronchial biopsy in mechanically ventilated patients. Crit Care Med 1997;25:440-446.

139. Weiss SM, Hert RC, Gianola FJ, et al: Complications of fiberoptic bronchoscopy in thrombocytopenic patients. Chest 1993;104:1025-1028.

146. Bechara R, Beamis J, Simoff M: Practice and complications of flexible bronchoscopy with biopsy procedures. J Bronchol 2005;12:139-142.

The complete list of references can be found at www.expertconsult.com.

13 Noninvasive Respiratory Monitoring

Amal Jubran | Martin J. Tobin

CHAPTER OUTLINE

Various devices are available for effective and noninvasive monitoring of the patient's gas exchange function, respiratory neuromuscular capacity, and respiratory mechanics. Such measurements are helpful in characterizing the pathophysiology of an underlying respiratory disorder, tracking the course of illness and the effects of treatment, minimizing the risk of complications, and determining the patient's readiness for the withdrawal of therapeutic interventions and support devices.

Advances in respiratory monitoring continue to occur in terms of technological improvements and in enhancing current understanding of the pathophysiology of respiratory failure.[1] It is estimated that 20% to 40% of patients in intensive care units (ICUs) are admitted solely for the purposes of monitoring and do not receive any treatment that is unique to the ICU.[2]

GAS EXCHANGE

The human eye is poor at recognizing hypoxemia.[3,4] With the availability of pulse oximetry, episodic hypoxemia has been found to be more common than was previously suspected, with an incidence ranging from 20% to 82%.[5] Patients experiencing hypoxemia have a threefold higher risk of death compared with patients who do not display desaturations.[6] Whether earlier detection and treatment of episodic hypoxemia can affect patient outcome is not known.

PULSE OXIMETRY

Pulse oximeters determine oxygen (O_2) saturation by measuring light absorption of arterial blood at two specific wavelengths, 660 nm (red) and 940 nm (infrared).[7,8] The ratio of absorbencies at these two wavelengths is calibrated empirically against direct measurements of arterial blood oxygen saturation ($Sa{O_2}$), and the resulting calibration algorithm is used to generate the pulse oximeter's estimate of arterial saturation ($Sp{O_2}$).[9] In addition to the digital readout of O_2 saturation, most pulse oximeters display a plethysmographic waveform, which can help clinicians distinguish an artifactual signal from the true signal (Fig. 13.1).

ACCURACY

The accuracy of commercially available oximeters in critically ill patients has been validated in several studies.[10] Compared with the measurement standard (multiwavelength oximeter), pulse oximeters have a mean difference (bias) of less than 1% and a standard deviation (precision) of less than 2% when $Sa{O_2}$ is 90% or above.[8] Although pulse oximetry is accurate in reflecting one-point measurements of $Sa{O_2}$, it does not reliably predict changes in $Sa{O_2}$. In 1085 simultaneous measurements of $Sa{O_2}$ and $Sp{O_2}$ in 41 ICU patients, changes in $Sa{O_2}$ correlated moderately with changes in $Sp{O_2}$ ($r = 0.6$), and the pulse oximeter tended to overestimate actual changes in $Sa{O_2}$.[11]

The accuracy of pulse oximeters deteriorates when $Sa{O_2}$ falls to 80% or less.[12] In critically ill patients, poor

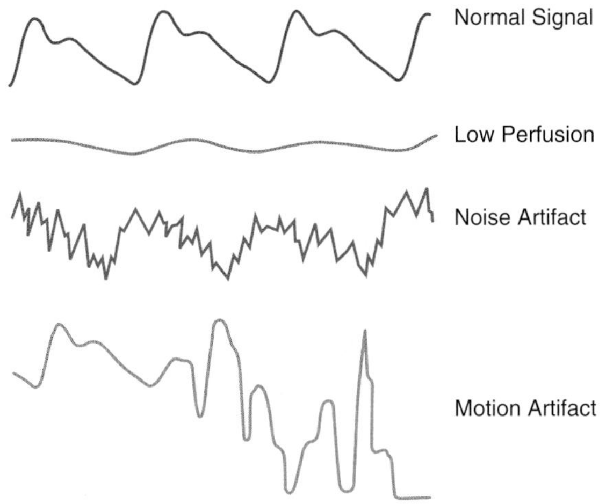

Figure 13.1 Common pulsatile signals on a pulse oximeter. *Top tracing,* Normal signal showing the sharp waveform with a clear dicrotic notch. *Second tracing,* Pulsatile signal during low perfusion showing a typical sine wave. *Third tracing,* Pulsatile signal with superimposed noise artifact giving a jagged appearance. *Bottom tracing,* Pulsatile signal during motion artifact showing an erratic waveform. (From Jubran A: Pulse oximetry. In Tobin MJ (ed): Principles and Practice of Intensive Care Monitoring. New York, McGraw-Hill, 1998, pp 261-287.)

Box 13.1 Limitations of Pulse Oximetry

- Physiologic limitations
  - Shape of oxyhemoglobin dissociation curve
- Interference from substances
  - Dyshemoglobins: carboxyhemoglobin, methemoglobin
  - Dyes
  - Nail polish
  - Ambient light
  - Skin pigmentation
- Limitation in signal processing
  - Low-perfusion state
  - Motion artifact
  - False alarms
- Limitation in knowledge of the technique

agreement between the oximeter and a CO-oximeter was observed, with bias ranging from −12% to 18%; and oximetry tended to systematically underestimate Sa_{O_2} when it was less than 80%.[13]

LIMITATIONS

Oximeters have a number of limitations that may lead to inaccurate readings (Box 13.1). Pulse oximeters measure Sa_{O_2}, which is physiologically related to arterial oxygen tension (Pa_{O_2}) according to the O_2 dissociation curve. Because the dissociation curve has a sigmoid shape, oximetry is relatively insensitive in detecting hypoxemia in patients with high baseline levels of Pa_{O_2}.[8,14]

Pulse oximeters use only two wavelengths of light; accordingly, they can discriminiate only two substances, oxyhemoglobin and reduced hemoglobin. Elevated carboxyhemoglobin and methemoglobin levels can therefore cause inaccurate oximetry readings.[15-18] Anemia does not appear to affect the accuracy of pulse oximetry.[19,20]

Intravenous dyes such as methylene blue, indocyanine green, and indigo carmine can cause falsely low Sp_{O_2} readings, an effect that persists for up to 20 minutes.[20] In critically ill patients requiring mechanical ventilation, nail polish—blue, white, purple, and black—has been shown not to affect the accuracy of Sp_{O_2} readings;[21] acrylic nails, however, may interfere with readings.[22] Falsely low and falsely high Sp_{O_2} readings occur with fluorescent and xenon arc surgical lamps.[23]

Skin pigmentation can affect the accuracy of pulse oximetry.[24,25] In critically ill patients,[12] bias plus precision was greater in black patients, 3.3 + 2.7%, than in white patients, 2.2 + 1.8%; also, a bias greater than 4% occurred more frequently in black patients (27%) than in white patients (11%).

Low-perfusion states, such as low cardiac output, vasoconstriction, and hypothermia, may impair peripheral perfusion, making it difficult for a sensor to distinguish a true signal from background noise. In patients experiencing hypothermia and poor perfusion during cardiac surgery, only 2 of 20 oximeters (Criticare CSI 503, Datex Satlite, Helsinki, Finland) provided measurements within +4% of the CO-oximeter value.[26] Measurements of Sp_{O_2} with a Biox 3700 oximeter had an associated bias greater than ±4% in 37% of patients receiving vasoactive therapy.[27]

Motion artifact is a frustrating problem, and it results in inaccurate readings and false alarms. Patient motion is a common reason for temporary or definitive abandonment of pulse oximetry in a particular patient. An innovative technological approach, termed *Masimo Signal Extraction Technology* (SET), was introduced to extract the true signal from artifact secondary to noise and low perfusion[28] (Fig. 13.2).

In 18 healthy volunteers, investigators compared the latest generation of pulse oximeters—Masimo SET (Irvine, CA), Nellcor OxismartXL (Pleasanton, CA), Philips Medical Systems FAST-Sp_{O_2} (Andover, MA), Respironics Novametrix MARSp_{O_2} (Wallingford, CT), and Siemens Oxisure (Danvers, MA)—with an older model, Nellcor N-200, under conditions of low perfusion and motion.[10] Of the five new-generation oximeters, Masimo SET and Nellcor OxismartXL outperformed the other three devices in reducing nuisance alarms and ensuring alarm reliability. These two oximeters also were found to have better protection against light interference than the other three devices.

Despite their popularity for continuous monitoring of O_2 saturation, pulse oximeters fail to provide valid data in a variety of settings.[29-31] In a prospective study in ICU patients, Sp_{O_2} signals accounted for almost half of a total of 2525 false alarms.[32] In 235 surgical ICU patients, a study revealed that false alarms from the pulse oximeter were secondary to low perfusion (21%), cardiac arrhythmias (9%), motion artifacts (8.4%), shivering (1.7%), and extubation (1.7%).[33]

An underrecognized and worrisome problem with pulse oximetry is that many users have a limited understanding of how the oximeter functions and the implications of the measurements obtained. One survey revealed that 30% of physicians and 93% of nurses thought that the oximeter measured Pa_{O_2}. Some clinicians did not recognize that Sp_{O_2} values in the high 80s represent seriously low values of Pa_{O_2}. Of special concern was the observation that some doctors and nurses were not especially worried about patients with

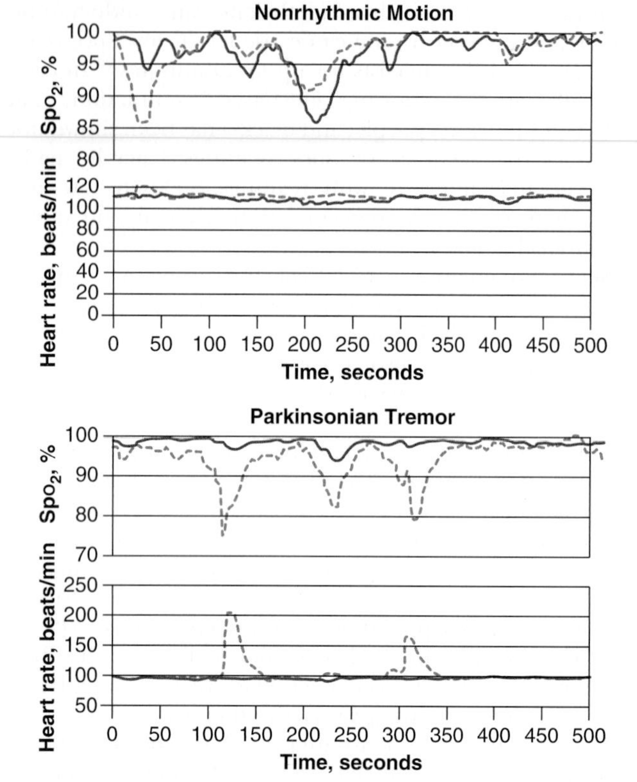

Figure 13.2 Pulse oximetry signals with motion artifact: *top panel,* recorded during nonrhythmic motion (i.e., gross arm motion); *lower panel,* recorded during parkinsonian tremor. *Red line* denotes Masimo Signal Extraction Technology (SET), aimed at minimizing spurious pulse oximetry readings due to motion artifact; *blue line* denotes conventional pulse oximetry. Spurious changes in measured oxygen saturation (Spo_2) less with Masimo SET than with conventional pulse oximetry. (From Dumas C, Wahr JA, Tremper KK: Clinical evaluation of a prototype motion artifact resistant pulse oximeter in the recovery room. Anesth Analg 1996;83:269-272.)

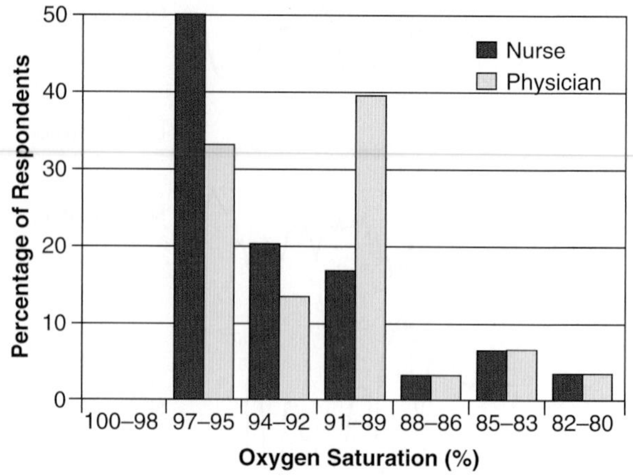

Figure 13.3 The lowest values for O_2 saturation measured by pulse oximetry (Spo_2) considered acceptable in a fit adult by a group of physicians and nurses. Spo_2 values less than 88% (equivalent to Pao_2 of less than 55 mm Hg) were considered acceptable by 27% of the respondents. The percentages represented by *bars* for each of the respondent groups add up to 100%. (Modified from Stoneham MD, Saville GM, Wilson IH: Knowledge about pulse oximetry among medical and nursing staff. Lancet 1994;344:1339-1342.)

Spo_2 values as low as 80% (equivalent to Pao_2 less than 45 mm Hg)[34] (Fig. 13.3). Another audit demonstrated that fewer than 50% of nurses and physicians were able to identify that motion artifact and arrhythmias can affect the accuracy of pulse oximetry.[35]

CLINICAL APPLICATIONS

With the introduction of pulse oximetry, hypoxemia (defined as an Spo_2 value less than 90%) is now detected more often in critically ill patients.[36] Changes in Spo_2 may not accurately reflect changes in Pao_2. Accordingly, caution is required in clinical decision making in critically ill patients based solely on pulse oximetry. Although pulse oximetry is a suitable way of measuring arterial oxygenation, it does not assess ventilation. Indeed, measurements of Spo_2 have been shown to be inaccurate in assessing abnormal pulmonary gas exchange, defined as an elevated alveolar-arterial O_2 difference.[5]

Pulse oximetry can assist with titration of fractional inspired oxygen concentration (Fio_2) in ventilator-dependent patients, although the appropriate Spo_2 target depends on a patient's pigmentation.[12] The Spo_2 target value that predicts a satisfactory level of oxygenation is 92% in white patients and 95% in black patients (Fig. 13.4).

Pulse oximetry has been evaluated as a means of screening for respiratory failure in patients with severe asthma.[37] Respiratory failure was unlikely in patients with Spo_2 greater than 92%. Of interest, this threshold value of 92% is the same target value that reliably predicted a satisfactory level of oxygenation during titration of Fio_2 in ventilator-dependent patients.[12]

The use of pulse oximetry compared with other vital signs in predicting hospital complications from pulmonary embolus has been investigated.[38] In 207 patients with documented pulmonary embolism, a room-air Spo_2 value obtained in the emergency department was the most important predictor of death: the mortality rate was 2% in patients with Spo_2 95% or greater versus 20% with Spo_2 less than 95%. When the threshold value was prospectively evaluated in 119 patients, in 10 of whom hospital complications developed, Spo_2 less than 95% had a sensitivity of 90%, specificity of 64%, and overall diagnostic accuracy of 67%. Although the number of patients with complications was low, these data suggest that pulse oximetry may be useful in predicting outcome in patients with pulmonary embolus.

Moller and associates[39] conducted the first prospective, randomized study of pulse oximetry on the outcome of anesthesia care in 20,802 surgical patients. Detection of hypoxemia (defined as an Spo_2 less than 90%) was 19-fold higher in the oximeter group than in the control group. Myocardial ischemia was more common in the control group than in the oximetry group, occurring in 26 and 12 patients, respectively. Pulse oximetry, however, did not decrease the rate of postoperative complications or mortality.

The lack of proven efficacy of pulse oximetry in the study of Moller and associates[39] was related to the sample size. These investigators concluded that it would take at least 500,000 patients to show a reduction in a rare event such as myocardial infarction and 1.9 million patients to show a reduction in anesthesia-related deaths. When

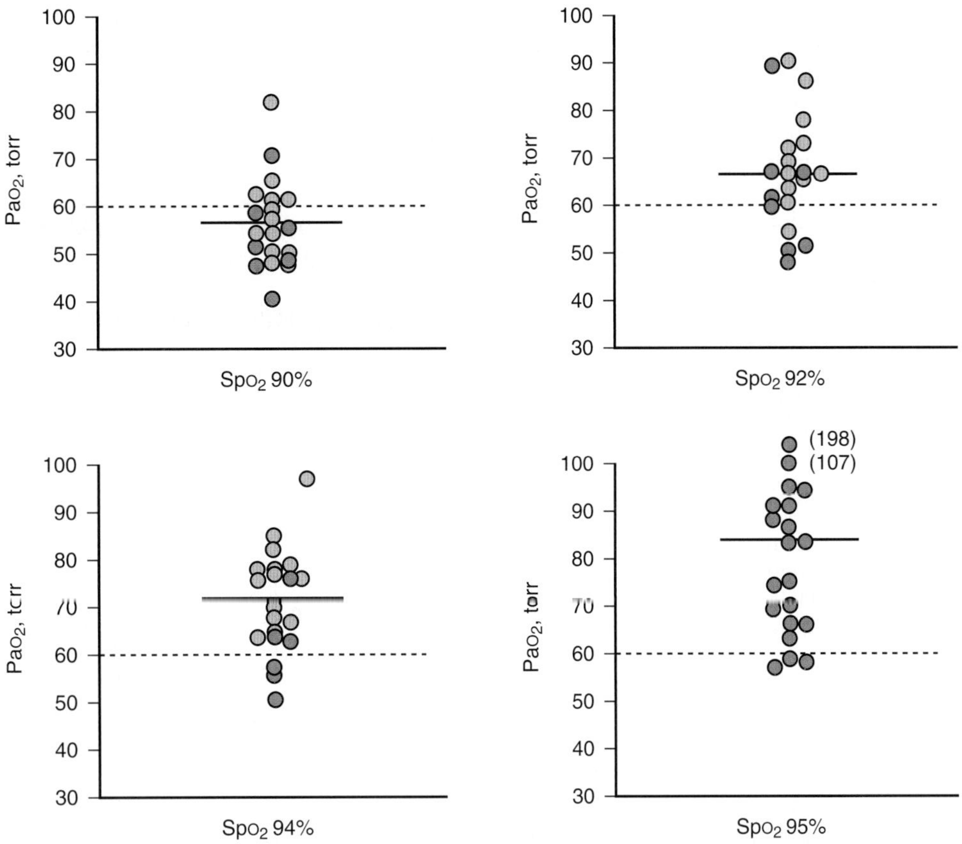

Figure 13.4 Arterial oxygen tension (Pa_{O_2}) values at pulse oximetry O_2 saturation (Sp_{O_2}) values of 90%, 92%, 94%, and 95%. The inspired O_2 concentration (F_{IO_2}) was adjusted to achieve a particular steady-state Sp_{O_2} value in a group of 54 critically ill patients. The solid horizontal line represents the mean Pa_{O_2} value obtained at each Sp_{O_2} target. The orange and blue circles represent values obtained in white and black patients, respectively. In white patients, an Sp_{O_2} target of 92% resulted in a satisfactory level of oxygenation, whereas a higher Sp_{O_2} target, 95%, was required in black patients. (Modified from Jubran A, Tobin MJ: Reliability of pulse oximetry in titrating supplemental oxygen therapy in ventilator-dependent patients. Chest 1990;97:1420-1425.)

anesthesiologists in the study were surveyed,[40] 80% of them reported feeling more secure when they used a pulse oximeter. Of 104 anesthesiologists, 19 believed that the pulse oximeter helped them avoid serious complications (such as esophageal intubation, tracheal tube disconnection or displacement, anesthesia machine failure, and respiratory problems immediately after extubation). It is this mindset that has established pulse oximetry as an essential component of the standard of care despite a failure to achieve a level of proven efficacy with a *p* value of less than 0.05. The lack of concurrence between randomized trial proof of efficacy of pulse oximetry and its requirement as part of the standard of care has major ramifications for all monitoring techniques.[1]

COST EFFECTIVENESS

Studies evaluating the cost effectiveness of pulse oximetry have reported that fewer arterial blood gas (ABG) samples were obtained if Sp_{O_2} data were available to the caregivers.[41-43] The effect of implementing pulse oximetry in an ICU without any specific plan for its appropriate use was examined in 148 patients before the implementation of oximetry and 141 patients after its implementation.[44] The number of ABG samples decreased from 7.2 to 6.4 per patient per day—a reduction of only 10.3%, compared with average reductions of 39% in the previous studies.[5] This suggests that without explicit guidelines, the pulse oximeter was used in addition to, rather than instead of, blood gas sampling.

Pulse oximetry probably constitutes one of the most important advances in respiratory monitoring. The major challenge facing pulse oximetry is whether this technology can be incorporated effectively into diagnostic and management algorithms that improve the efficiency of clinical management in the ICU.

TRANSCUTANEOUS BLOOD GAS MONITORING

Transcutaneous measurements of O_2 tension (Ptc_{O_2}) are made by placing a heated Clark polarographic electrode directly on the skin and measuring the O_2 that diffuses from the blood to the skin.[45] This technique more commonly is used by neonatologists because neonatal skin is thin, so Ptc_{O_2} values approximate Pa_{O_2} values. In a multicenter study including 251 patients of various ages (range, 4 weeks to 60 years), the Ptc_{O_2}/Pa_{O_2} ratio was 1.05 in neonates and 0.93 in older patients when Pa_{O_2} was less than 80 mm Hg. This ratio, however, decreased to 0.88 in neonates and 0.74 in older patients when the Pa_{O_2} was greater than 80 mm Hg.[46] During low-perfusion states, Ptc_{O_2} measurements do not reflect changes in Pa_{O_2}. In critically ill patients, the $Ptco_2/Pao_2$ ratio decreased from 0.79 ± 0.12[5] when the cardiac index was greater than 2.2 L/minute/m^2 to 0.12 ± 12 when the cardiac index was less than 1.5 L/minute/m^2.[47]

Transcutaneous monitoring of the partial pressure of carbon dioxide ($Ptcco_2$) can be performed using a modified Severinghaus electrode. The underlying skin is heated to 44° C to enhance CO_2 diffusion through the skin. Heating also increases the local production of CO_2, with the result that transcutaneous Pco_2 values usually are higher than arterial Pco_2 ($Paco_2$) values.[47] Because of greater diffusibility of CO_2 compared with O_2 through the skin, the correlation of $Ptcco_2$ with $Paco_2$ usually is good: $r = 0.93$.[46]

The accuracy of $Ptcco_2$ as a surrogate measure for $Paco_2$ was evaluated in 50 critically ill patients in a medical ICU.[48] Of the 189 paired measures of Pco_2 obtained, 21 were excluded from analysis because of profound skin vasoconstriction. Of the available 168 measurements, mean difference between $Paco_2$ and $Ptcco_2$ was −0.2 ± 4.6 mm Hg; correlation between two measurements was 0.92. A strong correlation was observed between changes in $Paco_2$ and $Ptcco_2$ ($r^2 = 0.78$) (Fig. 13.5). These data suggest that transcutaneous Pco_2 may be reliable in monitoring changes in $Paco_2$, provided that no major vasoconstriction is present.

CAPNOGRAPHY

The carbon dioxide concentration at the end of a tidal breath—end-tidal CO_2—can be employed as a continuous, indirect measure of $Paco_2$. In intubated patients with respiratory failure, correlation between end-tidal CO_2 and $Paco_2$ was good ($r = 0.78$).[49] The correlation between changes in end-tidal CO_2 and changes in $Paco_2$ from baseline, however, was considerably weaker ($r = 0.58$). Change in end-tidal CO_2 incorrectly indicated the direction of change in $Paco_2$ in 43% of patients being weaned from mechanical ventilation after cardiac surgery.[50]

Capnometry commonly is used in detecting esophageal intubation[51-53] (Fig. 13.6). When the trachea of a patient with an intact pulmonary circulation is intubated, end-tidal CO_2 is recorded. When, however, the endotracheal tube is erroneously placed in the esophagus, end-tidal CO_2 will be zero. Monitoring of end-tidal CO_2 has been compared with three other methods—auscultation, negative-pressure testing using a self-inflating bulb, and transillumination—for verifying tracheal tube placement.[54] Monitoring of end-tidal CO_2 was found to be the most reliable.

RESPIRATORY NEUROMUSCULAR FUNCTION

AIRWAY OCCLUSION PRESSURE

Measuring airway pressure 0.1 second after initiation of an inspiratory effort against airway occlusion ($P_{0.1}$) provides a

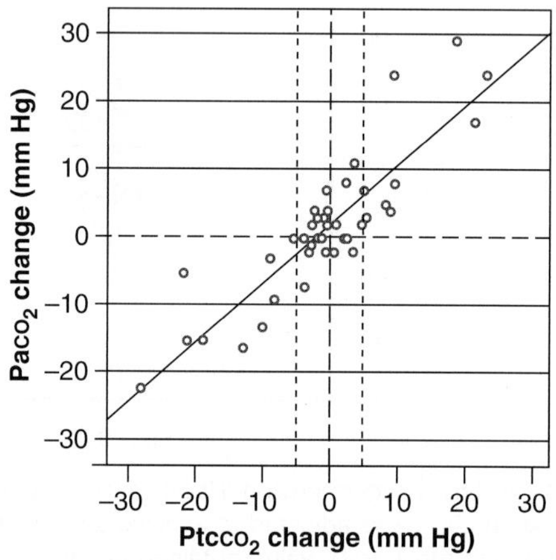

Figure 13.5 Change in transcutaneous Pco_2 ($Ptcco_2$) versus change in arterial Pco_2 ($Paco_2$) in 40 samples. The solid line represents the linear regression equation ($R^2 = 0.78$); *broken lines* represent $Ptcco_2$ values at 0, +5, and −5 mm Hg. Note that a mismatch between changes in $Ptcco_2$ and $Paco_2$ (transcutaneous changes were positive although arterial changes were negative, or vice versa) occurred in 8 of the 40 values (22%). (Modified from Rodriguez P, Lellouche F, Aboab J, et al: Transcutaneous arterial carbon dioxide pressure monitoring in critically ill adult patients. Intensive Care Med 2006;32: 309-312.)

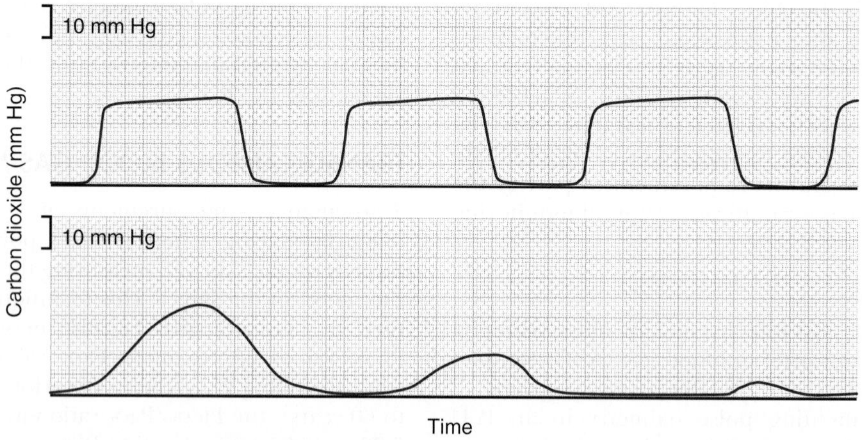

Figure 13.6 End-tidal CO_2 tracing and esophageal intubation. *Upper panel*: End-tidal CO_2 tracing in a patient in whom an endotracheal tube was inserted correctly in the trachea. During inhalation, end-tidal CO_2 is 0 mm Hg. During exhalation, the CO_2 tracing rises steeply, attains a near plateau, and then quickly returns to the baseline. *Lower panel*: End-tidal CO_2 tracing in a patient in whom an endotracheal tube was erroneously inserted in the esophagus. The expected shape of the CO_2 tracing has been replaced by small transient rises in the CO_2 tracing, which progressively decrease with each squeeze of the Ambu bag.

measure of respiratory drive. In ventilator-dependent patients, $P_{0.1}$ has been shown to correlate significantly with the work of breathing during pressure-support ventilation ($r = 0.87$).[55] By taking advantage of the decrease in airway pressure to open the demand valve during triggering, investigators have demonstrated that commercially available ventilators can measure $P_{0.1}$ accurately.[56] Several studies[56-58] have indicated that an elevated $P_{0.1}$ predicted weaning failure, but the threshold separating success from failure differed among the studies.[59]

MAXIMAL INSPIRATORY AIRWAY PRESSURE

Maximum inspiratory pressure (Pimax), a global measure of inspiratory muscle strength, is measured using a one-way valve that allows exhalation but prevents inhalation.[60,61] Pimax is one of the standard measurements employed to determine a need for the continuation of mechanical ventilation. Values that are more negative than −30 cm H_2O are considered to predict weaning success; values that are less negative than −20 cm H_2O are predictive of weaning failure. These criteria, however, frequently are falsely positive and falsely negative.[62]

BREATHING PATTERN

Rapid shallow breathing is a common respiratory pattern in patients who fail a trial of weaning from mechanical ventilation,[63] and this can be quantitated in terms of the frequency–to–tidal volume ratio (f/V_T). The higher the f/V_T, the more pronounced the rapid, shallow breathing and the greater the likelihood of unsuccessful weaning. An f/V_T above 100 breaths per minute per liter suggests that a trial of weaning is unlikely to be successful.[62] When prospectively evaluated, f/V_T was found to be superior to nine other weaning predictors: sensitivity was 0.97, specificity 0.64, positive predictive value 0.78, and negative predictive value 0.95.[60]

The usefulness of f/V_T in predicting weaning outcome was challenged. Using a meta-analysis, an American College of Chest Physicians (ACCP) Task Force concluded that f/V_T was unreliable.[64,65] In their evaluation of published reports on f/V_T, the Task Force ignored the important influence of pretest probability on the interpretation of test results. The implications of pretest probability are greater for weaning than for many clinical situations because weaning involves a sequence of three diagnostic tests: measurement of predictors, followed by a weaning trial, followed by an extubation trial. The undertaking of three diagnostic tests in a sequential manner poses an enormous risk for the occurrence of test referral and spectrum bias. The introductions of such biases will, in turn, increase the pretest probability.[66,67] Indeed, the mean pretest probability of weaning success was 75% in the studies included in the meta-analysis. When data from studies included in the Task Force meta-analysis were entered into a bayesian model with pretest probability as the operating point, the observed posttest probabilities were closely correlated with the values predicted by the original study on f/V_T: $r = 0.86$ for positive predictive value and $r = 0.82$ for negative predictive value.[68]

It has been suggested that measurements of f/V_T at 30 minutes into a weaning trial more accurately predict outcome than measurements in the first minute.[69,70] Although it is true that including data for the first 30 seconds or so may be unrepresentative, this does not mean that it takes 30 minutes to establish a steady state.

Jubran and colleagues[70] studied the time required for f/V_T to reach a point of equilibration in 17 weaning failure and 14 weaning success patients. The median time (plus interquartile range) to reach +10% of the final value of f/V_T was 2 (1 to 2) minutes in both the weaning success and the weaning failure patients (Fig. 13.7). Within 2 minutes of the onset of the T-tube trial, 77% of the weaning failure patients and 73% of the weaning success patients had reached +10% of the final value of f/V_T. As indicated by these data, a reasonable strategy is to commence measurement of f/V_T at 60 seconds after removal of the ventilator and then continue the measurement for another 60 seconds.

Continuous recording of breathing pattern provides an important approach for assessing the ability of the respiratory controller to maintain or adjust its response over time.[71] Simple measurements, such as coefficients of variation, indicate that healthy subjects display considerable variation in tidal volume and respiratory cycle time from one breath to the next.[72] Signal analysis techniques reveal that this variability is composed of random and nonrandom fractions.[73-78] The predominantly random character of the variability makes it possible for the respiratory system to engage in tasks other than gas exchange. A smaller fraction of variability is nonrandom; moreover, tidal volume and

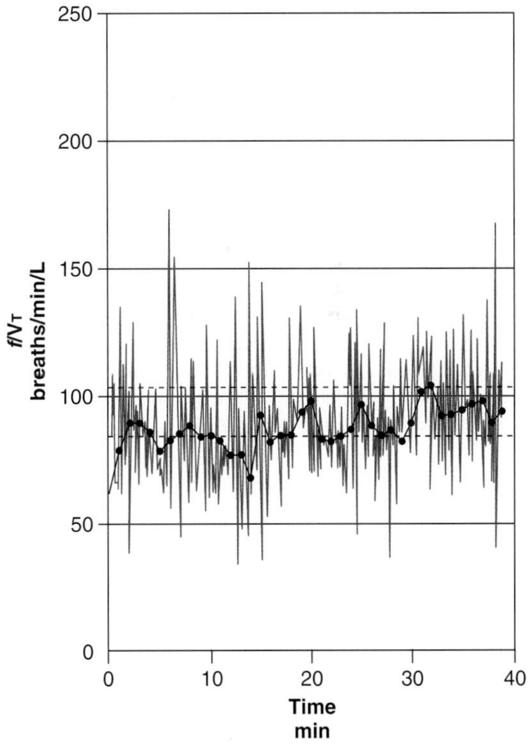

Figure 13.7 Time-series plot of frequency–to–tidal volume ratio (f/V_T) during a T-tube trial of spontaneous breathing in a weaning failure patient. *Black dots* represent 1-minute averages. The *solid line* indicates the average value of f/V_T of the final minute of the trial. The *dashed horizontal lines* indicate +10% of the final minute values of f/V_T. The time taken to reach +10% of the final value of f/V_T was 2 minutes. (From Jubran A, Grant BJ, Laghi F, et al: Weaning prediction: Esophageal pressure monitoring complements readiness testing. Am J Respir Crit Care Med 2005;171:1252-1259.)

respiratory cycle time of one breath are significantly related to those of the preceding breath.[73,74,76,77] When healthy subjects are faced with external chemical or mechanical loads, however, the random fraction decreases significantly.[74,76,77] This decrease in random variability may lessen the freedom of the respiratory system to undertake behavioral tasks.[76,77,79]

Using autocorrelation analysis and fast-Fourier transformation, Brack and associates[80] showed that patients with restrictive lung disease display a marked decrease in breath-to-breath variability of breathing. The random fraction of variability was approximately 1/27 of that found in healthy subjects, and the nonrandom correlated fraction was as much as three times higher in the patients. Slight variations from the average resting tidal volume caused large increases in dyspnea in the patients, but not in the healthy subjects[80] (Fig. 13.8). In patients undergoing a weaning trial, Wysocki and coworkers[81] noted a higher gross variability of breathing

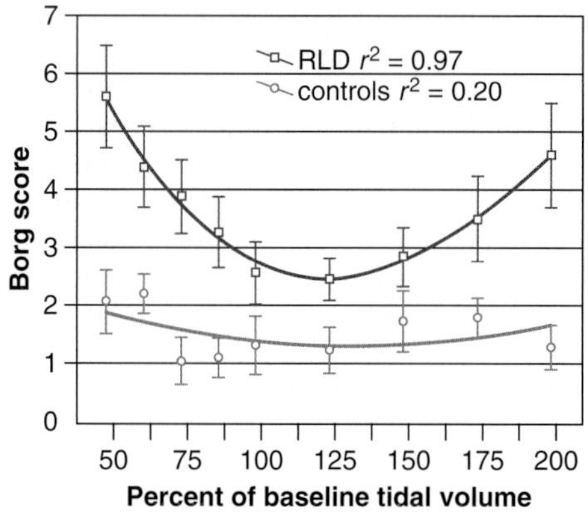

Figure 13.8 The relationship between variation in tidal volume and dyspnea (Borg score) in patients with restrictive lung disease and in control subjects. Dyspnea scores were higher in the patients than in the control subjects ($P < 0.01$, ANOVA); dyspnea varied with tracked volume in the patients ($P < 0.05$, ANOVA) but not in the control group. The regression between dyspnea and tidal volume was parabolic in the patients ($y = 10.3 - 0.12x + 0.0005x^2$; $P < 0.0001$), but not in the control subjects ($y = 2.76 - 0.02x + 0.00008x^2$; $P = 0.5$). *Bars* represent ± SEM. ANOVA, analysis of variance; SEM, standard error of the mean. (From Brack T, Jubran A, Tobin MJ: Dyspnea and decreased variability of breathing in patients with restrictive lung disease. Am J Respir Crit Care Med 2002;165:1260-1264).

(quantitated in terms of coefficient of variation) in patients who were successfully weaned than in patients who failed the trial. These data suggest that an increase in the ability to vary breathing may be associated with a favorable weaning outcome.[82]

CHANGES IN END-EXPIRATORY LUNG VOLUME

Alterations in the end-expiratory level of signal from an inductive plethysmograph can provide a measurement of the change in functional residual capacity provided that motion artifact is absent[83,84] (Fig. 13.9). Inductive plethysmography has been used to estimate a patient's level of auto-PEEP (positive end-expiratory pressure).[49] By noting the level of external PEEP at which end-expiratory lung volume increased, a close estimate of the patient's original level of auto-PEEP can be obtained. An attractive feature of this technique is that it does not disturb expiration, unlike the occlusive technique, in which foreshortening of expiratory time is unavoidable.[85]

RESPIRATORY MECHANICS

Measurements of respiratory mechanics in a relaxed ventilator-dependent patient can be obtained using the technique of rapid airway occlusion during constant-flow inflation.[86] Rapid airway occlusion at the end of a passive inflation produces an immediate drop in both airway pressure (Paw) and transpulmonary pressure (PL) from a peak value (Ppeak) to a lower initial value (Pinit), followed by a gradual decrease until a plateau (Pplat) is achieved after 3 to 5 seconds[87,88] (Fig. 13.10). Pplat on the Paw, PL, and Pes tracings represents the static end-inspiratory recoil pressure of the total respiratory system, lung, and chest wall, respectively.

ELASTANCE (COMPLIANCE)

The end-inspiratory airway occlusion method is used clinically to measure the static compliance, or its reciprocal, elastance, of the respiratory system (Est,rs) according to the following equation[89]:

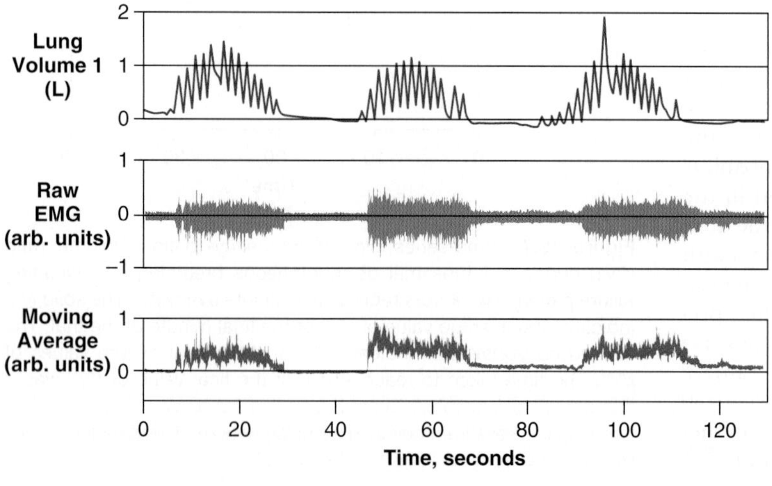

Figure 13.9 Changes in lung volume measured by inductive plethysmography (*top tracing*), raw electromyographic signal of scalene muscle activity (EMG) (*middle tracing*), and moving time average (*bottom, integrated signal*) during three consecutive cycles of Cheyne-Stokes breathing in a representative patient. Note the repeated increases in end-expiratory lung volume with each hyperpnea. (From Brack T, Jubran A, Laghi F, Tobin MJ: Fluctuations in end-expiratory lung volume during Cheyne-Stokes respiration. Am J Respir Crit Care Med 2005;171:1408-1413.)

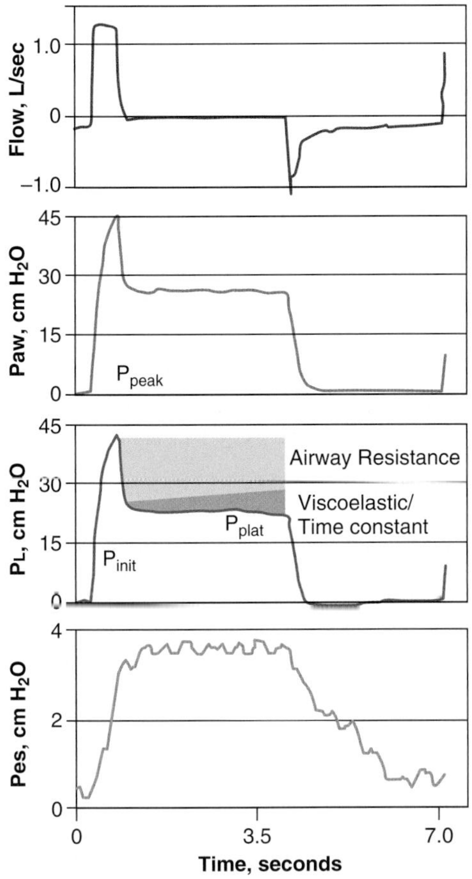

Figure 13.10 Flow (inspiration upward), airway pressure (Paw), transpulmonary pressure (PL), and esophageal pressure (Pes) tracings in a representative patient during passive ventilation. An end-inspiratory occlusion produced a rapid decline in both Paw and PL from a peak value (Ppeak) to a lower initial pressure (Pinit), followed by gradual decrease to a plateau pressure (Pplat). Pplat on the Paw, PL, and Pes tracings represents the static end-inspiratory recoil pressures of the total respiratory system, lung, and chest wall, respectively. Using this technique, total resistance can be partitioned into ohmic airway resistance and tissue resistance, which reflects the viscoelastic properties (stress relaxation) and time-constant inhomogeneities within the respiratory tissues. (Modified from Jubran A, Tobin MJ: Passive mechanics of lung and chest wall in patients who failed and succeeded in trials of weaning. Am J Respir Crit Care Med 1997;155:916-921.)

$$\text{Est,rs} = \text{Pplat} - \text{PEEPtot}/\text{V}_\text{T}$$

where Pplat is plateau pressure obtained after occlusion of the airway, PEEPtot is the sum of external and intrinsic PEEPs if present, and V_T is tidal volume (see Fig. 13.10).

Mechanical ventilation in itself can produce or aggravate lung injury in patients with acute respiratory distress syndrome (ARDS).[90-92] Injury may be decreased by minimizing alveolar overdistention. To avoid lung injury, ideally the alveolar volume should be monitored, but that is not possible. Alveolar volume is reflected by peak alveolar pressure, which can be assessed indirectly by measuring the plateau pressure during an end-inspiratory hold maneuver. It has been recommended that plateau pressure not exceed 32 cm H_2O.[93,94]

A new era of ventilatory management began in 1990, when a report demonstrated that lowering tidal volume caused a 60% decrease in the expected mortality rate among patients with ARDS.[95] Subsequently, randomized trials were undertaken.[96-99] In 861 patients, the ARDS Network investigators reported a 22% difference in mortality rates with use of a tidal volume of 6 mL/kg versus 12 mL/kg.[100] It is now generally accepted that the use of high tidal volumes in patients with ARDS is associated with high mortality rates.[93,101] Whether the use of low tidal volumes implies a survival advantage is controversial.[101-103]

PRESSURE-VOLUME CURVES

A pressure-volume curve of the respiratory system in a paralyzed patient can be constructed by measuring the airway pressure as the lungs are progressively inflated with a 1.5- to 2-L syringe. A lower inflection point and an upper inflection point may be seen on the pressure-volume curve.[104] The lower inflection point is thought to reflect the point at which small airways or alveoli reopen, corresponding to closing volume. In patients with acute lung injury, investigators have recommended that PEEP be set at a pressure slightly above the lower inflection point.[105]

When an "open-lung approach," consisting of use of a lower tidal volume (less than 6 mL/kg) with PEEP individually titrated to be consistently above the inflection point on the pressure-volume curve, was compared with a conventional approach, consisting of use of tidal volume of 12 mL/kg and a low PEEP level, the mortality rate was significantly reduced in the group managed with the new approach.[96,106]

A National Institutes of Health (NIH)-sponsored trial of high versus low PEEP, however, failed to demonstrate a significant survival advantage for patients randomized to the high PEEP group.[107] Several methodologic considerations cast doubt on the conclusions of the investigators.[108] First, baseline characteristics of the two groups were not balanced; the low PEEP group patients had higher Pa_{O_2}/F_{IO_2} ratios and were younger than patients in the high PEEP group. Second, PEEP-induced recruitment was estimated by improvement in oxygenation. It is well known that changes in oxygenation depend not only on recruitment but also on cardiac output.[109] Thus, oxygenation may have improved without any lung recruitment. Third, recruitment potential was not stratified, so that patients who were not likely to benefit were assigned to both groups.[110]

The importance of individualizing PEEP in ventilator management in patients with ARDS was confirmed in a Spanish trial. One group of patients was randomized to a treatment group in which PEEP was titrated to 2 cm H_2O above the lower inflection point. The mortality rate was lower in these patients than in control group patients who did not receive customized titration of PEEP.[111]

RESISTANCE

Airway resistance can be measured in ventilator-dependent patients using the technique of rapid airway occlusion during constant-flow inflation[86,87,89,112] (see Fig. 13.10).

Measurements of airway resistance are helpful in assessing the response of patients to bronchodilator therapy. In a

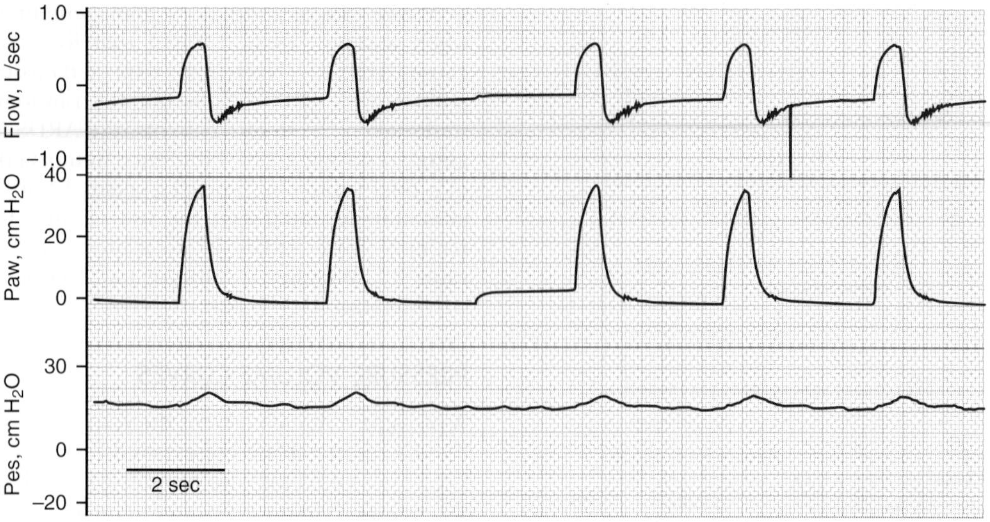

Figure 13.11 Recordings of flow, airway pressure (Paw), and esophageal pressure (Pes) in a patient receiving controlled mechanical ventilation. After the third breath, the airway was occluded at end-expiration using the end-expiratory hold function on the ventilator. During the period of zero flow, pressure in the alveoli and in the ventilator circuit equilibrates, and the plateau pressure reflects auto- or intrinsic positive end-expiratory pressure (PEEPi), indicated by the *arrow.*

study in ventilator-dependent patients with chronic obstructive pulmonary disease (COPD), a significant decrease in airway resistance occurred after giving 4 puffs, with no further effect after the addition of 8 and 16 puffs (cumulative doses of 12 and 28 puffs).[113,114]

INTRINSIC POSITIVE END-EXPIRATORY PRESSURE

The static recoil pressure of the respiratory system at end-expiration may be elevated in patients receiving mechanical ventilation.[89] This positive recoil pressure, or intrinsic PEEP (static PEEPi), can be quantified in relaxed patients using an end-expiratory hold maneuver on a mechanical ventilator immediately before the onset of the next breath[11,115] (Fig. 13.11), or as a change in Paw required to reduce expiratory flow to zero and initiate lung inflation by the ventilator (dynamic PEEPi). In patients with COPD, dynamic PEEPi is lower than static PEEPi; this discrepancy is attributed to the presence of time-constant inequalities.[116,117]

PEEPi poses a significant inspiratory threshold load that has to be fully counterbalanced by increasing inspiratory muscle effort in order to generate a negative pressure in the central airway and trigger the ventilator. Thus, PEEPi adds to the triggering pressure such that the total inspiratory effort needed to trigger the ventilator is the set trigger sensitivity plus the level of PEEPi. This is one of the factors that may account for the not infrequent observation of a patient who is unable to trigger a ventilator despite obvious respiratory effort[118-123] (Fig. 13.12).

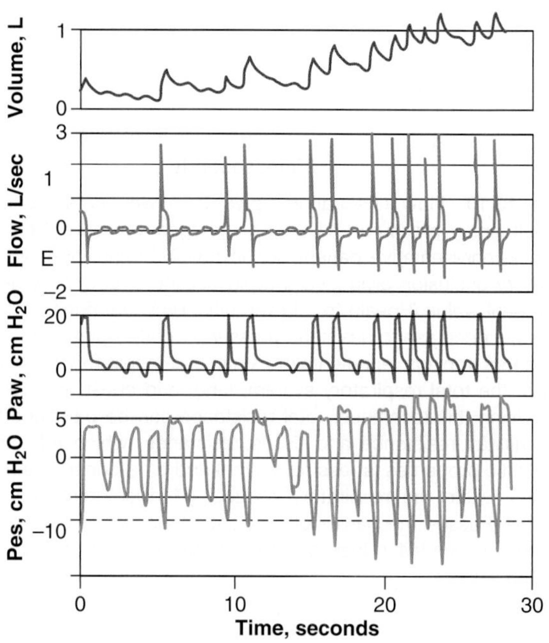

Figure 13.12 Recordings of tidal volume, flow, airway pressure (Paw), and esophageal pressure (Pes) in a patient with chronic obstructive pulmonary disease receiving pressure support ventilation. Approximately half of the patient's inspiratory efforts do not succeed in triggering the ventilator. Triggering occurred only when the patient generated a Pes less than 8 cm H_2O (indicated by the *dashed line*), which was equal in magnitude to the opposing elastic recoil pressure. (From Tobin MJ, Jubran A: Pathophysiology of failure to wean from mechanical ventilation. Schweiz Med Wochenschr 1994;124: 2139-2145.)

In a study of ventilator-dependent patients, Leung and colleagues[120] reported that ineffective triggering occurred with all assisted modes of mechanical ventilation. The ineffective or wasted efforts were significantly related to resistance ($r = 0.85$), elastance ($r = -0.61$), and static PEEPi ($r = 0.77$). A decrease in the magnitude of inspiratory effort at a given level of assistance was not the cause—indeed, effort was 38% higher during nontriggering attempts than during the triggering phase of attempts that successfully opened the inspiratory valve. Significant differences, however, were observed in the breaths before the triggering and nontriggering attempts. Breaths before nontriggering attempts were associated with shorter respiratory cycle time and expiratory time and higher static PEEPi compared with the

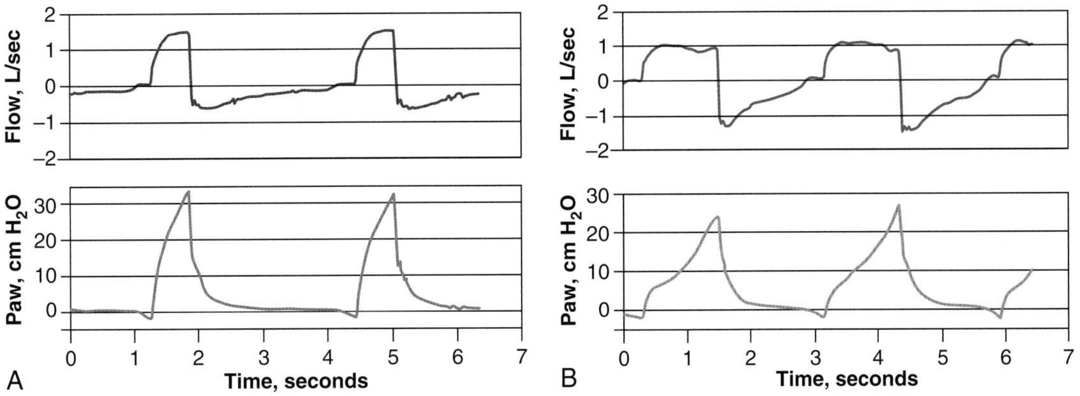

Figure 13.13 Flow and airway pressure (Paw) during assist-control ventilation at different flow rates: 60 L/minute (**A**) and 30 L/minute (**B**). **A,** The small negative phase coupled with the smooth rise and convex appearance of the Paw waveform indicates that the patient is making a slight inspiratory effort to breathe. **B,** The more pronounced negative phase together with excessive scalloping of the Paw waveform indicates that the patient is making a strenuous effort to breathe as a result of the inadequate flow setting. (From Jubran A, Tobin MJ: Monitoring during mechanical ventilation. In Tobin MJ (ed): Principles and Practice of Mechanical Ventilation. New York, McGraw-Hill, 2006, p 1051.)

breaths before triggered attempts. These findings suggest that ineffective triggering resulted not from a decrease in the magnitude of effort but rather from inspiratory efforts that were premature and insufficient to overcome the elevated elastic recoil pressure associated with dynamic hyperinflation.

AIRWAY PRESSURE PROFILE

A continuous recording of airway pressure provides helpful information about the amount of respiratory work being performed by a patient receiving ventilator assistance. Ideally the waveform should show a smooth rise with a convex appearance during inspiration.[1,124] By contrast, a prolonged negative phase with excessive scalloping of the tracing reflects increased inspiratory effort; this pattern indicates unsatisfactory sensitivity and inappropriate flow settings (Fig. 13.13). A "bump" on the airway pressure tracing observed while the ventilator is still pumping gas in the patient may reflect recruitment of expiratory muscles (Fig. 13.14).

Use of a flow setting that does not meet a patient's ventilatory demands will cause inspiratory effort to increase. Sometimes the flow is increased to shorten the inspiratory time and increase the expiratory time. An increase in flow, however, can cause immediate and persistent tachypnea; if this happens, the resulting decrease in expiratory time may lead to increased PEEPi.[125,126] In general, however, an increase in inspiratory flow does not lead to an increase in PEEPi[126] (Fig. 13.15).

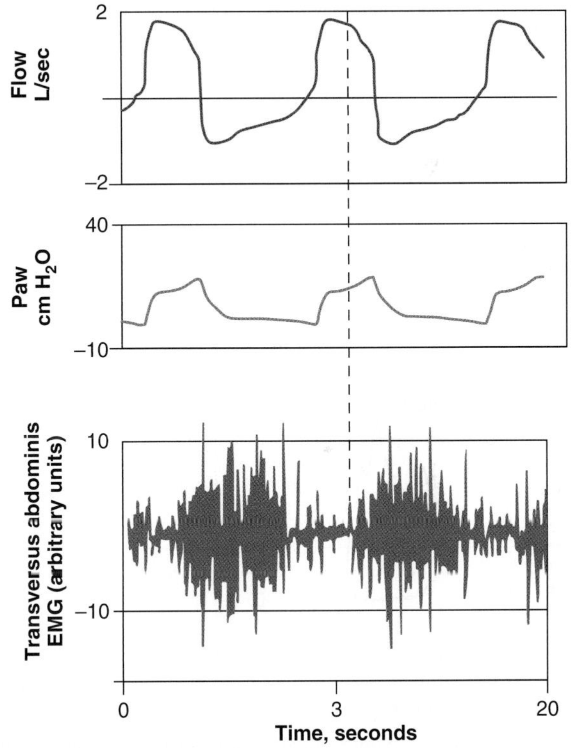

Figure 13.14 Recordings of flow (*top*) and airway pressure (Paw; *middle*) and transversus abdominis electromyogram (EMG; *bottom*) in a critically ill patient with chronic obstructive pulmonary disease receiving pressure support of 20 cm H_2O. The onset of expiratory muscle activity (*vertical dotted line*) occurred when mechanical inflation was only partly completed. (From Parthasarathy S, Jubran A, Tobin MJ: Cycling of inspiratory and expiratory muscle groups with the ventilator in airflow limitation. Am J Respir Crit Care Med 1998;158: 1471-1478.)

FLOW-VOLUME CURVES

Flow-volume curves may be helpful in indicating a need for endotracheal suctioning. In 50 intubated patients, Jubran and Tobin[127] found that the presence of a sawtooth pattern strongly suggested the presence of secretions (positive predictive value, 94%), and the absence of this pattern suggested that secretions are unlikely to be present (negative predictive value, 77%) (Fig. 13.16). Clinical examination had much higher false-positive and false-negative rates (42% and 43%, respectively) than the flow-volume curves (12% and 14%, respectively). The usefulness of a sawtooth pattern for detecting secretions was confirmed by Guglielminotti and colleagues[128] in a study of 62 patients who were receiving pressure support or assist-control ventilation.

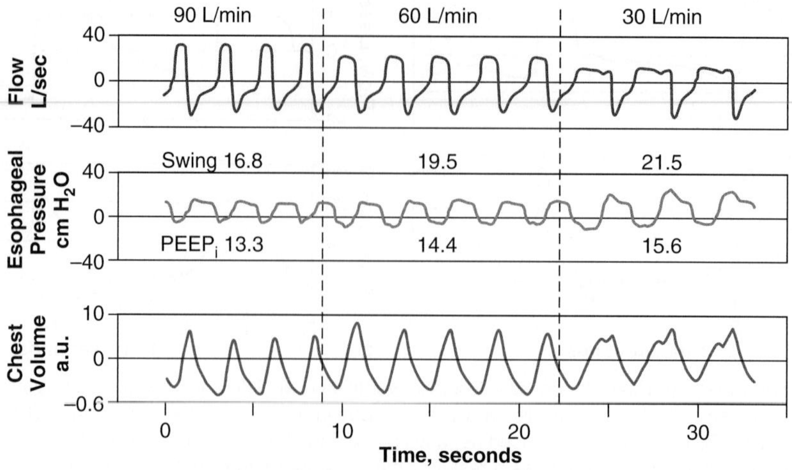

Figure 13.15 Continuous recordings of flow, esophageal pressure (Pes), and the sum of rib cage and abdominal motion in a patient with chronic obstructive pulmonary disease receiving assist-control ventilation at a constant tidal volume. As flow increased from 30 L/minute to 60 and 90 L/minute (from *right* to *left*), frequency increased (from 18 breaths per minute to 23 and 26 breaths per minute, respectively), PEEPi decreased (from 15.6 cm H_2O to 14.4 and 13.3 cm H_2O, respectively), and end-expiratory lung volume also fell. Increases in flow from 30 L/minute to 60 and 90 L/minute also led to decreases in the swings in Pes from 21.5 cm H_2O to 19.5 and 16.8 cm H_2O, respectively. a.u., arbitrary units; PEEPi, intrinsic positive end-expiratory pressure. (From Laghi F, Segal J, Choe WK, Tobin MJ: Effect of imposed inflation time on respiratory frequency and hyperinflation in patients with chronic obstructive pulmonary disease. Am J Respir Crit Care Med 2001;163:1365-1370.)

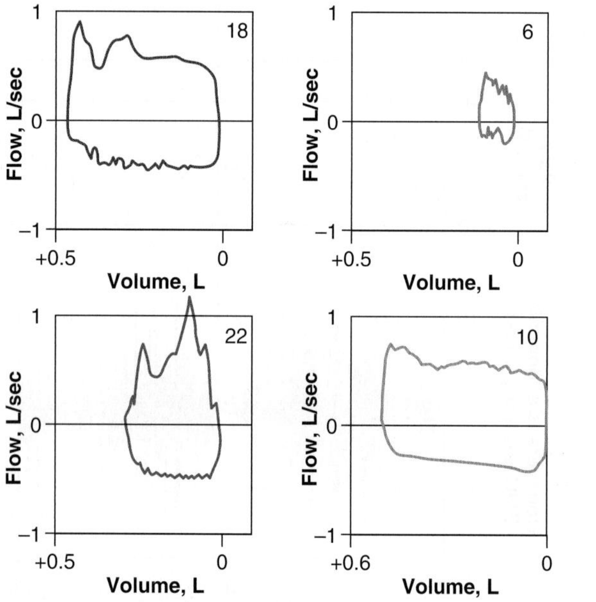

Figure 13.16 Flow-volume curves obtained in four patients with secretions. Note the presence of a sawtooth pattern on both the inspiratory and expiratory flow-volume curves. (The numbers to the *upper right* in each grid are the original patient numbers.) (From Jubran A, Tobin MJ: Use of flow-volume curves in detecting secretions in ventilator-dependent patients. Am J Respir Crit Care Med 1994;150: 766-769.)

KEY POINTS

- Roughly 20% to 40% of patients in an ICU are admitted mainly for the purpose of monitoring.
- Pulse oximetry can accurately measure oxygen saturation at levels of 90% or above; its accuracy deteriorates when the saturation falls to 80% or less.
- Inaccurate readings from pulse oximetry can occur as a result of interference from substances or from problems in signal processing.
- Hypoxemia is detected more frequently in patients monitored with pulse oximetry than in patients in whom this modality is not used.
- Transcutaneous monitoring of PCO_2 may be reliable in monitoring changes in arterial PCO_2 in the absence of major vasoconstriction.
- Measuring airway pressure at 0.1 second after initiating an inspiratory effort against an occluded airway is closely associated with increased work of breathing during mechanical ventilation.
- One-time measurements of breathing pattern (frequency and tidal volume) are helpful in predicting weaning outcome; continuous measurements of breathing pattern can provide information about the function of the respiratory controller.
- Measurements of respiratory mechanics in a ventilator-dependent patient can be easily performed at the bedside using the rapid airway occlusion technique.
- Continuous recordings of airway pressure can provide useful information about the respiratory work performed by a patient receiving mechanical ventilation.
- Flow-volume curves may be helpful in indicating a need for endotracheal suctioning.

SELECTED REFERENCES

1. Jubran A, Tobin MJ: Monitoring during mechanical ventilation. In Tobin MJ (ed): Principles and Practice of Mechanical Ventilation, 3rd ed. New York, McGraw-Hill, 2012, pp 1136-1165.
5. Jubran A: Pulse oximetry. In Tobin MJ (ed): Principles and Practice of Intensive Care Monitoring. New York, McGraw-Hill, 1998, 261-287.
39. Moller JT, Pedersen T, Rasmussen LS, et al: Randomized evaluation of pulse oximetry in 20,802 patients: I—Design, demography, pulse oximetry failure rate and overall complication rate. Anesthesiology 1993;78:436-444.
46. Palmisano BW, Severinghaus JW: Transcutaneous Pco_2 and Po_2: A multicenter study of accuracy. J Clin Monit 1990;6: 189-195.
54. Knapp S, Kofler J, Stoiser B, et al: The assessment of four different methods to verify tracheal tube placement in the critical care setting. Anesth Analg 1999;88:766-770.
56. Conti G, Cinnella G, Barboni E, et al: Estimation of occlusion pressure during assisted ventilation in patients with intrinsic PEEP. Am J Respir Crit Care Med 1996;154:907-912.
62. Yang K, Tobin MJ: A prospective study of indexes predicting outcome of trials of weaning from mechanical ventilation. N Engl J Med 1991;324:1445-1450.
88. Polese G, Rossi A, Appendini L, et al: Partitioning of respiratory mechanics in mechanically ventilated patients. J Appl Physiol 1991;71:2425-2433.
104. Brochard L: Respiratory pressure-volume curves. In Tobin MJ (ed): Principles and Practice of Intensive Care Monitoring. New York, McGraw-Hill, 1998, pp 597-616.
124. Tobin MJ, Laghi F, Jubran A: Ventilator-induced respiratory muscle weakness. Ann Intern Med 2010;153:240-245.

The complete list of references can be found at www.expertconsult.com.

14 Tracheostomy

Yaakov Friedman | Sabine Sobek

CHAPTER OUTLINE

HISTORY

Most medications, devices, and surgical techniques employed in today's intensive care unit (ICU) have resulted from twentieth century medical advances. However, one of the most common surgical procedures, tracheostomy, has been described for nearly 6000 years. The terms *tracheostomy* and *tracheotomy* are derived from the Greek words *tracheia arteria,* translated "rough artery," and refer to the trachea being the vital conduit of air.[1] Tracheostomy means permanent opening (*stoma,* Greek for "mouth"), to be distinguished from the temporary nature of a tracheotomy (*tome,* "to cut"). Today the terms are used interchangeably for any artificial airway created in the trachea, with tracheostomy used more commonly.

McClelland divides the history of the tracheostomy into five periods beginning with "The Period of Legend" (2000 BCE to 1546 CE).[2] The first written reference to tracheostomy is in the sacred book of Hindu medicine, the *Rig Veda,* dated between 2000 BCE and 1000 BCE, and describes "the bountiful one, who without a ligature, can cause the windpipe to reunite when the cervical cartilages are cut across."[3,4] The earliest depictions of a tracheostomy being performed date back to about 3600 BCE and show two Egyptian kings undergoing a tracheostomy.[5,6] Homer referred to tracheostomy as a way of relieving choking persons by cutting open the trachea, and Alexander the Great is described to have used the point of his sword to open the trachea of one of his soldiers who was choking while eating.[2] The next successful tracheostomy was performed in the second century CE by Antyllus as documented 400 years later by Paul of Aegina, who wrote that the use of tracheostomy was encouraged in cases of upper airway obstruction and provided a technical description of the operation.[7] Mention of tracheostomy can be found in the Roman and Arabic literature, although during the Dark Ages of medicine and science the technique of tracheostomy (and virtually all other surgeries) was forgotten for nearly 1000 years.[6,8]

The second period, "The Period of Fear" (1536 to 1833),[2] starts with the Renaissance, when European physicians experimented with tracheostomy for trauma, aspirated foreign bodies, drowning, and Ludwig's angina. Fabricius of Aquapendente tells us that the timidity at that time was due partly to "lack of knowledge of anatomy, partly to fear of a loss of reputation, should the patient die after the operation." In his day, tracheostomy was known as the "scandal of surgery." About the same time, in 1546, the first definite account of a successful tracheostomy was recorded by Antonius Brasavola, who told of "opening the windpipe and saving the life of a patient near death from angina and an abscess which was obstructing the canalis pulmonis."[1,8] Over the next 2 centuries, opposition to tracheostomy diminished because of the interest in anatomy and autopsy, as evidenced by the drawings and writings of Leonardo da Vinci, Julius Casserius, and others.[6,9-11]

The clinical importance of tracheostomy became evident during sporadic diphtheria epidemics, and multiple publications of successful tracheostomies can be found in many European countries after 1620.[8] In 1730, Scottish surgeon George Martine treated upper airway obstruction resulting from diphtheria with tracheostomy. He also recommended the use of an inner cannula for ease of care and recognized that tracheal wounds heal spontaneously without the need for surgical repair.[8,12] In America, fear of tracheostomy was still quite prevalent, as evidenced in the well-known controversy surrounding the death of George Washington in 1799, when bloodletting won over relieving an epiglottitis-related upper airway obstruction with a tracheostomy.[6,13] Until 1825, during these first several thousand years in the history of tracheostomy, only 28 tracheostomies are verifiable.

After Napoleon Bonaparte's nephew died of diphtheria in 1807, a grand prize was offered for new insights into this disease and its treatment. This heralded the "Period of Drama," which lasted from 1833 to 1931. Based on subsequent research, especially by Bretonneau and his pupil Trousseau, tracheostomy became a relatively established procedure, particularly for croup and diphtheria. Before Bretonneau, tracheostomy had been known under many different names, including bronchotomy, laryngotomy, pharyngotomy, sectio epiglottis, scisio cannae, and incisio cannae pulmonis. In 1718 Heister had introduced the term *tracheotomy* and recommended that all other terms be discarded, but it was not until Bretonneau used this term in a paper describing a successful operation in 1825 for diphtheria that it gained widespread acceptance.[8,14] Trousseau described a series of 200 French children, most dying of diphtheria, in whom he reduced mortality rate from nearly 100% to 75% with tracheostomy.[15] American surgeon Thomas Shastid published an account of performing tracheostomies on children in the 1890s in a small Illinois town during a diphtheria epidemic.[16,17]

In the mid-1800s, Snow and Trendelenburg advocated tracheostomy for administration of inhaled anesthetics,[3,18] but endotracheal intubation, performed by MacEwan in 1878[19] and O'Dwyer in 1880,[20] and popularized by Bartholomay and Dufor in 1907 and Kelly in 1912, soon replaced tracheostomy as the route for delivering general anesthesia.[3,21] This put the performance of tracheostomy squarely in the hands of surgeons experienced in upper airway problems, most notably Chevalier Jackson, whose name became virtually synonymous with tracheostomy. In his hands, the rate of mortality attributable to tracheostomy decreased from 25% to less than 5%.[22]

The fourth period, the "Period of Enthusiasm" (1932 to 1965), was heralded by a revolutionary shift in the indications for the procedure and major advances in the technique. During this period the main sentiment was "if you think of tracheostomy, do it," without consideration of possible adverse outcomes. Up to then the main indication for tracheostomy was upper airway obstruction, mostly caused by severe croup and diphtheria, which practically disappeared as a result of the development of antibiotics and immunization. In the 1950s, with the poliomyelitis epidemic in Europe and North America, the need for positive-pressure ventilation (PPV) and tracheobronchial suctioning created new indications for tracheostomy.[23] At present, these are still the major indications for tracheostomy in the ICU, and they caused the number of tracheostomies performed at Massachusetts General Hospital to increase from fewer than 10 in 1947 to more than 150 in 1959. Before 1958, not a single tracheostomy was performed there for the sole purpose of providing PPV.[24]

In the mid-1960s the last period in the history of tracheostomy began, the "Period of Rationalization." With the coming of age of the use of the endotracheal tube (ET) even for prolonged ventilatory support, a discussion of the advantages and disadvantages of both methods has emerged and is ongoing, especially with the development of percutaneous tracheostomy (PT).

The exponential increase in tracheostomy in the 1950s and 1960s revived older controversies. In 1921, Chevalier Jackson discussed proper technique and complications.[25] He condemned the use of high tracheostomy, believing it caused laryngeal stenosis. For 50 years, this was the prevailing wisdom of neck surgery and airway maintenance. Jackson drew his conclusions, however, primarily from unsterile emergency tracheostomies performed by inexpert practitioners.[25] Laryngeal stenosis probably resulted from factors other than the site of incision, especially when performed with preexistent laryngeal disease.[26,27] Jackson's reputation made surgeons reluctant to perform high tracheostomies until the advent of cardiac surgery made them necessary to avoid contaminating median sternotomy incisions. In 1976, two cardiac surgeons, Brantigan and Grow, published the first large series of high tracheostomies and found few complications.[28] Acceptance of high tracheostomy permitted reintroduction of PT; a technique described 20 years earlier.

As previously described, when ICUs were developed, tracheostomy became one of the most frequently performed procedures in critically ill patients.[29] This created a need for a safe, cost-effective bedside procedure that would eliminate the necessity for transport of the patient from the ICU to the operating room, with its attendant risks, which are discussed subsequently.

In 1955, Shelden and associates[30] described the first PT, using a slotted needle to guide a cutting trocar into the trachea. This technique was abandoned after fatalities resulted from trocar lacerations of vital structures adjacent to the airway.[31,32] In 1969 Toye and Weinstein[33] described a modified Seldinger technique in which a splitting needle was inserted into the trachea, and through this a guidewire was placed. A single lead dilator was passed over the guidewire, the needle split away, and the tracheostomy tube placed. This technique had a 1% incidence of perioperative death and a 6% incidence of paratracheal insertion, which ultimately caused it also to be abandoned.[34]

In 1985, Ciaglia and colleagues,[35] drawing from experience with cricothyroidotomy, described a true Seldinger technique for quick and easy bedside tracheostomy: percutaneous dilational tracheostomy (PDT). In this technique, multiple curved dilators of gradually increasing size are placed over a guidewire, creating an opening for a tracheostomy tube.

Subsequently, several different versions of PT have been described. In 1988, Hazard and associates[36] had few complications using three straight dilators instead of Ciaglia's seven curved dilators. In 1989, Schachner and colleagues[37] reported a dilating forceps technique (Rapitrac), which is no longer available for use because of its high incidence of complications. In 1990, Griggs and coworkers[38] described passing a blunt-tipped modified Kelly forceps over a guidewire to allow dilation of an aperture adequate to place a tracheostomy tube (guidewire dilator forceps [GWDF] technique). This technique is similar to the Rapitrac, but with a lower incidence of complications. In 1999, Ciaglia developed a soft-tipped, tapered dilator (Blue Rhino, Cook Critical Care, Inc., Bloomington, IN) that was used to create a stoma via a single-step dilation.[39] This approach replaced the multiple dilations necessary in Ciaglia's original kit, theoretically reducing complications and the time necessary to perform PDT. Fantoni's translaryngeal tracheotomy technique was introduced in 1993 and modified in 1996,[40] in which a guidewire is directed in retrograde fashion from the trachea to the mouth over which a cuffed cone-cannula is placed. The cannula is drawn through the neck, and a cuffed tube is placed in the trachea over the cannula as it is removed. The PercuTwist, developed in 2002, uses a dilator with a threaded screw to allow the insertion of a 9-mm tracheostomy tube.[41] The latest modification of the Ciaglia technique of PDT was developed in 2005 and uses balloon dilatation to create the stoma (Blue Dolphin, Cook Critical Care, Inc., Bloomington, IN).[42,43]

THE ARTIFICIAL AIRWAY

In critical care medicine, regardless of the patient's diagnosis, there are four indications for placement of an artificial airway, which can be either an endotracheal or tracheostomy tube: (1) relieving airway obstruction, (2) providing mechanical ventilation (MV), (3) preventing aspiration in the unprotected airway, and (4) facilitating tracheobronchial toilet.[44,45]

Intubation and tracheostomies are performed not because of a specific disease, but because an indication is present as a result of disease. Patients do not need intubation because they have chronic obstructive pulmonary disease or have taken a drug overdose; rather, they require ventilatory support or cannot protect their airway. In examining the rationale for intubation or tracheostomy, clinicians working in the ICU should identify the patient as having an indication for an artificial airway, and before it is removed, there must no longer be an indication for an airway.

Although tracheostomy was considered the emergency airway of choice in the past, now endotracheal intubation is preferred for initial airway management. This is because more practitioners are familiar with endotracheal intubation (which requires less specialized equipment and training), and studies indicate that, in the emergency setting, endotracheal intubation has fewer life-threatening complications[46-48] such as bleeding and pneumothorax, which are extremely rare. Independent of esophageal placement, mortality rate from endotracheal intubation is 0.05%, but ranges from 1% to 2% for emergency tracheostomy.[29] Tracheostomy should be considered an elective or semielective procedure when the airway is already secured.

Occasionally, endotracheal intubation under direct laryngoscopic visualization is not the initial airway management of choice because of massive facial trauma, tracheal obstruction, or anomalous anatomy.[49,50] In such cases, endotracheal intubation sometimes can be facilitated through fiberoptic bronchoscopy.[51] When intubation is impossible even with bronchoscopy, or when bronchoscopy is unavailable, the preferred emergency airway procedure is cricothyroidotomy.[52,53] The primary role of tracheostomy is long-term airway care for patients who initially were treated with ETs or cricothyroidotomies, although reports of PT performed in an emergency setting have been published.[54-57]

TIMING OF TRACHEOSTOMY

The question as to when to replace an ET with a tracheostomy tube is a subject of much discussion, remaining highly controversial independent of technique. Beatrous[44] stated in 1968 that, "Timing is an aspect of tracheostomy that deserves much more emphasis than it is apparently receiving. Delay defeats the purpose of the operation."

The debate as to when to replace an ET with a tracheostomy tube centers on the advantages and disadvantages of the tracheostomy tube, as listed in Table 14.1.[58-126] Unfortunately there are very few definite studies confirming or refuting these advantages.

The decision as to when to perform a tracheostomy is more often based on personal preference of the treating physician than on data. For patients with an airway obstruction that cannot be relieved, tracheostomy is the treatment of choice because it is the only airway that can safely remain long term.[127,128] In most other situations the decision is not as straightforward as ultimately only 5% to 11% of patients on MV require placement of a tracheostomy tube.

Table 14.1 Advantages and Disadvantages of Tracheostomy

Advantages	Disadvantages
Protection from laryngeal injury[58-75,110,115]	Tracheal complications[29,69,71,74,102,103,109]
Security of airway[69,73-77]	Procedural risk[29,44,47,48,73,74,94,103-108]
Facilitation of weaning[74,78-92,116-121]	Risk of stoma infection[44,48,74,94,106]
Improved patient comfort and psychological well-being[74,93,94,122]	Risk of cannula displacement[29,48,74,106]
Earlier oral nutrition[95]	Delay in weaning and decannulation[85,109]
Possibility of speech[76,95-98]	Delay in ICU discharge[100,125]
Easier nursing care (mouth care, tracheal suctioning)[73,74,96-98]	Increased risk of pneumonia[29,74,109]
Improved patient mobility[73,74,111]	Poor stoma healing after decannulation[48,102]
Decreased sedation requirements[94,123]	Poor cosmetic results after decannulation[48,108]
Decreased risk of sinusitis and pneumonia[73,74,85,87,89,116-118,121]	Increased awareness of loss of voice, stoma pain, fear of procedures (e.g., suctioning)[113,114]
Earlier ICU discharge[86,87,89,91,92,99,116,118-120,121,124]	Fear and panic attacks after decannulation[113,114]
Earlier hospital discharge[89,116,117,124]	Increased mortality after ICU discharge with tracheostomy cannula in place[126]
Improved survival*[87,88,91,100,101,121]	

*Improved survival after tracheostomy has not been demonstrated in all studies (see text).
ICU, intensive care unit.

Nevertheless, those patients account for 26% of all ventilator days and 14% of hospital days.[101,125,129]

Although the need for tracheostomy sometimes can be predicted early in the ICU course (e.g., neurologic ICU patients with infratentorial lesions who have brainstem dysfunction[130] or a low Glasgow Coma Scale score[90,99]), in most situations this is not the case. Finding early clinical predictors that would identify patients who require a tracheostomy is most problematic in patients receiving MV.[131-134] Many studies from the early and mid-1990s attempted to establish criteria to satisfy the recommendations of the 1989 Consensus Conference on Artificial Airways in Patients Receiving Mechanical Ventilation, which stated that "the decision to convert to tracheotomy should be made as early as possible . . . to minimize the duration of translaryngeal intubation. Once the decision is made, the procedure should be done without undue delay."[135]

Unfortunately, good studies to determine optimal timing of tracheostomy are difficult to perform. Existing studies tend to be either retrospective reviews, which often include a large number of patients but are prone to bias, or randomized, controlled trials that are generally underpowered owing to the large number of patients required to detect significant outcome benefits.[129] Multiple publications address the question of timing of tracheostomy in a variety of patient populations.[85-92,115-120,124,136-138] Most are retrospective reviews of ICU databases in which timing of tracheostomy is retrospectively correlated with multiple outcomes. In these studies, the definition of "early" ranges from 3 to 21 days, and "late" ranges from 7 to 28 days, making it hard to draw any firm conclusions. It seems clear from these studies, however, that the procedural and short-term complications of tracheostomy are low, and that in general the outcome of patients with tracheostomy is at least no worse than that of patients managed with prolonged translaryngeal endotracheal intubation.

Some studies show a decrease in mortality rate in patients with tracheostomy.[100,101,120,125] However, one has to question if this difference is partly explained by the fact that patients with anticipated high mortality risk are not offered a tracheostomy. A frequent finding is that placement of a tracheostomy reduces time on MV,[86,87,89-92,101,116,118,119,121] but even this is not consistent. Other studies have shown no change[85,115,138] or even markedly prolonged times[100] on MV. This may reflect either a less aggressive approach to weaning after a potentially permanent airway has been placed or a selection bias reflecting higher early mortality rate in the patients not receiving a tracheostomy.

Randomized controlled trials of early tracheostomy versus late tracheostomy or prolonged translaryngeal intubation are rare. In 2004, Rumbak and associates[87] showed that early tracheostomy in critically ill medical patients decreased time on MV, ICU length of stay, and ventilator-associated pneumonia. Additionally, early tracheostomy decreased mortality rate by 50% despite well-matched baseline characteristics. They also evaluated the patients for the most feared complication of tracheostomy, tracheal stenosis, during the hospital course and at 10 weeks. No significant differences in the incidence or severity of stenosis were seen, although there was a trend favoring early tracheostomy.[87]

These findings conflict with the findings of several other randomized controlled trials. A trial by Sugerman and coworkers[72] showed no differences in any of the measured outcomes (ICU length of stay, death, and pneumonia). This study was significantly limited by incomplete data collection and physician bias. Another randomized controlled trial in trauma patients by Barquist and associates was prematurely terminated after the first interim analysis with only 60 patients enrolled due to lack of differences in the primary outcomes; ICU length of stay, ventilator-associated pneumonia, and ventilator days.[136]

A well-designed trial in France looked at multiple end points including death, pneumonia, duration of MV, complications, sedation requirements, and subjective patient comfort. There were no differences in any of the parameters, except in late laryngeal complications and patient discomfort. All patients who had an endotracheal as well as a tracheostomy tube during the course of their illness favored tracheostomy. Unfortunately, only 10% to 20% of eligible patients were actually enrolled in the trial and the study was grossly underpowered to detect any significant differences.[115] Finally, a study assessing the impact of early tracheostomy (6-8 days) on the risk of developing ventilator-associated pneumonia showed a statistically insignificant trend ($p = 0.07$) toward reduction in the incidence of pneumonia.[120] Another large trial showed no benefit of early tracheostomy except reduced use of sedatives.[123] Interpreting length of ICU and hospitalization data from these trials requires knowledge of post-tracheostomy disposition, which may vary depending on the country in which the study was performed. Specifically, the availability of long-term ventilator facilities might not be apparent.

An older trial in the 1970s by Stauffer and colleagues,[69] which is frequently quoted as an argument for prolonged translaryngeal intubation, found significantly more complications that were judged more severe in patients who underwent tracheostomy compared to patients with translaryngeal intubation. Most notably, the incidence of tracheal stenosis after tracheostomy was significantly higher (65% versus 19%). Nonetheless, they also found that patients treated with prolonged translaryngeal intubation followed by tracheostomy had significantly more laryngeal injury and an increased frequency of tracheal stenosis compared with patients who underwent tracheostomy after a short period of translaryngeal intubation.[69]

Conclusions from all these studies indicate that a tracheostomy should be offered only to patients anticipated to survive who require secure, long-term airway access. The timing of tracheostomy tube placement should be individualized and depends on three factors: (1) underlying disease, (2) indication for artificial airway, and (3) expected ultimate outcome. An article published in 2012 found that the hospital mortality rate of patients undergoing PDT was 30% with 14-day and 6-month mortality rates of 11% and 40%, respectively.[122] Predictors of poor short-term outcome were found to be older age, diagnosis of malignancy, cardiogenic shock, and presence of a ventricular assist device. A realistic discussion of prognosis therefore should be part of the informed consent prior to placement of a tracheostomy.

Despite several negative trials that were generally underpowered and with the emergence of bedside PDT, a recommendation for earlier tracheostomy still seems appropriate as the early complication rate in experienced hands is low and is likely outweighed by the probable benefits, especially

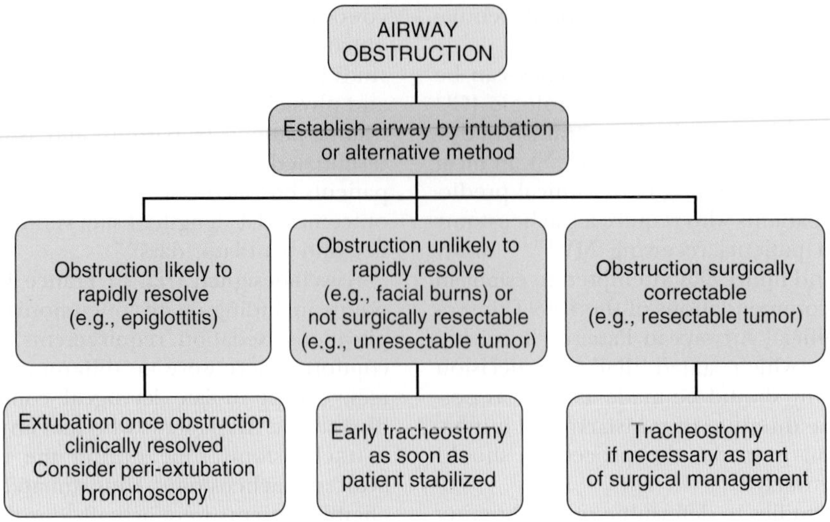

Figure 14.1 Timing of tracheostomy in airway obstruction.

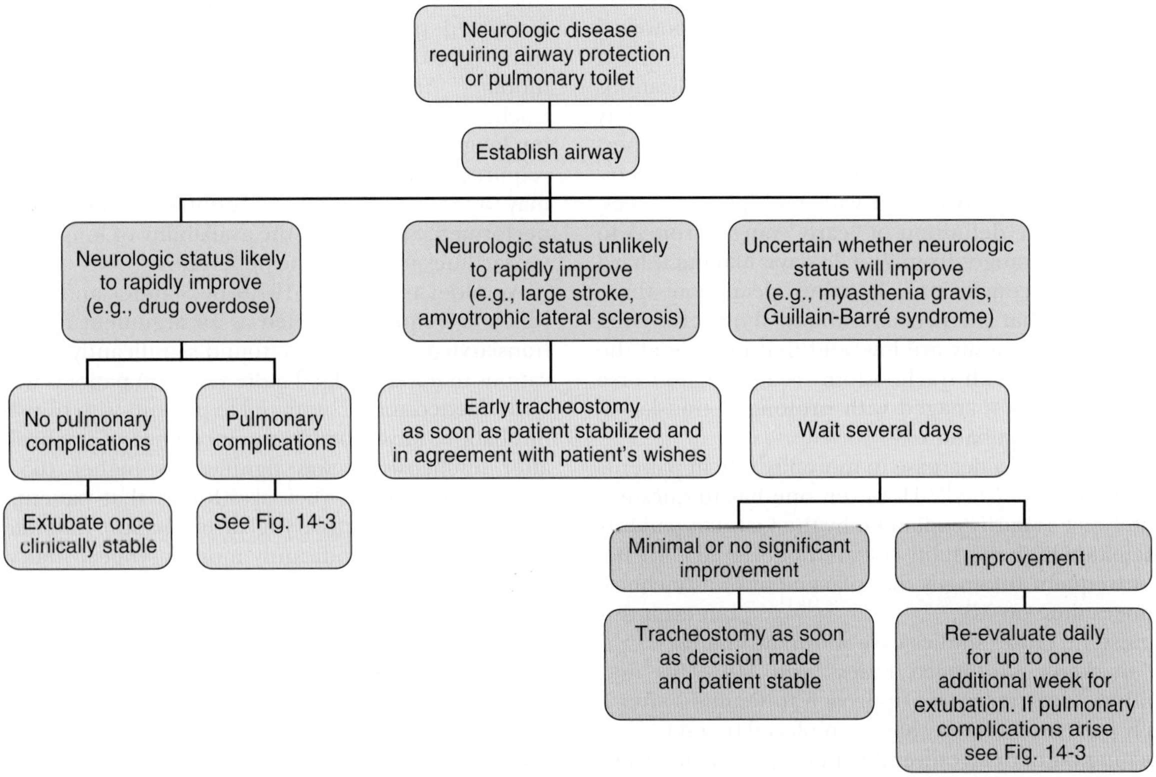

Figure 14.2 Timing of tracheostomy in neurologic disease.

patient comfort. Figures 14.1 through 14.3 provide suggested algorithms regarding the timing of tracheostomy placement based on whether the patient's pathologic condition is primarily upper airway obstruction, neuromuscular, or pulmonary.

UPPER AIRWAY OBSTRUCTION

In patients who have upper airway obstruction, the timing of tracheostomy depends on the likelihood of rapid resolution of the obstruction and whether surgical intervention is required (see Fig. 14.1).

NEUROMUSCULAR CONDITIONS

Many ICU patients intubated because of stupor, coma, or neuromuscular weakness (see Fig. 14.2) are susceptible to aspiration, as they may have laryngeal dysfunction and may not be able to generate an effective cough.[139] In most patients, the duration of the pathologic condition is predictable, either short (e.g., drug overdose) or long (e.g., large stroke, amyotrophic lateral sclerosis).[140-145] In some cases of postoperative weakness, cerebrovascular accident, and peripheral neuromuscular weakness (e.g., Guillain-Barré syndrome, myasthenia gravis), the course is uncertain.[139,146-149]

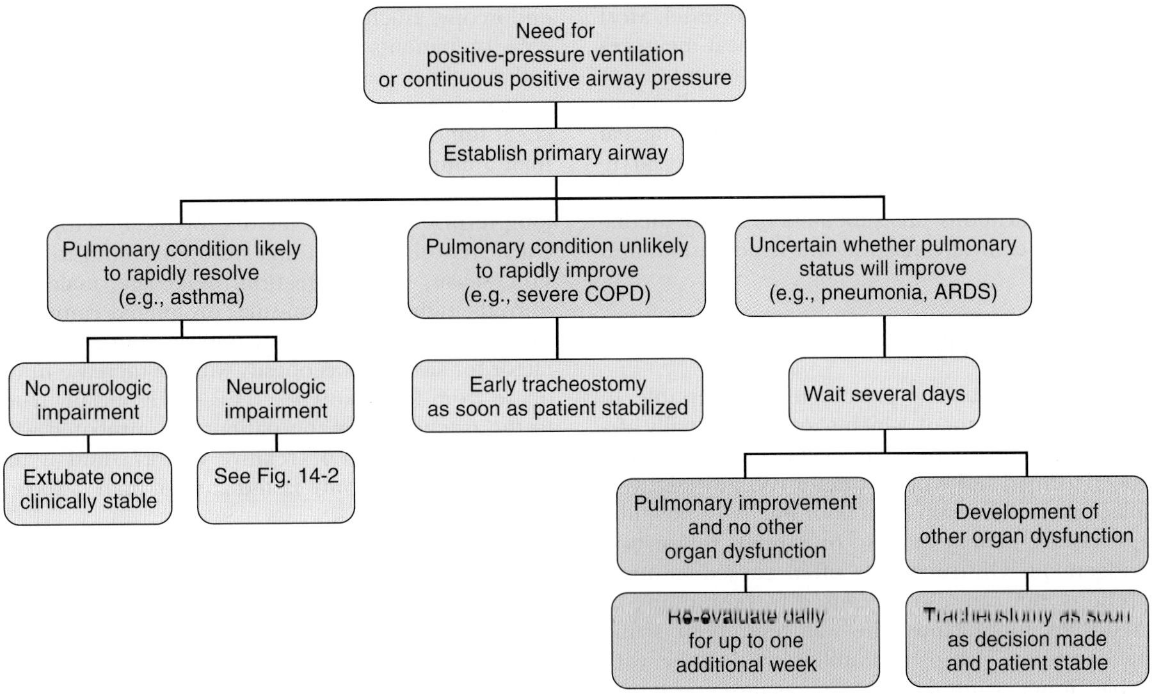

Figure 14.3 Timing of tracheostomy in pulmonary disease. ARDS, adult respiratory distress syndrome; COPD, chronic obstructive pulmonary disease.

A second factor involved in the decision to perform tracheostomy is the coexistence of pulmonary complications, such as atelectasis, pneumonia, or aspiration (see Fig. 14.3).

PULMONARY CONDITIONS

The spectrum of diseases for patients intubated because they require MV is so broad that firm rules regarding tracheostomy have not been established. The approach to the timing of tracheostomy in these situations is difficult because the duration of ventilatory support is frequently hard to predict. This is demonstrated in some randomized studies comparing early and late tracheostomy in which 50% to 75% of patients randomized to delayed tracheostomy did not undergo this procedure because of either death or extubation.[115,120,150] Despite this and multiple studies not supporting survival benefits or faster liberation from ventilator support but with data supporting improved patient well-being, it is advisable to consider early tracheostomy once the patient has stabilized, if the patient is expected to survive and needs a long-term airway, and a tracheostomy can be safely performed.

However, a recently published paper followed 73 ICU patients who received a tracheostomy and were transferred to a floor experienced in the care of patients with tracheostomies.[126] Patients who were not decannulated in the ICU had a significantly higher mortality rate compared to the patients who were decannulated prior to transfer (11% versus 26%). The only other factors associated with increased mortality rate were the presence of tenacious sputum at ICU discharge and a body mass index (BMI) greater than 30 kg/m^2. "The cause of in-ward deaths was cardiopulmonary arrest in 33% of ICU-decannulated patients, versus 90% of those discharged with a cannula in place ($p = 0.08$), most of which occurred overnight." The authors feel the most likely cause of death was respiratory arrest that was likely cannula related, suggesting suboptimal monitoring and care for nondecannulated patients after ICU discharge. This study, though very concerning, was a single-center, prospective, observational trial. Therefore, this finding may reflect an institutional problem rather than a problem inherent to the procedure. Nevertheless, this issue needs further investigation.

COMPLICATIONS OF TRACHEOSTOMY

Throughout the history of tracheostomy, complications have been the most scrutinized aspect. Complications have been categorized as occurring during performance of the tracheostomy (procedural), while the tube is in place (in situ), or after decannulation.[29,102,106] Older studies report a major complication rate of approximately 15% (range, 6% to 66%), with a mortality rate of approximately 1.5% (range, 0% to 5%).[29,47,48,69,71,102-107,151] More recent studies show generally lower complication rates ranging from 1.4% to 27%, and essentially negligible mortality rate.[152-158] A recent multicenter review showed that major procedural complications are rare and are only dependent on operator experience, but not surgical technique or location of the procedure.[157]

PROCEDURAL COMPLICATIONS

The most common serious procedural complications are pneumothorax (0.9% to 5%) and severe hemorrhage (5%).[44,47,48,71,103,105,151] Pneumothorax usually results from violation of the pleural space as it ascends into the neck. Operative hemorrhage is usually venous, originating from the anterior jugular venous system, the thyroid gland isthmus, and very rarely may be arterial from an aberrant vessel. Most of the time bleeding can be controlled by local measures alone, but occasionally will require surgical intervention for hemostasis.[156] Other serious but very rare complications (<1%) include tube misplacement, tracheoesophageal perforation, aspiration, thyroid laceration, recurrent laryngeal nerve damage, and cardiopulmonary arrest.[29,48,151,152,156] Less serious complications are subcutaneous and mediastinal emphysema, clinically insignificant hypotension, and desaturation.[152-154,157]

IN SITU COMPLICATIONS

After a tracheostomy tube is placed, it is susceptible to obstruction and displacement, which may be potentially life-threatening, especially if a problem occurs before a secure tract has been formed and is not promptly recognized.[29,48,106] Tube displacement may result from poor tracheostomy tube selection, excessive patient motion, or careless reinsertion after dislodgement. Obstruction is often caused by tenacious secretions, but can also be caused by positioning of the tracheostomy tube against the wall after poor sizing of the tracheostomy. Use of a double-cannula tube with a disposable inner cannula protects against occlusion by encrusted secretions,[8,159] though this may delay successful weaning because of the increased outer diameter of the tube.[160]

Increasing peak airway pressure, increased resistance during manual bag ventilation, or difficulty passing a suction catheter may indicate tube obstruction or displacement. Providing adequate humidity, adhering to suctioning and tracheostomy care protocols, and minimizing tube manipulation help avert this.[48,106,151]

Another common in situ complication is stomal infection, which occurs in 36% of all tracheostomies.[69] Trivial stomal infection can be treated topically.[48] Necrotizing wound infection can occur, and may extend into the mediastinum, causing life-threatening sepsis.[154,161] Many patients will have bacterial colonization of the tracheobronchial tree, especially with resistant gram-negative organisms (50% to 66%) making them more susceptible to develop nosocomial pneumonia.[29,103,127,162]

In contrast to intraprocedural venous hemorrhage, in situ hemorrhage usually results from the tracheostomy tube tip eroding into a major artery, generally the innominate (0.2% to 4%).[29,69] The resultant tracheoinnominate fistula will present as massive bleeding, sometimes heralded by smaller bleeds or a pulsating tracheostomy tube. Treatment consists of immediate tamponade and operative ligation, despite which tracheoinnominate fistula carries a 75% mortality rate.[29,48,163] Other in situ complications include mucosal ulceration, tracheal erosion, tracheal dilatation, and very rarely tracheoesophageal fistula.[48,69,106,164-168]

COMPLICATIONS AFTER DECANNULATION

The most important postdecannulation complication after tracheostomy is tracheal stenosis.[29,69,71,74,103,155-157,169] It can develop in three distinct areas: subglottic, at the stoma site, or at the cuff site. A mild degree of tracheal narrowing after decannulation at the site of the stoma is very common, and if patients are carefully evaluated with imaging and endoscopy, tracheal narrowing can be found in 30% to 75% of patients after tracheostomy.[69,158,169] Most patients with tracheal stenosis remain asymptomatic and require no treatment.[74] Symptoms generally occur when the tracheal lumen diameter is reduced by either 75% or to less than 5 mm.[103] Recent studies showed a risk of symptomatic stenosis in 0.6% and 10% of patients who were followed long term.[157,158,169] Risk factors for the development of tracheal stenosis at the stoma site were found to be hypotension, sepsis, stoma infection, older age, male sex, use of steroids, tight-fitting cannula, prolonged cannulation, and excessive motion. In a study published in 2012 another risk factor for stenosis was obesity with an increase in risk in the obese from 0.4% to 9.9%. This was especially true if prior to the tracheostomy the patient was intubated with an ET greater than size 7.5 (relative risk 27) and if intubation prior to tracheostomy lasted longer than 7 days (relative risk 2.5).[157]

Stenosis at the site of the cuff is related to mucosal pressure necrosis, exposing the tracheal rings. As the airway is often chronically colonized this will cause chondritis ultimately leading to tracheomalacia or tracheal stenosis. The introduction of the high-volume, low-pressure cuffs has decreased the incidence of this complication by a factor of 10.[170-174] Despite the use of low-pressure cuffs, Stauffer reported that about 20% of patients required excessive cuff pressures to achieve a seal, though the rate was similar in patients with endotracheal or tracheostomy tubes.[69] As has been shown, a low-pressure cuff does not guarantee a low pressure, especially in patients with high pulmonary inflation pressures. Therefore, cuff pressures should routinely be measured and maintained at the lowest appropriate level, ideally less than 25 mm Hg. Even this may not prevent tracheal injury because lateral wall pressure varies widely, is unmeasurable, and may compromise local tracheal blood supply.[166,174-176]

The question whether tracheostomy tubes cause more tracheal stenosis than ETs cannot be answered at this time as most patients who undergo tracheostomy were initially treated with translaryngeal intubation of variable duration, and often require the chosen airway device for a prolonged period. These confounding variables make it impossible to state with certainty if stenosis was caused by the endotracheal or tracheostomy tube unless it is at the site of the stoma. Subglottic stenosis, which is more commonly due to translaryngeal intubation, is more difficult to repair surgically.[110,177-179] Other late complications, which occur infrequently, include tracheocutaneous fistula, tracheomalacia, tracheal granulomas, vocal cord dysfunction, and cosmetic deformities.[102,152,180,181]

RISKS OF PATIENT TRANSPORT

A further risk for patients who are having a tracheostomy performed is related not to the procedure itself, but to transporting patients to the operating room. The incidence of harmful events in patients during transport is 33% to 68%,[182,183] with Waddell reporting that "one patient a month suffered major cardiorespiratory collapse or death as a direct result of movement."[184] To address this issue and to reduce tracheostomy complications, Ciaglia developed the technique of PDT in 1985.[35]

PERCUTANEOUS TRACHEOSTOMY

Many descriptive series and reviews have examined short-term and long-term complications of percutaneous tracheostomy (PT)[104,158,185-195] and prospective comparisons of PT with surgical tracheostomy (ST).[196-203] By virtue of these studies, PT has become an integral part of the care of critically ill patients, with PDT the most common PT performed today.[204,205] In many institutions PT is the procedure of choice when a tracheostomy is needed for an ICU patient.[195,206]

When reading and analyzing the literature related to PT, it is essential to know which of the currently available procedures of PT are being discussed: one of the PDTs (Ciaglia Blue Rhino, Blue Dolphin, or the Portex multiple straight dilator kit), Griggs' GWDF, Fantoni's translaryngeal tracheostomy, or Frova's PercuTwist[207] (see "History" section earlier).

It is important to realize that all PDT techniques are percutaneous tracheostomies, but not all PTs are PDTs.[207] Most PTs reported in the literature have been performed using the Ciaglia dilational technique (PDT),[104,152,188,194,195,208] followed by Griggs' GWDF technique.[208] There is evident confusion with respect to the different techniques of PT, as seen in an article on surgical airway management in the ICU in which the description of PDT is that "sequential dilators are used to enlarge a tract," but the picture of the commercial kit that "has the necessary instruments" for the procedure is one of the single-dilator Blue Rhino.[209] Confusion occurs when publications describe PT performed using Portex kits (Keene, NH), but fail to clarify which of the kits that Portex makes for PT was used. One, manufactured in the United States, is made for the Ciaglia PDT technique using three straight dilators. The other is made in Europe for the Griggs GWDF technique.[38] Finally, confusion regarding technique of PT is especially evident in most published meta-analyses, with only two that compared studies of only one technique of PT (namely PDT) and ST,[210,211] and the others comparing at least two different techniques of PT to ST.[152,212-214]

Each of these techniques has its own particulars with respect to technique and complication rates. When evaluating PT techniques or comparing PT with ST, the technique that is being used must be specified.[207] This was not done in many studies of PT[207,212-214] and significantly affected the conclusions[215] of the meta-analysis of PT versus ST by Dulguerov and coworkers.[152]

Clear knowledge of the technique and complication rates of the different types of PT will allow an informed judgment as to which of the techniques should be chosen to be performed. Based on the fact mentioned earlier that most reports of PT are of Ciaglia's dilational technique, predominantly using curved dilators (either single or multiple), the most popular technique of PT seems to be PDT. In most studies that compared PT with ST, PDT was used.[196-203] One compared translaryngeal tracheostomy versus ST,[216] and two others compared GWDF technique versus ST.[217,218]

Reports by van Heerden and associates,[219] Nates and colleagues,[220] and Fikkers and coworkers[221] have compared short-term outcomes using the Griggs GWDF technique versus PDT. Van Heerden and associates[219] showed no difference in complications, Nates and colleagues[220] showed a significantly higher incidence of bleeding using the GWDF technique, and Fikkers and coworkers[221] showed a higher rate of minor procedural and postdecannulation complications in GWDF technique. Cantais and associates[222] compared GWDF technique with translaryngeal tracheostomy, finding a higher rate of serious complications in the translaryngeal tracheostomy group. Byhahn and colleagues compared PercuTwist with PDT (single dilator)[223] and found more patients in whom insertion of the cannula was difficult/impossible with the PercuTwist. Montcriol and coworkers[224] found PercuTwist to take significantly longer than GWDF technique.

In an attempt to reduce the chance of injury to the posterior tracheal wall, and to speed up the procedure, Ciaglia developed the gradually tapered soft Blue Rhino dilator in 1999.[39] Two randomized comparisons of multiple-dilator PDT with the single-dilator Blue Rhino PDT[39,225] showed a shorter procedure duration for the single-dilator PDT. Also, no intervention was required despite a statistically higher incidence of tracheal ring fracture in the single-dilator group in one study.[39] In the multiple-dilator group, there were two injuries to the posterior tracheal wall and one pneumothorax.[39] The latest development in PDT uses balloon dilation and is a true single-step procedure.[42,43] Cianchi and associates[43] found that balloon dilation took significantly longer than the single-dilator PDT and that limited intratracheal bleeding was more frequent after balloon dilation.

TECHNIQUE

The technique of PDT can be learned by attending a training course or observing the procedure, followed by assisting and performing PDT under supervision until proficiency is attained, which usually occurs after performing 10 to 20 procedures.[203] The operator's initial efforts should be performed under supervision of an experienced operator using bronchoscopic guidance,[153] in an already intubated patient. It is important to remember that there is a learning curve with this procedure. Complications are more likely to occur early in the practitioner's experience with PDT.[226]

Initially, PDT was thought to be contraindicated in emergencies, in children, in obese patients, and in patients who had a previous tracheostomy, uncorrectable coagulopathies, or severe anatomic neck deformities,[35] but its performance has been described in all of these groups except children younger than 14 years old.[54,56,57,185,186,189,195,227-232] We believe PDT remains absolutely contraindicated in young children and patients with certain severe anatomic neck deformities (e.g., fused, anterior flexed neck, overlying neck mass). An emergent PDT to establish an airway should be done only by practitioners with significant experience in the procedure.

Prior to PDT, the patient is placed on 100% oxygen, given glycopyrrolate, intravenous sedation, and a paralytic agent, and positioned supine with the neck hyperextended. The first or second tracheal interspace is identified, and the ET is positioned so that the end of the tube is proximal to the intended tracheostomy site.

The ET is usually positioned by either palpating the ET cuff to identify the tube position,[233] or using bronchoscopic guidance.[104,187,234] Besides facilitating proper tube positioning, using the bronchoscope allows direct visualization of needle insertion, ensuring midline placement and intratracheal insertion of the tracheostomy tube.[104] Marx and Ciaglia[235] who originally recommended nonendoscopic ET positioning, later recommended use of bronchoscopy. Recently, Mallick and colleagues[236] prospectively compared capnography and bronchoscopy to confirm tracheal placement, and Jackson and coworkers[237] retrospectively compared PDT with and without bronchoscopy and found no difference in complications. Other authors[232,233,238,239] do not routinely use bronchoscopy to perform PDT and recommend its use for training and in selected patients with difficult airways, which has been our experience.

The skin is anesthetized with1% lidocaine with epinephrine to prevent bleeding, a small localization needle is introduced into the tracheal lumen, and 3 to 5 mL of lidocaine injected. If a bronchoscope is not used, the ET should be gently rotated and oscillated to ensure that it was not impaled by the needle, after which a 15-gauge needle is inserted through which a guidewire is passed, and the needle removed. To ensure midline placement of the tracheostomy tube the head must remain midline throughout the procedure and the trachea fixed during dilation and tube insertion.

A 1-cm midline vertical or horizontal incision is made and a short punch dilator inserted to enlarge the tract from skin to trachea. A guiding catheter is placed over the guidewire, which remains in place for the duration of the procedure to add stiffness and facilitate passage of the dilator(s), which should be inserted at a right angle to the patient's neck. Dilation of the tract may be performed with multiple curved dilators,[35] three straight dilators,[36,233] a single tapered dilator (Blue Rhino),[39] or an expanding balloon (Blue Dolphin).[42,43] The tract is dilated until an appropriately sized tracheostomy tube (that was previously loaded on a curved obturator) can be inserted (Figs. 14.4 to 14.6, see online video of the technique of PDT). The obturator, guidewire, and guiding catheter are removed; the inner cannula is inserted; and the cuff is inflated. Breath sounds, returned tidal

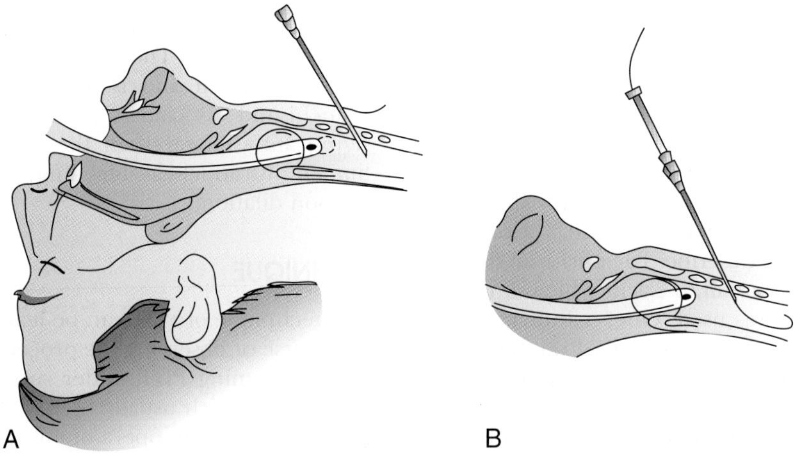

Figure 14.4 **A,** Insertion of a 15-gauge needle into the trachea. **B,** Guidewire is inserted through the needle into the trachea. (From Friedman Y, Franklin C: The technique of percutaneous tracheostomy. J Crit Illness 1993;8:289. Copyright © Margulies Medical Art, Miami, FL.)

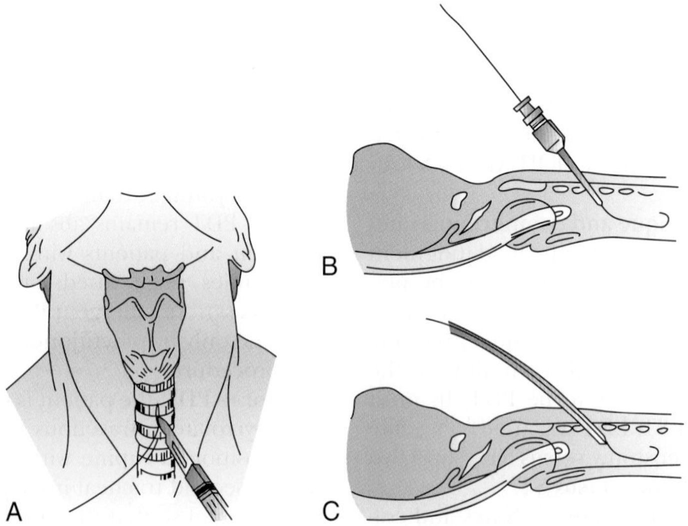

Figure 14.5 **A,** A vertical incision is made in the skin. **B,** A punch dilator is inserted. **C,** A plastic guiding catheter is introduced over the guidewire. (From Friedman Y, Franklin C: The technique of percutaneous tracheostomy. J Crit Illness 1993;8:289. Copyright © Margulies Medical Art, Miami, FL.)

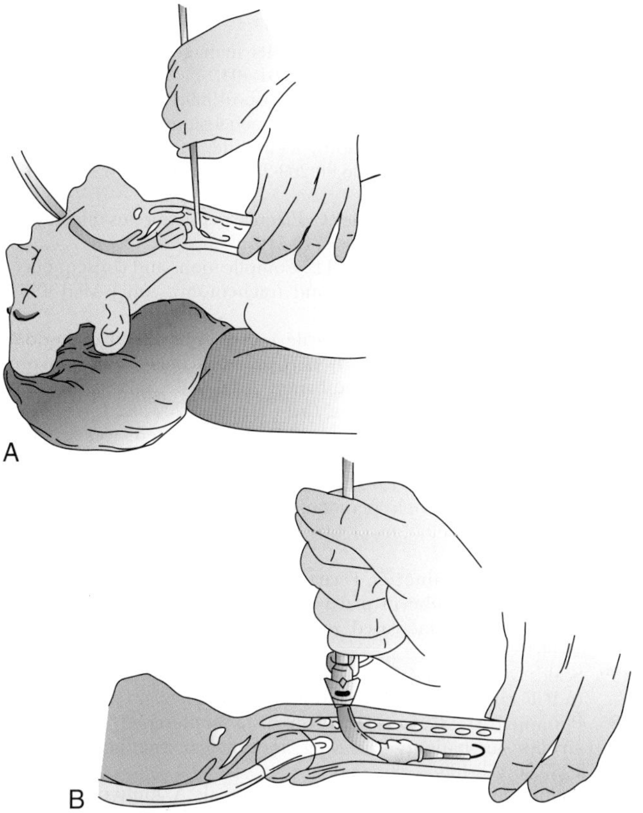

Figure 14.6 **A,** The dilator is inserted over the guidewire-guiding catheter assembly. **B,** Placement of the tracheostomy tube obturator assembly. (From Friedman Y, Franklin C: The technique of percutaneous tracheostomy. J Crit Illness 1993;8:289. Copyright © Margulies Medical Art, Miami, FL.)

volume, and cuff pressure must be checked before the tracheostomy is secured. A chest film should be obtained to verify tube position and the absence of barotrauma. In experienced hands, the procedure can be performed in less than 5 minutes.

PERCUTANEOUS DILATIONAL TRACHEOSTOMY VERSUS SURGICAL TRACHEOSTOMY

As mentioned previously, it seems that the Ciaglia PDT has become the benchmark for PT. Although other techniques have been described, none has been as widely accepted,[33,37,38,40,41,195,208,232] and some are no longer available.[33,37] Kits currently available to perform PDT contain a single tapered dilator (Cook Blue Rhino, three straight dilators [Portex], or equipment for balloon dilation [Cook Blue Dolphin]). At this point in the history of PT, PDT is the technique that should be the focus of discussion.

Nonrandomized, observational studies of PDT show short-term and long-term complication rates (e.g., mortality, paratracheal insertion, bleeding, infection, and tracheal stenosis rates),[35,36,104,153,158,185-193,195] that are comparable to or lower than those in similar studies of ST.[44,47,69,71,74,102-106,108,109] The largest observational study[195] of PDT followed 1000 patients and had an overall complication rate of only 1.4% (1.2% in normal risk and only 1.7% even in high-risk patients). The authors concluded that PDT "should be considered the gold standard in patients requiring elective tracheostomy in the ICU."

However, using these articles to justify use of PDT over ST is probably not appropriate, as they are from different eras and there are differences in technique and equipment. Also, complications may have been defined or selected differently. Thus, it is important to examine the prospective trials of PDT versus ST,[196-203,240,241] which presumably used the same definitions and procedures in both groups. The two latest and largest of these studies found that there was a shorter time to PDT once the decision was made to perform a tracheostomy.[202,241] Additionally, Silvester and associates[202] found a lower incidence of postoperative infection and a trend toward a better cosmetic sequelae in PDT, and Beltrame and colleagues[241] found that PDT was faster to perform. Others showed a lower incidence of minor in situ complications of PDT.[196,197,199]

There have been several meta-analyses comparing PT versus ST.[152,210-214] As mentioned previously, only two[210,211] examined studies that used only one technique of PT, namely PDT. The others had as many as four different techniques of PT, which will likely affect the results and conclusions of the analyses.[152,212-214] The largest single-technique meta-analysis of Freeman and coworkers[211] showed that PDT had less procedural and in situ bleeding, a lower stomal infection rate, and lower overall postoperative complications.

Finally, a recent evidence-based analysis of PT versus ST found 13 studies of PT that reached a type II level of evidence. Of the nine that used PDT, eight were prospective studies and one was a meta-analysis. Six had complication rates that favored PDT and two favored ST. However, the authors of this analysis raised several issues: (1) that the findings of improved outcomes of PDT were based on significant reduction of minor complications, but there were no differences in major complications; (2) that the patient selection was biased in favor of PDT by excluding high-risk patients; and (3) that there was no consistent long-term follow-up.[242]

What can be said is that PDT has been shown to have a shorter procedure time than ST.[196,197,241] It has also been shown to have less delay from the time the decision to perform the tracheostomy was made until the procedure was performed.[202,215,241] Some data suggest that this may shorten ICU stay and time on the ventilator (see Table 14.1). Bedside PDT eliminates the need for transport to the operating room, reducing the morbidity and mortality rates for intrahospital transport[182-184] and has been shown to be more cost-effective than ST because of decreased utilization of resources.[201]

Although the complication rate of PDT has not been shown conclusively to be lower than that of ST, it appears at least as low and may be lower. The convenience and ease of performing PDT afford flexibility in managing patients. In addition, PDT offers the advantage of avoiding the inherent morbidity and mortality risks of patient transport to the operating room and decreasing cost. Although there will always be indications for ST, either at the bedside or in the operating room, PDT seems to be a reasonable alternative that intensivists, anesthesiologists, and surgeons can and should learn to perform.

KEY POINTS

- Artificial airways are placed for one of the following indications: relieving obstruction, providing MV, preventing aspiration, or tracheobronchial toilet.
- Tracheostomy usually is performed as a replacement for a previously established airway. Whenever possible, tracheostomy should be performed in a controlled setting with an artificial airway already in place.
- As a long-term airway, a tracheostomy has several advantages over an ET (e.g., protection from laryngeal injury, airway security, patient comfort and mobility, and easier nursing care). More data are needed to determine if tracheostomy facilitates weaning, allows earlier ICU discharge, or has fewer long-term complications.
- Patients who require a tracheostomy must be identified as early as possible, and the procedure must be performed without delay to minimize the duration of translaryngeal intubation.
- Complications from tracheostomies can be procedural, in situ, or late and range from 1.4% to 27%. The mortality rate for tracheostomy is less than 1%.
- PDT is an alternative to ST. Complications, morbidity, and mortality rates are comparable with those of ST. As more practitioners become familiar with PDT, it may become the procedure of choice for ICU patients.
- Several significantly different techniques of PT have been described with different complication rates. Practitioners need to be clear about which technique of PT is being used or discussed.

SELECTED REFERENCES

2. McClelland RMA: Tracheostomy: Its management and alternatives. Proc Roy Soc Med 1972;65:401-404.
22. Jackson C: Tracheotomy. Laryngoscope 1909;19:285-290.
29. Heffner JE, Miller KS, Sahn SA: Tracheostomy in the intensive care unit: Part 1. Indications, technique, management. Part 2. Complications. Chest 1986;90:269-274 (Part 1), 1986;90:430-436 (Part 2).
35. Ciaglia P, Firsching R, Syniec C: Elective percutaneous dilatational tracheostomy. Chest 1985;87:715-719.
69. Stauffer JL, Olson DE, Petty TL: Complications and consequences of endotracheal intubation and tracheotomy. Am J Med 1981; 70:65-76.
87. Rumbak MJ, Newton M, Truncale T, et al: A prospective, randomized, study comparing early percutaneous tracheotomy to prolonged translaryngeal intubation (delayed tracheotomy) in critically ill medical patients. Crit Care Med 2004;32:1689-1694.
100. Kollef MH, Ahrens TS, Shannon W: Clinical predictors and outcomes for patients requiring tracheostomy in the intensive care unit. Crit Care Med 1999;27:1714-1720.
104. Kost KM: Endoscopic percutaneous dilatational tracheotomy: A prospective evaluation of 500 consecutive cases. Laryngoscope 2005;115:1-30.
126. Hernandez Martinez G, Fernandez R, Sanchez Casado M, et al: Tracheostomy tube in place at intensive care unit discharge is associated with increased ward mortality. Respir Care 2009;54: 1644-1652.
129. Scales DC, Kahn JM: Tracheostomy timing, enrollment and power in ICU clinical trials. Intensive Care Med 2008;34:1743-1745.
135. Plummer AL, Gracey DR: Consensus conference on artificial airways in patients receiving mechanical ventilation. Chest 1989;96:178-180.
157. Halum SL, Ting JY, Plowman EK, et al: A multi-institutional analysis of tracheostomy complications. Laryngoscope 2012; 122:38-45.
195. Kornblith LZ, Burlew CC, Moore EE, et al: One thousand bedside percutaneous tracheostomies in the surgical intensive care unit: Time to change the gold standard. J Am Coll Surg 2011;212: 163-170.
207. Friedman Y: Percutaneous tracheostomy: What technique is it? Crit Care Med 2001;29:1289-1290.
242. Pappas S, Maragoudakis P, Vlastarakos P, et al: Surgical versus percutaneous tracheostomy: An evidence-based approach. Eur Arch Otorhinolaryngol 2011;266:323-330.

The complete list of references can be found at www.expertconsult.com.

Chest Tube Thoracostomy

15

Vincent E. Lotano

CHAPTER OUTLINE

Chest thoracostomy chest tubes can be lifesaving. Decisions regarding chest tubes can be confusing, however, and chest tubes can be dangerous if placed when not indicated or by inexperienced personnel without proper supervision. The technique, indications, and potential complications of chest tubes should be well known to health care personnel working in the intensive care unit (ICU), as should management after placement. A nonfunctioning or malpositioned chest tube provides misleading information to the managing clinicians.

HISTORY

Hippocrates drained an empyema using a metal tube.[1] Playfair developed underwater seal drainage of chest tubes in 1875.[2] Credit for the invention of the chest tube is usually given to Hewett,[3] who in 1876 devised a system of continuous drainage of the empyema cavity using a rubber catheter that drained into a glass jar filled with a weakly antiseptic solution.[4] Use of the chest tube was not widely adopted, however, until the 1917 influenza epidemic.[5] Closed tube thoracostomy drainage of the pleural space after thoracotomy was first reported by Lilienthal in 1922.[6]

ANATOMY AND PHYSIOLOGY OF THE PLEURAL SPACE

The pleural space is the interface between the chest wall and the lung and represents a critical component of pulmonary function. The visceral and parietal pleurae are composed of a single layer of mesothelium. The blood supply of the parietal pleura is of systemic origin (intercostal vessels), whereas the blood supply of the visceral pleura is of pulmonary origin (pulmonary artery and veins). The bronchial arteries may contribute significantly to the blood supply of the visceral surface.[7]

Both pleural surfaces are lined by an extensive lymphatic network that ultimately drains into the thoracic duct via the mediastinal (visceral) and intercostal (parietal) lymph nodes. There are extensive communications between lymphatics above and below the diaphragm.

Pleural fluid may originate from three sources—parietal capillaries, visceral capillaries, or interstitium. Starling's law of transcapillary exchange governs the movement of fluid across the pleural space. The pressure in the capillaries of the visceral pleura is less than that in the parietal capillaries because it drains into the pulmonary venous bed. The net hydrostatic pressure (35 cm H_2O) favors movement of fluid from the parietal pleura to the pleural space (Fig. 15.1). This pressure is derived from the subtraction of −5 cm H_2O (pleural pressure) from 30 cm H_2O (parietal hydrostatic pressure). This net hydrostatic pressure is opposed by the net oncotic pressure (29 cm H_2O), which is derived from the subtraction of 5 cm H_2O (pleural oncotic pressure) from 34 cm H_2O (plasma oncotic pressure). A gradient of 6 cm H_2O (34 − 29 cm H_2O) favors pleural fluid formation.[8] The pleural lymphatics prevent the accumulation of this pleural fluid. Stomas, unique to the parietal pleura, facilitate communication between the pleural space and the capillaries. It is estimated that this mechanism allows clearance of 20 mL of pleural fluid per hour per hemithorax in a 70-kg human.[9,10] The lymphatic network clears protein from the pleural space; smaller molecules can be directly absorbed by the pleural capillaries. Intercostal and diaphragmatic muscle activity influences the rate of lymphatic flow. Hypoventilation and anesthesia reduce lymphatic flow and the rate of absorption of protein.[11]

DRAINAGE SYSTEMS

The original three-bottle system has been compartmentalized into a plastic unit that is easily transportable and readily pressure-adjustable, consisting of a trap bottle, a water-seal bottle, and a manometer bottle (Fig. 15.2). The trap bottle collects the pleural fluid. The water-seal bottle prevents air from returning to the pleural space during the negative pleural pressure phase on inspiration. The manometer bottle uses the distance below its fluid line to generate a negative pressure when suction is applied. For example, 20 cm of water generates a −20 cm H_2O pressure.[12] Modern collection and suction systems use a single compartmentalized system (Fig. 15.3).

INDICATIONS AND CONTRAINDICATIONS

SIMPLE PNEUMOTHORAX

Pneumothorax is defined as air that has entered the pleural space, either spontaneously or as a result of traumatic tears in the pleura after chest injury or after invasive procedures. Treatment of pneumothorax entails removing air from the pleural space, reexpanding the underlying lung, and preventing recurrence.[13] If the patient is clinically stable, the treatment depends on the size of the pneumothorax and whether or not the patient is mechanically ventilated. If the pneumothorax is small, and the patient is not mechanically ventilated, the pneumothorax can be observed. If the pneumothorax is large, or the patient is mechanically ventilated, a chest tube should be placed.[14] A large pneumothorax is defined as being greater than 15% to 20%.[15] Needle aspiration has also been described as a consideration for treatment of spontaneous pneumothorax. However, a repeat chest radiograph must be obtained to assure no recurrence in which case a chest tube would be required.[16]

If an occult pneumothorax is identified, which is a pneumothorax found incidentally on computed tomography (CT) scan without evidence clinically or on chest radiograph, observation may be an option. The optimal management remains controversial with regard to tube placement; however, two retrospective reviews demonstrate safe observation without tube placement in patients requiring positive-pressure ventilation.[17,18]

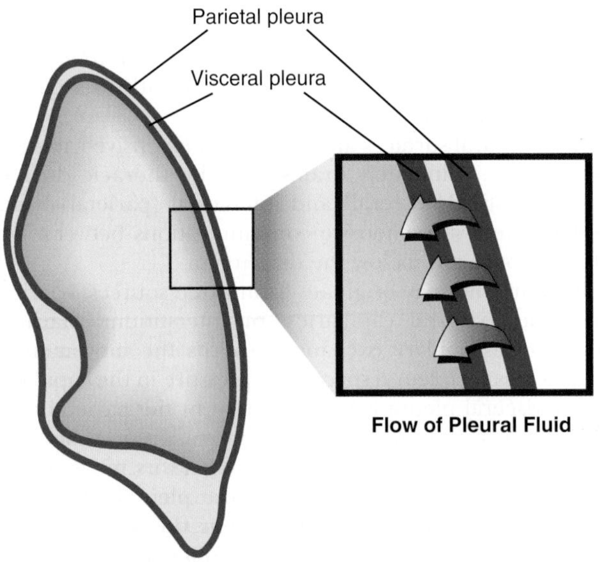

Figure 15.1 The direction of fluid movement across the pleural space is shown, moving from the parietal through the visceral pleural surface where transport into the lymphatic system occurs.

TENSION PNEUMOTHORAX

Tension pneumothorax is a life-threatening clinical situation that requires emergent and immediate treatment (Fig. 15.4). Air collects and builds up pressure in the chest cavity through a tear in the lung or bronchial tree. Air enters the chest with each mechanical or spontaneous breath, with no route for escape. Initially, the affected lung simply collapses, but as tension increases, the diaphragm flattens, and the mediastinum is shifted toward the contralateral side.[19] The contralateral lung is compressed, further decreasing effective ventilation. The great vessels also are compressed, and venous return is reduced drastically. This reduction in venous return results in rapid and disastrous cardiopulmonary collapse.[20] The diagnosis is ideally made on a clinical basis, and treatment is initiated without waiting for radiographic confirmation. Any tension pneumothorax should have immediate large-bore needle decompression. A readily available large-bore angiocatheter is preferentially inserted in the second intercostal space at the midclavicular line. A rush of pleural air under pressure confirms the diagnosis and location. After decompression (conversion to a simple pneumothorax), the catheter is left in until a tube thoracostomy has been placed.[21]

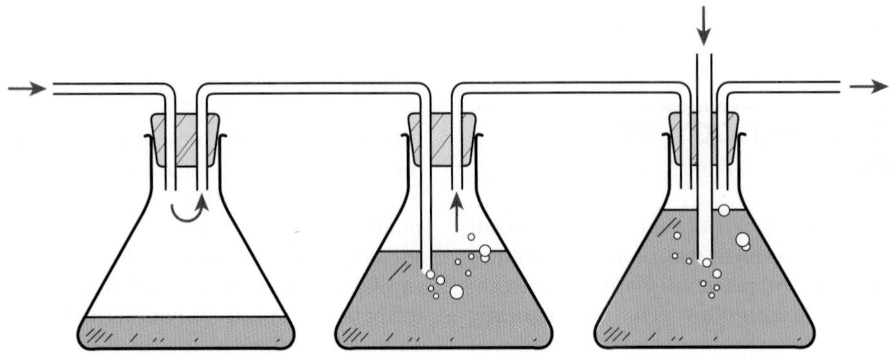

Figure 15.2 Three-bottle system consisting of (from *left to right*) trap bottle, water-seal bottle, and manometer bottle.

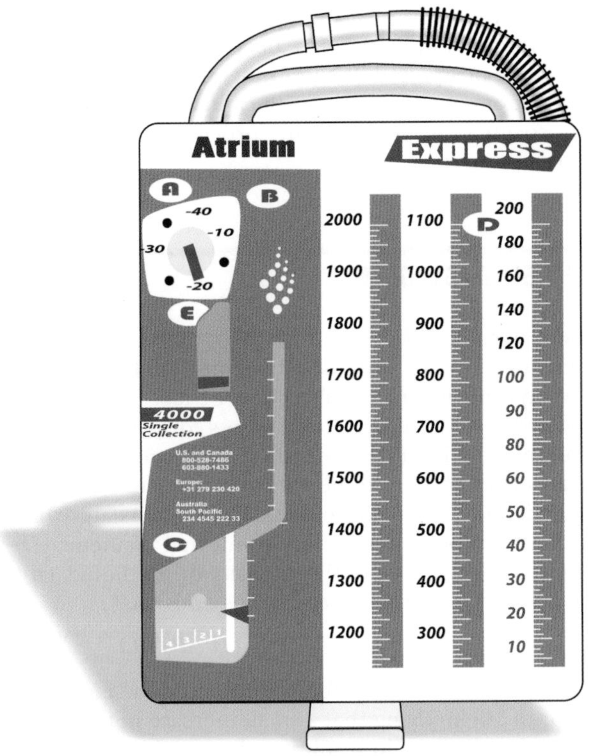

Figure 15.3 Modern drainage system.

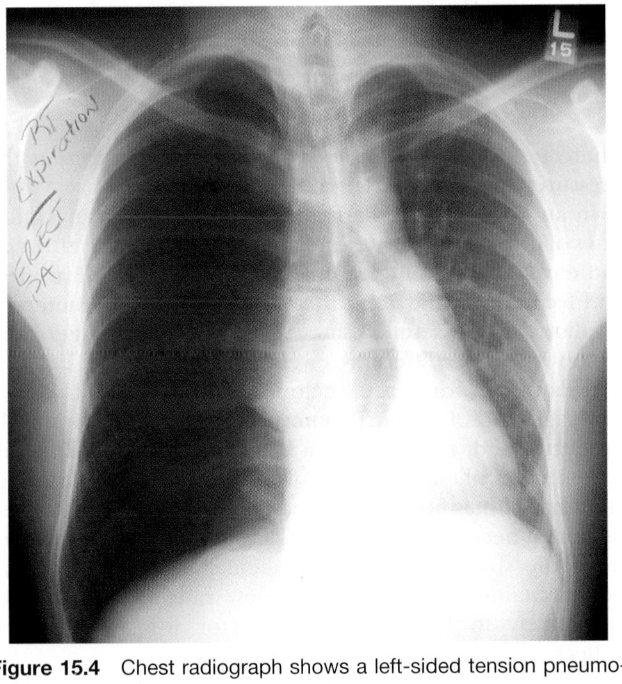

Figure 15.4 Chest radiograph shows a left-sided tension pneumothorax with mediastinal shift to the right.

PLEURAL EFFUSIONS

Pleural effusions, both transudative and exudative, are frequently seen in the ICU. The incidence of pleural effusions in the ICU varies with screening methods, from approximately 8% for physical examination to more than 60% for routine ultrasound.[22,23] Several factors contribute to the occurrence of pleural effusions in ICU patients. Large amounts of intravenous fluid are often administered during the first few days to patients admitted for shock. Pneumonia also is common as a reason for ICU admission and as a complication of mechanical ventilation. Heart failure, atelectasis, hypoalbuminemia, and liver disease are present in many ICU patients. In surgical ICUs, cardiac or abdominal surgery is often followed by specific, large, protracted pleural effusion; in multiple-injury patients, hemothorax is possible.[24] The criteria of Light and colleagues,[25] which are based on the ratio of protein or lactate dehydrogenase levels in the pleural fluid and blood, differentiate exudates from transudates with a negative predictive value of 96% and a sensitivity of 98%.[24]

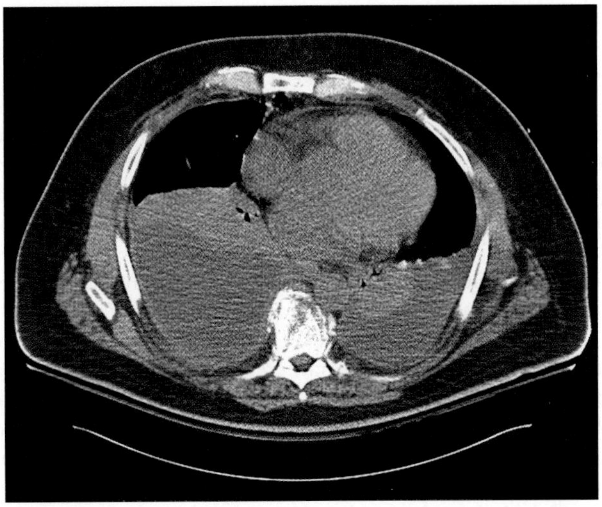

Figure 15.5 An empyema is shown in the right pleural space. Note the thickened pleura surrounding the collection, characteristic of this diagnosis.

Provided that basic rules are followed, thoracentesis is safe in ICU patients.[22] A chest tube may be placed for large or symptomatic pleural effusions. The optimal drainage duration for uninfected pleural effusions has not been established. A reasonable approach may be to remove the chest tubes when drainage decreases to less than 200 mL/day.[26]

In the evaluation of a parapneumonic effusion or empyema, if the thickness of the pleural fluid is more than 10 mm on a decubitus radiograph, or if the pleural fluid is of similar depth and loculated, the pleural fluid should be examined to determine the stage of the effusion. Drainage of an infected pleural space is required to achieve source control as a key component of treatment (Fig. 15.5). If the fluid is removed completely and does not reaccumulate, no additional therapy need be directed toward the effusion. At the time of the initial therapeutic thoracentesis, the pleural fluid should be sent for Gram stain and culture and analysis of leukocyte, lactate dehydrogenase, glucose, and pH levels. Indicators of a poor prognosis from the pleural fluid include positive Gram stain or culture, glucose less than 60 mg/dL, lactate dehydrogenase more than three times the upper limits of normal for serum, or pH less than 7.20.

If the therapeutic thoracentesis removes all of the pleural fluid and the fluid recurs, the next step is guided by the initial pleural fluid findings. If none of the poor prognostic indicators is present, no invasive procedures are indicated if the patient is doing well clinically. If any of the poor prognostic indicators were present at the initial thoracentesis, a second therapeutic thoracentesis should be performed, and the pleural fluid should be reanalyzed. If the pleural fluid accumulates a third time, a small chest tube should be inserted into the pleural space, unless none of the poor prognostic factors were present at the time of the second thoracentesis.[27] If the patient shows signs of systemic infection, and fluids have been inadequately drained, an open thoracotomy and drainage may be required.[28,29]

When a hemothorax is suspected, the essential management, along with appropriate resuscitation, is intercostal drainage. This achieves two objectives: first, to drain the pleural space, allowing expansion of the lung, and second, to allow assessment of rates of continuing blood loss. After satisfactory resolution of hemothorax managed with intercostal drainage alone, the drain should not be removed too promptly. Other circumstances permitting, the patient should be mobilized fully with adequate thoracic physiotherapy. These measures should allow optimal drainage of the pleural cavity.[30] Complete drainage of blood also prevents empyema and fibrothorax.[31]

Pneumomediastinum is usually a self-limited entity (Fig. 15.6). It follows alveolar rupture into the pulmonary interstitium and is produced by an acute episode of high intrathoracic pressure. The differential diagnosis includes cardiac, pulmonary, musculoskeletal, and esophageal causes. Spontaneous pneumomediastinum is usually a self-limited clinical entity.[32] Coupled with positive-pressure ventilation or subcutaneous emphysema, however, cautious observation is recommended owing to the possibility of a pneumothorax leading to tension pneumothorax.

There is no good evidence to support prophylactic chest tubes with high levels of positive end-expiratory pressure. These tubes may be difficult to place and may create more issues. A patient on high positive end-expiratory pressure should be closely observed for any evidence of pneumothorax. If this should occur, a chest tube should be placed at that time.

Contraindications to chest tube placement are mainly relative. The most common would be coagulopathy. If the draining indication is less than urgent and can be delayed until the coagulopathy can be corrected, the procedure should be postponed. If chest tube placement is emergently needed, one must proceed with caution and actively correct the coagulation issues while proceeding with the tube thoracostomy.

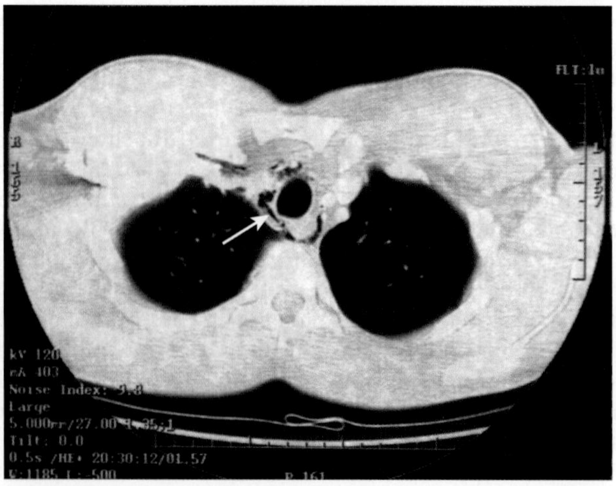

Figure 15.6 Pneumomediastinum (*arrow*). The pneumomediastinum occurred during a forceful singing period.

CHEST TUBE SIZE

There is some difference of expert opinion as to optimal chest tube size for various indications. Medicine in general is always moving in the direction of less invasive, smaller, more focused and direct treatments for issues that require some type of intervention. Chest drainage is no different. In an effort to determine the best size tube, two laws are quoted. The first is Poiseuille's law, which states that flow through a tube depends on the internal diameter (D) and length (L) of the tube, the viscosity of the liquid (η), and the pressure difference between its ends (ΔP):

$$\text{Flow rate} = (\pi/128)\,(D^4 \Delta P/\eta L)$$

If the diameter of the tube is doubled, flow increases by a factor of 16, implying that a small increase in the size of the drainage tubes would result in substantial improvements in the flow rates.[33]

Another formula key to chest tube size selection is the flow rate of the air or the liquid that can be accommodated by the tube. The Fanning equation determines the flow of moist gas with turbulent flow characteristics through a chest tube:

$$v = p^2 r^5 P/fl$$

where v is the flow, r is the radius, l is the length, P is the pressure, and f is the friction factor.[12,34-36]

In an in vitro study, Park and coworkers[37] measured flow rates of different viscosity fluids (serous, blood, pus) through catheters of different diameters, ranging from 6F to 18F, and found that flow rates increased for larger catheters as predicted by Poiseuille's law. At catheter sizes larger than 7F, however, the differences were small.

Reports on drainage techniques suggest that before drainage of a collection, diagnostic needle aspiration should be performed, initially with a 22-gauge needle and, if this is unsuccessful, subsequently with a 20-gauge or 18-gauge cannula.[38] It has been postulated that if pus can be aspirated by such a needle, it should be drainable through a catheter twice the size (i.e., >6F).[39] As such, if drain patency can be maintained, the maximum flow rate of the catheter is unlikely to be the limiting factor for most pleural collections.[33]

Given the variety of liquids and accompanying pleural debris that may be drained by a chest tube, no single formula exists for flow of these many materials. The principal determinants of airflow through a tube, bore and length, are logically key determinants of flow for various pleural liquids, including blood and pus. Chest tube selection must take into account not only what material is being drained but also its rate of formation. Ongoing production of more viscous fluids requires a larger bore tube than for a similar volume of air produced.[40]

In our institution, we have had good success with small tubes placed under radiologic guidance into empyema cavities. These small catheters also have complemented larger tubes that have drained most of the chest but have left small residual pockets, which would be difficult to access blindly with large, less flexible tubes.[41]

TECHNIQUE OF INSERTION

When inserting a chest drain for the first time, regardless of the technique, the procedure should be proctored by an experienced supervisor whenever possible. The procedure can be lifesaving or life-threatening, depending on how it is done. Many things should be verified before any skin incision or needlestick is performed. The patient should be well informed as to what is going to happen and why and must give consent. The chest radiograph should be present at the procedure, and the date, patient's name, and affected side should be confirmed by the operator and one other health care professional. Next, all instruments should be confirmed to be present at the procedure. Someone should be available to get additional items needed during the procedure and to reassure the patient during the procedure.

Mild sedation or anxiolysis is typically needed before the procedure, and intravenous access is essential for the ability to give intravenous pain medication. If the procedure is done carefully and with good local anesthesia, there is usually minimal to no need for intravenous sedation. Coagulation parameters (i.e., prothrombin time, partial thromboplastin, and platelets) should be confirmed to be normal or, if abnormal, adequate for coagulation (typically platelet count 50,000/μL and international normalized ratio ≤1.5 IU). Most hospitals have closed tube thoracostomy trays premade; however, the components that should be available are as follows[42]:

1. Skin antiseptic solution
2. Sterile drapes
3. Syringes—10 mL × 3
4. Needles—21-gauge, 23-gauge, 25-gauge
5. Local anesthesia—1% or 2% 10 mL lidocaine
6. Scalpel—No. 11 or 15 blade
7. Sutures—2-0 silk (to anchor tube) and 3-0 nylon (to close site when tube is removed if desired)
8. Heavy scissors
9. Drain sponge dressings and 4 × 4 dressings
10. Curved hemostat clamps
11. Clamp for chest tube
12. Underwater seal collection system
13. Sterile chest tube—sizes 24F and 32F (depending on what is found to be drained; blood or pus should be 32F, air or fluid can be 24F)
14. Syringes or specimen cups for culture

The patient should be positioned supine with the head of the bed elevated to 30 degrees and the arm held behind the head or abducted to 90 degrees if placement behind the head is impossible. Mark the site of insertion with indelible marker so it is not removed with the skin preparation.

Insertion should be in the "safe triangle" illustrated in Figure 15.7. This is the triangle formed by the anterior border of the latissimus dorsi, the lateral border of the pectoralis major muscle, a line superior to the horizontal level of the nipple, and an apex below the axilla. The most common position for chest tube insertion is in the midaxillary line, through the safe triangle. This position minimizes risk to underlying structures such as the internal mammary artery and avoids damage to muscle and breast tissue resulting in scarring. A more posterior position may be chosen if suggested by the presence of a loculus, although this site is more uncomfortable for the patient, and there is a risk of the drain kinking.[43]

The patient should be prepared and draped in sterile fashion with a wide field (Fig. 15.8), and the operator should be wearing sterile gown, gloves, hat, and mask. Local

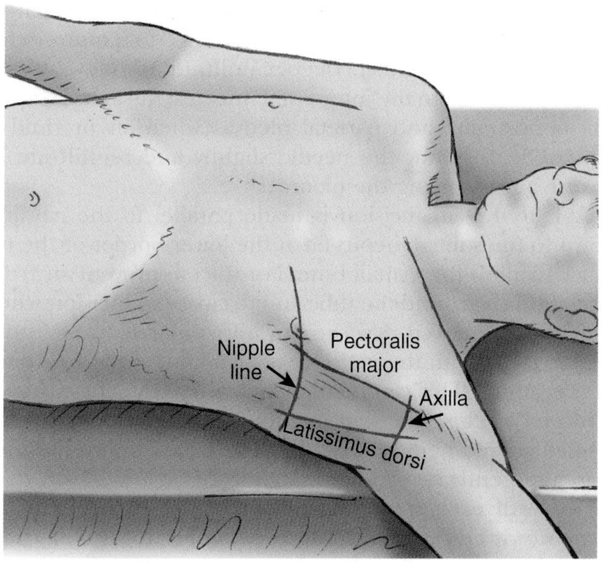

Figure 15.7 Position of patient and safe triangle for identification of injection site.

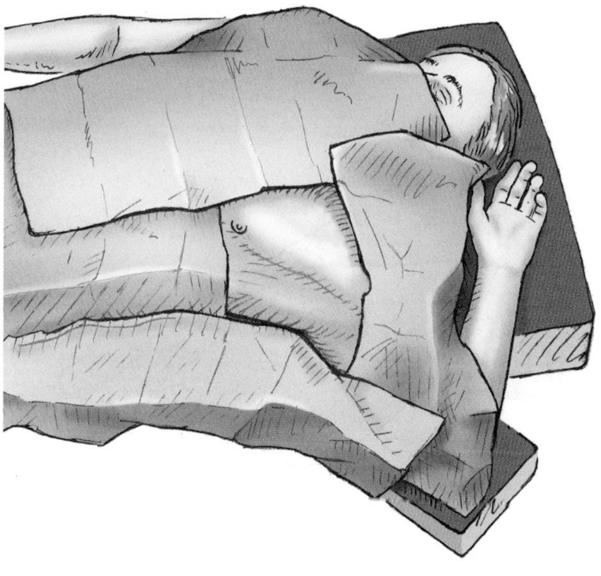

Figure 15.8 Prepared field for chest tube placement.

anesthesia should be instilled with a 23-gauge or 25-gauge needle making a skin wheal and allowing 2 to 5 minutes for anesthetic to take effect. Deeper infiltration follows with a 21-gauge needle to the intercostal muscles, the area over the rib, periosteum, and parietal pleura (when air or fluid is aspirated, withdraw the needle slightly and reinfiltrate to ensure anesthetizing the pleura).[42]

A 1- to 1.5-cm incision is made parallel to the rib and down to the subcutaneous fat at the lower border of the rib space to allow for a small tunnel or tract to prevent air from being drawn around the tube and to close the incision when the tube is removed. A vertical or horizontal mattress suture is placed through the incision, tying a knot at the free ends of the suture. This can be used later when the chest tube is removed to close the skin incision. A tract is created using a small curved hemostat by inserting it closed into the incision and gently spreading. It should be removed and reinserted with each spreading maneuver.[44] This needs to be done slowly and carefully to prevent pain; this is done multiple times continuously using gentle forward pressure toward the upper border of the rib at the intercostal space to be entered. The right hand opens and closes the instrument, and the left hand is placed close to the tip to prevent plunging into the chest (Fig. 15.9). When the intercostal muscle has been dissected, the pleura is entered. There is a rush of air or fluid. When possible, a gloved finger should be inserted into the chest cavity to ensure there are no adhesions between the lung and the chest wall. This is most important if the patient has had a history of multiple chest tubes or thoracic surgery.

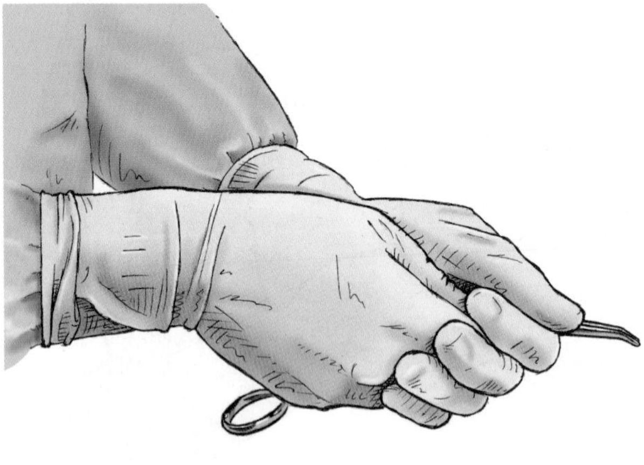

Figure 15.9 Position of hands on hemostat or clamp to minimize iatrogenic injury.

Before beginning the procedure, the tube should be prepared and placed on the sterile field within easy reach. A closed clamp may be passed through the distal hole and out the end of the tube to facilitate placement (Fig. 15.10). This technique may be easier than trying to open the clamp in the intercostal space to advance the chest tube. The tube can then be passed over the clamp in a Seldinger-type technique. Another method is to place the tube in the clamp prior to insertion into the chest. The tube should be positioned against the outside curve of the clamp (see Fig. 15.10). When placed, the tube should be clamped at the distal end to prevent leakage. The tube should be connected to the tubing in a sterile fashion. The clamp can then be removed. Reexpansion of a longstanding pneumothorax may be painful, and reexpansion should be done slowly with use of intermittent clamping. This also is true for chronic pneumothorax and pleural effusions to avoid reexpansion pulmonary edema. Onset of coughing may be a sign of onset of reexpansion pulmonary edema, at which point the clamp should be reapplied. Reexpansion pulmonary edema is discussed later in the section on complications. The tube should be anchored in place with heavy silk suture, and sterile dressings should be applied. A chest radiograph should be obtained and reviewed.

MANAGEMENT OF THORACOSTOMY TUBES

A malfunctioning chest tube can be more dangerous than no chest tube at all. Tension pneumothorax may not be considered as a cause of hypotension if a drainage catheter is in the pleural space; however, if the catheter is not functioning properly, a tension pneumothorax may still be present. In the ICU, especially in the presence of positive-pressure ventilation, a chest tube should be assessed as frequently as any vital sign, ensuring that the tube is patent and draining. If a moderate or large air leak suddenly stops, the tube should be assessed immediately to ensure the tube is not kinked or plugged.

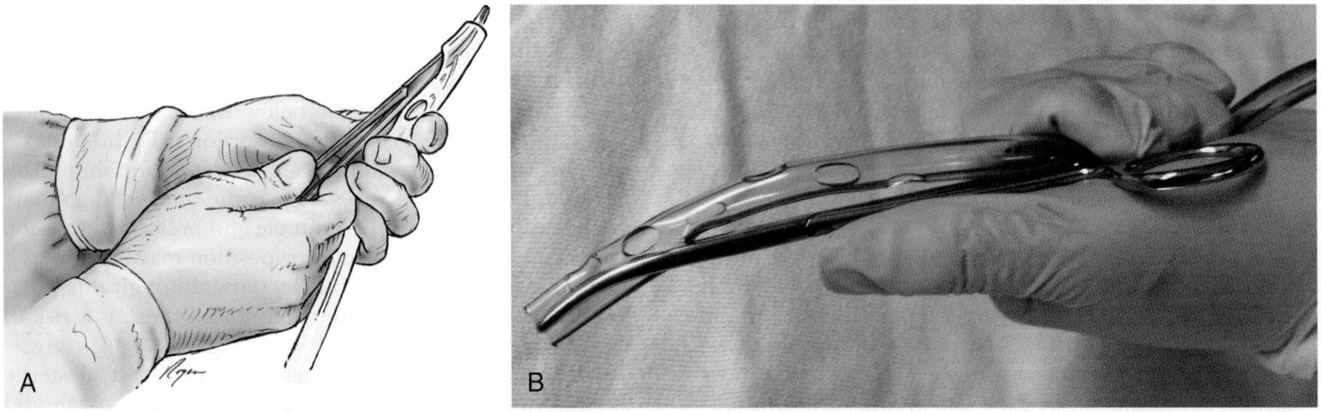

Figure 15.10 Insertion of clamp through distal hole of chest tube to facilitate proper placement of chest tube.

When a thoracic drain has been placed, a chest radiograph should be obtained immediately and reviewed. This is done to confirm placement and assess success of intervention. The amount and character of the drainage or air leak or both should be assessed. A chest radiograph should be done every day for as long as the tube is in place.[45,46] There is an ongoing debate as to whether to place a tube to water seal or suction when an air leak is present. In two studies of postoperative patients, it was shown that water seal was superior to suction in stopping air leak.[47,48] In the presence of a large air leak, however, if the pneumothorax increases or a subcutaneous emphysema develops, the tube should be placed back to suction (usually 20 cm H_2O), and a chest radiograph should be immediately obtained. If there is no air leak for 24 hours, and the drainage is less than 2 mL/kg/day, it is safe to remove the tube.[49] One protocol option begins with thoracostomy tubes placed to 20 cm H_2O suction immediately after insertion.[45] Tubes are usually assessed for air leak and drainage. Suction is continued if an air leak is present, or if the drainage is greater than or equal to 200 mL in 24 hours. If these criteria are not met, the tubes are placed to water seal. Chest radiographs are not obtained routinely on water seal or before removal. If no air leak is present after 6 hours on water seal, the tube is removed.[50] If a tube is nonfunctioning, it should be removed. If one chooses to place the tube to water seal before removal, a chest radiograph obtained 3 hours after water seal excludes development of a clinically significant pneumothorax.[51]

Clamping a chest drain before removal may be necessary. If an air leak is small and intermittent, clamping followed by chest film may help determine if the patient is likely to develop a pneumothorax after removal.[52] The house staff and nursing staff must be fully informed, however, so the tube can be immediately unclamped if there is any respiratory difficulty. Clamping of the chest tube in the face of massive hemothorax (1500 mL on placement) also has been advocated; however, in a study creating hemothorax spontaneously in piglets, chest tube clamping did not decrease hemorrhage or mortality rate but worsened gas exchange without improving hypotension.[53]

There are no data to support prophylactic antibiotic use for chest tube placement in the ICU in nontrauma patients. In traumatic hemothorax, multiple factors, including the condition under which the tube is inserted (emergent or urgent), the mechanism of injury, retained hemothorax, and ventilator care, contribute to development of pleural space infection. The incidence of empyema ranges between 0% and 18% and is decreased with the use of prophylactic antibiotics. Administration of antibiotics for longer than 24 hours does not reduce this risk further.[54]

Obtaining a chest film after removal of a chest tube has been standard practice at most institutions. Timing usually ranges from 6 to 24 hours after the tube is removed. Two retrospective studies and one prostpective study concluded that it is unnecessary to obtain routine chest radiographs after chest tube removal.[55-57] Other authors advocate obtaining a single upright chest radiograph 24 hours after chest tube removal to evaluate for recurrence of hemothorax or pneumothorax.[56] In a mechanically ventilated patient, a chest film should be obtained after chest drain removal. A study by Pizano and colleagues[58] of 214 patients undergoing positive-pressure ventilation concluded that the number of clinically significant pneumothoraces after chest tube removal seems to be small. The concern persists, however, regarding expansion of a small pneumothorax into a tension pneumothorax. Failure to diagnose a large and expanding pneumothorax could lead to a life-threatening situation. Pizano and colleagues[58] supported obtaining a chest film within 3 hours after chest tube removal. It also seemed safe to remove a chest tube from patients undergoing positive-pressure ventilation if standard removal criteria were met.[58,59]

Routine milking and stripping of chest tubes is performed primarily in postoperative cardiac surgical patients. The data do not support routine milking and stripping unless there is clot in the tubing. A significant negative pressure can be generated in the chest during the procedure and could be detrimental. Few such complications are cited in the literature, however.[60]

Postplacement chest radiograph may raise the question of placement in the fissure of the lung, potentially compromising function. This may lead to manipulation to change position. Chest tubes appearing to be in the pleural fissure on plain radiograph function as effectively, however, as tubes located elsewhere in the pleural space.[61,62]

The positioning of the tubing connecting the chest tube to the drainage system is important. In one study, three tubing positions were studied: straight, coiled, and dependent loop (allowing fluid to collect in a dependent loop with the loop left alone in some, and periodically lifted and drained at 15-minute intervals in others). It was found that the dependent loop left alone did not drain adequately. The straight and coiled positions were optimal for drainage of fluid. If the dependent loop cannot be avoided, lifting and draining it every 15 minutes would maintain adequate drainage.[63]

Removal of a chest tube is associated with pain. In one study, 4 mg of intravenous morphine was given 20 minutes before removal versus 30 mg of intravenous ketorolac given 60 minutes before removal. Either of these regimens was found to reduce pain substantially during chest tube removal without causing adverse sedative effects.[64] Another study compared topical lidocaine-prilocaine cream (EMLA) versus intravenous morphine. The investigators found that topical EMLA cream was more effective, but it had to be applied 3 hours before chest tube removal.[65]

Removal of the chest tube must be timed with the breathing pattern of the patient. Some authors advocate removal at end inspiration, whereas others recommend removal at end expiration. The reason some advocate end inspiration is that when the tube is removed the patient may gasp from the pain and may be more likely to suck in air through the site. In one study, a similar rate of postremoval pneumothorax was found. Both methods were found to be safe.[66] There are two ways to close the sites after the tube has been removed. If sutures were placed, they are tied down. If no sutures were placed, an occlusive dressing must be made with 4 × 4 dressings and tape and petroleum jelly gauze.

COMPLICATIONS

Complications of chest tube placement include improper positioning, bleeding, nerve damage, injury to diaphragm or abdominal organs, mechanical problems, pain, and bronchopleural fistula. There are multiple case reports identifying issues including atrial fibrillation, pleurocutaneous fistula, extrathoracic herniation of a lung bulla, chylothorax, and neuropathies.[67-76] Any structure or organ in the chest or upper abdomen can be damaged or perforated with chest tube insertion. The heart, lung, aorta, vena cava, pulmonary artery, nerves, liver, spleen, and stomach all are vulnerable. Damage is more likely to occur with the use of a trocar, but can occur if the clamp dissecting through the intercostal space is not controlled by the operator. A sudden thrust into the chest, especially in a small chest, can easily reach the mediastinum.

Reexpansion pulmonary edema is a rare and potentially lethal complication of tube placement for pneumothorax, pleural effusion, and severe atelectasis (Fig. 15.11).[77] The estimated mortality rate is 20%.[78] Onset of symptoms is often immediate, but can be delayed 24 hours.[78] Severe coughing heralds the development of pulmonary edema. The patient becomes tachypneic and tachycardic as hypoxia increases. The patient does not respond to oxygen therapy because blood is shunted past fluid-filled alveoli. Rarely, bilateral or contralateral edema develops.[79] The pathophysiology is complex. Multiple factors contribute to a capillary bed with increased permeability. An inflammatory response occurs when the lung reexpands. This response is believed to be secondary to expansion-related mechanical injury to the alveolar-capillary membrane and reperfusion injury as blood flow returns to the now fully expanded lung.[80] Patients 20 to 39 years old are more susceptible.[81] The duration of pneumothorax also has been implicated in the incidence of reexpansion pulmonary edema.[82] Early case series found that spontaneous pneumothorax was present an average of 14 days with a minimum of 3 days before edema would develop.[83] The severity of the pneumothorax may be more predictive than its duration in developing pulmonary edema. In the series by Matsuura and coworkers,[81] no patient with a pneumothorax less than 30% of the lung field developed pulmonary edema. Seventeen percent of patients with total collapse and 44% of patients with tension pneumothorax had this complication. Some authors support slow reexpansion by lower negative pressure as beneficial, whereas others support the idea that it is not so much the degree of negative pressure as the rate of reexpansion that is important.[82] In clinically stable patients with a large (30% of the lung field) primary pneumothorax, the American College of Chest Physicians recommends either small-bore (≤14F) catheter or 16F to 22F chest tube placement.[14] Connection to a Heimlich valve or a water-seal device is recommended. If the lung fails to reexpand, suction is deemed appropriate.

The mainstay of therapy remains oxygenation, a low threshold for mechanical ventilation with positive end-expiratory pressure, diuresis if it can be tolerated, and hemodynamic support. Reexpansion pulmonary edema usually resolves in 24 to 72 hours.[80]

IMAGING

Areas in the chest that require chest tube drainage may be loculated owing to adhesions from pneumonias or multiple chest tube placements, making it difficult and dangerous to place a drain blindly into the chest. The use of ultrasound or CT guidance can be invaluable.[84] Ultrasound and CT also can be used to verify location of tubes previously placed. In one study, 51 pigtail catheters placed under radiologic guidance (CT or ultrasound) were reviewed, with an overall success rate of 88%. The specific success rates were 92%, 85%, and 91% for loculated pleural effusion, pneumothorax, and empyema, respectively. Complications were few and minor.[85]

A chest radiograph should be performed immediately after chest drain placement, but the position of the tube may still be in question. CT has proved to be useful when this occurs (Fig. 15.12). Placement locations such as

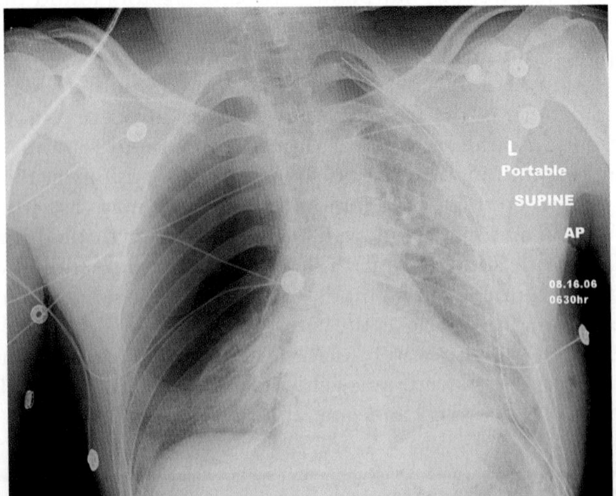

Figure 15.11 Chest radiograph shows reexpansion pulmonary edema on left and giant blebs on right.

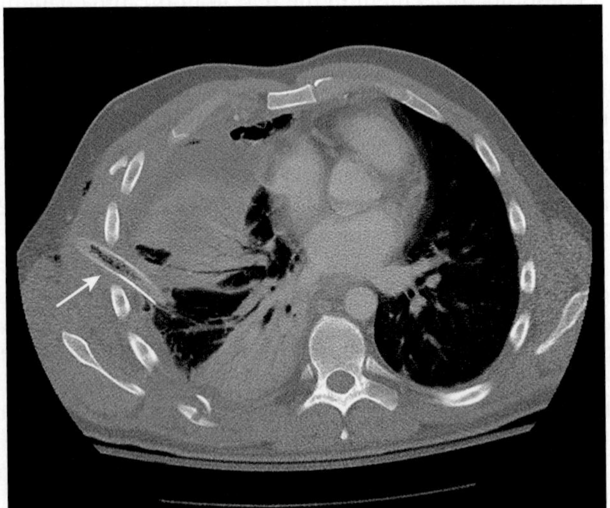

Figure 15.12 Computed tomography scan shows a loculated pleural effusion with chest tube location (indicated by *arrow*).

intraparenchymal, intrafissural, mediastinal, chest wall, and abdominal may be identified.[86] In a study in which CT revealed 28 malpositioned chest tubes among 76 tubes placed in 54 patients, frontal chest radiograph revealed only 6 of the 28.[87]

KEY POINTS

- Chest tube selection must take into account not only what material is being drained but also its rate of formation.
- When inserting a chest drain for the first time, the procedure should be proctored by an experienced supervisor.
- The chest radiograph should be present at the procedure, and the date, patient's name, and affected side should be confirmed by the operator and one other health care professional.
- Insertion should be in the "safe triangle."
- In the ICU, especially in the presence of positive-pressure ventilation, a chest tube should be assessed as frequently as any other vital sign.
- There are no data to support prophylactic antibiotic use for chest tube placement in the ICU in nontrauma patients.
- The mainstay in therapy for reexpansion pulmonary edema remains oxygenation, a low threshold for mechanical ventilation, diuresis (if tolerated), and hemodynamic support.
- CT has proved to be extremely accurate in evaluating the position of a chest tube.

SELECTED REFERENCES

67. Maritz D, Wallis L, Hardcastle T: Complications of tube thoracostomy for chest trauma. S Afr Med J 2009;99(2):114-117. Erratum in S Afr Med J 2009;99(3):130.
68. Hsu KF, Wang HB, Hsieh CB: Refractory atrial fibrillation following tube thoracostomy. Can Med Assoc J 2010;182(3):280. Epub 2010 Feb 1.
69. Menger R, Telford G, Kim P, et al: Complications following thoracic trauma managed with tube thoracostomy. Injury 2012;43(1):46-50. Epub 2011 Aug 11.
70. Lin MT, Shih JY, Lee YC, Yang PC: Pleurocutaneous fistula after tube thoracostomy: Sonographic findings. J Clin Ultrasound 2008;36(8):523-525.
71. Okur E, Tezel C, Baysungur V, Halezeroglu S: Extrathoracic herniation of a lung bulla through a tube thoracostomy site. Interact Cardiovasc Thorac Surg 2008;7(6):1210-1211. Epub 2008 Sep 23.
72. Limsukon A, Yick D, Kamangar N: Chylothorax: A rare complication of tube thoracostomy. J Emerg Med 2011;40(3):280-282. Epub 2008 Aug 30.
73. Iribhogbe PE, Uwuigbe O: Complications of tube thoracostomy using advanced trauma life support technique in chest trauma. West Afr J Med 2011;30(5):369-372.
74. Rosing JH, Lance S, Wong MS: Ulnar neuropathy after tube thoracostomy for pneumothorax. J Emerg Med 2010. [Epub ahead of print].
75. Shaikhrezai K, Zamvar V: Hazards of tube thoracostomy in patients on a ventilator. J Cardiothorac Surg 2011;6:39.
76. Kesieme EB, Dongo A, Ezemba N, et al: Tube thoracostomy: Complications and its management. Pulm Med 2012;2012:256878. [Epub 2011 Oct. 16.]

The complete list of references can be found at www.expertconsult.com.

16 Intracranial Monitoring

Alan R. Turtz

CHAPTER OUTLINE

In general, chapters on intracranial monitoring focus on intracranial pressure (ICP). This chapter expands the scope of discussion to include the intracranial monitoring of pressure, cerebral blood flow (CBF), and brain tissue oxygenation.

INTRACRANIAL PRESSURE MONITORING

The history of ICP monitoring dates to 1891, when Quincke measured the cerebrospinal fluid (CSF) pressure via a lumbar puncture.[1] Soon afterward, Cushing showed that as ICP increases and approaches systemic arterial pressure in an animal model, hypertension, bradycardia, and respiratory changes become evident.[2] The use of continuous ICP monitoring was first described by Guillaume and Janny[3] using an intraventricular catheter in 1951. Nine years later, Lundberg[4] published the first systematic observations of ICP and its response to medical and physiologic interventions. Using ventricular catheters, he showed the clinical value of direct ICP monitoring and described pressure waveforms, of which the Lundberg A wave has the most practical importance in the intensive care unit (ICU). These A, or plateau, waves are characterized by a steep increase in ICP to 60 to 80 mm Hg lasting 2 to 5 minutes or longer, followed by a rapid decrease to near initial baseline pressures. This represents a pathologic response to decompensation of pressure controlling mechanisms.[4-6] Since these early investigations, CSF pressure and ICP measurement have been developed and refined further.

An ICP monitor is an invaluable research and clinical tool, contributing to the understanding of intracranial pathologic conditions and the assessment of therapeutic interventions. ICP monitoring can be used for patients with intracerebral hemorrhage, Reye syndrome, hepatic encephalopathy, encephalitis, stroke, hydrocephalus, near-drowning, and subarachnoid hemorrhage, but most of the clinical experience with ICP monitoring involves traumatic brain injury (TBI). In severe TBI, it is important to know if ICP is elevated. Early signs and symptoms of increased ICP include headache, lethargy, nausea, and vomiting. In critically ill patients, these clinical signs may be nonspecific and unreliable.[6] In addition, the positive trend toward early intubation and sedation, if not pharmacologic paralysis, eliminates the neurologic assessment of a patient with the exception of pupils. Even papilledema, a hard physical sign of increased ICP, is rarely seen acutely in patients with TBI.[7] Computed tomography (CT) is arguably the most useful diagnostic tool in patients with TBI, but may not reliably determine the ICP.

ICP monitoring in severe TBI has become routine because it facilitates rational management, provides prognostic information, and improves outcomes.[8-11] ICP monitoring can provide crucial information relative to cerebral perfusion pressure (CPP); detect the development or enlargement of a mass lesion, such as contusion or hematoma; facilitate the estimation of intracranial compliance; and be the only parameter to follow in a pharmacologically paralyzed patient, apart from the pupillary examination. It is rarely justifiable to treat a patient for intracranial hypertension empirically without a mechanism for measuring the effect of treatment, such as a clinical examination or ICP.

There are well-defined guidelines for the use of ICP monitoring in TBI, which include patients with an abnormal CT scan and a Glasgow Coma Scale score of 8 or less after cardiopulmonary resuscitation. An abnormal CT scan is defined as one that reveals hematomas, contusion, edema, or compressed cisterns. It also is recommended to consider monitoring head-injured patients with a Glasgow Coma Scale score of 8 or less even if the head CT scan is negative if two of the following three criteria are met on admission: age older than 40, systolic blood pressure less than 90 mm Hg, or signs of posturing (Fig. 16.1).[12]

Although ICP monitoring can be a useful tool in the ICU, this technology has limitations. It is crucial not to assign undue weight to a normal ICP if other clinical information suggests otherwise. ICP does not always increase in the

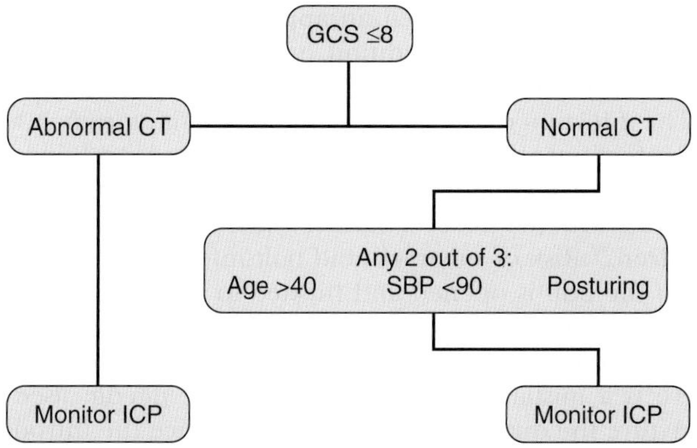

Figure 16.1 Indications for intracranial pressure (ICP) monitoring. CT, computed tomography; GCS, Glasgow Coma Scale; SBP, systolic blood pressure. (From Brain Trauma Foundation, American Association of Neurological Surgeons, Joint Section on Neurotrauma and Critical Care: Management and prognosis of severe traumatic brain injury: Part I. Guidelines for the management of severe traumatic brain injury. J Neurotrauma 2000;17:47-69.)

presence of midline shift.[13,14] More specifically, a temporal lobe mass can herniate over the tentorial edge and cause brainstem compression without a concomitant increase in ICP.[15,16] Likewise, there is not good correlation between supratentorial and infratentorial pressures,[17] so it is imperative to remember that patients with a posterior fossa mass can deteriorate rapidly without a significant increase in ICP measured in the supratentorial compartment.[6]

ICP waveform analysis includes systolic and diastolic pressures with superimposed respiratory variation; however, the mean pressure is of practical importance. A normal adult mean ICP is 10 mm Hg or less with transient physiologic elevations above this value seen in a head-down position or during a Valsalva maneuver (see discussion of secondary injury in Chapter 67).[6] The Association for the Advancement of Medical Instrumentation developed standards for ICP monitoring devices that require a pressure range from 0 to 100 mm Hg, an accuracy of ±2 mm Hg in the range of 0 to 20 mm Hg, and a maximal error of 10% between 20 mm Hg and 100 mm Hg.[18] There are four basic types of clinically useful monitoring systems: ventricular catheter, subarachnoid bolt, fiberoptic device, and catheter tip strain gauge.

VENTRICULAR CATHETER

A ventriculostomy is the gold standard for ICP monitoring. It can be inserted through a twist drill craniostomy at the bedside and can also be used to drain CSF or for the estimation of intracranial compliance. The catheter is connected to a fluid-filled system, which is connected to an external transducer. The transducer converts the measured pressure to an electrical signal, which provides a waveform and numerical value displayed on a monitor through a signal processor. A three-way stopcock is used to divert CSF from the monitor to a drainage bag if needed. This setup allows the catheter to be zeroed as frequently as necessary with the transducer positioned at the level of the center of the brain, which generally corresponds to the external auditory meatus. This system has the potential to be opened and contaminated and infected. The most significant risk of a ventriculostomy is infection; rates of 27% have been cited,[10,19-22] although most reported rates are in the 1% to 10% range.[21,23-26] Infection rates are similar regardless of procedure location (ICU or the operating room).[20,21,27] Tunneling the catheter subcutaneously to a distant skin exit site seems to reduce the infection risk. Other risk factors for infection include irrigation of the catheter or drainage system and the presence of intraventricular blood.[20,21,28] Duration of monitoring also may be a risk factor for infection. Some studies have found an increase in infection rates when ventriculostomies were left in for longer than 5 days,[20,21,25] but more recent data reveal no significant reduction in infection rates when catheters were replaced before the fifth day.[29] Likewise, other investigators have found no significant relationship between duration of monitoring and rate of daily infection for 2 weeks.[30] The literature on the role of prophylactic antibiotics during external CSF drainage is also variable.[20,26,28,31] A Brain Trauma Foundation Level III recommendation discourages routine ventricular catheter exchange as well as prophylactic antibiotics for ventricular catheter placement.[32] Antibiotic-impregnated catheters have been shown to reduce infection rates[33] and are being used routinely in some centers.

Hemorrhage at the time of placement occurs about 1% to 2% of the time and only rarely needs to be surgically evacuated.[6,25,34] A more common problem with placement is difficulty in accessing small, compressed, or shifted ventricles, resulting in malposition and a poor waveform. Although a ventriculostomy is generally considered to be the most precise and accurate method of measuring ICP,[35] malfunction occurs if the ventriculostomy becomes clogged with air, blood, or debris, or if the ventricles are collapsed around the fenestrations in the catheter tip.

In addition to its primary use as an ICP monitor, a ventriculostomy is commonly used in the ICU as a drain for patients with TBI or hydrocephalus. Common causes of acute hydrocephalus in an adult ICU include cerebellar stroke or hemorrhage, intraventricular hemorrhage, and aneurysmal subarachnoid hemorrhage. A common and often debated concern regarding CSF drainage with a ventriculostomy is that it can cause subfalcine herniation in the presence of a hemispheric mass or upward herniation of the cerebellum in the presence of an infratentorial lesion.[36] Under these circumstances, we believe that surgical decompression of the primary mass also should be considered. Another potential risk of ventricular catheter insertion is aneurysmal rebleeding[37] after an acute subarachnoid hemorrhage. Our group's opinion is that the benefit of treating hydrocephalus with high ICP far outweighs the small, potential risk of aneurysmal rebleeding, and we have a low threshold for placing a ventriculostomy in these patients.

If a ventriculostomy is primarily used for drainage of CSF, adequate spontaneous CSF resorption must be restored before the catheter can be safely removed. CSF resorptive capacity must be gauged according to the CSF drainage rate. Adjusting the height of the drainage system drip chamber controls the rate of external CSF drainage and the ICP that must be exceeded before drainage occurs. It can be assumed that 1 cm of CSF equals 1 cm H_2O. The height of the drip chamber is measured from the same external anatomic landmark as the ICP transducer, ranging from 0 to 20 cm (approximately 15 mm Hg) above the external auditory meatus in usual circumstances.

To reduce the amount of external CSF drainage, the drip chamber is usually raised by incremental amounts every 12 to 24 hours. As this is done, CSF resorptive mechanisms are gradually challenged. If CSF resorption is insufficient, most of the CSF continues to drain through the ventriculostomy, but if CSF resorption is sufficient, little CSF drains externally. When CSF resorption seems to be sufficient, CSF drainage is stopped, and ICP is monitored for 24 hours or more to confirm that spontaneous CSF resorption is adequate and ICP will not increase to dangerous levels.

We generally manage ventriculostomies for hydrocephalus by leaving the reservoir open to drain at a specific height above the ear and close it every hour for an ICP reading. In hydrocephalus, the ICP should never be significantly higher than the gradient the patient is draining against (i.e., the height of the drip chamber). We also specify our drainage gradient in millimeters of mercury to correlate the drip chamber to the monitor and manually correlate the height of the CSF column in the drainage system with the monitor as a system check at least daily. A typical order may read: "leave ventriculostomy open to drain at 15 mm Hg (20 cm CSF) above the ear and monitor ICP every hour." ICP readings with the drain open are inaccurate, and the drainage port needs to be temporarily clamped when measuring an ICP. Likewise, the drain should be clamped and placed to monitor when changing position or during transport to avoid overdrainage, which may cause ventricular collapse and possibly subdural bleeding.

SUBARACHNOID BOLT

The subarachnoid bolt technique for ICP monitoring was developed because of concern about the infection rate associated with ventriculostomies, and because small ventricular size after head trauma often makes catheter insertion difficult.[38] A subarachnoid bolt is a self-tapping metal or plastic tube that is screwed into a twist drill craniostomy at the bedside. The dura at the base of the bolt is perforated with a spinal needle to allow CSF to fill the bolt, which is connected to pressure tubing filled with preservative-free (nonbacteriostatic) saline that leads to an external transducer leveled to the ear. In contrast to a ventriculostomy, the subarachnoid bolt is only a monitoring instrument; CSF is not withdrawn from it. It usually provides a reliable ICP waveform and pressure reading, but is susceptible to error if the dural perforations become obstructed with blood or debris, or if brain swelling obliterates communication with CSF. Uncapping the bolt to flush debris with 0.2 mL of preservative-free saline solution can restore accurate ICP readings and is unlikely to cause dangerous ICP elevation.[39] The subarachnoid bolt tends to underestimate ICP, particularly when ICP is elevated.[39,40] Because the subarachnoid bolt measures the local ICP at the surface of the hemisphere, it can be inaccurate if a pressure gradient is present between the left and right supratentorial compartments.[19] The existence of compartmental pressure differences has been debated, but such gradients can occur between the left and right hemispheres or the supratentorial and infratentorial compartments and sometimes are only transient.[19,41-43] This is an important phenomenon to consider, and if a discrepancy exists between an apparently normal ICP and the patient's clinical condition or CT scan or both, treatment of elevated ICP may be warranted.

The infection risk for subarachnoid bolts is extremely low, and infections are nearly always superficial and rarely involve the brain or meninges.[20] No local or systemic infection was reported with the use of subarachnoid bolts in 124 comatose children.[44] Risk of subarachnoid bolt infection is increased when the bolt is opened and flushed to improve the waveform.[20] Subarachnoid bolts are rarely associated with brain injury; however, intracerebral hematoma may occur[45] if there is a mishap with the drill, or if the needle used to puncture the dura is passed too deeply. Since the introduction of fiberoptic catheters, subarachnoid bolts are being used less often.

FIBEROPTIC INTRACRANIAL PRESSURE MONITORS

Fiberoptic ICP monitors use miniature transducers that are coupled via fiberoptic cables to an external instrument. These monitors can be placed at the bedside through a standard twist drill craniostomy or through a smaller opening made with a 2.71-mm bit. The transducer is incorporated into the end of a tube and can be used alone or in combination with a ventriculostomy. Fiberoptic systems operate by projecting light through an optic fiber to a miniature, displaceable mirror in the catheter tip.[46] The amount of light reflected to a collecting optic fiber depends on the mechanical displacement of the mirror, which is a function of ICP. Fiberoptic devices can be inserted into the lateral ventricle, the brain parenchyma, or the subdural space. The greatest advantage of fiberoptic catheters is that they do not require fluid coupling for pressure transduction, which avoids the problems of waveform dampening and artifacts from poor coupling. Because they do not require fluid coupling, there also is less opportunity for contamination. The mechanism that does the actual pressure transduction is what is inserted into the patient; the system functions independent of head position, and the monitor is zeroed once before it is placed. This feature also is a disadvantage because the transducer cannot be recalibrated to zero after insertion. System accuracy compared with a ventriculostomy has been shown in the subdural space, brain parenchyma, and ventricles, although the parenchymal fiberoptic pressures may consistently exceed ventriculostomy pressures by nearly 10 mm Hg.[47-49] The fiberoptic device has an average daily drift of ±0.6 mm Hg. Over a 5-day period, there is an average drift of 2.1 mm Hg with a maximal drift of ±6 mm Hg. This drift over time may be enough to necessitate replacement if ICP monitoring is required for more than 5 days.[6,49,50]

Complications with the use of fiberoptic catheters relating to hemorrhage[51,52] and infection[51] have been reported, but our experience is that clinically relevant problems are unusual, particularly with intraparenchymal monitors. We do exercise caution, however, in patients with coagulopathy.

CATHETER TIP STRAIN GAUGE

The catheter tip strain gauge consists of a miniaturized solid-state pressure sensor mounted in a titanium case at the tip of a long, thin, flexible nylon tube. The transducer tip contains a silicon microchip with diffuse piezoresistive strain gauges that connect to tiny wires that travel the length of the tube. This is a small wire with a diameter of 1.2 mm that can be placed at the bedside. It can be incorporated into a ventricular catheter and used in any intracranial space. This device is accurate with a low daily drift range between −0.125 mm Hg and +0.110 mm Hg. It shares many of the advantages and disadvantages of fiberoptic devices,[6,53,54] but we have found it more cumbersome to place and secure through a bedside twist drill craniostomy.

CEREBRAL BLOOD FLOW MONITORING

The primary objective concerning the ICU management of brain-injured patients is the prevention and management of secondary injury in an effort to prevent ischemia. We typically monitor ICP and mean arterial blood pressure continuously, which allows us to calculate CPP. Under normal circumstances, knowing the CPP allows a good estimation of CBF, which is a more direct measure of blood supply to the brain. In head injury, the relationship between CPP and CBF is less predictable. An ideal intracranial monitor would provide direct, continuous measurements of regional and global CBF at the bedside.

Measuring CBF outside the ICU began with Kety and Schmidt in 1948 and more recently has been done with xenon-enhanced CT,[55,56] but these methods only give snapshots of CBF and do not allow for continuous monitoring at the bedside.[57] Continuous monitoring techniques in the ICU are classified as direct or indirect. Direct and continuous monitoring of CBF at the bedside includes laser Doppler flowmetry and thermal diffusion.

The laser Doppler flow sensor (1.5 mm diameter), which emits a monochromatic light, is placed into the white matter through a burr hole. The sensor measures the volume or concentration of red blood cells and their velocity and generates a flow signal. Although laser Doppler flow does allow continuous measurements of perfusion, the sample volume is small (1 mm^3), and only relative changes can be determined. Laser Doppler flow provides a qualitative estimate of regional CBF displayed in arbitrary units.[58] A quantitative estimate of regional CBF can be acquired with the thermal diffusion method.[59] With this technique, a probe with two small thermistors is inserted into the brain to measure the tissue's ability to dissipate heat, and a microprocessor converts this into CBF displayed in the standard units of mL/100 g/minute.[57]

An indirect method for measuring blood flow at the bedside is transcranial Doppler ultrasound, which measures mean blood flow velocity in the basal cerebral vessels.[60] Although not equivalent to volume flow, changes in CBF can be inferred from changes in blood flow velocity.[61] Continuous transcranial Doppler monitoring is still cumbersome, however, because of problems of probe fixation to the head and computer interfacing.[57] Another indirect way of continuously monitoring CBF at the bedside is by measuring jugular venous bulb oxygenation.

Normal mean CBF is 50 to 60 mL/100 g/minute with higher flow in the gray matter and lower flow in the white matter. When hemoglobin is fully saturated with oxygen, arterial blood carries approximately 20 mL of oxygen per deciliter to the brain. The oxygen content of venous blood draining the brain varies and depends primarily on how much oxygen the brain extracts. Normal internal jugular hemoglobin oxygen saturation ranges from 55% to 69%, and the normal difference between the arterial and jugular venous oxygen content (arteriojugular difference [$AJDO_2$]) is 6.3 ± 2.4 mL/dL. Stated differently, under normal circumstances, the brain extracts 6.3 ± 2.4 mL/dL of oxygen from the arterial blood to meet the metabolic needs of the brain.

Normally, the cerebral metabolic rate of oxygen ($CMRO_2$) is coupled to CBF; as demand increases, supply increases, and vice versa. In head injury, there may be a problem with supply (i.e., CBF may be compromised). If there is inadequate CBF to meet the metabolic demands of the brain, more oxygen is extracted from the available blood. Under this circumstance, the difference between blood going into the brain and blood coming out of the brain increases; $AJDO_2$ increases as the oxygen saturation in the jugular vein decreases.

$AJDO_2$ is proportional to $CMRO_2$ or inversely proportional to CBF or both.[62-65] Assuming that the $CMRO_2$ is constant, an increase in the amount of oxygen extraction as reflected by a decrease in jugular oxygen saturation (increased $AJDO_2$) implies that CBF has been compromised. Conversely, if $AJDO_2$ decreases and metabolism remains constant, we can infer an increase in CBF (i.e., hyperemia). Measuring jugular bulb oxygen can be a useful way to monitor a patient who requires hyperventilation for ICP control (see Chapter 66). Hyperventilation is a powerful tool for reducing ICP and enhancing CPP, but at the expense of increasing cerebrovascular resistance, with the consequent reduction of blood in the brain. The goal of treatment is to prevent ischemia, the ultimate and proximate cause of secondary injury. There is an obvious conflict when attempting to prevent ischemia by reducing the amount of blood delivered to the brain. $AJDO_2$ is sensitive to changes in cerebrovascular resistance; jugular vein monitoring may reveal inappropriate reductions of CBF as a result of hyperventilation.[62]

Most of the data concerning jugular bulb monitoring come from the trauma literature. In a prospective study of 353 patients with severe TBI, Cruz[66] found that outcome at 6 months was significantly better in the patients who had monitoring and management of cerebral extraction of oxygen along with CPP compared with the patients undergoing monitoring and management of CPP alone.

Increased $AJDO_2$ also can be detected during the early phases of head injury when CBF is pathologically reduced. Typically, the patient is being rescued at the scene, transported, and triaged during this early phase of injury, when CBF is low and ventilation is not carefully titrated. Hyperventilation is frequently used during this vulnerable period, often empirically and sometimes inadvertently.[62,67] Complicating this scenario is superimposed hypotension and hypoxia, which can occur during the early phases of resuscitation and later in the ICU.[68-70] Despite its usefulness, there are significant limitations to this monitoring technique. Measurements can be done by intermittent sampling, which is accurate but is limited by intermittent information, or continuous monitoring of oxygen saturation using fiberoptic catheters, which require careful maintenance and have reliability issues.[63,71]

It is easier to use the oxygen saturation of the venous blood in the jugular, rather than direct measurements of oxygen content, but because the percentage of oxygen saturation in the jugular bulb depends on hemoglobin concentration, it cannot be used independently for estimating the relationship between $CMRO_2$ and CBF. If the patient is anemic, more oxygen may be extracted from the available blood, even under conditions of normal CBF. When measuring oxygen saturation, $AJDO_2$ needs to be calculated, taking the hemoglobin concentration into consideration. Also, $AJDO_2$ is an overall estimate of the global relationship between CBF and $CMRO_2$ and cannot differentiate focal abnormalities. In addition, there is a limit to how much oxygen can be extracted from the available blood. If maximal extraction is reached, and CBF continues to deteriorate, the $AJDO_2$ does not continue to increase. Under this circumstance, $AJDO_2$ appears stable despite a progressively worsening situation. Other pitfalls in monitoring $AJDO_2$ are observed under conditions in which oxygen extraction itself is impaired, such as in cases of mitochondrial dysfunction or a large stroke in which oxygen is not extracted at all.[62]

Several important technical factors are associated with $AJDO_2$ monitoring. The side chosen (right or left jugular bulb) is important and can be affected by the side of the brain with the most injury whether or not it is the side of dominant venous drainage.[72-74] How high the tip of the catheter is positioned is another consideration and requires x-ray confirmation.[75] The speed at which samples are drawn also may affect the results.[76] Complications are uncommon and include carotid puncture[63,77] and subclinical internal jugular vein thrombosis.[77]

Ultimately, jugular bulb monitoring is geared toward the assessment of global CBF and cerebral oxygenation and can be useful in guiding therapeutic hyperventilation.[78,79] In severe TBI, there is enough evidence to recommend its use for titrating the level of hyperventilation;[80] however, some clinicians find jugular bulb monitoring to be cumbersome, to be prone to artifact, and to have other potential problems with poor data quality.[81-83] Because of all of the problems involved with this technique, monitoring of $AJDO_2$ has not been universally accepted as a useful tool in the routine management of head-injured patients. There remain strong arguments for and against the use of jugular bulb monitoring.[66,84]

BRAIN TISSUE OXYGENATION MONITORING

Oxygen tension in brain tissue is as close to a gold standard of cerebral oxygenation as we have at the bedside. Brain tissue oxygen tension can be directly measured using a small flexible microcatheter (<0.5 mm in diameter) that is usually inserted into the frontal white matter and fixed onto a special bolt. The normal brain tissue oxygen tension is approximately 40 mm Hg.[85-89] Cerebral oxygen tension is generally reflective of CBF and local oxygen extraction. In this sense, brain tissue oxygen tension may represent the "pool of oxygen" in brain tissue.[57,90,91] Changes in brain tissue oxygen tension can be used to monitor evolving disturbances of tissue metabolism.[81,92-94]

Ischemic damage seems to correlate to a brain tissue oxygen tension less than 8 to 10 mm Hg as measured by a Licox catheter (Integra Neuroscience, Plainsboro, NJ).[81] A meta-analysis of three studies including 158 patients with severe TBI found overall cerebral hypoxia, defined as a monitored brain tissue oxygen tension less than 10 mm Hg, was associated with worse outcome and increased mortality rate.[95] Another study treated 70 severe head injury patients with management directed to maintaining brain tissue oxygenation greater than 25 mm Hg in addition to conventional ICP and CPP management. The results were compared with 53 matched, historical controls treated with conventional management only. The mean daily ICP and CPP and the frequency of episodes of ICP greater than 20 mm Hg and CPP less than 60 mm Hg were similar in both groups. Forty percent of patients with management guided by only ICP and CPP had a favorable outcome compared with 70% of patients with management guided by brain tissue oxygenation.[96] Additional studies demonstrate a relationship between brain tissue oxygen tension, ICP, and outcome. Recent[97,98] guidelines suggest a treatment threshold of less than 15 mm Hg,[99] but the author's preference is to consider treatment at values less than 20 to 25 mm Hg, and a recent study demonstrated a relationship between mortality rate and values less than 29 mm Hg.[100]

Local cerebral hypoxia in the presence of normal ICP, CPP, and mean blood pressure may be caused by insufficient arterial oxygenation,[92] a mismatch between supply (CBF) and demand ($CMRO_2$),[101] or hyperventilation-induced hypocapnia.[92,102] Hyperventilation can decrease brain tissue oxygen tension because of decreased CBF, which can negate the perceived benefit of improving ICP and CPP.[81,93,102-108] Hyperventilation has a particular risk of causing cerebral hypoxia when P_{CO_2} is less than or equal to 30 mm Hg, or within the first 24 hours[104,105] because of a further reduction of an already reduced CBF.[109] Brain tissue oxygen tension has been shown not to be independently influenced by increases in CPP greater than 60 mm Hg,[83,93,108] which supports more recent evidence suggesting that maintaining a CPP greater than 60 mm Hg may be unnecessary,[110,111] and is consistent with current guidelines to keep CPP in the range of 50 to 70 mm Hg in severe TBI.[112]

When strategically placed, these monitors are very sensitive in detecting local tissue hypoxia at the tip of the probe. An inherent problem with this technique (as with all focal monitors) is that placement of the probe into the area of interest becomes important.[57] There are rational arguments as to the best region to monitor. Brain tissue oxygen tension values close to a contusion are smaller relative to a region that looks normal on a CT scan.[113] Some authors recommend monitoring the zone surrounding a contusion because of its high risk of tissue death. Other authors place the probes in uninjured brain with the idea being that a reduction in the brain tissue oxygen tension in the uninjured hemisphere is reflecting a diffuse decrease in arterial oxygenation, an increase in ICP, a decrease in CPP, overaggressive hyperventilation, or some other global event.[81]

SUMMARY

Most intracranial monitoring techniques are employed for circumstances involving increased ICP, and ICP monitoring has proved to be useful, reliable, and straightforward. As such, ICP monitoring has become a standard of care and is widely used. It is much more difficult to obtain continuous, clinically useful information with CBF monitoring methods, and these methods have found limited use outside academic institutions. Brain tissue oxygen monitoring is a relatively new technique with mounting evidence to justify continued use, with the hope of providing additional information to the clinician charged with managing the complicated, dynamic pathophysiologic processes of brain-injured patients.

KEY POINTS

- The primary objective concerning ICU management of brain-injured patients is the prevention and management of secondary injury in an effort to prevent ischemia.
- ICP monitoring should be considered for patients with TBI with a Glasgow Coma Scale score of 8 or less.
- ICP monitoring in severe TBI has become routine because it facilitates rational management, provides prognostic information, and improves outcomes.
- It is crucial not to assign undue weight to a normal ICP if other clinical information suggests otherwise.
- A normal adult mean ICP is 10 mm Hg or less with transient physiologic elevations above this value, and normal CPP is generally 60 to 80 mm Hg.
- Ventriculostomies and fiberoptic intraparenchymal monitors are the mainstays of ICP monitoring devices.
- Oxygen tension in brain tissue is as close to a gold standard of cerebral oxygenation as we have at the bedside.

KEY POINTS (Continued)

- Local cerebral hypoxia in the presence of normal ICP, CPP, and mean blood pressure may be caused by insufficient arterial oxygenation, a mismatch between supply (CBF) and demand ($CMRO_2$), or hyperventilation-induced hypocapnia.
- Hyperventilation has a particular risk of causing cerebral hypoxia when PCO_2 is less than or equal to 30 mm Hg, or within the first 24 hours.
- Maintain CPP in the range of 50 to 70 mm Hg in severe TBI.

SELECTED REFERENCES

8. Copez JJ, Meagher RJ, Narayan RK: When and how should I monitor intracranial pressure? In Valadka AB, Andrews BT (eds): Neurotrauma. New York, Thieme, 2005, pp 53-57.
11. Farahvar A, Gerber L, Chiu YL, et al: Increased mortality in patients with severe traumatic brain injury treated without intracranial pressure monitoring. J Neurosurg 2012;117(4): 729-734; available at http://thejns.org/doi/abs/10.3171/2012.7.JNS111816.
12. Brain Trauma Foundation, American Association of Neurological Surgeons, Joint Section on Neurotrauma and Critical Care: Management and prognosis of severe traumatic brain injury: Part I. Guidelines for the management of severe traumatic brain injury. Indications for intracranial pressure monitoring. J Neurotrauma 2000;17:47-69.
33. Harrop J, Sharan A, Ratliff J, et al: Impact of a standardized protocol and antibiotic-impregnated catheters on ventriculostomy infection rates in cerebrovascular patients. Neurosurgery 2010; 67:187-191.
81. Kiening KL, Sarrafzadeh AS, Stover JF, et al: Should I monitor brain tissue Po_2? In Valadka AB, Andrews BT (eds): Neurotrauma. New York, Thieme, 2005, pp 62-67.
97. Oddo M, Levine J, Mackenzie L, et al: Brain hypoxia is associated with short-term outcome after severe traumatic brain injury independently of intracranial hypertension and low cerebral perfusion pressure. Neurosurgery 2011;69:1037-1045.
99. Brain Trauma Foundation: Brain oxygen monitoring and thresholds. J Neurotrauma 2007;24(Suppl 1):S65-S70.

The complete list of references can be found at www.expertconsult.com.

17 Gastrointestinal Endoscopy

Fedele J. DePalma | Adam B. Elfant

CHAPTER OUTLINE

HISTORY

The first documented endoscopic foray into the human body was performed by Philip Bozinni in the early 1800s, when he used a speculum fitted with a candle and mirror to examine the urinary tract.[1] The first gastroscopy was performed in 1868 by German physician Adolf Kussmaul, with a rigid metal tube passed carefully down a patient's esophagus into his stomach. In 1932, Rudolph Schindler, in collaboration with a German engineer, Georg Wolff, developed a semiflexible instrument with a flexible distal shaft. Although this device was hailed as the first safe workable gastroscope, it was not without limitation, including incomplete visualization of the esophagus and stomach, patient discomfort, and absence of photographic documentation.[2] Fiberoptics were introduced into the endoscope in 1957 by Basil Hirschowitz, and in the 1960s and 1970s further advancements were made with endoscope length, improved visualization, and greater control. Video cameras and monitors were subsequently incorporated into endoscopic technology, allowing others to view what was previously available only to the endoscopist.

Early experience with rigid and semiflexible proctosigmoidoscopes and colonoscopes was disappointing because of the tortuous nature of the sigmoid and colon, and early fiberoptic instruments fared no better. Bergein Overholt made adjustments in torque and control to develop a prototype flexible fiberoptic instrument in 1963.[3] The first total colonoscopy was performed in Sardinia, Italy, in 1965. Luciano Provenzale and Antonio Revignas instructed a patient to swallow a piece of polyvinyl tubing, which ultimately emerged from the anus. They attached a side-viewing gastroscope and gently pulled it through the entire colon to the cecum.[3] Further refinements were carried out in England, the United States, and Japan, and in 1969 Hiromi Shinya performed the first polypectomy, removing a 1.5 cm pedunculated polyp from the sigmoid colon of a 70-year-old Chinese gentleman.[4] Shortly thereafter, colonoscopy became a routine procedure performed by gastroenterologists and other health care providers all over the world.

Endoscopic cannulation of the duodenal ampulla was first accomplished in Chicago by William S. McCune and colleagues in 1968 and is considered the first reported case of endoscopic retrograde cholangiopancreatography (ERCP).[5] Sphincterotomy was performed in 1974 facilitating removal of two common bile duct stones[6] and ushering in a new era of therapeutic pancreaticobiliary endoscopy. Today, ERCP remains an invaluable procedure in evaluating and treating diseases of the pancreas and biliary tract.

The first ultrasound examination within the gastrointestinal (GI) lumen was performed by physician John Julian Wild and electrical engineer John Reid in 1956, when they developed the transrectal ultrasound probe.[7] The incorporation of ultrasound into a standard endoscope occurred in 1976, when Lutz and Rosch passed an ultrasound probe through an accessory port of an endoscope. Further improvements were achieved by Strohm and colleagues and Eugene DiMagno and coworkers, who introduced their own prototype echoendoscopes in 1980. The first endoscopic ultrasound (EUS)–guided fine-needle aspiration was performed on submucosal lesions of the stomach in 1991 by Giancarlo Caletti.[8]

ENDOSCOPIC EQUIPMENT

Today's endoscopes have a control section that is grasped with the left hand and allows for scope control and passage of therapeutic instruments. An insertion tube extends from the bottom of the control section and is grasped with the right hand and passed into the patient. Buttons on the control section allow for suction, insufflation, and washing of the lens. Channel ports distal to the hand controls on the control section allow for the passage of various accessories. Four-way deflection of the distal endoscope tip is performed through manipulation of the angulation control knobs, which are attached to a series of wires that run the length of the insertion tube. The distal end of the insertion tube, either forward viewing (i.e., endoscope, colonoscope) or side viewing (duodenoscope), contains lenses for illumination and imaging and channel openings for air, water, suction, and passage of instruments.

EUS equipment differs from the standard endoscope in that an ultrasound transducer is incorporated into the distal end of the insertion tube. The transducer emits sound waves that are directed at adjacent tissues and deflected back to the transducer. Individual tissues have different acoustic qualities. Radial and linear echoendoscopes are currently available. Interventional procedures, such as fine-needle aspiration and injections, may be performed safely with the latter echoendoscope.[9]

All video endoscopes have an image sensor called a charge-coupled device (CCD) mounted at the tip of the endoscope, which transmits an image to a video processor for display. Advances in CCD technology have resulted in the current high-resolution or high-definition (HD) endoscopes, which produce signal image resolutions that range from 850,000 pixels to more than 1 million pixels, allowing for detailed inspection of the GI mucosa.[10]

The wireless video capsule is a small disposable unit containing a small camera, short focal length lens, light source, two batteries, and a radio telemetry transmitter.[11] There are presently three types of video capsules: an esophagus-specific capsule incorporating two CCD chips oriented at 180 degrees, a small bowel video capsule employing a single CCD chip with an 8-hour battery capacity, and experimental colonic video capsules utilizing time-sensitive deactivation and reactivation of the illumination and telemetry elements in order to preserve battery power during small bowel transit. Accessory devices have allowed endoscopic advancement of activated video capsules into the small intestine of patients who have dysfunctional esophageal and gastric motility or altered upper GI anatomy due to prior surgery. The capsule is activated by removal from a magnetic holder, and battery life is approximately 8 hours. Two frames per second are captured by the camera and transmitted to a data recorder that is carried by the patient. Data are downloaded from the recorder to a personal computer and interpreted. Handheld devices have also recently been developed to allow real-time monitoring of video capsule images.

ANESTHESIA

Choice of anesthesia is based on patient profile, the endoscopic procedure, and preference of the endoscopist, anesthesiologist, and patient. Essential patient information includes prior adverse events from anesthesia, current medications, pertinent medical history, cardiopulmonary status, age, allergies, body habitus, and social history. Patients with alcohol or narcotic dependency may require high doses of opiates and benzodiazepines. Agents such as propofol may facilitate their sedation. Pregnancy should be excluded in any woman of childbearing age. The level of sedation also depends on the endoscopic procedure. Flexible sigmoidoscopy and esophagogastroduodenoscopy (EGD) may require minimal or moderate sedation, whereas more complex and lengthier procedures, such as ERCP and EUS, may require deep sedation or even general anesthesia. Table 17.1 illustrates the different depths of sedation as defined by The American Society of Anesthesiologists Task Force.[12]

Regardless of the type of sedation, cardiopulmonary status should be monitored at all times. Standard equipment should include a pulse oximeter, continuous electrocardiogram, and cyclical blood pressure monitoring. Personnel trained in airway support should always be present. The cardiopulmonary complication rate is 0.005% for EGD and 0.01% for colonoscopy.[13]

Four drug types are commonly used in GI endoscopies: pharyngeal anesthesia, benzodiazepines, opiates, and propofol. Pharyngeal anesthetics, such as lidocaine, benzocaine, and tetracaine, are used to suppress the gag reflex during upper GI tract procedures. These agents, applied by spray or gargling, are active for approximately 1 hour. Potential risks include aspiration owing to loss of gag reflex and, rarely, methemoglobinemia.[14]

Benzodiazepines, such as midazolam and diazepam, are used to induce relaxation and amnesia by binding to

Table 17.1 Levels of Sedation and Anesthesia

Anesthesia Management Component	Minimal Sedation (Anxiolysis)	Moderate Sedation (Conscious Sedation)	Deep Sedation/ Analgesia	General Anesthesia
Responsiveness	Normal response to verbal stimulation	Purposeful response to verbal or tactile stimulation	Purposeful response after repeated or painful stimulation	Unarousable even with painful stimulus
Airway	Unaffected	No intervention required	Intervention may be required	Intervention often required
Spontaneous ventilation	Unaffected	Adequate	May be inadequate	Frequently inadequate
Cardiovascular function	Unaffected	Usually maintained	Usually maintained	May be impaired

Adapted from Gross JB, Bailey PL, Connis RT, et al. Practice guidelines for sedation and analgesia by non-anesthesiologists. Anesthesiology 2002;96:1004-1017.

receptors of the postsynaptic γ-aminobutyric acid neurons. Both have similar properties, with the latter possessing a longer half-life and milder amnestic properties.[15] Onset of action occurs in 1 to 2.5 minutes with intravenous midazolam and 8 minutes with diazepam.[16] Adverse reactions include respiratory depression and hypotension. Overdoses can be reversed with flumazenil, although caution should be used because seizures secondary to acute withdrawal may occur.

Opiates such as fentanyl and meperidine are used for analgesia and sedation. A synergistic effect occurs when opiates are given concurrently with intravenous benzodiazepines. Fentanyl has a rapid onset (1.5 minutes) with a short duration of action (0.5 to 1 hour), whereas meperidine has an onset of 5 minutes and lasts 3 to 5 hours.[16] Common adverse reactions include respiratory depression, hypotension, constipation, nausea, and vomiting. Overdosage can be reversed with naloxone, an opioid antagonist. Long-term opiate users may experience acute withdrawal symptoms with naloxone. Serotonin syndrome may occur if monoamine oxidase inhibitors are used with meperidine.

Propofol, an ultra-short-acting anesthetic agent, has been increasingly used in recent years.[17] Propofol has a rapid onset of action, deeper levels of sedation, and faster recovery time compared with narcotics and benzodiazepines.[18] Propofol use during colonoscopy has been shown to carry a lower risk of cardiopulmonary complications compared with traditional agents.[19] Controversies exist as to its cost-effectiveness and the requirement that it be administered exclusively by an anesthesiologist.

ESOPHAGOGASTRODUODENOSCOPY

EGD is one of the most commonly performed procedures in the world and has become the primary tool for evaluating the esophagus, stomach, and proximal portion of the duodenum. EGD is performed for a wide variety of indications and has a diagnostic and therapeutic role (Box 17.1). There are relatively few contraindications to upper endoscopy (Box 17.2).

EGD is a safe procedure. Perforation occurs in approximately 0.05% to 0.70% of patients,[20] with the higher incidence in patients undergoing therapeutic intervention (i.e., biopsy, dilation, mucosal resection). Bleeding may occur as a result of Mallory-Weiss tears, cautery injury, or sclerotherapy injection and after biopsy or polypectomy.

Prior to undergoing elective EGD, patients should be fasting for at least 6 hours. Motility agents, such as erythromycin, may be beneficial in clearing the stomach of blood or food.[21] In situations of possible airway compromise, elective intubation is reasonable. A 20% incidence of aspiration pneumonia was initially demonstrated after emergent EGD for upper GI bleed.[22] A subsequent retrospective study of 220 patients failed to show any significant difference in post-EGD pulmonary infiltrates, witnessed aspiration, cardiopulmonary complications, or in-hospital mortality rate.[23] Despite the lack of a conclusive double-blinded randomized trial, endotracheal intubation may be appropriate in patients with active hematemesis, altered mental status, unstable cardiopulmonary function, or agitation. Alternatives to intubation may include pre-endoscopy lavage, overtube placement, or the use of large-caliber endoscopes for suction.

Before administration of anesthesia, patients should be in the left lateral position, with the head elevated and

Box 17.1 Indications for Esophagogastroduodenoscopy

Persistent upper abdominal symptoms despite appropriate therapy
Upper abdominal symptoms associated with signs or symptoms suggesting serious organic disease (anorexia, weight loss) or new-onset symptoms in patients >50 years of age
Dysphagia or odynophagia
Esophageal reflux symptoms (persistent or recurrent despite appropriate therapy)
Persistent vomiting of unknown cause
Familial adenomatous polyposis syndromes
Confirmation and specific histologic diagnosis of radiologically shown lesions
- Suspected neoplastic lesions
- Gastric or esophageal ulcer
- Upper tract stricture or obstruction

Gastrointestinal bleeding
- Active or recent bleed
- Suspected bleed (chronic blood loss, iron deficiency anemia)

Sampling of tissue or fluid
Documentation or treatment of varices (banding, sclerotherapy)
Assessment of acute injury after caustic ingestion
Treatment of bleeding lesions such as ulcers, tumors, vascular abnormalities (electrocoagulation, heater probe, laser photocoagulation, injection therapy)
Removal of foreign bodies
Removal of selected polypoid lesions
Dilation of stenotic lesions
Placement of feeding or drainage tubes (percutaneous endoscopic gastrostomy, percutaneous endoscopic jejunostomy)
Management of achalasia (botulinum toxin, balloon dilation)
Palliative treatment of neoplasms (laser, multipolar electrocoagulation, stent placement)
Surveillance for malignancy in patients with premalignant conditions (Barrett's esophagus)

Adapted from American Society of Gastrointestinal Endoscopy: Appropriate use of gastrointestinal endoscopy. Gastrointest Endosc 2012;75:1127-1131.

Box 17.2 Contraindications to Esophagogastroduodenoscopy

Risk to patient's health or life judged to outweigh most favorable benefits of procedure
Conditions in which adequate patient cooperation or consent cannot be obtained
Perforated viscus—known or suspected

Adapted from American Society of Gastrointestinal Endoscopy: Appropriate use of gastrointestinal endoscopy. Gastrointest Endosc 2012;75:1127-1131.

supported by a pillow. Monitoring devices for vital signs, electrocardiogram, and pulse oximetry are attached, supplemental oxygen should be administered, and a bite guard should be placed in the mouth.

In addition to diagnostic capabilities, therapeutic interventions may be performed during upper endoscopy, particularly in the setting of GI hemorrhage. Several modalities are available for treating GI bleeding, including thermal cautery, electrocautery, needle injection, rubber band ligation, mechanical clips, laser therapy, argon plasma coagulation, and tissue adhesives.

Thermal cautery probes deliver predetermined pulses of heat (250° C) to an endoscopic catheter tip, which is transferred to tissue on contact.[24] Thermal probe coagulation can be applied to peptic ulcers, vascular lesions, and Mallory-Weiss tears. Another option for contact thermal coagulation is monopolar or bipolar electrocautery. With electrocautery, electrical current flows from electrode tip through contacted tissue. Monopolar cautery requires attaching an electrical ground to the patient and may cause extensive burn injuries and tissue stickiness. Monopolar cautery is typically not used for hemostasis, but serves a role in snare polypectomy. Bipolar cautery consists of two active electrodes incorporated into a single catheter probe, allowing electrical current to pass from one electrode through the tissue and back to the other electrode. Consequently, bipolar cauterization allows for improved control of coagulation depth.

Injection therapy for nonvariceal and variceal bleeding is performed with sclerotherapy injector needles. Solutions commonly employed are epinephrine in saline (1:10,000) and sclerosing agents, such as polidocanol and ethanolamine. Epinephrine reduces bleeding by vasoconstriction, vessel tamponade, and platelet aggregation.[25,26] The potential exists for systemic side effects from submucosal injections because plasma epinephrine levels can transiently increase four to five times above basal levels.[27] To date, only a single case of hypertension and ventricular tachycardia after epinephrine injection has been reported.[28] Sclerosing agents achieve hemostasis through inflammation and sclerosis and have been employed in peptic ulcer hemorrhage and variceal bleeding. Mediastinitis, perforation, stricture formation, and infection are among the reported complications.[29]

Injector needles are also used in nonbleeding situations. Polyps and superficial tumors can be raised with submucosal injection of saline or epinephrine prior to polypectomy. This technique reduces the likelihood of postpolypectomy hemorrhage or perforation.[30] Lesions requiring surgery can be tattooed with ink to facilitate localization by the surgeon.

Rubber band ligation is an effective tool for hemostasis. The delivery system is loaded onto the endoscope tip, and current models allow for deployment of multiple rubber bands before reloading. For variceal bleeding, endoscopic variceal ligation has become the treatment of choice and is superior to endoscopic sclerotherapy in speed of variceal eradication, decreased risk of recurrent bleeding, and fewer complications.[31] Other uses of banding include gastric varices, peptic ulcers, Dieulafoy's lesions, postpolypectomy hemorrhage, and internal hemorrhoids.

Metal clips, or endoclips, have been used successfully for GI bleeding,[32] closure of perforations,[33] anastomotic leaks,[34] and prevention of postpolypectomy bleeding.[35] The potential for significant tissue injury is small as only the mucosal and submucosal layers are involved in the grasping.[36] The procedure may be technically challenging if massive bleeding is present, or the angle of approach is tangential to the lesion.[37]

Laser therapy, utilizing neodymium:yttrium-aluminum-garnet (Nd:YAG) or argon, is delivered through probes passed via the endoscope to treat bleeding lesions and for tumor ablation. Nd:YAG and argon lasers differ in the width and depth of tissue effect, with the former having the greater effect.[38] Advantages of laser therapy include improved accuracy and not requiring direct contact with the desired target.

Argon plasma coagulation is a noncontact method of hemostasis that delivers argon gas through a catheter probe. The argon gas is ionized, delivering thermal energy to adjacent target tissue. Large areas and tissue not in direct view, due to the tangential arcing nature of the argon gas, can be treated rapidly. Clinical uses include adjunctive ablative therapy after piecemeal resection of colonic polyps, radiation proctopathy, GI vascular lesions, bleeding peptic ulcers, Barrett's esophagus ablation, and palliation of GI malignancies.[39,40]

Tissue adhesives constitute a newer class of agents for GI hemostasis. The major types of tissue adhesives are fibrin sealants and cyanoacrylate. Fibrin sealants form a coagulum through the interaction of fibrinogen, factor XIII, and thrombin.[41] Extensively used in the surgical fields for tissue adhesion, hemostasis, and wound care, fibrin sealants also have been used endoscopically in bleeding peptic ulcers,[42] variceal bleeding,[43] and GI fistulas.[44] Cyanoacrylate is synthetic glue that rapidly polymerizes into a solid complex when in contact with water or blood.[45] Cyanoacrylate has been used with success for esophageal and gastric varices.[46,47] A serious complication of tissue adhesives is embolization and infarction.[48]

In addition to hemostasis, upper endoscopy is routinely employed for other therapeutic situations. Foreign object ingestion and food bolus impaction occur commonly. Although most foreign bodies pass spontaneously, up to 20% of cases may require endoscopic intervention. Various types of endoscopy, ranging from rigid to flexible, and equipment (Box 17.3) are available for foreign body retrieval. An overtube is available for airway protection and

Box 17.3 Devices Used for Foreign Body Retrieval

- Overtube
- Pronged forceps
- Tooth forceps
- Nets
- Baskets
- Retrieval loops
- Magnetic extractors

Adapted from Nelson DB, Bosco JJ, Curtis WD, et al: The ASGE technology status evaluation report: Endoscopic retrieval devices. American Society for Gastrointestinal Endoscopy. Gastrointest Endosc 1999;50:932-934.

frequent esophageal intubations. Retrieval should be performed within 24 hours or more urgently if the ingested object is sharp, is a disc battery, or is causing the patient pain or difficulty in handling secretions. If it is not possible to remove the object endoscopically and it is less than 2.5 cm, the object can be gently maneuvered into the stomach, from which spontaneous passage usually occurs.[49] Unsuccessful removal or obstruction requires surgical evaluation.

Esophageal narrowing is a common reason for recurrent food impaction. Narrowing may occur from benign conditions, such as peptic strictures and Schatzki's rings, or malignancy compressing the lumen. Endoscopic dilation can be performed on anatomic narrowings of the esophagus, pylorus, and anastomotic strictures. Four types of dilators are currently available: tip-weighted push bougies (Maloney or Hurst), wire-guided dilators (Savary-Gilliard or American), through-the-scope dilating balloons, and clear optical dilators that allow direct endoscopic visualization. Dilation also is indicated in patients with achalasia, although recurrence is common, and clinical efficacy is decreased with subsequent dilations.[50] In general, endoscopic dilation increases the risk of perforation, with reported rates between 0.1% and 0.4%.[51]

Endoscopic stenting with endoprosthesis can be performed in a wide variety of clinical scenarios. Stenting is performed for fistulas, anastomotic leaks,[52] and malignant and nonmalignant perforations.[53,54] In addition, malignant obstructive lesions of the esophagus, stomach, duodenum, and colon can be stented for palliation. Stents vary in size, in material (plastic or metal mesh), and by the presence or absence of a covering. Complications include increased reflux if the gastroesophageal junction is involved, bleeding, perforation, and stent migration.

Photodynamic therapy involves pretreatment of a desired target lesion with an injected photosensitizing agent, which is subsequently activated by the application of a light source. The activated photosensitizer achieves an excited state with reactive oxygen radicals that result in cellular injury.[55] In addition to high-grade dysplasia of Barrett's esophagus and esophageal cancer, photodynamic therapy has been employed for neoplasms throughout the GI tract, including the stomach, bile duct, pancreas, and colon.[56]

Radiofrequency ablation of the distal esophagus has been developed as a treatment for high-grade dysplasia in Barrett's esophagus. The HALO system (Barrx Medical, Inc., Sunnyvale, CA) consists of a balloon that contains 60 separate 250-μm electrodes circumferentially oriented on its outer surface, with electrodes separated by a distance of 250 μm. Immediately adjacent electrodes function as bipolar devices that deliver heat to the mucosa at a controlled depth. Radiofrequency energy is delivered through the electrodes, which causes superficial tissue destruction circumferentially over a length of 3 cm. A 90-degree model allows for more focal ablation.[57]

Percutaneous endoscopic gastrostomy (PEG) tube placement is a common procedure for gastroenterologists. The purpose of PEG tube placement is to improve quality of life, shorten hospitalization, prevent aspiration, improve nutritional and functional status, and prolong survival.[58] Controversy exists as to whether PEG tube placement is beneficial in patients with terminal anorexia-cachexia syndromes or in permanent vegetative states.[59,60] In addition to providing nutritional support, PEG placement has been used for long-term gastric decompression and recurrent gastric volvulus management. Placement is contraindicated if the anterior abdominal wall cannot be brought into contact with the anterior gastric wall, such as in morbid obesity and significant ascites. Complications, although infrequent, include wound infection, necrotizing fasciitis, peritonitis, septicemia, peristomal leakage, device dislodgement, bowel perforation, and fistula formation.[60] Possible implantation metastasis in patients with head and neck cancer also has been reported.[61] Pneumoperitoneum is seen in 40% of cases, but most are asymptomatic and eventually resolve.[62]

WIRELESS CAPSULE ENDOSCOPY

Wireless video capsule endoscopy (VCE) is a safe, noninvasive method for visualizing the entire small bowel. The capsule examination typically is performed in an ambulatory setting. Preparation involves an overnight fast. Although data are conflicting, a bowel preparation has been shown to improve visualization and result in a higher rate of capsules reaching the small intestine.[63,64] Metoclopramide also may be beneficial in ensuring a complete small bowel evaluation before expiration of the battery life.[65] After swallowing the pill, the patient can leave the outpatient office, resume nonstrenuous daily activity, and eat 4 hours later. The data recorder is returned after 8 hours.

Common indications for VCE are evaluating obscure GI bleeding, suspected Crohn's disease, small intestinal tumors and polyps, diarrhea, malabsorption disorders, and abdominal pain.[66,67] VCE has been shown to be superior to push enteroscopy and small bowel barium radiography in detecting sources of obscure GI bleeding.[68] Superiority also was shown when VCE was compared with double-balloon enteroscopy.[69] A major limitation of VCE is the inability to perform therapeutic interventions.

In general, VCE is a safe procedure. Contraindications for VCE include swallowing disorders, known or suspected GI obstruction, stricture, fistula, pregnancy, and possibly cardiac pacemakers or implantable defibrillators. (Although listed as a contraindication by the manufacturer, more recent studies have shown no interference with cardiac pacemakers and implantable defibrillators by VCE.[70,71]) The capsule does not reach the cecum within recording time in 16% of cases. Abdominal x-ray study should be performed to evaluate for capsule retention, which occurs in 1.9% of all examinations, usually secondary to an anatomic abnormality, and may require endoscopic or surgical removal.[72,73] A patency system similar in size to a video capsule, but dissolvable if retained in the body, may be useful in screening high-risk patients for possible small bowel stenosis.[74] Patients with swallowing disorders or delayed gastric emptying can have the capsule endoscopically placed into the small bowel.

A variation of the small bowel video capsule exists to evaluate the esophagus. Although similar in design to the small bowel capsule, the esophageal video capsule incorporates a camera at each end, with each camera taking 7 frames per second for a total of 14 frames per second.[11] Fasting time is only 2 hours, and the examination time is less than 1 hour. The patient ingests the pill in a supine position and is gradually raised to an upright position at 2-minute intervals. The esophageal video capsule can be used to evaluate for Barrett's disease, esophageal varices, and complications of gastroesophageal reflux disease.

ENTEROSCOPY

With increasing use of wireless capsule endoscopy, the need for direct visualization and therapeutic intervention in the small bowel is growing. Until recently, deep enteroscopy had been accomplished through push enteroscopy, with or without incorporation of an overtube; through intraoperative enteroscopy performed with a surgeon's assistance during laparotomy; or through a Sonde enteroscope. These techniques are limited in that they are invasive, do not allow for examination of the entire small bowel, or do not permit therapeutic intervention to be undertaken. More recently, alternative endoscopic approaches have been developed to overcome these limitations.

Double-balloon enteroscopy uses two balloons, one at the tip of an enteroscope, and the other at the end of an overtube backloaded onto the enteroscope. Using alternating inflation and deflation of the balloons during sequential advancement of the scope and the overtube, the double-balloon enteroscope is progressively advanced through the small bowel. Utilizing both oral and anal intubation, evaluation of the entire small bowel is possible. Single-balloon enteroscopy, like double-balloon enteroscopy, incorporates a backloaded overtube with a balloon at the tip. Unlike the double-balloon enteroscope, the tip of the scope is deflected to anchor the scope against the bowel wall and permit advancement of the overtube. After advancement, the balloon on the overtube can be inflated, the intestine pleated over the overtube, and the scope advanced once again. Severe complications from double-balloon enteroscopy are described in 1% to 1.7% of patients, with pancreatitis being the most common (0.3%), and bleeding and perforation also encountered.[75] Fewer data are available regarding the complications of single-balloon enteroscopy.[76]

Spiral enteroscopy was developed with the potential advantages of decreased time and increased control in examining the small bowel. The enteroscope is advanced into the small bowel by continuous rotation of the raised helix-fitted overtube, which pleats the small bowel mucosa over the overtube. An inner sleeve allows the independent motion of the overtube during advancement and withdrawal.[77] Spiral enteroscopy has demonstrated a complication rate of 0.4% with perforation found to be the leading severe complication.[76]

Several studies have been performed comparing various combinations of each of the three modalities. Studies comparing single- and double-balloon enteroscopy have consistently demonstrated that double-balloon enteroscopy offers deeper penetration into the small bowel. Studies are conflicting, however, on whether there is any difference in diagnostic and therapeutic outcomes.[78-80] Spiral enteroscopy offers shorter procedure time when compared to balloon-assisted enteroscopy but no apparent difference in diagnostic yield.[81]

COLONOSCOPY

The colonoscope is used by general practitioners, surgeons, and gastroenterologists to evaluate the colon and distal ileum. A shorter version, the flexible sigmoidoscope, is available for sigmoid examination. Colonoscopy has replaced the routine sigmoidoscopy and barium studies as the gold standard for large bowel evaluation. Indications range from colorectal screening and evaluation of anemia to therapeutic interventions such as polypectomy and palliative stenting (Box 17.4). Relative contraindications to colonoscopy are acute diverticulitis, and suspected perforation.

Before colonoscopy, the patient should be on a clear liquid diet with subsequent fasting after bowel preparation. Several bowel preparations are commercially available, including polyethylene glycol, sodium-free polyethylene glycol, low-volume polyethylene glycol with bisacodyl, and tablet sodium phosphate.[82] Nausea, vomiting, and abdominal discomfort are common side effects among all bowel preparations. Sodium phosphate, owing to inducement of rapid volume changes, is contraindicated in patients with serum electrolyte abnormalities, advanced hepatic dysfunction, renal failure, recent myocardial infarction, unstable angina, congestive heart failure, ileus, malabsorption, and ascites.[82] A recent meta-analysis demonstrated that the use of a split-dose polyethylene glycol for bowel preparation before colonoscopy significantly improved the number of satisfactory bowel preparations, increased patient compliance, and decreased nausea compared with the full-dose polyethylene glycol.[83] Inadequate bowel preparation has been attributed to failure to follow preparation instructions; later colonoscopy start time; inpatient status; procedural indication of constipation; use of tricyclic antidepressants;

Box 17.4 Indications for Colonoscopy

- Evaluation of abnormal imaging study
- Evaluation of unexplained gastrointestinal bleeding
  - Hematochezia
  - Melena
  - Presence of fecal occult blood
- Unexplained iron deficiency anemia
- Screening and surveillance for colonic neoplasia
- Chronic inflammatory bowel disease
- Clinically significant diarrhea of unexplained origin
- Intraoperative identification of a lesion not apparent at surgery (polypectomy site, location of a bleeding site)
- Treatment of bleeding from lesions such as vascular malformations, ulceration, neoplasia, and postpolypectomy site (electrocoagulation, heater probe, laser, or injection therapy)
- Foreign body removal
- Excision of polyp
- Decompression of acute megacolon or sigmoid volvulus
- Balloon dilation of stenotic lesions
- Palliative treatment of stenosing or bleeding neoplasms (laser, electrocoagulation, stenting)
- Marking a neoplasm for localization during surgery

Adapted from American Society of Gastrointestinal Endoscopy: Appropriate use of gastrointestinal endoscopy. Gastrointest Endosc 2012;75:1127-1131.

male gender; and history of cirrhosis, stroke, or dementia.[84] Patients undergoing flexible sigmoidoscopy usually do not require complete bowel purgation. An enema before the procedure usually is sufficient to clear the distal colon.

Complete colonoscopic examination is achieved in approximately 94% of patients.[85] Advanced age, female gender, body mass index less than 25 kg/m^2, diverticular disease in women, and a history of constipation or reported laxative abuse in men are predictors of a technically difficult colonoscopy.[86] In general, complications from diagnostic colonoscopy are rare. Hemorrhage and perforation occur in 0.001% to 0.008% and 0.005% to 0.14% of patients, respectively.[87,88] Interventional procedures, such as polypectomy, can increase the risk of bleeding and perforation to 2% and 0.3%.[89] There is a theoretical risk of colonic explosion during cautery from accumulation of colonic gases, usually as a result of a carbohydrate-based bowel preparation such as mannitol.[90]

Polypectomy is one of the most common interventions during colonoscopy. Pedunculated or sessile polyps may be removed with biopsy forceps, snare cautery, or argon plasma coagulation. As noted earlier, complications may be reduced with submucosal injection of saline or epinephrine.

Common causes of colonic hemorrhage include diverticulosis, postpolypectomy bleeding, vascular malformations, and hemorrhoids. Diverticular and postpolypectomy bleeding may be controlled with epinephrine injection, heater probe, electrocautery, or metallic clips. Band ligation also may be effective in hemostasis of postpolypectomy bleeds. Vascular malformations may be ablated with heater probe, electrocautery, laser, argon plasma coagulation, and metallic clips. Hemorrhoidal bleeds are effectively controlled with elastic band ligation, either with a rigid proctoscope or with a flexible video endoscope.[91]

Anastomotic strictures may occur from inflammatory bowel disease or postsurgical resection. These strictures can be dilated with balloon dilators or managed with self-expanding metallic stents.[92] Endoluminal stenting may be used as palliation or as a bridge to surgery for near obstructive malignant lesions.[93] Laser therapy is another option for tumor ablation.[94]

Colonic decompression and placement of temporary rectal tubes is indicated in patients with sigmoid or cecal volvulus and acute pseudo-obstruction. Foreign objects also may be removed endoscopically.

ENDOSCOPIC RETROGRADE CHOLANGIOPANCREATOGRAPHY

ERCP is used to evaluate and treat diseases of the pancreas, bile ducts, gallbladder, and liver. With the advent of highly diagnostic alternative modalities, such as magnetic resonance imaging and EUS, the role of ERCP has slowly evolved into a therapeutic rather than diagnostic tool (Box 17.5).[95] The procedure is performed under anesthesia with the patient lying on the left side or prone. Significant coagulopathy should be corrected if sphincterotomy is to be performed. Antibiotic prophylaxis is indicated in patients undergoing ERCP for suspected biliary obstruction where incomplete drainage is anticipated or in patients with sterile pancreatic fluid collections that communicate with the pancreatic duct. Patients undergoing EUS with aspiration of a cystic lesion along the GI tract and patients undergoing percutaneous feeding tube placement are also recommended to receive antibiotic prophylaxis.[96] Glucagon may be beneficial to reduce peristalsis of the small bowel, facilitating cannulation of the bile duct. Secretin may be administered to assist in identification of the papilla of Vater in the setting of ulceration, scarring, or malignancy, or the minor papilla in cases of pancreas divisum.

Box 17.5 Indications for Endoscopic Retrograde Cholangiopancreatography

- Treatment of choledocholithiasis
- Treatment of biliary pancreatitis
- Evaluation and treatment of recurrent pancreatitis
- Evaluation and treatment of ascending cholangitis
- Tissue sampling of suspected biliary and pancreatic malignancies
- Diagnosis of ampullary tumors
- Malignant and benign biliary stricture management (sphincterotomy, dilation, stent placement)
- Photodynamic therapy
- Diagnosis and treatment of biliary and pancreatic duct injury and leak
- Pancreatic pseudocyst (stent)
- Stent removal
- Biliary manometry
- Endoscopic sphincterotomy in type I sphincter of Oddi dysfunction
- Endoscopic sphincterotomy in type II sphincter of Oddi dysfunction with manometry-confirmed pressure >40 mm Hg

Adapted from Adler DG, Baron TH, Davila RE, et al: ASGE guideline: The role of ERCP in diseases of the biliary tract and pancreas. Gastrointest Endosc 2005;62:1-8.

After oral intubation, the side-viewing duodenoscope is advanced into the second portion of the duodenum, where the papilla of Vater is located, and the papilla is subsequently cannulated. Visualization of the common bile duct or pancreatic duct is achieved with injection of contrast dye and radiographic fluoroscopy. Biliary obstruction, usually secondary to choledocholithiasis, may be treated with ERCP. Stone extraction is successful in 90% of cases.[97] Techniques for stone extraction involve biliary sphincterotomy or balloon sphincteroplasty, followed by stone removal by soft balloon or wire basket. Large stones may be fragmented before removal with mechanical, laser, or electrohydraulic lithotripsy. Inadequate bile drainage may require biliary stenting to prevent ascending cholangitis.

Bile duct stenting is used to alleviate obstruction caused by malignant and benign disorders and to treat bile duct injuries and leaks.[98] Pancreatic stents are used for pancreatic duct disruptions[99] and pseudocysts that communicate with the pancreatic duct.[100] Stents vary in diameter, length, material (plastic, metallic, and biodegradable), and occlusion rates.

Malignant and benign strictures may be dilated with hydrostatic balloons. ERCP also is used to obtain brush cytology, fine-needle aspiration, or biopsy specimens of a suspected malignancy. Sensitivity is typically low, ranging from 30% with brushings to 60% with all three methods combined.[101] Reports of photodynamic therapy for nonresectable cholangiocarcinoma have been described.[102] Manometry, the measurement of biliary and pancreatic sphincter pressures, may be used to evaluate sphincter of Oddi dysfunction, postcholecystectomy pain, and idiopathic pancreatitis.

Choledochoscopes and pancreatoscopes are small endoscopes that can be passed through a duodenoscope channel port into the common bile duct or pancreatic duct. This placement allows direct visualization of the duct lumen. Direct visualization of vasculature within a biliary stricture may help differentiate benign from malignant lesions.[103]

ERCP carries a substantial morbidity risk. Pancreatitis is the most common complication, occurring in 7% of cases.[104] Although the benefits of prophylactic administration of gabexate mesylate are controversial,[105,106] pancreatic stenting of high-risk patients seems to be efficacious.[107] Stenting decreases papillary hindrance to pancreatic duct drainage. Other reported complications include hemorrhage, cholangitis, and perforation.[108]

ENDOSCOPIC ULTRASOUND

EUS, a combination of endoscopy and ultrasonography, is used for evaluation of luminal walls and structures adjacent to the GI tract. Dedicated ultrasound endoscopes with linear or radial viewing can be used. In addition, high-frequency ultrasound probes that can be passed through the channel port of standard endoscopes are commercially available.[109]

A common application of EUS is to evaluate benign and malignant mucosal and submucosal lesions. EUS is employed routinely for detection and staging of esophageal, gastric, ampullary, pancreaticobiliary, colorectal, and lung neoplasms. EUS also is used to evaluate chronic pancreatitis and biliary disorders, such as calculi. In general, EUS is an extremely sensitive tool and is often superior to computed tomography or magnetic resonance imaging for diagnosis and staging of neoplasia.[110] An advantage of EUS over these noninvasive modalities is the ability to perform therapeutic interventions when needed. Fine-needle aspiration can be done with EUS, which also can be used for pseudocyst drainage, celiac plexus blocks, cholangiography, pancreatography, and tumor ablation.[111]

Preparation of the patient is similar to that for standard endoscopy. Complications from instrumentation vary, depending on the clinical scenario. Perforation rates, usually cervical esophageal in origin, occur in 0.03%.[112] Despite the low risk of bacteremia after EUS fine-needle aspiration, prophylactic antibiotics are recommended for pancreatic cystic lesions and perhaps the perirectal space. Pancreatitis, hemorrhage, and bile peritonitis also have been reported.[113]

ENDOSCOPY IN THE PREGNANT PATIENT

Endoscopy in the general population is commonplace and widely regarded as safe. Endoscopy during pregnancy, however, raises the unique concern of fetal safety and is generally avoided when possible. Potential risks of endoscopy include teratogenesis or premature induction of labor from medications, hypoxemia, and hemodynamic fluctuations, all of which could cause fetal harm. Also, a lack of quality research into the safety of these procedures during pregnancy adds to the uncertainty of performing endoscopic procedures in this population.[114]

In controlled studies, no differences were seen between pregnant and nonpregnant patients undergoing EGD[115] or in fetal outcomes regardless of a history of EGD during pregnancy.[116] Gross acute upper GI bleeding, dysphagia associated with involuntary weight loss, and suspected GI mass have all been suggested as acceptable indications for EGD in the pregnant patient. Data surrounding colonoscopy during pregnancy are less robust, limited to small studies, case series, and case reports, and therefore accurate estimation of risk is not possible. Colonoscopy should be considered for unknown colonic mass or stricture, severe uncontrolled colonic hemorrhage, as an alternative to surgery in colonic pseudo-obstruction, and when required before colonic surgery.[114]

ERCP is associated with unique risks that must be appreciated when considering performing the procedure on a pregnant patient. Procedural time is often longer and increased doses of anesthetic medications are required as compared to EGD. ERCP also places the patient at risk for postprocedural complications including bleeding and perforation from sphincterotomy and post-ERCP pancreatitis. ERCP during pregnancy also introduces a theoretical risk from fetal radiation exposure during fluoroscopy. Despite these risks, it is felt that ERCP can safely be performed during pregnancy as the literature has consistently demonstrated a high maternal success rate, a low procedural complication rate, and generally favorable fetal outcomes.[114] Additionally, although estimates of fetal radiation exposure vary, with careful technique, doses of radiation can be limited to less than the 5 rad threshold often used to minimize risk of fetal anomalies or pregnancy loss.[117] Indications for ERCP during pregnancy include choledocholithiasis with obstructive jaundice, ascending cholangitis, or gallstone pancreatitis, or in the presence of biliary or pancreatic ductal injury.[114]

When considering GI endoscopy in the pregnant patient the physician must ultimately weigh the risks of performing the procedure to the fetus against the benefits to the mother. Guidelines exist offering suggestions to help minimize these risks, such as limiting procedures to patients with strong indications, choosing medications that are safe during pregnancy, close involvement of obstetric staff, and performance of the procedure by an experienced endoscopist. In situations in which therapeutic intervention is necessary, endoscopy may offer a safe alternative to surgery.[118]

KEY POINTS

- Endoscopy serves a diagnostic and a therapeutic role in the management of patients.
- Informed consent must be obtained before any elective endoscopic procedure.

Continued on following page

KEY POINTS (Continued)

- Perforation and bleeding are the major complications of endoscopy. Although standard endoscopy is generally low risk, interventional procedures increase the rate of complications. A benefit versus risk analysis must be done before any procedure.
- Cardiopulmonary decompensation is a possible complication of anesthesia.
- Endoscopy is the most effective technique to identify and control GI hemorrhage.
- Endoscopy plays a crucial role in the palliative care of patients with GI tract malignancy.
- ERCP has evolved into a therapeutic tool for treating pancreaticobiliary disease.
- Endoscopy in the pregnant patient can be done safely but should be limited to patients with strong indications.

SELECTED REFERENCES

10. Varadarajulu S, Banerjee S, Barth B, et al: GI endoscopes. Gastrointest Endosc 2011;74:1-6.
15. Lichtenstein DR, Jagganath S, Baron T, et al: Sedation and anesthesia in GI endoscopy. Gastrointest Endosc 2008;68:815-926.
21. Hwang JH, Fisher, DA, Ben-Menachem T, et al: The role of endoscopy in acute non-variceal upper GI hemorrhage. Gastrointest Endosc 2012;75:1132-1138.
76. May A: How to approach the small bowel with flexible enteroscopy. Gastroenterol Clin North Am 2010;39:797-806.
104. Anderson MA, Fisher L, Jain R, et al: Complications of ERCP. Gastrointest Endosc 2012;75:467-473.
114. Cappell M: Risks versus benefits of gastrointestinal endoscopy during pregnancy. Nat Rev Gastroenterol Hepatol 2011;8:610-634.

The complete list of references can be found at www.expertconsult.com.

18 Continuous Renal Replacement Therapy

Amay Parikh | Lakhmir S. Chawla

CHAPTER OUTLINE

Acute kidney injury (AKI) is common and serious. The incidence of AKI in hospitalized patients ranges from 5% to 7% and is rising rapidly.[1-4] In a multinational study of critically ill patients, the prevalence of AKI requiring dialysis was 5.7% with a mortality rate of 60.3%.[5] In addition, patients with AKI have a higher risk for developing other nonrenal comorbid conditions,[6] and when present in conjunction with other conditions, AKI is associated with higher mortality rate.[7-9] The use of renal replacement therapy (RRT) for treatment of AKI has been ongoing over the last 60 years.[10] According to Hoste and Schurgers, 200 to 300 patients per 1 million population per year develop AKI and are treated with RRT.[11] Despite this, these patients still have a mortality rate of 50% to 60%.[11] Advances and optimization of RRT could benefit the high mortality rate associated with AKI.

The establishment of continuous renal replacement therapy (CRRT) evolved as a treatment for the hemodynamically unstable patient unable to undergo standard intermittent hemodialysis (IHD). Although world trends for CRRT use show an increase in utilization, the majority of the world continues to treat AKI with IHD.[12] Although CRRT offers many theoretical advantages such as better fluid balance, hemodynamic management, and renal recovery, the superiority of CRRT over IHD for RRT in the intensive care unit (ICU) remains controversial.[13]

This chapter first reviews the physiologic principles behind the multifaceted aspect of CRRT before moving onto the technical aspects and clinical issues. We also discuss possible technical complications and ethical considerations in the use of CRRT.

PHYSIOLOGIC PRINCIPLES

Dialysis uses a semipermeable membrane to alter the molecular composition and concentration of blood to restore the body back toward homeostatic balance. Blood flows along one side of the semipermeable membrane and a wash solution, dialysate, flows on the opposite side of the membrane (Fig. 18.1). Dialysis relies upon two physical forces—*diffusion* and *convection*—either in isolation or in combination (Fig. 18.2). In *diffusion*, the net movement of solute is directly dependent on the diffusivity of the solute and solvent, permeability of the membrane, surface area across the membrane, and concentration gradient. Other membrane characteristics also play a role: thickness, pore size, and electrostatic charge. In order to maximize the concentration gradient between the blood and dialysate, the dialysate runs countercurrent to the flow of blood. Any substance that is in higher concentration in the blood than the dialysate flows "down" its concentration gradient and leaves the blood and flows into the dialysate. Conversely, any solute that is in higher concentration in the dialysate (e.g., bicarbonate) will leave the dialysate, cross the semipermeable

HEMODIALYSIS

Indications

- Metabolic acidosis that is refractory to medical treatment
- Electrolyte abnormalities, such as hyperkalemia, that are refractory to medical treatment
- Intoxication with dialysable drugs (e.g., salicylates, lithium)
- Volume overload that is refractory to diuretics
- Uremia and its complications (encephalopathy, pericarditis, bleeding)

In patients with chronic kidney disease:

- Glomerular filtration rate 10–15 mL/min/1.73m^2
- Weight loss, anorexia, loss of appetite
- Any of the sequelae of impaired renal function listed above

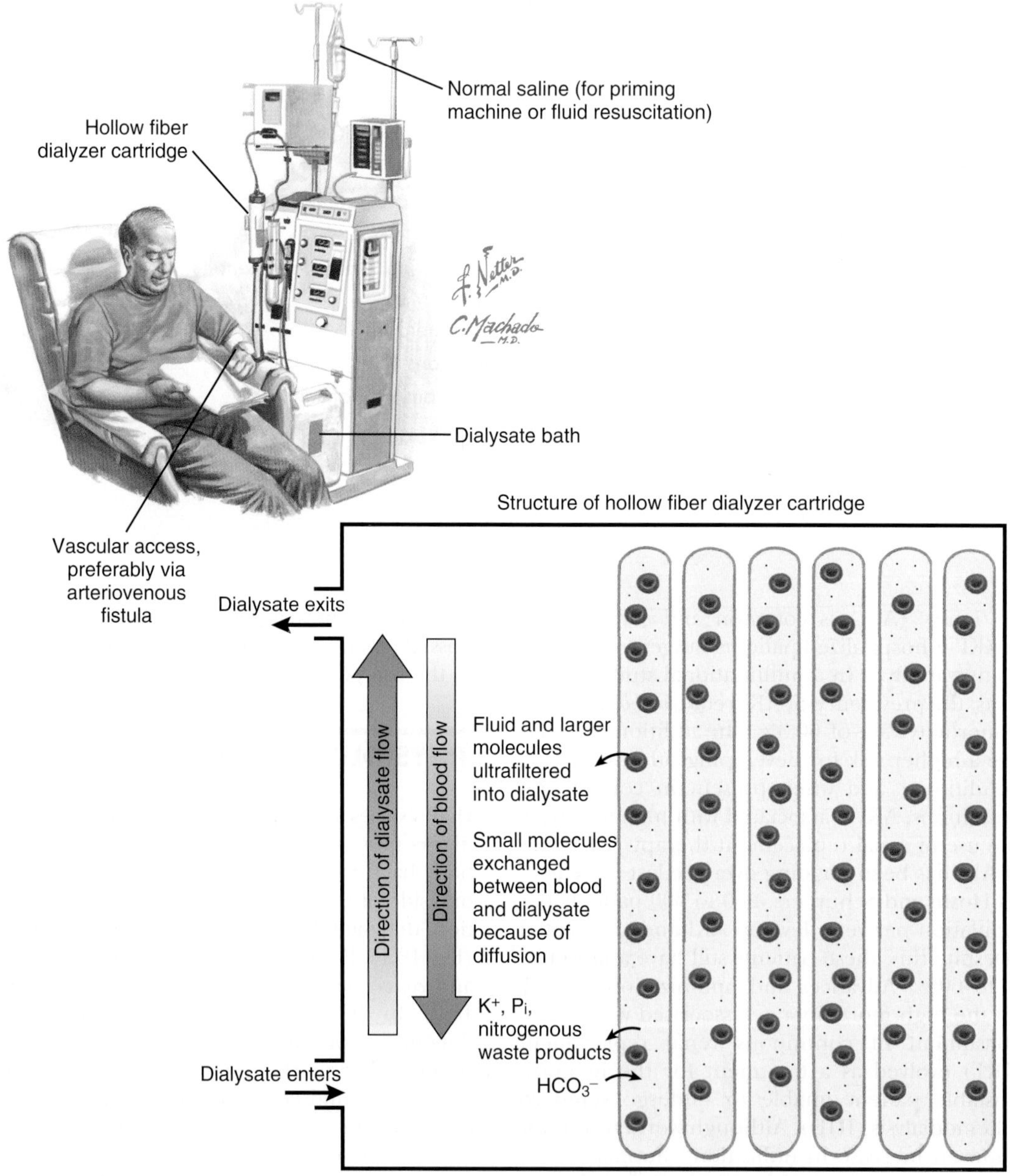

Figure 18.1 Hemodialysis and the filter at a microscopic level. Netter illustration from www.netterimages.com @ Elsevier Inc. All rights reserved. (Netter Plate 10-9 Membrane and Dialysis).

membrane, and enter the blood. The movement of molecules down their concentration gradient from one solution to another continues until equilibrium is achieved in both the blood and dialysate. Diffusion is more efficient in the clearance of small-molecular-weight substances (less than 500 daltons [D]). This is particularly useful in correcting the imbalance in small molecule electrolytes (e.g., K, Ca, Mg, PO_4) (see Fig. 18.1). Thus, thoughtful manipulation of dialysate allows the clinician to decide what will be removed from the blood and what will be added to the blood during a dialysis session.

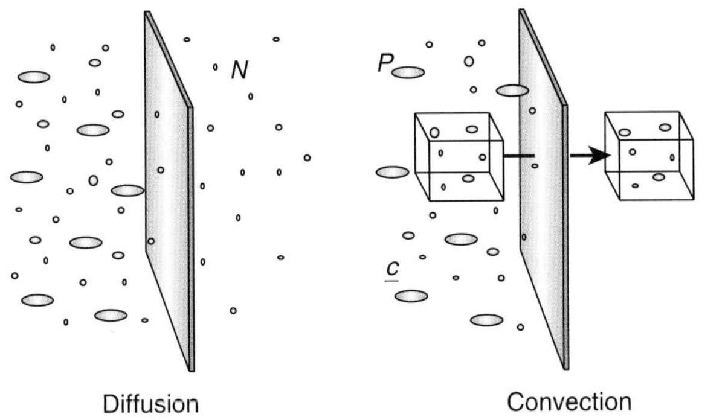

Figure 18.2 Diffusion and convection are schematically represented. During diffusion, the solute flux (Jx) is a function of the solute concentration gradient (dc) between the two sides of the semipermeable membrane, the temperature (T), the diffusivity coefficient (D), the membrane thickness (dx), and the surface area (A), according to the following equation: Jx = DTA (dx/dx). Convective flux of solute (Jf) requires instead a pressure gradient between the two sides of the membrane (transmembrane pressure, or TMP), which moves a fluid (plasma water) with its crystalloid content in a process called ultrafiltration (which is also dependent on the membrane permeability coefficient, or Kf). Colloids and cells will not cross the semipermeable membrane, depending on the pores' size. Jf = Kf × TMP and TMP = Pb − Pd − π where Pb is the blood hydrostatic pressure, Pd is the hydrostatic pressure on the ultrafiltrate side of the membrane, and p is the oncotic pressure. From Ronco, C. In Critical Care Nephrology, 2/E. Phila., WB Saunders, 2008. (Fig. 210-001).

In convection, solutes move across a membrane in response to or following solvent flux or drag: solutes are moving along with the solvent containing them (Fig. 18.3). This is similar to a wave pushing seashells onto the shore. *Solvent drag* is limited only by the pore size or electrostatic charge of any semipermeable membrane that is applied across the passage of the solution. In convection, the concentration of a solute is similar on either side of the membrane. Convection is more efficient at the clearance of large-molecular-weight substances (500-5000 D). Convective removal of plasma water from blood across a large-pore, semipermeable membrane results in an *ultrafiltrate* with a solute composition equivalent to plasma water.

Fluid removal is termed *ultrafiltration* (UF). UF utilizes hydrostatic pressure, which is applied across a semipermeable membrane. This is a form of convective removal of solute. The clearance of molecules in UF is dependent on the volume of fluid removed. It may be applied in isolation (in volumes usually <5 L/day) or in combination with other blood clearance techniques, such as dialysis. Table 18.1 reviews the commonly used terms in CRRT.

One other form of clearance of the blood is through a process called *adsorption*. This refers to molecules in the blood sticking or adhering to the semipermeable membrane. This process is dependent on the molecules contained in the blood and the composition of the semipermeable membrane. Adsorption is usually time dependent (i.e., as

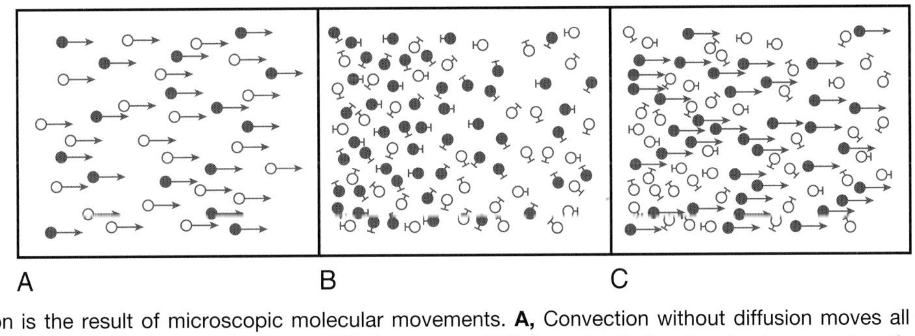

Figure 18.3 Diffusion is the result of microscopic molecular movements. **A,** Convection without diffusion moves all molecules equally and does not result in separation. **B,** Unhindered ordinary diffusion causes initially separated molecules to move together. **C,** Forced diffusion, provided by an external force, separates molecules when the force acts differently on different molecular types. From Ronco, C. In Critical Care Nephrology, 2/E. Phila., WB Saunders, 2008. (Fig. 209-001).

Table 18.1 Modalities of Continuous Renal Replacement Therapy (CRRT)

Feature	SCUF	CVVH	CVVHD	CVVHDF
Method of clearance	Convection	Convection	Diffusion	Convection and diffusion
Middle molecular size clearance	+	+++	+	+++
Replacement fluid	None	Present	None	Present
Dialysate	None	None	Present	Present
Effluent composition	Ultrafiltrate	Ultrafiltrate	Dialysate + ultrafiltrate	Dialysate + ultrafiltrate

CVVH, continuous venovenous hemofiltration; CVVHD, continuous venovenous hemodialysis; CVVHDF, continuous venovenous hemodiafiltration; SCUF, slow continuous ultrafiltration.

the semipermeable membrane is used over time, it will become saturated with a given molecule). The process begins anew when the membrane is changed (approximately every 72 hours). Some inflammatory cytokine clearance occurs through this process.[14]

MODALITIES

The various modalities of CRRT are depicted in Table 18.1 and Figure 18.4.

When UF only is employed on a continuous basis, this is termed slow continuous ultrafiltration (SCUF). This modality would be considered in patients with volume overload, for example, in congestive heart failure (CHF) or anasarca from nephrotic syndrome or liver disease.

Dialysis may also be performed on an intermittent basis (IHD or sustained low-efficiency dialysis [SLED]) (see Fig. 18.1) or a continuous basis (Figs. 18.4 and 18.5). When performed continuously, this is known as continuous venovenous hemodialysis (CVVHD). The "venovenous" refers to the access employed and will be discussed in a later section.

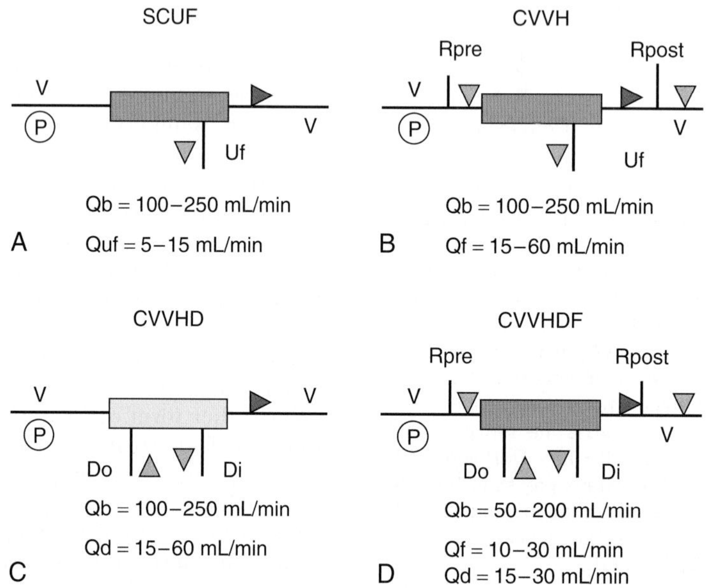

Figure 18.4 Schematic representation of the most common continuous renal replacement therapy (RRT) setups. **A,** Slow continuous ultrafiltration (SCUF). **B,** Continuous venovenous hemofiltration (CVVH). **C,** Continuous venovenous hemodialysis (CVVHD). **D,** Continuous venovenous hemodiafiltration (CVVHDF). See text for specifications. Dark triangles represent blood flow direction; light triangles indicate the flow of dialysate/replacement solutions. Di, dialysate in; Do, dialysate out; P, pump; Qb, blood flow; Qd, dialysate solution flow; Qf, replacement solution flow; Quf, ultrafiltration flow; Rpost, replacement solution postfilter; Rpre, replacement solution prefilter; Uf, ultrafiltration; V, vein. From Ronco, C. In Critical Care Nephrology, 2/E. Phila., WB Saunders, 2008. (Fig. 210-002).

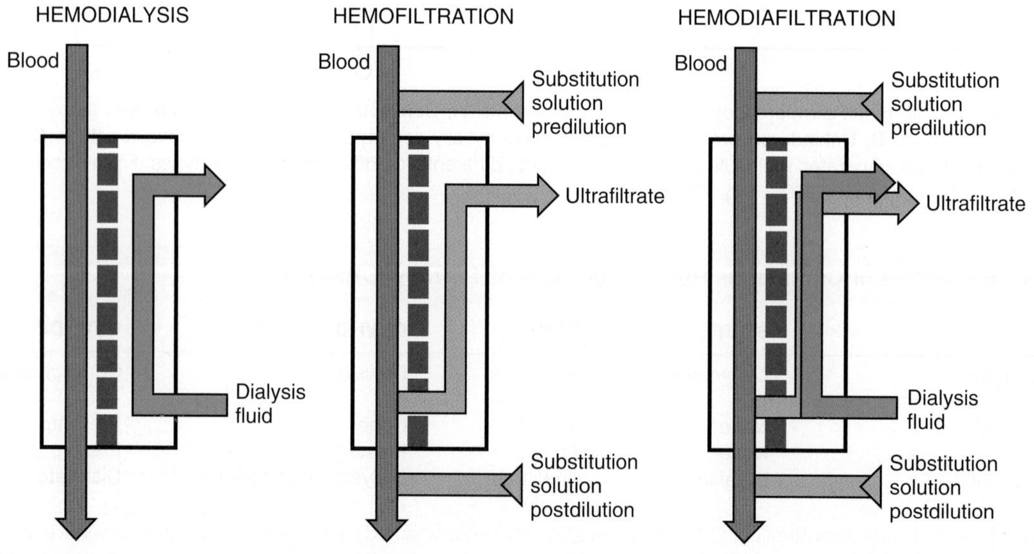

Figure 18.5 Schematic representation of different renal replacement modalities: hemodialysis, hemofiltration, and hemodiafiltration. From Ronco, C. In Critical Care Nephrology, 2/E. Phila., WB Saunders, 2008. (Fig. 215-001).

As described earlier, this is a diffusion-based process that primarily provides small molecule clearance.

Hemofiltration (HF) relies on convective removal of plasma solute, in high fluid volumes, across a semipermeable membrane (see Fig. 18.5). Hydrostatic pressure is applied across the semipermeable membrane as a positive pressure on the blood side of the membrane or a negative pressure on the fluid collection side, or both. Fluid lost through this process is restored with replacement fluid in either a predilutional mode (before the filter containing the semipermeable membrane) or in a postdilutional mode (after the filter). The composition of the effluent fluid created by this system of plasma water exchange (*hemofiltrate*) depends on the membrane *sieving coefficient* for that particular solute and that particular semipermeable membrane. The sieving coefficient is expressed in terms of the ratio of the solute concentrations of the hemofiltrate to the plasma and is a function of membrane thickness, pore size, and electrostatic charge (Fig. 18.6). Hemofiltration is more efficient in middle-molecular-weight compound clearance, but less so for smaller solutes. When performed on a continuous basis, this is known as continuous venovenous hemofiltration (CVVH).

Finally, *hemodiafiltration* (HDF) combines both diffusive and convective solute removal (see Fig. 18.5). When performed continuously, this is known as continuous venovenous hemodiafiltration (CVVHDF). Dialysate is used in this configuration and runs countercurrent to the blood.

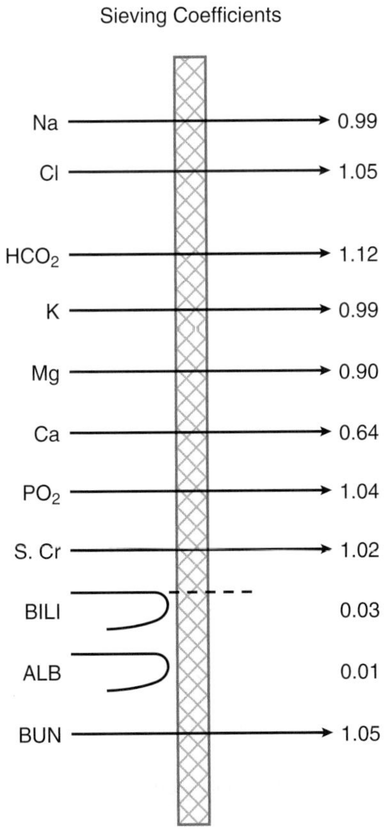

Figure 18.6 In vivo measured sieving coefficients for various serum contents during hemofiltration with a noncuprophane membrane. From Ronco, C. In Critical Care Nephrology, 2/E. Phila., WB Saunders, 2008. (Fig. 019-001).

Concurrently, replacement solution is infused either prefilter or postfilter. This allows for both efficient low-molecular-weight and enhanced middle-molecular-weight clearances. This modality has been employed for sepsis and multiorgan failure, in which removal of cytokine mediator substances is thought to be important.[15]

Figure 18.4 illustrates the mechanics of each of these modalities. Any modality may be described according to its frequency (I [intermittent] versus C [continuous]) and technique (H or HF [hemofiltration], HD, HDF, or UF) as shown in Table 18.2. To date, no one modality has been shown to be superior to the others. Continuous techniques are additionally described according to their vascular access: arteriovenous (AV) or venovenous (VV) (see later discussion under "Access"). Much debate has occurred regarding the superiority of intermittent therapies versus the continuous therapies. To date, the continuous therapies have not been shown to be superior in clinical outcomes to the intermittent therapies. Although the intermittent therapies (IHD and SLED) may be less costly, the continuous modalities allow for hemodynamic stability, enhanced fluid removal, and delivered dose of dialysis.[16]

PRINCIPLES OF ULTRAFILTRATION

Achieving fluid balance by removal is the most frequently requested application for dialytic intervention and is considered the simplest form of continuous therapy. Fluid is drawn from the blood space across a semipermeable membrane. The fluid removed, or ultrafiltrate, has the characteristics of plasma water. With knowledge of the sieving coefficients of a particular membrane for various solutes, the ultrafiltrate can be used to determine the composition of serum and can help avoid an excessive number of blood draws.

In prescribing UF, a specific volume of fluid loss should be determined, with the UF rate (Q_F) set to achieve that loss over a set time frame. It cannot be overemphasized that this form of therapy is by nature *slow*. The steady, constant loss of fluid at a rate that does not exceed the plasma-refilling rate gives this form of therapy its hemodynamic stability. If extremely rapid UF in a short time frame is the therapeutic intent, intermittent forms of pump-driven UF are more efficient and therefore the treatment of choice.

The artificial membranes usually employed have a high UF coefficient (K_{Uf}), allowing water to pass quite freely. Any pressure difference between the blood side and the ultrafiltrate side of the filter results in fluid passage. Higher pressures in the blood compartment of the filter result in net fluid flow from the blood to the ultrafiltrate compartment. This flow is enhanced by applying negative pressures to the ultrafiltrate compartment through gravity or by pumped mechanical suction. This pressure should be held constant and not be subject to rapid variations. If transmembrane pressures are too high, membrane rupture and blood loss may result.

Common UF rates range from 100 to 400 mL/hour. Larger amounts may be obtained if there is a need for rapid fluid removal. Automated continuous machines control UF through a volume-driven system, establishing a fixed loss of a determined amount of fluid from the system over a given time period (usually on an hourly basis).

Table 18.2 Commonly Used Forms of Extracorporeal Renal Replacement Therapy

Therapy	Definition	Use	Specific Techniques
Ultrafiltration	Plasma water removal, usually <5 L/d	Fluid overload High delivery in CRF AKI CHF	SCUF CVVUF IUF
Hemodialysis	Diffusion-based process using dialysate and semipermeable membrane	Azotemia Acid-base disturbance Electrolyte balance Volume control	CVVHD IHD SLED
Hemofiltration	Convection-based process using plasma water exchange methods across semipermeable membrane	Azotemia Acid-base disturbance Electrolyte balance Volume control Cytokine removal ARDS, AKI, CHF, MOF	CVVH IH
Hemodiafiltration	Combining diffusion and convection (10-L exchanges) for small and middle molecular loss	Azotemia Volume control Cytokine removal ARDS, AKI, CHF, MOF	CVVHDF IHDF

AKI, acute kidney injury; ARDS, acute respiratory distress syndrome; ARF, acute renal failure; CHF, congestive heart failure; CRF, chronic renal failure; CVVH, continuous venovenous hemofiltration; CVVHDF, continuous venovenous hemodiafiltration; CVVUF, continuous venovenous ultrafiltration; IH, intermittent hemofiltration; IHD, intermittent hemodialysis; IHDF, intermittent hemodiafiltration; IUF, intermittent ultrafiltration; MOF, multiple organ failure; SCUF, slow continuous ultrafiltration; SLED, sustained low-efficiency dialysis.

The blood flow rate (Q_B) has a significant effect on any UF system. During UF, plasma water is removed from the blood as it moves through the dialysis filter, thereby increasing the viscosity of blood in the filter. If the viscosity increases excessively, the system will clot. Therefore, whenever UF is being prescribed, an appropriate Q_B must be prescribed in order to accommodate the prescribed UF.

Careful attention should be given to the amount of access recirculation. Rates greater than 15% are associated with a greater incidence of clotting. This tendency is more evident at higher UF rates (>300 mL/hour), at which the returning blood tends to have a higher hematocrit, creating a more viscous, afferent blood flow.

PRINCIPLES OF HEMOFILTRATION

As more fluid removal is performed, additional fluid may be needed to replace that which is lost. This is termed hemofiltration or plasma water exchange. Fluid replacement can be delivered into the blood circuit either prefilter, before UF has occurred (predilutional hemofiltration), or after fluid has been removed by the filter (postdilutional hemofiltration).

In predilutional hemofiltration, ultrafiltrated fluid reflects the mixture of blood and replacement solution. To use ultrafiltrate as a surrogate for blood sampling (see previous discussion) would be problematic because correction has to be made for the degree of dilution and for the electrolytic composition of the replacement fluid. Because the oncotic pressure of blood is reduced within the filter, a greater rate of fluid removal is possible at the same transmembrane hydrostatic pressure. This increased rate of fluid removal is offset by dilution of plasma solute. In other words, the overall mass transfer of uremic toxins is reduced, and higher rates of fluid exchange are required to compensate. It is common to have exchange rates of 30 to 40 L/day. Predilutional hemofiltration may also be used for patients with high hematocrit levels in an effort to reduce clotting episodes.

Postdilutional fluid replacement has the advantage of being easier to perform, with lower rates of fluid exchange compared with the predilutional system. One problem with this form of replacement is the increased oncotic pressures at the venous end of the filter. With high rates of exchange or high degrees of access recirculation, blood viscosity may be increased to the extent that clotting may occur. Therefore, fluid exchange rates may be dictated by such factors as hematocrit, blood flow, and access recirculation. Table 18.3 compares predilutional and postdilutional CVVH.

The end point of hemofiltrative therapy is determined by the balance between solutes removed with the ultrafiltrate and those replaced with the substitution fluid. A blood pump is used to increase blood flow and allow higher filtration rates. Infusion pumps are used for the delivery of replacement solution.

The system should be kept below a filtration fraction of 15% in postdilution and 30% in predilution hemofiltration for efficient operation and a lower risk of clotting.

PRINCIPLES OF HEMODIALYSIS

In hemodialysis (HD), the flow of dialysate is countercurrent to that of blood to maximize transmembrane concentration differences across all blood concentrations and at all levels of the filter. Blood flow (100 to 300 mL per minute)

Table 18.3 Comparison of Pre- and Postdilution Techniques for Continuous Venovenous Hemodiafiltration/Hemofiltration

Feature	Predilution	Postdilution
Clearance	Less clearance per milliliter	High small solute clearance per milliliter
Efficiency	Reduced efficiency by 10-15% and reduced filtration fraction	
Ultrafiltration rate limitations	Ultrafiltration rate not limited	Ultrafiltration rate limited by blood pressure and hemoconcentration
Blood viscosity	Low viscosity of the blood	High viscosity of the blood and increased risk of clotting

is maintained well above the usual dialysate flow rates (15 to 30 mL per minute). By contrast, in IHD, blood, rather than dialysate flow, is the limiting factor in diffusive clearance. Clearance of low-molecular-weight substances (e.g., urea, creatinine) is "flow-dependent" because there is little resistance to transmembrane movement posed by the porous membrane. Substances of larger molecular weight (e.g., β_2-microglobulin, vitamin B_{12}) are relatively slow in crossing the dialyzer membrane and are "membrane-dependent" molecules. Using the high-flux membrane characteristics generally employed with continuous therapies, substances with molecular weights (masses) of 20,000 to 30,000 D are transferred at rates that have an inverse relationship to their molecular weights.

Electrolytes, urea, and creatinine easily cross membranes at a rate that is directly proportional to membrane surface area, temperature, and concentration difference, and inversely proportional to viscosity, distance from the membrane, and molecular size. Changing the concentration of various elements in the dialysate alters solute balance. Balance is achieved, however, only between transferable particles. Protein-bound solutes are not subject to the concentration gradients that drive the molecular transport across the membrane. This concept is the basis for altered drug kinetics when patients are subjected to continuous supportive therapy.

In CVVHD, dialysate flow rates remain the most influential factor in determining urea clearance.[17] Dialysate usually is delivered via pumps at rates of 15 to 40 mL per minute. Given adequate blood flow through the circuit, one can see why the limiting factor for flow-dependent transfer is the relatively low dialysate flow rate. Blood flow and filter membrane have limited effects on the diffusion of molecules compared with the potential of dialysate flow changes.

In addition to the diaysate inflow, the dialysate outflow also must be controlled. By setting the outflow rate higher than dialysate inflow rates, one can create a negative transmembrane pressure promoting UF across the dialysis membrane. This difference in flow is used to establish the rate of UF. An increase or decrease in this flow difference would increase or decrease the rate of fluid loss. Dialysate flow is external to and independent of blood flow, and therefore, one may see continued dialysate flow in a system with virtually no blood flow. Although decreases in hemofiltration flow rates may indicate system clotting, dialysate flow rate changes have no predictive value for clotting and may continue despite blood-side occlusion.

Table 18.4 Clinical Considerations in Continuous versus Intermittent Renal Support in the Intensive Care Unit

	Method of Delivery	
Condition/Feature	Intermittent	Continuous
Hemodynamic instability	No/yes	Yes
High fluid requirements	No/yes	Yes
High potassium generation	Yes	No
High catabolism	Yes	Yes/no
Peripheral vascular disease	Yes	Yes/no
Global cardiac dysfunction	No/yes	Yes
Septic shock	No/yes	Yes
APACHE II score >25	No/yes	Yes

APACHE II, Acute Physiology and Chronic Health Evaluation II [disease severity classification system].

Box 18.1 Nonrenal Indications for Continuous Renal Replacement Therapy (CRRT)

- Lactic acidosis - with ongoing production
- Crush injury - Myoglobin removal
- Tumor lysis syndrome
- Temperature control
- Massive volume overload
- High ammonia
- Removal of toxins with high intracellular concentrations (e.g., Li^+)
- Maintenance of cerebral perfusion pressure (CPP) (suggested by some evidence)

CONTINUOUS RENAL REPLACEMENT THERAPY VERSUS INTERMITTENT THERAPY

The clinical presentation and circumstances may favor either intermittent or continuous therapies (Table 18.4). There are many theoretical benefits that may favor the use of CRRT over intermittent forms of therapy, such as improved hemodynamic stability, faster resolution of fluid overload, and increased dialysis dose delivery (Table 18.5). Box 18.1 lists some nonrenal indications for using CRRT.

Table 18.5 Intermittent and Continuous Forms of Renal Replacement Therapy

	Modality		
Feature	IHD	SLED	CRRT
Setting	Hemodynamically stable	Hemodynamically unstable	Hemodynamically unstable Increased intracranial pressure
Advantages	Rapid removal of low-molecular-weight substances and toxins Time when not receiving treatment may be used for diagnostic or therapeutic procedures Reduced anticoagulation exposure Low cost	Hemodynamic stability Time when not receiving treatment may be used for diagnostic or therapeutic procedures Decreased anticoagulation requirements	Easy control of fluid balance Hemodynamic stability Continuous removal of toxins
Disadvantages	Hypotension with rapid fluid removal Dialysis disequilibrium with risk of cerebral edema Technically complex	Slower clearance of toxins Technically complex	Slower clearance of toxins May require anticoagulation Patient immobilization Hypothermia Increased costs

CRRT, continuous renal replacement therapy; IHD, intermittent hemodialysis; SLED, sustained low-efficiency hemodialysis.

Box 18.2 Disadvantages of Continuous Renal Replacement Therapy (CRRT)

Anticoagulation
No rapid removal of electrolytes
Limited role in overdose
Hypothermia (masks a true fever)
Electrolyte depletion: K^+, PO_4^{3-}, Ca^{2+}, Mg^{2+}
Bleeding and thrombosis complications
Minimal removal of protein-bound substances
Membrane adsorption
Negative balance of selenium, copper, thiamine, Mg^{2+}, Ca^{2+}

Box 18.3 Indications for Renal Support

- Fluid control
- Electrolyte balance
  - Hyperkalemia
  - Hyponatremia
  - Hyperphosphatemia
  - Hypermagnesemia
- Acid-base control
  - Metabolic acidosis
  - Mixed acidosis/alkalosis
  - Severe metabolic alkalosis
- Azotemia
- Uremic symptoms
  - Gastrointestinal upset
  - Obtundation
- Uremic signs
  - Pericarditis
  - Neuropathy
- Other
  - Toxin removal

However, clinical trials demonstrating an evidence-based assessment of these potential advantages are still lacking.

Hemodynamic stability is one of the most important advantages for the use of CRRT over intermittent modalities. Slower removal of solute and fluid from the intravascular space by continuous techniques should allow adequate time for refilling from the interstitium and intracellular space, theoretically minimizing therapy-induced hypotension. There are longer term implications for renal recovery, with IHD-related hemodynamic instability potentially predisposing to recurrent renal injury. The data from rigorous, comparative studies seem to lead to varying conclusions, however.

Continuous therapies are able to deliver a higher dose of clearance compared to intermittent therapies. The concept of dose will be covered later in this chapter. Intermittent therapy may have to be provided at a high frequency to produce equivalent levels of solute removal.

Definitive data to support many of the suspected advantages of CRRT are still lacking. In fact, Box 18.2 lists some of the disadvantages of CRRT. Interpretation of much of the published data has been hampered by retrospective analysis, the use of historical control groups, incomplete randomization, incomplete descriptions of patient populations and dialysis dose delivery, and study group–control group heterogeneity.

In the absence of a solid evidence base, how should one decide between prescribing continuous or intermittent therapy? The basic indications for delivering renal support remain unchanged (Box 18.3) and range from the most frequent request for fluid balance to more esoteric requirements such as toxin removal. Common considerations in choosing to apply intermittent or continuous support are listed in Table 18.3, being mindful of numerous relative advantages and disadvantages of each (see Table 18.5).

Hybrid therapies that combine CRRT and IHD techniques are described in the literature as extended daily dialysis, SLED, or prolonged daily intermittent RRT. These therapies use standard IHD equipment to apply lower solute clearances and UF rates for prolonged periods and aim to combine the desirable features of each modality—reduced rate of UF for improved hemodynamic stability, low efficiency solute removal to minimize solute disequilibrium, longer treatment duration to achieve prescribed dialysis dose, and intermittency for the convenience of diagnostic and therapeutic procedures during scheduled downtime.

Sustained low-efficiency dialysis is typically performed with low blood flows of about 200 mL per minute and dialysate flows of 100 to 300 mL per minute. Clearance is predominantly diffusive; however, available systems may also combine diffusive and convective clearance via HDF. Overall, hybrid therapy provides a high dose of dialysis with minimal urea disequilibrium and good control of electrolytes, with survival similar to that predicted by a variety of illness severity scores.

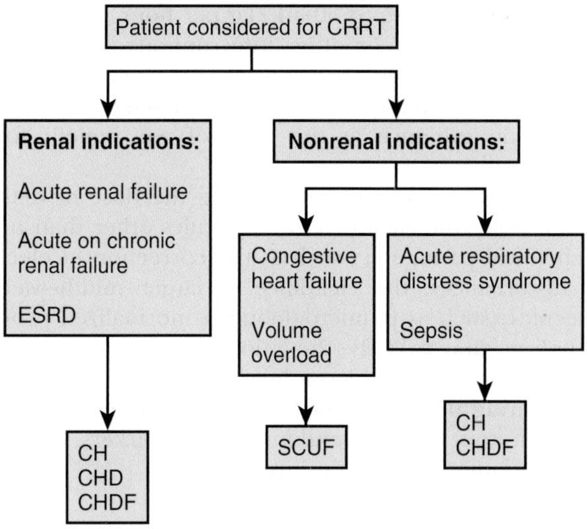

Figure 18.7 Algorithm for the choice of modality in continuous renal replacement therapy (CRRT). CH, continuous hemofiltration; CHD, continuous hemodialysis; CHDF, continuous hemodiafiltration; ESRD, end-stage renal disease; SCUF, slow continuous ultrafiltration. From Ronco, C. In Critical Care Nephrology, 2/E. Phila., WB Saunders, 2008. (Fig. 019-008).

CONTINUOUS HEMODIALYSIS VERSUS CONTINUOUS HEMOFILTRATION

Deciding between the forms of dialytic therapy is dependent on a number of factors: rate of catabolism, mean arterial pressure with resultant blood flow rates, UF rates required or desired, and access choice. The patient's primary diagnosis also influences which modality is chosen, as some data suggest an improved outcome with the use of hemofiltration in some patients with multiple organ failure. Therapy effect on such vastly differing substances as urea and creatinine, molecules of "middle" molecular weight (β_2-microglobulin, vitamin B_{12}), cytokines (tumor necrosis factor-α, interleukins), and hormones (endothelin, angiotensin) is the subject of intense research on potential differences in therapy choice and its influence on patient outcome.

Assuming a flawless period of therapy delivered by all modalities, urea clearance would have a great influence on therapy choice. Circuit variations, anticoagulation, "downtime" of the differing techniques, clotting frequency, and blood and dialysate flow rates all should be considered in the choice. Interruptions to therapy decrease overall treatment effectiveness.

Blood urea nitrogen and creatinine are frequently used as indicators of the need for renal support. Urea or creatinine appearance rates can be used as a gauge of the *quantity* of therapy required. Patients with high urea generation rates should receive HD. The only influence on urea removal in hemofiltration is fluid *exchange* rates; the increased need for fluid removal carries with it a need for greater differences in fluid exchanges, limiting the replacement volume. Given a maximal UF rate dictated by the system's blood flow rate (maximal filtration fraction) and by the patient's hematocrit level, solute clearances are restricted and may be inadequate for that particular patient's needs. Selection of HD allows for the UF rates needed without compromising solute clearance because dialysate flow rates are generally not as limited.

The influence of the dialysate rate on dialyzer clearance is depicted in Figure 18.7. The higher the rate, the more effective the urea clearance, until one reaches a rate approximating the effective plasma flow of the system. The stability of continuous therapies lies in their low rates of exchange over a longer period. The increase in clearance rates must be balanced against the desire to provide stable therapy. If one desires a high rate of removal in a short time, then an intermittent therapy should be employed.

A drawback to diffusive methods of delivery is the relatively low removal rates of the higher-molecular-weight substances. As noted earlier, convection provides greater clearance for substances 5000 to 20,000 D. HD may have limitations when the goal of therapy is targeted toward these larger molecules. This may be the basis for the early reports of improved outcome with patients who were subjected to HDF techniques. The suggested advantage comes from the removal of cytokines and the influence on endotoxin adsorption.

Figure 18.7 depicts an approach to determining the modality of CRRT based on the patient presentation.

PRESCRIPTION VARIABLES

DOSE

Dose in RRT refers to how much of a measure of the quantity of a representative marker solute is removed from a patient. The concept of dose is used to gauge the adequacy of a given treatment. Urea clearance has been the standard molecular marker for IHD. Urea is chosen as an easily measured surrogate for low-molecular-weight products of metabolism. Measuring total urea in the effluent fluid and continuous plasma urea concentration could allow calculation of clearance. However, this is cumbersome and approximations of dose are instead estimated from flow rates of dialysate.

The current recommendation for a minimum dose of RRT supports the delivery of at least 20 mL/kg per hour of CVVH, CVVHD, or CVVHDF. Usually this will require a prescribed dose of 25 to 30 mL/kg per hour (if expecting treatment downtime or other interruptions in treatment, see "Prescribed Versus Delivered Dose"). Although higher doses of dialysis might be beneficial in selected patients, there is no evidence at this time of any benefit for a higher dose.

Other approaches for determining the dose of dialysis include using the clearance of molecules other than urea. Biochemical parameters such as the correction of electrolyte disturbances, the clearance of larger middle-weight molecules (such as β_2-microglobulin), normalized protein catabolism ratio (nPCR), the anion gap, or the strong ion gap have been suggested as a "marker." Clinical parameters of measuring dialysis include fluid balance, improvement and respiratory function, and nutritional markers. However, all of these markers remain investigational.

PRESCRIBED VERSUS DELIVERED DOSE

It is recommended that the prescription of dialysis should exceed that which is calculated to be adequate because there is a difference between what is prescribed and what is actually delivered. In a number of cases the delivered dose of dialysis is much smaller than what is prescribed.[18,19] This can be due to interruptions in treatment due to hemodynamic instability, patient testing, circuit clotting, access recirculation, or other reasons why a patient may need to be disconnected from a machine.

TECHNICAL CONSIDERATIONS

CIRCUITS AND MATERIAL

ACCESS

Access for CRRT is accomplished through a central venous catheter. Vascular access is typically venovenous (VV), as opposed arteriovenous (AV). Intermittent techniques may be either AV (through AV fistulas or grafts) or VV (through venous catheters). The afferent limb of the blood circuitry is termed "arterial" regardless of whether this is truly arterial blood (AV) or not (VV). The returning, efferent limb is termed "venous." AV fistulas or grafts in general may not be utilized as this would require needles to be continuously placed in the fistula or graft, which may damage it.

Several venous catheters are available; the double-lumen design is the most popular because of ease of insertion and good flow characteristics (Figs. 18.8 and 18.9).[20] Catheter failure, either from poor flow or clotting, is the most common cause of therapy underdelivery.[21] System clotting and resistance to blood flow are some of the most frequent manifestations of catheter failure.

The most common sites for dialysis catheter placement are the femoral and internal jugular approaches. Femoral access requires the patient to remain in bed with no more than a 30-degree bend between trunk and leg.[22] The internal jugular and subclavian approaches allow for mobilization, but carry with them the risk of pneumothorax or other intrathoracic trauma during placement. Femoral catheters shorter than 20 cm from hub to tip are associated with higher degrees of access recirculation. Catheters at least 24 cm in length may produce improved flow rates, presumably because their tip reaches the inferior vena cava.[23] Use of the subclavian vein also includes the long-term risk of subclavian venous stenosis with repeated access and should be avoided. If a patient is to require an AV fistula in the future for end-stage renal disease, subclavian stenosis will delay maturation of the AV fistula placed on the same side.

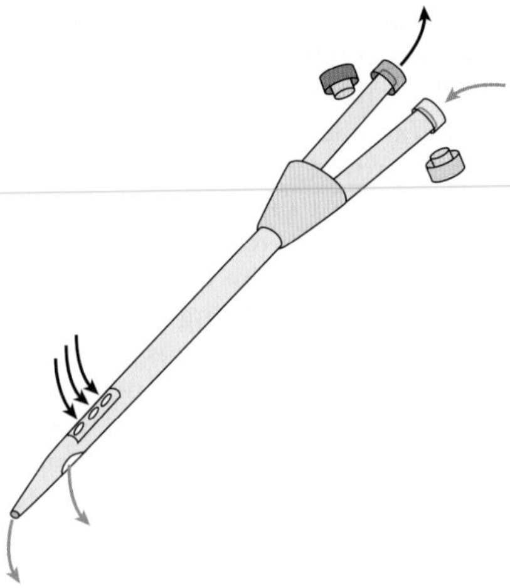

Figure 18.8 Double-lumen polyurethane central venous catheter for short-term use. From Ronco, C. In Critical Care Nephrology, 2/E. Phila., WB Saunders, 2008. (Fig. 222-006).

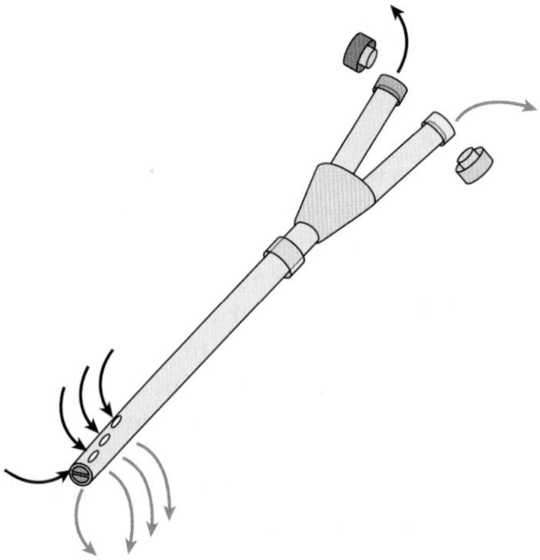

Figure 18.9 Double-lumen silicone (2D) central venous catheter for long-term use in action. From Ronco, C. In Critical Care Nephrology, 2/E. Phila., WB Saunders, 2008. (Fig. 222-007).

TUBING

Long tubing for blood transport increases exposure of blood to nonbiologic surfaces, which cools the blood and increases the risk of clotting. The presence of sampling ports, entry ports, and stopcocks may create blood turbulence. Negative preblood pump pressures can easily introduce air into the circuit from a dysfunctional afferent limb of a catheter and would carry the risk of air embolism were it not for the presence of an air trap in the efferent limb of the circuit.

MEMBRANE

The details of membrane technology are beyond the scope of this chapter; however, the key highlights will be presented here.

The prevalent filter design in CRRT is hollow-fiber. The design consists of a blood compartment and a dialysate compartment, with respective inflow and outflow ports, separated by a semipermeable membrane. The hollow-fiber dialyzer consists of a tubular casing containing thousands of narrow capillary fibers through which blood flows between the arterial and venous header—two small spaces at either end of the filter where blood collects before and after running through the capillary fiber bundle. The capillaries, whose walls constitute the semipermeable membrane, are bathed in dialysate fluid, usually running in countercurrent fashion to blood flow.

The hollow-fiber design allows for the maintenance of systemic blood pressure. However, if clots form at the arterial header, a large surface area of membrane for electrolyte exchange may become unavailable.

Membranes may be made from (1) cellulose (e.g., cuprophane), (2) substituted cellulose (the free hydroxyl groups of cellulose, thought to activate complement, are bound to other substances, e.g., acetate in cellulose acetate membranes), (3) cellulosynthetic material (synthetic material incorporated with the cellulose polymer, e.g., Hemophan), and (4) synthetic material (made of noncellulosic materials, e.g., polysulfone, polyacrylonitrile [PAN], polyamide, and polymethyl methacrylate). A caveat for the use of the PAN filter is the concurrent use of angiotensin-converting enzyme inhibitors; the highly negatively charged membrane tends to bind and activate Hageman factor XII, with subsequent generation of bradykinin—a potential cause for anaphylactic reactions during long-term IHD with PAN. Administration of angiotensin-converting enzyme inhibitors may compound the problem because of their propensity to increase bradykinin production. The asymmetrical design of the polyamide membrane is well suited for UF and hemofiltration, but not for diffusion. PAN and cellulose acetate may have a better structure for diffusive therapies.

FLUIDS

Solutions of fluid take the form of either dialysate or replacement fluid. When hemofiltration is performed, replacement fluid composition dictates the resultant concentration of electrolytes. Similarly, knowing the composition of dialysate is important to determine to what equilibrium the electrolytes will settle. The sieving coefficients for relevant electrolytes and blood components are listed in Figure 18.6. Elements with a negative charge that are small enough to cross the membrane do so at greater than unity. This apparent active transport is actually accomplished through a dynamic process similar to the Gibbs-Donnan effect seen in stagnant fluid balance. Because negatively charged proteins are unable to cross the membrane, chloride and bicarbonate move against a concentration gradient to maintain electrical neutrality. The exaggerated loss of these elements must be reflected in the replacement solution used.

Calcium and magnesium levels should be monitored closely, and replacement should be initiated at an early stage. Because therapy is effective in removing phosphate and generally fluids do not contain phosphate, deficiencies develop, requiring supplementation. In general, these electrolytes are monitored every 12 hours.

As a general rule, to avoid undue hemoconcentration, the filtration rate for postdilutional hemofiltration should be no more than 15% of plasma flow through the filter. A 30% filtration fraction may be allowed in predilutional techniques.

Most fluids either contain lactate or bicarbonate at the base buffer. Other substances have also been considered, for example, the use of acetate or citrate. The use of citrate has an added advantage of being an anticoagulant. Acetate, although previously used extensively in long-term HD, may give rise to vasodilation, myocardial depression, and increased oxygen consumption.[24] As a result acetate should be avoided for CRRT.

Lactate undergoes hepatic conversion to bicarbonate on an equimolar basis. Although more stable than bicarbonate, there are numerous theoretical disadvantages to its use in CRRT. Although bicarbonate-based and lactate-based solutions can correct acidosis, bicarbonate is preferred because lactate-buffered fluids may require intravenous bicarbonate supplementation to achieve the same bicarbonate level.[25] The metabolism of exogenous lactate may be impaired in critical illness, with accumulation giving rise to a paradoxic metabolic acidosis.[26] Hyperlactatemia carries with it potential negative hemodynamic effects and metabolic complications, including increased protein catabolism and reduced adenosine triphosphate regeneration.[27] Complications of lactate overload are more likely to develop in patients with liver impairment and poor peripheral perfusion, particularly with high-volume treatment. Lactate intolerance is defined arbitrarily as a greater than 5 mmol/L increase in lactate levels during therapy.

Bicarbonate, although the more physiologic anion, also has specific drawbacks. It exists in solution with other ions in a state of equilibrium under specific physical conditions of temperature and pressure:

$$CO_2 + H_2O \leftrightarrow H_2CO_3 \leftrightarrow H^+ + HCO_3^-$$

When CO_2 outgassing from the solution occurs (e.g., delivering bicarbonate using an open-top container), overall bicarbonate concentration may be reduced. Additionally, calcium and magnesium can precipitate out as insoluble carbonate compounds when sterilized with the buffer. Many bicarbonate-based solutions are produced with lower concentrations of both cations to help ameliorate this problem, with final mixing of the electrolyte and bicarbonate solutions just before use. A novel adaptation has electrolyte and bicarbonate solutions housed and sterilized in separate chambers of the same bag. A connecting valve is broken just before use to mix the two fluids. A final caveat to the use of bicarbonate is its apparent predilection to bacterial growth—at least in liquid bicarbonate concentrates used in long-term dialysis.

From the data available, although it seems that lactate-based substitution or dialysate fluids may be used safely in many patients, they should be avoided in patients with lactic acidosis or hyperlactatemia and in patients with hepatic failure. Bicarbonate-buffered solutions should be used in these cases.

ANTICOAGULATION

Circuit clotting is the most frequent cause of therapy interruption in CRRT. Various factors may account for the hypercoagulable state in a patient receiving CRRT.[28] Anticoagulation during CRRT is necessary to preserve the life of the extracorporeal circuit, to maximize the CRRT dose, and to minimize blood loss caused by clotting during CRRT. The ideal anticoagulant should have no effect on systemic hemostasis, no increase in hemorrhagic risk, only be limited to the extracorporeal circuit, optimize filter performance in circuit life, have a short half-life, be easily monitored, be easily reversible, and be inexpensive.[29] Options for anticoagulation of the circuit include using no anticoagulation, unfractionated heparin, low-molecular-weight heparin, citrate, and in rare circumstances thrombin antagonists or prostaglandins. Box 18.4 lists current strategies to prevent circuit clotting. According to a world survey, 44% of those surveyed preferred unfractionated heparin for anticoagulation.[30]

The option of no anticoagulation is usually used in patients with intrinsic coagulopathies such as hepatic failure or low platelet count. Circuits are usually primed with saline or heparin. Intermittent normal saline flushes may be used as well. The rates of filter clotting using this method vary widely. The mean filter life lies between 16 and 70 hours if the patient is coagulopathic. In cases of severe coagulopathy, shorter filter life may be seen. The disadvantages of no anticoagulation include the need for increased UF, the risk of dialyzer fiber rupture, and the extra nursing workload.[31] The hemoconcentration induced by high UF volumes in CVVH and CVVHDF promotes clotting but may be minimized by predilutional fluid replacement. This comes at the price, however, of the inefficiency of ultrafiltering a mixture of just-infused replacement fluid and plasma, the proportions of which are important considerations in the CRRT prescription.

Unfractionated heparin works by inactivating factors Xa and IIa. The molecular weights of unfractionated heparins range from 5 to 30 kDa. The half-life of unfractionated heparin is 90 minutes; however, this may be increased up to 3 hours in renal failure. The use of unfractionated heparin involves infusing continuous heparin at the arterial site of the circuit. Usually a bolus of 2000 to 5000 IU of heparin is used. Continuous infusion of heparin ranges between 5 and 20 units/kg per hour. In general, an activated partial thromboplastin time (aPTT) goal ranges between 34 and 45 seconds (1.5-2.0 times the normal). The reported circuit patency of this ranges between 20 and 40 hours. The advantages of using unfractionated heparin include the fact that it is effective, widely available, involves simple monitoring (i.e., aPTT), is easily reversed with protamine, is inexpensive, and has a short half-life. The disadvantages of the use of unfractionated heparin include systemic bleeding, unpredictable kinetics, aPTT not being a reliable predictor for bleeding, heparin resistance due to low antithrombin levels, and heparin-induced thrombocytopenia (HIT).

HIT may develop during heparin therapy.[32] HIT begins with heparin exposure stimulating the formation of heparin-platelet factor 4 antibodies, usually 5 to 12 days after starting therapy. This triggers the release of procoagulant platelet particles. Both thrombosis and thrombocytopenia ensue and cause significant vascular complications. The prevalence of HIT varies among several subgroups, with greater incidence in surgical as compared with medical populations. HIT must be acknowledged for its intense predilection for thrombosis and suspected whenever thrombosis occurs after heparin exposure. In CRRT, this is manifested as recurrent filter clotting. The treatment of HIT mandates the cessation of all heparin exposure and the institution of an antithrombotic therapy, most commonly using a direct thrombin inhibitor. Current "diagnostic" tests, which primarily include functional and antigenic assays, have more of a confirmatory than diagnostic role in the management of HIT. Platelet aggregation studies are highly specific but lack sensitivity, so if they and heparin-induced platelet activation tests yield negative results, an enzyme-linked immunosorbent assay should be performed. Direct thrombin inhibitors are appropriate, evidence-based alternatives to heparin in patients with a history of HIT.

Direct thrombin inhibitors such as recombinant hirudin (lepirudin), danaparoid, and argatroban have been used in response to HIT.[33,34] Bleeding resulting from overdosage of lepirudin or argatroban may be treated with the administration of fresh-frozen plasma. Hemofiltration with high-flux dialyzers also can reduce the plasma levels of hirudin.

Citrate regional anticoagulation works by chelating free calcium in the extracorporeal circuit and prevents the activation of calcium-dependent procoagulants. The anticoagulant effect of citrate is measured by ionized calcium levels. Anticoagulation is reversed by a calcium infusion. Normal blood levels of citrate are approximately 0.05 mmol/L. The bleeding time for a patient with citrate levels of 4 to 6 mmol/L can be infinite. Levels of 12 to 15 mmol/L are required for storing blood products for transfusion therapy. Citrate levels are usually performed in another facility or reference laboratory. Citrate has a plasma half-life of 5 minutes and is rapidly metabolized by the liver, kidney, and muscle cells. The extracorporeal clearance of citrate is the same as that of urea. The sieving coefficient ranges between 0.87 and 1.0. The clearance of citrate is the same for both CVVH and CVVHD.[35] The advantage of using citrate is that

Box 18.4 Current Strategies to Prevent Continuous Renal Replacement Therapy Circuit Clotting

- Heparin
  - Standard, prefilter
  - Regional
  - Low dose, prefilter
  - Systemic
- Low-molecular-weight heparin
- Citrate
- No anticoagulation
  - Saline solution flushes
  - No intervention
- Prostacyclin
- Hirudin
- Heparin bonding
- Serine protease inhibitors

it is regional and avoids bleeding complications. It also doubles as a buffer. It is more effective than heparin in studies,[36,37] and it does not cause thrombocytopenia. Two early trials have shown that the use of citrate for regional anticoagulation yields no additional bleeding risk and leads to longer filter life.[36,37] The largest citrate randomized controlled trial used citrate for anticoagulation in a postdilutional CVVH modality with blood flows of 220 mL per minute and citrate concentration of 3 mmol/L.[38] The study showed a lower mortality rate in patients receiving citrate regional anticoagulation. It is hypothesized that citrate inhibits leukocytes esterase, which may yield immunologic benefits. The major disadvantage of citrate stems from its metabolic complications and the complex protocols that are involved in its administration. Metabolic consequences of citrate use include metabolic alkalosis from citrate overdose or toxicity, metabolic acidosis in a setting of severe liver disease or hypoperfusion, hypernatremia from hyperosmolar citrate solutions (4% sodium citrate), and hypocalcemia and hypercalcemia from inappropriate calcium supplementation. The risk factors for citrate toxicity include liver disease, nursing or pharmacy errors leading to overdose, shock liver, and severe hypoperfusion states. The detection of citrate toxicity then becomes extremely important. One should expect citrate toxicity when noticing a rising anion gap, worsening metabolic acidosis, a falling systemic ionized calcium, escalating calcium infusion requirements, or a total calcium/systemic ionized calcium ratio greater than 2.5 : 1.[39] Strategies to manage citrate toxicity include decreasing the citrate infusion rate, decreasing the blood pump speed, and increasing the dialysate flow rate.

The decision as to which citrate protocol to use depends on the available citrate solutions, the method of citrate delivery, and the CRRT circuit options. Available commercial citrate solutions include concentrations of sodium citrate between 1.32% and 4%. Regional citrate anticoagulation may be performed using 4% trisodium citrate or with ACD-A solution (anticoagulant citrate dextrose solution, form A) containing 3% combined trisodium citrate (2.2 g/100 mL), citric acid (0.73 g/100 mL), and dextrose (2.45 g/100 mL) (Baxter-Fenwal Healthcare Corp., Deerfield, IL). ACD-A solution is preferred over trisodium citrate for routine regional citrate anticoagulation because it is less hypertonic and commercially prepared, potentially reducing mixing errors and the complications associated with overinfusion. Regional citrate anticoagulation protocols differ in the type of citrate preparation used, the mode of dialysis, and the ability to customize dialysis solutions. There is a fixed relationship between the blood flow in citrate delivery. The titration of citrate delivery should be based on the ionized calcium level. The amount of citrate delivered to achieve a blood citrate concentration of 4 mmol/L depends on the blood flow.[40]

In a typical circuit (Fig. 18.10) arterial blood leading from the patient is first infused with citrate, which chelates the free ionized calcium. This blood then enters the filter where a calcium-free dialysate is used. Postfilter ionized calcium is monitored and used to titrate the citrate rate to ensure anticoagulation. The goal is to keep the ionized calcium at less than 0.35 mmol/L. The returning blood combines with the venous blood in the body, which normalizes the ionized calcium and prevents systemic anticoagulation. Calcium is

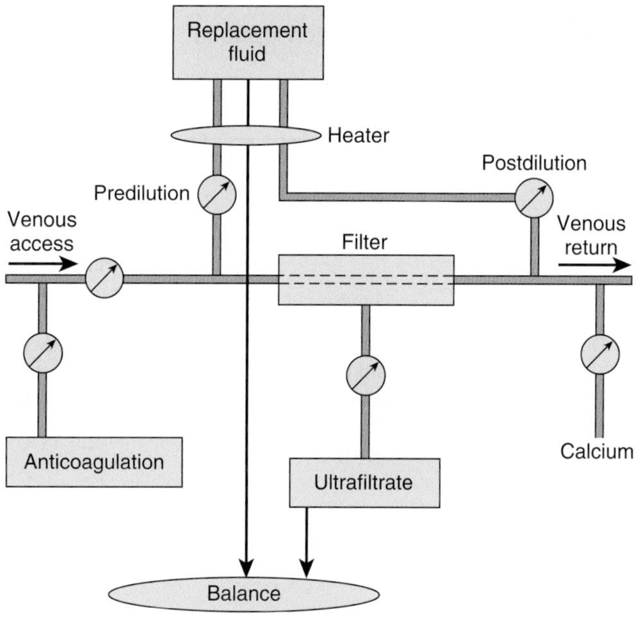

Figure 18.10 Schematic presentation of the continuous venovenous hemofiltration (CVVH) circuit. The circuit has a heater, a balance, and six pumps: a blood pump, an ultrafiltrate pump, two pumps for replacement (predilution and postdilution), an anticoagulation pump, and a calcium pump, to be used for citrate anticoagulation. From Ronco, C. In Critical Care Nephrology, 2/E. Phila., WB Saunders, 2008. (Fig. 248-001).

infused through a separate central line to replace the calcium lost in the ultrafiltrate. Citrate is metabolized primarily in the liver to bicarbonate and the bound calcium is released. For CVVH, citrate may or may not be a component of the replacement fluid.

A number of citrate protocols have been published. Protocols vary based on the number of fluid solutions utilized and commercial versus hospital specific fluid options. Published protocols include those from Massachusetts General Hospital,[41] Gainesville,[42] University of Alabama at Birmingham,[43] Sunnybrook,[44] and San Diego.[45]

Low-molecular-weight heparins (such as enoxaparin, dalteparin, and nadroparin) have also been examined for their effect on circuit life.[46] Prostacyclin (prostaglandin I_2), a potent, short-acting, endogenous inhibitor of platelet aggregation, has also been studied.[47]

Clinical experience with various agents and strategies influence choice. Table 18.6 reviews the advantages and disadvantages of each anticoagulation option.

THERAPEUTIC CONSIDERATIONS

PATIENT SELECTION

The question as to whether a patient needs renal replacement therapies is often difficult. There is no consensus as to the indication to start RRT, the criteria to start RRT, or the appropriate time for initiation of RRT. The conventional indications include volume overload, metabolic acidosis, hyperkalemia, uremia, azotemia without uremic manifestations, and drug overdose. The risks of dialysis include

Table 18.6 Anticoagulation Options

Feature	None	Heparin (Unfractionated)	Low-Molecular-Weight Heparin	Citrate
Advantages	Reduced risk of bleeding	Widely available Commonly used Short half-life Available reversal agent Monitoring accomplished with routine tests (aPTT) Low cost	Reduced risk of HIT Predictable kinetics (weight-based dosing) Monitoring not required	Strict regional anticoagulation—reduced risk of bleeding
Disadvantages	Risk of blood loss and clotting of system Microthrombi in filter may decrease efficiency	Narrow therapeutic index—risk of bleeding Heparin resistance HIT	Risk of accumulation in kidney failure If monitoring required, then a nonroutine test is necessary (anti-factor Xa) Incomplete reversal by protamine May be more expensive than unfractionated heparin	Overdose may be fatal Citrate may accumulate in patients with hepatic dysfunction and shock, which may result in metabolic acidosis and hypocalcemia Metabolic complications (acidosis, alkalosis, hypernatremia, hypocalcemia, hypercalcemia) Increased complexity requires a strict protocol

aPTT, activated partial thromboplastin time; HIT, heparin-induced thrombocytopenia.

hypotension, complications of placing vascular access, and air embolism (extremely rare). Additional risks and complications are listed in Box 18.5 Patients in the ICU may have a number of conditions that impact the decision to initiate and prescribe RRT. In general, if patients have insufficient renal function, CRRT can be utilized to provide organ support much in the way that the ventilator is used to provide pulmonary support. Potential indications for renal support include nutrition, fluid removal in CHF, cancer chemotherapy, the treatment of respiratory acidosis in acute respiratory distress syndrome (ARDS), and fluid management in multiorgan failure.[48]

TIMING OF INITIATION AND DISCONTINUATION

The use of the traditional biomarkers such as creatinine may delay the initiation of RRT. As a result, criteria such as RIFLE (risk, injury, failure, loss of kidney function, end-stage renal disease) have been used to grade the severity of one's AKI. It is known that the net fluid balance affects the outcomes of critically ill patients; fluid overload itself may be a marker of more severe disease. The difficulty in answering the question as to when to initiate RRT is that we will never know whether those who received dialysis would have recovered renal function if they had not received the therapy. There is no prospective randomized controlled trial to answer this question.

Dialysis is discontinued when the signs of renal recovery are apparent. This often takes the form of increased urine output, the decrease in biomarkers, or improvement in the patient's clinical status. CRRT may be switched to intermittent forms when the patient is hemodynamically stable and daily fluid balance would afford intermittent treatments (usually no more than 2 L positive per day). However, as with the initiation of dialysis there is no consensus as to when the therapy should be discontinued.

RENAL RECOVERY

Recovery of renal function may manifest quite differently, depending on whether the patient was supported with intermittent or continuous techniques. Patients receiving CRRT may not show the typical signs of renal recovery because often their fluid balance is close to their premorbid weight. A decrease in the baseline serum creatinine without a change in the CRRT prescription may be the first sign of renal improvement. Urine creatinine and sodium may be more helpful in assessing patients receiving continuous rather than intermittent therapy. Recognizing these differences helps avoid extending therapy beyond what is needed and aids in hastening recovery when it has begun.

PHARMACOKINETICS DURING CONTINUOUS RENAL REPLACEMENT THERAPY

Altered drug kinetics is an important aspect of CRRT management, with some agents being cleared in significant quantities. Depending on membrane pore size, the passage of substances with molecular weights of 20,000 to 30,000 D is possible and may accommodate most drugs. As the clearance of drugs is limited to the free, non–protein-bound fraction, the degree of plasma protein binding dictates

Box 18.5 Possible Complications of Continuous Renal Replacement Therapy

Access

- Distal arterial insufficiency
- Embolism (air, thrombus, foreign body)
- Early
  - Early thrombosis
  - Infection
  - Hematoma (local/retroperitoneal)
- Late
  - Angiocutaneous fistula
  - Stenosis
  - Aneurysm (pseudo/real)
  - Loss of potential long-term intermittent hemodialysis arteriovenous fistula/graft site

Blood Pump

- Air embolism
- Blood loss

Lines

- Disconnection/hemorrhage
- Infection
- Thrombosis
- Kinking

Kidney

- Clotting
- Membrane rupture
- Backdiffusion of pyrogens from contaminated dialysate
- Membrane hypersensitivity reaction

Therapy

- Overanticoagulation/citrate intoxication
- Electrolyte abnormalities (see Table 18-7)
- Amino acid losses
- Fluid imbalance
- Hypothermia

whether dialysis or filtration would result in significant removal. Pharmacokinetics also is highly dependent on the drug's volume of distribution. Also, if the contribution of alternative elimination pathways to overall drug clearance is significant, then the clinical relevance of extracorporeal removal may be minimal.

A drug with low protein binding, a low volume of distribution, and low clearance by alternative pathways is one that would be cleared significantly by CRRT. Vancomycin and the aminoglycosides are good examples, and such agents require dosage adjustments if administered during continuous therapy.

Body clearance of drugs without significant tubular secretion or reabsorption is a linear function of creatinine clearance. Estimation of drug clearance by dialytic modalities is a more complex proposition and has to take account of dialysate and blood flow rates; the molecular weight of the drug; and membrane surface area, thickness, and composition. Nomograms used in the prediction of dialytic drug clearance may be used,[49] but these provide only a general guideline. The impact of molecular weight differs between dialytic techniques and may be lower in CVVHD, which usually uses high flux membranes at a low dialysate flow rate (Q_D). Under these circumstances, the Q_D may approximate Q_F in the previous equations.[50] Drug clearance during CVVHDF may be estimated by combining calculations of filtrative removal with calculations of dialytic removal, but the complex interplay between convection and diffusion is not fully appreciated by this approach.

A final confounder of pharmacokinetic predictability is the impact of membrane adsorption of the drug, which may be substantial with PAN/AN69 materials and may vary depending on the frequency of filter changes. Such filters that remain in situ for long enough can start to release their adsorbed drug back into the circulation. In adjusting dosing of a drug that is significantly cleared by CRRT, a choice must be made either to shorten the dosing interval (to maintain plasma levels) or to increase the dose (to optimize peak concentrations) depending on that agent's mode of action. Formulas have been developed to estimate adjustments of dose and dosing interval.[50,51]

Published data do exist to help guide drug dosing during CRRT, but they come from a variety of sources and are often not standardized. The use of aids to estimate dose, such as those detailed previously, is required.

COMPLICATIONS OF THERAPY

Perhaps the most frequent problems encountered are electrolyte derangements (Table 18.7). With the use of hemofiltration, as we have seen earlier, the replacement solution determines the final electrolyte outcome. The replacement solution must reflect the sodium, chloride, and bicarbonate concentrations that one would like to achieve in patient serum and the relative loss via the hemofilter. The substance's particular sieving coefficient can be used to determine therapeutic losses, following the formula:

$$[\ ]_s \times S_{coef} \times Q_F$$

where $[\ ]_s$ is the incoming blood concentration of the substance, S_{coef} is its sieving coefficient, and Q_F is the UF rate (see Fig. 18.6). Not only the actual replacement fluid, but *all* fluid must be taken into consideration. Frequently, drug vehicles with water or hypotonic hyperalimentation solutions are calculated in the fluid exchange, but not in the electrolyte balance. The resultant loss of sodium (in the hemofiltrate) and the replacement with hypotonic solution produce a true hyponatremia. The exaggerated loss of bicarbonate and chloride also produces variations if these balances are not considered in the total composition delivered to the patient.

Ionized calcium, magnesium, and phosphate also are lost during continuous hemofiltration and HD. This is a different situation from that of intermittent therapies, where these substances are usually retained and need to be subject to a limited intake. It is not unusual for patients to require the addition of magnesium, calcium, and phosphate to cover therapeutic losses and establish normal plasma levels. Serum levels should be checked frequently (up to every 12 hours), and replacement should be calculated as noted earlier.

Table 18.7 Common Electrolyte Problems During Continuous Renal Replacement Therapy with Their Solutions

Problem	Solutions
↓ Na^+	1. Change all fluid infusions to 0.9% saline or equivalent. 2. Increase dialysate sodium (add NaCl). 3. Ensure adequate sodium delivery in replacement solution.
↓ HCO_3^-	1. Ensure adequate HCO_3^- concentration in dialysate/replacement. 2. With lactate-based solutions, consider change to HCO_3^- base (especially in liver failure or shock). 3. Increase HCO_3^- in TPN.
↓ Ca^{2+}	1. Increase Ca^{2+} in TPN. 2. Add Ca^{2+} to dialysate/replacement (if HCO_3^- base, may need to add elsewhere). 3. Ensure adequate oral Ca^{2+} intake if appropriate.
↓ PO_4^{2-}	1. Pay close attention to antacid use (acts as gastrointestinal PO_4^{2-} binder; may need to be stopped). 2. Increase PO_4^{2-} in TPN.
↓ Mg^{2+}	1. Increase Mg^{2+} in TPN. 2. Add Mg^{2+} to dialysate/replacement (if HCO_3^- base, may need to add elsewhere). 3. Supplement as MgCl or $MgSO_4$.
↑/↓ K^+	1. Avoid repeated bolus therapy if ↓ K^+. 2. Adjust K^+ in dialysate/replacement. 3. If ↑ K^+ uncontrolled, add intermittent therapy. 4. May need addition or discontinuation of K^+ binder therapy.

TPN, total parenteral nutrition.

Continuous HD procedures also require frequent electrolyte monitoring. Serum values generally reflect the dialysate concentration of that particular solute. Establishing a potassium floor of 4 mEq/L merely requires that the dialysate concentration of potassium also be set at 4 mEq/L. Common electrolyte problems seen in patients receiving continuous therapies are listed in Table 18.7. Box 18.5 lists other possible complications.

ETHICAL CONSIDERATIONS

Bioethical issues related to CRRT have been widely discussed. Many times the use of dialysis involves the decision of tapering aggressive interventions. Oftentimes, the kidney appears to be the last organ in the chain of multiorgan failure. From the family's perspective the use of dialysis is usually not a predefined life-sustaining measure. The use of dialysis is often a source of conflict of attitudes between the treating teams of the patient. The decision to initiate dialysis should be a discussion between the treating team, the one prescribing CRRT, and the patient and caregivers. This can either be a long-term treatment for a short-term test case in the setting of longstanding chronic disease or set an advance illness. The discontinuation or withdrawal many times is the decision of the entire team.

NONRENAL APPLICATION OF CONTINUOUS THERAPIES

The hemodynamic stability of continuous renal therapies has contributed to their use in situations in which fluid loss is desired but patient status has restricted more standard dialytic or other therapeutic interventions. The ability to manipulate a continuous extracorporeal blood circuit also has opened wide opportunities to assess a variety of different nonrenal applications (Fig. 18.11). The basic circuit has been incorporated into liver assist devices (currently undergoing clinical testing), and the ability to either warm or cool circulating blood has applications in clinical and experimental medicine. The adsorptive nature of different membrane types and structures also has been the focus for potential therapeutic interventions.

Perhaps the most frequently cited area of use has been isolated UF for the treatment of CHF. Several studies have described the utility of UF for the removal of extravascular lung water in models subjected to pulmonary damage or fluid overload.

The sieving and adsorptive qualities of the continuous extracorporeal circuit have found their way into the manipulation and eventual management of patients with sepsis or systemic inflammatory response syndrome. Numerous experimental studies have touted the ability of various membranes either to remove or to adsorb various cytokines. Tumor necrosis factor-α, interleukin 1, interleukin 6, and interleukin 8 have been the most studied, but endothelin, lipopolysaccharide fragments, and C3a and C5a also have been identified. High-volume zero-balance hemofiltration has been the focus of several animal experiments, in which control of systemic inflammatory response syndrome has been noted.

Clinical translation of this approach consistently has failed to confirm bench findings for many reasons. Extracorporeal removal of inflammatory mediators may be negligible in relation to endogenous turnover. Extracorporeal treatment was usually initiated within a short time frame after induction of experimental sepsis; this is almost impossible to achieve in the real world. Potentially beneficial substances, such as interleukin 10, water-soluble vitamins, and elements such as zinc or selenium, also may be cleared. As a result, clinical application of these techniques has been viewed with some caution.

The adsorptive qualities of specific membranes (AN-69, PAN) have been the most accepted mode of clinical attempts at cytokine control. Although early data seem to point to an impact in lowering blood cytokine levels, a cumbersome and costly exchange of circuit filters, with saturation seen at 2 to 4 hours, brings into question the practicality of this approach.

SUMMARY

The use of continuous extracorporeal therapies in the management of AKI has added another therapeutic option to the armamentarium of clinicians caring for an increasingly

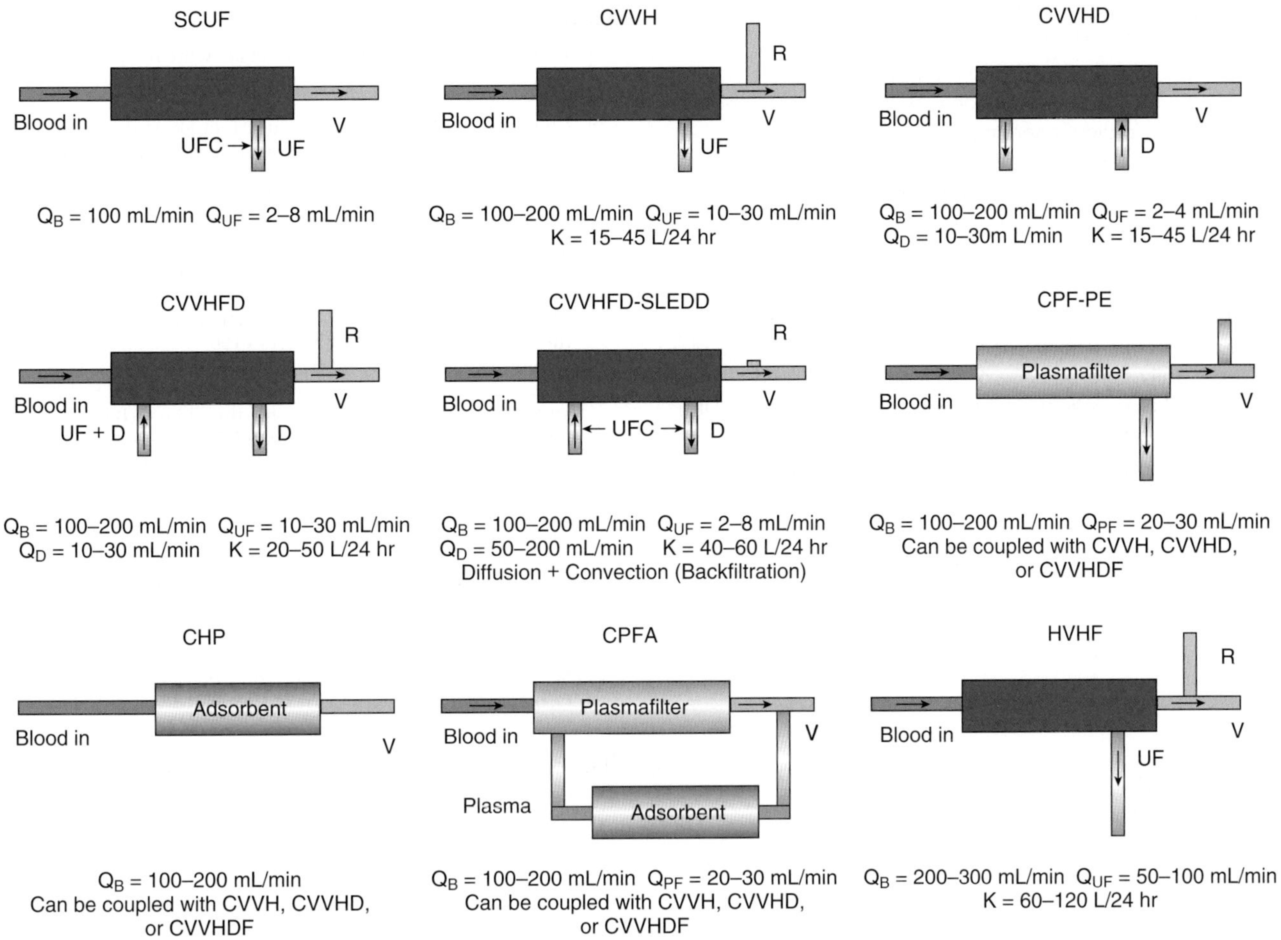

Figure 18.11 Modalities of CRRT. Techniques available today for renal replacement in the intensive care unit. CHP, continuous hemoperfusion; CPF-PE, continuous plasmafiltration–plasma exchange; CPFA, coupled plasmafiltration-adsorption; CVVH, continuous venovenous hemofiltration; CVVHD, continuous venovenous hemodialysis; CVVHDF, continuous venovenous hemodiafiltration; CVVHFD, continuous venovenous high-flux dialysis; D, dialysate; HVHF, high-volume hemofiltration; K, clearance; QB, blood flow; QD, dialysate flow; QPF, plasmafiltrate flow; QUF, ultrafiltrate flow; R, replacement; SCUF, slow continuous ultrafiltration; SLEDD, sustained low-efficiency daily dialysis; UF, ultrafiltration; UFC, ultrafiltration control system. From Ronco, C. In Critical Care Nephrology, 2/E. Phila., WB Saunders, 2008. (Fig. 240-006).

complicated ICU population. The heterogeneity of the ICU AKI experience warrants the availability and use of the appropriate form of renal support as dictated by the individual patient's condition, allowing the patient to derive the greatest potential benefit. Applying these various tools in a rational and cost-effective manner is the true challenge for physicians who practice intensive care medicine.

KEY POINTS

- CRRT holds many theoretical advantages over intermittent modalities, including maintenance of hemodynamic stability, enhanced fluid removal, and increased dialysis dose delivery. Despite these benefits, there has yet to be a clear outcome advantage with this form of therapy.
- The role of therapy application (diffusion versus convection) may be decided less on the character of the therapy and more on the potential for membrane clearance: larger molecules (convection) and smaller molecules (diffusion).

KEY POINTS (Continued)

- A typical CRRT prescription would include the following elements: blood flow 250 to 300 mL per minute; dialysate or replacement flow rate 20 to 25 mL/kg per hour; and UF rate as determined by the daily fluid balance goal of the patient. Owing to treatment interruptions, the patient may not receive the prescribed dose.
- Central venous access is necessary for CRRT and is best accomplished by a dialysis catheter placed preferably in the internal jugular or femoral vein.
- A variety of bicarbonate-based and lactate-based solutions are available commercially. Close evaluation of the various components helps identify the appropriate composition for the particular patient need. In general, potassium concentrations of 4 mEq/L

Continued on following page

KEY POINTS (Continued)

are used to maintain or raise a patient's serum potassium. Concentrations of 0 or 2 mEq/L are used to lower a patient's serum potassium.

- Many different strategies currently are available to help prevent clotting of the extracorporeal circuit: heparin, citrate, and argatroban are the most commonly used.
- There is no clear consensus as to when to start or stop CRRT. Criteria for discontinuation of CRRT include hemodynamic stability, recovery of renal function, and a net daily fluid balance of no more than 2 L (to ensure that a patient may receive HD without large UF requirements).
- CRRT affects the pharmacokinetics of many drugs prescribed in critical care practice. Knowledge of the extracorporeal prescription and individual properties of the drug helps determine appropriate dosing during ongoing continuous treatment.
- Ethical issues must be considered prior to offering, initiating, and discontinuing CRRT.

SELECTED REFERENCES

5. Uchino S, Kellum JA, Bellomo R, et al: Acute renal failure in critically ill patients: A multinational, multicenter study. JAMA 2005;294(7):813-818.
9. Chertow GM, Burdick E, Honour M, et al: Acute kidney injury, mortality, length of stay, and costs in hospitalized patients. J Am Soc Nephrol 2005;16(11):3365-3370.
16. Parikh A, Shaw A: The economics of renal failure and kidney disease in critically ill patients. Crit Care Clin 2012;28(1):99-111.
17. Bellomo R: Do we know the optimal dose for renal replacement therapy in the intensive care unit? Kidney Int 2006;70(7):1202-1204.
21. Vijayan A: Vascular access for continuous renal replacement therapy. Semin Dial 2009;22(2):133-136.
30. Uchino S, Bellomo R, Morimatsu H, et al: Continuous renal replacement therapy: A worldwide practice survey. The beginning and ending supportive therapy for the kidney (B.E.S.T. kidney) investigators. Intensive Care Med 2007;33(9):1563-1570.
42. Munjal S, Ejaz AA: Regional citrate anticoagulation in continuous venovenous haemofiltration using commercial preparations. Nephrology (Carlton) 2006;11(5):405-409.
43. Tolwani AJ, Prendergast MB, Speer RR, et al: A practical citrate anticoagulation continuous venovenous hemodiafiltration protocol for metabolic control and high solute clearance. Clin J Am Soc Nephrol 2006;1(1):79-87.
47. Davies H, Leslie G: Anticoagulation in CRRT: Agents and strategies in Australian ICUs. Aust Crit Care 2007;20(1):15-26.
49. Schetz M: Drug dosing in continuous renal replacement therapy: General rules. Curr Opin Crit Care 2007;13(6):645-651.

The complete list of references can be found at www.expertconsult.com.

19

Use of Sedatives, Analgesics, and Neuromuscular Blockers

Curtis N. Sessler | Katie M. Muzevich

CHAPTER OUTLINE

Critically ill patients often experience unpleasant sensations including pain, anxiety, dyspnea, and other forms of distress.[1-4] This is particularly true for mechanically ventilated patients who make up a significant proportion of intensive care unit (ICU) patients. The ICU environment, and ICU care in general, is widely regarded as not ideally suited to patient comfort. For example, most patients may have surgical incisions and often have a variety of indwelling tubes and vascular catheters. Further, sleep disruption is common, sound and light levels are often excessive, and patient communication and mobility are impaired. Core principles of ICU care are to provide comfort to our patients and to relieve their suffering.[5-8] Although nonpharmacologic interventions can improve patient comfort,[9] clinicians have relied upon administration of analgesic and sedative medications to reduce the sensation of pain and anxiety, to control agitation, and to enhance tolerance of the ICU environment.[10-12] However, clinical experience and research over the past decade have demonstrated the hazards associated with excessive or unnecessarily prolonged sedation and the importance of accurately achieving targeted analgesia and sedation.[13-17] Newly revised clinical practice guidelines from the Society of Critical Care Medicine (SCCM)[6] and other recent guidelines and reviews on sedation and analgesia[18-23] highlight the importance of adopting a management approach that is patient-focused and strives to use the lowest effective dose of medications. The past decade has also brought a greater appreciation for the importance that development of delirium in the ICU has for long-term outcomes including downstream cognitive dysfunction.[6,24-29] The topic of ICU delirium is reviewed in detail elsewhere in this textbook (Chapter 72). Finally, the use of neuromuscular blocking agents (NMBAs) to achieve therapeutic paralysis is undergoing reevaluation, particularly for optimizing management of acute respiratory distress syndrome (ARDS).[30-33] The use of sedatives, analgesics, and NMBA in managing critically ill patients is reviewed in this chapter.

Surveys and clinical reports indicate that the majority of ICU patients experience pain, dyspnea, or other forms of distress and receive sedative and analgesic medications.[10-12,34] Some of the key terms and definitions related to patient distress and neurobehavioral abnormalities in ICU patients are presented in Box 19.1.[35] Much of the discomfort is related to various stressors. In one case series, being in pain, being unable to sleep, and having tubes in the nose or mouth were the most prominent stressors reported by recovering ICU patients.[4] Clearly, providing relief from these and other issues is an important goal of analgesic and sedative therapy. Consequences of suboptimal analgesia and sedative therapy can include problems related to inadequately controlled pain and anxiety or excessive sedation. Agitation, defined as "excessive motor activity associated with internal tension," is perhaps the most widely recognized manifestation of uncontrolled anxiety or pain and is a problem because it can result in dramatic events, such as self-removal of important tubes and catheters, or even violence directed toward care providers. Overt agitation is a common occurrence among critically ill patients with rates as high as 20% of patient-shifts and nearly three quarters of patients during ICU stay.[35-38] Self-removal of critical indwelling tubes and vascular catheters is the most common manifestation of overt agitation, placing the patient in peril from loss of an

Box 19.1 Terms for Patient Distress and Neurobehavioral Abnormalities in the Critically Ill

Agitation: Excessive motor activity associated with internal tension. The motor activity usually is nonpurposeful but may be irrationally purposeful and counterproductive.
Anxiety: A sustained state of apprehension with accompanying autonomic arousal in response to a real or perceived threat.
Apprehension: The subjective experience of dread and foreboding.
Autonomic arousal: Stimulation of the sympathetic and parasympathetic nervous systems and the autonomically controlled humoral axes. Autonomic arousal is manifested physically by tachycardia, systolic hypertension, hyperventilation, and diaphoresis.
Cognitive dysfunction: Reduced memory and analytical skills, confusion, and impaired judgment.
Coma: A state of unarousable unresponsiveness.
Defensive withdrawal: A physical and psychological reaction to an unpleasant situation manifested by avoidance, reduced responsiveness, and hypervigilance.
Delirium: An acute, potentially reversible impairment of consciousness and cognitive function that fluctuates in severity. Manifestations include apprehension, agitation, cognitive distortion, abnormal thought processes (including hallucinations), and impairments of short-term memory, arousal, and attention.
Distress: A global term for suffering, strain, or misery affecting the body or the mind.
Dyspnea: The experience of difficulty or distress in breathing.
Obtundation: Pathologic drowsiness, often accompanied during wakefulness by reduced attention and interest in the environment.
Pain: An unpleasant sensory or emotional experience associated with either actual or potential tissue damage that typically leads to evasive action.
Patient-ventilator asynchrony: An erratic breathing pattern in mechanically ventilated patients characterized by suboptimal matching of patient respiratory drive and mechanics with ventilator function.
Stress response: Reactions of the body and the mind to threats or forces of a deleterious nature that tend to upset physiologic homeostasis.
Stupor: A sustained state of spontaneous unarousability interruptible only by vigorous, direct external stimulation.

Modified with permission from Sessler CN, Grap MJ, Brophy GM: Multidisciplinary management of sedation and analgesia in critical care. Semin Respir Crit Care Med 2001;22:211-225.

artificial airway and positive-pressure ventilation, abrupt cessation of infusion of critical medications such as vasopressors, and the risk and discomfort associated with reinsertion of tubes and lines.[39] In prospective studies, device removal rates range widely from 22 to 157 events per 1000 patient-days[40,41] and have an associated added cost.[42] Documentation of patient agitation has become commonplace with the broad use of scales that address both sedation and agitation.[43] In addition to device removal and care provider assault, agitation is often accompanied by an intense stress response with catecholamine surge resulting in tachycardia, hypertension, and tachypnea.[44,45] Withdrawal of continuous infusion sedative and analgesic medications to promote awakening is associated with a two- to fourfold increase in circulating catecholamines[46] and can produce evidence of withdrawal that peaks within 6 hours.[47] Adrenergic stress response has been linked to hypercoagulability, glucose intolerance, increased catabolism, immunosuppression, sleep disturbance, and delirium. Further this can precipitate adverse events such as myocardial ischemia, increased intracranial pressure (ICP), tachyarrhythmias, and complications of uncontrolled hypertension in susceptible individuals.[48] Finally, it is also worth considering that overt agitation can be a marker for extreme distress that has a cause that may be life-threatening or that could be rapidly resolved upon recognition and management.[21,35,36] Endotracheal tube malposition or obstruction, severe chest pain from myocardial ischemia, and tension pneumothorax are examples of conditions for which severe agitation in the nonverbal patient may be an important clue to an urgent dangerous situation. In fact, agitation was a common clinical antecedent prior to cardiopulmonary arrest in one study.[49]

Although the primary effect of analgesic and sedative medications is the relief of pain, anxiety, agitation, and related problems, such relief is usually accompanied by reduced level of consciousness. Excessive and unnecessarily prolonged impaired sensorium is associated with additional complications—as a result of excessively deep sedation (i.e., pressure sores or nerve compression from reduced movement), or as a result of sedation-related delayed recovery from critical illness and mechanical ventilation with higher rates of complications and interventions related to longer ICU length of stay (LOS). Further, long-term neuropsychological consequences of ICU sedation are increasingly recognized.[25] Accordingly, it is critical to take a structured approach to managing analgesia and sedation, which includes carefully examining the specific patient-focused goals of therapy, using validated tools for evaluation and monitoring, and implementing management that explicitly targets using the lowest effective dose of the best analgesic and sedative medications for the specific patient. Some important components for analgesia and sedation management gleaned from prior reviews and current clinical practice guidelines are listed in Box 19.2.[6,19-23]

Analgesia and sedation are most effective when they are patient-focused because each patient and circumstances have unique features that may influence the response to therapy. Some of the predisposing and precipitating conditions that can contribute to the development of anxiety, pain, and delirium are noted in Figure 19.1.[19,35] For example, a variety of underlying medical conditions—such as alcohol or substance abuse,[50] psychiatric disorders, and chronic pain—can influence the likelihood of developing anxiety, pain, or delirium and can affect the response to therapy.[37] Further, inadvertent discontinuation of home medications such as opioids, benzodiazepines, or antipsychotic medications because of lack of awareness of their prior use is not uncommon with unscheduled ICU admissions and is an important reason to perform detailed medication reconciliation with patients and their family members. Although the notion that "ICU psychosis" is actually caused by the ICU is misleading, it is clear that excessive noise, light, and repeated

Box 19.2 Key Concepts for Management of Sedation and Analgesia

1. Develop a multiprofessional, structured approach for managing analgesia and sedation in your ICU. Utilize key user buy-in, education, protocols, order sets, ICU rounding checklists, and other tools to promote durable integration into patient care.
2. Perform patient assessment and optimize ICU environment:
   a. Identify predisposing and precipitating factors; manage correctable factors.
   b. Optimize patient comfort and tolerance of the ICU environment, including controlling light and noise and promoting sleep.
   c. Optimize mechanical ventilation settings for patient-ventilator synchrony.
   d. Provide preemptive analgesia to alleviate pain associated with painful procedures.
3. Regularly perform and document structured patient evaluation and monitoring:
   a. Establish and communicate treatment goals.
   b. Assess presence and severity of pain as well as response to therapy using self-report or a validated pain assessment tool.
   c. Assess level of sedation using a validated sedation scale as well as response to therapy.
   d. Assess presence and severity of agitation using a validated agitation scale.
   e. Identify delirium using a validated delirium assessment instrument.
4. Implement a structured, patient-focused management strategy:
   a. Select analgesic and sedative drugs based on patient needs and unique characteristics (such as alcohol or substance abuse), drug allergies, organ dysfunction (particularly renal or hepatic dysfunction), need for rapid onset or offset of action, anticipated duration of therapy, prior response to therapy, and published evidence.
   b. Focus first on analgesia, then sedation. Use opioids as primary analgesics, but consider adding adjunctive agents or interventions.
   c. Evaluate and manage severe agitation, including a search for causative factors, and perform rapid tranquilization.
   d. Identify delirium, correct precipitating factors, and administer appropriate medications to reduce the intensity and duration of delirium.
   e. Titrate analgesic and sedative drugs to a defined target, using the lowest effective dose and aiming for light level of sedation.
   f. Implement a structured strategy to avoid accumulation of medications/metabolites: utilize scheduled interruption of medications, or intermittent dosing, of analgesic and sedative drugs. Perform safety screen to select proper candidates for interruption of sedation.
   g. Link reductions in analgesic and sedative drugs to spontaneous breathing trials and to early mobilization.
   h. Avoid potential adverse effects of analgesic and sedative drugs; quickly identify and manage adverse effects that occur.
5. Recognize and take steps to ameliorate analgesic and sedative drug withdrawal during de-escalation of therapy.

ICU, intensive care unit.

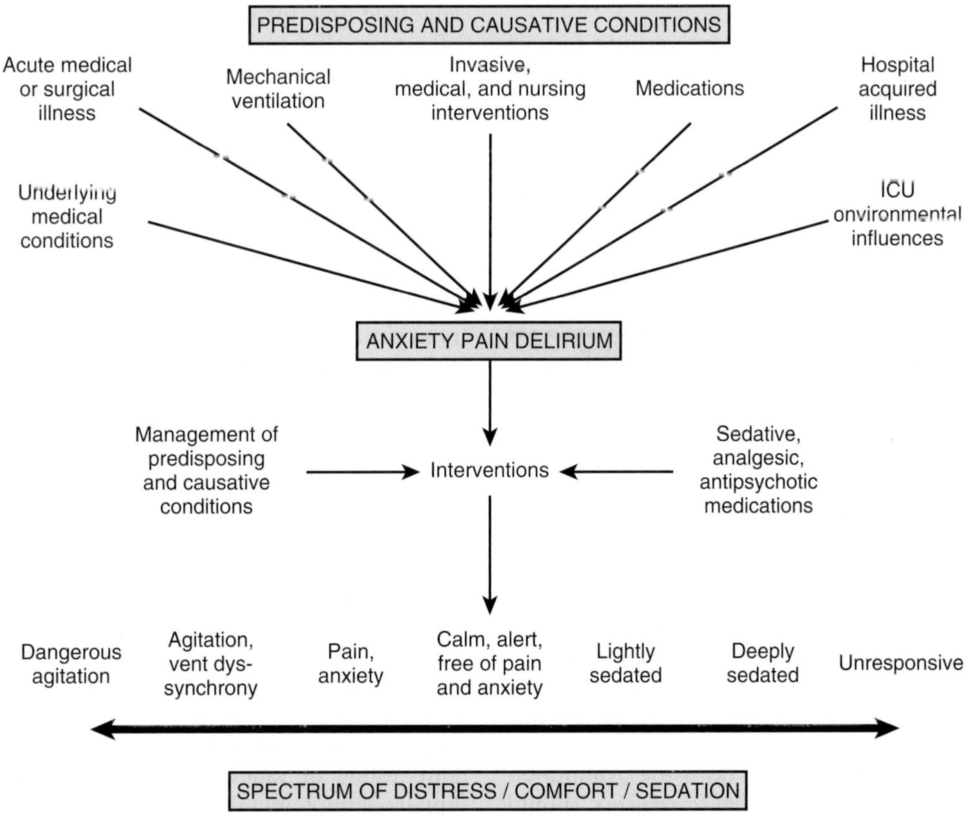

Figure 19.1 The spectrum of distress, comfort, and sedation. (With permission from Sessler CN, Varney K: Patient-focused sedation and analgesia in the ICU. Chest 2008;133(2):552-565.)

Box 19.3 Conditions and Medications Associated with Agitation and Delirium

Conditions

Central nervous system (CNS) disorders—stroke
Infections—sepsis, encephalitis
Withdrawal from sedative agent (alcohol, benzodiazepine, opioid, nicotine)
Medication intoxication (CNS stimulants)
Metabolic disorders (hypoglycemia, thyrotoxicosis)
Electrolyte disorders (hyponatremia, hypermagnesemia)
Poisoning
Hypoxia
Endotracheal tube or tracheostomy tube malposition or occlusion
Patient-ventilator asynchrony
Pneumothorax
Pain (cardiac/vascular/gut ischemia, headache, distended viscus—e.g., bladder, bowel, indwelling tubes/catheters/devices, poor body or limb position)
Sleep deprivation

Medications

Antibiotics
Anticholinergics
Anticonvulsants
Antihistamines
Benzodiazepines
Cardiovascular medications
Corticosteroids
Opioids
Nonsteroidal anti-inflammatory agents

patient awakening to check vital signs or perform tests at night contribute to fragmented sleep and can provoke anxiety and delirium.[51-53] Acute medical illness, surgical interventions, mechanical ventilation and the interface (i.e., tracheostomy tube, endotracheal tube, oronasal mask), and nursing interventions such as suctioning and turning can contribute to pain and discomfort.[3,4,54] A variety of conditions and medications have been associated with the development of delirium and agitation, as displayed in Box 19.3.[35]

PAIN MANAGEMENT IN THE INTENSIVE CARE UNIT

Pain is widely experienced in the ICU setting and can result from invasive procedures, surgery, and monitoring devices, as well as more direct stimuli from injury, inflammation, and immobility.[55] Treating pain is a core component of the caregivers' responsibility to relieve suffering and offers the physiologic benefits of relieving pain-induced altered glucose control, myocardial ischemia, immune system dysfunction, hypercoagulability, ventilator asynchrony, impaired ventilation, and disrupted sleep.[55] Mechanisms for these downstream effects include neurohormonal derangements, catecholamine release, and stress response.[55,56]

Effective treatment of pain begins with the assumption that pain is widely present and that caregivers should systematically evaluate each patient for the presence of pain and its intensity and characteristics, on a repetitive basis.[6,8,9,55] Caregivers tend to underrecognize pain and often fail to preemptively treat pain.[3,57] Accordingly, clinicians should err on the side of presuming pain is present—particularly when considering that it is far more effective to prevent and manage pain at an early stage than after it has become severe. Ideally, pain should be described in regard to location, duration, type, exacerbating and relieving factors, and intensity. Pain is sometimes conceptualized by subtypes, including somatic, visceral, and neuropathic, because manifestations and management can be different.[55] For example, somatic pain is typically dull and aching, often localized, and responds well to opioids and nonsteroidal anti-inflammatory agents (NSAIDs). In contrast, visceral pain is often cramping and colicky and may respond to anticholinergic therapy, although the burning and shooting neuropathic pain is often best treated with antidepressant and anticonvulsant agents.

Because pain is a subjective interpretation by an individual, the ability of that individual to convey the presence and magnitude of pain is of great value in guiding evaluation and management.[58] Detailed verbal communication by ICU patients is often limited; however, use of simple tools such as the numerical rating scale or a series of cartoon faces ranging from smiling to crying can facilitate communication by pointing or nodding in the nonverbal but cognitively intact patient.[59] A simple horizontal 0 to 10 numerical scale with enlarged font was judged to be most feasible and valid in one study of pain intensity rating scales.[60] Other techniques to enhance the use of self-reporting of pain include adding descriptive words to the numerical scale, carefully explaining the tool and correct use with each encounter, providing glasses and hearing aids if necessary, allowing adequate time for instructions and patient response.[58] Use of a scale that incorporates descriptive pictures, like the faces scale, can facilitate self-reporting of pain intensity regardless of potential language barriers.

Many ICU patients are cognitively impaired and self-reported pain intensity is not feasible. Accordingly, clinicians must rely upon observed behaviors that have been documented to correlate well with self-reported pain or to be associated with noxious stimuli.[54,57,61-63] Investigators have combined behaviors into structured assessment tools. Interestingly, much of the early work in pain assessment for noncommunicative ICU patients was in infants and young children, resulting in the development of the COMFORT scale,[64] the Face, Legs, Activity, Cry and Consolability (FLACC) observation tool,[65] and others. Subsequently a variety of pain assessment tools for nonverbal critically ill adults have been developed, validated, and thoroughly reviewed.[58,66,67] In the 2012 SCCM guidelines,[6] published pain observation tools for adults in the ICU were identified as the Critical-Care Pain Observation Tool (CPOT),[68] the Behavioral Pain Scale (BPS),[69] the Behavioral Pain Scale—Nonintubated (BPS-NI),[70] the Non-Verbal Pain Scale (NVPS),[71] the Pain Behavioral Assessment Tool (PBAT),[54,72] and the Pain Assessment, Intervention, and Notation (PAIN) tool.[73] Extensive psychometric testing was performed including examination of scale development, testing of reliability, and testing of validity, feasibility, and scale relevance or impact of implementation in ICU patient outcomes yielding

Table 19.1 Critical Care Pain Observation Tool (CPOT)

Indicator	Description	Observations	Score
Facial expression	No muscular tension observed	Relaxed, neutral	0
	Presence of frowning, brow lowering, orbit tightening, and levator contraction	Tense	1
	All of the above facial movements plus eyelids tightly closed	Grimacing	2
Body movements	Does not move at all (does not necessarily mean absence of pain)	Absence of movements	0
	Slow, cautious movements, touching or rubbing the pain site, seeking attention through movements	Protection	1
	Pulling tube, attempting to sit up, moving limbs/ thrashing, not following commands, striking at staff, trying to climb out of bed	Restlessness	2
Muscle tension	No resistance to passive movements	Relaxed	0
	Resistance to passive movements	Tense, rigid	1
	Strong resistance to passive movements; inability to complete them	Very tense or rigid	2
Compliance with the ventilator	Alarms not activated; easy ventilation	Tolerating ventilator or movement	0
	Alarms stop spontaneously	Coughing but tolerating	1
	Asynchrony: blocking ventilation; alarms frequently activated	Fighting ventilator	2
OR			
Vocalization (extubated patients)	Talking in normal tone or no sound	Talking in normal tone or no sound	0
	Sighing, moaning	Sighing, moaning	1
	Crying out, sobbing	Crying out, sobbing	2
Total, range			0-8

From Gelinas C, Fillion L, Puntillo KA, et al: Validation of the critical-care pain observation tool in adult patients. Am J Crit Care 2006;15(4):420-427; used with permission.

a maximum score of 25 and weighted score of 0 to 20. The CPOT had the highest weighted score of 14.7, followed by the BPS with 12.0,[6] and these two scales are recommended in the 2012 SCCM guidelines as the most valid and reliable behavioral pain scales for monitoring pain in adult medical, postoperative, and trauma ICU patients who are unable to self-report and in whom motor function is intact and behaviors are observable.[6] CPOT and BPS are displayed in Tables 19.1 and 19.2. Pain is often accompanied by changes in vital signs, with tachycardia, hypertension, and tachypnea being most common. However, changes in vital signs are inconsistently associated with pain, with many confounding factors that can mask anticipated changes—such as administration of beta blockers, as well as lack of specificity with many other causes of tachycardia, hypertension, and tachypnea.[74] Accordingly, 2012 SCCM guidelines recommend against the use of vital signs (or observational pain scales that include vital signs) alone for pain assessment in adult ICU patients.[6] However, it is acknowledged that vital signs may be an important cue to prompt further pain assessment.[6] Other potentially useful approaches include evaluating pain risk profile, use of surrogate (such as family members) report,[75] and performance of an analgesic trial.[3,55,58]

There are several important tenets for managing pain in the ICU. First, when initiating sedative treatment for mechanically ventilated ICU patients, analgesia should be the first step, followed by the addition of a sedative-anxiolytic agent. This "analgesia first" approach is suggested in the 2012 SCCM guidelines[6] as well as many expert reviews.[18-23,55] Second, the use of preemptive analgesia should be administered prior to the performance of interventions, such as chest tube removal, that are associated with having a high likelihood of producing pain.[6] It is more effective to prevent pain or manage it at an earlier and milder stage than after pain has become severe.

Table 19.2 Behavioral Pain Scale (BPS)

Item	Description	Score
Facial expression	Relaxed	1
	Partially tightened (e.g., brow lowering)	2
	Fully tightened (e.g., eyelid closing)	3
	Grimacing	4
Upper limbs	No movement	1
	Partially bent	2
	Fully bent with finger flexion	3
	Permanently retracted	4
Compliance with ventilation	Tolerating movement	1
	Coughing but tolerating ventilation for most of the time	2
	Fighting ventilator	3
	Unable to control ventilation	4

From Payen JF, Bru O, Bosson JL, et al: Assessing pain in critically ill sedated patients by using a behavioral pain scale. Crit Care Med 2001;29(12):2258-2263; used with permission.

Successful pain management in the ICU incorporates pharmacologic and nonpharmacologic treatment.[9] Parenteral opioids are the primary agents used to treat pain in the ICU setting, but use of selected nonopioid and atypical agents can enhance pain relief and may reduce adverse effects. The major parenteral opioids for continuous infusion in ICU patients—fentanyl, morphine, hydromorphone, and remifentanil (see Table 19.4)[9]—are generally considered to be equivalent in regard to analgesic potential as well as class-based adverse effects such as respiratory depression or reduced level of consciousness. Important differences among agents in regard to lipid solubility, volume of distribution (Vd), half-life, clearance, metabolism, and active metabolites have important effects on onset, peak, and offset of action, potency, and the influence of renal or hepatic dysfunction.[9] Some of the medication features that can influence opioid selection for a particular patient are noted in Table 19.3. For example, morphine sulfate is metabolized to several active metabolites, including morphine-6-glucuronide, which is as active as the parent compound and accumulates in renal failure, resulting in prolonged effects including analgesia but also somnolence and respiratory depression.[76] The rapid equilibration of fentanyl from plasma to lipid-rich brain tissue is responsible for its rapid onset of action but its high lipophilicity also contributed to large Vd and delayed offset of action after prolonged infusion. Remifentanil has a small Vd, and rapid clearance with metabolism by esterases, yielding a short half-life and rapid offset of action that is independent of renal and hepatic function.[77,78] Several opioids not listed deserve mention. Meperidine has the potential for neuroexcitatory adverse effects such as seizures[79] and is not recommended for ICU use.[6] Methadone can slow the development of tolerance to other opioid agents when coadministered but has unpredictable pharmacokinetics and is not administered by continuous infusion.[6] Methadone is also a potent precipitating agent for prolonging the rate-corrected QT interval (QTc).[80,81] Although opioids are most effective for pain management in the ICU patient, these agents have a well-documented propensity to produce adverse effects (AEs), which are reviewed, along with comments for each AE, in Table 19.4.[9,55] Comprehensive pain management should include awareness of the likely adverse effects and how best to avoid them and to recognize and manage them.

It is often advantageous to use the lowest effective dose of an opioid analgesic, particularly when intolerable side effects are present. Additionally, there are clinical settings in which a nontraditional approach may be more effective, safer, and better tolerated. Employment of alternative or complementary approaches such as adding nonopioid or atypical analgesic agents, use of epidural or other neuraxial alternatives to parenteral opioid, and use of complementary nonpharmacologic interventions should be considered in selected cases.[9]

NONOPIOID AND ATYPICAL AGENTS

The use of nonopioid medications is best approached from the perspective of differentiating neuropathic pain for which anticonvulsants, antidepressants, and other agents play a primary role versus non-neuropathic pain for which opioids are the first line of therapy and other agents are used to reduce opioid dosage and reduce side effects. There is compelling evidence that the addition of oral gabapentin or carbamazepine to opioids provides superior pain relief for neuropathic pain in ICU patients when compared to opioids alone,[82,83] and this use is strongly recommended in this setting in the 2012 SCCM guidelines.[6] Pharmacotherapy for neuropathic pain has been extensively studied in randomized controlled trials (RCTs) in non-ICU patients, and medications including tricyclic antidepressants, selective serotonin receptor inhibitors (SSRIs), serotonin and norepinephrine reuptake inhibitors (SNRIs), anticonvulsants, tramadol, dextromethorphan, ketamine, topical capsaicin, lidocaine patch or gel, cannabinoids, and other agents have shown efficacy, albeit often in trials with small sample size and with associated side effects.[84]

Nonopioid adjuvant therapy in non-neuropathic pain can help reduce the quantity of opioids administered and potentially decrease the incidence and severity of opioid-related side effects. Such agents have been extensively studied in various non–critically ill populations—primarily postoperative patients, with efficacy demonstrated in meta-analyses of RCTs for corticosteroids, NSAIDs, acetaminophen, ketamine, and others.[85-88] There is relatively limited research in ICU patients and most of the RCTs performed with ICU patients have been in the postoperative setting. Best studied in the ICU population are IV (intravenous) acetaminophen, cyclooxygenase inhibitors, and ketamine.[89-91] As a result of the limited evidence base in ICU patients, the 2012 SCCM guidelines generally support this approach as a weak recommendation for the addition of nonopioids for non-neuropathic pain.[6] The potential benefits as well as risks of nonopioids for ICU use are further discussed in reviews published in 2009.[9,55]

REGIONAL ANESTHESIA AND ANALGESIA

Although systemic administration of opioids for pain management in the ICU is typically by the IV route, regional approaches can offer advantages in selected cases.[9] Options for regional anesthesia and analgesia (RAA) include continuous epidural analgesia (CEA) and anesthesia (central neuraxial techniques) and continuous peripheral nerve or plexus block. With medication delivery in close proximity to the spinal cord or nerves, these techniques can promote parenteral opioid sparing, which is associated with less respiratory depression and gastrointestinal hypomotility and conveys other benefits. However, these techniques introduce new issues related to needle and catheter placement and maintenance, as well as physiologic alterations related to local anesthetic block and epidural drug delivery. Critically ill patients are often at higher risk for complications due to coagulopathy, thrombocytopenia, sepsis, and hemodynamic instability. Peripheral nerve blocks are particularly useful for anatomically localized pain such as limb injury or operation. However, of all the various RAA techniques, the greatest experience in ICU patients is with CEA.

Similar to other pain management issues, there is more published research to support the use of RAA in noncritical care settings, and most ICU studies focus on patient who are postoperative or have sustained injury. The recent evidence-based review undertaken to develop the 2012 SCCM guidelines provides the most relevant and current basis for use of

Table 19.3 Common Opioid Medications

Drug	Metabolism	Onset/Duration	Dosing	Titration	Advantages	Disadvantages
Fentanyl	CYP3A4	1-2 min/2-4 hr (longer in liver failure)	*Bolus:* 25-50 μg IV push *Maintenance:* 12.5-200 μg/hr continuous infusion	Increase/decrease in increments of 25-50 μg every 5-30 min as needed; may be used to attain goal RASS or goal pain score	Less hypotension than with morphine; short-acting, less accumulation with organ dysfunction than with other opiates	CYP3A4 inhibitors may increase fentanyl effect; tolerance develops over time
Hydromorphone	Hepatic	5-10 min/2-4 hr (longer in liver failure)	*Bolus:* 1-4 mg IV push *Maintenance:* 0.25-50 mg/hr (no real maximum dose)	Increase/decrease in increments of 1-4 mg every 15-30 min as needed; may be used to attain goal RASS or goal pain score	May be preferred in patients with tachyphylaxis to fentanyl; does not accumulate with renal dysfunction like morphine	Long-acting and very potent
Morphine	Conjugation; active metabolites that undergo renal excretion	5-10 min/2-4 hr (longer in liver failure and ESRD)	*Bolus:* 2-4 mg IV push *Maintenance:* 0.5-49 mg/hr	Increase/decrease in increments of 1-4 mg every 15-30 min as needed; may be used to attain goal RASS or goal pain score	May be preferred in patients with tachyphylaxis to fentanyl	Accumulates with renal and hepatic dysfunction; hypotension due to histamine release
Remifentanil	Plasma esterase	1-3 min/10-20 min	*Bolus:* 1 μg/kg over 1 min IV push *Maintenance:* 0.6-15 μg/kg/hr (use ideal body weight if more than 30% over ideal body weight)	Increase/decrease in increments of 1-2 μg/kg every 5-10 min as needed; may be used to attain goal RASS or goal pain score	No accumulation in hepatic or renal dysfunction	Can cause bradycardia and hypotension; may increase intracranial pressure

CYP3A4, cytochrome P-450 3A4; ESRD, end-stage renal disease; RASS, Richmond Agitation Sedation Scale.

Table 19.4 Common Opioid Adverse Effects

Potential Adverse Effect	Comment
Allergy	Rare; most common with morphine
Arrhythmias	QTc prolongation with methadone
CNS depression	Accumulation of active morphine metabolite in renal failure
Constipation	Start bowel regimen early if sustained opioid administration is likely Enteral naloxone is sometimes effective, but reverses analgesia
Cough	Most common with fentanyl and similar agents
Dry mouth	Use oral lubricants
Histamine release	Uncommon with fentanyl and similar agents Slow infusion rate Treat with combination of H_1 and H_2 agonists
Hyperalgesia	Paradoxic increase in pain sensitivity More common with short-acting opioids
Myoclonus	Consider reduced opioid dose or switch agent; hydrate
Nausea/vomiting	Administer antiemetic until tolerance develops
Neurotoxicity	Avoid meperidine—associated with highest incidence Can occur with morphine or hydromorphone, particularly at higher doses or in renal failure
Opioid dependency	Withdrawal symptoms can develop—usually coincide with clearance Prevent by tapering; reinstitute agent if withdrawal occurs
Pruritus	Consider naloxone, serotonic antagonists such as ondansetron
Rigidity	Most common with fentanyl and similar agents but can occur with any agent at high dose
Serotonin syndrome	Reported with meperidine and methadone Avoid concomitant serotonin reuptake inhibitor

CNS, central nervous system.
Adapted from Erstad BL, Puntillo K, Gilbert HC, et al: Pain management principles in the critically ill. Chest. 2009;135(4): 1075-1086; used with permission.

RAA in ICU patients.[6] Specific patient populations were examined, and only thoracic epidural anesthesia/analgesia for postoperative analgesia in patients undergoing abdominal aortic surgery received a strong recommendation as a superior alternative to IV opioids.[92] Interestingly, high-level evidence was also available to compare lumbar epidural analgesia to IV opioids in the same population and no benefit was demonstrated.[93] Patients with traumatic rib fractures are the other population for which benefit from RAA was demonstrated for ICU patients. Specifically, use of thoracic epidural analgesia was associated with superior pain control and reduced incidence of pneumonia—but more hypotension—compared to parenteral opioids,[94,95] and its use is supported as a weak recommendation in this setting.[6] The evidence was insufficient to recommend thoracic epidural analgesia for intrathoracic or nonvascular abdominal surgical procedures.[6] Similarly, the lack of high-quality research prevented a recommendation regarding the use of RAA for medical ICU patients.[6]

COMPLEMENTARY TECHNIQUES

Nonpharmacologic interventions such as music, relaxation, and provision of information can provide complementary pain relief and can be considered.[9,55,96-98] However, although they are low cost, easy to provide, and safe, they have a relatively weak body of evidence to support their routine use, and they are not "high impact," providing only limited opioid-sparing or pain intensity reduction capability.[9,55,96]

SEDATION MANAGEMENT

Sedative drugs have formed the cornerstone for patient comfort and tolerance of the ICU environment for decades by calming anxiety, providing amnesia, and controlling agitation. There have been changing paradigms from preferential use of moderate- to long-acting benzodiazepines[5] and acceptance of prolonged deep sedation a decade ago, to patient-focused sedation with careful monitoring, analgesia first, and more recently to an emphasis on the use of nonbenzodiazepine sedative agents and using the lightest level of sedation possible.[6] Management of sedation should be preceded by examining individual patient characteristics and effective pain control. It incorporates establishing the goals of sedative therapy, monitoring of the depth of sedation, selecting and administering the best agent(s) for the particular patient, and using protocolized management of sedation that includes structured elements to assure use of the lowest effective dose and lightest level of sedation. Common goals of therapy include relief of anxiety, control of frank agitation, promotion of patient-ventilator synchrony, and elimination of awareness when an NMBA is used. Monitoring of the depth of sedation is now routinely performed in most ICUs and is applied to titrate medications to a targeted level of consciousness and to avoid excessive or prolonged sedation.

Monitoring the depth of sedation is most commonly performed by observing patient behaviors, often after varying levels of stimulation, using a structured sedation scale.[43,67,99] The domain being tested is that of arousal or level of consciousness and typically ranges from alert to comatose. Ramsay and coworkers developed the first widely utilized sedation scale for ICU patients—a 6-level scale based upon response to the assessor's voice and to physical stimulation.[100] Subsequent scale development has introduced assessment of agitation, ranging from calm to combative. Useful features of sedation-agitation scales include multidisciplinary development; ease of administration, recall, and interpretation; well-defined discrete criteria for each level; sufficient sedation levels for effective drug titration; assessment of agitation; demonstration of good inter-rater reliability for relevant patient populations; and evidence of validity.[43] Recently the SCCM guideline task force performed a careful analysis of the sedation scales that have undergone validation analysis in ICU patients, including the Ramsay Sedation Scale (RSS),[100] the New Sheffield Sedation Scale,[101] the Observer's Assessment of Alertness/Sedation Scale (OAA/S),[102] the Sedation Intensive Care Score (SEDIC),[103] the Motor Activity Assessment Scale (MAAS),[104] the Adaption to the Intensive Care Environment (ATICE) tool,[105] the Minnesota Sedation Assessment Tool (MSAT),[106] the Vancouver Interaction and Calmness Scale (VICS),[107] the Sedation Agitation Scale (SAS)[108] and the Richmond Agitation Sedation Scale (RASS).[109] Of these, the RASS had the highest total weighted psychometric score (19 of 20 possible points), followed by the SAS (16.5 points), and these two instruments are recommended in the 2012 SCCM guidelines as the most valid and reliable sedation assessment tools for measuring quality and depth of sedation in adult ICU patients.[6] The RASS, developed by a multidisciplinary group led by Sessler, is displayed in Table 19.5.[109] The RASS incorporates assessment of arousal in response to 2 levels of stimulation (voice, physical), presence or absence of cognition, sustainability of response, and the presence and intensity of agitated behavior into a 10-level scale subcategorized with positive (agitation) and negative (sedation) values.[109] The SAS, developed by Riker and colleagues, is displayed in Table 19.6.[108] Both RASS and SAS have been extensively tested for inter-rater reliability and validity in a cross section of ICU populations, correlated with subjective and objective measures of sedation, and evaluated for ease of use in clinical settings.[6,67,108-112] The introduction of a sedation scale into clinical practice has been demonstrated to result in higher quality sedation with fewer hours of oversedation, as well as reduced utilization of sedative and analgesic drug doses, shorter duration of mechanical ventilation, and reduced use of vasopressors.[113,114] Structured assessment and management of agitation and pain were similarly associated with less agitation, quicker extubation, and fewer nosocomial infections.[115]

Table 19.5 Richmond Agitation Sedation Scale (RASS)

Score	Term	Description
+4	Combative	Overtly combative or violent; immediate danger to staff
+3	Very agitated	Pulls on or removes tube(s) or catheter(s) or displays aggressive behavior toward staff
+2	Agitated	Frequent nonpurposeful movement or patient-ventilator dyssynchrony
+1	Restless	Anxious or apprehensive, but movements not aggressive or vigorous
0	Alert and calm	
−1	Drowsy	Not fully alert, but demonstrates sustained (>10 sec) awakening, with eye contact, to voice
−2	Light sedation	Briefly (<10 sec) awakens with eye contact to voice
−3	Moderate sedation	Any movement (but no eye contact) to voice
−4	Deep sedation	No response to voice, but any movement to physical stimulation
−5	Unarousable	No response to voice or physical stimulation

Performed using a series of steps: observation of behaviors (score +4 to 0), followed (if necessary) by assessment of response to voice (score −1 to −3), followed (if necessary) by assessment of response to physical stimulation such as shaking shoulder and then rubbing sternum if no response to shaking shoulder (score −4 to −5).

From Sessler CN, Gosnell MS, Grap MJ, et al: The Richmond Agitation Sedation Scale: Validity and reliability in adult intensive care unit patients. Am J Respir Crit Care Med 2002;166:1338-1344; used with permission.

Table 19.6 Sedation Agitation Scale (SAS)

Score	Term	Description
7	Dangerous agitation	Pulling at endotracheal tube, trying to remove catheters, climbing over bedrail, striking at staff, thrashing side to side
6	Very agitated	Does not calm despite frequent verbal reminding of limits; requires physical restraints; biting endotracheal tube
5	Agitated	Anxious or mildly agitated; attempts to sit up; calms down to verbal instructions
4	Calm and cooperative	Calm, awakens easily, follows commands
3	Sedated	Difficult to arouse, awakens to verbal stimuli or gentle shaking but drifts off again, follows simple commands
2	Very sedated	Arouses to physical stimuli but does not communicate or follow commands; may move spontaneously
1	Unarousable	Minimal or no response to noxious stimuli; does not communicate or follow commands

From Riker RR, Picard JT, Fraser GL: Prospective evaluation of the Sedation-Agitation Scale for adult critically ill patients. Crit Care Med 1999;27(7):1325-1329; used with permission.

Objective measures of cerebral function have been developed to quantify the level of consciousness as reflected by the cortical electrical activity based upon processed electroencephalographic (EEG) signals.[67,116] Raw EEG signals are difficult to interpret, but proprietary mathematical algorithms have been developed and incorporated into commercially available devices to simplify interpretation of the power and frequency of the signal by converting this into a numerical display ranging from 0 (flat EEG) to 100 (fully alert). The Bispectral Index (BIS), Narcotrend Index (NI), Patient State Index (PSI), and State Entropy (SE) are examples of processed EEG monitors that have been used to assess level of consciousness in ICU patients.[6] The addition of assessing the "evoked potential" to an auditory signal (i.e., auditory evoked potentials [AEPs])—displayed as the Auditory Evoked Response Index [AAI]) incorporates measurement of latency and amplitude of the evoked electrical potential.[117] Collectively, these devices offer the advantage of continuous display of data, which can be used to rapidly detect unanticipated changes in level of consciousness, such as accidental cessation of propofol infusion.[67] However, validation studies of these objective tools against sedation scales and other parameters has yielded inconsistent results.[6,67,118] A particularly challenging problem has been filtering out electromyographic (EMG) signals generated by activity of muscles of the head that lie between the brain and the EEG electrodes.[119] Additionally, demonstration of added value to justify widespread use of this expensive monitoring technology when compared to routine sedation scale monitoring has been lacking in RCTs of ICU patients. Accordingly, the use of objective measures of brain function to assess the depth of sedation in noncomatose adult ICU patients who are not receiving NMBAs is not recommended in the 2012 SCCM guidelines.[6] There are unique clinical circumstances for which objective monitoring may be superior to routine clinical monitoring, including patients who are receiving NMBAs and the guidance of titration of anticonvulsant medications to achieve burst suppression.[6]

SEDATIVE DRUG THERAPY

Sedative medications are widely used in the ICU setting and although various agents can be administered by other routes, most are given IV—either by continuous infusion or intermittent bolus. Traditionally, benzodiazepines have formed the cornerstone of ICU sedation,[5] but recent clinical trial results and meta-analyses suggest that nonbenzodiazepines such as propofol and dexmedetomidine may be associated with better results such as less delirium and shorter ventilator time.[6] Benzodiazepines activate γ-aminobutyric acid (GABA) A receptors, producing anxiolytic, amnestic, sedating, and hypnotic effects.[6,120] Benzodiazepines cause respiratory depression and systemic hypotension—problems that are particularly prominent in the elderly. Although diazepam, midazolam, and lorazepam have been employed for ICU sedation over the years, diazepam is now used infrequently. Key pharmacokinetic and clinical features of midazolam and lorazepam are displayed in Table 19.7. Delayed offset of action is relatively common with these drugs for a variety of reasons including tissue saturation after prolonged administration, impaired metabolism due to hepatic dysfunction, and in the case of midazolam, accumulation of active renally cleared metabolites.[6,120,121] Continuous infusion of lorazepam can lead to accumulation of the diluent vehicle, propylene glycol, causing toxicity that is characterized by metabolic acidosis and acute kidney injury, and accompanied by development of an increased osmolal gap.[122,123]

Propofol is perhaps the most widely utilized agent administered for continuous IV sedation in the United States.[124] Propofol binds to GABA receptors as well as glycine, nicotinic, and muscarinic receptors producing effects similar to those from benzodiazepines.[6,125] Like benzodiazepines, propofol has no analgesic effects. Propofol is highly lipid soluble, quickly crossing the blood-brain barrier and rapidly redistributing into peripheral tissues. These features result in rapid onset and offset of action (see Table 19.7). However, prolonged administration can result in tissue saturation that can ultimately produce delayed offset of action. Similar to benzodiazepines, propofol commonly causes respiratory depression as well as systemic hypotension. Because propofol is dissolved in a lipid emulsion, higher rates of propofol infusion can produce hypertriglyceridemia and acute pancreatitis. Each milliliter of propofol solution contains 1.1 kcal of nutrition, and thus an infusion rate of about 40 mL/hour results in more than 1000 kcal of nutrition in 24 hours. Propofol infusion syndrome (PRIS) is an uncommon complication that is typically associated with prolonged infusion of high-dose propofol (i.e., >70 μg/kg/minute), although cases are reported at lower infusion rates or briefer administration. PRIS is characterized by metabolic acidosis, hypotension, cardiac arrhythmias, hypertriglyceridemia, and less commonly with acute kidney injury, rhabdomyolysis, liver dysfunction, and hyperkalemia.[6,126,127]

Dexmedetomidine is a selective α_2-receptor agonist with sedative properties similar to benzodiazepines and propofol, but has a number of unique features. In contrast to other sedatives, dexmedetomidine has analgesic properties and can be opioid-sparing; is sympatholytic, potentially producing prominent bradycardia as well as hypotension at higher doses; is associated with a more alert state relative to anxiolytic properties; and has minimal effect on respiratory drive.[128,129] It does not bind GABA receptors. Selected pharmacokinetic and clinical characteristics are displayed in Table 19.7. The most common adverse effects are hypotension and bradycardia. Hypotension can be particularly prominent when a loading dose is used—although hypertension can also occur. Clinical trial results suggest that when compared directly to midazolam, dexmedetomidine may be associated with lower prevalence of delirium.[130] The 2012 SCCM guidelines suggest that dexmedetomidine may be preferred over benzodiazepines in mechanically ventilated patients who have delirium and require continuous IV infusion of sedative medications.[6]

MANAGEMENT OF SEDATION

Sedative drug therapy is an important component of sedation and analgesia management as discussed earlier and outlined in Box 19.2. Careful selection and titration of sedative drugs are critical to achieve optimal patient comfort while avoiding the adverse impact of excessive or unnecessarily prolonged sedation. The use of structured approaches to sedation and analgesia via algorithms and protocols has

Table 19.7 Common Sedative Medications

Drug	Metabolism	Onset/Duration	Dosing	Titration	Advantages	Disadvantages
Lorazepam	Conjugation to inactive metabolite	5-20 min/6-8 hr (duration prolonged in elderly or those with cirrhosis or ESRD to 43-72 hr)	*Bolus:* 2-4 mg IV push *Maintenance:* 2-6 mg IV/PO every 4-6 hr (preferred); infusion 0.25-20 mg/hr	Infusion: Increase/decrease in increments of 0.5-2 mg every 10-60 min to attain goal RASS score	Long half-life allows for intermittent dosing; less accumulation with renal/hepatic dysfunction	Propylene glycol toxicity in patients with renal failure; accumulation common with continuous infusion
Midazolam	Cytochrome P-450 3A4; active metabolite renally excreted	5-10 min/1-4 hr (accumulates in ESRD/CHF/liver failure)	*Bolus:* 2-4 g IV push *Maintenance:* 0.5-25 mg/hr	Increase/decrease in increments of 1-2 mg every 5-60 min to attain goal RASS score	Short-acting in patients with preserved organ function or with bolus dosing; fast onset	CYP3A4 inhibitors may increase effect; accumulates with both renal and hepatic dysfunction; distributes to adipose tissue
Propofol	Conjugation	30-50 sec/3-10 min	*Maintenance:* 2.5-105 μg/kg/min	Increase/decrease in increments of 2.5-15 μg/kg/min every 1-15 min to attain goal RASS score	Short-acting; less delirium than with benzodiazepines	Hypotension, increased triglycerides, pancreatitis, propofol-related infusion syndrome, zinc depletion (with brand name only)
Dexmedetomidine	Hepatic via cytochrome P-450 and glucuronidation	Immediate onset only when bolus is given; ~3 hr to achieve full effect if bolus omitted/6 min (longer in liver failure)	(*Bolus:* 0.5-1 μg/kg, *rarely given* owing to hypotension/bradycardia) *Maintenance:* 0.2-1.5 μg/kg/hr	Increase by 0.1 μg/kg/hr no more often than every 30 minutes May titrate to effect (goal RASS score) OR until heart rate decreases by 10-20 beats/min Full effect will take ~3 hours to see If patient becomes hypotensive or bradycardic (HR <55), contact physician and stop infusion	Associated with less delirium than other agents; short-acting; little to no respiratory depression	Hypotension (especially with bolus dose and in fluid-resuscitated patients), bradycardia

CHF, congestive heart failure; ESRD, end-stage renal disease; HR, heart rate; RASS, Richmond Agitation Sedation Scale.

achieved a prominent place in ICU practice. There are several common themes. One theme is to tailor the sedation to the specific patient, including medication selection based upon sedation goals (such as rapid arousal), avoidance of side effects (such as hypotension), and consideration of elimination issues (such as avoiding midazolam in a patient with impaired renal function). Although all of the sedative drugs listed in Table 19.7 have a role in ICU sedation management, emerging evidence appears to favor using propofol or dexmedetomidine in preference to benzodiazepines in patients for whom continuous infusion sedation is needed—as suggested in the 2012 SCCM guidelines.[6] A recent meta-analysis limited to moderate or high-quality RCTs demonstrated slightly longer ICU LOS with benzodiazepines, in comparison to propofol or dexmedetomidine.[6] In a 2008 meta-analysis of 16 RCTs that compared propofol to alternative agents for moderate to long duration sedation (i.e., >2 days), propofol was associated with shorter duration of mechanical ventilation and shorter ICU LOS.[131] In a 2010 meta-analysis of 24 RCTs comparing dexmedetomidine to alternative agents, ICU LOS was shorter with dexmedetomidine and duration of mechanical ventilation was not significantly different.[132] Two recent studies deserve additional comment. A multicenter RCT comparing dexmedetomidine to midazolam by Riker and colleagues demonstrated that dexmedetomidine was associated with shorter time to extubation, lower prevalence of delirium, and fewer infections but no difference in ICU LOS, mortality rate, or sedation quality. Dexmedetomidine was less potent than midazolam and was associated with more bradycardia but less hypertension.[130] Jakob and coworkers recently reported two phase-3 multicenter RCTs that compared dexmedetomidine to midazolam and to propofol.[133] Patients randomized to dexmedetomidine had shorter duration of mechanical ventilation than with midazolam, but not with propofol. Patient interaction (communication, arousability, cooperation) was better with dexmedetomidine than with either other agent, but hypotension and bradycardia were more common.

A second major theme is to focus first on analgesia, as discussed earlier. The 2012 SCCM guidelines suggest that analgesia-first sedation be used in mechanically ventilated adult ICU patients.[6] Asking first about pain, before the patient has been sedated and cognitively impaired, is advantageous. Additionally, several RCTs have demonstrated analgesia-based sedation to be associated with shorter duration of mechanical ventilation in comparison to hypnotic-based sedation.[134-136] Finally, Strom and associates randomized mechanically ventilated adult ICU patients to bolus morphine (analgesia-based, limited sedation) versus morphine plus propofol for the first 48 hours, then midazolam (sedation + analgesia), and found shorter duration of mechanical ventilation and ICU LOS but threefold more agitation when sedative drugs were minimized.[16]

A third major theme is to strive for a light level of consciousness and to avoid accumulation of medications and their active metabolites, thus reducing the likelihood of delayed awakening. This approach is strongly recommended in the 2012 SCCM guidelines,[6] based in part on studies like those of Strom and associates.[16] The underlying rationale for this approach arises from the observation by Kollef and colleagues that use of continuous IV sedation and analgesia is associated with delayed recovery from respiratory failure and longer LOS.[13] Although a variety of sedation management strategies have been demonstrated to shorten the duration of mechanical ventilation, the most robust data support the use of a sedation protocol or the implementation of daily interruption of sedation.[6,20] In an early RCT, Brook and coworkers found the use of a nurse-implemented protocol that emphasized intermittent therapy to be associated with shorter duration of mechanical ventilation, reduced ICU and hospital LOS, and fewer tracheostomies compared to usual management.[14]

The following year, Kress and colleagues showed in an RCT that daily interruption of IV sedation (DIS) until the patient was alert or agitated and then restarting the medications at 50% of the original dose was accompanied by more rapid recovery from respiratory failure, as well as performance of fewer tests for unexplained altered mental status.[15] Interestingly, not all of the benefit could be attributable to reduced accumulation of medications or active metabolites because total propofol dosage was similar between groups although significantly less midazolam was used with daily interruption.[15] This prompted speculation that the DIS might also permit earlier identification of sufficient respiratory reserve for ventilator weaning—"wake up and breathe."[137] Girard and colleagues subsequently demonstrated that the strategy of combining DIS with performance of a spontaneous breathing trial (SBT) led to faster recovery from respiratory failure as well as reduced all-cause 1-year mortality rate compared to SBT alone.[138] Abrupt withdrawal of sedative (and sometimes analgesic) medications is accompanied by severalfold increases in circulating catecholamines as well as tachycardia and hypertension.[46] Experts have expressed concern that this unmasked stress response might be associated with cardiac ischemia.[139] In a prospective study, DIS was not accompanied by electrocardiographic or cardiac enzyme evidence of myocardial ischemia in at-risk patients.[46] Questions have also been raised as to potential impact of this abrupt withdrawal of medications designed to provide comfort on downstream neuropsychological disturbances such as posttraumatic stress disorder (PTSD).[139] An additional study by Kress and colleagues demonstrated no increase in subsequent PTSD and, actually, trends for better neuropsychological health months after daily interruption,[140] perhaps as a result of the added opportunities to establish concrete memories during awakening.[141] There are populations for whom complete cessation of IV sedatives and analgesics is probably unwise. Girard and colleagues incorporated a safety screen into their protocol and avoid performing DIS in patients (a) receiving sedative infusion for active seizures or alcohol withdrawal, (b) receiving escalating doses due to ongoing agitation, (c) receiving NMBA, (d) having evidence of myocardial ischemia within the past 24 hours, or (e) having elevated ICP.[138] It may be that alcoholic patients are at particular risk for poor tolerance of daily interruption because patients randomized to this intervention had worse outcomes compared to a protocol approach in an RCT conducted in an ICU with a high prevalence of patients with alcohol use disorders.[142]

A variety of other structured approaches have been examined in prospective trials, although many have utilized a less robust two-phase approach. Protocols that utilize an evidence-based nurse-implemented algorithm that seeks to minimize medication doses has been linked to shorter duration of mechanical ventilation,[143-148] shorter ICU and hospital LOS,[144,147,148] lower direct drug costs,[144,146] less opioid medication,[148] less medication-induced coma,[148] and lower 30-day mortality rate.[148] These interventions appear to be less effective in Australian ICUs, perhaps as a result of higher nurse : patient ratios.[149,150] Other algorithms apply active pharmacist input,[151] or focus on pain and agitation.[115] There are few multicenter RCTs that compare several approaches—more are needed. In a preliminary study,[152] Mehta and associates found DIS to be equivalent to a sedation protocol, setting the stage for a larger Canadian RCT. Carson and colleagues found continuous infusion propofol with DIS to be superior to intermittent lorazepam.[153]

In summary, a variety of structured approaches to sedation management are effective for speeding recovery from respiratory failure and critical illness. Practical considerations for establishing a sedation protocol include multidisciplinary development, integrating published algorithms into the local environment, and sustaining a durable approach despite the challenges of insufficient time and resources.[20] Finally, emphasis on protocolized light sedation brings additional opportunities such as linkage to SBTs[138] and to early mobilization,[154] but new challenges such as managing patient agitation[16] and consequences such as self-extubation.[138] The 2012 SCCM guidelines recommend using a multidisciplinary ICU team approach with provider education, preprinted protocols and order sets, and ICU rounds checklists to facilitate pain, agitation, and delirium management guidelines and protocols.[6]

NEUROMUSCULAR BLOCKING AGENTS

In contrast to analgesic and sedative medications, neuromuscular blocking agents (NMBAs) are administered relatively infrequently in the management of mechanically ventilated ICU patients. In an international study of mechanically ventilated patients, 13% of patients received NMBAs.[155] However, up to 55% of patients with ARDS in modern clinical trials receive an NMBA at some point in their management,[156] with even higher rates with interventions such as high-frequency oscillatory ventilation (HFOV).[157] The most common indication for an NMBA is to facilitate mechanical ventilation in particularly challenging scenarios such as severe status asthmaticus or ARDS. NMBAs can enhance oxygenation, reduce the risk of barotrauma, and improve synchronization of the patient and ventilator.[30,158] Additional data suggest that pulmonary and systemic inflammation may be reduced, although the mechanism(s) are not established.[159] Indications for use of NMBAs include facilitation of mechanical ventilation, control of ICP, management of status epilepticus, reduction of oxygen consumption from muscle rigidity or shivering, the presence of an open surgical abdomen, prevention of lactic acidosis in conditions such as tetanus or neuroleptic malignant syndrome, and empirically in patients with severe ARDS (Pao_2:Fio_2 ratio < 120 mm Hg). Lacking robust RCTs, it is noteworthy that previously published guidelines assigned a grade of C (weak) for the recommendation to use an NMBA for these indications.[30] Most use of NMBAs is driven by improving control of a particular problem such as patient-ventilator asynchrony or elevated ICP that persists despite use of less invasive measures.[30,31,160] However, results of a 2010 multicenter RCT support the empiric administration of cisatracurium to all patients with fulminant ARDS (Pao_2:Fio_2 < 120 mm Hg) who do not have contraindications.[32] The findings and limitations of this provocative study are discussed further.

COMPARISON OF AGENTS (TABLE 19.8)

The neuromuscular junction consists of a prejunctional motor nerve ending separated from a postjunctional membrane—or motor endplate—of skeletal muscle by a synaptic cleft. Acetylcholine (ACh) is released from vesicles in the prejunctional motor ending and bind nicotinic cholinergic receptors of the motor endplate, producing a change in membrane potential as a result of influx of sodium and efflux of potassium. Calcium is released from the sarcoplasmic reticulum, producing muscle action potential. Depolarizing NMBAs such as succinylcholine bind the receptors and cause the ion channel to remain open, producing depolarization and potentially causing sufficient potassium efflux to produce hyperkalemia. Additional depolarizations cannot occur until the agent diffuses from the receptors. Succinylcholine is the prototypical paralytic for rapid sequence intubation, due to its rapid onset and short duration of action.[161] However, it can precipitate malignant hypertension and can cause hyperkalemia, which can lead to fatal arrhythmias.[162] The cause of this adverse event is thought to be up-regulation of ACh receptors along the skeletal muscle membrane. Stimulation of these additional receptors by succinylcholine results in potassium efflux, leading to hyperkalemia. Hence, caution should be used when succinylcholine is considered for patients at risk for up-regulation of ACh receptors such as upper or lower motor denervation, chemical denervation (by muscle relaxants, drugs, or toxins), immobilization, infection, direct muscle trauma, muscle tumor, muscle inflammation, and burn injury. Furthermore, succinylcholine should be avoided in patients with renal dysfunction, as hyperkalemia is potentiated in this population. Additionally, succinylcholine has been associated with increases in intracranial and intraocular pressure and should be used with caution in patients with acute ocular or traumatic brain injury.[163]

The nondepolarizing agents are bulky molecules with ACh-like moieties that bind the ACh receptors without ion flow or depolarization. Broadly, the nondepolarizing NMBAs are divided into two structural classes, aminosteroidal and benzylisoquinolinium agents. The aminosteroidal NMBAs incorporate an ACh-like structure onto a steroid backbone.[164] Much like other steroidal drugs, elimination of the aminosteroidal agents is organ dependent. Pancuronium, the first aminosteroidal NMBA, antagonizes not only nicotinic ACh receptors, but also muscarinic receptors.[165] This results in vagal blockade and tachycardia, making it less ideal for patients with significant cardiac disease.[30] Compared to other aminosteroidal NMBAs, pancuronium has a long half-life, which allows for sustained neuromuscular blockade to be achieved with intermittent bolus dosing.[30] Because of the long half-life, organ-dependent metabolism, and production of active metabolites, pancuronium has a high propensity to accumulate in critically ill patients.

Table 19.8 Properties of Neuromuscular Blocking Agents

Property	Atracurium	Cisatracurium	Pancuronium	Rocuronium	Succinylcholine	Vecuronium
Mechanism of action	Nondepolarizing	Nondepolarizing	Nondepolarizing	Nondepolarizing	Depolarizing	Nondepolarizing
Class	Benzylisoquinolinium agent	Benzylisoquinolinium agent	Aminosteroidal agent	Aminosteroidal agent	Acetylcholine-like	Aminosteroidal agent
Onset	3-5 min	2-3 min	2-3 min	1-2 min	1-1.5 min	3-4 min
Duration	25-35 min	45-60 min	90-100 min	30 min	5-10 min	35-45 min
Renal elimination	<5%	<20% by renal and hepatic pathways combined	60-80%	30%	<10%	10-20%
Hepatic elimination	—	<20% by renal and hepatic pathways combined	15-40%	—	—	20-30%
Biliary excretion	—	—	5-10%	50%	—	40-75%
Hofmann elimination and ester hydrolysis	Yes	Yes	No	No	—	No
Plasma cholinesterase	No	No	No	No	Yes	No
Active metabolites	None (toxic metabolite laudanosine)	None	3-OH and 17-OH pancuronium	None	Succinylmonocholine (clinically insignificant depolarizing muscle relaxant properties)	3-Desacetylvecuronium
Bolus dosing	0.4-0.5 mg/kg	0.1-0.2 mg/kg	0.02-0.1 mg/kg	0.6-1 mg/kg	0.3-1.5 mg/kg	0.08-0.1 mg/kg
Continuous dosing	5-20 µg/kg/min	3 µg/kg/min (initial)	0.8-1.7 µg/kg/min	8-12 µg/kg/min	0.6-6 mg/kg/hr (not routinely recommended)	0.8-1.7 µg/kg/min
Histamine release	Yes (dose-dependent)	No	No	No	Yes	No
Vagal blockade tachycardia	No	No	Yes	At higher doses	None (actually can cause bradycardia from vagal stimulation)	No
Prolonged blockade	Rare	Rare	Yes	No	Yes (in patients with reduced plasma cholinesterase activity)	Yes

Newer aminosteroidal NMBAs, such as vecuronium and rocuronium, offer advantages over pancuronium as they do not antagonize muscarinic receptors. Vecuronium is an intermediate-acting aminosteroidal NMBA with both renal and hepatic elimination. It offers utility both for procedural and sustained paralysis, but like pancuronium, can accumulate in patients with organ dysfunction. Rocuronium has the fastest onset and shortest duration of action of the aminosteroidal NMBAs, making it ideal for rapid sequence intubation in circumstances when succinylcholine is contraindicated. Like all aminosteroidal NMBAs, it exhibits organ dependent clearance; however, when used intermittently for procedural paralysis, this is rarely of clinical significance.

In contrast to the aminosteroidal NMBAs, benzylisoquinolinium agents are nonsteroidal agents that are degraded by plasma esterase and Hofmann degradation.[164,165] Atracurium was the first benzylisoquinolinium NMBA and was advantageous in that it was an intermediate-acting paralytic with organ-independent clearance. However, atracurium causes significant histamine release and thus must be used with caution in patients with hypotension or shock. Additionally, patients with organ dysfunction are at increased risk of seizures when atracurium is used for sustained paralysis due to accumulation of a toxic metabolite, laudanosine.[31] Cisatracurium is the cis-cis isomer of atracurium and represents approximately 15% of the atracurium conformation.[164] Like atracurium, cisatracurium undergoes clearance via plasma esterase and Hofmann degradation but is devoid of histamine release and toxic metabolites.

MONITORING

Monitoring of the patient during chemical paralysis is performed to ensure safety and effectiveness of the intervention. Goals of monitoring include achieving the targeted depth of sedation to accomplish therapeutic goals while reducing the likelihood of undesired prolonged paralysis or acute quadriplegic myopathy (AQM) and also avoiding other potential complications. Different targets for NMBAs may vary from merely reduced spontaneous movement or better synchronization of spontaneous breathing with mechanical ventilation to apnea for fully passive ventilation or complete cessation of all skeletal muscle activity. Accordingly, observation of limb and respiratory muscle activity as well as review of graphic display of ventilator data should be performed to confirm the therapeutic target is reached. Testing of deep tendon reflexes may be helpful as they disappear as 100% blockade is reached. Monitoring the depth and duration of paralysis is important in order to optimize neuromuscular blockade for each individual patient and to avoid complications of therapy.[30,31,160,166] Such monitoring typically includes clinical evaluation as well as an objective measure of the extent of blockade using peripheral nerve stimulation (PNS) testing by evaluating the response to "train-of-four" (TOF) stimulation. In TOF testing, four equal brief electrical charges are delivered every 0.5 second from a nerve stimulator device that is attached to leads placed on the skin overlying a superficial nerve that innervates an easily observed muscle. The most common placement is over the ulnar nerve with observation of contraction of the adductor pollicis muscle or over the facial nerve with observation of contraction of the orbicularis oculi muscle. It is estimated that if less than 75% of receptors are blocked, the four muscular contractions are equal in intensity and that once more than 90% of receptors are blocked no contractions occur. A common safety goal is for titration of the NMBA so that one to three muscle contractions are present, thus potentially avoiding excessive dosing. It is worth considering, however, that clinical effectiveness (such as patient-ventilator synchrony) is sometimes achieved while TOF reveals all four contractions. In contrast, in order to achieve apnea or complete cessation of muscular activity, TOF of zero may be necessary. In this circumstance, periodically decreasing the NMBA infusion rate until TOF of one or more may be necessary to avoid excessive dosing.

Despite the intuitive value of monitoring the depth of NMBA dosing, clinical trials that compare PNS monitoring to clinical monitoring alone have not consistently demonstrated added value. In one RCT, Rudis and coworkers demonstrated more rapid recovery to four of four TOF contractions and to spontaneous breathing as well as fewer episodes of delayed recovery when vecuronium infusion was titrated to achieve one of four TOF contractions in comparison to patients with clinical monitoring alone.[167] Patients with impaired renal function had the slowest recovery. In contrast, PNS monitoring did not lead to better outcomes in prospective trials of patients who received atracurium[168] or cisatracurium.[169] Further, intentional dosing of cisatracurium to achieve TOF of zero only marginally prolonged the recovery time.[170] Finally, no PNS monitoring was performed in the 2010 placebo-controlled RCT in which 178 patients received a 48-hour cisatracurium infusion and there was no difference in the rate of ICU paresis compared to the placebo group.[32] Unfortunately, maintenance of TOF more than zero does not guarantee AQM will not occur. Most reported cases developed despite documented appropriate TOF results. Accordingly, although the 2002 SCCM guidelines recommended that all patients receiving NMBA should be assessed both clinically and by TOF monitoring (grade B recommendation) with a goal of adjusting the degree of NMBA to achieve 1 to 2 twitches (grade C recommendation), the validity of this recommendation is most compelling when vecuronium infusion is used but less so for atracurium or cisatracurium given subsequent published reports.[30] Monitoring of patients who are receiving NMBAs should also address prevention and early detection of venous thromboembolism (VTE), pressure ulcers, corneal ulcers, patient awareness, and inadequately controlled pain and anxiety.

COMPLICATIONS

The primary safety concerns with NMBAs are for prolonged paralysis due to persistent drug effect or from AQM. Both circumstances result in significant weakness and are considerations in the broad differential diagnosis of weakness in the ICU patient. Causes of weakness range widely from severe electrolyte disturbances like hypermagnesemia or hypophosphatemia to critical illness polyneuropathy, steroid myopathy, or Guillain-Barré syndrome. A variety of factors can increase the risk for prolonged recovery from NMBAs, including organ dysfunction and resulting impaired clearance of the parent compound, accumulation of active

Box 19.4 Drugs That Potentiate or Antagonize the Actions of Nondepolarizing Neuromuscular Blocking Agents (NMBAs)

Drugs That Potentiate the Action of Nondepolarizing NMBAs

Local anesthetics
Lidocaine
Antimicrobials (aminoglycosides, polymyxin B, clindamycin, tetracycline, vancomycin, amphotericin B, colistin)
Antiarrhythmics (procainamide, quinidine)
Magnesium
Calcium channel blockers
β-Adrenergic blockers
Immunosuppressive agents (cyclophosphamide, cyclosporine)
Dantrolene
Diuretics (furosemide, bumetanide, ethacrynic acid)
Lithium carbonate
Corticosteroids
Inhaled anesthetics (enflurane, halothane, isoflurane, methoxyflurane, nitrous oxide)
Acetylcholinesterase inhibitors

Drugs That Antagonize the Actions of Nondepolarizing NMBAs

Phenytoin
Carbamazepine
Theophylline
Ranitidine

Modified from Murray MJ, Cowen J, DeBlock H, et al: Clinical practice guidelines for sustained neuromuscular blockade in the adult critically ill patient. Crit Care Med 2002;30(1):142-156; and Warr J, Thiboutot Z, Rose L, et al: Current therapeutic uses, pharmacology, and clinical considerations of neuromuscular blocking agents for critically ill adults. Ann Pharmacother 2011;45(9):1116-1126.

metabolites, drug-drug interactions, and other medical conditions. Drugs that potentiate or antagonize the actions of nondepolarizing NMBAs are listed in Box 19.4. There is also considerable variability in duration of effect among NMBAs. The aminosteroids are eliminated by a combination of renal clearance and hepatic metabolism to a number of compounds, some of which are active and are eliminated in the urine. Accordingly, dysfunction of liver or kidneys is associated with prolonged paralysis.[31,171] Resolution of paralysis is not predictable with vecuronium, particularly with prolonged infusion.[171,172] This contrasts sharply with the benzylisoquinoliniums with recovery times of about 1 hour, even despite prolonged infusion[169] and with higher doses.[170] Perhaps most instructive is a prospective head-to-head comparison of vecuronium and cisatracurium in ICU patients in which average recovery time was fivefold longer with vecuronium.[173] Close monitoring of depth of sedation using TOF PNS appears to reduce the incidence of prolonged paralysis with vecuronium[167] but is of less certain value with atracurium or cisatracurium.[168,169]

AQM is a potentially devastating form of NMBA-related weakness in which the muscle weakness can be severe and quite protracted.[30] AQM is characterized by weakness of the limb and trunk muscles with sparing of the extraocular muscles as well as preserved sensory function and cognition. Understanding of the mechanisms underlying AQM have evolved from suspicion that myonecrosis alone was responsible to that of altered muscle membrane properties with loss of motor protein myosin and myosin-associated thick filament proteins. Work by Larsson and associates has demonstrated that a combination of myofibrillar protein degradation plus down-regulation of protein synthesis at the transcriptional level is prominent.[174] Key predisposing factors for ICU-acquired weakness appear to be functional denervation—such as from NMBAs and corticosteroids. The argument has been made that prolonged deep sedation may be another source of immobilization.[33] Additional risk factors for ICU-acquired polyneuropathy and myopathy include sepsis and other forms of systemic inflammation, hyperglycemia, malnutrition, and prolonged immobility. Although both aminosteroid and benzylisoquinolinium agents have been linked to AQM in case reports, it is noteworthy that in the relatively limited prospective clinical trial literature of NMBA in ICU patients, AQM is described in about 5% of patients who received vecuronium but none of the more than 200 patients who were administered atracurium or cisatracurium infusion.[169] Further, in the largest multicenter RCT of cisatracurium versus placebo, there was no difference in the incidence of ICU-acquired weakness.[32] Finally, some experts consider the causality of NMBA—particularly short-duration NMBA—for producing ICU-acquired weakness to be far from certain.[33]

EVOLVING ROLE IN ACUTE RESPIRATORY DISTRESS SYNDROME

NMBAs have been utilized for years to optimize gas exchange in patients with severe ARDS. Numerous RCTs demonstrate and other observational studies indicate that as many as one half of ARDS patients receive at least intermittent NMBA, with the most common indication being refractory hypoxemia. Sustained increases in $Pa{O_2}$:$F{IO_2}$ ratio have been demonstrated in small RCTs.[158,159] Interestingly, preliminary studies also have demonstrated lower levels of proinflammatory cytokines in bronchoalveolar lavage fluid and circulating blood in patients randomized to cisatracurium, in contrast to placebo.[159] In 2010, Papazian and coworkers published the results of a French multicenter RCT in which 340 patients with severe ARDS ($Pa{O_2}$:$F{IO_2}$ < 150 mm Hg) were randomized to receive a 48-hour infusion of cisatracurium or placebo.[32] Patients randomized to cisatracurium had better outcomes including lower rate of death at 28 days and trends for lower rates of death in the ICU and the hospital, more ventilator-free days and organ failure–free days, and fewer barotraumas. Post hoc analysis showed that the mortality rate benefit was limited entirely to the patients with most profound hypoxemia ($Pa{O_2}$:$F{IO_2}$ < 120 mm Hg), although the relationship of other key outcomes to baseline oxygenation was not reported. Impressively, there was no difference in rates of ICU paresis, and limb weakness was identical for cisatracurium and placebo groups. A number of methodologic issues are worth noting, including no use of PNS for monitoring, use of very deep sedation (Ramsay Sedation Score = 6), use of ketamine for sedation in 20%

of patients, open label use of cisatracurium in 56% of placebo patients, the use of very modest PEEP despite severe hypoxemia, and the high barotrauma for placebo patients. Clinicians are eager for additional RCTs to confirm the findings.

SUMMARY AND CONCLUSIONS

The use of analgesic and sedative medications in the ICU setting is widespread and, although often viewed as a component of "supportive care" of critically ill patients, clearly can impact major outcomes. Accordingly, adopting a thoughtful, structured, and multidisciplinary approach to managing analgesia and sedation is important and centers around reasoned medication selection, close monitoring, and employing strategies to use the lowest effective dose. Similarly, NMBA administration can be of critical importance in managing selected clinical situations and should be guided by monitoring and limiting use to the shortest duration possible.

KEY POINTS

- A combination of non-pharmacological and pharmacological interventions can be useful to enhance tolerance of discomfort of invasive procedures, postoperative pain, and sleep deprivation common to the ICU experience.
- Adopting a patient-focused approach to managing sedation and analgesia that strives to minimize the depth and duration of reduced consciousness is associated with better outcomes.
- Development of delirium in the ICU is associated with worse outcomes, including impaired cognitive function after discharge.
- Agitated behavior is a common occurrence associated with adverse consequences including self-removal of critical tubes and lines and excessive adrenergic stress response.
- Identification of delirium or agitation should prompt a search for predisposing and precipitating medical conditions and medications.
- Self-reporting using standardized tools is the best method to detect and quantify pain; however, observation of characteristic behaviors can be helpful in the patient who is unable to self-report.
- Routine use of a validated sedation-agitation scale such as RASS or SAS promotes better communication, more precise sedative drug titration, and timely detection and grading of agitation.
- Recent research supports the use of non-benzodiazepines in preference to benzodiazepines when continuous infusion sedation is required.
- Targeting a more alert state for mechanically ventilated ICU patients is associated with better outcomes including shorter duration of mechanical ventilation, fewer tests, and shorter ICU length of stay.

KEY POINTS (Continued)

- Neuromuscular blocking agents (NMBAs) are administered infrequently to ICU patients, most often to facilitate the earlier stages of mechanical ventilation in severe ARDS or status asthmaticus.
- Safe and effective use of NMBA requires prevention of undetected pain and awareness in the paralyzed patient, prevention of adverse consequences of paralysis such as corneal damage or nerve injury from inappropriate positioning, prophylaxis against deep venous thrombosis, and monitoring to avoid excessive dosing.

SELECTED REFERENCES

5. Jacobi J, Fraser GL, Coursin DB, et al: Clinical practice guidelines for the sustained use of sedatives and analgesics in the critically ill adult. Crit Care Med 2002;30(1):119-141.
6. Barr J, Fraser GL, Puntillo K, et al: Clinical practice guidelines for the management of pain, agitation, and delirium in adult patients in the intensive care unit. Crit Care Med 2013;41(1):263-306.
9. Erstad BL, Puntillo K, Gilbert HC, et al: Pain management principles in the critically ill. Chest 2009;135(4):1075-1086.
14. Brook AD, Ahrens TS, Schaiff R, et al: Effect of a nursing-implemented sedation protocol on the duration of mechanical ventilation. Crit Care Med 1999;27(12):2609-2615.
15. Kress JP, Pohlman AS, O'Connor MF, Hall JB: Daily interruption of sedative infusions in critically ill patients undergoing mechanical ventilation. N Engl J Med 2000;342(20):1471-1477.
19. Sessler CN, Varney K: Patient-focused sedation and analgesia in the ICU. Chest 2008;133(2):552-565.
20. Sessler CN, Pedram S: Protocolized and target-based sedation and analgesia in the ICU. Crit Care Clin 2009;25(3):489-513.
22. Honiden S, Siegel MD: Analytic reviews: Managing the agitated patient in the ICU: Sedation, analgesia, and neuromuscular blockade. J Intensive Care Med 2010;25(4):187-204.
23. Patel SB, Kress JP: Sedation and analgesia in the mechanically ventilated patient. Am J Respir Crit Care Med 2012;185(5):486-497.
30. Murray MJ, Cowen J, DeBlock H, et al: Clinical practice guidelines for sustained neuromuscular blockade in the adult critically ill patient. Crit Care Med 2002;30(1):142-156.
31. Warr J, Thiboutot Z, Rose L, et al: Current therapeutic uses, pharmacology, and clinical considerations of neuromuscular blocking agents for critically ill adults. Ann Pharmacother 2011;45(9):1116-1126.
32. Papazian L, Forel JM, Gacouin A, et al: Neuromuscular blockers in early acute respiratory distress syndrome. N Engl J Med 2010;363(12):1107-1116.
58. Puntillo K, Pasero C, Li D, et al: Evaluation of pain in ICU patients. Chest 2009;135(4):1069-1074.
130. Riker RR, Shehabi Y, Bokesch PM, et al: Dexmedetomidine vs midazolam for sedation of critically ill patients: A randomized trial. JAMA 2009;301(5):489-499.
133. Jakob SM, Ruokonen E, Grounds RM, et al: Dexmedetomidine vs midazolam or propofol for sedation during prolonged mechanical ventilation: Two randomized controlled trials. JAMA 2012;307(11):1151-1160.
138. Girard TD, Kress JP, Fuchs BD, et al: Efficacy and safety of a paired sedation and ventilator weaning protocol for mechanically ventilated patients in intensive care (Awakening and Breathing Controlled trial): A randomised controlled trial. Lancet 2008;371(9607):126-134.

The complete list of references can be found at www.expertconsult.com.

20 Principles of Drug Dosing in Critically Ill Patients

Quinn A. Czosnowski | Todd A. Miano

"All things are poison, and nothing is without poison; only the dose permits something not to be poisonous."

—PARACELSUS, SIXTEENTH CENTURY PHYSICIAN

CHAPTER OUTLINE

The pharmacologic effect of a drug is the result of complex interactions between its physiochemical characteristics and the biologic systems of the human body. The amount of drug given with each dose and the frequency of dosing are two of the most critical determinants of successful pharmacotherapy. Indeed, these factors are often the only differences between lifesaving effects and life-threatening toxicity. Dosing regimens are based on an understanding of these interactions and are designed to maximize the beneficial effects of drug exposure while minimizing risk of toxicity. When selecting a dosing regimen the clinician must be able to answer the following questions: What serum concentrations will be produced by the dose administered? How will the concentration change over time? Answers to these questions are provided by the science of pharmacokinetics (PK), which tells us what the body does to drugs: absorption, distribution, metabolism, and excretion. However, understanding PK alone is not sufficient to design optimal dosing regimens. Other important questions remain: What concentration is needed to produce the desired effect? What concentration has the potential to produce toxicity? These questions are answered by the science of pharmacodynamics (PD), the study of what drugs do to the body. Understanding PD allows the clinician to relate specific serum concentrations to pharmacologic effects. The use of both pharmacokinetic and pharmacodynamic principles enables the clinician to maximize therapeutic efficacy while minimizing toxicity.

An additional level of complexity exists in critically ill patients. The majority of pharmacokinetic and pharmacodynamic information available has been obtained from studies in healthy volunteers and other non–critically ill populations. Critically ill patients differ from those often studied because they frequently experience hepatic and renal dysfunction, receive aggressive fluid resuscitation, and require vasoactive medications to maintain adequate organ perfusion. These physiologic alterations can dramatically alter dose response and vary greatly from patient to patient and even from day to day in the same patient. In addition, patients also frequently have significant comorbid conditions, such as chronic kidney disease, cirrhosis, and heart failure, which affect dose response.

GENERAL PHARMACOKINETIC PRINCIPLES

The pharmacokinetic profile of a drug is a mathematical model that describes the determinants of drug exposure. A complete model provides quantitative estimates of drug absorption, distribution, metabolism, and excretion after

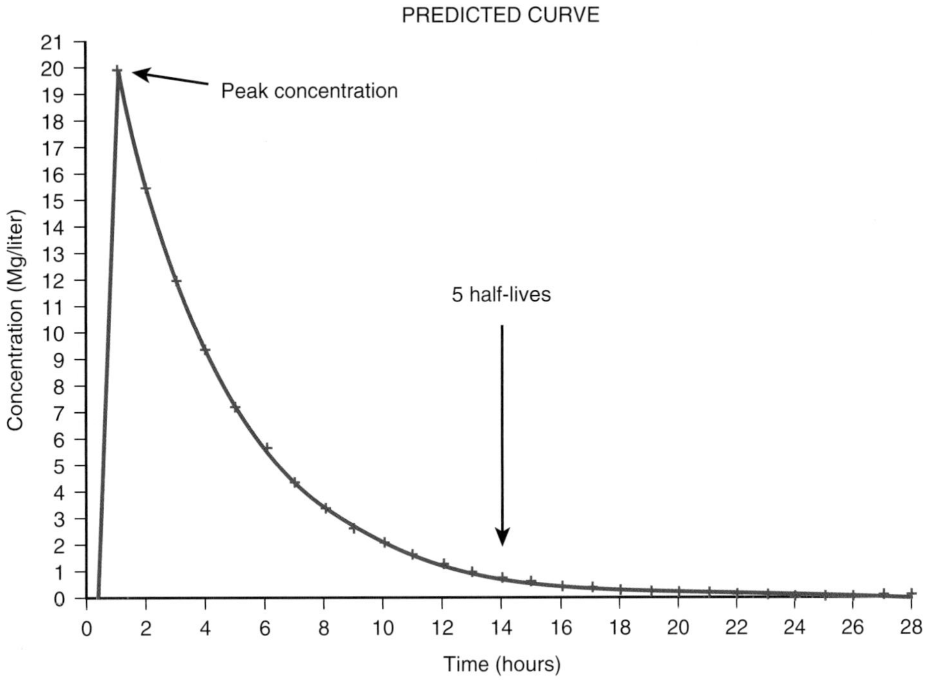

Figure 20.1 Concentration vs. time curve following a single 200-mg intravenous dose of tobramcyin in a 50-kg female. Note: Peak concentration determined by Vd and the size of dose given. Time course of elimination is determined by clearance and Vd. Approximately 90% of dose is eliminated after 5 half-lives.

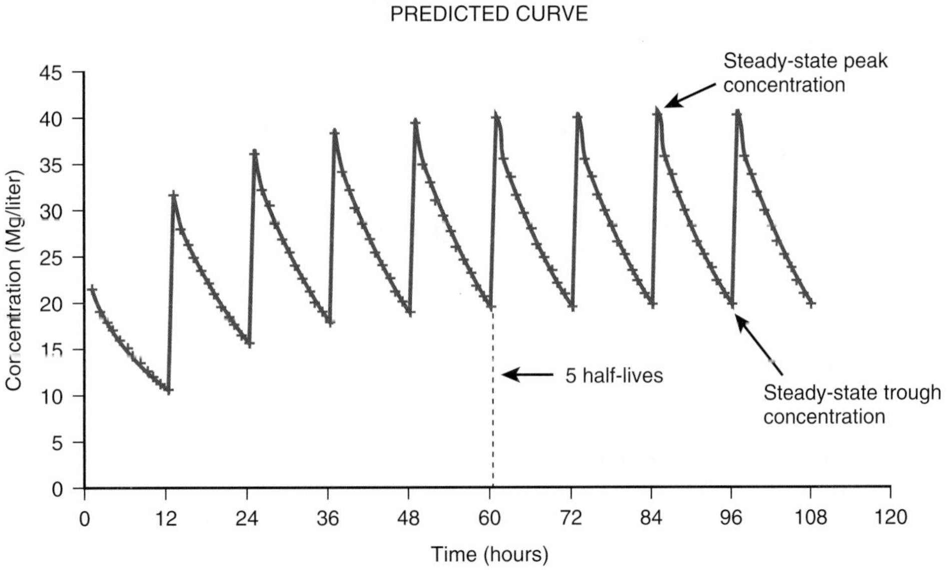

Figure 20.2 Concentration vs. time curve demonstrating accumulation after repeated dosing of 750 mg vancomycin every 12 hours in a 50-kg patient. Note: Dosing regimens are based upon steady-state concentrations. Therapeutic drug monitoring should be conducted when regimens have reached steady state, which occurs after 5 to 7 half-lives.

single doses, in addition to the extent of serum and tissue accumulation after multiple doses. Figure 20.1 depicts the concentration-time curve for a single intravenous (IV) dose of tobramycin. The curve allows for estimation of the maximum concentration achieved by the dose in addition to the time course of drug elimination. If dosing is repeated before elimination is complete, accumulation occurs and will continue until the system reaches "steady state," at which time the rate of administration is in equilibrium with the rate of elimination (Fig. 20.2). The definition of common PK terms can be found in Table 20.1.

ABSORPTION

The first step in modeling exposure is to quantify the relationship between drug dosage administered and the amount

Table 20.1 Basic Pharmacokinetic Parameters

Parameter	Definition	Notes
Volume of distribution (Vd)	$Vd = \frac{\text{Dose (mg)}}{\text{peak concentration (mg/L)}}$	Size of distribution compartment Quantifies the degree to which drug distributes into tissue
Area under the concentration-time curve (AUC)	$AUC = \frac{\text{Dose (mg/hour)}}{\text{Cl (L/hour)}}$	Total drug exposure produced by administered dose
Clearance (Cl)	$Cl = \frac{\text{Dose (mg/hour)}}{\text{AUC (mg/L/hour)}}$	Volume of blood cleared of drug per unit time
Elimination rate constant (Ke)	$Ke = \frac{\text{Cl (L/hour)}}{\text{Vd (L)}}$	The rate of drug elimination from the body per unit of time Relates clearance (liters cleared per hour) and Vd (volume to be cleared). This value is inversely related to drug half-life.
Bioavailability (F)	$F = \frac{AUC_{PO}/dose_{PO}}{AUC_{IV}/dose_{IV}}$	Percentage of dose that reaches systemic circulation Varies by route: Intravenous—100% Oral, subcutaneous, transdermal—variable: 0-100% Value expressed as a percentage of exposure relative to intravenous administration

of drug that reaches the systemic circulation. This relationship is known as the drug's bioavailability. IV administration provides 100% bioavailability, whereas this value can be considerably less for other routes. Oral ingestion is the most common route of administration in the general population and remains useful in many critically ill patients. Bioavailability through oral administration is usually less than 100% and is a function of two main factors: (1) absorption, which is the intrinsic ability of the drug to cross the gastrointestinal tract, and (2) presystemic metabolism, also known as the first-pass effect, which occurs primarily in the liver, and to a lesser extent in the intestinal lumen. Drugs that undergo extensive hepatic metabolism may have large first-pass effects and thus low bioavailability compared to IV administration. Similarly, drugs that are poorly absorbed will have low bioavailability.

Factors that determine absorption from the gastrointestinal (GI) tract include drug characteristics such as lipid solubility, ionization, and molecular size, in addition to physiologic factors such as gastric emptying rate, intestinal blood flow, motility, gastric and intestinal pH, gut wall permeability, and whether the dose is administered during the fasted or fed state.[1] Most drugs are orally absorbed through passive diffusion; although carrier-mediated absorption can also be important. The most important sites of absorption are the upper and lower segments of the small intestine.[2] The stomach regulates absorption through gastric emptying but is not an important site for absorption. Similarly, little drug absorption occurs in the colon with the exception of extended-release products.[1] Drugs with low oral bioavailability will require larger doses administered orally to produce equivalent exposure to that obtained from IV administration. Some drugs (e.g., vancomycin) have such poor bioavailability after oral administration that they cannot be used to treat the same disease processes as the IV formulations. Bioavailability is an important consideration when converting between oral and IV routes. For example, a patient who takes furosemide 80 mg orally at home would need only 40 mg given intravenously because this drug has 50% bioavailability on average. Other routes of administration include subcutaneous (SC) and intramuscular injection, transdermal absorption, buccal absorption, and inhalation. Many drugs that are available as IV preparations are amenable to SC and intramuscular administration. However, some IV drugs have characteristics that preclude administration by routes other than large-bore catheters. These drugs include those with very basic or acidic pH, or those that act as vesicants and therefore need diluents added to maintain solubility. Drugs with adequate lipid solubility are amenable to transdermal and buccal administration.

DISTRIBUTION

After reaching the systemic circulation an administered dose then distributes throughout the body to produce a peak concentration. The relationship between the dose administered and the peak concentration observed after accounting for bioavailability is termed the *volume of distribution* (Vd). Vd estimates the size of the compartment into which the drug distributes. Total plasma volume in the average adult is 3 to 4 L.[1] However, the Vd for most drugs is much greater than this value. The discrepancy between plasma volume and a drug's Vd is accounted for by the extent that drugs concentrate in various tissues. The main determinants of Vd are the drug's lipid solubility, degree of protein binding, and extent of tissue binding.[1] High lipid solubility increases Vd through improved passage across cell membranes. Avid tissue binding also increases Vd as this concentrates drug outside the vascular space. Conversely, because only unbound drug can cross cell membranes and bind to tissue, high protein binding decreases Vd.

The simplest conceptualization of Vd is to view the body as a bucket—one large compartment where drug rapidly equilibrates between plasma and tissue and has uniform distribution (Fig. 20.3A). The one-compartment assumption is useful for drugs with small to intermediate Vds, such as aminoglycoside antibiotics, because these drugs have

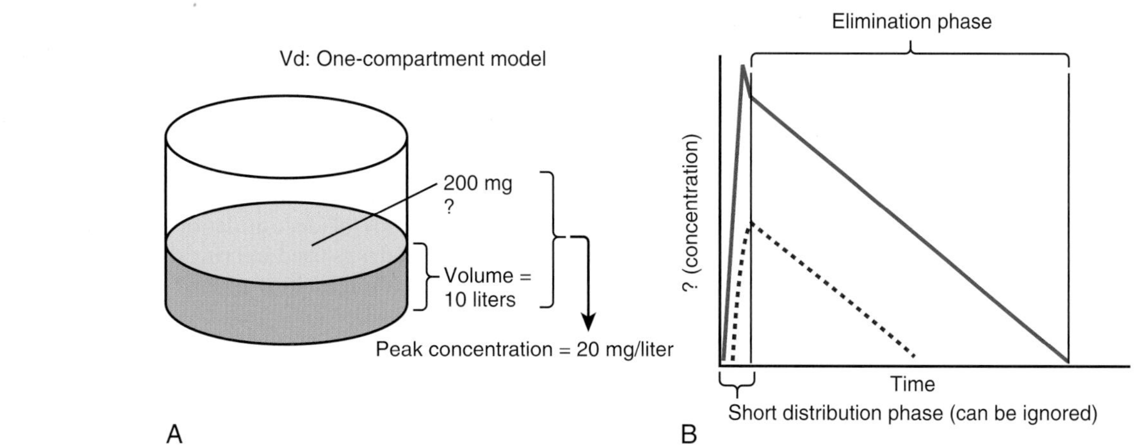

Figure 20.3 One-compartment model of drug distribution when drug rapidly distributes between plasma and tissue. **A,** Volume of distribution (Vd) defines the relationship between dose and peak concentration. **B,** Concentration vs. time curve for one-compartment model on a logarithmic scale. Solid line represents serum concentration. Dashed line represents tissue concentration. Note that tissue concentrations increase during the distribution phase. Because target receptors are frequently within tissues, the time course of the dashed line determines the onset and duration of effect.

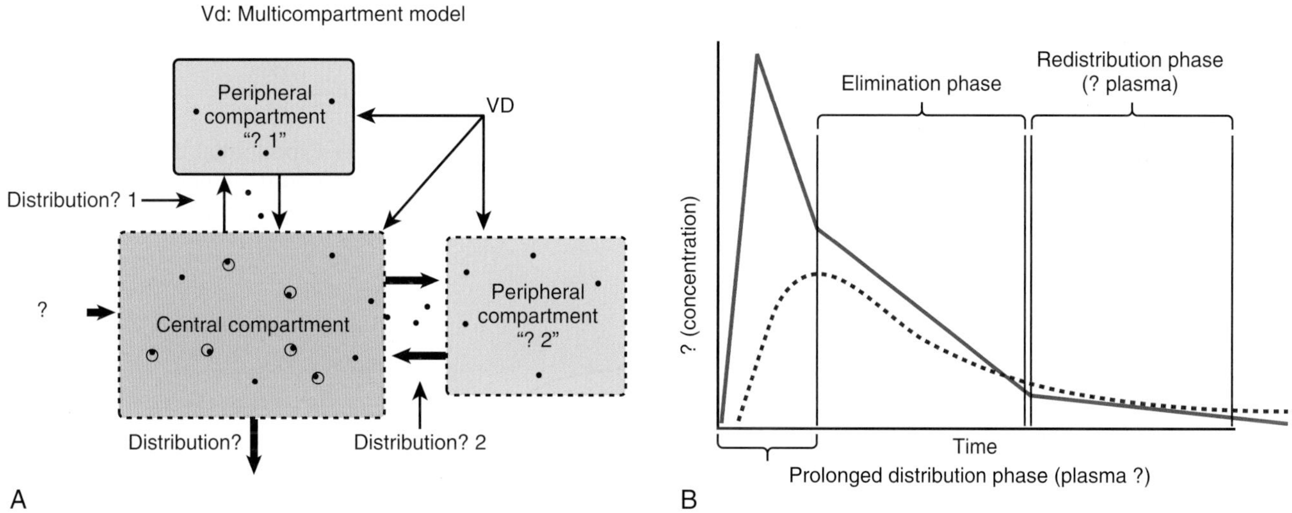

Figure 20.4 Multicompartment model of drug distribution when drug requires a longer period of time to achieve equilibrium between plasma and tissue. **A,** Depiction of a multicompartment model of volume of distribution (Vd). Drug enters the central compartment (serum) and then distributes into peripheral compartments (tissues). Total drug Vd is the sum of the individual compartments. Drug must then distribute back into serum to be eliminated. White circles represent serum protein molecules. Black circles represent drug molecules. **B,** Concentration vs. time curve for one-compartment model on a logarithmic scale. Solid line represents serum concentration. Dashed line represents tissue concentration. Note that tissue concentrations increase during the distribution phase. Large Vd drugs require prolonged distribution phases to saturate the peripheral compartments. The large Vd also results in a prolonged redistribution phase, which prolongs drug half-life.

a short distribution phase owing to their limited tissue penetration. Drugs with large Vds, such as fentanyl and amiodarone, require longer periods of time to achieve equilibrium between serum and tissue and thus have a prolonged distribution phase. As a result, the one-compartment assumption fails to accurately describe large Vd drugs. An alternative is to view the body as multiple compartments: a central compartment composed of blood, extracellular fluid, and highly perfused tissues; and one or more peripheral compartments composed of tissue beds with lower perfusion and drug binding affinity (Fig. 20.4A). The number of peripheral compartments required will be determined by the differential distribution rate in each tissue. Two-compartment models adequately describe most large Vd drugs; however, a three-compartment model can be useful for agents that act in the central nervous system because of slower distribution as a result of the blood-brain barrier.

CLEARANCE

Drug elimination begins immediately upon entry into the body and can be divided into two main components: metabolism and excretion. Metabolism occurs mainly in the liver via enzymatic degradation, although it occurs to lesser extents in other tissues such as the kidney, lung, small intestine and skin and via enzymes found in the serum. Nonenzymatic metabolism also occurs in the serum, as is the case for cisatracurium, which undergoes spontaneous degradation in the serum through ester hydrolysis. Excretion occurs primarily in the kidney, bile, and feces. Some drugs are eliminated predominantly by a single mechanism. For example, more than 95% of elimination for the aminoglycoside antibiotics occurs through excretion in the kidneys. Other drugs, such as ceftriaxone, are removed through multiple pathways. Regardless of pathway, the degree of protein binding exhibited by a drug is an important determinant of elimination rate, as only unbound drug can be eliminated from the serum.

The rate of drug removal via all routes of elimination is termed *clearance,* which is expressed as the volume of plasma cleared per unit of time. This value is assumed to be constant for most drugs. Defining total body clearance in terms of volume has important implications. If the *volume of blood cleared per unit of time* is constant, it then holds that the *amount of drug cleared per unit of time* must change in proportion to serum concentration. An increase in the rate of drug administration will lead to an increase in serum concentration, which in turn leads to commensurate increases in the rate of drug removal. Serum and tissue concentrations will accumulate until the rate of elimination is in equilibrium with the rate of administration, at which time the system is said to be at "steady state" (Figs. 20.2 and 20.5). Accumulation follows a linear pattern for most drugs, meaning that increases in dose are always matched by proportional increases in elimination, thus producing proportional changes in serum concentration (see Fig. 20.5). Drugs that follow this pattern of accumulation are said to have first-order kinetics. However, some drugs exhibit saturable elimination. These drugs follow linear accumulation until the saturation point for elimination is reached. Once elimination is saturated, small changes in dose can produce substantial increases in concentration (see Fig. 20.5). Drugs that follow this pattern of accumulation have zero-order kinetics. Examples of drugs used in critically ill patients that have saturable elimination include phenytoin, heparin, propranolol, and verapamil.

HALF-LIFE

Once clearance is known the clinician can estimate the time needed for a given dose to be eliminated. Elimination time is commonly expressed in terms of half-life, which is the period of time required for the amount of drug to decrease by 50%. Half-life is calculated from the elimination rate constant:

$$\text{ke} = \frac{\text{clearance (liters/hour)}}{\text{volume of distribution (liters)}}$$

ke can be further transformed into half-life:

$$t_{1/2} = \frac{0.693}{\text{ke}}$$

For any system that follows exponential decay, half-life can be used to estimate the amount of elimination that has occurred: after 5 half-lives more than 90% is eliminated.

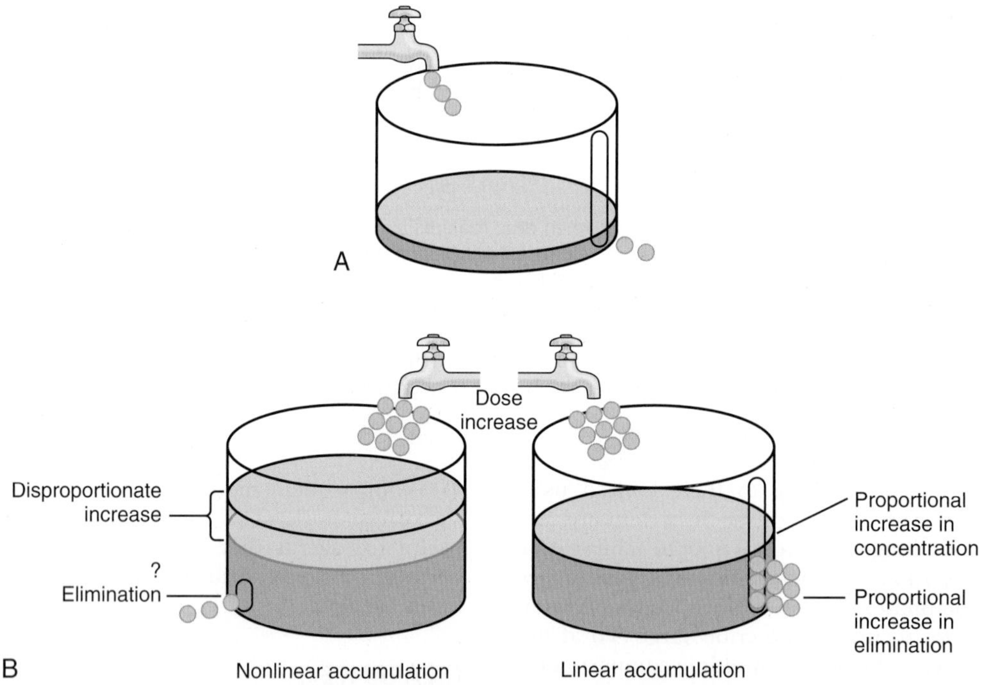

Figure 20.5 Pharmacokinetic principle of linear and nonlinear drug elimination. **A,** Faucet and bucket representation of drug elimination. Faucet represents drug input rate. The channel in the side of the bucket represents drug elimination pathways. At steady state drug input is in equilibrium with drug elimination. **B,** The effect of a dose increase. On the right is an example of first-order kinetics. The channel allows for elimination to increase in proportion to the dose increase, producing proportional changes in drug level. On the left is an example of zero-order kinetics, in which elimination is constant after the saturation point. Here, the elimination channel is saturated at low input rates, producing a disproportionate increase in drug level.

Elimination approaches 100% after 7 half-lives. The time required for a dosing regimen to reach steady state is also an exponential function and thus can be estimated using half-life. This "5-7" rule of thumb is useful at the bedside. Dosing regimens approach maximal effects after 5-7 half-lives. Similarly, drug effects are usually completely dissipated after 5-7 half-lives. Using this rule, it can be predicted that drugs with long half-lives may take several days to produce target effects. This is less than ideal in the critically ill population when effective treatment is needed rapidly. As a result, loading doses are frequently used to hasten the time to steady state. Loading doses can be calculated by multiplying the target steady-state peak concentration by the patient's Vd. Recommendations for effective loading doses of most long half-life drugs are provided in the package labeling as applicable.

It is important to note that the time needed to eliminate a given dose is not only dependent on the clearance rate, but also on the drug's Vd. It is intuitive that half-life will be affected by changes in elimination pathways (e.g., renal failure). However, changes in Vd can have equally important effects on half-life, which can lead to higher than expected drug accumulation independent of changes in drug clearance. This effect has important implications for critically ill patients in whom Vd can be significantly altered.

MODELING THE CONCENTRATION-TIME CURVE

When estimations of bioavailability, Vd, and clearance are available, the concentration-time curve can be modeled. As discussed earlier, the one-compartment model is useful for hydrophilic drugs with small Vd. Figure 20.3B depicts serum concentration-time curve of a one-compartment model drug after IV administration plotted on a logarithmic scale. The initial peak concentration can be estimated using Vd and the size of the dose. The peak is followed by a short distribution phase, during which time drug is removed from the plasma through distribution to tissue in addition to being eliminated. After distribution is complete, the curve is defined by a second phase when drug is removed from plasma via elimination only. The time course of this phase can be estimated using half-life. The transition from distribution to elimination phase can be seen as a change in slope of the concentration curve. This is known as a bi-exponential pattern of decay. Because the distribution phase is short (usually 15-30 minutes) it can usually be ignored when performing calculations.

Conversely, large Vd drugs are more accurately represented using a two-compartment model (Fig. 20.4B). The important difference between one-compartment and two-compartment models is the significance of the distribution phase, which is much longer for drugs following a two-compartment model. As in the one-compartment model, the transition between distribution and elimination phases can be seen. However, a third phase is also evident near the end of the curve. This redistribution phase is a result of slow release of drug from the tissues back into the serum. This slow tissue release, known as the "context-sensitive half-life," is responsible for the increased duration of pharmacologic effect seen after continuous infusions of highly lipophilic drugs such as fentanyl, midazolam, and propofol.

PHARMACODYNAMICS

As described in preceding sections, PK allows the clinician to estimate serum and tissue concentrations produced from dosing regimens. For example, a clinical pharmacist can use pharmacokinetic calculations to determine that 200 mg of tobramycin given as a 30-minute IV infusion will produce a peak concentration of 20 mg/L and will have an elimination half-life of 5 hours (see Fig. 20.1). Unfortunately, this information alone is not sufficient to guide dosing. From this example it is obvious that PK gives no information regarding whether these concentrations are appropriate. The clinician must still determine whether the peak concentration will be effective in treating the patient's infection while also determining the risk of nephrotoxicity associated with this level. This is when the study of pharmacodynamics (PD), which defines the relationship between drug concentration and effect, becomes important.

Although PD concepts are important for all dosing decisions, PD parameters have been best defined for antibiotics in part because the effect of interest (bacterial killing) can be readily measured through in vitro and in vivo studies. Therefore, the PD portion of this chapter will focus on antibiotics. However, the basic concepts can be applied to all drugs. Minimum inhibitory concentration (MIC) was the first PD parameter to show utility in predicting the effectiveness of antibiotic regimens. The MIC of an antibiotic is the minimum concentration needed to inhibit bacterial growth in vitro. It is intuitive from this that effective dosing regimens in humans would produce concentrations above this value. Less intuitive is determining how much higher the MIC concentrations need to be and for how long. Decades of research into these questions have elucidated additional PD parameters that help to optimize antibiotic dosing (Fig. 20.6). Interest in PD dose optimization has resurged in recent years in response to the convergence of increasingly drug-resistant bacteria with the lack of novel compounds in

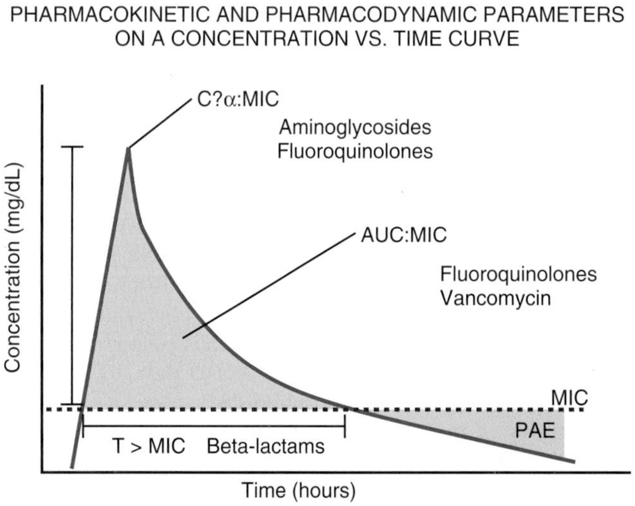

Figure 20.6 Pharmacokinetic and pharmacodynamic parameters on a concentration vs. time curve. This figure depicts how drug concentration relates to bactericidal effect for various antimicrobial agents.

the drug development pipeline to treat these dangerous pathogens.[3] Consequently, it is more important now than ever to maximize the effectiveness of the agents currently in use.

Two main factors determine the PD profile of an antibiotic: the dependence of effect on concentration and the persistence of effect after dosing. Antibiotics are first classified by the extent to which the rate of bacterial killing increases in response to increases in concentration. Some antibiotics show a robust dose response, whereas others do not. This relationship was elucidated in the neutropenic murine thigh infection model, when the effect of increasing antibiotic concentration on bacterial killing was examined.[4] In repeated studies, the model showed that increasing concentration substantially increases both the magnitude (change from baseline) and the rate (change over time) of bacterial killing for aminoglycoside antibiotics such as tobramycin and the fluoroquinolone antibiotics such as ciprofloxacin. However, the same effects are not observed for the β-lactam classes of antibiotics. Although small concentration effects are observed in some models, the effect is saturated at a relatively low concentration (4-5 times the MIC). The difference in effect is related to the location of each agent's target receptor. Both aminoglycoside and fluoroquinolone antibiotics have receptor targets that are intracellular. Penetration of these antibiotics into the cell is enhanced by high concentrations. As a result, the activity of these agents can be predicted by the ratio of the peak concentration achieved by a given dose to the MIC of the organism. Accordingly, these agents are classified as concentration-dependent antibiotics. Conversely, β-lactams inhibit the formation of bacterial cell wall via inhibition of penicillin-binding protein (PBP). This protein is located on the bacterial cell surface, allowing effective binding at lower concentrations. In fact, in vitro analyses have shown that nearly all available PBP targets become saturated at concentrations that are four to five times the bacteria's MIC.[5] Above this level, the action of β-lactams is relatively independent of concentration, making the duration of time that concentrations remain above the MIC the parameter most predictive of effect.

Another important observation from in vitro models is the persistent inhibition of bacterial growth after drug concentration falls below the MIC. This phenomenon, known as the postantibiotic effect (PAE), is common to all antibiotics, although the magnitude varies depending on the specific antibiotic and pathogen being analyzed. PAE is usually prolonged (3-6 hours) for agents that inhibit nucleic acid and protein synthesis such as the aminoglycosides.[4] Most cell wall active agents such as the β-lactams have a short PAE for gram-positive bacteria and complete absence of PAE against gram-negative bacteria. As a result, bacterial regrowth occurs immediately as concentration falls below the MIC.[4] Carbapenems are an exception to this as they are cell wall active agents and have a prolonged PAE.

Synthesis of these data allows antibiotics to be grouped according to their pattern of concentration dependence and persistent effects. The first pattern is that of concentration dependence combined with prolonged PAE. Activity of agents following this pattern is predicted by peak:MIC ratio and is optimized by giving large doses less frequently. The second pattern is one of time dependence combined with short PAE. Activity of agents that follow this pattern is predicted by time above the MIC (T > MIC) and is optimized by giving smaller doses more frequently. A third pattern is that of concentration dependence with short PAE. The lack of significant PAE renders both peak:MIC and T > MIC relationships as important predictors of effect. As a result, activity is best predicted by total antibiotic exposure and is quantified by the AUC:MIC ratio, where AUC is the area under the curve. The fourth and final pattern is one of time-dependent killing combined with moderate to prolonged PAE. The presence of PAE renders these agents less dependent on T > MIC, making AUC:MIC the most predictive parameter.

It is important to note that most PD analysis is based on total drug concentrations in the serum. However, only free drug concentrations that reach the site of action will affect bacterial killing. Thus, total drug concentrations in the serum may not always reflect antibiotic activity. This likely is not a concern for small Vd drugs with negligible protein binding, such as aminoglycoside and many β-lactams. These agents achieve rapid equilibration between serum and tissue and free concentrations are similar to total concentrations. However, total serum concentration may not be ideal for drugs with high protein binding or those with a large Vd. Tissue level analysis may offer better predictions for these drugs. However, owing to the greater difficulty in performing such analysis, their availability is limited.

β-LACTAMS

Alexander Fleming first discovered penicillin in 1928, marking the dawn of the antibiotic era. It was more than 2 decades later when Harry Eagle first noted that penicillin's effect could be modulated by dosing regimen. Specifically, he observed that penicillin's ability to kill bacteria was dependent on the amount of time that the drug was maintained at or above the bacteria's MIC.[6] Later experiments confirmed time above MIC (T > MIC), as the PD index that predicts bacterial killing for penicillin and other β-lactam agents.[4] The T > MIC required for optimal response varies among the different β-lactams and is likely related to differences in the rate of bacterial killing and presence of PAE. Cephalosporins require the highest T > MIC (50-70%), followed by the penicillins (30-50%) and the carbapenems (20-40%). The importance of T > MIC has gained increasing attention in the last decade as a result of increasing bacterial resistance. Resistant bacteria have elevated MICs, making it more difficult to achieve adequate T > MIC (Fig. 20.7). In addition, PK studies conducted in critically ill patients have shown that standard β-lactam dosing regimens may produce unacceptably low serum concentrations, resulting in diminished T > MIC.[7,8] Although failure to achieve adequate T > MIC has been shown to predict outcome in numerous animal models,[9] there have been relatively few data in humans until recently. One study of patients with gram-negative bacteremia found mortality rates to double as the MIC increased from 4 mg/L to 8 mg/L in patients who were treated with cefepime.[10] The importance of this finding is magnified when one considers that an MIC of 8 mg/L is considered to be within

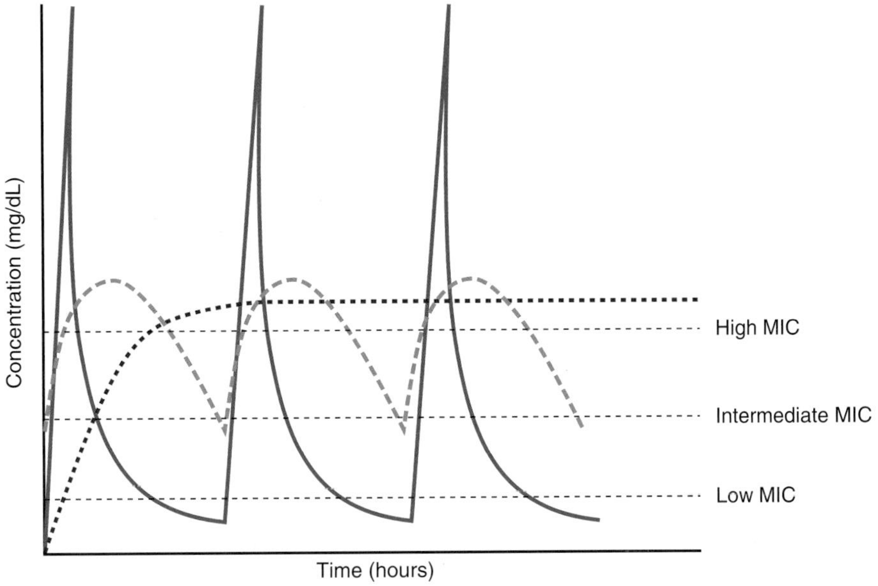

Figure 20.7 Impact of increasing minimum inhibitory concentration on ability to achieve pharmacodynamic goals and impact of differing dosing regimens. Solid lines represent standard, short infusion administration. Dashed-dotted line represents extended infusion administration. Dashed line represents continuous infusion.

the susceptible range for cefepime. A similar increase in mortality rate was found in patients with bacteremia due to *Pseudomonas aeruginosa:* the relative risk of 30-day mortality was increased nearly fourfold when standard doses of piperacillin were used to treat isolates with elevated MICs to piperacillin.[11] Although serum concentrations were not measured in these studies, the data provide indirect evidence that links reduced T > MIC to poor clinical outcome. In another study of gram-negative infection treated with cefepime, actual T > MIC was calculated using serum concentration data. The study showed that likelihood of achieving bacterial eradication was significantly correlated with T > MIC.[12]

The inability to achieve adequate T > MIC has led to the investigation of alternative dosing regimens. Simple dose escalation strategies are hampered by increasing the risk for toxicity. One alternative is to change the shape of the concentration-time curve using continuous or extended infusions. As seen in Figure 20.7, extending the infusion duration changes the shape of the concentration-time curve to promote longer T > MIC. Several PK studies have confirmed that these alternative dosing strategies can increase T > MIC without increasing the size of the dose. One study found that T > MIC following a 2-g dose of meropenem was increased 15% by extending the infusion duration from 0.5 hour to 3 hours.[13] Although there are no outcome data in humans comparing extended infusions to continuous infusions, PK studies suggest a similar probability of target attainment.[14]

An additional theoretical consideration when comparing the extended and continuous strategies is the risk of selecting resistant bacteria. Mathematical modeling of bacterial growth dynamics suggests that a constant rate of bacterial killing creates more opportunity for generating resistant mutants than does a fluctuating kill rate.[15] This effect has been demonstrated in an in vitro model of ceftazidime continuous infusion, when maintenance of steady-state serum concentrations slightly above the bacteria's MIC resulted in the emergence of resistant bacteria subpopulations.[16] This has led some investigator to recommend serum concentration monitoring if continuous infusions are used, with adjustment of the infusion rate to ensure steady-state concentrations are adequate.[17] Although extended infusions produce more consistent concentrations compared to standard infusions, they produce greater fluctuation compared to continuous infusion. Extended infusions also possess the logistical advantage of less infusion time and therefore greater IV access. This is of particular benefit in patients who require multiple vasoactive and nutritional infusions.

Despite having sound PK/PD rationale, the clinical benefit of extended or continuous infusion strategies has yet to be documented in randomized clinical trials.[18] Most available trials have important methodologic limitations. Although extended infusions increase T > MIC compared to standard infusions, the benefit is of greatest importance for bacterial isolates with elevated MICs because standard doses already provide optimal T > MIC when MIC is low. The benefit of extended infusions is also a function of the patient's renal function. Nicasio and associates recently found 3-hour infusions of cefepime increased T > MIC compared to standard 0.5-hour infusions but the effect was limited to patients with preserved renal function (creatinine clearance [CrCl] 50-120 mL/minute).[19] This effect modification is due to the prolonged half-life of cefepime in renal dysfunction, leading to higher trough concentrations and increased T > MIC. In light of these considerations, it is likely that the benefit of extended infusion strategies is greatest in patients with preserved renal function who are infected with high MIC pathogens, such as *P. aeruginosa* and *Acinetobacter baumannii.*

AMINOGLYCOSIDES

Aminoglycosides are broad-spectrum gram-negative agents that have been in clinical use since the 1960s. These agents quickly developed a reputation for having poor effectiveness and a high rate of nephrotoxicity compared to β-lactam agents. However, much of the initially dismal results observed with these agents are likely related to an inadequate knowledge of their PD profile. At the time, PD data available from β-lactam studies demonstrated T > MIC to be the important factor predicting efficacy.[6] As a result, early dosing strategies used small (1-2 mg/kg) doses given every 8 to 12 hours and little attention was paid to peak concentrations. The importance of achieving an adequate peak:MIC ratio was first described in patients by Moore and colleagues, who found that the likelihood of having a positive clinical response was greater than 90% when peak concentrations were 8 to 10 times the infecting organism's MIC.[20] A later study found that time to defervescence and normalization of leukocytosis was greater than 90% when peak:MIC ratio was 10 or greater.[21] These data suggest that achieving high peak aminoglycoside concentrations is fundamental to successful treatment. In recognition of this, clinicians began to monitor peak aminoglycoside levels and adjust dosing regimens to ensure optimal peak:MIC ratios.

Aminoglycosides also exhibit a prolonged PAE. The duration of PAE in neutropenic animal models varies from 1 to 8 hours and is a function of the peak:MIC ratio.[22] Higher ratios produce longer PAE. In addition, data suggest that PAE may be enhanced in patients with an intact immune system.[4] Based on the combination of concentration-dependent activity and a prolonged PAE the efficacy of these agents could be maximized by giving large doses less frequently. This strategy is known as extended interval dosing (EID). Because aminoglycosides have short half-lives, the drugs are completely cleared from serum near the end of a 24-hour dosing interval in patients with normal renal function. Although the absence of drug may be concerning for the regrowth of bacteria, this is prevented by the PAE. In addition, a drug-free period near the end of the dosing interval minimizes the phenomenon known as adaptive resistance. Primarily described in *P. aeruginosa* infection, *adaptive resistance* refers to the diminished rate of bacterial killing after initial exposure to aminoglycosides.[23] This effect is caused by up-regulation of membrane-bound efflux pumps, which decrease the amount of drug that reaches the site of action inside the cell.[23] When the bacteria are free from drug exposure for a sufficient amount of time the adaptive resistance is lost and the bacteria will become fully sensitive again. Thus, in addition to achieving high peak:MIC ratios, EID may also allow for the reversion of adaptive resistance and greater bactericidal effect.

A wide variety of doses have been utilized in EID strategies. However, the most common are 5 to 7 mg/kg for gentamicin and tobramycin and 15 to 20 mg/kg for amikacin.[24] These doses were chosen based directly on PK/PD relationships. EID assumes that patients have a Vd that is within the normal range (0.25-0.3 L/kg). When given to patients who meet this assumption, the doses will produce peak concentrations that range from 16 to 24 mg/L and will achieve target peak:MIC ratios for isolates with an MIC up to 2 mg/L.[25] EID is also designed to achieve a drug-free period of at least 4 hours at the end of the dosing interval.[25] Because aminoglycosides are cleared renally, dosing frequency is based on renal function assessment using estimated CrCl. To achieve an adequate drug-free interval, doses are given every 24 hours for patients with CrCl greater than 60 mL/minute, every 36 hours with CrCl 40 to 59 mL/minute, and every 48 hours with CrCl less than 40 mL/minute.[25] If aminoglycosides are used in renal dysfunction it is important that they still be dosed on weight owing to their peak:MIC dependent activity. EID of aminoglycosides has not been adequately studied in some patient populations (i.e., cystic fibrosis, thermal injury, pregnancy). The lack of validation data leads to the exclusion of these patients from EID nomograms, with the alternative being to use traditional dosing. However, based on our knowledge of the optimal PD parameter and the increased clearance seen in these populations, traditional dosing strategies may result in higher failure rates.

The benefit of EID has been studied in many small clinical trials and the results summarized in multiple meta-analyses. The conclusion from these studies is that EID produces similar efficacy to traditional dosing that is guided by close monitoring of peak concentrations.[26] However, most trials employed combination therapy with a β-lactam agent with activity against the infecting pathogen, potentially masking the effect of aminoglycoside dosing strategy.

As mentioned earlier, the use of aminoglycosides is limited by their propensity to induce nephrotoxicity. Nephrotoxicity is the result of accumulation in the epithelial cells of the proximal renal tubule. Of great importance is the fact that the rate of accumulation is saturable at relatively low concentrations in the tubule lumen.[27] This means that toxicity is not concentration dependent but rather time dependent. The implication is that high peak concentrations are just as safe as low peak concentrations. Once saturated, the rate-limiting step of tissue accumulation becomes the duration of exposure. Because EID produces a drug-free period near the end of the dosing interval, it reduces the amount of time drug can accumulate, potentially reducing toxicity. In vivo studies have confirmed that EID reduces renal accumulation.[28] It has been shown that a threshold of accumulation is needed before nephrotoxicity is produced and that this threshold is typically reached after 5 to 7 days of therapy.[29] Importantly, using EID prolongs the time to toxicity but the risk is not abolished. Once the duration of therapy exceeds 1 week, toxicity increases substantially regardless of dosing strategy. Duration of therapy was found to be a significant risk factor for toxicity in a cohort of elderly patients receiving once-daily aminoglycoside therapy.[30] The incidence of nephrotoxicity was only 3.9% in the 51 patients who received aminoglycoside therapy for less than 7 days compared to 30% in the 37 patients who received 8 to 14 days of therapy, and 50% of 8 patients receiving more than 14 days.

The aminoglycosides serve as a good example of how understanding PD principles can optimize the use of antibiotics. Concentration-dependent activity, prolonged PAE, adaptive resistance, and saturable renal accumulation characterize these agents. The use of EID takes best advantage of these characteristics. Regardless of dosing strategy, using the shortest duration of therapy possible is essential to minimizing the risk of toxicity.

VANCOMYCIN

Methicillin-resistant *Staphylococcus aureus* (MRSA) remains one of the most important pathogens causing infection in critically ill patients.[31] Vancomycin has been the drug of choice for treating this pathogen for nearly 50 years. It inhibits cell wall formation in gram-positive bacteria in a similar fashion to the action of β-lactams. However, vancomycin binds a different receptor and produces a slower bactericidal effect. This slow bactericidal activity likely explains the slower symptom resolution and higher failure rates with vancomycin compared to β-lactams in the treatment of MRSA infections.[32] The current breakpoint for vancomycin susceptibility against *Staphylococcus* species is an MIC of 2 mg/L.[33] In recent years, studies have identified MIC to be an important indicator of response to vancomycin therapy, which serves as a good example of how MIC can modify the ability of dosing regimens to achieve PD targets.[34]

It was unclear for many years which PD parameter correlated best with vancomycin activity. Because vancomycin, like the β-lactams, inhibits cell wall formation, one might presume T > MIC to be the best parameter. This assumption is supported by in vitro models showing that bacterial killing rate is concentration independent once above the MIC.[35] Other models show total drug exposure, as measured by the 24-hour AUC, to be more important for clinical response. In a study of patients with lower respiratory tract infection, Moise-Broder and coworkers found the AUC:MIC ratio to predict clinical response better than T > MIC.[36] They found a sevenfold increased probability of clinical cure and a decreased time to bacterial eradication when the AUC:MIC ratio was at least 400. No correlation with outcome was found for T > MIC. The discrepancy between vancomycin PD targets identified with in vitro models and human data underscores the importance of understanding the role of protein binding and tissue penetration. This is especially important for critically ill patients who can have altered tissue permeability and serum protein concentrations. Despite these limitations, total AUC:MIC ratio seems to be the best predictor of vancomycin activity and provides a parameter that can be easily monitored at the bedside.

Vancomycin dosing guidelines published in 2009 state that an AUC:MIC ratio of 400 or greater is the most appropriate PD target and that vancomycin trough concentrations should be monitored as a surrogate for AUC.[37] The guidelines recommend targeting steady-state trough concentrations of 15 to 20 mg/L for infections difficult to treat such as endocarditis, osteomyelitis, bacteremia, meningitis, and pneumonia. These troughs will achieve an AUC:MIC ratio of 400 or greater for pathogens with an MIC less than 1 mg/L. It is important to note that the success of this trough target is dependent on pathogen MIC. Mathematical simulations show that trough concentrations of 15 to 20 mg/L are unable to achieve target AUC:MIC ratios when the pathogen MIC is greater than 1 mg/L.[38] These simulations are supported by a recent meta-analysis that found a 64% relative increase in mortality risk when comparing high MIC (>1.5 mg/L) isolates to low MIC (<1.5 mg/L) isolates.[34] Although most MRSA isolates still have an MIC of 1 mg/L or less, many institutions have documented gradual increases in the number of isolates with MIC greater than 1 mg/L over the past decade.[39]

MRSA isolates with a high MIC represent a currently unsolved therapeutic dilemma. An intuitive solution would be to increase target trough concentration in hopes of achieving target AUC:MIC. Steady-state troughs of 25 to 30 mg/L would reliably achieve AUC:MIC ratios greater than 400 against an MIC of 2 mg/L. This strategy would likely be unfeasible, however, as recent data have linked high troughs with increased risk of nephrotoxicity. One observational study showed the risk to increase when the initial trough concentration was greater than 20.[40] This finding is in agreement with data from a recent randomized clinical trial comparing vancomycin to linezolid for treatment of pneumonia.[41] The rate of nephrotoxicity was increased in patients who receive vancomycin compared to linezolid (18.2% vs. 8.4%, respectively). In addition, a dose response was observed in the vancomycin arm: toxicity was observed in 37% of patients with initial trough greater than 20 mg/L, 22% when initial trough was 15 to 20 mg/L, and 18% when initial trough was less than 15 mg/L. Although these data use trough concentration to assess the dose:response relationship, trough is closely correlated with peak concentration and total AUC. Consequently, it is unclear which parameter is most closely associated with toxicity. An observational study showed continuous IV (CIV) infusions of vancomycin to have a slower rate of onset of nephrotoxicity compared to intermittent IV (IIV) infusion despite having similar cumulative doses in the two groups.[42] This study suggests that toxicity may be related to high peak concentrations, although more data are needed to verify these findings. The only randomized clinical trial to date of this strategy found no difference in safety or efficacy of continuous versus intermittent IV vancomycin.[43] Consequently, until more data are available, targeting troughs above 15 to 20 mg/L or the use of high-dose CIV infusions cannot be recommended.

Another option for treating high MIC isolates is to use alternative agents with activity against MRSA (i.e., linezolid, daptomycin, telavancin, and ceftibiprole). However, to date no agent has definitively been shown to provide improved outcome compared to vancomycin in the general treatment of MRSA. Additionally, few data are available that compare agents specifically in patients with high MIC isolates, and cross-resistance between vancomycin and alternative agents has been noted.[44]

THE EFFECT OF CRITICAL ILLNESS ON PHARMACOKINETICS AND PHARMACODYNAMICS

Understanding the basic concepts of PK and PD is essential to providing safe and effective drug therapy. However, the physiologic derangements found in critically ill patients can significantly alter PK/PD relationships, which can lead to both exaggerated and diminished pharmacologic response with standard dosing regimens. Consequently, the ICU clinician must integrate a thorough understanding of critical illness physiology with PK/PD principles to provide appropriate drug therapy. A summary of these changes can be found in Table 20.2.

The systemic inflammatory response syndrome (SIRS) is present to some degree in nearly all critically ill patients.

Table 20.2 Pharmacokinetic Changes during Critical Illness

Parameter	Relevant Critical Illness Physiology	Effect on Pharmacokinetics
Absorption	Reduced mesenteric and subcutaneous blood flow during shock	Reduced peak concentration and AUC
	Delayed gastric emptying	Delayed onset of effect
	Reduced GI motility	Variable
Distribution	Capillary leak and fluid resuscitation	Increased Vd for hydrophilic drugs
	Reduced albumin concentration	Increased Vd for drugs highly bound to albumin
	Increased AAG concentration	Decreased Vd for drugs highly bound to AAG
	Decreased tissue binding	Decreased tissue binding
Clearance	SIRS response producing increased blood flow to liver and kidneys	Increased drug clearance
	Acute kidney injury and acute liver injury	Decreased drug clearance
	Reduced albumin concentration	Increased drug clearance for drugs highly bound to albumin
	Increased AAG concentration	Decreased clearance for drugs highly bound to AAG

AAG, α_1-acid glycoprotein; AUC, area under the curve; GI, gastrointestinal; SIRS, severe inflammatory response syndrome; Vd, volume of distribution.

Common insults such as sepsis, trauma, surgery, the acute respiratory distress syndrome, and pancreatitis all produce SIRS. Salient features of SIRS are increased heart rate, decreased arterial vascular tone, and increased vascular membrane permeability.[45] Without adequate fluid resuscitation the result is low intravascular volume, inadequate preload, and subsequent low cardiac output. As a result, blood flow to organs such as the liver and kidneys can be compromised, leading to decreased drug clearance and serum and tissue accumulation. This physiology is commonly seen in patients admitted with sepsis when adequate resuscitation has not yet occurred. Fluid resuscitation restores preload and increases cardiac output. Because of increased heart rate and low systemic vascular resistance, patients with resuscitated SIRS or sepsis frequently have hyperdynamic physiology in which organ blood flow can be higher than normal.[46] Consequently, drug clearance will also be higher than normal. This change is of special concern in patients with sepsis as it may lead to increased antibiotic clearance, suboptimal PD achievement, and worse treatment response.[47] Low serum levels of cephalosporin antibiotics have been documented in septic patients given standard doses.[7] In addition, the need for increased dosing frequency has been documented for trauma patients treated with vancomycin.[48] Although there are no clinical trial data examining this issue, there is a physiologic rationale to administer higher doses or extended infusions of β-lactams and other renally cleared drugs to patients with hyperdynamic physiology.[47] This is likely most pertinent during the first 48 to 72 hours of treatment for patients with sepsis. Importantly, sepsis also frequently leads to organ dysfunction including acute liver and kidney injury. As a result, dosing decisions need to be reassessed daily. Careful assessment of renal and hepatic clearance is required and must be combined with prudent judgment of the risk-benefit ratio of each individual drug. Clinicians may err on the aggressive side of dosing decisions for drugs with a wide therapeutic index such as the β-lactam antibiotics. Conversely, the risk-benefit ratio may support more conservative dosing decisions for drugs that have serious dose-related toxicity such as antiarrhythmic agents and anticoagulants.

The amount of fluid resuscitation required to maintain intravascular volume in patients with SIRS can be significant. Early goal-directed therapy of sepsis frequently results in patients having a net gain of more than 10 L of fluid during treatment.[49] Significant increases in fluid balance are not limited to sepsis, but are also found in postsurgical patients, trauma patients, and patients with ARDS.[50,51] These changes in fluid balance combined with the capillary leaks produced by SIRS can have significant effects on the Vd of hydrophilic drugs. The aminoglycoside antibiotics serve as a prototypical example. The average Vd of aminoglycosides is 0.25 L/kg in non–critically ill patients.[52] This value is compared to an average of 0.36 L/kg in general surgical and 0.75 L/kg in medical ICU populations, respectively.[53,54] In addition to being significantly increased, there can be a great deal of variability in Vd among patients. In a general surgical population aminoglycoside Vd has been reported to range from 0.14 L/kg to 0.67 L/kg. These increases in Vd result in decreased peak concentrations with a given dose. Owing to the linear kinetics of aminoglycosides a doubling of Vd will decrease peak concentration by one half. Thus, in EID of tobramycin a typical 5 mg/kg dose in a patient with a Vd of 0.25 L/kg would result in a peak of 20 mg/L, although a patient with a Vd of 0.5 L/kg would have a peak of 10 mg/L. The patient with the smaller Vd (0.25 L/kg) would achieve the target peak:MIC ratio of 10 for treatment of a *Pseudomonas aeruginosa* isolate with an MIC of 2 mg/L. However, the patient with the Vd of 0.5 L/kg would achieve a suboptimal peak:MIC ratio of 5.

A seemingly obvious solution to the previous dilemma would be to administer 10 mg/kg of tobramycin to the patient with a larger Vd. Indeed, this would achieve a peak of 20 mg/L and target peak:MIC ratio. However, there is an additional consequence of increased Vd that limits the feasibility of dose escalation. As discussed earlier in the PK section, drug half-life is a function of both clearance and Vd. Thus, increases in Vd also increase half-life.

Consequently, the time required to clear a given dose will be increased *independent of clearance*. Again, because aminoglycoside PK is linear, a doubling of Vd results in a doubling of half-life. Failure to recognize the effect of Vd on half-life would lead the ICU clinician to choose an incorrect dosing interval, which would lead to excess drug accumulation and toxicity. Although the consequences of Vd on peak concentration and half-life are readily apparent for the aminoglycoside antibiotics, it is an important consideration for all drugs used in critically ill patients.

In addition to changes in organ blood flow and volume status, critically ill patients also have altered serum protein concentrations, which can have important effects on drugs that are highly protein bound. The two most important serum proteins that contribute to drug binding are albumin, which binds mostly to acidic drugs, and α_1-acid glycoprotein (AAG), which binds mostly to basic drugs. A variety of factors contribute to altered serum protein concentration, including malnutrition, hemodilution, and the acute phase response.[55] Interestingly, the acute phase response has a variable effect on these proteins: albumin decreases while AAG increases.[56] A change in serum protein concentration alters the unbound fraction of drug in the serum. Determination of the effects of altered free drug fraction requires consideration of the following: only the free fraction produces pharmacologic effects; only the free fraction is available to distribute into tissues; and only the free fraction is available to be cleared from the body. Increased free fraction produces increased Vd and clearance. The net effect of these changes is a lower total serum concentration with relatively unchanged absolute free concentration.[57] Because only free drug concentration can bind to target receptors, the change in protein binding *does not* alter pharmacologic response. As a result, dose adjustments are unnecessary. This is the case for most drugs that are highly protein bound. However, there is a short list of drugs for which changes in protein binding can produce clinically important changes when the drugs are given IV. Such drugs have a high extraction ratio (see discussion under "Hepatic Disease") and a narrow therapeutic index.[57] Examples relevant to ICU practice include midazolam, haloperidol, fentanyl, lidocaine, milrinone, diltiazem, and nicardipine. Decreased serum protein concentration can result in exaggerated free drug exposure, prolonged duration of effect, and increased risk of adverse events. Increased serum protein concentration would produce the opposite: reduced free drug exposure with possible inadequate response. This result would be important for drugs highly bound to AAG, such as lidocaine.[56] Unfortunately, there are few data available in critically ill patients that examine the effect of altered protein binding on PK/PD relationships in critically ill patients.

It is perhaps most important to consider the effects of altered protein concentration when monitoring serum concentrations to guide dosing decisions. As described earlier, altered protein binding changes the relationship between *total serum concentration* and pharmacologic effect, although the relationship between *free drug concentration* and effect frequently remains unchanged. As a result, using total serum concentration to guide dosing in critically ill patients can lead to erroneous dose adjustments and potential toxicity or therapeutic failure. Although the use of free drug concentration monitoring has been limited mostly to the antiepileptic phenytoin, it may also be useful for other highly protein bound drugs classes, including immunosuppressants and antibiotics.[57-59]

SPECIAL CONSIDERATIONS REGARDING ROUTES OF ADMINISTRATION

Although oral administration is useful in critically ill patients, the route may not always be appropriate. Physiologic changes such as decreased mesenteric blood flow, altered GI motility, gastric acid suppression, and gut wall edema can alter the rate and extent of absorption from the GI tract.[60] The hemodynamic response to hypotension involves shunting blood flow away from mesenteric circulation, substantially limiting a drug's access to the systemic circulation.[61] Hepatic blood flow may be preserved in the short term owing to the "hepatic buffer" response but is often decreased with prolonged states of low systemic perfusion.[62] Low hepatic blood flow will limit hepatic metabolism and result in increased bioavailability of drugs with a large first-pass effect. The net effect of these derangements can be highly unpredictable but often lead to diminished bioavailability. Slow gastric emptying, which occurs in 50% to 60% of critically ill patients, delays the onset of absorption and often results in lower peak serum concentrations.[63,64] Despite these changes, the overall exposure as measured by the AUC is not significantly different compared to healthy volunteers.[65] Impaired small intestine motility also slows the rate of absorption. However, because residence time in the GI tract will be increased, bioavailability may actually increase for poorly absorbable drugs such as furosemide and ampicillin.[2] Carrier-mediated absorption may be limited independent of changes in motility or blood flow as a result of dysfunctional membrane transporters.

There are limited data that describe the effectiveness of oral administration in critically ill patients. Some studies, conducted in patients tolerating enteral feeding, show absorption to be adequate for drugs with normally high bioavailability such as fluconazole and ciprofloxacin.[66,67] However, other studies show unpredictable and sometimes inadequate absorption.[68] Given this variability and the absence of a useful parameter to monitor GI function at the bedside, the IV route is preferred in patients with hemodynamic instability. The oral route should be reserved for patients who are clinically stable and tolerating enteral feeding. When transitioning medications from IV to oral, it is helpful to begin with agents that have easily measurable effects, such as cardiovascular agents.

The SC route is also used in critically ill patients, most commonly for insulin administration and pharmacologic venous thromboembolism (VTE) prophylaxis. Unfortunately, few studies examine the PK of SC administration in critically ill patients. The available data are limited to a few small studies of the low-molecular-weight heparins. Dorffler-Melly and associates compared anti–factor Xa activity produced by prophylactic doses of enoxaparin in three groups: non-ICU patients, ICU patients, and ICU patients receiving vasopressors. Peak anti–factor Xa activity was decreased by

60% in patients receiving vasopressors.[69] In another study, only 28% of patients on vasopressors achieved the target anti–factor Xa level after receiving 3000 IU of certoparin daily.[70] Although these data are provocative, the clinical importance of low anti–factor Xa levels is unclear. Some reports have correlated low levels with thrombosis, whereas others have not.[71,72] Despite this uncertainty, recent investigations have begun to examine the effect of higher doses and use of the IV route for VTE prophylaxis.[73,74] Not surprisingly, the data show that increased doses lead to increased drug exposure and higher anti–factor Xa levels. Although higher levels may decrease thrombosis risk, they may also increase bleeding risk. As such, outcome data from large clinical trials are needed before such strategies can be recommended.

DRUG-DOSING CONSIDERATIONS IN SELECT CRITICAL CARE POPULATIONS

RENAL DISEASE

Acute kidney injury (AKI) is a common occurrence in the ICU. Using a consensus definition, rates of AKI range from 10% to 30% in the general ICU population, and 40% to 60% in patients with severe sepsis and septic shock In addition, approximately 5% will require some form of hemodialysis.[75] This frequency is an important concern for drug dosing because renal elimination is one of the two primary routes of drug clearance. Therefore, it is important for ICU practitioners to understand the basic approach to renal drug dosing.

ASSESSING RENAL FUNCTION

Accurate assessment of renal function is imperative to make appropriate dosing decisions. This assessment may include a measurement or estimate of the glomerular filtration rate (GFR). Inulin is the gold standard for the assessment of renal function.[76] However, owing to limited availability and high cost, it is rarely used outside a research setting. In its place creatinine is frequently used as a marker for renal function as it is produced at a fairly constant rate and is largely removed by glomerular filtration. The most reliable method that employs creatinine is via a timed urine creatinine collection. A 24-hour collection is ideal to account for changes that may occur in volume status, hemodynamics, or organ function throughout the day. However, a 24-hour collection period has multiple opportunities for error and is often impractical because a practitioner must wait longer than 24 hours to assess a patient's renal clearance. As a result, shorter durations of collection have been examined. Unfortunately, the results are varied, with some investigators demonstrating poor correlation with collections less than 8 hours and others showing good correlation with collections as short as 2 hours.[77,78] Consequently, the ideal duration of collection is unclear. In addition, it is important to note that timed urine collections are not free from bias in critically ill patients. One report found both a 30-minute and 24-hour urine creatinine collection to be significantly biased compared to inulin clearance.[79] Despite this limitation direct measurement of urine creatinine can still be useful to make dosing decisions in patients who are receiving narrow therapeutic index drugs or are at the extremes of age or weight.

Although direct measurement is ideal, most practitioners use equations to estimate renal clearance due to inherent limitations in the collection process. Equations exist to estimate both the GFR and also CrCl. Table 20.3 lists the two most commonly used equations and considerations for their use.[80-82] There has been much clinical debate as to the optimal equation to use for drug dosing. Historically the most frequently used method has been the Cockcroft-Gault (CG) equation, which provides an estimate of CrCl. This choice is primarily due to the fact that most available dosing recommendations are based on PK studies that estimated renal function with the CG equation.[83] More recently, the Modification of Diet in Renal Disease (MDRD) equation has become widely used clinically as an estimate of GFR. It has been primarily used for staging of kidney disease, and at one time recommendations were to avoid using it for drug dosing. This proscription was largely based on the fact that numerous studies have compared the CG and MDRD

Table 20.3 Commonly Used Equations to Estimate Renal Clearance

Equation	Estimated Parameter (units)	Formula	Considerations
Cockcroft-Gault	CrCl (mL/min)	(140 − age) BW/(SCr • 72) • (0.85 if female)	Inaccurate in patients with acutely changing renal function Ideal weight parameter is controversial in obese patients
Reexpressed MDRD (four-variable)	GFR (mL/min/1.73 m^2)	175 • $SCr^{-1.154}$ • $age^{-0.203}$ • (0.742 if female) • (1.21 if AA)	Inaccurate in patients with acutely changing renal function Must be individualized for body surface area by multiplying estimated GFR × (estimated BSA/1.73 m^2) Little information available in obese, elderly, or hepatic disease patients

AA, African American; BSA, body surface area; BW, body weight (in kg); CrCl, creatinine clearance; GFR, glomerular filtration rate; MDRD, Modification of Diet in Renal Disease [Study]; SCr, serum creatinine.

equations and have shown discordance between drug-dosing recommendations derived from the two equations.[82] Despite these data, in 2009 the National Kidney Disease Education Program suggested that either equation could be used for drug dosing purposes.[83] Many practitioners continue to use the CG equation because of its ease of use, because of its familiarity, and because many dosing recommendations were derived from this equation. Several other less frequently used equations to estimate CrCl or GFR can be found in more detailed reviews on estimating renal clearance.[76]

Regardless of which approach to renal function assessment is used, it is important to remember that all have limitations. Because changes in serum creatinine are delayed in comparison to changes in actual renal function, calculations based on this marker will be unreliable in rapidly changing renal function. These equations will overestimate renal function when creatinine is increasing and may underestimate renal function when creatinine is decreasing. Other patient populations that require specific considerations are patients at the extremes of weight and elderly patients. Both CG and MDRD equations have varied results in patients older than 65 years of age. The MDRD equation has been shown to overestimate kidney function in elderly patients, and the CG equation may either overestimate or underestimate renal clearance.[84,85] Obese patients also present problems when determining renal clearance for the purposes of drug dosing. The MDRD equation has been shown to underestimate renal clearance in obese patients, and the CG equation overestimates renal clearance in obese patients when the total body weight (TBW) is used.[86] To date no estimating equation has been validated for use in the obese patient population. If an estimating equation is to be used, some data suggest the weight selected should be based on the degree of obesity. A study by Pai and colleagues suggests using TBW in overweight patients (BMI [body mass index] < 30 kg/m^2), adjusted body weight (ABW) in obese patients (BMI 30 to <40 kg/m^2), and lean body weight (LBW) in morbidly obese patients (BMI ≥ 40 kg/m^2).[87]

As a result of the inherent limitations of renal function assessment in critically ill patients, many renal dose adjustment decisions are done with a fair deal of uncertainty. Accordingly, it is essential for the clinician to have a clear understanding of the risks of toxicity associated with excessive dosing as well as the consequences of therapeutic failure associated with underdosing. In some instances aggressive dose reduction may potentially be detrimental. The best example of a situation in which a dose reduction may be delayed is in patients receiving antibiotic therapy. Antibiotics work by a number of different PD parameters as discussed previously, but all require that the concentration at the site of the infection exceed the MIC of the bacteria. Underdosing of antibiotics can have serious implications including selection of resistant organisms and increased morbidity and mortality rates. This is of special concern for patients with severe sepsis and septic shock. Moreover, most antibiotics have relatively wide therapeutic windows; thus, the risk of toxicity is frequently low, even with excessive dosing. In this scenario it may be reasonable to err on the side of higher doses. Therefore, many practitioners will deliver at least one normal dose of an antibiotic before adjusting based on renal function. On the other end of the spectrum are narrow therapeutic index drugs (i.e., digoxin, lidocaine) that may result in toxicity relatively quickly if changes in renal clearance are not considered. In patients with poor or worsening renal function many of these narrow therapeutic index drugs should be avoided. If use is unavoidable the lowest starting dose should be utilized with frequent toxicity monitoring and assessment of serum concentrations.

DOSING IN RENAL REPLACEMENT THERAPY

Several factors contribute to drug clearance in patients receiving renal replacement therapy (RRT). They can generally be broken down into dialysis, drug, and patient factors. The two methods by which dialysis can remove drugs are diffusion and convection. Diffusion is a passive process during which substances move down a concentration gradient across a dialysis filter. It is the more effective method of drug removal during RRT and is influenced by dialysis filter surface area and composition.[88] Convection is an active process during which drugs are removed through pressure gradients. Convection removes a smaller percentage of drug and is more dependent on dialysis factors including flow rates and the sieving coefficient of the drug.[89] However, sieving coefficients are not readily available for most drugs, and therefore the fraction of unbound drug is often used to assess the likelihood of drug clearance.

The three main drug factors that affect clearance are molecular weight, protein binding, and Vd. Drugs with molecular weights exceeding 1000 daltons are not effectively removed by low flux dialysis membranes. However, they may be removed to a larger degree by "high flux" dialysis membranes.[89] Similar to endogenous clearance mechanisms, clearance by RRT is inversely related to the degree of protein binding and Vd. Because large Vd (>1.5 L/kg) drugs distribute well into tissue, there is limited drug in the serum to be removed, whereas small Vd drugs (<0.7 L/kg) reside primarily in the serum, increasing the likelihood of removal. Other drug factors that may impact clearance are water solubility and plasma clearance. Patient factors include those that affect protein binding (i.e., pH, serum albumin, other drugs, disease states), Vd (volume status, fluid resuscitation), and concomitant organ function.[89,90]

A number of different methods of RRT may be used in critically ill patients including both intermittent and continuous durations. Because intermittent hemodialysis (IHD) is the most commonly used form of dialysis, drug clearance data are more readily available. As a result, most drug information references will provide dosage recommendations for IHD. Continuous renal replacement therapy (CRRT), on the other hand, provides a number of challenges as there is a lack of pharmacokinetic studies with many drugs. The data that do exist often differ from study to study and are highly dependent on a number of differences including filter composition and surface area, duration of procedure, pre- or postreplacement fluid administration, and flow rates of blood, dialysate, and ultrafiltrate.[88,90] Therefore, it is important that practitioners evaluate these characteristics for similarities and differences with their patients before applying any dosing recommendation. An in-depth review of the types of RRT and degree of drug removal is beyond the scope of this chapter, but several references are available that provide this information.[90,91] However, the general degree of drug removal is as follows: continuous venovenous hemodiafiltration > continuous venovenous hemodialysis > continuous venovenous hemofiltration > slow extended daily dialysis > intermittent hemodialysis.[90]

Once a dosing recommendation has been made in patients receiving CRRT it is important to continue monitoring patients for changes in their dialysis prescription and residual renal function. Dialysis flow rates and ultrafiltration rates often change on a daily basis and can result in alterations in drug clearance. Although CRRT implies that a patient is receiving treatment for 24 hours per day this is frequently not the case. In fact, the reported mean daily stop times for CRRT range from 3 to 8 hours per day owing to a number of reasons including filter clotting, radiologic procedures, catheter exchange, patient mobilization, and surgery.[92,93] As discussed previously, because it is difficult to estimate drug clearance in patients receiving RRT, careful assessment of the risk-benefit ratio between effectiveness and toxicity is required.

HEPATIC DISEASE

The liver serves as the primary site for drug metabolism, and therefore, drug dosing is an important consideration in any patient with hepatic disease. Hepatic drug clearance (CL_H) is an extremely complex process, dependent on hepatic blood flow (Q_H) and the hepatic extraction ratio (E_H). The hepatic extraction ratio depends on Q_H, intrinsic clearance of unbound drug (CL_{int}), and the fraction of unbound drug in blood (f_u).[94] The following equations can be used to estimate CL_H:

$$CL_H = Q_H \bullet E_H$$

$$CL_H = Q_H \bullet (f_u \bullet CL_{int})/(Q_H + f_u \bullet CL_{int})$$

Most data regarding changes in drug clearance are in patients with cirrhosis and therefore do not necessarily apply to acute changes in liver function. Few data are available in patients with acute hepatic dysfunction, making assessments and recommendations in this patient population difficult. Drugs can be categorized as either high or low extraction ratio drugs. Elimination of high extraction ratio drugs is limited by hepatic blood flow and is less sensitive to changes in drug protein binding or enzyme activity (i.e., CL_{int}). After absorption from the GI tract the first stop for all drugs is the liver. High extraction ratio drugs undergo presystemic metabolism commonly referred to as the hepatic first-pass effect. This results in significantly decreased bioavailability and serum drug concentrations. In patients with decreased hepatic blood flow the first-pass effect is decreased, leading to increased serum concentrations and potentially more adverse effects. This effect is most pronounced in drugs that normally have low bioavailability after oral administration.

Low extraction ratio drugs are more sensitive to changes in drug protein binding and enzyme activity (i.e., CL_{int}) and are affected to a lesser degree by changes in blood flow. Plasma protein binding of drugs is decreased in hepatic disease due to a number of reasons including decreased protein production (albumin, AAG) and accumulation of endogenous compounds, which inhibit protein binding. As mentioned previously, this decrease in protein binding can increase free drug exposure for certain drugs, increasing the risk of adverse effects. Intrinsic hepatic clearance is the ability of the liver to clear unbound drug from the blood. It is highly dependent on the activity of metabolic enzymes and hepatic transporters. These processes may be altered in chronic liver disease, resulting in decreased drug metabolism. The two phases of hepatic metabolism are phase 1 (i.e., hydrolysis, oxidation, reduction) and phase 2 (i.e., acetylation, glucuronidation, sulfation). The cytochrome P-450 family of enzymes is responsible for approximately 75% of drug metabolism and is classified as phase 1 reactions.[95] Phase 1 metabolism is dependent on molecular oxygen and is thought to be more sensitive to changes that result in decreased oxygen delivery such as to shunting, sinusoidal capillarization, and reduced liver perfusion.[94,96] Although data demonstrate that enzyme activity is decreased with increasing disease severity, the decreases are variable and nonuniform across the different CYP450 isoenzymes. Although phase 2 metabolism was historically thought to be spared in patients with liver disease, recent data suggest that it is impaired in patients with advanced cirrhosis as well.[94]

ASSESSING HEPATIC FUNCTION

Unfortunately, owing to the complexity of hepatic elimination there are few data to guide drug dosing recommendations in these patients. One of the primary reasons is that a simple method to quantify liver function does not exist. Liver transaminases (i.e., aspartate aminotransferase [AST], alanine aminotransferase [ALT]) are markers of hepatocellular injury and do not reflect synthetic function. Although international normalized ratio (INR) and albumin reflect synthetic capacity they do not adequately capture the complex process of drug metabolism. Although scoring systems have been developed to assess severity of liver disease, no score has been developed for the sole purpose of drug dosing. Although not designed for drug dosing, the Pugh modification of the Child-Turcotte scoring system has been shown to predict changes in drug clearance that occur in hepatic disease.[97] The scoring system can be found in Table 20.4.[97] The utility of this score has led to the Food and Drug Administration (FDA) recommendation that it be used to categorize degree of liver impairment in patients enrolled in hepatic PK studies completed during drug development.[98] There are several limitations to its use in the ICU

Table 20.4 Child-Pugh Classification of Liver Disease

Indicator	1 point	2 points	3 points
Albumin (g/dL)	>3.5	2.8-3.5	<2.8
Prothrombin time (seconds > control)	<4	4-6	>6
Total bilirubin (mg/dL)	<2	2-3	>3
Encephalopathy (grade)	None	1 or 2	3 or 4
Ascites	None	Slight	Moderate

Total score: 5-6 points, mild/group A; 7-9 points, moderate/group B; 10-15 points, severe/group C.

setting. Unlike equations used in renal disease the Child-Pugh scoring system does not quantify the ability of the liver to metabolize specific drugs. Moreover, it has not been validated in patients with acute liver dysfunction. In addition, it may be influenced by factors in critically ill patients that are not related to liver dysfunction (i.e., depressed albumin from the acute phase response). Despite these limitations, it is still the most useful tool to assess hepatic function at the bedside. Another scoring system, primarily used for prioritizing liver transplantation recipients, is the Model for End-Stage Liver Disease (MELD) score. It has not been adequately studied for drug dosing, and therefore, recommendations should not be made based on the score.

DOSING IN HEPATIC DISEASE

In critically ill patients with chronic hepatic disease it is important that a Child-Pugh score be calculated to assess the degree of liver impairment. Dosing recommendations based on Child-Pugh score are included in the package labeling for many medications and should be referenced when available. When there are no recommendations based on Child-Pugh score, a decision must be made based on clinical judgment. Some general considerations include avoiding drugs metabolized by the CYP450 system in favor of drugs that undergo phase 2 metabolism (i.e., glucuronidation) or renal elimination. If all available choices undergo phase 1 metabolism, then consider the agent with the shortest duration of action. Because the first-pass effect may be reduced in the setting of hepatic dysfunction consider reduced doses of high extraction ratio drug (i.e., drugs which normally have low bioavailability) when using the oral route of administration. Reduce maintenance doses of low hepatic extraction ratio drugs (i.e., drugs with good bioavailability). Although there are few data to support a specific dose reduction with most medications, a reduction of at least 50% is probably warranted in patients with severe disease. A number of valuable references provide more detailed dosing recommendations on a number of medications, and they should be consulted prior to making dosing decisions in these patients.[99-102]

OBESE PATIENTS

Approximately 30% of adults in the United States are considered obese.[103] Available data suggest upward of 25% of all patients admitted to ICUs can be categorized as obese, with 6% to 7% of patients being morbidly obese.[104,105] These alterations in body weight present potential pharmacokinetic challenges with many drugs that have not been adequately studied in this population.

PHARMACOKINETIC ALTERATIONS IN OBESITY

The two primary pharmacokinetic parameters, Vd and clearance, may be altered in obese patients. The increase in adipose tissue seen in obesity may lead to an increase in Vd for highly lipophilic drugs. This can result in two important changes: a decrease in peak concentration and an increased half-life (see previous discussion of half-life under "General Pharmacokinetic Principles"). The result may be a reduced response to initial doses and an increase in time to reach steady state. The effects of obesity on clearance are less clear. Some studies have shown increased renal and hepatic blood flow in obese individuals, which should lead to increased clearance. In addition, there is evidence of glomerular hyperfiltration in obese patients.[106] Less clear is how clearance changes with increasing degrees of obesity and how clearance correlates with different body weight parameters. Leading hypotheses related to these questions include the following: (1) Obese individuals exhibit higher absolute clearance than normal weight comparators, (2) clearance does not increase in a linear fashion with TBW, and (3) clearance and LBW are linearly correlated. Unfortunately, not all drugs are affected to the same degree by obesity, and therefore, pharmacokinetic considerations must be made on a drug-drug basis.[106,107]

DOSING CONSIDERATIONS

The first step in determining a drug dosage for an obese patient is deciding what weight to use. This presents a significant challenge as the ideal weight parameter to use for drug dosing varies among agents. Drugs may be dosed based on ideal body weight (IBW), ABW, TBW, LBW, or body surface area (BSA) (Table 20.5).[108-110] TBW may be appropriate for very lipophilic drugs, as Vd increases in a nearly linear fashion with body weight.[106] Drugs with moderate lipophilicity do not distribute completely into adipose tissue and as a result TBW-based recommendations may lead to overdosing of hydrophilic drugs. The ideal weight to use may also vary based on the patient's degree of obesity, which is often assessed using BMI or percentage of ideal body weight (% IBW). Obesity is frequently defined using BMI, with the commonly accepted definition being a value greater than 30 kg/m^2. However, dosing recommendations based on BMI are frequently unavailable.

Because hydrophilic drugs do not distribute well into adipose tissue other adjustment factors are often used. LBW can be a useful predictor of pharmacokinetic behavior of drugs that are highly water soluble as it accounts for nonfat cell mass and intercellular connective tissue. The term IBW was based on historical data that compared the relative mortality rate of people of different height-weight combinations. It has frequently been used as a surrogate for LBW in

Table 20.5 Equations to Determine Body Size Indicators

Descriptor	Equation
Body mass index (kg/m^2)	TBW/height $(m)^2$
Body surface area (m^2) (Mosteller formula)	$\sqrt{\left[\frac{(\text{height (cm)} * \text{TBW})}{3600}\right]}$
Ideal body weight (kg)	*Men:* 50 kg + 2.3 kg/inches of height over 5 feet *Women:* 45 kg + 2.3 kg/inches of height over 5 feet
Adjusted body weight (kg)	0.4[TBW – IBW] + IBW
Lean body weight (kg)	*Men:* [1.1 • TBW] – 120[TBW/height (cm)]^2 *Women:* [1.07 • TBW] – 148[TBW/height (cm)]^2
Percentage of IBW (%)	(TBW/IBW) • 100

IBM, ideal body weight (in kg); TBW, total body weight (in kg).

many pharmacokinetic studies due to ease of use.[111] Some lipophilic drugs that have an increased Vd in obese patients are dosed based on ABW. Different correction factors have been used to calculate ABW, but the most common factor is 0.4. The equations to calculate these values are listed in Table 20.5.

As with renal and hepatic disease it is imperative to assess the risk-benefit ratio with each drug prior to making any dosing decisions in obese patients. Some drugs have been studied using different weight parameters and it is always beneficial to know this information prior to deciding on a drug dose. A list of commonly used ICU medications and weight parameters that should be used is provided in Table 20.6.[107,112-125] Perhaps more concerning is the uncertainty regarding the effect of obesity on the PK/PD of drugs that use fixed doses.

Another consideration should be the safety profile of a particular drug. When using wide therapeutic index drugs

Table 20.6 Optimal Weight Parameter to Use in Dosing Selected Agents in Obese Individuals

Medication	Weight to Use	Special Considerations
Anticoagulants		
Unfractionated heparin (UFH)	TBW	If TBW is used, some practitioners suggest a dose-capping strategy, or the substitution of ABW in morbidly obese patients (BMI >40 kg/m^2) Doses should be adjusted in accordance with TDM
Low-molecular-weight heparin (LMWH)	TBW	TDM in patients >190 kg Prophylaxis: higher-than-normal dose warranted VTE: Dose capping not warranted ACS: Dose capping based on PI
Fondaparinux	TBW	VTE: <50 kg: 5 mg SC daily; 50-100 kg: 7.5 mg SC daily; >100 kg: 10 mg SC daily
Argatroban	TBW	PI dosing up to 140 kg
Lepirudin	TBW	PI recommends dose capping at 110 kg
Bivalirudin	TBW	PI dosing up to 152 kg
Antimicrobials		
Acyclovir	IBW*	Nephrotoxicity, neurotoxicity are dose-limiting side effects
Aminoglycosides	ABW	TDM should be used to adjust dosing
Colistimethate	IBW*	Nephrotoxicity, neurotoxicity are dose-limiting side effects
Daptomycin	TBW	CK should be checked weekly to assess for toxicity
Vancomycin	TBW	TDM should be used to adjust dosing
Antiepileptics		
Phenytoin	*LD:* ABW *MD:* IBW	LD should be capped at 2 g; MD should be based on IBW and adjusted by levels
Neuromuscular Blocking Agents		
Succinylcholine	TBW	Dosing based on TBW leads to better conditions for intubation
All others	IBW*	Most data suggest prolonged duration of action with use of TBW to determine dose TOF monitoring and clinical assessment should be used to guide doses in patients requiring continued paralysis
Sedatives		
Benzodiazepines	*Bolus:* TBW *MD:* IBW	A less aggressive bolus dose may be warranted in a nonintubated patient in the ICU
Dexmedetomidine	TBW	Has been studied in patients weighing up to 285 kg
Propofol	*Bolus:* IBW *MD:* TBW	Data suggest TBW best correlates with Vd and Cl; however, owing to risk of hypotension with bolus dosing and ability to rapidly titrate, it may be appropriate to use IBW for bolus dosing
Thrombolytics		
Alteplase	TBW	AMI: 100 mg standard dose PE: 100 mg standard dose Acute ischemic stroke: 0.9 mg/kg, with total dose capped at 90 mg

*IBW should be used unless the patient's TBW is less than the IBW. In that case, TBW should be used.

ABW, adjusted body weight; ACS, acute coronary syndrome; AMI, acute myocardial infarction; CK, creatine kinase; Cl, clearance; IBW, ideal body weight; LD, loading dose; MD, maintenance dose; PE, pulmonary embolism; PI, package insert; TBW, total body weight; TDM, therapeutic drug monitoring; TOF, train-of-four; Vd, volume of distribution; VTE, venous thromboembolism.

a more aggressive initial approach may be appropriate. This is often the case with β-lactam antibiotics, although a more conservative approach may be warranted with narrow therapeutic index drugs that are dosed based on weight (i.e., phenytoin, sedatives, and digoxin). If therapeutic drug monitoring is available for an agent, it should be used to monitor for achievement of goals, and doses should be based on these valuable data. If therapeutic drug monitoring (TDM) is not available then it may be appropriate to administer small doses of an agent with frequent redosing based on response rather than administering one large dose.

DOSING CONSIDERATIONS WITH SPECIFIC AGENTS IN OBESITY

Antimicrobials

Using the appropriate weight to dose antimicrobial drugs is extremely important, as underdosing may lead to therapeutic failures and overdosing may lead to toxicity (i.e., nephrotoxicity with aminoglycosides or acyclovir). Unfortunately, data are limited for many commonly used antimicrobials. Aminoglycosides are one of the most widely studied antibacterial drugs in obese patients owing to their narrow therapeutic index and widespread availability of serum concentrations. Studies suggest increased aminoglycoside Vd (9-58%) and renal clearance (15-91%) in obese patients.[122] Their hydrophilic structure and small Vd suggest incomplete adipose distribution, and in fact studies have identified ABW as the optimal weight parameter.[122] Because both clearance and Vd exhibit substantial variability in obese patients it is extremely important that therapeutic drug monitoring be used to optimize aminoglycoside dosing in this cohort.

As with aminoglycosides, numerous studies in the literature evaluate vancomycin kinetics in obesity. These studies demonstrate variable changes in Vd and increased clearance in obesity.[122] Current vancomycin guidelines recommend that patients should be dosed on TBW with adjustments in dosing regimen based on therapeutic drug monitoring.[37] However, this is somewhat controversial as patients weighing more than 100 kg would receive loading doses exceeding 2 g. These are substantially larger than what has been used in the past, and in light of the uncertainty regarding nephrotoxicity with increasing trough level, some clinicians may not be comfortable with this aggressive approach to loading doses. However, with the AUC:MIC ratio being the pharmacodynamic parameter that best correlates with clinical efficacy, weight-based dosing with TDM should be used to optimize therapy.

Other available antimicrobials that are dosed based on weight include acyclovir, colistimethate sodium, daptomycin, and sulfamethoxazole/trimethoprim (SMX/TMP). Acyclovir is a relatively hydrophilic drug, and therefore IBW should be used for dosing in obese patients.[112,126] Nephrotoxicity has been reported in obese patients who receive acyclovir dosed on TBW.[127] Data regarding the optimal dosing weight for colistimethate sodium are limited. However, one recent study suggests using IBW unless the patient's TBW is less than IBW.[128] Currently available data with daptomycin suggest dosing based on TBW.[129] However, patients must be monitored for elevations in creatine kinase (CK) on a weekly basis as rhabdomyolysis would be the primary adverse effect of concern. There are insufficient data to make a recommendation on dosing of the lipophilic antibiotic SMX/TMP in obese patients. If available and high-dose SMX/TMP therapy is necessary, therapeutic drug monitoring should be used to guide dosing.

Several antibiotic classes are not normally dosed based on weight, including penicillins, cephalosporins, carbapenems, and fluoroquinolones. There are relatively few pharmacodynamic data in obese patients for these classes. However, these drugs are generally well tolerated and therefore it is probably reasonable to use aggressive dosing strategies in these patients (i.e., maximal studied doses or less aggressive adjustment for renal dysfunction). This approach may not be prudent in patients at increased risk of particular adverse effects such as seizures with imipenem or rate-corrected QT interval (QTc) prolongation with fluoroquinolones.

Sedatives

Benzodiazepines, dexmedetomidine, and propofol are the most commonly used sedatives in the ICU. The benzodiazepines are highly lipophilic compounds that have significantly increased Vd and clearance in obese patients.[130] Because they demonstrate an increased Vd the use of TBW has been suggested for bolus doses of benzodiazepines. However, the risk of respiratory depression in patients without an advanced airway is an important consideration. Because the parenteral benzodiazepines all have relatively rapid onset the use of smaller doses based on IBW repeated every 5 to 15 minutes is a reasonable approach in patients without an advanced airway. In one study midazolam half-life was increased nearly threefold in obese patients.[119] This effect increases the risk of accumulation, oversedation, and delirium in obese patients, especially with continuous infusions. When benzodiazepines must be used, intermittent doses based on IBW are preferred.

Although propofol is a highly lipophilic compound, available data do not demonstrate changes in Vd or clearance in obese patients. This information would suggest that TBW should be used for maintenance doses in this patient population.[124,131] However, propofol is associated with several significant adverse effects including hypotension with bolus dosing and the life-threatening propofol-related infusion syndrome (PRIS) with high doses or extended durations of infusion. Owing to the hemodynamic complications associated with propofol an initial bolus based on IBW followed by additional small doses might be reasonable. Because it is a short half-life drug it can be rapidly titrated to effect. High doses and the risk of PRIS represent a more complicated therapeutic dilemma. One of the recognized risk factors is a dose of propofol exceeding 83 μg/kg/minute.[132] It is not known how dosing based on TBW vs. IBW would affect the development of PRIS. Therefore, these patients should be closely monitored for symptoms of PRIS including metabolic acidosis, lactate, hyperkalemia, rhabdomyolysis, an elevated CK, or cardiac failure. If these symptoms develop, they should have propofol stopped immediately.[132] Pharmacokinetic data for dexmedetomidine in critically ill patients is not readily available. However, dexmedetomidine has been studied in patients up to 285 kg using TBW and the manufacturer provides dosing recommendations based on TBW for patients weighing up to 185 kg.[125] If TBW is used, then it is important that the dose be titrated to effect with monitoring for hypotension and bradycardia.

Anticoagulants

Anticoagulant dosing in obesity presents challenges because overdosing may result in bleeding complications and underdosing can result in worsening of thrombosis. Weight has been reported to be the single best predictor of unfractionated heparin (UFH) requirements with numerous weight-based nomograms being published.[133] TBW is frequently used for UFH dosing in nonobese and non–morbidly obese patients. However, the exact weight parameter that should be used in morbid obesity (BMI > 40 kg/m^2) is unclear. When TBW is used in morbid obesity there is a higher rate of supratherapeutic activated partial thromboplastin time (aPTT).[134,135] Despite the potential for higher than anticipated aPTTs several studies reported no difference in major bleeding events or rates of primary event recurrence when UFH was dosed on TBW.[136,137] Owing to the lack of prospective data in this patient population some practitioners recommend dosing on an ABW or a dose-capping strategy if TBW is used.[134,138] This decision may be influenced by the indication and risk for bleeding with practitioners using a more aggressive approach in the treatment of VTE and a less aggressive dosing approach for atrial fibrillation or acute coronary syndrome (ACS). Regardless of what weight is used for the bolus dose, the subsequent infusion should be adjusted based on therapeutic drug monitoring.

Unlike UFH there has been significantly more research on the ideal weight parameter for low-molecular-weight heparins (LMWHs) with TBW being identified as the best predictor of LMWH requirements.[121] Pharmacodynamic data for LMWHs are available in patients weighing up to 190 kg.[139] Because of the limited data in patients more than 190 kg some practitioners recommend a dose-capping strategy at this weight. Although a dose-capping strategy may seem prudent, there are no data to suggest this will limit bleeding risk while still achieving the therapeutic goal. With this in mind a more prudent approach is to use TBW for VTE treatment doses in patients weighing more than 190 kg combined with TDM to avoid excessive exposure. If TDM is used, an anti–factor Xa level should be checked 4 hours after the third dose of a LMWH. Because VTE doses are not weight based, current guidelines recommend using an increased fixed dose of LMWH in obese patients.[118] However, specific recommendations are not made regarding dose adjustments largely because of variability in the available data. Several available reviews provide a more detailed discussion of the available anticoagulants for prophylaxis, VTE, and ACS in the obese patient population.[121,123,140]

ELDERLY PATIENTS

Current estimates from the administration on aging predict that by 2050 approximately 20% of the U.S. population will be older than 65.[141] As a result elderly patients will make up a larger percentage of ICU admissions. These patients frequently have multiple chronic diseases and are at increased risk for polypharmacy. Unfortunately, prior to 1990 drug companies were not required to study drugs in elderly patients. This leads to a lack of dosing recommendations that are specific to the elderly patient population.

As individuals age a number of physiologic changes occur that lead to significant pharmacokinetic alterations. Drug absorption may be decreased as a result of changes in gastric pH, gastric emptying, splanchnic blood flow, and GI motility. Half-life and Vd may be increased for lipophilic drugs as a result of increases in body fat and decreases in lean body mass. Hydrophilic drugs will have increased serum concentrations because of decreases in total body water. The free fraction of highly protein bound drugs is increased as a result of decreases in serum protein production. Decreases in hepatic blood flow and hepatic mass may result in decreased hepatic first-pass effect and potentially decreased phase 1 metabolism. Age-related decreases in renal blood flow and GFR may result in impaired renal drug elimination.[142] Unfortunately, these changes vary among patients, making drug dosing especially challenging.

In an effort to minimize polypharmacy and adverse drug effects several criteria have been developed to screen medication therapy in elderly patients. The most commonly cited are the Beers' criteria, originally developed in 1991 and updated in 2012.[143] The most recent version includes 53 medications or medication classes divided into 3 categories. A newer set of recommendations that are gaining popularity are the STOPP (Screening Tool of Older Persons' potentially inappropriate Prescriptions) criteria. They consist of 64 medications or medication classes divided into 10 categories. Both criteria have been validated and at least one should be used in the evaluation of the appropriateness of medications in elderly patients. In addition to the use of screening criteria drug therapy should be started at a low dose and carefully titrated until the lowest effective dose is achieved.

PREGNANCY

Pregnancy is a dynamic state with physiologic changes occurring throughout gestation. These changes include alterations in cardiovascular, pulmonary, GI, renal, and hepatic function that may result in clinically significant changes in drug PK.[144] Pregnant patients are frequently excluded from PK trials, limiting data that describe PK/PD and fetal adverse effect profiles for many drugs commonly used in critically ill pregnant patients. An in-depth discussion of all drug classes in pregnancy is beyond the scope of this chapter. There are several good review articles in the literature for specific drugs or disease states that should be reviewed prior to using the agents in pregnancy.[145,146]

PREGNANCY PHARMACOKINETIC CHANGES

Pregnancy results in multiple physiologic changes that affect absorption, distribution, metabolism, and elimination of various drugs. Absorption may be decreased due to a reduction in GI motility and an increased gastric pH. However, these changes are minimal and therefore are unlikely to significantly alter outcomes. Distribution is potentially increased due to changes in volume (up to 50% increase in blood volume) and decreases in protein binding (up to 30% decreases in albumin). These changes may lead to either lower or higher concentrations of free drug in the serum depending on the properties of the agent administered. Pregnancy increases hepatic blood flow and has variable effects on CYP enzymes. Available data suggest an increased activity of CYP26, CYP2C9, CYP2A6, and CYP3A3 and a decrease in the activity of CYP1A2 and CYP2C19. Renal elimination increases throughout gestation with an 80% increase in renal plasma flow during the second trimester, leading to a 50% increase in GFR. Consequently, pregnant women will often require higher doses of drugs with renal elimination; however, this requirement will change throughout pregnancy.[147]

The more important drug-related concern in pregnant women is the risk for the medications to affect fetal development. The system commonly used to evaluate teratogen risk in the United States is the FDA category system. Pregnancy categories include A (controlled clinical studies in humans showing safety), B (animal studies show no risk AND human data lacking), C (animal studies show risk AND human data lacking), D (human data show risk, benefit > risk), and X (animal or human data show significant risk, risk > benefit). In 2008 the FDA proposed major revisions to the drug labeling for pregnancy and lactation. The proposed changes are designed to provide better information when making prescribing decisions. Once the changes are approved they will replace the old pregnancy categories. However, at the time of this writing they are still under review.

In a best-case scenario we would use only category A drugs in critically ill pregnant women. However, because pregnant women are a protected research population they are frequently excluded from clinical trials; therefore, few drugs are listed as category A for pregnancy. Many agents that are category B or C can often be used safely in pregnancy. If available, category A, B, or C drugs should be used. However, if the indicated drug is category D and there are no alternatives, a careful risk-benefit assessment must be undertaken. Many antiepileptic drugs (AEDs) are pregnancy category D, making acute seizure management challenging in pregnancy. Levetiracetam is a pregnancy category C drug and is preferred over other agents. Out of the many AEDs that are category D drugs, valproic acid is believed to have the highest fetal risk and therefore should be avoided.[148] Category X drugs are contraindicated in pregnancy. Table 20.7 lists some commonly used ICU drugs and their pregnancy categories.[149-153]

BURN INJURY

Two phases of burn injury have significant effects on PK and PD. The first 48 hours following injury are characterized by hypovolemia, edema, hypoalbuminemia, and decreases in GFR. The second phase occurs beyond 48 hours and is a hyperdynamic state. During this hyperdynamic phase patients will have increased renal and hepatic blood flow, altered serum protein production, and insensible drug losses through exudate leakage resulting in altered binding, distribution, and clearance.[154]

The pharmacokinetic changes seen with burn injury vary from patient to patient, making drug dosing recommendations difficult. A 2008 review article discusses the available pharmacokinetic data.[154] As with other disease states, therapeutic drug monitoring should be used if available to determine drug doses. Because significant changes in serum proteins are common, the use of levels that detect free drug concentrations are preferred. If free levels are not available, clinicians must be aware that a total level in the therapeutic range does not necessarily reflect an appropriate drug dose. In these situations physical and laboratory assessment to evaluate therapeutic efficacy and adverse effects is warranted. If TDM is not available and the agent is a wide therapeutic index drug, then using maximal drug dosing is acceptable to ensure therapeutic effect.

HYPOTHERMIA

The process of cooling patients to mild hypothermia (32-34° C) has been studied for a number of different conditions including traumatic brain injury, spinal cord injury, stroke, cardiac surgery, and cardiac arrest.[155] It is most frequently used after cardiac arrest and is currently a recommended treatment in comatose adult patients following out-of-hospital ventricular fibrillation cardiac arrest. In addition, the guidelines from the American Heart Association suggest it may be beneficial for other cardiac arrest patients including in-patients and those with nonshockable rhythms.[156] With the increasing prevalence of hypothermia for cardiac arrest and the potential for use in other indications it is important to understand the impact hypothermia has on drug PK.

Hypothermia results in multiple physiologic changes that may impact the kinetics and dynamics of certain agents. Available literature report varied effects of hypothermia on drug absorption, distribution, drug target affinity, and time to onset.[157] However, hypothermia has been repeatedly shown to decrease drug clearance. This is especially true for drugs that undergo hepatic metabolism via the CYP450 system. Midazolam is one of the most studied drugs in hypothermia because of its frequent use as a sedative and metabolism by CYP3A4 and CYP3A5. One study in traumatic brain-injured patients cooled to less than 35° C demonstrated a fivefold increase in midazolam serum concentrations and a 100-fold decrease in clearance compared to a group of normothermic patients.[158] Data from healthy volunteers predicted an 11% decrease in midazolam clearance for every 1° C decrease in temperature below 36.5° C.[159] This is an important consideration, as it may result in a prolonged duration of pharmacologic effect, even after rewarming. Similar results have been reported for other drugs metabolized by the CYP450 family of enzymes.[160]

Although hypothermia has been shown to alter the clearance of drugs metabolized by the CYP450 family of enzymes, there are fewer data on the impact of hypothermia on toxicity. Pending further research it is important for ICU practitioners to recognize drugs that are metabolized by the liver and to monitor drug levels when possible and other markers of drug efficacy (i.e., sedation scores).

PHARMACOGENETICS

Pharmacogenetics is the study of genetic polymorphisms between patients, and pharmacogenomics takes a genome-wide approach in the study of drug response polymorphisms. The first reports of genetic polymorphisms affecting drug response were published in the 1950s. One of these early reports involved prolonged apnea after succinylcholine administration in patients with a variant of the enzyme responsible for succinylcholine metabolism.[161] It has become

Table 20.7 Medications Commonly Used in the Intensive Care Unit (ICU)* and Associated Pregnancy Risk

	Pregnancy Risk Category		
Drug Class	Category A, B, or C†	Category D‡	Category X§
Anticoagulants	*Preferred:* LMWH *Second line:* UFH *Only for use in patients with HIT:* Fondaparinux Argatroban Bivalirudin Lepirudin		Warfarin
Antiepileptics—IV drugs only	Lacosamide Levitiracetam	Phenobarbital Phenytoin Valproic acid	
Antihypertensives—IV drugs only	*Preferred:* Labetalol Hydralazine *Second line:* Nicardipine	Nitroprusside Enalaprilat	
Antimicrobials‖	*First line:* Amphotericin B Carbapenems Cephalosporins Penicillins *Second line:* Fluoroquinolones Vancomycin	Aminoglycosides Amikacin Gentamicin Tobramycin Fluconazole Metronidazole Nitrofurantoin Sulfamethoxazole-trimethoprim Voriconazole	
Sedatives	Propofol Dexmedetomidine	Lorazepam Midazolam	
Miscellaneous	Furosemide	Amiodarone Spironolactone Nonsteroidal anti-inflammatory drugs	HMG-CoA reductase inhibitors Spironolactone

*This list is not all-inclusive. The risk-benefit ratio must be weighed before any drug is used in pregnant patients.
†Human data show no risk or low risk or are lacking.
‡Human data show risk, but risk may outweigh benefit.
§Contraindicated.
‖Antimicrobials should not be withheld because of pregnancy, especially if alternatives are associated with worse infection-related outcomes.
HIT, heparin-induced thrombocytopenia; HMG-CoA, β-hydroxy-β-methylglutaryl–coenzyme A; IV, intravenous; LMWH, low-molecular-weight heparin; UFH, unfractionated heparin.

an area of increasing interest with variants identified that cause alterations in metabolism, transport, and drug interactions.[162] Unfortunately, to date few studies have assessed the impact of polymorphisms on agents commonly used in the ICU. A 2010 review discusses some of the genetic polymorphisms that are most likely to impact drug therapy in the ICU.[163] As this area of research continues to grow and more data become available it is likely that pharmacogenetics will have a significant impact on care of the critically ill patient.

Genetic variations in metabolism are some of the best understood genetic polymorphisms. Variations have been described for both phase 1 and phase 2 reactions. These variations may result in patients becoming extensive or poor metabolizers and may result in increased toxicity or decreased efficacy. The majority of research has focused on the cytochrome P-450 family because it is responsible for approximately 75% of all drug metabolism. Within the CYP family most research has focused on 2D6, 2C19, and 2C9. The most studied of these enzymes is 2D6, with variants being associated with increased serum concentrations of carvedilol, metoprolol, and flecainide although decreased response is observed with codeine and tramadol. Variants in CYP2C9 are associated with increased dose response to warfarin and variants in CYP2C19 are associated with decreased efficacy of clopidogrel and the proton pump inhibitors.[163] Other metabolizing enzymes that have variant alleles include *N*-acetyltransferase 2 and thiopurine *S*-methyltransferase. Slow acetylators of hydralazine, procainamide, and sulfamethoxazole are at an increased risk of immune-related toxic conditions such as systemic lupus erythematosus. On the other hand, slow acetylators of isoniazid are at increased risk of neurotoxicity, and rapid acetylators have an increased risk of hepatitis.

Even though a number of commonly used ICU drugs are metabolized by these enzymes, prescribing based on pharmacogenetics and phenotyping is still uncommon. The reasons are multifactorial and are in part due to the lack of data showing improved outcomes and the expenses associated with the tests. In fact, guideline statements recommended against routine pharmacogenetic screening prior to the use of clopidogrel or warfarin.[164,165] Until further data are available these recommendations are unlikely to change. Based on current studies there isn't much of a role for routine pharmacogenetic testing in critically ill patients. However, as more data become available it may become a standard of care in the ICU.

PRINCIPLES OF THERAPEUTIC DRUG MONITORING

As discussed previously, most of the currently available drugs have few clinical trial data in critically ill patients. This

Table 20.8 Therapeutic Monitoring for Commonly Used Drugs*

Drug	Type/Timing of Level	Therapeutic Concentration	Notes
Antiepileptics			
Phenobarbital	*Trough:* 0-30 minutes before dose	20-40 µg/mL	Phenobarbital is a long-half-life drug (36-125 hours), so a significant amount of time will be required to achieve steady state after a dosage adjustment
Phenytoin	*Trough:* 30 minutes before dose *Peak:* 1 hour after loading dose in setting of status epilepticus	Free level: 1-2 µg/mL Total level: 10-20 µg/mL	Free levels should be checked in patients with decreased albumin or renal disease or in the presence of displacers (e.g., valproic acid)
Valproic acid	*Trough:* 30 minutes before dose	50-100 µg/mL	Some patients may require levels from 100 to 150 µg/mL to achieve efficacy but are at increased risk for adverse effects
Antimicrobials			
Aminoglycosides			
Traditional dosing	*Peak:* 30 minutes after dose *Trough:* 30 minutes before dose	Gentamicin/tobramycin peak (µg/mL) 5-10 Gentamicin/tobramycin trough (µg/mL) 1-2	Peak goals vary depending on indication/source of infection Amikacin goals are 3× gentamicin/tobramycin goals
High-dose extended-interval dosing	*Two random levels:* between 6 and 14 hours after dose	Gentamicin/tobramycin peak (µg/mL) 15-25 Gentamicin/tobramycin trough (mg/L) <1	Peak goals for doses of 5-7 mg/kg/day of gentamicin/tobramycin Amikacin dose and goals are 3× the gentamicin/ tobramycin goals
Vancomycin	*Trough:* 30-60 minutes before dose	10-20 µg/mL	Trough goal dependent on severity and location of infection Some data suggest a goal AUC/MIC of ≥400
Cardiac			
Digoxin	*Random level*: at least 6 hours after dose	Heart failure: 0.5-0.8 ng/mL Rate control: <2 ng/mL	Rates of adverse effects increased significantly above 2 ng/mL For rate control, the lowest effective dose that achieves effect should be used
Immunosuppressants			
Cyclosporine	*Trough*: 12 hours after dose	100-400 ng/mL	Goal dependent on indication and time since initiation
Tacrolimus	*Trough*: 12 hours after dose	5-20 ng/mL	Goal dependent on indication and time since initiation

*If patient presents with symptoms of drug failure or toxicity, it may be reasonable to check serum concentration for all drugs before steady state is attained.

AUC, area under the curve; MIC, minimum inhibitory concentration.

lack of information leads to the extrapolation of data from non–critically ill patients, which may lead to therapeutic failure or toxicity. In this situation TDM can play an important role. Simply put, TDM is the development of a drug-dosing protocol based on static serum concentrations. The goal of this approach is to maximize therapeutic efficacy while minimizing the potential adverse effects associated with supratherapeutic concentrations. Unfortunately, TDM is not appropriate for all medications, and several factors must be assessed before TDM can be performed in any medication.

Several factors make a medication appropriate for TDM: (1) An assay is available that is accurate, specific, and can be conducted in a timely manner, (2) adequate pharmacokinetic data exist for the drug and they show significant interindividual variability, (3) there is a narrow range between therapeutic and toxic effects and these effects are proportional to the serum concentrations, (4) the therapeutic and toxic ranges are clearly defined, and (5) a constant pharmacologic effect is seen over time.[166]

After the decision is made to check a serum concentration, several factors must be evaluated as they are likely to influence the interpretation of the data. These factors include but are not limited to the time, duration, dose, and route of drug administration; the time the samples were drawn in relation to the previous and subsequent doses; whether the assay measures free or total (bound plus unbound) drug; patients' concomitant disease states; and the response to therapy and presence of adverse effects. Failure to consider these variables may lead to misinterpretation of the data. Although the data obtained through TDM can be extremely helpful, the practitioner must not forget to compare the results to the clinical presentation of the patient. This is important because not all patients are the same and what is therapeutic in one patient may be toxic in another even if the serum concentrations are the same. This variability makes assessing the patient's response to therapy even more important.

In general we reserve TDM for drugs that are associated with an increased risk for toxicity due to a narrow therapeutic index. The optimal time to monitor serum drug concentrations is highly dependent upon the drug being used and the patient's clinical presentation. However, after any dosage change a drug should reach steady state (5-7 drug half-lives) before a serum concentration is checked. There are some exceptions to this rule, for example, after a loading dose of phenytoin or valproic acid in a patient who does not appear to respond or after the first dose of an aminoglycoside if a high-dose extended-dosing nomogram is being used. The other situation when serum concentrations may be checked at different intervals is in a patient who has changing organ function. Table 20.8 lists some drugs that have clearly defined therapeutic concentrations and for which TDM is commonly utilized.[52] Several medications are not included in this table because serum drug concentrations are not routinely monitored but markers of their efficacy are monitored (i.e., heparin, LMWHs, direct thrombin inhibitors). In addition, there are a number of other medications for which TDM may become more prevalent in the future but TDM is not currently the standard of care. Some potential examples include β-lactam antibiotics, levetiracetam, and mycophenolate mofetil.

CONCLUSION

In order to maximize the efficacy and minimize toxicities associated with medications it is important for practitioners to understand the basic principles of PK and PD. This knowledge becomes even more important in critically ill patients who undergo a number of physiologic changes and have a number of disease states that result in altered drug responses. All medication regimens in critically ill patients should be individualized based on knowledge of a drug's kinetics and dynamics along with an understanding of the impact the patient's comorbid conditions will have on these parameters. In addition, therapeutic drug monitoring should be utilized if available, particularly with narrow therapeutic index drugs. Through the vigilant use of this knowledge practitioners can maximize therapeutic outcomes in their patients while minimizing toxicity.

KEY POINTS

- Most drug-dosing recommendations are based on studies in healthy volunteers and often do not account for the pharmacokinetic and pharmacodynamic alterations seen in critically ill patients.
- Alterations in drug absorption, distribution, metabolism, and clearance are common in critically ill patients, and failure to modify drug dosages based on these changes may result in increased drug toxicity or treatment failure.
- The pharmacodynamic parameter that determines efficacy varies among drug classes as demonstrated by the different targets to maximize bacterial kill among aminoglycosides (concentration dependent, peak:MIC ratio), β-lactams (time dependent, T > MIC), and vancomycin (time and concentration dependent, AUC/MIC).
- Physiologic changes seen with critical illness may alter the rate and extent of medication absorption from the GI tract, making IV administration the preferred route in patients with hemodynamic instability.
- Commonly encountered factors in critically ill patients that impact drug PK and PD include renal disease, hepatic disease, obesity, advanced age, pregnancy, thermal injury, and hypothermia.
- Current data do not support routine pharmacogenetic testing for critically ill patients; however, as more data become available it may become a standard of care for some medications.
- When available, patient-specific PK based on appropriately timed serum concentrations (i.e., therapeutic drug monitoring) should be used to minimize toxicity and maximize the efficacy of drug therapy.

SELECTED REFERENCES

4. Craig WA: Pharmacokinetic/pharmacodynamic parameters: Rationale for antibacterial dosing of mice and men. Clin Infect Dis 1998;26:1-10; quiz 1-2.
37. Rybak M, Lomaestro B, Rotschafer JC, et al: Therapeutic monitoring of vancomycin in adult patients: A consensus review of the American Society of Health-System Pharmacists, the Infectious Diseases Society of America, and the Society of Infectious Diseases Pharmacists. Am J Health Syst Pharm 2009;66:82-98.
82. Nyman HA, Dowling TC, Hudson JQ, et al: Comparative evaluation of the Cockcroft-Gault Equation and the Modification of Diet in Renal Disease (MDRD) study equation for drug dosing: An opinion of the Nephrology Practice and Research Network of the American College of Clinical Pharmacy. Pharmacotherapy 2011;31:1130-1144.
90. Heintz BH, Matzke GR, Dager WE: Antimicrobial dosing concepts and recommendations for critically ill adult patients receiving continuous renal replacement therapy or intermittent hemodialysis. Pharmacotherapy 2009;29:562-577.
94. Verbeeck RK: Pharmacokinetics and dosage adjustment in patients with hepatic dysfunction. Eur J Clin Pharmacol 2008;64: 1147-1161.
107. Hanley MJ, Abernethy DR, Greenblatt DJ: Effect of obesity on the pharmacokinetics of drugs in humans. Clin Pharmacokinet 2010;49:71-87.
142. Klotz U: Pharmacokinetics and drug metabolism in the elderly. Drug Metab Rev 2009;41:67-76.
147. Anderson GD: Pregnancy-induced changes in pharmacokinetics: A mechanistic-based approach. Clin Pharmacokinet 2005;44: 989-1008.
157. van den Broek MP, Groenendaal F, Egberts AC, Rademaker CM: Effects of hypothermia on pharmacokinetics and pharmacodynamics: A systematic review of preclinical and clinical studies. Clin Pharmacokinet 2010;49:277-294.
163. Empey PE: Genetic predisposition to adverse drug reactions in the intensive care unit. Crit Care Med 2010;38:S106-S116.
166. Spector R, Park GD, Johnson GF, Vesell ES: Therapeutic drug monitoring. Clin Pharmacol Ther 1988;43:345-353.

The complete list of references can be found at www.expertconsult.com.

PART 2

CRITICAL CARE CARDIOVASCULAR DISEASE

Circulatory Shock

21

Anand Kumar | Ulug Unligil | Joseph E. Parrillo

CHAPTER OUTLINE

INTRODUCTION

The syndrome of shock in humans is often the final pathway through which a variety of pathologic processes lead to cardiovascular failure and death. As such, it is perhaps the most common and important problem with which critical care physicians contend. The importance of shock as a medical problem can be appreciated by the prominence of its three dominant forms. Cardiogenic shock related to pump failure is a major component of the mortality associated with cardiovascular disease, the leading cause of death in the United States with almost 800,000 deaths annually.[1] Similarly, hypovolemic shock remains a major contributor to early mortality from trauma, the most common cause of death in those between the ages of 1 and 45 (approximately 200,000 cases annually.[1,2] Finally, despite improving medical and surgical therapy, overall mortality coded as septicemia has increased from the 13th to the 11th most frequent cause of death in the United States.[1,3] Most current estimates suggest that there are more than 100,000 cases of septic shock annually in the United States alone.[4,5] In addition, all forms of shock increase the probability of other major comorbidities such as serious infection, acute respiratory distress syndrome (ARDS), and multiple organ dysfunction syndrome (MODS).

Additional online-only material indicated by icon.

This chapter provides an overview of circulatory shock with an emphasis on the common elements and important differences in the pathophysiology and pathogenesis of the various forms of the syndrome. This focus on common elements of different forms of shock will continue through sections on systemic shock hemodynamics, microvascular dysfunction, mechanisms of cellular injury, oxygen supply dependency, compensatory responses, diagnostic approach/evaluation, and management/therapy.

HISTORY

Despite recognition of a posttraumatic syndrome by Greek physicians such as Hippocrates and Galen, the origin of the term *shock* is generally credited to the French surgeon Henri Francois Le Dran who, in his 1737 "A Treatise of Reflections Drawn from Experience with Gunshot Wounds," coined the term *choc* to indicate a severe impact or jolt.[6] An inappropriate translation by the English physician Clarke, in 1743, led to the introduction of the word *shock* to the English language to indicate the sudden deterioration of a patient's condition with major trauma.[6] It was Edwin A. Moses,[7] however, who began to popularize the term, using it in his 1867 "A Practical Treatise on Shock after Operations and Injuries." He defined it as "a peculiar effect on the animal system, produced by violent injuries from any cause, or from violent mental emotions." Prior to this definition, the rarely used term *shock* referred in a nonspecific sense to the immediate and devastating effects of trauma, not a specific posttrauma syndrome. Although not entirely accurate by today's standards, his definition was one of the first to separate the syndrome involving the body's response to massive trauma from the immediate, direct manifestations of trauma itself.

By the late 1800s, two theories of traumatic shock physiology dominated. The first, based on observations by Bernard, Charcot, Goltz, and others, was proposed by Fischer in 1870.[8-10] He suggested that traumatic shock was caused by generalized "vasomotor paralysis" resulting in splanchnic blood pooling. The corollary was that total circulating blood volume is preserved in shock. The second dominant theory, articulated by Mapother in 1879, suggested that decreased cardiac output in traumatic shock is caused by intravascular volume loss due to extrusion of plasma through the vessel wall from the intravascular space to the interstitium.[11] He proposed that this was a consequence of the failure of "vasodilator nerves" in traumatic shock and subsequent generalized arteriolar vasoconstriction. With the 1899 publication of "An Experimental Research into Surgical Shock" (perhaps the first experimental studies of shock), George W. Crile provided scientific data supporting a variation of the vasomotor paralysis theory.[12] After documenting the importance of decreased central venous pressure and venous return in experimental shock due to hemorrhage and demonstrating the potential for intravascular volume replacement as therapy, he proposed that traumatic shock was caused by exhaustion of the overstimulated "vasomotor center" and subsequent generalized relaxation of large vessels (veins) leading to decreased ventricular filling and cardiac output.

Further advances in shock research were substantially driven by military concerns. During World War I, Walter B. Cannon and other physiologists/physicians studied the early clinical response to battlefield trauma. Their work eventually led to the publication of the classic monograph "Traumatic Shock" in 1923.[13] Cannon and his colleagues were the first to relate trauma-associated hypotension in a large group of patients to a fall in blood volume, loss of bicarbonate, and accumulation of organic acids. Others, using dye dilution techniques, demonstrated that severity of shock was directly related to the decrease in intravascular volume.[14] Clinical data from war casualties also suggested the importance of reduced blood flow (independent of blood pressure) in shock.[15] The observation that blood in the capillaries of victims of massive trauma was hemoconcentrated compared to venous blood would lead to the practice of resuscitating trauma patients with dried pooled plasma rather than whole blood in the early part of World War II.[16]

Although work originating from the battlefields of World War I clearly linked traumatic shock associated with substantial, obvious bleeding to a loss of circulating blood volume, the origin of traumatic shock in the absence of defined hemorrhage was unclear. The accepted explanation for this phenomenon remained a variation of the vasomotor paralysis theory of shock. It was postulated that nonhemorrhagic, posttraumatic shock ("wound shock") was caused by the liberation of "wound toxins" (histamine or other substances), which resulted in *neurogenic* vasodilation and peripheral blood pooling. However, after the war, Blalock and others demonstrated in animal models that nonhemorrhagic traumatic shock was due to the loss of blood and fluids into injured tissue rather than circulating toxins resulting in stasis of blood within the circulation.[17]

Additional advances occurred during World War II. Using injured subjects from the European front, Henry Beecher confirmed that hemorrhage and fluid loss leading to metabolic acidosis was a major cause of shock.[18] In the first use of indicator dye techniques in humans for studying blood flow, Cournand and Richard, in 1943, demonstrated that cardiac output was typically reduced in shock.[19] They also reinforced Blalock's findings regarding nonhemorrhagic "wound shock" in trauma patients by demonstrating that circulating blood volume was reduced in such patients through loss of fluid into damaged tissues. The importance of maintaining intravascular volume in traumatic and hemorrhagic shock was supported by the well-known cardiovascular physiologist, Carl J. Wiggers, who published a landmark series of studies[20] in the 1940s using a standardized animal model, which showed that prolonged hypovolemic shock resulted in a resuscitation-resistant state that he termed *irreversible shock.* He defined it as a condition resulting from "a depression of many functions but in which reduction of the effective circulating blood volume is of basic importance and in which impairment of the circulation steadily progresses until it eventuates in a state of irreversible circulatory failure." Aggressive fluid support became the standard of resuscitation for trauma and shock.

Subsequently, the Korean War fueled the research that demonstrated the relationship of acute tubular necrosis (ATN) and acute renal failure (ARF) to circulatory shock.[21] In addition, studies of battlefield casualties clearly demonstrated the relationship between early resuscitation and survival.[21] During the Vietnamese conflict, with the widespread use of ventilator technology, the dominant research concern became postshock infection and "shock lung" (ARDS), a concern that has evolved to the present interest in shock-related MODS.

DEFINITIONS AND CATEGORIZATION OF SHOCK

The definition of shock has evolved in parallel with our understanding of the phenomenon. As noted, until the late 1800s, the term *shock* was used to indicate the immediate response to massive trauma, without regard to a specific posttrauma syndrome. The definition consisted of descriptions of its obvious clinical signs. In 1895, John Collins Warren[22] referred to shock as "a momentary pause in the act of death," which was characterized by an "imperceptible" or "weak, threadlike" peripheral pulse and a "cold, clammy sweat."

Subsequently, with the introduction of noninvasive blood pressure monitoring devices, most clinical definitions of shock added the requirement for arterial hypotension. In 1930, Blalock[8] included arterial hypotension as one of the required manifestations of shock when he defined it as "peripheral circulatory failure resulting from a discrepancy in the size of the vascular bed and the volume of the intravascular fluid." Simeone,[23] as recently as 1964, suggested that shock exists when "the cardiac output is insufficient to fill the arterial tree with blood under sufficient pressure to provide organs and tissues with adequate blood flow."

Current technology, which allows for the assessment of perfusion independent of arterial pressure, has shown that hypotension does not define shock. The emphasis in defining shock is now on tissue perfusion in relation to cellular function. According to Fink,[24] shock is "a syndrome precipitated by a systemic derangement of perfusion leading to widespread cellular hypoxia and vital organ dysfunction." Cerra[25] has emphasized supply/demand mismatch in his definition: "a disordered response of organisms to an inappropriate balance of substrate supply and demand at a cellular level."

The appropriate definition of shock varies with the context of its use. For paramedical personnel, a definition that incorporates the typical clinical signs of shock (arterial hypotension, tachypnea, tachycardia, altered mental status, and decreased urine output) may suffice. For the physiologist, shock may be defined by specific hemodynamic criteria involving alterations of ventricular filling pressures, venous pressures, arterial pressures, cardiac output, and systemic vascular resistance. Similarly, in the appropriate context, shock could also be defined by alterations of biochemical/bioenergetic pathways or intracellular gene expression. For the physician, however, we find the most appropriate definition to be "the state in which profound and widespread reduction of effective tissue perfusion leads first to reversible, and then, if prolonged, to irreversible cellular injury."

Effective tissue perfusion, as opposed to tissue perfusion per se, is an important issue. Effective tissue perfusion may be reduced by either a global reduction of systemic perfusion (cardiac output) or by increased ineffective tissue perfusion due to a maldistribution of blood flow or a defect of substrate utilization at the subcellular level (Box 21.1).

CLASSIFICATION

Although hypovolemic shock associated with trauma was the first form of shock to be recognized and studied, by the early 1900s it became broadly recognized that other clinical conditions could result in a similar constellation of signs and symptoms. Sepsis as a distinct cause of shock was initially proposed by Laennec (1831) and subsequently supported by Boise (1897).[26,27] In 1934, Fishberg and colleagues introduced the concept of primary cardiogenic shock due to myocardial infarction.[28] Later the same year, Blalock developed the precursor of the most commonly used classification systems of the present.[29] He subdivided shock into four etiologic categories: hematogenic or oligemic (hypovolemic), cardiogenic, neurogenic (e.g., shock after spinal injury), and vasogenic (primarily septic shock). Shubin and Weil, in 1967, proposed the additional etiologic categories of hypersensitivity (i.e., anaphylactic), bacteremic (i.e., septic), obstructive, and endocrinologic shock.[30] However, as the hemodynamic profiles of the different forms of shock were uncovered, a classification based on cardiovascular characteristics, initially proposed in 1972 by Hinshaw and Cox,[31] came to be accepted by most clinicians. The categories include (1) hypovolemic shock, due to a decreased circulating blood volume in relation to the total vascular capacity and characterized by a reduction of diastolic filling pressures and volumes; (2) cardiogenic shock related to cardiac pump failure due to loss of myocardial contractility/functional myocardium or structural/mechanical failure of the cardiac anatomy and characterized by elevations of diastolic filling pressures and volumes; (3) extracardiac obstructive shock involving obstruction to flow in the cardiovascular circuit and characterized by either impairment of diastolic filling or excessive afterload; and (4) distributive shock caused by loss of vasomotor control resulting in arteriolar and venular dilation and (after resuscitation with fluids) characterized by increased cardiac output with decreased systemic vascular resistance. We have adapted these categories into an etiologic/physiologic classification of shock that is summarized in Figure 21.1 and Box 21.2. This figure and box represent our current understanding of the causes and typical hemodynamic features of different forms of shock.

Despite this hemodynamic-based categorization system, it is important to note the mixed nature of most forms of clinical shock. Septic shock is nominally considered a form of distributive shock. However, prior to resuscitation with

Box 21.1 Determinants of Effective Tissue Perfusion in Shock

Cardiovascular Performance (Total Systemic Perfusion/Cardiac Output)

Cardiac Function

Preload
Afterload
Contractility
Heart rate

Venous Return

Right atrial pressure (dependent on cardiac function)
Mean circulatory pressure
  Stressed vascular volume
  Mean vascular compliance
Venous vascular resistance
  Distribution of blood flow

Distribution of Cardiac Output

Intrinsic regulatory systems (local tissue factors)
Extrinsic regulatory systems (sympathetic/adrenal activity)
Anatomic vascular disease
Exogenous vasoactive agents (inotropes, vasopressors, vasodilators)

Microvascular Function

Pre- and postcapillary sphincter function
Capillary endothelial integrity
Microvascular obstruction (fibrin, platelets, white blood cells, red blood cells)

Local Oxygen Unloading and Diffusion

Oxyhemoglobin affinity
  RBC 2,3 DPG
  Blood pH
  Temperature

Cellular Energy Generation/Utilization Capability

Citric acid (Krebs) cycle
Oxidative phosphorylation pathway
Other energy metabolism pathways (e.g., ATP utilization)

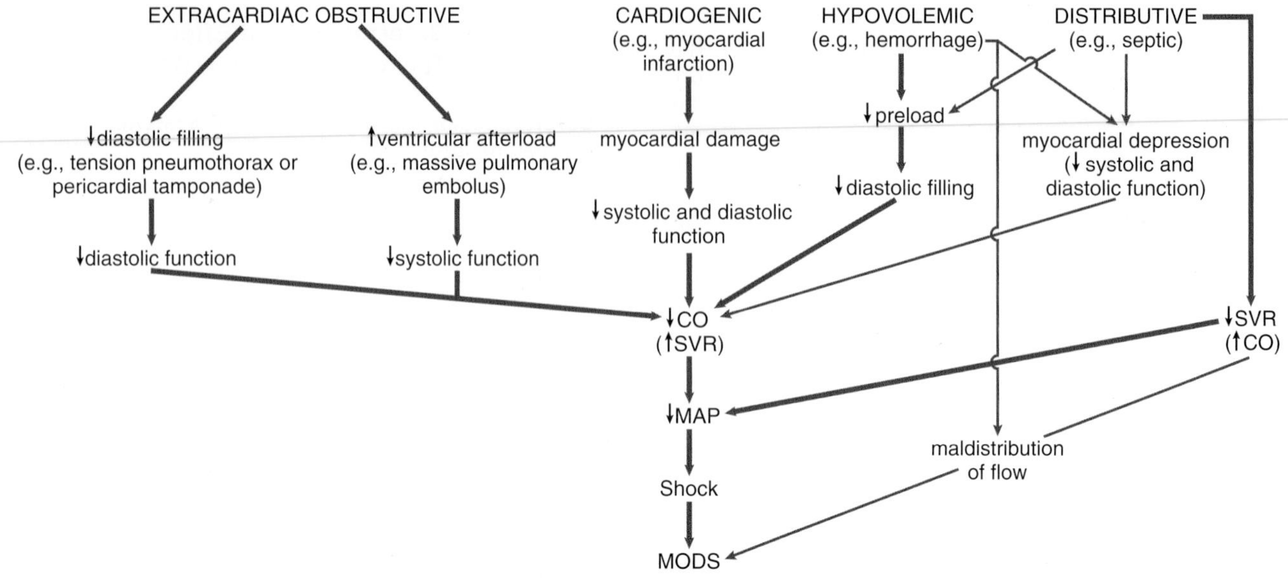

Figure 21.1 The interrelationships among different forms of shock. For cardiogenic, hypovolemic, and obstructive shock, hypotension is primarily due to decreased cardiac output with systemic vascular resistance rising secondarily. With distributive (particularly septic shock), hypotension is primarily due to a decrease in systemic vascular resistance with a secondary increase of cardiac output. In many forms of shock, the hemodynamic characteristics are influenced by elements of hypovolemia, myocardial depression (ischemic or otherwise), and vascular dysfunction (which may affect afterload). Dominant pathophysiologic pathways are denoted by heavier lines. CO, cardiac output; SVR, systemic vascular resistance; MAP, mean arterial blood pressure; MODS, multiple organ dysfunction syndrome.

fluids, a substantial hypovolemic component may exist due to venodilatation and third-spacing. In addition, depression of the myocardium in human septic shock is well documented (see Fig. 21.1).[32-34] Similarly, hemorrhagic shock in experimental models has been linked to both myocardial depression[35,36] and vascular dysfunction (see Fig. 21.1).[37,38] Cardiogenic shock typically presents with increased ventricular filling pressures. However, many patients have been aggressively diuresed prior to the onset of shock and may have a relative hypovolemic component. In addition, systemic vascular resistance (SVR) is only inconsistently increased in cardiogenic shock, suggesting that an inflammatory element may exist under some circumstances. Finally, shock from any cause may cause a deterioration of the coronary perfusion pressure, the difference between mean arterial pressure (MAP) and the higher of left ventricular diastolic pressure or the right atrial pressure, resulting in some degree of myocardial ischemia and myocardial dysfunction.[39] Thus, although four categories of shock exist based on hemodynamic profile, clinical shock states tend to combine components of each.

HYPOVOLEMIC SHOCK

Hypovolemic shock may be related to dehydration, internal or external hemorrhage, gastrointestinal fluid losses (diarrhea or vomiting), urinary losses due to either diuretics or kidney dysfunction, or loss of intravascular volume to the interstitium due to decrease of vascular permeability (in response to sepsis or trauma). In addition, venodilatation due to a number of causes (sepsis, spinal injury, various drugs and toxins) may result in a relative hypovolemic state (see Box. 21.2, Fig. 21.1). Hemodynamically, hypovolemic shock is characterized by a fall in ventricular preload resulting in decreased ventricular diastolic pressures and volumes (Table 21.1). Cardiac index (CI) and stroke volume index (SVI) are typically reduced. In addition to hypotension, a decreased pulse pressure may be noted. Due to a decreased output and unchanged or increased metabolic demand, mixed venous oxygen saturation (MVo_2) may be decreased and the arteriovenous oxygen content difference widened. Clinical characteristics include pale, cool, clammy skin (often mottled); tachycardia (or if severe shock, bradycardia)[7,40]; tachypnea; flat, nondistended peripheral veins; decreased jugular venous pulse; decreased urine output; and altered mental status.

A number of factors may influence the development and hemodynamic characteristics of hypovolemic shock in humans. Studies in animals and humans have demonstrated a clear relationship between the degree of circulating blood volume loss and clinical response.[41-44] Acute loss of 10% of the circulating blood volume is well tolerated, with tachycardia the only obvious sign. CI may be minimally decreased despite a compensatory increase in myocardial contractility. SVR typically increases slightly, particularly if sympathetic stimulation augments mean arterial pressure (MAP). Compensatory mechanisms begin to fail with a 20% to 25% volume loss. Mild to moderate hypotension and decreased CI may be present. Orthostasis (with a blood pressure decrease of 10 mm Hg and increased heart rate of 20 to 30 beats/minute) may become apparent. There is a marked increase in SVR and serum lactate may begin to rise. With decreases of the circulating volume of 40% or more, marked hypotension with clinical signs of shock is noted. CI and tissue perfusion may fall to less than half normal. Lactic acidosis is usually present at this stage and predicts a poor outcome.[45,46] The case fatality rate can exceed 50% in hemorrhagic shock associated with trauma.[47]

The rate of loss of intravascular volume and the preexisting cardiac reserve is of substantial importance in the

Box 21.2 Classification of Shock

Hypovolemic (Oligemic)

Hemorrhagic
Trauma
Gastrointestinal
Retroperitoneal
Fluid depletion (nonhemorrhagic)
External fluid loss
Dehydration
Vomiting
Diarrhea
Polyuria

Interstitial Fluid Redistribution

Thermal injury
Trauma
Anaphylaxis

Increased Vascular Capacitance (Venodilatation)

Sepsis
Anaphylaxis
Toxins/drugs

Cardiogenic

Myopathic

Myocardial infarction
Left ventricle
Right ventricle
Myocardial contusion (trauma)
Myocarditis
Cardiomyopathy
Postischemic myocardial stunning
Septic myocardial depression
Pharmacologic
Anthracycline cardiotoxicity
Calcium channel blockers

Mechanical

Valvular failure (stenotic or regurgitant)
Hypertropic cardiomyopathy
Ventricular septal defect

Arrhythmic

Bradycardia
Sinus (e.g., vagal syncope)
Atrioventricular blocks
Tachycardia
Supraventricular
Ventricular

Extracardiac Obstructive

Impaired diastolic filling (decreased ventricular preload)
Direct venous obstruction (vena cava)
Intrathoracic obstructive tumors
Increased intrathoracic pressure (decreased transmural pressure gradient)
Tension pneumothorax
Mechanical ventilation (with positive end-expiratory pressure [PEEP] or volume depletion)
Decreased cardiac compliance
Constrictive pericarditis
Cardiac tamponade
Acute
Post MI free wall rupture
Traumatic
Hemorrhagic (anticoagulation)
Chronic
Malignant
Uremic
Idiopathic

Impaired Systolic Contraction (Increased Ventricular Afterload)

Right Ventricle

Pulmonary embolus (massive)
Acute pulmonary hypertension

Left Ventricle

Saddle embolus
Aortic dissection

Distributive

Septic (bacterial, fungal, viral, rickettsial)
Toxic shock syndrome
Anaphylactic, anaphylactoid
Neurogenic (spinal shock)
Endocrinologic
Adrenal crisis
Thyroid storm
Toxic (e.g., nitroprusside, bretylium)

development of hypovolemic shock. As an example, whereas an acute blood loss of 1 L in a healthy adult may result in mild to moderate hypotension with a reduced pulmonary artery occlusion pressure (PAOP) and central venous pressure (CVP),[42] the same loss over a longer period of time may be well tolerated due to compensatory responses such as tachycardia, increased myocardial contractility, increased red blood cell 2,3-diphosphoglycerate (2,3 DPG), and increased fluid retention. On the other hand, a similar slow loss may lead to substantial hemodynamic compromise in a person with a limited cardiac reserve, even while the person's PAOP and CVP remain elevated.

Hypovolemic shock represents more than a simple mechanical response to loss of circulating volume. It is a dynamic process involving competing adaptive (compensatory) and maladaptive responses at each stage of development. Thus, although intravascular volume replacement is always a necessary component of resuscitation from hypovolemia or hypovolemic shock, the biologic responses to the insult may progress to the point where such resuscitation is insufficient to reverse the progression of the shock syndrome. Patients who have sustained a greater than 40% loss of blood volume for 2 hours or more may be unable to be effectively resuscitated.[37,41,44] A series of inflammatory mediator, cardiovascular, and organ responses to shock are initiated, which supersede the importance of the initial insult in driving further injury.

CARDIOGENIC SHOCK

Cardiogenic shock results from the failure of the heart as a pump (see Box 21.2, Fig. 21.1). It is the most common cause

Table 21.1 Hemodynamic Profiles of Shock*

Diagnosis	CO	SVR	PWP	CVP	$S\bar{V}O_2$	Comments
Cardiogenic shock						
Caused by myocardial dysfunction	↓↓	↑	↑↑	↑↑	↓	Usually occurs with evidence of extensive myocardial infarction (>40% of left ventricular myocardium nonfunctional), severe cardiomyopathy, or myocarditis
Caused by a mechanical defect						
Acute ventricular septal defect	LVCO ↓↓ RVCO > LVCO	↑	nl or ↑	↑↑	↑ or ↑↑	If shunt is left to right, pulmonary blood flow is greater than systemic blood flow; oxygen saturation "step-up" (≥5%) occurs at right ventricular level; ↑ $S\bar{V}O_2$ is caused by left to right shunt
Acute mitral regurgitation	Forward CO ↓↓	↑	↑↑	↑ or ↑↑	↓	Large V waves (≥10 mm Hg) in pulmonary wedge pressure tracing
Right ventricular infarction	↓↓	↑	nl or ↑	↑↑	↓	Elevated right atrial and right ventricular filling pressures with low or normal pulmonary wedge pressures
Extracardiac obstructive shock						
Pericardial tamponade	↓ or ↓↓	↑	↑↑	↑↑	↓	Dip and plateau in right and left ventricular pressure tracings. The right atrial mean, right ventricular end-diastolic, pulmonary artery end-diastolic, and pulmonary wedge pressures are within 5 mm Hg of each other
Massive pulmonary emboli	↓↓	↑	nl or ↓	↑↑	↓	Usual finding is elevated right-sided heart pressures with low or normal pulmonary wedge pressure
Hypovolemic shock	↓↓	↑	↓↓	↓↓	↓	Filling pressures may appear normal if hypovolemia occurs in the setting of baseline myocardial compromise
Distributive shock						
Septic shock	↑↑ or nl, rarely ↓	↓ or ↓↓	↓ or nl	↓ or nl	↑ or ↑↑	The hyperdynamic circulatory state (↑ CO, ↓ SVR) associated with distributive forms of shock usually depends on resuscitation with fluids; before such resuscitation, a hypodynamic circulation is typical
Anaphylaxis	↑↑ or nl, rarely ↓	↓ or ↓↓	↓ or nl	↓ or nl	↑ or ↑↑	

*The hemodynamic profiles summarized in this table refer to patients with the diagnosis listed in the left column who are also in shock (mean arterial blood pressure < 60-65 mm Hg).

CO, cardiac output; CVP, central venous pressure; LV, left ventricular; nl, normal; PWP, pulmonary wedge pressure; SVR, systemic vascular resistance; $S\bar{V}O_2$, mixed venous oxygen saturation; ↑↑ or ↓, mild to moderate increase or decrease; ↑↑ or ↓ ↓, moderate to severe increase or decrease.

Modified from Parrillo JE: Septic shock: Clinical manifestations, pathogenesis, hemodynamics, and management in a critical care unit. In Parrillo JE, Ayers SM (eds): Major Issues in Critical Care Medicine. Baltimore, Williams & Wilkins, 1984.

of in-hospital mortality in patients with Q-wave myocardial infarction.[48,49] Hemodynamically, cardiogenic shock is characterized by increased ventricular preload (increased ventricular volumes, pulmonary wedge pressure [PWP] and CVP) (see Table 21.1). Otherwise hemodynamic characteristics are similar to those for hypovolemic shock (see Table 21.1). In particular, both involve reduced CI, SVI, and ventricular stroke work indices with increased SVR. Due to inadequate tissue perfusion, the MVO_2 is substantially reduced and the arteriovenous oxygen content difference increased. The degree of lactic acidosis may predict mortality.[50] Clinically, the specific signs of shock are similar. However, signs of congestive heart failure (volume overload) are typically present in cardiogenic shock. The jugular and peripheral veins may be distended. An S3 and evidence of pulmonary edema are usually found.

Cardiogenic shock is most commonly due to ischemic myocardial injury with a total of 40% of the myocardium nonfunctional.[49,51-53] Such damage may involve a single large myocardial infarction or may involve accumulation of damage from multiple infarctions. In addition, viable but dysfunctional "stunned" myocardium may temporarily contribute to cardiogenic shock postinfarction. Cardiogenic shock usually involves an anterior myocardial infarction with left main or proximal left anterior descending artery occlusion. Historically, the incidence of cardiogenic shock due to Q-wave infarction has ranged from 8% to 20%.[48,54-56] Although several large studies demonstrate lower incidence rates (4% to 7%) when patients receive thrombolytic interventions,[55,57-60] retrospective community studies suggest no overall decrease in the incidence of postinfarction cardiogenic shock or cardiogenic shock mortality (70% to 90%) in the first decades following the introduction of this therapy.[48] Further, no trials have demonstrated that thrombolytic therapy reduces mortality rates in patients with established cardiogenic shock.[60,61] In contrast, several major studies suggest that mortality of infarction-related cardiogenic shock may be improved by emergent angioplasty.[56,62-64] Accordingly, data suggest a reduction in the incidence of acute infarction-related cardiogenic shock to <2% in 2003 in association with widespread use of emergent percutaneous coronary intervention.[62] This intervention has also been associated with a reduction of cardiogenic shock mortality risk from 60% to 84% to 43% to 47% in two large analyses.[56,62]

Mortality is better for cardiogenic shock due to surgically remediable cardiac lesions. Mitral valve failure may be associated with rupture or dysfunction of chordae or papillary muscles due to myocardial ischemia or infarction, endocarditis, blunt chest trauma, or prosthetic valve deterioration and is characterized by "v" waves of greater than 10 mm Hg on a PAOP tracing. Ischemic papillary muscle rupture frequently occurs 3 to 7 days after an infarct in left anterior descending coronary artery territory and may be preceded by the onset of a mitral regurgitant murmur.[65] Mortality is high in the absence of surgical therapy.[65] Acute aortic valve failure is most commonly due to endocarditis but may involve mechanical failure of prosthetic valves, or aortic dissection. Ventricular septal defects caused by myocardial infarction may also result in the abrupt onset of cardiogenic shock and can be diagnosed by a 5% step up in hemoglobin oxygen saturation between the right atrium and the pulmonary artery (due to left-to-right shunting of blood through the septum).[66] As with ischemic papillary muscle rupture, rupture of the intraventricular septum is most frequently seen with occlusions of the left anterior descending artery, a few days after infarction.[66]

The pathophysiology of cardiogenic shock due to a right ventricular infarction and failure is different from other forms of cardiogenic shock. Although some degree of right ventricular involvement is seen in half of inferior myocardial infarctions, only the largest 10% to 20% result in right ventricular failure and cardiogenic shock.[67] These infarctions usually involve part of the left ventricular wall as well. Isolated infarctions of the right ventricle are rare.[67,68]

Because therapy of this form of shock requires fluid resuscitation and inotropes (rather than vasopressors), differentiation from other causes of cardiogenic shock is crucial. Conditions compromising right ventricular function such as cardiac tamponade, restrictive cardiomyopathy, constrictive pericarditis, and pulmonary embolus are also included in the differential diagnosis. Each of these conditions may present with some of the typical clinical and hemodynamic findings of right ventricular infarction including Kussmaul's sign, and pulsus paradoxus with elevation and equalization of CVP, right ventricular systolic pressure, pulmonary artery diastolic pressure, and PAOP. Prognosis in this form of cardiogenic shock is distinctly better than that of cardiogenic shock due to left ventricular infarction[69,70]; however, an inferior infarction with right ventricular injury has a substantially worse prognosis than such an infarction without significant right-sided involvement.[71]

As with hypovolemic shock, a number of interactions may complicate the development of cardiogenic shock. Optimal cardiac performance in patients with impaired myocardial contractility may occur at substantially higher than normal PAOP (i.e., 20 to 24 mm Hg). Yet patients who develop cardiogenic shock are frequently initially treated with diuretics and may have a degree of hypovolemia (relative to their optimal requirements). Thus, patients should not be diagnosed with cardiogenic shock unless hypotension (MAP < 65 mm Hg) and reduced cardiac output (CI < 2.2 L/min/m^2) coexist with an elevated ventricular filling pressure.[72] Cautious fluid challenge may be required (in the absence of overt pulmonary edema) to increase the filling pressures to an optimal range. Other interactions include increased right ventricular ischemia due to decreased right coronary perfusion pressure (MAP decreased while right ventricular end-diastolic pressure is increased) and increased right ventricular afterload due to pulmonary hypertension. Right ventricular ischemia may also lead to right ventricular dilatation, septal shift, and impairment of left ventricular function.

Other causes of cardiogenic shock include acute myocarditis, end-stage cardiomyopathy, brady- or tachyarrhythmias, hypertrophic cardiomyopathy with obstruction, and traumatic myocardial contusion (see Box 21.2).

OBSTRUCTIVE SHOCK

Extracardiac obstructive shock results from an obstruction to flow in the cardiovascular circuit (see Box 21.2, Fig. 21.1). Pericardial tamponade and constrictive pericarditis directly impair diastolic filling of the right ventricle. Tension pneumothorax and intrathoracic tumors indirectly impair right ventricular filling by obstructing venous return. Massive pulmonary emboli (two or more lobar arteries with >50% of the vascular bed occluded), nonembolic acute pulmonary hypertension, large systemic emboli (e.g., saddle embolus), and aortic dissection may result in shock due to increased ventricular afterload.

The characteristic hemodynamic/metabolic patterns are, in most ways, similar to other low output shock states (see Table 21.1). CI, SVI, and stroke work indices are usually decreased. Because tissue perfusion is decreased, the MVo_2 is low, the arteriovenous oxygen content difference increased, and serum lactate frequently elevated. Other hemodynamic parameters are dependent on the site of the obstruction. Tension pneumothorax and mediastinal tumors may obstruct the great thoracic veins, resulting in a hemodynamic pattern (decreased CI and elevated SVR) similar to hypovolemia (although distended jugular and peripheral veins may be seen). Cardiac tamponade typically causes increased and equalized right and left heart ventricular diastolic pressures, pulmonary artery diastolic pressure, CVP, and PAOP. In constrictive pericarditis, right and left ventricular diastolic pressures are elevated and within 5 mm Hg of each other. Mean right and left atrial pressures may or may not be equal as well. Massive pulmonary embolus will result in right ventricular failure with elevated pulmonary artery and right heart pressures whereas PAOP remains normal. A systemic saddle embolus or aortic occlusion due to dissection causes peripheral hypotension and signs of left ventricular failure including an elevated PAOP. Clinical signs are similarly dependent on the site of the obstruction.

As with other forms of shock, the time course of development of the insult has a substantial impact on the clinical response. Ischemic rupture of the left ventricular free wall (usually 3 to 7 days after myocardial infarction) leads to immediate cardiac tamponade and shock with as little as 150 mL blood in the pericardium.[73-75] Survival requires emergency surgery.[74,75] Similar situations may develop with bleeding into the pericardium after blunt chest trauma or thrombolytic therapy. Pericardial tamponade due to malignant or inflammatory pericardial effusions usually develop much more slowly. Although shock may still develop, it usually requires substantially more pericardial fluid (1 to 2 L) to cause critical failure of right ventricular diastolic filling.[73] No large reliable studies examining mortality rates with and without therapy in these conditions are available due to the small numbers of cases.

A similar time course–dependent risk is seen with major pulmonary emboli. In those without preexisting cardiopulmonary disease, a massive embolus involving two or more lobar arteries and 50% to 60% of the vascular bed[76,77] may result in obstructive shock. However, if recurrent smaller pulmonary emboli result in right ventricular hypertrophy, a substantially larger total occlusion of the pulmonary vascular bed may be required to cause right ventricular decompensation. Analyses have suggested that the presence of shock due to pulmonary embolus (regardless of underlying chronic cardiopulmonary dysfunction) indicates a three- to sevenfold increase in mortality risk with the majority of deaths occurring within an hour of presentation.[78,79] An analysis of more than 70,000 unstable (hemodynamic instability or ventilator-requiring) patients with pulmonary embolus in the national inpatient sample shows that mortality in untreated patients is approximately 47%.[80] Systemic thrombolysis is associated with a substantial reduction in mortality to 15%. Where available, catheter-directed therapy may be even more efficacious with a lower risk of serious hemorrhage.[81] Shock due to pulmonary embolism is an indication for urgent thrombolytic or catheter-directed intervention.

DISTRIBUTIVE SHOCK

The defining feature of distributive shock is loss of peripheral resistance. Septic shock is the most common form and has the greatest impact on intensive care unit (ICU) morbidity and mortality.

Hemodynamically, distributive shock is characterized by an overall decrease in SVR (see Table 21.1). However, resistance in any specific organ bed or tissue may be decreased, increased, or unchanged. Initially, CI may be depressed and ventricular filling pressures decreased. After fluid resuscitation, when filling pressures are normalized or increased, CI is usually elevated. Due to hypotension, left and right ventricular stroke work indices are normally decreased. MVo_2 is increased above normal. Concomitantly, arteriovenous oxygen content difference is narrowed despite the fact that oxygen demand is usually increased (particularly in sepsis). The basis of this phenomenon may be that because total body perfusion (CI) is increased, perfusion is not effective in that either it does not reach the necessary tissues or the tissues cannot utilize the substrates presented. As a reflection of this inadequate "effective" tissue perfusion, lactic acidosis may ensue. Clinical characteristics of resuscitated distributive shock include, in contrast to the other forms of shock, warm, well-perfused extremities, a decreased diastolic blood pressure, and an increased pulse pressure. Nonspecific signs of shock include tachycardia, tachypnea, decreased urine output, and altered mentation. In addition, evidence of the primary insult may exist (urticaria for anaphylaxis, spinal injury for neurogenic shock, and evidence of infection in septic shock).

Septic shock (shock due to infection) and sepsis-associated multiple organ failure are the most common causes of death in ICUs of the industrialized world. As many as 800,000 cases of sepsis are admitted every year to American hospitals (comparable to the incidence of first myocardial infarctions) with half of those developing septic shock and about half of those (200,000) dying.[82] Since the 1970s there has been a progressive increase in the incidence of and total deaths from sepsis and septic shock.[5] The total toll of septic deaths is comparable to deaths from myocardial infarction and far exceeds the impact of illnesses such as AIDS or breast cancer.[82,83]

Septic shock is caused by the systemic activation of the inflammatory cascade. Numerous mediators including cytokines, kinins, complement, coagulation factors, and eicosanoids are activated or systemically released, resulting in profound disturbances of cardiovascular and organ system function[84] (Table 21.2). These mediators, particularly tumor necrosis factor α (TNFα), interleukin-1β (IL-1β), platelet activating factor (PAF), and prostaglandins are thought to mediate reduced peripheral vascular resistance seen in septic shock.

Loss of vascular autoregulatory control may explain some of the typical metabolic findings of sepsis and septic shock. An early theory postulated the existence of microanatomic shunts between the arterial and venous circulations. During sepsis, these shunts were said to result in decreased SVR and increased MVo_2.[85] However, although microanatomic shunting has been noted in localized areas of inflammation, systemic evidence of this phenomenon in sepsis and septic shock is lacking.[85-89] "Functional" shunting due to defects of microcirculatory regulation in sepsis has also been suggested.[90,91] Overperfusion of tissues with low metabolic requirements would increase MVo_2 and narrow the arteriovenous oxygen content difference. Relative vasoconstriction of vessels supplying more metabolically active tissues would result in tissue hypoxia and lactate production due to anaerobic metabolism. Observations that some capillary beds may be occluded by platelet microaggregates, leukocytes, fibrin deposits, and endothelial damage support this theory.[86,90,92] Additional support comes from studies that demonstrate evidence of oxygen supply–dependent oxygen consumption in sepsis.[93-97] A third theory suggests that circulating mediators cause an intracellular metabolic defect involving substrate utilization, which results in bioenergetic failure (decreased high-energy phosphate production) and lactate production.[98,99] Increased mixed venous oxygen saturation could then be explained by perfusion, which is increased in excess of tissue oxygen utilization capability. However,

Table 21.2 Inflammatory Mediators in Sepsis and Septic Shock

Mediator	Major Reported Effects
Pro-inflammatory Cytokines	
Tumor necrosis factor-α (TNFα)	Stimulates release of interleukin-1, interleukin-6, interleukin-8, platelet-activating factor, leukotrienes, thromboxane A_2, prostaglandins; may be able to stimulate macrophages directly to promote its own release Stimulates production of polymorphonuclear cells by bone marrow; enhances phagocytic activity of polymorphonuclear cells Promotes adhesion of endothelial cells, polymorphonuclear cells, eosinophils, basophils, monocytes, and, occasionally, lymphocytes by inducing increased expression of adhesion molecules Activates common pathway of coagulation and complement system Directly toxic to vascular endothelial cells; increases microvascular permeability Acts directly on hypothalamus to produce fever Reduces transmembrane potential of muscle cells and depresses myocardial contractility Decreases arterial pressure, systemic vascular resistance, and ventricular ejection fraction; increases cardiac output
Interleukin-1β (IL-1β)	Stimulates release of TNF, interleukin-6, interleukin-8, platelet-activating factor, leukotrienes, thromboxane A_2, prostaglandins; may also be capable of stimulating its own production Activates resting T cells to produce lymphocytes and other products; supports B-cell proliferation and antibody production; is cytotoxic for insulin-producing B cells Promotes adhesion of endothelial cells, polymorphonuclear cells, eosinophils, basophils, monocytes, and, occasionally, lymphocytes by inducing increased expression of adhesion molecules Promotes polymorphonuclear cell activation and accumulation Increases endothelial procoagulant activity Acts synergistically with TNF; enhances tissue cell sensitivity to TNF Depresses myocardial contractility Acts directly on hypothalamus to produce fever
Interleukin-2	May promote release of TNF and interferon-gamma Decreases arterial pressure, systemic vascular resistance, and ejection fraction; increases cardiac output
Interleukin-4	Enhances lymphocyte adhesion to endothelial cells Induces antigen expression on macrophages Synergistically increases TNF- or interleukin-1-induced antigen expression on endothelial cells, but inhibits the increased expression of adhesion molecules by TNF, interleukin-1, or interferon-gamma
Interleukin-6	Induction of hepatic acute phase protein response Induces myelomonocytic and terminal B lymphocyte differentiation; activates T cells/thymocytes May contribute to septic myocardial depression Inhibits TNF production
Interleukin-8	Chemotactic for both neutrophils and lymphocytes; induces tissue infiltration of both Inhibits endothelial-leukocyte adhesion; decreases the hyperadhesion induced by those molecules
Interleukin-17	Induces synthesis of TNF-α, IL-1β, IL-6, G-CSF, GM-CSF, TGF-β, and other chemokines
Interleukin-18	Initiates cell-mediated immune response Increases secretion of interferon-γ
Interferon-γ	Promotes release of TNF, interleukin-1, interleukin-6 (possibly due to its ability to augment effects of endotoxin on macrophages); augments production of adhesion molecules May act synergistically with TNF to produce cytotoxic and cytostatic activity; interacts with other cytokines in variable ways Encourages polymorphonuclear cell activation and accumulation; enhances the phagocytic activity of polymorphonuclear cells Promotes macrophage activation, macrophage microbicidal function, and expression of cellular receptors for TNF-α
Macrophage migration inhibitory factor (MIF)	Increases TNF-α and TLR4 expression Activates T-lymphocytes Increases mortality in experimental peritonitis
High-mobility group box protein-1 (HMGB1)	Possesses both cytokine and intracellular signaling activity May generate late organ failure of sepsis Impairs vascular endothelial integrity

Continued on following page

Table 21.2 Inflammatory Mediators in Sepsis and Septic Shock (Continued)

Mediator	Major Reported Effects
Anti-inflammatory Cytokines	
Interleukin-4	Induction of differentiation of naïve helper T cells to Th2 cells
Interleukin-10	Down-regulation of macrophage function, leading to decreased TNF-α release
Interleukin-1 receptor antagonist (IL-1RA)	Antagonistic blockade of IL-1β
Transforming growth factor β1 (TGFβ)	Broad immunomodulatory activity (protective in endotoxic shock) Inhibition of effect of proinflammatory cytokines on a variety of tissues Suppression of macrophage pro-inflammatory responses Interference with phagocytic activation
Endothelial Factors	
Endothelin 1	Strongly promotes vasoconstriction
Nitric oxide	Mediates vascular smooth muscle relaxation and arteriovenular dilatation in septic shock May be responsible for septic myocardial depression Involved in leukocyte/macrophage antimicrobial activity
Arachidonic Acid Pathway Factors and Metabolites	
Phospholipase A_2	Releases arachidonic acid (the precursor of eicosanoids such as leukotrienes, prostaglandins, and thromboxanes) Decreases arterial pressure, systemic vascular resistance, and ventricular ejection fraction; increases cardiac output
Leukotrienes	Promote neutrophil chemotaxis and adhesion of neutrophils to endothelium (neutrophils have specific receptors for leukotriene B_4) Increase vascular permeability, either directly or through interaction of neutrophils and endothelial cells Decrease coronary blood flow and myocardial contractility
Thromboxane A_2	Produces vasoconstriction of vascular beds; secondarily promotes release of endothelium-derived relaxing factor and may stimulate prostacyclin production Causes platelet aggregation and neutrophil accumulation Increases vascular permeability; enhances permeability of both single- and double-unit membranes Produces pulmonary bronchoconstriction
Prostaglandin E_2	Inhibits interleukin-1 production Low concentrations stimulate TNF release; higher concentrations suppress TNF production at a dose-dependent level Causes vasodilation and increased blood flow Has a beneficial effect on tissue perfusion and may thereby decrease the severity of tissue damage Acts synergistically with prostacyclin to increase the effects of serotonin and bradykinin on vascular permeability
Prostacyclin (prostaglandin I_2)	Inhibits platelet aggregation and adhesion Causes vasodilation and increased blood flow; in early sepsis, exerts a beneficial effect on tissue perfusion Produces smooth muscle relaxation
Others	
Platelet-activating factor	Stimulates release of TNF, leukotrienes, thromboxane A_2 Promotes leukocyte activation and subsequent free-radical formation Encourages platelet aggregation leading to thrombosis Markedly alters microvascular permeability, thereby promoting microvascular fluid loss Exerts a negative inotropic effect on the heart; lowers arterial blood pressure
Complement fragment C3a	Causes mast cell degranulation and vasodilatory mediator release
Fragment C5a	Causes smooth muscle contraction and mucous secretion Causes mast cells to degranulate and release vasodilatory mediators Promotes TNF release Enhances polymorphonuclear cell activation, migration, adherence, and aggregation Induces capillary leakage May decrease systemic vascular resistance and produce hypotension

Adapted from Bone RC: The pathogenesis of sepsis. Ann Intern Med 1991;115:457.

animal studies using nuclear magnetic resonance (NMR) spectroscopy demonstrate that high-energy phosphates are not depleted in septic animals as is expected in all of these theories.[100-102] According to these and other studies, cellular ischemia is not the dominant factor in metabolic dysfunction in sepsis.[100-106] Rather, circulating mediators may result in cellular dysfunction, aerobic glycolysis, and lactate production in the absence of global ischemia.[101] This position is weakened by data suggesting that increased lactate in septic shock is also associated with decreased pH (which would not be expected in aerobic glycolysis)[101] and, to some extent, by studies that support the existence of oxygen supply–dependent oxygen consumption in sepsis.[94-97]

The trigger for systemic activation of the inflammatory cascade is the presence of gram-negative bacilli in 50% to 75% of cases of septic shock. Gram-positive bacteria account for most of the remainder, but infection with fungi, protozoa, and viruses can also result in septic shock.[107-109] Investigations suggest a surprising commonality of signaling mechanisms in septic shock via Toll-like receptors from a broad range of etiologic agents.[110-114] Despite aggressive supportive care and antibiotic treatment, mortality is 50% overall and may exceed 70% for gram-negative septic shock.[107] Of those succumbing to septic shock, approximately 75% are early deaths (within 1 week of shock), primarily due to hyperdynamic circulatory failure.[115] Late mortality is usually due to MODS.[115]

More than any other form of shock, distributive and, particularly, septic shock involves substantial elements of the hemodynamic characteristics of other shock categories (see Fig. 21.1, Table 21.1). As noted, all forms of distributive shock involve decreased mean peripheral vascular resistance. Prior to fluid resuscitation, distributive shock also involves a relative hypovolemic component. The first element of this relative hypovolemia is an increase of the vascular capacitance due to venodilatation. This phenomenon has been directly supported in animal models of sepsis[116-120] and is reinforced by the fact that clinical hypodynamic septic shock (low cardiac output) can usually be converted to hyperdynamic shock (high cardiac output) with adequate fluid resuscitation.[115,121,122] Relaxation of vascular smooth muscle is attributed to a number of the mediators known to circulate during sepsis. These same mediators also contribute to the second cause of hypovolemia in sepsis, third-spacing of fluid to the interstitium due to a loss of endothelial integrity. In addition, a number of studies have demonstrated that human septic shock is characterized by myocardial depression (biventricular dilatation and decreased ejection fraction).[32-34] Circulating substances such as TNFα, IL-1β, platelet activating factor (PAF), leukotrienes, and, most recently, interleukin-6 (IL-6) have been implicated in this process.[123-130]

Anaphylactic shock is a form of distributive shock caused by the release of mediators from tissue mast cells and circulating basophils. Anaphylaxis, an immediate hypersensitivity reaction, is mediated by the interaction of IgE antibodies on the surface of mast cells and basophils with the appropriate antigen. Antigen binding results in the release of the primary mediators of anaphylaxis contained in the basophilic granules of mast cells and basophils. These include histamine, serotonin, eosinophil chemotactic factor, and various proteolytic enzymes.[131] Subsequently, a number of secondary lipid mediators are synthesized and released including PAF, bradykinin prostaglandins, and leukotrienes (slow-reacting substance of anaphylaxis).[131] An anaphylactoid reaction (clinically indistinguishable from anaphylaxis) results from the direct, nonimmunologic release of mediators from mast cells and basophils and can also result in shock.

Anaphylaxis is triggered by insect envenomations (*Hymenoptera* bees, hornets, and wasps) and certain drugs, especially antibiotics (beta-lactams, cephalosporins, sulfonamides, vancomycin).[131] In addition, less frequently, heterologous serum (e.g., tetanus antitoxin, snake antitoxin, antilymphocyte antisera), blood transfusion, immunoglobulin (particularly in IgA-deficient patients), and egg-based vaccine products have been implicated.[131] Anaphylactoid reactions can be caused by a wide range of medical agents including ionic contrast media, protamine, opiates, polysaccharide volume expanders such as dextran and hydroxyethyl starch, muscle relaxants, and anesthetics.[131]

The hemodynamic features of anaphylactic shock are very similar to those for septic shock and include elements of hypovolemia (due to interstitial edema and venodilatation) and myocardial depression.[132-136] Cardiac output and ventricular filling pressures may be reduced until patients are fluid resuscitated.[136,137] In addition to typical findings of shock, patients may demonstrate urticaria, angioedema, laryngeal edema, and severe bronchospasm.

Neurogenic shock involves the loss of peripheral vasomotor control due to dysfunction or injury of the nervous system. The classic example is shock associated with spinal injury. A similar phenomenon is active in vasovagal syncope and spinal anesthesia, but such conditions are self-limited and transient. The major cause of shock in spinal injury appears to be loss of venous tone resulting in increased venous capacitance. Arteriolar tone may also be affected, resulting in increased cardiac output after fluid resuscitation.

Adrenal crisis (see also Chapter 59) is an uncommon cause of shock, which can be difficult to diagnose as it occurs in patients with other active disease processes and the clinical features may mimic infection. It is a life-threatening emergency that requires prompt diagnosis and management.

Adrenal crisis is caused by a deficiency of adrenal production of mineralocorticoids and glucocorticoids. It may occur de novo in patients with critical illness or may occur against a background of occult adrenal insufficiency. In the critical care setting, the most common cause of de novo acute adrenal insufficiency is bilateral adrenal hemorrhage in association with overwhelming infections (classically meningococcal, but frequently gram-negative bacteria), human immunodeficiency virus infection, or anticoagulation.[138,139] In addition, fungal infections such as histoplasmosis, blastomycosis, and coccidioidomycosis and malignant infiltration of the adrenals may cause acute adrenal insufficiency in ICU patients.[139] In some patients, steroid production remains adequate for the baseline state despite adrenal disease. Once stressed, however, the adrenal response is inadequate, leading to decompensation and adrenal crisis. Stressors may be relatively innocuous or may be severe. A febrile illness, infection, trauma, surgery, dehydration, or any other intercurrent illness may trigger the crisis. Abrupt cessation of glucocorticoid therapy or replacement may also result in adrenal crisis.

Symptoms are generally nonspecific and may include anorexia, nausea, vomiting, diarrhea, abdominal pain, myalgia, joint pains, headache, weakness, confusion, and agitation or delirium.[139,140] Fever (often out of proportion to any minor infection) is almost always present, and hypotension, initially due to hypovolemia, is frequent.[139] The initial hemodynamic pattern may resemble hypovolemic shock (if shock is due only to adrenal crisis). With volume resuscitation, a high output, vasopressor-refractory shock may become apparent.[141,142]

Shock due to adrenal crisis may be masked by or contribute to shock due to other concomitant critical illnesses, particularly septic shock. Thus, if vasopressor-refractory shock occurs in patients potentially predisposed to adrenal insufficiency, a cortisol level and rapid adrenocorticotropic hormone (ACTH) stimulation test must be performed and the patient given glucocorticoids and other therapy.

An unrecognized "relative" adrenal insufficiency has been implicated in the pathogenesis of human septic shock.[143-147] In this circumstance, sepsis is associated with a suboptimal adrenal response with an improvement in cardiovascular parameters or outcome with "stress" dose corticosteroid administration.[143,145,146,148,149] One randomized controlled trial has suggested that prospective "stress dose" therapy with a combination of hydrocortisone (50 mg intravenous every 6 hours) and fludrocortisone (50 μg oral/nasogastric daily) for 7 days improved outcome in nonresponders to corticotropin challenge.[150] Unfortunately, confirmatory randomized trials have failed to reproduce this finding.[151,152]

COMPENSATORY RESPONSES TO SHOCK

Shock is usually not a discrete condition occurring abruptly after injury or infection. With the onset of hemodynamic stress, homeostatic compensatory mechanisms engage to maintain effective tissue perfusion. At this time, subtle clinical evidence of hemodynamic stress may be apparent (tachycardia, decreased urine output), but overt evidence of shock (hypotension, altered sensorium, metabolic acidosis) may not. Therapeutic interventions have a high probability of preventing ischemic tissue injury and initiation of systemic inflammatory cascades during this early compensated stage. Adaptive compensatory mechanisms fail and organ injury ensues if the injury that initiates shock is too extensive or progresses despite therapy. As the duration of established shock increases, therapy is less likely to be effective in preventing organ failure and death.

Various sensing mechanisms involved in physiologic compensatory responses exist to recognize hemodynamic and metabolic dyshomeostasis (Fig. 21.2). Low-pressure right atrial and pulmonary artery stretch receptors sense volume changes. A decrease in circulating volume (or an increase of venous capacitance) results in an increase in sympathetic discharge from the medullary vasomotor center.[153,279,280] Aortic arch, carotid, and splanchnic high pressure baroreceptors sense early blood pressure changes close to the physiologic range.[153,279,280] An increase of sympathetic discharge from the medullary vasomotor center results from a small to moderate decrease in blood pressure associated with early shock. However, once mean arterial pressure falls below about 80 to 90 mm Hg, aortic baroreceptor activity is absent. Subsequently, carotid baroreceptor response is eliminated as mean pressure falls below 60 mm Hg. As blood pressure falls further, carotid and aortic chemoreceptors, sensitive to decreased P_{O_2}, increased P_{CO_2}, and increased hydrogen ion concentrations (decreased pH), dominate the response. These receptor complexes, active only when mean blood pressure is less than approximately 80 mm Hg, are of minimal relevance during physiologic states.[153] During shock, they make a substantial contribution to increases of sympathetic tone.

During severe shock, the most powerful stimulus to sympathetic tone is the central nervous system ischemic response.[153] The lower medullary chemoreceptors for this response (thought to be sensitive to increased CO_2 associated with decreased cerebral perfusion) become active when mean blood pressure falls below 60 mm Hg. Sympathetic stimulation provided by these receptors peaks at mean pressures of 15 to 20 mm Hg and results in maximal stimulation of the cardiovascular system.[153] The Cushing response to increased intracranial pressure is an example of activation of this reflex under different circumstances.

Other mechanisms also play a role in the compensatory response to shock. Vasopressin release is regulated by alterations of serum osmolality. During effective hypovolemia due to intravascular volume loss or increased vascular capacitance, low-pressure, right atrial stretch receptors can override osmolar control of vasopressin response to result in the retention of body water.[153,281] Similarly, during hypovolemia and shock, the juxtaglomerular apparatus in the kidneys responds to decreased perfusion pressure by renin release.[153]

All compensatory responses to shock, whether hemodynamic, metabolic, or biochemical, support oxygen delivery to vital organs. These responses are similar (to varying extents) for different classes of shock and can be broken down into four components: (1) preserving mean circulatory pressure (a measure of venous pressure) by either maintaining total intravascular volume or increasing stressed volume (i.e., increasing venous tone), (2) optimizing cardiac performance, (3) redistributing perfusion to vital organs, and (4) optimizing the unloading of oxygen at the tissues (Box 21.3, Fig. 21.E3).

Mean circulatory pressure and venous return are sustained in early shock by a number of mechanisms. Acutely, total intravascular volume is supported by alterations of capillary hydrostatic pressure as described by Starling.[282] Sympathetic activation results in precapillary vasoconstriction. In combination with initial hypotension, this results in decreased capillary hydrostatic pressure.[282] A decrease in capillary hydrostatic pressure enhances intravascular fluid shift due to maintained plasma oncotic pressures. Transcapillary fluid influx following the removal of 500- to 1000-mL blood volumes in humans can be as high as 2 mL/minute with full correction of intravascular volume by 24 to 48 hours.[283] The intravascular volume may also be supported by the osmotic activity of glucose generated by glycogenolysis. Increased extracellular osmolarity results in fluid redistribution from the intracellular to the extracellular space.

Intravascular volume is also conserved by decreasing renal fluid losses. Renal compensatory mechanisms are of limited value in acute shock but can have more impact in the subacute phase. Decreased renal perfusion associated with reduced cardiac output and afferent arteriolar

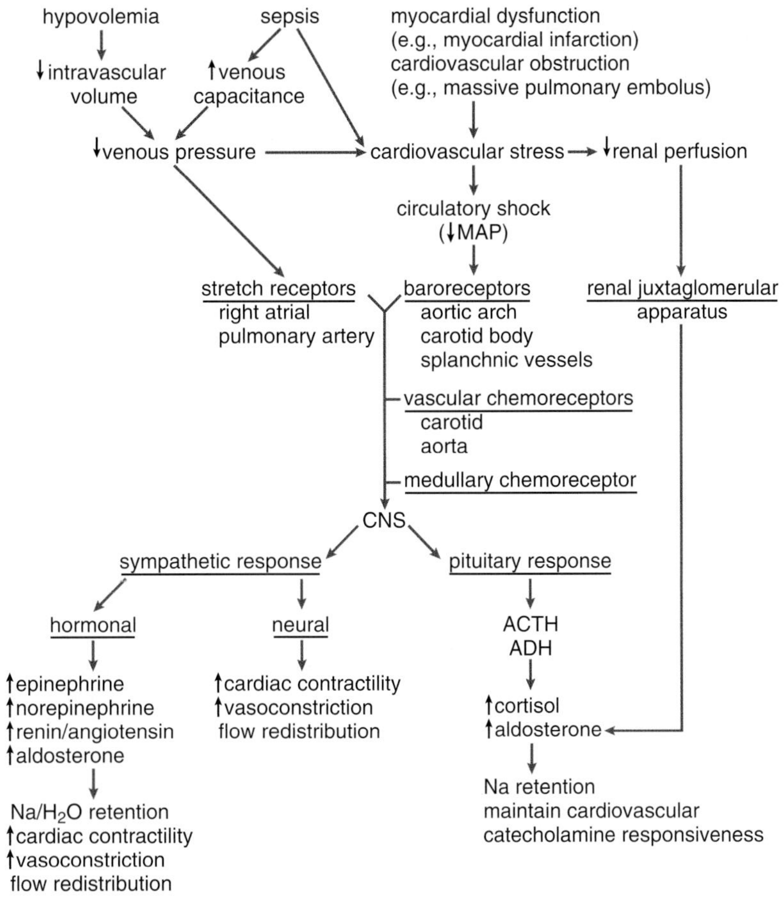

Figure 21.2 Neurohormonal response to shock. During early cardiovascular stress, the neurohormonal response may be limited to increased activity of the juxtaglomerular apparatus and stimulation of right atrial and pulmonary artery low-pressure mechanoreceptors. With further hypotension, high-pressure vascular baroreceptors, vascular chemoreceptors, and the medullary chemoreceptor are sequentially stimulated, resulting in augmented neurohormonal activity with increased pituitary hormone (ACTH and ADH) release and increased sympathetic outflow from the central nervous system. Volume retention, increased venous tone, increased cardiac contractility, and blood flow redistribution to vital organs results.

constriction results in a fall in glomerular filtration rate and urine output. In addition, decreased renal perfusion pressure, sympathetic stimulation, and compositional changes in tubular fluid[153] result in renin release from the juxtaglomerular apparatus. Renin release leads to the adrenal cortical release of aldosterone (via angiotensin II), which increases sodium reabsorption in the distal tubules of the kidney in exchange for potassium or hydrogen ion.[153] Angiotensin II also exerts a powerful direct vasoconstricting effect (particularly on mesenteric vessels) while increasing sympathetic outflow and adrenal epinephrine release. As noted, vasopressin (antidiuretic hormone) release occurs through activation of right atrial low pressure. Angiotensin II augments this release by increasing sympathetic outflow. The release of vasopressin from the posterior pituitary results in water retention at the expense of osmolarity. Hyponatremia can result. Vasopressin, like angiotensin II, also results in vasoconstriction, particularly of the splanchnic circulation.

Finally, increased sympathetic activity and release of adrenal epinephrine results in systemic venoconstriction, particularly of the venous capacitance vessels of the splanchnic circulation. This supports mean circulatory pressure and venous return by increasing stressed volume.

Increased sympathetic nervous system activity accounts for most of the enhancement of cardiac performance during shock. Local release of norepinephrine by sympathetic nerves and the systemic release of epinephrine result in the stimulation of cardiac alpha and beta-adrenergic receptors resulting in increases of heart rate and contractility that optimize cardiac output and support blood pressure. Angiotensin II may also exert direct as well as indirect (sympathetic stimulation) inotropic effects on myocardium. Improved cardiac function also results in decreased right atrial pressure, which tends to increase venous return.

Redistribution of blood flow during shock has already been discussed. Increased sympathetic vasoconstrictor tone, systemic release of epinephrine from the adrenals, vasopressin, endothelin, and angiotensin II cause vasoconstriction in all sensitive vascular beds including the skin, skeletal muscle, kidneys, and splanchnic organs.[154] Dominant autoregulatory control of blood flow spares brain and heart blood work from these effects. Redistribution of flow to these vital organs is the effective result.

The effects of decreased delivery of oxygen to the tissues during shock can be attenuated by local adaptive responses. Hypoperfusion and tissue ischemia will result in local acidosis due to decreased clearance of CO_2 and anaerobic metabolism. Local acidosis decreases the affinity between oxygen and hemoglobin at the capillary level.[153] The resultant rightward shift of the oxyhemoglobin dissociation curve allows

Box 21.3 Cardiovascular/Metabolic Compensatory Responses to Shock

Maintain Mean Circulatory Pressure (Venous Pressure)

Volume
Fluid redistribution to vascular space (increased total vascular volume)
- From interstitium (Starling effect)
- From intracellular space (osmotic)

Decreased renal fluid losses
- Decreased glomerular filtration rate (GFR)
- Increased aldosterone
- Increased vasopressin

Pressure
Decreased venous capacitance (increased stressed volume)
- Increased sympathetic activity
- Increased circulating (adrenal) epinephrine
- Increased angiotensin
- Increased vasopressin

Maximize Cardiac Performance

Increased contractility
Sympathetic stimulation
Adrenal stimulation

Redistribute Perfusion

Extrinsic regulation of systemic arterial tone
Dominant autoregulation of vital organs (heart, brain)

Optimize Oxygen Unloading

Increased RBC 2,3 DPG
Tissue acidosis
Pyrexia
Decreased tissue Po_2

Table 21.3 Organ System Dysfunction in Shock

Central Nervous System	Encephalopathy (ischemic or septic) Cortical necrosis
Heart	Tachycardia, bradycardia Supraventricular tachycardia Ventricular ectopy Myocardial ischemia Myocardial depression
Pulmonary System	Acute respiratory failure Acute respiratory distress syndrome
Kidney	Prerenal failure Acute tubular necrosis
Gastrointestinal System	Ileus Erosive gastritis Pancreatitis Acalculous cholecystitis Colonic submucosal hemorrhage Transluminal translocation of bacteria/antigens
Liver	Ischemic hepatitis "Shock" liver Intrahepatic cholestasis
Hematologic System	Disseminated intravascular coagulation Dilutional thrombocytopenia
Metabolic	Hyperglycemia Glycogenolysis Gluconeogenesis Hypoglycemia (late) Hypertriglyceridemia
Immune System	Gut barrier function depression Cellular immune depression Humoral immune depression

greater unloading of oxygen from hemoglobin for a given Po_2. Tissue ischemia is also accompanied by decreased tissue Po_2 (relative to normal), which further augments the unloading of oxygen. Pyrexia associated with sepsis may also contribute to a rightward shift of the oxyhemoglobin dissociation curve, whereas hypothermia is associated with a leftward shift. For that reason, maintenance of normothermia during resuscitation from shock helps to optimize oxygen unloading.

ORGAN SYSTEM DYSFUNCTION DUE TO SHOCK (TABLE 21.3)

CENTRAL NERVOUS SYSTEM

Central nervous system neurons are extremely sensitive to ischemia. Fortunately, the central nervous system vascular supply is highly resistant to extrinsic regulatory mechanisms. Although cerebral perfusion is clearly impaired in shock, flow remains relatively well preserved until the later stages.[284,285] Absent primary cerebrovascular impairment, cerebral function is well supported until mean arterial pressure falls below approximately 50 to 60 mm Hg.[286] Eventually, irreversible ischemic injury may occur to the most sensitive areas of the brain (cerebral cortex). Before this fixed injury, an altered level of consciousness, varying from confusion to unconsciousness, may be seen depending on the degree of perfusion deficit. Disturbances of acid/base/electrolytes may also contribute. Electroencephalographic (EEG) recordings demonstrate nonspecific changes compatible with encephalopathy. Sepsis-related encephalopathy may occur at higher blood pressures (due in part to the effects of circulating inflammatory mediators) and is associated with increased mortality.[287]

HEART

The major clinically apparent manifestations of shock on the heart are due to sympathoadrenal stimulation. Increased heart rate, in the absence of disturbances of cardiac conduction, is almost universally present. Vagally mediated paradoxical bradycardia may seen on occasion in severe hemorrhage.[40] In patients predisposed to myocardial ischemia or irritability, catecholamine-driven supraventricular tachycardias and ventricular ectopy with ischemic electrocardiogram (ECG) changes are not common. Like the brain, the blood supply to the heart is autoregulated. This, in combination with the resilient nature of myocardial tissue, renders it resistant to sympathetically driven vasoconstriction and shock-related hypoperfusion injury. Overt necrosis does not typically occur, although evidence of cellular injury may be present.

Most forms of shock are associated with increased contractility of healthy myocardium. Regardless, shock can have a substantial impact on myocardial contractility and compliance. Hypotension during cardiogenic (and other forms of shock) is associated with decreased coronary artery perfusion pressure. In patients with coronary artery disease or increased filling pressures, decreased coronary artery perfusion pressure may lead to overt ischemia. Further, circulating myocardial depressant substances contribute to myocardial depression in septic[229] and hemorrhagic[230] shock. This has been linked to decreased beta adrenoreceptor affinity and density as well as potential defects of intracellular signal transduction involving nitric oxide, G proteins, cAMP, and cGMP.[126] Circulating depressant substances may also be present during cardiogenic shock.[232]

RESPIRATORY SYSTEM

Early alterations of pulmonary function seen during acute circulatory shock are primarily related to changes in central drive or muscle fatigue. Increased minute volume occurs as a result of augmented respiratory drive due to peripheral stimulation of pulmonary J receptors and carotid body chemoreceptors as well as hypoperfusion of the medullary respiratory center. This results in hypocapnia and primary respiratory alkalosis.[153,288] With increased minute volume and decreased cardiac output, the V/Q ratio increases. Unless arterial hypoxemia complicates shock, pulmonary resistance is initially unchanged or minimally increased. Coupled with an increased workload, respiratory and diaphragmatic muscle impairment due to hypoperfusion (manifested by decreased transmembrane electrical potential) may lead to early respiratory failure.[289] Adult respiratory distress syndrome (ARDS) due to inflammatory or free radical injury to the alveolar capillary cell layers following established shock may develop as a late cause of respiratory failure.

KIDNEY

Acute renal failure is a major complication of circulatory shock with associated mortality rates between 35% and 80%.[290] Although initial injury manifested by decreased urine output occurs, other clinical manifestations of renal dysfunction (increased creatinine, urea, and potassium) may not be noted for 1 to 3 days. Once hemodynamic stabilization has been achieved, it becomes apparent that urine output does not immediately improve and both serum creatinine and urea continue to rise. The single most common cause of acute renal failure is renal hypoperfusion resulting in acute tubular necrosis (ATN). The most frequent cause of renal hypoperfusion is hemodynamic compromise from septic shock, hemorrhage, hypovolemia, trauma, and major operative procedures. ATN that occurs in the setting of circulatory shock is associated with a higher mortality than in other situations.

Part of the reason for the kidney's sensitivity to hypoperfusion has to do with the nature of its vascular supply. The renal vascular bed is moderately autoregulated. Increases of efferent arteriolar tone can initially maintain glomerular perfusion despite compromise of renal flow.[291] Renal hypoperfusion does not become critical until relatively late in shock when maximal vasoconstriction of renal preglomerular arterioles[291] results in cortical, then medullary, ischemic injury.

Decreased urine output in shock can pose a diagnostic dilemma, as it can be associated with both oliguric ATN and hypoperfusion-related prerenal failure without ATN. Indices suggestive of the latter include a benign urine sediment, a urine sodium concentration <20 mEq/L, fractional urine sodium excretion <1%, urine osmolality >450 mOsm/L, and a urine/plasma creatinine ratio >40. Useful markers of acute renal failure due to ATN include hematuria and heme granular casts, a urine sodium concentration >40 mEq/mL, fractional excretion of urine sodium to >2%, urine osmolarity <350 mOsm/L, and a urine:plasma creatinine ratio <20.[292] Of note, ATN caused by circulatory shock may be associated with urine sodium <20 mEq/L and fractional excretion < 1% if the acute renal injury is superimposed upon chronic effective volume depletion as may be seen with cirrhosis and congestive heart failure.[293]

GASTROINTESTINAL SYSTEM

The gut is relatively sensitive to circulatory failure. The splanchnic vasculature is highly responsive to sympathetic vasoconstriction. Typical clinical gut manifestations of hypoperfusion, sympathetic stimulation, and inflammatory injury associated with shock include ileus, erosive gastritis, pancreatitis, acalculous cholecystitis, and colonic submucosal hemorrhage. Enteric ischemia produced by circulatory shock and free radical injury with resuscitation may breach gut barrier integrity with translocation of enteric bacteria and antigens (notably endotoxin) from the gut lumen to the systemic circulation, resulting in the propagation and amplification of shock and MODS.[294,295]

LIVER

Like the gut, the liver is highly sensitive to hypotension and hypoperfusion injury. "Shock liver," associated with massive ischemic necrosis and major elevations of transaminases, is atypical in the absence of extensive hepatocellular disease on very severe insult.[296] Centrilobular injury with mild increases of transaminases and lactate dehydrogenase is more typical. Transaminases usually peak within 1 to 3 days of the insult and resolve over 3 to 10 days. In either case, early increases in bilirubin and alkaline phosphatase are modest. Despite the production of acute phase reactants in early circulatory shock, synthetic functions may be impaired with decreased generation of prealbumin, albumin, and hepatic coagulation factors. After hemodynamic resolution of shock, evidence of biliary stasis with increased bilirubin and alkaline phosphatase can develop, even though the patient is otherwise improving. Postshock MODS involves similar hepatic pathology.

HEMATOLOGIC SYSTEM

Hematologic manifestations of circulatory shock tend to depend on the nature of shock. Disseminated intravascular coagulation (DIC), characterized by microangiopathic hemolysis, consumptive thrombocytopenia, consumptive coagulopathy, and microthrombi with tissue injury, is most commonly seen in association with septic shock. Because it is due to simultaneous systemic activation of coagulation and fibrinolysis cascades, it can be differentiated from the coagulopathy of liver failure by determination of endothelial cell–produced factor 8 (normal or increased with hepatic dysfunction). In the absence of extensive tissue injury/trauma, hemorrhagic shock is rarely associated with DIC.[297] Dilutional thrombocytopenia is the most common cause of coagulation deficits after resuscitation for hemorrhage.[298]

METABOLIC ALTERATIONS

Metabolic alterations associated with shock occur in a predictable pattern. Early in shock, when hemodynamic instability triggers compensatory responses, sympathoadrenal activity is enhanced. Increased release of ACTH, glucocorticoids, and glucagon and a decreased release of insulin results in glycogenolysis, gluconeogenesis, and hyperglycemia.[281,299] An increased release of epinephrine results in skeletal muscle insulin resistance sparing glucose for use by glucose-dependent organs (heart and brain). Late in shock, hypoglycemia may develop, possibly due to glycogen depletion or failure of hepatic glucose synthesis. Fatty acids are increased early in shock but fall later as hypoperfusion of adipose containing peripheral tissue progresses. Hypertriglyceridemia is often seen during shock as a consequence of catecholamine stimulation and reduced lipoprotein lipase expression induced by circulating TNFα.[299] Increased catecholamines, glucocorticoids, and glucagon also increase protein catabolism, resulting in a negative nitrogen balance.[299]

IMMUNE SYSTEM

Immune dysfunction, frequent during and after circulatory shock and trauma, rarely has immediate adverse effects but likely contributes to late mortality. Underlying mechanisms of immune dysfunction include ischemic injury to barrier mucosa (particularly of the gut), leading to anatomic breaches (colonic ulceration) and potential mucosal translocation of bacteria and bacterial products; parenchymal tissue injury due to associated trauma, inflammation, ischemia or free radical injury; and direct ischemic or mediator (immunosuppressant cytokines, corticosteroids, prostaglandins, catecholamines, endorphins)-induced dysfunction of the cellular and humoral immune systems.[300,301] In particular, macrophage function is adversely affected during trauma and circulatory shock. A decrease in antigen presenting ability impairs the activation of T and B lymphocytes. Associated with this defect are a decrease in Ia antigen expression, a decrease in membrane IL-1β receptors, and the presence of suppressor T-lymphocytes. Phagocytic activity of the reticuloendothelial system is also compromised, partially due to an acute decrease in fibronectin levels. Suppression of T lymphocyte immune function is manifested by decreased responsiveness to antigenic stimulation and a decreased helper:suppressor ratio. Decreased production of IgG and IgM suggests B cell suppression. Nonspecific immune suppression is expressed as decreased neutrophil bactericidal function, chemotaxis, opsonization, and phagocytosis.

Resuscitation agents used in shock may also substantially depress immune function. For example, red blood cell transfusion used in traumatic hemorrhagic shock and in support of oxygen transport in septic shock[302] has been shown to suppress immune function and lead to increased infections (and improved allograft survival).[303,304] Similarly, dopamine, used for hemodynamic support in shock, has been shown to suppress pituitary production of prolactin (required for optimal immune function), thereby suppressing T-cell proliferative responses.[305] Thus, dopamine may contribute, along with stress-induced increases in immunosuppressive glucocorticoids, to T-cell anergy seen in critically ill patients.

All of these factors may contribute to the propensity of critically ill patients to develop ongoing organ system dysfunction as well as a variety of infections during the postshock phase. It is notable that one third to one half of patients with shock die late in their course following resolution of the acute shock phase.

DIAGNOSTIC APPROACH AND EVALUATION

Shock is always a life-threatening emergency. Diagnosis, evaluation, and management must often occur virtually simultaneously. The diagnosis must be made as early as possible while shock is well compensated. Once marked hypotension and hypoperfusion are present, mortality increases. Because early recognition and treatment are key to survival, the diagnosis is primarily a clinical one. Laboratory and imaging studies are useful for confirming the diagnosis and determining the specific shock etiology. However, therapy of shock should never be delayed in order to accommodate these studies. The initial diagnosis of shock can and should be made strictly on clinical signs and symptoms.

Because shock is the common end point of a variety of insults, evaluation and management for all forms of shock involve a common approach (Box 21.4).

CLINICAL EVALUATION

Impending shock is characterized by the typical compensatory response to cardiovascular stress. Tachycardia, tachypnea, and oliguria (<0.5 mL/kg/h) are usually present. Cool extremities are seen in hypodynamic shock. The blood pressure may be elevated or normal with maximal sympathetic stimulation. With progression, however, blood pressure falls, whereas pulse pressure narrows (except in the case of distributive shock). Frank hypotension (mean arterial pressure <60 to 65 mm Hg in adults) may ensue. The chronic level of blood pressure must be considered. Normotension in a normally hypertensive patient may denote a critical degree of hypoperfusion. With further progression anuria may develop, extremities may become mottled and dusky (except in distributive shock), and the sensorium may become clouded. It is important to note that clinical parameters can underestimate initial resuscitative requirements in critically ill subjects including those with septic shock.[306-309]

Other clinical manifestations of shock are useful for attempting to differentiate the etiology. Hypovolemic shock is characterized by decreased jugular venous pressure. Cardiogenic shock may evidence elevated jugular venous pressure with hepatojugular reflux, an S3, an S4, and regurgitant heart murmurs. Obstructive shock signs usually depend on the nature of the obstruction. Pulmonary embolus may be characterized by dyspnea and right-sided evidence of heart

Box 21.4 General Approach to Shock: Initial Diagnosis and Evaluation

Clinical (Primary Diagnosis)

Tachycardia, tachypnea, cyanosis, oliguria, encephalopathy (confusion), peripheral hypoperfusion (mottled extremities), hypotension (systolic blood pressure < 90 mm Hg)

Laboratory (Confirmatory)

Hemoglobin, WBC, platelets
PT/PTT
Electrolytes, arterial blood gases
Ca, Mg
BUN, creatinine
Serum lactate
ECG

Monitoring

Continuous ECG and respiratory monitors
Arterial pressure catheter
Central venous pressure monitor (uncomplicated shock)
Venous oximetry*
Pulmonary artery flotation catheter*
- Cardiac output
- Pulmonary artery occlusion pressure
- Central or mixed venous oxygen saturation (intermittent or continuous)

Oximetry*
Echocardiogram (functional assessment)*

Imaging

Chest x-ray
X-ray views of abdomen*
Computerized axial tomogram (CT scan)—abdomen or chest*
Echocardiogram (anatomic and functional assessment)*
Pulmonary perfusion scan*

*Optional.

failure. Cardiac tamponade may demonstrate Kussmaul's sign, a pulsus paradoxus and distant heart sounds. Septic shock in the absence of neutropenia usually exhibits a focus of infection along with fever, chills, and warm extremities. Patients with septic shock and neutropenia often have no clinically apparent focus. Elderly patients may present with little more than unexplained hyperventilation and hypotension.

LABORATORY STUDIES

Laboratory data are used to confirm the diagnosis of shock and to help clarify the etiology. Leukocyte count is frequently elevated early in shock due to demargination of neutrophils. Leukopenia may be found in sepsis and late shock. Hemoglobin concentration is variably affected depending on the etiology of shock. For example, nonhemorrhagic hypovolemic shock and septic shock with extravasation of intravascular water to the interstitium may result in an apparent erythrocytosis. Platelet count increases acutely with the stress of circulatory shock, but with progression of sepsis or resuscitation of massive hemorrhage, thrombocytopenia may occur. Arterial blood gases and electrolytes may demonstrate a nonanion gap acidosis if hypovolemic shock is associated with excessive diarrhea and metabolic alkalosis if associated with vomiting. An anion gap acidosis, often due to elevated levels of lactic acid, usually reflects prolonged inadequate tissue perfusion. Serum creatinine and blood urea nitrogen (BUN) are rarely changed after the acute onset of shock, even if renal injury is present. With slower onset of shock—for example, in sepsis—increased creatinine is common and early resolution is an excellent marker of effective resuscitation and survival. Markers of renal function can also be helpful diagnostically. An isolated increased BUN with anemia and normal creatinine may suggest gastrointestinal bleeding. An arterial blood gas will help to determine the adequacy of oxygenation and give evidence of acid base disturbances. An electrocardiogram (ECG) is critical for the diagnosis of ischemic cardiac injury either as a primary cause of cardiogenic shock or secondary to hypotension associated with shock of another etiology.

Lactate levels (particularly serial determinations) are of use in assessment of prognosis. Substantial data suggest that lactate levels, as a marker of tissue oxygen debt, can predict outcome in shock.[45,46,310-314] The utility of lactate assessment is limited by the fact that it is a relatively late marker of tissue hypoperfusion.[315,316] Significant tissue ischemia and injury are present by the time it is elevated. In addition, the liver clears lactate. Liver failure may markedly increase elevated lactate levels during hypoperfusion. Conversely, normal hepatic clearance may obscure limited lactate production by ischemic tissues. Glycolysis and alkalosis will also nonspecifically increase lactate levels.[317,318] However, since in the appropriate setting, arterial lactate levels beyond 2 mEq/L are associated with increased mortality,[46,50,312,313,319] such levels should be considered to represent tissue ischemia in the absence of another clearly defined etiology. The adequacy of resuscitation of shock can also be assessed using serial changes of systemic lactate.[314,319,320] Resolution of elevated lactate, however, may lag following the implementation of effective resuscitation.[321]

Central venous oxygen saturation can also be used to assess the prognosis and efficacy of resuscitation in shock states including septic shock.[302,309,322,323] However, central venous saturation, which has been suggested to represent a reliable marker of resuscitation efficacy in sepsis,[302] does not appear to correlate well with lactate clearance in some sepsis studies, perhaps reflecting elements other than oxygen debt in those conditions.[320] Poor correlation with mixed venous oxygen saturation has also been noted in septic shock.[324]

IMAGING

A chest radiograph is useful in ruling out pneumonia as a source of septic shock, pulmonary edema as a manifestation of cardiogenic shock, tension pneumothorax, pericardial tamponade, and so on. Although abdominal views may be helpful on occasion, intra-abdominal processes resulting in shock are usually clinically apparent. Computerized axial tomograms may be helpful in directing management in specific instances (occult internal hemorrhage, aortic dissection, pulmonary embolus). Similarly, transthoracic and transesophageal echocardiography can diagnose with great accuracy the specific repairable cardiac or aortic lesions associated with shock and can be highly suggestive of other important diagnoses including hemodynamically significant pulmonary embolus. Pulmonary perfusion scans are useful for confirming massive pulmonary embolism. Other imaging modalities have less of a role in the evaluation of acute shock.

INVASIVE HEMODYNAMIC MONITORING

All patients suspected of having circulatory shock should have an indwelling arterial pressure catheter placed. Blood pressure assessment by manual sphygmomanometry or automated noninvasive oscillometric techniques may be inaccurate during shock due to marked peripheral vasoconstriction.[325] In addition, neither technique supplies continuous monitoring of the rapidly changing hemodynamic status of unstable patients. Further, an arterial catheter allows ready access for arterial blood gas samples and other laboratory tests. In most cases, a peripheral site, such as the radial artery, is utilized. However, given the potential for disparity of pressures between central and peripheral sites,[326] if marked peripheral vasoconstriction due to either sympathetic stimulation or exogenous catecholamines obscures the peripheral pulses, a central site such as the femoral artery may be preferred.

Central venous pressure monitoring is frequently used during the perioperative period to assess the intravascular volume status in patients without critical illness. Because of the relatively stable hemodynamic status of these patients and the questionable benefit of pulmonary artery catheterization in these patients, such an approach is adequate. Similarly, CVP monitoring for otherwise healthy patients being resuscitated for hypovolemic shock may provide useful data. In the appropriate clinical context, CVP monitoring may also occasionally be useful in differentiating among different forms of shock (e.g., low CVP in hypovolemic shock, high CVP in cardiac tamponade). As a rule, though, CVP monitoring is inadequate for the hemodynamic assessment of critically ill patients, particularly those with shock. A number of studies have conclusively shown that central venous pressure does not accurately estimate left ventricular preload in critically ill patients.[327,328]

The use of the flow-directed balloon-tipped pulmonary artery catheters with thermodilution cardiac output determination capability has been the standard of practice for the hemodynamic assessment of circulatory shock. Their use is supported by a number of studies that demonstrate that experienced physicians cannot accurately determine cardiac filling pressures or cardiac output based on clinical evaluation alone.[329,330] In addition to cardiac output determination, pulmonary artery catheters provide continuous monitoring of central venous and pulmonary artery waveforms and pressures. Pulmonary artery occlusion pressure (as an estimate of left ventricular end-diastolic pressure and volume) and waveform can be obtained intermittently. Waveform analysis may be useful in cardiovascular diagnoses of cardiac tamponade, restrictive cardiomyopathy, congestive heart failure, ventricular hypertrophy, and mitral or tricuspid regurgitation. These devices also allow withdrawal of blood from the pulmonary artery, enabling the determination of MVo_2 in order to verify sufficient oxygen delivery during hypodynamic shock. In addition, they can demonstrate evidence of right heart and pulmonary artery oxygen saturation "stepups" for the diagnosis of left-to-right shunts associated with cardiac anatomic abnormalities such as ventricular septal defect. In shock, the flow-directed balloon-tipped pulmonary artery catheter is useful for etiologic classification, determination of optimal management, and to follow the response to therapy. Typical hemodynamic profiles of different forms of shock have been described in Table 21.1.

The utility of pulmonary artery catheterization has been questioned. In a case-matched study, researchers suggested that increased resource utilization and mortality were associated with the use of pulmonary artery catheters in the ICU.[331] A series of randomized studies performed since then have reported on the role of the pulmonary artery catheter (PAC) in the setting of major noncardiac surgery,[332] congestive heart failure (CHF),[333] sepsis and adult respiratory distress syndrome (ARDS),[334] acute lung injury,[335] and in the general ICU setting.[336,337] In the perioperative management of patients undergoing major noncardiac surgery, the use of a PAC did not impact mortality and was associated with a greater incidence of pulmonary embolism.[332] In critically ill patients diagnosed with CHF, management directed with the use of a PAC did not influence mortality but resulted in more in-hospital adverse events.[333] Another study comparing the use of a PAC versus central venous monitoring in acute lung injury found no difference in organ failure or mortality.[335] A large trial evaluating the role of the PAC in the management of patients with ARDS secondary to sepsis also found no significant differences in mortality if a PAC was utilized or not.[334] Two randomized studies of general ICU patients similarly concluded that the use of PAC among critically ill patients neither increased nor decreased mortality.[336,337] Most, although not all, meta-analyses have shown no consistent benefit with the PAC.[338-341] These studies failing to show a lack of clinical benefit have been paralleled by other studies questioning some of the basic premises of PAC utility. Several studies have shown a lack of correlation between PAOP/CVP and ventricular volumes in the critically ill.[342,343] One study has even demonstrated that PAOP and CVP fail to predict ventricular filling volume, cardiac performance, or the response to volume infusion in normal volunteer subjects.[344] Despite these data, no studies have examined the use of pulmonary artery catheters in cases of shock specifically. Nonetheless, the use of the PAC in the United States has decreased dramatically since the 1990s.[345]

One parameter that a pulmonary artery catheter uniquely provides is mixed venous oxygen saturation. This measure may assess the adequacy of resuscitation of low output states prior to the presence of anaerobic metabolism (as signified by increased lactate). MVo_2 rises with increases of perfusion above requirements and falls, with increasing oxygen extraction ratio, as perfusion becomes inadequate (Fig. 21.3). Normal MVo_2 falls within the 65% to 75% range. During myocardial infarction, saturations of less than 60% are found with congestive heart failure, and less than 40% with cardiogenic shock.[323] Lactate accumulation and supply-dependent oxygen consumption begin to appear as saturation levels fall below 30% to 40%.[346,347] MVo_2 is especially useful in determining whether low cardiac outputs indicate supply-dependent oxygen consumption (MVo_2 low) or normally depressed metabolic demands (normal MVo_2). Due to the maldistribution of perfusion in distributive shock (or

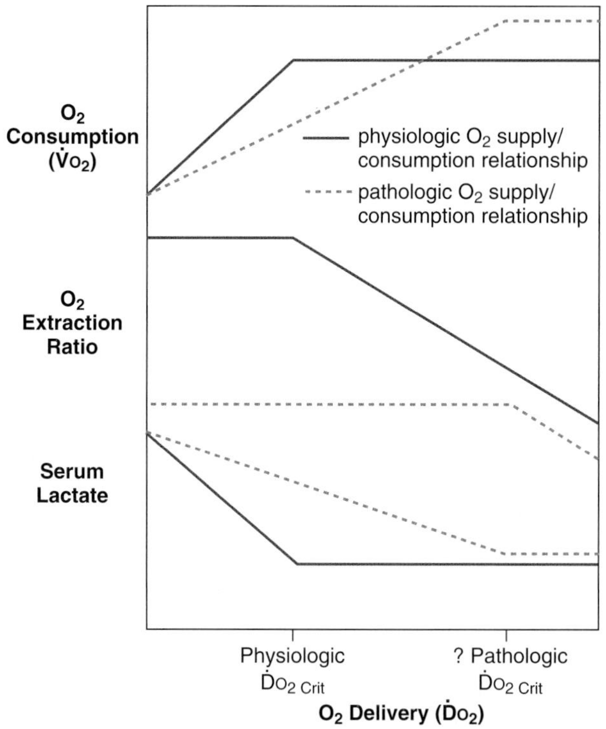

Figure 21.3 Oxygen supply–dependent oxygen consumption in shock. Physiologic supply–dependent oxygen consumption is characterized by a biphasic relationship between oxygen delivery (DO_2) and oxygen consumption (VO_2). The inflection point defines the physiologic critical oxygen delivery (DO_{2crit}). Below this DO_{2crit}, VO_2 is linearly dependent on DO_2, the oxygen extraction ratio is maximal, and lactate (indicating anaerobic metabolism) is produced. Above the physiologic DO_{2crit}, VO_2 is independent of DO_2, the oxygen extraction ratio varies to maintain a constant VO_2, and lactate is not produced.

substrate utilization defect in septic shock) and left-to-right shunting in cardiogenic shock associated with ventricular septal defects, MVO_2 is not useful in assessment in those conditions. Central venous oxygen saturation ($cSVO_2$) has been proposed as an alternate way to examine the adequacy of resuscitation.[302,309]

Oxygen delivery and oxygen consumption variables can also be determined using pulmonary artery catheter–derived data. Although such global perfusion data appear to have prognostic significance for large groups of the critically ill, their utility is controversial when applied to individual patients.

Modifications to the standard pulmonary artery flotation catheter allow continuous monitoring of MVO_2 or determination of right ventricular ejection fractions and volumes. Although both innovations have been utilized for clinical research purposes and each theoretically offers unique insights into shock, they have no defined role at this time in clinical shock management.

ANCILLARY MONITORING TECHNIQUES

OXIMETRY

Because oxygen delivery is dependent on arterial oxygen saturation, pulse oximetry should, in theory, provide useful data during circulatory shock. However, limitations of the technique include the fact that ambient light sources, dyshemoglobinemias (methemoglobin, carboxyhemoglobin), lipemia, and hypothermia can affect results.[348] Motion artifact may generate a false signal.[349] Shock-associated vasoconstriction also impairs signal aquisition. One study has shown that a cardiac index less than 2.4 L/min/m^2 is associated with signal loss.[350] Although these problems limit the utility of pulse oximetry in the acute management of circulatory shock, the technique may be more helpful during postresuscitation monitoring. At this time, sequential arterial blood gases provide more reliable data during acute shock.

Transcutaneous and transconjunctival oxygen tension measurement are newer noninvasive techniques used for determining tissue oxygen tension, which show some promise in the management of patients at risk for or following the resuscitation of circulatory shock. In the absence of shock, transcutaneous probes reflect arterial oxygenation.[351] A number of studies, however, have suggested that if arterial oxygen tension is stable, the devices may be of use in assessing global or regional changes in perfusion and oxygen metabolism.[352-355] Global hypoperfusion due to low output shock (as well as local vasoconstriction) results in decreased transcutaneous oxygen tension and a decreased ratio of transcutaneous to arterial oxygen tension.[353] Decreased transcutaneous oxygen tension, seen early in hemorrhagic shock, may precede hypotension.[354,355] Decreases in transconjunctival oxygen tension predict hemodynamic collapse in perioperative patients[352] and death in patients with cardiogenic shock.[355] Transcutaneous and transconjunctival measurement of oxygen tension may also be useful in assessing the adequacy of tissue perfusion during resuscitation from hypodynamic shock.[356,357]

As anaerobic glycolysis with lactate generation is paralleled by the production of hydrogen ions during hypodynamic shock, noninvasive measurement of tissue pH may provide an attractive, metabolism-based assessment of adequacy of tissue oxygenation/perfusion. Because the stomach is easily accessible, may reflect overall splanchnic perfusion during shock,[358] and splanchnic perfusion is known to be altered early in shock,[359] most clinical work has focused on gastric mucosal pH. Studies suggest that gastric intramucosal pH correlates closely with systemic and organ oxygen consumption, organ failure, and outcome in critically ill humans.[360,361] Normalization of gastric mucosal pH has been suggested as one appropriate target during resuscitation of circulatory shock.[362] Limited evidence suggests such an approach may be associated with improved survival.[363] However, further supportive studies are required before this can be accepted as an appropriate therapeutic target.

Near infrared spectroscopy (NIRS) is an innovative technique able to noninvasively monitor regional tissue blood flow, oxygen delivery, and oxygen utilization. Although several investigators have claimed the ability to examine mitochondrial oxidation state (particularly the redox state of cytochrome aa3, the terminal portion of the electron transport chain), these measurements may actually reflect only tissue oxygenation.

Normal tissue oxygenation is the ultimate expression of normal cardiopulmonary function. Any major perturbation of cardiopulmonary status including incipient shock should ultimately express decreased tissue oxygenation. Because peripheral tissue perfusion is, as part of normal compensatory mechanisms, among the first to become restricted during cardiovascular stress, peripheral tissue oxygenation may serve as an excellent marker of cardiovascular stress. Near-infrared light is known to pass through biologic tissues such as skin and muscle. By illuminating a tissue with a known amount of incident light, the amount recovered depends on the degree of absorption by chromophores within the tissue and the amount of scattering. Only three chromophores are known to absorb light in the near-infrared wavelength spectrum: hemoglobin, myoglobin, and cytochrome aa3. All three are known to vary their absorption of near-infrared light depending on whether they are in an oxygenated or deoxygenated/reduced state. By monitoring these parameters, NIR spectroscopy is a unique tool that allows for real-time assessment of the adequacy of tissue perfusion during both the resuscitation and ongoing management of patients with shock. Studies in both animals and humans have suggested the potential utility of this technique in assessment of shock including hypovolemic/traumatic[364-369] and septic.[370,371]

The application of advanced echocardiography techniques to the ICU environment as intermittent monitoring tools may represent one of the most exciting developments in critical care management. A number of factors have hastened this development. These include questions regarding the safety and efficacy of routine pulmonary artery catheter utilization; the availability of relatively inexpensive, portable echocardiography systems; the application of advanced software algorithms to analyze data; and the development of new, high-resolution echocardiographic techniques including transesophageal and contrast echocardiography. The confluence of these factors has resulted in a substantial increase in the use of echocardiography in the ICU assessing hemodynamic instability and shock. In addition to its long-recognized ability to detect anatomic lesions (pericardial tamponade, pericardial effusion, septal defects, valvular disease, aortic dissection), new techniques allow for the assessment of cardiac output, stroke volume, preload (ventricular volumes), intravascular volume status (inspiratory inferior caval collapse), pulmonary artery pressures, systolic contractility (ejection fraction), diastolic function, and regional motion abnormalities at baseline and under stressed conditions.[372] The utility for diagnosis of hemodynamically significant pulmonary embolism has also been established.[373] The widespread dissemination of echocardiographic skills among the next generation of intensivists has allowed for a substantial reduction in the use of invasive monitoring techniques including pulmonary artery catheterization.

MANAGEMENT AND THERAPY

Patients suspected to be in circulatory shock should be managed in an intensive care unit with continuous ECG monitoring and close nursing support. Those whose etiologic diagnosis is in doubt, whose hemodynamic instability does not quickly resolve with intravenous fluids, or who are medically complicated should undergo invasive hemodynamic monitoring with arterial and pulmonary artery catheters. Laboratory tests, as mentioned earlier, should be performed at or before admission.

Management of shock can be divided into specific therapy for the triggering injury and general therapy of the shock syndrome. Examples of specific therapy include antibiotics and drotrecogin-alfa (activated) for treatment of septic shock, blood transfusion for hemorrhagic shock, thrombolysis for acute myocardial infarction or massive pulmonary embolus, and pericardial aspiration for pericardial tamponade. Specific therapy for different etiologies of shock will be discussed in their separate chapters.

AIMS

Because the shock syndrome shares many characteristics across different etiologies, the general management of shock is similar in all cases. The basic goal of circulatory shock therapy is the rapid restoration of effective perfusion to vital organs and tissues prior to the onset of cellular injury. Because effective tissue perfusion depends on both sufficient cardiac output and adequate driving pressure, therapy of shock requires maintenance of an appropriate cardiac index and mean blood pressure (Box 21.5). However, because for brief periods marked hypoperfusion is better tolerated than severe hypotension, the first specific resuscitative aim, support of blood pressure (>60 to 65 mm Hg in a baseline normotensive patient), may initially take priority over the second specific aim, maintenance of cardiac index. Finally, maintaining perfusion sufficiently high that arterial lactate concentration remains under 2.2 mmol/L is a generally accepted approach to avoiding anaerobic metabolism and ischemic tissue injury (see Box 21.5). The practice of targeting oxygen delivery to specified supranormal oxygen delivery goals or to evidence of supply-independent oxygen consumption in the ICU has been substantially discredited by clinical studies.[374-377] However, early targeting (<6 hr post presentation) to a central venous oxygen saturation ($cSVo_2$) of >70% using a defined protocol with fluids, blood transfusion, and dobutamine support has been shown to improve outcome in severe sepsis and septic shock.[302] This approach has not been validated in other forms of shock.

Box 21.5 General Approach to Shock: Immediate Goals

Hemodynamic

- MAP > 60 to 65 mm Hg (higher in the presence of coronary artery disease)
- CVP = 8 to 12 mm Hg/PAOP = 12 to 15 mm Hg (may be higher for cardiogenic shock)
- CI > 2.1 L/min/m^2

Optimization of Oxygen Delivery

- Hemoglobin > 9 g/dL; > 7 g/L postshock is sufficient
- Arterial saturation > 92%
- MVO_2 > 60%, $SCVO_2$ > 70%
- Normalization of serum lactate (to < 2.2 mM/L)

Reverse Organ System Dysfunction

- Reverse encephalopathy
- Maintain urine output > 0.5 mL/kg/hr

It is of note that one of the major achievements in shock therapy since the early 2000s has been the recognition that the speed of implementing supportive and specific therapies may be critical to an improvement in outcomes. This concept of a "golden hour" has long been recognized in the context of specific and resuscitative therapy of trauma-induced hypovolemic shock with blood products and surgical management[378,379] and then cardiogenic shock due to myocardial infarction with emergent primary angioplasty or thrombolysis.[380] A similar rapid treatment paradigm has been established for thrombolytic therapy for obstructive shock due to massive pulmonary embolus.[78,79,381] Similarly, rapid fluid resuscitation (<6 hours)[302] and antimicrobial therapy (<1 hour)[107] have been shown to be key to maximizing survival in cases of severe sepsis and septic shock. The accelerated provision of effective therapy probably accounts for reports of improved clinical outcomes with medical emergency response teams.[382-384] Variation in the baseline provision of effective therapy likely accounts for the inconsistent results seen with such teams.[385] The importance of early aggressive resuscitative and specific therapy of all shock states cannot be sufficiently emphasized.

RESUSCITATION

The universal basics of resuscitation underlie the initial management of circulatory shock. Because many patients with circulatory shock may have accompanying trauma and a decreased level of consciousness, the ventilatory status of the patient must be secured. This may involve tracheal intubation or mechanical ventilation, if necessary. Oxygen should be provided at a sufficiently high concentration to supply an arterial oxygen saturation of greater than 90% to 92%. Unintubated patients may require high flow (30 to 45 L/min) or rebreathing oxygen delivery systems, as many patients will have unusually high minute ventilation volumes. Intubated patients should initially receive full ventilatory support in order to decrease systemic oxygen demand. Given that pulmonary infiltrates (aspiration, pneumonia, or ARDS) are common, positive end-expiratory pressure (PEEP) may be necessary to ensure adequate oxygenation. Potential adverse hemodynamic effects from positive pressure ventilation (related primarily to decreased venous return) may be seen but can be minimized by fluid loading so that the patient is euvolemic or modestly hypervolemic.

Depending on the clinical situation, pain management may be necessary. Again, potential adverse hemodynamic effects may be seen if intravascular volume is inadequate because all measures result in some degree of venodilatation either directly or by decreasing sympathetic tone. Two- to 4-mg intravenous boluses of morphine are recommended. During circulatory shock, clearance of morphine by the liver may be impaired due to hepatic hypoperfusion. Besides relieving pain, analgesia should also decrease systemic oxygen consumption.

Management of lactic acidosis developing during circulatory shock is problematic. Bicarbonate therapy may have adverse effects on intracellular pH even while improving the pH of the extracellular fluid. Further, even when pH is extremely low, bicarbonate therapy does not improve systemic hemodynamics in shock associated with acidosis.[386] In addition, increasing serum pH may adversely affect the oxyhemoglobin dissociation relationship. The optimal approach to the management of lactic acidosis is to improve organ and systemic perfusion so that anaerobic metabolism is limited and the liver and, to a lesser extent, kidneys can clear the accumulated lactate. If this is not effective, restricting the use of sodium bicarbonate to situations in which pH is less than 7.1 to 7.15 may be appropriate.

Initial management of circulatory shock should almost always include a crystalloid fluid challenge. In the absence of invasive monitoring with a pulmonary artery catheter, the only practical exception is if clinical evidence strongly suggests ventricular filling pressures are already elevated. This is usually limited to clinical situations involving cardiogenic shock and marked pulmonary edema. Even then, if pulmonary edema is manageable, crystalloid challenge may be appropriate. The volume of the challenge is variable. Large volumes, on the order of 1 to 2 L given rapidly (0.5 to 1 L every 10 to 15 minutes), are frequently used in hemorrhagic and septic shock. One hundred– to 200-mL boluses may be used during cardiogenic shock. If shock does not resolve promptly after the initial fluid challenge, patients should undergo a more detailed invasive (central venous catheter) or noninvasive (echocardiographic) assessment. As previously discussed, a central role for pulmonary artery catheterization in shock is now questioned and highly controversial.

Although aggressive fluid resuscitation is well accepted in the therapy of shock, emerging data support more limited resuscitation in some contexts. Resuscitation to hypotensive targets (target systolic blood pressure 80 to 100 mm Hg) has been recommended in hemorrhagic shock due to penetrating trauma based on data showing improved survival using this approach.[387,388] In addition, a limited fluid resuscitation protocol for 7 days has been shown to improve the number of ventilator- and ICU-free days in acute lung injury without increasing the prevalence of shock or the mortality rate.[389] A more limited early fluid resuscitation has also been shown to be associated with improved survival in children with shock associated with infection in under-resourced settings.[390]

In addition, substantial controversy exists regarding the appropriate use of crystalloid and colloid fluids after initial resuscitation attempts. The basis of this controversy lies with the differing oncotic properties of the fluids. Crystalloid fluids (such as normal saline and lactated Ringer's solution) contain sodium chloride in a quantity that closely matches extracellular fluid. No large molecules are present. Thus, such fluids distribute into the extracellular space. Colloids, in addition, contain albumin or large osmotically active carbohydrates (hydroxyethyl starch, dextran), which may be held within the intravascular space resulting in an increase of the plasma oncotic pressure. It has been suggested that in shock associated with microvascular changes of permeability (such as sepsis), colloid fluids will remain in the intravascular space, leading to decreased tissue edema and noncardiogenic pulmonary edema.[391] However, the limited human studies available suggest that although radiographic infiltrates may appear more severe with crystalloid resuscitation of sepsis, gas exchange is comparable to colloid resuscitation.[41]

Importantly, it has been proposed that colloids may provide better outcomes in the resuscitation of shock due to the rapidity and persistence of volume expansion compared to crystalloid infusion.[41,392] However, clinical studies for the most part have not supported this contention. Meta-analyses have largely failed to demonstrate the clinical outcome superiority of crystalloids compared to either albumin or synthetic colloids.[393] In fact, one meta-analysis of randomized, controlled studies examining the effect of fluid administration in critically ill patients with burn injury, hypovolemia, or hypoalbuminemia suggested increased mortality in patients treated with colloids.[394] In one large, randomized study of albumin versus normal saline, a trend toward improved outcomes with albumin in severe sepsis and saline in trauma failed to reach significance.[395] More recently, a substantial body of literature has shown that synthetic colloids increase the risk of renal injury and death, particularly in sepsis and septic shock.[396-398] An increased risk of renal injury/dialysis requirement and risk of death was shown for hydroxyethyl starch versus Ringer's solution therapy in two large randomized trials of sepsis.[397,398] There are some data, though, that suggest colloid resuscitation may clear lactate more quickly and result in less renal injury than crystalloid in penetrating trauma.[399] Given the much higher costs of colloids and the higher risk of renal injury and death with synthetic colloids, resuscitation of shock should generally focus on crystalloid solutions unless speed of resuscitation is paramount (i.e., there is acute major trauma or massive hemorrhage). In those settings, colloidal solutions may be initially favored until blood is available.

With respect to hemoglobin, one randomized trial has suggested that a hemoglobin level of 70 g/L is sufficient for most patients in the ICU (other than those with a high severity of illness or acute coronary syndrome).[400,401] Although several other studies have pointed out the potential risks associated with blood transfusion in the ICU setting,[402-405] no study has directly examined hemoglobin requirements during shock. The only study to (indirectly) examine blood transfusion in shock suggested that early augmentation of hematocrit to >30% during septic shock as part of a protocol to drive central venous oxygen saturation to >70% was associated with improved survival.[302] For that reason, it is reasonable to recommend that a hemoglobin of 90 to 100 g/L be maintained during acute shock.

Once intravascular volume is optimized, the next line of therapy of circulatory shock usually involves inotropes and vasopressors. Alternately, vasopressors may be occasionally required for brief periods of blood pressure support in extremely hypotensive patients prior to the initiation of fluid infusion.

Four major classes of agents are used clinically for inotropic or vasopressor support: sympathomimetics, phosphodiesterase inhibitors, cardiac glycosides, and vasopressin (anti-diuretic hormone) (Table 21.4). Sympathomimetics (catecholamines) may activate cardiac beta-1 and alpha adrenoreceptors, peripheral vascular alpha or beta-2 receptors, and vascular dopaminergic receptors. Cardiac beta-1 adrenoreceptors augment heart rate and myocardial contractility by increasing activity of adenylate cyclase resulting in increased generation of cyclic adenosine monophosphate (AMP).[406] Alpha receptors act through phospholipase C production of inositol triphosphate and diacylglycerol.[407-409] Peripheral vascular alpha receptors cause vasoconstriction, whereas peripheral beta-2 adrenoreceptors induce a mild vasodilatation. Cardiac alpha adrenoreceptors contribute to increased contractility (but not heart rate) when stimulated.[407,409] Dopaminergic adrenoreceptors, mediating dilatation, are found in the arterial vessels supplying vital organs (including the heart, brain, kidneys, and splanchnic organs).[410] Phosphodiesterase inhibitors such as amrinone and milrinone augment cardiac contractility by inhibition of cyclic AMP degradation. They also relax vascular smooth muscle.[411] Despite a long history of digitalis use in the management of congestive heart failure and data suggesting hemodynamic benefit in sepsis,[412] cardiac glycosides are rarely used for the acute management of circulatory shock due to their narrow therapeutic index and long half-life. Uncontrolled studies have shown that endogenous vasopressin concentrations may be relatively deficient in shock states and that infusion of vasopressin (which has little effect in healthy, normotensive subjects) can have a profound pressor effect during vasodilatory shock.[413-416]

Norepinephrine, an endogenous catecholamine, exerts both powerful inotropic (cardiac alpha and beta-1 adrenoreceptors) and peripheral vasoconstriction effects (alpha adrenoreceptors). It is currently the favored catecholamine for the initial management of shock. It can be used for persistent hypotension despite high-dose dopamine during septic and obstructive shock. It should generally be used only transiently in cardiogenic shock because it may dramatically reduce forward flow. Similarly, it should not be required during hemorrhagic shock except for extremely brief periods of blood pressure support pending volume infusion. Infusion rates of 2 to 20 μg/min are commonly used, but if necessary, higher rates may be tried. Suggestions that there is clinical utility in the concomitant use of "low"-dose dopamine with norepinephrine to generate sparing of pressor and shock-associated renal injury have been refuted.[417-419]

Dopamine has fallen out of favor as the initial vasopressor used for circulatory shock. A central and peripheral nervous system neurotransmitter and the biologic precursor of norepinephrine, it stimulates three different receptors: vascular dopaminergic, cardiac $\beta 1$, and vascular α. In addition, a part of dopamine's myocardial effects is mediated by the release of endogenous norepinephrine. Dose-dependent maximal stimulation of each of dopamine's target receptors has been suggested to result in different typical hemodynamic responses at different infusion rates. At infusion rates of less than 4 to 5 μg/kg/min, dopaminergic effects have been said to dominate, but studies suggest this has little clinical relevance (although in the past it was the theoretical basis for the use of low-dose dopamine for renal protection).[418,419] Vascular DA2 receptors vasodilate the renal, mesenteric, myocardial, and cerebral vascular beds. In addition, renal DA1 receptors mediate a mild natriuresis.[420] β-adrenoreceptor-mediated cardiac inotropic effects have been suggested to dominate at doses below approximately 10 μg/kg/min with α-adrenoreceptor vasopressor effects more prominent at doses over 10 μg/kg/min.[410] It is important to note, however, that dopaminergic and cardiac adrenergic effects are not suppressed at higher doses but rather that additional effects are seen. In addition, there is substantial inter-individual variation in response with some showing substantial vasopressor or inotropic responses at low infusion rates. For management of circulatory shock, dopamine

Table 21.4 Relative Potency of Intravenously Administered Vasopressors/Inotropes Used in Shock*

		Cardiac		Peripheral Vasculature			
	Dose	Heart Rate	Contractility	Vasoconstriction	Vasodilation	Dopaminergic	Typical Clinical Use
Dopamine	1-4 μg/kg/min 5-10 μg/kg/min 11-20 μg/kg/min	1+ 2+ 2+	1-2+ 2+ 2+	0 1-2+ 2-3+	1+ 1+ 1+	4+ 4+ 4+	All shock
Norepinephrine	2-20 μg/min	2+	2+	4+	0	0	Refractory shock
Dobutamine	1-20 μg/kg/min	1-2+	3+	1+	2+	0	CHF; cardiogenic, obstructive and septic shock
Dopexamine†	0.5-6 μg/kg/min	2+	1+	0	3-4+	4+	CHF; cardiogenic shock
Epinephrine	1-8 μg/min	4+	4+	4+	3+	0	Refractory shock or anaphylactic shock
Phenylephrine	20-200 μg/min	0	1+	4+	0	0	Neurogenic or septic shock
Isoproterenol	1-8 μg/min	4+	4+	0	4+	0	Cardiogenic shock (bradyarrhythmia), torsades de pointes, ventricular tachycardia
Vasopressin	0.04-0.10 U/min (start 0.01-0.04 U/min; titrate up 0.02-0.04 U/min every 20-30 min)	0	0	4+	0	0	Vasodilatory (e.g., septic) shock
Milrinone	37.5-75 μg/kg bolus over 10 min; 0.375-0.75 μg/kg/min infusion	1+	3+	0	2+	0	CHF; cardiogenic shock

*The 1-4+ scoring system represents an arbitrary quantitation of the comparative potency of different vasopressors/inotropes.
†Not clinically released in the United States. CHF, congestive heart failure.

is often started at 5 μg/kg/min and increased rapidly (5 μg/kg/min every 2 or 3 minutes) to a maximum of 20 μg/kg/min until the target blood pressure is reached. If vasopressor effects are inadequate at these infusion rates, a norepinephrine infusion is begun.

Dobutamine, which is structurally derived from isoproterenol, is a racemic mixture of two synthetic stereoisomers. In combination, the stereoisomers increase myocardial contractility through alpha and beta-1 cardiac adrenoreceptors.[421,422] Weak arteriolar vasodilatory effects are mediated through the dominance of beta-2 adrenoreceptor-mediated vascular relaxation over alpha-adrenoreceptor-mediated vasoconstriction in the arterial circulation. Evidence suggesting that dobutamine induces vasoconstriction in the systemic venous bed (resulting in increased mean circulatory pressure and the augmentation of venous return/cardiac output) implies that alpha-adrenoreceptor-mediated effects may be dominant in small capacitance vessels.[167,421,422]

Although its hemodynamic effects are otherwise similar to isoproterenol, dobutamine has been reputed to exert minimal chronotropic effects.[422,423] This attribute has been questioned[424] and may have been based on the selection of congestive heart failure patients with beta-adrenoreceptor down-regulation and other potential alterations of adrenoreceptor signal transduction.[423,425] Dobutamine's powerful inotropic effect is due to a combination of its direct effect on myocardial contractility, its afterload reducing effect, and alpha-adrenoreceptor-mediated venoconstriction.[422,423] In contrast to dopamine, it causes a reduction in filling pressures and a greater increase in cardiac output at equivalent doses.[426,427] In addition, although it increases myocardial oxygen demand (like dopamine), myocardial perfusion is also augmented (in contrast to dopamine[428]). The most well-accepted use of dobutamine in circulatory shock relates to cardiac etiologies.[422,423] Once blood pressure is corrected, dobutamine may be used to increase cardiac performance and decrease elevated ventricular filling pressures associated with cardiogenic pulmonary edema. In this setting dobutamine may in fact increase blood pressure. Alternately, if myocardial damage is extensive, vasodilatory properties may dominate, resulting in hypotension. Dobutamine may also be of use in obstructive shock pending definitive intervention and can be used to augment low CI occasionally seen in fluid-resuscitated septic shock. Our own experience suggests that maintenance of a PAOP of at least 15 mm Hg is required during dobutamine infusion in order to avoid hypotension in patients with septic shock. Its use for augmenting oxygen delivery in septic shock has been substantially abandoned.[429,430]

Epinephrine is occasionally used when other inotrope/vasopressors have failed to support blood pressure or cardiac output in circulatory shock. It is the first-line agent for management of anaphylactic shock. In addition, it is used to support myocardial contractility postcardiopulmonary bypass.[431] Epinephrine stimulation of alpha, beta-1, and beta-2 receptors results in increases of myocardial contractility that are more pronounced than with any other inotrope. Nanogram/kg/min infusion rates result in significant increases in cardiac output.[431] Epinephrine is also frequently used in septic shock refractory to other inotropes/vasopressors. Effects attributable to impaired myocardial perfusion (chest pain, arrhythmias, ST depression) in patients with known coronary artery disease are usually limited to patients receiving more than 120 ng/kg/min.[432] Although the usual infusion rate is 1 to 8 μg/min, higher rates can be used with the potential for increasing toxicity.

Milrinone, a bipyridine phosphodiesterase inhibitor, increases intracellular concentrations of cyclic AMP by blocking cyclic AMP breakdown.[411] Although some controversy has existed regarding the relative contributions of increased myocardial contractility and decreased vascular tone with respect to the apparent inotropic properties of phosphodiesterase inhibitors, data confirm the presence of substantial increases of myocardial contractility[433]; these agents also produce substantial vasodilatation. The most accepted use for milrinone in the intensive care unit is in the management of congestive heart failure, cardiogenic shock, and postcardiopulmonary bypass myocardial dysfunction.[411] Experimental animal studies suggest phosphodiesterase inhibitors may exert beneficial hemodynamic effects in sepsis by augmenting cardiac output and increasing oxygen delivery without increasing consumption.[434] Occasional clinical reports suggest a potential management role in catecholamine-refractory septic shock.[435]

Phenylephrine is a synthetic catecholamine that is unique in its almost pure alpha-adrenergic agonist effects. Its most common uses are intraoperatively to counteract the vasodilatory effects of anesthetics and in septic shock where its lack of beta-adrenergic activity may help limit deleterious increases in heart rate seen with other agents. Isoproterenol is another synthetic catecholamine with dominant beta-1 and beta-2 activity. Its previous indications for use have largely been supplanted by dobutamine. Due to its powerful chronotropic effects, it can be useful in the management of bradyarrhythmias and torsades de pointes ventricular tachycardia (for overdrive pacing), but otherwise it has no specific role in the management of circulatory shock.

Vasopressin levels in septic shock have been shown to be significantly suppressed.[413] Studies have shown that intravenous infusion of vasopressin into patients with septic shock results in a profound pressor response.[414] This profound pressor response occurs despite the absence of such an effect with even larger amounts of vasopressin in normotensive patients. Investigators have also documented efficacy in other vasodilatory shock states with refractory hypotension including milrinone-induced shock in severe heart failure,[436] postcardiotomy vasodilatory shock,[437] unstable brain dead organ donors,[438] and late phase hemorrhagic shock.[416] Vasopressin (0.1 to 1 U/mL in normal saline or D5W) may be initiated at 0.02 to 0.04 U/min and titrated up every 20 to 30 minutes to 0.1 to 0.12 U/min. Few patients will respond with higher doses. It is of note that in large doses, vasopressin may produce bradycardia, minor arrhythmias, premature atrial contraction, heart block, peripheral vascular constriction or collapse, coronary insufficiency, decreased cardiac output, myocardial ischemia, and myocardial infarction. In patients with coronary artery disease, even small doses of the drug can precipitate angina. At the upper end of dosing, a significant subset of patients may develop digital, mesenteric, or myocardial ischemia, so it is imperative to use the minimal amount of vasopressin possible to achieve desired blood pressure goals. Published data suggest vasopressin can be used for up to 4 to 6 days if necessary. A randomized, blinded study of vasopressin treatment of septic shock has shown that the addition of vasopressin (versus norepinephrine) to open label vasopressors offered no overall advantage.[439] Because of the limited experience with this compound and the relatively longer half-life of the drug, vasopressin should be utilized only after hemodynamic stabilization with standard agents (catecholamines) has been attempted.

CONCLUSION

Although the syndrome of shock ultimately involves common late pathologic elements, the early pathophysiologic processes underlying different conditions resulting in circulatory shock are both diverse and complex. Our concepts of shock, which once focused on broad cardiovascular physiologic mechanisms, have more recently centered on issues of microvascular function and cellular metabolism. In the future, this focus may evolve toward questions of altered cellular gene expression in a variety of tissues. Advances in therapy have developed in parallel to these changes in our understanding of shock pathophysiology. Early work on the therapy of shock concentrated on correcting hemodynamic derangements through the use of vasopressors and inotropes. Clinical trials over decades have centered on anticytokines such as anti-TNFα and various novel resuscitative compounds. The most advanced experimental therapies involve the direct manipulation of gene expression via antisense oligonucleotides and transcription factor inhibitors. Despite these advances, however, many questions remain. Only ongoing basic research and clinical trials will answer them.

KEY POINTS

- Shock is the final pathway through which a variety of pathologic processes lead to cardiovascular failure and death.
- Shock is the state in which the profound and widespread reduction of effective tissue perfusion leads to cellular injury. The inability of cells to obtain or utilize oxygen in sufficient quantity to optimally meet their metabolic requirements is common to all forms of shock. Hypotension alone does not define shock.
- Based on hemodynamic characteristics, shock is categorized as hypovolemic, cardiogenic, extracardiac obstructive, or distributive.
- Although one hemodynamic categorization dominates, most forms of clinical shock involve some cardiovascular characteristics of several categories.
- The clinical picture of shock is dependent on the etiology, the magnitude of the injury or insult, and the degree of physiologic compensation. Physiologic compensation is determined by the time course of the development of shock and the preexisting cardiovascular reserve.

KEY POINTS (Continued)

- The systemic hemodynamic aspects of shock can be described by the interactive contributions of cardiac and vascular function to blood pressure and cardiac output.
- Physiologically, blood pressure is dependent on cardiac output and vascular resistance; cardiac output is not dependent on blood pressure.
- Failure to maintain the blood pressure required for autoregulation during hypodynamic circulatory shock indicates a severe reduction in cardiac output.
- In a closed cardiovascular circuit, cardiac output as determined by heart rate, preload, afterload, and contractility equals venous return as determined by venous pressure (mean circulatory pressure), right atrial pressure, and venous resistance. Total systemic perfusion is therefore dependent on cardiac-vascular interactions.
- In addition to sufficient cardiac output at sufficient pressure, effective perfusion requires normal local and systemic microvascular function resulting in the appropriate distribution of cardiac output.
- During hypovolemic and other forms of hypodynamic shock, extrinsic blood flow regulatory mechanisms overwhelm the autoregulatory response of most vascular beds. Blood flow to vital organs such as the heart and brain is relatively well preserved due to dominant autoregulatory control.
- During distributive shock, particularly septic shock, organ blood flow is disturbed at higher mean arterial pressures, suggesting a primary defect of microvascular function.
- Cellular dysfunction and organ failure in shock involves the interactions of cellular ischemia, circulating or local inflammatory mediators, and free radical injury.
- All compensatory responses to shock support oxygen delivery to vital tissues. The mechanisms include support of venous pressure, maximization of cardiac function, redistribution of perfusion to vital organs, and optimization of oxygen unloading.
- Circulatory shock may be associated with encephalopathy, adult respiratory distress syndrome, acute tubular necrosis, ischemic hepatitis or intrahepatic cholestasis, thrombocytopenia, immunosuppression, and multiple organ dysfunction syndrome.
- Because early recognition and treatment are the keys to improved survival, the diagnosis of shock is primarily based on clinical criteria. Laboratory and radiologic data are used to confirm the diagnosis and to help clarify etiology.
- Clinically, shock is characterized by physiologic compensatory responses including tachycardia, tachypnea, oliguria, and signs of physiologic decompensation, particularly hypotension.

Continued on following page

KEY POINTS (Continued)

- Shock should be managed in an intensive care unit with continuous monitoring and close nursing support. Patients whose etiologic diagnosis is in doubt, whose hemodynamic instability does not quickly resolve with intravenous fluids, or who are medically complicated should undergo noninvasive (echo) or invasive hemodynamic monitoring with arterial and centrally placed catheters. Pulmonary artery catheters remain a reasonable option in some cases.
- The basic goal of therapy of circulatory shock is the restoration of effective perfusion to vital organs and tissues prior to the onset of cellular injury.
- The specific aims of resuscitation of shock include support of mean blood pressure above 60 to 65 mm Hg, maintenance of a cardiac index greater than 2.1 $L/min/m^2$, and restriction of arterial lactate concentrations to less than 2.2 mmol/L.

SELECTED REFERENCES

5. Martin GS, Mannino DM, Eaton S, Moss M: The epidemiology of sepsis in the United States from 1979 through 2000. N Engl J Med 2003;348:1546-1554.
38. Thiemermann C, Szabö C, Mitchell JA, Vane JR: Vascular hyporeactivity to vasoconstrictor agents and hemodynamic decompensation in hemorrhagic shock is mediated by nitric oxide. Proc Natl Acad Sci U S A 1993;90:267-271.
63. Hochman JS, Sleeper LA, Webb JG, et al: Early revascularization in acute myocardial infarction complicated by cardiogenic shock. SHOCK Investigators: Should we emergently revascularize occluded coronaries for cardiogenic shock [see comments]. N Engl J Med 1999;341:625-634.
79. Wood KE: Major pulmonary embolism: Review of a pathophysiologic approach to the golden hour of hemodynamically significant pulmonary embolism. Chest 2002;121:877-905.
107. Kumar A, Roberts D, Wood KE, et al: Duration of hypotension before initiation of effective antimicrobial therapy is the critical determinant of survival in human septic shock. Crit Care Med 2006;34:1589-1596.
151. Sprung C, Annane D, Keh D, et al: Hydrocortisone therapy for patients with septic shock. N Engl J Med 2008;358:111-124.
239. Kilbourn RG, Gross SS, Jubran A, et al: N-methyl-L-arginine inhibits tumor necrosis factor-induced hypotension: Implications for the involvement of nitric oxide. Proc Natl Acad Sci U S A 1990;87:3629-3623.
302. Rivers E, Nguyen B, Havstad S, et al: Early goal-directed therapy in the treatment of severe sepsis and septic shock. N Engl J Med 2001;345:1368-1377.
331. Connors AF Jr, Speroff T, Dawson NV, et al: The effectiveness of right heart catheterization in the initial care of critically ill patients. JAMA 1996;276:889-897.
335. Wheeler AP, Bernard GR, Thompson BT, et al: Pulmonary-artery versus central venous catheter to guide treatment of acute lung injury. N Engl J Med 2006;354:2213-2224.

The complete list of references can be found at www.expertconsult.com.

22 Cardiogenic Shock

Steven M. Hollenberg | Joseph E. Parrillo

CHAPTER OUTLINE

Cardiogenic shock is the syndrome that ensues when the heart is unable to deliver enough blood to maintain adequate tissue perfusion. Acute myocardial infarction (MI) is the leading cause, but other potential etiologic factors need to be considered.[1,2] Without prompt diagnosis and appropriate management, morbidity and mortality rates are substantial, approaching 60% for all age groups.[2,3] Rapid evaluation and prompt initiation of supportive measures and definitive therapy in patients with cardiogenic shock may improve both early and long-term outcomes.

DEFINITION

The clinical definition of cardiogenic shock includes decreased cardiac output and evidence of tissue hypoxia in the presence of adequate intravascular volume. The diagnosis of circulatory shock (Box 22.1) is made at the bedside by the presence of hypotension along with a combination of clinical signs indicative of poor tissue perfusion, including oliguria, clouded sensorium, and cool, mottled extremities. Hemodynamic criteria include sustained hypotension (systolic blood pressure < 90 mm Hg for at least 30 minutes) and a reduced cardiac index (<2.2 L/min/m^2) in the presence of elevated filling pressures (pulmonary capillary occlusion pressure > 15 mm Hg).[4] Cardiogenic shock is diagnosed after documentation of myocardial dysfunction and exclusion or correction of factors such as hypovolemia, hypoxia, and acidosis.

EPIDEMIOLOGY

Pump failure due to cardiogenic shock has long been known to carry a high mortality rate. The seminal article outlining prognosis after MI was a single center series of 250 patients reported by Killip in 1967.[5] Killip divided patients into four classes as follows:

Killip class I: no evidence of congestive heart failure
Killip class II: presence of an S_3 gallop and/or bibasilar rales
Killip class III: pulmonary edema (rales greater than halfway up the lung fields)
Killip class IV: cardiogenic shock

Nineteen percent of the 250 patients were in class IV at presentation, and their mortality rate was 81%.[5]

With the advent of right-sided heart catheterization, Forrester and Swan defined hemodynamic subsets after MI analogous to the clinical subsets outlined by Killip.[4] Subset I consisted of patients with normal pulmonary capillary wedge pressure (PCWP) and cardiac output, subset II consisted of patients with elevated PCWP and normal cardiac output, subset III consisted of patients with normal PCWP and decreased cardiac output, and subset IV consisted of patients with elevated PCWP and decreased cardiac output.[4]

Despite advances in management of heart failure and acute MI, the mortality rate of patients with cardiogenic shock has remained high.[2,6-8] Data suggest an increase in

Box 22.1 Diagnosis of Cardiogenic Shock

Clinical Signs

Hypotension
Oliguria
Clouded sensorium
Cool and mottled extremities

Hemodynamic Criteria

Systolic blood pressure < 90 mm Hg for > 30 min
Cardiac index < 2.2 L/min/m²
Pulmonary artery occlusion pressure > 15 mm Hg

Box 22.2 Causes of Cardiogenic Shock

Acute Myocardial Infarction

Pump failure
- Large infarction
- Smaller infarction with preexisting left ventricular dysfunction
- Infarct extension
- Reinfarction
- Infarct expansion

Mechanical complications
- Acute mitral regurgitation due to papillary muscle rupture
- Ventricular septal defect
- Free wall rupture
- Pericardial tamponade

Right ventricular infarction

Other Conditions

End-stage cardiomyopathy
Myocarditis
Myocardial contusion
Prolonged cardiopulmonary bypass
Septic shock with severe myocardial depression
Left ventricular outflow tract obstruction
- Aortic stenosis
- Hypertrophic obstructive cardiomyopathy

Obstruction to left ventricular filling
- Mitral stenosis
- Left atrial myxoma

Acute mitral regurgitation (chordal rupture)
Acute aortic insufficiency

survival in the 1990s, coincident with the use of reperfusion strategies.[7-9] Cardiogenic shock, however, remains the most common cause of death in hospitalized patients with acute MI.

INCIDENCE

Accurate determination of the precise incidence of cardiogenic shock is difficult because patients who die of MI prior to reaching the hospital generally do not receive this diagnosis.[6,10-13] Nonetheless, estimates from a variety of sources have been fairly consistent. The Worcester Heart Attack Study,[6] a community-wide analysis, found an incidence of cardiogenic shock of 7.5%, an incidence that remained fairly stable from 1975 to 1997.[6,9] The incidence was similar in the randomized GUSTO (Global Utilization of Streptokinase and Tissue Plasminogen Activator for Occluded Coronary Arteries) trial (7.2%),[14] in other multicenter thrombolytic trials,[10-12] and in patients with ST-segment elevation MI in the National Registry of Myocardial Infarction (NRMI) database from 1995 to 2004 (8.6%).[7] More recently, however, the incidence of cardiogenic shock has fallen from about 8% to about 6% of MIs, with most of the change resulting from a decrease in cardiogenic shock developing after initial presentation, supporting the notion that early revascularization strategies are an important contributor to the decline.[3]

ETIOLOGY

The most common cause of cardiogenic shock is left ventricular failure in the setting of an extensive acute MI, although a smaller infarction in a patient with previously compromised left ventricular function may also precipitate shock. Cardiogenic shock can also be caused by mechanical complications such as acute mitral regurgitation, rupture of the interventricular septum, or rupture of the free wall—or by large right ventricular infarctions. In a report of the SHOCK (**SH**ould we emergently revascularize **O**ccluded **C**oronaries for shoc**K**) trial registry of 1160 patients with cardiogenic shock,[2] 78.5% of patients had predominant left ventricular failure, 6.9% had acute mitral regurgitation, 3.9% had ventricular septal rupture, 2.8% had isolated right ventricular shock, 1.4% had tamponade or cardiac rupture, and 6.5% had shock resulting from other causes.

Other causes of cardiogenic shock include myocarditis, end-stage cardiomyopathy, myocardial contusion, septic shock with severe myocardial depression, myocardial dysfunction after prolonged cardiopulmonary bypass, valvular heart disease, and hypertrophic obstructive cardiomyopathy (Box 22.2). An important consideration is that some cardiogenic shock may have an iatrogenic component. Early diagnosis of impending shock or of patients at high risk for development of shock is essential, both to speed intervention and to avoid therapies that may worsen hemodynamics. In many cases of cardiogenic shock in the setting of MI, the diagnosis is not made until the patient has been triaged and admitted to an inpatient setting. Patients may have received early beta blockade or angiotensin-converting enzyme inhibition, therapies that may impact hemodynamics substantially.

Patients may have cardiogenic shock at initial presentation, but most do not; shock usually evolves over several hours,[15,16] suggesting that early treatment may potentially prevent shock. In fact, some data indicate that early thrombolytic therapy may decrease the incidence of cardiogenic shock.[17] In the SHOCK trial registry, 75% of patients developed cardiogenic shock within 24 hours after presentation, with a median delay of 7 hours.[2] Results from the GUSTO trial were similar;[13] among patients with shock, 11% were in shock on arrival and 89% developed shock after admission.

Risk factors for the development of cardiogenic shock in MI generally parallel those for left ventricular dysfunction and the severity of coronary artery disease. Shock is more likely to develop in patients who are elderly, are diabetic, and have anterior MI.[5,15,18,19] Patients with cardiogenic shock are also more likely to have histories of previous infarction, peripheral vascular disease, and cerebrovascular disease.[18,19] Decreased ejection fractions and larger infarctions (as evidenced by higher cardiac enzymes) are also predictors of the development of cardiogenic shock.[18,19] Analysis from the GUSTO-3 trial has identified age, lower systolic blood pressure, heart rate, and Killip class as significant predictors of the risk for development of cardiogenic shock after presentation with acute MI.[20] Use of a predictive scoring system derived from this study may be useful in identifying patients at high risk for the development of cardiogenic shock and targeting such patients for closer monitoring.[20]

Cardiogenic shock is most often associated with anterior MI. In the SHOCK trial registry, 55% of infarctions were anterior, 46% were inferior, 21% were posterior, and 50% were in multiple locations.[2] These findings were consistent with those in other series.[21] Angiographic evidence most often demonstrates multivessel coronary disease (left main occlusion in 20% of patients, three-vessel disease in 64%, two-vessel disease in 23%, and one-vessel disease in 13% of patients).[22] The high prevalence of multivessel coronary artery disease is important because compensatory hyperkinesis normally develops in myocardial segments that are not involved in an acute MI, and this response helps maintain cardiac output. Failure to develop such a response, because of previous infarction or high-grade coronary stenoses, is an important risk factor for cardiogenic shock and death.[16,23]

PATHOGENESIS

SYSTEMIC EFFECTS

Cardiac dysfunction in patients with cardiogenic shock is usually initiated by MI or ischemia. The myocardial dysfunction resulting from ischemia worsens that ischemia, creating a downward spiral[24] (Fig. 22.1). When a critical mass of ischemic or necrotic left ventricular myocardium fails to pump, stroke volume and cardiac output decrease. Myocardial perfusion, which depends on the pressure gradient between the coronary arterial system and the left ventricle and on the duration of diastole, is compromised by hypotension and tachycardia, exacerbating ischemia. The increased ventricular diastolic pressures caused by pump failure reduce coronary perfusion pressure, and the additional wall stress elevates myocardial oxygen requirements, further worsening ischemia. Decreased cardiac output also compromises systemic perfusion.

When myocardial function is depressed, several compensatory mechanisms are activated, including sympathetic stimulation to increase heart rate and contractility and renal fluid retention to increase preload. These compensatory mechanisms may become maladaptive and can actually worsen the situation when cardiogenic shock develops. Increased heart rate and contractility increase myocardial oxygen demand and exacerbate ischemia. Fluid retention and impaired diastolic filling caused by tachycardia and ischemia may result in pulmonary congestion and hypoxia. Vasoconstriction to maintain blood pressure increases

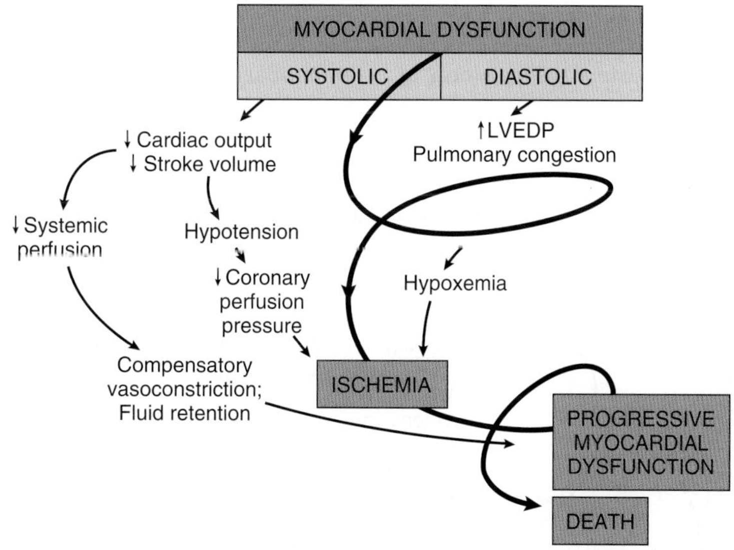

Figure 22.1 The "downward spiral" in cardiogenic shock. Cardiac dysfunction is usually initiated by myocardial infarction or ischemia. When a critical mass of left ventricular myocardium fails to pump, stroke volume and cardiac output decrease. Myocardial perfusion is compromised by hypotension and tachycardia, exacerbating ischemia. The increased ventricular diastolic pressures that result from pump failure further reduce coronary perfusion pressure, and the additional wall stress elevates myocardial oxygen requirements, also worsening ischemia. Decreased cardiac output also compromises systemic perfusion, which can lead to lactic acidosis and further compromise of systolic performance. When myocardial function is depressed, several compensatory mechanisms are activated, including sympathetic stimulation to increase heart rate and contractility and renal fluid retention to increase preload. These compensatory mechanisms may become dysfunctional and can actually worsen the situation when cardiogenic shock develops by increasing myocardial oxygen demand and afterload. Thus, myocardial dysfunction resulting from ischemia worsens that ischemia, setting up a vicious cycle that must be interrupted to prevent patient demise. LVEDP: left ventricular end-diastolic pressure. (Modified from Hollenberg SM, Kavinsky CJ, Parrillo JE: Cardiogenic shock. Ann Intern Med 1999;131:49.)

myocardial afterload, further impairing cardiac performance and increasing myocardial oxygen demand. This increased demand, in the face of inadequate perfusion, worsens ischemia and begins a vicious cycle that will end in death if not interrupted (see Fig. 22.1). The interruption of this cycle of myocardial dysfunction and ischemia forms the basis for the therapeutic regimens for cardiogenic shock.

Not all patients fit into this classic paradigm. In the SHOCK trial, the average systemic vascular resistance (SVR) was not elevated, and the range of values was wide, suggesting that compensatory vasoconstriction is not universal. Some patients had fever and elevated white blood cell counts along with decreased SVR, suggesting a systemic inflammatory response syndrome.[25] This has led to an expansion of the paradigm to include the possibility of the contribution of inflammatory responses to vasodilation and myocardial stunning, leading clinically to persistence of shock (Fig. 22.2).[25] Supporting this notion is the fact that the mean ejection fraction in the SHOCK trial was only moderately decreased (30%), suggesting that mechanisms other than pump failure were operative.[25] Immune activation appears to be common to a number of different forms of shock. Activation of inducible nitric oxide synthase (iNOS) with production of nitric oxide and peroxynitrate has been proposed as one potential mechanism.

MYOCARDIAL PATHOLOGY

Cardiogenic shock is characterized by both systolic and diastolic myocardial dysfunction.[16,26] Progressive myocardial necrosis has been observed consistently in clinical and pathologic studies of patients with cardiogenic shock.[16,27] Patients who develop shock after admission often have evidence of infarct extension, which can result from reocclusion of a transiently patent infarct artery, propagation of intracoronary thrombus, or a combination of decreased coronary perfusion pressure and increased myocardial oxygen demand.[18,19] Myocytes at the border zone of an infarction are more susceptible to additional ischemic episodes; therefore, these adjacent segments are at particular risk.[28] Mechanical infarct expansion, which is seen most dramatically after extensive anterior MI, can also contribute to late development of cardiogenic shock.[18,29]

Ischemia remote from the infarct zone may be particularly important in producing systolic dysfunction in patients with cardiogenic shock.[23,30] Patients with cardiogenic shock usually have multivessel coronary artery disease,[2,16] with limited vasodilator reserve, impaired autoregulation, and consequent pressure-dependent coronary flow in several perfusion territories.[31] Hypotension and metabolic derangements thus have the potential to impair the contractility of noninfarcted myocardium in patients with shock.[32] This can limit hyperkinesis of uninvolved segments, a compensatory mechanism typically seen early after MI.[23,30]

Myocardial diastolic function is also impaired in patients with cardiogenic shock. Myocardial ischemia causes decreased compliance, increasing the left ventricular filling pressure at a given end-diastolic volume.[33,34] Compensatory increases in left ventricular volumes to maintain stroke volume further increase filling pressures. Elevation of left ventricular pressures can lead to pulmonary edema and hypoxemia (see Fig. 22.1).

In addition to abnormalities in myocardial performance, valvular abnormalities can contribute to increased pulmonary congestion. Papillary muscle dysfunction caused by ischemia is common and can lead to substantial increases in left atrial pressure; the degree of mitral regurgitation may be lessened by afterload reduction. This mechanism is distinct from complete rupture of the papillary muscle, a mechanical complication that presents dramatically, with pulmonary edema and cardiogenic shock.

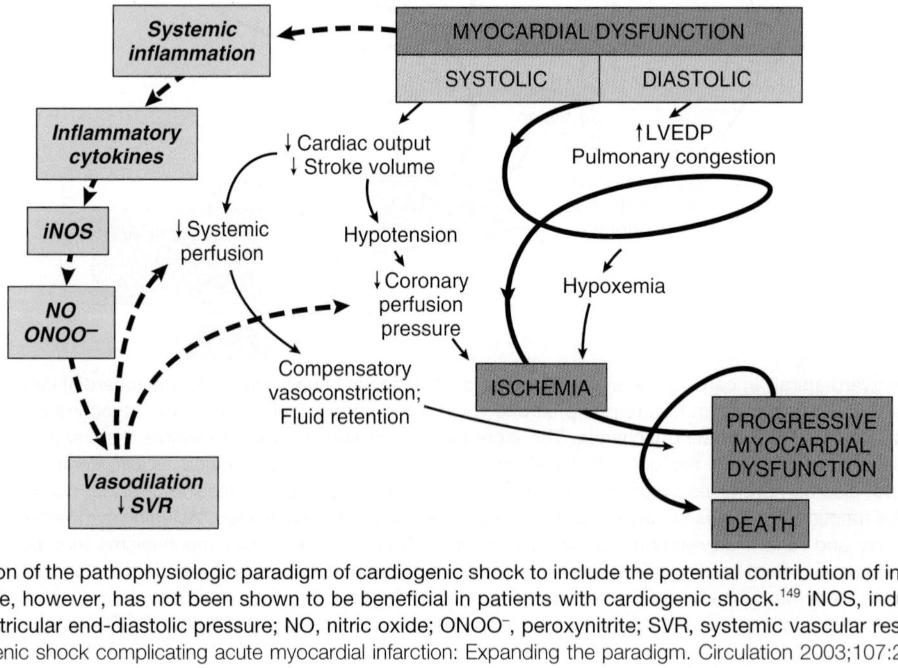

Figure 22.2 Expansion of the pathophysiologic paradigm of cardiogenic shock to include the potential contribution of inflammatory mediators. Inhibition of nitric oxide, however, has not been shown to be beneficial in patients with cardiogenic shock.[149] iNOS, inducible nitric oxide synthase; LVEDP, left ventricular end-diastolic pressure; NO, nitric oxide; ONOO⁻, peroxynitrite; SVR, systemic vascular resistance. (Adapted from Hochman JS: Cardiogenic shock complicating acute myocardial infarction: Expanding the paradigm. Circulation 2003;107:2999.)

CELLULAR PATHOLOGY

Tissue hypoperfusion and consequent cellular hypoxia lead to anaerobic glycolysis, with depletion of adenosine triphosphate and intracellular energy reserves. Anaerobic glycolysis also causes accumulation of lactic acid and resultant intracellular acidosis. Failure of energy-dependent ion transport pumps decreases transmembrane potential, causing intracellular accumulation of sodium and calcium and myocyte swelling.[35] Cellular ischemia and intracellular calcium accumulation can activate intracellular proteases.[36] If the ischemia is severe and prolonged enough, myocardial cellular injury can become irreversible, with the classic pattern of myonecrosis: mitochondrial swelling, accumulation of denatured proteins and chromatin in the cytoplasm, lysosomal breakdown, and fracture of the mitochondria, nuclear envelope, and plasma membrane.[35,36]

Accumulating evidence indicates that apoptosis (programmed cell death) may also contribute to myocyte loss in MI.[28,36,37] Although myonecrosis clearly outweighs apoptosis in the core of an infarcted area, evidence for apoptosis has been found consistently in the border zone of infarcts after ischemia and reperfusion and sporadically in areas remote from the ischemia area.[28,37] Activation of inflammatory cascades, oxidative stress, and stretching of myocytes have been proposed as mechanisms that activate the apoptotic pathways.[36,37] Although the magnitude of apoptotic cell loss in MI remains uncertain, inhibitors of apoptosis have been found to attenuate myocardial injury in animal models of postischemic reperfusion; these inhibitors may also have therapeutic potential for myocyte salvage after large infarctions.[37]

REVERSIBLE MYOCARDIAL DYSFUNCTION

A key to understanding the pathophysiology and treatment of cardiogenic shock is to realize that large areas of nonfunctional but viable myocardium can also cause or contribute to the development of cardiogenic shock in patients after MI (Fig. 22.3). This reversible dysfunction can be described in two main categories: stunning and hibernation.

Myocardial stunning represents postischemic dysfunction that persists despite restoration of normal blood flow; eventually, however, myocardial performance recovers completely.[38] Originally defined in animal models of ischemia and reperfusion,[39] stunning has been recognized in the clinical arena.[38,40] Direct evidence for myocardial stunning in humans has been found using positron emission tomography (PET) scanning in patients with persistent wall motion abnormalities after angioplasty for acute coronary syndromes; perfusion measured by ^{13}N-ammonia was normal in the presence of persistent contractile dysfunction.[41] The pathogenesis of stunning has not been conclusively established but appears to involve a combination of oxidative stress,[42] perturbation of calcium homeostasis, and decreased myofilament responsiveness to calcium.[38,43,44] In addition to these direct effects, data from studies in isolated cardiac myocytes suggest that circulating myocardial depressant substances may contribute to contractile dysfunction in myocardial stunning.[45] The intensity of stunning is

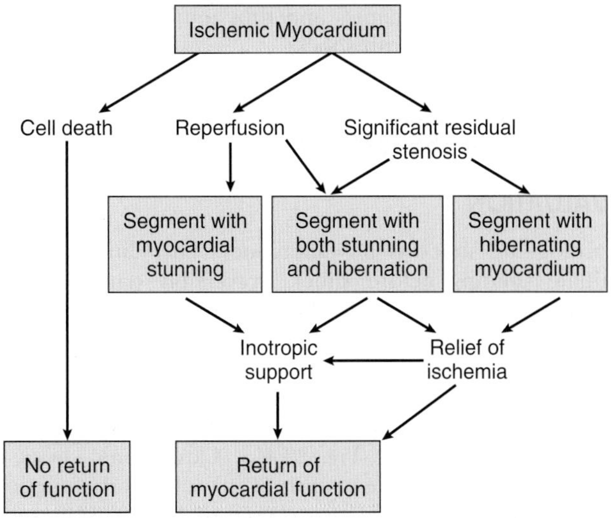

Figure 22.3 Possible outcomes after myocardial ischemia. After myocardial ischemia, either necrosis or reversible dysfunction may occur. Myocardial stunning represents postischemic dysfunction that persists despite restoration of normal flow. These segments respond to inotropes and will recover function if supported. Hibernating myocardium is a state of persistently impaired myocardial function at rest due to residual stenosis; function can be restored to normal by relieving ischemia. Repetitive episodes of stunning can coexist with or mimic myocardial hibernation. The concept that stunned or hibernating segments can recover contractile function emphasizes the importance of measures to support hemodynamics in patients with cardiogenic shock. (Modified from Hollenberg SM, Kavinsky CJ, Parrillo JE: Cardiogenic shock. Ann Intern Med 1999;131:50.)

determined primarily by the severity of the antecedent ischemic insult.[38]

Myocardial hibernation comprises segments with persistently impaired function at rest due to severely reduced coronary blood flow; inherent in the definition of hibernating myocardium is the notion that function can be normalized by improving blood flow.[46-48] Hibernation can be seen as an adaptive response to reduce contractile function of hypoperfused myocardium and restore equilibrium between flow and function, thereby minimizing the potential for ischemia or necrosis.[49] Revascularization of hibernating myocardium can lead to improved myocardial function,[50] and improved function appears to translate into improved prognosis.[51,52]

Although hibernation is conceptually and pathophysiologically different from myocardial stunning, the two conditions are difficult to distinguish in the clinical setting and may in fact coexist.[38,52] Repetitive episodes of myocardial stunning can coexist with or mimic myocardial hibernation.[38,46,53] Consideration of myocardial stunning and hibernation is vital in patients with cardiogenic shock because of their therapeutic implications. Hibernating myocardium improves with revascularization, and stunned myocardium retains inotropic reserve and can respond to inotropic stimulation.[38] In addition, the fact that the severity of the antecedent ischemic insult determines the intensity of stunning[38] provides one of the rationales for reestablishment of patency of occluded coronary arteries in patients with cardiogenic shock. Finally, the notion that some myocardial tissue may recover function emphasizes the importance of measures to support hemodynamics and thus minimize myocardial necrosis in patients with shock.

CLINICAL ASSESSMENT

EVALUATION

Cardiogenic shock is an emergency. The clinician must initiate therapy before shock irreversibly damages vital organs; at the same time, he or she must perform the clinical assessment required to understand the cause of shock and to target therapy to that cause. A practical approach is to make a rapid initial evaluation on the basis of a limited history, physical examination, and specific diagnostic procedures (Fig. 22.4).[24] Cardiogenic shock is diagnosed after documentation of myocardial dysfunction and exclusion of alternative causes of hypotension such as hypovolemia, hemorrhage, sepsis, pulmonary embolism, tamponade, aortic dissection, and preexisting valvular disease.

Patients with shock are usually ashen or cyanotic and can have cool skin and mottled extremities. Cerebral hypoperfusion may cloud the sensorium. Pulses are rapid and faint and may be irregular in the presence of arrhythmias. Jugular venous distention and pulmonary rales are usually present, although their absence does not exclude the diagnosis. A precordial heave resulting from left ventricular dyskinesis may be palpable. The heart sounds may be distant, and third or fourth heart sounds are usually present. A systolic murmur of mitral regurgitation or ventricular septal defect may be heard, but these complications may occur without an audible murmur.

An electrocardiogram should be performed immediately; other initial diagnostic tests usually include chest radiography and measurement of arterial blood gas, electrolytes, complete blood count, and cardiac enzymes.

Echocardiography is an excellent initial tool for confirming the diagnosis of cardiogenic shock and ruling out other causes of shock (Box 22.3); therefore, early echocardiography should be routine. Echocardiography provides information on overall and regional systolic function, and can rapidly diagnose mechanical causes of shock such as papillary muscle rupture and acute mitral regurgitation, acute ventricular septal defect, and free wall rupture and tamponade.[54,55] Unsuspected severe mitral regurgitation is not uncommon. In some cases, echocardiography may reveal findings compatible with right ventricular infarction.

Box 22.3 Role of Echocardiography in Cardiogenic Shock

Evaluate overall systolic performance
Delineate regional wall motion abnormalities
Rule out mechanical causes of shock
  Papillary muscle rupture
  Ventricular septal rupture
  Free wall rupture
  Tamponade
Diagnose right ventricular infarction

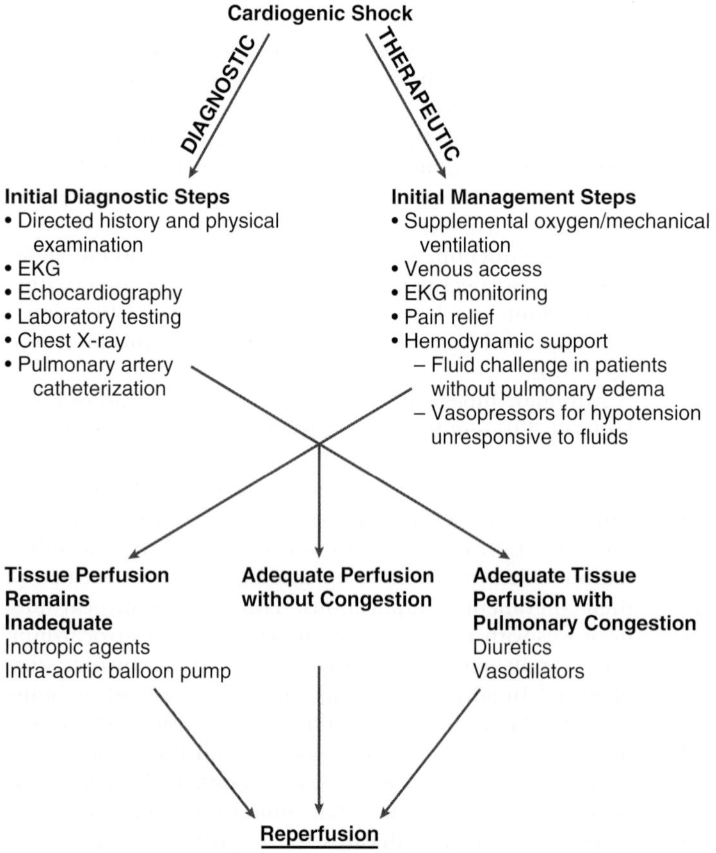

Figure 22.4 An approach to the diagnosis and treatment of cardiogenic shock caused by myocardial infarction. Right ventricular infarction and mechanical complications are discussed in the text. CABG, coronary artery bypass grafting; IABP, intra-aortic balloon pumping. (Modified from Hollenberg SM, Kavinsky CJ, Parrillo JE: Cardiogenic shock. Ann Intern Med 1999;131:51.)

Invasive hemodynamic monitoring can be quite useful to exclude volume depletion, right ventricular infarction, and mechanical complications.[16,35] The hemodynamic profile of cardiogenic shock includes a pulmonary capillary occlusion pressure greater than 15 mm Hg and a cardiac index less than 2.2 L/min/m^2. It should be recognized that optimal filling pressures may be greater than 15 mm Hg in individual patients due to left ventricular diastolic dysfunction. Right-sided heart catheterization may reveal an oxygen step-up diagnostic of ventricular septal rupture or a large v wave that suggests severe mitral regurgitation. The hemodynamic profile of right ventricular infarction includes high right-sided filling pressures in the presence of normal or low occlusion pressures.[56,57]

Coronary angiography is usually performed as a precedent to revascularization, and will be considered later.

INITIAL MANAGEMENT

Maintenance of adequate oxygenation and ventilation are critical; intubation and mechanical ventilation are often required, if only to reduce the work of breathing and facilitate sedation and stabilization before cardiac catheterization. Central venous and arterial access, bladder catheterization, and pulse oximetry are routine. Electrolyte abnormalities should be corrected. Hypokalemia and hypomagnesemia are predisposing factors to ventricular arrhythmias, and acidosis can decrease contractile function. Relief of pain and anxiety with morphine sulfate (or fentanyl if systolic pressure is compromised) can reduce excessive sympathetic activity and decrease oxygen demand, preload, and afterload. Arrhythmias and heart block may have major effects on cardiac output, and should be corrected promptly with antiarrhythmic drugs, cardioversion, or pacing. Cardiology consultation has been shown to be associated with improved outcomes in patients with MI and is strongly indicated in the setting of cardiogenic shock.[58] In addition, measures proven to improve outcome after MI, such as nitrates, beta blockers, and angiotensin-converting enzyme inhibitors,[59] have the potential to exacerbate hypotension in cardiogenic shock and should be stopped until the patient stabilizes.

THERAPY

Following initial stabilization and restoration of adequate blood pressure, tissue perfusion should be assessed (see Fig. 22.4). If tissue perfusion remains inadequate, inotropic support or intra-aortic balloon pumping (IABP) should be initiated. If tissue perfusion is adequate but significant pulmonary congestion remains, diuretics may be employed. Vasodilators can be considered as well, depending on the blood pressure.

The initial approach to the hypotensive patient should include fluid resuscitation unless frank pulmonary edema is present. Patients are commonly diaphoretic and relative hypovolemia may be present. In the original description of hemodynamic subsets in MI, approximately 20% of patients had low cardiac index and low PCWP; most had reduced stroke volume and compensatory tachycardia.[60] Some of these patients would be expected to respond to fluid infusion with an increase in stroke volume, although the magnitude of such a response depends on the degree of ischemia and cardiac reserve.

Fluid infusion is best initiated with predetermined boluses titrated to clinical end points of heart rate, urine output, and blood pressure.[61] Ischemia produces diastolic as well as systolic dysfunction, and thus elevated filling pressures may be necessary to maintain stroke volume in patients with cardiogenic shock. Patients who do not respond rapidly to initial fluid boluses or those with poor physiologic reserve should be considered for invasive hemodynamic monitoring. Optimal filling pressures vary from patient to patient; hemodynamic monitoring can be used to construct a Starling curve at the bedside, identifying the filling pressure at which cardiac output is maximized. Maintenance of adequate preload is particularly important in patients with right ventricular infarction.

When arterial pressure remains inadequate, therapy with vasopressor agents, titrated not only to blood pressure but to clinical indices of perfusion and mixed venous oxygen saturation, may be required to maintain coronary perfusion pressure. Maintenance of adequate blood pressure is essential to break the vicious cycle of progressive hypotension with further myocardial ischemia. Norepinephrine is preferable to dopamine for hypotension in this situation. Dopamine acts as both an inotrope (particularly 3-10 μg/kg/minute) and a vasopressor (10-20 μg/kg/minute). Norepinephrine (0.02-1.0 μg/kg/minute) acts primarily as a vasoconstrictor, has a mild inotropic effect, and increases coronary flow. A recent randomized trial comparing norepinephrine and dopamine in 1678 patients with shock found no significant difference in 28-day mortality rate in the overall trial, but a prespecified subgroup analysis did find increased mortality rate with dopamine in the 280 patients with cardiogenic shock.[62] Phenylephrine, a selective α_1-adrenergic agonist, may be employed to support blood pressure when tachyarrhythmias limit therapy with other vasopressors, although it does not improve cardiac output. Vasopressin, which causes vasoconstriction, has a neutral or slightly depressant effect upon cardiac output, and increases vascular sensitivity to norepinephrine, may be added to catecholamines if needed.

In patients with inadequate tissue perfusion and adequate intravascular volume, cardiovascular support with inotropic agents should be initiated. Dobutamine, a selective β_1-adrenergic receptor agonist, can improve myocardial contractility and increase cardiac output without markedly changing heart rate or SVR; it is the initial agent of choice in patients with systolic pressures greater than 90 mm Hg.[63-65] Dobutamine may exacerbate hypotension in some patients and can precipitate tachyarrhythmias. Phosphodiesterase inhibitors such as milrinone increase intracellular cyclic adenosine monophosphate (cAMP) by mechanisms not involving adrenergic receptors, producing both positive inotropic and vasodilatory actions. Milrinone has fewer chronotropic and arrhythmogenic effects than catecholamines.[66] In addition, because milrinone does not stimulate adrenergic receptors directly, its effects may be additive to those of the catecholamines.[67] Milrinone, however, has the potential to cause hypotension and has a long half-life; in patients with tenuous clinical status, its use is often reserved for situations in which other agents have proved ineffective.[16] Standard administration of milrinone calls for a loading dose followed by an infusion, but most clinicians eschew the loading dose in patients with marginal blood pressure.

Levosimendan, a calcium sensitizer, has both inotropic and vasodilatory properties and does not increase myocardial oxygen consumption. Levosimendan reduces the calcium-binding coefficient of troponin C by stabilizing the conformational shape, which enhances myocardial contraction with lower intracellular calcium concentrations.[68] Several relatively small studies have shown hemodynamic benefits with levosimendan in cardiogenic shock after MI,[69] one suggesting a better hemodynamic effect than dobutamine,[70] but survival benefits with use of levosimendan have not been shown in either cardiogenic shock or acute heart failure.[71] Levosimendan has the potential to cause hypotension and thus should be used with some caution in patients with cardiogenic shock. Levosimendan is not available in the United States.

Infusions of vasoactive agents need to be titrated carefully in patients with cardiogenic shock to maximize coronary perfusion pressure with the least possible increase in myocardial oxygen demand. Invasive hemodynamic monitoring can be extremely useful in allowing optimization of therapy in these unstable patients, because clinical estimates of filling pressure can be unreliable;[72] in addition, changes in myocardial performance and compliance and therapeutic interventions can change cardiac output and filling pressures precipitously. Optimization of filling pressures and serial measurements of cardiac output (and other parameters, such as mixed venous oxygen saturation) allow for titration of the dosage of inotropic agents and vasopressors to the minimum dosage required to achieve the chosen therapeutic goals. This control minimizes the increases in myocardial oxygen demand and arrhythmogenic potential.[61,73]

Diuretics should be used to treat pulmonary congestion and enhance oxygenation. Vasodilators should be used with extreme caution in the acute setting owing to the risk of precipitating further hypotension and decreasing coronary blood flow. After blood pressure has been stabilized, however, vasodilator therapy can decrease both preload and afterload. Sodium nitroprusside is a balanced arterial and venous vasodilator that decreases filling pressures and can increase stroke volume in patients with heart failure by reducing afterload.[74] Nitroglycerin is an effective venodilator that reduces the pulmonary capillary occlusion pressure and can decrease ischemia by reducing left ventricular filling pressure and redistributing coronary blood flow to the ischemic zone.[75] Both agents may cause acute and rapid decreases in blood pressure and dosages must be titrated carefully; invasive hemodynamic monitoring can be useful in optimizing filling pressures when these agents are used.

THROMBOLYTIC THERAPY

Although it has been demonstrated convincingly that thrombolytic therapy reduces mortality rates in patients with acute MI,[10,76-78] the benefits of this therapy in patients with cardiogenic shock are less certain. It is clear that thrombolytic therapy can reduce the likelihood of subsequent development of shock after initial presentation.[14,76,77,79] This is important because most patients develop cardiogenic shock more than 6 hours after hospital presentation.[2,14]

Nonetheless, no trials have demonstrated that thrombolytic therapy reduces mortality rate in patients with established cardiogenic shock. The numbers of patients are small because most thrombolytic trials have excluded patients who have cardiogenic shock at presentation.[80] In the GISSI (Gruppo Italiano per lo Studio della Streptochinasi Nell'Infarto Miocardico) trial,[10,80] 30-day mortality rates were 69.9% in 146 patients with cardiogenic shock who received streptokinase and 70.1% in 134 patients receiving placebo. The International Study Group reported a mortality rate of 65% in 93 patients with shock treated with streptokinase and a mortality rate of 78% in 80 patients treated with recombinant tissue plasminogen activator (rt-PA).[12] In the GUSTO trial,[13] 315 patients had shock on arrival; mortality rate was 56% in patients treated with streptokinase and 59% in patients treated with rt-PA.[14,81]

The failure of thrombolytic therapy to improve survival in patients with cardiogenic shock may seem paradoxical in light of evidence that the absolute reduction in mortality rate with thrombolytics is greatest in those at highest risk at presentation. The meta-analysis performed by the Fibrinolytic Therapy Trialists (FTT) Collaborative Group demonstrated a reduction in mortality rate from 36.1% to 29.7% when thrombolytic therapy was used in patients with initial systolic blood pressures less than 100 mm Hg. In patients with initial heart rates greater than 100 beats per minute the mortality rate decreased from 23.8% to 18.9%.[82] However, most patients in these subgroups did not meet criteria for cardiogenic shock.

Consideration of the efficacy of thrombolytic therapy once cardiogenic shock has been established makes the disappointing results in this subgroup of patients easier to understand. The degree of reperfusion correlates with outcome,[79,83] and reperfusion has been shown to be less likely for patients in cardiogenic shock.[21,83,84] When reperfusion is successful, mortality rate has been shown to be significantly reduced.[21] The lower rates of reperfusion in patients with shock may explain some of the disappointing results in this subgroup in the thrombolytic trials.

The reasons for decreased thrombolytic efficacy in patients with cardiogenic shock include hemodynamic, mechanical, and metabolic factors. Decreased arterial pressure limits the penetration of thrombolytic agents into a thrombus.[85] Passive collapse of the infarct artery in the setting of hypotension can also contribute to decreased thrombolytic efficacy, as can acidosis, which inhibits the conversion of plasminogen to plasmin.[85] Two small studies support the notion that vasopressor therapy to increase aortic pressure improves thrombolytic efficacy.[86,87]

INTRA-AORTIC BALLOON PUMPING

IABP reduces systolic afterload and augments diastolic perfusion pressure, increasing cardiac output and improving coronary blood flow.[88,89] These beneficial effects, in contrast to those of inotropic or vasopressor agents, occur without an increase in oxygen demand. IABP is efficacious for initial stabilization of patients with cardiogenic shock.[90,91] Small randomized trials in the prethrombolytic era, however, failed to show that IABP alone increases survival.[92,93] IABP alone does not substantially improve blood flow distal to a critical coronary stenosis.[94]

IABP is probably not best used as an independent modality to treat cardiogenic shock. It may, however, be an essential support mechanism to allow definitive therapeutic measures to be undertaken. In the GUSTO trial, patients who presented with shock and had early IABP placement showed a trend toward lower mortality rates, even after exclusion of patients who underwent revascularization.[13,95] A similar trend was seen in the SHOCK trial registry, although it did not persist after adjustment for age and catheterization.[2] Several observational studies have also suggested that IABP can improve outcome in patients with shock, although revascularization procedures are a confounding factor in these studies.[96-99] IABP has been shown to decrease reocclusion and cardiac events after emergency angioplasty for acute MI.[100,101] The TACTICS trial randomized 57 patients with MI complicated by hypotension or cardiogenic shock to IABP or placebo in conjunction with fibrinolysis; the trial was terminated early due to difficulties with enrollment and was thus underpowered.[102] Although there was no difference in the primary end point of 6-month mortality rate (34% versus 43%, $p = 0.23$), patients presenting in Killip class III or IV heart failure showed a trend toward benefit with IABP (39% versus 80%, $p = 0.05$).[102]

REVASCULARIZATION

Pathophysiologic considerations and extensive retrospective data favor aggressive mechanical revascularization for patients with cardiogenic shock due to MI. Emergency percutaneous revascularization is the only intervention to date that has been shown to consistently reduce mortality rates in patients with cardiogenic shock.

DIRECT CORONARY ANGIOPLASTY

Reestablishment of brisk (TIMI [Thrombolysis in Myocardial Infarction] grade 3) flow in the infarct-related artery is an important determinant of left ventricular function and survival after MI.[79] Direct percutaneous transluminal coronary angioplasty (PTCA) can achieve TIMI grade 3 flow in 80% to 90% of patients with MI[103-105] compared with rates of 50% to 60% 90 minutes after thrombolytic therapy.[79,106] In addition to improving wall motion in the infarct territory, increased perfusion of the infarct zone has been associated with augmented contraction of remote myocardium, possibly due to recruitment of collateral blood flow.[23]

Use of angioplasty in patients with cardiogenic shock grew out of its use as primary therapy in patients with MI.[21,107-117] Observational studies from registries of randomized trials, most notably the GUSTO-1 trial, have also reported improved outcomes in patients with cardiogenic shock selected for revascularization,[14,84,118] and these findings have also been confirmed in reports from NRMI.[119]

RANDOMIZED STUDIES

Prompt revascularization is the only intervention that has been shown consistently to reduce mortality rates in cardiogenic shock. In the landmark SHOCK trial, patients with shock caused by left ventricular failure complicating ST-segment elevation myocardial infarction (STEMI) were randomized to emergency revascularization ($n = 152$), accomplished by either coronary artery bypass grafting (CABG) or angioplasty, or initial medical stabilization ($n = 150$). IABPs were used in 86% of patients in both groups. The landmark "Should We Emergently Revascularize Occluded Coronaries for Cardiogenic Shock" (SHOCK) study [120,121] was a randomized, multicenter international trial that assigned patients with cardiogenic shock to receive optimal medical management—including IABP and thrombolytic therapy—or to cardiac catheterization with revascularization using PTCA or CABG.[120] The trial enrolled 302 patients and was powered to detect a 20% absolute decrease in 30-day all-cause mortality rates. Mortality rate at 30 days was 46.7% in patients treated with early intervention and 56% in patients treated with initial medical stabilization, but this difference did not quite reach statistical significance ($p = 0.11$).[120] It is important to note that the control group (patients who received medical management) had a lower mortality rate than that reported in previous studies; this may reflect the aggressive use of thrombolytic therapy (64%) and balloon pumping (86%) in these control subjects. These data provide indirect evidence that the combination of thrombolysis and IABP may produce the best outcomes when cardiac catheterization is not immediately available. At 6 months, mortality rate in the SHOCK trial was reduced significantly (50.3% compared with 63.1%, $p = 0.027$),[120] and this risk reduction was maintained at 12 months (mortality rate 53.3% versus 66.4%, $p < 0.03$) (Fig. 22.5).[121] Encouragingly, this 13% absolute improvement in survival remained stable at both 3 and 6 years of follow-up.[122] In addition, most survivors have good functional status.[123]

Subgroup analysis showed a substantial improvement in mortality rates in patients younger than 75 years of age at both 30 days (41.4% versus 56.8%, $p = 0.01$) and 6 months

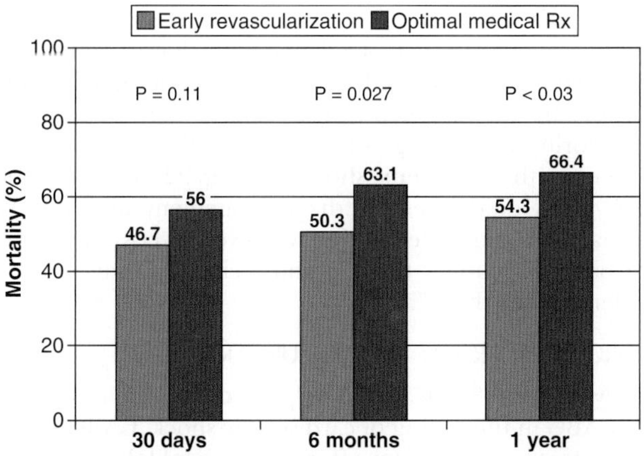

Figure 22.5 Mortality rates in the randomized SHOCK trial at 30 days, 6 months, and 1 year in the early revascularization and optimal medical management groups. (Data from Hochman JS, Sleeper LA, Webb JG, et al: Early revascularization in acute myocardial infarction complicated by cardiogenic shock. N Engl J Med 1999;341:625-634; and Hochman JS, Sleeper LA, White HD, et al: One-year survival following early revascularization for cardiogenic shock. JAMA 2001;285:190-192.)

(44.9% versus 65.0%, $p = 0.003$).[120] For patients older than 75, no benefit of revascularization was demonstrated in the SHOCK trial, although this was a small subgroup, and further analysis suggested baseline differences so that the elderly patients randomized to medical therapy appeared to have been a lower-risk group.[124] In the SHOCK trial registry, elderly patients treated with early revascularization had better outcomes than those treated medically, suggesting that it is possible to select elderly patients who will benefit from aggressive treatment.[125]

The SMASH (Swiss Multicenter Trial of Angioplasty for Shock) trial was independently conceived and had a very similar design, although a more rigid definition of cardiogenic shock resulted in enrollment of sicker patients and a higher mortality rate.[126] The trial was terminated early due to difficulties in patient recruitment for two different reasons: Early on, several centers declined to participate because it was felt that it would not be ethical to undertake early invasive evaluation in such extremely ill patients, and then, after publication of several encouraging studies documenting the superiority of percutaneous coronary intervention (PCI) over thrombolysis for acute MI, many centers felt that it had become unethical *not* to proceed to early evaluation and revascularization.[127] In the SMASH trial, although the patient numbers were very small (55 patients in all), an absolute reduction in 30-day mortality rate similar to that seen in the SHOCK trial was observed (69% mortality rate in the invasive group versus 78% in the medically managed group, RR [relative risk] = 0.88, 95% CI [confidence interval] = 0.6-1.2, p = NS [not significant]).[126] This benefit was also maintained at 1 year.

When the results of both the SHOCK and SMASH trials are put into perspective with results from other randomized, controlled trials of patients with acute MI, an important point emerges: Despite the moderate *relative* risk reduction (for the SHOCK trial, RR 0.72, CI 0.54-0.95; for the SMASH trial, RR 0.88, CI, 0.60-1.20) the *absolute* benefit is important, with 9 lives saved for 100 patients treated at 30 days in both trials, and 13.2 lives saved for 100 patients treated at 1 year in the SHOCK trial. This latter figure corresponds to a number needed to treat of 7.6, one of the lowest figures ever observed in a randomized, controlled trial of cardiovascular disease. In our judgment, these data strongly support the superiority of a strategy of early revascularization in most patients with cardiogenic shock (see Fig. 22.4). In the latest ACC/AHA guidelines for the management of acute MI, primary coronary intervention was given a class I indication for patients younger than 75 and a class IIa indication for patients older than 75.[128]

CORONARY ARTERY BYPASS SURGERY

Analysis of the SHOCK trial helps to define the indications for CABG in the setting of cardiogenic shock. CABG should be the first line of therapy offered in cases of left main artery disease or triple-vessel disease as well as in cases in which the patient has sustained mechanical complications necessitating surgical repair. In patients with multivessel disease in the SHOCK trial, complete revascularization was achieved more frequently (87% versus 23%). Long-term mortality rates were similar in the CABG and PCI groups despite worse coronary anatomy and more diabetes in the surgical group.[129]

OTHER CAUSES OF CARDIOGENIC SHOCK

RIGHT VENTRICULAR INFARCTION

Right ventricular infarction occurs in up to 30% of patients with inferior infarction and is clinically significant in 10%.[130] Patients present with hypotension, elevated jugular venous pressure, and clear lung fields. The diagnosis is made by identifying ST-segment elevation in right precordial leads or by characteristic hemodynamic findings on right-sided heart catheterization (elevated right atrial and right ventricular end-diastolic pressures with normal to low pulmonary artery occlusion pressure and low cardiac output). Echocardiography can demonstrate depressed right ventricular contractility.[57] Patients with cardiogenic shock on the basis of right ventricular infarction have a better prognosis than those with left-sided pump failure.[130] This difference may be due in part to the fact that right ventricular function tends to return to normal over time with supportive therapy,[131] although such therapy may need to be prolonged.

Supportive therapy for patients with right ventricular infarction begins with maintenance of right ventricular preload with fluid administration. In some cases, however, fluid resuscitation may increase pulmonary capillary occlusion pressure but may not increase cardiac output, and overdilation of the right ventricle can compromise left ventricular filling and cardiac output.[131] Inotropic therapy with dobutamine may be more effective in increasing cardiac output in some patients, and monitoring with serial echocardiograms may also be useful to detect right ventricular overdistention.[131] Maintenance of atrioventricular synchrony is also important in these patients to optimize right ventricular filling.[57] For patients with continued hemodynamic instability, IABP may be useful, particularly because elevated right ventricular pressures and volumes increase wall stress and oxygen consumption and decrease right coronary perfusion pressure, exacerbating right ventricular ischemia.

Reperfusion of the occluded coronary artery is also crucial. Restoration of normal flow by direct angioplasty resulted in dramatic recovery of right ventricular function and a mortality rate of only 2%, whereas unsuccessful reperfusion was associated with persistent hemodynamic compromise and a mortality rate of 58%.[132] Prompt revascularization of patients with right ventricular infarction is a class I recommendation in the American College of Cardiology/American Heart Association (ACC/AHA) guidelines for the treatment of acute MI.[133]

ACUTE MITRAL REGURGITATION

Ischemic mitral regurgitation is usually associated with inferior MI and ischemia or infarction of the posterior papillary muscle, which has a single blood supply, usually from the posterior descending branch of a dominant right coronary artery.[134] Papillary muscle rupture typically occurs 2 to 7 days after acute MI and presents dramatically with pulmonary edema, hypotension, and cardiogenic shock. When a papillary muscle ruptures, the murmur of acute mitral regurgitation may be limited to early systole because of rapid equalization of pressures in the left atrium and left ventricle.

More importantly, the murmur may be soft or inaudible, especially when cardiac output is low.[135]

Echocardiography is extremely useful in the differential diagnosis, which includes free wall rupture, ventricular septal rupture, and infarct extension with pump failure. Hemodynamic monitoring with pulmonary artery catheterization may also be helpful. Management includes afterload reduction with nitroprusside and IABP as temporizing measures. Inotropic or vasopressor therapy may also be needed to support cardiac output and blood pressure. Definitive therapy, however, is surgical valve repair or replacement, which should be undertaken as soon as possible because clinical deterioration can be sudden.[135,136] Although mortality rate is 20% to 40%, survival and ventricular function are improved compared with medical therapy.[137]

VENTRICULAR SEPTAL RUPTURE

Patients who have ventricular septal rupture have severe heart failure or cardiogenic shock, with a pansystolic murmur and a parasternal thrill. The hallmark finding is a left-to-right intracardiac shunt ("step-up" in oxygen saturation from right atrium to right ventricle). On pulmonary artery catheter tracing, it can be difficult to distinguish ventricular septal rupture from mitral regurgitation, because both can produce dramatic v waves. The diagnosis is most easily made with echocardiography.

Rapid stabilization, using IABP and pharmacologic measures followed by operative repair, is the only viable option for long-term survival. Because perforations are exposed to shear forces, the rupture site can expand abruptly. Repair can be technically difficult owing to the need to suture in areas of necrosis. Surgical mortality rate is 20% to 50%, especially for serpiginous inferoposterior ruptures, which typically are less well circumscribed than anteroapical ruptures. Right ventricular function is an important determinant of outcome in this setting. Timing of surgery has been controversial, but guidelines now recommend that operative repair should be undertaken early, within 48 hours of the rupture.[59] Placement of a septal occluding device may be helpful in selected patients.

FREE WALL RUPTURE

Ventricular free wall rupture usually occurs during the first week after MI; the classic patient is elderly, female, and hypertensive. The early use of thrombolytic therapy reduces the incidence of cardiac rupture, but late use may increase the risk, particularly in older patients.[138] Free wall rupture presents as a catastrophic event with a pulseless rhythm. Salvage is possible with prompt recognition, pericardiocentesis to relieve acute tamponade, and thoracotomy with repair.[139]

MYOCARDIAL DYSFUNCTION AFTER CARDIOPULMONARY BYPASS

Transient depression of ventricular contractility is common after cardiopulmonary bypass, and can represent a significant clinical problem. The differential diagnosis includes inadequate operation, cardiac tamponade (which may be localized and difficult to detect), and increased right ventricular afterload, but most cases likely result from myocardial stunning. The heart is rendered globally ischemic during aortic cross-clamping and then reperfused, and because demonstrable myocardial necrosis is rare, stunning can be implicated. Stunning after bypass has been documented in a study in which an ultrasonic probe was left on the epicardial surface for 2 to 3 days in 31 patients following bypass surgery; left ventricular wall thickening fell after surgery, reached a nadir at 2 to 6 hours, and subsequently improved, usually returning to baseline by 24 to 48 hours.[140]

The degree of myocardial dysfunction after cardiac surgery is variable, and may depend on the cardioplegia solution, the method of administration (antegrade or retrograde), the mode of administration (continuous or intermittent), and the temperature of the solution and of the patient during surgery.[38] In the clinical setting, transient depression of ventricular contractility is common and usually reversible within 24 to 48 hours. The depression of contractility can be severe to cause cardiogenic shock. In this event, therapy with inotropic agents, vasodilators, and IABP is necessary. Occasionally, even a left ventricular assist device may be employed.[40] Better understanding of the mechanisms of post–cardiopulmonary bypass myocardial dysfunction may lead to better preventive and therapeutic approaches.

MYOCARDITIS

Acute myocarditis can be benign and self-limited or fulminant, with severe congestive heart failure or atrial and ventricular arrhythmias. After acute myocarditis, patients can recover completely, or they can have severe left ventricular dysfunction. In some patients with acute inflammatory myocarditis, an aberrant immune response occurs, with continuing inflammation, and this can result in the eventual development of a dilated cardiomyopathy.

Evidence exists that some patients with myocarditis will benefit from immunosuppressive therapy, but how to identify which patients should be treated remains controversial. A trial initiated at the National Institutes of Health randomized 102 patients with dilated cardiomyopathy, no significant coronary artery disease, and ejection fraction less than 35% to oral prednisone or placebo.[141] The prospectively defined end point, an increase in radionuclide-measured ejection fraction of more than 5 percentage points, was observed in 53% of patients treated with prednisone compared to only 27% of control subjects at 3 months ($p < 0.05$), but the improvement did not persist at 9 months when patients were switched to alternate-day prednisone therapy.[141] Another clinical trial of immunosuppressive therapy for myocarditis showed no improvement in mean ejection fraction with immunosuppression, although the admission criteria in this trial were quite restrictive, the therapeutic regimens heterogeneous, and the incidence of definitive myocarditis uncertain.[142] We advocate consideration of corticosteroids in patients with myocarditis who do not respond to conventional heart failure therapies.

Although it might seem that patients with fulminant myocarditis might be the best candidates for immunosuppressive therapy, a recent series confounds this notion by reporting excellent long-term survival in patients with

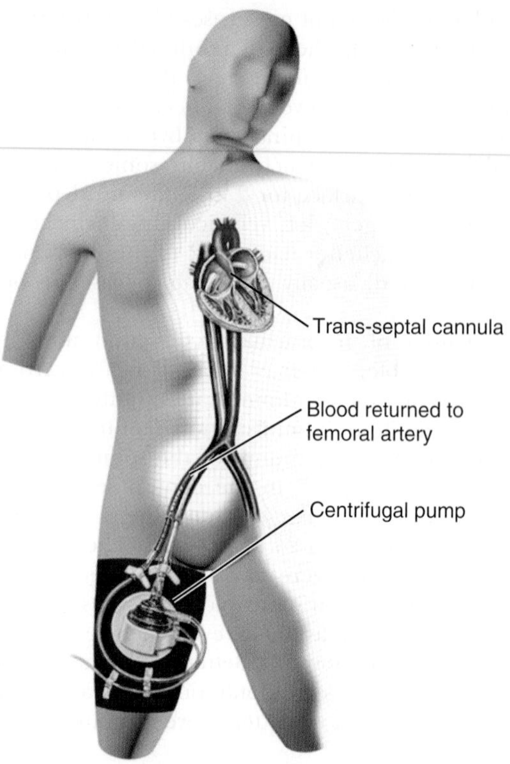

Figure 22.6 The TandemHeart percutaneous left ventricular assist device in situ. Blood is removed from the left atrium using a catheter placed from the femoral vein across the interatrial septum and pumped into the femoral artery. (Image courtesy of CardioAssist, Pittsburgh, PA.)

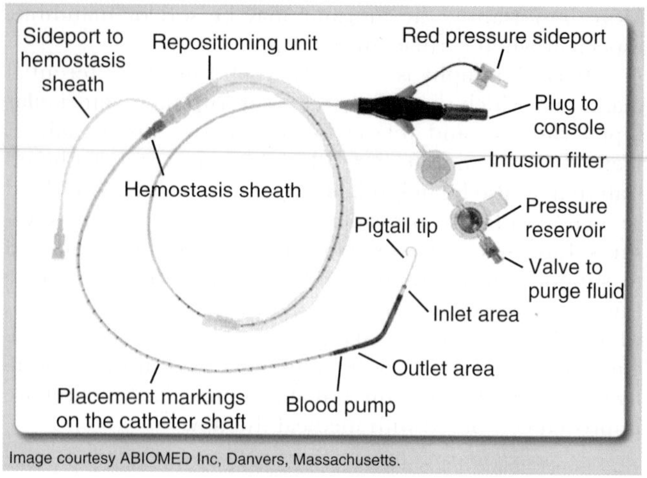

Figure 22.7 The Impella catheter when placed across the aortic valve (*left*). The inflow port is positioned within the left ventricle, and the outflow port is just above the valve. Impella catheter with introducer and sheath (*right*). (Images courtesy of Abiomed, Danvers, MA.)

myocarditis and a fulminant course.[143] Patients with acute myocarditis without a fulminant course had a much worse prognosis in this series,[143] pointing up the need for further research to identify subgroups of patients with dilated cardiomyopathy who may benefit from adjunctive therapies.

LEFT VENTRICULAR ASSIST DEVICES

In patients with potentially reversible causes of myocardial dysfunction, aggressive cardiovascular support with a combination of inotropic agents and intra-aortic balloon counterpulsation may be required for hours or days to allow sufficient time for recovery. If these measures fail, mechanical circulatory support with left ventricular assist devices (LVADs) can be considered.[144] Mechanical support with LVADs can interrupt the downward spiral of myocardial dysfunction, hypoperfusion, and ischemia in cardiogenic shock, allowing time for recovery of stunned or hibernating myocardium.

Percutaneously implanted LVADs are used in situations of cardiogenic shock, during high-risk percutaneous interventions, in postcardiotomy shock, and in fulminant myocarditis. Two currently approved devices, the TandemHeart (Fig. 22.6) and the Impella (Fig. 22.7), can be placed in the cardiac catheterization laboratory. The TandemHeart device is a bypass system with inflow of oxygenated blood from the left atrium and outflow to the femoral artery using a centrifugal flow pump; it can provide blood flow up to 5 L/minute. The Impella device is inserted across the aortic valve and pumps blood from a distal port from within the ventricle out to the ascending aorta through a proximal port of the device; there are two versions, one capable of pumping 2.5 L/minute, and one with a larger diameter that can provide up to 5 L/minute, although the actual flow is dependent on afterload. The inflow cannula with its pump is under fluoroscopic guidance. The device sits across the aortic valve. These devices augment cardiac output and blood pressure while decreasing myocardial oxygen demand. Both devices offer the potential for near-complete cardiac support but do require adequate right ventricular function. Known complications of percutaneous LVAD use include limb ischemia and bleeding.

Two recent trials compared the use of IABP to the TandemHeart for patients with cardiogenic shock,[145,146] and another compared use of the Impella to IABP therapy;[147] the results of these trials were combined in a meta-analysis that included 100 patients.[148] Hemodynamic benefits for the percutaneous LVADs compared with IABP were shown, with higher cardiac indices and mean arterial pressures as well as lower PCWPs. However, LVAD use showed no mortality rate benefit over IABP at 30 days.[148]

For patients with end-stage heart failure and refractory shock, a variety of surgically placed assist devices can be employed for circulatory support. These devices retrieve blood from the left ventricular apex and use a pumping device, either continuous or pulsatile, to return the blood into the ascending aorta. Full consideration of these devices is beyond the scope of this chapter; in cardiogenic shock, they are usually used as a bridge to recovery or transplantation, although in other contexts they may be used as destination therapy.

CONCLUSION

Cardiogenic shock remains a prevalent and dangerous syndrome that requires accurate and efficient diagnosis. Mortality rates in patients with cardiogenic shock have improved but remain frustratingly high. Its pathophysiology involves a downward spiral in which ischemia causes myocardial dysfunction, which in turn worsens ischemia. Areas of nonfunctional but viable myocardium can also cause or contribute to the development of cardiogenic shock. Expeditious coronary revascularization is crucial, and the randomized multicenter SHOCK trial[120] has provided important data that help clarify the appropriate role and timing of revascularization in patients with cardiogenic shock. The potential for reversal of myocardial dysfunction with revascularization provides the rationale for supportive therapy to maintain coronary and tissue perfusion until more definitive revascularization measures can be undertaken. Application of a thorough understanding of the essentials of pathophysiology, diagnosis, and treatment of cardiogenic shock can allow for expeditious management and improved outcomes.

KEY POINTS

- Cardiogenic shock is a state of inadequate tissue perfusion due to cardiac dysfunction. Acute MI is the leading cause.
- The pathogenesis of cardiogenic shock is a "downward spiral" in which MI or ischemia causes myocardial dysfunction and compromised myocardial perfusion, exacerbating ischemia.
- Large areas of nonfunctional but viable myocardium (either stunned, hibernating, or both) can also cause or contribute to the development of cardiogenic shock in patients after MI.
- The challenge in initial management of cardiogenic shock is that evaluation and therapy must begin simultaneously. The clinician must perform the clinical assessment required to understand the cause of shock while initiating supportive therapy before shock causes irreversible damage.
- Thrombolytic therapy alone has less efficacy in patients with cardiogenic shock than in other settings; this is due to a combination of hemodynamic, mechanical, and metabolic factors.
- IABP alone has not been shown to decrease mortality rate in cardiogenic shock, but it may be an essential support mechanism to allow definitive therapeutic measures to be undertaken.
- Pathophysiologic considerations and extensive retrospective data favor aggressive mechanical revascularization for patients with cardiogenic shock due to MI. Results of the recent SHOCK study support

KEY POINTS (Continued)

a strategy of early revascularization in most patients with cardiogenic shock.

- Other acute mechanical causes of low cardiac output must be excluded. If present, urgent surgery may be required.
- In patients with potentially reversible causes of myocardial dysfunction (including severe myocarditis), aggressive cardiovascular support with a combination of inotropic agents and intra-aortic balloon counterpulsation may be required for hours or days to allow sufficient time for recovery.

SELECTED REFERENCES

2. Hochman JS, Boland J, Sleeper LA, et al: Current spectrum of cardiogenic shock and effect of early revascularization on mortality. Results of an International Registry. Circulation 1995;91:873-881.
3. Goldberg RJ, Spencer FA, Gore JM, et al: Thirty-year trends (1975 to 2005) in the magnitude of, management of, and hospital death rates associated with cardiogenic shock in patients with acute myocardial infarction: A population-based perspective. Circulation 2009;119:1211-1219.
24. Hollenberg SM, Kavinsky CJ, Parrillo JE: Cardiogenic shock. Ann Intern Med 1999;131:47-59.
25. Hochman JS: Cardiogenic shock complicating acute myocardial infarction: Expanding the paradigm. Circulation 2003;107:2998-3002.
61. Hollenberg SM, Ahrens TS, Annane D, et al: Practice parameters for hemodynamic support of sepsis in adult patients: 2004 update. Crit Care Med 2004;32:1928-1948.
62. De Backer D, Biston P, Devriendt J, et al: Comparison of dopamine and norepinephrine in the treatment of shock. N Engl J Med 2010;362:779-789.
120. Hochman JS, Sleeper LA, Webb JG, et al: Early revascularization in acute myocardial infarction complicated by cardiogenic shock. N Engl J Med 1999;341:625-634.
121. Hochman JS, Sleeper LA, White HD, et al: One-year survival following early revascularization for cardiogenic shock. JAMA 2001;285:190-192.
128. Kushner FG, Hand M, Smith SC Jr, et al: 2009 Focused Updates: ACC/AHA Guidelines for the Management of Patients With ST-Elevation Myocardial Infarction (updating the 2004 Guideline and 2007 Focused Update) and ACC/AHA/SCAI Guidelines on Percutaneous Coronary Intervention (updating the 2005 Guideline and 2007 Focused Update): A report of the American College of Cardiology Foundation/American Heart Association Task Force on Practice Guidelines. Circulation 2009;120:2271-2330.
148. Cheng JM, den Uil CA, Hoeks SE, et al: Percutaneous left ventricular assist devices vs. intra-aortic balloon pump counterpulsation for treatment of cardiogenic shock: A meta-analysis of controlled trials. Eur Heart J 2009;30:2102-2108.

The complete list of references can be found at www.expertconsult.com.

23 Septic Shock

Stephen Trzeciak | R. Phillip Dellinger | Joseph E. Parrillo

CHAPTER OUTLINE

OVERVIEW

This chapter pertains to pathophysiology, assessment, and management of septic shock, the most severe and overt manifestation of the septic condition. This discussion will specifically focus on cardiovascular and hemodynamic aspects. Other critically important elements of sepsis pathophysiology, assessment, and management (i.e., beyond the cardiovascular and hemodynamic aspects) will be addressed in a separate chapter (see Chapter 25, Sepsis and Multiple Organ Dysfunction). This chapter is also focused specifically on the adult patient with septic shock, as principles and evidence may differ in important ways in the pediatric population.

HISTORICAL PERSPECTIVE

The word *sepsis* originated from the Greek language. *Sepsis* was synonymous with putrefaction and pertained to the bacteria-mediated decomposition of organic matter.[1] The term persisted for more than 2700 years with essentially unchanged meaning.[2] In the twentieth century, our modern understanding of the term *sepsis* became rooted in a disease in which the clinical manifestations were attributed to severe infection and the release of pathogenic bacterial products into the patient's bloodstream.[3,4]

The term *shock* comes from the French word "choquer," meaning "to collide with." This is particularly appropriate terminology for shock due to sepsis, given our modern understanding of the sepsis pathophysiology, whereby the body's host defenses essentially collide with the invading microorganism, triggering a profound proinflammatory host response.[1]

CONTEMPORARY DEFINITIONS

Shock is defined as a failure of the cardiovascular system to maintain effective tissue perfusion. If effective tissue perfusion is not promptly restored, cellular dysfunction and acute organ failure may occur and may become irreversible, leading to acute organ system failure. When shock develops because of a systemic inflammatory response to infection, it is termed *septic shock.* The American College of Chest Physicians (ACCP) and the Society of Critical Care Medicine (SCCM) first published consensus conference definitions for sepsis syndromes more than 20 years ago,[5] and these definitions were revisited and further developed by international consensus in 2003.[6] *Septic shock* was defined as infection-induced hypotension (systolic blood pressure <90 mm Hg [or a drop of >40 mm Hg] plus signs of tissue hypoperfusion despite adequate fluid resuscitation). The concurrent presence of clinical signs of tissue hypoperfusion (e.g., metabolic acidosis, encephalopathy, acute lung injury, oliguria, acute kidney injury, peripheral extremity discoloration, or impaired capillary refill) is an integral component of making the diagnosis of septic shock, because baseline blood pressure can vary among patients, and patients with lower baseline blood pressure may tolerate an arterial pressure lower than the values stated here without being in circulatory shock. The overarching purpose and major impact of the efforts to establish the contemporary definitions given here was the promotion of uniformity in inclusion criteria for sepsis clinical trials.[7]

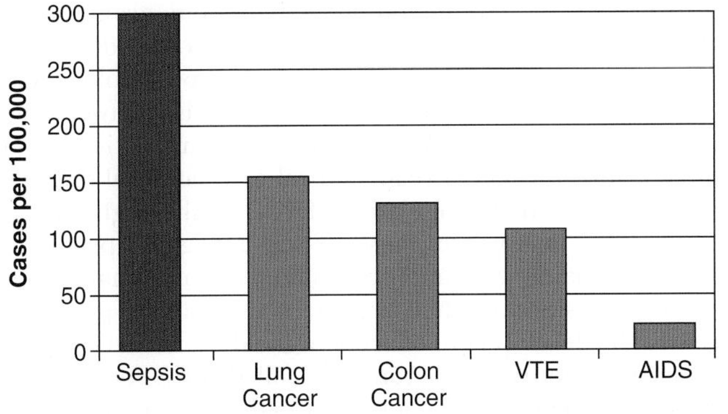

Figure 23.1 Incidence (cases per 100,000 population) of severe sepsis in the United States compared to four high-profile diseases.[8-11] AIDS, acquired immune deficiency syndrome; VTE, venous thromboembolic disease.

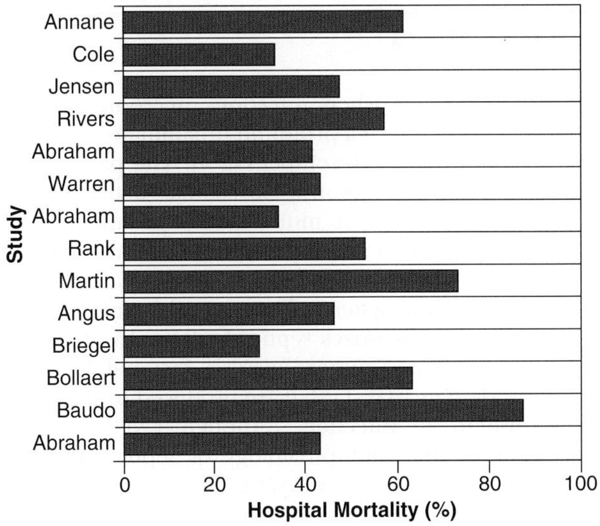

Figure 23.2 A compilation of septic shock mortality rates taken from the placebo arms of sepsis clinical trials published over the past decade (listed by first author). (Adapted from Dellinger RP: Cardiovascular management of septic shock. Crit Care Med 2003;31(3):946-955.)

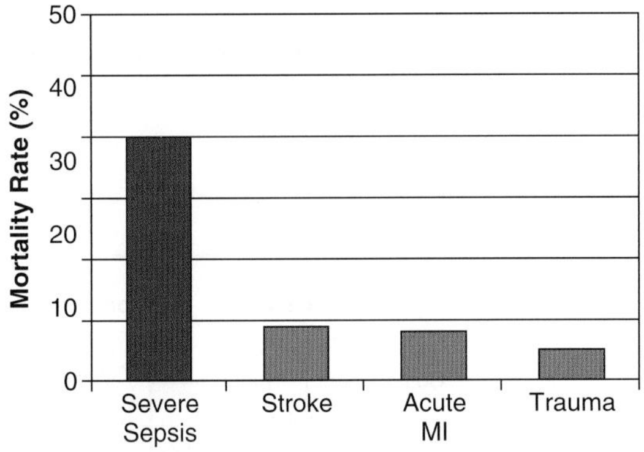

Figure 23.3 Mortality rate of severe sepsis in the United States compared to three diseases that are treated aggressively with time-sensitive interventions.[8,15-17] MI, myocardial infarction.

EPIDEMIOLOGY

Severe sepsis (sepsis plus acute organ system dysfunction) is a common and deadly disease with major public health implications. Although heterogeneity of definitions of sepsis has historically made the incidence of severe sepsis and septic shock difficult to precisely measure, estimates of the incidence have been possible. Using the International Classification of Diseases (ICD)-9 codes for infection and organ dysfunction, Angus and coworkers estimated that 751,000 cases of severe sepsis occur in the United States every year.[8] Figure 23.1 displays the incidence of severe sepsis in the United States compared to other common diseases. The incidence of severe sepsis currently exceeds the incidence of lung and colon cancer, venous thromboembolic disease, and acquired immune deficiency syndrome (AIDS),[8-11] and the incidence is projected to increase by 1.5% per year, resulting in more than 1 million cases of severe sepsis annually by the year 2020.[8] The incidence of sepsis and septic shock is known to be increasing because of a longer lifespan for patients with severe chronic medical conditions that predispose them to acquiring sepsis. This includes an increase in the number of immunocompromised patients in the community, number of infections caused by resistant organisms, increased use of intravascular catheters, and aging of the population.[8]

Sepsis is the leading cause of death among critically ill patients[12] and is responsible for as many deaths annually in the United States as acute myocardial infarction.[8] Figure 23.2 displays control arm mortality rates in septic shock clinical trials.[1] In a recent large multicenter registry study, septic patients with both arterial hypotension and severe lactic acidosis experienced a 46% mortality rate, whereas the mortality rate for arterial hypotension or severe lactic acidosis alone was 37% and 30%, respectively.[13] Overall, severe sepsis in general ranks as the tenth leading cause of death in the United States, with 215,000 deaths annually and an estimated 30% in-hospital mortality rate.[8,14] Figure 23.3 displays the mortality rate for severe sepsis compared to other high-profile diseases that may require critical care (acute ischemic stroke, acute myocardial infarction, and trauma).[8,15-17] The apparent disparity in mortality rates across these diseases may be explained in part by differences in the conventional approach to treatment, as acute ischemic stroke, acute myocardial infarction, and trauma are all typically treated with aggressive interventions in a time-sensitive fashion. Similar to the "golden hour" concept for trauma care that was first recognized more than 30 years ago[18] we are now beginning to understand that early aggressive interventions for sepsis can also have an impact on outcome.

It is also important to recognize that, in addition to a high mortality rate, severe sepsis and septic shock are associated with serious risk of morbidity among survivors.[19,20] A systematic review of the literature found that sepsis survivors had substantially diminished quality of life and a sharply reduced long-term survival after typical short-term (i.e., 28-day) outcomes are assessed.[19] Among older adults, severe sepsis has been associated with major persistent cognitive impairment and functional disability that could have a substantial impact on those patients' ability to live independently.[20] Taken together, even among patients who survive the sepsis insult, the development of severe sepsis or septic shock can represent a pivotal event in the trajectory of a patient's life.

PATHOGENESIS

Septic shock results when infectious microorganisms in the bloodstream induce a profound inflammatory response causing hemodynamic decompensation. The pathogenesis involves a complex response of cellular activation that triggers the release of a multitude of proinflammatory mediators. This inflammatory response causes activation of leukocytes and endothelial cells, as well as activation of the coagulation system. The excessive inflammatory response that characterizes septic shock is driven primarily by the cytokines tumor necrosis factor-alpha (TNF-α) and interleukin 1 (IL-1) that are produced by monocytes in response to an infection. Although TNF-α and IL-1 are central to the pathophysiology of septic shock and act synergistically to induce hypotension in experimental models, a number of other vital mediators are also known to play a major role, including high-mobility group box 1 (HMGB1) protein.[21] Another important recent advance in our understanding of septic shock pathophysiology has been identification of the close link that exists between the proinflammatory response of septic shock and activation of the coagulation system (e.g., clinical or subclinical disseminated intravascular coagulation [DIC]).[22] Although the systemic inflammatory response of sepsis triggers profound macrocirculatory and microcirculatory changes that impair tissue perfusion, another important mechanism playing a role in the development of acute organ dysfunction in septic shock is apoptosis (programmed cell death). Accelerated apoptosis is known to be a critical pathogenic event in this disease. In addition, certain genetic polymorphisms are becoming recognized as major determinants of susceptibility to infection, as well as risk of death from septic shock. Key steps in the pathogenesis of septic shock are shown in Figure 23.4.

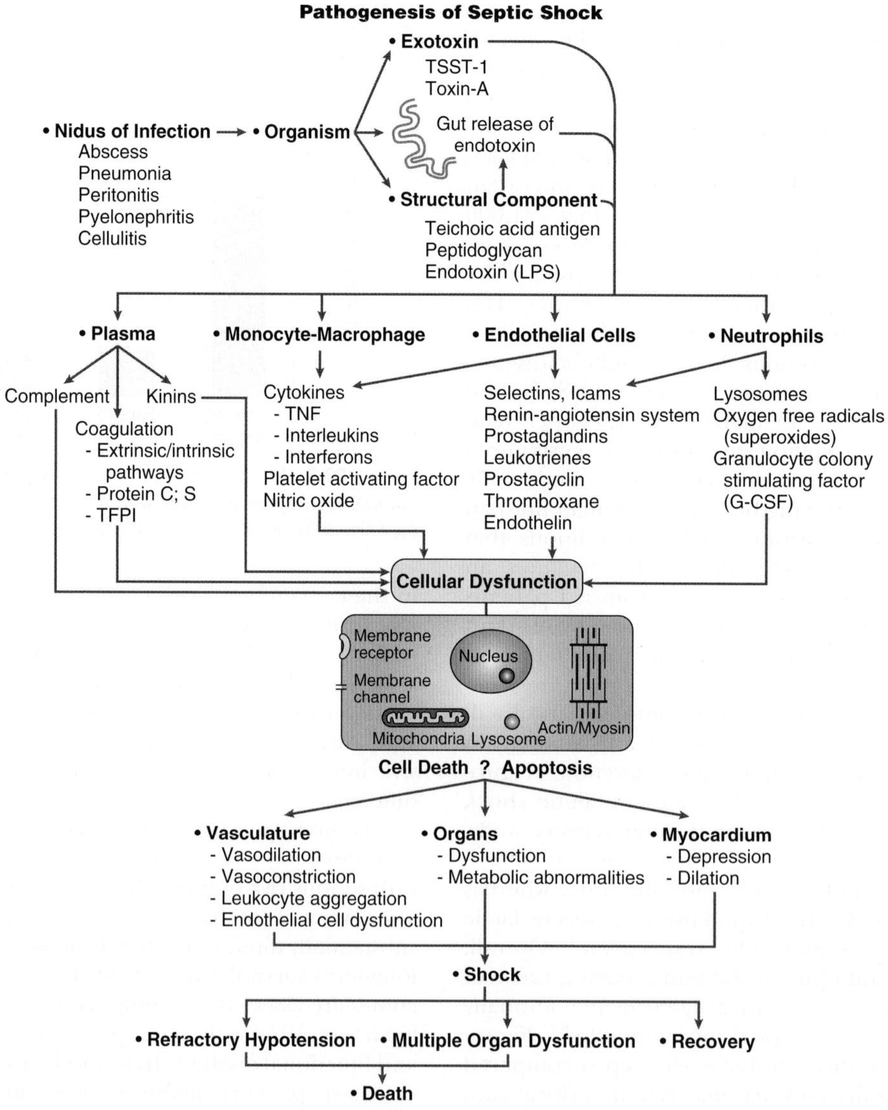

Figure 23.4 Pathogenetic sequence of the events in septic shock. LPS, lipopolysaccharide; TFPI, tissue factor pathway inhibitor; TNF, tumor necrosis factor; Toxin A, *Pseudomonas aeruginosa* toxin A; TSST-1, toxic shock syndrome toxin 1. (Data from Parrillo JE: Pathogenetic mechanisms of septic shock. N Engl J Med 1993;328:1471-1477.)

CLINICAL PRESENTATION

Patients with septic shock will typically manifest signs of systemic inflammation including fever or hypothermia, tachycardia, tachypnea, and elevation or reduction of the white blood cell count. Although the absence of arterial hypotension does not necessarily exclude the possibility of subclinical tissue hypoperfusion,[23] the hallmark of septic shock is arterial hypotension despite adequate volume resuscitation requiring vasoactive drugs for hemodynamic support. Other signs of potential tissue hypoperfusion may include lactic acidosis, oliguria, encephalopathy, or diminished capillary refill in the extremities. Patients with septic shock typically have multiple organ system dysfunctions; clinical evidence of other organ system dysfunction may range from subtle abnormalities to overt organ failure. Multiorgan system involvement in sepsis may include cardiovascular, respiratory, renal, central nervous system, hepatic, metabolic, or hematologic dysfunction. Respiratory system dysfunction manifests as acute lung injury or, in the most extreme cases, the acute respiratory distress syndrome (ARDS). Sepsis-induced renal dysfunction typically manifests with oliguria and may progress to acute renal failure requiring dialysis. Central nervous system dysfunction will manifest as encephalopathy, which may range from mild cognitive impairment to overt coma. Cholestasis is a common manifestation of hepatic dysfunction in sepsis, but in the presence of severe shock, ischemic hepatitis ("shock liver") may occur. Metabolic derangements of septic shock include a loss of glycemic control (hyper- or hypoglycemia) as well as metabolic acidosis. Septic shock is commonly associated with a consumptive coagulopathy, which is likely present in almost all patients at least subclinically,[24] but may also manifest clinically with thrombocytopenia, prolongation of the prothrombin time, or in the most severe cases, overt DIC.

The multiple organ dysfunction associated with septic shock is not only a critical event in the pathogenesis of this disease, but is also closely linked with mortality rate.[8,25,26] There is an approximate 20% increase in septic shock mortality rate with each additional organ system that fails.[8] *Early* evidence of organ failure is an especially strong predictor of death.[26,27] Early improvement in organ function (e.g., 0-24 hour improvement in the Sequential Organ Failure Assessment [SOFA] score[28,29]) is closely related to sepsis survival, whereas later improvement after the first 24 hours has little predictive value.[27] These data, garnered largely from observational studies as well as placebo arms of interventional trials, support the concept that aggressive therapy for sepsis to reverse (or prevent the development of) acute organ system failure within the first 24 hours is closely associated with eventual outcome.

HEMODYNAMIC PROFILE OF SEPTIC SHOCK

The hemodynamic profile of septic shock is the most complex hemodynamic profile of all shock etiologies (Fig. 23.5). What sets septic shock apart from other causes of circulatory shock is the fact that there may be multiple different mechanisms of circulatory shock occurring simultaneously.[1,30] Septic shock may have features of (1) hypovolemic shock (poor cardiac filling secondary to severe systemic capillary leak and increased venous capacitance), (2) cardiogenic shock (infection-induced myocardial depression), and (3) distributive shock (arteriolar vasodilation with tissue hypoperfusion in the face of an adequate cardiac output).[1]

HYPOVOLEMIA

The release of proinflammatory mediators into the circulation causes injury to the integrity of the endothelial cell surface throughout the systemic microvasculature, resulting in severe capillary leak and extravasation of fluid into tissues. Venodilation also compromises venous return. These are major factors in producing hypovolemia in the patient with septic shock. The septic shock patient may have a markedly decreased cardiac preload, especially in the initial phase of therapy. Aggressive resuscitation with intravenous volume expansion modulates the hemodynamic profile of septic shock and allows the patient to achieve a hyperdynamic (i.e., high cardiac output) state.[1] The combination of a decreased preload and myocardial depression means that in the early phase of sepsis resuscitation, patients may initially be hypodynamic (i.e., low cardiac output) prior to receiving adequate volume resuscitation. Capillary leak is an ongoing process in the course of septic shock therapy, and therefore hypovolemia may recur later in the course of the disease, even after adequate cardiac filling has been initially achieved. Fluid balance (input of intravenous fluids and output of urine) is an unreliable parameter for assessing adequacy of fluid resuscitation in septic shock.

MYOCARDIAL DYSFUNCTION

Septic shock is associated with depression of biventricular function with a decrease in the ejection fraction. Ventricular dilation occurs as a compensatory mechanism and raises end-diastolic volume so that stroke volume can be preserved, taking advantage of the Starling principle. When myocardial dysfunction occurs, a high cardiac output can still be achieved in many circumstances because of biventricular dilation, tachycardia, and arteriolar dilatation, as long as the patient is adequately volume resuscitated and does not have a severe cardiac suppression (related either to previously existing cardiac dysfunction or overwhelming sepsis-induced suppression of cardiac systolic function).[30] The most important inflammatory mediators that induce myocardial depression are TNF-α, IL-1, and perhaps nitric oxide.[31,32] Coronary blood flow is typically normal or increased in septic shock.[33] Although coronary blood flow can be diminished by severe arterial hypotension that compromises coronary perfusion pressure (especially if there is preexisting coronary artery disease), myocardial ischemia does not appear to be the causative factor of the depression in myocardial performance. It has been reported that nearly half of patients with septic shock will have echocardiographic evidence of some degree of depression of systolic function, even in the absence of preexisting cardiac disease.[34] However, myocardial depression is typically not the predominant feature of the septic shock hemodynamic profile.[30]

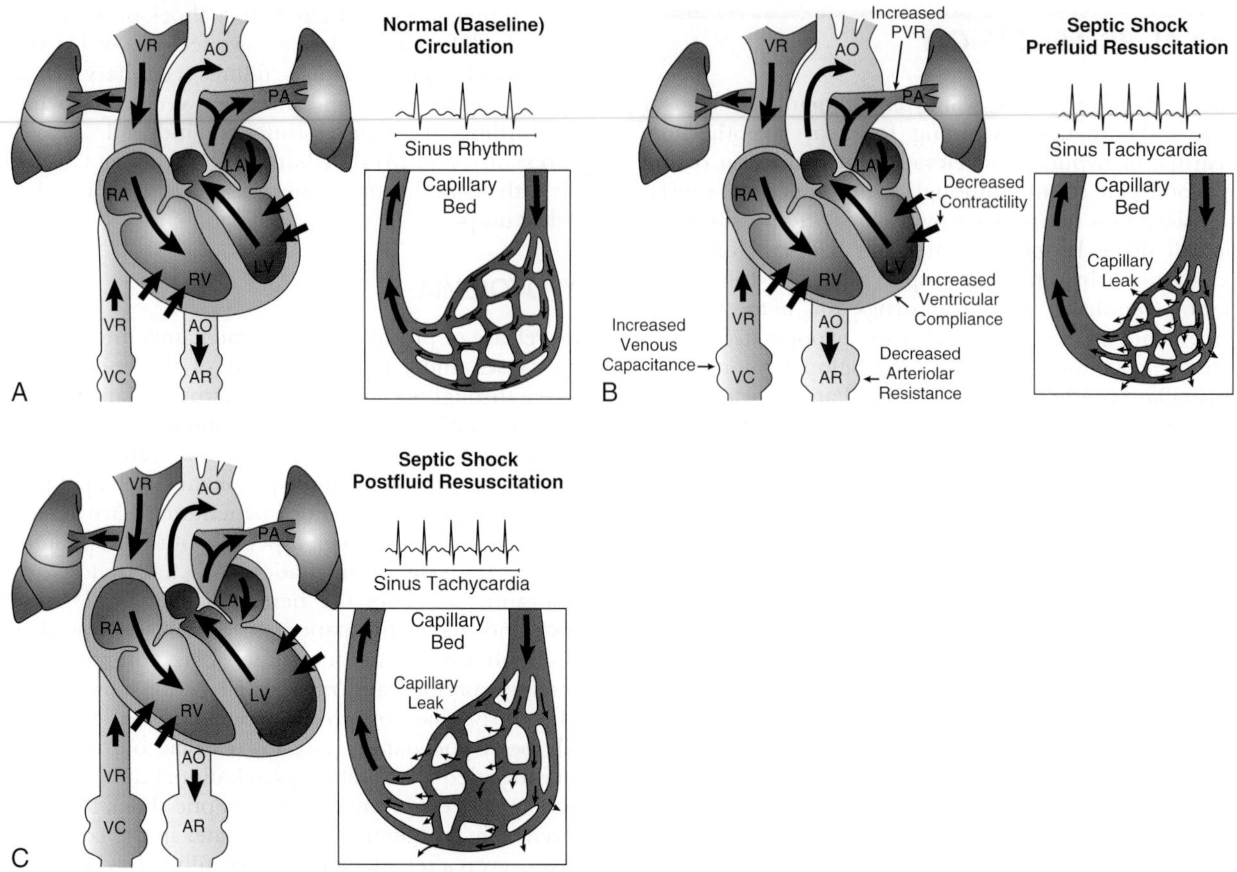

Figure 23.5 Cardiovascular changes associated with septic shock and the effects of fluid resuscitation. **A,** Normal (baseline) state. **B,** In septic shock, left ventricular blood return is reduced owing to a combination of capillary leak (*inset*), increased venous capacitance (VC), and increased pulmonary vascular resistance. The stroke volume is further compromised by a sepsis-induced decrease in left and right ventricular (RV) contractility. Tachycardia and increased left ventricular compliance serve as countermeasures to combat low cardiac output, the latter by increasing left ventricular preload. However, cardiac output remains low to normal. Finally, a decrease in arteriolar (systemic vascular) resistance allows a higher stroke volume at any given contractility and left ventricular filling state, but also the potential for severe hypotension, despite restoration of adequate left ventricular filling. **C,** Aggressive fluid resuscitation compensates for capillary leak, increased venous capacitance, and increased pulmonary vascular resistance by reestablishing adequate left ventricular blood return. Decreased arteriolar resistance (AR), tachycardia, and increased left ventricular compliance compensate for decreased ejection fraction. Ejection fraction increases as left ventricular filling increases. The net result is that after adequate volume resuscitation, most patients with severe sepsis have a high cardiac output and low systemic vascular resistance state. AO, aorta; LA, left atrium; LV, left ventricle; RA, right atrium; VR, venous return; →, blood flow (cardiac output); ⇒, contractility. (From Dellinger RP: Cardiovascular management of septic shock. Crit Care Med 2003;31(3):946-955.)

For the majority of patients, aggressive intravascular volume expansion to restore adequate cardiac filling pressures will be enough to achieve a reasonable cardiac output.

DISTRIBUTIVE SHOCK

Septic shock is characterized by peripheral maldistribution of blood flow to tissues such that tissue hypoperfusion abnormalities can persist despite a normal or high cardiac output. This is called "distributive shock."[30] This maldistribution of blood flow may occur at both microcirculatory and macrocirculatory levels. The role of microcirculatory dysfunction is discussed in detail in the next section of this chapter. At the level of the macrocirculation, the autoregulation of blood flow within any single organ system in a normal host can typically maintain effective tissue perfusion over a wide range of systemic pressures (usually ranging from a mean arterial pressure [MAP] of 50 mm Hg to 150 mm Hg). However, there is heterogeneity of blood flow distribution throughout the body in septic shock due to preferential shunting of blood flow to vital organs (e.g., the brain and myocardium). The gastrointestinal tract may be the earliest organ system to experience tissue hypoperfusion in septic shock, as blood is shunted away from the splanchnic circulation in order to preserve blood flow to the brain, myocardium, and skeletal muscles. Ischemic injury to the gastrointestinal tract may be a source of ongoing systemic inflammation in septic shock.

The three components of the hemodynamic profile of septic shock are displayed in Figure 23.6.

MICROCIRCULATORY AND MITOCHONDRIAL DYSFUNCTION

After restoration of adequate cardiac filling pressures and achievement of optimal cardiac output in patients with septic shock, tissue dysoxia may still occur via a number of

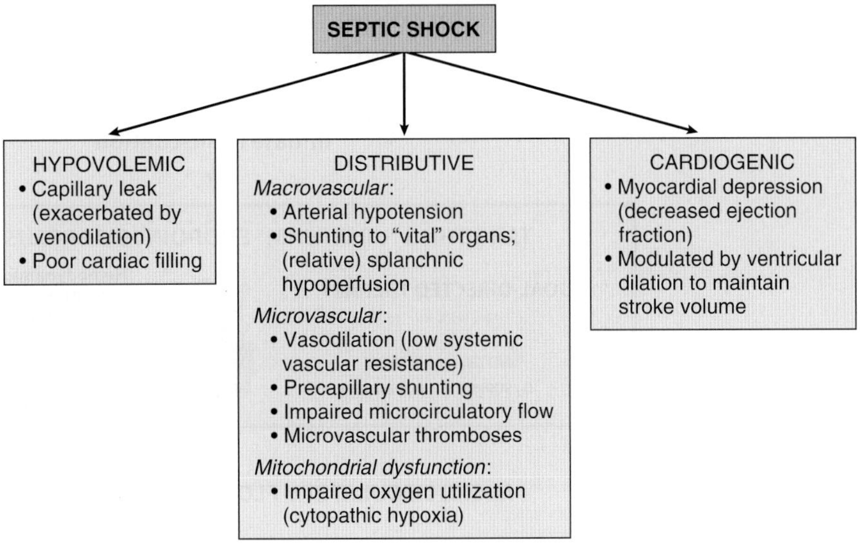

Figure 23.6 Major components of the hemodynamic profile in septic shock. (From Trzeciak S, Parrillo JE: Septic shock. In Society of Critical Care Medicine 8th Adult Critical Care Refresher Course. Chicago, Society of Critical Care Medicine, 2004.)

pathogenic mechanisms. These mechanisms of tissue dysoxia in the face of a normal or a supranormal cardiac output may be due to either (1) microcirculatory dysfunction or (2) mitochondrial dysfunction. These pathogenic mechanisms impair the way in which individual cells can either receive or utilize oxygen, respectively.

MICROCIRCULATORY DYSFUNCTION

Microcirculatory dysfunction is a pivotal element of the pathogenesis of septic shock.[35-38] Although the macrocirculation (heart and large arteries) regulates the global distribution of blood flow throughout the body, it is the microcirculation that controls the delivery of blood flow to tissues. Using intravital videomicroscopy, experimental models of sepsis have demonstrated impaired microcirculatory flow velocity, "stopped-flow" microvessels, increased heterogeneity of regional perfusion, and low density of perfused capillaries.[39-42] These derangements can cause marked alterations of oxygen transport including impaired tissue oxygen extraction.[43] With the advent of new investigational videomicroscopy techniques, it is now possible to study the microcirculatory network in human subjects with septic shock. Microcirculatory failure appears to be one of the critical pathogenic events in sepsis that is associated with acute multiorgan dysfunction and death.[35-38] As these alterations of microcirculatory flow in sepsis can occur in the *absence* of global hemodynamic perturbations (i.e., absence of low arterial pressure or low cardiac output),[36,42,44] derangements of small vessel perfusion are largely a function of intrinsic events in the microcirculation.

The causes of microcirculatory flow alterations in sepsis (Fig. 23.7) are multifactorial and include endothelial cell dysfunction, increased leukocyte adhesion, microthrombi formation, rheologic abnormalities, altered local perfusion pressures due to regional redistribution of blood flow, and functional shunting.[39,45] The proinflammatory cytokines released in sepsis cause diffuse endothelial cell activation, which is associated with neutrophil activation, expression of endothelial adhesion molecules (i.e., integrins and selectins), and localization of white blood cells to areas of

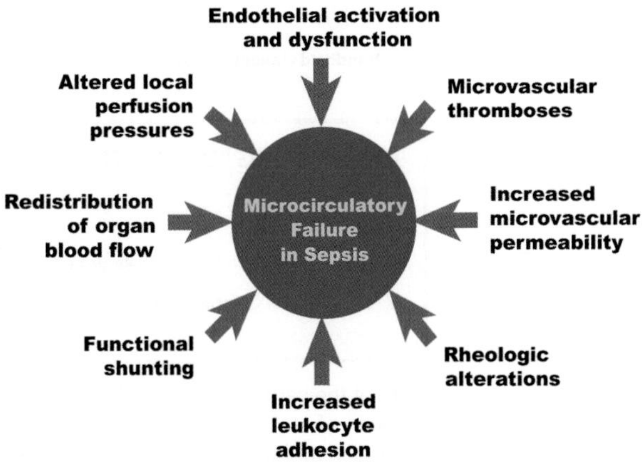

Figure 23.7 Causes of microcirculatory failure in sepsis. (Adapted from Spronk PE, Zandstra DF, Ince C: Bench-to-bedside review: Sepsis is a disease of the microcirculation. Crit Care 2004;8(6):462-468.)

microvascular injury. Pan-endothelial cell injury increases microvascular permeability with the influx of proinflammatory cells into the tissues; this is hypothesized to be an important pathogenic step in the development of acute system organ dysfunction in sepsis. Leukocyte adhesion of white blood cells to the microvessel endothelial surface (primarily in the postcapillary venule) further impedes microcirculatory blood flow. The endothelial injury also triggers the activation of the coagulation cascade via expression of tissue factor on the microvascular endothelium, resulting in fibrin deposition and microvascular thrombosis that may further impair microcirculatory flow. All of these mechanisms collectively contribute to microcirculatory failure in septic shock.[37,39]

Although septic shock research has classically been focused on macrocirculatory hemodynamic parameters that reflect the distribution of blood flow globally throughout the body, a functional microcirculation is another critical component of the cardiovascular system that is necessary for *effective* blood flow to tissues. This conceptual framework is depicted in Figure 23.8. Although a shift of research focus

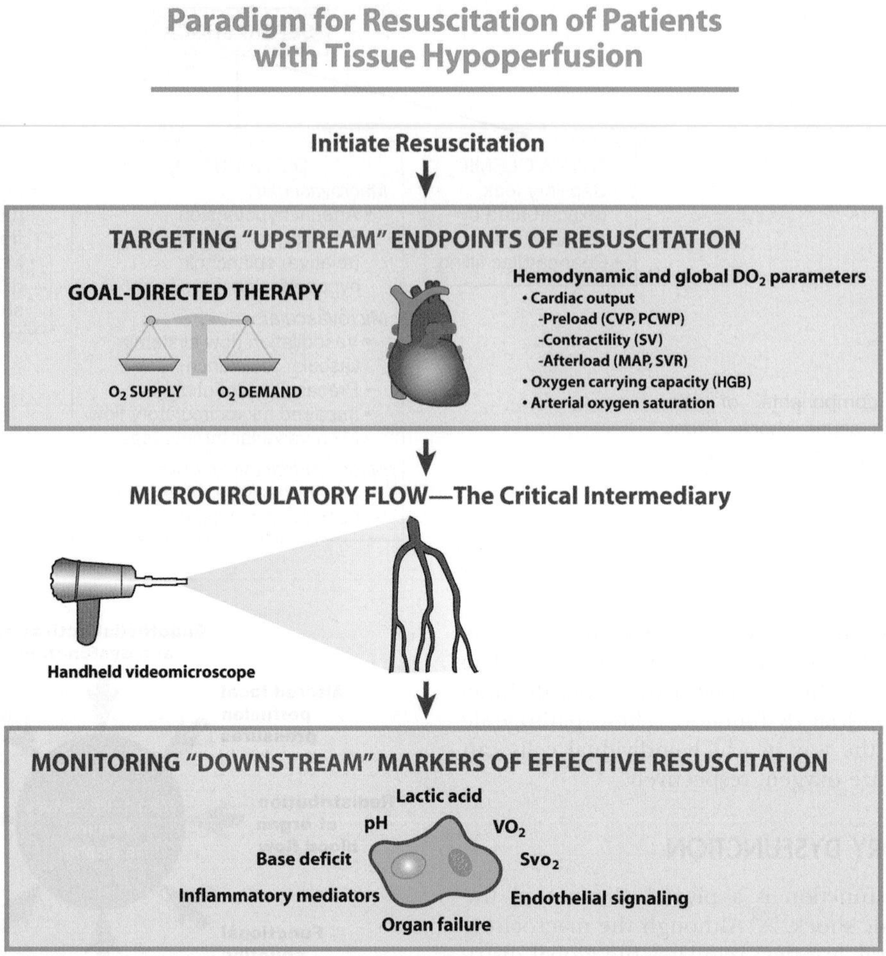

Figure 23.8 New paradigm of the cardiovascular profile of septic shock featuring the importance of the microcirculation. Conventional resuscitation targets the optimization of macrocirculatory (i.e., "upstream") hemodynamic parameters, with the monitoring of "downstream" surrogates of tissue perfusion to determine the effectiveness of resuscitation. The microcirculation is the critical intermediary. Although the macrocirculation (heart and large arteries) regulates the global distribution of blood flow throughout the body, an intact and functional microcirculation is necessary for the effective delivery of blood flow to tissues. Intrinsic microcirculatory dysfunction can be a pivotal pathogenic event in the development of sepsis-associated tissue hypoperfusion. Using new videomicroscopy techniques, microcirculatory flow can now be studied in human subjects with septic shock. CVP, central venous pressure; DO_2, oxygen delivery; HGB, hemoglobin; MAP, mean arterial pressure; PCWP, pulmonary capillary wedge pressure; SV, stroke volume; $S\bar{v}O_2$, mixed venous oxygen saturation; SVR, systemic vascular resistance; VO_2, oxygen consumption.

from global hemodynamic parameters to indices of microvascular perfusion could potentially be viewed as a major change of direction for septic shock research, the microcirculation likely represents a logical next frontier in the evolution of our understanding of circulatory failure in shock states.[37,46] Although there are currently no therapies to specifically target microcirculatory dysfunction in sepsis, going beyond optimization of macrocirculatory hemodynamics and developing new innovative strategies to reverse microcirculatory failure could (in the future) potentially represent a cutting edge method to augment tissue perfusion in sepsis.

MITOCHONDRIAL DYSFUNCTION

There is strong evidence that cellular utilization of oxygen can be markedly impaired in septic shock.[47] Bioenergetic failure can occur even after effective restoration of blood flow to tissues has been achieved, and this has been termed "cytopathic hypoxia." Despite the current absence of therapies to reverse cytopathic hypoxia, this phenomenon does have some relevance for clinical practice, as impaired cellular oxygen extraction and utilization can manifest clinically with acute organ system failure in the setting of markedly elevated values for mixed (or central) venous oxygen saturation. This venous hyperoxia likely reflects bioenergetic failure and identifies a population at exceptionally high risk of death.[48] Cytopathic hypoxia has been associated with acute organ dysfunction, but the extent to which this does or does not represent a cause-and-effect relationship has not yet been fully elucidated.

Microcirculatory and mitochondrial dysfunction likely coexist in septic shock. Both of these pathogenic mechanisms can impair tissue oxygen delivery and utilization, but the relative contribution of either mechanism is difficult to discern and may vary considerably.

MANAGEMENT OF SEPTIC SHOCK

OVERVIEW AND MANAGEMENT GUIDELINES

The Surviving Sepsis Campaign (SSC) first published comprehensive international consensus guidelines for sepsis management in 2004.[49,50] The SSC guidelines have been updated over time as the best evidence for sepsis management continues to evolve. The critical care practitioner should be familiar with the concepts in the SSC guidelines and is referred to the most recent update for a comprehensive review including evaluation of the strength of evidence for each recommendation.[50a] The SSC guidelines writing committee comprised representatives from numerous medical professional societies that relate to the care of the septic patient, and these medical professional societies have endorsed the guidelines.

The treatment recommendations in the SSC guidelines are intended to provide guidance for clinicians. However, treatment decisions must be individualized to the patient, and the recommendations cannot replace a clinician's decision-making capability when he or she is presented with a patient's unique set of clinical data. In addition, resource limitations in some institutions may prevent physicians from accomplishing some treatment recommendations. Thus, the SSC guidelines are intended to represent "best practice" recommendations for the management of sepsis rather than standard of care.

GENERAL PRINCIPLES

The patient with septic shock should be brought to a critical care area as quickly as possible to facilitate rapid resuscitation and optimal hemodynamic support. Continuous electrocardiographic monitoring and pulse oximetry are useful tools in the management of critically ill patients with sepsis.[51,52] In addition, a variety of more invasive devices may be of use. The arterial catheter has two functions: It allows frequent blood sampling and continuous assessment of arterial pressure. The pulmonary artery catheter (PAC) can provide data such as cardiac filling pressures, cardiac index, and systemic vascular resistance. The data gathered from the PAC can be useful for titrating vasoactive medications in septic shock. Although indications for PAC utilization are controversial and are often debated, it is important to recognize that the PAC represents a tool for guiding therapy rather than being a therapeutic intervention in itself. Monitoring venous oxygen saturation (either mixed venous oxygen saturation [$S\bar{v}O_2$] or central venous oxygen saturation [$ScvO_2$]) can yield information on the oxygen supply/demand relationship, especially in the early resuscitation phase of septic shock therapy.[23] A markedly low value for either $S\bar{v}O_2$ or $ScvO_2$ indicates a significant imbalance in the oxygen supply/demand relationship, and likely indicates a need for augmenting global oxygen delivery.

Metabolic parameters to monitor the effectiveness of resuscitation and cardiovascular support are limited; however, measurement of blood lactate can provide important information. In 1964, Weil first proposed the utilization of blood lactate levels as a surrogate of adequacy of tissue perfusion.[53] It is important to realize, however, that elevation of blood lactate does not necessarily indicate ineffective tissue perfusion, as metabolic derangements and altered cellular metabolism may cause hyperlactatemia and can be responsible for the elevation of blood lactate observed in sepsis. Despite this, blood lactate levels still have prognostic value in septic patients. Regardless of the cause of lactate elevation in sepsis, markedly elevated blood lactate (e.g., lactate ≥4 mmol/L) signals an increased risk of death.[54-58]

ANTIBIOTIC THERAPY AND SOURCE CONTROL

Early administration of empiric antibiotic therapy and expeditious source control to eliminate any nidus of infection are imperative in the management of septic shock. Appropriate antibiotics given early may substantially improve the likelihood of survival.[59,60] A choice of antibiotics is usually empiric because the organism is not yet identified when antibiotics must be delivered. Failure to include antibiotic coverage for what is later identified to be the offending organism has been associated with increased risk of death;[61] therefore, broad-spectrum antibiotics are necessary as soon as septic shock is identified. Kumar and associates performed a large-scale multicenter retrospective study of patients with septic shock and found a linear association between the duration of hypotension prior to first dose of antibiotic administration and risk of death.[62] One recent prospective emergency department (ED)–based study from Puskarich and colleagues found higher survival rates if antibiotics were administered prior to shock onset compared to after shock onset, but in contrast to the Kumar data the authors did not find a measurable effect of incremental time to administration of antibiotics on survival.[63] One potential reason to explain these results is that the Kumar study was a heterogeneous population and the therapeutic interventions (e.g., early resuscitation and hemodynamic support) that the patients received were not standardized, whereas all the patients in the Puskarich study were ED patients treated according to a standardized early resuscitation protocol.

The SSC currently recommends that intravenous antimicrobial therapy be started as soon as possible, preferably within an hour of recognition of septic shock. Even though a 1-hour time window is deemed desirable, the SSC acknowledges that longer time frames are common in real-world clinical practice, and practice surveys verify that a 1-hour window is currently not standard of care.[13] One reason for this could be the fact that sepsis often mimics other disorders, and the diagnosis of sepsis as the cause of the illness is often not obvious at the time of initial presentation. As such, the need for antimicrobial agents in the treatment of the patient may also not be immediately obvious. Once the diagnosis is made (or strongly suspected), antimicrobial therapy should be started promptly. Initial empiric antimicrobial selection should be broad enough to cover all likely pathogens based on clinical circumstances. In patients with septic shock, de-escalation or restriction of antibiotic therapy as a strategy to reduce the development of antimicrobial resistance is not recommended until after a causative organism has been identified or after the patient's condition has markedly improved.

Pertaining to source control, the SSC recommends that a specific anatomic diagnosis of infection requiring consideration for emergent source control (e.g., laparotomy for intra-abdominal source) be sought and diagnosed or excluded as rapidly as possible. Thus, imaging studies, if needed, should be performed as soon as possible to make the diagnosis. One important caveat to this is the inherent hemodynamic instability and overall severity of illness in septic shock that may make invasive procedures or transport of patients outside the intensive care unit for imaging studies potentially unsafe. Balancing potential risks and benefits in that scenario is very important. When a procedure for source control is found to be necessary, the surgical drainage should be undertaken for source control as soon as feasible following successful initial resuscitation. Specifically, the SSC recommends that this occur within the first 12 hours after the diagnosis is made. One exception to this may be necrotizing pancreatitits with suspected infection, for which a delayed approach to surgical management (i.e., intravenous antimicrobial therapy only at first, in addition to supportive care) may be preferred.

EARLY RESUSCITATION

One of the initial goals in the early management of a patient with septic shock is effective resuscitation to restore adequate tissue perfusion and decrease the risk of organ system injury. A number of hypotheses have been developed to explain the relationship between shock and the development of organ failure in critical illness. One hypothesis suggests that organ failure during critical care occurs as a consequence of inadequate oxygen delivery. Based on this hypothesis, a number of investigators have suggested that patients should be resuscitated to supranormal goals of systemic oxygen delivery in an attempt to prevent organ failure and improve outcome. The concept of supranormal oxygen delivery refers to the use of fluid resuscitation and inotropic drugs to drive up the oxygen delivery to achieve a predefined target. Several studies have examined this concept, although it is important to recognize that some studies have been performed in heterogeneous populations of critically ill patients rather than sepsis populations. The earliest clinical trials in perioperative high-risk surgery patients demonstrated an outcome benefit.[64,65] Subsequently, however, numerous trials of supranormal oxygen delivery in critically ill patients failed to demonstrate any benefit. In the largest of these studies, Gattinoni and coworkers found no difference in survival or organ failure in a large number of critically ill patients when comparing patients resuscitated to supranormal end points to those receiving standard care.[66] In a study by Hayes and associates, increasing oxygen delivery to supranormal levels with the use of high-dose dobutamine was associated with a reduction in survival.[67] A meta-analysis concluded that supranormal oxygen delivery in critically ill patients was not beneficial[68] and this concept largely fell out of favor in the 1990s.

For goal-oriented hemodynamic optimization to be beneficial, it has become clear that *timing* is critical. In contrast to the trials in perioperative high-risk surgery patients, subjects in the Gattinoni study were randomized much later, up to 72 hours after initial presentation.[66] In a meta-analysis of critically ill patients that stratified studies by severity and the timing of interventions (early versus late), an outcome benefit was identified in the subset of patients with a high severity of illness and early initiation of interventions.[69] A recent meta-analysis, this time specifically focused on patients with sepsis, found that quantitative resuscitation (i.e., early hemodynamic optimization targeting predefined quantitative end points of resuscitation) was associated with lower mortality rate in sepsis patients, but only if applied early, defined as less than 24 hours after presentation.[70] These data suggest that quantitative resuscitation in the treatment of severe sepsis and septic shock can in fact be beneficial—in the right patient.

This early intervention concept was the rationale behind the study of early goal-directed therapy (EGDT) for severe sepsis and septic shock by Rivers and colleagues.[23] EGDT is a type of quantitative resuscitation for septic patients that involves targeting central venous oxygen saturation ($Scvo_2$) as a monitor of the adequacy of oxygen delivery. In a single-center randomized controlled trial of 263 ED patients with severe sepsis and septic shock, Rivers and colleagues targeted predefined end points of resuscitation including central venous pressure (CVP) 8 to 12 mm Hg, MAP 65 mm Hg or greater, and $Scvo_2$ 70% or greater in the ED. The authors reported that the EGDT protocol was associated with a 16% absolute risk reduction for mortality rate (30.5% vs. 46.5%). This study was an important contribution to the literature in showing that early interventions in the resuscitation phase of therapy can be associated with a significant improvement in long-term survival for patients with sepsis.

Recently, a multicenter ED-based randomized trial from Jones and associates compared lactate clearance (defined as a decrease by ≥10% in the serum lactate concentration) versus $Scvo_2$ as an end point of sepsis resuscitation.[71] Among 300 patients with sepsis-induced tissue hypoperfusion, the authors found that lactate clearance was noninferior to $Scvo_2$ for the primary outcome of all-cause in-hospital deaths. These data suggest that, in addition to ensuring adequate cardiac preload and arterial blood pressure, lactate clearance has potential as a resuscitation target in sepsis-induced tissue hypoperfusion.

The data are conflicting as to what therapeutic interventions are typically needed beyond intravascular volume expansion and vasopressor agents in the early resuscitation of patients with sepsis. In the Jones trial, after aggressive administration of intravenous crystalloid to achieve a CVP of 8 to 12 mm Hg and vasopressor agents to achieve an arterial pressure of 65 mm Hg or greater in a stepwise resuscitation algorithm, very few patients required additional therapies for augmentation of oxygen delivery to achieve either lactate clearance or $Scvo_2$ goals (i.e., only 7% required packed red blood cell transfusion and 3% required inotropes). In contrast, 64% of patients in the EGDT ($Scvo_2$ targeted) arm in the Rivers study were treated with blood transfusions and 14% were treated with inotropic support. The Rivers data would suggest that packed red blood cell transfusions and inotropes are commonly required therapies for optimization of oxygen delivery in sepsis resuscitation, whereas the Jones trial (and multiple other recent observational clinical studies) suggests that these additional therapies are rarely required to achieve resuscitation goals. Although the optimal end points of quantitative resuscitation for sepsis remain controversial, it is generally accepted that the earlier the therapeutic interventions are delivered, the greater the capacity for benefit. Therefore, the resuscitation phase of therapy appears to be an important window of opportunity for impact on outcome.

Currently, the SSC recommends the following end points for quantitative resuscitation: CVP 8 to 12 mm Hg, MAP 65 mm Hg or greater, urine output 0.5 mL/kg/hour or greater, and $Scvo_2$ 70% or greater (or mixed venous oxygen saturation [$S\bar{v}O_2$] ≥ 65%). Although arterial pressure and urine output are routinely monitored in critical care practice, targeting CVP and central or mixed venous oxygen saturation necessitates invasive hemodynamic monitoring. If invasive hemodynamic monitoring is not yet in place (or is not established for any reason), aggressive empiric resuscitation should still be performed because it is possible that empiric resuscitation can optimize cardiac filling pressure and oxygen delivery even if the specific values for CVP or central/mixed venous oxygen saturation are not recorded. The SSC also recommends targeting resuscitation to lactate normalization as soon as possible in patients with elevated serum lactate levels, especially if $Scvo_2$ values are not available. Targeting both $Scvo_2$ at 70% or greater and lactate normalization as a combined end point is also an option if both are available.

The SSC acknowledges limitations with utilizing static ventricular pressure estimates (e.g., CVP) for assessing intravascular volume status in septic shock patients. Specifically, measuring CVP in a range that is typically thought to be normal (or even high) does not necessarily exclude the possibility of preload-dependent cardiac output, especially in patients with preexisting chronically elevated cardiac filling pressures (e.g., cardiomyopathy or pulmonary artery hypertension). However, a markedly low value for CVP can be helpful in that it can reliably indicate the presence of hypovolemia in patients with circulatory shock. Targeting dynamic measures of fluid responsiveness during resuscitation and perhaps volumetric indices (e.g., pulse pressure variation, stroke volume variation) may eventually prove to be advantageous, but these newer techniques of intravascular volume assessment have not yet been widely adopted in practice and require future research.

The SSC also acknowledges that achievement of quantitative resuscitation goals can be challenging in routine clinical practice. Although some centers have been successful in implementing programs for quantitative resuscitation,[72] a recent large multicenter observational study of the translation of SSC recommendations to clinical practice found that clinicians currently achieve all recommended end points of resuscitation less than 50% of the time.[13] The reasons for this are likely multifactorial but may include the fact that from a practical standpoint the provision of quantitative resuscitation at the bedside can be relatively resource intensive, and some institutions may not have the necessary infrastructure to provide this service consistently at the present time.

CARDIOVASCULAR SUPPORT

The main goal of cardiovascular support in septic shock is to use intravascular volume expansion and vasoactive agents to help restore and maintain effective tissue perfusion. The main components of cardiovascular support in septic shock can be grouped into three separate and distinct categories: volume resuscitation, vasopressor therapy, and inotropic support. The goal of volume resuscitation is to optimize cardiac filling in order to augment cardiac output. Although many vasoactive drugs have both vasopressor and inotropic activity, this distinction is made on the basis of intended goals of therapy. Vasopressor activity primarily raises the arterial pressure, whereas inotropic activity augments myocardial contractility and raises cardiac output.

VOLUME RESUSCITATION

Aggressive intravascular volume expansion is another cornerstone of septic shock management and is the best initial therapy for the cardiovascular instability of sepsis. The initial hypotension observed in many patients with sepsis-induced cardiovascular instability may be reversed with volume infusion alone. A reasonable approach to initial volume resuscitation in the adult patient is the rapid administration of 2 to 3 L of crystalloid solution (e.g., 0.9% NaCl or lactated Ringer's solution). If (after initial volume infusion) the hemodynamic instability has resolved, further aggressive resuscitation may be unnecessary and the patient may be relegated to a somewhat higher maintenance fluid.

Because there is no proven benefit of colloid therapy over crystalloids in resuscitation,[73] the SSC currently recommends initiating volume resuscitation with crystalloid for patients with septic shock and suspicion of hypovolemia. The SSC-recommended volume of crystalloid is a minimum of 30 mL/kg fluid challenge. If there is hemodynamic improvement with this initial fluid challenge, clinicians may continue repeated fluid challenges to see if further hemodynamic improvement occurs. The SSC further suggests consideration of the addition of albumin infusion to initial crystalloid resuscitation if the initial crystalloids are judged to be ineffective. The SSC recommends against the use of synthetic hydroxyethyl starches in volume resuscitation because these agents have been associated with increased risk of acute kidney injury.

If a PAC is in place, the target for pulmonary capillary wedge pressure in a patient without preexisting cardiopulmonary disease is likely in the range of 12 to 15 mm Hg;[74] however, it is imperative to remember that the "optimal" cardiac filling pressure may vary widely from patient to patient. One prudent strategy of volume resuscitation (rather than targeting a predefined cardiac filling pressure) would be to continue fluid bolus administration until the cardiac index fails to rise with additional intravascular volume expansion, indicating optimization of cardiac preload. An extremely high left ventricular filling pressure should be avoided because it could contribute to pulmonary capillary leak and cause impairment of oxygenation if the patient has concomitant acute lung injury. In the absence of a PAC to guide therapy, and if a patient has persistent hypotension refractory to an initial 30 mL/kg crystalloid intravascular volume infusion, it would be prudent to continue administering fluid boluses in attempts to raise the arterial pressure (unless the patient is manifesting clinical signs that pulmonary edema is developing, [e.g., increasing supplemental oxygen requirement]).[75] Decisions on aggressiveness of fluid resuscitation should be made with consideration of oxygenation status. Patients with minimal supplemental oxygen requirements can be more aggressively fluid resuscitated with minimal concern for deleterious effects of intravascular volume expansion, but more cautious fluid administration is required in patients requiring higher FIO_2 to maintain adequate oxygenation. Because the intravascular volume that optimizes stroke volume may produce worsening of oxygenation in patients with acute lung injury, intubation and mechanical ventilation may be required in order to assure adequate tissue perfusion.

VASOPRESSOR THERAPY

In addition to fluid administration, pharmacologic support of blood pressure is frequently necessary in both the initial resuscitation and subsequent support of patients with septic shock. These agents are, after fluids, the next most important interventions for the initial management of the hemodynamically unstable patient. Restoration of adequate arterial pressure is the end point of vasopressor therapy. The SSC recommends targeting a MAP of 65 mm Hg; however, blood pressure does not always equate to systemic blood flow, and the precise MAP to target may not necessarily be the same for all patients. LeDoux, Astiz, and coworkers demonstrated that, in septic shock patients treated with norepinephrine to maintain target MAP, MAPs of 65, 75, and 85 mm Hg achieved equivalent indices of tissue perfusion.[76] In an observational study of patients with septic shock Varpula and associates found that an area under the curve of 65 mm Hg was the best predictor of positive outcome and showed that among multiple hemodynamic variables, a MAP above 65 mm Hg was the best predictor of a favorable outcome.[77] It is notable that a MAP of 65 mm Hg may be inadequate for a patient with preexisting poorly controlled essential hypertension and associated vascular disease. Similarly, it should be recognized that in some patients it is possible to have arterial pressures lower than 65 mm Hg without tissue hypoperfusion. It is hypotension in the presence of tissue hypoperfusion that merits therapy with vasopressor agents. End points of resuscitation such as arterial pressure should be combined with assessment of regional and global perfusion. Other bedside indicators of persistent tissue hypoperfusion (besides hypotension) include oliguria, encephalopathy, poor capillary refill, and metabolic acidosis. Thus, even though the SSC recommends targeting a MAP of 65 mm Hg for most patients, the optimal MAP should be individualized based on the clinical considerations noted here.

The appropriate use of vasopressors may require accurate assessment of a patient's cardiovascular status with invasive hemodynamic monitoring. However, in the earliest stage of therapy, it is common to institute vasopressor therapy when invasive monitoring data is not immediately available if a patient remains hypotensive despite adequate intravascular volume expansion. If the MAP remains low (e.g., <65 mm Hg) with evidence of ongoing tissue hypoperfusion despite adequate fluid resuscitation, vasopressor therapy is indicated. In some circumstances, patients with sepsis may require vasopressor support even if hypovolemia has not yet been resolved. Below a threshold blood pressure, autoregulation of blood flow in vascular beds may be lost and linearly dependent on blood pressure; thus the administration of vasopressor agents to achieve a minimal perfusion pressure and maintain adequate flow is reasonable as an emergency measure in some situations while fluid resuscitation is ongoing.

INDIVIDUAL VASOACTIVE AGENTS

Multiple different vasoactive agents including norepinephrine, epinephrine, vasopressin, dopamine, and phenylephrine can achieve arterial pressure goals in the management of patients with septic shock. The different catecholamine agents have different effects on α- and β-adrenergic receptors. The hemodynamic actions of these receptors is well described: α-adrenergic receptors promote vasoconstriction, but β_1-adrenergic receptors increase heart rate and myocardial contractility and β_2-adrenergic receptors cause peripheral vasodilation. Given the differential effects of vasopressor drugs upon adrenergic receptors, these different agents have different effects upon arterial pressure and systemic blood flow. In this context, the quintessential question as to which catecholamine is the best initial choice for treating septic shock is best framed as a question of which agent is most appropriate for a given therapeutic strategy in an individual patient, and is largely dependent upon that individual patient's hemodynamic status. Rather than a "one size fits all" strategy, vasoactive agents should be carefully selected based on the intended goals of therapy.

Vasoactive agents and their characteristics are summarized in Table 23.1. The selection of one of these drugs over the other as a first-line agent is a controversial and an often debated subject in the field of critical care medicine. Both norepinephrine and dopamine will effectively raise the

Table 23.1 Vasoactive Agents Commonly Used for Hemodynamic Support in Sepsis

Agent	Typical Dose	Chronotropic Effects	Inotropic Effects	Vasoconstriction
Dopamine	6-20 μg/kg/min	++	++	+/++ (dose-dependent)
Epinephrine	1-10 μg/min	++	++	++
Norepinephrine	2-30 μg/min	+	+	++
Phenylephrine	20-200 μg/min	–	–	++
Vasopressin	0.01-0.03 U/min	–	–	++
Dobutamine	2-15 μg/kg/min	++	++	–

From Trzeciak S, Parrillo JE. Septic shock. In Society of Critical Care Medicine, 8th Adult Critical Care Refresher Course. Chicago: Society of Critical Care Medicine, 2004, used with permission.

blood pressure and the cardiac index, but the rise in cardiac index will be greater with dopamine. Dopamine, however, may cause or exacerbate tachycardia or dysrythmias.[78] Norepinephrine is a more potent drug than dopamine in achieving a target MAP.[1] Information from five randomized trials (n = 1993 patients with septic shock) comparing norepinephrine and dopamine does not support the routine use of dopamine in the management of septic shock.[79]

Epinephrine is a potent α- and β-adrenergic agent that increases MAP by vasoconstriction and also increases the cardiac index. Although epinephrine is a potent agent in raising the arterial pressure, the chief concern with the use of epinephrine has been the potential for impaired splanchnic perfusion.[80-82] A large-scale randomized controlled trial comparing epinephrine to norepinephrine plus dobutamine reported no difference in vasopressor withdrawal, organ failure, and mortality rate. There was also no difference in the rates of serious adverse events. The authors concluded that there is no difference in efficacy and safety for epinephrine versus norepinephrine plus dobutamine in the management of septic shock.[83]

Vasopressin is an agent that has both vasoconstriction and antidiuretic properties. Vasopressin constricts vascular smooth muscle directly via V_1 receptors, and may also increase the responsiveness of the vasculature to endogenous or exogenous catecholamines.[84,85] Normally, endogenous vasopressin levels are very low, and there is essentially no vasoconstriction effect in a normal host. However, in septic shock vasopressin levels are initially extremely elevated. In prolonged septic shock, a relative vasopressin deficiency can develop. It has been postulated that this relative vasopressin deficiency may be the result of the depletion of the pituitary stores or the downregulation of vasopressin production by the pituitary via the effects of nitric oxide.[84] Exogenous administration of low-dose vasopressin can have a dramatic hemodynamic response in this scenario, rapidly restoring arterial pressure.[86,87] A large randomized clinical trial compared vasopressin to norepinephrine in 776 subjects with vasopressor-dependent septic shock. Patients were randomized to vasopressin (0.03 U/minute) or norepinephrine (15 μg/minute). For the group as a whole (intent-to-treat analysis) there was no difference in the primary end point of 28-day mortality rate. It appears that vasopressin (up to 0.03 U/minute) may be equally safe and effective as norepinephrine in patients with septic shock after fluid resuscitation.[88] Doses of vasopressin higher than 0.04 U/minute are not recommended due to concerns of coronary, digital, and mesenteric ischemia.

Phenylephrine is a pure vasoconstrictor with α-adrenergic effects alone. Although one potential advantage of using phenylephrine is that it will not cause or exacerbate tachycardia, the increase in peripheral resistance may produce a deleterious lowering of cardiac output. Phenylephrine may be useful in select patients with severe dysrhythmias associated with catecholamine infusion because it has no β-adrenergic effects, as well as in patients with refractory hypotension in the presence of a known high cardiac index.

The SSC recommends norepinephrine as the first-line vasopressor agent in septic shock. The SSC further recommends the addition of either epinephrine or vasopressin (0.03 U/minute) if a second vasopressor agent is needed to support the blood pressure.

INOTROPIC SUPPORT

Inotropic support may be required for patients with septic shock. In the context of severe sepsis-induced myocardial depression, or if the patient has severe preexisting myocardial dysfunction, an inotrope may be necessary to augment cardiac output (typically in combination with a drug that is supporting the MAP). The SSC recommends that dobutamine be the inotrope selected. When used beyond early quantitative resuscitation (first 6 hours of therapy) inotropic therapy is guided by measurements of cardiac index. A reasonable goal for inotropic therapy would be a cardiac index of 3.0 L/minute/m^2 or greater.

CORTICOSTEROIDS

Administering high doses of steroids (30 mg/kg of methylprednisolone) failed to show an outcome benefit in septic shock in large-scale randomized controlled trials in the 1980s.[89,90] These studies used large doses of steroids over a short time period in an attempt to blunt the proinflammatory response of sepsis. In contrast, an alternative strategy of administering low-dose (i.e., "stress" or "physiologic" dose) steroids appeared to be promising in multiple small studies in the 1990s.[91,92] Despite the fact that septic shock patients typically have elevated serum cortisol levels, it was identified that some patients with septic shock may have "relative adrenal insufficiency," as evidenced by failure to mount a significant elevation of serum cortisol in response to intravenous adrenocorticotropic hormone (ACTH) stimulation. Relative adrenal insufficiency in the context of septic shock may predispose a patient to persistent cardiovascular failure that is refractory to conventional hemodynamic support therapies, and administration of exogenous low-dose steroids could help achieve shock reversal. On the other hand, administration of exogenous steroids could be associated with deleterious effects such as immunosuppression or myopathy.

In 2000, Annane and colleagues performed an observational study focusing on the ability to respond to an ACTH stimulation test in septic shock.[93] The highest 28-day mortality rate (75%) was observed in patients who did not increase serum cortisol level greater than 9 μg/dL. Being a "nonresponder" was a better predictor of death than an initially low cortisol value. In a randomized controlled trial by the same investigators in 2002, 300 severely ill (persistent hypotension despite fluid resuscitation and vasopressor initiation) septic shock patients were randomized to 7 days of hydrocortisone plus fludrocortisone versus placebo.[94] The study found that in the 229 nonresponders administration of low-dose steroids was associated with an improvement in time to shock reversal and mortality rate. Patients who responded appropriately to ACTH stimulation test did not demonstrate a benefit with low-dose steroids.

The concept of low-dose steroid administration was further tested in a multicenter randomized controlled trial (CORTICUS).[95] This study found no difference in the primary outcome measure of mortality rate between those treated with steroids compared to placebo. However, it is notable that (1) in contrast to the Annane study in which all subjects had vasopressor-refractory septic shock, the CORTICUS study tested a more diverse patient population with overall lower severity sepsis, and (2) randomization in the Annane study occurred within 8 hours of developing shock as opposed to CORTICUS, which randomized subjects up to 72 hours after shock onset. Despite the fact that low-dose steroids do not appear to improve outcome in diverse, less severely ill populations of patients with sepsis, patients with vasopressor-unresponsive septic shock likely benefit. In summary, although steroid therapy should not be used in all patients with septic shock, it could be considered in those with persistent circulatory shock despite the administration of vasopressor agents.

The SSC recommends that intravenous hydrocortisone not be administered to septic shock patients if fluid resuscitation and vasopressor agents can restore an adequate arterial pressure. If arterial pressure cannot be successfully restored and maintained, the SSC suggests intravenous hydrocortisone at a maximum dose of 200 mg per day. The SSC does not recommend the use of an ACTH stimulation test to identify candidates for steroid therapy, but rather using bedside clinical criteria such as the presence of vasopressor-refractory shock. The SSC does not recommend the addition of fludrocortisone to hydrocortisone when steroids are administered. Hydocortisone should be tapered off when vasopressor agents are no longer required.

SUMMARY

Successful management of the patient with septic shock continues to be a major clinical and public health challenge, as evidenced by persistently high mortality rates associated with this disease. The principal goals of sepsis therapy remain early identification, early empiric antibiotic therapy and infection source control, aggressive resuscitation, and effective cardiovascular support. The hemodynamic profile of septic shock is the most complex of all shock profiles and may be characterized by simultaneous hypovolemia, myocardial depression, and peripheral vascular dysfunction. Clinicians should define goals and end points of hemodynamic support in individual patients, titrate therapies to those end points, and evaluate the effectiveness of their interventions based on improving indices of tissue perfusion.

KEY POINTS

- Septic shock is a clinical syndrome resulting from a systemic infection that triggers an excessive inflammatory response and produces cardiovascular instability.

KEY POINTS (Continued)

- The initial management of the patient with septic shock is aggressive resuscitation and cardiovascular support, as well as early empiric administration of broad-spectrum antibiotics.
- Initial cardiovascular support is achieved with aggressive intravascular volume expansion.
- Vasopressors are administered to patients who remain hypotensive despite fluid administration. Although the selection of vasopressors must be individualized, norepinephrine is typically considered a first-line agent.
- End points of resuscitation should be physiologic values that reflect adequacy of regional and global perfusion. Clinicians should define goals and end points of hemodynamic support, titrate therapies to those end points, and evaluate the results of their interventions on improving indices of tissue perfusion.

SELECTED REFERENCES

1. Dellinger RP: Cardiovascular management of septic shock. Crit Care Med 2003;31:946-955.
2. Geroulanos S, Douka ET: Historical perspective of the word "sepsis." Intensive Care Med 2006;32:2077.
3. Schottmueller H: Wesen und Behandlung der Sepsis. Inn Med 1914;31:257-280.
4. Vincent JL, Abraham E: The last 100 years of sepsis. Am J Respir Crit Care Med 2006;173:256-263.
5. American College of Chest Physicians/Society of Critical Care Medicine Consensus Conference: Definitions for sepsis and organ failure and guidelines for the use of innovative therapies in sepsis. Crit Care Med 1992;20:864-874.
6. Levy MM, Fink MP, Marshall JC, et al: 2001 SCCM/ESICM/ACCP/ATS/SIS International Sepsis Definitions Conference. Crit Care Med 2003;31:1250-1256.
7. Trzeciak S, Zanotti-Cavazzoni S, Parrillo JE, Dellinger RP: Inclusion criteria for clinical trials in sepsis: Did the American College of Chest Physicians/Society of Critical Care Medicine consensus conference definitions of sepsis have an impact? Chest 2005; 127:242-245.
8. Angus DC, Linde-Zwirble WT, Lidicker J, et al: Epidemiology of severe sepsis in the United States: Analysis of incidence, outcome, and associated costs of care. Crit Care Med 2001;29:1303-1310.
9. American Heart Association: Heart disease and stroke statistics—2004 update. Dallas, American Heart Association, 2004.
10. Center for Disease Control and Prevention: Cases of HIV infection and AIDS in the United States by race/ethnicity, 1998-2002. Rockville, MD, CDC, 2003.

The complete list of references can be found at www.expertconsult.com.

24 Cardiac Tamponade

Zoltan G. Turi | Sajjad A. Sabir

CHAPTER OUTLINE

FUNDAMENTALS OF TAMPONADE

Cardiac tamponade is a condition characterized by an increase in pressure external to the heart resulting in impaired filling of the cardiac chambers. In the typical scenario, as fluid in the pericardium accumulates, cardiac output falls. The diagnosis represents a continuum from mild tamponade with subtle diagnostic findings to a critical clinical setting with imminent mortality.[1] The variability in presentation, including diagnostic findings and course, and the morbidity and mortality associated with treatment make this a particularly challenging clinical problem in critical care medicine.

PERICARDIAL ANATOMY

The pericardium consists of a visceral and a parietal pericardial segment, the former being composed of a single layer of cells that adhere to the cardiac epicardial surface.[2,3] The parietal pericardium is the structure responsible for the clinically relevant features of tamponade; it is a relatively noncompliant structure composed of collagen and elastin and normally is less than 2 mm thick. The mechanical properties of the pericardium—in particular, those reflected by its pressure-volume curve (Fig. 24.1)—are responsible for the clinical features seen in cardiac tamponade.

The pericardium extends from the lower third of the superior vena cava to the apex of the heart. It is attached to the sternum, the diaphragm, and the great vessels. Because it extends beyond the heart border, trauma to not only the heart but also the great vessels approaching the heart borders can lead to cardiac tamponade.[4]

PHYSIOLOGY

Cardiac tamponade is a result of decreased transmural pressure, typically from the accumulation of fluid in the pericardial space (Fig. 24.2). Other causes of "tamponade-like physiology" are related to extrinsic compression of the heart,[5] although these pathologic processes should be separated from those causing constriction rather than true tamponade. Differentiating these two distinct physiologic entities, constriction and tamponade, is essential to diagnosis and management.

The fluid accumulating in the pericardial space can be blood, serous fluid, purulent material, clot, or rarely gas. As fluid accumulates, the pericardium stretches, until it reaches a point (see Fig. 24.1) at which its degree of compliance is exhausted, so that it has become largely inelastic. At this point, any further increase in intrapericardial fluid is associated with a decrease in intracardiac chamber volume, because the total volume of pericardial fluid, heart muscle, and the cardiac chambers becomes fixed by pericardium no longer able to stretch. This in turn results in decreased filling of the heart and consequently decreased stroke volume. To maintain cardiac output, an early compensatory mechanism is an increase in heart rate. Subsequent adaptations to maintain blood flow to central end organs (heart, brain, kidneys) are venous pressure rise, peripheral vasoconstriction, increase in ejection fraction, and selective shunting of blood to preserve flow to the essential end

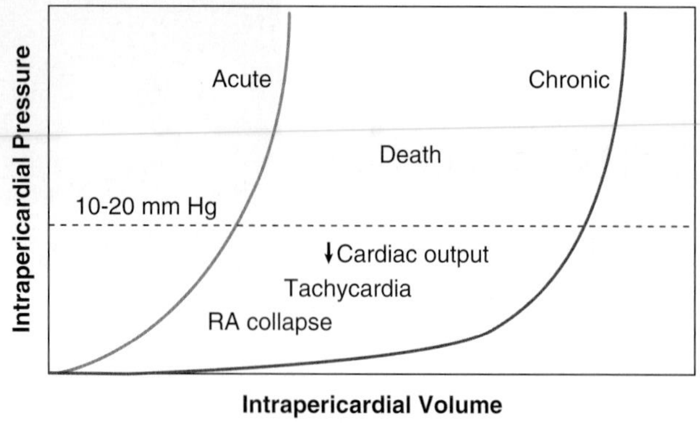

Figure 24.1 Pressure-volume curves for normal pericardium on the *left* and compliant pericardium on the *right*. In the setting of rapid onset of effusion in the normal pericardium, low volumes, typically starting from less than 50 mL, lead to a rise in pressure that exceeds the limit of pericardial stretch, with early onset of tamponade physiology. With more compliant pericardium, a result of chronic stretching, critical extramural pressures do not result until substantially higher volumes are achieved, in some cases more than 1 L.

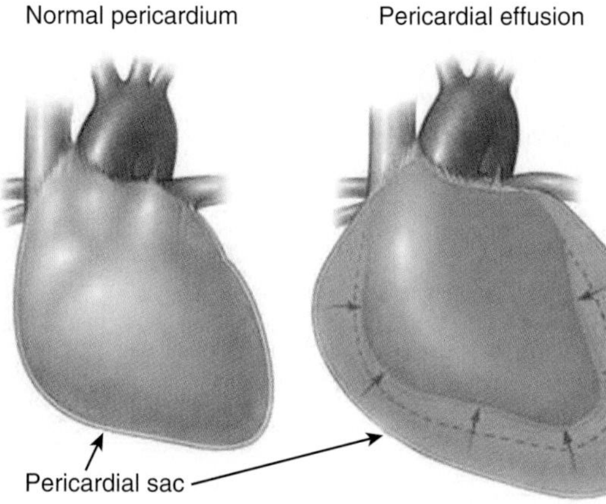

Figure 24.2 The pericardium surrounding the heart in a normal physiologic setting and in tamponade. The pericardium can be seen to extend to the proximal great vessels. Note the large amount of effusion in the image on the *right,* consistent with chronic pericardial stretch, which leads more slowly to tamponade. (From Holmes DR Jr, Nishimura R, Fountain R, Turi ZG. Iatrogenic pericardial effusion and tamponade in the percutaneous intracardiac intervention era. JACC Cardiovasc Interv 2009;2(8):705-717.)

organs. Venous pressure increase is accomplished by fluid retention and peripheral venoconstriction. In severe tamponade, equalization of right atrial, right ventricular diastolic, pulmonary diastolic, pulmonary artery wedge, and intrapericardial pressures occurs. Both pulmonary and systemic arterial and pulse pressures fall. Tamponade is a continuum, ranging from a primarily echocardiographic finding of right-sided chamber collapse to shock and pulseless electrical activity.

PERICARDIAL PRESSURE

The normal pericardium contains a small amount of fluid, typically in a range of 20 to 50 mL, resulting in no more than 5 mm of separation between the visceral and the parietal pericardial surfaces. Pressure in the normal pericardium reflects intrathoracic pressure, which in turn reflects atmospheric pressure, with variation influenced by respiration. During inspiration, the pressure falls a few millimeters below atmospheric pressure (by convention, 0 mm Hg); during expiration, it falls a few millimeters above. The difference between intracardiac and intrapericardial pressures, the transmural pressure, in turn distends or compresses the cardiac chambers. Because intrapericardial mean pressure in patients breathing unassisted typically is the same as atmospheric pressure, whereas right atrial pressure is normally in the range of 2 to 8 mm Hg, the latter is the typical range of net right atrial transmural pressure. When intrapericardial pressure rises to the level of right atrial pressure, the right atrium collapses, a typical feature of early cardiac tamponade, though this nonspecific finding can be seen with hypovolemia alone.

The normal parietal pericardium, because of its limited compliance, limits abrupt expansion of the heart as a whole.[6] Thus, in the setting of right ventricular infarction, for example, acute dilation of the right ventricle is at the cost of left ventricular volume decrease—a ventricular interdependence phenomenon similar to that illustrated in Figure 24.3. Acute chamber enlargement resulting from other etiologic conditions or disorders, such as abrupt volume loading or sudden onset of severe valvular regurgitation, is impeded by the constraint of pericardium that has reached the limits of its intrinsic elasticity. Because right-sided heart filling occurs preferentially with inspiration, when negative intrathoracic pressures result in increased venous return and higher right-sided chamber volume, left ventricular stroke volume and hence systolic blood pressure tend to fall as left atrial and left ventricular volumes decrease. This exaggerates the normal respiratory variation, and systemic pressure falls with inspiration to a level at which pulsus paradoxus, defined by convention as a greater than 10 mm Hg decrease in systolic pressure, is seen. In addition, decreased intrathoracic pressure has a disproportionate effect on the pulmonary venous circulation, which is not exposed to the high pericardial pressures; hence, a disproportionate fall during inspiration in the pulmonary vein to left atrial gradient further exacerbates the decrease in left atrial filling.[7] The fall in systolic pressure is not in fact a paradox but rather an exaggeration of normal respiratory variation of approximately 3%[8] with associated inspiratory decrease in left ventricular stroke volume. With severe tamponade, total elimination of pulse pressure can be seen with individual heartbeats, as in the example in Figure 24.4.

The inability to dilate further means that additional volume beyond the intrinsic stretch limit of the pericardium, such as from bleeding into the pericardial sac, results in increasing compression of heart chambers as volume expands in the pericardial space. Because the right-sided chambers have the lowest intracardiac pressures, in particular the right atrium, those are the first chambers showing collapse, in particular in diastole, when the tricuspid valve is open and the right atrium can decompress into the right ventricle. With a progressive increase in intrapericardial pressure, compression of the right ventricle in diastole occurs during pressure equalization with the right atrium. Eventually, as intrapericardial pressure continues to rise, compression of the left-sided chambers ensues.

In contrast with acute tamponade physiology, in which hemodynamic decompensation may occur after only a

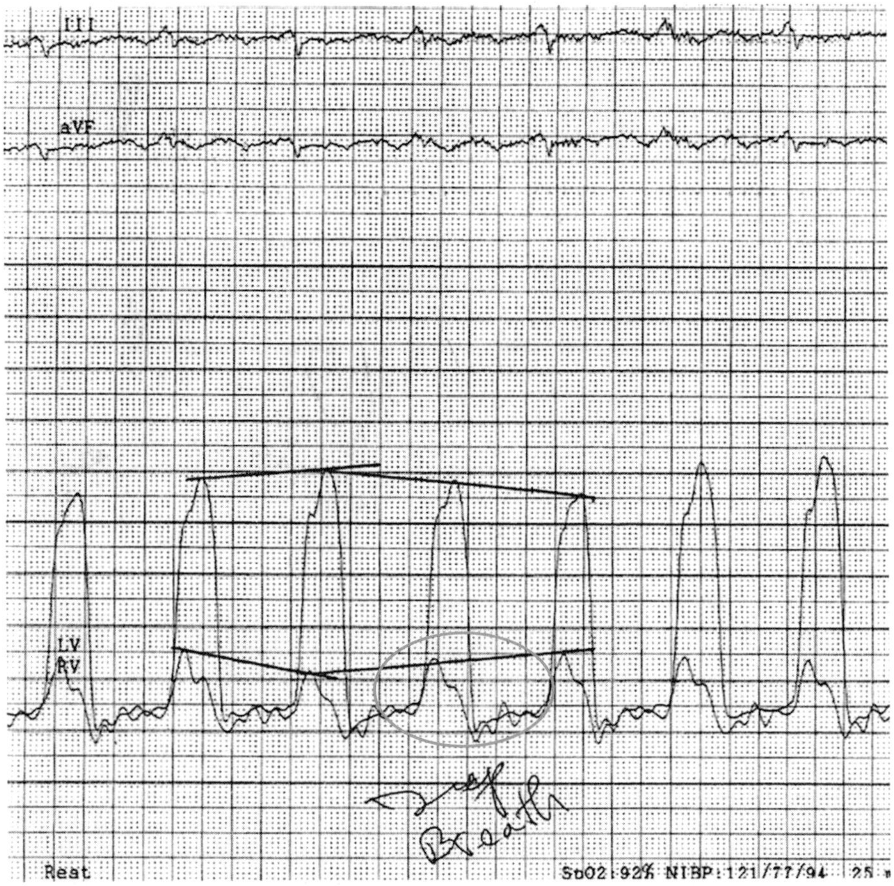

Figure 24.3 Hemodynamic tracings from a patient with ventricular interdependence (200–mm Hg scale). With inspiration, left ventricle (LV) systolic pressure falls as right ventricle (RV) systolic pressure increases. Because of ventricular interdependence, the right ventricular and left ventricular systolic pressures trend in opposite directions (lines connecting peak systolic pressures diverge during phases of the respiratory cycle). Diastolic pressures in both ventricles are essentially identical *(green oval)*. Absence of pulsus paradoxus and preserved systolic pressure make this physiology consistent with constriction rather than tamponade. The patient had a clot in the pericardial space after prior cardiac trauma.

modest accumulation of fluid, generally in the range of 100 to 200 mL, chronic pericardial effusion results in a gradual increase in distensibility of the pericardium. With increasing compliance, large amounts of fluid can accumulate at low pressure without decreasing transmural pressure or compressing the cardiac chambers (see Fig. 24.1). Even in chronic low pressure–high volume tamponade, a limit of distensibility is eventually reached that results in similar pathophysiology as with acute tamponade, in some cases only after a liter or more of fluid has accumulated. Once the steep portion of the pressure-volume curve is reached, it is important to appreciate that with accumulation of another 50 to 100 mL of pericardial fluid, hemodynamic decompensation can occur rapidly, with similar outcomes as in patients who suffer from acute tamponade, such as is seen with penetrating trauma, coronary artery perforation, aortic dissection, or cardiac rupture.

ETIOLOGY

Pericardial effusions generally can be characterized as transudate or exudate, infectious or bloody, with tamponade occurring with variable frequency depending both on the rapidity of fluid accumulation and, to a somewhat lesser degree, on characteristics of the effusion and physiology determined by its etiology. Transudates are characteristic of congestive heart failure, radiation, and uremia; exudates are characteristic of infections, malignancy, and connective tissue disorders. Laboratory testing may help differentiate exudates from transudates; pericardial and serum protein, albumin, lactate dehydrogenase (LDH), cholesterol, and glucose should be obtained,[9] although some of the differentiating characteristics applicable to pleural effusions may not be discriminatory in pericardial effusions.[10] In addition, pericardial fluid total and differential cell count, Gram stain, aerobic and anaerobic culture, and mycobacterial and fungal evaluation should be performed along with cytology when malignancy is considered. Molecular techniques can be useful in diagnosing otherwise occult infections.[11] Amylase is reserved for cases where pancreatic disease or esophageal rupture are part of the differential diagnosis.

Conditions predisposing to slow accumulation such as heart failure, myxedema, chronic renal failure, and connective tissue disorders in general are less likely to cause acute tamponade, whereas those associated with rapid development, such as malignancy, infection (including bacterial, fungal, and human immunodeficiency virus related), or particularly hemorrhage, commonly result in abrupt

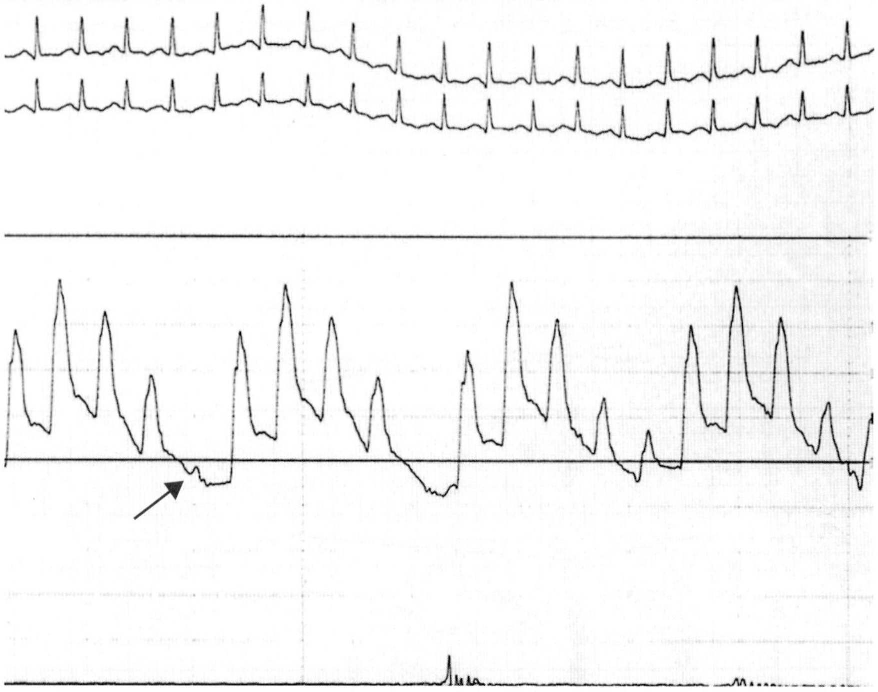

Figure 24.4 Hemodynamic tracing of systemic pressure in cardiac tamponade, 100–mm Hg scale. Systolic pressure variation is nearly 40 mm Hg, and pulse pressure is markedly reduced during inspiration. Note the complete obliteration of the systemic pressure during deep inspiration in the beat highlighted by the *arrow*. Because of low stroke volume, cardiac output is being maintained to some extent by a high heart rate (146 beats per minute).

hemodynamic deterioration. The effect of inflammation in decreasing compliance of the pericardium exacerbates the hemodynamic effects of effusions associated with pericarditis.[12] The potential etiologic disorders are highly variable, with significant influence of demographics and geography, so that tamponade secondary to tuberculous pericardial effusion in immune-compromised patients is a not uncommon presentation in Africa,[13] whereas in industrialized nations malignant effusions are a far more common cause.[14] Large and usually benign pericardial effusions are seen frequently after heart transplantation, possibly immune mediated.[15] Large pleural effusions can cause sufficient compression of the heart that tamponade physiology occurs.[16] The most common etiologic disorders are listed in Table 24.1; more detailed discussion of the various causes is presented later in the chapter, organized by the hospital setting in which presentation typically is seen.

HISTORY AND PHYSICAL EXAMINATION

Dyspnea is the most common symptom of tamponade, although its etiology sometimes is unexplained and it usually is not associated with significant concomitant pulmonary vascular congestion. It is likely to be secondary to decreased cardiac output and encroachment on lung volume by the expanding pericardium as well as any simultaneous pleural effusions. The patient may describe a sensation of fullness in the chest or abdomen and dysphagia, associated with venous engorgement and passive congestion, stretching of the richly innervated pericardium, and occasionally vagal stimulation.[17] Because most patients with tamponade have comorbid conditions accounting for their effusion, additional signs and symptoms are likely to be related to pericarditis, malignancy, or other concomitant conditions.

The hallmarks of cardiac tamponade on physical examination relate to features associated with venous hypertension, low cardiac output, and effects of the layer of fluid between the heart and the chest wall. In patients with tamponade, the general appearance changes substantially during progressive increase in pericardial pressure. Because tamponade represents a continuum, some patients with early tamponade physiology look well, whereas patients with more advanced tamponade show features of a low-output state, with clinical manifestations reflecting the high catecholamine levels required to maintain cardiac output. They become progressively more anxious and agitated and less communicative and may be struggling to breathe. Patients may complain of chest pain associated with pericardial irritation, not infrequently radiating to the neck, jaw, or shoulder[18]; if venous congestion is acute, patients may experience pain from stretching of Glissen's capsule around the liver.

PULSUS PARADOXUS

The physical examination in significant tamponade can include Beck's triad, described in 1935 by the surgeon C. S.

Table 24.1 Etiology of Cardiac Tamponade

Causative Disorder/Condition	Frequency (%)
Most Common*	
Idiopathic	23
Malignancy	22
Iatrogenic	18
Acute myocardial infarction	8
Purulent (including tuberculous)	8
Renal failure	3
Miscellaneous	**18**
Aortic dissection	
Myxedema	
Trauma	
Connective tissue disorders	
Radiation therapy	

*Frequency of common etiologies of tamponade is based on 119 cases in Barcelona, Spain. Other relatively common causes of effusion include congestive heart failure, hypoalbuminemia, coagulopathy, and postcardiotomy and Dressler's syndromes. Etiologies of tamponade will be dependent on geography and patient demographics and also will be strongly influenced by the presence of oncology, trauma, or dialysis units. For a comprehensive list of tamponade etiologies based on prior data, see Box 6.1.

Data from Sagrista-Sauleda J, Merce J, Permanyer-Miralda G, et al: Clinical clues to the causes of large pericardial effusions. Am J Med 2000;109:95-101.

Beck.[19] This entity features jugular venous distention, decreased arterial pressure, and a small, quiet heart. As described earlier, pulsus paradoxus is the result of cardiac chamber interdependence and a decrease in left ventricular chamber volume with inspiration. It can be detected at the bedside by auscultation of Korotkoff sounds, identifying the highest and lowest pressures at which sounds are first heard during inspiration and expiration; alternatively, a simpler and more useful technique is to palpate the radial artery pulse with the cuff inflated to the maximum pressure at which the pulse appears and then to lower the cuff pressure in increments of 10 mm Hg to detect the pressure at which pulses are continuously noted throughout the respiratory cycle. In the patient whose systolic pressure is shown in Figure 24.4, simple palpation of the radial pulse would detect the loss of pulse pressure in the beat flagged by the red arrow. It is important to recognize that although pulsus paradoxus is a classic feature of severe tamponade, as a diagnostic feature it is of limited sensitivity and specificity.

Various thresholds other than the relatively arbitrary 10 mm Hg threshold have been proposed to increase specificity, including a 10% decrease, rather than a 10 mm Hg fall.[20] A drop in *systolic* pressure greater than 50% of the *pulse* pressure also has been proposed.[1] Use of a 15 or 20 mm Hg fall in pressure by physical examination is a less sensitive but far more specific finding for tamponade but may result in delayed diagnosis. Pulsus paradoxus may be present in other conditions that result in an exaggerated decrease in systolic pressure with inspiration, such as massive pulmonary embolism, severe chronic obstructive pulmonary disease (which also can feature constrictive physiology because of limited expansion of the heart in the setting of hyperexpanded lungs),[20] and right ventricular infarction.[21] Furthermore, other features of the systemic blood pressure and pulse are important to consider. With a progressive decrease in cardiac filling overall, a decline in systemic pressure (regardless of phase of the respiratory cycle) as well as a decrease in pulse pressure (the difference between systolic and diastolic pressures) occurs, reflecting decreasing stroke volume and decreasing cardiac output. Thus, it may be impossible to palpate radial artery pulsations; with severe tamponade, the patient is likely to feel cool and clammy, a finding consistent with severe peripheral vasoconstriction.

Tachycardia is almost invariable, except for comorbid conditions associated with a decrease in heart rate, such as electrical conduction disturbances, severe hypothyroidism, or aggressive β-blockade. Tachycardia is a compensatory mechanism for decreased stroke volume, is also caused by high catecholamine levels, and may result from pericardial irritation of the sinus node that stimulates a higher heart rate. On occasion, acute bradycardia may be seen in tamponade, sometimes the first finding after hemorrhage into the pericardial sac. Although a well-preserved systolic pressure and a wide pulse pressure are uncommon in tamponade, neither a low pressure nor a narrow pulse pressure is completely specific. Further, early in the course of tamponade, acute surge in catecholamine levels may result in hypertension rather than shock; in addition, patients with tamponade in the setting of renal disease and chronic hypertension appear to present more often with elevated systolic pressures.[22]

Box 24.1 Tamponade Settings in Which Pulsus Paradoxus May Not Be Present

- Nonrestrictive (large) atrial septal defect
- Severe aortic insufficiency
- Loculated effusion
- Left ventricular hypertrophy and other causes of elevated left ventricular diastolic pressure
- Shock due to hypovolemia, or profound circulatory collapse with tamponade
- Severe left ventricular dysfunction
- Low-pressure tamponade
- Right ventricular hypertrophy or other cause of impaired right ventricular filling
- Positive-pressure ventilation
- Arrhythmias

The pulsus paradoxus may be absent in conditions in which ventricular interdependence is masked[23] (Box 24.1), such as a nonrestrictive atrial septal defect, in which inspiration also increases left atrial filling, or aortic insufficiency, in which left ventricular filling in diastole is increased by regurgitation from a high-pressure source: the aorta. Localized tamponade may have some general tamponade features (such as decreased stroke volume) but may not result in ventricular interdependence—hence, the clinical picture may be that of a sick patient with tamponade but without pulsus paradoxus. Markedly elevated left-sided heart diastolic pressures in severe left ventricular hypertrophy and other disease states may exceed the elevated right atrial and intrapericardial pressures in tamponade, decreasing the effect of inspiration on the interdependence of the right and left sides of the heart. An example in which both pulse pressure and pulsus paradoxus would be insensitive markers of tamponade is aortic dissection that combines aortic insufficiency with tamponade, in which a wide pulse pressure may be seen in some patients with partial compensation, and in which pulsus paradoxus, as discussed, may be masked. By contrast, conditions resulting in impaired right ventricular filling, such as right ventricular hypertrophy in severe pulmonary hypertension, also may result in the absence of a pulsus paradoxus[24]; furthermore, in settings such as cor pulmonale, the dramatic elevation in right-sided diastolic pressures will delay onset of the otherwise highly sensitive and early finding of right atrial and right ventricular diastolic collapse until tamponade is severe.[25] A substantial number of case reports describe physiologic conditions in which the classic findings for tamponade are not seen or are attributable to other etiologic disorders.[26]

VENOUS PRESSURE

Because impairment of right-sided filling is usually the first manifestation of increasing pericardial pressure, high jugular venous pressure manifested by prominent venous pulsations may be the earliest finding on physical examination, occurring with increasing intrapericardial and right atrial pressures. Jugular venous distention may, however, be simultaneously absent because venoconstriction, a common finding with acute tamponade, makes detection of elevated venous pressures difficult. It also will be masked by low-volume tamponade, including volume-depleted states such as trauma, when, in addition to hemorrhage into the pericardium, significant blood loss has occurred. Other settings in which venous distention may not be observed are post-dialysis in patients with uremic pericardial effusions, and excessive diuresis, sometimes as part of treatment for symptoms of congestive heart failure when the cause of elevated filling pressures has not been appreciated.[27] In general, lack of venous engorgement in tamponade, particularly when the latter is acute, is not uncommon. Thus, prominent jugular venous distention may suggest an alternative diagnosis, such as severe right-sided heart failure. Increased venous pressure with inspiration, Kussmaul's sign, is a feature of constriction, reflecting increased venous return to the thorax without increased right atrial filling, because the latter is constricted by the pericardium. This is in contrast with tamponade, in which negative intrathoracic pressure is transmitted through the pericardial effusion, and results in increased right-sided heart filling with decrease in venous pressure. Because these findings are difficult to differentiate in most acutely ill patients, much of the subsequent description about right atrial pressure is based on catheter based hemodynamic findings rather than the physical examination.

The Y descent, in contrast with pericardial constriction, in which it is prominent, typically is limited or absent (Fig. 24.5). Unlike in pericardial constriction, filling of the right ventricle (and hence emptying of the right atrium) is impaired throughout the cardiac cycle, because extrinsic compression by pericardial fluid results in elevated diastolic pressures in the right ventricle when rapid filling would otherwise occur. Because the pericardium allows additional atrial expansion during ventricular ejection (when ventricular volume decreases), the X descent is typically the more prominent negative pressure wave seen. The classic square

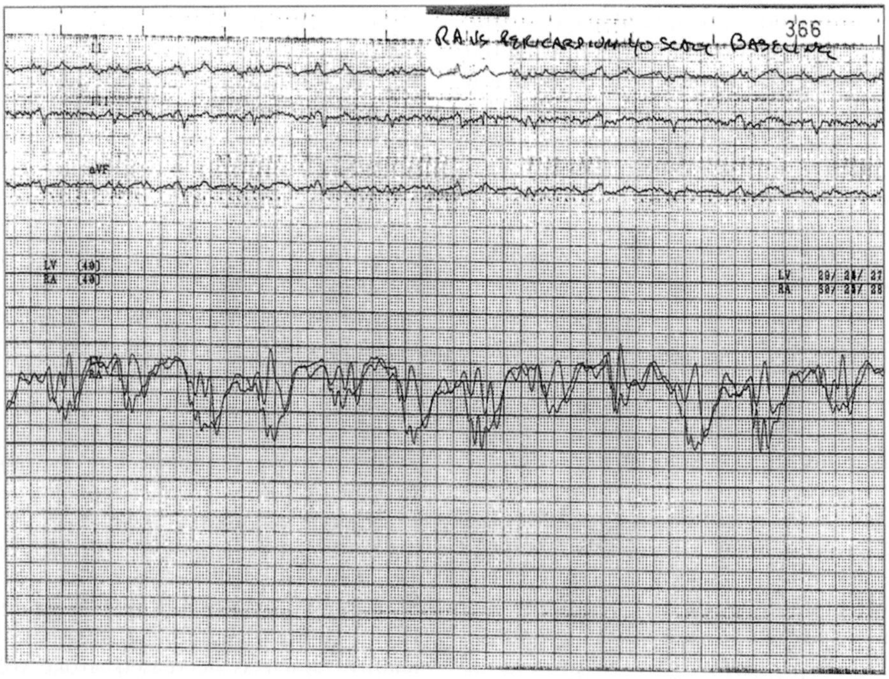

Figure 24.5 Hemodynamic tracings showing right atrial (RA) and intrapericardial pressures (incorrectly labeled LV) on a 40–mm Hg scale. Note the equivalence of pressures as well as the high mean pressure, 27 mm Hg, consistent with tamponade and hemodynamic decompensation. The Y descent is nearly absent.

root sign seen in the right ventricular pressure tracing in constriction is absent in tamponade.

In contrast with acute tamponade, with chronic effusion persistent elevation in pericardial pressure leads to a parallel rise in central and peripheral venous pressure, as well as fluid retention with elevated intravascular volume. Venous congestion as well as peripheral edema and end-organ signs of chronic venous hypertension, such as passive congestion of the liver, become more common in this setting.

CARDIAC AND CHEST EXAMINATION

The quiet heart in Beck's triad relates to several features that tend to muffle the intensity of heart sounds. First, the insulating effects of pericardial fluid on sound waves tend to decrease the sound volume transmitted to the chest wall. Second, low stroke and filling volumes tend to decrease the forces that cause the sounds generated by heart valve closure, with low pulse pressure in both the aortic and the pulmonary arteries. Because the S3 gallop is created by rapid ventricular filling, a phenomenon absent in tamponade, it would not be expected, nor would an S4, because the hemodynamic characteristics of late diastolic atrial emptying that causes the fourth heart sound are not seen.[1] A pericardial friction rub, if pericarditis is involved, may be heard. Except in severe tamponade, the pericardium around the apex of the heart may contain relatively little fluid, and left ventricular contraction typically is vigorous unless underlying left ventricular dysfunction also is present. Hence, a palpable point of maximal impulse may be felt.

A particular feature that differentiates tamponade from decompensated congestive heart failure is the typical presence of clear lungs in the case of the former. Although both right and left atrial pressures are markedly elevated, flow into the pulmonary circulation is limited, and the pressure-volume curve for the pulmonary vascular system is not affected.

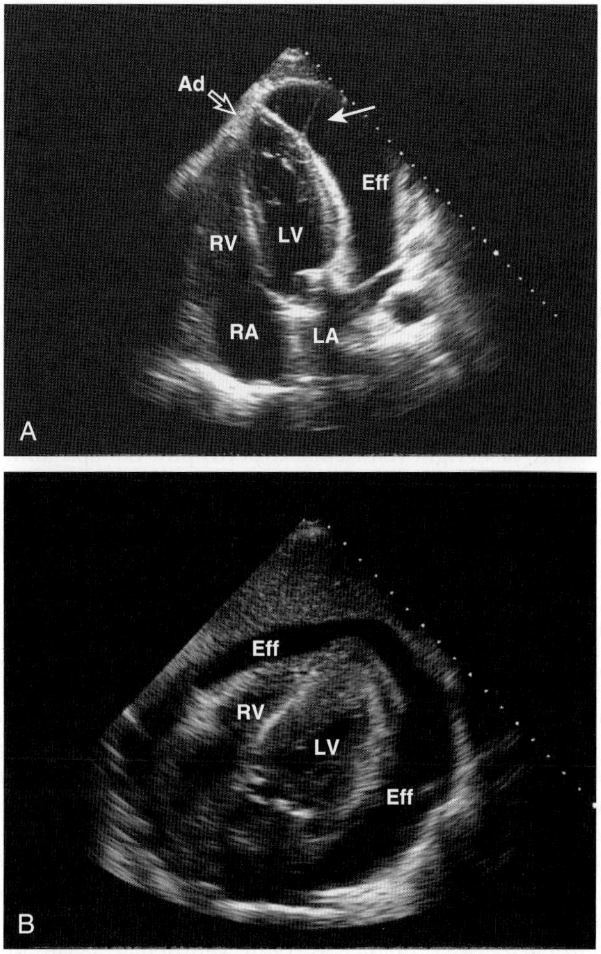

Figure 24.6 Echocardiographic images of two types of pericardial effusions. **A,** A large posterior pericardial effusion, with relatively little fluid anterior to the heart or at the apex. The apex is adherent to the pericardial surface. The *arrow* points to a fibrous strand. This is a fairly typical appearance of a chronic postcardiotomy effusion. Needle access would be problematic. **B,** By contrast, this effusion is circumferential, with somewhat more fluid behind the left ventricle, a largely gravitational effect. Leaning the patient forward 20 to 30 degrees would facilitate pericardiocentesis, although the patient was not significantly hemodynamically compromised. Ad, adhesion; Eff, effusion; LA, left atrium; LV, left ventricle; RA, right atrium; RV, right ventricle.

DIAGNOSTIC TESTS

ECHOCARDIOGRAPHY

Echocardiography is the most easily accessible and accurate means for the timely diagnosis of tamponade and remains the diagnostic modality of choice.[28] Besides evaluating presence and degree of chamber collapse, the echocardiogram is useful for assessing the amount and location of effusion in the pericardial space, for characterizing the fluid, and for judging the hemodynamic effect. Cardiac tamponade represents an echocardiographic continuum, from a small accumulation of fluid with at most subtle clinical findings, to large, usually circumferential[29] accumulations with resultant cardiogenic shock. Until effusions are at least moderate in size, fluid may be shifted by gravity to a location primarily posterior to the heart, because most patients are recumbent during echocardiography (Fig. 24.6).

Several echocardiographic features have been described in tamponade that result from an increase in intrapericardial pressure. These include exaggerated late diastolic right atrial collapse, early diastolic right ventricular collapse, significant respiratory variation in Doppler inflow velocities across the tricuspid and mitral valves, a plethora of the inferior vena cava, exaggerated expiratory flow reversal of the hepatic veins, and blunted diastolic flow of the inferior vena cava (IVC) during expiration.[30] Because the right-sided cardiac chambers are more compliant, thin walled, and at relatively low pressure, the increase in intrapericardial pressure results in the collapse of these chambers first.

Immediately after atrial contraction, the right atrial volume is at its lowest, whereas right ventricular volume is at its maximum; total pericardial volume in cardiac tamponade is relatively fixed. The increase in ventricular filling during diastole increases pericardial pressure, which prevents expansion of the right atrium during atrial relaxation (late ventricular diastole).[31] Persistence of right atrial collapse for more than one third of the cardiac cycle is a useful marker for early tamponade physiology. This phenomenon is best appreciated from the apical or subcostal four-chamber views (see Fig. 8.43 in Chapter 8).

The right ventricle, conversely, is more vulnerable to collapse during early diastole, when its pressure is at its lowest as it expands following closure of the pulmonic valve. The right ventricular outflow tract is the more compressible area of the right ventricle and hence tends to collapse first.[30] With increasing intrapericardial pressure, the collapse extends to the right ventricular free wall, which is best appreciated on parasternal long or short axis views (see Figure 8.44 in Chapter 8). This is a more specific finding for tamponade than right atrial collapse, as the latter can occur in the setting of hypovolemia alone. However, right ventricular diastolic collapse may not be seen in conditions that result in significantly elevated right ventricular diastolic pressure or in right ventricular hypertrophy. Collapse of the higher-pressure left-sided chambers, particularly the left ventricle, is uncommon, but, when seen, is highly specific for tamponade. Collapse of the left atrium is not uncommon in the immediate postcardiac surgery period, frequently a result of loculated effusion causing regional tamponade.[32]

Although cardiac chamber collapse is a highly sensitive marker and typically seen before clinical manifestations of tamponade, a number of other findings are more specific. As discussed previously, pulsus paradoxus results from exaggerated ventricular coupling. The ventricular interdependence (Fig. 24.7) can be appreciated on echocardiography by demonstration of marked respiratory variation of Doppler flow across the atrioventricular or semilunar valves (see also Figs. 8.43 and 8.44 in Chapter 8). During inspiration, the drop in intrathoracic pressure results in increased right ventricular (RV) filling. As right ventricular cavity size increases during diastole, the increased intrapericardial pressure impairs expansion of the right ventricular free wall, and continued RV filling is accomplished only by diastolic expansion of the interventricular septum. The consequent bulging of the interventricular septum into the left ventricular (LV) cavity during diastole results in marked reduction in LV compliance and inspiratory filling.[12,33] These filling changes are reflected in a marked inspiratory increase in tricuspid valve Doppler inflow velocities with simultaneous inspiratory decrease in mitral valve inflow velocities.

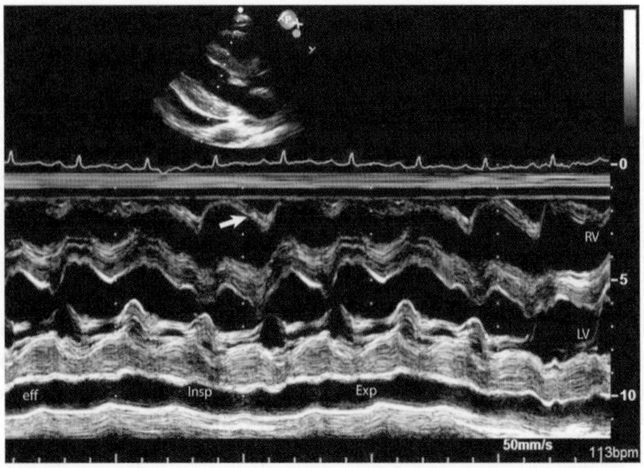

Figure 24.7 Classic findings for ventricular interdependence in cardiac tamponade. See the legend for Figure 8.45 in Chapter 8.

Reciprocal changes are noted during expiration. A corollary to these respiratory changes is noted in the hepatic vein and vena cava flow patterns. Normal vena cava flow into right atrium occurs during both ventricular systole and diastole. In tamponade, already impaired diastolic flow is further compromised in expiration by the exaggerated ventricular interdependence. This hemodynamic effect manifests on Doppler as blunted diastolic caval flow during expiration with increased expiratory flow reversal in the Doppler flow pattern of hepatic veins[34] (Fig. 24.8). Although it is expected that in tamponade the IVC will be dilated and nonreactive,[35] a plethora of the IVC can be seen in any condition causing elevation of right atrial pressure, including positive pressure ventilation in an intubated patient.

Portable echocardiography, performed at the bedside, in the emergency room, or in critical care units, is highly reliable in cardiac tamponade.[36,37] However, adequate training in basic technique and fundamental anatomy is essential to avoid misdiagnosis. Epicardial fat can be confused with effusion,[38] and isolated or coexistent pleural effusions, mediastinal masses, and atelectasis can confound the diagnosis as well.[39] It is important to assess the heart from as many echo windows as possible for small but opportunistic loculated accumulations of fluid, for the presence of clot, fibrinous "strandlike" material or masses, and for compression from processes outside the pericardium, such as a mediastinal hematoma and pleural effusion, all of which will significantly impact management.

X-RAY STUDIES

The classic "water bottle" configuration of the heart is due to a large pericardial effusion and therefore occurs only if the pressure-volume curve has altered sufficiently through chronic accumulation to allow significant increase in pericardial volume. It is a misconception that a normal-sized heart excludes tamponade; in acute tamponade the heart size can be expected to appear normal or minimally enlarged.[12] With marked enlargement of the cardiac silhouette, the finding is nonspecific and not readily distinguishable from cardiomegaly, although in tamponade pulmonary vascular congestion is usually not seen, whereas prominence of the vena cava may be noted. Other modalities such as computed tomography (CT) scanning and magnetic resonance imaging (MRI) show large effusions and can demonstrate chamber collapse. In addition, characterization of pericardial thickness and of the pericardial fluid to differentiate between blood and fluid of different densities can be useful. Although CT and MRI show primarily anatomy rather than physiology, they can identify chamber collapse, characterize soft tissue, and demonstrate reflux into the azygous vein, a useful sign of tamponade.[40] CT scanning can provide information supplemental to that seen on echocardiography, including identification of extracardiac disease lesions,[41] and can provide additional sensitivity for the detection of loculated effusions.[42] Coronary sinus compression on CT is an early and specific indicator of tamponade.[43]

ELECTROCARDIOGRAPHY

The classic electrocardiographic features include low voltage, a result of poor transmission of electrical activity

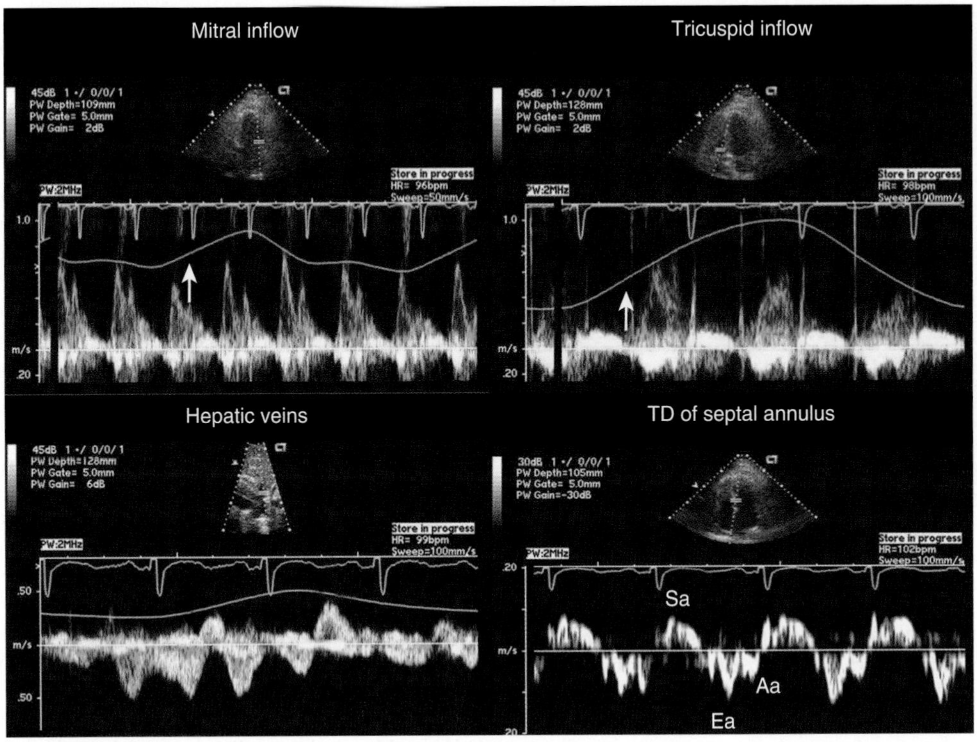

Figure 24.8 Pulsed Doppler signal of hepatic vein showing reduced forward flow *(arrows)* and increased diastolic flow reversal during expiration (E) in tamponade. I, inspiration.

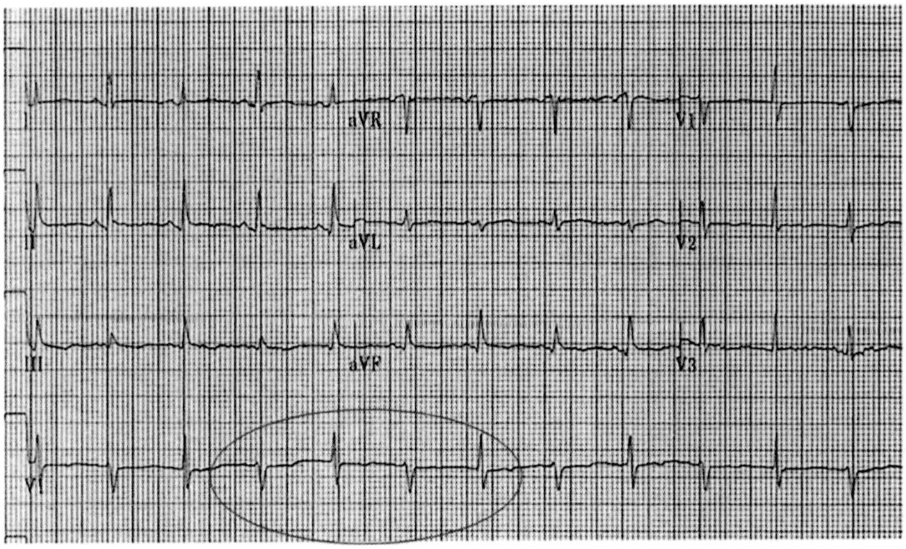

Figure 24.9 Electrocardiogram demonstrating classic electrical alternans in a patient with pericardial tamponade. Note the change in amplitude of the R wave in lead V1 *(red oval).* Similar findings are seen throughout the limb and precordial leads shown.

across the fluid in the pericardial space, and electrical alternans, an insensitive but relatively specific finding for tamponade generated by swinging of the heart in the fluid-filled chamber (Fig. 24.9). Electrical alternans typically is seen only with large effusions in the later stages of tamponade, although the finding is related more to fluid volume and the ability of the heart to swing within the pericardial space. It may involve alternans of both QRS complexes and P waves. Thus, tamponade with adhesions (Fig. 24.10), loculation, or masses that restrict heart motion may not manifest the alternans phenomenon.

OVERALL ASSESSMENT

In general, the severity of tamponade can be judged by the extent of hypotension, tachycardia, and pulsus paradoxus on physical examination and confirmed by findings on echocardiography.[44] Mild tamponade features no hypotension or tachycardia, and no pulsus, with mild RV collapse by echo. Patients with moderate tamponade have preservation of systemic pressure, but have tachycardia, some degree of pulsus paradoxus, and clear RV collapse on echo. Severe

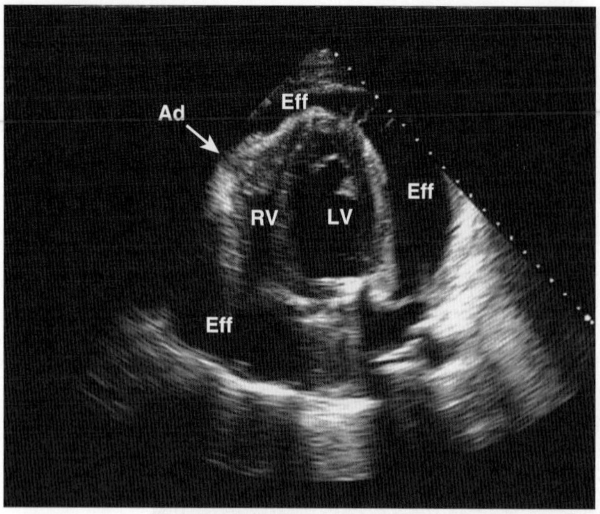

Figure 24.10 Echocardiogram showing pericardial tamponade with right-sided collapse, adhesion of the right ventricle to the pericardium *(arrow),* and fibrous strands of early adhesions seen at the 1 o'clock position near the apex of the left ventricle. Even if the effusion accumulates further, electrical alternans would be less likely because of lack of mobility of the heart. Ad, adhesion; Eff, effusion; LV, left ventricle; RV, right ventricle.

tamponade is associated with tachycardia, shock, profound pulsus paradoxus, and chamber collapse with a swinging heart on ultrasound.[21] Hemodynamic findings correlate with increasing pericardial pressure at each stage of tamponade,[45] initially less than right atrial or pulmonary wedge pressure, then equilibrating with right but less than left atrial pressure, and in severe tamponade equilibrating with both.

SPECIAL SYNDROMES IN TAMPONADE

Although most cases of tamponade have at least some of the classic features, there are several important variants. Loculated effusions that compress the heart primarily in one region are typically postsurgical, although they may be due to neoplasms or a number of other etiologies; they are discussed in the section on postcardiac surgery cases that follows. There are also a number of conditions where pulsus paradoxus does not occur or is masked, summarized in Box 24.1.

EFFUSIVE CONSTRICTIVE DISEASE

This phenomenon is an important-to-recognize condition occurring in less than 10% of patients with tamponade,[46] but up to 40% in some series. Hospitals with disproportionately high populations of oncology patients, because of tumor metastases or postradiation pericardial involvement, or tuberculosis, will have a higher percentage of tamponade patients with this diagnosis. The syndrome can occur after acute pericarditis of multiple etiologies and may even be transient.[47] The classic features of tamponade are seen on presentation, and a history of malignancy should increase the suspicion of prepericardiocentesis.

Effusive constrictive disease is a setting in which careful hemodynamic monitoring is very helpful for accurate diagnosis. Monitoring of intrapericardial and right atrial or wedge pressure during pericardiocentesis demonstrates findings as seen in Figure 24.11. In general, with relief of tamponade intrapericardial hypertension resolves, and classic respiratory variation is seen in most patients, whereas right atrial pressure remains elevated though lower than prior to the pericardiocentesis. The Y descent becomes prominent because of the elimination of high transmural pressures that restrict filling during early diastole in tamponade, unmasking classic constrictive physiology. Figure 24.12 shows echocardiographic images in a typical patient with this syndrome.

LOW- AND HIGH-PRESSURE TAMPONADE

Low-pressure tamponade has been defined as featuring hypotension secondary to pericardial effusion but with low venous and intrapericardial pressures, most commonly in the setting of hypovolemia resulting from dehydration or blood loss. A more formal definition, based on a single site experience, was described by Sagrista-Sauleda and colleagues[48] as an intrapericardial pressure less than 7 mm Hg, with a post-pericardiocentesis right atrial pressure less than 4 mm Hg and equalization of intrapericardial and right atrial pressures before pericardiocentesis. Importantly, 20% of their patients with cardiac tamponade met these criteria (and 10% of their patients with large pericardial effusions), suggesting that low-pressure tamponade, previously the subject primarily of case reports and small series, may be more common than previously appreciated. Because of low pressures, there is a lack of features such as pulsus paradoxus or jugular venous distention, with only 24% demonstrating these classic findings, making the diagnosis significantly more difficult. Fluid challenge may result in more typical findings.

Patients with chronic hypertension in whom tamponade develops occasionally have high blood pressure despite tamponade physiology, presumably because of an exaggerated systemic pressure response to the catecholamine storm associated with tamponade.[49] In this setting, injudicious use of the usual medications to lower blood pressure can result in profound hemodynamic compromise.

SETTINGS IN WHICH TAMPONADE IS SEEN

THE EMERGENCY ROOM

The primary cause of tamponade in the emergency room relates to hemopericardium, although the complete range of medical etiologies can be seen in this setting. Trauma[50] includes gunshot and stab wounds, as well as penetrating and crush wounds to the chest, including those related to automobile accidents. Penetrating wounds are significantly more likely to result in tamponade than crush injuries.[51] Medical presentations with acute hemopericardium include aortic dissection with tamponade, postmyocardial infarction rupture, or leaking thoracic aneurysm, situations in which pericardiocentesis may lead to further hemodynamic

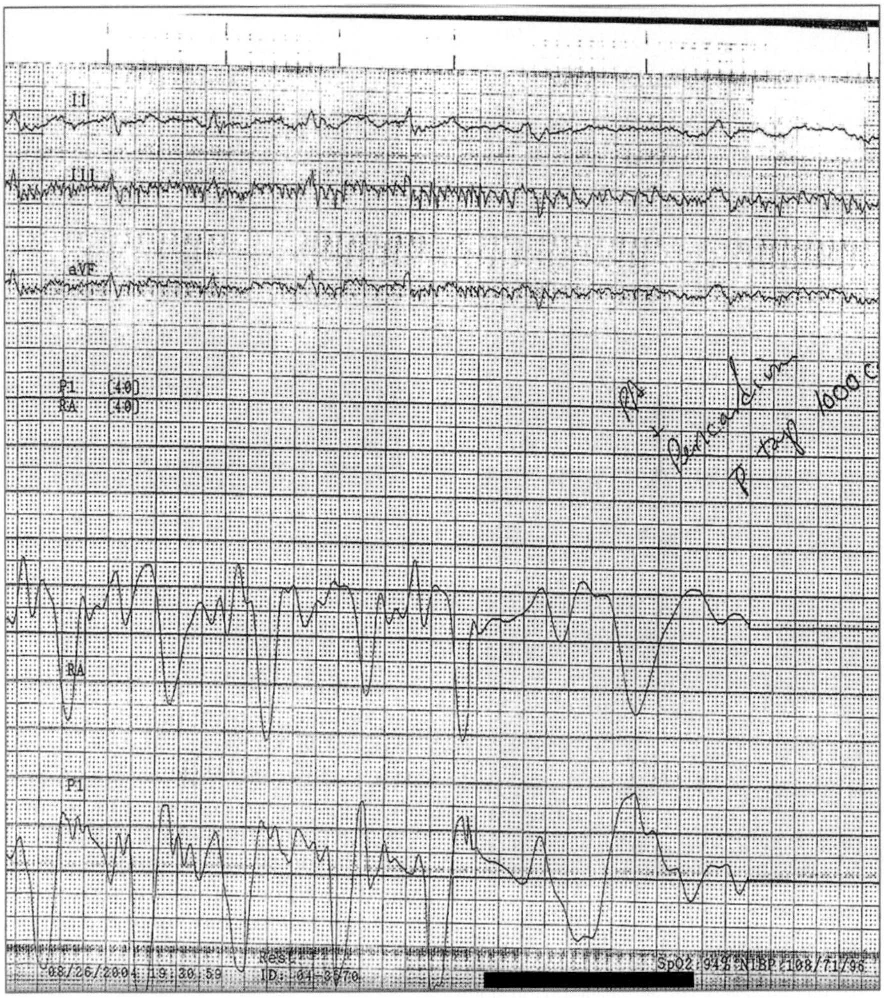

Figure 24.11 Hemodynamic tracings (40–mm Hg scale) obtained 1 hour after those seen in Figure 24.5. After pericardiocentesis of 1 L of fluid, the pericardial pressure has achieved a mean equivalent to atmospheric pressure (0 mm Hg by convention), while right atrial pressure remains elevated near 22 mm Hg. This is physiology consistent with effusive-constrictive disease. On removal of the effusion, the hemodynamics, including the newly seen steep Y descent, are classic for constriction. This patient had a malignant pericardial effusion. P, intrapericardial pressure; RA, right atrium.

decompensation,[52,53] as well as hemopericardium secondary to overanticoagulation. In general, acute hemopericardium may be associated with continued hemorrhage as well as clot in the pericardium; the latter makes complete drainage difficult. Clot alone can compress the heart and cause tamponade-like physiology. The clinical presentation of acute intrapericardial hemorrhage is typically shock, and jugular venous distention may or may not be present because of venoconstriction and hypovolemia as previously described. Use of echocardiography in the emergency room in patients with unexplained dyspnea is an important diagnostic tool.[54]

THE CARDIAC CATHETERIZATION AND ELECTROPHYSIOLOGY LABORATORIES

Perforation of the heart, including coronary arteries and cardiac chambers, during invasive cardiac procedures has become an increasingly important cause of pericardial tamponade.[55] Common scenarios include electrophysiology procedures, where relatively stiff catheters are placed in the relatively thin-walled structures of the right heart, including the right atrium, right ventricle, and the coronary venous system including the coronary sinus. Anticoagulation, when required for electrophysiology procedures, such as those involving left atrial ablation, raises the risk substantially. Perforation of coronary arteries occurs in particular with atheroablation devices such as those used for rotational atherectomy, directional atherectomy and lasers, with guidewires used in chronic total occlusions or injudiciously manipulated distal to the target lesion, and with oversized balloons and stents.[56] Even with normal sizing, settings such as myocardial bridges or ruptured balloons are associated with vessel perforation or rupture. A third setting is transseptal puncture, a resurgent technique because of burgeoning technologies requiring left atrial access[57] but associated with a significant risk of tamponade.[58] Besides left-sided ablations, mitral valvuloplasties, and percutaneous circulatory bypass (with its intake source in the left atrium), transseptal puncture is required for a number of techniques under development, including left atrial appendage occlusion and percutaneous mitral valve repair. The risk of pericardial effusion and tamponade with these interventions

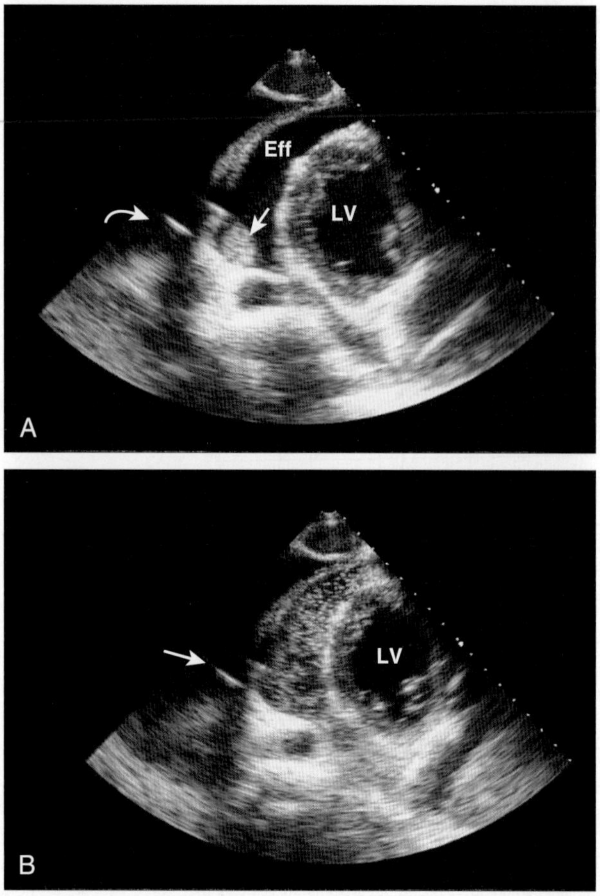

Figure 24.12 Echocardiographic images from a patient with effusive-constrictive disease. **A,** Tamponade. *Curved arrow* points to needle in pericardial space; *straight arrow* points to tumor mass. The pericardium is thickened. **B,** Agitated saline has been injected through the needle *(arrow)* to confirm entry into the pericardial space. Eff, effusion; LV, left ventricle.

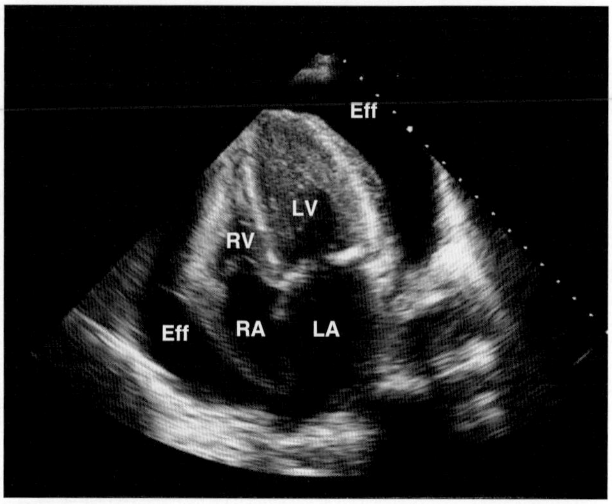

Figure 24.13 Echocardiogram showing large circumferential pericardial effusion in myxedema. Severe tamponade is rare. Eff, effusion; LA, left atrium; LV, left ventricle; RA, right atrium; RV, right ventricle.

contributes significantly to their overall morbidity and mortality.[55] However, and somewhat counterintuitively, electrophysiologists now frequently anticoagulate prior to transseptal puncture or perform the procedure in patients already on full oral anticoagulation.[59] This practice is driven by fear of thromboembolism rather than tamponade, the former an important complication of left-sided ablations in particular, which can be long procedures, and associated with clot inducing char formation. Other endovascular procedures associated with tamponade include myocardial biopsy and central venous line placement, pacemaker lead extraction, as well as erosion of devices implanted across the atrial septum or in the left atrial appendage.[60]

The potentially catastrophic setting of free perforation during coronary interventions is usually readily diagnosable during the procedure, with free flow in the pericardium seen during coronary injection, sometimes before the patient shows any signs of hemodynamic deterioration. This is readily treatable with balloon occlusion of the coronary artery at the perforation site, pericardiocentesis if necessary, and excluding the fenestration with a covered stent. However, lower-grade perforations that result in pooling of contrast or small adventitial craters can be more subtle. It is essential to discontinue anticoagulation on such patients and consider heparin reversal, and to ensure that personnel responsible for postprocedure management monitor the patient closely for hypotension and tachycardia. With transseptal punctures, hypotension at any time during the case, but especially after anticoagulation is administered, should raise the possibility of tamponade. A quick and relatively specific finding in the catheterization laboratory is straightening and lack of motion of the left heart border on anteroposterior fluoroscopy associated with hypotension (and sometimes reflex bradycardia); rapid intervention is essential in these patients. Hypotension after the procedure should raise the possibility that left atrial access involved a "stitch perforation" whereby the needle exited the right atrium and then entered the left atrium through the pericardial space; this mishap is possible with low punctures and frequently manifests only when catheters are removed from the fenestration at the end of the procedure. In patients who have had pacemaker placement, tamponade can develop acutely or after considerable delay as in the case of lead erosion.[61]

CRITICAL CARE UNITS AND MEDICAL WARDS

Tamponade in the critical care unit typically is due to complications of myocardial infarction, concomitant sepsis with purulent pericarditis, or hemorrhage into the pericardium because of anticoagulation (either iatrogenic or endogenous) or, most commonly, is secondary to neoplasms. In myocardial infarction, tamponade can be acute, secondary to massive or limited rupture, or somewhat more insidious in onset as part of Dressler's syndrome, with hemodynamic compromise sometimes exacerbated by anticoagulation. Tamponade also can be iatrogenic, in particular, secondary to placement of various lines through the venous or arterial circulation. Uncommon causes of tamponade, even with pericardial effusions of sometimes significant size, are viral pericarditis, congestive heart failure, uremia, myxedema (Fig. 24.13), and connective tissue disorders.

In patients with malignancy, several possible causes of tamponade are seen, including tumor involvement in the pericardium, postradiation pericarditis, graft-versus-host disease, and direct or indirect complications of therapy.[62] Patients with malignancies also are at increased risk for infectious pericarditis, coagulopathies or thrombocytopenia with secondary hemorrhage, and hypothyroid- and hypoalbuminemia-related effusions. AIDS and other immunosuppressed patients similarly are predisposed to infectious tamponade, as well as pericardial tumor involvement, including that from lymphoma. The mechanisms of pericardial effusion in cancer are varied but include direct spread to the pericardium from primary tumors such as lung, mediastinal, and esophageal cancer; hematogenous spread such as with lymphomas; and obstruction of the lymphatic drainage of the heart by tumors in the mediastinum.

Tamponade after cardiac surgery is an important phenomenon, usually occurring as a result of hemorrhagic effusion. Early postoperative tamponade is not uncommon and is important to recognize as a cause of hypotension because it has been reported to occur with a frequency of 5% to 10%, although this generally is thought to be in the 1% range in the modern era.[63] Moderate to large pericardial effusions that do not cause hemodynamic compromise have been much more common.[64] Delayed tamponade after heart surgery, with onset on average at 2 to 3 weeks postoperatively but as late as 6 months or more, occurs in less than 1% of patients but is disproportionately more common in patients undergoing valve surgery, probably related to postoperative anticoagulation in this cohort.[65,66] Delayed tamponade probably is a variant of the more common postcardiotomy syndrome.

Late tamponade typically is due to loculated effusion resulting from formation of adhesions (see Figs. 24.6 and 24.10) during recovery from surgery. Such adhesions can cause decreased cardiac output if they compress the left side of the heart, and in some cases pulmonary edema occurs if obstruction to inflow results. A variety of clinical problems related to increased right-sided heart pressure occur when tamponade involves the right side, including a clinical picture that resembles superior vena cava syndrome; several case reports have described right-to-left shunting across a patent foramen ovale as well.[67] Pericardiectomy to prevent postoperative tamponade has an uncertain risk-benefit ratio but does appear to decrease the incidence of hemodynamic compromise.[68]

Patients on dialysis present a special diagnostic and management problem. With underdialysis, volume overload can exacerbate chronic fluid accumulation in the pericardial space. Hypotension during or after dialysis may be secondary to inadequate intravascular volume and diminished venous pressure and needs to be avoided as well.

MANAGEMENT

Pericardial tamponade is life threatening, requiring difficult diagnostic and, in particular, management decisions. When hemodynamics do not suggest significant compromise and effusion is small to moderate in volume, intervention frequently is not necessary and may involve increased risk to the patient, whereas late intervention may be fatal. Typically, the risk associated with pericardiocentesis is inversely related to the volume of accumulated fluid and also is related to the location of the effusion. Thus, relatively small effusions, early in the course of tamponade, usually are located primarily posteriorly because of gravity-dependent accumulation. Waiting until the effusion is large and occupies significant volume anteriorly decreases the risk of percutaneous drainage but increases the possibility of decompensation and death before intervention. Frequent monitoring of hemodynamics and the application of sound clinical judgment are essential, but an optimal algorithm does not exist. Comorbid conditions such as endogenous or extrinsic anticoagulation may substantially confound the situation.[69] The clinical decision to drain the effusion percutaneously or to send the patient for thoracotomy will be a function of the clinician's assessment of risk of the former versus the potential advantages of surgery in obtaining pericardial tissue and providing a pericardial window as well. If the percutaneous approach is chosen, performing pericardiocentesis in the cardiac catheterization laboratory has significant advantages. However, the benefit of positioning the pericardial effusion anteriorly, for increased safety during needle entry into the pericardial space, requires that the patient's chest be elevated during the procedure, which typically can be accomplished only to a 20- or 30-degree angle on most catheterization tables because of the image intensifier unless the table has tilt capabilities. A moribund patient frequently needs pericardiocentesis performed at the bedside without fluoroscopic guidance, sometimes without adequate hemodynamic monitoring, and at times without echocardiographic monitoring—all of which are associated with increased risk of failed pericardiocentesis and adverse cardiac events. Patients with severe tamponade are often anxious and hypoxic; sedation is hazardous as is intubation, though the latter is at times necessary. As a result of associated positive intrathoracic pressure, intubation may cause abrupt hemodynamic deterioration because it decreases venous return to the heart.[2] Cardiopulmonary resuscitation using chest compression is unlikely to be effective; immediate pericardiocentesis or thoracotomy are ordinarily the only possibilities for survival. Further discussion of percutaneous interventions for tamponade can be found in Chapter 6.

Little in the way of medical treatment is clearly therapeutic for tamponade. Volume expansion in relatively acute tamponade will support right-sided filling in patients with low circulatory volumes, such as are seen in trauma.[70] Patients with chronic tamponade typically have considerable fluid retention, and additional hydration is unlikely to be of benefit. Pressors may be modestly helpful, but for patients with preserved cardiac function, catecholaminergic drugs provide only modest augmentation of cardiac output; patients with hemodynamically important tamponade are usually already maximally catecholamine stimulated. Vasodilator therapy is less clearly beneficial, and drugs that decrease preload, such as nitrates and nitroprusside, should be avoided if the patient is hypotensive. Reversal of anticoagulation is essential, both to stop bleeding into the pericardial space and to decrease the risk of trauma to the heart or major blood vessels during pericardiocentesis (e.g., coronary arteries, hepatic vessels). The introduction of direct thrombin inhibitors may affect this portion of the management algorithm because they are not reversible with vitamin K, and there are anecdotal reports of tamponade occurring after the introduction of oral versions of these agents[71] as well as failed pericardiocentesis during percutaneous coronary intervention associated with bivalirudin administration.[72] Antibiotic therapy in the setting of purulent pericarditis and tamponade is not expected to acutely relieve hemodynamic decompensation in most settings; postdrainage treatment, including local infusion of drugs, is discussed in Chapter 6. A targeted approach for patients with malignant pericardial disease includes the use of sclerosing agents combined with antineoplastic drugs infused into the pericardial space, sometimes combined with radiation; a variety of such management strategies continue to be applicable for some cancer patients.[73] Leaving an indwelling drain is controversial because of the associated risk of infection, although there is some evidence that it can decrease the risk of recurrent tamponade.[74] An excellent review of the clinical approach to pericardial disease in general has been published by the European Society of Cardiology.[75]

ACKNOWLEDGMENT

The author wishes to acknowledge Priscilla Peters for kindly providing Figures 24.6, 24.7, 24.8, 24.10, 24.12, and 24.13.

KEY POINTS

- Pericardial tamponade represents a continuum, ranging from effusions associated with little or no hemodynamic compromise to hemodynamic collapse.
- The primary physiologic feature of tamponade is impairment of cardiac chamber filling due to high intrapericardial pressure, with a resultant decrease in cardiac output.
- Acute tamponade occurs after a relatively limited accumulation of fluid in the setting of a nondistensible pericardium.
- Chronic tamponade may involve a pericardial effusion of 1 L or more; because hemodynamic decompensation occurs in the steep part of the pressure-volume curve, accumulation of a small amount of additional fluid can result in substantial hemodynamic deterioration.
- Pulsus paradoxus is seen in a variety of conditions besides cardiac tamponade and is absent despite

KEY POINTS (Continued)

tamponade in a number of settings. A large pericardial effusion and right ventricular collapse, a 10 to 20 mm Hg or larger decrease in systolic pressure with inspiration, and a significant decline in pulse pressure combined are specific for tamponade.

- Right atrial pressure, except in settings such as hypovolemia, usually is significantly elevated, but jugular venous distention may not be seen with acute tamponade.
- Despite markedly elevated right and left atrial pressures, pulmonary vascular congestion usually is not seen.
- Persistent high right atrial pressure after fluid drainage suggests effusive-constrictive disease, most commonly associated with malignancy but also seen with infection and acute pericarditis.
- Management of pericardial tamponade involves determining the optimal timing and method of intervention. Fluid and drug therapy constitute modest adjunctive care only.

SELECTED REFERENCES

1. Hancock EW: Cardiac tamponade. Med Clin North Am 1979;63:223-237.
2. Little WC, Freeman GL: Pericardial disease. Circulation 2006;113:1622-1632.
3. Spodick DH: Macrophysiology, microphysiology, and anatomy of the pericardium: A synopsis. Am Heart J 1992;124:1046-1051.
6. Watkins MW, LeWinter MM: Physiologic role of the normal pericardium. Annu Rev Med 1993;44:171-180.
12. Spodick DH: Acute cardiac tamponade. N Engl J Med 2003; 349:684-690.
18. Khandaker MH, Espinosa RE, Nishimura RA, et al: Pericardial disease: Diagnosis and management. Mayo Clin Proc 2010;85: 572-593.
21. Goldstein JA: Cardiac tamponade, constrictive pericarditis, and restrictive cardiomyopathy. Curr Probl Cardiol 2004;29:503-567.
46. Sagrista-Sauleda J, Angel J, Sanchez A, et al: Effusive-constrictive pericarditis. N Engl J Med 2004;350:469-475.
55. Holmes DR Jr, Nishimura R, Fountain R, Turi ZG: Iatrogenic pericardial effusion and tamponade in the percutaneous intracardiac intervention era. JACC Cardiovasc Interv 2009;2:705-717.
75. Maisch B, Seferovic PM, Ristic AD, et al: Guidelines on the diagnosis and management of pericardial diseases executive summary; the task force on the diagnosis and management of pericardial diseases of the European Society of Cardiology. Eur Heart J 2004;25: 587-610.

The complete list of references can be found on www.expertconsult.com.

25

Severe Sepsis and Multiple Organ Dysfunction

Sergio L. Zanotti-Cavazzoni | R. Phillip Dellinger | Joseph E. Parrillo

CHAPTER OUTLINE

INTRODUCTION

The term *sepsis* is derived from the Greek word *sepsin,* which means "to make putrid." The relationship between infection and sepsis has been recognized for many years. However, the precise mechanisms by which infection results in sepsis, severe sepsis, septic shock, or multiple organ dysfunction remain to be fully elucidated. Improvements in our understanding of this syndrome have led to the development of novel therapeutic strategies and have increased our appreciation for the complex interactions that exist in sepsis between pathogens and the host response to infection. Despite these advances, severe sepsis remains one of the most significant causes of morbidity and mortality in patients admitted to the intensive care unit (ICU).[1] In this chapter we will discuss the current definitions, epidemiology, and pathogenesis of severe sepsis and multiple organ dysfunction. In addition, we will review current management options and discuss an approach to treatment based on pathophysiology.

DEFINITIONS

For many years the term *sepsis* was loosely applied in clinical practice and was used to describe a very heterogeneous patient population. In recognition of this problem, a consensus conference was convened to create standardized definitions and formulate a blueprint to guide future research in sepsis.[2] The term *systemic inflammatory response syndrome* (SIRS) was introduced. SIRS can occur in response to a variety of severe clinical insults and is defined by the presence of two or more of the following conditions: (1) temperature > 38° C or < 36° C, (2) heart rate > 90 beats per minute, (3) respiratory rate > breaths per minute or a $Paco_2$ < 32 mm Hg, and (4) white blood cell count > 12,000 cells/mm^3. *Sepsis* occurs when SIRS is caused by infection. *Severe sepsis* is sepsis with associated organ dysfunction, hypoperfusion, or hypotension. Hypoperfusion and perfusion abnormalities may include, but are not limited to, lactic acidosis, oliguria, or an acute alteration in mental status. *Septic shock* is defined by the presence of sepsis-induced hypotension (systolic blood pressure < 90 mm Hg or a reduction ≥ 40 mm Hg from baseline in the absence of other causes for hypotension), despite adequate fluid resuscitation along with the presence of perfusion abnormalities.[2] The introduction of these definitions created a common language that was especially helpful in designing and defining populations for clinical trials.[3] On the other hand, criticism of these definitions pointed out that they were too sensitive and were not useful when applied clinically to individual patients.[4] In 2001 a second consensus conference with a broader representation was convened to revisit these definitions.[5] The conference recommended keeping the 1992 definitions unchanged secondary to lack of new evidence to support new definitions. However, the consensus conference recommended expanding the diagnostic criteria for sepsis in an effort to enhance recognition at the bedside (Box 25.1). In addition, the Predisposition Insult infection Response Organ dysfunction (PIRO) system for staging sepsis was proposed. This staging system is still relatively new and further development and research will be needed prior to its implementation in clinical practice. Examples and

Table 25.1 The PIRO System for Staging Sepsis

Domain	Present	Future
Predisposition	Premorbid conditions, age, and sex	Genetic polymorphism in components of the inflammatory response (e.g., TNF)
Insult infection	Culture and sensitivity of pathogens; identification of possible target for source control	Assays of specific microbial products and gene transcript profiles
Response	SIRS, other signs of sepsis, septic shock, C-reactive protein	Markers of activated inflammation or impaired host responsiveness
Organ dysfunction	Organ dysfunction as number of failing organs or composite scores	Measure of cellular response to insult-apoptosis, cytopathic hypoxia, cell stress

SIRS, systemic inflammatory response syndrome; TNF, tumor necrosis factor.
Adapted from Levy M, Fink MP, Marshall JC, et al: 2001 SCCM/ESICM/ACCP/ATS/SIS International Sepsis Definitions Conference. Crit Care Med 2003;31:1250-1256.

Box 25.1 Diagnostic Criteria for Sepsis

Infection, documented or suspected, plus some of the following findings:

Temperature > 38.3° C or > 36° C
Heart rate > 90 min or > 2 SD above normal value for age
Arterial hypotension (SBP < 90 mm Hg, MAP < 70 or an SBP decrease > 40 in adults or < SD below normal for age)
Mixed venous oxygen saturation (SvO_2) > 70%
Cardiac index > 3.5 L/min/M^2
Tachypnea
Decreased capillary refill or mottling
Altered mental status
Significant edema or positive fluid balances
Hyperglycemia in the absence of diabetes
WBC count > 12,000 μL or < 4000 μ
Normal WBC with > 10% immature forms
Plasma C-reactive protein > 2 SD above the normal value
Plasma procalcitonin > SD above the normal value
Hyperlactatemia (> 1 mmol/L)
Evidence of organ dysfunction:
Arterial hypoxemia (PaO_2/FiO_2 < 300)
Acute oliguria
Creatinine increase > 0.5 mg/dL
Coagulation abnormalities (INR > 1.5 or a PTT > 60s)
Ileus
Thrombocytopenia
Hyperbilirubinemia

INR, international normalized ratio; MAP, mean arterial pressure; PTT, partial thromboplastin time; SBP, systolic blood pressure; SD, standard deviation; WBC, white blood cell.

possible measures for the future in each domain are shown in Table 25.1.

EPIDEMIOLOGY

Severe sepsis constitutes a major health care problem.[6-8] Estimates of the incidence of severe sepsis in the United States report that approximately 750,000 cases occur per year (3 cases per 1000 population).[6] Almost 70% of these cases receive care in a high dependency unit (ICU, intermediate care unit, or coronary care unit).[6] The incidence of severe sepsis and septic shock has increased over time both in North America and in Europe.[6-8] The incidence of severe sepsis is projected to increase by 1.5% every year.[6] These increases in incidence are attributed to an aging population with a growing number of patients with a compromised immune system, infected with resistant pathogens, and undergoing prolonged, high-risk surgical interventions.[8] Severe sepsis is more frequent with increased age, in males, and in nonwhite patients.[6,8] Before the mid-1980s, gram-negative bacteria were the most common pathogens responsible for severe sepsis. Over the years an increase in cases from gram-positive bacteria has been reported, and today gram-positive bacteria are the predominant pathogens in severe sepsis.[8] The incidence of sepsis resulting from fungal organisms has increased substantially since the 1990s.[8] The most common sites of infection include the respiratory system, the bloodstream, and the genitourinary tract.[6,7,9]

Although mortality for severe sepsis and septic shock has decreased over time, severe sepsis still kills one in four patients affected worldwide.[6,7,10,11] Mortality increases with age in black men and with increased number of failing organs.[8] Over time the hospital length of stay for patients with sepsis has decreased, and the number of discharges to nonacute medical care facilities has increased.[8] In addition to causing high morbidity and mortality, severe sepsis has a significant economic impact. Estimates report an average cost per patient of $22,000, representing on annual impact to the health care system in excess of $16.5 billion in the United States alone.[6]

PATHOPHYSIOLOGY

Severe sepsis is the result of complex interactions between infecting organisms and the host response. Important components of this host response in the early phases of sepsis include the immune system, activation of the inflammatory cascade, and alterations in hemostasis. In later stages of sepsis, organ failure, immunosuppression, and apoptosis play an important pathophysiologic role. Both characteristics of the infecting organism and of the host response influence the outcome of sepsis. Virulence factors, high burden of infection, and resistance to antibiotics are all organism characteristics associated with increased risk of severe sepsis. There is a growing body of literature suggesting that host responses might be influenced by genetic polymorphisms.[12-17] This might explain why some patients develop severe sepsis to a particular pathogen and others do not. We will further discuss some of the relevant components of the host response in severe sepsis.

ROLE OF THE IMMUNE SYSTEM IN THE EARLY PHASES OF SEPSIS

The immune response to infection takes place through the actions of two pathways: the innate immune system and the adaptive immune system. The goal of the innate immune system is to provide protection in the first minutes to hours after an infectious challenge. Although initially thought to be a nonspecific response, research has demonstrated that the innate immune system recognizes pathogens by means of pattern-recognition receptors (Toll-like receptors [TLRs], Table 25.2). Toll-like receptors bind to highly conserved structures on microorganisms, which are not easily altered by microbes to evade detection and are present on broad groups of organisms.[18] Our current understanding of TLRs suggests that the immune cells use different TLRs to detect several features of an organism and based on the composite information gained generate a tailored response to the invading pathogen.[18] Activation of Toll-like receptors by microorganisms stimulates signaling pathways that increase production of pro-inflammatory cytokines such as tumor necrosis factor (TNF-α), interleukin-1β (IL-1β), and nuclear factor-κB (NF-κB), as well as anti-inflammatory cytokines such as interleukin-10 (IL-10).[18,19] Toll-like receptor activation also results in up-regulation of microbial killing mechanisms, such as the production of reactive nitrogen species.[20] Toll-like receptors play a pivotal role in initiating the innate immune response and are important regulators of the adaptive immune response to infection. Recognition of these proteins and their functions expanded our understanding of the pathophysiology of sepsis and has provided a new target for therapeutic interventions.[21]

The adaptive immune system amplifies the response initiated by the innate immune system with a higher degree of specificity. In addition to their interactions with the innate immune system, microorganisms stimulate specific cell-mediated and humoral adaptive immune responses. Two types of lymphocytes, B cells and T cells, play an important role in the adaptive immune response. Adaptive immune responses (humoral and cellular) require days to develop. However, they are amnestic through the generation of memory T and B lymphocytes and, in the case of reexposure to the same pathogen, can elicit a faster response. CD4 T cells are divided into two types: type 1 helper T-cell (Th1) and type 2 helper T-cell (Th2). Factors such as type of organism, site of infection, and burden of infection influence the response elicited by T cells. In general, Th1 cells secrete pro-inflammatory cytokines (TNF-α and interleukin-1β) and Th2 cells secrete anti-inflammatory cytokines (interleukin-4 and interleukin-10).[22] B lymphocyte cells are responsible for releasing immunoglobulins in response to microorganisms. These immunoglobulins bind to organism-specific antigens and enhance recognition and destruction by other immune cells (natural killer cells and neutrophils). Several other cell types are involved in the adaptive immune response to infection (Fig. 25.1).

Table 25.2 Role of TLRs in Pathogen Rcoognition and Pathophysiology of Human Disease

Toll-like Receptor	Pathogen or Disease State
TLR1	Lyme disease
	Neisseria meningitidis
TLR2	*Mycobacterium tuberculosis*
	Chagas disease
	Leptospirosis
	Fungal sepsis
	CMV viremia
TLR3	Many
TLR4	Gram-negative bacteria
	Septic shock
	Chlamydia trachomatis
	Chlamydia pneumoniae
	Certain viruses
	Mycobacterium tuberculosis
TLR5	Flagellated bacteria (e.g., *Salmonella*)
TLR7	Viral infections
TLR8	Viral infections
TLR9	Bacterial and viral infections
TLR10	Unknown

ROLE OF INFLAMMATION

For many years the prevailing theory has been that sepsis is the result of an uncontrolled inflammatory response.[1,2] This paradigm was based on extensive animal experimentation with models of inflammation that may not necessarily reflect human disease. Animal models of sepsis that utilized large doses of endotoxin or bacteria created a "cytokine storm" that when blocked resulted in improvements in mortality. However, in human sepsis most patients have a complex host response that includes activation of both pro-inflammatory and anti-inflammatory cascades. Early death from overwhelming inflammation is not the norm, and most patients who die develop complications related to immunosuppression, apoptosis, and multiorgan failure later in the course of the disease. These differences may partially explain why so many anti-inflammatory compounds worked in animal models yet failed to improve mortality in human clinical trials. The interplay between pro-inflammatory cytokines, anti-inflammatory cytokines, and cytokine inhibitors is a dynamic process that influences the host response to sepsis. Pro-inflammatory cytokines such as TNF-α and IL-1β increase early in sepsis and have overlapping and synergistic effects in further stimulating the inflammatory cascade.[23] Pro-inflammatory cytokines activate monocytes, macrophages, and neutrophils; stimulate neutrophil margination; and increase gluconeogenesis. In addition, pro-inflammatory cytokines have an important role in the development of clinical abnormalities such as

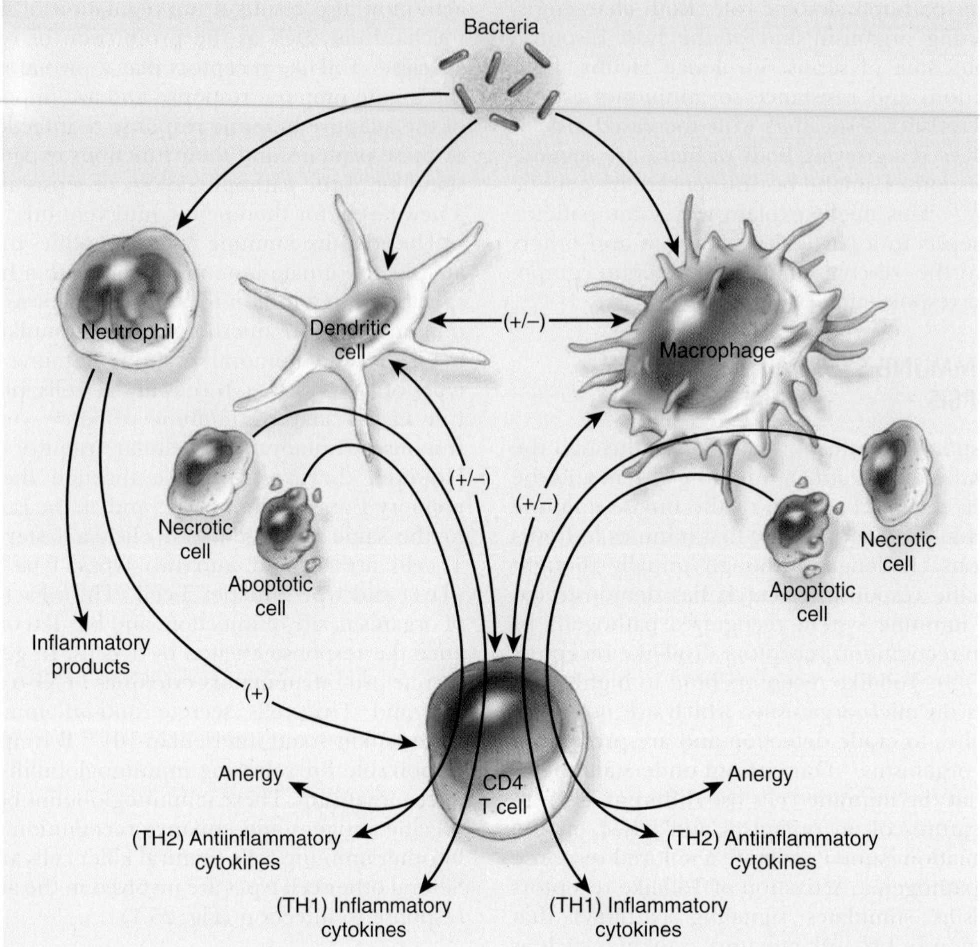

Figure 25.1 Response of immune cells to infection. The immune response to pathogens involves various types of cells. Crosstalk exists between the different cell lines of the immune system (dendritic cells, macrophages, lymphocytes, and neutrophils). The + sign represents up-regulation, and the – sign down-regulation. Many interactions on the figure have both + and – signs, representing the possibility of either up-regulation or down-regulation, depending on a variety of factors. (Adapted from Hotchkiss RS: The pathophysiology and treatment of sepsis. N Engl J Med 2003;348:138-150, Figure 1, p 140.)

fever, hypotension, capillary leakage with decreased intravascular volume, and myocardial depression.[23] More recently, pro-inflammatory cytokines such as macrophage migration inhibitory factor (MIF) and high mobility group 1 protein (HMG-1) have received attention as downstream mediators of inflammation and potential therapeutic targets.[24-27] The role of anti-inflammatory cytokines in sepsis is still not fully understood. Current understanding suggests that sepsis-induced multiorgan failure and death may be caused in part by a shift to an anti-inflammatory phenotype and by apoptosis of key immune cells.[28,29] This shift is driven in part by increased levels of anti-inflammatory cytokines and results from a shift in helper T-cell populations (from Th1 to Th2).[30] Inflammation plays an important role in the host response to sepsis. It is now apparent that simple therapeutic strategies that block specific pro-inflammatory cytokines are insufficient to modulate this response.[31,32] As our understanding of the intricate relationship between pro-inflammatory and anti-inflammatory responses increases, we might become more successful in modulating these to improve patients' outcomes.

ALTERATIONS OF HEMOSTASIS

Another important factor in the pathophysiology of sepsis is the alteration of the hemostatic balance. In sepsis this balance is altered by an increase in procoagulant factors paired with a decrease in anticoagulant factors (Fig. 25.2). Under normal conditions the intraluminal vascular surface has anticoagulant properties. During sepsis, stimulation from cytokines promotes expression of tissue factor on endothelial cells, monocytes, and neutrophils.[33,34] Tissue factor triggers the extrinsic coagulation pathway by activating factor VII. Activation of the extrinsic pathway leads to the formation of thrombin. The intrinsic pathway is triggered by activation of factor XI and leads to amplification of the coagulation cascade with further formation of thrombin. Excessive coagulation is normally counterbalanced by several anticoagulant factors. Anticoagulant factors such as antithrombin III, activated protein C, protein S, and tissue factor pathway inhibitor are decreased in sepsis.[35] These circumstances push the hemostatic balance toward the procoagulant state. Activation of the coagulation cascade leads

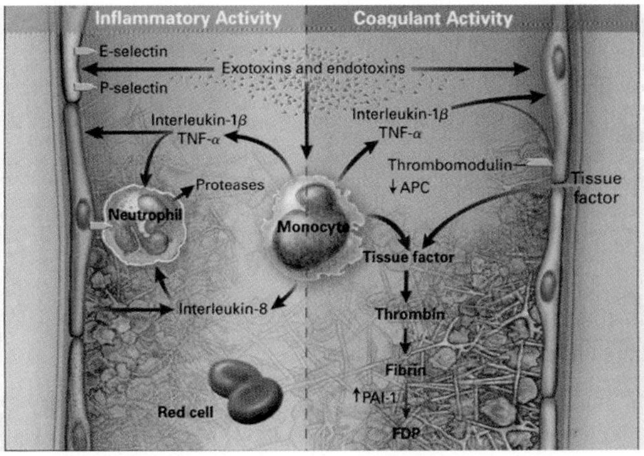

Figure 25.2 Relationship between inflammatory and coagulation systems in sepsis. Monocytes are activated by endotoxins and exotoxins from bacteria and release tumor necrosis factor-alpha (TNF-α) and interleukin-1β (IL-1β). TNF-α and IL-1β activate the inflammatory cascade via neutrophils and the production of other proinflammatory cytokines, and, in combination with tissue factor, they also activate the coagulation cascade, with production of fibrin and fibrin degradation products (FDP). APC, activated protein C. (Adapted from Matthay MA: Severe sepsis: A new treatment with both anticoagulant and anti-inflammatory properties. N Engl J Med 2001;344:759-762, Figure 1A, p 761.)

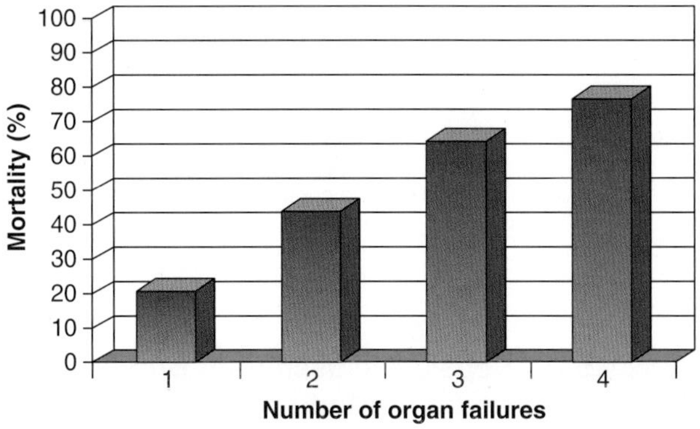

Figure 25.3 Relationship between number of organ failures and mortality. As the number of organ failures rises, mortality from severe sepsis progressively increases. With four organ failures, for example, mortality approaches 80%. (Data from Angus D, Linde-Zwirble WT, Clermont G, et al: Epidemiology of neonatal respiratory failure in the United States: Projections from California and New York. Crit Care Med 2001;29:1303-1310.)

to a consumption of coagulation factors. The clinical expression of this phenomenon is disseminated intravascular coagulation (DIC). Disseminated intravascular coagulation is characterized by a consumptive coagulopathy, which can result in an increased risk of bleeding but more commonly in sepsis causes damage by increasing the risk of thrombosis. In sepsis the excessive formation of fibrin from thrombin compounded by the suppression of fibrinolysis and the impairment of anticoagulant pathways leads to widespread formation of microthrombi. It has been proposed that these microthrombi lead to microcirculatory alterations and play an integral role in the pathogenesis of organ failure.[36,37]

MANAGEMENT

Severe sepsis is a medical emergency. When one considers its morbidity and the relationship between number of organ failures and mortality (Fig. 25.3), it makes sense to treat patients emergently and institute therapies that can prevent the progression of organ failure and improve outcomes in a time-sensitive fashion. Several therapies for severe sepsis have a potential time-sensitive effect on outcome (e.g., when instituted early have a higher likelihood of improving outcomes than when instituted with time delays) (Box 25.2). Although severe sepsis is associated with a higher mortality than other diseases considered medical emergencies, such as trauma, acute ischemic stroke, and acute myocardial infarction, it is still not treated with the same degree of urgency. This may be secondary to difficulties in recognizing severe sepsis early and a lack of understanding its consequences and their therapeutic implications by physicians outside the intensive care unit.

Recognizing these problems, the Society of Critical Care Medicine (SCCM), the European Society of Intensive Care Medicine (ESICM), and the International Sepsis Forum

Box 25.2 Potential Time-Sensitive Therapeutic Interventions

- Antimicrobial treatment
- Goal-directed resuscitation
- Mechanical ventilation
- Glucose control

(ISF) created the Surviving Sepsis Campaign (SSC). The SSC conglomerates experts in the field of sepsis from around the world and currently counts with the endorsement of 29 international medical societies and the Institute for Healthcare Improvement (www.ihi.gov). The campaign has aimed to improve standards of patient care, secure funding for research, and ultimately reduce the mortality of severe sepsis worldwide. To achieve these goals, the SCC has published evidence-based practice guidelines and consensus recommendations for the management of patients with severe sepsis.[38,39,39a] These guidelines were first published in 2004 and revised in 2008, and a second revision for 2012 is currently in press. To increase the impact of these clinical guidelines at the bedside, the SCC created the sepsis bundles.[40] The *sepsis resuscitation bundle* should be implemented over the first 6 hours after recognition of a patient with severe sepsis, and the *sepsis management bundle* should be implemented over the first 24 hours of admission to the hospital. A number of nonrandomized studies have shown that compliance with the bundles and application of their clinical recommendations in the form of protocols can improve patient outcomes.[41-43] More important, the publication of phase 2 of the SSC international performance improvement program demonstrated the significant impact compliance with the sepsis bundles has on reducing mortality in severe sepsis.[44] This large prospective study evaluated the implementation of a multifaceted intervention to facilitate compliance with selected guideline recommendations in the intensive care unit, emergency department, and wards of hospitals from around the world. Data from 15,022

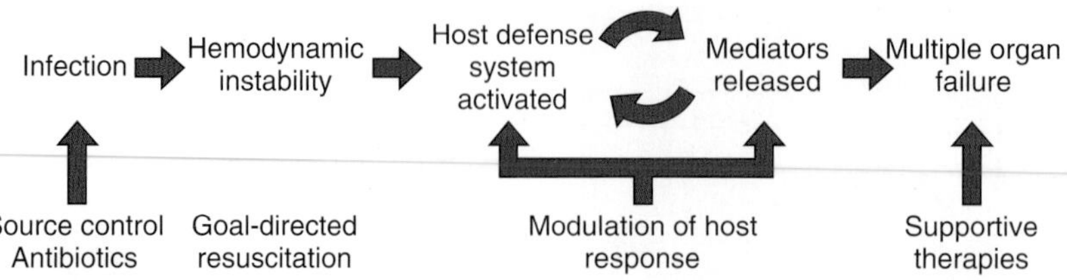

Figure 25.4 Approach to treatment of severe sepsis.

Box 25.3 Sepsis Resuscitation Bundle (to be started immediately and completed within 3 hours)

- Serum lactate measured*
- Blood cultures obtained prior to antibiotic administration
- Minimize time to administration of broad-spectrum antibiotics with a maximum of 3 hours from ED triage and 1 hour for non-ED ICU admissions
- In the event of hypotension or lactate > 4 mmol/L (36 mg/dL) deliver an initial minimum of 30 mL/kg of crystalloid (or colloid equivalent)

*A normal lactate level does not exclude severe sepsis.
ED, emergency department; ICU, intensive care unit.

Box 25.4 Septic Shock Bundle (to be started immediately and completed within 6 hours)

- Apply vasopressors for hypotension that does not respond to initial fluid resuscitation to maintain mean arterial pressure (MAP) ≥ 65 mm Hg.
- In the event of persistent arterial hypotension despite volume resuscitation (septic shock) or initial lactate > 4 mmol/L (36 mg/dL):
  - Achieve a central venous pressure (CVP) of ≥ 8 mm Hg.
  - Achieve central venous oxygen saturation ($ScvO_2$) of ≥ 70%.

subjects at 165 sites were analyzed to determine the compliance with bundle targets and association with hospital mortality. Compliance with the entire resuscitation bundle increased from 10.9% to 31.3% by the end of 2 years ($p <$ 0.0001). Compliance with the entire management bundle started at 18.4% and increased to 36.1% by the end of 2 years ($p = 0.008$). This increase in compliance was associated with a decrease in unadjusted hospital mortality from 37% to 30.8% ($p = .001$). The adjusted odds ratio for mortality improved the longer the site participated in the SSC.[44] Based on emerging data and recently published studies, the last revision of the guidelines recommends dropping the management bundle and dividing the resuscitation bundle into two parts:[39a]

- Initial resuscitation bundle
  - To be initiated immediately upon identifying patients with severe sepsis and septic shock
- Septic shock bundle
  - To be initiated immediately and completed within 6 hours for patients with septic shock

The complete new bundles are shown in Box 25.3 and Box 25.4. The optimal treatment of severe sepsis is a dynamic and constantly evolving process. We will discuss current treatment recommendations based on up-to-date clinical data. However, as new research emerges it is likely that new therapies will be described, and treatment recommendations presented in this chapter may need to be modified.

Like in other medical emergencies the first priority in treating patients with severe sepsis should be assessing and optimizing the "ABCs": airway, breathing, and circulation. In conjunction with initial stabilization of physiologic abnormalities, one should initiate appropriate diagnostic interventions to assess potential sources of infection and severity of organ dysfunction. Therapeutic interventions for severe sepsis should be implemented quickly and in conjunction. For the sake of discussion we will approach the treatment of severe sepsis based on pathophysiologic abnormalities produced by the syndrome (Fig. 25.4). We will discuss in further detail management of the infectious insult, hemodynamic optimization, modulation of the host response, and finally supportive therapies.

INFECTION MANAGEMENT

Severe sepsis is initiated by an infectious insult. Therefore, infection management constitutes one of the cornerstones of treatment in these patients. Infection management consists of source control and the administration of appropriate empiric antimicrobials that are effective against presumed causative pathogens. Administration of appropriate antibiotics is a time-sensitive intervention. Administration of antibiotics is often delayed, and this can result in worse outcomes.[45] Delays in appropriate antibiotic administration are much more likely to result from system failures (e.g., order not written by physician, delay from pharmacy, etc.) than from bacteriologic resistance.[46] Current guidelines recommend that appropriate antibiotics be administered to patients with severe sepsis within 1 hour of diagnosis.[39] Results from a retrospective study in a large group of septic shock patients suggests that every hour appropriate antibiotics are delayed after the onset of hypotension, the odds ratio for mortality increases in a stepwise manner.[47] Additional studies have shown increased mortality with delays in appropriate antibiotic administration.[43,44,48,49] One study done in patients in the emergency department showed that if antibiotics were given prior to the onset of shock, mortality was significantly decreased.[50] However, among patients who received antibiotics after shock recognition, mortality did not change with hourly delays in antibiotic administration.[50] The goal should be to administer appropriate antibiotics as soon as possible in patients with severe sepsis. To accomplish this objective, hospitals must examine their particular dynamics and devise systems to optimize antibiotic administration.

Studies in patients with sepsis have reported an incidence of positive blood cultures in the range of 20% to 50%.[8,51-53] Considering the growing need for broad-spectrum empirical regimens and the need to narrow down antimicrobial regimens in order to decrease resistance, obtaining blood cultures prior to the administration of antibiotics is essential. In most cases, one must start antibiotics without bacteriologic confirmation of the causative pathogen. Studies have demonstrated that the appropriateness of initial antibiotic therapy has a significant impact on patient outcomes.[54,55] In one prospective cohort study of critically ill patients, inadequate initial antibiotic therapy was associated with a statistically significant increase in all-cause and infection-related hospital mortality.[56] Factors associated with administration of inadequate antibiotics included prior administration of antibiotics, bloodstream infections, increasing acute physiology and chronic health evaluation (APACHE II) scores, and decreasing age.[56] If one considers the detrimental effect on mortality, it is apparent that in patients with severe sepsis, one cannot afford to miss potential causative organisms when empirically selecting an antimicrobial regimen. The choice of antibiotics should be based on the following factors:

- Probable pathogens based on clinical diagnosis and source of infection (pneumonia, bloodstream infection, abdominal source, etc.)
- Site where infection was acquired (community versus hospital acquired)
- Results obtained from diagnostic tests such as Gram stains
- Resistance patterns of local and hospital bacterial flora
- Patient comorbidities, drug allergies, and previous antibiotic exposure

Initial empiric anti-infective therapy should include one or more drugs that have activity against likely pathogens and that penetrate the presumptive site of infection in adequate concentrations. Recently used anti-infective drugs in a particular patient should be avoided as the likelihood of resistance increases. Clinicians should also consider whether candidemia is a likely pathogen based on the presence of predisposing risk factors. When indicated, empirical antifungal therapy should take into account local flora and previous exposure of the patient to azole drugs. Recent Infectious Disease Society of America (IDSA) guidelines recommend either fluconazole or an echinocandin.[57] Empiric use of echinocandin is preferred in critically ill patients, those exposed to azole drugs, and in settings where infection with *C. glabrata* is suspected or documented. Initial antibiotic therapy for severe sepsis should be broad in spectrum and progressively narrowed as microbiologic data become available. In culture-negative patients, the de-escalation of antibiotics may become challenging. In these cases, clinical evolution can be used to guide decisions. A detailed discussion of specific antibiotic regimens is beyond the scope of this chapter; the reader is referred to other chapters in the textbook and to the synopsis in Table 25.3.

The term *source control* refers to measures implemented to control the source of infection. Source control interventions can be divided into three broad categories: (1) drainage of an abscess, (2) debridement/drainage/incision of infected tissue, and (3) removal of an infected foreign body.[58] Attention to identifying potential sources amenable to source control measures should be part of the initial evaluation of patients with sepsis. The timing of intervention depends on several factors. When source interventions are simple, such as removal of an infected central venous catheter, they should be implemented immediately. In cases of unstable patients were surgery might be required, delaying source control while optimizing hemodynamic status may be appropriate. Finally, in cases such as necrotizing fasciitis, in which delays carry a significant risk of increasing mortality, one must proceed to surgery as early as possible. Examples of specific source control measures in patients with sepsis are shown on Table 25.4.

HEMODYNAMIC OPTIMIZATION

Severe sepsis is associated with a host of hemodynamic abnormalities. These abnormalities can ultimately lead to sepsis-induced tissue hypoperfusion if not addressed early and aggressively. The hemodynamic profile of severe sepsis and septic shock is initially characterized by components of hypovolemic, cardiogenic, and distributive shock.[59] In the initial phases of resuscitation, addressing the hypovolemic component is most important. Early in sepsis, increased capillary leak and increased venous capacitance will result in effective hypovolemia with decreased venous return to the heart. Low intravascular volume paired with sepsis-induced myocardial depression will result in a decrease in stroke volume (SV). Administration of intravascular fluids can alter this early phase of sepsis characterized by hypovolemia, tachycardia, and depressed cardiac output. Initial steps in hemodynamic optimization for patients with severe sepsis should include evaluation for signs of sepsis-induced tissue hypoperfusion. Signs of global hypoperfusion such as hypotension, tachycardia, oliguria, delayed capillary refill, altered mentation, increased blood lactate, and low mixed venous oxygen saturation are helpful when present to establish tissue hypoperfusion. However, these signs are not always sensitive and they must be complemented with assessment of indices of regional hypoperfusion. Patients with severe sepsis should have good venous access. Central venous access is preferred as it can also be used for hemodynamic monitoring.

The importance of early intervention in patients with sepsis-induced tissue hypoperfusion has been highlighted by the results of an early goal-directed therapy (EGDT) clinical trial by Rivers and colleagues.[60] In this study, patients with sepsis-induced hypoperfusion (lactate > 4 mmol or hypotension after fluids) were randomized to receive either standard resuscitation or an early goal-directed (EGDT) protocol during the first 6 hours of admission to the emergency department. In both groups, end points of resuscitation included central venous pressure (CVP) ≥ 8 to 12 mm Hg, mean arterial pressure (MAP) ≥ 65 mm Hg, and urine output ≥ 0.5 mL/kg/hr. To achieve these goals,

Table 25.3 Antibiotic Selection for Sepsis Based on Site of Infection

Site	Bacteria	First-Line Agent	Second-Line Agent
Abdominal			
Primary peritonitis	Enterobacteriaceae *S. pneumoniae* *Enterococcus faecalis*	Third-generation cephalosporins: —Cefotaxime —Ceftriaxone	Quinolones Imipenem-cilastatin Piperacillin-tazobactam
Secondary peritonitis	Aerobic gram-negatives *Bacteroides fragilis* *Enterococcus* species *P. aeruginosa* *Candida* species	Imipenem-cilastatin or imipenem-cilastatin ± aminoglycoside	Antipseudomonal β-lactam Third-generation cephalosporin ± metronidazole Quinolone ± metronidazole Third-generation cephalosporin ± Aminoglycoside ± Amphotericin B
Tertiary peritonitis	*Enterococcus* species *Candida* species *Staphylococcus epidermidis*	Imipenem-cilastatin ± aminoglycoside ± amphotericin B	Antipseudomonal β-lactam Third-generation cephalosporin ± Aminoglycoside ± Amphotericin B
Genitourinary	Gram-negatives	Quinolones Third-generation cephalosporins	
Intravascular			
Catheter related	*S. aureus* *S. epidermidis* Gram-negatives	Vancomycin ± extended-spectrum cephalosporin ± aminoglycoside	
Lung			
Early: community acquired	*Streptococcus pneumoniae* *Legionella* species *Mycoplasma pneumoniae* *Chlamydia* species *Staphylococcus aureus* *Haemophilus* species *Klebsiella* species	Third-generation cephalosporins plus macrolide: Ceftriaxone Cefotaxime Ceftizoxime	Quinolones
Late: Nosocomial	*Pseudomonas aeruginosa* *S. aureus (MRSA)* *Enterobacter* species *Klebsiella* species *Escherichia coli* *Acinetobacter* species	Antipseudomonal β-lactam plus vancomycin ± aminoglycoside	Antipseudomonal β-lactam ± Quinolone Imipenem-cilastatin ± Aminoglycoside Fourth-generation cephalosporin

Table 25.4 Source Control Techniques

Drainage	Intra-abdominal abscess Thoracic empyema Septic arthritis Pyelonephritis, cholangitis
Debridement	Necrotizing fasciitis Infected pancreatic necrosis Intestinal infarction Mediastinitis
Device removal	Infected vascular catheter Urinary catheter Colonized endotracheal tube Infected intrauterine contraceptive device
Definitive control	Sigmoid resection for diverticulitis Cholecystectomy for gangrenous cholecystitis Amputation for clostridial myonecrosis

patients were treated with intravenous crystalloids and vasopressors. The EGDT group had as an additional end point, central venous oxygen saturation ($Scvo_2$) ≥ 70%, which was continuously measured from a subclavian or jugular central venous catheter. $Scvo_2$ was used as an index for oxygen delivery. If $Scvo_2$ was < 70% after reaching targets for CVP and MAP, patients received packed red blood cells for a hematocrit ≤ 30, or dobutamine infusion if the hematocrit was ≥ 30. Patients in the EGDT group received more fluids, dobutamine, and transfusions in the first 24 hours. In-hospital mortality was significantly lower in the EGDT group when compared to the standard therapy group (30.5% versus 46.5%, respectively, [p = 0.009]). Observational studies published after the Rivers study have demonstrated a strong association between improved clinical outcomes and maintenance of MAP ≥ 65 mm Hg as well as central venous oxygen saturation ($Scvo_2$) of ≥ 70%.[61] Furthermore, several more recent studies have showed improved outcomes with the use of protocolized quantitative resuscitation in severe sepsis and sepsis-induced tissue hypoperfusion.[42,62-65] Although the specific merits of each individual intervention within a quantitative resuscitation or EGDT protocol can be discussed, the results of these studies strongly support early intervention with predefined hemodynamic settings and protocolized care.

As stated before, the initial step in optimizing hemodynamics in patients with severe sepsis is aggressive fluid resuscitation. Although experts agree on the value of early and aggressive volume replacement, controversy persists over the optimal type of fluid. This debate revolves around the use of crystalloids (saline, Ringer's lactate) versus colloids (albumin, hydroxyethyl starches). A large meta-analysis evaluated data from 56 trials and found no difference in mortality between crystalloids and colloids when used for initial fluid resuscitation.[66] Three randomized studies did not find a difference in mortality when starches (heta-, hexa-, or penta-) where compared to other fluids. However, these studies did report a significant increase in acute kidney injury with the use of starches.[67-69] The Saline versus Albumin Fluid Evaluation (SAFE) study prospectively randomized 7000 critically ill patients to receive 4% albumin or 0.9% saline for fluid resuscitation.[70] There were no significant differences between groups in mortality and other secondary outcomes. A subgroup analysis conducted in patients with sepsis revealed a trend toward improved outcomes in patients treated with albumin, although this difference did not achieve statistical significance. We believe that achieving end points of resuscitation is more important than the type of fluid utilized. In North America consideration for cost differences has made crystalloids the initial fluid of choice for resuscitating patients with severe sepsis. However, based on emerging data it seems appropriate to add albumin to the initial fluid resuscitation regimen in severe sepsis and septic shock.

Patients with severe sepsis may present with significant intravascular volume depletion. Aggressive fluid boluses are usually required to restore tissue perfusion. It is recommended that patients receive at least 20 to 30 mL/kg of crystalloid initially.[39,71] This may be supplemented with more fluids based on markers of perfusion in repeated boluses of 300 to 500 mL.[71] Current guidelines recommend achieving the following hemodynamic end points of resuscitation during the first 6 hours of treatment: CVP ≥ 8 to 12 mm Hg, mean arterial pressure (MAP) ≥ 65 mm Hg, urine output ≥ 0.5 mL/kg/h, and central venous oxygen saturation ($Scvo_2$) $\geq 70\%$.[39,72] For further discussion on the pathophysiology and treatment of hemodynamic abnormalities in sepsis, the reader is referred to Chapter 23.

MODULATION OF THE HOST RESPONSE

Over the years, research efforts in severe sepsis have been heavily involved with therapies targeted at modulating the host response. Several pathways and mechanisms have been studied in clinical trials (Table 25.5). Unfortunately, very little success has been found in these endeavors. Initial attempts were aimed at blunting the inflammatory response with nonspecific agents such as high-dose glucocorticoids and ibuprofen.[73-75] Another unsuccessful strategy involved the use of antibodies directed at endotoxin in patients with gram-negative sepsis.[76-81] However, the area that received the greatest attention was modulation of the inflammatory cascade by targeting specific pro-inflammatory cytokines such as tumor necrosis factor (TNF-α) and interleukin-1β (IL-1β). Multiple clinical trials enrolling thousands of patients tested compounds directed at specific pro-inflammatory cytokines, among them TNF monoclonal antibody, interleukin-1 receptor antagonist, and soluble TNF receptor.[82-89] Unfortunately, none of these compounds improved survival of patients with severe sepsis in randomized studies. The failure of these therapies led to a reappraisal of the pathophysiology, potential therapeutic targets, and clinical trial design in severe sepsis. As the role of the coagulation cascade and its crosstalk with inflammation in sepsis was recognized, a series of new clinical trials took place. Three large trials studied the effects of anticoagulants in severe sepsis (Box 25.5).

Antithrombin III (AT III) is a progressive inhibitor of thrombin and factor Xa.[90] Studies showed that AT III supplementation attenuated the systemic inflammatory response in patients with severe sepsis.[91] A large (n = 2314)

Table 25.5 Pathways and Mediators of Sepsis, Potential Treatments, and Results of Randomized, Controlled Trials (RCTs)*

Pathway	Mediators	Treatment	Results of RCTs
	Lipopolysaccharide (endotoxin)	Antilipopolysaccharide[9]	Negative
Proinflammatory pathway	TNF-α	Anti-TNF-α[13,14]	Negative
	Interleukin-1β	Interleukin-1-receptor antagonist[15]	Negative
	Prostaglandins, leukotrienes	Ibuprofen,[16] high-dose corticosteroids[17]	Negative
	Bradykinin	Bradykinin antagonist[18]	Negative
	Platelet-activating factor	Platelet-activating factor acetyl hydrolase[19]	Negative
	Proteases (e.g., elastase)	Elastase inhibitor	Negative
	Nitric oxide	Nitric oxide synthase inhibitor[21]	Negative
Procoagulant pathway	Decreased protein C	Activated protein C[5]	Negative
	Decreased antithrombin III	Antithrombin III[23]	Negative
	Decreased tissue factor-pathway inhibitor	Tissue factor-pathway inhibitor[24]	Negative
Antiinflammatory	TNF-α receptors	TNF-α receptors[13]	Negative

*Studies cited in table may be found in the complete list of references for this chapter provided online.
TNF, tumor necrosis factor.
Adapted from Russell, JA: Management of sepsis. N Engl J Med 2006; 355:1699-1713.

Box 25.5 Supportive Care for Patients with Sepsis and Septic Shock

- Mechanical ventilation
- Deep vein thrombosis prophylaxis
- Gastrointestinal ulcer prophylaxis
- Nutrition
- Glucose control
- Sedation

multicenter, double-blinded, placebo-controlled trial evaluated the safety and efficacy of AT III in adult patients with severe sepsis.[92] At 28 days there was no difference in mortality between the treatment group and the placebo group (38.9% versus 38.7%, respectively). Patients who received AT III had a higher risk of bleeding (relative risk > 1.7). A subgroup analysis of patients not receiving concomitant heparin showed a trend (statistically nonsignificant) toward reduced mortality at 28 and 90 days with AT III. This specific subgroup of patients with severe sepsis may warrant further investigations. Tissue factor pathway inhibitor (TFPI) has been show to modulate the extrinsic pathway in preclinical models of severe sepsis. Recombinant human TFPI (tifacogin) was evaluated in clinical trials of patients with severe sepsis. Although the results of a phase II trial suggested a trend toward improved mortality, a large phase III trial, the OPTIMIST (Optimized Phase III Tifacogin in Multicenter International Sepsis Trial) study failed to show a mortality benefit in patients treated with this compound.[93,94] Patients treated with tifacogin had a higher risk of bleeding complications irrespective of their baseline international normalized ratios (INRs).[93] Studies evaluating different dosing regimens and the application of this drug in patients with pneumonia are still being conducted. Finally, recombinant human activated protein C (rhAPC) was evaluated in clinical trials. A landmark study, the protein C worldwide evaluation in severe sepsis (PROWESS) trial, demonstrated improved 28-day survival in patients with severe sepsis treated with rhAPC.[95]

The phase III randomized, double-blind, placebo-controlled, multicenter international study, PROWESS trial evaluated the efficacy of drotrecogin alfa (activated) in patients with severe sepsis.[95] This study enrolled 1690 patients and was terminated early after an interim safety analysis found a significant reduction in mortality in the treatment group compared to placebo (24.7% versus 30.8%, respectively [$p = 0.005$], relative and absolute risk reductions of 19.4% and 6.1%, respectively). Patients treated with drotrecogin alfa (activated) showed a trend toward a higher incidence of bleeding (3.5% versus 2%; $p = 0.06$). Subgroup analysis demonstrated that patients at higher risk of death as measured by APACHE II scores (APACHE II ≥ 25) and number of organ failures (two or more organ failures) had an increased benefit from the drug. Effects on mortality seemed to be lost in low-severity patients. Based on this study, the Food and Drug Administration (FDA) approved the use of drotrecogin alfa (activated) in adult patients with severe sepsis with a high risk of death. Angus and colleagues reported, after long-term follow-up, that those patients who were treated with drotrecogin alfa (activated) had an increased median survival (9 months) compared to patients treated with placebo.[96] Once again, beneficial effects of the drug seemed to be greatest in patients with a higher severity of disease. Two additional phase IV studies were published post the FDA's approval of the drug. The ENHANCE trial was a single-arm open-label study that enrolled 2375 patients with severe sepsis.[97] ENHANCE evaluated the use of drotrecogin alfa (activated) in a more routine clinical setting beyond the restrictions of a controlled randomized study. In this study, the effect of the drug on mortality was similar to PROWESS (25.3% in ENHANCE versus 24.7% in PROWESS). The risk of bleeding during infusion was higher when compared to PROWESS (3.6% versus 2.4%). However, the higher rate of postinfusion bleeding observed in the ENHANCE population (3.2% versus 1.2%) suggests a higher incidence of background bleeding. A second phase IV trial, the ADDRESS study, was a randomized, blinded, placebo-controlled trial that evaluated the efficacy of the drug in severe sepsis in patients judged prospectively by the enrolling clinician to have a low risk of death (APACHE II score < 25 or single organ failure based on regulation requirements in countries of study entry).[98] This study enrolled 2646 patients and found that treatment with the drug offered no mortality benefit when compared to placebo in a low-risk-of-death population. Serious bleeding events were similar to those reported in PROWESS. There was significant criticism from several academic experts on the approval of drotrecogin alfa (activated) based on one single positive prospective randomized trial that was terminated prematurely because of positive results. Additionally critics argued that the drug was associated with a higher risk of bleeding when used in the clinical setting and that it was approved for a population that had not been prospectively evaluated in randomized trials (based on the post hoc analysis of the APACHE II quartiles). The publication of the PROWESS SHOCK trial, showing no benefit of drotrecogin alfa (activated) in patients with septic shock (mortality 26.4% in patients given drotrecogin alfa [activated] versus 24.2% in patients receiving placebo) led to the worldwide withdrawal of the drug from the market.[99] The choice to withdraw was a voluntary decision by Eli Lilly and Company and was likely heavily influenced by business calculations. Drotrecogin alfa (activated) has important biologic effects that could be helpful in modulating the host response in severe sepsis. It is very probable that we do not know how best to select patients who would benefit from this drug. In the future, we should consider ways to improve our process in drug development from clinical trial design to regulatory approval. Furthermore, it seems that more sophisticated selection of patients will be instrumental in future studies evaluating new agents designed to modulate the host response to sepsis.[100]

SUPPORTIVE THERAPIES

As with other critical illnesses, patients with severe sepsis require various supportive therapies (see Box 25.5). These therapies are general supportive measures that prevent complications associated with critical illness. Improvement in these therapies over the years probably plays a role in the historical decrease in mortality observed in several disease processes such as severe sepsis and acute respiratory distress syndrome (ARDS). Patients with severe sepsis often present with tachypnea and hypoxemia. Mechanical ventilation is often utilized for support. Studies in patients with ARDS have demonstrated that ventilation strategies utilizing low tidal volume (6 mL/kg) are associated with significantly lower mortality than ventilation with more traditional tidal volumes (12 mL/kg).[101] This is most likely due to a decrease in ventilator-induced lung injury. Several meta-analyses have suggest decreased mortality in patients with established ARDS who are treated with a volume and pressure limited ventilator strategy.[102,103] Current guidelines recommend the use of a protective lung strategy (low tidal volume; inspiratory plateau pressure < 30 cm H_2O) in mechanically ventilated patients with severe sepsis.[39] Goals for oxygen saturation should be an $Sao_2 \geq 90\%$. This can be achieved by increasing the fraction of inspired oxygen (Fio_2) and/or application of positive end-expiratory pressure (PEEP). In patients with sepsis-induced ARDS who do not have evidence of tissue hypoperfusion, a conservative approach to fluid management is recommended.[104] Patients on mechanical ventilation who are clinically improving should be evaluated on a daily basis for weaning from mechanical ventilation. Patients with severe sepsis on mechanical ventilation should be managed with appropriate sedatives and analgesics. For a detailed discussion, the reader is referred to Chapter 19.

Patients with severe sepsis should receive prophylaxis for the development of deep vein thrombosis (DVT). In the absence of contraindications, patients should receive pharmacologic DVT prophylaxis. Treatment with low-dose unfractioned heparin (UFH), adjusted-dose UFH, or low-molecular-weight heparin (LMWH) is recommended.[105] Treatment for DVT prophylaxis with UFH or LMWH is not contraindicated during infusion of drotrecogin alfa (activated). Stress ulcer prophylaxis is recommended for all patients with severe sepsis. Histamine-2 receptor antagonists are more effective than sucralfate in decreasing bleeding risk and transfusion requirements.[106] Proton pump inhibitors have not been assessed in a direct comparison with histamine-2 receptor antagonists but do demonstrate equivalency and ability to increase gastric pH.[105]

Severe sepsis is a catabolic state. Metabolic alterations in patients with severe sepsis include breakdown of proteins, carbohydrates, and lipids; negative nitrogen balance; and hyperglycemia with insulin resistance. As with other critically ill patients, those with severe sepsis require adequate nutritional support. Enteral nutrition offers several advantages including lower cost, preservation of gastric mucosa integrity, decreased incidence of infections, and avoidance of parenteral nutritional catheters and their potential complications.[107] In patients who cannot tolerate enteral nutrition, parenteral nutrition should be utilized.[108] Immunomodulation through nutritional supplements has been proposed in patients with severe sepsis but remains experimental at this point.

Hyperglycemia and insulin resistance are commonly present in patients with severe sepsis. This phenomenon is a common feature of the metabolic response to critical illness and stress and has been described after major surgery, in trauma, acute myocardial infarction, and several other disease states. Furthermore, there is a growing body of literature suggesting that hyperglycemia related to critical illness is associated with poor outcomes.[109-113] Proposed mechanisms for this deleterious effect include impaired neutrophil function, increased risk of infection, poor wound healing, and procoagulant state as a consequence of hyperglycemia.[114] Treatment of critical illness–related hyperglycemia with insulin has been proposed to modulate these effects and improve patient outcomes. Van den Berghe and associates studied the effects of tight glycemic control on outcomes in a population of mechanically ventilated surgical critical care patients.[115] In this study, patients were randomized to receive intensive insulin therapy (target blood glucose 80-110 mg/dL) or standard therapy (target blood glucose 180-200 mg/dL). Patients treated with the intensive insulin regimen had significant improvements in overall ICU mortality rates (4.6% versus 8.0%). This benefit in mortality was more pronounced among patients who stayed in the ICU longer than 5 days (10.6% versus 20.2%, $p = 0.005$). In addition, intensive insulin therapy was associated with a 46% reduction in bloodstream infections, a 44% reduction in the incidence of critical illness polyneuropathy, a 41% decrease in the need for renal replacement therapy, and a 50% reduction in number of transfused units of packed red blood cells. The same group reported the results of a similar study in medical intensive care unit patients.[116] In this clinical trial, intensive insulin was not associated with improved mortality when compared to standard therapy. Intensive insulin therapy was associated with decreased mortality in patients who remained in the ICU > 3 days, but it was associated with increased mortality in those who remained in the ICU < 3 days. Prospective identification of these patient groups was difficult. Studies published more recently have not found the same benefit in mortality with intensive insulin therapy.[69,117-119] The NICE-SUGAR study, a large randomized trial with > 6000 patients, found that intensive glucose control increased mortality among adults in the ICU.[120] In this study, a blood glucose target of 180 mg or less/dL resulted in lower mortality than did a target of 81 to 108 mg per deciliter.[120] Two questions remain germane to the glycemic control issue: First, what is the downside of tight glycemic control? Second, what level of glucose should we target? The biggest downside to tight glycemic control probably relates to the risk of hypoglycemia and the morbidity/mortality this could cause in critically ill patients. In both studies by Van den Berghe and colleagues, hypoglycemia was more common in the intensive insulin group than in the standard group (surgical study: 5.2% versus 0.7% and medical study: 18.7% versus 3.1%, respectively).[115,116] In subsequent studies, the incidence of hypoglycemia was consistently higher. As an example in the NICE-SUGAR study, severe hypoglycemia (blood glucose level, ≤40 mg/dL) was reported in 6.8% of the patients in the intensive-control group and in 0.5% of the patients in the conventional-control group ($p < 0.001$).[120] Concerns for the effects of hypoglycemia on ICU patients are well founded. However, it does not appear that short-term hypoglycemia that is quickly recognized and treated carries deleterious consequences.[121] There is no clear answer with respect to what glucose level we should target in patients with severe sepsis. It is important to note that the studies that showed benefit with tight glycemic control compared intensive insulin therapy to high controls (180-200 mg/dL), whereas those that did not demonstrate benefit compared

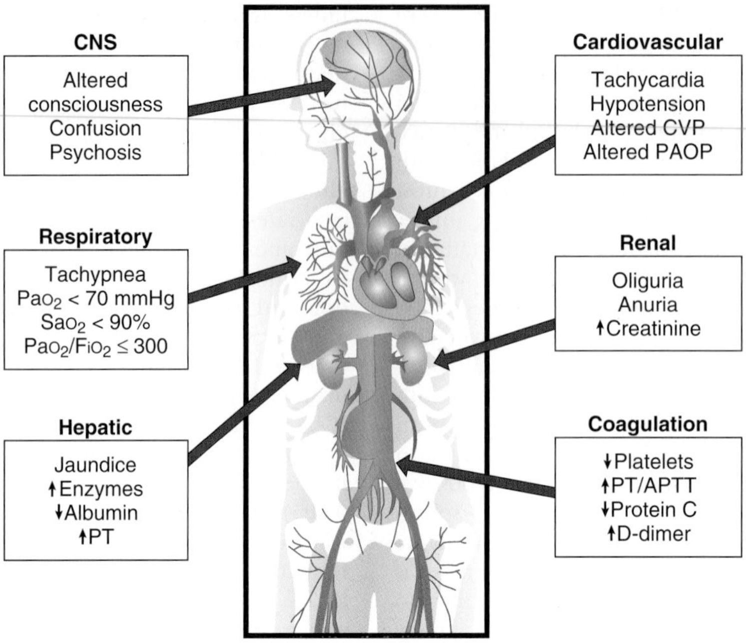

Figure 25.5 Identification of organ failure in severe sepsis. Clinical and laboratory criteria to identify organ failure are shown for each organ system. APTT, activated partial thromboplastin time; CNS, central nervous system; CVP, central venous pressure; PAOP, pulmonary artery occlusion pressure; PT, prothrombin time. (Adapted from Balk RA: Pathogenesis and management of multiple organ dysfunction or failure in severe sepsis and septic shock. Crit Care Clin 2000;16:337-352.)

intensive insulin therapy to moderate controls (108-180 mg/dL). Considering the current available evidence, it is recommended that glucose be kept < 180 mg/dL in patients with severe sepsis. To minimize the risk of hypoglycemia, patients on intensive insulin regimens should have frequent blood glucose monitoring.

MULTIPLE ORGAN DYSFUNCTION

Multiple organ dysfunction is a common complication of sepsis. Multiple organ dysfunction syndrome (MODS) occurs when two or more organ systems fail sequentially or at the same time in a patient with sepsis. Various organs, such as the brain, heart, lung, kidney, and liver, can be affected in patients with severe sepsis. Often these organs are distant from the site of primary insult, and development of organ failure occurs as a response to complicated interactions and pathophysiologic events. Metabolic and hematologic dysfunctions are also common with severe sepsis and MODS. MODS significantly contributes to higher mortality. Studies have shown that mortality in patients with severe sepsis increases in parallel with increases in number and severity of organ failures.[122,123] Russell and associates evaluated the pattern of organ dysfunction in early sepsis and its relationship with mortality.[124] In this study, clinically significant pulmonary dysfunction, although common early in sepsis, was not associated with 30-day mortality. Early dysfunction of other organs and, particularly, worsening neurologic, coagulation, and renal dysfunction over the first 3 days were associated with significantly higher 30-day mortality.

Recognition of early organ dysfunction is important because it is likely that early intervention can affect outcomes. The clinical manifestations of MODS for individual organs are summarized in Figure 25.5. The cornerstones of treatment for MODS are based on appropriate treatment for the underlying cause (sepsis) and on early organ-specific support interventions. As discussed previously, early implementation of therapies directed at control of infection, hemodynamic support, and modulation of the host response are key to improving organ dysfunction and patient outcomes. Perhaps the single most important aspect relates to early and aggressive hemodynamic support. As demonstrated in the study by Rivers and colleagues, goal-directed interventions instituted in the first 6 hours of presentation to the hospital have a tremendous impact on long-term organ function and survival.[60] We further discuss some salient features of the pathophysiology of MODS and the use of scoring systems. For a more detailed discussion on organ-specific supportive therapies, the reader is referred to other chapters in this textbook.

PATHOPHYSIOLOGY OF MULTIPLE ORGAN DYSFUNCTION SYNDROME IN SEPSIS

The mechanisms that result in the development of MODS in patients with sepsis are still not fully understood. Additionally, the reason that some patients develop MODS and others do not remains unknown. However, new insights into the pathophysiology of severe sepsis have led to a better understanding of potential mechanisms leading to MODS. In patients in whom MODS develops, the host response to infection becomes sustained and uncontrolled, leading to a complex interaction of inflammatory, anti-inflammatory, and procoagulant cascades culminating in the development of organ failure. A key determinant of organ failure seems to be tissue hypoperfusion. Our current knowledge seems to point out two important mechanisms in the development of sepsis-induced tissue hypoperfusion: microvascular dysfunction and cytopathic hypoxia.

In early unresuscitated sepsis, tissue hypoperfusion is to a great extent driven by decreased intravascular volume and the resulting drop in cardiac output (hypovolemic shock).[54] Despite aggressive volume resuscitation, however, many patients still show evidence of tissue hypoperfusion, probably secondary to vasodilation and maldistribution of blood flow (distributive shock).[71] Furthermore, a subset of patients with normalized macrovascular hemodynamic parameters (e.g., blood pressure, CVP, and cardiac output) can still show evidence of sepsis-induced tissue hypoperfusion.[125] New technology has allowed investigators to evaluate the microcirculatory flow in patients with severe sepsis.[126] Redistribution of capillary blood flow has been demonstrated in both animal models and clinical sepsis.[36,37] The importance of this finding has been highlighted by studies demonstrating that functional (impaired blood flow) and structural (shunting, redistribution) abnormalities in microcirculation are associated with death and organ failure in patients with severe sepsis and septic shock.[37,127]

In the early phases of sepsis, decreased oxygen delivery (DO_2) can result in tissue hypoperfusion. However, in late sepsis there is evidence of impaired tissue oxygen utilization even after optimization of DO_2.[128] The inability of cells to use oxygen in the face of adequate DO_2 in sepsis has been termed *cytopathic hypoxia.*[128] Development of cytopathic hypoxia is closely linked to mitochondrial dysfunction. The inability of the mitochondria to use oxygen to produce energy in the form of adenosine triphosphate leads to impaired cellular function. Proposed mechanisms that result in cytopathic hypoxia in sepsis include diminished delivery of pyruvate into the mitochondria, inhibition of mitochondrial enzymes, and activation of poly-(adenosine phosphate-ribosyl) polymerase (PARP).[129] The exact mechanisms leading to organ failure in sepsis remain unidentified. Organ failure in sepsis is reversible in patients who survive. Furthermore, in patients who do not survive, there is no histopathologic evidence of tissue damage.[28] Hotchkiss and associates have described extensive lymphocyte apoptosis in sepsis and have proposed this mechanism as an important driver of the impaired immune response seen in late sepsis and MODS.[130,131] Finally, multiple organ failure has been hypothesized to be an adaptive metabolic response to overwhelming inflammation in sepsis.[132] The hypothesis holds that multiple organ failure induced by sepsis is primarily a functional abnormality that serves as a protective reactive mechanism and that the decline of organ function is triggered by a decrease in mitochondrial activity. This decrease in mitochondrial activity leads to a reduction in cell metabolism and occurs as a consequence of humoral and mediator-induced changes.[118]

ORGAN DYSFUNCTION SCORING SYSTEMS

Severity of illness scoring systems have been developed and applied in the ICU to describe patient populations. These scoring systems have been useful in predicting expected mortality and comparing different patient populations. The use of general outcome prediction models, such as the APACHE, the Mortality Probability Model (MPM), and the second Simplified Acute Physiologic Score (SAPS), is discussed in detail in Chapter 74. Therefore, this discussion is limited to scoring systems used to specifically assess organ dysfunction.

It is recognized that the risk of death for patients with severe sepsis is directly related to the number of dysfunctional organs. Organ dysfunction scoring systems have been developed as a tool for the clinician to characterize the severity of illness and follow the clinical evolution of patients with sepsis. The more commonly used systems are the Sequential Organ Failure Assessment (SOFA), the Logistic Organ Dysfunction System, and the Multiple Organ Dysfunction Score. Perhaps the most commonly used is the SOFA score (Table 25.6). It was initially described by Vincent and colleagues to assess the incidence of organ dysfunction

Table 25.6 The Sequential Organ Failure Assessment Score

	0	1	2	3	4
Respiratory: PaO_2/FiO_2 ratio	> 400	≤ 400	≤ 300	≤ 200[c]	≤ 100[c]
Coagulation: platelets (× 10^3 μL^{-1})	> 150	≤ 150	≤ 100	≤ 50	≤ 20
Liver: bilirubin (mg dL^{-1})	< 1.2	1.2-1.9	2-5.9	6-11.9	> 12
Cardiovascular: hypotension	No hypotension	MAP < 70 mm Hg	Dop ≤ 5 or Dob any dose	Dop > 5, Epi ≤ 0.1 or Nor ≤ 0.1	Dop ≥ 50, Epi > 0.1 or Nor > 0.1
Central nervous system: GCS	15	13-14	10-12	6-9	< 6
Renal: creatinine (mg dL^{-1}) or daily urine output (mL)	< 1.2	1.2-1.9	2-3.4	3.5-4.9 or < 500	> 5 or < 200

MAP, mean arterial blood pressure; Nor, norepinephrine; Dop, dopamine; Dob, dobutamine; Epi, epinephrine; FiO_2, fraction of inspired oxygen; GCS, Glasgow Coma Scale score.

Adapted from Vincent JL, de Mendonca A, Cantraine F, et al: Use of the SOFA score to assess the incidence of organ dysfunction/failure in intensive care units: Results of a multicenter, prospective study. Working group on "sepsis-related problems" of the European Society of Intensive Care Medicine. Crit Care Med 1998;26:1793-1800.

in critically ill patients.[123] Using the SOFA scores in patients with severe sepsis, these researchers found that mortality rates were lowest in patients without organ dysfunction (9%) and rose progressively with the number of organ dysfunctions (one organ, 22%; two organs, 38%; three organs, 69%; ≥ four organs, 83%).[123] The type of organ dysfunction also affects mortality. Hebert and coworkers[106] used logistic aggression analysis of the results of a simple multiple system organ failure score to determine the odds ratio for death for specific organ system dysfunctions. This study showed that the adjusted odds ratios (OR) for covariates most predictive of mortality were hematologic (OR = 6.2), neurologic (OR = 4.4), hepatic (OR = 3.4), cardiovascular (OR = 2.6), and age (OR = 1.05). It is important to remember that there are caveats when employing organ dysfunction scores for the management of individual patients with severe sepsis. Most important, organ dysfunction is not a static process and it changes over time. Levy and colleagues reported that changes in SOFA score over the first 24 hours were associated with outcomes in patients with severe sepsis. Improvement in cardiovascular, renal, or respiratory failure over the first 24 hours was associated with lower mortality.[133] On the other hand, worsening SOFA scores for these organ systems were associated with higher mortality (an approximately 60% mortality rate). Finally, how these scores change over time in response to therapeutic interventions is probably of greater value than an initial organ dysfunction score.

KEY POINTS

- Sepsis is the result of a systemic inflammatory response to infection. *Severe sepsis* is defined as sepsis with organ failure.
- The pathophysiology of severe sepsis is complex and involves alterations in the immune system, the inflammatory response, and the coagulation cascade.
- Severe sepsis is common and is associated with high morbidity and mortality.
- Severe sepsis is a medical emergency. Institution of time-sensitive therapeutic interventions is a key factor in modulating and improving outcomes.
- The cornerstones for treatment of sepsis are management of the infection, hemodynamic support, modulation of the host response, and general supportive care.
- Infection management includes the early administration of appropriate antibiotics and institution of source control measures.

KEY POINTS (Continued)

- Hemodynamic support consists of early and aggressive fluid resuscitation and maintenance of predefined hemodynamic end points. Studies have shown that early goal-directed therapy for hemodynamic support can improve mortality in patients with severe sepsis.
- To maximize patient outcomes, appropriate supportive therapy must be provided in the ICU: protective lung ventilation, proper nutrition, prophylaxis against DVT, and glucose control.
- Multiple organ dysfunction syndrome (MODS) occurs when failure of two or more organs develops in a patient with severe sepsis.
- Treatment of MODS is based on treatment of the underlying insult and organ-specific supportive measures.

SELECTED REFERENCES

5. Levy MM, Fink MP, Marshall JC, et al: 2001 SCCM/ESICM/ACCP/ATS/SIS International Sepsis Definitions Conference. Crit Care Med 2003;31:1250-1256.
6. Angus DC, Linde-Zwirble WT, Lidicker J, et al: Epidemiology of severe sepsis in the United States: Analysis of incidence, outcome, and associated costs of care. Crit Care Med 2001;29:1303-1310.
39a. Dellinger RP, et al. Surviving sepsis campaign: International guidelines for management of severe sepsis and septic shock, 2012. Crit Care Med 2013 Feb;41:580. (http://dx.doi.org/10.1097/CCM.0b013e31827e83af) Accessed on May 10, 2013.
44. Levy MM, Dellinger RP, Townsend SR, et al: The Surviving Sepsis Campaign: Results of an international guideline-based performance improvement program targeting severe sepsis. Crit Care Med 2010;38:367-374.
47. Kumar A, Roberts D, Wood KE, et al: Duration of hypotension before initiation of effective antimicrobial therapy is the critical determinant of survival in human septic shock. Crit Care Med 2006;34:1589-1596.
60. Rivers E, Nguyen B, Havstad S, et al: Early goal-directed therapy in the treatment of severe sepsis and septic shock. N Engl J Med 2001;345:1368-1377.
70. Finfer S, Bellomo R, Boyce N, et al: A comparison of albumin and saline for fluid resuscitation in the intensive care unit. N Engl J Med 2004;350:2247-2256.
99. Ranieri VM, Thompson BT, Barie PS, et al: Drotrecogin alfa (activated) in adults with septic shock. N Engl J Med 2012;366:2055-2064.
118. Investigators CS, Annane D, Cariou A, et al: Corticosteroid treatment and intensive insulin therapy for septic shock in adults: A randomized controlled trial. JAMA 2010;303:341-348.
119. Preiser JC, Devos P, Ruiz-Santana S, et al: A prospective randomised multi-centre controlled trial on tight glucose control by intensive insulin therapy in adult intensive care units: The Glucontrol study. Intensive Care Med 2009;35:1738-1748.

The complete list of references can be found on www.expertconsult.com.

Hypovolemic Shock

26

A. B. J. Groeneveld

CHAPTER OUTLINE

Although hypovolemic shock has been recognized for more than 100 years, Wiggers[1] in 1940 first offered a definition of hypovolemic shock that has remained significant until now: "Shock is a syndrome resulting from depression of many functions, but in which the reduction of the effective circulating blood volume is of basic importance, and in which impairment of the circulation steadily progresses until it eventuates in a state of irreversible circulatory failure." Today, hypovolemic shock can be defined as an acute disturbance in the circulation leading to an imbalance between oxygen supply and demand in the tissues, caused by a decrease in circulating blood volume, mostly caused by trauma and hemorrhage.[2] An oxygen debt develops when uptake no longer matches the demand for oxygen and leads to cellular ischemia and ultimately cell death. The condition is life threatening and, if left untreated, becomes irreversible after a certain period. Rapid and adequate resuscitation is mandatory to save lives. Conversely, hypovolemic shock carries a relatively favorable prognosis, if rapidly and adequately recognized and treated.

Hypovolemic shock can occur outside and inside the hospital, in trauma or surgery complicated by excessive loss of blood, but also in the course of burns, gastrointestinal hemorrhage, diarrhea, uncontrolled diabetes mellitus, addisonian crisis, and other conditions (Box 26.1). Some other types of shock, including septic, anaphylactoid, cardiogenic, and burn shock, may be accompanied by hypovolemia. The types of shock not primarily caused by hypovolemia are beyond the scope of this chapter.

PATHOGENESIS AND PATHOPHYSIOLOGY

During hypovolemic shock, the loss of circulating blood volume amounts to 15% to 80%. Hypotension ensues when this loss exceeds about 40% and is thus a relatively late and insensitive symptom. The prior hydration status, severity and type of injury, coagulation status, and resuscitation efforts determine the amount of blood lost after trauma. The severity of shock is determined mainly by the speed, duration, and severity of the loss of circulating volume. The pathophysiology of hypovolemic shock concerns primary events, directly relating to the loss of circulating blood volume, and secondary mechanisms, evoked to compensate for this decline, and concerns all components of the circulation. The factors are dealt with together in a general discussion and in a more focused discussion on tissue and organ perfusion and function during hypovolemic shock.

CIRCULATORY CHANGES

GENERAL CHANGES

Because hypovolemia results in a decrease in preload of the heart and low filling pressures or volumes, the cardiac output decreases.[3-9] After unloading of the baroreceptor and activation of the sympathetic nervous system, tachycardia ensues, although some patients may respond with transient sympathetic inhibition and vagal nerve–mediated

Box 26.1 Causes of Hypovolemic Shock

Loss of Blood

Internally—rupture of vessels, spleen, liver; extrauterine pregnancy

Externally—trauma; gastrointestinal, pulmonary, uterine, renal blood loss

Loss of Plasma

Burn wounds; gastrointestinal losses (diarrhea, ileus, pancreatitis)

Loss of Fluids and Electrolytes

Gastrointestinal and renal losses (uncontrolled diabetes mellitus, adrenocortical insufficiency)

bradycardia during a sudden, severe loss of circulating blood volume.[3,10-16] Tachycardia partially compensates for the decrease in stroke volume. A moderate decrease in cardiac output can be recognized from a decline in pulse pressure, orthostatic hypotension, and fall in regional perfusion indices.[8,17,18] Hypovolemia results in wider than usual swings in central venous pressure (CVP) and arterial blood pressure during the respiratory cycle of spontaneous and mechanical ventilation because of increased sensitivity of the underfilled heart in the ascending part of the cardiac function curve to fluctuations in venous return associated with varying intrathoracic pressure.[19,20] Although activation of the sympathetic nervous system and resulting arterial vasoconstriction during a moderate decrease in cardiac output prevent a severe reduction in arterial blood pressure, a further decrease in cardiac output leads to hypotension and shock.[8,10] Systemic vascular resistance increases early after development of hypovolemic shock but may decrease in the later stages of shock, and this may herald irreversibility and death. The increase in resistance (and heart rate) may be transiently attenuated after an imbalance between sympathetic and vagal activity, possibly associated with release of opioids within the central nervous system and into the systemic circulation.*

Shock is characterized by an oxygen debt in the tissues.[9,24-26] In the presence of sufficient oxygen, aerobic combustion of 1 mol of glucose yields 38 mol of energy-rich adenosine triphosphate (ATP), which can be hydrolyzed to provide energy for the vital and metabolic functions of the cell.[27] In the absence of oxygen, glucose taken up by cells cannot be combusted because of insufficient uptake of pyruvate into the mitochondrial tricarboxylic acid cycle having a reduced turnover rate. Partly inactivated pyruvate dehydrogenase may play a role in the latter reductions. Pyruvate is converted into lactate, and the lactate-to-pyruvate ratio increases, concomitantly with a reduction in mitochondrial redox potential.[24,27-29]

Anaerobic glycolysis in the cytosol ultimately yields, per mol of glucose, 2 mol of ATP.[27] Hydrolysis of ATP yields hydrogen ions (H^+) that lead, when buffers are exhausted, to intracellular and ultimately to extracellular metabolic acidosis.[30] These mechanisms form the basis of the so-called lactic acidosis during hypovolemic shock, whereby the lactate level in arterial blood is elevated above the normal 2 mmol/L associated with acidosis, and constitutes a useful measure of the oxygen debt in the tissues.[26,27,31-34] Nevertheless, the energy deficit and lactate production in the cells in response to a lack of oxygen can be limited and organ function can be improved by supplying pyruvate and pyruvate dehydrogenase activators, such as dichloroacetate.[27,29,35-37] Intracellular acidosis may otherwise protect ischemic cells from dying.[36]

The specificity of elevated lactate-to-pyruvate levels for an oxygen debt in the tissues has been doubted.[27,38] Aerobic glycolysis is probably linked to the membrane Na^+/K^+-ATPase and stimulation of β_2-receptors during sympathetic activation. Catecholamine (epinephrine) secretion may temporarily increase, rather than decrease, ATPase activity, and augment glycolysis and circulating lactate levels in tissues such as skeletal muscle, without a lack of oxygen and reduced ATP resources, during development and resuscitation from hypovolemic shock.[38,39] Conversely, adrenergic antagonists may reduce lactic acidosis during hypovolemic shock.[38] Epinephrine may increase glycogenolysis. Together, increased glycolytic fluxes independent of oxygen uptake may lead to equal elevations of pyruvate and lactate in the tissues, without the acidosis resulting from ATP hydrolysis with an oxygen debt.[27] This situation may partly explain why the extent to which changes in the lactate level parallel changes in the anion gap or bicarbonate/base excess concentration during shock and resuscitation is controversial, and why elevated lactate levels sometimes may fail to predict an increase in oxygen uptake during an increase in oxygen delivery.[40-42] This also may explain in part the discrepancies in the course of oxygen-related variables and lactate levels during catecholamine treatment of shock when attempting to boost oxygen delivery.[42]

The lactate level in blood is determined by production, distribution, and elimination.[27] Produced lactic acid in the presence of oxygen may be converted via pyruvate to glucose or oxidized. Bicarbonate is then released. The liver plays a central role in this process, so that the elimination of lactate and clearance from plasma is impaired in case of liver ischemia or prior hepatic disease, even though renal uptake may increase.[27,43,44] Nevertheless, changes in the lactate level in blood, rather than absolute values, mainly reflect changes in production and are a fair measure for the course of shock and the response to therapy, even in the presence of liver disease.[27,45] Although not beyond doubt, the origin of lactate in hypovolemic shock can be skeletal muscle, lung, and gut, particularly if severe liver ischemia, hypoxia, and acidosis in shock attenuate the hepatic uptake of lactate delivered by the gut through the portal vein.[27,43,44,46-48] The respiratory muscles also may contribute to lactic acidosis in a spontaneously breathing patient because, first, the respiratory muscles may demand a share of the cardiac output at the cost of other tissues, and, second, this share may be insufficient to meet oxygen demands of the diaphragm, which may be increased in view of hyperventilation.[33,49-52]

Notwithstanding the aforementioned limitations, an increase in the lactate level in blood and a decrease in the bicarbonate content/base excess or pH and an increase in the anion gap may be fair predictors of morbidity (multiple organ failure [MOF]) and mortality, whereas clearance of

*3, 6, 10, 11, 13, 16, 21–23

lactic acidosis usually indicates a better outcome. A decrease in the blood lactate level during resuscitation from hypovolemic shock is usually a favorable sign and associated with survival, whereas an increase in the lactate level and progressive acidosis usually are associated with morbidity and mortality, even though successful resuscitation may transiently increase the lactate level because of washout of lactate from ischemic tissues.* The mentioned variables may thus serve as guides for resuscitation.

OXYGEN BALANCE

Because insufficient uptake of oxygen relative to demand in the tissues during shock is central, insight into the factors that determine oxygen uptake in shock is important.[25,27] Oxygen delivery is determined by the cardiac output and the content of oxygen in arterial blood, that is, the arterial blood hemoglobin concentration and the saturation of hemoglobin with oxygen. The oxyhemoglobin dissociation curve determines the saturation of hemoglobin with oxygen for a given partial pressure of oxygen (Po_2) in blood. During hypovolemic shock, a decrease in hemoglobin concentration, oxygen saturation, or both aggravates the effect of a decrease in cardiac output in compromising oxygen delivery to the tissues. Cardiac output is determined by preload, afterload, contractility, and heart rate.[7]

During a decrease in oxygen delivery with hypovolemic shock, the body maintains sufficient uptake of oxygen only if the extraction of oxygen increases, and the arteriovenous oxygen content gradient widens, resulting in a decrease in oxygen saturation of venous blood.† Associated with a decrease in oxygen delivery, tissue Po_2 declines, and its heterogeneity increases, possibly indicating focal ischemia.‡ The decline in tissue Po_2 may be even greater than the decrease in draining venous blood because of some increase in microvascular oxygen shunting at low blood flows.[68,69] In animals, it has been shown that the increase in oxygen extraction to compensate for a decrease in oxygen delivery is maximum (but not 100%) if oxygen delivery decreases to less than 8 to 15 mL/kg per minute, that is, the critical oxygen delivery (Fig. 26.1).§ Although the critical oxygen delivery may vary widely among studies, following differences in species, basal oxygen needs, and methods to decrease oxygen delivery, data obtained in patients suggest that the critical oxygen delivery in humans may also amount to approximately 8 mL/kg per minute.[58,64] During a decrease in oxygen delivery below this critical value in hypovolemic shock, oxygen uptake decreases to less than tissue demand, cellular ischemia ensues, and the body must rely on anaerobic metabolism to meet energy requirements.¶ Blood lactic acidosis, lacticacidemia, results. Conversely, oxygen uptake is supply-dependent if oxygen delivery is lower than the critical value and blood lactate levels are elevated, whereas oxygen uptake may not be supply-dependent if the lactate level in blood is normal.| Treatment of hypovolemic shock, by infusing fluids and blood, is aimed at an increase in

*27, 31, 32, 40, 45, 53–57
†6, 9, 21, 22, 26, 33, 39, 44, 58–67
‡30, 44, 48, 59, 68, 69
§6, 22, 27, 39, 60–62, 65, 66
¶9, 25, 33, 39, 58, 59, 61, 64–66, 70
|27, 32, 42, 58, 64, 70

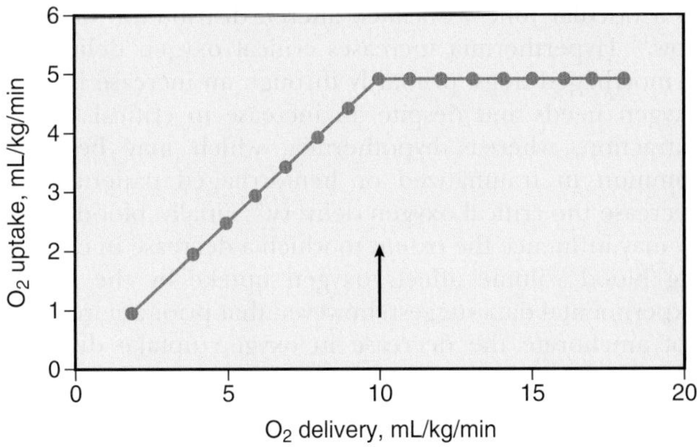

Figure 26.1 Relationship between oxygen uptake and oxygen delivery during progressive hypovolemia. *Arrow* indicates the critical oxygen delivery.

cardiac output and the oxygen content of blood and in oxygen delivery above the critical value so that oxygen uptake increases to meet body requirements and the lacticacidemia decreases.*

The critical oxygen delivery is a function of the body oxygen needs and the capability of the body to extract oxygen during a decline in delivery. The body oxygen needs may increase during hypovolemic shock, as a consequence of increased respiratory muscle activity and increased levels of catecholamines in the blood after activation of the sympathetic nervous system, but downregulation of the metabolic stimulant effect of catecholamines has been described.† The critical extraction of oxygen is a function of the adaptation of regional blood flow to tissue needs, the number of perfused capillaries and of diffusion distances, and the exchange surface area for oxygen.[63,75] During a reduction in oxygen delivery, however, oxygen uptake is limited by convective transport of oxygen to the tissues, rather than by diffusion of oxygen to respirating mitochondria.[76]

In experimental animals, a change in hemoglobin affinity for oxygen, by altering the storage duration of reinfused blood, hardly changes the critical oxygen extraction, but changes in acid-base status that affect the position of the oxyhemoglobin dissociation curve may have some effect on the oxygen extraction capabilities of the body.[60,76] Acid infusion may increase slightly, and base infusion may reduce oxygen extraction during supply-limited oxygen uptake.[76] Nevertheless, hypercapnia may decrease critical oxygen extraction and increase critical oxygen delivery because of blood flow redistribution.[77] A leftward shift of the oxyhemoglobin dissociation curve may impair maximum oxygen extraction during a reduction in oxygen delivery and may increase mortality rate in experimental animals with hypovolemic shock.[60] Although the oxyhemoglobin dissociation curve may shift to the left in critically ill patients, for example, after transfusion of old, stored blood,[78] the effect on oxygen uptake is unclear.

The effect of changes in body temperature is twofold: Changes are accompanied by changes in total body oxygen needs and by changes in critical oxygen extraction, probably

*9, 27, 31–33, 42, 71–73
†13, 14, 33, 39, 50, 74

by a vascular tone–associated altered distribution of blood flow.[61] Hyperthermia increases critical oxygen delivery in hemorrhaged dogs, primarily through an increase in body oxygen needs and despite an increase in critical oxygen extraction, whereas hypothermia, which may be more common in traumatized or hemorrhaged patients, may decrease the critical oxygen delivery.[61] Finally, blood viscosity may influence the extent to which a decrease in circulating blood volume affects oxygen uptake by the tissues. Experimental data suggest, however, that prior anemia does not ameliorate the decrease in oxygen uptake during a decrease in oxygen delivery with hypovolemic shock, indicating that the convective transport of oxygen is the major determinant of oxygen uptake when delivery is impaired, even though prior hemodilution may increase oxygen extraction capabilities and decrease critical oxygen delivery.[6,70]

Taken together, these factors may influence the extent to which oxygen uptake decreases during reduced delivery and how far oxygen delivery should be enhanced during resuscitation from hypovolemic shock. The critical oxygen delivery varies among tissues. The oxygen needs of the kidney may decline during a decrease in renal oxygen delivery because a decrease in renal perfusion may lead to a reduction in glomerular filtration and to a reduction in energy-consuming tubular resorption.[63] In contrast, during progressive hypovolemia, the gut may experience supply dependency of oxygen uptake earlier than nongut tissue, partly because of a higher critical oxygen delivery (higher needs and less extraction of oxygen) and partly because of redistribution of blood flow away from the gut mucosa after more intense vasoconstriction in gut than in nongut tissue.* Clinically, this may result in nonocclusive bowel ischemia. Respiratory muscles may also have a higher critical oxygen delivery than the body as a whole during progressive hemorrhage.

Concomitant with an increased arteriovenous oxygen extraction during a decrease in oxygen delivery, the arteriovenous gradient of the carbon dioxide (CO_2) content widens.[8,52,81] The latter is associated with an increase in tissue and venous partial pressure of carbon dioxide (Pco_2) relative to arterial Pco_2 and a decrease in venous pH exceeding the decrease in pH in arterial blood.[44,52,68] This widening of gradient is caused by the Fick principle and a greater decline in cardiac output than in oxygen uptake and CO_2 production in the tissues because of inhibited oxidative metabolism. Nevertheless, the oxygen uptake usually decreases more than CO_2 production, leading to an increase in respiratory quotient.[49,65] This increase is likely to be caused by buffering of lactic acid by bicarbonate in the tissues and effluent blood, a shift toward glucose instead of fat use for residual oxidation in ischemic tissues, or a combination of both. The end-tidal expiratory CO_2 fraction decreases in association with a reduction in oxygen uptake and CO_2 production for a given ventilation.[65] Conversely, a decrease in arterial Pco_2 during a decline in CO_2 production versus ventilation may be attenuated by an increase in deadspace ventilation resulting from a decrease in pulmonary blood flow/ventilation ratio.[49] An increase in deadspace ventilation leads to widening of the gap between the arterial and expiratory Pco_2.[49]

It has been suggested that the severity and duration of the oxygen debt accumulated during hypovolemic shock is a major determinant of survival in animals[3,6] and in patients with trauma/hemorrhage and after major surgery.[26,42,82] After trauma and hemorrhage, the defect in circulating blood volume and tissue oxygenation may be greater in patients who develop acute respiratory distress syndrome (ARDS) and MOF than in patients without these complications.* In patients undergoing major surgery, the oxygen debt during and after surgery may relate directly to the development of postoperative organ damage (i.e., MOF) and demise.[73,82] Conversely, a high oxygen delivery and uptake during resuscitation may be associated with survival, whereas values that may be too low for elevated tissue demands are believed to contribute to ultimate demise, at least in animals with hypovolemic shock and critically ill patients after trauma or major surgery.† An increase of oxygen delivery and oxygen uptake to supranormal values has been suggested to improve survival further, although the latter debate has not been settled yet.‡ Extensive ischemic mitochondrial damage may limit an increase in oxygen consumption during resuscitation and reperfusion.

MACROCIRCULATION

During loss of blood volume, various mechanisms come into play that may counteract the resultant decrease in cardiac output and tissue oxygenation. First, a decrease in cardiac output during hypovolemic shock results in a redistribution of peripheral blood flow.§ This redistribution is partly the result of regional autoregulation to maintain blood flow, in which endothelial cells and production of endogenous partly gaseous vasodilators, including endothelial nitric oxide synthase–derived nitric oxide (NO), heme oxygenase–derived carbon monoxide, hydrogen sulfide, and metabolic by-products in the tissues including CO_2, potassium, and adenosine, may play a central role.[86-94] Endothelium-derived NO relaxes underlying smooth muscle in the vessel wall, via stimulation of guanylate cyclase and cyclic guanosine monophosphate (cGMP), which can be inhibited by methylene blue.[87,88,95,96] Carbon monoxide also acts via cGMP.[91] Some authors describe that inhibition of endothelial NO synthase ameliorates early hypotension and even the mortality risk during bleeding.[92] When NO is released, the reactivity to endogenous and exogenous vasoconstrictors may be diminished, even early in hypovolemic shock.[92,97] Other authors describe endothelial injury and dysfunction in various organs with diminished endothelium and NO-dependent vasorelaxation, which could be overcome by L-arginine and other NO donors, including ATP-$MgCl_2$, pentoxifylline, or heparin, so that blockade of endothelial NO synthase–derived NO may be detrimental.[87-89,97,98]

The opposing vasoconstricting factors include catecholamines, liberated by the activated sympathetic nervous system and the adrenal medulla; direct sympathetic stimulation of the vessel wall; angiotensin II, liberated through

*4, 22, 63, 74, 79, 80

*2, 40, 42, 45, 83, 84
†9, 25, 26, 42, 45, 55, 67, 73, 82, 83
‡9, 25, 26, 40, 42, 67, 83
§3, 63, 74, 79, 80, 85

an activated renin-angiotensin-aldosterone system; and vasopressin, released by the pituitary in hypovolemic shock.* Endothelin is an endothelium-derived potent vasoconstrictor, released on catecholamine stimulation or hypoxia, and its release may contribute to vasoconstriction, particularly in hepatic and renal vascular beds.[100,101] Finally, a decrease in cardiac filling may reduce cardiac secretion of atrial natriuretic peptides, reducing the vasodilating and diuretic effect of these factors.[102] Levels may also increase as a consequence of diminished renal clearance.[103,104]

Depending on the degree that the mechanisms are operative, the general result of the interplay is that blood flow to intestines, skeletal muscle, and skin is diverted toward vitally more important organs, such as heart and brain, so that the increase of overall peripheral resistance during hypovolemic shock is distributed differently among various organs, with greater increases in gut, skeletal muscle, and skin than in heart and brain.† The kidney also is a target for hypovolemic shock; renal perfusion may be maintained during mild hypotension after hypovolemia, but it rapidly decreases if severe hypotension supervenes, and the decrease may exceed that in other organs.‡ In hypovolemic human volunteers, this redistribution of blood flow accords with the patterns described.[74]

The redistribution of blood flow results in a greater share of oxygen delivery going to organs with high metabolic demand, such as heart and brain, than tissues with less metabolic demands, including skin, skeletal muscle, kidney, gut, and pancreas.§ The redistribution is probably necessary to optimize the uptake of delivered oxygen to the tissues and partly accounts for the increase in oxygen extraction during a decrease in oxygen delivery.[63,75] In dogs, the ability of the body to extract oxygen diminishes with α-receptor blockade of sympathetic activity, suggesting that redistribution of blood flow aided by the sympathetic nervous system is a major determinant of critical oxygen extraction.[63]

MICROCIRCULATION

Vasoconstriction after activation of the sympathetic nervous system during hypovolemia (hemorrhage) occurs in the arteries and medium-sized arterioles but not in terminal arterioles, which may even dilate, as judged from vital microscopy studies in animals.¶ Relatively spared terminal arteriolar blood flow is presumably caused by vasodilating metabolic responses to a decline in nutrient blood flow. Nevertheless, capillary flow usually diminishes, and heterogeneity, both in space and time, increases, particularly in irreversible shock and independent of cardiac output.| Traumatic/hypovolemic shock may induce expression of adhesion molecules on primed neutrophils and vascular endothelium and this, together with a reduced flow rate, may promote adherence of neutrophils to endothelium.[95,111-119] This adherence may impair red blood cell flow, particularly in capillaries and postcapillary venules.‖ Other authors suggest that capillary leukostasis is pressure-dependent and not receptor-dependent and reversible when perfusion pressure has been restored.[121] Finally, endothelial cells may swell and may hamper capillary red and white blood cell flow.[95,98,110,122] The microcirculation can be visualized, even in humans, by buccal or sublingual orthogonal polarization spectroscopy and side stream dark-field imaging.[123]

Vasoconstriction is not confined to arteries, but also occurs in the venous vasculature, more in large than in small venules and particularly in the splanchnic area, and, again, this is largely mediated by increased activity of the sympathetic nervous system and vasopressin and angiotensin II release.[5,12,68,108] Because most of the circulating blood volume is located in small venules, splanchnic venoconstriction results in a decrease in compliance and less volume for a given intravascular pressure in the venous system, increasing return of blood to the heart.[5,7] Hence, partitioning circulating volume in stressed and unstressed portions now favors the former. During hypovolemic shock, the precapillary to postcapillary resistance increases, resulting in a decrease in capillary hydrostatic pressure and in fluid resorption from the interstitial space as opposed to normal filtration from capillary to interstitium, even though interstitial hydrostatic pressure decreases.[4,5] This is accompanied by diminished transport of protein from blood to interstitium.[124]

Cellular water is mobilized, unless, at a later stage, the cell swells following Na^+ overload.[21,98,110,125-129] Studies on fluid volumes in hypovolemic shock are not equivocal, but generally suggest that the interstitial and cellular compartments are depleted in defense of the circulating blood volume to promote venous return to the heart.[5,7,125,126] Mobilization of fluid from the interstitial and cellular compartment can be promoted by plasma hyperosmolarity, through an increase in the glucose concentration.[130,131] Chronically starved rats with depleted glycogen stores more rapidly die of hypovolemic shock than fed ones, and this can be prevented by prior glucose infusion.[130] In addition, the lymphatics may show increased pumping ability, increasing return of fluid into the systemic circulation independently of the reduced capillary fluid filtration rate.[132] Lymphatic return of interstitial protein and fluid may contribute to repletion of circulating protein and fluid volume.[132]

Hemorrhage and hypovolemic shock lead to a decrease in hematocrit and a decrease in plasma proteins through transfer of fluid (and protein) from the interstitial to the intravascular space.[4,5,124] Refilling of the intravascular space diminishes in time after a sudden decrease in circulating volume, when a decline in colloid osmotic pressure, associated with hypoproteinemia, and an increase in hydrostatic pressure accomplish a new steady state in capillary exchange through readjustment of the pericapillary hydrostatic and colloid osmotic pressures, which determine fluid and protein transport.[5] Conversely, hypoproteinemia can promote transcapillary fluid transport and expansion of the interstitial space, if hydrostatic pressure returns toward normal (e.g., during crystalloid fluid resuscitation).[126,133-136] During a sudden decrease in circulating blood volume by hemorrhage, some time is needed before the decrease in hematocrit and of proteins in blood is completed, and this decrease is aggravated by nonsanguineous fluid

*3, 10–14, 74, 81, 99
†3, 10, 12, 14, 15, 21, 22, 29, 63, 74, 85, 105
‡3, 14, 63, 74, 86, 106
§6, 14, 22, 63, 80, 105, 107
¶4, 46, 69, 79, 108, 109
|46, 69, 75, 79, 95, 110
‖46, 79, 95, 112, 114, 120

resuscitation.[126,134,137] Finally, increased sympathetic discharge results in contraction of the spleen, releasing red blood cells into the circulation and defending a fall in hematocrit.[14]

CELLS

During hypovolemic shock, the oxygen lack in the tissues causes a decline in the mitochondrial production and concentration of high-energy phosphates in the tissues because of greater breakdown than production of these compounds.[24,29,46,138,139] This decline is a function of the severity and duration of regional hypoperfusion relative to oxygen demand. The decrease in the redox status and high-energy phosphates during experimental hypovolemic shock is more pronounced in some tissues (diaphragm, liver, kidney, and gut) than in others (heart and skeletal muscle), so regional lactate production may vary.*

A decrease in high-energy phosphates heralds irreversible cell injury during ischemia, whereas a less severe decline may result only in prolonged programmed cell death—apoptosis. In animals with hypovolemic shock and in critically ill patients, the circulating levels of ATP can be diminished, and ATP degradation products, including adenosine, inosine, hypoxanthine, and xanthine, can be elevated, suggesting breakdown of ATP following a lack of oxygen in the tissues.[28,29,56,141,142] Conversely, reperfusion is associated with restoration of energy charge, depending on the effect of ischemia, the oxygen demand, and the level of reperfusion. The intravenous administration of energy in the form of ATP-$MgCl_2$ may help tissues (kidney, liver, heart, gut) to recover from ischemia and resume function, independently of the vasodilating effects of the compound.[24,128,143,144] Also, pretreatment with coenzyme Q_{10}, involved in the respiratory chain reactions in mitochondria, has a beneficial effect during hypovolemic shock and resuscitation, at least in dogs.[81] Nevertheless, part of the mitochondrial dysfunction after trauma and hypovolemic shock has been suggested to be independent of a lack of oxygen.[53] Near-infrared spectroscopy, which can be applied in animals and patients, may indeed reveal normal absorption spectra for tissue oxyhemoglobin and low mitochondrial cytochrome *aa*3 redox status.[53,123,145]

About 60% of the energy produced by respirating mitochondria is needed to fuel the Na^+/K^+ pump of the cell, through which the gradient in electrolyte concentrations and electrical potential over the cell membrane are controlled.[24] When ATP becomes insufficient because of a decline in production associated with lack of oxygen and production of protons increases, the Na^+/K^+ pump is inhibited and the Na^+/H^+ exchanger is activated, and this results, together with a possibly selective increase in cell membrane permeability for ions, in an influx of Na^+ into and efflux of H^+ and K^+ out of the cell, leading to cellular uptake of fluid.† Measurement of membrane potentials of skeletal muscle and liver in experimental animals has shown that hypovolemic shock rapidly decreases the transmembrane potential (a less negative inner membrane potential), associated with electrolyte and fluid shifts across the cell membrane.‡ A decrease in activity of the Na^+/K^+ pump may contribute to hyperkalemia because of potassium exchange between cells, interstitial fluid, and vascular space.[38,46,111,125] Finally, calcium (Ca^{2+}) influx into cells and their mitochondria inhibits cellular respiration and ultimately contributes to cellular damage and swelling, particularly during resuscitation, and this can be prevented by administration of Ca^{2+} antagonists.* Because of cellular influx, the plasma-free Ca^{2+} levels may decrease in experimental and human hypovolemic shock.[127,149,150] Intracellular lysosomes lose their integrity so that proteolytic enzymes are released and contribute to cell death.[4,24,107,151] These enzymes eventually may reach the systemic circulation and may damage remote organs.[4,24,107,151]

As has become apparent in past years, the cellular response to stress, such as heat and tissue hypoxia, involves the expression of certain genes, coding for synthesis of the so-called heat-shock proteins, which play an important role in protecting the cells against stress.[152-155] The clinical significance of these molecular cellular changes is unknown. The response may be partially responsible, however, for the decreased susceptibility to and tissue injury by hemorrhagic shock in animals with a prior challenge by endotoxin or other forms of preconditioning.[113,156]

ORGAN PERFUSION AND FUNCTION IN SHOCK

HEART

According to Starling's law of the heart, a change in preload, approximated by the end-diastolic volume and determined by the venous return of blood to the heart, directly results in a change in stroke volume, defining myocardial function.[7] The relationship between end-diastolic filling pressure and volume reflects compliance. Apart from preload, cardiac output also depends on afterload, which is approximated by the end-systolic volume of the heart, and contractility, reflected by the peak systolic pressure-to-volume relationship (maximal elastance).[7,55,157] A diminished response of the stroke work by the heart, that is, the product of stroke volume and arterial blood pressure, to an increase in preload during resuscitation from hypovolemic shock may indicate diminished cardiac contractility that is associated with a worse outcome (e.g., caused by preexisting cardiac disease, hypovolemic shock itself, myocardial contusion, or combinations).[4,55,158,159] The effect of hypovolemic shock on myocardial function in animal models is controversial. Depending on models, methods, and definitions of cardiac dysfunction, some authors describe a decrease, but others describe an unchanged function of the left side of the heart.† The latter can be explained if a decrease in contractility of the heart is masked by the inotropic effect of catecholamines and other positive inotropic substances, such as endothelin, liberated during hypovolemic shock, even though receptor-mediated catecholamine responses may decline.[4,23,100,160]

Although coronary blood flow may be defended, and the oxygen demands of the heart may decrease associated with a decrease in filling (preload) and arterial blood pressure (afterload) during initial hypovolemic shock, hypotension

*24, 38, 46, 106, 139, 140
†24, 46, 111, 125, 127, 146, 147
‡24, 46, 111, 125, 127, 146

*24, 125, 127, 139, 148, 149
†4, 127, 157, 158, 160, 161

may become so severe that coronary vasodilation to compensate for a decline in perfusion pressure becomes exhausted, so that myocardial oxygen delivery decreases to less than the oxygen needs of the heart and ischemia ensues, particularly if tachycardia is present.[3,21,140,161-163] This sequence leading to ischemia may occur primarily in endocardium because of more rapidly exhausted vasodilation in endocardium than epicardium and redistribution of blood flow from the inner to the outer layer of the heart.[140] The subendocardium may become ischemic, and patchy necrosis may ensue. Because of regional transmural and intramural differences in vasodilator reserve, myocardial ischemia may be heterogeneously distributed and associated with a diminished redox state, lactate production, and creatine phosphate breakdown.[140,164] Ischemia ultimately may contribute to a decrease in myocardial contractility during hypovolemic shock. Smooth muscle–dependent and, particularly, endothelium-dependent coronary vasomotion may be impaired after hypovolemic shock.[89,165] Myocardial edema and compression of capillaries with resultant impairment of diffusion and extraction of oxygen may also contribute to a decrease in regional coronary blood flow, regional myocardial ischemia, and decreased myocardial function in hemorrhaged animals.[127,131,140,161]

Hypovolemic shock may induce a decrease in left ventricular compliance and relaxation.[160,161] The diastolic dysfunction may be particularly pronounced during resuscitation from hypovolemic shock.[157,160,161] Postischemic failure (stunning) also may play a role during resuscitation, at least temporarily. Ischemia-reperfusion of the heart results in accumulation of intracellular Ca^{2+}.[127] This may impair mitochondrial and sarcoplasmic reticulum function and contribute to impaired cardiac function after hypovolemic shock.[127,160] In dogs, the administration of Ca^{2+} blockers may prevent such deterioration during resuscitation from hypovolemic shock.[127] Finally, systemic release or intramyocardial production of negative inotropic substances and inflammatory mediators such as tumor necrosis factor (TNF)-α, interleukin (IL) 6 and platelet activating factor, oxidant damage, metabolic acidosis, diminished adrenoreceptor density, and resultant diminished sensitivity of the heart to circulating catecholamines may contribute to myocardial dysfunction during hypovolemic shock.* Pentoxifylline may improve endothelial and myocardial function.[166] Reversibility of dysfunction is associated with survival.[161]

The clinical evidence for myocardial dysfunction during hypovolemic shock is scarce.[46,55,163] Nevertheless, it is conceivable that severe hypotension reduces the balance between oxygen delivery and demand of the heart because many patients with hypovolemic shock may be elderly with coronary artery disease, compromising coronary vasodilation. Some may have preexisting impaired function while on beta blockers. For a patient with hypovolemic shock, a decrease in left ventricular compliance, contractility, or both may imply that a relatively high filling pressure would be needed to restore cardiac output during fluid resuscitation.[55,71,161,163,171] The averaged optimal pulmonary capillary wedge pressure (PCWP), that is, the pressure above which cardiac output does not increase further, may not be elevated in patients with hypovolemic shock (i.e., 12 to 15 mm Hg), although in some patients, abnormally elevated filling pressures may be needed to increase cardiac output, or cardiac output does not increase at all during fluid resuscitation.[55,71,171,172] A diminished function of the heart may hamper restoration of oxygen delivery to the tissues during resuscitation necessary for survival.[9,45,55,159,160] Myocardial dysfunction may thus be greater in nonsurvivors than in survivors. There may be some electrocardiographic or enzymatic evidence for myocardial ischemia and injury, and some patients may experience a myocardial infarction as a complication of severe hypovolemic shock after hemorrhage.[163,173]

LUNG

Hypovolemic shock often induces an increase in ventilatory minute volume, resulting in tachypnea or hyperventilation and a decrease in arterial P_{CO_2}.[33,49,50,52,174] Unless complicated by pulmonary abnormalities, these changes are, at least initially, not the result of hypoxemia but an increase in dead-space ventilation following a decrease in pulmonary perfusion so that a higher minute ventilation is necessary for a given CO_2 production to eliminate CO_2 from the blood and to maintain a normal P_{CO_2} in arterial blood.[33,49,50] Minute ventilatory volume may increase further if a decrease in P_{CO_2} is necessary to compensate for metabolic acidosis after accumulation of lactate in the blood.* The imbalance between increased demands of the diaphragm and reduced blood flow in shock may finally lead to respiratory muscle fatigue and a subsequent decline in ventilatory minute volume.[50]

Hypovolemic shock caused by trauma and hemorrhage and followed by extensive transfusion therapy of red blood cell concentrates can be complicated by pulmonary edema and impaired gas exchange.[51,175-180] In some patients, fluid overloading, overtransfusion, and an elevated filtration pressure (PCWP) may be responsible: transfusion-associated circulatory overload (TACO). In others, pulmonary edema may be due to a pulmonary vascular injury, however, and increased vascular permeability at a relatively low PCWP, indicating noncardiogenic permeability edema or ARDS.[51,174,177,178] The reaction to diuretics may help to differentiate between hydrostatic and permeability edema of the lungs. The latter seems relatively rare in polytransfused, polytraumatized patients unless associated with complications, but other studies suggest that about 30% of patients with severe trauma/hemorrhage, particularly if polytransfused, may develop ARDS.[177,178,180,181]

Experimental studies are at variance concerning alterations in capillary permeability of the lungs during hypovolemic shock and resuscitation.[4,133,174,182,183] According to some investigators, hypovolemic shock following bleeding and transfusion mildly increases transvascular filtration of fluid and proteins and results in accumulation of interstitial fluid as a consequence of increased permeability,[182] but other authors do not observe such changes.[131,133,182,184] In other animal studies, however, traumatic/hypovolemic shock resulted in extensive morphologic changes of the lung,

*11, 23, 36, 107, 149, 161, 164, 167–170

*27, 32, 33, 49, 50, 52, 174

with endothelial and interstitial edema, accumulation of degranulated neutrophils, and scattered fat emboli, which may resemble the pulmonary changes after traumatic/hypovolemic shock in humans.[156,174,185-187] As measured by the transvascular albumin flux in the lungs, almost 80% of patients with multiple trauma may show increased pulmonary vascular permeability in the disease course.[51] This leak ultimately may contribute to pulmonary edema, impaired mechanics, and gas exchange.[51] As suggested by animal experiments, among others, several factors may play a role, including release of proinflammatory mediators (TNF-α) and priming and activation of blood neutrophils after ischemia-reperfusion, contusion or ischemia-reperfusion of the lungs themselves, pulmonary microemboli of neutrophils, platelets and fat particles from the medulla of fractured long bones and pelvis, and neutrophilic antibodies or humoral or cellular breakdown products and released cytokines in long-stored and transfused blood products (transfusion-related acute lung injury, TRALI).* Translocated endotoxin may also play a role.[185] Finally, aspiration of foreign material or gastric contents and posttraumatic pneumonia and sepsis may contribute to the development of ARDS in trauma patients. When pulmonary edema has developed, active resorption by alveolar cells becomes necessary for clearance. This process is cylic AMP–dependent and can be disturbed by inducible nitric oxide synthase (iNOS)–derived NO and peroxynitrite and enhanced by expression of heme oxygenase, which may mitigate lung injury in animal models.[156] How this translates clinically is unclear.

BRAIN

Classically, brain perfusion and microcirculation are considered to be relatively spared during progressive hypovolemia because of the extensive autoregulatory capacity of cerebral arteries.[15,189] In case of autoregulation impairment after neurotrauma, however, brain perfusion may decrease, and subsequent reperfusion may contribute to secondary cerebral damage during hypovolemic shock and resuscitation. Hemorrhagic shock and resuscitation per se may also impair autoregulatory capacity of brain vessels, however, because of endothelial dysfunction and diminished NO-dependent vasodilator reactivity, so that the brain may experience an oxygen debt and subsequent metabolic and functional deterioration.[29,88]

KIDNEY

Hypovolemic hypotension is an important risk factor for acute kidney injury and failure after trauma.[138] During a decrease in cardiac output following progressive hemorrhage, renal blood flow can be maintained because of renal vasodilation, so that the kidneys may not participate in the systemic vasoconstriction that characterizes hypovolemic shock.[3] Vasodilating prostaglandins are released in the kidney through activation of the cyclooxygenase pathway of arachidonic acid metabolism in response to ischemia, increased sympathetic activity, and angiotensin II, so that renal vasodilation during the early phase of hemorrhage can be blocked by prostaglandin synthesis inhibition, resulting in a profound decrease in blood flow even if accompanied by an increase in arterial blood pressure.[3] When blood pressure decreases during progressive hypovolemia, the renal vessels constrict, impairing blood flow to the kidneys more than to other organs.† This is partly caused by a baroreflex-mediated increase in sympathetic activity; activation of the renin-angiotensin-aldosterone system; and release of catecholamines, angiotensin II, endothelin, and vasopressin.[13,14,74] During prolonged hypovolemic shock, sympathetic inhibition may protect against renal ischemia.[14] This propensity for vasoconstriction is thus partly offset if NO and other factors with vasodilatory actions are released intrarenally.[4,86] Inhibition of NO synthesis increases blood pressure, however, and increases renal perfusion and glomerular filtration during hypovolemic shock.[86] In another study, endothelium-dependent renal vasodilation was impaired after hypovolemic shock.[87]

Renal ischemia results in a decrease in glomerular filtration (prerenal renal failure) that is less than the decline in blood flow so that the filtration fraction often increases.[138] The latter is caused by greater constriction of efferent than of afferent arterioles in glomeruli, in which high levels of circulating angiotensin II are probably involved. The decrease in glomerular filtration together with an increase in tubular resorption of electrolytes and fluids, mediated by increased levels of antidiuretic hormone released by the pituitary and decreased levels of atrial natriuretic peptides through low atrial filling, results in oliguria or anuria (<0.3 mL/kg/hour) and a low sodium content of urine.[138]

The decrease in renal perfusion during hypovolemic shock is often accompanied by redistribution of blood flow from outer to inner cortex and medulla, which is already borderline hypoxic even in the normal state.[127] If long-lasting and severe, the cortical kidney becomes ischemic, despite a decrease in oxygen needs associated with fewer energy needs for tubular resorption in the presence of less filtration, so that the levels of high-energy phosphates decline.[138,139] Severe and prolonged renal ischemia and metabolic deterioration finally result in acute kidney injury and failure with morphologic changes, particularly in proximal tubules and medullary segments (acute tubular necrosis) when an increase in renal perfusion does not immediately restore filtration and diuresis, but rather injures renal structures (reperfusion injury), limiting a return of blood flow and glomerular filtration during resuscitation.[129,138,185,186] This is often recognized by a persistent oliguria and a gradual increase in creatinine and urea levels in blood. In addition, the plasma levels and urinary excretion of biomarkers of injury and dysfunction may increase.[104]

GUT

During hypovolemic shock, blood flow from stomach to colon is redistributed to other organs, and this may be primarily mediated by elevated sympathetic activity and increased levels of vasopressin and angiotensin II even though vascular reactivity to the latter may diminish.‡ Vasoconstriction may overwhelm NO and other vasodilating mechanisms, and endothelium-dependent vasodilation may

*51, 117, 174, 175, 180, 183, 185, 187–191

†3, 14, 74, 85, 86, 106, 139

‡3, 13, 14, 22, 79, 80, 97, 105, 139, 152, 192, 193

be impaired after oxidant endothelial injury.[194] Gut ischemia is aggravated further by the countercurrent mechanism in mucosal (villous) blood flow, promoting diffusional shunting of oxygen from arteries to veins, bypassing tissues. Other studies reported that gut mucosal blood flow may be relatively spared during hypovolemia, however.[75,105] Portal blood flow decreases, and portal blood levels of lactate increase after gut ischemia.[27,48,195]

Gastric mucosal ischemia may result in diminished energy-consuming acid production and may predispose to mucosal stress ulceration.[192,196] Microscopic studies in experimental animals show damage of gastric mucosa, villous epithelium in small bowel, and mucosa of the large bowel after hypovolemic shock.[114,192,197-199] Gastric mucosal ischemia-reperfusion injury after bleeding may be aggravated by gastric acid itself, neutrophils, inflammatory mediators, endothelin, reactive oxygen species (ROS), and proteases.[198,200] Bowel ischemia and mucosal damage during hypovolemic shock in the dog may ultimately lead to leakage of fluid from the bloodstream to the bowel lumen, instead of normal resorption of luminal fluids.[115,197] Diarrhea may contribute to intravascular volume depletion during severe and prolonged hypovolemic shock, at least in animals.

Gut mucosal ischemia, energy depletion, injury, and inflammation may compromise the barrier function of the mucosa, enhancing the likelihood that bacteria and endotoxins in intestinal lumen (large bowel) translocate through the damaged gut wall to lymph nodes, portal venous blood, or both.* The gut epithelial (lumen to plasma) permeability for small molecules also is increased. Indigenous flora, generated toxic ROS, cytokines, Ca^{2+} overload, iNOS, peroxynitrite, phospholipase A_2 activation, and activated and adhering neutrophils during ischemia and reperfusion probably all play a role in the injury, promoting hyperpermeability and translocation.[199,203] Mucosal injury and translocation can be inhibited by compounds targeted against these factors.[199] Impaired detoxifying capacity of the Kupffer cells of the liver because of ischemia or preexistent liver disease may contribute further to bacteria and endotoxins reaching the systemic circulation and contributing to progression of shock by triggering an inflammation cascade, ultimately resulting in release of vasoactive substances.[4,204,205] This translocation has been shown to contribute to the lethality of hypovolemic shock in experimental animals because clearance or blockade of translocated bacteria and endotoxins is associated with survival, and germ-free animals survive an episode of bleeding more often and longer than ones with normal intestinal flora.[4,143,203,205] Finally, it has been shown that the absorptive capacity of the gut for carbohydrates, amino acids, and lipids decreases during hypovolemic shock.[148,195] Although enteral feeding during hypovolemic shock and after resuscitation may increase metabolic demands of the gut, there is experimental evidence that luminal application of nutrients, particularly of enterocyte-fueling glutamine, induces an increase in small vessel blood flow, ameliorates damage, and diminishes the likelihood for translocation of endotoxins and bacteria during resuscitation from hemorrhage.[206]

In humans, hypovolemia leads to a decline in hepatosplanchnic perfusion.[74] Stomach mucosal lesions may be common after prolonged hypovolemic shock, but overt bleeding is a relatively rare event, particularly in a rapidly, adequately resuscitated patient.[207] Agents that decrease energy-demanding gastric acid production may protect against stress ulcers during mucosal ischemia.[196] The gut is usually quiescent during hypovolemic shock in humans. Ileus is often present, and the patient is managed expectantly until bowel sounds return and enteral feeding is likely to be tolerated. Occasionally, a bowel infarction and perforation may complicate hypovolemic shock as a consequence of nonocclusive ischemia.[148] Gut absorptive capacity may decrease,[148] perhaps caused by gut ischemia. The adequacy of gastrointestinal blood flow can be monitored in humans with the help of a balloon catheter in the stomach (or gut), in which fluid or air is installed, or sublingually or buccally with help of a sensor (tonometry).* The mucosal P_{CO_2} thus measured decreases, and the mucosal-to-blood P_{CO_2} gradient increases, during a decrease in mucosal blood flow relative to demand. An increase of this gradient may occur at an earlier stage than an increase in heart rate or decrease in arterial blood pressure during progressive hypovolemia, constituting an early and sensitive sign of shock.[208] Gastrointestinal tonometry can be used as a guide for resuscitation.† The clinical occurrence and significance of translocation of intestinal bacteria and endotoxins to mesenteric lymph nodes and the bloodstream are unclear, although the capacity of the human gut wall to resorb orally administered small molecules, including lactulose relative to mannitol, may increase, indicating epithelial barrier dysfunction.[54,204,205,211-214]

LIVER

Liver microvascular and sinusoidal perfusion decline during hypovolemic shock because of diminished portal and hepatic arterial blood flow, roughly in proportion to the decrease in cardiac output so that in contrast to the gut there is no angiotensin II–mediated selective vasoconstriction in the hepatic arterial bed.‡ Endogenous mechanisms, including release of NO, carbon monoxide, and hydrogen sulfide in the absence of endothelial dysfunction, may counteract a decrease in perfusion, which is promoted by thromboxane A_2 and endothelin.[91,155] A decrease in blood flow may result in liver ischemia, a decrease in high-energy phosphate contents and clearance function as evidenced by insufficient capacity to clear indocyanine green from blood and a decrease in the bile excretion rate.§ The capacity to clear gut-derived endotoxin, cytokines and lactate also may decrease, and the ischemic liver produces lactate.[43] Hepatic ischemia may result in a diminished capacity for metabolism of drugs such as lignocaine[219] and for gluconeogenesis from lactate and amino acids, contributing to hypoglycemia in the late stage of hypovolemic shock.[12,139] Inflammation of the liver causes cytokine expression; hepatic sinuses become filled with adherent neutrophilic aggregates, lining cells may swell, and microcirculatory failure and centrilobular necrosis/apoptosis may ensue with leakage of enzymes

*142, 185, 186, 199, 201–203

*40, 54, 68, 92, 106, 123, 139, 166, 196, 208–211
†40, 54, 92, 106, 123, 139, 166, 196, 208–211
‡95, 106, 139, 144, 149, 166, 215–217
§28, 44, 91, 95, 142, 144, 149, 215–218

into the circulation.* ROS and NO-derived and toxic peroxynitrite and damage of endoplasmatic reticulum and mitochondria may be involved. Clinically, bilirubin and transaminases may be transiently elevated in blood, abnormalities attributed to ischemic hepatitis.[222,223] A clinically useful measure of hepatic oxygen debt is an increase in the plasma ratio of β-hydroxybutyrate to acetoacetate (ketone body ratio), which occurs concurrently with a decrease in the hepatic mitochondrial redox state.[28,91,95,223]

SPLEEN

The spleen contracts during hypovolemic shock, probably caused by increased sympathetic activity, and this results in release of red blood cells into the circulation.[3,14] Changes in hematocrit during the early phase of bleeding probably underestimate the severity of plasma losses. The spleen also releases stored platelets.

PANCREAS

The pancreas is severely ischemic during hypovolemic shock.[107] Ischemic pancreatitis may lead to autodigestion of acinar cells and liberation of pancreatic lysosomal enzymes into the systemic circulation, including proteases and factors with negative inotropic properties on the heart, although the latter factors may also come from ischemic gut.[4,107,166] Ligation of the pancreatic duct may be beneficial in experiments by preventing gut injury and barrier failure, among others.[224]

HORMONES AND METABOLISM

As mentioned before, a severe decrease in cardiac output resulting in a decrease in arterial blood pressure during hypovolemic shock results in activation of the sympathetic nervous system through the baroreceptor reflex and liberation of norepinephrine from nerve endings and epinephrine from adrenal medulla so that circulating levels of these catecholamines increase.[11-13,74,81,99] The insulin secretion by the pancreas is inhibited, and glucagon secretion is enhanced by high circulating norepinephrine levels.[99] The renin-angiotensin-aldosterone system is activated, and the pituitary secretion of vasopressin/antidiuretic hormone and opioids increases.[11-13,23,99] The pituitary response to stress further includes an increase in adrenocorticotropic hormone (ACTH) with resultant corticosteroid release by the adrenal cortex, unless limited by the so-called relative adrenal insufficiency following hypoperfusion-induced adrenal damage.[12,99,152] These factors may be essential for survival because prior adrenalectomy decreases survival of animals subjected to hypovolemic shock, and steroid repletion is protective in this respect.[12] This protective effect can be attributed to, among others, less overactivation of the sympathetic nervous system and increased sensitivity of the heart and vasculature to circulating levels of catecholamines.[12]

Finally, the secretion of atrial natriuretic peptides by the myocardium declines in response to hypovolemia and diminished wall stress of the atria. These factors, among others, result in tachycardia and a diminished renal excretion of water and salt to restore circulating blood volume. Endogenous opioids could play a role in maintaining shock by their vasodilating and myocardial depressant properties, however.[11,13,23] Administration of the opioid antagonist naloxone and its derivatives augment arterial blood pressure in hypovolemic shock.[13,23,143,225] Similarly, thyrotropin-releasing hormone depresses the opioid system and increases arterial blood pressure, cardiac function, and survival during hypovolemic shock in animals.[23] Thyroid hormone may have a similar effect.[226]

During trauma, hypovolemic shock, and cellular ischemia, intermediary metabolism undergoes profound changes, partly caused by an altered hormonal milieu.[99] The early hyperglycemic response to traumatic/hypovolemic shock is the combined result of enhanced glycogenolysis, caused by the hormonal response to stress and elevated epinephrine, cortisol, and glucagon levels; increased gluconeogenesis in the liver, partly mediated by glucagon; and peripheral resistance to the action of insulin, the secretion of which may be diminished shortly after onset of shock but may be enhanced later after shock.[24,47,99,129] This resistance is most likely the result of an altered hormonal milieu—the increase in circulating epinephrine and cortisol levels. During the late, irreversible stage of hypovolemic shock, however, hypoglycemia supervenes, at least in animal models, because glycogen stores may be depleted and the capacity for gluconeogenesis by the liver may decrease because of ischemia.[12,24,47,111,130]

Increased gluconeogenesis in the liver, and to a lesser extent in the kidneys, follows increased efflux of amino acids such as alanine and glutamine from the muscle to the liver because of breakdown of muscle protein.[99,222] The latter is evidenced by increased urinary losses of nitrogen and a negative nitrogen balance.[99,222] Amino acid metabolic changes may contribute to the immunodepression of trauma. Lactate produced in muscle also can be converted to glucose in the liver.[99] Finally, fatty acid metabolism undergoes profound changes, with depressed lipolysis, ketogenesis, and combustion of fatty acids during shock and an increase in the resuscitation phase.[99,222] Some investigators regard a deranged intermediary metabolism of primary importance for the eventual outcome of shock, whereas others merely consider these changes a result of the shock process itself.[222]

INFLAMMATORY AND IMMUNOLOGIC CHANGES

Activation of the xanthine-oxidase system and formation of uric acid from the ATP breakdown products hypoxanthine and xanthine during reperfusion could liberate ROS, which damage vascular endothelium and parenchymal cell membranes through peroxidation of lipids.* The release of ROS during ischemia-reperfusion may activate macrophages and attract neutrophils, partly mediated by release of cytokines via activated nuclear factor-κB (NF-κB).[194,228] The interaction of ROS fueled by oxygen and NO may further play a role in inflammation and vascular tone after perfusion.[90,228] ROS scavengers may inhibit formation of toxic

*95, 166, 185, 186, 216, 220, 221

*117, 188, 198, 199, 227, 228

peroxynitrite via NO, and ROS and may inhibit breakage of DNA single strands and activation of poly(ADP-ribose) polymerase, which contributes to cellular injury.[90,92,221] Some time after hypovolemic shock and resuscitation, iNOS may become active particularly in the gut and liver; circulating NO breakdown products may increase and inhibition of the excessive NO release may ameliorate hemodynamic changes, organ inflammation, and neutrophil accumulation and function, partly via less peroxynitrite formation, unless inhibition leads to a decrease in cardiac output.[90,92,155,220] Increased iNOS-derived NO also may be prevented and treated by corticosteroids or ACTH fragments.[93,229]

Proinflammatory mediators may be expressed locally in a variety of organs in response to hemorrhagic shock, including heart and lungs, and this is partly under control of α-sympathoadrenergic and neuroimmune stimuli, toll-like receptor 4, NF-κB, hypoxia-inducible factor, glycogen synthase kinase-3β, and other factors involved in cell signaling.[228,230-233] During and after hemorrhage, hypovolemic shock, and resuscitation, macrophages, including lung macrophages and Kupffer cells in the liver, may release cytokines, including TNF-α, IL-1, IL-6, and IL-8. This inflammatory response is attenuated when reperfusion takes place in hypoxic, rather than normoxic, conditions.[234] The response can be ameliorated by blockade of NF-κB, administration of the macrophage-inhibitor pentoxifylline, or ATP-$MgCl_2$ increasing hepatic blood flow.*

Ischemia per se and the immune consequences of gut barrier injury may play a role in Kupffer cell responses. The reperfused gut, together with the liver, may be a source of systemically released cytokines, as suggested by animal experiments and observations in humans after trauma, and translocated endotoxin may play a role.† During reperfusion after resuscitation, cytokines may induce and amplify the inflammatory response to ischemia and may induce further local and remote organ damage with circulatory changes.[166,187,236,240,241] Spillover of mediators into the mesenteric lymph or portal and systemic circulations during reperfusion of prior ischemic gut may have deleterious effects on remote organs by inducing neutrophil activation and adherence, which may contribute to a lung vascular injury with increased permeability.[185,186,188,240,241] Circulating levels of proinflammatory cytokines may be of predictive value for remote organ damage, including ARDS, after trauma in patients.[230,237,238] Endotoxin binding or antibodies and cytokine antibodies may ameliorate remote tissue damage after bleeding, hypovolemic shock, and resuscitation.[185,186]

Trauma and shock/resuscitation have also been shown to activate the complement and the arachidonic acid systems.[151,242-245] Complement activation may yield potent vasodilating and leukoattractant substances and contribute to remote inflammatory organ damage (ARDS). Ischemia may generate phospholipase A_2, catalyzing arachidonic acid metabolism into prostaglandins via the cyclooxygenase pathway, releasing thromboxane A_2 and prostacyclin, and into leukotrienes via the lipoxygenase pathway.[10,151,243] Thromboxane A_2, released from platelets, neutrophils, and cell membranes, has potent vasoconstricting properties and promotes aggregation of platelets and neutrophils, whereas prostacyclin has vasodilating properties and inhibits platelet and neutrophil aggregation.[243] Leukotrienes have vasoconstricting properties, increase capillary permeability, and attract neutrophils.[151] Vasoconstricting prostaglandins may be involved in tissue damage during ischemia-reperfusion, and vasodilating prostaglandins may be involved in the vasodilated state of terminal hypovolemic shock.[10,242] Another lipid mediator that may be released is platelet-activating factor, but the precise action of this mediator is unclear.[149,170]

The interplay of these factors may result in endothelial activation throughout the body and an inflammatory reaction, ultimately involving attraction, activation, and endothelial adherence of neutrophils, as shown in animal models of hypovolemic shock after bleeding and ischemia-reperfusion.* Neutrophils release vasoconstricting, platelet-aggregating, and damaging thromboxane A_2 and may inhibit vasodilating prostacyclin, via secreted ROS and proteases such as elastase.[117,228,238,244,246] Neutrophil aggregation and secreted activation products also may also play a role in the reperfusion injury by impairing resumption of small vessel blood flow, even in the presence of a seemingly adequate cardiac output and arterial blood pressure.† In humans, the activation of neutrophils after trauma, with increased adhesion molecule expression and propensity for degranulation, is associated with morbidity after trauma, such as development of MOF and predisposition to sepsis.[115-117,233,237,247] After initial leukopenia (neutropenia) following trapping of leukocytes in the microcirculation, activation of the pituitary-adrenal axis and release of corticosteroids and catecholamines during hypovolemic shock result in an increase of circulating neutrophils following demargination and release from bone marrow, together with eosinopenia and lymphocytopenia.[46,112-115,216] A tertiary decrease of circulating neutrophils in patients with a downhill course may be explained by microcirculatory sequestration.[115] The hemodynamics, organ function, and survival of rats with hypovolemic shock/resuscitation are improved if rats are made neutropenic before the challenge, and this may relate to improved regional and capillary blood flow.[112,243] A monoclonal antibody against or antagonists of neutrophil-endothelial adhesion molecules decrease reperfusion injury in lungs, liver, stomach, and intestines after hypovolemic shock or ruptured aortic aneurysm and may improve survival, at least in animal models.[114,117,118,187,228] This does not impair host defense against subsequent bacterial infections.[114]

However, neutrophils may later become downregulated after initial stimulation by circulating proinflammatory and anti-inflammatory mediators.[111,229,248] Neutrophil dysfunction is evidenced by a diminished potential to migrate and to digest and kill bacteria, perhaps in the presence of an inhibited respiratory burst.[111,188,247,248] In hemorrhaged mice, the infusion of granulocyte colony-stimulating factor or IL-6 after hemorrhage may partly prevent neutrophil defects and protect against death from subsequent pulmonary sepsis.[248] Also, the opsonization function of macrophages, that is, the

*166, 186, 187, 193, 216, 230, 235–237
†54, 193, 204, 205, 238–241

*10, 113, 114, 116, 151, 166, 188, 198, 216, 228, 240, 242, 244
†46, 79, 95, 112, 114, 206, 243

reticuloendothelial system, is depressed so that removal from the circulation of fibrin, cell aggregates, and bacteria by the liver is at least transiently impaired.* This may relate to the appearance after hypovolemic/traumatic shock of substances in blood that depress reticuloendothelial system function or to a decrease of the α_2-glycoprotein fibronectin in plasma, a substance that aids the reticuloendothelial system in opsonization.[4,167,236,249,251] This deficiency may contribute to development of MOF and might be reversed by infusion of plasma cryoprecipitate.[251] Hypovolemic shock and gut-derived factors may blunt the increase in bone marrow cytopoiesis after soft tissue trauma and endotoxin and contribute to susceptibility to sepsis.[252,253]

Hemorrhagic/hypovolemic shock and subsequent resuscitation depress the immune system by suppressing the function of not only neutrophils but also lymphocytes and macrophages; this depresses humoral and cellular immune responses, decreasing antigen presentation and delayed hypersensitivity to skin test antigens and increasing susceptibility to sepsis.† Part of this may be mediated via neuroimmune modulation and resulting efferent sympathetic, adrenergic, and vagal stimulation.[37,93] In patients, the immune defect correlates with the extent and severity of trauma and the degree of blood resuscitation required, but animal experiments document that hemorrhage/resuscitation per se depresses immune function, although trauma and blood transfusions may only be synergistic in this respect.[236,250,254,255,258] Priming of immune cells may explain in part the increased sensitivity to endotoxin and sepsis after hypovolemic shock, although other authors have described that prior hypovolemic shock and priming decreased the immune response and increased the tolerance to endotoxin or sepsis.[114,184,187,259] Hemorrhage decreases the capability of lymphocytes to proliferate and to produce lymphokines (IL-2) in response to mitogens, an effect that seems dependent on an energy or NO deficit or on Ca^{2+} influx in these cells after ischemia because the defect can be overcome by administration of Ca^{2+} influx blockers.[236,250,254,255,258] Increased macrophage production of cytokines during hypovolemic shock and resuscitation may be followed by decreased ability of the cells to release mediators such as TNF-α and to express HLA-DR, upon challenges, and to process and present antigens to lymphocytes. This may relate to a cellular energy deficit, accumulation of Ca^{2+}, and enhanced prostaglandin E_2 synthesis.‡ The immunodepression after hypovolemic shock and predisposition to sepsis may finally include the release by Kupffer cells, among others, of anti-inflammatory mediators, such as IL-10 and soluble receptors (receptor antagonists) for previously released proinflammatory cytokines, and this may relate to sepsis-induced MOF and increased risks of morbidity and mortality in trauma patients.[250,260] Otherwise, the immunologic consequences of trauma, hemorrhage, and hypovolemic shock depend on numerous additional factors, including gender and other genetic influences.[230,247,250] Men may exhibit more immunodepression after trauma/hemorrhage than women. The clinical implication may be that men are more susceptible than women to microbial infections after trauma.[261]

Circulating coagulation factors and platelet counts may decrease after hypovolemic shock and resuscitation, whereas fibrin products may increase. This is the consequence of coagulation activation and fibrinolysis inhibition by endothelial activation, tissue injury, and inflammatory responses, even though dilution after fluid resuscitation may heavily contribute.[181,237,262] Disseminated intravascular coagulation (DIC) and fibrin deposits, if insufficiently removed by the fibrinolytic system, are believed to contribute to a decrease in plasma coagulation factors and to widespread microvascular organ dysfunction.[181,237,263] Proinflammatory responses, some resuscitation fluids, hypothermia, and acidosis may contribute to DIC and the coagulation defect of severe hemorrhagic/traumatic shock.[237,264]

*4, 24, 167, 236, 249, 250
†2, 111, 235, 236, 247, 248, 250, 253–257
‡166, 235, 236, 247, 250, 256

REPERFUSION AND IRREVERSIBLE SHOCK

Reperfusion of various organs, including the heart, gut, skeletal muscle, brain, kidneys, and liver, after a transient episode of ischemia, as occurs during hypovolemic shock, results in the so-called reperfusion injury, which limits the possibility for resumption of microvascular tissue blood flow and function of organs, particularly of the liver, even if cardiac output and arterial blood pressure have been restored to normal value.* Redistribution of blood flow during hypovolemia may be only partly attenuated by reperfusion.

Reperfusion after a certain period of shock and diminished oxygen uptake results in an increase in oxygen uptake above baseline levels, provided that oxygen delivery and cellular function are adequate.[42,62,73,99] This repayment of the oxygen debt is largely determined by the increased demands for oxygen to resynthesize ATP from adenosine and phosphates and to rebuild the lost energy stores. This repayment is determined by the extent to which mitochondria are damaged during ischemia and the availability of substrates to resynthesize high-energy phosphates and restore cellular contents of these compounds because the substrates needed for synthesis may have been washed out, necessitating de novo synthesis.[24,142,143] Resuscitation may not completely restore energy levels, the activity of the Na^+/K^+ pump, and the membrane potential of skeletal muscle and liver necessary to remove accumulated fluid and Na^+ in the cell.[125,127,142]

Reperfusion not only results in resumption of oxygen delivery but also of Ca^{2+} to the tissues. This Ca^{2+} may be taken up by cells and may contribute to the reperfusion injury by damaging cell organelles, inhibiting mitochondrial respiration, and activating proteases and prostaglandin synthesis.[127,129,148,149] Reperfusion injury of heart, gut, kidneys, and liver after resuscitation from hypovolemic shock in animals may be prevented in part by administration of Ca^{2+} influx blockers independently of their vasodilating effects, suggesting that Ca^{2+} overload is partly responsible for the reperfusion injury.[127,129,148,149] Finally, endothelial damage and swelling and cellular aggregation may hamper the regional regulation of blood flow during resuscitation from

*79, 114, 144, 149, 166, 199, 206, 215, 228, 265, 266

hypovolemic shock.[79,95,110,122] Neutrophil-mediated endothelial injury may increase capillary permeability and contribute to fluid losses during resuscitation.[112,178,179,228,267] Conversely, the intravenous administration of energy in the form of ATP-$MgCl_2$ or adenosine-regulating compounds may help tissues to recover from ischemia and resume function, independently of the vasodilating effects of the compounds, by providing energy, improving the microcirculation, and reducing cell swelling to promote survival.* Nevertheless, the ability of organs or the whole body to increase oxygen uptake during reperfusion above normal may be associated with survival in experimental animals with hypovolemic shock and in hypovolemic patients after trauma or major surgery, whereas inability may be associated with ultimate demise.[9,73,82] Also, ischemic preconditioning may protect against hemorrhagic shock and reperfusion-induced tissue injury.[156]

If shock syndrome with hypotension and subnormal oxygen uptake persists after optimal fluid repletion and attempts at reperfusion with inotropic and vasoactive drugs, the condition can be regarded as irreversible and terminal.[4,9] The term *irreversible shock* has been mainly used in animal experiments, however, in which reinfusion of the shed blood after a certain period is unable to reverse the shock syndrome.[4,268] Various factors may play a role.[4] First, vascular decompensation may contribute to a further decrease in blood pressures and may include diminished constrictive reactivity, dilation of arterioles, and insensitivity to circulating or exogenous catecholamines.[97,108] The decline in vascular resistance may be partly caused by metabolic vasodilation in ischemic and acidotic tissues, overcoming vasoconstrictive influences.[4,10,108] Other factors that may be involved include dysfunction of vascular smooth muscle after induction of iNOS and resultant increased production of vasodilating NO in the vessel wall, acidosis and activation of low ATP-activated K^+ channels, histamine release, and prostaglandin-induced neurotransmission failure.† Circulating levels of NO breakdown products, nitrate and nitrite, may be elevated already early after hemorrhage in animals and trauma in humans, although other authors described low levels in humans.[269] iNOS upregulation and NO production may be prevented by NO blockers, corticosteroids, or ACTH fragments.[92,93,229] Finally, central cerebral or humoral mechanisms may contribute to the irreversible hemorrhagic shock, and this may relate to endogenous opioids, thyrotropin-releasing hormone, or macrophage-derived cannabinoids.[13,23,270]

The decrease in arterial vascular resistance may be particularly pronounced in the tissues, showing most intense vasoconstriction during hypovolemic shock, including gut and skeletal muscle, offsetting the redistribution of blood flow during hypovolemic shock and increasing blood flow to these organs at the expense of blood flow to vital tissues.[10,22] In contrast, venous compliance and resistance increase, leading to peripheral pooling of blood and a decrease in venous return to the heart.[4,166] The latter changes may be particularly pronounced in the splanchnic region.[166] During prolonged or irreversible hypovolemic shock, capillary hydrostatic pressure may increase after arteriolar vasodilation and venular constriction, resulting in a decrease in the precapillary-to-postcapillary resistance ratio and promoting fluid filtration into the interstitium.[4,5] Capillary permeability also may increase, resulting in a high capillary hydraulic conductance and a decrease in the reflection coefficient for plasma proteins. Increased permeability for proteins increases capillary filtration for a given intravascular hydrostatic pressure and promotes the formation of edema.[178,267] The increase in permeability may be the consequence of endothelial damage and loss of protective glycocalyx by ischemia-reperfusion, possibly involving ROS and proinflammatory mediators.[271] It may contribute further to a decline in circulating blood volume.[5,267] Cells may swell, and this may diminish circulating blood volume further.[4,125,127-129] Expansion of the cellular and interstitial fluid volume at the expense of the intravascular volume is manifested by a preterminal increase of the hematocrit.[4,5,126]

Irreversible hypovolemic shock may contribute to MOF and death of patients.[2,207] An inflammatory response to ischemic tissue and patchy necrosis/apoptosis may contribute to organ damage and dysfunction and thereby to the irreversibility of hypovolemic shock.[4,114,228] Reperfusion injury may aggravate organ damage and contribute to irreversible shock.[114,228,266] The pump function of the heart may diminish after a decrease in systolic contractility and compliance, and this may contribute to irreversibility of shock during resuscitation.[158] Myocardial dysfunction may contribute to the development of pulmonary alveolar edema if aggressive fluid infusion in attempts to increase cardiac output results in an elevated PCWP.[4] Diminished function of the heart may hamper restoration of oxygen delivery and uptake to the tissues during resuscitation.[9,45,157,158] Damage of the gut mucosa may cause translocation of luminal bacteria and endotoxins from gut lumen to systemic circulation, at least in experimental animals, and the resultant sepsis may contribute to the irreversibility of hypovolemic shock.*

CLINICAL FEATURES

CAUSES

One of the most frequent causes of hypovolemic shock is blood loss after trauma (see Box 26.1), including blood loss during or after major surgery.[2] Ruptured aortic aneurysm and gastrointestinal hemorrhage are other frequent causes of hypovolemic shock. Upper gastrointestinal bleeding can be caused by peptic ulcer disease, reflux esophagitis, variceal bleeding, erosive gastritis (stress ulcer), or aortoduodenal fistula after vascular surgery. Lower gastrointestinal bleeding can result from diverticular disease, carcinomas, or polyps in the colon. Sometimes, massive hemoptysis resulting from a tumor, tuberculosis, fungal infection, or bronchiectasis can be the cause of hypovolemic shock. Hematuria as a result of a tumor or trauma is a rare cause of hypovolemic shock. During multiple trauma, blood loss is essential in causing hypovolemic shock, but trauma itself can activate various mediator systems, with resultant release

*24, 128, 143, 144, 158, 230
†10, 29, 92, 93, 96, 97, 139, 229, 242

*4, 185, 197, 199, 202–205, 214

of vasoactive substances that contribute to the development of shock. In contrast to pure hypovolemic shock, cardiac output can be elevated, and peripheral vascular resistance is often decreased in cases of multiple trauma.[25]

In trauma patients, external blood loss can be accompanied by internal, invisible blood loss after renovascular trauma or major fractures (e.g., fractures of pelvis or femur). After blunt abdominal trauma, splenic or hepatic ruptures and perforations of hollow viscera are possible. Blunt chest trauma can be accompanied by an aortic rupture, tension pneumothorax, hemothorax or hemopericardium, and tamponade. Femoral artery injury (after puncture) can lead to massive retroperitoneal hematoma. Nonmechanical causes of hypovolemic shock include uncontrolled diabetes mellitus and acute adrenocortical insufficiency, causing severe renal fluid losses. Acute and severe vomiting following obstruction of the gastric outlet or gut, diarrhea, and burn wounds result in loss of plasma water.

SIGNS AND SYMPTOMS

Hypovolemic shock warrants an early diagnosis, avoiding delay in initial treatment. As soon as possible after admission of the patient, fluid resuscitation should begin via a large-bore catheter in a peripheral vein or a percutaneously inserted central venous catheter. During initial fluid resuscitation a history is taken and a brief but thorough physical examination is performed. The latter serves to establish rapidly the cause and severity of shock. Extensive manipulation of a fractured spine or extremity should be avoided. The history of a patient in hypovolemic shock is mainly determined by its cause. The patient may complain of thirst, diaphoresis, and shortness of breath. The patient's mental state is usually normal unless shock is severe and the patient becomes apathetic or confused. With less severe cases, the patient is anxious, and with more severe cases, the patient is apathetic.

For a clinical diagnosis of shock, hypotension and clinical signs of organ ischemia should be present. Arterial blood pressure and clinical signs are relatively insensitive for small blood losses (Table 26.1).[208] This sensitivity can be improved by using the shock index, calculated from heart rate divided by systolic blood pressure.[18] The clinician can recognize shock from a decrease in systolic blood pressure to less than 90 mm Hg or a decrease of more than 40 mm Hg below preshock levels, with a reduction in pulse pressure. Hypotension may be so severe that blood pressure is unrecordable noninvasively. There can be a large gradient between invasively and noninvasively measured arterial blood pressure and between central and radial artery pressure during shock and drug-induced vasoconstriction.[272] Hypotension may become particularly marked when the patient sits or stands versus when the patient is supine (orthostatic hypotension).[8,17,18] Postural dizziness, tachycardia, and hypotension are reliable and early signs of hypovolemia, whereas dryness of mucous membranes and axillae, decreased turgor, supine hypotension, and other signs have less diagnostic value.[17,18]

Tachycardia may be absent in case of prior use of beta blockers. Elderly patients may have atrial fibrillation and a high ventricular response. Occasionally, bradycardia is present, particularly when vagally mediated fainting supervenes.[16] The peripheral veins are collapsed, and the jugular venous pressure is low. Conversely, an elevated jugular venous pressure should warn the clinician of associated obstruction of the circulation, following pneumothorax, pericardial tamponade, and others, or of pump failure following myocardial contusion or infarction. The respiratory cycle–induced changes in stroke volume and in systolic arterial blood pressure and CVP are exaggerated.[20] Although dependent on tidal volume and respiratory compliance, these variations in a mechanically ventilated patient may constitute fair indices of hypovolemia, so high variations may predict an increase in cardiac output upon fluid loading.[19] Noninvasive, pulse contour–based techniques are suitable for these purposes. Fluid responsiveness also can be predicted by an increase in blood pressure and decrease in stroke volume and pressure variations during leg raising or similar maneuvers. The body temperature may decrease, particularly in elderly patients. The gradient between the ambient and toe temperature may be a fair index of peripheral blood flow and a measure for the severity of hypovolemic shock because a reduction in skin blood flow (cold, clammy skin) is an early and ominous sign of shock in view of selective cutaneous vasoconstriction.[123] Other signs of hypovolemic shock include tachypnea, oliguria/anuria, diaphoresis, cold and clammy skin with diminished capillary refill, and peripheral cyanosis.

The clinical diagnosis of hypovolemic shock is not difficult in the presence of hypotension and visible loss of

Table 26.1 Clinical Classification of Severity of Posthemorrhagic Hypovolemic Shock

Feature	Class I	Class II	Class III	Class IV
Blood loss				
mL	<750	750-1500	>1500-2000	>2000
%	<15	15-30	>30-40	>40
Heart rate (beats/min)	<100	>100	>120	>140
Blood pressure	Normal	Normal	Decreased	Decreased
Pulse pressure	Normal	Decreased	Decreased	Decreased
Respiratory rate	14-20	20-30	30-40	>40
Urinary output (mL/h)	>30	20-30	5-15	Negligible
Mental status	Slightly anxious	Mildly anxious	Anxious, confused	Confused, lethargic
Fluid replacement (mL/h)	Crystalloid	Crystalloid/colloid	Crystalloid and blood	Crystalloid and blood

blood volume, as occurs during trauma (e.g., fractures), gastrointestinal or pulmonary hemorrhage, burn wounds, and diarrhea. Internal hemorrhage after a ruptured aortic aneurysm, blunt abdominal trauma, or hemothorax is difficult to diagnose except when the history of the patient and obvious physical signs, including dullness on thoracic percussion and abdominal distention and tenderness, point to potential internal bleeding. In the case of upper gastrointestinal blood loss, one should look for signs of chronic liver disease, including palmar erythema, spider nevi, and portal hypertension (ascites), because they could predict variceal bleeding as a cause of hypovolemic shock. Brown discoloration of the palms of the hands and mucosal membranes may point to adrenocortical insufficiency, and a smell of acetone in expiratory breath may point to uncontrolled (ketoacidotic) diabetes mellitus.

DIAGNOSTIC APPROACH

GENERAL

The diagnostic workup of a patient with hypovolemic shock should not hamper initial resuscitation. After the history and physical examination, the necessity for further diagnostic procedures depends on the underlying cause of shock.

If trauma and external blood loss are the cause of shock, control of external bleeding, crossmatching of blood, and infusion of fluids and blood components have a higher priority than further diagnostic procedures. Treat first what kills first. Blunt chest trauma can be complicated by aortic rupture, tension pneumothorax, hemothorax or hemopericardium, and tamponade. A chest radiograph can be useful to diagnose these conditions. After blunt abdominal trauma, splenic or hepatic ruptures are possible, and an abdominal tap and analysis of the fluid can be performed to exclude or establish intra-abdominal bleeding or hollow organ perforation.[273,274] This diagnostic procedure has been largely replaced, however, by imaging, if time permits, with help of so-called focused assessment sonography for trauma (FAST) or computed tomography of the abdomen in the emergency department. This helps in selecting patients for explorative laparotomy in order to avoid negative surgery or for percutaneous coiling.[273,274] The abdominal viscera show characteristic lesions in hemorrhagic shock with low filling of large veins, decreased perfusion of some organs, wall thickening, submucosal edema, and enhancement of the gut.[275] A ruptured abdominal aortic aneurysm can be diagnosed via ultrasonography or angiography if the patient's condition allows the use of such an invasive, time-consuming procedure. The usefulness of emergency aortic clamping or balloon tamponade for massive abdominal hemorrhage is controversial.[276] In the case of gastrointestinal hemorrhage, diagnostic procedures also are performed after initial resuscitation, including gastroscopy for upper gastrointestinal bleeding, sigmoidoscopy for lower gastrointestinal bleeding, and angiography. Introduction of a nasogastric tube (and early intubation) can be useful to aspirate blood, diagnose bleeding, prevent aspiration during vomiting, and follow the course of bleeding.

LABORATORY INVESTIGATIONS

At admission of a patient with suspected hypovolemic shock, blood samples should be taken to determine the hemoglobin/hematocrit and leukocyte and platelet counts; electrolyte, creatinine, and lactate concentrations; arterial blood gases and pH; and blood typing (crossmatching). Immediately after hemorrhage, the hemoglobin content and hematocrit of blood are normal, but they decrease in time with refilling of the plasma compartment, as does the protein content.* A high hemoglobin content and hematocrit can be encountered during pure loss of plasma (water), as occurs during burn wounds or severe diarrhea. Acute hypovolemic shock may be accompanied by slight leukopenia followed by leukocytosis.[46,111,112,248,253] If coagulation disorders are suspected (therapy with anticoagulants, liver disease, bleeding tendency), platelet counts and coagulation tests should be performed. Transient thrombocytopenia may ensue if shock is severe and massive amounts of whole blood are lost and rapidly replaced by erythrocyte concentrates or nonsanguineous fluids (i.e., through dilution). Isolated thrombocytopenia without DIC may thus occur.

The concentrations of electrolytes (sodium, potassium, chloride) in blood are essentially normal unless the concentrations in the fluid lost deviate from those in plasma (hypertonic and hypotonic dehydration) and resuscitation fluids and shock is accompanied by severe metabolic acidosis. In the latter example, potassium leaves the cell, potentially leading to hyperkalemia.[111,125] More often, however, less severe forms of shock are accompanied by hypokalemia because of adrenergic receptor–stimulated Na^+/K^+-ATPase. Saline fluid loading or overloading can result in hyperchloremic metabolic acidosis. Adrenocortical insufficiency may result in hyponatremia, hyperkalemia, and hyperchloremic acidosis, caused by changes in urinary excretion induced by mineralocorticoid deficiency. In a patient with liver disease, the corresponding abnormalities can be found in laboratory studies. In the case of uncontrolled diabetes mellitus, hyperglycemia and glucosuria are observed. As previously mentioned, the glucose concentrations in blood can be elevated in early shock and, occasionally, depressed in late shock. Finally, the concentration of unbound Ca^{2+} in blood may diminish during hypovolemic shock after cellular uptake and polytransfusion of red blood cell concentrates if they contain calcium-binding citrate as an anticoagulant.[127,150]

During hypovolemic shock, metabolic acidosis, often associated with an elevated lactate level in blood, is common and of prognostic significance, although the decrease in bicarbonate and base excess may not parallel the increase in lactate.[27,31-33,38,41] The pH can be subnormal after lactic acidosis and a decrease in the bicarbonate content, even if ameliorated by hyperventilation and a decrease in P_{CO_2}.[27,32,33,49,50] The lactate level in blood can be determined rapidly and followed frequently (every 2 hours). The lactate level and its course during treatment also is of prognostic significance during shock because during successful treatment the lactate level decreases and the bicarbonate concentration and pH increase, whereas an unchanged or even increased lactate level during resuscitation is usually

*126, 132, 133, 137, 182, 183, 277, 278

associated with morbidity, including sepsis, MOF, and death.[27,31,32,56] An elevated anion gap, the difference between the sodium on the one hand and the sum of the bicarbonate and chloride concentrations in blood on the other hand, can be a first sign of lactic acidosis, although, as previously mentioned, elevated lactate levels may not be associated with acidosis in the absence of an oxygen debt.[27] The serum creatinine concentration is initially normal. The urea content increases following prerenal renal insufficiency, catabolism, or breakdown of blood in the gut during gastrointestinal hemorrhage. In the urine, the osmolarity is increased.

The sodium content is low, together with a low fractional excretion of sodium (FE_{Na}),[138] calculated as the quotient of urinary (U) and plasma (P) sodium (Na) and creatinine (creat) concentrations:

$$FE_{Na} = (U_{Na}/P_{Na})/(U_{creat}/P_{creat})$$

In case of acute renal injury (acute tubular necrosis), the urinary sodium content and fractional excretion are increased.[138] This increased sodium also occurs during adrenocortical insufficiency. Prior diuretic therapy may invalidate this diagnostic tool, however, whereas the fractional excretion of urea may not be affected by diuretics.[104] Tubular injury may be tracked from increased urinary excretion of biomarkers, which may help predict the need for renal replacement therapy.[104]

Miscellaneous abnormalities may include elevated levels of nitrate and nitrite, the stable breakdown products of NO.[269] Transient elevations of bilirubin, alkaline phosphatase, γ-glutamyltransferase, and transaminases in blood may be severe and denote ischemic liver damage.[222,223] Elevations of creatinine kinase may be caused by skeletal muscle, cardiac, gut, or, less likely, brain damage. Elevated troponin concentrations may specifically indicate cardiac injury.[163,173]

MONITORING

Noninvasive monitoring of arterial blood pressure to judge the course of shock and its response to treatment suffices for some patients with hypovolemic shock. Nevertheless, there may be substantial differences between the invasive and noninvasive readings of arterial blood pressure, favoring arterial catheterization and invasive monitoring. Urinary output should be measured hourly in patients with shock to judge the adequacy of treatment because transition of oliguria to a diuresis exceeding 40 mL/hour is an indicator of adequate renal perfusion. The gradient between toe and body temperature and capillary refill time can be used as noninvasive indices of peripheral perfusion.[123]

Unless hypovolemic shock is rapidly reversed by initial infusion of fluids, there is often a need for hemodynamic and respiratory monitoring in the intensive care unit for a patient with hypovolemic shock. The goal of monitoring is to document the course of shock and its reaction to treatment. Complications can be diagnosed in an early phase so that action can be rapidly undertaken, if necessary. Respiratory monitoring is meant to detect, at an early stage, respiratory insufficiency and muscle fatigue, which are caused by an imbalance in oxygen supply to demand and which may necessitate intubation and mechanical ventilatory support.[50]

Arterial blood pressure can be monitored invasively via a catheter in the radial, axillary, or femoral artery, introduced percutaneously using the Seldinger technique, under aseptic conditions. Percutaneous insertion of a double-lumen or triple-lumen central venous catheter may be useful but does not allow for more rapid fluid infusion than through two peripheral cannulas. The internal jugular, subclavian, or femoral vein may be used for that purpose. This also permits monitoring of CVP and oxygen saturation and a measure of total body oxygen supply-to-demand ratio and predictor of fluid responsiveness. Pressures in the lesser circulation (pulmonary arterial pressure and PCWP) can be measured with the help of a balloon-tipped pulmonary artery catheter inserted percutaneously and advanced under pressure monitoring until the inflated balloon wedges in a pulmonary artery side branch. This catheter also allows for thermodilution measurement of cardiac output and obtaining mixed venous blood for blood gas analysis.[73,279] Together with arterial blood measurement of oxygen variables, this allows the calculation of oxygen delivery, extraction, and uptake.[9,25,73] These calculations may contribute to judging the severity of shock and its response to treatment.[6,9,25,73]

The CVP reflects the filling pressure of the right ventricle, and the PCWP reflects the left atrial pressure and, in the absence of mitral valve disease, the filling pressure of the left ventricle.[19] Under certain circumstances, however, including ventilation with positive end-expiratory pressure or measurement above the level of the left atrium, when the measured pressure is more influenced by alveolar than by venous pressure, the CVP and PCWP may overestimate true (i.e., transmural) right and left atrial pressures. The response of filling pressure and cardiac output to fluid loading, as measured with the central venous or pulmonary artery catheter, is an index of myocardial function and can be useful to assess fluid responsiveness, particularly in case of preexistent and prognostically unfavorable cardiac disease.* Measurement of PCWP is important if function or compliance of the left ventricle is altered (e.g., in case of preexistent heart disease), when the CVP may underestimate PCWP.[55,71] Conversely, the CVP may overestimate PCWP in cases of severe pulmonary hypertension and right ventricular failure. It has been suggested that changes in CVP during fluid loading do not predict changes in PCWP.[71] The intensity and speed of therapy can be guided by the response of filling pressures and cardiac output, as measured with the use of the central venous or pulmonary artery catheter.[9,19,31,42,55]

These measurements also can help to time, choose, and dose concomitant therapy with inotropic or vasopressor agents. Together with the plasma colloid osmotic pressure, the PCWP determines filtration of fluid across pulmonary capillaries according to the Starling equation. Monitoring of the PCWP during infusion of fluids may prevent pulmonary edema because infusion can be guided by the filling pressures of the heart. Taken together, data obtained with the pulmonary artery catheter are useful if the hypovolemic origin of shock is not immediately apparent in complicated cases, as in patients with preexistent cardiac disease.[9,25,73] Data obtained with the catheter are of diagnostic value in complicated forms of shock because hypovolemic shock is

*19, 20, 55, 71, 159, 171

characterized by low filling pressures and cardiac output and a high peripheral vascular resistance. These characteristics may serve to differentiate from other types of shock. The indications for insertion may also include a high risk for shock in patients undergoing major surgery and shock of unknown origin when clinical judgment fails to recognize severe hypovolemia.

Difficulties during treatment also may constitute indications for pulmonary artery catheterization, including hypovolemic shock unresponsive to liberal fluid repletion in the absence of a low jugular venous pressure or CVP and hypovolemic shock together with preexistent cardiac disease unresponsive to fluid repletion if a large discrepancy between CVP and PCWP is suspected and if vasoactive drugs are considered. Monitoring the PCWP may help to lessen the risk for pulmonary edema during fluid loading. Contraindications for pulmonary artery catheterization include those for central venous catheterization. The complications of the technique are discussed elsewhere. Although the use of pulmonary artery catheters is hotly debated because of lack of direct evidence that they help to increase survival, there are some indications that therapy guided by variables collected with the catheter improves the outcome of selected critically ill patients after trauma or surgery.[9,25,73,280] Nevertheless, the exact hemodynamic and metabolic resuscitation goals are difficult to define, so the usefulness of the pulmonary artery catheter is difficult to prove.[9,26,42,67,280]

As an alternative to invasively inserted catheters, various less invasive or even noninvasive (pulse contour–based) systems have been developed that circumvent some of the problems associated with filling pressures as preload indicators and predictors of responsiveness of cardiac output to fluid loading.[19,20,281] Among others, the transpulmonary thermodilution technique with detection of thermal changes after central venous injection of cold dextrose 5% in water in the iliac artery allows for calculation of cardiac output, global end-diastolic volume, and extravascular lung water—measures of cardiac preload, pulmonary fluid filtration, and edema.[281] Assessment of cardiac volumes can be helpful to judge function, similar to echocardiography.[157,281] The latter technique also evaluates filling or injury of large vessels, suspected cardiac contusion, and pericardial tamponade.[282] The diameter (changes) of the large veins can be used as an indicator of filling status. The use of pulse-contour techniques for beat-to-beat evaluation of arterial pressure curve–derived stroke volume, as well as pulse pressure and stroke volume variations invoked by the respiratory cycle to guide fluid treatment in mechanically ventilated patients, remains controversial.[20,281] The esophageal Doppler flow probe with which flow time, stroke volume, and cardiac output can be estimated is somewhat operator dependent.

Developments in monitoring the circulation of a patient in hypovolemic shock further include continuous monitoring of central venous or mixed venous oxygen saturation with the help of the fiber-optic technique introduced via catheters, allowing for the continuous evaluation of the oxygen supply-to-demand ratio; right ventricular end-diastolic volume monitoring as an index of filling status; and measurement of tissue blood flow, Po_2, Pco_2, and oxygenation by electrodes and optic techniques.* Venous O_2 saturations may indeed help to guide fluid resuscitation in clinical practice because a low saturation increases upon adequate fluid challenges in fluid-responsive patients. Tissue Po_2 decreases and Pco_2 increases during regional perfusion failure, and these events (in skin, conjunctiva, muscle, or bladder) are probably early signs of hypovolemia following redistribution of blood flow before hypotension ensues and have be used as guides to treatment.* The adequacy of gastrointestinal blood flow can be judged noninvasively with the help of a tonometer balloon catheter in the stomach (or gut) or with help of a sensor sublingually or buccally, in which fluid or air is instilled, and the Pco_2 is measured to calculate the mucosal-to-blood Pco_2 gradient, as explained previously.† Fluid treatment guided by the adequacy of gastrointestinal mucosal perfusion as judged by tonometry could improve the outcome of hemorrhaged trauma patients compared with resuscitation based on standard hemodynamic variables alone.[40,123,209,211]

Monitoring the end-tidal CO_2 fraction, determined by and directly related to the blood flow–dependent tissue CO_2 production, and the gradient to arterial Pco_2, determined by blood flow–dependent dead-space ventilation, can help to judge the response to resuscitation.[49,65] Hydrostatic pressure measurements in the urinary bladder may reflect the measurements in the abdominal compartment and may help to identify intra-abdominal hypertension and abdominal compartment syndrome developing during extensive fluid resuscitation.[285] This may impair gut and renal perfusion with subsequent dysfunction and warrant decompression laparotomy.[285]

APPROACH TO MANAGEMENT

GENERAL

Treatment of shock cannot be delayed, so in practice diagnosis and treatment are done simultaneously. Treatment of hypovolemic shock is aimed at the restoration of the circulation and treatment of the underlying cause. Box 26.2 describes some general guidelines, but we do not specifically address burn wound shock requiring a special approach. The main therapeutic goal in hypovolemic shock is to restore circulating blood volume and to optimize oxygen delivery so that oxygen uptake plateaus (see Fig. 26.1) and meets tissue needs.[72,286] Optimization of cardiac output, stroke work, and tissue oxygenation and maintenance of arterial blood pressure are physiologically reasonable resuscitation targets for patients.[42] Optimization does not imply maximization above levels adequate for tissue needs.[26,67] Studies by some investigators have suggested that supranormal rather than normal oxygen delivery and consumption may be associated with survival from severe trauma or hemorrhage, including a ruptured aortic aneurysm, and that therapeutic targeting at these values (with oxygen delivery >600 mL/minute/m^2 and oxygen consumption >170 mL/minute/m^2) improves the outcome of severe trauma in humans.[9,25,40,42,83] These concepts are highly controversial, however. In any case, resuscitation based on blood pressure

*30, 44, 48, 53, 59, 68, 123, 145, 209, 283, 284

*8, 44, 48, 59, 68, 123

†40, 54, 68, 92, 106, 139, 166, 196, 208, 210, 211

Box 26.2 Guidelines for Treatment of Hypovolemic Shock

1. Insert large-bore intravenous catheter; perform laboratory investigations (crossmatching, hemoglobin/hematocrit, platelet count, electrolytes, creatinine, arterial blood gas analysis and pH, lactate, coagulation parameters, transaminases, albumin). Watch for need to supply oxygen, intubation, or artificial ventilation (so that arterial Po_2 > 60 mm Hg and oxygen saturation > 90%).
2. Resuscitation with fluids is done primarily with crystalloids, sometimes colloids. At >25% loss of blood volume, give erythrocyte concentrates; at >60% loss, also give fresh frozen plasma (e.g., after about three erythrocyte concentrates and earlier in case of massive bleeding or disturbed coagulation). In case of polytransfusions (>80% loss) and platelet counts <50 (<100 in massive and intracranial bleeding) × 10^9/L, platelet suspensions should be given. Massive red blood cell transfusion is preferably performed via microfilter. Also consider antifibrinolytics and fibrinogen.
3. Diagnose and treat underlying cause, concomitantly with guideline 2.

alone probably does not fully restore tissue oxygenation, particularly in the case of myocardial dysfunction after shock and resuscitation.[42,55]

Adequate resuscitation from hypovolemic shock should result in an increase in oxygen delivery and uptake, a decrease in lactate levels, and amelioration of metabolic acidosis.* Concomitantly with the increase in cardiac output, arterial blood pressure increases, but normal levels may not be necessary to aim at during resuscitation.[71,72,172] Indeed, successful resuscitation in terms of a restored cardiac output and arterial blood pressure may poorly reflect effective recovery of tissue perfusion, even though reversal of oliguria is considered a favorable return of renal perfusion.† Animal experiments have suggested that early circulatory optimization also ameliorates inflammatory changes after trauma/hemorrhage. In attempts to restore oxygen delivery, hypoxemia should be prevented or corrected, although recent evidence suggests that hypoxic resuscitation ameliorates proinflammatory responses to reperfusion as compared to normoxic resuscitation.[234] The arterial oxygen saturation, important for the oxygen content of delivered blood, usually exceeds 90% if the Po_2 is greater than 60 mm Hg. If arterial Po_2 is less than 60 mm Hg, supplemental oxygen can be given through a nasal cannula or mask, but hyperoxemia should be avoided. The patient should be intubated and artificially ventilated in case of impending respiratory insufficiency from whatever cause. Prophylactic positive end-expiratory pressure in attempts to prevent the development of ARDS in at-risk patients, including patients with traumatic/hemorrhagic shock, is useless.

For the initial stabilization of trauma patients in shock with severe abdominal trauma or bleeding from lower extremities, passive leg raising or Trendelenburg positioning has been used, but a large benefit on preload-augmented tissue oxygen delivery has been doubted.[8,19,20,287] The pneumatic antishock garment can be applied as a temporary, immediately lifesaving procedure to (1) stop the hemorrhage and splint pelvic and lower extremity fractures for transportation of the patient after inflation, (2) mobilize blood volume by exerting external pressure on the leg and abdomen, and (3) redirect flow toward vital organs such as the heart and brain.[288-290] Use of the garment and hypertonic saline may act synergistically.[288] The disadvantages of the procedure include aggravation of pressure-dependent and uncontrolled bleeding and ischemia of intra-abdominal organs. Deflation should be gradual to prevent lethal hypotension after return into the circulation of vasoactive substances and lactic acid from ischemic tissue.[288,289] The use of the pneumatic antishock garment has greatly declined in recent decades. Spontaneous breathing against an inspiratory threshold or decreasing expiratory pressure during mechanical ventilation may increase venous return and has been studied experimentally.[291] Measures to establish a way to the bloodstream for infusing fluids include insertion of a large-bore catheter in a peripheral vein or, if cannulation of peripheral veins seems impossible because of collapse, a catheter in a central (i.e., jugular/subclavian) vein. The latter catheter also allows monitoring of CVP. The intraosseous route for administration of hypertonic fluids is particularly useful in traumatized children with hypovolemic shock.[292] To this end, a marrow screw is inserted in the sternum or tibia. Fluids can be given by gravity or pressure.

Further treatment of hypovolemic shock depends on the underlying cause. Immediate surgery is warranted in case of extensive trauma and ongoing internal or external blood loss. Massive intra-abdominal bleeding after blunt or penetrating injury may warrant attempts for control by drug therapy with vasopressin, aortic clamping, or preferably, coiling during a radiologic examination prior to laparotomy for insufficient control. Gastrointestinal hemorrhage can be stopped by conservative treatment, including histamine-2 receptor blockade and endoscopic electrocoagulation or laser coagulation of bleeding peptic ulcers, or coiling of bleeding vessel during angiography. Bleeding varices can be treated by continuous infusion of vasopressin or somatostatin, a Sengstaken-Blakemore balloon tube, endoscopic injection sclerotherapy or banding, or transjugular intrahepatic portosystemic shunt. Surgery is rarely necessary in the institutional presence of experienced intervention radiologists. Apart from fluids, uncontrolled diabetes mellitus necessitates continuous intravenous infusion of insulin (about 6 U/hour). Acute adrenocortical insufficiency warrants administration of steroids (hydrocortisone 100 mg two to four times daily).

RESUSCITATION STRATEGIES

The speed with which shock can be reversed depends on the delay from onset to treatment and the severity of shock, as estimated from the clinical condition and hemodynamic status. The speed of fluid infusion can be guided by the clinical condition of the patient, heart rate and blood pressure, diuresis, and determinations every 2 hours of the arterial blood lactate level and acid-base balance.[31] Repeated assessment of jugular venous pressure, auscultation of the

*9, 26, 27, 31–33, 42, 67, 71–73, 83, 172
†30, 79, 111, 129, 144, 149, 166, 215

lungs, and arterial blood gases are indicated to prevent overhydration and pulmonary edema. If a central venous or pulmonary artery catheter is in place, a fluid challenge protocol can be used (Table 26.2).[31] Monitoring of central venous or PCWP or preload volumes allows for rapid infusion of solutions and evaluation of the response of oxygen delivery and uptake to resuscitation.[9,25,31,73] When in doubt, predicting fluid responsiveness in the patient, for instance with cardiac failure on mechanical ventilation, by passive leg raising and other tests that reversibly challenge the circulation can be helpful to further guide fluid therapy and avoid harmful fluid overloading.[19,20]

The usefulness of immediate and vigorous resuscitation in the course of uncontrolled bleeding (e.g., after penetrating vascular trauma) has been challenged in recent years.[279,293-295] Studies have shown that infusion of substantial amounts of nonsanguineous fluids and increasing pressure-dependent bleeding lead to dilution of blood components, coagulation disturbances, and increased mortality risk unless the bleeding is controlled before resuscitation.[279,290,294,295] The clinical implication is that resuscitation perhaps should not take place, at least not vigorously, at the scene of the accident when bleeding cannot be controlled and transport to the hospital where the bleeding can be controlled is practicable. This may apply not only to trauma patients but also to patients with a ruptured abdominal aneurysm. Authors have proposed slow (low volume) rather than rapid (early and large volume) infusion rates and controlled hypotensive resuscitation (e.g., with help of vasodilators) at least as long as bleeding is uncontrolled.[290,293,294,296-298] The value of this type of resuscitation in humans with hyperoncotic/hypertonic solutions, including acetate with vasodilating and buffering properties, is debatable.[210,279,298] Also, the levels of hypotension that are safe remain unclear.[299] Conversely, early vasopressor therapy by vasopressin, for instance, may benefit patient outcomes more than large-volume infusions.[300] The treatment of massive bleeding by blood products requires an institutional protocol. Closed-loop control of fluid therapy may become clinically applicable in the near future.[301]

Table 26.2 Fluid Therapy

Timing	CVP (cm H_2O*) (Guided by)	PCWP (mm Hg) (Guided by)	Infusion
Start	<8	<10	200 mL/10 min
	<12	<14	100 mL/10 min
	= 12	= 14	50 mL/10 min
During infusion	↑ >5	↑ >7	Stop
After 10 min	= 2	= 3	Continue
	2 > ↑ = 5	3 > ↑ = 7	Wait 10 min
	↑ >5	↑ >7	Stop
After waiting	Still ↑ >2	Still ↑ >3	Stop
10 min	↑ = 2	↑ = 3	Repeat

*10 cm H_2O = 7.3 mm Hg.
CVP, central venous pressure; PCWP, pulmonary capillary wedge pressure.
Adapted from Weil MH, Henning RJ: New concepts in the diagnosis and fluid treatment of circulatory shock. Anesth Analg 1979;58:124.

FLUIDS

During hypovolemic shock, the repletion of intravascular volume is of primary importance to restore cardiac output and oxygen transport to the tissues before repletion of the interstitial and intracellular fluids.* Available fluids are described in Tables 26.3 to 26.5. Electrolyte solutions (the crystalloid fluids) are shown in Table 26.3, and high-molecular-weight solutions (the colloid fluids) are shown in Tables 26.4 and 26.5. In the first group, the hypertonic fluids (i.e., fluids with a higher osmolarity than plasma) are presented. Among the colloid solutions are solutions with a higher colloid osmotic pressure than plasma—the hyperoncotic solutions. Hypertonic and hyperoncotic solutions are plasma expanders because they are able to mobilize cellular and interstitial fluid during resuscitation and to expand plasma volume rapidly.

Table 26.6 shows how the volume of the various compartments is replenished during fluid resuscitation. Because infusion of glucose 5% hardly increases intravascular volume, this solution has no place in resuscitation from hypovolemic shock. Lactated Ringer's solution containing

*9, 25, 31, 33, 69, 71–73, 172, 209, 286, 294, 302–304

Table 26.3 Crystalloid Fluids

Fluid	Na^+ (mmol/L)	K^+ (mmol/L)	Cl^- (mmol/L)	Ca^{2+} (mmol/L)	Glucose (mmol/L)	Lactate (mmol/L)	HCO_3^- (mmol/L)	Osmolarity (mOsm/L)
Glucose 5%					278			278
NaCl 0.65%	111		111					222
NaCl 0.9%	154		154					308
NaCl 3%	513		513					1025
NaCl 7.5%	1283		1283					2567
NaCl 30%	5000		5000					10,000
Ringer's lactate	130	4	110	3		27		275
$NaHCO_3$ 1.4%	167						167	334
$NaHCO_3$ 4.2%	500						500	1000
$NaHCO_3$ 8.4%	1000						1000	2000

Table 26.4 Pharmacology of Colloid Fluids

Name	Component (g/L)	Na^+ (mmol/L)	K^+ (mmol/L)	Cl^- (mmol/L)	Ca^{2+} (mmol/L)	Glucose (mmol/L)	Lactate (mmol/L)	Osmolarity (mOsm/L)
Natural Colloids								
Albumin 5%	50	130-160		130-160				308
Albumin 25%	240 g with globulins 10 g	130-160		130-160				1500
Plasma protein fraction 5%	Albumin 44 g with globulins 6 g	130-160	<2			167		290
Gelatin								
Urea-gelatin + electrolytes	35	145	5.1	145	6.25			391
Modified gelatin + electrolytes	30	152	5	100			30	320
Dextran (MW)								
Dextran 40 + glucose 5%	50					278		278
Dextran 40 + NaCl 0.9%	50	154		154				310
Dextran 40 + glucose 5%	100					278		278
Dextran 40 + NaCl 0.9%	100	154		154				310
Dextran 70 + glucose 5%	60					278		278
Dextran 70 + NaCl 0.9%	60	154		154				310
Starch (MW)								
Hydroxyethyl starch (130) + NaCl 0.9%	60	154		154				310
Hydroxyethyl starch (200) + NaCl 0.9%	60/100	154		154				310
Hydroxyethyl starch (450) + NaCl 0.9%	60	154		154				310
Pentastarch (264) + NaCl 0.9%	100	154		154				354

MW, molecular weight in thousands.

K^+ should not be used during renal insufficiency because of the danger of inducing hyperkalemia. Infusion of lactate-containing solutions during lactic acidosis may be controversial because the capacity of the liver to regenerate bicarbonate from lactate may be impaired.[33] Nevertheless, infusion of lactate-containing solutions such as lactated Ringer's for resuscitation from hypovolemic shock generally does not substantially increase lactate levels, worsen acidosis, or adversely affect outcome.[305] However, racemic Ringer's lactate may be proinflammatory and proapoptotic as compared to normal saline and only L-lactate containing solutions are therefore currently recommended.[191] Adverse effects of overzealous fluid administration of any type include promotion of pulmonary edema and ascites formation with subsequent aggravation of abdominal compartment syndrome.[285,286]

The natural colloids consist of albumin and plasma solutions. Albumin is an effective colloidal solution for intravascular volume repletion, and its intravascular half-life is approximately 16 hours.* For the artificial colloids, the volume-expanding effect and the duration of action generally increase with increasing in vivo molecular weight (Table 26.7). About one third of the hyperoncotic fluids with high molecular weight (dextran 70 and hydroxyethylstarch) may still be in the circulation after 24 hours, whereas dextran 40 is retained for approximately 3 hours. Dextrans and gelatins are perhaps equally effective in restoring circulating volume.[309,310] The latter substances might increase tissue blood flow in the microcirculation. Dextrans are currently less often used than gelatins and starches and institutional

*9, 25, 135, 137, 172, 303, 304, 306–308

Table 26.5 Biology of Colloid Fluids

Type	Molecular Weight	Colloid Osmotic Pressure (mm Hg)	Maximum Dose (mL/kg/24 h)	Anaphylactoid Reactions	Coagulation	Diuresis
Albumin	69,000					
5 g/L		20	—	Rare	—	(↓)
25 g/L		100	—	Rare	—	(↓)
Dextran						
Dextran 40	40,000					
50 g/L		27	40	Rare	↓	↓
100 g/L		170	20	Rare	↓	↓
Dextran 70	70,000					
60 g/L		59	20	Rare	↓	↓
Gelatin	35,000					
35-40 g/L		26-30	20	Rare	—	—
Starch						
Hydroxyethylstarch, 60 g/L	130,000	36	33	Very rare	(↓)	(↓)
Hydroxyethylstarch, 60 or 100 g/L	200,000	25	20	Very rare	(↓)	(↓)
Hydroxyethylstarch, 60 g/L	450,000	30	20	Very rare	(↓)	(↓)
Pentastarch, 100 g/L	264,000	55		Very rare	(↓)	(↓)

↓, decrease; (↓), risk for decrease.

Table 26.6 Changes in Volume of Body Compartments During Infusion of Fluids

Compartment	Glucose 5%	NaCl 0.9%	Hypertonic NaCl	Normal COP Colloids	High COP Colloids
Intravascular	↑	↑	↑↑	↑↑	↑↑↑
Interstitial	↑↑	↑↑	↓	—	↓
Intracellular	↑↑↑	—	↓	—	↓

COP, colloid osmotic pressure.

Table 26.7 Distribution of Artificial Colloids 24 Hours After Intravenous Infusion in Normal Volunteers

Colloid	Half-life (h)	Concentration in Blood (%) Plasma*	Urine*	Extravascular*	Overall Survival
Dextran 40	2.5	18	60	22	144 h
Dextran 70	25.5	29	38	33	4-6 wk
Gelatins	3.5	13	65	21	168 h
Hydroxyethylstarch 130 or 200	2.5	7	60	33	96 h
Hydroxyethylstarch 450	25.5	38	39	23	17-26 wk

*Percent total dose administered.

Adapted from Mishler JM: Systemic plasma volume expanders: Their pharmacology, safety, and clinical efficacy. Clin Haematol 1984; 13:75.

and geographic habits largely determine the choice among fluids.

The starch compounds have gained wide interest for the resuscitation of hypovolemic shock.* These colloids are at least as effective as albumin but less expensive.[135,136,172,308,312] Because the molecular range of the starch compounds varies enormously, the pharmacokinetics are complex.[311] Nevertheless, about 40% of the infused hetastarch (molecular weight >200) still remains in the circulation after 24 hours because 30% of the infused substance may have a half-life of 67 hours. Ninety percent of smaller starch is cleared in 24 hours. The duration of the volume-expanding effect of the starches depends not only on molecular range and concentration but also on the so-called substitution

*62, 136, 170, 303, 304, 308, 311

grade, which is the number of hydroxyethyl groups per glucose unit, and the substitution type, the ratio of C2 to C6 hydroxyethylation.[311] A high molecular weight, high substitution grade, and high C2/C6 ratio retard breakdown by plasma amylase and prolong intravascular retention. The residual starch compounds are partly excreted by urine and partly taken up by the reticuloendothelial system. Accumulation may also occur in dendritic cells of the skin and the liver and in the renal tubules, with subsequent adverse effects. Starch compounds may increase the amylase level in blood and may confound the diagnosis of acute pancreatitis. Experimental evidence shows that some starch compounds, particularly in the 100,000 to 300,000 D molecular weight range, have the advantage in sealing the capillary endothelium in case of increased permeability after ischemia or trauma, diminishing fluid and protein filtration and preventing edema.[136,179,311,312]

In the resuscitation of hypovolemic shock (e.g., after trauma or burns), the use of hypertonic solutions with sodium concentrations greater than 0.9% also has gained wide interest.* The solutions essentially consist of hypertonic sodium chloride, to which colloids have often been added. The combinations include NaCl 7.5% with dextran 70 (6%/10%), NaCl 7.2% with dextran 60 (10%), and NaCl 7.5% with hydroxyethylstarch 6%.[33,62,122,314-317] Hypertonic solutions usually result, at a much lower infusion volume than isotonic solutions (small volume resuscitation), in a rapid hemodynamic improvement, that is, an increase in cardiac output and in oxygen delivery and uptake and arterial blood pressure in experimental animals and patients with traumatic/hypovolemic shock.† Infusion of rapidly acting hypertonic saline, particularly if combined with hyperoncotic colloids, increases survival in bleeding animals compared with infusion of either component or other isotonic or hypertonic (nonelectrolyte) solutions.[316] Clinical trials also have shown some value of hypertonic solutions in the initial treatment of hypovolemic shock after burns and trauma with uncontrolled bleeding.[119,286,314,316,317] The use of hypertonic saline solutions, however, warrants close monitoring of plasma sodium levels to prevent excessive hypernatremia and hyperosmolarity.[313-316]

The hypertonic fluids primarily act through resorption of interstitial and cellular fluid volume and expansion of the plasma volume.[7,131,314] It has been calculated that only 4 mL/kg 7.5% saline solution can increase circulating plasma volume by 8 to 12 mL/kg body weight. A hyperosmolarity-induced increase in cardiac contractility may also contribute to the increase in cardiac output, although this effect has been doubted.[318] Other potential mechanisms include activation of pituitary and pulmonary osmoreceptors, leading to release of vasopressin and vagal afferent-mediated venoconstriction, and hyperosmolarity-induced arterial vasodilation.[7,62,313,314] Infusion of hypertonic sodium combined with hyperoncotic colloid solutions more rapidly and completely increases cardiac output and arterial blood pressure, and the effects last longer than those produced with infusion of hypertonic or colloid solutions alone.[313-317] During infusion of hypertonic saline, particularly if combined with hyperoncotic colloid solutions, the distribution of peripheral oxygen delivery is reversed to a more favorable pattern with preferential perfusion of vital organs, including gut and kidney.[62,313] The increase in oxygen uptake in bled dogs was less rapid and complete during resuscitation with hypertonic saline plus hydroxyethylstarch, however, than during infusion of relatively large volumes of the latter.[33,62]

The hypertonic solutions may also ameliorate immunodepression, the translocation of bacteria, and susceptibility to sepsis after hypovolemic shock in rodents.[201,319] Hypertonic solutions (plus dextrans) restore capillary blood flow and organ function during resuscitation better than isoosmotic fluids because of their ability, among others, to reduce endothelial cell swelling, adhesion molecule expression, neutrophil activation and adherence, and cellular apoptosis compared with normotonic crystalloids such as racemic Ringer's lactate.[191,320] Hypertonic solutions may also prevent lung injury after hemorrhage/resuscitation, probably via these mechanisms.[95,119,122,319]

*33, 62, 119, 122, 201, 210, 286, 292, 303, 313–317
†33, 62, 131, 210, 292, 313–317

FLUID CONTROVERSIES

The choice between available fluids should be guided by the estimated extent and type of fluid losses; their composition and localization; and the properties of infusion fluids, their distribution over body compartments, and, perhaps, the associated costs, which are high for albumin, intermediate for artificial colloids, and low for crystalloid solutions.[131,302-304] Nevertheless, the use of various solutions for resuscitation from hypovolemic shock is hotly debated, partly because the importance of the colloid osmotic pressure for resuscitation and prevention of pulmonary edema is uncertain.[302] Also, the relative merits and detriments (i.e., safety) of natural and artificial colloids remain unclear.[302,321]

Capillary filtration depends on the pericapillary hydrostatic and the colloid osmotic pressure gradient, according to the Starling equation. If at a given permeability an imbalance in pressures augments capillary filtration of fluids, a decrease in interstitial colloid osmotic pressure, an increase in interstitial hydrostatic pressure (which also depends on the compliance of the interstitium), and increased lymph flow can either alone or in combination partially prevent gross accumulation of interstitial fluid (edema). The colloid osmotic pressure of plasma is primarily determined by the plasma albumin content and normally measures about 24 mm Hg.[31,126,137,322] The pressure can be estimated from albumin and protein concentrations in plasma, but infusion of artificial colloid solutions invalidates this calculation, so proper assessment of plasma colloid osmotic pressure necessitates direct measurement.[137,323] Because of a decrease in circulating plasma protein levels, hypovolemic shock results in a decrease in plasma colloid osmotic pressure.* During hypoproteinemia and a reduced plasma colloid osmotic pressure, fluid filtration for a given hydrostatic pressure increases until the pericapillary colloid osmotic pressure gradient decreases and a new steady state, often at increased lymph flow, has been achieved.[133,135,136] Evoking safety mechanisms such as a reduced interstitial colloid osmotic pressure and increased lymph flow may keep the

*31, 126, 133, 134, 137, 182, 183

interstitium relatively dry, and these mechanisms may be more effective in the lung than in the systemic circulation.[133] During hypoproteinemia, the hydrostatic pressure needed to invoke pulmonary edema decreases, however, because of more rapid exhaustion of safety mechanisms.[135,324] Conversely, increased lung water caused by an elevated hydrostatic pressure can be ameliorated by colloid infusion.[324]

For a given increase in hydrostatic pressure, the infusion of crystalloids decreases the plasma colloid osmotic pressure and tends to enhance, if insufficiently compensated by a decrease in the pericapillary colloid osmotic pressure gradient, pulmonary and systemic fluid filtration and interstitial fluid expansion more than infusion of albumin/colloids, which maintain plasma colloid osmotic pressure.* Crystalloid solutions replenish not only the intravascular but also the interstitial space by increased filtration, whereas colloid fluids tend to primarily fill the former compartment, at least initially.[131,278] Widening of the intravascular-to-interstitial colloid osmotic pressure gradient may prevent increased fluid filtration, but the effect may be transient when some colloids have been filtered along with fluids into the interstitium and a new steady state of perimicrovascular pressure and draining lymph flow has been established.[136] The mechanism may form the basis for the well-known observation that colloid solutions yield a twofold to threefold greater expansion of the intravascular space than crystalloids and that the latter have greater tendency for edema formation for a given amount of fluid infused, so less colloid than crystalloid is probably needed for resuscitation to similar hemodynamic end points in hypovolemic shock.† In some clinical trials, colloids proved to be superior to crystalloids in resuscitation from hypovolemic shock,[137,172,309] in terms of both the speed and the extent of correction of the hemodynamic abnormalities. Conversely, this may also explain the observations of some investigators that during resuscitation from hypovolemic shock pulmonary edema can be prevented in part if the intravascular filtration pressure (i.e., the gradient between plasma colloid osmotic and PCWP) is kept greater than approximately 6 mm Hg, with an elevated risk for pulmonary edema, particularly in case of increased permeability, if the gradient is less than approximately 3 mm Hg, and that resuscitation with colloids less often induces evidence for pulmonary edema than infusion of crystalloids during hypovolemic shock.‡

If the permeability for proteins increases and the reflection coefficient decreases, the hydraulic conductance of the capillary membrane also increases.[133] Increased permeability for proteins increases capillary fluid filtration for a given intravascular hydrostatic pressure and promotes the formation of edema.[308] During increased permeability, the filtration of fluids and expansion of the interstitial fluid space depend more than normally on hydrostatic pressures and less on colloid osmotic pressures because the colloid osmotic pressure gradient is decreased.[133] The differences between the types of solutions in fluid filtration and formation of edema in the lung and peripheral tissues diminish.[326] This may explain in part why some clinical studies did not find a predictive value of the colloid osmotic pressure-PCWP gradient for pulmonary edema and lack of a difference between fluid types for formation of pulmonary edema and impaired gas exchange during resuscitation from hypovolemic shock.[302,307] Moreover, an increase in CVP increases the back-pressure for lymph flow. Careful animal studies on hypovolemic shock combined with a lung vascular injury showed, however, that colloids are more effective than crystalloids in restoring the circulation and that the former increased lung water less than the latter unless permeability was severely increased.[308,326] This can be explained by the fact that even in case of increased permeability the reflection coefficient is not zero, and that the pericapillary colloid pressure gradient still exerts some influence on the transcapillary movement of fluids.

Clinical studies on the colloid/crystalloid controversy may be difficult to interpret because of differences in patient populations and end points between fluid types.[302,321] Lack of similar end points used for resuscitation may partly explain why infusion of colloid solutions increased the risk for pulmonary failure compared with infusion of crystalloids because colloids, owing to their greater intravascular volume-repleting effect, tend to increase hydrostatic filtration pressure in the lung more rapidly than crystalloid fluids even though colloid osmotic pressure is maintained or increases during infusion of the former and decreases with the latter.[306] The importance of a difference in hydrostatic pressure for the risk of pulmonary edema would be accentuated in case of increased permeability.[306] Finally, pulmonary mechanics, gas exchange, and radiographic changes used to evaluate the effects of fluid infusions in many studies may not accurately reflect changes in lung water.[52,172,306-308]

There are safety concerns with artificial colloids, particularly in the presence of other risk factors for organ damage.[304,321] Potential disadvantages of (artificial) colloid over crystalloid solutions include inhibition of the coagulation system; the risk for anaphylactoid reactions; inhibition of renal salt and water excretion; renal injury; and perhaps, at least for albumin, depression of myocardial function, possibly owing to binding of Ca^{2+}, although this has not been seen in all studies.[171,172,321,327] Of all artificial colloids, dextrans affect coagulation most adversely, independently of hemodilution, by interfering with coagulation factors and diminishing thrombocyte and red blood cell aggregation.[327] The gelatins may also have some intrinsic effects on coagulation, whereas the anticoagulant effects of hydroxyethyl starches probably relate, in addition to hemodilution, to less endothelial release of von Willebrand factor.[290,311,327] Anaphylactoid reactions to artificial colloids are extremely rare and vary from slight fever and skin reactions to life-threatening anaphylactic shock. Starch compounds elicit these reactions less often than dextrans and gelatins.[311] Large-molecular-weight starches may accumulate in subcutaneous tissues and may cause pruritus, even for weeks after administration.[311] However, resuscitation of trauma patients with hydroxyxethyl starch may result in less endothelial damage, renal injury, and pulmonary dysfunction than resuscitation with gelatins.[179] Nevertheless, the renal damaging effect of starch is probably greater than that of gelatins in patients with prior risk factors for acute kidney injury.[321] Hence, colloids may contribute to the development of acute kidney injury and failure, particularly in the case of

---

*31, 126, 133–137, 172, 183, 303, 307, 324
†25, 135, 137, 172, 307–309, 325
‡31, 134, 137, 172, 303, 308, 309, 322, 323

overadministration, which may otherwise be more frequent with artificial colloids than with albumin/plasma solutions, which can be monitored by measurements of plasma albumin concentrations. As opposed to albumin/plasma, infusion of colloid solutions is often bound to a maximum (see Table 26.5). Side effects may be more frequent with artificial colloids than with albumin/plasma infusion even though the latter carries a very low risk of anaphylactoid reactions and disease transmission. Crystalloid and artificial colloid solutions may activate neutrophil-endothelial interactions and depress macrophage and immune functions more than albumin does.[191,321,328,329] In contrast to lactated Ringer's solution, Ringer's ethyl pyruvate solution has favorable anti-inflammatory and cell-protecting actions.[29,37]

If used in the resuscitation from hypovolemic shock, artificial colloids may still be preferred over natural colloids because the latter are more expensive and less available, even though albumin and plasma solutions are effective volume expanders. There is some evidence that the type of fluids infused during hypovolemia may influence the extent and speed with which oxygen uptake is restored: infusion of colloid (plasma/albumin) solutions in hypovolemic postoperative and trauma patients may increase uptake of oxygen for a given increment in plasma volume and oxygen delivery more rapidly than infusion of crystalloids and may thereby improve outcomes.[9,25,330] This is thought to result in part from increased diffusion distances for oxygen in the tissues subsequent to tissue edema, evoked by massive crystalloid infusion.[9,25,307] Administration of nonbuffered (unbalanced) crystalloid solutions such as normal saline carries the risk of hyperchloremic metabolic acidosis, which can be avoided in part by infusion of buffered (balanced) solutions such as Ringer's lactate.[325] Nevertheless, meta-analyses suggest, at least in some groups, a slightly increased mortality risk after resuscitation with artificial colloids.[302,321,331,332] In the SAFE study comparing albumin and saline for resuscitation in the intensive care unit, a slight but nonsignificant increase in mortality rate was observed in the (neuro)trauma subgroup treated by albumin infusions, although animal studies suggest some beneficial and anti-inflammatory effects of albumin resuscitation from hemorrhagic shock.[333]

BLOOD PRODUCTS AND SUBSTITUTES

Resuscitation with blood components may restore tissue oxygen delivery and energy metabolism more rapidly, completely, and persistently than resuscitation with crystalloid during hemorrhage and hypovolemic shock, although this is controversial.[162,305] Nevertheless, it has been suggested that infusion of sodium salts may be essential, and that addition of saline to blood improves survival from hypovolemic shock after hemorrhage because of correction of both the intravascular and the interstitial volume deficits.[313]

In the treatment of hypovolemic shock following ongoing hemorrhage, infusion of red blood cells in the form of erythrocyte concentrates, or packed red blood cells, remains crucial.[277,286,334] This is achieved by autotransfusion from uncontaminated areas during surgery, if possible; by infusion of blood group O Rh-negative donor blood in emergency situations; or by infusion of typed and stored/anticoagulated donor blood. The position of the oxyhemoglobin dissociation curve of old, stored blood is shifted to the left.[60,78] Although this theoretically may impair the delivery and uptake of oxygen in the tissues, the effects of these changes in animal experiments are usually limited and clinical repercussions are unclear.[60,76] Transfusion of substantial amounts of erythrocyte concentrates is preferentially accomplished through a microfilter to avoid alloimmunization and infusion of neutrophils and other cellular aggregates, which develop in time during storage of blood and which may lodge in the lung, promote pulmonary injury, and impair gas exchange, leading to TRALI.[175-177] Today, prior leukocyte-reduced red blood cell concentrates are often used, but it is controversial whether this is associated with less risk. Excluding multiparous women who may have become sensitized to allogenic leukocytes and may carry leukocyte antibodies contributing to TRALI is another strategy applied in some countries. Also, humoral mediators released in stored blood or during infusion might be responsible in part for pulmonary vascular injury after massive transfusion of blood.[180,190] Nevertheless, massive transfusion may remain a risk factor for bacterial sepsis, ARDS, and MOF, independently from bleeding and severity of hypovolemic shock.* Finally, transfusion of blood components and plasma carries a small risk of transmitting infectious diseases and depressing immune function.[305,329]

Because loss of blood also leads to loss of coagulation factors and platelets, and blood concentrations are diluted further during nonsanguineous fluid resuscitation, replenishing plasma levels by infusion of fresh frozen plasma and platelets is usually required to help stop ongoing bleeding.[262] Fresh frozen plasma should not be used solely for the treatment of hypovolemia, even though plasma may diminish endothelial hyperpermeability through restoration of glycocalyx.[262,271] The strategy of blood products infusion has undergone some changes in the last decade, in which studies suggest optimal hemostasis and outcome when fresh frozen plasma units are infused at a 1:1 ratio with packed red blood cell concentrates and random donor platelet units at a 1:3 to 1:5 ratio.[334,337,338] If, during resuscitation, the clotting times are prolonged by a factor of 1.5 or more, more fresh frozen plasma can be given, and if platelet counts decrease to less than 50 to 100 $\times 10^9$/L, platelets can be transfused, particularly in case of intracranial or life-threatening bleeding. The value of prophylactic administration of coagulation factors in a polytransfused, traumatized patient to prevent further bleeding after initial hemostasis is unclear, however. Supplementation of Ca^{2+} may be necessary only if more than 12 to 20 units of packed red blood cells, anticoagulated with Ca^{2+}-binding citrate, have been given if rapidly transfused and particularly if liver function is impaired.[150] Further treatment is guided by ionized Ca^{2+} determinations in plasma. Fibrinogen concentrates are increasingly used with increasing evidence that fibrinogen plays an important role in coagulation and that primary hyperfibrinolysis is common in trauma patients, as revealed by thrombelastometry.[334,337] Antifibrinolytic drugs, such as tranexaminic acid, given prior to fibrinogen concentrates are useful adjuncts.[339] The exact place of recombinant factor VIIa, a potent procoagulant, in the treatment of refractory bleeding has not been settled yet.[286,340] The factor stops

*84, 175–177, 180, 181, 190, 335, 336

bleeding and saves blood transfusion, but cost-effectiveness is unclear. Adverse effects include a tendency for thromboembolic events.[340] The bleeding tendency of trauma is also aggravated by hypothermia and acidosis, but it is unclear whether aggressive treatment of hypothermia or acidosis substantially ameliorates coagulation disturbances and to what extent DIC contributes.[181,264,337] The importance of the latter also remains somewhat unclear, and treatment may consist of infusion of antithrombin III concentrates or, in case of severe bleeding, of fresh frozen plasma and platelets.[181]

To overcome some of the problems associated with donor or autologous red blood cell transfusions, investigators have intensively searched for safe and effective hemoglobin substitutes applicable in humans.[230,286,341-343] These substitutes include chemical oxygen carriers, hemoglobin modifications, and liposome/vesicle-encapsulated hemoglobin.[344] The chemical hemoglobin modifications have been designed to prevent or limit the renal toxicity of free hemoglobin. They include polymerized, modified, cross-linked, and recombinant hemoglobins.[34,345] The use of hemoglobin substitutes has been under clinical investigation. Some nonrecombinant substitutes seemed to increase arterial and, particularly, pulmonary arterial blood pressure more than accounted for by fluid loading, but some compounds have more adverse effects than others.[346] This may relate to the property of hemoglobin to scavenge NO or release endothelin and platelet-activating factor, or combinations, and the use of these solutions is therefore still not without hazard.[346] Diaspirin cross-linked hemoglobin may beneficially influence intracranial hemodynamics during resuscitation from hypovolemic shock.[296] A clinical trial on diaspirin-cross-linked hemoglobin in trauma failed to improve survival over resuscitation with saline, however.[341] The use of hemoglobin substitutes such as perfluorocarbons has not yet reached the stage of widespread, routine clinical practice, although they may effectively carry oxygen in humans and may improve resuscitability from hypovolemic shock following bleeding in animals compared with nonhemoglobin-based solutions.[341-343,347] Further research is ongoing.

ACIDOSIS AND OPTIMAL HEMATOCRIT

The underlying idea for partial correction of metabolic acidosis is that acidosis is detrimental for, among others, myocardial function by increasing pulmonary artery pressure and right ventricular afterload, impairing catecholamine sensitivity, and diminishing adrenergic receptors and intracellular Ca^{2+} transport necessary for contraction, even if masked by increased sympathetic activity.[36,168] Metabolic acidosis may increase the tendency for life-threatening ventricular arrhythmias and may lessen defibrillation thresholds and vascular tone.[27] The need for treatment of metabolic (lactic) acidosis (e.g., by intravenous administration of buffer solutions) remains unclear.* Administration of sodium bicarbonate may carry the risk for aggravation of intracellular acidosis in the tissues because bicarbonate releases CO_2 during buffering and CO_2 more rapidly traverses the cell membrane than the bicarbonate ion.* Alkali therapy with sodium bicarbonate carries the risks of shifting the oxyhemoglobin dissociation curve to the left and impairing tissue oxygenation, a decrease in ionized Ca^{2+}, and causing hypernatremia and osmolarity, although the consequences of these theoretical drawbacks are unclear.[27,36,44] Albeit not beyond doubt, experimental and clinical studies suggest that the administration of buffers such as sodium bicarbonate is not harmful, even though the hemodynamic and metabolic effects of the solution may not surpass those obtained by saline infusion.† In many institutions, small doses of alkali buffers such as sodium bicarbonate (50 to 100 mL of a 4.2%, 0.5 mmol/mL solution) are still given to treat metabolic (lactic) acidosis if arterial pH is less than 7.2 and acidosis persists despite optimal cardiovascular resuscitation.[27,36] During sodium bicarbonate infusion, the patient should be hyperventilated to prevent hypercapnia in arterial blood and bicarbonate doses should be guided by the arterial blood acid-base status to prevent alkalosis and diminished oxygen release after overadministration.[27,44,348] Prevention of hypercapnia may obviate increased CO_2 diffusion and aggravation of intracellular acidosis.[27,36] The value of buffers, including bicarbonate/carbonate, that do not generate CO_2 and prevent aggravation of intracellular acidosis is still controversial.[27,35,348,349] Dichloroacetate is a stimulator of pyruvate dehydrogenase, and the drug may ameliorate lactate accumulation and postresuscitation organ dysfunction, but there is probably no benefit for patient outcome.[27,35,36]

The hematocrit is the main determinant of blood viscosity, and the latter determines, together with the geometric features of the vascular bed, the blood flow in the microvasculature.[120] Experimental studies suggest that during normovolemic hemodilution normal oxygen delivery is achieved at a range of hematocrit values from 12% to 65% for the heart; 30% to 65% for the brain; 30% to 55% for liver, intestine, and kidney; and 30% to 60% for the whole body because adaptations in vessel diameter and changes in blood flow in this hematocrit range are able to compensate for changes in oxygen content, maintaining a normal oxygen delivery.[85,120,265,350] The optimal hematocrit for the whole body may not conform to the regional optimal hematocrit.

Because blood is a non-newtonian fluid, so that blood viscosity depends not only on hematocrit but also on blood flow velocity (shear stress), there may be differences along the vascular profile in blood viscosity, with propensity for red blood cell aggregation in postcapillary venules, where flow velocity is lower than in arterioles, particularly during hypovolemic shock.[4,120] Increased blood viscosity in postcapillary venules may contribute to impaired tissue perfusion during hypovolemic shock.[4] Conversely, the volume status, myocardial function, and vascular tone contribute to blood viscosity so that, for example, the optimal hematocrit for oxygen delivery is lower during hypovolemia than hypervolemia.[21,120,350] Finally, red blood cell deformability is decreased in hemorrhagic shock, contributing to increased viscosity.[224]

*27, 35, 36, 44, 52, 348, 349

*27, 35, 36, 52, 348, 349
†27, 35, 36, 44, 348, 349

Taken together, it is hard to generally define the optimal hematocrit for oxygen delivery to the body during hypovolemic shock, even though hematocrit-induced changes in the rheologic properties of blood may contribute to hemodynamic changes in critically ill patients.[21,120,350,351] Most, but not all, authors believe, however, that mild hemodilution (hematocrit approximately 0.30) may benefit delivery and uptake of oxygen in the tissues and promote survival of critically ill patients with hypovolemia, whereas severe hemodilution or hemoconcentration may be detrimental.* A low hematocrit in the course of hypovolemic shock after major surgery may warrant red blood cell replacement, whereas a high hematocrit may necessitate infusion of nonsanguineous fluids.[9,352] Mild hemodilution may benefit resumption of red blood cell flow and oxygen uptake after prior ischemia.

VASOACTIVE DRUGS

Generally, catecholamines do not have a place in the treatment of hypovolemic shock unless they are used to bridge a period in which infusion fluids are not yet available, or if adequate fluid resuscitation has proved insufficient to reverse hypotension (irreversible shock) and to increase oxygen delivery to the point that tissue needs are met.† Persistent hypotension despite normovolemia can be caused by a low cardiac output following myocardial dysfunction or by peripheral vasodilation. Data obtained with advanced hemodynamic monitoring may help to identify these abnormalities, which can be important for choosing among the available vasopressor and inotropic drugs, which have widely differing receptor affinities and hemodynamic effects.[9,45]

Treatment with the drugs is best guided by the prevailing hemodynamic profile and aims at optimization of the circulation toward values associated with survival.[9,42,45] Drugs are given as a continuous intravenous infusion, preferably via a central vein. The initial dose is low, and often combinations of drugs are used. The use of catecholamines should be judicious and carefully guided by hemodynamic parameters to reach predefined hemodynamic goals.[9] β-Adrenergic drugs increase cardiac output by inotropic (β_1) or vasodilating (β_2) properties.[9,353] Dopaminergic compounds may preferentially increase splanchnic and renal perfusion, glomerular filtration, and diuresis.[66,284] Dobutamine, having vasodilating β_2 properties, may exert greater effects on delivery and uptake of oxygen than dopamine at a lower PCWP.[9,353] A decrease in the arterial blood pressure concomitantly with a decreased wedge pressure after dobutamine infusion may warrant additional fluid repletion.[9] Drugs with α-adrenergic activity, such as norepinephrine, increase arterial blood pressure, but this increase may not lead to a decrease in cardiac output because they may increase venous return to the heart by decreasing venous compliance.[7] The vascular reactivity to vasoconstrictors may diminish in the late phase of shock, but norepinephrine remains the agent of first choice in the (bridging to definitive) treatment of hypovolemic shock after fluid loading.[354] The use of adrenergic drugs is not without hazards. They may enhance the metabolic demands of the body so that the oxygen supply-to-demand ratio is not favorably influenced even if oxygen delivery is enhanced.[355] Particularly, epinephrine may increase lactic acid levels independently of oxygen balance.[38] Low-dose dopamine has been shown, at least in bled dogs, to impede oxygen extraction by the gut during a decrease in oxygen supply, probably associated with transmural distribution of blood flow.[66] Finally, vasoconstricting vasopressin and methylene blue, a guanylate cyclase inhibitor, have been tried to overcome intractable hypotension in this phase.[96,300] Vasopressin has also been used in the initial management of uncontrolled hemorrhagic shock to safeguard arterial pressure for vital organ (e.g., cerebral) perfusion without overzealous fluid administration that may dilute coagulation factors and promote further bleeding.[300]

*9, 21, 73, 120, 176, 265, 351, 352
†9, 42, 45, 209, 284, 353

BRAIN INJURY AND RESUSCITATION

Hypovolemia and a decreased mean arterial blood pressure are considered as major threats for cerebral perfusion in brain injury. The latter may create intracranial hypertension following edema, bleeding, and contusion so that perfusion is more dependent on pressure than normal. Small volume resuscitation from hypovolemia with hypertonic (and hyperoncotic) solutions could increase mean arterial blood pressure at a small increase in plasma volume and could, by virtue of hypertonicity, decrease cerebral edema and intracranial pressure. The solutions are highly suitable for treatment of multiple trauma that includes the brain.[314,315] Conversely, too much normotonic, certainly hypotonic, and perhaps albumin solutions may aggravate cerebral edema, but too little fluids and under-resuscitation with resulting hypotension and hypoperfusion may do the same. Vasopressor drugs such as vasopressin may be useful adjuncts in the initial treatment of hemorrhagic hypotension plus brain injury.

IN PRACTICE

In practice, the different types of fluids, including isotonic and hypertonic crystalloid and iso-oncotic or hyperoncotic colloid solutions, are often combined in the resuscitation from hypovolemic shock (see Box 26.2). For resuscitation of hypovolemic shock following hemorrhage, typed blood is often not immediately available, even though a blood sample for crossmatching has been sent to the blood bank as soon as possible after admission. If shock is severe and warrants immediate infusion of blood, type O Rh-negative erythrocyte concentrates can be safely used. In the absence of blood, resuscitation should begin with nonsanguineous fluids. During hypovolemic shock, initial resuscitation is often begun with hypertonic or isotonic (balanced) crystalloids, supplemented with colloid solutions, and finally accomplished through infusion of erythrocyte concentrates and plasma (Fig. 26.2).

In the case of uncontrolled diabetes mellitus, profound diarrhea, and acute adrenocortical insufficiency with loss of plasma water and electrolytes, the infusion of crystalloid solutions usually suffices. These solutions restore intravascular, interstitial, and intracellular (in case of diabetes

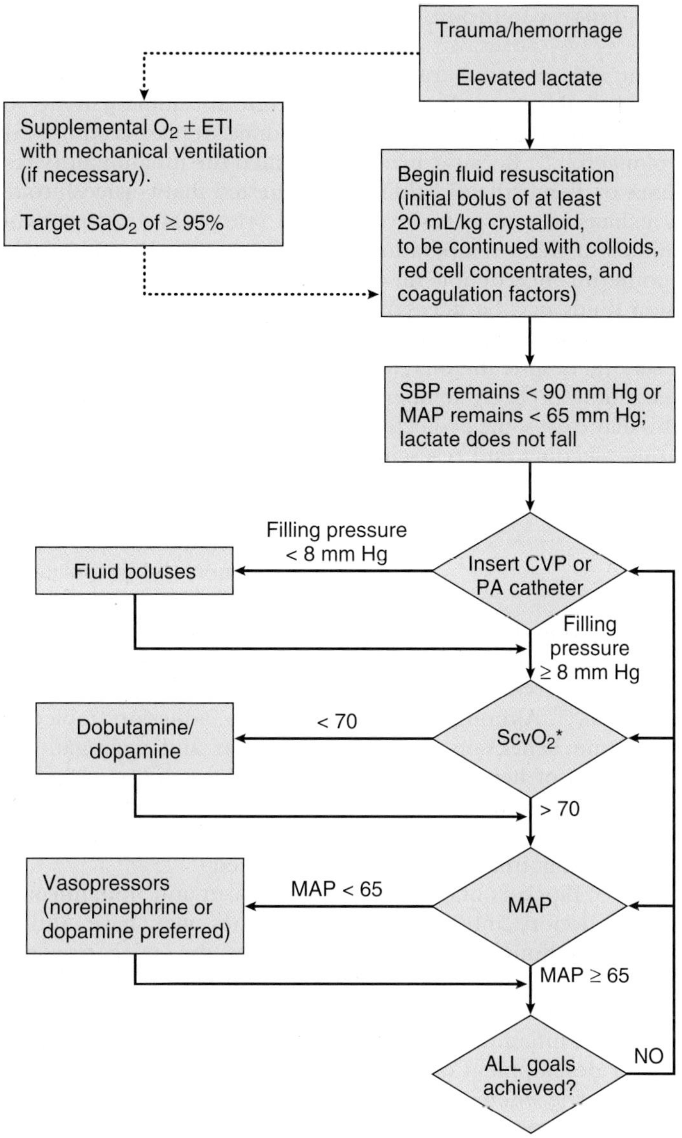

*If pulmonary artery catheter is used a mixed venous O_2 saturation is an acceptable surrogate, and 65% would be the target.

Figure 26.2 Hypovolemic shock management protocol. CVP, central venous pressure; ETI, endotracheal intubation; MAP, mean arterial pressure; PA, pulmonary artery; SaO_2, oxygen saturation; SBP, systolic blood pressure; $ScvO_2$, central venous oxygen saturation.

mellitus) fluids. Changes in the electrolyte concentrations in blood have to be corrected through adaptation of the type and composition of the infusion fluid; in the case of hypokalemia (and in the presence of diuresis), potassium should be supplemented.

SUPPORTIVE CARE

A vomiting patient in hypovolemic shock should be protected against aspiration of gastric contents by early intubation. The value of specific measures for prevention of hemorrhagic gastric mucosal stress ulceration remains controversial.[207] After resuscitation from shock, attention also should be paid to the nutritional status of the patient.[222] It should be judged whether enteral or parenteral nutrition is necessary to improve nitrogen balance and energy intake.[356] Although enteral feeding during hypovolemic shock and after resuscitation may increase metabolic demands of the gut, luminal application of nutrients such as glutamine may induce an increase in mucosal blood flow, ameliorate damage, and diminish the likelihood for translocation of endotoxins and bacteria and of septic complications.[148,206] In addition, there is some evidence that early enteral feeding favorably influences organ function after hemorrhage and reperfusion, in contrast to (early) parenteral feeding, which may have adverse effects even though earlier meeting caloric requirements.[148] The value of selective decontamination of the digestive tract or luminal absorption of endotoxin to prevent sepsis and its harmful sequelae originating from the gut is still controversial in multiple trauma, although such measures may inhibit the cytokine response to hypovolemic shock in animals.[357]

When treating pain in a patient with extensive trauma, morphinomimetics are cautiously applied because the drugs may have adverse circulatory effects during hypovolemic shock and half-life may be prolonged.[11,358] Because many resuscitated patients after trauma or hemorrhage exhibit hypothermia, partly caused by exhausted energy reserves and infusion of substantial amounts of room temperature infusion fluids, and because hypothermia may denote more severe illness, rewarming infusion fluids may be necessary during resuscitation, and this may prevent some organ dysfunction and perhaps promote survival despite the increase in oxygen demand with an elevation in body temperature.[56,217,264] In contrast, there also may exist some protective effect of mild hypothermia during bleeding and resuscitation, particularly when accompanied by brain injury, at least in experiments.

MISCELLANEOUS THERAPIES

A wide array of experimental drugs has been tried in animal experiments to improve the hemodynamics, ameliorate inflammation, and increase survival rates from hypovolemic shock and resuscitation.[230] Although many experimental drugs have shown some benefit in animal models of hypovolemic shock, in terms of hemodynamics during shock and after resuscitation and ultimate survival, there are now clinical trials ongoing or showing a benefit of such interventions in humans, including treatment with immune-enhancing factors.[24,93,118,230,359] Blockers of NO synthesis (L-arginine analogs) and NO donors, inhibitors of activated K^+ channels (oral antidiabetic, sulfonylurea drugs), Na^+/H^+ exchanger (amiloride, benzamide), and poly(ADP-ribose) polymerase have been tried in animal experiments to overcome vascular unresponsiveness, inflammation, and organ dysfunction early or late after development of hypovolemic shock.* ATP-$MgCl_2$ may provide energy to cells, improve the microcirculation, reduce cell swelling, protect tissues from injury, and promote organ function and survival during hypovolemic shock and resuscitation.[24,128,143,144] Ca^{2+}-entry blockers have been used to prevent intracellular accumulation of Ca^{2+} and further damage of ischemic cells during resuscitation from hypovolemic shock.† Opiate antagonists or inhibitors such as naloxone, ACTH, and thyrotropin-releasing hormone been shown to increase arterial blood pressure, decrease inflammation, and improve survival.‡ Sedatives and analgesic drugs such as dexmedetomidine and ketamine may have anti-inflammatory properties and are tissue protective.[360] Other vasoactive agents, including thyroid hormone, glucagon, and angiotensin inhibitors, with a preferential effect on splanchnic blood flow also may have beneficial effects in hypovolemic shock.[105,225,226]

Experimental models indicate that pretreatment with xanthine oxidase inhibitors (allopurinol) or scavengers of ROS or antioxidants including lazaroids may ameliorate microvascular hemodynamics and membrane injury of organs such as the heart and gut and improve survival after resuscitation from hypovolemic shock, although some of these compounds may have greater effects than others.* A study in trauma patients with elevated lipid peroxidation products in plasma showed that superoxide dismutase ameliorated the inflammatory response and MOF.[239] It has been suggested that corticosteroids prevent lysosomal disruption and release of toxic proteases, prevent NO synthesis, and ameliorate the hemodynamic changes and promote survival during hypovolemic shock in animals.[92,167,229,268] Cortisol treatment may increase the vascular sensitivity for catecholamines, particularly in patients in whom adrenal cortisol secretion is low relative to severity of disease, the so-called relative adrenal insufficiency. It may also decrease respiratory infections in the hospital course.[361] Intravenously administered ACTH fragments may have an adrenal-independent central opioid-inhibiting effect, which may help to prevent vascular decompensation and treat hypotension, even clinically.[93] Drugs such as pentoxifylline and complement inhibitors may prevent neutrophil-mediated endothelial injury, dysfunction, and downregulation of NO synthesis after bleeding and resuscitation, diminishing endothelium-dependent vasodilation.[118,215] Pentoxifylline may ameliorate not only macrophage cytokine generation, but also adhesion molecule expression and neutrophil activation and aggregation and may improve red blood cell deformability. Administration of pentoxifylline or other methylxanthines may ameliorate reperfusion injury, at least in the rat gut and liver, and survival may be enhanced.[79,166,206,230,319]

Heparin and nonanticoagulant heparin sulfate or other analogues may have anti-inflammatory effects and may improve the microcirculation, and administration may partly protect various tissues, including the liver and gut, against reperfusion injury after hypovolemic shock by bleeding.[250,363] Protease inhibitors, such as aprotinin, may also have beneficial effects. Administration of female hormones or inducers such as dehydroepiandrosterone or testosterone depletion after trauma/hemorrhage and resuscitation partly protects animals from microcirculatory organ dysfunction and immunosuppression, and a wide variety of mechanisms has been implicated.[218] The potential of other immunologic and hormonal agents to treat immunosuppression has also been shown.[218,250,362] Further drug developments include anticytokine strategies and tissue protective agents interfering with cell stress, apoptosis, or necrosis, such as erythropoietin.[216] Mesenchymal stem cells are under investigation.

COMPLICATIONS AND PROGNOSIS

As previously indicated, hypovolemic shock may adversely affect the function of various organs. Even after successful resuscitation from hypovolemic shock, some patients may develop dysfunction of various organ systems (MOF), as evidenced by ARDS, acute kidney injury and failure, hyperbilirubinemia, diminished motility and resorptive capacity of the bowel, ischemic colitis, anoxic brain damage, severe

*92, 93, 139, 147, 221, 230
†49, 127, 129, 230, 235, 238, 257
‡11, 13, 23, 24, 228, 230

*194, 198, 199, 227, 228, 230

muscle loss, and complications such as acalculous cholecystitis, ischemic perforation of the bowel, and DIC with a bleeding tendency.* The pathogenesis of the syndrome in humans is still unclear and probably multifactorial, so polytransfusions, ischemia, reperfusion injury, inflammatory reactions, and metabolic changes all may play a role, as previously mentioned.[180,190,228] Hemorrhagic (hypovolemic) shock after trauma may be complicated on days 1 to 3 after the trauma by the systemic fat embolism syndrome, with low platelets and petechiae, fever, acute lung and brain injury, and retinal abnormalities. Prevention and treatment of such complications involves stabilizing fractures, preventing intramedullary pressure, and otherwise being merely supportive. Therapy of the MOF syndrome is also supportive and aimed at the replacement of organ function, prevention and treatment of infections, adequate nutrition, and circulatory support.[222] During development of ARDS, the disturbed gas exchange does not respond to liberal oxygen therapy, so intubation and mechanical ventilation are often required for oxygen delivery to the tissues. Further treatment is aimed at diminishing pulmonary edema by judicious manipulation of the hydrostatic pressure in the lungs and the colloid osmotic pressure of plasma (e.g., with help of diuretics), avoiding a decrease in oxygen transport to the tissue. In the case of acute kidney injury and failure, attempts can be made to treat fluid overloading by promoting diuresis with help of diuretics if arterial blood pressure is adequate. If unsuccessful, renal replacement therapy (e.g., by continuous arteriovenous or venovenous hemofiltration) may be necessary.[365] There is also some suggestion that the technique, when large ultrafiltration fluid volumes are used, allows for some removal of harmful proinflammatory mediators from the circulation and contributes to hemodynamic stabilization and organ function independently of renal replacement therapy.[365]

As mentioned, hemorrhage, shock, and resuscitation after trauma may transiently alter immune responses. Together with wounds, this may predispose to susceptibility for bacterial infection and sepsis. Sepsis is a common complication of trauma and is believed to contribute to the development of MOF, including ARDS, in patients ultimately dying.[2,205] Because trauma itself may result in fever and leukocytosis, the recognition of bacterial infection and sepsis in trauma patients is difficult; recognition is aided by infection markers such as circulating C-reactive protein and procalcitonin. Suspected or proven infection should be treated by appropriate antibiotics and drainage, if needed. Despite cardiovascular supportive measures, MOF carries a mortality rate approaching 100% if more than three to four systems fail.[82,205,270]

CONCLUSION

Hypovolemic shock is a life-threatening condition necessitating prompt diagnosis and therapy to prevent MOF and death. Despite new insights into pathophysiology and new horizons for treatment, the main principles of management remain the rapid and complete repletion of circulating blood volume and treatment of the underlying cause.

*2, 40, 82, 205, 239, 263, 364

KEY POINTS

- Hypovolemic shock is an acute disturbance in the circulation leading to an imbalance between oxygen supply and demand in the tissues caused by a decline in circulating blood volume.
- Changes in the blood lactate or bicarbonate level reflect the severity and course of shock and roughly predict outcome.
- Compensatory mechanisms evoked during hypovolemic shock attempt to defend vital organ perfusion and function.
- Hypovolemic shock leading to ischemia-reperfusion triggers an inflammatory response. The syndrome also is characterized by a diminished immunologic defense.
- The most frequent cause of hypovolemic shock is trauma.
- The main principles for treatment of hypovolemic shock are rapid and complete repletion of circulating blood volume and treatment of the underlying cause. In principle, vasoactive drugs have no place in the treatment of hypovolemic shock.
- Advanced hemodynamic monitoring is indicated in case of difficulties in diagnosis, treatment of hypovolemic shock, or both.
- During treatment of hypovolemic shock, repletion of circulating blood volume and oxygen delivery to the tissues is more rapid with infusion of colloid than of crystalloid fluids unless the latter are hypertonic. On the other hand, synthetic colloids have more (severe) adverse effects and their safety is currently hotly debated. Infusion of concentrates of red blood cells and fresh frozen plasma is indicated in the case of blood loss.
- The pathogenesis of MOF after hypovolemic shock is multifactorial. The main preventive measure is a rapid restoration of tissue oxygen balance.

SELECTED REFERENCES

1. Wiggers CJ: Present status of shock problem. Physiol Rev 1942;22:74.
17. McGee S, Abernethy WB, Simel DL: Is this patient hypovolemic? JAMA 1999;281:1022.
72. Kaufman BS, Rackow EC, Falk JL: The relationship between oxygen delivery and consumption during fluid resuscitation of hypovolemic and septic shock. Chest 1984;85:336.
91. Pannen BHJ, Köhler N, Hole B, et al: Protective role of endogenous carbon monoxide in hepatic microcirculatory dysfunction after hemorrhagic shock in rats. J Clin Invest 1998;102:1220.
104. Trof RJ, Di Maggio F, Leemreis J, Groeneveld AB: Review: Biomarkers of acute renal injury and renal failure. Shock 2006;26:245.
123. De Lima A, Bakker J: Noninvasive monitoring of peripheral circulation. Intensive Care Med 2005;31:1316.
161. Chatpun S, Carbales P: Cardiac systolic function recovery after hemorrhage determines survivability during shock. J Trauma 2011;70:787.

172. Rackow EC, Falk JL, Fein IA, et al: Fluid resuscitation in circulatory shock: A comparison of the cardiorespiratory effects of albumin, hetastarch, and saline solutions in patients with hypovolemic and septic shock. Crit Care Med 1983;11:839.
236. Chaudry IH, Ayala A, Ertel W, Stephan RN: Hemorrhage and resuscitation: Immunological aspects. Am J Physiol 1990; 259:R663.
281. Trof RJ, Beishuizen A, Cornet AD, et al: Volume-limited versus pressure-limited hemodynamic management in septic and non-septic shock. Crit Care Med 2012:40:1177.

The complete list of references can be found at www.expertconsult.com.

27

Traumatic Shock and Tissue Hypoperfusion: Nonsurgical Management

David J. Dries

CHAPTER OUTLINE

In 1934, Blalock suggested four categories of shock: hypovolemic, vasogenic, neurogenic, and cardiogenic.[1,2] In more recent clinical practice, additional categories of shock have been proposed.[3] Hypovolemic shock, the most common, results from reduction in circulating blood volume. Volume loss may be loss of whole blood, plasma, or extracellular fluid or a combination of all three. Vasogenic shock occurs as a result of changes in the resistance of vessels so that a normal blood volume fails to occupy the available space. Neurogenic shock (spinal shock) is a form of vasogenic shock in which spinal anesthesia or spinal cord injury leads to vasodilation. Septic shock is another form of vasogenic shock in which there is increased capacitance. A decrease in peripheral arterial resistance, a decrease in venous capacitance, and a peripheral arteriovenous maldistribution occur. Cardiogenic shock results from failure of the heart as a pump. Obstructive shock results from mechanical obstruction to cardiac function, as seen with tamponade, tension pneumothorax, or massive pulmonary embolism.[4]

Traumatic shock includes several components of the conditions mentioned previously.[5] Hypovolemia caused by blood loss is compounded by neurogenic, cardiogenic, or obstructive shock plus the vasogenic component of maladaptive mediator cascades initiated by tissue injury. Traumatic shock involves hemorrhage in combination with soft tissue trauma and fractures. As a result, study of pure hemorrhagic shock may have limited relevance to the pathophysiologic condition of traumatic shock. Most studies have shown significant differences in the biologic condition of traumatic shock compared with that of pure hemorrhagic shock based on the activation of mediator cascades.[2]

Conflicting observations in literature are due at least in part to the assumption that hemorrhagic shock and traumatic shock are identical insults.[2,3] Pulmonary complications after simple hemorrhage are uncommon in clinical practice, but pulmonary dysfunction is a common comorbid condition after major trauma with attendant soft tissue or long bone injury.[2,6] Activation of mediator systems is far more intense with traumatic shock than with pure hemorrhage.[7] Conflicting data regarding changes in cytokine levels after a traumatic insult are likely due to the fact that systemic cytokine levels do not reflect local production of these mediators. Measurement of tissue levels of mediator production may be necessary to determine accurately whether there is upregulation of various mediator systems after trauma or hemorrhage.

Soft tissue injury alone upregulates mediator systems.[2,8] A small animal study with closed femur fractures showed Kupffer cell activation 30 minutes after injury.[9] Another study assessed the effects of skeletal muscle injury in combination with hemorrhage in a porcine model of hemorrhagic shock. To reach a given physiologic end point (reduction in cardiac index and oxygen delivery), hemorrhage of 40% of the blood volume was required in a pure hemorrhagic shock model. If skeletal muscle injury was added, hemorrhage of only 29% of blood volume was necessary to reach the same end point.[2,10] The ability to maintain cardiac function after hemorrhage was impaired in this study by superimposition of a soft tissue injury, emphasizing the difference between hemorrhagic shock and traumatic shock. A synergy in activation of neuroendocrine and inflammatory mediator systems is likely when traumatic injury and hemorrhagic shock are present. More recent work describing coagulation changes occurring with injury emphasizes the danger of combined injury and hypoperfusion of soft tissue in failure of appropriate coagulation response.[11]

CLASSIC NEUROENDOCRINE RESPONSE

The essential homeostatic response to acute blood loss is preservation of cerebral and cardiac perfusion with maintenance of normal blood pressure as sensed by carotid body and aortic arch receptors. Peripheral vasoconstriction and curtailment of fluid excretion are seen. Cardiac contractility and peripheral vascular tone also are altered. Pain, hypoxemia, acidosis, infection, changes in temperature, and availability of substrates such as glucose affect this response. A decrease in blood volume alone without hypotension may activate the hypothalamic-pituitary axis. The magnitude of neuroendocrine response depends not only on the volume of blood loss, but also the rate at which blood loss occurs. This response may be modified by patient age, prescribed medications, preexisting illness, and the use of ethanol or other drugs. With spinal cord transection, operative intervention below the level of injury does not produce typical activation of the hypothalamic-pituitary axis. Similarly, consciousness is unnecessary for activation of this response because it may occur under anesthesia.[2,12-16]

The initial effect seen with hemorrhage is sympathetic vasoconstriction. Capacitance of the circulatory system is reduced, and aortic arch or carotid sinus baroreceptors respond to changes in blood pressure by modulation of sympathetic tone.[2,17] Atrial receptors respond to changes in vascular wall stretch and pressure. Afferent vagal fibers carry signals leading to loss of tonic inhibition of heart rate and immediate activation of thoracolumbar sympathetic outflow with norepinephrine release from postganglionic sympathetic fibers. As blood loss increases, so does the role played by arterial baroreceptors. Another part of this hormonal response is corticotropin-releasing factor secreted by the hypothalamus, vasopressin release, and growth hormone-releasing factor release.[12]

The clinician sees cool extremities in response to these changes associated with hypovolemia. Venous capacitance also decreases, resulting in accelerated venous return to the heart. Selective arterial vasoconstriction maintains blood flow to the heart and brain until compensation fails. Intense triggering of sympathetic signals is activated when arterial blood pressure decreases to less than 50 mm Hg and is maximally stimulated when systolic blood pressure is less than 15 mm Hg.[2] Although metabolic vasoregulation in the heart and brain helps avoid local vasoconstriction, blood flow to other tissues decreases dramatically. Renal blood flow may be reduced to 5% to 10% of normal with acute hypovolemia. Flow to the splanchnic circulation, skin, and skeletal muscle also decreases. These vasoconstrictor responses are mediated by epinephrine and norepinephrine from the adrenal medulla and local sympathetic activity at the vasculature. With increases in acidosis and hydrogen ion concentration, coronary vasodilation occurs as opposed to constriction of arteries in skeletal muscle and the splanchnic circulation.[3,18,19]

Multiple endocrine responses are seen with trauma and associated hypovolemia. Plasma levels of glucagon, growth hormone, cortisol, and corticotropin (adrenocorticotropic hormone) increase.[2,3,5] The renin-angiotensin-aldosterone axis is stimulated with release of vasoconstrictive angiotensin II. Vasopressin release also occurs after hemorrhage, resulting in water absorption in the distal tubule of the kidney. Vasopressin induces splanchnic vasoconstriction. Research suggests that with prolonged hemorrhage, vasopressin depletion may occur, and supplements of this hormone by clinicians may be warranted. Growth hormone and glucagon promote gluconeogenesis, lipolysis, and glycogenolysis. Catecholamines that inhibit insulin release and hyperglycemia and increase blood osmolarity are thought to shift fluid from cells and the interstitium into the intravascular space. More recent data associate hyperglycemia in the setting of injury with adverse outcome, however. The cellular mechanism for this response remains unclear. Loss of fluid or salt through the kidneys also is limited by these hormonal effects, which serve to conserve the circulating blood volume.[18,20-22]

Compensated acute hypovolemia occurs when the aforementioned mechanisms are sufficient to avoid widespread cellular injury and organ decompensation.[2] If volume loss continues, or resuscitation is inadequate, a cycle of decline occurs with regional perfusion defects leading to tissue and microcirculatory changes. Progression from compensated to decompensated and irreversible shock is often defined in retrospect. Frequently, a patient with acute irreversible hemorrhage has been hypotensive for an extended period and cannot be resuscitated despite fluid administration and use of vasoactive drugs.[23] Presumed mechanisms in this situation include microcirculatory failure with loss of vasomotor response and integrity of the vascular bed. Patients with subacute but ultimately irreversible shock can be resuscitated initially, but progressive organ injury and end-organ dysfunction follow.

INFLAMMATION IN SHOCK AFTER INJURY

In addition to blood loss, extensive research suggests that trauma may be considered an inflammatory disease.[24-27] It has been shown that a variety of mediators and indicators of inflammatory response are elevated in severely injured patients. For many of these factors, it could be shown that they were significantly elevated in patients eventually dying compared with survivors, and that prediction of outcome is possible with a significant degree of accuracy. Peak inflammatory activity as measured by plasma values has been noted within hours of injury. Although it cannot at present be decided which of these parameters may play a direct pathophysiologic role in development and promotion of inflammatory response and consecutive organ dysfunction, and which is an indicator of this reaction, inflammatory mediators may reflect pathophysiologically relevant disturbances set off by tissue injury and blood loss with consecutive ischemia and reperfusion incidents.[28]

Shock after trauma differs from pure hypovolemic shock in that effects of release of mediators by tissue injury are superimposed on hypovolemia. It also is clear that not all damage after shock is the result of tissue hypoxia, and that much of cellular damage follows reperfusion and subsequent inflammation. Loci of this inflammatory response are the wound, with activation of macrophages and production of proinflammatory mediators, and the microcirculation, with activation of blood elements and the endothelium.[28,29]

CELLULAR ENERGETICS

With blood loss, classic circulatory variables, such as systolic blood pressure, remain normal or supranormal until 30% of blood loss occurs.[2,30] With progressive cellular hypoxia, mitochondria still may be able to metabolize oxygen.[2] Nonetheless, with significant hypovolemia, total oxygen available to tissue is severely reduced, causing anaerobic metabolism, which is energy inefficient because one molecule of glucose is no longer able to contribute to resynthesis of 32 mol of adenosine triphosphate but only to 2 mol. Glucose must reach cells through the circulation, which is critically reduced. In addition, the end product is no longer carbon dioxide, which can be eliminated by ventilation, but lactic acid and hydrogen ions, leading to metabolic acidosis. Acidosis drives cellular swelling with loss of extracellular fluid volume into the cells. Lactate finally is metabolized by the liver, which also is hypoxic. Transcapillary refill and lymph flow direct interstitial fluid to increase the circulating blood volume, but ultimately capillaries are damaged by hypoxia and the action of activated neutrophils, which increases interstitial edema. Finally, autoregulation of microcirculation is destroyed, leading to fluid sequestration and sludging in the microvasculature. These factors are responsible for increased diffusion distance for oxygen from capillaries to the mitochondria, which further impairs oxygen extraction. Tissue hypoxia also is the most potent stimulus for proinflammatory activation of macrophages and release of vasoactive or arachidonic acid metabolites, such as prostaglandins and thromboxane. Hypovolemia, shock, and any other cause of brain hypoxia also are detrimental to recovery, particularly in patients with head injury because these conditions induce secondary brain damage.

IMMUNE MEDIATOR CASCADES

Although a variety of initiating events may occur, the subsequent inflammatory response is qualitatively similar.[2] Local activation of the complement cascade produces anaphylatoxins, which are strong attractants and stimulants of neutrophils. Local endothelium expresses endothelial leukocyte adhesion molecules, which attract the neutrophil population. Activated neutrophils also express adhesion molecules, leading to aggregation, margination in the vascular endothelium, and migration through vessel walls at the area of injury. This inflammatory response produces a respiratory burst with formation of oxygen radicals and synthesis of proteolytic enzymes (elastase). Local release of bradykinin, histamine, and prostaglandin induces local vasodilation and increased capillary permeability from macromolecules, resulting in a protein-rich exudate. Local phagocytes release messenger molecules, such as granulocyte-macrophage colony-stimulating factor and macrophage colony-stimulating factor, which activate the bone marrow to produce more inflammatory cells. Neutrophils injure otherwise healthy tissues.[2,31-34]

In a slower response, the monocyte population is attracted to the site of injury, where it differentiates to macrophages and contributes to the inflammatory process by phagocytosing and killing bacteria or disposing of necrotic tissue or both. Macrophages are activated further by triggers such as hypoxia or C5a, macrophage-activating factor, and interleukin (IL)-1-like activity from neutrophils. On stimulation, macrophages release a variety of classes of secretory products, which may be proinflammatory (proteolytic enzymes, oxygen radicals, IL-1, IL-6, tumor necrosis factor) or anti-inflammatory (IL-10, prostaglandin E_2). Macrophage mediators such as prostaglandin E_2, tumor necrosis factor, IL-1, IL-2, and IL-6 provide systemic signals adapting metabolic and defense mechanisms. Macrophages take several days after activation to develop full inflammatory capacity. They also may release nitric oxide and cytotoxic radicals. In the setting of injury, this local inflammatory process spills over to cause an exaggerated systemic response with inflammatory damage to otherwise healthy cells and organs distant to the site of injury. Secondary infection may occur in the compromised host, leading to generalized inflammation and multiorgan dysfunction (Box 27.1).[2,35,36]

NEUROIMMUNE RESPONSE TO TRAUMA

More recent work examines the link between the autonomic nervous system and modulation of immune response during traumatic injury. Anatomic interactions with immune-competent cells have been identified, and functional consequences of this interaction in the host are now being examined. Integrated hemodynamic, metabolic, behavioral, and immune responses allowing host adaptation are the stress response.[37-41]

Box 27.1 Inflammatory Mediators Associated with Development of Multiple Organ Dysfunction Syndrome in Injured Patients*

First 24 Hours

Thromboxane B_2
C3a
Terminal cytolytic complement complex
C-reactive protein
Elastase
Tumor necrosis factor-α
Interleukin 6
Lipofuscin
Lactate
Antithrombin III

Days 2-5

Elastase
Interleukin 6
Lipofuscin
Soluble intercellular adhesion molecule 1

Day >8

Elastase
Interleukin 1
Interleukin 6
Neopterin
Lipofuscin
Tumor necrosis factor-α if sepsis

*A variety of inflammatory mediators are associated with soft tissue injury, bony injury, and blood loss associated with various forms of trauma. The time course of mediator appearance in limited studies done to date is suggested in this box. In experimental models and limited clinical data, the presence of soft tissue or bony injury in addition to hemorrhage accelerates and magnifies the production of these mediators over clinical and experimental models in which hemorrhage alone is seen.

From Goris RJ: Pathophysiology of shock in trauma. Eur J Surg 2000;166:100-111.

Catecholamines are neurotransmitters that affect immune response humorally through circulating adrenal-derived epinephrine and locally through neuronal release of norepinephrine. There is anatomic evidence of central nervous system (CNS)–lymphoid organ connection through autonomic and sensory fibers and immune tissues, including bone marrow, thymus, spleen, and lymph nodes.[37] This sympathetic innervation of lymphoid organs is found across species and has been confirmed by immunohistochemistry. In bone marrow, myelinated and nonmyelinated fibers are distributed with vascular plexuses where they influence hematopoiesis and cell migration. In the lungs, noradrenergic nerve fibers supply tracheobronchial smooth muscle and glands. In addition, nerve fibers have been shown throughout the different compartments of the bronchus-associated lymphoid tissue forming close contact with mast cells, cells of the macrophage/monocyte lineage, or other lymph node cells. In the thymus, noradrenergic nerve fibers have been localized in the subcapsular, cortical, and corticomedullary regions associated with blood vessels and intralobular septa branching into cortical parenchyma where they reach to thymocytes.[37,42]

The functional effects of catecholamines on cells of the immune system have been confirmed in human volunteers. In addition, relevance of this control mechanism and the implications for dysregulation have been shown by rapid systemic release of IL-10 and the high incidence of infection in patients with sympathetic storm from accidental or iatrogenic brain trauma.[37] Although detrimental effects of sustained and exaggerated sympathetic nervous system activation on cardiovascular and metabolic homeostasis have long been recognized, attention is now directed to the likelihood of immune dysregulation as well.

The neuroimmune axis is a bidirectional network composed of descending pathways linking the CNS to peripheral immune tissues and a parallel afferent arm linking the immune system with the CNS. The integrity of this loop allows for communication between the CNS and peripheral immune system integrating neuronal and immune signals in the periphery and in the CNS. Cells from the immune system express functional receptors and signal transduction pathway components for several neuroendocrine mediators allowing functional cellular responses to agonist stimulation. Similarly, cells in the CNS are capable of synthesizing, secreting, and responding to inflammatory and immune molecules. There is considerable evidence that the peripheral immune system can signal the brain to elicit a sickness response during infection, inflammation, and injury. Peripheral immune molecules such as cytokines influence CNS action through mechanisms including entry into the brain through a saturable transport mechanism or through areas that lack the blood-brain barrier. Afferent neurons of the vagus nerve also are activated (Fig. 27.1).[43-45]

Severe trauma is characterized by the classic activation of the sympathetic nervous system and the recently recognized contribution of the inflammatory and neuroimmune response to injury.[37] The sympathetic nervous system has significant anatomic and functional interaction with cells of the immune system and plays an important role in control of the magnitude of early inflammatory response to injury by ensuring expression of adequate cytokine balance.[37] Sympathetic neural pathways exert direct effects on cells of the immune system, affecting cytokine expression, lymphocyte function, and cytotoxic activity. In return, the inflammatory mediators released communicate with the CNS through stimulation of sensory and vagal afferents or by crossing the blood-brain barrier through active transport mechanisms and pathways allowing access to hypothalamic-pituitary structures. Immune-derived mediators, such as cytokines and chemokines, can modulate neurotransmission affecting activation of descending autonomic and neuroendocrine pathways.[37]

ACUTE COAGULOPATHY AFTER TRAUMA

HISTORICAL PERSPECTIVE

Hemorrhagic shock accounts for a significant number of deaths in patients arriving at hospital with acute injury. Patients with uncontrolled hemorrhage continue to die despite adoption of new surgical techniques with improved

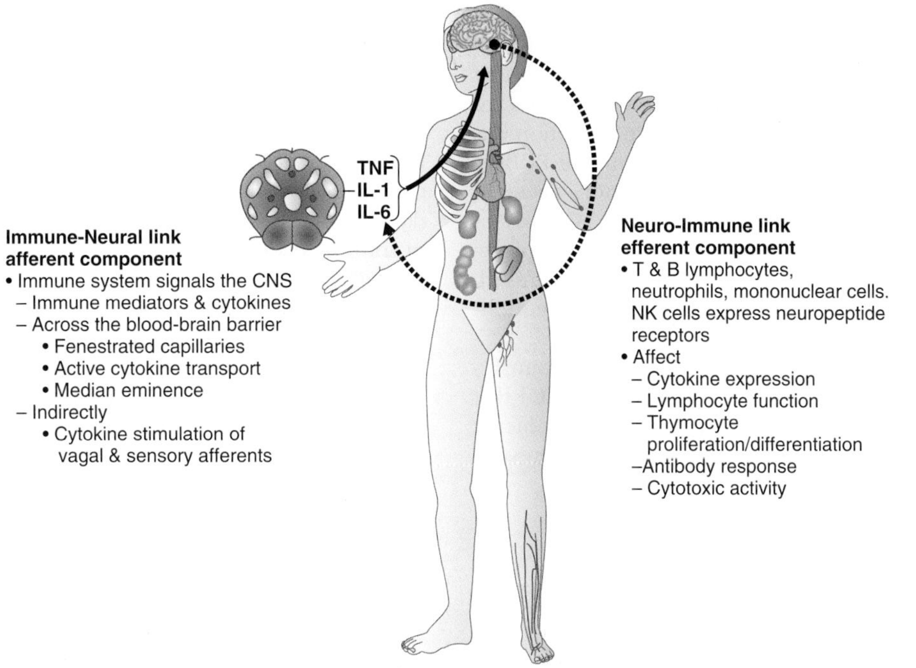
TNF
IL-1
IL-6
Immune-Neural link
afferent component
• Immune system signals the CNS
– Immune mediators & cytokines
– Across the blood-brain barrier
• Fenestrated capillaries
• Active cytokine transport
• Median eminence
– Indirectly
• Cytokine stimulation of vagal & sensory afferents
Neuro-Immune link
efferent component
• T & B lymphocytes, neutrophils, mononuclear cells. NK cells express neuropeptide receptors
• Affect
– Cytokine expression
– Lymphocyte function
– Thymocyte proliferation/differentiation
–Antibody response
– Cytotoxic activity

Figure 27.1 Endocrine, neurologic, and immunologic response to injury is linked through afferent and efferent arcs as described in the text and drawn in this figure. Patients sustaining blunt injury or soft tissue loss in addition to hemorrhage show clinical evidence of increased cytokine and inflammatory mediator production with acceleration of the process described here. The best clinical data in support of this pair of arcs come from patients with traumatic brain injury. CNS, central nervous system; IL-1, interleukin 1; IL-6, interleukin 6; NK, natural killer; TNF, tumor necrosis factor. (From Molina PE: Neurobiology of the stress response: Contribution of the sympathetic nervous system to the neuroimmune axis in traumatic injury. Shock 2005;24:3-10.)

transport and emergency care.[46,47] Coagulopathy, occurring even before resuscitation, contributes significantly to the morbidity associated with bleeding.[48,49] Recognition of the morbidity associated with bleeding and coagulation abnormality dates to the Vietnam conflict. At that time, standard tests including prothrombin time (PT) and partial thromboplastin time (PTT) correlated poorly with effectiveness of acute resuscitation efforts. Similar work in the late 1970s was performed in civilian patients receiving massive transfusion. Again, PT, PTT, and bleeding time were only helpful if markedly prolonged.[50,51]

Studies in the 1970s and 1980s provided additional detail regarding the limitation of simple laboratory parameters and factor levels.[51,52] In a study of multiple patients requiring massive transfusion, platelet counts fell in proportion to the size of transfusion although factors V and VIII correlated poorly with the volume of blood transfused. Where coagulopathy appeared, patients seemed to respond to platelet administration. In subsequent studies, patients receiving a large number of blood products were followed for microvascular bleeding. Moderate deficiencies in clotting factors were common, but they were not associated with microvascular bleeding. Microvascular bleeding was associated with severe coagulation abnormalities such as clotting factor levels less than 20% of control values. In statistical analysis, clotting factor activities less than 20% of control levels were predicted by significant prolongation of PT and PTT. These earlier investigators also suggested that empiric blood replacement formulas available at the time were not likely to prevent microvascular bleeding because consumption of platelets or clotting factors did not consistently appear and simple dilution caused by resuscitation fluids frequently did not correspond to microvascular bleeding.[52]

The attention of the American trauma community was drawn to coagulopathy after trauma with the description of the "bloody vicious cycle" by the Denver health team over 20 years ago.[48] These investigators noted the contribution of hypothermia, acidosis, and hemodilution associated with inadequate resuscitation and excessive use of crystalloids. Subsequent work extended these observations describing early coagulopathy that could be independent of clotting factor deficiency.[53] In a more recent trial, early coagulopathy was noted in the setting of severe injury, which was present in the field, prior to emergency department arrival and initiation of fluid resuscitation. Coagulopathic patients were at increased risk for organ failure and death.

In a study questioning historical transfusion practice emphasizing administration of packed red blood cells (PRBCs) in the setting of massive trauma, Hirshberg and coworkers, using clinical data, developed a computer model designed to capture interactions between bleeding, hemodynamics, hemodilution, and blood component replacement during severe hemorrhage. Resuscitation options were offered in this model and their effectiveness evaluated.[54] After setting thresholds for acceptable loss of clotting factors, platelets, and fibrinogen, the authors modeled behavior of coagulation during rapid exsanguation without clotting factor or platelet replacement. The PT reached a critical level first followed by fibrinogen and platelets. If patients were resuscitated with small amounts of crystalloid, leaving overall blood volume reduced, the effective life of components in the coagulation cascade was increased. More aggressive fresh frozen plasma (FFP) replacement in the patient with significant bleeding was supported by this model. The optimal ratio for administration of FFP to PRBCs in this analysis was 2:3. Delayed administration of FFP led to critical clotting factor deficiency regardless of subsequent administration of FFP. Fibrinogen depletion was easier to correct. After administration of 5 units of PRBCs, the hemostatic threshold for fibrinogen was not exceeded if a FFP-to-PRBC ratio of 4:5 was employed. Analysis of platelet dilution demonstrated that even if platelet replacement was delayed until 10 units of PRBCs were infused, critical platelet dilution was prevented with a subsequent platelet-to-PRBC ratio of 8:10.[54]

The essential message of this work is that massive transfusion protocols, emphasizing PRBCs, in existence when this study was performed provide inadequate clotting factor replacement during major hemorrhage and neither prevent nor correct dilutional coagulopathy.

RECENT STUDIES

Brohi and coworkers from the United Kingdom helped to reinvigorate discussion of coagulopathy after injury by adding new coagulation laboratory techniques to previous clinical observations.[55] After reviewing over 1000 cases, patients with acute coagulopathy after injury had higher mortality rates throughout the spectrum of Injury Severity Scores (ISS). Contrary to historical teaching that coagulopathy was a function of hemodilution with massive crystalloid resuscitation, these authors noted that the incidence of coagulopathy increased with severity of injury but not necessarily in relationship to the volume of intravenous fluid administered to patients. Brohi and others helped to reemphasize the observation that acute coagulopathy could occur before significant fluid administration, which was attributable to the injury itself and proportional to the volume of injured tissue. Development of coagulopathy was an independent predictor of poor outcome. Mediators associated with tissue trauma including humoral and cellular immune system activation with coagulation, fibrinolysis, complement, and kallikrein cascades have been associated with changes in hemostatic mechanisms similar to those identified in the setting of sepsis.[55-57]

Factors contributing to coagulopathy in the setting of injury have been further reviewed.[58] Hypothermia relates to development of coagulopathy by reduction in platelet aggregation and decreased function of coagulation factors in nondiluted blood. Patients with temperature reduction below 34° C had elevated PT and PTT. Coagulation, like most biologic enzyme systems, works best at normal temperature. Similarly, acidosis occurring in the setting of trauma as a result of bleeding and hypotension also contributes to clotting failure. Animal work shows that a pH less than 7.20 is associated with hemostatic impairment. Platelet dysfunction and coagulation enzyme system changes are noted when blood from healthy volunteers is subjected to an acidic environment.[59,60]

We are now seeing that with or without hypothermia and acidosis, posttraumatic coagulopathy may develop in a significant number of patients. Although dilution-driven coagulopathy must be considered, loss of clotting factors has been associated with exaggerated inflammation in association with injury.

Hess and coworkers, as part of an international medical collaboration, developed a literature review to increase awareness of coagulopathy independent of crystalloid administration following trauma.[57] The key initiating factor is volume of tissue injury. Patients with severe tissue injury but no physiologic derangement, however, rarely present with coagulopathy and have a lower mortality rate.[61,62] Tissue damage initiates coagulation as endothelial injury at the site of trauma leads to exposure of subendothelial collagen and activation of the coagulation cascade.

Hyperfibrinolysis is seen as a direct consequence of the combination of tissue injury and shock. Endothelial injury accelerates fibrinolysis because of direct release of tissue plasminogen activator.[57,63] Tissue plasminogen activator expression by endothelium is increased in the presence of thrombin. Fibrinolysis is accelerated because of the combined effects of endothelial tissue plasminogen activator release with ischemia and inhibition of plasminogen activator inhibitor in shock. Although hyperfibrinolysis may focus clot propagation on sites of actual vascular injury, with widespread insults, this localization may be lost.

A number of important cofactors must be present to stimulate coagulopathy in the setting of injury.[57] Shock is a dose-dependent cause of tissue hypoperfusion. Elevated base deficit has been associated with coagulopathy in as many as 25% of patients in one large study. Progression of shock appears to result in hyperfibrinolysis. One mediator implicated in coagulopathy after injury is activated protein C. Immediate postinjury coagulopathy is likely a combination of effects caused by large volume tissue trauma and hypoperfusion (Fig. 27.2).[57]

As will be discussed later, equivalent ratios of FFP, PRBCs, and platelets are now considered for management of significant hemorrhage with coagulopathy after injury. Hypothermia and acidemia must be controlled to reduce their impact on enzyme systems.[64] Similar to sepsis, cross-talk has been noted between coagulation and inflammation systems with injury. Activation of coagulation proteases may induce inappropriate inflammation with activation of cascades such as complement and platelet degranulation.[65,66] Trauma patients are initially coagulopathic with increased bleeding. This condition may progress to a hypercoagulable state, putting them at risk for thrombotic events. This late thrombotic state bears similarities with coagulopathy of severe sepsis and depletion of protein C. Injured and septic patients share a propensity toward multiple organ failure and prothrombotic states.[67,68]

FLUID THERAPY

Warmed isotonic electrolyte solutions are recommended for initial resuscitation of traumatic shock by the Committee on Trauma of the American College of Surgeons. This type of fluid provides transient intravascular expansion and stabilizes the intravascular volume by replacing accompanying fluid losses into the interstitial and intracellular spaces. Lactated Ringer's solution is the initial fluid of choice. Normal saline is the second choice. Normal saline has the potential to cause hyperchloremic acidosis. This complication is more likely if renal function is compromised (Table 27.1).[69]

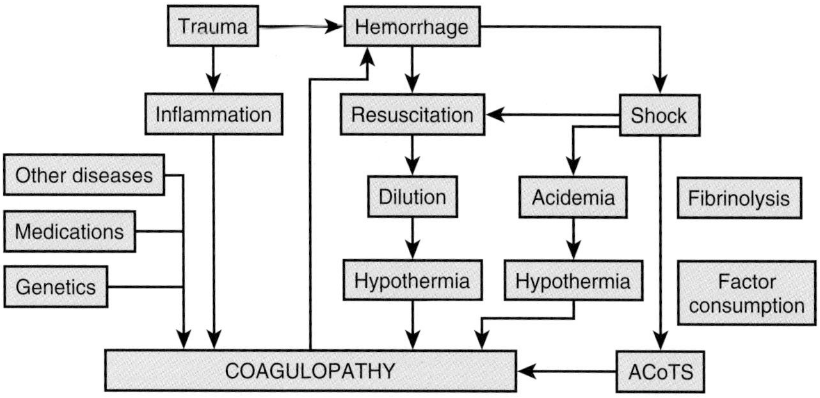

Figure 27.2 A diagram showing some of the mechanisms leading to coagulopathy in the injured. Trauma can lead to hemorrhage, which can lead to resuscitation, which in turn leads to dilution and hypothermia causing coagulopathy and further hemorrhage. This is classic "dilution coagulopathy." Hemorrhage can also cause shock, which causes acidosis and hypothermia that in turn lead to coagulopathy, the "fatal triad." Trauma and shock can also cause the acute coagulopathy of trauma shock (ACoTS) associated with factor consumption and fibrinolysis. Coagulopathy is further associated with trauma-induced inflammation and modified by genetics, medications, and acquired diseases. (From Hess JR, Brohi K, Dutton RP, et al: The coagulopathy of trauma: A review of mechanisms. J Trauma 2008;65:748-754.)

Table 27.1 Estimated Fluid and Blood Losses Based on Initial Clinical Presentation*

Clinical Finding	Class I	Class II	Class III	Class IV
Blood loss (mL)	≤750	750-1500	1500-2000	>2000
Percent blood loss by shock categories	<15%	15-30%	30-40%	>40%
Pulse rate (beats/min)	<100	>100	>120	>140
Blood pressure	Normal	Normal	Decreased	Decreased
Pulse pressure	Normal or increased	Decreased	Decreased	Decreased
Respiratory rate	14-20	20-30	30-40	>35
Urine output (mL/h)	>30	20-30	5-15	Negligible
Central nervous system/mental status	Slightly anxious	Mildly anxious	Anxious, confused	Confused, lethargic
Fluid replacement (3:1 rule)	Crystalloid	Crystalloid	Crystalloid and blood	Crystalloid and blood

*This is the standard approach to resuscitation of shock after injury as described in the Advanced Trauma Life Support course promulgated by the Committee on Trauma of the American College of Surgeons. The crystalloid of choice used in resuscitation is lactated Ringer's solution. Clinical parameters are used to estimate the degree of blood loss, and fluid resuscitation begins with 1-2 L of lactated Ringer's solution given through large-bore peripheral intravenous lines. When the response to resuscitation is limited or transient, O-negative or type-specific blood is added to resuscitation while the cause of shock is sought and additional treatment is given.

From American College of Surgeons Committee on Trauma: Advanced Trauma Life Support for Doctors, 7th ed. Chicago, American College of Surgeons, 2004, pp 69-85.

An initial warm fluid bolus is given rapidly—usually 1 to 2 L for an adult and 20 mL/kg for a child.[45] Patient response is observed during this initial fluid resuscitation, and subsequent therapeutic decisions are based on this response. The required amount of fluid and blood is difficult to predict on initial evaluation of the patient. A rough guideline promulgated by the American College of Surgeons for the total amount of crystalloid volume acutely required is 3 mL of crystalloid fluid to replace each 1 mL of blood loss, allowing for restitution of plasma volume lost into interstitial and intracellular spaces. It is most important, however, to assess patient response to fluid resuscitation and evidence of adequate end-organ perfusion as measured by urine output and level of consciousness, rather than provide fluid based on a specific formula. If the amount of fluid required to restore or maintain adequate end-organ function exceeds the previously mentioned estimates, careful reassessment of the situation and exploration for unrecognized injuries, bleeding, or other causes of shock are necessary (Table 27.2).

In clinical practice, large volume resuscitation with lactated Ringer's solution has become common in trauma care.[70] However, recent military and laboratory work features a growing concern about tissue edema from large volume resuscitation. In recent decades, a persisting picture of acute lung injury due to increased filtration across pulmonary microcapillaries with pulmonary inflammation emerged. This process would later be called the acute respiratory distress syndrome.[71] Other observations included increased interstitial fluid of gut and heart tissues, abdominal compartment syndrome, extremity compartment syndrome in uninjured extremities, and pericardial effusion.[72,73]

Hemorrhage is a multifactorial disease; circulatory and inflammatory effects of hemorrhagic shock occur simultaneously. Unfortunately, laboratory studies have repeatedly shown that the choice of resuscitation fluid may worsen hemorrhage-induced cellular dysfunction, immune modulation, and inflammation. Fluids affect neutrophil activity by

Table 27.2 Responses to Initial Fluid Resuscitation*

Factor	Rapid Response	Transient Response	No Response
Vital signs	Return to normal	Transient improvement, recurrence of decreased blood pressure and increased heart rate	Remain abnormal
Estimated blood loss	Minimal (10-20%)	Moderate and ongoing (20-40%)	Severe (>40%)
Need for more crystalloid	Low	High	High
Need for blood	Low	Moderate to high	Immediate
Blood preparation	Type and crossmatch	Type-specific	Emergency blood release
Need for operative intervention	Possibly	Likely	Highly likely
Early presence of surgeon	Yes	Yes	Yes

*The Advanced Trauma Life Support course advocates ongoing evaluation of patient response to initial fluid administration. Patients with no response frequently require emergent blood transfusion and transfer to the operating room. Patients with transient response also frequently require operative intervention. Most patients, particularly in centers seeing blunt injury, respond rapidly to an initial 1-2 L of crystalloid and are cleared to proceed to more detailed imaging to determine internal injuries after normalization of clinical parameters.

From American College of Surgeons Committee on Trauma: Advanced Trauma Life Support for Doctors, 7th ed. Chicago, American College of Surgeons, 2004, pp 69-85.

changing life span, activation, and gene expression. Resuscitation fluids also enhance inflammatory cascade through upregulation of cellular receptors and proinflammatory mediators. The choice of fluid also affects cellular gene expression, apoptotic cell death, and extracellular matrix integrity.[70,74-76]

ISOTONIC CRYSTALLOIDS

Of isotonic crystalloids, lactated Ringer's solution has been most extensively studied to determine its role in hemorrhage-induced immune dysfunction, inflammation, and management of ischemia and reperfusion injury. Lactated Ringer's solution has been shown to upgrade vascular endothelial adhesion molecules and to increase expression of CD11b and CD18 binding sites on neutrophils. Neutrophil oxidative burst is also stimulated by lactated Ringer's solution. In other organs, Ringer's lactate has been found to increase apoptosis in the bowel, the liver, and the lung with multiple cell types affected including macrophages, endothelial cells, epithelial cells, and smooth muscle cells.[70,77]

Despite laboratory findings about the dangers of lactated Ringer's solution, it remains the fluid of choice in many centers and the recommended fluid of the Advanced Trauma Life Support (ATLS) protocol. Efforts have been made to examine why lactated Ringer's solution is cytotoxic and identify ways to improve it. Traditionally, lactated Ringer's solution came in racemic form; laboratory work implicates the D-isomer of lactate as its primary toxic component.[78] The D-isomer was found to increase neutrophil oxidative burst, enhance apoptosis, and drive inflammation. The L-isomer of lactate may confer immune protection through attenuation of neutrophil activation, alteration of leukocyte gene expression, and reduction in apoptosis.[79,80]

COLLOIDS

Hyperoncotic colloid solutions have also been studied in resuscitation roles for traumatic hemorrhage. The natural colloid albumin does not induce neutrophil oxidative burst and may confer a protective immunologic effect by decreasing neutrophil expression of adhesion molecules.[81] At present, albumin sees little application in resuscitation at the scene of injury but has been investigated in critical care practice.

An artificial colloid, 6% hetastarch, has been found to have a number of deleterious resuscitation effects in animal models including increased neutrophil oxidative burst and pulmonary apoptosis. Beneficial effects include decreased neutrophil migration. At present, natural and artificial colloids have failed to show clinical benefits in comparison with crystalloid solutions.[82,83] Laboratory concerns and lack of a positive clinical outcomes mandate argue against the use of colloids in early resuscitation of hemorrhagic shock.

Recent reviews suggest important differences in safety among colloids. Examination of data comparing colloids with crystalloids must take into account materials employed. When albumin was used as a reference, the incidence ratio for anaphylactoid reactions was 4.51 after administration of hydroxyethyl starch, 2.32 after dextran, and 12.4 after gelatin. Artificial colloid administration was consistently associated with coagulopathy and clinical bleeding, most frequently in cardiac surgery patients receiving starches. Albumin had the lowest rate of total adverse events and serious adverse events.[84] Although albumin is isolated from human plasma, no evidence of viral disease transmission has been consistently identified. Life-threatening anaphylactoid reactions were infrequent for all colloids. Hydroxyethyl starch, as compared with albumin, more than quadrupled the incidence of anaphylactic reactions, whereas dextran more than doubled them. The incidence of these reactions in recipients of gelatin was greater by an order of magnitude than after albumin infusion. Because artificial colloids are derived from nonhuman source materials, they may be recognized as foreign and are more likely to provoke this immune-mediated response. The foreign nature of artificial colloids also may hinder metabolic clearance and promote tissue deposition. On the basis of extensive evidence, albumin is the safest colloid for consideration in resuscitation of traumatic shock.[84] Although factors such as desirability of anticoagulant activity may favor other artificial colloids, this is not true in the setting of injury.[85-87]

Multicenter data comparing albumin and saline for fluid resuscitation were obtained in Australia and published in 2004.[88] Nearly 7000 patients were randomly assigned to administration of 4% albumin or normal saline for intravascular fluid resuscitation procedures. Mortality rate and the incidence of single and multiple organ dysfunction were comparable in the two groups. Subset analysis suggests, however, poorer outcomes in the setting of injury. In the subgroup of 140 patients included with principal diagnoses of trauma, a treatment effect seemed to favor administration of saline. In this trial, the increased relative risk of death among patients with trauma compared with patients without trauma resulted from an excess number of deaths among patients who had trauma with brain injury. The difference in mortality rates between albumin and saline groups among patients with trauma involving brain injury must be viewed cautiously because the number of involved subjects is small. In the Australian trial, patients with traumatic brain injury constituted only 7% of the study population, and the excess number of deaths in the albumin group was 21. Other parameters that could be helpful in evaluation of the impact of albumin in the setting of brain injury, such as functional neurologic status, were not provided. In contrast with the experience in trauma, the Australian trial suggests some evidence of treatment benefit favoring administration of albumin in patients with severe sepsis. Given contemporary resuscitation technology, factors influencing the choice of resuscitation for critically ill patients include specific clinician concerns, treatment tolerance, safety, and cost.

HYPERTONIC SALINE

Increased transmembrane sodium gradient caused by hypertonic saline generates intravascular volume expansion similar to hyperoncotic colloids and superior to conventional isotonic crystalloids such as lactated Ringer's solution and normal saline. Animal models suggest that hypertonic saline solutions dilate precapillary arterioles and shunt oxygen to vital organs.[89,90] Hypertonic saline solutions also have fewer proinflammatory properties than other clinical crystalloids and colloids. Hypertonic saline does not induce expression of inflammatory cytokine receptor genes in multiple studies and blunts hemorrhage-induced increase in plasma levels of proinflammatory cytokines, IL-10, and granulocyte-macrophage colony-stimulating factor. Hypertonic saline also does not increase apoptotic cell death in liver, lung, or bowel.[70]

What about the impact of hypertonic saline and associated hypernatremia on head injury?[91] Studies in experimental animals and humans suggest that hypertonic saline may be highly effective in treating head injury, either alone or associated with hemorrhagic hypotension. Tissue swelling in a closed cranium threatens to cause major pressure-induced brain damage or death, and concomitant hemorrhage hypotension reduces cerebral oxygen delivery, resulting in a secondary ischemic insult. Historical data suggest a twofold higher incidence of adverse outcomes in patients with brain injury combined with hypotension. Early data suggest that patients treated with hypertonic saline with dextran are more likely to survive to discharge than individuals treated with standard resuscitation care.[92,93]

Despite laboratory data suggesting that hypertonic saline may be an effective tool in resuscitation-induced injury, mixed clinical data have not led to widespread utilization of this material.

HYPERTONIC-HYPERONCOTIC FLUIDS

Mixture of hypertonic saline with dextran has been the most extensively tested hypertonic-hyperoncotic fluid.[70] Use of combinations of hypertonic saline and dextran suggests that this material is effective in expanding plasma volume, restoring hemodynamics, and improving microcirculatory perfusion. In the laboratory, hypertonic saline and dextran solutions blunt hemorrhage-induced inflammatory response by neutrophils and, in clinical trials, decreased adhesion molecule expression.[94] As with hypertonic saline solutions, there has been concern that hypertonic saline mixed with dextran could accelerate hemorrhage, increase mortality rate, and cause hypernatremia and hyperchloremia.[95] Despite multiple clinical trials comparing hypertonic saline and dextran solutions to more traditional resuscitation products, no improvement in mortality rate or change in the pattern of organ failure is seen.[96]

Mechanisms by which hypertonic/hyperoncotic resuscitation may be effective in models of head injury and hemorrhage show reduction in water content in noninjured portions of the brain with reduction in intracranial pressure and cerebral edema. In a large animal model, when hypertonic saline was compared with a synthetic colloid, colloid alone had no effect on brain water content.[97,98]

The optimal crystalloid/nonblood colloid resuscitation fluid or regimen has yet to be defined. Hypertonic solutions remain on the horizon of opportunity owing to rapid expansion of plasma volume and improvement of hemodynamics, expanding the therapeutic window until patients may be transported to definitive treatment. Optimally, resuscitation as applied clinically and studied in the preclinical setting must be titrated to desired physiologic and metabolic performance objectives.

CRYSTALLOIDS VERSUS COLLOIDS

Plasma and blood were the fluid replacements of choice in traumatic shock until the early 1960s, when a variety of investigators showed the need to replace the extracellular fluid deficit with crystalloid solutions. These observations were followed by a variety of clinical studies comparing colloid, typically albumin, solutions with crystalloids, typically lactated Ringer's solution. Consistent with early studies, colloids, when given on an equal volume basis, more effectively increase cardiac output and oxygen transport. Another finding of this early work was the need to give crystalloids in far greater quantities than colloids to achieve consistent hemodynamic objectives.[99,100]

Later studies from the Vietnam era compared resuscitation of patients who were given whole blood and crystalloids with patients given whole blood plus 5% albumin. Fluid infusion volumes were far higher in the patients given crystalloid solutions. There was no evidence of pulmonary edema, and patients treated with crystalloids seemed to fare better than patients treated with resuscitation containing albumin. Albumin seemed to have less effect on restoration of renal function with suggestion of detrimental effects in pulmonary response, myocardial contractility, and coagulation. Large animal models suggested that pulmonary compromise could relate to increased capillary permeability to albumin. Increased losses of albumin to the heart, kidneys, liver, and brain also were reported.[99,101] More extensive studies in injured patients supported reservations regarding the use of albumin. Evaluation of patients randomly selected to receive 150 g of albumin per day intraoperatively and postoperatively noted poorer outcomes than in patients receiving lactated Ringer's solution. Both groups received whole blood and FFP. Patients treated with albumin required greater ventilator support and had poorer oxygenation.[99,102,103] In another carefully conducted trial of patients with multiple trauma, no differences in cardiopulmonary function between patients resuscitated with lactated Ringer's solution and patients given 5% albumin and lactated Ringer's solution were identified.[104] Normal cardiac index was used as a therapeutic end point. To maintain adequate cardiac output, patients who received crystalloids required far more resuscitation volume than patients treated with albumin. These authors concluded that cardiac output was an appropriate end point for resuscitation, and that no advantage was accrued based on the type of fluid employed. A clear cost advantage of crystalloids was identified.[99]

Guyton and Lindsey[105] examined the effect of colloid oncotic pressure on pulmonary edema. They observed that reducing the serum protein level lowered the threshold of left atrial pressure at which pulmonary edema could occur. Zarins and colleagues[106] subsequently showed that a low colloid oncotic pressure alone did not cause an elevation in extravascular lung water. Because of the remarkable efficiency of pulmonary lymphatics, arterial blood gases, shunt fraction, and lung compliance were unchanged despite a 14% increase in body weight caused by infusion of lactated Ringer's solution to keep high pulmonary artery occlusion pressures. No pulmonary edema was created despite the presence of ascites and marked peripheral edema. Demling and coworkers[107] confirmed these findings with a chronic lung lymph fistula in sheep. Holcroft and coworkers[108] produced pulmonary edema in baboons during resuscitation from hemorrhage by continuously administering large volumes of lactated Ringer's solution sufficient to elevate pulmonary artery occlusion pressures 15 mm Hg above baseline levels. With cessation of infusion, filling pressure rapidly returned to normal.

BLOOD COMPONENT THERAPY

Despite work from multiple groups suggesting that simple replacement of PRBCs was not a sufficient answer for the most severely injured patient, particularly in the setting of coagulopathy, the concept of combination blood component replacement remained outside the mainstream of trauma care for over 20 years.[48,52,109] It took armed conflicts and experience in a multinational group of trauma centers to bring awareness of the need for multiple blood component therapy in massive bleeding to the level of general trauma practice.

The 1970s and 1980s saw several groups propose resuscitation of significant hemorrhage with combinations of blood components. Kashuk and Moore proposed multicomponent blood therapy in patients with significant vascular injury.[48] In a study of patients with major abdominal vascular injury, Kashuk and coworkers noted frequent deviation from a standard ratio of 4:1 or 5:1 for units of PRBCs to units of FFP. The ratio was 8:1 in nonsurvivors and 9:1 where overt coagulopathy was noted. Fifty-one percent of patients in this series were coagulopathic after vascular control was obtained. Using multivariate analysis, Ciavarella and coworkers from the Puget Sound Blood Center and Harborview Medical Center proposed aggressive supplementation of platelets in the setting of massive transfusion. These investigators noted that platelet counts below $50 \times 10^9/L$ correlated highly with microvascular bleeding in trauma and surgery patients. Fibrinogen repletion was also emphasized. Guides to resuscitation included fibrinogen level, PT, and PTT. Supplemental FFP or cryoprecipitate was recommended for low fibrinogen levels.[52] Lucas and Ledgerwood, summarizing extensive preclinical and clinical studies, suggested administration of FFP after 6 units of PRBCs had been infused. Additional FFP was recommended for every five additional PRBC transfusions. Monitoring included platelet count, PT, and PTT after each 5 units of PRBCs are administered. Platelet transfusion is generally unnecessary unless the platelet count falls below 50,000.[109]

Rhee and coworkers, using the massive database of the Los Angeles County Level I Trauma Center, examined transfusion practices in 25,000 patients.[110] Approximately 16% of these patients received a blood transfusion. Massive transfusion (≥10 units of PRBCs per day) occurred in 11.4% of transfused patients. After excluding head-injured patients, these authors studied approximately 400 individuals. A trend toward increasing FFP use was noted during the 6 years of data that were reviewed (January 2000 to December 2005). Logistic regression identified the ratio of FFP to PRBC use as an independent predictor of survival. With a higher ratio of FFP:PRBC, a greater probability of survival was noted. The optimal ratio in this analysis was an FFP:PRBC ratio of 1:3 or less. Rhee and coworkers provide a large retrospective data set demonstrating that earlier more aggressive plasma replacement can be associated with improved outcomes after bleeding requiring massive transfusion. Ratios derived in this massive retrospective data review support the observations of Hirshberg and coworkers.[54] Like the data presented by Kashuk and coworkers in another widely cited report, this retrospective data set suggests improved clinical outcome with increased administration of FFP.[111]

Another view of damage control hematology comes from Vanderbilt University Medical Center in Nashville, Tennessee. This group implemented a trauma exsanguination protocol involving acute administration of 10 units PRBC with 4 units FFP and 2 units platelets. In an 18-month period, 90 patients received this resuscitation and were compared to a historical set of control subjects. The group of patients receiving the trauma exsanguination protocol as described by these investigators had lower mortality rates, higher blood product use in initial operative procedures, and more frequent use of products in the initial 24 hours, though overall blood product consumption during hospitalization was decreased.[112]

The strongest multicenter civilian data report examining the impact of plasma and platelet administration along with red blood cells on outcome in massive transfusion comes from Holcomb and coworkers.[113] These investigators report over 450 patients obtained from 16 adult and pediatric centers. Overall survival in this group is 59%. Patients were gravely ill as reflected by an admission base deficit of −11.7, pH 7.2, Glasgow Coma Scale score of 9, and a mean ISS of 32. Examination of multicenter data reflects an improvement in outcome as the ratio of FFP to PRBCs administered approaches 1. FFP, however, is not the sole solution to improved coagulation response in acute injury. These workers also examined the relationship of aggressive plasma and platelet administration in these patients. Optimal outcome in this massive transfusion group was obtained with aggressive platelet as well as plasma administration. Worst outcomes were seen when aggressive administration of plasma and platelets did not take place. When either FFP or platelets were given in higher proportion in relationship to PRBCs intermediate results were obtained. Not surprisingly, the cause of death that was favorably affected was truncal hemorrhage.

A summary statement comes from Holcomb and a combination of military and civilian investigators.[56,57] These workers identify a patient group at high risk for coagulopathy and resuscitation failure due to hypothermia, acidosis, hypoperfusion, inflammation, and volume of tissue injury. In the paradigm proposed by these writers, resuscitation begins with prehospital limitation of blood pressure at approximately 90 mm Hg preventing renewed bleeding from recently clotted vessels. Intravascular volume resuscitation is accomplished using thawed plasma in a 1:1 or 1:2 ratio with PRBCs. Acidosis is managed by use of THAM (tromethamine) and volume loading with blood components as hemostasis is obtained. A massive transfusion protocol for these investigators included delivery of packs of 6 units of plasma, 6 units of PRBC, 6 units of platelets, and 10 units of cryoprecipitate in stored individual coolers. These coolers are supplied until discontinuation by the trauma team. Even in causalities requiring resuscitation with 10 to 40 units of blood products, Holcomb and coworkers found that as little as 5 to 8 L of crystalloid are utilized during the first 24 hours, representing a decrease of at least 50% compared to standard practice. The lack of intraoperative coagulopathic bleeding allows surgeons to focus on surgical hemorrhage. The goal is arrival of the patient in intensive care unit (ICU) in a warm, euvolemic, and nonacidotic state. International normalized ratio (INR) approaches normal and edema is minimized. Subjectively, patients treated in this way are more readily ventilated and easier to extubate than patients with a similar blood loss treated with standard crystalloid resuscitation and smaller amounts of blood products. Holcomb and others suggest that massive transfusion will be required in 6% to 7% of military patients and 1% to 2% of civilian trauma patients.

END POINTS

THE PROBLEM

Severely injured trauma patients are at high risk of developing multiple organ failure or death. Initial treatment priorities include appropriate fluid administration and rapid hemostasis.[114,115] Inadequate tissue oxygenation leads to anaerobic metabolism and tissue acidosis. Depth and duration of shock are associated with cumulative oxygen and metabolic debt. Resuscitation is incomplete until the metabolic debt is paid, and tissue acidosis is eliminated with restoration of aerobic metabolism. Many patients seem to be adequately resuscitated based on normalization of vital signs but have occult hypoperfusion and ongoing tissue acidosis (compensated shock). These individuals are at risk for later organ dysfunction and death.[69]

As stated in the Advanced Trauma Life Support protocol, the standard of care remains restoration of normal blood pressure, heart rate, and urine output.[69] When these parameters remain abnormal (uncompensated shock), the need for additional resuscitation is obvious. After normalization of these parameters, however, many trauma patients still have evidence of inadequate tissue oxygenation or gastric mucosal ischemia. Recognition of this state and its reversal are crucial to reduce the risk of organ dysfunction or death. The optimal marker of adequate resuscitation in injury remains unclear.[116]

Not all patients can be managed in the same way. More recent literature describing management of neurologic trauma suggests poor outcome with any degree of hypotension during prehospital care, resuscitation, or subsequent in-hospital course. Episodes of hypotension and hypoxia were associated with poor neurologic outcome in a review of more than 700 patients from the Traumatic Coma Data Bank with a Glasgow Coma Scale score less than 9. In this large study, patients without hypotension or hypoxia had a 27% risk of death and a 51% chance of favorable recovery. In the presence of hypotension, with or without hypoxia, the risk of death increased to 65% to 75%. Contrary to the needs of patients with penetrating trauma in whom early aggressive resuscitation may lead to increased bleeding, hypotension should be avoided in head-injured patients. Resuscitation parameters specific to various types of injury have not been reported.[117-119]

OXYGEN DELIVERY PARAMETERS

Shoemaker and various coworkers provided early stimulus to optimization of hemodynamic management in high-risk surgical patients by examining hemodynamic profiles of survivors of surgical shock states versus patients who died.[120] Survivors had significantly higher oxygen delivery and cardiac index values than nonsurvivors. Values correlating with survival included cardiac index greater than 4.5 L/minute/m^2, oxygen delivery greater than 600 mL/minute/m^2, and oxygen consumption equal to or greater than 170 mL/minute/m^2. These initial observations led to a series of articles from this group suggesting reduction in resource consumption and improvement in morbidity and mortality rates with resuscitation to supranormal oxygen delivery parameters. Initial augmentation of oxygen delivery came with volume loading followed by dobutamine and blood transfusions as needed to a hemoglobin level of 14 g/dL.[121-124]

Attempts by other investigators to replicate these findings met limited success. Moore and coworkers used a resuscitation protocol aimed at maximizing oxygen delivery and found no benefit with resuscitation to achieve supranormal oxygen delivery.[116,125] A variety of studies suggested that patients failing to reach resuscitation goals were at increased risk for multiple organ failure. Other workers noted that patients who did not obtain supranormal oxygen delivery values were at high risk of developing organ failure regardless of treatment strategy.[126,127] Obtaining hemodynamic and oxygen transport parameters seems to be more predictive of survival than useful as a goal for resuscitation, particularly if fluid administration is adequate.

In addition to conflicting outcomes in oxygen transport trials, technical concerns have been raised.[116] These studies cannot be totally blinded. Patients in control groups often obtain similar physiologic end points to those in treatment groups. Other aspects of care were sometimes inconsistent, and entrance criteria varied among investigators. There also is potential mathematical coupling of oxygen delivery and consumption because both are calculated values that share many of the same measured variables.[117] Some clinicians argue that the pathologic relationship between oxygen delivery and consumption trials cannot be accepted with confidence, unless oxygen consumption is measured directly. Finally, use of traditional oxygen delivery and consumption as resuscitative end points requires a pulmonary artery catheter and special expertise for operation and insertion. Routine use of pulmonary artery catheterization or central venous catheters has not been a part of acute trauma resuscitation or emergency medical management.[69,116,117]

LACTATE

As an indicator of shock, blood lactate has proved accurate at assessing severity, predicting mortality risk, and assessing response to resuscitation in the hands of various workers.[116,117] At the cellular level, the explanation is based on oxygen transport principles. With shock and inadequate oxygen delivery, mitochondrial respiration is impaired. The primary cellular fuel, pyruvate, is shunted from its normal aerobic path (conversion by pyruvate dehydrogenase to acetyl coenzyme A and subsequent entry into the tricarboxylic acid cycle) to the anaerobic pathway (conversion to lactate by lactate dehydrogenase). Anaerobic metabolism makes inefficient use of cellular substrate, and high-energy phosphate stores are rapidly depleted. During cellular ischemia, lactate is released into the bloodstream and ultimately converted to glucose in the liver and kidney via the Cori cycle. Because it directly reflects anaerobic metabolism, lactate is thought to serve as a mirror of global hyperperfusion because increasing lactate levels indicate increasing oxygen debt.[117,128]

Initial and peak lactate levels and duration of increased lactate concentration correlate with development of multiorgan dysfunction after trauma.[116] In a study of trauma patient resuscitation, patients normalizing lactate levels at 24 hours survived, whereas patients who normalized lactate levels between 24 and 48 hours had a 25% mortality rate; patients who did not normalize by 48 hours had an 86% mortality rate.[129] Theoretically, severity of metabolic acidosis secondary to tissue hyperperfusion should be reflected in lactate levels, anion gap, and base deficit. This is not a consistent finding among investigators studying trauma resuscitation.[130,131] In addition, although lactate levels are rapidly available, conclusive data tying specific lactate levels and targets to improved resuscitation outcomes are unavailable.

BASE DEFICIT

Inadequate oxygen delivery to tissues leads to anaerobic metabolism. The degree of anaerobiosis is proportional to the depth and severity of hemorrhagic shock, which should be reflected in lactate and base deficit. Arterial pH is not as useful because compensatory mechanisms attempt to normalize this parameter. Serum bicarbonate levels offer better correlation with base deficit (removal or addition of base in the blood).[116,132,133]

Similar to lactate, base deficit has been carefully studied.[116] A greater base deficit has been associated with blood pressure reduction, increased blood loss, and transfusion requirements. A series of studies by Davis and coworkers link base deficit to resuscitation requirements and end-organ dysfunction, such as acute respiratory distress syndrome, renal failure, and coagulopathy. Cytokine and adhesion molecule changes also have been found to parallel changes in base deficit.[134-140]

Base deficit may vary with patient populations. Concern remains in older patients that base deficit is nonspecific and may reflect metabolic acidosis due to a variety of causes, including renal dysfunction and diabetes.[116,117] Similar to temporal changes in lactate, base deficit variation over time may add to the value of this parameter.[132] Patients with elevated base deficit also showed impaired oxygen use reflected in lower oxygen consumption. The timing of base deficit measurement also is important. One study suggested that the worst base deficit in the initial 24 hours was predictive of mortality rate along with blood pressure and estimated blood loss.[138] Some workers debate whether alcohol intoxication may worsen base deficit for similar levels of injury severity and hemodynamics after trauma. In a large database survey, use of alcohol did not change significant predictive value of admission lactate and base deficit.[141,142] Resuscitation with normal saline (hyperchloremic metabolic acidosis) or lactated Ringer's solution (accumulation of D-lactate) may increase base deficit independent of injury severity. Acidosis associated with hyperchloremia is associated with lower mortality rate than that from other causes, particularly anaerobic metabolism.[116,143] Base deficit levels and time to normalization of base deficit are similar to data for lactate in that correlation has been established with the need for resuscitation and risk of organ dysfunction and death after injury. Specific thresholds for outcome have not been determined, however, and there are no multicenter data that conclusively show that using base deficit as an end point for resuscitation improves survival.[116]

GASTRIC MUCOSAL pH

As systemic perfusion decreases, blood flow to vulnerable organs (brain and heart) is maintained at the expense of other organs (skin, muscle, kidneys, and intestines). Detection of subclinical ischemia to these organs may allow identification of patients requiring additional resuscitation despite normalized vital signs.[116,144] Gastric tonometry is based on the finding that tissue ischemia leads to an increase in tissue partial pressure of carbon dioxide (P_{CO_2}) and subsequent decrease in tissue pH. Because CO_2 diffuses readily across tissues and fluids, the P_{CO_2} of gastric secretions rapidly equilibrates with that in gastric mucosa. For elevation in gastric pH values to be accurate, it is important to withhold gastric feedings and suppress gastric acid secretion. To perform gastric tonometry, a semipermeable balloon is attached to a special nasogastric tube and placed in the stomach. The balloon is filled with saline, and CO_2 is allowed to diffuse into the balloon for a specific time. P_{CO_2} in the saline is then measured. Continuous CO_2 measuring electrodes are sometimes employed. Intramucosal pH is calculated from the Henderson-Hasselbalch equation. The difference between intragastric P_{CO_2} and arterial P_{CO_2}, or the intramucosal pH, correlates with the degree of gastric ischemia.[145]

In studies of a small number of trauma patients, patients with low intramucosal pH (≤7.32) were more likely to develop complications or die.[146-148] Patients with normal intramucosal pH fared well. Correlation to other parameters has not been rigorously studied. A larger trial examined the value of intramucosal pH and the gastric mucosal-arterial CO_2 gap (difference between intragastric P_{CO_2} and arterial P_{CO_2}). Ability to predict multiple organ dysfunction and death was maximized with intramucosal pH less than 7.25 and CO_2 gap greater than 18 mm Hg. Similar to studies using blood lactate and base deficit, time course for changes in CO_2 gap or intramucosal pH may be important. Ivatury and associates[149,150] compared changes in intramucosal pH with oxygen transport values. Although intramucosal pH changes paralleled improvement in oxygen transport, delay in achieving intramucosal pH was more predictive of organ system failure than oxygen transport parameters. The gap between gastric mucosal and arterial P_{CO_2} was similarly predictive. After resuscitation, changes in mucosal pH were an early predictor of complications.

Newer fiber-optic technologies increase the ease of gastric mucosal pH assessment.[151] Although this parameter may be predictive of early resuscitation failure, accepted thresholds for failure and outcome data do not support widespread use to guide initial resuscitation after injury (Fig. 27.3).

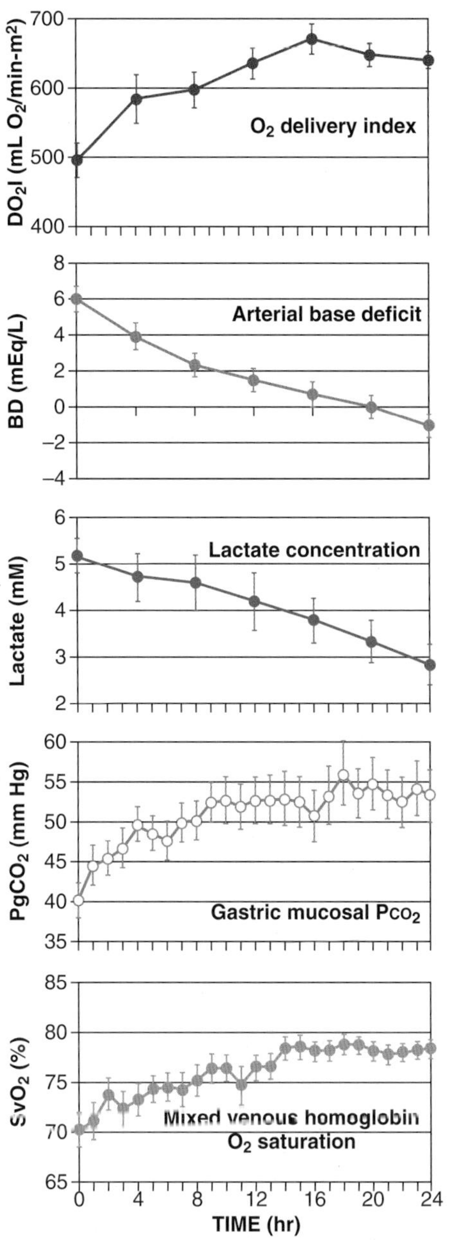

Figure 27.3 Changes in oxygen transport parameters, biochemical indicators of resuscitation success, and local acid-base changes as reflected in gastric mucosal P_{CO_2} are described here. These collected data from McKinley and coworkers suggest the correlation between these common resuscitation parameters. Not all investigators or specific patient groups have complete correspondence among all resuscitation indices, however. (From McKinley BA, Valdivia A, Moore FA: Goal-oriented shock resuscitation for major torso trauma: What are we learning? Curr Opin Crit Care 2003;9:292-299.)

NEAR-INFRARED SPECTROSCOPY

Measurement of skeletal muscle oxyhemoglobin levels by near-infrared spectroscopy offers a noninvasive measurement for evaluating adequacy of resuscitation from normalization of tissue oxygenation.[116,117,145,152] This technology allows simultaneous measurement of tissue partial pressure of oxygen (P_{O_2}), P_{CO_2}, and pH. In human volunteers, cerebral cortex and calf oxygen saturation as measured by near-infrared spectroscopy decreased in proportion to blood loss. Oxygenation index (oxygenated hemoglobin—deoxygenated hemoglobin) also decreased. Studies in injury suggest correlation of tissue oxygen saturation with systemic oxygen delivery, base deficit, lactate, and gastric mucosal P_{CO_2}.[153]

This technology provides information regarding mitochondrial function. Normally, tissue oxyhemoglobin levels reflecting local oxygenation are tightly coupled to cytochrome function, reflecting mitochondrial oxygen

Box 27.2 Adrenal Insufficiency

Check adrenal function in patients who fail to respond to resuscitation.[a-c] Adrenal insufficiency, a rare occurrence in the general population (<0.01%), is seen in 28% of seriously ill patients and 60% of severely injured trauma patients in contemporary series.[d] Severe illness and stress activate the hypothalamic-pituitary-adrenal axis and stimulate the release of corticotropin (adrenocorticotropic hormone) from the pituitary, which stimulates release of cortisol from the adrenal cortex. This action is an essential component of general adaptation to illness and contributes to maintenance of cellular and organ homeostasis.[a,c]

Although a growing body of literature reviews adrenal insufficiency in critical illness with an emphasis on sepsis, we have seen a significant incidence of adrenal insufficiency, reflected by low serum cortisol levels, in severe injury with or without direct trauma to the brain.[e,f] We suspect adrenal insufficiency in patients who are young and otherwise healthy and require vasoactive drugs in addition to large amounts of resuscitation fluid. Our approach to making the diagnosis of acute adrenal insufficiency is a spot cortisol level. Although a variety of treatment protocols for hormonal replacement exist, we provide 50 mg of hydrocortisone every 6 hours or 100 mg of hydrocortisone every 8 hours for 5 days. Consistent with the treatment threshold reported by Marik and Zaloga,[b,f] we treat if a random cortisol concentration is less than 25 μg/dL. Severely injured patients have been reported to have random cortisol levels greater than 30 μg/dL.[d] Although outcome data are unavailable to suggest the value of adrenal replacement in critically stressed young trauma patients, we have seen the effectiveness of this intervention repeatedly in our own practice.

[a]Cooper MS, Stewart PM: Corticosteroid insufficiency in acutely ill patients. N Engl J Med 2003;348:727-734.
[b]Marik PE, Zaloga GP: Adrenal insufficiency in the critically ill: A new look at an old problem. Chest 2002;122:1784-1796.
[c]Burchard K: A review of the adrenal cortex and severe inflammation: Quest of the "eucorticoid" state. J Trauma 2001;51:800-814.
[d]Offner PJ, Moore EE, Ciesia D: The adrenal response after severe trauma. Am J Surg 2002;184:649-654.
[e]Rivers EP, Gaspari M, Saad GA, et al: Adrenal insufficiency in high-risk surgical ICU patients. Chest 2001;119:889-896.
[f]Marik PE, Zaloga GP: Adrenal insufficiency during septic shock. Crit Care Med 2003;31:141-145.

consumption. In preliminary studies, when patients showed change in mitochondrial function, even in the absence of abnormality in systemic oxygen transport, multiple organ failure was more likely.[154] Nonetheless, at this time, work in this area is preliminary, and a role for this technology in management of traumatic shock has not been defined.

ADRENAL INSUFFICIENCY

Adrenal insufficiency is reviewed in Box 27.2.

CLINICAL STRATEGIES

Clinical observations of shock in injury have been made for hundreds of years, but the optimal treatment continues to be debated.[115] Early observations are attributed to Paré, Le Dran, Latta, and Gross.[155,156] Crile and Henderson were among the first to attribute the hemodynamic instability of shock to decreased intravascular volume and to propose therapy based on restoration of intravascular volume with administration of intravenous fluid.[115,156] During the First World War, physiologists Cannon and Bayliss observed patients in clinical shock.[6] These observers noted that patients with crush injuries despite absence of obvious blood loss also developed signs and symptoms of shock.[157,158] Cannon later suggested the concept of deliberate hypotension in the treatment of wounds to the torso during war with the intent of minimizing internal bleeding until the time at which operative intervention could control the hemorrhage.[159,160] In later studies, other authors reported laboratory models of ongoing arterial hemorrhage and concluded that regardless of the means used to increase blood pressure, either fluid resuscitation or vasopressor, bleeding would increase, with subsequent death.[161,162]

Current guidelines for the treatment of hypotension secondary to hemorrhage after trauma recommend rapid infusion of crystalloid solutions to restore blood pressure.[69,160] This premise is based in part on clinical studies and laboratory data showing that hemorrhagic shock in animals produced with controlled blood loss was reversible when blood loss was replaced with two to three times that volume of a crystalloid solution.[163-165] Although controlled hemorrhage is a well-defined laboratory model, resuscitation of a patient with multiple injuries and active or uncontrolled bleeding may represent very different pathophysiology.[115]

In 1950, Wiggers[166] developed a standard hemorrhagic shock model in dogs. He and others showed that severe hypotension over several hours produced a condition in which infusion of withdrawn blood restored arterial pressure only temporarily.[115] After intervals ranging from 30 minutes to 3 hours, arterial pressure declined again. Additional infusions of blood were followed by progressively poorer recovery and more rapid development of circulatory failure, ultimately resulting in the demise of the animal. This decompensation point in shock, defining a time at which reinfusion of shed blood could not resuscitate the animal, led to the concept of irreversible shock.[167] The approach to resuscitation of cellular, organ, and organism changes after hemorrhagic shock using the Wiggers model has been applied to all types of injury based in part on the elegant experiments of Shires and colleagues[163] and a series of other investigators.[69,70]

EARLY LIMITED RESUSCITATION

ANIMAL STUDIES

Several large animal studies explored the use of varying degrees of fluid resuscitation in animals receiving injuries leading to uncontrolled hemorrhagic shock. Bickell and coworkers[168] created infrarenal aortotomy using a stainless steel wire in 16 anesthetized Yorkshire swine weighing 23 to 40 kg, which had been instrumented with pulmonary artery and carotid artery catheters. When the wire was pulled, a 5-mm aortotomy with subsequent intraperitoneal hemorrhage followed. Animals were alternately assigned to an untreated control group or a treatment group receiving 80 mL/kg of lactated Ringer's solution as an intravenous bolus. The volume of blood loss and mortality rate were significantly increased in animals treated with lactated Ringer's solution relative to the untreated control group. All control animals survived, whereas animals treated with lactated Ringer's solution died in less than 2 hours. Volume of hemorrhage identified in treated animals exceeded 2 L, whereas control animals lost on average less than 800 mL of blood.

Several observations may be made in relation to this widely cited report. First, mortality rate in the control group was low, leading one to question the severity of injury in the animal model. Second, fluid resuscitation administered, although consistent with replacement of two to three times the volume loss in blood with crystalloid, far exceeds standard resuscitation for a human patient of comparable weight. In addition, the rapidity of fluid administration may have served to diminish further any potential positive impact of fluid administration in this model of injury. The effect seen was reproduced, however, with other types of fluid administration in a comparable injury model. Other large animal studies of hypotensive resuscitation used graded resuscitation protocols.[169,170]

Stern and coworkers[169] examined a swine model combining femoral artery hemorrhage via a catheter to a mean arterial pressure of 30 mm Hg with subsequent intra-abdominal aortic laceration producing a 4-mm tear and uncontrolled intraperitoneal hemorrhage. Three groups of animals were resuscitated to mean arterial pressures of 40 mm Hg, 60 mm Hg, and 80 mm Hg. No untreated control group was employed. Resuscitation was begun when the pulse pressure of each animal reached 5 mm Hg. Animals were resuscitated with saline at 6 mL/kg/minute to a maximum of 90 mL/kg, after which resuscitation fluid was changed to shed blood at 2 mL/kg/minute to a maximal volume of 24 mL/kg. Animals were observed for 60 minutes or until death. As noted previously, mortality rate was significantly higher in animals receiving the most aggressive resuscitation compared with less aggressively treated groups. Animals resuscitated most aggressively had higher volumes of intraperitoneal hemorrhage than the two other experimental groups. In addition, oxygen delivery, which was monitored in these animals, was significantly greater in the group resuscitated to a mean arterial pressure of 60 mm Hg than in the two other experimental groups. Similar observations were made in a second report from this same group in a study by Kowalenko and colleagues.[170]

Clinical and preclinical studies focused on early limitation of crystalloid resuscitation and hemorrhagic shock focus on penetrating torso trauma but do not address initial care of patients with head injury, the leading cause of traumatic death in the United States. Historically, when shock accompanies head injury, the incidence of adverse outcome doubles. Because of the vulnerability of the injured brain to even brief periods of reduced perfusion, guidelines for the management of head injury state that delayed resuscitation cannot be considered applicable in head trauma.[118] Nonetheless, in a large animal model using a standard cerebral injury along with uncontrolled hemorrhage secondary to aortotomy, there was no evidence of increased secondary cerebral ischemia with delayed resuscitation. Conventional resuscitation with lactated Ringer's solution resulted in signs of increased secondary brain injury.[171]

CLINICAL STUDIES

Martin and coworkers[172] provided preliminary data in patients on the effect of aggressive versus delayed prehospital resuscitation of uncontrolled hemorrhagic shock after penetrating injury. These workers evaluated the effect of delaying fluid resuscitation until surgical intervention could control the source of hemorrhage on outcome of hypotensive trauma victims. Injury severity was similar in standard resuscitation and delayed resuscitation groups. The rate of survival to hospital discharge was 69% in the delayed resuscitation group and 56% in the standard resuscitation group. The difference between these groups did not reach statistical significance owing to small sample size.

Much attention has been directed to resuscitation of patients after injury after a report from Bickell and associates[173] that appeared in the *New England Journal of Medicine.* The authors reported a prospective clinical trial of adults with penetrating truncal trauma who were hypotensive in the field as indicated by a systolic blood pressure less than 90 mm Hg. Patients were randomly assigned to placement of intravascular catheters with standard prehospital and trauma center fluid resuscitation using lactated Ringer's solution or an experimental group in which vascular catheters were placed but intravenous fluids were not administered until patients reached the operating room. Patients were excluded from this trial if they were noted to have a field revised trauma score of zero consistent with cardiopulmonary arrest or had sustained fatal gunshot wounds to the head with neurologic injury that precluded long-term survival.[28] In addition, patients with penetrating truncal injury who did not require operation were excluded. After 1069 patients were screened during the 37 months of this study, 598 patients were enrolled—309 in an immediate resuscitation group receiving standard fluids according to Advanced Trauma Life Support protocols and 289 in a delayed resuscitation group, which did not receive intravenous fluids until reaching the operating room.[69]

The immediate and delayed resuscitation groups were well matched with respect to age, gender, and anatomic injury as measured by the ISS, Revised Trauma Score (physiologic response to injury), and systolic blood pressure.[174,175] Field response times for prehospital providers in this trial were short, averaging 30 minutes or less. The trauma center interval (i.e., the interval in the hospital before operation) was surprisingly long—44 minutes in the immediate resuscitation group and 52 minutes on average in the group receiving delayed resuscitation. Prehospital fluid administration averaged less than 900 mL in the immediate resuscitation group versus less than 100 mL in the delayed resuscitation cohort. Fluid administration in the trauma center before operation averaged greater than 1600 mL of fluid in the immediate resuscitation group, whereas the delayed resuscitation patients averaged 283 mL of fluid received. Operative blood loss between the study groups was not different. Among the 289 patients who received delayed fluid resuscitation, 203 (70%) survived and were discharged from the hospital. Of the 309 patients who received immediate fluid resuscitation, 193 (62%) survived (P = 0.04). Patients in the delayed resuscitation group displayed a trend toward reduced postoperative complications, including acute respiratory distress syndrome, sepsis syndrome, acute renal failure, coagulopathy, wound infection, and pneumonia, compared with patients in the immediate resuscitation group ($P = 0.08$).

A subgroup analysis from this study was reported at a subsequent meeting of the American Association for the Surgery of Trauma. When Wall and coworkers[176] examined major subgroups in the patient population reported by Bickell and colleagues, a statistical difference in hospital survival could be shown only in patients who had sustained penetrating cardiac injury.[115] Patients with major vascular injury, solid organ injury requiring operation, or noncardiac thoracic injury had comparable survival in the immediate and delayed resuscitation groups.

Although these early clinical studies represent a remarkable accomplishment in design, organization, and data analysis, many questions remain unanswered. None of the studies reported was blinded, and a randomization scheme was not employed. In the trial of Bickell and colleagues, in which the difference in mortality rate rested in a difference in survival of a small number of patients in the experimental groups, 22 patients in the delayed resuscitation group were given intravenous fluids in violation of study design.[173] Although these individuals were appropriately included in an intent-to-treat analysis, the impact of selected fluid administration on study outcome is unclear. The authors also have been criticized for excluding patients *after* randomization because of injuries considered too minor (no operative therapy) or too severe (revised trauma score of zero). Exclusion of these patients may invalidate the statistical approach employed and increase the difficulty of the clinician seeking guidance from this work. Finally, time spent in the trauma center by these hypotensive patients with injuries requiring operation was surprisingly long. Although the resuscitation groups described differed statistically in vital signs and hematologic parameters, it is unclear whether the differences observed had clinical significance.

We await additional data on the military approach to resuscitation, which requires innovation and effectiveness in austere environments.[177] Contemporary recommendations include limitation of fluid administration unless systolic blood pressure is less than 80 to 85 mm Hg or is rapidly falling. Another clinical indicator for fluid resuscitation is decreasing mentation without evidence of head injury. Key assessment parameters are mental status and the presence of a radial pulse. In many settings, no fluids are administered in the presence of a strong radial pulse and normal mentation. Pulse deterioration or decreasing level of consciousness are indicators for intervention. When fluids are given, a number of small-volume colloids with high tonicity or colloids in combination with hypertonic saline are being investigated. Even early hospital resuscitation is designed to emphasize the use of blood products and minimize crystalloids and nonblood colloids in the setting of major injury.

CLINICAL PATHWAY—EARLY RESUSCITATION

In all of the preclinical and clinical work described, the mechanism of injury and survival remains unclear. Among considerations are the impact of fluid resuscitation on early clot formation in the setting of uncontrolled hemorrhage.[115,169] Other workers suggest that rapidity in resuscitation of pulse pressure may relate to mechanical disruption of initial thrombus.[169] Fluid resuscitation may contribute to dilution of clotting factors in the setting of exaggerated bleeding in uncontrolled hemorrhage.[115,160] The data to support these observations are limited. Coagulopathy proportional to volume of injured tissue and severity of shock may be seen even before resuscitation fluids are provided.[11]

Despite provocative preclinical and clinical data, there is insufficient evidence to propose practice guidelines or make recommendations. "Uncontrolled" hemorrhage itself remains undefined. This problem is best seen as injury with blood loss occurring in the absence of surgical or mechanical hemostasis or the "control" provided by regulated blood removal through a vascular cannula. It is unclear whether a vascular injury after a torso gunshot wound and a shattered spleen after an automobile crash are different in this regard. The bottom-line message from all of the studies is that elevation of the blood pressure to normal or supranormal levels results in resumption of bleeding from the uncontrolled site, and rebleeding leads to recurrent shock and death of the experimental animal. Other work shows that animals subjected to shock could be successfully resuscitated at lower than "normal" mean arterial pressures if the bleeding site was controlled as part of the resuscitation program. Shock victims resuscitated with electrolyte solutions are subject to progressive hemodilution, and this may lead to death. The lessons that clinicians should learn from this body of data are as follows.[69,115,145,11]

1. Operation to control bleeding is part of resuscitation.
2. Blood pressure levels are convenient but possibly misleading end points for shock resuscitation in that resuscitation to normal or supranormal pressures may be harmful if the effort delays operation to control bleeding or the pressure elevation causes rebleeding. Better end points (e.g., tissue oxygenation or other metabolic parameters) are needed.
3. Blood loss is increased in the setting of significant soft tissue insults combined with shock. Early administration of blood products should stimulate use of a balanced administration strategy with PRBCs, FFP, and platelets given in equal proportions.
4. Resuscitation of traumatic shock, similar to fluid management of a burned patient, requires repeated observation, judgment, and skill and cannot be accomplished by recipe or formula.

The clinical trials that have sought to extend the previously described experimental concepts into the realm of patient care have dealt primarily with blood loss secondary to penetrating injury because this clinical condition is as close a simulation to a pure hemorrhage model as is available in clinical medicine. It is useful to emphasize that multiple blunt injury, multiple wounds, and extensive soft tissue trauma are not similar to pure hemorrhage models in that occult blood and fluid losses and other inflammatory factors exist that make the quantitation of injury severity difficult.

MANAGEMENT OF TRAUMATIC SHOCK IN THE INTENSIVE CARE UNIT

Before admission to the ICU, resuscitation is directed at maintaining blood pressure and reducing heart rate through volume loading with crystalloid and blood products. Relatively simple clinical end points are employed.[69] *This approach should be adequate for 95% of injured patients.* On admission to the ICU, severely injured patients may receive a central venous catheter or a pulmonary artery catheter to monitor hemodynamics and refine further the direction of resuscitation.[178] A series of early reports by Shoemaker and coworkers proposed that supranormal oxygen delivery (600 mL/minute/m^2) and resuscitation to a plateau oxygen consumption were appropriate clinical end points. Although observations of improved hemodynamic response in survivors of injury make intuitive sense, driving injured patients to supranormal hemodynamic performance was not associated with improvement in clinical outcome.[116,122-125] Reduced goals for oxygen delivery (500 mL/minute/m^2) are proposed among end points for support of patients receiving pulmonary artery catheter monitoring.[179-181]

In a series of studies characterizing resuscitation of injured patients in the ICU, Moore and coworkers used the pulmonary artery catheter to describe response to fluid administration. Criteria identifying patients considered for placement of a pulmonary artery catheter and need for ICU resuscitation include major injury (two or more abdominal organs, two or more long bone fractures, complex pelvic fractures, flail chest, or major vascular injury), blood loss (anticipated need for >6 units PRBC during the first 12 hours after hospitalization), and metabolic stress (arterial base deficit > 6 mEq/L during the first 12 hours after hospital admission). A trauma victim older than 65 years with any two of the previous criteria also warrants consideration for pulmonary artery catheter insertion and ICU resuscitation. Patients with these criteria who also incurred severe brain injury, defined as Glasgow Coma Scale score less than or equal to 8 in the trauma ICU and abnormality on brain computed tomography scan, were not resuscitated by protocol during development of this approach unless assessed by the attending neurosurgeon to be at low risk of secondary brain injury with these procedures.[180,181] In my practice, I find that the brain, similar to other organs, benefits from aggressive resuscitation (Table 27.3).

A sequential approach to shock resuscitation using a pulmonary artery catheter is advocated by Moore with McKinley and coworkers.[178,179] This approach includes a series of interventions including administration of PRBC and lactated Ringer's solution to optimize cardiac index and pulmonary capillary wedge pressure as described in a classic Starling curve. Milrinone, dobutamine, and norepinephrine are used as vasoactive agents as necessary to provide mean arterial pressure greater than 65 mm Hg and oxygen delivery index greater than 500 mL/minute/m^2. These patients require large volumes of protocol-directed shock resuscitation (approximately 15 L for oxygen delivery index >500 mL/minute/m^2). Significant urine output volumes also should be expected. This large net positive balance suggests unrecognized ongoing blood loss or extreme fluid shifts between intravascular, interstitial, and intracellular compartments, or both, for severely injured patients (Fig. 27.4).

The protocol-driven approach described has provided a variety of observations.[182] First, even elderly patients respond

Table 27.3 Summary of Protocol for Resuscitation of Shock Resulting from Major Torso Trauma*

Intervention	Threshold	Method
Transfuse (PRBC)	DO_2I <500 mL/min/m^2; hemoglobin <10 g/dL (age ≥65 years, <12 g/dL)	1 g hemoglobin/dL/unit PRBC; bolus transfusion; then hemoglobin analysis (bedside); then calculate DO_2I
Volume load (LR)	DO_2I <500 mL/min/m^2; hemoglobin ≥10 g/dL (age ≥65 years, ≥12 g/dL); PCWP <15 mm Hg (age ≥65 years, <12 mm Hg)	1-L LR bolus infusion (age ≥65 years, 0.5 L); then measure PCWP; then calculate DO_2I
Starling curve (NS)	DO_2I <500 mL/min/m^2; hemoglobin ≥10 g/dL (age ≥65 years, ≥12 g/dL); PCWP ≥15 mm Hg (age ≥65 years, ≥12 mm Hg)	0.5- or 0.25-L NS bolus infusion; then measure PCWP and CI: CI-PCWP optimal if ΔCI ≤–0.3; ΔPCWP ≤+4 with two consecutive boluses; then calculate DO_2I
Inotrope	DO_2I <500 mL/min/m^2; hemoglobin 10 g/dL (age ≥65 years, ≥12 g/dL); CI and PCWP optimized	Milrinone, 0.1-µg increments to 0.8 µg/kg/min, or dobutamine, 2.5-µg increments to 20 µg/kg/min; calculate DO_2I
Vasopressor	DO_2I <500 mL/min/m^2; MAP <65 mm Hg	Norepinephrine, 0.05-µg increments to 0.2 µg/kg/min; measure MAP; calculate DO_2I

*Details of the resuscitation protocol used by McKinley and coworkers are given. Selected drugs for inotropic and vasopressor support are listed. Patients also are treated to age-appropriate hemoglobin levels and given fluid infusion based on a volume loading protocol until filling pressures and DO_2I are optimized.

CI, cardiac index; CWP, capillary wedge pressure; DO_2I, oxygen delivery index; LR, lactated Ringer's solution; MAP, mean arterial pressure; NS, normal saline; PCWP, pulmonary capillary wedge pressure; PRBC, packed red blood cells.

Modified from McKinley BA, Kozar RA, Cocanour CS, et al: Normal versus supranormal oxygen delivery goals in shock resuscitation: The response is the same. J Trauma 2002;53:825-832.

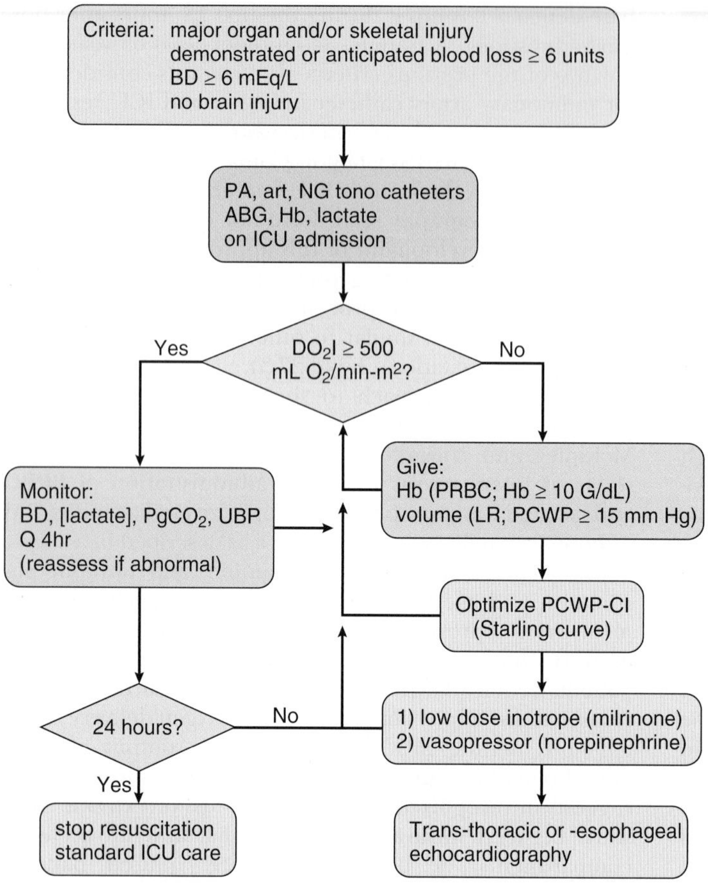

Figure 27.4 A few patients require additional aggressive resuscitation in the ICU. Frequently, these patients require insertion of a pulmonary artery catheter. This protocol is the most widely reported strategy for crystalloid and blood administration in stabilization of these patients coming from a series of articles published by McKinley, Moore, and associates. ABG, arterial blood gas; BD, base deficit; CI, cardiac index; DO_2I, oxygen delivery index; Hb, hemoglobin; ICU, intensive care unit; LR, lactated Ringer's solution; NG, nasogastric; PA, pulmonary artery; PCWP, pulmonary capillary wedge pressure; $PgCO_2$, transgastric oxygen; UBP, urinary bladder pressure. (From Marr AB, Moore FA, Sailors RM, et al: Preload optimization using "Starling curve" generation during shock resuscitation: Can it be done? Shock 2004;21:300-305.)

to ICU resuscitation after injury.[180] In general, the maximal oxygen delivery response is less than that of younger patients, and elderly patients have a greater requirement for inotropic support.[183] Second, a Starling curve generation approach is feasible and reliably improves hemodynamic resuscitation from major trauma. Supranormal resuscitation is neither necessary nor desirable in the management of patients with trauma associated with shock.[178] Third, aggressive resuscitation, particularly in the setting of ongoing bleeding, increases the risk of elevated intra-abdominal pressure and abdominal compartment syndrome.[184] Preload-driven resuscitation may cause bowel edema with subsequent venous obstruction, declining cardiac output, decreased urinary output, and compromise of systemic oxygenation. Finally, although many end points for interventions for goal-directed resuscitation in critical injury exist, systemic oxygen transport is the current state of the art in the most severely injured patients and is the basis for future development of clinical processes for resuscitation of shock caused by major trauma (Fig. 27.5).[182]

The utility of the pulmonary artery catheter in the management of patients with severe injury is suggested by a study using data obtained in the National Trauma Data Bank.[185] From more than 450,000 records, 53,000 patients were reviewed. These patients were admitted between January 1994 and December 2001. Patients survived more than 48 hours and underwent at least one diagnostic or therapeutic procedure. The patients were 16 to 90 years old and distinguished by ISS and initial base deficit. Approximately 2000 patients who had insertion of a pulmonary artery catheter during hospitalization were compared with 51,000 patients who did not. Logistic regression analysis was used to develop a model that examined mortality rate after injury. Factors included in the model were use of a pulmonary artery catheter, age, emergency department base deficit, ISS, comorbid conditions, mechanism of injury, and specific injury patterns as identified by the Abbreviated Injury Scale. Overall, patients managed with a pulmonary artery catheter were older and had a higher ISS, greater emergency department base deficit, and higher mortality rates (29.7% with pulmonary artery catheter versus 9.8% without pulmonary artery catheter). Patients with spine, abdominal, chest, or head injury and patients with at least one Abbreviated Injury Scale score equal to or greater than 3 were more likely to be managed with a pulmonary artery catheter.

Pulmonary artery catheter use was associated with increased mortality rate in all subgroups of ISS, emergency department base deficit, and age. As age, base deficit, and ISS increased, however, the risk of death associated with pulmonary artery catheter use decreased, and an apparent benefit of pulmonary artery catheter use emerged. In contrast, less severely injured trauma patients (ISS 16 to 24) and severely injured patients without high admission base deficit (>–5) had increased mortality rate associated with pulmonary artery catheter placement regardless of age.

Although these observations come from a large database, retrospective study design and subgroup analysis are not optimal for definitive hypothesis testing. Finally, neither timing of placement for pulmonary artery catheters nor cause of death and specific relationship to placement of the

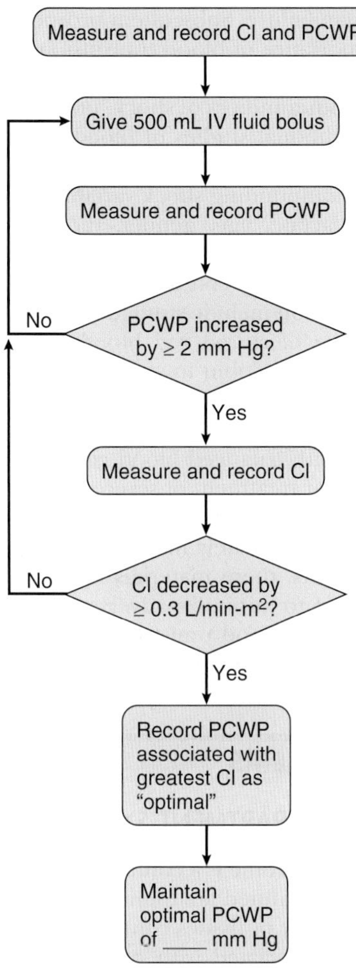

Figure 27.5 This simple algorithm describes a Starling curve protocol for optimization of filling pressures as a part of resuscitation of severely injured patients in the critical care unit where a pulmonary artery catheter is employed. CI, cardiac index; PCWP, pulmonary capillary wedge pressure. (From Marr AB, Moore FA, Sailors RM, et al: Preload optimization using "Starling curve" generation during shock resuscitation: Can it be done? Shock 2004;21:300-305.)

pulmonary artery catheter could be conclusively examined by analysis of the National Trauma Data Bank. Nonetheless, these data suggest that injured patients may derive benefit from pulmonary artery catheter-guided resuscitation to avert complications related to persistent perfusion deficits. Further focused examination of patients with risk factors for poor outcome is warranted.[185]

MASSIVE TRANSFUSION

Independent of mechanism of injury, hemorrhagic shock consistently is the second leading cause of early death among injured patients, with only CNS injury consistently more lethal.[186] Primary CNS injury is devastating and has a high rate of prehospital mortality; prevention is the best strategy.[187] Hemorrhagic shock accounts for 30% to 40% of trauma deaths and is more amenable to interventions to reduce mortality and morbidity rates.[186] In addition, approximately 25% of CNS injuries are complicated by hemorrhagic shock.[188,189] Hemorrhage contributes to death during the prehospital period in 33% to 56% of cases, and exsanguination is the most common cause of death among individuals found dead on arrival of emergency medical services personnel.[47] Hemorrhage accounts for the largest proportion of mortality rates occurring within the first hour of trauma center care and greater than 80% of operating room deaths after major trauma.[186,190] Although the need for massive transfusion (defined as administration of ≥10 units of PRBC in <24 hours) is probably necessary in only 3% of patients in busy trauma centers, this intervention can be lifesaving, and preliminary data suggest that early aggressive administration of blood products reduces morbidity and mortality rate and decreases overall product use.[191]

Numerous general observations can be made.[191-193] Most patients receiving massive transfusion are treated initially with crystalloid fluids followed by non-cross-matched type O red blood cells. Plasma therapy is typically delayed while waiting for blood typing and plasma to thaw. Platelets frequently are not given until patients have multiple units of PRBCs. Coagulopathy is common and difficult to correct. Plasma and platelets are inadequately used and greater emphasis is needed on plasma and platelet administration.

A typical massive transfusion protocol begins in the emergency department when the senior trauma practitioner orders transfusion of O-negative PRBC and invokes an organization-specific massive transfusion protocol.[193,194] This is followed by administration of 4 to 6 additional typed or O-negative units of PRBC and a similar number of units of FFP and platelets. Therapy continues with containers sent from the blood bank, each containing red blood cells, plasma, and platelets. Goals are normalization of the PT and elevation of the platelet count to 50 to 100 × 10^9/L. The fibrinogen level is checked after 6 to 12 units of PRBC, and cryoprecipitate is given if the fibrinogen level is less than 1 g/L. This triggers administration of 10 units of cryoprecipitate. Once a common component of massive transfusion strategies, recombinant activated factor VII has been deemphasized in both military and civilian practice.[195-198]

Major trauma centers have developed transfusion protocols to address rapid blood loss and trauma-associated coagulopathy. This strategy has demonstrated improved survival in severely injured trauma patients. Although many centers have implemented massive transfusion protocols, a standardized initiation policy has not been defined. Frequently, activation of massive transfusion protocols is provider dependent and variability exists among high-volume centers.

A number of scoring systems have been developed to rapidly predict the patient requiring massive transfusion.[199-201] Of these scores, the ABC (assessment of blood consumption) score, which incorporates penetrating mechanism of injury, positive ultrasound examination of the abdomen in the emergency department, arrival systolic blood pressure of 90 mm Hg or less, and arrival heart rate of 120 beats/minute or more, has been reported and validated in large patient sets. Although multiple more sophisticated criteria have been proposed, having an ABC score of two criteria or greater correctly classified the patient requiring massive transfusion in up to 85% of cases. Other investigators point out that hypotension and evidence of coagulopathy are the strongest predictors of massive transfusion. Additional data from military and civilian practice is awaited to bring further clarity to appropriate transfusion triggers.

TRANEXAMIC ACID

Tranexamic acid is a derivative of amino acid lysine that inhibits fibrinolysis by blocking binding sites on plasminogen. This agent has been used in a variety of surgical trials and has been demonstrated to reduce blood transfusion requirement. The massive CRASH-2 study, incorporating over 20,000 patients, evaluates tranexamic acid as a means to address fibrinolysis occurring as a component of coagulopathy after trauma.[202,203] CRASH-2 was conducted in over 250 hospitals and 40 countries. Over 20,000 patients with significant bleeding or at risk for significant bleeding were assigned within 8 hours of injury to either tranexamic acid or matching placebo. All-cause mortality rate was significantly reduced with tranexamic acid. Specific risk of death due to bleeding was also significantly reduced. This remarkable outcome was accomplished without a significant increase in thrombotic events. Subsequent analysis of the CRASH-2 data, however, reveals that greatest efficacy came when treatment was initiated within 3 hours after injury. In fact, treatment after 3 hours seemed to increase the risk of death due to bleeding. A recent review of military experience with tranexamic acid, the MATTERs trial, also demonstrates improved outcomes with early administration of this inexpensive drug shortly after injury. This military experience with tranexamic acid suggests improvement in outcome in patients receiving as little as 1 unit of PRBCs. Incremental risk with administratin of tranexamic acid was not demonstrated.[204]

The role for tranexamic acid in trauma systems where massive transfusion protocols incorporate FFP containing all indigenous antifibrinolytic elements in plasma remains unclear. In developed trauma systems, the best place for tranexamic acid may actually be in the prehospital environment as this material can readily be maintained in helicopter and road transport programs. Prehospital administration of blood products, especially plasma, is uncommon in civilian settings; thus, tranexamic acid offers an early opportunity to manage coagulopathy.[205] Opportunities for use of this promising material in the critical care setting are being defined.

RISKS OF EARLY RED BLOOD CELL TRANSFUSION

Blood transfusion in trauma has been identified as an independent predictor of multiple organ failure, systemic inflammatory response syndrome, increased postinjury infection, and increased mortality rate in multiple studies.[206] Cumulative risks have been related to the number of units of PRBC transfused, increased storage time of transfused blood, and possibly the presence of leukocytes in donor blood. Many authors have concluded that blood transfusion in an injured patient should be minimized whenever possible.[207]

Large single-institution data sets examined the impact of blood transfusion in postinjury multiple organ failure.[136,208,209] Variables identified as early independent predictors of multiple organ failure included age older than 55 years, ISS equal to or greater than 25, and greater than 6 units of PRBC in the first 12 hours after admission. Base deficit greater than 8 mEq/L in the first 12 hours and lactate greater than 2.5 mol/L also were independent predictors of multiple organ failure. Subsequent prospective work confirmed the importance of blood transfusion as an independent risk factor for postinjury multiple organ failure after controlling for other indices of shock, including base deficit and lactate. Additional studies of blood product use after injury associate blood transfusion with increased mortality rate. Potential confounding shock variables, including base deficit, serum lactate, age, gender, race, Glasgow Coma Scale score, and ISS, were controlled in this analysis.

Factors contributing to complications associated with red blood cell transfusion include storage time, increased endothelial adherence of stored red blood cells, nitric oxide binding by free hemoglobin in stored blood, donor leukocytes, host inflammatory response, and reduced red blood cell deformability.[205,210] Nonetheless, transfusion of an injured patient with balanced blood component therapy is the only option for treatment of severe hemorrhagic shock. Although other hemoglobin-based oxygen carriers hold great promise and ultimately may provide better outcomes for injured patients, these materials have not come to be used. In an effort to minimize adverse events, attempts to minimize the use of blood transfusion in injury are appropriate outside major hemorrhage.

SPECIAL PROBLEMS

ABDOMINAL COMPARTMENT SYNDROME

A compartment syndrome is a condition in which increased pressure within a confined anatomic space adversely affects function and viability of tissues contained within. Confined anatomic spaces associated with compartment syndromes are fascial spaces of the extremities, the globe as in glaucoma, and the cranial cavity as in epidural or subdural hematoma. Abdominal compartment syndrome is a condition in which sustained pressure within the abdominal wall, pelvis, diaphragm, and retroperitoneum adversely affects the function of the gastrointestinal tract and related extraperitoneal organs. Abdominal compartment syndrome is receiving increasing recognition as a complication of massive resuscitation after trauma, burns, or other surgical procedures (Box 27.3). Operative decompression is frequently required. Pressures around 5 to 7 mm Hg in the peritoneal cavity are normal. Short-duration pressure increases frequently occur with coughing, Valsalva maneuvers, defecation, and weightlifting. Intra-abdominal pressure can be nonpathologically increased in obese individuals. Elevated intra-abdominal pressure is a common finding among critically ill medical and surgical patients.[211-213]

A more recent consensus conference on abdominal compartment syndrome has created improved definitions in relation to abdominal compartment syndrome (Table 27.4). For standardization, intra-abdominal pressure should be expressed in mm Hg and measured at end expiration with the patient supine after ensuring that abdominal muscle contractions are absent. The transducer is zeroed at the midaxillary line. The current reference standard for intra-abdominal pressure measurement is pressure measured via an indwelling urinary drainage catheter within the bladder. The recommended technique for measuring intra-abdominal pressure is to clamp the urinary catheter and

Box 27.3 Risk Factors for Intra-abdominal Hypertension and Abdominal Compartment Syndrome

- Acidosis (pH < 7.2)
- Hypothermia (core temperature < 33° C)
- Polytransfusion (>10 units packed red blood cells/24 hours)
- Coagulopathy (platelets < 55,000/mm^3 *or* activated partial thromboplastin time 2× normal or higher *or* prothrombin time < 50% *or* international standardized ratio > 1.5)
- Sepsis (American-European Consensus Conference definitions)
- Bacteremia
- Intra-abdominal infection or abscess
- Peritonitis
- Liver dysfunction or cirrhosis with ascites
- Mechanical ventilation
- Use of positive end-expiratory pressure (PEEP) or the presence of auto-PEEP
- Pneumonia
- Abdominal surgery, especially with tight fascial closures
- Massive fluid resuscitation (>5 L colloid or crystalloid/24 hours)
- Gastroparesis, gastric distention, or ileus
- Volvulus
- Hemoperitoneum or pneumoperitoneum
- Major burns
- Major trauma
- High body mass index (>30)
- Intra-abdominal or retroperitoneal tumors
- Prone positioning
- Massive incisional hernia repair
- Acute pancreatitis
- Distended abdomen
- Damage control laparotomy
- Laparoscopy with excessive inflation pressures
- Peritoneal dialysis

From Malbrain ML, Cheatham ML, Kirkpatrick A, et al: Results from the International Conference of Experts on Intra-abdominal Hypertension and Abdominal Compartment Syndrome, I: Definitions. Intensive Care Med 2006;32:1722-1732.

Table 27.4 Consensus Definitions List

Definition 1	IAP is the steady-state pressure concealed within the abdominal cavity.
Definition 2	APP = MAP − IAP.
Definition 3	FG = GFP − PTP = MAP − 2 × IAP.
Definition 4	IAP should be expressed in mm Hg and measured at end expiration in the complete supine position after ensuring that abdominal muscle contractions are absent and with the transducer zeroed at the level of the midaxillary line.
Definition 5	The reference standard for intermittent IAP measurement is via the bladder with a maximal instillation volume of 25 mL sterile saline.
Definition 6	Normal IAP is approximately 5-7 mm Hg in critically ill adults.
Definition 7	IAH is defined by a sustained or repeated pathologic elevation in IAP ≥12 mm Hg.
Definition 8	IAH is graded as follows: grade I, IAH 12-15 mm Hg; grade II, IAP 16-20 mm Hg; grade III, IAP 21-25 mm Hg; grade IV, IAP > 25 mm Hg.
Definition 9	ACS is defined as a sustained IAP >20 mm Hg (with or without an APP <60 mm Hg) that is associated with new organ dysfunction/failure.
Definition 10	Primary ACS is a condition associated with injury or disease in the abdominopelvic region that frequently requires early surgical or interventional radiologic intervention.
Definition 11	Secondary ACS refers to conditions that do not originate from the abdominopelvic region.
Definition 12	Recurrent ACS refers to the condition in which ACS redevelops after previous surgical or medical treatment of primary or secondary ACS.

ACS, abdominal compartment syndrome; APP, abdominal perfusion pressure; FG, filtration gradient; GFP, glomerular filtration pressure; IAH, intra-abdominal hypertension; IAP, intra-abdominal pressure; MAP, mean arterial pressure; PTP, proximal tubular pressure.

From Malbrain ML, Cheatham ML, Kirkpatrick A, et al: Results from the International Conference of Experts on Intra-abdominal Hypertension and Abdominal Compartment Syndrome, I: Definitions. Intensive Care Med 2006;32:1722-1732.

instill a maximal volume of 25 mL of sterile, room-temperature saline into the bladder with the patient in the supine position. After zeroing a transducer and a stabilization period of at least 30 to 60 seconds, the mean intra-abdominal pressure can be read on a bedside monitor or as the height of the fluid column in urinary drainage tubing.

Intra-abdominal hypertension is defined by a sustained or repeated intra-abdominal pressure greater than 12 mm Hg or an abdominal perfusion pressure less than 60 mm Hg, where abdominal perfusion pressure = mean arterial pressure − intra-abdominal pressure. Abdominal compartment syndrome is present when organ dysfunction occurs as a result of intra-abdominal hypertension. Abdominal compartment syndrome is further defined by sustained or repeated intra-abdominal pressure greater than 20 mm Hg or abdominal perfusion pressure less than 60 mm Hg in association with new-onset single or multiple organ system failure. In contrast to intra-abdominal hypertension, abdominal compartment syndrome is not graded but rather considered as an "all or none" phenomenon.[213,214]

Intra-abdominal hypertension has a variety of physiologic effects. In experimental preparations, animals die as a result of congestive heart failure as abdominal pressure passes a critical threshold. Increased intra-abdominal pressure decreases cardiac output and left and right ventricular stroke work, while increasing central venous pressure, pulmonary artery wedge pressure, and systemic and pulmonary vascular resistance. Abdominal decompression reverses these changes. As both hemidiaphragms are displaced upward with increased intra-abdominal pressure, decreased thoracic volume and compliance are seen. Decreased volume within the pleural cavity causes atelectasis and decreases alveolar clearance. Pulmonary infections also may result. Ventilated patients with abdominal hypertension require increased airway pressure to deliver a fixed tidal volume. As the diaphragm protrudes into the pleural cavity, intrathoracic pressure increases with reduction in cardiac output and increased pulmonary vascular resistance. Ventilation and perfusion abnormalities result, and blood gas measurements show hypoxemia, hypercarbia, and acidosis.[215]

Elevation in intra-abdominal pressure also causes renal dysfunction. Inadequate renal perfusion pressure and renal filtration gradient have been proposed as critical factors in the development of renal insufficiency associated with elevated intra-abdominal pressure. The filtration gradient is the mechanical force across the glomerulus and equals the difference between glomerular filtration pressure and proximal tubular pressure. In the presence of intra-abdominal hypertension, proximal tubular pressure may be assumed to equal intra-abdominal pressure. Glomerular filtration pressure may be estimated as mean arterial pressure minus intra-abdominal pressure. Changes in intra-abdominal pressure may have a greater impact on renal function and urine production than changes in mean arterial pressure. Oliguria is thought to be one of the first signs of intra-abdominal hypertension. Control of intra-abdominal pressure leads to reversal of renal impairment. Oliguria may be seen with intra-abdominal pressure of 15 to 20 mm Hg. Deterioration in cardiac output plays a role in diminished renal perfusion, but even with maintenance of cardiac output, impairment of renal function persists in intra-abdominal hypertension.[211,216-218]

Other organs affected by increased intra-abdominal pressure include the liver, where hepatic blood flow has been shown to decrease with abdominal hypertension.[219,220] It may be assumed that hepatic synthesis of acute-phase proteins, immunoglobulins, and other factors of host defense may be impaired by reduced hepatic blood flow. Other gastrointestinal functions may be compromised by increased intra-abdominal pressure. Splanchnic hypoperfusion may begin with an intra-abdominal pressure of 15 mm Hg. Reduced perfusion may create changes in mucosal pH, translocation, bowel motility, and production of gastrointestinal hormones. Finally, intracranial hypertension is seen with chronically increased intra-abdominal pressure. Intracranial hypertension has been shown to decrease when intra-abdominal pressure is reduced in morbidly obese patients and in intracranial injury.

Operative decompression is the method of choice for treatment of patients with intra-abdominal hypertension and associated evidence of organ dysfunction. After decompression, improvements in hemodynamics, pulmonary function, tissue perfusion, and renal function have been shown in a variety of clinical settings. To prevent hemodynamic decompensation during decompression, intravascular volume should be restored, oxygen delivery should be normalized, and hypothermia and coagulation defects should be corrected. The abdomen should be opened in patients with adequate venous access and controlled ventilation. Adjunctive measures to combat reperfusion washout from by-products of anaerobic metabolism include acute use of vasoconstrictor agents to avoid sudden changes in blood pressure. After decompression of the abdomen, the fascial gap is left open using one of a variety of temporary abdominal closure methods.

In a recent report, Cheatham and Safcsak review their experience with percutaneous, ultrasound-guided drainage of ascitic fluid contributing to abdominal hypertension and abdominal compartment syndrome.[221,222] These investigators suggest that in patients with significant fluid accumulation creating abdominal hypertension, percutaneous drainage can avoid the need for decompressive laparotomy with its associated morbidity and occasional complications. Additional reports from other centers are required. To date, apart from the large experience described previously, percutaneous control of fluid accumulation to manage abdominal hypertension and compartment syndrome is limited to case reports.

EXTREMITY COMPARTMENT SYNDROME

The numerous causes of extremity compartment syndrome include complications of open and closed fractures, arterial injury, temporary vascular occlusion, snakebite, drug abuse, burns, physical exertion, and gunshot wounds. The most common cause of compartment syndrome is muscle injury leading to edema, which is correlated to the amount of tissue damage. Pressure is increased within the closed fascial space first by intracellular swelling followed by hematoma formation if a fracture is present. Because extremities, particularly at the calf, are composed of relatively unyielding fascial compartments, circulatory compromise occurs as tissue pressure increases with resulting ischemia and tissue damage. Leakage of intracellular fluid follows, and a further increase in intracompartmental pressure is seen.[223]

When extremity injuries produce complete ischemia, skeletal muscle that is deprived of oxygen may survive for 4 hours without irreversible damage. Total ischemia of 8 hours' duration produces irreversible change. Peripheral nerves conduct for 1 hour after onset of total ischemia and can survive for 4 hours with only neurapraxic damage. After 8 hours, axonotmesis and irreversible damage occur. Ischemia caused by reduction or cessation of blood flow occurs when the perfusion gradient to a muscle compartment falls below a critical level. Perfusion is related to the compartment pressure. When intracompartmental blood pressure is 25 mm Hg, tissue perfusion in injured tissues is substantially decreased.[223-225]

Fasciotomy should be performed when intracompartmental pressure approaches 25 mm Hg, or if an extremity has been completely ischemic for 6 hours, the patient's clinical condition is worsening, substantial tissue injury is present, or tissue pressure is increasing.[225] Prophylactic treatment is valuable because fasciotomy does not reverse changes caused by initial extremity injury but can prevent changes resulting from secondary ischemic insults.

Pain, pallor, paralysis, paresthesias, and pulselessness are the classic hallmarks of extremity compartment syndrome. If treatment is not initiated until all of these signs are present, poor results are obtained. Pain and aggravation of pain by passive stretching of the muscles in the involved compartment is the most sensitive clinical finding. Assessment of pain is useful when patients are conscious and can respond cognitively to examination. In unconscious patients at risk for compartment syndrome, tissue pressure measurements may be the only objective criteria for diagnosis. Measurement of compartment pressures is obtained in all extremity compartments at risk and proximal and distal to any fractures. The highest pressure noted should serve as the basis for determining the need for fasciotomy.

PELVIC FRACTURES

Substantial blunt force is required to disrupt the pelvic ring. The extent of injury is related to the direction and magnitude of force applied. Associated abdominal, thoracic, and head injuries are common. Force applied to the pelvis can cause rotational displacement with opening or compression of the pelvic ring. Other types of displacement seen with pelvic fractures are vertical with complete disruption of the ring and the posterior sacroiliac complex.[226]

Patients with pelvic ring injuries are easily divided into two groups on the basis of clinical presentation—patients who are hemodynamically stable and patients who are hemodynamically unstable.[226] There is a dramatic difference in mortality rates between pelvic fracture patients who are hypotensive and patients who are hemodynamically stable. Hemodynamic stability and biomechanical pelvic instability are separate though related issues, which tends to confuse the clinical picture. The source of bleeding may be multifactorial and not directly related to the pelvic fracture itself. Blood loss secondary to pelvic fracture that contributes to hemodynamic instability is a significant risk factor, however. Early fracture diagnosis and stabilization using external skeletal fixation are crucial in the acute phase of patient management.[227] Treatment of the patient also is directed by response to initial fluid resuscitation. Retroperitoneal bleeding in a pelvic fracture usually arises from a low-pressure source—the cancellous bone at the fracture site or adjacent venous injury. Significant retroperitoneal arterial bleeding occurs in approximately 10% of patients. Clinical evidence has suggested that provisional fracture stabilization using external fixation devices or even wrapping the fractured pelvis in a bed sheet can control low-pressure venous bleeding. Continued, unexplained bleeding after provisional fracture stabilization suggests an arterial source. Angiography with embolization of the involved vessel is indicated. Therapeutic angiography also may be required after abdominal exploration if a rapidly expanding or pulsatile retroperitoneal hematoma is encountered.[228]

KEY POINTS

- Shock after trauma is not the same as simple hemorrhage. Blood loss is combined with an inflammatory component.
- Because of inflammation associated with hemorrhage, the rate and amount of resuscitation are increased after injury compared with hemorrhage outside the setting of trauma.
- The classic neuroendocrine response leading to conservation of salt and water in traumatic shock can be linked to neuroimmune feedback loops, which modulate inflammatory response.
- Although flaws in present crystalloid resuscitation preparations exist, a clear benefit of routinely available colloids has not been shown.
- A variety of metabolic and oxygen transport end points for resuscitation have been identified. In general, these end points change in a consistent fashion after injury. None of the available resuscitation end points is sufficient to limit or guide therapy after injury at this time.
- Resuscitation to supranormal oxygen transport parameters does not improve outcome after injury. A staged approach using a pulmonary artery catheter, which should be necessary in less than 5% of injured patients, may be helpful.
- Although massive transfusion reduces overall blood product requirements in patients with rapid blood loss, limited resuscitation and blood product conservation are seen as appropriate in many injured patients.

SELECTED REFERENCES

11. Dries DJ: The contemporary role of blood products and components used in trauma resuscitation. Scand J Trauma Resuscitation Emerg Med 2010;18:63.
46. Kashuk JL, Moore EE, Sawyer M, et al: Postinjury coagulopathy management: Goal directed resuscitation via POC thrombelastography. Ann Surg 2010;251:604-614.
47. Sauaia A, Moore FA, Moore EE, et al: Epidemiology of trauma deaths: A reassessment. J Trauma 1995;38:185-193.
56. Holcomb JB, Jenkins D, Rhee P, et al: Damage control resuscitation: Directly addressing the early coagulopathy of trauma. J Trauma 2007;62:307-310.
57. Hess JR, Brohi K, Dutton RP, et al: The coagulopathy of trauma: A review of mechanisms. J Trauma 2008;65:748-754.
61. Brohi K, Cohen MJ, Ganter MT, et al: Acute traumatic coagulopathy: Initiated by hypoperfusion: Modulated through the protein C pathway? Ann Surg 2007;245:812-818.
88. Finfer S, Bellomo R, Boyce N, et al: SAFE Study Investigators: A comparison of albumin and saline for fluid resuscitation in the intensive care unit. N Engl J Med 2004;350:2247-2256.
112. Cotton BA, Gunter OL, Isbell J, et al: Damage control hematology: The impact of a trauma exsanguination protocol on survival and blood product utilization. J Trauma 2008;64:1177-1183.
113. Holcomb JB, Wade CD, Michalek JE, et al: Increased plasma and platelets to red blood cell ratios improves outcome in 466 massively transfused civilian trauma patients. Ann Surg 2008;248:447-458.
115. Dries DJ: Hypotensive resuscitation. Shock 1996;6:311-316.

The complete list of references can be found at www.expertconsult.com.

28 Anaphylaxis and Anaphylactic Shock

Marilyn T. Haupt | Bala K. Grandhi

CHAPTER OUTLINE

The term *anaphylaxis* refers to a life-threatening event, allergic in nature, which may result from IgE- or non-IgE-mediated mast cell degranulation. The clinical manifestations of severe anaphylaxis are often explosive in onset and may lead to upper airway obstruction, respiratory failure, and circulatory shock. Milder symptoms can also develop. The term *anaphylactoid reaction*, which referred to a non-IgE-mediated reaction, is no longer being used. A recent National Institutes of Health (NIH) consensus conference defined anaphylaxis as one of the following three scenarios.[1]

1. Acute onset of a reaction (minutes to hours) with involvement of the skin, mucosal tissue, or both *and at least one of the following*: (a) respiratory compromise (b) or reduced blood pressure or symptoms of end-organ dysfunction;
2. Two or more of the following that occur rapidly after exposure to a *likely* allergen for that patient—involvement of the skin/mucosal tissue, respiratory compromise, reduced blood pressure or associated symptoms, and persistent gastrointestinal symptoms; or
3. Reduced blood pressure after exposure to a *known* allergen (adapted from Sampson and colleagues[1]).

The IgE-mediated anaphylactic response is classified as a type I reaction according to the Gell and Coombs classification. The IgE-mediated anaphylactic reaction has clinical features similar to other, milder type I reactions, such as allergic rhinitis, hives, urticaria, and allergic asthma. IgE-mediated anaphylactic reactions are characterized by a well-defined immunologic sequence of events that involves antigen-specific and IgE-specific effector cells. When stimulated, these cells release a variety of inflammatory mediators.[2] The effector cells consist of mast cells and basophils, which are based primarily in tissues and in the circulating blood volume. Severe anaphylaxis rapidly progresses to a generalized systemic reaction. Agents that produce well-documented IgE-mediated anaphylactic reactions include medications such as beta lactam antibiotics, biologic agents, nonsteroidal anti-inflammatory drugs (NSAIDs), foods (peanut and other legumes, nuts from trees [walnuts, almonds, etc.], milk, and egg), Hymenoptera venoms (honey bees, yellow jackets, hornets, wasps, and fire ants), natural rubber latex, occupational allergens, and seminal fluid prostate-specific antigen (Table 28.1).

Immune-mediated IgE-dependent or IgE-independent and non-immune-mediated mast cell degranulation-mediated anaphylactic reactions have similar clinical features. Agents capable of producing direct mast cell degranulation include NSAIDs, opiates, ciprofloxacin, and physical factors, (cold, heat, exercise). Patients who are taking beta blockers or ACE inhibitors may develop severe anaphylaxis to an inciting agent and are less likely to respond to first-line agents.[3-6]

In idiopathic anaphylaxis, the pathophysiology and triggering events are unknown. Idiopathic anaphylaxis is a diagnosis of exclusion. It is mostly seen in adults and adolescents. About half these patients have concomitant atopic disease. They respond to treatment with corticosteroids and antihistamines.[7,8] Special testing like serum tryptase, C4 levels may be necessary to exclude conditions such as systemic mastocytosis, hereditary angioedema, and acquired C1 inhibitor deficiency.

Factitious anaphylaxis is a type of Munchausen syndrome. Patients with this disorder typically have an acute crisis that resembles anaphylaxis because of intentional self-exposure

Table 28.1 Agents Frequently Associated with Immune and Nonimmune Types of Anaphylaxis

Category	Examples
Antibiotics	Penicillin and penicillin analogues, β-lactam antibiotics, cephalosporins, tetracyclines, erythromycin
Nonsteroidal anti-inflammatory drugs	Salicylates, ibuprofen, indomethacin
Narcotic analgesics	Morphine, codeine, meprobamate
Local anesthetics	Procaine, lidocaine, cocaine
General anesthetics	Thiopental
Muscle relaxants	Suxamethonium, tubocurarine, pancuronium
Blood products and antisera	Red blood cell, white blood cell, and platelet transfusions; gamma globulin; rabies, tetanus, diphtheria antitoxin; snake and spider antivenom
Diagnostic agents	Iodinated radiocontrast agents
Foods	Eggs, milk, nuts, legumes (peanuts, soybeans, kidney beans), fish, shellfish
Venoms	Bees, wasps, hornets, fire ants, scorpions, snakes
Enzymes and other biologic agents	Acetylcysteine, pancreatic enzyme supplements, chymopapain
Extracts of potential allergens used in desensitization	Pollen, food, venom extracts
Chemotherapeutic agents	Cisplatin, cyclophosphamide, daunorubicin, methotrexate
Insulin	Pork, beef, and human insulin
Other drugs	Protamine, chlorpropamide, parenteral iron, iodides, thiazide diuretics

to an allergen. These reactions may be attributed to an unknown allergen or a well-defined allergen such as bee venom.

Anaphylaxis may progress to shock, multiple organ failure, and death. Early recognition and rapid implementation of treatment is lifesaving. It is essential that patients with anaphylaxis be accurately diagnosed so that management can proceed as quickly as possible. Because these severe reactions may continue despite appropriate treatment, and because a recurrence of symptoms after an initial favorable response may occur, patients with severe life-threatening anaphylaxis should be admitted to the hospital or intensive care unit (ICU) for continued monitoring.

HISTORY AND INCIDENCE

Allergic emergencies have been described in humans since ancient times.[9-11] At the turn of the twentieth century, a more detailed description of these events was reported by two French physiologists, Portier and Richet.[12] They coined the term anaphylaxis, which originates from the French word *anaphylactique*, which means "reverse protection." It was believed that these reactions were in contrast to the attenuated or tachyphylactic reactions that commonly protect subjects from reintroduced antigens such as viruses. More recent research defining the role of IgE; the interactions between IgE, antigen, mast cells, basophils, and eosinophils; and the biochemical mediators from these cells has clarified the events leading to clinical anaphylaxis.[2,13-15]

The true incidence of the various types of anaphylactic reactions is difficult to determine because these reactions are often spontaneous and unpredictable and are clinically similar to other acute reactions. Lifetime prevalence of anaphylaxis due to all triggers is estimated to be 0.05% to 2%.[16] Estimates of the incidence of the most commonly reported episodes are possible, however. In the United States, penicillin alone probably accounts for several hundred fatalities each year.[17-19] Anaphylaxis to the cephalosporins also is commonly reported.[20] It has been estimated that among patients with an allergic reaction to a penicillin, there is a 3% to 7% rate of allergic reaction to a cephalosporin. Reports of anaphylactic reactions to the newer β-lactam antibiotics are accumulating.[21]

Insects, especially those of the Hymenoptera order, which includes bees, wasps, hornets, and fire ants, account for numerous immediate hypersensitivity reactions. About 3% of adults and 1% of children are affected and the anaphylaxis can be fatal at the first sting. About 50 people experience fatal reactions to insect stings every year in the United States, and about half of them do not have a prior sting exposure.[22-24] Fire ants are aggressive insects from South America that now reside in the southern United States. In some areas, they have been known to sting 58% of the residents yearly and account for serious allergic reactions.[25]

Snake bites account for probably a dozen or so anaphylactic deaths per year in the United States. Snake bites may be associated with typical anaphylactic symptoms and other problems related to the enzymes, proteins, and peptides in venom. Local tissue necrosis, coagulation problems, hemolysis, and neurologic transmission defects have been described. In the United States, most anaphylactic reactions to snake bites are caused by pit vipers. These snakes include rattlesnakes, water moccasins, and copperheads.[26,27]

Food-induced anaphylaxis is probably the most common cause of anaphylaxis and accounts for 30% of fatalities. Peanuts (legumes) and typical nuts from trees account for 90% of fatal cases. Additional common food antigens include fish, soybeans, egg whites, and shellfish.[28] Biphasic reactions are much more common in food-induced anaphylaxis than in other types of anaphylaxis and have been reported in 25% of fatal cases.[29-31]

Iodinated contrast agents account for approximately 125 deaths per year[32] and lead to clinical symptoms similar to anaphylaxis. Life-threatening reactions are extremely rare, with an incidence of 0.1%.[33,34] With the advent of low osmolar iodinated contrast agents, the risk of anaphylaxis to contrast agents has decreased drastically.[35]

Latex, used in surgical gloves, balloons, condoms, rubber bands, and many other products, may produce anaphylaxis.[36,37] The use of universal precautions as a result of the acquired immunodeficiency syndrome epidemic has increased the number of reactions to latex in health care workers. Children with spina bifida and genitourinary tract abnormalities are especially susceptible to latex-induced anaphylaxis because of frequent exposure to latex-containing bladder catheters and other products.

Anaphylactic reactions during anesthesia have been described and typically are associated with hypotension and cardiopulmonary arrest. One review suggests that most cases of intraoperative anaphylaxis are from muscle relaxants (e.g., suxamethonium, tubocurarine, pancuronium).[38] Latex, protamine, and blood products also may cause intraoperative anaphylaxis.

Anaphylaxis and other types of IgE-mediated allergic reactions tend to occur in susceptible, genetically predisposed individuals. The reason for the genetic inheritance of sensitivity to the antigens that produce anaphylaxis continues to be speculative. A popular theory is that type I reactions, when confined to an area of parasitic invasion (e.g., intestinal tract), facilitate the killing and removal of parasites and confer a survival advantage to individuals capable of mounting a type I response. Various clinical and laboratory observations support this view.[39-41] The sites of IgE synthesis in laboratory subjects correspond to the sites of entry of many parasites. These sites include the lymphoid tissue of the respiratory tract, the gastrointestinal tract, and the skin. Eosinophils, cells that migrate to the site of antigen introduction in anaphylaxis, elaborate mediators that are toxic to the outer parasitic covering.

When type I reactions to antigen are no longer restricted to local areas because of genetically determined or acquired factors, the release of mediators becomes generalized. Problems typical of a systemic response include increased microvascular permeability, loss of intravascular volume, abnormal vascular reactivity (especially vasodilation), and impaired pulmonary gas exchange. Local IgE-mediated reactions become decompensatory when systemic involvement ensues.

PATHOGENESIS AND PATHOPHYSIOLOGY

IMMUNOLOGIC MECHANISMS LEADING TO MAST CELL AND BASOPHIL ACTIVATION AND MEDIATOR RELEASE

When an antigen to which an individual has previously been sensitized is reintroduced, a sequence of events is initiated that leads to mediator release (Fig. 28.1). At least several weeks are required between the initial exposure to antigen and a subsequent exposure for clinical manifestations of anaphylaxis to occur. The antigen may be introduced through the skin, respiratory tract, or gastrointestinal tract. Antigen also may be introduced intravenously, usually in association with drug administration. Although most venoms are injected subcutaneously, some may access the circulation through an intravascular route.

In most cases of anaphylaxis, when antigen is reintroduced into the host, it encounters IgE, previously synthesized by plasma cells in response to a previous introduction of antigen. IgE, similar to other immunoglobulins, is composed of two heavy chains and two light chains linked by disulfide bonds. Two portions of the molecule have well-defined functions. The Fab portion of the molecule recognizes and binds antigen. The Fc portion of the molecule binds reversibly to receptors on the surface of mast cells and basophils (Fig. 28.2).

The combination of reintroduced antigen with antigen-specific IgE sets the stage for a sequence of biochemical and cellular events that produce the clinical syndrome of anaphylaxis. The bivalent antigen cross-bridges two IgE molecules (see Fig. 28.1). Cross-bridging facilitates the approximation of Fc surface receptors on mast cells and basophils, triggering the release of mediators from intracellular granules and membrane-based phospholipids. The systemic release of these mediators leads to the pathophysiologic

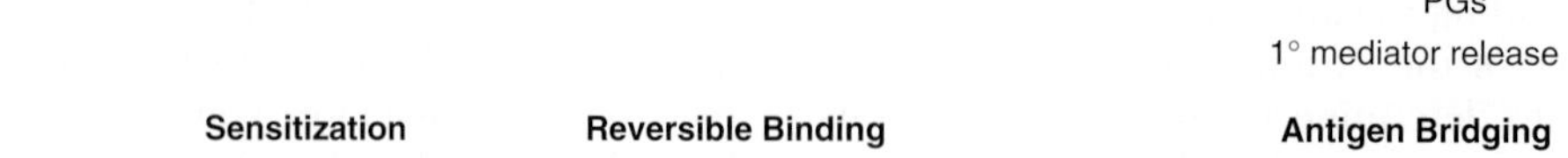

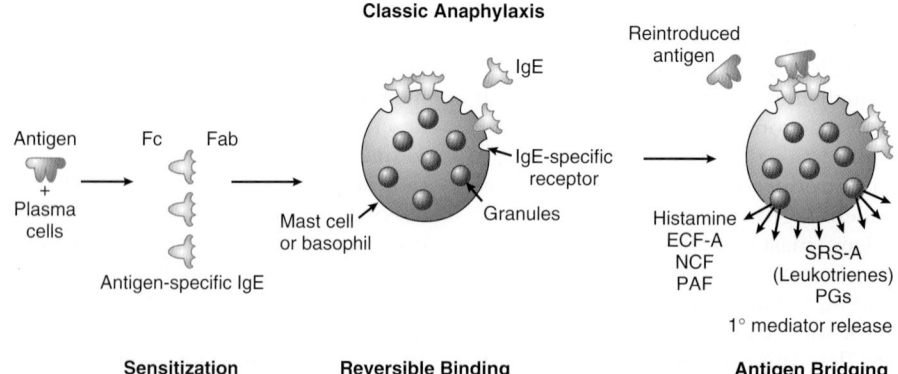

Figure 28.1 The sequence of events leading to mediator release starts with sensitization (initial introduction of a bivalent antigen) and synthesis of antigen-specific IgE. IgE then reversibly binds to mast cells or basophils. When antigen is reintroduced, two cell-bound IgE molecules are linked by the bivalent antigen in a process called *cross-linking*. Cross-linking facilitates the approximation of Fc surface receptors on the mast cell and basophil and initiates a sequence of intracellular biochemical reactions that culminate in mediator release. ECF-A, eosinophil chemotactic factor of anaphylaxis; NCF, neutrophil chemotactic factor; PAF, platelet-activating factor; PGs, prostaglandins; SRS-A, slow-reacting substance of anaphylaxis.

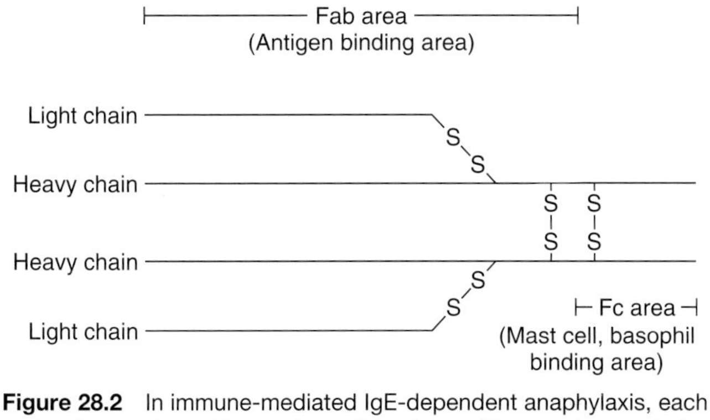

Figure 28.2 In immune-mediated IgE-dependent anaphylaxis, each molecule consists of four polypeptide chains. Two are heavy chains (epsilon [ε]) and are unique to the IgE class of immunoglobulins. Light chains are either kappa (κ) or lambda (λ) chains and may be found in other types of immunoglobulins.

changes that produce the clinical manifestations of anaphylaxis.

Clinical reactions similar to anaphylaxis mediated by immunoglobulins of the IgG class have been described. IgG molecules may combine with antigens, producing an antigen-antibody complex that activates complement. Activation of complement generates C3a and C5a, also known as *anaphylatoxins* because they stimulate mediator release from mast cells and basophils. IgG-mediated reactions are considered type III reactions according to the classification of Gell and Coombs or may be referred to as *Arthus* reactions. These reactions may characterize IgA-deficient individuals who exhibit sudden reactions to blood transfusions. These individuals may develop an antibody of the IgG class to the IgA in the transfused blood product.[42,43] This combination of IgG and IgA antibody activates complement, generates C3a and C5a, and produces a sudden reaction typical of anaphylaxis. Because approximately 1 in 700 individuals is IgA deficient, numerous people are susceptible to this type of blood transfusion reaction.[43] The anaphylactic responses to protamine may be IgG-, IgE-, or non-immune-mediated.[44-46]

NONIMMUNOLOGIC EVENTS LEADING TO MEDIATOR RELEASE

The mediators released during nonimmune reactions originate from mast cells and basophils and are identical to the mediators of immune-mediated anaphylaxis. The direct activation of surface receptors on mast cells and basophils by antigen may be responsible for mediator release in these reactions. Iodinated contrast agents, opiates, and highly charged polyionic antibiotics seem to activate surface receptors directly. Physical stimuli, including heat, cold, and hyperosmolar stimuli, also are capable of stimulating mast cells and basophils. Exercise-induced anaphylaxis may be associated with the stimulation of mast cells through cooling of the airways. Other possible mechanisms include complement activation without immune complex mediation (old preparations of propafol with cremophor diluent),[47] direct mast cell degranulation (merperidine),[48] and direct activation of the kinin-kallikrein pathway, resulting in the generation of bradykinin, C3a, and C5a (oversulfated chondroitin sulfate in heparin products).[49]

CELLULAR CHARACTERISTICS OF ANAPHYLAXIS

Despite the release of similar mediators during anaphylaxis, mast cells and basophils differ in several ways. Mast cells are more abundant than basophils and generally reside in the connective tissue of subcutaneous and submucosal areas. Basophils characteristically circulate in the blood.[50] Despite these differences in location and number, functional differences between the two cell types have not been clearly identified. Both types of cells have receptors for the Fc portion of IgE, and both have granules that bind basic dyes. In addition, the granules of both cells contain histamine and various other mediators that participate in the anaphylactic response.

Eosinophils are commonly identified in the tissues and plasma of patients with both immune- and non-immune-mediated anaphylactic reactions. These cells typically migrate to the site of antigen introduction. They are attracted by a variety of chemotactic factors, including factors derived from mast cells and basophils, antigen-antibody complexes, histamine, and complement. The granules of eosinophils stain with acidophilic dyes and contain a variety of biochemical mediators that are toxic to helminthic parasites. Substances that inactivate leukotrienes and histamines also are elaborated. Eosinophils function as modulators of the inflammatory response triggered by mast cell and basophil activation.[51,52]

Platelets and polymorphonuclear leukocytes also may be involved in the anaphylactic response. These cells respond to mast cell–derived and basophil-derived chemotactic factors and to tissue injury. They release a variety of mediators that may be responsible for recurrent and late-phase reactions (see the following discussion).

BIOCHEMICAL MEDIATORS OF ANAPHYLAXIS

The biochemical mediators of anaphylaxis are divided into *primary* and *secondary* mediators. Mediators directly released from mast cells and basophils are termed *primary mediators* (Table 28.2). Secondary mediators are released from other cell types in response to primary mediator release (Table 28.3). Primary mediators are subdivided further into *preformed* and *newly synthesized* mediators. Preformed mediators are formed and stored in the intracellular granules of mast cells and basophils. Newly synthesized mediators are derived from the metabolism of arachidonic acid, a phospholipid derived from cell membrane.

Histamine is a well-characterized primary mediator stored and released from the granules of mast cells and basophils. Histamine stimulates H_1 and H_2 receptors located on the surfaces of vascular and bronchial smooth muscle cells. Stimulation of H_1 receptors leads to precapillary arteriolar dilation, contraction of postcapillary venules, and formation of intracellular gaps between capillary endothelial cells. By increasing capillary hydrostatic pressure and permeability, these changes initiate the movement of plasma into the interstitial space. In the lung, H_1 receptor stimulation is associated with bronchial smooth muscle contraction. H_2 receptor stimulation leads to vasodilation, enhanced mucus

Table 28.2 Physiologic Effects of Primary Mediators of Anaphylaxis Derived from Mast Cells and Basophils

Mediator(s)	Physiologic Effect(s)
Histamine	
H_1-receptor stimulation	Bronchial smooth muscle contraction Increased vascular permeability Cardiac arrhythmias Increased mucus secretion Vasoactive effects (vasodilation, vasoconstriction)
H_2-receptor stimulation	Increased vascular permeability Increased mucus and gastric acid secretion Activation of inhibitory lymphocytes
H_3-receptor stimulation	Inhibition of histamine synthesis and release
Platelet-activating factor	Increased vascular permeability Bronchospasm Aggregation and activation of platelets Attraction of neutrophils and eosinophils
Eosinophil chemotactic factors	Attraction of eosinophils
Neutrophil chemotactic factors	Attraction of neutrophils
Arachidonic acid metabolites	
Prostaglandin D_2	Bronchoconstriction Potentiates leukocyte migration
Prostaglandin E_2	Bronchodilation
Prostaglandin F_2	Bronchoconstriction
Leukotriene C_4, leukotriene D_4, leukotriene E_4	Bronchoconstriction Increased vascular permeability
Leukotriene B_4	Attraction of neutrophils and eosinophils
Enzymes	
Hydrolytic enzymes	Degradation of parasitic and host tissue
Proteases	Degradation of parasitic and host tissue Interaction with complement components, coagulation cascade, and kinin system
Tryptase	Generation of complement anaphylatoxins, inhibition of fibrinogen
Carboxypeptidase	Deactivation of complement anaphylatoxins
Oxidative enzymes	
Superoxide dismutase	Inactivation of oxygen and associated cytotoxic effects
Peroxidase	Inactivation of cytotoxic effects of hydrogen peroxide
Heparin	Anticoagulant activity May assist in the repair of injured tissues
Adenosine	Bronchospasm Regulates mast cell degranulation
Serotonin	Vasoactive effects

Table 28.3 Secondary Mediators of Anaphylaxis and Physiologic Effects

Mediator(s)	Physiologic Effect(s)
Neutrophil, platelet, and eosinophil-derived mediators	Permeability, coagulation changes, proteolysis
Activated complement system	
C3a and C5a	Contract bronchial smooth muscle; increase vascular permeability; attract neutrophils, macrophages, and monocytes
C6-C9	Membrane damage
Activated coagulation cascade	Intravascular coagulation, permeability changes, tissue injury
Activated kinin system (bradykinin)	Increases vascular permeability

secretion, increased heart rate and myocardial contractility, increased gastric acid secretion, and inhibition of T cells. The vasoactive and cardiac effects of H_2 receptor stimulation primarily contribute to the clinical manifestations of anaphylaxis.

The family of arachidonic acid metabolites known as *leukotrienes* consists of newly synthesized primary mediators that function as potent vascular permeability agents and bronchoconstrictors. Arachidonic acid metabolism via the cyclooxygenase pathways produces prostaglandins with bronchoconstrictive effects—prostaglandin D_2 and prostaglandin F_2. Other mediators that are released are tryptase, carboxypeptidases, and proteoglycans.

The primary mediator release from mast cells and basophils sets the stage for involvement by secondary mediators. Secondary mediators include products of enzyme-dependent cascading biochemical pathways. In addition, secondary mediators may be derived from other involved cells, such as neutrophils, platelets, and eosinophils.

BIOCHEMICAL AND PHARMACOLOGIC REGULATION OF MEDIATOR RELEASE

The biochemical regulation of mediator release provides a rationale for the pharmacologic therapy of anaphylaxis. The release of primary mediators is thought to be modified by intracellular levels of cyclic adenosine monophosphate (cAMP) and cyclic guanosine monophosphate (cGMP) and calcium and other bivalent cations. Pharmacologic agents that affect the intracellular levels of these modulators and inhibit mediator release are often used in the treatment of anaphylaxis (Box 28.1).

β_2-Adrenergic agonists increase intracellular levels of cAMP by activating adenylate cyclase. This increase in cAMP subsequently inhibits the release of mediators. The methylxanthines aminophylline and theophylline also increase cAMP levels through the inhibition of phosphodiesterase. Because cGMP antagonizes the action of cAMP, agents that decrease cGMP inhibit mediator release. Anticholinergic drugs decrease cGMP levels and may have a role in the treatment of anaphylaxis.

Mediator release from mast cells and basophils is associated with an influx of calcium. Although calcium blocking agents theoretically may be useful in the treatment of anaphylaxis, clinical experience with use of these agents for this condition is lacking. Conversely, calcium administration may be harmful in anaphylaxis because of its association with enhanced mediator release. Other bivalent cations, such as magnesium and manganese, also enhance mediator release. Multiple tyrosine kinases are activated and regulate by exerting either stimulatory or inhibitory actions on the signal transduction cascade.[53-55] Sphingosine-1-phosphate has been identified recently as one of the mediators that serves as a modulator in the mast cell. In addition, it is now labeled as a circulating mediator in anaphylaxis.[56]

Box 28.1 Intracellular Regulation of Mediator Release by Pharmacologic Agents

Inhibit Release

By increasing cAMP

β-Adrenergic drugs (e.g., epinephrine)
Phosphodiesterase inhibitors (e.g., aminophylline, theophylline)

By decreasing cGMP

Anticholinergic drugs (e.g., ipratropium)

Enhance Release

By decreasing cAMP

β-Adrenergic blocking agents
α-Adrenergic drugs

By increasing cGMP

Cholinergic drugs

cAMP, cyclic adenosine monophosphate; cGMP, cyclic guanosine monophosphate.

PATHOPHYSIOLOGIC EFFECTS OF MEDIATORS

The numerous mediators released during anaphylactic crisis have many physiologic effects that have been studied extensively in the laboratory. Although it is difficult to determine the specific actions of each mediator in anaphylaxis, the cumulative effects of mediator release have been described in the clinical setting. These effects include abnormalities secondary to increased vascular permeability; vascular resistance changes, primarily vasodilation; and bronchospasm. Autopsies of fatal cases of anaphylaxis reveal edema of the lungs, upper airway (including the larynx and epiglottis), skin, and viscera. Pulmonary congestion is typical in fatal anaphylaxis, and light microscopy often reveals fluid-filled pulmonary alveoli.[57] In another series of fatal cases of anaphylaxis, acute pulmonary emphysema was observed in almost half of cases.[58] This condition is characterized by hyperextended alveoli and thinning of the alveolar septum. Because of the association of acute pulmonary emphysema with laryngeal edema, these fatalities were thought to be caused by upper airway obstruction, with alveolar rupture resulting from forced exhalation against the obstruction.

Cardiac abnormalities, including arrhythmias, reduced contractility, and myocardial ischemia, have been described in anaphylaxis but seem to be uncommon.[59] These abnormalities may be secondary to the effects of histamine and other mediators on the myocardium. Other contributing factors include circulatory shock, hypotension, increased adrenergic tone, and drugs used to treat anaphylaxis.

LATE-PHASE OR BIPHASIC REACTIONS

Both immune-mediated and non-immune-mediated anaphylactic reactions may be followed by late-phase reactions (also termed *biphasic reactions*). These reactions typically occur 6 to 12 hours after the initial reaction as a result of the migration of mast cells, basophils, and polymorphonuclear leukocytes into areas of antigen introduction. A secondary wave of mediator release and recurrence of symptoms may be observed.[60-62]

CLINICAL AND HEMODYNAMIC FEATURES

The constellation of clinical signs and symptoms in anaphylaxis may vary widely for individuals; however, severe, rapidly progressive symptoms after exposure to antigen are characteristic. The portal of entry for the antigen, the rate of absorption, and the degree of hypersensitivity to the antigen also influence the clinical presentation. Current research is focusing on the role of genetic factors as well. Gastrointestinal symptoms, including nausea, vomiting, abdominal cramps, and diarrhea, may precede more generalized clinical manifestations after ingestion of an antigen. Inhalation of an antigen may be associated with nasal coryza, a sensation of tightness or a lump in the throat, hoarseness, stridor, wheezing, and dyspnea. Introduction of antigen through the skin may produce local pruritus, urticaria, and swelling before progression to systemic symptoms.

The most life-threatening reactions are usually explosive in nature, often occurring within minutes of exposure to the antigen. Victims of these reactions have been noted to describe a feeling of impending doom before more defined symptoms develop. Generalized cutaneous abnormalities include erythema, urticaria, and flushing. Swelling of the periorbital and perioral areas is characteristic. Upper and lower airway abnormalities are common and especially dangerous. Swelling of the posterior pharynx, uvula, tonsils, and vocal cords may develop rapidly. Auscultation of the chest may reveal generalized wheezing and prolongation of expiration. Auscultatory and radiographic signs of pulmonary edema are characteristic of severe episodes. Signs of circulatory shock include hypotension, oliguria, and lactic acidosis from intravascular volume depletion. In some instances, such as the intravenous injection of venom or a drug, circulatory shock may develop without preceding cutaneous and respiratory abnormalities. The clinical features of anaphylaxis may respond quickly to treatment or, in the most severe cases, may last for several hours to several days. An initial favorable response to treatment may be followed by a late-phase reaction—a recurrence of symptoms resulting from a second wave of mediator release approximately 6 to 12 hours after the initial reaction.[60,62]

Hemodynamic descriptions of human anaphylaxis are limited to detailed studies of a few cases. The loss of circulating plasma volume is characteristic and is associated with hemoconcentration, hypotension, tachycardia, decreased cardiac filling pressures, and decreased cardiac output.[63,64] Vasodilation, associated with a decrease in systemic vascular resistance, may contribute to the reduction in venous return and cardiac output. When oxygen delivery decreases to levels below systemic oxygen demands, anaerobic metabolic pathways are activated, and lactic acidosis emerges.[65] Decreases in myocardial contractility seem to be minimal in studies of human anaphylaxis using routine hemodynamic monitoring. This is supported by the observation that most patients with anaphylaxis respond favorably to fluid therapy and do not require inotropic support.[63-67] In a few case reports, reduced myocardial contractility has been observed in association with myocardial ischemia and infarction.[68-73] Some of these adverse cardiac effects have been associated with epinephrine administration, but in some cases they also have been noted before pharmacologic treatment.[68-73]

Laboratory studies provide more detailed descriptions of the hemodynamic features of anaphylaxis. After antigenic challenge in primates, a transient increase in cardiac output is observed and is followed by decreases in arterial pressure, right and left ventricular filling pressures, and peripheral vascular resistance.[74] The transient increase in cardiac output has been attributed to vasodilation-induced left ventricular unloading or an increase in cardiac contractility or both. Elevated plasma levels of epinephrine, norepinephrine, and histamine have been shown in laboratory animals and humans and may contribute to this increase in contractility.[75,76] Cardiac output eventually decreases when hypotension and shock become established. In human and canine models of anaphylaxis, a reduction in venous return has been observed secondary to vasodilation and pooling of blood in the splanchnic circulation.[77-79] Loss of plasma volume from increased vascular permeability is probably a contributing factor.

When pulmonary edema fluid is sufficiently copious to be sampled from the airway of patients with anaphylaxis, albumin concentrations and oncotic pressures are nearly identical to plasma values. These findings and the association of pulmonary edema with low pulmonary artery wedge pressures suggest that the pulmonary edema in anaphylaxis is noncardiogenic and secondary to increased microvascular permeability.[63] Although transient pulmonary hypertension and increased pulmonary vascular resistance have been observed in primates immediately after antigen challenge,[74] it is unknown whether pulmonary hypertension characterizes human anaphylaxis.

Hemodynamic characteristics of human anaphylaxis are determined by generalized vasodilation and increased vascular permeability, which lead to venous pooling of blood and loss of circulating plasma volume. Permeability edema develops in the lung. Changes in cardiac contractility are not typical of human anaphylaxis; however, reduced contractility may characterize patients who exhibit signs of myocardial ischemia or infarction, especially in association with epinephrine therapy.

MANAGEMENT

INITIAL MANAGEMENT

The initial assessment of a patient with suspected anaphylaxis should be brief and specific because immediate therapeutic interventions are required. Because a variety of conditions may appear similar to anaphylaxis (Box 28.2), it is important to rule out these events quickly. Vasovagal episodes are among the most common conditions confused with anaphylaxis. Bradycardia, pale skin, and diaphoresis in an acutely ill patient are suggestive of a vasovagal attack, in contrast to the tachycardic, flushed appearance typical of anaphylaxis.

When it is strongly suspected that the patient is experiencing a severe or potentially severe anaphylactic episode, the following steps should proceed rapidly (Fig. 28.3): (1) assurance of a patent airway, (2) removal of toxin at the site of introduction or an attempt to delay the systemic absorption of toxin or both, (3) establishment of intravenous access for fluid therapy, and (4) initiation of pharmacologic support with epinephrine (Box 28.3). A team approach is

Box 28.2 Conditions That Mimic Anaphylaxis

- Vasovagal episodes
- Acute pulmonary events
  - Acute asthmatic attacks
  - Acute pulmonary edema
  - Pulmonary embolus
  - Spontaneous pneumothorax
  - Foreign body aspiration
- Acute cardiac events
  - Supraventricular tachycardias
  - Acute myocardial infarction/ischemia
- Drug overdoses
- Insulin shock
- Carcinoid attacks

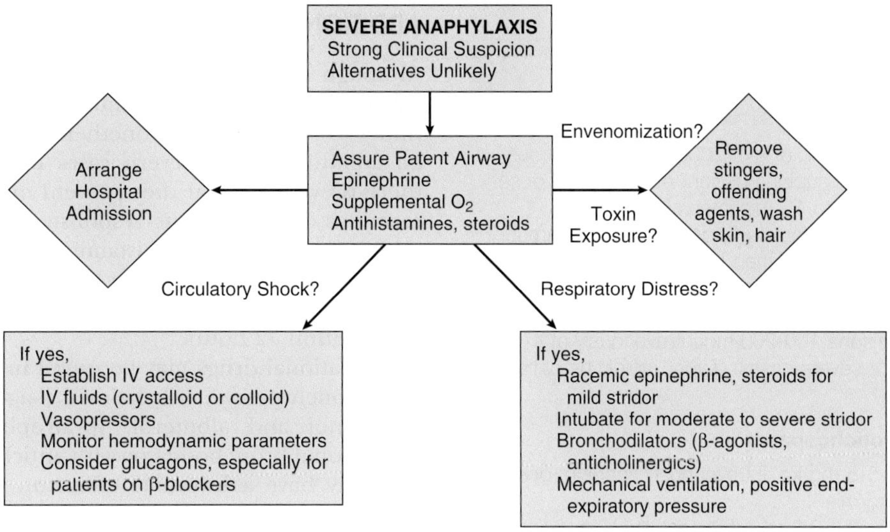

Figure 28.3 Overview of the clinical management of severe anaphylaxis.

essential in severe cases of anaphylaxis because assessment and interventions must proceed rapidly and, if possible, simultaneously.

Admission to the hospital is required for all patients experiencing severe anaphylaxis. Hospital personnel should have advanced airway skills and be capable of managing hemodynamic instability. Although symptom recurrence is uncommon in patients who respond favorably to treatment,[79] hospital admission and monitoring is recommended for all patients with severe anaphylaxis because of the potential for late-phase reactions, which may be severe and may occur 12 hours after the initial attack. While in the hospital, the patient should be monitored for signs of circulatory shock, respiratory failure, and upper airway obstruction. Blood pressure, urine output, and heart and respiratory rate require frequent evaluation.

The electrocardiogram should be monitored continuously during the acute period because anaphylaxis has been associated with serious arrhythmias and cardiac ischemia. In addition, drugs used to treat anaphylaxis and circulatory shock may precipitate cardiac problems. When signs of circulatory shock and impaired pulmonary gas exchange develop, advanced hemodynamic monitoring is required. As with other types of circulatory shock, fluid therapy, inotropic and vasopressor therapy, and optimization of ventilatory support require titration under hemodynamic guidance to maintain organ perfusion, pulmonary gas exchange, and systemic oxygen delivery.

Close attention to the airway is essential because laryngeal edema is an important cause of morbidity and death. Frequent assessment for hoarseness, stridor, and upper airway obstruction is required for patients whose airways are not protected with an endotracheal tube. The head and neck should be positioned to prevent airway obstruction by the tongue. If inspiratory stridor develops, endotracheal intubation should be attempted. Because intubation may be difficult in the presence of laryngeal edema, skilled personnel capable of performing difficult endotracheal intubations and emergency surgical airways should be available.

If intubated patients are unable to breathe spontaneously or have labored respirations, mechanical ventilation should be initiated. Positive end-expiratory pressure and other advanced ventilatory techniques are often necessary when hypoxemia, pulmonary edema, and decreased pulmonary compliance develop. In nonintubated patients, 6 to 8 L per minute of oxygen through a facemask is recommended.[80]

The site of antigen introduction should be identified. If the patient is unconscious or unaware of the site of antigen introduction, a thorough search of skin surfaces should proceed. Retained stingers from *Hymenoptera* may be found and require complete and immediate removal. Delaying venomization from an extremity using a constricting band or local application of epinephrine or suctioning venom are controversial practices. However, immobilization is recommended. Thorough washing of the skin should follow exposure to antigen that has contacted the skin surface.

The mainstay of pharmacologic therapy for anaphylaxis is epinephrine. Epinephrine is of proven efficacy in reversing the bronchoconstriction and hypotension associated with anaphylaxis. The β-adrenergic effects of epinephrine inhibit mediator release by increasing intracellular levels of cAMP. In addition, β-adrenergic stimulation reverses bronchospasm, increases myocardial contractility, and increases heart rate. The α-adrenergic vasoconstrictive properties of epinephrine may increase diastolic pressure and enhance coronary flow.

All medical personnel should be aware that two dilutions of epinephrine are commonly available: 1 mg/mL or 1 : 1000 dilution and 0.1 mg/mL or 1 : 10,000 dilution. For the initial treatment of anaphylaxis, most authorities recommend that 0.3 to 0.5 mg of the 1 : 1000 solution (0.3 to 0.5 mL) be given intramuscularly. This dose may be repeated at 5- to 15-minute intervals if symptoms do not improve. In children, the recommended dose is 0.01 mg/kg not to exceed 0.5 mg.

Fluid therapy is an essential component of anaphylaxis treatment. Adults should receive 1 to 2 L of normal saline

Box 28.3 Pharmacologic Approach to the Acute Management of Anaphylaxis

Give epinephrine 0.3-0.5 mL of a 1:1000 solution intramuscularly with patient in a supine position. An additional dose may be repeated in 5- to 15-min intervals.

If patient remains in shock despite fluids and initial intramuscular epinephrine treatment, then intravenous epinephrine at the rate of 2-10 μg/min should be administered and titrated to effect.

Administer hydrocortisone 100-200 mg intravenously at 4- to 6-hour intervals (for severe cases). Taper rapidly as patient improves.

For Persistent Bronchospasm

Give aminophylline 5-6 mg/kg intravenously loading dose, then 0.4-0.9 mg/kg/min.

Give metaproterenol 0.2-0.3 mL (5% solution) in 2.5 mL normal saline solution administered by nebulization; repeat every 3-4 hours as needed.

Give ipratropium bromide aerosol (2 puffs) inhaled and repeated at 2-hour intervals.

Provide intravenous fluids according to degree of hemoconcentration or, in more severe cases, hemodynamic factors. Normal saline, Ringer's lactate, 5% human serum albumin. Hydroxyethyl starch should be avoided.

For Hypotension and Shock

For continued hypotension and other signs of circulatory shock start with an epinephrine drip.

- Epinephrine drip at 2-10 μg/min

One of the following vasopressors may added for persistent hypertension:

- Norepinephrine drip 4-8 mg in 1 L normal saline at 4-8 μg/min
- Dopamine drip 200 mg in 0.5 L normal saline at 5-16 μg/kg/min

The following may be given if no contraindications:

- Diphenhydramine 25-50 mg orally or intravenously at 4-hour intervals

as soon as possible for severe anaphylaxis. Fluids reverse the intravascular volume deficits typical of anaphylaxis. Both crystalloidal and colloidal fluids are effective. Clinicians should be aware that two to three times as much crystalloid is required compared with colloid to achieve comparable intravascular volume repletion. However, colloid may trigger another anaphylaxis reaction by itself. Reversal of hemoconcentration is a reasonable resuscitative goal for patients who are stable and responding favorably to treatment. In unstable patients with wide fluctuations in vital signs and worsening pulmonary function, fluid therapy should be administered in the ICU with advanced hemodynamic monitoring capability.

If hypotension and other signs of circulatory shock persist after the initial administration of epinephrine and fluids, then intravenous epinephrine is recommended. Bolus doses are no longer recommended because of dosing errors and side effects.[81] The initial dose for intravenous epinephrine infusion is 2 to 10 μg per minute, titrated to effect on blood pressure.[82] Sometimes patients may need an additional vasopressor along with epinephrine.

ADDITIONAL THERAPEUTIC OPTIONS

Although the role of epinephrine in anaphylaxis is established, the role of antihistamines and corticosteroids continues to be debated.[80] Nonetheless, corticosteroids should be administered in severe cases of anaphylaxis because there is evidence that they prevent or attenuate late-phase reactions, increase tissue responsiveness to β-agonists, and inhibit the synthesis of histamine. Methylprednisolone or hydrocortisone may be given for 72 hours and can then be rapidly tapered off because almost all the biphasic reactions occur within 72 hours.[83,84]

Inhalational drugs may be useful in patients with persistent bronchospasm. Inhalational β-agonists include metaproterenol and albuterol. Ipratropium bromide is an inhalational bronchodilator with anticholinergic properties and may have a favorable effect on mediator release by decreasing cGMP levels. This agent may be used in combination with inhalational β-agonists.

Laryngeal edema, if mild, may respond to nebulized racemic epinephrine. Localized vasoconstriction from the α-adrenergic properties of these drugs minimizes edema formation in the larynx and adjacent areas. Racemic epinephrine may be administered by nebulization (0.5 mL of a 2.25% solution diluted in 3.5 mL distilled water). Intravenous corticosteroid therapy also may be useful in this condition. Severe laryngeal edema associated with respiratory distress or stridor should always be treated with intubation of the trachea.

Several other agents have been used in cases of human anaphylaxis or in laboratory models of anaphylaxis with apparent success. Glucagon, a pancreatic hormone that increases intracellular cAMP levels by activating adenylate cyclase, was effective in a case report of a patient with anaphylaxis who was receiving beta-blocker therapy.[85,86] Current research focuses on understanding mast cell and basophil biology, targeting tyrosine kinases, and developing antibodies to IgE.[87,88]

Arrangements must be made for patients who have experienced anaphylaxis to receive follow-up care by a physician experienced in the management of acute allergic events. Skin testing may be required to identify the inciting agent. Instructions in self-treatment after antigen exposure are necessary. Autoinjectors of epinephrine 0.15 mg and 0.30 mg (1:1000) and oral antihistamines for patients to self-administer are available.

PROPHYLAXIS AND IMMUNOTHERAPY

If a patient must be treated with a drug that has previously produced severe allergic symptoms or anaphylaxis and no alternative exists, premedication should be implemented. Most authorities recommend premedication with H_1 and H_2 blockers and corticosteroids. Several studies have confirmed that premedication with these agents decreases anaphylactic reactions to radiocontrast media.[89-91] In very high risk patients, some authorities believe that epinephrine or isoproterenol should be included as premedication.[92] Because fatal anaphylaxis has been described in patients who received premedication, it is preferable, if clinically possible, to avoid all antigens associated with anaphylaxis.

Methods to desensitize individuals immediately before administration of a drug have been described in detail, especially for penicillin,[93] aspirin,[94] and insulin.[95] These techniques, which involve exposure to antigen in 20- to 30-minute increments, may be unsuccessful, however, and occasional fatalities have been reported.[96-98]

Long-term desensitization may be useful in patients who have experienced anaphylaxis to antigens that are difficult to avoid, especially foods and venoms. This type of immunotherapy involves initial injection of a minute dose of antigen followed by gradual increases in dose at weekly or biweekly intervals according to the patient's tolerance.[99,100] A non-IgE-blocking antibody forms and decreases the reactivity of mast cells and basophils to antigen.

Education and acute and long-term desensitization should be the responsibility of physicians experienced in the management of immediate hypersensitivity disorders. The critical care physician is responsible for ensuring the referral of patients who have experienced anaphylaxis to the care of appropriately trained specialists.

KEY POINTS

- Classic anaphylaxis is an IgE-mediated allergic reaction (type I) with acute systemic manifestations.
- Nonimmune and IgE-independent anaphylactic reactions are clinically identical to classic anaphylaxis and respond similarly to treatment.
- Mediators derived from mast cells and basophils are responsible for the major pathophysiologic effects of anaphylaxis.
- Eosinophils also release mediators that modulate the inflammatory response of anaphylaxis.
- Mediators from polymorphonuclear leukocytes and platelets are responsible for late-phase reactions after the initial anaphylactic event.
- Histamine, leukotrienes, and prostaglandins are important biochemical mediators of anaphylaxis. Release of these mediators is associated with increased vascular permeability and bronchial smooth muscle constriction.
- Pharmacologic agents that increase cAMP levels inhibit mediator release and may be beneficial in anaphylaxis.
- Agents that decrease cGMP levels (e.g., anticholinergic drugs) also inhibit mediator release.
- Fatal anaphylaxis is often associated with upper airway obstruction from laryngeal edema.
- The initial presentation of a patient with anaphylaxis depends on the portal of entry of the antigen and may include a local skin reaction and respiratory, upper airway, and gastrointestinal symptoms.
- Late-phase reactions may occur 6 to 12 hours after the initial anaphylactic event and are associated with a recurrence of symptoms.

KEY POINTS (Continued)

- Hemodynamic characteristics of anaphylaxis include tachycardia, hypotension, decreased cardiac filling pressures, and decreased systemic vascular resistance.
- The mainstays of anaphylaxis management are to (1) ensure airway patency, (2) remove or delay the absorption of toxins, (3) establish access for fluid therapy, and (4) initiate pharmacologic support with epinephrine.
- Corticosteroids should be given in severe cases to prevent late-phase reactions.
- Antihistamines (H_1 and H_2 blockers) are routinely given if there are no contraindications.
- Inhaled β-agonist agents, aminophylline, and inhaled anticholinergic agents may be given for continued bronchospasm.
- All patients who have experienced anaphylaxis should be referred to an appropriately qualified specialist for follow-up. These patients may require allergy testing, desensitization, and premedication strategies.

ACKNOWLEDGMENT

The authors would like to thank Ravi Chandra Gutta, MD, for his assistance in reviewing and critiquing this manuscript.

SELECTED REFERENCES

1. Sampson HA, Munoz-Furlong A, Campbell RL, et al: Second symposium on the definition and management of anaphylaxis: Summary report—Second National Institute of Allergy and Infectious Disease/Food Allergy and Anaphylaxis network symposium. J Allergy Clin Immunol 2006;117:391-397.
3. Simons FER: Anaphylaxis: Recent advances in assessment and treatment. J Allergy Clin Immunol 2009;124:625-636.
16. Lieberman P, Camargo CA Jr, Bohlke K, et al: Epidemiology of anaphylaxis: Findings of the American College of Allergy, Asthma and Immunology Epidemiology of Anaphylaxis Working Group. Ann Allergy Asthma Immunol 2006;97:596-602.
18. Park MA, Li JT: Diagnosis and management of penicillin allergy. Mayo Clin Proc 2005;80:405.
53. Peavy RD, Metcalfe DD: Understanding the mechanisms of anaphylaxis. Curr Opin Allergy Clin Immunol 2008;8:310-315.
81. Simons KJ, Simons FE: Epinephrine and its use in anaphylaxis: Current issues. Curr Opin Allergy Clin Immunol 2010;10:354.
82. Lieberman P, Nicklas RA, Oppenheimer J, et al: The diagnosis and management of anaphylaxis practice parameter: 2010 update. J Allergy Clin Immunol 2010;126:477.
83. Tole JW, Lieberman P: Biphasic anaphylaxis: Review of incidence, clinical predictors, and observation recommendations. Immunol Allergy Clin North Am 2007;27:309-326.
88. Thomas M, Crawford I: Best evidence report: Glucagon infusion in refractory anaphylactic shock in patients on beta-blockers. Emerg Med J 2005;22:272.
91. Tramer MR, von Elm E, Loubeyre P, et al: Pharmacologic prevention of serious anaphylactic reactions due to iodinated contrast media: Systemic review. BMJ 2006;333:675.

The complete list of references can be found at www.expertconsult.com.

29 Severe Heart Failure

Fredric Ginsberg | Joseph E. Parrillo

CHAPTER OUTLINE

DEFINITION, EPIDEMIOLOGY, AND STAGING OF HEART FAILURE

Heart failure can be defined as an inability of the heart to provide cardiac output adequate to meet the metabolic demands of the body at a normal filling pressure. The term *heart failure* commonly refers to a syndrome of signs and symptoms caused by excessive salt and fluid retention, increased left and right ventricular filling pressures, and decreased cardiac output. Heart failure is a progressive illness with a high mortality rate. Death can occur either at the end of progressive worsening of the heart failure syndrome or suddenly and unexpectedly in patients who appear clinically stable. Appropriate therapies for heart failure, involving medications, revascularization, and devices, have the potential to reverse the processes that cause heart failure and thus improve cardiac performance, which can result in stabilization of the patient's symptoms, enhance functional status, and improve chances for survival.

Heart failure is a very common illness; 5.8 million Americans are affected.[1,2] It is estimated that 1% of the population of Americans over the age of 65 are affected by heart failure, and 20% of hospital admissions in patients over age 65 are due to heart failure.[3] Men and black Americans are affected more frequently. In 2008 670,000 new cases of heart failure were diagnosed in the United States, where there are nearly 1 million hospital discharges, 658,000 visits to the emergency department, over 3.4 million ambulatory outpatient visits, and 6.5 million hospital days annually for patients with a primary diagnosis of heart failure.[1,2] Over 56,000 people in the United States died in 2007 with heart failure as the primary cause. The treatment of heart failure incurs a very large economic burden on the U.S. health care system. Estimated direct and indirect cost of heart failure in 2010 was $29 billion. The majority of this cost was related to the treatment of patients hospitalized with heart failure.

Epidemiologic data showed significant increases in both the incidence and prevalence of heart failure in the U.S. population in the 1990s,[3] likely influenced by the aging of the population, a high prevalence of hypertension, and improved treatment and survival of patients with ischemic heart disease.[4] However, there is evidence that hospitalizations for heart failure have declined during the past decade. In the United States, the rate of hospitalization for heart failure declined from 2845 per 100,000 patient-years in 1998 to 2007 per 100,000 person-years in 2008, a decline of 29%.[5]

Patients hospitalized with acute heart failure are usually elderly, with a mean age in the early 70s. In the United States, roughly 80% of patients will have a previous history of heart failure,[6] and in European studies one third of patients had a new diagnosis of heart failure.[7] From 40% to 55% of patients will have normal or relatively normal left ventricular systolic function. This occurs more commonly in women than in men. Coronary heart disease is present in 50% to 60% of patients and hypertension in 72% of patients. Comorbid conditions are common, including renal disease in 30% of patients, diabetes mellitus in 43%, and chronic obstructive pulmonary disease (COPD) in roughly 30%.[6-8]

In the American College of Cardiology/American Heart Association Guidelines for the diagnosis and management of chronic heart failure, four stages in the development of heart failure are recognized (Fig. 29.1). This staging system emphasizes the progressive nature of left ventricular dysfunction and heart failure, and describes evidence-based guidelines for therapy for each stage.[4] It is important to realize that heart failure may be preventable. Several common medical conditions place patients at high risk for developing left ventricular dysfunction and the heart failure syndrome. Attention to and appropriate management of these conditions may prevent the development of heart failure. In addition, in patients who have left ventricular

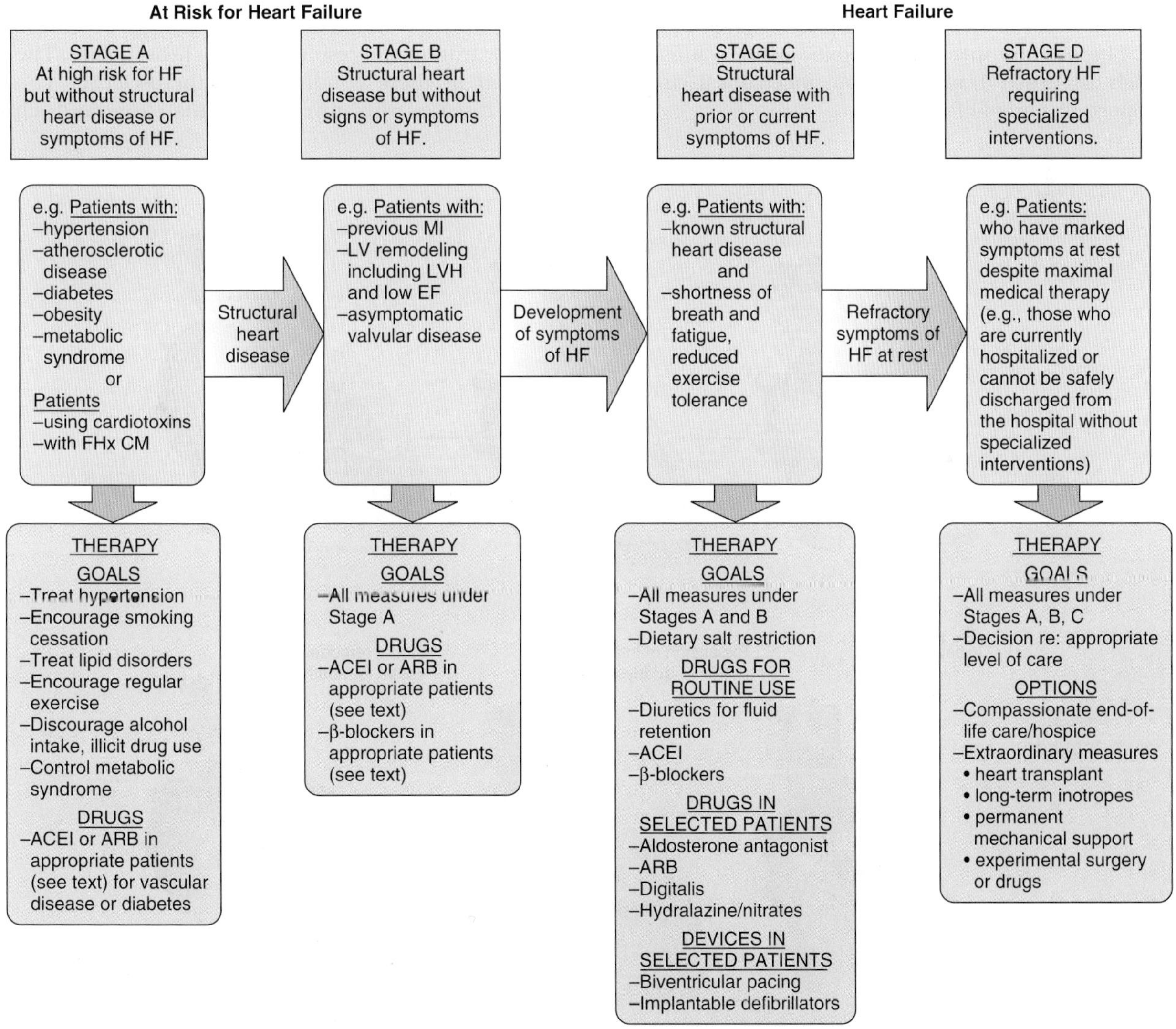

Figure 29.1 Stages in the development of heart failure and recommended therapy by stage. ACEI, angiotensin-converting enzyme inhibitor; ARB, angiotensin receptor blocker; EF, ejection fraction; FHx CM, family history of cardiomyopathy; HF, heart failure; LV, left ventricular; LVH, LV hypertrophy; MI, myocardial infarction. (Redrawn from Hunt S, Abraham WT, Chin M, et al: ACC/AHA 2005 Guideline Update for the Diagnosis and Management of Chronic Heart Failure in the Adult—Summary Article. A report on the American College of Cardiology/American Heart Association Task Force on Practice Guidelines (Writing Committee to Update the 2001 Guidelines for Evaluation and Management of Heart Failure): Developed in collaboration with the American College of Chest Physicians and the International Society for Heart and Lung Transplantation: Endorsed by the Heart Rhythm Society. Circulation 2005;112:1825-1852.)

dysfunction but who have not yet developed heart failure, appropriate therapy can improve prognosis and prevent the development of severe heart failure.

Stage A represents patients at high risk for heart failure but without structural heart disease or symptoms of heart failure. These patients include those with hypertension, atherosclerotic heart disease, diabetes, obesity, or the metabolic syndrome; those exposed to cardiotoxic medications; and those with a family history of cardiomyopathy. About 75% of patients who develop heart failure have antecedent hypertension.[2] Stage B patients have structural heart disease but without signs or symptoms of heart failure. This group includes patients who have suffered a myocardial infarction, those with abnormal left ventricular ejection fraction but no symptoms of heart failure, and those patients with asymptomatic valvular heart disease. Stage C patients have structural heart disease with prior or current symptoms of heart failure, such as shortness of breath, fatigue, and reduced exercise tolerance. Lastly, stage D patients have refractory symptoms of heart failure at rest despite maximal medical therapy. They require specialized or extraordinary interventions such as cardiac transplantation, mechanical circulatory support, or end-of-life care.

PATHOPHYSIOLOGY

Heart failure can be due primarily to left ventricular systolic dysfunction or diastolic dysfunction, although both abnormalities are often present together. Right ventricular dysfunction may accompany left ventricular dysfunction or may be the primary problem. Systolic heart failure results from inability of the heart to expel blood normally owing to depressed left ventricular contraction. The left ventricle is often dilated. There is loss of myocytes and fibrosis, resulting in reduced left ventricular ejection fraction. Diastolic heart failure is caused by a reduction in left ventricular compliance, which leads to impaired diastolic filling, higher left ventricular diastolic pressure, and elevated pulmonary capillary wedge pressure (PCWP). Diastolic heart failure is also called heart failure with preserved ejection fraction (HFpEF) or heart failure with normal ejection fraction (HFnEF) (Fig. 29.2A and B).

Numerous conditions may cause damage to left ventricular myocardium and result in systolic heart failure. The most common of these conditions is atherosclerotic coronary artery disease with myocardial infarction and chronic

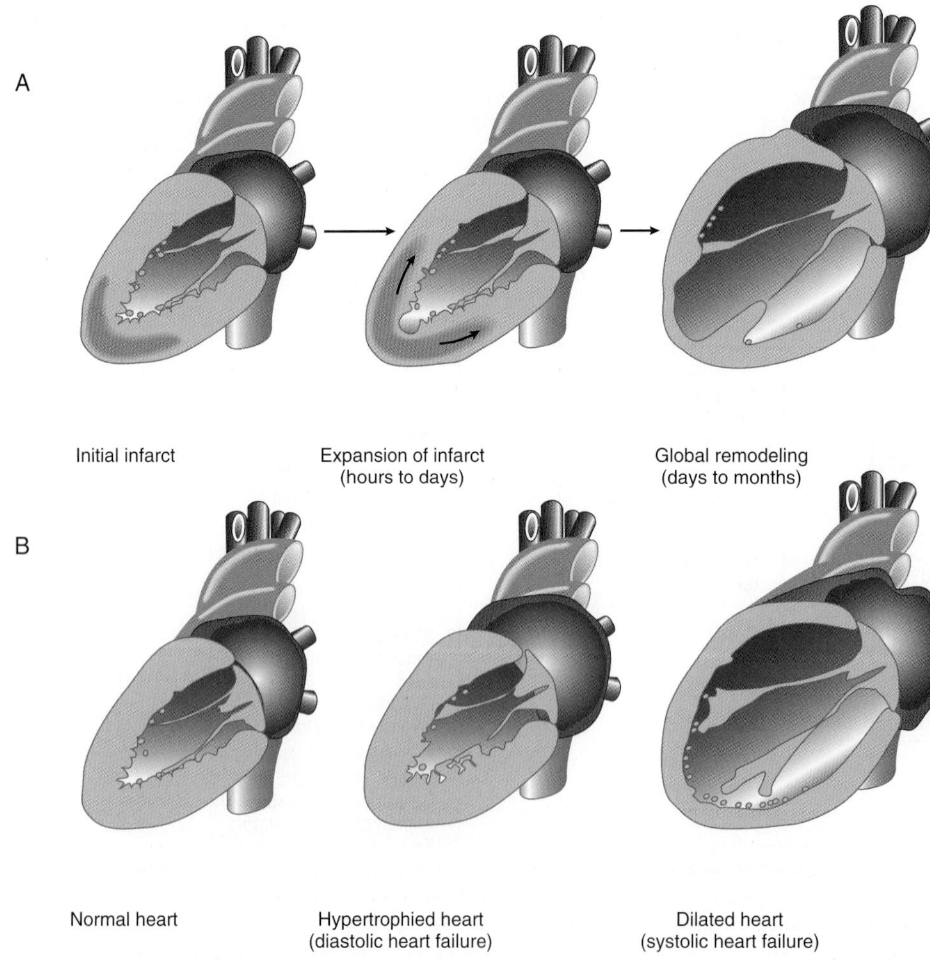

Figure 29.2 **A,** Left ventricle (LV) remodeling after acute myocardial infarction, resulting in a dilated LV with global systolic dysfunction. **B,** Ventricular remodeling in diastolic and systolic heart failure. Note differences in LV morphology in diastolic versus systolic heart failure. (Redrawn from Jessup M, Brozena S: Heart failure. N Engl J Med 2003;348:2007-2018.)

myocardial ischemia. Other common causes include hypertension; familial and idiopathic cardiomyopathy; viral myocarditis; valvular heart disease, such as aortic stenosis, aortic insufficiency, and mitral regurgitation; peripartum cardiomyopathy; transient apical ballooning syndrome (takotsubo cardiomyopathy); and cardiomyopathy due to cardiotoxic cancer chemotherapy. Less common causes are alcoholic cardiomyopathy, diabetic cardiomyopathy, and a cardiomyopathy seen in some patients with hyperthyroidism or severe obesity.[9-11]

After myocardial damage and loss of myocytes occur, a process known as ventricular *remodeling* is initiated. This remodeling results in dilation of the ventricular chamber, a change in ventricular geometry from ellipsoid-like to a more spherical shape, worsening of left ventricular contractile force, and reduction in ventricular ejection fraction.[3,12] In addition, the change in left ventricular geometry often leads to an increase in the size of the mitral annulus and altered physical relationships of the mitral valve structures. This results in increasing mitral regurgitation and worsening of the heart failure syndrome (see Fig. 29.2).

Remodeling is mediated by a series of maladaptive systemic responses, commonly termed *neurohormonal activation*. Two major systems involved in neurohormonal activation are the renin-angiotensin-aldosterone system and the sympathetic nervous system. Activation of the renin-angiotensin-aldosterone system leads to elevated levels of renin, angiotensin II, and aldosterone, which has deleterious consequences on cardiac function and hemodynamics.[3,12] These effects include salt and fluid retention, endothelial dysfunction, vasoconstriction, myocyte hypertrophy, myocardial fibrosis, and myocyte apoptosis (programmed cell death). Sympathetic nervous system activation is in part mediated via decreased cardiac output, which results in tachycardia, increased myocardial oxygen consumption, and peripheral vasoconstriction.[13] Renal effects of sympathetic nervous system activation lead to further activation of the renin-angiotensin-aldosterone system. Increased circulating norepinephrine levels also contribute to myocyte injury and death. Arrhythmias become common. A detrimental positive feedback loop is established, causing progressive deterioration in left ventricular structure and performance over time with progressive worsening of chronic heart failure.

Conditions commonly associated with diastolic heart failure include hypertension, left ventricular hypertrophy, and acute coronary ischemia. Diastolic heart failure is common in elderly populations, especially in women, likely due to progressive diastolic compliance abnormalities seen with aging. Uncommon conditions leading to diastolic heart failure include infiltrative and restrictive cardiomyopathies, such as amyloid cardiomyopathy, and chronic constrictive pericarditis.

DIAGNOSIS

Heart failure is a clinical diagnosis, determined after evaluation of a patient's symptoms and physical examination and supported by results of ancillary testing, such as chest x-ray and echocardiography. Typical symptoms of heart failure include shortness of breath at rest or with exertion, cough, swelling, orthopnea, and paroxysmal nocturnal dyspnea, which are due to pulmonary or systemic venous congestion. Fatigue, anorexia, and change in mental status are symptoms that may be caused by low cardiac output. Physical examination often reveals pulmonary rales; elevated jugular venous pressure; signs of cardiomegaly; cardiac murmurs, especially mitral regurgitation and third heart sound (S_3) gallop; hepatic enlargement; and ascites and edema. An S_3 gallop and elevated jugular venous pressure are the most specific signs of heart failure; absence of rales is not infrequent in patients with acute heart failure, and chest radiograph may not show obvious congestion.[14] Manifestations of more severe heart failure include marked dyspnea at rest, possibly resulting in respiratory failure, cyanosis, cool extremities, reduced urine output and altered mental state. A careful evaluation for the presence of pulsus paradoxus is important if cardiac tamponade is suspected. However, these signs and symptoms are not specific for heart failure, and coexisting conditions such as obesity, chronic lung disease, and deconditioning can add uncertainty to the clinical diagnosis. Heart failure is often both underdiagnosed and overdiagnosed in outpatient and emergency department settings.

Studies have shown that serum assays of B-natriuretic peptide (BNP) and N-terminal pro-BNP are very helpful in improving the accuracy of diagnosing heart failure. BNP is a 32–amino acid peptide produced by cardiac myocytes in response to pressure-induced wall stretch and tension.[15] Physiologic actions of BNP include arterial and venous dilation and natriuresis. A study of 1530 patients presenting to the emergency department with dyspnea showed that knowledge of BNP serum levels resulted in improved accuracy of the diagnosis of heart failure when compared to clinical judgment alone, from an initial range of 65% to 74%, up to 81% accuracy.[16] BNP levels above 100 pg/mL had a sensitivity of 90% and a specificity of 76% for the diagnosis of heart failure and were very useful for discriminating patients with dyspnea due to uncomplicated lung disease who had BNP values below 100 pg/mL.[17] Patients with BNP values below 100 pg/mL were very unlikely to have heart failure as the cause of dyspnea. Levels between 100 and 400 pg/mL can be seen in dyspneic patients with cor pulmonale, pulmonary hypertension not due to left ventricular failure, and acute pulmonary embolism. Heart failure is the likely diagnosis when levels are above 400 pg/mL. It should be emphasized that BNP levels should always be used in conjunction with all other clinical data to arrive at the correct diagnosis.

Evaluating BNP levels in heart failure patients in the emergency department was shown to decrease the need for hospitalization and decrease the need for intensive care unit (ICU) admissions, without affecting 30-day mortality rates.[18] Total hospital stay was shortened by 3 days, cost of treatment was significantly reduced, and time to initiation of definitive therapy in the emergency department was shortened by 30 minutes.

BNP levels correlate with disease severity, as values are higher in patients with more severe heart failure and with worse left ventricular systolic function. Higher levels also have been correlated with a poorer prognosis, and can predict an increased rate of functional deterioration and a higher mortality rate.[19] In a study of 114 patients admitted to the hospital with class IV heart failure, of all variables evaluated, predischarge BNP level was most strongly associated with death or readmission within 6 months, with BNP levels greater than 350 pg/mL having impressive sensitivity and specificity.[20] BNP levels may also be elevated in patients with diastolic heart failure, those with renal failure, and stable patients with chronic left ventricular systolic dysfunction with compensated heart failure. BNP levels may initially be low in patients with "flash" pulmonary edema, as they may present to the hospital more quickly than the time required for significant rises in serum BNP to occur.

Serum levels of N-terminal (NT) pro-BNP can also be used for the diagnosis of heart failure. A precursor hormone, pro-BNP, is cleaved to form BNP and NTpro-BNP, which is physiologically inactive. NTpro-BNP has a longer half-life than BNP. It is cleared from the serum by the kidneys, so levels are higher in patients with coexisting renal disease. Levels of NTpro-BNP rise significantly in older populations. A cut off level of NTpro-BNP below 300 pg/mL yielded a negative predictive value of 98% for exclusion of the diagnosis of heart failure.[21,22] The diagnosis of heart failure is very likely at levels over 450 pg/mL for patients under age 50, above 900 pg/mL in patients between 50 and 75 years old, and above 1800 pg/mL in patients over the age of 75.

PROGNOSIS IN ACUTE HEART FAILURE

Hospitalization for acute heart failure is associated with a poor prognosis. In-hospital mortality rate is high, reported at 4% to 8%. There is a 9% mortality rate at 60 to 90 days, and a 1-year mortality rate of 29%.[1,6,7,23-25] The 90-day rehospitalization rate is around 30%, although only half of these rehospitalizations are caused by heart failure. In a European heart failure database, in-hospital mortality rate was 6.9%, 12-week readmission rate was 24%, and total mortality rate at 12 weeks was 13.5%.[8] Randomized trials of pharmacologic therapy reported an annual mortality rate of 10% in patients with class II-III symptoms and 20% to 50% in class IV patients. In the most severe chronic heart failure group, patients awaiting cardiac transplantation, 1-year mortality rate was 75% with 2-year mortality rate of 92%.[26] More recent data indicate a decline in the risk-adjusted inpatient mortality rate, from 5.5% in 2000 to 2.8% in 2007. Similar reductions were seen in both sexes and across all age groups.[27] The prognosis for patients with cardiogenic shock due to acute myocardial infarction continues to be poor. Mortality rate remains 40% to 50% even with aggressive supportive therapy and emergency revascularization strategies.[28]

Several clinical factors have been shown to identify patients with a poorer prognosis and include lower left ventricular ejection fraction, low blood pressure on admission, and higher PCWP. In the United States ADHERE database registry of 62,275 admissions for heart failure, blood urea nitrogen (BUN) greater than 43 mg/dL, admission systolic blood pressure under 115 mm Hg, and creatinine level greater than 2.75 mg/dL were the three factors that indicated a poor prognosis for patients admitted with acute heart failure. The presence of an elevated BUN was associated with a fourfold increase in hospital mortality rates to 8.35%. The presence of all three factors yielded an in-hospital mortality rate of 19.8%[24] (Box 29.1).

Box 29.1 Factors Indicating a Poor Prognosis in Acute Heart Failure

- Hypotension (systolic blood pressure <115 mm Hg on admission)
- Presence of coronary artery disease
- Elevated blood urea nitrogen and serum creatinine
- Hyponatremia
- Low left ventricular ejection fraction
- Poor functional capacity
- Elevated serum biomarkers—B-natriuretic peptide, troponin
- Anemia
- Diabetes mellitus

Adapted from Nieminen MS, Bohm M, Cowie MR, et al: Executive summary of the guidelines on the diagnosis and treatment of acute heart failure. The Task Force on Acute Heart Failure of the European Society of Cardiology. Eur Heart J 2005;26:384-416.

Other factors associated with increased mortality rates include hyponatremia, higher serum BNP level, and elevation of serum troponin.[6,29,30] In ADHERE, higher levels of serum BNP on admission were associated with a higher in-hospital mortality rate, ranging from 1.9% in the lowest quartile to 6.0% in the highest quartile (BNP over 1730 pg/mL). The ability of BNP to predict prognosis was present even after multivariate adjustment for coexisting conditions, and was also true for patients with normal and abnormal left ventricular ejection fraction.[31] Serum troponin is elevated in 6% to 10.4% of patients admitted with acute heart failure (with serum creatinine <2.0 mg/dL). Troponin elevation was associated with a lower blood pressure, lower ejection fraction, and longer hospital length of stay. Hypothetical mechanisms of troponin release in chronic heart failure include ischemia, cytokine activation, oxidative stress, and apoptosis. Hospital mortality rate was 8.0% in troponin-positive patients and 2.7% if troponin-negative. The ability of troponin elevation to predict mortality rate also was independent of other variables and was true even in patients with nonischemic causes of heart failure.[32]

The coexistence of kidney disease significantly worsens the prognosis of patients with heart failure. Kidney disease aggravates the tendency to volume overload and heart failure decompensation, and heart failure often worsens renal function. This complex interaction of severe heart failure and worsening kidney function is called the *cardiorenal syndrome*. In addition, high-dose diuretic therapy may also temporarily worsen renal function. There is increasing evidence that elevated systemic venous pressure causing renal venous congestion plays an important role in the pathogenesis.[33] In a retrospective study of patients with acute heart failure who had right-sided heart catheterization, elevated central venous pressure was associated with reduced glomerular filtration rate (GFR) and higher all-cause mortality rate. These findings were independent of the measured cardiac output.[34] Up to 50% of patients hospitalized with heart failure demonstrate a GFR less than

60 mL/minute/m^2, and renal function may worsen in up to 30% of patients admitted with heart failure.[35] Patients at particular risk for developing worsening renal function are those with lower left ventricular ejection fractions, lower blood pressure, diabetes mellitus, a history of hypertension, and older age. These patients have longer hospital stays and higher readmission and mortality rates. A meta-analysis of 16 large studies of heart failure patients revealed that 29% of heart failure patients had moderate to severe impairment of renal function. These patients had more than 100% increased relative mortality risk. Any degree of renal impairment had an approximately 50% increased relative mortality risk.[36] The best treatment strategy for these patients is not clear, as patients with significant renal impairment have generally been excluded from large randomized pharmacologic heart failure trials.

ACUTE HEART FAILURE SYNDROMES

INITIAL EVALUATION AND THERAPY

Acute heart failure is defined as the rapid onset of severe symptoms of heart failure, usually within hours to several days. Acute heart failure can occur with predominant systolic or diastolic dysfunction. Acute heart failure is often life-threatening and requires urgent diagnostic and therapeutic interventions, often simultaneously.[23] Acute myocardial ischemia is a common cause and should always be considered in the differential diagnosis of this syndrome.

Several distinct clinical syndromes of acute heart failure can be identified[23] (Table 29.1).

1. Acute worsening or decompensation of chronic heart failure symptoms, either in the setting of known chronic cardiovascular illness or de novo. These patients do not have shock or pulmonary edema. This is the most common presentation of acute heart failure requiring admission to hospital, occurring in approximately 70% of patients with acute heart failure.
2. Acute pulmonary edema with normal blood pressure, often caused by acute myocardial infarction or acute coronary ischemia.
3. Acute pulmonary edema associated with elevated blood pressure, often in the setting of chronic severe hypertension and chronic kidney disease. Pulmonary edema accounts for roughly 25% of acute heart failure admissions.
4. Cardiogenic shock with heart failure, usually due to acute myocardial infarction. This syndrome is the most severe presentation of acute heart failure and is associated with high in-hospital mortality rates. This accounts for about 5% of acute heart failure cases.
5. "High cardiac output heart failure" often induced by sepsis, hyperthyroidism, or cardiac arrhythmia. This type is the least common presentation, occurring in a small percentage of patients.

Table 29.1 Acute Heart Failure Syndromes

Syndrome	Onset	Signs and Symptoms	Hemodynamics
Acute decompensated heart failure	Days weeks	Weakness Dyspnea Rales Third heart sound (S_3) gallop Edema	↑ PCWP ↓ CI Normal or ↑ RAP ↑ SVR
Acute pulmonary edema, normal BP	Abrupt-days	Severe dyspnea Diffuse rales Cyanosis S_3 gallop	↑↑ PCWP Normal or ↓ CI Normal RA Normal or ↑ SVR
Acute pulmonary edema with hypertension	Acute	Severe dyspnea Diffuse rales	↑↑ PCWP Normal CI Normal RAP ↑↑ SVR
Cardiogenic shock	Acute	Hypotension Cyanosis Lethargy Cool, clammy	↑↑ PCWP ↑ RAP ↓↓ CI ↑ SVR
High-output heart failure	Days-weeks	Dyspnea Rales	↑ PCWP ↑ CI ↓ SVR
RV failure	Days-weeks	Hypotension Edema Ascites	Normal or ↑PCWP ↑↑ RAP ↓↓ CI

BP, blood pressure; CI, cardiac index; PCWP, pulmonary capillary wedge pressure; RAP, right atrial pressure; RV, right ventricular; SVR, systemic vascular resistance; ↑, increased; ↑↑, markedly increased; ↓, reduced; ↓↓, markedly reduced.

Adapted from Nieminen MS, Bohm M, Cowie MR, et al: Executive summary of the guidelines on the diagnosis and treatment of acute heart failure. The Task Force on Acute Heart Failure of the European Society of Cardiology. Eur Heart J 2005;26:384-416; and Gheorghiade M, Zannad F, Sopko G: Acute heart failure syndromes. Circulation 2005;112:3958-3968.

6. Acute right ventricular failure, occurring with acute right ventricular myocardial infarction, massive pulmonary embolism, or cardiac tamponade.

Symptoms of acute heart failure are similar to those of chronic heart failure but are more severe. Symptoms of tissue hypoperfusion, such as fatigue, weakness, confusion, nausea, and anorexia, may be subtle but are important to recognize as they may herald impending cardiogenic shock. Chest pain may indicate acute coronary ischemia.

Physical examination often shows pulmonary rales and wheezes, an S_3 gallop, and elevation of jugular venous pressure. Peripheral pulses are weak and thready with diminished cardiac output states. A low cardiac output is reliably predicted by a low "proportional pulse pressure," which is calculated by the pulse pressure (systolic blood pressure minus diastolic blood pressure) divided by systolic blood pressure. A ratio below 0.25 predicts a cardiac index below 2.2 L/minute/m^2.[37,38] The skin may be cool and clammy and there may be evidence of cyanosis. Peripheral edema and ascites may indicate concomitant right ventricular failure of longer duration. Chest radiography is done urgently. An electrocardiogram (ECG) is needed to assess for signs of ischemia and infarction, and to evaluate for arrhythmia. Cardiac rhythm needs to be monitored continuously. Laboratory examination includes evaluation of hemoglobin and hematocrit, electrolytes, renal and liver function, thyroid profile, and cardiac biomarkers (troponin I or troponin T) to look for evidence of myocardial necrosis. BNP level assists in the diagnosis of heart failure in patients presenting with dyspnea, and can be followed serially to assess effectiveness of therapy. Pulse oximetry helps to assess oxygenation and pulmonary function. An arterial line is helpful in managing patients with hypotension or cardiogenic shock. Urgent two-dimensional echocardiography is essential to evaluate left ventricular size and function, right ventricular function, valve function, and the presence of pericardial effusion. Doppler echocardiographic assessment of valve stenosis and regurgitation and of hemodynamics is invaluable.

When patients are admitted to hospital with acute decompensation of chronic systolic heart failure, the specific reason for a patient's deterioration must be searched for and corrected when possible (Box 29.2). Environmental factors such as excessive salt and fluid intake or alcohol consumption are common. Patient adherence to outpatient therapies must be assessed, as heart failure regimens often involve numerous medications. Emotional and physical stressors should be corrected when feasible.

Concomitant administration of medications for noncardiac conditions can have detrimental effects. A partial listing includes corticosteroids and nonsteroidal anti-inflammatory drugs (NSAIDs). These drugs can cause fluid retention and can aggravate hypertension. NSAIDs also interfere with the beneficial renal effects of angiotensin-converting enzyme (ACE) inhibitors and can interfere with the action of loop diuretics.[39] The use of NSAIDs has been reported to increase the risk of hospitalization for heart failure by tenfold in patients with a history of heart failure.[8] Metformin and thiazolindinediones can contribute to water retention and aggravate the symptoms and signs of heart failure. Cancer chemotherapies can cause myocardial damage. Cardiac toxicity due to anthracycline chemotherapy is well described. Tyrosine-kinase inhibitors, a newer class of cancer chemotherapy, are also being recognized as agents that can aggravate heart failure and cardiomyopathy.[40] Cardiac medications such as calcium channel blockers and antiarrhythmic drugs can also have direct negative effects on left ventricular contractility. Calcium channel blockers are generally contraindicated in patients admitted with acute decompensated heart failure.[23] Type 1A and 1C antiarrhythmic drugs are also contraindicated in patients with abnormal left ventricular systolic function.

Acute and chronic extracardiac conditions may also cause heart failure decompensation. Pulmonary embolus, infectious illnesses, and sepsis occur commonly. Anemia, blood loss, and thyroid disease need to be assessed and corrected. Renal failure often has etiologic factors similar to those of heart failure (e.g., hypertension, vascular disease), and worsening renal function will often aggravate heart failure. Obstructive sleep apnea can lead to exacerbation of heart failure symptoms and can be effectively treated. Influenza and pneumococcal vaccines should be administered to patients to prevent the cardiac decompensation associated with respiratory infections.

Lastly, coexistent cardiovascular illness can aggravate heart failure. Acute or chronic coronary ischemia should always be suspected, evaluated, and corrected with revascularization strategies when appropriate. Uncontrolled

Box 29.2 Causes of Acutely Decompensated Heart Failure

Environmental Causes

Excess salt and fluid intake
Excess alcohol consumption
Medication noncompliance or misunderstanding
Emotional or physical stress

Adverse Medication Effects

Calcium channel blockers
Antiarrhythmic agents (types 1A, 1C)
Nonsteroidal anti-inflammatory drugs (NSAIDs)
Corticosteroids
Metformin, thiazolidinediones
Cancer chemotherapy

Cardiovascular Conditions

Acute ischemia/infarction
Pulmonary embolism
Uncontrolled hypertension
Arrhythmia
Worsening valvular regurgitation
Endocarditis

Extracardiac Illness

Sepsis, infection, hypoxia
Renal failure, urinary obstruction
Thyroid disease
Anemia, blood loss
Obstructive sleep apnea
Bilateral renal artery stenosis
Worsening of chronic lung disease

hypertension and cardiac arrhythmias (most commonly atrial fibrillation and ventricular arrhythmias) frequently accompany left ventricular dysfunction. Worsening valve regurgitation, endocarditis, and bilateral renal artery stenosis are other examples of conditions that can lead to heart failure exacerbations that are treatable.

There are few controlled-trial data to arrive at evidence-based guidelines for the treatment of acute heart failure. Many recommendations are based on small studies, experience, observation, and a general consensus of opinion.[41] The goals of initial therapy are to improve symptoms, optimize blood pressure, lower PCWP, and improve cardiac output. Treatments to reverse or prevent myocardial injury are instituted, and a search for reversible causes of heart failure needs to occur. Optimization of other comorbid conditions is important, including hyperglycemia, renal disease, and pulmonary function.

Initial therapy includes supplemental oxygen and assessment of the need for ventilatory assistance with noninvasive positive airway pressure ventilation or endotracheal intubation. Noninvasive ventilation improves oxygenation and pulmonary compliance and decreases work of breathing. Endotracheal intubation may be required for patients with severe hypercapnia, acidosis, and respiratory muscle fatigue. The use of continuous oxygen administration alone was prospectively compared with the use of continuous positive airway pressure ventilation (CPAP) and noninvasive intermittent positive pressure ventilation (NIPPV) in 1069 patients who presented with acute cardiogenic pulmonary edema. No difference among these therapies was noted in the primary end point of death at 7 days, or in the secondary end point of death plus endotracheal intubation at 7 days. Noninvasive ventilation did result in more rapid improvement in dyspnea, tachycardia, hypercapnia, and acidosis. There was no difference in safety or efficacy between CPAP and NIPPV.[42]

Initial medical therapy includes intravenous morphine, which acts as a vasodilator and often reduces heart rate. Intravenous loop diuretics, such as furosemide, offer rapid and effective symptom relief and are almost always prescribed. Intravenous vasodilators are very useful, especially in patients with severe hypertension; intravenous nitroglycerin and intravenous nitroprusside are used most commonly. Beta blockers should be given early to patients with heart failure and ischemic chest pain, hypertension, or tachyarrhythmias. They should be used with caution in patients with severe heart failure and should be withheld initially in the presence of hypotension, shock, bradycardia, or heart block. Calcium channel blocking agents are generally contraindicated in the acute setting.

Treatment of arrhythmias is essential. Rapid atrial fibrillation is a common problem in these patients. In the Euroheart Failure Study, 9% of patients hospitalized with acute heart failure had atrial fibrillation during the hospitalization, and 42% had a history of paroxysmal atrial fibrillation.[43] Other studies report atrial fibrillation in 25% to 30% of hospitalized heart failure patients.[36] Control of the ventricular response to atrial fibrillation is vitally important, especially in patients with diastolic heart failure. This control can be achieved rapidly with the use of intravenous beta blockers such as metoprolol or esmolol, parenteral digoxin, or intravenous amiodarone. Intravenous diltiazem can be used in patients whose left ventricular systolic function is known to be normal or near normal.

INDICATIONS FOR INVASIVE HEMODYNAMIC MONITORING

Placement of a pulmonary artery (PA) catheter enables the clinician to accurately measure PCWP, cardiac output, and mixed venous oxygen saturation. It can also help assess the effectiveness of therapy. Whether to *routinely* use PA catheters to assess and manage patients with acute heart failure has been long debated. The ESCAPE trial evaluated the routine use of PA catheterization in patients hospitalized with acute exacerbation of chronic heart failure and left ventricular systolic dysfunction.[44] There was no difference in the primary end point of days alive out of the hospital during 6 months after discharge in groups managed with or without a PA catheter. There were no significant adverse effects with PA catheter use in this study. There were no subgroups identified in which use of the PA catheter was beneficial. However, there was a trend noted in improving the initial diuresis, with less deterioration of renal function, in the PA catheter group. The authors concluded that there was no indication for the *routine* use of PA catheters in the setting of acute heart failure.

However, a PA catheter is often essential for the management of patients with acute severe heart failure. Findings on physical examination are often insensitive indicators of hemodynamic status. Indications for PA catheter use include cardiogenic shock, differentiating pulmonary from cardiac causes of dyspnea, hemodynamic assessment if one is unsure of the diagnosis or severity of heart failure by clinical assessment, worsening renal function, guiding parenteral vasodilator therapy, and in patients who are not improving with initially prescribed therapy.[37] PA catheter placement is also necessary as part of the evaluation for cardiac transplantation or the implantation of a ventricular assist device (VAD) (Box 29.3).

Consecutive patients with severe heart failure were evaluated and classified according to hemodynamic measurements of PCWP and cardiac index. Patients were described as "dry" with average PCWP less than 17 mm Hg, or "wet" with PCWP reading of 29 mm Hg on average. The patients were also described as "warm" versus "cold," based on a cardiac index of greater than 2.1 L/minute/m^2 versus an

Box 29.3 Indications for Invasive Hemodynamic Monitoring with a Pulmonary Artery Catheter in Acute Heart Failure

1. Cardiogenic shock
2. Cardiac or pulmonary cause of dyspnea not certain
3. Uncertainty regarding severity of heart failure
4. Worsening renal function during heart failure therapy
5. Guiding parenteral vasodilator therapy
6. Deteriorating heart failure status despite appropriate therapy
7. Evaluation prior to cardiac transplantation

index of less than 1.6 L/minute/m^2. The severity of symptoms and findings on physical examination did not predict the hemodynamic status as defined by invasive monitoring. In addition, the hemodynamic picture did not predict the response to therapy and survival was similar in all four groups, except that patients with higher cardiac output and lower PCWP had slightly better outcomes than patients with low cardiac output and high PCWP.[45]

Tailoring pharmacologic therapy to hemodynamic measurements is often helpful and necessary to determine precise measurements of cardiac output and left ventricular filling pressure, in order to guide intensive intravenous drug therapy. Aggressive therapy tailored to the response in hemodynamic measurements has been advocated as an effective method to obtain more rapid and sustained improvement in patients with the most severe heart failure.[46] When PCWP is reduced to less than 16 mm Hg, and right atrial pressure is reduced to less than 8 mm Hg, most patients will improve acutely and for the remainder of their hospitalization. Additional hemodynamic goals include reducing systemic vascular resistance to less than 1200 dynes × sec/cm^5, raising cardiac index to greater than 2.6 L/minute/m^2, and maintaining systolic blood pressure over 80 mm Hg. PCWP can be lowered to a normal value of 10 to 12 mm Hg in many patients with significant left ventricular dysfunction without untoward effects.[46,47] In a group of patients referred for cardiac transplantation, a combination of aggressive parenteral therapy, targeted to optimal hemodynamics, followed by conversion to appropriate oral therapy, resulted in clinical improvement so that 30% of these patients were able to be removed from transplant lists.[46]

Box 29.4 Goals of Therapy During Hospitalization for Acute Heart Failure

Clinical Changes

- Decreased dyspnea and orthopnea, improved exercise tolerance
- Improved pulmonary function and oxygenation
- Diuresis
- Decreased body fluid weight and edema
- Systolic blood pressure maintained >80 mm Hg

Laboratory Data

- Normalized serum electrolyte levels
- Optimized renal function
- Decreased serum B-natriuretic peptide levels

Hemodynamics

- Pulmonary capillary wedge pressure <16 to 18 mm Hg
- Right atrial pressure <8 mm Hg
- Normalized cardiac index

Improve Prognosis

- Treatment of ischemia
- Evidence-based pharmacologic therapy initiated
- Evaluation for use of device therapy (cardiac resynchronization therapy, implantable cardioverter defibrillator)

Adapted from Nieminen MS, Bohm M, Cowie MR, et al: Executive summary of the guidelines on the diagnosis and treatment of acute heart failure. The Task Force on Acute Heart Failure of the European Society of Cardiology. Eur Heart J 2005;26:384-416.

PHARMACOLOGIC MANAGEMENT OF ACUTE HEART FAILURE

Goals of treatment of heart failure can be defined as short-term, to relieve dyspnea and reverse acute hemodynamic decompensation, and long-term, to prevent rehospitalization, improve functional status, and prolong survival. Additional goals include preserving renal function, preventing arrhythmias, and preventing myocardial necrosis in patients with ischemic and nonischemic disease. Pharmacologic therapies to prevent or attenuate chronic remodeling should be instituted or strengthened prior to discharge from the hospital, as these have been shown to improve long-term survival (Box 29.4).

Pharmacologic treatment of heart failure is aimed at achieving these goals by improving fluid balance and reversing the neurohormonal activation responsible for the progressive decline in left ventricular function. Therapy usually involves combinations of multiple medications. Several drugs have been shown to improve symptoms and functional capacity, decrease the need for repeated hospitalizations, and improve mortality rates.

Careful serial assessment of patients is mandatory to guide pharmacologic therapy. Signs of heart failure on physical examination are important to follow, including daily weights, pulmonary rales, the presence of an S_3 gallop, jugular venous pressure, urine output, and pulse oximetry.

Table 29.2 Loop Diuretics Used for the Treatment of Acute, Severe Heart Failure

Agent	Oral Dose	Initial IV Dose (mg)	Maximum IV Bolus Dose (mg)
Bumetanide	0.5-1.0	1.0	4-8
Furosemide	20-40	40	160-200
Torsemide	10-20	10	100-200

IV, intravenous.

INTRAVENOUS DIURETICS

Although no randomized clinical trials exist, the use of loop diuretics is supported by a long history of clinical success. These agents increase renal excretion of salt and water. The onset of action of intravenous bolus furosemide is 30 minutes, and the drug peaks at 1 to 2 hours. The half-life of the medication is 6 hours, so twice daily dosing is usually required.[39] Other loop diuretics often used are bumetanide and torsemide (Tables 29.2 and 29.3). Several small clinical trials suggested that a constant infusion of a loop diuretic resulted in superior diuresis when compared to intermittent bolus dosing,[48,49] although other studies did not confirm this.[50] A large, randomized controlled study was performed

Table 29.3 Treatment of Refractory, Diuretic-Resistant Heart Failure

To Loop Diuretic, add:	Dose
Hydrochlorothiazide	25-50 mg once or twice daily
or metolazone	2.5-5.0 mg once or twice daily
or spironolactone	12.5-50 mg once daily

in patients hospitalized with acute decompensated heart failure who were taking a high dose of furosemide prior to admission. Patients were randomized within 24 hours of admission to bolus dosing or constant infusion, and usual daily outpatient dose (given intravenously) versus high dose (2.5 times their usual daily dose). No significant differences were noted in predefined outcomes between bolus and infusion administration. However, the high-dose group had better relief of dyspnea and more fluid and weight loss than the lower-dose group; also, 23% of the high-dose group had a significant deterioration in renal function, but at 60 days there was no difference in renal function between the two groups.[51]

An association between high-dose loop diuretics and a worse prognosis has been observed. There is concern that this may be mediated by further activation of the renin-angiotensin-aldosterone system by loop diuretics. However, in a retrospective analysis utilizing propensity matching, hospital mortality rate was not different between low-dose and high-dose diuretic groups.[52] It is likely that poorer outcomes associated with high-dose diuretics is not due to the drug itself but reflects a greater severity of heart failure illness with concomitant renal disease.[53]

Whatever initial dose of diuretic is chosen, subsequent dosing should be titrated to the response of the patient's fluid status and symptoms. Dosage reduction should be considered as the clinical status improves. Hypokalemia, alkalosis, and hypomagnesemia are frequent side effects of loop diuretics and can potentiate the occurrence of arrhythmias. Electrolyte levels must be carefully monitored during aggressive diuretic therapy.

Patients with chronic heart failure with or without renal dysfunction may exhibit resistance to loop diuretics, defined as an acute reduction in diuretic efficacy after repeated loop diuretic dosing. With chronic loop diuretic use, there is an increase in sodium reabsorption in the distal nephron and stimulation of aldosterone release. In edematous states there is delayed oral absorption of the drug. With renal dysfunction there may be reduced levels of drug delivered to the renal tubule. This resistance is associated with a poorer prognosis.[23] Diuretics that act distally in the renal tubule, such as metolazone or hydrochlorothiazide, or aldosterone blockers such as spironolactone can be added.[4] Combination diuretic therapy induces a greater diuresis than simply increasing the dose of loop diuretic further. The response may be delayed for 48 to 72 hours. Combining diuretics often augments diuresis even in the setting of significant chronic kidney disease, and a good response can be expected in over 70% of patients. Particular attention must be given to following potassium, sodium, chloride, and magnesium levels when combination diuretic therapy is prescribed[54] (Table 29.4).

Table 29.4 Continuous Intravenous (IV) Infusion of Loop Diuretics

Diuretic	Dose
Bumetanide	1 mg IV load, then 0.5-2 mg/hr infusion
Furosemide	40 mg IV load, then 10-40 mg/hr infusion
Torsemide	20 mg IV load, then 5-20 mg/hr infusion

Adapted from Nieminen MS, Bohm M, Cowie MR, et al: Executive summary of the guidelines on the diagnosis and treatment of acute heart failure. The Task Force on Acute Heart Failure of the European Society of Cardiology. Eur Heart J 2005;26:384-416.

VASOPRESSIN INHIBITORS

The use of novel diuretics, vasopressin inhibitors, has been evaluated in clinical trials of treatment of acute heart failure.[55] Vasopressin is a hormone synthesized in the hypothalamus; its major effect is to control free water clearance. It acts through V1a receptors in vascular smooth muscle and myocardium, leading to peripheral and coronary vasoconstriction, myocyte hypertrophy, and positive inotropy. Vasopressin also acts through V2 receptors at the renal tubule collecting ducts to cause free water retention and hyponatremia. Levels of vasopressin are increased in patients with chronic heart failure, and higher vasopressin levels correlate with worse heart failure severity. Vasopressin release is stimulated by changes in serum osmolality and cardiac output and leads to further vasoconstriction and retention of free water.[56] Inhibition of vasopressin's effects would have theoretic benefits in patients with heart failure.[57] In contrast to loop diuretics, inhibition of vasopressin theoretically would not cause hypotension or neurohormonal activation, and would not aggravate cardiac arrhythmias due to electrolyte depletion.

Conivaptan is a vasopressin antagonist that inhibits V1a and V2 receptors. Tolvaptan and lixivaptan are antagonists selective for the V2 receptor. These medications increase urine volume and free water excretion, with a rise in the serum sodium concentration. The use of conivaptan in patients with class III-IV heart failure was associated with increased urine output, and decreases in PCWP and right atrial pressure, without changes in cardiac output.[8] Oral use of tolvaptan was associated with fluid loss and diuresis without change in heart rate, blood pressure, or serum creatinine.

In a large, multicenter, placebo-controlled randomized trial called EVEREST, tolvaptan was administered to patients hospitalized with heart failure. There were no adverse consequences on heart rate, blood pressure, or serum electrolytes and there was more rapid improvement in dyspnea and signs of heart failure when compared to usual therapy.[58] Hyponatremia improved. Hemodynamic effects included rapid reduction in PCWP and right atrial pressure.[59] However, at 10-months follow-up after hospitalization, there was no improvement in mortality rates or readmission rates.[60] Vasopressin inhibitors are approved for treatment of severe hyponatremic states but are not approved for use in heart failure.

Table 29.5 Comparison of Hemodynamic Effects of Parenteral Vasodilators and Inotropic Agents

Hemodynamic Measure	Nitroprusside	Nesiritide	Dobutamine	Milrinone
Mechanism of action	Balanced vasodilator	Vasodilator, natriuretic	β_1-Adrenergic receptor stimulator	Phosphodiesterase inhibitor
Heart rate	–	–	Slight ↑	Slight ↑
Arrhythmia	–	–	+	+
Mean right atrial pressure	↓	↓	↓	↓↓
Left ventricular end-diastolic pressure	↓↓	↓↓	↓	↓↓
Mean arterial pressure	↓	↓	–	↓
Systemic vascular resistance	↓↓	↓↓	↓	↓↓
Cardiac index	↑	↑	↑↑	↑↑
dP/dt (inotropy)	–	–	↑↑	↑
Hypotension	+	+	Occasionally	+
Direct Na^+ excretion	–	+	–	–
Other considerations	Increased cyanide and thiocyanate levels with prolonged infusion	Serum B-natriuretic peptide level cannot be followed during infusion	Difficult to use in patients receiving long-term beta-blocker therapy	More vasodilator response at higher doses

–, minimal or no effect; +, positive effect; ↑ or ↓, mild increase or decrease, respectively; ↑↑ or ↓↓, moderate increase or decrease, respectively.

PARENTERAL VASODILATORS (TABLE 29.5)

Intravenous vasodilator therapy is often added to diuretic therapy to obtain more rapid improvement in severe heart failure. A clear indication for vasodilators is in patients with severe hypertension and pulmonary edema. Their use should also be considered in patients who are not responding to intravenous diuretics combined with standard oral therapies. Blood pressure response to these medications needs to be carefully monitored because hypotension is a common effect. Improvement in hemodynamics has been obtained with aggressive intravenous vasodilator therapy using intravenous nitroprusside, intravenous nitroglycerin, or nesiritide. The choice of agents depends on matching the patient's clinical picture and hemodynamics with the predicted effects of each vasodilator.[61,62]

NITROGLYCERIN

Intravenous nitroglycerin is an effective systemic and coronary vasodilator. It is very useful in heart failure due to acute coronary ischemia, as it improves coronary blood flow. Intravenous nitroglycerin lowers preload and PCWP, thereby reducing pulmonary congestion, without increasing oxygen demand. It is also an arterial dilator at high doses but is less effective at reducing afterload than nitroprusside. Dosage ranges between 5 and 200 μg/minute. A major limitation of the use of intravenous nitroglycerin is the rapid development of tolerance to the drug's effect, often occurring after only 24 hours of therapy. Prescribing a "nitrate-free" period during the daily dosage regimen has been advocated to limit the development of tolerance, but this option is not feasible in patients receiving parenteral therapy. Oral or topical nitrates may be added to chronic heart failure therapy with beta blockers and ACE inhibitors if blood pressure allows, but nitrates have not been shown to improve long-term prognosis.

NITROPRUSSIDE

Intravenous sodium nitroprusside is a powerful venous and arterial dilator. It is a drug of choice in treating hypertension-related heart failure with pulmonary edema and severe heart failure due to acute mitral regurgitation. The use of nitroprusside requires hospitalization in the ICU and invasive monitoring with a PA catheter and arterial line. This drug causes a significant reduction of afterload and preload, leading to decreased right atrial pressure, decreased systemic vascular resistance, decreased mean systemic blood pressure, decreased PCWP, and increased cardiac index in patients with heart failure and left ventricular dysfunction. Limitations of nitroprusside use include inducing a coronary "steal" syndrome in patients with active coronary ischemia.[39] In addition, toxic metabolites can accumulate with more prolonged administration. In patients with significant hepatic dysfunction, thiocyanate levels rise, and in patients with renal dysfunction, cyanide is generated. Dosage range is 0.3 to 5.0 μg/kg/minute.

NESIRITIDE (B-NATRIURETIC PEPTIDE)

Human BNP can be manufactured by recombinant DNA technology and is available as an intravenous medication, nesiritide, for heart failure therapy. BNP is a hormone produced by ventricular and atrial myocytes in response to stretch from cardiac chamber dilatation. Hemodynamic effects include venous and arterial dilation, coronary vasodilation, and natriuresis. Reduction in PCWP and right atrial pressure exceeding the effects of intravenous nitroglycerin, when compared directly, was reported.[61] It is not proarrhythmic and does not induce tolerance.[63] It may potentiate the effects of loop diuretics. Significant hypotension may limit its use in some patients.[39] Because the hypotensive effects of nesiritide are less marked than nitroprusside, nesiritide can be used without invasive hemodynamic monitoring and can be initiated in emergency department settings. Nesiritide is initiated as an intravenous bolus dose of 2 μg/kg followed by infusion of 0.01 μg/kg/minute.

Nesiritide was compared to dobutamine in patients with severe heart failure. Nesiritide infusion was associated with less tachycardia and ventricular arrhythmia.[64] Other nonrandomized studies suggested a trend toward improved survival and lower rehospitalization rates with nesiritide.[63] A meta-analysis of three randomized trials of nesiritide suggested a slight increase in mortality rates in patients given nesiritide versus a placebo control group, possibly mediated through an adverse effect on renal function.[65,66] A retrospective review of patients receiving intravenous vasoactive medications for acute heart failure indicated mortality rates, adjusted for clinical variables, were equivalent for patients receiving nitroglycerin or nesiritide. Patients who received intravenous nesiritide or intravenous nitroglycerin had a lower in-hospital mortality rate compared with patients who received dobutamine or milrinone.[67]

In view of these conflicting results of retrospective analyses, a randomized, placebo-controlled international study, called ASCEND-HF, was performed to evaluate the effect of nesiritide on relief of dyspnea, mortality rate, and renal function in patients hospitalized with acute heart failure; 7141 patients were enrolled. Over 90% of patients received loop diuretics and 15% received vasodilator therapy. Patients who received nesiritide had slightly better relief of dyspnea at 6 and 24 hours, although this did not meet a prespecified significant improvement in dyspnea score. There was no significant difference in hospital mortality rates, 30-day mortality rate, or death or rehospitalization at 30 days. There was no significant worsening of renal function in the nesiritide group. Hypotension was significantly more common in the nesiritide goup (26.6%) compared with control group (15.3%). The authors concluded that nesiritide was not useful for routine use in the management of patients with severe heart failure.[68]

Nesiritide should be used only in patients admitted to hospital with acute decompensated heart failure, to relieve dyspnea at rest when more conventional therapies have proved to be ineffective. This medication should not be used to replace diuretics, to enhance renal function, or to improve diuresis. It should not be used as an intermittent infusion in an outpatient setting.

ANGIOTENSIN-CONVERTING ENZYME INHIBITORS

ACE inhibitors are of limited use as parenteral therapy in patients with acute severe heart failure in the urgent setting. Enalaprilat is an intravenous bolus formulation that can be used in patients with chronic heart failure who are taking chronic oral ACE inhibitor therapy and who are unable to take oral medication. The maximal action occurs 1 to 4 hours after administration, with a 6-hour duration of action.

INOTROPIC DRUGS (SEE TABLE 29.5)

DOBUTAMINE

Dobutamine is a potent β_1-agonist. It also has β_2- and α-agonist properties. Its major effects are increased myocardial contractility and increased cardiac output. It increases myocardial oxygen demand. It also has venodilator properties. At doses of 2.5 to 15 μg/kg/minute, dobutamine will lower systemic vascular resistance and PCWP and cause a slight increase in heart rate. Higher doses are associated with vasoconstriction.

In patients with heart failure, β-receptors may be chronically downregulated. Therefore, the effects of dobutamine may be attenuated in chronic heart failure patients. Dobutamine may be detrimental in patients with active coronary ischemia or following myocardial infarction due to increased myocardial oxygen demand and oxygen consumption. Ventricular arrhythmias are associated with dobutamine use.[64] Tolerance to the effects of dobutamine has been demonstrated in patients with infusions lasting more than 24 hours, due theoretically to induction of β-receptor downregulation.[69]

MILRINONE

Milrinone is an inhibitor of myocyte phosphodiesterase. This leads to increased intracellular cyclic adenosine monophosphate and calcium. It is an inotropic agent that acts "downstream" from the β-receptor. Hemodynamic effects include reduction of right atrial pressure and reduction in pulmonary and systemic vascular resistance. In heart failure, stroke volume and cardiac output are increased with a slight fall in mean systemic arterial pressure. Milrinone acts as a coronary vasodilator, and there is no net increase in myocardial oxygen consumption. Arterial blood pressure and PCWP tend to be lowered more than with dobutamine, and milrinone's action is more prolonged. There is no tolerance or attenuation of its effect. Milrinone is started as a bolus dose 50 to 75 μg/kg, with a maintenance infusion of 0.375 to 0.75 μg/kg/minute. Doses need to be reduced in patients with renal failure. Its use is limited in patients with hypotension.

CONSIDERATIONS REGARDING THE USE OF INOTROPES

Inotropic drugs are used in patients with reduced LV systolic function and low cardiac output with persistent symptomatic hypotension and signs of end-organ hypoperfusion or cardiogenic shock. Clinically, this is often manifest as systolic blood pressure less than 90 mm Hg, narrow pulse pressure, cool and clammy extremities, anorexia, obtundation, and oliguria. Hemodynamic findings that may lead to use of inotropes include cardiac index less than 2.0 L/minute/m^2, PCWP greater than 20 mm Hg, and right atrial pressure greater than 10 mm Hg.[70]

The choice of milrinone versus dobutamine depends on the specific clinical circumstances.[71] Dobutamine tends to cause a slight rise in heart rate and has little effect on mean arterial pressure, whereas milrinone often lowers systemic arterial pressure due to more prominent lowering of systemic vascular resistance.[72,73] Patients who do not respond to dobutamine may have a favorable response to milrinone. In the setting of acute heart failure, milrinone is used more often then dobutamine in view of its more potent vasodilator properties. In addition, its effects are not primarily mediated through β-receptors, which is an important consideration in patients receiving concomitant beta-blocker therapy. However, dobutamine has a much shorter half-life than milrinone, so dobutamine-induced hypotension can be more rapidly reversed by discontinuing the drug, making dobutamine a somewhat safer drug in the acute setting. Several studies have been done evaluating the usefulness of routine inotropic therapy, comparing milrinone or dobutamine with placebo. The consistent conclusion has been that inotropic agents are not useful for routine use in patients with decompensated heart failure, and in fact may worsen short-term prognosis. The use of a 48-hour infusion of milrinone was evaluated as routine therapy in patients admitted with class III-IV heart failure, when inotropic therapy was not felt to be essential. When compared to standard therapy without milrinone, no improvement in symptom relief, hospital length of stay, or rehospitalization rate within 60 days was demonstrated.[74] Milrinone was associated with an increased incidence of hypotension and atrial arrhythmias. In the FIRST study of class III-IV heart failure patients, an average 14-day infusion of dobutamine was associated with an *increased* risk of morbid events and higher short-term mortality rates.[75] No clinical studies have shown improved short-term or medium-term outcomes with inotropic therapy. The use of inotropic agents has been consistently associated with a *worse* prognosis for survival.[39] These negative outcomes with inotropic agents are felt to be related to their propensity to stimulate sympathetic nervous system activation, increasing myocardial oxygen demand, exacerbating serious cardiac arrhythmias, increasing myocardial ischemia, and furthering myocyte loss. Stimulation of chronic hibernating myocardium may also result in myonecrosis.

If use of an inotrope is necessary, the shortest duration of therapy should be attempted (i.e., less than 72 hours). Current ACC/AHA Guidelines for evaluation and management of chronic heart failure indicate that long-term intermittent infusions of a positive inotropic drug as therapy for symptomatic systolic dysfunction is *contraindicated*.[4] Continuous intravenous infusion of an inotropic drug can be used as a bridge to therapy with mechanical circulatory assist devices or cardiac transplantation. Continuous inotrope infusion can also be recommended for palliation of symptoms in patients with refractory end-stage heart failure (stage D). These patients will have been deemed poor candidates for more advanced therapies. In this setting, quality of remaining life takes precedence over prolonging life. In one report of patients with refractory end-stage heart failure, median survival of patient on continuous inotrope infusion was 3.4 months, with 26% of patients surviving to 6 months.[76] The decision to use inotropic agents in this circumstance is one that should be carefully individualized.

VASOPRESSORS

DOPAMINE

Dopamine effects include increased renal blood flow (at low doses, 1-5 μg/kg/minute), increased myocardial contractility and chronotropy through stimulation of β-receptors (doses of 3-7 μg/kg/minute), and vasoconstriction at higher doses (5-20 μg/kg/minute). Dopamine is a less useful agent for treatment of heart failure because its effects result in tachycardia, coronary vasoconstriction, increased afterload, and increased oxygen consumption. Dobutamine generally will lead to a greater rise in cardiac output than dopamine. Dopamine can be used when significant hypotension is part of the hemodynamic picture, when it is necessary to restore adequate arterial pressure for end-organ perfusion. Although dopamine at low doses is frequently used as add-on therapy to inotropic agents in an attempt to increase renal blood flow and augment diuresis, no controlled trials have demonstrated dopamine's usefulness in this setting. No significant benefit of "renal dose dopamine" has been shown in preventing acute renal failure in high-risk patients or in the treatment of established renal failure.[69]

NOREPINEPHRINE

Norepinephrine is a sympathomimetic agent with strong α-agonist and weak β-agonist effects. In patients with heart failure, norepinephrine's main effect is to raise blood pressure by increasing systemic vascular resistance with little effect on cardiac output. It will increase myocardial oxygen demand. Its use in the setting of heart failure is restricted to patients with the most severe hypotension, unresponsive to dopamine, or in patients with complicating illnesses such as sepsis.[69] Norepinephrine should be weaned and discontinued as early as possible. Dosage range is 0.2 to 1 μg/kg/minute.

Norepinephrine and dopamine were compared in a randomized controlled trial of 1679 patients with shock, 280 (16.7%) of whom had cardiogenic shock. In the entire group, there was no difference in survival at 28 days if patients were treated with norepinephrine or dopamine. However, in the subgroup with cardiogenic shock (a predefined subgroup analysis), dopamine use was associated with a significantly increased mortality rate. In addition, in the entire group, dopamine was associated with significantly higher rates of arrhythmia (24% versus 12.4% with norepinephrine), especially atrial fibrillation, which led to stopping the vasopressor more frequently. There was also a higher rate of severe arrhythmia with dopamine (6.1%) compared with norepinephrine (1.6%).[77] Based on the results of this study, norepinephrine is the preferred vasopressor in patients with cardiogenic shock.

An algorithm for the approach to the evaluation and therapy of acute heart failure is presented in Figure 29.3.

ULTRAFILTRATION

A new approach to the treatment of acute heart failure is venovenous ultrafiltration. This process removes iso-osmolar extracellular fluid via a convection process and is not associated with changes in serum electrolytes.[78] Anticoagulation is utilized during the process. Newer ultrafiltration systems utilize peripheral arm veins, and central venous access is not required. In a study of 40 patients admitted with heart failure, usual care for heart failure with diuretic therapy was compared with usual care combined with ultrafiltration. At 24 hours, average fluid loss with diuretic therapy was 2838 mL, compared with 4650 mL with ultrafiltration. Weight loss and improvement in dyspnea was similar with the two therapies. Ultrafiltration was not associated with significant changes in heart rate or blood pressure.[79] In another study, 20 patients with acute decompensated heart failure with renal insufficiency and diuretic resistance were treated with an 8-hour course of ultrafiltration. Over 24 hours, an average of 8650 mL of fluid was removed, with an

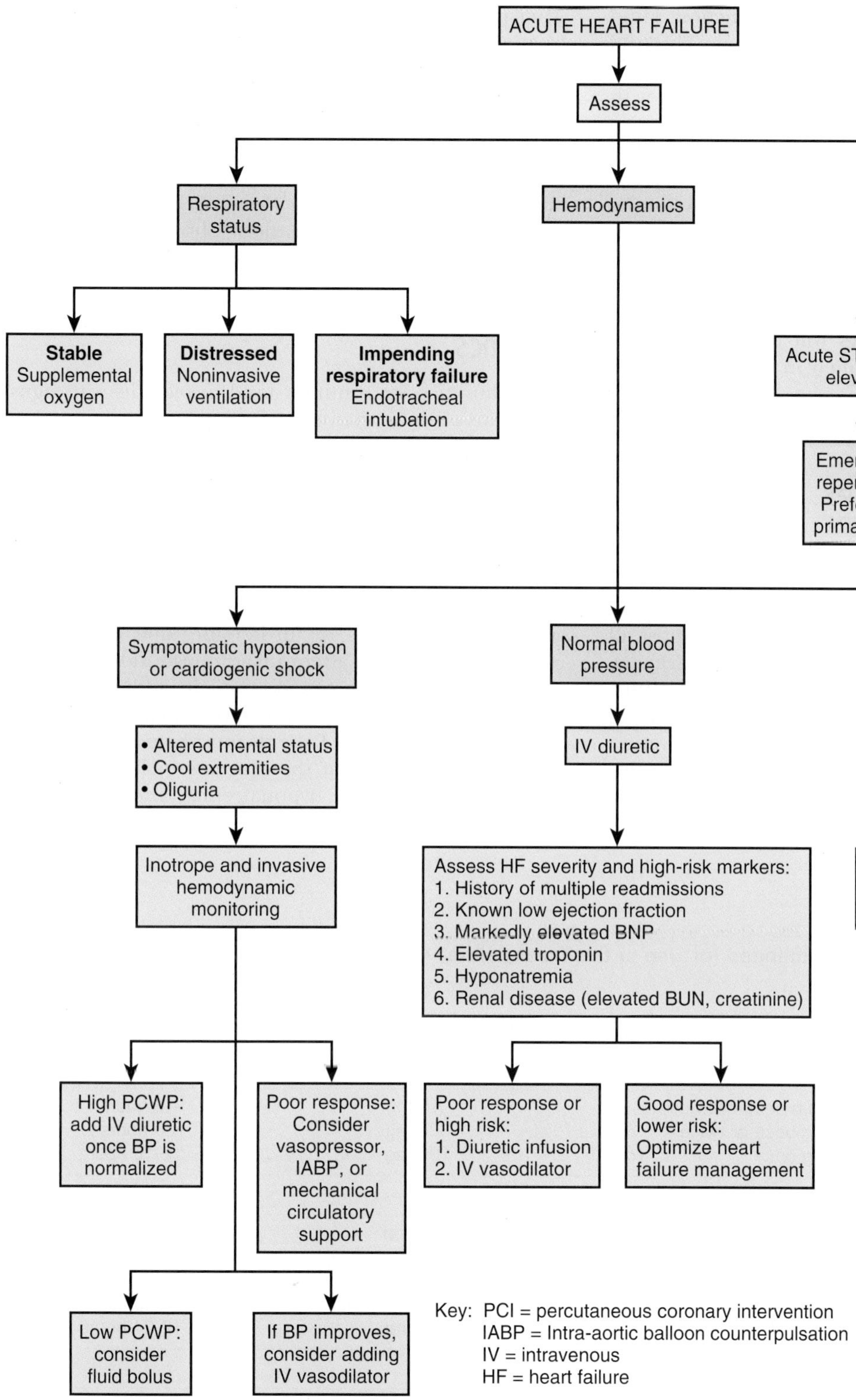

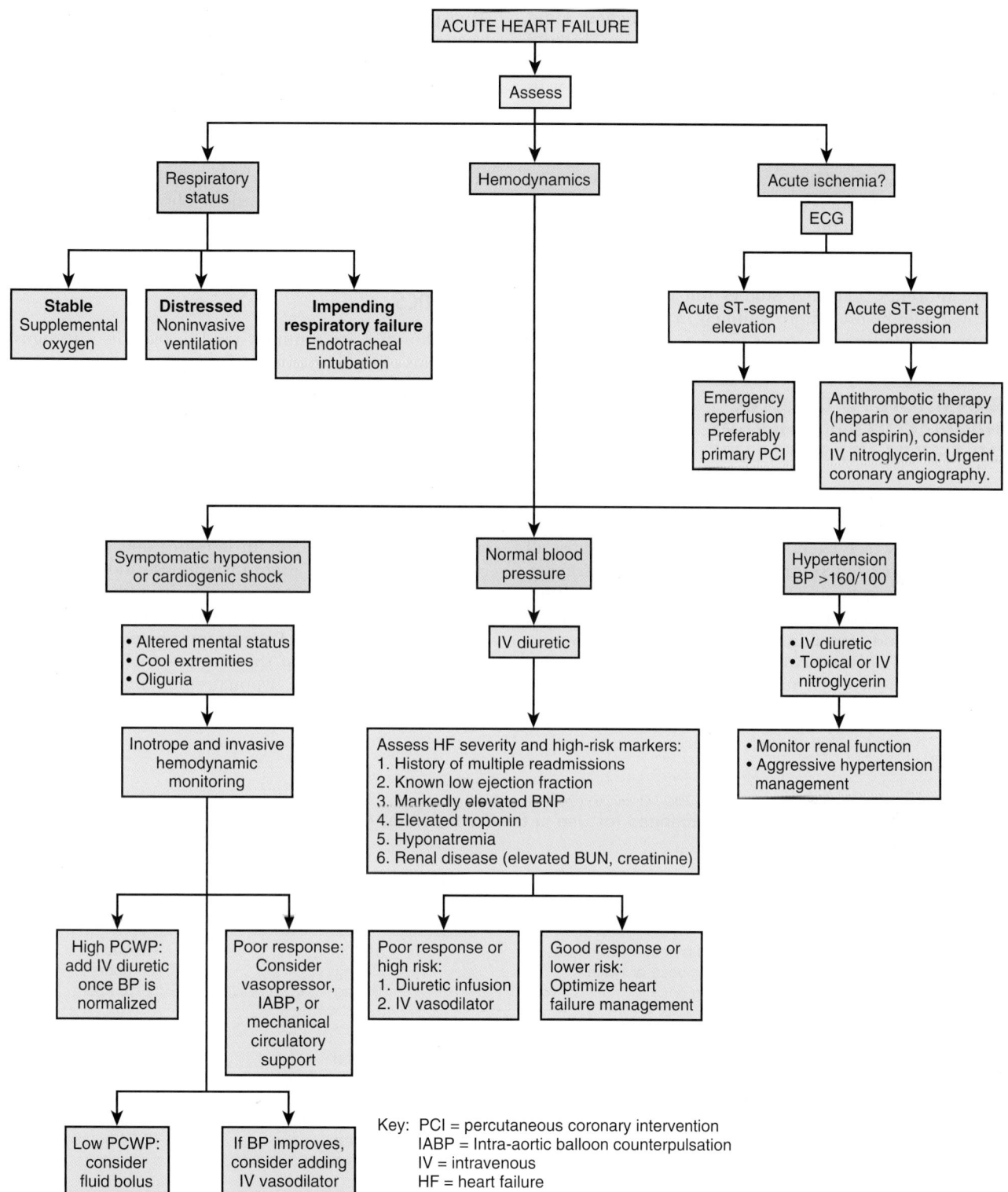

Figure 29.3 Algorithm for the treatment of acute heart failure. (Adapted from Pang PS: Acute heart failure syndromes. Emerg Med Clin North Am 2011;29:675-688.)

average weight loss of 6 kg during hospitalization. Renal function remained stable, and there was no associated hypotension.[78]

The UNLOAD trial investigated the use of ultrafiltration compared to intravenous diuretic therapy in 200 patients admitted with acute decompensated heart failure. Ultrafiltration was associated with more rapid weight loss and fluid loss. At 90 days, there were fewer rehospitalizations for heart failure in the ultrafiltration group, without change in mortality rates. There was no difference with respect to renal function in the two groups.[80]

A trial was conducted that compared ultrafiltration with standard intravenous diuretic therapy in patients admitted to hospital with acute decompensated heart failure, persistent congestion, and worsening renal function. Fluid was removed with UF at a rate of 200 mL per hour. This trial showed worse outcomes with ultrafiltration at 96 hours of therapy. Renal function worsened with UF and did not with diuretics. Total weight loss was unchanged between the two groups. Serious adverse effects were more common in the UF group, mainly renal failure, bleeding, and catheter-related complications. There was no difference between the two groups in symptom relief, mortality, or rehospitalization at 60 days.[80a] At this time, ultrafiltration is reserved for the relief of severe congestion in patients who are refractory to aggressive diuretic therapy and should not be used to replace diuretics.[81] Further studies will determine if this therapy should be used more routinely in the management of acute heart failure.

TRANSITION TO CHRONIC PHARMACOLOGIC THERAPY FOR SEVERE HEART FAILURE

The medical treatment of chronic systolic heart failure is based on results of many large, randomized, placebo-controlled trials (see later) and is indicated for almost all causes of chronic left ventricular dysfunction. Pharmacologic agents should be started when left ventricular dysfunction is first diagnosed. Therapy is aimed at optimizing fluid balance and reversing the neurohormonal activation responsible for left ventricular remodeling and progressive decline in left ventricular function.[82] Long-term prognosis is directly related to the process of "reverse remodeling." After patients have improved with acute therapies, medical treatments are instituted to address the long-term goals of improvements in functional status, exercise tolerance, and survival. Standard drug regimens combine several classes of medication, all of which have been shown in large, randomized controlled trials to reduce mortality rate, reduce the rate of rehospitalization, and decrease the risk of sudden arrhythmic death. Doses of these medications are optimized during hospitalization. Chronic adherence with these medications is more consistent when they are initiated in-hospital.

DIURETICS

Loop diuretics are routinely used in patients with signs or symptoms of fluid retention.[4] Diuretics are continued once patients are euvolemic to prevent reaccumulation of fluid. A flexible dosing schedule, based on daily weights and close telephone contact with a heart failure treatment team member, can be very effective in maintaining a euvolemic state while reducing the frequency of side effects.

Furosemide is the most common loop diuretic used. Bumetanide or torsemide may be helpful in patients with suboptimal responses to furosemide, due to their more consistent absorption after oral administration. Metolazone or a thiazide diuretic can be used in addition to a loop diuretic in patients with more severe heart failure due to their synergistic effects. Patients must be periodically monitored for side effects of these agents including azotemia, hypokalemia, alkalosis, hyponatremia, and hypomagnesemia (Table 29.6).

Table 29.6 Oral Diuretics Recommended for Use in the Treatment of Fluid Retention in Chronic Heart Failure

Drug	Initial Daily Dose(s)	Maximum Total Daily Dose	Duration of Action
Loop Diuretics			
Bumetanide	0.5-1.0 mg once or twice	10 mg	4-6 hours
Furosemide	20-40 mg once or twice	600 mg	6-8 hours
Torsemide	10-20 mg once	200 mg	12-16 hours
Thiazide Diuretics			
Chlorothiazide	250-500 mg once or twice	1000 mg	6-12 hours
Chlorthalidone	12.5-25 mg once	100 mg	24-72 hours
Hydrochlorothiazide	25 mg once or twice	200 mg	6-12 hours
Indapamide	2.5 mg once	5 mg	36 hours
Metolazone	2.5 mg once	20 mg	12-24 hours
Potassium-Sparing Diuretics			
Eplerenone	12.5 mg once	20 mg	24 hours
Spironolactone	12.5-25 mg once	50 mg*	2-3 days
Triamterene	50-75 mg once	200 mg	7-9 hours

*Higher doses may occasionally be used with close monitoring of serum creatinine and potassium levels.

Adapted from Hunt S, Abraham WT, Chin M, et al: ACC/AHA 2005 Guideline Update for the Diagnosis and Management of Chronic Heart Failure in the Adult—Summary Article. A report on the American College of Cardiology/American Heart Association Task Force on Practice Guidelines (Writing Committee to Update the 2001 Guidelines for Evaluation and Management of Heart Failure): Developed in collaboration with the American College of Chest Physicians and the International Society of Heart and Lung Transplantation: Endorsed by the Heart Rhythm Society. Circulation 2005;112:1825-1852.

Table 29.7 Inhibitors of the Renin-Aldosterone System and Beta Blockers Commonly Used for the Treatment of Patients with Heart Failure and Low Ejection Fraction

Drug	Initial Daily Dose(s)	Maximum Dose(s)
Angiotensin-Converting Enzyme Inhibitors		
Captopril	6.25 mg 3 times	50 mg 3 times
Enalapril	2.5 mg twice	10-20 mg twice
Fosinopril	5-10 mg once	40 mg once
Lisinopril	2.5-5 mg once	20-40 mg once
Perindopril	2 mg once	8-16 mg once
Quinapril	5 mg twice	20 mg twice
Ramipril	1.25-2.5 mg once	10 mg once
Trandolapril	1 mg once	4 mg once
Angiotensin Receptor Blockers		
Candesartan	4-8 mg once	32 mg once
Losartan	25-50 mg once	50-100 mg once
Valsartan	20-40 mg twice	160 mg twice
Aldosterone Antagonists		
Spironolactone	12.5-25 mg once	25 mg once or twice
Eplerenone	25 mg once	50 mg once
Beta blockers		
Bisoprolol	1.25 mg once	10 mg once
Carvedilol	3.125 mg twice	25 mg twice (50 mg twice for patients weighing >85 kg)
Metoprolol succinate extended-release	12.5-25 mg once	200 mg once

Adapted from Hunt S, Abraham WT, Chin M, et al: ACC/AHA 2005 Guideline Update for the Diagnosis and Management of Chronic Heart Failure in the Adult—Summary Article. A report on the American College of Cardiology/American Heart Association Task Force on Practice Guidelines (Writing Committee to Update the 2001 Guidelines for Evaluation and Management of Heart Failure): Developed in collaboration with the American College of Chest Physicians and the International Society of Heart and Lung Transplantation: Endorsed by the Heart Rhythm Society. Circulation 2005;112:1825-1852.

BETA BLOCKERS (TABLE 29.7)

Catecholamine levels are increased in heart failure, and higher levels correlate with worse disease severity. Catecholamines have direct negative effects on the myocardium including induction of myocyte hypertrophy and apoptosis.[13] Clinically, these effects are evident as left ventricular dilatation, increased ischemia, increased peripheral vasoconstriction, and cardiac arrhythmia.

Beta blockers interfere with catecholamine-mediated activation of cardiac β-receptors and thereby attenuate β-receptor-mediated increases in heart rate and oxygen consumption. Sympathetic nervous system–mediated effects on remodeling can be prevented or attenuated. In addition, carvedilol blocks β-receptors and also α-receptors, which mediate vasoconstriction and increased cardiac contractility.

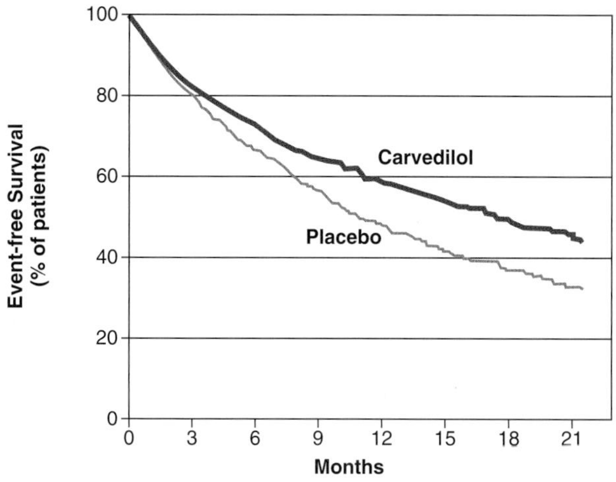

No. of Patients at Risk								
Placebo	1133	767	513	377	262	154	88	55
Carvedilol	1156	789	559	431	318	208	122	81

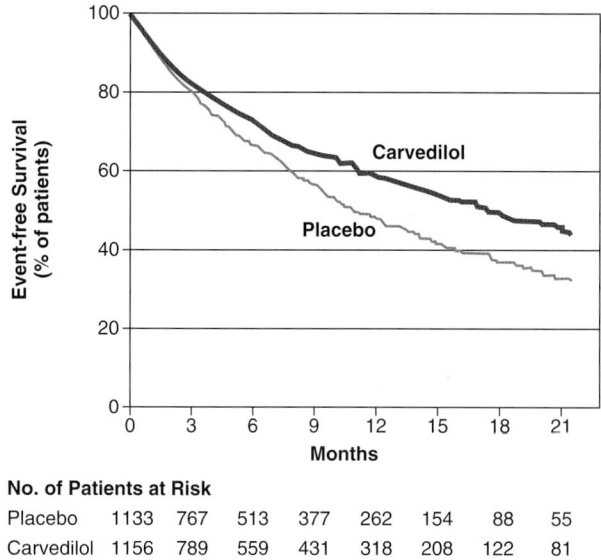

Figure 29.4 All-cause mortality rate in patients with class III to class IV heart failure, ejection fraction less than 25%, demonstrating significant survival benefit with carvedilol. (Redrawn from Packer M, Coats A, Fowler M, et al: Effect of carvedilol on survival in severe chronic heart failure. N Engl J Med 2001;344:1651-1658.)

Multiple large trials using beta blockers in thousands of patients with chronic heart failure, or in post–myocardial infarction patients with ejection fractions below 40%, have demonstrated significant and consistent reductions in the need for repeat rehospitalization for heart failure. Mortality rates are also significantly improved. The BHAT study showed a relative 26% reduction in mortality rates at 2 years in post–myocardial infarction patients treated with propranolol.[83,84] The CIBIS II trial using bisoprolol showed a 34% relative risk reduction in hospitalizations and mortality rates at 16 months of therapy.[85] The MERIT-HF study showed a relative reduction of 33% in these end points at 12 months using metoprolol succinate.[86] Patients with more severe heart failure, symptom class III-IV, with severely reduced ejection fractions below 25% were studied in the COPERNICUS trial. These patients began therapy with carvedilol during hospitalization. At mean follow-up of 10.4 months, a 35% relative mortality rate reduction was seen, with improvement in mortality rates beginning as early as 3 weeks after initiation of therapy[87] (Fig. 29.4). In these trials, beta blockers were not discontinued more frequently than placebo for perceived side effects, and there was no increased risk of heart failure exacerbation due to beta-blocker therapy when compared to placebo, even in the early phases of drug administration.[88] Several trials with carvedilol have shown an approximate 6% absolute increase in left ventricular ejection fraction after a minimum of 2 years of therapy.[89]

Beta blockers should be started for treatment of heart failure and left ventricular dysfunction when patients are stable. Beta blockers should be instituted early, once patients are deemed euvolemic, and titrated up to maximal recommended doses (e.g., metoprolol succinate 200 mg daily or carvedilol 25 mg twice daily) or maximally tolerated doses. They are useful in patients with ischemic and nonischemic cardiomyopathy. Beta blockers should be instituted in patients who appear compensated and stable off this medication, as these patients have a high likelihood of disease progression to symptomatic heart failure within 12 months. Beta blockers are recommended for left ventricular dysfunction even in the absence of symptoms (stage B patients). This therapy should be combined with other recommended heart failure pharmacologic therapy. Contraindications to beta-blocker use include severe bradycardia or bronchospastic lung disease.

For patients who are already taking beta-blocker therapy and who are hospitalized with acute decompensation of heart failure, beta blockers should be continued. Withdrawal of this medication was associated with higher short-term mortality rates and more frequent rehospitalizations for heart failure in several observational studies.[90] In patients with a severe heart failure exacerbation, reduction of the chronic dose by 50% can be considered. Beta blockers should only be stopped in the presence of symptomatic hypotension, cardiogenic shock, severe bradycardia, or heart block. If beta blockers are temporarily withheld, they should be reinstituted prior to discharge unless there are ongoing specific contraindications.[91,92]

ANGIOTENSIN-CONVERTING ENZYME INHIBITORS (SEE TABLE 29.7)

These agents act to counteract the effects of activation of the renin-angiotensin system by blocking the conversion of angiotensin I to angiotensin II, inhibiting the deleterious effects of angiotensin II and aldosterone. Many studies have shown benefits of ACE inhibitor therapy in post–myocardial infarction patients as well as patients with cardiomyopathy and heart failure. The SOLVD trial using enalapril in patients with class II-III heart failure and ejection fractions below 35% showed a 10% relative risk reduction in mortality rate at 3.5 years.[93] Enalapril given to patients less ill, with asymptomatic left ventricular dysfunction (ejection fractions under 35%) in the companion SOLVD trial showed a reduction in the clinical diagnosis of heart failure and a statistically significant reduction in heart failure hospitalizations at 3 years.[94] A meta-analysis performed of 32 trials involving 7105 patients, using captopril, enalapril, ramipril, quinapril, or lisinopril, found that ACE inhibitors reduce the risk of death and hospitalization due to heart failure.[95] These results indicate that the positive effects of ACE inhibitors are likely to be a class effect, and not specific to a particular agent.

Side effects of these agents include cough, worsening renal function in patients with underlying renal disease or renal artery stenosis, angioneurotic edema, and hyperkalemia. The dose of ACE inhibitors should be increased as renal function and blood pressure allow. Studies have shown that medium doses of ACE inhibitors, when compared to low doses, significantly reduce hospitalization rates for heart failure. However, higher doses given routinely do not significantly reduce cardiovascular events further.[96] Additional improvement in symptoms and mortality rates is thus best achieved by adding on beta blocker and other heart failure therapy rather than increasing ACE inhibitors to the highest doses.[97]

In a study of class II-III chronic heart failure patients over age 65, with an ejection fraction of less than 35%, the importance of first beginning heart failure therapy with an ACE inhibitor or a beta blocker was studied. The primary end point was time to death or hospitalization for heart failure. Initiation of the beta blocker bisoprolol was not inferior to the strategy of starting therapy with the ACE inhibitor enalapril. There was also no difference in safety.[98]

ANGIOTENSIN RECEPTOR BLOCKERS (SEE TABLE 29.7)

Angiotensin receptor blockers (ARBs) work to counter the effects of angiotensin II at the tissue level by blocking angiotensin II receptors. Multiple studies have shown benefits of these medications in patients with heart failure. Large numbers of patients in controlled trials have been studied, and these drugs have been as well studied as the ACE inhibitors. ARBs have been used as a substitute for ACE inhibitors or given in combination with ACE inhibitors and beta blockers.

The RESOLVD trial, using candesartan in heart failure patients with a mean ejection fraction of 27%, showed equivalent mortality rates and similar exercise tolerance and functional class to patients treated with enalapril at 3.5 years.[99] ELITE II, a study using losartan compared with captopril in patients with ejection fractions under 40%, showed no difference in mortality rates or congestive heart failure admissions. Losartan was better tolerated because of the lower incidence of problematic cough.[100] The ValHeft 2001 trial showed that valsartan as a substitute for ACE inhibitor therapy was associated with a relative 33% risk reduction in mortality rate when compared with placebo.[101] In CHARM, candesartan was prescribed for patients with ejection fractions under 40%. A 17.5% relative risk reduction in cardiovascular death and congestive heart failure admissions was seen when this ARB was used as a substitute for ACE inhibitors.[102] When candersartan was added to therapy with ACE inhibitors and beta blockers, a small 10% relative risk reduction was seen, without increased mortality rates.[103]

ARBs are an appropriate choice for patients who cannot be maintained on ACE inhibitors because of side effects such as cough. Patients with angioneurotic edema during ACE inhibitor therapy have often been successfully treated with ARBs without developing this complication.[104,105] Adding ARB therapy onto ACE inhibitors and beta blockers may achieve a small additional benefit, at the risk of more renal dysfunction and hyperkalemia.

ALDOSTERONE ANTAGONISTS (SEE TABLE 29.7)

Aldosterone antagonists counteract the salt and water retention caused by aldosterone. In addition, aldosterone is felt to be involved in the progressive myocardial fibrosis that occurs as part of the remodeling process. In the RALES trial, the aldosterone antagonist spironolactone was given to patients with severe, class III-IV heart failure with ejection fraction below 35%. A 24% relative risk reduction in mortality was seen in treated patients over 2 years, with reduced cardiovascular death and reduced need for rehospitalization[106] (Fig. 29.5). Thus, these agents are effective at

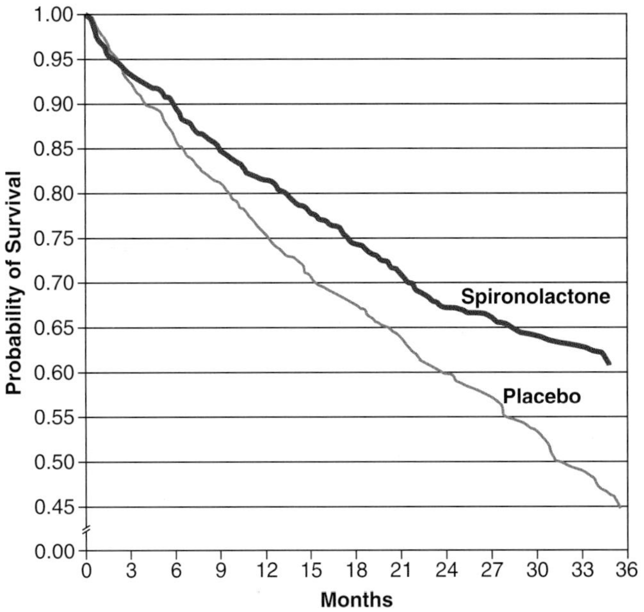

No. at Risk

Placebo	841	775	723	678	628	592	565	483	379	280	179	92	36
Spironolactone	822	766	739	698	669	639	608	526	419	316	193	122	43

Figure 29.5 Kaplan-Meier analysis of the probability of survival among patients in the placebo group and patients in the spironolactone group, treated for class III to class IV heart failure and left ventricular dysfunction. The risk of death was 30% lower among patients in the spironolactone group than among patients in the placebo group ($P < 0.001$). (Redrawn from Pitt B, Zannad F, Remme W, et al: The effect of spironolactone on morbidity and mortality in patients with severe heart failure. N Engl J Med 1999;341:709-717.)

improving outcomes in patients with the most severe chronic heart failure. Aldosterone antagonists are contraindicated in patients with renal insufficiency and creatinine levels over 2.5 mg/dL (or GFR under 30 mL/minute) or in patients with baseline potassium levels over 5.0 mmol/L. Spironolactone should be initiated at low doses, such as 12.5 mg daily or every other day, especially in elderly patients.

An analysis of a large Canadian health care database showed a substantial increase in the frequency of spironolactone use after the RALES study was published. This increased use was temporally associated with a two- to threefold increased rate of hospitalization for hyperkalemia.[107] This highlights the need for careful monitoring of serum electrolytes after aldosterone blockers are initiated.

Eplerenone is an aldosterone blocker similar to spironolactone except that it has less antiandrogen effects and thus is free of the side effect of gynecomastia in men. It has been found to be effective in treating heart failure following acute myocardial infarction (see later). More recently, it was also found to be very effective in patients with chronic heart failure. In EMPHASIS-HF, a placebo-controlled randomized study of 2737 patients with LV ejection fraction below 35% and class II heart failure, eplerenone was added to therapy with ACE inhibitors and beta blockers, at a target dose of 25 to 50 mg daily. Mean follow-up was 21 months. Eplerenone reduced the occurrence of the primary end point of cardiovascular death plus hospitalization for heart failure from 25.9% to 18.3% ($P < 0.001$), and with improvement in other clinical end points. Serious hyperkalemia that necessitated drug discontinuation occurred in only 1.1% of patients.[108]

Aldosterone blockade appears to result in beneficial effects in heart failure independent of its potassium sparing and diuretic effects.[109] Aldosterone blockers are an important therapy for heart failure and should be routinely added to ACE inhibitors and beta blockers in patients with symptomatic heart failure with low left ventricular ejection fraction.

COMBINATION HYDRALAZINE/ ISOSORBIDE DINITRATE

Combination therapy with the vasodilators hydralazine and isosorbide dinitrate (ISDN) was associated with improvement in mortality rate when compared to placebo in one study in the era prior to the advent of ACE inhibitors and beta-blocker therapy for heart failure.[110] A retrospective analysis of this study suggested that African-American patients may have benefited preferentially. To evaluate this finding prospectively, the A-Heft study enrolled over 1000 self-described African-American patients with class II-IV heart failure and ejection fractions below 45%. The use of the combination of hydralazine with ISDN, titrated to a dose of 75 mg hydralazine plus 40 mg ISDN given three times daily, was associated with a 40% relative risk reduction in mortality at 10 months and a 33% relative risk reduction in first hospitalization for heart failure. This therapy was added on to treatment with beta blockers, ACE inhibitors, and spironolactone.[111] Hydralazine-ISDN is approved for treatment of African-American patients with heart failure and left ventricular systolic dysfunction.

DIGOXIN

Digoxin works by inhibiting the myocyte sodium-potassium pump, leading to increased intracellular calcium levels and increased inotropy. It also has vagotonic effects. However, digoxin is a relatively weak inotropic agent. The use of digoxin in heart failure was studied in large numbers of patients in the Digitalis Investigation Group (DIG) trial. A decreased need for rehospitalization for heart failure was seen with this therapy. However, there was no improvement in overall mortality rate.[112] A post-hoc analysis of this data concluded that patients with lower serum digoxin levels (0.5-0.9 ng/dL) did have lower mortality rates and lower rates of heart failure hospitalization when compared to those with levels greater than 0.9 ng/mL.[113]

Digoxin is indicated only for patients with symptomatic heart failure, stages C and D.[4] It is also useful in heart failure patients with atrial fibrillation to help control the ventricular rate. Digoxin is not useful in the setting of acute heart failure, and it should be avoided in patients with hyopkalemia, bradycardia, or heart block.

CORONARY HEART DISEASE AND HEART FAILURE: SPECIAL CONSIDERATIONS

Coronary artery disease can lead to acute heart failure via several different mechanisms. Acute ischemia leads to impaired myocardial relaxation, acute diastolic dysfunction, and sudden elevation of left ventricular filling pressure. Acute ischemia can also cause "stunning," defined as myocardial dysfunction due to severe and prolonged ischemia without infarction, which may persist for days or weeks after normal blood flow is restored but which eventually recovers function. Acute myocardial infarction may cause myocardial necrosis and acute left ventricular systolic dysfunction due to loss of contractile tissue. Papillary muscle ischemia, infarction, and rupture result in acute, severe mitral regurgitation and acute heart failure. Infarction, necrosis, and rupture of the intraventricular septum result in left-to-right shunting and acute heart failure with cardiogenic shock. Chronic ischemia can cause myocardial dysfunction and systolic heart failure without infarction, a process termed "hibernation." Often, acute myocardial ischemia is superimposed on a ventricle impaired by chronic ischemia and infarction, so multiple mechanisms are usually present in patients with chronic coronary disease presenting with acute heart failure.[23,114]

In a European observational study of acute heart failure complicating acute coronary syndromes (ACS) in patients without previous history of heart failure, 13% of ACS patients presented with heart failure on admission.[115] Heart failure developed later during hospitalization in an additional 5.6% of patients. The incidence of acute heart failure of 15.6% was identical in patients with ST-segment elevation myocardial infarction and non–ST-segment elevation myocardial infarction. Eight percent of patients with unstable angina developed heart failure. Prognosis for these patients was poor, with in-hospital mortality rates of 12% for patients with heart failure on admission and 17.8% if heart failure developed during the hospitalization. This represents a three- to fourfold increase in mortality rates compared with patients with ACS without heart failure.

Several important points need to be stressed regarding acute heart failure and ACS. Acute heart failure may develop even without evidence of significant left ventricular systolic dysfunction on echocardiography and without acute necrosis documented by myocardial enzyme determinations. The majority of patients with ACS and heart failure do not have left ventricular systolic dysfunction at discharge, and only a minority of these patients develop chronic heart failure. These patients not only have high in-hospital mortality rates but also have a high rate of morbidity and mortality after discharge, with 8.5% additional mortality rate at 6 months and 6-month rehospitalization rate of 24%.[114]

Early aggressive pharmacologic and interventional reperfusion strategies are indicated and should always be considered in these patients. Acute treatment should include intravenous diuretics, intravenous nitroglycerin, and beta-blocker therapy. Intra-aortic balloon counterpulsation should be used in patients with signs and symptoms of continued ischemia despite aggressive medical therapies or who have cardiogenic shock. Urgent coronary angiography is indicated to determine the most appropriate reperfusion strategy.[114]

ACUTE HEART FAILURE FOLLOWING MYOCARDIAL INFARCTION

In a large registry of 5573 consecutive patients with acute myocardial infarction, 42% of patients had heart failure or left ventricular systolic dysfunction during hospitalization.[116] These patients tended to be older, were more commonly women, and were more likely to have had previous myocardial infarction or coronary bypass surgery. Comorbid conditions were present more commonly, including peripheral arterial disease, hypertension, diabetes mellitus, or previous stroke. In-hospital mortality rate for these patients was 13%, versus 2.3% for patients with acute myocardial infarction but without heart failure or left ventricular dysfunction. Mortality rate ranged 13% to 21% for patients with lung congestion and left ventricular ejection fraction below 40%. Other complications also occurred more commonly in these patients, including atrial and ventricular arrhythmias, reinfarction, and stroke (Figs. 29.6 and 29.7).

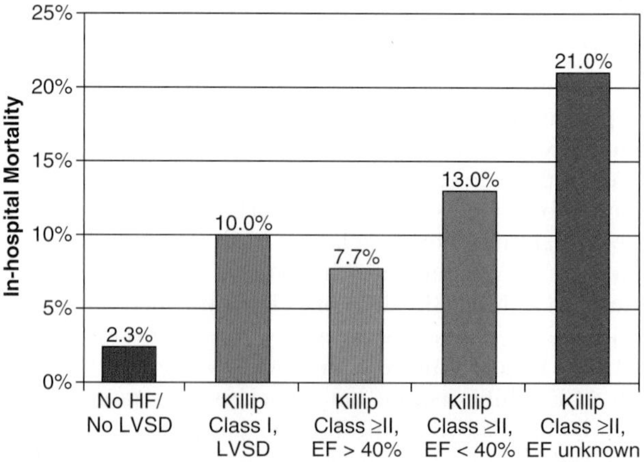

Figure 29.6 In-hospital mortality rate in patients admitted with acute myocardial infarction, according to presence of heart failure and left ventricular (LV) ejection fraction. EF, ejection fraction; HF, heart failure; Killip class I, patients without evidence of heart failure on physical examination; Killip class II, patients with evidence of heart failure on physical examination; LVSD, LV systolic dysfunction. (Redrawn from Velazquez EJ, Francis GS, Armstrong PW, et al: An international perspective on heart failure and left ventricular systolic dysfunction complicating myocardial infarction: The VALIANT Registry. Eur Heart J 2004;25:1911-1919.)

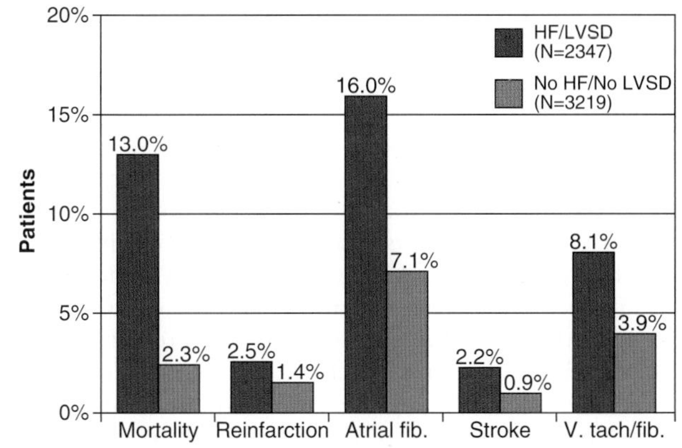

Figure 29.7 In-hospital clinical events among patients with and without heart failure (HF) or left ventricular systolic dysfunction (LVSD) ($P < 0.001$ for all events except reinfarction). Atrial fib, atrial fibrillation; V. tach/fib, ventricular tachycardia/ventricular fibrillation. (Redrawn from Velazquez EJ, Francis GS, Armstrong PW, et al: An international perspective on heart failure and left ventricular systolic dysfunction complicating myocardial infarction: The VALIANT Registry. Eur Heart J 2004;25:1911-1919.)

In patients with acute heart failure due to acute myocardial infarction, rapid reperfusion is the cornerstone of therapy and may be achieved with thrombolytic therapy, acute coronary angioplasty, or urgent coronary artery bypass surgery. In the GRACE Study, revascularization therapies were associated with a lower mortality rate in patients with ACS and acute heart failure.[115]

In patients who develop heart failure or significant left ventricular systolic dysfunction following myocardial infarction, a number of pharmacologic therapies have been shown in large placebo-controlled randomized studies to improve mortality rate and reduce repeat hospitalization. Beta blockers should be part of standard post–myocardial infarction therapy in these patients. In the CAPRICORN study, the use of carvedilol led to a significant 23% relative risk reduction.[117] SAVE was the first trial to show that the use of an ACE inhibitor, captopril, was beneficial in post–myocardial infarction patients with ejection fractions below 40%.[118] There was a 5% absolute mortality rate reduction after 42 months of follow-up. In AIRE, treatment with the ACE inhibitor ramipril, started 3 to 10 days after myocardial infarction in patients with heart failure, resulted in a significant mortality rate benefit at an average of 15 months of follow-up.[119] Another trial showed that treatment with the ACE inhibitor trandolapril following myocardial infarction and an ejection fraction below 35% resulted in a significantly improved survival at 2 to 4 years of follow-up.[120] In VALIANT, a high dose of the ARB valsartan was as effective as an ACE inhibitor in improving survival and reducing cardiovascular morbidity.[121]

Therefore beta blockers and ACE inhibitors should be started early and continued long term in patients with reduced left ventricular ejection fraction following acute myocardial infarction. ARBs are recommended in those patients who are intolerant to ACE inhibitors.

Aldosterone blockers have also been shown to be effective in improving prognosis in patients with heart failure or left ventricular dysfunction following myocardial infarction and are recommended for these patients. The EPHESUS study showed that eplerenone significantly reduced all-cause mortality rates and repeat hospitalizations at 16-month follow-up.[122] Reduction in mortality rate and sudden cardiac death was noted as early as 30 days after initiation of eplerenone.[123]

HEART FAILURE WITH PRESERVED LEFT VENTRICULAR EJECTION FRACTION (DIASTOLIC HEART FAILURE)

Heart failure can occur in patients with normal or relatively normal left ventricular systolic function. It is now recognized that in up to 50% of patients hospitalized with acute heart failure, the primary cardiac abnormality is diastolic dysfunction. There is no consistent definition or diagnostic test for diastolic heart failure. The European Society of Cardiology has proposed that this diagnosis can be applied to patients who present with clinical signs and symptoms of heart failure, who have normal left ventricular systolic function, and who have abnormal parameters of diastolic filling as demonstrated on Doppler echocardiography or invasive evaluation of diastolic function. A more practical definition includes the presence of heart failure and normal systolic function in the absence of primary valve disease.[82,124]

Diastolic heart failure occurs due to impairment of left ventricular filling and abnormal left ventricular relaxation. Pathophysiology includes myocyte hypertrophy, increased amounts of collagen in extracellular matrix, increased wall stiffness and wall thickness, abnormal left ventricular geometry with increased left ventricular mass-to-volume ratio, fibrosis, and impaired compliance. There is impaired left ventricular filling at normal left atrial pressures, and thus an increase in left ventricular filling pressure is necessary to maintain cardiac output. This leads to chronic pulmonary venous hypertension and pulmonary congestion. Patients with diastolic heart failure usually demonstrate normal indices of left ventricular systolic performance and contractility.[125-128]

Diastolic heart failure is a common entity. The reported frequency of diastolic heart failure in the general heart failure population varies according to the definition of diastolic heart failure used. Some reports include patients with mildly abnormal systolic function (i.e., ejection fraction over 40%), whereas others restrict inclusion to patients with ejection fraction above 50%. Prevalence is also affected by the demographics of study populations, including age of patients, inpatient and outpatient status, the proportion of African Americans and women studied, and whether patients were evaluated at an academic referral center or a community-based setting.[124] In the general population of Olmsted County, Minnesota, moderate to severe diastolic dysfunction was seen in 7% of echocardiogram studies.[2] The prevalence of diastolic heart failure in population-based studies was 3.1% to 5.5% of patients over age 65.[124] The prevalence of diastolic heart failure may be increasing.[129] As compared with patients with systolic heart failure, patients with diastolic heart failure tend to be older, are more commonly women, and have a higher prevalence of hypertension and a lower incidence of coronary artery disease. In various studies, up to 50% of hospital admissions for heart failure in the United States are for patients with diastolic heart failure. In an international observational database of 4953 hospitalizations for heart failure, 25% of patients had a left ventricular ejection fraction over 45%.[130] Up to 73% of patients with diastolic heart failure are women, with an incidence of hypertension or hypertensive heart disease of 64% to 78%. Reported incidences of concomitant diabetes (33-46%) and coronary artery disease (26-43%) are also high. Other common comorbid conditions include atrial fibrillation, abnormal renal function, and obesity.[131-134]

Patients who present with heart failure due to diastolic dysfunction have a history and physical examination indistinguishable from patients with systolic heart failure. Presenting blood pressure may be higher, and acute "flash" pulmonary edema may be more common. Common exacerbating factors include severe hypertension, medication noncompliance, myocardial ischemia, and valve dysfunction. In one study, no precipitating factors could be identified in 50% of these patients.[129]

The prognosis of patients with diastolic heart failure is serious. Mortality rate is probably not as high as in patients with systolic left ventricular dysfunction and heart failure, although one study found similar adjusted and nonadjusted mortality rates at 30 days and 1 year for hospitalized patients with heart failure and left ventricular ejection fraction less than 40% or greater than 50%.[135] In-hospital mortality rate is around 4%,[106] or four times age-matched control subjects.[131,136] Annual mortality rate is variable and likely depends on the frequency of comorbid conditions in the cohort of patients studied; it has been reported in the range of 1.3% to 17.5%.[127] Readmission rates are as high as 50% at 1 year. Factors that identify patients with a worse prognosis include renal dysfunction, worse functional class, male gender, and advanced age.[136]

Unlike systolic heart failure, there are no placebo-controlled randomized studies that have demonstrated effective therapy for diastolic heart failure. The CHARM-Preserved Study compared the use of the ARB candesartan with placebo in treating patients with heart failure and preserved systolic function. After an average 3-year follow-up, the mortality rate from cardiovascular cause or admission for heart failure was similar in the two groups. There was a modest impact on preventing hospitalizations due to heart failure in patients treated with candesartan.[137] The I-PRESERVE trial utilizing irbesartan in over 4000 patients with heart failure and left ventricular ejection fraction over 45% showed no beneficial effect on mortality rates or heart failure rehospitalizations.[138]

Several basic recommendations are widely agreed upon. Effective treatment of underlying conditions, such as hypertension, diabetes mellitus, and coronary artery disease, is essential. Lowering systolic blood pressure will lower mean left atrial pressure. Control of elevated blood glucose may help to retard myocardial fibrosis by lessening cross-linking of myocardial collagen. Control of myocardial ischemia is important, although there are no convincing controlled data that revascularization will reliably prevent recurrences of diastolic heart failure. Maintenance of sinus rhythm and avoidance of tachycardia are also important. Medical therapy of diastolic heart failure is primarily focused on alleviating symptoms. Diuretics are effective at improving pulmonary congestion. Lower doses of diuretics are generally utilized, as high doses often lead to volume depletion and hypotension in these patients with small left ventricular cavities. Long-acting nitrates are also useful to decrease left ventricular filling pressure, pulmonary venous pressure, and dyspnea.

Beta blockers can be useful to reduce heart rate and thus improve diastolic filling time. They are also effective medications for hypertension and coronary ischemia. Similarly, calcium channel blockers may improve symptoms of diastolic heart failure by treating hypertension and ischemia and improving diastolic relaxation. The use of ACE inhibitors and ARBs is helpful to lower blood pressure, reduce myocardial fibrosis, and block the adverse effects of the activation of the renin-angiotensin system. In a retrospective study of patients hospitalized with heart failure and ejection fraction greater than 40%, patients who were prescribed an ACE inhibitor had better quality of life scores, improved functional class, and lower adjusted mortality rate.[133] Aldosterone antagonists such as spironolactone or eplerenone treat hypertension and may reduce left ventricular hypertrophy and fibrosis.[113] Therapy with positive inotropic drugs or digoxin are not useful in patients with diastolic heart failure[4,139,140] (Table 29.8).

ACUTE MYOCARDITIS AND HEART FAILURE

Myocarditis is defined as inflammation of heart muscle and is an uncommon cause of acute heart failure. Patients with acute myocarditis can develop severe left ventricular dysfunction and acute heart failure. In a minority of cases, myocarditis can present with fulminant heart failure and cardiogenic shock, with a high mortality rate.[141,142] A large body of experimental animal data indicates that viral myocarditis results in activation of immune mechanisms, which can also result in chronic dilated cardiomyopathy and chronic heart failure.[141]

An infectious cause of myocarditis is common. Viral agents such as enterovirus and adenovirus have been implicated as causative agents by serologic data and examination of cardiac cell geomes. The protozoan *Trypanosoma cruzi* is the etiologic agent in Chagas' disease, a form of myocarditis that can lead to chronic heart failure, endemic in Central and South America. Immune mechanisms are pathogenic in the myocarditis due to giant cell arteritis and the myocarditis associated with progressive systemic sclerosis, systemic lupus erythematosus, and polymyositis.

Myocarditis is a diagnosis made on clinical grounds and should be suspected in patients who present with new-onset heart failure, with or without antecedent flu-like symptoms. Chest pain may be present. Elevated leukocyte count, elevated erythrocyte sedimentation rate, elevated creatinine kinase and troponin levels, and ECG changes suggestive of myocardial ischemia or infarction may be seen but are not always present. Endomyocardial biopsy may be used to aid in the diagnosis of myocarditis. However, histologic findings of both inflammation and myocyte necrosis in biopsy specimens have been very insensitive in making the diagnosis and have a high degree of interobserver variability. In patients suspected of having myocarditis on clinical grounds, only 10% to 67% of patients have had positive biopsies in reported series.[141,142] Cardiac magnetic resonance imaging

Table 29.8 Recommendations for Treatment of Patients with Heart Failure and Normal Left Ventricular Ejection Fraction

Recommendation	Class*	Level of Evidence†
Physicians should control systolic and diastolic hypertension in accordance with published guidelines.	I	A
Physicians should control ventricular rate in patients with atrial fibrillation.	I	C
Physicians should use diuretics to control pulmonary congestion and peripheral edema.	I	C
Coronary revascularization is reasonable in patients with coronary artery disease in whom symptomatic or demonstrable myocardial ischemia is judged to be having an adverse effect on cardiac function.	IIa	C
Restoration and maintenance of sinus rhythm in patients with atrial fibrillation might be useful to improve symptoms.	IIb	C
The use of β-adrenergic blocking agents, angiotensin-converting enzyme inhibitors, angiotensin II receptor blockers, or calcium antagonists in patients with controlled hypertension might be effective to minimize symptoms of heart failure.	IIb	C
The use of digitalis to minimize symptoms of heart failure is not well established.	IIb	C

*I: There is evidence or general agreement that therapy is beneficial, useful, and effective; IIa: there is conflicting evidence about the usefulness of therapy, but the weight of the evidence is in favor of efficacy; IIb: there is conflicting evidence about the usefulness of therapy, and use is less well established by evidence/opinion.

†A: Data are derived from multiple randomized clinical trials or meta-analysis; C: only consensus opinion of experts, case studies, or standard of care.

Adapted from Hunt S, Abraham WT, Chin M, et al: ACC/AHA 2005 Guideline Update for the Diagnosis and Management of Chronic Heart Failure in the Adult—Summary Article. A report on the American College of Cardiology/American Heart Association Task Force on Practice Guidelines (Writing Committee to Update the 2001 Guidelines for Evaluation and Management of Heart Failure): Developed in collaboration with the American College of Chest Physicians and the International Society of Heart and Lung Transplantation: Endorsed by the Heart Rhythm Society. Circulation 2005;112:1825-1852.

has more recently been shown to be an important tool in the diagnosis of myocarditis.[143,144]

Pharmacologic management of heart failure due to myocarditis is similar to the management of heart failure from other causes. Diuretics, ACE inhibitors, and beta blockers should be prescribed. Many patients will experience significant spontaneous improvement in left ventricular function during the first 6 months after diagnosis. The use of corticosteroids and other immunosuppressive drugs is controversial. Early studies suggested a small improvement in left ventricular ejection fraction with the use of corticosteroids.[145] Other studies suggest targeting immunosuppressive drugs to patients with signs of immune activation.[146] The Myocarditis Treatment Trial showed no significant benefit with immunosuppressive therapy, although there are several procedural problems with this study.[147] We generally recommend a 1- to 3-month trial of corticosteroids and azathioprine in patients with myocarditis and left ventricular dysfunction who are not improving spontaneously after 1 to 2 months with conventional heart failure therapies or who continue to worsen acutely. If the immunosuppressive regimen produces an improvement in ejection fraction, it can then be tapered over a 6- to 12-month period.[142]

Myocarditis with acute, severe heart failure and cardiogenic shock is termed fulminant myocarditis. These patients often require treatment with intravenous vasodilators and inotropes and may be candidates for implantation of a VAD as a bridge to recovery or transplantation. When supported aggressively, most patients will recover fully with normal ventricular function, and fulminant myocarditis has a good late prognosis. Therefore, aggressive supportive therapy, including the use of VADs, is indicated, even in gravely ill patients.[148] Cardiac transplantation may be necessary for patients who do not improve.

DEVICE THERAPY: IMPLANTED CARDIOVERTER-DEFIBRILLATORS AND CARDIAC RESYNCHRONIZATION THERAPY

Sudden death is a frequent occurrence in heart failure patients, especially in patients with cardiomyopathy due to coronary artery disease. Sudden death is presumed to be due to sustained ventricular arrhythmia in the majority of cases. It is estimated that 30% of patients with heart failure and ejection fractions under 30% die suddenly. The implanted cardioverter-defibrillator (ICD) is standard therapy and is indicated for both secondary prevention of life-threatening ventricular arrhythmias as well as primary prevention of sudden cardiac death in patients with severe left ventricular systolic dysfunction. This therapy is supported by the results of several large, randomized controlled trials.

Prophylactic antiarrhythmic drug therapy aimed at preventing sudden arrhythmic cardiac death has been shown to be ineffective and may even worsen prognosis. In the Cardiac Arrhythmia Suppression Trial (CAST), patients with coronary artery disease, a history of myocardial infarction, and frequent premature ventricular contractions on baseline Holter monitoring had an increased mortality rate when treated with the antiarrhythmic drugs encainide or flecainide, despite good suppression in frequency of arrhythmia on follow-up Holter monitoring.[149] This adverse effect on mortality rate is presumed due to the known potential for these drugs to worsen arrhythmia ("proarrhythmia"). Therefore, class IA and IC antiarrhythmic drugs quinidine, procainamide, disopyramide, flecainide, and propafenone are not useful for prevention of sudden death and are contraindicated in patients with heart failure and left ventricular systolic dsyfunction.

Amiodarone was also studied for primary prevention of sudden death, as the propensity for proarrhythmia is less than with type I antiarrhythmics; 675 patients with heart failure and ejection fractions below 40% were randomized to treatment with amiodarone or placebo, with no survival difference between the two groups at 45 months.[150] There was a trend toward reducing mortality rates with amiodarone in patients with nonischemic cardiomyopathy. In another study, 1486 post–myocardial infarction patients with ejection fractions under 40% were randomized to amiodarone or placebo with no difference in mortality rates in 21 months, although there was a suggestion of a reduction in deaths due to arrhythmia.[151] Unlike the findings in CAST, there was no observed increased risk of death with amiodarone. Thus, this medication is not helpful in the prevention of sudden cardiac death, but it is considered safe for treatment of supraventricular arrhythmias in heart failure patients.

IMPLANTED CARDIOVERTER-DEFIBRILLATOR THERAPY

The ICD was compared to antiarrhythmic drugs for secondary prevention of sudden cardiac death in the AVID study. These patients had been resuscitated from cardiac arrest or survived ventricular tachycardia associated with syncope and had ejection fractions under 40%. In the study 1016 patients were randomized to receive an ICD or antiarrhythmic drugs (over 90% received amiodarone). There was a statistically improved survival rate with ICD therapy at 1, 2, and 3 years of follow-up.[152] In two other studies of similar patients, a nonsignificant reduction in rates of all-cause mortality and arrhythmic death was seen with the ICD when compared to amiodarone,[153,154] and increased mortality rate was seen with propafenone therapy (a class IC antiarrhythmic).[154] Published guidelines recommend ICDs as first-line therapy, in preference to antiarrhythmic drugs, in patients with ischemic and nonischemic cardiomyopathy who have survived a cardiac arrest or an episode of sustained ventricular tachycardia.[82]

ICD therapy has also been evaluated as primary prevention of arrhythmic death in patients with coronary heart disease and previous myocardial infarction with left ventricular dysfunction, without symptomatic clinical arrhythmias, and also in patients with nonischemic cardiomyopathy. In MADIT I, post–myocardial infarction patients with ejection fractions below 35% and asymptomatic nonsustained ventricular tachycardia on monitoring were studied with electrophysiologic testing. Patients were enrolled in this study if they had inducible ventricular tachycardia not suppressed with antiarrhythmic therapy. At 2 years of follow-up, total mortality rate was significantly reduced from 39% in the medically treated group (standard medical therapy with or without amiodarone) to 15% in the ICD group.[155] In the MUSTT study, a similar cohort of patients showed an improvement in mortality rate from 55% in patients treated with medication to 24% in patients treated with ICDs at 5 years.[156] In MADIT II, the patient population was extended to include patients with a history of myocardial infarction and ejection fractions of less than 30%. Importantly, in this study, neither ventricular arrhythmias seen on monitoring nor those induced at electrophysiologic study were necessary for inclusion. A statistically significant improvement in total mortality rate was seen in patients treated with ICDs, from 19.8% to 14.2% at 4 years[157]. It should be noted that class IV heart failure patients were not included in any of these studies.

The Sudden Cardiac Death Heart Failure Trial (SCD-HeFT) enrolled patients with functional class II and III heart failure with left ventricular ejection fractions under 35%. This study differed from MADIT I and II in that a greater number of patients (48%) had nonischemic cardiomyopathy. Primary prevention of sudden cardiac death was compared among standard heart failure pharmacologic therapy, standard therapy combined with amiodarone, and standard therapy plus an ICD. After a mean follow-up of 45.5 months, mortality rate was improved from 29% in the medical group and 28% in the amiodarone group to 22% in the ICD group, which was statistically significant. This improvement was particularly notable in class II heart failure patients.[158] Benefits of ICD therapy were seen in patients with both ischemic and nonischemic cardiomyopathy. In the DEFINITE study, the use of the ICD as primary prevention was evaluated in 458 patients with nonischemic cardiomyopathy who had ventricular arrhythmia seen on routine monitoring. After a mean follow-up of 29 months, total mortality rate was not significantly reduced (17.5% with placebo vs. 12% in ICD, $P = 0.08$) but prevention of sudden death was significantly reduced.[159] A meta-analysis of all studies in which ICDs were used as primary prevention in patients with nonischemic cardiomyopathy indicated a statistically significant 31% relative risk reduction in favor of ICDs.[160]

Thus, the approved use of ICD therapy for prevention of sudden cardiac death has been extended to prophylactic primary prevention therapy in patients with symptomatic heart failure, class II-III and left ventricular ejection fractions under 35% due to both ischemic as well as nonischemic cardiomyopathy.[82]

CARDIAC RESYNCHRONIZATION THERAPY

In many patients with heart failure, there is abnormal timing and coordination of systolic motion of the intraventricular septum and left ventricular free wall, termed dyssynchrony. This often coexists with His-Purkinje conduction system disease, with marked QRS prolongation on ECG.[161] In fact, left bundle branch block pattern with long QRS duration is associated with an increase in all-cause mortality rate in heart failure patients. Pacemaker therapies have been developed to correct left ventricular dyssynchrony, delivering timed pacing to both intraventricular septum and left ventricular free wall. This is termed biventricular pacing or cardiac resynchronization therapy (CRT). Standard dual-chamber transvenous leads are placed in the right atrium (in the absence of chronic atrial fibrillation) and right ventricle. The left ventricular free wall is paced via a third electrode passed through the coronary sinus into an epicardial lateral cardiac vein. Alternatively, a left ventricular lead can be placed directly on the epicardium of the lateral wall of the left ventricle via thoracoscopy. The pacemaker is programmed to coordinate timing of septal stimulation via the right ventricle with left ventricular lateral wall stimulation[161,162] (Fig. 29.8).

In the MIRACLE trial, 453 patients with ejection fractions under 35% and class III-IV heart failure and QRS duration greater than 130 ms were treated with standard medical therapy or resynchronization therapy plus medical therapy. At 6 months of follow-up, CRT resulted in a statistically significant improvement in 6-minute walking distance, quality of life score, and functional class, with fewer hospitalizations for recurrent heart failure.[161] No significant mortality rate improvement was noted during a relatively short follow-up period. There was an 8% rate of unsuccessful left ventricular lead placement and a 1.2% incidence of serious complications of implantation of the pacemaker device, including coronary sinus dissection or perforation. A meta-analysis of three major resynchronization trials in 1634 patients concluded that chronic resynchronization therapy was associated with a statistically significant 51% reduction in death from progressive heart failure.[163]

In the CARE-HF study, resynchronization therapy (without ICD) was evaluated in 813 patients with class III-IV heart failure due to left ventricular systolic dysfunction, with ejection fraction under 35% and QRS duration greater than 150 ms or QRS duration greater than 120 ms with signs of dyssynchrony on echocardiography. The primary end point of all-cause mortality rate plus unplanned hospitalization from cardiovascular causes was reduced from 55% in medically treated patients to 39% in resynchronization patients ($P <$ 0.001). All-cause mortality rate was reduced from 30% to 20% with resynchronization therapy ($P < 0.002$). Mean follow-up was 29.4 months. Measures of quality of life were improved, and ejection fractions improved.[164] Thus, resynchronization therapy alone, without an ICD, can reduce mortality rates as well as improve symptoms in chronic heart failure patients.

Devices combining biventricular pacing and ICD capabilities were evaluated in patients with systolic heart failure and low ejection fraction. These patients often have indications for both devices. The rationale is to decrease morbidity and mortality rates associated with progressive heart failure as well as decrease mortality rates associated with sudden life-threatening ventricular arrhythmia. Biventricular pacing does not interfere with appropriate ICD detection and termination of ventricular arrhythmias.[165] The COMPANION trial enrolled 1520 patients with advanced heart failure, functional class III-IV, in sinus rhythm, who had the ECG finding of QRS duration greater than 120 ms. Therapies compared were best pharmacologic heart failure therapy, best therapy along with biventricular pacing, and best therapy along with combination biventricular pacing and ICD. Successful implantation occurred in 87% to 91% of patients in the latter two groups, with a procedural mortality rate of 0.5% to 0.8%. The primary end points of death from any cause or hospitalization for any cause, followed over 12 months, were 68% in the drug therapy group and 56% in both device groups, a significant difference. One-year rates of death or hospitalization due to cardiovascular cause were 60% in the drug group, with a relative risk reduction of 25% in the biventricular pacing group and 28% in the biventricular pacing/ICD group. The authors concluded that there was a significant reduction in heart failure hospitalizations with biventricular pacing, and there was an additional significant reduction in mortality rate when ICD therapy was added. Improvement occurred in both patients with ischemic and those with nonischemic cardiomyopathy.[166]

CRT was then studied in class II and III heart failure patients with ejection fraction below 30%; 1798 patients with QRS duration greater than 120 ms during native conduction, or 200 ms during ventricular pacing, were treated

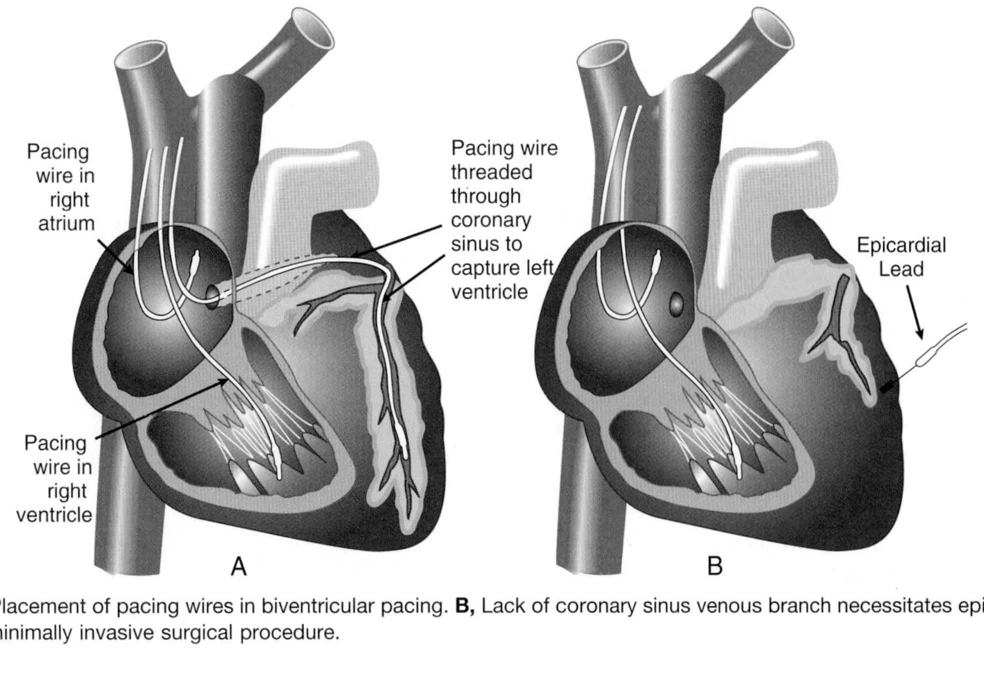

Figure 29.8 **A,** Placement of pacing wires in biventricular pacing. **B,** Lack of coronary sinus venous branch necessitates epicardial placement of third lead via minimally invasive surgical procedure.

with an ICD alone or with ICD plus CRT. At a mean follow-up of 40 months, there was a significant improvement with CRT in the primary end point of all-cause mortality rate plus hospitalization for heart failure (33.2% with CRT-ICD versus 40.3% with CRT alone, $P < 0.001$). Therefore, CRT has been successfully extended to class II heart failure patients with low ejection fraction.[167]

Currently, devices combining CRT with ICD are recommended for patients with left ventricular systolic dysfunction with ejection fraction under 35%, QRS duration 120 ms or greater on ECG, in sinus rhythm, and class II-IV heart failure symptoms despite optimal medical therapy. These devices provide both symptomatic benefit and improve survival in patients with heart failure.

MECHANICALLY ASSISTED CIRCULATORY SUPPORT: VENTRICULAR ASSIST DEVICES

It is estimated that over 100,000 patients in the United States have advanced functional class IV heart failure. These patients have a very poor short-term prognosis, even with appropriate pharmacologic and device therapy.[168] Cardiac transplantation offers an effective therapy for many patients with end-stage heart failure and is currently associated with a 1-year survival rate of over 80%. However, the pool of donor hearts is currently less than 3000 per year in the United States, and it is not increasing.[169,170] There is a role for mechanically assisted circulatory support in these patients utilizing VADs, which support or replace the function of the failing heart. VADs provide normal cardiac output and flow to vital organs.

Patients with heart failure who may benefit from VAD therapy are those with the worst prognosis, such as patients with refractory cardiogenic shock. In patients with chronic heart failure, factors that indicate a very poor prognosis include inability to wean from parenteral inotropic drugs, persistent class IV symptoms despite optimal medical and device therapy, progressive cardiorenal dysfunction precluding the use of ACE inhibitors, and hypotension preventing the use of ACE inhibitors or beta blockers.[168] Peak oxygen consumption of less than 12 mL/kg/minute on cardiopulmonary stress testing is also a poor prognostic indicator. Specific acute clinical circumstances in which VADs can be considered include cardiogenic shock following acute myocardial infarction or cardiac surgery, fulminant myocarditis, or severe postpartum cardiomyopathy.[171] A classification system to define the severity of heart failure illness and the urgency of the need for mechanically assisted circulatory support has been adopted (Fig. 29.9).

There are five clinical scenarios for the use of mechanical circulatory assistance:

1. VADs can be used as a bridge to cardiac transplantation. A mortality rate of 30% has been reported in patients listed for and awaiting heart transplantation, so VADs may enable many patients to survive to obtain transplantation.
2. VADs can be used as a "bridge to decision." These patients have urgent need for support but have severe medical conditions exacerbated by heart failure that make transplantation an initial poor option. These medical conditions may improve after a period of improved circulation with a VAD so that transplantation may become feasible.
3. VADs may be used as a bridge to definitive surgical therapy, such as in patients with severe ischemic heart disease who require coronary revascularization, which may lead to recovery of myocardial function.
4. A small minority of patients may require VAD therapy as a bridge to recovery, when improvement in cardiac function with nonsurgical approaches is expected. An example of this is patients with acute fulminant myocarditis.[148] In addition, there have been case reports of patients with subacute cardiomyopathy and severe heart failure who received VAD support for months and had improvement in left ventricular function such that the VAD was removed and patients survived without cardiac transplantation.[172] However, only 5% to 10% of patients with chronic heart disease will improve sufficiently for VAD removal.
5. Finally, current VADs have a low incidence of pump failure and can be used as long-term support, or "destination therapy."

Catheter-based pumps can be used for acute hemodynamic support and can provide cardiac output up to 3.5 L/minute.[171] These systems are implanted percutaneously and provide circulatory support for several days. The TandemHeart device (CardiacAssist, Pittsburgh, PA) requires placement of a catheter via a transatrial septal puncture. The Impella pump (Abiomed, Danvers, MA) is entirely intracorporeal and pulls blood from the left ventricle and pumps through the catheter tip in the aorta at a flow of 2.5 L/minute.[173]

The first VADs to be used were large extracorporeal devices, inserted via a midline sternotomy, that provided pulsatile flow. Because there were many moving parts, there was a high incidence of pump failure. Current VADs are smaller, are placed intracorporeally, and provide continuous, nonpulsatile flow. These have significantly improved long-term durability and are suitable for long-term support. Battery packs are small and wearable, so patients with VADs have freedom of movement and can participate in rehabilitation and normal daily activities (see Fig. 29.10). These devices do require systemic anticoagulation and antiplatelet therapy. A study comparing continuous flow VADs with pulsatile flow devices was reported in 2009; 200 patients were studied who had advanced heart failure and were ineligible for cardiac transplantation. The continuous flow device was associated with improved 2-year survival, fewer adverse events, fewer rehospitalizations, and improved quality of life. The incidence of pump failure requiring VAD replacement was reduced by 87%.[174] The Heart Mate II continuous flow VAD was approved for use in 2008 and was approved to be used as destination therapy in 2010.

A very important issue in VAD therapy is appropriate patient selection. Hemodynamic indications for use include persistent hypotension with systolic blood pressure less than 80 mm Hg, PCWP greater than 20 mm Hg, and cardiac index less than 2 L/minute/m^2 despite maximal pharmacologic support. Patient characteristics that define a worse prognosis with VAD therapy include older age, malnourishment (low albumin), renal dysfunction (i.e., serum

INTERMACS profile descriptions	Time frame for intervention
Profile 1: Critical Cardiogenic shock	
Patient with life-threatening hypotension despite rapidly escalating inotropic support, critical organ hypoperfusion, often confirmed by worsening acidosis and/or lactate levels. *"Crash and burn".*	Definitive intervention needed within hours.
Profile 2: Progressive decline	
Patient with declining function despite intravenous inotropic support, may be manifest by worsening renal function, nutritional depletion, inability to restore volume balance *"Siding on inotropes".* Also describes declining status in patients unable to tolerate inotropic therapy.	Definitive intervention needed within few days.
Profile 3: Stable but inotrope dependent	
Patient with stable blood pressure, organ function, nutrition, and symptoms on continuous intravenous inotropic support (or a temporary circulatory support device or both), but demonstrating repeated failure to wean from support due to recurrent symptomatic hypotension or renal dysfunction *"Dependent stability".*	Definitive intervention elective over a period of weeks to few months.
Profile 4: Resting symptoms	
Patient can be stabilized close to normal volume status but experiences daily symptoms of congestion at rest or during ADL. Doses of diuretics generally fluctuate at very high levels. More intensive management and surveillance strategies should be considered, which may in some cases reveal poor compliance that would compromise outcomes with any therapy. Some patients may shuttle between 4 and 5.	Definitive intervention elective over period of weeks to few months.
Profile 5: Exertion intolerant	
Comfortable at rest and with ADL but unable to engage in any other activity, living predominantly within the house. Patients are comfortable at rest without congestive symptoms but may have underlying refractory elevated volume status, often with renal dysfunction. If underlying nutritional status and organ function are marginal, patient may be more at risk than INTERMACS 4 and require definitive intervention.	Variable urgency, depends upon maintenance of nutrition, organ function, and activity.
Profile 6: Exertion limited	
Patient without evidence of fluid overload is comfortable at rest and with activities of daily living and minor activities outside the home but fatigues after the first few minutes of any meaningful activity. Attribution to cardiac limitation requires careful measurement of peak oxygen consumption, in some cases with hemodynamic monitoring to confirm severity of cardiac impairment. *"Walking wounded".*	Variable, depends upon maintenance of nutrition, organ function, and activity level.
Profile 7: Advanced NYHA II	
A placeholder for more precise specification in future, this level includes patients who are without current or recent episodes of unstable fluid balance, living comfortably with meaningful activity limited to mild physical exertion.	Transplantation or circulatory support may not currently by indicated.
Modifiers for Profiles	
TCS-Temporary Circulatory Support – can modify only patients in hospital (other devices would be INTERMACS devices) includes IABP, ECMO, TandemHeart, Levitronix, BVS 5000 or AB5000, Impella.	Possible Profiles to Modify 1,2,3 in hospital.
A-Arrhythmia – can modify any profile. Recurrent ventricular tachyarrhythmias that have recently contributed substantially to clinical compromise. This includes frequent ICD shock or requirement for external defibrillator, usually more than twice weekly.	Any profile.
FF-Frequent Flyer – can modify only outpatients, designating a patient requiring frequent emergency visits or hospitalizations for diuretics, ultrafiltration, or temporary intravenous vasoactive therapy.	3 if at home, 4,5,6. A frequent flyer would rarely be profile 7.

Figure 29.9 A classification of heart failure syndromes, with level 1 representing the most critical illness with an urgent need for mechanically assisted circulatory support. Levels 1 through 5 include patients with New York Heart Association (NYHA) class IV heart failure. Levels 5 and 6 describe patients with advanced NYHA class III heart failure. (From Stevenson LW, Pagani FD, Young JB, et al: INTERMACS profiles of advanced heart failure: The current picture. J Heart Lung Transplant 2009;28:535-541.)

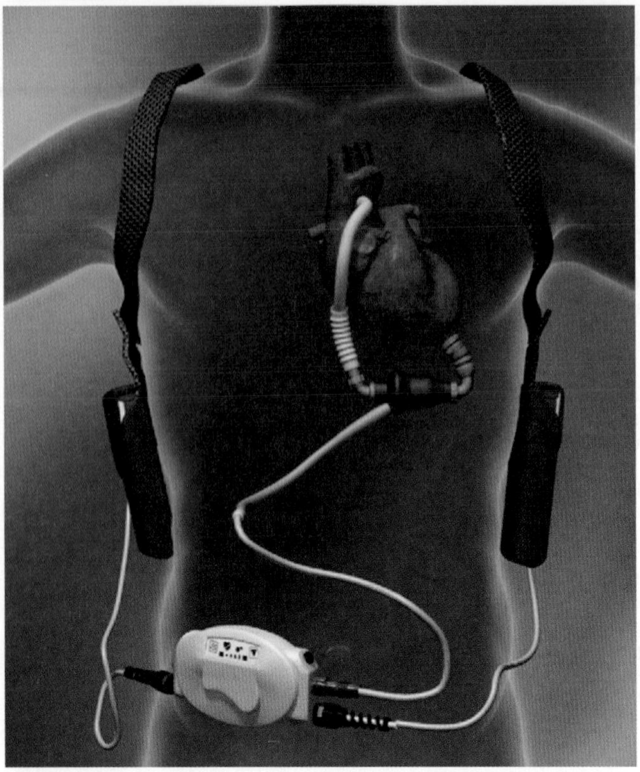

Figure 29.10 A continuous flow left ventricular assist device. The axial, continuous flow device is implanted within the chest and is attached to an external power source. (From Pagani FD, Miller LW, Russell SD, et al: Extended mechanical circulatory support with a continuous-flow rotary left ventricular assist device. J Am Coll Cardiol 2009;54:312-321.)

creatinine >3.0 mg/dL or BUN >51 mg/dL), hepatic dysfunction (elevated transaminase, bilirubin, and international normalized ratio), coagulopathy, neurologic deficits, low mean pulmonary artery pressure (reflecting right ventricular dysfunction), and anemia.[168,175] Contraindications to the use of VADs include severe chronic obstructive pulmonary disease, need for hemodialysis, aortic insufficiency, or aortic valve mechanical prosthesis.[168] Risk scores have been developed to attempt to define appropriate patient selection but need prospective validation. The major complications of VAD therapy include right ventricular failure, sepsis, thromboembolic complications including stroke, and bleeding often associated with an acquired von Willebrand factor deficiency. In patients who were deemed at lower risk, there was a 93.7% survival rate to hospital discharge and 81.2% 1-year survival rate. The highest risk patients had only 13.7% hospital survival rate and 10.7% 1-year survival rate.[175]

VADs are more frequently being used as long-term or "destination therapy." The REMATCH trial compared the pulsatile flow VAD as destination therapy with standard optimal heart failure medical therapy in 129 patients with class IV heart failure, ejection fraction less than 25%, and initial dependence on intravenous inotropes. This study showed improved survival and quality of life in patients treated with first-generation VADs. Survival rate at 1 year was 52% with a VAD as compared with 25% with medical therapy, but 2-year survival rate with VAD support was only 23% (compared with 8% for medical therapy).[176] The prognosis with current VAD technology is significantly better. In 2011, there were approximately 1500 VAD implants in the United States, virtually all of which were continuous flow devices: 23.7% were used as a bridge to transplant, 40.5% were used to determine transplant candidacy, and 34% were implanted as destination therapy. A classification system can be used to define short-term prognosis and suitability for VAD implantation[177] (see Fig. 29.9). Of patients receiving VADs, 14% had critical cardiogenic shock at the time of implant, 41.4% were failing continuous intravenous inotrope therapy, 27.7% were stable on inotrope therapy, and 12.1% had severe class IV symptoms at rest but were out of hospital. Current actuarial 1-year survival rate in all VAD recipients is 80%, with 2-year survival rate of 70%.[178]

With refinements in design and technologic improvements, long-term mechanical support of the failing left ventricle is now feasible for indefinite periods of time, especially as the incidence of infectious and thromboembolic complications are reduced. Newer VAD designs will incorporate totally implanted systems without external drive lines, which will significantly reduce the incidence of infectious complications.

KEY POINTS

- The diagnosis of heart failure is based on clinical findings and is supported by laboratory evidence, including serum natriuretic peptide levels and imaging with chest radiography and echocardiography.
- Factors that identify heart failure patients with a poorer prognosis include elevated BUN and creatinine, low systolic blood pressure, hyponatremia, markedly elevated BNP, and elevated serum troponin.
- When patients with chronic heart failure are admitted to hospital with acute decompensation, it is important to determine the reason for the acute change in status in order to attempt to reduce the risk of future episodes of decompensation and rehospitalization.
- The natural history of chronic heart failure with left ventricular systolic dysfunction involves progressive worsening of cardiac function and heart failure, which can be stabilized or improved with appropriate pharmacologic therapy, which includes beta blockers, angiotensin-converting enzyme inhibitors (or angiotensin receptor blockers), and aldosterone antagonists.
- Therapy with intravenous inotropes should be used only when heart failure is complicated by signs of systemic end-organ hypoperfusion or cardiogenic shock.
- Acute ischemia due to coronary artery disease should always be considered as a potential etiologic factor in patients presenting with acute heart failure. When ischemia is identified, aggressive revascularization therapies should be strongly considered to improve prognosis.
- Primary diastolic LV dysfunction, with normal LV systolic function, is a common cause of acute heart

KEY POINTS (Continued)

failure and is more often seen in elderly patients, hypertensive patients, and women.
- Devices that combine cardiac resynchronization ("biventricular pacing") with an internal cardioverter-defibrillator improve heart failure symptoms and improve survival in heart failure patients with low LV ejection fraction and prolonged QRS complex on ECG.
- As technology and design continue to improve, fully implanted mechanical ventricular assist devices will be used more often to support critically ill patients and will be used as long-term therapy to support patients with the most severe and refractory heart failure.

SELECTED REFERENCES

5. Chen J, Normand ST, Wang Y, Krumholz, HM: National and regional trends in heart failure hospitalization and mortality rates for Medicare beneficiaries, 1998-2008. JAMA 2011;306:1669-1678.
14. Pang, P: Acute heart failure syndromes: Initial management. Emerg Med Clin North Am 2011;29:675-688.
35. Mullens W, Abrahams Z, Francis GS, et al: Importance of venous congestion for worsening of renal function in advanced decompensated heart failure. J Am Coll Cardiol 2009;53:589-596.
51. Felker GM, Lee KL, Bull DA, et al: for the NHLBI Heart Failure Clinical Research Network: Diuretic strategies in patients with acute decompensated heart failure. N Engl J Med 2011;364:797-805.
80. Constanzo MK, Guglin ME, Saltzberg MT, et al: Ultrafiltration versus intravenous diuretics for patients hospitalized for acute decompensated heart failure. J Am Coll Cardiol 2007;49:675-683.
87. Packer M, Coats A, Fowler M, et al: Effect of carvedilol on survival in severe chronic heart failure. N Engl J Med 2001;344:1651-1658.
106. Pitt B, Zannad F, Remme W, et al: The effect of spironolactone on morbidity and mortality in patients with severe heart failure. N Engl J Med 1999;341:709-717.
134. Yancy CW, Lopatin M, Stevenson LW, et al: Clinical presentation, management, and in-hospital outcomes of patients admitted with acute decompensated heart failure with preserved systolic function. J Am Coll Cardiol 2006;47:76-84.
164. Cleland JAF, Danbert J, Erdmann E, et al: The effect of cardiac resynchronization on morbidity and mortality in heart failure. N Engl J Med 2005;352:1539-1549.
174. Slaughter MS, Rogers JG, Milano CA, et al: for the HeartMate II Investigators: Advanced heart failure treated with continuous-flow left ventricular assist device. N Engl J Med 2009;361:2241-2251.

The complete list of references can be found at www.expertconsult.com.

30 Acute Coronary Syndromes and Acute Myocardial Infarction

Steven Werns

CHAPTER OUTLINE

DEFINITIONS

Acute coronary syndrome (ACS) refers to "any constellation of clinical symptoms that are compatible with acute myocardial ischemia."[1] Therefore, the ACS spectrum encompasses unstable angina (UA), non–ST segment elevation myocardial infarction (NSTEMI), and ST segment elevation myocardial infarction (STEMI). The presence or absence in the blood of either troponin or the MB fraction of creatine kinase (CK-MB) determines the distinction between a diagnosis of either UA or myocardial infarction (MI). (For convenience, these and other relevant abbreviations are listed in Table 30.1.) An expert consensus document titled the "Third Universal Definition of Myocardial Infarction" was published in 2012 by a joint task force of the European Society of Cardiology, the American College of Cardiology Foundation (ACCF), the American Heart Association (AHA), and the World Heart Federation.[2] The clinical diagnosis of an acute MI was defined as a rise or fall of cardiac biomarkers (preferably troponin) with at least one value above the 99th percentile of the upper reference limit (URL) together with evidence of myocardial ischemia with at least one of the following: symptoms of ischemia, ECG changes indicative of new ischemia (new ST-T changes or new left bundle branch block), development of pathologic Q waves in the electrocardiogram (ECG), or imaging evidence of new loss of viable myocardium or new regional wall motion abnormality.[2] Definitions also exist for the diagnosis of an acute MI in three other circumstances: sudden death, after percutaneous coronary intervention (PCI), and after coronary artery bypass graft (CABG) surgery.[2]

The increased sensitivity of troponin compared with CK-MB and the new criteria for the diagnosis of acute MI dictate that many patients who were classified as having UA by the old criteria are now given a diagnosis of acute MI. Among 1851 patients who were enrolled in a prospective study, 538 patients received a diagnosis of acute MI based on dynamic changes in troponin T, compared with only 427 patients when CK-MB was used to diagnose acute MI, representing a 41% increase.[3] A retrospective analysis of 2181 patients with suspected ACS and no ST segment elevation found that the prevalence of acute MI ranged from 9.7% to 22% based on differing troponin-based definitions, compared with 7.8% based on CK-MB alone.[4] Meier and colleagues[5] studied 493 consecutive patients with suspected ACS. Of those, 224 patients had elevated CK-MB, and an additional 51 patients had normal CK-MB but elevated troponin I. The latter group was characterized by a greater incidence of comorbid conditions and higher 6-month mortality. Among 29,357 patients with non–ST segment elevation ACS who were enrolled in a registry called "Can Rapid Risk Stratification of Unstable Angina Patients Suppress Adverse Outcomes with Early Implementation of the ACC/AHA Guidelines?" (CRUSADE), 18% of patients were CK-MB negative and troponin positive.[6] The risk of in-hospital death was significantly increased among troponin-positive patients regardless of CK-MB status.

The Global Registry of Acute Coronary Events (GRACE) is a prospective observational registry of 26,267 patients with ACS who were admitted to 106 hospitals in 14 countries.[7] (A list of eponyms in use for various cardiac registries and drug trials is provided in Table 30.2.) Among the 10,719 patients (10.4%) with both CK-MB and troponin data, 1110 patients without elevation of CK-MB were diagnosed with acute MI by virtue of elevated troponin. Patients who were troponin negative had similar 6-month mortality regardless

Table 30.1 Cardiac Critical Care Abbreviations

ACC	American College of Cardiology
ACCF	American College of Cardiology Foundation
ACE	angiotensin-converting enzyme
ACS	acute coronary syndrome
ACT	activated clotting time
AF	atrial fibrillation
AHA	American Heart Association
APSAC	anisoylated plasminogen-streptokinase activator complex
aPTT	activated partial thromboplastin time
ARB	angiotensin receptor blocker
AVB	atrioventricular block
BMS	bare metal stent
BNP	brain natriuretic peptide
CABG	coronary artery bypass grafting
CAD	coronary artery disease
CHF	congestive heart failure
CI	confidence interval
CK-MB	MB* fraction of creatine kinase
CT	computed tomography
DES	drug-eluting stent
ECG	electrocardiogram
EF	ejection fraction
ESC	European Society of Cardiology
GP	glycoprotein
HDL	high-density lipoprotein
IABP	intra-aortic balloon pump
ICH	intracranial hemorrhage
ICU	intensive care unit
ICD	implantable cardioverter-defibrillator
INR	international normalized ratio
IRA	infarct-related artery
LAD	left anterior descending (artery)
LBBB	left bundle branch block
LDL	low-density lipoprotein
LMWH	low-molecular-weight heparin
LVEF	left ventricular ejection fraction
MI	myocardial infarction
MR	mitral regurgitation
MRI	magnetic resonance imaging
NNT	number needed to treat
NO	nitric oxide
NSAIDs	nonsteroidal anti-inflammatory drugs
NSTEMI	non-ST segment elevation myocardial infarction
NTG	nitroglycerin
PA	pulmonary artery
PCI	percutaneous coronary intervention
PCWP	pulmonary capillary wedge pressure
RCA	right coronary artery
rPA	reteplase
RVMI	right ventricular myocardial infarction
SK	streptokinase
STEMI	ST segment elevation myocardial infarction
tPA	tissue plasminogen activator
UA	unstable angina
UFH	unfractionated heparin
VF	ventricular fibrillation
VSR	ventricular septal rupture
VT	ventricular tachycardia

*Muscle-brain.

of CK-MB status, but patients who were CK-MB negative and troponin positive had a twofold greater hospital case-fatality rate.

The advent of highly sensitive troponin assays has contributed to further changes in the detection of acute MI in patients with myocardial ischemia.[8-10] Bonaca and colleagues[8] conducted a prospective study of the prognostic value of a sensitive assay for cardiac troponin I in 4513 patients with non–ST segment elevation ACS who were enrolled in a randomized trial of ranolazine versus placebo. Patients with low-level increases of serum troponin I (0.04 mcg/L to < 0.1 mcg/L) had a significantly higher risk of death at 12 months (6.4% versus 2.4%, $p = 0.005$). Another study found that implementation of a sensitive assay for troponin I in patients with suspected ACS increased the detection of MI by 29%, identified patients who were at the highest risk of recurrent MI and death, and was associated with improved clinical management that resulted in fewer deaths and admissions with recurrent MI.[9]

ST SEGMENT ELEVATION MYOCARDIAL INFARCTION

CLINICAL MANIFESTATIONS

CLINICAL HISTORY

The initial differentiation of ACS from other causes of chest pain is based on the chest pain history, physical examination, presence of risk factors for CAD, and the ECG. Certain chest pain characteristics are associated with decreased or increased likelihoods of ACS.[11] The feature that was found to be associated with the highest risk of a diagnosis of ACS is radiation of pain to one or both shoulders or arms. A prospective study of patients who presented to an emergency department for evaluation of chest pain determined that pain relief by nitroglycerin is not a useful indicator of the presence or absence of ACS.[12] Nitroglycerin relieved chest pain in 35% of patients with active CAD, compared with 41% of patients without active CAD ($p > 0.2$).[12]

Another literature review included 15 studies published from 1989 to 2002 that identified symptoms of ACS.[13] Chest pain was the most common symptom among both men and women, but atypical symptoms were common, especially among women. Compared with men, women with ACS were significantly more likely to report back and jaw pain, nausea, vomiting, dyspnea, indigestion, and palpitations. A significant fraction of patients with acute MI do not complain of chest pain at the time of presentation.[14-16] A total of 1674 U.S. hospitals contributed patients to the National Registry of Myocardial Infarction (NRMI) 2.[14] Among 434,877 patients with confirmed MI who were enrolled in the NRMI-2 registry between June 1994 and March 1998, 142,445 (33%) did not have chest pain at the time of presentation to the hospital. There were several notable differences between the groups who presented with and without chest pain. Only 23% of patients without chest pain had ST segment elevation on the initial ECG, compared with 47% of the patients with chest pain. The group of patients who presented without chest pain was older (74 versus 67 years) and had a higher proportion of women (49% versus 38%). A subsequent analysis of 1,143,513 patients who were enrolled in

Table 30.2 Cardiac Drug Trial and Registry Eponyms

4S	Scandinavian Simvastatin Survival Study
ACUITY	Acute Catheterization and Urgent Intervention Triage Strategy
AIMI	AngioJet Rheolytic Thrombectomy in Patients Undergoing Primary Angioplasty for Acute Myocardial Infarction
AIRE	Acute Infarction Ramipril Efficacy
APRICOT	Antithrombotics in the Prevention of Reocclusion in Coronary Thrombolysis
ASPECT-2	Antithrombotics in the Secondary Prevention of Events in Coronary Thrombosis-2
ASSENT	Assessment of Safety and Efficacy of a New Thrombolytic
BHAT	Beta-Blocker Heart Attack Trial
CADILLAC	Controlled Abciximab and Device Investigation to Lower Angioplasty Complications
CAPRICORN	Carvedilol Post-Infarct Survival Control in LV Dysfunction
CARE	Cholesterol and Recurrent Events Trial
CAST	Cardiac Arrhythmia Suppression Trial
CLARITY	Clopidogrel as Adjunctive Reperfusion Therapy
COMMIT	Clopidogrel and Metoprolol in Myocardial Infarction Trial
CREATE	Clinical Trial of Reviparin and Metabolic Modulation in Acute Myocardial Infarction Treatment Evaluation
CRISP AMI	Counterpulsation to Reduce Infarct Size Pre-PCI Acute Myocardial Infarction
CRUSADE	Can Rapid Risk Stratification of Unstable Angina Patients Suppress Adverse Outcomes with Early Implementation of the ACC/AHA Guidelines
CURE	Clopidogrel in Unstable Angina to Prevent Recurrent Events
DANAMI	Danish Multicenter Randomized Study on Fibrinolytic Therapy versus Acute Coronary Angioplasty for Acute Myocardial Infarction
DAVIT-II	Danish Verapamil Infarction Trial
Early ACS	The Early Glycoprotein IIb/IIIa Inhibition in Non-ST-Segment Elevation Acute Coronary Syndrome
EPHESUS	Eplerenone Post-Acute Myocardial Infarction Heart Failure Efficacy and Survival Study
EXTRACT	Enoxaparin and Thrombolysis Reperfusion for Acute Myocardial Infarction Treatment
FRISC	Fast Revascularization during Instability in Coronary Artery Disease
GISSI	Gruppo Italiano per lo Studio della Sopravvivenza nell'Infarto Miocardico
GRACE	Global Registry of Acute Coronary Events
GUSTO	Global Utilization of Streptokinase and t-PA for Occluded Coronary Arteries
HINT	Holland Interuniversity Nifedipine/Metoprolol Trial
HORIZONS-AMI	Harmonizing Outcomes With Revascularization and Stents in Acute Myocardial Infarction
ICTUS	Invasive versus Conservative Treatment in Unstable Coronary Syndromes
ISIS	International Study of Infarct Survival
LATE	Late Assessment of Thrombolytic Efficacy
LIPID	Long-Term Intervention with Pravastatin in Ischemic Disease Trial
MDPIT	Multicenter Diltiazem Postinfarction Trial
MERLIN	Middlesbrough Early Revascularization to Limit Infarction
MILIS	Multicenter Investigation of the Limitation of Infarct Size
MITI	Myocardial Infarction Triage and Intervention
NRMI	National Registry of MI
OASIS	Organization for the Assessment of Strategies for Ischemic Syndromes
OAT	Occluded Artery Trial
OPTIMAAL	Optimal Trial in Myocardial Infarction with the Angiotensin II Antagonist Losartan
PAMI	Primary Angioplasty in Myocardial Infarction
PAMI-II	Second Primary Angioplasty in Myocardial Infarction
PLATO	Study of Platelet Inhibition and Patient Outcomes
PROVE IT	Pravastatin or Atorvastatin Evaluation and Infection Therapy
PURSUIT	Platelet Glycoprotein IIb/IIIa in Unstable Angina: Receptor Suppression Using Integrilin Therapy
REACT	Rescue Angioplasty versus Conservative Treatment or Repeat Thrombolysis
RITA-3	Randomized Intervention Trial of Unstable Angina
SAVE	Survival and Ventricular Enlargement
SHOCK	Should We Emergently Revascularize Occluded Coronaries for Cardiogenic Shock?
SMILE	Survival of Myocardial Infarction Long-Term Evaluation
SWORD	Survival With Oral d-Sotalol
TACTICS	Treat Angina with Aggrastat and Determine Cost of Therapy with an Invasive or Conservative Strategy
TIMACS	Timing of Intervention in Acute Coronary Syndrome
TIMI	Thrombolysis in Myocardial Infarction
TRACE	Trandolapril Cardiac Evaluation
TRANSFER-AMI	Trial of Routine Angioplasty and Stenting after Fibrinolysis to Enhance Reperfusion in Acute Myocardial Infarction
TRITON-TIMI 38	Trial to Assess Improvements in Therapeutic Outcomes by Optimizing Platelet Inhibition with Prasugrel-Thrombolysis in Myocardial Infarction 38
VALIANT	Valsartan in Acute Myocardial Infarction
VANQWISH	Veterans Affairs Non-Q Wave Infarction Strategies in Hospital
WARIS II	Warfarin, Aspirin, Reinfarction Study

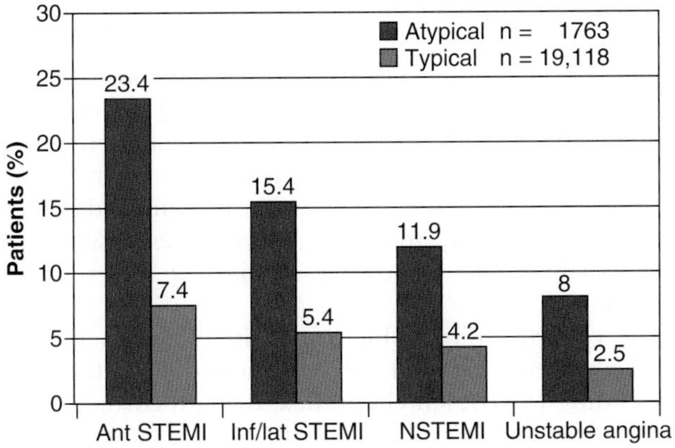

Figure 30.1 In-hospital mortality rate in subgroups with acute coronary syndrome (ACS) according to presenting symptoms. Ant, anterior; Inf/lat, inferior or lateral; NSTEMI, non-ST segment elevation myocardial infarction; STEMI, ST segment elevation myocardial infarction. (From Brieger D, Eagle KA, Goodman SG, et al: Acute coronary syndromes without chest pain, an underdiagnosed and undertreated high-risk group: Insights from the Global Registry of Acute Coronary Events. Chest 2004;126:461-469.)

the registry found that the proportion of patients who presented without chest pain was significantly higher for women than men (42% versus 30.7%; $p < 0.001$).[16] The gender differences in clinical presentation without chest pain diminished with increasing age.[16]

The absence of chest pain has a major impact on hospital management and outcomes, even among patients who present with ST segment elevation.[14-16] A report from the GRACE registry compared 6385 patients with STEMI and typical symptoms with 541 patients whose presenting symptoms did not include chest pain.[15] Patients without chest pain were significantly less likely to receive reperfusion therapy (i.e., fibrinolysis or primary PCI, β-blockers), and aspirin. Perhaps as a consequence of undertreatment, hospital mortality was significantly greater among patients with STEMI and no chest pain than among patients with chest pain (18.7% versus 6.3%; $p > 0.001$) (Fig. 30.1).

There is a longstanding belief that diabetes is associated with silent myocardial ischemia and painless MI due to autonomic neuropathy. Nevertheless, in the NRMI 2 registry, only 33% of the patients with painless MI had diabetes mellitus, and in the GRACE registry, only 32% of patients with painless ACS had diabetes.[14,15]

PHYSICAL EXAMINATION

The initial physical examination provides important prognostic information in patients with acute MI. Killip and Kimball published their classic study in 1967.[17] Among 250 patients with acute MI, 81 patients (33%) had no heart failure (Killip class I), 96 (38%) had mild heart failure (Killip class II), 26 (10%) had pulmonary edema (Killip class III), and 47 (19%) had cardiogenic shock (Killip class IV). Respective mortality rates were 6%, 17%, 38%, and 81%. Although the overall mortality for acute MI has decreased since 1967, the Killip class on admission remains a powerful predictor of outcome among patients treated with reperfusion therapy.[18,19] DeGeare and coworkers[19] performed an analysis of 2654 patients with acute MI who were enrolled in three primary angioplasty trials. Patients in Killip class IV were excluded. Increasing Killip class was associated with an increased need for intra-aortic balloon counterpulsation and a greater incidence of renal failure, major arrhythmias, and major bleeding. After controlling for confounding variables, the Killip class on admission remained a multivariate predictor of both in-hospital and 6-month mortality.

The physical examination also may provide clues to the diagnosis of causes of chest pain other than ACS. A pericardial friction rub may be audible in patients with pericarditis. Aortic dissection may be associated with diminished or absent pulses. Both diagnoses are important to exclude because they are contraindications to fibrinolytic therapy.

DIAGNOSTIC APPROACH

The American College of Cardiology Foundation/American Heart Association Task Force on Practice Guidelines has published detailed recommendations for the diagnosis and management of patients with ACS.[1,20-24] Conditions for which there is evidence, general agreement, or both that a given procedure or treatment is useful and effective are categorized as Class I[1,20] (not to be confused with Killip class I). Conditions for which there is conflicting evidence or divergence of opinion are categorized as Class II. The weight of evidence or opinion is in favor of usefulness or efficacy for Class IIa conditions, whereas usefulness or efficacy is less well established for Class IIb conditions. Class III conditions are those for which there is evidence or general agreement that a procedure/treatment is not useful or effective and may be harmful in some cases.

ELECTROCARDIOGRAM

The ACC/AHA Guidelines for the Management of Patients with ST-Elevation Myocardial Infarction include three Class I indications for an ECG.[20] The first is that all patients with chest discomfort or other symptoms suggestive of STEMI should have a 12-lead ECG within 10 minutes of arrival in the emergency department (and it should be interpreted by an experienced physician). The second is that serial ECGs should be performed at intervals of 5 to 10 minutes in patients with a nondiagnostic initial ECG if the patient remains symptomatic and there is a high clinical suspicion of STEMI. The third is that right-sided ECG leads should be obtained to screen for right ventricular MI in patients with inferior STEMI.

The electrocardiographic diagnosis of acute MI in the presence of a left bundle branch block (LBBB) is problematic.[25,26] Angiographic studies have demonstrated a low prevalence of acute MI among patients with a new LBBB.[27-30] Analysis of the Mayo Clinic's primary PCI database found that only 12 of 36 patients with a new LBBB and clinical symptoms suspicious for an MI met troponin criteria for an MI, resulting in emergency activation of the cardiac catheterization laboratory for a false-positive diagnosis of acute MI in two thirds of patients with a new LBBB.[28]

Sgarbossa and associates[31] devised an algorithm for the diagnosis of acute MI in patients with LBBB that used three electrocardiographic criteria: ≥ 1 mm ST segment elevation concordant with the QRS complex; ≥ 1 mm ST segment depression in leads V_1, V_2, or V_3; and ≥ 5 mm ST segment elevation discordant with the QRS complex. Several subsequent studies investigated the utility of the so-called Sgarbossa criteria.[26,29] A study that enrolled 83 patients with LBBB and symptoms suggestive of acute MI found that the ECG algorithm based on the Sgarbossa criteria had a sensitivity of only 10%.[26]

Patients with an acute MI who present with an LBBB that is new or of indeterminate age have a worse prognosis than patients without an LBBB. A bundle branch block was present on the admission electrocardiogram in 4% of the patients with a suspected acute MI who were included in a meta-analysis of nine trials that randomized 58,600 patients to either a control group or fibrinolytic therapy.[32] Mortality at 35 days for patients who were randomized to the control groups was greater among patients who presented with a bundle branch block (23.6%), compared with patients who had ST segment elevation in the anterior leads (16.9%) or inferior leads (8.4%), or ST segment depression 13.8%).[32] Fibrinolytic therapy was associated with a 25% reduction in mortality among patients who presented with a bundle branch block on ECG.[32] The publication did not provide information regarding the age of the bundle branch block or whether the meta-analysis was limited to patients with an LBBB or also included patients with a right bundle branch block.[32] Among 3053 patients with an acute MI who were enrolled in the Primary Angioplasty in Myocardial Infarction (PAMI) trials, an LBBB was an independent predictor of in-hospital death (odds ratio 5.53; 95% confidence interval [CI] 1.89 to 16.1; $p = 0.002$).[33]

Patients with LBBB and acute MI frequently have no chest pain at the time of presentation. Chest pain was not reported by 47% of the 29,585 patients with LBBB and acute MI who were enrolled in the National Registry of Myocardial (NRMI) 2 registry.[34] Patients who presented without chest pain were less likely to receive aspirin or a β-blocker and four times less likely to receive reperfusion therapy (odds ratio 0.25).[34] This may explain why patients with acute MI and LBBB who presented without chest pain had a 47% greater in-hospital mortality rate than patients who presented with chest pain (27% versus 18%; $p < 0.001$).[34]

A new or presumably new LBBB in patients with symptom onset within the prior 12 hours was designated as a Class I indication for either fibrinolytic therapy or primary percutaneous coronary intervention (PCI) in the guidelines for the management of acute MI that were issued by the American College of Cardiology/American Heart Association Task Force on Practice Guidelines in 2004.[20] According to the most recent revision of the practice guidelines for ST elevation MI, a new or presumably new LBBB "should not be considered diagnostic of acute MI in isolation."[24] The risks of fibrinolytic therapy may be increased in patients with LBBB due to older age and a higher prevalence of hypertension. Therefore, the most prudent strategy in patients with LBBB and a suspected acute MI may be immediate coronary angiography, both to diagnose an acute coronary artery occlusion and to eliminate the risk of fibrinolytic therapy in patients who cannot benefit from it (i.e., patients with a non–ST segment elevation MI or a non-cardiac condition). A more detailed discussion of the management of patients with LBBB and suspected MI can be found in an excellent review article that was published in 2012.[25]

The ECG provides additional important information in patients with acute MI. Patients with acute inferior STEMI who have ST segment depression in the precordial leads have larger infarctions, more complications post-MI, and a higher mortality rate than patients without precordial ST segment depression.[35] The presence of Q waves in the infarct territory on the initial ECG is an independent predictor of greater 30-day mortality irrespective of the infarct location or time between symptom onset and administration of fibrinolytic therapy.[36] Nevertheless, substantial myocardial salvage is possible despite Q waves on the initial ECG.[37]

The electrocardiographic leads with ST segment elevation have been correlated with occlusions of the left anterior descending (LAD), left circumflex, or right coronary arteries.[38,39] The number of leads with ST segment elevation before reperfusion therapy and the degree of resolution of ST segment elevation after either fibrinolytic therapy or primary angioplasty confer useful prognostic information. The Gruppo Italiano per lo Studio della Sopravvivenza nell'Infarto Miocardico (GISSI) trial investigators reported that in-hospital mortality was directly related to the number of leads with ST segment elevation for both the patients treated with streptokinase and the control group.[40] Treatment with streptokinase significantly reduced in-hospital mortality among patients with ST segment elevation in four or more leads, but not among patients with ST segment elevation that was confined to two or three leads[40] (Fig. 30.2). Early ST segment recovery is associated with improved infarct zone wall motion[41] and greater myocardial salvage as assessed by technetium-99m sestamibi scintigraphy.[42] Also, resolution of ST segment elevation within 90 minutes after either primary angioplasty or fibrinolytic therapy identifies patients with lower mortality at 30 days and 1 year and 5 years after STEMI.[43-46] Continuous ECG monitoring is customary for the detection of arrhythmias and conduction abnormalities.

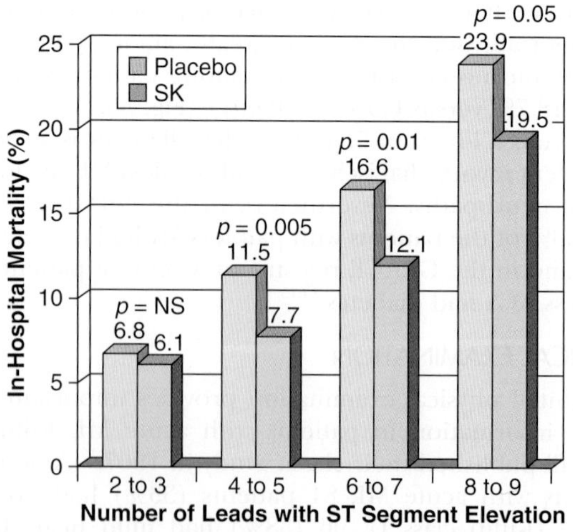

Figure 30.2 In-hospital mortality among patients randomized to the streptokinase (SK) and control groups in the Gruppo Italiano per lo Studio della Sopravvivenza nell'Infarto Miocardico (GISSI-1) trial. Treatment with streptokinase significantly reduced in-hospital mortality among patients with ST segment elevation in four or more leads, but not among patients with ST segment elevation that was confined to two or three leads. NS, not significant. (Data from Mauri F, Gasparini M, Barbonaglia L, et al: Prognostic significance of the extent of myocardial injury in acute myocardial infarction treated by streptokinase (the GISSI trial). Am J Cardiol 1989;63:1291-1295.)

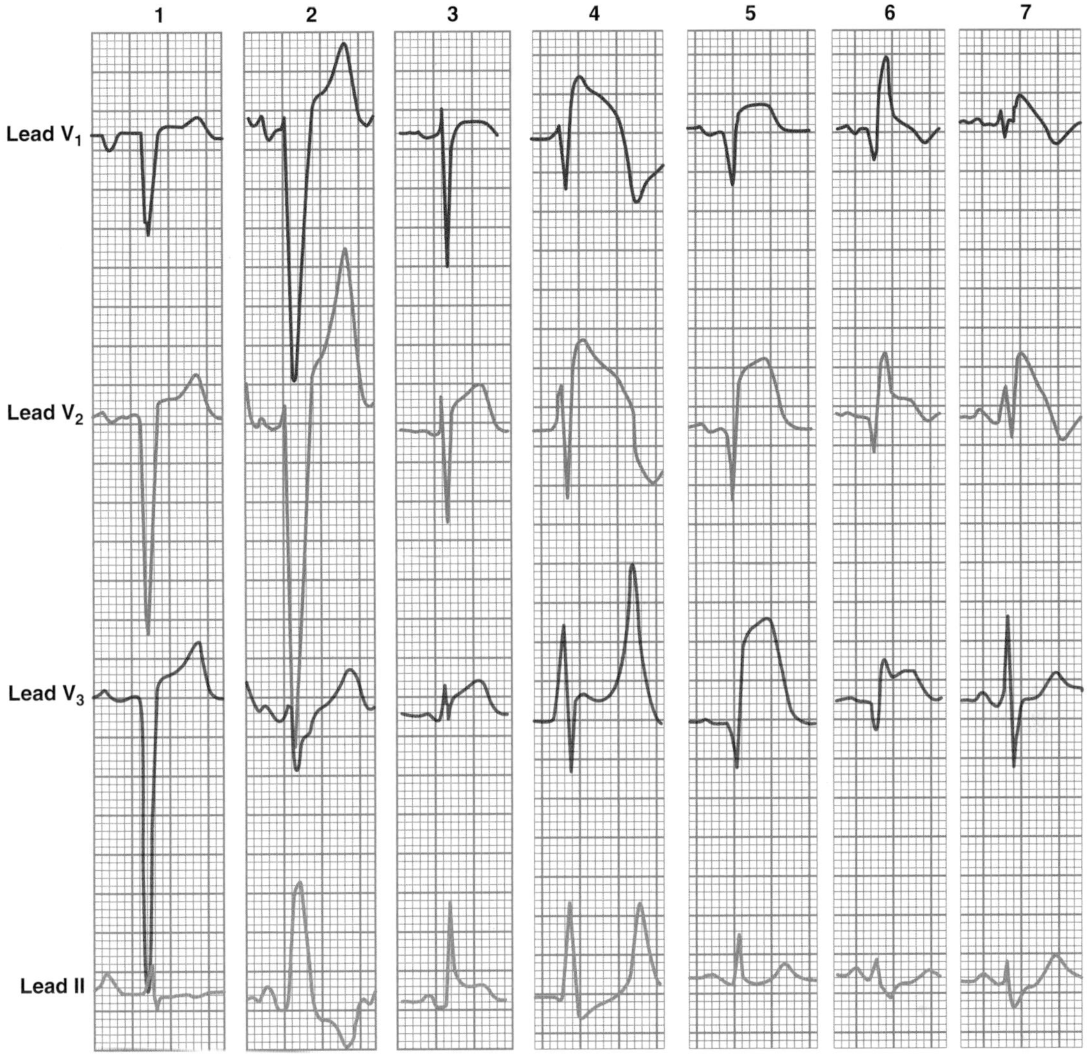

Figure 30.3 ST segment elevation in various conditions. *Tracing 1,* Left ventricular hypertrophy. *Tracing 2,* Left bundle branch block. *Tracing 3,* Acute pericarditis. *Tracing 4,* Hyperkalemia. *Tracing 5,* Acute anteroseptal infarction. *Tracing 6,* Acute anteroseptal infarction and right bundle branch block. *Tracing 7,* Brugada syndrome. (From Wang K, Asinger RW, Marriott HJ: ST segment elevation in conditions other than acute myocardial infarction. N Engl J Med 2003;349:2128-2135.)

It is important to recognize that ST segment elevation occurs in numerous conditions other than acute MI.[47] The list includes left ventricular hypertrophy, LBBB, acute pericarditis, hyperkalemia, Brugada syndrome, pulmonary embolism, and left ventricular apical ballooning syndrome (takotsubo cardiomyopathy)[47,48] (Fig. 30.3).

CARDIAC ENZYMES

Myocardial necrosis is accompanied by the release of several biochemical markers in circulating blood, including creatine kinase, myoglobin, troponins T and I, and lactate dehydrogenase. As noted previously, a typical rise and gradual fall of troponin or more rapid rise and fall of CK-MB are required to diagnose an acute, evolving, or recent MI.[2] The ACC/AHA guidelines, however, stress that decisions such as initiation of reperfusion therapy for patients with ST segment elevation and symptoms of STEMI should not be delayed until the results of serum cardiac biomarkers are available.[49]

Although troponin has become the preferred biomarker for myocardial necrosis, numerous other causes of an elevated troponin have been recognized, and several may be associated with chest pain or ST segment elevation.[50] An elevated troponin in patients with pulmonary embolism is associated with right ventricular dysfunction and an increased risk of hypotension and death.[51-53] Elevated cardiac troponin also has been reported in patients with acute pericarditis, and patients with ST segment elevation were more likely to have an elevated troponin.[54]

ECHOCARDIOGRAPHY

Echocardiography may be a useful diagnostic tool under a variety of circumstances. A transesophageal echocardiogram may be useful to differentiate STEMI from aortic dissection. Both transthoracic and transesophageal echocardiography are useful in patients with congestive heart failure (CHF) or hypotension to evaluate left and right ventricular function, to rule out cardiac tamponade, and to diagnose ventricular septal rupture or mitral regurgitation (MR). Mitral regurgitation is frequent among patients with uncomplicated MI. Color Doppler echocardiography was performed within 48 hours of admission in a series of 417 consecutive patients with acute MI.[55] Mild mitral regurgitation was present in 121 patients (29%), moderate mitral regurgitation in 21 (5%), and severe mitral regurgitation in 4 (1%).[55] Patients with any mitral regurgitation had higher 30-day and 1-year mortality rates, and mitral regurgitation was independently associated with increased 1-year mortality.[55] Echocardiography performed within 30 days after acute MI revealed mitral regurgitation in 50% of a cohort of 773 patients.[56] Cardiac auscultation did not detect a murmur in 54% of patients with mild and 31% of patients with moderate or severe mitral regurgitation.[56] Among 30-day survivors of an MI, during a mean follow-up period of 4.7 years moderate or severe mitral regurgitation detected by echocardiography within 30 days of MI was associated with a 55% increase in the relative risk (RR) of death independent of age, gender, left ventricular ejection fraction (EF), and Killip class.[56]

HEMODYNAMIC MONITORING

The value of pulmonary artery catheterization in critically ill patients has been questioned.[57] The evidence base regarding the impact of pulmonary artery catheters on outcome in patients with acute MI is limited to retrospective studies because pulmonary artery catheterization in patients with acute MI has not been evaluated in a prospective, randomized, controlled trial.[58-60] Cohen and associates[60] performed a retrospective analysis of pulmonary artery catheterization in patients with ACS who were enrolled in two large international randomized clinical trials, Global Utilization of Streptokinase and t-PA for Occluded Coronary Arteries (GUSTO) IIb and GUSTO III. The study compared the outcomes in 735 patients who received PA catheters with those in 25,702 patients who did not. Except for patients with cardiogenic shock, mortality at 30 days was significantly greater among patients who received pulmonary artery catheters, both before and after adjustment for baseline differences and subsequent events that may have prompted insertion of a pulmonary artery catheter.

According to the ACC/AHA Guidelines, the Class I indications for pulmonary artery catheter monitoring are (1) progressive hypotension that either is unresponsive to fluid administration or is developing in a patient in whom fluid administration is contraindicated and (2) a suspected mechanical complication, such as a VSD or papillary muscle rupture, if an echocardiogram has not been performed.[20] Intra-arterial pressure monitoring is recommended for patients with systolic blood pressure less than 80 mm Hg, patients with cardiogenic shock, and patients receiving vasopressor and inotropic drugs.[20]

Access site bleeding is a major risk of central line insertion in patients who have received fibrinolytic drugs. The femoral route is preferred, and noncompressible sites, such as the subclavian vein, are relatively contraindicated.

DIAGNOSTIC CARDIAC CATHETERIZATION AND CORONARY ANGIOGRAPHY

Conditions other than STEMI can cause ST segment elevation. Pericarditis, for example, is a relative contraindication to fibrinolytic therapy because of the risk of intrapericardial bleeding and tamponade. Therefore, urgent coronary angiography and primary angioplasty if indicated would be preferable to intravenous fibrinolytic therapy if there is any suspicion of pericarditis. Similarly, diagnostic cardiac catheterization should be performed if clinical findings and noninvasive studies are unable to differentiate aortic dissection from acute MI.

Right heart catheterization and contrast ventriculography can provide useful diagnostic information in patients with suspected acute MI. Measurement of right heart pressures is useful in patients with suspected right ventricular MI and in patients with hypotension. Measurement of the oxygen content of blood in the right atrium and pulmonary artery is useful in patients with a suspected VSD. A contrast left ventriculogram provides an assessment of regional and global left ventricular function and the competence of the mitral valve. Left ventriculography was performed during the index cardiac catheterization in 1976 (95%) of 2082 patients with acute MI who were enrolled in the Controlled Abciximab and Device Investigation to Lower Angioplasty Complications (CADILLAC) trial.[61] Mild mitral regurgitation was present in 192 patients (9.7%), and moderate or severe mitral regurgitation was present in 58 patients (2.9%). Mitral regurgitation was not detected by physical examination in 50% of a cohort of 50 patients with acute MI and moderately severe or severe mitral regurgitation that was demonstrated by left ventriculography.[62]

Numerous studies have addressed the role of routine early angioplasty after fibrinolytic therapy.[63-68] A prospective cohort study of 21,912 patients with a first acute MI concluded that revascularization within 14 days of the acute MI was associated with a significant reduction in 1-year mortality (RR 0.47; 95% CI 0.37 to 0.60; $p < 0.001$).[63] Several randomized trials have shown beneficial effects of a routine invasive strategy immediately after fibrinolysis,[65] within 24 hours after fibrinolysis,[66] and 1 to 6 weeks after acute MI.[67] The most recent trials have provided support for the practice of routine early angioplasty after fibrinolytic therapy.[68-70] The Trial of Routine Angioplasty and Stenting after Fibrinolysis to Enhance Reperfusion in Acute Myocardial Infarction (TRANSFER-AMI) enrolled 1059 patients with a "high-risk" STEMI who received fibrinolytic therapy at centers that did not have the capability to perform PCI.[68] The patients were randomized to either "standard" treatment (including rescue PCI or delayed angiography) or immediate transfer to another hospital for PCI within 6 hours after fibrinolysis. The primary end point—the composite of death, reinfarction, recurrent ischemia, new or worsening congestive heart failure, or cardiogenic shock within 30 days—occurred in 11% of the patients who were assigned to routine early PCI, compared with 17.2% of the patients who were assigned to standard treatment (RR 0.64; 95% CI 0.47 to 0.87; $p = 0.004$). Borgia and colleagues[69] performed a meta-analysis of seven randomized, controlled trials that compared routine early PCI after successful fibrinolysis with PCI only for patients without evidence of reperfusion (rescue PCI). After a follow-up period of 30 days routine early PCI after successful fibrinolysis reduced the rates of reinfarction (odds ratio 0.55; 95% CI 0.36 to 0.82; $p = 0.003$), the combined end point of death and reinfarction (odds ratio 0.65; 95% CI 0.49 to 0.88; $p = 0.004$), and recurrent ischemia (odds ratio 0.25; 95% CI 0.13 to 0.49; $p < 0.001$). The benefits of early PCI persisted after 6 to 12 months of follow-up. D'Souza and associates[70] performed a meta-analysis of eight randomized trials that compared routine early PCI with ischemia-driven PCI after fibrinolysis in patients with STEMI. PCI within 24 hours after fibrinolytic therapy was associated with less re-infarction and recurrent ischemia.

The 2004 and 2007 Focused Update of the ACC/AHA Guidelines for the management of patients with STEMI include five Class I recommendations, two Class IIa recommendations, and one Class IIb recommendation for coronary angiography in patients with acute MI[20,21] (Box 30.1). Coronary angiography is recommended in survivors of STEMI who are candidates for revascularization therapy with spontaneous ischemia, intermediate-risk or high-risk findings on noninvasive testing, hemodynamic or electrical instability, mechanical defects, prior revascularization, or high-risk clinical features.

APPROACH TO MANAGEMENT

Figure 30.4 presents an algorithm for the treatment of acute STEMI.

GENERAL CONSIDERATIONS

Patients who present to the emergency department with an acute MI will usually be diagnosed and treated before admission to the intensive care unit (ICU). It is not unusual, however, for STEMI to occur in patients receiving ICU treatment for other conditions, such as gastrointestinal bleeding or respiratory failure, or undergoing surgical procedures. As in the patients who present to an emergency department (ED), prompt performance and interpretation of an ECG constitute a critical initial step in management. Continuous ECG monitoring for arrhythmias is routinely practiced. Patients usually are advanced from nothing-by-mouth (NPO [*nil per os*]) status to clear liquids to a low-fat, low-cholesterol diet as tolerated. Stool softeners should be employed to prevent the hemodynamic effects of constipation.

OXYGEN

The effects of supplemental oxygen on ischemic injury was studied by Madias and colleagues.[71] Seventeen patients with acute anterior MI who were not in cardiogenic shock underwent precordial ST segment mapping before and after inhalation of 100% oxygen for 1 hour. The mean arterial partial pressure of oxygen increased from 70 mm Hg on room air to 278 mm Hg during oxygen inhalation. During oxygen inhalation there was a 16% reduction in the sum of all ST segment elevation, with reversion to baseline after oxygen was discontinued. Two hundred patients with suspected acute MI were enrolled in a double-blind, randomized trial of supplemental oxygen versus compressed air.[72] No apparent benefit was observed for oxygen therapy, and the mortality rate was higher in the oxygen group than in the control group (9/80 versus 3/77; p = NS). A meta-analysis of 3 trials that enrolled 387 patients found that the pooled relative risk of death for patients who were treated with oxygen compared to air was 2.88 (95% CI 0.88 to 9.83).[21] Hyperoxia during inhalation of high concentrations of oxygen causes an increase in coronary vascular resistance and a decrease in coronary blood flow.[73]

Although supplemental oxygen is routinely administered to patients with STEMI, according to the ACC/AHA guidelines the only Class I indication for this intervention is an

Box 30.1 ACC/AHA Practice Guidelines for Invasive Evaluation after ST Segment Elevation Myocardial Infarction (STEMI)

Class I

1. Coronary arteriography should be performed in patients with spontaneous episodes of myocardial ischemia or episodes of myocardial ischemia provoked by minimal exertion during recovery from STEMI.
2. Coronary arteriography should be performed for intermediate- or high-risk findings on noninvasive testing after STEMI.
3. Coronary arteriography should be performed if the patient is sufficiently stable before definitive therapy for a mechanical complication of STEMI, such as acute MR, VSR, pseudoaneurysm, or left ventricular aneurysm.
4. Coronary arteriography should be performed in patients with persistent hemodynamic instability.
5. Coronary arteriography should be performed in survivors of STEMI who had clinical heart failure during the acute episode but subsequently demonstrated well-preserved left ventricular function.

Class IIa

1. It is reasonable to perform coronary arteriography when STEMI is suspected to have occurred by a mechanism other than thrombotic occlusion of an atherosclerotic plaque. Such mechanisms would include coronary embolism, certain metabolic or hematologic diseases, and coronary artery spasm.
2. Coronary arteriography is reasonable in STEMI patients with any of the following: diabetes mellitus, left ventricular EF less than 0.40, CHF, prior revascularization, or life-threatening ventricular arrhythmias.

Class IIb

1. Coronary arteriography may be considered as part of an invasive strategy for risk assessment after fibrinolytic therapy or for patients not undergoing primary reperfusion.

Class III

1. Coronary arteriography should not be performed in survivors of STEMI who are thought not to be candidates for coronary revascularization.

CHF, congestive heart failure; EF, ejection fraction; MR, mitral regurgitation; VSR, ventricular septal rupture.

Modified slightly from Antman EM, Anbe DT, Armstrong PW, et al: ACC/AHA guidelines for the management of patients with ST-elevation myocardial infarction: A report of the American College of Cardiology/American Heart Association Task Force on Practice Guidelines (committee to revise the 1999 guidelines for the management of patients with acute myocardial infarction). Circulation 2004;110:e82-e292; Antman EM, Hand M, Armstrong PW, et al: 2007 focused update of the ACC/AHA 2004 guidelines for the management of patients with ST-elevation myocardial infarction: A report of the American College of Cardiology/American Heart Association Task Force on Practice Guidelines (writing group to review new evidence and update the ACC/AHA 2004 guidelines for the management of patients with ST-elevation myocardial infarction). J Am Coll Cardiol 2008;51:210-247.

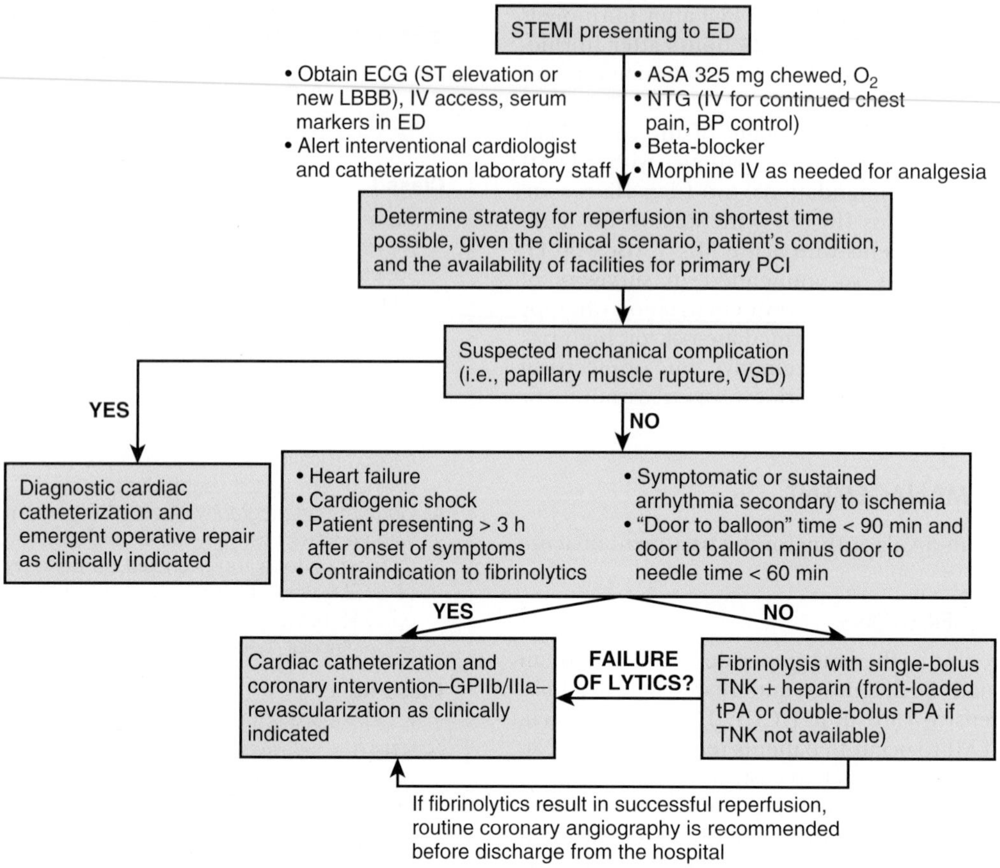

Figure 30.4 Algorithm for the treatment of acute ST segment elevation myocardial infarction (STEMI). *Note:* Nitroglycerin should be used with caution in patients with inferior wall myocardial infarction with possible right ventricular involvement. Nitroglycerin should be avoided altogether in hypotensive patients. ASA, acetylsalicylic acid (aspirin); BP, blood pressure; ECG, electrocardiogram; ED, emergency department; IV, intravenous; LBBB, left bundle branch block; MSO_4, morphine sulfate; NTG, nitroglycerin; PTCA, percutaneous transluminal coronary angioplasty; rPA, recombinant plasminogen activator (reteplase); TNK, tenecteplase; tPA, tissue plasminogen activator; VSD, ventricular septal defect.

arterial oxygen saturation less than 90%.[20] The guidelines also include a Class IIa indication: "It is reasonable to administer supplemental oxygen to all patients with uncomplicated STEMI during the first 6 hours."[20] Randomized, controlled trials of oxygen therapy in patients with STEMI are planned.[74]

ANALGESIA AND SEDATION

Relief of pain is an important goal in patients with acute MI. The 2007 Focused Update of the ACC/AHA 2004 Guidelines for the Management of Patients with ST-Elevation Myocardial Infarction included several recommendations regarding analgesic drugs.[21] According to the guidelines, morphine sulfate is the analgesic of choice for the management of pain associated with STEMI, and pain associated with STEMI is a Class I indication for intravenous morphine.[21] There are no published randomized trials of morphine therapy in patients with acute MI. An analysis of the CRUSADE registry, however, revealed that use of morphine was associated with a 50% higher mortality in patients with NSTEMI even after risk adjustment.[75] One proposed mechanism of morphine's adverse effect is opioid-induced cortisol deficiency.[76] Until additional data become available, it may be prudent to limit the use of morphine to patients with persistent pain despite treatment with nitrates and a β-adrenergic antagonist.

The abundant evidence that nonsteroidal anti-inflammatory drugs (NSAIDs) have adverse effects in patients with cardiovascular disease has been reviewed in great detail in multiple publications, including a scientific statement from the American Heart Association and a meta-analysis of 31 trials that enrolled 116,429 patients.[77-79] A Danish study of 58,432 patients who were hospitalized for a first-time acute MI between 1995 and 2002 found that treatment with either a selective cyclooxgyenase-2 inhibitor or a nonselective NSAID after discharge from the hospital significantly increased the risk of death.[80] A subsequent study by the same investigators found that even short-term treatment with NSAIDs was associated with an increased risk of death and recurrent MI in patients with a prior MI.[81] One possible explanation for the adverse cardiovascular effects of NSAIDs is inhibition of the clinical benefits of aspirin. An analysis of the Physicians' Health Study concluded that there was greater than a twofold increased risk of a first MI among healthy male U.S. physicians who were randomized to aspirin and also took other NSAIDs on > 60 days per year.[82] An important pharmacologic study demonstrated that inhibition of platelet aggregation by aspirin was blocked when ibuprofen was administered before aspirin.[83] The 2007 Focused Update of the ACC/AHA 2004 Guidelines for the Management of Patients with ST-Elevation Myocardial Infarction included two new recommendations regarding both nonselective and cyclooxygenase-2 selective NSAIDs: a Class I recommendation that patients routinely taking NSAIDs (except for aspirin) before a STEMI should have those agents discontinued at the time of presentation with STEMI; and a Class III recommendation that NSAIDs (except for aspirin) "should not be administered during hospitalization for STEMI because of the increased risk of mortality, reinfarction, hypertension, heart failure, and myocardial rupture associated with their use."[21]

NITRATES

The ability of sublingual or intravenous nitroglycerin to relieve chest pain in patients with acute MI is well documented.[84] The beneficial physiologic effects of nitrates include vasodilation of peripheral arteries and veins, causing reductions in pulmonary capillary wedge pressure (PCWP), mean arterial pressure, and peripheral vascular resistance, thereby decreasing left ventricular preload and afterload and myocardial oxygen demand.[85] Also, vasodilation of the coronary arteries may improve myocardial oxygen supply, especially in patients with a component of coronary spasm.[86] Severe hypotension and bradycardia have been observed after administration of either sublingual or intravenous nitroglycerin in patients with acute MI.[87] Patients with right ventricular MI may experience severe hypotension during administration of nitroglycerin because adequate right ventricular preload is required to maintain cardiac output. Nitroglycerin is contraindicated in patients who have taken phosphodiesterase inhibitors because they potentiate nitroglycerin-induced hypotension.[88]

There are two Class I indications for nitroglycerin in patients with STEMI. Sublingual nitroglycerin (0.4 mg) every 5 minutes for a total of three doses is recommended for relief of ischemic discomfort.[20] Intravenous nitroglycerin is indicated for relief of ongoing ischemic discomfort, control of hypertension, or management of pulmonary congestion.[20] It has been proposed that intravenous nitroglycerin may limit myocardial infarct size and expansion.[89] Two large clinical trials, however, were unable to demonstrate significant improvements in mortality by the prolonged administration of nitroglycerin after acute MI.[90,91] The GISSI-3 trial enrolled 19,394 patients with acute MI.[90] Patients who were randomized to treatment with nitroglycerin received intravenous nitroglycerin for 24 hours, followed by transdermal nitroglycerin for 6 weeks.[90] Nitroglycerin did not reduce the 6-week rate of death or clinical heart failure. The Fourth International Study of Infarct Survival (ISIS-4) enrolled 58,050 patients with suspected acute MI in a 2 × 2 × 2 factorial study that included randomization to isosorbide mononitrate 60 mg daily or placebo for 28 days.[91] No significant effect of nitroglycerin on mortality was found after 5 weeks or 1 year.

Several studies have investigated the effect of another nitrate, nitroprusside, on hemodynamics and outcome in patients with acute MI.[92-95] Intravenous nitroprusside reduced PCWP and increased cardiac index in patients with acute MI.[92,93] A comparison of intravenous nitroprusside with intravenous nitroglycerin in 10 patients with acute anterior MI demonstrated that ST segment elevation increased during infusion of nitroprusside, whereas it decreased during infusion of nitroglycerin.[92] Experimental data indicate that nitroprusside may exacerbate myocardial ischemia or injury by redistribution of myocardial blood flow from ischemic to nonischemic zones.[92] A Veterans Administration Cooperative Study enrolled 812 patients with acute MI and a PCWP greater than 12 mm Hg in a double-blind, randomized trial of nitroprusside infused for 48 hours.[95] Compared with the placebo group, mortality at 13 weeks was increased by nitroprusside in patients whose infusions started within 9 hours of the onset of pain. A smaller European trial randomized 328 patients with acute MI to infusion of nitroprusside or 5% glucose.[94] The trial was terminated when 1-week mortality in the control group was significantly greater than in the nitroprusside group (10.9% versus 3.1%; $p < 0.05$). The use of nitroprusside in patients with acute MI should probably be reserved for patients with severe hypertension that is unresponsive to treatment with intravenous nitroglycerin.

ASPIRIN

The Second International Study of Infarct Survival (ISIS-2) provided definitive evidence that aspirin reduces mortality in patients with acute MI.[96] The study used a 2 × 2 factorial design to randomize 17,187 patients to four treatment groups: streptokinase, aspirin 160 mg daily for 1 month, both, or neither. Aspirin reduced the rate of in-hospital reinfarction both in the patients who received streptokinase and in the patients who did not receive fibrinolytic therapy. At 35 days, the vascular-cause mortality rate was 9.4% among the patients in the aspirin treatment group patients, compared with 11.8% among those in the placebo group, representing a 23% reduction ($p < 0.00001$). Aspirin also significantly reduced all-cause mortality. Also, the combination of aspirin and streptokinase reduced mortality more than did either agent alone. The effects of the initial dose of aspirin on short-term outcomes after fibrinolytic therapy were tested by analyzing the outcomes of 48,422 patients with STEMI who were enrolled in two large clinical trials, Global Utilization of Streptokinase and Tissue Plasminogen Activator for Occluded Coronary Arteries (GUSTO) I and GUSTO III.[97] Compared with an initial dose of 162 mg, an initial dose of 325 mg was associated with a significant increase in moderate or severe bleeding in-hospital, but the rates of reinfarction and death at 24 hours, 7 days, and 30 days were not significantly different.[97] Nevertheless, the ACC/AHA Practice Guidelines for the Management of Patients with STEMI recommend that patients who present with acute STEMI who have not taken aspirin should receive 162 to 325 mg of non-enteric-coated aspirin, and the aspirin tablets should be chewed.[20] Also, the 2011 update of the guidelines for PCI include a Class IIa recommendation that "After PCI, it is reasonable to use 81 mg of aspirin per day in preference to higher maintenance doses."[98]

Reocclusion of a patent infarct artery after successful fibrinolytic therapy is associated with higher in-hospital mortality, reduced event-free survival after hospital discharge, and long-term impairment of regional and global left ventricular function.[99-102] There are conflicting opinions regarding aspirin's effect on reocclusion of an infarct artery.[103,104] The Antithrombotics in the Prevention of Reocclusion in Coronary Thrombolysis (APRICOT) study randomized 300 patients with an open infarct artery within 48 hours after fibrinolysis to three treatment groups: aspirin 325 mg daily, warfarin, or placebo.[105] Cardiac catheterization was performed 3 months later in 248 patients. The reocclusion rates were not significantly different: 32% (24/74) with placebo, 30% (24/81) with warfarin, and 25% (23/93) with aspirin. A pooled analysis of published studies estimated that the incidence of reocclusion after streptokinase or tissue plasminogen activator (tPA) is approximately 11% with aspirin, compared with 25% without aspirin.[103]

INHIBITORS OF THE PLATELET $P2Y_{12}$ RECEPTOR

The combination of aspirin with inhibitors of the platelet $P2Y_{12}$ receptor has been shown to be superior to aspirin alone in patients with a STEMI.[106-108] The Clopidogrel as Adjunctive Reperfusion Therapy (CLARITY) study enrolled 3491 patients who received fibrinolytic therapy for STEMI and randomized them to receive clopidogrel 75 mg daily or placebo in a double-blind fashion.[106] Coronary angiography performed at a median of 84 hours after randomization in each group demonstrated an occluded IRA in 18.4% of the placebo group patients, compared with 11.7% of the clopidogrel group patients ($p < 0.001$). PCI was performed during the index hospitalization in 1863 (53.4%) of the patients who were enrolled in the CLARITY trial.[108] The combined incidence of cardiovascular death, recurrent MI, or stroke from PCI to 30 days after randomization was significantly lower among patients who were treated with clopidogrel and aspirin compared with the patients who received aspirin alone (3.6% versus 6.2%; adjusted odds ratio 0.54; 95% CI 0.35 to 0.85; $p = 0.008$).[108] The Clopidogrel and Metoprolol in Myocardial Infarction Trial (COMMIT) randomized 45,852 patients with suspected acute MI to receive treatment with aspirin 162 mg daily plus clopidogrel 75 mg daily or placebo.[107] The in-hospital mortality rate was significantly lower for the clopidogrel group than for the placebo group (7.5% versus 8.1%; $p = 0.03$). The CLARITY study used a clopidogrel loading dose of 300 mg; the COMMIT study did not employ a loading dose.

A multivariate-weighted logistic regression analysis of the outcomes of 8429 STEMI patients who were enrolled in 26 randomized clinical trials concluded that pretreatment with a loading dose of clopidogrel before primary PCI was an independent predictor of coronary artery patency before PCI (odds ratio 1.51; 95% CI 1.31 to 1.74; $p < 0.0001$) and decreased mortality after PCI (odds ratio 0.57; 95% CI 0.38 to 0.85; $p = 0.0055$).[109] Among patients with STEMI who were enrolled in the Harmonizing Outcomes With Revascularization and Stents in Acute Myocardial Infarction (HORIZONS-AMI) trial and underwent primary PCI, a clopidogrel loading dose of 600 mg (n = 2158), compared with 300 mg (n = 1153) was associated with significantly lower 30-day rates of mortality, reinfarction, and stent thrombosis, and was an independent predictor of freedom from major adverse cardiac events at 30 days.[110]

Prasugrel, another inhibitor of the platelet $P2Y_{12}$ receptor, was studied in patients with ACS, including patients with STEMI, in the Trial to Assess Improvement in Therapeutic Outcomes by Optimizing Platelet Inhibition with Prasugrel-Thrombolysis in Myocardial Infarction (TRITON-TIMI) 38.[111,112] The trial randomized 3534 patients with STEMI who were undergoing either primary PCI (PCI within 12 hours of symptom onset) or secondary PCI (PCI between 12 hours and 14 days after symptom onset) to either prasugrel (60 mg loading dose and 10 mg/day maintenance dose) or clopidogrel (300 mg loading dose and 75 mg maintenance dose) for 6 to 15 months.[112] The primary end point of cardiovascular death, nonfatal MI, or nonfatal stroke, was significantly less frequent at both 30 days and 15 months among patients who were randomized to prasugrel compared with patients who were randomized to clopidogrel.[112]

Ticagrelor, an inhibitor of the platelet $P2Y_{12}$ receptor, was studied in patients with ACS, including patients with STEMI, in the Study of Platelet Inhibition and Patient Outcomes (PLATO).[113,114] The trial randomized 7544 patients with STEMI who were undergoing primary PCI to either ticagrelor (180 mg loading dose and 90 mg twice daily maintenance dose) or clopidogrel (300 mg loading dose and 75 mg maintenance dose) for 6 to 12 months.[114] Compared with clopidogrel, treatment with ticagrelor reduced several secondary end points, including MI (hazard ratio 0.80; $p = 0.03$), total mortality (hazard ratio 0.82; $p = 0.05$), and definite stent thrombosis (hazard ratio 0.66; $p = 0.03$); major bleeding was not significantly different (hazard ratio 0.98; $p = 0.76$).[114]

The 2007 and 2009 focused updates of the ACC/AHA Practice Guidelines for the Management of Patients with STEMI include several new recommendations regarding antiplatelet therapy (Box 30.2).[21,22] The Class I recommendations include the following: (1) clopidogrel 75 mg/day orally should be added to aspirin in patients with STEMI regardless of whether they undergo reperfusion with fibrinolytic therapy or do not receive reperfusion therapy. Treatment with clopidogrel should continue for at least 14 days. (2) A loading dose of a $P2Y_{12}$ inhibitor is recommended for STEMI patients for whom PCI is planned. The options include clopidogrel, prasugrel, and ticagrelor. Prasugrel is contraindicated in patients with a history of TIA or stroke and active pathologic bleeding. Also, prasugrel should not be administered to patients older than age 75 because of an increased risk of fatal and intracranial bleeding. Finally, the maintenance dose of prasugrel should be reduced to 5 mg daily in patients who weigh less than 60 kg.

ANTICOAGULANT THERAPY

The rationale for anticoagulant therapy in patients with STEMI includes promotion of infarct artery patency, and prevention of deep vein thrombosis, pulmonary embolism, left ventricular mural thrombus, and cerebral embolism. Left ventricular mural thrombus formation after acute MI occurs more commonly after anterior than nonanterior wall MI and is associated with an increased risk of systemic embolization.[115,116] Data conflict regarding the incidence of left ventricular thrombus in patients who receive reperfusion therapy. The GISSI-2 study, in which all patients received fibrinolytic therapy, observed left ventricular thrombi in 51 of 180 consecutive patients with a first anterior acute MI who underwent serial echocardiography within 48 hours after the onset of symptoms and before hospital discharge.[117] Another study, however, detected left ventricular thrombi in only 6.4% of patients with acute anterior MI who underwent echocardiography on days 1, 14, and 90 after MI.[118] A double-blind, randomized trial compared a 10-day course of high-dose subcutaneous UFH (12,500 units every 12 hours) with low-dose subcutaneous UFH (5000 units every 12

Box 30.2 ACC/AHA Practice Guidelines for Antiplatelet Therapy for Patients Undergoing PCI

Class I

1. Patients already taking daily aspirin therapy should take 81 mg to 325 mg before PCI.
2. Patients not on aspirin therapy should be given nonenteric aspirin 325 mg before PCI.
3. After PCI, use of aspirin should be continued indefinitely.
4. A loading dose of a $P2Y_{12}$ receptor inhibitor should be given to patients undergoing PCI with stenting. Options include the following:
   a. Clopidogrel 600 mg; the loading dose of clopidogrel for patients undergoing PCI after fibrinolytic therapy should be 300 mg within 24 hours and 600 mg more than 24 hours after receiving fibrinolytic therapy
   b. Prasugrel 60 mg
   c. Ticagrelor 180
5. The duration of $P2Y_{12}$ receptor inhibitor therapy should be as follows:
   a. In patients receiving a stent (BMS or DES) during PCI for ACS, $P2Y_{12}$ inhibitor therapy should be given for at least 12 months. Options include clopidogrel 75 mg daily, prasugrel 10 mg daily, and ticagrelor 90 mg twice daily.
6. In patients taking $P2Y_{12}$ receptor inhibitor therapy for whom CABG is planned and can be delayed, it is recommended that the drug be discontinued to allow for dissipation of the antiplatelet effect. The period of withdrawal should be at least 5 days in patients receiving clopidogrel or ticagrelor, and at least 7 days in patients receiving prasugrel, unless the need for revascularization or the net benefit of the of $P2Y_{12}$ receptor inhibitor outweighs the potential risks of excess bleeding.

Class IIa

1. After PCI, it is reasonable to use aspirin 81 mg per day in preference to higher maintenance doses.
2. If the risk of morbidity from bleeding outweighs the anticipated benefit afforded by a recommended duration of $P2Y_{12}$ inhibitor therapy after stent implantation, earlier discontinuation of $P2Y_{12}$ inhibitor therapy is reasonable.

Class IIb

1. Continuation of dual antiplatelet therapy beyond 12 months may be considered in patients undergoing DES implantation.

Class III

1. Prasugrel should not be administered to patients with a prior history of stroke or transient ischemic attack.

ACS, acute coronary syndrome; BMS, bare metal stent; CABG, coronary artery bypass graft; DES, drug-eluting stent; PCI, percutaneous coronary intervention

Modified from Levine GN, Bates ER, Blankenship JC, et al: 2011 ACCF/AHA/SCAI guideline for percutaneous coronary intervention: A report of the American College of Cardiology Foundation/American Heart Association Task Force on Practice Guidelines and the Society for Cardiovascular Angiography and Interventions. J Am Coll Cardiol 2011;58:e44-e122.

hours) in the prevention of left ventricular thrombus in 221 patients with acute anterior MI who did not receive fibrinolytic therapy.[119] Echocardiography 10 days after MI demonstrated left ventricular thrombi in 10 of 95 patients (11%) in the high-dose group and in 28 of 88 patients (32%) in the low-dose group ($p = 0.0004$). A meta-analysis of seven studies that enrolled 270 patients suggests that systemic anticoagulation in patients with mural thrombi reduces embolic complications.[115]

Clinical trials have evaluated both subcutaneous and intravenous unfractionated heparin (UFH) in patients with acute MI who were treated with various fibrinolytic agents. Randomized, controlled clinical trials have shown that adjunctive therapy with intravenous UFH increases the patency of the IRA after administration of tPA.[120,121] A meta-analysis that included 68,000 patients who were enrolled in randomized trials that compared UFH plus aspirin with aspirin alone showed that only 5 lives were saved per 1000 patients who received UFH in addition to streptokinase.[122] The meta-analysis was heavily influenced by two studies, GISSI-2[123] and ISIS-3,[124,125] that enrolled 62,067 patients who were randomly assigned to receive fibrinolytic therapy plus either aspirin alone or aspirin plus subcutaneous UFH. Another meta-analysis was limited to six randomized controlled trials that enrolled 1735 patients who received either intravenous UFH or no heparin after fibrinolytic therapy.[126] The analysis found that the addition of intravenous UFH to tPA or streptokinase had insignificant effects on mortality and reinfarction, but the risk of bleeding was significantly increased.[126]

Several randomized clinical trials[127-131] and meta-analyses[132,133] have been performed to compare low-molecular-weight heparin (LMWH) with placebo or UFH as adjuncts to fibrinolytic therapy in patients with STEMI. A meta-analysis of 16,943 patients who were enrolled in four randomized trials revealed that the end points of death or reinfarction at 7 days and at 30 days were significantly reduced by LMWH compared with placebo.[133] A meta-analysis of 7098 patients who were enrolled in six randomized trials revealed that LMWH, compared with UFH, reduced the rates of reinfarction during hospitalization and at 30 days, but the rates of death were not significantly different.[133] Neither meta-analysis included a subsequent trial, Enoxaparin and Thrombolysis Reperfusion for Acute Myocardial Infarction Treatment (ExTRACT)-TIMI 25, that compared enoxaparin, an LMWH, with UFH in patients with STEMI who received fibrinolytic therapy.[129,130] The study was a double-blind, randomized comparison of enoxaparin given subcutaneously twice daily until hospital discharge versus intravenous UFH for 48 hours in 20,506 patients with STEMI. A fibrinolytic agent was received by 99.7% of the patients: 55% received alteplase, 20% received streptokinase, 19% received tenecteplase, and 5.5% received reteplase. The primary end point, death or nonfatal recurrent MI through 30 days, occurred in 12% of patients in the UFH group and in 9.9% of patients in the enoxaparin group ($p < 0.001$). The rates of major bleeding at 30 days were 1.4% in the UFH group and 2.1% in the enoxaparin group ($p < 0.001$), but the rates of intracranial hemorrhage were not significantly different (UFH 0.7%, enoxaparin 0.8%; $p = 0.14$). The enoxaparin strategy significantly reduced the risk of nonfatal MI at 1 year (5.7% versus 6.8%;

hazard ratio 0.82; 95% CI 0.73 to 0.92; $p < 0.001$).[130] One of the mechanisms underlying the benefit of low-molecular-weight heparin compared with unfractionated heparin may be improved patency of the infarct artery after fibrinolytic therapy.[131]

Fondaparinux, a synthetic pentasaccharide, is a factor Xa inhibitor that binds antithrombin and inhibits factor Xa. The Organization for the Assessment of Strategies for Ischemic Syndromes (OASIS) conducted two trials to evaluate fondaparinux in patients with ACS[134] and STEMI.[135,136] The OASIS-6 trial was a randomized, double-blind comparison of fondaparinux 2.5 mg daily or control from days 3 through 9 in 12,092 patients with STEMI.[135] Forty-five percent of the patients received fibrinolytic therapy (streptokinase in 73%), 28.9% underwent primary PCI, and 23.7% did not receive any reperfusion therapy. The primary efficacy outcome, death or reinfarction at 30 days, was significantly lower in the fondaparinux group than in the control group (9.7% versus 11.2%; hazard ratio 0.86; 95% CI 0.77 to 0.96; $p = 0.008$). Also, fondaparinux significantly reduced the rates of death at day 9, day 30, and the end of the study (3 to 6 months). Significant heterogeneity in the effect of fondaparinux was observed in relation to the reperfusion strategy, with benefit observed in patients who received no reperfusion therapy or a fibrinolytic agent, but not in patients who underwent primary PCI. The rate of severe bleeding was not increased by fondaparinux.

A subgroup analysis of the OASIS-6 results was performed to compare the effects of fondaparinux with usual care (i.e., UFH or placebo) in patients with STEMI who did not receive any reperfusion therapy.[136] Fondaparinux significantly reduced the composite end point of death or recurrent MI, without an increase in severe bleeding or stroke, compared with UFH or placebo.[136]

The dose of fondaparinux must be adjusted in patients with renal insufficiency, but adjustment for body weight is not necessary. The anticoagulant effect of the drug cannot be monitored by conventional clotting tests, such as the activated clotting time or partial thromboplastin time. Also, the relatively long half-life of fondaparinux, 17 to 21 hours, conceivably may be viewed as an impediment to early sheath removal and ambulation after cardiac catheterization. Because of the risk of catheter thrombosis, fondaparinux should not be used as the sole anticoagulant during PCI, and an additional anticoagulant with antifactor IIa activity should be administered.[21]

Bivalirudin, a direct thrombin inhibitor, was compared with UFH plus glycoprotein IIb/IIIa inhibitors in 3602 patients with STEMI undergoing primary PCI in the HORIZONS-AMI trial.[137-139] Compared with UFH plus glycoprotein IIb/IIIa inhibitors, anticoagulation with bivalirudin was associated with a reduced rate of net adverse clinical events and major bleeding at 30 days and 1 year.[137,138] Also, treatment with bivalirudin was associated with both cardiac and all-cause mortality rates that were significantly lower after 30 days and 1 year.[137,138] Among the 477 patients who were classified as "high risk," the mortality rates at 1 year were 8.4% among patients treated with bivalirudin, compared with 15.9% among patients treated with UFH plus a glycoprotein IIb/IIIa inhibitor ($p = 0.01$).[139]

According to the updated recommendations for the use of anticoagulants as ancillary therapy to reperfusion therapy that were published in 2013,[24] "patients undergoing reperfusion with fibrinolytics should receive anticoagulant therapy for a minimum of 48 hours and preferably for the duration of the index hospitalization, up to 8 days or until revascularization if performed (regimens other than UFH are recommended if anticoagulant therapy is given for more than 48 hours because of the risk of heparin-induced thrombocytopenia with prolonged UFH treatment)." An activated partial thromboplastin time (aPTT) greater than 70 seconds during treatment with UFH was shown to be associated with a higher risk of death, stroke, and bleeding among patients who were enrolled in the GUSTO-1 trial.[140] Therefore, the ACC/AHA guidelines recommend adjustment of the dose of UFH to maintain an aPTT of 50 to 70 seconds. Also, the platelet count should be monitored daily during treatment with UFH because there is a 3% incidence of heparin-induced thrombocytopenia.[141] See Box 30.3 for recommendations regarding the doses of UFH, enoxaparin, fondaparinux, and bivalirudin.

FIBRINOLYTIC THERAPY

The dependence of myocardial necrosis on the duration of coronary occlusion was demonstrated using a canine model of MI.[142] The landmark angiographic study performed by DeWood and coworkers[143] confirmed the presence of coronary artery thrombi in patients with STEMI. Although these experimental and clinical observations provided a rationale for fibrinolytic therapy, the initial studies of fibrinolytic agents for acute MI preceded both findings. According to one review of the literature, the first reported use of fibrinolytic therapy for acute MI was in 1958.[144] By 1979, several multicenter studies of intravenous streptokinase had been performed, but the benefit of reperfusion therapy remained unproven, in part because the trial designs were flawed.[145,146]

Effect of Fibrinolysis on Survival

Four well-designed, multicenter randomized trials established that three fibrinolytic agents—streptokinase,[96,147] anisoylated plasminogen-streptokinase activator complex (APSAC) (i.e., anistreplase),[148] and tPA[149]—each reduced short-term and long-term mortality in patients with acute MI. The Fibrinolytic Therapy Trialists' Collaborative Group analyzed nine trials that randomized a total of 58,600 patients with suspected acute MI to a fibrinolytic therapy group or a control group.[150] The absolute risk of death increased with age, but absolute reductions in mortality were comparable among younger and older patients up to 75 years of age. Several trials had upper age limits for enrollment. The remaining trials enrolled 5788 patients 75 years or older and found no significant effect of fibrinolytic therapy on mortality at 35 days (25.3% for the control patients versus 24.3% for patients who received fibrinolytic therapy).[150]

The baseline ECG findings and the elapsed time between the onset of symptoms and the initiation of treatment were significant determinants of the impact of fibrinolytic therapy on mortality at 35 days[150] (Fig. 30.5). The greatest reduction in mortality was observed in patients who presented with either bundle branch block (BBB) (control 23.6% versus fibrinolytic 18.7%) or ST segment elevation in the anterior leads (control 16.9% versus fibrinolytic

Box 30.3 Dosing of Anticoagulant Drugs for Patients with STEMI

Anticoagulation to Support Primary PCI in STEMI

Class I

Bivalirudin

1. 0.75 mg/kg IV bolus, then 1.75 mg/kg/h infusion with or without prior treatment with UFH. Reduce infusion to 1 mg/kg/h with estimated creatinine clearance < 30 mL/min

UFH

1. With glycoprotein IIb/IIIa receptor antagonist planned: 50-70 U/kg IV bolus to achieve ACT 200-250 seconds
2. With no glycoprotein IIb/IIIa receptor antagonist planned: 70-100 U/kg IV bolus to achieve ACT 250-300 seconds

Anticoagulation in Patients Who Receive Fibrinolytic Therapy

Class I. Patients with STEMI undergoing reperfusion with fibrinolytic therapy should receive anticoagulant therapy for a minimum of 48 hours and preferably for the duration of the index hospitalization, up to 8 days or until revascularization if performed (regimens other than UFH are recommended if anticoagulant therapy is given for more than 48 hours because of the risk of heparin-induced thrombocytopenia with prolonged UFH treatment). Recommended regimens include the following:

a. UFH: initial intravenous bolus 60 U/kg (maximum 4000 U) followed by an intravenous infusion of 12 U/kg/hr (maximum 1000 U/hr) initially, adjusted to maintain the activated partial thromboplastin time at 1.5 to 2 times control (approximately 50 to 70 seconds)

b. Enoxaparin (provided the serum creatinine is less than 2.5 mg/dL in men and 2 mg/dL in women): for patients younger than 75 years of age, an initial 30 mg intravenous bolus, followed 15 minutes later by subcutaneous injections of 1 mg/kg every 12 hours; for patients at least 75 years of age, the initial bolus is eliminated and the subcutaneous dose is reduced to 0.75 mg/kg every 12 hours. Regardless of age, if the creatinine clearance (using the Cockroft-Gault formula) during the course of treatment is estimated to be less than 30 mL/min, the subcutaneous regimen is 1 mg/kg every 24 hours.

c. Fondaparinux (contraindicated if CrCl < 30 mL/min): initial dose 2.5 mg intravenously; subsequent subcutaneous injections of 2.5 mg daily starting the following day.

Anticoagulation in Patients Who Do Not Undergo Reperfusion Therapy

Class IIa. It is reasonable for patients with STEMI who do not undergo reperfusion therapy to be treated with anticoagulant therapy (non-UFH regimen) for the duration of the index hospitalization, up to 8 days.

ACT, activated clotting time; PCI, percutaneous coronary intervention; STEMI, ST-segment elevation myocardial infarction; UFH, unfractionated heparin

Data from Antman EM, Hand M, Armstrong PW, et al: 2007 focused update of the ACC/AHA 2004 guidelines for the management of patients with ST-elevation myocardial infarction: A report of the American College of Cardiology/American Heart Association Task Force on Practice Guidelines (writing group to review new evidence and update the ACC/AHA 2004 guidelines for the management of patients with ST-elevation myocardial infarction). J Am Coll Cardiol 2008;51:210-247; O'Gara PT, Kushner FG, Ascheim DD, et al: 2013 ACCF/AHA guidelines for the management of ST-elevation myocardial infarction: A report of the American College of Cardiology Foundation/American Heart Association Task Force on Practice Guidelines. J Am Coll Cardiol 2013;61:e78-e140.

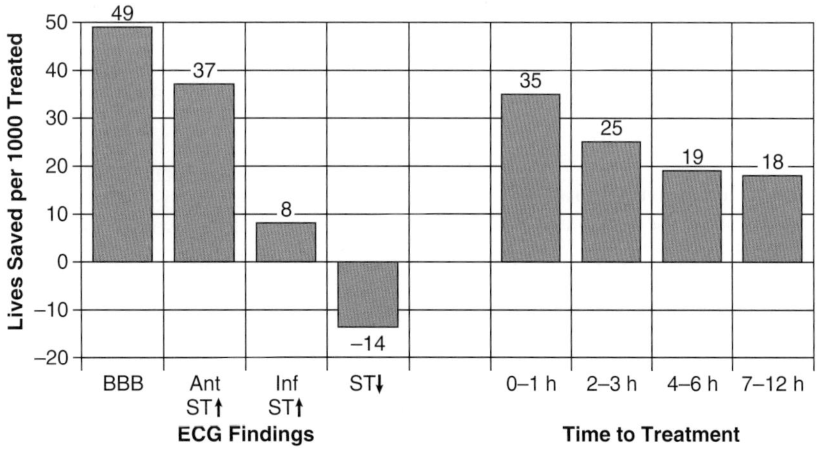

Figure 30.5 The impact of the presenting electrocardiogram (ECG) and the time to treatment on the 35-day mortality of 58,600 patients enrolled in nine randomized trials comparing streptokinase, APSAC (anistreplase), urokinase, or tissue plasminogen activator with placebo or control, expressed as the number of lives saved per 1000 patients who received fibrinolytic therapy. Ant ST, anterior ST segment elevation; APSAC, anisoylated plasminogen-streptokinase activator complex; BBB, bundle branch block; Inf ST, inferior ST segment elevation. (From Indications for fibrinolytic therapy in suspected acute myocardial infarction: Collaborative overview of early mortality and major morbidity results from all randomised trials of more than 1000 patients. Fibrinolytic Therapy Trialists' [FTT] Collaborative Group. Lancet 1994;343:311-322.)

13.2%).[150] Fibrinolytic therapy increased mortality among patients with ST segment depression on the baseline ECG.

A linear relationship between the absolute reduction in mortality and the delay from symptom onset to randomization was found among the 45,000 patients who presented with ST elevation or BBB on the ECG.[150] Fibrinolytic therapy significantly reduced mortality even among patients who received treatment 7 to 12 hours after the onset of symptoms, but patients who received treatment within the first hour after the onset of their symptoms received the greatest benefit. Patients who receive fibrinolytic therapy within the first hour after symptom onset have the greatest proportional mortality reduction,[151] as well as the highest incidence of so-called aborted MI, defined as maximal creatine kinase level up to twice the upper limit of normal and typical evolution of ECG changes.[152,153] A multicenter trial of fibrinolytic therapy reported that the baseline-adjusted mortality was significantly lower among the 13.3% of patients who had an aborted MI than among those who did not.[152]

Persistent occlusion of the IRA after acute MI is associated with left ventricular remodeling, resulting in increased left ventricular end-systolic volume, a major predictor of survival after acute MI.[154,155] Some evidence suggests that reperfusion later than 6 hours after the onset of symptoms has a favorable effect on ventricular remodeling, with less ventricular dilation observed after successful reperfusion than after no reperfusion therapy.[156,157] Several clinical trials have investigated the effects of fibrinolytic therapy on clinical events in patients who received treatment more than 6 hours after the onset of symptoms. A South American multicenter trial randomized 2080 patients within 7 to 12 hours after the onset of symptoms to receive streptokinase or placebo and found no significant difference in mortality rates in-hospital, after 35 days, and after 1 year.[158] The Late Assessment of Thrombolytic Efficacy (LATE) study randomized 5711 patients who presented with suspected acute MI between 6 and 24 hours after the onset of symptoms to receive tPA or placebo.[159] Treatment with tPA significantly reduced mortality among patients who received treatment within 12 hours of symptom onset: the 35-day mortality rate was 8.9% for the tPA group versus 11.97% for placebo, representing a relative reduction of 25.6% (95% CI 6.3% to 45%; $p = 0.0229$). Mortality at 35 days was not significantly reduced by the administration of tPA to patients who received treatment 12 to 24 hours after symptom onset.

The major causes of delayed fibrinolytic therapy for acute MI are failure of patients to seek medical care[160,161] and delays in administration of fibrinolytic therapy.[162,163] A retrospective review of data for 2409 patients hospitalized with acute MI in Minnesota in 1992 and 1993 reported that 40% of the patients delayed presentation to the hospital more than 6 hours after the onset of symptoms.[160] The ACC/AHA Practice Guidelines set a goal of initiating fibrinolytic therapy within 30 minutes of contact with the medical system.[20] Among 68,430 patients with STEMI who received fibrinolytic therapy and were enrolled in the NRMI-3 and NRMI-4 registries, only 46% of patients received a fibrinolytic drug within 30 minutes of arrival.[163] There was no significant improvement in the so-called door-to-needle time in the 1015 participating hospitals from 1999 to 2002.[163] A more recent study of 3219 patients with STEMI who received fibrinolytic therapy in 178 hospitals between 2007 and 2008 found that the "door-to-needle" time was ≤ 30 minutes in only 44.5% of patients.[164] Female gender and age > 75 were associated with longer door-to-needle times.[164] Prehospital administration of fibrinolytic therapy has been investigated as one approach to reducing the delay between symptom onset and reperfusion.[165-167] A meta-analysis of six randomized trials that compared prehospital with in-hospital fibrinolytic therapy for acute MI found that the time to fibrinolytic therapy and all-cause in-hospital mortality were significantly reduced by the prehospital administration of fibrinolytic drugs.[165]

Coronary Artery Patency after Fibrinolytic Therapy

Early angiographic studies investigated the rates of coronary reperfusion after intracoronary[168-170] or intravenous administration of fibrinolytic agents.[171] The Thrombolysis in Myocardial Infarction (TIMI) Study Group devised a grading system of coronary patency that has been adopted widely[171] (Box 30.4). Fibrinolysis was judged to be successful if an IRA that was occluded (TIMI grade 0 or 1) before treatment improved to either partial perfusion (TIMI grade 2) or complete perfusion (TIMI grade 3) 90 minutes after the fibrinolytic therapy began.[171] The first TIMI trial revealed that only 31% of occluded arteries were patent (TIMI grade 2 or 3) 90 minutes after intravenous streptokinase, compared with a 62% patency rate after a 3-hour intravenous infusion of tPA ($p < 0.001$).[172] Subsequent studies that examined the relationship between the TIMI grade flow and clinical outcome concluded that TIMI grade 3 flow, but not TIMI grade 2 flow, improves both in-hospital and long-term mortality after acute MI.[173,174] Therefore, the criteria for

Box 30.4 Definitions of Perfusion in the TIMI Trial

Grade 0 (no perfusion): There is no antegrade flow beyond the point of occlusion.

Grade 1 (penetration without perfusion): The contrast material passes beyond the area of obstruction but "hangs up" and fails to opacify the entire coronary bed distal to the obstruction for the duration of the cineangiographic filming sequence.

Grade 2 (partial perfusion): The contrast material passes across the obstruction and opacifies the coronary bed distal to the obstruction. However, the rate of entry of contrast material into the vessel distal to the obstruction or its rate of clearance from the distal bed (or both) is perceptibly slower than the rate of entry into or clearance from comparable areas not perfused by the previously occluded vessel (e.g., the opposite coronary artery or the coronary bed proximal to the obstruction).

Grade 3 (complete perfusion): Antegrade flow into the bed distal to the obstruction occurs as promptly as antegrade flow into the bed proximal to the obstruction, and clearance of contrast material from the involved bed is as rapid as clearance from an uninvolved bed in the same vessel or the opposite artery.

From Thrombolysis in Myocardial Infarction (TIMI) trial: Phase I findings. TIMI Study Group. N Engl J Med 1985;312:932-936.

evaluating fibrinolytic therapy were revised, and TIMI grade 2 flow is no longer considered a successful outcome.[175]

The GUSTO-I trial randomized 41,021 patients to four fibrinolytic strategies: streptokinase plus subcutaneous UFH, streptokinase plus intravenous UFH, accelerated tPA plus intravenous UFH, or a combination of streptokinase and tPA plus intravenous UFH.[176] Thirty-day mortality was lowest for the accelerated tPA-UFH regimen, 6.3%. A substudy of GUSTO-I included 2431 patients who underwent coronary angiography to assess patency of the IRA.[177,178] TIMI grade 3 flow was achieved 90 minutes after initiation of fibrinolytic therapy in 54% (157/292) of patients in the accelerated tPA-UFH group, compared with 31% of patients who received streptokinase plus UFH (176/576). Analysis of the relationship between patency at 90 minutes and mortality at 30 days regardless of treatment assignment revealed a significant difference between the mortality rate associated with grade 3 flow and the mortality associated with grade 0 or 1 flow (4.4% versus 8.9%; $p = 0.009$).

The relationship between time to treatment and the mortality reduction by fibrinolytic therapy may be a reflection of several factors. One is that earlier reperfusion achieves greater myocardial salvage.[179] Another factor is that time to treatment may influence the patency rate 90 minutes after administration of certain fibrinolytic drugs.[180] Patency of the IRA 90 minutes after administration of a nonfibrin-specific fibrinolytic drug, such as streptokinase, anistreplase, or urokinase, is lower when patients are first treated beyond 3 hours after the onset of symptoms than when the drugs are administered within 3 hours after onset.[172,180-182] After treatment with tPA or reteplase (rPA), fibrin-specific fibrinolytic agents, the rates of TIMI grade 3 flow are similar for patients who received treatment within 3 hours or at 3 hours or later after the onset of symptoms.[172,181,182] The time-dependent reperfusion efficacy is reflected by the rates of in-hospital mortality. A retrospective analysis of six angiographic trials that included 1174 patients found that in-hospital mortality among patients who received nonfibrin-specific drugs was twofold greater for patients treated more than 3 hours after symptom onset compared with patients treated within 3 hours.[182] Among patients who received tPA or rPA, in-hospital mortality did not differ for patients treated within 3 hours of symptom onset or later than 3 hours after symptom onset.

More sophisticated methodologies for assessing myocardial reperfusion have been devised, such as the TIMI frame count and TIMI myocardial perfusion grade.[183-185] Application of these methods demonstrated that even among patients with TIMI grade 3 flow after fibrinolytic therapy, clinical outcomes and survival are related to the speed of epicardial flow and the state of myocardial perfusion.[183,184] Therefore, a major goal of research has been to determine whether combinations of fibrinolytic and antiplatelet drugs might enhance myocardial reperfusion and achieve further reductions in mortality. Compared with full-dose tPA or rPA, a combination of a reduced dose of either tPA or rPA plus abciximab, a platelet glycoprotein IIb/IIIa (GP IIb/IIIa) inhibitor, was found to increase the rates of TIMI 3 flow at 60 and 90 minutes after administration.[186,187] Unfortunately, a difference in 30-day mortality between standard-dose rPA and half-dose rPA plus full-dose abciximab was not demonstrated by a large clinical trial, GUSTO-V, that enrolled 16,588 patients with evolving STEMI.[188]

Complications of Fibrinolytic Therapy

Intracranial hemorrhage and other hemorrhagic complications are the major risks associated with the administration of fibrinolytic therapy.[189,190] The NRMI-2 database accrued 71,073 patients who received tPA for acute MI from June 1, 1994, to September 30, 1996. Intracranial hemorrhage was confirmed by computed tomography (CT) or magnetic resonance imaging (MRI) in 625 patients (0.88%).[190] In-hospital mortality was 53%, and 25.3% of patients with intracranial hemorrhage who survived to hospital discharge had neurologic deficits. A multivariate analysis identified several risk factors that were significantly associated with an increased risk of intracranial hemorrhage: older age, female gender, systolic blood pressure greater than 140 mm Hg, diastolic blood pressure greater than 100 mm Hg, and history of stroke. An aPTT longer than 70 seconds was associated with an increased risk of hemorrhagic stroke in the GUSTO-I trial.[122] Bolus administration of fibrinolytic agents may be associated with an increased risk of intracranial hemorrhage compared with infusion.[191,192] Although phase II trials indicated a statistically nonsignificant reduction in the risk of intracranial hemorrhage, meta-analysis of phase III trials revealed a statistically significant 25% increase in the risk of intracranial hemorrhage with bolus fibrinolytic therapy.[192] According to the ACC/AHA guidelines, "The occurrence of a change in neurological status during or after reperfusion therapy, particularly within the first 24 hours after initiation of treatment, is considered to be due to intracranial hemorrhage until proven otherwise."[20] When intracranial hemorrhage is suspected, an emergency CT scan should be performed, and fibrinolytic, antiplatelet, and anticoagulant therapies should be discontinued until the diagnosis is ruled out. Cryoprecipitate or fresh frozen plasma should be given to replenish coagulation factors.[20] Protamine should be administered to patients who are receiving UFH. Neurosurgery to evacuate parenchymal hemorrhages or subdural hematomas may improve outcome.[100]

Among 40,903 patients enrolled in the GUSTO-I trial, 1.2% suffered severe bleeding, defined as bleeding that caused hemodynamic compromise that required treatment, and 11.4% experienced moderate hemorrhage, defined as bleeding that required transfusion but did not lead to hemodynamic compromise requiring intervention.[189] The most common sources of moderate and severe bleeding were procedure related. The rate of moderate or severe bleeding was 6% among patients who underwent no procedures, compared with 17% among patients who underwent coronary angiography, 43% among patients who received a PA catheter, and 50% among patients who received an intra-aortic balloon pump (IABP) or underwent coronary artery bypass surgery. Older age, lower body weight, and female sex were the three strongest independent predictors of hemorrhage. The risk of noncerebral bleeding was greater after streptokinase than after tPA, but the risk of intracranial hemorrhage was greater after tPA.

Patient Selection

The 2013 ACCF/AHA Guidelines for STEMI include one Class I indication for fibrinolytic therapy: in the absence of contraindications, fibrinolytic therapy should be given to patients with STEMI and onset of ischemic symptoms within the previous 12 hours when it is anticipated that primary PCI cannot be performed within 120 minutes of first medical contact.[24] The 2013 STEMI Guidelines also include one Class IIa recommendation for fibrinolytic therapy: in the absence of contraindications and when PCI is not available, fibrinolytic therapy is reasonable for patients with STEMI if there is clinical or ECG evidence of ongoing ischemia within 12 to 24 hours of symptom onset and a large area of myocardium at risk or hemodynamic instability.[24] There is a long list of absolute and relative contraindications to fibrinolytic therapy (Box 30.5). Special attention should be paid to factors that may increase the risk of intracranial hemorrhage, such as a history of such hemorrhage, recent closed head or facial trauma, uncontrolled hypertension, or ischemic stroke within the previous 3 months. PCI is preferable to fibrinolytic therapy in patients with an increased risk of intracranial hemorrhage. Active menstrual bleeding should not be considered a contraindication to fibrinolytic therapy.[194,195] The GUSTO-I trial included 12 menstruating women who received fibrinolytic therapy, 2 of whom required a transfusion for moderate vaginal bleeding.[195] Nontraumatic cardiopulmonary resuscitation also should not be considered a contraindication to fibrinolytic therapy.[194,196]

Box 30.5 Contraindications and Cautions for Fibrinolysis in ST Segment Elevation Myocardial Infarction

Absolute Contraindications

Any prior intracranial hemorrhage
Known structural cerebral vascular lesion (e.g., arteriovenous malformation)
Known malignant intracranial neoplasm (primary or metastatic)
Ischemic stroke within 3 months; *exception:* acute ischemic stroke within 4.5 hours
Suspected aortic dissection
Active bleeding or bleeding diathesis (excluding menses)
Significant closed head or facial trauma within 3 months
Intracranial or intraspinal surgery within 2 months
Severe uncontrolled hypertension (unresponsive to emergency therapy)
For streptokinase, prior treatment within the previous 6 months

Relative Contraindications

1. History of chronic, severe, poorly controlled hypertension
2. Severe uncontrolled hypertension on presentation (systolic blood pressure greater than 180 mm Hg or diastolic blood pressure greater than 110 mm Hg)
3. History of prior ischemic stroke more than 3 months earlier, dementia, or known intracranial pathology not covered in absolute contraindications
4. Traumatic or prolonged (beyond 10 minutes) CPR or major surgery (within 3 weeks)
5. Recent (within 2 to 4 weeks) internal bleeding
6. Noncompressible vascular punctures
7. For streptokinase/anistreplase: prior exposure (more than 5 days earlier) or prior allergic reaction to these agents
8. Pregnancy
9. Active peptic ulcer
10. Oral anticoagulant therapy

CPR, cardiopulmonary resuscitation; INR, international normalized ratio.

O'Gara PT, Kushner FG, Ascheim DD, et al: 2013 ACCF/AHA guideline for the management of ST-elevation myocardial infarction: A report of the American College of Cardiology Foundation/American Heart Association Task Force on Practice Guidelines. J Am Coll Cardiol 2013;61:e78-e140.

Increasing age is a risk factor for death and other adverse events after either primary PCI or fibrinolytic therapy for STEMI.[197] The risk of intracranial hemorrhage after fibrinolytic therapy also increases with advancing age.[190,198] Data are conflicting regarding the benefit or lack of benefit of fibrinolytic therapy in patients with STEMI who are older than 75. One analysis of a Medicare database that included 2673 patients aged 76 to 86 found that fibrinolytic therapy conferred a survival disadvantage, with a hazard ratio of 1.38 for 30-day mortality.[199] Fibrinolytic therapy was associated with a 13% reduction in the composite of 1-year mortality and cerebral bleeding in a cohort of 6891 patients 75 years and older with a first STEMI who were enrolled in a Swedish registry.[200] A study performed in the Netherlands randomized 87 patients with acute MI who were older than 75 to primary PCI or streptokinase.[201] The primary composite end point of death, reinfarction, or stroke at 30 days occurred in 4 (9%) patients in the PCI group, compared with 12 (29%) in the streptokinase group (RR 4.3, 95% CI 1.2 to 20; $p = 0.01$). After 1 year, mortality was significantly greater for the streptokinase group than for the PCI group (29% versus 11%; RR 3.4, 95% CI 1.0 to 13.5; $p = 0.03$). One caveat regarding the study is that the mean time from hospital admission to first balloon inflation was 59 ± 19 minutes (range 33 to 120 minutes)—considerably shorter than door-to-balloon times in the United States.

Many patients with acute MI have contraindications to fibrinolytic therapy or do not meet eligibility criteria for fibrinolytic therapy.[202,203] Contraindications such as recent surgery, trauma, or gastrointestinal bleeding would be relatively frequent in patients who develop an acute MI while already hospitalized for another illness. Analysis of patients with STEMI who were enrolled in the NRMI-2, -3, and -4 databases suggested that immediate mechanical reperfusion using either PCI or coronary artery bypass surgery reduced the risk of in-hospital death among patients with contraindications to fibrinolytic therapy.[204]

PERCUTANEOUS CORONARY INTERVENTION

Dr. Andreas Gruntzig performed the first balloon angioplasty of a coronary artery in 1977.[205] Dr. Peter Rentrop reported his initial experience with PCI for acute MI in 1979.[206,207] O'Neill and colleagues[208] published a randomized trial of PCI compared with intracoronary streptokinase for acute MI in 1986. The most recent meta-analysis identified 23 trials that randomly assigned a total of 7739 patients with STEMI to receive intravenous fibrinolytic therapy or undergo primary PCI, defined as PCI without previous or concomitant fibrinolytic therapy.[209] Numerous other randomized trials have been performed to investigate several other applications of PCI in patients with acute MI. Rescue PCI refers to PCI that is performed after unsuccessful fibrinolytic therapy. After successful fibrinolysis, PCI may be performed immediately, on a routine, deferred basis, or in a selective fashion (e.g., to treat inducible ischemia).

Primary Percutaneous Intervention

Myocardial salvage and long-term mortality are correlated with both the TIMI grade flow and the myocardial blush grade achieved after primary PCI for STEMI.[210-213] TIMI grade 3 flow is achieved in a high percentage of patients who undergo primary PCI for STEMI. The largest clinical trial of PCI compared with fibrinolytic therapy for acute MI was the Danish Multicenter Randomized Study on Fibrinolytic Therapy versus Acute Coronary Angioplasty in Acute Myocardial Infarction (DANAMI-2) study.[214-216] Immediate angiography was performed in 777 of the 790 (98%) patients who were randomized to undergo PCI. The initial angiogram showed TIMI grade 0 or 1 flow in 68% of patients, and grade 3 flow in 18%. PCI was attempted in 706 patients, resulting in postprocedural flow of TIMI grade 3 in 82%, grade 2 in 16%, and grade 0 or 1 in 2%. The Zwolle Myocardial Infarction Study Group reported the outcome of 1702 patients who underwent PCI for STEMI.[217] Successful PCI, defined as TIMI grade 3 flow and a residual lumen diameter less than 50%, was achieved more often during routine hours (8 a.m. to 6 p.m.) than during off-hours (6 p.m. to 8 a.m.) (96.2% versus 93.1%; $p < 0.01$).

Despite the presence of TIMI grade 3 flow, the myocardial blush grade, an indicator of myocardial perfusion, is abnormal in a majority of patients who undergo primary PCI for STEMI.[211,212] Among a cohort of 777 patients who underwent primary PCI for STEMI, normal myocardial blush (grade 3) was achieved in only 148 patients (19%), whereas 236 patients (30%) had blush grade 0 or 1.[211] Multivariate analysis showed that myocardial blush grade was an independent predictor of long-term mortality, with mortality after follow-up for 1.9 ± 1.7 years of 3% for grade 3, 6% for grade 2, and 23% for grade 0 or 1 myocardial blush ($p < 0.0001$).[211]

Distal embolization of thrombus[218] and microvascular "no reflow"[219] are two of the mechanisms of impaired myocardial perfusion after primary PCI. Distal embolization was observed in 27 of 178 patients (15%) who underwent primary PCI for STEMI.[218] Patients with distal embolization had lower left ventricular EFs at discharge from the hospital and higher long-term mortality. Microvascular obstruction detected by MRI is a prognostic marker for cardiovascular events after acute MI, even after controlling for infarct size.[219] Numerous clinical trials have been performed to investigate various mechanical methods of protecting the coronary microcirculation during PCI for ACS or acute STEMI.[220-231] Two different distal embolic protection devices, one that consists of a distal balloon occlusion and aspiration system and another that employs a filter, failed to improve myocardial reperfusion, reduce infarct size, or improve event-free survival in patients with acute MI.[224-226] A meta-analysis of 12 clinical studies concluded that the distal embolic protection devices had no significant effect on mortality.[229]

Use of the X-Sizer thrombectomy catheter (ev3, Inc., Plymouth, Minnesota) before coronary angioplasty or stenting appears to reduce distal embolization and improve epicardial flow, myocardial blush, and resolution of ST segment elevation, especially in patients with angiographic evidence of intraluminal thrombus.[220-222] The AngioJet Rheolytic Thrombectomy catheter (Possis Medical, Inc., Minneapolis, Minnesota) was evaluated in a multicenter, randomized study called the AngioJet Rheolytic Thrombectomy in Patients Undergoing Primary Angioplasty for Acute Myocardial Infarction (AIMI) study.[223] The AIMI trial randomized 480 patients within 12 hours of symptom onset of STEMI to PCI alone or PCI with adjunctive rheolytic thrombectomy. No significant differences were observed in myocardial perfusion blush or resolution of ST segment elevation. Infarct size measured by myocardial perfusion imaging was greater in the thrombectomy group, and major adverse cardiac events were more frequent in the thrombectomy group (6.7% versus 1.7%; $p = 0.01$).[223] A meta-analysis of five randomized trials concluded that adjunctive mechanical thrombectomy with either the AngioJet catheter or the X-Sizer catheter was associated with increased mortality compared with PCI alone (5.3% versus 2.8%; $p = 0.05$) in patient with acute MI.[229]

At least 16 clinical trials have been performed to test the effect of aspiration thrombectomy on clinical outcomes in patients with STEMI. The largest trial, the Thrombus Aspiration during Percutaneous Coronary Intervention in Acute Myocardial Infarction Study (TAPAS), was an open trial with a blinded evaluation of end points that randomized 1071 patients to either conventional PCI or thrombus aspiration using a 6 French aspiration catheter during PCI.[227,228] Thrombus aspiration resulted in improved myocardial blush grade and resolution of ST-segment elevation, and lower 1-year mortality.[227,228] Three of the four meta-analyses of randomized trials have concluded that adjunctive manual aspiration thrombectomy improves mortality in patients undergoing primary PCI for STEMI.[229-232] The 2009 Focused Updates of the ACC/AHA Guidelines for the Management of Patients with ST-Elevation Myocardial Infarction included a Class IIa recommendation for aspiration thrombectomy during PCI for STEMI.[22]

Abciximab, a GP IIb/IIIa inhibitor, has been reported to improve recovery of microvascular perfusion after PCI for acute MI.[233] An intracoronary bolus of abciximab reduced infarct size at 30 days by a small but significant amount in patients who underwent primary PCI for STEMI due to occlusion of the proximal or middle segments of the left anterior descending coronary artery.[234] On the basis of observations from small studies, intracoronary vasodilators, such as adenosine, frequently are employed to treat "no reflow" after PCI.[235-237]

Proponents of primary PCI and fibrinolytic therapy for acute MI have written excellent reviews of the advantages and disadvantages of both reperfusion therapies.[238,239] The evidence base supporting primary PCI for STEMI includes single-center series, multicenter randomized trials, large registries, and several meta-analyses. The Myocardial Infarction Triage and Intervention (MITI) Project Registry described a cohort of patients with acute MI who either underwent primary angioplasty (1050 patients) or received fibrinolytic therapy (2095 patients) at 19 hospitals in Seattle, Washington, between 1988 and 1994.[240] No significant difference in mortality was observed during hospitalization or long-term follow-up between the two groups. The MITI Registry included patients who received streptokinase, whereas a subsequent NRMI-2 report that was limited to patients who received tPA also found that in-hospital outcomes were similar for both methods of reperfusion.[241] Another cohort study of 20,683 Medicare beneficiaries with acute MI concluded that 30-day and 1-year mortality rates were lower among patients who underwent primary angioplasty than among patients who received fibrinolytic therapy.[242]

The DANAMI-2 trial did not show a significant difference between PCI and fibrinolytic therapy in the rates of death or stroke at 30 days, but the rate of reinfarction at 30 days was significantly lower: 1.6% for the PCI group compared with 6.3% for the fibrinolysis group ($p < 0.001$).[214] Although the 3-year mortality was not significantly different among low-risk patients, defined as a TIMI score of 0 to 4, the 3-year mortality among high-risk patients, defined as a TIMI score ≥ 5, was significantly lower for the patients who underwent PCI compared with the patients who received fibrinolytic therapy.[215] Published meta-analyses of PCI versus fibrinolytic therapy included DANAMI-2 and 22 other randomized trials.[209,243] The trials were rather heterogeneous in design: stents were used in 12 trials, GP IIb/IIIa inhibitors were used in 8 trials, and 5 trials compared fibrinolytic therapy with PCI performed after transfer from a referral hospital to a hospital that provides invasive cardiac services. The rates of short-term death, nonfatal reinfarction, stroke, and the combined end point of death, nonfatal reinfarction, and stroke were lower for PCI than fibrinolytic therapy. Another analysis pooled the individual patient 6-month follow-up data from 11 randomized trials of PCI versus fibrinolytic therapy for acute MI.[244] At 6 months, the mortality rates were 6.2% for PCI and 8.2% for fibrinolysis (RR 0.73; CI 0.55 to 0.98; $p = 0.04$). A meta-analysis of 11 randomized trials that enrolled 4320 patients with STEMI found that long-term mortality (≥ 1 year) was 24% lower among patients treated with primary PCI compared with patients treated with fibrinolytic therapy.[243] A meta-analysis of 12 observational studies that enrolled 54,571 patients with STEMI found that long-term mortality was not significantly reduced by primary PCI compared with fibrinolytic therapy.[243]

Analysis of patients enrolled in NRMI-2 showed that the in-hospital mortality was 28% lower among patients who underwent primary PCI at hospitals with the highest volume than among those who had PCI at hospitals with the lowest volume (adjusted RR 0.72; CI 0.60 to 0.87; $p < 0.001$).[245] Among 463 hospitals that performed primary PCI for STEMI and participated in NRMI-4, the hospitals with the greatest relative utilization of primary PCI, versus fibrinolytic therapy, for reperfusion had shorter door-to-balloon times and lower in-hospital mortality rates.[246] These data may have provided some of the rationale for the ACC/AHA Practice Guidelines regarding the performance of PCI for STEMI.[20] PCI should be performed in a cardiac catheterization laboratory that performs more than 200 PCI procedures per year, including at least 36 cases of primary PCI for STEMI. The operator should perform more than 75 PCI procedures per year.

Both the extent of myocardial salvage[179,247] and the mortality benefit[150,248,249] of fibrinolytic therapy and primary PCI are inversely related to the time elapsed between symptom onset and treatment. Among a cohort of 1791 patients with STEMI treated with primary PCI, the relative risk (RR) of death at 1 year increased by 7.5% for each 30-minute delay.[250] Several studies have analyzed the relationship between mortality and the so-called door-to-balloon time, defined as the duration of time between arrival at the hospital and the first balloon inflation.[249,251-253] Although some studies found that in-hospital mortality was not related to the door-to-balloon time,[251] most studies have shown that both in-hospital and late mortality are higher when door-to-balloon time is longer.[249,252,253] Among 2082 patients with acute MI who were enrolled in the CADILLAC trial, door-to-balloon time was an independent predictor of 1-year mortality in patients who presented within 2 hours after the onset of symptoms (n = 965; hazard ratio 1.24; 95% CI 1.05 to 1.46; $p = 0.013$), but not in patients who presented later than 2 hours (n = 944; hazard ratio 0.88; 95% CI 0.67 to 1.15; $p = 0.33$).[254]

The ACC/AHA Practice Guidelines set a goal of balloon inflation within 90 minutes of presentation, but observational studies indicate that this goal is seldom achieved.[163,255] Among 33,647 patients with STEMI who underwent primary PCI between 1999 and 2002 and were enrolled in the NRMI-3 and NRMI-4 registries, only 35% of patients received treatment within 90 minutes of arrival.[163] Krumholz and colleagues[256] analyzed the door-to-balloon times reported by hospitals to the Centers for Medicare & Medicaid Services from January 1, 2005, through September 30, 2010. Door-to-balloon time decreased from a median of 96 minutes in 2005 to a median of 64 minutes during the first three quarters of 2010.[256] The percentage of patients who had door-to-balloon times < 90 minutes increased from 44.2% to 91.4%.[256]

The time of day and day of week had significant effects on door-to-balloon times among 33,647 patients with STEMI who underwent primary PCI between 1999 and 2002 and were enrolled in the NRMI-3 and NRMI-4 registries.[257] Fifty-four percent of patients who underwent primary PCI were treated during off-hours (weekdays, 5 p.m. to 7 a.m. and weekends). Door-to-balloon times exceeded 90 minutes in 74% of patients who underwent PCI during off-hours, compared with 53% of patients treated during regular hours (weekdays, 7 a.m. to 5 p.m.) ($p < 0.001$). Treatment delays are far greater among patients who are transferred to another hospital to undergo primary PCI.[255] Among 4278 patients who underwent interhospital transfer for primary PCI during the period 1999 to 2002, the median total door-to-balloon time was 180 minutes.[255] Only 4.2% of patients underwent PCI within the benchmark of 90 minutes.[255] Analysis of 23 randomized trials that compared primary PCI with fibrinolytic therapy for STEMI indicated that PCI affords a mortality advantage only if the door-to-balloon time exceeds the door-to-needle time by less than 1 hour.[258]

Several approaches have been suggested to reduce the delay between symptom onset and reperfusion in patients treated by primary PCI. One approach that has been tested is performance of primary PCI at hospitals that have cardiac catheterization laboratories but lack on-site cardiac surgery.[259,260] One trial randomized patients with STEMI to undergo primary PCI (n = 225) or receive accelerated tPA (n = 226) at 11 community hospitals without on-site cardiac surgery.[260] The composite end point of death, recurrent MI, and stroke was significantly lower among patients treated with primary PCI than among those who received tPA, both 6 weeks after MI (10.7% versus 17.7%; $p = 0.03$) and 6 months after MI (12.4% versus 19.9%; $p = 0.03$). A subsequent study by the NRMI investigators compared the outcomes of 58,821 patients with STEMI who presented to 214 hospitals with on-site cardiac surgery with the outcomes of patients who presented to 52 hospitals without on-site cardiac surgery.[261] The patients who presented to hospitals without on-site cardiac surgery were less likely to receive guideline-recommended medications within 24 hours, and they were less likely to undergo acute reperfusion therapy, but there was no difference in mortality among patients who underwent primary PCI.[261] A meta-analysis of 11 studies that included 124,074 patients who underwent primary PCI for STEMI found that the in-hospital mortality for patients at hospitals without on-site cardiac surgery was not different from hospitals having on-site surgery (odds ratio, 0.96; 95% CI 0.88 to 1.05).[262] Another proposed strategy to reduce the delay between symptom onset and reperfusion is the diversion of patients with acute MI to a primary PCI hospital, instead of the current practice of transporting patients to the nearest emergency department.[238] A survey of 365 hospitals identified six strategies that were significantly associated with a faster door-to-balloon time.[263] The use of prehospital ECGs to diagnose and triage patients with a suspected STEMI is associated with a greater use of reperfusion therapy and shorter door-to-needle and door-to-balloon times.[264]

Late reocclusion after successful primary angioplasty is associated with decreased long-term survival.[265] The CADILLAC trial randomized 2082 patients with acute MI to undergo percutaneous transluminal coronary angioplasty (PTCA) or stenting.[266] Although stenting did not improve the myocardial blush score,[267] the angiographic rates of reocclusion of the IRA at 7 months was 5.7% after coronary stenting, compared with 11.3% after PTCA.[266]

At least 15 randomized clinical trials and at least 5 observational studies, plus numerous meta-analyses of those studies, have been performed to compare drug-eluting stents (DES) with bare metal stents (BMS) in patients with STEMI. The largest randomized trial enrolled 3006 patients with STEMI and found that compared with BMS, paclitaxel-eluting stents reduced angiographic evidence of restenosis and repeat revascularization for recurrent ischemia, without increasing the risk of stent thrombosis or death at 12 months.[268] Among 7217 patients who underwent PCI with stenting for acute MI in Massachusetts between April 1, 2003, and September 30, 2004, treatment with DES, compared with BMS, was associated with decreased rates of 2-year mortality and need for repeat revascularization.[269] On the other hand, the multinational GRACE registry reported that mortality from either 6 months to 2 years or from 1 to 2 years was significantly greater among 5093 STEMI patients who received DES, compared with BMS.[270] A meta-analysis of five observational studies found that STEMI patients treated with DES had a significantly lower mortality compared with patients who received BMS (odds ratio 0.65; 95% CI 0.53 to 0.80; $p < 0.001$).[271] A meta-analysis of 15 randomized, controlled trials that enrolled a total of 7867 STEMI patients concluded that compared with a BMS, a DES was associated with a reduction in target vessel revascularization, but an increased risk of very late stent thrombosis (> 1 year after PCI).[272] The apparent increased risk of very late stent thrombosis is consistent with both post-mortem and in vivo evidence of higher rates of incomplete stent apposition and uncovered stent struts among STEMI patients treated with DES compared with BMS.[273,274] Nevertheless, the 2009 Focused Updates of the ACC/AHA STEMI and PCI guidelines include a Class IIa recommendation that "It is reasonable to use a DES as an alternative to a BMS for primary PCI in STEMI."[22]

Rescue Percutaneous Coronary Intervention

Compared with TIMI grade 3 flow, TIMI grade 0 or 1 flow at 90 minutes after fibrinolytic therapy is associated with worse left ventricular function and increased mortality rates.[177,178] Compared with complete resolution of ST segment elevation, incomplete resolution of ST segment elevation after fibrinolytic therapy is associated with larger infarct size and greater short-term and long-term mortality.[42,44,275] Therefore, various angiographic or electrocardiographic criteria have been employed to define unsuccessful fibrinolysis and rescue PCI. A report from the TIMI 10B and TIMI 14 trials of fibrinolytic therapy defined rescue PCI as PCI performed between 90 and 150 minutes after the start of therapy for patients with TIMI 0 or 1 flow 90 minutes after the start of therapy.[276] The Middlesbrough Early Revascularization to Limit Infarction (MERLIN) trial defined failed fibrinolytic therapy as failure of the ST segment elevation in the worst lead to have resolved by 50% 60 minutes after the onset of fibrinolytic therapy.[277] The Rescue Angioplasty versus Conservative Treatment or Repeat Thrombolysis (REACT) trial's definition of rescue PCI was PCI performed within 12 hours after failed fibrinolytic therapy, defined as an ECG obtained 90 minutes after the start of fibrinolytic therapy that showed < 50% resolution of the ST segment in the lead showing the greatest ST segment elevation.[278] Thus, many of the patients who underwent PCI in the REACT trial would meet the TIMI group's definition of either adjunctive PCI, defined as PCI for patients with TIMI grade 2 or 3 flow, or delayed PCI, defined as PCI longer than 150 minutes after fibrinolytic therapy, rather than rescue PCI as defined by the TIMI group and other investigators.[276] Among patients enrolled in the TIMI 10B and 14 trials, the rate of TIMI grade 3 flow was significantly greater after adjunctive PCI than after rescue PCI (89% versus 78%, $p = 0.001$),[276] which might account for the REACT trial's 98% (106 of 108 patients) success rate for rescue PCI.[278]

There is conflicting information regarding the impact of rescue PCI on mortality. Among 150 patients who were enrolled in the TIMI 10B trial and had TIMI 0 or 1 flow 90 minutes after fibrinolytic therapy, 2-year mortality was significantly less among the patients who underwent rescue PCI (n = 120) than among those who did not (n = 30) ($p = 0.03$).[279] The randomized trials that compared rescue PCI with conservative therapy were insufficiently powered to detect an effect on mortality. Although differences in trial design and the definition of rescue PCI make it somewhat difficult to compare the results of various trials, at least two meta-analyses of the randomized trials have been published.[280,281] A pooled analysis of the short-term mortality (in-hospital or 30-day) among 942 patients who were enrolled in five randomized trials revealed that the risk of death was 36% lower among patients who were randomized to PCI (RR 0.64, 95% CI 0.41 to 1.00, $p = 0.048$).[280] Another meta-analysis included six trials that randomized 908 patients to rescue PCI or conservative therapy.[281] Rescue PCI was not associated with a reduction in all-cause mortality at 6 months (RR 0.69; 95% CI 0.46 to 01.05), but it was associated with significant reductions in the risk of heart failure and reinfarction, and an increased risk of stroke and minor bleeding.[281]

Perhaps as a result of the varying definitions used to define rescue PCI, the term *rescue PCI* was not employed in the 2009 Focused Updates of the STEMI and PCI practice guidelines.[22] Based on the results of the TRANSFER-AMI study, the guidelines recommend that high-risk STEMI patients who receive fibrinolytic therapy at a non-PCI-capable facility should be transferred immediately to a PCI-capable facility for diagnostic cardiac catheterization and PCI if appropriate. High-risk patients are defined as ≥ 2 mm of ST segment elevation in two anterior leads, or ≥ 1 mm ST segment elevation in inferior leads with at least one of the following: systolic blood pressure < 100 mm Hg, heart rate > 100/min, Killip class II or III, ≥ 2 mm of ST segment depression in the anterior leads, or ≥ 1 mm of ST segment elevation in right-sided lead V4 indicative of right ventricular involvement.[22]

SELECTION OF REPERFUSION STRATEGY

There is evidence that reperfusion therapy is underutilized in the United States.[282] The NRMI-2 registry included 84,663 patients with STEMI who presented to the hospital with diagnostic ECG changes on the initial ECG within 6 hours after symptom onset, and without contraindications to fibrinolytic therapy.[282] Despite their eligibility to receive reperfusion therapy, 24% received none (i.e., neither fibrinolytic therapy nor PCI). Age older than 75 years, female gender, lack of chest pain at presentation, and LBBB were independent predictors of failure to receive reperfusion therapy. Among patients enrolled in the NRMI-2 registry, patients in Killip class II or III were less likely to receive reperfusion therapy than patients in Killip class I.[283]

Patients who are candidates for reperfusion therapy and present initially to a PCI-capable facility should undergo cardiac catheterization with an intention of performing PCI within 90 minutes of arrival. Patients who are candidates for reperfusion therapy and present initially to a non-PCI-capable facility may be treated with fibrinolytic therapy or transferred to a PCI-capable facility for primary PCI. Transfer to a PCI-capable facility is favored for patients who have a high bleeding risk from fibrinolytic therapy, patients who present more than 4 hours after the onset of symptoms, and patients who present with high-risk features (≥ 2 mm of ST segment elevation in 2 anterior leads or ≥ 1 mm ST segment elevation in inferior leads with at least one of the following: systolic blood pressure < 100 mm Hg, heart rate > 100/min, Killip class II or III, ≥ 2 mm of ST segment depression in the anterior leads, or ≥ 1 mm of ST segment elevation in right-sided lead V4 indicative of right ventricular involvement).

Analysis of the NRMI-2 registry suggested that the risk of in-hospital death was reduced more by primary PCI than by fibrinolytic therapy in patients with CHF.[283] Thus, the ACC/AHA Practice Guidelines recommend primary PCI for patients with severe CHF or pulmonary edema (Killip class III) when the onset of symptoms is within 12 hours.[20] Primary PCI is considered reasonable (a Class IIa recommendation) for patients who present with severe CHF, persistent ischemic symptoms, or hemodynamic or electrical instability 12 to 24 hours after symptom onset.[20] As discussed subsequently, cardiogenic shock within 36 hours of acute MI is considered an indication for primary PCI.

PCI may be preferable to fibrinolytic therapy in patients with acute MI who are classified as high risk by virtue of a TIMI risk score of 5 or higher.[215] Among 1527 patients who were enrolled in the DANAMI-2 trial, no difference in mortality was observed between low-risk patients (TIMI score 0 to 4) who underwent primary PCI and those who received fibrinolytic therapy (8% versus 5.6%; $p = 0.11$) (Fig. 30.6).[215] The 3-year mortality rate was significantly lower in high-risk patients who underwent PCI than in patients who received fibrinolytic therapy (25.3% versus 36.2%; $p = 0.02$) (see Fig. 30.6).[215]

Acute MI in patients who have undergone previous CABG surgery frequently is due to thrombotic occlusion of saphenous vein bypass grafts, rather than occlusion of native coronary arteries.[284,285] Data are limited regarding the efficacy of intravenous fibrinolytic therapy in patients with previous CABG surgery, but in one small study, angiography revealed extensive residual thrombus in the presumed culprit vein grafts.[284] The Second Primary Angioplasty in Myocardial Infarction Trial (PAMI-2) included 58 patients with previous surgery who had either STEMI or NSTEMI.[285] The infarct-related vessel was a native coronary artery in 26 patients (45%) and a bypass graft in 32 patients (55%), including 31 saphenous vein grafts and 1 internal mammary artery graft. PCI was attempted in 72% of the bypass grafts, resulting in TIMI grade 3 flow in only 70.2% of the grafts, compared with 94.3% of native coronary arteries in patients without previous CABG surgery.

Patients presenting more than 12 hours after symptom onset are not considered candidates for fibrinolytic therapy but may benefit from primary PCI.[286] A trial that compared primary PCI with conservative therapy included 365 patients with acute STEMI between 12 and 48 hours after symptom onset.[286] Left ventricular infarct size measured by technetium Tc 99m sestamibi imaging 5 to 10 days after randomization was significantly smaller in patients managed using invasive strategies than in patients managed conservatively (8% versus 13%; $p < 0.001$). The Occluded Artery Trial (OAT) randomized 2166 stable patients with one- or two-vessel CAD and a total occlusion of the IRA 3 to 28 days after MI to medical therapy or PCI with stenting.[287] PCI did not reduce the occurrence of death, reinfarction, or CHF. Consequently, the following new Class III recommendation was included in the 2007 Focused Update of the ACC/AHA 2004 Guidelines for the Management of Patients with STEMI: "PCI of a totally occluded infarct artery greater than 24 hours after STEMI is not recommended in asymptomatic patients with one- or two-vessel disease if they are hemodynamically and electrically stable and do not have evidence of severe ischemia."[21]

PLATELET GLYCOPROTEIN ILB/IIIA RECEPTOR ANTAGONISTS

Numerous clinical trials have investigated the role of platelet GP IIb/IIIa inhibitors in patients with acute STEMI, either in conjunction with fibrinolytic agents or primary PCI.[288,289] One rationale of including a GP IIb/IIIa inhibitor in either pharmacologic or mechanical reperfusion strategies is that platelet inhibition may improve

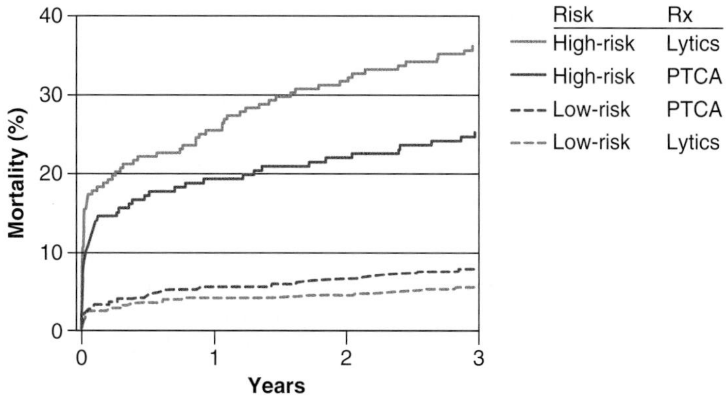

Number at risk

TIMI 0-4	Fx 556	533	531
	PA 578	546	540
TIMI ≥ 5	Fx 207	154	141
	PA 186	150	145

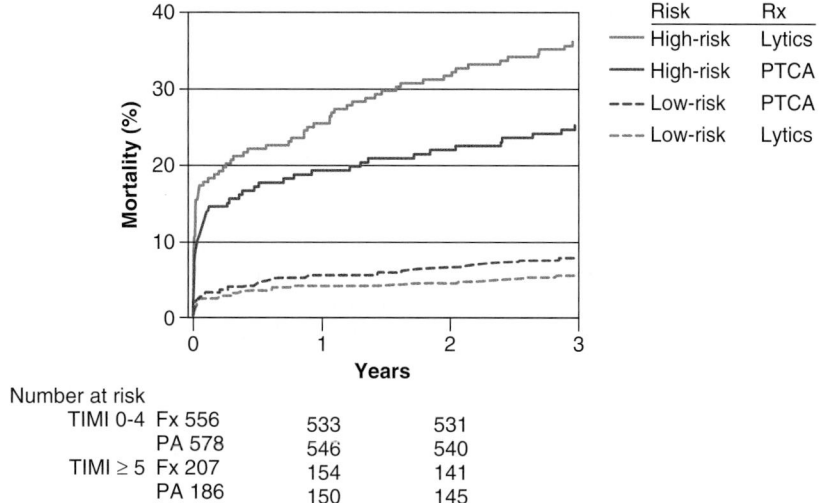

Figure 30.6 Mortality rates for low-risk patients *(dashed lines)* and high-risk patients *(solid lines)* who were randomized to receive fibrinolysis (Fx) *(blue lines)* or primary angioplasty (PA) *(red lines)* in the DANAMI-2 trial. Among 1134 patients who were classified as low risk by virtue of a TIMI risk score of 0 to 4, mortality after fibrinolysis and primary angioplasty was not significantly different. Among 393 patients with a TIMI risk score of 5 or higher, mortality was significantly lower after primary angioplasty compared with fibrinolysis. DANAMI, Danish Multicenter Randomized Study on Fibrinolytic Therapy versus Acute Coronary Angioplasty for Acute Myocardial Infarction; Fx, fibrinolytic therapy; PA, primary angioplasty; PTCA, percutaneous transluminal coronary angioplasty; TIMI, Thrombolysis in Myocardial Infarction study. (From Thune JJ, Hoefsten DE, Lindholm MG, et al: Simple risk stratification at admission to identify patients with reduced mortality from primary angioplasty. Circulation 2005;112:2017-2021.)

myocardial perfusion and enhance salvage of ischemic muscle by reducing distal embolization of platelet aggregates. Another proposed rationale is to achieve coronary artery patency using lower doses of fibrinolytic drugs. Although the addition of abciximab to either tPA[290] or rPA[187] has been shown to improve angiographic indices of myocardial reperfusion, combination therapy with abciximab and a fibrinolytic drug has not been shown to reduce mortality compared with fibrinolytic therapy alone. A trial that randomized 16,588 patients with acute STEMI to treatment with either standard-dose rPA or half-dose rPA plus full-dose abciximab showed no differences in either 30-day or 1-year mortality.[291] A meta-analysis of three fibrinolytic trials that included 23,166 patients who were randomized to receive either abciximab plus half-dose rPA or tenecteplase (TNK) versus full-dose rPA or TNK found that abciximab was associated with a significant reduction in the 30-day rate of reinfarction (2.3% versus 3.6%; $p < 0.001$), but 30-day mortality was 5.8% for both groups.[288] Therefore, there is no Class I indication for a combination of fibrinolytic agents with GP IIb/IIIa inhibitors in the ACC/AHA Practice Guidelines.[20]

Although at least 18 randomized trials have been performed to evaluate GP IIb/IIIa inhibitors in patients with acute STEMI who undergo primary PCI, it has been difficult to draw definitive conclusions for several reasons.[289] First, three different GP IIb/IIIa inhibitors have been studied, abciximab and the so-called small molecule inhibitors eptifibatide and tirofiban. Second, the agents have been studied in conjunction with various other antiplatelet, anticoagulant, and fibrinolytic regimens. Third, the timing of drug administration has varied from prehospital therapy to periprocedural treatment. Fourth, the trials have been underpowered to evaluate the effects on mortality.

The largest trial, HORIZONS-AMI, compared the combination of UFH and a GP IIb/IIIa inhibitor, either abciximab or eptifibatide, with bivalirudin in 3602 patients with STEMI who were treated with primary PCI.[137-139] Compared with UFH plus a GP IIb/IIIa inhibitor, treatment with bivalirudin was associated with a reduced rate of major bleeding and, among patients who were classified as "high risk," a lower 1-year mortality rate.[138,139]

A meta-analysis of 16 trials that enrolled a total of 10,085 patients with STEMI who underwent primary PCI concluded that GP IIb/IIIa inhibitors did not reduce the rates of mortality or reinfarction at 30 days.[289] A meta-analysis of 5 randomized trials (n = 2138 patients) that compared abciximab with the small-molecule GP IIb/IIIa inhibitors in STEMI patients undergoing primary PCI found no differences in outcome.[292] A meta-analysis that included 1662 patients who were enrolled in 11 randomized trials that compared early versus late administration of GP IIb/IIIa inhibitors before primary PCI concluded that early administration of abciximab improved survival compared with late administration.[293] A registry that enrolled 1086 patients who received abciximab also found that early administration of abciximab before transfer for PCI, compared with late administration, was associated with lower 1-year mortality among patients with a TIMI risk score ≥ 3.[294] A meta-analysis of 8 randomized trials that compared intracoronary with intravenous administration of GP IIb/IIIa inhibitors during primary PCI for STEMI found that intracoronary administration was associated with improved post-PCI blood flow and reduced mortality at 30 days.[295] The INFUSE-AMI trial, however, compared the effects of intracoronary abciximab with no abciximab in patients undergoing primary PCI for an anterior STEMI, and there was no significant difference in infarct size at 30 days measured by MRI.[234]

Based on these data, the 2009 focused update of the ACC/AHA Guidelines for the Management of Patients with STEMI included no Class I recommendations and two Class

II recommendations regarding the use of GP IIb/IIIa receptor antagonists in patients with STEMI.[22] A Class IIa recommendation is "It is reasonable to start treatment with glycoprotein IIb/IIIa receptor antagonists at the time of primary PCI (with or without stenting) in selected patients with STEMI." A Class IIb recommendation is "The usefulness of glycoprotein IIb/IIIa receptor antagonists (as part of a preparatory pharmacological strategy for patients with STEMI before their arrival in the cardiac catheterization laboratory for angiography and PCI) is uncertain."

β-BLOCKERS

β-Adrenergic blockers exert both antiarrhythmic and anti-ischemic effects. Experimental studies have shown that β-blockers increase the ventricular fibrillation threshold in ischemic myocardium,[296] and randomized clinical trials have demonstrated that early administration of intravenous followed by oral metoprolol reduces the incidence of ventricular fibrillation in patients with acute STEMI.[297,298]

Experimental studies have shown that β-blockers can limit the extent of myocardial infarction during coronary occlusion because they reduce heart rate, systemic arterial pressure, and myocardial contractility, thereby decreasing myocardial oxygen demand. Clinical data are conflicting, however, regarding the effects of β-blockers on infarct size in patients, with several studies showing reduced infarct size[299,300] and at least one showing no reduction.[301]

Numerous clinical trials have been performed to examine the effects of early or delayed β-blockade on short-term and long-term clinical outcomes in patients with acute MI. Both atenolol[302] and metoprolol[303] administered by intravenous infusion followed by oral administration reduced mortality in patients who did not receive fibrinolytic therapy. A pooled analysis of 27 randomized trials indicated that early β-blockade reduced mortality by 13% in the first week, and the mortality reduction benefit was greatest in the first 2 days.[304]

Subsequent trials have examined the impact of early intravenous β-blockade on the outcome of patients treated with fibrinolytic agents for acute STEMI.[305,306] In the TIMI II-B study, 1434 patients who received intravenous tPA for acute STEMI were randomized to immediate or deferred β-blockade.[305] The deferred blockade group received oral metoprolol beginning on day 6, whereas the immediate blockade group received intravenous metoprolol within 2 hours of initiation of tPA, followed by oral metoprolol. The incidence of reinfarction (2.7% versus 5.1%, $p = 0.02$) and recurrent chest pain (18.8% versus 24.1%, $p < 0.02$) at 6 days was lower in the immediate group. The GUSTO-I trial protocol recommended that patients without hypotension, bradycardia, or heart failure receive intravenous atenolol as soon as possible after enrollment, followed by oral atenolol daily.[306] Although adjusted 30-day mortality was significantly lower in patients who received atenolol, intravenous atenolol was associated with greater mortality compared with oral treatment alone (odds ratio 1.3; 95% CI 1.0 to 1.5; $p = 0.02$). Also, administration of intravenous atenolol was associated with increased risks of heart failure, shock, recurrent ischemia, and need for a pacemaker. The Clopidogrel and Metoprolol in Myocardial Infarction Trial (COMMIT) randomized patients with suspected acute MI to treatment with metoprolol (up to 15 mg intravenously, followed by 200 mg/day orally; n = 22,929) or placebo (n = 22,923).[298] Treatment was discontinued either at discharge from the hospital or on day 28 of the hospital stay; 93% of the patients had STEMI, and approximately 54% of the patients received a fibrinolytic agent. The risk of reinfarction during treatment was 18% lower among patients who received metoprolol (2% versus 2.5%; $p = 0.001$). The overall in-hospital mortality rates were 7.7% in the metoprolol treatment group and 7.8% in the placebo group (odds ratio 0.99; 95% CI 0.92 to 1.05; $p = 0.69$). Allocation to metoprolol was associated with a significant 22% reduction in death attributed to arrhythmia (1.7% versus 2.2%; $p = 0.0002$), but there was a 29% increase in death attributed to cardiogenic shock among the metoprolol treatment group (2.2% versus 1.7%; $p = 0.0002$).

At least 32 randomized trials including nearly 27,000 patients have been conducted to determine the effect of β-blockade on long-term survival after acute MI, and several meta-analyses have been published.[304,307,308] The Norwegian Multicenter Study Group randomized 1884 patients to receive double-blind treatment with either oral timolol or placebo beginning 7 to 28 days after acute MI.[309] The cumulative mortality rate at 33 months was 39% lower in the timolol group than in the placebo group (10.6% versus 17.5%; $p = 0.0005$), and the sudden-death rate at 33 months was reduced by 45% (7.7% versus 13.9%; $p = 0.0001$). After continued follow-up for up to 6 years, a significant difference in mortality was maintained.[310] The Beta-Blocker Heart Attack Trial (BHAT) demonstrated that treatment with propranolol beginning 5 to 21 days after acute MI also reduced mortality during an average follow-up period of 25 months.[311] A pooled analysis of 31 long-term trials found that β-blocker therapy was associated with a 23% reduction in the odds of death (95% CI 15 to 31).[308] According to that analysis, the calculated number of patients needed to treat (NNT) for 2 years with a β-blocker to avoid one death is 42, which is less than the calculated NNT for antiplatelet therapy, which is 153.[308]

The Carvedilol Post-Infarct Survival Control in LV Dysfunction (CAPRICORN) study is an important trial that was not available for inclusion in the pooled analyses discussed earlier.[312] The CAPRICORN study randomized 1959 patients with a left ventricular EF 40% or lower to carvedilol or placebo beginning 3 to 21 days after acute MI. Forty-six percent of the patients had received reperfusion therapy, and 97% had received an angiotensin-converting enzyme (ACE) inhibitor for at least 48 hours before randomization. After an average follow-up period of 1.3 years, a 23% reduction was found for all-cause mortality (12% versus 15%; hazard ratio 0.77; 95% CI 0.60 to 0.98; $p = 0.031$), identical to that reported in a meta-analysis of previous randomized trials.[308] The CAPRICORN trial supports the conclusion that β-blockade reduces mortality after acute MI even among patients who receive reperfusion therapy and ACE inhibitors for left ventricular dysfunction.

The 2007 Focused Update of the ACC/AHA 2004 Guidelines for the Management of Patients with ST-Elevation Myocardial Infarction includes several modifications of the 2004 guidelines and a new Class III recommendation.[21] The three Class I recommendations regarding oral β-blocker therapy are as follows: (1) oral β-blocker therapy should be initiated in the first 24 hours for patients who do not have any of the following: (a) signs of heart failure, (b) evidence of a low output state, (c) increased risk for cardiogenic shock (age > 70 years, systolic blood pressure < 120 mm Hg, sinus tachycardia > 110 bpm or heart rate < 60 bpm, and increased time since onset of symptoms of STEMI), or (d) other relative contraindications to β-blockade (PR interval > 0.24 seconds, second- or third-degree heart block, active asthma, or reactive airway disease); (2) patients with early contraindications within the first 24 hours of STEMI should be reevaluated for candidacy for β-blocker therapy as secondary prevention; and (3) patients with moderate or severe LV failure should receive β-blocker therapy as secondary prevention with a gradual titration scheme. There are Class IIa and III recommendations regarding intravenous β-blockade in patients with STEMI. The Class IIa recommendation states that it is reasonable to administer an IV β-blocker at the time of presentation to STEMI patients who are hypertensive and who do not have any of the following: (1) signs of heart failure, (2) evidence of low output state, (3) increased risk for cardiogenic shock (discussed earlier), or (4) other relative contraindications to β-blockade (discussed earlier). The Class III recommendations are that IV β-blockers should not be administered to STEMI patients who have any of the following: (1) signs of heart failure, (2) evidence of a low output state, (3) increased risk for cardiogenic shock, or (4) other relative contraindications to β-blockade.

ANGIOTENSIN-CONVERTING ENZYME INHIBITORS AND ANGIOTENSIN RECEPTOR BLOCKERS

Acute MI triggers neurohormonal activation that is characterized by elevated plasma renin activity and aldosterone, and plasma renin activity was found to be an independent predictor of cardiovascular mortality among patients who were enrolled in the Survival and Ventricular Enlargement (SAVE) trial.[313] ACE inhibitors have been shown to attenuate left ventricular enlargement after acute MI.[314] Multiple clinical trials have demonstrated that ACE inhibitors reduce mortality after acute MI. The GISSI-3 trial randomized 19,394 patients with acute MI, with or without ST segment elevation, to an oral lisinopril treatment group or an open control group within 24 hours of symptom onset.[90] Seventy-one percent of the patients received fibrinolytic therapy. Six-week mortality was 11% lower among patients in the lisinopril treatment group than it was for those in the control group (6.3% versus 7.1%; odds ratio 0.88; 95% CI 0.79 to 0.99). The ISIS-4 trial randomized 58,050 patients with acute MI to receive oral captopril or placebo within 24 hours of symptom onset.[91] Seventy-nine percent of the patients had ST segment elevation on the initial ECG, and 70% of eligible patients received fibrinolytic therapy, predominantly with streptokinase. Five-week mortality was 7% lower among patients who received captopril than among those in the control group (7.19% versus 7.69%; 95% CI 1 to 13; $p = 0.02$). The individual patient data from ISIS-4 and GISSI-3 were combined with the data from two other large trials, creating a database of 98,496 patients, who were randomized to ACE inhibitor treatment or control groups during the acute phase (0 to 36 hours) of acute MI.[315] Thirty-day mortality was 7% lower among patients who received an ACE inhibitor (7.1% versus 7.6%; 95% CI 2 to 11; $p = 0.004$). The absolute benefit of ACE inhibitor therapy was greater in patients with anterior MI.

Three additional trials have investigated the efficacy of ACE inhibitors in patients with left ventricular dysfunction or CHF: the SAVE study,[316] the Acute Infarction Ramipril Efficacy (AIRE) study,[317] and the Trandolapril Cardiac Evaluation (TRACE) study.[318] The SAVE study enrolled 2231 patients with an acute MI, no overt CHF, and a left ventricular EF 40% or lower as measured by radionuclide ventriculography.[316] The patients were randomized to double-blind treatment with captopril or placebo 3 to 16 days after acute MI. After an average follow-up period of 42 months, all-cause mortality was reduced by 19% (20% versus 25%; 95% CI 3 to 32; $p = 0.019$). The risk reduction was 22% among patients treated with fibrinolytic therapy (33% of the patients) compared with 17% among patients who were not. Captopril reduced the risk of recurrent MI by 25% (95% CI 5 to 40; $p = 0.015$).[319] The AIRE study enrolled 2006 patients with an acute MI and clinical or radiologic evidence of CHF.[317] The patients were randomized to double-blind treatment with ramipril or placebo beginning 3 to 10 days after acute MI. After average follow-ups of 15 months, all-cause mortality was reduced by 27% (17% versus 23%; 95% CI 11 to 40; $p = 0.002$). The TRACE study enrolled 1749 patients with an acute MI and an echocardiographic left ventricular EF 35% or lower.[318] The patients were randomized to double-blind treatment with trandolapril or placebo beginning 3 to 7 days after acute MI. The relative risk (RR) of death from any cause in the trandolapril group, as compared with the control group, was 0.78 (95% CI 0.67 to 0.91; $p = 0.001$). After follow-up for a minimum of 6 years, the life expectancy of patients was 4.6 years for patients who received placebo versus 6.2 years for those who were treated with trandolapril, a median increase of 15.3 months.[320] A pooled analysis of the data from individual patients who were enrolled in the SAVE, AIRE, and TRACE trials concluded that the mortality rate after a median treatment duration of 31 months was reduced from 29.1% in control patients to 23.4% in the ACE-inhibitor group (odds ratio 0.74; 95% CI 0.66 to 0.83; $p < 0.0001$).[321]

The Register of Information and Knowledge about Swedish Heart Intensive Care Admissions (RIKS-HIA) enrolled 105,225 patients with acute MI who were not treated with ACE inhibitors on admission.[322] The association between treatment with an ACE inhibitor at discharge from the hospital and the outcome at 1 year was evaluated using Cox regression analyses adjusted for medications at discharge and the propensity score. Among the entire cohort, treatment with an ACE inhibitor was associated with a 24% reduction in mortality (RR 0.76; 95% CI 0.73 to 0.80), but among patients without heart failure, a significant benefit was observed only in patients with renal dysfunction.

Two randomized clinical trials compared captopril with an angiotensin receptor blocker (ARB) in high-risk acute MI patients: the Optimal Trial in Myocardial Infarction with the Angiotensin II Antagonist Losartan (OPTIMAAL)[323] and the Valsartan in Acute Myocardial Infarction Trial (VALIANT).[324] The OPTIMAAL trial enrolled 5477 patients with acute STEMI who met any of the following entry criteria: symptoms or signs of CHF, left ventricular EF less than 35%, or new anterior Q waves. Fifty-four percent of the patients received fibrinolytic agents. The patients were randomized to double-blind treatment with either losartan, titrated to a target dose of 50 mg daily, or captopril, titrated to a target dose of 50 mg three times daily, within 10 days of symptom onset. After an average follow-up period of 2.7 years, no significant difference in all-cause mortality was found between the losartan and the captopril treatment groups (18% versus 16%; RR 1.13; 95% CI 0.99 to 1.28; $p = 0.07$). The prespecified criterion for noninferiority was not satisfied. The VALIANT trial enrolled 14,703 patients with acute MI complicated by clinical or radiographic signs of CHF or reduced left ventricular EF (≤ 35% by echocardiography or contrast ventriculography or ≤ 40% by radionuclide ventriculography), or both. Approximately 50% of the patients underwent reperfusion therapy; 35%, fibrinolytic therapy; and 15%, primary PCI. Within 10 days after the acute MI, the patients were randomly assigned to three treatment groups: valsartan monotherapy, captopril monotherapy, or the combination of valsartan and captopril. After an average follow-up period of 24.7 months, all-cause mortality was not significantly different for the three groups: valsartan 19.9%, captopril 19.5%, and the combination 19.3%. The investigators concluded that valsartan is at least as effective as captopril, because the criterion for noninferiority of valsartan relative to captopril was met.

Both aldosterone and angiotensin II, a potent stimulus of adrenal aldosterone production, are increased in patients with CHF despite chronic treatment with an ACE inhibitor. Aldosterone exerts numerous adverse cardiovascular effects, including increased myocardial collagen deposition and fibrosis and cardiomyocyte apoptosis.[325] Eplerenone, a selective aldosterone blocker, was studied in a multicenter, international, randomized, double-blind, placebo-controlled trial called the Eplerenone Post-Acute Myocardial Infarction Heart Failure Efficacy and Survival Study (EPHESUS).[326] The EPHESUS investigators enrolled 6632 patients with acute MI complicated by left ventricular dysfunction (EF less than 40%) plus either CHF or diabetes.[326] The patients were randomized to double-blind treatment with eplerenone or placebo beginning 3 to 14 days after acute MI. At the time of enrollment, 86% of the patients were taking an ACE inhibitor or ARB, and 75% were taking a β-blocker. During a mean follow-up period of 16 months, significantly fewer deaths occurred in the eplerenone group (478 of 3319 patients) than in the placebo group (554 of 3313 patients) (14.4% versus 16.7%; RR 0.85; 95% CI 0.75 to 0.96; $p = 0.008$). A reduction in the rate of sudden death from cardiac causes (RR 0.79; 95% CI 0.64 to 0.97; $p = 0.03$) also was observed. Serious hyperkalemia, defined as a serum potassium of 6 mmol/L or more, occurred in 5.5% of patients in the eplerenone group versus 3.9% of those in the placebo group ($p = 0.002$).

The ACC/AHA Practice Guidelines include the following Class I recommendations regarding inhibitors of the renin-angiotensin-aldosterone system: (1) ACE inhibitors should be started and continued indefinitely in all patients recovering from STEMI with LVEF less than or equal to 40% and for those with hypertension, diabetes, or chronic kidney disease, unless otherwise contraindicated; (2) ACE inhibitors should be started and continued indefinitely in patients recovering from STEMI who are not lower risk (lower risk defined as those with normal LVEF in whom cardiovascular risk factors are well controlled and revascularization has been performed), unless contraindicated; (3) the use of angiotensin receptor blockers is recommended in patients who are intolerant of ACE inhibitors and have heart failure or have had an MI with LVEF less than or equal to 40%; (4) it is beneficial to use angiotensin receptor blocker therapy in other patients who are ACE-inhibitor intolerant and have hypertension; (5) the use of aldosterone blockade in post-MI patients without significant renal dysfunction (serum creatinine less than 2.5 mg/dL in men and less than 2 mg/dL in women) or hyperkalemia (serum potassium ≥ 5 mEq/L) is recommended in patients who are already receiving therapeutic doses of an ACE inhibitor and β-blocker, have an LVEF of less than or equal to 40%, and have either diabetes or heart failure.[21] Intravenous ACE inhibitors should not be given within 24 hours of an acute MI because of the risk of hypotension.

ANTIARRHYTHMIC DRUGS

Both atrial and ventricular arrhythmias are common in patients with acute MI. The incidence of atrial fibrillation was 10.4% among 40,891 patients who were enrolled in the GUSTO-I trial.[327] Patients in whom atrial fibrillation developed after admission were more likely to have a stroke or die within 30 days after acute MI. Among patients enrolled in the TRACE study, which enrolled patients with an acute MI and a left ventricular EF less than 35%, atrial fibrillation occurred in 21% of patients and was associated with a 50% increase in adjusted mortality.[328] Intravenous β-adrenergic blockade is the preferred therapy for patients with sustained atrial fibrillation or atrial flutter that is not associated with hemodynamic compromise, whereas sustained atrial fibrillation or flutter that is associated with hemodynamic compromise is an indication for synchronized cardioversion. Intravenous amiodarone is indicated for treatment of atrial fibrillation that does not respond to electrical cardioversion or recurs after cardioversion. Sustained atrial fibrillation should be treated with anticoagulants.

The incidence of primary ventricular fibrillation, defined as that occurring within 48 hours of acute MI and in the absence of cardiogenic shock or severe CHF, was 4.7% among a cohort of 5020 patients hospitalized for an uncomplicated acute MI in Worcester, Massachusetts, during 11 1-year periods between 1975 and 1997.[329] The incidence of primary ventricular fibrillation in the GISSI-1 trial was not significantly different in the streptokinase and control groups (2.73% versus 2.93%; RR 0.93; 95% CI 0.75 to 1.15).[330] A meta-analysis of 15 randomized trials of fibrinolytic therapy for acute MI confirmed that the likelihood of this arrhythmia is not altered by fibrinolytic therapy, with an incidence of ventricular fibrillation during the first hospital day of 2.99% for both the fibrinolytic treatment and placebo groups.[331] There is evidence, however, that fibrinolytic therapy exerts a protective effect against secondary ventricular fibrillation, defined as ventricular fibrillation in patients with acute MI complicated by CHF or shock.[331,332] Thus, the meta-analysis of 15 fibrinolytic trials found that the odds ratio for the development of ventricular fibrillation at any time during hospitalization in the fibrinolytic treatment group was 0.83 (95% CI 0.76 to 0.90; $p < 0.0001$).[331]

Primary ventricular fibrillation is an independent predictor of in-hospital mortality whether it occurs early (up to 4 hours) or late (after 4 to 48 hours) after the onset of acute MI.[333] Among 9720 patients with a first STEMI who were enrolled in the GISSI-2 fibrinolytic trial, 356 of the 7755 patients who were in Killip class I at entry developed primary ventricular fibrillation.[333] Early primary ventricular fibrillation occurred in 302 patients (3.7%) and late primary ventricular fibrillation occurred in 54 patients (0.6%); 226 patients had ventricular fibrillation within 1 hour of the onset of acute MI symptoms. In-hospital mortality rates were 13% among patients with late primary ventricular fibrillation (RR 3.80; 95% CI 1.80 to 8.02) and 7% among patients with early primary ventricular fibrillation (RR 2.00; 95% CI 1.29 to 3.12), compared with 4% among patients in Killip class I on admission in whom ventricular fibrillation did not develop. The in-hospital mortality rate associated with primary ventricular fibrillation was much higher in the Worcester Heart Attack Study, with an overall case-fatality rate of 44%, although improved survival was observed in patients who had primary ventricular fibrillation in the 1990s.[329]

Among 11,712 patients enrolled in the GISSI-1 study, secondary ventricular fibrillation occurred in 311 patients (2.7%).[332] The incidence of secondary ventricular fibrillation within 24 hours of acute MI was similar among the patients treated with streptokinase and the control group, whereas streptokinase halved the frequency of secondary ventricular fibrillation later than 24 hours after admission (27/5860 versus 60/5852; RR 0.45; 95% CI 0.29 to 0.70). The protective effect of streptokinase was even greater among patients who were treated within 3 hours of symptom onset (9/3016 versus 39/3078; RR 0.23; 95% CI 0.12 to 0.45). In-hospital mortality was higher among patients with secondary ventricular fibrillation: 27.1% versus 17.3% for patients in Killip class II (RR 1.77; 95% CI 1.28 to 2.45) and 48.1% versus 35.3% for patients in Killip class III (RR 1.70; 95% CI 0.95 to 3.02). Secondary ventricular fibrillation did not affect in-hospital mortality among the patients in Killip class IV (67.9% with secondary ventricular fibrillation versus 71.9% without secondary ventricular fibrillation; RR 0.83; 95% CI 0.44 to 1.55).

Although primary and secondary ventricular fibrillation both are associated with an increased risk of in-hospital death, patients who survive to be discharged from the hospital after experiencing either type have a good prognosis. Among the patients who were enrolled in the GISSI-1 and GISSI-2 trials and had nonfatal primary ventricular fibrillation, 6-month mortality after hospital discharge among patients with the primary type was not significantly different from that in patients who did not have this arrhythmia.[333,334] In GISSI-2, patients who survived the hospital phase of an acute MI complicated by secondary ventricular fibrillation had a 1-year mortality of 10.4%, compared with 13.9% among patients who did not have secondary ventricular fibrillation (20/193 versus 322/2319; RR 0.72; 95% CI 0.44 to 1.15).[332]

Partly on the basis of the results of one double-blind, randomized study,[335] an editorial published in 1978 concluded that there was justification for routine prophylactic administration of lidocaine to all patients with acute MI to prevent primary ventricular fibrillation.[336] Subsequent studies of prophylactic lidocaine in acute MI, including more than 20 randomized trials and at least four meta-analyses, concluded that lidocaine reduces the incidence of ventricular fibrillation but increases mortality.[337] Therefore, according to the ACC/AHA Practice Guidelines that were published in 2004, prophylactic antiarrhythmic therapy is not recommended with use of fibrinolytic agents.[20] Also, the routine use of lidocaine is not indicated for suppression of isolated ventricular premature beats, couplets, runs of accelerated idioventricular rhythm, and nonsustained ventricular tachycardia. The guidelines favor intravenous amiodarone for treatment of sustained monomorphic ventricular tachycardia.

Although ventricular ectopy is a marker of an increased risk of sudden death in survivors of acute MI, trials of chronic, oral antiarrhythmic drugs have not shown beneficial effects. The Cardiac Arrhythmia Suppression Trial (CAST) I and CAST II found that treatment with the class IC drugs encainide and flecainide, or the class IA drug moricizine, increased mortality in survivors of acute MI.[338,339] *d*-Sotalol, a potassium channel blocker, also increased mortality among survivors of MI in the Survival with Oral *d*-Sotalol (SWORD) randomized trial.[340] Clinical trials of amiodarone, a class III antiarrhythmic drug, suggested that it may reduce the incidence of ventricular fibrillation or arrhythmic death among survivors of acute MI.[341,342]

The implantable cardioverter-defibrillator (ICD) has become the standard of care for the prevention of sudden death in survivors of acute MI.[343] There are two Class I indications for an ICD after STEMI: (1) an ICD is indicated for patients with ventricular fibrillation or hemodynamically significant sustained ventricular tachycardia later than 2 days after STEMI, provided that the arrhythmia is not judged to be due to transient or reversible ischemia or reinfarction. (2) An ICD is indicated for patients without spontaneous ventricular fibrillation or sustained ventricular tachycardia more than 48 hours after STEMI whose STEMI occurred at least 1 month previously, who have a left ventricular EF between 31% and 40%, demonstrated additional evidence of electrical instability (e.g., nonsustained ventricular tachycardia), and who have inducible ventricular fibrillation or sustained ventricular tachycardia on electrophysiology testing.[20]

CALCIUM ANTAGONISTS

No Class I indications are provided for calcium channel blockers in patients with acute MI because neither individual clinical trials nor analyses of the pooled results of multiple trials showed a reduction in mortality after acute MI.[307,344,345] A randomized study that compared diltiazem with placebo starting 3 to 15 days after acute MI found that diltiazem therapy was associated with an increased risk of cardiac events in patients with radiographic evidence of pulmonary congestion.[346] The same trial concluded that diltiazem increases the risk of late-onset CHF in patients with a left ventricular EF less than 40%.[347] Thus, there are two Class III recommendations for calcium channel blockers in acute MI: (1) Diltiazem and verapamil are contraindicated in patients with STEMI and associated systolic left ventricular dysfunction and CHF. (2) Nifedipine (immediate-release form) is contraindicated in the treatment of STEMI because of the reflex sympathetic activation, tachycardia, and hypotension associated with its use.[20]

LIPID-LOWERING AGENTS

Numerous trials have evaluated the effects of statins on coronary events in patients with acute and chronic CAD, but none of the trials restricted enrollment to patients with STEMI or provided subgroup analyses of the outcomes among patients with STEMI before enrollment. The Scandinavian Simvastatin Survival Study (4S) was the first clinical trial to demonstrate significant reductions in total mortality and coronary heart disease mortality by treatment with lipid-lowering therapy.[348] Seventy-nine percent of the patients had a history of MI. After a median follow-up period of 5.4 years, total mortality was 12% in the placebo group versus 8% in the patients who were randomly assigned to receive simvastatin (RR 0.70; 95% CI 0.58 to 0.85; $p = 0.0003$). Also, there was a 37% reduction in the risk of undergoing a myocardial revascularization procedure. The beneficial effects of statin therapy in patients with a history of MI were confirmed by two studies that randomized patients to receive pravastatin 40 mg daily or placebo: the Cholesterol and Recurrent Events (CARE) trial[349] and the Long-Term Intervention with Pravastatin in Ischemic Disease (LIPID) trial.[350] All patients who were enrolled in the CARE trial had a history of MI between 3 and 20 months before enrollment, and 64% of the patients enrolled in the LIPID trial had a history of MI between 3 and 36 months before enrollment.

A diagnosis of hyperlipidemia cannot be excluded during the first week after an acute MI because both total cholesterol and low-density lipoprotein (LDL) cholesterol decrease significantly during the first week after an acute MI.[351] There are numerous Class I recommendations for lipid management in patients who have had a STEMI. Although the current Class I guidelines recommend a target LDL cholesterol level less than 100 mg/dL, future guidelines may reflect data that support more aggressive treatment to achieve the goal of an LDL cholesterol level of less than 70 mg/dL.[352-354]

INTRA-AORTIC BALLOON COUNTERPULSATION

Several randomized trials have evaluated the utility of intra-aortic balloon counterpulsation in high-risk patients with acute MI not complicated by cardiogenic shock. The Second Primary Angioplasty in Myocardial Infarction (PAMI-II) investigators randomized 436 patients with a high-risk acute MI to insertion of an intra-aortic balloon pump (IABP) or no IABP after primary PCI.[355] The rates of reocclusion of the IRA, reinfarction, and mortality were not significantly different, and there was a higher incidence of stroke among patients who received an IABP (2.4% versus 0%; $p = 0.03$). Also, there was no enhancement of myocardial recovery at the time of hospital discharge or 6 weeks after discharge. The Counterpulsation to Reduce Infarct Size Pre-PCI Acute Myocardial Infarction (CRISP AMI) trial was a randomized trial to determine whether insertion of an IABP before primary PCI reduces infarct size in patients with an acute anterior STEMI without cardiogenic shock.[356] The mean infarct size, measured by cardiac magnetic resonance imaging 3 to 5 days after PCI was 42.1% of the left ventricle in the IABP group compared with 37.5% of the left ventricle in the control group ($p = 0.06$). Thus, the IABP has not been shown to be beneficial in patients with high-risk or anterior acute MI who undergo primary PCI. The use of the IABP in patients with cardiogenic shock is discussed in a subsequent section of this chapter and in the chapter on cardiogenic shock.

CORONARY ARTERY BYPASS GRAFT SURGERY

Randomized trials have not been performed to compare surgical reperfusion for acute MI with either conservative medical therapy or reperfusion by means of fibrinolytic therapy or PCI. A nonrandomized study compared the outcomes in 200 patients managed conservatively with those in 187 patients who underwent surgical reperfusion between 1972 and 1976.[357] In-hospital mortality was 5.8% among patients who underwent CABG surgery, compared with 11.5% among patients who did not undergo myocardial reperfusion ($p < 0.08$). Among the patients who underwent coronary bypass grafting within 6 hours from the onset of symptoms of acute MI, in-hospital mortality was only 2% (2/100), compared with 10.3% (9/87) among the patients who underwent surgery more than 6 hours after the onset of symptoms.

Although registry data indicate that CABG surgery within 24 hours of an acute STEMI is associated with a marked increase of in-hospital mortality,[358] emergency surgical revascularization should be considered in certain subsets of patients. Emergency CABG surgery is a reasonable option in patients with cardiogenic shock and coronary anatomy poorly suited for PCI (e.g., severe stenosis of the left main coronary artery). Among patients enrolled in the Should We Emergently Revascularize Occluded Coronaries for Cardiogenic Shock? (SHOCK) trial, survival rates were similar for CABG surgery and for PCI.[359] The 2011 ACCF/AHA Guideline for Coronary Artery Bypass Graft Surgery includes four Class I, two Class IIa, and two Class III recommendations regarding CABG in patients with acute MI[360] (Box 30.6).

Mortality after CABG surgery remains elevated during the first week after an acute MI.[358] Therefore, the 2004 ACC/AHA Practice Guidelines for the Management of Patients with ST-Elevation Myocardial Infarction recommended that patients who have been stabilized after STEMI and who have incurred a significant fall in LV function should have their surgery delayed to allow for myocardial recovery.[20]

An additional reason to delay surgery in stable patients is to permit recovery of platelet function in patients who have received a $P2Y_{12}$ inhibitor. Red blood cell transfusion of 4 units or more after CABG was an independent predictor of 1-year mortality among 1491 patients with ACS who underwent CABG.[361] There are conflicting data regarding the impact of $P2Y_{12}$ inhibitors on the risk of bleeding and transfusion after CABG. One retrospective analysis of 596 patients with ACS who underwent CABG found that exposure to clopidogrel within 5 days of surgery increased the risk of major bleeding and reoperation.[362] Among 1539 patients with ACS who were enrolled in the Acute Catheterization and Urgent Intervention Triage Strategy (ACUITY) trial and underwent CABG before discharge, CABG within 5 days of the last clopidogrel dose was not associated with higher rates of transfusion or major bleeding compared with the rates among patients who did not receive any clopidogrel before CABG.[363] Administration of clopidogrel within 5 days before CABG was associated with a modestly increased risk of red blood cell transfusion but was not significantly associated with reoperation for bleeding among 332 patients who were enrolled in the Duke Databank between January 1999 and December 2003.[364] According to the 2011 ACCF/AHA Guideline for CABG, clopidogrel and ticagrelor should be

Box 30.6 CABG in Patients with Acute MI

Class I

1. Emergency CABG is recommended in patients with acute MI in whom (1) primary PCI has failed or cannot be performed, (2) coronary anatomy is suitable for CABG, and (3) persistent ischemia of a significant area of myocardium at rest or hemodynamic instability refractory to nonsurgical therapy is present.
2. Emergency CABG is recommended in patients undergoing surgical repair of a postinfarction mechanical complication of MI, such as ventricular septal rupture, mitral valve insufficiency because of papillary muscle infarction or rupture, or free wall rupture.
3. Emergency CABG is recommended in patients with cardiogenic shock and who are suitable for CABG irrespective of the time interval from MI to onset of shock and time from MI to CABG.
4. Emergency CABG is recommended in patients with life-threatening ventricular arrhythmias (believed ischemic in origin) in the presence of left main stenosis greater than or equal to 50% or three-vessel CAD.

Class IIa

1. The use of CABG is reasonable as a revascularization strategy in patients with multivessel CAD with recurrent angina or MI within the first 48 hours of STEMI presentation as an alternative to a more delayed strategy.
2. Early revascularization with PCI or CABG is reasonable for selected patients older than 75 years of age with ST segment elevation or left bundle branch block who are suitable for revascularization irrespective of the time interval from MI to onset of shock.

Class III

1. Emergency CABG should not be performed in patients with persistent angina and a small area of viable myocardium who are stable hemodynamically.
2. Emergency CABG should not be performed in patients with no-reflow (successful epicardial reperfusion with unsuccessful microvascular reperfusion).

CABG, coronary artery bypass graft; CAD, coronary artery disease; MI, myocardial infarction; PCI, percutaneous coronary intervention; STEMI, ST segment elevation myocardial infarction

From Hillis LD, Smith PK, Anderson JL, et al: 2011 ACCF/AHA guideline for coronary artery bypass graft surgery: A report of the American College of Cardiology Foundation/American Heart Association Task Force on Practice Guidelines. J Am Coll Cardiol 2011;58:e123-e210.

discontinued for at least 5 days before surgery and prasugrel for at least 7 days to limit blood transfusions, while clopidogrel and ticagrelor should be discontinued for at least 24 hours in patients referred for urgent CABG.[360] Finally, the guideline includes a Class I recommendation that aspirin (100 mg to 325 mg) should be administered to CABG patients preoperatively.[360]

MANAGEMENT OF COMPLICATIONS

PERICARDITIS AND PERICARDIAL TAMPONADE

Pericarditis, defined as the detection of a pericardial friction rub, was diagnosed in 20% (141/703) of patients who were enrolled in the Multicenter Investigation of the Limitation of Infarct Size (MILIS).[365] The frequency of pericarditis was higher in patients with Q wave MI than in those with non–Q wave MI (25% versus 9%; $p < 0.001$). Pericarditis was associated with a lower admission left ventricular EF (42% versus 48%; $p < 0.001$) and a higher incidence of CHF (47% versus 26%; $p < 0.001$). Pericarditis was accompanied by pleuritic or positional chest pain in 70% of patients. Diagnostic electrocardiographic changes usually are absent in patients with infarction-associated pericarditis.[366] A prospective study of 423 patients with acute MI found that only 1 of the 31 patients with pericardial friction rubs had diagnostic ST segment changes.[366]

The GISSI investigators reported the frequency of pericardial involvement in patients who were enrolled in the GISSI-1 (n = 11,806) and GISSI-2 (n = 12,381) trials.[367] The incidence of pericardial involvement was lower among patients who received fibrinolytic therapy than among patients in the control groups (6.7% versus 12%). Earlier treatment with fibrinolytic therapy was associated with a lower risk of pericardial involvement. Although pericardial involvement was associated with a higher long-term mortality, it was not an independent prognostic factor because it was strongly associated with the extent of infarction as determined by ECG, peak creatine kinase, and echocardiography.

The ACC/AHA Practice Guidelines recommend aspirin for treatment of pericarditis after STEMI.[20] Colchicine or acetaminophen is recommended for patients who do not respond to aspirin. Corticosteroids and nonsteroidal anti-inflammatory drugs are discouraged because of an increased risk of scar thinning and infarct expansion. Finally, anticoagulation should be discontinued if a pericardial effusion is detected.

Hemorrhagic pericarditis and free wall rupture are two potential mechanisms of cardiac tamponade after acute MI. Among 102,060 patients with STEMI who were enrolled in seven randomized clinical trials and received fibrinolytic therapy, cardiac tamponade developed in 1018 patients (1%).[368] Among the patients with tamponade, 153 also had a ventricular septal rupture or acute mitral regurgitation, and 865 had isolated cardiac tamponade. The adjusted 30-day mortality among 7-day survivors with tamponade was significantly increased (hazard ratio 7.9; 95% CI 4.7 to 13.5; $p < 0.0001$). Pericardial tamponade accounted for 1.4% of patients with cardiogenic shock among 1422 patients with acute MI who were enrolled in either the SHOCK registry or the randomized trial.[369]

RECURRENT ISCHEMIA OR INFARCTION

Recurrent infarction (reinfarction) after an initial STEMI is relatively uncommon, but it often is an end point for clinical trials, because reinfarction is associated with increased morbidity and mortality.[370,371] Symptomatic recurrent MI during the index hospitalization occurred in 4.2% (836/20,101) of patients who were enrolled in four clinical trials of various fibrinolytic agents.[371] Recurrent MI occurred a median of 2.2 days after the initial MI and was associated with increased mortality rates at both 30 days (16.4% versus 6.2%; $p < 0.001$) and 2 years (hazard ratio 2.11, $p < 0.001$). In-hospital reinfarction occurred in 4.3% of patients (2258/55,911) a median of 3.8 days after fibrinolytic therapy in the GUSTO

I and GUSTO III trials.[370] The rates of reinfarction were 4.3% for alteplase, 4.5% for reteplase, and 4.1% for streptokinase ($p = 0.55$). Patients with in-hospital reinfarction had higher mortality at 30 days (11.3% versus 3.5%; odds ratio 3.5; $p < 0.001$) and from 30 days to 1 year (4.7% versus 3.2%; hazard ratio 1.5; $p < 0.001$).[370] Compared with patients who did not have reinfarction, patients with reinfarction had higher rates of CHF (31.9% versus 13.9%) and cardiogenic shock (15.9% versus 2.4%).

The frequency of recurrent ischemia or reinfarction after an initial STEMI depends on the modality of reperfusion and the adjunctive therapy employed. One of the purported advantages of primary PCI over fibrinolytic therapy is a decreased rate of reinfarction. The 30-day rates of reinfarction in the DANAMI-2 trial were 6.3% (49/782) among patients who were randomized to fibrinolytic therapy compared with 1.6% (13/790) among patients who were assigned to the angioplasty group ($p < 0.001$).[214] In a meta-analysis of 13 randomized trials of primary angioplasty versus fibrin-specific agents, the frequency of nonfatal reinfarction was 3% (74/2753) among patients randomized to angioplasty, compared with 6% (172/2757) among patients assigned to fibrinolytic therapy (odds ratio 0.42; 95% CI 0.31 to 0.55).[209]

There is evidence that coronary revascularization reduces the risk of reinfarction after fibrinolytic therapy. Among patients who were enrolled in four clinical trials of various fibrinolytic drugs, PCI or CABG surgery was performed during the index hospitalization in 26.1% (5238/20,039) of the patients and was associated with lower rates of both in-hospital recurrent MI (1.4% versus 4.7%, $p < 0.001$) and 2-year mortality.[371]

A variety of antithrombotic and antiplatelet therapies have been shown to reduce the risk of reinfarction after STEMI. In a trial that randomized 20,506 patients with STEMI to either enoxaparin or UFH as adjunctive treatment after fibrinolytic therapy, the rates of reinfarction at 30 days were 3% for the enoxaparin group (309/10,256) compared with 4.5% for the UFH group (458/10,223) (RR 0.67; 95% CI 0.58 to 0.77; $p < 0.001$).[131] A meta-analysis of 11 clinical trials found that administration of abciximab was associated with a reduction in the 30-day reinfarction rates among patients who underwent primary angioplasty (1% versus 1.9%; odds ratio 0.56; 95% CI 0.33 to 0.94; $p = 0.03$) and among patients who received fibrinolytic therapy (2.3% versus 3.6%; odds ratio 0.64; 95% CI 0.54 to 0.75; $p < 0.001$).[288]

Numerous clinical trials have investigated the effect of warfarin alone or in combination with aspirin on the risk of reinfarction and other events in patients with ACS, but most of the studies were not restricted to patients with STEMI, the target international normalized ratio (INR) has varied, and conflicting results have emerged.[372,373] The Warfarin Re-Infarction Study randomized 1214 patients to receive placebo or warfarin (target INR 2.8 to 4.8) after an average interval between the index MI and enrollment of 27 days.[374] Approximately 70% of patients had Q waves on the baseline ECG, most patients did not receive reperfusion therapy, and all patients were advised not to take aspirin or other antiplatelet drugs. During an average treatment period of 37 months, the rate of reinfarction was significantly reduced by warfarin compared with placebo (82/607 versus 124/607; RR 34%; 95% CI 19% to 54%; $p = 0.0007$).

The Antithrombotics in the Secondary Prevention of Events in Coronary Thrombosis-2 (ASPECT-2) study randomized 999 patients to receive one of three antithrombotic regimens: aspirin 80 mg daily, warfarin (target INR 3.0 to 4.0), or the combination of aspirin 80 mg daily and warfarin (target INR 2.0 to 2.5).[375] Patients were enrolled within 8 weeks of hospitalization for either UA (13%) or Q wave or non–Q wave MI. During a median follow-up period of 12 months, the primary composite end point of MI, stroke, or death was significantly less frequent for the two groups that received warfarin, but warfarin did not reduce the risk of MI, and it increased the risk of both major and minor bleeding.

The APRICOT-2 trial randomized 308 patients with a patent IRA within 48 hours after fibrinolytic therapy to receive either aspirin alone (80 mg daily) or aspirin plus warfarin for 3 months (target INR 2.0 to 3.0).[376] The rate of reinfarction during 3 months of follow-up was 2% (3/135) for combination therapy, compared with 8% (11/139) for aspirin alone ($p < 0.05$). The Warfarin, Aspirin, Reinfarction Study (WARIS II) randomly assigned 3630 patients who were hospitalized for an acute MI to one of three treatment groups: warfarin alone (with a target INR of 2.8 to 4.2), aspirin alone (160 mg daily), or the combination of aspirin 75 mg daily and warfarin (target INR 2.0 to 2.5).[377] Fibrinolytic drugs were administered to 53% to 55% of the patients in each group. During a mean observation period of 4 years, the rates of reinfarction were significantly less in both groups of patients who received warfarin: 9.7% (117/1206) for aspirin alone, 7.4% (90/1216) for warfarin alone (RR 0.74; 95% CI 0.55 to 0.998; $p = 0.03$), and 5.7% (69/1208) for aspirin plus warfarin (RR 0.56; 95% CI 0.41 to 0.78; $p < 0.001$). Another study that used a target INR of 1.5 to 2.5 found that the addition of warfarin to aspirin 81 mg daily did not reduce the rate of reinfarction compared with aspirin monotherapy (162 mg daily).[378] The combination of aspirin 80 mg daily with low, fixed-dose warfarin (1 mg or 3 mg) was not superior to aspirin 160 mg daily in patients with a recent STEMI or NSTEMI.[379] Thus, the clinical trials suggest that warfarin is superior to placebo, that the combination of aspirin and warfarin is superior to aspirin alone if the target INR is sufficiently high, and that the risk of major bleeding is increased by adding warfarin to aspirin. Also, the published data should not be extrapolated to patients who receive dual antiplatelet therapy (aspirin plus a thienopyridine) after either fibrinolytic therapy or coronary artery stenting, because most of the patients who were enrolled in the warfarin trials did not receive reperfusion therapy or a thienopyridine.

In the ISIS-2 trial, aspirin reduced the rate of in-hospital reinfarction both in the patients who received streptokinase and in those who did not receive fibrinolytic therapy. Higher platelet counts were associated with an increased risk of reinfarction among patients with STEMI for whom treatment consisted of aspirin plus a fibrinolytic drug.[380] The addition of clopidogrel to aspirin abolishes the increased risk of reinfarction as the platelet count increases.[380] In the CLARITY study, the rate of recurrent MI after fibrinolytic therapy was 4.1% among patients treated with clopidogrel and aspirin, compared with 5.9% among patients who received placebo and aspirin (representing a 31% reduction in odds).[106]

Clinical trials have demonstrated that β-blockers, ACE inhibitors, and statins also reduce the risk of reinfarction after acute MI, although most of the trials enrolled patients with both STEMI and NSTEMI, and subgroup analyses of outcomes in patients with STEMI were not published. Compared with metoprolol started 6 days after tPA for acute STEMI, metoprolol started within 2 hours of tPA was associated with lower rates of reinfarction (5.1% versus 2.7%; $p = 0.02$) and recurrent chest pain (24.1% versus 18.8%; $p < 0.02$) at 6 days.[305] The Norwegian Multicenter Study Group randomly assigned 1884 patients to double-blind treatment groups, to receive either oral timolol or placebo, beginning 7 to 28 days after acute MI.[309] The cumulative reinfarction rate at 33 months was 28% lower in the timolol group than in the placebo group (14.4% versus 20.1%; $p = 0.0006$). The CAPRICORN study randomized 1959 patients with a left ventricular EF of 40% or less to receive carvedilol or placebo beginning 3 to 21 days after acute MI. Forty-six percent of the patients had received reperfusion therapy and 97% had received an ACE inhibitor for at least 48 hours before beginning the study treatment. After an average follow-up period of 1.3 years, the rate of nonfatal MI was significantly lower in the carvedilol group than in the placebo group (3% versus 6%; hazard ratio 0.59; 95% CI 0.39 to 0.90; $p = 0.014$).

The GISSI 3 trial did not show an effect of lisinopril on the rate of reinfarction after 6 weeks.[90] Although the AIRE[317] and TRACE[318] trials failed to show a significant effect of ramipril or trandolapril on the long-term risk of reinfarction, the SAVE study[316,319] did observe a significant decrease in the reinfarction rate among patients who were randomly selected to receive captopril 3 to 16 days after acute MI. After an average follow-up period of 42 months, captopril reduced the risk of recurrent MI by 25% (95% CI 5% to 40%; $p = 0.015$).[319] Thus, ACE inhibitors may not reduce the short-term risk of reinfarction after acute MI, but they may decrease the long-term risk of reinfarction.

Numerous trials have evaluated the effects of statins on coronary events in patients with acute and chronic CAD, but none of the trials restricted enrollment to patients with STEMI and many of the trials pooled the data of patients with UA, NSTEMI, and STEMI. All patients who were enrolled in the CARE trial had a history of MI between 3 and 20 months before randomization; 61% were enrolled after a Q wave MI.[349] Although the mean interval from MI to enrollment was 10 months, during a median follow-up period of 5 years there was a significantly lower rate of nonfatal MI among patients who received pravastatin compared with patients who received placebo (6.5% versus 8.3%; RR 23%; 95% CI 4% to 39%; $p = 0.02$).[349]

Data are conflicting regarding the benefit of initiating statin therapy within 14 days of the onset of ACS. At least two meta-analyses of relevant randomized controlled trials have been published.[381,382] One analysis of 12 randomized trials concluded that statin therapy initiated within 14 days of hospital admission does not reduce the risk of death, MI, or stroke during the first 4 months after ACS.[381] Another meta-analysis of 13 randomized trials concluded that early statin therapy reduces death and cardiovascular events after 4 months of treatment.[382] A prospective cohort study using data from the Swedish Registry of Cardiac Intensive Care concluded that initiation of statin therapy before discharge was associated with a 25% reduction in 1-year mortality in hospital survivors of acute MI.[383]

Among a cohort of 2301 patients who suffered reinfarction after administration of fibrinolytic therapy in the GUSTO I and Assessment of Safety and Efficacy of a New Thrombolytic 2 (ASSENT 2) clinical trials, reinfarction was treated with repeat fibrinolysis (n = 864), with revascularization (n = 525), or conservatively (n = 835).[384] After adjustment for baseline characteristics, the 30-day mortality was significantly greater in the conservative group, 28%, compared with the repeat fibrinolysis group, 11% (odds ratio 2.2; 95% CI 1.5 to 3.1; $p < 0.001$) or the revascularization group, 11% (odds ratio 2.2; 95% CI 1.4 to 3.3; $p < 0.0001$). No significant difference was observed between the revascularization and repeat fibrinolysis groups.

The ACC/AHA Practice Guidelines provide several recommendations regarding the management of recurrent ischemia and reinfarction.[20] They recommend escalation of medical therapy with nitrates, β-blockers, and intravenous anticoagulation. Insertion of an IABP should be considered in patients with hemodynamic instability, poor left ventricular function, or a large area of myocardium at risk. Recurrent ischemic-type chest discomfort is a Class I indication for coronary angiography and PCI or CABG surgery in patients who are considered candidates for revascularization. There is a Class IIa recommendation for readministration of fibrinolytic therapy to patients with ischemic-type chest discomfort and recurrent ST segment elevation who are not considered candidates for revascularization or for whom coronary angiography and PCI cannot be implemented within 60 minutes of the onset of recurrent ischemia. A Class III recommendation regarding streptokinase states that it should not be readministered to patients who received a non-fibrin-specific fibrinolytic agent more than 5 days previously.

CONGESTIVE HEART FAILURE

Wu and colleagues[283] described the outcomes for patients with STEMI who were enrolled in the NRMI-2 database and had CHF on admission (Killip class II or III). A total of 36,303 of 190,518 patients with AMI (19.1%) had CHF on admission; 70.6% were in Killip class II and 29.4% were in Killip class III. Patients who presented with CHF were less likely to receive fibrinolytic therapy or undergo primary PTCA. CHF on admission was a strong independent predictor of in-hospital death (adjusted odds ratio 1.68; 95% CI 1.62 to 1.75).

Hasdai and associates[385] combined the data from four large randomized trials of fibrinolytic therapy for STEMI to describe the incidence, timing, and consequences of mild to moderate CHF in patients with STEMI. Excluding patients with cardiogenic shock, 17,949 of 61,041 (29.4%) patients had mild to moderate CHF. Among the cohort with mild to moderate CHF, 8.7% had CHF only at baseline, 57.6% had CHF only after admission, and 33.7% had CHF at baseline and after admission. The incidence of death was similar for patients without CHF and patients with CHF at baseline that resolved after admission. Patients with CHF that persisted from baseline or developed after admission had a four times greater risk of death at 30 days (8% versus 2%).

There is evidence that patients with STEMI complicated by CHF benefit from early revascularization. Analysis of an

Israeli database compared the outcomes of 629 patients with STEMI who presented in Killip class II or III CHF.[386] Mortality at 6 months was lower among patients who underwent PTCA or CABG surgery within 30 days compared with patients who were managed noninvasively (11.6% versus 27.4%; odds ratio 0.40; 95% CI 0.24 to 0.64; $p < 0.0001$). Analysis of the NRMI-2 registry suggested that the risk of in-hospital death was reduced more by primary PCI than by fibrinolytic therapy in patients with CHF.[283] Thus, the ACC/AHA Practice Guidelines recommend primary PCI for patients with severe CHF or pulmonary edema (Killip class III) when the onset of symptoms is within 12 hours.[20] Primary PCI is considered reasonable (a Class IIa recommendation) for patients who present with severe CHF, persistent ischemic symptoms, or hemodynamic or electrical instability 12 to 24 hours after symptom onset.[20]

It is important to recognize that CHF also is an important prognostic factor in patients with UA or NSTEMI.[387] Among a cohort of 13,707 patients with a confirmed diagnosis of ACS without prior CHF or cardiogenic shock at the time of presentation to the hospital, CHF (Killip class II or III) was present at hospital admission in 1778 patients (13%), and CHF developed later during hospitalization in an additional 869 patients (6.3%).[387] The incidence of CHF was similar in patients with STEMI (15.6%) or NSTEMI (15.7%) but less frequent in patients with UA (8.2%). CHF at the time of admission was associated with a fourfold increase in crude in-hospital mortality rates across all three ACS subsets. The cumulative 6-month mortality rate was greater among patients in whom CHF developed during hospitalization (25.3%) than among patients who had CHF at admission (20.7%) or patients who did not have CHF (5.9%).

ACE inhibitors, eplerenone, and β-adrenergic antagonists are believed to improve the long-term survival of patients with MI complicated by CHF.[388] The AIRE study showed that ramipril, initiated 3 to 10 days after acute MI, reduced all-cause mortality by 27% in patients with either STEMI or NSTEMI and clinical or radiologic evidence of CHF.[317] The EPHESUS study randomized patients with either STEMI or NSTEMI and left ventricular EF less than 40%, to eplerenone or placebo beginning 3 to 14 days after the acute MI.[326] Ninety percent of the patients had CHF, documented by the presence of pulmonary rales, a third heart sound, or evidence of pulmonary venous congestion on the chest radiograph. Concomitant medications included β-blockers in 75% of patients and an ACE inhibitor or angiotensin receptor blocker in 86%. At 30 days after randomization, eplerenone reduced the risk of all-cause mortality by 31% (3.2% versus 4.6%; RR 0.69; 95% CI 0.54 to 0.89; $p = 0.004$).[389] During a mean follow-up period of 16 months, the all-cause mortality rate was 14.4% in the eplerenone group and 16.7% in the placebo group (RR 0.85; 95% CI 0.75 to 0.96; $p = 0.008$).[326]

BHAT, a study that randomized patients to receive propranolol or placebo 5 to 21 days after acute MI, included 710 patients who had a history of CHF before enrollment.[390] After an average follow-up period of 25 months, propranolol reduced total mortality by 27% and sudden death by 47%. A retrospective analysis of the AIRE study was performed to determine the effects of β-blockade on the outcomes for patients with acute MI complicated by CHF.[391] β-Blocker treatment was an independent predictor of reduced risk of total mortality (hazard ratio 0.66; 95% CI 0.48 to 0.90). The CAPRICORN study showed that carvedilol, started 3 to 21 days after MI, reduced all-cause mortality by 33% in patients with a left ventricular EF of 40% or less.[312] Unfortunately, patients with acute MI complicated by CHF are less likely to receive a β-blocker than are patients without CHF.[392]

On the basis of the foregoing evidence, the ACC/AHA Practice Guidelines include eight Class I recommendations for patients with STEMI complicated by pulmonary congestion[20]: (1) an arterial oxygen saturation greater than 90% should be maintained using supplemental oxygen. (2) Morphine sulfate should be given. (3) Patients with a systolic blood pressure 100 mm Hg or higher should receive an ACE inhibitor, beginning with titration of a low dose of a short-acting drug such as captopril. (4) Patients with a systolic blood pressure of 100 mm Hg or higher should receive nitrates. (5) A loop diuretic should be administered to patients with volume overload. (6) Although β-blockade should be initiated before hospital discharge, β-blockers should not be administered acutely to patients with "frank cardiac failure evidenced by pulmonary congestion or signs of a low-output state." (7) Patients already receiving an ACE inhibitor who have a left ventricular EF less than 40% and either symptomatic CHF or diabetes should receive long-term aldosterone blockade unless hyperkalemia (serum potassium greater than 5 mEq/L) or significant renal dysfunction (serum creatinine greater than 2.5 mg/dL in men or greater than 2 mg/dL in women) is present. (8) Echocardiography should be performed urgently to evaluate left and right ventricular function and to exclude a mechanical complication.

In view of the fact that the relevant clinical trials included patients with both STEMI and NSTEMI, it is logical that treatment of NSTEMI patients with CHF should conform to the practice guidelines as discussed for STEMI patients with CHF. Figure 30.7 presents an algorithm for the emergency management of MI complicated by CHF or hypotension.

RIGHT VENTRICULAR DYSFUNCTION AND INFARCTION

Among 416 patients with acute MI who were enrolled in an echocardiographic substudy of the SAVE trial, right ventricular function was an independent predictor of mortality and the development of CHF.[393] The odds of cardiovascular mortality increased 16% for each 5% decrease in the percentage change in right ventricular cavity area from end diastole to end systole.

Occlusion of the right coronary artery (RCA) proximal to the acute marginal branches is the most frequent cause of right ventricular infarction, but occlusion of the LAD or a dominant left circumflex coronary artery also may result in right ventricular MI. Although autopsy studies have shown that anterior MI may be associated with a right ventricular infarction, right ventricular MI that is associated with hemodynamic compromise most commonly occurs in patients with an inferior MI because perfusion of the right ventricle occurs predominantly via the right ventricular branches of the RCA.[394,395] In a series of 125 patients with acute inferior MI who underwent emergency coronary angiography, echocardiography performed before coronary reperfusion demonstrated ischemic dysfunction of the right

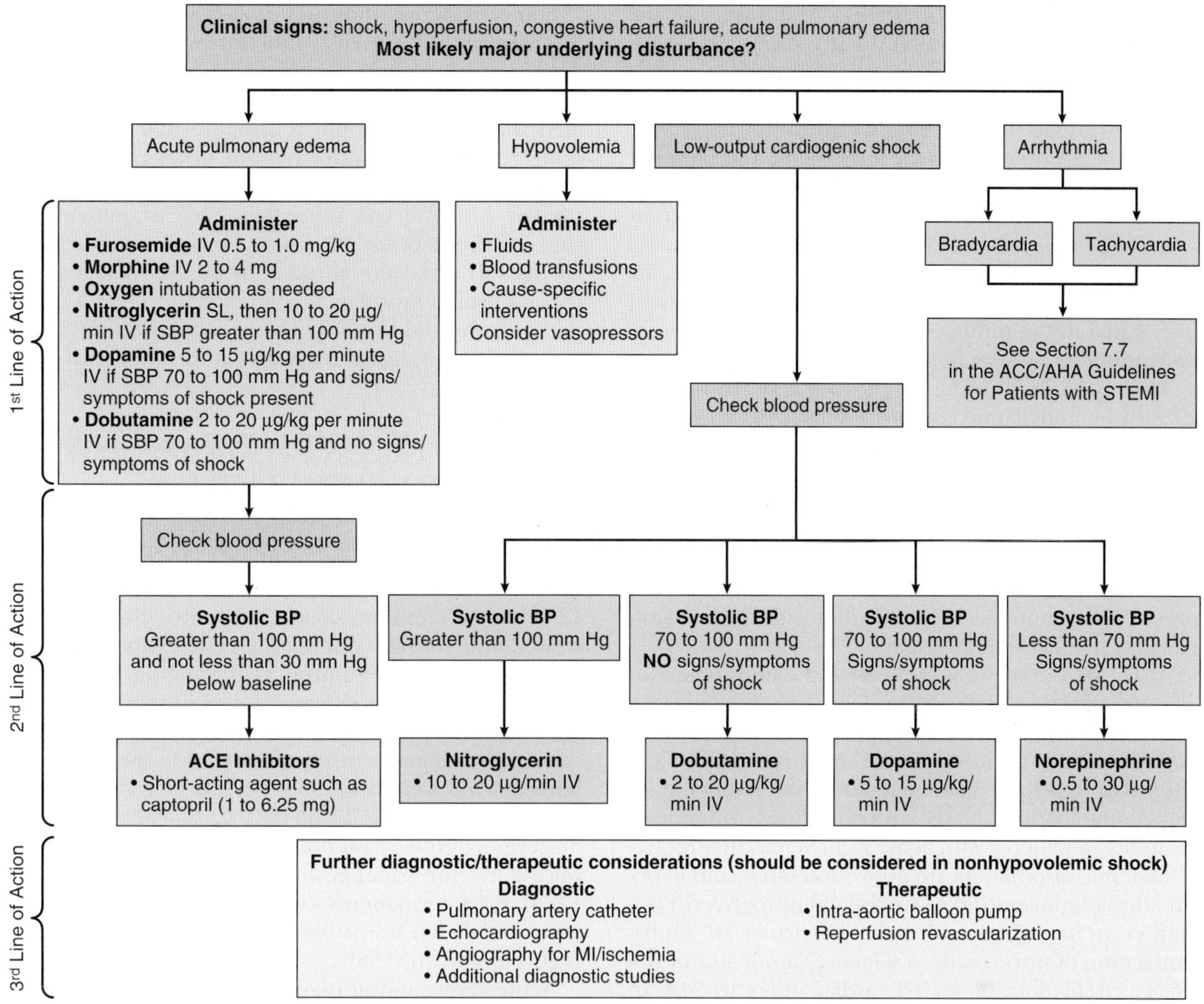

Figure 30.7 Algorithm for emergency management of complicated myocardial infarction (MI). ACE, angiotensin-converting enzyme; BP, blood pressure; IV, intravenous; SBP, systolic BP; SL, sublingual; STEMI, ST segment elevation myocardial infarction. (Data from Guidelines 2000 for cardiopulmonary resuscitation and emergency cardiovascular care: Part 7, the era of reperfusion: Section 1, acute coronary syndromes (acute myocardial infarction). Circulation 2000;102[Suppl I]:I-172-I-203.)

ventricle in 53 (42%) patients.[396] The RCA was the IRA in all patients with right ventricular MI, and depressed flow in the right ventricular branches was evident in each case. Right ventricular branch flow was preserved in patients without right ventricular MI.

Patients with inferior MI complicated by right ventricular infarction have an increased risk of major complications, including death, cardiogenic shock, and ventricular arrhythmias.[397] Cardiogenic shock during hospitalization occurred in 6.9% of a series of 491 patients with inferior MI complicated by right ventricular MI.[397] Patients with right ventricular infarction complicated by cardiogenic shock do not have a better prognosis than patients with cardiogenic shock associated with left ventricular failure.[398] Among a cohort of 1129 patients with acute inferior MI, there was no difference in left ventricular infarct size or function between patients with (n = 491) and patients without (n = 638) right ventricular MI, indicating that the increased risk of right ventricular MI is due to right ventricular dysfunction rather than greater left ventricular injury.[397] The impact of right ventricular MI on prognosis may depend on the patient's age.[399] Among a series of 798 consecutive patients with acute inferior MI, 296 (37%) satisfied electrocardiographic or echocardiographic criteria for right ventricular infarction.[399] Major complications (45% versus 19%, $p < 0.0001$) and in-hospital death (22% versus 6%, $p < 0.0001$) occurred more often in patients with than in those without right ventricular MI. The diagnosis of right ventricular MI increased the mortality risk in patients aged 65 or greater, but not among younger patients.

Although numerous electrocardiographic signs of right ventricular MI have been described, ST segment elevation in lead V_4R is the most reliable electrocardiographic indicator of this form of MI.[400] Zehender and associates[401] studied the diagnostic and prognostic value of ST segment elevation in V_4R in a series of 200 consecutive patients with acute inferior MI. ST segment elevation in lead V_4R was present on the initial ECG in 107 patients (54%). Based on the results of autopsy, coronary angiography, right ventriculography, nuclear scan, or invasive hemodynamic data, ST segment elevation in V_4R had 88% sensitivity, 78% specificity, and 83% diagnostic accuracy for right ventricular MI. ST segment elevation in V_4R was associated with an in-hospital mortality of 31%, compared with 6% among patients without

ST segment elevation in V_4R ($p < 0.001$). Multivariate analysis of clinical data confirmed that 0.1 mV or greater of ST segment elevation in V_4R was a strong independent predictor of in-hospital death (RR 7.7; 95% CI 2.6 to 23) and major complications (RR 4.7; 95% CI 2.4 to 9).

The triad of hypotension, clear lung fields, and elevated jugular venous pressure should raise a suspicion of right ventricular MI in patients with inferior STEMI, but the triad has a sensitivity of less than 25%.[402] The hemodynamic criteria that have been used to diagnose right ventricular MI are right atrial pressure greater than 10 mm Hg and equal or nearly equal to the pulmonary capillary wedge pressure, or a noncompliant pattern in the right atrium.[403] According to the ACC/AHA Practice Guidelines for STEMI, inferior STEMI with hemodynamic compromise is a Class I indication for recording lead V_4R and an echocardiogram to screen for right ventricular MI.[20] Echocardiographic signs of this disorder include right ventricular dilation, right ventricular asynergy, and abnormal interventricular septal motion.[403] Echocardiography also is valuable to exclude pericardial tamponade because both right ventricular MI and pericardial tamponade may manifest with hypotension and elevated jugular venous pressure.[404]

The ACC/AHA guidelines emphasize the importance of maintenance of right ventricular preload, reduction of right ventricular afterload, inotropic support of the right ventricle, maintenance of atrioventricular synchrony, and early reperfusion of the IRA.[20] Volume loading plus dobutamine, but not volume loading alone, has been shown to improve cardiac index in patients with acute right ventricular infarction.[405] Systemic vasodilators are poorly tolerated, and hypotension after administration of sublingual nitroglycerin is a common event in patients with right ventricular MI. Short-term inhalation of nitric oxide, a selective vasodilator of the pulmonary circulation, improved cardiac index by 24% in a series of 13 patients with right ventricular infarction and cardiogenic shock.[406] In patients with right ventricular MI complicated by cardiogenic shock and refractory low cardiac output and hypotension, insertion of a percutaneous ventricular assist device should be considered as a therapeutic option.[407]

The status of right atrial function is an important determinant of the hemodynamic consequences of right ventricular MI.[408] Hemodynamic compromise may result if the atrial contribution to ventricular filling is lost in patients with right ventricular MI. Therefore, high-grade atrioventricular block, other bradyarrhythmias, and atrial fibrillation are common causes of hypotension in patients with right ventricular MI. Ventricular pacing may not increase cardiac output in such patients, although atrial pacing and atrioventricular sequential pacing have been shown to improve cardiac output.[409,410] Atrial fibrillation associated with hemodynamic compromise is an indication for electrical cardioversion.

The elevated right atrial pressure in patients with right ventricular MI may cause refractory hypoxemia as a result of increased right-to-left shunting in patients with an atrial septal defect or patent foramen ovale.[406,411] Inhalation of NO reduced right-to-left shunting by 56% in a series of three patients with right ventricular MI.[406] Right-to-left shunting in patients with right ventricular MI also can be treated by percutaneous closure of the patent foramen ovale.[411]

Some evidence indicates that reperfusion of the IRA improves right ventricular function and clinical outcome in patients with MI. Successful PCI of an occluded RCA in patients with right ventricular infarction has been associated with improved right ventricular wall motion within 1 hour[412] and a reduction in right atrial pressure within 8 hours.[413] Three to 5 days after successful PCI, right ventricular function was normal in 95% of patients.[412] In a study of the data for 49 patients with shock and right ventricular MI who were enrolled in the SHOCK trial registry, the in-hospital mortality rate was found to be 65.2% among patients who did not undergo revascularization, compared with 42.3% among patients who underwent PCI or CABG surgery.[398]

MECHANICAL CAUSES OF CONGESTIVE HEART FAILURE OR LOW CARDIAC OUTPUT

Mitral Regurgitation

Among 1976 patients with acute MI who were not in cardiogenic shock and underwent cardiac catheterization within 12 hours of symptom onset, left ventriculography demonstrated mild mitral regurgitation in 192 patients (9.7%) and moderate or severe mitral regurgitation in 58 patients (2.9%).[61] By multivariate analysis, mild mitral regurgitation and moderate or severe mitral regurgitation were the two strongest independent predictors of 1-year mortality. The hazard ratios were 2.40 (95% CI 1.31 to 4.42; $p = 0.005$) for mild and 2.82 (95% CI 1.34 to 5.92; $p = 0.006$) for moderate or severe mitral regurgitation. The 1-year mortality rates were 2.9% for patients with no mitral regurgitation (n = 1726), 8.5% for patients with mild mitral regurgitation (n = 192), and 20.8% for patients with moderate or severe mitral regurgitation (n = 58).

Acute severe mitral regurgitation accounted for 6.9% of patients with cardiogenic shock among 1422 patients with acute MI who were enrolled in either the SHOCK registry or the randomized trial.[369] The median time from the onset of MI to shock was 12.8 hours.[414] In a postmortem series of 20 cases of papillary muscle rupture, the posteromedial papillary muscle was ruptured in 16 patients and the anterolateral papillary muscle was ruptured in four patients.[415] The greater tendency of the posteromedial papillary muscle to rupture is reflected by the distribution of the IRA in a series of 98 patients with acute mitral regurgitation and cardiogenic shock who were enrolled in the SHOCK studies. The location of the index MI was anterior in 34% of patients and nonanterior in 66%.[414]

The diagnosis of acute severe mitral regurgitation should be suspected in patients with acute onset of pulmonary edema or hypotension. The absence of a loud murmur does not exclude severe mitral regurgitation. The diagnosis can be confirmed by transthoracic or transesophageal echocardiography. The treatment of acute severe mitral regurgitation should include inotropic support, afterload reduction, an IABP, and emergency mitral valve surgery, but mortality is high despite surgical treatment. Among the patients with acute severe mitral regurgitation and cardiogenic shock who were enrolled in the SHOCK registry or the randomized trial, the in-hospital mortality rate was 40% among 43 patients who underwent valve surgery, compared with 71% among 51 patients who did not.[414]

Ventricular Septal Rupture

Among 41,021 patients with STEMI who were enrolled in the GUSTO-I trial, the incidence of ventricular septal rupture was only 0.2% (84/41,021 patients).[416] Acute ventricular septal rupture accounted for 3.9% of patients with cardiogenic shock among 1422 patients with acute MI who were enrolled in either the SHOCK registry or randomized trial.[369]

The clinical manifestations of ventricular septal rupture may include chest pain, dyspnea, and hypotension. A harsh holosystolic murmur may be audible. Cardiogenic shock occurred in 67% of patients in the GUSTO-I trial in whom ventricular septal rupture developed.[416] The diagnosis of ventricular septal rupture can be confirmed by Doppler echocardiography or right heart catheterization to measure the oxygen saturation in the right atrium, right ventricle, and pulmonary artery. The median time from MI to diagnosis of ventricular septal rupture was 16 hours among a series of patients with ventricular septal rupture and cardiogenic shock.[417] The electrocardiographic location of the MI was inferior in 26 patients, anterior in 22, both anterior and inferior in 3, and apico-lateral in 1 patient.[417] Only 35 of 55 patients underwent coronary angiography, and the IRA was identified in only 26 patients: the RCA in 12, the LAD in 11, and the left circumflex coronary artery in 3 cases.

The location of the IRA may be an important determinant of survival in patients with ventricular septal rupture.[416,418] Among a series of 25 patients with this diagnosis, mortality was greater among patients with inferior MI than among patients with anterior MI.[418] At least two factors may explain the differential outcome of patients with inferior and anterior MI complicated by ventricular septal rupture. First, the right ventricular volume overload caused by the left-to-right shunt may be less tolerated in the presence of ischemia or infarction of the right ventricle, both of which are more common with an inferior MI than an anterior MI. Second, histopathologic studies have shown that complex septal defects that are more difficult to repair surgically are more common in patients with an inferior MI.[419]

An IABP has been shown to decrease the shunt and increase systemic cardiac output in patients with ventricular septal rupture.[420] Therefore, vasodilator therapy and an IABP often are used to stabilize patients before surgical repair of the rupture. The overall in-hospital survival rate among patients with ventricular septal rupture in the SHOCK registry was only 13% (7/55).[417] Although six of the seven survivors underwent surgical repair, mortality was 81% (25/31) in the group of patients who underwent surgery. In the GUSTO-I trial, patients whose rupture was repaired surgically had better 30-day mortality (47%) than patients who received medical treatment (94%).[416] Percutaneous closure of acute ventricular septal rupture may be an option in the future.

Left Ventricular Free Wall Rupture

Rupture of the left ventricular free wall may manifest in any of several ways: pericardial tamponade with acute hemodynamic collapse and immediate death, gradual onset of tamponade and hypotension, or subacute formation of a pseudoaneurysm.[421] Although a 6% rate of cardiac rupture among patients with acute MI often is quoted, reports suggest that the rate probably is lower, at least among patients who receive reperfusion therapy. A total of 65 (1.7%) cases of cardiac rupture occurred among 3759 patients with STEMI who received fibrinolytic therapy and were randomized to receive either adjunctive heparin or hirudin.[422] The prevalence of cardiac rupture or pericardial tamponade was 2.3% (28/1190) among patients with cardiogenic shock in the SHOCK registry; 13 patients had both rupture and pericardial tamponade, 9 had tamponade alone, and 6 had rupture alone.[423]

It has been suggested that the incidence of cardiac rupture may be lower after primary PCI than after fibrinolytic therapy. The overall incidence of left ventricular free wall rupture was 2.5% (n = 34) among 1375 patients with STEMI who underwent primary PCI (55.4%) or fibrinolytic therapy (44.6%).[424] In a multivariate analysis, primary PCI was independently associated with a lower incidence of rupture, but no significant difference was observed in the incidence of rupture after primary PCI or fibrinolytic therapy (1.8% versus 3.3%; $p = 0.686$).

The timing of reperfusion therapy may affect both the risk and the timing of free wall rupture. Death from cardiac rupture appears to occur earlier in patients given fibrinolytic therapy than among patients who do not undergo reperfusion therapy.[425] Honan and associates[426] analyzed the relationship between the risk of cardiac rupture and the timing of fibrinolytic therapy for 58 cases of cardiac rupture among 1638 patients who were enrolled in four randomized trials that compared intravenous streptokinase with no fibrinolytic therapy (in the control group). The odds ratio of cardiac rupture increased significantly with increasing delay in the time to treatment. Regression analysis suggested that treatment within 7 hours after symptom onset reduces the risk of cardiac rupture, whereas treatment later than 17 hours after symptom onset increases the risk of cardiac rupture.[426] Thus, it was hypothesized that early fibrinolytic therapy reduces the risk of rupture by reducing the extent of myocardial necrosis, whereas late fibrinolytic therapy increases the risk of rupture by promoting hemorrhagic infarction.

The antemortem diagnosis of free wall rupture, pericardial tamponade, and left ventricular pseudoaneurysm usually is confirmed by an echocardiogram. An echocardiogram was obtained in 20 of the 28 patients in the SHOCK registry who had rupture or pericardial tamponade. A pericardial effusion was observed in 15 (75%) and a myocardial tear was detected in 39%.[423] Six patients underwent pericardiocentesis alone, and 21 had surgical repair of the rupture. The in-hospital survival rate was 39.3%.

CARDIAC ARRHYTHMIAS AND HEART BLOCK

Both atrial and ventricular arrhythmias are common in patients with acute MI. The incidence of atrial fibrillation was 10.4% among 40,891 patients who were enrolled in the GUSTO-I trial.[327] Among patients enrolled in the TRACE study, which enrolled patients with an acute MI and a left ventricular EF less than 35%, atrial fibrillation occurred in 21% of patients and was associated with a 50% increase in the adjusted mortality.[328] Management of atrial arrhythmias is discussed in another chapter.

The likelihood of primary ventricular fibrillation (occurring within 48 hours of acute MI and in the absence of cardiogenic shock or severe CHF) is not altered by fibrinolytic therapy, with an incidence of ventricular fibrillation during the first hospital day of 2.99% for both the fibrinolytic and placebo groups.[331] Some evidence, however, suggests that fibrinolytic therapy exerts a protective effect against secondary ventricular fibrillation (occurring in patients with acute MI complicated by CHF or shock).[331,332] Management of ventricular arrhythmias is discussed in Chapter 32.

The incidence of second-degree or third-degree AV block was 6.9% among 75,993 patients with STEMI who received fibrinolytic therapy and were enrolled in a database that combined four randomized clinical trials.[427] Inferior MI was the strongest independent predictor of AV block (odds ratio 3.3; 95% CI 3.1 to 3.5). In comparison with patients without AV block, adjusted mortality was greater at 30 days, 6 months, and 1 year among patients with AV block. The adjusted mortality odds ratios at 1 year were 2.4 (95% CI 2.2 to 2.6) for patients with AV block and inferior MI and 3.3 (95% CI 3.0 to 3.7) for patients with AV block and anterior MI.

Table 30.3 Grading of Angina Pectoris According to Canadian Cardiovascular Society Classification

Class	Description of Stage
I	"Ordinary physical activity does not cause . . . angina," such as walking or climbing stairs. Angina occurs with strenuous, rapid, or prolonged exertion at work or recreation.
II	"Slight limitation of ordinary activity." Angina occurs on walking or climbing stairs rapidly; walking uphill; walking or stair climbing after meals; in cold, in wind, or under emotional stress; or only during the few hours after awakening. Angina occurs on walking more than two blocks on the level and climbing more than one flight of ordinary stairs at a normal pace and under normal conditions.
III	"Marked limitations of ordinary physical activity." Angina occurs on walking one to two blocks on the level and climbing one flight of stairs under normal conditions and at a normal pace.
IV	"Inability to carry on any physical activity without discomfort—anginal symptoms may be present at rest."

Modified from Campeau L: Grading of angina pectoris. Circulation 1976;54:522-523 (Letter).

UNSTABLE AND NON–ST SEGMENT ELEVATION MYOCARDIAL INFARCTION

CLINICAL MANIFESTATIONS

DEFINITION

The ACC/AHA Practice Guidelines define *UA* as "an acute process of myocardial ischemia that is not of sufficient severity and duration to result in myocardial necrosis."[1] *NSTEMI* is defined as "an acute process of myocardial ischemia with sufficient severity and duration to result in myocardial necrosis."[1] Thus, NSTEMI is distinguished from UA by the detection of cardiac markers indicative of myocardial necrosis, such as troponin I or T, in patients with NSTEMI.

CLINICAL HISTORY

Criteria for the diagnosis of UA are based on the Canadian Cardiovascular Society (CCS) grading system[428] (Table 30.3). The three principal presentations of UA are angina that occurs at rest, new-onset CCS class III or IV angina, and angina that has increased from class I or II to class III or IV.[429]

The GRACE registry analyzed the presenting symptoms of 20,881 patients with STEMI, NSTEMI, or UA.[15] Among the patients with UA and NSTEMI, 5.7% and 12.3%, respectively, presented with symptoms other than chest pain. Patients with UA or NSTEMI who presented with atypical symptoms were less likely to undergo coronary angiography, PCI, or CABG surgery and were less likely to receive heparin, aspirin, or β-blockers. The absence of chest pain among patients with ACS was predictive of an increased risk of in-hospital death.

Several risk-stratification models have been developed to evaluate patients with suspected ACS. The TIMI risk score utilizes seven variables to calculate a score that is predictive of the risk of death and ischemic events in patients with suspected ACS.[430] Four of the seven variables are derived from the clinical history: age 65 years or older, at least three risk factors for CAD (family history of CAD, hypertension, hypercholesterolemia, diabetes, cigarette smoking), two or more anginal events within the previous 24 hours, and use of aspirin within the previous 7 days.[430] The GRACE risk score and a PURSUIT risk model also have been shown to have predictive power in patients with suspected ACS.[431,432]

PHYSICAL EXAMINATION

As in patients with STEMI, evidence of heart failure at the time of initial presentation has prognostic importance in patients with non–ST segment elevation ACS. In a database accrued from studies in 26,090 patients with UA or NSTEMI, heart rate, systolic blood pressure, and Killip class were independent predictors of mortality at 30 days and 6 months.[433] Patients in Killip class II, III, or IV constituted only 11% of the population but accounted for 30% of the deaths.

DIAGNOSTIC APPROACH

ELECTROCARDIOGRAM

The admission ECG has prognostic value in patients with ACS.[434,435] Although normal or nonspecific findings on the initial ECG confer a better prognosis than ST segment depression or elevation seen on the ECG, such findings do not predict a benign outcome in patients with suspected ACS.[435] The risk of death or reinfarction at 30 days or 6 months is similar in patients with ST segment elevation and in those with ST segment depression; the risk is lower among patients with isolated T wave inversion.[434] The GUSTO-IIb clinical trial enrolled 12,142 patients with symptoms of cardiac ischemia at rest and electrocardiographic signs of myocardial ischemia.[434] After adjustment for factors associated with an increased risk of death or reinfarction, the odds of death or reinfarction at 30 days were 1.68 (95% CI 1.36 to 2.08) in those with ST segment elevation and 1.62 (95% CI 1.32 to 1.98) in those with ST segment depression compared with those who had T wave inversion only on the admission ECG.[434]

The impact of invasive management on outcome in patients with ACS is predicted by the presence or absence of ST segment depression on the admission ECG. Among patients with ACS who were enrolled in the Fast Revascularization during InStability in Coronary Artery Disease (FRISC II) randomized trial comparing early invasive management and a noninvasive strategy, ST segment depression was present at enrollment in 45.5% of patients.[436] Among the patients who presented with ST segment depression, the invasive strategy reduced the risk of death or MI at 12 months from 18.2% to 12% (RR 0.66; 95% CI 0.50 to 0.88; $p = 0.004$). Mortality was reduced from 5.8% to 3.3% (RR 0.58; 95% CI 0.33 to 1.01; $p = 0.050$). Among the patients without ST segment depression, the corresponding rates of death or MI were 10.4% and 8.9% ($p = 0.36$), and the mortality rates were 2% and 1.2% ($p = 0.26$). A similar dichotomy was found in the Treat Angina with Aggrastat and Determine Cost of Therapy with an Invasive or Conservative Strategy (TACTICS)-TIMI 18 randomized trial of early invasive versus conservative strategies in patients with ACS.[437] Thus, according to the ACA/AHA Practice Guidelines for the management of patients with UA and NSTEMI, new or presumably new ST segment depression is a Class I indication for use of an invasive strategy.[1]

The magnitude[438,439] and the location[440] of ST segment depression also provide independent prognostic information in patients with UA and NSTEMI. Among 1846 patients who were enrolled in the TACTICS—TIMI 18 trial, the magnitude of ST segment depression was a predictor of unsuccessful medical therapy in patients who were randomized to the conservative strategy.[439] The magnitude of ST segment depression was an independent predictor of the extent of CAD among patients who were randomized to the early invasive strategy. After adjustment for baseline characteristics and the degree of troponin elevation, the benefit of an early invasive strategy was greater among patients with ST segment depression of 0.10 mV or greater, compared with patients with 0.05 to 0.09 mV of ST segment depression.

Among a cohort of 432 patients with a first NSTEMI, patients with ST segment depression in two or more lateral leads (I, aVL, V_5, or V_6) had lower left ventricular EFs, more frequent left main coronary artery or three-vessel CAD, and greater in-hospital mortality.[440] Although isolated T wave inversion on the admission ECG is associated with a better prognosis than ST segment depression or elevation, negative T waves in leads V_2 and V_3 are associated with critical stenosis of the proximal LAD and stunning of the myocardium supplied by the LAD.[441,442]

BIOCHEMICAL MARKERS

Biochemical markers such as troponin or CK-MB provide both diagnostic and prognostic information. As discussed, the distinction between NSTEMI and UA is based on the blood assays for biochemical markers of myocardial necrosis. Among 1404 patients with UA or NSTEMI who were enrolled in the TIMI IIIB trial, the mortality rate at 42 days was 3.7% (21/573) for patients with a baseline troponin I 0.4 ng/mL or greater, compared with 1% (8/831) for patients with a troponin I less than 0.4 ng/mL ($p < 0.001$).[443] There were significant increases in mortality with increasing levels of troponin I. An elevated troponin in patients with suspected ACS confers a greater risk of death or reinfarction even among patients without significant angiographic CAD.[444] Patients with ACS who have an elevated troponin, even if the elevation is minor, derive greater benefit from platelet GP IIb/IIIa inhibitors[445,446] or invasive management[447] than do patients without an elevated troponin.

Another biochemical marker that provides prognostic information is brain natriuretic peptide (BNP). An elevated BNP at the time of presentation or after hospital discharge in patients with ACS is an independent predictor of death or new-onset CHF during follow-up.[448,449]

CORONARY CT ANGIOGRAPHY

Several randomized trials have been performed to evaluate the utility of coronary CT angiography (CCTA) in "low-risk" patients with chest pain. Sixteen emergency departments enrolled 749 patients in a multicenter, randomized study called the Coronary Computed Tomographic Angiography for Systematic Triage of Acute Chest Pain Patients to Treatment (CT-STAT) trial.[450] The patients were randomized to either CCTA (n = 361) or rest-stress myocardial perfusion imaging (MPI) (n = 338). The time to diagnosis and costs of care were less in the patients who were randomized to CCTA.[450] A larger study randomized low to intermediate-risk patients with possible ACS, in a 2:1 ratio, to undergo CCTA or traditional care.[451] None of the 640 patients with a negative CCTA died or had an MI within 30 days.[451] A multicenter trial that randomized 1000 patients with suspected ACS but no ischemic electrocardiographic changes and a normal initial serum troponin found that patients evaluated by CCTA were discharged sooner than patients who underwent standard evaluation.[452] The patients who were randomized to CCTA, however, underwent more downstream testing and had greater radiation exposure.[452] The 2011 ACCF/AHA Focused Update of the Guidelines for the Management of Patients with UA or NSTEMI included a Class IIa recommendation that "In patients with suspected ACS with a low or intermediate probability of CAD, in whom the follow-up 12-lead ECG and cardiac biomarkers measurements are normal, performance of a noninvasive coronary imaging test (i.e., CCTA) is reasonable as an alternative to stress testing."[1]

APPROACH TO MANAGEMENT

Figure 30.8 presents an algorithm for the treatment of UA and non–ST segment elevation myocardial infarction. Specific components of management are discussed next.

ANTI-ISCHEMIC THERAPY

Nitrates

The Class I recommendations for anti-ischemic therapy in patients with UA or NSTEMI include nitroglycerin administered initially as a sublingual tablet or spray, followed by intravenous infusion. Although nitroglycerin often relieves

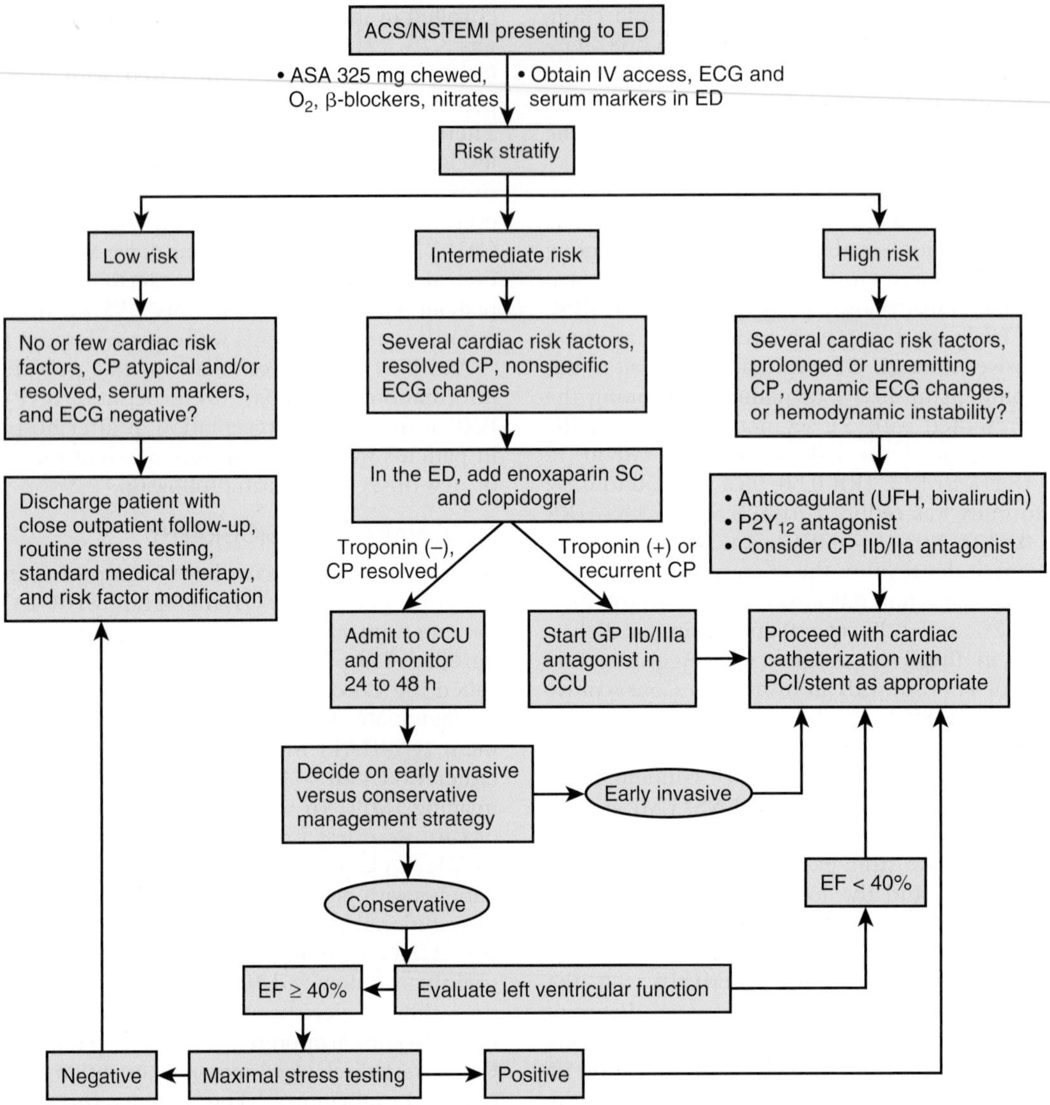

Figure 30.8 Algorithm for the treatment of unstable angina or non–ST segment elevation myocardial infarction. *Note:* Enoxaparin is not recommended for use in patients with known bleeding disorders or significant renal insufficiency (serum creatinine of 2 to 2.5 mg/dL or greater). ACS, acute coronary syndrome; ASA, acetylsalicylic acid (aspirin); CCU, critical care unit; CP, chest pain; ECG, electrocardiogram; ED, emergency department; EF, ejection fraction; IV, intravenous; NSTEMI, non–ST segment elevation myocardial infarction; PTCA, percutaneous transluminal coronary angioplasty; SC, subcutaneous. (From Antman EM, Anbe DT, Armstrong PW, et al: ACC/AHA guidelines for the management of patients with ST-elevation myocardial infarction: A report of the American College of Cardiology/American Heart Association Task Force on Practice Guidelines [committee to revise the 1999 guidelines for the management of patients with acute myocardial infarction]. Circulation 2004;110:e82-e292.)

chest pain in patients with ACS, nitrates have not been shown to reduce clinical events in patients with UA or NSTEMI. Abrupt cessation of intravenous nitroglycerin may be associated with rebound myocardial ischemia in patients with ACS.[453] After intravenous infusion of nitroglycerin for longer than 24 hours the development of tolerance may require an increase in the dose to maintain efficacy, but 200 μg/min usually is considered the maximum dose.

β-Blockers

The Class I recommendations for anti-ischemic therapy in patients with UA or NSTEMI include the administration of a β-blocker within the first 24 hours for patients who do not have signs of heart failure, evidence of a low output state, increased risk for cardiogenic shock, or other relative contraindications to β-blockade. Nevertheless, many patients who are eligible for a β-blocker therapy do not receive it, possibly because there are limited data regarding the efficacy of β-blockers in patients with UA or NSTEMI.[454] Clinical trials that evaluated β-blockers in patients with UA were not adequately powered to demonstrate reductions in mortality. A pooled analysis of randomized trials in patients with threatened or evolving MI concluded that β-blockers reduce the risk of MI by 13%.[455] A report from the GRACE registry analyzed the outcomes of 7106 patients with NSTEMI.[454] β-Blocker therapy was initiated within 24 hours of admission in 76% of patients without contraindications. After multivariable logistic regression analysis to adjust for presence of comorbidity, both in-hospital mortality (odds ratio 0.58; 95% CI 0.42 to

0.81) and 6-month mortality (OR 0.75; 95% CI 0.56 to 0.997) were lower among patients who received β-blockers than among patients who did not.

Calcium Antagonists

The Holland Interuniversity Nifedipine/Metoprolol Trial (HINT) found that nifedipine alone increased the risk of MI or recurrent angina, relative to placebo, by 24% in patients with UA.[456] Therefore, the ACC/AHA Practice Guidelines for UA and NSTEMI include a Class III recommendation for immediate-release dihydropyridine calcium antagonists in the absence of a β-blocker.

The Multicenter Diltiazem Postinfarction Trial (MDPIT) randomized 2466 patients to receive diltiazem or placebo 3 to 15 days after acute MI.[346] Approximately 70% of patients met ECG criteria for a Q wave MI, and 25% had non–Q wave MI. The percentage of patients with STEMI or NSTEMI was not reported. Total mortality rates for the two treatment groups were nearly identical, but treatment with diltiazem was associated with increased mortality in patients with either radiographic evidence of pulmonary congestion or a left ventricular EF less than 40%. Also, diltiazem was associated with an increased risk of late-onset CHF in patients with a left ventricular EF less than 40%.[347]

Gibson and colleagues[457] performed a post hoc subset analysis of the 817 patients with non–Q wave MI and no pulmonary congestion who were enrolled in two clinical trials: MDPIT and the second Danish Verapamil Infarction Trial (DAVIT-II).[457] The adjusted all-cause mortality was lower among patients who were given diltiazem or verapamil than among those who received placebo (RR 0.65; 95% CI 0.40 to 1.05). Nevertheless, calcium antagonists are not considered first-line therapeutic agents in patients with ACS and are reserved for patients with recurrent ischemia, but no severe left ventricular dysfunction, who have a contraindication to β-blockers.

Intra-aortic Balloon Counterpulsation

Intra-aortic balloon counterpulsation is believed to increase myocardial oxygen supply by increasing diastolic pressure and to reduce myocardial oxygen demand by afterload reduction of the left ventricle. The indications for an IABP in patients with ACS include refractory ischemia, hypotension, and cardiogenic shock, although this modality should be considered an adjunct to definitive therapies such as percutaneous or surgical myocardial revascularization.

ANTIPLATELET THERAPY

Aspirin

UA and NSTEMI are Class I indications for aspirin, which should be started as soon as possible and continued indefinitely. The recommendation is based on the results of four small randomized trials. A pooled analysis of the results concluded that aspirin reduces the risk of death or MI by 50% in patients with UA. The optimal dose of aspirin in patients with ACS is uncertain.[458] An aspirin dose of 75 mg/day reduced the risk of MI or death after 1 year in patients with UA or non–Q wave MI who were enrolled in a prospective, randomized, double-blind, placebo-controlled multicenter trial (RR 0.52; 95% CI 0.37 to 0.72).[459] Among 20,521 patients with ACS who were enrolled in the GUSTO IIb and Platelet Glycoprotein IIb/IIIa in Unstable Angina: Receptor Suppression Using Integrilin Therapy (PURSUIT) trials, an aspirin dose 150 mg or greater was associated with a lower risk of MI at 6 months, compared with an aspirin dose less than 150 mg (hazard ratio 0.79; 95% CI 0.64 to 0.98; p = 0.03).[460] The Clopidogrel in Unstable Angina to Prevent Recurrent Events (CURE) trial randomized 12,562 patients with ACS to aspirin plus clopidogrel 75 mg daily or aspirin plus placebo.[461] The study protocol recommended an aspirin dose of 75 to 325 mg and the dose was left to the discretion of the local investigator. In both arms of the study higher doses of aspirin were associated with an increased risk of major bleeding but clinical event rates were not reduced by higher doses of aspirin. PCI-CURE was a substudy of the CURE trial that consisted of the 2658 patients who underwent PCI.[462,463] A post hoc analysis of the patients who were enrolled in PCI-CURE found that the moderate-dose (101 to 199 mg) and high-dose (≥ 200 mg) aspirin groups had similar rates of cardiovascular death, MI, or stroke compared with the low-dose (≤ 100 mg) aspirin group, but high-dose aspirin was associated with an increased risk of major bleeding.[462,463]

The Clopidogrel and Aspirin Optimal Dose Usage to Reduce Recurrent Events–Seventh Organization to Assess Strategies in Ischemic Syndromes (CURRENT-OASIS 7) Trial was the first randomized trial to compare two different doses of aspirin in patients with ACS.[464,465] The primary results have been published in two complementary papers in the September 2, 2010, issue of the *New England Journal of Medicine (NEJM)* and the October 9, 2010, issue of *Lancet*.[464,465] The *NEJM* paper presents an analysis of the entire enrollment of 25,086 patients, including patients who did not undergo coronary angiography or PCI, whereas the *Lancet* paper describes a prespecified analysis of the 17,263 patients who underwent PCI. Among the entire cohort of 25,086 patients there was no significant difference between the higher dose of aspirin (300 to 325 mg daily) and the lower dose of aspirin (75 to 100 mg daily) with respect to the primary composite end point of cardiovascular death, myocardial infarction, or stroke at 30 days. Although the rates of major bleeding were 2.3% for both doses of aspirin, there was significantly less minor bleeding among the patients who received the lower dose of aspirin (4.4% versus 5%; hazard ratio 1.13; p = 0.04).

Based on an analysis of the PLATO trial, the label for ticagrelor, a platelet $P2Y_{12}$ receptor inhibitor, includes a "black box" warning that maintenance doses of aspirin reduce the effectiveness of ticagrelor. The most recent update of the practice guidelines for PCI includes a Class IIa recommendation that it is reasonable to prescribe a maintenance aspirin dose of 81 mg daily in preference to higher doses.[98]

Inhibitors of the Platelet $P2Y_{12}$ Receptor

Inhibitors of the platelet $P2Y_{12}$ receptor have been shown to improve outcomes in patients with UA or NSTEMI.[466,467] An open study that randomized patients with UA to ticlopidine or conventional therapy (excluding aspirin) demonstrated a 46% reduction in the risk of vascular death and nonfatal MI.[466] Clopidogrel has a more rapid onset of action and a better safety profile than ticlopidine. The CURE trial demonstrated that the combination of clopidogrel and aspirin, compared with aspirin alone, improved outcomes among patients with ACS without ST segment elevation.[467]

There is extensive evidence that platelet inhibition by clopidogrel is influenced by both drug interactions and certain genotypes that affect the metabolism of clopidogrel, a prodrug that is converted to an active metabolite by CYP2C19 activity, a hepatic cytochrome P450 enzyme.[468,469] Co-administration of clopidogrel and drugs that are metabolized by CYP2C19, such as some proton pump inhibitors, may inhibit the formation of clopidogrel's active metabolite, resulting in diminished platelet inhibition. On November 17, 2009, the United States Food and Drug Administration (FDA) issued a public alert regarding updated labeling of clopidogrel that included that following statement: "New data show that when clopidogrel and omeprazole are taken together the effectiveness of clopidogrel is reduced." There is also evidence, however, that proton pump inhibitors may be associated with an increased risk of adverse cardiovascular events in the absence of clopidogrel.[470] Concomitant use of proton pump inhibitors and thienopyridines was discussed in detail in an expert consensus document published by the American College of Cardiology Foundation, the College of Gastroenterology, and the American Heart Association.[471]

Genetic polymorphisms that affect CYP2C19 activity are common and are associated with variability in the bioavailability of clopidogrel's active metabolite, affecting platelet inhibition and clinical outcomes, including the risk of stent thrombosis. On March 12, 2010, the FDA approved a new label for clopidogrel that contained a "boxed warning" regarding the drug's decreased efficacy in patients with impaired capacity to convert clopidogrel to an active metabolite, prompting publication of a document by the ACCF/AHA.[472]

The drug interactions and genetic polymorphisms that affect clopidogrel's metabolism can be approached using several strategies. One potential strategy is to employ genetic testing to identify patients who are heterozygous or homozygous for loss-of-function alleles that impair metabolism of clopidogrel, but genetic testing is expensive and has not gained widespread acceptance. Another approach is alternative dosing regimens of clopidogrel. Numerous studies have found that a 600-mg loading dose of clopidogrel, compared with a 300-mg loading dose, reduces the risk of major adverse cardiovascular events after PCI without increasing the risk of major bleeding.[473] Also, increased loading and maintenance doses of clopidogrel produces greater platelet inhibition in patients who are heterozygous for the CYP2C19*2 loss of function allele.[474,475] High residual platelet activity during clopidogrel therapy is associated with an increased risk of ischemic events in patients with ACS who undergo PCI, but a randomized trial that compared standard- and high-dose clopidogrel regimens in patients with high residual platelet activity failed to show a reduction in the incidence of cardiovascular deaths, nonfatal MI, or stent thrombosis 6 months after PCI with drug-eluting stents.[476,477]

The CURRENT-OASIS 7 trial compared two regimens of clopidogrel in patients with ACS.[464,465] The double-dose patients received a clopidogrel loading dose of 600 mg and a daily maintenance dose of 150 mg on days 2 to 7, then 75 mg daily, whereas the standard-dose group received a loading dose of 300 mg followed by a daily maintenance dose of 75 mg. The frequency of major bleeding was greater among the patients who were randomized to the higher dose of clopidogrel. Although the double-dose regimen was associated with a reduction in cardiovascular events and stent thrombosis in ACS patients who underwent PCI, it is uncertain whether the higher maintenance dose that was administered for only 6 days provided any additional benefit beyond the documented benefit of the 600-mg loading dose.

A third approach is to prescribe other $P2Y_{12}$ inhibitors, such as prasugrel and ticagrelor. Cytochrome P450 genetic polymorphisms do not affect drug metabolite concentrations, inhibition of platelet aggregation, or clinical event rates in patients treated with prasugrel[478,479] or ticagrelor.[480] Also, compared with the combination of aspirin and clopidogrel, the combination of aspirin and ticagrelor reduced the risk of death in patients with ACS.[113] Thus, the combinations of clopidogrel, prasugrel, or ticagrelor with aspirin were included in the Class I recommendations for dual antiplatelet therapy in the 2012 ACCF/AHA Focused Update of the Guideline for the Management of Patients with UA/Non-ST-Elevation Myocardial Infarction.[23]

Whenever possible clopidogrel and ticagrelor should be discontinued at least 5 days before CABG surgery, and prasugrel should be stopped at least 7 days before CABG surgery, to attenuate the increased perioperative bleeding associated with inhibition of platelet $P2Y_{12}$ receptors.[97] Therefore, some practitioners prefer to withhold clopidogrel until the results of diagnostic cardiac catheterization are known, but this approach ignores the proven benefit of clopidogrel pretreatment in patients with ACS who undergo PCI[481] or CABG.[482] Also, CABG surgery can usually be deferred for 5 to 7 days, and percutaneous revascularization is more frequent than surgical revascularization in patients with ACS.[482] The CURE investigators concluded that the increased bleeding risk in patients who may require CABG surgery is outweighed by the overall reduction in ischemic events among all patients.[482] Also, among patients who were enrolled in the TRITON-TIMI 38 trial and underwent CABG, patients who were randomized to prasugrel had a lower rate of death after CABG, compared to the rate among patients who were randomized to clopidogrel, despite an increase in bleeding, platelet transfusion, and surgical reexploration for bleeding.[483] Thus, a policy of withholding $P2Y_{12}$ antagonists until after coronary angiography may harm more patients than a policy of starting a $P2Y_{12}$ antagonist upon admission to the hospital.

Platelet Glycoprotein IIb/IIIa Receptor Antagonists

Discontinuation of either UFH or LMWH in patients with UA is associated with a rebound increase in thrombin generation,[484] which may underlie the increase in death and MI that has been observed during the 12 hours after heparin is stopped in patients with ACS.[485,486] Compared with patients who were randomized to a placebo group, patients who were randomized to treatment with a GP IIb/IIIa antagonist, eptifibatide, experienced significantly fewer deaths and MIs during the 12 hours after heparin was terminated.[486]

A retrospective analysis of the PURSUIT trial found that treatment with eptifibatide was associated with improved outcome among patients in whom cardiogenic shock developed during hospitalization for ACS without persistent ST segment elevation.[487] Although randomization to eptifibatide treatment did not affect the occurrence of shock, patients with shock who received eptifibatide had significantly reduced adjusted odds of death at 30 days (odds ratio 0.51; 95% CI 0.28 to 0.94; $p = 0.03$). It is unlikely that improved outcome after PCI was responsible for the beneficial effect of eptifibatide because only 25% of the patients with shock in PURSUIT underwent PCI.

Boersma and colleagues[488] performed a meta-analysis of the individual patient data from six trials that randomized 31,402 patients with ACS without persistent ST segment elevation to a GP IIb/IIIa inhibitor treatment group (abciximab, eptifibatide, lamifiban, or tirofiban) or to a control group. Overall, there was a 9% reduction in the odds of death or MI at 30 days (10.8% versus 11.8%; odds ratio 0.91; 95% CI 0.84 to 0.98; $p = 0.015$).[488] The baseline troponin value was available in a subset of 11,059 patients (35% of the entire cohort). Among the 45% of patients with a troponin T or I level 0.1 ng/mL or greater, there was a 15% reduction in the odds of death or MI at 30 days compared with that for the control group (10.3% versus 12%; odds ratio 0.85; 95% CI 0.71 to 1.03). No risk reduction was observed among patients with negative troponins (GP IIb/IIIa inhibitor 7% versus control 6.2%; odds ratio 1.17; 95% CI 0.94 to 1.44). Another meta-analysis of the same six trials found that the impact of GP IIb/IIIa antagonists on outcome varied with the revascularization strategy.[489] The reduction of ischemic events was greater among patients who underwent PCI during the index hospitalization (odds ratio 0.82; $p = 0.01$) than among patients who were managed medically (odds ratio 0.95; $p = 0.27$).[489] The corresponding number of events prevented per 1000 patients treated was 20 for patients who underwent PCI compared with 4 for patients treated medically.

The Early Glycoprotein IIb/IIIa Inhibition in Non-ST-Segment Elevation Acute Coronary Syndrome (EARLY ACS) trial compared two strategies of GP IIb/IIIa administration in 9492 patients with ACS without ST-segment elevation who were assigned to an invasive strategy.[490] The patients were randomly assigned to either early eptifibatide beginning ≥ 12 hours before coronary angiography, or a matching placebo infusion with provisional, delayed use of eptifibatide after angiography. At 30 days the rate of death or MI was 11.2% in the early-eptifibatide group compared with 12.3% in the delayed eptifibatide group (odds ratio 0.89; 95% CI 0.79 to 1.01; $p = 0.08$). The rates of bleeding and red cell transfusion, but not severe bleeding, were significantly higher in the early-eptifibatide group.

Several Class I, II, and III recommendations for the use of platelet GP IIb/IIIa antagonists are included in the 2012 ACCF/AHA Focused Update of the ACC/AHA Guideline for the Management of Patients with UA/Non-ST-Elevation Myocardial Infarction.[23] Patients with definite UA/NSTEMI at medium or high risk and in whom an initial invasive strategy is selected should receive dual antiplatelet therapy on presentation: either a GP IIb/IIIa inhibitor (eptifibatide and tirofiban are preferred) or a $P2Y_{12}$ receptor inhibitor (clopidogrel or ticagrelor before PCI, and clopidogrel, prasugrel, or ticagrelor at the time of PCI) should be added to aspirin (Class I). For patients in whom an initial conservative strategy is selected, the guidelines recommend that patients with subsequent heart failure, serious arrhythmias, or recurrent symptoms or ischemia should undergo diagnostic angiography preceded by "upstream" administration of either a GP IIb/IIIa inhibitor (eptifibatide or tirofiban), clopidogrel, or ticagrelor in combination with aspirin and anticoagulant therapy (Class I). For patients in whom an initial conservative strategy is selected, the guidelines state that it is reasonable to add a GP IIb/IIIa inhibitor to aspirin and a $P2Y_{12}$ receptor inhibitor (clopidogrel or ticagrelor) before diagnostic angiography when there is recurrent ischemic discomfort (Class IIa). Among patients who are selected for an initial invasive strategy, upstream administration of a GP IIb/IIIa inhibitor before diagnostic angiography may be omitted in patients who are treated with both bivalirudin and at least 300 mg of clopidogrel at least 6 hours earlier than angiography or PCI (Class IIa). Upstream administration of a GP IIb/IIIa inhibitor is not recommended in UA/NSTEMI patients who are already receiving aspirin and a $P2Y_{12}$ receptor inhibitor and who are either at low risk for ischemic events or at high risk of bleeding (Class III). Finally, abciximab should not be administered to patients in whom PCI is not planned (Class III), presumably because the GUSTO IV ACS trial failed to show a benefit of abciximab among patients with ACS who did not undergo early coronary revascularization.[491]

GP IIb/IIIa antagonists increase the risk of bleeding, frequently involving the access site used for cardiac catheterization, but the risk of intracranial hemorrhage is not increased.[488] The meta-analysis discussed earlier found that the risk of major bleeding was 2.4% among patients who were randomized to a GP IIb/IIIa antagonist compared with 1.4% among control patients (odds ratio 1.62; 95% CI 1.36 to 1.94; $p < 0.0001$).[488] One preventable cause of bleeding is excess dosing of a GP IIb/IIIa antagonist, which occurred in 26.8% of patients with non–ST segment elevation ACS who were enrolled in the CRUSADE registry by 387 hospitals in 2004.[492]

A complete blood count including platelet count should be included in monitoring during administration of GP IIb/IIIa antagonists. A review of eight large placebo-controlled randomized trials, however, concluded that abciximab, but not eptifibatide or tirofiban, increases the incidence of thrombocytopenia.[493]

ANTITHROMBIN THERAPY

Unfractionated Heparin

At least seven randomized, placebo-controlled trials have compared UFH plus aspirin with aspirin alone in patients with UA, but none of them was adequately powered to detect a reduction in the rate of death or MI during hospitalization. A meta-analysis of six of the trials concluded that the addition of UFH to aspirin reduced the risk of death or MI during treatment by 33% (RR 0.67; 95% CI 0.44 to 1.02; $p = 0.06$).[494] Therefore, the ACC/AHA Practice Guidelines include intravenous UFH in the list of Class I recommendations for patients with UA or NSTEMI.[1] The guidelines also recommend daily measurement of hemoglobin or hematocrit and platelet count during treatment with UFH because of the increased risks of bleeding and thrombocytopenia. An analysis of patients who were enrolled in the CRUSADE registry in 2004 found that bleeding was related to excess dosing of UFH, which occurred in 32.8% of patients who received UFH.[492]

As discussed earlier, a rebound increase in thrombin generation with reactivation of UA has been observed after the discontinuation of UFH. One clinical trial observed an eightfold increase in death and a twofold increase in MI during the 12 hours after heparin was discontinued.[486] The rate of events during the 12 hours after heparin was terminated was significantly lower among patients who were randomized to treatment with eptifibatide than among patients in the placebo group.[486]

Low-Molecular-Weight Heparin

The FRISC study randomized 1506 patients with UA or non–Q wave MI to receive placebo or dalteparin, an LMWH, twice daily for 6 days, followed by once daily for 35 to 45 days.[495] A 63% reduction in the risk of death or MI occurred during the first 6 days (4.8% versus 1.8%; $p = 0.001$). Subsequently, 21,946 patients with non–ST segment elevation ACS have been enrolled in six randomized trials that compared enoxaparin, another LMWH, with UFH. A meta-analysis of the trials found no significant difference in death at 30 days for enoxaparin versus UFH (3% versus 3%; odds ratio 1.00; 95% CI 0.85 to 1.17).[496] A statistically significant reduction was observed in the combined end points of death and nonfatal MI at 30 days for enoxaparin versus UFH (10.1% versus 11%; odds ratio 0.91; 95% CI 0.83 to 0.99).

Although it had been hypothesized that the risk of bleeding would be less during treatment with LMWH than with UFH, the meta-analysis performed by Petersen and colleagues[496] found no significant difference between enoxaparin and UFH in the rates of blood transfusion or major bleeding at 7 days after initiation of the study treatment. The risk of bleeding during treatment with LWMH may be increased by excess dosing, which occurred in 13.8% of patients who were enrolled in the CRUSADE registry in 2004 and received LMWH.[492]

The current ACCF/AHA guidelines recommend the addition of anticoagulant therapy to antiplatelet therapy in patients with UA or NSTEMI as soon as possible after presentation.[23] Both UFH and enoxaparin received Class I recommendations for patients selected for either an invasive or conservative strategy.[23] Enoxaparin or fondaparinux is preferable to UFH in patients selected for an initial conservative strategy unless CABG is planned within 2 hours (Class IIa).[23]

DIRECT THROMBIN INHIBITORS

Direct thrombin inhibitors, such as hirudin and bivalirudin, have been evaluated in patients with ACS. The ACUITY trial was an open-label, randomized, multicenter trial that compared heparin plus a GP IIb/IIIa antagonist, bivalirudin plus a GP IIb/IIIa antagonist, and bivalirudin alone in patients with moderate-risk or high-risk non–ST segment elevation ACS who were undergoing an early invasive strategy.[497-499] NSTEMI was present in 59% of patients, and 41% had UA. Compared with patients who received a GP IIb/IIIa antagonist plus UFH or enoxaparin, patients who received bivalirudin alone experienced significantly less non-CABG-related major bleeding (3% versus 5.7%; RR 0.53; 95% CI 0.43 to 0.65). Compared with heparin plus a GP IIb/IIIa antagonist, bivalirudin alone resulted in a noninferior rate of the composite ischemia end point (7.3% versus 7.8%, respectively; RR 1.08; 95% CI 0.93 to 1.24; $p = 0.32$). Administration of bivalirudin plus a GP IIb/IIIa antagonist, as compared with heparin plus a GP IIb/IIIa antagonist, resulted in noninferior 30-day rates of the composite ischemia end point (7.7% versus 7.3%, respectively; RR 1.07; 95% CI 0.92 to 1.23; $p = 0.39$) and major bleeding (5.3% versus 5.7%, respectively; RR 0.93; 95% CI 0.78 to 1.10; $p = 0.38$). Bivalirudin is a Class I anticoagulant in patients with UA or NSTEMI who are selected for an invasive strategy.[1]

FACTOR XA INHIBITORS

Several factor Xa inhibitors, fondaparinux,[500] apixaban,[501] and rivaroxaban, have been studied in patients with ACS. The OASIS-5 trial compared fondaparinux with enoxaparin for a mean of 6 days in 20,078 patients with ACS.[500] The rate of major bleeding at 9 days was lower with fondaparinux than with enoxaparin (2.2% versus 4.1%; hazard ratio 0.52; $p < 0.001$). Also, the number of deaths at 30 days was significantly reduced by fondaparinux compared with enoxaparin (295 versus 352, $p = 0.02$). Fondaparinux is preferable to UFH or enoxaparin for patients with UA or NSTEMI who are selected to a conservative strategy and have an increased risk of bleeding (Class I).[23] Fondaparinux or enoxaparin are preferable to UFH in patients with UA or NSTEMI who are selected for an initial conservative strategy unless CABG is planned within 24 hours (Class IIa).[23] Because of the risk of catheter thrombosis, fondaparinux should not be used as the sole anticoagulant during PCI, and an additional anticoagulant with antifactor IIa activity should be administered.[21]

ANGIOTENSIN-CONVERTING ENZYME INHIBITORS

Little information is available regarding the administration of ACE inhibitors to patients with NSTEMI because most of the ACE inhibitor trials did not report subgroup analyses of patients with STEMI or NSTEMI. The Survival of Myocardial Infarction Long-Term Evaluation (SMILE) study enrolled 1556 patients with acute anterior MI who were not eligible for fibrinolytic therapy.[502] The patients were randomized to receive 6-week courses of placebo or zofenopril, an ACE inhibitor. Among the 526 patients with ECG criteria for NSTEMI, death or severe CHF occurred in 10.3% (28/273) of placebo patients and 3.6% (9/253) of zofenopril patients (RR reduction 65%; 95% CI 20% to 80%; $p = 0.003$).[503] The 1-year mortality rate also was significantly reduced by zofenopril (7.9% versus 15.8%; RR reduction 43%; 95% CI 14% to 57%; $p = 0.036$).

LIPID-LOWERING THERAPY

As discussed earlier, the 4S,[348] CARE,[349] and LIPID[350] trials have established the long-term benefits of starting statin therapy 3 months or later after hospitalization for an MI or UA. Analysis of the LIPID trial showed that initiation of pravastatin 40 mg daily 3 to 36 months after hospitalization for UA significantly reduced the risk of several end points, including death (RR 0.74; 95% CI 0.50 to 0.91; $p = 0.004$) and nonfatal MI (RR 0.67; 95% CI 0.51 to 0.88; $p = 0.004$).[504]

Data are conflicting regarding the benefit of early initiation of lipid-lowering therapy in patients with ACS. A retrospective analysis of the outcomes in 1616 patients with ACS concluded that statin pretreatment is associated with improved clinical outcome, whereas the discontinuation of statins after symptom onset is associated with an increased risk of death and nonfatal MI within 30 days.[505] An observational study that combined data from the GUSTO IIb and PURSUIT trials concluded that prescription of a lipid-lowering drug at hospital discharge was independently associated with a reduced risk of death at 6 months (hazard ratio 0.67; 95% CI 0.48 to 0.95; p = 0.023).[506] Another study of 12,365 patients with ACS concluded that there was no impact of early initiation of statin therapy on death, MI, or severe recurrent ischemia at 90 days.[507]

Numerous randomized trials have investigated the effects of statins on outcomes in patients with ACS. Compared with placebo, treatment with atorvastatin 80 mg daily beginning 24 to 96 hours after hospital admission reduced the rate of recurrent ischemic events at 16 weeks.[508] The Pravastatin or Atorvastatin Evaluation and Infection Therapy-Thrombolysis in Myocardial Infarction 22 (PROVE IT-TIMI 22) study compared atorvastatin 80 mg daily with pravastatin 40 mg daily started within 10 days of hospitalization for an ACS.[352] The primary end point was a composite of death, MI, UA, revascularization, and stroke. The rates for the primary end point at 2 years were 22.4% in the atorvastatin group and 26.3% in the pravastatin group, representing a 16% reduction in the hazard ratio in favor of atorvastatin (95% CI 5% to 26%; p = 0.005).

At least two meta-analyses of relevant randomized controlled trials have been performed to estimate the effects of early treatment with statins on short-term outcomes in patients with ACS.[381,382] One analysis of 12 randomized trials concluded that statin therapy initiated within 14 days of hospital admission does not reduce the risk of death, MI, or stroke during the first 4 months after ACS.[381] Another meta-analysis of 13 randomized trials concluded that early statin therapy reduces the rates of death and cardiovascular events after 4 months of treatment.[382]

INVASIVE VERSUS CONSERVATIVE MANAGEMENT

At least eight randomized trials have compared early invasive and early conservative management strategies for patients with ACS. Patients who are managed by an early conservative strategy undergo coronary angiography if evidence points to spontaneous recurrent ischemia or if results of stress testing are strongly positive despite medical therapy. Patients who are managed using an early invasive strategy undergo routine coronary angiography and coronary revascularization as indicated. Three relatively large trials demonstrated better short-term and long-term outcomes among patients randomized to the early invasive strategy compared with the early conservative strategy: FRISC II,[509-511] TACTICS-TIMI 18,[437] and the Randomized Intervention Trial of Unstable Angina-3 (RITA-3).[512,513] The FRISC II[509-511] and TACTICS-TIMI 18 trials randomized 2457 and 2220 patients, respectively, with UA or NSTEMI to either an early conservative or an early invasive strategy. Both trials found that the early invasive strategy was associated with a lower risk of death or MI at 6 months compared with the early conservative strategy: 9.4% versus 12.1% (RR 0.78; 95% CI 0.62 to 0.98; p = 0.031) for FRISC II and 7.3% versus 9.5% (odds ratio 0.74; 95% CI 0.54 to 1.00; $p < 0.05$) for TIMI 18. The early invasive strategy also was associated with a reduced rate of rehospitalization for ACS in both trials. After follow-up for 2 years in the FRISC II trial, patients who were randomized to the early invasive arm experienced lower rates of MI (9.2% versus 12.7%; RR 0.72; 95% CI 0.57 to 0.91; p = 0.005) and overall mortality (3.7% versus 5.4%; RR 0.68; 95% CI 0.47 to 0.98; p = 0.038).[511] The RITA-3 study randomized 1810 patients with non–ST elevation acute coronary syndromes to early invasive or early conservative treatment.[512,513] After a median follow-up period of 5 years, 142 (16.6%) patients randomized to the early intervention group and 178 (20%) patients assigned to the early conservative group died or had a nonfatal MI (odds ratio 0.78; 95% CI 0.61 to 0.99; p = 0.044). The death rates were 12% for the interventional group versus 15% for the conservative group (odds ratio 0.76; 95% CI 0.58 to 1.00; p = 0.054).

A meta-analysis of the 5-year outcomes of three large trials found that cardiovascular death or MI occurred in 14.7% (389 of 2721) of patients randomized to a routine invasive strategy versus 17.9% (475 of 2746) of patients who were randomized to a selective invasive strategy (hazard ratio 0.81, 95% CI 0.71 to 0.93; p = 0.002).[514] The absolute risk reductions for the combined end point of cardiovascular death or MI were 2%, 3.8%, and 11.1% for the low-, moderate-, and high-risk patients.

The early invasive strategy confers the greatest benefit in patients who are characterized by high-risk indicators such as ST segment depression[436,437] or elevated troponin.[447] Therefore, elevated troponin T or I and new or presumably new ST segment depression are included in a list of 13 high-risk indicators that warrant an early invasive strategy in patients with UA or NSTEMI (Box 30.7).[23] A meta-analysis of nine randomized trials that compared an invasive versus a conservative strategy in patients with non–ST segment elevation acute coronary syndromes included 1789 patients with diabetes mellitus.[515] Compared with the conservative strategy, the invasive strategy was associated with a 3.7% absolute risk reduction of nonfatal MI and a 5.1% absolute risk reduction of death, MI, or rehospitalization with ACS among patients with diabetes.[515] Consequently, diabetes is included in the list of 13 high-risk indicators that warrant an early invasive strategy in patients with non–ST segment elevation ACS.[23] An early conservative strategy may be selected for patients with a low TIMI or GRACE score and who lack the high-risk indicators listed in Box 30.7.

Several studies have attempted to determine the optimal timing of revascularization with PCI among patients with UA or NSTEMI who are selected for early invasive management. The Timing of Intervention in Acute Coronary Syndrome (TIMACS) trial randomly assigned 3031 patients with ACS without ST segment elevation to two groups: routine early intervention (coronary angiography ≤ 24 hours after randomization) or delayed intervention (coronary angiography ≥ 36 hours after randomization).[516] The median time to coronary angiography was 14 hours for the early-intervention group and 50 hours for the delayed-intervention group. Early intervention improved the primary composite end point of death, MI, or stroke at 6 months in the one third of patients who were at highest risk (hazard ratio 0.65; 95% CI 0.48 to 0.89), but not in the two thirds of patients at low or intermediate risk (hazard ratio 1.12; 95% CI 0.81 to 1.56). PCI was performed in 7749 patients with ACS without ST segment elevation who were enrolled in the ACUITY randomized trial.[517] Delay to PCI more than

Box 30.7 Initial Treatment Strategy: Invasive Versus Conservative Strategy

Invasive Strategy Preferred

1. Recurrent angina/ischemia at rest or with low-level activities despite intensive medical therapy
2. Elevated troponin T or troponin I
3. New or presumably new ST segment depression
4. Signs or symptoms of heart failure or new or worsening mitral regurgitation
5. High-risk findings from noninvasive testing
6. Reduced left ventricular function (LVEF less than 40%)
7. Hemodynamic instability
8. Sustained ventricular tachycardia
9. PCI within 6 months
10. Prior CABG surgery
11. High risk score (e.g., TIMI, GRACE)
12. Mild to moderate renal dysfunction
13. Diabetes mellitus

Conservative Strategy Preferred

1. Low risk score (e.g., TIMI, GRACE)
2. Patient or physician preference in the absence of high-risk features

CABG, coronary artery bypass graft; GRACE, Global Registry of Acute Coronary Events; LVEF, left ventricular ejection fraction; PCI, percutaneous coronary intervention; TIMI, thrombolysis in myocardial infarction.

From Jneid H, Anderson JL, Wright RS, et al: 2012 ACCF/AHA focused update of the guideline for the management of patients with UA/non-ST-elevation myocardial infarction (updating the 2007 guideline and replacing the 2011 focused update): A report of the American College of Cardiology Foundation/American Heart Association Task Force on Practice Guidelines. J Am Coll Cardiol 2012;60:645-681.

Table 30.4 ACCF/AHA Practice Guidelines: Recommendations for Revascularization with PCI and CABG in Patients with Unstable Angina/Non–ST Segment Elevation Myocardial Infarction

Extent of Disease	Treatment	Class
Left main disease,* candidate for CABG	CABG PCI	I III
Left main disease, not candidate for CABG	PCI	IIa
Three-vessel disease with LVEF < 0.5	CABG	I
Multivessel disease including proximal LAD with LVEF < 0.5 or treated diabetes	CABG PCI	I IIb
Multivessel disease with LVEF > 0.5 and without diabetes	PCI or CABG CABG	I I
Two-vessel disease with significant proximal LAD stenosis and either LVEF < 0.5 or ischemia on noninvasive testing	PCI	IIb
One- or two-vessel disease with or without significant proximal LAD stenosis but with a large area of viable myocardium and high-risk criteria on noninvasive testing	CABG or PCI	I
One-vessel disease with proximal LAD	CABG or PCI	IIa†
One- or two-vessel disease without significant proximal LAD stenosis with no current symptoms or symptoms that are unlikely to be ischemic and who have no ischemia on noninvasive testing	CABG or PCI	III†
Insignificant coronary stenosis	CABG or PCI	III

*≥ 50% diameter stenosis.

†Class/level of evidence IA if severe angina persists despite medical therapy.

ACCF, American College of Cardiology Foundation; AHA, American Heart Association; CABG, coronary artery bypass grafting; LVEF, ejection fraction; LAD, left anterior descending (artery); PCI, percutaneous intervention.

From Anderson JL, Adams CD, Antman EM, et al: 2011 ACCF/AHA focused update incorporated into the ACC/AHA 2007 guidelines for the management of patients with UA/non-ST-elevation myocardial infarction: A report of the American College of Cardiology Foundation/American Heart Association Task Force on Practice Guidelines. J Am Coll Cardiol 2011;57:e215-e367.

24 hours after presentation was associated with a significant increase in the mortality and MI rates at 30 days. A delay to PCI more than 24 hours after presentation was an independent predictor of both 30-day and 1-year mortality.

The ACCF/AHA Guidelines provide recommendations regarding the mode of coronary revascularization in patients with UA or NSTEMI[23] (Table 30.4). Coronary anatomy and left ventricular EF are two of the key factors that determine whether percutaneous or surgical revascularization is preferable in a patient with UA or NSTEMI. Although the guidelines do not specify a preference for PCI or CABG surgery in patients with a non–Q wave MI, periprocedural mortality was greater after CABG surgery than after PCI in the Veterans Affairs Non–Q-Wave Infarction Strategies in Hospital (VANQWISH) trial.[518] Thirty-day mortality was 11.6% after CABG surgery (11/95 patients), compared with 0% after PCI (0/98 patients).[518]

LONG-TERM MEDICAL THERAPY

Prescription of evidence-based medical therapy at the time of hospital discharge has a major impact on outcome in patients with ACS. Mukherjee and coworkers[519] calculated an appropriateness score based on the use of antiplatelet agents, β-blockers, ACE inhibitors, and lipid-lowering agents in patients with an indication for each class of drugs. The use of combination evidence-based medical therapies was independently associated with lower 6-month mortality among a cohort of 1358 patients with ACS (55% NSTEMI, 30% UA, and 15% STEMI). The odds ratio for death for prescription of all indicated medications versus none of the indicated medications was 0.10 (95% CI 0.03 to 0.42; $p < 0.0001$).

The ACCF/AHA guidelines for the management of patients with UA and NSTEMI include multiple Class I recommendations for long-term medical therapy (Box 30.8).[1] Aspirin 75 to 162 mg daily should be continued indefinitely.[23] Clopidogrel should be prescribed for at least 1 month, and ideally up to 1 year in patients treated medically without stenting. Patients who receive bare-metal stents should be treated with a $P2Y_{12}$ inhibitor for at least 1 month and ideally up to 1 year, whereas patients who receive drug-eluting stents should be treated with a $P2Y_{12}$ inhibitor for a minimum of 12 months.[98] β-Blockers are recommended for all patients without contraindications. ACE inhibitors are recommended for patients with CHF, left ventricular EF less than 40%, hypertension, or diabetes. Lipid-lowering agents are recommended for patients with an LDL cholesterol level greater than 100 mg/dL after dietary manipulation.

Box 30.8 Class I Recommendations for Long-Term Medical Therapy for Patients with Unstable Angina/Non–ST Segment Elevation Myocardial Infarction

1. For UA/NSTEMI patients treated medically without stenting, aspirin (75 to 162 mg/day) should be prescribed indefinitely; clopidogrel should be prescribed for at least 1 month and ideally up to 1 year.
2. β Blockers are indicated for all patients recovering from UA/NSTEMI unless contraindicated. Treatment should begin within a few days of the event, if not initiated acutely, and should be continued indefinitely. Patients recovering from UA/NSTEMI with moderate or severe LV failure should receive β-blocker therapy with a gradual titration scheme.
3. Angiotensin-converting enzyme inhibitors should be given and continued indefinitely for patients recovering from UA/NSTEMI with heart failure, LV dysfunction (LVEF less than 0.4), hypertension, or diabetes mellitus, unless contraindicated.
4. An angiotensin receptor blocker should be prescribed at discharge to those UA/NSTEMI patients who are intolerant of an ACE inhibitor and who have either clinical or radiologic signs of heart failure and LVEF less than 0.4.
5. Long-term aldosterone receptor blockade should be prescribed for UA/NSTEMI patients without significant renal dysfunction (estimated creatinine clearance should be greater than 30 mL/min) or hyperkalemia (potassium should be less than or equal to 5 mEq/L) who are already receiving therapeutic doses of an ACE inhibitor, have an LVEF less than or equal to 0.4, and have either symptomatic heart failure or diabetes mellitus.
6. The following lipid recommendations are beneficial:
   a. Lipid management should include assessment of a fasting lipid profile for all patients, within 24 hours of hospitalization.
   b. Statins, in the absence of contraindications, regardless of baseline LDL-C and diet modification, should be given to post-UA/NSTEMI patients, including postrevascularization patients.
   c. For hospitalized patients, lipid-lowering medications should be initiated before discharge.
   d. For UA/NSTEMI patients with elevated LDL-C (greater than or equal to 100 mg/dL), cholesterol-lowering therapy should be initiated or intensified to achieve an LDL-C of less than 100 mg/dL. Further titration to less than 70 mg/dL is reasonable.

ACE, angiotensin-converting enzyme; ACS, acute coronary syndrome; EF, ejection fraction; LDL, low-density lipoprotein.

Modified slightly from Anderson JL, Adams CD, Antman EM, et al: 2011 ACCF/AHA focused update incorporated into the ACC/AHA 2007 guidelines for the management of patients with UA/non-ST-elevation myocardial infarction: A report of the American College of Cardiology Foundation/American Heart Association Task Force on Practice Guidelines. J Am Coll Cardiol 2011;57:e215-e367.

KEY POINTS

- The ACSs—UA, NSTEMI, and STEMI—all share a common pathophysiology: erosion or rupture of an atherosclerotic plaque that precipitates either nonocclusive or occlusive coronary artery thrombosis.
- Patients with suspected STEMI should have an ECG performed and interpreted within 10 minutes of presentation, and serial ECGs should be performed at intervals of 5 to 10 minutes in patients with a nondiagnostic initial ECG and clinical findings strongly suggestive of STEMI. Right-sided lead tracings should be obtained to screen for right ventricular MI in patients with inferior STEMI.
- The two Class I indications for fibrinolytic therapy in patients with STEMI are (1) symptom onset within the prior 12 hours and ST elevation greater than 0.1 mV in at least two contiguous precordial leads or at least two adjacent limb leads and (2) symptom onset within the prior 12 hours and new or presumably new left bundle branch block.
- Fibrinolytic therapy should be initiated within 30 minutes of presentation.
- Intracranial hemorrhage should be ruled out in any patient with a change in neurologic status during or after fibrinolytic therapy.
- Nitrates are indicated for relief of ischemic discomfort in patients with STEMI, but large clinical trials did not demonstrate a reduction in mortality among patients who received nitroglycerin over prolonged periods after acute MI.
- Aspirin has been shown to reduce mortality in patients with acute MI or UA. Patients with STEMI should receive 162 to 325 mg of non-enteric-coated aspirin, and the aspirin tablets should be chewed.
- The addition of clopidogrel to aspirin has been shown to improve angiographic and clinical outcomes in patients with STEMI or ACS without ST segment elevation.
- A meta-analysis of 23 randomized trials concluded that the rates of short-term death, nonfatal reinfarction, stroke, and the combined end point of all three were lower for primary coronary intervention than for fibrinolytic therapy in patients with STEMI.
- Balloon inflation should occur within 90 minutes of presentation in patients with STEMI who undergo primary coronary intervention.

Continued on following page

KEY POINTS (Continued)

- Primary coronary intervention is preferable to fibrinolytic therapy in patients with STEMI under the following circumstances: the diagnosis of STEMI is uncertain, fibrinolysis is contraindicated, the door-to-balloon time is less than 90 minutes and the difference between the door-to-balloon and door-to-needle times is less than 60 minutes, and the patient is in Killip class III or IV (pulmonary edema or cardiogenic shock).
- In patients with acute MI, the early administration of β-blockers reduces the rate of reinfarction and chronic administration improves long-term survival.
- An ACE inhibitor should be administered orally within the first 24 hours of STEMI to patients with anterior infarction, pulmonary congestion, or left ventricular EF less than 40% in the absence of hypotension.
- An angiotensin receptor blocker should be administered to patients with STEMI who are intolerant of ACE inhibitors and have either CHF or a left ventricular EF less than 40%.
- Long-term aldosterone blockade should be prescribed for post-STEMI patients without significant renal dysfunction or hyperkalemia who are already receiving therapeutic doses of an ACE inhibitor, have a left ventricular EF of 40% or less, and have either diabetes or symptomatic CHF.
- Diltiazem and verapamil are contraindicated in patients with STEMI and associated systolic left ventricular dysfunction and CHF.
- Lipid-lowering therapy is indicated at the time of hospital discharge in all patients with STEMI.
- Patients with UA or NSTEMI should be treated with both an anticoagulant (UFH, enoxaparin, or fondaparinux) and at least dual antiplatelet therapy with aspirin and an antagonist of the platelet $P2Y_{12}$ receptor (clopidogrel, prasugrel, or ticagrelor).
- An early invasive strategy is favored in patients with UA or NSTEMI who have any of the following high-risk indicators: recurrent angina or ischemia despite intensive anti-ischemic therapy, elevated troponin, new or presumably new ST segment depression, recurrent angina or ischemia with CHF or new or worsening mitral regurgitation, a high-risk noninvasive stress test, left ventricular EF less than 40%, hemodynamic instability, sustained ventricular tachycardia, PCI within the past 6 months, prior CABG surgery, or a high risk score (TIMI, GRACE).

SELECTED REFERENCES

21. Antman EM, Hand M, Armstrong PW, et al: 2007 focused update of the ACC/AHA 2004 guidelines for the management of patients with ST-elevation myocardial infarction: A report of the American College of Cardiology/American Heart Association Task Force on Practice Guidelines (writing group to review new evidence and update the ACC/AHA 2004 Guidelines for the management of patients with ST-elevation myocardial infarction). J Am Coll Cardiol 2008;51:210-247.
23. Jneid H, Anderson JL, Wright RS, et al: 2012 ACCF/AHA focused update of the guideline for the management of patients with UA/non-ST-elevation myocardial infarction (updating the 2007 guideline and replacing the 2011 focused update): A report of the American College of Cardiology Foundation/American Heart Association Task Force on Practice Guidelines. J Am Coll Cardiol 2012;60:645-681.
47. Wang K, Asinger RW, Marriott HJ: ST-segment elevation in conditions other than acute myocardial infarction. N Engl J Med 2003;349:2128-2135.
68. Cantor WJ, Fitchett D, Borgundvaag B, et al: Routine early angioplasty after fibrinolysis for acute myocardial infarction. N Engl J Med 2009;360:2705-2718.
150. Indications for fibrinolytic therapy in suspected acute myocardial infarction: Collaborative overview of early mortality and major morbidity results from all randomised trials of more than 1000 patients. Fibrinolytic Therapy Trialists' (FTT) Collaborative Group. Lancet 1994;343:311-322.
287. Hochman JS, Lamas GA, Buller CE, et al: Coronary intervention for persistent occlusion after myocardial infarction. N Engl J Med 2006;355:2395-2407.
312. Dargie HJ: Effect of carvedilol on outcome after myocardial infarction in patients with left-ventricular dysfunction: The CAPRICORN randomised trial. Lancet 2001;357:1385-1390.
324. Pfeffer MA, McMurray JJ, Velazquez EJ, et al: Valsartan, captopril, or both in myocardial infarction complicated by heart failure, left ventricular dysfunction, or both. N Engl J Med 2003;349:1893-1906.
326. Pitt B, Remme W, Zannad F, et al: Eplerenone, a selective aldosterone blocker, in patients with left ventricular dysfunction after myocardial infarction. N Engl J Med 2003;348:1309-1321.
352. Cannon CP, Braunwald E, McCabe CH, et al: Intensive versus moderate lipid lowering with statins after acute coronary syndromes. N Engl J Med 2004;350:1495-1504.
356. Patel MR, Smalling RW, Thiele H, et al: Intra-aortic balloon counterpulsation and infarct size in patients with acute anterior myocardial infarction without shock. The CRISP AMI randomized trial. JAMA 2011;306:1329-1337.
464. The CURRENT-OASIS 7 Investigators. Dose comparisons of clopidogrel and aspirin in acute coronary syndromes. N Engl J Med 2010;363:930-942.

The complete list of references can be found at www.expertconsult.com.

31 Cardiac Arrhythmias

Richard Trohman | Shariff Attaya

CHAPTER OUTLINE

Management of serious cardiac arrhythmias is the shared responsibility of emergency specialists: critical care physicians, cardiologists, and electrophysiologists. The past 10 years have produced only modest changes in acute and subacute therapy of tachyarrhythmias. Antiarrhythmic drugs remain the mainstay of acute therapy for supraventricular arrhythmias and hemodynamically stable ventricular tachycardia. Temporary pacing remains the "gold standard" urgent/emergent therapy for symptomatic bradyarrhythmias. Permanent pacing is still the only option for treatment of chronic bradycardias. By contrast, dramatic improvement and change have occurred in the chronic therapy of tachyarrhythmias. Most supraventricular tachycardias can now be cured by catheter ablation. Patients with structural heart disease at risk for sudden cardiac death (SCD) and those resuscitated from hemodynamically unstable ventricular tachyarrhythmias now are managed with implantable defibrillators, with antiarrhythmic drugs used primarily as an adjunct for patients receiving frequent shocks.

Critical care physicians deal with a plethora of medical and surgical problems in their patients. Arrhythmias may be the primary abnormality or may be secondary to myocardial ischemia, electrolyte imbalance, or toxic/metabolic disturbances. Optimal management of arrhythmias requires expertise in electrocardiography and clinical pharmacology as well as knowledge of arrhythmia precipitants, including proarrhythmia caused by antiarrhythmic drugs.[1] The responsibility of the critical care physician is to facilitate transition from acute to chronic care by referring the patient with an arrhythmia to a cardiologist or an electrophysiologist. Therefore, the major emphasis of this chapter is on acute care of the patients with arrhythmias.

BRADYCARDIAS

Bradyarrhythmias usually present as either sinus node dysfunction (SND) or atrioventricular blockade (AV block). Bradyarrhythmias and indications and techniques for temporary cardiac pacing are reviewed extensively in Chapter 5. A brief overview is included here to highlight important issues for the intensivist.

SINUS BRADYCARDIA AND SINUS NODE DYSFUNCTION

Sinus bradycardia is generally defined as periods of sinus rhythm with rates less than 60 beats per minute. In the absence of symptoms, it usually is benign and requires no treatment. Sinus bradycardia is common in young adults (particularly the physically fit). Nocturnal rates of 35 to 40 beats per minute and pauses during sleep of 2 seconds or longer are not uncommon. Sinus arrhythmia (Fig. 31.1) is a normal variant in which there are respirophasic changes in the RR interval on electrocardiogram (ECG) (prolongation of RR intervals during expiration).

Sinus bradycardia may also be a manifestation of certain pathologic conditions such as increased intracranial pressure, oculocardiac reflex after ophthalmologic surgery, cervical and mediastinal tumors, hypothyroidism, hypothermia, gram-negative sepsis, Chagas' disease, depression, and anorexia nervosa. Sinus bradycardia is often seen after cardiac transplantation. Beta blockers, parasympathomimetic agents, calcium antagonists, amiodarone, and lithium commonly produce sinus bradycardia. Digoxin, in therapeutic doses, usually does not markedly affect the sinus node and is relatively safe to use in patients with SND.[2] Sinus bradycardia complicates 10% to 15% of acute myocardial infarctions and is most common with inferior infarcts. It also may be seen after successful thrombolysis. In the absence of hemodynamic compromise, it is associated with a more favorable prognosis than sinus tachycardia.[3]

Short-term pharmacologic enhancement of the sinus rate may be accomplished using atropine, catecholamines, or theophylline. Isoproterenol should be avoided in patients with ischemic heart disease and hypertrophic cardiomyopathy. No safe, reliable drug is available for long-term management of sinus bradycardia. Temporary pacing may suffice when the underlying condition is reversible. Permanent pacing should be employed to alleviate persistent bradycardia and symptoms.

Sinus bradycardia (with or without AV block) may occur during periods of autonomic instability. Examples include carotid hypersensitivity and neurocardiogenic syncope. These syndromes have cardioinhibitory (bradycardic), vasodepressor (vasodilatory), and mixed forms. Permanent pacing (which must include the ability to pace the right ventricle for heart block) is a well-established therapy for cardioinhibitory carotid sinus hypersensitivity. Neurocardiogenic syncope generally is a benign condition that usually can be managed without permanent pacemaker therapy. However, treatment for patients with frequent and severe cardioinhibitory spells, especially those in whom asystolic periods exceeding 5 seconds can be demonstrated clinically or during head-up tilt table testing, may include palliative pacemaker therapy.[4]

SND may manifest in a variety of ways, including persistent sinus bradycardia, sinus pause or arrest, sinoatrial (SA) exit block, and the bradycardia-tachycardia syndrome.

SA exit block occurs when an impulse from the sinus node is not conducted to the surrounding atrium. First-degree SA exit block results from intranodal conduction delay and is not manifest on surface ECG. Complete (third-degree) SA exit block will manifest as sinus arrest. Only second-degree SA exit block is uniquely manifest on surface ECG.

Type I second-degree SA exit block is characterized by progressive PP interval shortening before pauses that are less than two PP cycles in duration. In type II second-degree SA exit block, pauses are exact multiples of the basic PP interval. SA exit block usually is transient and often is reversible. Its presence should prompt a search for underlying causes such as enhanced vagal tone, acute myocarditis or infarction, or drug effect (as from digitalis).

Symptomatic SND virtually always requires permanent pacing. Patients with concomitant supraventricular tachycardias may require supplemental antiarrhythmic therapy. Drug therapy may aggravate the bradycardia and in many instances should be initiated after device placement. Catheter ablation may palliate or eliminate the tachyarrhythmia.

ATRIOVENTRICULAR BLOCK

The various forms of heart block are disturbances of impulse conduction. Heart block may be transient or permanent. The following paragraphs focus on disturbances of AV conduction.

In reality, first-degree AV block involves no AV block at all but is due to delayed conduction from the atria to the ventricles. Every atrial impulse is conducted to the ventricles in a delayed fashion such that the PR interval is greater than 200 ms. If the QRS complex on the surface echocardiogram is narrow, the delay nearly always is in the AV node. In the presence of a wide QRS complex, the delay may be in either the AV node or the His-Purkinje system.

Second-degree AV block is classified as Mobitz type I (Wenckebach), Mobitz type II, 2:1 AV block, or high-degree AV block. In Mobitz I (Wenckebach) block, PP intervals are constant, with gradual PR prolongation before failure of impulse conduction (nonconducted P wave) (Fig. 31.2). Although classic Wenckebach block involves simultaneous shortening of successive RR intervals before AV block,

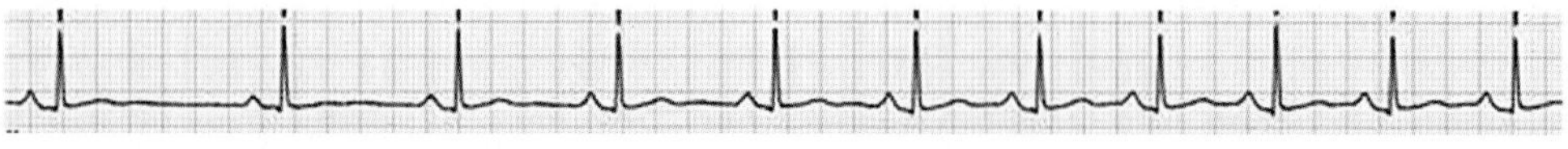

Figure 31.1 Sinus arrhythmia. A normal variant of sinus rhythm is sinus arrhythmia. Here, there are respirophasic changes in the RR interval on electrocardiogram (gradual prolongation of RR intervals during expiration).

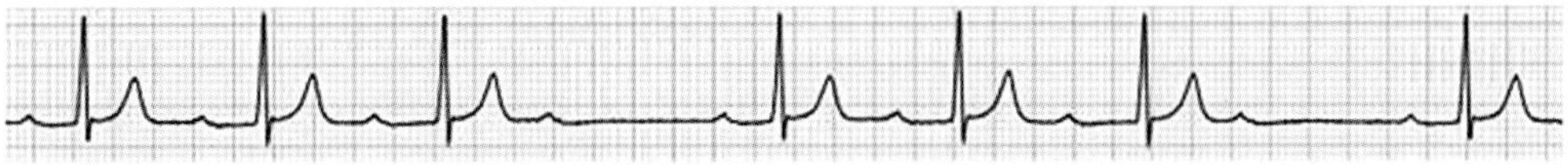

Figure 31.2 Second-degree atrioventricular block, Mobitz type I (Wenckebach). The PR interval progressively lengthens until a P wave is not conducted. The intervals may be fixed or variable. In this example, there are four P waves for every three QRS complexes.

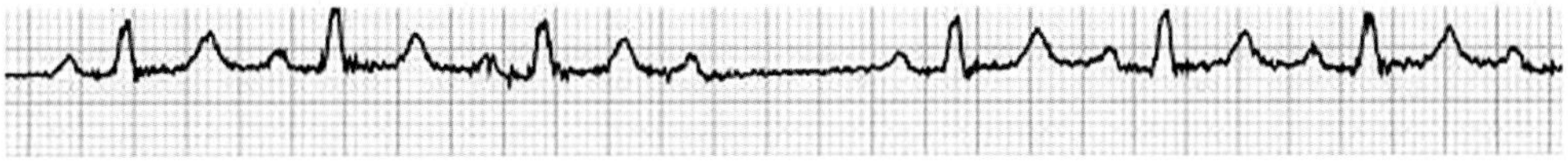

Figure 31.3 Second-degree atrioventricular block, Mobitz type II. There is a constant PR interval until a P wave is suddenly not conducted. Note the QRS is prolonged to approximately 120 ms.

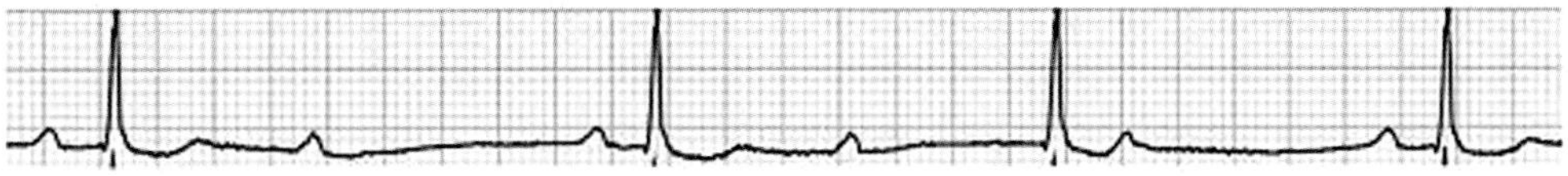

Figure 31.4 A 2:1 atrioventricular (AV) block. In the setting of AV block with a 2:1 interval, it is not possible to determine by surface electrocardiogram if the block is Mobitz type I or Mobitz type II. Narrow QRS complexes generally result from AV nodal block. Wide QRS complexes are compatible with block in either the AV node or His-Purkinje system.

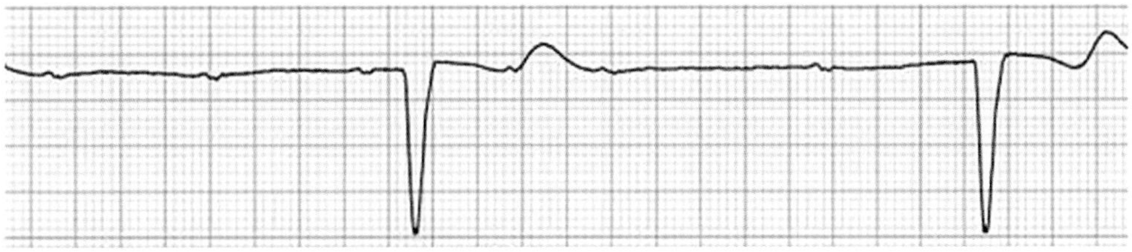

Figure 31.5 High-grade atrioventricular (AV) block. Two or more P waves are not followed by a QRS complex. In this example, there are three P waves for each QRS complex, an example of 3:1 high-grade AV block.

atypical alternations in RR intervals actually are more common. In younger people, Mobitz I AV block with normal QRS complexes generally is benign and does not progress to more advanced AV conduction disturbances. In older patients, the prognosis may be similar to that with Mobitz II block. Mobitz I second-degree AV block may accompany inferior myocardial infarction. The condition is benign, with a favorable prognosis, in the absence of hemodynamic compromise. The conduction disturbance usually is transient, and permanent pacing is not required.

Mobitz II AV block is characterized by sudden failure of atrial impulse conduction without prior PR prolongation (Fig. 31.3). This form of AV block frequently heralds development of complete AV block and Adams-Stokes syncope. Mobitz II second-degree AV block in the setting of anterior infarction is associated with pump failure and high mortality rates. Survivors should receive permanent pacemakers.

In general, the surface ECG allows the clinician to localize the site of AV block without the use of invasive electrophysiologic testing. Mobitz type I AV block with a narrow QRS almost always occurs at the AV node. Rarely, Mobitz I second-degree AV block may have an intra-His location. Mobitz I AV block with wide QRS complexes may occur in either the AV node or the His-Purkinje system. Mobitz II second-degree AV block (particularly in the presence of wide QRS complexes) localizes to the His-Purkinje system.

In general, atropine improves AV nodal conduction and carotid massage worsens it. These interventions typically have the opposite effect when AV block occurs in the His-Purkinje system. Atropine increases both atrial and ventricular rates in AV nodal block. Likewise, exercise (increased endogenous catecholamines) may reduce the extent of block. Precipitation of second-degree, high-grade, or complete AV block during exercise strongly suggests an infranodal site of block.

It is important to remember a few general rules to avoid common ECG misinterpretations of second-degree AV block. The 2:1 form of AV block may be nodal or infranodal. 2:1 block associated with narrow QRS complexes generally results from AV nodal block (Fig. 31.4). Wide QRS complexes are compatible with block in either the AV node or His-Purkinje system. If more than one P wave is not conducted to the ventricle, the term *high-grade AV block* is used (Fig. 31.5).

Complete AV block is diagnosed by the presence of independent atrial and ventricular activity on the ECG where the atrial rate is faster than the ventricular rate. When the atrial rhythm is sinus, AV dissociation is present, with the sinus rate exceeding the ventricular rate. The PP interval is constant. The RR interval is constant. The PR interval is variable in a random, nonrecurring pattern (Fig. 31.6). Complete AV block may also be present during all varieties of atrial tachycardia.

Complete AV block proximal to the His bundle results in a narrow QRS complex escape rhythm with rates of 50 to 60 beats per minute. Complete intra-His block may also result in a narrow QRS escape rhythm with ventricular rates less than or equal to 45 beats per minute.

Acquired complete AV block most commonly occurs distal to the His bundle, usually is secondary to a trifasicular conduction disturbance, is potentially life-threatening, and generally is irreversible. A wide QRS escape rhythm with ventricular rates less than 40 beats per minute is the rule. An exception is seen in the setting of inferior infarction, in which recovery of complete (narrow QRS) AV nodal block occurs in greater than 90% of patients (time to recovery 30 minutes to 16 days).[5]

Drug toxicity, coronary artery disease, and degenerative disease of the conduction system are the most common causes of AV block in adults. Surgery, electrolyte disturbances (such as hyperkalemia), endocarditis, myocarditis (Lyme carditis), tumors, myxedema, rheumatoid nodules, Chagas' disease, calcific aortic stenosis, polymyositis, amyloidosis, sarcoidosis, scleroderma, and vagotonic reflexes all may result in AV block. In truth, the number of factors and conditions that may result in AV block is nearly endless. "Hypervagal" responses (carotid hypersensitivity, neurocardiogenic syncope) may produce transient AV block (see later).[3]

Congenital complete AV block results from separation of the atrial musculature from the conduction system, or from nodoventricular disconnection. Mortality rate is highest in neonates, diminishes during childhood and adolescence, and then increases later in life. Patients may be asymptomatic for many years. It is difficult to predict prognosis in individual patients. Persistent ventricular rates less than 50 beats per minute correlate with the development of symptoms and syncope. Symptomatic patients and those patients with left ventricular dilatation should receive permanent pacemakers.

No reliable long-term pharmacotherapy exists for AV block. Transient AV nodal block may be managed with atropine. Infranodal block may be managed with (carefully titrated) isoproterenol until temporary or permanent pacing is established.

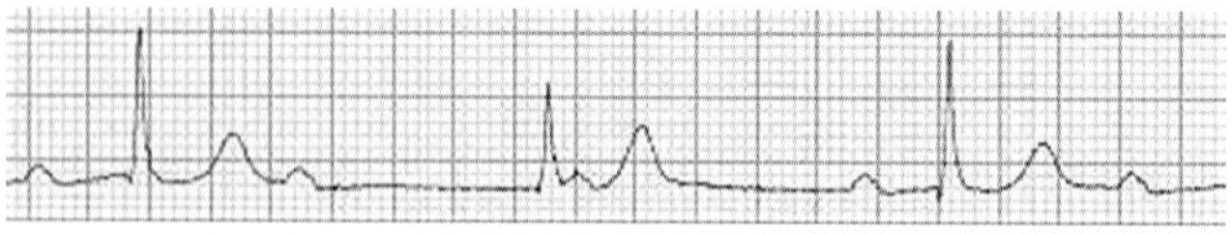

Figure 31.6 Complete heart block. The P waves and QRS complexes are regular, but they are not associated with one another.

JUNCTIONAL RHYTHM

When the sinus node does not depolarize the atrium for any reason (high vagal tone, SND), the cells near the AV junction (AV node, His bundle) may take over as the active pacemaker. Retrograde activation of the atrium, commonly manifest as negative P waves in the inferior leads (II, III, aVF), may be seen (Fig. 31.7). If the junctional rhythm goes faster than 60 beats per minute, it is termed an *accelerated junctional rhythm*. This is a common manifestation of digitalis toxicity.

VAGALLY MEDIATED SINUS ARREST, BRADYCARDIA, AND HEART BLOCK

The most common cause of nonconducted P waves during telemetry or Holter recordings is bradycardia-associated AV block. This manifests as sudden (usually nocturnal) block of one or more P waves with or without antecedent PR prolongation. This phenomenon is characterized by PP prolongation before AV block and is the result of transient increases in vagal tone. Vagally mediated sinus arrest, bradycardia, and heart block often occur in the intensive care unit (ICU) setting as a result of suctioning, gagging, femoral vessel compression (for hemostasis), and a variety of other triggers (Box 31.1). Vagal stimulation may lower blood pressure with or without significant bradycardia. Bradyarrhythmias and hypotension usually resolve when vagal stimulation ceases.

Box 31.1 Triggers for Vagally Mediated Heart Block

- Gagging reflexes such as with intubation or placement of a nasogastric tube
- Endotracheal suctioning and irrigation of the carina
- Distention of a visceral organ such as during colonoscopy or bladder irrigation
- Increased intrathoracic pressure as may occur with coughing or excessive tidal volumes on the ventilator
- Direct stimulation of the carotid body, which may occur with vascular surgery in this area
- Increased intracranial pressure and certain neurologic procedures
- Manual compression during femoral artery line removal
- Seizure-related
- Neurocardiogenic syncope or simple fainting in patients undergoing painful procedures or possibly in visitors to the intensive care unit

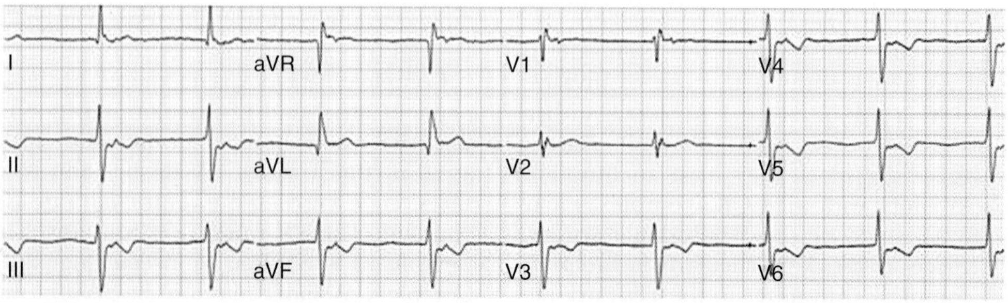

Figure 31.7 Junctional rhythm with retrograde P waves that are negative in the inferior leads.

Persistent bradycardia or hypotension mediated by vagal tone may require placing the patient in the Trendelenburg position, temporary saline infusion, or intravenous administration of atropine to fully resolve the episode.

SUPRAVENTRICULAR TACHYCARDIA

OVERVIEW

Tachyarrhythmias often occur in critically ill patients. Conditions such as hypoxemia, electrolyte imbalance, catecholamine excess (endogenous and exogenous), and other metabolic disturbances predispose patients (with or without preexisting arrhythmic substrates) to tachyarrhythmias. Intensivists must be prepared for acute management of supraventricular tachycardia. Knowledge of arrhythmia mechanisms, appropriate choices for acute pharmacotherapy, and indications for urgent or emergent direct current cardioversion are requisite.[6] We will discuss the mechanisms of supraventricular tachyarrhythmias, give an ECG-guided approach to their diagnosis, and cover specific treatments for these dysrrhythmias (pharmacologic and catheter ablation).

The substrate for most supraventricular tachycardias is present before ICU admission. Notable exceptions include atrial fibrillation (and flutter) after open-heart surgery and multifocal atrial tachycardia (MAT) (which may be transient, requiring no chronic therapy). Conditions such as hypoxemia, electrolyte imbalance, catecholamine excess (endogenous and exogenous), and other metabolic disturbances predispose patients (with or without preexisting arrhythmic substrates) to tachyarrhythmias.

PREMATURE ATRIAL CONTRACTIONS

Premature atrial, junctional, or ventricular beats are common in patients with or without structural heart disease and rarely result in significant alteration of cardiac output. They may occur as a result of enhanced sympathetic tone, metabolic stress, pericarditis, or direct mechanical irritation (as occurs with intracardiac catheters) and may result from the stimulant effects of caffeine, alcohol, intravenous inotropic support, or illicit drugs (such as cocaine). Atrial premature beats may be associated with aberrant conduction and confused with premature ventricular beats, or they may block in the AV node, creating a pause that may be confused with sinus arrest or SA exit block. Atrial premature beats may initiate reentrant supraventricular tachycardias or atrial fibrillation. Premature atrial contractions rarely require treatment, unless they trigger sustained supraventricular tachyarrhythmias.

PAROXYSMAL SUPRAVENTRICULAR TACHYCARDIA

Five types of paroxysmal supraventricular tachycardia (PSVT) are recognized: (1) AV nodal reentry tachycardia (AVNRT); (2) AV reentrant tachycardia (AVRT); (3) intra-atrial reentry; (4) automatic atrial; and (5) sinus node reentry. First-line chronic therapy for most supraventricular tachycardias is catheter ablation. The following discussion of therapy will be limited to acute pharmacologic management.

AVNRT is by far the most common and in the past accounted for 50% to 60% of PSVTs evaluated at referral centers.[7] The precise reentrant circuit is not defined; however, it is clear that the anterior and posterior AV nodal approaches and the perinodal atrial tissue are involved. In 76% to 90% of cases, antegrade conduction proceeds along the posterior (slow) AV nodal approach (pathway) and retrograde conduction along the anterior (fast) AV nodal pathway.[7,8] This is slow-fast AVNRT. Because retrograde conduction is so rapid, atrial and ventricular activation are virtually simultaneous. P waves are usually not visible on the surface ECG or may appear in the terminal portion of the QRS complex (pseudo R′ in lead V_1 or pseudo-S waves in the inferior leads). Atrial contraction on a closed AV valve may produce neck pounding.[9] Less common (so-called "unusual") variants (fast-slow, slow-slow, and slow–sort of slow) of AV nodal reentry also exist.[8]

AVNRT usually manifests after the age of 20 years[9] and is more common in women than in men. The typical heart rate in AVNRT ranges from 150 to 250 beats per minute. Palpitations, lightheadedness, and near-syncope may accompany an episode. True syncope is unusual. Neck pounding (see previously) is virtually pathognomonic,[8] but its absence does not exclude AVNRT.

Before catheter-based cures became routine, AVRT was the next most common (accounting for 30%) PSVT mechanism.[7] AVRT (also commonly referred to as orthodromic tachycardia) manifests (on average) at a somewhat earlier age than that typical for AVNRT. The antegrade limb of the circuit proceeds down the normal AV nodal His-Purkinje system. The retrograde limb uses an accessory pathway that usually is located along the mitral or tricuspid valve annulus. Because the accessory pathway conducts in only retrograde fashion, it is concealed (not seen on surface ECG).

Because AVRT proceeds normally antegradely, the QRS complex is generally narrow. The AVRT reentry circuit travels antegradely through the AV node and His-Purkinje system to the ventricles before retrograde activation of the atria occurs via the bypass tract. The extra time taken to travel by way of the ventricles creates a longer RP interval during tachycardia compared with that seen in AVNRT. Because AVNRT and AVRT activate periannular atrial tissue first, P waves (if visible on surface ECG) will be negative in the inferior leads. Upright P waves in these leads indicate atrial (or sinus) tachycardia. AVRT tends to go faster than AVNRT and is more prone to manifest with QRS alternans or left bundle branch block (LBBB) aberrancy.[10,11] A decrease in tachycardia rate on development of bundle branch block ipsilateral to the pathway is characteristic of AVRT. AV block is unusual during AVNRT and *excludes* the diagnosis of AVRT (which requires both atrial and ventricular participation). The presence of AV block strongly suggests the diagnosis of atrial tachycardia.

In the past, intra-atrial reentry, automatic atrial tachycardia, and sinus nodal reentry accounted for the remaining 8% to 10% of PSVTs.[7] Sinus node reentry rarely occurs as an isolated phenomenon.[12]

Approximately 50% of patients with intra-atrial reentry have evidence of structural heart disease.[13] This tachycardia is particularly prone to develop after surgery for congenital cardiac anomalies. Reentry occurs around structural barriers, such as suture lines. In patients without clear-cut structural disease, subtle changes such as scarring and fibrosis provide the substrate for reentry. Automatic atrial tachycardias occur along the crista terminalis, near the ostium of the coronary sinus, along the tricuspid and mitral annulus, in both atrial appendages, and within or in close proximity to the pulmonary veins. Automatic atrial tachycardias are exquisitely sensitive to catecholamines. Although these tachycardias may manifest in the absence of structural heart disease or obvious precipitants, they also are commonly associated with chronic lung disease, pneumonia, myocardial (atrial) infarction, and acute alcoholic binges. Amphetamine or cocaine abuse also may precipitate automatic atrial tachyarrhythmias.

Reentrant atrial tachycardias tend to be paroxysmal, whereas automatic forms are more likely to be incessant. In both, atrial rates less than 200 beats per minute are characteristic. Persistent elevation of the ventricular rate may result in a (reversible) tachycardia-mediated cardiomyopathy.

As noted, the presence of AV block during tachycardia provides strong evidence that the rhythm disturbance is atrial in origin. Negative P waves are not helpful in differentiating atrial tachycardia from AVNRT or AVRT. An inferior P wave axis with a negative P in lead I is diagnostic of left atrial tachycardia. An inferior P axis, a positive P in lead I, and a P wave morphology different from sinus rhythm can result only from atrial tachycardia.

Sinus node reentry may occur within the sinus node, the perinodal atrial tissue, or both. Although the mechanism may be difficult to prove clinically, most investigators agree that the P wave may be *nearly* identical to sinus rhythm, suggesting that the reentrant exit point may differ slightly from sinus pacemaker beats. Average rates generally are 130 to 140 beats per minute (range 80 to 200).

APPROACH TO PAROXYSMAL SUPRAVENTRICULAR TACHYCARDIA THERAPY

Acute management of PSVT should begin with attempts to slow or (transiently) interrupt AV nodal conduction. Vagal maneuvers (such as carotid sinus massage or Valsalva) may be tried first. Adenosine is the initial drug of choice for acute management of PSVT. An initial intravenous dose of 6 mg may be followed (2 minutes) later by 6 mg (if necessary), and 12 mg may be given (2 minutes) later if 6 mg is unsuccessful.

Adenosine should terminate more than 90% of AVNRT and AVRT. This agent also is effective in sinus node reentry. Adenosine also may terminate automatic atrial tachycardias, particularly those originating near the crista terminalis, where vagal innervation is rich. Termination may be transient because of adenosine's short half-life (10 seconds).

Intravenous verapamil (5 to 10 mg is injected over a period of 30 seconds, followed by an additional 5 mg, if necessary, after a 5- to 10-minute interval) or diltiazem (0.25 mg/kg, followed by an additional dose of 0.35 mg/kg, if necessary, after a 15-minute interval) usually is effective for PSVT termination when adenosine fails. AV block without arrhythmia termination (again) suggests the diagnosis of atrial tachycardia. Because of their longer half-lives, intravenous calcium channel blockers also may be effective for treatment of prompt tachycardia recurrence after initial success with adenosine.

Automatic atrial tachycardia is difficult to manage with pharmacotherapy. Precipitants should be treated or eliminated whenever possible. Beta blockers may slow atrial rate but rarely restore sinus rhythm. Adenosine may produce sinus rhythm; however, tachycardia may resume as soon as the drug is metabolized.[14] Vagal maneuvers may produce AV block but do not terminate these arrhythmias. Clinical successes have been obtained with class IC agents and amiodarone. Flecainide should be avoided in patients with coronary artery disease or significant left ventricular dysfunction. Intravenous flecainide is not available in the United States (see later). Amiodarone is available for intravenous administration. Intravenous amiodarone may result in hypotension (vasodilation) but usually does not exacerbate heart failure or cause proarrhythmia in the setting of preexisting left ventricular dysfunction.

Sinus node reentry may respond to vagal maneuvers, adenosine, verapamil, and digitalis (relatively slow onset of action limits acute application). Acute management of intra-atrial reentry is similar to that for atrial fibrillation in the absence of antegrade accessory pathway conduction (see later). Emergent or urgent direct current cardioversion is indicated when PSVT results in angina pectoris, congestive heart failure (CHF), or hypotension. Techniques for and limitations of direct current cardioversion are discussed later in the chapter. Automatic tachycardias (including MAT) do not respond to direct current cardioversion.

WOLFF-PARKINSON-WHITE SYNDROME AND ITS VARIANTS

The ECG pattern of Wolff-Parkinson-White syndrome (see "Electrocardiographic Patterns Intensivists Should Recognize"), short PR interval with preexcitation (delta wave), has a reported prevalence of 0.1% to 0.3% in the general population. It is twice as common in men as in women.

Classic Wolff-Parkinson-White syndrome occurs when the accessory AV pathway is capable of bidirectional conduction (AV and ventriculoatrial). Symptomatic presentation usually is during the teenage years or early adulthood. Pregnancy may exacerbate symptoms. The most common tachycardia is AV reentry (down the AV node and His-Purkinje system, up the bypass tract), identical to AVRT involving a concealed bypass tract. Approximately 25% of patients with a Wolff-Parkinson-White ECG pattern are incapable of retrograde conduction via the accessory pathway (and therefore do not have orthodromic AVRT). Asymptomatic patients generally have a benign prognosis; however, the initial presentation may be ventricular fibrillation (see later).[15]

Accessory pathways generally have conduction properties similar to those of myocardium. Decremental conduction, (AV conduction delay or block) which is characteristic of the AV node, is uncommon. Pathways may therefore be capable of very rapid antegrade (AV) conduction. In these instances, atrial fibrillation may be associated with irregular wide QRS tachycardia and ventricular rates in excess of 300 beats per minute (Fig. 31.8). Syncope or SCD (degeneration to ventricular fibrillation) may ensue. Intravenous ibutilide (1 mg infused over 10 minutes; a second 1-mg dose may be

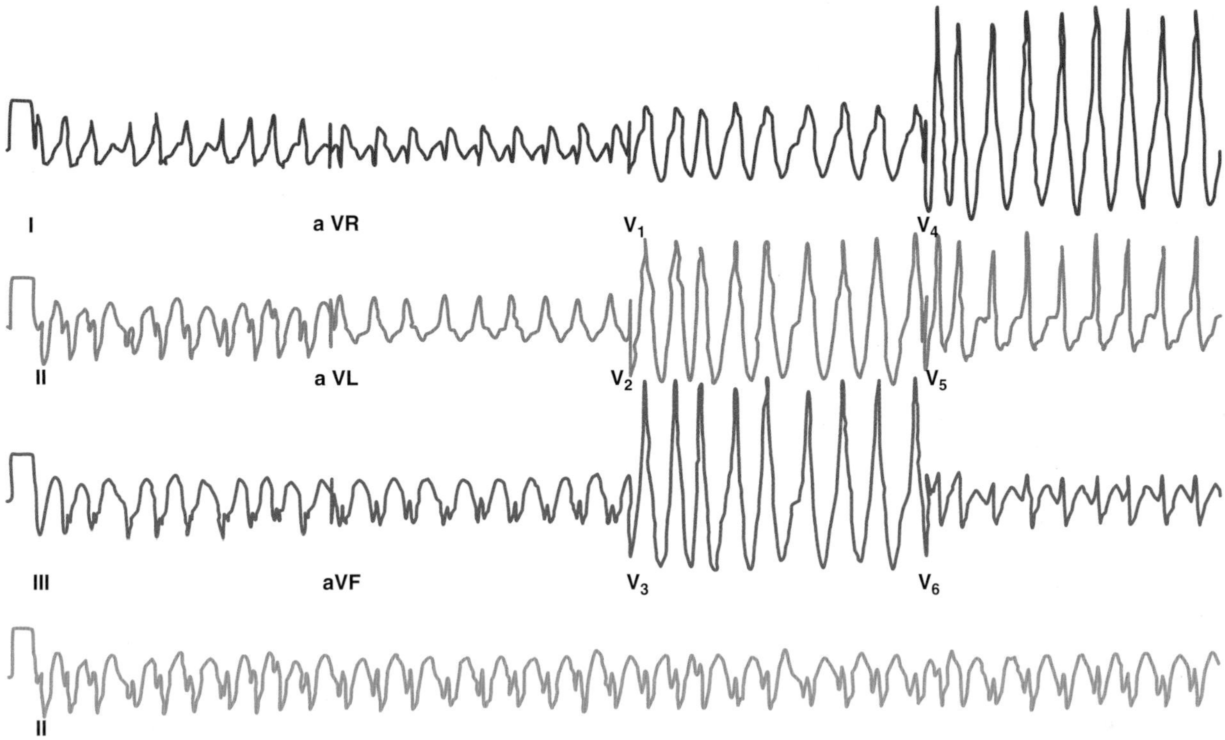

Figure 31.8 A 12-lead electrocardiogram (ECG) tracing from a patient with Wolff-Parkinson-White syndrome showing preexcited atrial fibrillation with rapid ventricular response. A rapid, "irregularly irregular" wide QRS tachycardia is present. Preexcited atrial fibrillation, as seen here, may degenerate to ventricular fibrillation. This ECG pattern should be promptly recognized by all practicing clinicians. I, II, III aVR, aVL, aVF, and V_1 to V_6 designate surface ECG leads. (From Trohman RG: Supraventricular tachycardia: Implications for the intensivist. Crit Care Med 2000;28(Suppl 10):N129-N135.)

given by infusion after a 10-minute wait, if necessary) also blocks antegrade accessory pathway conduction and is more likely to terminate acute episodes of atrial fibrillation or flutter (see later).[16]

Regular wide QRS tachycardia in patients with Wolff-Parkinson-White syndrome may have any of several mechanisms. Aberrancy resulting from right or LBBB (fixed or functional) may occur during orthodromic AVRT. As noted, bundle branch block ipsilateral to the accessory pathway may slow the tachycardia rate.

Antidromic tachycardia occurs when antegrade conduction proceeds via a free-wall accessory pathway, and retrograde conduction occurs over the normal His-Purkinje–AV nodal route. The ventricles are activated eccentrically beginning at the insertion of the accessory pathway. The resulting maximally preexcited wide QRS rhythm may be difficult to distinguish from ventricular tachycardia.

Although accessory pathways may be located anywhere along the AV groove, two variants with characteristic locations deserve mention. Paroxysmal junctional reciprocating tachycardia (PJRT) is a form of AV reentry that may be nearly incessant. The antegrade limb of the circuit is the normal AV conduction system. The retrograde limb is a concealed, decrementally conducting accessory pathway usually located posteroseptally. As noted earlier, incessant tachycardia may result in a tachycardia-mediated cardiomyopathy.

Atriofascicular pathways (Mahaim fibers) connect the right atrium and the right bundle branch. During sinus rhythm, preexcitation is minimal or absent. Typical Mahaim reentry travels antegradely down the bypass tract and retrogradely through the normal conduction system (usually beginning with the right bundle branch). A regular wide QRS typical LBBB pattern is seen.[17] These pathways conduct antegrade in a decremental fashion (retrograde accessory pathway conduction is absent) and occur much less frequently than typical AV accessory pathways. Patients with atriofascicular fibers frequently have multiple accessory pathways or AVNRT.[15,18]

ACUTE MANAGEMENT OF TACHYCARDIA ASSOCIATED WITH WOLFF-PARKINSON-WHITE SYNDROME

Acute tachycardia treatment depends on characteristics of its QRS complexes. A 12-lead ECG should be obtained whenever possible.

Orthodromic AVRT usually manifests with a narrow QRS complex (functional or fixed bundle branch block can widen the QRS). Treatment should begin with vagal maneuvers. If these do not terminate the tachycardia, intravenous adenosine is the initial drug of choice. These therapeutic interventions interrupt AVRT by creating transient AV nodal conduction block.

Treatment of wide QRS tachycardia should be directed at blocking conduction via the accessory pathway. Adenosine may terminate antidromic tachycardia (at the AV node), but it will not affect atrial tachyarrhythmias conducting rapidly across the accessory pathway. Because of its short half-life adenosine administration poses little risk, unless it precipitates atrial fibrillation.

Intravenous verapamil is contraindicated in the presence of wide QRS tachycardia. Its hypotensive effects may make patients hemodynamically unstable and contribute to the onset of ventricular fibrillation. Intravenous digoxin is not given to patients with Wolff-Parkinson-White syndrome and atrial fibrillation because it may (in approximately one third of patients) enhance antegrade accessory pathway conduction and may result in degeneration to ventricular fibrillation.

Patients whose supine systolic blood pressure is greater than 90 mm Hg can be given intravenous adenosine. It is administered in the same manner as described previously. Tachycardia termination suggests a supraventricular mechanism that includes the AV node as a requisite part of the circuit. Transient AV block suggests an atrial tachycardia. No response to adenosine suggests a ventricular origin.[19,20]

Direct current cardioversion should be available, preferably at the bedside, whenever treatment of a wide QRS tachycardia is undertaken. If, at baseline, the patient exhibits signs of hemodynamic compromise (angina, heart failure, or hypotension), drug therapy should be eschewed and direct current cardioversion employed to promptly restore sinus rhythm. If hemodynamic instability develops during drug therapy, direct current cardioversion should be performed immediately. Direct current cardioversion also should be the next elective therapy when pharmacotherapy is unsuccessful.

NONPAROXYSMAL ATRIOVENTRICULAR JUNCTIONAL TACHYCARDIA, PAROXYSMAL ATRIAL TACHYCARDIA WITH BLOCK, AND AUTOMATIC ATRIOVENTRICULAR JUNCTIONAL TACHYCARDIA

Nonparoxysmal AV junctional tachycardia occurs primarily in the setting of digitalis toxicity. It also is associated with cardiac surgery, myocardial infarction, and rheumatic fever. Hypokalemia may cause or exacerbate this arrhythmia. Sympathetic stimulation increases the tachycardia rate.

Digitalis toxicity also may precipitate atrial tachycardia (so-called paroxysmal atrial tachycardia with block) (Fig. 31.9). This tachycardia usually is managed by withholding digoxin and administering potassium. Lidocaine, phenytoin, and digoxin-specific antigen-binding fragments also may be used.

Automatic AV junctional tachycardia, also known (particularly in pediatrics) as junctional ectopic tachycardia, primarily affects children and infants. It often is incessant. In patients without congenital heart disease, it may manifest as a tachycardia-mediated cardiomyopathy.

This tachyarrhythmia results in marked hemodynamic deterioration after corrective surgery for congenital heart disease. It generally appears within 12 hours postoperatively and terminates within a few days if the patient survives. Digitalis, beta blockers, and class IA antiarrhythmics are ineffective in children. Amiodarone (which may suppress tachycardia or control its rate) should be administered when rates less than 150 beats per minute cannot be achieved by other means.[21] In adults, beta blockade may successfully control the rate. Adult automatic AV junctional tachycardia may be difficult to manage medically (Fig. 31.10). Recent reports suggest that catheter ablation can eliminate tachycardia while preserving AV conduction.[22-24]

MULTIFOCAL ATRIAL TACHYCARDIA

MAT is an automatic tachyarrhythmia. It is characterized by three or more morphologically distinct (nonsinus) P waves, atrial rates of 100 to 130 beats per minute, and variable AV block (Fig. 31.11).

MAT is commonly associated with respiratory disease and CHF. It has been reported in patients with cancer, lactic acidosis, pulmonary emboli, renal disease, and infection. Hypoxemia frequently is present. MAT may be exacerbated by digitalis or theophylline toxicity, hypokalemia, hypomagnesemia, and hyponatremia. These precipitants usually do not result in MAT if respiratory decompensation is absent. Although MAT is (in general) an uncommon arrhythmia, it is relatively common in the critical care setting. Treatment

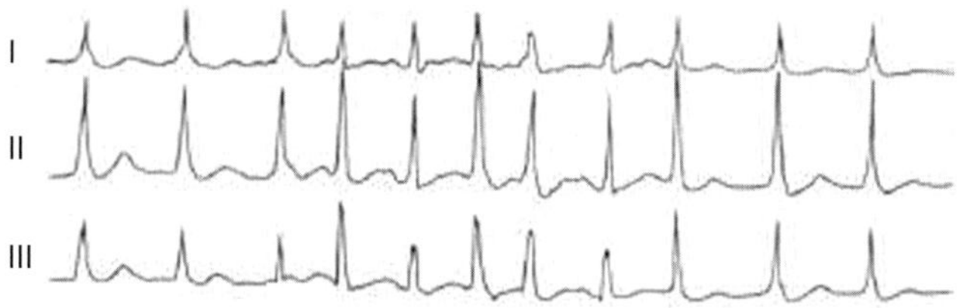

Figure 31.10 Atrioventricular (AV) junctional tachycardia. This rhythm strip demonstrates short bursts of tachycardia. The fifth and eighth beats are preceded by discernible P waves and are likely sinus in origin. AV junctional tachycardia can be difficult to manage medically. (From: Trohman RG, Haery C, Pinski SL: Focal radiofrequency catheter ablation of an irregularly irregular supraventricular tachycardia. Pacing Clin Electrophysiol 1999;22:360-362.)

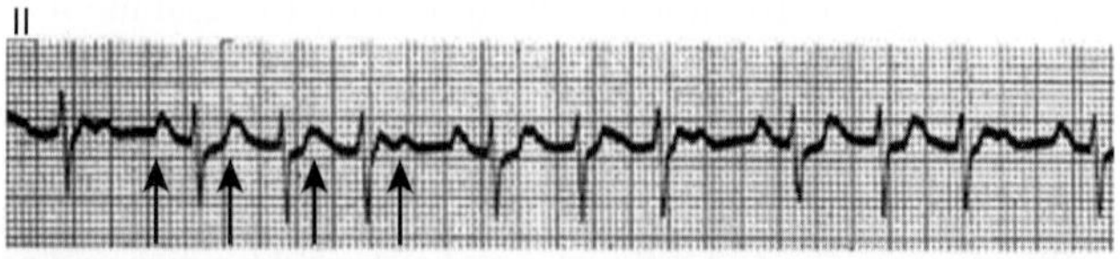

Figure 31.9 Atrial tachycardia with second-degree type I (Wenckebach) atrioventricular (AV) block. Atrial tachycardia with block can be seen in digitalis toxicity. In this example, second-degree type 1 AV block is seen. Atrial tachycardia or atrial fibrillation with complete heart block. The arrows show the P waves. (From Surawicz B, Knilans T: Chou's Electrocardiography in Clinical Practice: Adult and Pediatric, 6th ed. St. Louis, Elsevier, 2008.)

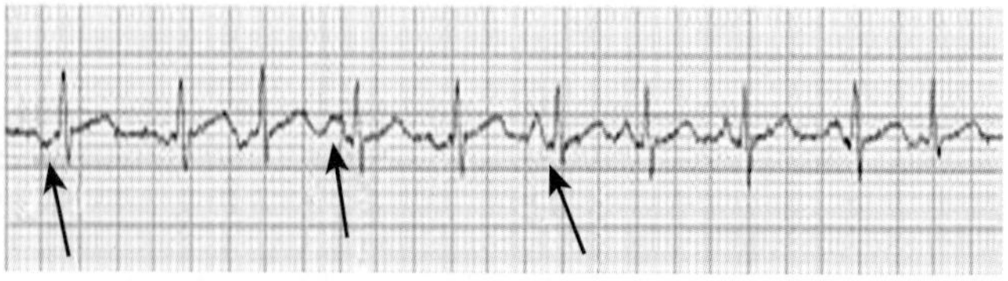

Figure 31.11 Multifocal atrial tachycardia is characterized by three or more morphologically distinct (nonsinus) P waves, atrial rates of 100 to 130 beats per minute, and variable atrioventricular block. Note the irregularity of the rhythm as well as the different P wave morphologic appearances (*arrows*) with different PR intervals.

of MAT usually is directed at elimination of the underlying precipitants. Metoprolol (used cautiously when bronchospasm is present) or verapamil may provide (atrial and ventricular) rate control and occasionally restore sinus rhythm.[25,26] Potassium and magnesium supplements may help suppress MAT. Amiodarone has also been useful in restoring sinus rhythm. MAT may, superficially, resemble atrial fibrillation. Careful examination of a 12-lead ECG may be required to distinguish between these two entities. Differentiation is important for proper patient management. As noted, MAT does not respond to direct current cardioversion and is not amenable to catheter ablation.

SINUS TACHYCARDIA

Sinus tachycardia usually is a normal reflex response to changes in physiologic, pharmacologic, or pathophysiologic stimuli such as exercise, emotional upset, fever, hemodynamic or respiratory compromise, anemia, thyrotoxicosis, poor physical conditioning, sympathomimetic or vagolytic agents, and abnormal hemoglobins.[27] The resulting increase in cardiac output usually is beneficial. Heart rate generally does not exceed 180 beats per minute, except in young patients, who may achieve rates higher than 200 beats per minute during vigorous exercise.[3] Tachycardia resolves when conditions return to baseline. The differential diagnosis for sinus tachycardia is presented in Table 31.1.

Sinus tachycardia is often present in ICU patients and sometimes is difficult to distinguish from other supraventricular tachycardias. When observed over time, sinus tachycardia will change its rate, with gradual acceleration and gradual deceleration. The P wave morphology of sinus tachycardia should be upright in leads I, II, aVF, and V_4 to V_6. Sinus tachycardia may slow transiently with vagal maneuvers or intravenous adenosine. If adenosine administration produces AV block, the P wave morphology can be clearly seen if a 12-lead ECG is run in rhythm strip mode. A negative P wave in (any of) leads I, II, aVF, and V_4 to V_6 excludes sinus tachycardia. P waves that are negative in lead I suggest a left atrial origin. Differentiation of "high" right atrial tachycardia waves from sinus tachycardia is more difficult. P-wave amplitude in the inferior leads may increase (normally) during sinus tachycardia. Comparison of the 12-lead P-wave morphology with that on an older 12-lead ECG tracing (if obtainable) when the patient was clearly in normal sinus rhythm may not result in an exact match.

ATRIAL FLUTTER

Although the precise reentrant circuit is unknown, typical atrial flutter traverses (with either counterclockwise or clockwise rotation) through an isthmus formed by the inferior vena cava, tricuspid valve, eustachian ridge, and coronary sinus ostia. Counterclockwise rotation is more common

Table 31.1 Differential Diagnosis of Sinus Tachycardia

Etiologic Category	Specific Disorders
Hemodynamic	Heart failure—systolic and diastolic heart failure caused by ischemic, valvular, or nonischemic myopathy
	Loss of circulating blood volume—gastrointestinal bleeding, anemia, shifts of intravascular fluid due to changes in colloidal osmotic pressure or inflammation
	Septic shock—dehydration
	Vascular shunts—intracardiac as well as aortovenous malformations, fistulas
	Pulmonary embolism
Metabolic and neurohumoral	Sepsis—infections and inflammatory conditions
	Hyperthyroidism
	Paget's disease of the bone
	Pheochromocytoma
	Carcinoid syndrome
	Beriberi heart disease
	Carcinoma
	Hyperpyrexia
	Acidosis
	Exercise
Pharmacologic	Sympathomimetic agents—isoproterenol, epinephrine, or dopamine
	Vagolytic agents, atropine, acopolamine
	Vasoldilators—nitrates, angiotensin-converting enzyme inhibitors, angiotensin receptor blockers, hydrazine, as well as centrally acting vasodilators
	Thyroid preparations, caffeine and nicotine
	Bronchodilators, including theophylline and terbutaline
	Anesthetic agents, including spinal anesthetics, causing peripheral vasodilation
	Drugs of abuse—amphetamines, cocaine, "ecstasy," cannabis
Neurologic/psychological	Pain
	Fear, anxiety, and hysteria
	Hyper-beta adrenergic phase of neurocardiogenic syncope
	Autonomic dysfunction such as with diabetes

and results in negative "flutter" waves in ECG leads II, III, aVF, and V_6. Atrial activity in lead V_1 is positively directed. Clockwise atrial flutter produces oppositely directed flutter waves in these leads. Atrial rates generally range between 250 and 350 beats per minute; however, slower rates may be seen in the presence of specific pharmacotherapy (which slows conduction within the circuit) or marked right atrial enlargement (presumably caused by a larger circuit).[28] Atrial flutter usually manifests with 2:1 AV block and ventricular rates of approximately 150 beats per minute.

Pharmacotherapy for (typical and atypical) atrial flutter is similar to that outlined for atrial fibrillation. Special care must be taken to avoid inadvertent precipitation of 1:1 AV conduction and subsequent hemodynamic deterioration. Radiofrequency ablation is first-line curative therapy for typical atrial flutter.

ATRIAL FIBRILLATION

Atrial fibrillation is the most important sustained supraventricular arrhythmia both in frequency and in potential for long-term sequelae. Atrial fibrillation and atrial flutter frequently coexist. More than 2 million people in the United States suffer from atrial fibrillation and this number is expected to rise as the population ages. The frequency of this arrhythmia increases dramatically after the age of 60.

Atrial fibrillation most often is associated with structural cardiac (diffuse atrial) disease. Unlike in typical atrial flutter, left atrial enlargement is more important than right atrial enlargement in the pathogenesis of atrial fibrillation.[29] The chaotic ECG appearance of this arrhythmia usually is the result of shifting reentrant circuits (multiple wavelet hypotheses). Atrial fibrillation may have focal triggers (usually in one or more pulmonary veins).[30] Causes of atrial fibrillation are listed in Box 31.2.

Box 31.2 Causes of Atrial Fibrillation

- Increased atrial pressure, secondary to:
  - Mitral or tricuspid valve disease
  - Myocardial disease (primary or secondary, leading to systolic or diastolic dysfunction)
  - Semilunar valve abnormalities (causing ventricular hypertrophy)
  - Intracardiac tumors or thrombi
- Atrial ischemia
  - Coronary artery disease
- Inflammatory or infiltrative atrial disease
  - Pericarditis
  - Amyloidosis
  - Myocarditis
- Age-induced atrial fibrotic changes
- Intoxicants and toxins
  - Alcohol
  - Carbon monoxide
  - Poison gas
- Increased sympathetic activity
  - Hyperthyroidism
  - Pheochromocytoma
  - Anxiety
  - Alcohol
  - Caffeine
  - Drugs
- Increased parasympathetic activity
- Primary or metastatic disease in or adjacent to the atrial wall
- Postoperative causes
  - Cardiac and pulmonary surgery
  - Overhydration
  - Pericarditis
  - Cardiac trauma
  - Hypoxia
  - Pneumonia
- Congenital heart disease
  - Particularly atrial septal defect
- Neurogenic causes
  - Subarachnoid hemorrhage
  - Nonhemorrhagic, major stroke
- Idiopathic

From Falk RH, Podrid PJ (eds): Atrial Fibrillation: Mechanisms and Management. New York, Raven Press, 1992.

ACUTE MANAGEMENT OF ATRIAL FIBRILLATION

Treatment of atrial fibrillation has three important components: (1) ventricular rate control; (2) restoration (and maintenance) of sinus rhythm; and (3) prevention of embolic phenomena.

Although atrial fibrillation is the most common sustained arrhythmia, there is no consensus on optimal atrial fibrillation management. In the critically ill, atrial fibrillation may be a "sign" (perhaps of disease severity) rather than an arrhythmic disease entity (as seen in noncritically ill patients with recurrent paroxysmal, persistent, and permanent atrial fibrillation). Critically ill patients are often in a hyperadrenergic state, which may increase ectopic triggers and shorten atrial refractoriness. This is likely the mechanism of atrial fibrillation in younger patients without chronic structural heart disease. In older patients with structural disease, increased adrenergic tone (and triggers) may precipitate atrial fibrillation when fibrosis has already created a suitable reentrant substrate.[31]

A logical approach to atrial fibrillation in the ICU requires the answers to the following questions:

1. Is the diagnosis of atrial fibrillation correct?
2. Are there causes/precipitants (see Box 31.2) that can be eliminated or corrected?
3. Is it necessary to restore and maintain sinus rhythm?
4. Is atrial fibrillation causing hemodynamic impairment (angina, heart failure, hypotension)?
5. What are the potential adverse effects of the various therapeutic options?[31]

It is important to carefully analyze a 12-lead ECG because, as previously noted, MAT may be misinterpreted as atrial fibrillation on a rhythm strip. The treatment of choice for MAT remains correction of precipitants such as hypoxemia, digitalis or theophylline toxicity, hypokalemia, or hypomagnesemia. Atrial fibrillation may, likewise, terminate (and be less likely to recur) when precipitants are removed or corrected.[31]

Atrial fibrillation that does not compromise the patient may not require aggressive therapy. Rate control strategies may suffice. Spontaneous atrial fibrillation termination may be difficult to distinguish from a clear-cut benefit of specific antiarrhythmic pharmacotherapy. Hemodynamic impairment should be treated with urgent or emergent direct current cardioversion.[31]

Serial direct current shocks are not appropriate for recurrent (within hours or days) paroxysms (self-terminating episodes) of atrial fibrillation. This scenario is relatively common in ICUs or after cardiac surgery. It is also important to avoid repetitive, futile shocks or delivery of direct current to an inadequately sedated patient because both of these may heighten the hyperadrenergic state and create or exacerbate a downward clinical spiral.[31-33] Restoration of sinus rhythm may be very difficult and impractical when a *severe* metabolic derangement or multisystem organ failure is present.[32]

Control of the ventricular rate (Table 31.2) is most frequently achieved using digoxin, beta blockers, calcium channel blockers (verapamil or diltiazem), or combinations of these agents. Verapamil should be administered cautiously to patients with significant left ventricular dysfunction. Although digoxin is effective in controlling rates at rest, exercise rate control is not often achieved. Digoxin remains appropriate therapy for patients with concomitant left ventricular dysfunction and CHF. Intravenous diltiazem is effective and well tolerated. Diltiazem may be administered by continuous intravenous infusion. The combination of efficacy, ease of parenteral delivery, and tolerance makes this agent an attractive option in the critical care setting.

A variety of agents may be used to restore sinus rhythm. Patients with adrenergically mediated atrial fibrillation should be managed initially with beta blockers. Sotalol and amiodarone are options in patients with atrial fibrillation refractory to beta blockade alone.

It has become relatively common to treat acute episodes with intravenous ibutilide. This unique class III agent prolongs action potential by blocking the rapid component of the delayed rectifier current.[34,35] This increase results in QT interval prolongation. Patients receiving intravenous ibutilide should be carefully monitored[34] (on telemetry for 4 to 8 hours) for development of torsades de pointes. Direct comparisons of intravenous procainamide and ibutilide have demonstrated clear superiority of ibutilide in conversion of atrial fibrillation and atrial flutter. Restoration of sinus rhythm with ibutilide occurred in 32% to 51% (atrial fibrillation) and 64% to 76% (atrial flutter) patients, compared with 0% to 5% (atrial fibrillation) and 0% to 14% (atrial flutter) after intravenous procainamide.[34,36,37] As a result of this data, use of procainamide for this indication has become passé. Ibutilide is suitable for acute cardioversion; however, prolonged intravenous or oral dosing is not available to prevent arrhythmia recurrence. Ibutilide may be administered safely to patients on concomitant antiarrhythmic agents.[38]

Intravenous amiodarone is (initially) primarily a calcium channel and beta blocker. It may be effective for rate control when other agents fail. The temptation to use intravenous amiodarone to restore sinus rhythm should be tempered by knowledge of its acute electrophysiologic effects. Its class I and, particularly, class III effects take time to occur, making this a poor choice for rapid conversion. Bolus treatment with intravenous amiodarone has been very disappointing (4% conversion) for acute conversion of atrial fibrillation. By contrast, in approximately 20% to 50% of patients with persistent atrial fibrillation (lasting longer than 24 to 48 hours), reversion to sinus rhythm is achieved with sustained administration (loading periods of up to 4 weeks) of oral amiodarone.[39] Intravenous amiodarone may result in less hypotension when used for rate control in the ICU than diltiazem.[40,41]

Table 31.2 Intravenous Drugs for Atrial Fibrillation

Drug	Acute Dose	Maintenance Dose	Comments
Drugs for Rate Control[*]			
Digoxin	1 mg over 24 h in increments of 0.25-0.5 mg	0.125-0.25 mg	Not very effective in high-catecholamine states; caution with renal disease
Esmolol[†]	0.5 mg/kg/min for 1 min	0.05-0.2 mg/kg/min	Short half-life; hypotension common
Verapamil	5-20 mg in 5-mg increments	5 to 10-mg boluses every 30 min *or* 0.005 mg/kg/min	Caution with left ventricular dysfunction
Diltiazem	20-25 mg *or* 0.25-0.35 mg/kg	10-15 mg/h	Well tolerated; may cause hypotension
Drugs for Cardioversion			
Procainamide	10-15 mg/kg at ≤50 mg/min	2-6 mg/min	May cause hypotension
Amiodarone[‡]	150 mg over 10 min, then 1 mg/min for 6 h	0.5 mg/min	May cause hypotension; many long-term side effects
Ibutilide	1 mg over 10 min A second dose may be given 10 min after the first	None	Prolongs QT; may cause torsades de pointes May lower energy requirement for direct current cardioversion

Adapted from Falk RH: Control of the ventricular rate in atrial fibrillation. In Falk RH, Podrid PJ (eds): Atrial Fibrillation: Mechanisms and Management. New York, Raven Press, 1992.

*Assumes no preexcitation.

†Metoprolol and propranolol also may be used.

‡Amiodarone also is effective for rate control.

Intravenous class IC agents (such as flecainide and propafenone) are the most effective drugs for converting atrial fibrillation of recent onset. Unfortunately, they are not available in the United States. Ibutilide is more effective than intravenous class IC agents for restoration of sinus rhythm in atrial flutter.[39] Electrical cardioversion remains the most effective way of restoring sinus rhythm in patients with atrial fibrillation. As noted, urgent electrical cardioversion should be contemplated for sustained tachycardias that precipitate angina, heart failure, or hypotension.

There are many pitfalls associated with acute atrial fibrillation management. Intravenous beta and calcium channel blockers may result in bradycardia, hypotension, and heart failure. Beta blockers may also aggravate or precipitate bronchospasm. Ibutilide may be proarrhythmic (torsades de pointes). Amiodarone is unlikely to be proarrhythmic in the absence of electrolyte abnormalities (hypokalemia, hypomagnesemia) or other drugs that have already prolonged the rate-corrected QT interval (QTc).[31,34,41]

In the absence of clear-cut evidence from randomized controlled trials, appropriate management should include treatment (or elimination) of potential precipitants and beta blockade (given the hyperadrenergic state of many ICU patients) as the initial pharmacotherapy of choice. If atrial fibrillation recurrence needs to be prevented and sinus rhythm maintained, institution of specific antiarrhythmic therapy (intravenous procainamide, intravenous or oral amiodarone, oral dofetilide, or sotalol) may be effective. We favor adding intravenous amiodarone. This recommendation is based on 100% bioavailability of the intravenous preparation (critically ill patients may not absorb oral drugs), amiodarone's noncompetitive β-antagonistic effects, its benefit in the perioperative period of cardiac surgery[42] (a time when endogenous and exogenous catecholamine levels are often high), and its efficacy in preventing atrial fibrillation recurrence.[31,41]

A recent meta-analysis of perioperative prophylactic amiodarone demonstrated decreased incidence of atrial fibrillation and flutter, ventricular tachyarrhythmias, stroke, and reduced length of stay after cardiac surgery.[42] Not all studies included used beta blockade, and the course of therapy was inconsistent among trials. The Prophylactic Oral Amiodarone for the Prevention of Arrhythmias That Begin Early after Revascularization, Valve Replacement, or Repair (PAPABEAR), a large randomized controlled trial, compared perioperative amiodarone with placebo and showed significant reduction in postoperative atrial tachyarrhythmias.[43] Toxicity risks were reduced because amiodarone was used for a short duration. Neither study demonstrated reduction in mortality rates. The data for perioperative amiodarone in cardiac surgery are compelling; however, incremental benefit beyond beta blockade alone remains unclear. It may still be reasonable to reserve amiodarone for postoperative atrial fibrillation in patients already receiving beta blockers and to limit use of amiodarone to 6 to 12 weeks postoperatively to prevent side effects.

Special Considerations for the Intensivist

As noted, patients in an intensive care setting frequently have active precipitants for reinitiation of atrial or ventricular arrhythmias. Such factors include hypoxemia, excess circulating (endogenous and exogenous) catecholamines, CHF, fever (sepsis), and pulmonary emboli, etc. Many of these conditions have overlapping features.

Digoxin, procainamide, dofetilide, and sotalol are excreted renally and must be carefully managed (or avoided) to prevent complications in patients with renal failure or insufficiency. Amiodarone is hepatically excreted and can be used safely in patients with renal insufficiency or renal failure on dialysis.

Prophylaxis against arrhythmia recurrence shares many of the limitations of acute therapy. Drugs administered orally may not be well absorbed, and intravenous agents (procainamide and amiodarone) may cause or exacerbate hypotension. These factors conspire to make prophylaxis against recurrence difficult.

Most digitalis toxicity–related supraventricular arrhythmias result in relatively slow heart rates and are reasonably well tolerated hemodynamically. Accelerated junctional rhythm and paroxysmal atrial tachycardia with block tend to terminate spontaneously after digoxin is stopped. Digitalis toxic ventricular tachycardia (classically bidirectional tachycardia) is more serious but often slow and hemodynamically well tolerated. Dilantin and lidocaine may be effective for control of digitalis-induced ventricular tachycardia. Digoxin antibodies can be used in cases in which watchful waiting or lidocaine is ineffective or ventricular tachycardia is poorly tolerated due to hemodynamic instability. Electrical cardioversion is contraindicated in the presence of digitalis toxicity. Refractory ventricular fibrillation may ensue.

The intensivist must balance complicated issues before undertaking direct current cardioversion. Strong effort should be focused on avoidance of low-yield attempts. Repeated doses of anesthesia and multiple shocks will ultimately result in further deterioration of critically ill patients. Optimal management of precipitants, careful choices, and monitoring of antiarrhythmic therapy, as well as a solid understanding of cardioversion and defibrillation techniques (see later), will maximize success. In some cases of atrial fibrillation, rapid ventricular rate cannot be controlled by pharmacotherapy. Radiofrequency ablation of the AV junction and permanent pacing may be required when medical therapy is ineffective.[44]

Anticoagulants for Stroke Prevention in Atrial Fibrillation. Prevention of embolic strokes remains the most important goal of therapy for atrial fibrillation. Anticoagulation plays a pivotal role in minimizing the risk of emboli (and strokes) during elective cardioversion of atrial fibrillation.[45] Classic recommendations for management of atrial fibrillation of more than 48 hours' duration include 3 weeks of therapeutic warfarin (to achieve a prothrombin time [PT]/international normalized ratio [INR] of 2.0-3.0) before direct current shock administration and (at least) 4 more weeks of warfarin after the procedure. Although emboli may be less frequent with atrial flutter,[45] it is clear that they occur,[46] and the recommendations are the same as for atrial fibrillation. Novel oral anticoagulants have recently been introduced for stroke prophylaxis in atrial fibrillation (see later).

Anticoagulation in the ICU. The intensivist rarely sees ideal candidates for classic anticoagulation. Outpatient preparation for an elective cardioversion would be an exception rather than the rule. Likewise, the intensivist sees many patients with recent or active bleeding (gastrointestinal, intracerebral) and a variety of coagulopathies that make anticoagulation absolutely or relatively contraindicated.

Short-term therapeutic anticoagulation with heparin before cardioversion (followed by warfarin in the usual manner) combined with transesophageal echocardiography (TEE) has gained acceptance as an alternative approach.[47] Data from the ACUTE trial suggested similar embolic rates (0.5% versus 0.8%) comparing conventional and TEE-guided approaches.[48]

TEE is useful for detecting left atrial thrombi. It provides an excellent, minimally invasive view of the left atrial appendage. Patients with obvious thrombi should be anticoagulated for up to 8 weeks and have demonstrable resolution of clot before cardioversion is attempted.[47]

The intensivist must carefully weigh the risks and benefits of anticoagulation for each individual patient. Difficult decisions about the safety of both short- and long-term anticoagulation may be compounded by concomitant disease processes. At times, TEE may be the only possible (partial) insurance against emboli. Negative results on TEE, however, do not constitute a guarantee against emboli, and the temptation to routinely substitute TEE for adequate anticoagulation should be avoided.

There are well-described risk factors that help the clinician balance the risk of anticoagulation and the risk of stroke from atrial fibrillation. The $CHADS_2$ and CHA_2DS_2-VASc (Congestive heart failure, Hypertension, Age ≥ 75 years [doubled risk weight], Diabetes mellitus, previous Stroke/transient ischemic attack [doubled risk weight], Vascular disease, Age 65 to 74 years, female Sex) risk scores as well as a novel bleeding risk score, HAS-BLED (Hypertension, Abnormal renal/liver function, Stroke history, Bleeding history or predisposition, Labile international normalized ratio, Elderly [≥65 years], Drugs/alcohol concomitantly) aid the clinician in balancing a patient's embolic stroke risk with the risk for bleeding.[49] Patients who are younger than age 65 years with normal hearts and "lone" atrial fibrillation (i.e., with none of the aforementioned risk factors) can be anticoagulated with aspirin 325 mg daily or perhaps not at all. Patients with 1 point should have individualized treatment, and patients with 2 points should be anticoagulated. Patients with rheumatic mitral stenosis or the presence of a prosthetic heart valve are among the highest risk for stroke and should be anticoagulated regardless of the $CHADS_2$ score.[50]

Until the last several years, warfarin has been the only oral anticoagulant used and approved for stroke prophylaxis in atrial fibrillation (as well as anticoagulation for mechanical heart valves and venous thromboembolism). Although warfarin has been proved effective, the need for frequent INR monitoring and its many interactions with other drugs and foods have made this agent cumbersome to use.

Recently, two classes of drugs, the direct thrombin (factor IIa) inhibitors and the factor Xa inhibitors (collectively termed "novel anticoagulants") have emerged as options for prophylaxis against stroke in patients with nonvalvular atrial fibrillation. As a majority of patients in atrial fibrillation are willing to consider switching to these medications, intensivists will undoubtedly encounter patients on these drugs and deal with issues that arise from their use.[51]

Dabigatran, a direct thombin inhibitor, is an oral anticoagulant dosed twice a day. The drug was studied in comparison to warfarin for reduction of strokes in patients with atrial fibrillation. The RE-LY trial found a decreased incidence of stroke with the 150 mg dose of dabigatran and similar risk of bleeding.[52] Dabigatran's half-life is 14 to 18 hours and it is recommended that it be stopped 2 to 3 days prior to an elective surgery (4 to 5 days seems more prudent). There is no specific antidote to this drug. Local measures may suffice for minor bleeding. Dialysis and dabigatran's relatively short half-life usually allow discontinuation of the drug to reverse the bleeding diathesis. The only current reversal option for dabigatran is emergency dialysis. Performing dialysis rapidly in unstable patients with bleeding or in those with large intracranial hemorrhage will present a very great challenge, even at level 1 trauma centers.[53]

In addition to thrombin (factor IIa), the coagulation factor Xa is a target for the novel anticoagulants. In the United States rivaroxaban and apixaban are approved for the treatment of atrial fibrillation, and additional drugs are being studied. The ROCKET-AF trial demonstrated that the once-daily drug rivaroxaban was noninferior to warfarin in reducing stokes with similar bleeding rates.[54] The AVERROES trial demonstrated apixaban was superior to aspirin in patients in whom warfarin was unsuitable.[55] Later, the ARISTOTLE trial demonstrated that apixiban was also superior to warfarin and caused less bleeding.[56] As with the direct thrombin inhibitors, there is no specific reversal agent for factor Xa inhibitors.

The factor Xa inhibitors have a shorter half-life and they are generally stopped the day prior to a surgery.[57] As mentioned, there has been little evidence to support any specific strategy of reversal of anticoagulation, and the rare nature of this problem makes randomized trials on the problem difficult to perform. Preliminary evidence suggests that prothrombin complex concentrate (PCC) immediately and completely reverses the anticoagulant effect of rivaroxaban in healthy subjects.[58] PCC improved laboratory parameters but did not reverse apixaban-induced bleeding in a rabbit model.[59]

DIRECT CURRENT CARDIOVERSION

Deep Sedation for Cardioversion

Direct current shocks should never be administered to a conscious patient. A high-energy shock delivered to an awake patient may result in lifelong emotional trauma and has been appropriately termed a calamity.[60]

Our preferred drug for deep sedation before cardioversion is propofol.[61] Dosing must be individualized. A bolus of 0.6 mg/kg usually is effective for routine elective cardioversion but may be excessive in a critically ill patient.[62] Propofol's adverse effects include apnea, bradycardia, hypotension, nausea, and pain and burning at the intravenous injection site that can be minimized by giving local lidocaine at the site. Overdose is treated with ventilation and oxygen, elevation of the legs, increasing flow rates of intravenous fluids, and administration of pressor agents and anticholinergic agents.

Regardless of who administers sedation, expert ability to manage the patient's airway must be immediately available. Electrophysiology laboratory nurses are often quite capable of administering deep sedation.[63] We recommend that an anesthesiologist be present for high-risk patients.

Technical Aspects

When the capacitors of a defibrillator charge, the device becomes capable of energy delivery (measured in watt-seconds or joules [J]). The energy is composed of voltage and current. Transthoracic current flow is partially determined by electrode placement. A variety of configurations has been employed. We have favored an anteroposterior (parasternal and left infrascapular) pathway for cardioverting atrial fibrillation and flutter and other atrial arrhythmias. This configuration provides the best vectors for energy delivery to the atria[64] (Fig. 31.12). We also have found it to be optimal for patients with an implantable cardioverter-defibrillator (ICD) and epicardial patches.[65]

Most problems with energy delivery have been eliminated with modern external defibrillators that deliver biphasic shocks. Devices with two different biphasic waveforms are available: rectilinear (Zoll Medical, Chelmsford, MA) and truncated exponential (Physiocontrol, Redmond, WA). Head-to-head comparisons have not found significant differences between these biphasic waveforms. Success rates for conversion of atrial fibrillation range from 87% to 100%.

Although it was common to recommend an initial monophasic energy of 100 J for atrial fibrillation (with initial success rates of 50%), we agree with Ewy and begin with 200 J.[64] An initial monophasic energy of 360 J for atrial fibrillation lasting longer than 48 hours also has been suggested.[64,66] A similar recommendation of 200 J also applies to biphasic waveforms, particularly for cardioversion in patients with atrial fibrillation of long duration.[47] Optimal monophasic energy delivery for cardioversion of atrial flutter was 100 J.[67] We generally use 100 J for biphasic cardioversion of atrial flutter as well.

R-wave synchronization should be ensured during cardioversion of arrhythmias with well-defined QRS complexes. Failure to do so may lead to shock delivery within the "vulnerable period" of the T wave and induction of ventricular fibrillation.

Determinants of Short- and Long-Term Success of Cardioversion

Transthoracic impedance influences current flow and procedural outcome. Current flow is inversely related to impedance. Impedance is influenced by a variety of factors. These factors include the phase of ventilation (impedance is lower with expiration than with inspiration), distance between electrodes, pressure on electrodes (air does not conduct well), effect of previous discharges (decreased impedance), time between discharges (waiting as long as 3 minutes may provide continued decreases in impedance), and patient body habitus (heavier weight or increased body mass index will decrease success).[64,68]

As noted, modern defibrillators have biphasic waveforms that are more effective per joule output than monophasic waveform defibrillators. Electrode size is also an important determinant of transthoracic impedance. Self-adhesive pads commonly are used in high-risk patients. They are easy to position precisely. Transthoracic impedance may be higher (70 to 100 ohms) with these pads compared with metal electrodes (50 ohms).[64] Optimal paddle size ranges from 8 to 12 cm. A conductive gel or paste must be used between the metal electrodes and the chest skin.[64] Smearing gel between paddles may deflect energy away from the heart.[69] A switch from from self-adhesive pads to paddles with pressure is a simple method to increase current delivered per shock and to promote procedural success.

Poor long-term success in cardioversion of atrial fibrillation relates to arrhythmia duration (longer than 1 year) and large left atrial diameter (greater than 5 cm). Untreated hyperthyroidism, mitral stenosis, or CHF increases the likelihood of recurrence. Use of concomitant antiarrhythmic drugs (especially amiodarone) may help maintain sinus

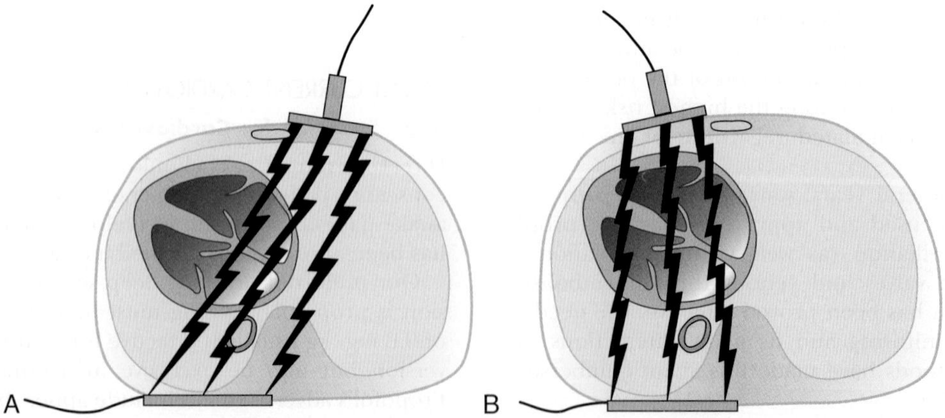

Figure 31.12 Anteroposterior electrode placement for cardioversion of atrial fibrillation and flutter. **A,** Right parasternal anteroposterior electrode placement. **B,** Left parasternal anteroposterior electrode placement. In each instance, the current vector transverses a critical mass of atrial myocardium. The right parasternal position has more of the right atrium between the electrodes and may be advantageous in patients with biatrial disease. The left parasternal position has a smaller interelectrode distance and less lung between electrodes. It has been advocated for patients with left atrial enlargement. (Adapted from Ewy GA: The optimal technique for electrical cardioversion of atrial fibrillation. Clin Cardiol 1994;17:79-84.)

rhythm. Atrial flutter recurrences are hard to prevent, even with pharmacotherapy. As mentioned earlier, typical atrial flutter should be eliminated with radiofrequency catheter ablation.

A BRIEF REVIEW OF ANTIARRHYTHMIC DRUGS

Initiation of chronic oral antiarrhythmic drug therapy for tachyarrhythmias usually is in the realm of practice of general cardiologists and electrophysiologists. Nevertheless, intensivists should be familiar with these agents, as well as current philosophies for their use. The older class IA drugs, including quinidine, procainamide, and disopyramide, now are rarely used because of the risk of QT prolongation and torsades de pointes, low efficacy rates, and poor noncardiac side effect profiles resulting in high discontinuation rates.[48,70] Antiarrythmic drugs in common use are described next.

Flecainide (class IC) is an excellent drug for treatment of all supraventricular tachycardias including atrial fibrillation. It is contraindicated in patients with coronary artery disease or significant left ventricular dysfunction (<40%). The typical starting dose is 100 mg given orally twice daily. The maximum recommended dose for paroxysmal supraventricular tachyarrhythmias is 300 mg/day. Potential adverse effects include proarrhythmia (incessant monomorphic ventricular tachycardia), exacerbation of CHF, and "organization" of atrial fibrillation to atrial flutter with a rapid ventricular response (1:1 AV conduction). Ventricular proarrhythmia is unlikely in the absence of significant structural heart disease (incidence approximately 2%). Flecainide has relatively few noncardiac side effects.

Propafenone (class IC) is an equally effective drug for control of supraventricular tachycardia and atrial fibrillation. Newly formulated sustained-release propafenone has more convenient twice-daily dosing, starting at 225 mg orally twice daily, titrated up to 425 mg twice daily if necessary. Sustained-release propafenone was safe and effective in a large outpatient trial (RAFT).[71] Side effects are similar to those of flecainide, with the addition of a "metallic taste in the mouth" (an unusual noncardiac side effect), which does not require drug discontinuation. Propafenone or flecainide can be beneficial on an outpatient basis in patients with paroxysmal atrial fibrillation who are in sinus rhythm when the drug is initiated.[72] Propafenone has mild β-blocking properties (more prominent in slow metabolizers) but usually not enough to rely on for AV blockade in atrial fibrillation or atrial flutter. Like flecainide, propafenone should not be used in patients with significant structural heart disease.

Sotalol (class III) generally is chosen for patients with coronary artery disease (or other structural heart disease), but can also be a first-line drug for atrial fibrillation in patients with no structural heart disease. It has β-blocking effects and blocks the rapid component of the delayed rectifier potassium current. Sotalol is renally excreted, and doses must be adjusted downward in patients with renal insufficiency. A 3% to 7% risk of torsades de pointes exists with sotalol, with this disturbance usually occurring in the first week of therapy. Other side effects include CHF, exacerbation of bronchospasm, bradycardia, and fatigue. The starting dose is 80 mg given orally twice daily, titrated up to 160 mg twice daily if necessary and as tolerated. Controversy exists over whether sotalol can be initiated as outpatient therapy. We recommend hospitalization with telemetry monitoring and daily 12-lead ECGs for safe initiation of sotalol.

Dofetilide (a class III agent) blocks the rapid component of the delayed rectifier potassium current. Similar to other class III drugs, it prolongs the QT interval and can cause torsades de pointes. In the United States, physicians must take a course and certify to use dofetilide. The drug is dispensed by a national registry system to ensure the physician writing the prescription is certified. Its main advantage is that it has a low proarrhythmia profile (with proper dosing) when used in patients with low ejection fractions. A second virtue is that it does not precipitate or aggravate CHF. The dosage range is 125 to 500 μg given twice daily, which is adjusted according to renal function and QT interval prolongation. Inpatient monitoring on a telemetry ward and frequent ECGs (obtained 2 hours after each dose) to monitor the QT interval are requirements for initiation of dofetilide therapy. The drug is, therefore, rather inconvenient to use. However, it is the only alternative to amiodarone for treatment of atrial fibrillation in patients with poor left ventricular function. Dofetilide usually is well tolerated, with few noncardiac side effects.

Amiodarone is a class III antiarrhythmic with sodium, potassium, and calcium channel blocking properties. In addition, it is a noncompetitive beta blocker and inhibits peripheral conversion of thyroxine (T_4) to triiodothyronine (T_3). It is considered the best atrial fibrillation rhythm control drug and generally regarded as the most effective antiarrhythmic agent for all tachyarrhythmias.[41] It is an excellent AV node–blocking drug. Even when the drug fails to achieve AF rhythm control, it usually will provide good rate control. Amiodarone has an extremely long half-life (a virtue for compliance, but a liability if side effects occur). Like dofetilide, it can be used in patients with low ejection fraction at risk of heart failure exacerbation. Amiodarone does not adversely affect survival and in some studies offered some protection against arrhythmia-related sudden death.[65-67] It can cause significant bradycardia but is associated with a very low incidence of ventricular proarrhythmia (less than 1%), despite the fact that it prolongs the QT interval. The drug requires an initial loading dose (regimens vary). A maintenance dose in the range of 200 mg (or less) per day usually can be achieved and is helpful in minimizing side effects. Occasionally, maintenance doses of 400 mg per day are required for tachycardia control. Amiodarone's long-term noncardiac side effects are significant and should limit its use in younger patients. Nevertheless, amiodarone is the most frequently prescribed specific antiarrhythmic drug in the United States. Side effects include pulmonary toxicity, polyneuropathy, photosensitivity, bradycardia, hepatic dysfunction, thyroid dysfunction, and ophthalmologic complications. Side effects are correlated with maintenance dose and duration of therapy. Baseline pulmonary function studies with diffusing capacity, chest radiograph, liver and thyroid function studies, and eye examination should be performed before or shortly after the drug is started. We recommend thyroid function tests, liver function tests, and a chest radiograph every 6 months

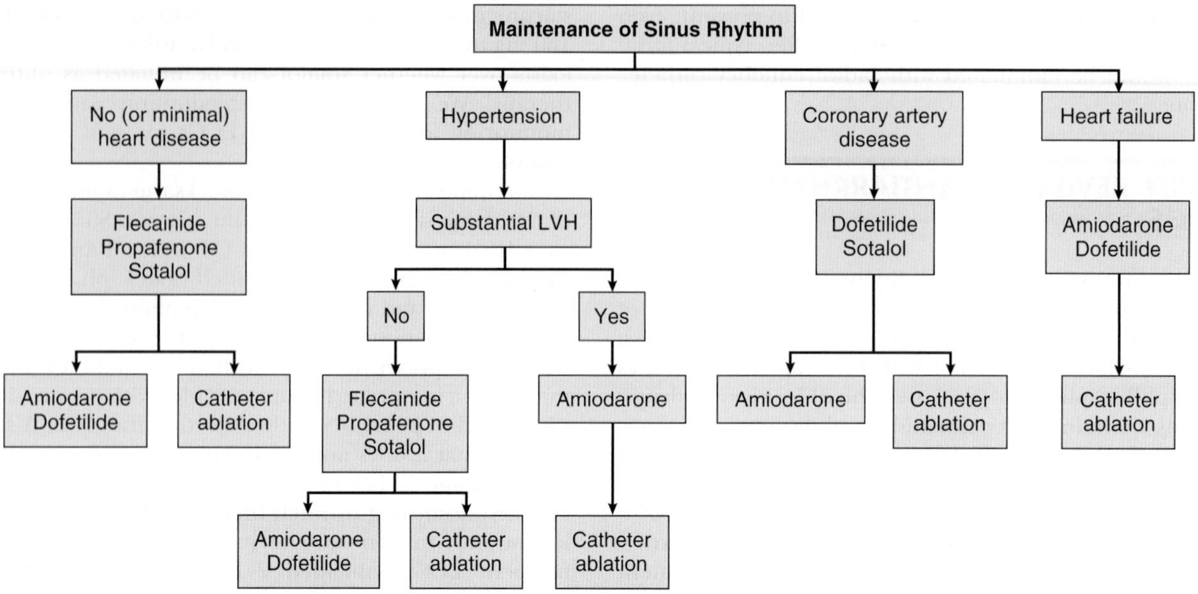

Figure 31.13 ACC/AHA/ESC 2011 guideline algorithm for oral antiarrhythmic drug therapy for maintenance of sinus rhythm in patients with atrial fibrillation. Although the figure suggests that dofetilide is a first-line agent for treatment of coronary artery disease, the text of the guidelines describes it as a second-line agent. LVH, left ventricular hypertension. (From Wann LS, Curtis AB, January CT, et al, writing on behalf of the 2006 ACC/AHA/ESC Guidelines for the Management of Patients With Atrial Fibrillation Writing Committee: 2011 ACCF/AHA/HRS focused update on the management of patients with atrial fibrillation (updating the 2006 guideline): A report of the American College of Cardiology Foundation/ American Heart Association Task Force on Practice Guidelines. J Am Coll Cardiol 2011;57:223-242.)

to look for signs of toxicity. It is particularly disturbing that pulmonary toxicity (which may be fatal) may be missed even with careful surveillance.

Dronedarone is a derivative of amiodarone developed for the treatment of atrial fibrillation and atrial flutter. Like amiodarone, dronedarone is a potent blocker of multiple ion currents, including the rapidly activating delayed-rectifier potassium current, the slowly activating delayed-rectifier potassium current, the inward rectifier potassium current, the acetylcholine activated potassium current, peak sodium current, and the L-type calcium current. Dronedarone also exhibits antiadrenergic effects. Dronedarone has been studied for maintenance of sinus rhythm and control of ventricular response during episodes of atrial fibrillation. Dronedarone reduces mortality rate and morbidity in patients with high-risk atrial fibrillation but may be unsafe in patients with persistent or permanent atrial fibrillation as well as individuals with severe heart failure.[73,74]

The AFFIRM trial randomized over 4000 patients to receive rate or rhythm control treatment strategies (plus warfarin sodium in both treatment groups). Because AFFIRM demonstrated no significant stroke, quality of life, or mortality rate differences with rhythm versus rate control, physicians must consider the risk-benefit ratio of antiarrhythmics to maintain sinus rhythm.[75-77] Patients with brief or minimally symptomatic recurrences of paroxysmal atrial fibrillation often do not require antiarrhythmic drugs. Patients with troublesome symptoms generally require suppressive antiarrhythmic therapy. Rate control and prevention of thromboembolism are appropriate in both situations.[50]

The 2011 ACC/AHA/ESC guidelines for the management of patients with atrial fibrillation recommend that antiarrhythmic drugs for rhythm control of paroxysmal atrial fibrillation be chosen using an algorithm (Fig. 31.13).[50] This algorithm takes into account whether or not the patient has structural heart disease, hypertension with or without "significant" left ventricular hypertrophy (echo wall thickness of 1.4 cm or greater), or coronary artery disease. If there is no structural heart disease, or minimal left ventricular hypertrophy only, the therapeutic agents of first choice are flecainide, propafenone, and sotalol. Second-line therapeutic options include amiodarone and dofetilide. If significant left ventricular hypertrophy is present, the treatment of first choice is amiodarone therapy. If coronary artery disease is present, the treatment of choice is sotalol (because of its β-blocking properties), with second-line therapies including dofetilide and amiodarone. If clinical heart failure is present, first-line agents are amiodarone and dofetilide.

Catheter ablation is recommended for patients with symptomatic paroxysmal atrial fibrillation refractory to or intolerant of at least one antiarrythmic medication. Catheter ablation is considered reasonable for symptomatic paroxysmal atrial fibrillation prior to initation of antiarrythmic drug therapy or symptomatic persistent atrial fibrillation refractory to or intolerant of at least one antiarrythmic medication. Catheter ablation may be considered for symptomatic persistent or longstanding persistent atrial fibrillation prior to initation of antiarrythmic drug therapy and for longstanding persistent symptomatic atrial fibrillation refractory to or intolerant of at least one antiarrythmic medication.[78]

VENTRICULAR ARRHYTHMIAS

The intensivist must be prepared to recognize and participate in the management of ventricular arrhythmias.

However, long-term management usually is prescribed by cardiologists and electrophysiologists. Therefore this section concentrates on the intensive care and emergency treatment of ventricular arrhythmias and only briefly addresses chronic therapy. The emergency treatment of cardiac arrest is covered in Chapter 1.

ARRHYTHMOGENESIS

Reentry is the most common mechanism for sustained ventricular arrhythmias. Three conditions are required for reentry. The first is the presence of two anatomically contiguous pathways separated by a central region of inexcitable tissue. Second, there must be unidirectional block in one of the pathways. Third, a zone of slow conduction also must be present to allow recovery and excitation of the region of block. Such conditions may be anatomically defined (as in the border zone of an old myocardial infarction scar) or result from functional disturbances in conduction and refractoriness.

Enhanced automaticity results in spontaneous impulse formation in cells that otherwise do not exhibit pacemaker activity. Diseased cardiac tissue is particularly susceptible to development of enhanced automaticity. This may result in rates faster than the normal pacemaker activity of the sinus node. Automatic cells (in the AV node, the His-Purkinje system, or the ventricles) may usurp the sinus node by means of enhanced automaticity if their depolarization is accelerated by drugs, sympathetic activity, or metabolic disturbances.

Triggered activity occurs when oscillations in membrane potential (called afterdepolarizations) reach the threshold for action potential formation, resulting in abnormal impulse formation. Early afterdepolarizations (EADs) result from delayed inactivation of inward ion currents during the plateau phase of the action potential. EADs appear to be important in the genesis of torsades de pointes (see later). Delayed afterdepolarizations (DADs) result from increased intracellular calcium. Digitalis toxicity is the classic example of DAD-induced triggered activity. Digitalis inhibits the Na^+-K^+ pump, thereby increasing intracellular Na^+, which in turn increases intracellular Ca^{2+} via the Na^+-Ca^{2+} exchange current.[79] Idiopathic outflow tract ventricular tachycardia may also result from DADs (cyclic AMP-mediated triggered activity).[80]

METABOLIC DISTURBANCES AND ISCHEMIA

Metabolic disturbances and ischemia are common in the critically ill. Patients may suffer from (synergistic or opposing) effects of multiple abnormalities. In the presence of partial predispositions, arrhythmias may not develop until patients are exposed to factors resulting in enhanced automaticity, delayed conduction, or changes in refractoriness.

Hypokalemia delays repolarization and prolongs action potential duration. This may lead to EADs and triggered arrhythmias. Hypomagnesemia and hypokalemia often coexist. Each is associated with QT prolongation and torsades de pointes. Repletion of Mg^{2+} is an important adjunct to the management of hypokalemia. Hypermagnesemia usually is not associated with arrhythmogenesis.

Hyperkalemia suppresses automaticity and slows conduction. The earliest ECG sign is peaked T waves. At high levels (usually 7.0 mEq/L or greater), marked QRS widening (sine wave morphology) may be seen, followed by cardiac arrest. Patients with renal insufficiency may be particularly susceptible. Cardiac effects of severe hyperkalemia may be lethal and require prompt intervention. The most rapid means of countering cardiac toxicity is intravenous administration of 10% calcium chloride. The ECG should be monitored to ensure that signs of hyperkalemia have been reversed. Calcium chloride, although effective emergently, does not lower serum potassium.

Sodium bicarbonate (usual dose 44 to 88 mEq) reduces serum potassium. Regular insulin (10 units) will result in redistribution of K^+ from the extracellular to the intracellular space but does not lower total body potassium stores. Insulin should be followed by 50 mL of 50% glucose.

Further treatment of hyperkalemia involves removal of potassium from the body. The most common method is administration of the cation-exchange resin sodium polystyrene sulfonate (Kayexalate). The usual dose is 50 g given two or three times daily. The most effective means of reducing body potassium is dialysis. Care must be taken to avoid precipitous reduction, especially in patients taking digitalis glycosides.[81] ECG patterns associated with electrolyte and metabolic disturbances are discussed in more detail later in this chapter.

Myocardial ischemia, from coronary artery disease, hemodynamic deterioration, or hypoxemia, can produce a variety of electrophysiologic effects. Acid-base disturbances and exogenous or endogenous catecholamines also can predispose affected patients to ventricular (often polymorphic) arrhythmias. The role of the sympathetic nervous system in arrhythmogenesis and electrical storm cannot be overemphasized.[79,82,83] Reentry, enhanced automaticity, and triggered activity may all be provoked.

In the absence of QT prolongation, ischemia is the most common cause of polymorphic ventricular tachycardia. Polymorphic ventricular tachycardia/ventricular fibrillation in the early phase (less than 48 hours) of an acute myocardial infarction does not require additional evaluation or treatment. Late polymorphic ventricular tachycardia/ventricular fibrillation complicating myocardial infarction usually occurs when severe heart failure or cardiogenic shock also has been problematic. The initial prognosis usually is determined by hemodynamic recovery rather than arrhythmias.

Ischemia is also a common cause of polymorphic ventricular tachycardia/ventricular fibrillation in the absence of acute infarction. A reduction in or withdrawal of catecholamines should be tried. Beta blockers should be titrated to tolerance. Intra-aortic balloon counterpulsation and acute revascularization should be considered. Pharmacologic therapy with amiodarone may be useful.

DIFFERENTIAL DIAGNOSIS OF WIDE QRS TACHYCARDIA

Wide complex tachycardia (WCT) may be supraventricular or ventricular in origin. Evaluation of WCT remains a common dilemma for clinicians. Numerous algorithms aid in arriving at the correct diagnosis. Unfortunately they are difficult to remember and an overreliance on algorithms may prevent clinicians from understanding the underlying arrhythmic mechanisms. Presence of AV dissociation is diagnostic of ventricular tachycardia. In general, supraventricular tachycardia with aberrancy will manifest with a typical bundle branch block pattern, whereas ventricular tachycardia will have more "bizarre" QRS complexes. Preexcited supraventricular tachycardias may be impossible to distinguish from ventricular tachycardia using ECG criteria alone. Algorithms (with good sensitivity and specificity) to help distinguish supraventricular tachycardia from ventricular tachycardia are summarized in Table 31.3.[83]

APPROACH TO VENTRICULAR ARRHYTHMIAS IN THE CRITICALLY ILL

New ventricular arrhythmias warrant an assessment of electrolytes, oxygenation, and acid-base status. Routine measurement of cardiac enzymes is not mandatory with the onset of each arrhythmia. The QT interval should be checked via 12-lead ECG. The 12-lead ECG also is useful in distinguishing monomorphic from polymorphic ventricular tachycardia. Dislodgement of intravascular catheters may result in mechanically induced arrhythmias. Catheter position may be confirmed by x-ray examination or fluoroscopy.

A comprehensive discussion of advanced cardiovascular life support (ACLS) is beyond the scope of this chapter. Current recommendations for management of adult cardiac arrest are discussed in Chapter 1 of this book and are summarized in recently published ACLS guidelines.[84]

SPECIFIC VENTRICULAR ARRHYTHMIAS

The occurrence of premature ventricular contractions (PVCs) and nonsustained ventricular arrhythmias in the ICU generally has little immediate importance. Reduction or withdrawal of exogenous catecholamines and elimination of metabolic disturbances often will decrease the frequency and severity of nonsustained ventricular tachycardia (NSVT). Acute antiarrhythmic drug therapy is rarely required unless symptoms of hemodynamic compromise occur.

The approach to NSVT that persists after recovery from acute illness depends on the underlying cardiac substrate. Asymptomatic persons without structural disease require no therapy. Patients with reduced left ventricular function (less than or equal to 35%) should be evaluated for ICD therapy.[85-87] Amiodarone, which has a neutral effect on mortality rates, may be used to suppress symptomatic NSVT in patients with significant structural heart disease.[85]

Acute management of sustained monomorphic ventricular tachycardia depends primarily on its hemodynamic stability. Unstable tachycardia should be treated promptly with direct current cardioversion. Stable arrhythmias may be treated with intravenous amiodarone or beta blockers. Although lidocaine remains an option, the International Cardiopulmonary Resuscitation (CPR) guidelines no longer recommend lidocaine as a first-line agent. Antitachycardia pacing may be considered in patients with transvenous or epicardial pacing leads. If these modalities are unsuccessful (or arrhythmia acceleration occurs), direct current cardioversion can be used to restore sinus rhythm. Electrical storm

Table 31.3 Electrocardiographic QRS Morphology Criteria Favoring Ventricular Tachycardia Over Supraventricular Tachycardia

Study	Morphology	Criteria Favoring Ventricular Tachycardia
Wellens et al, 1978[87a]	RBBB-like	Monophasic R in V_1
		qR, QS, RS in V_1
		rS, QS, qR in V_6
		R/S <1 in V_6 (S > R or QS in V_6)
		Left axis deviation
		QRS width >140 ms
Kindwall et al, 1988[87b]	LBBB-like	R in V_1 or V_2 >30 ms
		Any Q wave in V_6
		Onset of QRS to nadir of S ≥60 ms in V_1 or V_2
		Notching of downstroke of S in V_1 or V_2
Akhtar et al, 1988[87c]		Positive QRS concordance across the precordium
		Extreme left axis deviation (−90 to ±180 degrees)
	LBBB-like	Right axis deviation
		QRS >60 ms
	RBBB-like	QRS >140 ms
Brugada et al, 1991[87d]		Absence of RS complex in all precordial leads
		R to S interval >100 ms in ≥1 precordial lead
		Wellens' morphologic criteria in lead V_1 or V_6
Vereckei et al, 2008[87e]		Initial R wave in lead aVR
		Initial r or q wave >40 ms in lead aVR
		Notch on descending limb of negative onset, predominantly negative QRS in lead aVR
		$v_i/v_t \le 1$*

From Neiger JS, Trohman RG: Differential diagnosis of tachycardia with a typical left bundle branch block morphology. World J Cardiol 2011;3:127-134.

*Ventricular activation-velocity ratio (v_i and v_t = initial and terminal 40 ms, respectively, of QRS complex).

is defined as ventricular tachycardia or ventricular fibrillation occurring more than twice in 24 hours, usually requiring electrical cardioversion or defibrillation.[88] Although data are limited, beta blockade in conjunction with amiodarone appears to be the most effective therapy for electrical storm.[82,88]

Because the arrhythmic substrate usually is fixed (most commonly, coronary artery disease and prior myocardial infarction), recurrence rates may remain high even after elimination of "reversible" causes.[89,90] Although no definite guidelines exist in the presence of reversible causes, an ICD should be strongly considered in patients with left ventricular dysfunction (if comorbidity is not prohibitive). Electrophysiologic testing may be useful in patients with coronary artery disease but is much less reliable in patients with nonischemic cardiomyopathy.

Bundle branch reentry has been reported to account for up to 6% of the cases of monomorphic ventricular tachycardia.[91] This percentage may rise to 40% to 50% in patients with idiopathic dilated cardiomyopathy.[92] It has been our clinical experience that this arrhythmia is far less frequent. Nevertheless, bundle branch reentry should be considered in patients with marked left ventricular dysfunction (especially nonischemic), intraventricular conduction defects, and wide QRS tachycardia. It may appear after valve replacement surgery. The tachycardia circuit typically uses the right bundle branch as its antegrade limb and the left bundle branch as its retrograde limb. Tachycardia therefore manifests with classic LBBB morphology. Diagnosis and treatment may be accomplished during a single invasive electrophysiology session. The right bundle branch is easily ablated during sinus rhythm, permitting tachycardia cure without detailed mapping during hemodynamically unstable arrhythmias.[93,94] Although the postablation prognosis has been said to be favorable for patients with isolated bundle branch reentry, patients with residual inducible or spontaneous ventricular tachycardia should be offered ICD therapy. Patients with significant residual infranodal conduction delay (His-ventricular rates longer than 90 ms) after ablation should be considered for permanent pacing (usually with an ICD). It is appropriate to implant an ICD after ablation in patients with heart failure and ejection fractions less than 35%.

Optimal long-term management of patients with structural heart disease and sustained monomorphic ventricular tachycardia is to implant an ICD.[95,96] Hemodynamic stability does not predict a better long-term outcome.[95] Ablation generally is regarded as palliative and is used primarily to reduce shock frequency in patients with recurrent ventricular tachycardias.[97] However, substrate-based catheter ablation may reduce the ICD therapies in post-myocardial infarction patients who received ICDs for secondary prevention.[98]

The risk of recurrent polymorphic ventricular tachycardia/ventricular fibrillation is high, and the long-term prognosis is poor. Most patients, particularly those with left ventricular dysfunction, should have an ICD implanted if no contraindications exist. Idiopathic ventricular fibrillation may respond to catheter ablation if a single PVC focus (usually from the Purkinje system or the right ventricular outflow tract) is the consistent trigger.[99,100] Coronary artery spasm may result in ventricular fibrillation caused by myocardial ischemia. Recognition of this uncommon cause of cardiac arrest is critical. Ideal treatment for patients with coronary spasm and associated ventricular arrhythmias remains controversial. Titration of calcium channel blocker dose to prevent ergonovine-induced spasm eliminated arrhythmia in one small series.[101] Despite optimal medical therapy (nitrates and calcium channel blockers), this patient subgroup falls into a high-risk category of vasospastic angina and appears to be at greater risk for sudden death. Concomitant ICD implantation has been advocated to reduce this risk.[102]

LESS COMMON SUBSTRATES

Serious ventricular arrhythmias are uncommon in the absence of significant left ventricular dysfunction. A few specific entities should be readily recognized by the intensivist.

IDIOPATHIC VENTRICULAR TACHYCARDIA

Idiopathic ventricular tachycardias tend to originate in a "line of fire" from the right ventricular outflow tract (90%), left ventricular outflow tract, aortic cusps, and mitral annulus.[103] They often are facilitated by catecholamine infusion. The most common forms (right ventricular outflow tract tachycardia) have a typical, easily recognizable ECG pattern of LBBB with an inferior frontal lead axis (tall R waves in leads II, III, and aVF). These arrhythmias occur in the absence of apparent structural heart disease. Abnormalities may be detected using magnetic resonance imaging; however they do not definitely correlate with sites of arrhythmogenesis.[104,105] Very frequent episodes may result in a tachycardia-mediated cardiomyopathy.[106]

More than 90% of idiopathic ventricular tachycardias can be cured by catheter ablation (Figs. 31.14 and 31.15).[106,107] The most reliable method for localizing the site of origin is pace mapping. The 12-lead ECG will exactly match the spontaneous ventricular tachycardia QRS morphology at

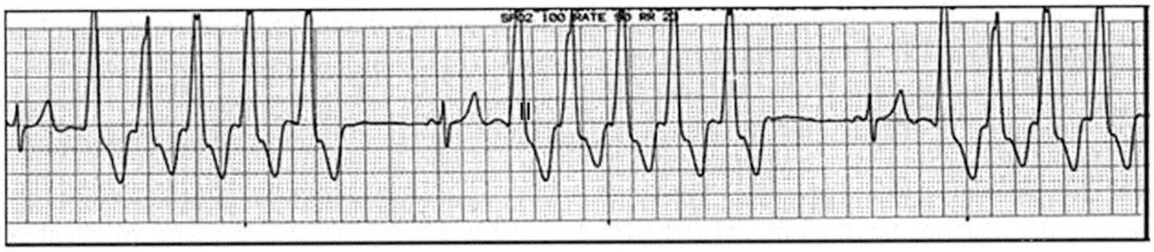

Figure 31.14 Nonsustained ventricular tachycardia from aortic cusp. An "idiopathic" ventricular tachycardia arising from the aortic cusp. (From Kakodkar S, Krishnan K, Awad S, et al: Reversible cardiomyopathy in an adolescent with idiopathic aortic cusp ventricular tachycardia. Pediatr Cardiol 2010;31(1):147-150.)

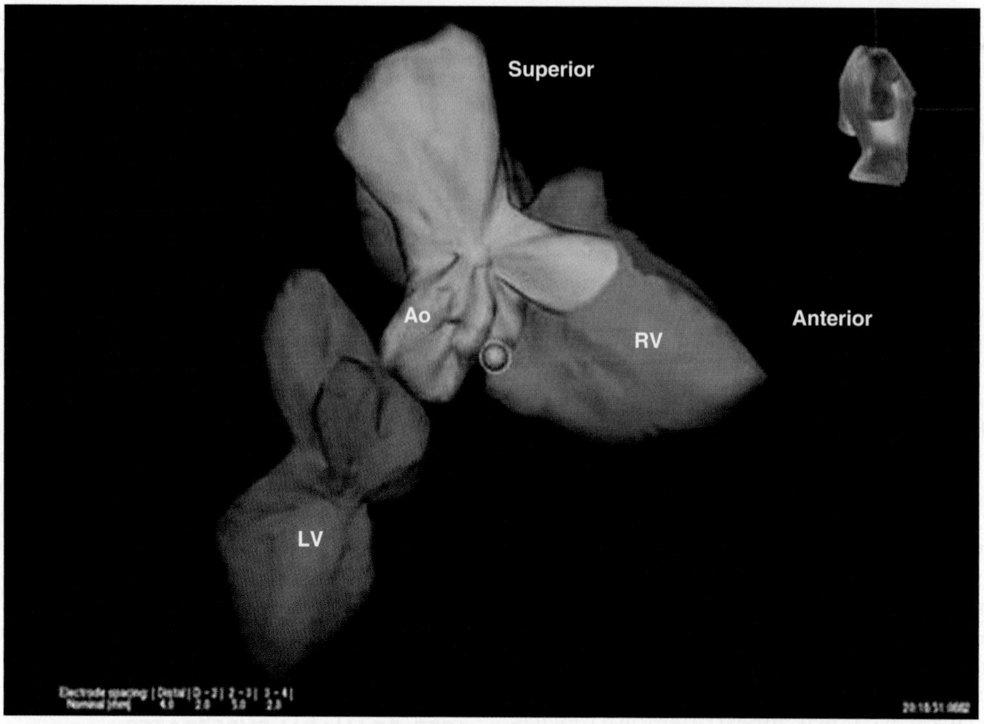

Figure 31.15 Mapping of a left ventricular outflow tract (LVOT) tachycardia. Using the EnSite system, a three-dimensional electroanatomic mapping was performed during the electrophysiology study. The nonsustained LVOT tachycardia originated from the noncoronary/right coronary cusp border. This arrhythmia was ablated successfully (ablation points shown as blue spheres). Ao, aorta; LV, left ventricle; RV, right ventricle. (From Kakodkar S, Krishnan K, Awad S, et al: Reversible cardiomyopathy in an adolescent with idiopathic aortic cusp ventricular tachycardia. Pediatr Cardiol 2010;31(1):147-150.)

the site of origin of the ventricular tachycardia. If a perfect 12/12-lead ECG pace map match can be obtained, the site is ablated. These tachycardias are adenosine-sensitive and thought to be the result of cyclic AMP–mediated DADs.[80] These arrhythmias may respond to treatment with adenosine and chronically to beta blockers or calcium channel blockers, which normally are ineffective in other ventricular tachycardias.

Another "idiopathic" left ventricular tachycardia manifests as a relatively narrow right bundle branch block (RBBB), left axis deviation tachycardia. The ECG and rhythm strip should be examined carefully for P waves. If the PP interval is slower and the P waves are dissociated, the diagnosis of ventricular tachycardia, rather than supraventricular tachycardia with aberrancy, is confirmed. This arrhythmia is verapamil-sensitive and can easily be ablated if necessary. The arrhythmia is due to macroentry in the terminal Purkinje fibers in the left distal third of the apical septum (Fig. 31.16). To ablate it, the lower third of the septum is mapped, looking for the sharpest, earliest Purkinje potential during ventricular tachycardia.[108] A second technique (also using Purkinje potentials) is equally effective.[109] This reentrant tachycardia is referred to by several different names, including fascicular ventricular tachycardia, verapamil-sensitive ventricular tachycardia, and Belhassen's ventricular tachycardia.

In patients with ventricular arrhythmias and obvious significant right ventricular disease, the diagnosis of arrhythmogenic right ventricular dysplasia (ARVD)/cardiomyopathy can be made. The left ventricle generally has milder abnormalities. ARVD typically occurs in young patients (80% of patients are diagnosed before the age of 40 years) and is an important cause of SCD in this population. It should, however, be emphasized that the overall risk of SCD is low (2% to 2.5% per year).[110]

Males are predominantly affected. ARVD is transmitted in an autosomal dominant pattern with variable penetrance (abnormal loci have been mapped to chromosomal regions 14q23, 1q42, 14q12, 2q32, 17q21, and 3p23).[110] Immunohistochemical analysis of endomyocardial biopsy samples revealing a diffusely reduced plakoglobin signal level appears to be a highly sensitive and specific test for ARVD.[111]

Ventricular arrhythmias in ARVD may be catecholamine dependent and are exacerbated during exercise tolerance testing in 50% of patients. Sotalol and amiodarone seem to be effective in ARVD. Catheter ablation has a palliative, complementary role. Arrhythmia recurrences at new foci may occur after apparent ablative success. Experience with ICDs in ARVD is limited. Patients resuscitated from cardiac arrest or those poorly responsive to (or intolerant of) antiarrhythmic drugs appear to be good candidates.[112]

The congenital long QT syndrome is a manifestation of a variety of ion channel mutations that result in prolonged ventricular repolarization. The three main features of congenital long QT syndrome are (1) prolongation of the rate-corrected QT interval (QTc); (2) cardiac arrest secondary to torsades de pointes (Fig. 31.17); and (3) QT prolongation, syncope, or sudden death in family members. Syncope often occurs in association with physical activity, emotional reactions, or acute arousal with auditory stimuli (the specific trigger in a variant of long QT syndrome, LQT2).[113,114] Beta blockers are the mainstay of treatment in patients with long

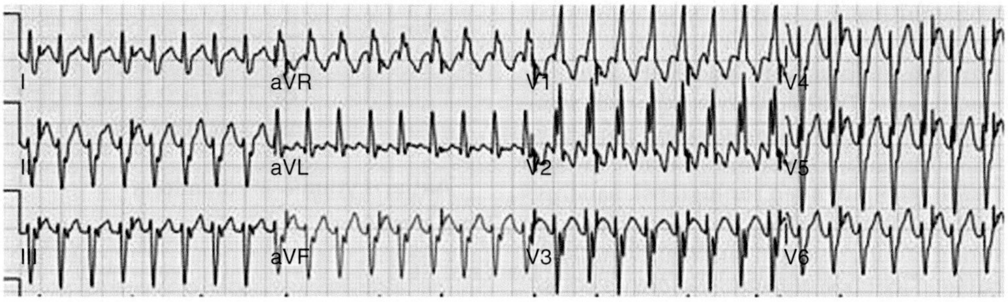

Figure 31.16 Verapamil-sensitive ventricular tachycardia in a 12-year-old.

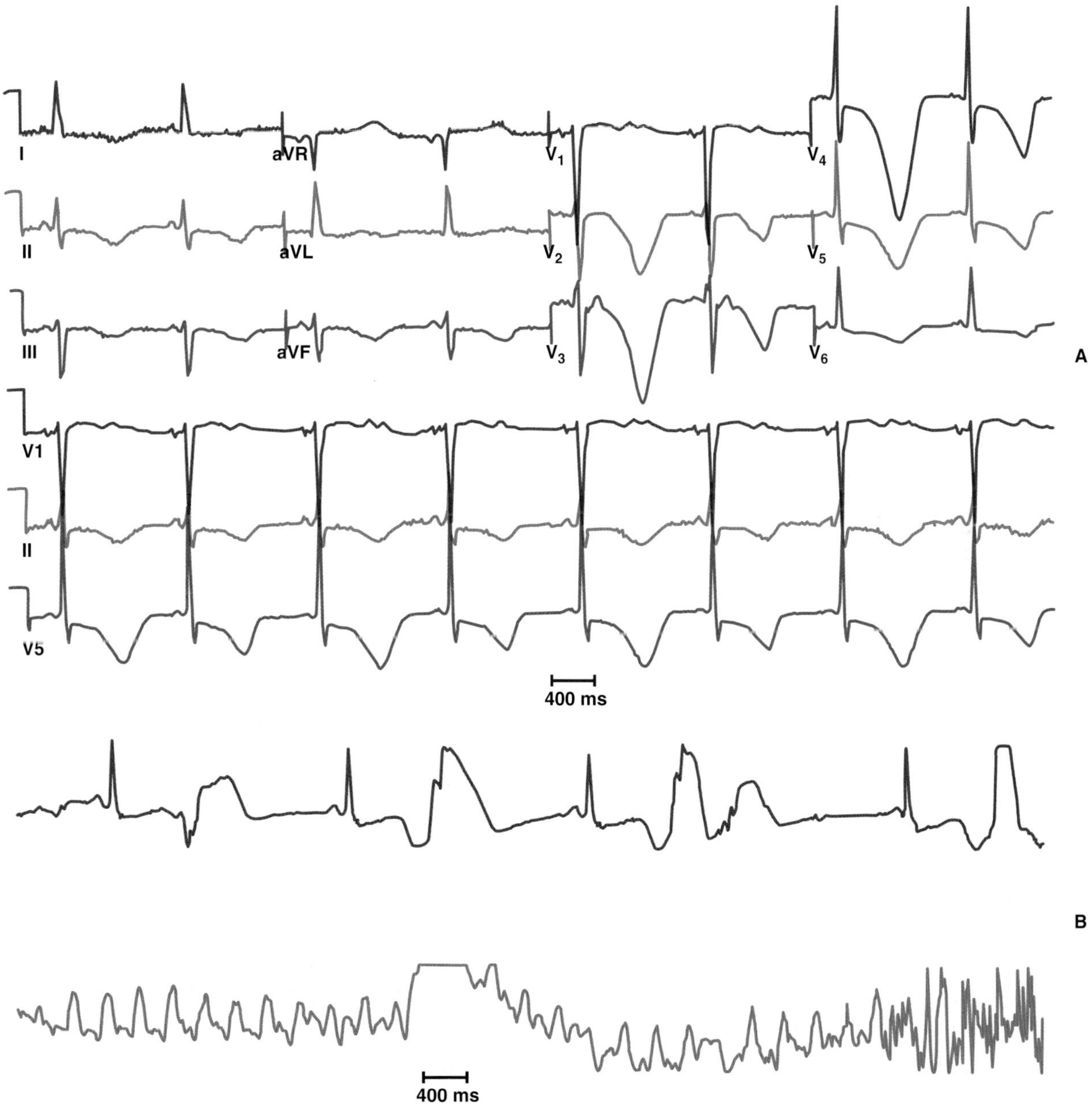

Figure 31.17 **A,** Marked QT prologation and T wave alternative is a harbinger of electrical instability. **B,** Increasing ventricular ectopy is followed by ventricular fibrillation. (Adapted from Trohman RG, Sahu J: Drug-induced torsades de pointes. Circulation 1999;99:E7.)

QT syndrome. Permanent pacing (ideally via an ICD) may be beneficial for patients in whom beta blockade is not effective or in whom excessive bradycardia develops. Limited experience has been reported with left cervicothoracic sympathetic ganglionectomy in patients with drug-refractory long QT syndrome and surgical expertise is available in only a few centers. ICDs are recommended for high-risk patients, including those with recurrent syncope on beta blockers, aborted SCD, a strong family history of sudden death, and the Jervell and Lange-Nielsen syndrome (homozygotes or compound heterozygotes with mutations in *KCNQ1* and *KCNE1*, resulting in abnormal I_{ks} ion current long QT syndrome and hereditary deafness).[115]

Although the short-term effects of gene-specific therapy (e.g., mexiletine or flecainide in patients with sodium channel abnormalities, potassium plus spironolactone in potassium channel defects) on the QT interval are encouraging,[116] long-term data are lacking regarding their ability to prevent arrhythmias in long QT syndrome. A trial of flecainide for another variant of the syndrome, LQT3, is ongoing.

QT prolongation may be acquired (most commonly caused by drug effects or toxic substances, electrolyte abnormalities, hypothermia, and central nervous system injury). Drug-induced QT prolongation usually is the result of I_{kr} ion current blockade.[35] Intensivists need to be particularly aware of the pharmacologic causes of QT prolongation (Box 31.3). Drug-induced torsades de pointes is managed initially with intravenous magnesium sulfate. Isoproterenol and temporary pacing increase ventricular rates, shorten QT intervals, and help prevent recurrent arrhythmias until the effects of the offending agent diminish.

The Brugada syndrome (first described in 1992) is characterized by RBBB with ST-segment elevation in leads V_1 to V_3, polymorphic ventricular tachycardia, and ventricular fibrillation.[117] Intensivists need to be particularly aware that febrile illnesses may trigger arrhythmic events.[118] Brugada syndrome has been linked to mutation in the sodium channel gene *SCN5A*. This mutation decreases sodium channel activity. It is inherited in an autosomal dominant pattern with variable penetrance. Males are more likely to be affected and have an increased risk of sudden death, probably related to a more prominent transient outward potassium current. The ECG abnormality originally was thought to be persistent; however, transient forms (in which the ECG may be normal for periods of time) have been described.[119] The electrocardiographic abnormalities may be unmasked by procainamide, flecainide, or ajmaline.

The cellular mechanism responsible for the ST-segment elevation is early repolarization of the ventricular epicardium as a result of rebalancing of currents at the end of phase I of the action potential. The transient outward potassium current (I_{to}) overwhelms inward currents. The action potential "dome" is abolished at some sites but not others. Propagation of the dome to sites where it is absent may result in so-called *phase II reentry,* the mechanism of arrhythmogenesis.[120] In this instance, diminished sodium channel activity facilitates loss of the action potential dome as a result of a negative shift in the voltage at which phase I begins. Different mutations in *SCN5A* appear to account for LQT3; however, a recent report suggests a genetic (and perhaps

Box 31.3 Drugs* Reported to Cause Prolongation of QT Interval or Torsades de Pointes/ Ventricular Tachycardia

Antiarrhythmic Medications

Class IA

Quinidine
Procainamide (metabolized to *N*-acetylprocainamide)
Disopyramide

Class III

Dofetilide
Ibutilide
Sotalol
Amiodarone

Class IV

Bepridil

Promotility Medications

Cisapride†

Antimicrobial Medications

Macrolides

Erythromycin
Clarithromycin

Fluoroquinolones

Sparfloxacin†

Antiprotozoals

Pentamidine

Antimalarials

Halofantrine
Chloroquine

Antipsychotic Medications

Phenothiazine neuroleptics

Thioridazine
Chlorpromazine
Mesoridazine

Butyrophenone neuroleptics

Droperidol
Haloperidol

Diphenylpiperidine neuroleptics

Pimozide

Miscellaneous Agents

Arsenic trioxide
Methadone

Vitamins, Supplements, and Herbal Preparations

Cesium
Licorice
Zhigancao

From Gupta A, Lawrence AT, Krishnan K, et al: Current concepts in the mechanisms and management of drug-induced QT prolongation and torsades de pointes. Am Heart J 2007;153:891-899.
*Partial listing.
†Unavailable or severely limited availability in the United States.

clinical) link between the Brugada syndrome and LQT3.[121] As with long QT syndrome, it appears that genetic heterogenicity exists in the Brugada syndrome.[122] In Japan and Southeast Asia, the Brugada syndrome may account for 40% to 60% of cases of idiopathic ventricular fibrillation. The ICD is the only effective therapeutic intervention against SCD.

Catecholaminergic polymorphic ventricular tachycardia (CMPVT) typically manifests in childhood as syncope or aborted cardiac arrest. Young boys have the worst prognosis (perhaps they are more sensitive to adrenergic stimulation). Beta blockers are the cornerstone of therapy, and dosing may be titrated according to exercise response. In 40% of patients, arrhythmia control will remain inadequate despite dose optimization during repeat exercise testing. ICDs are the therapeutic option of choice in these patients.[123]

Short-coupled torsades de pointes (SC-TdP) occurs in patients with structurally normal hearts and unremarkable ECG tracings (normal QT intervals). The coupling interval of the initiating beat is invariably less than 300 ms. It is a rare, potentially fatal disorder whose pathophysiology is unknown. The prognosis is poor, and effective pharmacologic therapy has not been identified. ICDs may be the best option. SC-TdP shares features with idiopathic ventricular tachycardia, and speculation that it may respond to catheter ablation if a single PVC focus (usually from the Purkinje system) is the consistent trigger is not unreasonable.[124,125]

Short QT syndrome (SQTS) is a heritable primary electrical disease characterized by an abnormally short QT interval (less than 300 ms) and a propensity to atrial fibrillation or SCD, or both. As in the long QT syndrome, more than one relevant genetic mutation has been identified. Shortening of effective refractory periods combined with increased dispersion of repolarization is the likely substrate for reentry and life-threatening tachyarrhythmias. The best form of treatment is still unknown, but prevention of atrial fibrillation has been accomplished with propafenone. Implantation of an ICD is recommended for prevention of SCD.[126,127]

Patients who experience electrical shock (including lightning strikes) sustain a wide spectrum of injuries with unique pathophysiologic characteristics that require special management. Patients with serious burns admitted to the ICU are trauma patients and should be treated accordingly. Initial prediction of outcome for patients who have experienced electrical shock is difficult, because the full degree of injury often is not apparent. SCD due to ventricular fibrillation is more common with low-voltage alternating current, whereas asystole is more frequent with electric shocks from direct current or high-voltage alternating current. Potentially fatal arrhythmias are more likely to be caused by horizontal current flow (hand to hand); current passing in a vertical fashion (from head to foot) more commonly causes myocardial tissue damage. Lightning strike is unique because it causes cardiac and respiratory arrest, resulting in a 25% to 30% mortality rate.[128]

Aggressive and prolonged CPR in patients who have experienced electrical shock is indicated for several reasons.[129] First, cardiac arrhythmias and prolonged respiratory arrest may be the only clinical problem, especially in patients struck by lightning. Second, as mentioned, patients who experience electrical shock commonly are young and have few or no comorbid conditions. These young patients may survive prolonged CPR with no or minor sequelae. It is important to remember that keraunoparalysis leading to autonomic dysfunction may masquerade as irreversible neurologic injury in patients who have been electrocuted. For practical purposes, guidelines for CPR as issued by the American Heart Association[84] still apply. The algorithm for asystole acknowledges that "atypical clinical features" need to be considered in deciding whether CPR should be continued after initial unsuccessful attempts.

If more than one person has been electrocuted at a scene of injury, standard triage practices need to be modified, especially in those struck by lightning. Most patients who do not experience cardiac or respiratory arrest will survive.[130] Thus, the usual triage principles should be reversed: First responders should focus initially on patients who appear clinically dead *before* patients who show signs of life are treated.

CARDIAC ARREST AND ELECTRICAL STORM

It is estimated that out of hospital sudden cardiac arrest (SCA) tragically ends over 300,000 lives in the United States[131,132] and is responsible for 3 million deaths worldwide each year.[133] Although the number of age-adjusted cardiovascular deaths has declined during the last 50 years, the proportion that are sudden has remained relatively constant (~50%).[134,135] SCA claims more lives each year than stroke, lung cancer, breast cancer, and AIDS combined.[136-138]

SCD is defined as natural death due to cardiac causes, foreshadowed by abrupt loss of consciousness, occurring within 1 hour of an acute change in cardiovascular status.[133,133] Unfortunately, SCA and SCD are nearly synonymous. Worldwide, survival after SCA is dismal (<1%). In the United States, mortality rate after SCA is about 95%.[134]

Merchant and colleagues[139] estimated the annual incidence of in-hospital cardiac arrest in the United States. Their calculation of approximately 200,000 annual victims provides pivotal perspective on the magnitude of this problem. Despite the similarity in annual incidence, out-of-hospital SCA is far more familiar to the medical community.[140]

Coronary artery disease is the primary cause (80%) of out-of-hospital SCA. Nonischemic cardiomyopathies account for 10% to 15%. The remaining 5% are related to valvular disease, inherited ion channel or receptor defects (long QT syndrome, Brugada syndrome, CMPVT, etc.), congenital heart disease, and other causes. Sadly, over 60% of SCA occurs as an initial clinical event or in patients with clinical disease characteristics suggesting relatively low risk.[133] Our risk stratification repertoire remains woefully inadequate for the vast majority of out-of-hospital SCA victims.[131,140,141]

In contrast, most in-hospital cardiac arrests result from preexisting conditions and are not due to sudden-onset cardiac arrhythmias. Progressive respiratory failure and shock are common precipitants. It has been suggested that this information be used to tailor better in-hospital cardiac arrest protocols.[142]

Ventricular fibrillation is the most frequently documented initial rhythm at the time of resuscitation from out-of-hospital cardiac arrest. In over 75% of cases the underlying cause is a ventricular tachyarrhythmia (ventricular fibrillation or pulseless ventricular tachycardia). Primary bradyarrhythmias (e.g., asystole) and pulseless electrical activity are less common.[143]

Interestingly, over 70% of in-hospital cardiac arrests present with asystole or pulseless electrical activity. Ventricular tachyarrhythmias are a far less common presentation (14%-24%).[142,144,145]

Out-of-hospital survival is linked directly to time between SCA onset and defibrillation or bystander CPR. Time to restoration of spontaneous circulation is also closely correlated with neurologic recovery. Brain damage begins in 4 to 6 minutes.[146] Studies of outcome as a function of initial rhythm recorded at the scene of out-of-hospital cardiac arrest demonstrate that bradyarrhythmias and asystole have the worst prognosis.[147,148]

Likewise, survival to hospital discharge is substantially increased when the first documented in-hospital cardiac arrest rhythm is "shockable" (pulseless ventricular tachycardia or ventricular fibrillation).[142] Shocks must take priority over CPR. Delayed defibrillation has been associated with a significantly lower probability of survival to hospital discharge.[149,150] Asystole often occurs late in an arrest (after energy stores required to generate ventricular fibrillation have been exhausted) and can be a surrogate for prolonged downtime.[140,148] Data exist suggesting that pulseless electrical activity portends a slightly better outcome compared to asystole.[140,145]

Children suffering in-hospital cardiac arrest have better survival to hospital discharge compared to adults. This is true (due to increased survival after pulseless electrical activity or asystole) despite a significantly lower prevalence of ventricular tachycardia/ventricular fibrillation as the initial rhythm in children suffering cardiac arrest.[146] For in-hospital cardiac arrest, adult survival rates range from roughly 15% to 21%.[142,144,145] In children, a survival rate of 27% has been reported.[142] Aggressive, prolonged CPR should be considered in young patients (particularly those with few or no comorbid conditions). Young patients may survive prolonged CPR with no or only minor sequelae.[128,140]

Electrical storm is defined as ventricular tachycardia or ventricular fibrillation occurring two times or more in a 24-hour period, usually requiring electrical cardioversion or defibrillation.[151] Small nonrandomized trials demonstrated amiodarone's safety and efficacy for recurrent drug-refractory sustained ventricular arrhythmias.[151,152] Intravenous amiodarone is more effective than lidocaine for out-of-hospital ventricular fibrillation resistant to shocks and epinephrine. More amiodarone-treated patients survive to hospital admission.[153] Fogel and associates demonstrated 80% 1-year survival rate in patients with recurrent hemodynamically unstable ventricular arrhythmias initially treated with intravenous amiodarone who were receiving oral amiodarone at discharge.[154] Patients with electrical storm following myocardial infarction treated with sympathetic blockade followed by oral amiodarone had significantly better short-term mortality rates compared with conventional antiarrhythmic drugs. Patients who received a combination of oral amiodarone and a beta blocker had the best outcomes.[82] Although limited data exist, beta blockade in conjunction with amiodarone appears to be the most effective therapy for electrical storm.[41]

Key objectives in post–cardiac arrest care include (1) optimizing cardiopulmonary function and vital organ perfusion; (2) transportation to a hospital or critical-care unit with a comprehensive post–cardiac arrest treatment system of care; (3) identification and intervention for acute coronary syndromes; (4) temperature control to optimize neurologic recovery; and (5) anticipation, treatment, and prevention of multiple organ dysfunction.[84]

The most important manifestations of the post–cardiac arrest syndrome are often neurologic. About 80% of patients remain comatose for longer than 1 hour after resuscitation, and less than 50% of admitted patients have a good neurologic recovery. *Targeted temperature management,* or *therapeutic hypothermia,* is an intervention intended to limit neurologic injury after resuscitation from cardiac arrest.[84] An Australian trial and a European multicenter trial suggested improved neurologic recovery and decreased mortality rate at 6 months after arrest.[155-157] A 2008 statement from the International Liaison Committee on Resuscitation (ILCOR) incorporated targeted temperature management into the comprehensive treatment bundle of therapy for the post–cardiac arrest syndrome.[158]

Several different methods are available for cooling in therapeutic hypothermia. Many techniques use commercially developed equipment specifically designed for targeted temperature management. The optimal regimen is still a matter of debate.[155]

Targeted temperature management has been used almost exclusively in patients with an out-of-hospital cardiac arrest due to ventricular fibrillation or pulseless ventricular tachycardia. There are no data from studies of sufficient quality to recommend this therapy in an adult who has had a cardiac arrest that is not due to a hemodynamically unstable ventricular tachyarrhythmia. Indications and contraindications for targeted temperature management after cardiac arrest are summarized in Box 31.4.[155]

CATHETER ABLATION OF CARDIAC ARRHYTHMIAS

Catheter ablation offers curative therapy for paroxysmal supraventriculat tachycardias (including those associated with the Wolff-Parkinson-White syndrome), atrial flutter, automatic atrial tachycardias, idiopathic ventricular arrhythmias, bundle branch reentrant ventricular tachycardias, and interfascicular ventricular tachycardias. Success rates in excess of 90% are common among experienced operators.

Catheter ablation is less successful in other (myocardial) ventricular tachycardias associated with structural heart disease and operator success rates are more likely to vary according to expertise and experience. It remains common to restrict these ablations to patients who fail combination therapy with an ICD and antiarrhythmic drugs (usually amiodarone).

As previously noted, catheter ablation may be considered as first-line *treatment* for some patients with atrial fibrillation. The 2012 HRS/EHRA/ECAS Expert Consensus Statement on Catheter and Surgical Ablation of Atrial Fibrillation

Box 31.4 Indications and Contraindications for Targeted Temperature Management in Comatose Patients after Cardiac Arrest

Patients for whom therapeutic hypothermia should be considered

- Adult patients successfully resuscitated from a witnessed out-of-hospital cardiac arrest of presumed cardiac cause (patients after in-hospital cardiac arrest may also benefit)
- Patients who are comatose (i.e., patients with a score on the Glasgow Coma Scale of less than 8 and patients who do not obey any verbal command at any time after restoration of spontaneous circulation and before initiation of cooling)
- Patients with an initial rhythm of ventricular fibrillation or nonperfusing ventricular tachycardia (patients presenting with other initial rhythms such as asystole or pulseless electrical activity may also benefit)
- Patients whose condition is hemodynamically stable (retrospective data suggest that patients in cardiogenic shock may also safely undergo hypothermia treatment)

Patients for whom therapeutic hypothermia should not be considered

- Patients with tympanic membrane temperature below 30° C on admission
- Patients who were comatose before the cardiac arrest
- Pregnant patients
- Patients who are terminally ill or for whom intensive care does not seem to be appropriate
- Patients with inherited blood coagulation disorders

Adapted from Holzer, M: Targeted temperature management for comatose survivors of cardiac arrest. N Engl J Med 2010;363: 1256-1264.

suggests that first-line ablation is reasonable for paroxysmal atrial fibrillation and may be considered for persistent or even longstanding persistent atrial fibrillation.[78]

Ablation should not be considered curative for atrial fibrillation, although some patients may be arrhythmia free without antiarrhythmic drugs for 5 or more years. Multiple procedures result in higher success rates than a single ablation session. Catheter ablation may also result in pharmacologic arrhythmia control that was not possible before ablation.

A variety of ablation techniques have been employed, although most operators focus primarily on electrically isolating the pulmonary veins (the most common source of triggering atrial ectopy). Linear left atrial lesions may be employed; however, gaps in these lines may create the substrate for reentrant atrial flutter. This limitation has reduced the popularity of linear lesions that were once favored as a routine portion of the procedure.

Other operators have targeted complex fractionated electrograms recorded during atrial fibrillation. The theory behind this technique is that "rotors" or wavelets of reentry (the substrate for atrial fibrillation) can be eliminated. One report has suggested that attacking complex fractionated electrograms adds little to pulmonary vein isolation for persistent atrial fibrillation.[159] A recent report that utilizes a special computer program to choose target sites has rekindled interest in this technique.[160]

Atrial fibrillation ablation success is highly dependent on careful patient selection. Patients with persistent or permanent atrial fibrillation, very large left atria, or age 75 years or older (similar success rates, complications more likely) are less likely to have an optimal outcome. Ideal candidates for catheter ablation of atrial fibrillation have symptomatic episodes of paroxysmal or persistent atrial fibrillation, have not responded to antiarrhythmic drugs, do not have severe comorbid conditions or significant structural heart disease, are younger than 65 to 70 years, have a left atrial diameter less than 50 to 55 mm, and have had persistent atrial fibrillation for less than 5 years.[161]

Although atrial fibrillation ablation is generally considered safe and effective, devastating complications may occur. The incidence of death associated with atrial fibrillation ablation is 0.1%. This is similar to the risk of death associated with ablation of regular supraventricular tachycardias. Cardiac tamponade is the most frequent fatal complication. Delayed development of an atrioesophageal fistula (10-16 days after procedure) is the second most frequent cause of death.[162] This complication is unique to ablation in the posterior left atrium.

PACEMAKERS AND IMPLANTABLE DEFIBRILLATORS

As a result of an aging population and expanded implantation indications, intensivists are increasingly likely to encounter patients with pacemakers or implantable defibrillators. Patients with these devices may be hospitalized for cardiac or noncardiac ailments.

The classic indication for permanent pacing is symptomatic bradycardia that is not due to a transient cause and is, therefore, unlikely to reverse. Most commonly, this occurs because of SND or AV blockade. Permanent pacing at rates greater than 70 beats per minute and rate-smoothing algorithms are useful to prevent drug-induced torsades de pointes. Pacing at 80 beats per minute may help prevent torsades de pointes and torsades de pointes "storm" in patients with congenital long QT syndrome.[4,163]

Magnet application to pacemakers may terminate slow reentrant atrial and ventricular tachycardias by creating a competitive, asynchronous paced rhythm that interrupts the reentrant circuit. If this maneuver is used, a defibrillator should be present in case underdrive pacing accelerates the arrhythmia.

Magnet application may also be useful for pacemaker identification and temporary inhibition of ICD tachyarrhythmia therapies. Three pacemaker companies make more than 90% of the pacemakers used in the United States. The device manufacturers have no standardized programmers, so the device brand must be known in order to bring the company-specific programmer to the patient. Medtronic pacemakers usually respond to magnet application by pacing at 85 beats per minute; Boston Scientific (formerly Guidant) devices at 100 beats per minute; and St. Jude devices at 98.6 beats per minute. Pacemakers will return to the programmed lower rate limit when the magnet is removed. Clinicians also can find out if a patient has a Medtronic pacemaker or implantable defibrillator by calling 1-800-MEDTRONIC; a Boston Scientific or Guidant device by calling 1-800-CARDIAC; and a St. Jude device by calling 1-800-PACEICD. Access to technical experts is also available via these telephone numbers.

The ICD has emerged as accepted therapy for primary and secondary prevention of sudden death.[164] Evidence-based results have demonstrated the clinical benefits of ICD therapy and indications for implantation have expanded rapidly over the past 10 years (Box 31.5).[165,166] Over 100,000 ICDs are implanted in the United States annually.[167]

Nevertheless, ICD therapy has associated risks including infection, inappropriate shocks, proarrhythmic potential, device malfunction, highly publicized manufacturer advisories, and procedural complications, which may adversely affect morbidity and quality of life.[166] Defibrillator implantation is not always psychologically benign. ICD specific adjustment disorders are not uncommon. Syndromes described include anxiety with secondary panic reaction; defibrillator dependence, abuse, or withdrawal; negative body image; and imaginary (phantom) shocks.[168] Recent problems with the Medtronic Sprint Fidelis and the St. Jude Riata and Riata ST transvenous high-voltage leads serve to emphasize the limitations of ICD therapy.[169,170]

Box 31.5 Implantable Cardioverter-Defibrillator (ICD) Indications

Class I

ICD therapy is indicated in patients:

Who are survivors of cardiac arrest due to ventricular fibrillation or hemodynamically unstable sustained VT after evaluation to define the cause of the event and to exclude any completely reversible causes

With structural heart disease and spontaneous sustained VT, whether hemodynamically stable or unstable

With syncope of undetermined origin with clinically relevant, hemodynamically significant sustained VT or ventricular fibrillation induced at electrophysiologic study

With LVEF less than or equal to 35% due to prior myocardial infarction who are at least 40 days past myocardial infarction and who are in NYHA functional class II or III

With nonischemic dilated cardiomyopathy who have an LVEF less than or equal to 35% and who are in NYHA functional class II or III

With LV dysfunction due to prior myocardial infarction who are at least 40 days past myocardial infarction, have an LVEF less than or equal to 30%, and are in NYHA functional class I

With nonsustained VT due to prior myocardial infarction, LVEF less than or equal to 40%, and inducible ventricular fibrillation or sustained VT at electrophysiologic study

Class IIa Indications

ICD implantation is reasonable:

For patients with unexplained syncope, significant LV dysfunction, and nonischemic dilated cardiomyopathy

LV, left ventricle; LVEF, left ventricular ejection fraction; NYHA, New York Heart Association; VT, ventricular tachycardia.

Our increasing risk stratification repertoire remains inadequate for the vast majority of SCA victims.[141] Some evidence suggests that only 35% to 51% of patients who are guideline eligible for an ICD receive one.[171,172] In contrast, a recent analysis of ICD recipients in the National Cardiovascular Data Registry—Implantable Cardiac Defibrillators Registry suggested that 22.5% did not meet evidence-based implantation criteria.[173] Patients are often referred for ICD replacement with little or no evidence of a well-informed discussion of the risks, expected benefits, and long-term goals of care.[166]

Investigators have raised important issues and asked pivotal questions such as the following: Who are we missing? Who are we overtreating? Who is best served by ICD therapy? Should all initial recipients receive replacement ICDs?[167,174]

Cardiac resynchronization therapy (CRT), or biventricular pacing, is an important therapeutic option with drug-refractory NYHA (New York Heart Association) class III or IV CHF, left ventricular ejection fraction at 35% or less, and a major left-sided conduction delay (QRS duration greater than 120 ms). Patients with RBBB and IVCD derive less benefit from CRT compared with those with a native LBBB. The underlying rhythm should be sinus or atrial fibrillation, with a slow enough ventricular response to allow continuous biventricular stimulation and capture. Biventricular pacing most frequently is used as part of an ICD system (CRT-D). Acute and chronic CHF contributes to the need for tachyarrhythmia treatment in ICD recipients. Although small trials (93 patients in total) have shown that biventricular pacing diminished ventricular arrhythmias, these results were not confirmed in larger trials.[4]

ELECTROCARDIOGRAPHIC PATTERNS INTENSIVISTS SHOULD RECOGNIZE

Intensivists encounter a variety of clinical conditions that have distinct manifestations on the surface ECG. Many of these patterns may be associated with significant brady- or tachyarrhythmias. Recognition of arrhythmic precipitants may be lifesaving in critically ill patients. In this section, we review important surface ECG patterns that are, or may be, associated with significant rhythm disturbances. Every intensivist should be able to recognize them.

ELECTROLYTE, ENDOCRINE, AND METABOLIC ABNORMALITIES

Electrolyte and metabolic abnormalities may affect cardiac depolarization or repolarization. The ECG may be the first clue that an electrolyte or metabolic abnormality is present.

Hyperkalemia is frequent in the critically ill, in particular in patients with impaired renal function. As the serum potassium increases, the ECG follows a characteristic stepwise pattern of derangement. The first sign of hyperkalemia on ECG is peaked T waves. Although there is no universal definition of "peaked," we agree with the definition of T waves greater than 10 mm in the precordium and 6 mm in the limb leads.[175] In addition to being peaked, the T waves typically appear narrow. At a potassium level of greater than 6.0 mmol/L, T-wave peaking is pronounced, the P wave will begin to lose amplitude, and the QRS complex begins to widen. At potassium levels greater than 7 mmol/L the P wave is no longer visible and QRS widening progresses. The ensuing ECG pattern is known as sinoventricular rhythm (Fig. 31.18).[176] Sine waves may become present as the widened QRS complex blends into the T wave (Fig. 31.19).[177] An abnormal ECG may be the initial sign of dangerous hyperkalemia and therapy should begin immediately to eliminate the hyperkalemia and stabilize the heart (calcium gluconate infusion).

Hypokalemia also results in characteristic ECG changes. The hallmark of hypokalemia is the U wave, an additional wave seen after the T wave (Fig. 31.20). As the hypokalemia becomes more severe, the U wave increases in amplitude, and T-wave amplitude will decrease. Eventually, the T wave and the U wave may fuse, giving the appearance of a widened T wave. This creates a prolonged QT interval, which may result in torsades de pointes. The risk of hypokalemia-induced arrhythmia is increased in patients receiving digitalis and during myocardial ischemia.[178]

Hypomagnesemia is usually associated with potassium depletion. ECG abnormalities seen are produced by hypokalemia. Hypermagnesemia is uncommon and usually associated with renal failure. Observed ECG changes result from concomitant electrolyte disturbances (hyperkalemia and hypocalcemia).[178]

The principal electrocardiographic feature of hypercalcemia is a shortening of the QT interval (Fig. 31.21).[176] This finding is not associated with arrhythmias. In contrast, patients with the rare SQTS have a QTc interval less than 360 ms (typically <300 ms) and a high risk of sudden death due to ventricular fibrillation (Fig. 31.22).[179] Patients often have permanent or paroxysmal atrial fibrillation and occasionally manifest depression of the PR interval. Tall, peaked T waves without flat ST segments and impaired rate-dependent QT shortening has been recorded.[180] SQTS appears to be inherited in an autosomal dominant pattern.

The principal finding in hypocalcemia is a prolongation of the QT interval. It should be noted that, unlike in hypokalemia, the T wave is normal sized and QT interval prolongation results from lengthening of the ST segment, not a broadening of the T wave due to fusion with a U wave. In severe hypocalcemia, PR and QRS intervals are frequently prolonged (Fig. 31.23).[176] Second-degree or third-degree AV block has been reported. J waves (see later) have occasionally been reported.[178]

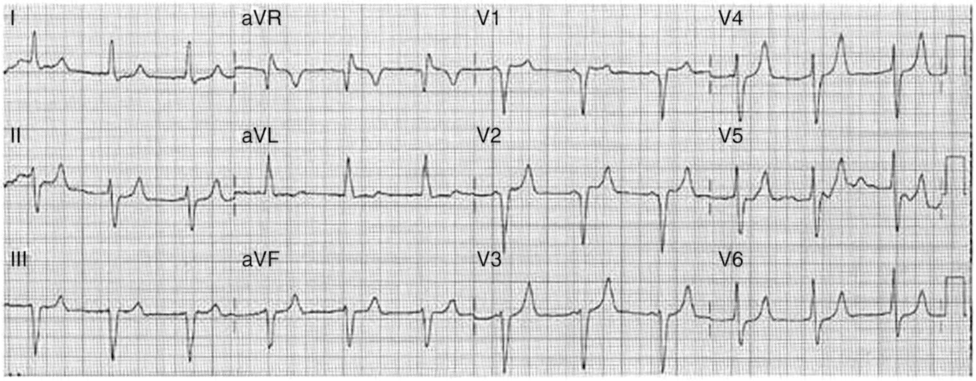

Figure 31.18 Sinoventricular rhythm. In severe hypokalemia, P waves are no longer visible. QRS widening also occurs. This rhythm is difficult to distinguish from an accelerated idioventricular rhythm. (From Baltazar RF: Basic and Bedside Electrocardiography. Philadelphia, Lippincott Williams & Wilkins, 2009.)

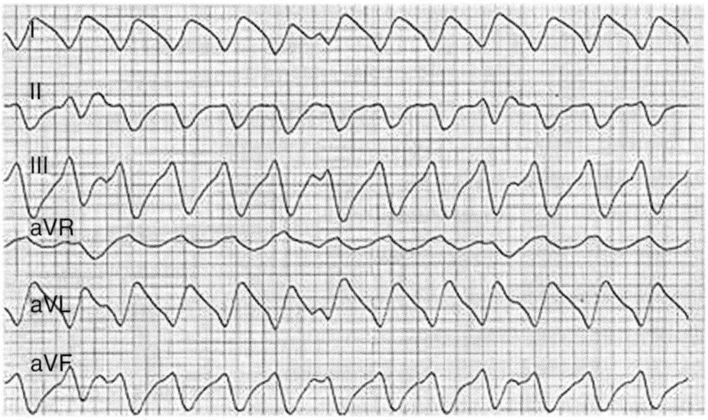

Figure 31.19 Sine waves seen in severe hyperkalemia. (From NEJM Image Challenge, http://www.nejm.org/action/showImageChallenge?ci=05032012, last accessed 6/13/12.)

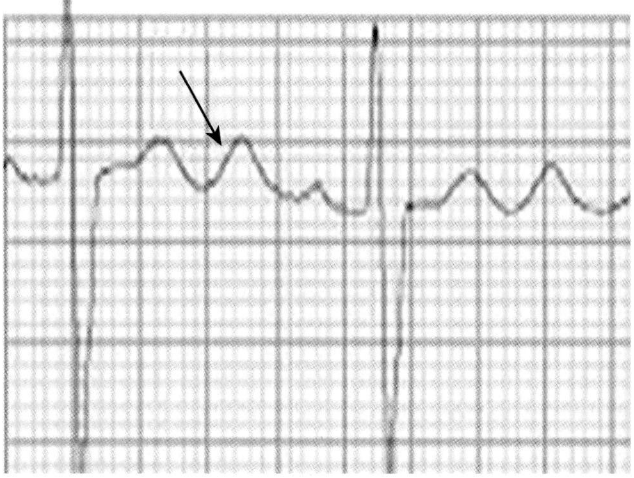

Figure 31.20 Hypokalemia. Prominent U waves are seen here (*arrow*).

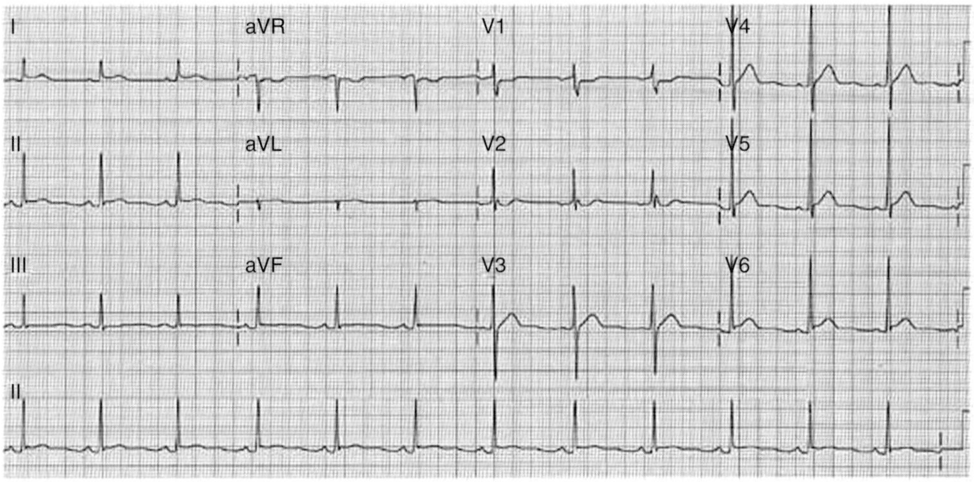

Figure 31.21 Hypercalcemia. A short QT segment is noted. This patient had a calcium level of 16 mg/dL. (From Baltazar RF: Basic and Bedside Electrocardiography. Philadelphia, Lippincott Williams & Wilkins, 2009.)

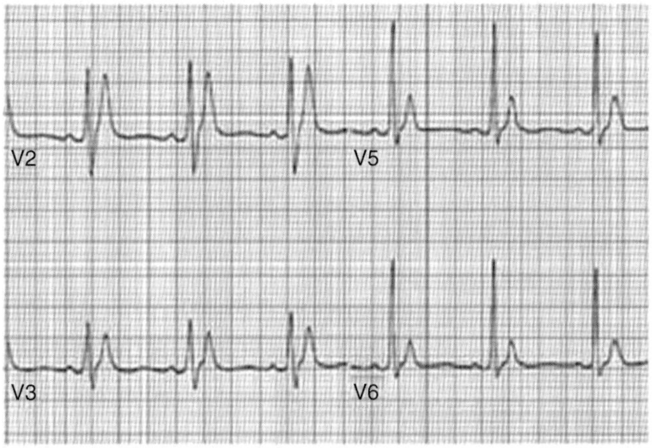

Figure 31.22 Patient with congenital short QT syndrome. (From http://www.shortqtsyndrome.org/dr_diagnosis.htm, last accessed 6/13/12.)

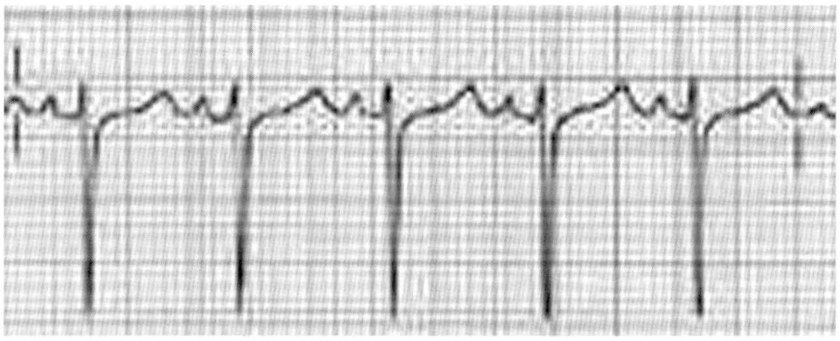

Figure 31.23 Hypocalcemia. A prolonged QT interval is the principal finding in hypocalcemia. Serum calcium is 7.2 mg/dL. (From Baltazar RF: Basic and Bedside Electrocardiography. Philadelphia, Lippincott Williams & Wilkins, 2009.)

In addition to electrolyte abnormalities, metabolic derangements can cause characteristic ECG findings. Hypothermia, both from accidental exposure as well as therapeutic cooling after cardiac arrest, has classic findings on ECG (Fig. 31.24).[181] As the core body temperature drops below 32° C, conduction becomes slower with slower sinus rates, prolonged PR and QT intervals, as well as junctional rhythms.[182] The finding of an Osborn or J wave is a hallmark of hypothermia. This wave appears as an upward deflection at the terminal portion of the R wave, before the J point. Additionally, the ECG baseline may have artifact or oscillations from shivering. Though classically associated with hypothermia, the Osborn wave may also be a sign of other conditions such as sepsis and diabetic ketoacidosis (which can be hypothermic conditions) as well as normothermic conditions such as neurologic insults and hypercalcemia.[183]

Hypothyroidism characteristically shows slowing of conduction and often has sinus bradycardia, low voltage, and prolonged PR and QT intervals as well as intraventricular conduction delays. Hyperthyroidism may cause sinus tachycardia and premature atrial complexes or may precipitate atrial fibrillation.

BRUGADA PATTERN

As mentioned earlier, the Brugada syndrome is characterized by an inherited disorder of sodium channels. Brugada pattern is characterized on the ECG by RBBB (complete or incomplete) morphology and abnormal repolarization characterized by ST-segment elevation in leads V_1 to V_3. Three distinct patterns have been identified. Type 1 features a "coved" type ST segment (more than 2 mm) elevation and a negative T wave. Type 2 features a "saddleback" ST-T configuration, recognized by two notches in the T wave. Type 3 can have a coved or saddleback morphology. This configuration is less specific for Brugada syndrome (Fig. 31.25).[184] A patient with any of the Brugada patterns and a history of cardiac arrest, syncope, or ventricular tachycardia should have an ICD implanted, as there is no effective drug therapy for this disease. It is not recommended that asymptomatic patients with the Brugada pattern on ECG receive a defibrillator, and clinical monitoring is advised instead. Should a patient suffer from electrical storm, isoproterenol is considered useful.[132]

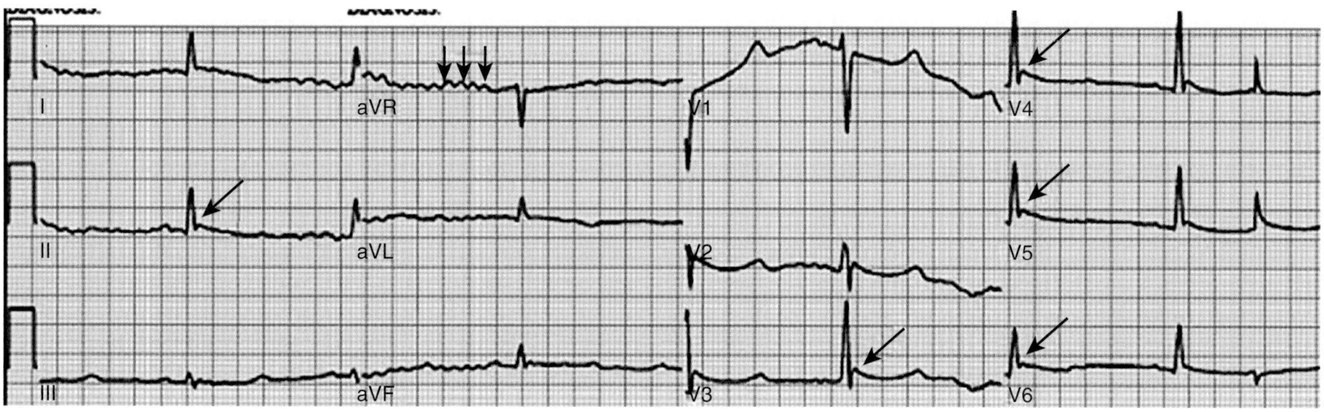

Figure 31.24 Osborn waves in hypothermia. Core body temperature of 27.1° C. Triple arrows show shivering artifact. The single arrows show Osborn waves (an upward deflection at the terminal portion of the R wave, before the J point). (From Sepehrdad R, Paulsen J, Amsterdam EA: The ECG that came in from the cold. Am J Med 2012;125(3):246-248.)

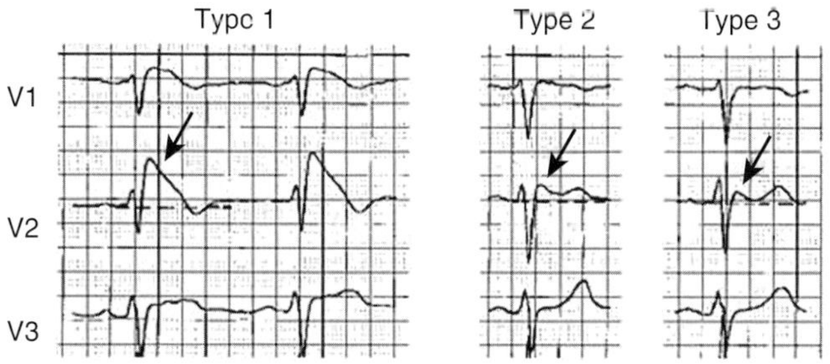

Figure 31.25 Brugada patterns type 1, 2, and 3. See text for details. (From Koonlawee Nademanee, Silvia G, Priori SG, et al: Proposed diagnostic criteria for the Brugada syndrome: Consensus report. Circulation 2002;106:2514-2519.)

LONG QT SYNDROMES

As mentioned previously, the congenital long QT syndrome is associated with SCD due to torsades de pointes. The three most common inherited forms (LQT1, LQT2, and LQT3) represent 75% of the inherited long QT syndrome. Each one of those subtypes has a specific mutation and an activity in which the arrhythmia (and hence syncope or cardiac arrest) is triggered. LQT1 is associated with events during exertion, LQT2 is associated with events occurring after hearing a sudden loud noise, and LQT3 is associated with events at rest or sleep. There are also ECG patterns associated with each of those three variants, though it should be noted that the clinical scenario will often correlate better than the ECG pattern to the specific gene mutation. The LQT1 has a broad T wave, the LQT2 has a bifid T wave, and the LQT3 has a long isoelectric segment and a narrow T wave. The LQT3 pattern appears somewhat similar to the ECG seen in hypocalcemia (Fig. 31.26).[185]

More commonly, however, intensivists will see patients with transient prolongations in their QT interval due to their illness, ingestion of medications, or antiarrhythmic drugs. These patients need to be monitored carefully for the development of torsades de pointes. In addition, an alternation in T wave amplitude can be seen. This is referred to as T wave alternans and represents a harbinger of worsening arrhythmias (Fig. 31.27). Dramatic QT

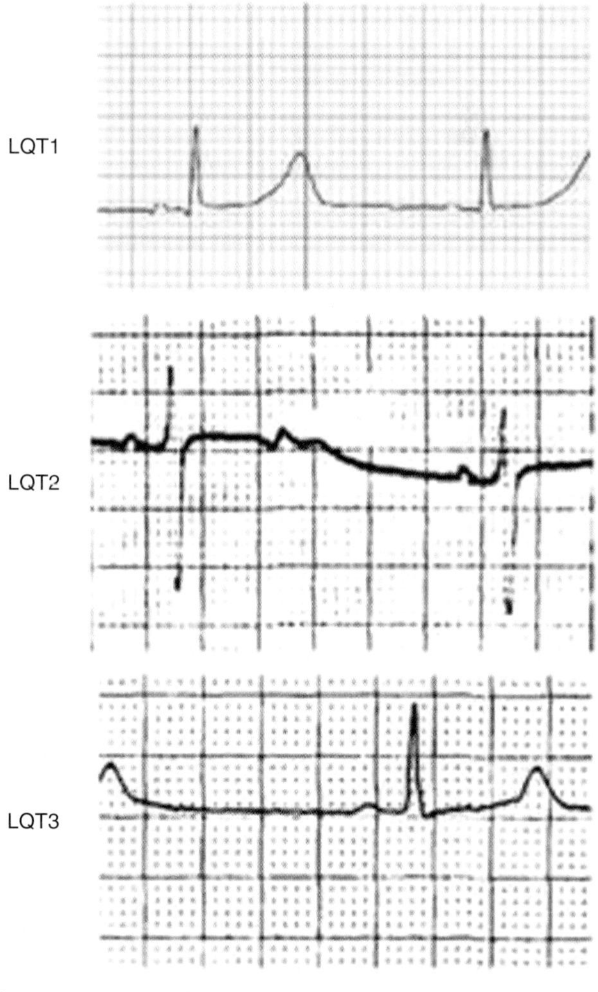

Figure 31.26 Long QT patterns based on genetic mutation. See text for details. (From Roden DM: Long-QT syndrome. N Engl J Med 2008;358:169-176.)

prolongation and T wave stroke may occur after cardiovascular accident.

TORSADES DE POINTES

The term *torsades* or *torsades de pointes* refers to a polymorphic ventricular tachycardia that appears to rotate around a horizontal axis, hence the name (from the French "twisting of the points") (Figs. 31.28 and 31.29).[34] The term torsades de pointes should be used only in the setting of the ventricular tachycardia seen with a prolonged QT interval (either acquired or congenital). It is important to differentiate this rhythm from other types of polymorphic ventricular tachycardia (as seen in ischemia) because the management is different. Urgent management of acquired long QT prolongation and torsades de pointes is typically intravenous magnesium sulfate and defibrillation for hemodynamic instability. As mentioned previously, isoproterenol and temporary pacing increase ventricular rates, shorten QT intervals, and help prevent recurrent arrhythmias until the effects of the offending agent diminish. Torsades de pointes is often initiated by a short-long-short sequence of a premature ventricular beat (short segment) followed by a compensatory pause (long segment). The long delay from the compensatory pause delays repolarization. As a result, the QT segment is prolonged after the compensatory pause, and it is more likely that the next depolarization will occur when the ventricle is vulnerable (R on T phenomenon).

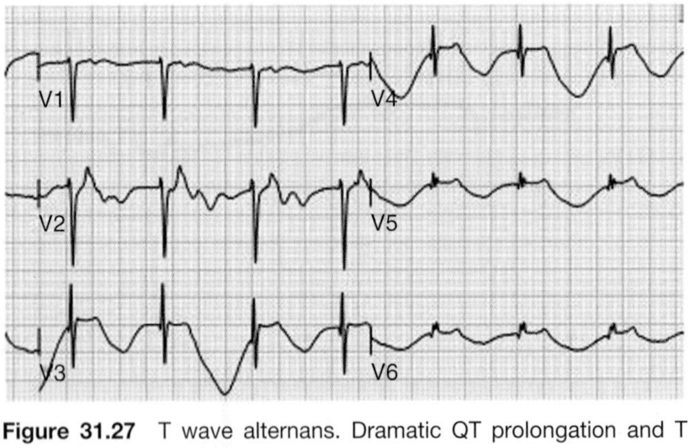

Figure 31.27 T wave alternans. Dramatic QT prolongation and T wave alternans after cardiovascular accident. T wave stroke is considered a harbinger of arrhythmias. A short run of torsades de pointes was subsequently noted.

WOLF-PARKINSON-WHITE PATTERN

As described previously, patients with Wolff-Parkinson-White syndrome can present in sinus rhythm or during an arrhythmia. There are three classic ECG patterns in this disorder depending on the patient's presenting rhythm. Patients in sinus rhythm with activation of the ventricle by both the normal AV node and His-Purkinje system as well as by the accessory pathway will have a fusion beat on their ECG. This beat manifests as a delta wave and short PR interval as part of the ventricle is activated (preexcited) by the accessory pathway (Fig. 31.30). Patients with Wolff-Parkinson-White pattern in sinus rhythm are asymptomatic and usually come to attention when presenting for other reasons, after an arrhythmia has broken, or on a routine ECG that incidentally detects the abnormality. T-wave inversion may develop after accessory pathway ablation (Fig. 31.31). This is a transient, reversible, repolariztion phenomenon and does not reflect myocardial ischemia.

Patients with an accessory pathway often present for the first time when they have palpitations. More often, the patients will present with an AVRT. In orthodromic AVRT, the conduction travels down the normal conduction system and retrograde up the accessory pathway. The QRS will be narrow (unless there is a preexisting or rate-related bundle branch block) and the delta wave will no longer be visible (the ventricle is entirely activated by the normal conduction pathway). In antidromic AVRT, the conduction will proceed antegrade down the accessory pathway and retrograde up the normal conduction system. There will be a wide complex regular tachycardia (maximal preexcitation).

Atrial fibrillation in a patient with Wolff-Parkinson-White must be recognized as it requires specific treatment, which

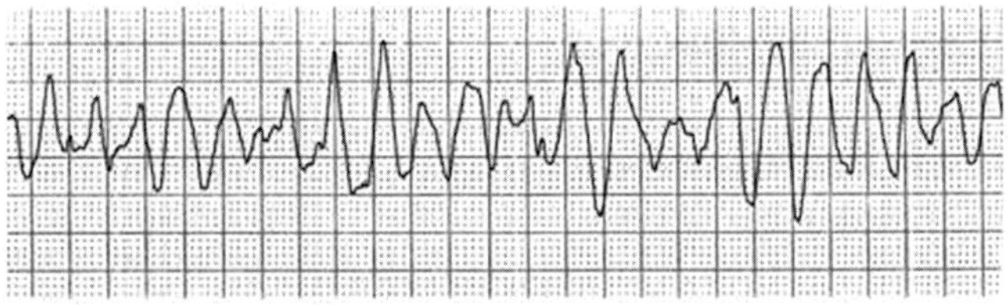

Figure 31.28 Torsades de pointes. The ventricular tachycardia on electrocardiogram appears to rotate around a horizontal axis, hence the name torsades de pointes, from the French "twisting of the points." (Adapted from Gupta A, Lawrence AT, Krishnan K, et al: Current concepts in the mechanisms and management of drug-induced QT prolongation and torsades de pointes. Am Heart J 2007; 153(6):891-899.)

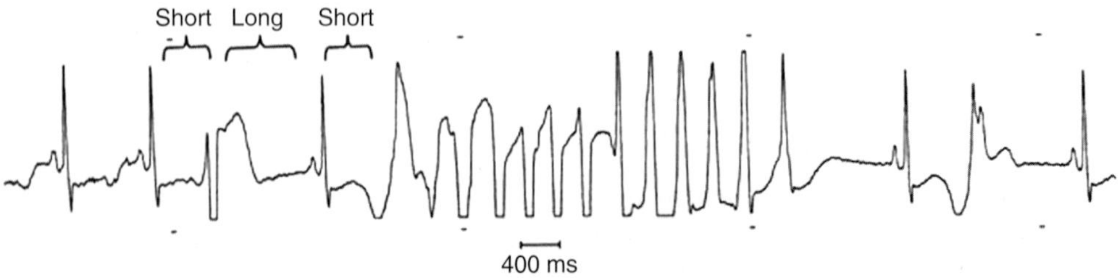

Figure 31.29 Torsades de pointes. An episode of torsades following a short-long-short sequence. (Adapted from Gupta A, Lawrence AT, Krishnan K, et al: Current concepts in the mechanisms and management of drug-induced QT prolongation and torsades de pointes. Am Heart J 2007;153(6):891-899.)

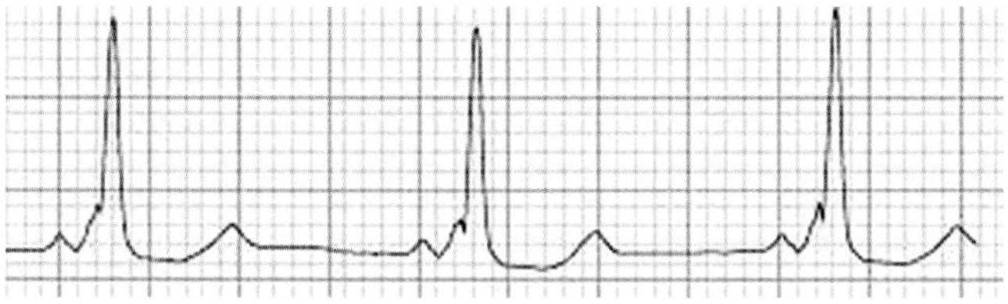

Figure 31.30 Wolff-Parkinson-White (WPW) pattern in sinus rhythm. In sinus rhythm, patients with a WPW pattern will have a delta wave, which is a fusion of normal conduction and conduction down the accessory pathway. The PR interval will be short as the accessory pathway will allow part of the ventricle to be activated earlier than the rest of the ventricle is activated by normal pathway.

is different from other forms of atrial fibrillation. The ECG shows an irregular rhythm with a delta wave. The ventricle is again being depolarized from both normal pathway as well as the accessory pathway. As mentioned earlier, AV nodal blocking agents, which are the mainstay of treatment in most cases of atrial fibrillation, may facilitate conduction down the accessory pathway. Decremental conduction (like the AV node) is rare in these accessory pathways and atrial fibrillation may be conducted very rapidly to the ventricles. There is a concern for triggering ventricular tachycardia or fibrillation, so drug therapies include ibutilide (which blocks the accessory pathway) or amiodarone (which blocks both the AV node and the accessory pathway). Additionally, both of these medications can convert atrial fibrillation back to sinus rhythm.

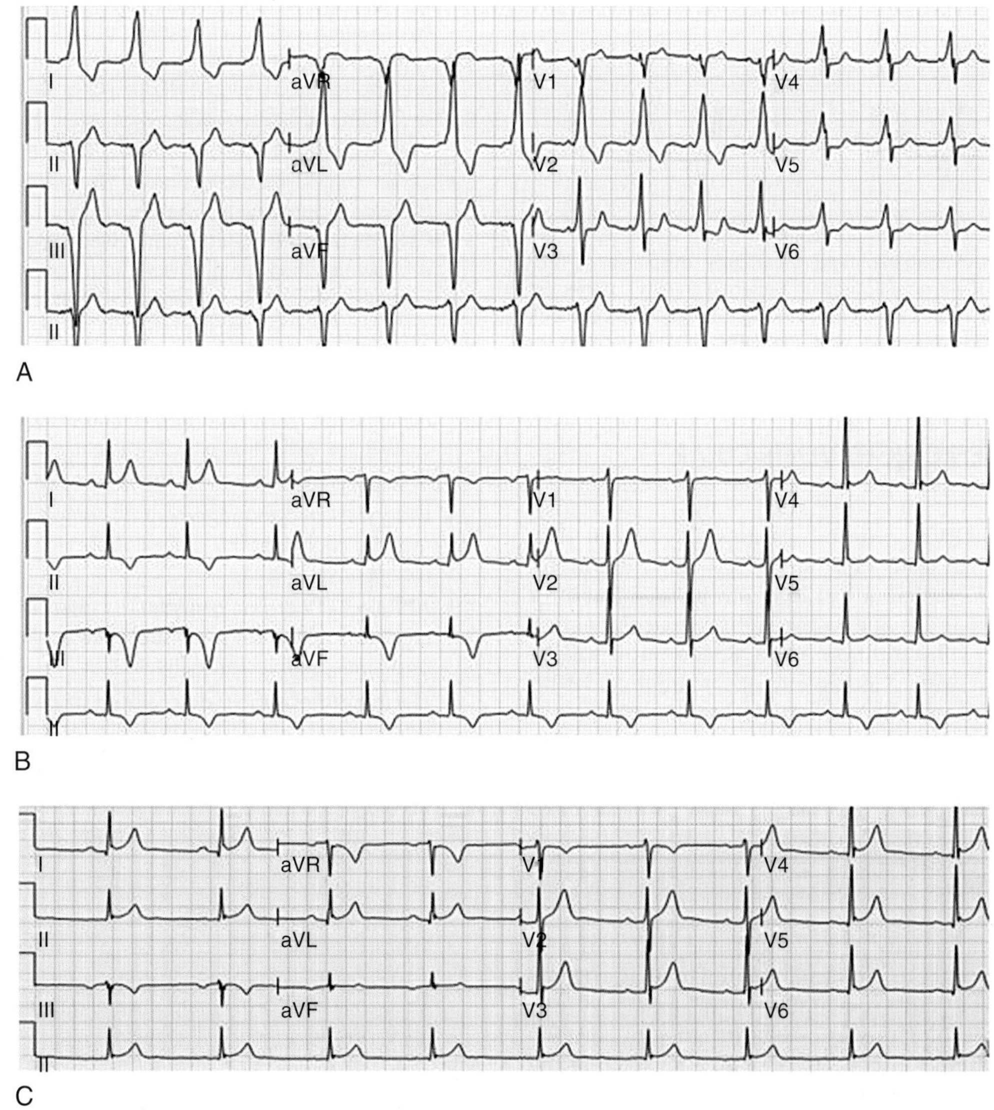

Figure 31.31 **A,** Memory T waves after ablation in Wolff-Parkinson-White (WPW) syndrome. Before procedure, note the delta wave. **B,** Memory T waves after ablation in WPW. After procedure, note the deep T-wave inversions. This is termed T-wave memory. **C,** Memory T waves after ablation in WPW syndrome. Normalization 1 week after ablation. Patients with WPW syndrome have an abnormal depolarization pattern, as evidenced by the delta wave. They also have repolarization abnormalities. Some of those repolarization abnormalities may become manifest after ablation of the accessory pathway. Here a patient with WPW syndrome had deep inverted T waves in the inferior leads after ablation of his accessory pathway. This pattern resolved 1 week later.

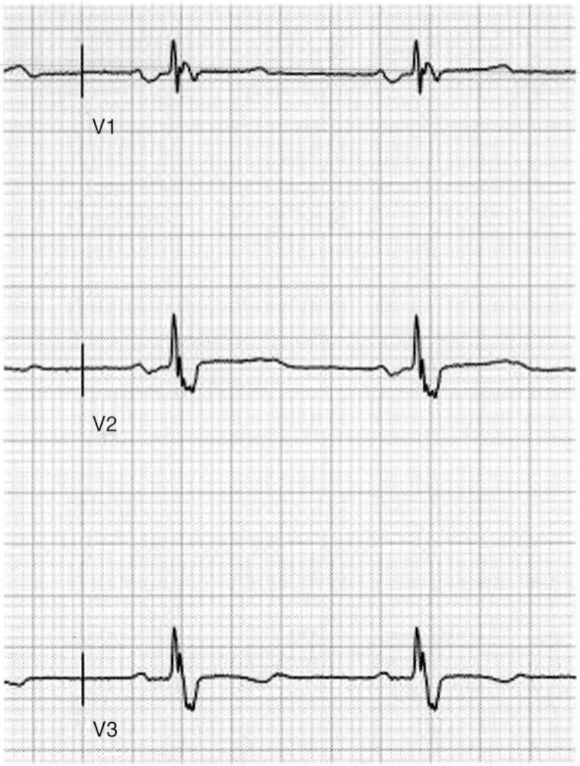

Figure 31.32 Arrhythmogenic right ventricular dysplasia (ARVD) with epsilon wave. Electrocardiogram in patient with ARVD. Note the T-wave inversion in V_3 and the incomplete right bundle branch block pattern. The upward deflection after the QRS in V_1 is termed an epsilon wave and is classic for ARVD.

ARRHYTHMOGENIC RIGHT VENTRICULAR DYSPLASIA

In patients with ARVD, inverted T waves may be noted in the right precordial leads (V_1, V_2, and V_3). In addition, an upward deflection, called an epsilon, may be seen just after the QRS complex and is due to late right ventricular activation (Fig 31.32).[186] In addition, the QRS duration will be prolonged, often with a complete or incomplete RBBB pattern. The ECG may be the initial clue to this disease. Ventricular tachycardia with a LBBB-like morphology (right ventricular origin) is often precipitated by catecholamines (e.g., exercise).

CONCLUSIONS

The intensivist must have a keen awareness of patterns, mechanisms, precipitants, and treatment of cardiac arrhythmias. The intensivist must remember that *all* antiarrhythmic therapies (pharmacologic and nonpharmacologic) have the potential for adverse effects. Reducing and eliminating arrhythmia precipitants may be safer and more effective than dramatic interventions. Antiarrhythmic drugs should be chosen carefully and the patient monitored closely. Direct current cardioversion should be used aggressively when the situation is emergent, cautiously when elective, and eschewed when futile. Ablation is effective therapy for most supraventricular tachycardias, idiopathic ventricular tachycardia, and bundle branch reentry and may be used as adjuvant therapy for patients with frequent appropriate ICD shocks. ICDs are the therapy of choice for primary and secondary prevention of SCD in patients with structural heart disease. Consultation with a cardiac electrophysiologist should be considered a routine part of the critical care physician's armamentarium.

KEY POINTS

- Intensivists managing arrhythmias must have expertise in electrocardiography, pharmacokinetics, pharmacodynamics, and bedside clinical acumen.
- All antiarrhythmic therapies (pharmacologic and nonpharmacologic) have the potential for adverse effects.
- Patients in an intensive care setting frequently have active arrhythmia precipitants. They include hypoxemia, excess circulating catecholamines, CHF, fever (sepsis), pulmonary emboli, electrolyte, and other metabolic disturbances. Reducing or eliminating arrhythmia precipitants may be safer and more effective than dramatic antiarrhythmic interventions.
- Direct current cardioversion of tachyarrhythmias should be used aggressively when emergent (angina pectoris, CHF, hypotension), cautiously when elective, and eschewed when futile. The critical care physician must carefully weigh the risks and benefits of direct current cardioversion for each patient.
- Left ventricular dysfunction is the most important predictor of cardiac death in patients with ventricular arrhythmias. Long-term management of sustained ventricular arrhythmias in the setting of structural heart disease is usually best accomplished with an ICD.
- Diagnosis and management of complex arrhythmias may be facilitated by consultation with a cardiac electrophysiologist.
- Ablation of cardiac arrhythmias often is first-line elective therapy for most supraventricular tachycardias and some ventricular tachycardias.
- Electrocardiographic data stored in permanent pacemakers and ICDs can easily be assessed to help the intensivist determine the patient's recent history and the frequency, rate, and duration of arrhythmias.
- Antiarrhythmic drugs can raise pacing and defibrillator thresholds and change supraventricular tachycardia and supraventricular tachycardia rates, necessitating device reprogramming.
- Intensivists encounter a variety of clinical conditions, which have distinct manifestations on the surface ECG. Recognition of arrhythmic precipitants may be lifesaving in critically ill patients.

SELECTED READINGS

6. Trohman RG: Supraventricular tachycardia: Implications for the intensivist. Crit Care Med 2000;28:N129-N135.
15. Blomstrom-Lundqvist C, Scheinman MM, Aliot EM, et al: ACC/AHA/ESC guidelines for the management of patients with supraventricular arrhythmias—executive summary. A report of the

American College of Cardiology/American Heart Association Task Force on Practice Guidelines and the European Society of Cardiology Committee for Practice Guidelines (writing committee to develop guidelines for the management of patients with supraventricular arrhythmias) developed in collaboration with NASPE-Heart Rhythm Society. J Am Coll Cardiol 2003;42: 1493-1531.

34. Gupta A, Lawrence AT, Krishnan K, et al: Current concepts in the mechanisms and management of drug-induced QT prolongation and torsades de pointes. Am Heart J 2007;153:891-899.
47. Fuster V, Ryden LE, Cannom DS, et al: ACC/AHA/ESC 2006 guidelines for the management of patients with atrial fibrillation: Full text: A report of the American College of Cardiology/American Heart Association Task Force on Practice Guidelines and the European Society of Cardiology Committee for Practice Guidelines (writing committee to revise the 2001 guidelines for the management of patients with atrial fibrillation) developed in collaboration with the European Heart Rhythm Association and the Heart Rhythm Society. Europace 2006;8:651-745.
50. Wann LS, Curtis AB, January CT, et al, writing on behalf of the 2006 ACC/AHA/ESC Guidelines for the Management of Patients With Atrial Fibrillation Writing Committee: 2011 ACCF/AHA/HRS focused update on the management of patients with atrial fibrillation (updating the 2006 guideline): A report of the American College of Cardiology Foundation/American Heart Association Task Force on Practice Guidelines. J Am Coll Cardiol 2011;57:223-242.
52. Connolly SJ, Ezekowitz MD, Yusuf S, et al: Dabigatran versus warfarin in patients with atrial fibrillation. N Engl J Med 2009;361: 1139-1151.
54. Patel MR, Mahaffey KW, Garg J, et al: Rivaroxaban versus warfarin in nonvalvular atrial fibrillation. N Engl J Med 2011;365: 883-891.
56. Granger CB, Alexander JH, McMurray JJV, et al: Apixaban versus warfarin in patients with atrial fibrillation. N Engl J Med 2011;365:981-992.
64. Ewy GA: The optimal technique for electrical cardioversion of atrial fibrillation. Clin Cardiol 1994;17:79-84.
72. Wann LS, Curtis AB, January CT, et al; 2006 Writing Committee Members, Fuster V, Rydén LE, Cannom DS, et al; ACCF/AHA Task Force Members, Jacobs AK, Anderson JL, Albert N, et al: 2011 ACCF/AHA/HRS focused update on the management of patients with atrial fibrillation (updating the 2006 guideline): A report of the American College of Cardiology Foundation/American Heart Association Task Force on Practice Guidelines. Heart Rhythm 2011;8(1):157-176.
78. Calkins H, Kuck KH, Cappato R, et al, Heart Rhythm Society Task Force on Catheter and Surgical Ablation of Atrial Fibrillation: 2012 HRS/EHRA/ECAS expert consensus statement on catheter and surgical ablation of atrial fibrillation: Recommendations for patient selection, procedural techniques, patient management and follow-up, definitions, end points, and research trial design: A report of the Heart Rhythm Society (HRS) Task Force on Catheter and Surgical Ablation of Atrial Fibrillation. Developed in partnership with the European Heart Rhythm Association (EHRA), a registered branch of the European Society of Cardiology (ESC) and the European Cardiac Arrhythmia Society (ECAS); and in collaboration with the American College of Cardiology (ACC), American Heart Association (AHA), the Asia Pacific Heart Rhythm Society (APHRS), and the Society of Thoracic Surgeons (STS). Endorsed by the governing bodies of the American College of Cardiology Foundation, the American Heart Association, the European Cardiac Arrhythmia Society, the European Heart Rhythm Association, the Society of Thoracic Surgeons, the Asia Pacific Heart Rhythm Society, and the Heart Rhythm Society. Heart Rhythm 2012;9(4):632-696.
128. Spies C, Trohman RG: Narrative review: Electrocution and life-threatening electrical injuries. Ann Intern Med 2006;145: 531-537.
132. European Heart Rhythm Association, Heart Rhythm Society, Zipes DP, Camm AJ, Borggrefe M, et al: American College of Cardiology; American Heart Association Task Force; European Society of Cardiology Committee for Practice Guidelines. ACC/AHA/ESC 2006 guidelines for management of patients with ventricular arrhythmias and the prevention of sudden cardiac death: A report of the American College of Cardiology/American Heart Association Task Force and the European Society of Cardiology Committee for Practice Guidelines (writing committee to develop guidelines for management of patients with ventricular arrhythmias and the prevention of sudden cardiac death). J Am Coll Cardiol 2006;48(5):e247-346.
141. Goldberger JJ, Cain ME, Hohnloser SH, et al: American Heart Association/American College of Cardiology Foundation/Heart Rhythm Society Scientific Statement on Noninvasive Risk Stratification Techniques for Identifying Patients at Risk for Sudden Cardiac Death. A scientific statement from the American Heart Association Council on Clinical Cardiology Committee on Electrocardiography and Arrhythmias and Council on Epidemiology and Prevention. J Am Coll Cardiol 2008;52:1179-1199.
158. Nolan JP, Neumar RW, Adrie C, et al: Post-cardiac arrest syndrome: Epidemiology, pathophysiology, treatment, and prognostication: A Scientific Statement from the International Liaison Committee on Resuscitation; the American Heart Association Emergency Cardiovascular Care Committee; the Council on Cardiovascular Surgery and Anesthesia; the Council on Cardiopulmonary, Perioperative, and Critical Care; the Council on Clinical Cardiology; the Council on Stroke. Resuscitation 2008;79: 350-379.

The complete list of references can be found at www.expertconsult.com.

32 Valvular Heart Disease in Critical Care

Zoltan G. Turi

CHAPTER OUTLINE

The profile of valvular heart disease in the critical care setting has evolved substantially over the past several decades. Aortic stenosis, mitral insufficiency, and aortic insufficiency are the most common valve diseases seen in the intensive care unit, but hypertrophic obstructive cardiomyopathy and mitral stenosis remain important entities as well. Patients with valvular heart disease in critical care units typically fall into one of two categories: (1) those who are critically ill because of valvular dysfunction or (2) those in whom valvular disease represents an important comorbid condition. Many patients present without prior diagnosis of heart valve disease, either because the progression has been insidious and the disease not previously diagnosed or because the onset has been acute. Improvements in technology and the ubiquitous availability of echocardiography have improved diagnosis, while clinician skills at integrating physical examination and other data have generally atrophied during this same time frame.

Rheumatic heart disease accounted for 50% or more of admissions for heart disease in the first half of the twentieth century, with congenital heart disease representing the other major indication for valve surgery through the 1960s.[1] With evolving technology and an increase in average life expectancy, heart valve surgery has shifted to valve repair, as well as replacement for a variety of acquired valvulopathies. The therapeutic armamentarium, once limited to minimal supportive medical therapy, then solely to valve replacement, has expanded to a variety of surgical repair techniques; a multitude of tissue and mechanical valve options for replacement; and, most recently, an expanding set of percutaneous interventions including percutaneous valve implantation and repair. In addition, various mechanical devices for temporary hemodynamic support are important adjuncts to the management of patients with valvular heart disease in the critical care setting.

Diagnosis of valvular heart disease in critical care units is challenging, with lack of a quiet environment for auscultation; comorbid conditions that affect physical findings; and stress, infection, or metabolic abnormalities that result in tachycardia and shorter intervals for evaluation of heart sounds. Patients in a low output state have softer heart sounds and murmurs as well. In addition, clinical reliance on physical examination has fallen, as has the ability to make accurate diagnosis of valve disease.[2] A delay in recognizing the presence of significant valve dysfunction continues to occur frequently, and some patients who have had prior routine medical outpatient care nevertheless present with undiagnosed valvular heart disease.[3] The currently accepted thresholds for mild, moderate, and severe valvular heart disease are shown in Table 32.1.

Table 32.1 Classification of Severity of Valvular Heart Disease Based on ACC/AHA Guidelines

A. Left-sided Valve Disease

Indicator	Mild	Moderate	Severe
Aortic Stenosis			
Jet velocity (m/sec)	<3.0	3-4	>4
Mean gradient (mm Hg)*	<25	25-40	>40
Valve area (cm²)	>1.5	1-1.5	<1
Valve area index (cm²/m²)			<0.6
Mitral Stenosis			
Mean gradient (mm Hg)*	<5	5-10	>10
Pulmonary artery systolic pressure (mm Hg)	<30	30-50	>50
Valve area (cm²)	>1.5	1-1.5	<1.0
Aortic Regurgitation			
Qualitative			
Angiographic grade	1+	2+	3-4+
Color Doppler jet width	Central jet, width <25% of LVOT	Greater than mild but no signs of severe AR	Central jet, width >65% LVOT
Doppler vena contracta width (cm)	<0.3	0.3-0.6	>0.6
Quantitative (cath or echo)			
Regurgitant volume (mL/beat)	<30	30-59	>60
Regurgitant fraction (%)	<30	30-49	>50
Regurgitant orifice area (cm²)	<0.1	0.1-0.29	>0.30
Additional essential criteria			
Left ventricular size		Increased	
Mitral Regurgitation			
Qualitative			
Angiographic grade	1+	2+	3-4+
Color Doppler jet area	Small, central jet (<4 cm² or <20% LA area)	Signs of MR greater than mild present, but no criteria for severe MR	Vena contracta width >0.7 cm with large central MR jet (area >40% of LA area) or with a wall-impinging jet of any size, swirling in LA
Doppler vena contracta width (cm)	<0.3	0.3-0.69	≥0.7
Quantitative (cath or echo)			
Regurgitant volume (mL/beat)	<30	30-59	≥60
Regurgitant fraction (%)	<30	30-59	≥50
Regurgitant orifice area (cm²)	<0.2	0.2-0.39	≥0.4
Additional essential criteria			
Left atrial size			Enlarged
Left ventricular size			Enlarged

B. Right-sided Valve Disease

Clinical Entity	Characteristic
Severe tricuspid stenosis	Valve area <1 cm²
Severe tricuspid regurgitation	Vena contracta width >0.7 cm and systolic flow reversal in hepatic veins
Severe pulmonary stenosis	Jet velocity >4 m/sec OR maximum gradient >60 mm Hg
Severe pulmonary regurgitation	Color jet fills outflow tract; dense continuous-wave Doppler signal with a steep deceleration slope

*Valve gradients are flow-dependent and when used as estimates of severity of valve stenosis should be assessed with knowledge of cardiac output or forward flow across the valve.

ACC/AHA, American College of Cardiology/American Heart Association; AR, aortic regurgitation; cath, catheterization; echo, echocardiography; LA, left atrial/atrium; LVOT, left ventricular outflow tract; MR, mitral regurgitation.

Modified from Bonow RO, Carabello BA, Chatterjee K, et al: ACC/AHA 2006 guidelines for the management of patients with valvular heart disease: A report of the American College of Cardiology/American Heart Association Task Force on Practice Guidelines (writing committee to revise the 1998 guidelines for the management of patients with valvular heart disease) developed in collaboration with the Society of Cardiovascular Anesthesiologists and endorsed by the Society for Cardiovascular Angiography and Interventions and the Society of Thoracic Surgeons. J Am Coll Cardiol 2006;48:e1-148.

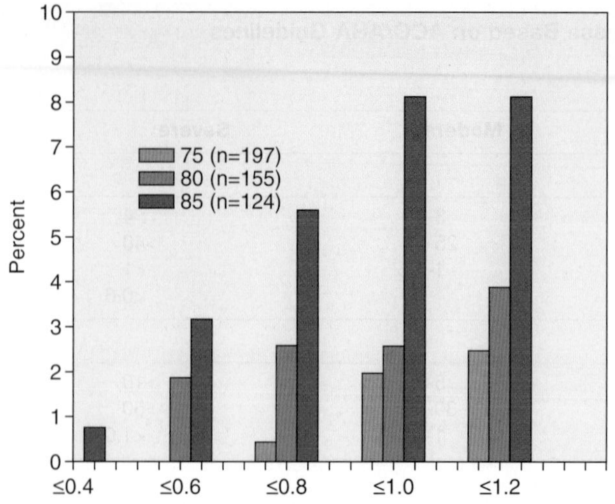

Figure 32.1 Doppler-derived estimates of aortic valve area at ages 75, 80, and 85 years from a randomized sampling of individuals in the general population. Bars represent percentages of individuals with valve areas at or below the thresholds on the abscissa (in cm^2). (Data from Lindroos M, Kupari M, Heikkila J, et al: Prevalence of aortic valve abnormalities in the elderly: An echocardiographic study of a random population sample. J Am Coll Cardiol 1993;21:1220-1225.)

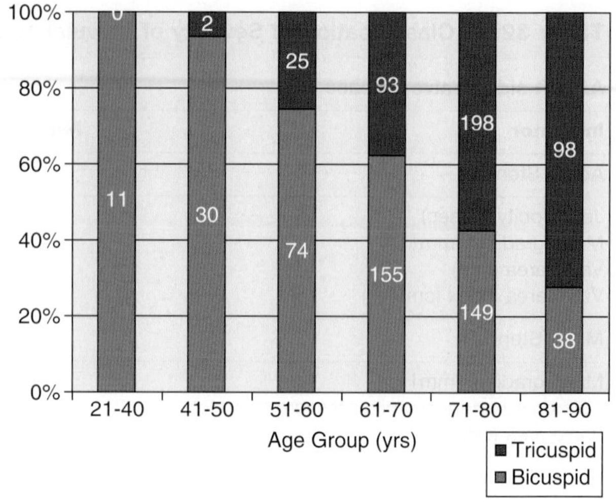

Figure 32.2 Distribution by age group of bicuspid versus tricuspid aortic valves in patients undergoing aortic valve replacement for aortic stenosis. (Modified from Roberts WC, Ko JM: Frequency by decades of unicuspid, bicuspid, and tricuspid aortic valves in adults having isolated aortic valve replacement for aortic stenosis, with or without associated aortic regurgitation. Circulation 2005;111:920-925.)

AORTIC STENOSIS

With the aging of the population, aortic stenosis (AS) has moved to the forefront in frequency of valvular heart disease encountered in older populations. The prevalence is surprisingly high; in patients 85 years of age, more than 8% of a random general population survey had Doppler-derived aortic valve area estimates of 1 cm^2 or less (Fig. 32.1),[4] which is consistent with severe AS by the 2006 American College of Cardiology/American Heart Association (ACC/AHA) guidelines.[5] Thus AS should be considered in the differential diagnosis of each elderly critical care patient with hemodynamic instability. The possibility of AS should be dismissed only after considering physical examination and electrocardiographic and, when applicable, echocardiographic and invasive findings, all of which have potential limitations in achieving accurate diagnosis as discussed subsequently.[6]

PATHOPHYSIOLOGY

AS represents a continuum, from hemodynamically insignificant congenital and atherosclerotic disease to end-stage decompensation secondary to severe valvular obstruction. The congenital pathway is typically secondary to a bicuspid aortic valve, the most common congenital cardiac anomaly if mitral valve prolapse is excluded, occurring in approximately 1.5% of the population[7] and originally described by Da Vinci in 1513.[8] The most common acquired anomaly is typically referred to as *degenerative disease,* an atherosclerotic process that represents a continuum from aortic valve sclerosis, which is not associated with a significant gradient, to a densely calcified aortic valve with severe outflow obstruction. Although the cause of aortic valve stenosis in patients undergoing aortic valve replacement (AVR) has shifted to calcific tricuspid aortic valve disease from bicuspid and rheumatic disease, this remains an age-related phenomenon, with a predominance of bicuspid aortic valve disease in patients younger than age 70 (Fig. 32.2).[9]

AORTIC VALVE SCLEROSIS

Aortic valve *sclerosis* is an important disease entity, although usually not because of hemodynamic considerations. Defined as calcification and thickening of the aortic valve without significant outflow obstruction (gradient <20 to 25 mm Hg), it is present in nearly 30% of the population older than age 65 and nearly 50% by age 85[10] and is associated with a 50% increase in 5-year cardiovascular mortality rate.[11] Its incidence is as high as 15-fold greater than aortic valve stenosis; the two diagnoses can be differentiated from one another by hemodynamics and physical examination findings discussed subsequently. In keeping with the primary atherosclerotic nature of aortic sclerosis, it is associated with increasing age, male gender, hypertension, smoking, elevated low-density lipoprotein and lipoprotein(a) levels, and diabetes.[10] The primary importance of aortic valve sclerosis is that it provides a window on the overall presence of vascular disease, in particular coronary artery disease.[12] Thus there should be a high index of suspicion of vascular disease in any patient with aortic valve sclerosis managed in the critical care setting.

Patients with aortic sclerosis do progress to aortic valve stenosis; a study of more than 2000 patients with valve thickening showed progression to severe AS in 2.5% over an average time interval of 7 years.[13] The fact that so-called degenerative disease of the aortic valve is absent in nearly half of octogenarians is also important to consider because it implies that it is not only aging but other factors that result in leaflet thickening, calcification, and stenosis. In the Helsinki Aging Study from which data are reflected in Figure 32.1, additional analysis demonstrated that not only age but also hypertension and low body mass index independently predicted calcification of the aortic valve, and age and serum ionized calcium were independently associated with valvular stenosis.[14] In general the process of sclerosis and then stenosis of the aortic valve appears, like atherosclerosis in general, to be an active inflammatory process, with deposition of lipoproteins, local inflammation with T lymphocyte and macrophage infiltration, fibroblast proliferation, and eventually osteoblast and bone formation.[15] Similar to other vascular disease, endothelial disruption likely leads to the initial lipid deposition in the leaflet tissues. The areas of early focal plaque formation appear at the loci of greatest stress: on the aortic side of the leaflets at the flexion points. Because bicuspid valves have greater mechanical stress, the average age at presentation of patients with bicuspid aortic valve stenosis is significantly lower than in the tricuspid aortic valve stenosis that is typically seen in an elderly population.[16]

An important element in understanding calcific AS is lack of commissural fusion; unlike rheumatic mitral valve stenosis, in which fusion of the commissures is the primary cause of obstructive disease, lack of mobility of the aortic valve leaflets is the primary cause of obstruction in AS. Rheumatic AS is associated with commissural fusion but is now a rare finding, even in countries where rheumatic heart disease is prevalent, and is usually associated with mitral valve involvement and typically aortic insufficiency as well. More obscure causes, such as unicuspid and quadricuspid aortic valve disease, are uncommon, although presentation can be delayed to adulthood. In the case of unicuspid aortic valves there is a strong association with AS,[17] whereas with quadricuspid aortic valves there is a high incidence of significant aortic insufficiency.[18]

Normal aortic valve area ranges from 3 to 4 cm^2. Significant resistance to outflow does not occur until the valve orifice is reduced more than 50%. Based on the simple hydraulic principle of Poiseuille's law, a 50% reduction in valve diameter results in approximately a 16-fold increase in resistance. In practice, as the resistance to outflow rises, the left ventricle is subject to pressure overload, resulting in compensatory hypertrophy. This in turn normalizes wall stress because the latter is proportional to chamber diameter times pressure divided by wall thickness (the LaPlace principle). The degree of wall thickness is variable: In patients with inadequate hypertrophic response, wall stress is inordinately high and there is early dilation and dysfunction.[19] In patients with a profound hypertrophic response disproportionate to valvular resistance, wall stress actually falls below normal and ejection fraction (EF) becomes supranormal,[20] a phenomenon that appears to be more common in women with AS. The EF for any degree of wall stress is predictable,[19] and patients who have disproportionately poor ejection phase indices (afterload mismatch) typically manifest left ventricular (LV) dysfunction beyond the depression that would be associated with high wall stress (Fig. 32.3),[21] a phenomenon described under low-gradient, low-output AS that follows.

LV hypertrophy, although it reduces wall stress, has several features that may be deleterious. With progressive hypertrophy, diastolic pressures may rise as LV compliance decreases, resulting in increased LV filling pressures. In addition, the myocardial supply-demand relationship is deleteriously affected by hypertrophy in this setting. With increased wall stress and increased wall mass, myocardial oxygen demand

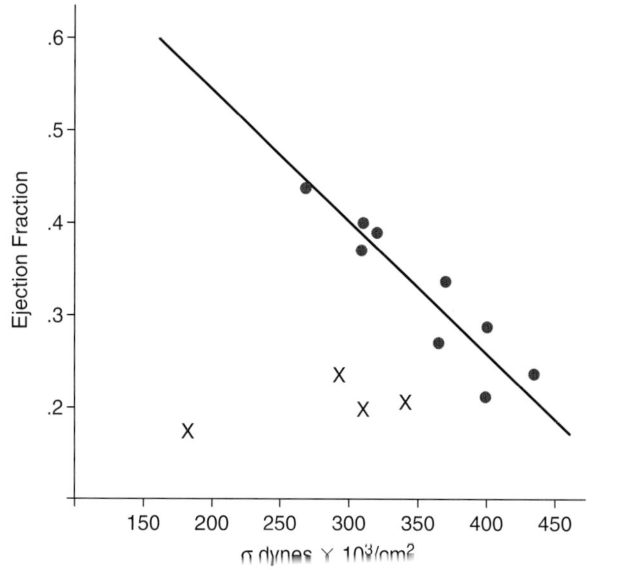

Figure 32.3 The relationship between ejection fraction and wall stress in patients with aortic stenosis. The patients (each represented by an "X") whose ejection fraction was disproportionately lower than the regression line had a poor overall outcome. In these patients ejection phase indices were depressed despite a low transvalvular gradient, a phenomenon suggesting intrinsic contractile dysfunction. (From Carabello BA, Green LH, Grossman W, et al: Hemodynamic determinants of prognosis of aortic valve replacement in critical aortic stenosis and advanced congestive heart failure. Circulation 1980;62:42-48.)

is increased; at the same time coronary flow reserve is decreased in AS,[22] and in later stages of the disease diastolic perfusion pressure is lowered. Because of abnormal flow reserve, conventional testing for ischemia in the setting of significant aortic valve stenosis has inadequate specificity to identify the presence or absence of hemodynamically significant concomitant coronary artery disease.[23]

Other features associated with AS that are important in the critical care setting include abnormal platelet function and decreased levels of von Willebrand factor,[24] with associated bleeding risk that improves with AVR. Another associated cause of bleeding is gastrointestinal angiodysplasia associated with aortic valve stenosis,[25] possibly exacerbated by the concomitant presence of von Willebrand syndrome.

The progression of AS is highly variable, but with the onset of moderately severe disease, the estimated mean decrease in valve area is on the order of 0.1 cm^2/year.[26] Certain demographics and noninvasive findings appear to predict the rate of progression, including age older than 50 years and moderate to severe valve calcification.[27] The issue of progression is particularly important in patients who are asymptomatic of the disease because AVR before it is necessary is undesirable but must be weighed against the risk of sudden death. The latter has been studied in a number of longitudinal studies and is rare if patients are followed prospectively. The patients who are most likely to require early intervention are those with peak Doppler systolic velocities greater than 4 m/second or who have a rapid increase in serial transvalvular Doppler velocity measurements.[26,27] This threshold has been confirmed by other series.[28] Once patients become symptomatic, with a classic triad of heart failure, angina, or syncope, hemodynamic deterioration can be rapid with significant associated mortality risk.[29]

DIAGNOSIS

PHYSICAL EXAMINATION

The hallmarks of the physical examination relate to the contour of the aortic pressure upstroke, with a low volume and delayed carotid upstroke (pulsus parvus et tardus), a late peaking systolic ejection murmur, and a diminished or absent aortic second sound. Figure 32.4 demonstrates the hemodynamics that manifest in an abnormal carotid pulse contour; unlike the brisk upstroke of LV pressure over time (dP/dt), the aortic pressure is slow to rise and of significantly lower volume. An ejection click may be present in young patients with congenital AS, but with increasing calcification of the valve, mobility decreases to a point at which an ejection click becomes unlikely. The aortic component of the second heart sound, reflecting deceleration and closure of the aortic valve, is diminished or absent in severe AS when the thickened aortic valve leaflets are poorly mobile, have little deceleration, and drift rather than snap shut. The murmur of AS is characteristically a crescendo-decrescendo murmur that is late peaking, consistent with the timing of the peak gradient as seen in Figure 32.4, and is typically best heard over the right upper sternum and clavicle. It reflects the high-velocity systolic jet directed into the ascending aorta. A second component, described by Gallavardin as a musical component, is best heard at the left lower sternal border. The latter confounds diagnosis because the murmur is suggestive of mitral regurgitation (MR), but in its true form it is purely secondary to aortic valve stenosis. Because handgrip raises resistance to LV ejection, the murmur should decrease if it is a true Gallavardin phenomenon, whereas when it is secondary to MR, it should increase.[30]

Unfortunately, none of these findings has sufficiently high sensitivity or specificity for AS or for differentiating moderate from severe disease.[3] Many patients with AS, particularly the elderly with stiff noncompliant vessels, will have a wide pulse pressure even with declining cardiac output and may have systolic hypertension. Hypotension may not be seen until late stages of the disease. The loudness of the murmur, which correlates to some degree with severity, is also not specific because body habitus and a variety of other factors affect the acoustics transmitted across the chest. Most importantly, in severe AS, as the cardiac output drops, the gradient generated decreases as well. In this setting the murmur may be quite soft, although sometimes still high pitched because of the high velocity across a tight constriction. A useful means of differentiating aortic sclerosis from stenosis is that in the former the systolic ejection murmur heard over the right sternum is typically midpeaking and mild to moderate in intensity, and it features a well-preserved aortic second heart sound. Although the physical findings described are variable, presence of the aortic second heart sound tends to exclude severe calcific AS.[31]

NONINVASIVE EVALUATION

In contrast to the physical examination, echocardiographic techniques have progressively improved over the past several decades and availability in the critical care setting in industrialized nations is ubiquitous. The characteristic echocardiographic features of AS are decreased valve leaflet mobility, calcification in all except congenital AS in adolescents and young adults, and an augmented Doppler velocity that generally allows accurate estimation of the gradient. In congenital bicuspid AS in young adults, when commissural fusion is dominant, a characteristic doming pattern is seen, but this disappears with progressive valve calcification. The severity of calcification correlates with extent of obstruction by middle age, and typically Doppler signal velocity with peak and mean pressure gradient and valve area by continuity equation provide an accurate overall assessment. However, the gradient is highly dependent on flow across the valve, and in low-output states the gradient may result in underestimation of severity of disease; in high-output states such as in patients with augmented cardiac output caused by inotropic stimulation, endogenous high catecholamine states, and sepsis, the gradient may be disproportionately higher than the severity of stenosis would suggest. The latest ACC/AHA guidelines describe the threshold for severe AS as antegrade

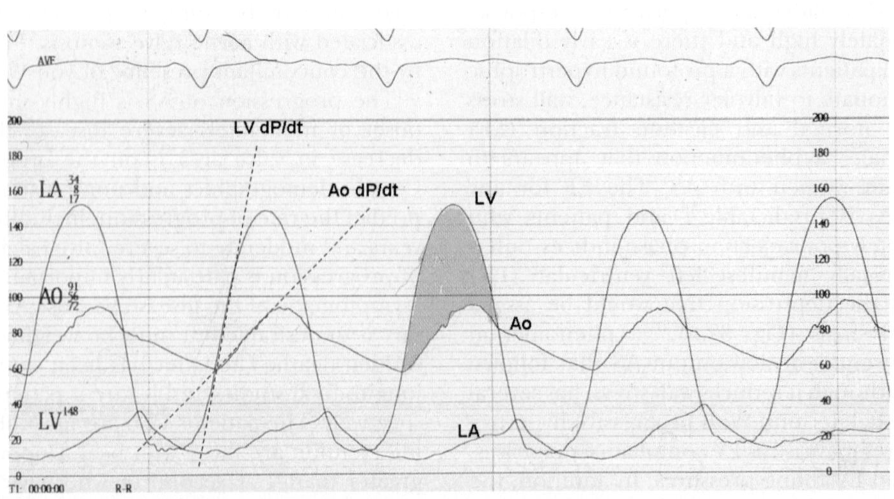

Figure 32.4 Left ventricular (LV), aortic (Ao), and left atrial (LA) pressure on 200 mm Hg scale, 100 mm/second paper speed. The aortic valve gradient is filled in yellow. The dramatic difference in the slope of left ventricular (LV dP/dt, *dashed blue line*) and aortic pressure upstroke (Ao dP/dt, *dashed red line*) and the low pulse pressure (≈30 mm Hg) in this patient with classic severe aortic valve stenosis is demonstrated.

jet velocity greater than 4 m/second, gradient greater than 40 mm Hg, and aortic valve area less than 1 cm^2, with the caveat that the gradient and jet velocity depend on the overall transvalvular flow[5] (see Table 32.1). Importantly, antegrade flow across the aortic valve does not equal cardiac output in patients with confounding conditions, including aortic insufficiency; thus, for example, a patient with mild to moderate AS and moderate aortic insufficiency may have a transvalvular gradient suggestive of severe AS. Finally, although most practitioners do not index the valve area, it is important to appreciate that in patients with large body surface areas, disease that might be considered moderate in smaller patients may be functionally severe.

Several caveats need to be considered before acceptance of noninvasive data in the critical care setting. Inadequate acoustic windows in some patients and difficulty in positioning patients on respirators and with multiple lines in place do limit echocardiographic imaging. Technical errors in recording and interpretation result in significant misdiagnosis: errors in recording angle, inadvertent imaging of MR jets instead of aortic outflow, assessing proximal velocity instead of the transvalvular signal, and selecting signals in the setting of arrhythmias that are not representative of mean heartbeats can all lead to skewed assessment of valve disease severity.[32] Further, a number of other potential confounding variables can lead to overestimation or underestimation of the severity of AS,[6,33] and valve area calculations by the continuity equation in a low-flow setting may be inaccurate.[34] Because the continuity equation depends on measurement of the LV outflow track dimension, which is prone to inaccuracy, another measure of AS severity, the dimensionless index (the ratio of blood flow velocity across the LV outflow track to that across the aortic valve), has been widely adopted.[35] A number of other techniques for determining the severity of AS supplement the most commonly used noninvasive tools, including three-dimensional echo, computed tomography,[36] and magnetic resonance imaging (MRI).[37] Overall, there has been a major a shift in the gold standard from catheter-derived to noninvasive-derived determination of AS severity, and cardiac catheterization is no longer indicated for hemodynamic assessment of aortic valve disease severity when noninvasive findings are unequivocal.[5]

The echocardiogram provides important additional information including severity of LV hypertrophy, LV function and size, and concomitant disease of other heart valves. The presence of regional wall motion abnormalities, in the absence of a conduction disturbance, suggests concomitant coronary artery disease. The electrocardiogram (ECG) in AS is typically abnormal and frequently features LV hypertrophy, with ST-segment abnormalities in the lateral leads typically described as a strain pattern.[38] Although occasionally mistaken for anterior ischemia or infarction, with loss of R voltage across the precordium and occasionally with narrow QS complexes, the ECG is not specific for severity of AS. With increasing calcification of the perivalvular tissues, heart block is seen, typically late in the course of the disease.

CARDIAC CATHETERIZATION

Cardiac catheterization is indicated in patients in whom the noninvasive data are equivocal, and coronary angiography is indicated in a range of settings identified in Box 32.1. The hemodynamics of AS are best recorded with a catheter or catheters placed simultaneously on either side of the aortic valve.[6,39] Unfortunately, most laboratories record femoral artery pressure in lieu of central aortic pressure or do a catheter pullback in lieu of simultaneous pressure tracings; both techniques can result in significant misinterpretation

Box 32.1 Indications for Cardiac Catheterization in Patients with Valvular Heart Disease

General Indications:

1. When noninvasive findings are inconclusive or discordant with clinical findings or inadequate imaging is obtained.
2. Right-sided heart catheterization when clinical decision making will be influenced by hemodynamics not otherwise obtainable.

Specific Indications for Coronary Angiography:

Class I

1. Before valve surgery or percutaneous balloon commissurotomy in patients with chest pain, other objective evidence of ischemia, decreased LV systolic function, history of CAD, or coronary risk factors.
2. In patients with apparently mild to moderate valvular heart disease but progressive angina, objective evidence of ischemia, decreased LV systolic function, or overt congestive heart failure.
3. Before valve surgery or percutaneous balloon commissurotomy in men 35 years and older, premenopausal women aged 35 years and older who have coronary risk factors, and postmenopausal women.

Class II

Surgery without coronary angiography is reasonable for patients requiring emergency valve surgery for acute valve regurgitation, aortic root disease, or infective endocarditis.

Class IIb

Coronary angiography may be considered for patients undergoing catheterization to confirm the severity of valve lesions before valve surgery without preexisting evidence of CAD, multiple coronary risk factors, or advanced age.

Class III

1. Coronary angiography is not indicated in young patients undergoing nonemergency valve surgery when no further hemodynamic assessment by catheterization is deemed necessary and there are no coronary risk factors, no history of CAD, and no evidence of ischemia.
2. Patients should not undergo coronary angiography before valve surgery if they are severely hemodynamically unstable.

Modified from Bonow RO, Carabello BA, Chatterjee K, et al: ACC/AHA guidelines for the management of patients with valvular heart disease: A report of the American College of Cardiology/American Heart Association Task Force on Practice Guidelines (writing committee to revise the 1998 guidelines for the management of patients with valvular heart disease) developed in collaboration with the Society of Cardiovascular Anesthesiologists and endorsed by the Society for Cardiovascular Angiography and Interventions and the Society of Thoracic Surgeons. J Am Coll Cardiol 2006;48:e1-148.

CAD, coronary artery disease; LV, left ventricular. Class refers to ACC/AHA Guidelines classification system.

of the severity of aortic valve disease.[40] A variety of other errors in catheterization laboratory pressure measurements makes the catheter-derived valve area generally more variable than desirable in all except a few laboratories, including inherent errors in estimating rather than measuring oxygen consumption and in assuming that the Gorlin constant (originally established for a limited subset of patients[41]) and the valve area itself remain constant under varying loading conditions.[34] In the catheterization laboratory as well, transvalvular flow may be underestimated if there is concomitant aortic insufficiency, resulting in overestimation of the severity of aortic valve disease.

LOW-GRADIENT, LOW-OUTPUT AORTIC STENOSIS

The critical care unit patient with a low to moderate gradient (typically <30 mm Hg) across the aortic valve in the setting of low cardiac output represents an important conundrum (and should be differentiated from the aortic *sclerosis* patient with low gradient not associated with depressed output). In general, the rules of hydraulics demonstrate that valve area is proportional to flow divided by the square root of the gradient.[41] Thus, when the valve area is fixed, increased flow is associated with an exponential rise in gradient when valve areas are less than 1 cm^2 (Fig. 32.5). When a patient in the critical care setting has depressed cardiac output and a low gradient across the aortic valve, there are two possible interpretations of these findings: either the patient has mild to moderate AS and poor LV function, or the patient has severe AS with a low EF appropriate to high wall stress (see Fig. 32.3) and secondary depression of cardiac output. In the case of the former, increasing flow results in better opening of the aortic valve, with only mild to moderate increase in gradient and an increase in the calculated valve area of 0.3 cm^2 or greater.[42]

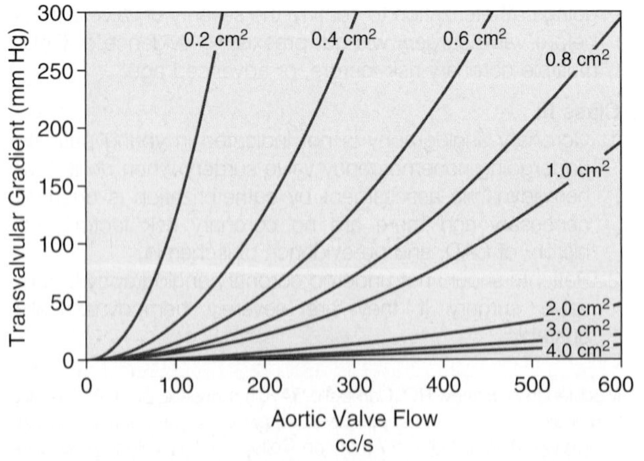

Figure 32.5 The relationship between transvalvular flow and transvalvular gradient for given valve areas. An exponential rise in gradient occurs when flow is increased with valve areas in the severe stenosis range (<1 cm^2). The curve demonstrates that change in gradient is proportional to the square of change in flow; thus doubling the flow rate results in a fourfold increase in gradient. (From Gorlin R, Gorlin SG: Hydraulic formula for calculation of the area of the stenotic mitral valve, other cardiac valves, and central circulatory shunts. Am Heart J 1951;41:1-29.)

In the latter case, a fixed obstruction to outflow exists and increasing transvalvular flow results in a dramatic increase in gradient. In addition to increasing flow across the valve in these patients, typically with dobutamine infusion,[43] the echocardiogram can be useful in several other ways[44]: valve calcification is suggestive of fixed outflow obstruction and, if severe, suggests that the underlying disease is severe AS rather than LV dysfunction. Preserved LV contractile reserve, with significant rise in stroke volume (>20%), peak velocity (>0.6 m/second), or mean transvalvular gradient (>10 mm Hg) at the time of dobutamine infusion is an additional useful marker. Lack of contractile reserve has been associated with lower operative survival rate[45] (6% vs. 33% in one study), although it should not be the sole parameter for the decision on whether or not to perform AVR: patients who survive may manifest significant recovery in LV function postoperatively.[46] Low contractile reserve should not preclude AVR in patients who do have severe fixed obstruction because their prognosis without surgery is abysmal.[47] One other variation of low-gradient low-output AS involves patients with small hypertrophied ventricles and preserved EF. This subset, sometimes called *high valvuloarterial impedance AS,* has low gradient because of low stroke volume; the burgeoning evidence base does show improved results with AVR.[48]

THERAPY

MEDICAL MANAGEMENT

Medical management is aimed solely at patient stabilization because pharmacologic intervention has never been shown to prolong life and can achieve modest hemodynamic improvement at best. In the critical care setting the approach to the patient with AS normally parallels treatment of corresponding degrees of heart failure, albeit with caution, because the normal therapeutic approach to heart failure can be deleterious or fatal in the setting of severe AS. The traditional heart failure therapies, in particular, diuretics and vasodilators, need to be used with care because reduction in preload can cause hypotension, decreased cardiac output, and a downward spiral into refractory shock. In patients with small-volume hypertrophic left ventricles, cardiac output is particularly preload dependent.

Atrial arrhythmias, in particular, atrial fibrillation (AF), can lead to abrupt and severe decompensation because of loss of the atrial contraction component of LV filling. Cardioversion in the critical care setting is particularly helpful in severely decompensated patients, and maintenance of sinus rhythm in patients who are otherwise suitable (e.g., left atrium <6 cm, recent onset of AF, and absence of clot in the left atrium by transesophageal echocardiography) should be a priority.

Despite the caveats, vasodilator therapy, including nitroprusside, has been used in the critical care setting in patients with severe LV dysfunction and severe AS.[49] In a select group of patients not dependent on inotropes, cardiac output rose significantly and there was overall hemodynamic improvement. Similarly, intra-aortic balloon pumping has been used, although there are only isolated case reports of efficacy.[50,51] As would be expected, both nitroprusside and intra-aortic balloon pumping result in afterload reduction and some increase in transvalvular flow along with some increase in aortic valve gradient.

Hemodynamic monitoring is essential for the pharmacologic management of decompensated severe AS patients in the critical care setting. Because of the dependence on preload, a fine threshold exists between optimal filling pressures and pulmonary edema. Vasodilator therapy as described earlier results in peripheral vasodilation, but because of the fixed obstruction to outflow it may not provide sufficient increase in stroke volume and cardiac output to maintain systemic blood pressure. Inotropic agents are frequently required, and patients with inadequate contractile reserve may show limited improvement. Beta blockers are relatively dangerous, although tachycardia is hemodynamically unfavorable, even in sinus rhythm. Beta blockade, if employed, should be used with great caution. Beta blockers decrease contractility and, in addition, an increase in heart rate may be the only remaining compensatory mechanism for low stroke volume because of the fixed resistance to outflow. Patients with severe AS can enter a "death spiral" in which hemodynamic recovery becomes impossible.

Lipid-lowering therapy and converting enzyme inhibitors have been the subject of substantial investigation,[52] although their role is in the chronic setting rather than during critical care. Two prospective randomized trials failed to show clear benefits of a statin[53,54] in slowing disease progression. Some preliminary evidence suggests potential benefits of angiotensin-converting enzyme (ACE) inhibitors in decreasing progression of aortic valve calcification,[55,56] but the available clinical data do not show slowing of AS progression.[57] Both lipid-lowering and converting enzyme inhibitors need to be tested in larger populations earlier in the course of aortic valve disease.

PERCUTANEOUS INTERVENTIONS

Balloon Valvuloplasty

Balloon aortic valvuloplasty is a temporizing measure for patients who are hemodynamically unstable and are at high risk for AVR. Although the procedure is therapeutic and indicated in congenital AS in children and young adults, the risk/benefit ratio in patients beyond their 20s is usually unfavorable. Because calcific AS is associated with open commissures and ossified leaflets, abrupt balloon inflation exerts its effect by improving leaflet compliance through the formation of multiple, usually microscopic, fracture lines in the calcified tissues. Stretching of the commissures is temporary, and any hemodynamic benefit of the latter resolves within hours. The leaflets lose their improved compliance within weeks to months, and the aortic valve area typically returns to baseline.

The acute hemodynamic results (Fig. 32.6) are poor compared with those of AVR, with a 50% reduction in gradient and an increase in aortic valve area of only 0.2 to 0.3 cm^2.[58] The in-hospital mortality rate was close to 10% in the National Heart, Lung and Blood Institute registry[59] and is substantially higher in patients with hemodynamic decompensation and multiorgan failure. Most valves have restenosed within a few months, with a recent series showing an 87% mortality rate after a median period of less than 7 months,[60] and no benefit for long-term outcomes has been

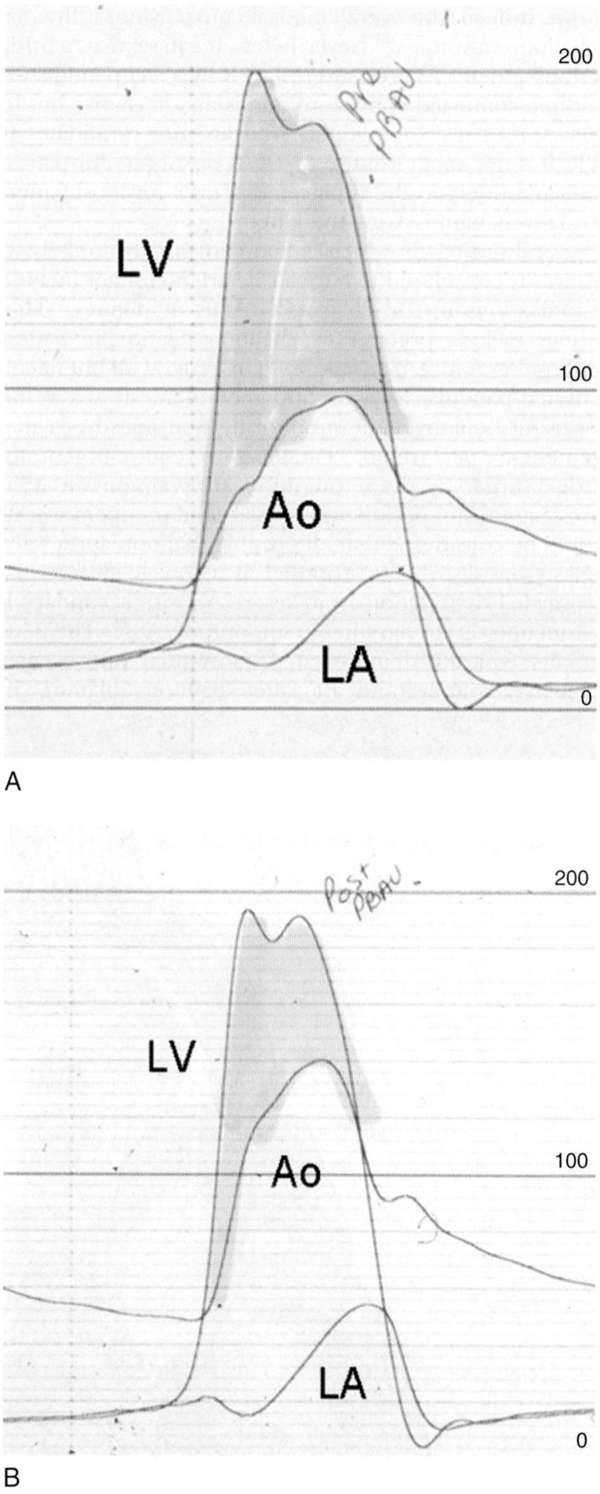

Figure 32.6 Hemodynamic response to percutaneous balloon aortic valvuloplasty. Tracings show before (**A**) and after (**B**) balloon dilation on 200 mm Hg scale. A successful 50% reduction in gradient occurs, but residual gradient remains 50 mm Hg, still in the severe category. The pulse pressure has increased from 60 mm Hg to 90 mm Hg, the peak aortic systolic pressure has increased to 140 mm Hg from 100 mm Hg, and the left ventricular pressure upslope can be seen to have improved dramatically. Ao, aorta; LA, left atrium; LV, left ventricle.

shown. Indeed, the overall clinical course is not influenced by balloon valvotomy.[61] Nevertheless, it can serve as a bridge to transcatheter AVR or surgical AVR in select patients with multiple comorbid conditions and is an alternative but low efficacy measure for patients who are not candidates for AVR. It is not an alternative to TAVR or surgery for patients who can undergo valve replacement, even for most patients at relatively high risk for the latter.

Several settings in which balloon aortic valvuloplasty was previously considered to have a role are no longer included as indications in the 2006 ACC/AHA guidelines.[5] These settings include preoperative balloon dilation in patients undergoing noncardiac surgery[62]; in general all but decompensated patients can withstand general anesthesia as long as careful hemodynamic monitoring and anesthesia management are performed.[63] Patients who require urgent noncardiac surgery in the setting of severe symptomatic AS do have a significant perioperative risk,[64] and preoperative AVR should be considered if at all possible. Balloon aortic valvuloplasty has also been proposed as a tool to differentiate myocardial dysfunction from severe AS with secondary LV dysfunction in low-gradient, low-output AS.[65] The latter patients typically demonstrated substantial improvement in stroke volume and EF after balloon dilation, but dobutamine stress testing is a far safer, less morbid screening tool.

Transcatheter Aortic Valve Replacement

Transcatheter aortic valve replacement (TAVR), a technology developed in the past decade, has revolutionized the treatment of AS. The procedure is of increasing importance in the critical care setting. Tissue valves are sewn to either balloon expandable or self-expanding stents, which are crimped onto a catheter and advanced across the stenotic native valve. Both balloon expandable (Fig. 32.7) and self-expanding technologies are widely available outside the United States. The landmark PARTNER (Placement of AoRtic TraNscathetER valves) study had two cohorts: PARTNER A enrolled high-risk but operable patients while PARTNER B enrolled patients deemed inoperable. PARTNER A randomized patients to surgical aortic valve replacement (SAVR) versus two types of TAVRs: transfemoral if the iliac and femoral vasculature was suitable for accommodating the large catheter shafts or transapical if not.[66] The results of TAVR and SAVR were similar, including mortality rate, stroke, and quality of life with published follow-up through 2 years; vascular complications were higher with TAVR and major bleeding and AF were higher

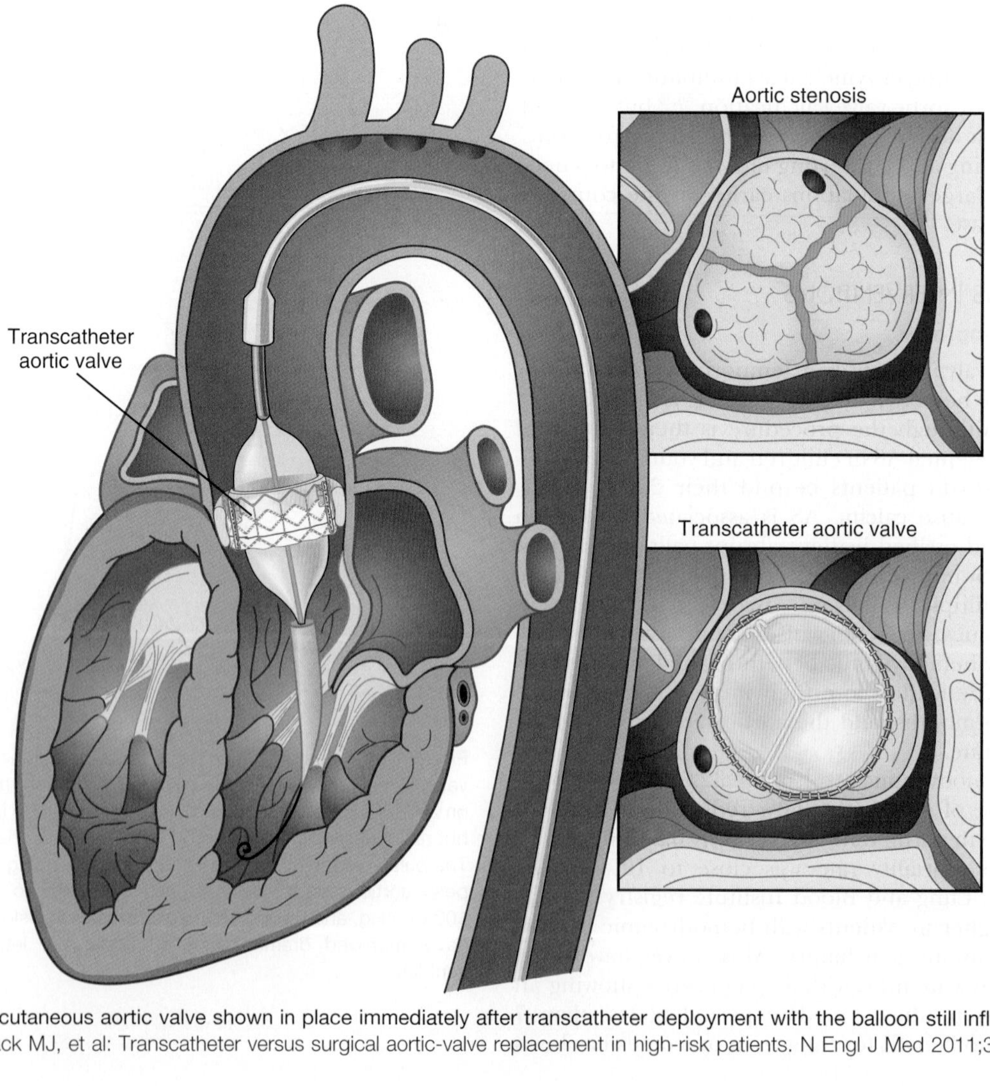

Figure 32.7 Percutaneous aortic valve shown in place immediately after transcatheter deployment with the balloon still inflated. (From Smith CR, Leon MB, Mack MJ, et al: Transcatheter versus surgical aortic-valve replacement in high-risk patients. N Engl J Med 2011;364:2187-2198.)

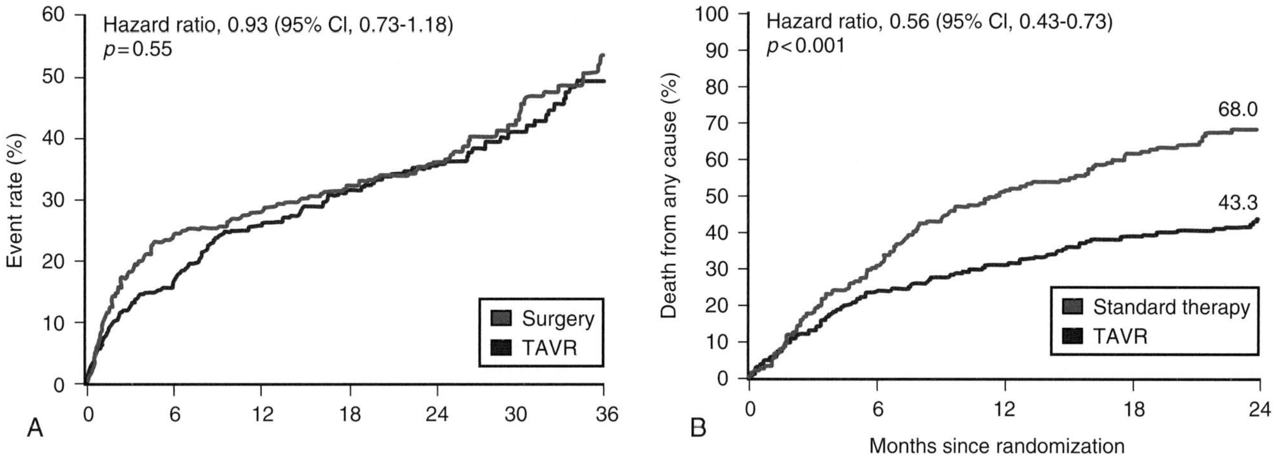

Figure 32.8 Results of the Placement of Aortic Transcatheter Valves (PARTNER) Trial. **A**, Death from any cause or stroke in the A cohort, the high-risk but operable patients who were randomized to surgical aortic valve replacement (n = 351) versus either transfemoral (n = 244) or transapical (n = 104) transcatheter deployment depending on the suitability of the femoral and iliac circulation. There were no differences in mortality rate or stroke. **B**, **Mortality in the B cohort, showing substantial survival advantage among the 179 patients undergoing transcatheter aortic valve replacement over the 179 patients treated with medical therapy.** (A from Smith CR, Leon MB, Mack MJ, et al: Transcatheter versus surgical aortic-valve replacement in high-risk patients. N Engl J Med 2011;364:2187-2198; B from Makkar RR, Fontana GP, Jilaihawi H, et al: Transcatheter aortic-valve replacement for inoperable severe aortic stenosis. N Engl J Med 2012;366:1696-1704.)

with SAVR[66] (Fig. 32.8A). PARTNER B randomized patients with suitable vasculature to transfemoral TAVR versus medical therapy.[67] Patients who received only medical therapy (with or without balloon valvuloplasty) had a 51% 1-year mortality rate compared to those inoperable patients randomized to TAVR who had a 31% 1-year mortality rate, an approximately 40% relative reduction (Fig. 32.8B). Thus, TAVR appears to be among the most dramatically successful of all modern cardiac interventions. However, it is noteworthy that the residual mortality rate in the inoperable TAVR patients remains very high, reflecting the severe comorbid conditions in patients who met inoperability criteria. There was also an initially higher stroke risk in the TAVR patients.[67] The risk of stroke in follow-up appears to be largely related to patient comorbid conditions that increase stroke risk, rather than the type of valve replacement.[68] The dramatic mortality risk benefit with TAVR in inoperable patients has been shown to continue through 2 years of follow-up; because the stroke risk is higher in the surviving medically treated population, the early excess stroke risk associated with TAVR largely resolves by 24 months.[69] Outside the United States, TAVR has been performed in some 70,000 patients; the Food and Drug Administration initially approved TAVR for inoperable patients based on the results of PARTNER B and subsequently approved the high-risk population treated in PARTNER A. A variety of investigational uses of the TAVR platform, such as valve-in-valve replacement for patients with bioprosthetic valve dysfunction (AS and aortic insufficiency) are being performed, primarily outside the United States[70]; the possibility that transcatheter valve-in-valve replacement will eventually supplant reoperation may change the algorithm for choice of tissue versus mechanical AVR.

The management of TAVR patients after valve replacement frequently takes place in the critical care unit. The higher rate of vascular complications associated with TAVR requires careful monitoring for limb ischemia, retroperitoneal hemorrhage, and a variety of other vascular complications.[71] Conduction disturbances, particularly after use of a self-expanding TAVR platform, occur in a significant percentage of cases, requiring permanent pacemaker placement.[72] A number of issues, such as the use of dual antiplatelet therapy and anticoagulation after TAVR remain to be fully investigated; most operators treat with dual antiplatelet therapy for periods ranging from 1 to 6 months; dual antiplatelet therapy plus anticoagulation for patients with AF is a combination with particularly high major bleeding risk, though the evidence base is incomplete, and many clinicians use only aspirin and warfarin in this setting.

Aortic Valve Replacement

AVR remains the treatment of choice for severe AS in patients who are considered to have reasonable operable risk. Class I indications are severe AS (valve area less than 1 cm^2) with symptoms or, regardless of symptoms, if patients have severe AS and are undergoing coronary artery bypass, are undergoing surgery of the aorta or other heart valves, or have LV dysfunction. A long list of class II indications generally focuses on patients who do not meet class I criteria but are thought to be at increased risk of rapid disease progression or hemodynamic compromise. In addition, patients with moderate AS who undergo other cardiac surgery generally have simultaneous AVR. Survival after AVR is excellent if LV function is preserved, with operative mortality rate in ideal candidates as low as 1%. In these patients, age-matched survival is not significantly different from patients without AS.[73] In the setting of LV dysfunction, however, postoperative life expectancy is relatively poor.[74] Nevertheless, conservative therapy for severe AS remains an undesirable alternative: A recent review of 453 patients treated without intervention despite severe AS had 1-year, 5-year, and 10-year survival rates of only 62%, 32%, and 18%, respectively,[75] with the worst survival in patients with renal failure, pulmonary hypertension, age older than 75 years, diminished EF, and congestive heart failure.

AORTIC INSUFFICIENCY

The overall prevalence of moderate or severe aortic insufficiency (AI) in the United States, as shown in the Framingham Offspring Study, ranged from 0.3% in the fifth decade of life to 2.2% for patients aged 70 to 83.[76] The frequency is age and male gender related. The diagnosis of AI is more difficult and the treatment issues in many ways more complex than for AS, with less of a clear dichotomy in the decision tree for valve replacement. AI needs to be considered in light of its acuity: Acute AI is usually associated with life-threatening comorbid conditions and the resultant acute regurgitation places great stress on the left ventricle and may itself be fatal. In contrast, chronic AI may evolve from clinically insignificant to requiring surgery over decades. Unlike AS, it is not primarily a disease of the aging process (although it does occur more frequently with increasing age) and is typically secondary to one of an extensive list of systemic or structural diseases that result in insufficiency of the aortic valve. Acute AI frequently requires urgent surgery, whereas chronic AI may be managed by watchful waiting and some limited options for medical therapy.

Box 32.2 Etiology of Acute and Chronic Aortic Insufficiency

Acute

Infective endocarditis
Aortic dissection
Trauma

Chronic

Dilation of the aorta
Systemic hypertension
Bicuspid aortic valve
Calcific degenerated aortic valve disease
Rheumatic aortic valve disease
Infective endocarditis
Myxomatous degeneration
Aortic dissection
Marfan syndrome
Trauma
Ankylosing spondylitis
Syphilis
Rheumatoid arthritis
Osteogenesis imperfecta
Giant cell aortitis
Ehlers-Danlos syndrome
Subaortic stenosis
Ventricular septal defect with cusp prolapse
Anorectic drug reaction

PATHOPHYSIOLOGY

Acute AI is generally associated with leaflet involvement by endocarditis or disruption of the aortic valve's annular structure by dissection or trauma. Chronic AI, by contrast, is caused by congenital valve abnormalities, most importantly bicuspid aortic valve disease, or by the degenerative process described earlier associated with AS. Conditions that distort the annulus and aortic root including systemic hypertension have been considered to be important causes of secondary AI, although the association between chronic AI and systemic hypertension remains to be confirmed.[76,77] Rheumatic AI, almost invariably associated with mitral valve involvement as well, remains prevalent in developing countries but is an uncommon cause of AI in industrialized nations.

In general, causes of AI (Box 32.2) have been divided into those that affect the leaflets primarily and those that affect the root and annulus. The former includes bicuspid and other aortic valve abnormalities, endocarditis, rheumatic aortic valve disease, the atherosclerotic process described earlier, connective tissue disorders, antiphospholipid syndrome (Libman-Sacks endocarditis), and toxicity from anorectic drugs.[78] The aortic root and annulus are affected by a variety of comorbid conditions that dilate the aortic root; Marfan and Ehlers-Danlos syndromes; osteogenesis imperfecta; chronic aortic dissection; syphilitic aortitis; connective tissue disorders; and, along with the valve leaflets, ankylosing spondylitis.

In isolated acute AI, the sudden onset of regurgitation imposes a large-volume load on the left ventricle in diastole prior to an adaptive process being in place. The abrupt rise in pressure is reflected by parallel development of left atrial and pulmonary vascular hypertension, frequently resulting in pulmonary edema. Because the compliance of a previously unaffected left ventricle is not sufficient to allow adequate dilation to absorb the regurgitant volume, the ventricle operates on the steep portion of its pressure-volume curve, with inadequate stroke volume to accommodate the high regurgitant flow. The effective (net) forward stroke volume (antegrade flow minus retrograde filling) is therefore low, compensated to some degree by tachycardia, but frequently insufficient to maintain normal cardiac output. This phenomenon is exaggerated in patients with preexistent LV hypertrophy in whom the ventricle is already operating on the steep portion of its pressure-volume curve, and particularly severe decompensation is seen when the left ventricle is small and hypertrophic. Critical care settings for the latter unfortunately include many of the common scenarios for acute AI including endocarditis in the setting of AS and aortic dissection in patients with hypertension and a dilated aortic root.[5]

Acute severe AI results in near approximation of aortic and LV pressures at end diastole, with consequent deleterious effects on coronary perfusion of the subendocardium (Fig. 32.9). Because coronary perfusion pressure is the difference between diastolic pressure in the aortic root and subendocardial pressure in the LV cavity, the decrease in aortic diastolic pressure and rise in subendocardial pressure that are hallmarks of acute AI can result in profound subendocardial ischemia, especially in patients with preexistent hypertrophy or patients with underlying coronary artery disease. In addition, because afterload and wall stress in this setting are increased, there is a rise in myocardial oxygen demand simultaneous with a fall in supply, occasionally leading to cardiogenic shock and death. Acute AI also results in early closure of the mitral valve as LV diastolic pressure rises above left atrial pressure, a phenomenon that has potential protective benefits for the pulmonary circulation.

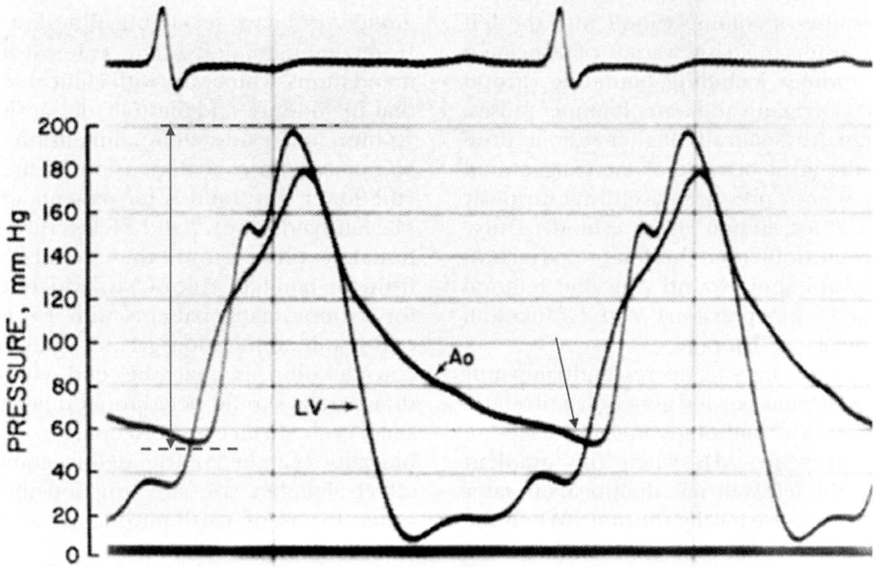

Figure 32.9 The hemodynamics of acute aortic insufficiency. The wide pulse pressure (150 mm Hg) difference between peak and minimum aortic pressure *(blue arrow)* and near diastasis of left ventricular and aortic pressure late in diastole *(red arrow)* are demonstrated. Ao, aorta; LV, left ventricle. (Modified from Grossman W: Profiles in valvular heart disease. In Baim D [ed]: Grossman's Cardiac Catheterization, Angiography and Intervention. Philadelphia, Lippincott Williams & Wilkins, 2006, p 654.)

In contrast, chronic AI features a host of adaptive processes by the left ventricle including progressive dilation, increased compliance, and hypertrophy. As with AS, hypertrophy results in lower wall stress but AI features an increase in afterload combined with progressive LV dilation and somewhat less hypertrophy, resulting in significantly higher wall stress than seen in compensated AS.[79] End-diastolic dilation of the left ventricle allows for larger stroke volumes to compensate for regurgitant fractions, which may be in the range of 50% or greater. With combined pressure and volume overload, unique among the valve disorders discussed in this chapter, LV adaptations allow for maintenance of normal overall function until ventricular remodeling and hypertrophy are no longer sufficient to maintain forward stroke volume and EF. With increasing wall stress and LV dilation, LV contractility is eventually impaired, at which point filling pressures begin to rise (or rise further) and patients become symptomatic. Coronary flow reserve in AI, as with AS, is impaired[80] and, combined with increased demand and the need for additional perfusion for a hypertrophic myocardium, may result in significant ischemia. The onset of symptoms may be abrupt, especially with new onset of atrial tachyarrhythmias or sudden increase in cardiac output demand such as with exertion or infection.

Although acute AI represents a relative or absolute medical emergency, chronic AI may have an insidious course over decades. Some insight into the rate of progression of chronic AI is provided by a meta-analysis incorporated into the most recent ACC/AHA guidelines.[5] In a review of nine admittedly heterogeneous studies incorporating nearly 600 primarily asymptomatic or mildly symptomatic patients with AI, average progression to symptoms with or without LV systolic dysfunction was 4.3% annually, and sudden death occurred in 0.2% annually.[5] Although this rate of progression is modest, patients do not necessarily develop symptoms before developing LV dysfunction or sudden death.[81] Age, end-systolic dimensions,[82] and rate of deterioration of end-systolic dimension and EF[83] are more sensitive tools for predicting outcome in chronic AI.

In contrast, in the setting of *symptomatic* AI that does not fall in the acute severe category, an annual mortality rate of 6% to 25% has been described, depending on severity of symptoms. By the 10-year follow-up, 75% had undergone AVR or died.[84]

DIAGNOSIS

PHYSICAL EXAMINATION

The hallmarks of *acute* severe AI include features consistent with congestive heart failure and low cardiac output including tachycardia, dyspnea, and signs of impaired cardiac output such as peripheral vasoconstriction. The wide pulse pressure that is a hallmark of AI may or may not be seen, in part because it is dependent on LV compliance. The classic AI murmur may not be heard because of the limited gradient between the aorta and left ventricle during diastole when LV diastolic pressures in some cases approach systemic diastolic pressures. Tachycardia and diminished effective forward flow in acute AI may offset the augmented systolic and wide pulse pressure seen in later stages of the disease, and these patients may have normal or occasionally diminished pulses, although more moderate acute AI may feature the more classic findings. Early closure of the mitral valve may result in a soft first heart sound, and distortions of leaflet anatomy may result in lack of a distinct aortic second heart sound. In some cases absence of a second heart sound in a patient presenting with cardiogenic shock may be the most prominent physical finding.[78]

The dramatic physical findings in *chronic* AI are among the most familiar to physicians and trainees. A wide pulse pressure results primarily because of increased stroke volume, which augments systolic pressure,[85] and low aortic diastolic pressures because of volume runoff into the left ventricle. This in turn results in a large variety of associated eponymous physical findings including bounding carotid and peripheral pulses (Corrigan's and water hammer pulses, respectively); Hill's sign (dramatically higher systolic pressure in the legs than the arms because of the exaggerated effect of harmonics on systolic pressure waveforms, variously described as having a 20 or 40 mm Hg threshold); Duroziez's sign (to and fro murmur over the femoral arteries); and Traube's sign ("pistol shot" sound over the femoral artery during simultaneous compression). With LV dilation, the apical impulse is displaced laterally.

The intensity of the classic diastolic decrescendo murmur heard over the left midsternal border generally correlates well with the severity of AI,[86] although in later stages of decompensation (or in acute AI), when the gradient between the aorta and the left ventricle disappears in later stages of diastole, the murmur typically shortens. When the murmur is better heard over the right (rather than left) sternal border, the cause of the AI may be secondary to a dilated aortic root rather than a primary leaflet abnormality.[87] Two other murmurs are frequently heard with moderate to severe AI: a systolic ejection murmur consistent with increased transvalvular flow and on occasion an Austin-Flint murmur. The latter is the apical diastolic rumble occasionally confused with mitral stenosis and thought to originate from vibration of the anterior mitral leaflet caused by the diastolic regurgitant jet originating at the aortic valve; it has been described only in the setting of severe AI.[87] In rheumatic AI, if a diastolic rumble is heard, mitral stenosis should be excluded. An S_3 gallop is most likely to be present when severe AI occurs in a setting of depressed LV function[88] but may merely reflect substantial volume loading; the finding is not specific.

NONINVASIVE EVALUATION

As with AS, noninvasive assessment has replaced cardiac catheterization for determining severity of AI. It provides both structural and physiologic information including visualization of the leaflets, annulus, and aortic root; semiquantitative assessment of the severity of AI; and characterization of LV size, hypertrophy, and function, as well as other structural heart disease. Transesophageal echocardiography has superior diagnostic sensitivity to transthoracic echo for certain parameters, in particular for detection of valvular vegetations.[89] A wide range of techniques for measurement of AI severity including width of the color Doppler jet compared with size of the LV outflow tract, width of the vena contracta, regurgitant volume, regurgitant fraction, and regurgitant orifice area are described in Chapter 8. The correlation of these parameters with severity of AI is listed in Table 32.1. Additional findings of importance are rate of jet velocity deceleration as diastasis is achieved between aortic and LV diastolic pressures and duration of diastolic flow reversal in the aorta.[90] In addition to echocardiography, cine MRI can assess severity of AI, size of chamber volumes, LV mass, wall thickness, and systolic function.[91] LV size and function have also been followed serially by radionuclide ventriculography.[92]

The size and function of the LV have been used to set thresholds at which AVR should be considered. The ACC/AHA guidelines[5] and the European Society of Cardiology guidelines[93] have set slightly different values for class I and II recommendations. The echocardiogram-based recommendations, which vary with clinical settings, use thresholds that include LV end-diastolic dimension greater than 70 to 75 mm and end-systolic dimension greater than 50 to 55 mm, aortic root dimension greater than 50 to 55 mm (the lower threshold is for patients with bicuspid valves or Marfan syndrome),[93] and EF less than 50%. As the observational data have grown, these numbers have shifted slightly from the familiar "rule of 55s," which recommended surgery for asymptomatic patients with EF less than 55% or LV end-systolic dimension greater than 55 mm. An important consideration is that the end-systolic and end-diastolic dimensions should be adjusted downward for patients with small body surface area. Keeping in mind that these threshold values can be confounded by comorbid conditions that affect chamber size and function including ischemic and other forms of cardiomyopathy, as well as multivalvular disease, is important.

The ECG was once an important tool in the serial assessment of patients with AI. Similar to AS, features of LV hypertrophy may be present. Progression of LV dilation and dysfunction were thought to correlate with development of an LV strain pattern, a phenomenon that has been confirmed.[94] As a result, the use of digitalis glycosides, which can cause a similar strain pattern, was discouraged in order to maintain relative specificity of the finding. Conduction disturbances remain an important feature, particularly heart block in the setting of endocarditis, discussed subsequently.

CARDIAC CATHETERIZATION

As with the other valvular diseases discussed in this chapter, cardiac catheterization is indicated only for patients with inconclusive noninvasive findings or when noninvasive findings are discordant with the rest of the clinical picture. Typical findings include a wide aortic pulse pressure and an exaggerated rise in LV diastolic pressure, reflecting continuous retrograde filling during diastole (see Fig. 32.9). Cardiac catheterization in this setting normally includes aortic root angiography; although the latter requires a significant dye load (typically 30 mL/second for 2 seconds) to be diagnostically accurate. The hallmark of severe AI is greater opacification of the left ventricle than the aorta. The indications for coronary angiography in this setting are listed in Box 32.1.

THERAPY

MEDICAL MANAGEMENT

In acute AI, medical therapy is targeted to stabilization pending AVR. Nitroprusside has been the standard for reducing peripheral vascular resistance and improving net forward flow across the aortic valve since the 1970s.[95] The use of arterial vasodilators is more complex when the patient is already hypotensive, and a combination of inotropes and afterload reduction should be considered. Although afterload reduction in this setting is highly beneficial, the otherwise optimal combination of afterload reduction and augmented pressure normally provided by intra-aortic balloon pumping in cardiogenic shock (see Chapters 7 and 30) is not a viable choice in AI. Counterpulsation during diastole increases the severity of AI with potentially catastrophic consequences; it represents an absolute contraindication to the intra-aortic balloon pump.

Besides vasodilator therapy, maneuvers to raise the heart rate may be helpful, especially in patients who are bradycardic or have a normal heart rate. Tachycardia disproportionately decreases the diastolic filling period, thereby decreasing the duration of regurgitation across the aortic valve. Both isoproterenol or electrical pacing to raise the heart rate have been used with therapeutic benefit.

In *chronic* AI, the evidence base is incomplete and somewhat controversial. The general consensus is that asymptomatic patients with mild to at most moderate AI with normal LV function who are not hypertensive do not require or benefit from vasodilator therapy.[81,83] Only when patients are not surgical candidates is vasodilator use in chronic AI a class I indication.[5] Class II indications are short-term treatment to optimize the patient's hemodynamic status prior to AVR and, more controversially, long-term therapy for asymptomatic patients with severe AI but preserved LV function. Two important studies with divergent results have been performed: One, using nifedipine, appeared to demonstrate some slowing of progression to need for AVR compared with patients on digoxin.[96] The second, a placebo-controlled study, failed to demonstrate clear benefits of vasodilator therapy with either nifedipine or an ACE inhibitor,[97] but there are concerns regarding the size of the study, dose of drug used, and modest severity of disease at baseline. Oral vasodilators that have been described as having potential therapeutic benefit include several dihydropyridine calcium channel blockers (nifedipine and felodipine), as well as hydralazine. The appropriateness of vasodilator therapy regardless of severity of disease is clearer in patients with systemic hypertension, in whom reduction of afterload has dual benefits. The dose of drug should be sufficient to show at least some reduction in systolic pressure. There is no evidence base to recommend other forms of medical therapy, such as nitrates or drugs commonly used to treat congestive heart failure to prevent progression of disease in chronic asymptomatic AI. In the critical care setting, however, inotropes and vasodilators are appropriate if patients have congestive heart failure or a low output state, or both.

AORTIC VALVE REPLACEMENT

Two factors primarily determine when a patient should be referred for valve replacement: the presence of symptoms and findings of LV systolic dysfunction.[5] Surgery results in superior long-term survival than medical therapy alone for symptomatic patients.[84,98] Similarly, patients with LV dysfunction have an inverse correlation between EF and mortality risk.[99] Three ACC/AHA class I indications for surgery, all for patients with severe AI, exist: (1) patients who have symptoms regardless of LV function; (2) patients with LV systolic dysfunction (EF less than or equal to 50%) regardless of symptoms; and (3) patients undergoing coronary bypass surgery or surgery on other heart valves or the aorta.

ACC/AHA class II indications use the thresholds defined by LV dimensions, again for patients with severe AI, using 55 mm as the end-systolic threshold and 75 mm as the end-diastolic threshold, but lowering those values by 5 mm when the rate of LV dilation is progressive or when patients have deteriorating exercise tolerance or an abnormal hemodynamic response to exercise. Patients with only moderate AI who are undergoing surgery on the aorta or coronary bypass are also considered to have class II indications.

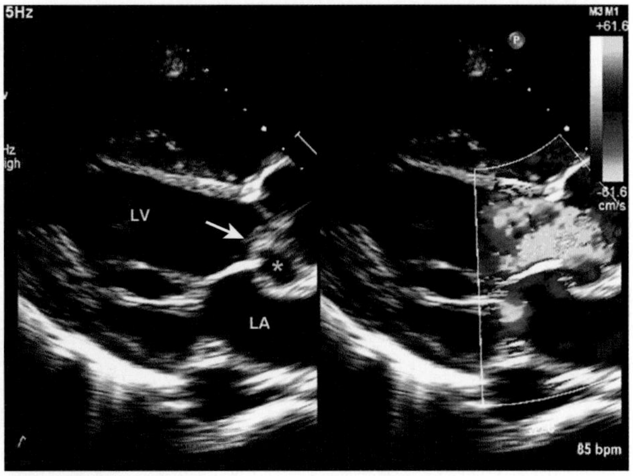

Figure 32.10 Vegetation *(arrow)*. On right is wide-open aortic insufficiency—the jet fills the outflow tract. Asterisk on left refers to walled-off echolucent abscess cavity. LA, left atrium; LV, left ventricle.

The question of whether it is ever too late to perform AVR in patients with AI has been raised.[85] Because the disease involves high afterload and wall stress, there is postoperative improvement in EF[100] even in patients with severe baseline LV dysfunction. In general there is substantial reversal of the physiologic adaptations required by chronic severe AI in the postoperative state.[101] Nevertheless, delay in referring patients for surgery is deleterious, with significant negative impact on outcomes[102]; the prognosis is adversely affected both by the severity and duration of LV dysfunction.[103] This includes a fourfold increase in operative mortality rate for patients with EF less than 35% (14%) compared with those with EF greater than 50% (3.7%). Thus the trend has been for earlier referral of symptomatic patients and more aggressive noninvasive monitoring for early detection of deterioration in LV function or dimensions.

Special consideration should be given to patients with acute aortic valve endocarditis. Deteriorating hemodynamics, as well as extension of infection as manifest by progressive heart block and ring abscess formation on echo (Fig. 32.10), are among several factors that mandate early surgery[104]; despite the semielective nature of the operation (with an operative mortality rate close to 10%) and the theoretical risk of an infected prosthesis, the long-term outcomes have been satisfactory, with 75% 10-year survival rate after hospital discharge.[105]

MITRAL REGURGITATION

Anatomically and physiologically, the mitral valve is the most complex of the heart valves, dependent for function on a complex interaction between leaflets, annulus, commissures, and the supporting apparatus consisting of chordae tendineae tethered to the papillary muscles (Fig. 32.11). Distortion or dysfunction of any of the elements and changes

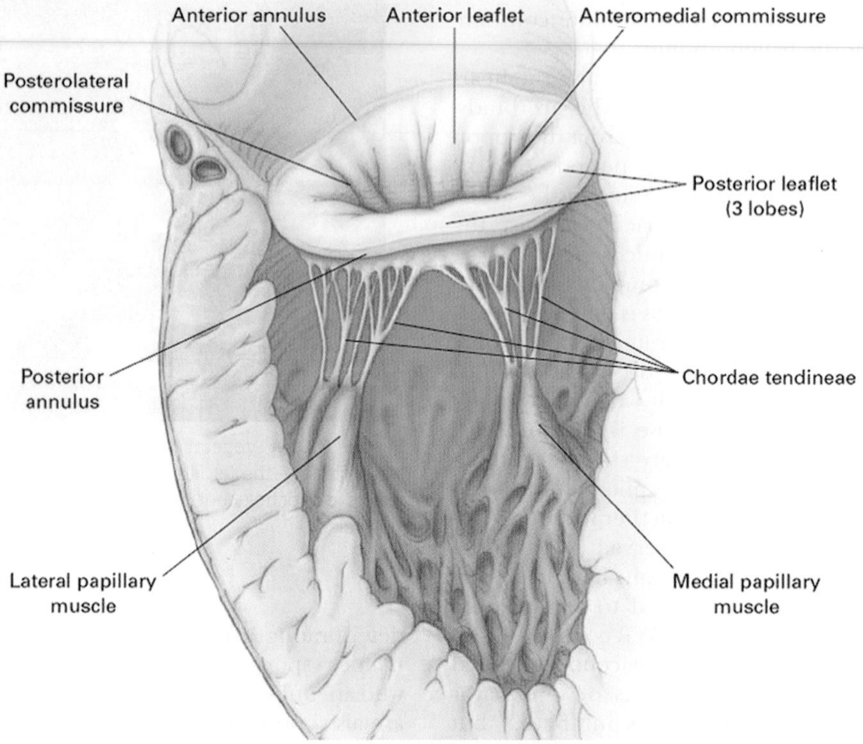

Figure 32.11 Structure of the mitral valve, its surrounding apparatus, and relationship to the left ventricle. Each component can contribute to the presence and extent of mitral regurgitation. (From Otto CM: Evaluation and management of chronic mitral regurgitation. N Engl J Med 2001;345:740-746.)

in function and geometry of the left ventricle and left atrium can all have a significant impact on flow across the mitral valve. In addition, unlike other valvulopathies, the mitral valve is highly dependent on the myocardial circulation. In contrast with the relatively passive nature of opening and closing of the aortic valve, mitral valve motion is an active process reflecting not just cyclic pressure variations but also tethering and dynamic interaction with the supporting apparatus. As with AI, mitral insufficiency (MR) has acute and chronic manifestations and chronic (rather than acute) insufficiency is more common. However, acute MR has a much larger variety of causes than acute AI and the overall incidence is higher. Data from the Framingham Offspring Study revealed a prevalence of moderate or greater MR from 0.9% of women in the fifth decade of life, to 11.2% of men between ages 70 and 83, and correlated with age, low body mass, and systemic hypertension.[76] As with AI, ventricular function predicts overall outcomes. Chronic MR can both cause and be the result of LV remodeling and heart failure and, when secondary to LV dysfunction, is associated with a significantly poorer overall prognosis than LV dysfunction without secondary MR.[106]

PATHOPHYSIOLOGY

Fundamental understanding of the pathophysiology of MR has expanded substantially in the past 2 decades. In particular, awareness of the role of the subvalvular apparatus in preserving LV function and data demonstrating the need for earlier referral to surgery have resulted in significant changes in clinical and surgical practice, leading to substantial improvement in outcomes.[107]

As with AI, MR results in volume overloading of the LV. Unlike AI, the afterload is not increased and overall LV ejection is enhanced rather than impaired by loading conditions, although in significant MR half or more of the ejection is retrograde into the left atrium. The incompetent mitral valve acts as a second pathway for blood ejection, which reduces afterload in a setting in which preload is increased, thus potentiating ejection via the Frank-Starling mechanism. The combination ultimately may raise EF to supranormal early in the course of the disease. As a result, patients with "normal" EF may already have significant impairment in LV function.[108] Adaptations to the volume loading include lengthening of the myocytes, which increases LV volume. Progressive MR eventually results in contractile dysfunction. Relatively early in the course of the disease, the sympathetic nervous system is activated as a compensatory mechanism to volume loading and decreased forward ejection.[109] Chronic high sympathetic tone results in secondary myocardial damage[110] and has been postulated as the rationale for potential benefit from beta blockade in chronic MR.[111] Over time, although some hypertrophy develops, the predominant response to volume overload without pressure overload is enlargement of chamber size. Extrapolating the LaPlace relationship, which is manifestly protective of wall stress in AS, the progressive expansion of LV dimensions in MR without similar compensatory hypertrophy results in increasing wall stress, which in turn results in increasing MR. In a similar manner, a second vicious circle is caused by the effect of MR on LV chamber size, which, as it enlarges, results in stretching of the annulus, further exacerbating MR.[112] Thus chronic MR can both cause and be the result of LV remodeling and heart failure.

The causes of MR vary by geography, with mitral valve prolapse being the most common in industrialized nations. Rheumatic MR remains common in developing countries. The causes of acute MR include ischemic MR, endocarditis, chordal rupture, papillary muscle dysfunction, and a variety of diseases affecting prosthetic valves (Box 32.3). The most likely causes of acute MR in the critical care setting are ischemia, including acute myocardial infarction and infectious endocarditis, and should be considered in any patient who develops sudden hemodynamic decompensation in the peri-infarction period or who has known endocarditis. Chronic MR is secondary to a variety of structural, degenerative, connective tissue, inflammatory, and ischemic disorders, as well as congenital abnormalities outlined in Box 32.3.

The classic teaching has been that acute MR secondary to ischemia was caused by papillary muscle dysfunction, most likely secondary to ischemia of the posteromedial papillary muscle, which is dependent on a single blood supply from the right coronary artery. The anterolateral papillary muscle typically has dual circulation from the left anterior descending and circumflex coronary arteries, specifically from a diagonal branch and a circumflex marginal branch. The source of papillary muscle circulation is in fact variable, and on occasion the anterior papillary muscle also has a single blood supply.[113] The role of impaired circulation to the papillary muscle as the cause of ischemic MR has been revisited,[114] and evidence to date suggests that ischemic MR is secondary to alterations in ventricular geometry and leaflet tethering rather than dysfunction caused solely by impaired circulation to the papillary muscle during ischemia,[115] although alterations in papillary muscle geometry can be seen in chronic ischemic MR.[116] The hemodynamics of dynamic, ischemic MR are shown in Figure 32.12.

Box 32.3 Etiology of Acute and Chronic Mitral Insufficiency

Acute

Mitral Annular Disorders

Infective endocarditis (with abscess)
Trauma (e.g., valve surgery)
Paravalvular leak
  Surgical—suture interruption
  Infection

Mitral Leaflet Disorders

Infective endocarditis (with perforation or vegetation interfering with coaptation)
Trauma
Atrial myxoma
Myxomatous degeneration
Systemic lupus erythematosus (Libman-Sacks lesions)

Chordal Rupture

Spontaneous
Myxomatous degeneration
  Mitral valve prolapse
  Marfan syndrome
  Ehlers-Danlos syndrome
Infective endocarditis
Acute rheumatic fever
Trauma

Papillary Muscle Disorders

Coronary artery disease
Acute global left ventricular dysfunction
Infiltrative diseases (amyloidosis, sarcoidosis)
Trauma

Primary Mitral Valve Prosthetic Disorders

Bioprosthetic cusp perforation
Bioprosthetic cusp degeneration
Mechanical failure (e.g., strut fracture)
Immobilized disk or ball

Chronic

Inflammatory

Rheumatic heart disease
Systemic lupus erythematosus
Scleroderma

Degenerative

Myxomatous degeneration (mitral valve prolapse)
Marfan syndrome
Ehlers-Danlos syndrome
Pseudoxanthoma elasticum
Calcification of mitral valve annulus

Infective

Endocarditis

Structural

Ruptured chordae tendineae
Spontaneous secondary to:
  Myocardial infarction
  Trauma
  Mitral valve prolapse
  Endocarditis
  Rupture or dysfunction of papillary muscle (ischemia or infarction)
Dilation of mitral valve annulus and left ventricular cavity
  Congestive cardiomyopathies
  Aneurysmal dilation of the left ventricle
Hypertrophic cardiomyopathy
Paravalvular prosthetic leak

Congenital

Mitral valve clefts or fenestrations
Parachute mitral valve abnormality in association with other congenital disorders

From Otto C, Bonow RO: Valvular heart disease. In Libby P, Bonow RO, Mann DL, Zipes DP (eds): Braunwald's Heart Disease. A Textbook of Cardiovascular Medicine. Philadelphia, WB Saunders, 2008, p 1657.

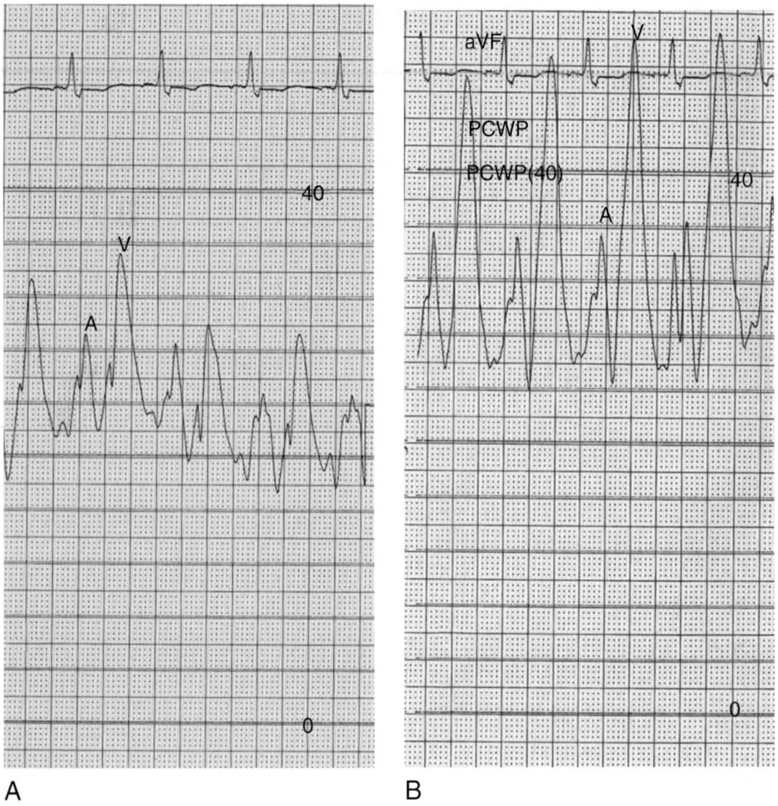

Figure 32.12 Dynamic mitral insufficiency in a patient with transient left ventricular dysfunction after recent acute myocardial infarction. The panel on the left demonstrates hemodynamics on a 40 mm Hg scale at baseline (**A**). Note elevated filling pressures at a mean of 24 mm Hg with V waves at average height of 32 mm Hg. The panel on the right (**B**) shows tracings recorded a few minutes later. Mean pulmonary capillary wedge pressure rose to 33 mm Hg with V waves to 48 mm Hg. A, A wave; PCWP, pulmonary capillary wedge pressure; V, V wave.

Analysis of thrombolysis in myocardial infarction data showed a 27% incidence of MR most commonly in the setting of anterior rather than inferior myocardial infarction, although these values vary widely by criteria and techniques used for screening, with the incidence ranging from 11% to 59%.[117] A Mayo Clinic review of more than 1300 acute myocardial infarction patients found moderate to severe MR in 12% and found it to be an independent predictor of both heart failure and survival.[118] It is associated with multivessel coronary artery disease, as well as prior infarction.[119]

Papillary muscle rupture is a rare but potentially catastrophic cause of flail leaflets and represents a surgical emergency.[120] In addition to the typical acute myocardial infarction setting, it may be secondary to trauma and isolated other causes such as postpartum Ehlers-Danlos syndrome.[121] Other causes of acute MR to consider (see Box 32.3) include spontaneous chordal rupture, infectious endocarditis with distortion of the valve leaflets or chordal rupture, and prosthetic valve dysfunction including paravalvular prosthetic valve leak. In patients with sudden onset of acute MR, retrograde flow is typically into a normal-sized and relatively noncompliant left atrium unless preexisting atrial hypertension has been present. The sudden volume loading immediately places the left atrium on the steep portion of its pressure-volume curve, which commonly causes acute pulmonary edema. As is the case with acute AI, the left ventricle is unable to adapt acutely and effective forward stroke volume is decreased. In the setting of myocardial infarction in particular, patients with acute MR may develop cardiogenic shock.

The classic hemodynamic response, a giant V wave, is shown in Figure 32.13. Differentiating a giant V wave from a prominent pulmonary artery pressure waveform can be difficult in the critical care setting, and repeated attempts to obtain a wedge pressure when the catheter is already in the wedge position may result in iatrogenic pulmonary artery hemorrhage.

DIAGNOSIS

PHYSICAL EXAMINATION

In acute MR the abrupt rise of left atrial pressure results from torrential retrograde flow, although the gradient between the left atrium and left ventricle may narrow substantially near the end of systole because of the substantial rise in left atrial pressure as shown in Figure 32.13. Thus the systolic murmur may decrease in intensity prior to the onset of the aortic second heart sound. A systolic thrill may be noted. The sudden and severe left atrial hypertension typically results in pulmonary edema with accompanying physical findings, as well as an increase in the pulmonic second sound and paradoxical splitting of the second heart sound. Because the adaptive mechanisms are not yet in place, features of LV volume overload are not seen, although a prominent precordial impulse, reflecting increased (albeit retrograde) ejection, may be noted. Unlike AI, the pulse pressure is not increased and may be reduced to reflect the lower forward stroke volume.

In chronic MR, precordial features of volume overload include a displaced point of maximal impulse and prominent precordial pulsation. An S_3 gallop is heard, especially

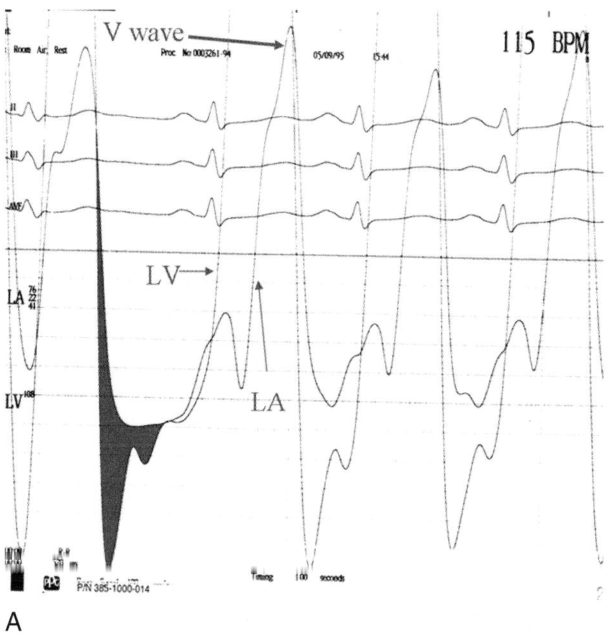

A

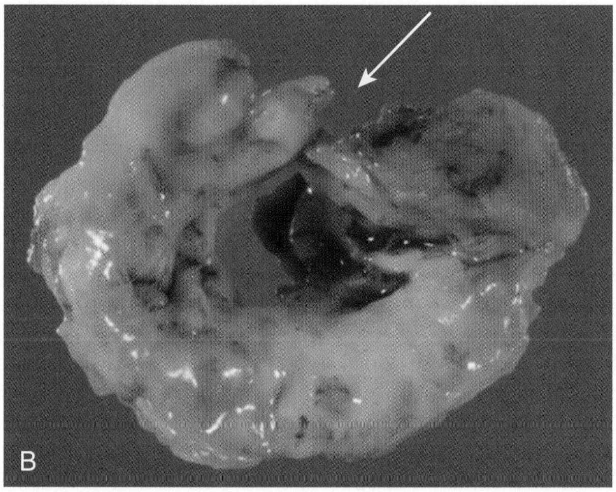

B

Figure 32.13 Hemodynamics (**A**) of severe MR (40 mm Hg scale) with giant V wave (to 70 mm Hg) late in systole. As LA pressure rises in acute severe mitral regurgitation, the gradient between the LV and LA pressure tracing is reduced and may result in a decrease in intensity of the murmur in late systole. The markedly thickened mitral valve (**B**) was excised from this patient after being torn *(arrow)* during balloon mitral commissurotomy. Elimination of mitral stenosis gradient *(area in A, filled in red)* is demonstrated. LA, left atrium; LV, left ventricle; MR, mitral valve insufficiency.

with marked dilation of the left ventricle,[88] and a diastolic flow murmur representing increased transvalvular flow (rather than mitral stenosis) may be present. The first heart sound may be soft, reflecting lack of brisk apposition of the mitral valve leaflets. The murmur of MR commences immediately following the first heart sound, reflecting the observation that a significant amount of regurgitation takes place during what would otherwise be isovolumic systole (which normally commences immediately following mitral valve closure). The murmur of chronic MR is characteristically blowing; may be medium or high pitched; is best heard at the apex; radiates to the axilla and left scapula (when severe); and extends throughout systole, reflecting the presence of a relatively high gradient throughout LV ejection.

The location of radiation can provide a clue to the affected leaflet: anteriorly directed jets result from posterior leaflet dysfunction, and conversely anterior leaflet prolapse results in a murmur best heard toward the patient's back. Because the Gallavardin phenomenon in AS mimics an MR murmur, it is important to differentiate these two when possible (AS and MR frequently occur concurrently, given the high LV systolic pressure with the former). The murmur of MR differs because it is holosystolic and increases rather than decreases with handgrip.

The intensity of the MR murmur reflects a number of phenomena relating to the size of the gradient, compliance of the left ventricle and left atrium, and contractility of the left ventricle but does not correlate well with extent of MR; thus, the murmur may be difficult to hear or inaudible, especially in the critical care setting.[122]

NONINVASIVE EVALUATION

Echocardiography provides visualization of the multiple structures responsible for causing MR including the valve leaflets, annulus, chordae tendineae papillary muscles, and left ventricle (see Fig. 32.11). Transesophageal echo provides superior imaging of the valve including assessment for vegetations in case endocarditis is suspected and better visualization of flail leaflets; it is particularly useful when the transthoracic views are incomplete or inadequate. In general, transesophageal echo is superior for fully assessing characteristics of the mitral regurgitant jet[123] and provides additional information in evaluating mitral valve morphology and motion. As with AI, Doppler methods allow assessment of the width of the regurgitant jet and size of the vena contracta, and semiquantitative measures of the regurgitant volume, regurgitant jet, and effective orifice area (see Table 32.1) are discussed in detail in Chapter 8. In patients presenting with acute heart failure and a hyperdynamic left ventricle, acute MR should always be considered.

CARDIAC CATHETERIZATION

Although the indications for cardiac catheterization (see Box 32.1) are similar to those for AS and AI, an additional consideration is included as a class I indication: to assess pulmonary artery pressures at rest and if necessary with exercise to evaluate appropriateness for surgery (see valve replacement indications later). The size of the V wave is not an accurate indicator of MR severity and is not used as a decision-making criterion for surgery because it may be unremarkable even in severe MR when there is high left atrial compliance. In addition, the size of the V wave is typically recorded by wedge rather than direct left atrial pressure, which can result in significant underestimation of the severity of MR (Fig. 32.14). Right heart catheterization and oxygen saturation sampling allow differentiation between the two most common causes of abrupt mechanical deterioration in acute MI: severe MR and ventricular septal defect. Both conditions can feature a large V wave because of sudden volume loading of a noncompliant left atrium: secondary to retrograde flow across the mitral valve in the case of acute MR and antegrade flow of shunted blood from the LV across the pulmonary circulation in the case of a ventricular septal defect.

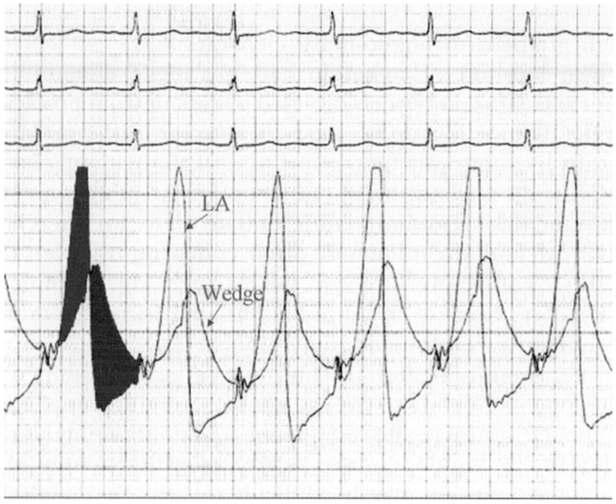

Figure 32.14 Underestimation of the left atrial V wave by pulmonary wedge pressure recording in the setting of severe mitral insufficiency (mitral regurgitation [MR]). The tracings show simultaneous left atrial and pulmonary artery wedge pressures in a patient with chronic severe MR because of paravalvular leak (40 mm Hg scale). The V wave on the wedge tracings is approximately 28 mm Hg, but on direct left atrial pressure the measurement obtained by transseptal puncture is 44 mm Hg. The gradients between wedge pressure and left atrial pressure during systole *(area filled in blue)* and during diastole *(area filled in red)* represent artifact because of damping and phase delay of pressure waveforms reflected across the pulmonary vascular bed. The effect of this damping is gross underestimation of the severity of the V wave and overestimation of any gradient between the left atrium (LA) and left ventricle; these in turn result in underestimation of severity of MR and overestimation of the severity of mitral stenosis when pulmonary wedge pressures are used. The mean of the two pressures is exactly the same.

THERAPY

MEDICAL MANAGEMENT

For acute, severe, symptomatic MR, the primary medical therapy consists of aggressive vasodilation with nitroprusside. It provides improved aortic flow, diminishes MR, and decreases left-sided filling pressures. In the setting of acute MR with shock, nitroprusside alone is usually considered undesirable because of poor end-organ perfusion if further hypotension is caused by the drug. Intra-aortic balloon pumping is highly effective in this setting[124] (see Chapter 7) because it lowers aortic impedance, improves cardiac output, and decreases regurgitant fraction at the same time as it restores blood pressure. A combination of an inotrope (typically dobutamine; a vasoconstrictor should be avoided) and nitroprusside can have similar salutary effects. When the acute MR is dynamic (i.e., occurs and resolves abruptly), the cause is frequently acute ischemia, and consideration should be given to evaluating the coronary circulation. In a small number of cases, acute coronary intervention has been documented to alleviate MR in the setting of acute ischemia.[125]

Therapy for chronic MR is more controversial. Because afterload is typically not increased, the benefits of afterload reduction are without clear physiologic foundation. As such, ACE inhibitors have consistently been shown not to be effective for chronic MR.[126-128] When concomitant systemic hypertension exists, physiologic benefits appear more convincing.[129] If patients have LV dysfunction superimposed on chronic MR, medical therapy with ACE inhibitors may be beneficial, and several studies have observed functional improvement with resychronization in this setting.[130] As with other valvular disorders, new-onset AF can result in abrupt hemodynamic deterioration and cardioversion should be considered with adjunctive pharmacotherapy to maintain sinus rhythm and rate control. Because of the sympathetic activation previously discussed, beta blockers appear to be beneficial[131,132] and may have additive benefit when used in combination with ACE inhibitors.[133] Both classes of drugs appear to be therapeutic when used after mitral valve repair.[134]

MITRAL VALVE SURGERY

Three types of surgeries are performed on the mitral valve: repair, replacement with preservation of the subvalvular apparatus and attachments, and replacement with transection of the chordae. Mitral valve repair has been consistently shown to improve outcomes compared with mitral valve replacement, both acutely and long term, with a fourfold lower operative mortality rate and a 30% improvement in 10-year survival rate.[135] With mitral valve replacement, patients who nevertheless have the chordal apparatus preserved have superior long-term outcomes compared with those who have the chords transected.[136] An additional benefit of repair is the avoidance of anticoagulation if patients are in sinus rhythm compared with replacement with a mechanical valve when anticoagulation is required.

In general, the timing of surgery for chronic MR should be prior to the onset of LV dysfunction. The most commonly used markers are symptoms and echocardiographic parameters including LVEF less than 60%.[5] Patients who develop class III or IV symptoms, even transiently, have a nearly 10-fold increase in annual mortality rate,[137] with evidence that early surgery in the setting of severe MR improves overall survival. The 60% threshold for surgery has been shown to correlate with postoperative LV function[138] as well as survival.[139] More recently the effective regurgitant orifice has been shown to be strongly predictive of 5-year mortality risk, with patients having an orifice of 40 mm^2 or greater having an odds ratio of death greater than 5:1 compared with patients with orifice size of 20 mm^2 or less.[140] Preoperative end-systolic diameter of 40 mm or less has also been associated with superior outcomes. Patients with AF in general have a worse prognosis,[141] although in large part because of embolic events rather than LV dysfunction, as do patients with pulmonary hypertension or right-sided heart failure, or both.[142] Mitral valve surgery, even in the setting of depressed EF, may result in postoperative return to normal function.[143] Comparison of long-term outcomes between operated and medically treated patients with asymptomatic MR has invariably favored the former,[140] although much of the data depend on nonrandomized registry data. In general, the key to improved function and outcomes is preserving the integrity of the submitral apparatus,[144] and comparison of successful repair versus replacement has indicated that high-volume institutions (>140 mitral operations/year) have the best results with nearly twice the rate of successful repair as low-volume institutions.[145]

A common teaching has been that repair or replacement of the mitral valve eliminates the "pop-off valve" represented by incompetent leaflets, resulting in dramatically increased afterload postoperatively. In turn, if significant preoperative LV dysfunction were present, the left ventricle would fail, with hemodynamic deterioration and subsequent death. In fact, careful investigation has demonstrated that postoperative deterioration of LV function was secondary to disruption of chordal integrity[146] and elimination of the favorable effects of the submitral apparatus on valvular-ventricular interaction rather than the elimination of a low-pressure decompression pathway. Afterload following mitral valve surgery with chordal transection does in fact increase, whereas patients subjected to mitral valve surgery with preservation of the chordal apparatus had decreased LV chamber volume and, in keeping with the LaPlace equation, reduced afterload.[147] Thus the recommendations regarding LVEF for surgery have changed dramatically, and successful repair of mitral valves in series of patients with EF less than 25% has been reported with operative risk of less than or equal to 5%.[148] The operative risk is in the 1% to 2% range for symptomatic patients with LV dysfunction but higher EF.[149] Similarly, the Society of Thoracic Surgeons database has reported mortality rates of approximately 5% with EF less than or equal to 30% but 3% with EF greater than 30%.[150] Propensity analysis of patients eligible for mitral valve repair who did or did not undergo the procedure has not shown a survival advantage in patients with mean EF less than 25%,[134] although a randomized trial has not been reported. Similarly, concomitant mitral valve surgery in patients undergoing coronary artery bypass graft (CABG) with moderate or greater MR did not clearly improve short-term survival.[151] Combining mitral valve surgery with a mesh placed around the heart to help prevent dilation and thus lower wall stress may have additional benefit for patients with MR and LV dysfunction.[149] Only in the setting of an EF of less than 30% or end-systolic dimension greater than 55 mm, as well as anatomy or surgical experience that suggests chordal preservation is unlikely, do the current guidelines recommend medical therapy alone.

In symptomatic acute severe MR, mitral valve surgery is a class I indication regardless of level of LV function. Both with infective endocarditis,[104] as well as with papillary muscle rupture, surgery is mandated to be performed with as little delay as possible.[152] However, the overall risk of mortality when MR accompanies acute myocardial infarction is substantially increased,[153] a phenomenon noted in patients undergoing emergent percutaneous intervention as well.[154] Chronic severe MR is much more complex, and the management algorithm is outlined in Figure 32.15.

FUTURE DIRECTIONS

A number of innovative technologies are being developed for percutaneous treatment of MR. The most extensively studied is based on a catheter-based edge-to-edge repair of the mitral leaflets designed to mimic a surgical procedure developed by Alfieri and colleagues.[155] The EVEREST (Endovascular Valve Edge-to-edge REpair STudy) II trial[156] compared 184 patients randomized to percutaneous versus 95 patients randomized to surgical mitral valve repair and had promising though somewhat nuanced results: although there was good safety profile and similar quality of life improvement, grade 2 or greater mitral insufficiency was present in nearly half the percutaneous repair patients at 1 year, compared with only 17% of the surgical repair patients. The surgical patients did have more adverse events, primarily blood transfusions. The surgical approach appeared clearly superior for patients with degenerative MR, with relative parity in outcomes in functional MR patients (those with structurally normal mitral valves, but typically dilatation of the mitral annulus). The Alfieri procedure is an uncommonly performed type of mitral valve repair, and as with most repair procedures typically involves placement of a prosthetic ring, an option not available with the percutaneous approach, and potentially a limitation of its long-term applicability as an isolated intervention.[157] In this context, it is worth noting that several percutaneous technologies are under development to constrict the coronary sinus that at least partially surrounds the mitral valve[158]; they thereby attempt to mimic the mechanical effects of a surgically placed mitral ring. For now, percutaneous edge-to-edge repair has had fair acceptance outside the United States and is being performed primarily in the setting of functional MR. A number of other technologies are under development.

HYPERTROPHIC OBSTRUCTIVE CARDIOMYOPATHY

Although a disease of the heart muscle rather than a primary valvular disorder, hypertrophic obstructive cardiomyopathy (HOCM) has important features of LV outflow obstruction and concomitant MR. The clinical presentation, physical examination, noninvasive and invasive findings, and overall management differ in general from AS or MR, and HOCM represents an important consideration for patients in critical care units,[159] where patients with a systolic murmur and hypotension, syncope, or exercise-induced cardiac arrest in particular should have HOCM included in the differential diagnosis.

PATHOPHYSIOLOGY

The hallmark of HOCM is dynamic obstruction of the LV outflow tract with eccentric hypertrophy; many variations exist, and obstruction is not always at the subvalvular level. Only approximately one fourth to one third of patients with hypertrophic cardiomyopathy (HCM) have a resting gradient of 30 mm Hg or greater.[160] HCM is found in approximately 0.2% of the population[161] and is defined as hypertrophy of the left ventricle that is not secondary to hypertrophic stimuli such as systemic hypertension or AS. Contrary to conventional wisdom, the majority of patients with HCM were found to have provokable gradients with exercise in a single large-volume center[162] (likely with some skewing from the nature of its referral population). The genetics of HCM have been studied extensively, and although complex, there is a familial association in a majority of patients. Although the clinical course may be generally benign in patients without risk factors for adverse events,[163] it is the most common cardiac cause of sudden death in young adults,[164] is associated with cardiac arrest in athletes,[165] and leads to heart failure, rhythm disturbances, and

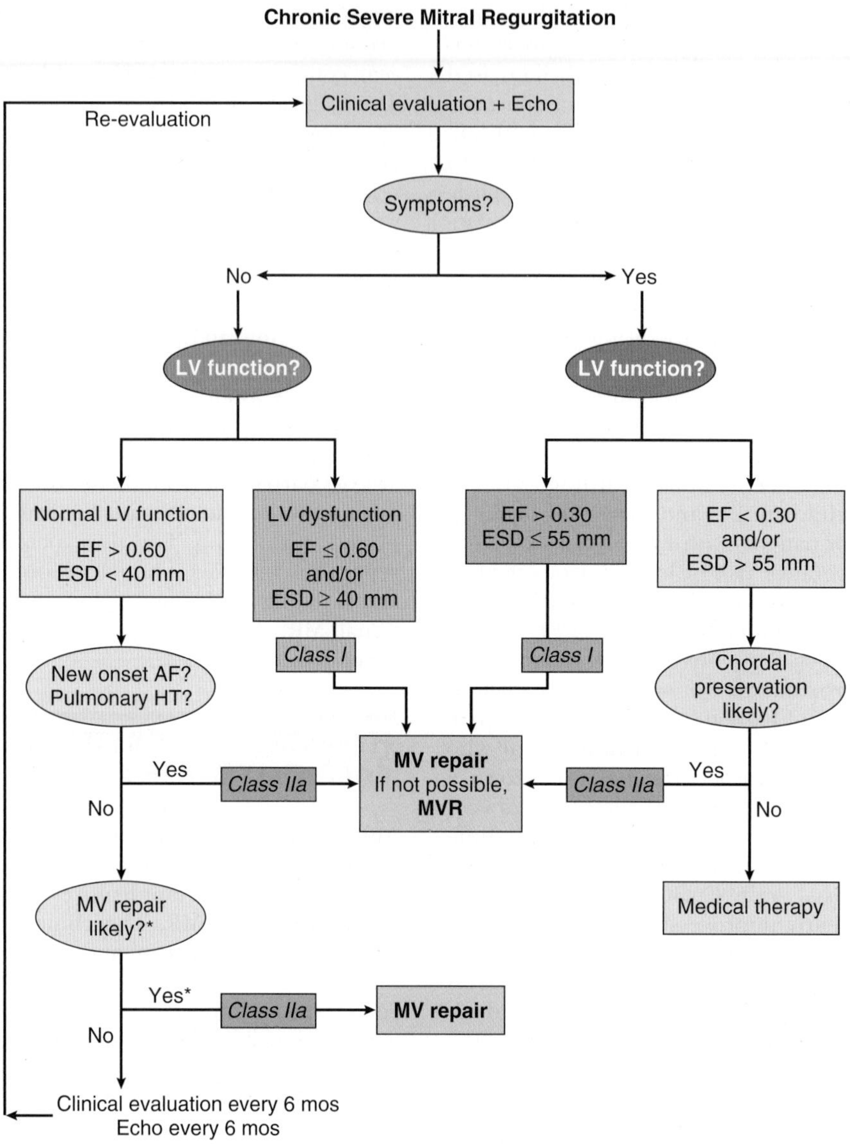

Figure 32.15 Algorithm for management of patients with chronic severe mitral regurgitation. *Mitral valve repair may be performed in asymptomatic patients with normal left ventricular (LV) function if performed by an experienced surgical team and if the likelihood of successful mitral valve (MV) repair is greater than 90%. AF, atrial fibrillation; EF, ejection fraction; ESD, end-systolic dimension; HT, hypertension; MVR, mitral valve replacement. (From Bonow RO, Carabello BA, Chatterjee K, et al: ACC/AHA 2006 guidelines for the management of patients with valvular heart disease: A report of the American College of Cardiology/American Heart Association Task Force on Practice Guidelines [writing committee to revise the 1998 guidelines for the management of patients with valvular heart disease] developed in collaboration with the Society of Cardiovascular Anesthesiologists and endorsed by the Society for Cardiovascular Angiography and Interventions and the Society of Thoracic Surgeons. J Am Coll Cardiol 2006;48:e1-148.)

occasional sudden death in older patients. The patients at high risk for sudden death, composing only about 10% to 20% of those within the HCM population, include those with prior cardiac arrest or sustained ventricular tachycardia, those with a family history of HCM and sudden death, hypotensive response to exercise, and severe LVH with wall thickness of 30 mm or greater.[166] A resting gradient across the outflow tract of more than 30 mm Hg alone predicts an increased risk of sudden death or development of moderate to severe congestive heart failure,[160] and there may be higher risk with very high gradients.[167] Because of impaired coronary flow reserve[168] and severe hypertrophy, myocardial ischemia is a potentially important factor in acute patient management; there is also an association between HOCM and myocardial coronary bridging.[169]

DIAGNOSIS

PHYSICAL EXAMINATION

The physical examination in HOCM features an abrupt early rise in systolic pressure followed by obstruction to LV outflow, resulting in a blunted pressure rise later in systole. This translates to the spike and dome pattern characteristic of HOCM on palpation of the carotid pulse. The typically hypertrophic septum (1.3 to 1.5 times the thickness of the posterior wall and typically 18 mm or greater in clinically significant HOCM) obstructs the outflow tract after initial ejection as LV volume decreases. Physiologic maneuvers or clinical states that lower LV volume abruptly such as standing, dehydration, or use of diuretics can substantially exacerbate the gradient and increase the intensity of the systolic ejection murmur characteristic of HOCM. Because the obstruction begins after the initial brisk ejection of blood from the ventricle, the onset of murmur is late after the first heart sound. It is best heard over the left base of the heart. In contrast to AS, the murmur typically does not radiate to the carotids, does not extend throughout systole, and decreases with squatting. The blunting of the carotid upstroke, so characteristic of AS, is not seen because of the vigorous early ejection.

NONINVASIVE EVALUATION

Abnormalities of mitral valve function are common. Systolic anterior motion of the mitral valve is associated with further obstruction[170]; in addition, MR is a typical secondary finding in HOCM. The ECG features LV hypertrophy, strain, and prominent Q waves in the inferior and precordial leads, with narrow QRS complexes being common. The echocardiogram is diagnostic for HOCM, providing both an anatomic basis and physiologic evidence of the degree of obstruction (Fig. 32.16).

CARDIAC CATHETERIZATION

Cardiac catheterization in HOCM may reveal the standard triad of the Brockenbrough-Braunwald-Morrow sign in the postextrasystolic heartbeat: increase in the gradient between the left ventricle and the aorta, decrease in systemic blood pressure, and narrowing of the pulse pressure (Fig. 32.17). Other stimuli that increase outflow obstruction and increase gradient are Valsalva maneuver and amyl nitrite inhalation, in addition to postextrasystolic potentiation.

THERAPY

MEDICAL MANAGEMENT

The management of critically ill patients with HOCM focuses on several core principles: optimizing LV volumes, specifically increasing preload while not decreasing afterload, decreasing contractility, and maintaining the patient in sinus rhythm. Thus the typical regimen of diuretics, vasodilators, and inotropes used in most patients presenting with congestive heart failure who do not have HOCM can severely exacerbate the outflow gradient and lead to further decompensation or death[171] (as can intra-aortic balloon pumping); somewhat counterintuitively in this setting, negative inotropes, in particular beta blockers, combined with volume loading can stabilize patients.[172,173] Other negative inotropes including verapamil and disopyramide appear to have favorable hemodynamic effects and may represent an alternative to beta blockade.[174] In the patient in shock, if vasopressors are required, agents such as phenylephrine, which are primarily peripheral vasoconstrictors, should be used rather than inotropic agents. Verapamil has negative inotropic benefits and some utility as an antiarrhythmic agent, as well as diastolic relaxation properties, and has been used successfully in both chronic therapy and acutely decompensated patients with HOCM.[175] Verapamil does have some potentially undesirable vasodilator properties

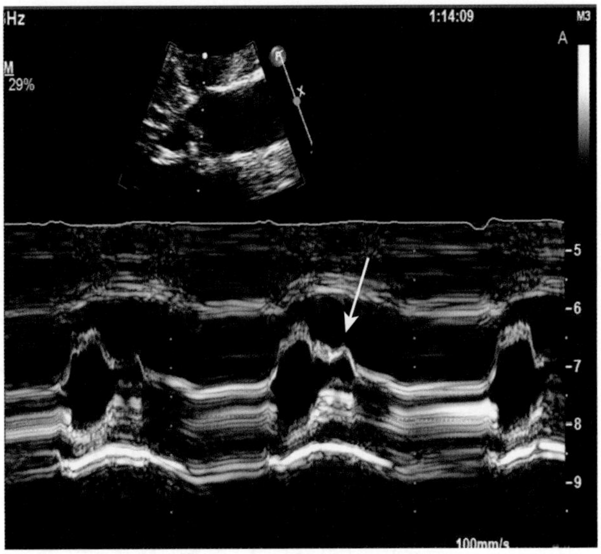

A

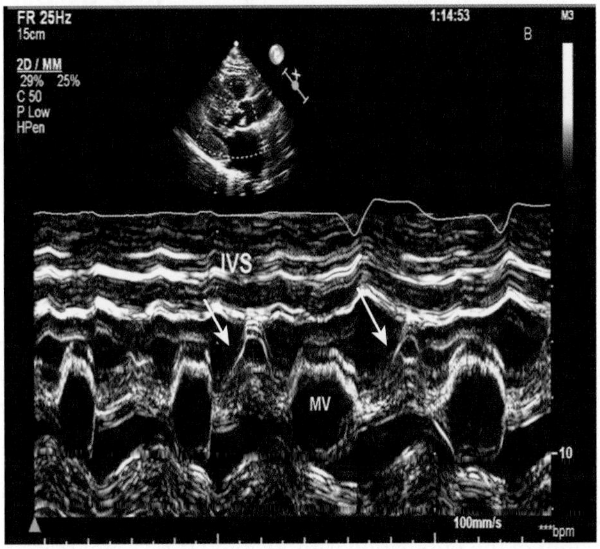

B

Figure 32.16 **A,** M-mode of hypertrophic obstructive cardiomyopathy with aortic valve opening showing the effect of midsystolic outflow obstruction; after initial normal opening, the aortic valve leaflets remain only partially separated because of diminished transvalvular flow *(arrow)*. **B,** Systolic anterior motion of the anterior mitral leaflet with apposition against outflow tract *(arrows)*. The severely hypertrophied septum on two-dimensional view is shown at the top of each panel.

and can cause synergistic depression of conduction and contractility in combination with beta blockade; the effects of combined therapy, if used, should be monitored closely.[176]

Patients with hypertrophic heart disease are highly dependent on the atrial contribution to cardiac output,[177] and patients with obstruction in particular depend on the additional LV filling from atrial contraction. AF is a cause of acute decompensation in HOCM patients, and cardioversion should be considered acutely. AF occurred in approximately one fourth of patients with HCM followed for 9 years and is predictive of heart failure–related death and stroke.[178] In terms of the latter, patients with HCM and

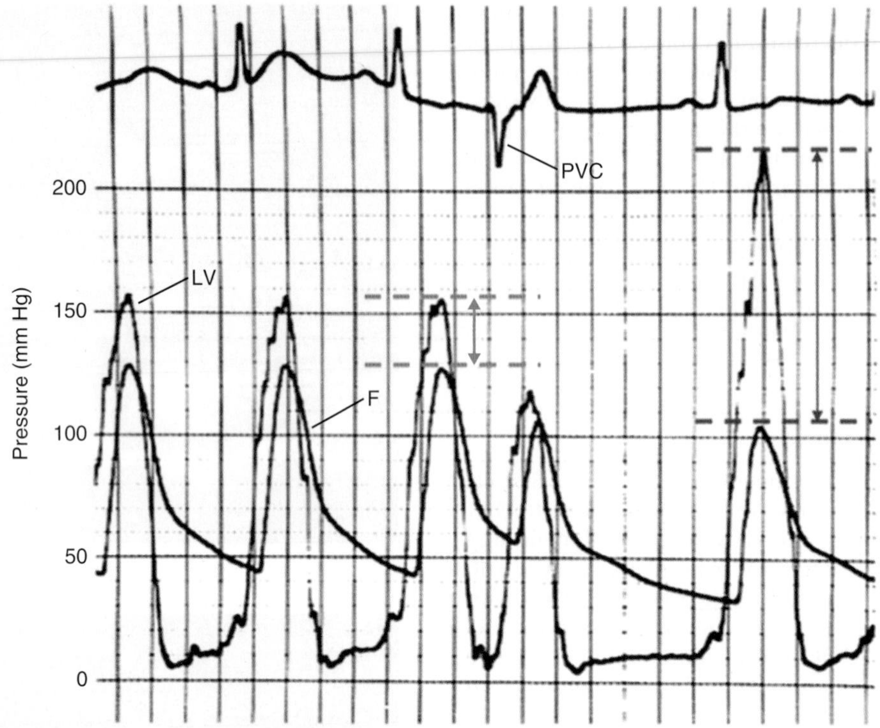

Figure 32.17 The Brockenbrough-Braunwald-Morrow sign. Dramatic exaggeration of the resting gradient in the postextrasystolic beat, with lower systemic pressure, and narrowed pulse pressure (difference between femoral systolic and diastolic pressure) are demonstrated—all hallmarks of dynamic outflow obstruction. *Dashed lines* represent left ventricle (LV) and aortic systolic pressures at rest *(green)* and after a premature ventricular contraction (PVC) *(red);* the gradient rises from a basal 30 mm Hg *(double-sided green arrow)* to approximately 130 mm Hg *(double-sided red arrow).* (Modified from Pollock SG: Pressure tracings in obstructive cardiomyopathy. N Engl J Med 1994;331:238.)

AF appear particularly predisposed to thromboembolic events[179]; anticoagulation has been shown to reduce the incidence significantly.[180] Left atrial size and function predict the onset of AF.[181] The Maze procedure and catheter ablation of left atrial pathways have been used successfully in small series to prevent recurrent AF.[182,183] Amiodarone has been particularly effective for the maintenance of sinus rhythm in the population with AF and HCM[184] and may also have additional efficacy in preventing sudden death in patients with episodes of nonsustained ventricular tachycardia.[185,186] Ventricular fibrillation appears to be the primary cause of sudden death and can be prevented with implantable defibrillators for either primary or secondary prevention, with activation of the devices in 5% to 11% of patients annually depending on indications for placement[187]; episodes of sustained ventricular tachycardia and a history of prior sudden death place patients in the highest risk category.

PERCUTANEOUS INTERVENTION OR SURGERY

Once patients develop refractory symptoms despite pharmacologic management and have significant obstruction to LV outflow, surgical myomectomy or alcohol septal ablation must be considered. The choice is controversial and depends on LV and coronary anatomy, comorbid conditions, severity of coexistent mitral valve or other potentially surgical heart disease, and a variety of other clinical issues; equivalence of outcomes with the less invasive percutaneous approach has not been demonstrated.[188] Typical thresholds for intervention are a resting peak instantaneous gradient of 50 mm Hg or more, although depending on degree of symptoms and provokability, a variety of other thresholds have been applied.[166] Mitral valve replacement can frequently be avoided, especially in patients without intrinsic mitral disease, in whom MR is largely abolished by myomectomy and relief of the outflow gradient.[189] In patients with intrinsic mitral valve disease or for a variety of other anatomic considerations, mitral valve surgery including use of low-profile prostheses is used.[166] Dual-chamber pacing, once considered therapeutically effective,[190] with theoretical benefit from asynchronous septal contraction and secondary reduction in outflow tract gradient, has not been shown to have clear therapeutic benefit in randomized clinical trials, with the most likely functional benefits occurring in a limited subset of elderly patients.[191]

MITRAL VALVE STENOSIS

Mitral valve stenosis (MS) is primarily a rheumatic disorder and, as such, has become increasingly uncommon in industrialized nations. Nevertheless, the disease remains prevalent in developing countries and a small but significant number of patients continue to present in the critical care setting throughout the world. Rheumatic MS involves disease of both the valve leaflets and submitral apparatus and may involve the valve ring as well (Fig. 32.18). Although MS is primarily caused by rheumatic deformity and scarring of the valve leaflets and subvalve with fusion of the commissures, a variety of disorders result in leaflet and annular calcification that also create obstruction between the left atrium and left ventricle. Most notably, mitral annular calcification, present in 6% of patients undergoing routine echocardiography,[192] is more prevalent in the elderly, women, smokers, and patients on dialysis (who have high parathyroid hormone levels). It may present with severe nonrheumatic mitral stenosis, although MR is a more common association.[192,193] A variety of uncommon other causes account for less than 1% of cases of MS.[194]

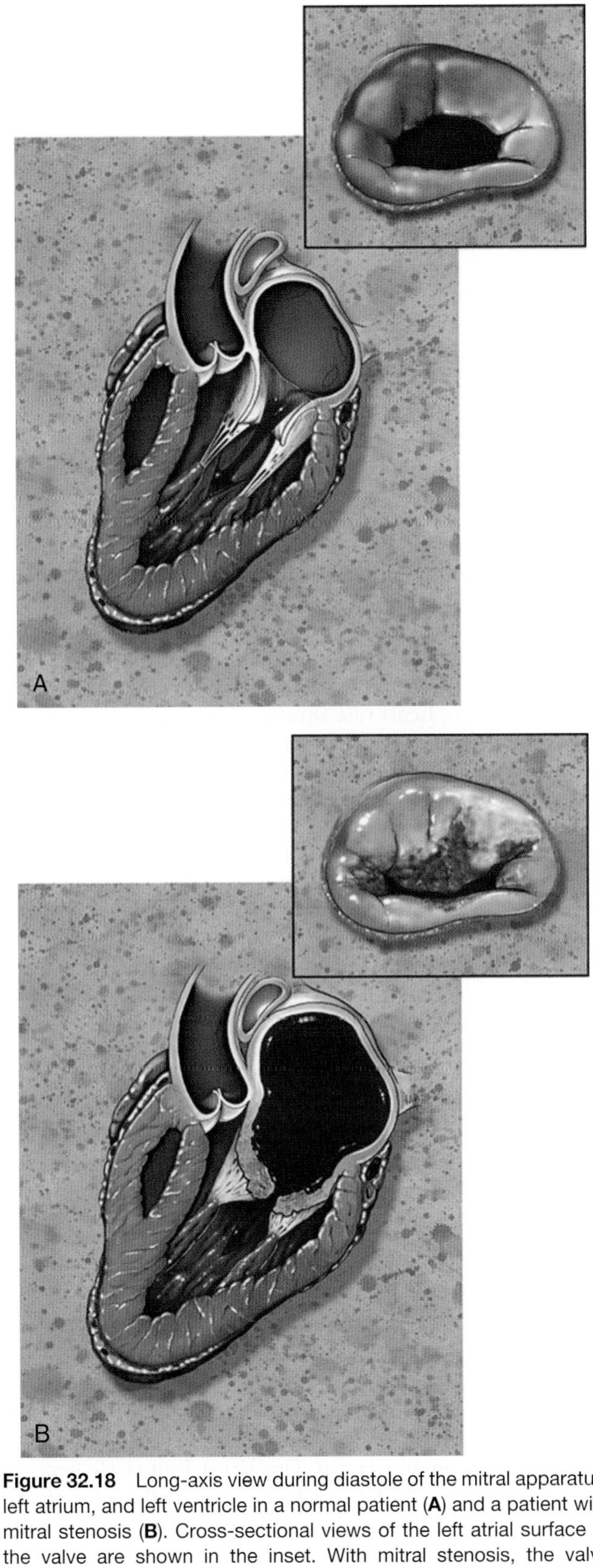

Figure 32.18 Long-axis view during diastole of the mitral apparatus, left atrium, and left ventricle in a normal patient (**A**) and a patient with mitral stenosis (**B**). Cross-sectional views of the left atrial surface of the valve are shown in the inset. With mitral stenosis, the valve opening is restricted with a characteristic doming appearance, the commissures are fused, the leaflets are thickened, the subvalvular apparatus is deformed, and some calcification is noted. The left atrium is enlarged. (From Turi ZG: Cardiology patient page. Mitral valve disease. Circulation 2004;109:e38-e41.)

PATHOPHYSIOLOGY

The physiologic hallmark of MS is obstruction to left atrial outflow resulting in rising left atrial and pulmonary pressures (the extent of the latter depends to a significant degree on left atrial compliance). The normal mitral valve is in the range of 4 to 6 cm^2, and patients typically do not become symptomatic until valve areas decrease significantly below 2 cm^2 (see Table 32.1). As valve area decreases, an additional pressure gradient is required to maintain transvalvular flow (see Fig. 32.5). Because antegrade flow is entirely during diastole, and the diastolic filling period shortens or lengthens disproportionately with increase or decrease in heart rate. respectively, the gradient is highly flow dependent. In MS, as with virtually all valvulopathies, cardiac output is potentially highly dependent on maintenance of sinus rhythm; because the influence on cardiac output is exaggerated by the need for active left atrial pumping across a stenotic orifice, atrial contraction is particularly important in MS. A frequent mode of presentation is acute congestive heart failure in a patient with MS who suddenly develops AF; the concomitant loss of atrial contraction and high ventricular rate with short diastolic filling period frequently results in pulmonary edema.

DIAGNOSIS

PHYSICAL EXAMINATION

The diagnosis of MS on physical examination is frequently missed, in part because it is uncommonly seen by most practitioners outside developing countries. Besides findings suggestive of congestive heart failure with a low output in the critical care setting, several findings correlate strongly with MS. A right ventricular lift may occur in patients with advanced and chronic pulmonary hypertension, and occasionally a palpable pulmonary second sound is felt. Both S_1 and P_2 are increased early in the course of the disease; with progressive deformity of the subvalvular apparatus, S_1 may become quite soft as mitral valve closure velocity decreases. The opening snap is preserved until the end stages of MS, and the severity of the disease correlates inversely with the length of time between S_2 and the opening snap. The diastolic rumble may not be heard if the patient is not placed in the lateral decubitus position and is difficult to hear in the critical care setting. Presystolic accentuation is the result of increased flow in late diastole caused by atrial contraction in patients in sinus rhythm. The diagnosis is often missed in both the outpatient and critical care settings,[195] and patients are sometimes treated for years for bronchitis, pneumonia, or asthma, when in fact the presentation is congestive heart failure with the underlying disease process being MS.

NONINVASIVE EVALUATION

The echocardiogram is the primary tool for diagnosis of MS. The typical hockey stick appearance of the rheumatic anterior mitral leaflet is caused by partial restriction of mobility (Fig. 32.19). Other important characteristics of the mitral leaflets are degree of thickening, mobility, and calcification, all of which, along with extent of subvalvular disease, help to address suitability for balloon dilation or commissurotomy rather than valve replacement.[196] It is important to differentiate rheumatic MS from severe nonrheumatic MS, as shown in Figure 32.19. Transesophageal echo provides the requisite sensitivity to detect left atrial thrombus prior to balloon commissurotomy or cardioversion. Severity of mitral stenosis is graded by physiologic and anatomic criteria: The former depend on Doppler interrogation of transvalvular flow, with peak velocity used to estimate the gradient; rate of decompression of the left atrial pressure, or pressure half time, correlates inversely with valve area. The valve area is frequently directly measured using planimetry of a cross-sectional view. Because these methods have potential for error, a number of alternative methodologies have been proposed,[197-199] although there is no agreement on a gold standard.[200] As with AS, a dramatic increase in gradient accompanies increased flow related to exercise or dobutamine infusion[201] (Figs. 32.20 and 32.21). Cardiac catheterization may be required if the noninvasive data are inconclusive; there is a tendency for the pulmonary wedge pressure/LV gradient to overestimate the severity of MS compared with left atrial/LV gradient measurement[202] (Fig. 32.22). Cardiac catheterization can also be used to assess pulmonary artery pressures and response to exercise if the clinical and noninvasive pictures are discordant.[5]

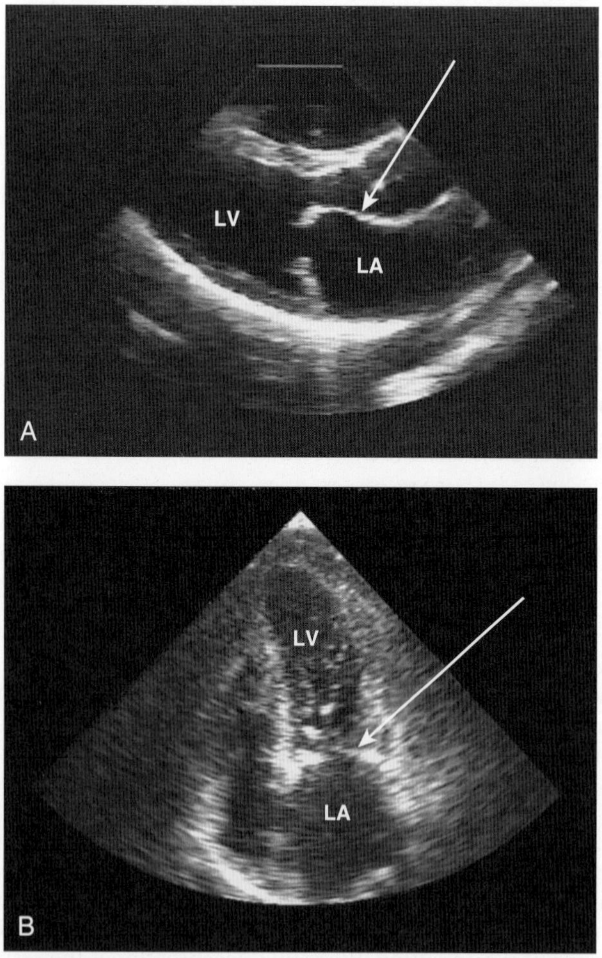

Figure 32.19 Two appearances of stenotic mitral valves. **A,** The parasternal long axis view shows typical rheumatic deformity with a hockey stick appearance of the anterior mitral leaflet *(arrow)*. **B,** The four-chamber view is from a patient with a significant gradient across the mitral orifice; this patient was on dialysis, did not have rheumatic heart disease, and demonstrated significant calcification of the mitral leaflets and annulus *(arrow)*. LA, left atrium; LV, left ventricle.

THERAPY

MEDICAL THERAPY

Medical therapy specifically aimed at improving hemodynamics in MS is basically twofold: slowing the heart rate and anticoagulation. In sinus rhythm, beta blockade is the preferred therapy; patients with significant bronchospasm or with coexistent, usually secondary, severe pulmonary hypertension with or without right-sided heart failure may not tolerate beta blockers. Diltiazem or low doses of beta blocker combined with diltiazem or verapamil are sometimes used in this setting. With combined therapy, care should be exercised that severe heart rate slowing or atrioventricular block does not occur, and verapamil may not be tolerated in right-sided heart failure. For the acutely decompensated patient with MS, diuretics, nitrates, inotropes (preferably agents that do not raise heart rate), and, to a lesser degree, arterial vasodilator therapy may all be beneficial.

Approximately 30% of patients with MS are thought to develop AF, with the risk increased by progressive increase in left atrial size. The risk of embolic events, especially stroke, is substantially higher than in AF patients without MS[203] (up to 15% in unanticoagulated patients), possibly in part because of a hypercoagulopathy and increased platelet activation associated with MS,[204] making the use of anticoagulation essential. It is not uncommon for the presenting finding to be an embolic event in a previously undiagnosed MS patient. Even in the setting of sinus rhythm,[5] if spontaneous echo contrast is seen in the MS patient or left atrial size is greater than 55 mm, anticoagulation may decrease stroke risk[204] and it should also be used in the sinus rhythm patient with prior embolic event or with left atrial thrombus detected by transesophageal echocardiography.

In the setting of new-onset AF and acute decompensation, cardioversion should be considered. Regardless of chronicity, heart rate slowing is essential; digoxin, beta blockers, diltiazem, or verapamil alone or in combination may be beneficial. Rate control only at rest is inadequate; many patients with low resting heart rates become tachycardic with minimal exercise. This is a vicious circle because the tachycardia may be a response to inadequate stroke volume; the tachycardia then lowers the diastolic filling period and further exacerbates the gradient. Control of tachycardia is important beyond its hemodynamic benefit; it also helps avoid tachycardia-induced cardiomyopathy.[205]

PERCUTANEOUS INTERVENTION OR SURGERY

Percutaneous balloon mitral valvuloplasty is equivalent or superior to surgery in patients with favorable valve

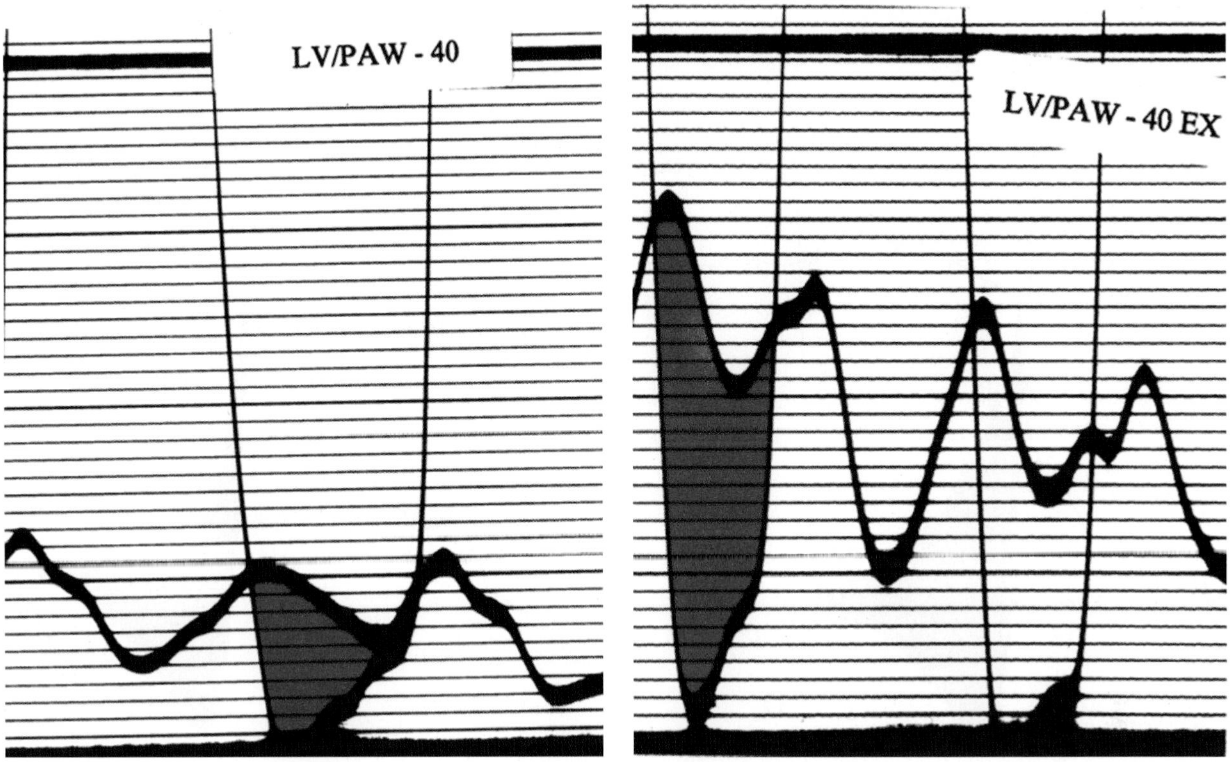

A B

Figure 32.20 Effect of exercise and increased heart rate on mitral valve gradient *(red)* in a patient with mitral valve stenosis (40 mm Hg scale). The left tracing (**A**) shows a mean gradient of approximately 5 mm Hg with diastasis late in diastole; with increased heart rate and cardiac output (**B**), the gradient rose to a mean of approximately 20 mm Hg, a fourfold increase. LV, left ventricle; PAW, pulmonary artery wedge.

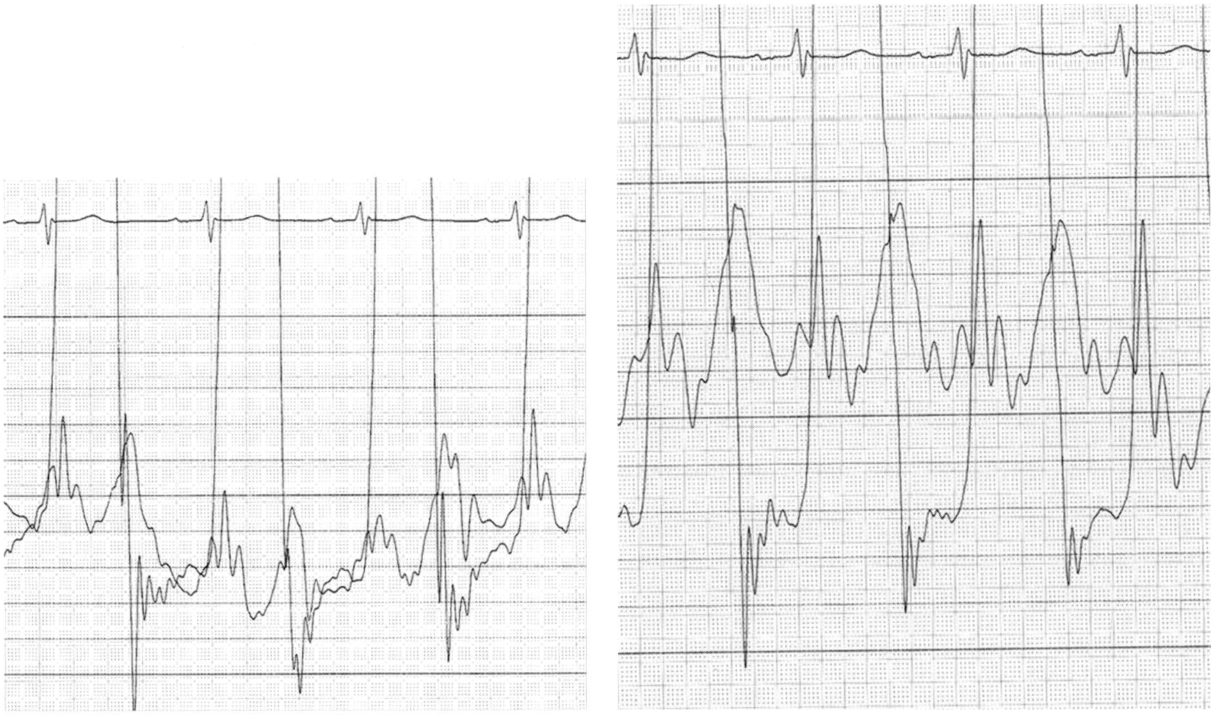

A B

Figure 32.21 Effect of dobutamine infusion on transmitral valve gradient (40 mm Hg scale). Effect in a patient whose gradient was nearly abolished at rest (**A**) and was augmented dramatically with infusion of dobutamine (**B**).

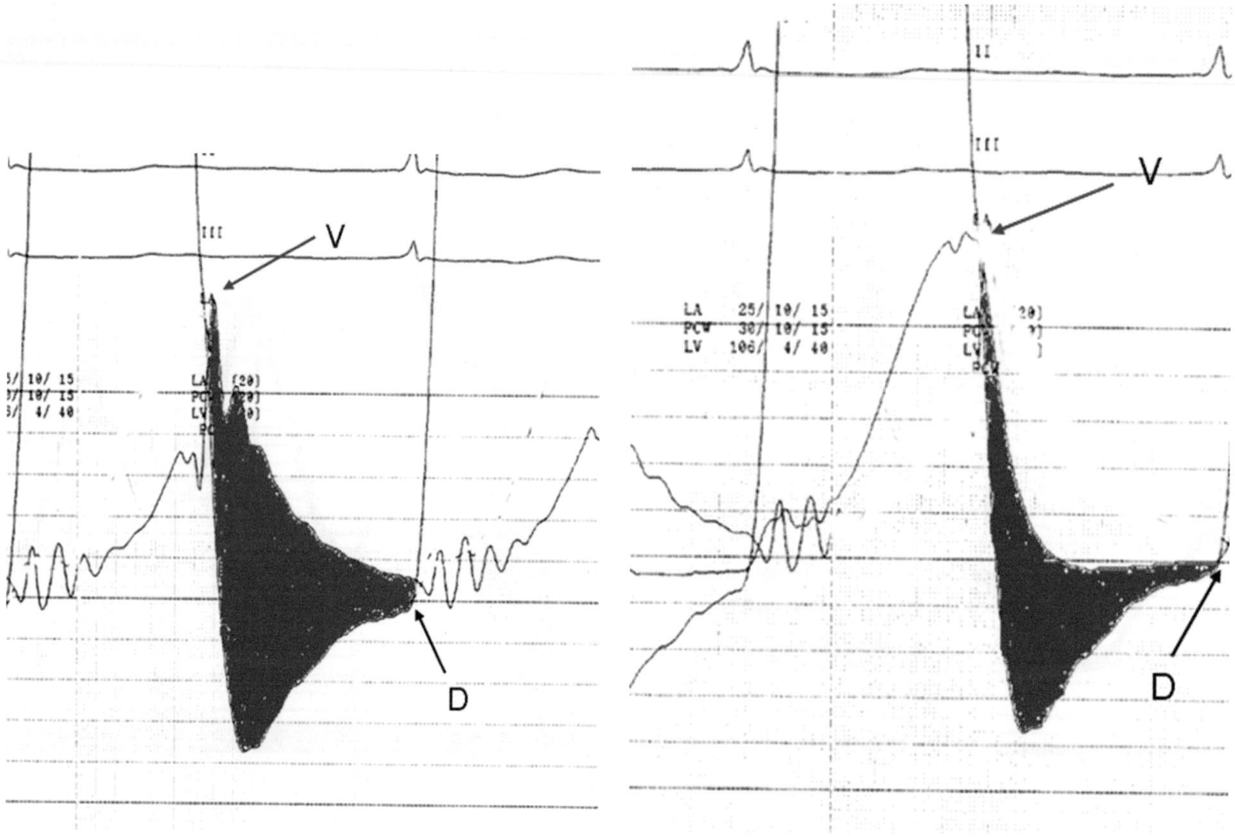

Figure 32.22 Effect of using pulmonary wedge pressure (**A**) or direct left atrial pressure (**B**) to assess gradient (*in red*) between the left atrium and left ventricle in mitral stenosis (40 mm Hg scale). Using the wedge pressure, the gradient appears to be approximately twice as great as when left atrial pressure is used. Rapid decompression of left atrial pressure is shown in the tracing on the right. The findings are consistent with mixed mitral stenosis and regurgitation, with the dominant physiology being secondary to mitral insufficiency. In both tracings, diastasis (D) is noted by end diastole, a feature not consistent with severe mitral stenosis except in marked bradycardia. The V wave height is similar in both tracings, unlike in Figure 32.12. The two tracings shown here were recorded a few seconds apart.

anatomy,[206,207] characterized by mild to moderate impairment of leaflet mobility, valve thickness, valve calcification, and subvalvular disease, the components of the Wilkins-Weyman echo score.[208] The scoring system has been shown to correlate with long-term outcomes.[209] Surgery should be reserved for patients with unfavorable anatomy, more than mild MR, or persistent thrombus in the left atrium despite anticoagulation.[5] The threshold for percutaneous or surgical intervention is a mitral valve area of 1.5 cm^2 or less. If patients are symptomatic and have favorable anatomy or if they are asymptomatic but have pulmonary hypertension (>50 mm Hg systolic at rest or >60 mm Hg with exercise), they have class I indications. Patients who have unfavorable anatomy and are functional class III or IV are considered to have a class II indication, especially if they are poor candidates for surgery. Asymptomatic patients with new-onset AF and favorable anatomy and symptomatic patients with mild MS (valve area >1.5 cm^2) who have pulmonary artery pressure greater than 60 mm Hg, wedge pressure 25 mm Hg or greater, or gradient 15 mm Hg or greater during exercise are also considered class II candidates.[5]

KEY POINTS

- Valvular heart disease in the critical care setting ranges from the primary cause of acute decompensation to a comorbid condition of varying degrees of clinical significance.
- Valvulopathy affects not only valve anatomy but also cardiac structure and function and overall hemodynamics; it is essential to consider all four elements in diagnosis and management.
- AS in the critical care setting requires careful titration of need to maintain cardiac output, avoid hypotension, and replace the aortic valve early if AS is the primary cause of symptoms.
- Low-gradient, low-output AS requires increasing cardiac contractility or transvalvular flow, or both, to differentiate severe AS from primary myocardial dysfunction.
- Acute aortic and mitral insufficiency in the decompensated patient benefits from vasodilator

KEY POINTS (Continued)

therapy; vasodilator treatment of chronic aortic and mitral insufficiency in asymptomatic patients does not have the benefit of a compelling evidence base.

- Intra-aortic balloon counterpulsation is useful in hemodynamically decompensated MR patients, is of some benefit in severely ill AS patients, but is contraindicated with HOCM and particularly in patients with AI.
- AF exacerbates hemodynamic deterioration in valvulopathies; if left atrial size is less than 6 cm and thrombus is not present, cardioversion and maintenance of sinus rhythm are highly beneficial.
- There are now only limited indications for prophylactic therapy with antibiotics for endocarditis prevention for the valvulopathies described in this chapter,[210] primarily the presence of prosthetic cardiac valves and a history of previous infectious endocarditis.

ACKNOWLEDGMENT

The author wishes to acknowledge Priscilla Peters for kindly providing Figures 32.10, 32.16, and 32.19.

SELECTED REFERENCES

5. Bonow RO, Carabello BA, Chatterjee K, et al: ACC/AHA 2006 guidelines for the management of patients with valvular heart disease: A report of the American College of Cardiology/American Heart Association Task Force on Practice Guidelines (writing Committee to Revise the 1998 guidelines for the management of patients with valvular heart disease) developed in collaboration with the Society of Cardiovascular Anesthesiologists endorsed by the Society for Cardiovascular Angiography and Interventions and the Society of Thoracic Surgeons. J Am Coll Cardiol 2006;48(3):e1-148.

15. Freeman RV, Otto CM: Spectrum of calcific aortic valve disease: Pathogenesis, disease progression, and treatment strategies. Circulation 2005;111(24):3316-3326.

66. Smith CR, Leon MB, Mack MJ, et al: Transcatheter versus surgical aortic-valve replacement in high-risk patients. N Engl J Med 2011;364(23):2187-2198.

67. Leon MB, Smith CR, Mack M, et al: Transcatheter aortic-valve implantation for aortic stenosis in patients who cannot undergo surgery. N Engl J Med 2010;363(17):1597-1607.

95. Miller RR, Vismara LA, DeMaria AN, et al: Afterload reduction therapy with nitroprusside in severe aortic regurgitation: Improved cardiac performance and reduced regurgitant volume. Am J Cardiol 1976;38(5):564-567.

97. Evangelista A, Tornos P, Sambola A, et al: Long-term vasodilator therapy in patients with severe aortic regurgitation. N Engl J Med 2005;353(13):1342-1349.

102. Tornos P, Sambola A, Permanyer-Miralda G, et al: Long-term outcome of surgically treated aortic regurgitation: Influence of guideline adherence toward early surgery. J Am Coll Cardiol 2006;47(5):1012-1017.

135. Enriquez-Sarano M, Schaff HV, Orszulak TA, et al: Valve repair improves the outcome of surgery for mitral regurgitation. A multivariate analysis. Circulation 1995;91(4):1022-1028.

159. Chockalingam A, Dorairajan S, Bhalla M, Dellsperger KC: Unexplained hypotension: The spectrum of dynamic left ventricular outflow tract obstruction in critical care settings. Crit Care Med 2009;37(2):729-734.

203. Carabello BA: Modern management of mitral stenosis. Circulation 2005;112(3):432-437.

The complete list of references can be found at www.expertconsult.com.

33 Acute Aortic Dissection

Frank Bowen | R. Phillip Dellinger

CHAPTER OUTLINE

INTRODUCTION

Thoracic aortic dissection (TAD) occurs with communication between the thoracic aorta lumen and wall with a separation of the thoracic aortic wall layers. Thoracic aortic dissection is to be contrasted with thoracic aortic aneurysm (TAA), which is defined as dilation of the thoracic aorta to a diameter of ≥1.5 times normal. Thoracic aortic aneurysm is a risk factor for TAD. Thoracic aortic aneurysm, although an important morbidity that may be associated with acute catastrophic leakage and death, is in and of itself not the acute emergency that is signified by a TAD. The international registry of acute aortic dissection reported an overall mortality of 27.4% with this condition. Surgical mortality was 26% for proximal (type A dissection) versus 58% for medical management and for distal (type B dissection), with 10.7% for medical management and 31% for surgical management.[1]

HISTORY

In 1819, Laenec introduced "aortic dissection" into the medical literature when he described an intimal tear distal to the aortic valve associated with a longitudinal space in the aortic wall postmortem.[2] An autopsy report in 1760 described aortic dissection and pericardial tamponade as the causes of death of King George II.[3] In 1863, Peacock reported a summary of findings in 80 patients with aortic dissection and classified the disease into three stages: intimal tear, propagation of the dissection with the potential for rupture, and recanalization of the lumen.[4] In 1896, Marfan described the aortic connective tissue abnormality now known to be associated with this entity.[5] In 1955, DeBakey treated a descending thoracic aortic dissection with resection and reapproximation of dissected layers with graph interposition.[6] In 1963, DeBakey and colleagues repaired an ascending aortic dissection complicated by aortic valvular insufficiency.[7]

TYPES OF TAD

The thoracic aorta is divided anatomically into the ascending portion, the transverse portion, and the descending portion.[8] The ascending aorta has two sections, the aortic root (valvular annulus and sinuses) and the tubular portion extending to the origin of the innominate artery. The transverse portion of the aorta is a short segment, and the brachiocephalic arteries come off this portion of the aorta. The descending thoracic aorta begins immediately distal to the left subclavian artery and extends to the diaphragm. The anatomic location of TAD has important clinical and prognostic implications. The most commonly used classification scheme for TAD is the Stanford System (Fig. 33.1), which has mostly replaced the first classification system, the DeBakey System (see Fig. 33.1). An advantage of the DeBakey System is that it does distinguish between dissections that are confined only to the ascending aorta (DeBakey type 2) and dissections that involve the entire aorta (DeBakey type 1). Using the Stanford System, which is more simplistic, any involvement of the ascending aorta classifies the dissection as a Stanford A, whereas lack of ascending aorta involvement classifies the dissection as a Stanford type B.

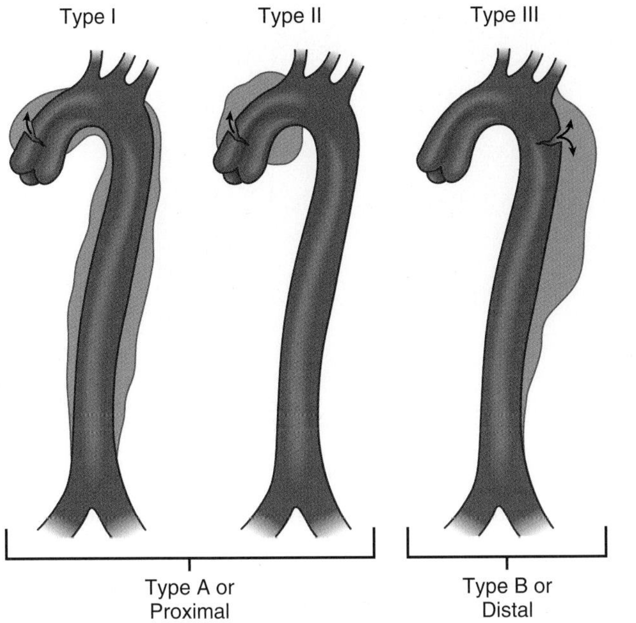

Figure 33.1 Pictorial representation of DeBakey 1, 2, and 3 as well as Stanford A and B classification of thoracic aortic aneurysms. (Used with permission. Braunwald E: Heart Disease: Textbook of Cardiovascular Medicine, 9th ed. Boston, WB Saunders.)

RISK FACTORS FOR THORACIC AORTIC DISSECTION

Multiple risk factors for TAD have been identified.[8] Men are at greater risk for developing TAD than women; approximately two thirds of patients with TAD are male.[9] The sex distribution is consistent across different classifications of aortic dissection. Women with TAD are more likely than men to have a history of hypertension. Women are older at the time of diagnosis of TAD when compared to men. The average age at diagnosis of TAD is 65 years and is younger for type A TAD than for type B TAD.[8] Specific risk factors for TAD are shown in Table 33.1. It is thought that the higher the blood pressure, the greater the probability of aortic dissection. In the presence of coarctation of the aorta, acute dissection typically occurs proximally rather than distal to the coarctation. The majority of patients with aortic dissection have hypertensive disease at the time of diagnosis.[10] It is thought that blood pressure control decreases the occurrence of aortic dissection. However, hypertension is not thought to be the sole cause of dissection in a given patient. Many think that pregnancy is an independent risk factor for aortic dissection, although analysis of the available data and the conclusions from these data is hampered by the small number of patients affected and coexisting additional predisposing factors such as hypertension.[11-13] In addition to blunt trauma, thoracic aortic dissection may be induced following establishing antegrade or retrograde arterial perfusion during cardiopulmonary bypass. Intra-aortic balloon counter-pulsation use may also trigger aortic dissection. There is increased risk of type A TAD after aortic valve replacement, especially with larger aortic diameters.[14] Finally, diagnostic angiography and cardiac catheterization may be complicated by aortic dissection (see Table 33.1).[14]

Table 33.1 Specific Risk Factors for Thoracic Aortic Dissection

Age and gender	Smoking	Trauma
Atherosclerosis	Aortitis	Pregnancy
Hypertension	Diabetes mellitus	Drug use*
Congenital cardiovascular defects†	Connective tissue syndromes‡	Aortic dilatation

*Cocaine, amphetamine, sildenafil.
†Bi-aortic value, aortic coarctation.
‡Marfan syndrome, Ehlers-Danlos syndrome, Turner syndrome, familial TAD.

PATHOPHYSIOLOGY

The aortic wall is composed of three layers: the innermost intima, the media (smooth muscle and elastic connective tissue), and the outermost adventitia. Hemodynamic stresses to the aortic inner walls can result from risk factors such as prolonged hypertension or inherently weakened connective tissue walls as seen in some connective tissue syndromes or a bicuspid aortic valve that alters the flow pattern of blood ejected out of the aorta. A dissection may be initiated by a tear or ulceration of the medial layer facilitated by degeneration from normal aging or compounded by the risk factors listed in Table 33.1. A classic aortic dissection is classified by an intimal tear into the media of the aortic wall, resulting in separation of the medial layer and formation of a false channel, allowing blood to flow into this channel. An intramural hematoma (IMH) can also be the trigger for a dissection when an accumulation of blood separates the medial layers; in this circumstance, the inciting entrance tear is lacking. IMH is more common in the elderly hypertensive patient's descending aorta. Finally, aortic ulcers can disrupt the aortic wall and result in aortic rupture or dissection. Patients with aortic ulcers are older than those with IMH. The false lumen of a TAD has the potential to extend both distally and proximally, potentially leading to obstruction of arterial origins from the aortic trunk, rupture back into the true vascular lumen (which can be lifesaving), extension into the pericardial sac with pericardial tamponade, or rupture into the pleural cavity with devastating hemorrhagic shock and death (Fig. 33.2A,B).

A thin adventitial wall facilitates external rupture of TAD. Predictors of continuing dissection offer the cornerstones of treatment strategy and include degree of sustained hypertension and upstroke surge pressure (slope of the pulse wave during systole or change in pressure over change in time [dpldt]). Primary aortic branches along the path of the dissection may become occluded, shear off, or remain in continuity with the true or false lumen. A branch itself may also dissect. Occurrence of the preceding entities combine to produce a wide variety of diverse signs and symptoms associated with thoracic aortic dissection.

Rupture is the most common cause of death during the early acute phase of TAD. The most frequent rupture route leading to death is into the pericardium causing tamponade. Compromise of arch vessels may lead to neurologic

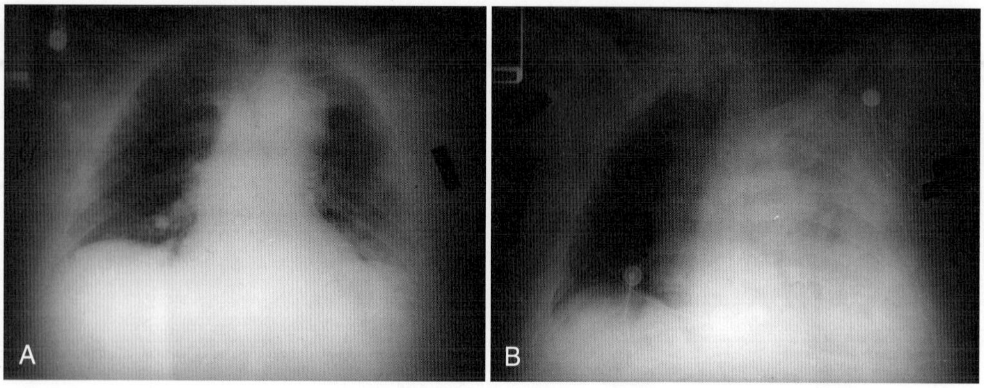

Figure 33.2 Chest radiograph with a widened mediastinum (**A**) with subsequent rupture of the thoracic aortic aneurysm into the left pleural space (**B**).

symptoms and injury. Death may also occur with involvement of the aortic root, producing primary ostial compromise and acute myocardial infarction or severe aortic regurgitation. Rarely, fistulas and high-degree heart block may be produced. The thin wall of any residual pseudoaneurysm following TAD tends to enlarge and over time is at high risk of rupture. Total thrombosis of the false lumen is rare, whereas distal reentry into the true lumen may help decompress the false lumen and increase the chance of survival. Postoperative false lumen patency is a predictor of late mortality.[15]

DIAGNOSIS

SYMPTOMS

The diagnosis of acute TAD is complicated by the infrequent occurrence of this clinical condition as well as the diagnostic difficulty and is particularly problematic because of the potential catastrophic outcome.[16] Typical symptoms of TAD are excruciating, severe at onset, pain of a sharp and tearing nature. The location of the pain (anterior chest, neck, jaw, inner scapular, and lumbar/abdominal) is linked to the location of the dissection. Symptoms, other than pain, include visceral symptoms (vomiting, diaphoresis, and syncope).

PHYSICAL EXAM

Although physical examination findings may be absent, if present, they are useful in directing the clinician's attention to this diagnosis.[16] Inequality of pulses in the upper extremity and a blood pressure differential of 20 to 30 mm Hg between the two extremities may be seen based on the location of the dissection. A new aortic regurgitation murmur occurs in a significant number of patients. Proximal dissection may also interfere with coronary artery blood flow, producing cardiogenic shock or rupture into the pericardium, producing pericardial tamponade. Pericardial tamponade would be supported by findings of jugular venous distention, muffled heart tones, tachycardia, and hypotension. Mass compression effects can produce findings such as superior vena cava syndrome, Horner syndrome, hoarseness, dyspnea, or dysphagia. Syncope is seen in 1 of 10 cases of TAD. Syncope likely results from acute cardiac dysfunction or vascular outflow obstruction of the carotid arteries. Vasovagal pain response may also be a potential etiology of syncope. When syncope is related to hypovolemic shock from rupture through the adventitia into the pleural space, the prognosis is grave.

IMAGING

CHEST RADIOGRAPH

The great majority of patients with thoracic aortic dissection has abnormalities on the chest radiograph. A normal chest radiograph may therefore help in decreasing the likelihood of aortic dissection. A study by Klompas looked at 1337 chest radiographs in patients with thoracic aortic dissection and reported abnormalities in 90% of patients.[17] The most common changes associated with dissection are abnormal aortic contour, widening of the mediastinum, pleural effusion, displacement of intimal calcification, abnormalities of the aortic knob, and displacement of the trachea or nasogastric tube to the right. In the absence of an abnormal aortic contour or mediastinal widening, a diagnosis of dissection is less likely.

COMPUTED TOMOGRAPHY

The most common diagnostic modality used for diagnosis of TAD is computed tomography (CT) (Fig. 33.3). A CT angiogram shows high sensitivity and specificity in diagnosis and exclusion of TAD. It is the optimal imaging modality for ruling out aortic dissection in patients with low clinical pretest probability. Limitations of this technique include use of ionizing radiation and contrast media, need for transfer to imaging station, and limited ability to access the aortic valve. Advantages are ready availability, turnaround time, delineation of entire aorta, and diagnosis of other disorders causing the patient's symptoms. Advances in CT angiographic techniques—such as spiral multidetection scanner technology that allows volume-rendered, three-dimensional reconstruction of a CT angiogram—are likely superior to magnetic resonance images (see Fig. 33.4 as an example of the technology).

ECHOCARDIOGRAPHY

Transthoracic echocardiography (TTE) should be performed early in the evaluation of any patient in whom the

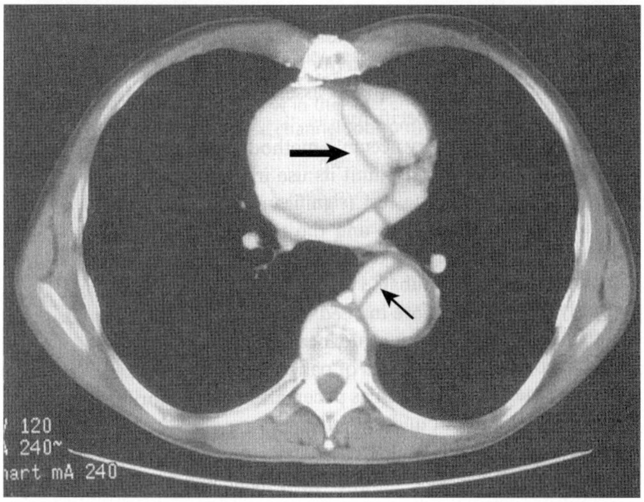

Figure 33.3 Computed tomographic angiogram demonstrating a thoracic aortic dissection. This Stanford type A dissection extends from the ascending aorta (large arrow pointing to the intimal flap) to the descending aorta (smaller arrow pointing to the latimal flap).

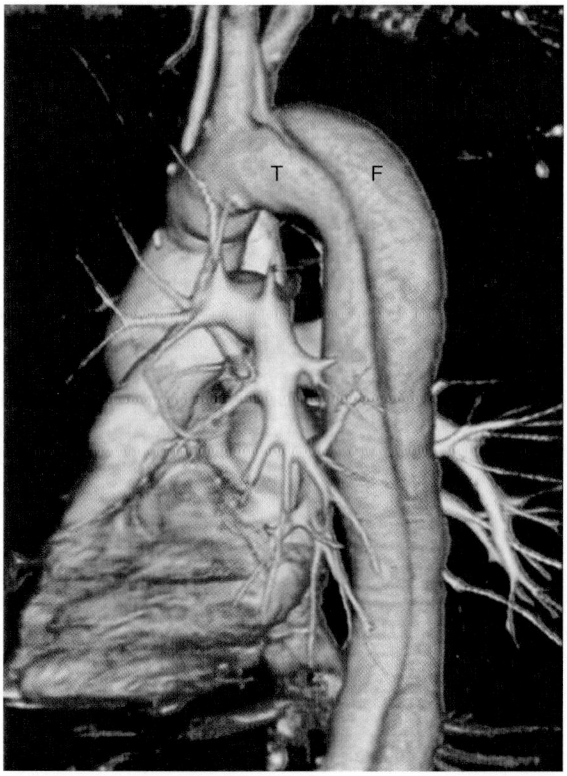

Figure 33.4 Volume-rendered enhanced image from computed tomographic angiography study showing true (T) and false (F) lumens in the descending thoracic aorta. (From Kapustin AJ, Litt HI: Diagnostic imaging for aortic dissection. Semin Thorac Cardiovasc Surg 2005; 17:219.)

diagnosis of ascending aortic dissection is entertained. If a pericardial effusion is present, signs of tamponade can be identified. TTE can help identify aortic dissection if multiple views are obtained—specifically, suprasternal, subcostal, and right parasternal views. The intimal flap may be identified within the lumen, with motion that is not synchronized

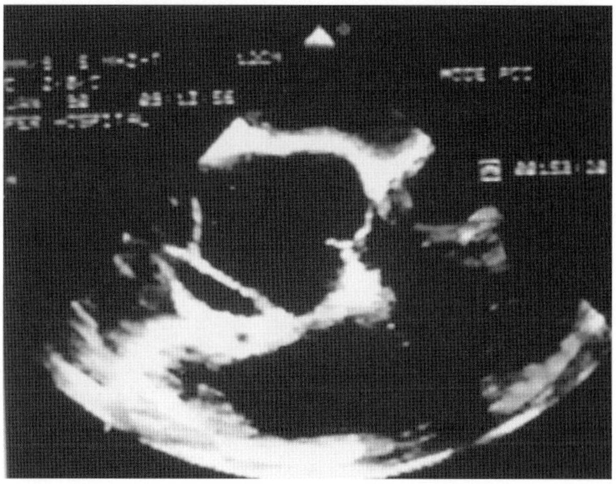

Figure 33.5 Transesophageal echocardiogram image showing intimal flap in the ascending aorta extending to the aortic annulus. (Courtesy of Priscilla Peters, Cooper University Hospital, Camden, N.J.)

with the surrounding structures. To minimize the chance of a false-positive result, the flap should be visualized in more than one view. The addition of color Doppler helps to identify flow artifacts (as opposed to an intimal flap) within the ascending aorta by demonstrating flow between the true and false channels at the site of an intimal tear and by showing a difference in the timing or direction of flow within the two lumens.[18] Color Doppler permits detection and quantification of aortic regurgitation. TTE is especially useful for diagnosing dissections involving the ascending aorta but is much less sensitive for descending dissections. If a dissection is not visualized in the patient with chest pain, finding regional wall motion abnormalitics may suggest the alternative diagnosis of coronary ischemia.

Transthoracic echocardiography (TEE) (Fig. 33.5) can be performed safely on most critically ill patients in a monitored setting.[19,20] To avoid precipitating hypertension, tachycardia, or gagging (straining) in a patient with suspected dissection, conscious sedation should be administered. Nearly all of the thoracic aorta can be visualized, including most of the arch. The area from the distal ascending aorta to the midarch, however, is difficult to evaluate with TEE because of interposition of the airway between the esophagus and the aorta.[21] The sensitivity of TEE for thoracic aortic dissection is close to 100%, but specificity is lower, owing primarily to reverberation artifacts that may be visualized within the ascending aorta, simulating an intimal flap.[22] Color flow Doppler with TEE may demonstrate flow through or on either side of the suspected intimal flap (Fig. 33.6). TEE is helpful for evaluating involvement of the coronary ostia and aortic valve. As with TTE, regional and overall ventricular wall motion can be evaluated and the presence of pericardial effusion can be determined.

AORTOGRAPHY

Once the gold standard for diagnosis of TAD, aortography fell into disfavor as the diagnostic study of choice owing to its invasive nature and a relatively high false-negative rate.[23] The sensitivity of aortography is lower than that of CT, and its specificity is no better. Reliance on iodinated contrast does not ensure direct visualization of a thrombosed lumen

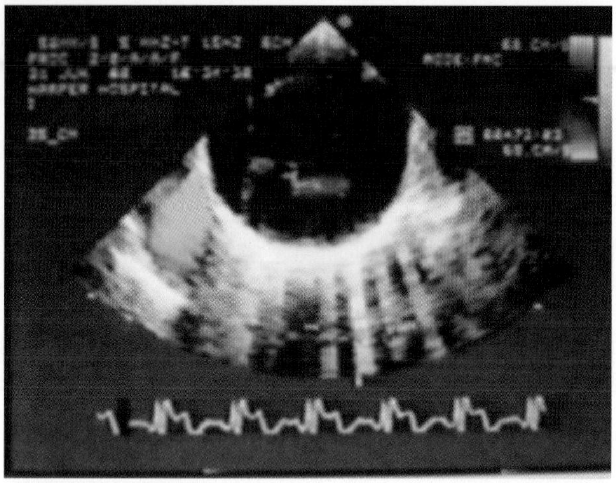

Figure 33.6 Image from a transesophageal echocardiogram revealing an intimal flap in the descending aorta. Color Doppler shows flow through two fenestrations in the flap. (Courtesy of Priscilla Peters, Cooper University Hospital, Camden, NJ.)

or intramural hematoma, or occasionally even confirm the presence of a second, false lumen.[24] Aortography has had a resurgence with the growth of endovascular intervention in the management of dissections where it facilitates stenting across intimal tears, fenestration of intimal flaps, and opening occluded branch vessels.[25,26]

MAGNETIC RESPONSE IMAGING (MRI)

The most reliable diagnostic finding with MRI is demonstration of two lumens separated by an intimal flap. Gadolinium-enhanced magnetic resonance angiography (MRA) allows the visualization of blood flow, which can be used to detect the presence and magnitude of aortic regurgitation or to demonstrate communication between the true and false lumens at the site of an intimal tear. An intimal flap can be identified in most cases, except when the false lumen is completely thrombosed. The diagnostic accuracy of MRI for aortic dissection approaches 100%.[27] Problematic is (1) that it cannot be performed in patients with pacemakers or defibrillators, aneurysm clips, or ferrous metal implants, (2) claustrophobia, and (3) life support equipment (ventilators, monitors, intravenous infusion pumps) with associated logistical issues. Image acquisition, despite advances in the technology, is more time consuming than with CT. Because it entails no radiation exposure, MRI may be an appropriate initial study in the stable patient[22] and for long-term follow-up evaluation.[22,28]

SUMMARY

Table 33.1 shows a comparison of diagnostic imaging modalities for evaluation of thoracic aortic dissection. The 2010 American Heart Association (AHA) guidelines for diagnosis of dissection give a class I recommendation for using either urgent transesophageal echo, MRI, or CT angiogram to determine a definitive diagnosis in patients with high clinical suspicion.[29] If the initial diagnostic test is negative in patients with high clinical suspicion, a second imaging modality should be completed. The diagnosis algorithm from the 2010 guidelines for the diagnosis and management of TAD is shown in Figure 33.7.

PERIOPERATIVE MANAGEMENT

GENERAL PRINCIPLES

Medical therapy is critical for survival with both type A and type B TAD.[30-33] Immediate initiation of medical therapy is imperative, both before surgical intervention for type A TAD and as definitive therapy for patients with type B TAD that is uncomplicated. The primary objectives of therapy are rapidly normalizing arterial blood pressure in hypertensive patients and reducing the force of left ventricular contractility in all patients. Following admission to the intensive care unit (ICU), vital signs are monitored continually; blood pressure should be compared between upper extremities, and the same for carotid pulses. Arterial line insertion is indicated. A radial arterial line on the side of higher blood pressure or a femoral arterial line is placed. For type B dissection, a right radial arterial line is preferred. Intravenous drugs are indicated for medical therapy. In order to limit shear force, which is propagating the dissection, it is important to control the rapidity of the rise of the systole, which is done by avoiding tachycardia (goal heart rate is 60 to 75 beats per minute), depressing contractility, and decreasing blood pressure. Because blood pressure is maintained at low normal, a Foley catheter is recommended in order to judge adequate tissue perfusion. Pain is a marker of continued dissection of a TAD, and subsiding of pain can be assumed to be a marker of halting of dissection. Medical therapy is the treatment of choice for uncomplicated type B TAD. It may also be successfully used in patients who are poor surgical candidates or in select patients with uncomplicated and stable type A TAD.

The mortality of nonoperative management of type A dissection may be up to 1% to 2% per hour in the early phase after symptom onset.[34] The goals of medical management should be stabilization, management of hypertension, and evaluation of neurologic and metabolic function while the operating room is being prepared for the patient. Most centers favor transport directly to the operating room after the surgical team has been mobilized to avoid any delay that would increase mortality. Exceptions to this rule are patients who may present with severe malperfusion that may preclude operative intervention (severe cerebral or visceral ischemia). These exceptions need to be thoroughly evaluated with CT scan and neurologic consultation if central nervous system issues are present. In the case of patients presenting with severe acidosis and elevated lactate levels, CT scan of the abdomen to evaluate for bowel infarction, which if present may make the patient inoperable, is indicated.

Postoperative management is heralded by the need to prevent hypertension. Life-long control of hypertension will be required. Most patients who undergo type A dissection repair will have evidence of residual dissection within the arch and descending aorta and a 15% risk for progressive aneurysmal dilatation. Blood pressure control over time reduces the incidence of late false channel aneurysm development and decreases the chance of redissection or rupture. Periodic evaluation of the status of the aorta over time following successful therapeutic intervention is needed and is typically done with CT scan. Following surgery, antihypertensive therapy is required immediately, as surgery does not

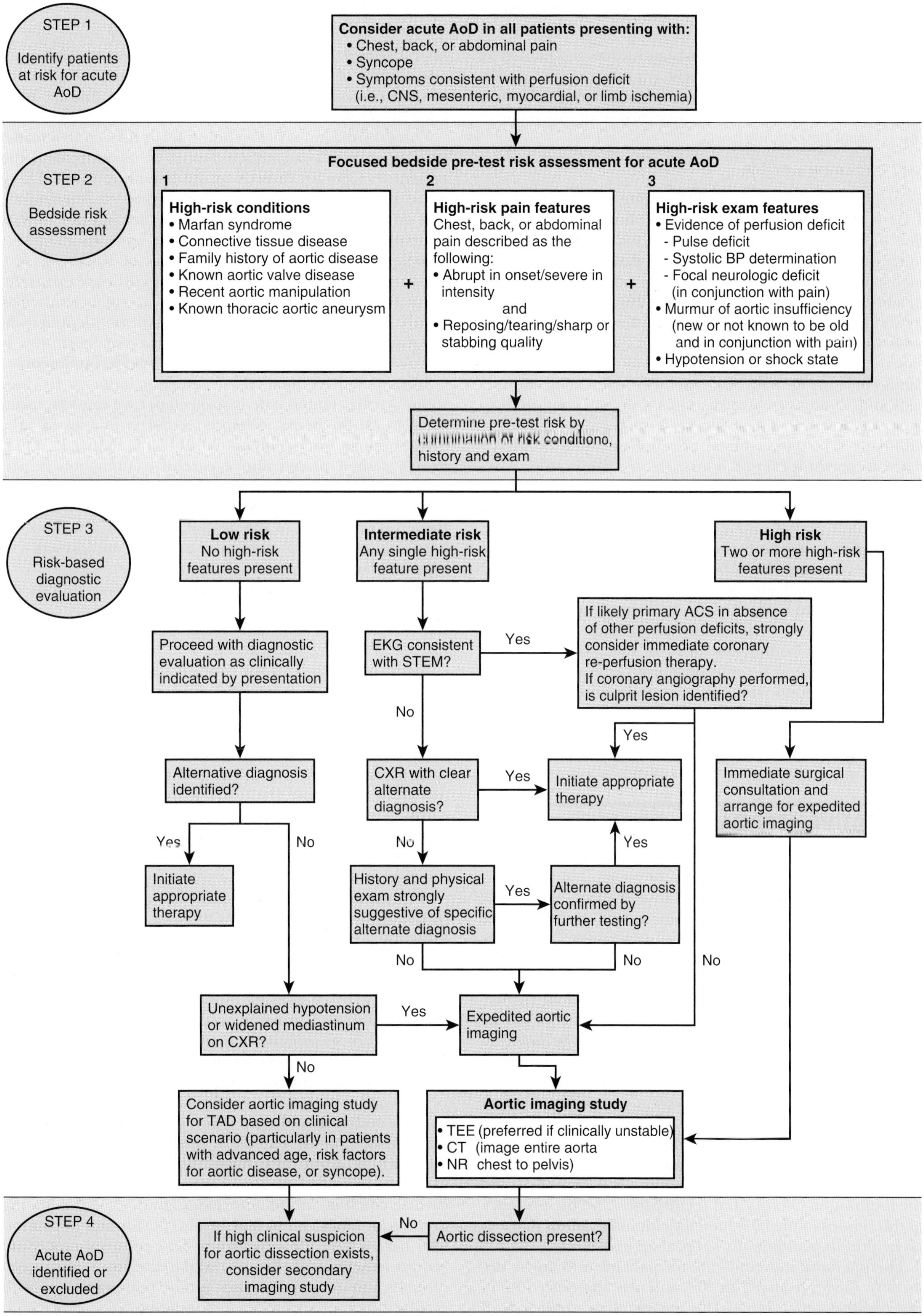

Figure 33.7 Algorithmic flow diagram approach to diagnosis or exclusion of aortic dissection. (Adapted with permission from Guidelines for the Diagnosis and Management of Patients with Thoracic Aortic Dissection. Circulation 2010;121:e266-e369.)

cure the false lumen that persists and leaves the patient at risk for descending thoracic aortic rupture. Signs of persistent pain, new left pleural effusion, or organ hypoperfusion may require a second endovascular procedure to stabilize the residual descending aorta.

SPECIFIC MEDICATIONS

Control of blood pressure and heart rate in the presence of TAD is essential.[35] Intravenous beta-blockers are the first line of therapy for aortic dissection and are immediately initiated to avoid tachycardia, which may occur with some medications chosen to lower blood pressure.[36] Beta-blockers, in addition to controlling heart rate, also depress contractility and lower blood pressure, both goals of therapy. Intravenous esmolol is the ideal drug as it is a quick onset and short-acting agent and can be titrated to effect. Intravenous diltiazem is an alternative to esmolol for decreasing contractility and avoiding tachycardia when there are contraindications to the use of beta-blockers, such as in the active asthmatic. This target blood pressure will then be anticipated to persist for 6 to 8 hours.

Nitroprusside is the vasodilator of choice for blood pressure control and is begun after the initiation of esmolol when blood pressure lowering is required. Nitroprusside acts by decreasing both preload and afterload. Because it may be associated with reflex tachycardia, it is only added after a beta-blockade is in place. Tachycardia should always be avoided in the presence of aortic dissection. Labetalol is an alternative choice to esmolol plus nitroprusside and is given as a loading dose of 10- to 40-mg boluses (based on degree of blood pressure response) q10 to 15 minutes until target blood pressure is reached or 300 mg is delivered.

Table 34.2 reviews drugs used in the medical therapy of acute TAD.

OPERATIVE APPROACH

ASCENDING AORTIC DISSECTIONS

Surgical intervention is indicated in all patients with proximal dissections, with the exception of patients with serious concomitant conditions that preclude surgery.[37] Stroke is the most common contraindication to surgery because there is real concern that anticoagulation (cardiopulmonary bypass) as well as reperfusion can result in further neurologic deterioration by converting the ischemic stroke to a hemorrhagic stroke. Every attempt must be made to perform a careful neurologic assessment prior to undertaking surgical intervention. Additional evidence of severe malperfusion (bowel ischemia) is also a contraindication to surgery.

Preoperative evaluation is essential to assess for the presence of aortic regurgitation, pericardial effusion, the extension of the dissection into the major aortic branches, and the localization of entry and reentry sites, and the presence of thrombosis in the false lumen yields information that can be helpful in planning the surgical approach.[38]

The operative mortality rate for patients with aortic dissections ranges from 5% to 10% and may approach 70% in cases with complications. The independent predictors of operative mortality include the presence of cardiac tamponade, the site of the tear, the time to operation, the presence of renal/visceral ischemia, renal dysfunction, and the presence of pulmonary disease.[39]

Once the diagnosis of ascending aortic dissection is made, cardiac surgical consultation should be obtained and the patient transported directly to the operating room. There is no indication for preoperative cardiac catheterization. Not infrequently patients will present with inferior cardiac ischemic changes (electrocardiogram leads II, III, AVF). Proximal disruption of the right sinus of Valsalva is very common and can result in right main coronary malperfusion. This will also become evident as right ventricular failure or inferior wall ischemia and will be identified on intraoperative TEE. Left main coronary malperfusion is almost uniformly fatal and is infrequently encountered.

Intraoperatively, general anesthesia is induced. In cases where cardiac tamponade is suspected, care must be taken to avoid cardiovascular collapse secondary to a loss of adequate preload when general anesthesia is induced. A TEE probe is then placed and a careful examination is performed. This should include evaluation of right and left ventricular function; extent of the intimal dissection from the sinus of Valsalva to the descending aorta; evaluation of aortic, mitral, and tricuspid valve function; and presence of a pericardial effusion.

Intraoperative planning should involve focus on two key elements: (1) restoration of competent aortic valvular function and (2) resection and reconstruction of all areas of disease in the ascending aorta.

Standard techniques for surgical reconstruction involve cardiopulmonary bypass with circulatory arrest. Arterial cannulation is performed in the femoral artery, innominate artery, or axillary artery. Venous cannulation is usually performed in the right atrium, and cardiopulmonary bypass is then initiated. A cross clamp is then applied across the ascending aorta, and the heart is arrested with retrograde cardioplegia. During this time the patient is then cooled for a period of circulatory arrest. During the cooling period, the ascending aorta is resected down to the sinotubular junction and the extent of dissection is evaluated.

Additionally the aortic valve is evaluated for leaflet pathology, and the sinus of Valsalva must be inspected to determine if this is the origin of the initial intimal tear. The right coronary ostium can frequently be disrupted from the intimal dissection, and if it cannot be reconstructed, coronary artery bypass grafting must be undertaken to prevent ischemia and myocardial infarction.

If there is no primary tear site in the sinus of Valsalva, most surgeons favor reconstruction of the aortic root with glue aortoplasty, and valve resuspension.[40] Indications for performing a full aortic root replacement with a valved conduit and a left and right coronary artery reimplantation (Bentall operation) include a tear through the sinus of Valsalva or an aortic valve that cannot be reconstructed. This can be performed with a mechanical valved conduit, pericardial conduit, or porcine heterograft.[40-44] Valve-sparing aortic root replacement may be also performed in patients who have a long life expectancy. This complex procedure requires resection of all aorta distal to the annulus, creation of neosinuses, and coronary artery reimplantation with reconstitution of aortic lumen continuity.[45]

Reconstruction of the distal aortic arch is performed while on circulatory arrest with the patient cooled to 15° to 25° C. Cerebral perfusion is often maintained during the circulatory arrest period and may be accomplished either antegrade (flow maintained in the axillary or innominate artery) or retrograde (flow through the superior vena cava). Current surgical practice favors the use of the antegrade techniques, as they improve cerebral oxygenation and increase the length that circulatory arrest can safely be performed without neurologic or systemic sequelae.

The distal aortic arch is frequently reconstructed with a glue aortoplasty (such as a hemiarch) or a total arch reconstruction with branch graft reconstruction if there is severe disruption at the level of the cerebral vasculature.

In addition, stent grafting of the distal thoracic aorta may be performed in an antegrade fashion while on a period of circulatory arrest (stented elephant trunk technique). This may stabilize the distal aorta, prevent future aneurysmal dilation, or facilitate a proximal endovascular landing zone for future endovascular therapy should that become necessary.[46]

Following reconstruction of the aortic arch, a Dacron graft is sewn to the distal arch and full cardiopulmonary bypass is reinitiated. The Dacron graft is then anastomosed to the sinus of Valsalva (or valve conduit), thus restoring continuity from the heart to the aortic arch. The patient is then rewarmed and weaned from cardiopulmonary bypass.

DESCENDING AORTIC DISSECTION AND ENDOVASCULAR THERAPY

Uncomplicated acute type B dissection is best managed medically. Approximately 15% of this type of dissection will develop aneurysmal degeneration and require surgical intervention within 5 years of the initial event. The indications for performing early surgery in patients with distal dissections are the rapid expansion of a dissecting aneurysm, rupture into the left chest, impending rupture, persistent and uncontrollable pain, or impairment of the blood flow to an organ or limb.[37,47-49] Open surgical repair carries extremely high morbidity and mortality, and endovascular stent grafting is the currently favored approach for the acute treatment of malperfusion.[50,51]

Organ malperfusion and ischemia in patients with aortic dissections are caused by encroachment on the aortic lumen that provides the blood supply to a branch vessel. The lumen supplying blood to the branch vessel may be the true lumen or the false lumen. A stent is deployed through the percutaneous approach within the lumen supplying the branch vessel to hold the lumen open by displacing the intimal flap toward and overcoming the pressure from the other lumen. To overcome the high pressures in the other lumen, a balloon fenestration procedure may be combined with the stent procedure.

The clinical success of endovascular stent placement for aortic dissection ranges from 76% to 100% with a reported 30-day mortality rate of up to 25%.[51-56] Data on the long-term follow-up of these patients are scarce.

The goals of treatment are coverage of the primary tear site, exclusion of the false lumen, restoration of blood flow to the true lumen, and restoration of organ perfusion and limb perfusion. Covered thoracic stent grafts are usually deployed from the left subclavian artery to the middle descending aorta. If the initial tear site begins at the origin of the subclavian artery, the proximal landing zone is advanced across the subclavian artery to the left common carotid. If there is evidence of a dominant vertebral system on CT scan, or clinical concern for left arm ischemia, a subclavian to carotid bypass graft can be performed via a separate neck incision. The use of intravascular ultrasound has also gained favor to ascertain that the graft is deployed correctly in the true lumen of the dissection.

About 13% of patients with aortic dissections receive stent-graft treatment, and this proportion is steadily increasing. With more data available and more advancement in operator expertise, stent graft placement may, in the future, become the standard treatment for most cases of distal aortic dissection, because waiting for the complications to occur may not be prudent given that the operative mortality rate in these situations approaches 70%.[54]

TREATMENT OF AORTIC INTRAMURAL HEMATOMA AND ATHEROSCLEROTIC AORTIC ULCER

The treatment of patients with both aortic intramural hematomas and atherosclerotic aortic ulcers is similar to that for patients with classic aortic dissections and depends on the aortic site involved. Both aortic intramural hematoma and atherosclerotic aortic ulcer are more common in the descending aorta and therefore are treated with aggressive medical therapy. Medical therapy should consist of the optimal control of blood pressure (BP), a decrease in aortic pulse dP/dt, as well as close long-term follow-up. Surgery is preferred for the treatment of patients with intramural hematomas and atherosclerotic aortic ulcers in the ascending aorta and aortic arch, and for patients with progressive dilatation and aneurysm formation of the aorta, irrespective of the site of involvement.[57-61] In a meta-analysis of 143 patients with aortic intramural hematomas, of whom 30 patients (21%) died, 20 deaths (67%) were due to aortic dissection or rupture.[62]

Interest has also grown in the use of endovascular treatment of type A aortic dissection with short segment stent grafting in high-risk patients.[63] Use of short segment grafts to cover an ascending tear is possible if the dissection is limited to the aorta just above the sinotubular junction and there is no associated valvular compromise. Placement may be performed retrograde or antegrade through the ventricle.

OUTCOMES AND PROGNOSIS

The rationale for surgical treatment of acute type A TAD is universally recognized. Patients with acute ascending aortic dissection treated medically fare far worse than those with dissection involving the descending aorta. Little controversy exists over the treatment of choice for the acute type B variety. For most patients, unless life- or limb-threatening vascular compromise is present, medical therapy is considered superior to surgical treatment.[64,65] If a complication such as rupture necessitating emergency surgery arises, however, the mortality rate is very high. Fortunately, this occurs infrequently. If operation is required for type B TAD within the first 2 weeks, mortality remains high.[66] Analysis of all early postoperative complications shows a much lower stroke rate for descending aorta repairs compared to repair of ascending dissections, although the incidence of pulmonary complications and spinal cord injury is higher.

SUMMARY

Aortic dissection is caused by a tear in the intima of the aorta that is propagated by the aortic pulse wave. The aortic pulse wave, or "shearing force," depends on a combination of myocardial contractility, heart rate, and BP. The risk factors for aortic dissection include advanced atherosclerosis, connective tissue diseases, and aortic coarctation. Dissections involving the area proximal to the left subclavian artery are considered to be type A, and when this area is not involved they are considered to be type B (involving the descending aorta only). Chest pain is the typical presenting symptom, and the classic chest radiographic finding is a widened mediastinum. Diagnosis is best made either with a contrast-enhanced CT scan or a transesophageal echocardiography. Dissection is usually diagnosed utilizing CT scanning with and without contrast enhancement, which demonstrates a grayish white false lumen predominantly filled with a clot alongside a bright white, dye-filled true aortic channel. Dissecting thoracic aortic aneurysms involving the arch and descending aorta that do not interfere with major vessel outflow are typically managed medically with BP control. Aneurysms involving the ascending aorta are typically surgically treated. Aneurysms of the ascending aorta may dissect proximally, producing a murmur of aortic insufficiency or acute pericardial tamponade. Distal migration may produce an obstruction of the major vascular outflow vessels or a rupture into the thorax. Occasionally, a leak may occur into the thorax, which on occasion is diagnosed in time to allow lifesaving surgery. The propagating force for a dissection is the change in pulse over the change in time or the maximum shearing force. This shearing force is minimized by a combination therapy of keeping the pulse in the low normal range, normalizing BP, and decreasing inotropy. Dissection of the aorta is a hypertensive emergency in which normalization of BP is indicated.

KEY POINTS

- Men are at greater risk for developing TAD than are women; approximately two thirds of patients with TAD are male.
- There is an increased risk of type A TAD after aortic valve replacement, especially with larger aortic diameters.
- Rupture is the most common cause of death during the early acute phase of TAD.
- The most common diagnostic modality used to diagnose TAD is computed tomography (CT).

KEY POINTS (Continued)

- Advances in CT angiographic techniques—such as spiral multidetection scanner technology that allows volume-rendered, three-dimensional reconstruction of the CT angiogram—are likely superior to magnetic resonance images.
- The primary objectives of therapy are rapidly normalizing arterial blood pressure in hypertensive patients and reducing the force of left ventricular contractility in all patients.
- Once the diagnosis of ascending aortic dissection is made, cardiac surgical consultation should be obtained and the patient should be transported directly to the operating room.
- In cases where cardiac tamponade is suspected, care must be taken to avoid cardiovascular collapse secondary to a loss of adequate preload when general anesthesia is induced.
- If there is no primary tear site in the sinus of Valsalva, most surgeons favor reconstruction of the aortic root with glue aortoplasty, and valve resuspension.

SELECTED REFERENCES

16. Upadhye S, Schiff K: Acute aortic dissection in the emergency department: Diagnostic challenges and evidence-based management. Emerg Med Clin North Am 2012;30:307-327.
17. Bushnell J, Brown J: Clinical assessment for acute thoracic aortic dissection. Ann Emerg Med 2005;46:90-92.
28. Kapustin AJ, Litt HI: Diagnostic imaging for aortic dissection. Semin Thorac Cardiovasc Surg 2005;17:214-223.
29. Hiratzka LF, Bakris GL, Beckman JA, et al: 2010 ACCF/AHA/AATS/ACR/ASA/SCA/SCAI/SIR/STS/SVM guidelines for the diagnosis and management of patients with Thoracic Aortic Disease. Circulation 2010;121:e266-e369.
30. Moon MR: Approach to the treatment of aortic dissection. Surg Clin North Am 2009;89:869-893.
31. Fattori R, Mineo G, Di Eusanio M: Acute type B aortic dissection: Current management strategies. Curr Opin Cardiol 2011;26:488-493.
32. Elefteriades JA: Thoracic aortic aneurysm: Reading the enemy's playbook. Curr Probl Cardiol 2008;33:203-277.
33. Feldman M, Shah M, Elefteriades JA: Medical management of acute type A aortic dissection. Ann Thorac Cardiovasc Surg 2009;15:286-293.
36. Elefteriades JA: Does medical therapy for thoracic aortic aneurysms really work? Are beta-blockers truly indicated? PRO. Cardiol Clin 2010;28:255-260.
45. Kallenbach K, Oelze T, Salcher R, et al: Evolving strategies for treatment of acute aortic dissection type A. Circulation 2004;110:II243-II249.
46. Uchida N, Katayama A, Tamura K, et al: Frozen elephant trunk technique and partial remodeling for acute type A aortic dissection. Eur J Cardiothoracic Surg 2011;40:1066-1071.
66. Gallo A, Davies RR, Coe MP, et al: Indications, timing, and prognosis of operative repair of aortic dissections. Semin Thorac Cardivasc Surg 2005;17:224-235.

The complete list of references can be found at www.expertconsult.com.

Hypertensive Crises

34

Sergio L. Zanotti-Cavazzoni

CHAPTER OUTLINE

INTRODUCTION

Hypertension is a common clinical disorder. Estimates indicate that almost 30% of the U.S. adult population suffers from elevated blood pressure.[1] Furthermore, one third of these patients are unaware of their diagnosis, and of those who are diagnosed and treated, only 34% have adequate control of their blood pressure.[2] Severe elevations in blood pressure, hypertensive crises, will occur in about 1% of patients with chronic hypertension.[1,3] Hypertensive crises constitute a clinical problem that the intensivist will encounter in the hospital setting. Unfortunately, a paucity of clinical studies evaluating optimal therapeutic strategies and a lack of consideration for key pathophysiologic aspects have led to common misunderstandings and pitfalls in the management of patients with hypertensive crises.

DEFINITIONS

According to the seventh report of the Joint National Committee (JNC) on Detection, Evaluation, and Treatment of High Blood Pressure, hypertension is classified into three stages: *prehypertension, stage 1,* and *stage 2* (Table 34.1).[3] The terms *malignant hypertension* and *accelerated hypertension* have been abandoned. These terms were utilized to describe severe elevations in blood pressure associated with advanced retinopathy (Keith-Wagener-Barker stages 3 and 4). Prognosis of these clinical entities has improved dramatically with the advent of effective drugs for hypertension. In addition, studies have demonstrated that retinopathy as measured by the Keith-Wagener-Barker classification does not correlate with severity of hypertension or outcomes.[4]

Hypertensive crises are defined as severe elevations in blood pressure. Although some authors have suggested a diastolic blood pressure (DBP) > 120 mm Hg, it is preferable to evaluate acute elevations of blood pressure within the context of each individual patient and the effects a given blood pressure has on organ function in that patient. For example, an acute raise in diastolic blood pressure to a value of 100 mm Hg can cause significant damage in a previously normotensive individual whereas a diastolic pressure of 130 mm Hg may be tolerated in a patient with a history of uncontrolled hypertension. As we will see, these patients will require different therapeutic approaches. To clarify these situations better, hypertensive crises have been traditionally classified into hypertensive emergencies and hypertensive urgencies.

A *hypertensive emergency* is a severe elevation in blood pressure associated with the presence of acute end-organ damage. Hypertensive emergencies require immediate control of blood pressure, within 1 to 2 hours, to prevent further organ damage. This will usually require the use of intravenous medications and invasive monitoring (arterial line) in a high-dependency unit such as the intensive care unit. The principal systems susceptible to acute end-organ damage from severe elevations in blood pressure include the central nervous, cardiovascular, and renal systems (Fig. 34.1). Several clinical situations are associated with hypertensive emergencies (Box 34.1). The absolute level of blood pressure and the time course of this elevation will determine the development of a hypertensive emergency. However, acute end-organ damage can occur at different blood pressure values in different patients. Therefore, it is more useful to define hypertensive emergencies with the presence of acute end-organ damage as opposed to specified numbers of systolic or diastolic blood pressure. In addition to

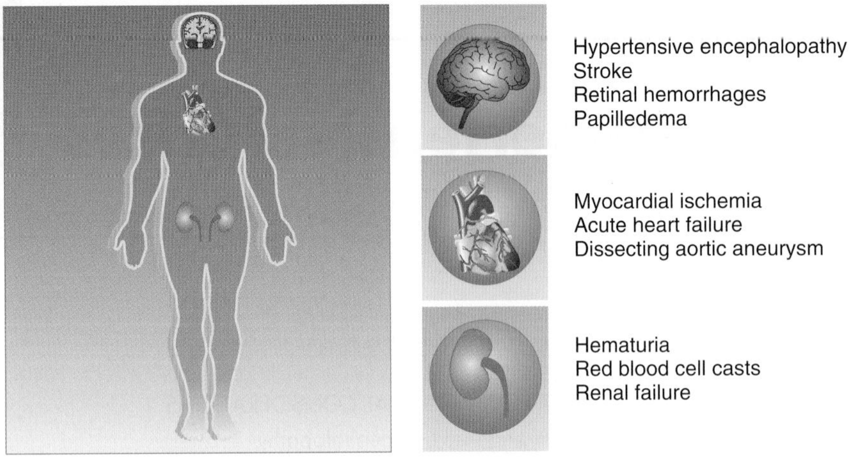

Figure 34.1 End-organ failure in hypertensive emergency.

Table 34.1 Classification of Hypertension (Joint National Committee [JNC] 7)

BP Classification	SBP (mm Hg)		DBP (mm Hg)
Normal	<120	and	<80
Prehypertension	120-139	or	80-89
Stage 1 hypertension	140-159	or	90-99
Stage 3 hypertension	≥160	or	≥100

BP, blood pressure; SBP, systolic blood pressure; DPB, diastolic blood pressure.

Box 34.1 Hypertensive Emergencies

- Hypertensive encephalopathy
- Cerebrovascular accident
- Acute aortic dissection
- Acute left ventricular failure
- Acute myocardial infarction
- Acute renal failure
- Preeclampsia/eclampsia
- Catecholamine excess states
- Postoperative hypertension

initiating immediate therapeutic interventions, patients with a hypertensive emergency may require further diagnostic evaluation to determine the cause of their elevated blood pressure. Depending on the population studied, 20% to 50% of patients presenting with a hypertensive emergency will have a secondary cause of hypertension identified.[5]

A *hypertensive urgency* occurs when severe elevations of blood pressure occur without evidence of acute end-organ damage. In hypertensive urgencies, the blood pressure can be lowered more gradually, over 24 to 48 hours. This can be accomplished usually with oral medications and does not require invasive hemodynamic monitoring in an intensive care unit. Hypertensive urgencies can be associated with chronic stable organ dysfunction, such as stable angina, chronic renal insufficiency, or previous cerebrovascular accident, without evidence of acute end-organ damage.

PATHOPHYSIOLOGY

The underlying pathophysiology of hypertensive crises is still not fully understood. The transition of mild hypertension or normotension to a hypertensive crisis is usually caused by an event that leads to an abrupt increase in blood pressure. Situations associated with this event may include cessation of hypertensive medications with potential rebound effects, consumption of illicit drugs, and severe pain, as well as several clinical syndromes. Blood pressure is determined by the product of cardiac output and systemic vascular resistance ($BP = CO \times SVR$). In most hypertensive crises, the initial rise in blood pressure is secondary to increased systemic vascular resistance. The rise in systemic vascular resistance is believed to be caused by humoral vasoconstrictors.[6] With the increase in blood pressure, mechanical stress on the arteriolar wall leads to endothelial damage and fibrinoid necrosis of the arterioles.[6,7] Vascular damage leads to loss of autoregulatory mechanisms, ischemia, and acute end-organ damage, which prompts further release of vasoconstrictors and initiates a vicious cycle (Fig. 34.2).[6,7]

APPROACH TO MANAGEMENT

Unfortunately there is a paucity of clinical trials to guide the clinician in the optimal management of patients with hypertensive emergencies. However, a systematic approach with consideration of underlying pathophysiology can help the clinician to avoid common pitfalls in the clinical management of patients with hypertensive crises. The most common pitfall in treating patients with hypertensive crises involves treating numbers without evaluating individual patients for acute end-organ damage. This usually is associated with inappropriate use of intravenous drugs with the potential for precipitous and harmful drops in blood pressure. A methodical approach to patients with severe elevations in blood pressure can help establish safe and effective

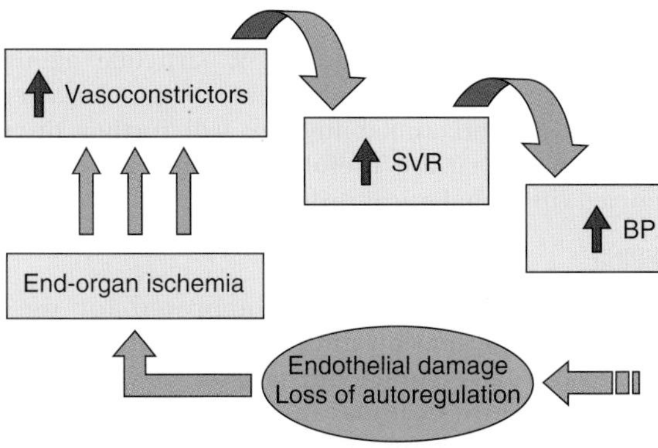

Figure 34.2 Pathophysiology of hypertensive emergency. Increase in humoral vasoconstrictors leads to increased systemic vascular resistance (SVR), which raises blood pressure. As blood pressure increases, endothelial damage results in loss of autoregulation and organ ischemia. Organ ischemia increases release of vasoconstrictors, and a vicious circle is initiated. BP, blood pressure.

treatment. To that effect, the clinician should address three fundamental questions:

1. Should the blood pressure be lowered acutely?
2. How much should the blood pressure be lowered?
3. Which medication should be used to lower the blood pressure?

SHOULD THE BLOOD PRESSURE BE LOWERED ACUTELY?

To answer this question, the clinician must determine if there is evidence of acute end-organ damage. In patients with hypertensive emergencies (the presence of acute end organ damage), the blood pressure should be lowered acutely to a safe target to prevent further end-organ damage. An organized approach in the evaluation of the patient is necessary. A focused history should determine a previous diagnosis of hypertension, medication history, use of illicit drugs or over-the-counter agents with potential hypertensive effects, and the presence of symptoms consistent with neurologic, visual, cardiac, or renal dysfunction. Physical examination should confirm vital signs. It is important to measure blood pressure adequately and in both upper extremities. Pulses should also be checked in all extremities, as inequalities in blood pressure or pulses can exist with aortic dissection. In addition, a thorough neurologic and cardiopulmonary examination should evaluate possible signs of end-organ failure such as altered mentation, new focal neurologic deficits, or cardiogenic pulmonary edema. A funduscopic examination of the eyes should be done to look for signs of acute papillary edema or new retinal hemorrhages. A set of simple diagnostic tests can complete the evaluation for acute end-organ damage. An electrocardiogram to rule out active ischemia and a chest x-ray to assess for pulmonary edema or signs of aortic pathology can help the clinician to evaluate the cardiopulmonary system. Abnormalities in blood urea nitrogen (BUN), creatinine, and the urinalysis (red blood cell [RBC] casts) suggest renal involvement. Additional tests may be indicated based on the individual characteristics of each case. An algorithm to establish the presence of

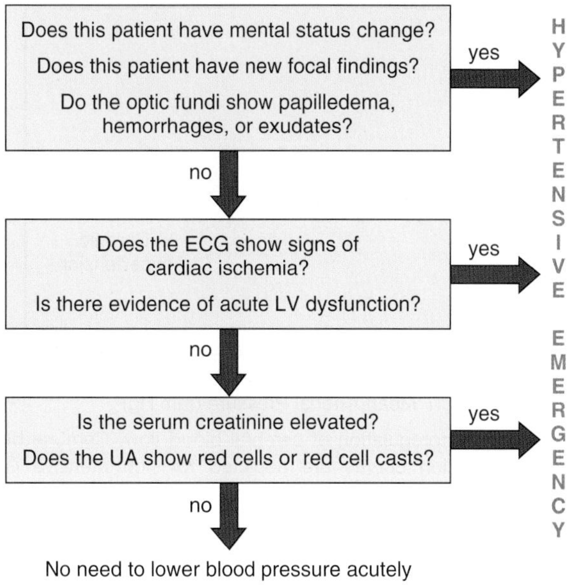

Figure 34.3 Evaluation algorithm for hypertensive emergency. Systematic evaluation for possible acute end-organ damage can proceed according to this scheme. If the answer to any of the questions is "yes," the patient has a hypertensive emergency and blood pressure should be lowered acutely. If the answer to all questions is "no," the patient does not have a hypertensive emergency and the blood pressure can be lowered gradually. ECG, electrocardiogram; LV, left ventricular; UA, urinalysis.

acute end-organ damage at the bedside when evaluating patients is presented in Figure 34.3.

If there is evidence of acute end-organ damage based on the clinical evaluation, the patient's blood pressure should be lowered acutely. However, if after a careful systematic clinical evaluation the exam and diagnostic tests do not show evidence of acute end-organ damage, the blood pressure does not require immediate reduction. It is important to emphasize that the presence or absence of acute end-organ damage and not the numerical value of the blood pressure should dictate the acuity with which blood pressure reduction should be achieved.

HOW MUCH SHOULD THE BLOOD PRESSURE BE LOWERED?

Once the decision to lower a patient's blood pressure acutely is made, the next step should be to establish a safe therapeutic target for the blood pressure reduction. The goals for treating hypertensive emergencies are to lower blood pressure to a level that prevents ongoing acute end-organ damage and at the same time avoid iatrogenic damage caused by precipitous falls in blood pressure causing hypoperfusion to organs. Understanding the autoregulation of blood pressure in normal states and in patients with chronic hypertension is essential to achieve these goals.

Different organs have the ability to autoregulate and maintain a constant blood flow through a range of mean arterial pressures (MAPs). Under normal conditions cerebral autoregulation will keep blood flow constant between MAPs of 60 to 150 mm Hg.[8] When the MAP drops, cerebral arteries will dilate, and if the MAP rises, they will constrict

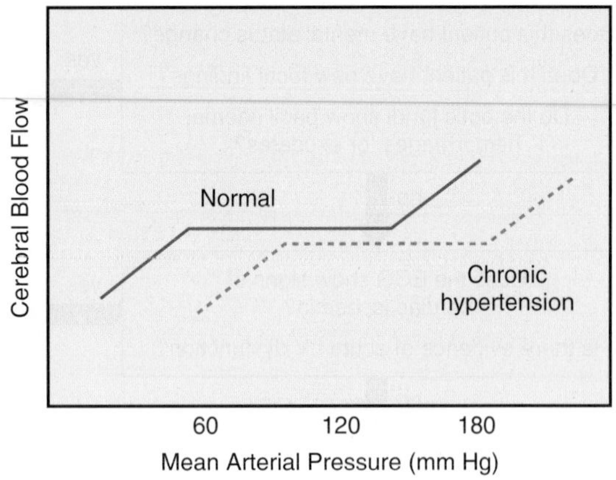

Figure 34.4 Autoregulation of cerebral blood flow. Cerebral blood flow autoregulation curves are depicted for normotensive *(solid purple line)* and chronic hypertensive *(dashed blue line)* states.

to maintain constant blood flow to the brain. Drops in the MAP below the lower limit of autoregulation will lead to hypoperfusion resulting in brain ischemia. Rises in the MAP above the higher limit of autoregulation will lead to acute end-organ damage from hypertension (hypertensive emergency). In the case of the brain, this may result in hypertensive encephalopathy. With chronic hypertension, compensatory functional and structural changes will occur in the vasculature.[9,10] These changes will shift the autoregulatory curve to the right.[11] The autoregulatory curve for cerebral blood flow in healthy individuals and in patients with chronic hypertension is shown in Figure 34.4. Hence, patients with chronic hypertension will have a higher tolerance to elevated blood pressures, as their autoregulatory curve is shifted to the right. This explains why many patients present with severely elevated blood pressure and no evidence of acute end-organ damage. However, rapid reductions of blood pressure to "normal" levels can fall below the lower autoregulatory capacity of the circulation in a chronically hypertensive patient. This phenomenon explains the hypoperfusion of vital organs and the development of renal failure or cerebral ischemia often seen when blood pressure is lowered too far or too fast.[12] Based on these principles, most experts would recommend that for most hypertensive emergencies the goal should be to lower MAP by 15% to 25% over a period of several minutes to hours, depending on the clinical situation.[13] Reduction of blood pressure to normal levels may be warranted in special situations such as those involving patients with aortic dissection or previously normotensive patients with a postoperative hypertensive emergency.

WHICH MEDICATION SHOULD BE USED TO LOWER THE BLOOD PRESSURE?

The ideal medication to treat a hypertensive emergency should have a rapid onset of action, high potency, immediate reversibility, no tachyphylaxis, and minimal or no adverse effects. Although there is no perfect medication, several agents with some of these characteristics are summarized in Table 34.2. There are a limited number of studies comparing agents in terms of clinical outcomes. With no clear outcome data the selection of a particular agent is based on the clinical scenario, pharmacologic characteristics of the drug, and availability. We will further discuss parenteral agents that are useful in treating hypertensive emergencies (in alphabetical order).

CLEVIDIPINE

Clevidipine is relatively new agent approved for use in treating severe hypertension during surgery. It is an ultrashort-acting calcium-channel antagonist. Clevidipine has vasoselective properties with a rapid onset of action and a very short half-life (<1 minute).[14] Clevidipine is metabolized by red blood cell esterases; therefore, its use is not affected in patients with renal and or hepatic failure. Clevidipine reduces blood pressure by a direct and selective effect on arterioles. It does not produce reflex tachycardia, and its effect on reducing afterload is often associated with increased cardiac output. Clevidipine is administered intravenously as a continuous drip. The initial dose is usually 1 to 2 mg/hour with adjustments as needed to obtain the desired response in blood pressure. The maintenance dose is usually 4 to 6 mg/hour; however, higher doses may be required in certain clinical situations. Small studies have compared clevidipine to nitroprusside for the treatment of severe hypertension in anesthetized patients undergoing surgery.[15,16] These studies showed that clevidipine had similar effects on blood pressure control with less effect on cardiac filling and heart rate. Although clevidipine has not been studied extensively in other clinical situations, its characteristics make it an attractive option for the treatment of hypertensive emergencies outside of the operating room. More recently it seems to have received increased attention in neurologic hypertensive emergencies.[17,18]

ESMOLOL

Esmolol is an ultra-short-acting cardioselective, beta-adrenergic agent that can be administered intravenously for the treatment of hypertensive emergencies.[19] Esmolol has a rapid onset of action (within 2 minutes), a short elimination half-life (approximately 9 minutes), and a rapid offset of action (within 15 to 30 minutes after stopping infusion).[20] Esmolol is rapidly metabolized by red blood cells and is not dependent on renal or hepatic function.[20] These properties enable easy titration of the drug and make it attractive in situations of a hypertensive emergency associated with intense adrenergic responses or tachycardia. This agent is available for intravenous (IV) use, both as a bolus and as a continuous infusion. The usual dose is 0.5 mg/kg as a loading dose, followed by a maintenance infusion of 25 to 300 μg/kg/min titrated to the patient's individual response.[20] Esmolol has been found to be effective in controlling postoperative hypertension and tachycardia in several clinical studies.[21-23] Esmolol has also been utilized successfully to treat hypertensive emergencies under other various clinical situations.[24,25] Esmolol seems to be more effective in situations where both blood pressure and tachycardia are present and there are no problematic issues with beta-blockade (severe systolic cardiac dysfunction or asthma). It is often used in conjunction with other agents to achieve a better response.

Table 34.2 Pharmacologic Agents Utilized in Treating Hypertensive Emergencies

Drug	Dosing	Elimination Half-Life	Onset of Action	Duration of Effect	Advantages	Disadvantages
Clevidipine	Initial dose 1-2 mg/hr with titration. Maintenance dose 4-6 mg/hr	Initial half-life 1 min	2-4 min	15 min	Rapid action, titratable, not metabolized by liver or kidney	Rapidly metabolized in pseudocholinesterase-deficient patients
Esmolol	200-500 µg/kg over 1-4 min, then 50 µg/kg/min for 4 min, and titer, then infuse 50-300 µg/kg/min	9 min	2 min	18-30 min	Easily titratable; cardioselectivity	Use with caution in patients with heart failure or asthma
Fenoldopam	Initial dose, 0.1 µg/kg/min with titration every 15 min, no bolus	5-10 min	5 min	30-60 min	Induces both a diuresis and natriuresis	Use with caution in patients with glaucoma
Labetalol	Bolus 20 mg, then 20-80 mg every 10 min for maximum dose 300 mg. Infuse at 0.52-2 mg/min	5 hrs	2-5 min	2-4 hrs	No reflex tachycardia	Use with caution is patients with asthma, heart failure, or bradycardia
Nicardipine	Initial dose, 5 mg/hr to maximum of 15 mg/hr	40-60 min	10-20 min	1-4 hrs	Minimal cardiodepressant effects; minimal dose adjustments required	Possible adverse effects include hypotension, headache, and flushing
Nitroprusside	Initial dose, 0.25 µg/kg/min, maximum dose 8-10 µg/kg/min	14 min	Within seconds	3-4 min	Immediate onset of effect	Hypotension; coronary steal; cyanide toxicity; light sensitivity; requires frequent monitoring

FENOLDOPAM

Fenoldopam is a selective dopamine agonist that causes systemic and renal vasodilation by stimulating dopamine-1 adrenergic receptors.[26,27] Fenoldopam is administered intravenously and has a rapid onset of action (5 minutes) and a short duration of action (30 to 60 minutes).[27] It is rapidly metabolized by conjugation in the liver to inactive metabolites that are excreted by the kidney. The plasma elimination half-life is approximately 5 to 10 minutes.[27] Fenoldopam is administered as a continuous infusion (without a bolus dose), at an initial dose of 0.1 µg/kg/min; this dose is titrated by 0.05 to 0.1 µg/kg/min based on desired effect up to a maximum dose of 1.6 µg/kg/min.[26] The most common adverse effects of the drug are related to its vasodilator properties and include hypotension, headache, reflex tachycardia, and flushing.[26] Fenoldopam also increases intraocular pressure and should be used with caution in patients with glaucoma.[28] Fenoldopam has been demonstrated to be safe and effective in postoperative hypertension.[29] Two clinical studies in severely hypertensive patients found fenoldopam to be comparable in efficacy to sodium nitroprusside.[30,31] Because of its effects on the renal vasculature and its ability to increase urine output, fenoldopam has been proposed as a renal protective drug. A number of small clinical studies report conflicting results in this respect. However, a meta-analysis found improved renal function and mortality in critically ill patients with acute kidney injury treated with fenoldopam.[32] In the setting of a hypertensive emergency, protective effects of fenoldopam on renal function have not been confirmed. However, because it does not affect renal function adversely and does not have increased toxicity in patients with renal failure, it may be a useful alternative to sodium nitroprusside in patients with hypertensive emergency and renal failure.

LABETALOL

Labetalol is a combined alpha- and beta-adrenergic receptor blocker that is currently approved for both oral and intravenous use in the treatment of hypertension. Labetalol lowers blood pressure by decreasing systemic vascular resistance by alpha1-blockade and at the same time counteracts the reflex tachycardia from vasodilation through its beta-blocker effect.[33,34] Labetalol reduces peripheral vascular resistance while maintaining cerebral, renal, and coronary blood flow. Unlike other beta-blockers, labetalol does not reduce cardiac output. When administered intravenously it has a rapid onset of action (2 to 5 minutes) with peak hypotensive effect occurring within 5 to 10 minutes and lasting 2 to 4 hours.[35] The drug is primarily metabolized by the liver and has a plasma elimination half-life of about 5 hours.[33] Labetalol is usually administered intravenously at a loading dose of 20 mg, followed by incremental doses of 20 to 80 mg every 10 minutes until the target blood pressure is achieved or a maximal dose of 300 mg has been reached. An alternative regimen is a continuous infusion starting at 1 to 2 mg/min and titrated upward to achieve a desired blood pressure end point. Adverse effects of labetalol include orthostatic hypotension, bronchospasm (should be avoided in asthma patients), heart failure, and significant bradycardia (should be avoided in the presence of sinus bradycardia or heart block greater than first degree). Labetalol has been shown to be effective in a wide range of clinical situations associated with hypertensive emergencies.[33,34,36-39]

NICARDIPINE

Nicardipine is a short-acting calcium channel antagonist that produces selective arteriolar dilation. Nicardipine decreases systemic vascular resistance, without producing reflex tachycardia while maintaining or increasing cardiac output.[40] Intravenous nicardipine has a rapid onset offset of action (the major effect lasts 10 to 15 minutes, and the plasma elimination half-life is 40 to 60 minutes), making it easily titratable when treating hypertensive emergencies.[41,42] An initial dose of 5 mg/hour is recommended, increasing the infusion rate by 2.5 mg/hour every 5 to 15 minutes (to a maximum rate of 15 mg/hour) until the desired hemodynamic response is achieved. Once the target blood pressure is achieved, the infusion rate can be reduced to 3 mg/hour and adjusted to maintain the desired end point. The drug is rapidly distributed throughout the body and is metabolized by the liver into inactive metabolites. Nicardipine should be avoided or used cautiously in patients with aortic stenosis, in patients with cardiomyopathy receiving beta-blockers, and in patients with impaired hepatic function. Several studies have documented the utility and safety of nicardipine in patients with hypertensive emergencies. Randomized studies have demonstrated that nicardipine has similar efficacy when compared to nitroprusside in the management of postoperative hypertension.[41,43]

NITROPRUSSIDE

For many years sodium nitroprusside was the standard intravenous drug administered for hypertensive emergencies, and it remains a viable alternative today. Nitroprusside is a potent balanced arterial and venous vasodilator that decreases both cardiac afterload and preload. Nitroprusside has a rapid onset of action (2 to 3 minutes) and a short serum half-life (1 to 2 minutes) and may be easily titrated.[44] Because of its potent effects on blood pressure, use of nitroprusside requires invasive hemodynamic monitoring (arterial line for continuous blood pressure monitoring). Nitroprusside is typically begun at 0.3 μg/kg/min and increased by 0.2 to 1 μg/kg/min every 3 to 5 minutes as needed until a maximum of 2 μg/kg/min. Cyanide and thiocyanate are metabolites of nitroprusside with potential toxic effects. Cyanide is released nonenzymatically from nitroprusside. Cyanide is converted to thiocyanate by the liver. Finally, the kidney excretes thiocyanate. The total dose of nitroprusside and the presence of liver or renal dysfunction increase the risk of toxicity. Cyanide toxicity can be associated with lactic acidosis, mental status changes, and hypotension. Signs of thiocyanate toxicity include delirium, headaches, nausea, abdominal pain, and muscular spasms.[45] To reduce possible toxicity, the duration of treatment with nitroprusside should be limited and the maintenance rate of infusion should not exceed 2 μg/kg/min. In patients requiring higher doses of nitroprusside, an infusion of thiosulfate is recommended to decrease the risk of toxicity.[46] Hydroxocobalamin has also been demonstrated to prevent and treat possible cyanide toxicity associated with the use of nitroprusside. Despite these concerns, nitroprusside has been utilized successfully in the treatment of hypertensive emergencies for many years, and with proper precautions toxicity is seldom encountered.

OTHER AGENTS

Several other agents have been used for treating severely elevated blood pressure. Many of them have been abandoned secondary to the emergence of safer and more efficacious alternatives. However, there are a few agents that despite some limitations compared to the drugs previously discussed may be useful in particular situations. Nitroglycerin directly interacts with nitrate receptors producing predominantly venous dilation. Because of its favorable effects on coronary perfusion and its ability to reduce preload, it is a drug well suited for treating hypertensive emergencies associated with myocardial ischemia or acute left ventricular failure.[47] Several clinical studies have shown the safety and efficacy of nitroglycerin for the treatment of hypertension after cardiac surgery.[48-50] Nitroglycerin is administered as a continuous infusion. The starting dose is 5 μg/min, and this dose can be titrated until a maximum of 200 μg/min is reached. Phentolamine is an α-adrenergic blocking agent that may be used for the management of catecholamine-induced hypertensive emergencies, such as pheocromocytoma.[51] Phentolamine is administered intravenously in 1- to 5-mg boluses. The effects are immediate and may last up to 15 minutes. This drug may cause arrhythmias and angina. One the blood pressure is controlled, a long-acting α-adrenergic blocking agent such as oral phenoxybenzamine can be started. Enalaprilat is an angiotensin-converting enzyme inhibitor (ACE inhibitor) that can be administered intravenously. Its onset of action is within 15 minutes and its duration of action is 12 to 24 hours.[52,53] The usual dose is of 1.25 mg IV every 6 hours, titrated by increments of 1.25 mg at 12- to 24-hour intervals to a maximum dose of 5 mg every 6 hours.[54] The degree of blood pressure reduction with enalaprilat correlates directly with the pretreatment levels of angiotensin II and plasma renin activity.[55] Enalaprilat is especially useful in hypertensive emergencies associated with scleroderma crises.[56] Hydralazine is a vasodilator that has been used in pregnancy-related hypertensive crises for many years. However, it has unpredictable effects on blood pressure and a long half-life. Nicardipine and labetalol are better choices for treating pregnant patients with hypertensive emergencies in the intensive care unit.

SPECIFIC CLINICAL CONSIDERATIONS

HYPERTENSIVE ENCEPHALOPATHY

When rises in mean arterial pressure exceed the upper limits of the cerebral blood flow, autoregulatory curve endothelial damage with extravasation of plasma proteins can lead to cerebral edema.[57] Hypertensive encephalopathy, the clinical manifestation of this phenomenon, is characterized

Box 34.2 Differential Diagnosis of Hypertensive Encephalopathy

Ischemic stroke
Intracerebral hemorrhage
Subarachnoid hemorrhage
Subdural hematoma
Epidural hematoma
Central nervous vasculitis
Brain mass
Seizure disorder
Central nervous system infection
Drug toxicity
Withdrawal syndrome

by headache, visual disturbances, confusion, and focal or generalized weakness. If untreated, hypertensive encephalopathy can lead to coma and death.[58] Magnetic resonance imaging has demonstrated that the majority of the cases involves the cortical regions of the brain.[59] However, hypertensive encephalopathy with brainstem involvement has also been described.[60,61] The differential diagnosis of hypertensive encephalopathy includes several neurologic syndromes (Box 34.2). These should be quickly ruled out with the use of imaging of the brain and other pertinent diagnostic tests. Treatment should be instituted immediately. The goal is to reduce the mean arterial pressure by 15% to 20% within the first 1 to 2 hours.[62] The hallmark of hypertensive encephalopathy is improvement of symptoms once the blood pressure is controlled. Caution should be taken not to cause worsening neurologic symptoms from hypoperfusion caused by lowering the mean arterial pressure excessively. Drugs suitable for treating hypertensive encephalopathy include nitroprusside, nicardipine, labetalol, and fenoldopam.

HYPERTENSIVE CRISIS IN CEREBROVASCULAR ACCIDENTS

Hypertension is common after both ischemic and hemorrhagic strokes. Extreme elevations in blood pressure have been associated with poor outcomes after ischemic and hemorrhagic stroke.[63,64] Significant elevations in blood pressure after strokes raise concerns for the potential development of reinfarction, cerebral edema, increased hemorrhage size, or hemorrhagic transformation of ischemic lesions. However, after acute stroke the cerebral vasculature's ability to autoregulate blood flow is impaired.[65] During this time period, flow to the brain is highly dependent on mean arterial pressure. Even modest reductions in blood pressure can compromise blood flow to the brain during this period with the potential for increased secondary neurologic damage. Optimal treatment of blood pressure during stroke is still not a settled debate. Current guidelines recommend withholding therapy for hypertension in the acute phase of ischemic strokes unless the patient will receive thrombolysis, there is evidence of concomitant acute end-organ damage, or excessive elevations in blood pressure are present (arbitrarily selected as systolic blood pressure > 220 or diastolic blood pressure >120 mm Hg).[66] For hemorrhagic strokes, current recommendations are to maintain MAP ≤ 130 mm Hg in patients with a history of hypertension and a MAP ≤ 100 mm Hg in patients who underwent craniotomy.[67] Current guidelines are summarized in Tables 34.3 and 34.4.

Table 34.3 Guidelines for Treatment of Hypertension in Ischemic Cerebrovascular Accidents

Clinical Parameter	Treatment
Patients *Not* Eligible for Thrombolysis	
SBP < 220 or DBP < 120 mm Hg	No treatment
SBP > 220 or DBP = 121-140 mm Hg	Labetalol or nicardipine to 10%-15% reduction
DBP > 140 mm Hg	Nitroprusside to 10%-15% reduction
	More labetalol or nicardipine
Patients Eligible for Thrombolysis	
Prior to Thrombolytics	
SBP > 185 or DBP > 110 mm Hg	Labetalol or nitroprusside
During or After Thrombolytics	
SBP = 180-230 or DBP 105-120 mm Hg	Labetalol
SPB > 230 or DBP = 121-140 mm Hg	Labetalol or nicardipine
DBP > 140 mm Hg	Nitroprusside

SBP, systolic blood pressure; DPB, diastolic blood pressure.

Table 34.4 Guidelines for Treatment of Hypertension in Hemorrhagic Cerebrovascular Accidents

Clinical Parameter	Treatment
SBP < 180 and DBP < 105 mm Hg MAP < 130 mm Hg	No treatment
SBP 180-230 or DBP 105-140 mm Hg MAP = 130-160 mm Hg	Labetalol, esmolol, nicardipine, enalaprilat
SBP > 230 or DBP > 140 mm Hg	Nitroprusside
Map > 160 mm Hg	Nicardipine + labetalol

MAP, mean arterial pressure; SBP, systolic blood pressure; DPB, diastolic blood pressure.

ACUTE AORTIC DISSECTION

Aortic dissection is a life-threatening complication of hypertension, caused by a tear in the intima of the aorta. This tear is then propagated by the aortic pulse wave. The aortic pulse wave (dP/dt) is dependent on myocardial contractility, heart rate, and blood pressure. The presenting symptom is usually severe sharp chest pain of abrupt onset. Chest x-ray may be associated with a widened mediastinum. The diagnosis is best made with contrast-enhanced computerized tomography or transesophageal echocardiography.[68] Aortic dissections are classified as type A (proximal to the left subclavian artery, involving the ascending aorta) or type B (distal to the left subclavian artery, involving the descending aorta).[69] The goal of treatment is rapid reduction of the pulsatile wave (dP/dt) and aortic stress. Both mean arterial pressure and cardiac output must be controlled in order to achieve this goal and prevent further propagation of the dissection in the aorta. In patients with aortic dissection, the mean arterial pressure and heart rate should be reduced to normal values as quickly as possible. Combining a vasodilator (nitroprusside, nicardipine, fenoldopam) with a beta-blocker (esmolol, metoprolol) is recommended.[70] All patients with aortic dissection need emergent cardiovascular surgical evaluation. Type A dissections usually require emergent surgery to prevent serious complications such as acute aortic insufficiency, hemopericardium, and cardiac tamponade.[71] Type B dissection is often managed medically. Indications for surgery in type B dissections include complications such as leak, rupture, and impaired flow to vital organs. See Chapter 33.

HYPERTENSIVE CRISES IN PREGNANCY

Hypertension is a common complication of pregnancy and is responsible for 18% of maternal deaths in the United States.[72] The spectrum of disease varies from mild increases in blood pressure to severe pregnancy-related syndromes with hypertensive emergencies such as preeclampsia and eclampsia.[73] Hypertension in pregnancy is defined as a systolic blood pressure ≥ 140 mm Hg or diastolic pressure ≥ 90 mm Hg. Preeclampsia is a pregnancy-specific condition defined by new onset hypertension, proteinuria (>300 mg/24 hours), and pathologic edema during gestation. Eclampsia is defined by the development of seizures or coma in a pregnant patient with preeclampsia. The challenge in pregnant patients with hypertensive crises is to lower the blood pressure in order to prevent maternal end-organ damage while minimizing acute changes in placental perfusion that could negatively impact the well-being of the fetus. Treatment of severe preeclampsia and eclampsia includes delivery of the fetus, magnesium sulfate for the prevention and treatment of seizures, and appropriate blood pressure control. The goal is to reduce the diastolic blood pressure to 100 mm Hg or the mean arterial pressure by 20%. Historically, hydralazine has been preferred in pregnant patients for its safety profile from a fetal perspective. However, data suggest it may not be the most effective or safe agent for this patient population.[74] For pregnant patients in need of acute lowering of blood pressure in the intensive care unit, drugs such as labetalol and nicardipine are probably better options.[75,76] Nitroprusside is reserved for refractory cases because of concerns for potential fetal cyanide toxicity. Finally, ACE inhibitors such as enalaprilat are contraindicated in the second and third trimester because of the increase in fetal and neonatal morbidity and mortality.

POSTOPERATIVE HYPERTENSION

Postoperative hypertension deserving of immediate intravenous treatment consideration has been arbitrarily defined as a systolic blood pressure > 190 mm Hg or a diastolic blood pressure > 100 mm Hg on two consecutive readings after surgery. Previous history of hypertension, high body mass index, age, and the grade of surgical stress are recognized risk factors for developing postoperative hypertension.[77] Severe increases in arterial blood pressure in the immediate postoperative period can result in serious complications such as heart failure, arrhythmia, myocardial ischemia, wound hemorrhage, and cerebral hemorrhage.[78] Considering the deleterious effects of prolonged postoperative hypertension, many authors have recommended aggressive treatment.[78] The goal of treatment is similar to other hypertensive emergencies: decrease blood pressure to safe levels and at the same time avoid complications related to hypotension. Although some clinicians feel that postoperative hypertension should be treated aggressively based on the potential for acute end-organ damage, others recommend evaluating for possible causes of hypertension such as pain, hypercarbia, hypoxemia, and urinary retention prior to initiating antihypertensive drugs. As most patients in the postoperative period are unable to take oral medications, even patients with no clear evidence of acute end-organ damage will receive intravenous medications. In patients with previous history of hypertension a reasonable goal is to reduce mean arterial pressure by 20%. In patients with no previous history of hypertension, the goal is to reduce blood pressure to normal levels. Clevidipine, nitroprusside, labetalol, and nicardipine have all been extensively studied in cardiac, vascular, and neurosurgical settings. Nitroglycerin is commonly used in postcoronary bypass surgery, and fenoldopam has been proposed for clinical settings with increased risk of renal ischemia.

CATECHOLAMINE-ASSOCIATED HYPERTENSIVE CRISIS

A hypertensive crisis related to excess catecholamines can result from several causes. Consumption of sympathomimetic agents (amphetamines, cocaine, phencyclidine, and certain diet pills), decongestants (ephedrine, pseudoephedrine), and other agents (atropine, alkaloids) can result in excessive catecholamine release and hypertension. Withdrawal from beta-blocker or alpha-blocking agents can cause a rapid surge in catecholamines and hypertension. In these cases, reinitiation of the particular drug may be sufficient to treat the elevated blood pressure. Additional causes include pheochromocytoma, autonomic dysfunction (i.e., Guillain-Barré syndrome) and ingestion of tyramine in conjunction with monoamine oxidase inhibitor therapy. As a general rule, in catecholamine-related hypertension the use of beta-blockers as initial therapy should be avoided. Loss of beta-adrenergically mediated vasodilation leaves alpha-mediated vasoconstriction unopposed and may cause further elevation in blood pressure. Pheochromocytoma is a rare tumor that produces excess catecholamine and can cause severe hypertension. Symptoms commonly associated with pheochromocytoma include headache, palpitations, diaphoresis, abdominal pain, anxiety, and hypertension. Some patients may present with orthostatic symptoms. For patients with a hypertensive emergency associated with pheochromocytoma, the drug of choice is phentolamine. Once blood pressure is controlled a beta-blocker can be added to control tachycardia. For less critical situations or after acute hypertension is controlled, the oral agent phenoxybenzamine can be used.

HYPERTENSIVE URGENCY

Hypertensive urgency refers to a clinical situation in which there is severe elevation of blood pressure without evidence of acute end-organ damage. This is a common clinical situation that is often mismanaged. Too often clinicians have the impulse to treat numbers and risk causing more damage to patients from precipitous drops in blood pressure. Despite markedly elevated blood pressure, patients with hypertensive urgency are at low risk of immediate complications. Morbidity from elevated blood pressure occurs over months to years. Therefore, it is more important to start patients with hypertensive urgency on a good long-term oral regimen and reduce their blood pressure gradually over 24 to 48 hours. One must avoid the use of medications that have the potential to produce abrupt drops in blood pressure and cause significant damage from hypoperfusion.[12,79] In this respect, practices such as the use of sublingual nifedipine in hypertensive urgency have been abandoned secondary to the potential hazards to patients.[80,81] Often, restarting a previously effective drug regimen is all that is needed to treat hypertensive urgencies. Physicians often feel compelled to treat elevated blood pressures immediately and feel a false sense of security if they see the numbers improve quickly. However, in the absence of acute end-organ damage this therapeutic strategy has a higher potential for causing damage and is not based on a clear scientific rationale.

KEY POINTS

- Hypertension is a common clinical disorder, with an estimated 30% of the U.S. adult population suffering from elevated blood pressure.
- A *hypertensive emergency* is a severe elevation in blood pressure associated with the presence of acute end-organ damage.

KEY POINTS (Continued)

- The treatment of a hypertensive crisis is guided by (1) whether the blood pressure should be lowered acutely, (2) how much it should be lowered, and (3) what medication should be used.
- The ideal medication to treat a hypertensive emergency would have a rapid onset of action, high potency, immediate reversibility, no risk of tachyphylaxis, and minimal or no adverse effects.
- Parenteral agents with specific indications in the treatment of hypertensive crises include clevidipine, esmolol, fenoldopam, labetalol, nicardipine, and nitroprusside.

SELECTED REFERENCES

3. National Heart L, and Blood Institute: Seventh report of the Joint National Committee on Prevention, Detection, Evalulation, and Treatment of High Blood Pressure (JNC VII). NIH 2003.
8. Strandgaard S, Paulson OB: Cerebral autoregulation. Stroke 1984;15:413-416.
18. Rivera A, Montoya E, Varon J: Intravenous clevidipine for management of hypertension. Integr Blood Press Control 2010;3: 105-111.
23. Gray RJ, Bateman TM, Czer LS, et al: Comparison of esmolol and nitroprusside for acute post-cardiac surgical hypertension. Am J Cardiol 1987;59:887-891.
30. Panacek EA, Bednarczyk EM, Dunbar LM, et al: Randomized, prospective trial of fenoldopam vs sodium nitroprusside in the treatment of acute severe hypertension. Fenoldopam Study Group. Acad Emerg Med 1995;2:959-965.
32. Landoni G, Biondi-Zoccai GG, Tumlin JA, et al: Beneficial impact of fenoldopam in critically ill patients with or at risk for acute renal failure: A meta-analysis of randomized clinical trials. Am J Kidney Dis 2007;49:56-68.
42. Wallin JD, Fletcher E, Ram CV, et al: Intravenous nicardipine for the treatment of severe hypertension: A double-blind, placebo-controlled multicenter trial. Arch Intern Med 1989;149: 2662-2669.
46. Hall VA, Guest JM: Sodium nitroprusside-induced cyanide intoxication and prevention with sodium thiosulfate prophylaxis. Am J Crit Care 1992;1:19-25; quiz 6-7.
67. Morgenstern LB, Hemphill JC 3rd, Anderson C, et al: Guidelines for the management of spontaneous intracerebral hemorrhage: A guideline for healthcare professionals from the American Heart Association/American Stroke Association. Stroke 2010;41: 2108-2129.
73. Vidaeff AC, Carroll MA, Ramin SM: Acute hypertensive emergencies in pregnancy. Crit Care Med 2005;33:S307-S312.

The complete list of references can be found at www.expertconsult.com.

35 General Principles of Postoperative Intensive Care Unit Care

Michael J. Hockstein | Laura S. Johnson

CHAPTER OUTLINE

Regionalization within a health care structure allows for more efficient control and use of limited resources. The intensive care unit (ICU) contains specially trained staff and a variety of support devices, such as mechanical ventilators, intra-aortic balloon pumps, ventricular assist devices, and dialysis machines, which in most cases cannot be used elsewhere. Optimally, the location of a patient is determined by matching the patient's needs with a location's resources and expertise.

Generally, the surgical ICU is where experience, staffing, skills, and technology converge to provide services that cannot be provided anywhere else within the hospital. Highly skilled nurses, often greater in number than the patients themselves, work intimately with intensivists and ancillary staff in an environment designed to stabilize, diagnose, and simultaneously treat the most acutely ill patients. ICU management by intensivists allows for improved staff and family satisfaction, reduced complication rates, lower costs, shorter length of stay, improved processes of care, and a morbidity and mortality risk advantage.[1-4] ICU systems focused on an environment of safety and compliance with evidence-based standards promote improvement in many outcome metrics.[5] Safe and efficient patient throughput allows for greater institutional procedural volume, which, when paired with surgeon procedural volume, has been shown to be associated with reduced mortality risk.[6]

Classic postoperative indications for ICU admission include advanced age or prolonged duration of the operation, both criteria without specifically defined thresholds. Other factors, such as the need for mechanical ventilation, volume resuscitation, or administration of vasoactive medications, make ICU care unavoidable. Monitoring of level of consciousness, airway, bleeding, pulses, rhythm, acidosis, urine output, and global perfusion also is facilitated by ICU admission. Identifying patients who may need postoperative ICU care can be difficult. Although there are scoring systems to assess risk and fatality (APACHE, SAPS, MPM, SOFA), it is difficult to apply these predictions to specific disease states or individual patients. Some prediction models utilize physiologic data for patients after admission to the ICU and have not been validated as preadmission screening tools.[7,8] Physicians may predict mortality risk even better than scoring systems.[9] In practice, most physicians do not use these tools to determine postoperative ICU admission. Admission criteria based on priority, diagnosis, and objective parameter models have been published by the Task Force of the American College of Critical Care Medicine and the Society of Critical Care Medicine.[10]

POSTOPERATIVE EVALUATION

Obtaining a comprehensive medical and surgical history is a fundamental step in understanding a patient in the surgical ICU. The medical record, traditionally written but now more commonly electronic, should contain all of the elements necessary to assemble the story up until the time of ICU admission, although deciphering a chart, particularly when it is long, requires time, patience, and detective skills. Data gathering usually begins by word of mouth from the providers delivering the patient. Effective "hand-off" is essential to maintain the continuity of care and to ascertain important operative events that may have escaped documentation. It is in fact a standard expected by The Joint Commission.[11] Certain questions are common to virtually all admissions:

1. How old is the patient?
2. What are the highlights of the medical/surgical history?
3. Was the operation elective or emergent?
4. What operation was performed, and what are the details of the surgery?
5. Are there any drains?
6. What are the current ventilator settings if the patient is intubated?
7. What medications is the patient receiving currently?
8. Where are the vascular access points? Were they placed under sterile conditions?
9. What was the intubation and anesthetic course like?
10. What were the complications, if any?

Age, comorbid conditions, and emergency operations all affect mortality risk. The details of the operation are key, often aided by diagrams in the chart. Resections, diversions, anastomoses, transplantations, use of prosthetic materials, and other surgical findings are some of the details that should be obtained. In addition, the type and location of each drain must be accounted for. Only by knowing where a drain is placed can a care provider know how to interpret the quantity and quality of the effluent. Each drain or wire must be labeled correctly. Also, the completion of wound closure must be ascertained (skin and fascia closed?). Finally, if the operation was incomplete or intentionally staged, the health care provider needs to inquire about intentions and timing of return to the operating room.

The significance of the anesthesia record should not be minimized. The details about trends in gas exchange, blood pressure, urine output, medications, and summary fluid balance should be reviewed. Always identify if the intubation was easy or difficult. Reviewing the ventilator settings that were used in the operating room sheds some light on any possible gas exchange difficulties and provides a first opportunity to make corrections. Tidal volumes in the operating room are often much larger than those used in the ICU. Identification of current medications and the purpose of each help to formulate short-term therapeutic strategies. Assessing the adequacy of intraoperative resuscitation begins with a review of the quantifiable gains and losses. Resuscitation fluids, blood products, urine output, cavity fluid, and blood losses should all be reviewed. Evaporative and extravascular (third space) losses may be more difficult to accurately quantitate. Major surgical procedures such as bowel resection can require 7 to 8 mL/kg/hour of resuscitation fluid and severe blunt or penetrating injury 10 to 15 mL/kg/hour to match these loses. Underresuscitation may occur in patients with congestive heart failure or anuric renal failure for fear of creating a state of uncorrectable fluid overload. What amounted to adequate resuscitation in the operating room may not be the case by the time the patient arrives in the ICU. A careful reassessment of the adequacy of resuscitation is necessary in virtually all postoperative ICU admissions. Typical postoperative maintenance intravenous fluid rates are 80 to 125 mL/hour, but can be substantially higher in the presence of ongoing intravascular volume loss. Isotonic fluids are the most appropriate maintenance fluids. It is useful to inquire about the last time the patient received narcotics, benzodiazepines, or paralytics and if reversal agents were given. Finally, any intraoperative laboratory values, particularly ones that require immediate attention, should be reviewed.

When time permits, attention should be directed back to the medical record. The clinician should scan the history and physical examination, progress notes, and consultations to develop a cohesive story line of events that led up to the operation. Did the illness have an impact on nutrition or functional state? How are other comorbid conditions or past operations related to the current presentation? The past medical history and the medication list should be scrutinized; the two are complementary. Inclusion of a disease in the past medical history and absence of an expected medication warrants further investigation (and vice versa). The medication list should be scanned in particular for antiseizure medications, bronchodilators, antihypertensives, antiarrhythmics, anticoagulants, diuretics, steroids, thyroid replacement, and insulin. It must be decided which medications must be continued in the immediate postoperative period and which can be temporarily delayed. If antibiotics were administered preoperatively, the clinician should identify what they were and how long had they been given and for what indication. In general, if administered preoperatively, bronchodilators, steroids, and insulin are resumed postoperatively. Long-acting antihypertensives should be avoided in the early postoperative period, and short-acting intravenous agents should be used to control hypertension. Diuretics should be avoided in the immediate postoperative period unless directed by invasive monitoring or required because of some other medical necessity. The use of early postoperative beta blockade in patients with coronary artery disease is encouraged if the overall hemodynamic performance allows. Most other medications can be safely delayed until the postoperative patient has shown satisfactory cardiopulmonary performance and stability.

Postoperative laboratory, imaging, and electrocardiogram studies should be selected on a case-by-case basis. Patients who have been moved from operating room table to bed and then transported for any distance are at risk for displacement of tubes and catheters. The admission chest radiograph allows for the evaluation of intravascular catheter and endotracheal, nasogastric, and thoracostomy tube positions in addition to visualization of the pleural, mediastinal, and parenchymal structures. Measurements of blood counts and chemistries are usually routine, but may be deemed unnecessary if preoperative or intraoperative values were unremarkable and the operation was uneventful. Laboratory abnormalities should be followed closely until a favorable trend is established. Patients at risk for perioperative myocardial injury or with new intraoperative arrhythmias should have an electrocardiogram and possibly cardiac enzyme determination.

The physical examination of the patient completes the initial postoperative evaluation. It starts as a cursory survey and concludes as a detailed examination. The examination should expose all parts of the patient that can be accessed, and the examiner should inspect and palpate the patient.

Box 35.1 Support for Adequate Clinical Perfusion

Mean arterial blood pressure >70 mm Hg
Heart rate <100 beats/minute
Warm, pink skin without cyanosis or mottling over the digits, thighs, or knees
Palpable pulses
Good capillary refill
Clear yellow urine >0.5-1 mL/kg/hour

Areas that are not under examination should be kept covered to preserve body temperature. If the bed sheets are being changed, it presents an opportunity to examine the back of the patient. An initial assessment of the vital signs, skin, pulses, and urine output provides preliminary insight into clinical perfusion (Box 35.1).

The endotracheal tube, if present, needs to be secured adequately. The health care provider should listen for obvious air leaks around the cuff. The presence of nasal or oral gastric tubes should be noted. All drainage tubes should be identified, and the quality and quantity of output should be scrutinized: Is it serous? Sanguineous? Bilious? Drainage from raw, inflamed surfaces is often serosanguineous. Frankly bloody drainage in quantities of more than 100 mL/hour suggests either surgical bleeding or coagulopathy. All intravascular catheters should be identified with the goal of determining which should be retained for use and which should be removed. Diagnostic catheters often remain unnoticed, and unused, particularly when in femoral vessels. Intravenous catheters not placed under sterile conditions should be removed immediately.

The neurologic examination may be suboptimal if the patient is still under the effects of anesthesia. Reducing or temporarily withholding narcotics and sedation can provide a window to complete a neurologic assessment. If further analgesia or sedation is still required, it may be resumed after the neurologic assessment. However, withholding sedation should not be done in the early postoperative course if it results in a state of competition with care (severe agitation, inability to oxygenate/ventilate, hemodynamic instability).

Intubation, general anesthesia, and mechanical ventilation can result in a variety of airway or parenchymal injuries. Breath sounds should be equal bilaterally. Asymmetry can be caused by atelectasis (possibly endotracheal tube malposition), pleural effusions, or pneumothorax and can be excluded by careful review of the chest radiograph. Examination of the respiratory system should include evaluation of thoracostomy tubes and the mechanical ventilator if present. Except in the case of pneumonectomy, thoracostomy tubes should be placed to suction pending demonstration of sustained lung inflation or resolution of significant drainage. The mechanical ventilator settings and airway pressures should be noted. Adjustments to mechanical ventilation may need to be made to accommodate shivering, metabolic abnormalities, and hypoxia in the early postoperative period. The clinician should ensure satisfactory initial oxygen saturation and avoid excessive tidal volumes. End-tidal carbon dioxide monitoring facilitates adjustment in ventilation and progress in weaning. Routine blood gas analysis is unnecessary but will be required to manage the more challenging derangements in gas exchange and acid/base disorders.

The cardiovascular examination is primarily directed at assessment of adequate clinical perfusion. Impressions from the initial survey of clinical perfusion plus any available data from invasive monitoring can be used to assess appropriate hourly maintenance fluid rate and the need for further volume resuscitation. Cardiac surgery patients may have mediastinal drains and pacing wires. The former should be connected to suction, and the quantity and quality of drainage should be scrutinized. Pacing wires should be tested for function on admission and can be capped if pacing is not needed. If a postoperative patient comes to the ICU with a permanent pacemaker or an implantable cardiac defibrillator, the device should be interrogated for mode and function at the earliest convenience.

In contrast to the lungs and heart, which can be imaged easily and whose function can be monitored objectively, the abdomen and its contents cannot be evaluated handily. The persistence of anesthesia or administration of narcotics can remove many of the signs and symptoms typically relied on to signal problems. Examination should focus on baseline location and quantity of pain, presence of abdominal distention, firmness to palpation, and quality and quantity of effluent from drains. Bleeding and progressive visceral edema can cause a rapid distention and loss of compliance of the abdomen, often before other findings occur, such as reduction in hemoglobin concentration, urine output, and blood pressure. Frequent follow-up examinations compared with baseline data may be the earliest way of recognizing an intra-abdominal catastrophe. The practitioner should be alert to abdominal distention with associated changes in clinical perfusion (such as low urine output) as a marker of abdominal compartment syndrome. Measurement and trending of bladder pressures can supplement other clinical findings in guiding decision making.

Knowing where the tip of each abdominal drain lies is necessary to evaluate the effluent. A drain lying outside the bowel or biliary system should not drain succus or bile. A drain that suddenly shows these fluids may herald loss of integrity of a surgical repair or de novo perforation. Unexplained or unexpected changes in the quantity of effluent from a drain also are notable.

Abdominal wounds are not always closed at the end of an operation. The clinician needs to determine if the skin or fascia has been left open and, if so, what kind of temporary closure is employed. If a temporary abdominal closure device is used, the quality and quantity of effluent from that device should be examined and documented. It is important to remember that temporary abdominal closure devices are not proof against abdominal compartment syndromes. The provider should be prepared to loosen the outer layers of an abdominal closure or dressing to provide temporary relief. Surgical or traumatic wounds, regardless of location on the body, should be examined for closure integrity, erythema, and induration.

Examination of pulses is important after vascular surgical procedures. Scheduled reassessments should document the presence and strength of pulses. Sudden reduction or loss of pulse signal can represent proximal vascular occlusion, a distal outflow obstruction, or increase in compartment pressures. Baseline cyanosis and mottling of extremities should be noted for subsequent comparison. In addition, a clinical examination (palpation) of the compartments should be performed to provide the practitioner a baseline for further comparison. Should the mechanism of injury increase the risk of muscle swelling and compartment syndromes, the practitioner can utilize invasive monitoring to measure compartment pressures, and should be prepared to pursue extremity fasciotomies.

Evaluation of a postoperative trauma patient in the ICU can be restricted by the presence of dressings and immobilizing casts and neck collars. Sometimes only toes or fingers are visible for examination. Postoperative admission to the ICU is a good opportunity to look for injuries missed during the initial evaluation and management period. In addition, the practitioner should be alert to potential iatrogenic injuries from intraoperative events; this would include electrical burns from ungrounded cautery circuits, infiltrated intravenous lines, and compression injuries from positioning in the operating room.

RECOVERY FROM ANESTHESIA

POSTOPERATIVE RESUSCITATION

ASSESSMENT

"Adequate resuscitation" is a state, often temporary, that allows for good clinical perfusion and physiologic stability. Patients with good clinical perfusion (expected heart rates, blood pressures, and urine outputs; absence of acidosis) may require no further resuscitation other than maintenance intravenous fluids. The correct maintenance fluid rate will be just enough to match intravascular losses out of proportion to that which is mobilizable from the interstitium but not so much as to needlessly expand the third space or interstium with edema. Subtle abnormalities in any of these parameters of perfusion may suggest a more serious physiologic derangement warranting further investigation and intervention. Resuscitation is the process of optimizing macroscopic and microscopic metabolic substrate delivery with the goal of avoiding an imbalance between supply and demand. The most fundamental concept is to ensure adequate oxygen delivery (Do_2) and meet the oxygen consumption ($\dot{V}o_2$) needs of tissues and organelles. Because the moment when $\dot{V}o_2$ exceeds Do_2 is difficult to determine, resuscitation "targets" serve as proxy markers of adequate Do_2. Resuscitation targets are reproducible, quantifiable values, such as pressures, outputs, metabolites, inflammatory mediators, or oxygen saturations, which represent therapeutic goals. Resuscitation targets provide an important opportunity for study and outcome validation. Despite the seemingly simple logic of employing resuscitation targets, few of these therapeutic goals have been shown to improve clinical outcome. Even routine data derived from a pulmonary artery catheter have not been shown to improve outcome in patients undergoing surgery with decompensated cardiogenic shock or acute lung injury.[12,13]

MANAGEMENT THEORY

Evaluation and optimization of blood pressure, filling pressures, Do_2, heart rate, and rhythm often occur simultaneously, particularly in unstable patients (Fig. 35.1). This may require ongoing volume resuscitation and support with vasopressors and inotropes. Restoration of "normal" blood pressure, heart rate, and urine output, however, do not ensure adequate Do_2 at the level of the microvasculature.[14] Overzealous resuscitation and supranormal Do_2 not only do not improve outcome but also may be detrimental.[15] Not all patients require the same type of resuscitation. Although the fundamental principles are the same, the particular resuscitation technique end points may differ among the different types of shock.[16,17] Crystalloid resuscitation may be appropriate in septic shock but detrimental in the early resuscitation of penetrating traumatic injury.[18,19] Even low-volume resucitation plays a role in the management of patients with penetrating traumatic injury or severe intraoperative hemorrhage.[20] Early goal-directed therapy with parameter-specific targets has not completely survived prospective validation. However, the principle of timely intervention remains a cornerstone for virtually all types of resuscitation. End points specific to particular mechanisms of injury can vary significantly.[21-23]

Targeted resuscitation strategies provide an orderly approach to resuscitation, monitoring, and outcome validation. In general, such strategies optimize cardiovascular performance and concurrently measure markers of adequate global Do_2 and $\dot{V}o_2$. Increased serum lactate concentration, decreased mixed venous oxygen saturation, and decreased central venous oxygen saturation are the proxy markers for inadequate global Do_2. However, normal values of mixed venous oxygen saturation and central venous oxygen saturation do not guarantee normal use of oxygen in the tissues, particularly at the regional level. Appropriate targets for microcirculatory resuscitation remain elusive. Noninvasive techniques have reduced the need to obtain physiologic data by the use of a pulmonary artery catheter.[24] Pulse and pressure wave analysis along with their derivitives (cardiac output and stroke volume variation) offer a less invasive way of measuring hemodynamic performance and predict volume responsiveness in the appropriate patient population.[25] Gastric tonometry, sublingual capnography, near-infrared spectroscopy, and orthogonal polarization spectral imaging are less mainstream technologies available to assess the effectiveness of resuscitation at the regional level.[26]

Resuscitation products should target the intravascular components that are inadequate, including red blood cell concentrates, platelets, coagulation factors, and acellular resuscitation fluids. Fluid type, bolus volume, and maintenance rate must be individualized. The optimal resuscitation fluid effectively should expand the intravascular space and minimize the inflammatory response (particularly in hemorrhagic shock[27,28]). All resuscitation fluids leak to some degree out of the intravascular space into the interstitium of the extracellular space. Hypotonic resuscitation fluids are inappropriate for volume resuscitation because of their inability to remain exclusively in the extracellular space. Volume per volume, hypertonic fluids cause more intravascular expansion than isotonic fluids. Hypertonic fluids yield no better outcomes than isotonic crystalloids, however, in the resuscitation of trauma patients.[29] Similarly, isotonic crystalloids are at least as efficacious or may be better than colloids to reach the same end points.[14] In trauma, burn,

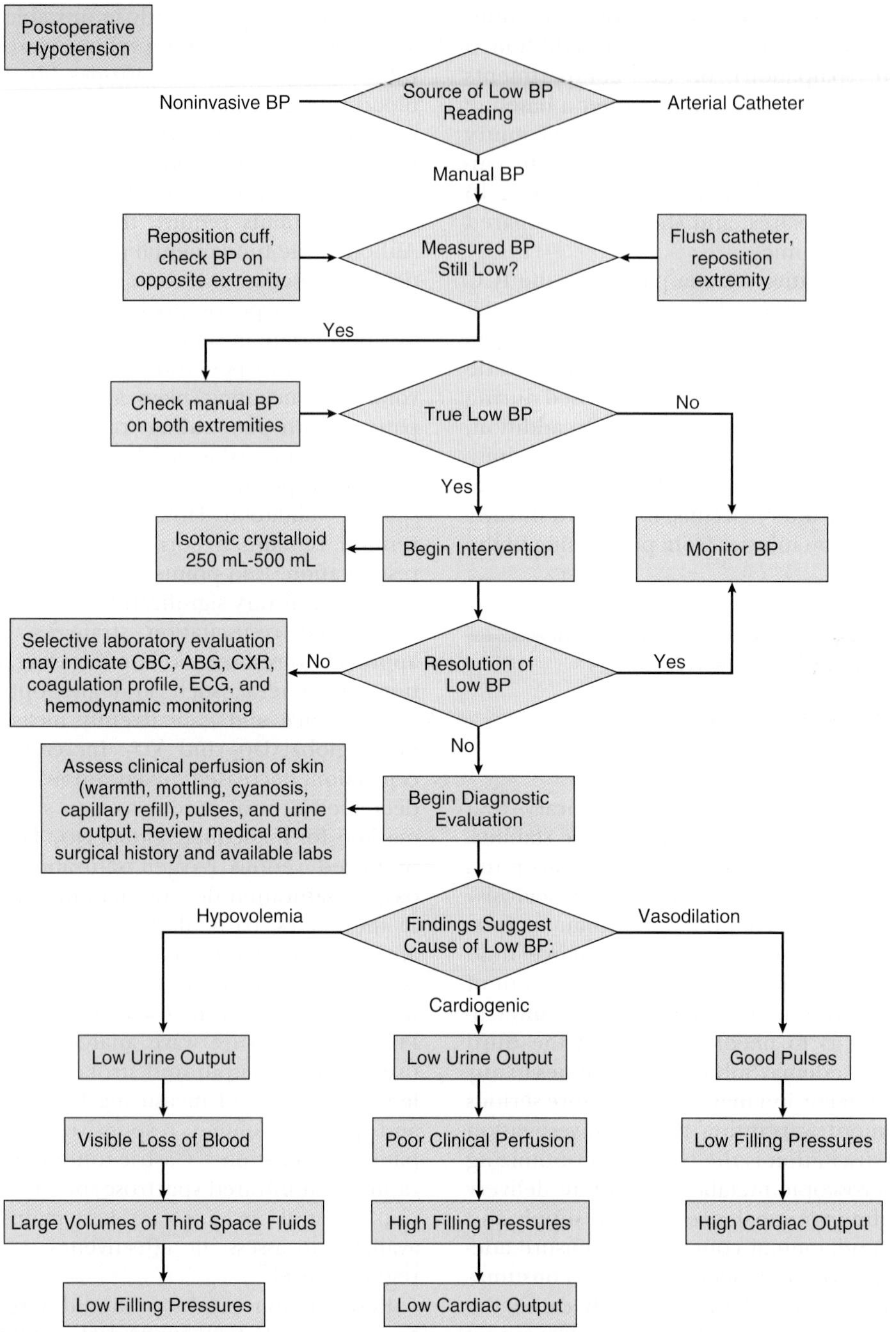

Figure 35.1 Approach to managing postoperative hypotension. ABG, arterial blood gases; BP, blood pressure; CBC, complete blood count; CXR, chest x-ray study; ECG, electrocardiogram.

and general surgery patients, resuscitation with colloids, as compared to crystalloids, has not been shown to reduce the risk of death.[30]

Metabolic consequences are associated with virtually all resuscitation fluids. Ringer's lactate can activate neutrophils and cause a potent inflammatory response.[31] Hypertonic saline and dextran combinations cause less of an inflammatory response but any mortality benefit is unproved.[32,33] Greater than 1 L of hypertonic saline typically results in the development of hypernatremia. Resuscitation exclusively with isotonic NaCl results in a hyperchloremic acidosis. Recent literature has suggested that hetastarch is associated with greater adverse events when compared to saline resuscitation.[34] Hetastarch can cause coagulopathy if greater than 1.5 L is given. All acellular resuscitation fluids, if given in sufficient quantities, cause dilutional anemia. As one can infer from this confusing and sometimes contradictory collection of recommendations, no single resuscitation fluid is satisfactory on its own.

TEMPERATURE CONTROL

Postoperative patients can come to the ICU with moderate to severe hypothermia. Heat is lost in the operating room as a result of vasodilation from volatile anesthetics, cool intravenous fluids and air temperature, large open surfaces, and evaporation. Excluding patients with potentially anoxic central nervous system injuries,[35] hypothermia complicates initial postoperative care by creating an in vivo coagulopathy, even when in vitro coagulation studies (normalized to 37° C) are normal. In trauma patients, reduction in enzyme activity and platelet function, leading to abnormal fibrin polymerization, occurs at temperatures less than 34° C.[36] Care must be taken when administering large volumes of cold blood products or even room temperature crystalloids. Fluid warming devices are available not only to prevent but also to treat hypothermia. All patients with postoperative hypothermia less than 36° C should be actively warmed with forced air blankets, and when normothermia has been achieved, patients should be kept covered to prevent heat loss. Active warming does not cause peripheral vasodilation and subsequent hypotension, and it does not paradoxically cause core cooling owing to heat exchange in cold extremities.

AWAKENING FROM ANESTHESIA

Before completing a successful resuscitation, sedation, analgesia, and anxiolysis should be maintained to facilitate patient comfort and to prevent interference with medical care (e.g., mechanical ventilation or motor activity jeopardizing airway, drains, and intravenous catheters). Selected agents should have minimal hemodynamic sequelae and relatively short duration of action so that frequent neurologic assessment can be performed. Daily interruption of continuous sedation has been shown to reduce ICU length of stay, duration of mechanical ventilation, and incidence of posttraumatic stress disorder.[37,38]

Narcotics such as fentanyl, morphine, and hydromorphone make ideal first-line analgesics. Delivered by continuous infusion and supplemented as needed, successful analgesia reduces pain-driven tachycardia and hypertension and facilitates cough and deep breathing. The sensation of anxiety is a potent dysphoric stimulus that can result in restlessness and interfere with care. Anxiety can be treated with short-acting intravenous benzodiazepines, such as lorazepam. Very short-acting benzodiazepines, such as midazolam, are less useful because of the dosing frequency necessary to prevent symptoms from returning. It is important not to use scheduled benzodiazepines to treat restlessness due to delirium. This practice can exacerbate delirium and worsen outcomes. Delirium can be identified using simple evaluation tools such as the Confusion Assessment Method for the ICU (CAM-ICU). Competitive restlessness due to delirium is best managed with atypical antipsychotics such as haloperidol, ziprazadone, and quetiepine.[39] Persistant restlessness, agitation, or delirium can compete with mechanical ventilation, confound hemodynamic stability, and impede the provision of care. If further reduction of level of consciousness is necessary, propofol or dexmedetomidine can be added and titrated to desired effect. Dexmedetomidine, a weak analgesic, can reduce narcotic requirements.[40] Propofol, however, has no intrinsic analgesic properties. In a patient who has serious pain, neither propofol nor dexmedetomidine should be used without the concurrent administration of a narcotic. The use of most agents mentioned can be limited by their tendency to reduce blood pressure and, in the case of dexmedetomidine, decrease heart rate.

When patients are resuscitated adequately, consideration can be given to awakening from residual sedation. On arrival to the surgical ICU or recovery room, unconsciousness, if present, is due to the residual effects of volatile anesthetics, narcotics, benzodiazepines, and paralytics. The effects of volatile anesthetics can persist for 20 to 60 minutes after their discontinuation, particularly if the agent is fat-soluble, the patient is obese, and the surgery was long. Paralytics can have longer than expected duration of action, and this should be suspected when a postoperative patient remains very weak (cannot perform a 10-second head lift) or does not move. A train-of-four twitch monitor can address this issue. Persistent chemical paralysis can be reversed with neostigmine and glycopyrrolate.

Reentry into consciousness may be accompanied by disorientation, anxiety, pain, and varying degrees of restlessness. In the absence of underlying encephalopathy, it is usually possible to get patients to follow commands, answer questions, and participate in the extubation process. The discomfort of an endotracheal tube can lead to unplanned self-extubation. It is important for the bedside care provider to maintain control of the recovery process by ensuring analgesia and anxiolysis. Small doses of narcotic or benzodiazepine or both can usually correct these problems without inducing further sedation and delay of extubation.[41] Patients with encephalopathy resulting from sepsis or shock may not recover a level of consciousness that allows participation in the weaning process. It is controversial whether such a patient should be extubated (avoiding the complications of prolonged extubation) or remain intubated until the ability to protect the airway is more certain. Dexmedetomidine can reduce restlessness without respiratory suppression and may be useful to facilitate extubation of a restless patient. Patients who require sedation for an extended time should receive doses of medication no higher than necessary to achieve the therapeutic target. Sedation scales, such as the Ramsay and Richmond Agitation Sedation Scale,[42] are useful to avoid oversedation and ultimately promote earlier liberation from mechanical ventilation.

POSTOPERATIVE EXTUBATION

Liberation from mechanical ventilation requires clinical readiness to begin weaning and demonstration of adequate physiologic reserve before extubation. Clinical readiness assesses completion of perioperative tasks at hand and questions any need for early return to the operating room. Resuscitation should be complete, hemostasis should be achieved, metabolic acidosis should be resolving, vasoactive support and gas exchange abnormalities should be minimized, anesthetic agents should be cleared, the ability to protect the airway should be present, and the patient should be awake and reasonably cooperative. These criteria have not been validated clinically, but similar consensus guidelines have been published.[43] Daily, if not more frequent, reassessment of clinical readiness is necessary to determine if it is reasonable to consider weaning.[44]

Patients who are ready clinically to progress to extubation should have an assessment of physiologic reserve. Having the patient breathe without mechanical assistance allows observation of respiratory rate, mechanical coordination of chest and abdomen, vital signs, end-tidal carbon dioxide concentration, and subjective comfort. If the patient was not mechanically ventilated preoperatively, the perioperative course has been uneventful, the patient is comfortable with stable vital signs, no tachypnea or respiratory muscle dyssynchrony is present, and there is no short-term plan to return to the operating room, the patient should begin spontaneous breathing trials and be evaluated for extubation.

Patients who do not achieve these basic criteria may require continued mechanical ventilation that maximizes patient comfort and unloads the respiratory muscles. These patients require a structured, evidence-based approach to ventilator weaning and assessment of adequate physiologic reserve. For more detailed information on weaning, refer to Chapter 43.

BEST PRACTICES

Achieving optimal outcomes should be pursued by providing optimal care. This is especially true for patients with longer length of stay. Effort should be expended pursuing interventions that have been shown to reduce complications, cost, morbidity, and mortality risk. Because a postoperative ICU patient is different in many ways from other ICU patients, some of these fundamental practices are applied with slight nuance and warrant additional mention.

PREVENTION OF VENOUS THROMBOEMBOLISM AND DEEP VENOUS THROMBOSIS

All postoperative ICU patients should be considered for venous thromboembolism (VTE) or deep venous thrombosis (DVT) prophylaxis. The risk of postoperative VTE depends upon both the type of procedure and modifying attributes such as age, prior VTE, history of cancer, obesity, or hypercoagulable state. Risk has been quantified and grouped based on the Modified Caprini Risk Assessment Model.[45] Low-risk general and abdominal-pelvic surgery patients should receive intermittent pneumatic compression (IPC) over no prophylaxis or anticoagulant-based prophylaxis. Moderate-risk general and abdominal-pelvic surgery patients should receive anticoagulant-based prophylaxis. Low-dose unfractionated heparin, low-molecular-weight heparin, or fondaparinux should be started in the absence of postoperative bleeding. High-risk general and abdominal-pelvic surgery patients should receive low-dose unfractionated heparin three times a day, low-molecular-weight heparin, or fondaparinux. The highest risk patients should receive mechanical prophylaxis via IPC devices, in addition to low-dose unfractionated heparin, low-molecular-weight heparin, or fondaparinux. In general surgery patients with a high risk of postoperative bleeding, mechanical prophylaxis should be the initial preventive modality until the risk of bleeding has decreased enough to allow for anticoagulant prophylaxis.[46]

Neurosurgical procedures or the use of neuraxial analgesia also require special consideration. Anticoagulant prophylaxis should not be in effect while epidural catheters are placed or removed and should be used with caution while an epidural catheter is in place. Patients undergoing intracranial surgery should receive mechanical prophylaxis with sequential compression devices. Anticoagulant prophylaxis should be added in neurosurgical patients at high risk for VTE/DVT beginning 24 hours postoperatively.

Trauma patients constitute an extremely heterogeneous group, making it difficult to study the strategies of VTE/DVT prophylaxis. There is disagreement in the literature about valid independent risk factors for VTE/DVT in trauma patients. Older age, spinal fractures, spinal cord injuries, traumatic brain injuries, prolonged mechanical ventilation, pelvic fractures, venous injuries, and multiple major operative procedures are often cited. In trauma patients, there are few large, prospective, randomized studies validating the efficacy of any method of VTE/DVT prevention.[47] Low-dose unfractionated heparin, which has proven efficacy in the general surgery population, is no better than absence of prophylaxis in a trauma patient.[48] Low-molecular-weight heparin given twice daily does offer a statistical benefit, however, in the prevention VTE/DVT in trauma patients.[49] Trauma patients without significant risks for bleeding should begin anticoagulant prophylaxis or postoperatively. Data are insufficient to make recommendations as to when anticoagulant prophylaxis in trauma patients with brain injury or liver or spleen fracture is safe. Waiting 24 hours after bleeding has ceased is a conservative time to delay.[50] In trauma patients at high risk for bleeding, mechanical prophylaxis can be used, although benefit is unproved. Note that IPCs cannot be applied to lower extremities with fractures, fasciotomies, or external fixators. Compression devices applied to the feet may be used as a substitute for IPC but have not been shown to be as efficacious as leg devices. In selected trauma patients expected to have prolonged immobilization or with significant risks for bleeding, inferior vena cava filters may be placed as VTE prophylaxis.[30] Inferior vena cava filters should not be used as a primary prophylactic strategy in trauma patients.[29] If available, removable filters should be considered, despite the low removal rates. In a trauma patient at high risk for VTE/DVT, the addition of mechanical prophylaxis to anticoagulant prophylaxis may be useful, but synergistic benefit is unproved.

STRESS ULCER PROPHYLAXIS

Stress-related mucosal disease (SRMD) is manifest as diffuse gastric mucosal petechiae, erosions (loss of epithelium, necrosis, and hemorrhage), and discrete ulcers. SRMD can progress to clinically significant bleeding resulting in hemodynamic instability and need for transfusion. It can develop as early as 24 hours after ICU admission. Patients at risk for SRMD include critically ill patients who require mechanical ventilation for greater than 48 hours; patients with coagulopathy, traumatic brain or spinal cord injury, or severe burns; and patients with a history of gastrointestinal bleeding or ulceration within the past year. Minor risks include sepsis, corticosteroids, and prolonged ICU admission.[51] The risk of clinically significant bleeding increases with the severity of illness, duration of mechanical ventilation, increased length of stay, and low intragastric pH. Hemodynamic compromise secondary to acute blood loss occurs in only a small percentage of patients with SRMD, but it is associated with a significantly increased mortality rate.[52]

Because of the morbidity and mortality rates associated with the complications of SRMD, it is important to identify patients at risk for SRMD and employ effective prophylaxis before bleeding occurs. Although early enteral nutrition has many benefits, the effects of enteral nutrition on SRMD are controversial and should not be used as a sole prophylactic strategy.[53] Pharmacologic prophylaxis targets mucosal protection or the suppression of acid secretion. Proton-pump inhibitors may be a good first choice for SRMD prophylaxis owing to degree of acid suppression, duration of action, lack of tolerance, and cost. Parenteral H_2 receptor antagonists may offer a cost advantage over proton-pump inhibitors. Prophylaxis with sucralfate is not preferred because of the efficacy profile of acid-suppression therapies and a higher rate of bleeding with sucralfate prophylaxis.

PREVENTING NOSOCOMIAL PNEUMONIA

The most significant risk for hospital-acquired pneumonia (HAP) in the postoperative patient is mechanical ventilation. Other significant risks include age more than 70 years, chronic lung disease, and depressed levels of consciousness. Though gastric acid suppression is also associated with an increased incidence of HAP, withholding ulcer prophylaxis can hardly be avoided in the patient mechanically ventilated for more than 48 hours.[54] Postoperative patients should be encouraged to take deep breaths, cough, ambulate, and use incentive spirometry. Semirecumbent body positioning, keeping the head of bed elevated more than 30 degrees, has been shown to reduce ventilator-associated pneumonia in mechanically ventilated patients.[55] Placing the bed in reverse Trendelenburg position can simulate this elevation without flexing the back, as could be difficult in trauma patients or patients with large open abdomens. Iatrogenic spread of bacteria that can cause pneumonia can be reduced by the enforcement of handwashing and by the use of appropriate barrier protection when performing procedures.[56] Before deflating the cuff of an endotracheal tube for tube removal or position change, ensure that secretions are suctioned clear from above the cuff.[36] Endotracheal tubes designed to provide drainage to the subglottic area above the tube's cuff have been shown to reduce the risk of ventilator-associated pneumonia.[57,58] The use of 0.12% chlorhexidine oral rinse has been associated with reductions in the rate of ventilator-associated pneumonia in surgical ICU patients and should be part of good oral hygiene.[59] Although there is evidence that selective digestive decontamination beyond the oropharynx also can reduce the risk of ventilator-associated pneumonia, it is unclear how the routine use of this technique would affect antimicrobial resistance.[60] The use of noninvasive ventilation in patients with exacerbations of chronic obstructive pulmonary disorder and congestive heart failure is associated with reductions in rates of nosocomial pneumonia, but there are few studies evaluating application of this technique in the management of postoperative respiratory failure.[61]

MANAGEMENT OF AGITATION AND DELIRIUM

Delirium is a major problem in postoperative ICU patients.[62] Previously believed to be an expected and unavoidable result of critical illness that resolves with clinical improvement, it is now known to be a significant marker of increased morbidity,[63] resource use, and long-term cognitive deficit. Delirium is an acute, variable change in mental status with inattention and either altered level of consciousness or disorganized thinking. Delirium can be hypoactive or hyperactive, the majority of patients being in the former group. Occurring in about 70% to 80% of ICU patients, delirium had been underdiagnosed until validated assessment tools such as the CAM-ICU became available.[64] Delirium is believed to be due to imbalances between the stimulatory and inhibitory neurotransmitters, particularly an increase in dopaminergic and decrease in γ-aminobutyric acid and cholinergic activity. Risk factors include age, preexisting dementia, sepsis, metabolic abnormalities, and medications. The use of benzodiazepines, narcotics, anticholinergics, and antipsychotics is associated with a substantial increase in risk. It is currently unclear whether prevention or treatment of delirium changes clinical outcomes such as fatality and long-term cognitive deficits.

Preventive strategies include avoidance of hypoxemia (Fig. 35.2), correction of metabolic disturbances, and adequate pain control. In addition, environmental normalization with minimization of unnecessary physical and auditory stimulation, restoration of sleep/wake cycles, frequent reorientation (particularly with family involvement), and early mobilization can help decrease rates of ICU delirium.[42] Pharmacologic treatment of delirium is suboptimal because the same medications intended to reduce disorganized thought may simultaneously increase sedation, prolonging the undesired state. Benzodiazepines may aggravate disorganized thought and should not be used to treat delirium. Haloperidol is the most commonly prescribed neuroleptic to treat delirium,[65] although its efficacy is yet to be validated. Other atypical antipsychotics such as olanzapine, quetiapine, ziprasidone, and risperidone have also recently gained popularity.[66,67] Until efficacy of any pharmacologic intervention is shown, medications should be used in the lowest doses possible for as brief a time as possible.

MANAGEMENT OF BLOOD GLUCOSE LEVEL

Hyperglycemia in a critically ill patient can be due to diabetes mellitus (established or new) or stress-induced release of counterregulatory mediators. It is associated with increased mortality risk after acute myocardial infarction, stroke, and severe traumatic brain injury. Hyperglycemia also is associated with reduced functional outcome after neurologic injury, the development of polyneuropathy in critically ill patients, increased rates of infectious complications in the postoperative period, and defective collagen formation in wound healing. Earlier studies[68-70] about the benefits of intensive insulin therapy had been published touting improved outcomes, but more contemporary evidence has shown results to the contrary.

Blood glucose less than 60 mg/dL occurs up to 32% of the time when intensive insulin strategies are utilized. Hypoglycemia can have a negative impact on mortality risk and neurologic outcome.[71] Identification of appropriate blood glucose target ranges and management techniques has required the prospective study of thousands (NICE-SUGAR)[72] of medical and surgical patients. From this data, and other meta-analyses, we can make some observations and logical management recommendations. Intensive insulin treatment, targeting a blood glucose of 80 to

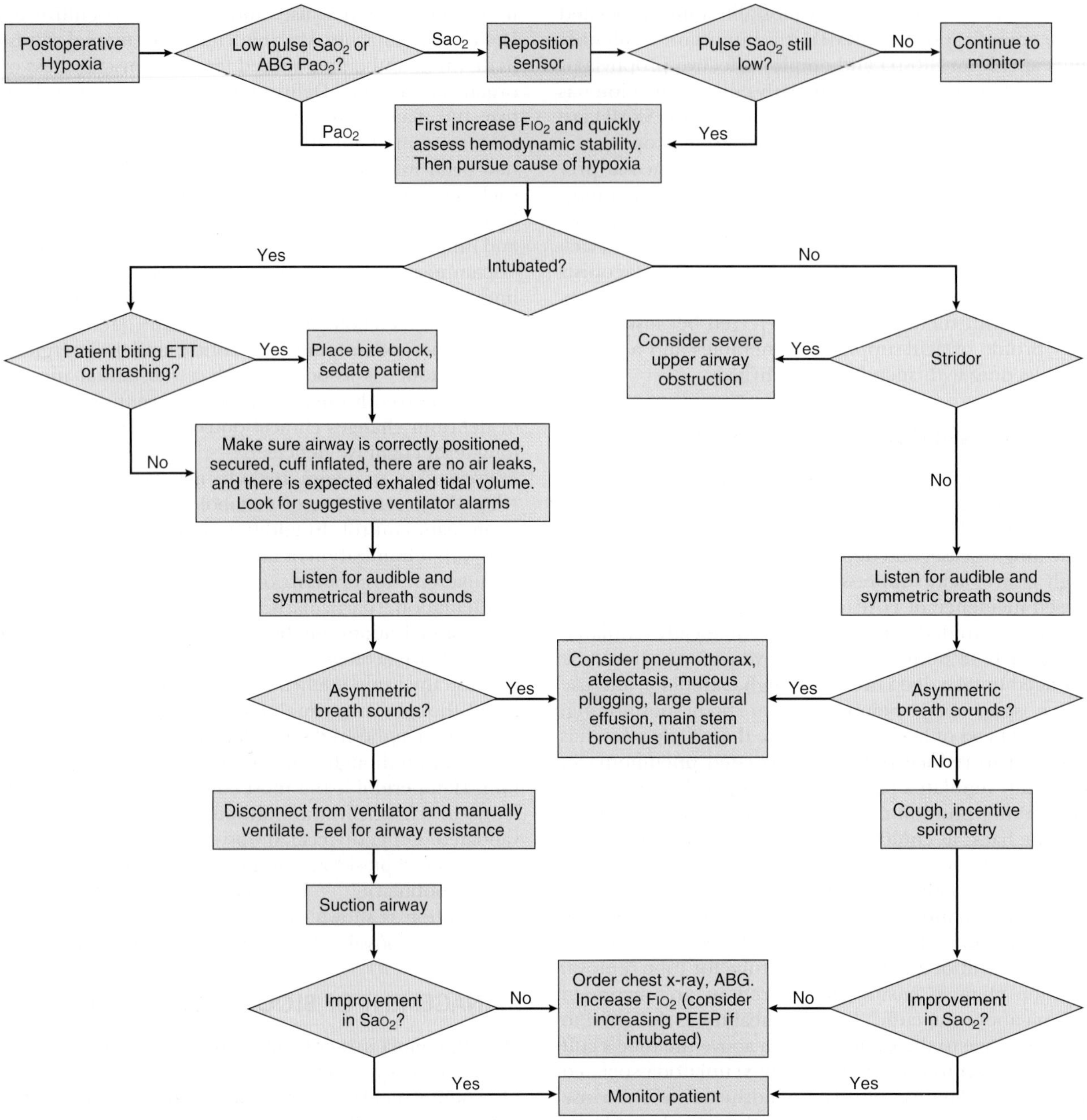

Figure 35.2 Approach to managing postoperative hypoxemia. ABG, arterial blood gas; ETT, endotracheal tube; F_{IO_2}, fraction of inspired oxygen; Pa_{O_2}, arterial oxygen tension; PEEP, positive end-expiratory pressure; Sa_{O_2}, arterial oxygen saturation.

110 mg/dL, increases the incidence of episodes of severe hypoglycemia and either has no effect on mortality risk or increases mortality risk when compared to more liberal blood glucose target ranges of 140 to 180 mg/dL and 180 to 200 mg/dL.

A rational approach to the management of blood glucose begins with minimizing causes of hyperglycemia such as unnecessary dextrose in intravenous fluids, choosing appropriate balances of carbohydrates and fats in the diet, and avoidance of overfeeding. Blood glucose targets in the 140 to 180 mg/dL range and an insulin regimen that minimizes hypoglycemia appear to be the most beneficial strategy.

Unreliable subcutaneous absorption, extreme or labile hyperglycemia, and inconsistent caloric intake are reasons to use short-acting, continuous intravenous insulin rather than slower-onset, longer-acting subcutaneous insulin. The treatment of hypoglycemia also needs to be considered an urgent therapy.

POSTOPERATIVE NUTRITION

Postoperative surgical patients are exposed to unique nutritional challenges as a result of the enhanced metabolic demands of wound healing and the abnormalities of bowel motility, anastomotic function, and swallowing. Nutritional support provides calories for metabolic processes, reduces catabolism of protein stores as an energy source, supplies substrate for anabolic processes, and provides an opportunity to reduce net protein losses in the face of ongoing protein catabolism. In an otherwise well-nourished postoperative patient, beginning nutritional support may be unnecessary, unless it is anticipated that oral intake at nutritional goal would be delayed for 7 days.[73] There are considerably fewer studies showing nutritional support strategies that work in the postoperative patient than ones that do not work.[74]

TIMING AND ROUTE

There are three routes of nutritional support—enteral nutrition (including nasogastric tube or postpyloric tube), parenteral nutrition, and oral feedings. With respect to outcomes, it is important to consider not only the route of administration but also the timing. Neither enteral nutrition nor parenteral nutrition seems to have an effect on *mortality* rates whether given preoperatively or postoperatively.[75] *Preoperative* nutritional support seems to benefit only severely malnourished patients by reducing complication rates.[76,77] Parenteral nutrition, which requires vascular access, is associated with complications related to non–catheter-related infection and catheter-related bloodstream infection. In addition to avoiding the complications associated with parenteral nutrition, enteral nutrition possibly reduces gut mucosal atrophy and up-regulates gut-associated immunity. In theory this protects against infections elsewhere by the common mucosal immune hypothesis.[78] In perioperative patients, sufficient evidence is lacking, however, to suggest that the effect of enteral nutrition on the gut barrier has any outcome advantage over parenteral nutrition.[79,80] Enteral nutrition has been shown to be associated with a lower risk of infection compared with parenteral nutrition.[81] Early enteral nutrition also has been shown to be associated with a shorter length of stay and lower incidence of infections compared with delayed enteral nutrition.[82] Enteral nutrition is the preferred route over parenteral nutrition because of the reduction in complications and cost. Early postoperative parenteral nutrition does not improve clinical outcomes and should be reserved only for patients who are unable to receive timely enteral nutrition.[83]

The combination of parenteral nutrition and early enteral nutrition has no advantage over early enteral nutrition alone in patients who are not malnourished.[84] Patients who are malnourished or are not expected to be tolerating enteral feedings at nutritional goal by about postoperative day 7 should begin parenteral nutrition. If otherwise adequately nourished postoperative ICU patients are expected to be tolerating enteral feedings at nutritional goal by postoperative day 7, early parenteral nutrition may not provide substantial benefit. Finally, patients who are able to tolerate enteral feedings but are unable to tolerate an amount equal to the nutritional goal require supplemental nutrition, typically parenteral nutrition.

When the decision is made to deliver enteral nutrition, tube feedings should be increased quickly in volume to reach nutritional goal. The initial destination for enteral nutrition is the stomach. Nothing about laparotomy itself precludes enteral nutrition with the return of bowel function (e.g., bowel sounds, flatus). Although bowel motility continues through surgery or returns shortly thereafter, gastroparesis is common postoperatively and may result in delayed gastric emptying. It may be recognized by abdominal distention, high daily nasogastric output (>500 mL/day), or high residual volume in the stomach (>300 mL). Gastroparesis has the potential to delay achieving delivery of adequate enteral nutrition and has resulted in a trend toward delivering enteral nutrition via a postpyloric route. There are recent data to suggest that postpyloric feedings in patients with severe traumatic brain injury reduces the incidence of overall and late pneumonia and in addition improves nutritional efficacy.[85] Other data suggest that there is no clinical benefit to postpyloric feeding with respect to incidence of pneumonia, ICU length of stay, mortality rate, or time to reach nutritional goal compared with the prepyloric route.[86] Evidence to demonstrate the clinical benefit of postpyloric to prepyloric feedings is possibly still equivocal. Gastroparesis often can be improved with prokinetic agents, such as metoclopramide or erythromycin.[87] It is reasonable to continue gastric enteral nutrition in the presence of gastric residual volumes of 150 to 300 mL as long as the patient is not experiencing nausea, vomiting, or progressive abdominal distention or has any evidence of functional gastric outlet obstruction or ileus. The nasogastric route of feeding is preferred, but if establishing stomach function is anticipated to be problematic, implantation placement of a jejunostomy feeding tube should be considered during laparotomy.

FEEDING CONSIDERATIONS IN GENERAL SURGERY PATIENTS

ESOPHAGUS

Patients requiring esophageal resection may present with some degree of malnutrition. It is important to resume nutritional support as soon as technically possible after the operation. These patients have fragile anastomoses in their chests, however, which usually have a suction catheter placed across the repair to decompress the postanastomotic structures. An oral diet is delayed to ensure mechanical integrity of the anastomosis. Some patients have a distal feeding tube placed at the time of surgery so that enteral nutrition does not need to be delayed. Patients who cannot receive oral or enteral nutrition by postoperative day 7 should be considered for institution of parenteral nutrition.

STOMACH

Gastric surgery may result in delayed gastric emptying. Vagal denervation can cause some degree of gastroparesis, and functional outlet obstruction may occur owing to edema at the site of anastomosis. Gastric enteral nutrition cannot be started until gastric emptying improves. If it seems that gastric enteral nutrition would be unacceptably delayed, a more distal enteral route should be secured, or parenteral nutrition should be started. Patients with new gastrostomies, whether placed percutaneously or via an open procedure, rarely have postoperative motility disturbances. It is common, however, to wait for 24 hours before the use of gastronomy feeding tubes.

SMALL AND LARGE INTESTINE

Postoperative ICU patients with manipulation, resection, or diversion of the bowel may have a transient ileus. Small bowel hypomotility, if present, resolves 6 to 8 hours after surgery, and some absorptive capacity is present even without normal peristalsis.[88,89] Large bowel hypomotility, if present, begins to resolve 24 hours postoperatively, heralded by the passage of flatus. Recognized postoperatively as abdominal distention on physical examination or a nonobstructed gas pattern on abdominal x-ray study, ileus usually resolves over 24 to 72 hours with conservative therapy including nasogastric suctioning. Refractory ileus in the absence of mechanical obstruction should suggest some unresolved inflammatory process. In the absence of such unresolved problems, ileus also can be improved with prokinetic agents. Neostigmine has been successful in decompressing acute colonic pseudo-obstruction.[90] The presence of enterotomy repairs, bowel anastomoses, or new ostomies should not be barriers to enteral nutrition with the return of bowel function.[91]

FISTULAS

Nutritional support in the presence of an enterocutaneous fistula is problematic because enteral nutrition can exacerbate fistula output. This output, particularly when high, can perpetuate or worsen malnutrition owing to the loss of nitrogen and also lead to significant losses of intravascular volume and total body water. With the exception of some colocutaneous fistulas, conservative therapy consists of bowel rest (nothing per mouth), parenteral nutrition, control of infection, correction of electrolyte disturbances, and local wound care.

PANCREATITIS

Acute pancreatitis is treated commonly in the surgical ICU. In mild acute pancreatitis, enteral nutrition has no effect on outcome and is recommended only in patients who cannot tolerate oral nutrition after 5 to 7 days.[92] In severe acute pancreatitis, the therapeutic pendulum has swung from bowel rest and parenteral nutrition back toward early enteral nutrition. Although no differences in mortality rate have been shown in severe acute pancreatitis between groups treated with enteral nutrition and parenteral nutrition, the early enteral nutrition group has significant reductions in stress response, infections, surgical interventions, and length of stay.[93,94] The theoretical benefit of feeding beyond the ligament of Treitz versus gastric feeding in patients with severe acute pancreatitis remains controversial in the available literature.

NUTRITION IN WOUND HEALING

Nutritional deficiencies can impede wound healing. Large open wounds are metabolically demanding and may be a source of substantial protein loss. Daily dietary goals of calorie and protein need to be increased accordingly. Deficiencies of vitamins and minerals (micronutrients) are infrequent, but should be suspected in malnourished (including unusual dietary habits) patients, elderly patients, and patients who have been receiving parenteral nutrition. Vitamin and mineral supplementation should accompany dietary calorie and protein in patients with deficiencies, but the benefit of pharmacologic doses of these micronutrients in the absence of deficiency is unproved. Vitamin A has been shown to antagonize the detrimental effects of corticosteroids on inflammation, epithelialization, and collagen synthesis. However, it does not lower infection rates or ameliorate impaired wound contraction associated with corticosteroid therapy.[95,96] Currently, vitamin A is not routinely used used to treat patients with corticosteroid-induced immunosuppression because evidence for benefit in clinical practice is lacking. Vitamin C is needed for hydroxylation of lysine and proline in collagen formation (see earlier discussion). The benefit of vitamin C supplementation in patients receiving a normal diet is not validated. Zinc is an essential trace mineral for protein synthesis, cell division, and protein synthesis; however, its supplementation has not been shown to be beneficial in patients who are not zinc deficient.[75] Glucosamine is required for the synthesis of hyaluronic acid, an abundant component of the extracellular matrix, but also lacks clinical validation of benefit.

WOUND HEALING AND CARE

PHYSIOLOGY AND BIOLOGY OF WOUND HEALING

Many tissues in the body respond to injury by undergoing a reparative process, which can be described histologically, biochemically, chronologically, or functionally. There are many ways to label these processes, but a simple and useful paradigm includes inflammatory, proliferative, and remodeling phases.[97,98] The process begins with hemostasis, inflammation, and generation of an extracellular matrix on which proliferating cells can attach. Wound healing is locally coordinated by cytokines and facilitated by systemically mobilized cellular elements and noncellular substrate. Ultimately, the normal healing process ends with collagen maturation. Collagen develops its tensile strength through intermolecular cross-linking of fibrils into larger and longer bundles. The collagen mass undergoes continual synthesis and degradation as weaker, randomly oriented collagen fibers are reorganized into stronger, linear, highly cross-linked bundles aligned toward mechanical stress placed on the wound. This remodeling process may last 6 to 12 months, with the tissue never fully recovering its original strength. In normal circumstances, these phases tend to be sequential with generous overlap between the end of one phase and the beginning of the next.

Surgical site infection (SSI), the presence of necrotic tissue, the presence of a foreign body, an immunocompromised state, ischemia, and poor surgical closure technique all can contribute to failed wound healing and possibly wound dehiscence. Wounds are classified by their native propensity for infection as clean, clean contaminated, contaminated, and dirty. Clean wounds are uninfected with little or no inflammation, and dirty wounds are those with gross contamination such as fecal matter. Clean-contaminated and contaminated wounds lie somewhere in the middle of this spectrum.[99] Although a clean or clean-contaminated surgical wound may be purposely closed by primary intention, a contaminated or dirty wound is left open to close slowly by granulation and wound contraction (secondary intention). Alternatively, a contaminated wound may be left open for several days prior to being closed (delayed primary closure) to prevent infection. The healing processes are similar in these various approaches to wound management. Successful healing of a closed surgical wound yields mechanical integrity by virtue of high tensile strength. Successful healing in an open wound may be measured by epithelialization with the promise of satisfactory mechanical integrity (scarring) over time. Understanding these interrelated processes facilitates logical wound care and helps to avoid diversions from normal wound healing.

EPITHELIALIZATION AND WOUND CARE

Development of an epithelial barrier begins within hours of injury. In partial-thickness wounds, the source of epithelial repopulation is remaining dermal structures, sweat glands, and hair follicles. Epithelial cells from the basal layers of the wound migrate across the underlying extracellular matrix, re-forming the characteristic basal to apical differentiation, until migration halts in the center of the wound because of contact inhibition. Wound coverage can be complete 24 to 48 hours after a clean surgical incision is closed by primary intention. At this time, no further wound protection is necessary, and skin cleansing with water is permitted. Bacteria, necrotic tissue, wound exudates, inflammatory cells, inflammatory mediators, and desiccation all retard re-epithelialization. Deeper or open wounds also show delayed epithelialization. Open wounds first must fill in with proliferating fibroblasts, capillaries, and a loose extracellular matrix made of collagen and proteoglycans (granulation tissue) before epithelialization can occur. Such tissue is of poor mechanical integrity.

The ability of epithelialization to occur from the margin of the wounds over the granulation tissue depends on the presence of adequate angiogenesis, absence of bacterial burden, the provision of a moist environment, and the removal of excess necrosis and proteinaceous exudates (which contain proteases and inflammatory mediators and support bacterial growth). With optimal circumstances, the maximal rate of epithelialization from the margins occurs at 1 to 2 mm/day. As the epithelial cells mature and stratification progresses, keratinization occurs.

Without moist, occlusive dressings over superficial wounds, eschar forms, delaying epithelialization. Only with clot proteolysis can the wound be resurfaced successfully. If the wound is kept moist with an occlusive dressing,[100] however, and accumulated exudates and necrotic tissue are removed frequently, epithelialization can occur. Small amounts of wound exudates and necrotic tissue can be removed with frequent, moist dressing changes and water irrigation; larger amounts may require surgical débridement. The optimal wound dressing provides a moist environment, has absorptive reserve to trap wound exudates, possesses bacteriostatic properties, and does not adhere to the wound. Large, open wounds may be dressed with moist gauze at the surface and reinforced with dry gauze packing (wet-to-dry dressing). Absorptive capacity is limited, however, and frequent dressing changes are required. Dressings made of hydrocolloids, materials that incorporate high-capacity absorptive materials into a self-adhering occlusive backing, are useful for open wounds of moderate size and allow for less frequent dressing changes. More recently, the vacuum-assisted closure has gained popularity for the management of large open wounds. Vacuum-assisted closure therapy is the combination of moderate suction applied above an absorptive surface, such as a towel or sponge, which is covered by an occlusive plastic drape. The application provides for increased blood flow, the promotion of angiogenesis, a reduction of wound surface area in certain types of wounds, and induction of cell proliferation. However, at this time, vacuum-assisted closure therapy has not been shown to reduce edema, improve bacterial clearance, or increase the speed of healing in chronic wounds.[101,102]

OPTIMIZING WOUND HEALING

The first rule of wound evaluation is "take off the dressing and look at the wound." Wounds should be evaluated at least daily or with each dressing change in the case of vacuum-assisted closure therapy for progression of healing and development of infection. Normally healing surgical incisions should be dry with a minimal dry eschar at the point of closure. The edges should have at most a 3- to 4-mm border of erythema and induration when fresh, which should resolve over about 1 week.

ANTIBIOTICS

The routine use of systemic antibiotics to aid wound healing, in the absence of actual SSI, should be avoided. Wound surfaces are typically colonized by bacteria, and this colonization is not detrimental to wound healing. An increased bacterial load, more than the typical colonization, may impede wound healing, however. Distinguishing between common colonization and an increased bacterial burden requires microbiologic confirmation. Simple swab cultures lack specificity, and quantitative tissue cultures revealing greater than 10^5 organisms per gram are necessary to identify true bacterial infection. Topical antibiotics are commonly applied to wound surfaces, but the benefits of topical antibiotics are not well documented.[72,103] The incorporation of silver into dressing materials adds bacteriostatic properties and may be useful to limit bacterial overgrowth in the wound.

SURGICAL SITE INFECTIONS

Infections of surgical incisions are referred to as *surgical site infections* (SSIs).[104,105] SSIs are *superficial* incisional SSIs when limited to skin and subcutaneous tissues above the fascia or *deep* incisional SSIs if extending below. Intracavitary SSIs are referred to as organ-space SSIs. The surgical site becomes inoculated either inward from the skin or outward from the structures beneath the incision. Most SSIs are caused by the gram-positive cocci found on the skin, such as *Staphylococcus aureus, Staphylococcus epidermidis,* and *Enterococcus* species. The type of operation also can influence the causative organisms of the SSI such that enteric aerobic gram-negative rods (*Escherichia, Enterobacter*) and anaerobic organisms (*Bacteroides*) are more likely after intestinal or head and neck surgery.[76]

Although it was once believed that mechanical bowel preparation would decrease postoperative infectious complication rates, this practice has not survived prospective validation.[106] The use of skin preparations, in addition to the use of narrow-spectrum "prophylactic" systemic antibiotics, has reduced the incidence of SSIs by decreaseing bacterial numbers. However, the administration of prophylactic antibiotics beyond 24 hours, even in the presence of colonic perforation or shock, does not contribute further to reducing the rate of SSIs.[107] In addition, prolonged use of prophylactic antibiotics may result in the emergence of multiple drug-resistant strains of organisms, *Clostridium difficile* colitis, nosocomial pneumonia, and catheter-related infections.[108] It is important to discontinue prophylactic antibiotics before the benefits of such therapy are overshadowed by the risks that their continuation brings with them.

A daily wound evaluation is necessary to identify early signs of wound infections. Nonpurulent drainage is not likely to be infected. Clear drainage from the wound may simply be escaping subcutaneous edema fluid or may signify seroma formation. However, wounds with an enlarging border of erythema and induration, without fluctuance or drainage, particularly when painful to palpation, suggest cellulitis or infection of deeper structures. Fluctuance and drainage may be from an abscess beneath the wound. Drainage that is turbid or frankly purulent should suggest true SSI. SSIs require opening of the incision for irrigation and drainage. Antibiotics may not be needed for uncomplicated SSIs, which respond to this intervention and local care.[76]

More complicated SSIs require systemic antibiotics directed at the likely pathogens. Culture of pus collected aseptically is useful to guide therapy, but simple swab cultures of the wound surface are of low specificity because of the presence of wound colonizers. Necrotizing SSIs can spread rapidly through soft tissues and involve the fascia (necrotizing fasciitis). Necrotizing soft tissue infections can have subtle findings at the skin surface (e.g., an advancing border of erythema), while forging a destructive path just below. Wounds that dehisce superficially or at the fascia should suggest aberration of normal wound healing. Dehiscence almost always requires surgical evaluation. When an abdominal wound has open skin, evaluation for status of the fascial closure is needed. The mechanical integrity can be evaluated by gently probing the closure with sterile cotton-tipped swabs. The edges of these wounds should show yellow fat or pink granulation. Dark gray, nonviable tissue should be obvious on inspection and should be debrided.

DRAINS

Few things in the postoperative patient are more puzzling and sometimes intimidating to the uninitiated than drains. Seemingly simple in construction and intuitive in purpose, the efficacy of these devices and their application is quite limited. A study of the history of drainage is a study in the evolution of medicine and surgery itself. The earliest description of drains shows their application for the removal of fluid from large cavities, such as the pleural space, abdomen, and bladder, and for the treatment of wounds.

Drains can be classified on many levels.[109] Drains with one end open to the atmosphere are known as "open" systems and constitute most early devices. Before the recognition of germ theory, it was not appreciated that open systems provided a free route for entrance of infectious agents into the body. Some open systems employed a filter at the open end to limit the ability of microorganisms to enter the system. "Closed" systems of drainage have no opening to the atmosphere directly; fluid collection terminates in a bag or canister.

Structurally, drains can be classified as "hollow" or "capillary." Hollow drains take on many shapes, but all have one or multiple internal lumens and have fenestrations throughout a portion of their length, sometimes including their ends. Fenestrations must be large enough to allow fluid and debris to enter, but not so large as to allow significant portions of tissue, such as omentum or intestine, to enter. Such migration into the drain has been the cause of drain failure, tissue adhesion, and organ injury. Capillary-type drains leverage the physical interaction that occurs between liquids and the walls of thin tubes and fibers. Structurally, capillary-type devices are made from tufts of thin fibers, fabrics (e.g., gauze), or thin tubes. Drains should be soft and flexible, but not so much that the lumen collapses with suction. Irritating materials, such as latex rubber, should be avoided (except in cases in which development of a fibrous tract is desired, such as in T-tube biliary drainage). Siliconized materials (Silastic) and polyvinyl chloride are commonly used in contemporary drainage systems.

Drains can be classified as "passive" or "active." Passive drains provide a route of low resistance to the body's exterior and are driven by capillary action and pressure gradients. Capillary-type drains are classified as passive drains. Active drains use an external source of negative pressure to establish a pressure gradient. Active drainage of deep recesses is classified as sump drainage. Sump drains were ultimately modified so that an additional lumen running alongside the primary lumen supplied atmospheric gas into the drainage site to prevent the intestine and omentum from occluding the fenestra.[110] Sump drains are used to drain the gastrointestinal tract and abscess cavities. Active drainage employing a closed system is used to obliterate potential spaces, particularly under skin/muscle flaps or other wounds.

Drains also are classified as therapeutic or prophylactic.[111] Therapeutic drainage is intended to remove necrotic debris, pus, or fistula drainage or to prevent premature closure of wounds. Prophylactic drainage is intended to prevent the accumulation of blood, pus, bile, pancreatic secretions, intestinal contents, and fluids. In the historical literature of medicine and surgery, it was noted that patients with ovariotomy developed accumulations of blood and fluid in the pelvis. It was believed that this fluid, in stagnation, would decompose and release toxins whose absorption resulted in fatal outcomes. In 1882, drains were used to "remove from cavities fluids liable to undergo putrefactive changes if retained and to cleanse such cavities by injection of disinfectants."[80]

The popularity of drainage in certain applications waxed and waned owing to its controversial effect on outcome, particularly mortality risk. When surgeons abandoned the use of abdominal drains during World War II, mortality rates decreased by 50% compared with those of World War I.[112] The use of prophylactic drains, particularly in abdominal surgery, was equally controversial. Capillary-based systems, which did more to prevent drainage of necrotic or purulent material than facilitate its removal, ultimately fell out of favor. Complications increased from the use of multiple or unnecessary drains and included ventral hernias, pain on removal, omental penetration of the drain's fenestrations, intestinal obstruction, adhesions (occasionally pulling omentum or bowel into the abdominal wall), fecal fistulas, and persistent sinus tracts. The pioneering surgeon Halsted believed that good surgical technique and obliteration of dead space obviated the need for drainage in nonseptic instances. He believed that drains "invariably produce some necrosis of tissue with which it comes in contact and enfeebles the power of resistance of tissues toward organisms. But given necrotic tissue plus infections, drains become almost indispensable."[80] Prophylactic drainage ultimately gave way to therapeutic drainage. In the 1920s, indications for drains included the "presence of free purulent material in considerable quantity . . . and the presence of an abscess sac."[80]

Currently, the indications for drainage include the following:

- Removal of cerebrospinal fluid (CSF) from the brain's ventricles or spinal cord for the purpose of reducing pressure in a closed space and improving perfusion pressure
- Removal of blood or fluid from the subdural space to prevent compression or shift of intracranial contents
- Closure of certain soft tissue wounds to minimize dead space and remove excess fluid and debris; often seen in neck surgery, breast surgery, and certain reconstructive procedures
- Drainage of the pleural space in the event of pneumothorax, hemothorax, or large pleural effusions
- Drainage of the pericardium to treat large pericardial effusions
- Drainage of abscess cavities; drains can be placed directly in the operating room or percutaneously with the guidance of imaging technologies
- Drainage of existing fistulas to create a controlled route of elimination; includes drainage of bile or pancreatic secretions, succus, or stool
- Surveillance drainage over the sites of complicated procedures involving the stomach, duodenum, pancreas, and rerouting anastomoses

Placement of surveillance drains is controversial because of the risk of creating a fistula by the drains themselves. However, in the event of a catastrophic breach in enteral integrity, such as the highly morbid duodenal stump "blowout," early identification and controlled drainage may be facilitated by placement of such a drain.

In general, the following questions must be answered for all drains:

1. What is the intended anatomic location of the drain?
2. How can location be confirmed?
3. What is the expected quantity and quality of the drain's output?
4. Is the drain functioning normally?
5. When should a drain be removed and according to what criteria?

Only by knowing the intended anatomic location of a given drain can a clinician determine the best way to confirm location and assess function. The visual location of a drain on physical examination does not ensure proper placement; a thoracostomy tube seen to penetrate the chest wall may not be in the pleural space, and a gastrostomy tube seen to penetrate the abdominal wall does not guarantee that the tip lies in the stomach. Sometimes the location of a drain cannot be confirmed, such as drains left in the peritoneum. This, short of advanced imaging techniques, leaves only assessment of quantity and quality of drain output as a guide to the drain's proper location and function. For these reasons, it is useful to know certain characteristics of specific drains.

The most common drains seen after neurosurgical procedures are the subdural drain and the ventriculostomy. The former drain is usually a Silastic drain left in the subdural space to drain blood or fluid after craniotomy. There is no way to confirm its location. These drains typically drain about 20 to 30 mL of serosanguineous fluid per hour until tapering off to minimal drainage after about 6 hours. Frankly bloody drainage, particularly when in higher volumes or persisting longer than a few hours, suggests active bleeding that requires correction of coagulopathy or neurosurgical intervention. The ventriculostomy tube, also made of Silastic, has its tip located in a lateral ventricle. The proper tip location can be confirmed by seeing a pulsatile waveform when the catheter has continuous pressure monitoring and by seeing CSF output. About 450 mL of CSF is produced a day; the volume of CSF drained depends on the height of the drainage system's external port relative to the height of the catheter's tip in the ventricle and the ability of the arachnoid granulations to reabsorb CSF. The fluid may be clear or sanguineous depending on the intracranial surgery performed. CSF that changes from clear or serosanguineous to frankly bloody suggests a serious problem, particularly in subarachnoid hemorrhage. Declining or absent CSF drainage or loss of a pulsatile waveform suggests tube occlusion by clot or malposition and requires neurosurgical attention.

Thoracostomy tubes are placed to drain pleural effusions and treat pneumothorax. Thoracostomy tubes can be inadvertently placed subcutaneously. Proper location is confirmed by chest radiograph. The tube may be intentionally positioned in many orientations; however, the most proximal "sentinel" hole should always lie within the pleural space, and the tube should not be kinked. A properly functioning, correctly located thoracostomy tube should show a cycling of intrapleural pressure with respiration when the drainage system is on "water seal." Absence of cycling may suggest tube occlusion or inappropriate location. Bubbling across the water seal suggests an air leak, but does not indicate the source of the leak. Persistence of the bubbles across the water seal when the thoracostomy tube is clamped close to the chest wall indicates a leak in the drainage system, not in the lung. Variable amounts of suction can be applied to the thoracostomy tube, particularly when draining an effusion or reinflating a lung after pneumothorax. Initial suction of −20 cm H_2O is appropriate in this clinical situation. Persistence of sanguineous drainage greater than 200 mL/hour for 2 to 3 hours after the correction of hypothermia and coagulopathy suggests surgical bleeding and requires attention. When fluid drainage has diminished to about 100 to 200 mL/day or air leaks have ceased, external suction can be removed, and the water seal alone can be used to prevent lung collapse. If effusions or pneumothorax do not return, as assessed on chest radiograph, the thoracostomy tube can be removed.

Nasogastric or orogastric tubes are used to decompress the stomach or provide a route for nutrition. Double-lumen sump tubes should never have the secondary port clamped; this secondary port prevents mucosal injury in the presence of suction. Inadvertent placement in the airways can be disastrous if enteral feedings are administered. Confirmation of gastric placement cannot be guaranteed by listening over the epigastrium during insufflation. Correct placement on radiograph is recognized by identifying the distal tip well below the diaphragm. Salivary and gastric output can be 0.75 to 1.5 L/day each. Continuous gastric suction can result in significant volume and chloride loss, leading to metabolic alkalosis. Gastric suction should be maintained until resolution of enteral obstructions or ileus. When the daily volume of gastric aspirate is less than 200 to 300 mL, gastric suction can be discontinued as long as nausea, vomiting, or abdominal distention does not result.

The color of gastric aspirate should be clear or yellow-green. Large volumes of bilious aspirate suggest the distal port of the drain is positioned beyond the pylorus. "Coffee grounds" or frank blood in the aspirate suggests bleeding in the stomach or duodenum. The stomach also can be accessed by placement of a surgical or percutaneous endoscopically assisted gastrostomy. These tubes infrequently migrate out of the stomach to lie in the peritoneum. Should acute abdominal pain or absence of typical gastric drainage occur in a patient with a recently placed gastrostomy, a radiographic contrast study of the gastrostomy should be done to exclude tube migration.

The liver produces 500 to 1500 mL of bile daily. Drainage of the common bile duct via a T-tube is used after complicated biliary surgery, often for obstruction. T-tubes are used less than in the past now that transhepatic catheter drainage and common bile duct stents/sphincterotomy are more commonplace. The drainage tube itself causes a modest inflammatory reaction resulting in the formation of a fibrous tract. The drainage system is closed, without suction, and terminates in a collection bag. Significant reduction or cessation of biliary output may suggest either obstruction or malposition of the T-tube or resolution of the obstruction.

With the exception of drains placed in abscess cavities and to control the direction of pancreatic and enteral fistula output, drains left in the abdominal cavity are seen less frequently than in the past. Drains left in the peritoneum should have relatively little output. Confirmation of their location is usually unnecessary. A change in the quality or quantity of drainage is important to note. New bile, succus entericus, or stool in a drain suggests a breach in the integrity of some part of the viscera and requires investigation or surgical attention.

Drains placed in subcutaneous spaces or areas of reconstruction are placed to gentle suction to obliterate potential spaces and remove excessive fluid and blood collection. Confirmation of absolute location is generally unnecessary. The quality of the fluid should be serous to serosanguineous in volumes less than 100 mL hourly for the first 3 to 6 hours postoperatively before tapering off. Frankly bloody drainage in higher volumes or of longer durations suggests surgical bleeding in the absence of coagulopathy.

ACKNOWLEDGMENTS

The authors wish the thank Sara Chaffee, MD; Maxwell A. Hockstein, BS; and Gary Ecelbarger, MS, RD, CNSC, for their assistance in research and editing.

KEY POINTS

- Optimally, the location of a patient in the ICU is determined by matching the patient's needs with a location's resources and expertise.
- The postoperative evaluation should include a thorough evaluation of the patient's medical and surgical history and a physical examination, which should encompass all parts of the patient that can be accessed by sight and touch.
- "Adequate resuscitation" is a state, often temporary, that allows for good clinical perfusion and physiologic stability. The most fundamental concept is to ensure adequate DO_2 and meet the $\dot{V}O_2$ needs of tissues and organelles.
- Resuscitation targets are reproducible, quantifiable values, such as pressures, outputs, metabolites, inflammatory mediators, or oxygen saturations, that represent therapeutic goals. Targeted resuscitation strategies optimize cardiovascular performance and concurrently measure markers of adequate global DO_2 and tissue use.
- Analgesics should be administered as the patient is resuscitated from anesthesia to facilitate comfort and avoid interference with medical care.
- Resuscitation should be complete, with hemostasis achieved, metabolic acidosis resolving, vasoactive support and gas exchange abnormalities minimized, anesthetic agents cleared, the ability to protect the airway present, and the patient awake and reasonably cooperative prior to initiating weaning from mechanical ventilation.
- Nutritional support is an important consideration in ICU patients due to the ongoing caloric demands of these complex patients. Early assessment of the available routes should be performed and the appropriate supplementation should be incorporated into the patient's daily care.
- Successful healing of a closed surgical wound yields mechanical integrity by virtue of high tensile strength. Successful healing in an open wound may be measured by epithelialization with the promise of satisfactory mechanical integrity (scarring) over time.
- The ability of epithelialization to occur from the margin of the wounds over the granulation tissue depends on the presence of adequate angiogenesis, the absence of bacterial burden, the provision of a moist environment, and the removal of excess necrosis and proteinaceous exudates (which contain proteases and inflammatory mediators and harbor bacterial growth).
- The first rule of wound evaluation is "take off the dressing and look at the wound." Wounds should be

KEY POINTS (Continued)

evaluated at least daily for progression of healing and for development of infection.

- Only by knowing the intended anatomic location of a given drain can a clinician determine the best way to confirm location and assess its function.

SELECTED REFERENCES

11. Petrovic MA, Martinez EA, Aboumatar H: Implementing a perioperative handoff tool to improve postprocedural patient transfers. Jt Comm J Qual Patient Saf 2012;38(3):135-142.
22. Dellinger RP, Levy MM, Carlet JM, et al: International Surviving Sepsis Campaign Guidelines Committee; American Association of Critical-Care Nurses; American College of Chest Physicians; American College of Emergency Physicians; Canadian Critical Care Society; European Society of Clinical Microbiology and Infectious Diseases; European Society of Intensive Care Medicine; European Respiratory Society; International Sepsis Forum; Japanese Association for Acute Medicine; Japanese Society of Intensive Care Medicine; Society of Critical Care Medicine; Society of Hospital Medicine; Surgical Infection Society; World Federation of Societies of Intensive and Critical Care Medicine. Surviving Sepsis Campaign: International guidelines for management of severe sepsis and septic shock: 2008. Crit Care Med 2008;36(1):296-327. Erratum in: Crit Care Med 2008;36(4):1394-1396.
30. Perel P, Roberts I: Colloids versus crystalloids for fluid resuscitation in critically ill patients. Cochrane Database Syst Rev 2012;6:CD000567.
37. Kress JP, Gehlbach B, Lacy M, et al: The long-term psychological effects of daily sedative interruption on critically ill patients. Am J Respir Crit Care Med 2003;168:1457-1461.
43. MacIntyre NR, Cook DJ, Ely EW, et al, American College of Chest Physicians; American Association for Respiratory Care; American College of Critical Care Medicine: Evidence-based guidelines for weaning and discontinuing ventilatory support: A collective task force facilitated by the American College of Chest Physicians; the American Association for Respiratory Care; and the American College of Critical Care Medicine. Chest 2001;120(6 Suppl): 375S-395S.
54. Herzig SJ, Howell MD, Ngo LH, Marcantonio ER: Acid-suppressive medication use and the risk for hospital-acquired pneumonia. JAMA 2009;301(20):2120-2128.
67. Banh HL: Management of delirium in adult critically ill patients: An overview. J Pharm Sci 2012;15(4):499-509.
71. Finfer S, Liu B, Chittock DR, et al, NICE-SUGAR Study Investigators: Hypoglycemia and risk of death in critically ill patients. N Engl J Med 2012;367(12):1108-1118.
85. Acosta-Escribano J, Fernandez-Vivas M, et al: Gastric versus transpyloric feeding in severe traumatic brain injury: A prospective, randomized trial. Intensive Care Med 2010;36:1532-1539.
102. Ubbink DT, Westerbos SJ, Evans D, et al: Topical negative pressure for treating chronic wounds. Cochrane Database Syst Rev 2008;(3):CD001898.

The complete list of references can be found at www.expertconsult.com.

36 Postoperative Management of the Cardiac Surgery Patient

David Anthony | Jose Diaz-Gomez | C. Allen Bashour | Robert Johnson

CHAPTER OUTLINE

This chapter will give the reader information on how to manage routine and complex cardiac surgery patients in the immediate and early postoperative period. The disproportionately small number of patients who undergo cardiac operations and have prolonged intensive care unit (ICU) stays often develop complications not unique to them but common to most ICU patients who have delayed recoveries or do not survive after a long ICU course. These ICU complications are covered elsewhere in this text. This chapter is divided by organ system into five broad areas (neurologic, cardiac, pulmonary, renal, transthoracic echocardiography) specific to these patients in this setting and includes a discussion of some miscellaneous topics.

NEUROLOGIC CARE

Despite improvements in cardiac surgery techniques and perioperative critical care, postcardiotomy neurologic complications remain a major cause of morbidity and death following cardiac surgery. A spectrum of neurologic complications is seen in the postoperative period. Complications can be classified as generalized (global deficit) or focal. Generalized deficits can be manifested as delayed awakening from general anesthesia, coma, or new onset of seizure. Focal deficits may be transient or permanent. Except in their most severe form, neurologic complications cannot be completely assessed until the patient returns to consciousness and is weaned from the ventilator. Focal abnormalities are usually evaluated by a computed tomography (CT) scan. A CT for nonfocal, cognitive dysfunction rarely yields new information that is helpful for patient management, and imaging studies most often show old, chronic changes such as atrophy or lacunar infarcts. The patient must be stable enough to withstand transport to the CT (if the institution does not have a portable scanner), which is usually not the case in the early postoperative period.

The risk factors for neurologic injury after cardiac surgery have been well elucidated, but effective risk modification to reliably prevent neurologic complications has been elusive. In certain operations, measures to reduce risk have been implemented and have become incorporated in perioperative management.[1,2] For example, patients with descending thoracic aortic operations are at significant intraoperative risk for spinal cord ischemia, as well as delayed injury (days postoperatively). These patients usually have a spinal drain placed preoperatively to reduce the risk of spinal cord injury. Spinal cord perfusion pressure (SCPP) is the difference between mean arterial pressure (MAP) and cerebrospinal fluid pressure (CSFP) (SCPP = MAP − CSFP); thus, lowering of CSFP will increase SCPP and potentially improve neurologic function as long as an adequate MAP is maintained.[3]

Neurologic complications are still considered one of the major risks associated with coronary artery grafting. The advanced age of bypass patients, high incidence of associated carotid occlusive disease, and increased aortic atheroembolic burden place older coronary artery bypass graft (CABG) patients at increased risk of central neurologic complications in the postoperative period.[4]

Other strategies for preoperative and intraoperative risk modification are becoming routine. They include selective use of preoperative carotid imaging, routine use of intraoperative transesophageal echocardiography (TEE) and epiaortic echocardiography, descending aortic cannulation with TEE guidance, aortic-no-touch technique, high-flow/high-pressure cardiopulmonary bypass (CPB), retrograde cerebral perfusion during circulatory arrest, carbon dioxide insufflation, intraoperative cerebral oxygen saturation monitoring, echocardiography de-airing, and maintenance of baseline perioperative blood pressure.[5,6] Early neurologic complications vary in clinical presentation from focal to global neurologic deficit such as seizures, ischemic encephalopathy, and coma. Several authors have classified these complications as type I (focal injury, stupor, and coma) and type II (seizures, neurocognitive dysfunction, and delirium).[7] This classification does not emphasize pathophysiologic mechanisms that could better inform preventive measures.[5,7] Regardless of the classification system used, overlap often exists.

In comparison to the other complications, focal neurologic deficits from stroke carry a mortality rate of up to 20% in the first postoperative month and prolong ICU and hospital lengths of stay.[8-10] In a mixed cardiac surgery patient population, the incidence of stroke varied among those patients having CABG, combined CABG and heart valve surgery, and ascending aorta repair.[11-13] The incidence of stroke depends on the surgical procedure (isolated CABG, 1.4-3.8%; combined CABG and valve, 7.4%; isolated valve, 4.8-8.8%; multiple valve, 9.7%; and aorta, 8.7%).[12]

Unfortunately, most of the known baseline patient variables associated with perioperative stroke are not modifiable. Despite the identification of many intraoperative variables that cause intraoperative stroke (macroembolism of debris, air embolism, hypoperfusion, hypoxemia, coagulation status), risk remains significant and continues in the early postoperative period. Although there was early enthusiasm for off-pump CABG as an operative technique to reduce stroke, in the most recent multicenter clinical trial the 30-day incidence of stroke was not significantly decreased compared with on-pump CABG.[14]

The majority of strokes are ischemic (62%); fewer are due to hypoperfusion (9%) or hemorrhage (<1%).[12] Hemorrhagic strokes are rare after cardiac surgery and the clinical presentation is notable for delayed awakening and coma despite discontinuing sedation or progressive clinical deterioration as intracranial pressure (ICP) increases. Hemorrhagic transformation is recognized in 20% of ischemic strokes.[10] Embolic strokes tend to present with acute hemiparesis and represent a compromise of specific cerebral artery area. Thrombotic or ischemic strokes are related to diminished blood flow with the most vulnerable areas being those between major cerebral artery perfusion territories (watershed areas).

Cardiac transplantation has a higher associated occurrence of neurologic complications than CABG.[15,16] Symptom onset for focal motor deficits in these patients usually occur after the second postoperative day, especially in patients receiving mechanical circulatory support or experiencing major postsurgical complications such as tamponade, severe cardiac dysfunction, prolonged CPB, or postoperative hepatic failure.

Predictive models may enable implementation of earlier interventions.[14] More than half of strokes are identified within the first day after CABG.[10] Because of associated morbidity and death, an objective neurologic evaluation by minimizing sedation in the first 2 postoperative hours is desirable. Weaning sedation should be initiated only when the risk of doing so is minimal (i.e., a normothermic, nonacidemic, nonagitated patient with minimal chest tube output).

Once a new focal neurologic deficit, seizure, or delayed awakening is documented, a noncontrast brain CT scan should be obtained immediately. The most important tomographic findings include loss of insular ribbon, loss of gray-white interface, loss of sulci, acute hypodensity, mass effect, and dense mean cerebral artery sign. Owing to the relative insensitivity of CT scans for diagnosing ischemia, early CT scans may be normal, despite areas of brain infarction.[17] Magnetic resonance imaging (MRI) may help identify these lesions.[17] MRI usually cannot be obtained safely in the early postoperative period because of the need to move the patient off the unit to a usually remote location and because non-MRI compatible pericardial pacing wires are routinely placed in cardiac surgery patients. MRI will document a new lesion in 26% to 50% of cases, but there is often lack of correlation with the neurocognitive deficit.[18,19] Brain CT scans are more sensitive in diagnosing large air embolism, which is often the cause of abnormal postoperative neurologic findings in these patients. In the patient with a focal deficit or persistent embolic events, transcranial Doppler, transthoracic echocardiography (TTE), or TEE can be used to help identify sources of recurrent cardiac or aortic embolization.

Stabilization of the patient who develops stroke after cardiac surgery is the most important initial intervention and includes continuation of cardiopulmonary support and tracheal intubation if the patient cannot protect the airway or has a Glasgow Coma Scale score less than 9. Secondary brain injury, which is additional brain injury due to the factors that initially caused an imbalance between oxygen supply and demand, should be prevented. The most important measures are prevention of hypoxemia, hypotension, hypercarbia, and hyperthermia.

From a ventilator standpoint, higher levels of positive end-expiratory pressure (PEEP) to maintain optimal oxygenation might be required. If the patient has documented intracranial hypertension and requires PEEP 10 cm H_2O or higher, ICP monitoring should be considered as high levels of PEEP and lung recruitment maneuvers may decrease cerebral perfusion. Increased PEEP may decrease cerebral perfusion pressure (CPP) by elevating ICP because CPP is the difference between MAP and ICP.

Although acute treatment of ischemic stroke is imperative, the traditional 3-hour time window for active stroke intervention and institution of thrombolytic therapy is often lost because the time of the last known normal is usually just before induction of anesthesia and duration of surgery usually exceeds 3 hours. Furthermore, intravenous administration of tissue plasminogen activator (tPA) is contraindicated in the immediate postoperative period because of the associated postoperative bleeding risk.

Intra-arterial administration of tPA is an alternative for acute treatment of ischemic stroke within 6 hours of clinical presentation. The safety and efficacy of intra-arterial urokinase and tPA in selected patients who presented ischemic stroke within 12 days after cardiac surgery have been demonstrated.[20] The mean time from operation to stroke was 4.3 days. Thrombolytic therapy was commenced within 3.6 hours. No operative intervention for bleeding was necessary and 38% of the patients had neurologic improvement. Mechanical clot retrieval is another acute stroke therapy in the first 8 hours since neurologic deficit. Patients who will likely benefit from this therapy include those with significant neurologic deficit and large vessel occlusion with core ischemia approximately less than 30% of the middle cerebral artery territory.

Anticoagulation therapy has not proved beneficial in the cardiac surgery patient with ischemic stroke. However, it should be considered in cases of basilar stenosis, internal carotid dissection, and suspected cardiac embolism and specifically with concurrent atrial fibrillation and stroke. In this circumstance, the risk of ongoing embolism to cerebral circulation may be considered higher than active bleeding after cardiac surgery. A hematology consult is recommended in cases of suspected hypercoagulable state as the cause of this disorder demands a more comprehensive workup and potentially may require lifelong anticoagulation therapy. Antiplatelet therapy should be initiated in all cardiac surgery patients with acute stroke, especially if thrombolytic therapy is contraindicated. Aspirin is usually prescribed. The dose ranges between 160 mg and 1300 mg per day. Combined antiplatelet therapy with clopidogrel is not recommended because of the significant risk of bleeding.

In cases of suspected perioperative air embolism (i.e., opening of heart chambers for valve repair or replacement), the patient should remain in the supine position to avoid further embolic phenomena. If tolerable, the patient should be maintained in Trendelenburg position and mechanical ventilator support with FIO_2 of 1.0 should be instituted. Measures to control intracranial hypertension (more common in intracranial hemorrhage) should be individualized after reassessment of brain CT imaging. Hyperventilation, as well as diuresis with mannitol or furosemide is recommended in the patient with intracranial hypertension.

In the cardiac surgery patient, coma is defined as prolonged unconsciousness after discontinuation of anesthetics, sedatives, and opioids and inability to show response to motor/verbal commands. A recent retrospective investigation found an incidence of delayed awakening in approximately 0.5% of all cardiac surgery patients.[21] However, the period of time in the immediate postoperative phase can be challenging as the necessity of adequate neurologic examination must be weighed against the patient's hemodynamic stability. If a specific diagnosis is not found, and there is concomitant severe heart failure, it portends a worse outcome.[21] Moreover, up to 20% of patients with postcardiotomy stroke present with delayed awakening and coma-like symptoms.[21]

Evaluation with brain CT is mandatory in these cases and it should occur as soon as the coma state has been recognized and reversible metabolic causes have been treated. The identified risk factors for delayed awakening after cardiac surgery in the aforementioned investigation included urgent cardiac surgery, elevated serum creatinine (Cr), and lower postoperative hemoglobin level.[21] Most of these patients had normal brain CT scan imaging and ultimately recovered consciousness after being comatose during the first 24 hours.[21] Although some investigators have proposed a role for altered renal excretion of sedatives in patients with postoperative renal failure or decreased oxygen delivery to the brain with anemia, the specific underlying mechanisms in these cases remain unclear.

Postoperative seizure is an independent predictor of permanent neurologic deficit and increased mortality risk.[22,23] A recent study showed seizures were a strong predictor of permanent neurologic deficit and increased mortality risk. It is important to remember that any neurologic injury can present initially as a seizure. The independent risk factors for postoperative seizures included deep hypothermic circulatory arrest, aortic calcification or atheroma, and critical preoperative state. Other specific risk factors for early seizures include perioperative administration of the antifibrinolytic tranexamic acid administration and preexisting renal insufficiency.

Tranexamic acid has proconvulsant properties and it is reasonable to hold the infusion of this agent in the early postoperative period if the patient presents with seizures. The most common proposed mechanism of seizures after cardiac surgery is focal or global ischemia from hypoperfusion (air or atheroembolism) or metabolic disorders. Early brain CT scan is essential because it may detect potential reversible causes of neurologic injury such as cerebral edema, intracranial bleeding, or emboli in a major cerebral artery.[10]

Delirium is considered a subtle category of brain injury in the postcardiotomy patient. The intensivist should include perioperative stroke in the differential diagnosis of perioperative psychomotor agitation or delirium in the ICU. A common missed diagnosis is drug and alcohol withdrawal in patients with acute delirium in the ICU.

CARDIOVASCULAR CARE

HEMODYNAMIC CHANGES

Patients undergoing CABG or valvular surgery often exhibit hemodynamic instability in the postoperative period. The pathologic remodeling secondary to preexisting cardiovascular disease, the inflammatory cascade initiated during CPB, and the changes in loading conditions and oxygen demand after surgical repair predispose these patients to hemodynamic perturbations following cardiac surgery. In the postoperative period, these patients frequently require pharmacologic support for maintenance of normotension and adequate cardiac output. In some cases of severe, refractory, cardiogenic shock, institution of mechanical ventricular support is required.

MEAN ARTERIAL PRESSURE

MAP is one of the most commonly measured and manipulated hemodynamic variables in the perioperative period. Although MAPs are routinely maintained in the 70 to 80 mm Hg range, target blood pressure may be altered based upon comorbid disease and the intraoperative course of events. Hypertensive patients with neurologic or renal disease may have altered autoregulatory curves, which require higher blood pressures for adequate end-organ function. Conversely, in patients with friable cardiac tissue, tenuous surgical repairs, or uncorrected aneurysmal disease lower MAPs may be desirable. Ideally, intraoperative manipulation of the blood pressure while observing the echocardiogram and changes in central venous (CVP) and pulmonary artery pressures (PAPs) will allow the practitioner to define optimal blood pressure.

HYPERTENSION

Cardiac surgical patients presenting in the postoperative period with hypertension should be evaluated for routine causes of acute postoperative hypertension and treated accordingly. Pain, residual neuromuscular blockade, hypoxemia, hypercarbia, hypothermia, or bladder distention may provoke hypertension. If these precipitants are ruled out, pharmacologic lowering of blood pressure with an infusion of a vasodilator, sodium nitroprusside, or nitroglycerin can be initiated. The rapid titratability and short duration of action of these medications is desirable as hemodynamic lability is commonplace. Alternatively, short-acting or ultrashort-acting dihydropyridine calcium channel blockers (e.g., nicardipine or clevidipine) have been used as they exert maximal effect in the peripheral arterial system with minimal impact on cardiac function.[24] While MAP is lowered, serial measurements of cardiac output and urine output should be recorded to assess the patient's tolerance of a lower blood pressure.

HYPOTENSION

With a reported incidence of 9% to 44%, hypotension is more common than hypertension following cardiac surgery.[25] Studies of off-pump CABG surgery compared to on-pump CABG surgery have demonstrated a significant increase in the incidence of hypotension in those patients exposed to CPB.[26] Some clinicians also associate the relatively common hypotensive response to more critically ill patients with prolonged medical management prior to surgery. Additionally, widespread use of angiotensin-converting enzyme inhibitors has been implicated as a potential contributor.[27] Regardless of the predisposing factors, postoperative hypotension demands prompt investigation and treatment.

From a physiologic standpoint, MAP = central venous pressure (CVP, mm Hg) + cardiac output (CO, L/minute) × systemic vascular resistance (SVR, $dyn \cdot s \cdot cm^{-5}$). A decrease in any of these parameters will reduce MAP. It is useful to consider the common causes of postoperative hypotension relative to these hemodynamic variables. Low CVP corresponds with hypovolemia. Decreased CO can occur as a consequence of cardiac insufficiency/cardiogenic shock or new-onset myocardial ischemia. Vasoplegia following CPB leads to a depressed SVR. Routine causes of hypotension in the acute postoperative period include hypovolemia, cardiac insufficiency/cardiogenic shock, vasoplegia following CPB, new-onset myocardial ischemia, and tamponade. Crucial to postoperative management is understanding the patient's intraoperative hemodynamics and immediate postbypass cardiac function.

The most readily correctable cause of hypotension is hypovolemia. Commonly boluses of crystalloid (500 mL to 1 L of 0.9% normal saline or lactated Ringer's solution) are administered and the patient's hemodynamic responses (MAP, CVP, PAP, and cardiac index [CI]) are evaluated. Colloid solutions can be used, but some concern exists when administering hetastarch solutions because of its effects on the coagulation cascade and potential contribution to a bleeding diathesis.[28]

A low preoperative ejection fraction (<35%), advanced age (>70 years old), and prolonged CPB times (>120 minutes) correlate with an increased risk of decreased cardiac output in the postbypass period.[29] Postoperatively, a depressed CI often manifests early, during separation from CPB in the operating room. The pattern observed on hemodynamic monitoring is a depressed CI (<2.2 L/minute/m^2), hypotension, normal or elevated SVR, and elevated filling pressures. Echocardiography demonstrates global ventricular hypokinesia. Patients will frequently require exogenous pharmacologic support to maintain a CI of greater than 2.2 L/minute/m^2. Epinephrine, dopamine, dobutamine, or milrinone may be initiated for inotropic support.[30] It is not uncommon for cardiac insufficiency to persist for several days following CPB.

Even after successful coronary revascularization, the astute practitioner must be vigilant for postoperative myocardial ischemia. During weaning from CPB, air may become entrained within the heart that is not effectively evacuated by the atrioventricular (AV) bypass vents. Some of this air may enter the coronaries and lead to cardiac arrest or ischemia. In addition, during chest closure, bypass grafts may become kinked, obstructing flow. During aortic or valvular surgery, graft material or sutures may inadvertently obstruct coronary ostia or may occlude native coronary flow. Although multiple patient monitors—electrocardiogram (ECG), pulmonary artery catheter, and echocardiography—can identify ischemia, studies have demonstrated new-onset wall motion abnormalities on echocardiography as the most sensitive and earliest indicator of malperfusion.[31,32] If ischemia is present, surgical revascularization or percutaneous coronary revascularization may be necessary for reestablishing flow.

For approximately 5% to 15% of patients, exposure to CPB will lead to a prolonged vasodilatory state or vasoplegia.[33] The classical pattern is normal biventricular function, normovolemia, and decreased SVR. In these patients, infusing additional volume will not increase MAP and will frequently decrease systemic pressure secondary to activation of the atrial stretch receptors. In patients who are adequately volume resuscitated, the most effective treatment is infusion of a vasopressor, commonly norepinephrine, phenylephrine, or vasopressin.[10] Patients requiring progressively increasing doses of vasopressors should be continually assessed for hypovolemia or anemia, as these problems might happen concurrently in the vasoplegic patient. Experimental evidence suggests that these patients may suffer from a relative vasopressin deficiency. As such, exogenous vasopressin added to one of the other aforementioned vasopressors has been used successfully to maintain an adequate MAP.[34]

TAMPONADE

Acute tamponade is a surgical emergency that demands immediate treatment. In the early postoperative period following cardiac surgery, tamponade may occur as a consequence of uncorrected coagulopathy or from chest tube obstruction. Classic signs of tamponade on physical examination include hypotension, pulsus paradoxus, diminished peripheral pulses, and oliguria. Invasive hemodynamic monitoring may demonstrate equalization of CVP, pulmonary artery (PA) diastolic, and PA systolic pressures as the pericardium fills and pericardial pressure exceeds intracardiac pressures. Echocardiographic signs include right atrial systolic collapse and right ventricular diastolic collapse.[35]

Unfortunately, although prompt recognition and treatment are crucial, many patients with tamponade fail to demonstrate classic physical examination findings. Depending upon the rate of accumulation, hypotension may be sudden and severe or may occur gradually over a period of hours. If decompensation is sudden and severe, emergent bedside reexploration is warranted. Otherwise, the patient may be taken to the operating room for emergent chest evacuation.

ARRHYTHMIAS

Postoperative arrhythmias are the most common complication after cardiac surgery with an overall reported incidence of 5% to 63%.[36] The most frequent arrhythmia is atrial fibrillation, which occurs in up to 40% of patients following bypass graft surgery and 60% of patients following combined CABG valve surgery.[36] Inflammation of the myocardium and mechanical disruption of the cardiac conduction system during surgery predispose cardiac surgical patients to bradyarrhythmias and heart block during the postoperative period. Accordingly, placement of temporary epicardial pacing wires in the ventricles and atria is routine.[37] Atrial wires will allow for AV synchrony during contraction, but removal of these wires from the more fragile atrial tissue may place the patient at an increased risk of atrial damage and tamponade.

Given the association of supraventricular arrhythmias with increased morbidity and length of stay, considerable research effort has focused on prevention and treatment.[38] In the postoperative period, 60% of arrhythmias manifest within the first 3 postoperative days.[38] For the patient with new-onset atrial fibrillation or flutter, the first step is to decide whether any hemodynamic instability is present. In the unstable patient, preparations should be made for immediate cardioversion according to Advanced Cardiac Life Support (ACLS) guidelines. In the hemodynamically stable patient, examination of the serum metabolic panel should be done for evidence of hypokalemia or hypomagnesemia with repletion of potassium or magnesium as necessary. If atrial fibrillation persists, the clinician must decide whether rate or rhythm control is preferred. Although rate control will limit tachycardia and myocardial oxygen consumption, it will not provide the benefit of atrial contraction and requires long term anticoagulation.

If rate control is deemed appropriate for the patient, the most common agents used include beta blockers (e.g., atenolol or metoprolol), calcium channel blockers (e.g., diltiazem or verapamil), and digoxin.[38] Care should be avoided when administering beta blockers to patients with severe chronic obstructive pulmonary disease (COPD) or reduced ejection fraction.

In patients with atrial fibrillation or flutter for less than 48 hours or with an echocardiogram devoid of intracardiac thrombus, rhythm control can be attempted. Prior to initiation of antiarrhythmic therapy, a 12-lead ECG should be examined for evidence of QT interval prolongation. The most common medications used for rhythm control include amiodarone, sotalol, procainamide, and ibutilide. In patients with decreased ejection fraction, amiodarone is the agent of choice. ECG monitoring should be performed during initiation and maintenance of rhythm control agents because any of these medications may provoke malignant arrhythmias. If medications fail to restore sinus rhythm and atrial fibrillation or flutter is less than 48 hours in duration, synchronized cardioversion with a biphasic defibrillator can be performed.

BLEEDING

If left untreated, hemorrhage and uncorrected coagulopathy can lead to devastating complications in the cardiac surgery patient. Excess bleeding occurs in 20% of cardiac surgical patients with approximately 5% requiring surgical reexploration.[39,40] Many factors contribute to this increased risk of hemorrhage. Preoperatively, patients are routinely on antiplatelet therapy and anticoagulant medications. Intraoperative exposure to CPB initiates contact activation of platelets with resultant thrombocytopathy and thrombocytopenia. In addition, the extracorporeal circuit exacerbates inflammation and amplifies fibrinolysis.[41]

Thromboelastography (TEG) and point-of-care (POC) testing are useful to guide blood product administration as the rapid rate of bleeding in the cardiac surgery patient outpaces the results obtained with standard laboratory testing.[42,43] In contrast to management of anemia in medical patients, transfusion of blood products in cardiac surgical patients is often determined by immediate clinical findings (e.g., intraoperative surgical field oozing, increased postoperative chest tube output, or hypotension). Increased rate of bleeding, greater than 500 mL over 2 hours, usually correlates with a source of bleeding that is amenable to surgical repair. Many institutions have established criteria upon which the surgical team will reexplore the patient for evacuation—chest tube output of greater than 500 mL within the first 2 postoperative hours requires surgical exploration. Initial evaluation of the bleeding cardiac surgery patient should focus on any abnormal physiologic parameters that may contribute to ongoing coagulopathy—severe acidemia, alkalemia, or hypothermia will impair hemostasis and should be corrected.

With the advent of cell-salvage technologies and increasing recognition of the adverse effects of red blood cell transfusion, there has been a decrease in the amount of blood given in the perioperative period.[44,45] Decisions regarding administration of red blood cells are based on patient-specific factors, including comorbid conditions and the adequacy of revascularization. Current American Society of Anesthesiology Practice Guidelines recommends transfusion of red blood cells when hemoglobin levels are less than 6 g/dL. Above this level, evidence of organ malperfusion and ischemia should be demonstrated prior to red blood cell transfusion.[46]

Given the deleterious effects of CPB circuitry on platelet quantity and function, hemorrhage that does not appear to have an overt surgical source often requires platelet transfusion. In a cardiac surgical patient with microvascular bleeding and normal physiologic parameters (normothermia, normal acid-base balance, etc.), platelet transfusion should be strongly considered. A platelet count greater than 100×10^9/L usually excludes thrombocytopenia as a contributing factor in the hemorrhagic cardiac surgical patient.[46]

Although intraoperative cell salvage has reduced the need for packed red blood cell transfusion, the washing of the blood during this process eliminates essential clotting factors.[47] Per American Society of Anesthesiology Guidelines, elevation of the prothrombin time (PT) greater than 1.5 times normal or elevation of the activated partial thromboplastin time (aPTT) greater than 2 times normal is an indication for fresh frozen plasma (FFP) transfusion. Although no specific algorithms exist for cardiac surgery, FFP administration is reasonable in the patient with normal platelet count and evidence of persistent bleeding.[46]

Pharmacologic options for reducing bleeding in the perioperative period include antifibrinolytic agents, desmopressin, and activated factor VII.[48-50] For maximal efficacy, antifibrinolytics should be started in the operating room prior to incision. Studies of desmopressin have demonstrated a reduction in blood loss, but no overall decrease in transfusion requirements. The newest hemostatic agent used for excess hemorrhage in the cardiac surgical arena is activated factor VII. Although approved for hemostatic control in hemophilia A or B patients, it has been successfully used off-label in cardiac surgery patients. Studies thus far have been encouraging, demonstrating decreased bleeding and transfusion requirements.[50,51]

PULMONARY CARE

Fluid overload is a common cause of poor gas exchange in the early postoperative period and can be readily assessed by reviewing intraoperative fluid balance and postoperative indicators of volume status. A positive intraoperative fluid balance greater than 4 L, and increased CVP and PA diastolic pressures are typical in fluid-overloaded patients. Pulmonary artery occlusion pressures do not have to be obtained or followed in this assessment. Unless early renal insufficiency has occurred, fluid-overloaded patients usually respond well to aggressive diuretic therapy with furosemide (intermittent dosing or a continuous infusion of up to 20 mg/hour).

Atelectasis is common in these patients and may not become clinically significant until after extubation when sedation and positive-pressure ventilation have been discontinued, especially in patients who are fluid overloaded. Atelectasis may lead to inadequate gas exchange, require better pain management, and mask continuous positive airway pressure (CPAP) while more aggressive diuresis is carried out. Adequate pain management is required to allow the patient to breathe deeply and perform incentive spirometry. Positive expiratory pressure therapy, EzPAP Positive Airway Pressure System (Smiths Medical), or other modalities employed by respiratory therapists early and continued until the patient is fully mobilized are imperative. If not prevented or treated early, atelectasis may lead to reintubation and possibly to pneumonia. Most lung dysfunction in the initial postoperative period is due to atelectasis, which usually responds well to higher PEEP levels.

A right mainstem intubation may lead to left-sided atelectasis and can be corrected early by careful inspection of the first postoperative chest radiograph when endotracheal tube position and position of mediastinal and plural chest drains as well as proper expansion of both lungs are determined. Bronchial obstruction by a mucous plug with lobar collapse commonly occurs, especially in the right lower lobe. Effective treatment usually requires removal of the plug either by aggressive pulmonary toileting or by bronchoscopy with bronchoalveolar lavage followed by a period of higher PEEP if the patient is still on ventilator support to reexpand the lung. Unless the plug is removed and the airway cleared, reexpansion is unlikely. Rarely, collapse of the right upper lobe may be seen in the case of superior lobe bronchus take-off directly from the trachea and occlusion there by the endotracheal tube. Review of the postoperative chest radiograph will usually lead to early diagnosis and treatment.

Simple pneumothorax may be seen on the first postoperative chest radiograph and may be corrected by increasing chest tube suction up to −20 cm H_2O in an optimally placed chest tube, or by placement of another chest tube usually in a more apical position. Postoperative pulmonary air leak from disruption of the visceral pleura in one or more areas may lead to tension pneumothorax if occult or unrecognized and chest tubes are removed prematurely.

Pleural effusions present after chest tubes have been removed are common but usually do not require removal by thoracentesis or chest tube thoracostomy unless they cause respiratory symptoms (Fig. 36.1). Hemothorax not due to ongoing postoperative bleeding is typically from bleeding that was not adequately drained by pleural or mediastinal chest tubes and does not usually require specific treatment.

Patients with baseline abnormal pulmonary function will usually manifest it to a worse degree postoperatively. Some patients, however, with preoperative cardiogenic pulmonary dysfunction improve often promptly after surgery (e.g., mitral stenosis, acute mitral regurgitation, or severe aortic stenosis).

Unanticipated, severe pulmonary dysfunction may be due to acute lung injury and is usually associated with inflammation and hemodilution related to CPB, particularly after long operations. After CPB, the lungs are especially susceptible to cytokine-mediated systemic reperfusion-inflammation injury due to the high blood flow they receive, or they may be injured by their own ischemia-reperfusion when there is no ventilation or pulmonary

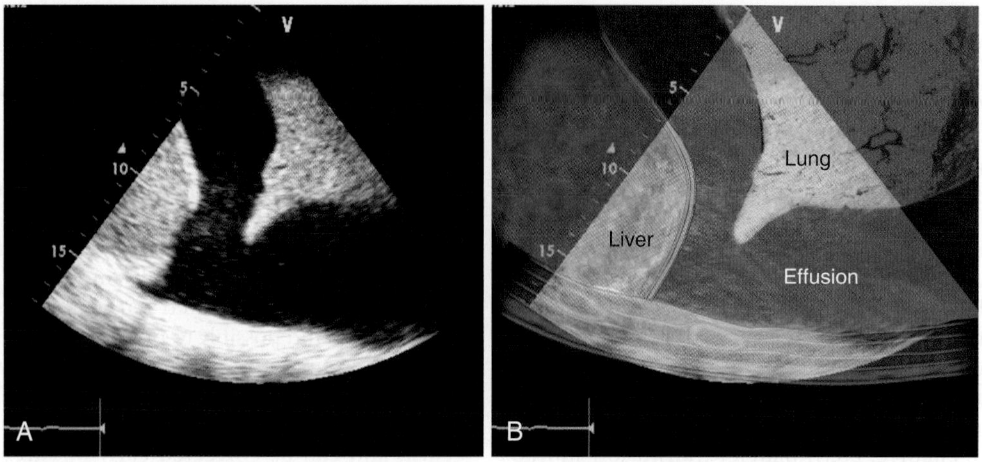

Figure 36.1 The examination of the pleura. Recognition of pleural effusion.

blood flow during CPB and oxygen delivery is by nonpulsatile bronchial flow only. Regardless of the mechanism, some pulmonary dysfunction is nearly universal.[52,53] Manifestations include decreased Pao_2/Fio_2 ratio, decreased pulmonary compliance, large alveolar-arterial gradients, and bronchoconstriction.

The management of these patients is similar to that for patients with acute respiratory distress syndrome. This requires adequate sedation and frequently muscle relaxation to better ventilate the patient by improving both coordination with ventilator cycles and chest wall compliance. Postinjury lung protective strategies include low tidal volume (6 mL/kg) delivered by pressure control ventilation. A low tidal volume minimizes volutrama and decreases minute ventilation, which results in hypercapnia that is acceptable as long as the pH remains greater than 7.25. A lower pH especially in postoperative cardiac surgery patients is not well tolerated because inotropes are less effective and arrhythmias more likely in the setting of severe acidemia. PEEP up to 20 cm of H_2O as hemodynamically tolerated may be required to wean Fio_2 levels below 60% to decrease the risk of free-radical–induced secondary lung injury. High PEEP may not be well tolerated in these patients due to impaired venous return and decreased cardiac output. Acute lung injury may occur as part of the systemic inflammatory response to CPB and does not typically progress to acute respiratory distress syndrome. With these lung-protective measures, more aggressive mechanical ventilation and muscle relaxation are not typically required and secondary lung injury is rare.

Postoperative diaphragm dysfunction may account for pulmonary problems in these patients. A paralyzed or palsied diaphragm may be suspected by finding an elevated hemidiaphragm on the first postoperative radiograph or after weaning from positive-pressure ventilation. Diaphragmatic dysfunction secondary to phrenic nerve injury (hypothermal, retractor stretch, or direct injury with mammary dissection) may prolong weaning or make weaning from ventilator support impossible.

Abdominal compartment syndrome from massive interstitial edema or retroperitoneal bleeding may occur after a long CPB time or intra-aortic balloon pump (IABP) insertion, respectively. In this case, the diaphragm is pushed into the thoracic cavity because of increased intra-abdominal pressure and excursion becomes minimal. Peak inspiratory pressures are high and it is difficult and often impossible to ventilate the patient adequately. Laparotomy and temporary expanded abdominal closure may be required to enable normal ventilation.

An increasing number of cardiac surgery patients are being successfully extubated in the operating room. The majority of patients who are not weaned and extubated in the operating room as part of an accelerated recovery protocol are candidates for extubation within 2 to 4 hours after ICU admission. Early postoperative conditions that mitigate against the initiation of ventilator weaning on arrival to the ICU after surgery are listed in Box 36.1.

A protocol-driven and respiratory therapist–managed reduction in initial postoperative intubation time has been achieved in many ICUs.[54] Some institutions use inclusion/exclusion criteria for selecting patients to be weaned under an accelerated recovery protocol.[55,56] Others employ a protocol wherein all patients are initially included, and a patient is excluded only when the patient does not meet the parameters for advancement. A practice that has been successful is to preoperatively select patients for accelerated recovery and make a final extubation decision in the operating room at the end of the case with input from both surgeon and anesthesiologist.

Tracheostomy is considered in patients who are difficult to separate from ventilator support. Tracheostomy reduces total mechanical ventilation time, shortens ICU and hospital stays, decreases the occurrence of pneumonia, reduces in-hospital mortality rate, and improves hospital resource utilization. It usually increases patient comfort and tolerance of mechanical ventilation and facilitates nursing care. It can improve communication and oral hygiene and make mobilization easier. It decreases the number of self-extubations and extubation-reintubation cycles, and decreases the requirement for sedation. Tracheostomy may also reduce upper airway injury including vocal cord ulceration, decrease dead space ventilation and airway resistance, and optimize work of breathing, thus facilitating separation from ventilator support, allowing for earlier transfer out of the ICU.

Although tracheostomy has conventionally been considered in patients who are ventilator dependent 2 weeks

Box 36.1 Early Postoperative Conditions or Criteria That Mitigate Against Initiation of Ventilator Weaning on Arrival in the ICU After Cardiac Surgery*

Primary Adverse Criteria

- Hemodynamic instability due to:
  - Atrial or ventricular arrhythmias
  - Low cardiac index
  - Hypotension, unexplained or uncontrolled
  - High level of inotropic or pressor support
- Ventilatory dysfunction
  - Low PaO_2/FiO_2 ratio
  - Difficult airway/intubation
- Excessive postoperative bleeding (>200-300 mL/hr)
- Hypothermia
- Mechanical ventricular assist
- Open sternum

Secondary Adverse Criteria

- Intra-aortic balloon pump counterpulsation support
- Long-standing pulmonary hypertension
- Operation for:
  - Acute myocardial infarction
  - Acute ventricular septal defect
  - Acute mitral regurgitation (papillary muscle rupture)
  - Descending aortic aneurysm

*Notably few of these are absolute contraindications to ventilator weaning, but they warrant consideration in the aggregate (see text).

FiO_2, fraction of inspired oxygen; ICU, intensive care unit; PaO_2, partial pressure of oxygen in arterial blood.

after cardiac surgery, there is little evidence to support this approach. Tracheostomy timing can be based on the determination at the end of the first ICU week of a patient's likelihood of successful weaning over the second week. If at that time successful weaning is considered unlikely, tracheostomy should be considered. Earlier tracheostomy (before the tenth postoperative day) in patients who require prolonged mechanical ventilation after cardiac surgery is associated with lower morbidity and mortality rates as well as decreased ICU and total hospital lengths of stay, and is not associated with an increased occurrence of mediastinitis.[57]

Venovenous extracorporeal membrane oxygenation and nitric oxide are two other modalities employed infrequently in selected patients with severe refractory respiratory failure after cardiac surgery. Nitric oxide has been used most effectively in patients with severe right ventricular dysfunction due to new-onset pulmonary hypertension to reduce right ventricular afterload. It is used under a protocol starting at 40 ppm and only continued if there is an immediate beneficial effect (reduction in pulmonary artery systolic pressure of 25% or greater). Weaning nitric oxide is usually first attempted within 24 hours of initiating it using PA pressure change as the weaning parameter and discontinued as soon as possible.

RENAL CARE

Despite significant research efforts and considerable focus on prevention and treatment, acute kidney injury (AKI) following cardiac surgery is associated with a significantly increased risk of morbidity and mortality. Although only 1% of patients will experience the most severe form of kidney injury and require some form of renal replacement therapy, this patient population has a 60% in-hospital mortality rate.[58] Risk stratification has identified several preoperative and postoperative risk factors for postoperative AKI—these include female gender, left ventricular ejection fraction (LVEF) less than 35%, exposure to angiographic contrast dye, duration of CPB, and low MAP during CPB.[59]

Causes of AKI are frequently divided into three distinct etiologic categories—prerenal, intrarenal, and postrenal. Although these aid in diagnostic evaluation, overlap may exist with multiple pathologic processes occurring in the same patient. Postrenal oliguria implies mechanical obstruction of the urologic system from the collecting ducts through the ureters. Diagnosis can be confirmed by Foley irrigation, renal and ureteral ultrasound, or computed tomographic scan of the abdomen and pelvis.

Prerenal causes occur when intravascular volume and cardiac output are insufficient to adequately perfuse the kidneys. In this state of ineffective circulating volume, the natural response of the kidneys is retention of blood volume and excretion of a small quantity of concentrated urine. If intravascular depletion or a depressed cardiac output persists, compensatory mechanisms may become overwhelmed. Thereafter, renal malperfusion becomes pathologic with the onset of acute tubular necrosis (ATN) and intrinsic renal injury.

Intrinsic renal failure refers to the state of direct damage to the kidney by ischemia or nephrotoxin exposure. The most common cause of intrarenal renal failure is ATN. This can result from prolonged periods of ischemia or exposure to nephrotoxic antibiotics, or contrast agents. Less commonly, certain medications (e.g., nafcillin or furosemide) can cause an inflammatory condition known as acute interstitial nephritis.

Initial evaluation of the patient with AKI should focus on the patient's preoperative risk factors, intraoperative course of events, exposure to nephrotoxic agents, and current hemodynamic and intravascular volume status. Laboratory parameters to assist in diagnosis of AKI include urine electrolytes, sodium (Na), Cr, blood urea nitrogen (BUN), and microscopic analysis of urine sediment. The fractional excretion of sodium (FeNa) or fractional excretion of BUN (FeBUN) is often used to distinguish prerenal causes of renal failure from intrarenal causes.

In the fluid-overloaded oliguric patient diuretics can be given to assess the patient's responsiveness and to remove excess volume. Although conversion from oliguric to nonoliguric renal failure through diuretics does not improve overall prognosis, it can improve oxygenation and hemodynamics.[60] If the patient is diuretic nonresponsive or has worsening electrolyte or acid-base imbalance, fluid overload with impairment of oxygenation or worsening heart failure, or has severe uremia, initiation of dialytic support should be considered. Several different dialysis modalities exist. In brief, continuous therapies offer more stable hemodynamics but do not clear as much solute or fluid per unit of time as intermittent dialysis.[61]

APPLICATIONS OF ECHOCARDIOGRAPHY AFTER CARDIAC SURGERY

The use of ultrasonography in the perioperative period has increased significantly over the past decade. In contrast to TEE usually performed by cardiologists and cardiothoracic anesthesiologists in the operating room, focused TTE is well suited for the postoperative period especially for unexplained hypotension and assessment of response to therapeutic interventions. Postoperative use of TTE can provide rapid and accurate diagnostic information in patients developing potentially life-threatening conditions. Although the image quality obtained in mechanically ventilated patients is usually better with TEE, TTE usually provides adequate views in postcardiotomy patients; and it is noninvasive, fast, performed at the bedside, reproducible, and focused on major cardiac and pleural space abnormalities.[62,63]

The use of TTE in periresuscitation (life support) care has two goals: (1) to assess the heart function, and (2) to identify treatable conditions. The focused echocardiographic evaluation in life support (FEEL) examination is briefly performed during cardiopulmonary resuscitation (CPR) with the primary objective of identifying potentially reversible causes of cardiopulmonary deterioration. The identification and appropriate management by TTE in the perioperative period of severe left ventricular dysfunction, pulmonary embolism, hypovolemia, or cardiac tamponade may be lifesaving.[64,65]

The recommended echocardiographic window to perform the FEEL examination is the subcostal view (Fig. 36.2). The FEEL examination may distinguish "true" pulseless electrical activity (PEA) from pseudo-PEA.[66] A recent publication demonstrated that in 35% of patients with an ECG diagnosis of asystole, 58% of those with PEA, coordinated cardiac motion was detected (pseudo-PEA) and associated with increased survival. Echocardiographic findings altered management in 78% of cases.[64]

In addition, FEEL protocol can facilitate the early detection of return of spontaneous circulation. One of the most common questions in the critically ill is the fluid responsiveness. Barbier and associates described the inferior vena cava (IVC) distensibility index in mechanically ventilated patients.[67] This index is based on change in size of IVC with respiration as it decreases with size with inspiration and increases with expiration:

$$\text{Distensibility index} = \frac{\text{IVC max (end expiration)} - \text{IVC min (end inspiration)}}{\text{IVC min (end expiration)}}$$

In this equation distensibility index is expressed as a percentage. A distensibility index greater than 18% predicts fluid responsiveness.

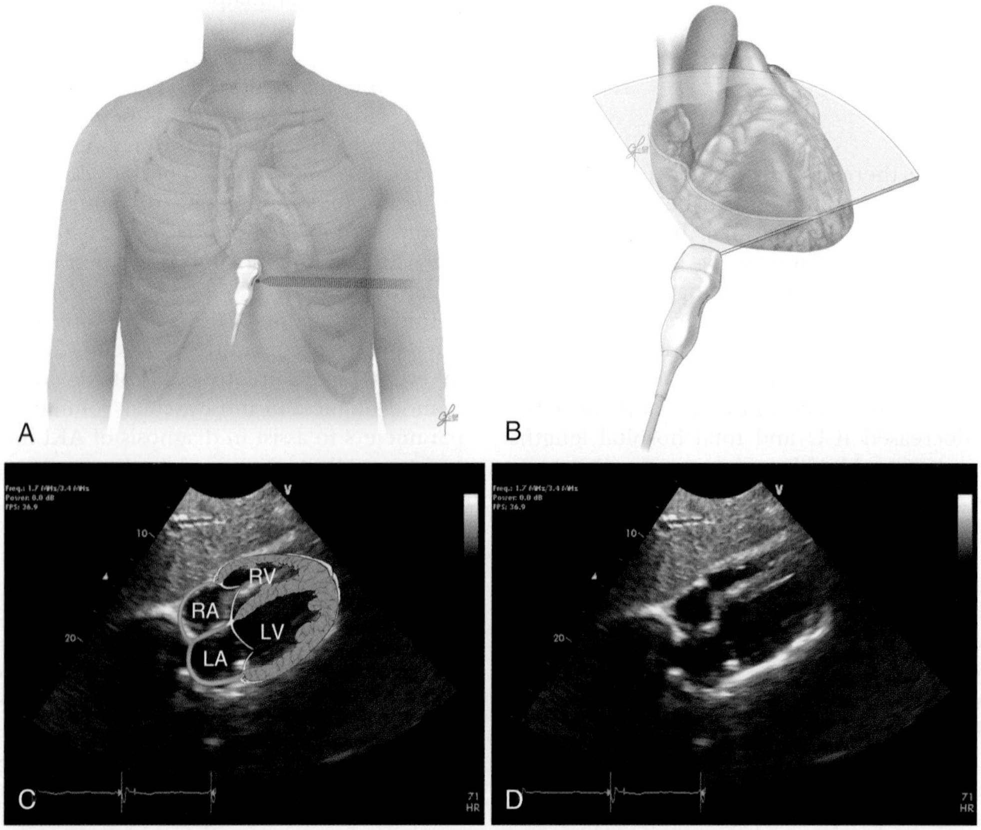

Figure 36.2 The FEEL examination—the subcostal view. **A,** Orientation of the probe in the epigastrium. **B,** Direction of the ultrasound beam. **C** and **D,** Identification of cardiac chambers.

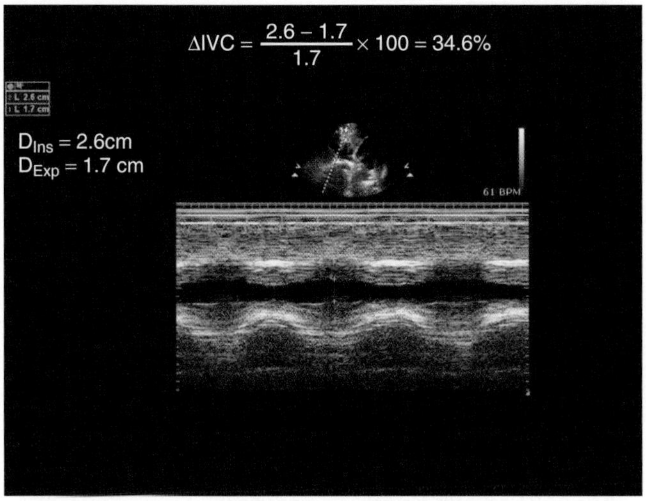

Figure 36.3 Inferior vena cava—diameter and distensibility index. Counterclockwise rotation from subcostal view (90 degrees). (Courtesy of Dr. Achi Oren-Grinberg: Beth Israel Deaconess Medical Center, Boston, MA.)

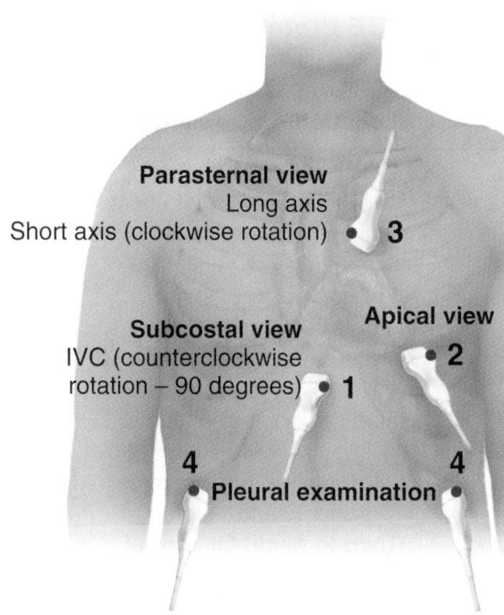

Figure 36.4 The focused assessed transthoracic echocardiography (FATE) protocol—transthoracic echocardiography views. 1, subcostal view; 2, apical view; 3, parasternal view; 4, pleural examination.

THE FATE EXAMINATION

The focused assessed transthoracic echocardiography (FATE) examination is a qualitative POC ultrasonography, which is ideal within the ICU. The FATE examination should include qualitative assessment of left and right ventricular function and intravascular volume status as minimum required information (Fig. 36.3). It supplements the critical care evaluation in the perioperative setting.[68,69] However, focused echocardiography does not replace a comprehensive echocardiogram performed per cardiology specialist whenever quantitative analysis or specific diagnoses such as endocarditis or valvular dysfunction are needed. Moreover, the correct application of this tool in postcardiotomy patients depends on the appropriate utilization of ultrasonography findings in the clinical context.[70]

The main goal of the FATE examination is to better characterize the state of shock/hypotension, volume status, and pleural disease:

Hypovolemia (measurement of IVC diameter and distensibility index)
Myocardial dysfunction (qualitative evaluation of the right and left ventricles, measurement of cardiac output and pulmonary pressures) including patients with acute respiratory failure
Pericardial effusion/tamponade (evaluation of tamponade physiology)
Pulmonary embolism (changes in acute right ventricular dysfunction)
Pulmonary edema (lines B, "comet tail" artifacts)
Pneumothorax (the sliding sign)

The appropriate process of applying FATE examination includes (a) acquisition of images, (b) recognition of normal anatomy of the heart, (c) fundamental knowledge of the more relevant diseases, and more importantly (d) applying findings to the clinical context.

ACQUISITION OF IMAGES

Bedside ultrasonography and acquisition of cardiac images are not exclusive of the comprehensive transthoracic examination. Moreover, the FATE examination must be considered an extension of the physical examination. Thus, before obtaining images with echocardiography it is important to keep in mind the position of the heart within the chest and the direction of the ultrasound beam (Fig. 36.4). In addition, thoracic ultrasonography offers better sensitivity and specificity than plain chest radiography. The evaluation of the pleurae mandate the knowledge of anatomic structures above and below both diaphragms. The acquisition of images can be very challenging in the postcardiotomy patient. Most of the time at least one view can be obtained and the goal of exclusion of important disease is achieved. Up to 40% of patients in the ICU have limited acquisition of echocardiography views. Although the TEE is an invasive technique, the unparalleled quality of ultrasonography examination is well known (Tables 36.1 and 36.2).

ROLE OF ULTRASONOGRAPHY IN POSTCARDIOTOMY TAMPONADE

Postcardiotomy surgery tamponade (PCST) is perhaps the most important diagnosis in the patient recovering from cardiac surgery. Its early recognition and intervention have a direct impact in patients' outcome. The process of diagnosing PCST begins with the identification of clinical signs and confirmation of the diagnosis with appropriate tools subsequently. A high index of suspicion should be maintained throughout the early postoperative cardiovascular ICU (CVICU) hours. Usually a progressive decrease of cardiac output after increased chest tube drainage and increased filling pressures occurs with PCST.[71]

Clinical signs such us Beck's triad (hypotension, distended neck veins, and diminished heart sounds) and pulsus paradoxus are neither sensitive nor specific of PCST.[72] Patients with other disorders such as constrictive

Table 36.1 The FATE Protocol: Technique

View	Location of Transducer	Probe Orientation Marker	Depth	Helpful Tips
Subcostal	2-3 cm below xiphoid process or RUQ if chest tubes are in place	~3 o'clock	15-25 cm	Hold the transducer from the top; apply angulations between 10 and 40 degrees Supine position
Subcostal–inferior vena cava	From the previous view, rotate transducer 90 degrees counterclockwise	~12 o'clock	16-24 cm	Keep right atrium to IVC junction on the screen Need to see the IVC merging into right atrium
Apical	Find the point of maximal impulse if feasible; otherwise, from anterior axillar line to nipple	~3 o'clock	14-18 cm	Ensure good contact with the rib (gentle pressure)
Parasternal–long axis	Third to fourth intercostal space	~11 o'clock	12-20 cm (up to 24 cm with pleural or pericardial effusion)	Ideally, left lateral decubitus position
Parasternal–short axis	Rotate 90 degrees clockwise from the parasternal–long-axis view, so ~2 o'clock	~2 o'clock	12-16 cm	*Aortic valve level:* Tilt transducer face slightly upward toward the patient's right shoulder *Mitral valve level:* Transducer is perpendicular to chest wall *Papillary muscle level:* Transducer faces slightly downward toward the patient's left flank

FATE, focused assessed transthoracic echocardiography; IVC, inferior vena cava; RUQ, right upper quadrant.

Table 36.2 Assessment of Structures with FATE Protocol

Assessment Focus	View(s)	Classification
Left ventricular (LV) function (qualitative)—"eyeballing": thickness of the myocardium	Parasternal–long-/short-axis view Apical view, subcostal view	Normal function Mild to moderate LV dysfunction Severe LV dysfunction Hyperdynamic
Right ventricular function	Parasternal–long-/short-axis view Apical view, subcostal view	
Pericardial space	Parasternal–long-/short-axis view Apical view, subcostal view	Pericardial effusion Tamponade physiology
Pleural effusion and pericardial effusion	Parasternal–long-axis view	
Inferior vena cava (IVC)	Subcostal view of the IVC	Diameter measurement: 2-3 cm from right atrium Normal diameter: 2.1 cm Respiratory phase variations, ideally on spontaneously breathing patients

FATE, focused assessed transthoracic echocardiography.

pericarditis, severe COPD, morbid obesity, and right ventricular infarction might present with pulsus paradoxus. In contrast, this sign can be absent in patients with atrial septal defect, regional tamponade, pulmonary hypertension, COPD with cor pulmonale, aortic insufficiency, and even positive-pressure mechanical ventilation.[72]

The various clinical presentations of PCST impose limitations to the FATE examination, especially posterior compartmented effusion. In addition, clotted and loculated blood is echo-dense, somewhat more challenging to diagnose, and could be mistaken for the myocardium itself. As a rapid screening tool it can very helpful if collapse of the right ventricle is noticed in the long-axis parasternal view or collapse of the right atrium/right ventricle, or left ventricle in the apical or subcostal views (Figs. 36.5 to 36.7). In addition, documentation of abnormally increased

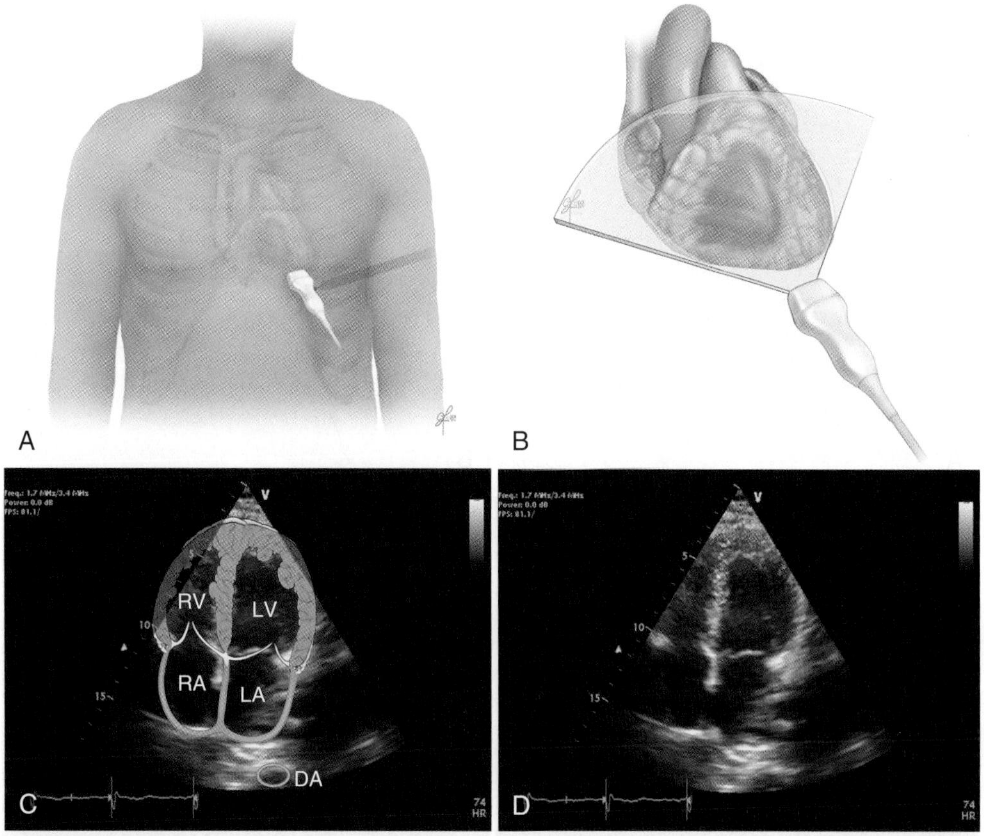

Figure 36.5 Apical view. **A,** Orientation of the probe in the apex. **B,** Direction of the ultrasound beam. **C** and **D,** Identification of cardiac chambers and heart valves.

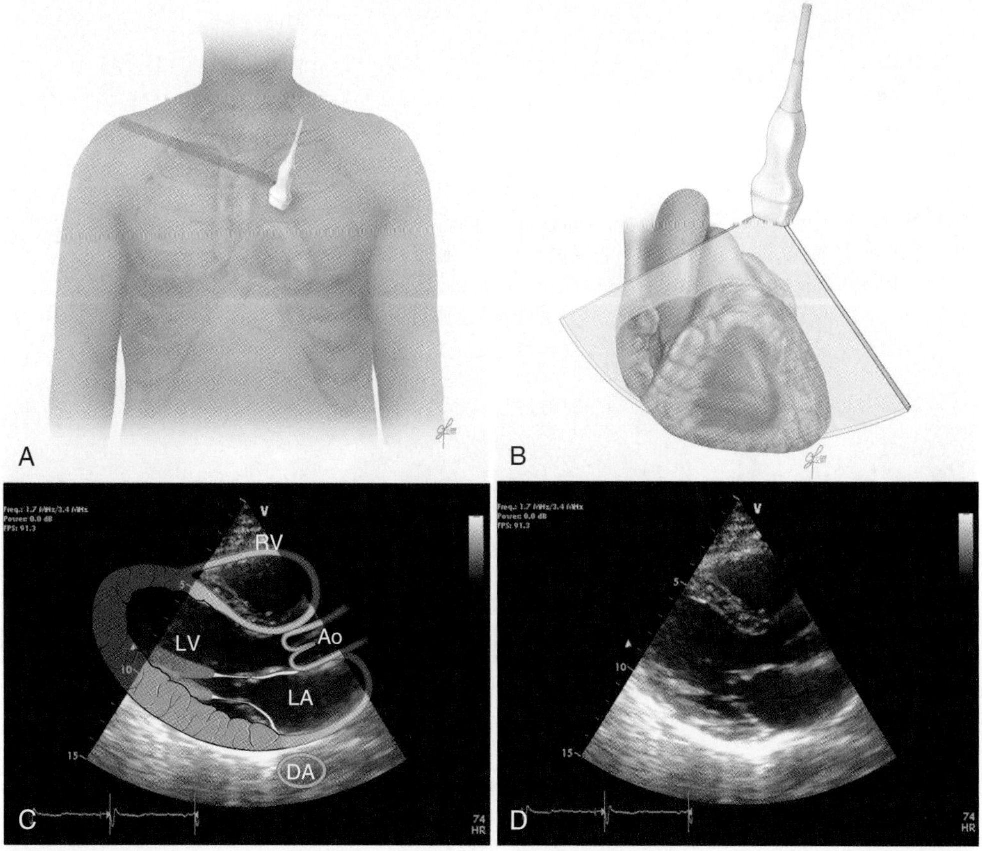

Figure 36.6 Parasternal—long axis view. **A,** Orientation of the probe in the apex. **B,** Direction of the ultrasound beam. **C** and **D,** Identification of cardiac chambers and heart valves.

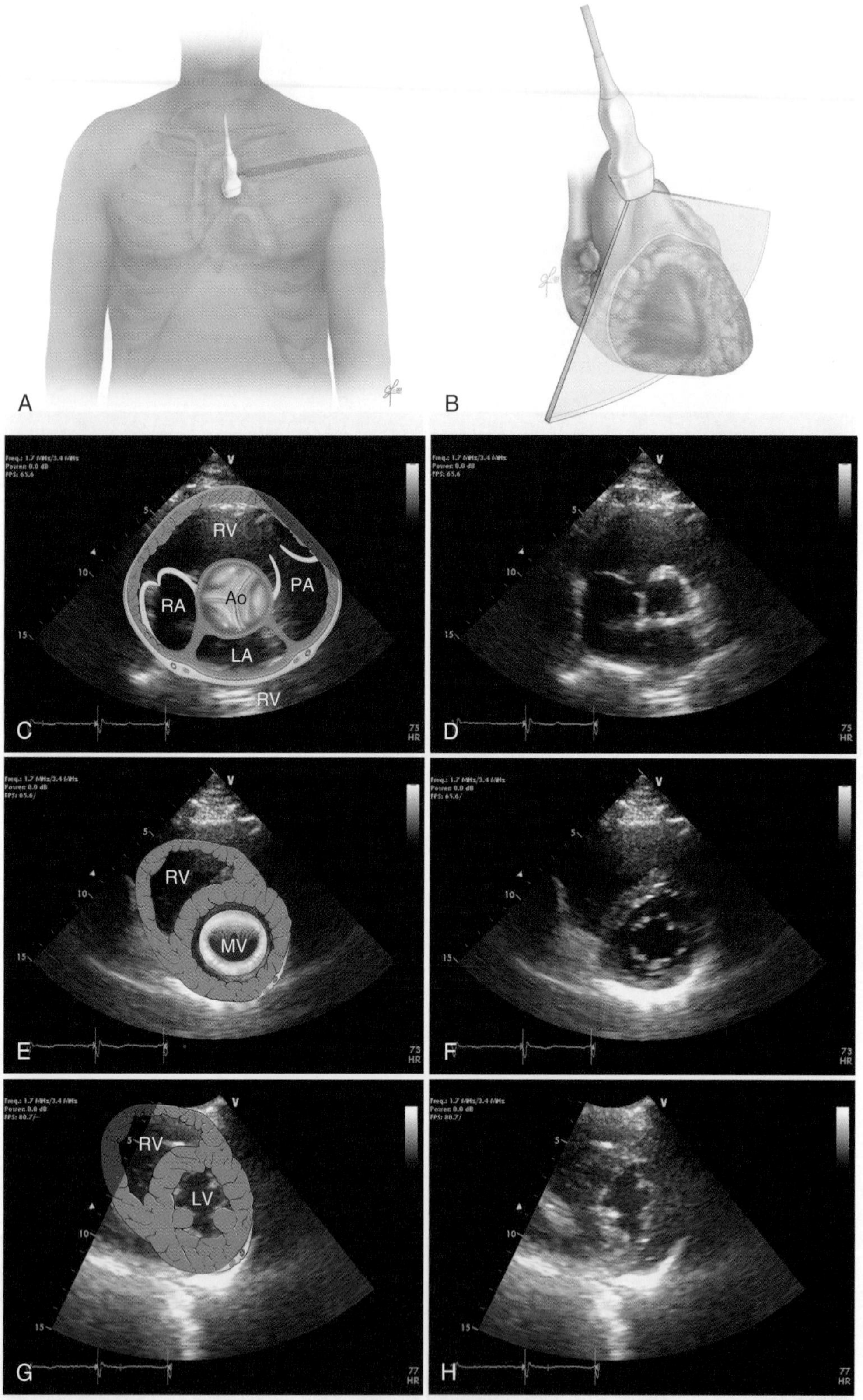

Figure 36.7 Parasternal—short axis view. **A,** Orientation of the probe in the left parasternal spaces. **B,** Direction of the ultrasound beam. **C** to **H,** Identification of cardiac chambers and heart valves.

Table 36.3 Echocardiographic Findings in Cardiac Tamponade

Typical	Atypical
Right atrium compression in early diastole*	Selective compression of the atria
Dilated inferior vena cava without respirophasic variability	Selective compression of right atrium
Echo-free space around the heart (circumferential pericardial effusion)	Bilateral atrial compression
Right ventricular diastolic collapse in the late diastole	Selective compression of right ventricle
Respirophasic variation of transmitral and transtricuspid flows	Selective compression of left ventricle
"Swinging heart" in the pericardial effusion	

*Right atrial collapse has higher sensitivity (68% vs. 60%) than right ventricular collapse but lower specificity (66% vs. 90%) in clinical tamponade. With hypovolemia this sign of tamponade might precede hemodynamic alterations.

diameter of the IVC (>2.5 cm) without variability with respiratory phases may help to distinguish from hemorrhagic shock in the setting of severe hypotension in the postoperative period.[73]

Transesophageal echocardiography is the definitive test whenever FATE examination has no conclusive findings to support PCST despite high suspicion of atypical presentation. The performance of echocardiographic evaluations should not delay an emergency surgical reexploration in the setting of postoperative shock.

The presence of acute bleeding into the pericardial space makes it appear as echolucent space. The presence of blood in the pericardium can be graded as small (0.5 cm), moderate (0.5-2 cm), or large (>2 cm). Right atrial systolic collapse that has duration greater than 30% of the entire systole is the most sensitive and specific sign of PCST. The best views to recognize this finding are subcostal or apical view on TTE and midesophageal four-chamber view by TEE. Doppler ultrasound can reveal a 35% increase respirophasic variation of the tricuspid/mitral E-wave velocity during spontaneous inspiration and a decrease of 25% in the mitral or left ventricle outflow track flow. Another important and helpful finding is the paradoxical movement of the interventricular septum (shift of the septum to the left ventricle in diastole and toward the right ventricle in systole) during spontaneous expiration and normalization in controlled ventilation (Table 36.3). Absence of right atrial collapse in cardiac tamponade is seen in severe pulmonary hypertension, RV dysfunction, COPD with cor pulmonale, and regional posterior tamponade.

RESCUE APPLICATIONS OF ECHOCARDIOGRAPHY

- The use of focused echocardiography in periresuscitation following cardiac surgery intends to identify the four treatable causes of cardiac arrest (severe ventricular dysfunction, pulmonary embolism, hypovolemia, and cardiac tamponade).
- The most useful echocardiography view in the setting of advanced cardiac life support is the subcostal. It can be performed after 5 cycles of CPR maneuvers.
- The identification of true PEA arrest has important prognostic implications as this subgroup of patients has worse prognosis in comparison to patients with pseudo-PEA (detection of coordinated cardiac motion).
- Post–cardiac surgery tamponade has various clinical presentations and may impose limitations to focused echocardiography, especially in those cases of posterior compartmented effusion.

MISCELLANEOUS CONSIDERATIONS

INTRA-AORTIC BALLOON PUMP WEANING

As noted elsewhere in this chapter, most patients with an IABP on arrival in the post–cardiac surgery unit have had the device percutaneously placed preoperatively in the catheterization laboratory. Appropriate management requires knowing the indication for its placement. In patients with unstable angina or left critical anatomy (usually a left main vessel obstruction, with or without proximal right coronary artery obstruction), the balloon often can be weaned as soon as the bleeding risks associated with removal are considered back to baseline. This may occur before extubation while the patient is still sedated. These are patients whose indication for IABP insertion has been corrected by the operation, and who do not require significant inotropic support, so the device is withdrawn in the early postoperative hours.

Less common and more challenging are the patients who had an IABP inserted for hemodynamic instability or cardiogenic shock preoperatively. In these patients, weaning from mechanical support may occur only after pharmacologic support (inotropes and vasopressors) has been weaned to a level that would allow them to be reinstituted or increased to support the patient after IABP removal. These are patients in whom a trial of ventilator weaning on IABP may be appropriate because the balloon unloads the afterload increases seen by a poor ventricle during awakening and ventilator weaning. In such patients, the IABP may be removed after extubation, but often ventilatory failure predominates, and the balloon weaning end points (minimal or no pharmacologic support) are reached well before extubation is an option. In these patients, mechanical support is weaned (decreasing the balloon augmentation ratio from 1:1 to 1:2 to 1:3, or by decreasing the balloon inflation volume). A normal response is to see the native (unloaded) systolic pressure increase as the MAP remains steady over 30 to 60 minutes. If these criteria are met, the balloon usually can be safely removed.

Patients who have an IABP placed intraoperatively may have had "prophylactic" mechanical support initiated, and, if on minimal pressor and inotrope support, with an anatomically corrective procedure, the device may be removed before extubation, as noted earlier. IABPs placed after CPB as an adjunct to weaning (see earlier) are frequently needed for days before successful weaning.

ROUTINE ORDER SETS

The post–cardiac surgery setting routinely makes good use of preprinted orders that, ideally, reflect a system-wide patient care pathway for the "typical" patient. It is important to review and revise these orders regularly to ensure that they remain appropriate in light of changes in accepted treatment principles and the institution's patient population. The review and revision of these order sets should include a review of patient care pathways or protocols. Protocol modifications should be part of a process involving surgeons, anesthesiologists, intensivists, nurses, respiratory therapists, pharmacists, infectious disease specialists, and nephrologists.

INTENSIVE CARE UNIT LENGTH OF STAY

Initial intubation time is associated with ICU length of stay. Most cardiac surgery patients can be extubated early and transferred out of the ICU within 24 hours. Rapid patient turnover is achieved in ICUs that use care pathways based on patient parameters and not the length of stay.[49] Patient-based parameters for a diuresis protocol would be based on a patient's weight relative to the preoperative weight, the BUN/Cr, and the CI/preload, not on time ("postoperative day 1"). When time-based parameters are used, they should be based on hours rather than days. Pacing wires might be removed routinely after any 12-hour period with no need for pacing or antidysrhythmic therapy, rather than "on postoperative day 2." Timing of chest tube removal may be based on volume and character of the drainage, rather than on an experientially derived time or postoperative day.

KEY POINTS

- Despite decreased overall mortality risk in coronary artery grafting, postoperative neurologic complications remain the major cause of morbidity and death. Among these complications, stroke portends the worse outcome.
- The most consistent pathophysiologic mechanism of stroke is embolism (>60%), followed by hypoperfusion and hemorrhage.
- Clinical presentation of postcardiotomy neurologic complications include altered consciousness and coma, focal neurologic deficit, and seizures.
- Brain CT scan is indicated at any time postcardiotomy patients present unexplained delayed awakening, new focal neurologic deficit, or seizure.
- Although brain MRI is not usually feasible in the early postoperative period following cardiac surgery, it provides better characterization of the cerebral ischemic lesions and it has a definite prognostic value.
- The most important initial interventions of patients suffering from postcardiotomy stroke include tracheal intubation (if the patient has a GCS score <9), mechanical ventilatory support, and aggressive treatment of hypoxemia, hypotension, hypercarbia, and hyperthermia.

KEY POINTS (Continued)

- Thrombolytic therapy is a feasible therapy in selected patients who present postcardiotomy stroke.
- Perioperative hemodynamic perturbations are common in cardiac surgical patients and depend on the patient's preoperative state, the nature of the surgical procedure, and the degree of intraoperative stunning.
- Optimal postoperative blood pressure should be determined in the context of the patient's comorbid conditions and the nature of the surgical procedure.
- Postoperative hypotension may be secondary to hypovolemia, cardiac insufficiency, vasoplegia, myocardial ischemia, or tamponade.
- Myocardial stunning and vasoplegia usually require exogenous pharmacologic support and improve over hours to days.
- Acute tamponade requires immediate recognition and treatment; unfortunately, classic physical examination signs may not manifest.
- The most common arrhythmia following cardiac surgery is atrial fibrillation, and clinicians must decide whether rate or rhythm control is preferable for their patients.
- Bleeding following cardiac surgery is relatively common and often requires transfusion of packed red blood cells, platelets, and FFP.
- Fluid overload is a common cause of poor gas exchange in the early postoperative period and can be readily assessed by reviewing intraoperative fluid balance and postoperative indicators of volume status.
- Atelectasis is common in these patients and may not become clinically significant until after extubation when sedation and positive-pressure ventilation have been discontinued, especially in patients who are fluid overloaded.
- Pleural effusions present after chest tubes have been removed are common but usually do not require removal by thoracentesis or chest tube thoracostomy unless they cause respiratory symptoms.
- Patients with baseline abnormal pulmonary function will usually manifest it to a worse degree postoperatively.
- Unanticipated, severe pulmonary dysfunction may be due to acute lung injury and is usually associated with inflammation and hemodilution related to CPB, particularly after long operations.
- Postoperative diaphragm dysfunction may account for pulmonary problems in these patients. A paralyzed or palsied diaphragm may be suspected by finding an elevated hemidiaphragm on the first postoperative radiograph or after weaning from positive-pressure ventilation.
- A protocol-driven and respiratory therapist–managed reduction in initial postoperative intubation time has been achieved in many ICUs

KEY POINTS (Continued)

- Earlier tracheostomy (before the tenth postoperative day) in patients who require prolonged mechanical ventilation after cardiac surgery is associated with lower morbidity and mortality rates as well as decreased ICU and total hospital lengths of stay, and is not associated with an increased occurrence of mediastinitis.
- Although AKI occurs in only 1% of cardiac surgery patients, it is associated with a 60% in-hospital mortality rate.
- Initial evaluation of the patient with AKI includes identification of patient-specific risk factors, estimation of intravascular volume status, and reduction of ongoing injury.
- Classification of AKI as prerenal, intrarenal, or postrenal has significant therapeutic and prognostic implications.
- Although diuretics may aid in removing excess volume, converting a patient from an oliguric to a nonoliguric state does not improve prognosis.
- Patients unresponsive to diuretic therapy who experience severe acid-base derangements, electrolyte abnormalities, or fluid overload impairing oxygenation, may require renal replacement therapy.

SELECTED REFERENCES

4. Roach GW, Kanchuger M, Mangano CM, et al: Adverse cerebral outcomes after coronary bypass surgery. Multicenter Study of Perioperative Ischemia Research Group and the Ischemia Research and Education Foundation Investigators. N Engl J Med 1996;335(25):1857-1863.
10. Filsoufi F, Rahmanian PB, Castillo JG, et al: Incidence, imaging analysis, and early and late outcomes of stroke after cardiac valve operation. Am J Cardiol 2008;101(10):1472-1478.
25. Levin MA, Lin HM, Castillo JG, et al: Early on-cardiopulmonary bypass hypotension and other factors associated with vasoplegic syndrome. Circulation 2009;120(17):1664-1671.
38. Echahidi N, Pibarot P, O'Hara G, et al: Mechanisms, prevention, and treatment of atrial fibrillation after cardiac surgery. J Am Coll Cardiol 2008;51(8):793-801.
41. Paparella D, Brister SJ, Buchanan MR: Coagulation disorders of cardiopulmonary bypass: A review. Intensive Care Med 2004; 30(10):1873-1881.
52. Clark SC: Lung injury after cardiopulmonary bypass. Perfusion 2006;21(4):225-228.
56. van Mastrigt GA, Maessen JG, Heijmans J, et al: Does fast-track treatment lead to a decrease of intensive care unit and hospital length of stay in coronary artery bypass patients? A meta-regression of randomized clinical trials. Crit Care Med 2006;34(6):1624-1634.
64. Breitkreutz R, Price S, Steiger HV, et al: Focused echocardiographic evaluation in life support and peri-resuscitation of emergency patients: A prospective trial. Resuscitation 2010;81(11):1527-1533.
69. Faris JG, Veltman MG, Royse C: Focused transthoracic echocardiography in the perioperative period. Anaesth Intensive Care 2011;39(2):306-307; author reply 7-8.
71. Carmona P, Mateo E, Casanovas I, et al: Management of cardiac tamponade after cardiac surgery. J Cardiothorac Vasc Anesth 2012;26(2):302-311.

The complete list of references can be found at www.expertconsult.com.

PART 3

CRITICAL CARE PULMONARY DISEASE

Acute Respiratory Failure

37

David P. Gurka | Robert A. Balk

CHAPTER OUTLINE

ACUTE RESPIRATORY FAILURE—TYPES 1 AND 2

Acute respiratory failure is defined as the inability of the respiratory system to meet the oxygenation, ventilation, or metabolic requirements of the patient.[1] Although the main function of the lungs appears to be related to gas exchange (i.e., oxygenation and ventilation), it should be remembered that the lung is a metabolically active organ as well.[1,2] Respiratory failure has been divided into two main types. Type 1 is hypoxemic respiratory failure, and type 2 is hypercapnic failure with or without hypoxemic respiratory failure.[2] More simply stated, type 1 respiratory failure is oxygenation failure and type 2 is ventilatory failure. Operationally, type 1 respiratory failure is defined by a partial pressure of oxygen in arterial blood ($Pa{O_2}$) less than 60 mm Hg and type 2 respiratory failure is defined by a partial pressure of carbon dioxide in arterial blood ($Pa{CO_2}$) greater than 50 mm Hg. The respiratory failure can be acute or chronic in nature, related to the onset and duration of the failure.[2,3] Some patients may present with an acute deterioration or worsening of their chronic respiratory dysfunction termed *acute-on-chronic respiratory failure.*[4]

Acute respiratory failure is commonly encountered in the intensive care unit (ICU) setting and may be the primary reason for the admission or a complication of the patient's medical condition(s) or treatment. Respiratory failure may be the result of a variety of causes, some of which may not directly involve the lungs or the respiratory muscles.[2] Like a chain composed of individual links representing the brain, peripheral nervous system, upper airway, lower airway, respiratory muscles, cardiovascular system, and lungs (Fig. 37.1),[2] respiratory failure may result when any of the links become sufficiently dysfunctional or weak. Like a chain, the body is only as strong as its weakest link, and respiratory failure may result when a component of the chain becomes sufficiently compromised. Common causes of hypoxemic and hypercapnic respiratory failure are listed in Box 37.1. This chapter reviews the basic mechanisms and clinical manifestations of type 1 and 2 respiratory failure and concludes with a more in-depth discussion of acute respiratory distress syndrome (ARDS), which includes clinical disorders in the type 1 category (ventilator management will be addressed in more depth in other chapters).

HYPOXEMIC RESPIRATORY FAILURE

BASIC MECHANISMS

Hypoxemic respiratory failure refers to the inability of the respiratory system to maintain satisfactory levels of oxygen in the arterial blood.[3] The five basic mechanisms of hypoxemia are listed in Box 37.2. Ventilation-perfusion abnormality is the most common.[2,3] Multiple mechanisms may be instrumental in the development of respiratory failure. Most of the abnormalities will improve with the administration of supplemental oxygen, except for a shunt abnormality in which the $Pa{O_2}$ continues to be low despite the administration of high levels of supplemental oxygen. The shunt may be either intracardiac (such as a right-to-left shunt through a patent foramen ovale) or intrapulmonary (as seen with pneumonia or ARDS).[5,6] A diffusion abnormality is infrequently the cause of hypoxemia in clinical practice and typically is only significant in the setting of tachycardia, high

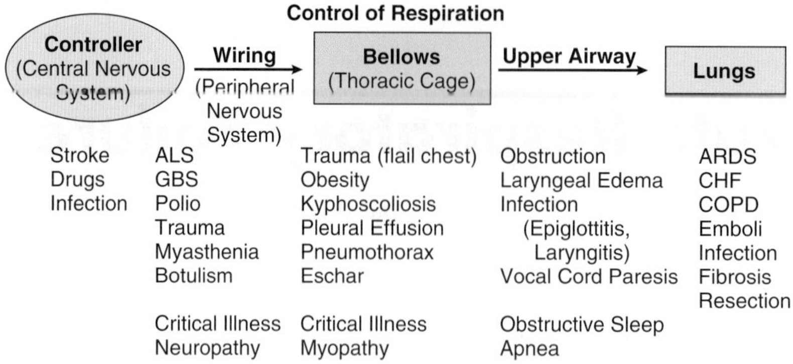

Figure 37.1 Control of respiration. ALS, amyotrophic lateral sclerosis; ARDS, acute respiratory distress syndrome; CHF, congestive heart failure; COPD, chronic obstructive pulmonary disease; GBS, Guillain-Barré syndrome; Myasthenia, myasthenia gravis or the Eaton-Lambert myasthenic syndrome.

Box 37.1 Common Causes of Hypoxemic and Hypercapnic Respiratory Failure

Brain

Bulbar poliomyelitis
Central alveolar hypoventilation
Cerebrovascular accident
Cerebral malignancy
Drug overdose (e.g., narcotic, sedative/hypnotic)
Elevated intracranial pressure
Encephalitis and meningitis
Pontine herniation
Postoperative anesthetic depression

Spinal Cord

Amyotrophic lateral sclerosis
Cervical cordotomy
Guillain-Barré syndrome
Poliomyelitis
Spinal cord trauma

Neuromuscular System

Acute intermittent porphyria
Botulism
Cholinergic crisis
Curariform drugs
Electrolyte disorders (e.g., hypophosphatemia, hypomagnesemia)
Hypokalemic periodic paralysis
Multiple sclerosis
Myasthenia gravis
Myxedema
Neuromuscular blocking antibiotics (e.g., polymyxin, streptomycin)
Organophosphate insecticides
Peripheral neuritis
Polymyositis
Respiratory muscle fatigue—critical illness polyneuropathy/polymyopathy
Tetanus

Upper Airway

Epiglottitis and laryngotracheitis
Large tonsils and adenoids
Obstructive sleep apnea
Postintubation laryngeal edema
Tracheal obstruction
Vocal cord paralysis

Thorax and Pleura

Chest wall burn with eschar formation
Chest wall trauma—flail chest
Kyphoscoliosis
Massive abdominal distention
Massive obesity
Muscular dystrophy
Large pleural effusion/pleural fibrosis
Pneumothorax
Rheumatoid spondylitis
Thoracoplasty

Cardiovascular System

Cardiogenic pulmonary edema
Left ventricular failure
Mitral stenosis
Biventricular failure
Fat embolism
Snake bite
Uremia
Volume overload
Pulmonary veno-occlusive disease

Lower Airway and Alveoli

Acute respiratory distress syndrome (ARDS)
Aspiration
Asthma
Atelectasis
Bronchiectasis
Bronchiolitis
Chronic obstructive pulmonary disease
Cystic fibrosis
Interstitial lung disease
Massive bilateral pneumonia
Near-drowning
Pancreatitis
Pulmonary contusion
Radiation lung injury
Sepsis
Smoke inhalation
Surgical resection of lung parenchyma

Box 37.2 Mechanisms of Hypoxemia

- Inadequate P_{AO_2}
  - Alveolar hypoventilation
  - Decreased F_{IO_2}
- $\dot{V}/\dot{Q}$ mismatch
- Shunt
  - Intrapulmonary
  - Intracardiac
- Diffusion abnormality
- Low $M\bar{V}O_2$

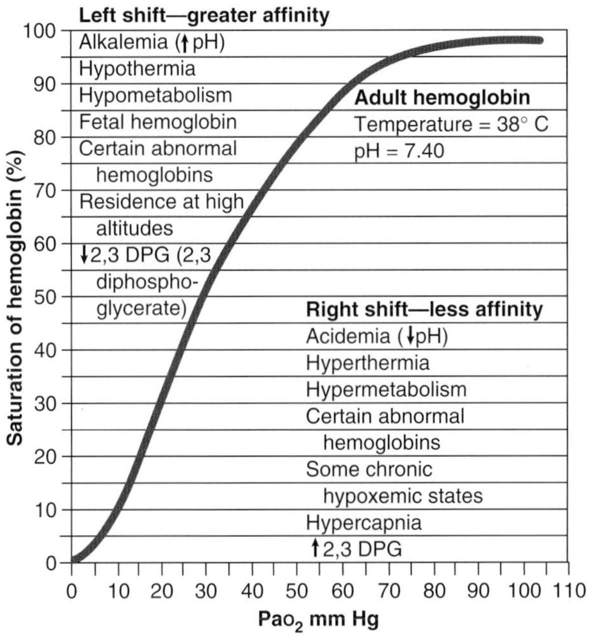

Figure 37.2 Oxyhemoglobin dissociation curve.

cardiac outputs, and when the diffusion capacity is below 25% of predicted.[3]

ASSESSMENT OF OXYGENATION

The hallmark of type 1 respiratory failure is hypoxemia, which is primarily assessed by the Pa_{O_2} of an arterial blood gas (ABG). An estimate of the patient's oxygenation status can be obtained by measuring the oxygen saturation using a pulse oximeter. An appreciation of the sigmoid shape of the oxyhemoglobin dissociation curve allows for a rough estimation of the Pa_{O_2} (Fig. 37.2). The curve will shift rightward or leftward in relation to changes in the pH, Pa_{CO_2}, temperature, and PO_4^{-2} concentration.[7] Determination of the ABG and knowledge of the exact F_{IO_2} allows for the calculation of the alveolar-arterial oxygen gradient[3] (A-a gradient) using the formula $P_{AO_2} - Pa_{O_2} =$ A-a gradient; thus,

$$P_{AO_2} = F_{IO_2}(P_B - P_{H_2O}) - Pa_{CO_2}/R$$

where

P_{AO_2}	Partial pressure of oxygen in the alveolus
Pa_{O_2}	Partial pressure of oxygen in the arterial blood
F_{IO_2}	Fraction of inspired oxygen
P_B	Barometric pressure
P_{H_2O}	Water vapor pressure at standard temperature and pressure
Pa_{CO_2}	Partial pressure of carbon dioxide in the arterial blood
R	Respiratory quotient (R = 0.8)

The A-a gradient is F_{IO_2} dependent and will increase as the F_{IO_2} increases. Because of this F_{IO_2} dependency, some have preferred to evaluate oxygenation abnormalities by calculating the Pa_{O_2}/P_{AO_2} ratio, which is independent of the F_{IO_2}.[3] For simplicity's sake, many individuals use the Pa_{O_2}/F_{IO_2} ratio as a measure of oxygenation abnormality. This value is used in the definition of ARDS and has gained wide-scale acceptance as a measure of abnormal oxygenation.[8] The shunt fraction or venous admixture can also be calculated while a patient breathes 100% oxygen and has reached steady-state oxygenation.

HYPERCAPNIC RESPIRATORY FAILURE

Hypercapnic respiratory failure can be the result of a variety of disorders as listed in Box 37.1.[9] Acute hypercapnic respiratory failure, also termed *acute ventilatory failure,* occurs when a patient's ABG reveals acute respiratory acidemia (pH <7.35) with a Pa_{CO_2} greater than 50 mm Hg. This definition is not generally applicable to patients with severe chronic obstructive lung disease or neuromuscular disorders who have developed a compensatory metabolic alkalemia in response to their chronic hypercapnia. However, these patients may have acute exacerbations or comorbid conditions that cause them to decompensate into *acute-on-chronic respiratory failure.*

In steady-state conditions the rate of CO_2 production ($\dot{V}_{CO_2}$) equals the rate of CO_2 elimination. Carbon dioxide elimination ($\dot{V}_{CO_2}$) is equal to the alveolar ventilation (V_A) multiplied by the partial pressure of carbon dioxide in the alveolar gas (P_{ACO_2}). Thus, the equation for carbon dioxide production is $\dot{V}_{CO_2} = V_A \times P_{ACO_2}$. In the pulmonary capillary, carbon dioxide is readily diffusible through the endothelial and epithelial cell membranes down a substantial concentration gradient of approximately 45 to 50 mm Hg (normal pulmonary arterial CO_2 [Pa_{CO_2}] versus essentially zero for the partial pressure of carbon dioxide in room air [P_{ICO_2}]) so that the alveolar and capillary blood partial pressures of CO_2 are equal ($P_{ACO_2} = Pa_{CO_2}$).

Not all respired air is effective alveolar ventilation because some of the total tidal ventilation (V_T) ventilates nonperfused areas or dead space (V_D) (both anatomic and pathologic). This relationship between tidal volume, dead space volume, and alveolar volume can be expressed as[3]:

$$V_T = V_A + V_D \text{ or } V_A = V_T - V_D$$

The minute ventilation (V_E) is equal to the sum of the dead space ventilation (V_D) and the alveolar ventilation (V_A): $V_E = V_D + V_A$. Combining and rearranging terms from these various equations yields the following relationship of carbon dioxide production and alveolar ventilation with the Pa_{CO_2}.[3]

$$PaCO_2 = \frac{\dot{V}CO_2}{VT - VD}$$

Therefore, elevated $PaCO_2$ can result from a combination of any of three clinical alterations: increased CO_2 production, decreased tidal ventilation, or increased dead space ventilation.[9] Increased CO_2 production arises from hypermetabolic states such as exercise, fever, sepsis, burns, trauma, excessive carbohydrate intake, and hyperthyroidism.[9] In isolation, these relatively common conditions rarely induce hypercapnic respiratory failure because the normal physiologic response to an elevated $PaCO_2$ is to increase minute (and therefore alveolar) ventilation to maintain eucapnia and a normal pH. Only those patients who are unable to increase their effective alveolar ventilation as a result of neuromuscular disorders affecting the muscles of respiration, the presence of excessive ventilation/perfusion ($\dot{V}/\dot{Q}$) mismatching, or increased dead space ventilation develop hypercapnic respiratory failure caused by elevated CO_2 production.

Ventilatory deficiencies, decreased tidal ventilation, and increased dead space ventilation that result in hypercapnic respiratory failure can be differentiated by using the A-a gradient equation. The $PAO_2 - PaO_2$ difference breathing room air is normally less than 10 to 15 mm Hg when simple alveolar hypoventilation is responsible for the hypoxemia noted on blood gas analysis. An increased $PAO_2 - PaO_2$ difference suggests a parenchymal lung process, usually associated with $\dot{V}/\dot{Q}$ abnormalities, to account for the additional hypoxemia in these patients with hypercapnic respiratory failure.

Decreased tidal volume hypoventilation can be caused by disorders affecting any component of the "neuromuscular sequence" starting in the central nervous system (CNS) and ending at the muscles of respiration (see Fig. 37.1). Among the more common causes are CNS depressants such as narcotics and sedatives, which diminish respiratory drive; cerebral vascular disorders, especially those that involve the brainstem, which impair the efferent signals to breathe; and disorders of neuromuscular transmission such as myasthenia gravis and the paraneoplastic Eaton-Lambert myasthenic syndrome (Box 37.3).[10,11] Abnormal respiratory mechanics can result from airflow obstruction, chest wall deformities, and loss of lung volume. Disorders that increase the respiratory load, such as a circumferential chest burn eschar or flail chest, or impair function of the respiratory muscles, such as kyphoscoliosis, will also lead to hypoventilation.

ASSESSMENT OF VENTILATION

The hallmark feature of inadequate ventilation is the presence of an elevated $PaCO_2$ with or without the presence of hypoxemia.[3,9] In the adult population the best method to detect an elevated $PaCO_2$ is with an ABG measurement. Noninvasive evaluation of ventilation in the critically ill adult, using end-tidal CO_2 ($PetCO_2$) measurements or transcutaneous CO_2 ($PtcCO_2$) determinations, is not as reliable as it is in the healthy adult or the neonate, respectively.[7]

CLINICAL MANIFESTATIONS

The risk factors for developing acute respiratory failure include the postoperative state, preexisting chronic illness, malnutrition, advanced age, morbid obesity, chronic bronchitis, and cigarette smoking. The clinical manifestations of respiratory distress may be subtle and nonspecific or may be obvious to even the untrained observer. The patient with respiratory distress may have an abnormal respiratory rate (too high or low) or display an irregular pattern of breathing. The patient with respiratory distress may evidence gasping ventilation, nasal flaring, or use of the accessory muscles of respiration. Intercostal retractions may be seen, and the patient may exhibit paradoxical respiratory movement. Typically, patients with acute respiratory failure, whether type 1 or type 2, will have altered heart rate and blood pressure. The majority will evidence a sympathetic response with tachycardia and hypertension, but patients may be hypotensive and bradycardic. Cardiac arrhythmias may be seen in both type 1 and type 2 respiratory failure. Patients with acute respiratory failure will usually be in distress and often appear apprehensive.[2,9] Many will be diaphoretic and have altered mental status or level of consciousness. Hypercapnic patients may demonstrate signs of a respiratory encephalopathy including somnolence, coma, asterixis, seizures, tremors, or myoclonic jerks. Papilledema and congested conjunctivae may be present. Type 1 respiratory failure patients may appear cyanotic.[9]

Box 37.3 Causes of Decreased Respiratory Muscle Strength or Endurance

Disorders of the phrenic nerve
- Guillain-Barré syndrome
- Poliomyelitis

Respiratory muscle atrophy

Disorders of neuromuscular transmission
- Myasthenia gravis
- Ventilator dependence
- Malnutrition
- Myopathy
- Critical illness polyneuropathy/myopathy

Altered diaphragmatic force-length relationship
- Dynamic hyperinflation and diaphragmatic flattening

ACUTE RESPIRATORY DISTRESS SYNDROME

Since the initial 1967 description of acute catastrophic respiratory failure in 12 patients who were subsequently declared to have the acute respiratory distress syndrome, there has been a great deal of research and clinical study attempting to understand the mechanism of injury and improve the outcome of these critically ill patients.[12-14] The hallmark of this disorder was the rapid onset of acute hypoxemic respiratory failure that was characterized by refractory hypoxemia despite the administration of high concentrations of supplemental oxygen; decreased pulmonary compliance; diffuse, bilateral pulmonary infiltrates; the absence of left-sided heart failure; and histologic evidence of alveolar damage with hyaline membrane formation, which was followed by fibrosis of the lung.[8,12,13] The subsequent 10 to 20 years of ARDS management were associated with extremely high mortality rates, at times approaching 90%, despite the provision of extremely aggressive supportive care.[15-20] Some of the initial clinical and basic investigations that attempted to improve the outcome of patients with ARDS were hampered by the lack of uniformly accepted definitions.[21-25] In 1994 an American-European Consensus Conference (AECC) defined acute lung injury (ALI) and ARDS in an attempt to eliminate confusion related to terminology for these conditions.[21,22] The definitions are clinically based and regard ALI as a continuum with the more severe oxygenation abnormalities reflective of ARDS. Among the main benefits of the uniform definition would be improved communication and enhanced clinical trial design.

The AECC definition of ALI and ARDS was challenged and there were noted discrepancies between the clinical and pathologic findings in individuals felt to have died with ARDS.[25] Esteban and colleagues[25] found that one third of the people who died with a clinical diagnosis of ARDS did not have histologic evidence of diffuse alveolar damage on postmortem examination. In addition, diffuse alveolar damage, the hallmark pathologic finding of ARDS, was evident in 10% of patients who died without a clinical diagnosis of ARDS. A subsequent study evaluated the sensitivity and specificity of the Murray Lung Injury Score, the AECC definition of ARDS, and a Delphi definition that incorporated oxygenation abnormality, X-ray findings, clinical onset, compatible clinical scenario, and absence of left-sided heart failure for ARDS.[26] The combination of Lung Injury Score greater than 2.5 with either the AECC definition or the Delphi definition of ARDS resulted in the best combination of sensitivity and specificity. Since its introduction, the AECC definition has been used by the vast majority of clinical trials evaluating new treatment strategies for patients with ARDS, particularly those conducted by the ARDS Network investigators, supported by the U.S. National Heart, Lung, and Blood Institute of the National Institutes of Health.[27-29] In 2011 experts from the European Society of Intensive Care Medicine, the American Thoracic Society, and the Society of Critical Care Medicine met in Berlin and proposed a new definition for staging ARDS as mild, moderate, or severe, based on the oxygenation impairment measured on a minimum of 5 cm H_2O positive end-expiratory pressure (PEEP) (10 cm H_2O for severe).[30] The new Berlin definition did not drastically differ from the prior AECC definition, but it clarified several important concepts:

1. Timing—patients with ARDS should be identified within 72 hours of a recognized risk factor and nearly all patients should be identified within 7 days.
2. Chest imaging—bilateral opacities consistent with pulmonary edema are seen on chest radiograph or chest computed tomography (CT) scan.
3. Origin of pulmonary edema—ARDS may be present in the setting of coexisting cardiogenic edema or volume overload if in the opinion of the treating physicians the respiratory failure is not fully explained by these conditions and there is a recognized risk factor for ARDS. In the absence of a recognized risk factor for ARDS there should be some objective assessment of cardiac function such as echocardiography or pulmonary capillary wedge pressure measurement.
4. Oxygenation—because PEEP can affect the $Pa{O_2}/F{IO_2}$ ratio there should be a minimum of 5 cm H_2O PEEP and 10 cm H_2O in those patients with severe ARDS ($Pa{O_2}/F{IO_2} < 100$).[30]

The Berlin definition for ARDS eliminates the use of the term "acute lung injury" to classify the severity of lung injury and defines mild ARDS as a $Pa{O_2}/F{IO_2}$ 300 or less but greater than 200, moderate ARDS as a $Pa{O_2}/F{IO_2}$ 200 or less but greater than 100, and severe ARDS as a $Pa{O_2}/F{IO_2}$ 100 or less, with morality rates associated with the different stages 27%, 32%, and 45%, respectively.[30]

To date there is no specific laboratory test that is pathognomonic for the diagnosis of ARDS.[8,21,27] All of the current definitions for ARDS require the presence of bilateral pulmonary infiltrates on chest imaging, but interpretation is not always straightforward.[21,31] When 21 experts were given 28 chest radiographs to evaluate for the presence of bilateral pulmonary infiltrates, they only agreed 43% of the time, and one third of the time five or more individuals differed in their interpretation.[29] The range of ALI/ARDS diagnoses was from 36% to 71%.[32]

RISK FACTORS

It has been recognized that ARDS may arise in association with a number of clinical conditions or risk factors, with sepsis being the most common (Box 37.4).[8,18,21,27,33-37] Various studies report that approximately 5% to 40% of septic patients will develop ARDS.[8,18,36] Shock (prolonged hypotension) and the systemic inflammatory response syndrome (SIRS) are also common risk factors. Other frequently encountered clinical risk factors include multiple emergency transfusions; aspiration injury; near-drowning; pancreatitis; trauma (particularly lung contusion, fat emboli from long bone fractures); burns; cardiopulmonary bypass; and disseminated intravascular coagulation (DIC). These clinical risk factors are synergistic, and when more than one of the clinical risk factors is present, the likelihood of ARDS is greater than just the sum of the collective risk factors.[8,17] The clinical risk factors associated with the development of ARDS appear to greatly influence the expected outcome. Whether ALI and ARDS arise from a direct pulmonary

Box 37.4 Common Clinical Risk Factors for ARDS

Sepsis and the systemic inflammatory response syndrome (SIRS)
Prolonged hypotension/shock
Trauma (long bone fractures, lung contusion, fat embolism)
Acid aspiration
Near-drowning
Multiple emergency blood product transfusions
Pancreatitis
Disseminated intravascular coagulation (DIC)
Post cardiopulmonary bypass
Burn injury

insult or from an extrapulmonary cause impacts the subsequent response to PEEP and ventilatory support (Box 37.5).[19] Age also has an impact on the likelihood for ARDS development.[30] Older individuals have a greater likelihood of developing ARDS from most of the risk factors noted earlier. In the setting of trauma the risk for ARDS seems to peak in the sixth and seventh decades and then declines.[38]

Negative pressure (postobstructive) pulmonary edema (NPPE or POPE) is a type of noncardiogenic pulmonary edema that can manifest as ARDS.[39] It is rare (five cases reported from a large tertiary medical ICU in 4 years),[40] can range in severity from mild hypoxemia treated with low-flow supplemental oxygen to profound hypoxemia requiring mechanical ventilation, and may even present as alveolar hemorrhage.[41-45] It is believed to be caused by increased vascular permeability resulting in alveolar and capillary damage from large levels of negative intrathoracic pressure generated by attempting to inspire against an occluded airway or airway obstruction.[46,47] This leads to a protein-rich alveolar exudate impairing gas exchange in mild-to-moderate cases and leaking of capillary blood into the alveoli in more severe circumstances. Most of the reported cases are related to surgical procedures: thyroidectomy,[48,49] septorhinoplasty,[50] tonsillectomy/adenoidectomy,[51] mandibular open reduction and internal fixation,[52] or cryosurgery for a tracheal obstruction.[53] Nonoperative conditions leading to NPPE have included laryngospasm,[54,55] occlusion of an endotracheal tube,[56,57] excessive tube thoracostomy suction pressure,[58] nonlethal hanging,[59] and even hiccups.[60,61] The common element is the rapid relief of a large airway occlusion. Patients often have no underlying cardiopulmonary disorders. NPPE may account for a small percentage of immediate postoperative extubation failures, particularly if an unrecognized mainstem intubation is present in an awake and spontaneously breathing patient. Clinical manifestations of hypoxemia and respiratory distress may be delayed up to 6 hours.[47] Therapy is supportive with supplemental oxygen and, if needed, positive-pressure ventilation (invasive or noninvasive).

Elevated intracranial pressures, either from traumatic brain injury or intracerebral hemorrhage, or status epilepticus can induce an ARDS-like clinical syndrome termed neurogenic pulmonary edema (NPE).[62,63] Although the exact mechanisms are not clear, an abrupt and massive release of catecholamines from injured neuronal tissues is thought to act directly on the lung parenchymal vasculature to promote a "capillary leak" of a protein-rich exudate as well as an increase in pulmonary vascular resistance[64] in addition to inducing a neurohumoral (takotsubo) cardiomyopathy.[65-67] The cardiomyopathy has the distinctive echocardiographic feature of ventricular apical ballooning and can persist for months.[68]

Box 37.5 Common Pulmonary and Extrapulmonary Causes of ARDS

Direct Pulmonary Causes

Pneumonia
Acid aspiration
Inhalational lung injury
Lung contusion
Chest trauma
Near-drowning

Extrapulmonary Causes

Sepsis—systemic inflammatory response syndrome
Shock—hypotension
Pancreatitis
Trauma (fat embolism)
Post cardiopulmonary bypass
Massive transfusion therapy
Burns
Elevated intracranial pressure (traumatic brain injury, intracerebral hemorrhage)

INCIDENCE AND PREVALENCE

The exact incidence and prevalence of ARDS has been variable and related to definitions used (Box 37.6).[8,38] Early reports suggested that there were 150,000 patients with ARDS each year in the United States.[8,33,36,69] This statistic led to an estimated incidence of 75 cases per 100,000 population. Proposed estimates have suggested that the incidence of ARDS ranges from 1.5 to 64 cases per 100,000 population.[38,69,70] A recent study evaluated the incidence and outcome of ALI in mechanically ventilated patients aged 15 or older cared for at 21 hospitals in and around King County, Washington, over a 15-month observation period.[38] The crude incidence of ALI was 78.9 per 100,000 person-years, and the incidence of ARDS was 58.7 per 100,000 person-years. On the basis of their results, the authors estimated the annual number of U.S. episodes was 332,100 cases of ARDS. The authors noted that increasing age was associated with an increased incidence and mortality rate in ARDS. A recent prospective observational study using the AECC definition and lung protective ventilatory support strategies in Spain (the ALIEN study) reported an incidence of 7.2 per 100,000 population per year for ARDS with an ICU and hospital mortality rate of 42.7% and 47.8%, respectively.[71]

Box 37.6 Incidence of ARDS

1985 Canary Island Conference: 1.5/100,000 person-years
1990 Utah: 4.8-8.3/100,000 person-years
1991 Berlin: 3/100,000 person-years
1995 Maryland: 10.5-14.2/100,000 person-years
1997 Sweden/Denmark: 13.5/100,000 person-years
2002 Australia: 28/100,000 person-years
2005 Seattle: 58.7-64/100,000 person-years

Adapted from Bersten AD, Edibam C, Hunt T, et al: Incidence and mortality of acute lung injury and the acute respiratory distress syndrome in three Australian states. Am J Respir Crit Care Med 2002;165:443-448; Rubenfeld GD, Neff MJ: Epidemiology of acute lung injury: A public health perspective. In Matthay MA (ed): Acute Respiratory Distress Syndrome. New York, Marcel Dekker, 2003, pp 40; and Rubenfeld GD, Caldwell E, Peabody E, et al: Incidence and outcomes of acute lung injury. N Engl J Med 2005;353:1685-1693.

CLINICAL MANIFESTATIONS

When ARDS becomes clinically apparent, the patient is usually noted to be in significant distress manifesting dyspnea, tachypnea, visible signs of respiratory distress, and increased work of breathing.[8,23,33,36] The typical presentation is manifest as an acute catastrophic complication in a patient who has one or more of the clinical risk factors for the development of this form of ARDS. The precipitating injury need not directly involve the pulmonary system.[8,36,72] Past definitions have emphasized the need to exclude patients with previous or known chronic pulmonary or cardiovascular diseases.[19-21,27] The AECC definition excluded patients with elevated left-sided heart filling pressures and chronic infiltrative lung disease as the cause of the radiographic or physiologic alterations, but the new Berlin definition will allow for the concomitant presence of ARDS and cardiac edema/volume overload as long as the predominant process is thought to be ARDS.[21,30]

The hallmark of ARDS is the presence of hypoxemia despite the administration of high concentrations of inspired oxygen, evidence of an increase in the shunt fraction, a decrease in pulmonary compliance, and an increase in the dead space ventilation.[8,24,30] The chest radiographic manifestation of ARDS is the presence of diffuse, bilateral pulmonary infiltrates with a normal cardiac silhouette. Recent reports have cautioned that even among trained experts there is often disagreement concerning the interpretation of the chest radiograph.[31,29,69,73] Chest CT has also demonstrated that the radiographic injury is not homogeneous and has a predominance in the dependent portions of the lung.[8,43] It is important to remember that ARDS is a clinical syndrome and the diagnosis is made clinically, not on the basis of a single radiograph, ABG analysis, or laboratory test.

PATHOLOGIC MANIFESTATIONS

Typically, type 1 alveolar cells compose the major gas exchange surface of the alveolus and are integral to the maintenance of the permeability barrier function of the alveolar membrane.[8] Type 2 pneumocytes are the progenitors of type 1 cells and are responsible for surfactant production and homeostasis.[8] During ARDS there is damage to the capillary endothelial and the alveolar epithelial cells.[8] Cellular injury and alteration of the normal barrier function results in a permeability defect that gives way to flooding of the alveoli with protein-rich fluid and inflammatory cells.[8,33,74] This results in the alteration of pulmonary mechanics, physiology, and gas exchange.[8,74] There is alteration of surfactant that results from damage to the type 2 pneumocyte and from the inactivation and dilution of alveolar surfactant from the protein and fluid that have entered into the alveolar space, respectively.[75,76] Surfactant dysfunction can lead to atelectasis and a further reduction in pulmonary compliance.[8,75-78] In addition, dysfunction of the alveolar epithelial cells can impair the resorption of fluid from the alveolar space, which augments the parenchymal injury process and gas exchange abnormalities.[8,79]

The observed pathologic findings in ARDS depend on the timing of the tissue sampling. During the initial stages of clinically evident lung injury there is histologic evidence of diffuse alveolar damage.[8] Histologic features of the injury include microthrombi composed of platelets and white blood cells within the capillary lumen, denudation of the alveolar epithelial lining cells, swelling of the capillary endothelial cells, interstitial and alveolar infiltration by polymorphonuclear leukocytes (PMNLs), and hyaline membrane formation within the alveoli.[8] Grossly, the lungs appear heavy and wet. Later, areas of type 3 collagen deposition with fibrosis will be present.[79] An intense inflammatory reaction involving PMNLs, activated monocytes, macrophages, and endothelial cells is present in the fibroproliferative phase of lung injury.[76,80,81] Pro- and anti-inflammatory molecules produced by these activated cells may be found in the circulating blood and bronchoalveolar lavage (BAL) fluid.[81-83] This phase may be followed by fibrosis, but this fibrosis does not appear to have the same permanence as typical fibrosis would have and may actually resolve over time in survivors of the injury.[84]

PATHOPHYSIOLOGY

ARDS may develop as a result of epithelial or endothelial cell injury.[8,13,85,86] Both sites of injury and cells are important for maintenance of normal barrier function and are capable of initiating an inflammatory response. In the majority of clinical settings the initial site of the ARDS involves the capillary endothelial cell, which may be the initial manifestation of a "panendothelial cell injury" resulting from SIRS.[83] Endothelial cell injury compromises the integrity of the vascular barrier and results in transudation of fluid and inflammatory mediators into the interstitial tissues and ultimately into the alveoli.[8,13] The frequent occurrence and early involvement of lung dysfunction as a component of multiple organ dysfunction/failure lends support to the hypothesis of a panendothelial cell injury as one of the target injuries in the setting of SIRS.[87]

The complex pathophysiologic processes that culminate in the production of ARDS involve a delicate balance between the body's proinflammatory and anti-inflammatory responses to the inciting clinical event.[83,87] The balance that exists between the various inflammatory molecules or mediators and the endogenous compensatory responses evoked by the inflammatory response will dictate whether or not lung injury and other forms of organ dysfunction will develop.[81] The ensuing interaction between SIRS and the compensatory anti-inflammatory response syndrome (CARS) will thus determine whether a patient successfully deals with an injury or is predisposed to develop organ dysfunction (excessive SIRS response) or immunosuppression and infectious complications (excessive CARS response).[83,87] This mixed antagonistic response syndrome (MARS) has tremendous impact on the fate of the critically ill patient.[87]

MANAGEMENT STRATEGIES

Basic management strategies for patients with ARDS are listed in Box 37.7.[8,18,21,23,33,36,88] Initial attention must be directed to providing lung protective ventilator support and identification of the predisposing underlying clinical risk factor(s) or condition(s), and there should be specific treatment directed at the underlying or predisposing disorder.[8,21-23] The recognition of sepsis and infection as frequent

Box 37.7 Basic Management Strategies for Patients with ARDS

Identify and treat underlying/predisposing cause of ARDS
Ventilatory support
- Lung protective ventilatory support strategy
- Application of PEEP (per ARDSnet protocol)

Restore and maintain hemodynamic function
- Conservative fluid replacement strategy using goal-oriented approach
- Vasopressor and inotropic support as needed to meet goals

Prevent complications of critical illness
- Stress ulcer (stress-related mucosal disease) prophylaxis
- Preventive strategies for PE and DVT
- Prevent infections such as ventilator-associated pneumonia (VAP)
- Control glucose and metabolic function
- Prevent development of multiple organ dysfunction/failure

Ensure adequate nutrition
Avoid oversedation and medication errors
Use of weaning protocol with spontaneous breathing trials when ready to wean
Cautious use of steroids for fibroproliferative phase (avoid if patient has received neuromuscular blocking drugs)

ARDS, acute respiratory distress syndrome; DVT, deep venous thrombosis; PE, pulmonary embolism; PEEP, positive end-expiratory pressure.

causes of ARDS should prompt an aggressive search for undiagnosed foci of infection and the administration of appropriate antimicrobial treatment and use of surgical drainage procedures as indicated.[15,17,89]

The cornerstone of supportive management is the provision of mechanical ventilatory support.[8,21-23] Recent experimental and clinical data report significant survival benefit from the use of lung protective ventilatory support strategies.[90,91] The primary goal of this support is to improve oxygenation and ensure that the lung is allowed to heal and avoid further injury. Use of nonprotective ventilatory support strategies may have a role in the persistent proinflammatory response and the development of multiple organ dysfunction syndrome (MODS) and multiple organ failure (MOF).[90-93]

MECHANICAL VENTILATION

See Chapter 11 for a more detailed discussion of mechanical ventilatory support in the management of patients with ARDS. Over the past 20 years there has been increasing recognition that the ventilatory support strategy used in the management of patients with ARDS may produce or augment lung injury or impair the healing process (Box 37.8).[94-98] Results of experimental animal studies demonstrated clinical, physiologic, and histologic abnormalities similar to those observed in patients with ARDS when animals with normal lungs were ventilated with large tidal volumes or were given high inflation pressures.[95-101] The alveolar overdistention produced by these ventilatory modes was felt to be the critical element in production of the lung injury.[95-98] Lung injury could result from the administration of large tidal volumes or the administration of positive pressure or negative pressure breaths that were sufficient to produce alveolar overdistention (termed *volutrauma*).[97-102] Other mechanisms that could potentially result in lung injury were the repetitive recruitment-derecruitment of distal airways (termed *atelectotrauma*) and alveoli or the disruption of alveoli resulting in translocation of organisms or air emboli.[97,98] Alveolar overdistention can also give rise to systemic inflammatory molecules that may contribute to the SIRS response and drive the development of MODS/MOF.[92,98] This has been termed *biotrauma*.[98] Interestingly, the lung injury produced by high inflation pressures or large tidal volumes in these experimental models could be ameliorated by the addition of therapeutic amounts of PEEP.[97,98] Subsequent human studies have evaluated the distribution of the radiographic lung injury in ARDS patients as determined by the use of CT scans of the chest and have noted the dependent nature of the injury.[74,103] The injury to the lungs was not diffuse and homogeneous as once believed. These dependent areas of injury comprised regions of alveolar flooding from the gravitational accumulation of lung water, areas of lung injury, and normal lung regions. The relatively normal ventral (nondependent) lung has been referred to as the "baby lung," and the injured (dependent) lung has been called the "sponge lung."[32,103] With the use of higher tidal volumes, PEEP, or high distending pressures, there was evidence of alveolar overdistention, particularly in the areas of normal lung. A multicenter trial of low versus traditional tidal volume ventilation in patients with ARDS demonstrated increased proinflammatory cytokines in the serum and BAL fluid of patients ventilated with the larger traditional tidal volumes, supporting the concept of biotrauma from alveolar overdistention.[92] Pulmonary barotrauma (pneumomediastinum, pneumopericardium, pneumoperitoneum, pneumothorax, subcutaneous emphysema, pulmonary interstitial emphysema, and air embolism) is a well-recognized complication of ventilatory support that has been reported in 7% to 15% of patients with ARDS.[104]

Box 37.8 Causes of Ventilator-Associated Lung Injury

Volutrauma
Atelectotrauma
Biotrauma
Barotrauma
Air embolism/translocation

The landmark study by NHLBI ARDS Network compared low tidal volumes (6 mL/kg of ideal body weight) against conventional tidal volumes (12 mL/kg of ideal body weight).[94] A protocol governed the use of PEEP according to the FIO_2 required to meet the oxygenation goals. A weaning protocol was used once the patient was on a reduced amount of ventilatory support. The trial was terminated after 861 patients were enrolled, following the determination of a significant (22% relative reduction) decrease in mortality rate associated with the use of low tidal volumes (39.8% vs. 31%; $P = 0.007$). A significant difference occurred between the low and high tidal volume groups in length of

Box 37.9 Potential Benefits of Hypercapnia in Patients with ARDS

↓ TNF-α release by alveolar macrophages
↓ PMNL-endothelial cell adhesion
↓ Xanthine oxidase activity
↓ NF-κB
↓ NOS activity
↓ Production of IL-8 and TOR from PMNLs

IL-8, interleukin 8; NOS, not otherwise specified; NF-κB, nuclear factor kappa-light-chain-enhancer of activated B cells; PMNL, polymorphonuclear leukocyte; TNF-α, tumor necrosis factor-alpha; TOR, toxic oxygen radicals.

From Kregenow DA, Rubenfeld GD, Hudson LD, Swenson ER: Hypercapnic acidosis and mortality in acute lung injury. Crit Care Med 2006;34:1-7.

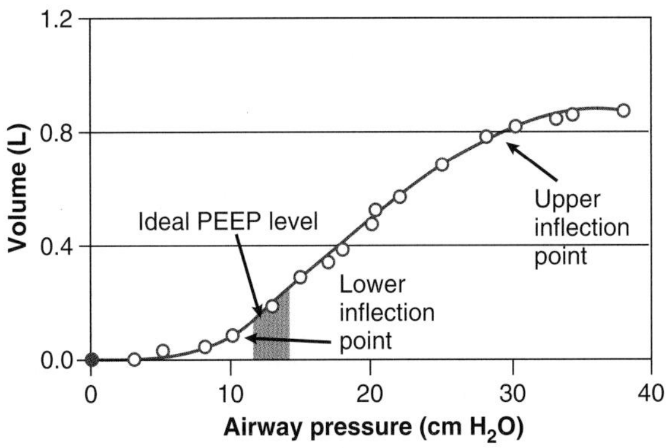

Figure 37.3 Pulmonary volume-pressure curve. PEEP, positive end-expiratory pressure. (Modified from Hospital Pulmonary Disease Board Review Manual 2000;7:7.)

stay, ventilator days, and development of MODS.[94] No difference occurred in the development of barotrauma between the two ventilator support strategies. On further analysis, this survival benefit was present irrespective of the patient's body mass index (BMI).[105]

The use of lower tidal volumes typically results in a controlled hypoventilation or permissive hypercapnia and can lead to hypercapnic acidosis.[106] Some experimental animal models of lung injury suggest that hypercapnic acidosis may be beneficial to the lung and produce less lung injury as measured by extravascular lung water (Box 37.9).[105] Other reports have detailed potentially harmful effects of hypercapnia on epithelial and endothelial barrier function, lung edema, edema clearance, inate immunity, and host defenses.[107]

PEEP is a major component of the ventilatory support strategy and may actually have a direct therapeutic role in the prevention of ventilator-induced lung injury (VILI), as noted in some of the experimental models of VILI.[8,96,108-117] PEEP is beneficial in the recruitment of atelectatic lung units and prevention of recruitment-derecruitment, and it increases the functional residual capacity (FRC), decreases the shunt fraction, and allows for a reduction to a less toxic FIO_2 while still maintaining adequate oxygen saturation and tissue oxygen delivery.[110,114-116,118] The application of the "right amount" of PEEP has recently taken on a more sophisticated approach. The ability to construct a pressure-volume curve to reflect the compliance of the patient's lung has allowed for the identification of both the lower and upper inflection points (Fig. 37.3).[117] Maintaining a PEEP level above the lower inflection point should potentially avoid the repetitive opening and closing of alveoli and the development of shear forces from the recruitment-derecruitment process, which may participate in the production or propagation of lung injury. If too much PEEP is applied, there may be overdistention of alveoli, which can potentiate volutrauma or barotrauma and have adverse consequences on pulmonary mechanics, hemodynamic function, and lung healing. Constructing pressure-volume curves to determine the "best PEEP" is a difficult undertaking and requires the patient to be heavily sedated or paralyzed and the use of a calibrated super syringe. Determining the precise lower inflection point on the inspiratory inflation curve is difficult, and the compliance curves may change (along with the inflection points) over time as the patient's lung compliance changes. To simplify the determination of PEEP, the ARDS Network ventilatory support protocol used a monogram for PEEP based on the FIO_2 requirements and the goal of maintaining a PAO_2 between 55 and 80 mm Hg.[94] For the protocol, end-inspiratory plateau pressure was kept lower than or equal to 30 cm H_2O and the pH was maintained in the 7.30 to 7.45 range. Despite the demonstrated significant improvement in mortality rates associated with this protocol, some felt that additional benefit could be seen with the use of higher levels of PEEP. A subsequent large, prospective, randomized controlled trial conducted by the ARDS Network evaluated the PEEP protocol from the initial trial (PEEP levels from 5 to 24 cm H_2O) versus higher levels of PEEP.[119] During the study there was a change to a higher PEEP strategy to ensure a difference in the amount of applied PEEP between the two treatment arms. No significant difference in deaths before discharge home, breathing without assistance by day 28, ventilator-free days, ICU-free days, organ failure–free days, or barotrauma was found.[119] Several studies have prospectively evaluated the benefits of higher versus lower PEEP strategies in the management of patients with ARDS, and a recent meta-analysis has failed to demonstrate a significant short-term mortality rate benefit associated with the use of higher PEEP.[119-123]

PEEP has the potential to have profound hemodynamic consequences in selected patients and clinical circumstances, and it is important to closely monitor patients with hemodynamic, echocardiographic, or other sophisticated monitors if there is a question of the adequacy of cardiac function when PEEP is applied.[6,109-111] Right-to-left shunting through a patent foramen ovale can occur in up to a third of patients with severe ARDS, and increasing PEEP may not produce the expected oxygenation benefits in these individuals.[124] The effect of PEEP may not be the same in the supine and prone positions. Apparently there is an enhanced ability to recruit alveoli when the patient is in the prone position as compared with the supine position when the patient is on the same amount of PEEP.[125] There may be a different responsiveness to the use of PEEP depending on whether the ARDS results from a direct pulmonary injury or a nonpulmonary process that gives rise to ARDS.[32]

Despite the survival benefits demonstrated by the use of the lung protective ventilatory support strategy, there has not been universal adoption of this technique of ventilatory support for all patients with ARDS. Reasons for this slower than expected incorporation into daily practice are many and varied and certainly go beyond lack of awareness. Young and coworkers[126] reported on the tidal volume used to ventilate ARDS patients at three large New England university hospitals. Prior to the publication and subsequent education of the ARDS Network results, the tidal volume averaged 12.3 mL/kg predicted body weight (9.8 mL/kg measured body weight). After the publication, the tidal volume dropped to 10.6 mL/kg predicted body weight (8 mL/kg measured body weight).

A multicenter French study has reported that the use of neuromuscular blockade with cisatracurium over the initial 48 hours of severe ARDS was associated with improved 90-day survival and longer time off ventilator support in contrast to conventional ventilator management.[127] A prior study by these investigators noted decreased inflammatory response associated with the use of neuromuscular blockade in patients with ARDS.[128] Although there is always a risk for prolonged neuromuscular weakness after use of neuromuscular blocking drugs, as well as in critical illness, there are many potential benefits in support of using neuromuscular blocking agents early in severe ARDS.[129] Some of these potential benefits include better patient-ventilator synchrony and interaction, less VILI (barotraumas, atelectrauma, biotrauma), better recruitment effect from administered PEEP, and decreased oxygen consumption.[129,130]

FLUID MANAGEMENT AND VASOACTIVE SUPPORT

There has been controversy regarding the approach to fluid management and oxygen delivery in the critically ill patient with ARDS.[131-142] Patients with ARDS often require aggressive management to restore and maintain appropriate hemodynamic function.[143-144] The SAFE trial demonstrated that resuscitation with saline is as beneficial as resuscitation with albumin in critically ill patients with shock.[145] Correcting shock and hemodynamic derangements in patients with ARDS is important because these are potential causes for the lung injury and may result in organ dysfunction/failure.[144] Several studies have reported increased survival associated with low pulmonary capillary occlusion pressure in the setting of ARDS.[131,133] Concern for compromised organ perfusion and predisposition to the development of organ system dysfunction and the development of MODS/MOF led to additional studies from the ARDS Network to evaluate a liberal versus conservative fluid replacement strategy (Fluid and Catheter Treatment Trial [FACTT] study).[146] In addition, this trial was designed to evaluate the utility and safety of using a pulmonary artery (PA) catheter to guide volume replacement as opposed to a central venous catheter.[147] The safety and potential benefits of using PA catheters in the critically ill has been an area of controversy since the 1990s.[148] In 1996, Connors and coworkers reported a lack of benefit and possible harm associated with the use of PA catheters in critically ill patients in the SUPPORT database.[149]

In a prospective, randomized controlled trial of PA catheters versus no PA catheters in the management of 676 adult patients with shock or ARDS, there was no difference in organ failure–free days, ventilator-free days, vasopressor-free days, or days in the ICU or hospital.[150] This trial did not have an algorithm to direct management based on the hemodynamic data obtained from the use of the PA catheter. The ARDS Network trial evaluated liberal versus conservative fluid management on the basis of the central venous catheter (central venous pressure [CVP]) data versus PA catheter (PA occlusion pressure [PAOP]) data in 1000 patients with established ARDS.[147] The use of a PA catheter did not significantly change 60-day survival or days of unassisted breathing in comparison with the use of a central venous catheter.[147] There was no difference between the groups in lung or renal function, use of vasopressors, renal replacement therapy, or hypotension. The PA catheter group did have twice as many catheter-related complications, predominantly in the form of arrhythmias, compared with the central venous catheter group.

The liberal fluid management arm of the FACTT study had an average net gain of almost 7 L over the first 7 days, whereas the conservative fluid management group averaged a loss of 136 mL over 7 days of cumulative fluid balance.[146] The use of the conservative fluid management strategy was associated with a significant improvement in oxygenation index and lung injury score and increased the number of ventilator-free days compared with the more liberal strategy. There was no difference in the development of shock or the need for renal replacement therapy between the two fluid management strategies.[146]

PREVENTION OF COMPLICATIONS OF CRITICAL ILLNESS

ARDS patients are also at risk for the complications that commonly complicate the course of the critically ill. Most of these complications are preventable, and prophylactic strategies should be employed whenever possible. Common complications include deep venous thrombosis and pulmonary embolism, stress-related gastrointestinal hemorrhage, ventilator-associated pneumonia (VAP) and nosocomial infections, metabolic abnormalities, critical illness polyneuropathy, and malnutrition.[151-155] Anticipation and prevention of these complications are vitally important. Prophylactic strategies to prevent stress-related mucosal disease and gastrointestinal bleeding using H_2 blockers, proton pump inhibitors, or possibly early enteral nutrition should occur in all patients unless otherwise contraindicated.[155,156] Deep vein thrombosis and pulmonary embolism prophylaxis should also be administered unless there are contraindications.[156] The use of enteral nutrition may be valuable in an attempt to prevent stress-related gastrointestinal bleeding and prevent translocation when normal barrier function of the gastrointestinal mucosa is compromised.[155,157-160] Nutritional support may also be important to maintain the proper level of immune function and potentially to prevent the development of malnutrition in the catabolic critically ill patient. The use of enteral formulas designed to enhance the immune response with increased amounts of arginine, glutamine, or selected fatty acids remains controversial. The use of enteral formulas with increased amounts of eicosapentaenoic acid and γ-linolenic acid has been shown to improve organ dysfunction and improve oxygenation in clinical trials but has not been demonstrated to improve survival in patients with ARDS.[161,162] The ARDS Network found that the use of twice daily enteral supplementation with ω-3 fatty acids, γ-linolenic acid, and antioxidants did not improve clinical outcome and was associated with a greater amount of diarrhea.[163] A subsequent (EDEN) randomized trial by the same investigators found that ARDS patients who received trophic (minimal enteral) feeding did just as well and had less gastric residual volume, vomiting, and constipation and a lower blood sugar and insulin requirement than the patients who received full enteral feeding over the first 6 days.[164] For those patients who do not tolerate enteral nutrition, waiting to provide parenteral nutritional support for up to 8 days was found to be well tolerated, was safer, had fewer complications, and was associated with a faster recovery in critically ill adult patients.[165]

A major goal of management should be the prevention of nosocomial or secondary infections/sepsis and multiple organ dysfunction/failure because these two conditions are currently responsible for the high mortality rate seen in patients with ARDS.[18,89,151-153] VAP is a frequent complication in critically ill ventilated patients. As previously mentioned, prevention of VAP should be a primary management goal for patients with ARDS. Detection of a complicating VAP can be difficult in the setting of the pulmonary radiographic infiltrates seen in patients with ARDS. Diagnosis of VAP and identification of the offending pathogen often require the use of bronchoscopy with BAL or protected specimen brushes coupled with semiquantitative culture analysis.[151,153] Recent data suggest that identifying the soluble triggering receptor expressed on myeloid cells (sTREM) may be beneficial in the detection of VAP but does not identify the specific etiologic organism.[166] European investigators have been enthusiastic about the technique of selective digestive decontamination (SDD) as a method to decrease nosocomial lung infections in the critically ill patient.[167] Keeping the head of the bed elevated above 30 degrees is also effective at preventing VAP.[156] Additional measures designed to decrease the development of VAP include continuous subglottic suction, coated endotracheal tubes, closed suction systems, and kinetic therapy.[156] Development of complications has been associated with increased morbidity rate, length of stay, cost of care, and possibly mortality rate.[155,156]

Pulmonary barotrauma has been reported to develop in approximately 7% to 15% of patients with ARDS.[104] When a pneumothorax is detected in a mechanically ventilated patient, prompt recognition and chest tube insertion are required to prevent the development of tension physiology.[104]

STRATEGIES TO IMPROVE OXYGENATION

In patients with severe ARDS and persistent hypoxemia various strategies have been developed in an attempt to improve oxygenation and lessen FIO_2 requirements. Included in these strategies are recruitment maneuvers, prone positioning, sighs, surfactant replacement therapy, partial liquid ventilation, inhaled nitric oxide, and enhanced edema clearance.[125,168-194] These techniques remain investigational at this time and should be subjected to rigorous evaluation to adequately determine their ability to improve outcome for patients with ARDS. Importantly, the use of higher tidal volumes (12 mL/kg ideal body weight) in the ARDS Network trial was associated with an improvement in oxygenation but a significantly decreased survival in patients with ARDS.[94]

Recruitment maneuvers represent an attempt to open the atelectatic distal airways and alveoli on the border of the collapsed flooded alveoli that compose the dependent area of radiographic lung injury.[98] Some experts believe that this maneuver should precede the provision of PEEP and ventilator support in the early phases of ARDS.[195] The maneuver is accomplished by increasing the PEEP to 35 to 50 cm H_2O and holding that level of pressure for 30 seconds. The ARDS Network attempted to define the value of a recruitment maneuver in 43 patients with ARDS by randomly assigning them to a recruitment maneuver with 35 to 40 cm H_2O for 30 seconds versus a sham recruitment maneuver.[179] The recruitment maneuver was assessed on the basis of a sustained improvement in oxygenation as judged by the ability to titrate PEEP/FIO_2 on the basis of the network algorithm and changes in lung compliance. There was no significant difference in the magnitude or duration of the oxygenation effect, compliance, or change in PEEP/FIO_2 titration. The group that received a recruitment maneuver did have a greater decrease in blood pressure during the maneuver. Other studies have reported that recruitment maneuvers are well tolerated from a hemodynamic standpoint and are not associated with increased cytokine release.[180]

Patients with ARDS may improve their oxygenation abnormalities when they are placed in the prone position.[168-175] This position may be more physiologic for most mammals and result in improved secretion removal, better ventilation/perfusion matching, and better aeration of the dorsal lung units.[172] The prone position may also prevent the heart from collapsing the left lower lobe and enhance the recruitment effects of PEEP by stabilizing the more flexible ventral chest wall.[172] Prone positioning may also unload the right ventricle in the setting of severe ARDS.[173] A number of trials have demonstrated an improvement in oxygenation during and after being placed in a prone position.[170-174] One prospective randomized trial designed to demonstrate survival advantage failed to do so.[175] A number of potential complications can result from the process of changing the patient from a supine to a prone position.[183,184] Included in the list of potential complications are tube/catheter malposition/problems, pressure sores, blindness, and difficulty with patient assessment and resuscitation.[183,184] Prone positioning should be considered in patients with low risk for such a position change who require high FIO_2 despite optimization of ventilator strategy.

INHALED NITRIC OXIDE

Inhaled nitric oxide is a bronchial and vascular smooth muscle dilator that also decreases platelet adherence and aggregation.[173,196] It has been shown to improve oxygenation by improving ventilation/perfusion relationships in the lung.[185,196,197] A reduction in PA pressure and pulmonary vascular resistance also occurs. These beneficial pulmonary effects are associated with minimal systemic effect from the inhaled nitric oxide because it is rapidly inactivated when the nitric oxide enters the circulation and is taken up by red blood cells. Multiple prospective, randomized, placebo-controlled clinical trials failed to demonstrate an improvement in survival despite the early improvement in oxygenation associated with the administration of inhaled nitric oxide.[191,193,194]

SURFACTANT REPLACEMENT THERAPY

Surfactant abnormalities are present in patients with ARDS related to decreased production, inactivation by alveolar proteins and proteolytic enzymes, and dilution by the alveolar fluid.[178] Theoretically, surfactant replacement should produce a survival benefit, just as it does in the infant respiratory distress syndrome.[177,178] Anzueto and colleagues[176] reported no difference in hemodynamic function, oxygenation, length of stay, duration of mechanical ventilation, and survival in 725 sepsis-induced ARDS patients who were prospectively randomized into a placebo-controlled trial of Exosurf (artificial surfactant) versus placebo. The researchers believe that the lack of associated surfactant proteins might account for the lack of efficacy. Trials are continuing to evaluate recombinant forms of surfactant replacement that include surfactant proteins.[177] A meta-analysis from a group of small trials evaluating recombinant surfactant protein C replacement in patients with ARDS noted an improvement in oxygenation but no survival benefit.[177] To date there has not been a survival benefit associated with the use of surfactant replacement therapy in adults with ARDS.[77,78,173]

ENHANCED EDEMA CLEARANCE

Accumulated fluid in the alveolus could potentially worsen the gas exchange, as well as produce adverse pulmonary mechanics with increased work of breathing. Recent strategies designed to improve edema clearance either using aquaporins or increasing the activity of the Na/K pump could potentially provide a benefit to patients with ARDS. The BALTI trial evaluated the use of intravenous β-agonist (salbutamol) in patients with ARDS and demonstrated a significant decrease in extravascular lung water at day 7.[186] The salbutamol-treated group also had lower end-inspiratory plateau pressures, and there was a trend toward a lower Murray Lung Injury Score. This group also had more supraventricular arrhythmias. A subsequent trial by the same investigators (BALTI-2) demonstrated increased 28-day mortality rate (risk ratio 1.47) with the use of intravenous salbutamol (albuterol).[187] The NHLBI ARDS Network investigators evaluated the use of nebulized salbutamol (albuterol 5 mg every 4 hours) and reported no change in ventilator-free days nor in in-hospital mortality rate.[188] The amount of edema in the lung can also be increased when there is a low oncotic pressure. To evaluate the potential benefit of infusing albumin and furosemide as opposed to furosemide alone to patients with ARDS, Martin and colleagues[190] conducted a randomized controlled trial in 40 hypoproteinemic patients with ALI. The albumin-infused group had an improvement in oxygenation, total protein, net fluid loss, increased number of shock-free days, and less hypotension. Although this is a small study, it does suggest a potential benefit of this maneuver in hypoproteinemic ARDS patients. Further investigation is necessary to determine the benefit of edema clearance strategies in the management of ARDS patients.

EXPERIMENTAL/INNOVATIVE THERAPIES

In an attempt to reduce the high mortality rate associated with ARDS, a number of experimental and innovative therapeutic approaches have been evaluated. A majority of these approaches target abnormalities that either produce or result from the systemic inflammatory response that is felt to be central to the pathogenesis of the injury. To date, none of these approaches has been demonstrated to offer significant benefit in well-conducted, prospective, randomized controlled, multicentered clinical trials. These approaches have included the early administration of high-dose corticosteroids, prostaglandin E_1, nonsteroidal anti-inflammatory drugs, antiendotoxin and anticytokine therapy, inhaled nitric oxide, surfactant therapy, antioxidant therapy, positional changes, and partial liquid ventilation.[169-174,177,185,191,192,198-234]

Many investigations in experimental animal models of ARDS have demonstrated benefit from pretreatment and early treatment with high-dose corticosteroids.[198-201] Similar benefit has been observed with a number of nonsteroidal anti-inflammatory agents in experimental animal models of lung injury.[202,210,211,235] Unfortunately, the use of anti-inflammatory strategies in humans with sepsis or ARDS has repeatedly failed to demonstrate significant benefit.[195,203,205,206,236,237] In fact, in subgroup analysis there was evidence of potential harm in patients with renal dysfunction who were administered high-dose methylprednisolone for treatment of severe sepsis and septic shock.[206] To further complicate this clinical situation, it has been demonstrated that a significant proportion of patients with septic shock and other critical illnesses have relative adrenal insufficiency as defined by the inability to elevate the plasma cortisol level more than 9 μg/dL after adrenocorticotropic hormone (ACTH) stimulation.[237] This relative adrenocortical deficiency has been implicated as a potential cause of the persistent shock state and impaired perfusion. However, these patients have not always been responsive to the administration of steroids, and the adrenergic hyporesponsiveness may be related to sepsis-induced nitric oxide production, desensitization, or downregulation of α- and β-adrenergic receptors.[237] Lower-dose, more physiologic steroid replacement may restore the α- and β-adrenergic responsiveness and potentially turn off the inflammatory reaction to allow for better healing and less injury.[237-239] Attempts to prevent the development of ARDS in high-risk patients with severe sepsis and septic shock with high-dose corticosteroids have not been shown to prevent the development of ARDS, improve the reversal of ARDS, or improve the outcome from ARDS.[206]

Steroid therapy has been shown to be beneficial in patients with severe *Pneumocystis jiroveci* (*carinii*) pneumonia and ARDS and possibly in patients with fat embolism.[198] In the patient with adrenal insufficiency, stress dose steroids should be administered. The use of corticosteroids to treat patients with established ARDS is controversial and is discussed later. Ibuprofen, a nonsteroidal anti-inflammatory drug, failed to significantly improve the outcome of patients with severe sepsis or septic shock and failed to prevent the development of ARDS in a prospective, randomized, placebo-controlled, multicentered clinical trial.[236]

A plethora of clinical trials have evaluated "antimediators" that have targeted the potential proinflammatory compounds that can be identified in the blood or BAL of patients at risk for or diagnosed with ARDS.[8,90,212,240,241] Despite encouraging results from preclinical experimental animal and early clinical studies, these innovative strategies have failed to demonstrate a significant survival benefit.[8,206,213,216-218,221-229] Attempts to change the inflammatory response by changing the ratio of omega 3/omega 6 fatty acids have evaluated the potential benefit of an enteral nutritional formula rich in eicosapentaenoic acid and γ-linoleic acid.[161] A large, multicentered, prospective, randomized trial demonstrated an improvement in lung injury score, oxygenation, and organ dysfunction as compared with an isocaloric, isonitrogenous enteral formulation.[161] Unfortunately, a survival benefit was not seen.

Pentoxifylline and lisophylline are xanthine derivatives that were felt to have utility in the management of sepsis and ARDS. Pentoxifylline is a rheologic agent that has the ability to inhibit toxic oxygen radical release, decrease platelet aggregation, decrease phagocytosis, diminish the response to platelet-activating factor (PAF) stimulation, and inhibit the release of tumor necrosis factor (TNF) into the systemic circulation. Clinical evaluation of this treatment strategy by the National Institutes of Health (NIH) ARDS Network found no significant benefit.[240]

ARDS may be produced or worsened by the elaboration of toxic oxygen radicals from the activated inflammatory cells.[8] The abundant production of toxic oxygen radicals may overwhelm the ability of the endogenous oxygen radical scavengers, superoxide dismutase (SOD), catalase, and the glutathione redux cycle. The administration of antioxidants such as *N*-acetylcysteine, procysteine, vitamin E, β-carotene, and vitamin C has been evaluated in the prevention and management of patients with ARDS.[143,233,242,243] No survival benefit was seen associated with the administration of *N*-acetylcysteine or procysteine versus control in patients with ARDS.[233]

PREVENTION

The ability to prevent the development of ARDS would be a welcome achievement that to date has been elusive. Two older trials demonstrated a significant reduction in the development of ARDS in surgical patients when ketoconazole, an imidazole thromboxane A_2 synthetase inhibitor, was administered to an at-risk population of patients.[244-245] However, when ketoconazole was evaluated by the ARDS Network in the treatment of patients with ARDS there was no benefit on survival.[246] The use of 3-hydroxy-3-methylglutaryl-coenzyme A reductase inhibitors (statins) as a prevention for ARDS was evaluated in an observational study of a large cohort of patients at risk for developing ARDS and was not found to decrease the development of ARDS or improve mortality rates, organ failure–free days, or ventilator-free days.[247]

FIBROPROLIFERATIVE PHASE

An improved understanding of the injury and repair phase of ARDS has resulted in the recognition of the late fibroproliferative phase.[8,81-84,248] This stage of the injury/repair process is characterized by replacement of damaged epithelial cells and accumulation of mesenchymal cells and connective tissue products in the airspaces and the intra-acinar microvessels.[79-81] Clinical manifestations include fever, leukocytosis, diffuse alveolar infiltrates on the chest radiograph, and persistent inflammatory mediators in the serum.[79-81] Gallium scans demonstrate an increase in pulmonary uptake, and BAL typically contains markers of inflammation and type 3 procollagen peptide.[79] Physiologic manifestations include the worsening of static pulmonary compliance, abnormal gas exchange, increased dead space ventilation, pulmonary hypertension, and lack of PEEP response.[248] This picture of persistent inflammation requires a dedicated approach to ensure that there is not an ongoing uncontrolled infectious process that has not been adequately addressed.[248] Once it is determined that this state is not the result of inadequately treated infection, therapy with corticosteroids is used by some experts.[248] Several anecdotal reports have suggested that this therapy may have potential efficacy in patients with a persistent inflammatory response.[198,248] A small, single-center, prospective, randomized, placebo-controlled, double-blind clinical trial in 24 patients with the fibroproliferative phase of ARDS demonstrated an improvement in survival, lung function, and organ system dysfunction.[249] This study has been criticized because it included the crossover of patients at day 10 and had a smaller study population than a previously reported uncontrolled trial from the same center.[249]

The use of steroid rescue for the patient with persistent ARDS or the fibroproliferative phase of ARDS was evaluated by the NIH-sponsored ARDS Network.[250] The study prospectively randomized 180 patients with ARDS for greater than or equal to 7 days into a placebo-controlled trial of methylprednisolone versus placebo. The primary efficacy outcome was alive at home at 60 days. Patients with septic shock, a defined need for corticosteroid therapy, disseminated fungal infection, or undrained abscess were excluded. The trial was conducted over 6 years and included a modification of the study protocol that included a reduction in the number of subjects from 400 to 180 and an increase in the inclusion $\mathrm{PaO_2/FiO_2}$ ratio. The use of methylprednisolone was associated with an early improvement in mortality rate, $\mathrm{PaO_2/FiO_2}$ ratio, blood pressure, ventilator, and ICU-free days. An increase in the white blood cell count and glucose level related to steroid administration occurred, along with a decrease in body temperature. No difference was measured in the primary efficacy end point and 60-day mortality rate, and no significant difference in 180-day outcome occurred between the two groups. The steroid treatment was not associated with an increase in serious infections. In fact, there was more pneumonia and septic shock seen in the placebo group than in the steroid-treated group. Unfortunately, the use of steroids was associated with more neuropathy and myopathy, but it is important to note that 30% of the steroid-treated patients were receiving neuromuscular blocking drugs.[250] Meduri and colleagues evaluated a low-dose prolonged methylprednisolone infusion in patients with early severe ARDS and noted a significant decrease in lung injury score and C-reactive protein level along with a decrease in ICU mortality rates, duration of mechanical ventilation, and multiple organ dysfunction scores.[251] The steroid infusion decreased levels of inflammatory biomarkers and coagulation.[252] The prolonged infusion strategy appeared to be safe and well tolerated, but this was a small study of 91 patients and the topic of steroid treatment in ARDS remains controversial; we eagerly await more definitive studies.

Macrolide antibiotics have been said to have important immunomodulatory properties that could prove to be beneficial in patients with ARDS. The ARDS Network has reviewed initial antibiotic data on 235 patients enrolled in the LARMA trial and found that 20% received a macrolide antibiotic within the first 24 hours of the trial.[253] These patients were more likely to have a pulmonary infection as a cause of ARDS. Of interest was the observation that the macrolide-treated patients had a 23% mortality rate compared to 36% mortality rate for nonmacrolide antibiotic regimens.[253] This interesting observation may warrant additional study.

The use of extracorporal membrane oxygenation (ECMO) was evaluated in the 1970s with dismal outcomes, but with refinements in the ability to provide extracorporal support in the operative and pediatric settings there has been an increased utilization of the technique in adult patients with severe oxygenation issues related to ARDS.[254-257] Improved catheters and understanding of the physiology of ECMO has brought the technique into more common use and was found to be associated with lower hospital mortality rate than non-ECMO support in ECMO referred patients with the severe 2009 influenza A (H1N1).[257] Significant improvement in outcome was also seen in a report from England, which contrasted treatment at a tertiary care referral center capable of ECMO versus treatment at a center that had only conventional support in patients with severe ARDS.[256] Because transfer to a center with ECMO capability did not necessarily lead to institution of ECMO, more stringent study is needed to clearly define the role for ECMO support in patients with significant oxygenation abnormalities associated with severe ARDS.

MULTIPLE ORGAN DYSFUNCTION/FAILURE

A frequent complication of an exaggerated proinflammatory state in the setting of sepsis, SIRS, and ARDS is the development of organ system dysfunction.[8,18,36,89,258] This dysfunction may involve single or multiple organs.[160,258] A recent consensus conference has suggested that the dysfunction of two or more organs such that normal homeostasis cannot be maintained in the setting of a systemic inflammatory response to a variety of insults is considered MODS.[259] This dysfunction may be partial or complete, reversible or irreversible.[160] A continuum of abnormalities ranging from dysfunction to failure for each organ is probable.[160] Unfortunately, as of this time there has been no consensus on the threshold that separates these two phenomena or the threshold between reversible and irreversible organ system dysfunction.[160]

MODS and MOF are the most common causes of death in the noncoronary ICU.[8,18,258,260,261] Many authorities consider ARDS as the earliest manifestation of an uncompensated systemic inflammatory process with excessive proinflammatory component.[87,172] One hypothesis for this injury suggests that in the absence of a direct injury to a specific organ, there must be multiple inflammatory insults to produce the clinically apparent MODS/MOF.[160] This hypothesis, called the "two-hit hypothesis,"[160] suggests that an initial sensitizing insult is followed within a specific period of time by a second insult that is capable of initiating a more profound proinflammatory response because the target cells have been upregulated or primed by the initial insult.[160] Multiple combinations of direct injury, ischemic injury, circulating humoral or inflammatory mediators, translocation of endotoxin or colonic bacteria, altered rheologic properties of the blood cells, or iatrogenic effects of the therapy administered may interact in the eventual production of MODS/MOF.[160]

PROGNOSIS

Recent studies report a significant reduction in the mortality rate from ARDS using lung protective ventilatory support and proper levels of PEEP.[8,83,241,243] Current trials report mortality rates in the range of 30% to 60% in comparison with 60% to 90% of the past.[8,94,262,263] The 30-day mortality rate seen in patients enrolled in the NIH-sponsored ECMO trial of the 1970s was 91% with both conventional and ECMO treatment.[262] Older reports from large tertiary referral centers documented mortality rates of 90% for patients with gram-negative septic shock and ARDS.[263] A large multicenter trial of inhaled surfactant in 725 patients with septic-induced ARDS demonstrated survival rates of 60% at 28 days in both the treatment and the control groups.[176] Today the mortality rate from ARDS appears to depend on the cause of the injury, the patient's underlying disease status, patient age, and institutional factors.[38,254] This improvement in mortality rate mandates the use of a concomitant control group as opposed to using historical control subjects in the assessment of new innovative therapeutic strategies.

The most common causes of death in patients with ARDS continues to be from MOF and recurrent sepsis.[3,8,16,36,260,261] Fewer than 20% of patients die because of the inability to adequately oxygenate or ventilate them.[260] The complexities of the balance between the proinflammatory and anti-inflammatory processes that encompass the pathophysiologic response of this injury direct the response from organ dysfunction secondary to an overzealous proinflammatory reaction to infectious complications. These complications result from the immune suppression of a predominant anti-inflammatory response.[83,264] When infection is present, the lung is a frequent site for the process and may be extremely difficult to diagnose.[35,89,151,152] Patients with pulmonary infections were found to typically have a septic clinical picture without definitive positive culture results.[35] On the other hand, in patients who were found to have positive blood cultures without antemortem identification of a specific site, the site of occult infection was commonly found to be in the abdomen at postmortem examination.[35] Predictors of high mortality rates from ARDS include the development of multiple organ dysfunction/failure, development of secondary sepsis, concomitant cancer, and the presence of cirrhosis or hepatic dysfunction.[16] A study evaluating predictors of mortality rate in patients with ARDS receiving lung protective ventilatory support reported that the oxygenation index (mean airway pressure $\times$ $F_{IO_2} \times 100 \div Pa_{O_2}$) was an independent predictor of mortality rate.[265]

After recovery from ARDS, the prognosis appears to be reasonably good. A recent report found that 80% of ARDS survivors discharged from the ICU were still alive 5 years later.[266,267] Although most ARDS survivors have initial abnormalities in pulmonary function quality of life, the majority return to near their baseline pulmonary function status within 3 to 6 months.[268,269] The major residual abnormality in pulmonary function is a restrictive pulmonary defect and a reduction in the carbon monoxide diffusion capacity.[268,269] These alterations may result in exercise desaturation in some patients or, more commonly, a decrease in timed walked distance.[268,269] When observed over the next 5 years, their pulmonary function did not improve a great deal after this initial improvement.[266,270] However, most patients continue to experience exercise limitation at 5 years, despite the fact that 65% have returned to work.[266]

Survivors of ARDS have been found to have a decreased health-related quality of life, increased respiratory symptoms, insomnia, depression, anxiety, and posttraumatic stress disorder.[271-274] ARDS survivors have been found to have a clinically significant reduction in their physical function and increased pulmonary symptoms in comparison with the matched survivors of critical illness.[271-277] Survivors of ARDS are also found to have long-term cognitive impairment, problems coping with their disability, and relationship strains.[274,275] Elderly patients, older than 70 years of age, seem to have worse outcomes with an increase in mortality rate compared with ARDS patients who are younger than 70 years of age.[273]

FUTURE CONSIDERATIONS

The growing knowledge of molecular biology and the elaborate mechanisms that govern a person's response to injury, repair, and cell death will likely have a major role in the management of patients with ARDS. Individuals with increased risk for ALI and ARDS development will no doubt be identified on the basis of their genetic profiles. This knowledge will likely affect future management. In years to come, scientists may potentially modify the genetic makeup or the biologic response of a susceptible individual by inserting selected genes or modifying the transcription or function of various regulatory proteins. Studies with mesenchymal stem cells have been conducted in rodents with lung injury and demonstrate potential promise for future therapy.[278]

SUMMARY

Acute respiratory failure is the inability of the respiratory system to meet the oxygenation (type 1 or hypoxemic failure) or ventilation (type 2 or hypercapnic failure) requirements of the patient. Hypoxemic respiratory failure is defined as a PaO_2 of less than 60 mm Hg and is the result of one of six potential mechanisms: low inspired FiO_2, hypoventilation, ventilation-perfusion mismatching, shunt, low $M\bar{v}O_2$ (pulmonary arterial oxygenation), or diffusion impairment. The exact cause may be elucidated by analysis of the alveolar-arterial oxygen gradient, response to the administration of supplemental oxygen, and the clinical context. Hypercapnic or ventilatory failure is defined as a $PaCO_2$ of greater than 50 mm Hg, generally with acidemia; it can be acute, chronic, or acute-on-chronic and is the result of one of three potential mechanisms: hypoventilation, increased dead space ventilation, or increased CO_2 production. Clinical manifestations can range from adrenergic sympathetic hyperactivity (tachycardia and hypertension) to tachypnea and respiratory distress to encephalopathy with somnolence. Therapy is with supplemental oxygen, assisted ventilation with or without high levels of PEEP, or both.

ARDS continues to have a significant morbidity and mortality rate despite the advances in understanding and management that have occurred over the past 4 plus decades. Major advances have occurred in our understanding of the pathogenesis and in our ability to adequately provide the required ventilatory support while the injury is allowed to heal. Attention has been directed toward lung protective ventilatory support, the use of local and systemic therapies, and attempts at prevention of injury in high-risk patient populations. Despite recent improvements in management and knowledge of the pathophysiologic alterations likely involved, the mortality rate continues to be unacceptably high. Recent improvements in prognosis have occurred, primarily in those patients younger than age 60. Remembering the systemic nature of the injury and developing effective preventive and reparative strategies is important as we look to the future of ARDS management. Repair of the acutely injured lung, whether from the initial event, the ventilator, or complicating infection, is an important target and may be more achievable than attempting to prevent the initial injury or intervene early enough to prevent the development of ARDS.

KEY POINTS

- Both type 1 and type 2 acute respiratory failure are common problems in the ICU and may represent the primary reason for ICU admission or be a complication arising in the critically ill patient.
- The ABG value is the cornerstone for the diagnosis and management of the patient with acute respiratory failure.
- The American-European Consensus Conference had operationally established definitions that identified a continuum of injury from ALI to the more severe form, ARDS. The degree of oxygenation abnormality distinguished the two. The New Berlin definition suggests that the degree of oxygenation abnormality when assessed on appropriate FiO_2 and PEEP has prognostic importance and defines mild, moderate, and severe ARDS with the elimination of ALI as a definitional term.
- The most common clinical risk factors for the development of ARDS include sepsis, SIRS, hypotension, shock, trauma, near-drowning, and aspiration injury.
- The pathophysiology of ARDS represents a complex interrelationship of anti-inflammatory and

Continued on following page

KEY POINTS (Continued)

proinflammatory responses, activation of the coagulation system, abnormal function of the microcirculation, and altered surfactant function. Alterations affect both the capillary endothelium and the epithelial lining cells.

- At this time the management of patients with ARDS is primarily supportive, but it is important to provide specific treatment directed at the underlying predisposing cause, use lung protective ventilation, and prevent complications of critical illness.
- The concept of VILI has now been supported by the results of recent clinical trials demonstrating a survival benefit associated with the use of lower tidal volumes to avoid alveolar overdistention.
- The proper amount of PEEP therapy is important in the management of patients with ARDS to avoid alveolar overdistention and the repetitive collapse and recruitment-derecruitment of alveoli and small airspaces.
- The use of steroids to treat the fibroproliferative phase of ARDS remains a controversial area. If there is no active untreated infectious process and there is a persistent inflammatory process in the lung, there may be a benefit associated with corticosteroid therapy; however, a recent multicenter trial conducted by the ARDS Network did not find a survival benefit at 60 days.
- Although the overall prognosis in ARDS has been improving, there is still a mortality rate that ranges from 30% to 60% and decreased overall health status and function persist for as far out as 5 years after recovery.

SELECTED REFERENCES

30. The ARDS Definition Task Force: Acute respiratory distress syndrome: The Berlin definition. JAMA 2012;307:2526-2533.
94. The Acute Respiratory Distress Syndrome Network: Ventilation with lower tidal volumes as compared with traditional tidal volumes for acute lung injury and the acute respiratory distress syndrome. N Engl J Med 2000;342:1301-1308.
119. The National Heart, Lung, and Blood Institute Acute Respiratory Distress Syndrome (ARDS) Clinical Trials Network: Higher versus lower positive end-expiratory pressures in patients with the acute respiratory distress syndrome. N Engl J Med 2004;351:327-336.
127. Papazian L, Forel JM, Gacouin A, et al: Neuromuscular blockers in early acute respiratory distress syndrome. N Engl J Med 2010;363:1107-1116.
146. The National Heart, Lung, and Blood Institute Acute Respiratory Distress Syndrome (ARDS) Clinical Trials Network: Comparison of two fluid management strategies in acute lung injury. N Engl J Med 2006;354:2564-2575.
147. The National Heart, Lung, and Blood Institute Acute Respiratory Distress Syndrome (ARDS) Clinical Trials Network: Pulmonary-artery versus central venous catheter to guide treatment of acute lung injury. N Engl J Med 2006;354:2213-2224.
163. Rice TW, Wheeler AP, Thompson BT, et al: Enteral omega-3 fatty acid, γ-linolenic acid, and antioxidant supplementation in acute lung injury. JAMA 2011;306:1574-1581.
250. The National Heart, Lung, and Blood Institute Acute Respiratory Distress Syndrome (ARDS) Clinical Trials Network: Efficacy and safety of corticosteroids for persistent acute respiratory distress syndrome. N Engl J Med 2006;354:1671-1684.
251. Meduri GU, Golden EM, Freire AX, et al: Methylprednisolone infusion in early severe ARDS: Results of a randomized controlled trial. Chest 2007;131:954-963.
267. Herridge MS, Tansey CM, Matte A, et al: Functional disability 5 years after acute respiratory distress syndrome. N Engl J Med 2011;364:1293-1304.

The complete list of references can be found at www.expertconsult.com.

Life-Threatening Asthma 38

S. Sujanthy Rajaram

CHAPTER OUTLINE

EPIDEMIOLOGY OF LIFE-THREATENING ASTHMA

In 2010, approximately 25.7 million Americans were diagnosed with asthma, including 7.1 million children. Prevalence of asthma in the United States was about 8.4% in 2010. Prevalence was higher among children, female adults of non-Hispanic black and Puerto Rican race or ethnicity, and those with family income below poverty level. In children prevalence was higher in boys than in girls. Populations at risk for asthma and asthma-related deaths include racial and ethnic minorities. African Americans have been reported to have a greater prevalence of asthma and greater likelihood of dying (190% higher death rate) from asthma compared with whites. The prevalence of asthma attacks is highest among Puerto Ricans.

Worldwide an estimated 300 million people suffer from asthma and this number is estimated to grow by more than 100 million by 2025. About 70% of asthmatics have allergies and 11% of cases are related to workplace conditions such as exposure to fumes, gases, or dust. Older asthmatic patients (≥60 years) tend to have severe or near-fatal asthma exacerbation compared to younger asthmatics (<60 years).[1-4]

TRIGGERS OF ACUTE ASTHMA

Common triggers for acute asthmatic attacks include air pollutants, respiratory tract infection, and allergen exposure. An association of panic-type anxiety and life-threatening asthma has been suggested. Box 38.1 contains a comprehensive list of precipitating factors.

MORTALITY RATES FOR ASTHMA

In the 1960s, a global alarm was sounded when sharp epidemic increases in asthma death rates were reported. Deaths approximately doubled in the United States from 1980 to 1995. After a long period of steady increase, asthma mortality and morbidity rates have continued to decline for the past decade.[3,5-7]

Box 38.1 Precipitating Factors for Severe Asthma

Atopy: Genetic factors (inherited predisposition to allergic diseases)
Environmental factors: Allergens—9% (e.g., dust mites, dogs, cats, cockroaches)
Upper respiratory tract infection—23%
Allergic rhinitis
Pneumonia—9%
Medications: Aspirin, nonsteroidal anti-inflammatory drugs; β-receptor blockers, angiotensin-converting enzyme inhibitors
Premenstrual worsening; postmenopausal hormone replacement therapy
Occupational asthma
Inhaled irritants (e.g., heroin, cocaine, smoking)
Reflux esophagitis
Sinusitis
Cold: viral infections
Exercise
Emotional stress; strong association with panic disorder
Tapering of steroids—3%
Noncompliance—32%

Data from references 14-16 and 121-123.

In patients 5 to 44 years old, death from asthma peaks in the summer months, although hospitalizations peak during the winter months. In older asthmatic patients, a different distribution is seen, with hospitalizations and mortality rates both peaking in the winter months. Older patients with asthma also have been shown to have fewer symptoms of dyspnea with methacholine-induced obstruction.[8]

Polynesians, African Americans, and black South Africans all have been reported to have higher asthma mortality rates. Likely reasons include genetic predisposition or poor management of severe asthma attacks because of reduced or delayed use of health care services and lower level of understanding. Self-medication also may play a role. Pendergraft and colleagues[9] reported that among 29,430 admissions in the United States with a primary diagnosis of asthma, 10.1% were admitted to intensive care units (ICUs), and 2.1% were intubated. The risk of in-hospital death was significantly higher in patients who were intubated and who had comorbid conditions. Near-fatal events occur in 2% to 20% of patients admitted to ICUs with acute severe asthma and in 2% to 4% of those intubated for respiratory failure. Risk factors for death from asthma are previous severe exacerbations with ICU admission or intubation, two or more hospitalizations within the past year, three or more emergency department visits in the past month, use of more than two canisters of short-acting β-agonist in the past month, and difficulty in perceiving or articulating asthma symptoms. African-American ethnicity, low socioeconomic status, urban residence, substance abuse, cigarette-smoke exposure, psychological factors (anxiety and depression), and comorbid problems such as cardiovascular diseases, chronic pulmonary diseases, and chronic psychiatric illnesses are other potential risk factors for death from asthma.

The strongest predictor of mortality risk from asthma is a prior episode of near-fatal asthma, estimated to be 15% to 22%. Asthma death rates per 1000 persons with asthma were 30% higher for females than males, 75% higher for blacks than whites, and seven times higher for adults compared to children. Adults over 65 years old had the highest death rate of 0.58 per 1000 persons with asthma.[9-13]

CLASSIFICATION

About 5% of asthma patients have "difficult asthma" (asthma difficult to control with maximal recommended doses of inhaled medications, in particular, inhaled corticosteroids). Most of these patients meet the criteria for severe asthma or may have chronic mild or moderate disease with acute exacerbations. Two clinical patterns of life-threatening asthma have been reported. A more serious type is the slow onset of life-threatening asthma characterized by onset over days to weeks, copious amounts of mucoid secretions with intense eosinophilic infiltration, and resistance to bronchodilator therapy. This pattern is described as "slow onset–late arrival," or type 1, and accounts for 80% to 85% of fatal asthma. Second is the sudden type of asthma characterized by onset over minutes to hours with acute bronchospasm, absence of large quantities of airway secretions with no mucous plugs but neutrophil infiltration of the submucosa, typically a marked response to bronchodilators, and quick recovery in most circumstances. This is described as "sudden asphyxic asthma," or the type 2 scenario of asthma death. Sudden-type asthma accounts for about 15% to 20% of fatal asthma.[14-16]

PATHOPHYSIOLOGY AND IMMUNOLOGY

The pathophysiologic processes leading to pulmonary function abnormalities in severe life-threatening asthma are bronchial smooth muscle contraction, bronchial inflammation–associated mucosal edema, and mucous plugging. Obstruction of airflow leads to low ventilation-perfusion areas and hypoxemia. Expiratory obstruction decreases forced expiratory volume in the first second (FEV_1). The hallmark of asthma is a decreased FEV_1/forced vital capacity (FVC) ratio. A severely asthmatic individual is unable to complete expiration because of expiratory airway resistance and tachypnea-induced limited expiratory time, leading to air trapping and an increasing functional residual capacity and a decreased FVC. The hyperinflation produces increased work of breathing. Edema and increased airway secretions also compromise inspiratory flow and, when combined with hyperinflation, often lead to high peak inspiratory pressures in a patient whose lungs are being mechanically ventilated. The cause of respiratory arrest in asthmatics is usually failure of the inspiratory muscles with ventilatory arrest.

Manthous and Goulding studied the effect of intravascular volume status on deadspace fraction in mechanically ventilated patients with severe asthma. They noted a mean increase in deadspace ventilation of 4.2% in response to intravascular volume expansion with 250 to 500 mL of normal saline solution.[17,18]

Characteristic findings of fatal asthma are airways showing infiltration with neutrophils and eosinophils, degranulated mast cells, sub–basement membrane thickening, loss of epithelial cell integrity, occlusion of bronchial lumen by mucus, hyperplasia and hypertrophy of bronchial smooth muscle, and hyperplasia of goblet cells. Asthma is an inflammatory response evidenced by the presence of cytokines that mediate inflammation and chemotactic chemokines in bronchoalveolar lavage fluid and pulmonary secretions. Some cytokines initiate inflammatory response by activating transcription factors, which act on genes that encode inflammatory cytokines, chemokines, adhesion molecules, and other proteins that induce and perpetuate inflammation. Adhesion molecules provide a mechanism for the adhesion of inflammatory cells to the endothelium and migration of these cells from the circulation into the lamina propria, epithelium, and the airway lumen itself.[19]

Busse and Lemanske described the immunology of allergic inflammation in asthma. IgE antibodies are linked to the severity of asthma. The release of cytokines depends on cross-linking of IgE by allergen. IgE antibodies are synthesized and released by B cells; briefly circulate in the blood; and bind to high-affinity IgE receptors on the surface of mast cells in tissues and peripheral blood basophils and low-affinity IgE receptors on lymphocytes, eosinophils, platelets, and macrophages.[20]

The early phase of asthma (usually resolves within 1 hour) is characterized by an inhaled allergen precipitating acute constriction of smooth muscles by release of histamines and leukotrienes from mast cells. A prolonged late phase (4 to 6 hours later) occurs as a result of cytokines and chemokines generated by resident inflammatory cells (mast cells, macrophages, epithelial cells) and recruited inflammatory cells (lymphocytes, eosinophils) and causes further obstruction of airflow. Numerous cytokines regulate the function of eosinophils and other cells in asthma. Interferon-γ is elevated in severe asthma during the acute phase. Data also suggest that interferon-γ contributes to the activation of eosinophils and likely augments inflammation. There are two types of helper $CD4^+$ T lymphocyte cells. Type 1 helper (T_H1) T cells produce interleukin (IL) 2 and interferon-γ, which are essential for cellular defense mechanisms. Type 2 helper (T_H2) T cells produce cytokines (IL-4, IL-5, IL-6, IL-9, and IL-13) that mediate allergic inflammation. Balance between the T_H1 and T_H2 type cytokine response contributes to the cause and evolution of atopic diseases, including asthma. The increasing prevalence of asthma in Western countries has led to the "hygiene hypothesis." The immune system in newborns is primarily T_H2 cells, and a timely and appropriate environmental stimulus is needed to create a balanced immune response. Alteration in the number of infections in early life, widespread use of antibiotics, adoption of the Western lifestyle, and repeated exposure to allergens may affect the balance between T_H1-type and T_H2-type cytokine responses and increase the likelihood of immune response by T_H2 cells and lead to asthma. Mild intermittent asthma is thought to be a T_H2 allergen-oriented reaction with adequate apoptosis and self-limiting inflammation, although severe persistent asthma is mediated by T_H1 cytokines with progressive loss of apoptosis leading to longer exacerbations, expanded memory cells, and persistent inflammation. Evidence continues to underscore the importance of immune factors in the development of asthma and resulting inflammatory process. This particular strategy and insight into the mechanisms of these processes would be important for future treatment of acute severe asthma.[19,21-25]

Airflow limitation in asthma is caused by bronchoconstriction, airway edema, airway hyperresponsiveness, and airway remodeling. Permanent structural changes can occur with airway remodeling, leading to poor response to therapy, including thickening of sub–basement membrane and subepithelial fibrosis, airway smooth muscle hypertrophy and hyperplasia, blood vessel proliferation and dilation (angiogenesis), and mucus gland hyperplasia and hypersecretion.[13]

ASTHMA GENETICS

Asthma and atopy are complex phenotypes that are influenced by genetic and environmental factors. About 79 genes have been associated with asthma or atopy phenotypes. The *ADAM33* gene has been associated with asthma. A locus on the short arm of chromosome 20 has been linked to asthma and bronchial hyperresponsiveness. If further investigations confirm that *ADAM33* is an asthma gene, future studies should enhance understanding of asthma and lead to new therapeutic targets. As Ober and Hoffjan described, such "molecular phenotyping" of patients with asthma and atopic diseases may generate informed decisions regarding treatment, laying the foundation for genomic medicine in the next decade.[26,27]

SYMPTOMS AND SIGNS

Wheezing may be expiratory and inspiratory and correlates with the degree of obstruction if adequate air movement is present. Absence of wheezing is an ominous finding in a severely distressed asthmatic patient because it implies minimal air movement and is a harbinger of respiratory arrest. Contraction of the sternocleidomastoid muscles and other accessory muscles indicates severe obstruction (FEV_1 < 1 L). Intense inspiratory effort leads to large swings in intrathoracic pressure and to an accentuated pulsus paradoxus (representing a decreased stroke volume during inspiration). Pulsus paradoxus is often appreciated during routine blood pressure measurement in acute severe bronchospasm because systolic blood pressure decreases dramatically during inspiration (this decrease is <10 mm Hg in normal individuals). A decrease of more than 15 mm Hg in a patient in an acute asthma episode is associated with severe reduction in FEV_1.[18,28,29]

Ominous signs and findings during an acute severe asthma episode include diaphoresis, inability to recline or talk, peak expiratory flow rate (PEFR) less than 60 L/minute, and use of accessory muscles. PEFR less than 25% predicted or personal best is defined as severe life-threatening asthma. In acute severe asthma, lung hyperinflation occurs secondary to increased expiratory airflow resistance, short expiratory time, high ventilatory demands, and increased postinspiratory activity of the inspiratory muscles. The presence of these factors in variable degrees does not allow the respiratory cycle to reach a static equilibrium volume at the end of expiration. Inspiration begins at a volume in which the respiratory system exhibits a positive elastic recoil pressure called intrinsic positive-end expiratory pressure (iPEEP), or auto-PEEP. This phenomenon is described as dynamic hyperinflation. Dynamic hyperinflation produces a significant decrease in systemic venous return to the heart, leading to a decrease in left ventricular diastolic filling. Also problematic is the increase in left ventricular afterload as a result of large negative intrathoracic pressure swings during inspiration. Pulmonary artery pressure also may be increased secondary to lung hyperinflation, resulting in increased right ventricular afterload. These events combine to produce pulsus paradoxus.[15]

Near-fatal asthma presents as raised $Paco_2$ requiring mechanical ventilation and is associated with high inflation pressures. Life-threatening asthma has any of the following features. Symptoms are altered mental status with confusion or coma, feeble respiratory effort, and exhaustion. Signs are cyanosis, silent chest, hypotension, bradycardia, oxygen saturation below 92% or Pao_2 less than 60 mm Hg, $Paco_2$ higher than 60 mm Hg, and FEV_1 below 30% predicted or personal best.[30]

All that wheezes is not asthma. Other entities to consider are upper airway obstruction and "cardiac asthma." Upper airway obstruction should be considered in patients at risk (e.g., tracheal stenosis in patients who were previously intubated) and when there is no response to therapy in a patient without history of asthma. If the patient's status would tolerate it, flow volume loops may be diagnostic. Likewise, wheezing that dissipates with intubation should make one suspect upper airway obstruction. Paradoxical vocal cord movement can stimulate asthma. Patients with acute left ventricular failure may wheeze as a result of interstitial fluid compression of bronchioles and edema-associated bronchiolar smooth muscle contraction.[31,32]

OBJECTIVE MEASUREMENT OF OBSTRUCTION

During an asthmatic attack, all indices of expiratory flow are significantly reduced, including FEV_1; FEV_1/FVC; PEFR; maximal expiratory flows at 75% (MEF_{75}), 50% (MEF_{50}), and 25% of vital capacity (MEF_{25}); and maximal expiratory flow between 25% and 75% of the FVC (MEF_{25-75}). With acute asthmatic crisis, high functional residual capacity, total lung capacity, and residual volume are observed.[15]

Although spirometry is the best objective measure of airway obstruction, a severely ill asthmatic patient is rarely able to perform the necessary full FVC maneuver. Objective assessment of airway obstruction in a severe asthmatic usually can be made by measuring the PEFR because this measurement requires patient cooperation only in the early part of the FVC maneuver. Because the greatest expiratory flow rates exist in early expiration, most patients are able to produce a reliable PEFR value. Normal expiratory flow rates vary considerably with age, sex, and height. In adults, a PEFR less than 100 to 125 L/minute implies severe obstruction to airflow. A severe exercebation of asthma is defined as an FEV_1 less than 40% or peak expiratory volume, less than 40% predicted, or less than 1 L. Values less than 25% are consistent with life-threteaning asthma. Failure to improve PEFR significantly with initial aggressive bronchodilator therapy is the best predictor of morbidity in a patient with acute severe asthma.[10]

LABORATORY AND RADIOGRAPHIC DATA

Asymmetrical breath sounds or chest pain should alert the physician to the possibility of pneumothorax and mandates an early chest radiograph. An increased white blood cell count may be produced by asthma alone in the absence of infection, β-receptor agonists, and theophylline shift of potassium intracellularly. Hypokalemia-induced dysrhythmias could occur after intensive bronchodilator therapy in elderly patients or in patients receiving other therapies that predispose to hypokalemia, such as steroidal and diuretic medications. Creatine phosphokinase (non-MB fraction) may be increased as a result of the strenuous activity of ventilatory muscles. Severe asthma may cause right-sided heart strain as shown on electrocardiogram; this resolves with clinical improvement. Arterial blood gas assessment adds little to the early management of acute asthma. The early stage of asthma usually reveals mild hypoxemia, hypocapnia, and respiratory alkalosis. A non–anion gap acidosis also may be observed in patients with severe asthma if several days of hyperventilation have led to renal compensation with bicarbonate wasting to compensate for the respiratory alkalosis. As the severity of obstruction increases, arterial carbon dioxide ($Paco_2$) normalizes and then increases as a sign of impending respiratory collapse. After initial therapy, arterial blood gases may be useful for decisions regarding hospital admission or tracheal intubation. Most asthma patients respond dramatically to initial therapy; arterial blood gases obtained when the patient is first seen are rarely predictive of outcome or useful clinically.[33]

Early attention should be directed toward aggressive therapeutic intervention. A normal $Paco_2$ level in a distressed asthmatic patient despite aggressive in-hospital therapy should alert the physician to respiratory fatigue and the danger of respiratory arrest. Respiratory acidosis may be preceded by a lactate-induced anion gap metabolic acidosis. This lactic acidosis is likely caused by a combination of failing inspiratory muscles, aggressive use of β-agonist therapy, and decreased liver perfusion resulting from increased intrathoracic pressure and blood flow diverted to the muscles of respiration. Lactic acidosis occurs more commonly in men and with administration of parenteral β-agonists.[34-36]

In patients with near-fatal asthma, high values for inflammation-related laboratory markers such as erythrocyte sedimentation rate (ESR), C-reactive proteins (CRP), and low nutritional status with low albumin levels were associated with poor prognosis. Exhaled nitric oxide is another biomarker of lung and airway inflammation. Elevated exhaled nitric oxide levels can be found in severe allergic asthma and may predict future exacerbations and steroid treatment response. Use of this biomarker is not recommended at this time and needs further evaluation.[37,38]

Box 38.2 Conditions Typically Requiring Hospitalization for a Patient with Severe Asthma

Acute respiratory acidosis despite aggressive bronchodilator therapy
Pneumonia
Pneumothorax
Initial PEFR <60 L/min (assumes full cooperation)
Inability to raise PEFR to 200 L/min despite aggressive therapy
FEV_1 or PEFR <25% of predicted and fails to improve by >10% after initial treatment
Inability to boost baseline bronchodilator regimen
Multiple visits to emergency department for severe asthma attack
History of tracheal intubation or ICU admission because of asthma

Admission to ICU

Respiratory distress
High pulsus paradoxus or falling pulsus in a patient with fatigue
Subjective sense of impending respiratory failure
Respiratory arrest
Altered mental status
Spo_2 90% despite supplemental oxygen
Rising $Paco_2$ coupled with clinical evidence of nonresolution

FEV_1, forced expiratory volume in the first second; ICU, intensive care unit; PEFR, peak expiratory flow rate.
Data from references 113 and 115.

INPATIENT ADMISSION DECISIONS

Conditions typically requiring hospitalization for a patient with severe asthma are listed in Box 38.2.

DRUG THERAPY (TABLE 38.1)

OXYGEN

If pulse oximetry confirms the presence of hypoxemia, oxygen should be given to maintain oxygen saturation at greater than 92%. A transient decrease in arterial oxygen tension has been shown in some patients after initiation of β-adrenergic agonist therapy in severe asthma. Mechanisms of this decrease relate to some combination of β_2-agonist-induced vasodilation in areas of decreased ventilation and increase in pulmonary blood flow resulting from a β_1-adrenergic inotropic and chronotropic effect. Saturation may decrease initially during bronchodilator therapy with β-agonists, which produce vasodilation and may increase intrapulmonary shunting. Studies in children suggest that aerosolized salbutamol administration may cause hypoxemia during acute episodes of asthma if the drug is administered without oxygen. Most published data show that salbutamol does not have a clinically important effect on oxygenation in asthmatic adults. This seems to be true for stable and acute asthma; however, these studies in adults exclude the most severe exacerbations more likely to be associated with marked hypoxemia. Because inhaled β-agonist should be given in this circumstance, the only clinical response is to treat any worsening of oxygenation that occurs with additional oxygen. Hyperoxia may be harmful and may be associated with hypercarbia due to regional release of hypoxic pulmonary vasoconstriction during asthma exacerbations.[5,39-42]

Moloney and colleagues showed that bronchoconstriction induced by dry air challenge can be prevented by humidifying inspired air. Humidification of inspired air should be achieved with a heated cascade humidifier. The use of heat and moisture exchangers is discouraged because they increase the deadspace and add to the expiratory airway resistance.[43]

β-ADRENERGIC THERAPY

INHALED β_2-SELECTIVE AGONISTS (ALBUTEROL OR SALBUTAMOL) AND SHORT-ACTING β-AGONISTS

Albuterol is the cornerstone of treatment for acute exacerbation in patients with acute asthma. Initial therapy in an acutely ill asthma patient, as recommended by the National Asthma Education and Prevention Program Update, is 2.5 to 5 mg of albuterol (0.5 to 1 mL of 0.5% solution in 5 mL of normal saline solution) by nebulization every 20 minutes for three doses (for optimal delivery, dilute aerosols to a minimum of 3 mL at gas flow of 6 to 8 L/minute), followed by 2.5 to 10 mg every 1 to 4 hours as needed, or 10 to 15 mg/hour continuously, with the titration based on response and severity of symptoms. Continuous nebulization should be considered in the most severe patients. Tachycardia and hypokalemia may occur with continuously nebulized albuterol. β_2-Selective agents delivered parenterally or orally lose much of the β_2 selectivity, which provides the rationale for inhalation treatment as the cornerstone of therapy.[25,32,39,40,43,44]

Adequate delivery of β-agonists can be accomplished by a metered-dose inhaler (MDI) with spacer during acute bronchospasm if proper technique is used and doses are increased. Four puffs of albuterol (0.36 mg) delivered with a spacer should be expected to be equipotent to 2.5 mg of albuterol by nebulization in patients with severe disease. It is advisable to deliver the β-agonist by nebulization in most acutely ill asthma patients because nebulization requires minimal coordination and cooperation of the patient and less bedside instruction and supervision by health care professionals. Many randomized controlled clinical studies over the last several decades have compared β-agonists delivered by MDIs or by nebulizer. Most studies show similar responses. Protocols typically include methods that ensure proper use of the MDI, however. Greater amounts of drug delivery are required with nebulized therapy to produce the same effect as that seen with an MDI with a spacer. To initiate therapy with nebulized albuterol and then switch to an MDI with spacer after the patient has improved and stabilized may be cost-effective. When aerosol β-agonists are delivered in intubated patients and patients receiving mechanical ventilatory support, much of the physiologic effect is lost as a result of deposition onto the endotracheal tube. Doubling the dose that would be used in a nonintubated patient is recommended.[45-47]

Table 38.1 Summary of Treatment for Life-Threatening Asthma

Treatment	Dose and Frequency	Comments
Oxygen	1-3 L/min by nasal cannula Goal is to maintain oxygen saturation (Spo_2) >92% Use heated cascade humidifier to avoid dry air–induced bronchoconstriction	Transient drop in O_2 tension with β-adrenergic therapy Avoid hyperoxia (may be associated with hypercarbia)
Bronchodilators		
β_2-Selective agonists: albuterol or salbutamol, levalbuterol	*Albuterol*: 2.5-5 mg (0.5-1 mL of 0.5% solution in 5 mL of normal saline) by nebulizer every 20 min for 3 doses total (for optimal delivery, dilute aerosols to a minimum of 3 mL at gas flow of 6-8 L/min), followed by 2.5-10 mg q1-4h as needed, or 10-15 mg/h continuously; titration based on response and severity of symptoms *Albuterol MDI*, delivered with a spacer (each spacer dose takes 1-2 min; 90 μg/puff), 4-8 puffs every 20 min for 4 h, then q4h as needed *Albuterol*: 5-7.5 mg by jet nebulizer (each treatment takes 15-20 min) *Levalbuterol* (0.63 mg/3 mL and 1.25 mg/3 mL nebulizer): 1.25-2.5 mg every 20 min for 3 doses total, then 1.25-5 mg q1-4h as needed, or 5-7.5 mg/h continuous nebulization *Levalbuterol MDI* (45 μg/puff): 4-8 puffs every 20 min for 4 h, followed by q1-4h as needed	Beta2-selective agonists are the cornerstone of therapy Continuous nebulization used for a majority of severely ill patients In study of continuous vs. intermittent therapy in severe exacerbations (excluding life-threatening asthma), no difference noted in pulmonary function improvement or need for hospitalization Lower frequency of side effects with continuous treatment Watch for hypokalemia, tremors, tachycardia, and lactic acidosis Oral or parenteral route: loss of β_2-selectivity MDI: 4 puffs of albuterol (0.36 mg) = 2.5 mg of albuterol nebulization Levalbuterol 0.63 mg = racemic albuterol 1.25 mg for efficacy and side effects *Intubated patients*: Nebulizers are less efficient in delivering doses to lower airways (6-10%) than MDIs (11%)
Epinephrine	*Subcutaneous epinephrine* dose for adults: 0.3-0.5 mL of a 1:1000 dilution (1 mg/mL), depending on age and weight; repeat every 20 min for 3 doses total	
Terbutaline	*Subcutaneous terbutaline*, 0.25 mg; repeat every 20 min for 3 doses total	Terbutaline is the parenteral agent of choice in pregnancy For refractory life-threatening asthma: intravenous epinephrine (high risk for cardiac events, infarction, and arrhythmias) or racemic epinephrine may be considered
Anticholinergics		
Ipratropium (for acute severe asthma warranting visit to emergency department)	*Ipratropium bromide*: 0.5 mg by nebulizer (0.25 mg/mL) every 20 min for 3 doses, then q2-4h as needed *Ipratropium MDI* (0.018 mg/puff): 4-8 puffs per treatment every 20 min for up to 3 h *Combinations*: Albuterol (2.5 mg/3 mL) + ipratropium (0.5 mg/3 mL): 3 mL every 20 min for 3 doses total, then as needed MDI delivering albuterol 90 μg + ipratropium 18 μg: 8 puffs every 20 min for up to 3 h	Ipratropium: Onset of action is slow (20 min), peak effectiveness at 60-90 min, no systemic side effects, improved lung function and reduced recovery time Use a handheld mouthpiece nebulizer (contamination of the ocular area with precipitation of narrow-angle glaucoma may occur if facemask is used for delivery of anticholinergic agent) Ipratropium may be combined with nebulized albuterol dose in the emergency room; no proven benefit shown in hospitalized patients
Corticosteroids: prednisone, prednisolone, methylprednisolone	40-80 mg/day in 1 or 2 divided doses until peak expiratory flow reaches 70% of predicted or personal best FEV_1 or PEFR <50%[16] Methylprednisolone 40 mg IV q6h OR Hydrocortisone 200 mg IV	No advantage of higher doses No advantage of IV therapy over oral if absorption and gut transit are not impaired Total steroid course: 3-10 days, <1 week; no need to taper steroids Inhaled steroids can be started at any time

Table 38.1 Summary of Treatment for Life-Threatening Asthma (Continued)

Treatment	Dose and Frequency	Comments
Heliox	Helium-oxygen mixture (80-20 or 70-30) Routine use cannot be recommended at this time	Improves O_2 and aerosolized medication delivery to distal lung Decreases flow turbulence and resistance Lower gas density facilitates exhalation, reduces air trapping and intrinsic PEEP Improves pulmonary function in subgroup of patients with most severe airflow obstruction
Magnesium sulfate	2 g IV given over 20 min; may repeat Monitor magnesium levels Avoid in renal insufficiency	Bronchodilatation from inhibition of the calcium channel and decreased acetylcholine release IV and inhaled or nebulized magnesium sulfate improves pulmonary function in acute severe asthma IV magnesium widely used as adjunct therapy

FEV_1, forced expiratory flow in 1 second; MDI, metered-dose inhaler; PEFR, peak expiratory flow rate.
Data from references 13, 16, 52, 111-115.

Aggressive inhaled selective β_2-agonist therapy is preferred to intravenous albuterol because the same end point usually can be achieved with less risk for toxicity. Intravenous albuterol (if available) may be considered as an alternative when patients with life-threatening asthma have failed to respond to inhaled therapy. Oral β_2-selective agents should not be used as primary treatment for patients with acute asthma because the therapeutic-to-toxicity ratio is less than with inhaled agents. Effects of corticosteroids and β_2-agonists on airflow obstruction may be additive.[48]

Levalbuterol, 0.63 mg, is equivalent to racemic albuterol, 1.25 mg, for efficacy and side effects. Levalbuterol is available as 0.63 mg/3 mL and 1.25 mg/3 mL nebulizer solutions. The recommended adult dose of levalbuterol is 1.25 to 2.5 mg every 20 minutes for three doses, then 1.25 to 5 mg every 1 to 4 hours as needed, or 5 to 7.5 mg/hour continuous nebulization.[25]

In outpatient settings, monotherapy with inhaled long-acting β-agonists (LABA, salmeterol, Formoterol) has been shown to increase severe and life-threatening asthma exacerbations and asthma-related deaths.[30]

SUBCUTANEOUS β-AGONIST THERAPY (EPINEPHRINE OR TERBUTALINE)

Subcutaneous β-agonist therapy has a disadvantageous therapeutic-to-toxicity ratio compared with inhaled β_2-selective agonists. Although there is no proven value of systemic therapy over aerosol therapy, rapid delivery of β-agonists to the airway may be beneficial in seriously ill asthmatic patients who are at imminent risk for respiratory arrest or in need of intubation and at low risk for β-agonist cardiac toxicity (young asthmatics). In this circumstance, a combination of inhaled and subcutaneously administered β-agonists may be useful. The subcutaneous epinephrine dose for adults is 0.3 to 0.5 mL of a 1:1000 dilution (1 mg/mL), depending on age and weight; it may be repeated in the initial management every 20 minutes for three times. An alternative subcutaneous β-agonist agent is subcutaneous terbutaline, 0.25 mg, which can be repeated every 20 minutes for three doses. When subcutaneous terbutaline is compared with subcutaneous epinephrine, equal cardiac side effects are seen. No clinical studies document benefit of subcutaneous terbutaline over subcutaneous epinephrine. Terbutaline is, however, the parenteral agent of choice in pregnancy. β_1-Adrenergic stimulators are given subcutaneously with caution to the elderly and to patients with documented or suspected coronary artery disease.[49,50]

Anecdotal reports have suggested the success of epinephrine administration through the endotracheal tube after respiratory arrest from asthma. Prospective trials are needed in this area. Despite the lack of confirmatory studies, in an asthma patient with respiratory arrest, it may be considered.[51]

CORTICOSTEROIDS

Corticosteroids are an essential part of in-hospital asthma therapy. The National Institutes of Health expert panel recommendation is intravenous methylprednisolone, 40 to 80 mg/day in one or two divided doses, until PEF reaches 70% of predicted or personal best. This is substantially lower dosage than the previous recommendations. Initial high-dose steroids with intravenous methylprednisolone 80 to 125 mg/day in divided doses (typically 40 mg every 6 hours) for the first 24 hours was recommended if the PEFR or FEV_1 remains less than 50% in severe asthmatics.[16] In hospitalized patients the use of higher than standard doses of prednisone (40-80 mg/day) offers no benefit. No differences in clinical effects between oral and intravenous forms of corticosteroid therapy have been proved. In acute severe asthma, intravenous steroids offer benefit with the possibility of early onset of action and peak effect. Some trials show improvement following initiation of steroids after a patient's condition was refractory to initial therapy. Others show benefit

Box 38.3 Potential Benefits of Corticosteroids in the Treatment of Asthma

Enhancement of β_2-receptor responsiveness by upregulating β_2-receptors on airway smooth muscle
Decrease in capillary basement membrane permeability; decrease vascular leak from endothelial cells
Decreased leukocyte attachment; decreased number of eosinophils, mast cells, and dendritic cells
Modulation of calcium migration intracellularly
Reduction in airway mucus production
Suppression of IgE receptor binding
Interruption of arachidonic acid inflammatory pathways
Decreased airway smooth muscle contraction, mucosal edema, and airway inflammation
Airway remodeling
Decreased cytokine and mediator production from epithelial cells

Data from references 13 and 52.

when corticosteroid therapy is initiated early in the course of an acute asthma episode. Most corticosteroid benefit is thought to be delayed for approximately 6 hours, although a potential for earlier beneficial effect has been postulated. The delay in effect may reflect the time necessary for steroids to induce upregulation of new β_2-receptors and reversal of β_2-receptor desensitization and downregulation. Some patients show corticosteroid resistance. Inhaled corticosteroids can be started any time during the exercebation. Total course of steroids can be 3 to 10 days and less than 1 week; there is no need to taper the dose.[13,16,52] Potential benefits of corticosteroids are listed in Box 38.3.

INHALED ANTICHOLINERGIC THERAPY WITH IPRATROPIUM

Although ipratropium achieves less bronchodilation at peak effect than β-agonists and less predictable clinical response, the effect is likely to be additive to albuterol. Most published evidence supports the addition of ipratropium to inhaled β-agonist therapy for acute asthma patients. It produces clinically modest improvement in lung function compared with albuterol alone. Addition of multiple high doses of ipratropium bromide in acute severe airflow obstruction in asthma patients in the emergency room has resulted in fewer hospital admissions. After admission to the hospital for acute severe asthma, clinical benefit from the addition of ipratropium is not detected in trials.[13,42,53,54]

The National Institutes of Health expert panel's recommended dose of ipratropium is 0.5 mg by nebulizer every 20 minutes for three doses, then every 2 to 4 hours as needed. Onset of action is slow (20 minutes), with peak effectiveness at 60 to 90 minutes and no systemic side effects. A handheld mouthpiece nebulizer system should be used for nebulization because contamination of the ocular area with precipitation of narrow-angle glaucoma may occur in susceptible individuals if a facemask is used for delivery of an anticholinergic agent. Ipratropium may be combined with the nebulized albuterol dose. The deposition of ipratropium may be enhanced, however, when it follows albuterol-induced bronchodilation. In a patient with severe asthma, ipratropium may produce a clinically significant response within minutes of administration, as opposed to the longer delay to response in chronic obstructive pulmonary disease patients with chronic stable disease. If ipratropium is delivered by MDI (0.018 mg/puff), 4 to 8 puffs per treatment is recommended.[13,40]

METHYXANTHINES: THEOPHYLLINE OR AMINOPHYLLINE

Although theophylline or aminophylline is an effective bronchodilator compared with placebo in patients with acute bronchospasm, inhaled β-agonists are accepted to be superior to theophylline as single agents for acute bronchospasm. Consensus opinion and meta-analyses support no significant additive clinical benefit with the addition of theophylline to a full course of inhaled β-agonists. Although a few studies have shown physiologic benefits evident at 24 or 48 hours, the addition of theophylline to high-dose inhaled β-agonist and corticosteroid therapy in patients with acute severe asthma seems to offer no clear-cut or substantial clinical benefit. Methylxanthines are infrequently used for acute asthma because of unpredictable pharmacokinetics and known side effects.[40,55-58] Because theophylline toxicity is a potential problem, the use of theophylline should be limited to patients with life-threatening asthma who fail to respond to other therapy.

MAGNESIUM SULFATE

Magnesium has multifactorial actions relative to potential reversal of bronchoconstriction, which is based on characteristics of inhibition of the calcium channel and decreased acetylcholine release. Hashimoto and colleagues[59] showed that 40% of asthmatic patients exhibited magnesium deficiency, and that low magnesium erythrocyte concentrations reflected decreased magnesium stores in patients with bronchial asthma.

A Cochrane meta-analysis concluded that use of intravenous magnesium sulfate improves pulmonary function and decreases hospital admissions in acute severe asthma, particularly in patients with severe exacerbations. Inhaled magnesium sulfate improves pulmonary function during acute exacerbations of asthma, although it fails to show alterations in clinically important outcomes, such as hospital admissions. Magnesium sulfate can improve pulmonary function modestly and when dosed appropriately has no significant side effect profile.

Traditionally, 2 g of magnesium sulfate is administered over 20 minutes. Repeat doses, if used, require careful monitoring of magnesium levels and assessment for clinical manifestations of toxicity. Magnesium therapy should be avoided in the presence of renal insufficiency.[59-61]

HELIOX

Heliox (mixture of helium and oxygen optimally effective at a 70 : 30 mix) has been shown to improve the delivery and deposition of nebulized albuterol. If a patient requires more than 30% oxygen, it cannot be used. Heliox may be useful in acute severe asthma refractory to conventional treatment. There are no data to support the use of heliox as the initial treatment for acute severe asthma. Heliox is available in mixtures of 60:40, 70:30, and 80:20. Helium is less dense than air and can be delivered through a tight-fitting nonrebreathing mask or, in an intubated patient, through the ventilatory circuit. Heliox results in decreased large airway resistance. One might anticipate that the role of heliox would be limited by the fact that heliox improves flow in large turbulent airways, and most of the obstruction in asthma is in the peripheral airways. Studies have nonetheless shown the ability of heliox to decrease inspiratory and expiratory resistance in severe asthma. Its potential to decrease PEEP not set on the ventilator (auto-PEEP) might be particularly useful. Heliox may augment carbon dioxide removal by facilitating carbon dioxide movement across the endothelial-epithelial barrier compared with the presence of a mixture of oxygen and nitrogen as the carrier gas. Heliox also has been shown to improve oxygenation, which may allow higher helium concentrations to be delivered.[62-64]

OTHER AGENTS

ANTIBIOTICS

Antibiotic therapy in an asthma patient is indicated only if bacterial infection is present. The Telithromycin, Chlamydophilia, and Asthma (TELECAST) study reported that, in patients presenting for unscheduled care because of an acute asthma exacerbation, treatment with telithromycin showed a significant improvement in FEV_1 over placebo at the end of a 10-day treatment period.[65] One of the primary efficacy end points, improvement in asthma symptom scores, was significantly greater in the telithromycin group than placebo. An editorial pointed out the possible anti-inflammatory effects of macrolides in the treatment of asthma but did not recommend this as standard therapy at this time.[66]

FLUIDS

If the patient is volume depleted, normal saline or lactated Ringer's solution is used to reestablish adequate intravenous volume. There is no evidence that excess volume replacement liquefies or facilitates loosening of secretions. Chest physiotherapy and other maneuvers to mobilize secretions physically also are not recommended. Nebulization of acetylcysteine is not indicated and may irritate the airways. Saline solution and acetylcysteine have been successfully used as part of bronchial lavage with fiberoptic bronchoscopy in patients with severe asthma.[67]

KETAMINE

Ketamine is an intravenous analgesic agent that has bronchodilator properties but may stimulate bronchial secretions and laryngospasm and may cause tachycardia, hypertension, delirium, dissociative state, and lowering of seizure threshold. So far no trials have been published to prove its effectiveness. When intubation of a severe acute asthmatic is required, in the absence of hypertension and known seizure disorder, ketamine seems to be an optimal induction agent. It also may be used in life-threatening situations when conventional therapy has failed.[40,68]

LEUKOTRIENE ANTAGONISTS

Leukotriene receptor antagonists (LTRAs: montelukast, zafirlukast) improve lung function and are often used in the management of chronic asthma, but their role in acute asthma is unclear. Significant improvement in pulmonary function within 10 minutes of intravenous administration of leukotriene antagonists was demonstrated in one study in patients with severe asthma exercebation.[69]

OMALIZUMAB (ANTI-IGE ANTIBODY)

Recombinant anti-IgE antibody (omalizumab) improves asthma control in severely allergic asthmatics, reducing inhaled steroids and rescue medication requirement and improving asthma-related quality of life. Its role in acute severe asthma is unstudied. The delay in onset of effect likely makes its impact less likely.[70]

Strunk and Bloomberg reported that patients likely to benefit from omalizumab are patients with evidence of sensitization to perennial aeroallergens who require high doses of inhaled corticosteroids that have a potential for adverse effects, patients with frequent exacerbations of asthma, and patients with severe disease-related noncompliance. Total IgE levels should be measured in all patients, and the recommended dose, 0.016 mg/kg body weight per international unit of IgE every 4 weeks, should be administered subcutaneously at 2- or 4-week intervals. Strunk and Bloomberg recommended adding omalizumab in a compliant patient with severe asthma after a trial of leukotriene modifiers or extended-release theophylline proved ineffective.[71]

NONTRADITIONAL THERAPY OF SEVERE BRONCHOSPASM (TABLE 38.2)

Asthmatic patients who fail to respond to conventional therapy should be considered for nontraditional therapy. Nontraditional treatment alternatives include intensification of β-agonist therapy beyond routinely recognized standards, general anesthetic agents, and bronchial lavage. Continuous intravenous albuterol has been used in Europe but is unavailable in the United States. It is unlikely that it adds any additional benefit over increasing the aggressiveness of treatment with inhaled bronchodilators. Intravenous isoproterenol and terbutaline have been used in children but are not recommended in adults.

In a patient with refractory severe asthma who is receiving mechanical ventilatory support, anecdotal success with isoflurane or halothane anesthesia, intravenous thiopental, and rectally administered ether has been reported. Intravenous ketamine has the potential for administration in the ICU and is likely the best alternative for anesthetic therapy. Que and Lusaya anecdotally showed significant improvement when using sevoflurane induction for emergency cesarean section in a woman with severe life-threatening asthma. Maternal and neonatal outcome were good. Propofol has been reported to relax smooth muscle in arteries and veins, and a bronchodilator effect has been suggested. A case series report showed temporally related improvement in severe asthmatic bronchospasm after propofol infusion.[72-80]

Table 38.2 Adjunct Therapies for Bronchospasm

Nontraditional Therapy for Severe Bronchospasm	Comments
Intravenous β_2-agonists	No data show any benefit in adding IV agent to nebulization Avoid IV isoproterenol owing to danger of myocardial toxicity Rapid bronchodilation in impending respiratory failure
Oral or IV leukotriene receptor antagonists (LTRAs): montelukast 10 mg oral daily, zafirlukast	Improves pulmonary function within 10 min Oral LTRAs can be added as an adjunct in severe asthma
Non-invasive positive-pressure ventilation (NPPV)	NPPV reduces the need for endotracheal intubation in severe asthma exacerbation
Inhaled nitric oxide (NO) (adding 15 ppm to the inspiratory circuit)	Rapid improvement in ventilated patients with asthma refractory to medical treatment
Omalizumab (anti-IgE antibody)	Role in acute asthma is unstudied Improves asthma control in allergic asthmatics
General anesthetic agents: isoflurane or halothane anesthesia IV thiopental, IV propofol, IV ketamine	Propofol relaxes the smooth muscles in arteries and veins and has bronchodilator effect
Plasma exchange (during pregnancy) Pumpless extracorporeal carbon dioxide removal Extracorporeal life support (ECLS)	Case reports of adjunct therapies; used as salvage therapy for life-threatening asthma
Glucagon	Rapid smooth muscle relaxant, short half-life; small study report
Nebulized DNase (dornase 2.5 mg via tracheal tube)	Case report of use in pregnant patient with rapid improvement
Bronchial lavage	Anecdotal reports: exacerbates auto-PEEP, decreases oxygenation

IgE, immunoglobulin E; IV, intravenous; PEEP, positive end-expiratory pressure.
Data from references 13, 84-86, 116-120.

Although anecdotal success has been reported, critically ill mechanically ventilated asthmatic patients are poor candidates for bronchial lavage because the procedure itself would exacerbate auto-PEEP and decrease oxygenation. The procedure is likely to produce a significant increase in auto-PEEP and worsening of hypoxemia. Anecdotal success has been shown with the use of plasma exchange in refractory life-threatening status asthmaticus in pregnancy. The measurement of preplasma and postplasma exchange complement factors and immunoglobulin revealed 50% elimination. Glucagon, a rapid-acting smooth muscle relaxant with a short half-life, also has been studied for potential benefit in acute severe asthma. In a small study of 21 glucagon-treated (0.03 mg/kg) patients and 25 placebo-treated patients, no differences were found. Successful bronchodilation was defined as a PEFR increase of 60 L/minute at 10 minutes. Standard bronchodilator therapy also was administered. Finally, rapid improvement in a mechanically ventilated asthma patient refractory to medical therapy was temporally related to addition of 15 ppm of inhaled nitric oxide to the inspiratory circuit.

Recent case reports suggest that extracorporeal carbon dioxide removal seems to be a valuable adjunct to mechanical ventilation for life-threatening asthma, and emergency extracorporeal life support (ECLS) as salvage therapy also has been reported.[81-86]

ACUTE SEVERE ASTHMA IN PREGNANCY

Asthma complicates 3% to 12% of pregnancies and is perhaps the most common serious medical problem to complicate pregnancy. Exacerbations occur in approximately 20% of all pregnant women with asthma, can occur any time during gestation, but tend to occur late in the second trimester. Acute attacks of asthma during labor are rare. Simultaneous management of the mother and the fetus is a challenge. The goal in approaching a pregnant patient with severe asthma is to prevent maternal hypoxemia.[16,87-89]

Studies of pregnancy-associated asthma reveal increased incidence of maternal and fetal complications, which include preeclampsia, perinatal fatality, low birth weight, and preterm infants. The risk of uncontrolled asthma is considered to outweigh any risk associated with the use of recommended medications for asthma. It is important that a physician skilled in the management of asthma be involved in the patient's care. Uterine contractions are common during asthma exacerbation and usually do not progress to preterm labor. When more than one β-adrenergic tocolytic agent is being administered simultaneously (systemically and inhaled), the possibility of excessive systemic effects should be considered. This is particularly true as it pertains to maternal and fetal tachycardia. One study compared perinatal outcomes in 259 pregnant women treated with inhaled β_2-adrenergic agonists with 101 pregnant women with asthma not treated with inhaled β_2-agonists and with 295 pregnant women without asthma and found no difference in rates of perinatal mortality, congenital malformations, preterm delivery, or delivery of low-birth-weight infants. There also were no differences in Apgar scores, rates of complications of labor or delivery, and postpartum bleeding. Oral steroid use was associated with an increased risk of preterm delivery, although it is difficult to separate the effect of the medication from the effect of exacerbation.[90,91]

Asthma exacerbations have the potential to lead to severe problems for the fetus. During pregnancy, asthma exacerbations should be managed aggressively. During pregnancy, acute severe asthma is treated initially with inhaled short-acting β-agonist by MDI or nebulizer, one to three doses in the first hour; oxygen; and if no response, oral systemic corticosteroids. If there is severe exacerbation of asthma (PEFR <50%), β-agonist could be given continuously or every 20 minutes, combined with inhaled ipratropium bromide. Fetal assessment and monitoring should be done until the patient is stabilized. To control asthma, there are limited data using leukotriene receptor antagonists in humans during pregnancy, although reassuring animal data are available. Studies and clinical evidence confirm safety of theophylline at recommended doses (to serum concentrations of 5 to 12 μg/mL) during pregnancy. There were higher levels of reported side effects and discontinuation of the medication, however. The experimental animal studies confirm the association of high-dose theophylline and adverse pregnancy outcomes in animals.[87-92]

MECHANICAL VENTILATION IN ASTHMA PATIENTS

INDICATIONS

Endotracheal intubation should be strongly considered at the time of presentation if the patient has central cyanosis, mental status changes, or a depressed level of consciousness. Inability to oxygenate or ventilate the lungs of an asthmatic patient adequately mandates tracheal intubation. A sustained respiratory rate greater than 40 breaths per minute may imply impending respiratory fatigue and mandates consideration of tracheal intubation. The decision to intubate patients is most frequently made based on clinical deterioration. Patients other than those intubated in association with cardiac arrest had an excellent prognosis.

An increasing arterial $Paco_2$ despite aggressive therapy is an ominous sign. Although an elevated $Paco_2$ is not an indication for intubation, an increasing $Paco_2$ despite aggressive therapy typically calls for intubation and mechanical ventilation. Nowak and colleagues showed that an elevated $Paco_2$ correlates with FEV_1 less than 25% of age-predicted values. Another sign of imminent respiratory failure is paradoxical breathing. Normally, as the diaphragm contracts, it moves caudad, and the abdomen moves out. When the diaphragm fails, it moves cephalad to fix the rib cage and assist the intercostal muscles of inspiration, and in that circumstance the abdomen moves in with inspiration. The intubation technique should be the one in which the operator feels most proficient. The largest endotracheal tube practical should be selected to decrease the degree of auto-PEEP.[93]

AEROSOL DELIVERY

Aerosol delivery in an intubated patient receiving mechanical ventilatory support poses a significant problem because the nebulized agent reaching the lung parenchyma is markedly reduced, with most of the agent deposited in the endotracheal tube, probably because of its 90-degree curve. It is important to connect the ventilator circuit nebulizer system as close to the patient as possible and to consider increasing the amount of active agent in each treatment, usually double the dose used in a nonintubated patient. An MDI with a spacer is generally accepted as being as effective in delivering bronchodilator medication in patients receiving mechanical ventilation as nebulized therapy, and it costs less. Either method may give varying delivery based on technique and ventilator and patient variables.[48]

SEDATION AND ANALGESIA

Sedation and analgesia are almost always required in preparation for intubation in a patient with a severe asthma episode. Sedation and analgesia generally should be avoided in nonintubated patients with asthma unless they are used as part of premedication for intubation. After the patient is intubated successfully and mechanical ventilation has been instituted, a combination of benzodiazepines or propofol and opioids should be administered during initial mechanical ventilator therapy.

NEUROMUSCULAR BLOCKADE

Some patients require neuromuscular blocking agents (NMBAs), especially early in their ventilatory course to control respiratory rate in the presence of life-threatening auto-PEEP and in some patients to facilitate intubation. Status asthmaticus patients receiving mechanical ventilation who are given corticosteroids and NMBAs are at risk for developing prolonged muscle weakness after discontinuation of NMBAs. This is particularly likely in patients with renal impairment, females, associated hypophosphatemia, and higher degrees of paralysis. Concomitant use of corticosteroids and NMBAs typically produces proximal and distal muscle weakness. Creatine kinase may be elevated, and myoglobinuria may be present. Steroid myopathy, by contrast, primarily involves proximal muscles, and the creatine kinase level is normal.[94]

If NMBAs are needed to initially stabilize the intubated, mechanically ventilated asthmatic (oxygenation, ventilation, and blood pressure), intermittent dosing should be used and they should be discontinued as soon as possible. In the rare patient who needs to be continuously paralyzed, infusions must be stopped every 4 to 6 hours to prevent accumulation and evaluation. A peripheral nerve stimulator should be used to limit paralysis to no less than a recording of one or two twitches in response to a train-of-four stimulus, as opposed to higher degrees of paralysis. The rationale for neuromuscular blockade is to control the respiratory rate, decrease chest wall stiffness, eliminate muscle loading from patient-ventilator dysynchrony and oxygen consumption, and lower the risk of barotrauma. These goals can often be achieved with a three-twitch or four-twitch response. If NMBAs are needed for longer than 24 hours, they should be discontinued daily to ensure patient arousal. Prolonged muscle paralysis may lead to a denervated state with an increased number of steroid receptors. The additive effect of NMBAs and steroids may be related to this finding. In patients with asthma, cisatracurium is the first-choice NMBA because it is eliminated by esterase degradation and spontaneous breakdown in the serum.[16,95-97]

INITIATING MECHANICAL VENTILATION

The strategy of mechanical ventilation is to avoid excessive airway pressures and reduce dynamic hyperinflation. To achieve this goal, it may be necessary to allow "controlled hypoventilation" or "permissive hypercapnia." Recommended initial ventilator settings are tidal volume of 8 mL/kg ideal body weight and a frequency of 10 to 14 breaths per minute, minute ventilation less than 10 L/minute, and expiratory time increased and targeted to avoid auto-PEEP and to achieve arterial oxygen saturation greater than 90%. If volume ventilation is used, peak inspiratory flow rates should be set at 60 to 80 L/minute with a decelerating waveform. The use of noncompressible tubing facilitates lowering of inspiratory time and adds to expiration time. Total volume is reduced to 6 mL/kg ideal body weight or less to achieve inspiratory plateau pressure (IPP) of 30 cm H_2O or less. The way to minimize hyperinflation is to minimize inspiratory time (inspiration-expiration ratio ≤ 1:3) while providing adequate oxygenation and ventilation, considering permissive hypercapnia in the latter case. Controlled mechanical ventilation may be required during initial ICU stay and requires heavy sedation and analgesia, or more typically sedation, analgesia, and muscle paralysis. Assisted controlled ventilation without heavy sedation or sedation/paralysis predisposes the patient to hyperinflation if the patient's breathing rate is high. Heavy sedation or sedation/paralysis reduces carbon dioxide production, facilitates measurement of end-inspiratory and end-expiratory pressures, and facilitates mechanical ventilation of severely asthmatic patients. Pressure-control ventilation is discouraged because of fluctuating high airway resistance and intrinsic PEEP. Keeping the peak alveolar pressures low (IPP of ≤30 cm H_2O) prevents overdistention of alveoli distal to the least obstructed airway.[98,99]

See Box 38.4 for a summary of general mechanical ventilation guidance in severe asthma with hyperinflation.

AUTO–POSITIVE END-EXPIRATORY PRESSURE

DEFINITION AND PREDISPOSING FACTORS

Auto-PEEP occurs when ventilator settings result in an inspiratory-to-expiratory ratio that does not allow adequate expiratory time for total exhalation of the delivered ventilator breath. Because airway obstruction increases expiratory time, mechanically ventilated asthma patients are at increased risk for auto-PEEP. After the first breath delivered in a setting conducive to auto-PEEP, the next breath is delivered before complete emptying of the first breath. With each subsequent breath that fails to empty completely, end-inspiratory and end-expiratory lung volumes increase, as do flow and pressure at end expiration. The increase in lung volume predisposes to the risk of barotraumas, and elevations of intrathoracic pressure decrease cardiac output.[100]

With volume ventilation, end-inspiratory lung volume and peak alveolar pressure increase until barotrauma occurs, the peak pressure limit alarm setting is exceeded, and total volume decreases, or equilibrium is reached. Equilibrium is established as a result of the distention-induced larger caliber of airways (reduced resistance to expiratory flow) and the increased lung recoil (caused by increased end-inspiratory lung volume), eventually allowing complete emptying of the delivered tidal volume. Equilibrium is reached, however, with significant end-expiratory flow still occurring when the next ventilator breath is delivered.

With pressure-control ventilation, the onset and worsening of acute PEEP decreases delivered tidal volume at the set applied pressure because tidal volume is determined by the ventilator system pressure that is constant and the intrathoracic pressure in the patient, which is increasing. The continued expiratory flow at end expiration represents positive pressure relative to atmospheric pressure. PEEP exists, even though it is not set on the ventilator (auto-PEEP). Auto-PEEP may be associated with significant increases in mean intrathoracic pressure. This condition may be accompanied by associated hypotension (decreased venous return to heart) and barotrauma (pneumothorax).

DIAGNOSIS AND TREATMENT

When there is no other obvious cause (e.g., tension pneumothorax), auto-PEEP should be suspected clinically in an intubated asthmatic patient who is hypotensive after institution of mechanical ventilation. A higher minute ventilation, likely to occur in assist control mode ventilation in an awake asthma patient, predisposes to auto-PEEP. Treatment of auto-PEEP is performed by decreasing total inspiratory time and is best accomplished by decreasing the rate; controlling and minimizing ventilator rate is the most important target of treatment of auto-PEEP. This requires heavy sedation in most cases and NMBAs in some, at least for a short time. Increasing expiratory time is a diagnostic and a therapeutic maneuver and the intervention of choice to treat auto-PEEP. Decreasing tidal volume also is effective but less efficient. Unless inspiratory flow rate was set inappropriately low (<80 L/minute), shortening the total inspiratory time by increasing flow rate is a less effective way of decreasing auto-PEEP and may hyperinflate areas of lung with short time constants for filling. The inspiratory-to-expiratory ratio is not a good barometer for risk for auto-PEEP. Absolute time of expiration for each breath and size of tidal volume are direct correlates of risk for and treatment of auto-PEEP. Auto-PEEP can be detected easily with graphic flow displays showing expiratory gas flow still present at the onset of the next inspiration.

Auto-PEEP can be measured with the occlusion technique or esophageal balloon technique. Occlusion of the expiratory and inspiratory circuit of the ventilator just before the onset of the next breath causes the pressure in

Box 38.4 Mechanical Ventilation Strategies[99,113]

- Goals: To control dynamic hyperinflation: use low tidal volume and respiratory rate (controlled hypoventilation with permissive hypercapnea)
- To reduce hyperinflation: use longer expiratory time and lower respiratory rate
- FIO_2 to maintain saturation ≥ 90%
- Maintain plateau pressure ≤ 30 cm H_2O
- Initiate tidal volume 8 mL/kg and may lower to 6 mL/kg
- Initial rate 10 to 12 breaths/min
- Inspiratory flow rate 80 to 100 mL/hour
- Accept lower than normal pH (permissive hypercapnia) as long as no contraindication (e.g., increased intracranial pressure)

Data from references 99 and 113.

the lungs and ventilator circuit to equilibrate. The displayed pressure represents the level of auto-PEEP. With the esophageal balloon technique, the negative deflection in esophageal pressure (representing pleural pressure) from the onset of inspiratory effort to the onset of inspiratory flow represents both the inspiratory muscle pressure necessary to counterbalance the end-expiratory elastic recoil of the respiratory system and the amount of auto-PEEP. Auto-PEEP (intrinsic positive end-expiratory pressure) is measured as the negative delflecton of the esophageal pressure (Pes) from the onset of inspiratory effort to the point of zero flow.

In the absence of an esophageal balloon device, the ability to reflect accurately the auto-PEEP–related pressure at the alveolar level in an intubated patient depends on a prolonged end-expiratory hold (3 to 4 seconds) and the absence of patient inspiratory or expiratory effort during measurement. This measurement is unlikely to be accurate unless the patient is heavily sedated or sedated/paralyzed. Unless full equilibration to a no-flow state is allowed at end inspiration with the system closed to the ventilator, the auto-PEEP level exerted at the alveolar level is typically underestimated. The typical end-expiratory hold used in clinical practice of 0.4 to 1 second is less likely to provide a reliable measurement.

INCREASED WORK OF BREATHING WITH AUTO–POSITIVE END-EXPIRATORY PRESSURE

Auto-PEEP in the presence of assisted ventilation modes (assist control and synchronized intermittent mandatory ventilation) implies that the patient must initiate gas flow by producing an inspiratory effort equal to not only the sensitivity setting of inspiratory triggering, but also the level of auto-PEEP. Extrinsic PEEP normally has no indication, however, in acute severe asthma during controlled mechanical ventilation. If it is not advantageous or possible to eliminate auto-PEEP in the patient with assisted ventilation modes, applying or increasing ventilator-set PEEP to a level slightly below total PEEP would decrease patient effort necessary to trigger the ventilator breath. Inappropriately set ventilator PEEP offers additional risks to the patient, and this approach is recommended only by health care professionals well schooled in the intricacies of mechanical ventilation.[98]

BAROTRAUMA

The risk for barotrauma in an intubated asthma patient correlates best with peak alveolar pressure as estimated by IPP. The amounts of measured auto-PEEP and peak inspiratory pressures are less reliable predictors. Peak inspiratory pressure, although correlating to some degree with IPP and end-inspiratory lung volume, also reflects resistance in the endotracheal tube and tracheobronchial tree, which may be considerable in the presence of a small endotracheal tube, airway secretions, mucosal thickening, and bronchoconstriction.

In a heavily sedated or sedated/paralyzed patient, IPP measurement is the best means for estimating peak alveolar pressure and the best indicator of hyperinflation and risk for barotraumas because closure of airways toward the end of expiration may lead to underestimation of hyperinflation. In the presence of normal chest wall and abdominal compliance factors, an IPP equal to or greater than 30 cm H_2O puts the patient at risk for exceeding maximal alveolar size (total lung capacity). Decreases in IPP are usually accomplished by using low tidal volumes and minimizing auto-PEEP. In a paralyzed patient, the collection of the total exhaled volume of gas obtainable with 20 to 60 seconds of apnea allows the measurement of end-inspired volume above apnea functional residual capacity. This volume may be 3 L despite the use of small tidal volumes.[101,102]

Because high IPP is reduced by lowering tidal volume, a reduction in the tidal volume directly decreases the risk for barotraumas, as does any maneuver that decreases auto-PEEP. If, after heavy sedation or sedation/paralysis, the IPP remains 30 cm H_2O or greater despite decreases in tidal volume to the lowest value that allows an acceptable pH, typically greater than or equal to 7.20, the use of bicarbonate infusion to allow acceptable pH with further reduction of tidal volume may be considered.[103]

The concept of reducing the tidal volume and accepting a higher $Pa{CO_2}$ and lower pH is called *permissive hypercapnia.* Permissive hypercapnia is relatively safe in asthma and well tolerated in the absence of contraindications, such as increased intracranial hypertension and pregnancy. Physicians are uncomfortable with allowing $Pa{CO_2}$ to become greater than 80 to 100 mm Hg, but several case reports described short durations of hypercapnia (>150 mm Hg) as well tolerated, and one report described $Pa{CO_2}$ of 200 mm Hg for 10 hours with no consequences reported. Permissive hypercapnia limits volutrauma and hemodynamic consequences of increased intrathoracic pressures. In normoxic states, acute hypercapnia has limited potential for inducing severe intracellular acidosis. If permissive hypercapnia results in pH less than 7.2, increased sedation and paralysis and methods of decreasing carbon dioxide production, such as reducing fever, overfeeding, and patient effort, should be considered. In the absence of tissue hypoperfusion or volume overload, iatrogenic compensation for acute respiratory acidosis with intravenous bicarbonate administration is appropriate. In severe acidosis, large amounts of bicarbonate may be necessary to elevate the pH substantially, potentially leading to volume overload.[104-107]

Permissive hypercapnia should be considered in the mechanically ventilated asthmatics with life-threatening asthma, severe hyperinflation, and inability to achieve a satisfactory IPP without producing an unacceptable acidemia. Permissive hypercapnia is well tolerated in most patients, even when $Pa{CO_2}$ is 90 mm Hg (12 kPa), as long as pH remains greater than or equal to 7.20. It should be avoided, however, in the presence of increased intracranial pressure and clinically significant myocardial dysfunction and during pregnancy to avoid fetal distress.

NON-INVASIVE POSITIVE-PRESSURE VENTILATION

Noninvasive positive-pressure ventilation (NPPV) is a safe treatment and can reduce the need for intubation in a selected group of patients with severe asthma and hypercapnia who fail to improve with initial medical management. Fernandez and colleagues further describe that the rationale for NPPV in severe asthma is its potential for improving alveolar ventilation, decreasing the risk of respiratory muscle fatigue. Mask continuous positive airway pressure (CPAP)

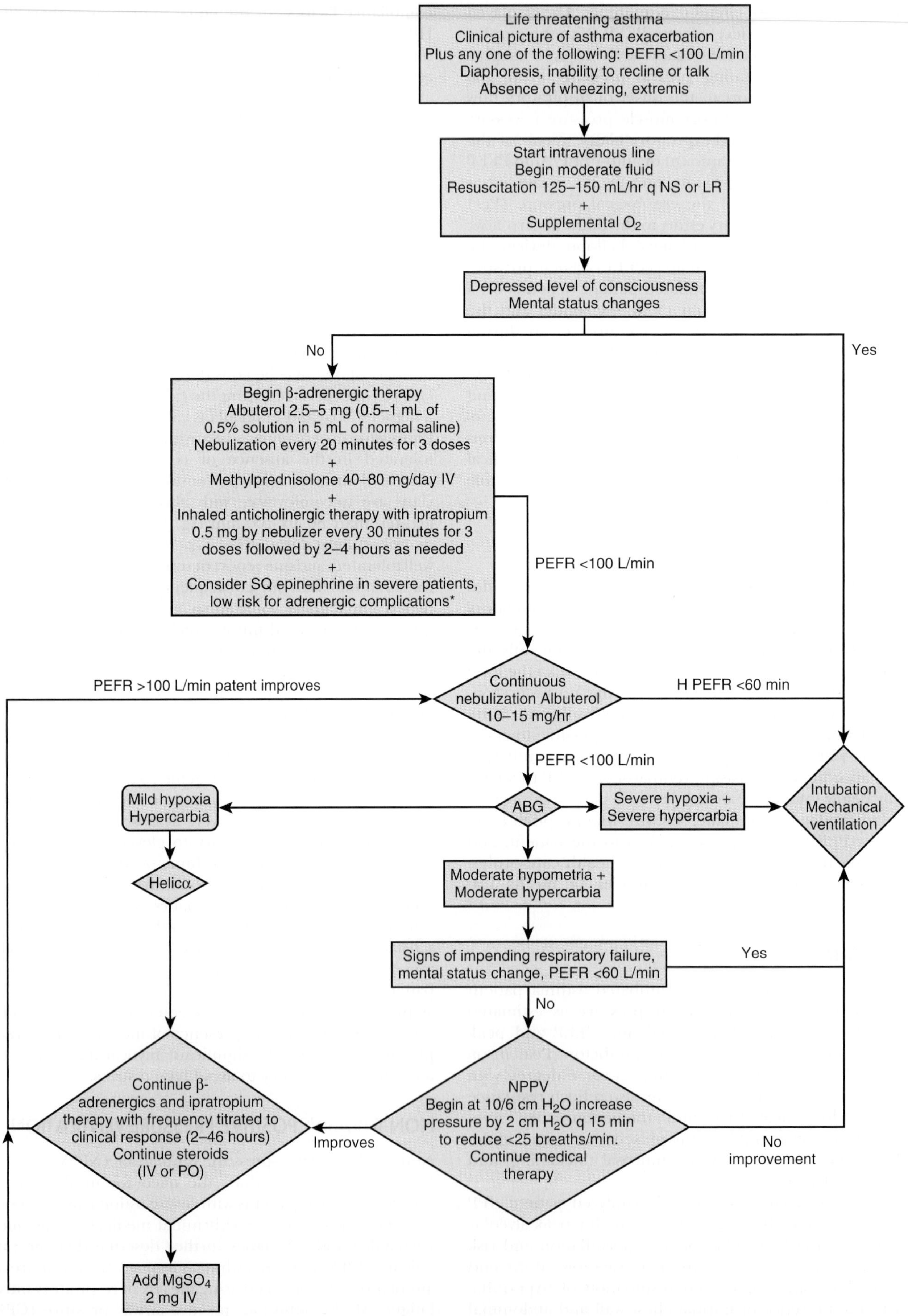

Figure 38.1 Approach to acute life-threatening asthma. *Check for hypokalemia and treat. ABG, arterial blood gas; LR, lactated Ringer's solution; NPPV, non-invasive positive-pressure ventilation; NS, normal saline; PEFR, peak expiratory flow rate.

Box 38.5 Contraindications for Non-invasive Positive-Pressure Ventilation

Uncooperative or obtunded patients
Hemodynamic instability
Cardiac or respiratory arrest
Encephalopathy
Facial surgery or deformity
High risk for aspiration
Nonrespiratory organ failure
Severe upper gastrointestinal bleeding
Unstable arrhythmia
Upper airway obstruction

From Stather DR, Stewart TE: Clinical review: Mechanical ventilation in severe asthma. Crit Care 2005;9:581-587.

produces bronchodilation and decreases the airway resistance, reverses atelectasis, and promotes removal of secretions. The work of the diaphragm and the inspiratory muscles is reduced, and intrinsic PEEP may be offset. In addition, CPAP decreases the adverse hemodynamic effects of large negative inspiratory swings in pleural pressure, which compromise right and left ventricular performance. NPPV potentially may enhance delivery of inhaled β-agonists. One study showed a small but statistically significant greater improvement in PEFR when NPPV was used for initial β-agonist delivery. A nonrandomized study by Meduri and associates reported a reduction in $Paco_2$ and improvement in dyspnea with the use of NPPV in 17 episodes of asthma with acute respiratory failure.[108-111]

CPAP, as opposed to NPPV, has been studied in asthmatic patients after induction of bronchospasm with aerosolized histamine. CPAP of 12 cm H_2O increased the minimal pleural pressure and decreased swings in transdiaphragmatic pressure. Although ventilation increased, the inspiratory work per liter decreased significantly, as did the pressure time product for the inspiratory muscles. Functional residual capacity increased slightly. The authors concluded that CPAP produced a load on the inspiratory muscles, improving their efficiency and decreasing the energy cost of inspiration. Despite the potential for benefit of NPPV or CPAP in selected patients in severe acute asthma, it should be used with caution pending controlled clinical trials. Ram and colleagues[112] also concluded in a Cochrane analysis that application of NPPV in status asthmaticus, despite some promising preliminary results, remains controversial. The need for endotracheal intubation in acute severe asthma has decreased after the introduction of NPPV as shown by a retrospective cohort study. If NPPV is used, initial setting should be an expiratory positive airway pressure (CPAP or PEEP) of about 5 cm H_2O and inspiratory pressure (or pressure support) of approximately 8 cm H_2O. If tidal volumes are shallow (<7 mL/kg), inspiratory pressure can be increased gradually by 2 cm H_2O every 15 minutes, to a goal to reduce the respiratory rate to less than 25 breaths per minute. Peak pressures greater than 15 to 20 cm H_2O rarely can be tolerated without mask leaks or discomfort or claustrophobia.[19] See Box 38.5 for contraindications for NPPV.[108-114]

Box 38.6 Complications of Acute Severe Asthma

Pneumothorax
Pneumomediastinum
Subcutaneous emphysema
Pneumopericardium
Tracheoesophageal fistula (mechanically ventilated patients)
Myocardial ischemia (coronary artery disease patients)
Mucous plugging and atelectasis
Theophylline toxicity
Lactic acidosis
Electrolyte disturbances—hypokalemia, hypophosphatemia, hypomagnesemia
Myopathy
Anoxic brain injury

From Papiris S, Kotanidou A, Malagari K, et al: Clinical review: Severe asthma. Crit Care 2002;6:30-44.

COMPLICATIONS OF ASTHMA

See Box 38.6 for complications of asthma.

APPROACH TO ACUTE LIFE-THREATENING ASTHMA

Figure 38.1 is an algorithm that shows the approach to acute life-threatening asthma.

KEY POINTS

- The cause of respiratory arrest in asthmatic patients is usually failure of the inspiratory muscles with ventilatory arrest.
- Ominous signs and findings in a patient with acute severe asthma, if not quickly reversed, include diaphoresis, inability to recline, inability to talk, increased $PaCO_2$, PEF less than 60 L/minute or FEV less than 25% of personal best or predicted values, and use of accessory muscles.
- Pathophysiology of asthma consists of three key abnormalities: bronchoconstriction, airway inflammation, and mucous impaction.
- The *ADAM33* gene is significantly associated with asthma.
- Inhaled β_2-agonists are the cornerstone of medical therapy for hospitalized severe asthmatics. The addition of steroids is recommended.
- Adequate delivery of β-agonists can be accomplished by use of an MDI with a spacer during acute bronchospasm if proper technique is used and doses are increased. It is advisable to deliver the β-agonist by nebulization in most acutely ill asthma patients

Continued on following page

Table 38.3 Treatments Not Recommended in Acute Severe Asthma

Intervention/Agent Not Recommended	Comments
Methylxanthines: aminophylline, theophylline	Not recommended in acute severe asthma Use only in patients not responding to standard treatment and refractory Possible treatment adjunct in patients with "steroid-resistant" asthma or those already taking a methylxanthine (Tf)
Antibiotics	Antibiotics indicated only in patients with evidence of pneumonia or sinusitis or fever and purulent sputum
Aggressive hydration	Assess fluid status and appropriate hydration in intubated patients
Chest physical therapy	Not beneficial and stressful to the patient
Mucolytics: acetylcysteine, potassium iodide	May worsen airflow obstruction or cough
Sedation	Avoid anxiolytics and sedatives in nonintubated patients
Long-acting β-agonists: salmeterol, formoterol	No data available on acute severe asthma

From National Heart, Lung, and Blood Institute and National Asthma Education and Prevention Program Expert Panel Report 3: Guidelines for the Diagnosis and Management of Asthma. Full report. NIH Publication No. 08-5846. Bethesda, MD, National Institutes of Health, 2007.

KEY POINTS (Continued)

because nebulization requires minimal coordination and cooperation of the patient and less bedside instruction and supervision by health care professionals.

- Larger doses and more frequent dosing intervals for inhaled β-agonist therapy are needed in acute severe asthma because of decreased deposition at the site of action (low tidal volumes and narrowed airways), alteration in dose-response curve, and altered duration of activity. Continuous nebulization is an option.
- Theophylline is not recommended for general use in hospitalized patients with acute asthma (Table 38.3). Intravenous magnesium is recommended for the most severe asthma attacks.
- Although there is no proven value of systemic therapy over aerosol therapy, rapid delivery of β-agonists to the airway may be beneficial in seriously ill asthmatic patients who are at imminent risk for respiratory arrest or need intubation and who are at low risk for β-agonist cardiac toxicity (young asthmatics). In these patients, a combination of inhaled and subcutaneously administered β-agonists in this circumstance may be useful.
- If NMBAs are used, attempts to withdraw these agents over the first 24 to 48 hours after intubation are advised.
- Auto-PEEP is treated by decreasing total inspiratory time. Increasing expiratory time is best accomplished by decreasing rate. Decreasing tidal volume also is effective. Prolonging expiratory time is a diagnostic and a therapeutic maneuver.
- The concept of reducing the tidal volume to decrease alveolar inflation and accepting a higher $PaCO_2$ and lower pH is called permissive hypercapnia and should be considered in asthma patients undergoing mechanical ventilation therapy with life-threatening asthma, severe hyperinflation, and high IPP.

SELECTED REFERENCES

13. National Heart, Lung, and Blood Institute and National Asthma Education and Prevention Program Expert Panel Report 3: Guidelines for the Diagnosis and Management of Asthma Full report. NIH Publication No. 08-5846. Bethesda, MD, National Institutes of Health, 2007.
16. Rodrigo GJ, Rodrigo C, Hall JB: Acute asthma in adults: A review. Chest 2004;125:1081-1102.
25. National Asthma Education and Prevention Program: Expert Panel Report: Guidelines for the Diagnosis and Management of Asthma: Update on Selected Topics 2002. NIH publication No. 02-5074. Bethesda, MD, National Institutes of Health, 2003, p 122.
37. Kim M, Cho Y, Moon H, Cho S: Factors for poor prognosis of near-fatal asthma after recovery from a life threatening asthma attack. Korean J Intern Med 2008;23(4):170-175.
40. American Heart Association Guidelines for Cardiopulmonary Resuscitation and Emergency Cardiovascular Care: Part 10.5: Near fatal asthma. Circulation 2005;112:1-142.
52. Manser R, Reid D, Abramson M: Corticosteroids for acute severe asthma in hospitalized patients. Cochrane Database Syst Rev 2001;(1):CD001740.
60. Rowe BH, Bretzlaff JA, Bourdon C, et al: Magnesium sulfate for treating exacerbations of acute severe asthma in the emergency department. Cochrane Database Syst Rev 2000; CD001490.
62. Rodrigo GA, Rodrigo C, Pollack CV, et al: Use of helium-oxygen mixture in the treatment of acute asthma: A systematic review. Chest 2003;123:891-896.
68. Stather DR, Stewart TE: Clinical review: Mechanical ventilation in severe asthma. Crit Care 2005;9:581-587.
70. Holgate ST, Chuchalin AG, Hebert J, et al: Efficacy and safety of a recombinant anti-immunoglobulin E antibody in severe allergic asthma. Clin Exp Allergy 2004;34:632-638.
92. Quick Reference from the Working Group Report on Managing Asthma during Pregnancy: Recommendations for Pharmacologic Treatment Update 2004. NIH publication No. 05-3279. Bethesda, MD, National Institutes of Health, 2004.
98. Oddo M, Feihl F, Schaller MD, et al: Management of mechanical ventilation in acute severe asthma: Practical aspects. Intensive Care Med 2006;32:501-510.
106. Mutlu GM, Factor P, Schwartz DE, et al: Severe status asthmaticus: Management with permissive hypercapnia and inhalation anesthesia. Crit Care Med 2002;30:477-480.
112. Ram FS, Wellington S, Rowe B, et al: Non-invasive positive pressure ventilation for treatment of respiratory failure due to severe acute exacerbations of asthma. Cochrane Database Syst Rev 2005;(3):CD004360.

113. Mannam P, Siegel MD: Analytic review: Management of life threatening asthma in adults. J Intensive Care Med 2010;25:3.
114. Murase K, Tomii K, Chin K, et al: The use of noninvasive ventilation for life threatening asthma attacks: Changes in the need for intubation. Respirology 2010;15:714-720.
115. Lugogo NL, MacIntyre NR: Life threatening asthma: Pathophysiology and management. Respir Care 2008;53(6):726-739.

The complete list of references can be found at www.expertconsult.com.

39 Chronic Obstructive Pulmonary Disease

Guillermo Domínguez-Cherit | Juan Gabriel Posadas-Calleja

CHAPTER OUTLINE

In 1997, the U.S. National Heart Lung and Blood Institute and the World Health Organization held an international workshop that led to the first Global Initiative on Obstructive Lung Disease (GOLD) report. The most recent iteration of the GOLD guidelines defines chronic obstructive pulmonary disease (COPD) as a preventable and treatable disease with some significant extrapulmonary effects that may contribute to the severity in individual patients. Its pulmonary component is characterized by chronic airflow limitation that is not fully reversible. The airflow limitation is usually both progressive and associated with abnormal inflammatory response of the lungs to noxious particles and gases.[1]

DEFINITIONS

Although controversies remain over the definition of exacerbation, how they should be monitored, and their underlying mechanisms, acute exacerbations of COPD (AECOPD) are major and increasingly recognized events in the disease course. They typically occur one to three times per year. Exacerbations are associated with an increase in economic burden[2] and a decline in health-related quality of life.[3] Those patients with more than two exacerbations per year have significantly worse health-related complications and decline in lung function than those with two or fewer exacerbations.[4] As mentioned before, there is no general agreement on the definition of AECOPD, but it has been defined according to the presence of specific signs and symptoms, worsening in symptoms, and the need for medical intervention, and each of these approaches has positive and negative connotations. It is well recognized, however, that the presence of increased shortness of breath, increased sputum volume, and increased purulence are the three specific symptoms that represent an exacerbation.[5]

BACKGROUND

COPD affects more than 200 million people worldwide and is the fourth leading cause of death. COPD is a disease that is both preventable and treatable. COPD is a major cause of morbidity and death in the world, with an increasing burden due to epidemiologic changes that expose more of the population to COPD risk factors. Although the major environmental risk for COPD is tobacco smoking, only 20% of smokers develop COPD. Indoor air pollution from burning biomass fuel is associated with increased risk of COPD in developing countries. In the United States, COPD is the fourth leading cause of death[6] and is exceeded only by heart attacks, cancer, and stroke.

COPD has had a similar effect on health and mortality rate throughout the developed and underdeveloped sectors of the world, and many of the important issues surrounding COPD in the United States apply elsewhere.[7]

The real prevalence is masked by the burden of undiagnosed COPD; when the British Lung Foundation "missing millions" campaign performed spirometry screening in 3802 adults, they found that the prevalence of COPD was 10.2% (4.4% having GOLD II or worse) with only a quarter having a prior diagnosis.[8]

PATHOPHYSIOLOGY

The main pathophysiologic feature in COPD is the limitation to expiratory flow.[9] Chronic expiratory flow limitation and hyperinflation are the mechanical hallmarks of COPD.[10] Expiratory airflow limitation results from many factors; among them, narrowing of the peripheral airways,[11] mucus hypersecretion,[12] and impaired ciliary clearance[13] are the most important factors.

Several mechanistic concepts have been implicated in the pathogenesis of COPD. First, the hallmark of COPD is development of exaggerated chronic inflammation in the lung in response to inhalation of cigarette smoke compared with smokers without lung disease.[14] Host factors including genetic susceptibility, epigenetic changes, and oxidative stress contribute by amplifying inflammation induced by cigarette smoke. Second, patients with deficiency of α_1-antitrypsin, the main inhibitor of neutrophil elastase, develop emphysema early in life owing to an increase in proteolytic activity.[15] Third, an imbalance between oxidants and antioxidants in the lungs of patients with COPD, resulting in excessive oxidative stress, not only amplifies airway inflammation in smokers but also induces cell death of structural cells in the lung. Disruption of the balance between cell death and replenishment of structural cells in the lung contributes to the destruction of alveolar septa, leading to emphysema.[16] Autoimmunity has been proposed as a late pathogenic event in the progressive course of the disease.

COPD is characterized by a specific pattern of inflammation involving increased numbers of $CD8^+$ T_C lymphocytes present only in smokers who develop the disease. These cells as well as neutrophils and macrophages release inflammatory mediators and interact with epithelial cells in the airways, lung parenchyma, and pulmonary endothelium; all these relationships and interactions produce structural changes in the lungs by activation of growth factors.[17] Changes in the airway architecture, endothelium, and lung parenchyma lead to the characteristic physiologic abnormalities and symptoms of COPD.

In acute exacerbations there is an increase in sputum neutrophil numbers as well as an increase in neutrophils in bronchial biopsies, which rarely are seen in the stable state.[18] Interestingly virally induced exacerbations are associated with increased expression of eosinophils in sputum. Viral infections induce the expression of chemokine (C-C motif) ligand 5 (CCL5) in airway epithelial cells,[19] CCL5 may act synergistically with $CD8^+$ cells to enhance the apoptosis of virally infected cells, thus leading to increased tissue destruction.[20] Also, an increase in the concentration of the elastolytic enzyme matrix metalloproteinase-1 during exacerbations is consistent with evidence of elastolysis, which may provide a causal link between exacerbations and accelerated decline in lung function.[21]

Data from patients with AECOPD that required mechanical ventilation indicates the presence of increased central drive, dyspnea, tachypnea, reduced tidal volume, and development of hypercapnic respiratory failure, but ventilation/perfusion match remains relatively preserved.[22] AECOPD appears to be characterized by increased central drive, decreased inspiratory capacity, and decreased inspiratory muscle force, perhaps secondary to dynamic hyperinflation. There is an association between increased serum levels of interleukin 6 (IL-6) and leukotriene B4 (LTB4) and the magnitude of dyspnea, respiratory rate, and inspiratory capacity, suggesting that it may be possible to detect serum changes that reflect the inflammatory burden of the exacerbation.[23]

Although hypercapnia depends on the severity of airflow limitation, there is considerable variability in the relationship of Pa_{CO_2} to forced expiratory volume in 1 second (FEV_1) and total lung resistance, best explained by contribution of dead space and minute ventilation. In stable COPD patients with severe airflow obstruction, shallow breathing is the main factor associated with CO_2 retention,[24] the diaphragm is less effective than in normal subjects, and with increasing airflow obstruction and hyperinflation, the contribution of the rib cage muscle to the generation of ventilatory pressure increases.[25] Abdominal muscles are recruited during expiration in patients with severe COPD, and the expiratory rise in gastric pressure is directly related to intrinsic positive end-expiratory pressure (PEEPi). During acute exacerbation, patients with severe airflow obstruction increase the inspiratory recruitment of the rib cage muscles relative to the diaphragm. This recruitment is associated with abdominal muscle contraction and a reduction in abdominal volume at end expiration, which contributes to PEEPi. Dynamic hyperinflation can be overestimated during chronic and acute airway obstruction if abdominal muscle function is not evaluated.[26]

The worsening gas exchange and the deterioration of the arterial blood gas values during acute exacerbations in patients with severe COPD can be explained by several factors. These factors are, in no particular order, respiratory muscle fatigue,[27] increases in dead space ventilation, and alveolar hypoventilation.[28] Minute ventilation may be normal early in an exacerbation, but the respiratory rate is generally increased. There is an associated increase in physiologic dead space that impairs CO_2 elimination and may result in acidemia.[29] The hypoxemia seen during exacerbations results from the combination of two factors: alveolar hypoventilation and, later, worsening of ventilation/perfusion matching. Increases in ventilation/perfusion heterogeneity are attributed to (1) a reduction in the effectiveness of hypoxic vasoconstriction as a protective mechanism as pulmonary artery pressure rises and vasodilatory inflammatory mediators are released, and (2) the failure to redirect perfusion away from inadequately ventilated regions because of the reduction in cross-sectional area of the pulmonary vascular bed.

Box 39.1 Clinical Signs of Acute Exacerbations of Chronic Obstructive Pulmonary Disease

Increasing cough
Worsening dyspnea
Increased sputum production
Purulent sputum

CLINICAL MANIFESTATIONS

Most COPD patients with acute exacerbations initially demonstrate some combination of increasing cough, worsening of dyspnea, increased sputum production, purulent sputum, or increase in viscosity of the sputum, rather than a deterioration noted by laboratory or respiratory function parameters (Box 39.1). Symptoms may come on slowly over several days or acutely, depending somewhat on the severity of the underlying disease. Often, patients have a history of upper respiratory tract infection. Patients generally appear in acute distress. Vital signs typically demonstrate tachycardia and tachypnea, and blood pressure can be reduced in response to the effect of PEEPi. Use of accessory inspiratory muscles may be seen with increasing severity of exacerbations. With inspiration, the diaphragm normally moves down as it contracts, forcing the abdominal contents out. With diaphragmatic fatigue, the diaphragm no longer functions as a primary muscle of inspiration but instead assists the intercostal muscles' inspiratory effort by fixing the rib cage. This action is associated with a rise in the diaphragm, and the abdomen moves in instead of out, as it does with normal inspiration. This sign is called *paradoxical breathing*[28] and it implies respiratory muscle fatigue and often imminent ventilatory failure and respiratory arrest.[29] Wheezing and other auscultatory findings of obstruction are also present. Cyanosis is an insensitive manifestation, but when seen, it denotes severe hypoxemia. Patients with severe acute CO_2 retention may present in coma.

PRECIPITATING FACTORS

The most common precipitant factor is respiratory infection, either bacterial or viral.[30,31] Air pollution can also precipitate exacerbations of COPD[32,33]; however, the cause of one third of AECOPD events cannot be identified. Some other conditions that can ether mimic or induce an exacerbation include pneumonia, arrhythmia, pneumothorax, pulmonary embolism,[34] and pleural effusion. Medication failure and lack of compliance have been shown also to lead to exacerbations.

INFECTIONS

Bacteria and viruses account for the vast majority of episodes of exacerbation. Respiratory viruses are associated with 30% of exacerbations with or without a superimposed bacterial infection.[35] Another study reported that up to 78% of the patients admitted into the hospital with severe AECOPD had evidence of viral or bacterial infection.[19]

Several studies have been conducted to investigate airway bacterial infections as etiologic factors involved in COPD exacerbations.[36-38] Bronchoscopic sampling of the distal airway has demonstrated the presence of pathogenic bacteria in 50% of exacerbations. Acquisition of new strains of bacterial pathogens has been associated with more than twofold increase in the risk of AECOPD.[39] At present, there appears to be an agreement that the major pathogens isolated from sputum during acute exacerbation are *Haemophilus influenzae, Streptococcus pneumoniae,* and *Moraxella catarrhalis*[40]; however, all of these bacteria can be isolated in patients during the stable phases of COPD.[41,42] Atypical bacteria, mostly *Chlamydia pneumoniae,* have been implicated in approximately 10% of acute exacerbations.[43,44] Other potential microorganisms that should be considered include other *Streptococcus* species, enteric gram-negative bacilli, and *Legionella.*[45] Bacterial colonization may be a factor increasing airway inflammation.[46] There is an association between bacterial colonization and increased markers of inflammation in sputum and in the frequency of exacerbations.[47]

Approximately 50% of AECOPD events are associated with upper respiratory tract virus infections. Infections with rhinovirus, respiratory syncytial virus, and influenza virus have been associated with AECOPD.[48] COPD patients with a history of frequent exacerbations may be more susceptible to respiratory viral infections. There is increasing recognition that many patients with exacerbations have concomitant viral and bacterial infection. Approximately a quarter of patients admitted to hospital with AECOPD have coinfection with viruses and bacteria, and those patients have more severe exacerbations.[48]

ENVIRONMENTAL FACTORS

Environmental factors are among noninfectious causes of COPD exacerbation that should be investigated as precipitating causes.[32,49,50] Epidemiologic studies have shown that hospital admissions with AECOPD increase slightly with a rise in atmospheric levels of sulfur dioxide, ozone, nitrogen dioxide, and particulates. There is convincing evidence that exposure to particulates with a 50% cutoff aerodynamic diameter of 10 μm is associated with increased hospital admissions for AECOPD.[51] Air pollution is implicated as a trigger of exacerbations[52]; however, a direct cause-and-effect relationship has been difficult to establish over the last 50 years.[53] From an epidemiologic viewpoint, definitive evidence exists regarding a role of air pollutants in the increased death rates seen in cities during periods of heavy pollution.[54] The recent dramatic increase in motor vehicle traffic has produced a relative increase in the levels of newer pollutants, such as ozone and fine-particulate air pollution. Elucidation of the mechanisms of the harmful effects of these pollutants should allow improved risk assessment for the patients with airway diseases who are susceptible to the effects of these air pollutants.

PULMONARY THROMBOEMBOLISM

Pulmonary thromboembolism (PTE) can precipitate acute COPD exacerbations through either impairment of gas exchange or increases in pulmonary vascular pressures.[55,56] Some evidence suggests that deep venous thrombosis occurs in more than 5 million people each year. More than 500,000 people eventually develop PTE, which is the primary cause of death in more than 100,000 patients annually in the United States.[57] The precise incidence of PTE in COPD is unknown. Studies in COPD patients have found pulmonary embolus in up to 50% of autopsies and in patients admitted to hospital with severe AECOPD of unknown cause; 25% had pulmonary embolism confirmed by spiral computed tomography (CT).[58] PTE risk factors inherent to COPD are sedentary lifestyle, right ventricular failure, right ventricular mural thrombi, and secondary polycythemia.[59] Patients with COPD have also been shown to have increased platelet aggregation and increased plasma β-thromboglobulin.[60]

Up to 30% of untreated thromboembolic patients die. The necessity of diagnosing PTE as the precipitating factor in acute COPD exacerbation is crucial. However, the diagnosis of PTE is extremely difficult in COPD exacerbation. Nonetheless, the approach to diagnosis is similar to that used with other patients.[61] Unfortunately, most patients with COPD have an indeterminate ventilation/perfusion scan, usually making this scan unhelpful in evaluation for PTE.[62] For patients with such indeterminate results (low or intermediate probability), noninvasive testing of the lower extremity should be conducted.[63-65] If positive results for deep venous thrombosis are obtained, anticoagulation therapy must be initiated. It has been proposed that use of newer D-dimer assays may also have a role as a diagnostic tool; however, even with a sensitivity of 98%, specificity is problematic, with a value of 39%.[66] When the diagnosis is still in doubt (intermediate-probability scan and negative leg study or low-probability scan and negative leg study with intermediate clinical probability of PTE), helical CT or conventional pulmonary angiography may be required. Even though the safety of pulmonary angiography in patients with cor pulmonale has been questioned, data from the Prospective Investigation of Pulmonary Embolism Diagnosis (PIOPED) study support both safety and accuracy in patients with COPD.[61] Helical CT has become an increasingly accepted technique and is the method of choice for direct visualization of pulmonary emboli (PE). The quantitative assessment of tissue perfusion may yield more important information for patient management than the direct visualization of emboli by CT alone. Enhanced multislice helical CT with thin collimation can be used to analyze precisely the subsegmental pulmonary arteries and may identify even more distal pulmonary arteries. Recent data suggest that spiral CT may be an alternative to angiography, particularly when results are not discordant with pretest clinical probability of PE and when combined with other tests that support CT findings (D-dimer, leg ultrasound, lung scanning), and may have adequate sensitivity and specificity in the COPD population.[62]

MEDICATION FAILURE OR NONCOMPLIANCE

Many acute COPD exacerbations can be explained in terms of inadequate pharmacologic therapy or noncompliance with pharmacologic therapy. These factors are likely underestimated causes of exacerbation in COPD patients. It is also possible that patients have toxic drug effects of cardiac, gastrointestinal, or metabolic nature. Certain pharmacologic drug interactions can precipitate toxicity or loss of effect of one drug, and the physician must ascertain whether newer medications for other conditions have recently been added to the patient's therapeutic regimen.[67,68]

OTHER CAUSES

Clinical decompensation in patients with stable COPD may also occur as a result of acute congestive heart failure (CHF) or cardiac arrhythmia. One study found that 27% of COPD patients die as a result of coronary disease,[69] likely related to risk factors such as smoking, diabetes mellitus, and vasculopathy. Heart failure may also lead to a symptomatic exacerbation of COPD; however, it may be difficult to differentiate the symptoms of CHF and those of AECOPD.[70]

Other causes of exacerbation include sleep-disordered breathing,[71-73] vocal cord paralysis, tumor or scarring from prior intubations, and the development of spontaneous pneumothorax.[74,75] Finally, pleural effusion can also produce respiratory deterioration, especially in patients with poor respiratory reserve.[76]

INITIAL MANAGEMENT

Because chronic airflow obstruction cannot be reversed, acute management of COPD is directed at reversible pathogenic mechanisms, including pulmonary infection, airway tissue inflammation, bronchoconstriction, and support of failing muscular function. Box 39.2 summarizes initial general management.

OXYGEN

Long-term oxygen treatment has been demonstrated to significantly reduce mortality rate in patients with COPD and severe resting arterial hypoxemia.[77] Oxygen therapy is indicated for patients with an arterial oxygen tension (Pa_{O_2}) of less than 55 mm Hg. The therapeutic goal is to maintain oxygen saturation greater than 90% during rest, sleep, and exertion, as it is now well established that such measures increase survival and that 24 hours is more effective than 12 hours. There is a clear rationale for the use of oxygen in severe COPD. Enhancing blood oxygenation by increasing the concentration of inspired oxygen compensates for a major physiologic consequence of COPD with hypoxemia. Oxygen remains the mainstay of initial therapy in most COPD exacerbations. Relief of hypoxemia, and

Box 39.2 General Management of Acute Exacerbations of Chronic Obstructive Pulmonary Disease

Adjust O_2 to Sp_{O_2} goal 88% to 92%
Initiate and maintain β-agonist and anticholinergic agents combined
Start prednisone 50 mg/day for 7 days
Start antibiotics if signs of infection

consequently of hypoxemic pulmonary vasoconstriction, decreases pulmonary vascular resistance, with variable effects on the ventilation/perfusion ratio.[78,79] Oxygen delivery may increase as a result of increases in oxygen arterial content and anticipated improved right-sided heart function. However, one study demonstrated that relief of hypoxemia did not increase cardiac output.[80]

Hypercapnia is well tolerated when it is chronic.[81-83] However, oxygen should be administered cautiously in patients who are chronically hypercapnic because it is known to lead to clinically significant rises in $Pa{CO_2}$ in select COPD patients as a result of changes in the physiologic dead space and perhaps suppression of the respiratory drive.[84,85] Acute increases in $Pa{CO_2}$ are more likely to occur in patients with elevated baseline $Pa{CO_2}$. A randomized study has shown that, although oxygen administration worsened hypercapnia and respiratory acidosis, these changes were well tolerated in most patients.[86] Oxygen therapy should not be withheld in acutely ill hypoxemic patients because tissue hypoxia can lead to acute organ dysfunction. However, oxygen should be initiated at a low $F{IO_2}$ and slowly titrated up as necessary with vigilant monitoring to document improvement and stabilization in $Pa{O_2}$, with special attention paid to maintaining the oxyhemoglobin between 88% and 92% or greater without producing dangerous falls in pH as a result of rises in CO_2. These dangerous rises in $Pa{CO_2}$ are typically associated with worsening mental status. Nasal cannulas or Venturi masks can be used to initiate a low $F{IO_2}$. Either nasal cannula at a flow rate of 1 L/minute or a Venturi mask initially at the lowest setting (25%) is appropriate for initiating oxygen in patients known or suspected to be chronic CO_2 retainers. However, in the presence of acute severe hypoxemia in patients with impending respiratory failure, high-flow oxygen therapy may be in the patient's best interest, regardless of the risk for CO_2 retention.[87]

DRUG TREATMENT

BRONCHODILATORS

Bronchodilator therapy has important roles in both the prevention and treatment of AECOPD. Bronchodilators are the primary treatment to alleviate patient symptoms, improve physiologic state, and prevent or reverse respiratory failure; however, its use has not been shown to improve survival. Systematic reviews have demonstrated that inhaled delivery of short-acting β_2-selective agonists and anticholinergic agents have greater effect on spirometry and is the therapy of choice for AECOPD over parenteral bronchodilators.[88] Bronchodilator treatment in acutely ill COPD patients has been shown to decrease inspiratory muscle loading, with an increase in FEV_1 and a decrease in functional residual capacity (FRC) and dynamic hyperinflation.[89] In mechanically ventilated patients, a reduction in expiratory resistance and dynamic hyperinflation (measured as a decrease in PEEPi) has been described.[90]

There is no evidence supporting the use of one inhaled β_2-selective agonist over another. There is no difference in outcome between β_2-agonist compared with ipratropium bromide and no evidence that the combination of these two drugs is any more effective in AECOPD; these results are in contrast with the greater efficacy of these combinations in stable COPD.[88] The widespread use of inhaled β-agonists has been accompanied by clinical concern of cardiac complications in elderly patients and those with coronary artery disease. However, in a study performed on clinically stable COPD or asthma patients with a history of myocardial ischemia, no ischemic events, or dysrhythmias, were observed when commonly used doses of salbutamol were administered.[91] To date, no clinical studies have evaluated the use of inhaled long-acting bronchodilators (either β_2-agonist or anticholinergic agents) with or without inhaled corticosteroids during AECOPD.

Several studies have suggested that the combination of β_2-agonists and anticholinergic agents prevent exacerbations, particularly long-acting agents.[92-96] It is possible that these agents reduce exacerbation frequency as a result of the effect on reduction of dynamic hyperinflation at rest and exercise,[97] as well as nonbronchodilator mechanisms, such as anti-inflammatory effect.[98]

Intravenous methylxanthines (theophylline or aminophylline) are considered second-line therapy, only to be used in selected cases when there is insufficient response to short-acting bronchodilators. Side effects of methylxanthines are significant and the clinical response is inconsistent.

CORTICOSTEROIDS

COPD is recognized as an inflammatory disorder, and the severity of airway inflammation correlates with the severity of the underlying COPD.[99] During exacerbations, there is a large increase in concentration of proinflammatory cells, including neutrophils. Systemic corticosteroids improve lung function significantly, shorten hospital stay, and reduce the risk for relapses as compared with placebo in patients with AECOPD.[100] In the ISOLDE trial, the median exacerbation rate was reduced by 25%, and there was also a reduction in the health status deterioration.[101] Systemic corticosteroids have been demonstrated to improve respiratory mechanics in mechanically ventilated patients, with a decrease in airway resistance and dynamic air-trapping.[102] A meta-analysis demonstrated that the use of systemic corticosteroids was associated with significant reduction in treatment failure, defined as either clinical deterioration, withdrawal from the study due to unsatisfactory clinical improvement, or relapse of exacerbation symptoms during the follow-up period. It also showed beneficial effects in reducing the length of hospitalization by a weighted mean of 1.42 days.[103]

Oral corticosteroids have beneficial effects in the management of AECOPD. Prednisolone, administered at 30 mg/day for 14 days, shortened the length of hospitalization by 2 days, improved FEV_1 by 60 mL/day, and accelerated recovery from symptoms.[104] The majority of patients with COPD probably requires only 2 weeks with oral corticosteroids and therapy for 8 weeks produced no incremental benefits above those achieved at 2 weeks.[105] One of the most important concerns regarding the use of corticosteroids in AECOPD is the possibility of confusing it with community-acquired pneumonia. Nevertheless, there is no evidence that corticosteroid use worsened the prognosis of community-acquired pneumonia if appropriate antibiotics are used; moreover, systemic corticosteroids may reduce morbidity and mortality rates in community-acquired pneumonia.[106]

The use of inhaled corticosteroids is associated with decrease in exacerbation events by 12% to 25%.[107] Studies involving inhaled corticosteroids and long-acting β_2-agonist showed reduction in exacerbation frequency to a greater extent than using either corticosteroid or long-acting β_2-agonist alone.[108,109] There is also a trend toward mortality rate reduction over 3 years of 17.5%, although without statistical significance.[110] There is no evidence that the addition of inhaled corticosteroids to systemic corticosteroids in AECOPD has any impact either in recovery or in mortality rate.

ANTIBIOTICS

Use of antibiotics in AECOPD remains a controversial topic, with some authors recommending antibiotic therapy and others not, maybe in part because of the heterogeneity of the population studied.[111,112] Compared with placebo, antibiotic use during AECOPD reduced treatment failures by 46%, defined as requiring additional antibiotics within the first 7 days or unchanged or deteriorated symptoms within 21 days. Antibiotics reduced treatment failures particularly in those patients who were hospitalized but not when they were used in ambulatory patients.[113] Three clinical trials involving 181 patients demonstrated that in-hospital mortality rate can be reduced by 78% with the use of antibiotics during AECOPD.[114,115] Patients who present with dyspnea and increased sputum volume or purulence or patients who require mechanical ventilation benefit from a 3- to 7-day course of oral or parenteral antibiotics.[116]

Although routine sputum cultures are recommended in all patients with AECOPD, invasive techniques (transtracheal aspirates,[117,118] bronchoscopic aspirates, or protected specimen brushing[5,119-123]) are not indicated. Exceptions include culture-negative community-acquired pneumonia not responding to therapy and ventilator-associated pneumonia (VAP).[124,125] Because many COPD patients have airway colonization by bacteria, without clinical signs of infection and exacerbation, there is no clear significance of a positive culture in a COPD patient; however, in the presence of exacerbation associated with an alteration in sputum character or quantity, potentially pathogenic organisms grown from sputum should be covered with an appropriate antibiotic.[126] Thus, the selection of empiric antibiotics to treat AECOPD should depend on the severity of underlying disease and severity of COPD exacerbation. Therapy for more severe exacerbations should include coverage for antibiotic-resistant bacteria, such as *Pseudomonas* or methicillin-resistant *Staphylococcus aureus*.

HEMODYNAMIC SUPPORT

FLUID MANAGEMENT

COPD patients often have chronic pulmonary hypertension, which may worsen with COPD exacerbation because of hypoxic vasoconstriction, dynamic lung hyperinflation, and in mechanically ventilated patients, PEEPi. This may lead to acute or worsening right ventricular failure. In one study, the prevalence of right ventricular failure in terminal COPD patients was 66% and the prevalence of left ventricular failure was only 6%.[127] As in other patients with right ventricular failure, hemodynamic stability is related to maintenance of mean arterial pressure. Mean systemic pressure can potentially be increased in these patients by increasing intravascular volume or by selectively improving compliance of the pulmonary vascular bed.[128] Intravenous fluid challenge is the initial step in hemodynamic support in the presence of hemodynamic compromise. Despite the presence of peripheral edema, diuretics should be avoided, given the potential to induce loss of intravascular volume, decreased venous return, decreased cardiac output, and hypotension.

Likewise, because pulmonary hypertension produces chronically elevated right ventricular pressures, fluid challenge could potentially worsen the hemodynamic status of patients with cor pulmonale. Overzealous fluid administration may raise right ventricular pressure to the point that it produces a shift in the interventricular septum and a reduction in left ventricular compliance and filling. Currently, no consensus or guidelines exist concerning invasive pulmonary artery catheterization in this group of patients; however, in patients remaining hypotensive after initial volume challenge or in patients with organ perfusion abnormalities and biventricular failure, invasive monitoring may be clinically useful.

INOTROPES AND VASODILATORS

In patients who remain hemodynamically unstable despite fluid therapy, adrenergic therapy is advised. Although some literature recommends adrenergic therapy for right ventricular failure using norepinephrine[129,130] or dobutamine,[131] we could find no controlled trials of adrenergic drug therapy in hemodynamically unstable COPD patients. However, pulmonary embolism patients have a hemodynamic derangement similar to that of COPD patients with right ventricular failure, and as such, dobutamine seems a reasonable choice in attempts to increase right ventricular function and increase cardiac output in the normotensive patient with decreased tissue perfusion. In the presence of hypotension, dobutamine would be used in combination with a combined inotrope vasopressor such as norepinephrine or dopamine. Nitroglycerine has been shown in one study to enhance right ventricular performance when added to dobutamine.[132] Nitroglycerine should be administered cautiously in patients who may have suboptimal right ventricle filling. Digoxin has no anticipated clinical utility in right ventricular failure, unless it is associated with left ventricular failure or arrhythmias that respond to digoxin.[133-135]

Although vasodilators have been used in clinical trials of COPD with right ventricular failure,[136-143] there is no consistent evidence of clinical outcome benefit. Inhaled nitric oxide, a selective pulmonary vasodilator with a short half-life and no systemic vasodilator properties, has shown variable results in patients with AECOPD.[144-148]

NUTRITIONAL SUPPORT

Chapter 82 deals with overall nutritional support of the critically ill patient. Highlights of some issues directly related to the COPD patient follow.

Malnutrition has been recognized as a factor that increases mortality rate[149,150] in COPD. Weight gain has been associated with decreased mortality rate.[151] Nutritional status tends to decline markedly during acute illness in COPD patients,[152-154] and patients may not recover to their previous nutritional state during convalescence, with recurrent exacerbations leading to a stepwise decline in nutritional status over time.[155] Recent studies have shown that skeletal muscle mass is directly related to muscle dysfunction in COPD patients.[156] Nutritional status has been correlated with weaning outcome.[157] Short-term studies of oral supplemental feeding or enteral feeding have demonstrated increases in body weight and improvement in immunologic markers and respiratory muscle function.[158-160] Nutritional support has been demonstrated to produce improvement in lung function in hospitalized patients with acute exacerbation of COPD.[161]

Special care must be taken to avoid overfeeding patients with COPD exacerbation because excess calories, particularly if carbohydrate rich, elevate total oxygen consumption and CO_2 production, which may complicate management in patients with hypercapnia.[162] In one study of mechanically ventilated patients, enteral nutrition was administered with a fixed carbohydrate content and an association between total caloric intake and CO_2 production when providing nutritional support to the COPD patient with acute respiratory failure (ARF) was noted. It has been recommended that enteral alimentation provide total calories from 1.25 to 1.3 times the resting energy expenditure of the patient with a respiratory quotient target of 0.7 to 0.8 and that carbohydrate calories be limited to 40% of total calories.[163]

NONINVASIVE MECHANICAL VENTILATION

ARF in the setting of AECOPD is characterized by the worsening of hypoxemia and a variable degree of carbon dioxide retention and acidemia. Worsening in ventilation/perfusion ratio ($\dot{V}/\dot{Q}$) mismatching is probably the leading mechanism in the occurrence of the hypoxemia by the enlargement of physiologic dead space and the rise of wasted ventilation.[164] The increase in airway resistance and the need of a higher minute ventilation may result in expiratory flow limitation, dynamic hyperinflation, and related PEEPi with subsequent increased inspiratory threshold load and dysfunction of the respiratory muscles, which may lead to their fatigue.[165] Dyspnea, right ventricular failure, and encephalopathy characterize severe AECOPD complicated by ARF. Arterial pH reflects the acute worsening of the alveolar ventilation, and, regardless of the chronic level of Pa_{CO_2}, it represents the best marker of the ARF severity.[166]

Those patients with severe AECOPD develop ARF requiring ventilatory support. The frequency of this support varies among series, being as high as 74%.[167] Ventilatory support may be of two types: invasive and noninvasive. Noninvasive ventilation (NIV) using nasal masks or facemasks has proved efficacious in ARF caused by COPD in several clinical studies, with success rates as high as 65% in some series.[168-170] As with invasive mechanical ventilation, the goals of NIV include respiratory muscle rest, ventilatory support during treatment of reversible conditions, and the correction of severe hypoxemia and hypercarbia.

Several prospective, randomized, controlled studies confirmed the clinical efficacy of NIV in the treatment of the ARF during AECOPD. Compared to standard medical therapy alone the application of NIV improves survival, reduces the need for endotracheal intubation and the rate of complications, and shortens length of stay in hospital and intensive care unit (ICU).[167,170,171]

INDICATIONS

Patients with mild exacerbation, with normal or mildly reduced pH (pH > 7.35) and without clinical signs of respiratory failure, do not appear to benefit from a trial of NIV.[172]

In patients with moderate ARF, characterized by pH levels between 7.25 and 7.30, NIV is indicated for a few hours per day (<12 hours/day) in order to prevent endotracheal intubation, with low failure rates (15% to 20%), and appear to have the greater benefit.[173]

In more severely ill patients (pH < 7.25), the rate of NIV failures is inversely related to respiratory acidosis. In this population, the use of NIV as an alternative to invasive ventilation does not affect the mortality rate or the duration of ventilatory support, but it is associated with a lower rate of complications (VAP, difficult weaning). Despite the elevated rate of failure, it is worth a short trial of NIV if no contraindication is present (decreased level of consciousness, cardiac or respiratory arrest, severe gastrointestinal bleeding, severe hemodynamic instability, facial surgery or trauma, upper airway obstruction, inability to clear secretions).[174]

IMPLEMENTATION OF NONINVASIVE POSITIVE-PRESSURE VENTILATION

NIV is usually delivered in assisted ventilation modality but no differences in success rate were found when applied in controlled ventilatory modality.[175] Leak is a constant feature of NIV and may affect triggering of the ventilator, delivered F_{IO_2}, and air humidification. As such, the choice of the interface is one of the crucial issues affecting NIV outcome; although facemask is the standard interface to deliver NIV in patients with ARF, poor mask tolerance, skin lesions, and leaks are reported among factors causing NIV failure and intubation requirement.[176]

The nasal mask has less dead space, causes less claustrophobia, minimizes potential complications in case of vomiting, and allows both expectoration and oral intake of fluids without the need to remove the mask. However, facemasks are preferable in severely dyspneic patients because the nasal resistance to breathing is decreased with combined nose and mouth air entry. Also, opening of the mouth during nasal noninvasive positive-pressure ventilation produces loss of tidal volume, which decreases effectiveness. In our opinion, the facemask is optimal for initial use in most patients with severe respiratory distress.

The use of pressure support ventilation (PSV) is the most common mode of ventilation for application of NIV. Nonetheless, bilevel positive airway pressure has become the preferred mode of NIV administration in COPD patients because it is generally as comfortable as PSV but produces greater improvement in gas exchange and reduces the work of breathing more effectively than PSV alone.[177-179] Specifically designed noninvasive bilevel ventilators will have a better leak tolerance and adjust trigger and cycle sensitivity to improve patient-ventilator synchrony.[180]

The goal of NIV is to provide ventilatory support to rest fatigued respiratory muscles while the underlying illness is treated. The use of adequate ventilatory support is important regardless of the ventilator and modality chosen to deliver NIV. When using pressure-cycled modes, the recommended approach is to start at low pressures for patient comfort and titrate the pressure support or inspiratory positive airway pressure (IPAP) to achieve a tidal volume of at least 6 mL/kg, improvement in clinical signs (RR < 25 beats per minute, reduced accessory muscle use), and patient comfort.[181] External PEEP, referred to as expiratory positive airway pressure (EPAP) in bilevel ventilators, may counteract PEEPi, and thus aid triggering, reduce oxygen consumption, and improve comfort. Although PEEPi can be as high as 15 cm H_2O in patients with severe AECOPD, EPAP levels higher than 5 cm H_2O are rarely tolerated or necessary. Therefore, slow titration to patient comfort is important to maximize the likelihood of NIV success. Improvements in pH, $Paco_2$, and level of consciousness at 60 minutes are predictors of success in patients on AECOPD who respond to NIV.[178]

The British Thoracic Society recommended that patients with ARF who respond to NIV be maintained as continuously as possible during the first 24 hours. If the respiratory status has stabilized, then the duration of ventilatory support can be reduced on subsequent days. Masks are removed for meals, conversation, comfort, and respiratory treatment as necessary.[182]

WEANING

Weaning from NIV may be accomplished either by progressively decreasing the levels of inspiratory positive-pressure support or by permitting the patient to be intermittently off NIV for increasing lengths of time. A combination of both strategies can also be used. In general, it is useful to wean patients by progressively increasing the period of spontaneous breathing without NIV. Once the acute process improves, many patients can be weaned relatively quickly. Unlike invasive ventilation, NIV can be reinstituted easily and quickly if the patient shows signs of fatigue or intolerance to spontaneous breathing. The use of nocturnal NIV may be needed during the early weaning period and may be continued at home in some patients.[183]

Some studies have analyzed weaning outcome in intubated patients with AECOPD, comparing NIV with conventional weaning methods. Results showed that NIV reduced weaning time, shortened intensive care days, decreased the incidence of nosocomial pneumonia, and improved 60-day survival rates.[184,185] NIV has also been used successfully in another study on patients with hypercarbia after extubation.[186] A meta-analysis concluded that, notwithstanding, the use of NIV to facilitate weaning, in mechanically ventilated patients, with predominantly COPD, is associated with promising but insufficient evidence of clinical benefit at present.[187]

INVASIVE MECHANICAL VENTILATION

Patients requiring immediate admission to the ICU are those who presented with severe dyspnea that responds inadequately to initial emergency therapy, with changes in mental status (confusion, lethargy, coma), persistent or worsening hypoxemia (Pao_2 < 40 mm Hg), and/or severe or worsening respiratory acidosis (pH < 7.25) despite supplemental oxygen and NIV, hemodynamic instability with the need of vasopressors, and the need for invasive mechanical ventilation.

Invasive ventilation is indicated for patients who are not suited for NIV or who failed NIV, respiratory or cardiac arrest, respiratory pauses with loss of consciousness or gasping for air, altered level of consciousness (from psychomotor agitation to coma), massive aspiration, persistent inability to remove respiratory secretions, severe hemodynamic instability without response to fluids and vasopressors, severe ventricular arrhythmias, and life-threatening hypoxemia in patients unable to tolerate NIV. Patients with AECOPD requiring invasive mechanical ventilation have a higher ICU mortality rate and in-hospital mortality rate when compared with nonventilated patients.[188]

INITIAL APPROACH AND MAINTENANCE

VENTILATION MODES

Mechanical ventilation of patients with AECOPD should be targeted to decrease excessive respiratory work. Patient-triggered ventilation modes, either assist-control or synchronized intermittent mandatory ventilation (SIMV), typically accomplish this goal. Special care must be taken; however, if these modes are not adequately adjusted to fit the characteristics of the patient, an increase in respiratory work will result.[189]

PSV has been extensively used and reviewed in the literature.[190,191] In AECOPD patients, PSV has been shown to decrease inspiratory effort as the applied pressure is increased; however, the response among patients varied significantly.[180] At higher levels of support pressure, many patients show an activation of the respiratory muscles during the late phase of inflation, with the potential to produce ventilation dyssynchrony. This may be more common in patients with longer time constants and those who require higher inspiratory flows delivered for longer periods.[192]

We recommend that ventilation be provided as total support during the initial phase of respiratory management (assist-control volume ventilation or high-level PSV).

INSPIRED OXYGEN

The goal of oxygenation should be to maintain an oxyhemoglobin saturation of at least 90% to 92%. In dark-skinned patients, pulse oximetry may overestimate oxyhemoglobin saturation, and in these patients, we recommend targeting pulse oximetry values of 95% to ensure adequate oxygenation. Although there is no clear-cut clinical evidence that allows determination of the Fio_2 threshold of concern for oxygen toxicity, based on animal studies of oxygen toxicity in normal lungs, attempts to lower Fio_2 to 0.6 or less by the end of the first 24 hours of mechanical ventilation is a reasonable goal.[193]

INTRINSIC POSITIVE END-EXPIRATORY PRESSURE

Before discussing ventilation settings in AECOPD complicated with ARF, a review of intrinsic PEEP (PEEPi, auto-PEEP, dynamic hyperinflation) is in order. The two primary pathophysiologic changes that contribute to the development of respiratory distress and ARF in patients with obstructive lung disease are increased expiratory airflow resistance and dynamic hyperinflation. In COPD, the alveolar attachments that normally keep the smaller airway open via radial traction are lost. This leads to airway narrowing and collapse especially during expiration. In AECOPD the already narrowed airways may be further compromised by increased secretions, mucosal swelling, and peribronchial inflammation. The time constant for lung emptying is prolonged and end-expiratory lung volume is dynamically increased. Therefore, the next inspiratory effort occurs before the expiratory phase is completed, leading to air-trapping, and the respiratory system is prevented from returning to its resting state at the end of the expiration and thus dynamic hyperinflation develops. Dynamic hyperinflation results in PEEPi.[194] Initially, PEEP is beneficial because it maintains the airways open, thereby reducing the airway resistance.

PEEPi is typically not detected on the pressure gauge of the ventilator because it is open to the atmosphere except for a very brief moment at the end of expiration. If the expiration port of the circuit is occluded at end expiration in a relaxed patient with a delay of next inspiration, the pressure inside the lungs and in the circuit will begin to equilibrate; if occlusion is sufficiently prolonged, PEEPi may be recorded.[195]

PEEPi has numerous hemodynamic and mechanical consequences. When PEEPi is excessive, barotrauma may occur. Hemodynamic consequences of PEEPi effect are more common with decreased venous return, decreased stroke volume, and hypotension. PEEPi also increases the work of breathing, which is represented by an increase of workload during spontaneous inspiration and by an increase in the threshold of ventilator triggering. PEEPi is treated by increasing expiratory time and decreasing the minute ventilation, as well as reducing the airflow resistance by bronchodilators and corticosteroids. This effect is achieved by decreasing the respiratory rate and tidal volume.

INSPIRATORY TRIGGERING SENSITIVITY SETTINGS

The setting of the optimal triggering threshold is more difficult in COPD patients, especially if dynamic lung hyperinflation exists. This is because the patient needs to generate a negative pressure equal to PEEPi before interfacing with the preset sensitivity on the ventilator. When PEEPi is high, the patient may exert significant inspiratory effort before the triggering threshold is reached, another cause of dyssynchrony. On the other hand, if the sensitivity of the ventilator has been placed at a very sensitive level, the ventilator may cycle inappropriately and can cause serious respiratory alkalosis, especially in the absence of significant PEEPi. Many ventilators have flow-triggered options, and although theoretically flow triggering may reduce patient effort, some reports failed to show differences when flow triggering is compared with newer pressure-triggering devices, even in COPD patients, although it is known that flow-triggered ventilators work better when the patient has elevated requirements of inspiratory flow.[196,197]

INSPIRATORY FLOW RATE

High inspiratory flow rate helps satisfy the demands of most dyspneic or tachypneic COPD patients; moreover, it decreases the likelihood of dynamic hyperinflation and PEEPi. This decreases inspiratory time and increases expiratory time, minimizing PEEPi. An improvement in gas exchange has been found when inspiratory flows were increased from 40 to 60 L/minute in COPD patients.[198]

TIDAL VOLUME

In patients with known or suspected PEEPi, smaller tidal volumes (6 to 8 mL/kg) may be necessary to prevent alveolar overdistention, dynamic hyperinflation, and barotrauma.

RESPIRATORY RATE

In the presence of PEEPi or in patients with high risk of developing PEEPi, elevations in respiratory rate must be avoided because expiratory time will be significantly decreased. Although SIMV with low spontaneous tidal volume may control minute ventilation, it has variable effects on PEEPi and may significantly increase respiratory workload. For these reasons, controlled mechanical ventilation with optimal sedation and even muscular paralysis may be the optimal approach.

POSITIVE END-EXPIRATORY PRESSURE

In the past, PEEP was avoided in patients with AECOPD because of the concern of worsening dynamic hyperinflation. It is now recognized that the application of extrinsic PEEP below 75% to 85% of PEEPi may facilitate ventilator triggering, because alveolar pressure now needs to be decreased to only below the level of the external PEEP, instead of below the level of atmospheric pressure, decreasing the work required to trigger the inspiration.[199,200]

The key points to optimize mechanical ventilation in AECOPD include recognition of the presence of worsening of expiratory airflow limitation and consequent dynamic hyperinflation, reducing the dynamic hyperinflation and PEEPi by providing the longest expiratory time possible, reducing patient ventilatory demands and minute ventilation and reducing the airway flow limitation with bronchodilators and corticosteroids, adjusting the minute ventilation to correct the pH but not the CO_2 to minimize hyperventilation, and keeping the plateau pressure below 30 cm H_2O to minimize barotrauma.

WEANING

In general, restoration of respiratory muscle function requires approximately 24 to 48 hours of mechanical ventilation.[201-203] Before weaning patients with AECOPD from mechanical ventilation, the premorbid condition that triggered ARF should be corrected and an adequate neuromuscular competency/workload ratio achieved. Therefore, the strategy for facilitating weaning from the ventilator should include an increase in inspiratory force and a decrease in the load on the respiratory system. See Chapter 43 for a comparison of various weaning techniques.

EXTUBATION TO NONINVASIVE VENTILATION

Earlier studies have supported the idea that NIV can facilitate weaning and improve outcomes in difficult-to-wean patients by avoiding the complications of prolonged intubation. There is evidence that the use of NIV as a method of

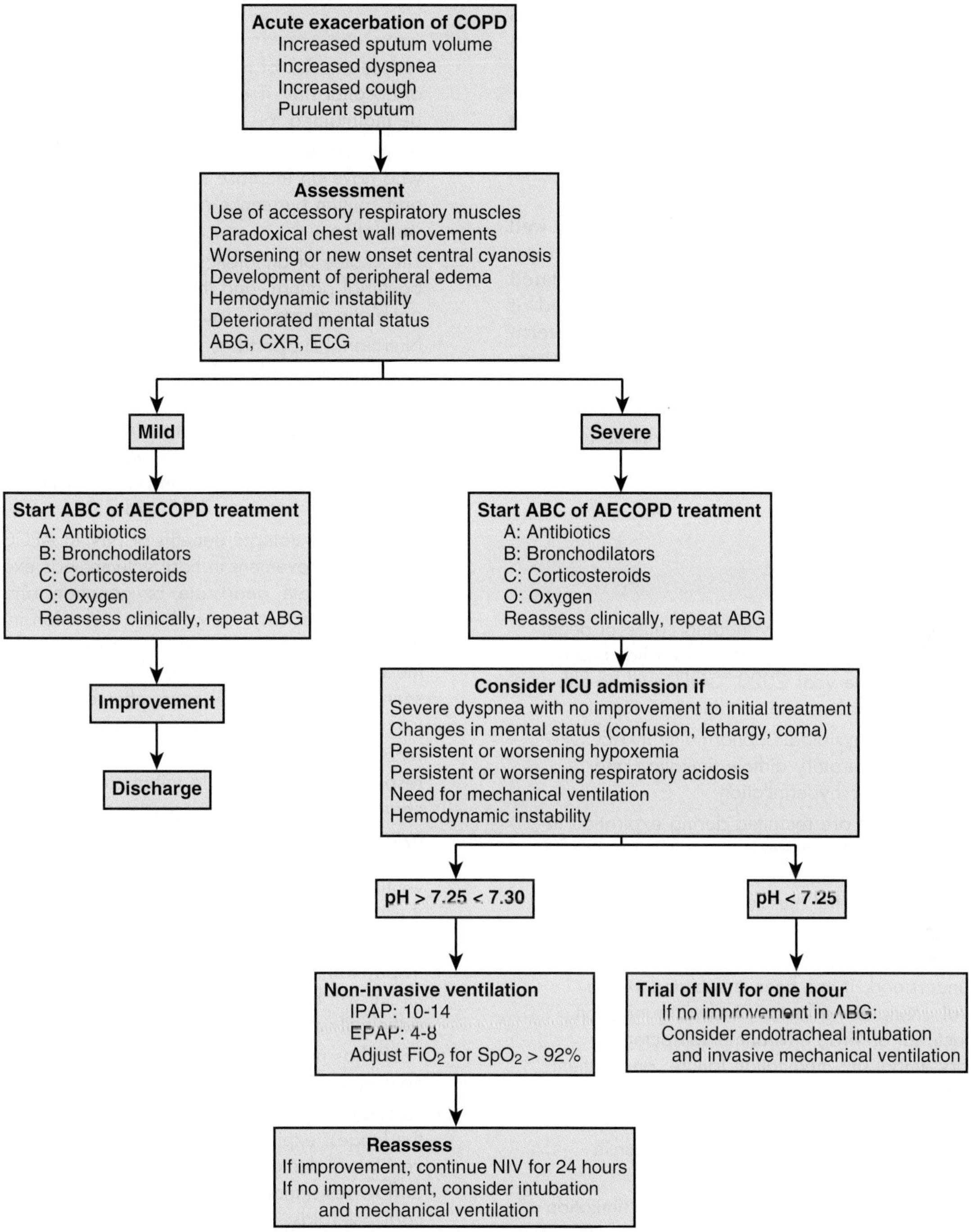

Figure 39.1 Management of acute exacerbations of chronic obstructive pulmonary disease.

weaning in patients with AECOPD and CHF resulted in shorter periods of intubation, decreased length of hospital and ICU stay, lower rate of nosocomial pneumonia, and improved ICU and 90-day survival.

Figure 39.1 is a suggested algorithm for the management of the AECOPD.

PROGNOSIS

The outcome for the patients with AECOPD with ARF depends on the severity of the COPD, the trigger for ARF, and avoidance of ICU complications. In patients who require mechanical ventilation for acute exacerbation, the overall in-hospital mortality rate is greater than 20%.[204] For elderly patients, the mortality rate is greater than 50%.[205] In a multicenter study of patients aged 65 or older, the mortality rate was 30% at hospital discharge, 41% at 90 days, 47% at 180 days, and 59% at 1 year. The time course and recovery following COPD exacerbation in a cohort of 101 patients with a mean FEV_1 of 41.9% has been reported.[206] Patients recorded daily morning peak expiratory flow rate (PEFR) following the onset of the exacerbation. Median recovery time for PEFR was 6 days. Recovery of PEFR to baseline values was complete in only 75.2% of exacerbations at 35 days, and 7.1% of exacerbations had still not returned to baseline at 91 days.[206]

TERMINAL CARE FOR THE END-STAGE PATIENT

All patients with severe end-stage COPD should be well educated about their prognosis and limitations of therapy. Some patients may elect not to be mechanically ventilated when the COPD is in the late stage and the likelihood of extubation is extremely low. Others may choose short-term ventilation only in the hope of a reversible cause. Others may choose long-term ventilation with tracheostomy and home or special facility mechanical ventilation. It is important that emotional and psychological support be given for the end-stage patient and his or her family.

KEY POINTS

- Worldwide, COPD is the only leading cause of death that still has a rising mortality rate, and it has been estimated that by the year 2020, COPD will be fifth among the most burdensome conditions to society.
- The fundamental physiologic abnormality in AECOPD is worsening of expiratory airflow limitation and consequent dynamic hyperinflation.
- Abdominal muscles are recruited during expiration in severe COPD patients. Dynamic hyperinflation can be overestimated during chronic and acute airway obstruction if abdominal muscle function is not evaluated.
- Although the precise cause of acute exacerbation is poorly understood, it has been associated with a number of precipitating factors, including infection, either bacterial or viral; environmental factors; pulmonary embolism; medication failure; and patient noncompliance.
- Acute increases in $PaCO_2$ with administration of supplemental oxygen are more likely to occur in patients with elevated baseline $PaCO_2$.
- The cornerstone of treatment of airway flow limitation in AECOPD is based on the ABCs: antibiotics, bronchodilators, and corticosteroids.
- A combination of inhaled short-acting β_2-agonists and inhaled anticholinergics is indicated during exacerbations to alleviate patient symptoms.
- When a metered-dose inhaler (MDI) is used for acute exacerbations, the addition of a spacing device, which enhances lower airway drug deposition, is indicated to ensure adequate drug delivery.
- In patients with severe respiratory distress, nebulizers are still the best option to ensure optimal drug delivery.
- Systemic corticosteroids shorten recovery time; improve lung function (FEV_1) and arterial hypoxemia; and

KEY POINTS (Continued)

reduce the risk of relapse, treatment failure, and length of hospital stay. Treatment with corticosteroids should be maintained for 10 to 14 days.

- Antibiotics should be given to patients with AECOPD who have an increase in dyspnea, sputum volume, and sputum purulence or who require mechanical ventilation.
- The choice of antibiotics should be based on the local bacterial pattern, and the recommended length of antibiotic therapy is usually 5 to 10 days.
- Nutritional support has been demonstrated to produce improvements in lung function in hospitalized patients with AECOPD.
- NIV reduces the rate of intubation and mortality rate in selected patients with ARF secondary to AECOPD. The highest benefit occurs in patients with moderate ARF with pH between 7.25 and 7.3.
- Potential physiologic benefits of NIV in AECOPD include improvement in tidal volume, gas exchange, respiratory rate, heart rate, oxygenation, and diaphragm activity, as well as a reduction in arterial CO_2 with a concomitant improvement in pH. When these beneficial responses occur, they are typically seen in the first several hours after beginning NIV.
- ICU admission for patients with AECOPD is recommended in patients with severe dyspnea that responds inadequately to initial emergency therapy, changes in mental status, persistent or worsening hypoxemia or persistent or worsening respiratory acidosis despite NIV, the need for mechanical ventilation, and hemodynamic instability.
- If the expiration port of the circuit is occluded at end expiration in a relaxed patient with a delay of next inspiration, the pressure inside the lungs and in the circuit will begin to equilibrate; if occlusion is sufficiently prolonged, PEEPi may be recorded.
- PEEPi has numerous hemodynamic and mechanical consequences.
- To reduce dynamic hyperinflation and PEEPi, provide the longest expiratory time possible, reduce patient ventilatory demand and minute ventilation, and reduce airflow resistance by using bronchodilators and corticosteroids.

SELECTED REFERENCES

28. Barbera JA, Roca J, Ferrer A, et al: Mechanisms of worsening gas exchange during acute exacerbations of chronic obstructive pulmonary disease. Eur Respir J 1997;10:1285.
31. Soler N, Torres A, Ewig S, et al: Bronchial microbial patterns in severe exacerbations of chronic obstructive pulmonary disease. Am J Respir Crit Care Med 1998;157:1498.
77. Eaton T, Lewis C, Young P, et al: Long term oxygen therapy improves health-related quality of life. Respir Med 2004;98:285.
85. Hanson CW III, Marshall BE, Frasch HF, et al: Causes of hypercarbia with oxygen therapy in patients with chronic obstructive pulmonary disease. Crit Care Med 1996;24:23.
131. Angle MR, Molloy DW, Penner B, et al: The cardiopulmonary and renal hemodynamic effects of norepinephrine in canine pulmonary embolism. Chest 1989;95:1333.

147. Yoshida M, Taguchi O, Gabazza EC, et al: Combined inhalation of nitric oxide and oxygen in chronic obstructive pulmonary disease. Am J Respir Crit Care Med 1997;155:526.
157. Bernard S, LeBlanc P, Whittom F, et al: Peripheral muscle weakness in patients with chronic obstructive pulmonary disease. Am J Respir Crit Care Med 1998;158:629.
188. Seneff MG, Wagner DP, Wagner RP, et al: Hospital and 1-year survival of patients admitted to intensive care units with acute exacerbation of chronic obstructive pulmonary disease. JAMA 1995;274:1852.
198. Connors AF, McCaffree DR, Gray BA: Effect of inspiratory flow rate on gas exchange during mechanical ventilation. Am Rev Respir Dis 1981;124:537.
200. Smith TC, Marini JJ: Impact of PEEP on lung mechanics and work of breathing in severe airflow obstruction. J Appl Physiol 1988; 65:1488.

The complete list of references can be found at www.expertconsult.com.

40 Hypoventilation and Respiratory Muscle Dysfunction

Franco Laghi

CHAPTER OUTLINE

Hypercapnic respiratory failure is conventionally defined as a state in which ventilation is insufficient to maintain an arterial tension of carbon dioxide (Pa_{CO_2}) of less than 45 mm Hg for the level of metabolic activity (measured by CO_2 production, $\dot{V}_{CO_2}$).[1] Under steady-state conditions, the relationship among Pa_{CO_2}, alveolar ventilation ($\dot{V}_A$), and $\dot{V}_{CO_2}$ is given by the equation:

$$Pa_{CO_2} = (\dot{V}_{CO_2}/\dot{V}_A) \times K$$

in which K (usually stated as 0.863) is a constant that converts measurement of $\dot{V}_{CO_2}$ from standard conditions to body temperature conditions. The term $\dot{V}_A$ represents the portion of minute ventilation ($\dot{V}_E$) that reaches the terminal gas exchange units and is calculated as

$$\dot{V}_A = \dot{V}_E - \dot{V}_D$$

where $\dot{V}_D$ equals dead space ventilation. A reduction in $\dot{V}_A$ may result from an inadequate $\dot{V}_E$ or an increase in $\dot{V}_D$ (resulting from an increase in true $\dot{V}_D$ or a functional increase in $\dot{V}_D$ secondary to lung regions with high ventilation-perfusion [$\dot{V}_A/\dot{Q}$] relationships).*

Hypercapnia is synonymous with alveolar hypoventilation for the patient's level of carbon dioxide production. Alveolar hypoventilation can result from decreased neuromuscular capacity and increased respiratory load (Fig. 40.1).[2] Isolated impairments in gas exchange—i.e., conditions in which the alveolar-arterial O_2 gradient* is increased—usually do not cause hypercapnia.[3] When gas exchange is impaired, however, the magnitude of neuromuscular derangements causing hypercapnia or the magnitude of increased respiratory loads causing hypercapnia is less than the corresponding derangements when gas exchange is normal. Conditions in which gas exchange contributes to hypercapnia are usually characterized by ventilation-perfusion inequality. When gas exchange is impaired total minute ventilation may actually be increased despite a concurrent decrease in alveolar ventilation.

DECREASED NEUROMUSCULAR CAPACITY

Disease states that may result in decreased neuromuscular capacity and thus in alveolar hypoventilation include

*Terminology of dead space is confusing. *Anatomic dead space* is made up of the conducting airways (nose, mouth, pharynx, larynx, trachea bronchi, and bronchioles). *Alveolar dead space* is made up of alveoli that receive some or no blood flow, which does not match ventilation (units with very high $\dot{V}_A/\dot{Q}$ ratio). *Physiologic dead space* is the sum of anatomic dead space and alveolar dead space.[1]

*The alveolar-arterial O_2 gradient (A-aD_{O_2}) is calculated as $P_{AO_2} - Pa_{O_2}$, in which P_{AO_2} (alveolar O_2 tension) can be estimated according to the simplified alveolar gas equation:

$$P_{AO_2} = F_{IO_2} \times (P_B - P_{H_2O}) - Pa_{CO_2}/R$$

where F_{IO_2} = fractional concentration of inspired O_2 (about 0.21 when breathing room air), P_B = barometric pressure (about 760 mm Hg at sea level), P_{H_2O} = water vapor pressure (usually taken as 47 mm Hg at 37° C), and R = respiratory exchange ratio of the whole lung. The respiratory exchange ratio (R) = CO_2 production/O_2 consumption ($\dot{V}_{CO_2}/\dot{V}_{O_2}$). R is normally about 0.8. In steady state, R is determined by the relative proportions of free fatty acids, protein, and carbohydrate consumed by the tissues. In this equation, it is assumed that alveolar P_{CO_2} and Pa_{CO_2} are the same (usually they nearly are). In healthy young subjects (≤30 years old) breathing air at sea level, A-aD_{O_2} is usually less than 10 mm Hg, but it increases to as much as 28 mm Hg in healthy 60-year-old subjects.[1]

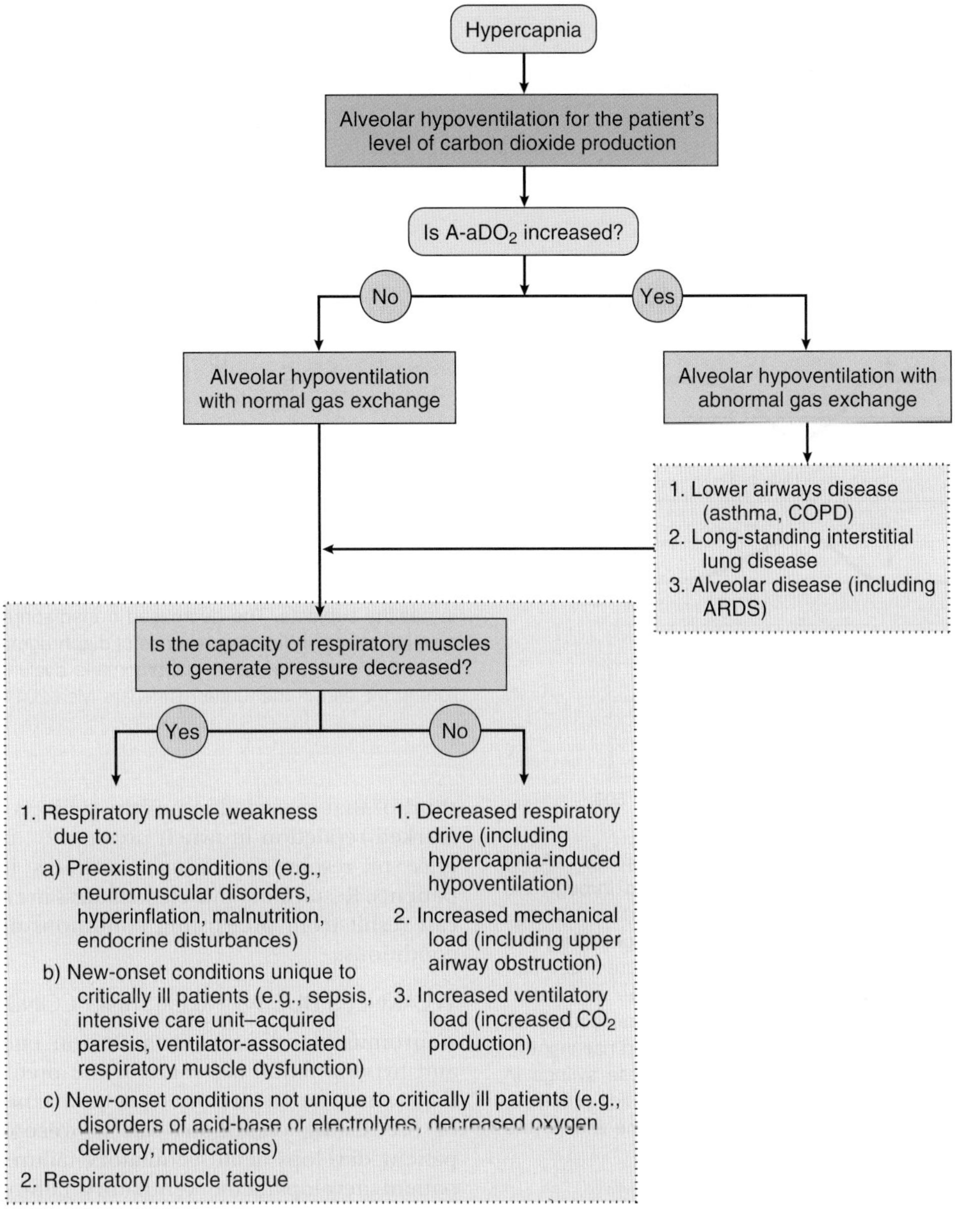

Figure 40.1 Diagnostic approach to critically ill patient with hypercapnia. A-aDO_2, alveolar-arterial difference in partial pressure of oxygen; ARDS, acute respiratory distress syndrome; COPD, chronic obstructive pulmonary disease.

conditions characterized by decreased respiratory center output and by respiratory muscle weakness and respiratory muscle fatigue.

DECREASED RESPIRATORY CENTER OUTPUT

Isolated decreases in respiratory drive can produce ventilatory failure without distress. Potential causes include sedative overdose,[1] hypothyroidism,[4] metabolic alkalosis,[5] semistarvation,[6] and central alveolar hypoventilation syndrome. The latter can be either idiopathic (i.e., primary alveolar hypoventilation, or Ondine's curse) or secondary to neurologic lesions, such as trauma, infection (poliomyelitis), infarction, and obesity hypoventilation syndrome.[4] In mechanically ventilated patients, decreases in respiratory drive are suspected when patients develop marked increases in P_{CO_2} despite relatively normal measurements of resistance and elastance and no apparent evidence of lower motor neuron disease.[7] Whether sleep deprivation decreases respiratory drive remains controversial.[8,9]

RESPIRATORY MUSCLE WEAKNESS

DETECTION OF RESPIRATORY MUSCLE WEAKNESS IN CRITICALLY ILL PATIENTS

Measurements of airway pressure during maximal voluntary inspiratory efforts are used to evaluate global inspiratory muscle strength.[10] In healthy subjects, maximum inspiratory airway pressure is usually more negative than −80 cm H_2O.[10] In mechanically ventilated patients recovering from an episode or acute respiratory failure, maximum inspiratory airway pressure can range from less negative than −20 cm H_2O to about −100 cm H_2O.[7,11,12] Values of maximal airway pressure during voluntary maneuvers depend greatly on a

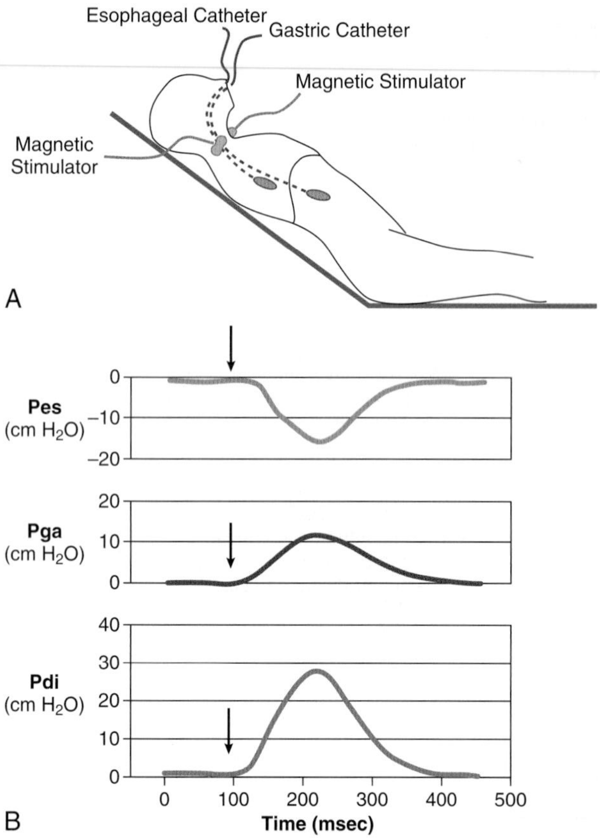

Figure 40.2 Recording of transdiaphragmatic twitch pressure. **A,** An esophageal balloon and a gastric balloon are passed through the nares. Magnetic stimulation of the phrenic nerves elicits diaphragmatic contraction. **B,** Continuous recordings of esophageal (Pes) and gastric pressures (Pga) and transdiaphragmatic pressure (Pdi)—calculated by subtracting Pes from Pga. Phrenic nerve stimulation (*arrows*) results in contraction of the diaphragm with consequent fall in intrathoracic pressure (negative defection of Pes) and rise in intra-abdominal pressure (positive deflection of Pga). These swings in pressure are responsible for the transdiaphragmatic twitch pressure. The smaller the transdiaphragmatic twitch pressure, the smaller the force generation capacity of the diaphragm.

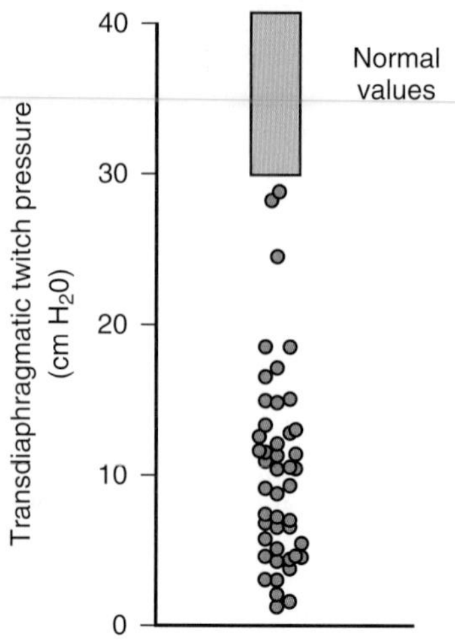

Figure 40.3 Transdiaphragmatic pressure in response to single stimulations (twitch stimulation) of the phrenic nerves recorded in ventilated patients recovering from acute respiratory failure. The boxed area represents the 95% confidence interval of values obtained in healthy subjects. The decreased transdiaphragmatic twitch pressure in patients indicates presence of diaphragmatic weakness. (From Laghi F: Ventilator-induced diaphragmatic dysfunction: Is there a dim light at the end of the tunnel? Crit Care Med 2011;39:903.)

level of motivation and comprehension of the maneuver (often not obtainable in critically ill patients).[13] Not surprisingly, in patients requiring short-term mechanical ventilation, measurements of maximum inspiratory airway pressure commonly do not differentiate between weaning success and weaning failure patients.[12-14]

In contrast to the voluntary nature of maximal voluntary inspiratory efforts, transdiaphragmatic pressures elicited by single stimulations of the phrenic nerves—or twitch pressure—are independent of patients' motivation and eliminate the influence of the central nervous system.[10] Activation can be achieved with either an electrical stimulator[15] or a magnetic stimulator,[15] though the latter is easier to use in mechanically ventilated patients (Fig. 40.2).[13,16,17]

In healthy volunteers, magnetic stimulation elicits twitch pressures that average 31 to 39 cm H_2O.[10] In patients with severe chronic obstructive pulmonary disease (COPD), twitch pressures average 19 to 20 cm H_2O.[18,19] The value of transdiaphragmatic twitch pressure in patients recovering from an episode of acute respiratory failure is about one third of that recorded in healthy subjects (Fig. 40.3).[20] This marked reduction in twitch pressure[16,17] indicates the presence of respiratory muscle weakness in most of these patients. Respiratory muscle weakness in critically ill patients can result from preexisting conditions or from new-onset conditions.

WEAKNESS DUE TO PREEXISTING CONDITIONS

Neuromuscular diseases, malnutrition, endocrine disorders, and hyperinflation are some of the preexisting conditions that can cause respiratory muscle weakness. The existence of preexisting conditions can be recognized before the patient develops acute ventilatory failure, at the time the patient develops acute ventilatory failure, or when acute ventilatory failure is already established.[4,21-24]

Neuromuscular Disorders

The capacity of the respiratory muscles to generate tension can be decreased in certain disorders, such as stroke, amyotrophic lateral sclerosis, spinal cord injuries, poliomyelitis, Guillain-Barré syndrome, neuropathies due to massive intoxications of arsenic[25] or thallium,[26] chronic inflammatory demyelinating polyneuropathy, axonopathy of acute intermittent porphyria, myasthenia gravis, acid maltase deficiency, and muscular dystrophies such as myotonic dystrophy (i.e., the most frequent adult form of muscular dystrophy).[4,27,28]

Hypercapnic respiratory failure usually occurs when respiratory muscle strength falls to 39% of the predicted normal value.[29] However, Gibson and associates[30] described several patients with neuromuscular disease who had a normal partial pressure of CO_2 despite decreases in respiratory muscle strength to less than 20% of predicted. Conversely, some patients with only moderate respiratory muscle weakness displayed hypercapnia (Fig. 40.4).[30] In other

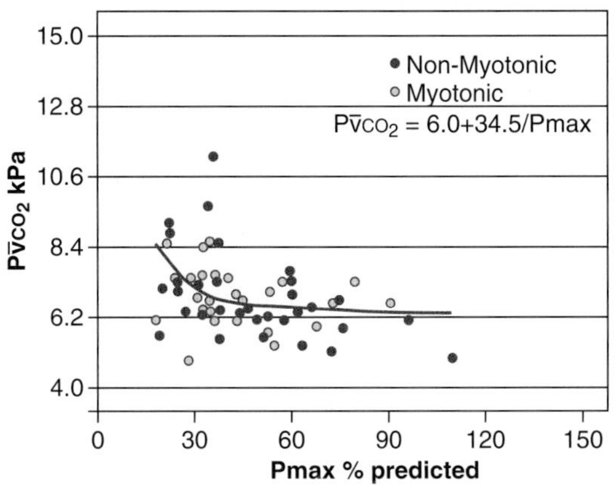

Figure 40.4 Relationship between muscle strength and mixed venous partial pressure of CO_2 ($P\bar{v}CO_2$) in patients with respiratory muscle weakness. Respiratory muscle strength is the arithmetic sum of maximum static inspiratory and expiratory mouth pressures (Pmax = PImax + PEmax). The open circles are patients with myotonic dystrophy, and the closed circles are patients with a variety of nonmyotonic muscle diseases. As respiratory muscle weakness became more severe $P\bar{v}CO_2$ rose, although considerable variability was observed among patients. The regression lines were similar in the myotonic and nonmyotonic patients. (From Gibson GJ, Gilmartin JJ, Veale D, et al: Respiratory muscle function in neuromuscular disease. In Jones NL, Killian KJ [eds]: Breathlessness. The Campbell Symposium. Hamilton, Ontario, Boehringer-Ingelheim, 1992.)

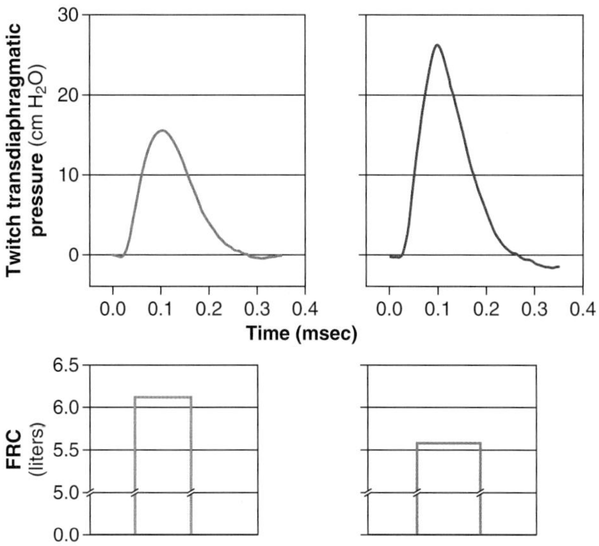

Figure 40.5 Twitch transdiaphragmatic pressure elicited by phrenic nerve stimulation (*upper panels*) and functional residual capacity (FRC) (*lower panels*) in a patient with severe emphysema before (*left*) and after (*right*) lung volume reduction surgery. The increase in transdiaphragmatic pressure after surgery was in part due to a decrease in the operating lung volume as demonstrated by the decrease in functional residual capacity. (Data from Laghi F, Jubran A, Topeli A, et al: Effect of lung volume reduction surgery on neuromechanical coupling of the diaphragm. Am J Respir Crit Care Med 1998;157:475.)

words, reductions in muscle strength do not consistently predict alveolar hypoventilation in this setting.

Hyperinflation

Hyperinflation is a common preexisting problem in patients with obstructive lung diseases such as COPD,[4] cystic fibrosis,[31] bronchiolitis,[32] and lymphangioleiomyomatosis.[4] The severity of preexisting hyperinflation commonly worsens in patients experiencing an exacerbation of COPD.[33] Hyperinflation has a number of adverse effects on inspiratory muscle function: the inspiratory muscles operate at an unfavorable position of the length-tension relationship (Fig. 40.5);[34] flattening of the diaphragm decreases the size of the zone of apposition with the result that diaphragmatic contraction causes less effective rib cage expansion.[4] Hyperinflation also has an adverse effect on the elastic recoil of the thoracic cage.[4] This means that the inspiratory muscles must work not only against the elastic recoil of the lungs but also against that of the thoracic cage. The functional consequences of dynamic hyperinflation are probably the main mechanisms of ventilatory failure in patients with COPD.[35] Hyperinflation can also occur de novo in patients with pneumonia, chest trauma, and acute respiratory distress syndrome (ARDS).[33,36] Impairment of inspiratory muscle function is less likely in patients with ARDS than in patients with obstructive lung disease because patients with ARDS breathe at a low lung volume despite dynamic hyperinflation.[36,37]

Malnutrition

Malnutrition is highly prevalent among critically ill patients requiring mechanical ventilation,[38,39] and it is associated with poor prognosis.[39] Malnutrition decreases muscle mass and respiratory muscle strength both in humans[40,41] and in laboratory animals.[42-44] Likely mechanisms contributing to decrease in respiratory muscle mass include proteolysis of myofibrillar proteins by the ubiquitin-proteasome proteolytic system (Fig. 40.6) and apoptosis.[4,45] Apoptosis can be triggered by local and circulating tumor necrosis factor-α and by release of cytochrome *c* from the mitochondria.[46,47]

In patients with COPD, inspiratory muscle strength is about 30% less in poorly nourished patients than in well-nourished patients with equivalent airway obstruction.[18] Similarly, malnourished patients with anorexia nervosa can present with reduced inspiratory muscle strength to 35% to 50% predicted,[41] impaired respiratory muscle endurance,[49] impaired hypercapnic ventilatory response,[49] and occasionally, with hypercapnia at rest.[41] In malnourished patients, inspiratory weakness,[41,48,49] fatigability,[48] and dyspnea[48] are partially reversible with nutritional support. The process is slow and, in laboratory animals, can take months of refeeding for muscle mass to return to normal values.[50] To date, it remains unclear whether malnutrition by itself can cause sufficient respiratory muscle weakness to produce hypoventilation. It is more likely for malnutrition to be a contributory factor and not a sole cause of hypercapnic respiratory failure.

Endocrine Disturbances

Endocrine disturbances such as hypothyroidism,[51] hyperthyroidism,[47,52-54] and acromegaly[55] can adversely affect respiratory muscle function. Proteolysis of myofibrillar proteins by the ubiquitin-proteasome proteolytic system[45] (see Fig. 40.6) is probably responsible for respiratory muscle catabolism and weakness of hyperthyroidism.[47] This mechanism is implicated in muscle wasting associated with acidosis, renal

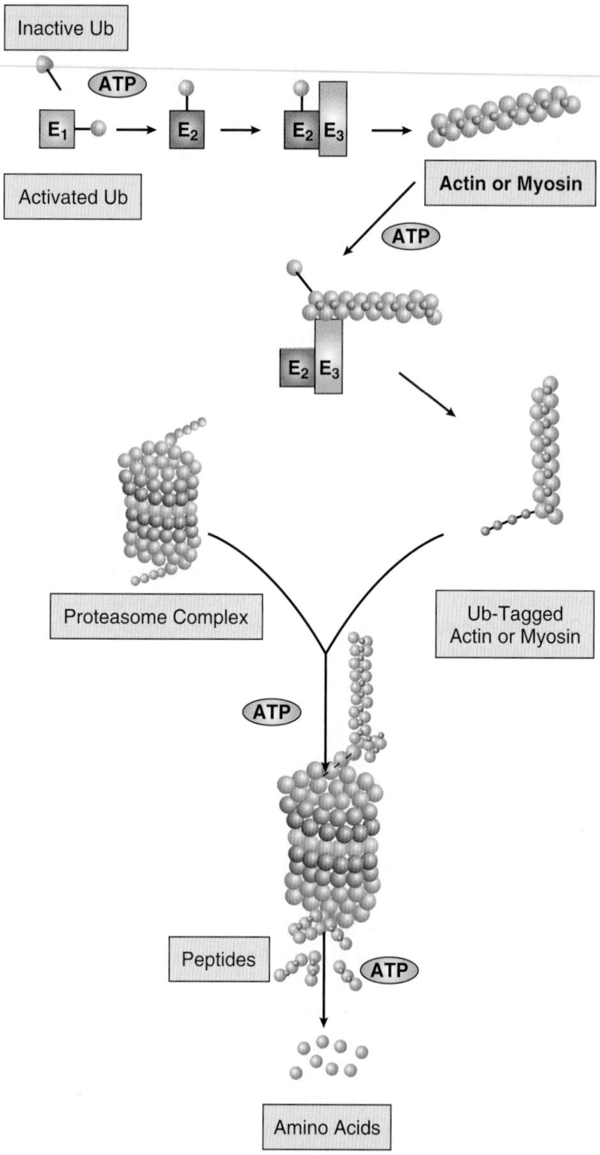

Figure 40.6 Ubiquitin-proteasome degradation of contractile proteins. The first step in degradation of actin and myosin is activation of ubiquitin (Ub) by a first enzyme, E_1—a process requiring adenosine triphosphate (ATP). Activated ubiquitin interacts with a second enzyme, E_2, a carrier protein. Ub and E_2 join a third enzyme, E_3. E_3 transfers activated Ub to actin and myosin. The cycle is repeated until a chain of Ub is bound to the contractile proteins. The chain of Ub binds to one end of a proteasome complex in a process requiring ATP. The Ub chain is subsequently removed (allowing reuse of Ub), and actin and myosin are unfolded and pushed into the core of the proteasome. Multiple enzymes within the core degrade actin and myosin into small peptides. The peptides are extruded from the proteasome and degraded to amino acids by peptidases in the cytoplasm. The ubiquitin-proteasome system degrades myofibrillar proteins only after they have been cleaved and released by other proteolytic pathways—i.e., the ubiquitin-proteasome pathway cannot degrade intact myofibrillar proteins. (From Laghi F, Tobin MJ: Disorders of the respiratory muscles. Am J Respir Crit Care Med 2003;168:10-48.)

failure, denervation, cancer, diabetes, acquired immunodeficiency syndrome (AIDS), trauma, and burns.[45] In contrast to other endocrine disturbances, respiratory muscle weakness is unusual in patients with Cushing syndrome.[56]

WEAKNESS DUE TO NEW-ONSET CONDITIONS

New-onset respiratory muscle weakness in critically ill patients may result from conditions that are unique to these patients. These conditions include ventilator-associated respiratory muscle dysfunction, sepsis-associated myopathy, and intensive care unit (ICU)-acquired paresis. New-onset respiratory muscle weakness can also result from conditions that are not unique to critically ill patients, including acid-base disorders, electrolyte disturbances, decreased oxygen delivery, and certain medications. Respiratory muscle weakness due to conditions that are unique to critically ill patients are often associated with alterations in respiratory muscle structure, although the others are not necessarily associated with alterations in muscle structure. Recovery from respiratory muscle weakness (if it occurs at all) is slow when the weakness is caused by alterations in muscle structure. In contrast, recovery of respiratory muscle weakness in conditions that are not necessarily associated with alterations in muscle structure is usually quick once the underlying triggering factor has been corrected.

Ventilator-Associated Respiratory Muscle Dysfunction

Since the late 1980s, several groups have studied the effect of mechanical ventilation on the muscles of laboratory animals.[57] A seminal study by Anzueto and colleagues[58] showed that 11 days of controlled mechanical ventilation (CMV) together with neuromuscular blocking agents produced a 46% decrease in respiratory muscle strength (Fig. 40.7). Subsequent studies have revealed that complete cessation of diaphragmatic activity with CMV—alone[59] or in combination with neuromuscular blocking agents[60]—results in atrophy and injury of diaphragmatic fibers (Fig. 40.8). Muscle fibers generate less force in response to stimulation, not simply because of their decreased bulk but even when normalized for cross-sectional area.[57] The decrease in diaphragmatic force ranges from 20% to more than 50%. The alterations in muscle function occur rapidly, within 12 hours of instituting mechanical ventilation,[61] and they appear to increase as ventilator duration is prolonged.[62,63]

Mechanical ventilation may also harm the respiratory muscles of patients. In 1988, Knisely and coworkers[64] reported that the cross-sectional area of diaphragmatic fibers in infants who had died after receiving mechanical ventilation for 12 or more days was much smaller than that in infants who had received mechanical ventilation for 7 days or less (Fig. 40.9). Fibers taken from extradiaphragmatic muscles were similar in the two groups. Twenty years later, Levine and associates[65] obtained biopsies of the diaphragm from 14 brain-dead organ donors who were maintained on CMV for 18 to 69 hours. They also obtained intraoperative biopsies of the diaphragms of eight control patients who had received CMV for 2 to 3 hours. Histologic measurements revealed marked diaphragmatic atrophy in the brain-dead patients. Compared with the control group, the mean cross-sectional areas of muscle fibers were decreased by more than 50%. A number of these results

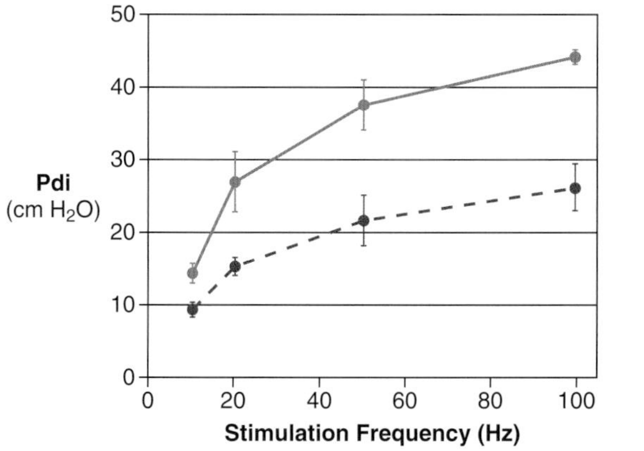

Figure 40.7 Transdiaphragmatic pressure (Pdi) response to phrenic nerve stimulation before (*solid line*) and after 11 days (*dashed line*) of mechanical ventilation. That the Pdi recorded after 11 days of mechanical ventilation shows a decreased response to all stimulation frequencies is suggestive of ventilator-associated diaphragmatic dysfunction (Modified from Anzueto A, Peters JI, Tobin MJ, et al: Effects of prolonged controlled mechanical ventilation on diaphragmatic function in healthy adult baboons. Crit Care Med 1997;25:1187.)

have been corroborated by Jaber and colleagues[63] and Hermans and coworkers,[66] who also reported a progressive decrease in diaphragmatic contractility of mechanically ventilated patients. The decrease in contractility correlated with the duration of ventilator support (Fig. 40.10).[63,66]

Biochemical and gene-expression studies in animals and humans[65,67] suggest that oxidative stress is probably one of the most proximal mechanisms in the biochemical cascade that leads to ventilator-induced muscle injury.[68] Oxidative stress decreases contractility by causing protein oxidation and by promoting protein catabolism[68]—including up-regulation of the autophagy-lysosome pathway.[69] The synergism between ventilator-induced muscle injury and oxidative stress has caused investigators to explore whether early administration of antioxidants might minimize muscle injury.[70-72] In a study of more than 200 critically ill patients—80% of whom required acute ventilator support—duration of mechanical ventilation was nearly 3 days shorter in those who completed a 10-day antioxidant supplementation protocol (vitamin E and vitamin C) than in those who completed a 10-day course of placebo.[73] Similar results have

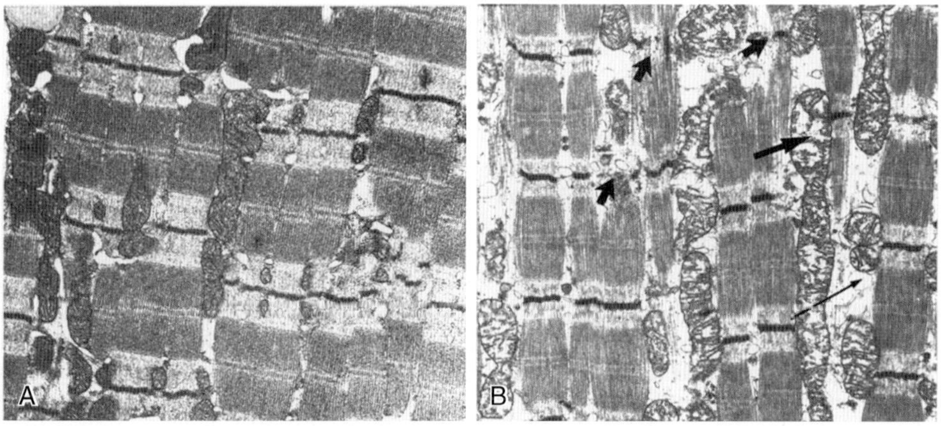

Figure 40.8 Electron microscopy of the diaphragm (longitudinal section) of a rabbit under control conditions (**A,** specimen processed with 1100-mOsm fixative) and after 3 days of controlled mechanical ventilation (**B,** specimen processed with 500-mOsm fixative). The control rabbit has an intact ultrastructure. The mechanically ventilated rabbit shows several areas of disrupted myofibrils (*short thick arrows*), the mitochondria are swollen (*long thick arrow*) and have abnormal cristae, and the intermyofibril space contains lipid droplets (*long thin arrow*), indicating decreased lipid uptake by the mitochondria. (From Laghi F, Tobin MJ: Disorders of the respiratory muscles. Am J Respir Crit Care Med 2003;168:10-48. Electron micrographs provided by Dr. Catherine S. H. Sassoon, Long Beach VA Hospital and University of California, Irvine, CA.)

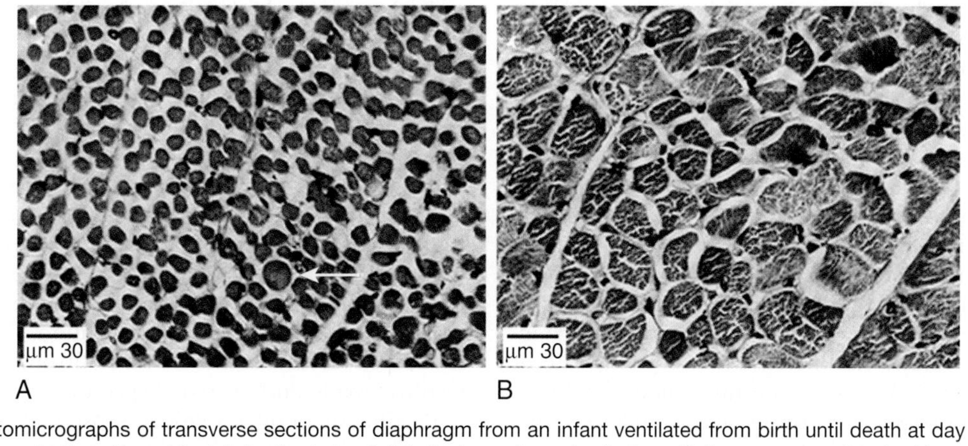

Figure 40.9 Photomicrographs of transverse sections of diaphragm from an infant ventilated from birth until death at day 47 (**A**) and from an infant ventilated from birth until accidental death at day 3 (**B**). Prolonged mechanical ventilation was associated with reduction in myofiber cross-sectional area. (The *yellow arrow* indicates a developing myofiber also known as Wohlfart myofiber.) (Modified from Knisely AS, Leal SM, Singer DB: Abnormalities of diaphragmatic muscle in neonates with ventilated lungs. J Pediatr 1988;113:1074.)

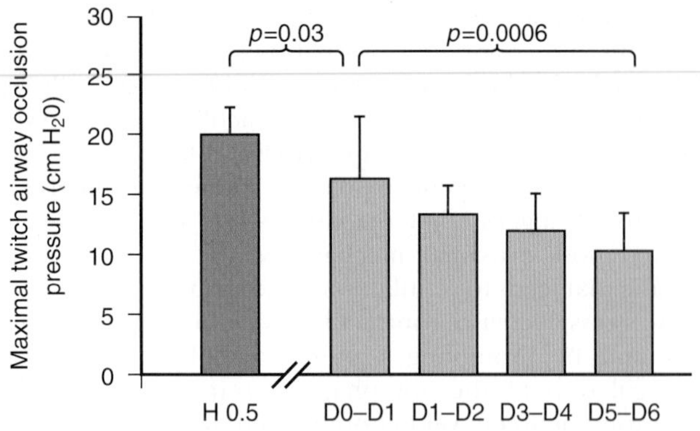

Figure 40.10 Twitch airway pressure elicited by magnetic stimulation of the phrenic nerves in six patients who received mechanical ventilation (MV) for 30 minutes (short-term MV; *open bar*) and in six patients who received MV for about 6 days (long-term MV; *solid bars*). On day 1 twitch airway pressure was already less in the long-term than in the short-term MV group. In addition, long-term MV was associated with a progressive decrease in twitch pressure over time—mean reduction of 32 ± 6% after 6 days of MV. H, number of hours of mechanical ventilation; D, number of days of mechanical ventilation. (From Jaber, Petrof BJ, Jung B, et al: Rapidly progressive diaphragmatic weakness and injury during mechanical ventilation in humans. Am J Respir Crit Care Med 2011;183:364-371.)

been reported in critically ill surgical patients requiring mechanical ventilation.[74] Whether the decrease in duration of mechanical ventilation was, at least in part, due to the potential positive effects of antioxidants on the respiratory muscles remains to be demonstrated. Of concern, however, was the report that administration of the antioxidant *N*-acetylcysteine (NAC) to critically ill patients with severe sepsis worsened sepsis-induced organ failure.[75]

In animal models, ventilator settings can affect the extent of ventilator-associated respiratory muscle dysfunction.[76-79] In rabbits, assist-control mechanical ventilation causes a nonsignificant decrease in diaphragm muscle contractility, which contrasts with the 48% decrease recorded with CMV.[76] Similar results have been obtained when comparing CMV to adaptive support ventilation in piglets[78] or when comparing CMV to pressure support in rats[79] or CMV to intermittent spontaneous breathing again in rats.[77] These observations raise the important question of whether maintenance of partial diaphragmatic activity or intermittent loading of the diaphragm could prevent the harm done to diaphragmatic function by mechanical ventilation.[80]

Considering that decrease in protein synthesis probably contributes to ventilator-associated respiratory muscle dysfunction,[81,82] it would seem biologically plausible that administration of anabolic factors—such as growth hormone—might be of benefit in ventilated patients. Unfortunately, when growth hormone has been administered to patients requiring prolonged mechanical ventilation, duration of mechanical ventilation was not decreased, nor was muscle strength increased.[83] Of concern was the report that recombinant growth hormone can increase the mortality rate of critically ill patients.[84] An even more fundamental point in regard to ventilator-associated respiratory muscle dysfunction has been raised recently by the preliminary data of Hooijman and associates.[85] These investigators measured the contractile properties of single diaphragmatic fibers obtained from nine brain-dead organ donors who had received CMV for 30 to 84 hours (case subjects) and from nine patients undergoing surgery for localized lung cancer (control subjects). In this preliminary study no difference was noted between the muscle fibers of the two groups of patients with respect to maximum force per unit area, calcium sensitivity of contractile force, and rate constant of redevelopment of force (Ktr). How to reconcile the preliminary results of Hooijman and associates[85] with previous data obtained on muscle strips from animal models and by phrenic nerve stimulation in patients remains to be determined.

Sepsis-Associated Myopathy

Sepsis, a common occurrence in critically ill patients, can produce ventilatory failure by causing respiratory muscle dysfunction and increased metabolic demands.[86] Septic animals develop failure of neuromuscular transmission (due to increased sarcolemmal electric potential)[87-89] and failure of excitation-contraction coupling.[86,90] Mechanisms responsible for failure of excitation-contraction coupling include the cytotoxic effect of nitric oxide and its metabolites, free radicals, ubiquitin-proteasome proteolysis, and possibly, decrease in nicotinic acetylcholine receptors.[91,92] Local dysregulation of the circulation and Krebs cycle may also contribute.[86]

Nitric oxide, a free radical that has a negative inotropic effect in the heart and skeletal muscle, is produced in large amounts during sepsis by a nitric oxide synthase inducible by lipopolysaccharide and several cytokines (Fig. 40.11).[93] Increased expression of inducible nitric oxide synthase in the diaphragm during sepsis is associated with morphologic evidence of widespread damage to the myofiber membrane, or sarcolemma (Fig. 40.12).[88] Diaphragmatic contractions enhance this sepsis-induced sarcolemmal injury,[94] while early mechanical ventilation decreases sarcolemmal injury and the associated diaphragmatic dysfunction.[95] The beneficial effects of resting the diaphragm with the use of mechanical ventilation are not coupled with a decrease in oxidative stress or with a decrease in the expression of inducible nitric oxide synthase in the muscle.[95] These observations suggest the existence of a detrimental interaction of two independent stressors (oxidative and biomechanical stresses) on the sarcolemma during sepsis.[95]

To determine whether the inducible nitric oxide synthase pathway contributes to impaired skeletal muscle contractility in humans, Lanone and coworkers[96] obtained samples of the rectus abdominis in 16 septic patients and 21 control subjects. The muscles of the patients had lower contractile force, and increases in inducible nitric oxide synthase expression (mRNA and protein) and activity. Immunohistochemical studies revealed the generation of peroxynitrite (a highly reactive oxidant formed by the reaction of nitric oxide with superoxide anion). Exposure of control muscles to the amount of peroxynitrite found in patients caused an irreversible decrease in force generation. These data suggest that sepsis decreases muscle force through the production of nitric oxide and its toxic byproducts.

Production of nitric oxide in sepsis may be protective and not solely deleterious.[94,97-99] In mice deficient in inducible[97] or constitutive (neuronal) nitric oxide synthase,[94] endotoxin caused a greater decline in diaphragmatic contractility

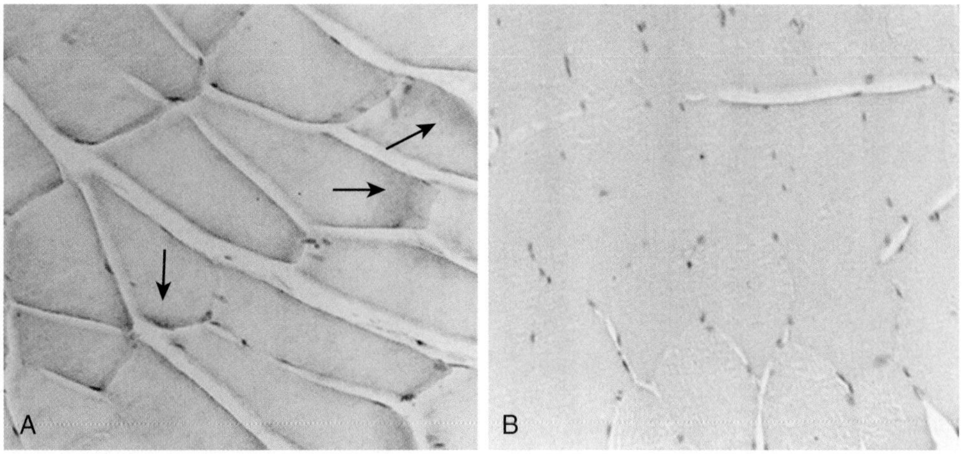

Figure 40.11 A, A sample of gastrocnemius muscle obtained from an adult Sprague-Dawley rat injected 12 hours earlier with *Escherichia coli* endotoxin (20 mg/kg). The section was stained with an antibody to inducible nitric oxide synthase. Positive staining (*brown coloration*, *arrows*) is evident inside the fibers. **B,** A sample of gastrocnemius muscle obtained from a rat injected 12 hours earlier with normal saline. No positive staining is evident. (From Laghi F, Tobin MJ: Disorders of the respiratory muscles. Am J Respir Crit Care Med 2003;168:10-48. Photomicrographs provided by Dr. Sabah N. Hussain, Royal Victoria Hospital, Montreal, Canada.)

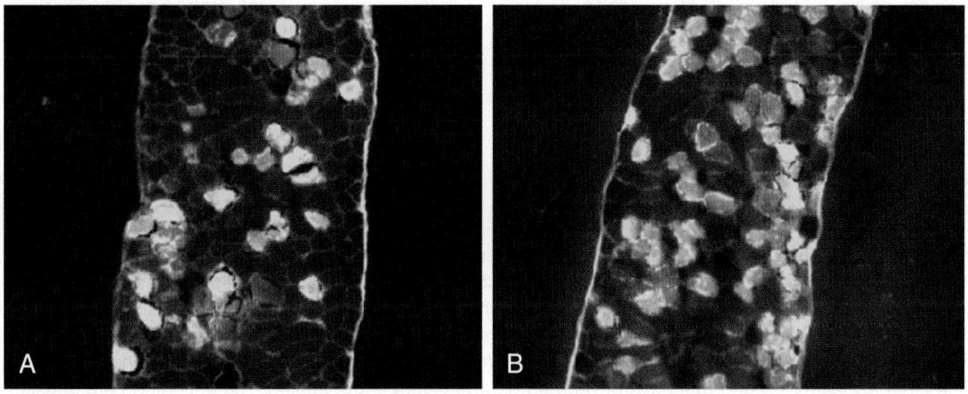

Figure 40.12 A, A strip of diaphragm obtained from a C57BL/6 mouse injected 12 hours earlier with normal saline. The strip was stimulated for 3 minutes (50 Hz, 300-ms duration) and then immersed for 90 minutes in Krebs solution containing a fluorescent probe, Procion orange 14 (0.15, wt/vol). **D,** A strip of diaphragm obtained from a C57BL/6 mouse injected 12 hours earlier with *Escherichia coli* endotoxin (20 mg/kg). Stimulation and staining were conducted as described in A. Sarcolemmal damage, indicated by yellow staining, was increased by endotoxin. (From Laghi F, Tobin MJ: Disorders of the respiratory muscles. Am J Respir Crit Care Med 2003;168:10-48. Photomicrographs provided by Dr. Sabah N. Hussain, Royal Victoria Hospital, Montreal, Canada.)

than in nondeficient mice. This finding contrasts with the observation that nitric oxide synthase inhibitors prevent muscle dysfunction in septic rats.[88,93,100] Although the results may be species-dependent,[94] the data underscore that nitric oxide has both antioxidant and pro-oxidant actions.[101]

In addition to nitric oxide and its derivatives, several other oxygen-derived free radicals (superoxide anion, hydroxyl radicals, hydrogen peroxide) contribute to the decreased contractility of the diaphragm in sepsis.[99,102-104] This increased expression of oxygen-derived free radicals in sepsis is accompanied with enhanced activity of the antioxidant enzyme superoxide dismutase[102] and with increased expression of the heme oxygenase-1 pathway.[104] The heme oxygenase-1 pathway is a powerful cellular system that protects against oxidative stress and contractile fatigue during sepsis.[104] Administration of an inhibitor (zinc protoporphyrin IX) or an inducer (hemin) of heme oxygenase activity respectively enhances or reduces the oxidative stress and contractile failure of the diaphragm in a rat model of sepsis.[104] In septic rats, decreased diaphragmatic contractility can also be improved by the administration of specific scavengers of superoxide ions, hydrogen peroxide, and hydroxyl radicals.[102]

Intensive Care Unit–Acquired Paresis

While cared for in the ICU, critically ill patients can develop muscle weakness and, occasionally, paralysis. Some of these patients have evidence for axonal degeneration and denervation atrophy (Fig. 40.13).[4] This constellation of findings is known as critical illness polyneuropathy (Table 40.1).[105] Cytokines[106] and low-molecular-weight neurotoxins[107] released during episodes of sepsis or when patients develop multiple organ failure are thought to be responsible for this axonal degeneration. Critical illness polyneuropathy has been considered one of the manifestations of multiple organ failure syndrome. Sepsis and multiple organ

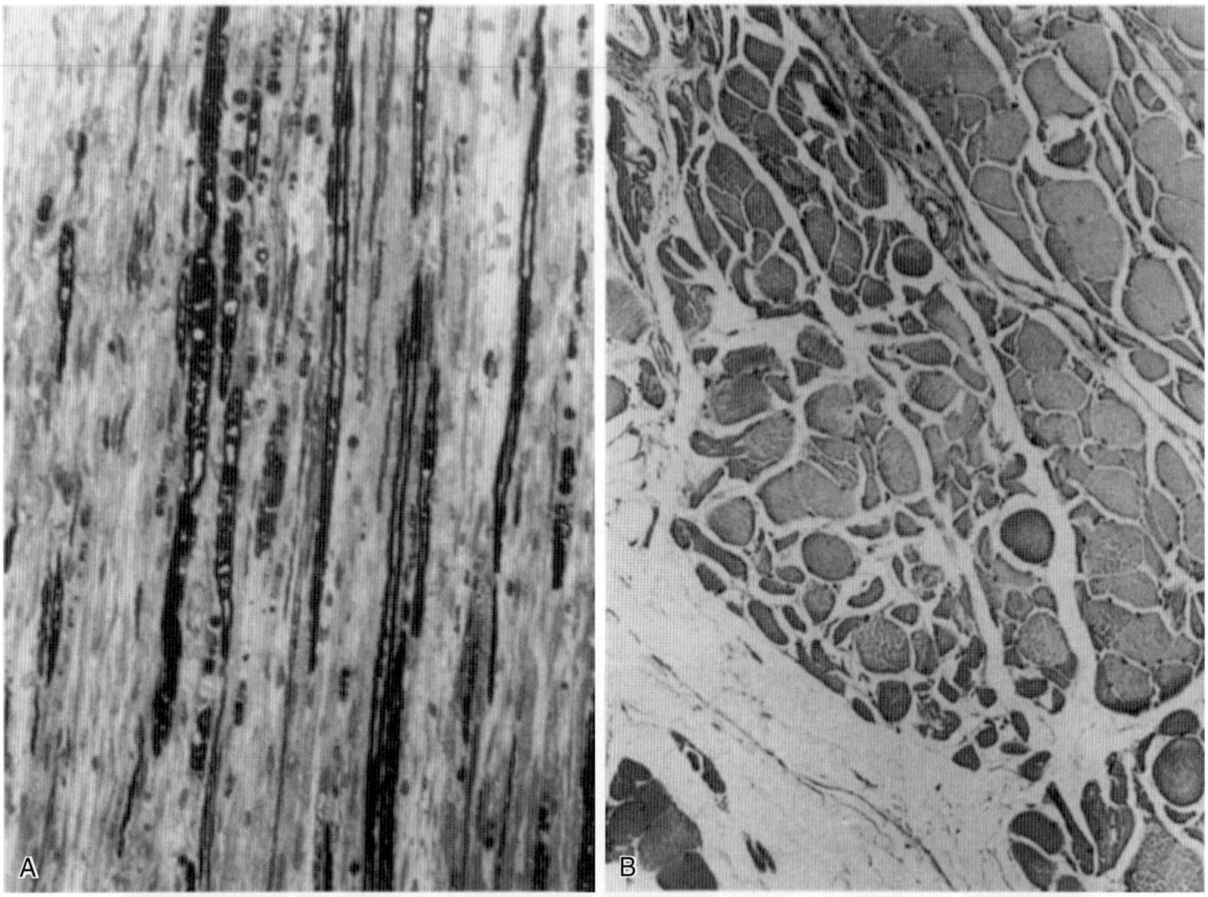

Figure 40.13 Transverse section of a peripheral motor nerve (deep peroneal nerve, **A**) and of a skeletal muscle (intercostal, **B**) in patients who developed profound weakness following a prolonged hospital course characterized by sepsis, multiple organ failure syndrome, and inability to wean from mechanical ventilation. **A,** The long thin dark structures seen in the left panel are myelin sheaths that contain axons. The axons are degenerating and dying. Following death, they disintegrate. The myelin surrounding the disintegrating axons collapses around the axonal debris to form ovoids of myelin—seen better on the lateral portions of the left micrograph. **B,** Amid muscle fibers that are normal in size and shape there are atrophic ones that appear small and that have developed contours with acute angles. These findings are consistent with denervation atrophy secondary to axonal degeneration, so-called critical illness polyneuropathy. (From Zochodne DW, Bolton CF, Wells GA, et al: Critical illness polyneuropathy. A complication of sepsis and multiple organ failure. Brain 1987;110:819.)

failure, though, are not essential prerequisites for the development of critical illness polyneuropathy.[108,109] Tight control of hyperglycemia may reduce the risk of polyneuropathy and the duration of mechanical ventilation.[110]

In other patients, rather than axonopathy, there is evidence of isolated myopathy (i.e., critical illness myopathy).[4] Patients developing isolated myopathy often have been treated with steroids and neuromuscular blocking agents (e.g., patients with status asthmaticus).[4] Muscle biopsies demonstrate a general decrease in myofibrillar protein content and a selective loss of thick filaments (myosin) within type I and type II fibers (Table 40.2 and Fig. 40.14). Animal models of critical illness myopathy suggest that medical denervation with paralytic agents cause an up-regulation of glucocorticoid receptors in the muscle.[111] If the animal subsequently receives high-dose corticosteroids, it will develop depletion of thick myosin filaments.[111] Although a decrease in thick-filament proteins may be important for prolonged weakness,[112] this decrease is probably not the cause of the acute paralysis,[113] particularly in patients with compound motor action potentials of low amplitude.[114] Impaired muscle membrane excitability is probably more important during the acute stage.[113,115]

In the last few years it has become increasingly apparent that critical illness neuropathy and myopathy often coexist.[106,109,115-118] It has become common to refer to patients who become weak while in the ICU as a result of acquired neuropathy or myopathy (not associated with a known disorder) as simply having ICU-acquired paresis.[115,116,118] In patients with ICU-acquired paresis duration of weaning from mechanical ventilation can be two to seven times longer than in patients without ICU-acquired paresis.[119]

The functional outcome of ICU-acquired paresis is not uniform. Approximately 50% to 60% of patients experience complete recovery (ability to breathe spontaneously and to walk independently) over a period of 2 weeks to 6 months or longer.[112,119,120] About 30% experience severe persistent disability with tetraparesis, tetraplegia, or paraplegia.[119] Other investigators report even worse outcome: only 2 of 10 patients left the hospital in one study.[117] Whether it is possible to prevent ICU-acquired paresis in patients recovering from severe acute illness, and whether that would result

Table 40.1 Examples of Electromyography (EMG) Findings in Respiratory Muscle Weakness

EMG Feature	Axonal Injury	Myelin Injury	Neuromuscular Conduction Defect	Myopathy
Compound muscle action potential (amplitude)*	Reduced	Normal to slightly reduced	Normal†	Normal
Sensory nerve action potential (amplitude)‡	Reduced	Normal to reduced	Normal	Normal
Conduction velocity	Normal to slightly reduced	Reduced	Normal	Normal
Spontaneous muscle depolarization§	Present	Absent	Absent	None to present
Amplitude of compound muscle action potential with stimulation at 3 Hz¶	Unchanged	Unchanged	Decreased	Unchanged
Motor unit activation	Decreased	Decreased	Normal	Increased

Examples of injuries and deficits: *axonal injury*, critical illness polyneuropathy; *myelin injury*, Guillain-Barré syndrome; *neuromuscular conduction defect*, myasthenia, prolonged neuromuscular blockade; *myopathy*, critical illness myopathy.

*Elicited by motor nerve stimulation.

†Decreased in Lambert-Eaton syndrome.

‡Elicited by sensory nerve stimulation.

§Spontaneous muscle depolarization (caused by denervation) is detected by presence of fibrillation potentials and positive sharp waves.

¶Repetitive nerve stimulation is performed to exclude neuromuscular transmission defects such as prolonged neuromuscular paralysis.

Although features of myopathy can be recorded by electromyographic studies, electromyography cannot always distinguish critical illness myopathy from critical illness polyneuropathy, and muscle biopsy may be needed.

From Laghi F, Tobin MJ: Disorders of the respiratory muscles. Am J Respir Crit Care Med 2003;168:10.

Table 40.2 Characteristics of Types of Muscle Fibers

Characteristic	Type I	Type IIa	Type IIx	Type IIb
Contractile Properties				
Velocity of shortening	+	++	+++	++++
Tetanic force	+	+	++	++
Endurance	++++	+++	++	+
Work efficiency*	+++	++	++	+
Histochemistry				
Mitochondrial volume density	+++	+++	++	+
ATP consumption rate	+	++	+++	++++
Oxidative enzymes	+++	+++	++	+
Glycolytic enzymes	+	++	+++	++++
Glycogen	+	++	++	+++
Capillary supply	+++	+++	++	+
Diameter	+	++	++	+++

*Amount of work performed per unit of adenosine triphosphate (ATP) consumed.

A single myosin heavy chain isoform typically is expressed within an adult skeletal muscle fiber. Fibers classified as type I, IIa, IIx, or IIb express myosin heavy chain isoform I (or slow), IIa, IIx, or IIb, respectively. Type IIx fibers have been reported in peripheral muscles of humans and animals and in the diaphragm of animals. Type IIx fibers have not been reported in the human diaphragm. More than one myosin heavy chain isoform is expressed in a few fibers (about 14% of adult rat diaphragm coexpresses myosin heavy chain isoforms IIb and IIx, and less than 1% coexpresses myosin heavy chain isoforms I and IIa).[226] Whereas the velocity of muscle contraction depends primarily on the myosin heavy chain isoform, the velocity of muscle relaxation is mainly determined by troponin C calcium binding and release and by calcium reuptake by the sarcoendoplasmic reticulum calcium-adenosine triphosphatase (SERCA). Several SERCA isoenzymes have been identified: SERCA 1 is expressed in type II fibers (fast calcium reuptake), and SERCA 2a is expressed in type I fibers (slow calcium reuptake).[227] The density of pumping sites largely accounts for different rates of calcium uptake in fast- and slow-twitch muscle fibers.[227] Despite this separation of tasks, velocity of contraction and velocity of relaxation tend to parallel each other: type II fibers contract and relax with a greater velocity than type I fibers. Slower velocity of relaxation allows fusion of repetitive twitches at lower frequencies of stimulation than with fast relaxations. Impairment of SERCA activity has been implicated in the development of fatigue and in disease states including heart failure and corticosteroid myopathy.

From Laghi F, Tobin MJ: Disorders of the respiratory muscles. Am J Respir Crit Care Med 2003;168:10.

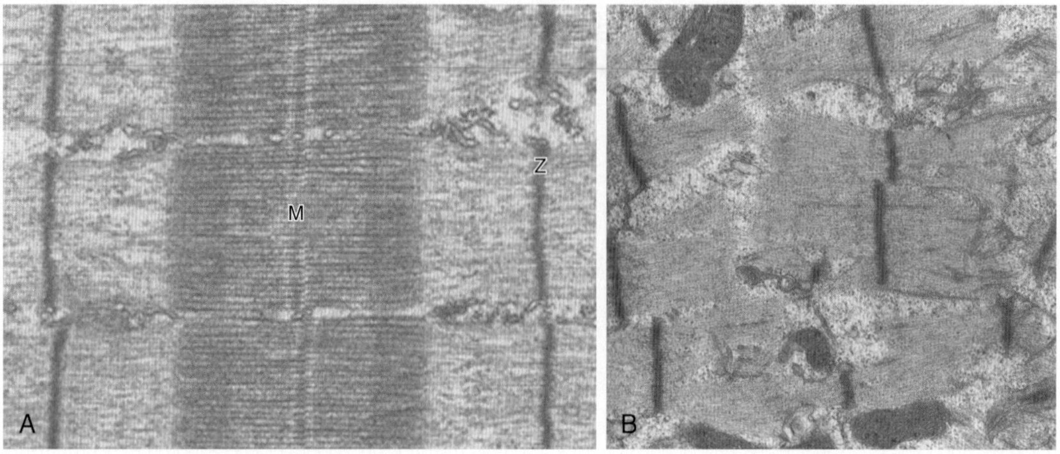

Figure 40.14 Electron micrographs of normal skeletal muscle (*right panel*) and skeletal muscle from a patient who received steroids and the neuromuscular blocking agent vecuronium during a hospitalization with status asthmaticus followed by flaccid quadriplegia. Compared with the normal structure, the patient developed extensive loss of thick (myosin) myofilaments and relative preservation of thin (actin) filaments. Muscle strength returned to normal 2 months after discontinuation of vecuronium. M, M-line formed by myosin filaments and M-line proteins; Z, Z-disk formed by a lattice of filaments that join the actin filaments of one sarcomere with the actin filaments of the adjacent sarcomere. (From Eisenberg BR: Can electron microscopy distinguish fiber types? In Bradley WG, Gardner-Medwin D, Walton JN [eds]: Recent Advances in Myology. Amsterdam, Excerpta Medica, 1975; and from Danon MJ, Carpenter S: Myopathy with thick filament (myosin) loss following prolonged paralysis with vecuronium during steroid treatment. Muscle Nerve 1991;14:1131.)

in shorter duration of mechanical ventilation remains unknown.

Acid-Base Disorders

Alkalosis, either metabolic or respiratory, does not affect skeletal muscle strength[121-123] and might improve endurance.[121] Whether acidosis, either metabolic or respiratory, impairs respiratory muscle function remains controversial. Because the contractile response to metabolic and respiratory acidosis is not necessarily the same,[124,125] metabolic acidosis and respiratory acidosis will be discussed separately.

Metabolic Acidosis. Until recently, there was little doubt that metabolic acidosis could decrease muscle contractility.[126,127] Purported mechanisms included reduction of actin-myosin cross-bridge activation by H^+ competitive inhibition of Ca^{2+} binding to troponin-C, reduced transition of actin-myosin cross-bridges from low- to high-force state, inhibition of myofibrillar adenosine triphosphatase (ATPase), inhibition of glycolytic rate, inhibition of maximal shortening velocity, and inhibition of sarcoplasmic ATPase with reduction of sarcoplasmic Ca^{2+} reuptake leading to reduced Ca^{2+} release from the sarcoplasmic reticulum.[128] Despite the biologic plausibility, investigators have reported no effect[125,129] or marginal effect[130] of metabolic acidosis on respiratory muscle function. Yanos and colleagues[125] assessed maximal transdiaphragmatic pressure elicited by tetanic stimulation of the phrenic nerves in seven anesthetized dogs during respiratory acidosis (pH 7.1) and during lactic acidosis (pH 7.1). They observed a fall in maximal diaphragm strength with respiratory acidosis (−18%, $p < 0.05$), but not with lactic acidosis (+3%). Similarly, when Coast and associates[130] exposed isolated diaphragm strips of rats to different concentrations of lactic acid they recorded decreases in force when the pH was lowered to 6.8—but only after the muscle strips were stressed with 75 contractions (25 Hz, 250-ms train duration, one train per second). Contractility was not affected when the pH was decreased to ~7.0 at rest, and following the set of 75 contractions when delivered at a pH of 7.1 and 7.2.[130] These negative results are in line with some—but not all[131,132]—recent investigations questioning the inhibitory role of metabolic acidosis on limb muscle contractility at physiologic temperatures.[133-136] For instance, Nielsen and colleagues[136] reported that metabolic acidosis (pH 6.80) counteracts the detrimental effects of increased extracellular K^+ concentrations (which occur with forceful contractions) on the excitability and force generation of the rat soleus muscle. In humans, Degroot and coworkers[134] measured intracellular H^+ concentration during sustained isometric foot plantar flexion. In contrast to what would be expected if acidosis caused decrease in contractility, Degroot and coworkers[134] reported a decrease in intracellular H^+ concentration during the first 10 seconds of exercise when force was declining and a rise in intracellular H^+ concentration immediately after exercise, when force partially recovered.[134] Whether severe metabolic acidosis in humans might impair skeletal function by causing a reduced central nervous system drive remains to be demonstrated.[126]

Acute Respiratory Acidosis. There are contrasting reports on the effect of acute respiratory acidosis on respiratory muscle contractility.[122,123,125,137] In anesthetized dogs, diaphragmatic contractility decreases pari passu with the severity of acute respiratory acidosis[122] (but has no effect on gastrocnemius muscle contractility).[125] Similarly, in healthy volunteers, acute increases of arterial carbon dioxide to 54 mm Hg (corresponding to a pH of about 7.29) reduces the capacity of the unfatigued diaphragm to generate pressure by 10% to 30% (Fig. 40.15).[123] Such reduction in pressure generation is even greater when arterial carbon dioxide is increased to 63 mm Hg (corresponding to a pH of about 7.22).[123] Acute respiratory acidosis can decrease respiratory muscle endurance,[123,138] and it can increase the extent of

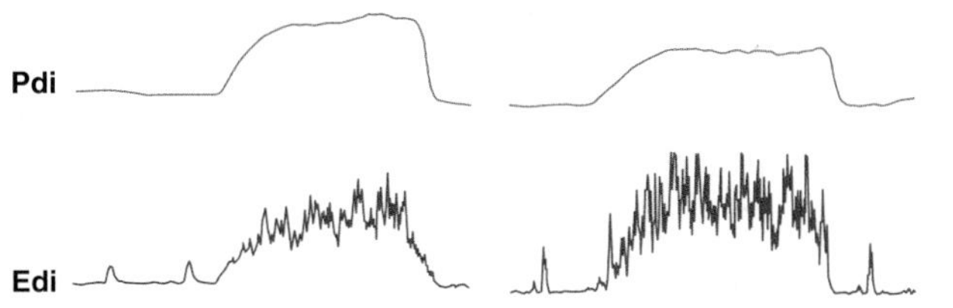

Figure 40.15 Transdiaphragmatic pressure (Pdi) and electrical activity of the diaphragm (Edi) during a voluntary isometric contraction in a healthy subject during normocapnia (*left panel*) and during acute hypercapnia (end-tidal CO_2, 7.5%, *right panel*). For a given Edi during hypercapnia the pressure output of the diaphragm was decreased. (From, Juan G, Calverley P, Talamo C, et al: Effect of carbon dioxide on diaphragmatic function in human beings. N Engl J Med 1984;310:874.)

diaphragmatic fatigue at the conclusion of 2 minutes of maximal voluntary ventilation.[139] Despite greater voluntary activation of the diaphragm,[140] hypercapnic patients with COPD generate lower maximal static inspiratory pressures than patients with normocapnia.[141,142]

A direct inhibitory effect of acute respiratory acidosis[122,123,125,138,139] on respiratory muscle contractility and respiratory muscle endurance could provide a potential mechanism for the rapid clinical deterioration that can occur with severe asthma and during COPD exacerbations.[123] Yet, the human data suggesting a direct deleterious effect of acute respiratory acidosis on respiratory muscle function[123,138,139,141] is not uniform. Some investigators report no change in diaphragmatic contractility[137,139] (but decrease in force of the adductor pollicis)[137] when acute respiratory acidosis causes a decrease in pH to about 7.16 to 7.27,[137,143] no change in the maximum relaxation rate of the diaphragm,[143] and no effect in the extent of diaphragmatic fatigue 20 to 90 minutes after loading.[139]

For several reasons it is difficult to reconcile the conflicting data on the effects of acute respiratory acidosis on respiratory muscle contractility reported in the literature. First, the nonsignificant decrease in diaphragmatic contractility of 12% (twitch pressure) recorded during acute hypercapnia in 12 healthy subjects in one study[137] raises the possibility of type II error. Second, it is impossible to state that more severe acidosis was responsible for the different results in human investigations considering the comparable pH values of the negative[137] and positive[123] studies. Third, it is unlikely that different frequencies of stimulation used to assess the respiratory muscles[123,137,139] are responsible for the contrasting results because, when present, acidosis-associated decrease in contractility is frequency independent.[122] Moreover, three additional considerations further cloud our understanding of any interaction (if present) between acute respiratory acidosis and respiratory muscle contractility. First, respiratory acidosis (pH 6.50-6.88) may actually enhance and not depress skeletal muscle contractility.[136,144] Second, it is unknown whether comorbid conditions, which often affect hypercapnic patients, such as sepsis, decreased cardiac function, and impaired respiratory mechanics could act synergistically with acute hypercapnia in worsening respiratory muscle function. Third, it is unknown whether equivalent levels of pH occurring as a result of acute- or acute-on-chronic respiratory acidosis may—or may not—have the same effect on respiratory muscle function.

Electrolyte Disturbances

Respiratory muscle function may be impaired by decreased levels of phosphate,[145] calcium,[146] magnesium,[147] and potassium.[148] Aubier and associates[145] studied the effects of severe hypophosphatemia (0.55 ± 0.18 mmol/L) on diaphragmatic function in eight patients with acute respiratory failure who were mechanically ventilated. Diaphragmatic function was quantified before and after phosphorus replacement therapy by recording transdiaphragmatic twitch pressure elicited by phrenic nerve stimulation. Correction of hypophosphatemia was accompanied by a significant increase in transdiaphragmatic twitch pressure—i.e., from 9.8 ± 3.8 cm H_2O before phosphate infusion to 17.3 ± 6.5 cm H_2O after phosphate infusion ($p < 0.001$). Changes in the serum phosphorus level and transdiaphragmatic pressure were well correlated ($r = 0.73$). These results strongly suggest that hypophosphatemia can impair the contractile properties of the diaphragm during acute respiratory failure.

The same investigators assessed the effects of hypocalcemia on diaphragmatic function in 12 anesthetized dogs.[146] A continuous infusion of the chelating agent ethylene glycol-bis(2-aminoethylether)-*N,N′*-tetraacetic acid (EGTA) was used to produce hypocalcemia. Over the 2 hours of observation, a progressive reduction in diaphragmatic force production paralleled the progressive reduction in ionized serum calcium.

Hypomagnesemia, a common occurrence in the ICU, can also cause respiratory muscle weakness. Dhingra and colleagues[147] reported improvements in maximal inspiratory and expiratory pressures in 17 hypomagnesemic patients following magnesium replacement therapy but not following placebo therapy.

Severe hypokalemia can be caused by several disorders including posthypercapnic alkalosis, renal tubular acidosis, primary hyperaldosteronism, gastrointestinal potassium losses, use of diuretics, thyrotoxic periodic paralysis, familial hypokalemic paralysis, β_2-adrenergic agonists, and licorice ingestion. When the serum potassium concentration decreases below 2.0 to 2.5 mEq/L, patients may develop muscular weakness (including respiratory muscle weakness) and arrhythmias. Hypokalemia-associated respiratory muscle weakness can result in respiratory failure and death.[148]

Decreased Oxygen Delivery

Laboratory animals with cardiogenic shock[149] or with septic shock[86,150] die of respiratory failure. Death is not caused by pulmonary disease per se but by an inability of the respiratory muscles to maintain adequate ventilation. This inability to maintain adequate ventilation is caused by insufficient oxygen delivery to the respiratory muscles.[4]

Whether the decrease in oxygen delivery to the respiratory muscles—or the respiratory centers—during shock is sufficient to decrease respiratory muscle performance and cause hypoventilation in patients, although likely,[151] remains to be determined. A nonrandomized study by Kontoyannis and coworkers[152] in 28 patients with cardiogenic shock provides support for the view that hemodynamic instability could decrease respiratory muscle performance in patients with shock. Compared with nonventilated patients, ventilated patients were weaned from an intra-aortic balloon pump more often, and their survival was greater.[152] These results are in line with the observation of Viires and associates[153] who reported decreased metabolic requirements of the diaphragm following institution of mechanical ventilation in dogs with cardiogenic shock.

Some hemodynamic situations that are less extreme than shock could still affect respiratory muscle performance, including failed attempts of spontaneous respiration during weaning from mechanical ventilation. Jubran and colleagues[154] investigated the importance of hemodynamic performance in determining weaning outcome in 8 ventilator-supported patients who failed a trial of spontaneous breathing and 11 patients who tolerated a trial and were successfully extubated. Immediately before the trial, mixed oxygen venous saturation was not different between the two groups. Mixed venous oxygen saturation progressively decreased over the course of the trial in the failure group, whereas it remained unchanged in the success group (Fig. 40.16, upper panel). Although the calculated oxygen demand was similar in the two groups, the manner in which it was met differed between them. In the success group, oxygen transport increased, mainly resulting from an increase in cardiac index; in the failure group, the increase in demand was met by an increase in oxygen extraction, resulting in a decrease in mixed venous oxygen saturation (Fig. 40.16, lower panel). Although increased, the oxygen extraction ratio at the end of the trial in the failure group was close to the ratio reported to signify the onset of anaerobic metabolism (0.60)[155] in only two patients, who had ratios of 0.50 and 0.56, respectively. The ability of the failure group to deal with respiratory muscle energy demands through aerobic pathways is probably related to the capacity of the diaphragm to achieve higher blood flow than most other skeletal muscles.[156] During loading, the diaphragm rapidly increases oxygen extraction to a plateau of about 55% to 65%; further increases in oxygen demand are achieved by increases in blood flow.[157,158] The diaphragmatic musculature appears to be extremely resistant to hypoxic stress, and animals can maintain a ventilation that is sufficient to avoid hypercapnia until phrenic vein P_{O_2} falls to 12 mm Hg.[156] Likewise, investigators have found that an oxygen tension of about 10 mm Hg in the phrenic vein is the threshold associated with the onset of diaphragmatic lactate production[159] and the development of fatigue.[160] The lowest mixed venous oxygen tension recorded by Jubran and colleagues[154] was 26 mm Hg, which is above the threshold for onset of diaphragmatic lactate production. This association needs to be interpreted with caution, however, because mixed venous blood contains effluents from many tissue beds other than the diaphragm. The investigation of Jubran and colleagues[154] is the first documentation that, when challenged by an increase in mechanical load,[7] the respiratory muscles of critically ill patients do not appear to switch from aerobic to anaerobic metabolism.

High variability in hemodynamic response during failure to wean has been reported by Zakynthinos and coworkers.[14] Similar to Jubran and colleagues,[154] Zakynthinos and coworkers[14] recorded a decrease in mixed venous oxygen saturation and an increase in oxygen consumption (met mainly by an increase in oxygen extraction) in 9 of 18 weaning failure patients. In the remaining 9 failures, however, mixed venous oxygen saturation and oxygen consumption were not affected by the weaning trial. It is unclear whether the absent interaction between weaning failure and oxygen consumption was due to depression of the respiratory centers, limited capacity to extract oxygen, or limited cardiac reserve.[161]

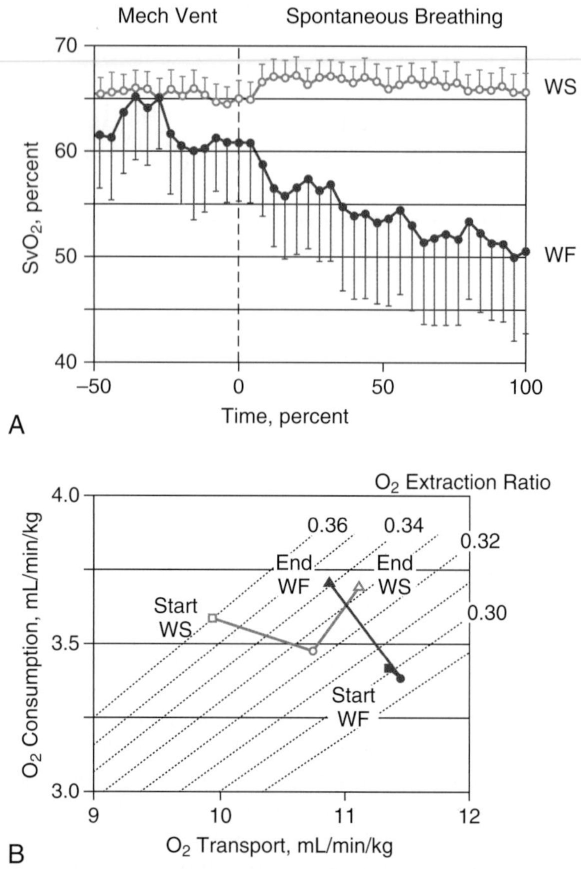

Figure 40.16 **A,** Mixed venous oxygen saturation ($S\bar{v}_{O_2}$) during mechanical ventilation and a trial of spontaneous breathing in 11 weaning success patients (WS, *open symbols*) and in 8 weaning failure patients (WF, *closed symbols*). During mechanical ventilation, $S\bar{v}_{O_2}$ was similar in the two groups ($p = 0.28$). Between the onset (*dashed line*) and the end of the trial, $S\bar{v}_{O_2}$ decreased in the failure group ($p < 0.01$), whereas it remained unchanged in the success group ($p = 0.48$). Over the course of the trial, $S\bar{v}_{O_2}$ was lower in the failure group than in the success group ($p < 0.02$). Bars indicate SE (standard error). **B,** Oxygen transport, oxygen consumption, and isopleths of oxygen extraction ratio in the success (WS, *open symbols*) and failure (WF, *closed symbols*) groups during mechanical ventilation (*squares*) and at the onset (*circles*) and end (*triangles*) of a spontaneous breathing trial. See text for details. (Modified from Jubran A, Marthu M, Dries E, et al: Continuous recordings of mixed venous oxygen saturation during weaning from mechanical ventilation and the ramifications thereof. Am J Respir Crit Care Med 1998;158:1763.)

Medications

Weakness can result from medications that have a direct myotoxic effect, such as blockade of myocyte glycoprotein synthesis and electron transport caused by inhibitors of the hydroxymethylglutaryl coenzyme A reductase or nucleoside analogs used in patients with human immunodeficiency virus.[162-165] Weakness can also result with neuromuscular blocking agents and aminoglycosides, which interfere with neuromuscular transmission.[166,167]

Paralysis, including the respiratory muscles, can persist after discontinuation of neuromuscular blocking agents.[167-169] Prolonged neuromuscular blockade has been defined as 2,[167] 4,[169] or 6 hours[168] of paralysis after discontinuation of neuromuscular blocking agents. Prolonged blockade is estimated to occur in 12% to 44% of patients receiving pancuronium or vecuronium for 1 or more days.[167-169] The risk with vecuronium is increased in patients with renal failure.[167,169] Accumulation of metabolites of the neuromuscular blocking agents is responsible for the prolonged blockade.[167] Recovery from prolonged neuromuscular blockade begins within 2 days of the last dose,[167,168] and this contrasts with the prolonged course of critical illness myopathy or neuropathy.[112,120,170,171] Train-of-four monitoring of the dose of a neuromuscular blocking agent with a peripheral nerve stimulator may hasten recovery.[169]

LIMITATIONS IN THE CURRENT CLASSIFICATION OF RESPIRATORY MUSCLE WEAKNESS

When one is studying respiratory muscle weakness leading to hypoventilation in critically ill patients it is necessary to bear in mind the current limited understanding of these conditions, as follows:

1. The distinction between preexisting conditions and new-onset conditions can be arbitrary.
2. Conditions that are preexisting (malnutrition and hyperinflation) can worsen during the course of an unrelated critical illness.
3. The nosologic designation is often unsatisfactory—see the nebulous distinction between ICU-acquired paresis and sepsis-associated myopathy or between ICU-acquired paresis and ventilator-associated respiratory muscle dysfunction.
4. Conditions in which respiratory muscle weakness is associated with muscle damage can display also some degree of muscle atrophy—see diaphragmatic atrophy in cases of ventilator-associated respiratory muscle dysfunction.
5. Laboratory specificity to differentiate the various conditions causing weakness in the ICU is limited.
6. In any given patient more than one mechanism may be responsible for respiratory muscle weakness.
7. Respiratory muscle weakness can be combined with depressed drive—for example, in the setting of hypercapnia-induced hypoventilation.

RESPIRATORY MUSCLE FATIGUE

Contractile fatigue occurs when a sufficiently large respiratory load is applied over a sufficiently long period.[15,172-180] Contractile fatigue can be brief or prolonged. Short-lasting fatigue results from accumulation of inorganic phosphate,[135,181,182] failure of the membrane electrical potential to propagate beyond T tubules,[183] and to a much lesser extent intramuscular acidosis.[184-186] Short-lasting fatigue appears to have a protective function, because it can prevent injury to the sarcolemma caused by forceful muscle contractions.[187] Long-lasting fatigue[173] is consistent with the development of, and recovery from, muscle injury (Fig. 40.17).[187,188]

Whether critically ill patients develop short-lasting or long-lasting contractile fatigue of the respiratory muscles is not clear. Patients who fail a trial of weaning from mechanical ventilation are at particular risk of developing fatigue because they experience marked increases in respiratory load.[7,11,33] The addition of a new injury to the respiratory muscles (secondary to the development of contractile fatigue) might be the ultimate determinant of whether or not some patients are ever successfully weaned. Circumstantial evidence of contractile fatigue in patients experiencing respiratory distress has been reported.[7,189-191] Because of technical limitations,[189-191] these early data did not provide proof of contractile fatigue.[10,192]

The most direct method for detecting fatigue in patients is to measure the transdiaphragmatic pressure (Pdi) elicited by phrenic nerve stimulation over time (see Fig. 40.2).[15,173]

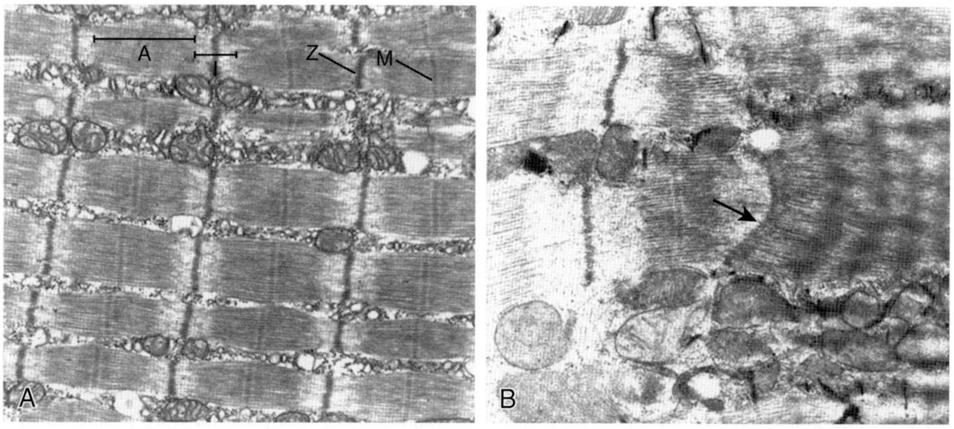

Figure 40.17 Electron micrographs of longitudinal sections from the costal diaphragm of a healthy control hamster (*left panel*) and a hamster exposed to 6 days of resistive loading (*right panel*). The left panel shows normal sarcomeres with distinct A-bands, I-bands, Z-bands, and M-lines that are aligned between adjacent myofibrils. The right panel shows load-induced damage recognizable by Z-band streaming (*arrow*) and disruption of sarcomeric structure (*right section of right panel*) with loss of distinct A-bands and I-bands. Z-band streaming is attributed to a loss of cytoskeletal protein elements such as desmin, α-actinin, and vimentin. Magnification for both micrographs: ×16,500. (From Laghi F, Tobin MJ: Disorders of the respiratory muscles. Am J Respir Crit Care Med 2003;168:10-48. Electron micrographs provided by Drs. David C. Walker and Darlene W. Reid, University of British Columbia, Vancouver, Canada.)

When employing this technique in critically ill patients, it is especially challenging to ensure that successive stimulations are all generated at the same end-expiratory lung volume, to ensure a constant degree of neural depolarization by the stimulator, and ensure that twitch potentiation (the transient increase in pressure that occurs with a recent forceful contraction) does not occur.[15,173] Controlling for these factors, Laghi and associates[13] studied 11 weaning-failure patients and 8 weaning-success patients before and after a T-tube trial. Twitch Pdi was 8.9 ± 2.2 H_2O before and 9.4 ± 2.4 H_2O after the trial in the weaning-failure patients (Fig. 40.18). The respective values in the weaning-success patients were 10.3 ± 1.5 and 11.2 ± 1.8 cm H_2O. Not a single patient developed a decrease in twitch Pdi. The absence of fatigue was surprising because 7 of the 9 weaning-failure patients had a tension-time index (the product of two fractions: [mean pressure per breath/maximum transdiaphragmatic pressure] × [inspiratory time/total time of respiratory cycle]) above the threshold reported to lead to task failure and fatigue (0.15).[193]

One of the most likely reasons that patients did not develop fatigue is that physicians reinstituted mechanical ventilation before there was enough time for its development. The relationship between tension-time index and the length of time that a load can be sustained until task failure follows an inverse-power function. Bellemare and Grassino[193] expressed the relationship as follows:

$$\text{time to task failure} = 0.1\,(\text{tension} - \text{time index})^{-3.6}$$

The increase in tension-time index over the course of the weaning trial[13] and predicted time to task failure[193] are shown in Figure 40.19. At the point that the physician reinstituted mechanical ventilation, patients were predicted to be an average of 13 minutes away from task failure. Moreover, the time to task failure was underestimated because diaphragmatic recruitment during maximal voluntary contractions was incomplete (Fig. 40.20).[13] In other words, patients display clinical manifestations of severe respiratory distress for a substantial time before they would develop fatigue. In an ICU setting, these clinical signs will lead attendants to reinstitute mechanical ventilation before fatigue has time to develop. Other factors that might have protected the respiratory muscles from contractile fatigue include development of dynamic hyperinflation (susceptibility to fatigue is greater when fatiguing protocols are conducted at optimal muscle length rather than when a muscle is shortened)[194] and activation of extradiaphragmatic muscles of respiration.[195]

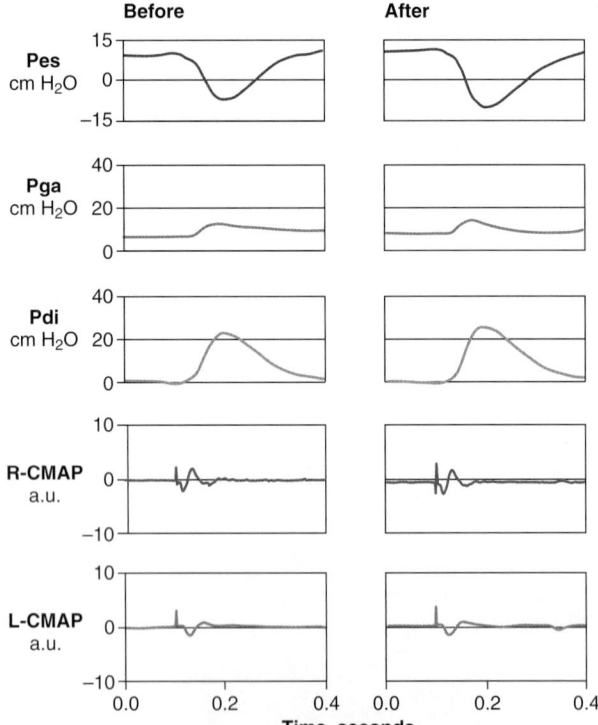

Figure 40.18 Esophageal pressure (Pes), gastric pressure (Pga), transdiaphragmatic pressure (Pdi), and compound motor action potentials (CAMP) of the right and left hemidiaphragms after phrenic nerve stimulation before (*left*) and after (*right*) a failed trial of weaning. The end-expiratory value of Pes and the amplitude of the right and left CAMPs were the same before and after the trial, indicating that the stimulations were delivered at the same lung volume and that the stimulations achieved the same extent of diaphragmatic recruitment. The amplitude of twitch Pdi elicited by phrenic nerve stimulation was equivalent before and after weaning. (From Laghi F, Cattapan SE, Jubran A, et al: Is weaning failure caused by low-frequency fatigue of the diaphragm? Am J Respir Crit Care Med 2003;167:120.)

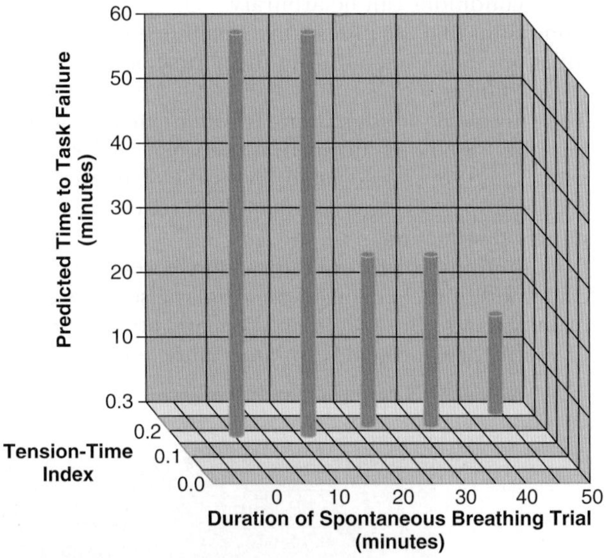

Figure 40.19 The interrelationship between the duration of a spontaneous breathing trial, tension-time index of the diaphragm, and predicted time to task failure in nine patients who failed a trial of weaning from mechanical ventilation. The patients breathed spontaneously for an average of 44 minutes before a physician terminated the trial. At the start of the trial, tension-time index was 0.17, and the formula of Bellemare and Grassino[193] (see text for details) predicted that patients could sustain spontaneous breathing for another 59 minutes before developing task failure. As the trial progressed, tension-time index increased and predicted time to the development of task failure decreased. At the end of the trial, tension-time index reached 0.26; that patients were predicted to sustain spontaneous breathing for another 13 minutes before developing task failure clarifies why patients did not develop a decrease in diaphragmatic twitch pressure. In other words, physicians interrupted the trial based on clinical manifestations of respiratory distress before patients had sufficient time to develop contractile fatigue. (From Laghi F, Tobin MJ: Disorders of the respiratory muscles. Am J Respir Crit Care Med 2003;168:10-48.)

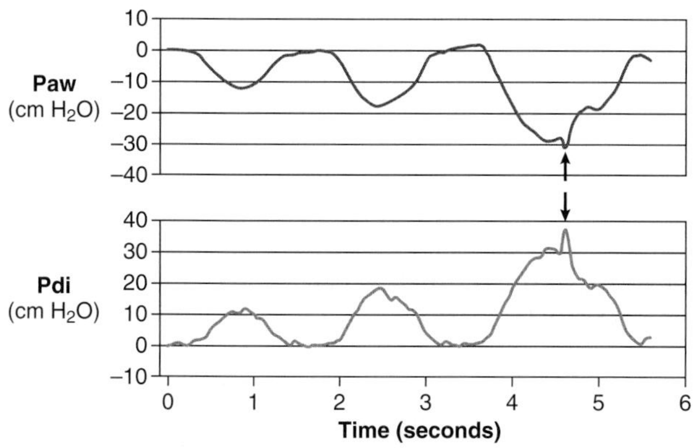

Figure 40.20 Continuous recordings of airway pressure and transdiaphragmatic pressure during airway occlusion in a patient with chronic obstructive pulmonary disease after an unsuccessful trial of spontaneous breathing. Phrenic nerve stimulation (*arrow*) during the maximal inspiratory effort resulted in a detectable superimposed twitch. That a twitch could be superimposed during the maximal effort indicates that diaphragmatic activation was incomplete.

Studies in animals[184,196-198] support the finding that patients do not develop long-lasting contractile fatigue of the respiratory muscles. Inspiratory loading in animals causes respiratory failure and acidosis before force output decreases or substrate is depleted in the diaphragm,[184,196-198] suggesting that central[199] and reflex mechanisms[200,201] affect the breathing pattern[185] and α-motor neuron firing rates[202] in response to loading. Two neural pathways may convey information from the respiratory muscles to the central nervous system.[203,204] One pathway transmits information from mechanoreceptors (Golgi tendon organs and muscle spindles)[200,205] in the dorsal column, relaying it to the brainstem and thalamus, before reaching the sensomotor cortex.[206] This pathway may participate in proprioceptive control of the respiratory muscles, integrating movements originating in the motor cortex.[199] The second pathway consists of vagal[198] and possibly phrenic nerve afferents (group IV phrenic afferent fibers)[200] that reach the amygdala after relaying in the brainstem and then projecting to the mesocortex (cingulated gyrus). This pathway may deal with respiratory nociception,[199,207] such as dyspnea (through the relay in the amygdala),[208] and with the ventilatory response to carbon dioxide (through the relay in the brainstem, ventral cerebellum, and limbic system).[199,207,209] In addition to these two pathways projecting to the central nervous system, there is evidence for the existence of a spinal pathway responsible for phrenic-to-phrenic reflex inhibition.[201] An increase in carbon dioxide during loading may also protect the respiratory muscles by decreasing reactive oxygen species production.[210]

Resistive breathing causes hypercapnia without affecting diaphragmatic force output or aerobic metabolism (assessed by ^{31}P nuclear magnetic resonance spectroscopy) in spontaneously breathing piglets.[7,185,211] The hypoxia combined with resistive breathing caused a decrease in diaphragmatic force and inadequate oxidative metabolism, as reflected by accumulation of inorganic phosphorus and decreased phosphocreatine.[185] Force output and oxidative metabolism returned to baseline values with normoxia despite persistent loading.[185] The investigators speculated that loading produces a decrease in central activation (to the point of ventilatory failure), which decreases metabolic demands and prevents peripheral fatigue; additional stress of hypoxia may overwhelm this defense mechanism and cause peripheral fatigue.[185] Hypoxemia can also induce degradation of myofibrillar proteins.[212]

Hypoxia impairs the respiratory centers at a higher oxygen tension than it impairs the respiratory muscles,[160,213] making it difficult to decipher the effects of hypoxemia on the respiratory muscles. Animals develop severe alveolar hypoventilation and respiratory arrest before the tension-generating ability of the diaphragm has begun to decrease.[160,213] As previously stated, it is unknown whether, in patients with shock,[151] decreases in oxygen delivery to the respiratory muscles[154,214] or respiratory centers can be sufficient to cause hypoventilation.

INCREASED LOAD

Increased respiratory load can result from increased mechanical load and increased ventilatory requirements.

INCREASED MECHANICAL LOAD

Patients in acute respiratory failure usually experience an increased mechanical load.* The patients typically have a 30% to 50% greater inspiratory resistance,[7,13,33] 100% greater dynamic elastance,[7,11] and 100% to 200% greater intrinsic positive end-expiratory pressure (PEEP)[7,11,13] than do similar patients who are not in acute respiratory failure. Inspiratory effort—quantified by calculation of the pressure time product of the inspiratory muscles—is almost equally divided in offsetting intrinsic PEEP, elastic recoil, and inspiratory resistance (Fig. 40.21).[7,211] Abnormal mechanics arise from bronchoconstriction, bronchial edema, pulmonary edema,[7] and lung inflammation.[215,216] Rapid shallow breathing can aggravate the abnormalities in lung elastance, intrinsic PEEP, and carbon dioxide clearance.[7,33] Expiratory muscle recruitment can also increase intrinsic PEEP and breathing effort.[218] In some patients, increased mechanical load results from upper airway obstruction. The upper airway, which encompasses the passage between the nares and carina, can be obstructed by functional or anatomic causes. Among the first are vocal cord paralysis and laryngospasm. Among the second are trauma, burn, infections, foreign bodies, and tumors. Functional and anatomic obstruction can occur postoperatively in patients with redundant pharyngeal soft tissue (sleep apnea) and loss of muscle tone related to postanesthetic state.[1] Upper airway obstruction is one of the most urgent and potentially lethal medical emergencies.[1] Complete airway obstruction lasting for as little as 4 to 6 minutes can cause irreversible brain damage.[1]

INCREASED VENTILATORY REQUIREMENTS

Increased ventilatory requirements can result from increased carbon dioxide production, increased dead space ventilation, and elevated respiratory drive. Carbon dioxide

*See References 7, 11, 13, 33, 211, and 215-217.

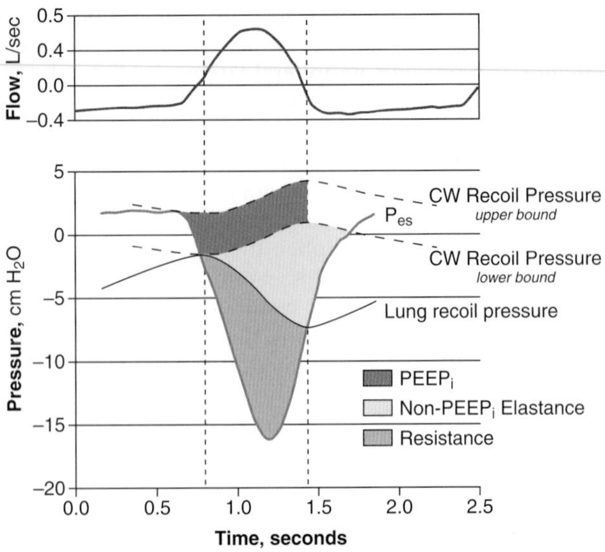

Figure 40.21 Quantification of inspiratory effort with pressure-time product of the inspiratory muscles. Flow (inspiration upward) and pressure tracings during spontaneous breathing. Recoil pressures of the chest wall (CW) and lung are calculated from dynamic elastances of the chest wall and lung, respectively, and lung volume. Upper bound inspiratory pressure-time product (PTP) is calculated using the integral of the difference between esophageal pressure (Pes) and upper bound CW recoil pressure from the onset of the rapid decrease in Pes to the transition from inspiratory to expiratory flow. The component of PTP due to intrinsic positive end-expiratory pressure (PEEPi) is computed using the integral of the difference between the upper and lower bounds of CW recoil pressure from the onset of rapid decrease in Pes to the transition from inspiratory to expiratory flow. The component of PTP due to non-PEEPi elastance is computed using the integral of the difference between lung recoil pressure and lower bound CW recoil pressure from the onset of inspiratory flow to the moment of transition from inspiratory to expiratory flow. The resistive fraction of PTP is computed using the integral of the difference between Pes and lung recoil pressure. The *vertical interrupted lines* represent points for zero flow. (From Jubran A, Tobin MJ: Pathophysiologic basis of acute respiratory distress in patients who fail a trial of weaning from mechanical ventilation. Am J Respir Crit Care Med 1997;155;906.)

production can increase as a result of sepsis,[86] fever, shivering, drugs (salicylates), lipogenesis,[219,220] and a shift in utilization of fuels from lipids (RQ = 0.7) to carbohydrates (RQ = 1.0).[221] An increase in carbon dioxide production can only be a contributory factor and not a sole cause of hypercapnic respiratory failure.[3]

The ratio of dead space to tidal volume is normally 0.30. The ratio increases up to 0.65 in patients with severe COPD,[222] ARDS,[223] and other severe lung diseases.[3] Patients can compensate for such an increase in dead space by doubling minute ventilation.[3] Such an increase in minute ventilation poses a minor challenge when respiratory mechanics and respiratory muscles are normal; for example, hypercapnia is uncommon with pulmonary vascular disease.[3] Accordingly, an increase in dead space ventilation should never be considered the primary mechanism responsible for hypercapnic respiratory failure unless there is a concurrent abnormality in the control of breathing, or in the mechanical load of the respiratory muscles or in their contractile performance.[3]

Stimulation of pulmonary irritant or J receptors, neurologic lesions, sepsis, and toxins can inappropriately increase respiratory drive. Whether an inappropriately heightened drive places sufficient stress on the respiratory muscle to cause respiratory muscle fatigue and, consequently, hypoventilation remains to be determined.

HYPERCAPNIA-INDUCED HYPOVENTILATION

Severe hypercapnia depresses the central nervous system and decreases respiratory motor output.[220] A vicious circle can arise, whereby hypercapnia causes depressed drive leading to more hypercapnia.[224,225] The possibility of hypercapnia-induced hypoventilation is supported by reports of successful resolution of hypercapnic respiratory failure in some patients following short-term infusion of the respiratory stimulant, doxapram.[224,225]

SUMMARY

A relative or absolute decrease in respiratory muscle output is responsible for alveolar hypoventilation and hypercapnic respiratory failure. The number of distinct clinical entities that result in hypercapnia is vast and often more than one disease process may coexist—e.g., hyperinflation-associated respiratory muscle weakness and ventilation-perfusion inequality in patients with COPD. The relative or absolute decrease in respiratory muscle output in patients with hypercapnia may stem from a decrease in respiratory drive, excess mechanical load on the respiratory muscles, and respiratory muscle weakness (see Fig. 40.1). Whether respiratory muscle fatigue is responsible for hypercapnic respiratory failure is an important issue that has yet to be resolved.

KEY POINTS

- Hypercapnia is synonymous with alveolar hypoventilation (for the patient's level of carbon dioxide production).
- A relative or absolute decrease in respiratory muscle output is responsible for alveolar hypoventilation.
- Isolated impairments in gas exchange usually do not cause hypercapnia.
- When gas exchange is impaired the magnitude of neuromuscular impairment or increased respiratory load conducive to hypercapnia can be less than the corresponding derangements when gas exchange is intact.
- Respiratory drive is elevated in many patients with acute ventilatory failure. This finding does not necessarily exclude the possibility that during episodes of ventilatory failure the central nervous system is not fully recruiting the respiratory muscles and may be contributing to CO_2 retention.

KEY POINTS (Continued)

- In critically ill patients, respiratory muscle weakness is probably responsible for a large number of cases of alveolar hypoventilation.
- Metabolic disturbances such as hypophosphatemia, hypomagnesemia, hypokalemia, and hypocalcemia can cause respiratory muscle weakness.
- Hyperinflation places the respiratory muscles in a mechanical disadvantage to generate the driving pressure of the respiratory system.
- Hyperinflation can occur during episodes of respiratory distress even in patients without history of airway disease (e.g., asthma or COPD).
- The role of respiratory muscle fatigue in causing hypercapnic respiratory failure remains to be determined.
- Severe hypercapnia can in itself be conducive to alveolar hypoventilation by depressing respiratory drive.
- It is still unclear whether respiratory or metabolic acidosis has a clinically relevant direct effect on respiratory muscle contractility.

SELECTED REFERENCES

4. Laghi F, Tobin MJ: Disorders of the respiratory muscles. Am J Respir Crit Care Med 2003;168(1):10-48.
7. Tobin MJ, Laghi F, Jubran A: Ventilatory failure, ventilator support and ventilator weaning. Compr Physiol 2012 Oct 1;2(4):;2:2871-2921.
13. Laghi F, Cattapan SE, Jubran A, et al: Is weaning failure caused by low-frequency fatigue of the diaphragm? Am J Respir Crit Care Med 2003;167(2):120-127.
63. Jaber S, Petrof BJ, Jung B, et al: Rapidly progressive diaphragmatic weakness and injury during mechanical ventilation in humans. Am J Respir Crit Care Med 2011;183(3):364-371.
65. Levine S, Nguyen T, Taylor N, et al: Rapid disuse atrophy of diaphragm fibers in mechanically ventilated humans. N Engl J Med 2008;358(13):1327-1335.
92. Callahan LA, Supinski GS: Sepsis-induced myopathy. Crit Care Med 2009;37(10 Suppl):S354-S367.
137. Mador MJ, Wendel T, Kufel TJ: Effect of acute hypercapnia on diaphragmatic and limb muscle contractility. Am J Respir Crit Care Med 1997;155(5):1590-1595.
141. Begin P, Grassino A: Inspiratory muscle dysfunction and chronic hypercapnia in chronic obstructive pulmonary disease. Am Rev Respir Dis 1991;143(5 Pt 1):905-912.
180. Yan S, Lichros I, Zakynthinos S, et al: Effect of diaphragmatic fatigue on control of respiratory muscles and ventilation during CO_2 rebreathing. J Appl Physiol 1993;75(3):1364-1370.
195. Parthasarathy S, Jubran A, Laghi F, et al: Sternomastoid, rib-cage and expiratory muscle activity during weaning failure. J Appl Physiol 2007;103:140-147.

The complete list of references can be found at www.expertconsult.com.

41 Nonpulmonary Causes of Respiratory Failure

Ramya Lotano

CHAPTER OUTLINE

INTRODUCTION

An estimated 20% of respiratory failure is a result of nonpulmonary causes such as disorders that affect the upper airway, chest wall, muscles of respiration, and nervous system. Hypoventilation is the primary pathophysiologic etiology of all of these disorders.[1]

HYPOVENTILATION

PATHOPHYSIOLOGY (FIG. 41.1)

Hypoventilation is defined as alveolar ventilation that is inappropriately low for metabolic demands. Alveolar (A) and arterial (a) $PaCO_2$ are elevated. Arterial pressure is decreased. Alveolar hypoventilation exists when arterial PCO_2 increases above the normal range of 37 to 43 mm Hg.[2-7]

Hypoventilation is associated with arterial hypoxemia (when breathing room air oxygen) and a raised arterial PCO_2. The rise in $PaCO_2$ as a result of hypoventilation can be calculated using the *alveolar ventilation equation*.[8] In a single-compartment lung model, alveolar PCO_2 and PO_2 are inversely related according to the alveolar air equation. An increase in alveolar PCO_2 is associated with an obligatory fall in alveolar PO_2. During hypercapnia, the alveolar minus arterial $P(A-a)O_2$ difference predicted by this model (while breathing room air) is "normal." Regarding the combination of hypercapnia and a normal $P(A-a)O_2$ difference as a requirement to diagnose nonpulmonary disorders associated with hypoventilation is common clinical practice. However, these disorders are also commonly complicated by microatelectasis, retention of secretions, and bronchopneumonia, which cause abnormal ventilation/perfusion inequality and increase the $P(A-a)O_2$ difference. Conversely, the $P(A-a)O_2$ difference has been shown to be an unreliable index of abnormal gas exchange in the presence of substantial hypercapnia. For these reasons, a normal $P(A-a)O_2$ difference is not helpful in differentiating pulmonary from nonpulmonary causes of respiratory failure. The alveolar partial pressure of oxygen is calculated with the formula:

$$PAO_2 = PIO_2 - PaCO_2\left(FIO_2 + \frac{1-FIO_2}{R}\right)$$

where FIO_2 is the inspired oxygen fraction (0.21 in all calculations) in the dry gas, PIO_2 is the inspired PO_2, and R is the respiratory exchange ratio (assumed to be 0.8). In other words, the flow of CO_2 molecules across the alveolar membrane per minute is divided by the flow of O_2 molecules across the membrane per minute. $PaCO_2$ is the ideal alveolar carbon dioxide tension.

This important equation indicates that the level of PCO_2 in alveolar gas and in arterial blood is inversely related to the alveolar ventilation.

This is true only if a steady state of alveolar ventilation and carbon dioxide production rate exists. In clinical

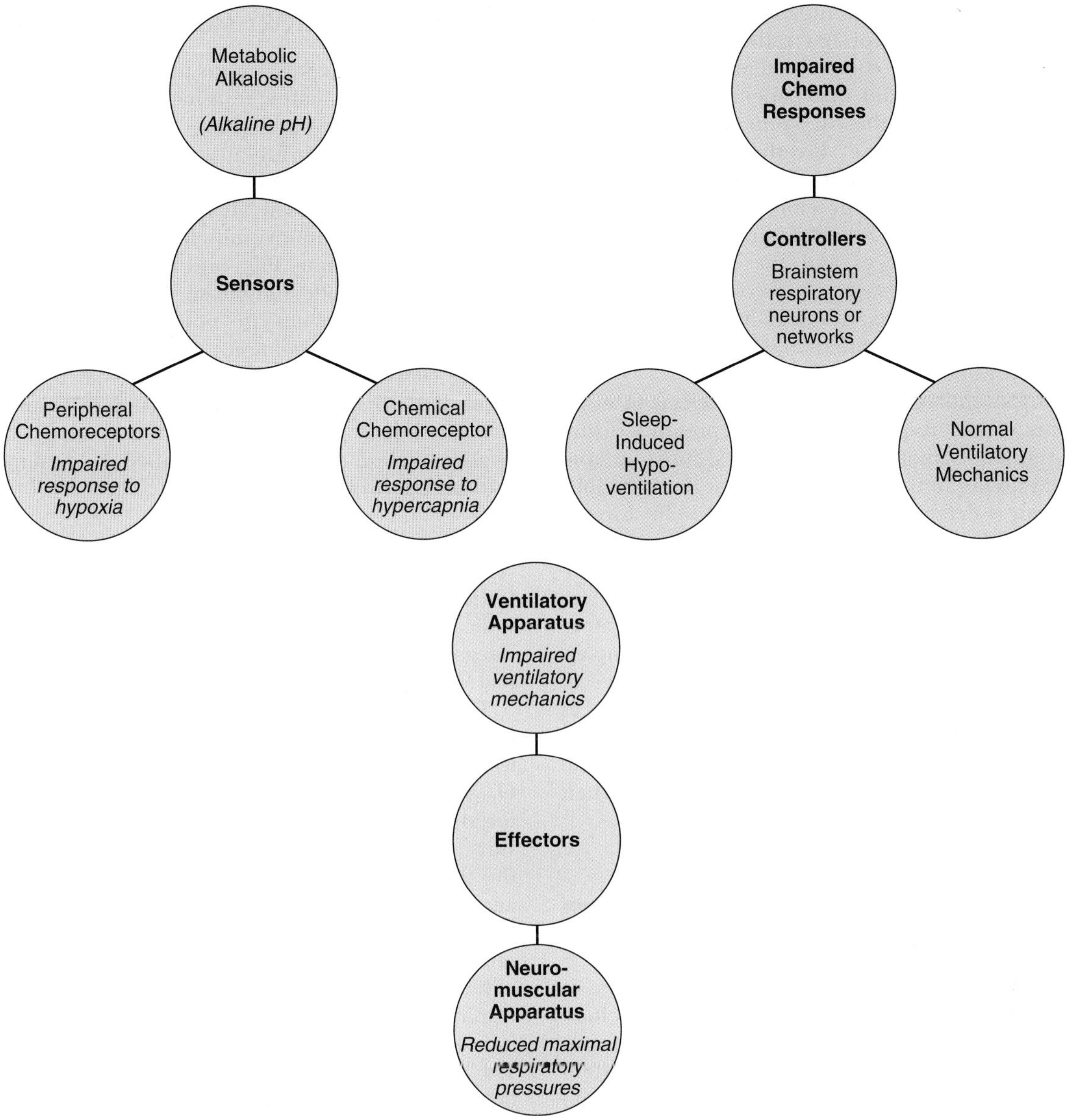

Figure 41.1 Mechanisms underlying chronic alveolar hypoventilation.

practice it is common to consider the combination of hypercapnia and a normal $P(A - a)O_2$ difference as a requirement to diagnose nonpulmonary disorders associated with hypoventilation.[9] However, hypoventilation-induced atelectasis causing abnormal gas exchange will result in an increase in $P(A - a)O_2$ difference.[10] In the presence of substantial hypercapnia, an abnormal alveolar-to-arterial oxygen difference may not rule out a nonpulmonary cause of hypoventilation.

MECHANISMS UNDERLYING CHRONIC ALVEOLAR HYPOVENTILATION (SEE FIG. 41.1)

Defects in the metabolic control system result in hypoventilation when abnormalities in blood gases and cerebral acid-base status are not sensed or if sensed do not produce an appropriate change in motor output of the medullary respiratory neurons. Patients with such defects fail to breathe normally in response to metabolic respiratory stimuli, but because the behavioral control system, respiratory motor pathways, and ventilatory apparatus are intact, they are capable of voluntarily driving respiration. As a result, patients with defects in the metabolic control system typically demonstrate normal ventilatory mechanics, but they have impaired responses to metabolic respiratory stimuli and often hypoventilate severely during sleep, when ventilation is critically dependent on the metabolic control system.[1,3,11-17] As a result of chronic hypoventilation, these patients have a primary respiratory acidosis leading to a secondary increase in extracellular bicarbonate ion concentration.[18,19]

In contrast, patients with a primary metabolic alkalosis may develop secondary hypoventilation as a compensatory response. This type of hypoventilation represents not a defect in respiratory control but rather an appropriate response of the metabolic control system to a disturbance in acid-base status. It is said that patients with metabolic alkalosis "shouldn't" breathe, in contrast to those with control defects, who "won't" breathe, and those with mechanical defects, who "can't" breathe. However, the degree of hypoventilation that develops in response to metabolic alkalosis depends on several factors, including associated electrolyte disturbances and the sensitivity of the peripheral chemoreceptors to the accompanying hypoxemia.[19,20] Therefore, patients with weak hypoxic responsiveness tend to hypoventilate more than do patients with brisk hypoxic responsiveness.

Chronic hypoventilation resulting from defects in effector elements of the respiratory system represents disturbances of ventilatory motor and mechanical function, and these defects do not in themselves mean that the metabolic control system is defective. Because the same effector elements also serve the behavioral control system, these patients are usually unable to breathe normally even when consciously attempting to do so. Hence, such defects are characterized either by reductions in the maximum inspiratory pressures that can be generated voluntarily or by impairment of lung volumes and flow rates.[21] In the presence of such neural or mechanical defects, coexisting disturbances in respiratory control are often difficult to identify because the neuromuscular or mechanical defect may preclude normal responses to chemical respiratory stimuli even when the control system is intact.[1]

ETIOLOGIC CLASSIFICATION

Plum and Leigh[22,23] described nonrespiratory causes of respiratory failure. Causes of hypoventilation include depression of the respiratory center by drugs such as morphine derivatives and barbiturates; diseases of the brainstem such as encephalitis; abnormalities of the spinal cord conducting pathways such as high cervical dislocation; anterior horn cell diseases including poliomyelitis that affect the phoenix nerves or supplying intercostal muscles; diseases of nerves to respiratory muscles (e.g., Guillain-Barré syndrome); diseases of the myoneural junction such as myasthenia gravis; diseases of the respiratory muscles themselves such as progressive muscular dystrophy; thoracic cage abnormalities (e.g., crushed chest); upper airway obstruction (e.g., thymoma); hypoventilation associated with extreme obesity (Pickwickian syndrome); and other miscellaneous causes such as metabolic alkalosis and idiopathic states.[2] In all these conditions the lungs are normal.

RESPIRATORY FAILURE FROM NEUROMUSCULAR DISEASE

Neuromuscular diseases are accompanied by variable degrees of involvement of the muscles of inspiration and expiration. The clinical manifestations reflect the compromise of both muscle groups.[24] Disorders of respiratory control and those of peripheral neuromuscular disease are shown in Tables 41.1 and 41.2, respectively.

TESTS OF RESPIRATORY MUSCLE STRENGTH

Respiratory muscle weakness is the hallmark of most neuromuscular disease. Simple tests measure maximal inspiratory and expiratory pressures (PI_{max} and PE_{max}). These tests are conducted by measuring airway pressures while requiring the patient to make maximal inspiratory and expiratory efforts against a closed airway at low or high volumes, respectively.[25] Respiratory muscle force is dependent on age, sex, and lung volume. PI_{max} and PE_{max} of greater than 60 to 80 cm H_2O exclude significant neuromuscular weakness. Abnormally low values are not diagnostic but indicate a need for further assessment.

The classic example of chronic alveolar hypoventilation secondary to brainstem disease is that seen in bulbar poliomyelitis or encephalitis. Secondary causes of alveolar hypoventilation are usually signified by features of the underlying disease.

TESTS OF RESPIRATORY CONTROL AND DRIVE

If the tests of pulmonary function testing are unremarkable, indicating no parenchymal, neuromuscular, or chest wall disease accounting for the patient's hypercapnia or abnormal ventilation, tests of respiratory control are indicated.

These tests include measurement of hypoxic and hypercapnic ventilatory responses (because ventilatory response to hypoxia and hypercarbia can be potentially hazardous, O_2 saturation and end tidal CO_2 tension should be monitored); analysis of breathing pattern; mouth occlusive pressure (measurement of maximal pressure generated during the first 0.1 second of normal inspiratory effort when the airway is occluded); and elastic and resistive load testing (by breathing through progressively narrower tubes while the sensation of dyspnea is measured by the Borg scale).

Electromyography permits more direct measurements of respiratory muscle strength. Respiratory muscle fatigue is indicated by paradoxical respirations or *respiratory alternans.* The mechanism consists of intermittent decreases or cessation of the contribution of the diaphragm to the inspiratory effort. It has been assumed that this pattern of muscle recruitment indicates diaphragmatic fatigue.[26]

CLINICAL RECOGNITION AND MANIFESTATIONS

Alveolar hypoventilation exists when arterial P_{CO_2} increases above the normal range. In clinically important hypercarbia, P_{CO_2} typically ranges from 50 to 70 mm Hg. Lethargy, confusion, and a depressed level of consciousness are seen as a result of hypercapnia. An increase in intracranial pressure and cerebral blood flow, as well as a decrease in myocardial contractility, occur.[2] The oxyhemoglobin dissociation curve shifts to the right, which leads to an increase in the release of oxygen to the tissues.

In the acute form, progressive weakness of respiratory muscles leads to rapid reduction in vital capacity followed by respiratory failure with hypoxemia and hypercarbia. Symptoms are those of acute respiratory failure including dyspnea, tachypnea, and tachycardia. In the chronic form,

Table 41.1 Disorders of Ventilatory Control*

Disorder	Associations	Mechanism
Metabolic alkalosis[54]	Maintenance of metabolic alkalosis for any length of time means that renal homeostatic mechanisms for HCO_3^- excretion have been disrupted.	Impaired autonomic control of ventilation. Voluntary control remains intact.
Ondine's curse[55,56] (congenital or acquired central alveolar hypoventilation)	Usually caused by congenital hypoventilation syndrome but can be from surgical incisions into the second cervical segment to relieve intractable pain.[57] Can also be seen in medullary infarction in an intermittent form.[58-60]	Impaired automatic control of ventilation. Voluntary ventilation remains intact. Classically, the patient "forgets to breathe" when asleep. Patient maintains relatively normal blood gas while awake.[3,61]
Carotid body resection[62]	Introduced in Japan in the 1940s as a treatment for asthma.[63,64] Also seen after bilateral endarterectomy for carotid vascular disease.	Depressed hypoxic ventilatory drive during exercise. Generally eucapnic at rest. Destruction of peripheral chemoreceptors.[65,66]
Cheyne-Stokes respiration[67,68]	Commonly associated with cardiac disease; can also be seen in neurologic disease sedation, sleep, altitude acclimatization.[69]	Delay between changes in ventilation and detection of the resulting arterial P_{CO_2} by the central chemoreceptors maintains a cyclic pattern of respiration.
Myxedema	In critically ill patients, laboratory differentiation between severe hypothyroidism and the euthyroid-sick syndromes is difficult and may require measurement of free hormone levels.	Respiratory muscle weakness. Depression of ventilatory drive.[70-72]
Starvation	Nutritional intervention can return muscle ventilatory function to normal levels. Furthermore, it seems likely that the ventilatory drive can be influenced by dietary intake of amino acids and glucose.	Decreased ventilatory drive, decreased respiratory muscle function, alterations of lung parenchyma and depressed lung defense mechanisms.
Drug effects	Opiates, barbiturates, benzodiazepines	Should be used judiciously in patients with preexisting hypoventilation.
	Medroxyprogesterone†	Increases ventilatory drive in normal males leading to about 5 mm fall in Pa_{CO_2}. Used in obesity hypoventilation syndrome.[73-75]
	Theophylline†	Increases hypoxic ventilatory response and prevents the fall in hypoxic ventilatory response.
	Acetazolamide†	Efficacy and side effects of long-term use are unknown. Small, crossover study reduced central apnea in patients with congestive heart failure.[76]

*Studies cited in this table may be found in the complete list of references for this chapter provided online.
†Effects used for treatment.

impairment of the respiratory muscles affects mechanical properties of the lungs and chest wall, decreases the ability to clear secretions, and eventually may alter the function of the central respiratory centers. Symptoms include orthopnea, fatigue, disturbed sleep, and hypersomnolence.[27]

Significant hypoxemia may coexist with chronic hypercapnia or occur with the onset of additional acute pulmonary disorders. The administration of supplemental oxygen is expected to worsen hypercapnia. Major processes that contribute are worsening of ventilation perfusion mismatching caused by an attenuation of hypoxic pulmonary vasoconstriction, a decrease in the binding affinity of hemoglobin for CO_2 (Haldane effect), and a decrease in minute ventilation. Importantly, the clinician must be aware that it is imperative to provide supplemental oxygen to maintain adequate tissue oxygenation. This precaution will avoid potentially life-threatening consequences; however, in the spontaneously breathing patient, the lowest F_{IO_2} that produces acceptable oxygenation should be chosen. The major adverse effect seen in patients with hypercapnia with use of supplemental oxygen is an abrupt discontinuation of oxygen leading to hypoxemia.[28-30]

When hypoventilation is not caused by decreased central nervous system drive, neuromuscular weakness, or bellows dysfunction, tachypnea is a relatively early manifestation that can be seen in association with near-normal maximum respiratory pressures.[31] Orthopnea that develops within seconds of lying down is a classic symptom of patients with diaphragmatic paralysis. The pathophysiology of dyspnea resulting from gravitational influences and the mechanical function of the diaphragm during water immersion, another manifestation of diaphragmatic paralysis, are discussed by

Table 41.2 Disorders of the Peripheral Neuromuscular System*

Site of Disease	Disease	Type of Respiratory Failure
Spinal Cord		
Space-occupying lesions	Syringomyelia	Chronic respiratory failure
	Multiple sclerosis[77]	Chronic respiratory failure
	Mass	Chronic respiratory failure
Anterior horn cell lesions	Poliomyelitis[5,16,78]	Chronic respiratory failure
	Amyotrophic lateral sclerosis	Chronic respiratory failure
Inhibiting neuronal blockade	Tetanus	Acute respiratory failure
Any level	Traumatic injury	Acute respiratory failure
Motor Nerves		
Peripheral Neuropathy		
	Phrenic nerve injury[54]	Acute/chronic respiratory failure
	Beriberi[79]	Chronic respiratory failure
	Guillain-Barré[80]	Chronic respiratory failure
	Critical illness polyneuropathy[81,82]	Chronic respiratory failure
	Lyme disease[83]	Chronic respiratory failure
	Diphtheria[84]	Acute respiratory failure
Neuromuscular Junction		
	Tick paralysis[85]	
	Organophosphate poisoning	Acute respiratory failure
	Botulism[86]	Acute respiratory failure
	Eaton-Lambert syndrome	Acute respiratory failure
	Myasthenia gravis[5,31]	Acute/chronic respiratory failure
Muscle Involvement		
Dystrophies	Muscular dystrophy[5,31,87-89]	Chronic respiratory failure
	Myotonic dystrophy[90,91]	Chronic respiratory failure
Myopathy	Polymyositis, dermatomyositis, and other collagen vascular diseases[92]	Chronic respiratory failure
	Malnutrition[93]	Chronic respiratory failure
	Thyroid, adrenal, pituitary glands	Chronic respiratory failure
	Metabolic acid-base, electrolyte[4,18-20]	Acute respiratory failure
Disorders of the Chest Wall	Obesity hypoventilation[4,94-96]	Acute/chronic respiratory failure
	Asphyxiating thoracic dystrophy[97]	Acute/chronic respiratory failure
	Fibrothorax[98]	Acute/chronic respiratory failure
	Thoracoplasty[98]	Acute/chronic respiratory failure
	Ankylosing spondylitis[98]	Acute/chronic respiratory failure
	Flail chest	Acute/chronic respiratory failure

*Studies cited in this table may be found in the complete list of references for this chapter provided online.

McCool and Mead.[32] Normal diaphragm contraction is associated with a downward movement of the diaphragm and outward movement of the abdomen. When subjects with diaphragmatic paralysis are observed in a supine posture, a paradoxical inward motion of the abdomen can be observed during inspiration. Because these patients are unable to develop transdiaphragmatic pressure gradients, the abdominal contents are drawn toward the chest by the inspiratory fall in pleural pressure generated by the accessory muscles of respiration.[33]

PATIENT MANAGEMENT

RESPIRATORY FAILURE

Respiratory failure is defined as a failure to maintain adequate gas exchange and is characterized by abnormalities of arterial blood gas tensions. *Type 1 failure* is defined by a $Pa{O_2}$ of less than 60 mm Hg with a normal or low $Pa{CO_2}$. *Type 2 failure* is defined by a $Pa{O_2}$ of less than 60 mm Hg and a $Pa{CO_2}$ of greater than 50 mm Hg. Respiratory failure can be acute, acute on chronic, or chronic. Although not always clear cut, this distinction is important in deciding on the location of patient treatment and the most appropriate treatment strategy, particularly in type 2 respiratory failure:

- *Acute* hypercapnic respiratory failure: the patient will have no, or minor, evidence of preexisting respiratory disease, and arterial blood gas tensions will show a high $Pa{CO_2}$, low pH, and normal bicarbonate.
- *Chronic* hypercapnic respiratory failure: evidence of chronic respiratory disease, high $Pa{CO_2}$, near normal pH, high bicarbonate.
- *Acute-on-chronic* hypercapnic respiratory failure: an acute deterioration in an individual with significant preexisting

hypercapnic respiratory failure, high $Paco_2$, low pH, high bicarbonate.[34]

ACUTE RESPIRATORY FAILURE CAUSED BY NEUROMUSCULAR DISEASE

Involvement of the inspiratory and expiratory muscle groups in neuromuscular disease occurs to variable degrees.[24,35] Inspiratory muscle fatigue occurs as muscle weakness progresses or because of excessive ventilatory demands, as in systemic infection. Respiratory rate increases as a usual response to preserve minute ventilation. Work of breathing is increased in tachypnea due to increased dead-space ventilation and by decreased relative time spent in expiration. Blood flow to respiratory muscles is compromised because this occurs primarily during expiration.[35] Weakness of inspiratory muscles predisposes to atelectasis because of reduced tidal volume and vital capacity. The elastic recoil of the stretched thoracic and lung tissue provides driving pressure for airflow. Therefore, expiratory muscle weakness has less impact on respiratory ventilation and mechanics. Essential function of the expiratory muscle is that of generation of an effective cough and clearance of secretions.

Respiratory clinical manifestations include tachypnea, abdominal paradox, respiratory alternans, and small tidal volume.

The risk of respiratory failure increases significantly when the vital capacity (VC) falls below 15 mL/kg, particularly if there is a clear downward trend. Serial measurements of vital capacity at the bedside are helpful in this situation.[36,37] Careful assessments of ability to protect airway, oxygenation, ability to ventilate, and chest radiographs are essential in determining need for assistance with ventilation.[38] Ideally, ventilatory support should be initiated in the setting of impending respiratory failure, when there has been a clear downward trend, rather than having to initiate after the development of cardiovascular instability. Noninvasive ventilation or endotracheal intubation with initiation of positive pressure ventilation is indicated at this time. An anticipatory approach avoids risks associated with emergent intubation and minimizes complications.[39-41]

Supportive care is an important factor. Nutritional support, psychological and emotional support, physical therapy, range of motion exercises to prevent joint malalignment, tendon shortening and skin care to prevent pressure sores, and prevention of thromboembolic disease should be initiated as soon as possible.

NONINVASIVE POSITIVE PRESSURE VENTILATION

In a patient with intact bulbar function, noninvasive ventilation should be the ventilatory support of choice because of its efficacy, convenience, and portability. A progression of underlying disease will ultimately require invasive ventilation.

Noninvasive ventilation (NIV) is widely used for acute and chronic respiratory failure via mask (Figs. 41.8, 41.9, 41.10, and 41.11). If arterial blood gas tensions do not improve, the level of support can be increased. If the aim is to abolish muscle effort completely, there is little to be gained by increasing the level of inspiratory pressure above 20 cm H_2O (chest wall deformity) or 25 cm H_2O (chronic obstructive pulmonary disease).[42,43] NIV is widely considered to be an effective treatment in patients with chronic ventilatory failure caused by chest wall deformity and neuromuscular disease.[44]

WHEN TO USE NONINVASIVE VENTILATION IN NONPULMONARY CAUSES OF RESPIRATORY FAILURE[45]

PATIENTS

- Chest wall deformity
- Neuromuscular disorder
- Decompensated obstructive sleep apnea (OSA)

BLOOD GASES

- Respiratory acidosis ($Paco_2 > 50$ mm Hg, pH < 7.35, or $H^+ > 45$ nmol/L) that persists despite maximal medical treatment and appropriate controlled oxygen therapy (patients with pH < 7.25 or $H^+ > 56$ nmol/L respond less well and should be managed in an intensive care unit)
- Low A-a oxygen gradient (patients with severe life-threatening hypoxemia are more appropriately managed by tracheal intubation)

CLINICAL STATE

- Sick but not moribund
- Able to protect airway
- Conscious and cooperative
- Hemodynamically stable
- No excessive respiratory secretions
- Few comorbidities

CONTRAINDICATIONS EXCLUDED

- Facial burns/trauma/recent facial or upper airway surgery
- Vomiting
- Fixed upper airway obstruction
- Undrained pneumothorax

PREMORBID STATE

- Potential for recovery to quality of life acceptable to the patient
- Patient's wishes considered

CONTRAINDICATIONS TO NONINVASIVE VENTILATION[34]

- Facial trauma/burns
- Recent facial, upper airway, or upper gastrointestinal tract* surgery
- Fixed obstruction of the upper airway
- Inability to protect airway*
- Life-threatening hypoxemia*
- Hemodynamic instability*
- Severe comorbidity*
- Impaired consciousness*
- Confusion/agitation*
- Vomiting

*NIV may be used despite the presence of these contraindications if it is to be the "ceiling" of treatment.

- Bowel obstruction*
- Copious respiratory secretions*
- Focal consolidation on chest radiograph*
- Undrained pneumothorax*

CHRONIC RESPIRATORY FAILURE

Prolonged mechanical ventilation is defined by the Centers for Medicare and Medicaid Services in the United States as greater than 21 days of mechanical ventilation for at least 6 hours per day.[46] Most patients requiring prolonged mechanical ventilation will have a tracheostomy (Fig. 41.12) placed to facilitate comfort, communication, and chronic ventilator facility or home ventilation placement. Common problems among patients undergoing prolonged mechanical ventilation are similar to those on short-term ventilation including the following:[47-50]

- Infections (e.g., pneumonia, line sepsis, *Clostridium difficile* colitis)
- Ileus
- Renal failure
- Pneumothorax
- Seizures
- Tracheal bleeding
- Laryngeal edema
- Development of tracheal granulation tissue
- Tracheoesophageal fistula formation
- Loss of airway patency because of unplanned extubation or decannulation

*NIV may be used despite the presence of these contraindications if it is to be the "ceiling" of treatment.

CHRONIC VENTILATORY-ASSIST DEVICES

Methods of chronic mechanical ventilation include noninvasive and invasive techniques (Tables 41.3 and 41.4). Ventilatory-assist devices have been used for chronic respiratory failure for decades. Initially, negative-pressure ventilators were used, but this approach was soon replaced by the

Table 41.3 Ventilatory-Assist Devices*

Mode of Ventilation	Example	Advantages	Disadvantages	Applications
Abdominal displacement	Pneumobelt (Fig. 41.2A through C)	Noninvasive	Requires sitting. Skin abrasions at points of contact.	Diaphragm paralysis or weakness, high cord lesions, mainly for daytime use. Typical settings rate 16-24; pressure 35-50 cm H_2O.
		Portable	Upper airway obstruction.	
	Rocking bed (Fig. 41.3)	Simplicity	Not portable.	Diaphragm paralysis or weakness, mainly for nocturnal use. Typical settings 12-16/min.
Diaphragmatic pacing (Fig. 41.4)			Motion sickness.	Intact phrenic nerve and diaphragm muscle; high cord lesion and central hypoventilation.
Expiratory aids[99]; manually assisted coughing ("quad" coughing), cough in-exsufflator percussionator				Peak cough flow augmentation in patients with expiratory muscle weakness.
Hayek oscillator (Fig. 41.5)				
Glossopharyngeal breathing				Postpolio and muscular dystrophy patients. Respiratory muscle weakness, but upper airway function is intact.
Negative-pressure ventilation	Pneumosuit (Fig. 41.6)	Portable	Difficulty applying suit. Cumbersome.	Typical settings: Pressure −20 to −40 cm H_2O.[101]
			Upper airway obstruction.	Rate 14.18.
	Chest cuirass	Allows speech and feeding	Fitting difficulties.	Typical settings: Pressure −20 to −40 cm H_2O.[101]
		Portable	Upper airway obstruction.	Rate 14-18.
	Iron lung (Fig. 41.7)	Reliable	Confining.	Second line for patients if nasal ventilation fails.
			Not portable.	Typical settings: Rate 12-14. Pressure −12 to −25 cm H_2O.

Table 41.3 Ventilatory-Assist Devices* (Continued)

Mode of Ventilation	Example	Advantages	Disadvantages	Applications
Positive-pressure ventilation			Upper airway obstruction	Mode of first choice. Nasal route preferred, oronasal or mouthpiece if nasal unsuccessful. Typical settings Rate 12-24; inspiratory pressure 10-20 cm H_2O Expiratory pressure 12-15 cm H_2O.
Volume-cycled	PLV-100 and 102 (Respironics, Inc.) Companion 2801 (Mallinckrodt, Inc.)	Allows tidal volume adjustment		
	LP 6 Plus	High/low airway pressure alarms		
	LP 10	Apnea alarms		
Pressure-cycled	Quantum PSV	Usually used noninvasively		
	BI-PAP S/T	Mandatory rate available		
	KnightStar 335			
	VPAP Adapt SV (ResMed Inc.)			Adaptive-servo[100] ventilator is designed specifically to treat central sleep apnea (CSA) in all its forms. Adapts to the patient's ventilatory needs on a breath-by-breath basis and automatically calculates a target ventilation. Adjusts the pressure support to achieve it.

*Studies cited in this table may be found in the complete list of references for this chapter provided online.

Table 41.4 Interfaces for Ventilatory-Assist Devices

Mode of Delivery	Example	Advantages	Disadvantages
Noninvasive	Nasal mask (Fig. 41.8)	Avoids tracheostomy complications Less claustrophobia	Mouth leak Patent nares required Nasal bridge ulceration Patient cooperation required
	Nasal pillows (Fig. 41.9)	Avoids tracheostomy complications	Mouth leak
	Oronasal mask (Fig. 41.10)	Avoids tracheostomy complications	Poor seal Aspiration risk Cannot speak
	Mouthpiece (Fig. 41.11)	Avoids tracheostomy complications	Increased secretions Cannot speak
Invasive	Tracheostomy (Fig. 41.12)	Allows suctioning	Surgical procedure required

use of volume-cycled ventilation delivered by a tracheostomy. Because this patient population was in a terminal stage without other treatment options, tracheostomy and chronic ventilation became the standard of therapy if the patient wanted to continue aggressive care.

Major ethical considerations surround the institution of chronic ventilatory support.[51] This issue is evolving rapidly because of the widespread availability of relatively inexpensive technology. Guidelines have been published regarding clinical indications and management strategies for the use of noninvasive positive pressure ventilation, although they are based on inadequate data.[52,53] The discussion about ventilatory assistance should occur before an emergent setting. Adequate and unbiased information should be given to

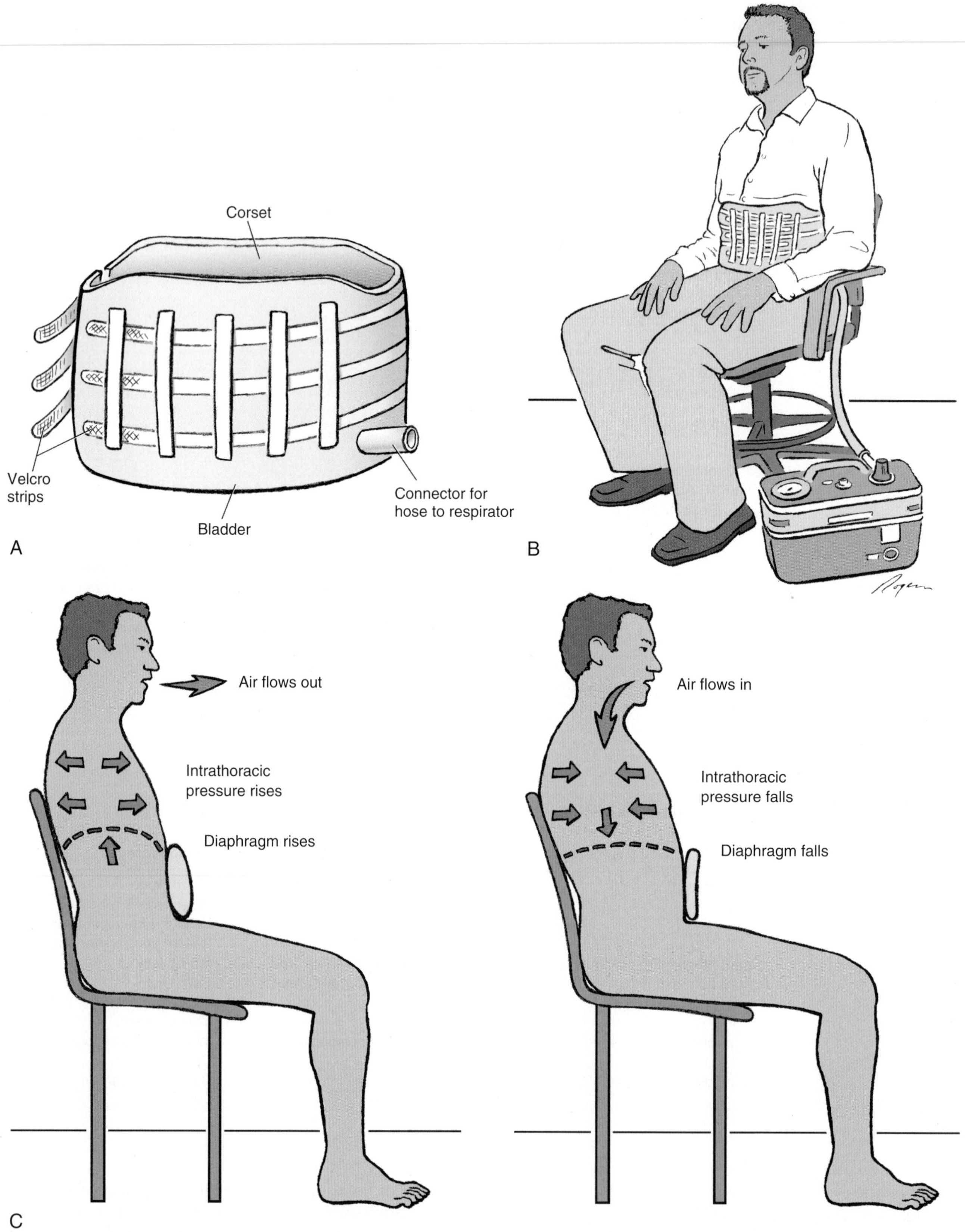

Figure 41.2 A-C, Pneumobelt. **B,** Pneumobelt connected to the Thompson Bantam positive pressure ventilator. The ventilator intermittently inflates a rubber bladder contained within the corset.

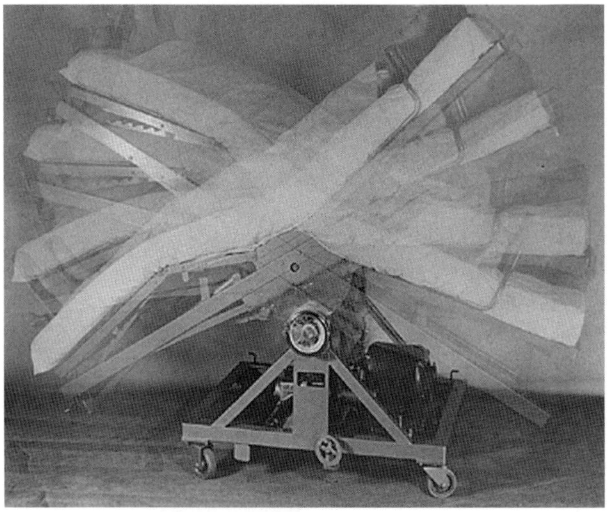

Figure 41.3 Rocking bed.

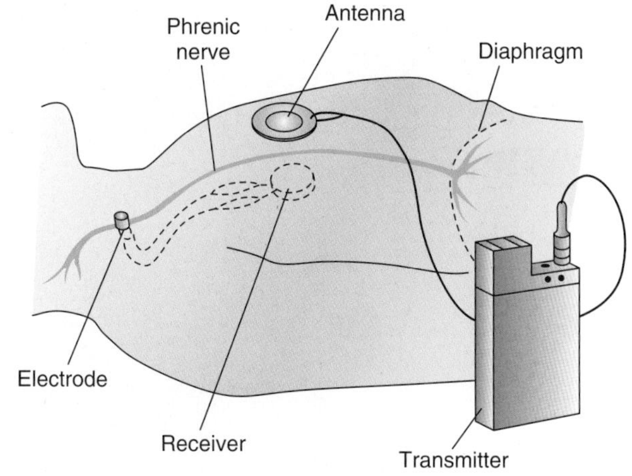

Figure 41.4 Diaphragmatic pacer.

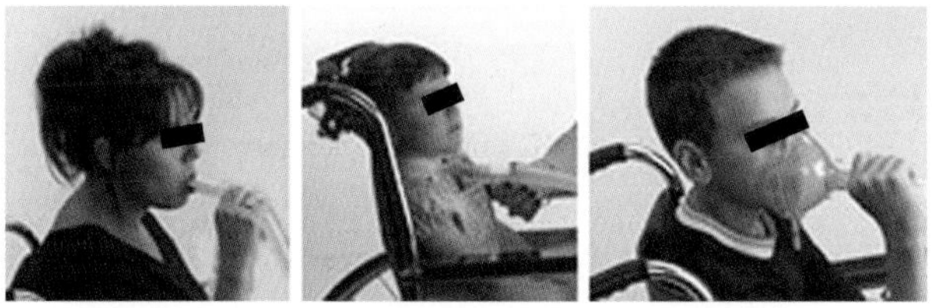

Figure 41.5 Patients using cough assist devices.

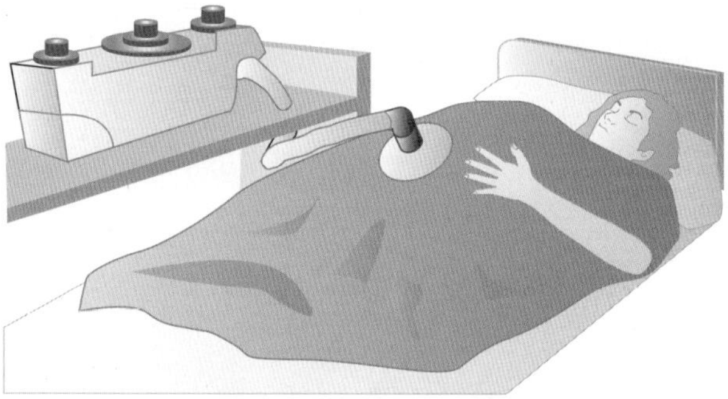

Figure 41.6 Pneumosuit.

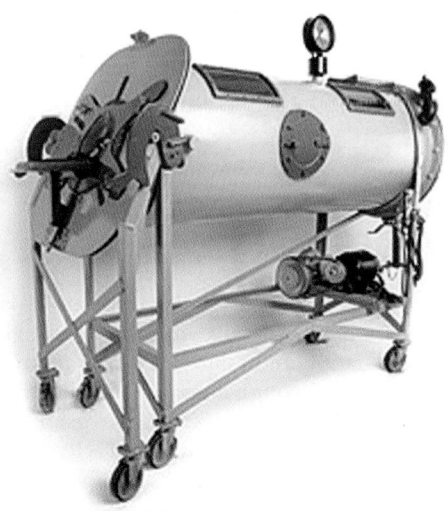

Figure 41.7 Iron lung.

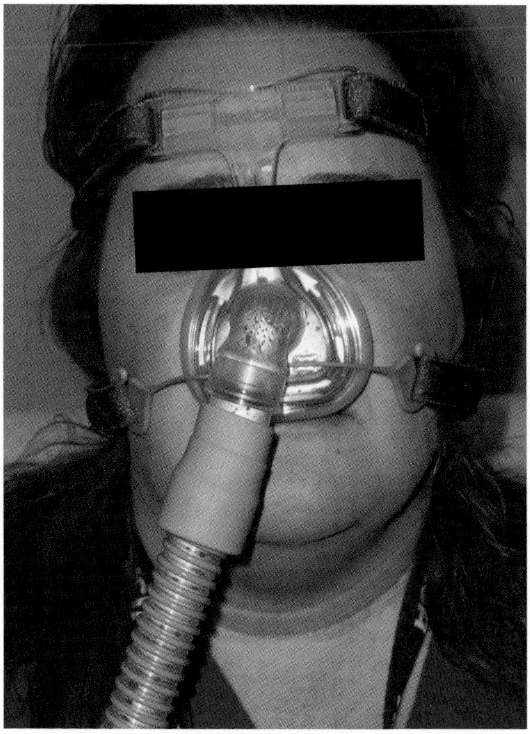

Figure 41.8 Nasal mask.

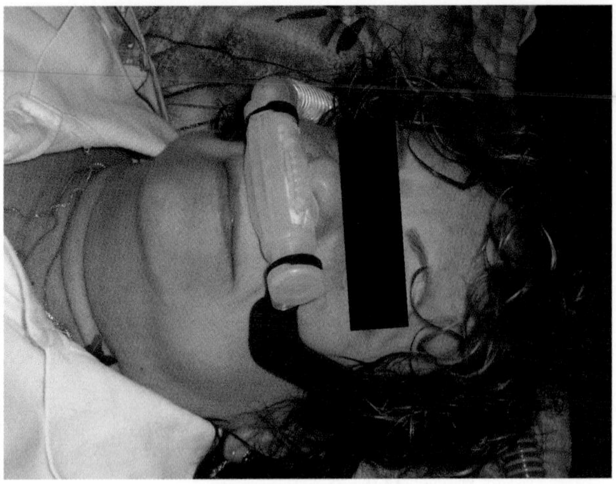

Figure 41.9 Nasal pillows.

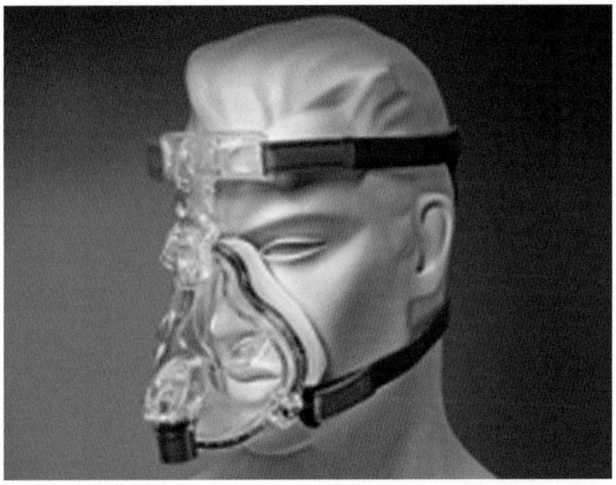

Figure 41.10 Oronasal mask. (Courtesy of Respironics, Murrysville, PA.)

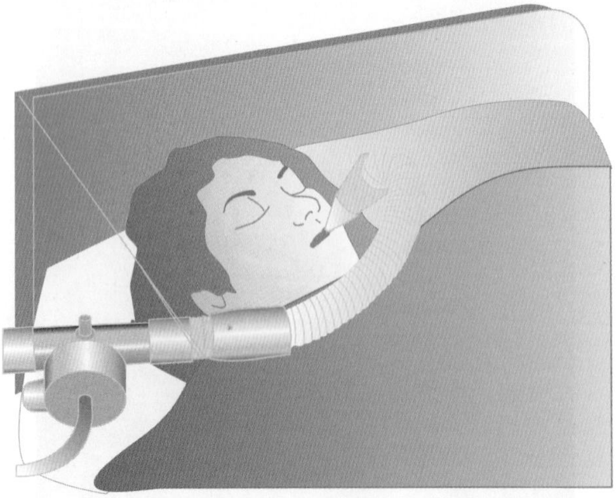

Figure 41.11 Mouthpiece.

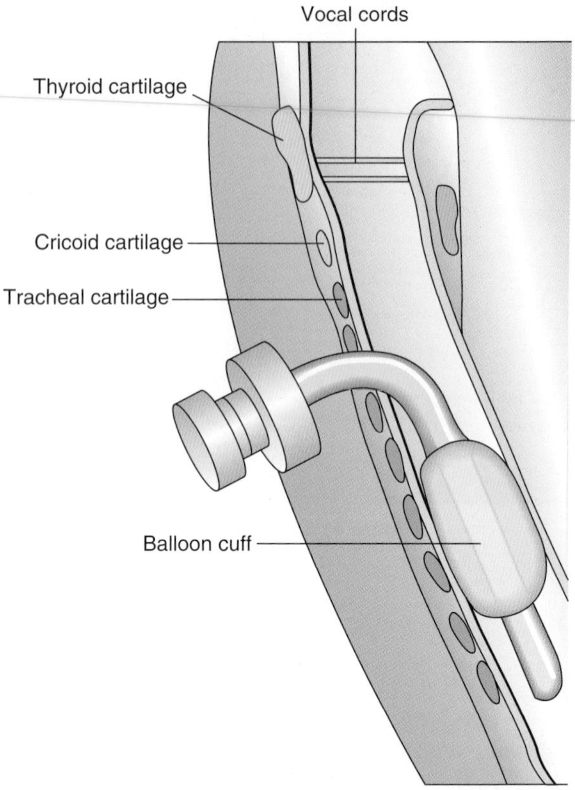

Figure 41.12 Completed tracheostomy.

patients so that they can make an informed decision. Different ventilatory methods and modes of delivery should be discussed with patients, including the possibility of foregoing any type of mechanical ventilation. Patient and caregiver quality of life and satisfaction have only recently been investigated in this population, and many unanswered questions remain. Management of the terminal phase can also be difficult.

MANAGEMENT OF AIRWAY SECRETION CLEARANCE

An understanding of neuromuscular respiratory pathophysiology and the modes of effective noninvasive cough support is key in the evaluation and management of neuromuscular diseases. A variety of cough-augmentation therapies or a combination of these therapies can be used to support cough.[102] Here are some examples of clearance device categories:

- Manual cough augmentation
- Hyperinflation maneuvers
- Functional electrical and magnetic stimulation
- Mechanical in-exsufflation therapy

KEY POINTS

- A normal $P(A - a)O_2$ difference should not be required as a diagnostic criterion for nonpulmonary causes of respiratory failure.
- The etiologic classification of nonpulmonary disorders causing respiratory failure consists of the following broad categories: disorders of ventilatory control, neuromuscular disorders, disorders of the chest wall, and upper airway obstruction.
- Clinical recognition of these disorders depends on familiarity with the physiologic consequences of chronic hypoxia and hypercapnia, the signs and symptoms of respiratory muscle weakness, and their effects on pulmonary function tests.
- An understanding of neuromuscular respiratory pathophysiology and the modes of effective noninvasive cough support is key in the evaluation and management of neuromuscular diseases.
- The approach to the management of acute respiratory failure does not differ in principle from the approach used for lung diseases.
- Noninvasive nocturnal ventilatory support has gained acceptance as a means of controlling diurnal hypercapnia and providing respiratory muscle rest.

SELECTED REFERENCES

1. Murray M, Nadel J: Murray and Nadel's Textbook of Respiratory Medicine, 4th ed. Philadelphia, Elsevier, 2005.
4. Rochester DF, Enson Y: Current concepts in the pathogenesis of the obesity-hypoventilation syndrome. Am J Med 1974;57:402-420.
9. Demers RR, Irwin R: Management of hypercapneic respiratory failure: A systematic approach. Respir Care 1979;24:328.
21. Jackson CE, Rosenfeld J, Moore DH, et al: A preliminary evaluation of a prospective study of pulmonary function studies and symptoms of hypoventilation in ALS/MND patients. J Neurol Sci 2001;191:75-78.
34. Wyatt J, Bellis F: British Thoracic Society guidelines on non-invasive ventilation. Emerg Med J 2002;19:435.
43. International Consensus Conferences in Intensive Care Medicine: Noninvasive positive pressure ventilation in acute respiratory failure. Am J Respir Crit Care Med 2001;163:283-291.
46. MacIntyre NR, Epstein SK, Carson S, et al: Management of patients requiring prolonged mechanical ventilation: Report of a NAMDRC consensus conference. Chest 2005;128:3937-3954.
52. Robert D, Willig TN, Leger P, Paulus J: Long-term nasal ventilation in neuromuscular disorders: Report of a consensus conference. Eur Respir J 1993;6:599-606.
53. Clinical indications for noninvasive positive pressure ventilation in chronic respiratory failure due to restrictive lung disease, COPD, and nocturnal hypoventilation: A consensus conference report. Chest 1999;116:521-534.
82. Latronico N, Peli E, Botteri M: Critical illness myopathy and neuropathy. Curr Opin Crit Care 2005;11:126-132.

The complete list of references can be found at www.expertconsult.com.

42 Pneumonia: Considerations for the Critically Ill Patient

Girish B. Nair | Michael S. Niederman

CHAPTER OUTLINE

Severe pneumonia with respiratory failure and sepsis is one of the commonest indications necessitating intensive care unit (ICU) admission. Pneumonia along with influenza was the eighth leading cause of death in 2009 alone. Pneumonia patients are managed in the ICU when severe forms of community-acquired pneumonia (CAP) are present or when a hospitalized patient develops life-threatening nosocomial pneumonia. Pneumonia patients admitted to the ICU usually have more severe disease, other comorbid medical conditions, and much higher mortality rate compared to the patients admitted to the wards.[1]

The incidence of pneumonia in hospitalized patients is directly related to the degree of underlying systemic illness and number of days on the ventilator.[2] The elderly account for a disproportionate number of critically ill patients with all forms of pneumonia, often because they commonly have comorbid illness, which predisposes them to more severe forms of infection, and their short- and long-term mortality rates are higher than those of younger patients.[3] Also, hospitalized patients receive therapeutic interventions that predispose them to pneumonia such as endotracheal intubation, nasogastric feeding, antibiotic therapy, and use of immunomodulatory medications. In 2005, there were more than 60,000 deaths in persons aged 15 years or older related to CAP in the United States.[4] The mortality rate from severe CAP is over 30% in patients admitted to the ICU.[5] Critically ill patients who develop ventilator-associated pneumonia (VAP) have a higher mortality rate compared with similar patients without VAP and incur USD $10,019 or more in additional hospital costs.[6]

With newer guidelines, there has been an emphasis on identifying patients with severe pneumonia early in the clinical course, facilitating early ICU admission, because this has been shown to decrease the mortality rate.[7] Different scoring systems such as the ATS/IDSA guidelines (developed by American Thoracic Society and Infectious Diseases Society of America), PIRO (Predisposition, Insult, Response and Organ dysfunction) scores for CAP, and Acute Physiology and Chronic Health Evaluation score (APACHE II) and VAP PIRO score for VAP are used for assessing the severity of illness in pneumonia patients. It is still uncertain whether the use of any scoring system can lead to decreased mortality rates and more favorable outcomes in the management of patients with pneumonia. There is also interest in using biomarkers, such as procalcitonin (PCT), to diagnose the severity and guide the use and duration of antimicrobial therapy in patients with severe CAP and VAP.[8-10]

The emergence of multidrug-resistant (MDR) microorganisms is an alarming problem in the ICU and considerable forethought is necessary in choosing the right antibiotic to be used in this setting. In the ICU, almost 90% of episodes of nosocomial pneumonia occur in patients who are being mechanically ventilated for other reasons. Recent directives by the Centers for Medicare and Medicaid Services (CMS) and the Institute for Healthcare Improvement have led to the belief that VAP is preventable and should be a "never event" during the hospital stay. This may have led to underreporting in many instances.[11] Many ICUs have incorporated ventilator bundles as a preventive strategy to minimize VAP, which may be an effective strategy, even if not being able to completely eliminate the problem.

The incidence of pneumonia in nursing homes varies from 0.3 to 2.3 episodes per 1000 resident care days with a 30-day mortality rate of 14.7%.[12] In the 2005 ATS guidelines on nosocomial pneumonia, patients with exposure to MDR organisms by virtue of being in contact with the health care environment prior to admission were defined as having health care–associated pneumonia (HCAP). This group included residents of a nursing home or long-term care facility; recipients of recent intravenous antibiotic therapy, chemotherapy, or wound care within the past 30 days; and chronic hemodialysis patients.[2] The focus in managing these patients was to empirically treat for MDR pathogens. However, recent studies have shown that the HCAP population has significant heterogeneity, and that treatment of all patients does not always need to include coverage for methicillin-resistant *Staphylococcus aureus* (MRSA) and drug-resistant gram-negative organisms.[13]

Pneumonia is unusual among medical illnesses because its pathogenesis, therapy, and prevention can be discussed, but there is tremendous controversy about how to best diagnose its presence. In this chapter we discuss the risk factors, pathogenesis, and recent advances in the treatment, complications, and various controversies that exist in the care of all forms of pneumonia patients in the ICU.

DEFINITIONS AND RISK FACTORS

Patients who are unable to mount an effective immune response are at increased risk of developing serious pneumonia. If the host defense mechanism is overwhelmed by the size of the inoculum, the virulence of the infecting microorganisms, or an excessive inflammatory response to infection, the patient can develop severe respiratory failure or sepsis. Depending on the time of onset and setting in which the infection developed, pneumonia is classified as community-acquired or nosocomial pneumonia, with specific definitions for VAP and HCAP among patients with nosocomial pneumonia (Box 42.1).

Box 42.1 Classification of Pneumonia

Community-Acquired Pneumonia (CAP)

An alveolar infection that develops in the outpatient setting or within 48 hours of admission to a hospital.

Nosocomial Pneumonia

Hospital-Acquired Pneumonia (HAP)

Pneumonia occurring ≥48 hours after hospital admission and not incubating at the time of admission.

Ventilator-Associated Pneumonia (VAP)

Pneumonia occurring ≥48 hours after endotracheal intubation and mechanical ventilation.

Health Care–Associated Pneumonia (HCAP)

Pneumonia in patients with one or more of the following risk factors for multidrug-resistant (MDR) bacteria: (1) hospitalization for ≥2 days in an acute care facility within 90 days before infection; (2) residence in a nursing home or long term care facility; (3) antibiotic therapy, chemotherapy, or wound care within 30 days before current infection; (4) hemodialysis treatment at a hospital or clinic; (5) home infusion therapy or home wound care; or (6) family member with infection due to MDR pathogen.

SEVERE COMMUNITY-ACQUIRED PNEUMONIA

Even though there is no uniform definition for severe pneumonia, patients who require ventilator support or vasopressor support are generally regarded as having severe pneumonia, but it is more challenging to define severe illness in patients who are not receiving these interventions. However, identifying patients with severe pneumonia is important for proper resource utilization, and outcomes can be improved if these patients are identified early, avoiding delayed admission to the ICU, which is in itself a poor prognostic factor.

Several prognostic scoring systems were developed to predict the mortality risk and guide the site of care decision. The pneumonia severity index (PSI) and the British Thoracic Society's CURB-65 score help with determining mortality risk for patients with CAP.[14] The PSI was developed to identify patients with a low risk of dying, placing all patients into five classes, based on the demographic characteristics, coexisting illnesses, physical examination findings, laboratory measurements, and radiographic findings. The ICU is most often used for patients in classes IV and V, who have a 30-day mortality risk of 4% to 10% and 27%, respectively.[15] However, the PSI score may overestimate severity of illness in patients with older age, while underestimating severity in young patients without comorbid conditions.[16] The complexity of the PSI contrasts with the simpler bedside scoring system, CURB-65. With this tool, 1 point is assigned each for the presence of confusion, blood urea nitrogen (BUN) greater than 7.0 mol/L (19.6 mg/dL), respiratory rate of 30 or more breaths/minute, systolic blood pressure 90 mm Hg or less, or diastolic blood pressure 60 mm Hg or less, and age 65 years or more.[17] Mortality rate increases proportionately with scores higher than 3 (score 3, 17%; score 4, 41.5%; and score 5, 57%).

Severe pneumonia and the host inflammatory response to infection are determined by several variables, including the identity of the pathogen, the timeliness and appropriateness of therapy, and patient variables. The latter include the genetic makeup of the individual, age, nutritional status, sex, and comorbid medical conditions. Although the PSI and CURB-65 score performed well to determine mortality risk, there is still a need to identify patients who will need ICU level of care at the earliest possible time point.[18,19] According to the 2007 ATS/IDSA guidelines, severe CAP is present if a patient requires invasive mechanical ventilation or vasopressors or has any three of the nine minor criteria (Box 42.2).[19] The PIRO score has also been used and is calculated within 24 hours of ICU admission with 1 point assigned for each of comorbid conditions (chronic obstructive pulmonary disease [COPD], immunosuppressed state), age older than 70 years, multilobar opacities on chest radiograph, shock, severe hypoxemia, acute renal failure, bacteremia, and acute respiratory distress syndrome (ARDS). Patients can be stratified into four classes: (1) low, 0 to 2 points; (2) mild, 3 points; (3) high, 4 points; (4) very high, 5 to 8 points. In patients admitted to the ICU, the PIRO score had a better performance than APACHE II and ATS/IDSA criteria to predict 28-day mortality rate.[18]

Severe pneumonia is a dynamic inflammatory process, and predicting which stable-appearing patients will require ICU care later is difficult. Hence, critically ill patients who do not have obvious need for ICU care, such as invasive respiratory/vasopressor support (IRVS), must satisfy certain minor criteria in order to be recognized. However, the predictive value of using just three minor criteria alone for making a decision to admit to the ICU is uncertain, and in one study, the use of four minor criteria improved the accuracy of predicting subsequent need for ICU care.[20,21] A recent prospective study from Scotland excluded patients with the two major ATS/IDSA criteria present on admission, and demonstrated that each of the nine minor criteria was associated with an increased risk of need for mechanical ventilation, need for vasopressor support, and 30-day mortality.[22]

Another system developed in Australia—SMART-COP—can assess the need for intensive respiratory or vasopressor support.[23] The SMART-COP was developed primarily to identify the need for IRVS. Different point scores were assigned to various parameters: low **S**ystolic blood pressure less than 90 mm Hg (2 points), **M**ultilobar pneumonia (1 point), low **A**lbumin level less than 3.5 g/dL (1 point), high **R**espiratory rate 25 to 30 breaths/minute (1 point), **T**achycardia higher than 125 beats/minute (1 point), **C**onfusion (1 point), poor **O**xygenation (2 points), and low arterial **p**H less than 7.35 (2 points). A score of more than 3 points identified 92% of patients requiring IRVS, with a specificity of 62.3%, outperforming PSI and CURB-65 scores to identify this specific end point.[23] The SMART-COP as well as the ATS/IDSA 2007 guidelines are the most accurate for predicting need for ICU care.[24]

Renaud and coworkers examined risk factors for early admission to the ICU among 6560 patients, who presented to the emergency department and did not require immediate respiratory or circulatory support.[25] They identified 11 criteria independently associated with ICU admission: male gender, age younger than 80 years, comorbid conditions, respiratory rate of 30 breaths/minute or higher, heart rate of 125 beats/minute or higher, multilobar infiltrate or pleural effusion, white blood cell count less than 3 or more than 20 g/L, hypoxemia (oxygen saturation <90% or arterial partial pressure of oxygen [Pa_{O_2}] <60 mm Hg), BUN of 11 mmol/L or higher, pH less than 7.35, and sodium less than 130 mEq/L. They used these criteria to develop the risk of early admission to ICU index (REA-ICU index), which stratified patients into four risk classes, with the risk of ICU admission on days 1 to 3 ranging from 0.7% to 31%.[25]

Recent data from the German Competence Network for the Study of CAP (CAPNETZ) Study Group demonstrated that serum biomarkers (PCT) can be used as good predictors for short- and long-term all-cause mortality rates in patients admitted with CAP.[26] A low level of PCT value in patients classified as high risk by PSI and CURB-65 scores predicted a low risk of dying, and probably a low need for ICU admission.[27] Ramirez and colleagues showed that the ATS/IDSA 2007 minor criteria had comparable predictive value with other scores, such as CURB-65 and SMART-COP, but that the use of biomarkers like PCT and C-reactive protein (CRP), along with minor criteria, helped in predicting the need for delayed ICU admission.[28] Pathophysiologic severity markers of severe sepsis, like **s**oluble **r**eceptor for **a**dvanced **g**lycation **e**nd products (SRAGE) along with severity scores have been examined in patients with CAP and are encouraging but need further studies for validation.[29]

Box 42.2 Severe Pneumonia: Diagnostic Criteria*

Major Criteria

Invasive mechanical ventilation
Use of vasopressors to maintain blood pressure

Minor Criteria

Respiratory rate ≥30 breaths/min
Multilobar infiltrates
New onset confusion/disorientation
Uremia (BUN >20 mg/dL)
Leukopenia (WBC count <4000 cells/μL)
Pa_{O_2}/F_{IO_2} ratio ≥250
Thrombocytopenia (platelet count <100,000 cells/μL)
Hypothermia (core temperature <36° C)
Hypotension requiring aggressive fluid resuscitation

*According to ATS/IDSA 2007 Guidelines.
ATS/IDSA, American Thoracic Society/Infectious Diseases Society of America; BUN, blood urea nitrogen; WBC, white blood cell.

RISK FACTORS FOR SEVERE FORMS OF COMMUNITY-ACQUIRED PNEUMONIA

Most patients with severe CAP (45-65%) have coexisting illnesses, and patients who are chronically ill have an increased likelihood of developing a complicated pneumonary illness (Box 42.3).[30] The most common chronic illnesses in these patients are respiratory disease such as COPD, cardiovascular disease, and diabetes mellitus. In addition, certain habits such as cigarette smoking and

Box 42.3 Risk Factors for Development of Severe Community-Acquired Pneumonia (CAP)

- Advanced age (>65 years)
- Comorbid illness: chronic respiratory illness (including COPD), cardiovascular disease, diabetes mellitus, neurologic illness, renal insufficiency, malignancy
- Cigarette smoking (risk for pneumococcal bacteremia)
- Alcohol abuse
- Absence of antibiotic therapy before hospitalization
- Failure to contain infection to its initial site of entry
- Immune suppression
- Genetic polymorphisms in the immune response

COPD, chronic obstructive pulmonary disease.

alcohol abuse are also quite common in those with severe CAP, and cigarette smoking has been identified as a risk factor for bacteremic pneumococcal infection.[31] Other common illnesses in those with CAP include malignancy and neurologic illness (including seizures). Milder forms of pneumonia may be more severe on presentation, if patients have not received antibiotic therapy prior to hospital admission. In addition, genetic differences in the immune response may predispose certain individuals to more severe forms of infection and adverse outcomes and may be reflected by a family history of severe pneumonia or adverse outcomes from infection.[32] Also, genetic variability of the pulmonary surfactant proteins A and D may affect clearance of microorganisms and the extent of the inflammatory response, influencing the severity and outcomes for patients with CAP, notably missense single nucleotide polymorphisms and haplotypes of SFTPA1, SFTPA2, and SFTPD.[33] Recent evidence also provides insights on the risk of developing pneumonia in patients taking inhaled corticosteroids. In a meta analysis of 18 randomized controlled trials with a total of 16,996 patients, inhaled corticosteroids were associated with a significantly increased risk of serious pneumonia when compared with placebo (relative risk [RR] 1.81; $P < 0.001$) or when the combination of inhaled corticosteroids and long-acting β-agonists was compared with long-acting β-agonists (RR 1.68; $P < 0.002$).[34] However, the mortality rate of patients developing CAP while on inhaled corticosteroids may actually be lower than in patients not receiving this therapy.

MORTALITY RISK FROM COMMUNITY-ACQUIRED PNEUMONIA

In a meta analysis of 33,148 patients with CAP, the overall mortality rate was 13.7%, but those admitted to the ICU had a mortality rate of 36.5%.[5] Eleven prognostic factors were significantly associated with different odds ratios (OR) for mortality rate: male sex (OR = 1.3), pleuritic chest pain (OR = 0.5), hypothermia (OR = 5.0), systolic hypotension (OR = 4.8), tachypnea (OR = 2.9), diabetes mellitus (OR = 1.3), neoplastic disease (OR = 2.8), neurologic disease (OR = 4.6), bacteremia (OR = 2.8), leukopenia (OR = 2.5), and multilobar infiltrates (OR = 3.1). In other studies, the clinical features that predict a poor outcome (Box 42.4) include

Box 42.4 Risk Factors for Poor Outcome from Community-Acquired Pneumonia (CAP)

Patient-Related Factors

- Male gender
- Absence of pleuritic chest pain
- Nonclassical clinical presentation (nonrespiratory presentation)
- Neoplastic illness
- Neurologic illness
- Age >65 years
- Family history of severe pneumonia or death from sepsis

Abnormal Physical Findings

- Respiratory rate >30 breaths/min on admission
- Systolic (<90 mm Hg) or diastolic (<60 mm Hg) hypotension
- Tachycardia (>125 beats/min)
- High fever (>40° C) or afebrile
- Confusion

Laboratory Abnormalities

- BUN >20 mg/dL
- Leukocytosis or leukopenia
- Multilobar radiographic abnormalities
- Rapidly progressive radiographic abnormalities during therapy
- Bacteremia
- Hyponatremia (serum sodium <130 mmol/L)
- Multiple organ failure
- Respiratory failure
- Hypoalbuminemia
- Arterial pH <7.35
- Pleural effusion

Pathogen-Related Factors

- High-risk organisms: type III pneumococcus, *Staphylococcus aureus*, gram-negative bacilli (including *Pseudomonas aeruginosa*), aspiration organisms, SARS coronavirus
- Possibly high levels of penicillin resistance (MIC of at least 4 mg/L) in pneumococcus

Therapy-Related Factors

- Delay in initial antibiotic therapy (more than 4-6 hours)
- Initial therapy with inappropriate antibiotic therapy
- Lack of clinical response to empiric therapy within 72 hours

BUN, blood urea nitrogen; MIC, minimum inhibitory concentration; SARS, severe acute respiratory syndrome.

advanced age (>65 years), preexisting chronic illness of any type, the absence of fever on admission, respiratory rate more than 30 breaths/minute, diastolic or systolic hypotension, elevated BUN (>19.6 mg/dL), profound leukopenia or leukocytosis, inadequate antibiotic therapy, need for mechanical ventilation, hypoalbuminemia, and the presence of certain "high-risk" organisms (type III pneumococcus, *S. aureus*, gram-negative bacilli, aspiration organisms, or postobstructive pneumonia). Timing of initial appropriate antibiotics is also important, with a delay in the initiation of appropriate antibiotic therapy of more than 4 hours being associated with increased mortality risk.[35-37] Other clinical features associated with an increased mortality risk include rapid radiographic progression during therapy, nonrespiratory clinical presenting symptoms, and the presence of HCAP risk factors.

Many studies suggest that early ICU admission confers a better outcome in patients with severe CAP than delayed admission. In a study comparing patients directly admitted to the ICU from the emergency department to those moved to the ICU within 3 days after admission, delayed-transfer patients had a higher 28-day mortality rate (23.4% vs. 11.7%; $p = 0.02$) and a longer median hospital length of stay (13 days vs. 7 days; $p < 0.001$).[38] In a study of 17,869 cases of CAP in the United Kingdom, only 5.9% needed ICU care, but early admission (within 2 days of hospitalization) appeared to be preferable and was associated with a lower mortality rate (46.3%) than was late admission (>7 days in the hospital, 57.6% mortality rate).[7] In patients with severe CAP, the expected mortality rate for those admitted to the ICU is 35% to 40%, but higher rates have been observed if the percentage of patients who are mechanically ventilated is higher than 60%, implying that the prognosis is worse if ICU care is first provided late in the course of illness, after the onset of overt respiratory failure.[7] Restrepo and colleagues noted that late admission to the ICU, more than 24 hours after presentation in patients with severe CAP, resulted in a higher mortality rate than did early admission (47.4% vs. 23.2%, $p = 0.02$; hazard ratio 2.6).[39]

PNEUMONIA ACQUIRED IN THE HOSPITAL

Hospital-acquired pneumonia (HAP) is the second most common nosocomial infection in the United States,[40] and current guidelines have emphasized the importance of the time of onset of the disease and the presence of risk factors for infection due to MDR pathogens in defining the approach to therapy. The major goals are early, appropriate antibiotic therapy in adequate doses and appropriate de-escalation of initial antibiotic therapy, based on microbiologic cultures and the clinical response of the patient.[2]

Early- and late-onset HAP and VAP are diagnosed 2 to 5 days, and more than 5 days, after hospitalization, respectively. The pathogens associated with early-onset HAP and VAP are a group of "core pathogens," including *Streptococcus pneumoniae, Haemophilus influenzae,* methicillin-susceptible *Staphylococcus aureus* (MSSA), and enteric gram-negative bacilli (*Escherichia coli, Klebsiella* species, *Proteus* species, and *Enterobacter* species). In contrast, late-onset HAP and VAP are caused by all the core pathogens, plus drug-resistant pathogens such as MRSA and MDR gram-negative bacilli (*Pseudomonas aeruginosa, Acinetobacter* species, *Enterobacter* species, and extended-spectrum β-lactamase [ESBL]–positive strains).

Unlike CAP, there are no well-studied scoring systems to assess disease severity in patients with HAP and VAP. Clinical studies have used surrogate markers such as the APACHE II, or the Sequential Organ Failure Assessment (SOFA) score as a measure of organ dysfunction and severity assessment.[41] The Clinical Pulmonary Infection Score (CPIS) was originally introduced for diagnoses in patients with VAP (described later in the text), but it has also been used to follow the response of VAP patients to therapy.[42] The value of APACHE II, SOFA score, and CPIS in the prediction of mortality risk during VAP episodes was assessed in a prospective observational study, which found that an APACHE II score greater than 16 (determined at the time of VAP diagnosis) was the only independent predictor of the mortality risk (OR 5; $p = 0.019$) in a logistic regression analysis.[43] In a prospective study by Lisboa and colleagues from Spain, including 441 patients with VAP in three multidisciplinary ICUs, the mortality risk in patients with VAP was assessed by a simple four-variable VAP PIRO score: comorbid conditions (COPD, immunocompromised state, heart failure, cirrhosis, or chronic renal failure); bacteremia; systolic blood pressure less than 90 mm Hg; and ARDS.[44] Patients were stratified into three levels of risk: (1) mild, 0 to 1 points; (2) high, 2 points (hazard ratio, 2.14); and (3) very high, 3 to 4 points (hazard ratio, 4.63). More recently, a newer and easier scoring system, the IBMP-10, was proposed and is based on the presence of **i**mmunodeficiency; (2) **b**lood pressure less than 90 mm Hg (systolic) or less than 60 mm Hg (diastolic); **m**ultilobar infiltrates noted on a chest radiograph; **p**latelet count less than 100,000/μL; and duration of hospitalization before the onset of VAP of more than **10** days.[45] IBMP-10 score was comparable to the APACHE II score in its ability to predict mortality risk in patients with VAP but needs further validation in prospective studies.

RISK FACTORS ASSOCIATED WITH NOSOCOMIAL PNEUMONIA

The 2005 ATS/IDSA guidelines characterized the predisposing factors for developing nosocomial pneumonia as modifiable and nonmodifiable. Mechanical ventilation (for > 2 days) is the most important risk factor for nosocomial pneumonia, but other identified risks include age older than 60, malnutrition (serum albumin < 2.2 g/dL), acute lung injury (ARDS), coma, burns, recent abdominal or thoracic surgery, multiple organ failure, transfusion of more than 4 units of blood, transport from the ICU, prior antibiotic therapy, elevation of gastric pH (by antacids or histamine-type 2 blocking agents), large volume aspiration, use of a nasogastric tube (rather than a tube placed in the jejunum or a tube inserted through the mouth), use of inadequate endotracheal tube cuff pressure, prolonged sedation and paralysis, maintaining patients in the supine position in bed, use of total parenteral nutrition (TPN) feeding rather than enteral feeding, and repeated reintubation.[2] When a patient is mechanically ventilated, the risk of pneumonia is greatest in the first 5 days (3% per day), and declines thereafter to a risk of 2% per day for days 6 to 10, and to a rate of 1% per day or lower after this.[46] Noninvasive ventilation for respiratory failure is associated with a much lower risk of pneumonia than endotracheal intubation.

The relation between pneumonia and ARDS is particularly interesting, because up to one third of all cases of ARDS may be the result of pneumonia, and in some series, pneumonia is the most common cause of acute lung injury. In addition, secondary nosocomial pneumonia is the most common infection complicating the course of established ARDS.[47,48] Seidenfeld and coworkers reported better survival in patients with ARDS in the absence of infection, but a subanalysis for pneumonia was not available.[48] In a study by Chastre and colleagues of 243 consecutive patients who required mechanical ventilation 48 or more hours, 55% of the ARDS patients developed VAP compared to 28% without ARDS ($p = 0.0005$).[49] Most patients who developed VAP had been treated with prior broad-spectrum antibiotics, and were infected with MDR pathogens (MRSA, nonfermenting gram-negative bacilli, and Enterobacteriaceae).

Pneumonia also presents a particular problem in the postoperative patient, particularly after elective thoracic, cardiac, or abdominal surgery. Other surgical groups that are at high risk for pneumonia include the victims of major trauma, particularly those suffering head injury and blunt chest trauma. When a patient has a pulmonary contusion, it may be very difficult to distinguish this process from secondary lung infection on the basis of clinical and radiographic findings.

MORTALITY RISK FROM VENTILATOR-ASSOCIATED PNEUMONIA

Mortality rates from VAP can be as high as 50% to 70%, and case-control studies have documented death directly attributable to the presence of pneumonia.[50] The patients with HAP often have other associated comorbid illnesses that predispose them to a high risk of dying, independent of the presence of pneumonia. Attributable mortality rate, defined as death directly related to infection and not due to underlying conditions, is challenging to measure, but older studies reported a higher mortality rate for patients with VAP than for similarly ill ventilated patients without VAP (52.4% with VAP, compared to 22.4% for patients without).[51] Recently, however, Bekaert and colleagues assessed the population-attributable risk of ICU VAP by taking into account the confounding that is caused by time-dependent severity-of-illness indicators.[52] They estimated that 4.4% (95% confidence interval, 1.6-7.0%) of the deaths in the ICU on day 30 and 5.9% (95% confidence interval, 2.5-9.1%) on day 60 were attributable to VAP. This corresponds to an ICU attributable mortality rate for VAP of about 1% on day 30 and 1.5% on day 60.

Antibiotic-resistant organisms may add to the mortality risk of VAP, not because of increased virulence, but rather because these organisms are often not anticipated, and when present, are often initially treated with ineffective antibiotic regimens.[53] The factor associated with the greatest impact on attributable mortality rate is the accuracy and timeliness of initial antibiotic therapy. Use of the wrong therapy, or delays in the initiation of therapy, are the most important predictors of VAP mortality rate.[54] Initial appropriate therapy (using an agent to which the etiologic pathogen is sensitive) can reduce mortality rate, but administration of correct therapy at a later date, after initially incorrect therapy, may not effectively reduce mortality rate.[54] The benefit of accurate empiric therapy may not apply to all patients, but may be greatest for those infected with *P. aeruginosa* or *S. aureus*[55] and for those without the most severe degree of multiple organ dysfunction at the time of therapy.[56] For some patients, even using the correct therapy does not reduce the risk of death if it is not given in adequate doses and if the therapy does not reach the site of infection.

Although a number of host and bacteriologic factors enhance the mortality risk of nosocomial pneumonia, development of a superinfection, as opposed to primary nosocomial pneumonia, is a particularly ominous finding. Rello and associates observed that pulmonary superinfection had a 67% mortality rate, whereas primary nosocomial pneumonia had a 38% mortality rate.[57] In earlier studies, Graybill and coworkers observed a 62% mortality rate with superinfection pneumonia, compared to a 40% mortality rate for primary nosocomial lung infection.[58] These data, as well as information from Fagon and colleagues, emphasize the important role of prior antibiotics in enhancing mortality risk, an outcome that is likely the result of secondary infection by more virulent pathogens.[59,60] As a result, antibiotic use has two pivotal roles in prognosticating outcome from nosocomial pneumonia: outcome is improved if the correct therapy is chosen, but if this therapy is followed by superinfection, then mortality risk is increased, generally because these infections involve difficult-to-treat drug-resistant organisms. Closely related to antibiotic resistance is the presence of bacteremia in patients with VAP, which is associated with increased mortality risk.[61]

When therapy is given, it is important to decrease the number and spectrum of antimicrobial therapy once culture data become available, referred to as "de-escalation." Several recent studies have demonstrated that the use of de-escalation is associated with lower mortality risk compared to escalation or compared to a strategy of making no effort to reduce antibiotic therapy.[62-64] The choice of how to administer a specific agent can also affect outcome, and one study of MRSA VAP found that the mortality risk with intermittent infusion of vancomycin was twice as high as when this agent was administered by continuous infusion.[65] Other risk factors for mortality (Box 42.5) include prolonged duration of ventilation, coma on admission, creatinine greater than 1.5, transfer from another ward to the ICU, the presence of certain high-risk pathogens (particularly an antibiotic-resistant organism such as *P. aeruginosa, Acinetobacter* spp., or *S. aureus*), bilateral radiographic abnormalities, age older than 60 years, ultimately fatal underlying

Box 42.5 Mortality Risk Factors for Nosocomial Pneumonia

Historical Data

Prior antibiotic therapy
Age >60 years
Underlying fatal illness
Prolonged mechanical ventilation
Inappropriate antimicrobial therapy
Transfer to the intensive care unit from another ward

Physiologic Findings

Respiratory failure
Coma on admission
Multiple system organ failure
APACHE II score rising to greater than 20 at 72 hours after diagnosis

Laboratory Findings

Serum creatinine >1.5 mg/dL
Gram-negative pneumonia, especially *Pseudomonas* or *Acinetobacter* infection
Infection with any drug-resistant pathogen
Bilateral radiographic abnormalities
Fungal pneumonia
Polymicrobial infection

APACHE II, Acute Physiology and Chronic Health Evaluation II [study].

condition, shock, prior antibiotic therapy, multiple system organ failure, nonsurgical primary diagnosis, and a rising APACHE II score during pneumonia therapy.[2,66]

HEALTH CARE–ASSOCIATED PNEUMONIA

The ATS/IDSA guidelines included HCAP as a form of nosocomial pneumonia because these patients were at risk for infection with MDR pathogens because of recent contact with the health care environment. HCAP includes patients who were hospitalized in an acute care hospital for 2 or more days within 90 days of the infection; those who reside in a nursing home or long-term care facility; individuals who received recent intravenous antibiotic therapy, chemotherapy, or wound care within the past 30 days; and those attending a hospital or hemodialysis clinic. Recent clinical investigations have shown that HCAP includes a diverse group of patients, with some at risk for MDR organisms and others not. In fact, many HCAP patients have been treated successfully with a monotherapy regimen or with regimens used for CAP.[13] Patients in the HCAP population who are at risk for MDR pathogens were those with severe illness or those with other risk factors including hospitalization in the past 90 days, antibiotic therapy in the past 6 months, poor functional status as defined by activities of daily living score, and immune suppression.

PATHOGENESIS

GENERAL OVERVIEW

The respiratory system has both innate and adaptive immunity, which helps prevent potentially harmful pathogens from adhering to the respiratory mucosa and proliferating. Multiple defense barriers in the conducting and gas exchange surfaces of the respiratory tract filter out invading pathogens. The combined effects of the physical, innate, and acquired host defense systems serve to recognize, localize, kill, and remove pathogens. The pathogens that reach the conducting airways are exposed to the soluble constituents in airway fluids. Multiple antimicrobial peptides, such as lysozyme (lytic to bacterial membranes); lactoferrin (which excludes iron from bacterial metabolism); IgA and IgG; and defensins are present in the airway mucosa and pathogens are expelled by the coordinated mucociliary system and cough reflex. Particles 1 µm and smaller reach the alveolar surface and interact with the alveolar macrophages and other components such as IgG, complement, surfactant, and surfactant-associated proteins. Bacteria are opsonized by IgG, complement, or surfactant proteins SP-A and SP-D and are ingested by alveolar macrophages. Pathogen recognition is mediated by toll-like receptors. They initiate local inflammatory response by releasing interleukins and cytokines and carry microbial antigens into the interstitium and to regional lymph nodes where they are taken up by specialized dendritic cells and presented to responding lymphocytes to initiate adaptive immune responses.[67]

Pneumonia develops when these host defenses are overwhelmed by the invading microorganisms (Fig. 42.1). This may occur because the patient has an inadequate immune response, often as the result of underlying comorbid illness, which can lead to anatomic abnormalities (endobronchial obstruction, bronchiectasis), disease-associated immune impairment, or therapy-induced dysfunction of the immune system (corticosteroids, endotracheal intubation).[2,68,69] Pneumonia can also occur in patients who have an adequate immune system if the host defense system is

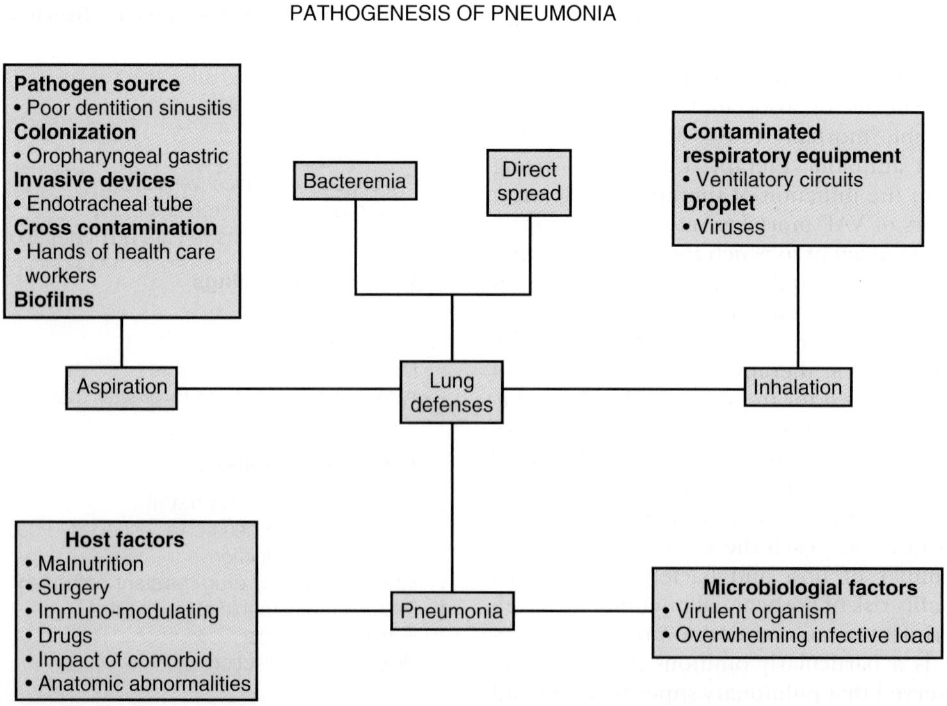

Figure 42.1 Different routes of entry for pathogenic organisms into the respiratory tract are shown. The innate and adaptive immune systems try to contain the infection while host and microbiologic factors modulate the lung's response to the pathogen.

overwhelmed by a large inoculum of bacteria (massive aspiration) or by a particularly virulent organism to which the patient has no preexisting immunity (such as an endemic virus) or to which the patient has an inability to form an adequate immune response. With this paradigm in mind, it is easy to understand why previously healthy individuals develop infection with virulent pathogens such as viruses (influenza), *Legionella pneumophila, Mycoplasma pneumoniae, Chlamydophila pneumoniae,* and *S. pneumoniae.* However, for chronically ill patients, it is possible for them to be infected not only by these virulent organisms but also by organisms that are not highly virulent. Owing to host defense impairments, organisms that commonly colonize these patients can cause infection as a result of an inadequate immune response. These organisms include enteric gram-negative bacteria (*E. coli, Klebsiella pneumoniae, P. aeruginosa, Acinetobacter* spp.) and fungi (*Aspergillus* and *Candida* spp.). There can also be genetic variations in the immune response, making some patients prone to overwhelming infection, due to an inadequate response, and others prone to acute lung injury, due to an excessive immune response.[32] In fact, the failure to localize the immune response to the respiratory site of initial infection may explain why some patients develop acute lung injury and sepsis as the inflammatory response extends to the entire lung and systemic circulation.[70]

ROUTE OF ENTRY

Bacteria can enter the lung via several routes, but aspiration from a previously colonized oropharynx is the most common way that patients develop pneumonia. Although most pneumonias result from microaspiration, patients can also aspirate large volumes of bacteria if they have impaired neurologic protection of the upper airway (stroke, seizure), or if they have gastrointestinal illnesses that predispose to vomiting. Other routes of entry include inhalation, which applies primarily to viruses, *L. pneumophila,* and *Mycobacterium tuberculosis;* hematogenous dissemination from extrapulmonary sites of infection (right-sided endocarditis); and direct extension from contiguous sites of infection. In critically ill hospitalized patients, bacteria can also enter the lung from a colonized stomach (spreading retrogradely to the oropharynx, followed by aspiration), from a colonized or infected maxillary sinus, from colonization of dental plaque, or directly via the endotracheal tube (from the hands of staff members). Studies have also shown that the use of nasal tubes (into the stomach or trachea), can predispose to sinusitis and pneumonia, but that a gastric source of pneumonia pathogens in ventilated patients is not common.[71,72]

COLONIZATION OF THE UPPER RESPIRATORY SYSTEM AND DIGESTIVE TRACT

Colonization of the upper respiratory and digestive tracts with pathogenic microorganisms is a major risk factor for the development of pneumonia.[73] Factors enhancing airway colonization include antibiotic therapy, endotracheal intubation, smoking, malnutrition, general surgery, dental plaque, and therapies that elevate the gastric pH.[74] The stomach can be the source of 30% of the enteric gram-negative bacteria that colonize the trachea of intubated patients, but it is difficult to decide if such colonization leads to pneumonia. In a recent multicenter randomized controlled study by Lacherade and colleagues, the use of intermittent subglottic secretion drainage resulted in a significant reduction in microbiologically confirmed VAP compared to control subjects (14.8% vs. 25.6%; $P = 0.02$),[75] without a significant difference in the duration of mechanical ventilation and hospital mortality rate. The findings suggest that interruption of gastric to oral to tracheal transmission of bacteria can help to prevent VAP. The importance of oral colonization in VAP pathogenesis was shown in a study by DeRiso and coworkers, which demonstrated that the use of the oral antiseptic chlorhexidine in 353 patients undergoing coronary artery bypass surgery significantly reduced the incidence of respiratory tract infections by 69%.[76] It has become difficult to separate colonization from infection in intubated patients, particularly with the recognition of ventilator-associated tracheobronchitis (VAT).[77] VAT patients have an infection, with clinical signs (fever, leukocytosis, and purulent sputum) and microbiologic findings (Gram stain with bacteria and leukocytes, with either a positive semiquantitative or a quantitative sputum culture) but the absence of a new infiltrate on chest radiograph. It remains uncertain if VAT can progress to VAP, or if the two events are independent of one another. If VAT is a precursor of VAP, then serial surveillance cultures of endotracheal aspirates could identify MDR pathogens for targeted antibiotic treatment when VAT is present, in an effort to prevent VAP.[78]

THE ROLE OF RESPIRATORY THERAPY EQUIPMENT AND ENDOTRACHEAL TUBES

The endotracheal tube bypasses the filtration and host defense functions of the upper airway and can act as a conduit for direct inoculation of bacteria into the lung. This route may be particularly important if bacteria form a biofilm and colonize the inside of the endotracheal tube itself.[79,80] This can occur if tracheobronchial organisms reach the endotracheal tube, a site where they are able to proliferate free from any impediment by the host defense system. Bacteria commonly do grow at this location in a biofilm, which promotes the growth of MDR organisms.[80] The biofilm represents a "sequestered nidus" of infection on the inside of the endotracheal tube, and particles can be dislodged every time the patient is suctioned. This is one of the mechanisms explaining the strong association between endotracheal intubation and pneumonia. Given the presence of biofilm in endotracheal tubes, it may be tempting to regularly reintubate patients and use a fresh tube, but this approach is not recommended because reintubation is itself a risk factor for VAP.[81] Afessa and colleagues reported that the use of the silver-coated tube reduced the mortality rate of patients who developed VAP despite having the silver tube in place, compared with the mortality rate of patients who developed VAP with a standard tube in place (14% vs. 36%; $P = 0.03$).[82] However, the overall mortality rate was high in patients with the silver tube, and the rate of death from respiratory failure was higher in the silver tube–treated patients than those with the standard tube (19% vs. 11%, $P = 0.02$), raising doubts on the impact of using the silver-coated tube on VAP patients. Other interventions, such as use of devices to remove biofilm from the tube interior and the coating of tubes with mimics of antimicrobial peptides (ceragenins), are in development to interrupt the pathogenesis of VAP.[83]

Just as a patient's own tracheobronchial flora can spread to the endotracheal tube and amplify to large numbers, a similar phenomenon can occur in respiratory therapy equipment and in ventilator circuits.[84,85] Ventilator circuit colonization has been studied and the greatest bacterial numbers are found at sites nearest to the patient, not the ventilator, suggesting that circuit contamination originates from the patient.[84] One highly contaminated site is the condensate in the tubing, and this material can inadvertently be inoculated into patients if the tubing is not handled carefully. Because condensate colonization occurs in 80% of tubings within 24 hours, it does not appear that frequent ventilator circuit changes are useful or even able to reduce the risk of pneumonia; in one study, tubing changes every 24 hours (rather than every 48 hours) served as a risk factor for pneumonia.[86] Although most patients have ventilator tubing changed every 48 hours, several studies have shown no increased risk of infection if tubing is never changed or changed infrequently.[87,88] The use of heat moisture exchangers may be one way to avoid this problem, but they have had an inconsistent effect on preventing VAP. In addition, frequent changes of heat moisture exchangers (i.e., every 24 hours) have not been shown to have an impact on the incidence of VAP, and heat moisture exchangers should be changed no more frequently than every 48 hours.[89]

Box 42.6 Epidemiologic Conditions and Related Specific Pathogens in Community-Acquired Pneumonia (CAP)

Chronic obstructive pulmonary disease: *Haemophilus influenzae, Pseudomonas aeruginosa, Legionella* species, *Streptococcus pneumoniae, Moraxella catarrhalis, Chlamydia pneumoniae*
Structural lung disease: *Pseudomonas aeruginosa, Burkholderia cepacia, Staphylococcus aureus*
Alcoholism: *S. pneumoniae,* oral anaerobes, *Klebsiella pneumoniae, Acinetobacter* species, *Mycoplasma tuberculosis*
Lung abscess: CA-MRSA, oral anaerobes, endemic fungal pneumonia, *M. tuberculosis,* atypical mycobacteria
Exposure to birds: *Chlamydophila psittaci, Histoplasma capsulatum*
Exposure to rabbits: *Francisella tularensis*
Exposure to farm animals or parturient cats: *Coxiella burnetii* (Q fever)
Hotel or cruise ship stay in previous 2 weeks: *Legionella* species
Travel to or residence in southwestern United States: *Coccidioides* species, hantavirus
Travel to or residence in Southeast and East Asia: *Burkholderia pseudomallei,* avian influenza virus, SARS coronavirus
Injection drug use: *S. aureus,* anaerobes, *M. tuberculosis, S. pneumoniae*
Bioterrorism: *Bacillus anthracis, Yersinia pestis, F. tularensis*

CA-MRSA, community-associated methicillin-resistant *S. aureus*; SARS, severe acute respiratory syndrome.

CLINICAL FEATURES

HISTORICAL INFORMATION

Pneumonia is generally characterized by symptoms of fever, cough, purulent sputum production, and dyspnea in a patient with a new or progressive lung infiltrate, with or without an associated pleural effusion. In nonventilated patients, cough is the most common finding and is present in up to 80% of all CAP patients, but is less common in those who are elderly, those with serious comorbid conditions, and individuals coming from nursing homes. Patients with CAP and an intact immune system generally have classic pneumonia symptoms, but the elderly patient can have a nonrespiratory presentation with symptoms of confusion, falling, failure to thrive, altered functional capacity, or deterioration in a preexisting medical illness, such as congestive heart failure.[90] The absence of clear-cut respiratory symptoms and an afebrile status have themselves been identified as predictors of an increased risk of death. Pleuritic chest pain is also commonly seen in patients with CAP, and in one study, its absence was also identified as a poor prognostic finding.[91] A recent study pointed out that nonsteroidal anti-inflammatory drugs prior to hospitalization were associated with a higher chance of developing pleuropulmonary complications (OR = 8.1).[92]

Certain clinical conditions are associated with specific pathogens in patients with CAP, and these associations should be evaluated when obtaining a history (Box 42.6).[19] For example, if the presentation is subacute, following contact with birds, rats, or rabbits, then the possibility of psittacosis, leptospirosis, tularemia, or plague, respectively, should be considered. *Coxiella burnetti* (Q fever) is a concern with exposure to parturient cats, cattle, sheep, or goats; hantavirus with exposure to mice droppings in endemic areas; and *Legionella* with exposure to contaminated water sources (saunas). Following influenza, superinfection with pneumococcus, *S. aureus* (including MRSA), and *H. influenzae* should be considered. With travel to endemic areas in Asia, the onset of respiratory failure after a preceding viral illness should lead to suspicion of a viral pneumonia, which could be severe acute respiratory syndrome (SARS) or avian influenza.[93] Endemic fungi (coccidioidomycosis, histoplasmosis, and blastomycosis) occur in well-defined geographic areas and may present acutely with symptoms that overlap with acute bacterial pneumonia. Clinicians should also be cognizant of the risk of bioterrorism and be able to detect clinical features of *Bacillus anthracis, Yersinia pestis,* and *Francisella tularensis.*

Nosocomial pneumonia often presents with less definitive clinical findings, particularly in those who are mechanically ventilated, in which the clinical diagnosis is made in patients with a new or progressive radiographic infiltrate, along with some indication that infection is present (fever, purulent sputum, or leukocytosis). In addition, some patients can have purulent sputum and fever, without a new infiltrate, and be diagnosed as having purulent tracheobronchitis, an infectious complication of mechanical ventilation (VAT) that may also require antibiotic therapy, but is not pneumonia.[2] In taking a history from a patient with nosocomial pneumonia, it is important to identify if there are risk factors present for drug-resistant organisms. For ventilated patients, these factors include prolonged ICU stay (≥5 days), recent antibiotic therapy, and the presence of HCAP risks.[2,60] In CAP patients, risk factors for drug-resistant pneumococcus include recent β-lactam therapy, exposure to a child in day care, alcoholism, immune suppression, and multiple medical comorbid conditions.[94,95]

PHYSICAL EXAMINATION

Physical findings of pneumonia include tachypnea, crackles, rhonchi, and signs of consolidation (egophony, bronchial breath sounds, dullness to percussion). Patients should also be evaluated for signs of pleural effusion. In addition, extrapulmonary findings should be sought to rule out metastatic infection (arthritis, endocarditis, meningitis) or to add to the suspicion of an "atypical" pathogen, such as *M. pneumoniae* or *C. pneumoniae,* which can lead to such complications as bullous myringitis, skin rash, pericarditis, hepatitis, hemolytic anemia, or meningoencephalitis. One of the most important ways to recognize severe CAP early in the course of illness is to carefully count the respiratory rate.[96,97] In the elderly, an elevation of respiratory rate can be the initial presenting sign of pneumonia, preceding other clinical findings by as much as 1 to 2 days and tachypnea is present in over 60% of all patients, being present more often in the elderly than in younger patients with pneumonia.[97] In addition, the counting of respiratory rate can identify the patient with severe illness, who commonly has a rate more than 30 breaths/minute. Gurgling sounds heard during quiet breathing or speech have been independently associated with HAP.[98] Overall, the clinical diagnosis of pneumonia has moderate sensitivity (79%) and specificity (66%),[99] and in general, definitive imaging studies are required in critically ill patients.

ETIOLOGIC PATHOGENS

COMMUNITY-ACQUIRED PNEUMONIA

The microorganisms causing CAP may vary according to geographic area and underlying patient risk factors. Even with extensive diagnostic testing, an etiologic agent is defined in only about half of all patients with CAP, pointing out the limited value of diagnostic testing, and the possibility that we do not know all the organisms that can cause CAP. The most common cause of CAP is pneumococcus (*S. pneumoniae*), an organism that is frequently (at least 40% of the time) resistant to penicillin or other antibiotics, leading to the term drug-resistant *Streptococcus pneumoniae* (DRSP). Fortunately, most penicillin resistance in the United States is still more commonly of the "intermediate" type (penicillin minimum inhibitory concentration, or MIC, of 0.1 to 1.0 mg/L) and not of the high-level type (penicillin MIC of 2.0 mg/L or more).[100] Pneumococcal resistance to other antibiotics is also common, including macrolides and trimethoprim-sulfamethoxazole, but the clinical relevance and impact on outcome of these in vitro findings is uncertain, and most experts believe that only organisms with a penicillin MIC of 4 mg/L or more are associated with an increased risk of death.[101] Recently, the U.S. definitions of resistance have changed for nonmeningeal infection, with sensitive being defined by a penicillin MIC of 2 mg/L or less, intermediate as an MIC of 4 mg/L, and resistant as an MIC of 8 mg/L or more. With these new definitions of resistance, very few pathogens will be defined as resistant, but those that are may affect outcome.

All patients with severe CAP should be considered to be at risk for DRSP, and in addition, those admitted to the ICU can have infection with atypical pathogens, which account for up to 20% of infections, either as primary infection or as copathogens. The identity of these organisms varies over time and geography. In some areas, *Legionella* is a common cause of severe CAP, although in others *C. pneumoniae* or *M. pneumoniae* predominate.[30] Other important causes of severe CAP include *H. influenzae, S. aureus,* which includes MRSA (especially after influenza), and enteric gram-negative organisms (including *P. aeruginosa*) in patients with appropriate risk factors (particularly bronchiectasis and steroid-treated COPD).

Recently, a toxin-producing strain of MRSA has been described to cause CAP in patients after influenza and other viral infections (Fig. 42.2). This community-acquired MRSA (CA-MRSA) is biologically and genetically distinct from the MRSA that causes nosocomial pneumonia, being more virulent and necrotizing, and associated with the production of the Panton-Valentine leukocidin (PVL).[102,103] Viruses can be a cause of severe CAP, including influenza virus, as well as parainfluenza virus and epidemic viruses such as coronavirus (which caused SARS) and avian influenza.[93] Viral pneumonia (SARS and influenza) can lead to respiratory failure, and occasionally tuberculosis or endemic fungi can result in severe pneumonia. Recent experience with the 2009 pandemic influenza A (H1N1) infection showed that critical illness was associated with severe hypoxemia and that multisystem organ failure occurred rapidly after hospital admission and mostly in young adults and pregnant patients.[104]

Unusual etiologic organisms should be considered, especially in patients who have epidemiologic risk factors for specific pathogens, as discussed earlier. In addition, certain "modifying factors" may be present that increase the likelihood of CAP caused by certain pathogens.[2] Thus, the risk factors for DRSP include β-lactam therapy in the past 3 months, alcoholism, age older than 65 years, immune suppression, multiple medical comorbid conditions, and contact with a child in day care.[94] Risk factors for gram-negative infections include residence in a nursing home, underlying cardiopulmonary disease, multiple medical comorbid conditions, probable aspiration, recent hospitalization, and recent antibiotic therapy. Many of these patients who are at risk for gram-negative infections would now be reclassified as having HCAP.[2,105]

Some ICU patients are at risk for pseudomonal infection, although others are not, and the risk factors for *P. aeruginosa* infection are structural lung disease (bronchiectasis), corticosteroid therapy (>10 mg prednisone/day), broad-spectrum antibiotic therapy for more than 7 days in the past month, previous hospitalization, and malnutrition.[2] Although aspiration has often been considered a risk factor for anaerobic infection, a study of severe CAP in

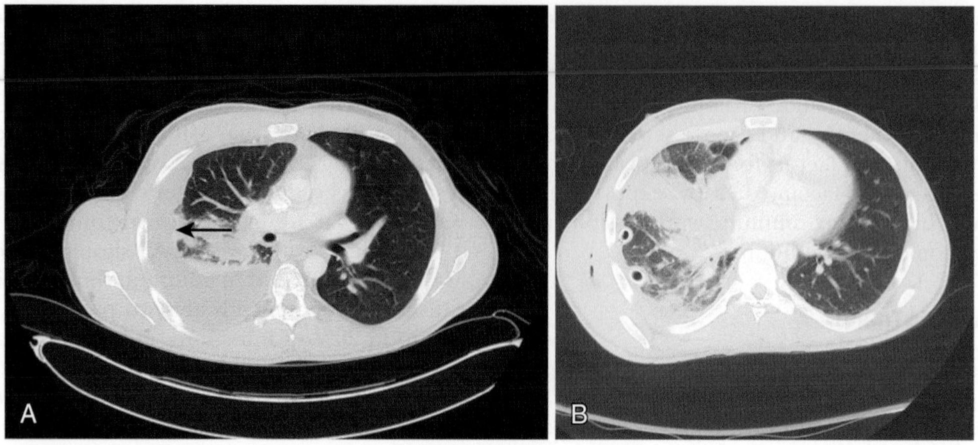

Figure 42.2 Computed tomography (CT) scan of the chest of a 25-year-old male admitted with right-sided pleuritic pain after recent influenza infection, showing empyema (**A**). A repeat CT scan after video-assisted thoracotomy showing intraparenchymal necrosis (**B**). Tissue culture grew community-acquired methicillin-resistant *Staphylococcus aureus*. Patient was treated with linezolid and had complete resolution of the infiltrate in a 1-month period.

elderly patients with aspiration risk factors found that this population was very likely to have gram-negative infection, and that, using sensitive microbiologic methods, anaerobes were uncommon.[106] Previous studies looking at microbiologic causes in patients admitted with CAP to the ICU have shown wide variation in the results, with a limitation being that not all microbiologic tests were applied systematically for all patients. A recent prospective observational study by Cillóniz and coworkers on 362 consecutive adult patients with CAP admitted to the ICU within 24 hours of presentation reported that 11% of all cases were polymicrobial, with *S. pneumoniae*, respiratory viruses, and *P. aeruginosa* being the commonest isolated pathogens.[107] Other studies have also shown a high frequency of multiple pathogens, including a mixture of bacterial and "atypical" pathogens, which may explain why most patients with severe CAP need to be treated empirically for both groups of organisms. Chronic respiratory disease and ARDS criteria were independent predictors of polymicrobial causes and inappropriate initial antimicrobial treatment was more frequent in the polymicrobial infection group compared with the monomicrobial infection group (39% vs. 10%, $P < 0.001$).

NOSOCOMIAL PNEUMONIA

All patients with this illness are at risk for infection with a group of bacteria referred to as "core pathogens," which include pneumococcus, *H. influenzae*, MSSA, and nonresistant gram-negative organisms (*E. coli, Klebsiella* spp., *Enterobacter* spp., *Proteus* spp., and *Serratia marcescens*). In addition, some patients are also at risk for infection with other organisms, depending on the presence of risk factors such as prolonged hospitalization (≥5 days), prior antibiotic therapy, recent hospitalization (within 90 days), recent antibiotic therapy, residence in a nursing home, or need for chronic care outside the hospital.[2,60] Patients with these risk factors can possibly be infected with MDR gram-positive and gram-negative organisms including MRSA, *P. aeruginosa* and *Acinetobacter* spp. Recognition of the multiple risk factors associated with these resistant pathogens has made it clear that patients with either early-onset or late-onset nosocomial pneumonia can be infected with MDR organisms. In addition, up to 40% of patients with VAP have polymicrobial infection, involving multiple pathogens.[108] In immunosuppressed patients uncommon pathogens such as *Aspergillus* species, *Candida* species, *L. pneumophila, Pneumocystis jiroveci, Nocardia* species, and viruses such as cytomegalovirus should be suspected.[74]

Most data on nosocomial pneumonia bacteriology come from patients with VAP, and the cause in nonventilated patients is presumed to be similar, based on the presence of risk factors for drug-resistant pathogens. In patients with VAP, infection with enteric gram-negative organisms is more common than infection with gram-positive organisms, although the frequency of MRSA infection is increasing in this population, as is infection with *Acinetobacter* spp.[109] In a recent prospective study comparing the clinical and microbiologic characteristics of 315 episodes of ICU-acquired pneumonia (VAP 52% vs. non-VAP 48%) the types of etiologic pathogens and outcome were similar regardless of whether pneumonia is or is not acquired during mechanical ventilation.[110]

HCAP patients have been included in the nosocomial pneumonia guidelines as being a group at risk for infection with MDR gram-positive and gram-negative organisms.[2] Although many ICU-admitted patients with this illness are infected with these organisms, one study of nursing home patients requiring mechanical ventilation for severe pneumonia showed that these organisms were not present if the patient with severe pneumonia had not received antibiotics in the preceding 6 months and was also of a good functional status (as defined by activities of daily living).[111] In approaching the bacteriology of nosocomial pneumonia, it is important to recognize that each hospital, and each ICU within a given hospital, can have its own unique flora and antibiotic susceptibility patterns, and thus therapy needs to be adapted to the organisms in a given institution, which can change over time.[112] In addition, it is especially important to know this information because antibiotic resistance is a common factor contributing to initially inappropriate empiric antibiotic therapy. Choosing the wrong empiric therapy has been a particular problem for organisms such as *P. aeruginosa, Acinetobacter* spp., and MRSA.[53] These highly resistant organisms can be present in as many as 60% of patients who develop VAP after at least 7 days of ventilation and who have also received prior antibiotic therapy.[2,60]

ISOLATION OF PATIENTS WITH PNEUMONIA

Patients with certain suspected pathogens should be placed in respiratory isolation to protect both the staff and other patients from infection with these organisms. This practice includes primarily airborne pathogens that spread via the aerosol route and includes any patient who is suspected of having tuberculosis, influenza, respiratory syncytial virus (RSV), or any other epidemic viral infection. Tuberculosis should be considered in any patient with a history of a preceding indolent pneumonia, and in those with severe pneumonia and a history of human immunodeficiency virus (HIV) infection or recent immigration from endemic areas of infection. Patients with MRSA and highly resistant gram-negative infections may need gown, glove, and mask precautions to avoid spread of these difficult-to-treat bacteria.

DIAGNOSTIC ISSUES

GENERAL CONSIDERATIONS

Therapy of severe pneumonia should be started empirically, and laboratory and imaging studies should be done to corroborate the diagnosis and identify the etiologic agent when possible. A specific causal diagnosis is obtained in less than 50% of patients with CAP and the major focus of diagnostic testing is to assess the severity of illness and allow early identification of pneumonia-related complications.[14] However, in most cases of VAP an etiologic agent can be demonstrated, but the presence of a positive culture cannot reliably distinguish infection from colonization.

RADIOGRAPHIC EVALUATION

In all forms of pneumonia, a chest radiograph is used to identify the presence of a lung infiltrate, but in some clinical settings, especially in suspected VAP, there can be noninfectious causes for the radiographic abnormality. A chest radiograph is used to identify complicated and severe illness, such as multilobar infiltrates, cavitation, or a loculated pleural effusion (suggesting an empyema). Chest radiographic patterns are generally not useful for identifying the cause of CAP, although hematogenous dissemination will have bilateral peripheral infiltrates, and aspiration most commonly involves the superior segment of the right lower lobe or posterior segment of the right upper lobe. Findings such as pleural effusion (pneumococcus, *H. influenzae, M. pneumoniae,* pyogenic streptococci) and cavitation (*P. aeruginosa, S. aureus,* anaerobes, MRSA, tuberculosis) can suggest certain groups of organisms. The chest radiograph may be suboptimal in patients with early infection, severe granulocytopenia, and bullous emphysema and in obese patients. In those instances, it is reasonable to repeat a chest radiograph in 24 to 48 hours.[19] A computed tomography (CT) scan of the chest has better sensitivity in diagnosing an infiltrate (Fig. 42.3), but routine CT scan has not been shown to be associated with improved outcomes. Thin-section CT cannot reliably distinguish bacterial pneumonias from other causes, especially in patients with

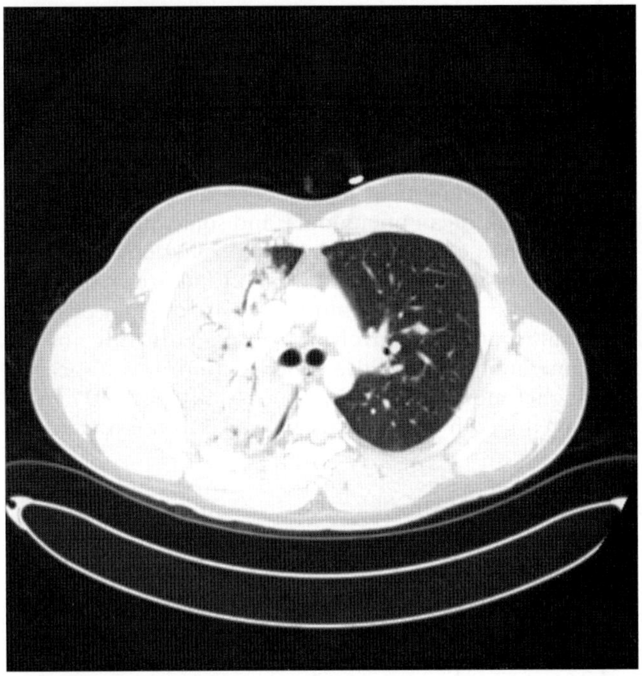

Figure 42.3 A 30-year-old male sanitation worker with severe community-acquired pneumonia in the right lung. He was treated with ceftriaxone and moxifloxacin with clinical resolution of symptoms.

underlying lung diseases or immunocompromised conditions except in cases of *Pneumocystis* pneumonia, which has a characteristic pattern.[113,114] Chest ultrasound is progressively being used to identify the safe site for sampling of the pleural fluid. In the ICU, radiographs are often done at the bedside, and are of such poor quality that pneumonia may be missed or confused with other diagnoses.

ROUTINE LABORATORY TESTS

A complete blood count, chemistry panel, and arterial blood gas analysis are necessary for all patients admitted to the ICU. Leukopenia is seen in patients with severe pneumonia and sepsis caused by pneumococcus or by gram-negative organisms. Both leukocytosis and leukopenia are associated with poor prognosis in patients with CAP[19] and with thrombocytosis and thrombocytopenia.[115] Hyponatremia (serum sodium <130 mEq/L) on admission is associated with poor outcome in CAP patients.[116] Elevated liver function tests can be seen in a variety of viral and bacterial pneumonias secondary to atypical agents such as *Legionella* spp. and *Mycoplasma* spp., Q fever, tularemia, and psittacosis, as well as in pneumococcal infection.

BLOOD CULTURE

The ATS/IDSA 2007 guidelines recommend that patients with severe CAP and patients with other risk factors, listed later, should have two sets of blood cultures. These results are more likely to be positive if the patient has not received antibiotics at the time of sampling or has any of the following risk factors: underlying liver disease, systolic blood pressure less than 90 mm Hg, fever less than 35° C or greater than 40° C, pulse greater than 125 beats/minute, BUN greater than 10.71 mmol/L (30 mg/dL), serum sodium less than 130 mmol, and leukocyte count less than 5000 or greater than 20,000 cells/mL.[117] Blood cultures should also be considered in patients with asplenia, cavitary infiltrates, or a history of ongoing alcohol abuse. The presence of bacteremia may not worsen prognosis but does allow identification of drug-resistant organisms, and most positive blood cultures in CAP reveal pneumococcus. However, in nosocomial pneumonia, the presence of bacteremia does not necessarily mean pneumonia, and some other extrapulmonary source of infection should be ruled out, especially if the organism present in the blood culture is different from the one in the respiratory tract. In a recent prospective, multicenter trial involving 689 patients with nosocomial pneumonia, a positive blood culture was associated with higher mortality rate (57.1% vs. 33%, $P < 0.001$) and a prolonged length of ICU stay compared to nonbacteremic patients.[61]

SPUTUM EXAMINATION

Sputum culture should be accompanied by a Gram stain to guide interpretation of the culture results but not to focus initial antibiotic therapy. In some situations, Gram stain can be used to broaden initial empiric therapy by enhancing the suspicion for organisms that are not covered in routine empiric therapy (such as *S. aureus* being suggested by the presence of clusters of gram-positive cocci, especially during a time of epidemic influenza). A good specimen contains fewer than 10 squamous epithelial cells and more than 25 polymorphonuclear cells per low-power field. The routine testing of expectorated sputum is not useful in the absence of a helpful Gram stain in patients with CAP. In ventilated patients the presence of pathogenic organisms in sputum culture is not diagnostic, because this finding cannot separate oropharyngeal and tracheobronchial colonization from parenchymal lung infection. In addition, some ventilated patients can have VAT, an illness with all the clinical features of pneumonia, but with no new lung infiltrate, and this illness may require antibiotic therapy and involve the same pathogens, present in high concentrations, as are present in VAP.[2]

INVASIVE CULTURES

Bronchoscopy is not indicated as a routine diagnostic test, but may be needed in some patients with severe forms of CAP to establish an etiologic diagnosis. In these patients, the results of diagnostic testing can often be used to focus the initially broad-spectrum empiric therapy to a simpler regimen.[118] In patients with HAP the sputum culture is often not reliable, and in an effort to make the diagnosis more secure, and to avoid the treatment of colonization and not infection, some investigators have used quantitative sampling of lower respiratory secretions collected either bronchoscopically (bronchoalveolar lavage, protected specimen brush) or nonbronchoscopically (endotracheal aspirate, nonbronchoscopic catheter lavage) in patients with suspected VAP. When quantitative cultures are collected, the presence of pneumonia is defined by the growth of bacteria above a predefined threshold concentration.[119,120] Although the results can guide therapy decisions, most clinicians use antibiotic therapy, regardless of quantitative culture data, in patients who have clinical signs of sepsis and suspected pneumonia. Regardless of whether quantitative cultures are used, all patients with suspected nosocomial pneumonia should have a lower respiratory tract culture collected prior to the start of antibiotic therapy. If this is not a quantitative culture, then a sputum or tracheal aspirate should be obtained and the findings reported "semiquantitatively" as light, moderate, or heavy growth of bacteria.[2,120] Unfortunately, a negative culture is difficult to interpret if the patient has had initiation or change in antibiotic therapy in the preceding 72 hours. If, however, either a quantitative or semiquantitative culture is negative, or does not show a highly resistant pathogen, and antibiotics have not been changed in the past 72 hours, then the therapy can often be stopped or focused to a narrower spectrum.[2,121] A number of studies have examined the ability of quantitative cultures to impact outcome in VAP, and in general, although results are conflicting, there is no consistent evidence that they improve patient outcome or lead to more de-escalation of antibiotics.[122]

URINARY ANTIGEN, SEROLOGIC, AND POLYMERASE CHAIN REACTION TESTING

Routine serologic testing is not recommended, and a serologic diagnosis of a specific pathogen is based on acute and convalescent blood serologic examinations showing a fourfold increase in titers. This type of testing is used for epidemiologic diagnosis of atypical agents such as *C. pneumoniae, C. psittaci, Coxiella burnetii* (Q fever), and *M. pneumoniae.* However, in patients with severe illness, the diagnosis of *Legionella* infection can be made by urinary antigen testing, which is the test that is most likely to be positive at the time of admission, but a test that is specific only for serogroup I infection.[19,123] Examination of concentrated urine for pneumococcal antigen may also be valuable. Urinary pneumococcal antigen has a sensitivity of 50% to 80% and specificity of over 90%. False-positive tests are seen in patients who had pneumonia within the previous 3 months. Polymerase chain reaction (PCR) assays are used for the detection of viruses (as was the case in the H1N1 epidemic) and other agents such as *M. tuberculosis.* Direct immunofluorescence or enzyme immunoassay is used for detection of viral antigens such as influenza, parainfluenza, RSV, and adenovirus. The impact of a positive test on management is still unclear, but a negative test is valuable in directing a focused antibiotic regimen.

ROLE OF BIOMARKERS

SERUM BIOMARKERS

Inflammatory biomarkers like CRP, PCT, midregional proadrenomedullin, midregional proatrial natriuretic peptide (MR-proANP), proarginine-vasopressin, proendothelin-1, and the interleukins have been used to distinguish bacterial infection from viral infection. Ramirez and associates showed that inflammatory biomarkers like PCT, CRP, tumor necrosis factor-α, and interleukin 6 levels were higher in patients admitted to the ICU, including those with delayed ICU admission, than those not needing ICU care.[28]

PCT is a "hormokine" (hormone with cytokine-like behavior), a peptide precursor of the hormone calcitonin, with a half-life of 25 to 30 hours. It is produced in response to bacterial microbial toxins and inhibited by virus-related cytokines. In patients with CAP, PCT levels on admission correlate with disease severity and identify high-risk patients with similar accuracy as the CURB-65 score and with a higher prognostic accuracy compared with CRP and leukocyte count.[27,124] In fact, if the PCT level on admission is low, prognosis is good, regardless of PSI class or CURB-65 score.[124] Serum levels tend to be high in patients with severe bacteremic CAP, and serial measurements help guide the duration of antibiotic therapy.[125] Luyt and colleagues reported that PCT levels decreased during the clinical course of VAP but were significantly higher from day 1 to day 7 in patients with unfavorable outcomes.[126] A recent prospective study by Bloos and colleagues on 175 patients with severe pneumonia admitted to the ICU (CAP, HAP, and VAP, equally distributed) showed that PCT levels were higher and remained persistently elevated in nonsurvivors compared to survivors.[127] The initial and maximum PCT levels correlated with maximum SOFA score and the initial PCT levels were higher in CAP than in VAP patients (median; 2.4 vs. 0.7 ng/mL, $P < 0.001$) but not significantly different from HAP patients (2.2 ng/mL), but patients with CAP were more severely ill, with a higher APACHE II score. In another multicenter, prospective, parallel-group study in the ICU setting, patients were randomly assigned in a 1:1 ratio to PCT-guided ($n = 311$ patients) or control ($n = 319$) groups and antibiotic regimens were instituted based on a protocol with predefined cutoff levels of PCT. There was no difference in mortality rate between PCT group and control group at day 28 (21.2% vs. 20.4%),[10] but patients in the PCT group had significantly more days without antibiotics than those in the control group (14.3 days vs. 11.6 days, $P < 0.0001$). This supports earlier data that a drop in PCT levels could be used to define when antibiotic treatment can be safely withdrawn.[9]

OPEN LUNG BIOPSY

This procedure is rarely needed unless there is persistence of infiltrates on imaging and suspicion for atypical organisms (such as *Aspergillus*, cytomegalovirus, *Cryptococcus* spp., *Nocardia*, and *Toxoplasma gondii*) is high in an immunocompromised host with progressive disease not responding to standard treatment regimens. Open lung biopsy is also useful if a pneumonia mimic (inflammatory lung disease, pulmonary hemorrhage, or malignancy) is suspected.

RECOMMENDED TESTING FOR COMMUNITY-ACQUIRED PNEUMONIA

The ATS/IDSA guidelines recommend that all CAP patients admitted to the ICU should have a chest radiograph, blood and lower respiratory tract (sputum, endotracheal aspirate, bronchoalveolar lavage, or bronchoscopic specimen) cultures, and *Legionella* and pneumococcal urine antigen testing. If the patient has a moderate-sized pleural effusion, this should be tapped and the fluid sent for culture and biochemical analysis. Those with a cavitary infiltrate on chest imaging should have fungal cultures and tuberculosis testing performed.

Severity assessment scores such as ATS/IDSA 2007 guidelines or SMART-COP can be used to determine the severity of the disease and serum biomarkers like PCT should be used to guide site of care decisions. In patients with no response to treatment or unrelenting high levels of biomarkers, further imaging or invasive diagnostic methods such as bronchoscopy and thoracentesis should be performed and an alternate diagnosis other than CAP should be considered. A suggested diagnostic/treatment approach is provided in Figure 42.4.

RECOMMENDED TESTING FOR NOSOCOMIAL PNEUMONIA

Nosocomial pneumonia is diagnosed when a patient has been in the hospital for at least 48 to 72 hours and then develops a new or progressive infiltrate on chest radiograph, accompanied by at least two of the following three: fever, leukocytosis, and purulent sputum. As mentioned, these clinical findings may be sensitive but not specific for infection, and efforts to improve the clinical diagnosis of pneumonia have involved the previously mentioned CPIS.[128] The CPIS uses six criteria (fever, purulence of sputum, white blood cell count, oxygenation, degree of radiographic abnormality, and presence of pathogens in the sputum), with each scored on a scale from 0 to 2, and pneumonia is diagnosed with a total score of at least 6 (out of a maximum of 12). The CPIS was modified by Singh and coworkers to include radiographic progression in order to improve diagnostic accuracy (Table 42.1).[129] The CPIS at 72 hours

Table 42.1 Modified Clinical Pulmonary Infection Score

Sign	0	1	2
Temperature (°C)	36.5-38.4	38.5-38.9	<36 or >39
White blood cell count (cells/μL)	4.0-11.0	<4.0 or >11.0	>500 band forms
Oxygenation (PaO_2/FiO_2)	>240 or ARDS		<240 and no ARDS
Radiographic findings	No infiltrate	Diffuse infiltrate	Localized infiltrate
Radiographic progression	No progression		Radiographic progression after CHF and ARDS excluded
Tracheal secretions	Absence of secretions	Nonpurulent	Purulent
Culture of tracheal aspirate	Pathogenic bacteria cultured: rare or light quantity or no growth	Pathogenic bacteria cultured: moderate or heavy quantity	Same pathogenic bacteria as on original Gram stain: add 1 point

ARDS, acute respiratory syndrome; CHF, congestive heart failure.

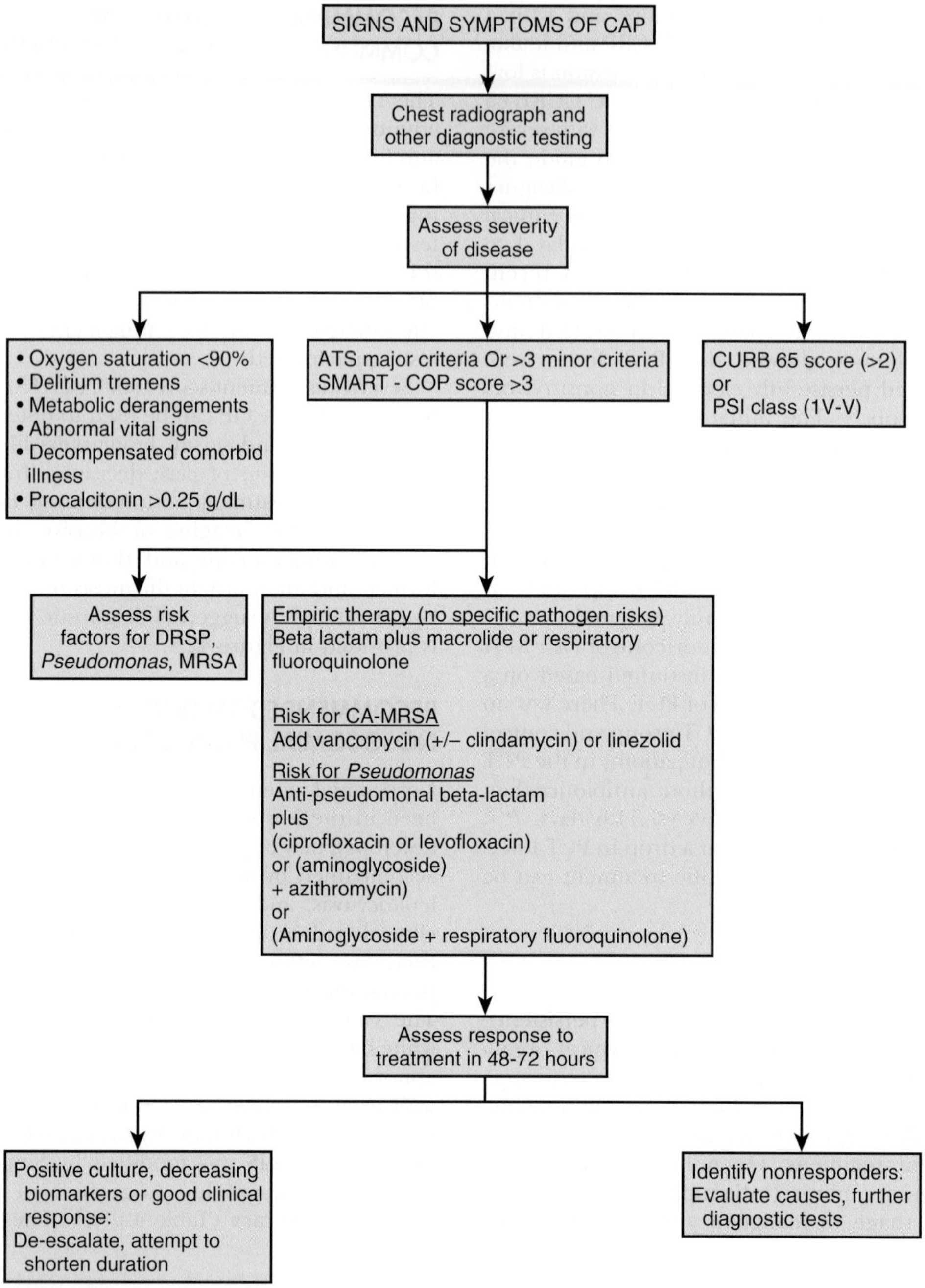

Figure 42.4 A suggested algorithm for diagnosis and management of community-acquired pneumonia in the intensive care unit setting.

was calculated on the basis of all seven variables and took into consideration the progression of the infiltrate and culture results of the tracheal aspirate specimen. A CPIS greater than 6 at baseline and at 72 hours was considered suggestive of pneumonia and indicated the need for a full course of antibiotic therapy. However, subsequent studies showed that CPIS has a low sensitivity and specificity for diagnosing VAP compared to quantitative cultures of bronchoalveolar lavage fluid, with considerable interobserver variability.[130] Thus, the use of CPIS remains controversial and has been most successfully used in guiding treatment decisions for patients with a low likelihood of VAP and in guiding the duration of therapy and defining the response to treatment.[42,131]

Many studies have documented that VAP is diagnosed more often clinically than can be confirmed microbiologically, and the diagnosis is further obscured by the fact that most mechanically ventilated patients are colonized by enteric gram-negative bacteria, and thus the finding of potential pathogens in the sputum has limited diagnostic value. Many patients with suspected nosocomial pneumonia can have other diagnoses, which can be suggested by the rapidity of the clinical response and by the nature of the clinical findings. These diagnoses include atelectasis and congestive heart failure (very rapid clinical resolution), or in the case of a lack of response to therapy, inflammatory lung diseases, extrapulmonary infection (sinusitis, central-line infection, intra-abdominal infection), or the presence of an unusual or drug-resistant pathogen. The ATS/IDSA guidelines for nosocomial pneumonia have recommended that all patients have a lower respiratory tract sample collected prior to starting therapy and that the technique and culture method be one that the clinician is expert at performing and interpreting. Lower respiratory tract cultures can be obtained bronchoscopically or nonbronchoscopically and can be cultured quantitatively or semiquantitatively. A suggested algorithm for diagnosis and treatment of nosocomial pneumonia is provided in Figure 42.5.

THERAPY

GENERAL CONSIDERATIONS

Timely initiation of appropriate antibiotics has significant mortality benefit for both severe CAP and VAP patients. The ATS and IDSA have developed algorithms for initial empiric therapy, based on the most likely etiologic pathogens in a given clinical setting.[2,19] If diagnostic testing reveals a specific etiologic pathogen, then therapy can be focused on

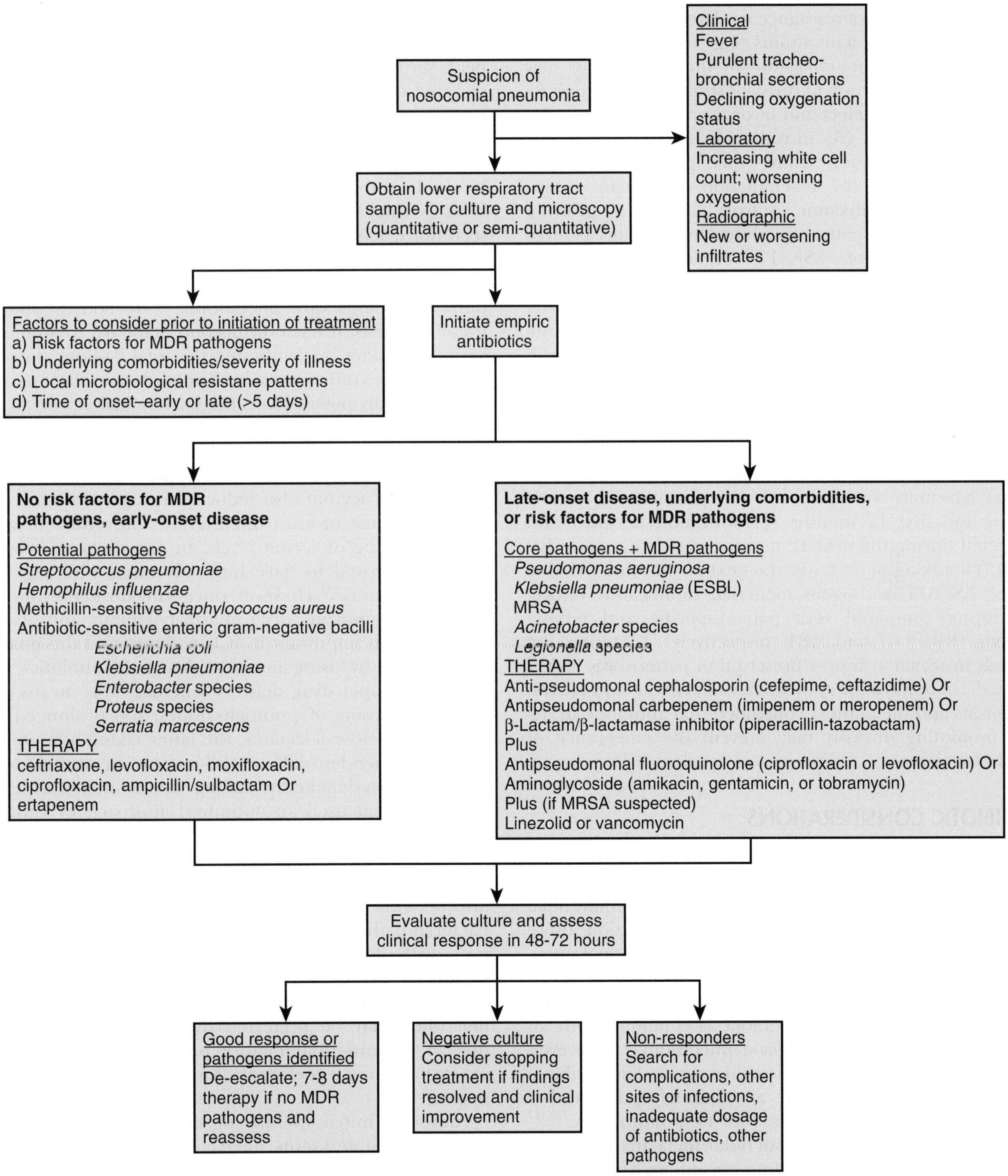

Figure 42.5 A suggested algorithm for the diagnosis and treatment of nosocomial pneumonia.

those results. De-escalation of antibiotics is valuable in the management of VAP because most patients are at risk for infection with MDR pathogens, requiring empiric broad-spectrum antibiotics, and this can lead to antibiotic overuse and further development of resistance if therapy is not adjusted once culture and clinical response data become available.[64]

MICROBIAL RESISTANCE

Patients in the ICU are at a high risk of developing infection, which is often due to antibiotic-resistant pathogens. The incidence of resistance is related to several factors: (1) induction of resistant strains (e.g., emergence of resistance during treatment because of the selection of new mutations), (2) selection of resistant strains (e.g., antimicrobial treatment may select and favor overgrowth of preexisting resistant flora), (3) introduction of resistant strains (e.g., cross-transmission from other patients or health care workers), and (4) dissemination of resistant strains (e.g., suboptimal infection control).[132] There is growing concern about MDR pathogens in the United States, belonging to the group of "ESKAPE" organisms (*Enterococcus faecium, S. aureus, K. pneumoniae, Acinetobacter baumanii, P. aeruginosa,* and *Enterobacter* species).[133,134] A recent prospective interventional study evaluated the effect of antimicrobial diversity on resistance caused by the ESKAPE pathogens in patients with VAP. The study was conducted over 44 months and examined three different antimicrobial strategies implemented consecutively: (1) a patient-specific period, when therapy was based on preexisting risk factors; (2) a 24-month scheduling period, in which antipseudomonal β-lactams were selected and prioritized quarterly during the first 12 months (prioritization periods) and restricted during the next 12 months (restriction periods); and (3) a mixing period over the next 10 months. VAP due to the ESKAPE pathogens increased significantly during scheduling compared with patient-specific and mixing periods (RR, 2.67 and 3.84, respectively).[135] During the periods in which a diverse prescription pattern was implemented, there was a lower incidence of VAP due to ESKAPE organisms and the authors concluded that antibiotic strategies promoting diversity may prevent the emergence of MDR organisms.

ANTIBIOTIC CONSIDERATIONS

All patients with severe pneumonia treated in the ICU should receive initial empiric combination therapy. The rationale for this approach is to provide broad antimicrobial coverage to assure appropriate therapy. In addition, there has been the hope that, in the therapy of nosocomial pneumonia, combination therapy could prevent the emergence of resistance during therapy and potentially provide synergistic activity if a β-lactam antibiotic is combined with an aminoglycoside (for *P. aeruginosa* pneumonia). However, only with bacteremic *P. aeruginosa* pneumonia has combination therapy (generally with an aminoglycoside and a β-lactam) been shown to be superior to monotherapy.[136,137] In the absence of bacteremia, an older meta analysis found no therapeutic benefit to adding an aminoglycoside to a β-lactam in critically ill patients, but the impact on appropriateness of therapy was not evaluated.[137] Currently, with the high prevalence of MDR pathogens in nosocomial pneumonia, combination therapy increases the likelihood of appropriate therapy, compared to monotherapy. In fact, in the Canadian Clinical Trials group study of VAP, even though combination therapy did not reduce mortality rates, compared to monotherapy, it led to appropriate therapy 84% of the time when MDR pathogens were present, compared to 11% of the time when these organisms were treated with monotherapy.[138]

One practical problem to using aminoglycosides is that they have a narrow therapeutic-to-toxic ratio and a high incidence of nephrotoxicity, particularly in elderly patients. When these drugs are used, it is important to achieve high peak serum levels to optimize efficacy, but to also avoid elevated trough levels, which correlate with toxicity. When peak serum levels have been monitored, levels of more than 7 μg/mL for gentamicin and tobramycin and more than 28 μg/mL for amikacin have been associated with more favorable outcomes.[139] One other limitation of aminoglycosides is their relatively poor penetration into bronchial secretions, achieving only 40% of the serum concentrations in the lung. In addition, antimicrobial activity is reduced at the low pH levels that are common in the bronchial secretions of patients with pneumonia.[140] To address some of these concerns, it has now become standard to administer aminoglycosides by combining the total 24-hour dose into a single dose, rather than in divided doses. This approach is theoretically possible because bactericidal activity of aminoglycosides is optimized by high peak concentrations, and once-daily dosing relies on the prolonged postantibiotic effect of aminoglycosides. This approach might not only improve efficacy but also reduce (or at least not increase) toxicity because of low trough levels, and reduce the need for monitoring of serum levels. In one meta-analysis, this approach proved to have little advantage with regard to efficacy or safety.[141] However, once-daily dosing is now standard, and optimizing drug pharmacokinetics and pharmacodynamics is important in ICU patients, and this goal can be achieved by using maximal doses of antibiotics while choosing proper drug delivery schemes. This means using once-daily dosing of aminoglycosides, and prolonged infusion of high-dose β-lactams, the latter taking advantage of the time-dependent killing of β-lactams, in contrast to the concentration-dependent killing by aminoglycosides. In one study that used an optimized approach to antibiotic dosing and delivery versus standard therapy, infection-related mortality rate was reduced (8.5% vs. 21.6%).[142]

Initial empiric therapy of CAP treated in the ICU should also be with a combination of agents, usually directed at bacterial pathogens and atypical pathogens. In severe CAP, even with documented pneumococcal bacteremia, dual therapy is associated with reduced mortality rate compared to monotherapy. In the selection of a second agent, a macrolide may be preferred over a quinolone, possibly due to its anti-inflammatory properties, with the main exception being a preference for quinolones if *Legionella* is suspected.

Although initial therapy of severe pneumonia usually requires multiple agents, once culture data are available, as part of a de-escalation strategy, monotherapy can often be used. Even patients with severe nosocomial pneumonia can be converted to monotherapy, provided that certain high-risk organisms are absent (*P. aeruginosa, Acinetobacter* spp., and MRSA), but the antibiotics that have been effective as monotherapy for severe VAP include imipenem, meropenem, doripenem, cefepime, ciprofloxacin, high-dose levofloxacin (750 mg daily), and piperacillin/tazobactam.[2,121,143-147] Circumstances in which monotherapy should not be used include the following: (1) in any patient with severe CAP, in which the efficacy of this approach has not been demonstrated; (2) in suspected or documented bacteremic infection with *P. aeruginosa;* (3) in the empiric therapy of VAP if the patient has risk factors for infection with MDR pathogens; and (4) if the patient has nosocomial pneumonia and both *S. aureus* and *P. aeruginosa* are identified in culture as the etiologic pathogens. Monotherapy of nosocomial infection should never be attempted with a third-generation cephalosporin because of the possibility of emergence of resistance during therapy as a result of production of chromosomal β-lactamases by the Enterobacteriaceae group of organisms.[9]

If *P. aeruginosa* is the target organism, then antibiotics with efficacy against this pathogen are needed. Antipseudomonal β-lactam antibiotics include the penicillins—piperacillin, azlocillin, mezlocillin, ticarcillin, and carbenicillin; the third-generation cephalosporins ceftazidime and cefoperazone; the fourth-generation cephalosporin cefepime; the carbapenems imipenem, doripenem, and meropenem; the monobactam aztreonam (which can be used in the penicillin-allergic patient); and the β-lactam/β-lactamase inhibitor combinations ticarcillin/clavulanate and piperacillin/tazobactam. Other antipseudomonal agents include the quinolone ciprofloxacin, high-dose levofloxacin (750 mg/day), and the aminoglycosides (amikacin, gentamicin, tobramycin).

In patients with suspected MRSA pneumonia, therapy should be with either vancomycin or linezolid (a bacteriostatic, oxazolidinone antibiotic). Early subgroup analysis of two prospective randomized, controlled trials suggested that linezolid led to higher cure and survival rates, compared to vancomycin in patients with documented MRSA VAP.[148] A subsequent prospective study of patients with suspected MRSA VAP, randomized to receive either linezolid, 600 mg, or vancomycin, 1 g every 12 hours, showed trends in favor of linezolid for bacteriologic cure and survival that were not statistically significant.[149] The comparison between linezolid and vancomycin has been evaluated by several meta analyses, which showed no definitive difference, except for a trend in favor of linezolid for clinical success.[150] Recently, a large multicenter trial comparing linezolid to optimally dosed vancomycin was completed, including nearly 400 patients with documented MRSA VAP and HCAP. In that trial, linezolid led to a significantly higher rate of clinical response than vancomycin, but no difference in mortality rate.[151] In the study, vancomycin caused more nephrotoxicity, a problem that has been increasingly common when trough levels are pushed above 15 mg/L. Telavancin is another agent that has been studied in MRSA VAP, but when compared to vancomycin, it had no clear advantage and a similar rate of nephrotoxicity but did lead to better clinical responses when MRSA was intermediately sensitive to vancomycin, with MIC values higher than 1 mg/L.[152] In fact, recent studies have shown that the frequency of MRSA with these higher MIC values is increasing, and this is further challenging the efficacy of vancomycin.[153] Tigecycline has efficacy against MRSA, but has not shown efficacy in VAP, although daptomycin is active against MRSA when it causes bacteremia but is inactivated by pulmonary surfactant, and thus cannot be used to treat pneumonia.

Acinetobacter spp. are inherently resistant to cephalosporins, penicillins, and aminoglycosides.[154] In the past, the most reliable therapy for these agents was a carbapenem, but now resistance to carbapenems is more common, necessitating the use of polymixin B and E (colistin). *Acinetobacter* is sensitive in vitro to tigecycline, but in a clinical trial, tigecycline monotherapy was inferior to imipenem in the therapy of VAP, including when *Acinetobacter* was present, and thus if this agent is used, it is probably best as part of a combination regimen, along with a carbapenem, sulbactam, colistin, or an aminoglycoside.[155]

ROLE OF CORTICOSTEROIDS

The fact that inflammatory markers such as IL-6, IL-8, and IL-10 are elevated in patients with severe CAP and decrease in the first few days of appropriate antibiotic therapy favored the possible use of immunomodulators and anti-inflammatory medications such as macrolides, or steroids as an adjunct to reduce the proinflammatory cytokines. One randomized controlled trial of 48 patients compared hydrocortisone infusion (240 mg/day) to placebo, and found that steroid therapy reduced mortality rates, length of stay, and duration of mechanical ventilation.[156] Subsequent studies have not consistently shown benefit for the use of corticosteroids as routine therapy in severe CAP. A meta analysis of available data concluded that there was no definite benefit but also no adverse consequences,[157] although a prospective randomized controlled trial showed a higher frequency of late clinical failure when steroids were used as adjunctive therapy in CAP.[158] Corticosteroids were also used as adjunctive therapy in patients with severe H1N1 pneumonia with ARDS, and were associated with an increased mortality rate, suggesting harm from their use.[159] Given the currently available data, corticosteroids should not be part of routine therapy of severe CAP. In special situations, however, steroids may have value. Patients with pneumonia and pneumococcal meningitis may benefit from adjunctive corticosteroid therapy (dexamethasone) if it is started prior to the initiation of antibiotic therapy, because it may lead to improved long-term neurologic outcomes.[160,161] Patients with *P. jiroveci* pneumonia also benefit from corticosteroid therapy, if the initial arterial oxygen tension is less than 70 mm Hg, by attenuating some of the inflammation that is induced by antibiotic killing of the organisms. In patients with pneumonia and refractory shock some investigators have considered using corticosteroids to treat relative adrenal insufficiency, but a large prospective randomized trial could not demonstrate benefit.[162]

NONPHARMACOLOGIC MEASURES

Adjunctive therapeutic measures are needed in some patients, including oxygen, chest physiotherapy (if at least 30 mL of sputum daily, and a poor cough response), mucolytic agents, and aerosolized bronchodilators.

COMMUNITY-ACQUIRED PNEUMONIA THERAPY ALGORITHM (SEE FIG. 42.4)

For ICU-admitted CAP patients, initial therapy should be directed at DRSP, *Legionella,* and other atypical pathogens in all patients, and for selected patients, enteric gram-negative and other organisms should also be targeted, based on epidemiologic risk assessment. Therapy falls into two categories, depending on whether the patient is at risk for *P. aeruginosa* (structural lung disease such as bronchiectasis, therapy with broad-spectrum antibiotics for more than 7 days in the last month, use of corticosteroids [more than 10 mg of prednisone daily], malnutrition, or HIV infection). In certain circumstances, such as pneumonia complicating influenza, therapy should also include empiric coverage for *S. aureus* (including MRSA).

MONOTHERAPY VERSUS COMBINATION THERAPY

In all treatment algorithms, no ICU-admitted CAP patient should receive empiric monotherapy, even with a quinolone.[95] In a study comparing levofloxacin to a β-lactam/quinolone combination, the single-agent regimen was not tested in patients with septic shock and was not optimally effective for those treated with mechanical ventilation.[163] Rodríguez and colleagues reported in a subset of patients with CAP and shock that combination therapy with either a β-lactam and a macrolide or a β-lactam and a quinolone had a 28-day survival advantage compared to patients receiving monotherapy with a quinolone or a β-lactam alone.[164] In contrast, another prospective observational study of 218 mechanically ventilated patients with CAP found that the use of a macrolide, but not a quinolone, was associated with reduced mortality rate.[165] Several other studies have specifically shown benefit for combination therapy in patients with documented pneumococcal bacteremia. In one study that examined data from 2209 Medicare patients with bacteremic pneumonia, the initial use of antibiotic with atypical pathogen coverage, particularly a macrolide, was independently associated with a decreased 30-day mortality risk (odds ratio [OR] = 0.76; $P = 0.03$).[166] This confirmed earlier data from a prospective study of bacteremic pneumococcal pneumonia patients, showing that combination antibiotic therapy (usually by adding a macrolide antibiotic) was associated with lower 14-day mortality rate compared to monotherapy (23.4 vs. 55.3%, $P = 0.0015$) for patients with severe illness.[167]

ATS/IDSA 2007 GUIDELINES

Recommended therapy for severe CAP, in the absence of pseudomonal risk factors, should be with a selected intravenous β-lactam (cefotaxime, ceftriaxone, ertapenem, a β-lactam/β-lactamase inhibitor combination), combined with either an intravenous macrolide or an intravenous antipneumococcal quinolone (levofloxacin or moxifloxacin). For patients with pseudomonal risk factors, therapy can be with a two-drug regimen, using an antipseudomonal β-lactam (imipenem, meropenem, piperacillin/tazobactam, cefepime) plus ciprofloxacin (the most active antipseudomonal quinolone) or levofloxacin (750 mg daily); or alternatively with a three-drug regimen, using an antipseudomonal β-lactam plus an aminoglycoside plus either an intravenous antipneumococcal quinolone (levofloxacin, or moxifloxacin) or a macrolide.[95,168] In patients with bacteremic pneumococcal pneumonia, particularly in those with severe illness, as discussed earlier, dual therapy including a macrolide has been associated with improved outcomes.[167]

In patients with risk factors for MRSA, vancomycin (and possibly clindamycin) or linezolid alone should be added to the regimen. Most experts recommend that CA-MRSA be targeted in patients with severe, necrotizing CAP including those with empyema, following a viral illness, particularly influenza. Optimal therapy has not been defined, and vancomycin alone may not be sufficient, and has led to clinical failure, presumably because it is not active against the PVL toxin production that accompanies CA-MRSA. For that reason, it may be necessary to add clindamycin to vancomycin or to use linezolid, because both of these latter agents can inhibit toxin production.[103]

TIMING OF ANTIBIOTICS

In addition to the antibiotic approach to therapy outlined previously, there are several other considerations in the management of severe CAP. These plans include providing the first dose of therapy as soon as possible and providing coverage in all patients for atypical pathogens using either a macrolide or a quinolone in the regimen, based on data that such an approach reduces mortality rate.[169-171]

DURATION OF TREATMENT

There is little information on the proper duration of therapy in patients with CAP, especially those with severe illness. Even in the presence of pneumococcal bacteremia, short durations of therapy may be possible, with a rapid switch from intravenous to oral therapy in responding patients. Generally, *S. pneumoniae* can be treated for 5 to 7 days if the patient is responding rapidly and has received accurate empiric therapy at the correct dose. The presence of extrapulmonary infection (such as meningitis), and the identification of certain pathogens (such as bacteremic *S. aureus,* and *P. aeruginosa*) may require longer durations of therapy. Identification of *L. pneumophila* pneumonia may require at least 14 days of therapy, depending on severity of illness and host defense impairments, although recent data have shown that quinolone therapy may be the best approach to management and that durations as short as 5 days with levofloxacin 750 mg may be effective.[172] Biomarkers, especially PCT, can be followed serially to guide duration of therapy for severe CAP. Although early studies of PCT did not involve patients with severe pneumonia, one large randomized controlled trial, including 326 ICU patients with CAP, showed that serial measurement of PCT, compared to standard care, led to a reduction in duration of therapy of 3.3 days.[10] The switch to oral therapy, even in severely ill patients, may be facilitated by the use of quinolones, which are highly bioavailable and achieve the same serum levels with oral therapy as with intravenous therapy.

NOSOCOMIAL PNEUMONIA THERAPY ALGORITHM (SEE FIG. 42.5)

In defining therapy for patients with nosocomial pneumonia, it is important to evaluate (a) time of onset of infection, (b) underlying comorbid conditions, (c) severity of disease—based on scoring systems, and (d) risk factors for MDR pathogens. Antibiotic therapy should be given at the first clinical suspicion of infection, and empiric therapy should be dictated by dividing patients into a group not at risk for MDR pathogens, and a group that is at risk. Those who are not at risk for MDR pathogens include patients with both early onset of infection, and no risks for HCAP such as recent hospitalization, treatment in a health care–associated facility (nursing home, dialysis center, etc.), and no history of recent antibiotic therapy in the past month. Patients with either late-onset infection or the presence of any of the other MDR risk factors are treated empirically for infection with MDR gram-negative and gram-positive pathogens. Not all HCAP patients are at risk for MDR pathogens, and those who are not can receive a narrow-spectrum regimen, similar to that used for CAP. The HCAP patient who is at risk for MDR pathogens is the patient with severe pneumonia and any additional MDR risk such as antibiotic therapy or hospitalization in the past 3 months, poor functional status, and immune suppression. MDR pathogens are not likely in HCAP patients with severe pneumonia who do not have any of these other risks present.[106]

CHOOSING THE APPROPRIATE REGIMEN

Patients who have no MDR risks can be treated for the "core pathogens" listed earlier, generally with a monotherapy regimen of a second- or nonpseudomonal third-generation cephalosporin, a β-lactam/β-lactamase inhibitor combination, ertapenem, or a quinolone (levofloxacin or moxifloxacin).[2] If the patient is penicillin-allergic, therapy can be with a quinolone or the combination of clindamycin and aztreonam. As mentioned earlier HCAP patients without MDR risks should also receive monotherapy, an approach that has been successful in this well-defined subgroup of individuals.

Patients at risk for MDR pathogens generally require combination therapy, rather than monotherapy, which is effective against the core pathogens, as well as MDR gram-negative organisms and MRSA. As discussed, combination therapy is necessary for this population because it provides broad-spectrum coverage, thereby minimizing the chance of initially inappropriate therapy.[173] The empiric therapy for patients at risk for MDR pathogens should include an aminoglycoside or quinolone (ciprofloxacin or high-dose levofloxacin) plus an antipseudomonal β-lactam (imipenem, meropenem, doripenem, piperacillin/tazobactam, aztreonam, or cefepime). Because most patients are at risk for a second ICU-acquired infection, it may be prudent to use an aminoglycoside for the first episode of infection, reserving the quinolone for any subsequent infection, because of concern about quinolone induction of multidrug resistance, which could limit subsequent therapy options.[174] In addition, the efficacy of quinolones against MDR gram-negative organisms in the ICU is not as good as in years past, making an aminoglycoside a more reliable empiric choice in most hospitals. In one study, when a quinolone was added to the best β-lactams, the combination was only minimally better than monotherapy, covering less than 85% of the gram-negative organisms, but when amikacin was added to the same β-lactams, coverage was over 95%.[175] Empiric therapy of MRSA is needed when the patient is at high risk for this pathogen because of a tracheal aspirate Gram stain showing gram-positive organisms or because of other risk factors. In this setting, a third drug should be added, either linezolid or vancomycin, but as discussed previously, recent data have suggested an advantage for linezolid in patients with documented MRSA VAP, because of higher clinical efficacy and a lower risk of nephrotoxicity.[151] When *Acinetobacter* spp. or ESBL-producing Enterobacteriaceae are present, therapy should be with a carbapenem if the pathogen is sensitive; if not, then therapy could be with colistin, or a combination of agents, including tigecycline with sulbactam, colistin, or an aminoglycoside.

In the selection of an empiric therapy regimen, it is also necessary to know which antibiotic the patient has recently received (within the past 14 days) and to choose an agent that is in a different class, because repeated use of the same class of antibiotic may drive resistance to that class, especially if the pathogen is *P. aeruginosa*.[176] Similar findings have been made for patients with bacteremic pneumococcal pneumonia and CAP, and repeat use of an agent within 3 months may mean that the patient is being treated with an agent to which pneumococcus is more likely to be resistant.[177] In addition, the recent use of quinolones may present a particular problem, because in the ICU, recent quinolone therapy may predispose to not only quinolone-resistant organisms but also to infection with MDR pathogens, extended-spectrum β-lactamase-producing gram-negative organisms, and MRSA.[178] For all patients with VAP, it is important to use the correct dose of antibiotic, and the recommended doses for patients with normal renal function appear in Box 42.7.

Although it is possible to use risk factors to identify the patient who is likely to be infected with MDR pathogens, it is important to realize that each hospital, and each ICU has its own unique organisms, and patterns of antimicrobial resistance, and that these patterns change over time. Therefore, it is necessary to monitor local patterns of resistance and to choose empiric therapy that is likely to be effective in a given clinical setting.[112] One other therapeutic concept that has been considered is that of "antibiotic rotation," an idea that means that the standard empiric regimens are intentionally varied over time to expose bacteria to different antibiotics and potentially minimize the selection pressure for resistance. In some studies, this approach has been effective in reducing the incidence of infection with resistant organisms.[179] One of the limitations of antibiotic rotation is that it may mean the use of the same regimen repeatedly in the same patient, and this may itself be a risk factor for selecting for resistance.[180] Currently, this approach is not widely used or recommended.

DURATION OF TREATMENT

There are limited data regarding the optimal duration of treatment for nosocomial pneumonia. Most patients in the past have received 10 to 14 days of treatment, although those infected with non-lactose-fermenting organisms such as *P. aeruginosa* have received 14 to 21 days of treatment.[74] If the lower respiratory tract cultures are negative, it may be possible to stop therapy (especially if an alternative diagnosis is suspected) or to shorten the duration of therapy. In addition, if cultures show that the initial empiric regimen was appropriate, and if the patient has a good clinical response (reflected by a drop in the CPIS or decreased

Box 42.7 Recommended Doses of Commonly Used Antibiotics for Critically Ill Patients

β-Lactams

Cefepime 1-2 g q8-12h
Ceftazidime 2 g q8h
Ceftriaxone 2 g once daily
Imipenem 1 g q8h or 500 mg q6h; can give by prolonged infusion
Meropenem 1 g q6-8h, but can use up to 2 g q6-8h by prolonged infusion
Doripenem 500 mg q8h, by 1- or 4-hour infusion (not approved for pneumonia)
Piperacillin-tazobactam 4.5 g q6h

Aminoglycosides

Gentamicin OR tobramycin 7 mg/kg/day
Amikacin 20 mg/kg/day

Anti-Staphylococcal Agents (MRSA)

Vancomycin 15 mg/kg q12h, aiming for a trough of 15-20 mg/L
Linezolid 600 mg q12h

Quinolones

Ciprofloxacin 400 mg q8h
Levofloxacin 750 mg once daily

Colistin (Polymyxin E)

9 million units/day in three divided doses

MRSA, methicillin-resistant *Staphylococcus aureus*.

levels of biomarkers), then it may be possible to reduce the duration of therapy to as little as 7 to 8 days, although this may not be possible if the etiologic pathogen is *P. aeruginosa* or MRSA.[181] One large study in ICU patients has shown that it is possible to reduce the duration of therapy for pneumonia, including nosocomial pneumonia, by following serial measurements of PCT. In this prospective, randomized, controlled trial, 295 patients with HAP were randomized to have therapy duration defined by clinical evaluation or a PCT algorithm, and with PCT guidance the duration of therapy was reduced by 2.3 days.[10]

DE-ESCALATION OF TREATMENT

Many patients with nosocomial pneumonia will get an initial empiric therapy that is broad spectrum, and thus it is important to consider de-escalation of the initial regimen as serial clinical and microbiologic data become available.[121] If the patient has received a broad-spectrum regimen and the cultures do not show MDR organisms, then the patient can finish therapy with any of 7 monotherapy regimens that have been documented to be effective for severe VAP, in the absence of MDR organisms: ciprofloxacin, doripenem, imipenem, meropenem, piperacillin/tazobactam, cefepime, and high-dose levofloxacin. If *P. aeruginosa* is present, combination therapy with a β-lactam and aminoglycoside should continue for no more than 5 days, after which the patient can be switched to monotherapy with an agent to which the organism is sensitive.[2] When de-escalation has been used, meaning either the switch to a more narrow-spectrum regimen, the use of fewer drugs, or both, mortality rate in VAP has been reduced, compared to when patients do not have de-escalation.[62,63,121] There are many unrealized opportunities for using this approach, including patients with *P. aeruginosa* infection and sensitive pathogens, and in those with a good clinical response and negative respiratory tract cultures.[121] Studies of de-escalation have found that the frequency of this practice varies from 22% to 74% of nosocomial pneumonia patients.[64] Factors associated with a higher rate of de-escalation are use of a protocol for when to narrow antibiotic therapy, use of initially appropriate therapy, the finding of a positive (rather than negative) respiratory tract culture, the use of an empiric broad-spectrum and multidrug regimen, and a low incidence of MDR pathogens in the ICU. The diagnostic method for pneumonia is not consistently related to the rate of de-escalation.

LOCALIZED TREATMENT

For selected patients who are infected with highly resistant organisms, and not responding to systemic antibiotics, it may be valuable to add aerosolized antibiotics (such as gentamicin, tobramycin, colistin, and ceftazidime). Aerosolized administration of antibiotics offers the advantage of achieving high concentrations of antibiotics at the site of infection, and as a result, it may be possible to overcome the problems of poor lung penetration of certain agents (aminoglycosides) and in addition, to provide the high levels of antibiotics that are needed to kill certain resistant organisms. Locally administered antibiotics are rarely absorbed, and systemic toxicity is minimized. In spite of these theoretical advantages, many efficacy questions remain to be answered by clinical trials. Aerosolized antibiotics are not usually recommended for routine treatment of pneumonia but may have a role as adjunctive therapy in patients with MDR organisms not responding to systemic therapy.[182] However, new data suggest that the use of adjunctive aerosolized amikacin, delivered with a special small-particle nebulizer, in patients with a high frequency of MDR gram-negative organisms causing VAP, may lead to an earlier clinical response, resulting in a shorter duration of systemic antibiotic therapy and a lower need to escalate antibiotic therapy.[183]

EVALUATION OF NONRESPONDING PATIENTS

Because pneumonia is a clinical syndrome, not all patients with this diagnosis actually have lung infection, or some may be infected with an unusual or nonsuspected pathogen. In addition, some patients can develop complications of the illness or its therapy, and all of these situations may lead to an apparent nonresponse to therapy.

With effective therapy, most patients with CAP become afebrile by day 3 to 5, and most have a clinical response by day 3. Similarly, even with VAP, most patients have some improvement, particularly in oxygenation, by day 3.[2,42] Nonresponding patients with either CAP or VAP should be evaluated for alternative diagnoses (inflammatory lung

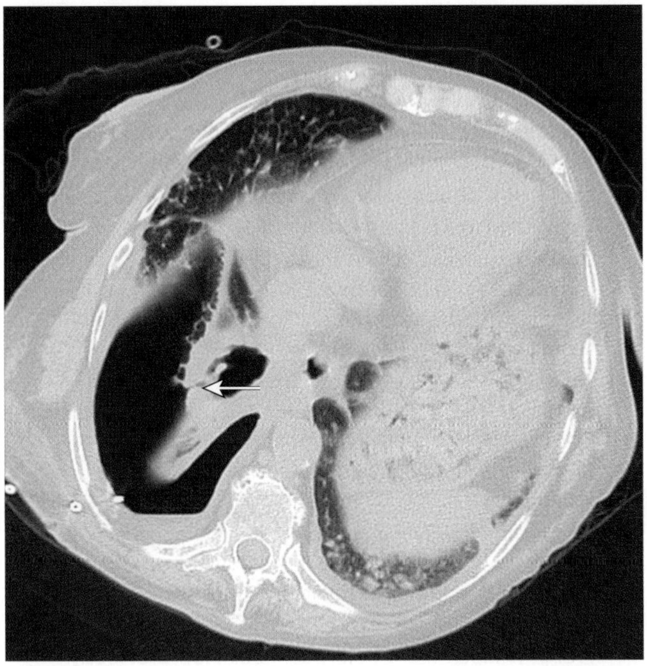

Figure 42.6 A representative computed tomography image of the chest from a 67-year-old woman with a history of chronic obstructive pulmonary disease and bronchiectasis, admitted with right lower lobe pneumonia and empyema complicated with a bronchopleural fistula (*bold arrow*). The pleural fluid grew *Streptococcus pneumoniae* and she was treated with video-assisted thoracoscopy and decortication.

disease, atelectasis, heart failure, malignancy, pulmonary hemorrhage, pulmonary embolus, a nonpneumonic infection); a resistant or unusual pathogen (including tuberculosis and fungal infection); a pneumonia complication (empyema, lung abscess, drug fever, antibiotic-induced colitis, bronchopleural fistula) (Fig. 42.6); or a secondary site of infection (central-line infection, intra-abdominal infection). The evaluation of a nonresponding patient should be individualized but may include CT scanning of the chest, pulmonary angiography, bronchoscopy, and occasionally open lung biopsy.

PREVENTION

COMMUNITY-ACQUIRED PNEUMONIA

Prevention through vaccination and smoking cessation assumes importance for all groups of patients, but especially for the elderly patient and those with comorbid conditions (COPD, cardiovascular disease, diabetes, cigarette smokers, alcoholism), who are at risk for both a higher frequency of infection and a more severe course of illness. Appropriate patients should be vaccinated with both pneumococcal and influenza vaccines. Even for the patient who is recovering from CAP, immunization while in the hospital is appropriate to prevent future episodes of infection, and the evaluation of all patients for vaccination need and the provision of information about smoking cessation are now performance standards used to evaluate the hospital care of CAP patients.

PNEUMOCOCCAL VACCINATION

All high-risk patients and patients older than 65 years should be vaccinated with the 23-valent polysaccharide vaccine. It should be considered in all patients with chronic illnesses such as congestive heart failure, COPD, diabetes, asthma, chronic liver disease, functional or anatomic asplenia, and alcoholism. It is also provided to cigarette smokers, and immunocompromised adults, although the efficacy is somewhat reduced in the latter group. Immunocompromised vaccine candidates include those with HIV infection, malignancy, immune-suppressing therapy (including corticosteroids), and chronic renal failure. In those who were initially vaccinated before the age of 65 years, revaccination is provided once after 5 years. In immunocompromised patients, revaccination is given 5 years after initial vaccination. If there is uncertainty about whether the patient has recently been vaccinated, it is probably best to give a pneumococcal vaccination, because repeat administration, even more often than recommended, is not generally associated with an adverse reaction.[184] In a study of 62,918 adults with CAP hospitalized across 109 centers in the United States, prior vaccination against pneumococcus showed improved survival, decreased chance of respiratory failure or other complications, and decreased length of stay compared with patients who did not receive vaccination.[185]

Hospital-based immunization is recommended, and one study found that among 1633 patients with pneumonia treated in the hospital, 62% had been hospitalized in the preceding 4 years.[186] In addition, 80% of these patients had a high-risk condition that would have qualified them to receive pneumococcal vaccine. Based on these observations, it seems likely that many cases of CAP could be prevented if pneumococcal vaccine was given to all hospitalized patients who qualify for the vaccine, regardless of why they are hospitalized.

INFLUENZA VACCINATION

Yearly influenza vaccine should be administered to all high-risk patients (adults 65 years of age and older, pregnant women, those with chronic comorbid medical conditions, and American Indians and Alaskan Natives) and persons who can transmit the infection to high-risk patients, such as health care workers and household members of high-risk patients.

NOSOCOMIAL PNEUMONIA

Although no single method is able to prevent nosocomial pneumonia reliably, multiple small interventions may have benefit, especially those focused on modifiable risk factors for infection. Recently, these interventions have been combined into "ventilator bundles," which have been demonstrated to reduce the incidence of VAP, if applied carefully.[187,188] Most of these bundles include multiple interventions, so it is difficult to know which individual manipulations are most valuable. Successful bundles have included interventions such as elevation of the head of the bed to 30 degrees (to avoid the risk of aspiration present with the supine position), daily interruption of sedation to attempt weaning, peptic ulcer disease prophylaxis, endotracheal tube suctioning (possibly with a closed suction system), hand washing, careful oral care (including oral chlorhexidine), and tight control of blood glucose.[40] In spite of the success of this approach, one recent randomized study has demonstrated a lack of benefit and feasibility of routine elevation of the head of the bed.[189] The efficacy of this approach has led to a movement to aim for "zero VAP" in all ICUs, but it remains uncertain if this goal is really achievable, and if hospitals that consistently report this result have simply changed the diagnostic criteria for VAP, because in many instances, the incidence of VAP has been reduced, without a reduction in associated outcomes such as mortality rate and ICU length of stay.

Other widely used measures in mechanically ventilated patients are avoidance of large inocula of bacteria into the lung (careful handling of ventilator circuit tubing), mobilization of respiratory secretions (frequent suctioning, use of rotational bed therapy in selected individuals), nutritional support (enteral preferred over parenteral), placing of feeding tubes into the small bowel (to avoid aspiration, which is more likely with stomach tubes), and avoidance of large gastric residuals when giving enteral feeding. In addition, any tube inserted into the stomach or trachea should be inserted through the mouth and not the nose, whenever possible, to avoid obstructing the nasal sinuses, and to prevent nosocomial sinusitis, which can lead to nosocomial pneumonia.[40] A specially adapted endotracheal tube that allows for continuous aspiration of subglottic secretions may interrupt the oropharyngeal to tracheal transfer of bacteria and reduce the incidence of pneumonia.[190] In addition, modifications of the endotracheal tube have been developed, including silver coating of the tube and a focus on maintaining endotracheal tube cuff pressure to avoid leakage of tracheal secretions to the lung, and both approaches have had some success. In addition, new devices to remove biofilm from the surface of the endotracheal tube are in development, but their clinical benefit is not yet defined. Because endotracheal intubation is a risk for pneumonia, noninvasive positive-pressure ventilation should be used whenever possible, and this approach is associated with a lower pneumonia risk than traditional mechanical ventilation. Early tracheostomy has been considered a potentially effective means of VAP prevention, but a large randomized trial did not confirm such a benefit.[191] There is no specific role for prophylactic systemic or topical antibiotics, but some data suggest that patients with coma due to stroke or head trauma and those who may have aspirated during an emergent intubation may benefit from a 24-hour course of systemic antibiotics.[192] The use of selective digestive decontamination (SDD), which involves the use of prophylactic systemic and topical (mouth and intestinal tract) antimicrobials, has been a controversial strategy for VAP prevention for many years. Although one large trial has recently reported benefit, there are many concerns with this approach, including the development of antibiotic resistance, and the possibility that the use of oral chlorhexidine and ventilator bundles may be just as effective as the entire SDD regimen.[193,194]

KEY POINTS

- Patients with severe CAP admitted to the ICU, as well as patients with VAP, continue to have a high mortality rate, despite initiation of multiple novel therapeutic and preventive strategies in the ICU.
- Delay in ICU admission in patients with severe CAP is associated with increased mortality risk.
- Scoring systems such as the ATS/IDSA 2007 definition for severe pneumonia and PIRO (predisposition, insult, response, and organ dysfunction) scores are useful for assessing the severity of illness in CAP patients.
- The use of biomarkers, such as procalcitonin, to diagnose the severity and guide the use and duration of antimicrobial therapy in patients with severe CAP and VAP is being adopted increasingly in various ICUs.
- *S. pneumoniae* is the most common pathogen causing severe CAP, and enteric gram-negative bacteria and *S. aureus* are the most common causes of nosocomial pneumonia.
- HCAP is much more heterogeneous than previously thought and not all patients require empiric broad-spectrum antibiotic therapy directed at multidrug-resistant pathogens.
- The most important risk factor for death in patients with VAP is inappropriate empiric antibiotic therapy; other mortality risk factors include respiratory failure, coma on admission, bilateral radiographic abnormalities, and infection with resistant organisms.
- Initiation of appropriate and early antibiotic therapy in patients with severe pneumonia is associated with increased survival.
- In choosing an antibiotic for a patient with severe pneumonia, history of recent antibiotic use and local antibiogram is crucial, and care should be taken to avoid using the same antibiotics prescribed in the recent past (3 months for a patient with CAP, and any agent prescribed in the last 2 weeks for a patient with VAP).
- Empiric broad-spectrum antibiotics are required for patients with severe pneumonia. However, patients should be reevaluated after 72 hours and efforts should be made to narrow the spectrum of therapy and the number of drugs based on microbiologic data and clinical response.
- Nonresponders should be evaluated for treatment failure or complications from infection.
- Use of hospital-based immunization practices has helped reduce the incidence of CAP, and use of "ventilator bundles" in the ICU is associated with a significant reduction in the incidence of VAP.

SELECTED REFERENCES

2. Niederman MS, Craven DE, Bonten MJ, et al: Guidelines for the management of adults with hospital-acquired, ventilator-associated, and healthcare-associated pneumonia. Am J Respir Crit Care Med 2005;171:388-416.
10. Bouadma L, Luyt CE, Tubach F, et al: Use of procalcitonin to reduce patients' exposure to antibiotics in intensive care units (PRORATA trial): A multicentre randomised controlled trial. Lancet 2010;375:463-474.
13. Brito V, Niederman MS: Healthcare-associated pneumonia is a heterogeneous disease, and all patients do not need the same broad-spectrum antibiotic therapy as complex nosocomial pneumonia. Curr Opin Infect Dis 2009;22:316-325.
14. Nair GB, Niederman MS: Community-acquired pneumonia: An unfinished battle. Med Clin North Am 2011;95:1143-1161.
19. Mandell LA, Wunderink RG, Anzueto A, et al: Infectious Diseases Society of America/American Thoracic Society consensus guidelines on the management of community-acquired pneumonia in adults. Clin Infect Dis 2007;44:S27-S72.
24. Niederman MS: Making sense of scoring systems in community acquired pneumonia. Respirology 2009;14:327-335.
50. Heyland DK, Cook DJ, Griffith L, et al: The attributable morbidity and mortality of ventilator-associated pneumonia in the critically ill patient. The Canadian Critical Trials Group. Am J Respir Crit Care Med 1999;159:1249-1256.
64. Niederman MS, Soulountsi V: De-escalation therapy: Is it valuable for the management of ventilator-associated pneumonia? Clin Chest Med 2011;32:517-534.
167. Baddour LM, Yu VL, Klugman KP, et al: Combination antibiotic therapy lowers mortality among severely ill patients with pneumococcal bacteremia. Am J Respir Crit Care Med 2004;170: 440-444.
181. Chastre J, Wolff M, Fagon JY, et al: Comparison of 8 vs 15 days of antibiotic therapy for ventilator-associated pneumonia in adults: A randomized trial. JAMA 2003;290:2588-2598.

The complete list of references can be found at www.expertconsult.com.

43 Weaning from Mechanical Ventilation

Martin J. Tobin

CHAPTER OUTLINE

Mechanical ventilation is often lifesaving, but it is associated with numerous complications.[1,2] Accordingly, it is imperative to disconnect patients from the ventilator at the earliest feasible time. Deciding the right time to initiate this disconnection process, usually referred to as *weaning*, is one of the greatest challenges in critical care medicine.[3] If a physician is too conservative and postpones the initiation of weaning, the patient is placed at an increased risk of life-threatening, ventilator-associated complications. Conversely, if weaning is begun prematurely, the patient may suffer cardiopulmonary or psychological decompensation of sufficient severity to set back a patient's clinical course.[4]

This chapter reviews the pathophysiology of weaning failure, weaning-predictor testing, different weaning techniques, and extubation.

PATHOPHYSIOLOGY OF WEANING FAILURE

After patients have been disconnected from the ventilator, up to 25% experience respiratory distress severe enough to necessitate the reinstitution of mechanical ventilation.[5,6] The pathophysiologic mechanisms of weaning failure can be divided into those occurring at the level of the respiratory control system, mechanics of the lung and chest wall, the respiratory muscles, the cardiovascular system, and gas-exchange properties of the lung.[7]

CONTROL OF BREATHING

Many weaning-failure patients develop hypercapnia. Accordingly, it had been thought that these patients experience an acute decrease in minute ventilation consequent to a decrease in respiratory center output.[3] Measurements of respiratory motor output, using mean inspiratory flow or airway occlusion pressure ($P_{0.1}$), have consistently revealed an increase, not a decrease, in respiratory drive in weaning-failure patients.[4,8,9]

Weaning-failure patients, however, exhibit marked abnormalities in respiratory timing, specifically marked shortening of inspiratory time (TI), which is coupled with shortening of expiratory time (TE). The decrease in both TI and TE means that respiratory frequency (f) is markedly elevated. The shortening of TI combined with a normal mean inspiratory flow (VT/TI) results in a marked decrease of tidal volume (VT).[8] This combination (elevated f and decreased VT) is referred to as rapid shallow breathing—now recognized as the physiologic hallmark of weaning failure (Fig. 43.1).[3]

RESPIRATORY MECHANICS

The most detailed study of respiratory mechanics during weaning trials was carried out by Jubran and Tobin.[10,11] Immediately before commencement of a trial of spontaneous breathing, patients who went on to tolerate or

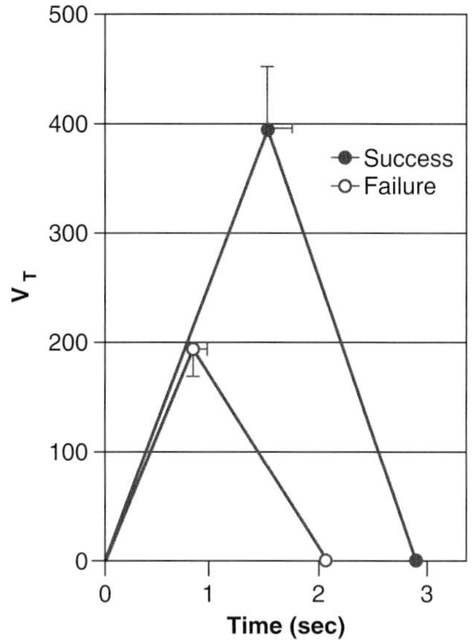

Figure 43.1 The mean respiratory cycle during spontaneous breathing in 7 weaning-failure patients and 10 weaning-success patients. The early termination of inspiratory time in the weaning-failure patients leads to a decrease in tidal volume (VT). The decrease in inspiratory time, coupled with a decrease in expiratory time, results in a faster respiratory frequency. Bars represent 1 SE. (Redrawn from Tobin MJ, Perez W, Guenther SM, et al: The pattern of breathing during successful and unsuccessful trials of weaning from mechanical ventilation. Am Rev Respir Dis 1986;134:1111-1118.)

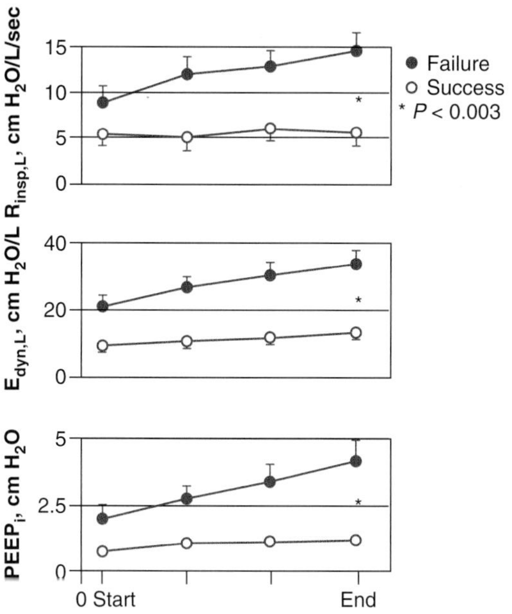

Figure 43.2 Inspiratory resistance of the lung (Rinsp,L), dynamic lung elastance (Edyn,L), and intrinsic positive end-expiratory pressure (PEEPi) in 17 weaning-failure patients and 14 weaning-success patients. Data displayed were obtained during the second and last minutes of a T-tube trial, and at one third and two thirds of the trial duration. Between the onset and end of the trial, the failure group developed increases in Rinsp,L ($P < 0.009$), Edyn,L ($P < 0.0001$), and PEEPi ($P < 0.0001$) and the success group developed increases in Edyn,L ($P < 0.006$) and PEEPi ($P < 0.02$). Over the course of the trial, the failure group had higher values of Rinsp,L ($P < 0.003$), Edyn,L ($P < 0.006$), and PEEPi ($P < 0.009$) than the success group. (Redrawn from Jubran A, Tobin MJ: Pathophysiologic basis of acute respiratory distress in patients who fail a trial of weaning from mechanical ventilation. Am J Respir Crit Care Med 1997;155:906-915.)

fail the trial showed little or no difference in detailed measurements of passive respiratory mechanics.[11] Resistance, elastance, and intrinsic positive end-expiratory pressure (PEEPi) were equivalent in the two groups.

Over the course of the trial, all of these variables became more abnormal in the weaning-failure patients than in the weaning-success patients (Fig. 43.2).[10] Respiratory resistance increased progressively, reaching about seven times the normal value at the end of the trial. Pulmonary elastance increased, reaching five times the normal value. Intrinsic PEEP more than doubled over the course of the trial. A similar pattern has been observed by other investigators.[12] The observation that respiratory mechanics were equivalent in weaning-success and weaning-failure patients immediately before a weaning trial but deteriorated immediately in the weaning-failure patients as soon as they began to breathe spontaneously indicates that some mechanism associated with the act of spontaneous breathing causes the worsening of respiratory mechanics that leads to weaning failure.

PATIENT EFFORT

To compensate for the marked worsening of respiratory mechanics, patients need to make a greater inspiratory effort. It had been thought that weaning-failure patients make weaker inspiratory efforts than do weaning-success patients.[7] On the contrary, direct measurements of work of breathing and pressure-time product[13,14] show that weaning-failure patients consistently make a greater inspiratory effort than do weaning-success patients (Fig. 43.3).[10,15]

RESPIRATORY MUSCLES

Numerous research groups have shown that maximal inspiratory pressure (PImax), a measure of respiratory muscle strength, does not discriminate between weaning-success and weaning-failure patients.[7] These findings led to the belief that respiratory muscle weakness is not an important determinant of weaning outcome. PImax, however, can misrepresent respiratory muscle strength because the values are heavily influenced by patient motivation and cooperation.[13] A more objective measure of diaphragmatic strength is obtained by stimulation of the phrenic nerves and recording the resulting transdiaphragmatic pressure (Pdi). Weaning-failure patients have twitch Pdi values below 10 cm H_2O, whereas values of 35 to 39 cm H_2O are observed in healthy subjects.[16] These data suggest that weaning-failure patients may have considerable muscle weakness.

Stimulation of the phrenic nerves and recording of the resulting Pdi also provides the most direct measure of diaphragmatic fatigue.[13] Laghi and coworkers[17] employed this technique in 11 weaning-failure and 8 weaning-success patients before and after a T-tube trial. No patient in either group exhibited a fall in twitch pressure. This result was surprising. Related analyses disclosed why. Failure patients became progressively distressed during the trial, leading

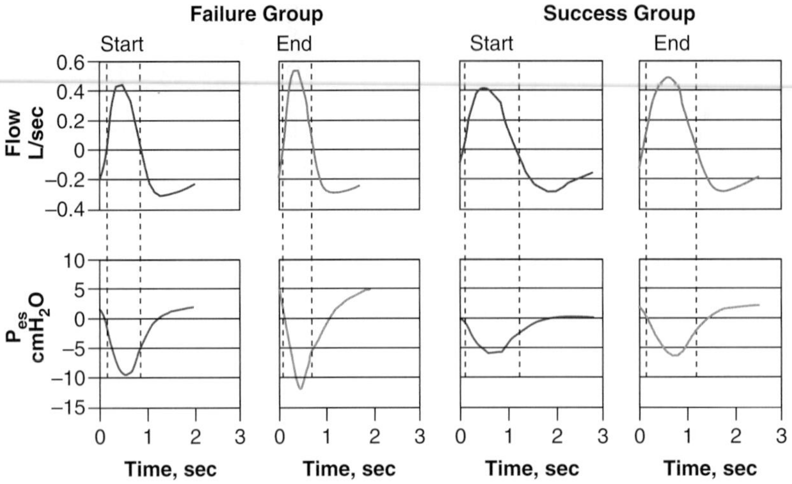

Figure 43.3 Ensemble average plots of flow and esophageal pressure (Pes) at the start and end of a T-tube trial in 17 weaning-failure patients and 14 weaning-success patients. At the start of the trial, the inspiratory excursion in Pes was greater in the failure patients, and it increased further by the end of the trial. To generate these plots, flow and Pes tracings were divided into 25 equal time intervals over a single respiratory cycle for each of the five breaths for each patient in the two groups. For a given patient, the five breaths from the start of the trial were then superimposed and aligned with respect to time, and the average at each time point was calculated. The group mean tracings were then generated by ensemble averaging of the individual mean from each patient. The same procedure was performed for breaths at the end of the trial. (Redrawn from Jubran A, Tobin MJ: Pathophysiologic basis of acute respiratory distress in patients who fail a trial of weaning from mechanical ventilation. Am J Respir Crit Care Med 1997;155:906-915.)

clinicians to reinstate ventilator support before patients had breathed long enough to develop fatigue (Fig. 43.4).[17,18] In other words, monitoring clinical signs of distress provides sufficient warning to avoid respiratory muscle fatigue.

CARDIOVASCULAR PERFORMANCE

During a weaning trial, patients can experience substantial increases in right and left ventricular afterload.[19,20] These afterload increases most likely result from associated increases in negative swings of intrathoracic pressure. At the completion of a weaning trial, the level of oxygen consumption is equivalent in weaning-success and weaning-failure patients. How the cardiovascular system meets the oxygen demand differs in the two groups of patients. In weaning-success patients, oxygen demand is met through an increase in oxygen delivery, mediated by the expected increase in cardiac output on discontinuation of positive-pressure ventilation.[20] In weaning-failure patients, oxygen demand is met through an increase in oxygen extraction; these patients have a relative decrease in oxygen delivery.[20] The greater oxygen extraction causes a substantial decrease in mixed venous oxygen saturation, contributing to the arterial hypoxemia that occurs in some patients.[20]

GAS EXCHANGE

Studies employing the multiple inert-gas technique have revealed that the ventilation-perfusion maldistribution and acute hypercapnia observed in weaning-failure patients is produced primarily by shallow breathing (low V_T).[7] About half of weaning-failure patients experience an increase in Pa_{CO_2} of 10 mm Hg or more over the course of a spontaneous breathing trial.[10] The hypercapnia is not usually a consequence of a decrease in minute ventilation. Instead, it results from rapid, shallow breathing, which causes an increase in dead space ventilation. In a small proportion of weaning-failure patients, primary depression of respiratory motor output may be responsible for the hypercapnia.[10]

WEANING-PREDICTOR TESTING

In randomized controlled trials (RCTs) of different weaning techniques, most patients who had received mechanical ventilation for a week or longer were able to tolerate ventilator discontinuation on the first day that weaning-predictor tests were measured.[5,6] Many of these patients probably would have tolerated extubation a day or so earlier. As such, one of the main sources of weaning delay is the failure of the physician to think that the patient just might come off the ventilator. Psychological research suggests that much of this delay in ventilator weaning results from clinicians being overconfident in their intuition that a patient is not ready for a weaning trial.[4] Another source of error is the failure of clinicians to pay close attention to pretest probability—they fail to recognize the importance of bayesian principles in clinical decision making. When taking care of a ventilator-supported patient, physicians should be mindful of these cognitive processes and employ compensatory tactics, specifically the use of screening tests, to spot a patient's readiness for weaning. By alerting an unsuspecting physician to a patient's readiness to tolerate unassisted ventilation—hours or days before he or she would otherwise order a spontaneous breathing trial—weaning-predictor tests circumvent the cognitive errors inherent in clinical decision making.[4]

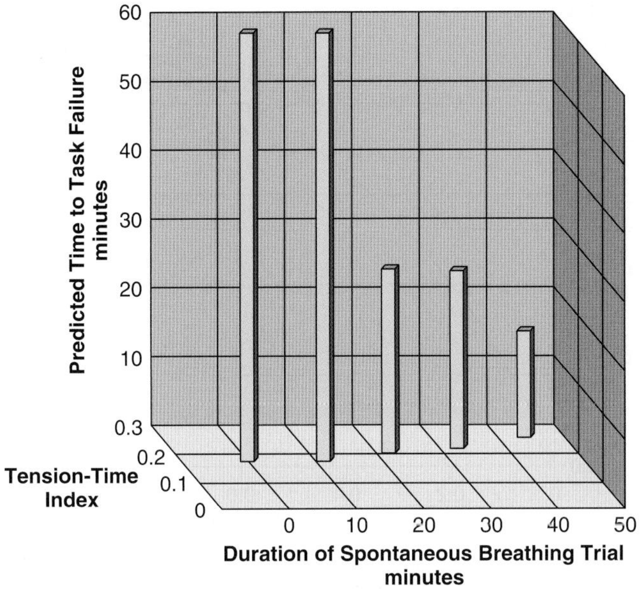

Figure 43.4 Interrelationship between the duration of a spontaneous breathing trial, tension-time index of the diaphragm, and predicted time to task failure in nine patients who failed a trial of weaning from mechanical ventilation. The patients breathed spontaneously for an average of 44 minutes before a physician terminated the trial. At the start of the trial, the tension-time index was 0.17, and the formula of Bellemare and Grassino[18] predicted that patients could sustain spontaneous breathing for another 59 minutes before developing task failure. As the trial progressed, the tension-time index increased and the predicted time to development of task failure decreased. At the end of the trial, the tension-time index reached 0.26. That patients were predicted to sustain spontaneous breathing for another 13 minutes before developing task failure clarifies why patients did not develop a decrease in diaphragmatic twitch pressure. In other words, physicians interrupted the trial on the basis of clinical manifestations of respiratory distress, before patients had sufficient time to develop contractile fatigue. (Redrawn from Laghi F, Tobin MJ: Disorders of the respiratory muscles. Am J Respir Crit Care Med 2003;168:10-48.)

PITFALLS IN USE OF WEANING-PREDICTOR TESTS

Physicians commonly view diagnostic testing in monolithic terms: a test is a test is a test. In reality, diagnostic testing has to satisfy two very different tasks: one is screening, the other is confirmation.[21] The characteristics of these test types differ, and a single diagnostic test rarely fulfills both functions.[21]

The fundamental job of a weaning-predictor test is screening.[4] Because the goal is to not miss anybody with the condition under consideration, a good screening test has a low rate of false-negative results; to achieve this goal, a higher false-positive rate is acceptable. Thus an ideal screening test has a high sensitivity.[4,21]

Weaning involves the use of three diagnostic tests in sequence: measurement of predictors, a weaning trial, and a trial of extubation.[4] The sequential nature of the testing gives rise to particular problems in studies undertaken to investigate the reliability of a predictor test. One is spectrum bias. This occurs when a new study population contains fewer (or more) sick patients than the population in which a diagnostic test was originally developed.[21,22] A second is test-referral bias. This occurs when the results of a test under evaluation are used to select patients for a reference-standard test, such as use of a weaning-predictor test to select patients for a reference-standard test (passing a weaning trial that leads to extubation).[21,22]

A third factor that affects studies of the reliability of a predictor test is base-rate fallacy.[22,23] Consider a diagnostic test for a disease that has a false-positive rate of 5% and false-negative rate of 0%, and the incidence of the disorder (under consideration) is 1 per 1000 persons. A randomly selected person undergoes diagnostic testing. The result comes back positive. What is the chance this person has the disease? More than 80% of physicians answer 95%. The correct answer is 1.96%.[23] Physicians who answer 95% are failing to take into account the pretest probability of the disorder. Thus they fall into the trap of base-rate fallacy.

Pretest probability is a physician's estimate of the likelihood of a particular condition (weaning outcome) before a diagnostic test is undertaken.[4] Post-test probability (typically expressed as positive or negative predictive value) is the new likelihood after the test results are obtained. A good diagnostic test achieves a marked increase (or decrease) in the post-test probability (over pretest probability). For every test in every medical subspecialty, the magnitude of change between pretest probability and post-test probability is determined by Bayes's theorem.[22] Three factors (alone) determine the magnitude of the pretest to post-test change: sensitivity, specificity, and pretest probability. Sensitivity and specificity are commonly assumed to remain constant for a test. In truth, test-referral bias, a common occurrence in studies of weaning tests, leads to major changes in sensitivity and specificity.[21] Likewise, major changes in pretest probability arise as a consequence of spectrum bias.[21] All of these factors need to be carefully considered when reading a study that evaluates the reliability of a weaning-predictor test.

RESPIRATORY FREQUENCY/TIDAL VOLUME RATIO

The ratio of respiratory frequency to tidal volume (f/V_T) is measured during 1 minute of spontaneous breathing (Fig. 43.5).[24] Measurements of f/V_T in the presence of pressure support or continuous positive airway pressure (CPAP) will result in inaccurate predictions of weaning outcome.[4] The higher the f/V_T ratio, the more severe the rapid, shallow breathing and the greater the likelihood of unsuccessful weaning. An f/V_T ratio of 100 best discriminates between successful and unsuccessful attempts at weaning.[24]

The initial evaluation of f/V_T was reported in 1991.[24] Since then, this test has been evaluated in more than 25 studies. Reported sensitivity ranges from 0.35 to 1.[22] Specificity ranges from 0 to 0.89.[22] At first glance, this wide scatter suggests that f/V_T is an unreliable predictor of weaning outcome. This was also the viewpoint of an Evidence-Based Medicine Task Force that undertook a meta-analysis of the studies.[25,26] The Task Force, however, failed to take into account test-referral bias and spectrum bias.[4] In consequence, the Task Force committed at least 15 major errors—any one of which was sufficient to scupper their conclusions.[27,28] In contrast, when data from the studies (included in the meta-analysis) were compared against the test characteristics in the original 1991 report, taking into

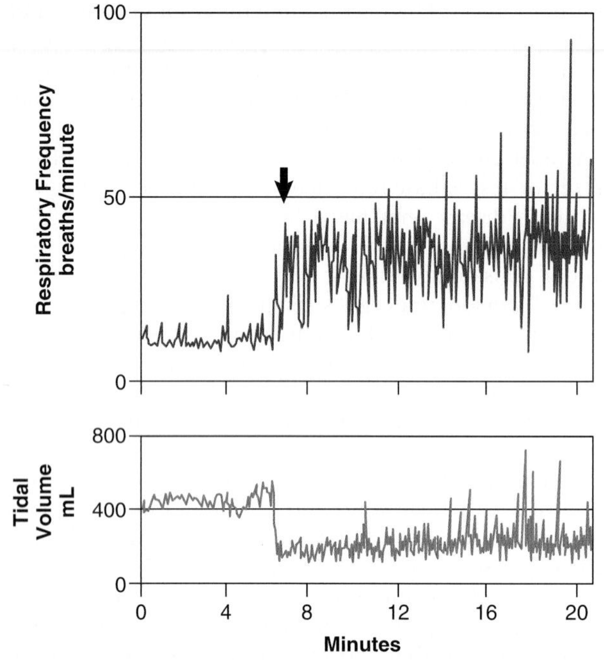

Figure 43.5 A time-series, breath-by-breath plot of respiratory frequency and tidal volume in a patient who failed a weaning trial. The arrow indicates the point of resuming spontaneous breathing. Rapid, shallow breathing developed almost immediately after discontinuation of the ventilator. (Redrawn from Tobin MJ, Perez W, Guenther SM, et al: The pattern of breathing during successful and unsuccessful trials of weaning from mechanical ventilation. Am Rev Respir Dis 1986;134:1111-1118.)

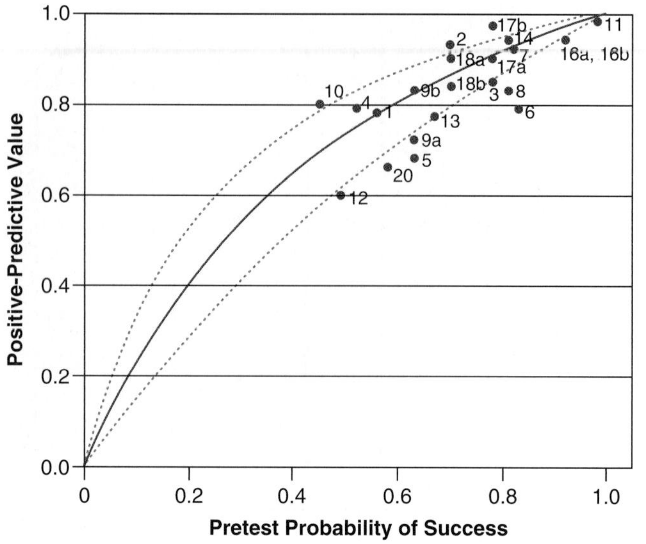

Figure 43.6 Positive predictive value (post-test probability of successful outcome) for f/VT plotted against pretest probability of successful outcome. The curve is based on the sensitivity and specificity originally reported by Yang and Tobin[24] and Bayes's formula for 0.01-unit increments in pretest probability between 0.00 and 1.00.[22] The lines represent the upper and lower 95% confidence intervals for the predicted relationship of the positive predictive values against pretest probability. The observed positive predictive value in a study is plotted against the pretest probability of weaning success (prevalence of successful outcome). (Redrawn from Tobin MJ, Jubran A: Variable performance of weaning-predictor tests: Role of Bayes' theorem and spectrum and test-referral bias. Intensive Care Med 2006;32:2002-2012.)

account bayesian pretest probability, the weighted Pearson correlation coefficient was 0.86 ($P < 0.0001$) for positive predictive value and 0.82 ($P < 0.0001$) for negative predictive value (Figs. 43.6 and 43.7).[22]

The primary job of a weaning-predictor test is screening, which requires a high sensitivity.[4,21] The average sensitivity in all of the studies on f/VT was 0.89, and 85% of the studies reveal sensitivities higher than 0.90.[22] This sensitivity compares well with commonly used diagnostic tests.[4]

The whole purpose of diagnostic screening is to perform a simple test at a time when a physician's pretest probability is low (less than 50%).[4] A screening test should be cheap, easy to perform, pose minimal risk to patients, and provide a quick answer. A spontaneous breathing trial that involves 30 to 120 minutes of monitored performance is the antithesis of a screening test. Yet, the Evidence-Based Medicine Task Force recommends that clinicians should start weaning with a spontaneous breathing trial (a confirmatory test), and use the initial few minutes of the trial as a screening test.[25] This is analogous to saying that when you suspect diabetes, start with a glucose tolerance test and then, as the test gets under way, ask the patient for a urine sample in order to do a dipstick.[29]

WEANING TRIALS

When a screening test is positive, the clinician proceeds to a confirmatory test.[21] The goal of a positive result on a

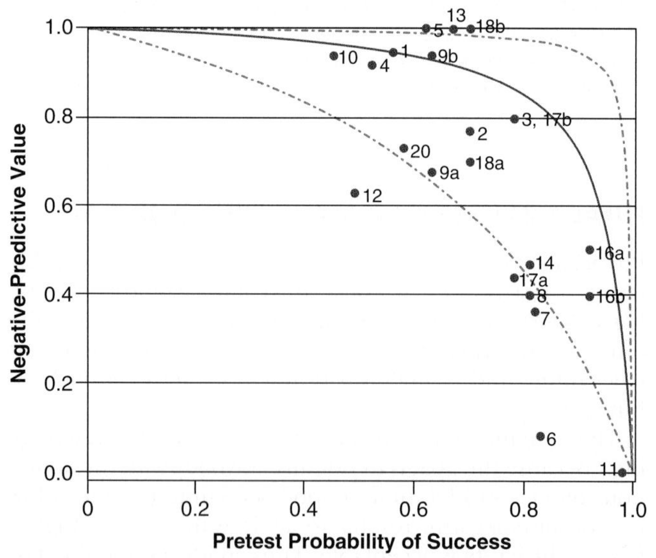

Figure 43.7 Negative predictive value (post-test probability of unsuccessful outcome) for f/VT. The curve, its 95% confidence intervals, and placement of a study on the plot are described in the legend of Figure 43.6. The observed negative predictive value in a study is plotted against the pretest probability of weaning success (prevalence of successful outcome). (Redrawn from Tobin MJ, Jubran A: Variable performance of weaning-predictor tests: Role of Bayes' theorem and spectrum and test-referral bias. Intensive Care Med 2006;32:2002-2012.)

confirmatory test is to rule in a condition[19]: The likelihood of a patient tolerating a trial of extubation is high. An ideal confirmatory test has a low rate of false-positive results (i.e., a high specificity).[21] Unfortunately, the specificity of a spontaneous breathing trial is not known. Indeed, its specificity will never be known because its determination would require an unethical experiment: extubating all patients who fail a weaning trial and counting how many require reintubation.[4]

MULTIPLE T-TUBE TRIALS

Of the four methods available for conducting a weaning trial, the use of repeated T-tube trials, several times a day, is the oldest method.[3] The patient receives an enriched supply of oxygen through a T-tube circuit. Initially 5 to 10 minutes in duration, T-tube trials are extended and repeated several times a day until the patient can sustain spontaneous ventilation for several hours. This approach has become unpopular because it requires considerable time on the part of intensive care staff.

INTERMITTENT MANDATORY VENTILATION

For many years, intermittent mandatory ventilation (IMV) was the most popular method of weaning.[3] With IMV, the mandatory rate from the ventilator is reduced in steps of 1 to 3 breaths per minute, and an arterial blood gas value is obtained about 30 minutes after each rate change.[30] Unfortunately, titrating the number of breaths from the ventilator in accordance with the results of arterial blood gases can produce a false sense of security. As few as two to three positive-pressure breaths per minute can achieve acceptable blood gas values, but these values provide no information regarding the patient's work of breathing (which may be excessive).[4] At IMV rates of 14 breaths per minute or fewer, patient inspiratory efforts are increased to a level likely to cause respiratory muscle fatigue.[31,32] Moreover, this occurs not only with the intervening spontaneous breaths but also with ventilator-assisted breaths. Consequently, use of IMV may actually contribute to the development of respiratory muscle fatigue or prevent its recovery.[7]

PRESSURE SUPPORT

When pressure support is used for weaning, the level of pressure is reduced gradually (decrements of 3 to 6 cm H_2O) and titrated on the basis of the patient's respiratory frequency.[33] When the patient tolerates a minimal level of pressure support, he or she is extubated. What exactly constitutes a "minimal level of pressure support" has never been defined.[34]

ONCE-DAILY T-TUBE TRIALS

The fourth method of weaning is to perform a single daily T-tube trial, lasting for 30 to 120 minutes. If this trial is successful, the patient is extubated. If the trial is unsuccessful, the patient is given at least 24 hours of respiratory muscle rest with full ventilator support before another trial is performed.[4]

COMPARISON OF WEANING METHODS

Until the early 1990s, it was widely believed that all weaning methods were equally effective, and the physician's judgment was regarded as the critical determinant.[3] The results of RCTs have revealed that the period of weaning is as much as three times as long with IMV as with trials of spontaneous breathing.[5,6] In a study involving patients with respiratory difficulties on weaning, trials of spontaneous breathing halved the weaning time as compared with pressure support[6]; in another study, the weaning time was similar with the two methods.[5] Performing trials of spontaneous breathing once a day is as effective as performing such trials several times a day but much simpler.[6] In patients not expecting to pose any particular difficulty with weaning, a half-hour trial of spontaneous breathing is as effective as a 2-hour trial.[35]

WEANING BY PROTOCOL VERSUS USUAL CARE

Six groups of investigators have undertaken RCTs comparing the use of protocols versus usual care in the management of weaning. Three groups—Namen and colleagues,[36] Randolph and associates,[37] and Krishnan and coworkers[38]—found that protocolized weaning was without benefit. Data from the other three studies are sometimes viewed as supportive of the superiority of protocolized weaning. The studies by Kollef and colleagues[39] and by Ely and associates,[40] however, contain internal-validity problems of such magnitude that the data cannot be accepted as valid evidence on which to base a claim that protocols per se expedite weaning. The third study, by Marelich and coworkers,[41] revealed no benefit in one of the two ICUs in the study. In summary, only half of one study out of six studies revealed valid support for protocolized weaning, with the remainder providing no evidence of benefit.

Tanios and colleagues[42] undertook an RCT to determine whether the inclusion of f/V_T in a weaning protocol influenced weaning time. In the f/V_T-protocol group, patients could proceed to a weaning trial (CPAP and pressure support) if—and only if—they had an f/V_T of less than 106. In the second study arm, clinicians did not follow the protocolized approach to weaning. The duration of weaning was longer in the f/V_T-protocol group than in the nonprotocol group.

The study has two major problems. First, the investigators assume that physicians managing patients in the control group did not calculate f/V_T. Physicians, however, are highly aware that respiratory frequency and tidal volume are key variables in deciding whether a patient will tolerate weaning and extubation.[3] Once this knowledge has crept into a physician's brain, it cannot be surgically extirpated at the point of commencing an RCT. To ensure that physicians did not employ breathing pattern in the decision making, Tanios and colleagues[42] would have had to have taken steps to hide or occlude the display of frequency and tidal volume on the bedside monitor and ventilator screen.

Second, f/V_T was one component in a weaning protocol. It is important to make a distinction between the use of a protocol in conducting a research study and its use in everyday clinical practice. In the research protocol of Tanios and colleagues,[42] patients who had an f/V_T of 105 or less progressed to a weaning trial, whereas patients with an f/VT of 106 or higher were returned to the ventilator. When conducting research, this is exactly how a protocol must be specified and followed. No flexibility is permitted. A competent clinician, however, would think it daft to slavishly comply with a protocol that decided an entire day of ventilator management on a one-unit difference in a single measurement of f/VT.[43] Rather, intelligent physicians customize knowledge to the particulars of each patient and are expected to outperform the inflexible application of a protocol—as has been shown in numerous studies of weaning protocols.

EXTUBATION

Decisions about weaning and decisions about extubation are commonly combined.[44] When a patient tolerates a weaning trial without distress, a clinician feels reasonably confident that the patient will be able to sustain spontaneous ventilation after extubation. Before removing the endotracheal tube, however, the clinician must also judge whether or not the patient will be able to maintain a patent upper airway after extubation.

Of patients who are expected to tolerate extubation without difficulty, approximately 10% to 20% fail and require reintubation.[5,6] The mortality rate among patients who require reintubation is more than six times as high as the mortality rate among patients who can tolerate extubation.[35] The reason for the higher mortality rate is unknown. It might be related to the development of new problems after extubation or to complications associated with reinsertion of a new tube. A more likely explanation is that the need for reintubation reflects greater severity of the underlying illness.[42]

Many physicians find it convenient to extubate a patient once he or she can breathe comfortably on a pressure support of about 7 cm H_2O and PEEP 5 cm H_2O based on the belief that such "minimal ventilator settings" are simply overcoming the resistance engendered by an endotracheal tube.[45] This claim ignores the inflammation and edema that develop in the upper airways after an endotracheal tube has been in place for a day or more. On removal of the tube, the mucosal swelling produces an increase in upper airway resistance. Straus and associates[46] demonstrated experimentally that the respiratory work dissipated against the supraglottic airway after extubation is almost identical to the work dissipated against an endotracheal tube before extubation. Thus, applying any level of pressure support causes physicians to underestimate the respiratory resistance a patient will encounter after extubation. The addition of a small amount of pressure support produces surprisingly large reductions in inspiratory work in ventilated patients: 5 cm H_2O decreases inspiratory work by 31% to 38% and 10 cm H_2O decreases work by 46% to 60%.[34,47] Independently, the addition of 5 cm H_2O of PEEP can decrease the work of breathing by as much as 40% in ventilated patients.[4] In the case of a patient who might experience cardiorespiratory difficulties after extubation, it is incumbent on a physician to ensure that the patient is able to breathe comfortably for about 30 minutes in the complete absence of pressure support or PEEP before removal of the endotracheal tube.[45]

CONCLUSION

In conclusion, to minimize the likelihood of either delayed weaning or premature extubation, a two-step diagnostic strategy is recommended: measurement of weaning predictors followed by a weaning trial. Because each step constitutes a diagnostic test, clinicians must be mindful of the scientific principles of diagnostic testing when interpreting the information generated by each step. The critical step is for the physician to contemplate the possibility that a patient *just might* be able to tolerate weaning. Such diagnostic triggering is assisted through the use of a screening test, which is the rationale for measurement of weaning-predictor tests. Importantly, one should not postpone this first step by waiting for a more complex diagnostic test, such as a T-tube trial. Many complex facets of pulmonary pathophysiology impinge on weaning management. Thus, weaning requires individualized care at a high level of sophistication.

KEY POINTS

- Most patients who fail a trial of weaning from mechanical ventilation do so because of a markedly increased respiratory load, which, in turn, is secondary to severe worsening of respiratory mechanics over the course of the weaning trial.
- Less common reasons for weaning failure include weakened respiratory muscles or impaired cardiovascular performance; primary abnormalities of the respiratory centers or intrapulmonary shunt are uncommon mechanisms of weaning failure.
- Several studies suggest that most patients weaned successfully could have tolerated the weaning attempts had they been initiated a day or more earlier. Such data emphasize the need for the early use of screening tests.
- The primary goal of a screening test is to not miss anybody with the condition under consideration; thus, the test should have a high sensitivity. The ratio of respiratory frequency to tidal volume (f/VT) has been evaluated in more than 25 studies; its average sensitivity is 0.89.
- Weaning involves the undertaking of three diagnostic tests in sequence. The sequential nature of the testing predisposes to the occurrence of test-referral bias and spectrum bias.
- Of the techniques used for a weaning trial, IMV has been repeatedly shown to be inferior to the use of T-tube trials or pressure support.
- Six randomized trials have evaluated the usefulness of protocols in the management of weaning. Three studies observed no benefit with the use of protocols. Two of the remaining three studies had major methodologic problems, leaving only one study supporting the use of protocols.

SELECTED REFERENCES

4. Tobin MJ, Jubran A: Weaning from mechanical ventilation. In Tobin MJ (ed): Principles and Practice of Mechanical Ventilation, 3rd ed. New York, McGraw-Hill, 2012, pp 1185-1220.
5. Brochard L, Rauss A, Benito S, et al: Comparison of three methods of gradual withdrawal from ventilatory support during weaning from mechanical ventilation. Am J Respir Crit Care Med 1994; 150:896-903.
6. Esteban A, Frutos F, Tobin MJ, et al: A comparison of four methods of weaning patients from mechanical ventilation. Spanish Lung Failure Collaborative Group. N Engl J Med 1995;332:345-350.
7. Tobin MJ, Laghi F, Jubran A: Ventilatory failure, ventilator support, and ventilator weaning. Compr Physiol 2012;2:1-51.
10. Jubran A, Tobin MJ: Pathophysiologic basis of acute respiratory distress in patients who fail a trial of weaning from mechanical ventilation. Am J Respir Crit Care Med 1997;155:906-915.
12. Vassilakopoulos T, Zakynthinos S, Roussos C: The tension-time index and the frequency/tidal volume ratio are the major pathophysiologic determinants of weaning failure and success. Am J Respir Crit Care Med 1998;158:378-385.
15. Laghi F, Cattapan SE, Jubran A, et al: Is weaning failure caused by low-frequency fatigue of the diaphragm? Am J Respir Crit Care Med 2003;167:120-127.
22. Tobin MJ, Jubran A: Variable performance of weaning-predictor tests: Role of Bayes' theorem and spectrum and test-referral bias. Intensive Care Med 2006;32:2002-2012.
24. Yang KL, Tobin MJ: A prospective study of indexes predicting the outcome of trials of weaning from mechanical ventilation. N Engl J Med 1991;324:1445-1450.
45. Tobin MJ: Extubation and the myth of "minimal ventilator settings." Am J Respir Crit Care Med 2012;185(4):349-350.

The complete list of references can be found at www.expertconsult.com.

44 Acute Pulmonary Embolism

Kenneth V. Leeper, Jr. | Michael Sterling

CHAPTER OUTLINE

Pulmonary venous thromboembolism (VTE) and deep venous thrombosis (DVT) are different manifestations of the same disease. Despite adequate VTE prophylaxis in the intensive care unit (ICU) the presence of a VTE event is a constant threat to critically ill patients. Although the critical care clinician may encounter the embolization of air, fat, infected clots, amniotic fluid, tumor, and inorganic substances, by far VTE will be the most common pulmonary embolic condition encountered. Critical care clinicians will encounter life-threatening pulmonary embolism (PE) ranging from hemodynamically stable patients with varying degress of right ventricular dysfunction (RVD) to acute massive PE, defined as hemodynamic shock from acute PE, which represents the most serious manifestation along the spectrum of venous thromboembolic disease.[1-3] According to population-based studies, the annual incidence of VTE in the United States has ranged from 200,000 to a recent estimate of 900,000 cases in which approximately 300,000 people die every year from acute PE.[4,5] More recently, in 2006, 467,000 patients were hospitalized with DVT and 247,000 patients were admitted with acute PE.[6] VTE is associated with a significant health care costs. Based on 2004 provider payments, the economic burden of VTE costs ranges between \$5.8 billion and \$7.8 billion.[7]

The mortality rate can exceed 58% in patients with acute PE presenting with shock, and most of these deaths occur within 1 hour of presentation.[1,2] Acute PE is the third most common cause of death among hospitalized patients, and

Additional online-only material indicated by icon.

with an aging population the number of people with VTE is expected to increase. For these reasons, the U.S. Surgeon General issued a "Call to Action" in 2008, identifying VTE as a major public health problem.[8]

The development of DVT occurs largely in the lower extremities and can result in the sequelae of PE, post-thrombotic syndrome, and chronic thrombotic pulmonary hypertension.[9] Venous thrombosis is associated with significant morbidity and mortality rates but can be prevented in most patients.[2,3]

In this chapter we will review the epidemiology, risk factors, diagnosis, risk assessment, and management of acute PE. In our discussion we will review VTE in special adult populations, VTE prophylaxis in the ICU, and long-term prognosis.

PREVALENCE OF VENOUS THROMBOEMBOLISM IN INTENSIVE CARE UNIT PATIENTS

ICU patients represent a heterogeneous population. In prospective screening studies for DVT, in the absence of thromboprophylaxis, the incidence of DVT in a medical-surgical ICU ranges from approximately 13% to 33%.[10-12] In an autopsy review of six studies of 436 critically ill patients the incidence of PE ranged from 7% to 27% (mean 13%); PE contributed or directly caused death in 0% to 12% (mean 3%) of the patients. It is important to note that in a majority of the patients there was no antemortem suspicion of fatal PE.[13]

Contemporary prevalence of VTE that are admitted to or occur in the ICU setting can be obtained from large VTE clinical trials. Approximately 10% of patients entered into the PIOPED-I (Prospective Investigation of Pulmonary Embolism Diagnosis) study for possible PE were hospitalized in a medical or surgical critical care unit.[14] In the recent international, multicenter EINSTEIN PE trial,[15] which randomized 4823 symptomatic PE patients to rivaroxiban or enoxaparin and a vitamin K antagonist, 600 patients (12.4%) required ICU admission. Finally, in the PROTECT trial (Prophylaxis for Thromboembolism in Critical Care Trial)[16] among 3764 critically ill patients enrolled in which a majority were on mechanical ventilator support and 40% were on vasopressor therapy, dalteparin and unfractionated heparin (UFH) were the agents used for VTE prophylaxis. The primary end point was proximal DVT presence. Using compression ultrasonography (CUS), 3.5% of the patients had proximal DVT on admission. The incidence of proximal DVT was 5.1% in the dalteparin group and 5.4% in the UFH group. The proportion of patients with pulmonary emboli was significantly lower with dalteparin (24 patients, 1.3%) than with UFH (43 patients, 2.3%).[16]

There is controversy over routine DVT screening in the ICU. As mentioned earlier, most ICU patients with DVT are asymptomatic and the clinical signs for DVT are nonspecific. CUS is time consuming and not cost effective. Efforts must be made to ensure adherence to current DVT prophylaxis guidelines. In ICU patients in whom these guidelines cannot not be fully implemented (intracranial, spinal, or leg injuries, or patients at increased bleeding risk) then routine CUS screening may be appropriate.[17-21]

RISK FACTORS

In the nineteenth century Virchow described stasis, vascular wall abnormalities, and hypercoagulability as general risk factors for the development of DVT.[22]

As illustrated in Table 44.1, patients admitted to the ICU possess multiple preexisting VTE risks factors on admission to the ICU, yet in the International Cooperative Pulmonary Embolism Registry (ICOPER) 20% of the patients had idiopathic or unprovoked PE.[3]

The interaction between patient-related and setting-related risk factors appears to be responsible for the development of the VTE.[23-25] Patient-related risk factors are usually acquired and are longstanding. Examples of patient-related risk factors are age, history of prior VTE, malignancy, neurologic and medical illnesses that result in immobility, cardiopulmonary disorders, collagen vascular disease, and vasculitis. In addition, patient-related factors may include genetic and acquired thrombophilia and hormone replacement therapy and oral contraceptive therapy. Setting-related risk factors are usually temporary. Examples of setting-related risk factors include hospitalizations, nursing home placement, and admission to the ICU.

Virchow has described several risk factors unique to the ICU setting that predispose patients to VTE events. In a prospective observational study of 93 medical-surgical ICU patients, the investigators identified several ICU-related factors that are associated with increased risk of VTE, including mechanical ventilation, immobility, femoral venous catheters, sedatives and paralytic drugs, and failure to prescribe VTE prophylaxis. Prolonged mobility in the ICU setting is the result of mechanical ventilation, sedative

Table 44.1 Selected Risk Factors for Venous Thromboembolism (VTE)

Genetic Risk Factors	Acquired Risk Factors	Triggering Risk Factors	ICU-Acquired Risk Factors
Antithrombin III deficiency	Age	Surgery	Sepsis
Protein S and C deficiency	Previous VTE	Pregnancy	Vasopressor use
Prothrombin gene mutation	Obesity	Estrogens	Central venous line
	Malignancy	Immobility	Platelet transfusions
	Antiphospholipid syndrome		Pharmacologic paralysis
	Collagen vascular disease		Use of recombinant factor VIIa

ICU, intensive care unit.

administration, and paralytic agents. These four factors (mechanical ventilation, immobility, sedation, and paralysis) may converge to greatly increase the risk of VTE.[26] Sedation and paralysis also predispose to other ICU complications including increased duration of mechanical ventilation, and critical illness polyneuropathy.[27,28]

DEEP VENOUS THROMBOSIS

It is estimated that as high as 95% of clinically significant pulmonary emboli originate from the deep veins of the lower extremity. The proximal deep veins of the leg are the most common sites of origin of clots that embolize to the pulmonary circulation. A general consensus suggests that clinically significant proximal DVTs and risk for PEs originate by proximal extension of calf DVT.[47,48] Venous thrombi are created in the setting of low flow and low shear stress. These thrombi consist of fibrin strands, red blood cells, and platelets. The thrombi form in the valve pockets of calf veins and extend to the proximal veins.[48] After the thrombosis is formed there is raised venous capillary pressure, which increases the transcapillary filtration and the pressure rate, resulting in edema. In approximately 50% of patients, venous outflow obstruction decreases within 3 months by lysis and recanalization.[49] Patients who have early edema are most likely to have residual thrombosis. Clots that continue to propagate have a greater risk to break apart and lead to embolization. This generally occurs more frequently in the first few days after clot formation. Clots that do not continue to propagate resolve by either fibrinolysis or organization. These processes generally occur within 7 days of clot formation.[49,50]

In general only 25% of patients with suspected DVT actually have it.[47] The detection of DVT in critically ill patients is hampered by the patient's inability to report symptoms and the unreliability of physical signs of DVT. CUS is noninvasive and highly sensitive and specific for the diagnosis of proximal lower extremity DVT.[51] Full compressibility of either the femoral or popliteal veins excludes proximal DVT[51] when compared to the gold standard demography; CUS has a sensitivity of 97% to 100% and a specificity of 98% to 99% for the detection of proximal thrombosis. Ultrasonography is less accurate in the diagnosis of distal calf vein thrombosis.[51,52] Whether high-risk critically ill patients should be systematically screened for DVT using CUS, given the high incidence of DVT and limitation of clinical examination, is unresolved.[13,17]

Upper extremity deep venous thrombosis (UEDVT) accounts for approximately 4% of the venous thromboembolic events.[53] Primary UEDVT makes up one third of all UEDVTs. Primary UEDVTs appear to be associated with inherited thrombophilic conditions, and the risk markedly increased to 14-fold when oral contraceptives were used.[54] Catheter UEDVTs are more associated with the placement of a central venous catheter, and these patients are more likely to be inpatients than outpatients, as demonstrated by a large registry.[55] In addition, patients with cancer have an increased occurrence of UEDVT when a central venous catheter is placed in these areas.[55] Catheter-related UEDVT may have a higher pulmonary embolic potential than primary UEDVT.[52]

PATHOPHYSIOLOGY

Nearly two thirds of patients who die from pulmonary thromboembolism die within 1 hour of presentation, but anatomically massive pulmonary emboli (>50% obstruction of the pulmonary circulation) are responsible for only half of the deaths. The term *major pulmonary thromboembolism* has been used to describe any pulmonary thromboembolus that results in a hemodynamically significant event.[1] In patients with pulmonary thromboembolism, hemodynamic presentation is an important predictor of survival. The Urokinase Pulmonary Embolism Trial (UPET) demonstrated that the presence of hemodynamic decompensation was associated with a sevenfold increase in mortality rate.[56] ICOPER confirmed these results by demonstrating a fourfold increase in mortality rate for those patients with hemodynamic instability.[3] Because of the associations between outcome from pulmonary thromboembolism and shock or hypotension, aggressive intervention in patients thought to have pulmonary thromboembolism has given rise to the term *golden hour,* during which timely diagnosis and treatment are paramount.[1]

HEMODYNAMIC CONSEQUENCES

The principal pathophysiologic effects of pulmonary thromboembolism result from the acute impaction of material into pulmonary circulation and the resulting vascular obstruction and humoral mediator release as depicted in Figure 44.1.[57] In nonthrombotic obstruction of the pulmonary vasculature, obliteration of 60% to 70% of the vascular tree is required to cause an elevation of the pulmonary artery pressure. In contrast, only 30% of the vascular tree must be obstructed in pulmonary thromboembolism for elevation of the pulmonary artery pressure to be achieved.[58,59] Therefore, factors other than simple mechanical obstruction of the pulmonary vascular system play a role in the elevation of the pressures in the pulmonary vasculature during pulmonary thromboembolism.

The production of platelet-derived vasoconstrictors may play a role in augmenting the increase in pulmonary vascular resistance (PVR) (Fig. 44.2).[57,58,60] Thromboxane A_2 (TxA_2) is a potent vasoconstrictor and is the end product of arachidonic acid metabolism. TxA_2 is produced by endothelial cells, and even in greater quantities by platelets in response to platelet aggregation. It has been demonstrated that there is increased production of TxA_2 in the early phase of PE, which contributes to the PVR elevation and may be attenuated by cyclooxygenase (COX) inhibition in animal models.[57] Serotonin (5-hydroxytryptamine) is one of the most potent pulmonary vasoconstrictors. Infusion of serotonin in an animal model can actually simulate the signs and symptoms of PE. Like TxA_2, platelets are the primary source of serotonin production in PE. Serotonin antagonism can reduce PVR.[57,60]

As shown in Figure 44.1, the degree of mechanical obstruction, the interplay of neurohumoral mediators, and the patient's underlying cardiopulmonary status will dictate the degree of RVD. A rapid rise in the pulmonary artery resistance produces a significant rise in right ventricular (RV) afterload, thereby causing RV dilatation. The dilation

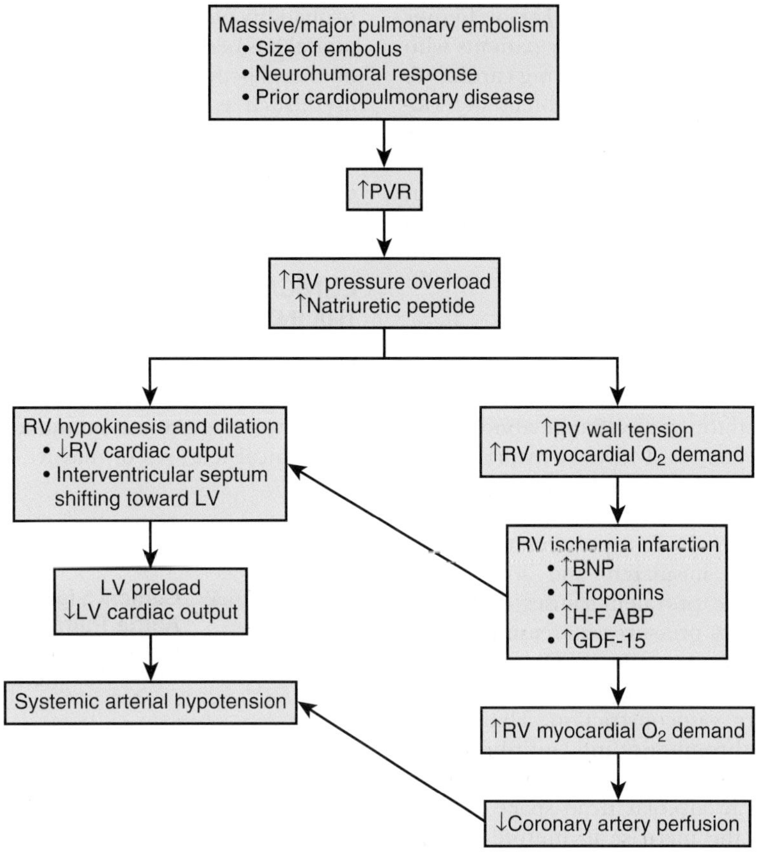

Figure 44.1 The pathophysiology of acute massive/major pulmonary embolism. GDF-15, growth differentiation factor-15; H-FABP, heart type fatty acid binding protein.

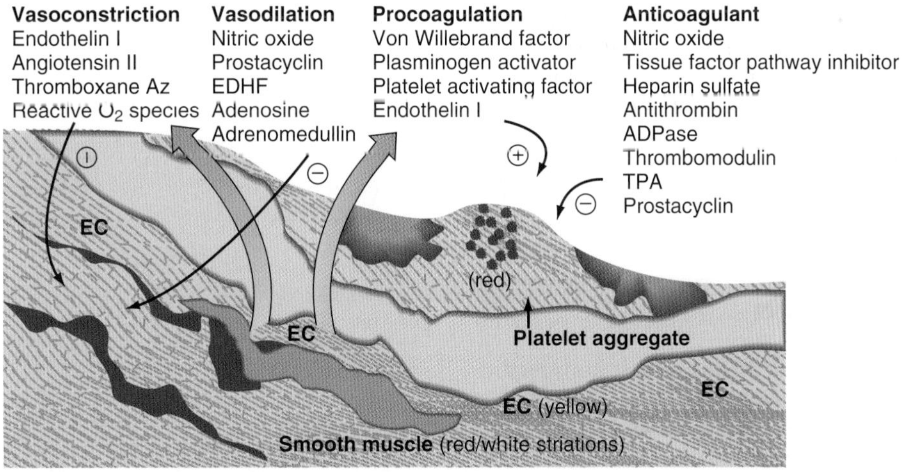

Figure 44.2 Platelet-derived vasoactive factors influencing pulmonary vascular resistance.

of the right ventricle results in shifting of the interventricular septum into the left ventricle, decreasing left ventricular (LV) preload.[61-63] Moreover, RV dilation potentially promotes an increase in constrictive forces by the pericardium, leading to reduced LV compliance. Decreasing LV preload and compliance subsequently lead to lowering of the cardiac output and systemic hypotension with resultant decrease in aortic perfusion pressure and decreasing right coronary perfusion pressure.[64,65] A compromised and burdened right ventricle is a direct result of oxygen demand outstripping oxygen supply, creating an ischemic environment for the right ventricle. The functional status of the cardiopulmonary system is very important in the initial hemodynamic presentation and is a major determinant of short- and long-term outcome.[66] In patients without cardiopulmonary disease the anatomic and humoral obstruction must be 75% or greater to cause a mean pulmonary artery pressure (MPAP) of 40 mm Hg or higher, which is not sustainable; even the previously healthy heart may proceed to cardiovascular collapse and fail.[66] Right atrial pressure (RAP) elevation occurs when the MPAP is 30 mm Hg or higher and obstruction exceeds 35% to 40%.[67] Many patients who have a pulmonary embolic event have underlying cardiopulmonary disease. In these patients cardiopulmonary deterioration (CPD) may occur with a lesser degree of vascular obstruction.[66] This is illustrated by the UKEP (Urokinase-Embolie Pulmonaire) Trial in which an initial presentation of shock with acute PE was seen in 56% of patients who had prior cardiopulmonary disease compared to 2% without cardiopulmonary disease. Obstruction of greater than 50% was uncommon.[68]

RESPIRATORY CONSEQUENCES

Hypoxemia is the most common gas exchange abnormality in patients. However, the Pa_{O_2} and alveolar-arterial (A-a) gradient have been reported to be normal in approximately 30% of patients with PE.[69] Figure 44.2 summarizes the gas exchange abnormalities as a result of the pulmonary embolic event. Ventilation-perfusion mismatch and low mixed venous oxygen levels are the prevalent causes of hypoxemia.[70,71] As pulmonary artery pressures increase, right-to-left flow across a patent foramen ovale (PFO) may occur. Endothelial damage may result from hypoxic exposure and further lead to pulmonary vasoconstriction. Hypoxemia may even promote a prothrombotic and antifibrinolytic effect.[57]

In acute PE an increase in alveolar dead space impairs CO_2 elimination; however, the increase in minute ventilation results in hypocapnia. In patients with massive PE there can be a paradoxical elevation of the Pa_{CO_2} as a result of a marked increase in dead space ventilation.[72] In PE patients because of an increase in alveolar dead space there is a reduction in alveolar CO_2 content, which can be detected by capnography by a reduction in the capnographic waveform area. In one study, PE patients significantly demonstrated a reduction in the capnographic waveform area when compared to patients without PE.[73] There is widening of the $P_{ET}CO_2$-Pa_{CO_2} gradient. Bedside $P_{ET}CO_2$ coupled with a Wells score has been shown to have a high negative predictive value.[74]

CLINICAL PRESENTATION

The signs and symptoms of acute PE are at best nonspecific. The presence of syncope, current DVT, hemoptysis, leg swelling, active cancer, surgery, leg pain, and shock each marginally increases the probability of PE. Further, the absence of dyspnea or tachycardia marginally reduces the probability of PE.[75]

Approximately 50% of patients with acute PE present to the emergency department. In the Emperor Registry, among 1880 documented PE patients from 22 U.S. emergency departments, the most common presenting signs and symptoms were dyspnea at rest (50%), pleuritic chest pain (39%), dyspnea with exertion (24%), and syncope, which occurred in 5% as the initial presentation of acute PE. Only 58 patients (3%) had systolic blood pressures of 90 mm Hg or lower on presentation.[76]

Clinical prediction rules have been used in the emergency department setting to determine the pretest probability of acute PE.[77] The most widely known prediction model has been the Wells score and it can allow for a dichotomous classification.[78,79] Other prediction scores have been used, such as the Geneva and the modified Geneva.[77,78] All prediction scores appear to have similar accuracy but are influenced by the local prevalence of PE. The clinical prediction scores are enhanced in identifying the patient with low probability of PE coupled with low D-dimer value.[79]

CLINICAL PRESENTATION ON ADMISSION TO THE INTENSIVE CARE UNIT

In patients admitted to the ICU with PE the clinical manifestations may be more demonstrative, as shown in Table 44.2. In the Urokinase Pulmonary Embolism Trial (UPET), the clinical features of massive PE were evaluated. Sudden

Table 44.2 Clinical Signs and Symptoms of Acute Pulmonary Embolism Potentially Requiring Intensive Care Unit Management

Clinical Variable	Frequency (%) Submassive PE	Massive PE	*p* Value
Symptoms	78	86	<0.01
Dyspnea	85	97	<0.01
Pleuritic pain	50	70	<0.01
Apprehension	20	44	<0.01
Altered mental status	4	17	<0.05
Diaphoresis	47	62	<0.01
Syncope	85	81	
Signs	51	50	
Tachycardia (heart rate >100 beats/min)	47	66	
Tachypnea (respiratory rate >20 breaths/min)	81	87	
Fever (>37.5° C)	51	50	
Deep venous thrombosis	47	39	
Cyanosis	3	24	<0.05
Other Signs			
Jugular venous distention			
Shock		12*	
Cardiac arrest (PEA)			

PE, pulmonary embolism; PEA, pulseless electrical activity.
*Adapted from Stein PD, Willis PW III, DeMets DL: History and physical examination in acute pulmonary embolism in patients without pre-existing cardiac or pulmonary disease. Am J Cardiol 1981;47;218-223.

unexplained onset of dyspnea was the most common symptom and was present in 80% of the patients. A majority of the patients had a well-defined risk factor. Tachypnea and tachycardia were present in 88% and 63% of the patients, respectively. Accentuated second heart sound was noted in 67%, and S_3 or S_4 gallop was present in 47%. Clinical shock was noted in 12%.[80] Syncope can occur. Retrosternal non-pleuritic chest pain may mimic the pain experienced with a myocardial infarction and represent demand ischemia of the right ventricle. The differential diagnosis of pulseless electrical activity (PEA) is massive PE and should be expected when there is a known major risk factor.

The signs and symptoms of submassive PE will depend upon the degree of RVD. Dyspnea may be progressive over the last 4 to 6 days. Chest pain can be either pleuritic or nonpleuritic in nature. If pulmonary infarction occurs as result of distal embolization, then hemoptysis may occur. From the PIOPED II database, 92% of patients with main or lobar pulmonary emboli had dyspnea or tachycardia in contrast to segmental emboli dyspnea and tachycardia, where 65% had these findings.[81,82]

Patients with massive PE and shock manifest systemic hypotension, poor perfusion of the extremities, tachycardia, and tachypnea. In addition, patients appear weak, pale, diaphoretic, oliguric, and develop altered mental status. The patient may be hypoxemic and require high flow oxygen or urgent intubation and mechanical ventilation. Varying degrees of RVD may be observed. The presence of jugular venous distention, with and without inspiratory collapse, RV heave, summation gallop, accentuated P_2, and presence of tricuspid regurgitation represent the impact the embolus has had on pulmonary vasculature and RV function. If a central line is placed via the subclavian or jugular route, the $Scvo_2$ is usually less than 65%.

RECOGNITION OF PULMONARY EMBOLISM DURING INTENSIVE CARE UNIT ADMISSION

When a patient is admitted to the ICU for a non-PE-related clinical diagnosis, the abrupt and unexplained occurrence of some combination of chest pain, dyspnea, tachypnea, hypotension, and hypoxemia should raise the suspicion of PE. Unexplained fever with and without mild leukocytosis could represent a possible VTE event.[83] Hemoptysis can occur as a result of small distal pulmonary emboli causing alveolar hemorrhage. If PE occurs while the critically ill patient or postoperative patient is on mechanical ventilation, the clinical suspicion and conformation can be difficult. An increase in minute ventilation dead space or an increase in supplemental oxygen may be clues to an embolic event. If the patient has end-tidal CO_2 (P_{ETCO_2}) monitoring an increase in the $Paco_2$-P_{ETCO_2} gradient may occur.[73]

DIAGNOSTIC TESTING FOR PULMONARY EMBOLISM

ARTERIAL BLOOD GAS MEASUREMENT

Hypoxemia and an increased alveolar-arterial gradient are usually seen in PE but can be normal in about 14% and are most likely the result of small embolic events.[84,85] The initial acid-base disturbance is a respiratory alkalosis, which may evolve to a metabolic (lactic) acidosis as hypotension and shock ensue. A linear relationship between PE severity and Pao_2 in patients without prior cardiopulmonary disease has been described. In the UPET and PIOPED trials 12% and 19% of patients, respectively, had Pao_2 80 mm Hg or greater.[86] Hypocarbia is usually present with acute PE because of hyperventilation, but hypercapnia can occur with large PEs producing increased dead space.[87,72]

CHEST RADIOGRAPHY

The chest radiograph is abnormal in most cases of PE; however, radiographic findings possess inadequate sensitivity to rule out PE. Common radiographic abnormalities include atelectasis, pleural effusion, parenchymal opacities, and elevation of a hemidiaphragm. Radiographic findings of pulmonary infarction often show a wedge-shaped, pleural-based triangular opacity with an apex pointing toward the hilus (Hampton hump). Focal oligemia or decreased vascularity has been known as the Westermark sign. These findings are suggestive of PE but are infrequently prospectively observed.[88,89] Radiographic findings of RVD may include a prominent central pulmonary artery (knuckle sign) and cardiomegaly. In one large prospective cohort of PE patients a normal chest radiograph was found in 24% of the patients.[89] A normal-appearing chest radiograph in a patient with severe dyspnea and hypoxemia, is suggestive of a pulmonary embolic event.

ELECTROCARDIOGRAPHY

In 1935 McGinn and White first described the association between acute PE and specific electrocardiogram (ECG) changes when they noted the $S_1Q_3T_3$ pattern in seven patients with acute cor pulmonale.[90] A normal ECG can occur with PE in a frequency ranging from 9% to 30%. The most common ECG abnormalities in the setting of PE are tachycardia and nonspecific ST-T wave abnormalities. The classic findings of right-sided heart strain and acute cor pulmonale are tall, peaked P waves in lead II (P pulmonale); right-axis deviation; right bundle branch block; and an $S_1Q_3T_3$ pattern. Only 20% of patients with proven PE have any of these classic ECG abnormalities.[91-93] T-wave inversion in the precordial leads representing subepicardial ischemia may be seen. The presence of this ECG finding is associated with increased degree of vascular obstruction and elevation of the pulmonary artery (PA) pressure.[94] The new onset of atrial fibrillation has been thought to be associated with a pulmonary embolic event. In a recent study the occurrence of atrial fibrillation did not in general increase the probability of PE.[95] However, if chest pain were the only symptom, the presence of atrial fibrillation increases the probability of PE (odds ratio [OR] 2.42, 95% confidence interval [CI] 0.97-6.07).

D-DIMER ASSAY

The serum D-dimer is a degradation product produced by plasmin-mediated proteases of cross-linked fibrin. D-dimer is measured by a variety of assays. These assays are categorized as quantitative, semiquantitative, qualitative rapid enzyme-linked immunosorbent assays (ELISAs); quantitative and semiquantitative latex; and whole-blood assays. The quanitative rapid ELISAs are the best assays to use in terms of sensitivity and likelihood ratio.[96] When clinical prediction scores indicate that the patient has a low or moderate pretest probability of PE, D-dimer testing is useful to further define the likelihood of PE. Negative results on a high-sensitivity D-dimer test in a patient with a low pretest probability of PE (Wells rule) are associated with a low likelihood of VTE and reliably exclude PE.[97] In a large prospective, randomized trial in patients with a low probability of PE who had negative D-dimer results, not performing additional diagnostic testing was not associated with an increased frequency of symptomatic VTE during the subsequent 6 months.[98]

D-dimer testing loses its ability to predict the likelihood of PE in older patients and in the presence of cancer, pregnancy, and various inflammatory or infectious disorders. If the pretest probability for PE is high, D-dimer testing should not be performed and objective testing should be done.[96]

Combining D-dimer results with measurement of the exhaled end-tidal ratio of carbon dioxide to oxygen (P_{ETCO_2}/P_{O_2}) can be useful for diagnosis of PE. Kline and colleagues demonstrated in moderate-risk patients a positive D-dimer (>499 ng/mL) and a P_{ETCO_2}/P_{O_2} less than 0.28 significantly increased the probability of finding segmental or larger PE on computed tomography (CT) multidetector-row pulmonary angiography.[99] In contrast, a P_{ETCO_2}/P_{O_2} greater than 0.45 predicted the absence of segmental or larger PE.

DUPLEX COMPRESSION ULTRASONOGRAPHY

Currently, DVT is largely diagnosed by duplex CUS. When using CUS, the ultrasonographic transducer pressed against veins shows they are easily compressed, but the muscular arteries are extremely resistant to compression. Where DVT is present, the veins do not collapse completely when pressure is applied using the ultrasonographic probe.[100-102]

Before an ultrasonographic scan can be considered negative, the entire deep venous system must be examined using centimeter-by-centimeter compression testing of every vessel. The risk of a DVT event following a single whole leg CUS in 3 months is 0.57% (95% CI 0.25-0.89).[103]

CUS is associated with a sensitivity of 97% for proximal DVT, 72% for distal DVT, and a specificity of 94%.[104] In a meta-analysis of the role of CUS in DVT, CUS alone had a sensitivity of 93.8% (92.0-95.3%) for proximal DVT, 56.8% (49.0-66.4%) for distal DVT, and specificity of 97.8% (97.0-98.4%).[105]

VENTILATION-PERFUSION NUCLEAR SCANS

The $\dot{V}/\dot{Q}$ scan has a limited role in the diagnosis of acute PE in the ICU, although its diagnostic accuracy is no different from that in non–critically ill populations.[106] Because of the advancing technology of CT scanning, the lung scan is used in the critical care units in special circumstances such as renal insufficiency or in the patient who is not intubated and capable of transport from the ICU to the nuclear medicine suite for a full view scan. If the institution has a portable lung scanner this can be used in the ICU but the number of images is reduced when compared to the standard $\dot{V}/\dot{Q}$ scan.

A high-probability scan, as shown in Figure 44.3, is sufficient diagnostic evidence of PE to begin anticoagulation therapy, and a normal $\dot{V}/\dot{Q}$ scan is considered sufficient evidence to exclude PE. However, the frequency of low- or intermediate-probability scans (indeterminate scans) can be as high as 50% to 70%, with a 10% to 50% probability of PE. Therefore, it is impossible to initiate anticoagulation therapy based on this indeterminate lung scan probability. In the first PIOPED study, only 40% of patients with PE had a high-probability $\dot{V}/\dot{Q}$ scan result, whereas another 40% of patients with PE had an indeterminate result and 14% had a low-probability result. A high-probability $\dot{V}/\dot{Q}$ scan had a positive predictive value of 88% in patients without prior history of PE. The combination of a high clinical probability with the high-probability lung scan resulted in a 96% positive predictive value. The negative predictive value of a low-probability scan was 88% and improved to 96% when combined with a low clinical probability. Thus, a low-probability scan with a low clinical probability score rules out PE as definitively as a normal scan. Finally, 39% of the patients had intermediate scans and 32% of these patients had angiographically proven PE.[14,107]

Preexisting cardiopulmonary disease diminishes the clinical utility of $\dot{V}/\dot{Q}$ scans by increasing the prevalence of nondiagnostic scans. Nondiagnostic scans are more likely to occur in patients with preexisting cardiopulmonary disease. Lung scans are not useful to either establish or rule out the diagnosis of PE in more than 80% of cases. A similar disadvantage of $\dot{V}/\dot{Q}$ lung scans is noted in critically ill patients with prior cardiopulmonary disease. Nevertheless, $\dot{V}/\dot{Q}$ lung scans can be performed in the critically ill, even if patients are receiving mechanical ventilation, and chest radiographic abnormalities can be used as a surrogate of ventilation defects. Despite the limited ventilation component under positive-pressure respiration, the perfusion component is not significantly affected by mechanical ventilation. $\dot{V}/\dot{Q}$ scans remain a useful tool in patients with contraindications to pulmonary angiography or CT angiography.[108,109]

MULTIDETECTOR COMPUTED TOMOGRAPHY SCAN OF THE CHEST

The PIOPED II study firmly established the role of CT pulmonary angiography (CTPA) and largely replaced ventilation-perfusion ($\dot{V}/\dot{Q}$) lung scintigraphy as the main imaging modality in suspected PE.[110] The technology is continually evolving and its use is widespread. As illustrated in Figure 44.4, CTPA provides direct visualization of emboli throughout the pulmonary arterial vasculature. The advantage of CTPA over pulmonary angiography and lung scan is the discovery of an alternative diagnosis when PE is not found on CTPA. In one study, an alternative diagnosis was established in 57% of patients who did not have a PE.[111] Currently, CTPA is the "gold standard" for PE diagnosis. A meta-analysis of 23 studies with 4657 patients with a negative CTPA who did not receive anticoagulation showed a 3-month rate of subsequent VTE of 1.4% (95% CI 1.1-1.8) and a 3-month rate of fatal PE of 0.51% (0.33-0.76), which compares favorably with the results noted after a normal "gold

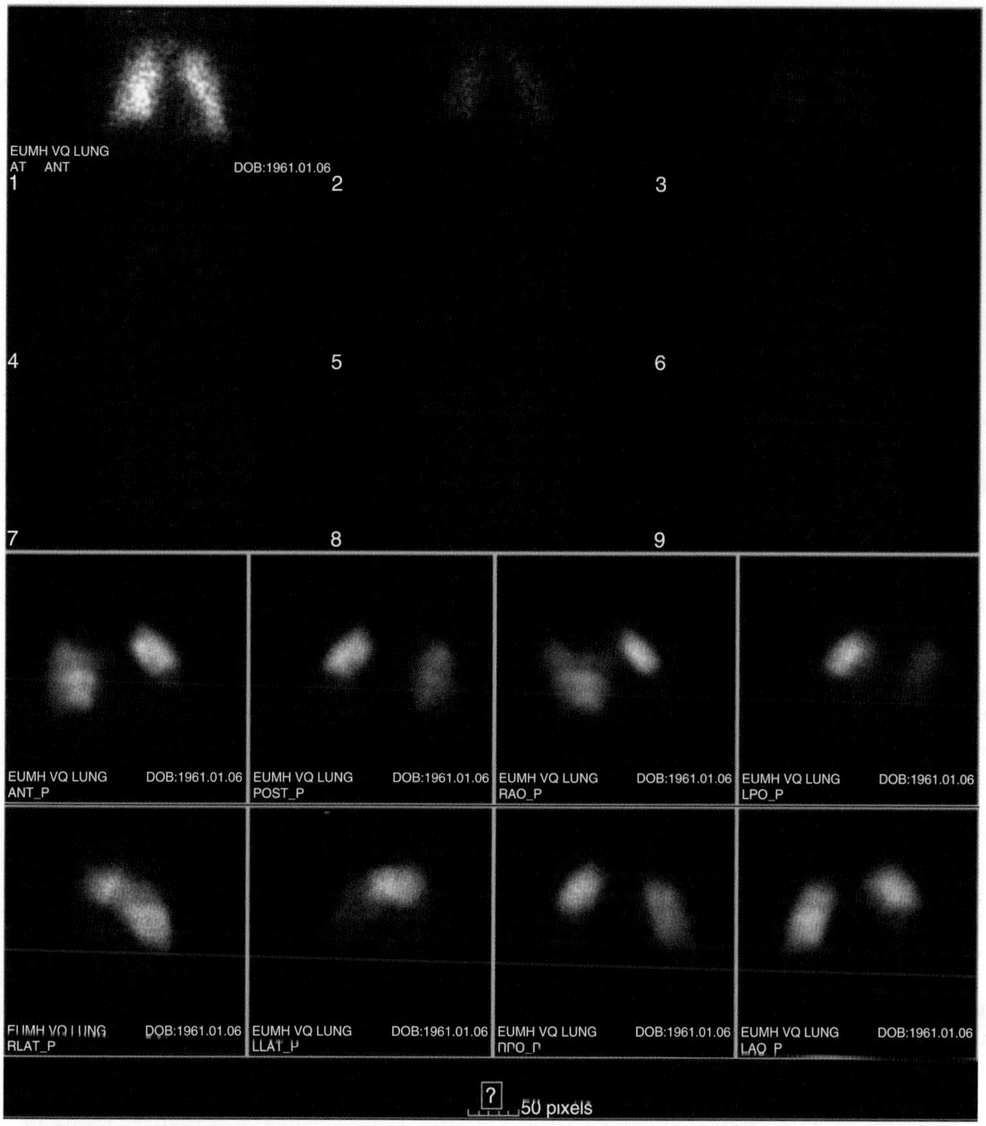

Figure 44.3 High-probability ventilation-perfusion lung scan in a patient with submassive pulmonary embolism and right ventricular strain. Large left lung perfusion defects with a right upper lobe apical perfusion defect are present. Ventilation is normal.

standard" invasive contrast pulmonary angiogram.[112] The increased use of CTPA raises concerns about the increased incidence of cancer attributable to radiation.[113] For this reason, combined use of CTPA and CT leg venography should not be performed because the latter adds little to diagnostic utility. In the PIOPED II trial, no patient with PE or DVT would have been undiagnosed if imaging of the pelvic and proximal leg veins had been omitted.[107,110]

MAGNETIC RESONANCE IMAGING

In the PIOPED II study, CT angiography of the chest, as many as 25% of patients had a contraindication for the test. Preexisting renal failure and pregnancy were the primary conditions that prevented this mode from being used as the primary test for the evaluation of PE.[110] Thus, gadolinium-enhanced magnetic resonance pulmonary angiography (MRA) could potentially be used to diagnose PE because it is devoid of radiation. The accuracy of this technique combined with magnetic resonance venography (MRV) has been studied in the prospective, multicenter PIOPED III accuracy study. The proportion of technically inadequate images ranged from 11% to 52% across the seven participating centers. Technically adequate MRA had a sensitivity of 78% and a specificity of 99%, whereas technically adequate MRA and MRV had a sensitivity of 92% and a specificity of 96%. However, 194 (52%) of 370 patients had technically inadequate results, which substantially restricts its clinical use.[114]

RISK STRATIFICATION

Death from an embolic event almost always results from hemodynamic deterioration due to an abrupt rise in pulmonary vascular resistance overwhelming the contractile power of the right ventricle. Progressive hemodynamic and respiratory deterioration characterizes the clinical presentation of major or massive PE and is seen in approximately 5% of PE patients.[2] Patients can be categorized as having submassive

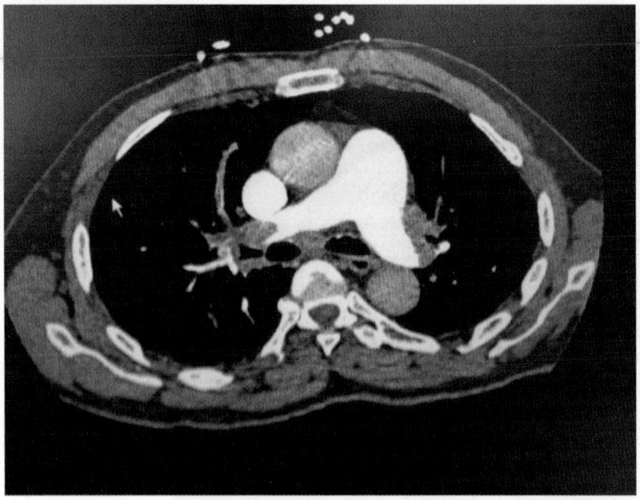

Figure 44.4 Extensive bilateral lobar pulmonary emboli.

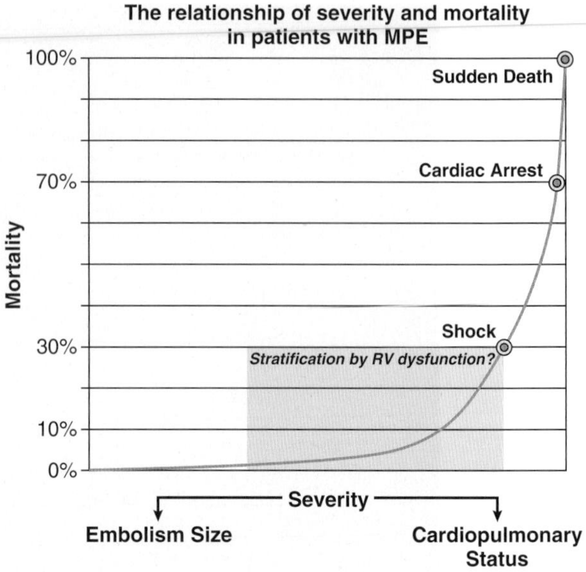

Figure 44.5 Pulmonary embolism mortality rate based on initial hemodynamic presentation.

PE. Risk stratification becomes important to identify this group of patients who present with relative hemodynamic stability but exhibit varying degrees of RVD. Risk stratification schemes in normotensive patients center on RV function assessment after an embolic event and identify patients who may be at risk for progressive hemodynamic deterioration. Approximately 50% of patients who are normotensive have varying degrees of RVD and 10% will die. The European Society of Cardiology recommends a classification of PE into high-risk and non–high-risk groups. The high-risk groups represent the massive or major PE presentations. The non–high-risk group is further subdivided into intermediate risk in which the mortality rate ranges between 3% and 15% and a low-risk group in which the mortality rate is less than 3%. Initial therapeutic interventions are greatly influenced by risk stratification that includes clinical scoring systems, laboratory data, and imaging.[115-117]

The presence of RVD is a predictor of the increased risk of embolic-related adverse events and mortality rates when compared with patients without RVD.[2] Patients who present with circulatory shock usually have severe RVD and have mortality rates up to 65%.[1,2,115] In PE patients with normal hemodynamics and evidence of RVD the mortality rates can range from 8% to 14%. Several registry studies have observed that the frequency of RVD in normotensive patients is approximately 40%.[116,117] In PE patients with initial normal hemodynamics and no RVD the mortality rate is low (0-3%).

CLINICAL AND HEMODYNAMIC PARAMETERS

The initial hemodynamic presentation of PE is the most powerful predictor of outcome, as illustrated in Figure 44.5. Arterial hypotension at the time of PE presentation is an early predictor of death. In the 2392 patients from the ICOPER study, the 90-day mortality rates were 52.4% in patients with systolic arterial blood pressures below 90 mm Hg, and 14.7% in those patients who had preserved arterial blood pressures. In addition, comorbid conditions increase the risk of adverse clinical events, even in the presence of anatomically small PE. In the ICOPER findings, age over 70, congestive heart failure, cancer, and chronic lung disease were identified as independent predictors of 3-month mortality risk, with approximately twofold increase in the risk of death.[2] In one study, altered mental status at presentation was associated with a sevenfold increase in risk of adverse outcome. Altered mental status most likely reflected decreased cardiac perfusion or hypoxia. In the same study the initial presentation of shock was associated with a threefold increase in risk of 30-day adverse outcome (death, secondary shock, or recurrent PE).[117]

Patients can be clinically risk stratified by the use of a clinical scoring system known as the Pulmonary Embolism Severity Index (PESI), which also has a simplified version.[118,119] This prognostic model was developed by Aujesky and colleagues (Table 44.3) using a large database of hospitalized PE patients from which they derived and validated a prediction rule that identified acute PE patients with low to high risk for fatal PE and adverse events. Using 11 variables of predictors, five distribution categories emerged looking at inpatient fatality, 30-day all-cause mortality rate, and the adverse outcomes of nonfatal cardiogenic shock or cardiopulmonary arrest. Class I to class III all-cause mortality rates ranged between 0% and 3.1%, although class IV to class V all-cause mortality rates were between 10% and 24%. This score has an excellent negative predictive value and readily identifies low-risk patients but suffers in the attempt to predict patients at high risk for adverse events.[119] A more simplied PESI score has been developed and has a high negative prediction value.[120]

In patients with symptomatic acute PE, the presence of DVT may have prognostic significance. In a prospective study by Jiménez and coworkers, among 707 patients diagnosed with acute PE, 51.2% had concomitant DVT and 10.9% had PE-specific fatality at a 3-month follow-up. Patients with PE with the presence of DVT at the time of diagnosis had an adjusted hazard ratio (HR) of 2.05% (95% CI 1.24 to 3.38) and PE-specific fatality-adjusted HR of 4.25 (95% CI 1.61 to 11.25). These findings were validated by a large international registry trial (RIETE) that again demonstrated a significant prediction of all-cause mortality rate

Table 44.3 Pulmonary Embolism Severity Index (PESI)

Scoring

Predictor	Points Assigned
Age	Age, in years
Male gender	+10
Cancer	+30
Heart failure	+10
Chronic lung disease	+10
Pulse >110 beats/min	+20
Systolic blood pressure <100 mm Hg	+30
Respiratory rate >30 breaths/min	+20
Temperature <36° C	+20
Altered mental status	+60
Arterial Sao_2 <90%	+20

Risk Classification

Class and Distribution	Score Range	Inpatient Mortality Rate (%)	30-Day Mortality Rate (%)	Nonfatal Cardiogenic Shock or Cardiopulmonary Arrest
Class I (19.4%)	<65	0.8	1.1	0.4
Class II (21.5%)	65-85	1.8	3.1	1.3
Class III (21.7%)	85-105	4.2	6.5	2.1
Class IV (16.4%)	106-125	5.9	10.4	1.9
Class V (21.0%)	<125	15.8	24.5	4.6

Adapted from Aujesky D, Obrosky DS, Stone RA, et al: Derivation and validation of a prognostic model for pulmonary embolism. Am J Respir Crit Care Med 2005;172:1041-1046.

and PE-specific mortality rate when the concomitant DVT was present during the acute embolic event. These results suggest that patients with symptomatic acute PE have an increase in all-cause mortality rate, PE-related death, and recurrent VTE over a 3-month period if at the time of PE a diagnosis of proximal DVT is also present.[121]

ELECTROCARDIOGRAM

Several studies have demonstrated that ECG signs of RV strain correlate with the presence of RVD.[122,123] A study by Punukollu and associates showed that T-wave inversion in leads V_1 to V_3 had a specificity of 88% and diagnostic accuracy of 81% for RVD in acute PE.[124] Daniel and colleagues developed an ECG scoring system based on typical features of acute PE such as presence of right bundle branch block (RBBB), T-wave inversions, and additional features of right-sided heart strain that predicted severe pulmonary hypertension (sPAP >50 mm Hg) with a specificity of 97.7% if the patient's "ECG score" is 10 or greater.[125] The ECG may also be a tool for risk stratification of normotensive acute PE patients. In a study by Vanni and coworkers among 306 patients with documented PE 130 (34%), patients demonstrated ECG findings of right-sided heart strain. In this study ECG findings of right-sided heart strain were defined as incomplete or complete RBBB, $S_1Q_3T_3$, or inverted T waves in the precordial leads V_1, V_2, and V_3. For this study only one of these ECG patterns had to be present. The investigators demonstrated that the presence of RV strain on the initial ECG was associated with clinical deterioration and death (HR 2.58) in normotensive PE patients.[122]

CARDIAC BIOMARKERS

Biomarkers are relied on in the risk stratification of patients with PE. Tests for biomarkers are widely available and there is usually a quick turnaround from the clinical laboratory. Caution must be taken on the interpretation of these biomarkers. It is important for the critical care clinician to understand the clinical issues that impact the interpretation of the biomarkers and understand the negative and positive predictive values.[115] Elevations of brain natriuretic peptide (BNP) and troponin occur in many patients with PE and correlate with magnitude of RVD.

ECHOCARDIOGRAPHY

The echocardiogram has become the main imaging modality to assess RV structure and function. In addition, pulmonary artery pressures can be estimated. Most hospitals in the United States have portable echocardiographic technology allowing for serial assessment of the impact of treatment on RVD. In hemodynamically stable patients with PE, 20% to 40% will have some echocardiographic finding of RVD.[116,117] Box 44.1 illustrates the echocardiographic finding of acute PE. Toosi and colleagues performed a quantitative risk assessment of various echocardiographic measurements of RVD in acute PE. For in-patient mortality rate the positive predictive values range between 11% and 20% and the negative predictive values are 97% to 100%.[140] The major drawback with the role of the echocardiographic definition of RVD of acute PE is that it lacks standardization. There is no clear agreement on which of the echocardiographic

Box 44.1 Echocardiographic Features of Acute Pulmonary Embolism

Global reduction of RV function
RV dilation
RV hypokinesis
McConnell's sign (free wall hypokinesis sparing of the apex)
Interventricular septal flattening
"D-shaped" LV resulting from paradoxical septal motion
RV/LV thrombus
Dilated inferior vena cava without inspiratory collapse
Pulmonary hypertension
Tricupid regurgitation with a jet velocity >2.6 m/sec
Patent foramen ovale (PFO)—result of increased pulmonary artery pressures

LV, left ventricle; RV, right ventricle.

findings predicts adverse outcomes and fatality in normotensive submassive PE. However, an echocardiographic finding of right ventricle/left ventricle ratio of greater than 0.9 was found to be an independent risk factor of in-hospital death (OR 2.7% CI 1.7-6.0) in a large registry trial.[141]

In the ICOPER study that included 1035 PE patients with systolic arterial pressure 90 mm Hg or higher, an echocardiogram was performed within 24 hours of PE diagnosis. The incidence of RVD was 39% (405 patients). The 30-day survival rates were lower in patients with RV hypokinesis (84%) compared with those without RV hypokinesis (91%), HR 1.94 (CI, 1.41-3.16; $p \leq 0.001$). The negative predictive value of 30-day mortality rate of echocardiographic confirmation of RVD was 91%. The positive predictive value was 16%.[2]

In the assessment of RVD, if cardiac biomarkers are elevated, how well does this correlate with RVD on transthoracic echocardiography? A study by Logeart and coworkers found that a BNP level of less than 100 pg/mL had a negative predictive value of 100% and TnI of less than 0.10 ng/mL had a negative predictive value of 67% for the presence of RVD on echocardiography. Combining a BNP of greater than 100 pg/mL and TnI of greater than 0.10 ng/mL had a positive predictive value of 80% for the presence of RVD by echocardiography.[142]

The echocardiogram can visualize free-floating right-sided heart thrombi. In the ICOPER study patients with this finding had a mortality rate of 21% compared with 11% in those without right-sided heart thrombi.[143] The detection of a patent forman ovale or atrial septal defect by echocardiography may be a warning finding for the development of paradoxical embolization, which is associated with a risk of stroke and increased mortality rate.[144]

For the evaluation of circulatory shock transesophageal echocardiography (TEE) is a useful diagnostic modality. In patients with massive PE who cannot undergo CTPA, when TEE is performed, it has a 60% to 80% sensitivity and a 95% to 100% specificity to diagnose acute PE. TEE has a 9% to 95% sensitivity and a 100% specificity in main pulmonary artery PE.[145] In patients with unexplained cardiac arrest or pulseless electrical activity (PEA), TEE has been shown to identify acute massive PE. In a small study of 25 patients with PEA, TEE demonstrated eight (36%) patients with massive PE.[146]

Echocardiography is an important diagnostic and prognostic tool in the management of patients with PE. Echocardiography also influences the therapeutic strategy based on cardiac hemodynamics and RV function. It is simple, quick, noninvasive, accurate, convenient, and safe, while providing critical information on the physiologic effects of PE on cardiac hemodynamics as well as RV size and function.

COMPUTED TOMOGRAPHY PULMONARY ANGIOGRAPHY

CT scans findings of right-sided heart dysfunction are illustrated in Figures 44.6A and B. The detection of RV enlargement by spiral chest CT has recently been evaluated in the risk stratification of patients with acute PE. Using measurements from a reconstructed CT four-chamber view, RV enlargement, defined as a ratio of RV to LV dimension of greater than 0.9, was a significant independent predictor of 30-day mortality rate.[146] In a recent multicenter study of 460 consecutive patients with multidetector CT confirmed PE a majority of the study cohort were hemodynamically stable and 50% had RVD at the time of diagnosis. Again, an RV/LV ratio of 0.9 or greater provided good correlation with RVD demonstrated by echocardiography. In addition, RVD found on multidetector CT was an independent risk factor for death and clinical deterioration. The investigators propose that multidetector CT scan potentially can be the single procedure, not only for diagnosis of PE but also for risk stratification. However, this assumption will require more validation studies.[112]

In hemodynamically stable patients with acute PE, assessing RV/LV ratio may be important in not only risk stratification but also the location of the emboli. In a recent multicenter study of 516 hemodynamically stable PE patients central localization of emboli was found to be an independent mortality risk factor, although distal localization was inversely associated with adverse events. Thus, anatomic findings by CT scan may be important in assessing risk in hemodynamically stable patients with pulmonary embolus.[147]

Table 44.4 summarizes the various risk modalities used in risk stratification of acute PE.

THE MANAGEMENT OF ACUTE PULMONARY EMBOLISM

PHARMACOLOGIC MANAGEMENT

The anticoagulation treatment for DVT and acute PE is essentially the same. Anticoagulation therapy does not dissolve the clot but prevents extension. Anticoagulation therapy indirectly decreases clot burden by allowing the natural fibrinolytic system to dissolve thrombus. When PE is suspected, if there is no contraindication, anticoagulation therapy should be started immediately while diagnostic studies are being performed.[148]

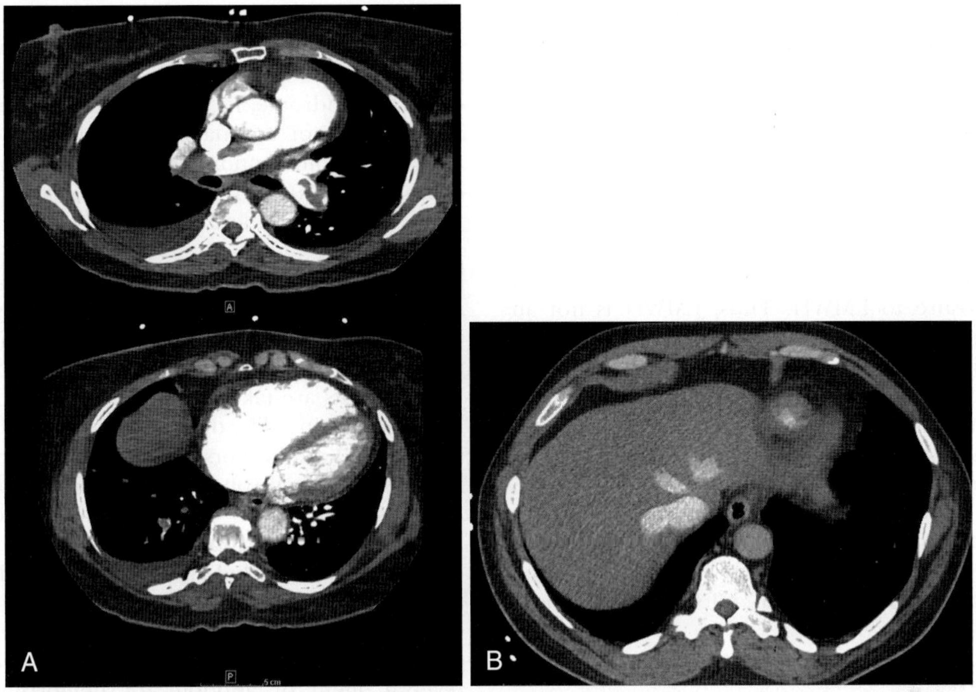

Figure 44.6 **A,** Computed tomography (CT) scan findings of major pulmonary emboli with right ventricular dysfunction (RVD). **B,** CT scan findings of RVD (RV/LV ratio >0.09). B Hepatic reflux of contrast indicated significant RVD.

Table 44.4 Risk Stratification Determination in Acute Pulmonary Embolism

Risk Stratification Test	RV Dysfunction Potentially Present
Compression ultrasonography	Presence of proximal DVT
Natriuretic peptide	BNP >90 pg/mL NT-proBNP >500 pg/mL
Cardiac troponins	TnT >0.1 ng/mL TnI >0.4 ng/mL
Transthoracic echocardiography	Apical four-chamber view: RV/LV ratio >0.9 Qualitative RV systolic dysfunction
Chest computed tomography pulmonary angiogram (CTPA)	Reconstructed four-chamber view: RV/LV ratio >0.9
Electrocardiogram	New complete or incomplete RBBB Anteroseptal ST-segment elevation or depression Anteroseptal T-wave inversion

BNP, brain natriuretic peptide; DVT, deep venous thrombosis; LV, left ventricle; RBBB, right bundle branch block; RV, right ventricle.

UNFRACTIONATED AND LOW-MOLECULAR-WEIGHT HEPARIN

Heparins act by binding to the natural anticoagulant antithrombin, thereby accelerating the inactivation of thrombin by antithrombin and several other activated coagulation factors This mechanism of action will prevent extension of the thrombus. UFH is usually administered as an initial bolus, followed by a continuous intravenous infusion. Because of a large individual difference in the binding of heparins to plasma proteins, the doses should be adjusted to the results of the activated partial thromboplastin time (aPTT) or the anti–factor Xa (anti-Xa) activity.[149]

The effectiveness of heparin therapy depends largely on achieving a critical therapeutic level of heparin within the first 24 hours of treatment. Nomogram dosing of heparin has been shown to achieve this goal.[150] The critical therapeutic level of heparin is 1.5 times the baseline control value or the upper limit of normal range of the aPTT. This level of anticoagulation is expected to correspond to a heparin blood level of 0.2 to 0.4 U/mL by the protamine sulfate titration assay and 0.3 to 0.6 by the anti-Xa assay.[151] If intravenous UFH is chosen, an initial bolus of 80 U/kg or 5000 U followed by an infusion of 18 U/kg/hour or 1300 U/hour should be given, with the goal of rapidly achieving and maintaining the aPTT at levels that correspond to therapeutic heparin levels. Fixed-dose and monitored regimens of subcutaneous UFH are available and are acceptable alternatives.[148,150]

Low-molecular-weight heparins (LMWHs) have many advantages over UFH. These agents have a greater bioavailability, can be administered by subcutaneous injections once or twice a day, and have a longer duration of anticoagulant effect. There is a lower risk of osteoporosis and immune-mediated thrombocytopenia.[152] A fixed dose of LMWH can be used and laboratory monitoring is not necessary except in clinical circumstances such as morbid obesity, low weight (<40 kg), pregnancy, and renal insufficiency.[153] Comparison trials between LMWH and UFH have demonstrated that LMWH is at least as effective and as safe as UFH, and there are no significant differences in recurrent thromboembolic events, major bleeding, or mortality risk between the two types of heparin.[154] Caution must be used when administering LMWH in patients with renal insufficiency. LMWH is primarily cleared by the kidneys. Therefore, monitoring anti-Xa activity should be performed in patients with impaired renal function. If the creatinine clearance is less than 30 mL/minute, UFH should be used.[155]

LMWH heparin has a significantly lower incidence of heparin-induced thrombocytopenia (HIT), yet HIT can still occur with exposure to LMWH. Thus, LMWH is not an anticoagulant substitute for the patient with HIT requiring VTE prophylaxis or thrombosis treatment.[156]

LMWH can be administered safely in an outpatient setting. This has led to the development of programs in which clinically stable patients with PE are treated at home, at substantial cost savings.[157] An international, open-label, randomized trial compared outpatient and inpatient treatment (both using the LMWH enoxaparin as initial therapy) of low-risk patients with acute PE and concluded that outpatient treatment was not inferior to inpatient treatment.[158]

FONDAPARINUX

Fondaparinux is a synthetic polysaccharide derived from the antithrombin binding region of heparin. Fondaparinux catalyzes factor Xa inactivation by antithrombin without inhibiting thrombin, and studies have shown that it is effective in the initial treatment and prophylaxis of the VTE. Fondaparinux has been shown to be just as effective and safe as UFH and enoxaparin.[159] Fondaparinux dosing is based upon various weight ranges. For patients weighing less than 50 kg, 5 mg once daily is recommended. Patients weighing 50 to 100 kg are given 7.5 mg, and those weighing greater than 100 kg receive 10 mg daily. HIT is rare with the use of fondaparinux because of this lack of interaction with platelet factor 4 (PF4).[148]

WARFARIN THERAPY

The anticoagulant effect of warfarin (Coumadin) is mediated by the inhibition of vitamin K–dependent factors, which are II, VII, IX, and X. Vitamin K antagonists (VKAs) include substances with a short (acenocoumarol), intermediate (warfarin, fluindione), or long (phenprocoumone) half-life. For this reason, and because of genetically induced metabolic variability, the variable vitamin K content of food, a narrow therapeutic index, and interactions with other drugs, the effect on coagulation must be closely monitored. The peak effect does not occur until 36 to 72 hours after drug administration and the dosage is difficult to titrate. Administration of heparins or fondaparinux should overlap during at least 5 days with that of VKAs. After 5 days the parenteral drug can be stopped when the anticoagulant concentration induced by the VKA has achieved international normalized ratio (INR) between 2.0 and 3.0.[148,160]

The current American College of Chest Physicians (ACCP) guidelines for warfarin therapy suggest that the target INR is 2.5 even in high-risk patients (e.g., antiphospholipid syndrome). Because of its lack of validation, the ACCP does recommend pharmacogenetic testing. Warfarin should be started on day 1 or 2 that heparin is started. Usually warfarin 10 mg is administered and INR is adjusted to target INR. There is an increased risk of bleeding when antiplatelet drugs (acetylsalicylic acid, clopidogrel) are administered along with warfarin. In patients with acute coronary syndrome, mechanical valves, or recent coronary artery bypass or coronary stents, there is a likely benefit from the combination. Nonsteroidal anti-inflammatory drugs (NSAIDs) also increase the risk of bleeding when taken with warfarin and should be avoided.[160]

NEW ORAL ANTICOAGULANTS

A new generation of anticoagulants is emerging with promising advantages over current therapy. These drugs have their effect on specific steps of the coagulation cascade. These agents are taken orally and do not require hematologic monitoring. The direct thrombin inhibitor dabigatran and factor Xa inhibitors rivaroxban, apixaban, and edoxaban are moving through the pipeline for Food and Drug Administration (FDA) drug approval. Rivaroxaban recently received U.S. FDA approval to expanded use of Xarelto (rivaroxaban) to include treating DVT or PE and to reduce the risk of recurrent DVT and PE following initial treatment. Two studies have demonstrated that rivaroxaban is as effective as warfarin.[15,161] A major drawback, there is no reversal agent or antidote for hemorrhage induced by rivaroxaban.[162]

DURATION OF ANTICOAGULATION THERAPY

A patient with a first thromboembolic event occurring in the setting of reversible risk factors, such as immobilization, surgery, or trauma, should receive warfarin therapy for at least 3 months. No difference in the rate of recurrence was observed in either of two studies comparing 3 versus 6 months of anticoagulant therapy in patients with unprovoked first events.[69,70] The current recommendation is anticoagulation for at least 3 months in these patients; the need for extending the duration of anticoagulation should be reevaluated at that time.[163]

The current ACCP guidelines recommend that all patients with unprovoked PE should undergo a risk-to-benefit evaluation to determine if long-term therapy is needed (grade 1C).[163] Long-term treatment is recommended for these patients who do not have risk factors for bleeding and in whom accurate anticoagulant monitoring is possible (grade 1A). Patients who have PE and preexisting irreversible risk factors, such as deficiency of antithrombin III, protein S and C, factor V Leiden mutation, or the presence of antiphospholipid antibodies, should be placed on long-term anticoagulation.

HEPARIN-INDUCED THROMBOCYTOPENIA

Thrombocytopenia is common in the ICU setting but rarely is it caused by HIT. Because heparin is a common drug used in the ICU setting, this entity frequently is included in the differential diagnosis of the thrombocytopenia. The downstream consequences of overdiagnosis can be problematic, especially if it produced breaches in treating patients with VTE or protecting them from VTE.

HIT is a transient prothrombotic disorder initiated by heparin. The main features of HIT are (1) thrombocytopenia resulting from immunoglobulin G–mediated platelet activation and (2) in vivo thrombin generation and increased risk of venous and arterial thrombosis.[164]

HIT may manifest clinically as an extension of the thrombus or formation of new arterial thrombosis. HIT should be suspected whenever the patient's platelet count falls to less than 100,000/μL or less than 50% of the baseline value, generally after 5 to 15 days of heparin therapy. The pretest probability for HIT can be determined by the application of the "4 Ts": (1) Thrombocytopenia, (2) Timing, (3) Thrombosis, and (4) no oTher explanation of thrombocytopenia. At low scores the probability of the presence of platelet-activating HIT antibiodies is low; at high scores there is a moderate probability of the presence of the antibodies.[164,165]

The diagnosis of HIT is based upon assays that detect the presence of platelet-activating antibodies. The PF4-dependent enzyme immunoassay (EIA) test may lead to overdiagnosis of HIT. However, a negative EIA essentially rules out HIT. The serotonin release assay (SRA) is more specific for HIT than the PF4-dependent EIA. EIA is measured in optical density units (OD) and the strength of this measurement is a strong predictor of a positive SRA and confirmed HIT. In a patient with thrombocytopenia in whom the OD of EIA was less than 1.5 units the thrombocytopenia was not caused by HIT.[164,165]

The treatment of patients who develop HIT is to stop all heparin products, including catheter flushes and heparin-coated catheters, and to initiate an alternative, nonheparin anticoagulant, even when thrombosis is not clinically apparent. Preferred agents include direct thrombin inhibitors, such as lepirudin or argatroban. Start warfarin while the patient receives an alternative, nonheparin anticoagulant and only when the platelet count has recovered to at least 100,000/μL (preferably to 150,000/μL).[148]

THROMBOLYTIC THERAPY

The goal of thrombolytic therapy, by accelerating the conversion of plasminogen to plasmin, is to promote clot lysis and unload the right ventricle by decreasing pulmonary vascular obstruction. Thrombolysis has demonstrated a more rapid resolution of pulmonary vascular obstruction with improvement of RV hemodynamics within 2 hours after initiation of infusion. However, the controversy regarding thrombolytic therapy is the unloading of the right ventricle associated with improved mortality rate. In the larger original thrombolysis trials, streptokinase and urokinase were compared with heparin alone at infusion rates of 24 and 12 hours, respectively. These studies demonstrated rapid reperfusion of the pulmonary vasculature, reduction in pulmonary resistance, and no difference in mortality rate when compared to heparin.[166,167]

Currently three thrombolytics have FDA approval in the United States for acute PE: streptokinase, urokinase, and alteplase. Streptokinase and urokinase are nonselective agents activating both circulating and clot-bound plasminogen. Both agents have significant limitations; streptokinase is antigenic and may cause hypotension. Alteplase (tissue plasminogen activator [tPA]) is fibrin specific and is the thrombolytic of choice for the management of PE.[168,169]

The current ACCP key recommendations for the use of thrombolytic therapy in acute PE are noted here:[163]

1. In patients with acute PE associated with hypotension (e.g., systolic blood pressure <90 mm Hg) without a high bleeding risk, we suggest systemically administered thrombolytic therapy (grade 2C—weak recommendation [suggestion]/low quality or very low quality evidence).
2. In most patients with acute PE not associated with hypotension, we recommend against systemically administered thrombolytic therapy (grade 1C—strong recommendation/low quality or very low quality evidence).
3. In selected patients with acute PE without hypotension and with a low bleeding risk in whom there appears to be a high risk of developing hypotension, we suggest administration of thrombolytic therapy (grade 2C—weak recommendation [suggestion]/low quality or very low quality evidence).
4. When a thrombolytic agent is used, we suggest short infusion times (e.g., a 2-hour infusion) (grade 2C—weak recommendation [suggestion]/low quality or very low quality evidence).
5. In patients with acute PE when a thrombolytic agent is used, we suggest administration through a peripheral vein. Central administration is not deemed necessary (grade 2C—weak recommendation [suggestion]/low quality or very low quality evidence). Incidence of major hemorrhage from systemic thrombolytic administration can be as high as 20%, including a 3% to 5% risk of hemorrhagic intracranial complications.

Currently, the thrombolytic that is recommended is tPA at a dose of 100 mg given intravenously over 2 hours. Once the tPA is started the UFH infusion is stopped. After the 2-hour infusion the heparin is restarted, without a loading dose, when the aPTT is less than 80 seconds after tPA is complete.

Contraindications to systemic thrombolytic therapy in acute PE include an intracranial neoplasm, recent (i.e., <2 months) intracranial surgery or trauma, active or recent internal bleeding during the prior 6 months, history of a hemorrhagic stroke, bleeding diathesis, severe uncontrolled hypertension (i.e., systolic blood pressure >200 mm Hg or diastolic blood pressure >110 mm Hg), nonhemorrhagic stroke within the prior 2 months, surgery within the previous 10 days, and thrombocytopenia (i.e., <100,000 platelets/mL). Thrombolytic therapy may cause moderate bleeding in menstruating women, but it has not been associated with major hemorrhage. Therefore, menstruation is not a contraindication to thrombolytic therapy.[170]

SUBMASSIVE PULMONARY EMBOLISM WITH HEMODYNAMIC STABILITY AND RIGHT VENTRICULAR DYSFUNCTION

In patients with acute PE who are normotensive but demonstrate some degree of RVD, the treatment is somewhat controversial and may depend upon the degree of RVD present to initiate aggressive steps to protect RV function. There is a spectrum of RVD and RV injury. If RVD is manifested by only RV wall dilation and not injury, then the outcome may be different when injury begins to occur. The normotensive patients with evidence of RV injury will require expedited protection of RV function.

ROLE OF THROMBOLYTIC THERAPY IN NORMOTENSIVE SUBMASSIVE PULMONARY EMBOLISM WITH RIGHT VENTRICULAR DYSFUNCTION

Patients with known or suspected PE must be treated initially with UFH infusion. It appears that RVD in normotensive PE patients is associated with an increased risk of short-term adverse events and death than in patients without RVD. A number of studies have suggested that thrombolytic therapy should be considered in these patients. In the Management Strategy and Prognosis of Pulmonary Embolism Registry, of 719 acute PE patients with normal systemic arterial blood pressure and echocardiographic evidence of RVD, 550 were treated with heparin alone and 169 patients received thrombolytic therapy. The subgroup analysis demonstrated that patients undergoing thrombolysis had a significantly lower in-house mortality rate at 4.1% in contrast to anticoagulation alone at 10.5%. PE recurrence was observed in 7.7% in the thrombolysis group and in 18.7% in patients receiving anticoagulation alone.[2] Although this study demonstrated differences in terms of mortality rates and PE recurrence between the two groups, it must be emphasized that this was a registry trial and not a randomized clinical investigation Therefore, it was subject to unavoidable selection bias.

An important study that attempted to determine whether normotensive patients with PE-induced RVD should receive thrombolytic therapy produced some very interesting conclusions. In a prospective trial (MAPPET-3 [Management Strategies and Prognosis of Pulmonary Embolism-3 Trial]) of 256 patients with PE, the investigators randomized patients to receive heparin plus either recombinant tissue plasminogen activator (rtPA) or placebo. This study used a combined end point of in-hospital death or clinical deterioration (escalation of therapy needed). Clinical deterioration was defined as a requirement for either a catecholamine infusion to treat hypotension or shock, secondary or "rescue" thrombolysis, endotracheal intubation, cardiopulmonary resuscitation, or emergency catheter or surgical embolectomy. Initially the study results seem to support the use of thrombolytic therapy. Patients treated with anticoagulation alone were more likely to die or require treatment escalation than those who received rtPA (24.6% vs. 11.0%; $p = 0.006$), and importantly, there was no difference in the incidence of major bleeding or intracranial hemorrhage between the two treatment groups. The difference between the two groups was due to a more frequent need for secondary emergency thrombolysis in the heparin group, although the overall mortality rate was not affected by thrombolysis.[171] One of the major problems with this study was the lack of a consistent definition of RVD. In this study various modalities were used to define RVD and included echocardiography, right-sided heart catheterization, and even ECG signs of RV strain. Nevertheless, this study has been the catalyst for a large multinational European trial currently under way to attempt to resolve the controversy surrounding the role of thrombolytic therapy in patients with PE who are normotensive but have RVD.

Based upon the current ACCP guidelines, normotensive PE patients who have RVD (from clinical, biomarker, and echocardiographic findings) and no contraindications to thrombolysis, systemic thrombolysis should be considered (grade 2C recommendation).

ROLE OF CATHETER-DIRECTED THERAPY IN NORMOTENSIVE SUBMASSIVE PULMONARY EMBOLISM WITH RIGHT VENTRICULAR DYSFUNCTION

Catheter-directed therapy (CDT) has the potential to locally reduce clot burden in the pulmonary artery by mechanically disrupting the clot or locally infusing low-dose thrombolytics or both. In hemodynamically stable patients with RVD who have right and left pulmonary PE or main pulmonary artery clot CDT may be considered. However, CDT provides an additional option in the treatment of patients with life-threatening PE and a possible alternative to surgical embolectomy and systemic thrombolysis, especially in patients who are poor surgical candidates and have relative contraindications to systemic thrombolysis. Bleeding risk appears to be lower in CDT administered thrombolysis compared to systemic thrombolysis.[172]

The three types of catheter-based interventions are (1) aspiration thrombectomy, (2) thrombus fragmentation, and (3) rheolytic thrombectomy. Each of these techniques has similar success rates in systematic reviews.[172]

The infusion of tPA can be accomplished unilaterally or bilaterally at a total dose rate of 1.0 to 2.0 mg/hour depending on the degree of clot burden. In patients who may be at greater risk for bleeding or may require prolonged infusions greater than 24 hours, fibrinogen levels should be monitored. When the fibrinogen level is decreased below 150 to 200 mg/dL the infusion should be reduced or discontinued.[172] The ACCP currently recommends that CDT be considered in selected highly compromised patients with PE who are unable to receive thrombolytic therapy because of bleeding risk. The decision to consider CDT therapy should be multidisciplinary in nature. Case-by-case assessment is based upon risk stratification findings and the patient's risk of systemic thrombolysis and status as a candidate for surgical management.

ROLE OF INFERIOR VENA CAVA FILTERS IN PATIENTS WITH SUBMASSIVE PULMONARY EMBOLISM WITH RIGHT VENTRICULAR DYSFUNCTION

The goal of the inferior vena cava (IVC) filter intervention is to present further potentially lethal embolic episodes from impacting on an already compromised right ventricle. The current IVC filters that are utilized are retrievable and usually placed by interventional radiology. There has been a marked increase in the use of IVC filters for treatment and prevention of the venous thromboembolic disease. Stein and colleagues showed that the use of IVC filters in the United States has increased from 2000 in 1979 to 92,000 in 2006.[174]

IVC filters are usually placed in patients with acute PE or DVT who develop active bleeding during anticoagulation and an existing contraindication to anticoagulation. IVC filters should also be considered in the following situations: (1) recurrent thromboembolism despite adequate anticoagulation, (2) the presence of a large free-floating caval thrombus, (3) chronic recurrent PE with pulmonary hypertension, and (4) patients who have had surgical embolectomy or pulmonary endarterectomy.[175]

The Greenfield filter was introduced in 1973, and subsequently many types of permanent IVC filters have been developed; these filters are usually placed under

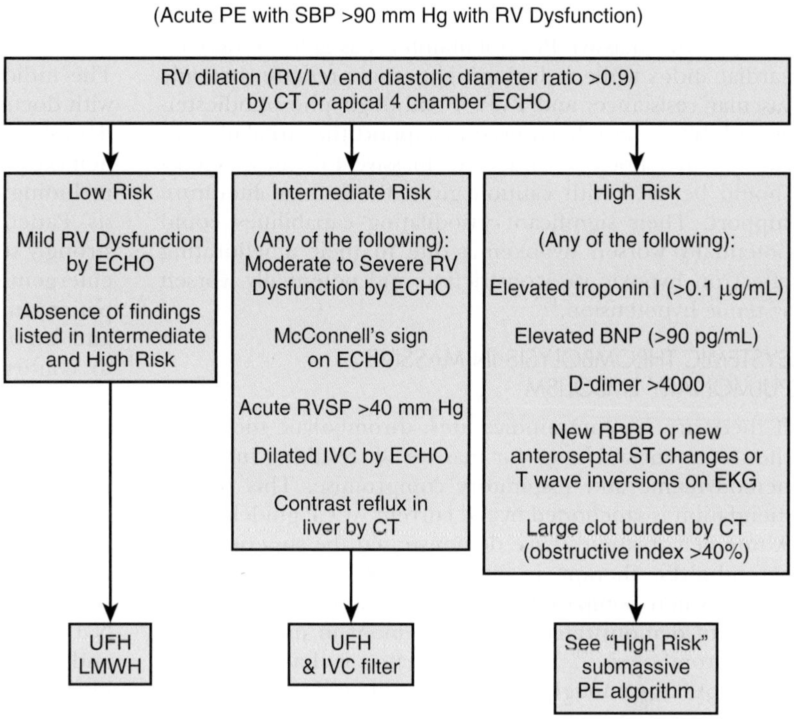

Figure 44.7 Submassive pulmonary embolus algorithm. BNP, brain natriuretic peptide; CT, computed tomography; ECHO, echocardiogram; IVC, inferior vena cava; LMWH, low molecular weight heparin; RBBB, right bundle branch block; RV, right ventricle; RVSP, right ventricular systolic pressure; UFH, unfractionated heparin.

fluoroscopic guidance.[176] Retrievable IVC filters offer an attractive alternative to the standard permanent filters. These retrievable filters are inserted in patients who may have transient contraindications to anticoagulation or patients who have increased bleeding risks (e.g., trauma patients and neurosurgical patients) or in whom the RV hemodynamics normalize. These filters should be removed within 3 months after implantation; unfortunately, these filters are not removed in "real world" practice.[175]

In patients with submassive PE and RVD who are normotensive the role of the retrievable IVC filter to prevent further embolization is controversial. In a small retrospective study adjunctive placement of an IVC filter, especially in patients with RV strain, resulted in no deaths. In patients who did not receive a filter the in-house mortality rate was 10.2%.[179] Prospective studies are needed to further explore the role of retrievable IVC filters in this patient population.

Figure 44.7 illustrates the therapeutic options available for the management of submassive PE in normotensive patients with RVD. In summary, the goals of these interventions are to reduce clot burden and to prevent further embolic impact on a compromised right ventricle.

MASSIVE PULMONARY EMBOLISM

RESPIRATORY SUPPORT

Although mechanical ventilation is often required in massive PE, the hemodynamic effects of mechanical ventilation may further aggravate the vicious circle of RVD and ischemia by augmenting RV afterload and further decreasing LV preload. Limiting the vasodilating hemodynamic effects of sedation and anesthesia needed for intubation is important. Intubating a patient with massive PE should not be prophylactic, and the risk versus benefit must be weighed carefully for each patient.[180]

HEMODYNAMIC SUPPORT IN MASSIVE PULMONARY EMBOLISM

Volume Resuscitation

Fluid should be administered in massive PE with caution. Fluid resuscitation may increase RV afterload precipitating RV failure as well as augment septal ballooning into the left ventricle, further decreasing cardiac output and worsening systemic hypotension. It is therefore recommended that small boluses of fluid (250-500 mL aliquots) be used initially to evaluate affect.[181,182]

Vasoactive Drugs

There are no randomized controlled studies among different vasoactive agents in massive PE. Norepinephrine (NE) which has both α-adrenergic and β-adrenergic effects, is superior to phenylephrine in a canine model of PE in terms of both improving cardiac output and improving myocardial perfusion.[183] NE has been shown to increase cardiac contractility and RV perfusion pressure, thus increasing coronary blood flow. Therefore, NE has become the most frequently used vasoactive agent for hemodynamic support of massive PE.[183,184] Dopamine, which possesses both β-adrenergic and, at sufficiently high doses, α-adrenergic agonist effects, appears to offer similar benefit. However, its use may be limited by the development of tachycardia.[185]

Inotropic Agents

Dobutamine, in combination with NE in the hypotensive patient, should be considered first-line therapy when treating cardiogenic shock secondary to a massive PE. In 10 patients with massive PE, dobutamine was able to increase cardiac index while reducing right atrial pressure, systemic vascular resistance, and PVR.[186] Although phosphodiesterase inhibitors have been used to support the circulation in cardiogenic shock secondary to massive PE, these agents should be used with caution given the lack of literature support. Their significant vasodilating capabilities could potentially worsen hypoxemia due to their ameliorating effect on hypoxic vasoconstriction and potentially worsen systemic hypotension.[187]

SYSTEMIC THROMBOLYSIS IN MASSIVE PULMONARY EMBOLISM

If there are no contraindications, thrombolytic therapy is the treatment of choice for massive PE resulting in severe hemodynamic and respiratory compromise. This recommendation is sanctioned by the current ACCP guidelines.[163] A number of studies have demonstrated the superiority of thrombolytic therapy in improving RV function (24-48 hours) when compared with heparin alone. The studies have not demonstrated an improvement in mortality rate with thrombolysis.[166,167,188-190] One reason is that the studies were not large enough for mortality rate to be an outcome measurement. A meta-analysis by Wan and colleagues demonstrated that patients with massive PE had a reduction in mortality rate and PE recurrence and adverse events when compared with heparin alone (19.0% to 9.4%; OR, 0.45; 95% CI, 0.22-0.92).[191] If thrombolytic therapy is given within 48 hours of the pulmonary embolic event there may be greater clinical improvement. However, thrombolysis may continue to be beneficial even in patients who have symptoms up to 2 weeks out from their initial PE symptoms.[192]

The thrombolytic agent usually given is tPA in a 2-hour infusion via peripheral venous line. UFH should not be given at the time with thrombolytic therapy. UFH should be restarted after the thrombolytic infusion is completed and when the aPTT is less than twice the normal value.

Massive PE can lead to cardiac arrest and the initial rhythm may include PEA and asystole. When cardiac arrest occurs, the mortality rate is in the range of 66% to 95%. Thrombolytic therapy given in boluses of 50 mg has been shown in case reports to be lifesaving.[193]

INFERIOR VENA CAVA FILTERS IN MASSIVE PULMONARY EMBOLISM

An observational study from an international registry that suggests that IVC filter placement in patients with massive PE (i.e., with hypotension) was associated with a reduction in combined end point of mortality rate and recurrent PE. This study cohort was small; however, it appears to be reasonable that IVC filters should be placed in patients with poor cardiopulmonary reserve.[194]

Unstable PE patients who are treated with standard anticoagulation therapy may benefit further with prophylactic placement of IVC filters. In a recent study by Stein and associates,[195] the mortality rate in 38,000 unstable patients treated with standard anticoagulant therapy alone was 51% compared with 33% in 12,850 who had vena cava filters in addition to anticoagulants. This represents a 35% decrease in the case fatality rate when vena cava filters are combined with standard anticoagulant therapy.

PULMONARY EMBOLECTOMY IN MASSIVE PULMONARY EMBOLISM

The indications for pulmonary embolectomy are patients with documented massive PE confirmed if possible by angiography (CTPA or pulmonary angiography) with persistent hemodynamic instability despite aggressive medical therapy including consideration of the local or systemic thrombolysis. Patients with refractory shock in which massive PE is strongly suspected should be transferred to a center where emergent surgical management for PE is performed. These patients must be urgently transferred to the operating room and on the operating table TEE should be performed to confirm the diagnosis. Despite these efforts, patients who present with cardiac arrest have a high surgical mortality rate.[195,196]

The mortality rate from pulmonary embolectomy ranges from 30% to 40%. There has been concern that medical therapy may delay definitive surgical therapy and may account for the high mortality rate. Among 1047 patients who underwent pulmonary embolectomy from 1961 to 1984 the average in-house mortality rate was 32%. Using the National Inpatient sample from 1999 to 2008, recently Stein and colleagues showed that the case fatality rates for unstable patients (shock or ventilator-dependent) with PE undergoing pulmonary embolectomy was 40% and in stable patients 24% with an overall case fatality rate of 28%. The case fatality rates were lower in patients with the primary diagnosis of PE who had few comorbid conditions. It was observed in both groups that patients with IVC filters had a lower case fatality rate than those who did not have filters.[197,198] More recently the surgical mortality rates for pulmonary embolectomy have decreased at specialized centers (Fig. 44.8, pulmonary embolectomy). A multidisciplinary approach appears to be the key to diagnosis, treatment, and postoperative care, translating to reduced mortality and morbidity rates.[199,200]

ENDOVASCULAR THERAPY IN MASSIVE PULMONARY EMBOLISM

In patients with massive PE who are not candidates for either pulmonary embolectomy or systemic thrombolysis, if there is institutional expertise for endovascular management, this should be considered. The goal is to convert a massive PE into a submassive PE with resultant improvement in the patient's hemodynamic and respiratory status. Initially CDT provides mechanical debulking of the clot, and if indicated because of persistent elevation of pulmonary artery pressures, infuse low-dose (3 mg/hour) tPA directly into the clot over a 12- to 24-hour period. CDT should be considered and the decision should be made quickly as part of a multidisciplinary discussion.[172-203] Complications of CDT are rare, but when they occur they can be serious. They include perforation of the pulmonary artery or perforation of the atrium or ventricle with pericardial tamponade. These interventions should be performed only by clinicians who are experienced in catheter-based intervention and within institutions that have defined protocols and multidisciplinary teams to manage these critically ill patients.

The management of high-risk submassive PE is summarized in Figure 44.9. For the normotensive patient with PE it is important to quickly risk stratify and identify the patient with RVD and large clot burden. If patients in this subset

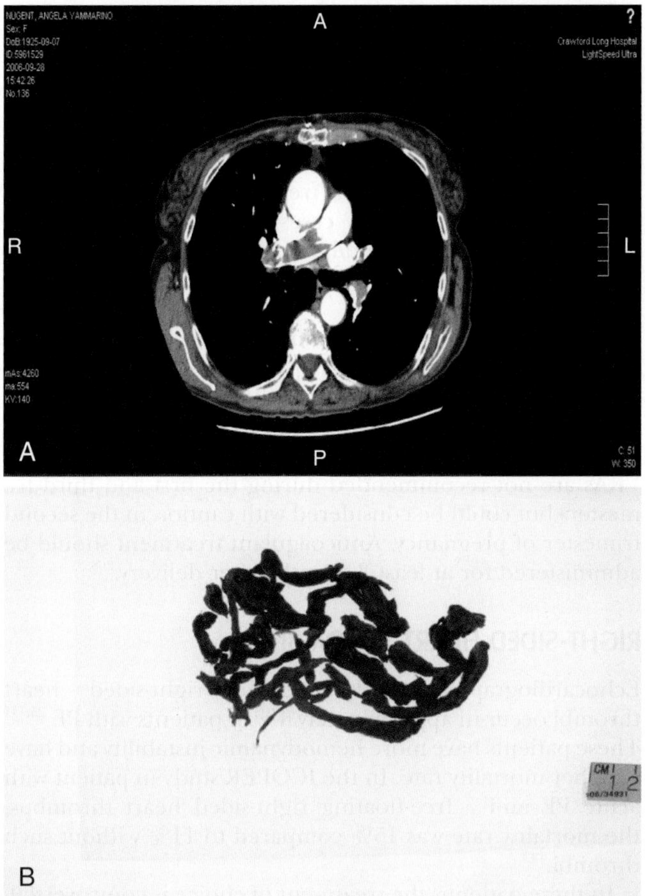

Figure 44.8 Large clot burden removed by pulmonary embolectomy.

manifest signs of RV injury with persistent elevations in troponin and echocardiographic evidence of RV overloading with impending RV failure, then systemic thrombolytic therapy, local thrombolytic therapy, and surgical management are management options to be considered. In the patient with massive PE, as with submassive PE with RVD, there must be multidisciplinary coordination between interventional cardiology and radiology and cardiothoracic surgery to quickly determine the best treatment approach. Both respiratory and hemodynamic support will allow some time to consider the various management options.

SPECIAL POPULATIONS

PREGNANCY

The incidence of PE during pregnancy ranges between 0.3 and 1 per 1000 deliveries.[204] PE is the leading cause of pregnancy-related maternal death in developed countries. In the United States, maternal death from PE ranks third after hemorrhage and hypertensive disorders.[105,206] There is a fivefold increased risk of VTE in the pregnant woman because of venous stasis, a prothrombotic state as a result of increased levels of coagulation factors, reduced protein S, and fibrinolytic activity.[207] The two major PE risk factors in pregnancy are a personal history of VTE and heritable thrombophilias.[208] The risk of PE is higher in the postpartum period, particularly after a cesarean section. The clinical features of PE are no different in pregnancy compared with the nonpregnant state. There have been no prospective trials that have validated existing prediction models to

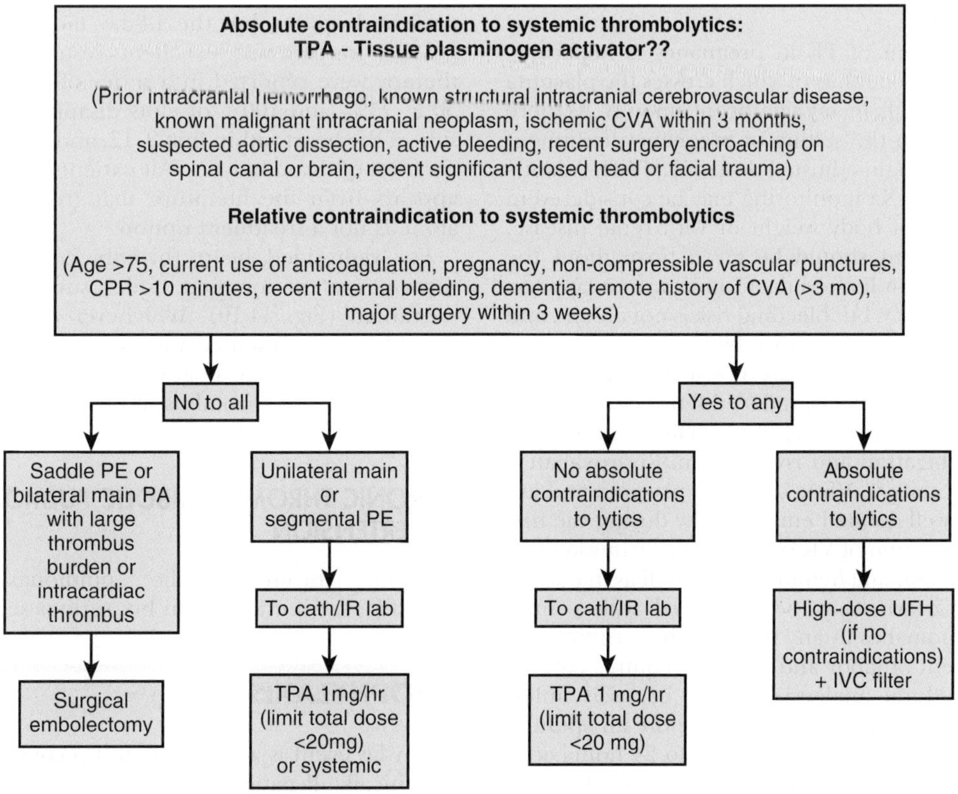

Figure 44.9 "High-risk" submassive pulmonary embolus with right ventricular injury algorithm.

exclude PE in pregnancy. It is been shown from a maternal death review that pregnant women who died from PE are over the age of 35, are obese (body mass index >30), and have chronic medical conditions.[209]

DIAGNOSIS OF PULMONARY EMBOLISM IN PREGNANCY

Although D-dimer may be elevated in pregnancy, leading to a high rate of false positives, a normal D-dimer value has the same exclusion value for PE in pregnant women as in other patients with suspected PE. However, it has been suggested that D-dimer testing is not recommended for evaluation of suspected VTE in pregnancy or the early postpartum period. Therefore, it should be measured even though the probability of a negative result is lower than in other patients with suspected PE.[207]

An elevated D-dimer assay should be followed by CUS of the lower extremities. If CUS demonstrates DVT, then anticoagulation can occur and thoracic imaging is not necessary. If CUS is negative and the diagnosis is still suspected, then thoracic imaging is warranted. It is important to note that the upper limit of radiation with regard to the danger of injury to the fetus is considered to be 50 mSv (50,000 mGy), and all radiologic tests (CT and $\dot{V}/\dot{Q}$) fall well below this limit.[208] In a pregnant or postpartum woman suspected of PE with a normal chest radiograph either a ventilation-perfusion scan or a perfusion scan alone will be sufficient. A normal lung scan essentially excludes the diagnosis of PE. Perfusion scanning compares favorably with CT as far as exposure of breast tissue to radiation is concerned.[209] If the chest radiograph is abnormal and the lung scan is nondiagnostic, then CTPA is recommended.

TREATMENT OF PULMONARY EMBOLISM IN PREGNANCY

The medical treatment of PE in pregnancy is heparin—either UFH or LWMH, neither of which crosses the placenta or is found in breast milk in any significant amount. As there are no specific data in the setting of pregnancy, treatment should consist of a weight-adjusted dose of LMWH. Adaptation according to anti-Xa monitoring may be considered in women at extremes of body weight or with renal disease. The heparin treatment should be given throughout the entire pregnancy. From limited data fondaparinux appears efficacious in pregnancy, but bleeding risk is not absent, and care is required when used as second-line therapy.[210]

The new oral anticoagulants are not to be used during pregnancy. Teratogenic effects, reduced fetal viability, hemorrhagic changes, and placental abnormalities have been found in both dabigatran and rivaroxaban. Rivaroxaban is secreted in breast milk.[210] VKAs cross the placenta and are associated with a well-defined embryopathy during the first trimester. Administration of VKAs in the third trimester can result in fetal and neonatal hemorrhage as well as in placental abruption. Warfarin may be associated with central nervous system anomalies in any trimester in pregnancy.[208]

The management of labor and delivery requires particular attention. Epidural analgesia cannot be used unless LMWH is discontinued at least 12 hours before an epidural approach. Treatment can be resumed 12 to 24 hours after withdrawal of the epidural catheter. In any case, close collaboration among obstetrician, anesthetist, and critical care physician is recommended. After delivery, heparin treatment may be replaced by anticoagulation with VKA. Anticoagulant treatment should be administered for at least 3 months after delivery. VKAs can be given even to breastfeeding mothers.[208] Thrombolytic therapy should be used when there is a life-threatening pulmonary embolic event. At the time of delivery, thrombolytic treatment should not be used except in extremely severe cases and if surgical embolectomy is not immediately available. Indications for IVC filters in pregnant women are similar to those in other patients with PE.

In summary, in pregnant women with a clinical suspicion of PE an accurate diagnosis is paramount, as a prolonged course of heparin is required. All diagnostic modalities, including CT scanning, may be used without significant risk to the fetus. LMWHs are recommended in confirmed PE; VKAs are not recommended during the first and third trimesters but could be considered with caution in the second trimester of pregnancy. Anticoagulant treatment should be administered for at least 3 months after delivery.[208]

RIGHT-SIDED HEART THROMBI

Echocardiographically documented right-sided heart thrombi occur in approximately 4% of patients with PE.[25,143] These patients have more hemodynamic instability and have a higher mortality rate. In the ICOPER study in patient with acute PE and a free-floating right-sided heart thrombus, the mortality rate was 15% compared to 11% without such thrombi.[143]

In these patients, the treatment of choice is controversial. Thrombolytic therapy or surgical embolectomy have both been used and there have been multiple reports of successful results. In the ICOPER, thrombolytic treatment was the preferred option, but the 14-day mortality rate was above 20%.[143] In contrast, excellent results with thrombolytic therapy were reported in a series of 16 patients, in which 50%, 75%, and 100% of clots disappeared from the right side of the heart within first 2, 12, and 24 hours after administration of thrombolytics. All patients survived 30 days.[211] It appears from the literature that treatment with heparin alone is not a treatment option.

For right-sided heart thrombi crossing the interatrial septum (patent foramen ovale) surgical embolectomy is warranted (Fig. 44.10). Whichever therapy is selected, it should be implemented without delay: in the presence of unequivocal echocardiographic visualization of a mobile right-sided heart thrombus, no further diagnostic tests are needed.[25,203,212,213]

CHRONIC THROMBOEMBOLIC PULMONARY HYPERTENSION

Chronic thromboembolic pulmonary hypertension (CTEPH) is an uncommon but serious sequela of PE.

PROPHYLAXIS

The VTE event is a common and recognized complication in critically ill patients. A VTE event can have dire consequences on the critically ill patient with preexisting

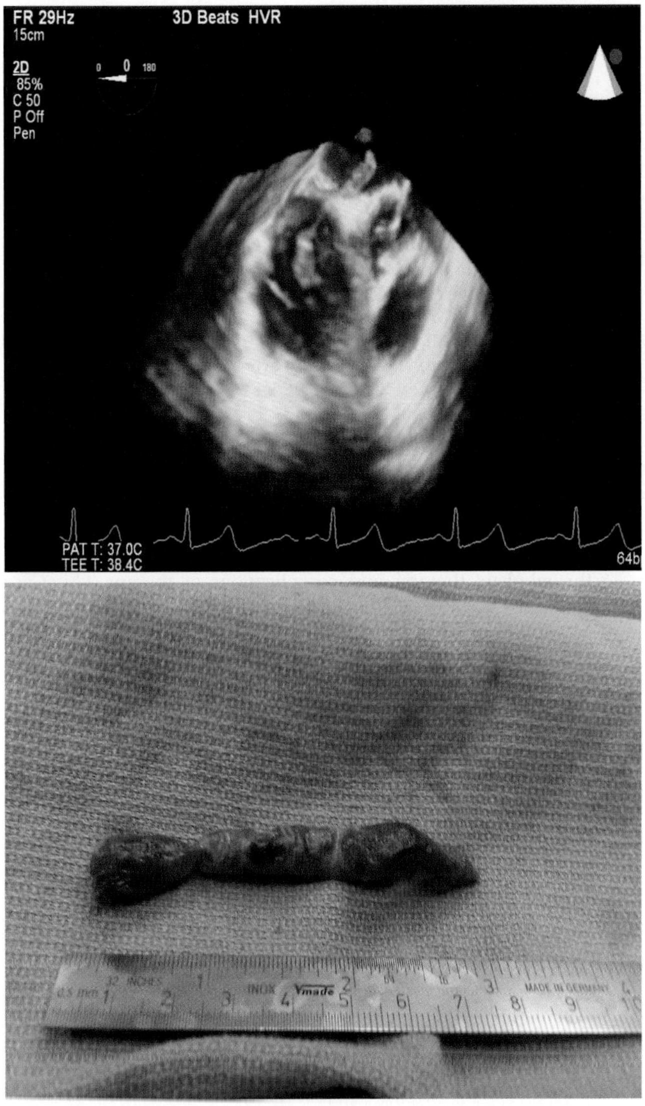

Figure 44.10 Embolism in transit through the patent foramen ovale and surgical removal. (Courtesy of Dr. Omar Lattouf–Emory University Cardiothoracic Surgery.)

cardiopulmonary compromise. All critically ill patients have significant risk factors for VTE and also are at higher risk for bleeding. Venous thromboembolic prophylaxis decreases the risk of VTE in ICU patients.[17-21] DVT prophylaxis is effective at reducing the risk of death. In several meta-analyses of surgical patients, prophylactic measures reduced the development of thromboembolic events by more than 50% and also the VTE-attributable mortality rate.[224]

Lack of adherence to evidence based VTE prophylaxis guidelines has been problematic on a national and international scale.[13,224] With the implementation of electronic medical admission order sets universal VTE prophylaxis can be achieved. Extended posthospitalization prophylaxis has been recommended in orthopedic surgical and medical patients. The advent of safe and effective prophylaxis strategies makes all critical care patients candidates for some form of preventive therapy on the basis of risk factors present in this population of patients. Several studies suggest that more than 85% of hospitalized patients are receiving some sort of DVT prophylaxis. VTE prophylactic measures are growing in ICUs with quality care initiatives targeting this intervention via bundled care pathways.[225,226]

The administration of prophylactic LMWH (or low-dose unfractionated heparin) can be administered to the majority of critically ill patients. Critically ill patients at high risk for clinically important bleeding should receive mechanical thromboprophylaxis until the bleeding risk decreases. Renal insufficiency is not a contraindication to the use of LMWH or low-dose unfractionated heparin.

LONG-TERM PROGNOSIS

Nearly 25% of patients with PE do not survive the first year after the diagnosis. A majority of these patients succumb to underlying conditions, such as cancer or chronic heart disease, rather than PE. After surviving the first year the patient continues facing bleeding complications from anticoagulation therapy, the risk of recurrent VTE, the development of cancer, and the development of CTEPH.[227]

KEY POINTS

- DVT and PE are different manifestations of the same disease and are associated with significant morbidity and mortality rates. The U.S. Surgeon General issued a "Call to Action" in 2008, identifying VTE as a major public health problem.
- It is important to identify patient-related and setting (ICU)-related risk factors for the development of VTE. ICU risk factors that are associated with massive PE are malignancy, cardiopulmonary disorders, and immobilization.
- Nearly two thirds of patients who die from pulmonary thromboembolism die within 1 hour of presentation, giving rise to the concept of the "golden hour" to accomplish both diagnosis and commence treatment. The principal pathophysiologic effects of pulmonary thromboembolism result from the impaction of clot in the pulmonary circulation with resulting vascular obstruction and humoral mediator release.
- Life-threatening PE, ranging from signs and symptoms of RVD to frank shock, are the major clinical presentations to the ICU.
- Risk stratification is useful in the assessment of submassive normotensive PE with RVD. RVD can be identified from clinical findings, ECG, cardiac biomarkers, and imaging modalities (echocardiogram and CTPA). The initial hemodynamic presentation of PE is the most powerful predictor of outcome. Central location of a thrombus is an independent risk factor for death.
- The cornerstone of pharmacologic management of VTE is heparin. Heparin therapy should be initiated, if there is no contraindication, as the diagnostic evaluation is being performed. UFH, LMWH, or fondaparinux followed by warfarin is currently the standard treatment for low-risk PE. New oral agents have been recently approved. Thrombolytic therapy, if

Continued on following page

KEY POINTS (Continued)

there are no contraindications, should be used in patients with massive PE and considered in patients with submassive PE with evidence of severe RVD.

- The management of the normotensive submassive PE patient centers on reducing RV afterload and preventing further insult to the right ventricle. Systemic and endovascular delivery of thrombolytic agents can reduce RV strain. The placement of a retrievable IVC filter can prevent further embolic impact on the RV.
- Supportive therapy for massive PE employs judious use of fluids to avoid further increases in RV strain. NE is the vasopressor of choice to maintain perfusion pressure. Dobutamine should be used to improve contractility. These temporizing measures will allow the critical care team to mobilize thrombolytic, endovascular, and surgical management strategies. All diagnostic modalities, including CT scanning, may be used without significant risk to the fetus in the pregnant woman. LMWHs are recommended in confirmed PE. Anticoagulant treatment should be administered for at least 3 months after delivery.
- Thrombolytic therapy or surgical intervention should be considered for right-sided heart thrombi. If a patent foramen ovale is present or right-sided heart thrombi cross the patent foramen ovale, surgery should be performed.
- CTEPH is more common than once thought and is best managed with pulmonary endarterectomy. It is important to identify these patients early.
- VTE prophylaxis strategies are necessary for nearly all critical care patients.
- Four years after PE the majority of patients will have either died or had recurrent PE, cancer diagnosis, arterial cardiovascular disease, or CTEPH. We must do more in following up these post-PE patients.

SELECTED REFERENCES

1. Wood KE: Major pulmonary embolism: Review of a pathophysiologic approach to the golden hour of hemodynamically significant pulmonary embolism. Chest 2002;121:877-905.

115. Stamm JA: Risk stratification for pulmonary embolism. Crit Care Clin 2012;28:301-321.

116. Sanchez O, Planquette B, Gosset-Wolmant M, et al: Triaging in pulmonary embolism. Semin Respir Crit Care Med 2012;33:156-162.

119. Aujesky D, Obrosky DS, Stone RA, et al: Derivation and validation of a prognostic model for pulmonary embolism. Am J Respir Crit Care Med 2005;172:1041-1046.

129. Klok FA, Inge CMM, Huisman MV: Brain type natriuretic peptide levels in the prediction of adverse outcome in patients with pulmonary embolism. A systematic review and meta-analysis. Am J Respir Crit Care Med 2008;178:425-430.

132. Becattini C, Vedovati MC, Agnelli G: Prognostic value of troponins in acute pulmonary embolism: A meta-analysis. Circulation 2007;116(4):427-433.

135. Jiménez D, Aujesky D, Moores L, et al: Combinations of prognostic tools for identification of high-risk normotensive patients with acute symptomatic pulmonary embolism. Thorax 2011;66:75-81.

148. Tapson V: Treatment of pulmonary embolism: Anticoagulation, thrombolytic therapy, and complications of therapy. Crit Care Clin 2010;27:825-839.

172. Kuo WT: Endovascular therapy for acute pulmonary embolism. J Vasc Interv Radiol 2012;23:167-179.

196. Dauphine C, Omari B: Pulmonary embolectomy for acute massive pulmonary embolism. Ann Thorac Surg 2005;79:1240-1244.

200. Kadner A, Schmidli J, Schonhoff F, et al: Excellent outcome after surgical treatment of massive pulmonary embolism in critically ill patients. J Thorac Cardiovasc Surg 2008;136:448-451.

214. Fedullo P, Kerr KM, Kim NH, Auger WR: Chronic thromboembolic pulmonary hypertension. Am J Respir Crit Care Med 2011;183:1605-1613.

The complete list of references can be found at www.expertconsult.com.

Pulmonary Hypertension

45

Rodrigo Cartin-Ceba | Mykola V. Tsapenko | Ognjen Gajic

CHAPTER OUTLINE

Pulmonary hypertension (PH) is a complex and heterogeneous pulmonary vascular disorder that leads to elevated pulmonary vascular resistance (PVR) and right ventricular failure. During recent years, multiple advances in the therapy and management of PH have been made; however, this disorder continues to cause significant morbidity and mortality. PH is defined by a resting mean pulmonary arterial pressure (mPAP) greater than 25 mm Hg, associated with PVR greater than 240 dynes • second • cm^{-5} (or >3 Wood units) measured by right-sided heart catheterization. It is very important for the intensivist to distinguish those patients who have chronic PH secondary to any of the five groups included in the clinical classification described in Box 45.1 from other conditions that are usually faced in the intensive care unit (ICU) that can cause an acute elevation in the PVR. The acute elevation of pulmonary artery (PA) pressure observed in critically ill patients can develop on top of preexisting chronic PH (acute on chronic). It can be transient without consequences, or it can be prolonged and progress to severe acute PH, leading to life-threatening complications that include refractory systemic arterial hypotension, severe hypoxemia, right ventricular dysfunction and failure, and ultimately cardiogenic or obstructive shock and death. The most common acute elevation of PA pressures in the ICU is seen in the setting of left-sided heart disease (elevated pulmonary venous pressure) or in patients with preexisting pulmonary vascular disease. It is also well recognized after cardiothoracic surgery, during sepsis, after pulmonary embolism (PE), and in acute respiratory distress syndrome (ARDS). Unfortunately, in most cases acute PH remains underdiagnosed and its treatment begins only after serious complications have been developed.

PATHOPHYSIOLOGY OF PULMONARY HYPERTENSION AND RIGHT VENTRICULAR FAILURE

DEVELOPMENT OF PULMONARY HYPERTENSION

In order to understand the pathophysiology of PH and before reviewing its current clinical classification, it is important to identify where the vascular insult originates. Conditions that raise the postcapillary pressure (pulmonary venous pressures) such as left-sided heart failure or mitral stenosis differ significantly from conditions that primarily affect the pulmonary arteries and arterioles such as idiopathic pulmonary artery hypertension (IPAH). The former causes a gradient between the PA diastolic and pulmonary capillary wedge pressure (PCWP) that is relatively small, with histopathologic changes in the arterial vessels that consist of mild medial hypertrophy and reversible intimal changes. In the latter, there is an increased pulmonary arteriovenous pressure gradient, and histologic changes on the

Box 45.1 Clinical Classification of Pulmonary Hypertension

1. Pulmonary arterial hypertension (PAH)
   1.1. Idiopathic PAH
   1.2. Heritable
      1.2.1. BMPR2
      1.2.2. ALK1, endoglin (with or without hereditary hemorrhagic telangiectasia)
      1.2.3. Unknown
   1.3. Drug- and toxin-induced
   1.4. Associated with:
      1.4.1. Connective tissue diseases
      1.4.2. HIV infection
      1.4.3. Portal hypertension
      1.4.4. Congenital heart diseases
      1.4.5. Schistosomiasis
      1.4.6. Chronic hemolytic anemia
   1.5 Persistent pulmonary hypertension of the newborn
   1′ Pulmonary veno-occlusive disease (PVOD) and/or pulmonary capillary hemangiomatosis (PCH).
2. Pulmonary hypertension owing to left heart disease
   2.1. Systolic dysfunction
   2.2. Diastolic dysfunction
   2.3. Valvular disease
3. Pulmonary hypertension owing to lung diseases and/or hypoxia
   3.1. Chronic obstructive pulmonary disease
   3.2. Interstitial lung disease
   3.3. Other pulmonary diseases with mixed restrictive and obstructive pattern
   3.4. Sleep-disordered breathing
   3.5. Alveolar hypoventilation disorders
   3.6. Chronic exposure to high altitude
   3.7. Developmental abnormalities
4. Chronic thromboembolic pulmonary hypertension
1′. Pulmonary hypertension with unclear multifactorial mechanisms
   5.1. Hematologic disorders: myeloproliferative disorders, splenectomy
   5.2. Systemic disorders: sarcoidosis, pulmonary Langerhans cell histiocytosis: lymphangioleiomyomatosis, neurofibromatosis, vasculitis
   5.3. Metabolic disorders: glycogen storage disease, Gaucher disease, thyroid disorders
   5.4. Others: tumoral obstruction, fibrosing mediastinitis, chronic renal failure on dialysis

ALK1, activin receptor-like kinase type 1; BMPR2, bone morphogenetic protein receptor type 2; HIV, human immunodeficiency virus.
From Simonneau G, Robbins IM, Beghetti M, et al: Updated clinical classification of pulmonary hypertension. J Am Coll Cardiol 2009; 54:S43-54.

pulmonary vasculature are more marked, including significant intimal hypertrophy with fibrosis, marked smooth muscle hypertrophy, vasoconstriction, adventitial proliferation, and thrombosis in situ.[1] These changes cause vascular flow obstruction and eventually lead to abnormal angiogenesis and formation of plexiform arteriopathy. Endothelial dysfunction also develops with an imbalance between vasodilation and vasoconstriction and between apoptosis and proliferation, mechanisms that are thought to play the most important role in the development of chronic progressive PH. Hypoxemic pulmonary vasoconstriction is an important determinant of arterial PH in patients with respiratory disorders.[1] In many types of PH, production of endogenous vasodilators (nitric oxide [NO] and prostacyclin) is impaired and production of vasoconstrictors (endothelin-1, thromboxane A) is increased.[1] That is why the common treatment strategy for PH is to achieve the balance in key molecular pathways by increasing available NO and prostacyclin, or reducing the effects of endothelin-1. Acute cases are characterized by sudden increase in pulmonary arterial pressure (PAP) as seen when mechanical obstruction with subsequent vasoconstriction develops during an acute PE. In ARDS, both hypoxemia and the accumulation of intravascular fibrin and cellular debris contribute to subsequent vascular obliteration and PH.[2] Endotoxin and vasoactive mediators related to pulmonary vasoconstriction also play significant roles in development of the PH during sepsis. Several animal studies have shown that endotoxin may cause not only systemic hypotension but also pulmonary biphasic hypertension, decrease in compliance, and increase in resistance of the respiratory system.[3] Those endotoxin-dependent hemodynamic and respiratory effects are mediated by excessive release of inflammatory mediators and imbalance in production of NO, prostanoids, and endothelin-1.[3,4] PH in endotoxemia is characterized by a constriction of proximal pulmonary arteries during the early phase followed by decreased compliance of distal pulmonary vasculature.[5] Endotoxin infusion can also dramatically affect right ventricular function: in the very early phase of endotoxemic shock, right ventricular-vascular coupling is preserved by an increase in right ventricular contractility. Later, myocardial oxygen consumption and the energy cost of right ventricular contractility are increased, which along with progressive endotoxin-induced PH lead to right ventricular dysfunction and failure.[6]

RIGHT VENTRICULAR FAILURE

The right ventricle (RV) differs from the left ventricle (LV) in morphologic appearance and functionality.[7] Despite the requirement for a similar cardiac output between the RV and LV, the bioenergetic requirement for right ventricular function is approximately 20% of the LV. The RV is thinner than the LV and its shape differs from that of the LV, having a crescent-shaped morphologic appearance. These differences reflect the low resistance, low impedance, and high compliance of the pulmonary circulation.[7] The high compliance allows quick adaptations to changes in preload; however, unlike the LV, the RV tolerates poorly the acute increases in afterload, which could lead to hemodynamic collapse.[8] It is important to emphasize these differences between the ability of the RV to adapt to sudden (acute) versus gradual (chronic) elevation of PAP. A normal RV can acutely adapt to high flow, but is barely able to tolerate any but very short acute high-pressure load.[9] The normal RV cannot acutely increase the mPAP to more than 40 mm Hg.[10] In chronic sustained elevation of afterload as seen in PH, the RV increases its wall thickness by hypertrophy of the muscle mass and assumes a more rounded shape (Fig. 45.1). Eventually and despite the compensatory right ventricular hypertrophy to the sustained long-term pressure overload, the RV dilates. Neurohormonal activation develops during

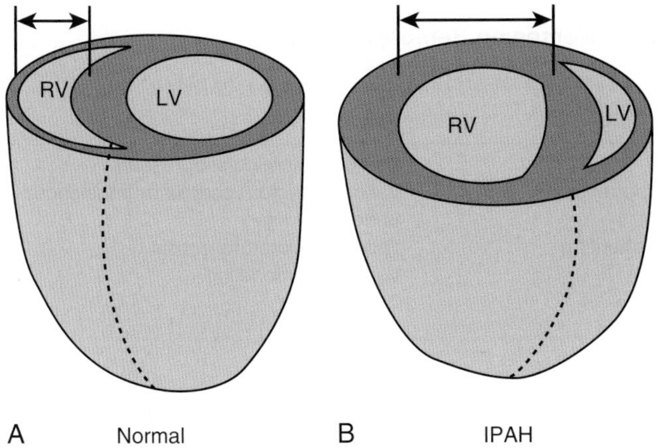

Figure 45.1 RV configuration in health (left, **A**) and pulmonary hypertension (right, **B**). IPAH, idiopathic pulmonary artery hypertension; LV, left ventricle; RV, right ventricle. (Modified with permission from Bogaard HJ: The right ventricle under pressure. Chest 2009;135: 794-804.)

the right ventricular dilatation and is an important mechanism in both acute and chronic right ventricular failure. The consequence of sympathetic hyperactivity is an increase in PVR with impedance of flow, causing right ventricular strain that impairs filling and causes right ventricular volume and pressure overload. Furthermore, the RV dilatation increases oxygen consumption and reduces contractility, which is going to decrease right ventricular perfusion, and a vicious circle develops that ultimately leads to death. Tricuspid regurgitation develops as a result of right ventricular dysfunction and defines a poor prognosis.[11] It is important also to mention the concept of functional interdependence between the RV and the LV. Anatomically, the superficial myocardial fibers encircle both ventricles, and both chambers are contained within the pericardium, sharing the interventricular septum.[12] During elevation of right-sided heart pressures, the interventricular septum shifts progressively to the left with subsequent development of left ventricular diastolic dysfunction that reduces the LV's cardiac output and coronary perfusion pressure.[8,13] A downstream adverse effect of right-sided heart failure is the development of systemic venous hypertension leading to concomitant visceral organ congestion and dysfunction. Regardless of the underlying cause of PH, the final common pathway for hemodynamic deterioration and death is right ventricular failure.

CLINICAL CLASSIFICATION OF PULMONARY HYPERTENSION

The classification of PH has presented different modifications since its first classification made in 1973 at a conference endorsed by the World Health Organization. The most recent classification of PH, described in Box 45.1, is based on causative diseases and was updated during the Fourth World Symposium on PH held in Dana Point, California.[14] For the intensivist, it is important to recognize two different scenarios: patients with chronic PH admitted to the ICU for an acute process that may or may not worsen the underlying PH and patients with no history of chronic PH who develop acute PH during their ICU stay secondary to various conditions. It is also important to distinguish between pulmonary arterial hypertension as seen in IPAH and pulmonary venous hypertension as seen in left ventricular failure. A classification of PH in the ICU is described in Box 45.2.

Box 45.2 Etiology of Pulmonary Hypertension in the Intensive Care Unit

Acute and Acute-on-Chronic Venous Pulmonary Hypertension

Pulmonary hypertension secondary to left ventricular dysfunction/failure with left atrial hypertension:
- Congestive heart failure, acute myocardial infarction, diastolic dysfunction, severe valvular disease (e.g., mitral regurgitation, mitral stenosis)
- Pulmonary venoocclusive disease (VOD)

Acute-on-Chronic Arterial Pulmonary Hypertension

Worsening of preexisting pulmonary hypertension, usually with respiratory or cardiovascular decompensation, by either of two mechanisms:
- Natural progression
- Precipitation by acute condition (e.g., sepsis/ARDS, PE, drugs)

Acute Arterial Pulmonary Hypertension

Without preexisting pulmonary hypertension:
- Massive PE
- ARDS, sepsis, drug-induced, others

ARDS, acute respiratory distress syndrome; PE, pulmonary embolism.
From Tsapenko MV: Arterial pulmonary hypertension in noncardiac intensive care unit. Vasc Health Risk Manag 2008;4:1043-1060.

ACUTE ON CHRONIC PULMONARY HYPERTENSION

Individuals with preexisting PH (i.e., IPAH or portopulmonary hypertension [group 1]) are particularly vulnerable to acute illnesses, which commonly result in rapid clinical deterioration and even death.[15] Besides the entities described in group 1 of the Dana Point classification, several other conditions that are associated with chronic PH and are more commonly encountered in the ICU include left ventricular heart failure (with or without preserved ejection fraction causing pulmonary venous hypertension; group 2); interstitial lung diseases, chronic obstructive pulmonary disease (COPD), chronic hypoventilation syndromes, and sleep disorder breathing (group 3); and chronic pulmonary thromboembolic disease (group 4). Several clinical factors faced during intercurrent critical illness can aggravate or unmask the hemodynamics of patients with preexisting PH and are outlined in Table 45.1. These patients with chronic PH can rapidly deteriorate and usually die from progressive right ventricular failure (49%), progressive respiratory failure (18%), or sudden cardiac death (17%). Cardiopulmonary resuscitation (CPR), even when attempted in the hospital

Table 45.1 Intensive Care Unit (ICU) Factors Associated with Worsening Hemodynamics in Pulmonary Hypertension

Pulmonary	Cardiac	Vascular
Hypercapnia	Volume overload	Use of systemic vasopressors
Hypoxemia	Pulmonary venous hypertension (left ventricle failure)	Vasoconstrictor/vasodilator imbalance
Acidosis	Increased right to left shunting	Endothelial injury
High airway pressure	Right ventricle strain	Vascular microthrombosis
Decreased compensatory capacity	Use of inotropes	Vascular remodeling

setting, is rarely successful. Only 6% of patients survived for more than 90 days and most of the survivors had identifiable causes of circulatory arrest that were rapidly reversible. The pulmonary blood flow is virtually absent in these patients during CPR. In 54%, cardiorespiratory arrest was associated with an intercurrent illness,[15] illustrating how preexisting PH adversely affects patients' compensatory capacity and ability to survive an acute illness.

ACUTE PULMONARY HYPERTENSION

Acute PH is caused by an abrupt increase in PVR. The prototype of this process is an acute PE; however, other conditions frequently seen in the ICU can also be associated with acute increase in PVR such as acute decompensated left ventricular failure, post cardiac surgery, ARDS, and sepsis.[16] Acute right ventricular failure develops in 61% of patients who present with massive PE that involves at least two lobar arteries. The mortality rate ranges from 3% in hemodynamically stable patients to 59% in unstable ones.[17,18] Hemodynamic instability in the setting of PE is defined as systolic blood pressure (SBP) less than 90 mm Hg or a drop in SBP greater than 40 mm Hg from baseline for more than 15 minutes that is not otherwise explained by hypovolemia, sepsis, or new arrhythmia.[18] The degree of shock inferred from the presence of metabolic acidosis, but not transthoracic echocardiography (TTE) findings, is the most powerful predictor of death in these patients.[17,19]

ACUTE RESPIRATORY DISTRESS SYNDROME AND SEPSIS

Right ventricular dysfunction as a complication of ARDS is more gradual than in patients with massive PE, usually occurring at least 48 hours after the beginning of respiratory support.[16] Evaluation of right ventricular function by TTE in a group of 75 ARDS patients submitted to protective ventilation demonstrated 25% incidence of acute right ventricular failure, resulting in detrimental hemodynamic consequences associated with tachycardia. However, those changes in heart function were reversible in patients who recovered; furthermore, it did not increase mortality rate.[16] Although the initial magnitude of PH was not an indicator of mortality rate, mPAP increased in nonsurvivors, but not in survivors when followed for 7 days.[20] Thus, development of PH in ARDS patients seems to be a sign of poor prognosis. In another cohort of 352 ARDS patients, both mortality rate and incidence of right ventricular failure were related to the level of plateau pressure during mechanical ventilation. In patients without acute cor pulmonale, the odds ratio of mortality for an increase in plateau pressure from 18–26 to 27–35 cm H_2O was 1.15 ($p = 0.635$); however, for patients with acute cor pulmonale, the odds ratio of mortality for an increase in plateau pressure from 18–26 to 27–35 cm H_2O was 3.32 ($p = 0.034$), suggesting that the threshold for a safe plateau pressure depends on the presence or not of acute cor pulmonale.[21] Importantly, the implementation of low tidal volume ventilation in patients with ARDS has significantly lowered not only mortality rates but also incidence of acute right ventricular failure in this patient population.[16] In addition to being the major risk factor for ARDS development, sepsis itself can sometimes lead to severe acute arterial PH.[22]

POSTSURGICAL PULMONARY HYPERTENSION

Some surgical interventions, in particular vascular, cardiac, and thoracic surgery, may cause acute elevation of mPAP either during the surgery or shortly after the intervention has been completed. This is particularly dangerous in patients with preexisting PH, because even short-lasting increased pressure overload to the RV could lead to profound decompensation with all downstream negative hemodynamic consequences. Preexisting PH is one of the major risk factors for morbidity and death in cardiothoracic surgery patients.[23] PH is a major determinant of perioperative morbidity and mortality rate in special situations such as heart and lung transplantation, pneumonectomy, and ventricular assist device placement.[24] The elevated PAP during and after surgery is thought to develop secondary to acute left-sided heart failure/dysfunction, or it can also be a consequence of pulmonary parenchymal and endothelial injury with activation of the systemic and pulmonary inflammatory response to cardiopulmonary bypass circulation or ischemia-reperfusion.[25] Protamine-mediated acute PH and right ventricular failure in the perioperative period are common complications of cardiopulmonary bypass circulation during open-heart operations.[26] PH can also develop later as a result of ARDS[27] or other complications (sepsis, PE, etc.) not directly related to either surgery or anesthesia.

INTEGRATED APPROACH TO THE DIAGNOSIS OF PULMONARY HYPERTENSION

When PH is suspected based on presentation, examination, and risk factors, a comprehensive and structured evaluation should be performed. Physical examination is usually variable and nonspecific. The presence of an accentuated pulmonary component of S_2, an early systolic click, and a midsystolic ejection murmur from turbulent pulmonary outflow should raise the suspicion. Left parasternal lift and an S_4 are signs of right ventricular hypertrophy. Distended jugular veins and hepatojugular reflux indicate high central venous pressure. Right ventricular S_3, hepatomegaly, ascites, systemic hypotension, peripheral edema, and cool extremities are all signs of right ventricular failure. A high level of suspicion is paramount in establishing a timely diagnosis of PH in order to initiate therapy. The diagnostic endeavor is aimed at making the diagnosis of PH and also in finding its cause. General guidelines for the evaluation of PH are described in detail in Figure 45.2. Chest radiographic findings are usually nonspecific but enlarged main and hilar PA shadows could be seen. RV enlargement best seen in the lateral views could also suggest PH. Moreover, the chest radiograph can also present findings of underlying primary lung disease such as emphysema or pulmonary fibrosis. Electrocardiography has a low sensitivity and specificity for the diagnosis of PH; however, evidence of right atrial enlargement, right axis deviation, and RV enlargement is suggestive of the disease. In many cases, PH remains undiagnosed and its treatment begins only after serious complications have developed. Some serologic markers, such as troponin and natriuretic peptides, are important for the evaluation of right ventricular dysfunction. Serum troponin may be elevated in patients with PH and has been associated with right ventricular overdistention and

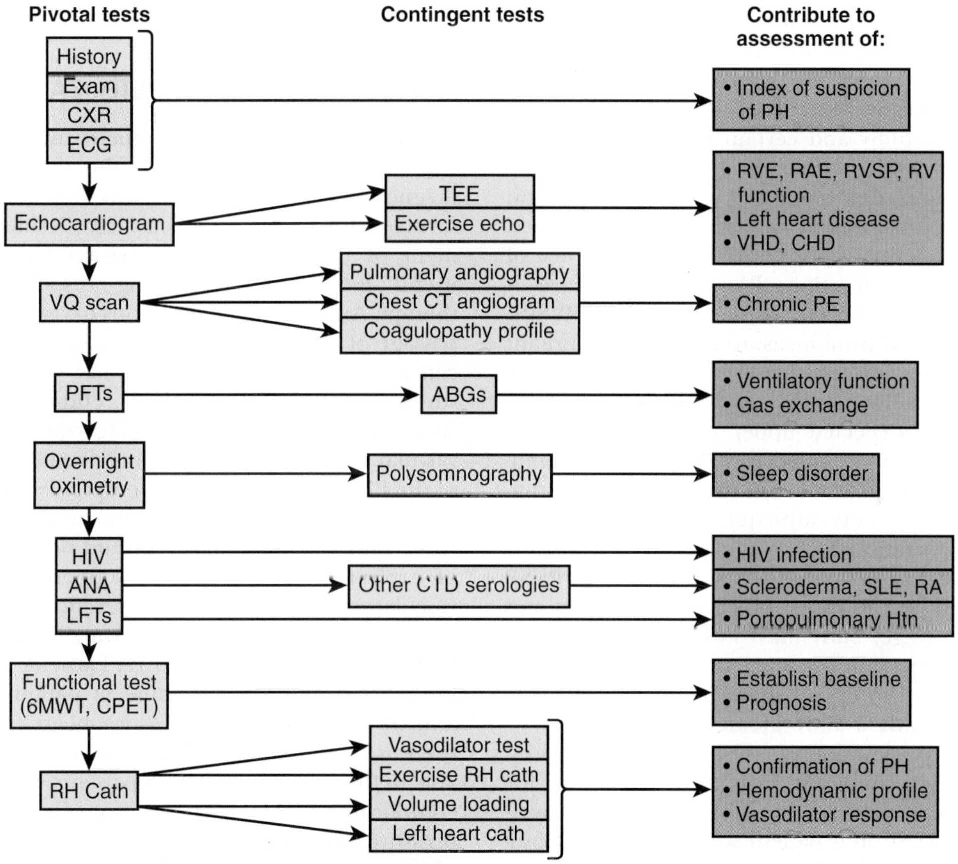

Figure 45.2 General guidelines for the evaluation of pulmonary hypertension: because the suspicion of PH may arise in various ways, the sequence of tests may vary. However, the diagnosis of PAH requires that certain data support a specific diagnosis. In addition, the diagnosis of IPAH is one of excluding all other reasonable possibilities. Pivotal tests are those that are essential to establishing a diagnosis of any type of PAH either by identification of criteria of associated disease or exclusion of diagnoses other than IPAH. All pivotal tests are required for a definitive diagnosis and baseline characterization. An abnormality of one assessment (such as obstructive pulmonary disease on PFT), does not preclude that another abnormality (chronic thromboembolic disease on $\dot{V}/\dot{Q}$ scan and pulmonary angiogram) is contributing or predominant. Contingent tests are recommended to elucidate or confirm results of the pivotal tests and need only be performed in the appropriate clinical context. The combination of pivotal and appropriate contingent tests contributes to assessment of the differential diagnoses in the right-hand column. It should be recognized that definitive diagnosis may require additional specific evaluations not necessarily included in this general guideline. 6MWT indicates a 6-minute walk test. ABGs, arterial blood gases; ANA, antinuclear antibody serologic test; CHD, congenital heart disease; CPET, cardiopulmonary exercise test; CT, computed tomography; CTD, connective tissue disease; CXR, chest x-ray; ECG, electrocardiogram; HIV, human immunodeficiency virus screening; Htn, hypertension; IPAH, idiopathic pulmonary artery hypertension; LFT, liver function test; PAH, pulmonary artery hypertension; PE, pulmonary embolism; PFT, pulmonary function test; PH, pulmonary hypertension; RA, rheumatoid arthritis; RAE, right atrial enlargement; RHC, right-sided heart catheterization; RVE, right ventricular enlargement; RVSP, right ventricular systolic pressure; SLE, systemic lupus erythematosus; TEE, transesophageal echocardiography; VHD, valvular heart disease; $\dot{V}/\dot{Q}$ scan, ventilation-perfusion scintigram. (From McLaughlin VV: Expert consensus document on pulmonary hypertension. J Am Coll Cardiol 2009;53:1573-1619.)

ischemia. Troponin I leak due to acute right ventricular strain from PE has been well studied and may predict mortality rate.[28,29] Elevated B-natriuretic peptide (BNP) is an important prognostic indicator and correlates strongly with PVR, cardiac output, and functional status in patients with PH.[30] A high level of plasma BNP, and in particular, a further increase in plasma BNP during follow-up, may have a strong independent association with increased mortality rates in patients with PH.[31] However, the significance of measuring BNP level in patients with PH in the acute setting remains unclear.

The most useful tools for the diagnosis and management of PH are echocardiography and right-sided heart catheterization.

ECHOCARDIOGRAPHY

Echocardiography is the most important and useful noninvasive study for screening of PH. It is very important for diagnosing and determining the degree and clinical significance of PH in critically ill patients. It can noninvasively visualize cardiac anatomy and certain intracardiac shunts and valvular abnormalities, estimate right atrial and pulmonary arterial pressures, determine the severity of right and left ventricular dysfunction and wall motion abnormalities, and reveal other potential causes of PH. In the absence of pulmonary outflow obstruction, PA systolic pressure is equivalent to right ventricular systolic pressure (RVSP), which can be calculated from measured systolic regurgitant tricuspid flow velocity and estimated right atrial pressure. PH by TTE is usually defined as RVSP greater than 35 mm Hg with the expected upper normal limit up to 40 mm Hg in older or obese subjects.[32] However, it has limitations and echocardiography has a 45% false-positive rate of diagnosis when patients subsequently undergo right-sided heart catheterization.[33]

Among 3790 healthy people who underwent TTE, RVSP was highly variable in the range of 15 to 57 mm Hg and was associated with age, body mass index (BMI), gender, wall thickness, and ejection fraction. An RVSP greater than 40 mm Hg was found in 6% of those older than 50 years and 5% of those with a BMI greater than 30 kg/m^2.[32] Therefore, not every elevation of RVSP indicates the presence of a pathologic condition. Possible explanations for mildly elevated RVSP detected by TTE include[34] (1) overestimation of the RVSP in a patient with true normal pulmonary pressure; (2) serendipitous observation of a transient pressure elevation in an otherwise healthy individual; (3) discovery of stable mild PH, and (4) discovery of early progressive PH.

Echocardiographic signs of significant PH include right ventricular dilation (D-shaped RV) and its hypertrophy (in sustained cases), septal dyskinesia and bowing into the LV during late systole to early diastole, RV hypokinesis, tricuspid regurgitation, right atrial enlargement, and a dilated inferior vena cava.[19,35,36] In patients with chronic PH, predictors of poor outcome include right atrial enlargement, septal bowing, and the development of a pericardial effusion.[37] Increased RV size combined with increased outflow resistance and reduced ejection fraction have been also described in acute right ventricular failure.[19] A specific pattern of right ventricular dysfunction in acute PE has been characterized by a severe hypokinesia of the RV mid-free wall, with normal contractions of the apical segment.[38]

Images may be suboptimal in critically ill patients because of limitations related to the patient's general condition, limited positioning, attached monitoring devices, wound dressings, or ventilatory support. Transesophageal echocardiography (TEE) may be more accurate and sensitive in critically ill patients than TTE, especially in acute diseases such as PE when acute PH is highly suspected.[39] Newly developed handheld ultrasound devices capable of TEE may sufficiently replace a standard cart-based TEE system in unstable critically ill patients.[40] Advanced Doppler echocardiographic techniques allow for comprehensive hemodynamic assessment of the patients with PH. A high correlation between PA catheter and Doppler echocardiography evaluations of cardiac output, transpulmonary gradient, and PVR were observed in patients with severe PH.[41]

RIGHT-SIDED HEART CATHETERIZATION

Invasive hemodynamic assessment using right-sided heart catheterization is considered the gold standard for the diagnosis of PH[35]; however, this procedure must be performed thoroughly and accurately. Besides direct measurement of the hemodynamic parameters, it also provides useful information regarding response to vasodilator therapy. Analysis of mixed venous oxygen saturations during passage of the PA on its way through the cardiac chambers can allow diagnosis of intracardiac shunts. A PCWP measurement reflects left ventricular end-diastolic (filling) pressure. Values less than 15 mm Hg rule out left ventricular, valvular, and pulmonary venous diseases as possible causes of the PH.[35] It is important to emphasize that misinterpretation of the PCWP is a common pitfall during right-sided heart catheterization and it should be measured at the end of expiration and in several segments of the pulmonary vasculature because pulmonary veno-occlusive disease can cause elevated wedge pressure only in affected segments.[42] In the ICU, placement of a PA catheter for diagnosis and monitoring is highly desirable in patients with severe PH and in patients with progressive heart failure.[43] Although there is a little doubt that the hemodynamic data are valuable in the care of critically ill patients with acute conditions complicated by PH, there are no data available on how PA pressure monitoring could affect management and outcome of these patients. Indeed, placing a PA catheter could be a challenging and dangerous procedure in such patient populations. Technical difficulties could be related to severe tricuspid regurgitation, right ventricular dilatation, elevated PAP, and decreased cardiac output. Complications of PA catheterization are particularly dangerous in patients with PH and right ventricular dysfunction/failure. Arrhythmias in response to PA catheterization can have potentially life-threatening consequences by decreasing cardiac output, or converting into fatal ventricular arrhythmias. Obtaining a PCWP may be technically difficult in patients with markedly elevated PAP and also carries a high risk of sometimes fatal pulmonary arterial rupture. Finally, the presence of tricuspid regurgitation can significantly decrease accuracy of cardiac output calculations by thermodilution. Theoretically, the Fick method may be more accurate, but in critically ill patients with increased pulmonary metabolism and high or very low cardiac output, its accuracy may not be optimal.[44]

MANAGEMENT OF ARTERIAL PULMONARY HYPERTENSION AND RIGHT VENTRICULAR FAILURE IN THE INTENSIVE CARE UNIT

GENERAL MANAGEMENT PRINCIPLES

In patients with preexisting PH, an acute illness can lead to significant hemodynamic changes with profound and refractory systemic arterial hypotension, mainly secondary to increased PVR associated with decreased cardiac output and decrease systemic vascular resistance (SVR). This would require tight hemodynamic monitoring and aggressive treatment with combinations of pulmonary vasodilators, inotropic agents, and systemic arterial vasoconstrictors to manage acute right ventricular dysfunction and failure and also to maintain coronary and end-organ perfusion.[45] The first step is to optimize the volume status and avoid volume overload. Then efforts should be made to achieve the following: improve cardiac output, reduce PVR (by using vasodilators with fewer systemic effects and $\dot{V}/\dot{Q}$ mismatch); treat reversible factors such as hypoxemia, acidosis, anemia; and maintain adequate SVR to ensure end-organ perfusion and adequate coronary filling pressures.[46] A general therapeutic approach to pulmonary hypertension in the ICU is outlined in Figure 45-3.

MONITORING

ICU monitoring of PH and right ventricular failure is of paramount importance. Besides the utilization of a PA catheter as outlined previously, serial TTE could also be useful for assessment of right ventricular function. Additionally, close attention should be made to monitoring end-organ function. Urinary output and serum creatinine should be used to monitor renal function. Liver function tests should also be followed closely for assessment of liver impairment, especially during severe right ventricular failure and development of passive liver congestion.

Previous studies have raised concerns and controversy regarding the use of PA catheters and their utility for invasive measurement of cardiac function in critically ill subjects with shock.[47,48] However, individuals with severe PH and right ventricular failure are probably best monitored by an invasive method to allow continuous measurement of key hemodynamic values such as cardiac index, mPAP, PVR, and Svo_2. General markers of tissue perfusion such as lactate

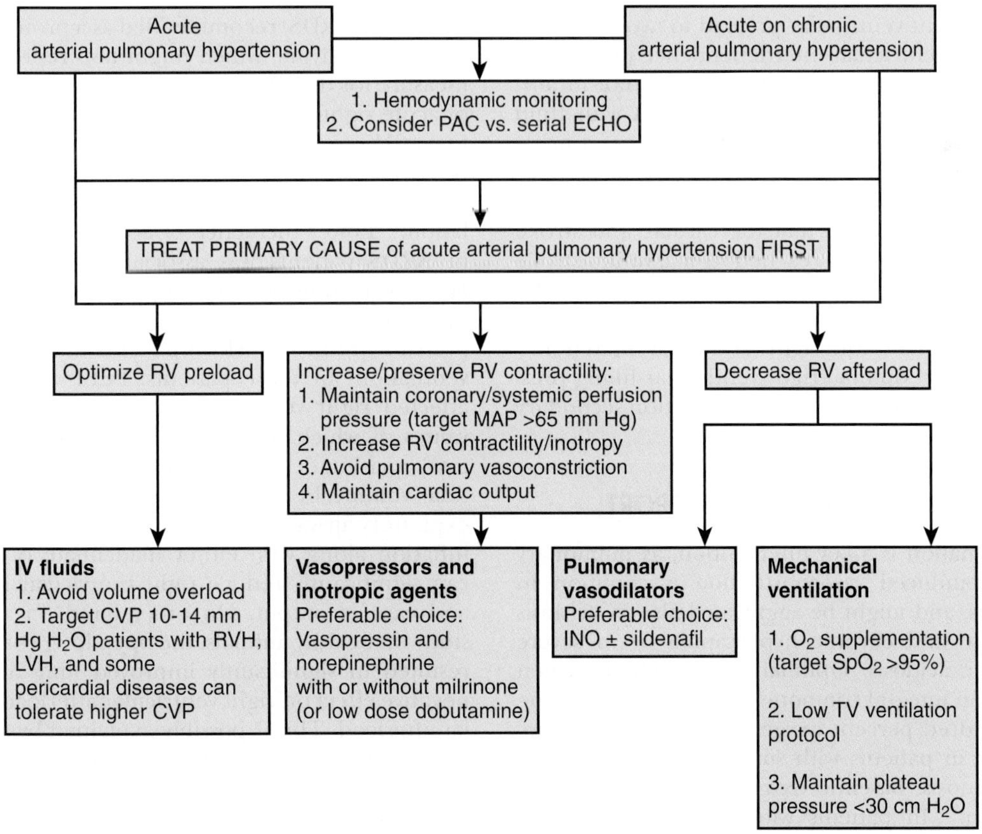

Figure 45.3 Therapeutic approach to pulmonary hypertension in the intensive care unit. CVP, central venous pressure; ECHO, echocardiogram; INO, inhaled nitric oxide; IV, intravenous; LVH, left ventricular hypertrophy; MAP, mean arterial pressure; PAC, pulmonary artery catheter; RV, right ventricle; RVH, right ventricular hypertrophy; Spo_2, oxygen saturation in the blood; TV, tidal volume. (From Tsapenko MV: Arterial pulmonary hypertension in noncardiac intensive care unit. Vasc Health Risk Manage 2008;4:1043-1060.)

levels and neurohormonal/myocardial markers such as natriuretic peptides and troponin can also be utilized for monitoring.

FLUID MANAGEMENT

Fluid management is a difficult task in these patients because both hypervolemia and hypovolemia can have severe effects on the overall hemodynamic status. With a normal RV, the right ventricular ejection fraction is usually dependent on right ventricular preload.[49] However, when right ventricular afterload is increased, even a relatively small increase in blood volume may result in right ventricular dysfunction. Right ventricular dysfunction can occur with volume expansion, despite constant PVR and a decrease in mPAP. Further observations have drawn the conclusion that high right ventricular filling pressure restores normal hemodynamics only if PVR is normal and right ventricular contractility is not markedly reduced.[50] In patients with PH, right ventricular dysfunction/failure can reduce left ventricular filling and lead to severe cardiogenic shock. Patients with cardiogenic shock secondary to right ventricular dysfunction usually have a very high (>20 mm Hg) right ventricular filling pressure.[51] In addition to decreased right ventricular contractility and cardiac output, right ventricular dilatation can further limit left ventricular filling via ventricular interdependence shifting of the interventricular septum toward the left ventricular cavity. Traditional practice with aggressive fluid resuscitation can thus worsen the patient's condition. The challenge in fluid management in those patients is to find the optimal right ventricular preload to avoid the detrimental effects of ventricular interdependence on left ventricular function. In the majority of cases (but not in all), right ventricular failure is generally associated with fluid overload and measures should be made to achieve a negative fluid balance.[52] Hemodynamic monitoring in patients with right ventricular failure due to acute right ventricular myocardial infarction showed that the cardiac and stroke indexes increased and the RV reached its maximum stroke work index when the filling pressure was 10 to 14 mm Hg. These values may be regarded as the optimal level of RV filling pressure in patients with right ventricular infarction.[53] There are no data on optimal right ventricular filling pressure in patients with right ventricular dysfunction secondary to acute PH.

OXYGENATION AND VENTILATORY SUPPORT

Adequate oxygenation is a key intervention, as pulmonary arterial hypoxic-induced vasoconstriction is common in these individuals, and might be aggravated also by acidosis as seen in acute and chronic hypercapnia or in severe shock with lactic acidosis. Optimal supplemental oxygen management is an integral component of PH therapy in the ICU.[54] One hundred percent oxygen is a selective pulmonary vasodilator in patients with sustained PH, regardless of primary diagnosis, baseline oxygenation, or right ventricular function.[55] In patients with ARDS, the vascular response to oxygen was different, and administration of 100% O_2 caused the intrapulmonary shunt to deteriorate owing to the collapse of unstable alveolar units with very low ventilation-perfusion ratios. This is in contrast to administration of 100% O_2 to patients with COPD, in whom only the dispersion of the blood flow distribution was changed, suggesting release of hypoxic pulmonary vasoconstriction.[56]

Hypercapnia has been shown to induce PH in animal models. There are no data on how it could affect acute PH in humans. However, a study on healthy volunteers revealed that human pulmonary vascular responses to hypercapnia and hypocapnia consist, respectively, of constriction and dilatation that take 1.5 to 2 hours to reach a steady level. The time courses for recovery in eucapnia are similar. Hypercapnia generated a rise in cardiac output by changing heart rate; hypocapnia produced a fall in cardiac output by changing stroke volume. The finding of marked vasodilatation in response to hypocapnia demonstrates that there is normally a substantial vascular tone in the human pulmonary circulation.[57]

The management of mechanical ventilation in patients with PH is often challenging due to the effects of positive airway pressure, in addition to the side effects of sedatives. Noninvasive ventilation should initially be considered; however, if intubation is required, careful attention must be paid to the effects of the sedatives on the hemodynamics and to the interaction of the patient with the ventilator. Controlled ventilation alters right ventricular function primarily by increasing right ventricular afterload during the lung inflation period.[58] Transpulmonary pressure (and related tidal volume), but not airway pressure itself, was the main determinant factor of right ventricular afterload during mechanical ventilation.[59] This supports low-volume strategy in ARDS, recommended as a protective measure for lung parenchyma, which might also represent a protective measure for the RV and pulmonary circulation.[59] Frequency of acute right ventricular failure in ARDS patients declined from 61% to 25% over the last 15 to 30 years, which could be explained in part by fundamental alterations in respiratory support and implementation of low tidal volume ventilation.[16] Lower incidence of acute right ventricular failure in ARDS patients was associated with lower (<27-30 cm H_2O) plateau pressures.[21] Right ventricular systolic function was generally negatively affected by positive end-expiratory pressure (PEEP) in ARDS patients undergoing mechanical ventilation. In those patients, PEEP titration significantly affected right ventricular outflow impedance, the lowest values of which were associated with the achieved better total quasi-static lung compliance (calculated by dividing tidal volume by the difference between plateau and end-expiratory airway pressures).[60] This suggests that lung hyperinflation along with either inadequate or excessive PEEP can significantly reduce right ventricular systolic function and cardiac output. On other hand, in an experimental study on healthy animals, the open lung concept ventilation resulted in significantly improved lung aeration with no negative effect on right ventricular afterload or left ventricular afterload. This is possibly explained by a loss of hypoxic pulmonary vasoconstriction due to alveolar recruitment. The reductions in the cardiac output and in the mPAP were the consequences of a reduced preload.[61] A clinical study in patients after cardiac surgery also found no evidence that ventilation, according to the open lung concept, affects right ventricular afterload.[62]

VASOPRESSORS AND INOTROPIC AGENTS

The choice of any particular agent in patients with PH should take into consideration its effects on PVR and cardiac output when used alone or in combination with other agents. Most traditional vasopressors and inotropes have not been studied in the setting of arterial PH and hemodynamic instability.

Dobutamine is the most commonly used inotropic agent in patients with PH. It augments myocardial contractility and reduces left ventricular afterload via peripheral vasodilatory effects. In low doses (up to 5 μg/kg/minute) dobutamine decreased PVR, lowered mean systemic arterial pressure, and slightly increased cardiac output[63]; at doses of 5 to 10 μg/kg/minute, dobutamine caused significant tachycardia and systemic hypotension without improving PVR.[63,64] In cases of systemic hypotension patients may require concomitant use of norepinephrine or other peripheral vasoconstrictors to maintain appropriate systemic perfusion pressures. A combination of inhaled nitric oxide (INO) and dobutamine infusion produced an additive effect on pulmonary circulation[63] with increased cardiac performance and improved oxygenation[65] and had no adverse effects on systemic hemodynamics. In an animal model of acute right ventricular failure secondary to acute PH, dobutamine was superior to norepinephrine in improving right ventricular function by optimizing pulmonary vasodilation and improving right ventricular contractility.[63]

Norepinephrine (NE) is widely used in critical care settings to treat hemodynamically unstable patients. It exerts significant inotropic effects via β_1-receptor agonism and α_1-receptor-mediated vasoconstriction. In addition to positive effects on cardiac output and systemic arterial pressure, NE is able to improve the right ventricular oxygen supply/demand ratio,[66] although it increases PVR and could worsen PH.[67] However, at a lower dose (<7 μg/minute), NE exerts more vasoconstrictive effect in systemic than in pulmonary circulation.[67] NE was superior to *phenylephrine* in restoring systemic arterial pressure, decreasing PVR, augmenting right ventricular myocardial blood flow, and improving cardiac output in animal models of acute PE.[68] In patients with chronic PH who developed systemic hypotension following induction of anesthesia, NE in contrast to phenylephrine decreased the ratio of PAP to systemic blood pressure without a change in cardiac index.[67] Experimental data also showed that α-adrenergic stimulation can cause a disproportionate rise in PVR,[69] which is implicated in the development of acute PH in critical illnesses. Besides this, phenylephrine also causes bradycardia with further adverse consequences on pulmonary and systemic hemodynamics.[70] These findings all make NE preferable over phenylephrine for the treatment of hypotension in patients with chronic PH.[67] Moreover, NE can be used successfully in combination with selective pulmonary vasodilators for the treatment of patients with acute and chronic PH.[45,71]

Dopamine produces dose-dependent dopaminergic, β- and α-adrenergic effects on cardiac output and vascular tone. In patients with chronic PH, dopamine infusion led to increased heart rate, mean pulmonary and systemic pressure, and cardiac index with concomitant fall of SVR.[72] However, administration of dopamine, similar to *epinephrine,* is associated with high risk of tachyarrhythmia, with potentially dramatic hemodynamic consequences in patients with severe PH.[70] In a small animal study of sepsis-induced PH, epinephrine infusion increased SVR and cardiac output and lowered PVR.[73] Isoproterenol is another agent that has positive inotropic and chronotropic effect, which in therapeutic doses increases cardiac output and produces pulmonary and peripheral vasodilation. In animals with acute PH, administration of isoproterenol did not reduce PAP, and instead produced significant tachycardia and was associated with arrhythmias.[74]

Vasopressin is an endogenous hormone with a weak noradrenergic vasopressor effect on the systemic vasculature and an ability to produce NO-mediated selective pulmonary vasodilation.[75] In healthy animals, a linear relationship was observed between vasopressin levels and SVR without significantly affecting PVR or any vascular compliance.[74] It was very effective (at a dose of 0.1 U/minute) in treating refractory low SVR hypotension concomitant with PH in postoperative patients.[76] Experimental data on the use of vasopressin in acute PH is controversial. In one setting, vasopressin infusion produced significant pulmonary vasodilation,[77] although at a higher dose (1.16 U/kg/hour) in another animal model it caused increased PVR and decreased cardiac output with a decrease in right ventricular contractility.[78] Studies of the coronary vasoconstriction and the inotropic effect of vasopressin are also controversial, and the effects appear to depend on the dose used and the model studied.[79] However, the use of vasopressin at a low dose (0.04 U/minute) produces favorable hemodynamic effects without substantial decline in cardiac output and pulmonary vasoconstriction,[79] which makes it a preferable agent for patients with PH.

Levosimendan (a myocardial and vascular calcium sensitizer) besides positive systemic hemodynamic effects also has pulmonary vasodilatory properties and positive inotropic effects on the RV. This makes it particularly effective in treatment of right ventricular dysfunction related to PH.[80,81] In this setting, it restored right ventricular function even better than dobutamine, mainly because of more efficient pulmonary vasodilation on top of similar inotropic effects. A pilot prospective randomized controlled study on patients with ARDS in association with septic shock showed that levosimendan improves right ventricular performance mainly through pulmonary vasodilator effects.[82] It was also effective in restoring right ventricular function in patients with cardiogenic shock following myocardial infarction.[83]

Milrinone is a selective phosphodiesterase-3 inhibitor with significant inotropic and vasodilatory effects in both pulmonary and systemic circulation. It is widely used alone or in combinations in patients with decompensated heart failure, particularly in those with nonischemic left ventricular systolic dysfunction,[84,85] and those after cardiac surgery.[1,86] In animal models of both acute and chronic PH, milrinone significantly reduced PVR and improved right ventricular function.[87,88] In combination with INO, milrinone produced additive pulmonary vasodilatation in acute PH.[89] In another animal model of PH, addition of sildenafil to milrinone produced more effective pulmonary vasodilation and increased right ventricular contractility without significant systemic hypotension. Cardiac output and right ventricular performance were significantly improved after milrinone alone or in combination with sildenafil, but not with sildenafil alone.[90] The systemic vasodilatory effects of milrinone along with its relatively long half-life are the major limiting factors against its utilization in conditions associated with systemic hypotension or hemodynamic instability. Systemic vasopressors (norepinephrine and low-dose vasopressin) were effective in the treatment of the milrinone-induced systemic hypotension. However, a milrinone-vasopressin combination was associated with better hemodynamics than milrinone-norepinephrine during the management of right ventricular failure.[91] In a volume-resuscitated pediatric patient with septic shock, a combination of catecholamines with milrinone improved cardiovascular function.[92] In animal models, nebulization of milrinone predominantly dilated pulmonary blood vessels, resulting in a reduced pulmonary-to-systemic vascular resistance ratio, improvement in hemodynamic and oxygenation profiles, and prevention of the pulmonary endothelial dysfunction.[93,94] Inhaled milrinone was superior to intravenous milrinone in patients with PH after mitral valve replacement surgery; demonstrating less systemic hypotension, more reduction in intrapulmonary shunt fraction, and improvement in Pao_2/Fio_2 ratio.[86]

PULMONARY VASODILATORS

Reduction of right ventricular afterload is an important part in the management of a patient with PH. Most pulmonary vasodilators can be subdivided according to their action on the pulmonary vasculature via either cyclic guanosine monophosphate, prostacyclin, or endothelin pathways.[1] Used in stable patients either as monotherapy or in combination, they were able to reduce mortality rates and improve multiple other clinical and hemodynamic outcomes.[95,96] Not all of them can be utilized in a critical care setting: the route of administration, half-life, and systemic effects could significantly affect the choice of the medication. Pulmonary vasodilators with longer half-lives or significant systemic hemodynamic effects can decrease organ perfusion pressure and reduce right coronary blood flow with further deterioration of right ventricular performance.

INHALED NITRIC OXIDE

INO is a potent vasodilator able to lower PAP and right ventricular oxygen demand.[88] This improves cardiac performance without altering right ventricular contractility and cardiac output in hemodynamically stable patients with a variety of causes of PH.[87,89,97] INO also dilates pulmonary vasculature in ventilated lung areas, thereby improving $\dot{V}/\dot{Q}$ match and oxygenation.[91] It has a very short half-life and almost no systemic vasodilatory effects, which is very important in the treatment of hemodynamically unstable patients. Multiple studies on INO utilization in ARDS patients showed improvement in oxygenation for 24 to 48 hours and variable improvement in mPAP.[92] A combination of INO and other interventions, such as PEEP and prone positioning, also had beneficial and additive effects on arterial oxygenation.[93] However, INO had no favorable impact on the duration of ventilatory support or mortality rate in this patient population.[93,98] In cardiac surgery patients with a history of PH, INO was associated with lower heart rates, higher RV ejection fraction, and a lower requirement for vasopressor agents compared to milrinone.[99] INO has been successfully used and it was associated with improved outcomes in critically ill postoperative patients who developed severe PH or right ventricular failure.[95,100] A combination treatment of INO with other pulmonary vasodilators (milrinone, sildenafil, etc.) has been successfully used in management of acute PH in different conditions.[89,101] Besides its high applicability in many acute conditions, INO could be delivered in spontaneously breathing individuals by face mask or even nasal cannula as it was shown in pediatric practice.[102] INO treatment is associated with some side effects including methemoglobinemia[91,96] and NO_2 formation.[103] Abrupt withdrawal of INO has been associated with rebound PH, a significant drop in Pao_2, and life-threatening hemodynamic deterioration.[96,104] Close monitoring and gradual discontinuation are important to prevent and detect rebound PH.

PROSTANOIDS

Prostaglandin E_1 and prostacyclin are able to produce significant pulmonary vasodilatation and lower mPAP. They also possess antithrombotic, antiproliferative, and anti-inflammatory properties. Intravenous prostacyclin is highly effective in cases of severe PH and is also associated with a significant survival benefit.[105,106] Prostacyclin and its analogs (iloprost, epoprostenol, and treprostinil) in inhaled forms are as effective as intravenous forms in patients with chronic PH in different clinical settings.[107,108] All prostanoids have relatively long half-lives and can significantly affect systemic hemodynamics, which limits their use in critically ill or hemodynamically unstable patients.

In the ICU setting, inhaled prostaglandins have been used to treat severe sustained PH and intractable hypoxia, but were associated with systemic hypotension. Inhaled iloprost effectively decreased mPAP and improved RV performance immediately after separation from cardiopulmonary bypass.[109] Inhaled iloprost was also successfully used in the treatment of acute right ventricular dysfunction in the setting of preexisting PH in heart transplant recipients during weaning from cardiopulmonary bypass circulation and was not associated with significant systemic side effects. Intravenous prostacyclin (prostaglandin I_2 [PGI_2]) in combination with norepinephrine and dopamine was effective in the treatment of protamine-mediated acute PH and right ventricular failure in the setting of open heart surgery.[110] Inhaled prostacyclin showed different effects on oxygenation and pulmonary hemodynamics in patients presenting with primary pulmonary ARDS (reduction in Pao_2/Fio_2) compared with an extrapulmonary cause of ARDS (increase in Pao_2/Fio_2 along with a decrease in mPAP). Despite the observation that RV ejection fraction increased on INO, but not with PGI_2, both INO and PGI_2-aerosol showed beneficial effects on RV performance and may prove helpful in the treatment of acute PH.[104]

PHOSPHODIESTERASE-5 INHIBITORS

Sildenafil is a specific phosphodiesterase-5 inhibitor with sustained pulmonary vasodilatory effect and the ability to lower PVR and mPAP and to increase cardiac output in patients with different forms of chronic PH,[111,112] including patients with PH secondary to congestive heart failure.[101] In the chronic setting, it is highly effective alone or in combination with other pulmonary vasodilators: epoprostenol,[113] iloprost,[114,115] BNP,[116] and INO.[117] It was able to improve central hemodynamics and right ventricular function in ventilated patients with PH who required dobutamine administration.[118] Its ability to augment and prolong the hemodynamic effects of other pulmonary vasodilators has been successfully used to minimize rebound PH after INO discontinuation,[119] in weaning from intravenous vasodilators in patients after cardiac surgery[101] as well as in chronic PH therapy,[103] and in severe right ventricular dysfunction related to chronic PH.[119] In an animal model of another specific phosphodiesterase-5 inhibitor, zaprinast was more effective than milrinone in the management of acute PH, causing dose-dependent pulmonary vasodilation without significant systemic hypotension.[120] Intravenous zaprinast may also increase the efficacy and prolong the duration of action of INO; however, its efficacy in lung injury models was uncertain: nonselective vasodilation induced by intravenously administered zaprinast not only worsens gas exchange but also abolishes the beneficial effects of INO.[120] Subthreshold doses (which did not reduce mPAP) of zaprinast and sildenafil in patients with acute lung injury associated with PH improved responsiveness to INO.[121]

Calcium channel blockers have been used in hemodynamically stable patients with PAH who demonstrated a pulmonary vascular response to acute vasodilator challenge.[42] There are limited data on utilization of calcium channel blockers in critically ill patients with acute PH. Acute administration of nifedipine did not cause pulmonary vasodilatation, and in contrast led to increased right ventricular end-diastolic pressure and decreased right ventricular contractility.[106] Prolonged half-life and negative inotropic effects, which may precipitate fatal worsening of right ventricular failure, limit the use of calcium channel blockers in treatment of acute PH.

Endothelin receptor antagonists appear to be highly effective in the treatment of PH in the outpatient settings.[42] They have not been adequately studied in acute care settings. In an animal model, pretreatment with bosentan completely abolished endotoxin-induced acute PH and changes in pulmonary compliance and resistance.[3] Currently, the only possible implication in critically ill patients would be weaning or conversion from inhaled or intravenous pulmonary vasodilators to oral medication (bosentan and ambrisentan). There also seems to be a role for ambrisentan in the management of portopulmonary hypertension patients awaiting liver transplantation.[122]

Natriuretic peptides (atrial natriuretic peptide [ANP] and BNP) have diuretic and vasorelaxing properties and are able to counteract the renin-angiotensin system.[123] In patients with right ventricular failure, they produced dose-related pulmonary vasodilatation without worsening oxygen saturation or systemic hemodynamic and exerted favorable neurohormonal effects by suppressing aldosterone. BNP significantly attenuated the mPAP and acute hypoxic pulmonary vasoconstriction in otherwise healthy individuals,[124] but had no effect on mPAP or PVR in patients with PH. Use of nesiritide in hemodynamically unstable and hypotensive patients is limited, mainly because of reduction of SVR and resulting profound systemic hypotension.[125]

Nitroprusside and nitroglycerin both can cause significant pulmonary vasodilation similar to that of INO. However, nitroprusside has a longer half-life and can cause acute reduction of SVR leading to systemic hypotension, limiting its use in hemodynamically unstable and hypotensive patients.[87] A significant venodilator effect of nitroglycerin decreases right ventricular preload leading to adverse consequences in patients with right ventricular failure. Inhaled nitroglycerin may be a safer therapeutic option without adverse effect on systemic hemodynamic parameters.[126]

Intravenous *adenosine* is a pulmonary vasodilator with a very short half-life (6-10 seconds) and can be effective for short-term lowering of PVR.[105] In the setting of acute PH, adenosine infusion may help lower mPAP without systemic hypotension, which can reverse the clinical state of shock by achieving pulmonary vasodilatation.[127] At higher doses (70 to 100 mg/kg/minute) it caused systemic vasodilation.[113] Adenosine is also successfully used to treat persistent PH of the newborn.[128]

Dipyridamole inhibits phosphodiesterase-5 and thromboxane synthase, which explains its strong vasodilatory effect on pulmonary circulation. Dipyridamole can lower PVR, augment INO-induced pulmonary vasodilation,[114] acutely attenuate the adverse hemodynamic effects of rapid withdrawal of INO therapy, and attenuate excessive hypoxic pulmonary vasoreactivity. In pediatric patients with PH, dipyridamole was as effective as INO, but caused significant systemic vasodilatation.[115] Intravenous dipyridamole was used in acute management of PH in combination either with INO or intravenous nitroglycerin,[129] as well as for diagnostic purposes to identify reversibility of PH in potential cardiac transplant recipients with heart failure in whom a pulmonary vasodilator response to inhalation of INO alone was not observed.[130]

OTHER THERAPIES AND MECHANICAL CARDIOVASCULAR SUPPORT

The observations of survival advantage in patients with PH and a patent foramen ovale suggested that an intra-atrial right-to-left shunt could decompress the RV and increase left ventricular preload, thereby increasing systemic blood flow and improving systemic oxygen transport despite arterial oxygen desaturation. Atrial septostomy has been developed as an alternative/bridge treatment and applied in patients with lack of response to medical therapy in the absence of other surgical treatment options. It has substantial morbidity and mortality rates in critically ill patients with severe right ventricular failure.[131] With growing experience, procedure-related death rates have been reduced to 5.4%, and the most suitable patient group has been identified among patients with a mean right atrial pressure between 10 and 20 mm Hg.[132] Acute right ventricular failure after orthotopic heart transplantation was successfully managed by decompression of the RV through the patent foramen ovale of the donor heart and inhalation of iloprost.[133] Both pericardiectomy and creation of atrial septal defects have been used in extreme cases of acute right ventricular failure secondary to acute myocardial infarction.[134] Decompression of the RV through the septostomy may potentially be an effective alternative in the management of severe acute PH in the ICU setting. The defect could be subsequently closed using a transcatheter septal occlusion device after the patient's condition has been stabilized.

The treatment of choice for PH secondary to chronic thromboembolic disease is pulmonary thromboendarterectomy, which can be performed when organized thrombus is in the proximal vessels[135]; significant hemodynamic improvement has been reported after such intervention.

Mechanical support for the RV with RV-assist devices (RVAD) could be a reasonable option for reversible cases or as a bridge to final treatment (transplantation). In cases of acute right ventricular failure after heart transplantation, use of RVADs, extracorporeal membrane oxygenation (ECMO), femoral vein–to–femoral artery roller, or centrifugal pumps may facilitate hemodynamic stability until the transplanted heart has recovered or until a new heart has been found for retransplantation.[136] These devices could be successfully applied in other cases of potentially reversible acute PH and right ventricular failure. Intra-aortic balloon counterpulsation (IABP) has long been the mainstay of mechanical therapy for cardiogenic shock; however, not every patient has a hemodynamic response to IABP.[134] In patients with acute PH and right ventricular failure associated with systemic hypotension, IABP could improve coronary and peripheral perfusion and augment left ventricular performance with an acute decrease in afterload.[137]

The use of extracorporeal life support, such as venoarterial ECMO, and pumpless lung assist devices have become the preferred bridging strategy for patients with severe right ventricular failure[52] who are candidates for transplantation. Heart-lung and lung transplantation has been an option for the therapy of select patients with end-stage PH for the past 25 years. Currently, approximately 4% of the approximately 1700 single lung, double lung, and combined heart and lung transplants annually performed worldwide in adults are for the primary indication of PH.[138] Their long-term outcomes are comparable with patients with other primary indications for transplant.[138]

PROGNOSIS

Despite significant advances made in the therapy of PH, this condition continues to have a poor survival both in the chronic and in the acute setting. The final common pathway is development of right ventricular failure and subsequent multiorgan failure. The natural history of chronic PH was well documented by the National Institutes of Health (NIH) Registry in which 194 patients with IPAH were enrolled in a multicenter observational study from 1981 through 1985.[139] The estimated median survival in this registry was 2.8 years with 1-, 3-, and 5-year survival rates of 68%, 48%, and 34%, respectively. Studies from other countries, including Japan, India, and Mexico, have shown similar results, with a median survival estimate of 2 to 3 years. More recently, two large registries have provided more contemporary data regarding prognosis of patients with chronic PH. The French Registry recently characterized survival and important prognostic indicators in PH patients. This registry demonstrated that the survival of PH patients has improved compared to the predicted survival based on the NIH Registry, although it still remains suboptimal with 1-, 2-, and 3-year survival rates of 85.7%, 69.5%, and 54.9% for incident cases.[140] In a recent large United States–based registry (REVEAL registry), important prognostic variables found to be predictors of outcome in this study included cause of PH, functional class, gender, exercise tolerance, and hemodynamics that reflect right ventricular function.[141] Prognosis is also influenced by an underlying cause; for example, in PH associated with scleroderma, its prognosis appears to be worse than for IPAH, and the untreated 2-year survival rate may be as low as 40%.[142] The presence of PH and associated right ventricular failure in the ICU is associated with worse outcomes. In the settings of both COPD and ARDS, the presence of right ventricular failure contributes significantly to shortened survival.[143] The 3-year survival rate in patients with severe airflow obstruction and a PVR three to four times normal is less than 10% to 15%.[143,144] Death from PH depends mainly on the state of the RV, and patients with symptoms of severe right-sided heart dysfunction, such as syncope, and hemodynamic evidence of impaired right ventricular function, such as reduced cardiac output or mixed venous saturation and elevated right atrial pressure, usually surrender to the disease within 1 to 2 years.[139] It is very important to discuss the prognosis and the possibility of transplantation in addition to end-of-life care with these patients and their family members before they present to the ICU. It is also very important to take into account the limitations of current therapies and the complexity of this lethal disease.

KEY POINTS

- PH is a complex and heterogeneous pulmonary vascular disorder that leads to elevated PVR and RV failure; it is defined by a resting mPAP greater than 25 mm Hg and associated with a PVR greater than 240 dynes · second · cm^{-5} (or >3 Wood units) measured by right-sided heart catheterization.
- It is important to identify where the vascular insult originates: conditions that raise the postcapillary pressure (pulmonary venous pressures) such as left-sided heart failure or mitral stenosis differ significantly from conditions that primarily affect the pulmonary arteries and arterioles such as IPAH.
- For the intensivist, it is important to recognize two different scenarios: patients with chronic PH admitted to the ICU for an acute process that may or may not worsen the underlying PH, or who can progress to severe acute PH, leading to life-threatening complications that include refractory systemic arterial hypotension, severe hypoxemia, right ventricular dysfunction and failure, and ultimately cardiogenic or obstructive shock and death; and patients with no history of chronic PH who develop acute PH during their ICU stay secondary to various conditions such as PE or ARDS.
- A meticulous and comprehensive evaluation to determine the cause of PH is very important in order to clarify the prognosis and guide the treatment, which should be directed toward improving gas exchange and hemodynamics.

KEY POINTS (Continued)

- The choice of any particular vasopressor agent in patients with PH should take into consideration its effects on PVR and cardiac output when used alone or in combination with other medications.
- In hemodynamically unstable patients with preexisting PH, use of norepinephrine infusion with or without low-dose vasopressin infusion should be initiated to maintain satisfactory end-organ and coronary perfusion.
- Most of conventional pulmonary vasodilators were not tested in critical care settings. Some inhaled agents (INO, short-acting prostanoids) and infusible inotropic agents (dobutamine, milrinone) were able to alleviate PH in critically ill patients. However, they can cause significant systemic hypotension and should be used with caution in hemodynamically unstable patients.
- Mechanical support for the RV with RVAD, extracorporeal life support such as venoarterial ECMO, and pumpless lung assist devices could be reasonable options for reversible cases or used as a bridge to final treatment (transplantation). Heart-lung or lung transplantation should be considered in selected patients with severe PH.

SELECTED REFERENCES

1. Humbert M, Morrell NW, Archer SL, et al: Cellular and molecular pathobiology of pulmonary arterial hypertension. J Am Coll Cardiol 2004;43:13S-24S.
7. Greyson CR: The right ventricle and pulmonary circulation: Basic concepts. Rev Esp Cardiol 2010;63:81-95.
14. Simonneau G, Robbins IM, Beghetti M, et al: Updated clinical classification of pulmonary hypertension. J Am Coll Cardiol 2009;54:S43-S54.
42. McLaughlin VV, Davis M, Cornwell W: Pulmonary arterial hypertension. Curr Probl Cardiol 2011;36:461-517.
45. Tsapenko MV, Tsapenko AV, Comfere TB, et al: Arterial pulmonary hypertension in noncardiac intensive care unit. Vasc Health Risk Manage 2008;4:1043-1060.
46. Price LC, Wort SJ, Finney SJ, et al: Pulmonary vascular and right ventricular dysfunction in adult critical care: Current and emerging options for management: A systematic literature review. Crit Care 2010;14:R169.
52. Hoeper MM, Granton J: Intensive care unit management of patients with severe pulmonary hypertension and right heart failure. Am J Respir Crit Care Med 2011;184:1114-1124.
68. Hirsch LJ, Rooney MW, Wat SS, et al: Norepinephrine and phenylephrine effects on right ventricular function in experimental canine pulmonary embolism. Chest 1991;100:796-801.
105. McLaughlin VV, Genthner DE, Panella MM, Rich S: Reduction in pulmonary vascular resistance with long-term epoprostenol (prostacyclin) therapy in primary pulmonary hypertension. N Engl J Med 1998;338:273-277.

The complete list of references can be found at www.expertconsult.com.

46 Massive Hemoptysis

Janice L. Zimmerman | Raul Sanchez

CHAPTER OUTLINE

Hemoptysis varies in amount from intermittent blood-streaked sputum to massive arterial bleeding with asphyxiation or exsanguination. Massive hemoptysis is defined as the expectoration of blood from the respiratory tract in life-threatening quantities. Clinical definitions of massive hemoptysis focus on selected quantities of coughed blood between 200 and 1000 mL over 24 hours or less, with greater than 600 mL being the most common criterion.[1] Quantification of the amount of coughed blood is unreliable, often subjective, and fails to account for blood remaining in the lungs. The adverse clinical effects of hemoptysis such as impaired gas exchange, airway obstruction, or hypotension may be more relevant for defining a life-threatening condition.[2]

Fortunately, massive hemoptysis is rare and accounts for 4% to 18.5% of all cases of hemoptysis in recent studies.[3-5] Incidence studies are problematic because of the use of variable definitions. Although mortality rates as high as 71%[6] were reported in the past, mortality rates in recent studies of massive hemoptysis range from 0% to 38%.[2,3,7]

This chapter focuses on the most common causes of massive hemoptysis, clinical manifestations, and options for management.

ANATOMIC CONSIDERATIONS

The lung is unique among the visceral organs in that it receives a dual blood supply from different circulations. Because hemoptysis can occur from either the pulmonary or bronchial circulation, an anatomic understanding of these systems is important.

PULMONARY CIRCULATION

The pulmonary artery bifurcates into left and right main pulmonary arteries after it leaves the right side of the heart. The pulmonary circulation is a low-pressure system, but pulmonary artery pressures may rise to approach systemic pressures in pulmonary parenchymal and pulmonary vascular diseases. Nevertheless, pulmonary hypertension alone rarely causes hemoptysis.

Prospective angiographic studies for hemoptysis in which both pulmonary and bronchial circulations have been imaged do not exist. Bleeding from the pulmonary arterial circulation accounts for less than 10% of massive hemoptysis cases and has been noted in a variety of destructive pulmonary lesions including tuberculosis, lung abscess, and aspergillosis.[2,8] Aneurysms of the pulmonary artery, arteriovenous malformations (AVMs), and pulmonary artery rupture have also been reported.

BRONCHIAL CIRCULATION

Bleeding from the higher pressure bronchial circulation has been estimated to cause 88% of the cases of massive and submassive hemoptysis.[9] The bronchial arteries arise from the descending aorta with considerable anatomic variation.

The one or two bronchial arteries that supply each lung in the majority of individuals[10] arise from the area near the first and second intercostal arteries. Particularly on the right side, the bronchial arteries may arise directly from the proximal first intercostal artery. The arteries course along the trachea, major bronchi, and bronchioles and have terminal communications with the pulmonary capillaries or pulmonary venules. The small-vessel bronchial supply to the trachea and major bronchi drains into the azygos vein with direct communication to the superior vena cava. Aneurysmal dilation of bronchial arteries (Dieulafoy's vascular malformation) has been noted in some patients with hemoptysis, and it can occasionally be visualized endobronchially and noted on bronchial arteriography.[11]

A direct anastomotic communication between the bronchial and pulmonary arterioles has been sought to explain the preservation of lung parenchyma after injuries to the pulmonary vascular supply. Anatomic studies have found that intermeshing of pulmonary and bronchial capillary networks is the most common anastomotic arrangement that prevents pressurization of the pulmonary arterioles with systemic pressures.[12] However, in chronic inflammatory diseases of the airways, anatomic anastomoses have been found that allow direct pressurization of the pulmonary artery with systemic pressures.[13] The extent to which these vascular communications are related to hemoptysis remains unknown.

Bronchial arteries vasodilate in the presence of cholinergic, β_2-adrenergic, and some nonadrenergic, noncholinergic agonists. Although the effect of β_2-agonists on the course of hemoptysis remains unstudied, the balance between improved mucociliary clearance of blood affected by β_2-agonists and detrimental bronchial artery dilation should be considered.[14] Other physiochemical maneuvers can influence bronchial blood flow—cold air causes blanching of the human airway,[15] humidified air decreases bronchial blood flow compared with dry gas,[16] and increased alveolar pressure decreases bronchial blood flow by applied pressure at the capillaries.[12]

NONBRONCHIAL SYSTEMIC COLLATERAL CIRCULATION

In diseases of the lung associated with inflammation, neovascularization of the lung parenchyma can occur. Although proliferation of the bronchial circulation is the most common mechanism to extend the vascular supply, an extensive network of systemic arteries may neovascularize the lung after crossing the pleural space. This most commonly occurs in diseases that produce pleural scarring, such as in aspergillomas and cystic fibrosis (CF). Anatomically these collateral vessels commonly arise from the intercostal, subclavian, axillary, and phrenic arteries. However, nonbronchial collaterals have also been described from the internal mammary, thyrocervical, carotid, and even the coronary arteries. Suspicion that these vessels may be involved is heightened by recurrence of hemoptysis after bronchial artery embolization (BAE), the presence of pleural disease, and the absence of bronchial arteries supplying an area of lung parenchyma on initial bronchial arteriography.

PULMONARY VENOUS ABNORMALITIES

Bleeding from the pulmonary veins is most likely in cardiac disease such as mitral stenosis or mitral regurgitation. Focal varices of the pulmonary veins that are occasionally visualized on chest radiography, but are best identified on the venous phase of pulmonary arteriography, have been described.[17,18]

CAUSES OF HEMOPTYSIS

Bronchiectasis, tuberculosis or its sequelae, lung cancer, and aspergilloma (mycetoma) account for the largest proportion of massive hemoptysis cases. However, almost any of the many causes of hemoptysis (Box 46.1) can become massive on rare occasions. Clues to specific diagnoses are obtained by history, physical examination, chest radiography, and chest computed tomography (CT). Additionally, it is important to consider the demographics of the patient population when considering the cause of hemoptysis. For example, there is a predominance of causes related to infectious diseases (i.e., mycobacterial or parasitic) and their long-term complications in individuals from developing and impoverished countries. In contrast, malignancies and bronchiectasis are more common causes of massive hemoptysis in developed countries.

BRONCHIECTASIS

Bronchiectasis is characterized by abnormal dilation of the bronchi with altered mucociliary clearance, persistent bacterial colonization, chronic inflammation of the bronchial mucosa, and submucosal neovascularization that predisposes to hemoptysis. Hemoptysis in bronchiectasis can present as a single life-threatening episode but is more commonly heralded by intermittent blood streaks intermixed with purulent sputum. In patients without a previous diagnosis, the evaluation can be difficult because chest radiography can be normal or alveolar filling with blood can obscure abnormalities. Diagnosis can usually be confirmed with high-resolution chest CT. Suspicion of the diagnosis warrants broad-spectrum antibiotics to cover the multiple organisms causing infection in addition to management of the hemoptysis.

Bronchiectasis is the usual cause of massive hemoptysis in patients with CF and occurs in approximately 4.1% of patients during their lifetime.[19] Massive hemoptysis is more common in patients over the age of 18 years and has been associated with pancreatic insufficiency, *Staphylococcus aureus* colonization, reduced lung function, and diabetes.[19] Although *Pseudomonas aeruginosa* remains the predominant pathogen associated with decline in lung function, its presence does not translate into an increased incidence of hemoptysis. Origin of the bleeding is most often upper lobe bronchial or systemic arteries. These patients are difficult to treat because of minimal pulmonary reserve in the majority of patients at the time of hemoptysis. Guidelines for treatment of massive hemoptysis in CF patients recommend empiric antibiotic coverage to include *S. aureus*, discontinuation of nonsteroidal anti-inflammatory drugs,

Box 46.1 Causes of Focal Pulmonary Hemorrhage

Iatrogenic Disorders
Bronchoscopy
Lung biopsy
Pulmonary artery catheterization
Transtracheal aspiration
Radiofrequency ablation
Brachytherapy

Infectious Disorders
Lung abscess
Mycetoma
Necrotizing pneumonia (*Staphylococcus aureus,* gram-negative aerobes, *Legionella,* Actinomyces species, *Stenotrophomonas, Kytococcus sedentarius,* Leptospira species, Yersinia pestis, Francisella tularensis)
Parasitic infection (paragonimiasis, amebiasis, ascariasis, clonorchiasis, echinococciasis, hookworm infestation, strongyloidiasis, trichinosis, schistosomiasis)
Parenchymal fungal infection (aspergillosis, mucormycosis, coccidioidomycosis, histoplasmosis, maduromycosis, botryomycosis)
Tuberculosis (active or inactive)
Viral tracheitis
Herpetic tracheobronchitis

Interstitial Lung Diseases
Lymphangioleiomyomatosis
Sarcoidosis
Tuberous sclerosis
Pneumoconiosis
Langerhans cell granulomatosis

Miscellaneous Disorders
Amyloidosis
Bronchogenic cyst
Broncholithiasis
Bronchopleural fistula
Thoracic endometriosis
Foreign body
Tracheopathia osteoplastica
Lipoid pneumonia
Organophosphate aspiration
Chronic pancreatitis

Neoplastic Disorders
Bronchial adenoma
Lung cancer
Tracheal tumors (mucoepidermoid, squamous cell, adenoid cystic, glomus)
Pulmonary blastoma
Pleuropulmonary angiosarcoma
Sarcoma (synovial, myofibroblastic)
Clear cell tumor
Metastatic disease (prostate, renal, breast, ovarian)
Tracheobronchial schwannoma

Pulmonary Airway Diseases
Bronchiectasis
Bronchitis
Granulomatous tracheobronchitis (ulcerative colitis, Crohn's disease, Wegener's granulomatosis)
Cystic fibrosis
Bullous emphysema

Traumatic Injury
Blunt chest trauma
Penetrating injury
Ruptured bronchus
Lightning injury
Thoracic splenosis

Vascular Disorders
Pulmonary embolism, infarction
Systemic cholesterol emboli
Intralobar sequestration
Pulmonary artery aneurysms
Behçet's disease, Hughes-Stovin syndrome, traumatic pseudoaneurysms
Acquired arteriovenous malformations
Osler-Weber-Rendu syndrome (hereditary hemorrhagic telangiectasia)
Takayasu's arteritis
Aortic aneurysms
Trachea–innominate artery fistulas
Scimitar syndrome
Vena cava-bronchial
Dieulafoy's disease of bronchus
Ventriculopulmonary fistulas
Hemangioma (sclerosing, cavernous, tracheal)

discontinuation of airway clearance therapies, discontinuation of aerosolized hypertonic saline, and use of BAE to control bleeding.[20] Although inhaled tobramycin and dornase alfa use were associated with a lower hemoptysis incidence,[19] consensus was not reached on whether to discontinue these therapies in massive hemoptysis.[20]

TUBERCULOSIS

The resurgence of tuberculosis in many parts of the world and the prevalence of global travel mandate consideration of the disease whenever hemoptysis occurs. Hemoptysis can occur with active cavitary disease or as late sequelae of lung destruction causing bronchiectasis. Hemoptysis has also been reported in miliary tuberculosis, although the mechanism is unknown. The pathologic lesion that causes hemoptysis in tuberculosis is often Rasmussen's aneurysm, a small aneurysm of the pulmonary circulation positioned within a cavity wall. Bleeding from the bronchial circulation can also complicate bronchial erosions in active tuberculosis, and study of both circulations is occasionally necessary when resection for local disease is not possible. Although all patients suspected of having hemoptysis secondary to tuberculosis should be placed in respiratory isolation, active pulmonary tuberculosis is found in only a third of such cases. Post-tuberculous bronchiectasis requires antibacterial therapy.

LUNG MALIGNANCY

Lung cancer is associated with hemoptysis in 20% to 30% of cases and may be the presenting manifestation.[21] Although the clinical course of hemoptysis is often that of chronic blood-streaked sputum, massive hemoptysis may occur as a terminal event. Massive hemoptysis is most commonly associated with squamous cell type[22]; cavitation within the carcinoma[23]; and central endobronchial position, occasionally with invasion into the pulmonary arteries. The blood supply to most lung carcinomas is derived from diffuse neovascularization from the bronchial circulation, making BAE effective in some cases.

Other less common cancers can bleed when found in the lung. Kaposi sarcoma has a high incidence of bloody pleural effusions and hemoptysis. Angiosarcomas are vascular tumors that may bleed continuously from small tumor sites.[24] Choriocarcinomas may bleed profusely, particularly after initiation of chemotherapy. Metastatic disease including renal, ovarian, and breast cancer have rarely been associated with hemoptysis.

Massive hemoptysis may also result from interventions that treat lung malignancies. Endobronchial brachytherapy has resulted in massive, fatal hemoptysis and was found to be associated with direct contact of the brachytherapy applicator and tracheobronchial walls near great vessels.[25] Radiofrequency ablation of lung neoplasms has been associated with massive bleeding due to intraparenchymal hemorrhage and pulmonary artery pseudoaneurysm.[26,27]

LUNG ABSCESS

Lung abscesses are commonly found in parenchymal areas prone to aspiration. The indolent course of these infections allows time for hypertrophy of the bronchial circulation within the walls of the abscess cavity. Additionally, these cavities may enlarge and erode into major pulmonary arteries and other thoracic vessels, including the aorta.[28] With either of these abnormalities, bleeding can be massive and recurrent. Although the abscesses are focal and amenable to surgery, the patient who chronically aspirates because of alcoholism or dementia may have other contraindications for surgery.

CHRONIC BRONCHITIS

Chronic bronchitis rarely causes massive hemoptysis, but it is a frequent cause of mild hemoptysis. The pathologic lesions responsible for bleeding are likely dilated bronchial arteries that are eroded during active inflammation of the airways.[29] A comprehensive management approach is required to treat hemoptysis and ensure that other lesions such as lung cancer are not present.

OTHER PULMONARY INFECTIONS

Although hemoptysis can complicate any bacterial or fungal pneumonia, massive hemoptysis is rare unless tissue necrosis is present. Tissue necrosis is a hallmark of anaerobic, staphylococcal, and actinomycotic[30] pneumonias but can occur with many different bacterial causes. Septic pulmonary emboli, particularly from staphylococcal species, have a high incidence of concomitant lung cavitation.[31] Mycotic pulmonary artery aneurysms may also be hidden within pneumonias and can be diagnosed by pulmonary arteriography or multidetector CT angiography.[32]

Hemoptysis is particularly common in fungal pneumonias that invade the vasculature. Invasive *Aspergillus* can be found in nonimmunosuppressed patients with chronic obstructive pulmonary disease (COPD)[33] but is more commonly found in the persistently neutropenic patient. A characteristic radiographic pattern of cavitation and hemoptysis follows the recovery of neutrophils and should be anticipated in at-risk patients.[34,35] The use of prophylactic surgery to resect areas of infarcted lung tissue has been advocated[36,37] because of the high mortality rate associated with medical management of the hemoptysis. However, such surgery remains high risk, and controlled trials have not been performed. Although more rare, invasive pulmonary mucormycosis[38] may produce similar findings. Hemoptysis complicates primary coccidioidal infections in 15% of cases and may approach a 50% incidence in patients with chronic coccidioidal cavities. Histoplasmosis, cryptococcosis, and blastomycosis can also cause hemoptysis. Frequent and sometimes massive hemoptysis can occur with the parasitic diseases paragonimiasis,[39] echinococcosis,[40] strongyloidiasis, and ancylostomiasis.

PULMONARY EMBOLISM

Hemoptysis occurs in approximately 30% of patients with thrombotic pulmonary emboli. Characteristically, hemoptysis is mild and requires no specific therapy. Hemoptysis usually implies some degree of pulmonary infarction with potential disruption of either vascular supply. The suspicion for pulmonary emboli is increased in the presence of risk factors for thrombosis, multicentric bleeding, and pleuritic chest pain. Paradoxically, this cause of hemoptysis must be treated with anticoagulants to prevent propagation of venous thromboemboli. The incidence of worsening hemoptysis after heparin or thrombolytics has not been documented. Nonthrombotic emboli have also been associated with hemoptysis. Septic emboli usually respond to antibiotics alone.

ASPERGILLUS FUNGUS BALLS

Hemoptysis occurs in more than half of patients with pulmonary *Aspergillus* fungus balls.[41] The cavity walls are richly vascularized by branches of the bronchial circulation, and enlargement of these cavities may also extend into large branches of the pulmonary artery. The mechanism of hemoptysis is likely multifactorial from secondary bacterial invasion of the fungal cavity, microinvasion of the cavity wall by *Aspergillus* (semi-invasive aspergillosis), or less commonly by truly invasive disease. Therapy of hemoptysis depends on the underlying cause for the cavitary lung disease.

Systemic antifungal therapy remains controversial because there is not a well-defined means to diagnose semi-invasive disease.[42,43] Intracavitary amphotericin B, however, instilled via a transthoracic catheter has proved successful at dissolution and sclerosis of the cavity with control of hemoptysis and is a viable option in patients who are poor surgical candidates.[44,45] Alternatively, antifungal therapy with ketoconazole,[46] miconazole,[47] or amphotericin B[48] has been given endobronchially for fungus ball dissolution and hemoptysis control, but these techniques are effective in less than half of patients.[49] External beam radiotherapy of 3.5 Gy given once per week has been used as an adjunctive measure in nonoperable patients.[50]

Surgery remains the therapy of choice in patients with adequate pulmonary reserve due to the recurrent nature of hemoptysis. Simple aspergilloma (no abnormality in surrounding lung) has an excellent response to surgical resection, most commonly a lobectomy. Complex aspergilloma with surrounding pleural and parenchymal involvement usually requires pneumonectomy and is associated with variable success.[51] Fungus balls complicating sarcoidosis usually occur in patients with bilateral upper lobe cavitary disease (stage IV), in which underlying lung function prohibits resection.

CARDIOVASCULAR CAUSES

Mitral stenosis is one of the most common cardiac abnormalities that can present with hemoptysis.[52] The risk of hemoptysis is likely related to the elevation of pulmonary venous pressure and the rapidity with which the stenosis developed. Clinical examination may reveal an opening snap or diastolic murmur. An echocardiogram should be obtained for definitive diagnosis.

Other causes of increased pulmonary venous pressure, such as mitral regurgitation or severe congestive cardiomyopathy, may also produce hemoptysis that usually presents with radiographic pulmonary edema and a prodrome of pink frothy sputum. Fibrosing mediastinitis,[53] pulmonary veno-occlusive disease,[54] and congenital pulmonary venous stenosis[55] are less common causes of pulmonary venous congestion.

Rarely, hemoptysis will occur from systemic venous hypertension in severe biventricular heart failure by azygous vein hypertension and dilation. Because the azygous vein drains the trachea and major bronchi, the submucosal dilated venous plexus of the trachea can be friable and produce major hemoptysis.

INTERSTITIAL LUNG DISEASE

Only a few interstitial lung diseases are prone to hemoptysis. Lymphangioleiomyomatosis (LAM) is a disease of smooth muscle proliferation around pulmonary lymphatics, airways, and vasculature. Any of the triad of hemoptysis, pneumothorax, and chylothorax should suggest the diagnosis in a woman of childbearing age.[56] The airway granulomas of sarcoidosis have also been associated with hemoptysis, although the presence of traction bronchiectasis may be a more common cause. Additionally, the erosion of calcified hilar lymph nodes into the vasculature can produce hemoptysis. Other interstitial lung diseases that cause hemoptysis usually have diffuse alveolar hemorrhage.

BRONCHOLITHIASIS

Broncholithiasis is an infrequent cause of hemoptysis. The typical patient usually has an established diagnosis of mediastinal calcification from granulomatous disease. Previous infections of histoplasmosis, sarcoidosis, or tuberculosis are most common. Broncholithiasis is diagnosed by bronchoscopy when any degree of lymph node calcification is visualized in the bronchial lumen. Symptoms of cough, chest pain, airway obstruction, and hemoptysis can be seen. Lithoptysis, coughing out a broncholith, can also confirm the diagnosis.

Therapy of hemoptysis involves broncholith removal. Broncholith removal by rigid or flexible bronchoscopy is usually successful when the broncholith is free. When broncholiths are partially embedded in the airway wall, removal is best facilitated by rigid bronchoscopy[57] or by thoracic surgery. Surgical options include lymph node resection with or without bronchoplasty or lobectomy. One surgical series had a 34% complication rate and a 15% rate of recurrent or persistent disease.[58]

DIFFUSE ALVEOLAR HEMORRHAGE

Diffuse alveolar hemorrhage (DAH) most commonly presents abruptly and may or may not be associated with frank hemoptysis. The early manifestations are often confused with other alveolar filling processes such as pulmonary edema, bacterial pneumonia, or the acute respiratory distress syndrome (ARDS). Consideration of DAH is prompted by the presence of diffuse infiltrates on chest radiograph, the presence of systemic manifestations of vasculitis, the association of hemoptysis, hypoxemic respiratory failure, and the common finding of anemia.[59] Unfortunately, the many causes of DAH are often differentiated on the basis of laboratory tests that may not be routine in many hospitals. Furthermore, specific therapy is often not initiated until a definitive diagnosis has been established by biopsy.

The differential diagnosis of DAH is listed in Box 46.2. Although some of these diseases have no specific therapy, establishing a diagnosis and instituting supportive care help to avoid unnecessary diagnostic and therapeutic maneuvers. Many of the vasculitides are stabilized only with aggressive immunosuppressive therapy, which would not be appropriate for infectious diseases that can present with the same features in a chest radiograph.

Bronchoscopy with transbronchial biopsy and bronchoalveolar lavage (BAL) are usually performed in a patient with unknown pulmonary infiltrates in the intensive care unit (ICU) if respiratory compromise is not severe. Although often not sufficient to establish a specific diagnosis, finding a bloody lavage, hemosiderin-laden macrophages, and the lack of specific pathogens can presumptively yield a diagnosis of DAH. The diagnosis of DAH is best made by quantitation of hemosiderin in alveolar macrophages obtained by BAL. A Prussian blue stain is graded by the methods of Kahn and colleagues[60]; hemosiderin scores above 100 are virtually diagnostic of alveolar hemorrhage. Hemosiderin-laden macrophages may not appear in BAL fluid until 48 to 72 hours after acute hemorrhage, resulting in a low sensitivity for hemosiderin scores in this setting.[61]

Box 46.2 Causes of Diffuse Alveolar Hemorrhage

Immunologic Diseases

Anti–glomerular basement membrane antibody disease (Goodpasture's syndrome)
Vasculitides associated with circulating or in situ immune complexes
- Systemic lupus erythematosus
- Mixed connective tissue disease
- Schönlein-Henoch purpura
- Essential mixed cryoglobulinemia
- Tumor-related vasculitis
- Endocarditis-related vasculitis
- Polyarteritis nodosa
- Systemic necrotizing vasculitis

Vasculitides associated with antineutrophil cytoplasmic antibodies
- Wegener's granulomatosis
- Microscopic polyangiitis
- Idiopathic necrotizing crescentic glomerulonephritis

Rapidly progressive glomerulonephritis
Associated with other connective tissue diseases, pathophysiology unknown
- Rheumatoid arthritis
- Progressive systemic sclerosis
- Behçet's disease

Associated with other renal diseases
IgA nephropathy
Diabetic nephropathy
Associated with precipitating antibodies to milk (Heiner's syndrome)
Idiopathic pulmonary hemosiderosis
Primary antiphospholipid antibody syndrome

Chemical or Drug-Related Causes

Amiodarone
D-Penicillamine
Isocyanates
Nitrofurantoin
Retinoic acid
Trimellitic anhydride
"Crack" cocaine
Sirolimus
Everolimus
Propylthiouracil-induced vasculitis
Erlotinib
Bevacizumab
Gemcitabine
Infliximab

Transplant-Related Causes

Bone marrow transplant
Renal transplant
Lung transplant

Bleeding Diathesis

Thrombocytopenia
Leukemia with diffuse alveolar damage
Viral pneumonia
Bacterial or fungal sepsis
Radiation
Chemotherapy toxic to lung
Blast counts >80,000/μL
Extrinsic anticoagulants/thrombolytics
Warfarin overdose
Tissue plasminogen activator
Platelet glycoprotein IIb/IIIa inhibitors
Coagulopathies
Cirrhosis
DIC

Infections

Legionnaires' disease

Pulmonary Venous Hypertension

Mitral stenosis
Mitral regurgitation
Pulmonary capillary hemangiomatosis
Pulmonary veno-occlusive disease
Fibrosing mediastinitis
Congenital heart disease

Diffuse Lung Injury

Negative-pressure pulmonary hemorrhage
Breath-hold diving
Postictal neurogenic pulmonary edema

DIC, disseminated intravascular coagulation; IgA, immunoglobulin A.

IMMUNOLOGIC LUNG DISEASE

The differential diagnosis of DAH is narrowed significantly if renal abnormalities are present. Although pulmonary-renal syndromes can often be stabilized with high-dose corticosteroids alone pending further evaluation, directed therapy depends on the measurement of specific autoantibodies and evaluation of a renal biopsy. Alveolar hemorrhage is a hallmark of anti–glomerular basement membrane (GBM) antibody disease (Goodpasture's disease). This disease is 75% male-predominant and follows a flulike prodrome in 30% of patients. Pulmonary hemorrhage is the initial manifestation in 90%, and an abnormal urinalysis is found in 80%. An iron-deficiency anemia from sequestration of iron within pulmonary alveolar macrophages is commonly associated with the disease. The IgG antibodies reacting to a component of type IV collagen are found in linear deposits on the basement membrane of both alveoli and glomeruli and are circulating in 90% of cases.[62] In the appropriate clinical setting, the presence of circulating anti-GBM antibodies is sufficient to make a diagnosis without biopsy and institute plasmapheresis with or without plasma exchange for severe pulmonary or renal disease. After initial stabilization, corticosteroids and immunosuppressive medications will usually prevent further antibody production. Treatment with rituximab is also an option for patients intolerant of or refractory to standard therapy.[63]

Steroids alone are usually sufficient to treat alveolar hemorrhage associated with the immune complex vasculitides. These disorders are usually associated with hypocomplementemia and an elevated titer of antinuclear antibody. Systemic lupus erythematosus (SLE) is the most frequent of the immune complex disorders causing alveolar hemorrhage. SLE rarely presents with alveolar hemorrhage without other manifestations of active disease. Although the alveolar hemorrhage of SLE usually occurs from acute lupus pneumonitis, the high incidence of pneumonia, congestive heart failure, and aspiration in these patients makes a presumptive diagnosis problematic. Lupus pneumonitis usually stabilizes on 1 to 1.5 mg/kg/day methylprednisolone.

DAH also complicates other connective tissue diseases and systemic vasculitides with or without immune complex deposition. Mixed connective tissue disease, cryoglobulinemia, polyarteritis nodosa, progressive systemic sclerosis, rheumatoid arthritis, Behçet's disease, endocarditis and tumor-related vasculitis, Schönlein-Henoch purpura, and systemic necrotizing vasculitis have all been described in association with DAH. Specific diagnosis depends on the nonpulmonary features of disease presentation.

Alveolar hemorrhage is an unusual manifestation of Wegener's granulomatosis.[64] The classic triad of renal dysfunction, upper airway disease, and pulmonary infiltrates is present in less than 20% of patients at presentation; however, pulmonary infiltrates are present in 45%.[65] The pulmonary findings are characterized by nodules that may cavitate, lobar infiltrates that are often transient, upper airway obstruction from the granulomatous inflammation that follows airway ulceration, prominent interstitial markings with or without hilar and mediastinal adenopathy, or alveolar hemorrhage. Antineutrophil antibodies against proteinase 3 in cytoplasmic granules (c-ANCA) are found in the serum of 85% to 90% of patients with active Wegener's granulomatosis and are 97% specific for the diagnosis.[66]

Among the many causes of rapidly progressive crescentic glomerulonephritis (RPGN) are small-vessel vasculitides such as microscopic polyangiitis that are associated with pulmonary hemorrhage in a third of patients.[67] Therapy of these vasculitides and Wegener's granulomatosis usually includes corticosteroids and immunosuppressive therapy. In patients with life-threatening respiratory failure, extracorporeal membrane oxygenation (ECMO) has proved lifesaving in patients with ANCA-positive vasculitides and SLE awaiting onset of systemic therapy.[68,69] Use of recombinant factor VIIa has also been reported in this setting.[70,71]

IDIOPATHIC PULMONARY HEMOSIDEROSIS

Idiopathic pulmonary hemosiderosis is characterized by repetitive episodes of hemorrhage that occur without obvious precipitating factors. Open lung biopsy fails to demonstrate immune complexes, and no other organ system is affected. Therapy with corticosteroids and occasionally cyclophosphamide has been attempted, although no controlled trials have been performed.

IMMUNOCOMPROMISED HOST

DAH complicates autologous and allogeneic bone marrow transplantation in up to 21% of cases.[72,73] Risk factors include age younger than 40 years, the presence of underlying solid tumors, renal insufficiency, and severe mucositis. The typical presentation is characterized by onset near the time of leukocyte recovery and is heralded by high fever and diffuse pulmonary infiltrates that prompt BAL. Typically the lavage fluid appears progressively bloody over serial aliquots, and no pathogenic organisms are recovered on bacterial, fungal, or viral culture. Mortality rate has been reported from 80% to 100% despite aggressive supportive care[72,74] but may be improved with corticosteroid therapy.[75] The optimal dosage and duration of corticosteroid treatment remain controversial, but standard regimens include 1 g/day methylprednisolone administered for 3 days and thereafter tapered over 2 months.[75] The use of recombinant factor VIIa in patients with life-threatening DAH refractory to steroids has been reported.[71] More recent reports reveal a favorable prognosis in patients with early (first 30 days) versus late DAH and autologous versus allogeneic transplants with an overall mortality rate of 48%.[73]

A similar syndrome characterized by fever and pulmonary infiltrates has been noted in 5% of transplant patients, but hemoptysis is rare. Pulmonary capillaritis following lung transplant also can result in DAH. Hemoptysis is seen in up to 25% of cases, with fulminant respiratory failure seen in 18%.[76] This form of acute allograft rejection appears less responsive to corticosteroid therapy than acute lung rejection but has a more favorable response to plasmapheresis. No long-term adverse effects on allograft function are apparent.

BLEEDING DIATHESIS

Although hemoptysis may occur with intrinsic coagulopathies, extrinsic anticoagulants and antiplatelet agents, thrombocytopenia, and fibrinolytics, patients at risk should undergo bronchoscopy to exclude other lesions such as neoplasm. Usually, the disorders of hemostasis are not in themselves solely responsible for hemoptysis, and bleeding can usually be ascribed to the combined presence of another cause, often as insignificant as an upper respiratory infection.

Leukemia patients may be particularly susceptible to DAH when chemotherapy-induced thrombocytopenia is combined with diffuse alveolar damage from other causes. Viral infections, sepsis, radiation, chemotherapy agents with pulmonary toxicity, and leukostasis from blast counts exceeding 80,000 cells/mm^3 may all produce diffuse alveolar damage in leukemia.[77] Therapy is directed toward correction of thrombocytopenia and supportive care of lung injury.

DRUG-INDUCED ALVEOLAR HEMORRHAGE

Hemoptysis due to drug-induced alveolar hemorrhage is rare and may result from therapeutic medications, illicit drugs, and other agents. Implicated agents include crack cocaine,[78] amiodarone,[79] nitrofurantoin,[80] D-penicillamine,[81] retinoic acid,[82] propylthiouracil,[83] infliximab,[84] inhaled resins containing trimellitic anhydride,[85] and various chemotherapeutic agents.[86-89]

VASCULAR ABNORMALITIES

Almost all blood vessels that course through the thoracic cavity have been associated with fistula formation to an airway with resultant hemoptysis. Often this occurs in the setting of endovascular infection, inflammation, congenital or acquired stenoses, aneurysms of these vessels, or chest surgery. Some of the rare vascular-to-airway fistulas that have been described include (1) carotid artery to trachea in a patient with occult laryngeal cancer[90]; (2) various abdominal arterial supplies to pulmonary sequestrations[91]; (3)

syphilitic aneurysms of the ascending aorta and other thoracic arteries to pulmonary parenchyma[92]; (4) coronary artery bypass grafts to pulmonary parenchyma or bronchial artery[93,94]; (5) splenopulmonary shunt in portal hypertension following splenectomy[95]; (6) left ventricular pseudoaneurysms[96] to pulmonary parenchyma; and (7) vena caval–bronchial fistulas.[97] Several of the more common bronchovascular communications deserve comment.

AORTOBRONCHIAL FISTULAS

Dissecting aortic aneurysms are often of subacute or chronic duration with variable degrees of inflammation around the dissection. As an aneurysm enlarges it may cause lung compression, pleural adhesions, and dissection of blood into the pulmonary parenchyma. Particularly in situations in which an aortic graft has been previously placed, aortic graft infection may also be present. The net result is an often stuttering course of hemoptysis marked by sudden large bleeds. Therapy is surgical, although these operations are difficult in the presence of graft infections and prior operations.

PULMONARY ARTERY ANEURYSMS

Aneurysms of the pulmonary artery remain rare causes of hemoptysis.[98] Mycotic aneurysms are commonly caused by *Mycobacterium tuberculosis*, syphilis, *S. aureus*, and streptococcal species. Poststenotic dilation may occur in congenital pulmonary artery strictures. Structural vascular abnormalities such as those found in Marfan syndrome can also affect the pulmonary arteries.

Behçet's disease, characterized by oral ulcers, uveitis, arthritis, and cutaneous vasculitis, is the only common large-vessel vasculitis that affects the pulmonary arteries.[99] These multiple aneurysms may resolve with high-dose corticosteroid therapy or cyclophosphamide.[100,101]

An idiopathic syndrome characterized by fatal hemoptysis from pulmonary artery aneurysms, associated with fever and recurrent superficial and deep venous thromboembolism, was originally reported in 1959 by Hughes and Stovin.[102] Although infection and angiodysplasia have been proposed as possible causes of the aneurysms, the current consensus is that vasculitis is the primary process.[103]

ARTERIOVENOUS MALFORMATIONS

Pulmonary arteriovenous malformations (PAVMs) present with progressive hypoxemia, paradoxical emboli, or bleeding complications including hemoptysis or hemothorax.[104] Although the majority of these lesions are likely congenital telangiectasias that enlarged over years,[105] acquired arteriovenous malformations (AVMs) have been noted after chest surgery and trauma and have been associated with actinomycosis, schistosomiasis, cirrhosis, and metastatic carcinoma.[106] The hereditary Osler-Weber-Rendu disease (OWR) is associated with hemorrhagic telangiectasias in many organ systems. Approximately 15% of OWR patients have pulmonary arteriovenous aneurysms,[107] and up to 36% of patients with a single PAVM and 57% of patients with multiple PAVMs have OWR.[108] Bronchial artery telangiectasias with bleeding[109] have also been described, although the pathogenic relationship to pulmonary artery telangiectasias remains speculative. Treatment of PAVMs, particularly if hemoptysis has developed, is to obliterate the lesion with BAE.[110]

TRAUMA

Hemoptysis following major trauma requires emergent thoracic surgical consultation and management. Although some cases will be simple lung contusions that manifest as a focal radiographic abnormality on chest radiograph with blood-streaked sputum present, approximately 15% of thoracic trauma victims with hemoptysis need early exploration. The majority of cases with hemoptysis need bronchoscopy to localize bleeding and exclude a tracheobronchial rupture, which can be clinically silent for weeks. The most common reason for emergent thoracotomy remains pulmonary hemorrhage. Pneumonorrhaphy (suture repair of the lung) is preferred for minor injuries; lobectomy and pneumonectomy, performed for more severe injuries, carry mortality rates of 55% and 89%, respectively.[111]

Lung laceration is common after penetrating pulmonary injury. However, it can also occur after blunt thoracic trauma in which sheer forces of acceleration or deceleration leave intraparenchymal lacerations involving airways or vasculature. Continued bleeding into the lung can present with rupture into the pleural space (hemothorax), intraparenchymal hematoma formation, or hemoptysis. Thoracic splenosis is a rare and remote event from the time of trauma. In this condition, splenic tissue is transported across the diaphragm after penetrating injury, where it becomes functional and vascularized within the lung. Hemoptysis may thereafter occur spontaneously.

VASCULAR MONITORING CATHETERS

Use of pulmonary artery catheters has decreased significantly and complications causing hemoptysis occur rarely. Pulmonary artery catheters should be inflated in the proximal pulmonary circulation for 20 seconds or less to obtain pulmonary artery occlusion pressures. More distal and prolonged inflation can cause fatal pulmonary artery dissection, pseudoaneurysm formation, or pulmonary artery rupture.[112,113] Endovascular damage may predispose to thrombus formation and pulmonary infarction. Preventive measures include placement of the catheter at an insertion distance when full inflation is required to obtain an occlusion pressure, slowly inflating the balloon (never inflating against resistance), full inflation of the balloon to prevent the catheter tip from projecting beyond the balloon, and daily monitoring of catheter position with chest radiography.

If hemoptysis occurs with a pulmonary artery catheter in place, rapid diagnosis and treatment are required. Risk factors for pulmonary artery rupture include concomitant anticoagulation, cardiopulmonary bypass, balloon migration, hypothermia, advanced age, and pulmonary hypertension.[113] Surgical resection of the involved lobe or angiographic ablation of the involved pulmonary artery has been successful in decreasing the incidence of recurrent and often fatal hemoptysis. Other successful interventions for acute conditions have included proximal reinflation of the pulmonary artery catheter to stop blood flow to the pulmonary artery segment that is bleeding; high levels (18 mm Hg) of positive end-expiratory pressure to decrease the pulmonary artery to bronchial pressure gradient; resumption of cardiopulmonary bypass for patients in cardiac surgery; and operative banding of the pulmonary artery, which can be unclamped 48 hours later.[113,114]

MANAGEMENT

The primary principles of managing massive hemoptysis are airway and lung protection, localization of the bleeding source, and control of hemorrhage. Assessments and interventions are frequently performed empirically because the cause of hemoptysis may not be known at the time of presentation. Therapy to control minor and moderate hemoptysis can usually proceed along diagnostic paths. The inability to determine when and whether an individual patient's hemoptysis will worsen suggests that all patients with an estimated blood loss of more than 200 mL should be hospitalized in a unit in which airway support can be rapidly provided if necessary.

Massive hemoptysis should be managed within a framework of expeditious therapy to stabilize and resuscitate the patient. Figure 46.1 is a suggested algorithm for management. A multidisciplinary collaborative approach involving intensivists, pulmonologists, interventional radiologists, and thoracic surgeons is optimal to improve outcomes.[7] The urgency and aggressiveness of management are influenced by the rate of bleeding. The study by Crocco and colleagues[6] (Table 46.1) demonstrated that the incidence of death was 71% in patients with 600 mL of hemoptysis in less than 4 hours, compared with 22% and 5% mortality rate if 600 mL of hemoptysis occurred in 4 to 16 hours and 16 to 48 hours, respectively. Sputum containers should be placed at the bedside of patients who are not intubated to allow measurement of blood loss and an estimate of the bleeding rate. High bleeding rates, hemodynamic instability, and severe oxygenation failure signal the need for rapid evaluation and treatment. A critical care setting is optimal for patients with massive hemoptysis.

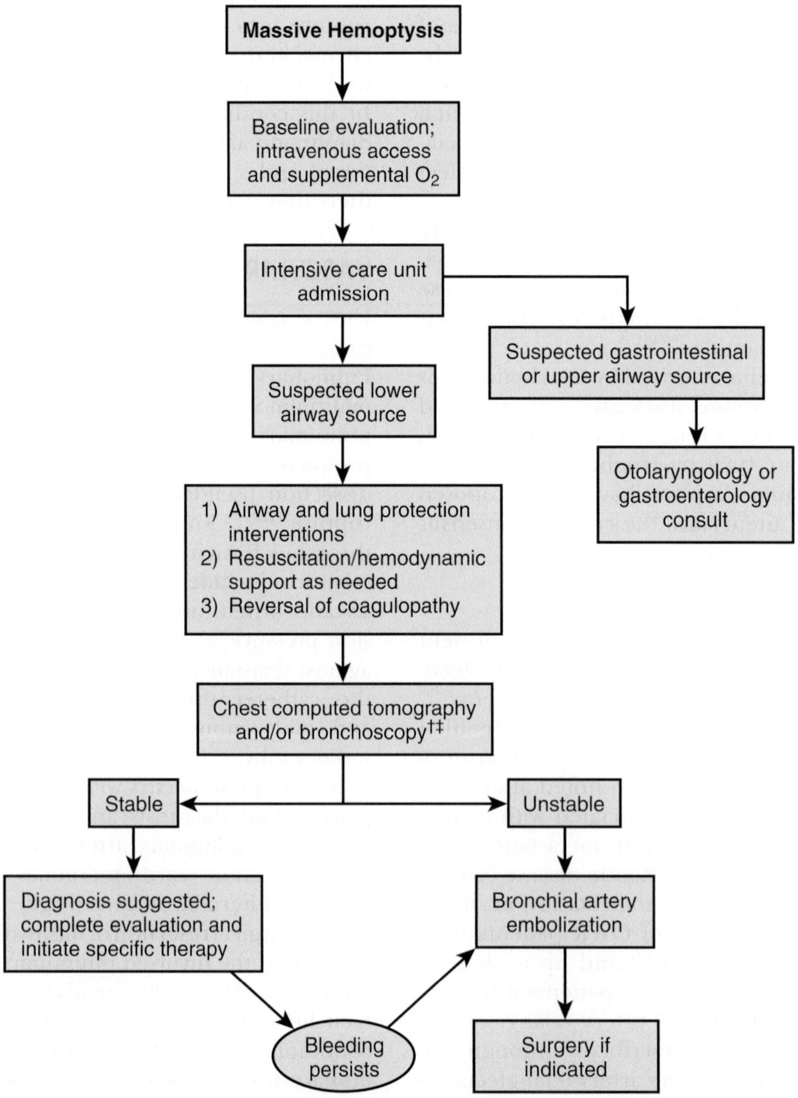

Figure 46.1 Massive hemoptysis. *History and physical examination, complete blood count, coagulation studies, type and cross-match, chest radiograph, arterial blood gas. †Local availability and patient stability should guide choice; computed tomography preferred in initial evaluation in stable patient. ‡Local measures including topical vasoconstrictors, bronchial blockers, laser photocoagulation, electrocautery, and hemostatic agents can be used endobronchially.

Table 46.1 Mortality Associated with Rate of Bleeding

	Operable					
	Surgical Management		No Surgery		Nonoperable	
Blood Loss	No. of Patients	Deaths	No. of Patients	Deaths	No. of Patients	Deaths
600 mL in <4 hr	11	4 (36%)	6	6 (100%)	11	10 (91%)
600 mL/4-16 hr	10	1 (10%)	3	1 (33%)	5	2 (40%)
600 mL/16-48 hr	11	1 (9%)	0	0	10	0

In addition to the management steps outlined later, laboratory studies should be obtained, including complete blood count, coagulation studies, and type and cross-match for possible blood transfusion. An arterial blood gas measurement may be needed to assess ventilation and acid-base status, although pulse oximetry is usually adequate to assess oxygenation. Additional studies may be needed to investigate possible causes of hemoptysis such as infection or vasculitis. The hemodynamic status of the patient should be evaluated and fluids or blood administered for hypotension or evidence of impaired oxygen delivery. Antibiotics may be indicated if there is suspicion of active infection.

AIRWAY AND LUNG PROTECTION

Patency of the airway and the ability to protect the airway should be assessed as soon as hemoptysis is noted. All patients should be provided with supplemental oxygen as needed to maintain adequate oxyhemoglobin saturation. Patients with mild to moderate amounts of hemoptysis usually do not require intubation but intubation in massive hemoptysis is usually needed to facilitate diagnostic and therapeutic interventions as well as to provide support for oxygenation and ventilation. Additional steps may be needed to prevent contamination of the unaffected lung from blood and to preserve respiratory function.

PATIENT POSITIONING

If the source of bleeding is localized to one lung, the patient with massive bleeding should be positioned with the bleeding side down to keep bleeding contained to one lung. Once the airway is secured, the optimal patient position is more controversial. Clotting of blood in a dependent lung has the potential to tamponade the bleeding, yet clotted blood in the proximal airway can result in lung collapse and atelectasis. Furthermore, if the pulmonary circulation is bleeding, it can be influenced by gravity by placing the bleeding segment higher than other areas of the chest. By converting that segment to a zone 1 condition in which alveolar pressure is higher than pulmonary artery pressure, bleeding may be decreased.

ENDOTRACHEAL INTUBATION

Endotracheal intubation is often difficult in patients with active bleeding. Orotracheal intubation is preferred to allow use of a larger endotracheal tube (preferably 8 mm inner diameter or larger) in order to facilitate suctioning, ventilation, and bronchoscopy. The orotracheal route also allows for selective mainstem bronchial intubation if needed.

If the patient's physical examination, chest radiograph, and other imaging studies readily identify the bleeding lung, specific interventions to protect the airway to the normal lung can be attempted. Mechanisms to localize ventilation to one lung using a single-lumen endotracheal tube include selective intubation of one of the mainstem bronchi and selective endobronchial tamponade with a bronchial blocker (see later discussion).

Selective bronchial intubation is easiest in a patient with a bleeding left lung. Because of the leftward displacement of the carina in most individuals, an endotracheal tube advanced blindly will almost always intubate the right main bronchus. Unfortunately, the right upper lobe bronchus is so close to the carina that a right mainstem intubation may also cause right upper lobe atelectasis. The ability to ventilate and oxygenate a patient with the right lower and right middle lobes alone depends on the underlying cardiopulmonary reserve. Intubation of the left main bronchus is facilitated by placing the patient in a right lateral decubitus position to shift the mediastinum rightward. Angulation of the endotracheal tube curvature toward the left and progression of the tube over a coudé catheter may be helpful. Selective mainstem intubations can be facilitated by a bronchoscope.

DOUBLE-LUMEN ENDOTRACHEAL TUBES

Devices utilized for single-lung ventilation have also been applied to the management of hemoptysis.[115] A double-lumen endotracheal tube is an alternative to a single-lumen endotracheal tube for airway management in massive hemoptysis. Successful placement of this type of endotracheal tube requires training and experience.[116] The independent isolation of each mainstem bronchus allows for single-lung ventilation and isolation of the unaffected lung from blood contamination when bleeding is localized to one lung. The smaller suction ports of each independent lumen can cause difficulty in suctioning blood. Endobronchial evaluation requires a pediatric bronchoscope or double-lumen tube removal once bleeding has been controlled. Proximal airway masses may preclude placement of a double-lumen endotracheal tube.

LOCALIZATION OF BLEEDING

Localization of bleeding facilitates diagnostic and therapeutic efforts regardless of the amount of hemoptysis. Because blood in the mouth can originate from the gastrointestinal tract or from diverse sites in the sinuses, nasal airway, or upper airway proximal to the larynx, an initial evaluation is needed to confirm that bleeding is from the lung. One series of hemoptysis patients found an upper airway source of bleeding in 10%.[117] The characteristics of the expectorated blood and clinical presentation of the patient often

Table 46.2 Features of Hemoptysis and Patient Presentation

Hemoptysis Feature	Clinical Presentation
Blood usually bright red	Often dyspneic
Portion of blood usually frothy	Hypoxemia
Alkaline pH	
Blood usually mixed with sputum	Preceding cough common
Alveolar macrophages may be present in sputum smear	Anemia and melena uncommon

help in differentiating hemoptysis from upper airway or gastrointestinal sources (Table 46.2). A pH assessment of the blood (low pH expected in gastric hemorrhage) and observation of expectorated sputum can be performed at the bedside.

CHEST RADIOGRAPH

All patients with hemoptysis need a baseline evaluation that consists of a physical examination and chest radiograph. The chest radiograph may suggest specific diagnoses and help in localization of bleeding. However, blood filling the alveoli can obscure an underlying pulmonary pathologic condition and present with bilateral infiltrates, making localization of the bleeding site problematic.

CHEST COMPUTED TOMOGRAPHY

The importance of chest CT in the diagnosis of acute hemoptysis and localization of bleeding has increased with advances in technology. In a series of 80 patients with massive hemoptysis, emergency high-resolution computed tomography (HRCT) was not only equivalent to bronchoscopy in localizing bleeding (70% vs. 73%), but it was more efficient than bronchoscopy for identifying the cause of bleeding (77% vs. 8%). Findings on HRCT also directly affected treatment in more than 30% of patients in this study.[118] HRCT also allows the adequate prediction of nonbronchial systemic arterial supply, which can be the cause of bleeding in massive hemoptysis and a significant cause of recurrent bleeding after successful BAE.[119] Contrast enhancement increases the yield by identifying vascular abnormalities (i.e., thoracic aneurysm or AVMs) that would allow for more timely surgical referral.

Use of multidetector CT angiography to visualize the bronchial and nonbronchial systemic vasculature has been found to increase the number of pulmonary artery vaso-occlusions and reduce the number of urgent surgical resections compared to single-detector helical CT.[120] In CF patients with massive hemoptysis, electrocardiographically synchronized, prospectively triggered multidetector CT angiography of the aorta accurately predicted the location of ectopic bronchial arteries. The use of this technique was felt to decrease the BAE radiation dose and contrast volume and likely reduced table time compared to a conventional complete aortogram.[121]

CT modalities including multiplanar reconstruction and endobronchial simulation (i.e., virtual bronchoscopy) will likely increase the diagnostic yield of chest CT even further as these techniques become more available. Chest CT, except in unstable patients, should therefore be performed in patients prior to bronchoscopy and BAE to efficiently guide management.

BRONCHOSCOPY

Although the diagnostic yield of bronchoscopy remains low in hemoptysis due to causes other than endobronchial carcinoma, it remains a vital tool in the management of acute massive hemoptysis in unstable patients. Localization of bleeding can facilitate immediate interventions for hemorrhage control including appropriate patient positioning, selective intubation, endobronchial tamponade, endobronchial infusions, laser photocoagulation, and guidance for BAE or surgical resection. Recent studies, however, have suggested that patients with lateralizing radiography and known causation who are candidates for BAE do not need prior bronchoscopy unless bronchoscopic airway management is necessary.[20,122,123] This strategy can avoid delays in definitive therapy, reduce cost, and avoid the risk of airway compromise from sedation associated with bronchoscopy.

During massive hemoptysis the rigid bronchoscope has some advantages over flexible fiberoptic instruments. Ventilation is secured through the bronchoscope lumen, suctioning is not impeded, and visualization is less likely to be significantly impaired. The flexible instrument has advantages of subsegmental localization of bleeding and visualization of the upper lobes. Because the two bronchoscopes have complementary properties, they are often used together. The rigid bronchoscope is used to secure ventilation and localize the bleeding lung; the flexible scope passed through the rigid scope allows for further definition of the bleeding site and diagnosis.

HEMORRHAGE CONTROL

EXPECTANT THERAPY

Cough suppression has been recommended for the majority of patients with massive hemoptysis with moderate doses of codeine being most commonly used. Although no prospective study has evaluated the efficacy of cough suppression on patient outcome, the large swings in intrathoracic pressure that occur with coughing are likely to be detrimental.

The additional factor that must be considered in cough suppression is the necessary removal of blood clots that can cause endobronchial obstruction. Particularly when a central airway lesion is responsible for bleeding, the suctioning necessary to remove blood clots may be associated with rebleeding and perpetuation of a vicious cycle. Blood clots left unsuctioned, however, may cause atelectasis, which is detrimental to patient weaning from the ventilator. Although endobronchial streptokinase (1000 IU/mL; total dose 30,000 to 80,000 IU) has been used for dissolution of central blood clots,[124] airway stabilization can usually be obtained with serial bronchoscopies and suctioning alone.

ENDOBRONCHIAL TAMPONADE

Acute lung bleeding may be amenable to control by endobronchial tamponade with balloon-tipped devices known as bronchial blockers.[125-128] Several types of devices are available: Fogarty vascular embolectomy catheter, a single-lumen endotracheal tube with an enclosed moveable bronchial blocker, and a wire-guided bronchial blocker.[129] Regardless of the selected device, experience is required for successful placement and safe utilization.[116] The blocker is directed to the bleeding bronchus under guidance of fiberoptic bronchoscopy. By advancing the blocker to the smallest subsegment to which bleeding can be visualized, bleeding can be contained and diagnostic workup can continue. Other balloon catheters can also be used for this purpose,[130] although they must be carried to the bleeding site on the outside of the bronchoscope by the bronchoscopic shuttle technique.[131] Multiple catheters can be placed if hemoptysis is multifocal and catheters can be left in place for 24 to 48 hours until bleeding is controlled.[128]

ENDOBRONCHIAL INFUSIONS

Although a variety of agents have been infused into the airway through the bronchoscope to control bleeding, no studies directly compare the agents with each other or with other modalities of therapy. Nevertheless, the potential advantage of these agents is their administration during bronchoscopy for localization of bleeding. Thrombin and fibrinogen-thrombin mixtures have been used in some sites to provide a hemostatic clot in the area of bleeding with good success.[132,133] Commercial fibrinogen is not available in the United States for patient use. Oxidized regenerated cellulose mesh, a biodegradable cellulose fabric, is an alternative procoagulant used in patients with massive hemoptysis and showed a 98% success rate in a series of 57 patients.[134] Once deployed in the area of hemorrhage, it absorbs blood, swelling into a gelatinous mass that promotes tamponade and coagulation. Endobronchial sealing with *n*-butyl cyanoacrylate, a biocompatible glue with prothrombotic properties, has also been used with success in small case series.[135]

Topical vasoconstrictors including iced saline,[136] epinephrine,[137] and vasopressin or vasopressin derivatives[138,139] have also been used effectively for airway bleeding in anecdotal reports. The likely mechanism is vasoconstriction of bronchial arteries. These may be a safe, effective alternative in patients without access to BAE or surgery, or in unstable patients in need of a temporizing intervention until definitive therapy is available.

LASER PHOTOCOAGULATION

The neodymium:yttrium aluminum garnet (Nd:YAG) or argon plasma laser has been used successfully for airway carcinoma with persistent hemoptysis. Recognizing that carcinomatous bleeding is usually progressive and can be life threatening, aggressive photocoagulation of the endobronchial site may provide the only possibility for palliation after chemotherapy and radiation have been exhausted. Success has been reported in approximately 60% of cancer patients with hemoptysis.[140] Appropriate training, however, is imperative to ensure appropriate patient selection and to avoid catastrophic complications such as tracheal fire or vessel perforation.[141]

BRONCHIAL ARTERY EMBOLIZATION

Bronchial artery embolization (BAE) was first described in 1974 to control massive hemoptysis in the nonsurgical patient.[142] Subsequent studies on safety and efficacy have confirmed immediate, safe control of hemoptysis in 79% to 100% of a variety of patients, resulting in early use of BAE in the management strategy.[143-151] The technique for BAE localizes the bronchial arteries supplying the lobe that is bleeding. A formal bronchial arteriogram is performed to ensure that there is no communication to the anterior spinal artery, to determine whether a vascular pathologic condition is present, and to ensure that the bleeding area of lung parenchyma is served by the vessel. Only rarely will vascular extravasation indicative of bleeding be observed, usually in massively bleeding patients. Angiographic signs that suggest a source of bleeding include hypertrophied/enlarged/tortuous bronchial arteries with parenchymal hypervascularity, bronchial artery aneurysms, and bronchial artery to pulmonary vein or pulmonary artery shunting.[152] Angiographic technique usually begins with injection of contrast agent in the descending aorta just below the left subclavian artery to identify bronchial arteries supplying the majority of the lung and phrenic arteries supplying the lung bases. Identification of anomalous origins of the bronchial arteries may require a full arch aortogram in some patients.[153] For pathologic conditions of the lower lung, a selective phrenic artery injection is used if the entire lung is not visualized by bronchial injections. Rarely, these lower injections may demonstrate a pulmonary sequestration. For pathologic conditions of the upper lung zone, a unilateral subclavian artery injection is done to exclude nonbronchial systemic collateral arteries.

No studies have evaluated the optimal embolization material for control of hemoptysis. Gelatin sponge particles, polyvinyl alcohol particles, or liquid polymers (e.g., *n*-butyl cyanoacrylate) with a predetermined polymerization time have all been used with success.[154] Velour, polyurethane particles of varying size, metal coils, protein macroaggregates, and fibrinogen-thrombin mixtures[155] have also been instilled. Combinations of materials are used in a significant number of patients.[150,156] Liquid sclerosants, such as absolute alcohol or Gelfoam powder, should be used with caution because they may pass into the smallest vessels at the bronchial surface, producing bronchial necrosis.[157]

Significant complications of BAE are rare when appropriate technique is employed. Chest pain, dysphagia, and fever are the most common complications. The most devastating complication is spinal cord infarction resulting from embolization of the anterior spinal artery, which arises from the bronchial artery circulation in approximately 5% of normal patients. However, with proliferation of the bronchial artery circulation, as occurs in CF, communication to the anterior spinal artery may be found in up to 55% of cases.[158] By performing high-quality bronchial arteriograms to define vascular anatomy and avoiding the anterior spinal artery by wedging the angiography catheter distal to its takeoff (or by avoiding the vessel altogether), a safe procedure can almost always be ensured. The recent introduction of microcatheter technology (i.e., "superselective" catheterization) allows achievement of a more distal, safe catheter position and has greatly reduced the number of aborted procedures and complications arising from anterior spinal artery embolization.

Recurrent hemoptysis is common after BAE and can occur immediately, in the first several weeks to months (early), or after several years (late). Immediate recurrence of hemoptysis in the first few days after BAE may occur in approximately 10% of patients[144] and may be due to several causes. For the patient who continues to bleed during the procedure, the appropriate blood vessel usually has not been embolized. Other common causes include bleeding from nonbronchial systemic or pulmonary vessels, particularly if not evaluated initially, and lysis of the hemostatic plug in the embolized bronchial artery. Recurrence of hemoptysis in the first several months after BAE may be related to incomplete embolization, although later recurrence at 1 to 2 years may be related to neovascularization or recanalization related to inflammation or disease progression.[159] Reporting of outcomes varies considerably in BAE studies but early recurrence of bleeding may occur in 3.5% to 26% of patients.[145,147,149,150] Late recurrence of bleeding may occur in 10% to 40% of patients.[143,145,146,149,150] The incidence of recurrence is not uniform in all lung diseases, and higher recurrence rates are noted in *Aspergillus* fungus balls, bronchiectasis, tuberculosis, and lung cancers.* Use of superselective embolization, which provides less of a stimulus for neovascularization, may improve recurrence rates.[161] BAE can be considered a palliative intervention for the acute cessation of massive hemoptysis that allows for a more controlled evaluation of the patient for potentially curative interventions.

SURGERY

A significant question in control of massive hemoptysis is whether conservative management techniques including endobronchial tamponade and BAE are better than emergent surgery in improving outcomes. Given the high success rates of BAE and low associated morbidity and mortality rates, more conservative techniques are now considered first-line therapy over emergent surgery. The proportion of patients with massive hemoptysis who undergo emergent or urgent surgery often is not reported, but recent studies found 12% to 14% of patients required surgical intervention.[151,162] Although perioperative and hospital mortality rates were high in past experience, more recent studies report a mortality rate of less than 15%.[162-165] The outcome of surgery is likely influenced by the cause and severity of hemoptysis, patient comorbid conditions, extent of lung resection, and experience of the surgical team. Absolute indications for surgery do not exist, but patients with vascular disruptions (e.g., leaking aortic aneurysm, AVMs, pulmonary artery rupture, chest trauma); focal fungal disease, tuberculosis, or bronchiectasis; or failed BAE or early recurrence of bleeding after BAE should be considered for urgent surgery in the setting of massive hemoptysis.[148,160] Mycetomas, active tuberculosis, and bronchiectasis represent a large majority of the causes of hemoptysis in surgical reports.

Important issues in the assessment of a patient for thoracic surgery include the underlying cardiopulmonary reserve, precise localization of bleeding, and the focality of the patient's disease. Unfortunately, the safety of the large intrathoracic pressure swings involved with bedside spirometry in a massively bleeding patient has not been established. Because alveolarized blood can produce significant chest restriction on spirometry, a functional assessment is often obtained on the basis of premorbid exercise tolerance.

Patients with fibrosis and adhesions between the lung and chest wall, commonly seen in tuberculosis, fungal disease, and bronchiectasis, have significant surgical risks because they often require pneumonectomy. Physiologic lung exclusion, in which the bronchus and pulmonary artery of the involved lobe or lung are surgically interrupted, leaving the pulmonary veins intact, appears to be a viable alternative in such patients. In a series of 20 patients, Dhaliwal and colleagues[166] reported control of bleeding in all patients with no fatality and no significant morbidity. Video-assisted thoracoscopic procedures may be successful in some patients.[167]

The decision regarding surgery for massive hemoptysis is a difficult one that often must be made rapidly, without all desired clinical information available. The availability of BAE and endobronchial tamponade may provide time for a reasoned decision to be made regarding surgery in all but the most rapidly bleeding patients.

OTHER THERAPIES

As new devices and interventions are developed for the management of other pulmonary and nonpulmonary conditions, some may be adapted to treat massive hemoptysis. Covered self-expanding stents have been used to occlude a bleeding site in a patient not treatable by BAE or surgery.[168,169] Recombinant activated factor VII has been used to control hemoptysis in DAH[70,170] and focal bleeding associated with community-acquired pneumonia,[171] thoracic trauma,[172] and CF.[173] Recombinant activated factor VII is not approved for use in hemoptysis, and clinicians must weigh adverse effects, thrombotic risk, and availability of other interventions when considering this treatment option.

KEY POINTS

- The adverse clinical effects of hemoptysis such as impaired gas exchange, airway obstruction, and hypotension are relevant for defining a life-threatening condition.
- Bleeding from the higher pressure bronchial circulation (rather than the pulmonary circulation) causes almost 90% of the cases of massive hemoptysis.
- Massive hemoptysis is more common with bronchiectasis, tuberculosis or its sequelae, lung cancer, and aspergilloma than with chronic bronchitis, pneumonia, and pulmonary emboli.
- DAH should be considered as a potential cause of hemoptysis in the presence of diffuse infiltrates on chest radiograph, systemic manifestations of vasculitis, hypoxemic respiratory failure, and anemia.
- The primary principles of managing massive hemoptysis are airway and lung protection, localization of the bleeding source, and control of hemorrhage.
- A multidisciplinary collaborative and organized approach to managing massive hemoptysis is needed to improve outcomes.

*See references 9, 143, 148-150, 159, 160.

KEY POINTS (Continued)

- Orotracheal intubation with a larger endotracheal tube (preferably 8-mm inner diameter or larger) is preferred for airway protection in massive hemoptysis to facilitate suctioning, ventilation, and bronchoscopy.
- Chest CT, except in unstable patients, should be performed in many patients prior to bronchoscopy and BAE to efficiently guide management.
- BAE is a safe and effective technique to control bleeding in massive hemoptysis and should be used as the initial therapeutic modality in most patients.
- Patients with vascular disease; focal fungal disease, tuberculosis, or bronchiectasis; or failed BAE or early recurrence of bleeding after BAE should be considered for urgent surgery of massive hemoptysis if they have sufficient cardiopulmonary reserve.

SELECTED REFERENCES

1. Jean-Baptiste E: Clinical assessment and management of massive hemoptysis. Crit Care Med 2000;28:1642.
2. Sakr L, Dutau H: Massive hemoptysis: An update on the role of bronchoscopy in diagnosis and management. Respiration 2010;80:38.
20. Flume PA, Mogayzel PJ, Robinson KA, et al: Cystic fibrosis pulmonary guidelines, pulmonary complications: Hemoptysis and pneumothorax. Am J Resp Crit Care Med 2010;182:298.
59. Lara AR, Schwarz MI: Diffuse alveolar hemorrhage. Chest 2010;137:1164.
116. Campos JH, Hallam EA, Van Natta T, Kernstein KH: Devices for lung isolation used by anesthesiologists with limited thoracic experience. Anesthesiology 2006;104:261.
148. Chun J-Y, Belli A-M: Immediate and long-term outcomes of bronchial and non-bronchial systemic artery embolisation for the management of haemoptysis. Eur Radiol 2010;20:558.
149. Daliri A, Probst NH, Jobst B, et al: Bronchial artery embolization in patients with hemoptysis including follow-up. Acta Radiol 2011;52:143.
152. Kalva SP: Bronchial artery embolization. Tech Vasc Intervent Radiol 2009;12:130.
156. Wang GR, Ensor JE, Gupta S, et al: Bronchial artery embolization for management of hemoptysis in oncology patients: Utility and prognostic factors. J Vasc Intervent Radiol 2009;20:722.
162. Andréjak C, Parrott A, Bazelly B, et al: Surgical lung resection for severe hemoptysis. Ann Thorac Surg 2009;88:1556.

The complete list of references can be found at www.expertconsult.com.

47 Pneumothorax and Barotrauma

Robert C. Hyzy | Rommel Sagana

CHAPTER OUTLINE

Additional videos for this topic are available online at expertconsult.com.

DEFINITION AND HISTORY

Pneumothorax is defined as air in the pleural space because of a break in the visceral or parietal pleura. The term *pneumothorax* was used for the first time in 1803.[1] Laennec[2] gave the first clinical description of pneumothorax in 1819; however, the first chest radiograph demonstrating this entity was not published until 1901.[3] Definitive therapy became available with the advent of tube thoracostomy in 1876.[4] It was thought to be always associated with tuberculosis until 1932 when "spontaneous pneumothorax in the apparently healthy" was first described.[5]

Spontaneous pneumothorax can be classified as primary or secondary. Primary spontaneous pneumothorax (PSP) occurs in patients with no apparent underlying lung disease. Secondary spontaneous pneumothorax (SSP) occurs in association with a known underlying lung disease such as chronic obstructive pulmonary disease (COPD).[6] Nonspontaneous causes of pneumothorax include traumatic and iatrogenic (Table 47.1).

INCIDENCE

The incidence of PSP in men varies geographically, from 7.4 per 100,000 population per year in the United States to 37 per 100,000 population per year in the United Kingdom. In women, the incidence is substantially less, ranging from 1.2 per 100,000 population per year in the United States to 15.4 per 100,000 population per year in the United Kingdom.[7] The reason for these differences is not known. In a study that evaluated 1199 patients with pneumothorax that included 865 male patients and 334 female patients, 60.3% of the pneumothoraces were spontaneous, 33.6% were traumatic, and 6.1% were iatrogenic.[8]

The estimates of the incidence of recurrent PSP range from 20% to more than 50% with most recurrences occurring within the first year.[9]

Table 47.1 Classification of Pneumothorax

Type	Etiology
Primary spontaneous pneumothorax (PSP)	No underlying lung disease (but blebs/bullae commonly present)
Secondary spontaneous pneumothorax (SSP)	Associated with underlying lung disease (e.g., chronic obstructive pulmonary disease, cystic fibrosis, AIDS with emphysema)
Traumatic iatrogenic pneumothorax	Related to trauma to the thorax Secondary to transthoracic or transbronchial lung biopsy (10% risk), central venous catheterization, supraclavicular nerve block

From Grundy S, Bentley A, Tschopp JM: Primary spontaneous pneumothorax: A diffuse disease of the pleura. Respiration 2012;83:185-189.

PATHOPHYSIOLOGY

EMPHYSEMA-LIKE CHANGES

PSP occurs in patients with no previously known lung disease. It is important to note, however, that this does not mean there is no underlying pathologic process. A finding of abnormal pleura is very common in PSP if looked for carefully.[10] Abnormalities seen in PSP are summarized in Table 47.2 and include blebs and bullae, which are otherwise known as emphysema-like changes (ELCs). These areas of weakness of the visceral pleura are prone to rupture, allowing air to leak into the pleural space. Abnormalities can be visualized radiographically with high-resolution computed tomography (CT) scans and macroscopically at thoracoscopy.[10,11] High-resolution CT imaging reveals these defects in approximately 80% of PSP patients. The literature is mixed as to whether the presence of or extent of ELCs is directly related to the risk of recurrence. Some case series suggest that there is no association,[12,13] although others suggest the presence of contralateral blebs/bullae is a risk factor for future pneumothorax.[14,15] The only clear conclusion that can be drawn is that there is a direct association between the presence of ELCs and the occurrence (but not necessarily recurrence) of a pneumothorax (Table 47.2 and Fig. 47.1).

PLEURAL POROSITY

ELCs are not the sole cause of PSP. Air leak has been described in areas where no ELCs are seen, leading to the concept known as "pleural porosity."[16,17] When evaluated with fluorescein-enhanced autofluorescence, areas of high-grade abnormality in the visceral pleura were frequently visualized separate from any area of abnormality seen with white light at thoracoscopy in patients with PSP. High-grade abnormalities were not seen in control patients.[18] Areas of fluorescein leak (i.e., areas of potential air leak) were visualized in only a small proportion of PSP, but these areas were noted to be distinct from areas of ELC. When studied with electron microscopy, the linings of some resected areas of ELC have been shown to be almost completely absent of mesothelial cells and have abnormal pores present[19] (Fig. 47.2).

Table 47.2 Pathologic Changes Associated with Primary Spontaneous Pneumothorax (PSP)

Pathologic Abnormality	Description
Emphysema-like changes (ELCs) (i.e., blebs/bullae)	Macroscopically visible areas of weakness on visceral pleura Occasionally seen to be the site of air leak Present in approximately 80% of cases Often bilateral
Fluorescein enhancement	Represents areas of pleural/subpleural abnormality not visible with white light autofluorescence Often present at sites distinct from ELC in lungs of patients with PSP and not in those of control subjects Provides evidence of diffuse pleural porosity
Distal airway inflammation	Inflammatory infiltration with lymphocytes and macrophages within walls of bronchioles Associated fibrotic changes and compensatory emphysema

From Grundy S, Bentley A, Tschopp JM: Primary spontaneous pneumothorax: A diffuse disease of the pleura. Respiration 2012;83:185-189.

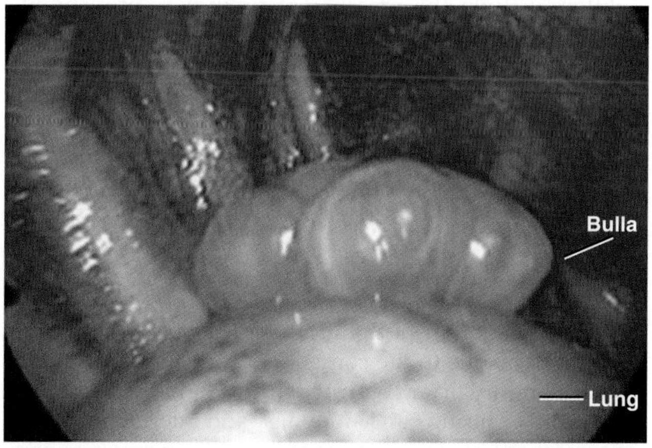

Figure 47.1 Large bulla at the apex of the left lung in a 12-year-old boy with recurrent primary spontaneous pneumothorax. (From Noppen M, De Keukelieire T: Pneumothorax. Respiration 2008;76: 121-127.)

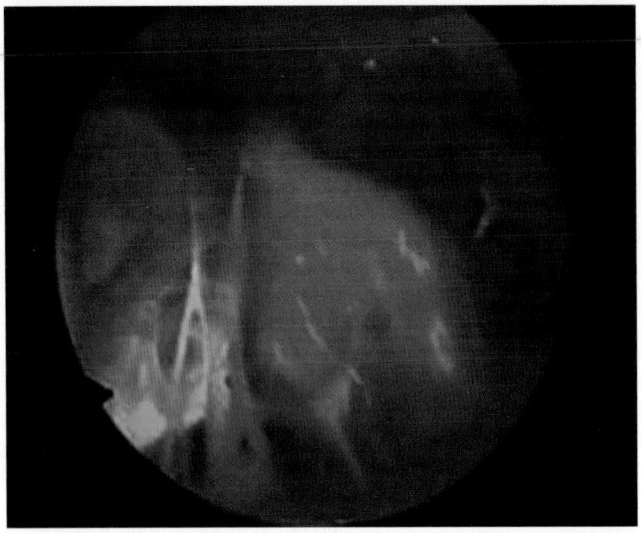

Figure 47.2 Air leak identified by fluorescein-enhanced autofluorescence thoracoscopy in a 27-year-old man with recurrent primary spontaneous pneumothorax. The air leak was situated at the base of a highly vascularized, severe malformation of the apex of the lung. (From Noppen M, De Keukelieire T: Pneumothorax. Respiration 2008;76: 121-127.)

DISTAL AIRWAY INFLAMMATION

Pathologic findings suggest an inflammatory cause to the formation of ELCs. Chronic distal airway inflammation with lymphocyte and macrophage infiltration alongside fibrotic changes and compensatory emphysema can be seen microscopically in areas of lung tissue from patients with PSP.[20] In a different study, the presence of respiratory bronchiolitis (RB) was seen in close to 90% of patients with PSP who underwent surgical resection in a different study.[21] However, all these patients in this study were smokers, and smoking is a recognized cause of RB. It has been proposed that distal airway inflammation associated with PSP leads to obstructive gas trapping and consequent increases in distal airway pressure, which possibly causes air leak into the pleural space.[22]

SMOKING

Cigarette smoking is a significant risk factor for PSP. It is thought to be due to the consequences of airway inflammation leading to airway obstruction with a check valve phenomenon, causing air trapping and development of pneumothorax.[22] The lifetime risk is 12% in smokers compared to 0.1% in nonsmokers. Risk is also directly related to the amount of cigarette smoking. Compared to nonsmokers, the relative risk of PSP in men was seven times higher in light smokers (1-12 cigarettes per day), 21 times higher in moderate smokers (13-22 cigarettes per day), and 102 times higher in heavy smokers (>22 cigarettes per day). For women, the relative risk was 4, 14, and 68 times higher in light, moderate, and heavy smokers, respectively.[23] Cessation of smoking appears to reduce the risk of recurrence,[9] and continued smoking increases the risk of recurrence.[24]

RB, a form of airway inflammation associated with cigarette smoking, may contribute to the development and recurrence of PSP. In a study with 115 patients with PSP who underwent video-assisted thoracoscopic surgery (VATS), pneumothorax recurrence rates were higher in patients with extensive rather than nonextensive RB for both nonoperative and postoperative pneumothorax.[25]

GENETICS

Familial inheritance of pneumothorax describing the clustering of PSP in certain families has been published. Autosomal dominant, autosomal recessive, polygenic, and X-linked recessive inheritance mechanisms have been proposed.[26-28] Birt-Hogg-Dubé (BHD) is an autosomal dominant cancer disorder that predisposes patients to benign skin tumors and renal cancer. It is associated with pleuropulmonary blebs and cysts that lead to PSP.[29] In one study of 198 patients with this syndrome, 48 patients (24%) had a history of pneumothorax.[30] The gene responsible for this familial cancer syndrome (*FLCN*) has been mapped to chromosome 17p11.2.[31,32] Other mutations of *FLCN* have been associated with spontaneous pneumothorax and bullous lung disease in the absence of Birt-Hogg-Dubé syndrome.[33]

Patients with Marfan syndrome are tall, and pneumothorax is a common pulmonary complication. Marfan syndrome is caused by the mutation in *FBN1* gene on chromosome 15. This gene is responsible for the formation of 10- to 12-nm microfibrils in the extracellular matrix of connective tissue. It is hypothesized that familial spontaneous pneumothorax is caused by a connective tissue disorder that exhibits mendelian inheritance and *FBN1* has been postulated as the causative gene.[34]

CLASSIFICATION

SPONTANEOUS PNEUMOTHORAX

PRIMARY SPONTANEOUS PNEUMOTHORAX

PSP is classically seen in previously healthy young men with an asthenic body habitus. The incidence of PSP rises with increasing height among adults of both sexes, more so in men. For those 76 inches or taller, the rate was 200 per 100,000 person-years.[35] It is hypothesized that individuals with tall stature and low body mass index combined with smoking are predisposed to develop ELCs owing to the pressure gradient between the lung base and the apex, resulting in increased alveolar distending pressures at the apex.[36] Smoking, as previously described, greatly increases the risk of PSP. Smoking increases the relative risk of developing spontaneous pneumothorax about ninefold in women and 22-fold in men, and there is a statistically significant dose-response relationship between smoking and spontaneous pneumothorax.[37]

SECONDARY SPONTANEOUS PNEUMOTHORAX

SSP has been described in a large variety of diseases including COPD with emphysema, cystic fibrosis (CF), tuberculosis, lung cancer, human immunodeficiency virus (HIV)-associated *Pneumocystis jiroveci* pneumonia, followed by more rare but "typical" disorders such as lymphangioleiomyomatosis (LAM) and histiocytosis X (Box 47.1). Because lung function in these patients is already compromised, SSP

Box 47.1 Frequent and/or Typical Causes of Primary Spontaneous Pneumothorax

Airway disease
- Emphysema
- Cystic fibrosis
- Severe asthma

Infectious lung disease
- *Pneumocystis jiroveci* (formerly *P. carinii*) pneumonia
- Tuberculosis
- Necrotizing pneumonia

Interstitial lung disease
- Idiopathic pulmonary fibrosis
- Sarcoidosis
- Histiocytosis X (Langerhans cell histiocytosis)
- Lymphangioleiomyomatosis

Connective tissue disease
- Rheumatoid arthritis, scleroderma, ankylosing spondylitis
- Marfan syndrome
- Ehlers-Danlos syndrome

Malignant disease
- Lung cancer
- Sarcoma

From Noppen M, De Keukelieire T. Pneumothorax. Respiration 2008;76:121-127.

often presents as a potentially life-threatening disease requiring immediate action, as opposed to PSP, which is more of a nuisance than a dangerous condition. The general incidence is almost similar to that of PSP.[38]

Chronic Obstructive Pulmonary Disease

COPD is the most common cause of SSP, with nearly 70% of SSP attributed to COPD.[39] The peak incidence of SSP from COPD typically occurs later in life averaging 60 to 65 years of age.[40] The clinical presentation of pneumothorax in COPD is often atypical—pain may be absent, anxiety and breathlessness may predominate and be out of proportion to the collapsed lung, and the classic sign of hyperresonance may not be helpful because of the underlying emphysema. The air leak in these patients is usually large, and the tissues are slow to heal, so it is weeks before the tubes can be taken out.[41]

Pneumothorax in Drug Abusers

When the peripheral veins of chronic abusers of drugs become obliterated because of a sclerotic or infectious process, the individual may attempt to use larger veins in the groin or neck. Attempted subclavian or supraclavicular ("pocket shot") injection of drugs in the street setting has led to unilateral or bilateral pneumothoraces.[42-44] Douglas and Levison[45] found that the incidence of pneumothoraces is equal in both sexes and that it is less of a problem in teenagers and in addicts older than 40 years of age. It was also noted that although most drug users describe using small (21- or 22-gauge) needles, a large, complete, or tension pneumothorax usually develops.

Pneumothorax in HIV-Infected Patients

Pneumothorax is an uncommon but potentially fatal complication of HIV infection. The first report of spontaneous pneumothorax in patients with acquired immunodeficiency syndrome (AIDS) was in 1984.[46] With the diagnosis of AIDS, a patient's risk of sustaining a nontraumatic pneumothorax increases to 450 times that of the general population.[47] It has since been described in a generalized HIV-infected population.[48,49] Pneumothorax complicated 1.2% of all hospital admissions in a cohort of 599 HIV-infected patients followed over 3 years in a prospective observational study. There was also an associated increase in in-hospital mortality rate (31% versus 6%) for patients without pneumothorax.[48]

A high incidence (2-9%) of pneumothorax has been reported in patients with AIDS and *Pneumocystis carinii* pneumonia (PCP).[50-52] *Pneumocystis carinii,* which was thought to be a protozoan, has been renamed as *Pneumocystis jiroveci* and is now classified as an archiascomycetous fungus.[53] Causes of pneumothorax in HIV-infected individuals include *P. jiroveci*[54-57] along with other infectious agents such as *Mycobacterium tuberculosis, M. avium intracellulare,* pulmonary cytomegalovirus, *Pneumococcus* organisms,[54] or pulmonary toxoplasmosis.[54] Pneumothorax has also been described in HIV-infected individuals from Kaposi sarcoma.[58]

The cause of pneumothorax in patients with PCP is unclear. Several investigators believe that extensive tissue invasion within the alveolar interstitium in severe PCP is an important factor in causing necrosis and subsequent pneumothorax. Several observations highlight this point. The most common sites of tissue invasion with PCP are the alveolar septa, pleurae, and vasculature.[59] Tissue invasion could cause necrosis as a result of direct tissue injury by toxins from *Pneumocystis,*[59] infarction from vascular compromise,[60,61] or as a result of the host inflammatory response.[62]

The administration of aerosolized pentamidine has been implicated in the pathogenesis of cavitation, cyst formation, and pneumothorax,[50,63,64] but the biologic basis for this relationship is unknown. No direct toxic action of pentamidine on the lungs has been described, so an indirect effect may be present. Cavitation due to PCP may occur primarily in the upper lobes and periphery because aerosolized pentamidine is preferentially delivered to the proximal parenchyma of the lower lobes. Inadequate deposition of pentamidine in the periphery of the lung could allow a chronic, low-grade infection with *Pneumocystis* to persist, leading to peripheral lung destruction and pneumatocele formation. Increased survival time of AIDS patients due to prophylaxis could allow for development of these lesions.[50]

Several other risk factors for AIDS-related pneumothorax have been identified. In addition to previous or active infection of *P. jiroveci* and aerosolized pentamidine, cigarette smoking and the presence of pneumatoceles on chest radiograph are risk factors.[65] The association between cigarette smoking and AIDS-related pneumothorax could be explained by subclinical obstructive disease preventing adequate deposition of aerosolized pentamidine in the lung periphery, resulting in subpleural *Pneumocystis* infection.[65] Pulmonary tuberculosis also appears to increase the risk of pneumothorax in AIDS.[66]

Catamenial Pneumothorax

In most cases, catamenial pneumothorax is related to pelvic or thoracic endometriosis.[67,68] Catamenial pneumothorax occurs typically within 24 to 72 hours after onset of menstruation. It is often recurrent and more common than previously thought. Two mechanisms have been described for pneumothorax related to endometriosis. The most common is the movement of endometrial implants to the diaphragm, preferentially to the right side because of the recognized peritoneal circulation up from the pelvis to the right side. These implants then create channels or "holes" through the diaphragm that allow the implants or air to move into the chest. The second and much less frequent cause of endometrial implants causing *pneumothorax* in the chest is through the venous implants that lodge into the lung itself.[69] Clinical manifestations of thoracic endometriosis include chest pain, dyspnea, and hemoptysis. Treatment for the prevention of recurrence is indicated after a first episode of catamenial pneumothorax because recurrences are frequent.[38]

Cystic Fibrosis

SSP occurs in approximately 6% of all patients with CF and this number increases to 16% to 20% among those who survive to age 18.[70,71] SSP from CF is usually due to rupture of apical subpleural cysts. The risk of pneumothorax is inversely proportional to the forced expiratory volume in 1 second (FEV_1). Other factors associated with an increased risk of pneumothorax include infection with *Pseudomonas aeruginosa*, *Burkholderia cepacia* complex, or *Aspergillus* species. A previous history of massive hemoptysis also increases risk.

NONSPONTANEOUS PNEUMOTHORAX

TRAUMATIC PNEUMOTHORAX

Pneumothorax ranks second to rib fractures as the most common sign of chest trauma. It occurs in up to 50% of chest trauma victims.[72] Most are caused by a penetrating injury, but closed chest trauma causing alveolar rupture from thoracic compression, fracture of a bronchus, and esophageal rupture have also been reported.[73,74] Traumatic pneumothorax can be classified as open, closed, tension, or hemopneumothorax. A tension pneumothorax should be managed immediately by decompression with a large-bore needle usually in the second anterior interspace in the midclavicular line. Open pneumothorax should have a moist sterile gauze pack placed over the open wound, followed by a chest tube. Hemopneumothorax (20% of trauma patients) requires insertion of a large-bore (28-36F) chest tube.[38]

Occult pneumothorax may be present in half of blunt abdominal trauma patients, many of which are undetected by chest radiograph.[75-79] CT of the chest should therefore always be performed in these patients. Most surgeons and emergency physicians will place a chest tube in occult and nonoccult pneumothoraces. Studies suggest, however, that clinically stable patients and those who do not have an enlarging pneumothorax may be treated conservatively, ultimately requiring chest tube placement in about 10% of cases.[80]

TRAUMATIC IATROGENIC PNEUMOTHORAX

Iatrogenic pneumothorax occurs most often following transthoracic needle biopsy (24%), subclavian vein catheterization (22%), thoracentesis (20%), transbronchial lung biopsy (10%), pleural biopsy (8%), and positive-pressure ventilation (7%).[81] Diagnosis of iatrogenic pneumothorax is often delayed. Small and asymptomatic iatrogenic pneumothorax, however, often do not need any treatment and resolve spontaneously. In larger or symptomatic pneumothoraces, simple manual aspiration or placement of a small catheter or chest tube attached to a Heimlich valve is usually sufficient.[82] Larger tubes may be necessary in patients with emphysema or when the patient is placed on a mechanical ventilator.

PULMONARY BAROTRAUMA DURING MECHANICAL VENTILATION

Pulmonary barotrauma (PBT) refers to alveolar rupture due to elevated transalveolar pressure (the alveolar pressure minus the pressure in the adjacent interstitial space). PBT was previously estimated to range between 3.8% and 41.7% of patients undergoing mechanical ventilation.[83] The rate in actuality may be lower because low tidal volume ventilation is becoming more common. Consequences of barotrauma include pneumothorax, pneumomediastinum, pneumoperitoneum, and subcutaneous emphysema.

Positive-pressure ventilation increases transalveolar pressure, which can cause alveolar rupture.[84] Alveolar rupture allows air from the alveolus to enter the pulmonary interstitium where it can dissect along the perivascular sheaths toward the mediastinum. This can lead to pneumothorax, pneumomediastinum, pneumoperitoneum, or subcutaneous emphysema[85,86] (Fig. 47.3). Bronchopleural fistula,

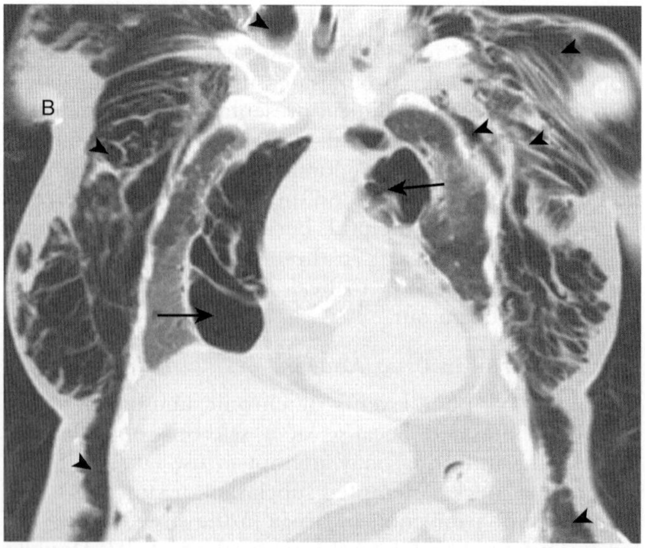

Figure 47.3 Chest computed tomography revealing extensive subcutaneous emphysema (*arrows*) from the lower neck to the upper abdomen and pneumomediastinum (*thick arrows*). (From Lai JI, Po-Chou L, Wang WS, et al: Barotrauma related extensive pneumothorax, pneumomediastinum, and subcutaneous emphysema in a patient with acute respiratory distress syndrome with low tidal volume. Postgrad Med J 2010;86:567-568.)

tension pneumothorax, tension lung cyst, and subpleural air cyst have also been reported but are less common.[87]

In a multicenter prospective cohort study of 5183 mechanically ventilated patients, the incidence of PBT was 3%.[88] Asthma, chronic interstitial lung disease, and acute respiratory distress syndrome (ARDS) were identified as independent risk factors for barotrauma. Other studies have also demonstrated that acute lung injury (ALI) and ARDS are independent risk factors for PBT.[89,90] Elevated peak and plateau pressures have been identified as risk factors.[91,92]

Neither open lung strategies using high levels of positive end-expiratory pressure (PEEP) nor recruitment maneuvers have been shown to increase the risk of barotrauma.[93,94]

Clinical Presentation

The clinical presentation of PBT can vary. With pneumothorax, patients may complain of dyspnea or chest pain. Physical findings can include tachycardia, tachypnea, hypertension, or oxyhemoglobin saturation accompanied by unilateral reduction of breath sounds. If a tension pneumothorax develops, there may be hypotension and tracheal deviation. Patients with pneumomediastinum may complain of dyspnea and chest or neck pain. Other findings include tachycardia, tachypnea, and hypertension. A crunching sound may be heard during auscultation. Rarely, hypotension from decreased venous return and cardiac output may occur if tension pneumomediastinum develops.[95] Pneumoperitoneum may manifest itself as abdominal pain. Other physical findings include abdominal distention, tenderness, and tympany. Rarely, abdominal compartment syndrome may develop if the pneumoperitoneum progresses to a tension pneumoperitoneum.[96] Subcutaneous emphysema generally presents as painless soft tissue swelling. It typically appears in the upper chest, neck, and face. Compression of the affected areas can reveal crepitus. A rare consequence of severe subcutaneous emphysema is compartment syndrome.[97]

Diagnosis

The diagnosis of pneumothorax is suspected when a patient presents with the symptoms and signs described earlier, then confirmed with a portable chest radiograph. An upright chest radiograph has the highest diagnostic yield for pneumothorax, although diagnosis in the intensive care unit (ICU) may be difficult as most patients are semirecumbent or supine.[98] In a fully upright chest radiograph, a pneumothorax appears as a radiolucent collection between the visceral and parietal pleurae in the superior portion of the chest. In contrast, when a patient is supine, free air collects in the anterior chest, displacing the costophrenic angle inferiorly, often creating a "deep sulcus" sign. The deep sulcus sign refers to a unilateral increase in the apparent size of the costophrenic angle (Fig. 47.4).

Bedside ultrasound is being used more readily in the ICU to rapidly diagnose pneumothorax. Utilizing the M-mode, the absence of "lung sliding" is indicative of the presence of a pneumothorax[99] (Video 47.1).

Tension pneumothorax is diagnosed clinically when a patient presents with unilateral absence of breath sounds, a shift of the trachea in the direction away from the absent breath sounds, and hemodynamic compromise in the appropriate setting. Immediate intervention is indicated as there is seldom time for a radiographic evaluation. Rapid clinical improvement following empiric aspiration of a suspected tension pneumothorax is diagnostically definitive. Subsequently, a tube thoracostomy is placed for ongoing management.

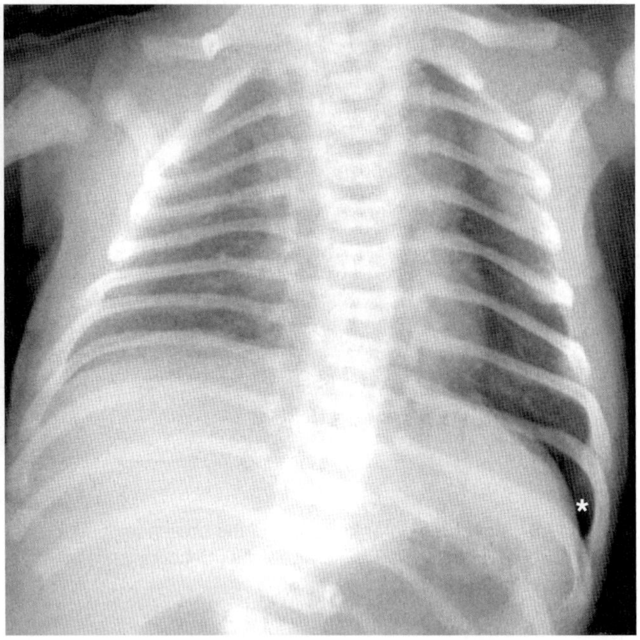

Figure 47.4 Supine chest radiograph of a neonate illustrates the deep sulcus sign with abnormal deepening and lucency of the left lateral costophrenic angle (*). (From Kong A: The deep sulcus sign. Radiology 2003;228(2):415-416.)

Pneumomediastinum frequently coexists with pneumothorax. It is usually diagnosed with a portable chest radiograph. It typically appears as radiolucent streaks in the mediastinum (Fig. 47.5).

Pneumoperitoneum is diagnosed with a chest radiograph less than one third of the time. A suspected pneumoperitoneum is best evaluated by chest CT.[100] The patient should remain in position for 5 to 10 minutes before the radiograph is taken. This allows time for air to collect in a sufficient volume to be detected radiographically. Pneumoperitoneum may be identified on a supine abdominal radiograph (see Fig. 47.5). Free air accumulates anteriorly when the patient is supine and on a chest or abdominal radiograph may present in several ways. Gas appearing on both sides of the bowel wall is referred to as Rigler's sign. Gas outlining the peritoneal cavity is known as the football sign. Gas outlining the medial umbilical folds is called an inverted V sign. Gas may also outline the falciform ligament or localize in the right upper quadrant.[101]

Subcutaneous emphysema is often found by identifying crepitus during physical examination. On chest radiograph of areas of tissue swelling, it can appear as radiolucent streaks throughout the subcutaneous tissue and muscle (see Fig. 47.5).

Prevention

To prevent barotrauma, it is generally recommended that plateau airway pressure be maintained at or below 35 cm H_2O. Plateau pressure is the most indicative of the alveolar

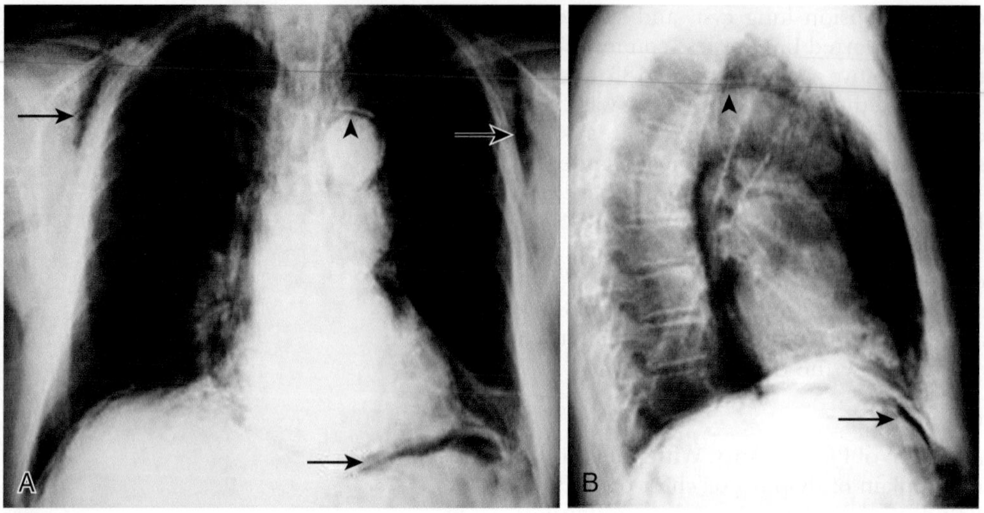

Figure 47.5 Chest radiographs revealing the presence of subcutaneous emphysema, pneumomediastinum, and pneumoperitoneum (*arrows*). (From Alexiou K, Sakellaridis T, Sikalias N, et al: Subcutaneous emphysema, pneumomediastinum and pneumoperitoneum after unsuccessful ERCP: A case report. Cases J 2009;2:120.)

pressure and therefore is the measure of greatest concern for the prevention of PBT. Lower plateau airway pressures have been associated with a lower incidence of PBT. A threshold pressure appears to exist at 35 cm H_2O, above which there is a higher incidence of barotrauma. A meta-analysis of 14 clinical trials demonstrated a strong relationship between PBT and a plateau airway pressure greater than 35 cm H_2O or a static compliance less than 30 mL per cm H_2O.[102] There have not been direct comparisons between management targeting a plateau airway pressure or peak airway pressure. Peak airway pressure is likely a less reliable predictor of PBT given the conflicting data.[103-109]

Management

The best treatment for PBT is early recognition, and immediate attempts should be made to reduce plateau airway pressure.[83] This may require lowering the tidal volume or PEEP, as well as increasing sedation, administering neuromuscular blockade, or advancing treatment of the underlying condition. In cases of pneumothorax while on a mechanical ventilator, there is no high-quality evidence that supports routine insertion of chest tubes for all patients. However, more than 30% of pneumothoraces in mechanically ventilated patients progress to tension pneumothoraces, indicating that these patients must be monitored closely. Treatment for mechanically ventilated patients who develop a pneumomediastinum, pneumoperitoneum, or subcutaneous emphysema is generally supportive unless there is evidence of tension pneumomediastinum or compartment syndrome from pneumoperitoneum or subcutaneous emphysema.[95]

Prognosis

PBT appears to be associated with increased mortality rate, even though barotrauma is not a direct cause of death in most patients. In a multicenter prospective cohort study, patients with barotrauma had a significantly higher mortality rate (51% versus 39%), a longer length of ICU stay (median 9 versus 7 days), and a longer duration of mechanical ventilation (median 6 versus 4 days) than patients without barotrauma.[88] Mortality rate may be related to the severity of the PBT. In one retrospective cohort study of 1700 mechanically ventilated patients, the mortality rate approached 100% when PBT caused a large (>500 mL per breath) bronchopleural fistula.[109] High-frequency jet ventilation is FDA (Food and Drug Administration) approved for the management of large bronchopleural fistulas, but this may be outweighed in some patients by increased plateau airway pressure (alveolar pressure), decreased oxygenation, or worse hypercapnia.[110]

PNEUMOTHORAX AFTER FIBEROPTIC BRONCHOSCOPY AND NEEDLE BIOPSY OF THE LUNG

Multiple literature reviews have documented the relative safety of fiberoptic bronchoscopy (FOB) with transbronchial biopsy. One review of more than 9000 such procedures found that the rate of pneumothorax was 1.9%.[111] An immediate postbronchoscopic chest radiograph rarely provides clinically useful information, and in FOB without transbronchial biopsy an immediate postbronchoscopy radiograph is not necessary.[112,113] Another study in 2006 concluded that in asymptomatic patients, routine radiograph after transbronchial biopsy is not necessary.[114] It was determined that certain patient populations should have routine radiographs performed after FOB with transbronchial biopsy: comatose or mentally retarded patients, patients receiving positive-pressure ventilation, patients with severe respiratory compromise as a result of disease or surgery, patients with bullous disease, patients who complain of chest pain, and outpatients. Pneumothorax after bronchoalveolar lavage without biopsy is extremely rare. The complication of pneumothorax after transbronchial needle aspiration is also low.[115]

Pneumothorax is the most common complication of needle aspiration or biopsy of the lung. It has been reported to occur in 17% to 26.6% of patients.[116-119] The chest tube insertion rate is much lower, ranging from 1% to

14.2%.[116-119] Risk factors for the development of biopsy-related pneumothorax include the presence of COPD, the absence of a history of ipsilateral surgery, small lesion size, a long needle path, and repeated pleural puncture.[116-121] Enlarging or symptomatic pneumothorax can be managed by manual aspiration or placement of a small-caliber chest tube.[120]

Delayed pneumothorax after percutaneous fine-needle aspiration has been reported. A study by Choi and colleagues[122] reported on their series of 458 patients who had undergone transthoracic needle biopsy. A follow-up chest radiograph was obtained immediately and at 3, 8, and 24 hours after the biopsy procedure. A pneumothorax that developed after 3 hours was defined as delayed pneumothorax. Pneumothorax developed in 100 of the 458 patients (21.8%), and delayed pneumothorax developed in 15 patients (3.3%). Female gender and absence of emphysematous changes correlated with an increased rate of delayed pneumothorax.

PNEUMOTHORAX AFTER THORACENTESIS

According to a 1998 National Center for Health Statistics study,[123] physicians perform an estimated 173,000 thoracenteses annually in the United States. Iatrogenic pneumothoraces resulting from thoracentesis increase morbidity rate, mortality rate, and length of hospitalization. Previous reports indicated chest tube insertion may be required in up to 50% of cases with a mean duration of placement of approximately 4 days.[124,125] Gordon and colleagues[126] performed a systematic review and meta-analysis of 24 studies reporting pneumothorax rates after thoracentesis involving 6605 thoracenteses. The overall pneumothorax rate was 6%. In cases in which pneumothorax developed, 34.1% required chest tube placement. Statistically significant risk factors for developing thoracentesis included performing thoracentesis as a therapeutic procedure as opposed to as a diagnostic procedure; the presence of cough, dyspnea, or chest pain during the procedure; and witnessing the aspiration of air during the procedure.[126] Although not statistically significant, other possible predictors included the need for two or more needle insertions and concurrent mechanical ventilation.[126] Ultrasonography guidance,[127-129] more experienced operators,[130] and fewer needle passes conferred lower complication rates,[131] which paralleled findings from central venous catheter insertion studies. Various mechanisms may explain the pneumothoraces that occur after thoracentesis: the lung may be punctured at the time of needle entry or after the fluid has been withdrawn, or a small amount of air may be drawn into the chest during aspiration or along the needle track if high negative intrapleural pressure develops.[132]

PNEUMOTHORAX RESULTING FROM NASOGASTRIC FEEDING TUBES

Small-bore Silastic feeding tubes are being used with increasing frequency for short- and long-term enteral hyperalimentation. The first reported case of pneumothorax as a complication of passing a narrow-bore feeding tube was in 1978.[133] This once rare complication has now become more common.[134-136] Narrow-bore feeding tubes are particularly likely to give rise to pneumothorax because of the tube's small diameter (2.7 mm), self-lubricating properties, and wire stylet. These factors allow undetected entry of the tube into the tracheobronchial tree, perforation of pulmonary tissue, and lodging in the pleural cavity.[137] Other factors that increase the risk of a misplaced feeding tube include the presence of an endotracheal or tracheostomy tube (these may increase pulmonary passage of the tube by preventing glottis closure and perhaps by inhibiting swallowing), altered mental status, denervation of airways, esophageal stricture, enlargement of the heart, and neuromuscular weakness.[138] The clinical signs commonly used to determine correct placement of the feeding tube may be misleading. Normally, to confirm the correct placement of a feeding tube in the stomach, a small amount of air is injected. This produces a characteristic gurgle in the left upper quadrant of the abdomen, but a "pseudoconfirmatory gurgle" with a feeding tube in the chest has been reported.[139] Aspiration of large amounts of fluid through the tube is also taken to be a test of correct placement into the stomach, but delayed aspiration of a large quantity of undigested feeding solution from the pleural space, mistaken for gastric contents, has been reported.[140]

PNEUMOTHORAX AFTER PERCUTANEOUS DILATIONAL TRACHEOSTOMY

Percutaneous dilational tracheostomy (PDT) was first described in 1985 by Ciaglia and colleagues.[141] A case series described subcutaneous emphysema and pneumothorax as complications after percutaneous tracheostomy in a series of 326 cases.[142] Their review of the literature showed that the incidence of subcutaneous emphysema was 1.4% and that of pneumothorax was 0.8%. Findings associated with pneumothorax included difficult PDT and the use of a fenestrated cannula.

SPECIAL SITUATIONS

PNEUMOTHORAX EX VACUO

Pneumothorax after partial resolution of total bronchial obstruction,[143] as a complication of lobar collapse,[144] and after therapeutic thoracentesis for malignant effusions[145] has been described. Acute lobar collapse results in a sudden increase in negative pleural pressure surrounding the collapsed lobe. Although the parietal and visceral pleural surfaces remain intact, the gas originating from the ambient tissues and blood is drawn into the pleural space, producing a pneumothorax called *pneumothorax ex vacuo*. Recognition of this type of pneumothorax is crucial because managing it requires relieving the bronchial obstruction rather than inserting a chest tube. The diagnosis of trapped lung requires documentation of chronicity and absence of pleural inflammation, pleural malignancy, or endobronchial lesion. The pathognomonic radiographic sign of a trapped lung is the pneumothorax ex vacuo, characterized as a small to moderate-sized air collection after evacuation of effusion.[146]

SPORT-RELATED PNEUMOTHORAX

Pneumothorax as a result of blunt trauma from contact sports is a recognized but underreported event. Several cases of pneumothorax or pneumomediastinum sustained during a contact sport have been described in the literature.[147,148] In a large case series, Kizer and MacQuarrie[149] identified 20 patients who had sustained a spontaneous or traumatic air leak while engaged in an outdoor sport.

BAROTRAUMA UNRELATED TO MECHANICAL VENTILATION

Although the term *barotrauma* has traditionally been used to describe the development of extra-alveolar air while on mechanical ventilation, in other instances it may be due to increased intra-alveolar pressure, causing air to leak out of the alveoli. PBT of ascent is a well-known complication of compressed air diving. Pulmonary edema and hemorrhage occur when lung volume decreases below residual volume. As a diver ascends and transalveolar pressure exceeds 20 to 80 mm Hg, overexpansion injury in the form of alveolar rupture can occur.[150-152] Divers who hold their breath as they ascend and those with obstructive airway diseases, such as asthma or COPD, are at increased risk.[153]

Pneumothorax is a relatively uncommon complication in divers, developing in only approximately 10% of those with evidence of barotrauma. Patients with a history of spontaneous pneumothorax, bullae, or cystic lung disease are at increased risk of pneumothorax and should be cautioned against diving.[154]

Pneumothorax develops when gas ruptures from the lung parenchyma into the pleural space. If this occurs at a significant depth, the pleural gas expands as the diver ascends (as described by Boyle's law) and can result in a tension pneumothorax. Manifestations include dyspnea, chest pain, tachycardia, hypotension, cyanosis, distended neck veins, tracheal deviation, hyperresonance to percussion, unilateral decrease in breath sounds, and accompanying subcutaneous emphysema in approximately 25% of cases.

If a pneumothorax results in severe hypoxemia or hemodynamic compromise, immediate pleural decompression is required. This is usually accomplished by inserting a large-bore needle into the second intercostal space in the midclavicular line of the affected hemithorax, followed by tube thoracostomy.

TENSION PNEUMOTHORAX

With a tension pneumothorax, the pleural pressure in the affected hemithorax exceeds atmospheric pressure, specifically during expiration. This is usually the result of a "check valve" mechanism that facilitates the ingress of gas into the pleural space during inspiration but blocks the escape of gas from the pleural space during expiration. The results are the accumulation of gas leading to a buildup of pressure within the pleural space. There is eventual respiratory failure from compression of the contralateral normal lung followed by circulatory collapse with hypotension and subsequent traumatic arrest with pulseless electrical activity (PEA) due to obstruction of venous return to the heart.

The classic signs of a tension pneumothorax are deviation of the trachea away from the side with the tension, an increased percussion note, and a hyperexpanded chest that moves little with respiration. Radiographically, tension pneumothorax shows a distinct shift of the mediastinum to the contralateral side and flattening or inversion of the ipsilateral hemidiaphragm (Fig. 47.6). Clinically unstable patients should undergo immediate needle decompression

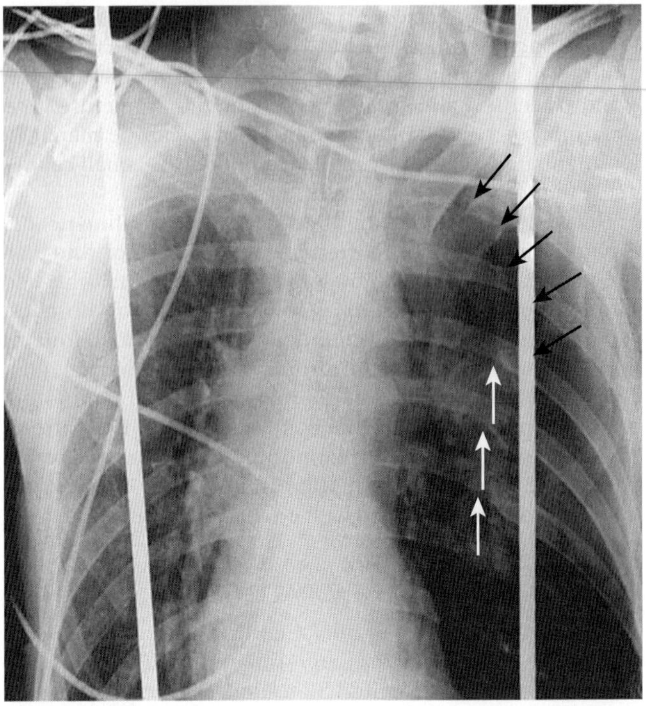

Figure 47.6 Chest radiograph of a left tension pneumothorax in a trauma patient. Note the mediastinal shift to the right, widened rib spacing, and posterior rib fractures on the left. A flattening of the left hemidiaphragm is also present (not shown). (From Barton E: Tension pneumothorax. Curr Opin Pulm Med 1999;5(4):269.)

followed by chest tube insertion. Decompression is performed by advancing a standard 14- or 16-gauge intravenous catheter into the pleural space at the junction of the midclavicular line and the second or third intercostal space. The needle is advanced until air can be aspirated into a syringe connected to the needle. The needle is withdrawn and the cannula is left open to air. An immediate rush of air out of the chest indicates the presence of a tension pneumothorax. The maneuver essentially converts a tension pneumothorax into a simple pneumothorax. A chest tube can then be placed.

CLINICAL FEATURES

PSP usually occurs when the patient is at rest.[155] Patients are typically in their early 20s when presenting with PSP, which is rare after age 40. Chest pain and dyspnea are the two main symptoms associated with the development of pneumothorax. One series evaluated 39 patients who presented with one of the two symptoms and 64% of them had both.[156] The pain is generally reported as ipsilateral, which usually resolves spontaneously within 24 hours.[40] The degree of dyspnea depends on the size of the pneumothorax and the condition of the underlying lung. Cough, malaise, orthopnea, and hemoptysis may also be presenting symptoms.

Physical examination can be normal in small pneumothoraces. Possible physical findings when a large pneumothorax is present include decreased chest excursion on the affected side, diminished breath sounds, and hyperresonant percussion. There may also be subcutaneous emphysema.

Labored breathing accompanied by hemodynamic compromise (tachycardia or hypotension) suggests a possible tension pneumothorax, which necessitates emergency decompression. Tension pneumothorax occurs due to the presence of a ball-valve mechanism; air enters the pleural cavity but cannot escape. As a result, positive pressure builds up. As the tension continues to increase, the diaphragm is flattened, the mediastinum is shifted to the opposite side, and ultimately cardiopulmonary collapse results.

Hypoxemia is common because collapsed and poorly ventilated portions of lung continue to receive significant perfusion. However, hypercapnia is unusual because underlying lung function is relatively normal and adequate alveolar ventilation can be maintained by the contralateral lung.[157] Acute respiratory alkalosis may be present if pain, anxiety, or hypoxia is substantial.

In certain situations, the symptoms of pneumothorax may have an atypical presentation and therefore require a high index of suspicion. During a transbronchial biopsy, a patient may complain of pleuritic chest pain followed by dyspnea. A pneumothorax after a subclavian vein catheterization may present with progressive dyspnea and an alteration of vital signs. In a mechanically ventilated patient, the initial presentation may include hypotension, new-onset respiratory distress, unilateral decrease in breath sounds, a decrease in static and dynamic compliance, and worsening oxygenation.[41,158,159]

Simultaneous bilateral pneumothoraces is a rare condition because, in humans, the left and right pleural spaces are completely separated. Patients can develop a persistent pleuro-pleuro channel after undergoing a median sternotomy, mediastinal surgery, or heart or heart-lung transplant surgery. This condition has been dubbed "iatrogenic buffalo chest" because the North American buffalo is one of few mammals that have communicating pleural spaces.[160] A unilateral thoracic procedure in this situation has been described to cause bilateral pneumothoraces[161,162] and "shifting pneumothorax."[163] Simultaneous bilateral spontaneous pneumothorax (SBSP) has been described in a case series with 12 patients.[164] Of the 12 patients, 5 had no underlying lung disease. In 7 patients, SBSP was secondary to pulmonary metastases, histiocytosis, undefined interstitial pulmonary disease, tuberculosis, pneumonia, and COPD.

ELECTROCARDIOGRAPHIC FEATURES

The presence of a pneumothorax may lead to distinct electrocardiographic changes, which can be mistaken for myocardial ischemia or infarction. Most findings have been described for left-sided pneumothorax. Poor R wave progression in the anterior precordial leads with a decrease in R wave from V_4 to V_5, rightward shift of frontal axis, diminution of precordial R voltage, decrease in QRS amplitude, and precordial T-wave inversion have all been described.[165-167] The absence of ST-segment elevation and a significant Q wave and reversal of electrocardiographic changes in the sitting position suggest pneumothorax. In right-sided pneumothorax, there is a loss of S wave in lead V_2 and prominent R-wave voltage, which may mimic posterior wall myocardial infarction.[168]

DIAGNOSTIC IMAGING MODALITIES

RADIOGRAPHIC SIGNS

Chest radiography and CT are the first-line imaging modalities used to identify a pneumothorax. The main feature of a pneumothorax on a chest radiograph is a white visceral pleural line. This line separates the visceral pleura from the parietal pleura by a collection of gas (Fig. 47.7). A pneumothorax may be identified using an upright, supine, or lateral decubitus chest radiograph. The lateral decubitus view is the most sensitive, and the supine view is the least sensitive.

UPRIGHT CHEST RADIOGRAPH

In an upright patient with a pneumothorax, most pleural gas accumulates in an apicolateral location. The visceral pleural line appears either straight or convex toward the chest wall. As little as 50 mL of pleural gas may be seen on a chest radiograph.[169] Although there is generally a loss of lung volume with a pneumothorax, the collapsed lung preserves its translucency because hypoxic vasoconstriction diminishes the blood flow to the collapsed lung. The value of obtaining an expiratory chest radiograph has been overstated. Inspiratory and expiratory upright chest radiographs detected pneumothorax with equal sensitivity.[170]

SUPINE CHEST RADIOGRAPH

In a supine patient with a pneumothorax, most pleural gas accumulates in a subpulmonary location. A "deep sulcus" sign occurs when gas outlines the anterior pleural reflection, the costophrenic sulcus, and the anterolateral border

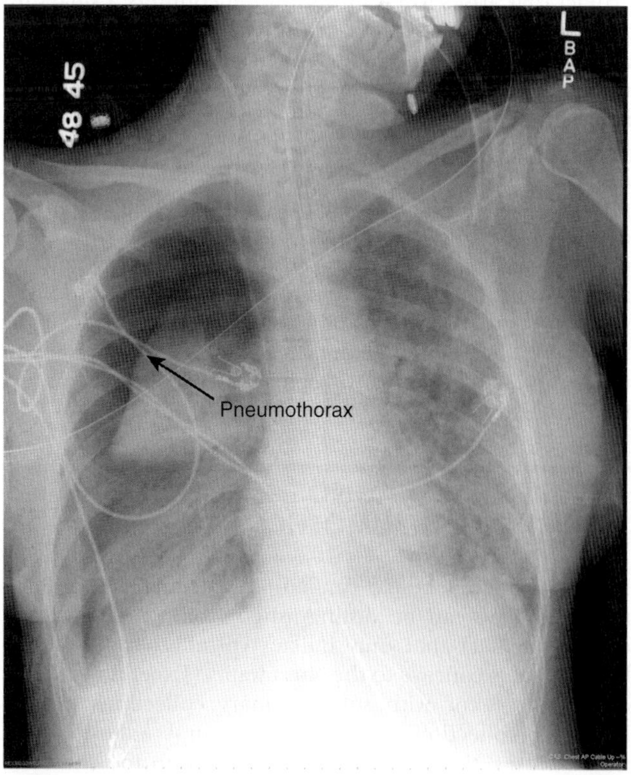

Figure 47.7 Radiograph of right lung pneumothorax. Arrow points to collapsed lung.

of the mediastinum (see Fig. 47.4). Rarely, pleural gas can accumulate in the phrenicovertebral sulcus. The visceral pleural line may be seen at the lung base and has a concave contour. Around 500 mL of pleural gas is needed in order to definitively diagnose pneumothorax on a supine chest radiograph.[169]

LATERAL DECUBITUS CHEST RADIOGRAPH

A pneumothorax is most easily detected with a lateral decubitus view. Most pleural gas in this position accumulates in the nondependent lateral location. The visceral pleural line appears as a straight or convex linc toward the chest wall. As little as 5 mL of pleural gas may be visible on a lateral decubitus view.[169]

COMPUTED TOMOGRAPHY

CT scanning is the most accurate imaging modality for the detection of pneumothorax although it is generally not the initial option. This method can identify small amounts of intrapleural gas, atypical collections of pleural gas, and loculated pneumothoraces. Complex pleural disease such as pleural effusion and cystic lung disease is optimally displayed by CT scanning.[171]

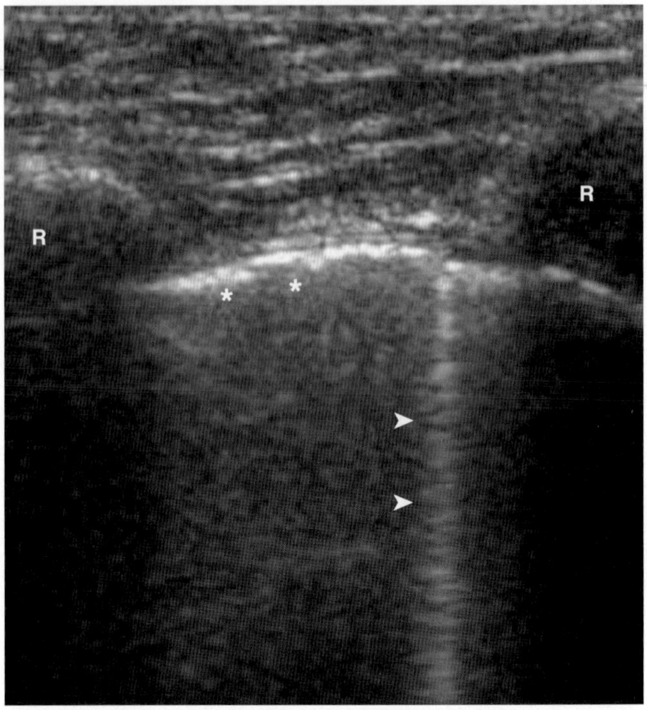

Figure 47.8 Rib shadows (R) are visible as bright reflectors with distal shadow. The pleura (* *) is a bright echogenic line beneath the ribs. Comet tail artifacts (*arrows*) arise from normal pleura reflecting sound waves. (From Mt. Sinai Emergency Ultrasound Division Tutorials. Accessed at http://sinaiem.us/tutorials/pneumothorax.)

PULMONARY ULTRASONOGRAPHY

Ultrasound was first used to detect pneumothorax in a horse in 1986 and then in humans shortly thereafter.[172] In a normal lung, the visceral and parietal pleurae are adjacent, and ultrasound shows shimmering or sliding at the pleural interface during respiration.[173] The absence of "lung sliding" indicates a pneumothorax. Comet tails are an ultrasound artifact that arises when ultrasound encounters a small air-fluid interface (Fig. 47.8). The presence of "sliding lung" and "comet tail" artifacts appear to reliably rule out pneumothorax (Video 47.1). The presence of a "lung point" sign is nearly 100% specific for the detection of pneumothorax. Here the visceral pleura is seen to be intermittently coming into contact with the chest wall during inspiration. The lung point sign may also be helpful in determining the actual size of the pneumothorax (Fig. 47.9). A review of four prospective studies found the sensitivity and specificity of ultrasound for pneumothorax to range from 86% to 98%, which was superior to supine chest radiography (sensitivity 28-75%).[174] A small pneumothorax may be missed with ultrasound, and patients with blebs or scarring may have a false-positive finding.[175]

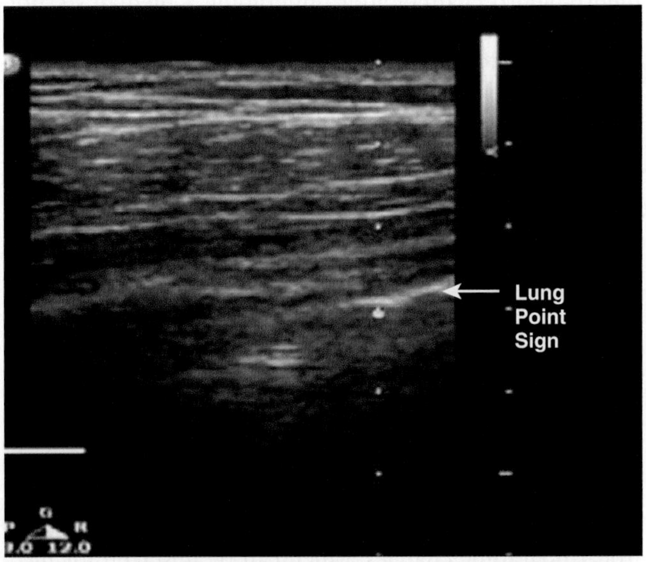

Figure 47.9 Lung point sign. B-mode depicting the lung point: Sliding lung touching the chest wall. (From Husain LF, Hagopian L, Waymen D, et al: Sonographic diagnosis of pneumothorax. J Emerg Trauma Shock 2012;5:76-81.)

DIFFERENTIAL DIAGNOSIS: CONDITIONS MIMICKING PNEUMOTHORAX

Large subpleural bullae can mimic a loculated pneumothorax. Bullae can be distinguished from pneumothorax due to the fact that only bullae typically have a medial border that is concave to the chest wall.[176] Exceptions to this distinction occur with subpulmonary collections of gas, loculated collections of gas, and pleural adhesions. In trauma cases, the stomach can herniate into the chest following rupture of the left hemidiaphragm, and a gas-filled stomach may be mistaken for a loculated pneumothorax. This can be disastrous if drainage with a thoracostomy tube is attempted. A skinfold can generally be distinguished from a pneumothorax by careful evaluation of the radiograph. Skinfolds generally extend beyond the rib cage, stop short of the ribs, and gradually increase in opacity with an abrupt dropoff at the edge of the image. Blood vessels often extend beyond the skinfold.[177]

MANAGEMENT

Figure 47.10 represents an algorithmic approach to the management of pneumothorax.

MANAGEMENT OF THE FIRST EPISODE OF PNEUMOTHORAX

Initial management is directed at removing air from the pleural space followed by preventing recurrence. Approaches for the management of the initial episode include observation, supplemental oxygen, simple aspiration of the pneumothorax, and tube thoracostomy. The choice of therapy in a given patient depends on various factors such as size of the pneumothorax, whether the pneumothorax is primary or secondary, the condition of the lungs, the clinical stability of the patient, the outcome of the patient, and whether the pneumothorax has occurred in a special setting. Various guidelines for managing pneumothorax have been published.[178,179]

ESTIMATING THE SIZE OF A PNEUMOTHORAX

Determining the size of a pneumothorax is difficult. The average interpleural distance (AID) approximates the size of a pneumothorax from a frontal chest radiograph by taking the sum of the distances in millimeters between the ribs and the visceral pleura at the apical, midthoracic, and basal levels and then dividing the sum by three. Another method is called the Light Index. It uses the following calculation to estimate the size of a pneumothorax:

$$\% \text{ pneumothorax} = 100 - \left(D_L^3/D_H^3 \times 100\right)$$

D_L is diameter of the collapsed lung **cubed.**
D_H is diameter of hemithorax on collapsed side **cubed.**

Both methods express the size of the pneumothorax as a percentage, although the Light method better correlates with the amount of pneumothorax gas removed by suction.[180,181]

These methods are difficult to apply and tend to underestimate the size of a pneumothorax. As a result, some clinicians tend to describe a pneumothorax as large or small rather than utilize percentages. The American College of Chest Physician guidelines defines a small pneumothorax as less than 3 cm in apex-to-cupola distance.[178] British Thoracic Society guidelines define a pneumothorax as small if the distance from chest wall to visceral pleural line is less than 2 cm. They define a large pneumothorax if the distance from the chest wall to the visceral pleural line is 2 cm or greater.[179]

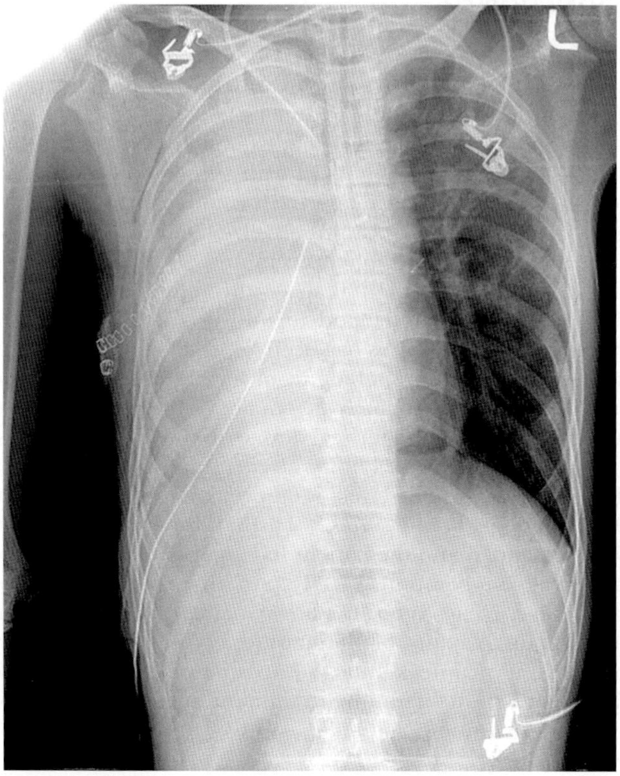

Figure 47.10 Reexpansion pulmonary edema. (From Tung YW, Lin F, Yang MS, et al: Bilateral developing reexpansion pulmonary edema treated with extracorporeal membrane oxygenation. Ann Thorac Surg 2010;89:1268-1271.)

TREATMENT OPTIONS

SUPPLEMENTAL OXYGEN

The choice of treatment depends on patient characteristics and clinical circumstances. Patients who are clinically stable and are having their first PSP can be observed with administration of supplemental oxygen if their pneumothorax is small (≤2 to 3 cm between the lung and chest wall on a chest radiograph).[182] Supplemental oxygen is used to facilitate reabsorption of pleural air, and its importance should not be underestimated. The absorption of gas depends in part on the gradient between the partial pressure in the capillaries and that in the pleural space. On room air, the net gradient is only 54 mm Hg, whereas it exceeds 550 mm Hg when the patient is on 100% oxygen.[180] A normal rate of reabsorption is 1.25% of the volume of the hemithorax per 24 hours.[7] The rate of reabsorption increases sixfold if humidified 100% oxygen is administered.[183] Therefore, hospitalized patients with any type of pneumothorax who are not subjected to aspiration of air or tube thoracostomy should be treated with supplemental oxygen at high concentrations.[184]

REMOVAL OF AIR FROM PLEURAL SPACE

In a patient whose pneumothorax is large (more than 20-25%), progressive, tension type, or symptomatic or who has an underlying chronic lung disease, is on a ventilator, or has a recurrent pneumothorax, the pleural space air should be removed. Several therapies have been developed for this purpose.

ASPIRATION

Simple aspiration is most easily accomplished by using a commercially available thoracentesis kit. An 18-guage needle with an 8 to 9F catheter is inserted in the second intercostal space in the midclavicular line. Once the catheter is inserted into the pleural space, the catheter is threaded deeper into the pleural space, and then the needle is withdrawn. Air is manually withdrawn through the indwelling catheter until no more can be aspirated. If the lung has not expanded after 4 L have been aspirated, then it is assumed there is a persistent air leak. Thoracoscopy should then be performed. A chest tube should be inserted if thoracoscopy is not readily available.

Once no further air can be aspirated, one of two methods may be approached.[185] A closed stopcock can be attached and the indwelling catheter secured to the chest wall. After 4 hours, a chest radiograph should be obtained and if there is adequate lung expansion, the catheter can be removed. Following another 2 hours of observation, another chest radiograph should be performed. If the lung remains expanded on this chest radiograph, the patient can be discharged.[186] Alternatively, the catheter can be left in place and attached to a Heimlich (i.e., one-way) valve. The patient can then be discharged with follow-up within 2 days.[178,187] One advantage of aspiration over tube thoracostomy is that the patient need not be hospitalized whether the catheter is removed after aspiration or left attached to the Heimlich valve. There is a lower morbidity rate compared to tube thoracostomy and the procedure is better tolerated. Outcomes have been found to be similar between thoracostomy and aspiration. In a meta-analysis of three randomized, controlled trials (194 patients) that compared aspiration versus tube thoracostomy, aspiration resulted in shorter hospitalization stays and similar clinical outcomes.[188] In another randomized trial, 137 patients who had a first episode of PSP were assigned to receive manual aspiration versus tube thoracostomy. The groups had similar rates of immediate (62 versus 68%) and 1-week success (89 versus 88%). Aspiration was associated with a shorter hospital stay (1.8 versus 4 days).[189]

TUBE THORACOSTOMY

If necessary, most patients with PSP can be managed with a small chest tube (≤22F) or chest catheter (≤14F).[190,191] In the absence of trauma and with good aseptic technique, prophylactic antibiotics are not recommended.[192] The preferred location for insertion of the chest tube is via an incision at the fourth or fifth intercostal space in the anterior or midaxillary line.[193-195] In men, this corresponds to the nipple line and in women, to the inframammary crease. It is important to direct the tube anteriorly because the tube tends to track between the lobes in patients who have complete fissures. If this happens, the tube may get walled off by the lung and cease functioning. The second intercostal space in the midclavicular line has been suggested as an alternative site for tubes, but this requires placement through the pectoralis muscle. This chest tube site is more painful for the patient and the tube is more difficult to dress and manage. Once an insertion site is identified, the tube is inserted using blunt dissection and secured in place.

The chest tube can then be connected to a water seal device, with or without suction and left in position until the pneumothorax resolves. Once the air leak has resolved, the lung has fully expanded, and the pleural air removed, then the chest tube can be removed in a sequential fashion. The chest tube can generally be removed if there is no visible air leak present and air does not accumulate when suction is removed. If there is any question as to whether an air leak has resolved, a "clamp trial" can be performed. This involves clamping the chest tube and performing a chest radiograph repeated at intervals (e.g., 2, 6, and then 12 hours). If air does not reaccumulate, the tube can be removed.

PERCUTANEOUS PNEUMOTHORAX CATHETERS AND THORACIC VENTS

Alternatives to tube thoracotomy involve using small-lumen catheters or thoracic vents (one-way valve feature). Small catheter tubes have the advantages of ease of insertion, good response, and low incidence of complications. Liu and colleagues reported that in their study using pigtail catheters in 50 patients versus traditional chest tubes in 52 patients that the pigtail drainage was no less effective than the traditional chest tube.[196] Complications can include catheter failure from kinking, malposition, inadvertent removal by the patient, and occlusion of the tube or valve by pleural fluid. A thoracic vent can also be used to manage a simple pneumothorax.[197,198] It is inserted in the second intercostal space in the midclavicular line. This device has the advantages of a urethane tube that does not kink, a self-contained one-way valve, and a unique signal diaphragm that reflects pleural pressure. This device is not suitable for use in patients who are expected to have large-volume or protracted air leaks.

THORACOSCOPY

VATS is an effective treatment of PSP.[199-201] Pleurodesis is created by pleural abrasion or a partial parietal pleurectomy. When necessary, an endoscopic stapler can be used to resect bullae.[202-205]

PERSISTENT AIR LEAK AND BRONCHOPLEURAL FISTULA

If a lung is at least 90% inflated but an air leak is present after 3 days, more aggressive treatment may be warranted. The simplest approach is to attach the chest tube to a unidirectional flutter valve such as a Heimlich valve. This allows rapid discharge of the patient with subsequent outpatient follow-up. An alternative approach is to perform an autologous blood patch.[206,207] This involves withdrawing blood from the patient's peripheral vein and aseptically infusing the blood into the pleural space through the chest tube. The ideal amount of blood to infuse is not known. The range in different series has been 24 to 200 mL. After infusion of the blood, the tubing from the chest tube is draped over a hook approximately 60 cm above the patient's head and then down to a water seal device on the floor. The chest tube is then removed 24 hours after cessation of the air leak. The most serious side effect is empyema, which occurred in 9% of patients in one series.[208] Lastly, if the lung is less than 90% expanded and the patient has a persistent air leak, the preferred intervention is VATS. An air leak persisting for more than 7 days is termed a *bronchopleural fistula* and can occur in up to a third of pneumothorax cases.[209] After 7 days of a persistent air leak, tube thoracostomy is deemed to have failed and more definitive treatment such as surgery or pleurodesis can be planned.

RECURRENCE PREVENTION

Once the initial episode of pneumothorax has resolved, the decision to prevent future pneumothoraces must be made. Different recurrence rates have been reported in the literature; from 20% to 52% after the first PSP.[210-212] In the following groups of patients, further management against recurrence is recommended: recurrent pneumothorax, patients with chronic air leak, patients with large bullae, patients who live in remote areas, and patients in which a recurrence could be a hazard (e.g., airline personnel or divers). The following are established risk factors for recurrence: more than one previous episode, COPD, air leak for more than 48 hours after first episode, and large cysts seen on radiograph. The following are possible risk factors for recurrence: nonoperative management of first episode (versus tube drainage) and tube drainage for only 24 hours during first episode (versus 3 to 4 days). Further management in these high-risk groups is aimed at preventing recurrence. Therapies to prevent recurrence include chemical pleurodesis, VATS, or surgical thoracotomy.

CHEMICAL PLEURODESIS

In patients who are unable or unwilling to undergo VATS, pleurodesis (adhesion of visceral and parietal pleura) can be done by introducing the sclerotic agent via the chest tube. Tetracycline had been used for pleurodesis,[213] but sterile tetracycline is no longer available. As a result, intrapleural instillation of doxycycline has been used as an alternative for pleurodesis.[214] Intrapleural doxycycline can be painful, so it is recommended that patients be premedicated with analgesics or anxiolytics. Talc slurry, which is composed of finely powdered magnesium silicate, can also be used for pleurodesis.[215-217] Recurrence rates after treatment vary between 5% and 8%. Controversy exists whether talc should be used as a sclerosant in young, otherwise healthy individuals due to safety concerns and fear of long-term complications. Intrapleural injection of talc for malignant pleural effusions has been associated with development of ARDS in 1% to 2% of patients.[218] Extensive pleural thickening and calcifications were reported in another patient years after treatment.[219] However, several studies support the safety of talc pleurodesis for prevention of recurrent pneumothorax.[215,220,221]

VIDEO-ASSISTED THORACOSCOPIC SURGERY PLEURODESIS

VATS is effective not only in the treatment of spontaneous pneumothorax but also in the prevention of recurrent pneumothorax.[222,223] The rate of recurrence is less than 5% after VATS with bleb/bullae resection and pleurodesis. Mechanical pleurodesis with dry gauze, chemical pleurodesis with talc, and laser ablation of the parietal pleura are among the techniques used.

SURGICAL THORACOTOMY

Surgical management for the first episode of spontaneous pneumothorax is indicated under the following circumstances: 3% to 4% of patients have a persistent leak resulting from a large fistula that needs to be closed surgically; about 5% of patients have frank hemothorax and surgical intervention is required to control the bleeding; and a trapped lung that fails to reexpand may require decortication.

The indications for open thoracotomy are the same as those for VATS. Thoracoscopy has virtually replaced open thoracotomy in the management of spontaneous pneumothorax due to shorter hospitalizations and less postoperative pain.[224,225] Thoracotomy is recommended only if thoracoscopy is unavailable or has failed.

MANAGEMENT UNDER SPECIAL CIRCUMSTANCES

SECONDARY SPONTANEOUS PNEUMOTHORAX

Patients with SSP should be hospitalized owing to their diminished pulmonary reserve from their underlying lung disease. Patients with a small pneumothorax (≤2 cm between the lung and chest wall on a chest radiograph) who are clinically stable may be observed. Patients with a large pneumothorax or who are clinically unstable should have a chest tube placed. Tube thoracotomy is generally preferred over needle aspiration because it is more likely to be successful. In one trial, tube thoracostomy was more likely to have the pleural air completely evacuated than with needle aspiration (93% versus 67%).[226] About 80% of patients with SSP will have lung expansion and cessation of their air leak within 7 days after tube thoracostomy.[227,228] Patients who are on mechanical ventilation or who are at risk for a large air leak should be managed with a 24 to 28F chest tube. A smaller chest tube (16 to 22F) is preferred for most other patients. The chest tube should be connected to a water seal device with or without suction. In general, the chest tube should remain in place until a procedure is performed to prevent a recurrent pneumothorax. Patients who decline preventive interventions can have their chest tube clamped 12 hours after the last evidence of an air leak. A chest radiograph should be done 24 hours after the last evidence of an air leak, and if the pneumothorax has not recurred, the chest tube can be removed.

PNEUMOTHORAX IN HIV-INFECTED PATIENTS

Because the majority of pneumothoraces in HIV-infected patients occurs in association with *P. jiroveci*, all HIV-infected patients who present with a pneumothorax should undergo a diagnostic evaluation for *P. jiroveci* infection. *P. jiroveci* pneumonia–related pneumothorax is complicated by a virulent form of necrotizing subpleural lesions, which result in diffuse air leaks that are refractory to standard treatment.[229] Asymptomatic patients with a small pneumothorax (less than 15-20%) may be observed. Symptomatic patients and those with a larger pneumothorax will need chest tube thoracostomy and those with a persistent air leak will likely need additional therapy with video-assisted thoracoscopy for stapling and pleurodesis. Patients who are poor operative candidates may benefit from bedside pleurodesis.

PNEUMOTHORAX IN CYSTIC FIBROSIS

Pleurodesis as an initial step in the management of pneumothorax in CF is considered contraindicated because it results in extensive pleural adhesions that jeopardize subsequent lung transplantation.[230] If initial tube thoracostomy does not bring resolution of air leak within 5 days, blebectomy should be performed. If blebectomy is unsuccessful, a definitive pleural ablative procedure should be considered.

CATAMENIAL PNEUMOTHORAX AND PNEUMOTHORAX COMPLICATING PREGNANCY

The initial episode is managed in the usual manner. Recurrences, which occur 72 hours before or after menstrual flow, are managed by pleurodesis or hormonal treatment.[231] Therapeutic options include oral contraceptive pills, danazol, progestational agents, and gonadotropin-releasing hormone (GnRH) analogs.[69] Thoracotomy should be considered if the patient is unable to take ovulation-suppressing drugs, has a recurrent pneumothorax while on drugs, or wants to become pregnant. Pneumothorax complicating pregnancy is managed in the usual way, but due to the fact that there is a high rate of recurrence during parturition, thoracotomy with resection of blebs if present should be considered.[232]

PNEUMOTHORAX IN AIR TRAVELERS

The volume of gas is inversely proportional to the pressure at which it is exposed. As barometric pressure falls in the aircraft cabin during ascent, trapped air in any noncommunicating body cavity, such as in a lung bleb or bulla, will expand. Regulatory government agencies, such as the Federal Aviation Administration, have requirements specifying that commercial aircraft cabins be pressurized to simulate an altitude (so-called cabin altitude) of approximately 8000 ft (2438 m). It is estimated that the volume of air in a noncommunicating body cavity will increase by approximately 38% upon ascent from sea level to the maximum "cabin altitude" of 8000 feet (2438 m).[233] For patients who develop signs and symptoms of a pneumothorax in-flight, administration of supplemental oxygen is the most important intervention. For patients in respiratory distress, emergency landing at the nearest airport will allow prompt evaluation and insertion of a chest tube, if needed. The optimal length of time to wait after resolution of a pneumothorax is unknown.[234] For patients with a prior pneumothorax, the decision regarding air travel must be made on an individual basis. One must take into consideration the likelihood of recurrence and how well the patient would tolerate a subsequent pneumothorax. A patient with relatively normal lung parenchyma could be permitted to fly 2 weeks after resolution of an iatrogenic pneumothorax. In a patient with severe bullous emphysema, limited cardiopulmonary reserve, and a prior spontaneous pneumothorax, air travel may be contraindicated.

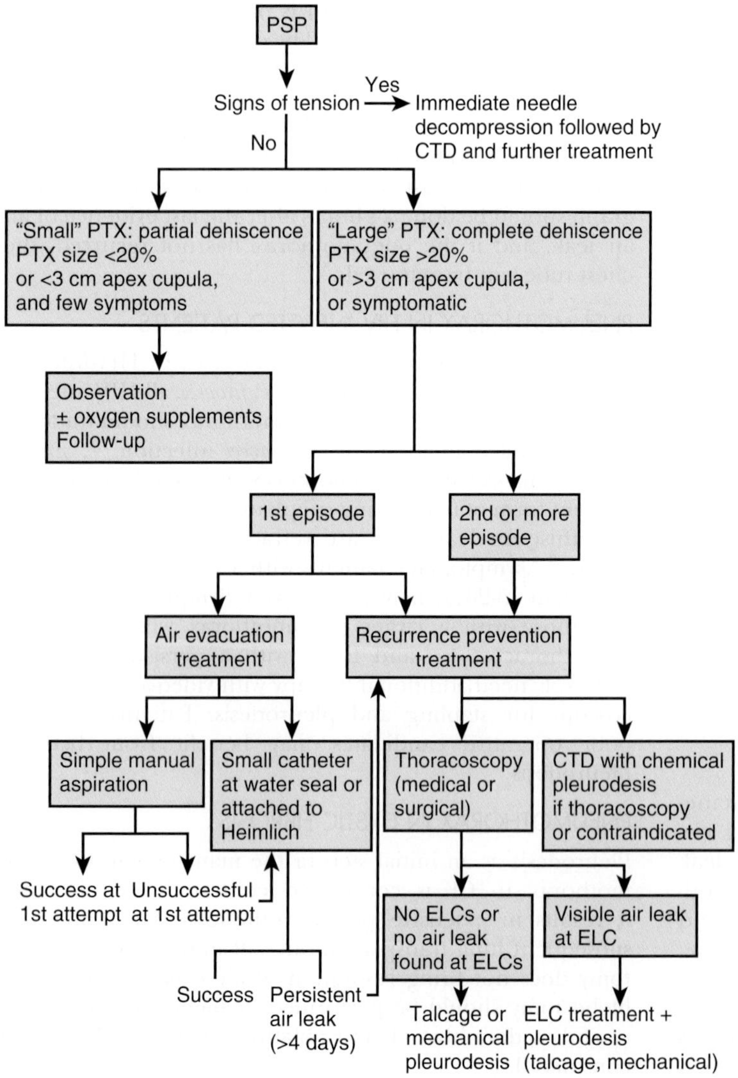

Figure 47.11 An algorithmic approach to the treatment of primary spontaneous pneumothorax.* After informed consent or in certain patient groups (aircraft personnel, divers).** Staple bleb/bullectomy, electrocoagulation, ligation. CTD, chest tube drainage; ELCs, emphysema-like changes; PTX, pneumothorax. (From Noppen M, De Keukeleire T: Pneumothorax. Respiration 2008;76:121-127.)

PNEUMOTHORAX IN LYMPHANGIOLEIOMYOMATOSIS

Lymphangioleiomyomatosis (LAM) is a rare and often fatal disease that affects predominantly women of childbearing age. The normal architecture of the lung is distorted by multiple small cysts, ranging from 0.1 cm to several centimeters in diameter, with progressive decline in lung function. Spontaneous pneumothorax occurs in 50% of cases. It is often recurrent, can be bilateral, and may necessitate pleurodesis.[235,236] Because of the morbidity and cost associated with multiple recurrences, recommendations include definitive intervention at the time of the initial pneumothorax. Pleurodesis in these cases does not preclude successful transplantation.[237]

COMPLICATIONS RELATED TO MANAGEMENT

Reexpansion pulmonary edema may occur after rapid reexpansion of a collapsed lung in patients with a pneumothorax. It is typically unilateral[238] (Fig. 47.11). The pathophysiologic mechanism is unknown. The incidence of reexpansion pulmonary edema initially appeared to be related to the rapidity of lung reexpansion and to the severity and duration of lung collapse. However, a study examining development of reexpansion pulmonary edema following thoracentesis found that it was independent of the volume of fluid removed and pleural pressures, and recommended that even large pleural effusions be drained completely as long as chest pain or end-expiratory pleural pressure less than −20 cm H_2O does not develop.[239] Patients typically present soon after the inciting event, although presentation can be delayed for up to 24 hours in some cases. The clinical course varies from isolated radiographic changes to complete cardiopulmonary collapse. Mortality rates as high as 20% have been described.[240] Treatment is generally supportive. Supplemental oxygen is administered and, if necessary, mechanical ventilation is used. The disease is usually self-limited.

KEY POINTS

- PSP occurs primarily in tall, thin, previously healthy young men, most of whom are smokers. Chest radiograph often shows apical subpleural blebs or bullae. Rupture of these bullae is *not* related to physical activity but may be related to changes in atmospheric pressure. COPD is the most common cause of secondary pneumothorax. Presentation of pneumothorax in COPD is often atypical and causes excessive morbidity and mortality rates.
- A high incidence of pneumothorax occurs in HIV-infected patients, related to PCP and the mechanical ventilation and bronchoscopy that are commonly required in these patients. In this group of patients, pneumothorax is frequently bilateral, recurrent, and unresponsive to conservative therapy.

KEY POINTS (Continued)

- Traumatic pneumothorax, which occurs as a result of a penetrating injury, may occur with closed chest trauma.
- Pneumothorax is a common complication of mechanical ventilation. Interstitial emphysema is a harbinger of this complication. High peak and mean airway pressures, PEEP, use of volume-cycled ventilators, intubation of right mainstem bronchus, chronic airway obstruction, and aspiration pneumonia increase the incidence.
- Simultaneous bilateral pneumothoraces and "shifting pneumothoraces" are rare but interesting conditions that may develop because of persistent pleuropleural communication called *iatrogenic buffalo chest.*
- An immediate postbronchoscopy chest radiograph is rarely useful but should be done in certain groups of patients (e.g., comatose, mentally retarded, ventilated, or with respiratory compromise).
- Pneumothorax induced by a misplaced small-bore feeding tube is not uncommon. Clinical signs may be misleading.
- A visceral pleural line with absence of lung markings peripherally is the classic radiographic sign of pneumothorax. When the chest radiograph is obtained in the supine position, the signs are very different.
- Pulmonary ultrasonography is a promising technique for detection and exclusion of pneumothorax, especially in critically ill patients.
- PBT refers to alveolar rupture due to elevated transalveolar pressure. The clinical presentation can vary, ranging from absent symptoms with subtle radiographic findings to respiratory distress or cardiac arrest due to a large tension pneumothorax. Prevention is critical and limiting plateau pressures to less than 30 cm H_2O may be an effective approach.
- The approach to management of a pneumothorax is dictated by the clinical condition rather than merely the size of the pneumothorax, which is best estimated by CT scan of the chest. Expectant therapy is recommended for a small PSP in a stable patient. Reabsorption of air is hastened by 100% oxygen.
- Air can be removed by simple aspiration, a small-lumen catheter, or tube thoracostomy. Unstable patients with large secondary pneumothorax must be managed with tube thoracostomy.
- Tension pneumothorax is a medical emergency and requires a high clinical suspicion followed by prompt thoracostomy if the patient is clinically stable. However, in an unstable patient, needle decompression followed by chest tube placement may be required.
- Definitive management of recurrent pneumothorax or persistent leak can be done by open thoracotomy or video-assisted thoracoscopy associated with pleurodesis, pleural abrasion, parietal pleurectomy, or bullectomy. In patients unsuitable or unwilling for

Continued on following page

KEY POINTS (Continued)

surgery, chemical pleurodesis via a chest tube may be done.

- Pneumothorax tends to recur in patients with CF. Blebectomy, without stripping the pleura, is recommended in these patients so that they may remain transplant candidates. Pleurodesis should not be done in these cases because adhesion development jeopardizes subsequent lung transplantation.
- Pneumothorax in pregnancy is managed in the usual manner initially. In view of the high recurrence rates during parturition, thoracotomy with resection of blebs should be considered.

SELECTED REFERENCES

6. Grundy S, Bentley A, Tschopp JM: Primary spontaneous pneumothorax: A diffuse disease of the pleura. Respiration 2012;83:185-189.
10. Noppen M: Spontaneous pneumothorax: Epidemiology, pathophysiology and cause. Eur Respir Rev 2010;19:217-219.
17. Baumann MH: Management of spontaneous pneumothorax. Clin Chest Med 2006;27:369.
83. Burns KE, Adhikari NK, Slutsky AS, et al: Pressure and volume limited ventilation for the ventilatory management of patients with acute lung injury: A systematic review and meta-analysis. PLoS One 2011;6(1):e14623.
99. Vezzani A, Brusasco C, Palermo S, et al: Ultrasound localization of central vein catheter and detection of post procedural pneumothorax: An alternative to chest radiography. Crit Care Med 2010;38:533.
126. Gordon CE, Feller-Kopman D, et al: Pneumothorax following thoracentesis. Arch Intern Med 2010;170(4):332-339.
174. Wilkerson RG, Stone MB: Sensitivity of bedside ultrasound and supine anteroposterior chest radiographs for the identification of pneumothorax after blunt trauma. Acad Emerg Med 2010;17:11.
178. Baumann MH, Strange C, Heffner JE, et al: Management of spontaneous pneumothorax. An American College of Chest Physicians Delphi Consensus Statement. Chest 2001;119:590.
179. MacDuff A, Arnold A, Harvey J, British Thoracic Society Pleural Disease Guideline Group: Management of spontaneous pneumothorax: British Thoracic Society Pleural Disease Guideline 2010. Thorax 2010;65(Suppl 2):18.
180. Light RW: Pneumothorax. In Light RW (ed): Pleural Diseases, 3rd ed. Baltimore, Williams & Wilkins, 1990, p 242.
190. Benton IJ, Benfield GF: Comparison of a large and small-caliber tube drain for managing spontaneous pneumothoraces. Respir Med 2009;103:1436.

The complete list of references can be found at www.expertconsult.com.

48 Toxic Gas, Fume, and Smoke Inhalation

John F. Fraser | Dirk M. Maybauer | Marc O. Maybauer

CHAPTER OUTLINE

INTRODUCTION

EPIDEMIOLOGY

The global burden of disease represented by inhalation injuries continues to grow. Industrialization of developing nations results in increased morbidity and mortality. Inhalation injury can be defined as "an injury due to the inhalation of thermal and/or chemical irritants" and comprises both acute and chronic exposures.

Chronic exposure to inhalation of atmospheric pollution may damage the lung over decades, predisposing to infection, pulmonary fibrosis, or cancer.[1] The World Health Organization estimates that more than a billion people, mainly in developing countries, develop airway and pulmonary inflammation resulting from inhaled smoke from indoor cooking fires, forest fires, and burning of crops.[2] In the industrial world, chronic inhalation injury may be due to cigarette smoking or occupational exposure (e.g., asbestos). This aspect of inhalation injury will not be further discussed in this textbook, and readers are referred to other resources.[3]

Acute smoke inhalation results in approximately 23,000 injuries and 5000 to 10,000 deaths per year in the United States alone. Among industrial countries, the United States has one of the highest incidences of smoke inhalation injuries.[4] The ensuing pulmonary derangements, which follow burn and smoke inhalation injuries, are major contributors to morbidity and mortality in fire victims. The pathophysiology of the injury is multifaceted and induces distant organ dysfunction (Fig. 48.1). The consequences of the profound airway inflammation are heightened by pulmonary shunting and augmented microvascular pressure gradient, resulting in hypoxemic respiratory failure.[5] Although survival from burn injury continues to improve, this is not mirrored in inhalation management. The acute lung injury caused by smoke inhalation and pneumonia has a major negative impact on mortality figures in patients with burn injuries. Inhalation injury alone increases mortality in burn victims by approximately 20% and pneumonia increases the rate by approximately 40%, with a maximal increase of approximately 60% when both are present.[6] The mainstay of treatment of the smoke inhalation sufferer remains optimal respiratory support with airway toilet, adequate fluid resuscitation, early and aggressive surgical interventions, and precise antimicrobial interventions. Continued research into this systemic process is needed to stop smoke inhalation injury being the major cause of death in fire victims.[7]

HISTORY

Inhalation injuries, both of toxins and smoke, have been recorded in the history books for several thousand years and have been used with enmity from the outset. Thucydides records the Spartans burning pitch, naphtha, and sulfur to produce sulfur dioxide while attacking Athenian cities in 423 BC.[8] The fifteenth century brought incendiary devices filled with sulfa and belladonna.[9]

The history of toxic gases other than smoke tends to run hand in hand with military conflict, and it wasn't until the

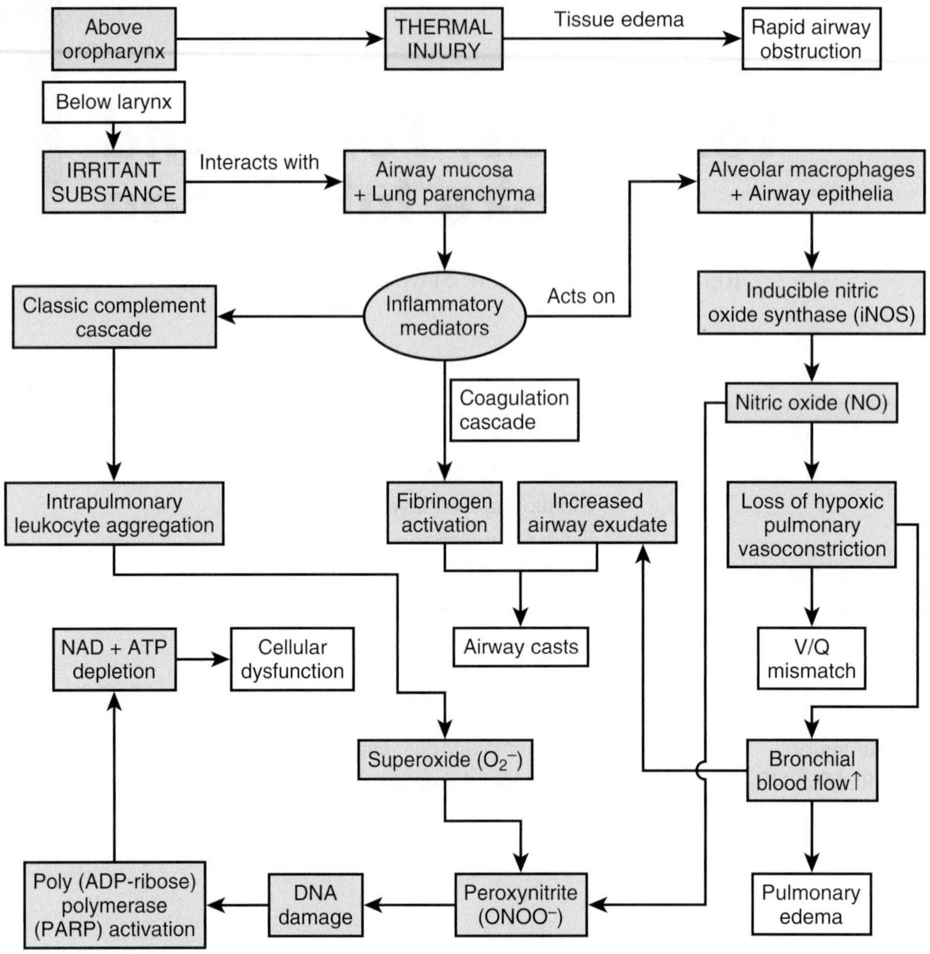

Figure 48.1 Pathophysiology of acute smoke inhalation injury.

First World War that the increased usage sparked off once more, where at least 14 different toxic respiratory agents were used. The years 1914-1915 marked the modern nascence of inhalation warfare when France released chloroacetone and Germany released thousands of liters of chlorine gas in Belgium, at Ypres. More than 1 million casualties were attributed to the use of chemical agents during that war, with sulfur gas being anointed as the "king of battle gases."[10]

The 1925 Geneva Protocol signed by many countries pledged never to use gas warfare again.[9] Sadly, this has not been adhered to, with Italy being accused of using mustard gas against Abyssinia in Ethiopia. The Chinese suffered gas inhalation at the hands of the Japanese during the Second World War, and the Kurds were victim to similar agents during the attacks by Iraq through the 1980s.[11] Sarin gas poisoning was used in Japan in the mid-1990s. In 1994 and 1995, inhaled biochemical weapons have been used for terrorism acts like the sarin gas attacks in Japan.[12] Cyanide (CN) may be considered one of the most likely agents of chemical terrorism, as it is capable of causing mass incapacitation and casualties and can cause mass confusion, panic, and social disruption. In addition, cyanide possesses all attributes of an ideal terrorist weapon: it is plentiful, readily available, and easily obtainable because of its widespread use in industry and laboratories.[13] Although military interest in biochemical warfare diminished following World War II, there was an understanding of the devastation possible with nuclear weapons; terrorist organizations understand the fear, panic, and collapse of infrastructure that could be realized through the release of such a substance in a busy city. It seems likely that there are many areas of the world where such agents are, or can be, manufactured in great quantities.[9]

Equally, smoke inhalation has a long record in history, with the first recording by Pliny in the first century AD. He described the execution of prisoners over greenwood smoke, and it seems he may have died through toxic smoke inhalation himself during the eruption of Vesuvius in 79 AD. More recently, two much more industrial occurrences highlighted the problems of smoke inhalation. The Cocoanut Grove fire of 1942 resulted in the deaths of 491 people who were trapped in a burning building. The number of patients who sustained burns was minimal, and it was then that the realization hit that smoke alone could kill as easily, if not more so, than cutaneous burns.[14] More than 2000 burn/smoke casualties resulted after the chain of fires and explosions that rippled through refineries and factories in Texas City, Texas, in the 1940s.[15] The understanding of smoke and carbon monoxide (CO) inhalation in enclosed spaces was further highlighted in the fire at the MGM Grand Hotel in Las Vegas in 1980 and the Stardust Nightclub fire in Dublin in 1981. Again, the small number of burn injuries was swamped by the deaths resulting from smoke and CO.[16]

Cyanide's independent role became clear in the 1980s, particularly after the aircraft fire at Manchester International Airport, Manchester, UK, in 1985 where the majority (87%) of the 54 individuals who died had potentially lethal levels of cyanide in their blood, as opposed to only 21% of these victims having carboxyhemoglobin (COHb) levels exceeding 50%. This event highlighted that different combustants produce different inhalants, and depending on the environment, these may be more lethal than carbon monoxide, which had been regarded as the primary toxic threat.[4] Hence, the determinants of inhalants are both environment and material being combusted. It is therefore a mixed toxicology following smoke inhalation.

The terrorism attacks on September 11, 2001, on the World Trade Center in New York were associated with a high incidence of inhalation injuries. Among the 790 injured survivors, 49% suffered from inhalation injury caused by toxic compounds in the smoke and dust.[17,18] Industrial catastrophes, biochemical warfare, and terrorism will continue to occur. This chapter's aim is to help physicians diagnose and then manage patients with inhalation injuries.

PATHOGENESIS OF INHALATION INJURY

TOXIC SMOKE COMPOUNDS

Smoke is a heterogeneous compound. Each fire produces different toxic features relating to the material combusted and the environment in which the fire occurs, specifically oxygen content. Hence, each patient suffering smoke inhalation may represent a new condition with a possibility of many different inhalants.[19] The components of smoke that cause damage are as follows:

- Heat.
- Particulates, deposited in the airways according to their size, with substances smaller than 1 µm in diameter able to reach the alveolar zone suspended in air. At that site, these chemically laden particles increase airway resistance and cause cell lysis and irritation while diminishing pulmonary surfactant production and efficacy.[19]
- Systemic toxins, such as carbon monoxide and cyanide, which adversely affect oxygen transport by erythrocytes and utilization by mitochondria.[20]
- Respiratory irritants are implicated in the high mortality rates. Water-soluble gases such as ammonia and hydrogen chloride react with water contained in mucous membranes and produce strong alkalis and acids, which elicit profound inflammatory reactions, which rapidly induce systemic changes via the dense alveolar-capillary interphase. Lipid-soluble irritants (e.g., oxides of nitrogen, phosgene, and aldehydes) exert their effects more slowly as they dissolve into the cellular membrane.[21]

HEAT

Burns to the nasal and oropharyngeal mucosa are common in fire-exposed victims, but it is rare to encounter thermal injury below the vocal cords. This is because the oropharynx acts as an effective "heat sink," with the thermal energy of the heated air dissipating into the cells they pass by, causing rapid cell injury, necrosis, and swelling of the upper airway (Fig. 48.2). This can result in upper airway obstruction, which can be fatal before the sequelae of pulmonary burn become apparent. Super-heated steam is an exception, where the oropharynx cannot absorb all the thermal energy, and hence airway burn occurs in this situation.[22]

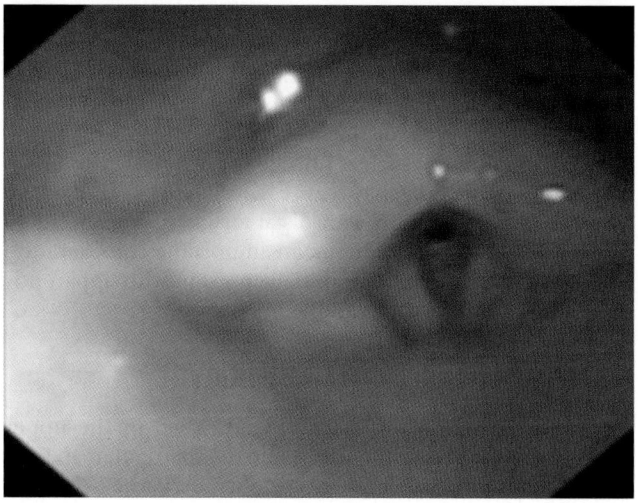

Figure 48.2 Swollen hyperemic epiglottis and narrowed laryngeal opening.

SYSTEMIC TOXINS

Systemic toxins are products of incomplete combustion and include carbon monoxide and hydrogen cyanide. Carbon monoxide intoxication, together with heat incapacitation and a hypoxic environment, is the most common immediate cause of death from fire.[20] Carbon monoxide is an odorless, colorless gas that binds to erythrocyte hemoglobin with about 250 times the affinity of oxygen. The resulting COHb molecule is unable to transport oxygen, thus impairing oxygen delivery to the tissue and shifting the oxygen-dissociation curve to the left.[23] Furthermore, at the tissue level, carbon monoxide competes with, and inhibits, oxygen binding to the cytochrome oxidase system of enzymes, inhibiting the aerobic metabolism chain and thus incapacitating cellular respiration.[21] Hence, CO paralyzes oxygen carriage in the blood and subsequent utilization in the tissue (see Table 48.2, presented later in the chapter). Thermal decomposition of nitrogen-containing polymers in oxygen-poor environments produces smoke containing hydrogen cyanide, inhibiting electron transport and cellular respiration.[19]

AIRWAY INJURY

Although the inhaled gases as described earlier can cause significant and fatal alterations in physiology, the chief mediator of the pathophysiology of smoke inhalation is particulate matter. Carbonaceous particles (soot) impregnated with a multitude of toxins reach the alveolar level suspended in air.[24] The chemicals associated with these particles vary depending on the products combusted but commonly include aldehydes from cellulose-based materials such as wood and paper; nitrogen oxides from fabric combustion;

halogen acids and sulfur dioxide from rubber; ammonia from wool, silk, and polyurethane; and phosgene from polyvinyl chloride.[22] Water-soluble compounds are readily soluble in airway mucus and interact freely with tissue at more proximal levels of the respiratory system. Less water-soluble compounds (such as phosgene) penetrate the airway mucosa deeply and may cause severe delayed damage through late interaction with distal airway tissues, up to 48 hours after exposure. This is an important consideration when treating patients who initially present with apparently mild clinical effects after smoke inhalation.[22]

PULMONARY PARENCHYMAL INJURY

Although thermal injury is mostly adsorbed in the upper airway, the other components of smoke—particulate materials, systemic toxins, and respiratory irritants—descend to the lung and trigger a cascade of events, resulting in pulmonary edema, bronchiolar obstruction, cell death, and ventilation/perfusion (V/Q) mismatch.[19]

Of paramount importance is the cascade of inflammatory mediators activated by the interaction of irritant substances with the airway mucosa and lung parenchyma. Intrapulmonary leukocyte aggregation following activation of the classic complement cascade releases even more chemokines and cytokines, leading to the production of free radicals of oxygen and nitrogen[25] from nitric oxide synthase (NOS)–triggered nitric oxide (NO) and peroxynitrite ($ONOO^-$) production. The vasodilation induced by NO rapidly increases bronchial blood flow and decreases the degree of the protective hypoxic pulmonary vasoconstriction in poorly ventilated areas of the lung, resulting in V/Q mismatch.[26] This also intensifies the spread of irritants from the pulmonary to systemic circulation. NO also combines with superoxide (O_2^-) produced in large quantities by activated neutrophils to form $ONOO^-$. This reactive nitrogen species leads to DNA damage and subsequent activation of poly (Adenosine diphosphate ribose [ADP-ribose]) polymerase, an important enzyme in DNA repair. This activation and subsequent action requires a large amount of chemical energy in the form of adenosine triphosphate (ATP) and Nicotinamide adenine dinucleotide (NAD), the depletion of which causes necrotic cell death of deprived energy-dependent tissues.[25] The combination of these effects contributes to tissue injury and increased pulmonary vascular permeability, leading to decreased diffusion, edema, and V/Q mismatch. Furthermore, neutrophils are sequestered from the systemic circulation to the intrapulmonary compartment and are activated, and fibrinogen release by inflammatory mediators causes airway cast formation and widespread plugging. These casts obstruct a number of the smaller airways, and subsequent efforts to mechanically ventilate this inhomogeneous lung can induce ventilator-induced barotrauma as normal lung is overdistended, whereas other regions collapse, and atelectasise. The further tissue injury is heightened with biotrauma of ventilation, and the production of chemokines leads to a potent accumulation of damage.[21]

Much of the study of smoke inhalation injuries in animal models has focused on aspects of this pathophysiologic sequence. Attempts to manipulate and alter the chain of effects experimentally have reinforced these theories and suggested exciting treatment targets. Nevertheless, experimental treatments have yet to deliver specific therapeutic modalities that improve the course of smoke inhalation injury.[5]

DIAGNOSTICS AND TREATMENT

INITIAL PREHOSPITAL RESCUE

The first priority at the injury scene is rescue of the victim from the source of fire to minimize the exposure time. This is usually the responsibility of firefighters.[4] The patient must be assessed as a trauma patient and not merely as the victim of an isolated burn or smoke inhalation injury. Standard early management of severe trauma (EMST) protocols must be observed, including stabilization of the neck. Following the immediate administration of a high flow of O_2 to reduce COHb levels, a primary survey must then follow to assess accompanying injuries such as burns or trauma with simultaneous estimation of the extent of smoke inhalation. In addition, it is important to determine whether the victim has been exposed to an explosion and to assess the possibility of blast injury to the lung. If possible, information about comorbidities should be obtained. Standard cardiopulmonary monitoring (electrocardiogram, pulse-oximetry, and noninvasive blood pressure) and intravenous access should be established.[27] Carbon monoxide poisoning can result in an erroneously high Sao_2 reading due to the light absorption of the classic "cherry red" hemoglobin in smoke inhalation. After these basic measures, the safety of the airway must be assessed. The risk of rapidly developing airway edema has to be taken into account even if no dyspnea is present, but it must be balanced by the real risks faced by endotracheal intubation itself in an unstable, potentially hypoxic patient with possible neck injuries. In the authors' opinion, endotracheal intubation that is entirely prophylactic is ill advised. Nevertheless, the airway with early edema is likely to worsen, particularly if significant fluid resuscitation is required for burn injury, and hence repeated and thorough assessment of the airway is mandatory. Patients with evidence of stridor or heat and smoke inhalation injury combined with extensive face or neck burns may mandate early intubation. In the case of oral burn without inhalation injury, an airway secured early represents the safest approach. However, victims with smoke inhalation injury but no facial or neck burns can be carefully observed and can be intubated later, if necessary.[28] The patient's head should be elevated to 45 degrees to minimize facial and airway edema. In the field, fluid resuscitation can be minimized to reduce the risk of airway compromise if the necessary skills or equipment are not readily available for intubation. Nebulized adrenaline or corticosteroids may be used in the hope of minimizing upper airway edema, although there is no conclusive evidence for the efficacy of these treatment strategies.[29] Bronchospasm is frequently observed, and the nebulized administration of bronchodilators, such as β2-agonists, will reduce this effect, while improving respiratory mechanics by decreasing airflow resistance and peak airway pressures in ventilated patients. This results in improved dynamic compliance. In addition, β2-agonists provide anti-inflammatory properties, represented by a decrease in inflammatory mediators such as histamine, leukotrienes, and TNF-α. Finally, β2-agonists are associated with improved airspace fluid clearance and stimulation of mucosal repair.[30-32]

After initial stabilization of the patient, information about the type of fire and combustible materials involved, whether the fire occurred in an enclosed space, and the estimated duration of exposure should be sought. In cases of presumed specific intoxication, appropriate therapies should begin.[21] Diagnosis of such intoxications is impossible in the field, but a high degree of suspicion must be maintained if the combustion materials and enclosed space lead the treating practitioner to assume risk of CO or CN. All patients should be immediately administered 100% O_2 from a high-flow facemask to reduce the CO binding to Hb. Specific therapies exist to treat the toxicity of carbon monoxide and cyanide, which aim to reduce the serum levels of these substances. Depending on the Glasgow Coma Scale, the severity of injury, and the symptoms, the patient's condition may mandate intubation and mechanical ventilation with an Fio_2 of 1.

Patients with the possibility of cyanide intoxication require standard supportive care, which may be augmented with specific antidote therapy—the choice of which is the more efficacious remains controversial. Amyl nitrate and sodium thiosulfate are used to oxidize hemoglobin to methemoglobin, which preferentially binds cyanide. In contrast to these antidotes, hydroxycobalamin (vitamin B12a) actively binds CN by forming cyanocobalamin, which is directly excreted via the kidney. Because it does not produce methemoglobin, hydroxocobalamin is safe to use in the preclinical setting. Accordingly, it represents the active compound of the "Cyanokit," which is used in the prehospital management of smoke inhalation injury in Europe with a reported reduction of mortality[33] (Table 48.1).

AIRWAY MANAGEMENT

Clinical suspicion of inhalation injury of the upper airway is aroused by the presence of certain risk factors such as history of exposure to fire and smoke in an enclosed space or a period of unconsciousness at the accident scene, burns including the face and neck, singed facial or nasal hair, altered voice, dysphagia, oral or nasal soot deposits, or carbonaceous sputum. The most immediate threat from inhalation injury is upper airway obstruction due to edema (see Fig. 48.2). Early intubation is recommended when this complication threatens and the patient was not intubated on scene.[34] However, exposure to smoke does not always lead to severe injury, and in the absence of overt evidence of respiratory distress or failure it may be difficult to identify patients who will experience progressive inflammation and ultimately require intubation of the trachea. When intubating in the field, optimal technique to secure a difficult airway is a contentious issue. Experienced operators may attempt to preserve spontaneous breathing, which allows patients to maintain their own reflexes even when intubation is not possible. Others may elect to perform a rapid sequence induction, which provides better intubating conditions but oblates all of the patient's own airway reflexes. Attention should be given to gastric residuals during enteric feeding after admission to the burn intensive care unit. In addition, the development of sepsis can slow gastric

Table 48.1 Treatment Strategies for Acute Smoke Inhalation

Current	Under Investigation
Rescue victim from source	Activated protein C
High flow 100% O_2	Anti-inflammatory drugs — Methylprednisolone — Phenytoin
Body check	Nitric oxide synthase inhibitors
Intravenous access	Antioxidants — Gamma-tocopherol — 21-aminosteroid
± Intubation	Endothelin-I-receptor antagonist tezosentan
If upper airway edema: — Nebulized adrenaline — Nebulized corticosteroids	P-selectin blockade
If bronchospasm: — Nebulized alpha2-agonists	Nebulized deferoxamine-pentastarch complex
If elevated COHb: — High-flow 100% O_2 — Hyperbaric oxygen	Mechanical ventilation — High-frequency percussive ventilation — Airway pressure release ventilation — Volumetric diffuse ventilator
If cyanide intoxication: — Amyl nitrate — Sodium thiosulfate — Hydroxocobalamin Cyanokit	Extracorporeal membrane oxygenation
Mechanical ventilation	Arteriovenous carbon dioxide removal
Low tidal volume	
Nebulized heparin	Pulmonary decontamination with nebulized amphoteric chelating agents
Nebulized *N*-acetylcysteine	

Table 48.2 Carboxyhemoglobin Concentration and Related Symptoms

COHb [in %]	Symptoms
<20	Slight headache and dilation of peripheral blood vessels
21-40	Severe headache and pulsating in temporal blood vessels, vertigo, dizziness, nausea and vomiting, circulatory collapse
41-60	Symptoms as above, syncope, tachycardia, hyperventilation, intermittent seizures, cyanosis, coma, shock, Cheyne-Stokes respiration
61-80	Coma, intermittent seizures, impaired heart and lung function, weak pulses, slow breathing, death within hours
>81	Death occurs within minutes

emptying, which can result in retained fluids in the stomach and risk of aspiration.[27]

A patient with a compromised airway has evolved to maintain the airway at all costs. This primitive survival instinct is neutered if paralyzing agents or heavy sedation is administered and the safe airway can rapidly become unsalvageable. Intubation of a spontaneously breathing patient, while being more technically challenging, is safer, as the patient will keep breathing at all costs. In terms of anesthetic airway management, the most profound and clinically significant effect of burn injuries on drug response relates to muscle relaxants. Burn injuries influence responses to both succinylcholine and the nondepolarizing muscle relaxants. In burned patients, sensitization to the muscle relaxant effects of succinylcholine can produce exaggerated hyperkalemic responses severe enough to induce cardiac arrest, though this tends to occur 24 to 48 hours post injury, rather than immediately.[35] However, recommendations regarding the safe use of succinylcholine after burn injury cannot be given. Various authors recommend avoidance of succinylcholine at intervals ranging from 24 hours to 21 days post burn injury,[36] but it seems clear that the hyperkalemic response associated with burn does not occur in the first day and hence the drug can be used with standard precautions at this stage.

An increase in the numbers of acetylcholine receptors and the proliferation of these receptors away from the neuromuscular junction have been suggested as common mechanisms explaining both reduced sensitivity to nondepolarizing relaxants and the exaggerated hyperkalemia that may follow succinylcholine administration in burned patients. Resistance is apparent by 7 days post injury and peaks by approximately 40 days. Sensitivity returns to normal after approximately 70 days. In contrast to other nondepolarizing neuromuscular blockers, mivacurium dosage requirements in pediatric patients appear to be unchanged by burn injury.[37]

Preoxygenation may be more difficult in the smoke inhalation victim, and relative loss of mandibular mobility may impair airway manipulation, making bag-mask ventilation difficult. The swelling and distortion of the mouth and mandibular aspect of the airway may make preoxygenation and direct laryngoscopy difficult or impossible. Preoxygenation with small aliquots of anxiolysis and analgesics (such as 0.5- to 1-mg increments of midazolam and 25- to 50-μg blouses of fentanyl IV) with sequential direct spraying of lignocaine to the oropharynx and then subsequently under direct vision of the larynx/epiglottic area is technically difficult but safe in experienced hands. Fiberoptic intubation with nebulized or directly sprayed lignocaine spray while maintaining spontaneous ventilation is equally safe but requires a substantial level of skill with the bronchoscope. However, pediatric patients are unable to cooperate and must be adequately sedated. Because deep sedation and full anesthesia cause collapse of pharyngeal tissues and airway obstruction, they are unsuitable for fiberoptic intubation in patients whose airway would be difficult to manage with a mask.[38]

Agents that may prove useful to facilitate fiberoptic intubation include the ultra-short-acting remifentanil. The novel alpha-2-adrenergic agonist dexmedetomidine, which provides sedation, anxiolysis, and analgesia with much less respiratory depression than other sedatives,[39] may be considered, though further data are required until its widespread use is adopted. Ketamine remains a very useful drug, as it provides some analgesia and facilitates a degree of spontaneous breathing while allowing dissociative anesthesia, However, airway secretions may be copious and the clinician must always be aware of this.

Securing an endotracheal tube in a patient with facial burns presents a variety of problems. Tape or ties across damaged or grafted skin can worsen tissue loss or induce graft failure. A useful technique to avoid these problems involves the use of a nasal septal tie.

The use of a laryngeal mask airway (LMA) has also been successful for airway management during burn surgery for children.[40] In the acute phase or in the intensive care unit, the LMA serves as a rescue device when endotracheal intubation fails, but it must be replaced with a definitive airway as soon as is practically possible, as gastroparesis is common in the burn patient.

MONITORING AND INVESTIGATIONS

Damages to the airway and lung from inhalation injury often develop with a latency of several hours and are affected by other injuries and degree of fluid resuscitation required. Nevertheless, airway management and the oxygenation status of the patient, regardless of intubation status, need to be frequently reevaluated; such is the dynamic nature of smoke inhalation injury.[22] After stabilization of cardiopulmonary hemodynamics and pulmonary gas exchange, the assumed diagnosis of smoke inhalation injury needs to be verified. However, as no uniform criteria are available, diagnosis of smoke inhalation injury has a subjective component based on history, physical examination with supporting imaging, and blood gas assays. Bronchoscopic examination of the airway represents the gold standard to detect a pathognomonic mucosal hyperemia with soot staining below the larynx being diagnosed (Fig. 48.3). Although chest radiographs are mandatory and may reveal injuries consistent with trauma—that is, fractured ribs, pneumothorax, and pulmonary contusion—they provide little information acutely as to the degree of smoke inhalation. Specific changes that may be seen related to the smoke inhalation

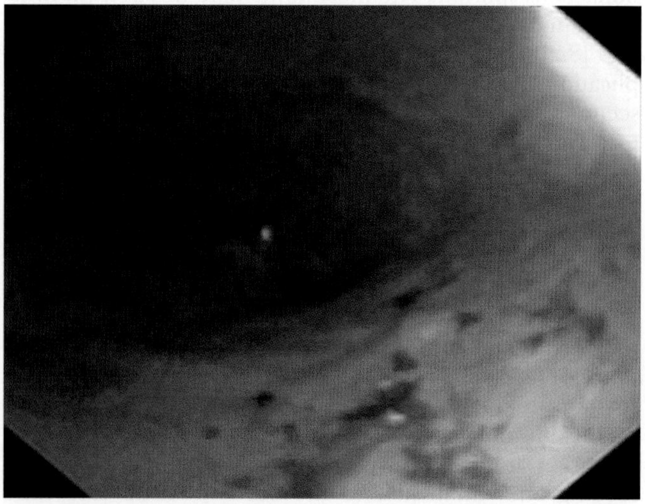

Figure 48.3 Soot staining in the hyperemic trachea.

include signs of diffuse atelectasis, pulmonary edema, or bronchopneumonia.[41]

A uniform algorithm for assessing inhalation injury or a reliable indicator of progressive respiratory failure in patients with smoke inhalation injury has not yet been established. This failure is largely explained by the extreme heterogeneity of the clinical presentation. In addition, the delay in the manifestation and development of acute lung injury (ALI) as a consequence of systemic inflammatory response syndrome (SIRS), initiated by accompanying burns or trauma, complicates the evaluation of the isolated effects of smoke inhalation. Frequent blood gas and sputum analyses are useful to monitor patients with smoke inhalation injury.[28] In addition, inexplicably high lactate levels, despite adequate fluid resuscitation, will be helpful for the diagnosis of CN poisoning. In a study by Pham and colleagues,[42] cyanide poisoning in the canine model showed two phases of injury. The first (compensated) phase had a mechanism consistent with a traditional global oxygen consumption defect. The second (decompensated) phase had a mechanism consistent with heart failure. This heart failure was due to bradycardia. The systolic blood pressure remained relatively constant, whereas diastolic blood pressure decreased by 19%. Cardiac output, heart rate, and DO_2 increased to a maximum of 6%, 10%, and 10%, respectively, at 40 minutes, after which they declined to a low of 32%, 28%, and 30% below baseline, respectively. Stroke volume remained constant. Oxygen consumption initially increased by 5% and then decreased to 24% below baseline. The oxygen extraction ratio (OER) initially declined to 35% below baseline and then increased throughout the rest of the study. In clinical practice, serial venous blood gases may unmask cytopathic hypoxia, by insufficient O_2 extraction, that may be seen as increased central venous ($Scvo_2$) or mixed venous (Svo_2) oxygen saturations.

FLUID RESUSCITATION

Optimal fluid management is critical to the survival of the victim of a major thermal injury, with additional or isolated inhalation injury, and when septic complications occur. Modern fluid resuscitation formulas originate from experimental studies in the pathophysiology of burn shock. Fluid resuscitation in the patient with thermal injury has been recognized as an essential aspect of the care since the first studies were published in 1905.[43] The improvement in outcome with cutaneous burns can be related to the development of a protocol based on providing adequate fluid resuscitation to allow optimal organ function while minimizing the physiologic cost associated with over-resuscitation.

Burn shock is both hypovolemic shock and cellular shock and is characterized by specific hemodynamic changes including decreased cardiac output, extracellular fluid, plasma volume, and oliguria. As in the treatment of other shock forms, the primary goal is to restore and preserve tissue perfusion in order to avoid ischemia. However, in burn shock, resuscitation is complicated by obligatory burn edema, and the voluminous transvascular fluid shifts that results from a major burn are unique to thermal trauma.[44] Blalock may have been the first to the postulate mechanism, where he induced burn to one side of mongrel dogs and assessed the weight changes in both burned and unburned tissue, demonstrating that burn tissue edema correlated to the drop in blood pressure and was similar in composition to plasma.[45] Although the exact pathophysiology of the postburn vascular changes and fluid shifts is still unclear, major components of burn shock are the increase in total body vascular permeability and the changes in microcirculation. Fluid resuscitation is aimed to support the patient throughout the initial 24-hour to 48-hour period of hypovolemia and has existed since the early 1950s.

Cope, in his seminal paper following the Cocoanut Grove disaster, was the first to report the increased fluid requirement seen in patients with smoke inhalation injury.[46] This observation has been confirmed by multiple other papers, despite the lack of thermal injury below the larynx; hence fluid loss seems unlikely. One theory, which concurs with much of the known pathophysiology, relates to inflammatory excess seen postsmoke inhalation. Approximately 28% of all neutrophils reside in the human lungs, and this percentage increases postinhalation insult. As described earlier, it is well recognized that the particulate and chemical nature of inhalation injury induces neutrophil activation and the release of numerous cytokines, proteases, and free radicals. This further recruits neutrophils from the systemic circulation, and the local inflammatory state rapidly becomes systemic due to the vast alveolo-capillary interphase transporting these mediators and modulators of vasodilatation to distant organs. The up-regulation is not only in number but also in responsiveness to endotoxin.[21,47] Regardless of mechanism, numerous authors have reported that smoke inhalation per se increased the fluid requirement substantially.[48-50]

Although under-resuscitation in thermal and smoke inhalation injury is known to induce organ failure and death, there are growing concerns with over-resuscitation, where the "fluid creep" can induce increased extravascular water content, resulting in compartment syndrome in extremities or in the abdomen.[51] Even after thousands of patients have been saved by fluid resuscitation, resuscitation formulas are still controversially discussed, depending on advantages and disadvantages for the individual patient. Crystalloid solutions, such as lactated Ringer's solution (sodium concentration 130 Meq/L), are the most popular resuscitation fluids currently utilized. Crystalloid formulas are the "Parkland formula" (which recommends 4 cc/kg/% total body surface area (TBSA) burn in the first 24 hours, with half of the amount administered in the first 8 hours) and the "Modified Brooke formula" (which recommends 2 cc/kg/% TBSA burn). Colloid formulas (Evans, Brooke, Slater), the Dextran formula (Demling), and hypertonic saline formulas (Monafo, Warden) are also in use.[44,52-54]

Concerns with colloid administration in the resuscitation of early burns began with Goodwin's work in the 1980s,[55] where it was suggested that there was a lack of benefit over crystalloid and potential pulmonary harm, and grew substantially in the late 1990s, but more recent work suggests that concerns of increased capillary leak particularly in the lungs are overplayed, and the pendulum seems to be swinging back toward the judicious use of colloid to minimize the risk of abdominal compartment syndrome (ACS). A randomized controlled trial (RCT) by O'Mara compared plasma to crystalloid in burn resuscitation and showed that colloid resulted in less ACS but no demonstrable improvement in outcome.[56]

Early studies in fluid resuscitation post smoke inhalation suggest a mean fluid requirement of 5.8 mL/kg/% TBSA burn for optimal outcomes, but more recent studies suggest the figure may be lower than originally expected.[49]

Hypertonic salt (HTS) solutions have been known for many years for effectiveness in the treatment of burn shock by fluid sparing effects and a reduction of volume load in the early phase of injury.[57] Rapid infusion leads to serum hyperosmolarity and hypernatremia, reducing the shift of fluids from intravascular to interstitial areas, which may prevent edema formation and the need for escharotomy.[58,59] The use of HTS, however, is controversial because although there may be beneficial effects, other studies have demonstrated an increase in mortality with HTS treatment of major burns.[60]

Part of the dubiety regarding the exact volume required relates to the lack of consensus of scoring severity of inhalation injury. The extent of cutaneous burn can be readily assessed. Such a scoring system for inhalation injury is lacking, and inhalation can be mild moderate or severe. In a 3-year retrospective review by Gamelli's group, numerous demographic and injury-related factors, including bronchoscopic scoring, failed to determine which patients with inhalation injury required increased fluid resuscitation. From its 80-patient cohort, the group postulated that a Pao_2/Fio_2 ratio of <350 may be the best early determinant of which patients would require excess fluid resuscitation.[61]

In addition to hypovolemia, the risk of infection in smoke inhalation patients is extraordinarily high. Shirani and coworkers[6] have shown that inhalation injury alone increased the mortality of burn patients by a maximum of 20%, and pneumonia by a maximum of 40%, with a maximum increase of approximately 60% when both are present. These data indicate that inhalation injury with additional septic complications such as pneumonia has significant, independent, additive effects on burn mortality and that these effects vary with age and burn size. The presence of inhalation injury and sepsis increases the fluid requirements for resuscitation from burn shock after thermal injury.[48] Chen and coworkers[62] have demonstrated that HTS confers beneficial effects on burn shock, reduces bacterial translocation, and enhances host defenses by several mechanisms in the treatment of burn shock and sepsis. It is of high interest to further investigate HTS in animal models and later on in humans. Future studies with HTS alone and in combination with already established resuscitation formulas are needed to find a risk/benefit ratio for such a treatment. HTS may have the potential to improve resuscitation strategies and outcome in burn care, but it cannot be recommended at the present time due to a lack of evidence.[63]

Despite the treatment of septic complications following inhalation injury, the gradual shift toward less fluid in both burn and smoke inhalation may relate to the changes in the intensive care unit (ICU) modalities of care—including point-of-care devices to assess oxygenation, less injurious ventilation, and more rapid debridement of burn tissue.[64]

Debates and ongoing research on fluid resuscitation may last for decades, but they are needed to improve outcomes in this patient population. However, in the authors' experience it is worthwhile to start fluid resuscitation using the "Modified Brooke formula" (which recommends 2 cc/kg/% TBSA burn) to closely monitor urine output (0.5 to 1 cc/kg/h recommended) and to increase fluid administration up to a rate that will maintain the recommended urine output. This strategy may prevent initial over-resuscitation in many patients, decreasing edema formation, and will suit the increased needs of patients with inhalation injury who may need up to 6 to 8 cc/kg/h to maintain adequate organ perfusion. Excessive fluid administration beyond a urine output of 1 cc/kg/h is ill advised.

Although protocols should not be abandoned, a routine and recurrent assessment of the patient with inhalation injury would be essential to minimize physiologic injury as a result of fluid resuscitation, whether too little or too much.

TREATMENT OF CARBON MONOXIDE INTOXICATION

Current treatment recommendations of CO poisoning begin with cessation of exposure, immediate administration of 100% oxygen, and supportive care.[65] The rationale of hyperbaric oxygenation therapy (HBOT) is based on its ability to rapidly displace CO from hemoglobin, thus reducing the duration of the hypoxemic state. Administration of 100% oxygen at 3 atmospheres reduces the CO half-life from 250 minutes in room air to 30 minutes.[28] Besides this efficiency, its use remains controversial due to the questioned correlation between COHb levels and outcomes. This may also be explained with limited access to the patient during HBOT, which has major impact on the treatment quality of combined burn injuries.[28] A Cochrane database review of six randomized controlled trials did not reveal a beneficial effect of HBOT compared to standard treatment in respect to neurologic sequelae.[66] However, the results should be interpreted with care, as concerns have been raised regarding design and analyses in all the included trials. In summary, all patients with CO intoxication should be immediately treated with 100% oxygen. Although data do not support its routine use, HBOT may be considered in stable patients with severe neurologic symptoms and high COHb concentrations (>50%), but no major burns and severe pulmonary injury.[47]

TREATMENT OF CYANIDE INTOXICATION

Hydrogen cyanide in fire smoke is an underappreciated threat and one of the most common poisonings in patients who suffer smoke inhalation.[67] Its lipophilicity and lack of dissociation allow it to penetrate through mucous membranes with ease, resulting in a myriad of symptoms within minutes, and possible death if the dose is large enough.[68] Patients may describe a burning, dry throat with inexplicable feelings of anxiety. Clinical signs range from a patient presenting with tachypnea, confusion (and the classic almond breath fetor) to unconsciousness, cardiovascular collapse, and death, generally from respiratory arrest (see Table 48.3).[20] The key for the receiving clinician is to have a high index of suspicion in such a patient, as there is no immediately available lab test. Blood gas analysis may reveal an inexplicably high lactate in the absence of CO poisoning or other trauma. However, CN poisoning frequently coexists with significant CO poisoning, and hence may be overlooked.[4,69] For adequate treatment of CN poisoning

Table 48.3 Hydrogen Cyanide Concentration in Air and Related Symptoms

HCN [ppm]	Symptoms
0.2-5	Odor threshold
10	Occupational exposure limit
18-36	Slight symptoms, headache
45-54	Will be tolerated for 30-60 minutes
100	Death within 1 hour
110-135	Death within 30-60 minutes
181	Death within 10 minutes
280	Immediate death

following smoke inhalation injury, several antidotes are available: The "CN antidote kit" includes amyl nitrite, thiosulfate, and sodium nitrite.[70] Because these substances are methemoglobin generators, which may additionally impair oxygen transport, they should be only used in case of proven diagnosis (increased plasma levels of CN) and under continuous monitoring in the intensive care unit, particularly in episodes of poisoning with CO simultaneously.[28] Methemoglobin chelates CN to form cyanmethemoglobin. As cyanmethemoglobin dissociates, free CN is converted to thiocyanate by liver mitochondrial enzymes (rhodanese) using thiosulfate as a substrate. Thiocyanate is then excreted into the urine.[71] In contrast to these antidotes, hydroxocobalamin, a vitamin B12 derivative, actively binds CN by forming cyanocobalamin, which will be directly excreted by the kidneys.[33] Data are growing regarding the safety and efficacy of hydroxocobalamin. Prospective observational studies reveal that empiric administration of hydroxocobalamin was associated with survival among 67% of patients who were confirmed post administration to have had cyanide poisoning. A randomized controlled trial in pigs assessed the efficacy of hydroxocobalamin versus sodium thiosulfate in the treatment of acute cyanide toxicity. The study indicated that in severe poisoning (CN administered to hypotension to 50% of baseline blood pressure), hydroxocobalamin was safe, efficacious, and resulted in much improved survival. Worryingly, sodium thiosulfate failed to reverse cyanide-induced shock. The authors concluded that only hydroxocobalamin was effective.[72] In case of intoxication with 1 mg CN, the recommended dose is 50 mg/kg hydroxocobalamin.[73] Because of the avoidance of methemoglobin production, hydroxocobalamin can be used safely in the preclinical setting. Accordingly, hydroxocobalamin represents the active compound of the "Cyanokit," which is used in the prehospital management of smoke inhalation injury in Europe with a reported improvement in mortality.[33]

Aggressive restoration of cardiopulmonary function augments the hepatic clearance of CN via the enzyme rhodanese and has been reported to be successful in severe CN poisoning (blood levels 5.6 to 9 mg/L) as well as after ingestion or smoke inhalation, even without the use of antidotes.[74-76] Hydroxocobalamin has been used safely and successfully by emergency personnel in out-of-hospital settings and may represent a new option in cases of suspected or confirmed cyanide poisoning in the field.[77] Therefore, the standard care of CN poisoning should combine the aggressive supportive therapy with current data supporting the use of hydroxocobalamin as the optimal specific therapy.[47]

BRONCHOSCOPY

Within each burn center, diagnostic as well as treatment options are determined by the availability of resources (such as 133Xe scans, fiberoptic bronchoscopy, or 24-hour/day anesthesia staff coverage) and local tradition. A clear diagnosis proving smoke inhalation has occurred allows for the planning and delivery of therapeutic interventions.[41] Inhalation injury can be diagnosed with confidence based on clinical presentation and bronchoscopic findings. Changes observed with bronchoscopy include erythema, lesion, erosion, ischemia, or necrosis of the mucous membrane, as well as small to significant edema, blisters, and unidentified damage of the lung parenchyma when the changes in the lower respiratory tract are below the reach of the fiberoptic scope, which can be used for inspection of the upper (oropharynx) and main (trachea and bronchi) respiratory tract[78] (see Figs. 48.2 and 48.3).

Early prediction of which patients are vulnerable to resuscitation stresses, increased pulmonary complications, respiratory failure, and mortality is complex and frequently not possible. Many attempts to identify prognostic indicators for patients with smoke inhalation injuries have been made.[79,80] It has been difficult to identify reliable indicators of progressive respiratory failure in patients with smoke inhalation injury. Most of these studies have involved small numbers of patients and assessed a small number of clinical features. Prognostic estimations will ultimately rely on a system that allows quantification of the severity of inhalation injury.[41] Many observational studies have compared outcomes with various grading systems.[61,78,81,82] These grading systems often combine bronchoscopic findings with a small number of other clinical findings. However, it has been recognized that proximal injury observed by bronchoscopy is frequently greater than the peripheral, parenchymal injury. Masanes and colleagues[83] found that inhalation injury could be diagnosed by fiberoptic bronchoscopy in some burn patients who were otherwise asymptomatic. Liffner and colleagues [82] found that their scoring system for grading the severity of bronchoscopic evidence of inhalation injury did not correlate with the development of acute respiratory distress syndrome (ARDS). Similarly, although it is generally recognized that inhalation injury increases fluid resuscitation needs in burn patients, Endorf and Gamelli found no correlation of severity of bronchoscopic findings with fluid resuscitation requirements.[61] In a review article, Woodson concluded that a consensus may be facilitated when a clinical variable or constellation of variables is identified that is reliably related to the development of respiratory failure or other complications in patients who have inhaled smoke.[41] A large multicenter study combining the experience of several institutions is more likely to identify such a correlation. However, consensus in diagnosis and quantification of inhalation injuries may await a theoretic advance with identification of a mediator or marker of cell injury or cell death that reliably and in some concentration-dependent way correlates with pulmonary or systemic complications of inhalation injury. A widely accepted grading system for inhalation injury severity is presently not available. However, a randomized controlled multicenter trial to validate a standardized scoring system for inhalation injury that can be used to both quantify injury severity and predict mortality after inhalation injury is warranted.[41]

MECHANICAL VENTILATION

Since the advent of positive pressure ventilation, there has been an understanding that this therapeutic maneuver can paradoxically cause harm as well as save lives. Numerous studies have tried to identify optimal ventilatory strategies, positive end-expiratory pressure (PEEP) levels, and modes. An open lung strategy with low-tidal-volume ventilation has been shown to be associated with improved outcome and reduced duration of ventilation.[84] In keeping with the ARDSnet data, low tidal volumes are mandated to minimize ventilator-induced lung injury (VILI).[85] An open lung strategy is advised due to the decrement of surfactant in this population, but no study has shown an improved outcome with higher levels of PEEP. The frequent casts that occur post smoke inhalation result in areas of collapsed alongside open lung, and application of PEEP may result in tidal hyperinflation in areas of the lung, whereas there is an inability to aerate the collapsed area of lung. Hence, frequent airway toilet with mucolytics is essential to minimize VILI. Newer modalities such as electrical impedance tomography to assess breath-to-breath changes have demonstrated the rapid changes in ventilatory inhomogeneities seen post smoke inhalation.[86] A number of specific modalities have been suggested specific to the ventilatory idiosyncrasies associated with smoke inhalation.[87]

An alternative to the classic ARDSnet low tidal volume ventilation in patients with ARDS may be high-frequency oscillation. A meta-analysis to determine the clinical and physiologic effects of high-frequency oscillation compared with conventional ventilation in patients with ARDS displayed improved survival and it is unlikely to cause harm. As ongoing large multicenter trials will not be completed for several years, these data help clinicians who currently use or are considering this technique for patients with ARDS.[87]

The volumetric diffusive ventilator (VDR) is a pneumatically powered, pressure-limited ventilator that stacks oscillatory breaths to a selected peak airway pressure by means of a sliding venture called a Phasitron, resulting in low tidal volumes. Exhalation is passive and a level of continuous positive airway pressure (CPAP) can be selected. In addition, VDR reestablishes the physiologic diffusive gas exchange, whereas standard ventilation modes induce a convective gas exchange.[88] A prospective clinical analysis revealed an improved gas exchange and a decrease in peak pressures.[89] A retrospective study in 330 patients with inhalation injury even reported a lower mortality rate.[90] Although these studies compared the VDR to high-volume ventilatory strategies, data regarding a comparison with modern low-tidal volume ventilation are still lacking. This may represent one reason why VDR is not universally accepted. Another factor might be that the VDR differs from other ventilators and, therefore, requires special training. In addition, tidal and minute volumes cannot be monitored, and humidified air as well as nebulized saline are necessary to prevent airway desiccation.[47]

As in conventional long-term ventilation of patients, common complications must be considered. Mosier and associates[91] documented that patients with combined thermal and inhalation injury requiring urgent intubation or prolonged ventilation have a high incidence of bacterial bronchial contamination. Inhalation injury creates a damaged tracheobronchial mucosa, and early intubation provides a portal for bacterial contamination. In patients with smoke inhalation that necessitated urgent intubation, a 50% incidence of ventilator-associated pneumonia (VAP) has been described.[92]

The use and timing of tracheostomy in burn patients elicit a great deal of passionate discussion but very little solid data. Burn survivors with TBSA >60% are more likely to undergo repeated surgery and have burns to the head and neck region, therefore increasing the requirement for tracheostomy. However, an association has been demonstrated between tracheostomy and high prevalence of chest infection in patients with inhalation injury, greater burn size, and prolonged mechanical ventilation.[93] The authors would advise caution in overinterpreting this study, as association does not infer causation, and sicker patients tend to be ventilated for longer periods, resulting in a higher incidence of both tracheostomy and VAP. The tracheostomy allows for less sedation, earlier mobilization, and a more comfortable method of ventilation for a long-term patient.

NEBULIZATION TREATMENTS

As described previously, smoke-inhalation injury causes a destruction of the ciliated epithelium that lines the tracheobronchial tree. Casts produced from these cells, polymorphonuclear leukocytes, and mucus can cause upper-airway obstruction, contributing to pulmonary failure.[21] In the early 2000s, it was proposed that a combination of aerosolized heparin and a mucolytic agent, *N*-acetylcysteine, can ameliorate cast formation and reduce pulmonary failure secondary to smoke inhalation. In a study of 90 consecutive pediatric burn patients at the Shriners Burns Hospital at Galveston, Texas, who had bronchoscopically diagnosed inhalation injury requiring ventilatory support, 5000 units of heparin and 3 mL of a 20% solution of *N*-acetylcysteine aerosolized every 4 hours the first 7 days after the injury resulted in a significant decrease in reintubation rates, in incidence of atelectasis, and in mortality for patients treated with the regimen when compared with controls, and this practice has ever since been part of the ventilation protocol at this institution.[94]

NONVENTILATORY PULMONARY TREATMENTS

Extracorporeal membrane oxygenation (ECMO) is used in specialized centers for neonatal, pediatric, and adult respiratory and cardiac failure. It requires a highly skilled team of intensivists and perfusionists, and echocardiographic support is essential for optimal usage of this modality.[95] The goal of ECMO is to support gas exchange, allowing the intensity of mechanical ventilation to be reduced and thus decreasing the potentially injurious effects of ventilator-induced lung injury until recovery. Furthermore, ECMO may be considered the definitive rescue therapy for refractory life-threatening hypoxemia, as pulmonary gas exchange is not required. Our group performed a systematic review of the literature to collect all available clinical data in order to elucidate the role and present evidence of ECMO on severe hypoxemic respiratory failure resulting from burn and smoke inhalation injury.[96] Only a small number of clinical trials with a limited number of patients were available. The data suggested a higher ECMO therapy survival than nonsurvival rate of burn patients suffering acute hypoxemic respiratory failure. ECMO run times of less than 200 hours correlate with higher survival compared to 200 hours or more, and scald burns show a tendency of higher survival than flame burns. However, based on the low number of studies and patients, as well as the low grade of evidence of these studies, there are currently inadequate data to support the use of ECMO in burn or smoke inhalation injury. Even though the reports are promising, especially in the pediatric burn population, this review highlighted the lack of evidence for the use of ECMO in this setting. ECMO in adult respiratory failure is controversial, as early randomized trials showed poor outcomes[97-99] and use has been limited to highly specialized centers. Nevertheless, ECMO technology and expertise have improved. More recently, the Conventional Ventilation or ECMO for Severe Adult Respiratory Failure trial[100] and selected case series have shown improved outcomes, with survival of 75% to 85% in refractory respiratory failure.[101,102] Therefore, randomized controlled trials on patients with burn and smoke inhalation injury are warranted to provide definitive recommendations and to further advance this therapeutic option in patients where other ventilatory modalities have failed. Currently, there are large animal studies assessing the efficacy of ECMO in severe smoke inhalation, with promising results.[103]

EXPERIMENTAL TREATMENTS

Against the background of the current literature, there has been a remarkable increase in our knowledge about the pathogenesis of smoke inhalation injury. There are several promising therapeutic approaches, including the nebulization of β2-agonists, antioxidants, or anticoagulants as well as the use of different ventilation modes.[104-112] However, as has been highlighted, smoke inhalation may begin as a single organ injury, but rapidly becomes systemic. Hence, although treatment paradigms may focus on smoke inhalation, it is more frequently a mixed insult of smoke and burn, smoke and pneumonia, smoke and toxicology, and smoke and trauma. Even isolated smoke inhalation generally induces distant organ dysfunction rapidly post injury. Hence, it is unlikely that a single "magic bullet" will be found for this condition, and the clinician is best equipped with a comprehensive understanding of the complex pathophysiology and multitudinous clinical presentations of smoke inhalation injury. The treatment can then be patient and inhalation specific, with a systemic rather than organ-specific approach to these patients (see Table 48.1).

KEY POINTS

- Smoke inhalation represents a huge burden of disease in patients with and without burn injury.
- Early signs may be mild so a high index of suspicion must be maintained, particularly in burn victims from an enclosed environment.
- Prophylactic control of the airway should be considered in patients with worsening symptoms.
- Concomitant poisoning with carbon monoxide or cynaide should be considered where an enclosed smoke inhalation occurs, and definitive treatment should be considered early.
- Bronchoscopy is a more useful tool than chest radiograph to determine severity of inhalation injury.
- Injurious ventilatory parameters can exacerbate the acute and late phase lung injury.
- Despite a great deal of research, exemplary critical care management is the only process that improves outcome in smoke inhalation management.

SELECTED REFERENCES

22. Toon MH, Maybauer MO, Greenwood JE, et al: Management of acute smoke inhalation injury. Crit Care Resusc 2010;12:53-61.
33. Fortin JL, Giocanti JP, Ruttimann M, Kowalski JJ: Prehospital administration of hydroxocobalamin for smoke inhalation-associated cyanide poisoning: 8 years of experience in the Paris Fire Brigade. Clini Toxicol 2006;44(suppl 1):37-44.
46. Cope O, Moore FD: The redistribution of body water and the fluid therapy of the burned patient. Ann Surg 1947;126:110-145.
47. Rehberg S, Maybauer MO, Enkhbaatar P, et al: Pathophysiology, management and treatment of smoke inhalation injury. Expert Rev Respir Med 2009;3:283-297.
56. O'Mara MS, Slater H, Goldfarb IW, Caushaj PF: A prospective, randomized evaluation of intra-abdominal pressures with crystalloid and colloid resuscitation in burn patients. J Trauma 2005;58:1011-1018.
61. Endorf FW, Gamelli RL: Inhalation injury, pulmonary perturbations, and fluid resuscitation. J Burn Care Res 2007;28:80-83.
66. Juurlink DN, Buckley NA, Stanbrook MB, et al: Hyperbaric oxygen for carbon monoxide poisoning. Cochrane Database Syst Rev 2005;CD002041.
69. Eckstein M, Maniscalco PM: Focus on smoke inhalation—the most common cause of acute cyanide poisoning. Prehosp Disaster Med 2006;21:s49-s55.
73. Borron SW, Baud FJ, Barriot P, et al: Prospective study of hydroxocobalamin for acute cyanide poisoning in smoke inhalation. Ann Emerg Med 2007;49:794-801, e791-e792.
76. Clark CJ, Campbell D, Reid WH: Blood carboxyhaemoglobin and cyanide levels in fire survivors. Lancet 1981;1:1332-1335.
104. Maybauer MO, Maybauer DM, Fraser JF, et al: Combined recombinant human activated protein C and ceftazidime prevent the onset of acute respiratory distress syndrome in severe sepsis. Shock 2012;37:170-176.
110. Maybauer MO, Maybauer DM, Fraser JF, et al: Recombinant human activated protein C attenuates cardiovascular and microcirculatory dysfunction in acute lung injury and septic shock. Crit Care 2010;14:R217.

The complete list of references can be found at www.expertconsult.com.

49 Immunologic Lung Disease in the Critically Ill

Gregory A. Schmidt | Lakshmi Durairaj

CHAPTER OUTLINE

Immunologic lung disease can arise in any anatomic compartment of the lung. Examples include the airways in bronchiolitis obliterans, the parenchyma in idiopathic pulmonary fibrosis (IPF), and blood vessels in vasculitis. In each instance these illnesses may prove severe enough to merit intensive care unit (ICU) management for diagnosis and treatment. Immunologic lung diseases tend to share three features during critical illness. First, restrictive lung physiology is generally present, so the risk of lung overdistention and associated ventilator-induced lung injury is real. Second, pulmonary hypertension may complicate management of the circulation. Finally, infection due to immunocompromise and drug-induced lung injury must be considered throughout critical illness, because these infections represent common and potentially treatable precipitants of crisis. Early recognition and treatment of immunologic lung diseases and their complications are essential to avoid permanent lung damage or death.

The focus of this chapter is immunologic lung disease. The emphasis is on those disorders that are likely to present to the medical intensivist. Asthma and neuromuscular diseases are covered elsewhere in this book and are not reviewed here.

CLINICOPATHOLOGIC CONSIDERATIONS DURING MECHANICAL VENTILATION

The lungs of patients with immunologic diseases, in particular, interstitial lung diseases such as IPF and connective tissue lung diseases, exhibit restrictive physiology with decreased lung volumes, decreased parenchymal compliance, and a loss of functional capillary beds leading to a reduction in the diffusing capacity.[1] In this manner the functionally smaller lungs (baby lungs) of these patients resemble the lungs of patients with the acute respiratory distress syndrome (ARDS). This concept is supported by computed tomography (CT) findings of heterogeneous disease involvement in the lungs of patients with both IPF and ARDS. This parallel can be used as a framework for managing tidal volumes during mechanical ventilation of patients with immunologic lung disease and respiratory failure. If large tidal volumes (or excessive inflation pressures) are used, relatively normal areas of lung will be overdistended, potentially exacerbating lung injury. Limiting tidal volumes to 6 mL/kg predicted body weight in patients with acute lung injury (ALI) or ARDS saves lives.[2] Similar data are not available regarding safe parameters for ventilating patients with chronic restrictive lung diseases, but limiting tidal volumes to roughly 6 mL/kg (and raising the rate accordingly) carries little risk. Moreover, retrospective analysis of mechanically ventilated patients without ALI/ARDS suggests that large tidal volumes may produce ALI (odds ratio 1.3 for each milliliter above 6 mL/kg predicted body weight).[3] Because there is little evidence that intrinsic positive end-expiratory pressure (PEEP) plays a physiologically important role in respiratory failure in patients with interstitial lung disease, rapid ventilatory rates are tolerated.[1] This approach may allow ventilation without resorting to permissive hypercapnia, which may aggravate pulmonary hypertension.[4,5] As in the ARDS lung, it seems likely that nonfunctional, diseased lung units exist alongside those with essentially normal function. However, unlike the acutely injured lung, atelectatic lung units available for recruitment through the use of elevated end-expiratory pressure are rare in conditions such as IPF. There is probably little clinical advantage to using high PEEP in patients with restrictive lung diseases; in fact, high levels of PEEP may be detrimental by overdistending the lung, as well as by contributing to cor pulmonale, as described later. In a cohort of ventilated patients with interstitial lung disease, high PEEP during the first 24 hours of mechanical ventilation was one of the independent determinants of death.[6] Although it is likely that high PEEP served as a marker (rather than a cause) of severity in this study, high PEEP should nevertheless be applied cautiously to minimize harm.

Another clinicopathologic process to consider in the ventilatory management of the patient with immunologic lung disease is pulmonary hypertension. Pulmonary artery pressures are chronically elevated in advanced stages with lung fibrosis, and this pressure increases further with the increased cardiac output that accompanies exercise, fever, and hypercarbia.[5,7] Pulmonary hypertension may eventually lead to cor pulmonale because of increased right ventricular afterload.[8] Mechanical ventilation may interact adversely with pulmonary hypertension. Positive-pressure ventilation alone impairs right-sided heart function, and this effect is exaggerated by PEEP.[9] PEEP increases afterload by increasing pulmonary vascular resistance.[10] The resulting increase in wall tension decreases right ventricular perfusion, which leads to myocardial ischemia.[10,11] Right ventricular ischemia may cause further dysfunction and dilation of the right side of the heart, in addition to diastolic dysfunction of the left ventricle (through ventricular interdependence), producing a cycle of progressively deteriorating circulatory function.[8] Thus, it is important to minimize further increases in pulmonary artery pressure and to maintain adequate systemic pressure to preserve perfusion of the right ventricle. Additionally, adequate oxygenation is essential to prevent reflex increases in pulmonary artery pressure and to maintain peripheral oxygen delivery. Finally, hypercapnia, which tends to raise pulmonary artery pressures, should generally be avoided. Because predicting the degree of pulmonary hypertension clinically is difficult—and the need to avoid increases in pulmonary artery pressures is so important—we advocate liberal use of echocardiography. Other forms of monitoring, such as central venous saturation measurement or pulmonary artery catheterization, might also be useful. When acute-on-chronic cor pulmonale compromises the circulation, dobutamine or norepinephrine is often helpful.[12] Inhaled nitric oxide or inhaled prostacyclin probably plays some role, at least to buy time in the critically impaired patient.[13,14] The role of newer pulmonary vasodilators such as bosentan and sildenafil in patients with acute cor pulmonale is unclear.

Rescue therapies such as extracorporeal membrane oxygenation or pumpless extracorporeal lung assist devices may be of benefit in selected cases when used early.[15,16] Data on noninvasive mechanical ventilation in immunologic lung disease is limited. Two small studies show that noninvasive ventilation can be used to avoid intubation and risk for ventilator-associated pneumonia with comparable or better short-term survival.[17,18]

IDIOPATHIC PULMONARY FIBROSIS

Idiopathic pulmonary fibrosis is a disorder of unknown cause characterized by inflammation of the lower respiratory tract that usually leads to irreversible scarring. Current and former smokers are at increased risk, and there may be an inherited susceptibility to develop this disease.[19-21] IPF most commonly presents as an outpatient illness with the insidious onset of exertional dyspnea and cough. On examination of the lungs, coarse crackles are found and clubbing of the fingers is characteristic.[21] Chest radiographs may show a spectrum of findings from peripheral reticular densities to end-stage honeycombed lung.[21] Alveolar infiltrates are unusual unless the patient has a concurrent lung cancer, pneumonia, or heart disease. The lung CT findings most closely associated with a pathologic diagnosis of IPF are lower-lung honeycombing and upper-lung irregular lines.[22] The histologic examination of IPF reveals *usual interstitial pneumonitis,* which is characterized by inflammation, fibroblastic foci, areas of fibrosis, and remodeling of the lung parenchyma. The pulmonary fibrosis appears to follow collapse of involved alveoli.

Death in patients with IPF is most often directly attributable to progression of the underlying disease, even when the disease is only of moderate severity.[21,23] Nevertheless, the clinician should seek treatable complicating conditions before making the difficult decision to withhold mechanical ventilatory support. Other causes of respiratory failure in IPF include infection, congestive heart failure, bronchogenic carcinoma, pulmonary embolism, and pneumothorax. Left ventricular failure is often found in association with IPF. These patients often have many of the risk factors (e.g., smoking, hyperlipidemia) that are associated with the development of atherosclerosis. For this reason, left ventricular failure may result from ischemic heart disease. Two other factors that may contribute to left ventricular failure in these individuals are systemic arterial hypertension and right ventricular failure. Hypoxemia may exacerbate these effects. A search for potentially treatable left ventricular failure should be considered in the deteriorating IPF patient.

Patients with IPF have about a 14-fold excess risk of developing lung cancer.[24] These malignancies are difficult to detect on an already abnormal chest radiograph and often cause rapid deterioration in the IPF patient. Treatment options for malignancy are often limited by poor pulmonary reserve. However, the diagnosis of lung cancer may greatly alter therapeutic planning. Furthermore, relieving airway obstruction and postobstructive infection may significantly palliate dyspnea.

Pulmonary embolism can also cause rapid deterioration and respiratory failure in IPF patients. Ventilation/perfusion scans often reveal nonsegmental perfusion defects and inhomogeneous areas of poor ventilation as a result of the IPF alone, so the utility of these scans in diagnosing pulmonary emboli is limited.[25] Pulmonary angiography or helical CT scanning should be considered if it can be performed safely.[25] We recommend empiric long-term anticoagulation for individuals with advanced IPF and severe pulmonary hypertension who are suspected of having pulmonary embolism but for whom a diagnostic evaluation is not feasible.[26]

Pulmonary infection is difficult to document in patients with end-stage IPF and is a frequent cause of rapid decline. Many end-stage patients who die of respiratory failure have an infection as the inciting event. Only subtle changes on the chest radiograph are present in most of these patients. CT scanning may show alveolar infiltrates. Strong consideration should be given to the use of antibiotics in all IPF patients who suffer an acute respiratory decline. Bronchoalveolar lavage (BAL) or protected brush specimens from the distal airway may identify specific bacterial pathogens. Often the organism is not identified, and broad-spectrum antibiotics are used. The end-stage fibrotic lung has grossly distorted airways and multiple cystic airspaces, so this empiric coverage should be designed to also cover anaerobic organisms. In our experience, long courses of antibiotics are frequently required to adequately treat respiratory infections in IPF. We use 10 to 14 days of intravenous antibiotics followed by a prolonged course of oral therapy (6 to 12 weeks) aimed at treating anaerobic organisms.

An important factor to consider in patients with advanced IPF who develop respiratory failure is that this disease is largely irreversible. Although many exciting new therapies are under investigation, current treatments are largely ineffective in reversing the decline in lung function.[27-29] Most patients with IPF who are in respiratory failure do not respond to corticosteroid therapy.[30] Cytotoxic therapy, such as cyclophosphamide, azathioprine, or cyclosporine, has not been shown to alter survival.[31,32] Mortality rate after ICU admission is high, raising the question of appropriateness of mechanical ventilation in most cases, with the exception of perioperative support or as a bridge to lung transplantation.[31,33-35] In a review of nine studies examining 135 patients with IPF ventilated in the ICU, the aggregate hospital mortality rate was 87% and the mortality rate within 3 months after discharge was 94%.[36] If patients are young, have early disease, or may be diagnosed with interstitial lung disease other than IPF, an open lung biopsy should be considered to exclude alternative treatable diseases. Recently, lung transplantation has become a viable option for some patients with end-stage IPF. It is imperative that physicians caring for these patients familiarize themselves with the referral protocols and policies of their respective regional transplant centers.

HAMMAN-RICH SYNDROME

Hamman-Rich syndrome, more recently called *acute interstitial pneumonia* (AIP), is a rapidly progressive interstitial pneumonia of unknown cause first described by Hamman and Rich.[37] The mean age of patients is 50 to 60 years, with a broad range and perhaps an increased risk for men.[37,38] The patients often describe a prodromal viral-like respiratory illness typically followed by subacute progressive dyspnea, fever, and nonproductive cough.

AIP usually evolves over 1 to 3 months, and in some instances, it appears within 1 to 2 weeks after the onset of symptoms. Signs of right-sided heart failure may exist, and diffuse or basilar crackles may be found on auscultation of the lung. Diffuse, bilateral interstitial infiltrates are characteristic on chest radiograph. The findings on CT scan include diffuse, patchy alveolar ground glass infiltrates and pleural effusion in one third of the cases.[39] Honeycombing may be present in subacute cases. Laboratory studies may show a leukocytosis with neutrophilia. Hypoxemia may be profound. Pulmonary function tests in patients without respiratory failure show a restrictive defect, generally without evidence of airway obstruction.[38]

For many years experts believed that this disease was simply a rapidly progressive form of IPF; now this disease is felt to be more related to ARDS. The pathologic features of AIP are characterized by diffuse, active fibrosis, with proliferating fibroblasts and minimal collagen. These findings appear acute and relatively uniform in age and resemble the organizing stage of diffuse alveolar damage as seen in ARDS.[40]

The prognosis of acute interstitial pneumonitis is poor, with only about a 40% short-term survival rate. Although the short-term mortality rate is similar to that for acute exacerbation of IPF, AIP survivors have near complete recovery of lung function in contrast to those with IPF.[41,42] Supportive care may involve ventilatory support. Antibiotics to treat possible underlying infection and corticosteroids to treat inflammation have been used in many cases, but the efficacy of these treatments is not proved.[38] In one small series, early efforts to exclude infection combined with lung-protective ventilation and high-dose corticosteroid therapy led to success in 8 of 10 patients.[43] We recommend rigorous exclusion of an infectious cause including open lung biopsy, if necessary, before considering any immunosuppressive therapy.

ALVEOLAR HEMORRHAGE SYNDROMES

Perhaps the most striking immunologically mediated lung diseases are those that present with alveolar hemorrhage. These disorders require prompt diagnosis and management. We limit our comments here to the disorders that most commonly present as alveolar hemorrhage: Goodpasture's syndrome, Wegener's granulomatosis (WG), microscopic polyangiitis (MPA), catastrophic antiphospholipid syndrome (CAPS), systemic lupus erythematosus (SLE), and idiopathic pulmonary hemosiderosis. Box 49.1 provides a more complete list of disorders that can lead to alveolar hemorrhage.

An essential goal of managing patients with alveolar hemorrhage is prompt diagnosis of the underlying disorder (Fig. 49.1). The first step is to document alveolar hemorrhage. The classic triad of hemoptysis, anemia, and diffuse infiltrates on chest radiograph strongly suggests alveolar hemorrhage, yet many patients with significant alveolar hemorrhage do not have hemoptysis.[44] Consequently, the absence of hemoptysis does not exclude the presence of alveolar hemorrhage. Thus, diffuse pulmonary infiltrates, respiratory distress, and anemia associated with clinical evidence of glomerulonephritis or other conditions associated with vasculitis should arouse suspicion for alveolar hemorrhage, even in the absence of hemoptysis.

Before any specific therapy is instituted, it is important to document the presence of alveolar hemorrhage. Other processes that result in diffuse alveolar filling must be excluded, such as inflammatory exudate from infection, cardiogenic pulmonary edema, and ARDS. In addition, one should

Box 49.1 Causes of Immune/Idiopathic Alveolar Hemorrhage

Goodpasture's syndrome
Wegener's granulomatosis
Other systemic vasculitides/collagen
Vascular diseases
  Microscopic polyangiitis
  Catastrophic antiphospholipid antibody syndrome
  Systemic lupus erythematosus
  Schönlein-Henoch purpura
  Behçet's disease
  Essential mixed cryoglobulinemia
  Rheumatoid arthritis
  Progressive systemic sclerosis
  Mixed connective tissue disease
Alveolar hemorrhage and glomerulonephritis unrelated to Goodpasture's syndrome, vasculitis, or collagen vascular disease*
Thrombotic thrombocytopenic purpura
Membranoproliferative glomerulonephritis
Immunoglobulin A nephropathy
Diffuse endocapillary proliferative glomerulonephritis
Focal proliferative glomerulonephritis
Alveolar hemorrhage resulting from drugs or chemicals
  D-Penicillamine
  Trimellitic anhydride
  Isocyanates
  Nitrofurantoin
  Amiodarone
  Propylthiouracil
  Infliximab
Idiopathic pulmonary hemosiderosis

*Idiopathic alveolar hemorrhage with pauci-immune necrotizing or crescentic glomerulonephritis is classified as nonspecific systemic vasculitis (presumptive).

Adapted from Leatherman JW: Diffuse alveolar hemorrhage in immune and idiopathic disorders. In Lynch JP III, De Remee R (eds): Immunologically Mediated Pulmonary Diseases. Philadelphia, JB Lippincott, 1991.

exclude hemorrhage from airway sources such as cancer, bronchitis, bronchiectasis, or excessive anticoagulation or an endogenous coagulation defect. Perhaps the most valuable test for documenting alveolar hemorrhage is bronchoscopy with BAL. Blood-tinged lavage fluid or frank blood in the airways is usually present.[45] Another test that can be used involves staining alveolar macrophages retrieved by lavage for hemosiderin. Normal individuals will have few hemosiderin-laden macrophages in BAL, but the intensity of staining and percentage of cells staining positive have been found to be predictive of alveolar hemorrhage.[46,47] We feel, however, that this test is of questionable clinical value. If patients have sufficient acute bleeding to cause infiltrates on chest radiograph, this should be seen easily in the lavage fluid. If the only evidence for hemorrhage is the presence of hemosiderin-laden macrophages, we would propose that the acute infiltrates are the result of another cause. Similarly, the negative predictive value of this test can be questioned because it may take up to 48 hours for intracellular hemosiderin accumulation after an acute bleed.[48] Documentation of an elevated diffusion capacity for carbon monoxide (DLCO) is also a means of evaluating for alveolar hemorrhage but is not practical during active bleeding or critical illness.[49,50] Bowley and coworkers demonstrated the usefulness of this measure as a sensitive index of recurrent alveolar hemorrhage in patients undergoing treatment.[50]

Treatment consists of supportive care including mechanical ventilation, prevention of infections and organ damage and immunosuppressive therapy directed at the underlying process. Rescue therapies such as recombinant factor VIIa and extracorporeal membrane oxygenation have been reported to be successful in anecdotal cases of refractory alveolar hemorrhage.[51-55] Survival following alveolar hemorrhage due to immunologic lung disease tends to be better compared to patients with alveolar hemorrhage from thrombocytopenia or sepsis.[56]

GOODPASTURE'S SYNDROME

Goodpasture's syndrome accounts for 20% to 30% of the cases of alveolar hemorrhage.[57] This disease is a classic pulmonary-renal syndrome with a high mortality rate from alveolar hemorrhage or renal failure if untreated. Anti–basement membrane antibody is a universal finding in this disease. Antibody deposition along the glomerular basement membrane (GBM) undoubtedly contributes to the renal pathologic examination of this disease; however, other cofactors, in addition to anti-GBM antibody, may be necessary for alveolar hemorrhage to develop. A higher incidence of alveolar hemorrhage has been reported in smokers with anti-GBM antibody disease.[58] Experimental studies also showed that exposure to 100% oxygen in animals with circulating anti–basement membrane antibody resulted in alveolar hemorrhage, whereas unexposed animals did not develop lung disease.[59] Genetic studies have shown a strong association with HLA-DRB alleles.[60,61]

A 2:1 male-female ratio exists with a median age of 21 years in patients with Goodpasture's syndrome.[62,63] Alveolar hemorrhage is the most common presentation of Goodpasture's syndrome. Evidence of renal involvement is usually present; however, some patients may only have microscopic hematuria.[57] Untreated, Goodpasture's syndrome carries a mortality rate approaching 100%, the cause of death being equally divided between uremia and alveolar hemorrhage.[63] With prompt dialysis, plasma exchange, and immunosuppression, however, the acute mortality rate of the disease is about 10%, with diffuse alveolar hemorrhage being the most common cause of early death.[64]

The evaluation of patients suspected of having Goodpasture's syndrome should include confirmation of alveolar hemorrhage, evaluation for renal disease, and testing for anti–basement membrane antibody. Circulating anti–basement membrane antibody can be demonstrated in more than 95% of patients through radioimmunoassay or enzyme-linked immunosorbent assay (ELISA).[65] Kidney biopsy should also be considered to confirm the diagnosis and to document the extent of glomerular loss. The characteristic glomerular lesion shows strong linear deposition of immunoglobulin G (IgG) along glomerular capillaries.[57] Other histologic features include segmental, necrotizing, crescentic glomerulonephritis indistinguishable from that found in other forms of vasculitis. Walker and colleagues[66] demonstrated that patients with greater than 85% crescents

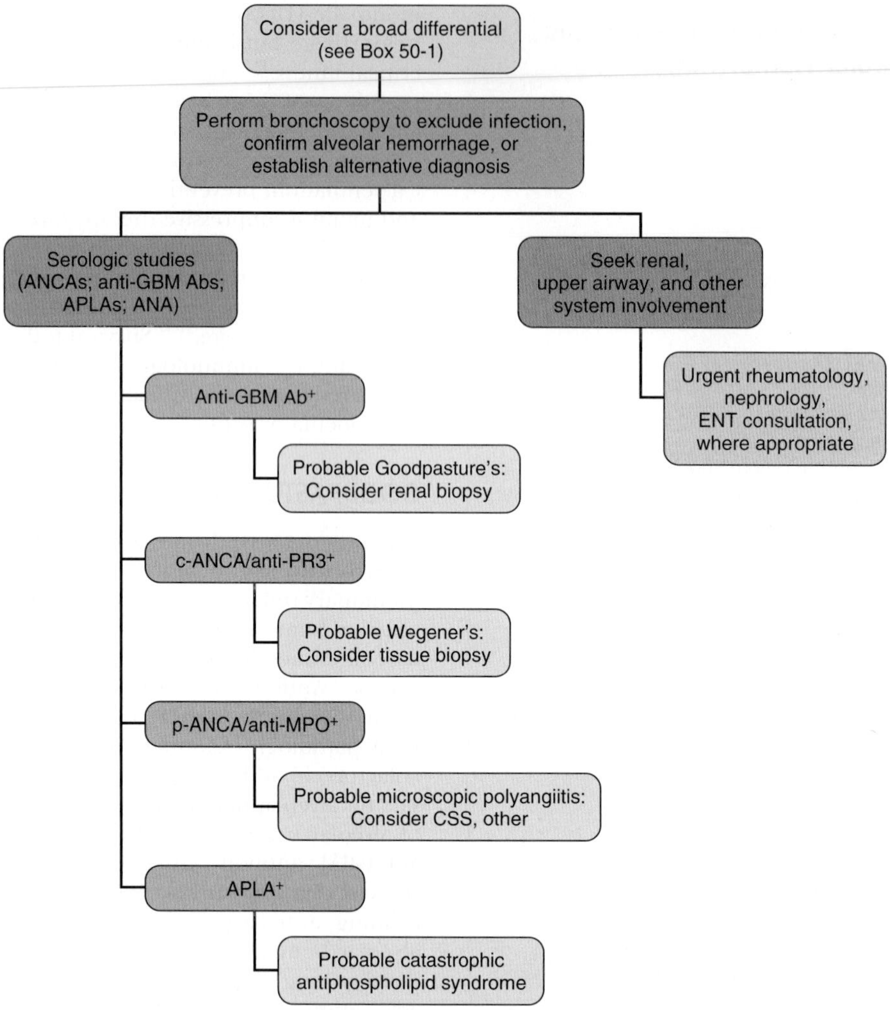

Figure 49.1 Diagnosis and management of alveolar hemorrhage syndromes. ANA, antinuclear antibodies; ANCA, antineutrophil cytoplasmic antibody; anti-GBM Abs, anti–glomerular basement membrane antibodies; anti-MPO, antimyeloperoxidase antibodies; anti-PR3, antiproteinase antibodies; APLAs, antiphospholipid antibodies; CSS, Churg-Strauss syndrome; ENT, ear, nose, and throat.

on biopsy were significantly less likely to regain renal function. Lung biopsy is rarely necessary and often nonspecific.

Treatment consists of dialysis, plasma exchange, and immunosuppressive therapy. Immunosuppression usually includes both cyclophosphamide and corticosteroids.[67] Dialysis should be performed early to reverse uremic platelet dysfunction and to prevent fluid overload because both factors may perpetuate alveolar hemorrhage. Mechanical ventilation may be necessary to provide respiratory support, as well as to facilitate clearing blood from the airways. When mechanical ventilatory support is used, efforts should be made to select lung-protective tidal volumes and to minimize the fraction of inspired oxygen. We also aggressively treat possible respiratory infection because it may precipitate and perpetuate alveolar hemorrhage. If the patient has received drugs that impair platelet function, such as aspirin, we also administer platelets in cases of life-threatening hemorrhage. Alveolar hemorrhage generally responds within 1 to 3 days to this treatment.[68] In refractory cases, there has been anecdotal response to mycophenolate or to anti-CD20 antibody. Once the patient has recovered, the importance of maintenance immunosuppression in preventing recurrent alveolar hemorrhage cannot be overemphasized.[57,68,69]

WEGENER'S GRANULOMATOSIS

Another form of vasculitis that commonly presents as alveolar hemorrhage is WG. This disorder is characterized by a granulomatous vasculitis involving the upper and lower airways and is associated with rapidly progressive renal failure. WG represented 15% of the cases of alveolar hemorrhage in a series reported by Leatherman.[57] The incidence of pulmonary hemorrhage in this disorder is reported to vary between 12% and 30%.[70,71] Clinical findings that may suggest a diagnosis of WG include nodules visible on a chest radiograph and evidence of upper airway involvement including chronic otitis media, sinusitis, nasal septal perforation, and tracheal stenosis.[72] Eye involvement with either proptosis or extraocular muscle entrapment may occur.[72] Skin lesions may include petechiae, palpable purpura, ulcers, vesicles, papules, and subcutaneous nodules.[70] Musculoskeletal findings include myalgias, arthralgias, and pauciarticular or migratory arthritis. Neurologic manifestations include sensorineural deafness, mononeuritis multiplex, and cranial nerve palsies.[70,72] Subglottic tracheal stenosis or obstruction can occur in these patients and should be considered before endotracheal intubation is undertaken. In up to 10% of patients, tracheostomy may be required to manage the airway at some time during the course of their illness.[72]

Laboratory findings in WG include leukocytosis, anemia, thrombocytosis, and an elevated erythrocyte sedimentation rate. A valuable laboratory test is the antineutrophil cytoplasmic antibody (ANCA), which detects IgG directed at a variety of neutrophil and monocyte antigens. Clinically important ANCAs are of two types: antiproteinase 3 antibodies (anti-PR3) and antimyeloperoxidase antibodies (anti-MPO). When serum containing these antibodies is applied to neutrophils and stained by indirect immunofluorescence, anti-PR3 produces a cytoplasmic pattern of staining (c-ANCA), whereas anti-MPO produces a perinuclear or nuclear pattern (p-ANCA). Both anti-PR3 (seen almost exclusively in WG) and anti-MPO (which may be seen in pauci-immune rapidly progressive glomerulonephritis, Churg-Strauss syndrome, and MPA) can be measured more directly by ELISA. The sensitivity of ANCA has been reported to be 80% to 96% in patients with active generalized (e.g., having renal involvement) WG, and generally these patients have both c-ANCA and anti-PR3 positivity. In the ANCA-associated systemic vasculitides, which include WG, alveolar hemorrhage has been found in patients who have tested positive for either c-ANCA or p-ANCA (see "Microscopic Polyangiitis" later). More recently, the presence of an immunoglobulin M (IgM) isotype of ANCA has been strongly associated with alveolar hemorrhage; conversely, patients lacking IgM ANCA may have a low risk for alveolar hemorrhage.[73] Frequently the diagnosis of WG relies on tissue examination. Biopsies of upper airway lesions are probably acceptable in nonemergent situations when diagnosis can be delayed. However, in the case of severe alveolar hemorrhage, there is frequently an emergent need for diagnosis so that effective treatment can be instituted. An open lung biopsy often provides the diagnosis. Potential infectious causes, especially mycobacterial and fungal pathogens, can also be excluded. Fauci and coworkers have developed a scheme of major and minor criteria for WG on the basis of histologic diagnosis. Three major pathologic manifestations were identified including parenchymal necrosis, vasculitis, and granulomatous inflammation[74]; however, in 18% of biopsies, less distinctive histologic features were the predominant findings. If definitive tissue biopsy cannot be obtained, a WG with alveolar hemorrhage diagnosis should be based on the histologic finding of a small vessel vasculitis or crescentic glomerulonephritis, together with compelling clinical evidence of WG consisting of cavitary pulmonary nodules or characteristic upper airway involvement.[57] Moreover, the presence of a positive c-ANCA test can help to confirm the diagnosis.

The recommended treatment for alveolar hemorrhage resulting from WG includes high-dose corticosteroids and cyclophosphamide.[57,75] We recommend that patients who are critically ill receive intravenous methylprednisolone at doses up to 1 g daily for the first 3 days in addition to cyclophosphamide at 3 to 5 mg/kg for 3 to 5 days. After this period, the prednisone dosage is reduced to 1 mg/kg/day and cyclophosphamide is continued at 1.5 mg/kg/day. Most patients respond favorably to this regimen, but the mortality rate remains substantial, often because of renal failure or sepsis. Plasma exchange or intravenous immunoglobulin may be useful in patients with life-threatening diffuse alveolar hemorrhage or when disease persists despite corticosteroids and cyclophosphamide.[76] Other rescue therapies include rituxan,[77] trimethoprim-sulfamethoxazole, anti–tumor necrosis factor antibodies, and antilymphocyte antibodies. The supportive measures described earlier for alveolar hemorrhage in Goodpasture's syndrome also apply to this disease.

MICROSCOPIC POLYANGIITIS

Microscopic polyangiitis is a systemic, small-vessel vasculitis. Symptoms may begin subtly with weeks to months of fever, weight loss, malaise, and myalgias. ICU admission is often precipitated by life-threatening diffuse alveolar hemorrhage, and MPA is probably the most common vasculitis to present this way. Renal failure caused by crescentic, rapidly progressive, focal segmental necrotizing glomerulonephritis can predate ICU admission or be recognized concurrently but eventually develops in nearly all cases without treatment. Joint and skin manifestations are occasionally seen, as well as peripheral nerve and gastrointestinal involvement. Most patients will have positive ANCA with specificity for MPO (p-ANCA), although some will be c-ANCA positive. Some patients initially suspected of having MPA will ultimately develop granulomatous upper airway disease, and the diagnosis is changed to WG.

Treatment requires high-dose corticosteroids and cyclophosphamide in the same doses as for WG. Intravenous immunoglobulin may be effective in difficult cases. Factor VIIa has also been tried, and the rescue therapies described earlier for WG may also be effective. For the patient with respiratory failure caused by alveolar hemorrhage, ventilator guidelines for ALI/ARDS should be followed. Once a patient survives the acute alveolar hemorrhage, there are reasonable prospects for long-term survival, although this depends to a large degree on whether renal function recovers. Pulmonary fibrosis is often present before, during, and after the initial diagnosis of MPA.[78]

CATASTROPHIC ANTIPHOSPHOLIPID SYNDROME

The term *antiphospholipid syndrome* was coined to describe patients with systemic thrombosis or recurrent fetal loss having increased antiphospholipid antibodies in the circulation. A subset presenting with widespread vascular thrombosis and a fulminating clinical course, often involving respiratory failure, was subsequently called the *catastrophic antiphospholipid syndrome* (CAPS).[79] This syndrome can occur in those without a recognized rheumatologic disease but also in those with SLE or other diseases.

CAPS generally has been considered a noninflammatory thrombotic disease leading to widespread ischemia and necrosis, producing multiorgan failure and death. More recently, however, cases of alveolar hemorrhage have been described in the setting of antiphospholipid syndrome in which thrombosis was not evident clinically or pathologically. These authors proposed that a nonthrombotic mechanism for pulmonary capillaritis and alveolar hemorrhage should be sought.[80]

Infections, trauma, procedures, drugs, and malignancy have been implicated as precipitating factors. Clinically there is often evidence of widespread arterial and venous occlusions. The renal, pulmonary, and central nervous systems are most often affected. Multiple pulmonary manifestations have been reported including pulmonary thromboembolism, pulmonary hypertension, and ALI in addition to diffuse alveolar hemorrhage. Serologic findings include elevated titers of anticardiolipin antibody or the lupus anticoagulant. Increased β_2-glycoprotein I has been linked to CAPS.[81]

Treatment generally involves immunosuppression along the lines of treatment for other immune alveolar hemorrhage syndromes. Plasmapheresis may be effective.[82] The role for anticoagulation in the acute setting of alveolar hemorrhage is uncertain, but we recommend first establishing control of bleeding with immunosuppressive therapy and plasmapheresis and then later instituting antithrombotic treatment.

SYSTEMIC LUPUS ERYTHEMATOSUS

In patients with SLE, a wide variety of lung lesions are found. Histologic evidence of alveolar hemorrhage can be found in 40% of patients at autopsy.[83] Massive alveolar hemorrhage is uncommon, being reported in only 5% of patients in one series of 99 patients with SLE and lung involvement.[84] Although massive alveolar hemorrhage may be the presenting manifestation of SLE, this is uncommon.[85,86] The clinical presentation of alveolar hemorrhage in SLE is similar to that in other alveolar hemorrhage syndromes; however, fever as high as 39° C to 40° C may be a prominent feature.[84] At the time of alveolar hemorrhage, patients often manifest other typical clinical findings of SLE, particularly nephritis, highlighting the systemic nature of this disease.[87]

The cause of alveolar hemorrhage in SLE is not entirely clear. In some patients, antiphospholipid antibodies, as discussed earlier, may play a role.[88] Pathologic studies of open lung biopsies have not always demonstrated immune complex deposition.[83,86] Patients with SLE often show a microscopic angiitis on biopsy.[85,87] Considerable clinical overlap between the alveolar hemorrhage syndrome and acute lupus pneumonitis exists.[83,87] Because treatment of both lesions is similar, we recommend separating these two pulmonary manifestations on clinical grounds without the need for open lung biopsy, as long as infection has been adequately excluded.

Infection is the most important factor to exclude in diagnosing alveolar hemorrhage in the patient with SLE. At least half of the patients with SLE who present with infiltrates should be expected to have an infectious cause.[83] Because many of these patients are receiving immunosuppressive therapy and because SLE is associated with impaired cellular immunity, the differential diagnosis for infectious agents is broad and includes bacterial, fungal, mycobacterial, viral, and parasitic pathogens. Bronchoscopy with lavage and transbronchial biopsies are the logical procedures used to search for an infectious cause. Open lung biopsy may be necessary in some cases.

Mortality rate from SLE-associated alveolar hemorrhage is variable in small series, ranging from about 20% to more than 85%.[57,86,87] Many patients develop respiratory failure, and the need for mechanical ventilation is associated with an increased mortality risk.[87] This high risk for respiratory failure is multifactorial, with contributions from alveolar hemorrhage, a high prevalence of underlying atelectasis, and diaphragmatic weakness.[89,90] We recommend treating these patients with both high-dose corticosteroids and cyclophosphamide in a regimen similar to that used for WG.

IDIOPATHIC PULMONARY HEMOSIDEROSIS

The diagnosis of idiopathic pulmonary hemosiderosis is, by definition, one of exclusion. The syndrome is typically an illness that presents in infancy or childhood.[91] The disease is characterized by recurrent episodes of alveolar hemorrhage, although often these episodes may be subclinical.[92] There have been familial clusters of cases.[93,94] Some cases of unexplained alveolar hemorrhage with onset during adulthood have been reported. The specific treatment of this illness is not clear. Most patients do well during the acute episode with supportive care alone, but there may be a short-term benefit from corticosteroid therapy. Long-term corticosteroid treatment has been described in some cases.

CRYPTOGENIC ORGANIZING PNEUMONIA

Cryptogenic organizing pneumonia (COP), also termed *idiopathic bronchiolitis obliterans with organizing pneumonia* (BOOP), frequently presents as an acute illness with respiratory failure. This disease often responds well to therapy without residual respiratory deficit, if timely diagnosis and treatment are undertaken. COP presents throughout adult life and shows no particular demographic associations.[95] The presenting symptoms include cough, dyspnea, or both in more than two thirds of cases. Flulike symptoms are present in 14%, and patients usually present with subacute symptoms within 3 months.[96,97] Examination of the lung reveals dry crackles in 50% to 75% of cases. Wheezing and finger clubbing are rarely seen. Up to 12% of patients can be expected to present with a normal physical examination.

The chest radiograph most often shows patchy alveolar infiltrates scattered throughout all lung fields. Interstitial infiltrates and nodular densities may be seen.[97] Some reports suggest that interstitial densities on chest radiograph may be associated with a worse prognosis.[98] High-resolution computed tomography (HRCT) of the chest shows predominantly subpleural or peribronchial areas of airspace consolidation, small nodules, or both in almost all cases.[99] These changes are not pathognomonic for COP, but the HRCT images may be useful for directing biopsies to abnormal areas. The results of physiologic testing characteristically reveal a restrictive ventilatory defect with reduced lung volumes. Obstructive flow defects are seen only in smokers.[97] The DLCO is frequently abnormal, out of proportion to the other pulmonary function tests.[96] Resting and exercise-induced hypoxemia are almost always present.

BAL usually shows increased cellularity. An increased percentage of lymphocytes, neutrophils, or eosinophils may exist, but this finding does not help distinguish COP from other lung diseases.[97] The diagnosis is difficult to make from a transbronchial lung biopsy because the tissue samples obtained are often not large enough.[96] Transbronchial biopsy is, however, useful to rule out other disorders, especially infections. The gold standard for diagnosis is the open lung biopsy.[96] Findings include patchy areas of intraluminal polyps of granulation tissue and constrictive bronchiolitis, organizing inflammation within the alveolar ducts, interstitial mononuclear cell infiltrate of variable density, alveolar space foam cells, and the absence of honeycombing or extensive interstitial fibrosis.[100]

COP may be associated with systemic diseases, certain inhalational exposures, or a drug reaction. A viral cause is hypothesized for at least a proportion of the cases of idiopathic COP.[101] An association between COP and connective tissue diseases, especially rheumatoid arthritis (RA), exists.[102] COP has also been reported in association with human immunodeficiency virus infection, radiation therapy, and smoking freebase cocaine.[103-105] Thus, it appears that COP may appear secondary to a variety of pulmonary insults and may represent an aberrant healing process in the distal airspace.

The mortality rate of COP is about 5%.[96] Typically, prednisone is used to treat this disease at a dose of 1 mg/kg/day. For the critically ill patient in the ICU, higher doses of parenteral corticosteroids can be used. Additional immunosuppression with cyclophosphamide is usually not required in COP and is associated with a high rate of complications.[106,107] When respiratory failure develops, the ventilatory management of COP is similar to that in patients with IPF, except that chronic pulmonary hypertension and right ventricular failure are less of a problem.

CONNECTIVE TISSUE DISEASES

Rheumatologic disorders affect the lungs in a variety of ways. Alveolar hemorrhage is discussed earlier. Interstitial fibrosis, vasculitis, pulmonary hypertension, and respiratory muscle weakness are mechanisms by which the patient with connective tissue disease may develop respiratory failure. In a recent study of 66 patients with connective tissue disease and respiratory failure, the most common underlying diagnoses were SLE, RA, and vasculitis.[108] Pneumonia was the leading cause of respiratory failure, followed by pulmonary edema and alveolar hemorrhage. The hospital mortality rate in this cohort was 62%. This section focuses on those rheumatologic disorders most likely to be encountered in an ICU.

LUPUS PNEUMONITIS

SLE is a systemic disorder characterized by widespread inflammation of serosal surfaces, skin, connective tissues, kidney, lung, and other organ systems. The characteristic finding of SLE is the presence of circulating autoantibodies, particularly antinuclear antibodies, and immune complexes. Pleuropulmonary involvement is common.[109] For the purposes of this discussion, we define *lupus pneumonitis* as any acute presentation of respiratory disease and pulmonary infiltrates, associated with SLE, that is neither infection nor frank alveolar hemorrhage (see previous discussion). Matthay found acute presentation of lung disease in 11% of patients hospitalized for SLE.[110] In 50% of these patients, lupus pneumonitis was the presenting manifestation of SLE, which is distinctly unusual in SLE-associated alveolar hemorrhage.[87]

The patients typically have dyspnea, cough, and pleuritic chest pain. Fever and tachypnea are also frequently present. The chest radiograph characteristically shows bilateral basilar or diffuse infiltrates, but unilateral infiltrates may be present and atelectasis may be a prominent feature. An accompanying pleural effusion is often present.[109-111] Cyanosis and basilar rales are often found on physical examination. The arterial blood gas frequently shows severe hypoxemia. Histopathologic findings on open lung biopsy are variable and may include areas of desquamative or unusual interstitial pneumonia, COP, and microscopic alveolar hemorrhage. Pulmonary infarction is associated with anticardiolipin antibody, and focal atelectasis from respiratory muscle weakness can be seen.[111-113] The rapidity of clinical deterioration can be alarming. The mortality rate for patients who present with the characteristic clinical features of lupus pneumonitis can be up to 50% despite treatment.[110,113] The treatment of these patients usually includes high-dose corticosteroids. Cyclophosphamide and azathioprine have been used in cases of progressive disease.[111-113] In patients with acute, severe neurologic lupus, cyclophosphamide was more effective than high-dose corticosteroids.[114] We recommend the initial use of both cyclophosphamide and high-dose corticosteroids in a regimen similar to that used to treat vasculitis (see previous discussion). Before initiating immunosuppressive therapy, it is essential to exclude infection with bronchoscopy or open lung biopsy. Maintaining a high suspicion for infection in the patient who is unresponsive to immunosuppression or who shows clinical deterioration despite treatment is also important.

RHEUMATOID ARTHRITIS

RA is a disease of subacute and chronic inflammation characterized by erosive arthritis that is usually symmetrical, affecting mainly the peripheral joints. A positive rheumatoid factor is present in at least 75% of cases. RA, like SLE, has a variety of associated pleuropulmonary manifestations that can present during the course of illness.[109] It is important for the intensivist to recognize the spectrum of lung disease associated with RA because many of the findings on chest radiograph can be ascribed to relatively benign disease.[115] Moreover, even moderately severe chronic pulmonary disease may go undetected because it is obscured by musculoskeletal limitations. Two of the more common forms of rheumatoid involvement that present with severe lung disease are interstitial fibrosis and COP.

Interstitial fibrosis is a relatively common finding in patients who have RA. In the overwhelming majority of patients, this is an incidental finding and is asymptomatic.[116]

The clinical course of RA-associated interstitial lung disease is typically much more benign than that seen in IPF; however, a subset of patients presents with fulminant interstitial lung disease associated with RA.[117] Like IPF, the physical examination frequently shows Velcro-like rales, and the chest radiograph in the more severe cases typically shows diffuse bilateral reticular or reticulonodular infiltrates.[117]

Patients with RA are generally admitted to the ICU with sepsis rather than complications of the arthritis itself.[118] Most of these patients have been treated previously with corticosteroids or other immunosuppressive regimens. Airway management may be particularly challenging because many RA patients have limited mouth opening, atlantoaxial instability, or cricoarytenoid arthritis. Fiberoptic intubation is a necessary skill for safely managing patients with RA and ventilatory failure.

RA is the most common connective tissue disease to present with COP. This illness typically presents with a subacute onset of dyspnea. The presentation and pathologic features of COP associated with RA are indistinguishable from those of idiopathic COP.[119] Diagnosis usually requires an open lung biopsy to define the histologic features. In a few patients the diagnosis is made by transbronchial biopsy. Bronchoscopy should be undertaken before immunosuppressive therapy to rule out infection. Treatment of this disorder is identical to the treatment of COP, but the prognosis for RA-associated COP appears to be worse.[120] For this reason, we consider cyclophosphamide earlier to treat this disease when it does not respond rapidly to corticosteroids.

PROGRESSIVE SYSTEMIC SCLEROSIS

Progressive systemic sclerosis (PSS) and the related disorder, the CREST (calcinosis, Raynaud's phenomenon, esophageal dysmotility, sclerodactyly, telangiectasis) syndrome, are disorders characterized by fibrosing inflammation of the skin with variable visceral involvement. Patients with PSS and CREST develop interstitial lung disease that histopathologically resembles the lung fibrosis associated with RA and IPF.[121] The prevalence of pulmonary fibrosis detected by chest radiograph is approximately 36% in PSS and 20% in CREST.[122] The clinical presentation is indistinguishable from other secondary causes of pulmonary fibrosis. Many of these patients also have chronic aspiration resulting from esophageal dysfunction, which can precipitate and exacerbate pulmonary inflammation and fibrosis.[123]

The diagnosis of lung disease in PSS and CREST usually does not require an open lung biopsy. Pulmonary function tests characteristically reveal a restrictive ventilatory defect with low lung volumes.[124] The detection of circulating autoantibodies may be helpful in diagnosing these diseases.[109] Anticentromere antibody presence is associated with a lower incidence of pulmonary fibrosis in CREST.[125,126] Anti-SCL-70 antibody presence is associated with a higher incidence of pulmonary fibrosis.[127] Bronchoscopy can be used to evaluate for an infectious process and to look for vegetable matter or lipid-laden macrophages, which may suggest chronic aspiration. Treatment of interstitial lung disease associated with PSS or CREST with cyclophosphamide has been shown to be effective in the National Institutes of Health Scleroderma Lung Study by improving physiology, relieving dyspnea, and enhancing quality of life. Nevertheless, the prognosis remains poor. The role of steroids is unproved.

Pulmonary hypertension is another common manifestation of lung involvement in PSS and the CREST syndrome. This can occur without evidence of other lung disease, but it is often associated with interstitial disease. When accompanying interstitial lung disease, pulmonary hypertension is often more prominent than one would expect from the degree of interstitial lung disease alone. The prevalence of pulmonary hypertension in PSS has been found to be about 33%. In CREST the prevalence of pulmonary hypertension is at least as high.[128] The cause of pulmonary hypertension in these disorders is not well understood. Some experts have speculated that early in the course of disease there is a period of vascular reactivity associated with Raynaud's phenomenon.[129] This period is hypothesized to be followed by a period of increased pulmonary pressures associated with local hypoxia.[130] Finally, there is vascular remodeling with intimal thickening and loss of capillary beds.[131]

The patient with pulmonary hypertension may present with exertional dyspnea or impending respiratory failure, but pulmonary hypertension may also be asymptomatic.[128] Physical findings include those features commonly associated with PSS or CREST. Findings suggestive of cor pulmonale may be present, including jugular venous distention with prominent "a" waves, loud or palpable S_2, left parasternal lift, and an S_4 gallop that increases with inspiration. Although approximately 88% specific, the physical examination is only about 63% sensitive to identifying definite pulmonary hypertension in PSS.[128] The single best marker of underlying pulmonary hypertension is a low DLCO. When the DLCO is below 40% to 55% of predicted normal values, pulmonary hypertension is likely to be present.[128,132] The sensitivity of this finding, irrespective of the presence of interstitial lung disease, is about 87% with a specificity of 88%.[128,132] The electrocardiogram may show right bundle branch block, right ventricular hypertrophy, or right atrial enlargement. Echocardiography is highly specific for pulmonary hypertension if a Doppler gradient analysis of tricuspid regurgitation suggests pulmonary hypertension.[133] The gold standard has been pulmonary artery catheterization with documentation of an elevated pulmonary artery pressure and a normal pulmonary capillary wedge pressure.

Early intervention with vasodilating agents may alter the course of pulmonary hypertension by preventing progression that is dependent on high pulmonary artery pressures or by ameliorating angiogenesis or fibrosis. Bosentan, the dual endothelin receptor inhibitor, has been found effective in clinical trials of subjects with pulmonary hypertension including those with scleroderma.[134] Other treatments such as prostanoids, endothelin receptor blockers, and sildenafil may play a role in chronic management of the patient with pulmonary hypertension. In the acute ICU setting, treatment of acute-on-chronic cor pulmonale generally involves seeking treatable precipitants, infusing rapidly acting vasoactive drugs such as dobutamine, and giving short-acting pulmonary vasodilators such as inhaled nitric oxide or inhaled prostacyclin. In mechanically ventilated patients, tidal volumes should be limited to reduce the potential for superimposing ALI.

HYPERSENSITIVITY PNEUMONITIS

Hypersensitivity pneumonitis, in the majority of cases, does not result in an illness that requires critical care management. The cases that do present acutely are important to identify because these patients respond well to treatment. Furthermore, identifying an inciting exposure can prevent serious relapse or progression to chronic lung disease. Acute and subacute hypersensitivity pneumonitis are the most likely forms of this illness to result in admission to the ICU. The cause of hypersensitivity pneumonitis involves exposure to an airborne agent (Table 49.1).[135] Associated symptoms include malaise, myalgia, fever, nonproductive cough, and dyspnea.[136] The patient's history may reveal an onset of symptoms within 4 to 6 hours of the exposure to a previously sensitized antigen.[137] The physical examination frequently reveals diffuse basilar lung crackles. The chest radiograph findings vary from normal to nodular or diffuse fluffy infiltrates. A predilection for involvement of the lung bases exists.[138] This is in contrast to the upper lung zone predominance seen in chronic hypersensitivity pneumonitis. The HRCT scan in the acute phase shows diffuse airspace consolidation that evolves to a fine nodular or reticulonodular pattern over the course of days to weeks. Laboratory studies generally show a leukocytosis with a leftward shift in neutrophils. Eosinophilia is variably present, usually at low levels.[136] A polyclonal gammopathy may be present. Specific serum precipitins should be interpreted only as evidence of exposure, not as definitive evidence of disease. Rheumatoid factor may be present in as high as 50% of cases.[136,137] Pulmonary function tests usually show restrictive defects with maintenance of expiratory flow rates.[139]

BAL nearly always shows increased cellularity.[140] In the acute phase of illness, within 24 to 48 hours of the onset of symptoms, BAL typically shows a predominance of neutrophils; as the illness progresses, BAL shows a predominance of lymphocytes, up to as high as 80%.[141-143] Most of the lymphocytes are suppressor/cytotoxic (CD8, suppressor cytotoxic; CD4, helper) T cells. The presence of many foamy macrophages in the BAL is also highly suggestive of hypersensitivity pneumonitis. Histopathologic examination of transbronchial biopsies or open lung biopsy shows an inflammatory process involving both the airspaces and the interstitium. A mononuclear cell infiltration with many lymphocytes exists. Foamy histiocytes and plasma cells can frequently be seen. Interstitial, often poorly formed, noncaseating granulomas may be present.[135,139]

The differential diagnosis of acute hypersensitivity pneumonitis should include other causes of interstitial pneumonitis such as COP or AIP (Hamman-Rich syndrome). Organic dust toxic syndrome also occurs under similar environmental exposures as hypersensitivity pneumonitis but represents an acute response to inhaled bacterial and fungal cell wall products.[144] This illness tends to be more acute, resolves spontaneously, and often appears in case clusters because the response is not a specific allergic hypersensitivity. Atypical community-acquired pneumonia should also be considered in the critically ill patient. BAL and transbronchial biopsies are helpful in evaluating for an infectious cause. After the diagnosis of hypersensitivity pneumonitis is made, treatment usually includes corticosteroids and environmental counseling to avoid repeated exposure.

Table 49.1 Hypersensitivity Pneumonitis (HSP) (Extrinsic Allergic Alveolitis): Reported Associations

Disease	Source of Particles
Farmer's lung	"Moldy" hay, grain, silage
Bird fancier's, breeder's, or handler's lung	Avian droppings or feathers
Humidifier or air conditioner lung	Contaminated water in humidification and air conditioning systems
Chemical worker's lung	Polyurethane foam, varnishes, lacquer
Bagassosis	"Moldy" bagasse (sugar cane)
Malt worker's lung	Moldy barley
Mushroom worker's lung	Mushroom compost
Sequoiosis	Redwood sawdust
Maple bark disease	Maple bark
Woodworker's lung	Oak, cedar, mahogany dusts; pine and spruce pulp
Cheese washer's lung	Moldy cheese
Suberosis	Cork dust
Sauna taker's lung	Contaminated sauna water
Pituitary snuff taker's lung	Heterologous pituitary snuff
Coffee worker's lung	Coffee beans
Miller's lung	Infested wheat flour
Fish meal worker's lung	Fish meal
Furrier's lung	Animal pelts
Lycoperdonosis	*Lycoperdon* puffballs
Compost lung	Compost
Wood trimmer's disease	Contaminated wood trimmings
Thatched roof disease	Dried grasses and leaves
Streptomyces albus HSP	Contaminated fertilizer
Cephalosporium HSP	Contaminated basement (sewage)
Detergent worker's disease	Detergent
Japanese summer house HSP	House dust? Bird droppings
Potato riddler's lung	"Moldy" hay around potatoes
Tobacco worker's disease	Mold on tobacco
Hot tub lung	Mold on ceiling
Winegrower's lung	Mold on grapes
Laboratory worker's HSP	Laboratory rat
Tapwater lung	Contaminated tapwater
Pauli's HSP	Laboratory reagent
Woodman's disease	Oak and maple trees

Adapted from Richerson HB, Bernstein IL, Fink JN, et al: Guidelines for the clinical evaluation of hypersensitivity pneumonitis. Report of the Subcommittee on Hypersensitivity Pneumonitis. J Allergy Clin Immunol 1989;84:839.

DRUG-INDUCED RESPIRATORY FAILURE

Drug-induced interstitial lung disease is a common complication of a variety of drugs including antibiotics and novel molecular targeted agents. Pathologic examination can include interstitial pneumonitis (interferons, methotrexate), acute eosinophilic pneumonia (SSRIs, sulfamides), alveolar hemorrhage (abciximab, allopurinol, retinoic acid), BOOP (minocycline, nitrofurantoin), and diffuse alveolar damage (bleomycin, cyclophosphamide, gemcitabine). Diagnosis is challenging as there are no pathognomonic findings in lung biopsy. Bronchoscopy might be helpful when there is eosinophilic predominance in the lavage and a clinical correlation. We recommend empirically withholding the offending agent when a patient presents with any of abovementioned forms of lung disease unless a compelling alternative diagnosis such as an infection has been identified. This complication often resolves when the offending agent is discontinued, but steroids are commonly used in the ICU setting to hasten recovery. The pneumotox.com website is a comprehensive resource that has an ever-evolving list of drugs that have been implicated in lung disease.[145]

SUMMARY

Patients with immunologic lung diseases can present with fulminant respiratory failure requiring care in an ICU. These conditions require a high index of suspicion because they may mimic many atypical pneumonia syndromes.[146] An efficient management strategy must include a rapid diagnosis; aggressive supportive care; and, often, therapy with immunosuppressive agents. Patients with an established diagnosis may already have received potent corticosteroids or cytotoxic therapy and are at great risk of opportunistic infection that can mimic a flare of their underlying immunologic lung disease.[107,147] In addition, although in many cases immunomodulatory therapies have greatly altered the course of these diseases, treatment remains nonspecific and involves considerable toxicity. Indeed, in some series up to half of disease-related deaths can be attributed to treatment toxicity including infections and secondary malignancies.[70] Supportive management generally entails lung-protective ventilation and, in appropriate patients, surveillance for pulmonary hypertension.

KEY POINTS

- Immunologic lung disease may present with fulminant respiratory failure. Appropriate diagnosis requires a high index of suspicion combined with a thorough history and physical examination.
- Pulmonary infection may mimic, exacerbate, or result from the treatment of any immunologic lung disease. Lower airway sampling through BAL, parenchymal brushing, or biopsy may be required to exclude infectious causes.

KEY POINTS (Continued)

- Respiratory failure as a manifestation of end-stage IPF portends a grave prognosis. Looking for potentially treatable causes of impaired lung function such as infection, myocardial ischemia, heart failure, pulmonary embolic disease, and malignancy is important.
- When respiratory failure complicates IPF or fibrosis associated with connective tissue diseases, lung-protective ventilatory strategies should be used and the potential role of concurrent pulmonary hypertension should be considered.
- Bronchoscopy with lavage sampling of the distal airspace is a valuable tool in the documentation of alveolar hemorrhage and the exclusion of infection.
- Prompt institution of anti-inflammatory therapy after diagnosing COP or hypersensitivity pneumonitis may result in little or no long-term pulmonary dysfunction.

SELECTED REFERENCES

1. Nava S, Rubini F: Lung and chest wall mechanics in ventilated patients with end stage idiopathic pulmonary fibrosis. Thorax 1999;54(5):390-395.
6. Fernandez-Perez ER, et al: Ventilator settings and outcome of respiratory failure in chronic interstitial lung disease. Chest 2008;133(5):1113-1119.
8. Schulman DS, Biondi JW, Matthay RA, et al: Differing responses in right and left-ventricular filling, loading and volumes during positive end-expiratory pressure. Am J Cardiol 1989;64(12): 772-777.
15. Petzoldt M, Braune S, Bittmann I, Kluge S: Rescue therapy with a pumpless extracorporeal lung assist device in a patient with acute interstitial lung disease and severe refractory hypercapnia. Respir Care 2012;57(2):293-297.
23. Martinez FJ, Safrin S, Weycker D, et al: The clinical course of patients with idiopathic pulmonary fibrosis. Ann Intern Med 2005;142(12):963-967.
56. Rabe C, Appenrodt B, Hoff C, et al: Severe respiratory failure due to diffuse alveolar hemorrhage: Clinical characteristics and outcome of intensive care. J Crit Care 2010;25(2):230-235.
67. Levy JB, Turner AN, Rees AJ, et al: Long-term outcome of anti-glomerular basement membrane antibody disease treated with plasma exchange and immunosuppression. Ann Intern Med 2001;134(11):1033-1042.
82. Waterer GW, Latham B, Waring JA, et al: Pulmonary capillaritis associated with the antiphospholipid antibody syndrome and rapid response to plasmapheresis. Respirology 1999;4(4): 405-408.
97. King TE Jr, Mortenson RL: Cryptogenic organizing pneumonitis. The North American experience. Chest 1992;102(1 Suppl): 8S-13S.
142. Semenzato G, Chilosi M, Ossi E, et al: Bronchoalveolar lavage and lung histology. Comparative analysis of inflammatory and immunocompetent cells in patients with sarcoidosis and hypersensitivity pneumonitis. Am Rev Respir Dis 1985;132(2):400-404.

The complete list of references can be found at www.expertconsult.com.

PART 4

CRITICAL CARE INFECTIOUS DISEASE

50 Nosocomial Infection in the Intensive Care Unit

Dennis G. Maki | Constantine Tsigrelis

CHAPTER OUTLINE

Intensive care units (ICUs) have contributed greatly to the survival of patients with trauma, shock states, and other life-threatening conditions[1-3] but are associated with a greatly increased risk of nosocomial (hospital-acquired) infection. Rates of nosocomial infection in patients requiring more than 1 week of advanced life support within an ICU are three to five times higher than in hospitalized patients who do not require ICU care.[4-8] Infection, usually nosocomial, is the most common cause of death, directly or indirectly, of patients who survive the early period after major trauma or full-thickness burns and is the most commonly identified cause of multiple-organ dysfunction syndrome.[9-11]

Although most of this book focuses on the diagnosis and management of critically ill patients in the ICU, nosocomial infections are clearly one of the most common and serious complications of ICU care and are usually a consequence of invasive monitoring or life support therapies. Thus, they are greatly preventable, and it is appropriate that measures to prevent nosocomial infections be addressed.

Published guidelines for prevention are now available, based increasingly on randomized trials that have established the efficacy of specific control measures. Knowledge and technology of asepsis with regard to surgery and high-risk medical devices are now sufficiently advanced that, if applied consistently, the risk of nosocomial infection can be greatly reduced.[12-15]

INCIDENCE AND PROFILE

DEFINITIONS

Obtaining meaningful data on rates of nosocomial infection that can form the basis for comparisons within a hospital and, especially, among hospitals and that can also be used

Additional online-only material indicated by icon.

to monitor secular trends and document the efficacy or lack of efficacy of control measures must begin with clear, unambiguous definitions. Although there are no standardized definitions for infection at specific sites that are universally accepted by clinicians or investigators, the Centers for Disease Control and Prevention (CDC) has published definitions for the purpose of surveillance of nosocomial infection within hospitals, which most U.S. centers and an increasing number of hospitals around the world have adopted (Box 50.1).[16,17] For research purposes, more stringent definitions for specific infections will usually be necessary,[18] especially for pneumonia.[19]

INCIDENCE

The incidence of hospital-acquired infection is most commonly expressed as the number of infections per 100 patients hospitalized and is highest in burn units[7,20] and surgical ICUs,[5-7,20-23] with intermediate risk in medical ICUs,* and lowest risk in coronary care units.[4,7,8,20]

Recognizing that the risk of nosocomial infection within ICUs is heavily influenced by the length of stay and that the length of stay ranges widely among ICUs in the same hospital and among different hospitals, the CDC has advocated the use of rates expressed per 1000 patient-days to permit more meaningful intrainstitutional and, especially, interhospital comparisons.[25-27] Furthermore, recognizing the powerful influence of exposure to invasive devices on susceptibility to infection[28,29] and the great variation in use of devices among different ICUs in the same hospital and among different hospitals, the CDC has further recommended surveillance of device-associated nosocomial infections expressed as infections per 1000 device-days.[25] Representative rates of device-associated nosocomial infection in U.S. hospitals, which can be used for intrahospital and interhospital comparisons, are shown in Table 50.1.[25-27] In the future, device-associated infection rates will be sought in accreditation reviews by the Joint Commission on the Accreditation of Healthcare Organizations (JCAHO)[30] as this influential organization continues to move toward measurement of patient outcomes as the most effective way to improve patient care in the United States.

Table 50.1 Rates of Device-Related Nosocomial Infection in U.S. Hospital Intensive Care Units (ICUs), Expressed per 1000 Device-Days

Type of Infection	Type of ICU	Rate (No. of Cases Per 1000 Device-Days) 2002-2004*	2006-2008†	2010‡
Catheter-associated urinary tract infection	Burn	6.7	7.4	4.7
	Trauma	6.0	5.4	3.2
	Surgical	4.4	4.3	2.4
	Medical	5.1	4.3	2.1
	Coronary	4.5	4.8	1.9
Ventilator-associated pneumonia	Burn	12.0	10.7	5.8
	Trauma	15.2	8.1	6.0
	Surgical	9.3	4.9	3.1
	Medical	4.9	2.3	1.2
	Coronary	4.4	2.1	1.3
Central line–associated bloodstream infection	Burn	7.0	5.5	3.5
	Trauma	7.4	3.6	1.9
	Surgical	4.6	2.3	1.2
	Medical	5.0	2.3	1.5
	Coronary	3.5	2.0	1.3

*Data from National Nosocomial Infections Surveillance System. National Nosocomial Infections Surveillance (NNIS) System Report, data summary from January 1992 through June 2004, issued October 2004. Am J Infect Control 2004;32:470-85.

†Data from Edwards JR, Peterson KD, Mu Y, et al. National Healthcare Safety Network (NHSN) report: data summary for 2006 through 2008, issued December 2009. Am J Infect Control 2009;37:783-805.

‡Data from Dudeck MA, Horan TC, Peterson KD, et al. National Healthcare Safety Network (NHSN) Report, data summary for 2010, device-associated module. Am J Infect Control 2011;39:798-816.

PROFILE AND SECULAR TRENDS

Approximately 40% of endemic nosocomial infections within ICUs are catheter-related urinary tract infections, and 25% are pneumonias—most associated with endotracheal intubation and mechanical ventilatory support. Up to 10% of patients hospitalized in a medical-surgical ICU for more than 72 hours acquire a nosocomial bloodstream infection, most commonly from an intravascular device.[25,31,32] Postoperative surgical site infections, *Clostridium difficile* infection, nosocomial sinusitis, and nosocomial meningitis account for the remainder.[4-8,25,33-37]

Nearly 50% of nosocomial infections in the ICU are caused by aerobic gram-negative bacilli, especially *Pseudomonas aeruginosa, Escherichia coli,* and *Klebsiella pneumoniae,* and 35% are caused by gram-positive cocci, most commonly coagulase-negative staphylococci, *Staphylococcus aureus,* and enterococci (Fig. 50.1).[38,39] Almost 15% are caused by *Candida* species.[38,39] Filamentous fungi such as *Aspergillus* and *Zygomycetes* are being increasingly encountered in patients with hematologic malignancy or those who received solid organ transplants.[40-42] *Legionella* species account for up to 10% of nosocomial pneumonias in centers that make efforts to diagnose *Legionella* infections.[43]

The microbial profile of infections at individual sites in ICU patients is shown in Table 50.2.[39] There has been an unrelenting increase in nosocomial infections caused by intrinsically resistant organisms, especially *P. aeruginosa, Acinetobacter* species, and other resistant gram-negative bacilli; coagulase-negative staphylococci, *S. aureus,* enterococci; and *Candida.*[31,38,39,44,45] Moreover, the incidence of infection caused by organisms with *acquired* resistance, especially methicillin-resistant *S. aureus* (MRSA); enterococci resistant to vancomycin (VRE), ampicillin, or both drugs; and gram-negative bacilli resistant to extended-spectrum β-lactams and fluoroquinolones, has increased even more sharply over the past several decades (Fig. 50.2).[39,46] The recent emergence of carbapenem-resistant *K. pneumoniae*

*See references 4, 5, 7, 20, 23, 24.

Box 50.1 Definitions for Health Care–Associated Infection of the Centers for Disease Control and Prevention (CDC)

Primary Bloodstream Infection*

1. Patient has a recognized pathogen cultured from one or more blood cultures (does not include organisms considered common commensals—see below) AND the organism cultured from blood is not related to an infection at another site

OR

2. Patient has common commensal organisms (e.g., coagulase-negative staphylococci [including *S. epidermidis*], diphtheroids [*Corynebacterium* spp. not *C. diphtheriae*], *Bacillus* spp. [not *B. anthracis*], *Propionibacterium* spp., viridans group streptococci, *Aerococcus* spp., and *Micrococcus* spp.) cultured from two or more blood cultures drawn on separate occasions AND at least one of the following signs or symptoms: fever (>38° C), chills, or hypotension AND signs and symptoms and positive laboratory results are not related to an infection at another site

Clinically Defined Pneumonia

1. For any patient, two or more serial chest radiographs with at least one of the following: new or progressive *and* persistent infiltrate, consolidation, or cavitation

AND at least *one* of the following:
- Fever (>38° C or >100.4° F) with no other recognized cause
- Leukopenia (<4000 WBCs/μL) or leukocytosis (12,000 WBCs/μL)
- For adults >70 years of age, altered mental status with no other recognized cause

AND at least *two* of the following:
- New onset of purulent sputum or change in character of sputum, increased respiratory secretions, or increased suctioning requirements
- New onset of worsening cough, dyspnea, or tachypnea
- Rales or bronchial breath sounds
- Worsening gas exchange (e.g., O_2 desaturation [e.g., $PaO_2/FIO_2 \le 240$]), increased oxygen requirements, or increased ventilation demands

Laboratory-Defined Pneumonia

1. Fulfillment of criteria listed above for clinically defined pneumonia,

AND at least one of the following:
- Positive growth in blood culture not related to another source of infection
- Positive growth in culture of pleural fluid
- Positive quantitative culture from minimally contaminated lower respiratory tract specimen (e.g., bronchoalveolar lavage [$\ge 10^4$ CFUs/mL] or protected specimen brushing [$\ge 10^3$ CFUs/mL]) (NOTE: an endotracheal aspirate is not a minimally contaminated specimen)
- ≥5% bronchoalveolar lavage–obtained cells contain intracellular bacteria on direct microscopic examination (e.g., Gram stain)
- Histopathologic examination shows at least *one* of the following findings as evidence of pneumonia:
  - Abscess formation or foci of consolidation with intense neutrophil accumulation in bronchioles and alveoli
  - Positive quantitative culture of lung parenchyma
  - Evidence of lung parenchyma invasion by fungal hyphae or pseudohyphae

Symptomatic Urinary Tract Infection

Must meet at least *one* of the following three criteria:

1. Patient had an *indwelling urinary catheter in place* at the time of specimen collection or onset of signs or symptoms

AND at least *one* of the following signs or symptoms with no other recognized cause:
- Fever (>38° C)
- Suprapubic tenderness
- Costovertebral angle pain or tenderness

AND *one* of the following findings:
- A positive urine culture of $\ge 10^5$ CFUs/mL with no more than two species of microorganisms (cultures reported as "mixed flora" do not meet UTI criteria)
- A positive urine culture of $\ge 10^3$ and $<10^5$ CFUs/mL with no more than two species of microorganisms, AND at least *one* of the following findings: positive dipstick for leukocyte esterase or nitrite, pyuria (i.e., urine specimen with ≥10 WBCs/μL of unspun urine or ≥3 WBCs/high-power field of spun urine), or microorganisms seen on Gram stain of unspun urine

OR

2. Patient had indwelling urinary catheter *removed within the 48 hours prior* to specimen collection or onset of signs or symptoms

AND at least *one* of the following signs or symptoms with no other recognized cause:
- Fever (>38° C)
- Urgency, frequency, dysuria, or suprapubic tenderness
- Costovertebral angle pain or tenderness

AND *one* of the following findings:
- A positive urine culture of $\ge 10^5$ CFUs/mL with no more than two species of microorganisms (cultures reported as "mixed flora" do not meet UTI criteria)
- A positive urine culture of $\ge 10^3$ and $<10^5$ CFUs/mL with no more than two species of microorganisms, AND at least *one* of the following findings: positive result on dipstick testing for leukocyte esterase or nitrite, pyuria (see above), or microorganisms seen on Gram stain of unspun urine

OR

3. Patient did not have an indwelling urinary catheter in place at the time of, or within 48 hours prior to, specimen collection or onset of signs or symptoms

AND at least *one* of the following signs or symptoms with no other recognized cause:
- Fever (>38° C) in a patient who is ≤65 years of age
- Urgency, frequency, dysuria, or suprapubic tenderness
- Costovertebral angle pain or tenderness

AND *one* of the following findings:
- A positive urine culture of $\ge 10^5$ CFUs/mL with no more than two species of microorganisms (cultures reported as "mixed flora" do not meet UTI criteria)
- A positive urine culture of $\ge 10^3$ and $<10^5$ CFUs/mL with no more than two species of microorganisms, AND at least *one* of the following findings: positive result on dipstick testing for leukocyte esterase or nitrite, pyuria (see above), or microorganisms seen on Gram stain of unspun urine

*All intravascular device-related bloodstream infections are classified with primary bloodstream infections.
CFUs, colony-forming units; FIO_2, fraction of inspired oxygen; PaO_2, arterial oxygen tension; UTI, urinary tract infection; WBCs, white blood cells.
Data from Centers for Disease Control and Prevention. NHSN Patient Safety Component Manual. Available at http://www.cdc.gov/nhsn/TOC_PSCManual.html. Accessed April 3, 2012.

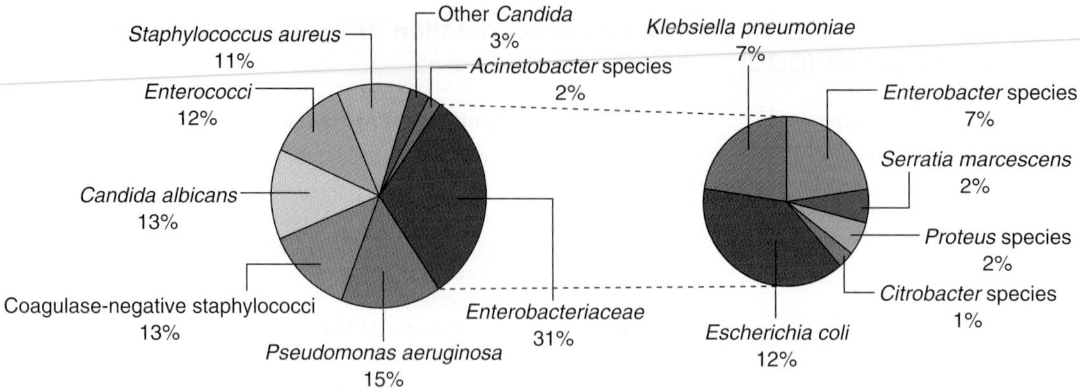

Figure 50.1 Microbiology of nosocomial infection in the intensive care unit (ICU). Based on 13,317 infections occurring in ICU patients in 97 participating U.S. hospitals in the Centers for Disease Control's National Nosocomial Infections Surveillance System (NNIS), January 1992 through July 1997. (Data from Richards MJ, Edwards JR, Culver DH, Gaynes RP: Nosocomial infections in medical intensive care units in the United States. National Nosocomial Infections Surveillance System. Crit Care Med 1999;27:887-892.)

Table 50.2 Profile of Nosocomial Infections in the Intensive Care Unit (ICU)

Infection	Major Pathogen(s)	Risk Factors
Urinary tract infection	*Escherichia coli* *Pseudomonas aeruginosa* *Klebsiella pneumoniae* Other gram-negative bacilli *Enterococcus* spp.	Urinary catheter Monitoring of urine output Other urologic manipulation or bladder irrigations Renal transplantation Diabetes Female > male
Pneumonia	*Staphylococcus aureus* *P. aeruginosa* *Acinetobacter* spp. *Enterobacter* spp. *K. pneumoniae* Other gram-negative bacilli	Tracheostomy Endotracheal tube, reintubation Nasogastric tube Intracranial pressure monitoring Stress ulcer prophylaxis with histamine H_2 blocker or antacids Immunosuppression Granulocytopenia
Surgical site infection	*S. aureus* Coagulase-negative staphylococci Enterococci *E. coli* and other gram-negative bacilli *Bacteroides fragilis* and other bowel anaerobes *Candida* spp.	Trauma, especially penetrating abdominal injury Gastrointestinal or radical gynecologic surgery Prolonged operation Immunosuppressive therapy Granulocytopenia Hepatic transplantation
Intravascular device–related bacteremia	Coagulase-negative staphylococci *S. aureus* *Enterococcus* spp. Gram-negative bacilli	Central venous catheter in place >5 days Heavy colonization of insertion site skin Femoral vein insertions Catheter guidewire exchanges
Contaminated infusate	*Enterobacter* spp. *S. marcescens* *Citrobacter* spp. *P. cepacia* or *Xanthomonas maltophilia*	
Antibiotic-associated diarrhea or colitis	*Clostridium difficile*	Prolonged antibiotic therapy, especially with clindamycin or broad-spectrum β-lactams Enteral tube feeding
Candidemia	*Candida* spp.	Broad-spectrum, prolonged antimicrobial therapy Mucosal or urinary colonization Central venous catheter Hyperalimentation Renal failure

Modified from Maki DG: Nosocomial infection. In Parrillo JE (ed): Current Therapy in Critical Care Medicine, 2nd ed. Philadelphia, BC Decker, 1991.

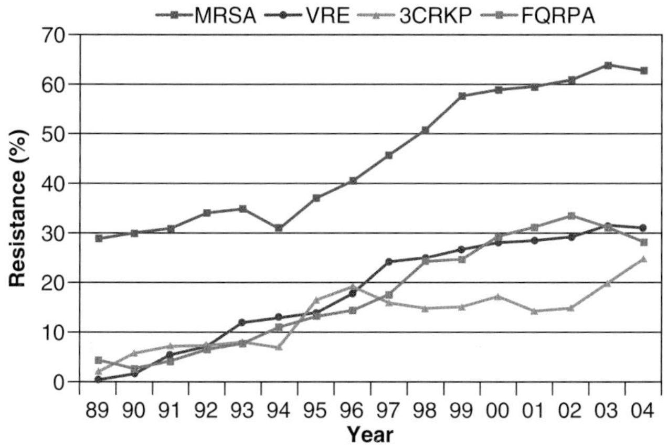

Figure 50.2 Temporal trends in the proportion of isolates resistant to antibiotics among pathogenically important bacteria in U.S. intensive care units (ICUs), National Nosocomial Infections Surveillance System (NNIS) 1989-2004. FQRPA, *Pseudomonas aeruginosa* resistant to fluoroquinolones; MRSA, methicillin-resistant *Staphylococcus aureus*; 3CRKP, *Klebsiella pneumoniae* resistant to third-generation cephalosporins; VRE, vancomycin-resistant enterococcus. (From Centers for Disease Control and Prevention: Trends in antibiotic resistance in National Nosocomial Infections Surveillance (NNIS) system hospitals, 1989-2004. Available at http://www.cdc.gov/ncidod/dhqp/pdf/ar/ICU_RESTrend1995-2004.pdf. Accessed January 15, 2007.)

has become a significant problem as there are limited therapeutic options to treat this pathogen.[39,47]

Nosocomial infections acquired in the ICU clearly differ from infections acquired in non-ICU patient care units within the same institutions. Overall rates are two to three times higher, and rates of ventilator-associated pneumonia (VAP) and primary bacteremia—most of which originate from intravascular devices—are 10 times higher. A far greater proportion of ICU-acquired infections are caused by antibiotic-resistant bacteria because the intensive antimicrobial therapy characteristic of modern-day ICUs grossly distorts patients' microflora. Moreover, more than half of all nosocomial epidemics now occur among the 10% of hospitalized patients confined to an ICU.[20,31] Finally, the risk of occupationally acquired infection among health care workers (HCWs), particularly by bloodborne viruses and herpes simplex virus (HSV), is highest among ICU personnel, as contrasted with those who work in non-ICU patient care units (see Protection of Health Care Workers in the Intensive Care Unit later).

MORBIDITY AND ECONOMIC IMPACT

Nosocomial infections have a considerable impact on morbidity and mortality rates and are estimated to affect more than 2 million patients in U.S. hospitals annually.[48] Table 50.3 summarizes major studies that have examined mortality, length of stay, and costs associated with the major nosocomial infections in U.S. hospitals.[2-19] Nosocomial infections have been ascribed by the National Institute of Medicine to be responsible for more than 80,000 hospital deaths each year and in 1995 resulted in more than $5 billion in excess health care costs.[48] Considering that nosocomial infections acquired by ICU patients account for nearly half of all infections in most hospitals, progress in reducing the incidence of infection acquired within ICUs could produce substantial economic benefits.

GENERAL INFECTION CONTROL MEASURES

HOSPITAL INFECTION CONTROL PROGRAMS

Beginning in the late 1960s, scattered U.S. hospitals began to establish infection control programs to conduct surveillance, to develop infection control policies, and especially to try to implement control measures more consistently.[116] In 1976 JCAHO added to its requirements for hospital accreditation the establishment of a formal infection control program.

In the early 1970s the CDC undertook determining the effectiveness of nosocomial infection surveillance and control programs in the United States through the auspices of the Study of the Efficacy of Nosocomial Infection Control (SENIC). The goals of SENIC were to determine the extent to which infection control programs had been adopted by U.S. hospitals and to ascertain how much these programs had reduced rates of nosocomial infection. SENIC was launched by a survey of all U.S. hospitals to determine the characteristics of infection control programs and was completed in 1975-1976 by a review of more than 339,000 patient medical records in 338 randomly selected hospitals.[117]

The SENIC found that hospitals reduced their nosocomial infection rates by approximately 32% if their surveillance and infection control program included four components: (1) emphasis on both surveillance and an infection control program, (2) at least one full-time infection control practitioner for every 250 beds, (3) a trained hospital epidemiologist, and (4) surveillance of surgical wound infections with feedback of wound infection rates to practicing surgeons.[118] However, the relative importance of each component varied for the four major types of nosocomial infections (surgical wound infections, urinary tract infections, bloodstream infections, and pneumonia).[118,119] SENIC suggests that nearly one third of all nosocomial infections are in theory preventable, whereas a 1983 survey of surveillance and control programs in a random sample of U.S. hospitals found that failure to implement all essentials of the program, particularly to have an adequate number of infection control practitioners or a trained hospital epidemiologist or to disseminate wound infection rates to surgeons, was greatly limiting the potential for prevention: U.S. hospitals were estimated to be preventing only 9% of all infections.[120]

It is hoped that surveillance and control programs will continue to evolve. Prevention of nosocomial infections is a major priority of the U.S. Public Health Service,[121] JCAHO,[30] and the Institute of Medicine.[122] With the shift to prospective-payment reimbursement, hospitals now have a powerful financial incentive to reduce their rates of nosocomial infection,[123] and it can be anticipated that efforts to prevent hospital-acquired infections will assume ever greater importance.

Table 50.3 Estimated Extra Days, Extra Charges, and Deaths Associated with Nosocomial Infections in U.S. Hospitals as Reported in Major Studies

Infection	Description	Average Extra Days in Hospital or ICU per Infection	Average Extra Charges or Costs per Infection ($)	Excess Mortality	
				Unadjusted	Attributable
Surgical Site Infection					
Kirkland et al, 1999[610]	CABG, vascular surgery, abdominal surgery, orthopedic surgery	6.5	3,089	NR	4.3%
Whitehouse et al, 2002[611]	Orthopedic surgery	14	17,708	NR	0.0%
Hollenbeak et al, 2000[612]	Deep chest infection after CABG	20	20,012	NR	19.4%
McGarry et al, 2004[613]	All major surgical procedures; only *Staphylococcus aureus* infections included	13	53,625	NR	16.8%
Herwaldt et al, 2006[614]	All major surgical procedures	NR	3,021	1.2%	0%
Ventilator-Associated Pneumonia					
Fagon et al, 1993[615]	Medical and surgical patients	13	NR	NR	27.1%
Heyland et al, 1999[616]	Medical and surgical patients	4.3	NR	NR	5.8%
Bercault et al, 2001[617]	Medical and surgical patients	5	NR	NR	27.4%
Rello et al, 2002[618]	Medical and surgical patients	11	40,000	NR	0%
Warren et al, 2003[619]	Medical and surgical patients	25	11,897	16%	NR
Cocanour et al, 2005[620]	Trauma patients	15	57,158	NR	0%
Bloodstream Infection					
Pittet et al, 1994[269]	Surgical patients	24	40,000	NR	35%
Digiovine et al, 1999[270]	Medical patients	10	34,508	NR	4%
Warren et al, 2006[621]	Medical and surgical patients	7.5	11,971	23%	NR
Catheter-Associated Urinary Tract Infection					
Bryan et al, 1984[475]	Medical and surgical patients	NR	NR	NR	12%
Tambyah et al, 2002[478]	Medical and surgical patients	NR	589	NR	NR

CABG, coronary artery bypass grafting; NR, not reported.
Studies cited in table (column 1) may be found in the complete list of references for this chapter provided online.

JCAHO mandates that all hospitals have an active program for the surveillance, prevention, and control of hospital-acquired infections, which begins with an institutional infection control committee with representation from the major clinical services and hospital departments including the institution's ICUs. The most essential members of the infection control program are the infection control practitioner(s), usually registered nurse(s), and the hospital epidemiologist, usually a physician with training in infectious diseases or microbiology, who implement the policies developed by the committee, educate hospital personnel about nosocomial infection control, and investigate suspected outbreaks (Box 50.2).

Surveillance of nosocomial infections is the cornerstone of an effective infection control program and offers numerous potential benefits[119,124]: (1) It permits determination of baseline (expected) infection rates, assisting recognition of outbreaks and evaluation of new policies and control measures; (2) it identifies institutional problems that require attention, permitting focused infection control efforts and education; (3) it provides reliable data that can be disseminated to individual departments, increasing awareness and involvement of individual staff members; (4) it increases the visibility of the infection control staff on patient care units, providing an opportunity for consultation and ad hoc education; and (5) it facilitates the earliest discovery of patients with communicable infections, permitting timely institution of isolation precautions to limit spread. Because total surveillance (of all infections) is labor intensive, most hospitals now focus their surveillance efforts on infections that are associated with high morbidity (e.g., nosocomial pneumonia), that greatly increase health care costs (e.g., post–cardiac surgery sternotomy infections), that are caused by antibiotic-resistant organisms with potential for spread (e.g., MRSA, *C. difficile*), or that are highly preventable (e.g., intravascular device-related bloodstream infections).[119,125]

The 1990s were characterized by major efforts by hospitals to apply the numerous facets of health care principles of quality improvement developed by industry. Hospital infection control programs had been working on quality improvement[126] but, influenced by JCAHO, were probably too heavily focused on process, namely, policies and procedures, rather than documenting outcome vis-à-vis reduced infection rates. Infection control programs in most U.S.

Box 50.2 Facets of a Hospital Infection Control Program

- Active infection control committee, with representation from major departments and services including the intensive care units (ICUs)
- Surveillance of nosocomial infections, especially in each ICU
- Comprehensive and regularly updated institutional policies and procedures for prevention of nosocomial infection:
  - Surveillance of nosocomial infections
  - Isolation and universal precautions
  - Sterilization and disinfection
  - Indications for and management of invasive procedures and devices:
    All types of intravascular catheters
    Hemodynamic monitoring
    Tracheostomy and endotracheal intubation
    Mechanical ventilation and other respiratory therapy
    Bronchoscopy and gastrointestinal endoscopy
    Anesthesia and the operating room
    Hemodialysis
    Intra-aortic balloon pumps
    Cardiopulmonary bypass
    Intracranial pressure monitoring
- Antimicrobial stewardship program
- Guideline for investigation of an epidemic
- Strong liaison with clinical microbiology laboratory
  - Representation on the infection control committee
  - Laboratory-based surveillance
  - Monitoring and reporting of trends in antimicrobial susceptibility
  - Retaining important isolates
  - Microbiologic support of all infection control activities
  - Subtyping of isolates for investigations or studies
- Educational programs for new employees, periodic updates dealing with nosocomial infection control
- Active employee health department:
  - Free immunizations (hepatitis B, measles, mumps, rubella, varicella, pertussis, influenza A)
  - Tuberculin screening
  - Postexposure protocols
- Quality assurance review of implementation of infection control policies and practices

Modified from Maki DG: Nosocomial infection. In Parrillo JE (ed): Current Therapy in Critical Care Medicine, 2nd ed. Philadelphia, BC Decker, 1991.

hospitals are now closely allied with their institutional quality improvement departments.[126,127]

Hospital infection control programs are also regulated by the Occupational Safety and Health Administration (OSHA) in terms of institutional standards and programs to protect HCWs from bloodborne pathogens[128] and tuberculosis[129]; the Environmental Protection Agency[130] has also published regulations in terms of disposal and tracking of medical waste—only a small fraction of which is truly biohazardous.[131]

Finally, it is essential that all health care personnel working in an ICU receive training in the epidemiology and control of nosocomial infections. This may be most important for house officers in teaching hospitals, who commonly enter the ICU with only the most rudimentary knowledge of asepsis but have hands-on contact with numerous patients each day. ICU physicians and nurses must be especially familiar with their hospitals' guidelines for the management of invasive devices, particularly intravascular catheters of all types,[132] urinary catheters,[133,134] endotracheal tubes,[135] and tracheostomies.[135] Moreover, all physicians need to be made aware that broad-spectrum antimicrobial therapy greatly increases the risk of superinfection by antibiotic-resistant bacteria and *Candida*, as well as *C. difficile.*

ROLE OF THE MICROBIOLOGY LABORATORY

Accurate and timely diagnostic microbiology is as essential for nosocomial infection control as it is for the clinical management of patients' infections. Although many infections can be diagnosed on the basis of clinical criteria alone, cultures and other laboratory tests allow infections to be diagnosed with much greater certainty, and certain infections such as bacteriuria, bacteremia, and fungal and viral infections cannot be diagnosed without cultures or other laboratory tests (see Box 50.1).[16,17] Moreover, accurate antimicrobial susceptibility testing of clinical isolates is the only means of monitoring trends in antibiotic resistance of hospital organisms.[136] Most importantly, identifying the microbial cause of nosocomial infections allows epidemiologic tracking of individual pathogens within the hospital, especially those that are commonly spread from patient to patient such as *S. aureus*, beta-hemolytic streptococci, enterococci, and the numerous gram-negative bacilli.

From an organizational standpoint, the institutional infection control program and clinical microbiology laboratory must have a close working relationship (see Box 50.2) to assist surveillance, which must be strongly laboratory based,[119,137] and to permit the detection and resolution of potential problems. The laboratory director or a senior member of the laboratory staff should be a permanent member of the infection control committee.

The primary role of the clinical microbiology laboratory in any infection control program is to provide up-to-date clinical microbiologic data for use in the surveillance of nosocomial infections and identification of potential outbreaks.[137] Protocols should be developed to ensure that laboratory staff immediately contact infection control personnel after the isolation of certain important pathogens such as MRSA or vancomycin-resistant enterococci (VRE) or the appearance of new resistance patterns in endemic organisms such as resistance of *Klebsiella* species to third-generation cephalosporins and carbapenems, or *P. aeruginosa* to aminoglycosides, fluoroquinolones, and carbapenems. Sifting through these data can be time consuming, and developing electronic information systems that streamline this process is essential to improving the efficiency of the infection control program. Commercial software programs that can automate this process are now available. Many of these programs automatically collate microbiologic data, provide rudimentary geographic information, and perform basic statistical analyses that can assist in the surveillance of nosocomial infections and identification of potential outbreaks.[138,139]

Reporting cumulative summaries of antimicrobial susceptibility data (antibiograms) is another essential responsibility of the clinical microbiology laboratory.[140,141] When implemented appropriately, the timely dissemination of antibiograms helps guide the choice of empiric antimicrobials, pending the results of clinical cultures, and provides valuable data to help the infection control department monitor institutional antimicrobial resistance trends and identify potential outbreaks.[142] The Clinical and Laboratory Standards Institute—formerly the National Committee for Clinical Laboratory Standards—recommends that institutional antibiograms be updated at least annually and has recently published standards for their content and format.[143] Automated electronic systems for collating and disseminating nearly real-time antibiograms along with antibiotic-use decision support exist and, when implemented properly, have been effective in improving antimicrobial utilization within the hospital setting.[144,145]

Monitoring of sterilizers with spore tests, environmental sampling, and advanced microbiologic support for epidemiologic investigations are additional responsibilities expected of most clinical microbiology laboratories, although some university hospital programs have dedicated personnel within their infection control programs who perform these activities.[137]

The clinical microbiology laboratory is a key resource in the investigation of a suspected outbreak. One of the first and foremost actions when a nosocomial outbreak is suspected is to immediately retrieve all available isolates of the putative epidemic pathogen for possible subtyping.[146] The need to move rapidly becomes apparent when it is realized that most hospital laboratories discard cultures as soon as the isolates have been fully characterized. All blood isolates should be routinely saved for at least 1 year.[146] Laboratory personnel must be requested to save clinical isolates of any unusual organisms that are encountered for the first time or clusters of any organism and to inform infection control personnel of the findings and availability of the isolates.

The rapid evolution of molecular microbiology has revolutionized epidemiologic investigation of nosocomial outbreaks. Molecular-based tests for the rapid diagnosis of bacterial,[147] viral,[78,148] and fungal[149] infections are now routinely available in most hospital-based and reference laboratories. Modern molecular tests can reliably detect minute numbers of organisms, allowing direct testing of clinical samples without the need for culture. In modern-day clinical virology, molecular tests based on polymerase chain reaction (PCR) for amplification of the pathogen's DNA or RNA have supplanted tissue cultures and now allow rapid diagnosis of infections that would otherwise often not be identifiable by classic methods.

The availability of molecular subtyping systems has greatly strengthened investigations of outbreaks, as well as research on the epidemiology of nosocomial infections.[150,151] The antimicrobial susceptibility pattern (antibiogram) or the detailed biochemical profile (biotype) is often useful for the initial epidemiologic subtyping of many bacteria and may be adequate for identifying an epidemic caused by an unusual pathogen. However, if an epidemic organism is a common species such as *S. aureus*, it can be difficult or even impossible to know with certainty that an outbreak derives from a common source using these techniques because they lack sufficient discriminatory power.[150]

The new molecular techniques of subtyping such as plasmid profile typing by agarose gel electrophoresis or the use of restriction endonuclease digests with pulsed-field electrophoresis (DNA fingerprinting)[150] are now available in most infection control research laboratories but should be adaptable by many hospital laboratories. Genetic probes promise even more powerful tools for investigating outbreaks, particularly those caused by antibiotic-resistant organisms.[147]

Although molecular-based tests offer several advantages over traditional microbiologic techniques, they are not a panacea. A number of molecular diagnostic assays (e.g., analyte specific reagents [ASRs]) marketed for clinical practice do not require approval by the U.S. Food and Drug Administration.[147] In the absence of published data on their accuracy and precision, the results of these tests must be interpreted with caution and should always undergo extensive inhouse validation before widespread adoption. Moreover, the exquisite sensitivity of many of these tests renders them more susceptible to false-positive results as a consequence of environmental contamination[152,153] and mandates stringent quality control practices and procedures.

ARCHITECTURAL AND ENVIRONMENTAL ISSUES

The role of the inanimate environment on the transmission of nosocomial infections has been a subject of intense debate for decades. It has been shown that hospital surfaces are almost universally contaminated by potentially pathogenic bacteria such *S. aureus*,[154] enterococcus,[155] and gram-negative bacilli such as *Acinetobacter baumanii*.[156] Prior to the 1970s, infection control personnel routinely sampled hospital surfaces. Despite this level of surface colonization, early studies found that the inanimate environment—surfaces, walls, and even air—does not contribute materially to the occurrence of most nosocomial infections,[157] other than invasive infections caused by airborne *Aspergillus* and other filamentous fungi in seriously immunocompromised patients.[40,41]

Although inanimate surfaces may rarely be involved in the direct transmission of infection to patients, more recent evidence suggests that surfaces may well play an important role in the nosocomial acquisition of pathogenic bacteria, indirectly, through contact with HCWs' hands and equipment (see Fig. 50.3). This indirect route of infection is of particular importance in the ICU, where all patients are heavily exposed to invasive devices and have a high risk of infection. In the ICU the inanimate environment may become a reservoir for the transmission of resistant nosocomial organisms such as MRSA,[158,159] *C. difficile*,[83,160] VRE,[155,161] and gram-negative bacilli such as *Klebsiella* spp., *Acinetobacter* spp., and *Enterobacter* organisms.[162,163] Studies have shown that enhanced surface decontamination with hypochlorite-containing cleaning solutions has been necessary to terminate outbreaks caused by *C. difficile*[164] and *Acinetobacter baumanii*.[156]

Although the ICU environment cannot be made microbe free, certain organizational, architectural, and environmental issues must be addressed with the design or remodeling of an ICU. The capacity to systematically improve the care of critically ill patients and prevent nosocomial infection requires a structural foundation on which the processes of care can be optimized (i.e., make it easy for HCWs to do it right and difficult to do it wrong). Accountability for compliance with critical policies and procedures and ongoing assessment of outcomes needs to be built into the administrative structure of the ICU.

An ICU must be adequately staffed to allow the processes of care to be carried out but also assure a high level of compliance with essential infection control measures such as hand hygiene and barrier isolation. Adequate staffing cannot be overemphasized; numerous studies have found greatly increased rates of nosocomial infection when ICUs are staffed suboptimally or when staffing requirements are met with temporary personnel who are unfamiliar with ICU infection control policies and procedures.[165,166] In a large nosocomial outbreak of *Enterobacter cloacae* infection in a neonatal ICU, Harbarth and colleagues[167] found that infection rates during periods of understaffing were strikingly higher than during periods with adequate levels of staffing (relative risk [RR] = 6, 95% confidence interval [CI] = 2.2 to 16.4). The effects of understaffing are likely multiple; however, erosion of basic hygienic practices with excessive patient-to-staff ratios likely explains much of this phenomenon.[168]

Many of the published recommendations for ICU architectural design[169] are empiric, and evidence that they reduce rates of nosocomial infection is, by and large, lacking. Although more research is necessary before specific features of ICU design achieve a level of evidence sufficient for an evidence-based guideline, certain facets of the ICU layout deserve attention:

- ICUs should be located in areas that limit traffic flow to essential ICU personnel.
- ICU facilities should be designed with ICU professionals in mind, ensuring appropriate space, resources, and environment for day-to-day operations.[169] Recognizing the growing variety and complexity of life support equipment required for the care of many patients, each cubicle or room should provide a minimum of 11 m^2 per bed.[170] The area should be large enough to accommodate the bed and all equipment yet allow immediate access to the patient at all times from both sides of the bed. Adequate space must also be provided for storage of nursing supplies. Facilities for disposal of biohazardous waste (e.g., bedpan flushers); for cleaning, reprocessing, and storage of ICU equipment; and for storage of housekeeping supplies should be separate from patient care areas. Single-patient rooms may increase the likelihood of handwashing being done and improve compliance with isolation practices, reducing the risk of cross-infection. For example, Mulin and colleagues[171] found that converting from an open unit to single rooms in their ICU greatly reduced rates of patient colonization with *A. baumanii*, and Shirani and colleagues[172] found that renovation of their burn unit to include separate bed enclosures reduced rates of nosocomial infection by 48%.[172]
- Materials used for fixtures, furniture, and other surfaces should be smooth and easy to clean; surfaces made of porous materials foster bacterial colonization.[173]
- An adequate number of sinks must be available for convenient handwashing by ICU personnel. Ideally, a sink should be located at the *entrance* of each cubicle or patient room to encourage handwashing by all entering personnel who will have contact with the patient or the immediate environment.[174,175] Separate sinks should be used for cleaning and reprocessing contaminated equipment. Sinks and sink drains are normally contaminated by pseudomonads,[176] although their role in the epidemiology of nosocomial infection is as yet unclear. However, sinks should be designed to minimize aerosol formation and splashback.
- All ICUs should be equipped with one or more class A isolation rooms, which include an anteroom for gowning and handwashing and the necessary modifications (negative pressure, roofline exhaust) to permit it to be used for patients with tuberculosis or other airborne infections such as chickenpox, measles, disseminated HSV infection, or a highly contagious emerging pathogen such as the severe acute respiratory syndrome (SARS) human coronavirus. If an ICU treats bone marrow transplant patients or other patients with prolonged severe granulocytopenia, positive-pressure isolation rooms using high-efficiency particle-arrest (HEPA) filters should be available. Isolation rooms for patients with infections transmitted by the respiratory route or to protect profoundly granulocytopenic patients must be kept closed to maintain control over the direction of airflow.
- A centralized, filtered air-handling system that provides at least six room exchanges per hour is essential.[170,177] Ideally, each patient's room should have the capacity of being set at positive or negative pressure with respect to the rest of the unit; if it cannot be, the room should be maintained permanently at positive pressure.

A variety of microorganisms including bacteria, mycobacteria, fungi, and parasites can be isolated from hospital water and have been implicated in endemic and epidemic nosocomial infections.[178] Many of these outbreaks were caused by bacteria typically thought of as "water" organisms such as *P. aeruginosa*,[176] *Stenotrophomonas maltophilia*,[179] and *A. baumanii*[16,180,181]; however, the most important and epidemiologically linked hospital water pathogen is the *Legionella* group.[182]

Nosocomial legionellosis was first described in 1979,[183] and it is estimated that up to 50% of cases of legionellosis are acquired in the health care setting,[184] with a mortality rate that approaches 30%.[185] Contamination of hospital potable water remains underappreciated despite studies showing that *Legionella* species can be recovered from 12% to 70% of hospital water systems,[186] and a number of studies in which nosocomial cases were identified only when specific diagnostic and surveillance methods were employed.[187,188] Characteristics of hospital water systems that are associated with *Legionella* contamination include piping systems with dead-ends that facilitate stagnation, large-volume water heaters that result in inefficient heating of hospital water, sediment buildup, water heater temperatures less than 60° C and tap water temperatures less than 50° C, maintaining water pH greater than 8 and receiving municipal water untreated with monochloramine.[189-191]

Despite the ubiquity of water systems colonized with *Legionella* species and studies demonstrating a correlation between the level of colonization and risk of infection, the CDC does not recommend routine surveillance of hospital water systems,[184] although this stance is controversial.[186] Researchers from Pittsburgh, Pennsylvania, and the Allegheny County Health Department have recommended a more proactive stepwise approach that involves initial surveillance of hospital water for *Legionella* contamination, regardless of the presence or absence of institutional nosocomial legionellosis, followed by continued surveillance based on the level of water contamination found or the presence of institutional legionellosis.[186]

Legionella species are resistant to chlorine and heat, making it challenging to eradicate them from contaminated hospital water systems.[191] Attempts to hyperchlorinate hospital water have been partially successful if chlorine levels are continuously maintained between 2 and 6 parts per million at all times but produce rapidly accelerated corrosion of water pipes and are expensive.[192] Thermal eradication is feasible, using a "heat-and-flush" method to raise water tank temperatures to greater than 70° C and distal water sites to greater than 60° C for short periods of time.[193] Although effective, superheating is labor intensive and there is the constant fear that patients or health care personnel may sustain scald injuries if they wash or shower with tap water during a flushing period. The use of technologies such as instantaneous steam heat for incoming water[193] and ultraviolet light[194] are technically feasible with newer hospital water systems but may be incompatible with older hospital water systems.

Perhaps the most attractive, effective, safe, and cost-efficient method for *Legionella* eradication may be the use of continuous copper-silver ionization systems to sterilize hospital water systems. These systems have been well studied over the past decade and have proved to be highly effective for reliably eradicating *Legionella* contamination of hospital water and, most importantly, for eliminating nosocomial legionellosis in institutions when other interventions have failed.[195] In our own institution (Maki DG), two clusters of nosocomial legionellosis prompted a retrospective review that identified 10 cases over an 11-year period. Surveillance of the hospital water system found that 75% of all samples contained low levels of *L. pneumophila*, which were shown to be clonally related to the 10 cases of nosocomial legionellosis. Installation of a continuous copper-silver ionization system led to complete eradication of *Legionella* from water samples, and no further cases of nosocomial legionellosis have been identified at our institution since 1995, among 255,000 patients hospitalized.

RELIABLE STERILIZATION PROCEDURES, CHEMICAL DISINFECTANTS, AND ANTISEPTICS

Reliable sterilization, disinfection, and antisepsis embrace virtually all measures aimed at prevention of nosocomial infection. *Critical* objects, which are introduced directly into the bloodstream or into other normally sterile areas of the body, such as surgical instruments, cardiac catheters, and implanted devices, must be reliably sterile and sterilized with steam, gas, hydrogen peroxide gas, or chemical sterilization. *Semicritical* items, which come into contact with intact mucous membranes, such as fiberoptic endoscopes, endotracheal tubes, or ventilator circuit tubing, can be decontaminated between patients by pasteurization or the use of high-level chemical disinfection with glutaraldehyde, peracetic acid, hydrogen peroxide, ethyl alcohol, or hypochlorite. *Noncritical* items, which normally come into contact only with intact skin, such as blood pressure cuffs or electrocardiograph electrodes, require hygienic cleansing or low-level disinfection with an iodophor, hypochlorite, quaternary ammonium or phenolic disinfectants, or alcohol.[196,197] The lone exception to this classification scheme is devices that pose a risk of transmitting prion-related diseases, including Creutzfeldt-Jakob disease (CJD) and variant CJD (vCJD).[198,199] Prions are not readily inactivated by conventional disinfection and sterilization procedures.[196,199] As a result, devices that pose a risk for transmission of prion-related diseases should undergo special sterilization procedures after cleaning that involve sodium hydroxide followed by low-temperature autoclaving (121° C) or high-temperature autoclaving (132° C for 1 hour or 134° C for ≥18 minutes).[197,199] Despite concerns that procedures involving semicritical items such as endoscopes and bronchoscopes may pose a risk for transmission of prion-related infections, there has not been a single report of CJD or vCJD associated with these devices. As a result, current guidelines recommend that only critical items and semicritical items that have come in contact with neurologic tissue (e.g., brain [including dura mater], spinal cord, eye, and pituitary tissue) should undergo special prion inactivation sterilization procedures.[197,199,200]

Numerous epidemics of gram-negative infection have been described in association with respiratory therapy equipment,[97,98] diagnostic equipment such as bronchoscopes and endoscopes,[98,102-104] and solutions used for cutaneous antisepsis.[201,202] Most of these outbreaks were traced to improper procedures or malfunction of automated systems used for the disinfection and sterilization of medical devices, although a number of epidemics in years past arose as a result of extrinsic contamination of solutions used for cutaneous antisepsis.[201,202] For these reasons, the importance of strict adherence to recommended policies and procedures for cleaning and reprocessing medical equipment used in the ICU cannot be overemphasized.

Endoscopes and bronchoscopes are essential diagnostic and therapeutic instruments in the ICU. Although most postendoscopy nosocomial infections are caused by inoculation of colonizing mucosal flora into normally sterile, vulnerable anatomic sites during the procedure, numerous epidemics have been traced to contaminated endoscopes.[98,102-104] Following use for bronchoscopy, endoscopes are typically contaminated with 6×10^4 colony-forming units per milliliter (CFUs/mL).[203] All endoscopes are considered semicritical medical devices by the Spaulding classification and therefore require high-level disinfection following use.[200] In order to ensure their safe use, flexible endoscopes should be reprocessed with the following procedures: (1) physical cleaning to reduce microbial bioburden and remove organic debris; (2) high-level disinfection—glutaraldehyde and automated chemical sterilizing systems that use peracetic acid are most commonly used in the United States—with adequate contact time between the disinfectant and device surface; (3) following disinfection, rinsing with sterile or filtered tap water to remove disinfectant residue; (4) flushing of all channels with 70% to 90% ethyl or isopropyl alcohol; and (5) drying with forced air.[200] Devices used with endoscopes that violate mucosal barriers, such as biopsy forceps, need to be reprocessed as critical medical items with full sterilization.[200] Other devices used in the delivery of respiratory care are also considered semicritical under the Spaulding classification and therefore should be reprocessed in a manner similar to endoscopes prior to reuse.[135]

Iodophors (e.g., 10% povidone-iodine), until recently, have been the most common agents used for cutaneous disinfection in North America. However, a large, prospective, randomized trial of cutaneous antiseptics used for drawing blood cultures showed that chlorhexidine was superior to 10% povidone-iodine and was associated with a more than twofold reduced rate of contaminated blood cultures (odds ratio [OR] = 0.40, 95% CI 0.21 to 0.75, $p = 0.004$).[204] Moreover, a meta-analysis examining the impact of different cutaneous antiseptic agents found that chlorhexidine was superior to povidone-iodine for both the prevention of intravascular catheter colonization and catheter-related bloodstream infection.[205] On the basis of these and other recent studies,[206,207] chlorhexidine-containing solutions are the preferred cutaneous antiseptics for insertion of intravascular devices in the ICU.[132] Whatever agent is used, it is essential that it be applied with vigorous scrubbing for a minimum of 1 minute to allow adequate time for germicidal activity.

HAND HYGIENE

The major reservoir of nosocomial infection in the ICU is infected or colonized patients, and the major mode of spread of most nosocomial bacterial pathogens, many viruses, and even *Candida* from patient to patient is by transient carriage on the hands of medical personnel (see Fig. 50.3). Studies of hand carriage of nosocomial pathogens by ICU personnel, using a simple rinse technique to quantify the transient flora,[208] have shown that, on average, approximately 60,000 CFUs (or 4.6 logs) are recovered from the hands of ICU personnel randomly sampled (Table 50.4). Nearly half of persons cultured at any point in time will be found to be carrying gram-negative bacilli, and 10% will be carrying *S. aureus*.[209] Serial culturing has shown that all ICU personnel, at various times, carry gram-negative bacilli and that nearly two thirds carry *S. aureus*. Carriage of both gram-negative bacilli and *S. aureus* is typically transient: sampling persons every other day over a prolonged period has shown *S. aureus* or the same gram-negative species in consecutive cultures only 16% of the time; prolonged carriage of a single gram-negative species seems to be rare—but has been reported.[210]

Hygienic handwashing before undertaking invasive procedures, handling open wounds, or having manual contact with high-risk patients (e.g., newborns or patients in ICUs) or after touching a source or object likely to be contaminated has been recognized since the time of Semmelweis and Lister as one of the most basic and important infection control measures. Despite universal acknowledgment of handwashing as a cornerstone of nosocomial infection control programs, compliance rates much above 50% have been difficult to achieve, and handwashing rates among HCWs have ranged from 9% to 50% in numerous observational studies.[168,211,212] Recent investigations have undertaken to better understand the reasons for poor compliance in the face of the compelling evidence that hand hygiene is essential for prevention of nosocomial infection,[168] identifying cutaneous irritation, inconvenient sink location,

Table 50.4 Studies of Microorganisms Carried on the Hands of Hospital Personnel Working in a Neurosurgery Unit*

Study Parameter	All Microorganisms	Gram-Negative Bacilli	*Staphylococcus aureus*
Mean $\log_{10}$ CFUs ± SD, recovered from persons' hands†	4.59 ± 0.69	1.04 ± 0.44	0.44 ± 0.44
(range of individuals' means)	(3.31-5.76)	(0.29-1.93)	(0-1.45)
% all cultures positive	100	44.5	11.2
% all personnel with at least one positive culture†	100	100	64

*At the University of Wisconsin Hospital.
†Based on 6 to 34 cultures obtained at random times from each of 25 employees working in the unit over a 4-month period.
CFUs, colony-forming units; SD, standard deviation.
From Maki DG: Control of colonization and transmission of pathogenic bacteria in the hospital. Ann Intern Med 1978;89:777-780.

time constraints, high workload, and understaffing. Of concern, risk factors for noncompliance with hand hygiene include being a physician (rather than a nurse); working in an ICU; and paradoxically, engaging in patient-care activities with a high risk of cross-transmission.[168] Interventions to redress these deficiencies have included targeted education; feedback; convenient location of sinks and hand hygiene agents; use of alternative, less irritative hand hygiene agents; hand care lotions or creams[213]; and patient education.[214]

Studies done with working hospital staff have shown that hygienic handwashing with an antiseptic-containing agent reduces the count of microorganisms on the hands of the user far more effectively than handwashing with a nonmedicated soap.[208] Repeated use of some antiseptics such as chlorhexidine has a cumulative suppressive effect on the transient hand flora. Routine use of an antiseptic-containing handwashing agent could, in theory, enhance the effectiveness of the handwashing that is done. Moreover, if an agent that exhibits prolonged antimicrobial activity, such as chlorhexidine, is used, it might also confer protection against contaminants acquired between handwashings.[208] However, antiseptic-containing handwashing agents are more expensive and often more irritating to the skin. Irritation can result in dermatitis and, paradoxically, increased colonization by gram-negative bacilli.[215]

Clearly, antiseptic-containing soaps are more effective in removing microorganisms from the hands of users, but will routine use of these agents for hygienic handwashing reduce the incidence of nosocomial infection in patients? Discontinuation of hexachlorophene for handwashing by personnel and bathing of infants in the United States in 1973 was followed by a marked upsurge in *S. aureus* infections in nurseries,[216] and use of chlorhexidine-containing handwashing agents was considered an essential measure for control of hospital outbreaks caused by multiply resistant *Klebsiella*[217] and MRSA.[218,219] However, since Semmelweis's study, few studies have prospectively evaluated the efficacy of antiseptic-containing handwashing agents for reducing endemic nosocomial infections, particularly infections caused by gram-negative bacilli.[215,220]

In 1982 a comparative sequential trial of three handwashing agents—a nonmedicated tissue soap, 10% povidone-iodine (Betadine Scrub), and 4% chlorhexidine (Hibiclens)—was undertaken in the trauma-surgical ICU of the University of Wisconsin Hospital.[215] Each agent was used exclusively for approximately 6 weeks, during which time hand cultures of ICU personnel were done at random and surveillance of infection in patients was carried out. Risk factors for infection in patients hospitalized during the use of each agent were comparable: Nearly two thirds of the patients in each period required ventilatory support and hemodynamic monitoring, and almost all had urinary catheters. The incidence of nosocomial infection in all groups was expectedly high, but it was 30% lower during the use of the two antiseptic-containing handwashing agents than during the use of the nonmedicated soap ($p < 0.001$). Povidone-iodine was irritating to the hands of most staff, and chlorhexidine had a slightly drying effect but was well tolerated, comparable with the nonmedicated soap.

In a similar study at the University of Iowa Hospital, Massanari[220] did not find significant differences in the rates of nosocomial infection when nonmedicated soap was used exclusively as compared with alternating cycles during which 4% chlorhexidine (Hibiclens) was used in surgical ICUs; however, the incidence of infection in the medical ICU was 50% lower during use of chlorhexidine ($p < 0.05$).

In the largest multiple-crossover prospective study—1894 adult patients in three ICUs—of the relative efficacy of antiseptic-containing handwashing agents used by personnel in ICUs, Doebbeling and colleagues[221] found that the use of 4% chlorhexidine (Hibiclens) was associated with a 30% reduction in nosocomial infections (OR = 0.73), as contrasted with rates when a 60% alcohol hand-rinsing agent (Cal-Stat) was used. Both regimens were well tolerated.

Recently, alcohol-based waterless hand rubs have become the agents of choice for hand hygiene and are now universally used in U.S. hospitals because of their convenience and broad-spectrum activity.[214] Alcohols have the most rapid and pronounced bactericidal action and greatly reduce the time needed for hand disinfection. A vigorous 1-minute rubbing with a sufficient volume of alcohol to wet the hands completely has been shown to be highly effective at reducing the density of skin flora.[222] Ethanol and iso- and *n*-propanol are the constituents of most commercially available alcohol-based hand rubs; at equal concentrations, *n*-propanol is most effective and ethanol the least. However, all have limited efficacy with gross soilage so that visibly soiled hands should always be washed with antiseptic soap and water.[174] Moreover, at least 3 mL of an alcohol-based rub is necessary to completely coat the hands and achieve optimal degerming. The use of alcohol hand rubs or gels will be augmented by making conveniently located calibrated dispensers widely available. However, many HCWs prefer individual containers that can be carried in a pocket, which makes it difficult to ensure that an adequate volume is used with each application.

Few trials have been conducted to evaluate the efficacy of alcohol-containing hand rubs for reducing nosocomial infection. Most are quasi-experimental before-after studies, and most have shown a short-term reduction in nosocomial infection rates with use of alcohol-containing hand rubs.[175,223,224]

The major factor limiting acceptance of alcohol products for hand antisepsis in the past was desiccation and irritation of skin. This is now obviated by incorporating emollients into alcohol-based hand rubs, which has enhanced acceptance by HCWs and may augment antibacterial activity by slowing the evaporation of alcohol.[225] A recent randomized clinical trial in 50 ICU HCWs compared a conventional 2% chlorhexidine gluconate wash with water to a waterless alcohol-based hand rub (61% ethanol with emollients) and showed that use of the waterless alcohol-based product produced significantly less skin scaling and irritation[226]; unfortunately, degerming was not assessed.

A recent review describes in detail the various hand hygiene agents available and their spectrum of activity.[214] Recommendations for hand hygiene by the CDC have been published (Table 50.5),[174] emphasizing hand

Table 50.5 Recommendations for Routine Hand Hygiene from the Centers for Disease Control and Prevention (CDC) Guideline

Recommendation	Level of Evidence*
• When hands are visibly dirty or contaminated with proteinaceous material or are visibly soiled with blood or other body fluids, wash hands with either a nonantimicrobial soap and water or an antimicrobial soap and water.	IA
• If hands are not visibly soiled, use an alcohol-based hand rub or, alternatively, wash hands with an antimicrobial soap and water, for the following situations:	IB
◦ Before direct contact with patients	
◦ Before putting on sterile gloves when inserting a central vascular catheter	
◦ Before inserting a urinary catheter, peripheral vascular catheter, or other invasive procedure not requiring surgery	
◦ After contact with patient's intact skin (e.g., while taking a pulse or blood pressure or lifting the patient)	
◦ After contact with body fluids, mucous membranes, nonintact skin, and wound dressings if hands are not visibly soiled	
◦ Moving from a contaminated body site to a clean body site during patient care	
◦ After contact with inanimate objects (e.g., medical equipment) in the immediate vicinity of the patient	
◦ After removing gloves	
• Before eating and after using a restroom, wash hands with a nonantimicrobial soap and water or with an antimicrobial soap and water.	IB
• Antimicrobial-impregnated wipes are not a substitute for using an alcohol-based hand rub or antimicrobial soap.	IB
• If exposure to *Bacillus anthracis* is suspected or proved, wash hands with nonantimicrobial soap and water or antimicrobial soap and water.	II

**Categorization of recommendations*: IA: strongly supported for implementation and strongly supported by well-designed experimental, clinical, or epidemiologic studies. IB: strongly recommended for implementation and supported by certain clinical or epidemiologic studies and by strong theoretical rationale. IC: required for implementation, as mandated by federal or state regulation or standard. II: suggested for implementation and supported by suggestive clinical or epidemiologic studies or by strong theoretical rationale. NR (no recommendation/unresolved issue): practices for which insufficient evidence or no consensus exists about efficacy.

Data from Boyce JM, Pittet D: Recommendations of the Healthcare Infection Control Practices Advisory Committee and the HICPAC/SHEA/APIC/IDSA Hand Hygiene Task Force. MMWR Recomm Rep 2002;16:1-45.

antisepsis with an antiseptic-containing soap or detergent or an alcohol-based hand rub (1) before and after direct contact with patients or the environment and equipment in the immediate vicinity of the patient and (2) before performing invasive procedures such as insertion of an intravascular device or urinary catheter. Use of skin care products—lotions or creams—to minimize irritant contact dermatitis associated with frequent handwashing and improve compliance with hand hygiene practices is highly recommended.

Institutional commitment is essential to improve compliance with recommended hand hygiene practices. The CDC guideline recommends that institutions (1) monitor and record adherence to hand hygiene by ward or service; (2) provide feedback to HCWs about their performance; and (3) monitor the volume of alcohol hand rubs used per 1000 patient-days.[174]

Clearly, further studies are necessary, particularly large comparative trials in which rates of nosocomial infection, rather than levels of cutaneous colonization, are used as the index of comparison. In the meantime the available data indicate that routine use of a chlorhexidine-containing product or alcohol-containing product will be more effective than use of a nonmedicated soap for hand hygiene in the high-risk areas of the hospital, such as ICUs, where cross-infection is most likely to occur.

ISOLATION PRECAUTIONS FOR COMMUNICABLE INFECTIONS

Isolation, the use of special precautions in the care of infected patients, is the only means of curtailing the spread of contagious microorganisms and preventing epidemics, especially in ICUs, where the risk of cross-infection is highest. Although requiring all persons entering an infected patient's room to wear gloves and a gown, possibly even a mask, may seem ritualistic and almost archaic, each aspect of the isolation procedure is directed at interrupting a potential mode of spread and is based on the known epidemiology of the infecting organism.[227] To be maximally effective, however, isolation procedures require compliance by each person coming into contact with the patient, including physicians. Isolation is also indicated, usually for the entirety of hospitalization, for all patients infected or known to be colonized by antibiotic-resistant nosocomial pathogens such as MRSA, multidrug-resistant gram-negative bacilli, or VRE; in such cases, isolation has been shown to be effective in reducing endemic infections[228,229] (Figs. 50.3 and 50.4) and in controlling outbreaks.[229]

ISOLATION SYSTEMS

Most U.S. hospitals subscribe to one of two CDC isolation systems developed by panels of experts. The simplest system,

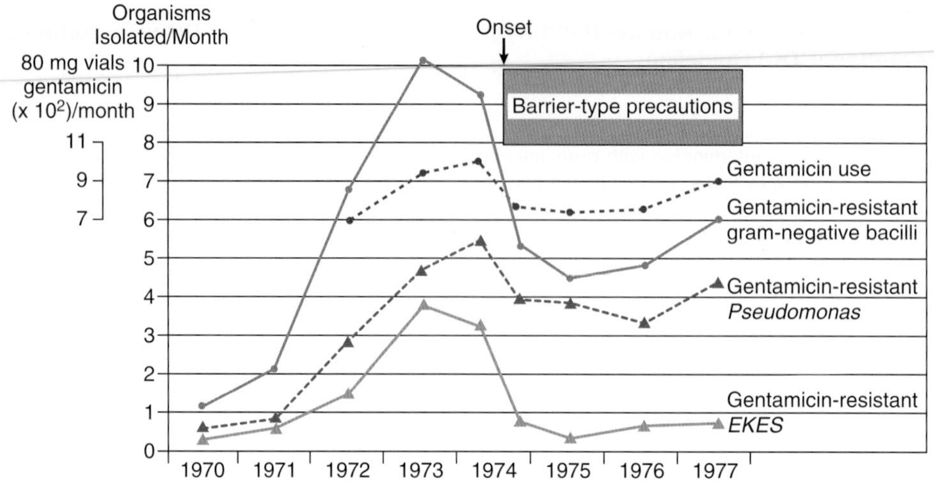

Figure 50.3 Impact of implementing barrier-type precautions (gown and gloves) with patients known to be colonized or infected by gram-negative bacilli resistant to gentamicin. Frequency of infections by gentamicin-resistant gram-negative bacilli and gentamicin use at Michael Reese Medical Center, 1970-1977. Data are plotted as the monthly average, and the averages for the first 7 and last 5 months of 1974 are plotted separately to demonstrate the effect of barrier-type precautions implemented in August 1974. *EKES, Escherichia coli, Klebsiella pneumoniae, Enterobacter* species, and *Serratia* species. (From Weinstein RA, Nathan C, Gruensfelder R, et al: Endemic aminoglycoside resistance in gram-negative bacilli: Epidemiology and mechanisms. J Infect Dis 1980;141:338-345.)

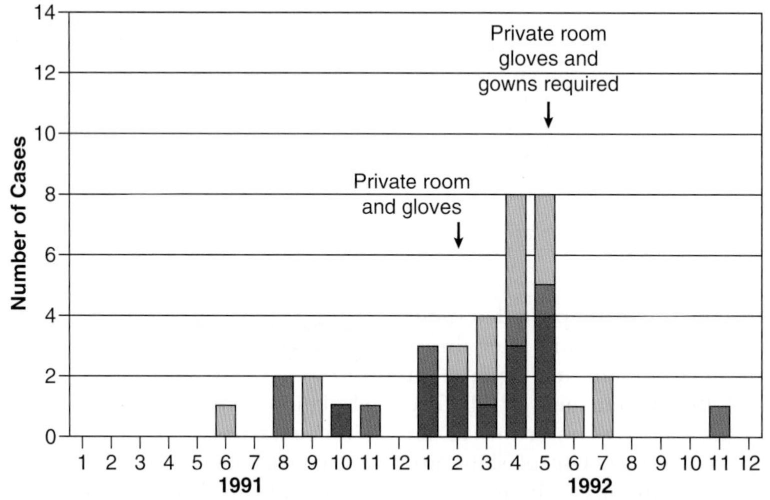

Figure 50.4 Impact of specific control measures on an institutional outbreak of vancomycin-resistant *Escherichia faecium.* Cases, by date of first positive culture for the epidemic strains (from January 1991 to December 1992). Number of cases = case patients in the intensive care unit (ICU) at time of first positive culture for the epidemic strain × other patients with previous exposure to the ICU × case patients never in the ICU. (From Boyce JM, Opal SM, Chow JW, et al: Outbreak of multidrug-resistant *Enterococcus faecium* with transferable vanB class vancomycin resistance. J Clin Microbiol 1994;32:1148-1153.)

category-specific isolation precautions, issued by the CDC in 1970,[227] groups diseases in seven categories by infections for which similar precautions are indicated: wound and skin precautions, enteric precautions, discharge precautions, blood precautions, respiration isolation, strict isolation, and protective isolation. Guidelines for *disease-specific* isolation precautions, issued in 1983,[230] consider each infectious disease individually, so only those precautions indicated to interrupt transmission of that specific disease are used. Disease-specific precautions minimize unnecessary isolation procedures; however, they are more complicated and may be implemented most effectively by a computerized system.

An alternative, simpler system, *body substance isolation,* has gained adherents and focuses on the isolation of potentially infectious body substances, such as blood, feces, urine, sputum, wound drainage, and other body fluids, of all patients through the use of simple barrier precautions—primarily gloves, gowns, plastic aprons, and masks or goggles. These barriers should be used when potentially infectious secretions are likely to soil or splash the clothing, skin, or face of the HCW.[231] Body substance isolation provides sufficient flexibility to augment the basic precautions taken with each patient, as needed, and adds private rooms with masks for infections transmitted by the airborne route. A criticism of this simpler system has been the reduced emphasis on handwashing when gloves are removed.[232]

The most recent CDC guideline[177] separates basic precautions into (1) *standard precautions* designed for the care of all patients in hospitals, regardless of their diagnosis or presumed infection status, and (2) additional *transmission-based precautions* designed for the care of specified patients who are known or suspected to be infected with highly transmissible or epidemiologically important pathogens. Standard precautions synthesize the major features of universal blood and body fluid precautions and are designed to reduce the risk of transmission of microorganisms from patient to patient and from patient to HCW, from both recognized and unrecognized sources of infection in the hospital. Transmission-based precautions are divided into three subgroups on the basis of the mode of transmission: contact precautions, droplet precautions, and airborne precautions. Contact precautions are recommended with multidrug-resistant bacteria that can be acquired by contact with the colonized patient or environmental surfaces or objects. Droplet precautions provide additional measures for transmission by large-particle droplets, such as during suctioning or bronchoscopy. Airborne precautions are added to standard precautions for the care of patients with tuberculosis and other microorganisms transmitted by the airborne route. In general, transmission-based precautions usually specify a private room—always for airborne precautions.

SPECIAL ISSUES IN THE ICU

An environmental issue pertaining to isolation may be most relevant in the ICU, namely, the greater potential for fomites or environmental surfaces to contribute to the spread of nosocomial infection, especially with antibiotic-resistant microorganisms. Although previous studies have not been able to demonstrate that the inanimate hospital environment, particularly surfaces, walls, or floors, contribute materially to the occurrence of nosocomial infection,[157,158] accumulating evidence suggests that this may not necessarily be true for ICUs, where uniform exposure to invasive devices makes patients unduly susceptible. A number of careful studies of the epidemiology of ICU-acquired infection with resistant organisms such as MRSA,[158,159] *C. difficile,*[83,160] and VRE[155,161,233] have shown heavy contamination of the inanimate environment immediately contiguous to the patient by strains implicated in nosocomial infections occurring in patients. Even if gloves are being worn as part of protective isolation or universal precautions, the possibility of transmission of microorganisms from the environment to patients on the gloved hands of HCWs is real. Prolonged wearing of gloves in the ICU, which is common, may increase the risk of nosocomial cross-infection, expanding the epidemiologic role of the inanimate environment with certain pathogens such as MRSA or VRE.[233]

Similarly, the use of common stethoscopes, sphygmomanometers, or electronic thermometers with multiple patients provides further opportunity for organisms to spread. Although stethoscopes are commonly contaminated by nosocomial organisms,[234] their role in cross-infection is less clear.[234] On the other hand, spread of VRE[235] and *C. difficile*[236] has been traced to contamination of electronic thermometers. All surfaces contiguous to the ICU patient should be wiped down with the general hospital disinfectant at least daily, and each ICU patient should have a dedicated stethoscope and sphygmomanometer. The use of electronic temperature measuring devices on multiple patients within an ICU bears reevaluation, unless stringent efforts are made to assure reliable decontamination of the device after each use.

As discussed, many nosocomial infections appear to derive from organisms carried on the hands of ICU personnel, who during the working day have contact with multiple patients. To improve nursing care and reduce the risk of cross-infection, ICUs must have an adequate number of staff. Although the optimal nurse/patient ratio for patients in an ICU is not known, increased rates of infection and outbreaks have occurred when nurses have been assigned to multiple critically ill patients who require complicated nursing care.[166] One-to-one nurse/patient ratios may significantly reduce the risk of cross-infection.

To contain the spread of certain resistant organisms in the ICU (e.g., MRSA, VRE), cohort nursing is strongly recommended. In cohort nursing, the care of patients known to be infected (or colonized) by the organism is provided by nurses (and respiratory therapists) who will not provide care during that shift for noninfected patients, and the nursing care of noninfected patients is restricted to personnel who will not have contact with infected patients, except in an emergency. Cohorting of patients known to be colonized or infected with MRSA is widely practiced but has not been adequately studied. In one recent prospective study, the authors found that there was no evidence of increased transmission of MRSA when patients were not cohorted.[237]

TUBERCULOSIS

The upsurge in tuberculosis since 1985, particularly the numerous nosocomial outbreaks caused by multidrug-resistant strains,[73-75,238,239] demonstrates the importance of isolation precautions to prevent the spread of tuberculosis within hospitals, especially within ICUs.[129] Guidelines[129] reemphasize the importance of air control by mandating the use of private negative-pressure rooms, combined with the use of ultraviolet lights or ventilatory modifications in which all air exiting the room is either filtered or exhausted directly to the roofline, away from hospital intake vents. Isolation room doors must be kept closed to maintain control over the direction of airflow, and all persons who enter a room in which tuberculosis isolation precautions are in effect must wear a disposable particulate respirator such as a dust-mist mask or a HEPA-filter mask. Gowns and gloves usually are not indicated. All ICUs should have one or more negative-pressure isolation rooms for the care of patients requiring respiratory isolation for tuberculosis and other airborne infections such as chickenpox or disseminated herpes zoster, disseminated HSV infection, or emerging, highly contagious airborne infections such as SARS. To reduce the risk of contaminating a ventilator or discharging *M. tuberculosis* into the environment, when mechanically ventilating a patient with suspected or confirmed pulmonary tuberculosis, a bacterial filter capable of filtering particles as small as 0.3 μm, with a filter efficacy of greater than 95%, should be placed on the patient's endotracheal tube or at the expiratory side of the breathing circuit of a ventilator.[129] ICU patients with tuberculosis not requiring mechanical ventilation should wear a surgical mask if leaving the negative-pressure isolation rooms for radiographic or other procedures.[129]

STANDARD PRECAUTIONS

The world epidemic of AIDS and evidence that more than 1 million persons in the United States are silent carriers of the human immunodeficiency virus (HIV) have engendered great concern among HCWs regarding the risk of exposure to HIV in the workplace. In 1987 the CDC and the Department of Labor issued detailed guidelines for *Universal Blood and Body Fluid Precautions*[240,241] to prevent exposure of HCW workers and patients to potentially hazardous blood or body fluids. Universal precautions were based on the concept that all blood and body fluids that might be contaminated with blood should be treated as infectious because patients with bloodborne infections can be asymptomatic or unaware they are infected. The relevance of universal precautions to other aspects of disease transmission was recognized, and in 1996 the CDC expanded the concept and changed the term to *Standard Precautions*.[242] Standard precautions integrate and expand the elements of universal precautions into a standard of care designed to protect health care personnel and patients from pathogens that can be spread by blood or any other body fluid, excretion, or secretion. Standard precautions apply to contact with (1) blood; (2) all body fluids, secretions, and excretions (except sweat), regardless of whether they contain blood; (3) nonintact skin; and (4) mucous membranes.

Gloves are recommended for venipunctures, insertion of intravascular devices, and whenever it can be anticipated that the hands could become contaminated by blood or another high-risk body fluid. If there is potential for splatter or contamination of clothing, a gown is added. When there is potential for aerosolization of body fluids, such as during surgery, intubation, endoscopy, or insertion of an arterial catheter, a mask and eye shielding are included. Because the vast majority of occupationally related HIV infections have involved needle sticks or other sharps injuries, every effort must be made to avert such injuries that could result in percutaneous inoculation of HIV or other bloodborne viruses.[240,243]

Because prophylactic use of barrier precautions appears to be of some benefit for the prevention of nosocomial infection[172,244,245] and all U.S. hospitals are currently mandated to follow standard precautions, it has been suggested that the use of gloves for all patient contacts, as is now common in many U.S. hospitals, should implicitly reduce the risk of nosocomial infection in general. However, this has not been demonstrated and there is concern that standard precautions might paradoxically increase the risk of nosocomial cross-infection.[246] In most U.S. hospitals it is still common to observe ICU personnel, many of whom routinely wear gloves for all patient contacts to protect themselves, put on gloves, touch heavily contaminated areas (e.g., an open wound or tracheostomy), and then, without removing the gloves, proceed to write in the patient's chart, answer the telephone, or care for another patient. This occurs because the health care providers have forgotten that although the gloves may protect themselves, the gloves must be immediately discarded after use to prevent cross-contamination of hazardous pathogens to other vulnerable sites on the same patient or transmission to other patients or the ICU environment. Before the era of AIDS and universal precautions, health care professionals were oriented toward protecting the patient and likely to wash their hands when exposed to potential contamination. Now the focus is centripetal, and many HCWs unfortunately view all precautions as measures to protect themselves. Thus prolonged wearing of gloves can result in heavy contamination of the gloves[247] and increase the risk of nosocomial cross-infection among patients.[233,248] It also puts the HCW at increased risk of dermatitis and allergic reactions to glove material.[249] Standard precautions do not obviate the need for designated isolation precautions for patients with communicable infections. The greatly expanded use of gloves as part of standard precautions in hospitals must now be accompanied by educational programs on how to use gloves effectively and in a manner that will not jeopardize patients. Staff must be strongly encouraged to wash their hands after removing gloves, especially after performing a bloody procedure, because blood often penetrates defects in gloves and can be found on the hands of the wearer.[250] Moreover, if the gloved HCW has had hands-on contact with a patient colonized by MRSA or VRE, the process of removing the gloves will result in contamination of the hands of the HCW by these organisms up to one third of the time.

ANTIBIOTIC STEWARDSHIP

There is a world crisis in antibiotic resistance (see Fig. 50.2),[251,252] which reflects in greatest measure the heavy use of systemic antibiotics worldwide over the past 30 years, especially in hospitals. Antimicrobial therapy has its greatest ecologic impact in the close confines of the ICU. Most nosocomial outbreaks caused by antibiotic-resistant microorganisms[253,254] have occurred in patients hospitalized in an ICU. Antibiotic pressure, which promotes the exchange of genes encoding drug resistance by a variety of transfer mechanisms (Fig. 50.5),[255] has been shown to be the single most important factor predisposing patients to nosocomial infection with resistant organisms. Modern-day ICUs are the breeding grounds for the multiply resistant bacteria that are now being encountered in hospitals throughout the world: MRSA; VRE; extended-spectrum β-lactamase-producing and carbapenemase-producing *K. pneumoniae* and *E. coli*, *Enterobacter*, *Serratia*, *Citrobacter*, and *P. aeruginosa* resistant to fluoroquinolones, aminoglycosides, or extended-spectrum β-lactams.[47,58-61,251] Broad-spectrum antimicrobial therapy is the root cause of antibiotic-associated diarrhea and colitis caused by *C. difficile*.[83]

Clearly, antimicrobials are widely overused and misused; more than 75% of patients in U.S. ICUs, other than coronary care units, receive antimicrobial agents, whereas studies indicate that more than half of hospitalized patients receiving antimicrobial therapy have no evidence of infection or clear justification to be receiving antibiotics.[256] Moreover,

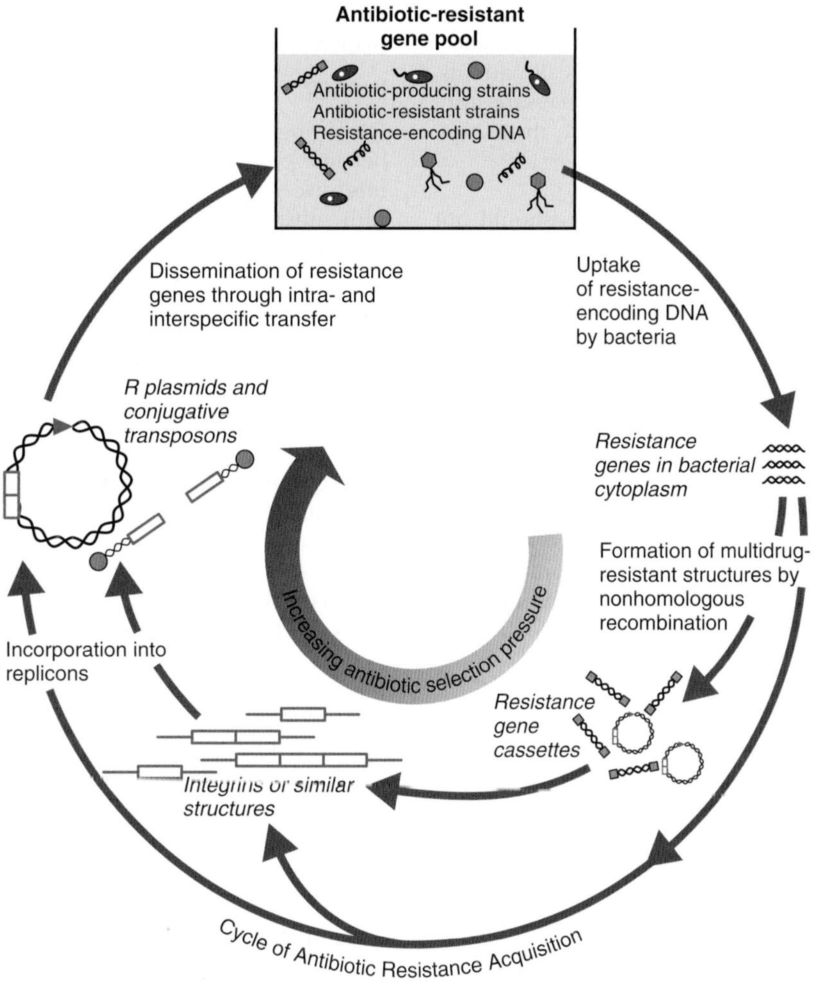

Figure 50.5 Schematic depicting the route by which antibiotic-resistant genes are acquired by bacteria in response to selection pressure of antibiotic use. The resistance gene pool represents all potential sources of DNA encoding antibiotic-resistant determinants in the environment; this includes hospitals, farms, or other microenvironments where antibiotics are used to control bacterial development. After uptake of single- or double-stranded DNA by the bacterial host, the incorporation of the resistance genes into stable replicons (DNA elements capable of autonomous replication) may occur by several different pathways that have not yet been identified. The involvement of integrins, as shown here, has been demonstrated for a large class of transposable elements in the *Enterobacteriaceae*. The resulting resistance plasmids could exist in linear or circular form in bacterial hosts. The final step in the cycle, dissemination, is brought about by one or more gene transfer mechanisms. (From Davies J: Inactivation of antibiotics and the dissemination of resistance genes. Science 1994;264:375-382.)

within ICUs, a high proportion of the antibiotics used are broad-spectrum/extended-spectrum penicillins, third- and fourth-generation cephalosporins, carbapenems, aminoglycosides, fluoroquinolones, or vancomycin. Greater efforts must be directed to improving the use of systemic antibiotics, especially within ICUs.

JCAHO now mandates that hospitals periodically review their use of antimicrobial agents through the use of antimicrobial audits.[30] Such audits should scrutinize the need for antimicrobial therapy—clear evidence of infection or clear justification for prophylactic use, the appropriateness of the regimen selected, and monitoring for therapeutic efficacy and side effects during therapy.[257] Educational programs and institutional guidelines for antimicrobial use that permit the hospital staff to construct guidelines and policies based on local needs and judgments, aided by published criteria, have been shown to materially improve antimicrobial use within the hospital.[256,258] Other important methods for controlling antimicrobial use include a restricted formulary, the policies of the clinical microbiology laboratory on reporting of susceptibility testing, and automatic stop orders for surgical prophylaxis.[256] Many institutions also place expensive or the most broad-spectrum drugs (e.g., third- and fourth-generation cephalosporins, extended-spectrum penicillins [e.g., piperacillin-tazobactam], carbapenems, aminoglycosides, fluoroquinolones, vancomycin, linezolid, fluconazole, echinocandins, lipid formulations of amphotericin B, ganciclovir, etc.) on a restricted list, requiring physicians who wish to use the agents to justify their use to a representative of the institutional antibiotic review committee.[259] Such programs greatly reduce use of restricted antibiotics and are gaining ever-wider acceptance.

Excellent resources,[260-262] including other chapters in this book (Chapters 20, 51, 52), are available to guide the selection and use of anti-infective drugs in critically ill patients. However, several principles can reduce unnecessary antimicrobial therapy and improve the use of the drugs that are given:

1. Fever without other indications of infection should not mandate automatically beginning antimicrobial therapy in an ICU patient.
2. Unless antimicrobial therapy is being given for surgical prophylaxis, it is most likely being given for the treatment of suspected or proved infection. Gram-stained smears, cultures, and other appropriate diagnostic tests, as indicated, should be done without fail before beginning antimicrobial therapy for treatment of presumed infection in an ICU patient.
3. Whenever antimicrobial therapy is begun, the reason should be documented in the patient's record (e.g., "for the treatment of pneumonia," "for surgical prophylaxis").
4. When possible, a single drug and the most narrow-spectrum drug or drugs should be used, especially if the infecting organism or organisms are known at the outset.
5. The need for continued antimicrobial therapy should be reassessed daily. If cultures identify the infecting microorganism or microorganisms, therapy should be modified, aiming for the most narrow-spectrum drug or drugs likely to be effective. If diagnostic studies are negative after 48 to 72 hours and the patient is not exhibiting signs of sepsis, antibiotic therapy should be discontinued, unless the patient is profoundly granulocytopenic.
6. Beyond monitoring for efficacy and adverse drug effects such as hypersensitivity or organ toxicity, it is essential that monitoring include surveillance for superinfection by resistant bacteria or *Candida* and for *C. difficile* infection.
7. Surgical antimicrobial prophylaxis should not extend beyond 24 hours postoperatively[263,264] and in most operations can be limited to a single dose.[263]

NOSOCOMIAL INFECTIONS AND SPECIFIC INFECTION CONTROL MEASURES

As noted earlier, most nosocomial infections, especially in immunologically competent patients and in ICUs, are causally related to surgical operations or exposure to invasive devices of various types (see Tables 50.1 and 50.2). Comprehensive guidelines for the prevention of infection with procedures or devices that pose the greatest risk (urinary catheters,[133,134,265] endotracheal intubation and mechanical ventilatory support,[135] intravascular catheters and infusion therapy,[132] hemodialysis,[266] and surgery[263]) have been published and can form the basis for institutional policies and procedures. Health care professionals working in ICUs are obligated to be informed about prevention of infection associated with the procedures they perform and the devices with which they work daily.

INTRAVASCULAR DEVICE–RELATED BLOODSTREAM INFECTION

IMPACT

Obtaining and maintaining reliable vascular access has become one of the most essential features of modern-day intensive care. Unfortunately, vascular access is associated with substantial and generally underappreciated potential for producing iatrogenic disease, particularly bloodstream infection (BSI) originating from infection of the percutaneous intravascular device (IVD) used for vascular access (i.e., IVD-related BSI), often referred to as "line sepsis." Nearly 60% of all nosocomial bacteremias derive from vascular access in some form,[18] and it is estimated that more than 500,000 IVD-related bloodstream infections occur in the United States each year.[267,268] Early studies found that IVD-related BSIs are associated with excess attributable mortality rate ranging up to 35%[269]; however, subsequent case-control studies have not consistently found excess mortality rates, especially of this magnitude.[270-272] This controversy aside, all studies examining the impact of IVD-related BSI on patient outcomes have found that IVD-related BSIs are associated with increased length of hospitalization and excess health care costs, averaging $30,000 per case.[269-272]

IVD-related BSIs are largely preventable. The goal must not be simply to identify and treat these infections but rather to prevent them. By drawing on existent knowledge of the pathogenesis and epidemiology of IVD-related BSI, rational and effective guidelines for prevention can be formulated.

DEFINITIONS

IVDs are associated with both local and systemic infection. The CDC has published definitions for IVD-related infection (see Box 50.1).[16,17] These definitions are useful for the purposes of surveillance but rely heavily on the construct, central venous catheter–associated BSI, which implicitly assumes that each primary BSI (i.e., a BSI without an identifiable local infection) originates from a central venous catheter (CVC). This practice results in an overestimation of the true risk of CVC-related infection because not all primary BSIs originate from a central venous device; some are secondary BSIs deriving from unrecognized postoperative surgical site or intra-abdominal infections or nosocomial pneumonias or originate from other vascular devices such as peripheral venous catheters or arterial catheters used for hemodynamic monitoring.

By applying molecular subtyping techniques[110,273,274] to the results of semiquantitative or quantitative cultures of the removed IVD and blood cultures or the results of cultures of blood drawn through the IVD and a separate concomitant percutaneous peripheral blood culture, it is now possible to reliably determine whether an IVD was the source of a nosocomial BSI. Using these new diagnostic techniques allows the formulation of simple but more rigorous definitions for IVD-related infection (Table 50.6), which we believe bear consideration as the standard for randomized trials and epidemiologic studies of IVD-related infection.[18] Recently published guidelines have outlined clinical definitions of IVD-related BSI similar to those listed

Table 50.6 Proposed Definitions for Intravascular Device (IVD)-Related Colonization, Local Infection, and Bloodstream Infection (BSI) Based on Microbiologic Confirmation of the IVD as Source

IVD colonization	(i) A positive semiquantitative* (or quantitative†) culture of the implanted portion or portions of the IVD; (ii) absence of signs of local or systemic infection.
Local IVD infection	(i) A positive semiquantitative* (or quantitative†) culture of the removed IVD or a positive microscopic examination or culture of pus or thrombus from the cannulated vessel; (ii) clinical evidence of infection of the insertion site (i.e., erythema, induration, or purulence); but (iii) absence of systemic signs of infection and negative blood cultures, if done.
IVD-related BSI	*If the IVD is removed:* (i) A positive semiquantitative* (or quantitative†) culture of the IVD or a positive culture of the catheter hub or infusate (or positive microscopic examination or culture of pus or thrombus from the cannulated vessel) AND one or more positive blood cultures, ideally percutaneously drawn, concordant for the same species, ideally by molecular subtyping methods; (ii) clinical and microbiologic data disclose no other clear-cut source for the BSI. *If the IVD is retained:* (i) If quantitative blood cultures are available, cultures drawn both from the suspect IVD and a peripheral vein (or another IVD) are both positive and show a marked step up in quantitative positivity (fivefold or greater) in the IVD-drawn culture; (ii) clinical and microbiologic data disclose no other clear-cut source for the BSI. OR (i) If automated monitoring of incubating blood cultures is available, blood cultures drawn concomitantly from the suspect IVD and a peripheral vein (or another IVD) show both are positive, but the IVD-drawn blood culture turns positive more than 2 hours before the peripherally drawn culture; (ii) clinical and microbiologic data disclose no other clear-cut source for the BSI.

*Roll plate of cannula segment(s) >15 colony-forming units (CFUs).

†Sonication culture of cannula segment(s) ≥10^3 CFUs/mL.

Modified from Crnich CJ, Maki DG: The role of intravascular devices in sepsis. Curr Infect Dis Rep 2001;3:497-506.

Table 50.7 Clinical, Epidemiologic, and Microbiologic Features of Intravascular Device–Related Bloodstream Infection

Nonspecific	Suggestive of Device-Related Etiology
Fever	Patient unlikely candidate for sepsis (e.g., young, no underlying diseases)
Chills, shaking rigors*	Source of sepsis inapparent, no identifiable local infection
Hypotension, shock*	Intravascular device in place, especially central venous catheter
Hyperventilation, respiratory failure	Inflammation or purulence at insertion site
Gastrointestinal*	Abrupt onset, associated with shock
Abdominal pain Vomiting Diarrhea	Bloodstream infection caused by staphylococci (especially coagulase-negative staphylococci), *Corynebacterium, Candida, Trichophyton, Fusarium,* or *Malassezia* species†
Neurologic*	Very high-grade (>25 CFUs/mL) candidemia
Confusion Seizures	Cluster of cryptogenic infusion-associated bloodstream infections caused by *Enterobacter cloacae, Pantoea agglomerans,* or *Serratia marcescens**†
	Sepsis refractory to antimicrobial therapy or dramatic improvement with removal of cannula and infusion*

*Commonly seen in overwhelming gram-negative sepsis originating from contaminated infusate, peripheral suppurative phlebitis, or septic thrombosis of a central vein.

†Conversely, bacteremia caused by streptococci, aerobic gram-negative bacilli, or anaerobes is unlikely to derive from an intravascular device.

Modified from Maki DG, Mermel LA: Infections due to infusion therapy. In Bennett JV, Brachman PS (eds): Hospital Infections, 4th ed. Boston, Lippincott-Raven, 1998.

in Table 50.7, although molecular subtyping methods are not recommended for routine clinical diagnosis of IVD-related BSI.[275]

RECOGNITION AND DIAGNOSIS

Clinical Features

Recent evidence-based guidelines provide the best current information on the evaluation of the ICU patient with fever or other signs of sepsis.[34] Before any decision regarding initiation of antimicrobial therapy or removal of an IVD, the patient must be thoroughly examined to identify all plausible sites of infection including VAP, catheter-associated urinary tract infection, surgical site infection, IVD-related BSI, *C. difficile* infection, and other infections.[34]

Despite the challenge of identifying the source of a patient's signs of sepsis,[34] several clinical, epidemiologic, and microbiologic findings point strongly toward an IVD as the source of a septic episode (Table 50.7).[267] Patients with an abrupt onset of signs and symptoms of sepsis without any identifiable local infection such as pneumonia or surgical site infection should prompt suspicion of infection of an IVD. The presence of inflammation or purulence at the catheter insertion site is now uncommon in patients with IVD-related BSI.[276] However, if inflammation, especially any purulence, is seen in combination with signs and symptoms of sepsis, it is highly likely the patient has IVD-related BSI and should prompt removal of the device. Finally, recovery of certain microorganisms in multiple blood cultures, such as staphylococci, *Corynebacterium* or *Bacillus* species, or *Candida* or *Malassezia,* strongly suggests infection of an IVD.

Blood Cultures

Starting anti-infective drugs for suspected or presumed infection in the critically ill patient without first obtaining blood cultures from two separate sites, at least one of which is drawn from a peripheral vein by percutaneous venipuncture, is indefensible. The volume of blood cultured is essential to maximize the sensitivity of blood cultures for diagnosis of bacteremia or candidemia: in adults, obtaining at least 20 mL, ideally 30 mL, per drawing (each specimen, containing 10 mL or 15 mL, inoculated into aerobic and anaerobic media) significantly improves the yield as compared with obtaining only 5 mL at each drawing and culturing a smaller total volume.[277,278] In adults, if at least 30 mL of blood is cultured, 99% of detectable bacteremias should be identified.[277,279] Similar operating characteristics are achieved in the pediatric population using a weight-based graduated volume approach to blood cultures.[280] Standard blood cultures drawn through CVCs provide excellent sensitivity for diagnosis of BSI but are less specific than cultures obtained from a peripheral vein.[281,282] If the patient has a long-term multilumen catheter, it may be reasonable to obtain a specimen from each lumen of the catheter because studies have found discordance (≈30%) among cultures obtained from different lumens of the same catheter.[283]

Every effort must be made to prevent introduced contamination when drawing blood cultures because a single contaminated blood culture has been shown to prolong hospitalization by 4 days and increase the costs of hospitalization by $4100 to $4400.[284,285] Tincture of iodine, isopropyl alcohol, chlorhexidine, or povidone-iodine combined with alcohol rather than povidone-iodine alone should be used for skin antisepsis prior to venipuncture for blood cultures, recognizing that studies have shown significantly reduced rates of contamination with use of these agents.[204,285,286] Up to 30% of blood cultures positive for coagulase-negative staphylococcus represent true infection[287,288]; however, the majority of single positive cultures represent contamination,[288] a finding that should reemphasize the need to obtain cultures from *two* separate sites whenever BSI is suspected.

Cultures of Removed Intravascular Devices

Removal and direct culture of the IVD has historically been the gold standard for confirming the presence of IVD-related BSI, particularly with short-term IVDs. Studies have shown that culturing catheter segments semiquantitatively on solid media[289] or quantitatively in liquid media (e.g., removing the adherent organisms by sonication[290]) provides superior sensitivity and specificity for diagnosis of IVD-related BSI, with a strong correlation between high colony counts and line sepsis. Growth of greater than or equal to 15 CFUs from a catheter segment by semiquantitative culture or growth of greater than or equal to 10^3 CFUs from a catheter cultured after sonication with accompanying local inflammation or signs of sepsis indicates local catheter infection. Significant growth in the absence of local or systemic inflammation suggests colonization of the device; if continued vascular access is necessary, a new device should be placed in a new location rather than replacing it with a new one in the same location by guidewire exchange.

Although recent studies[291] have suggested that quantitative methods (e.g., sonication) are superior to the semiquantitative methods (e.g., roll plate), other studies have shown them to be equivalent.[292,293] Because hub contamination progressing to intraluminal colonization is the primary route of infection for long-term devices (e.g., devices in place >10 days), quantitative techniques may be superior to semiquantitative techniques in detecting infections from these types of devices because they remove organisms from both the internal and external surface of catheters.[293] In contrast, semiquantitative methods may be preferred over quantitative methods in cases of suspected infection related to a short-term device (e.g., devices in place <10 days) because the primary route of infection in this setting is caused by extraluminal ingress of skin organisms at the catheter insertion site and the semiquantitative method is simple, less expensive, and allows identification of the infecting organisms a day earlier.

Direct and impression Gram stains[294] or acridine orange stains[293] of intravascular segments of removed catheters have shown excellent correlation with quantitative techniques for culturing catheters and can permit rapid diagnosis of catheter-related infection.

To rigorously identify the mechanism of IVD-related BSI in prospective studies, it is necessary to culture all potential sources of microorganisms at the time of catheter removal (Fig. 50.6): skin of the insertion site, each catheter hub, infusate from each lumen, as well as implanted catheter segments. If the results of these cultures appear to link a BSI with microorganisms isolated from one or more portions of the device by phenotypic criteria, efforts then need to be made to conclusively establish concordance, beyond speciation and antimicrobial susceptibility pattern, using one or more molecular subtyping systems such as multilocus enzyme electrophoresis, plasmid profile, or restriction-enzyme digestion of genomic DNA analyzed by pulsed-field electrophoresis.[273,274,278,295]

Diagnosis of Infection with Implanted Long-Term Intravascular Devices

The methods described earlier require removal of the device for confirmation of IVD-related BSI. This can pose formidable challenges to management with long-term, surgically implanted IVDs such as Hickman and Broviac catheters, cuffed and tunneled hemodialysis catheters, and subcutaneous central venous ports. Only 15% to 45% of

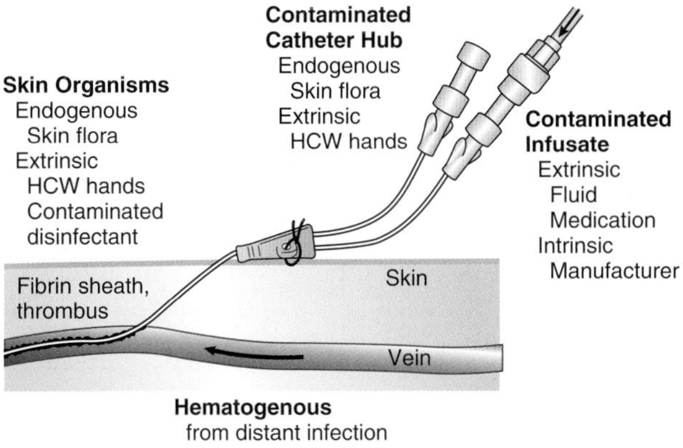

Figure 50.6 Potential sources of infection of a percutaneous intravascular device (IVD): the contiguous skin flora, contamination of the catheter hub and lumen, contamination of infusate, and hematogenous colonization of the IVD from distant, unrelated sites of infection. HCW, health care worker. (From Crnich CJ, Maki DG: The promise of novel technology for the prevention of intravascular device-related bloodstream infection. I. Pathogenesis and short-term devices. Clin Infect Dis 2002;34:1232-1242.)

long-term IVDs that are removed for suspected infection are truly colonized or infected at the time of removal.[296-299] To avoid unnecessary removal of IVDs, methods have been developed to diagnose IVD-related BSI while allowing the device to remain in place: (1) paired quantitative blood cultures drawn from the IVD and percutaneously from a peripheral vein[293] and (2) differential time to positivity (DTP) of paired standard blood cultures, one drawn from the IVD and the other from a peripheral vein.[300]

If a laboratory has available an automated quantitative system for culturing blood (e.g., Isolator lysis centrifugation system, Wampole Laboratories, Cranbury, NJ), quantitative blood cultures drawn through the IVD and concomitantly by venipuncture from a peripheral vein (or another IVD) can permit the diagnosis of IVD-related bacteremia or fungemia to be made with sensitivity and specificity in the range of 80% to 95%,[293] without removal of the catheter, if empiric antimicrobial therapy has not yet been initiated. IVD-drawn cultures demonstrating 5- to 10-fold higher concentrations of microorganisms per milliliter, as compared with counts of the same microorganism obtained in a culture drawn from a peripheral vein, confirm the presence of IVD-related BSI.

The differential-time-to-positivity (DTP) of paired blood cultures, one drawn through the IVD and the second, concomitantly from a peripheral vein, has also been shown to reliably identify IVD-related BSI of long-term IVDs if the blood culture drawn from the IVD turns positive 2 or more hours before the culture drawn peripherally. In studies of patients with long-term IVDs, the sensitivity and specificity of DTP ranged from 82% to 94% and 88% to 91%, respectively.[293,300] The performance of DTP in short-term IVDs has recently been examined, with disappointing results,[301] a finding that is not entirely unexpected given the predominant extraluminal route of infection with these devices.

Detection of Contaminated Infusate

To diagnose infection caused by contaminated infusate, a sample of IV fluid, aspirated from the line, should be cultured quantitatively and qualitatively[289]; concordance with positive peripheral blood cultures, without another identifiable source for the patient's BSI, definitively implicates infected infusate as the cause of the BSI. Anaerobic culture techniques are not necessary unless blood or another biologic product is involved.

INCIDENCE

Prospective studies, in which every attempt was made to conclusively identify the presence of an IVD-related BSI, show that every type of IVD carries some risk of causing BSI; however, the magnitude of risk varies greatly, depending on the type of device (Table 50.8).[302] The device that poses the greatest risk of IVD-related BSI today is the CVC in its many forms (see Table 50.8): short-term, noncuffed, single-lumen or multilumen catheters inserted percutaneously into the subclavian or internal jugular vein have shown rates of catheter-related BSI in the range of 3% to 5% (2 to 3 per 1000 IVD-days).[302] Far lower rates of infection have been encountered with surgically implanted cuffed Hickman or Broviac catheters and subcutaneous central venous ports (1 and 0.2 per 1000 IVD-days, respectively).[302] Contrary to popular belief, peripherally inserted central catheters (PICCs) used in inpatients and arterial catheters are associated with rates of catheter-related BSI approaching those seen with short-term, noncuffed, and nontunneled, multilumen CVCs—up to 2.1[303] and 3.4[304] BSIs per 1000 IVD-days, respectively.

PATHOGENESIS AND RISK FACTORS

Two major sources of IVD-related BSI exist: (1) colonization of the IVD, *catheter-related infection,* and (2) contamination of the fluid administered through the device, *infusate-related infection.*[267] Contaminated infusate is the cause of most *epidemic* IVD-related BSIs; in contrast, catheter-related infections are responsible for most *endemic* IVD-related BSIs.[18]

In order for microorganisms to cause catheter-related infection, they must first gain access to the extraluminal or intraluminal surface of the device, where they can adhere and become incorporated into a biofilm that allows sustained infection and hematogenous dissemination.[305] Microorganisms gain access to the bloodstream by one of three mechanisms (see Fig. 50.7): (1) skin organisms invade the percutaneous tract, probably assisted by capillary action, at the time of insertion or in the days following; (2) microorganisms contaminate the catheter hub (and lumen) when the catheter is inserted over a percutaneous guidewire or later manipulated; or (3) organisms are carried hematogenously to the implanted IVD from remote sources of local infection such as pneumonia.

With short-term IVDs (e.g., in place <10 days) such as peripheral IV catheters; arterial catheters; and noncuffed, nontunneled CVCs, most device-related BSIs are of cutaneous origin, from the insertion site, and gain access extraluminally, occasionally intraluminally at insertion with the guidewire.[306,307] In contrast, contamination of the catheter hub and luminal fluid is the predominant mode of invasive

Table 50.8 Rates of Intravascular Device (IVD)–Related Bloodstream Infection (BSI) Caused by Various Types of Devices Used for Vascular Access in Adults

					Rates of IVD-Related BSI			
					Per 100 Devices		Per 1000 IVD-days	
Device	**Studies, *n***	**Catheters, *n***	**IVD-days, *n***	**BSIs, *n***	Pooled Mean	95% CI	Pooled Mean	95% CI
Peripheral intravenous catheters	11	10,910	28,720	13	0.1	0.1-0.2	0.5	0.2-0.7
Arterial catheters	14	4,366	21,397	37	0.8	0.6-1.1	1.7	1.2-2.3
Short-term, nonmedicated central venous catheters	79	20,226	322,283	883	4.4	4.1-4.6	2.7	2.6-2.9
Pulmonary artery catheters	13	2,057	8143	30	1.5	0.9-2.0	3.7	2.4-5.0
Hemodialysis catheters:								
Temporary, noncuffed	16	3,066	51,840	246	8.0	7-9	4.8	4.2-5.3
Long-term, cuffed, and tunneled	16	2,806	373,563	596	21.2	19.7-22.8	1.6	1.5-1.7
Peripherally inserted central catheters (PICCs):	15	3,566	105,839	112	3.1	2.6-3.7	1.1	0.9-1.3
Long-term, tunneled, and cuffed central venous catheters	29	4,512	622,535	1013	22.5	21.2-23.7	1.6	1.5-1.7
Subcutaneous venous ports	14	3,007	983,480	81	3.6	2.9-4.3	0.1	0-0.1

Modified from Maki DG, Kluger DM, Crnich CJ: The risk of bloodstream infection in adults with different intravascular devices: A systematic review of 200 published prospective studies. Mayo Clin Proc 2006;81:1159-1171.

infection with *long-term* IVDs (e.g., in place >10 days) such as cuffed Hickman- and Broviac-type catheters, subcutaneous central ports, and PICCs.[308,309]

Also important is recognizing that infusate (parenteral fluid, blood products, or IV medications) administered through an IVD can also occasionally become contaminated and produce device-related BSI. Contaminated fluid is fortunately an infrequent cause of endemic infusion-related infection with most short-term IVDs; it is, however, an important cause of BSIs with arterial catheters used for hemodynamic monitoring and long-term IVDs such as Hickman or Broviac catheters, cuffed hemodialysis CVCs, and subcutaneous central venous ports.[307,310,311]

Most nosocomial epidemics of infusion-related BSI have been traced to contamination of infusate by gram-negative bacilli, introduced during its manufacture (intrinsic contamination) or during its preparation and administration in the hospital (extrinsic contamination).[146,312] If an epidemic is suspected, the epidemiologic approach must be methodical and thorough yet expeditious, directed toward establishing the bona fide nature of the putative epidemic infections (i.e., ruling out "pseudoinfections")[246] and confirming the existence of an epidemic; defining the reservoirs and modes of transmission of the epidemic pathogens; and most importantly, controlling the epidemic quickly and completely. Control measures are predicated on accurate delineation of the epidemiology of the epidemic pathogen. The essential steps in dealing with a suspected nosocomial outbreak have recently been reviewed (and are discussed later).[267]

In recent years the factors associated with an increased risk of IVD-related BSI have become better delineated (Table 50.9). Prolonged hospitalization and severity of illness clearly influence the risk, and clinical states such as granulocytopenia, AIDS, and bone marrow transplantation have been associated with fourfold to sixfold increased rates of IVD-related BSI.[313,314] However, the features of the IVD, its insertion, and its maintenance appear to have far greater impact on the overall risk of infection. In 289 patients, Merrer and colleagues[315] found that insertion of an IVD in the femoral versus the subclavian vein was associated with a greatly increased risk of infection (20 versus 3.7 BSIs per 1000 IVD-days, $p < 0.001$) and thrombotic complications (21.5% versus 1.9%, $p < 0.001$).[315] Moreover, Robert and colleagues[316] found that patients with primary BSI were more likely to have received care during times when there was a lower nursing-to-patient ratio and a higher proportion of temporary ("float") nurses rather than the full-time nursing staff.[316]

MICROBIOLOGY

Figure 50.7 summarizes the microbial profile of IVD-related BSI from 159 published prospective studies.[317] As might be expected from knowledge of the pathogenesis of these infections, skin microorganisms account for the largest proportion of these infections.

Table 50.9 Risk Factors for Intravascular Device–Related Bloodstream Infection with Short-Term Use

Risk Factor (with No. of Studies)	Relative Risk or Odds Ratio
Underlying Disease	
AIDS (2)	4.8
Neutropenia (2)	1-15.1
Gastrointestinal disease (1)	2.4
Surgical service (1)	4.4
ICU/CCU placement (3)	0.4-6.7
Extended hospitalization (3)	1-6.7
Other intravascular devices (2)	1-3.8
Systemic antibiotics (3)	0.1-0.5
Active infection at another site (2)	8.7-9.2
High APACHE III score (1)	4.2
Mechanical ventilation (1)	2-2.5
Transplant recipient (1)	2.6
Features of Insertion	
Difficult insertion (1)	5.4
Maximal sterile barriers (1)	0.2
Tunneling (2)	0.3-1
Insertion over a guidewire (8)	1-3.3
Insertion Site	
Internal jugular vein (6)	1-3.3
Subclavian vein (5)	0.4-1
Femoral vein (2)	3.3-4.8
Defatting insertion site (1)	1.0
Use of a multilumen catheter (8)	–6.5
Catheter Management	
Routine change of IV set (2)	1.0
Staffing in SICU (nurse-to-patient ratio) (1)	
1:2	61.5
1:1.5	15.6
1:1.28	4.0
1:1	1.0
Inappropriate catheter usage (1)	5.3
Duration of catheterization >7 days (5)	1-8.7
Colonization of catheter hub (3)	17.9-44.1
Parenteral nutrition (2)	–4.8

AIDS, acquired immunodeficiency syndrome; APACHE III, Acute Physiology and Chronic Health Evaluation III; CCU, critical care unit; ICU, intensive care unit; IV, intravenous; SICU, surgical intensive care unit.

Modified from Safdar NS, Kluger DM, Maki DG: A review of risk factors for catheter-related infection caused by percutaneously inserted, noncuffed central venous catheters: Implications for preventive strategies. Medicine 2002;81:466-479.

TREATMENT

Treatment of IVD-related BSI is discussed in Chapter 54 (Specific Infections with Critical Care Implications), under "Device-Related Endovascular Infections."

STRATEGIES FOR PREVENTION

Recommendations for the prevention of IVD-related BSIs were recently published by the Hospital Infection Control Practices Advisory Committee (HICPAC).[132] Table 50.10 summarizes the recommendations of the 2011 HICPAC guideline for the prevention of IVD-related BSI and scores each recommendation on the basis of the quality of the available scientific evidence. It must be reaffirmed that measures for prevention of any nosocomial infection must, wherever possible, be based on the best understanding of pathophysiology and epidemiology and, whenever possible, controlled clinical trials.

At-Device Insertion

1. *Choice of catheter and site of device insertion:* Obviously, the choice of IVD inserted into a patient will be guided primarily by that patient's particular needs (e.g., hemodialysis versus fluid administration). However, the astute clinician can mitigate much of the risk associated with vascular access by choosing the best device for the task at hand and inserting the IVD in a location associated with the least risk of infection. Studies suggest that multilumen IVDs are associated with a higher risk of infection than single-lumen catheters.[318] That said, if a patient has need for multiple infusions, inserting several single-lumen catheters will pose greater risks than a single multilumen catheter.

   To date, there have been no randomized studies designed to evaluate the optimal location for placement of short-term CVCs. However, the data accumulated from numerous observational studies suggest that the lowest risk of IVD-related BSI is seen with subclavian vein insertion and the highest risk with femoral vein insertion, with an intermediate level of risk associated with jugular vein insertions.[307,315]

   The femoral vein is often used for central venous access, especially on nonsurgical services, because of the ease of cannulation and the lower risk of mechanical complications from insertion (i.e., bleeding or pneumothorax). Unfortunately, prospective studies evaluating the risk of femoral vein device placement have shown that CVCs placed in the femoral vein are more likely to be colonized at the time of removal than catheters placed in the internal jugular vein (RR = 4.7, CI = 2 to 8.8, p = 0.0001)[319] and are associated with an increased risk of IVD-related BSI when compared with CVCs placed in the subclavian vein (4.4% versus 1.5%, p = 0.07).[315] Furthermore, prospective studies have found higher rates of catheter-related deep vein thrombosis with femoral catheters, in the range of 7% to 25%.[314,315] In general, we believe femoral access should be used only if emergent access is required, the inexperience of the operator limits placement in the upper body, or there is a contraindication to placement in the upper body (no available sites, an extensive burn, or severe coagulopathy). If a short-term CVC must be placed in the femoral vein or artery, we believe it is important that the catheter insertion site be located at least 2 inches (5 cm) below the inguinal crease or an intertriginous area, which is heavily colonized with bowel organisms and yeasts; this also allows a more secure protective dressing to be affixed.

   In contrast to short-term CVCs, observational studies of hemodialysis catheters have not been able to confirm a lower rate of infection with catheters inserted in the subclavian vein as compared with those inserted in the internal jugular vein,[320] although there is still excess risk

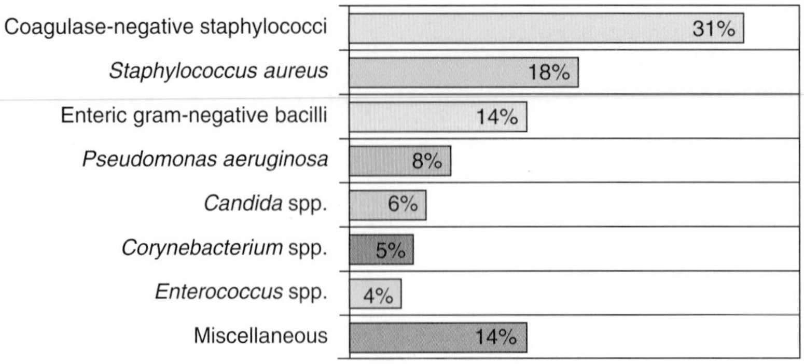

Figure 50.7 Microbial profile of intravascular device–related bloodstream infection based on an analysis of 159 published prospective studies. (Modified from Maki DG, Kluger DM, Crnich CJ: The microbiology of intravascular device-related (IVDR) infection in adults: An analysis of 159 prospective studies and implications for prevention and treatment. In Abstracts and Proceedings from the 40th Annual Meeting of the Infectious Disease Society of America. Chicago, Infectious Disease Society of America, 2002.)

Table 50.10 Summary of CDC/HICPAC Guideline Recommendations for Prevention of Intravascular Device (IVD)-Related Bloodstream Infection (BSI) in Adults

Recommendation	Strength*
General Measures	
• Educate health care personnel regarding indications for IVD use, proper procedures for IVD insertion/maintenance, and infection control measures. Periodically assess knowledge of and adherence to guidelines. Designate only trained personnel who demonstrate competence in IVD insertion/maintenance.	IA
• Ensure adequate nursing staffing levels in ICUs.	IB
• Use "bundles," whereby multifaceted strategies are bundled together to improve compliance with evidence-based recommended practices.	IB
Hand Hygiene, Aseptic Technique, and Maximal Sterile Barrier Precautions	
• Perform hand hygiene and maintain aseptic technique, before and after inserting, replacing, accessing, repairing, or dressing an IVD.	IB
• Use maximal sterile barrier precautions during insertion of CVCs, PICCs, or guidewire exchange: mask, cap, sterile gown, sterile gloves, sterile full-body drape.	IB
• Use minimum of cap, mask, sterile gloves, and small sterile fenestrated drape during insertion of peripheral arterial catheters.	IB
• Use maximal sterile barrier precautions during insertion of axillary or femoral artery catheters.	II
• Don new sterile gloves before handling new catheter during guidewire exchange.	II
Use either clean or sterile gloves when changing the dressing on IVDs.	IC
IVD Insertion	
• Use subclavian site for nontunneled CVC placement, rather than jugular or femoral (IB) (except avoid subclavian site for patients on dialysis or with advanced kidney disease—IA).	See text
• Avoid femoral vein for central venous access.	IA
• Weigh risks against benefits of placing CVC at recommended site to reduce infectious complications versus risk for mechanical complications (e.g., pneumothorax).	IA
• Use radial, brachial, or dorsalis pedis sites for peripheral arterial catheters, rather than femoral or axillary.	IB
• Prepare clean skin with >0.5% chlorhexidine preparation with alcohol before insertion of CVCs and peripheral arterial catheters and during dressing changes; can use tincture of iodine, an iodophor, or 70% alcohol, in patients with a contraindication to use of chlorhexidine.	IA
• Use sutureless securement device to reduce risk of infection.	II
• Use sterile sleeve to protect pulmonary artery catheters during insertion.	IB
• Use either sterile gauze or sterile, transparent, semipermeable dressing to cover catheter site.	IA
IVD Maintenance	
• Promptly remove any IVD that is no longer essential.	IA
• Replace gauze dressings on short-term CVC sites every 2 days.	II
• Replace transparent dressings on short-term CVC sites at least every 7 days.	IB
• Replace dressing if it becomes damp, loosened, or visibly soiled.	IB
• Monitor IVD insertion site when changing dressing or by palpation through intact dressing on regular basis; dressing should be removed to examine site if local or systemic signs of infection are present.	IB
• Do not use systemic antibiotic prophylaxis; and do not use topical antibiotic ointments on IVD exit sites, except for dialysis catheters.	IB
• Use a 2% chlorhexidine wash for daily skin cleansing.	II

Table 50.10 Summary of CDC/HICPAC Guideline Recommendations for Prevention of Intravascular Device (IVD)-Related Bloodstream Infection (BSI) in Adults (Continued)

Recommendation	Strength*	Recommendation	Strength*
• Replace administration sets in continuous use no more frequently than at 96-hour intervals but at least every 7 days (IA). When blood, blood products, or fat emulsions are given, replace tubing within 24 hours of initiating the infusion (IB). With propofol infusions, replace tubing every 6 or 12 hours, when the vial is changed (IA).	See text	• Do not use guidewire exchanges to replace a non-tunneled catheter suspected of infection; a new device should be placed in a new location.	IB
• Change needleless IV catheter system components at least as frequently as the administration set, but no more frequently than every 72 hours (for needleless connectors, do not change more frequently than every 72 hours or according to manufacturers' recommendations).	II	• When adherence to aseptic technique cannot be ensured (e.g., with insertion of catheter during a medical emergency), replace the catheter as soon as possible (i.e., within 48 hours).	IB
• Minimize contamination of needleless IV catheter systems by scrubbing the access port with an appropriate antiseptic (chlorhexidine, povidone-iodine, an iodophor, or 70% alcohol) and accessing the port only with sterile devices.	IA	**Technology**	
• Replace peripheral IV lines every 72-96 hours.	IB	• Use chlorhexidine–silver sulfadiazine or minocycline-rifampin–impregnated CVC in patients whose catheter is expected to remain in place >5 days, if the rate of IVD-related BSI is not decreasing after successful implementation of a comprehensive strategy to reduce rates of such infections.	IA
• Do not routinely replace CVCs, PICCs, hemodialysis catheters, pulmonary artery catheters (IB), or arterial catheters (II), solely for prevention of infection.	See text	• Use chlorhexidine-impregnated sponge dressing for temporary short-term catheters if the IVD-related BSI rate is not decreasing despite adherence to basic prevention measures.	IB
• Do not remove CVCs or PICCs solely because of fever unless IVD infection is suspected, but replace catheter if purulence is seen at the exit site, especially if the patient is hemodynamically unstable and IVD-related BSI is suspected.	II	• Use prophylactic antibiotic lock solution *only* in patients with long-term IVDs who have continued to experience IVD-related BSIs despite consistent application of infection control practices.	II

CVC, central venous catheter; ICU, intensive care unit; IV, intravenous; PICC, peripherally inserted central venous catheter.

Data from O'Grady NP, Alexander M, Burns LA, et al: Healthcare Infection Control Practices Advisory Committee (HICPAC). Guidelines for the prevention of intravascular catheter-related infections. Clin Infect Dis 2011;52(9):e162-93.

*Taken from CDC/HICPAC system of weighting recommendations based on scientific evidence: IA, strongly recommended for implementation and strongly supported by well-designed experimental, clinical, or epidemiologic studies. IB, strongly recommended for implementation and supported by some experimental, clinical, or epidemiologic studies and a strong theoretical rationale; or an accepted practice (e.g., aseptic technique) supported by limited evidence. IC, required by state or federal regulations, rules, or standards. II, suggested for implementation and supported by suggestive clinical or epidemiologic studies or a theoretical rationale.

associated with femoral vein placement.[321] More importantly, prospective studies of catheters used for hemodialysis have demonstrated a significant risk of great vein thrombosis and stenosis in catheters inserted into the subclavian vein that approaches 40% to 50% as compared with rates of 0% to 10% with catheters inserted into the internal jugular vein.[322,323] On the basis of these data, internal jugular vein insertion is preferable to subclavian vein insertion for central access for hemodialysis.

2. *Barrier precautions:* Hand hygiene with an antiseptic-containing preparation, either conventional handwashing with chlorhexidine (2% to 4%) or with a waterless alcohol rub or gel,[174] must always precede the insertion of an IVD and should also precede subsequent handling of the device or its administration set.[132] A new pair of disposable, nonsterile gloves, using a "no-touch" technique, is adequate for the placement of peripheral IV catheters in most patients; however, sterile gloves should be used during insertion in high-risk patients such as those with granulocytopenia. Sterile gloves are strongly recommended for placement of all other types of IVDs that are associated with a 1% or higher risk of associated bacteremia, specifically arterial catheters and all types of centrally placed devices including PICCs.[132]

Studies have shown that the use of maximal barriers including a long-sleeved, sterile surgical gown, mask, cap and large sterile drape, and sterile gloves significantly reduces the risk of CVC-related BSI (0.08 BSIs with maximal barriers versus 0.5 BSIs per 1000 IVD-days without maximal barriers, $p = 0.02$).[324] The use of maximal barriers has further been shown to be highly cost effective.[324] Considering that of all IVDs, CVCs are most likely to produce nosocomial BSI, a strong case can be made for mandating maximal barrier precautions during the insertion of all central IVDs.[132] They are not necessary, however, for arterial catheters used for hemodynamic monitoring, during which sterile gloves and a sterile fenestrated drape will suffice, because using maximal sterile barrier precautions does not appear to reduce the risk of arterial catheter-related BSI.[325] However, recently published guidelines for the prevention of IVD-related BSI[132] recommend that in addition to a using a minimum of a cap, mask, sterile gloves, and a small sterile fenestrated drape during the insertion of all peripheral arterial catheters, maximal sterile barrier precautions be used for axillary and femoral artery catheter insertion (see Table 50.10), although the evidence to support this recommendation is not strong.[326]

3. *IV teams:* Good technique is also essential. Studies have shown that the use of special IV therapy teams, consisting of trained nurses or technicians who can assure a consistent and high level of aseptic technique during catheter insertion and in follow-up care of the catheter, have been associated with substantially lower rates of catheter-related BSI and are cost effective.[327,328] But even if an institution does not have an IV team, it can greatly reduce its rate of IVD-related BSI by formal education of nurses and physicians and stringent adherence to IVD care protocols.[329,330]
4. *Cutaneous antisepsis:* Given the evidence for the importance of cutaneous microorganisms in the pathogenesis of short-term IVD-related infections, measures to reduce colonization of the insertion site would seem of the highest priority, particularly the choice of chemical antiseptics for disinfection of the site. Nine randomized, prospective trials comparing a chlorhexidine-containing antiseptic to either povidone-iodine or alcohol for preparation of the skin prior to insertion of a short-term IVD have been reported.[205-207,331] In the largest study to date, a randomized trial in 1050 CVCs and arterial catheters placed in a university hospital ICU, cutaneous antisepsis with 1% tincture of chlorhexidine showed a highly significant reduction in IVD-related BSIs compared with an iodophor (RR = 0.35, $p < 0.01$).[331] More recently, a meta-analysis that examined results from eight of the nine aforementioned studies found that use of chlorhexidine was associated with a nearly 50% reduction in the risk of IVD-related compared with povidone-iodine (RR = 0.49, 95% CI = 0.28 to 0.88).[205]

Insertion Site Care and IVD Maintenance

1. *IVD dressings:* IVDs can be dressed with sterile gauze and tape or with a sterile transparent, semipermeable, polyurethane film dressing. The available data suggest that the two types of dressings are equivalent in terms of their impact on IVD-related BSI with peripheral IVs and short-term CVCs.[332-334] In contrast, results from studies of arterial catheters have found that polyurethane dressings greatly increase the risk of IVD-related BSI.[332,335] As a result, polyurethane dressings should probably not be used on arterial catheters until future studies confirm their safety.
2. *Topical antimicrobial ointments:* In theory, application of a topical antimicrobial agent to the catheter insertion site should confer some protection against microbial invasion. Clinical trials of a topical combination antibacterial ointment containing polymyxin, neomycin, and bacitracin with peripheral IVs have shown marginal benefit,[336] but the use of polyantibiotic ointments has been associated with a fivefold increased frequency of *Candida* infection, limiting their utility.[336,337] One recent double-blind, placebo-controlled, randomized clinical trial in hemodialysis patients with permanent tunneled cuffed dialysis catheters showed that the use of topical bacitracin, gramicidin, and polymyxin B at the catheter exit site as compared with topical placebo was associated with a reduction in catheter-related bacteremia (0.63 versus 2.48 per 1000 IVD-days, $p = 0.0004$) and mortality rate (3 versus 13 deaths, $p = 0.004$), without an increase in *Candida* infection.[338]

   The topical antibacterial mupirocin, which is active primarily against gram-positive organisms, was shown in one study to significantly reduce colonization of internal jugular catheters without increasing colonization by *Candida* spp.,[339] and a study by Sesso and colleagues[340] showed significant reductions in hemodialysis catheter colonization (3.17 versus 14.27 per 1000 IVD-days, $p \leq 0.001$) and *S. aureus* IVD-related BSIs (0.71 versus 8.92 BSIs per 1000 IVD-days, $p \leq 0.001$).[340] Unfortunately, resistance of *S. aureus*[341] and coagulase-negative staphylococci[342] rapidly emerges during wide-scale mupirocin use,[343] which contravenes its use as a topical agent for the prevention of IVD-related BSI at this time.[132]

   Three prospective studies of topical povidone-iodine ointment applied to central venous catheter sites have failed to show a statistical benefit to its use,[336,344,345] but a single comparative trial in subclavian hemodialysis catheters showed that the use of topical povidone-iodine ointment was associated with a fourfold reduction in the incidence of IVD-related *S. aureus* BSI.[346]

   Based on these data, if a topical agent is to be used with hemodialysis catheters, either an iodophor or topical bacitracin, gramicidin, and polymyxin B (not currently available in the United States) may be most desirable.[132]
3. *Replacement of the device:* Studies have shown that peripheral IVs may be safely left in place for up to 96 hours if the patient and the insertion site are monitored closely.[347] Studies have suggested that the duration of peripheral catheterization may be prolonged even further,[348] but viewing reports of increasing nosocomial *S. aureus* bacteremias linked to prolonged peripheral venous catheterization,[349] more studies are required before this can become considered acceptable routinely.

   Scheduled replacement of short-term, noncuffed, nontunneled CVCs has long been practiced in many centers; however, some studies have called this practice into question.[350] Moreover, a meta-analysis found no benefit to routine replacement of short-term CVCs.[351] On the basis of these data, there appears to be no indication for scheduled replacement of short-term CVCs that are functioning well and show no clinical signs of infection.
4. *Guidewire exchanges of CVCs:* The management of CVCs that must be replaced, either because of mechanical

malfunction or suspected infection, deserves special attention. Replacement of CVCs by guidewire exchange is associated with a reduced risk of mechanical complications[350,351]; however, it is also associated with an increased risk of the newly placed CVC becoming infected and causing CVC-related BSI.[350] As a result, if circumstances necessitate guidewire exchange for placement of a new catheter (e.g., the patient has limited sites for access, is morbidly obese, or is at high risk of mechanical complications because of underlying coagulopathy), the same strict aseptic technique, which includes full barrier precautions, must be used. However, the tip or intracutaneous segment(s) of the removed CVC should routinely be sent for culture to determine whether the insertion tract is colonized. If it is, the newly inserted CVC should be promptly removed and a new CVC placed percutaneously in a new site. If the tract is not colonized, the newly exchanged CVC can remain in the old insertion site.

Although small studies have found some utility of guidewire exchange in the management of CVCs suspected of being infected,[352,353] we believe that, in the absence of randomized studies demonstrating its safety, guidewire exchange generally should not be performed if there is suspicion of IVD-related BSI, especially if there are signs of local infection such as purulence or erythema at the insertion site or signs of systemic sepsis without a source. In these cases the old catheter should be removed and cultured, and a new catheter should be inserted in a new site.

5. *Replacing the delivery system:* Whereas most infusion-related BSIs are caused by infection of the device used for vascular access, infusate can occasionally become contaminated and cause endemic BSIs.[307,354] If an infusion runs continuously for an extended period, the cumulative risk of contamination increases, and there is further risk that contaminants can grow to concentrations that could produce BSI in the recipient of the fluid. For more than 25 years, most U.S. hospitals have routinely replaced the entire delivery system of patients' IV infusions at 24- or 48-hour intervals[355] to reduce the risk of BSI from extrinsically contaminated fluid. Prospective studies indicate that IV delivery systems need not be replaced more frequently than every 72 to 96 hours, including infusions used for total parenteral nutrition or any infusions in ICU patients[347,356]; extending the duration of use can permit cost savings to hospitals.[356]

Four clinical settings might be regarded as exceptions to using 72 hours as an interval for routine set change[356]: (1) administration of blood products, (2) administration of lipid emulsion, (3) arterial pressure monitoring, and (4) suspicion of an epidemic of infusion-related BSI. In these circumstances, it may be most prudent for administration sets to be changed routinely at 24- or 48-hour intervals.

Arterial infusions used for hemodynamic monitoring appear to be more vulnerable to becoming contaminated during use and producing endemic[354] or epidemic septicemia,[99] caused by gram-negative bacilli. If the infusion for hemodynamic monitoring is set up so that the fluid flows continuously through the system, thus eliminating a blind stagnant column of fluid, extrinsic contamination appears to be greatly reduced and may even eliminate the need to replace the administration set, transducer assembly, and other components of the system at frequent intervals.[357,358] If disposable transducers are used, there appears to be no need to replace the transducer assembly and other components of the delivery system more frequently than every 4 days,[357] and it may be safe to replace them even less frequently.[358]

6. *Anticoagulation:* Thrombus formation on an intravascular device is associated with an increased risk of infection.[359,360] Two prospective studies have been performed to examine the efficacy of warfarin anticoagulation for reducing rates of IVD-associated thrombosis with long-term IVDs.[361,362] Both studies found that use of warfarin in a dose of 1 mg/day was associated with significantly reduced rates of thrombosis with long-term IVDs, although no data were provided on rates of IVD-related BSI.

The use of prophylactic heparin for reducing rates of IVD-related thrombosis and infection has been evaluated in a meta-analysis.[363] Examining a variety of different administration techniques in 14 randomized controlled studies, Randolph and colleagues[363] concluded that systemic heparinization significantly reduced the risk of IVD-associated thrombosis (RR = 0.43, CI = 0.23 to 0.78) and device colonization (RR = 0.18, CI = 0.06 to 0.6) but failed to show a reduction in IVD-related BSIs. Heparin-bonded pulmonary artery catheters may be less prone to IVD-related BSI than nonheparinized catheters.[307,364,365]

On the basis of these studies, low-level anticoagulation with warfarin is warranted for long-term IVDs as long as there is no contraindication (bleeding diathesis, brain tumor, or predilection to falls) and the INR (international normalized ratio) is maintained below 1.6.[361] For short-term IVDs, the use of low-dose subcutaneous heparin is more appropriate; it is commonly given to patients with CVCs or arterial lines as part of ICU thromboembolism prophylaxis.

Novel Technology

Despite compliance with recommended guidelines, many centers continue to have high rates of IVD-related BSI. Novel technology holds much promise (Box 50.3). Innovative technologies designed to reduce the risk of IVD-related BSI have proved not only to be effective but also to reduce health care costs, both with short-term and long-term IVDs.[305,366]

1. *Novel securement devices:* In a randomized trial of a novel sutureless device for securing noncuffed vascular catheters (StatLock, Venetec International), premature loss of pediatric PICCs caused by accidental extrusion and PICC-associated thrombosis was significantly reduced,[367] and in two additional trials the incidence of catheter-related BSI was significantly reduced with the use of the novel securement device, both in adults and children with PICCs.[367,368]

The promise of this device for reducing infection may derive from elimination of a festering skin suture wound contiguous to the newly inserted catheter and minimizing to-and-fro movement of the catheter, which may

Box 50.3 Novel Technology for Prevention of Intravascular Device (IVD)-Related Bloodstream Infection That Has Been Examined in Randomized Clinical Trials

- Sutureless securement devices
  - Topical antimicrobials/antiseptics
  - Topical anti-infective creams or ointments
  - Polymyxin-neomycin-bacitracin polyantibiotic ointment
  - Bacitracin, gramicidin, and polymyxin B ointment
  - Povidone-iodine ointment
  - Mupirocin ointment
- Dressings
  - Transparent, polyurethane film dressings
  - Hyperpermeable polyurethane dressings
  - Hydrocolloid dressings
  - Chlorhexidine-impregnated sponge dressings
- Innovative IVD design
  - Cuffed and tunneled central venous catheters
  - Subcutaneous central venous ports
  - Attachable silver-impregnated cuffs
- Anti-infective-coated catheters
  - Benzalkonium chloride–impregnated catheters
  - Chlorhexidine–silver sulfadiazine–coated catheters
  - Cefazolin-coated catheters
  - Minocycline-rifampin–coated catheters
  - Silver-impregnated catheters
- Anti-infective catheter hubs
  - Iodinated chamber
  - External povidone-iodine–saturated sponge cap
- Anti-infective lock solutions for long-term IVDs
  - Gentamicin
  - Vancomycin
  - Vancomycin-ciprofloxacin
  - Trisodium citrate–gentamicin
  - Minocycline–ethylenediaminetetraacetic acid (EDTA)
  - Ethanol
  - Taurolidine
- Scheduled (prophylactic) thrombolysis with urokinase

Modified from Crnich CJ, Maki DG: The promise of novel technology for the prevention of intravascular device-related bloodstream infection. I. Pathogenesis and short-term devices. Clin Infect Dis 2002;34:1232-1242, 1362-1368.

promote invasion of the tract by cutaneous microorganisms through capillary action.[369]

2. *Novel dressings:* Studies of polyurethane dressings, which contain antiseptics such as povidone-iodine or ionized silver, have been disappointing. However, on the basis of demonstrated superiority of chlorhexidine for cutaneous disinfection of access sites, a novel chlorhexidine-impregnated sponge dressing has been developed (Biopatch, Johnson and Johnson Medical, Inc.). It maintains a high concentration of the antiseptic on the insertion site under the dressing. The largest study to date found that use of the chlorhexidine-impregnated sponge dressing was associated with a 60% reduction in catheter-related BSI (RR = 0.37, $p = 0.01$).[370] Although there were no adverse side effects associated with the use of this dressing in this trial in adults, a pediatric trial found that 15% of low-birth-weight neonates developed local dermatotoxicity.[371]
3. *Anti-infective impregnated catheters:* Intravascular devices directly coated or impregnated with antimicrobials or antiseptics have been intensively studied over the past several decades. Eighteen randomized trials evaluating the efficacy of chlorhexidine-silver-sulfadiazine–impregnated or minocycline-rifampin–impregnated CVCs have been published in full article or abstract form since 1994.[273,274,295,372,373]

   Of the 16 published studies that examined the effect of antimicrobial-impregnated CVCs on rates of CVC-related BSI, 12 found either a statistically significant reduction or a strong trend toward a reduction in rates of CVC-related BSI.[372,373] Aggregate analysis of the 15 studies that compared antimicrobial-impregnated CVCs with nonimpregnated CVCs,[372,373] encompassing a total of 4250 CVCs, shows that antimicrobial-impregnated CVCs are associated with a 40% reduction in CVC-related BSI (61 BSIs/2129 devices vs. 101 BSIs/2118 devices, OR 0.60, 95% CI = 0.44 to 0.82, $p = 0.001$), a result remarkably similar to the findings of three published meta-analyses.[305,374,375]

   Finally, two rigorous and sophisticated economic analyses have found that antimicrobial-impregnated CVCs are cost effective.[376,377] Veenstra and colleagues showed that antimicrobial-impregnated CVCs remained cost effective even if the cost of a CVC-related BSI was as low as $687 per case; cost savings were $196 per antimicrobial-impregnated CVC when a more realistic cost of a CVC-related BSI of $9738 was used in the analysis.[376] Shorr and colleagues[377] showed that use of antimicrobial-impregnated CVCs was associated with a cost savings of $9600 per CVC-related BSI prevented and that $165 to $280 would be saved for every patient who received an antimicrobial-impregnated CVC.

   On the basis of this large body of data, two national advisory panels have recommended the use of antimicrobial-impregnated CVCs in clinical settings where, despite rigorous application of other preventive interventions, rates of IVD-related BSI remain unacceptably high (i.e., ≥3.3 BSIs per 1000 IVD-days).[132,378]
4. *Antimicrobial lock solutions:* Given the importance of hub contamination and intraluminal colonization in the genesis of IVD-related BSI with long-term IVDs, intraluminal instillation of an antibiotic or antiseptic solution has the potential to reduce the risk of BSI associated with these devices. Six randomized, prospective trials have examined a vancomycin-containing antibiotic lock solution for the prevention of IVD-related BSI, the largest of which found that use of a vancomycin or vancomycin/ciprofloxacin lock solution reduced the risk of IVD-related BSI nearly 80% ($p = 0.005$), with no evidence that the use of the lock solution promoted colonization or infection by vancomycin-resistant bacteria or fungi.[379,380] Yet concern about the emergence of resistance with prophylactic antibiotic-containing lock solutions has limited their wider acceptance to date. However, the use of prophylactic antibiotic lock solution is considered

acceptable in the 2011 HICPAC Guideline if a patient with an essential long-term IVD has continued to experience recurrent IVD-related BSIs despite consistent application of infection control practices.[132]

Various other prophylactic lock solutions have been studied as a means of preventing IVD-related BSI including trisodium citrate/gentamicin,[381] minocycline/ethylenediaminetetraacetic acid (EDTA),[382] ethanol,[383] and taurolidine-containing solutions.[384] Concerns about increased IVD complication rates[384] and drug-related toxicity[381] associated with the use of certain types of lock solutions, combined with the limited number of patients who have been studied while receiving these agents, precludes their routine use at this time.

5. *Catheter hubs:* A novel catheter hub that contains a chamber filled with iodinated alcohol has been shown to be effective in preventing colonization of IVDs in an animal model.[385] Use of this same hub model in some clinical studies has demonstrated significantly lower rates of IVD colonization compared with IVDs with control hubs.[386,387] One clinical trial has also demonstrated reduced rates of IVD-related BSIs with use of this hub (4% versus 16%, $p < 0.01$). A subsequent study also showed a reduction in hub-related IVD-related BSIs (1.7% versus 7%, $p < 0.049$), but overall rates of IVD-related BSIs in both groups were similar.[387] Another study was unable to find any benefit with regard to IVD colonization or IVD-related BSI with use of the novel hub.[388] This device is not yet available in the United States and until further studies more conclusively demonstrate its benefit, its use cannot be recommended at this time.

VENTILATOR-ASSOCIATED PNEUMONIA

INCIDENCE AND IMPACT

Hospital-acquired pneumonia (HAP) is defined as pneumonia that develops more than 48 hours after hospitalization.[389] VAP is a subset of HAP and is defined as pneumonia that occurs more than 48 to 72 hours after initiating mechanical ventilation.[389] Nearly 300,000 episodes of HAP occur in U.S. hospitals each year.[390] More than 90% of HAPs occur in patients undergoing mechanical ventilation, and 10% to 20% of mechanically ventilated patients will develop VAP.[391] Incidence rates of VAP are highest in trauma, burn, neurosurgical, neurologic, and surgical ICUs (see Table 50.1).[25] VAP increases length of hospitalization by 6.1 days and health care costs by $10,019 when compared with matched control subjects who had not developed VAP.[391] More importantly, VAP is associated with more nosocomial deaths than is infection at any other site[392]—at least 50,000 deaths in U.S. centers annually—and increases hospital mortality rate at least twofold in affected individuals.[391]

PATHOGENESIS

In the normal nonsmoking host, multiple host defense mechanisms contribute to protection against pneumonia.[393] The respiratory tract above the vocal cords is normally heavily colonized by bacteria, but unless the person has chronic bronchitis or has had respiratory tract instrumentation, the lower respiratory tract is normally sterile; although healthy adults aspirate frequently during sleep, the lower airways and pulmonary parenchyma of healthy, nonsmoking persons without lung disease are remarkably free of microbial colonization.[394] The major defense mechanisms include anatomic airway barriers, the cough reflex, mucus,[395] and mucociliary clearance.[396] Below the terminal bronchioles, the cellular and humoral immune systems are essential components of host defense.[397] Alveolar macrophages and leukocytes remove particulate matter and potential pathogens, elaborate cytokines that activate the systemic cellular immune response, and act as antigen-presenting cells to the humoral arm of immunity.[398] Immunoglobulins and complement opsonize bacteria and bacterial products within the respiratory tract, assisting phagocytosis.

In the mechanically ventilated patient, numerous factors conspire to compromise host defenses: Critical illness, comorbid conditions, and malnutrition impair the immune system.[399,400] Endotracheal intubation thwarts the cough reflex; compromises mucociliary clearance; injures the tracheal epithelial surface; and provides a direct conduit for bacteria from the mouth, hypopharynx, and stomach to gain direct access to the lower respiratory tract.[401] Moreover, the cuff of the endotracheal tube allows pooling of oropharyngeal secretions in the subglottic region, forming an ideal medium for microbial growth, which periodically leaks around the cuff into the trachea. It would probably be more accurate pathogenically to rename VAP as "endotracheal intubation–related pneumonia." This combination of impaired host defenses and continuous exposure of the lower respiratory tract to large numbers of potential pathogens through the endotracheal tube puts the mechanically ventilated patient at great jeopardy of developing VAP.

In order for microorganisms to cause VAP, they must first gain access to the normally sterile lower respiratory tract, where they can adhere to the mucosa and produce sustained infection. Microorganisms gain access by one of four mechanisms (Fig. 50.8): (1) aspiration of microbe-laden secretions, either from the oropharynx directly or, secondarily, by reflux from the stomach into the oropharynx, then into the lower respiratory tract[402-404]; (2) inhalation of contaminated air or medical aerosols[405]; (3) direct extension of a contiguous infection such as a pleural space infection[406]; or (4) hematogenous carriage of microorganisms to the lung from remote sites of local infection such as an IVD-related BSI.[407]

Although numerous epidemics of VAP have been caused by contaminated aerosols or medical respiratory devices,[97,98,103] the preponderance of evidence suggests that most endemic VAPs derive from aspiration of oropharyngeal organisms[41,408]:

- The oropharynx of critically ill patients is rapidly colonized with the pathogens that cause VAP, especially aerobic gram-negative organisms and *S. aureus*.[399]
- Studies in which multiple anatomic sites are cultured simultaneously over time have shown that the pathogenic microorganisms implicated in VAP are usually first recovered from the oropharynx and later from the tracheobronchial tree and stomach.[402-404,409] Moreover, heavy oropharyngeal colonization is a powerful independent

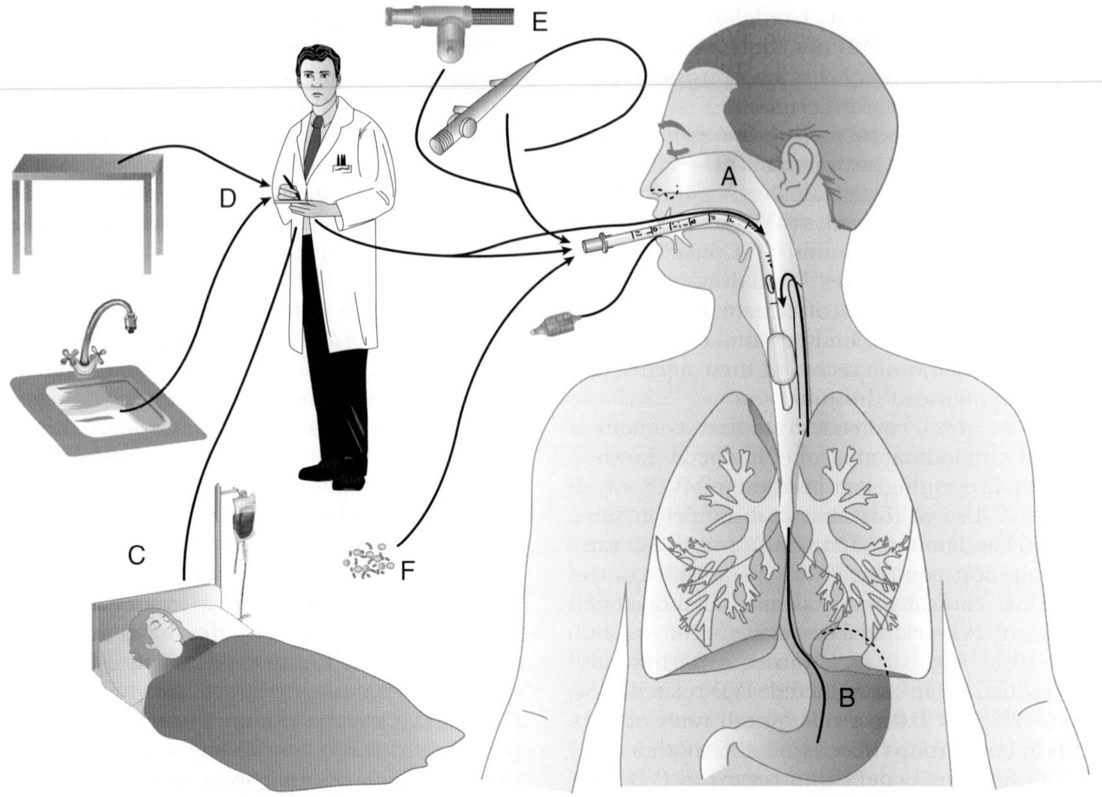

Figure 50.8 Routes of colonization/infection in mechanically ventilated patients. Colonization of the aerodigestive tract may occur endogenously (**A** and **B**) or exogenously (**C** through **F**). Exogenous colonization may result in primary colonization of the oropharynx or may be the result of direct inoculation into the lower respiratory tract during manipulations of respiratory equipment (**D**), during use of respiratory devices (**E**), or from contaminated aerosols (**F**). (From Crnich CJ, Safdar NS, Maki DG: The role of the intensive care environment in the pathogenesis and prevention of ventilator-associated pneumonia. Respir Care 2005;50:813-836.)

predictor of subsequent tracheobronchial colonization and VAP.[404]

- Reducing oropharyngeal colonization with topical antimicrobials and antiseptics has been shown to significantly reduce the risk of VAP.[410-413]

By this route, aspiration of oropharyngeal contents containing a large microbial inoculum overwhelms host defenses already compromised by critical illness and the presence of an endotracheal tube, readily leading to the development of VAP.

MICROBIOLOGY

Pathogens causing VAP may be part of the host's endogenous flora at the time of hospitalization or may be acquired exogenously after admission to the health care institution from the hands, apparel, or equipment of HCWs; hospital environment; and use of invasive devices (see Fig. 50.9). The normal flora of the oropharynx in the nonintubated patient without critical illness is composed predominantly of viridans streptococci, *Haemophilus* species, and anaerobes. Salivary flow and proteins (immunoglobulin, fibronectin) are the major host factors maintaining the normal flora of the mouth (and dental plaque). Aerobic gram-negative bacilli are rarely recovered from the oral secretions of healthy patients.[414] During critical illness, especially in ICU patients, the oral flora shifts dramatically to a predominance of aerobic gram-negative bacilli and *S. aureus*.[399] Bacterial adherence to the orotracheal mucosa of the mechanically ventilated patient is assisted by reduced mucosal IgA and increased protease production, exposed and denuded mucous membranes, elevated airway pH, increased numbers of airway receptors for bacteria because of acute illness, and antimicrobial use.

Early-onset VAP, which manifests within the first 4 days of hospitalization, is most often caused by community-acquired pathogens, such as *S. pneumoniae* and *Haemophilus* species (Fig. 50.9).[415] However, the microbial spectrum of VAP shifts to typical nosocomial pathogens with increasing lengths of mechanical ventilation and exposure to broad-spectrum antimicrobials (see Fig. 50.10).[415] That the preponderance of episodes of VAP have a late onset is supported by the fact that the most common pathogens recovered from mechanically ventilated patients with pneumonia are *P. aeruginosa*, *S. aureus*, and the Enterobacteriaceae (Fig. 50.10).[415,416] VAP is polymicrobial in up to 20% to 40% of cases. The role of anaerobic bacteria in VAP is not well defined.

DIAGNOSIS

Hospitals participating in the CDC's National Healthcare Safety Network (NHSN) use a standardized definition for clinically defined HAP[16,17] (see Box 50.1) on the basis of clinical criteria developed empirically more than 3 decades ago[417]: (1) systemic signs of infection—fever, tachycardia,

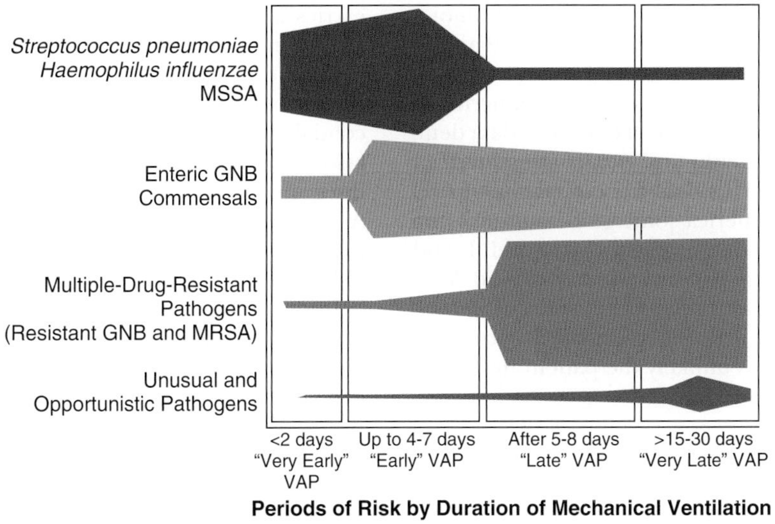

Figure 50.9 Microbial causes of ventilator-associated pneumonia based on increasing length of mechanical ventilation. The relative importance of each microbial category is indicated by the thickness of the bars as they progress through each stage from left to right. GNB, gram-negative bacilli; MRSA, methicillin-resistant *S. aureus*; MSSA, methicillin-susceptible *S. aureus*; VAP, ventilator-associated pneumonia. (From Park DR: The microbiology of ventilator-assisted pneumonia. Respir Care 2005;50:742-765.)

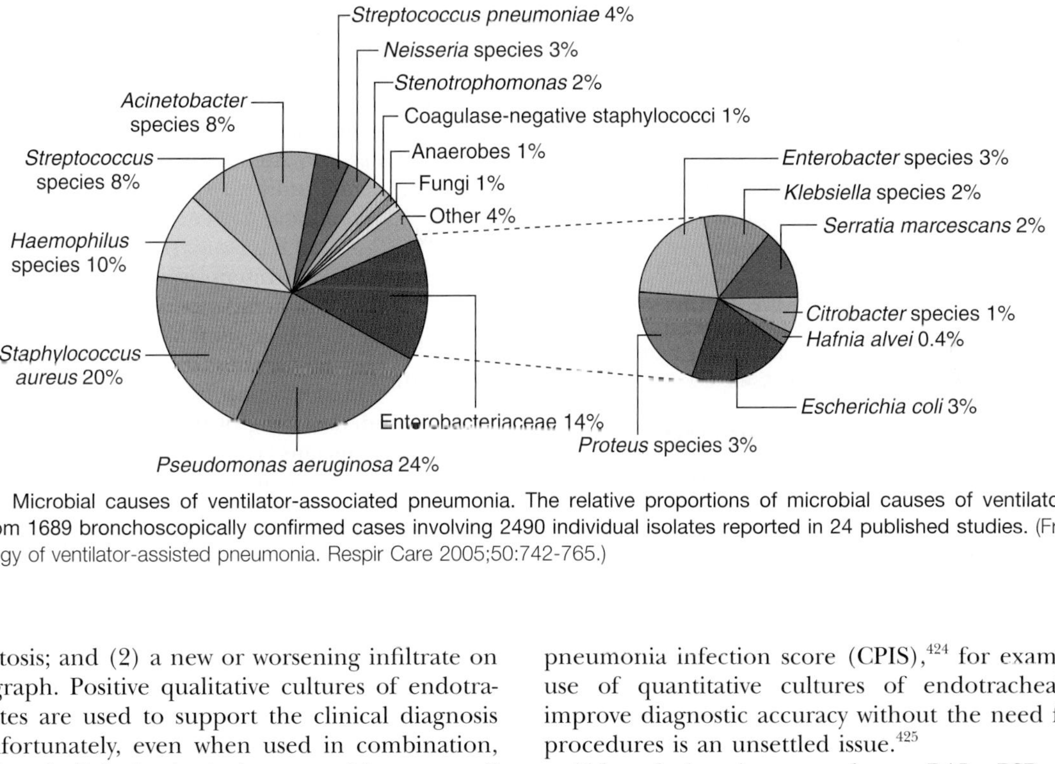

Figure 50.10 Microbial causes of ventilator-associated pneumonia. The relative proportions of microbial causes of ventilator-associated pneumonia from 1689 bronchoscopically confirmed cases involving 2490 individual isolates reported in 24 published studies. (From Park DR: The microbiology of ventilator-assisted pneumonia. Respir Care 2005;50:742-765.)

and leukocytosis; and (2) a new or worsening infiltrate on chest radiograph. Positive qualitative cultures of endotracheal aspirates are used to support the clinical diagnosis of HAP. Unfortunately, even when used in combination, the specificity of clinical criteria is poor, with an overall diagnostic accuracy of approximately 60% in published studies.[418,419]

Laboratory-defined HAP (see Box 50.1) relies on more specific criteria. Most experts have advocated routine use of invasive procedures when VAP is suspected—bronchoalveolar lavage (BAL), cultures of protected specimen brush (PSB) samples obtained by bronchoscopy, or blind (mini)-BAL, on the grounds that these diagnostic techniques have comparable sensitivity, greater specificity, and superior accuracy than clinical criteria alone.[416,420-423] Whether more rigorous clinical criteria such as the clinical pneumonia infection score (CPIS),[424] for example, or the use of quantitative cultures of endotracheal aspirates improve diagnostic accuracy without the need for invasive procedures is an unsettled issue.[425]

Although invasive procedures—BAL, PSB, and mini-BAL—are clearly more specific than clinical criteria, their impact on patient outcomes is much less clear.[426,427] Fagon and colleagues[426] found that patients with suspected VAP who were managed using an invasive diagnostic approach—bronchoscopic-guided PSB or BAL—had a significantly reduced 14-day mortality rate, reduced antibiotic-days, and reduced 28-day mortality rate on multivariate analysis, compared with patients managed using a clinical diagnostic approach (hazard ratio [HR] = 0.65, 95% CI = 0.46 to 0.91, $p = 0.01$).[426] However, Heyland and colleagues[427] found in a large multicenter Canadian trial that 28-day mortality rate and targeted antimicrobial use were identical among patients randomized to an invasive versus a clinical diagnostic approach. This study has been criticized for its exclusion of subjects at high risk for infection with antimicrobial-resistant pathogens.[428] In the absence of definitive data demonstrating the superiority of either approach, the American Thoracic Society–Society of Critical Care Medicine–Infectious Disease Society of America joint guideline acknowledges that both diagnostic approaches are useful and acceptable when evaluating patients with suspected VAP. This puts great weight on an initial Gram stain of a deep tracheal aspirate; however, if no microorganisms are seen, it can be concluded that it is unlikely the patient has bacterial VAP.[389]

RISK FACTORS

A number of independent risk factors have been shown to increase the likelihood of developing VAP (Table 50.11).[135,416] In general, these risk factors can be categorized as (1) factors that increase the likelihood or duration of mechanical ventilation, (2) factors that increase colonization of the oropharynx and gastric mucosa, (3) factors that increase the likelihood of aspiration, and (4) host factors that increase susceptibility to infection.

Prolonged mechanical ventilation, or reintubation, or both are the most powerful predictors of developing VAP. Cunnion and colleagues[429] found that mechanical ventilation in excess of 24 hours was associated with a 12-fold increased risk of developing VAP, and Trouillet and associates found that ventilation longer than 7 days was associated with a sixfold increased risk.[430] Emergent reintubation also carries a high risk of aspiration and was associated with a sixfold increased risk of VAP in a retrospective study.[431]

Poor dental hygiene increases the bacterial burden in the oropharynx and is an independent risk factor for nosocomial pneumonia.[432] Likewise, a high gastric pH (>5) is associated with greatly increased bacterial colonization of the gastric contents,[433] as well as an increased risk of VAP.[434] A number of studies have found that exposure to antacids or H_2-blockers is associated with an increased risk of VAP,[56] although this has not been a universal finding.[435]

Depressed levels of consciousness, nasogastric tubes, and endotracheal tubes are ubiquitous in the ICU and all increase a patient's risk of aspiration. That an altered level of cognition is associated with an increased risk of aspiration is supported by surveillance data showing increased rates of VAP in trauma and neurosurgical ICUs.[25] Joshi and colleagues[436] found that the use of a nasogastric tube was an independent predictor of VAP in a multivariate analysis (OR 6.5, 95%; CI 2.1 to 19.8). Finally, as noted, endotracheal tubes allow pooling of hypopharyngeal secretions that can leak around the cuff directly into the trachea, and a supine position appears to increase the risk of aspiration around the cuff.[437]

Host factors also contribute to an increased risk of developing VAP (see Table 50.11). Conditions such as advanced age, increased severity of illness, and the postsurgical state are rarely modifiable. However, poor nutritional status,[403] oversedation,[438] transfusion therapy,[439] and exposure to broad-spectrum antimicrobials[430] are associated with an increased risk of VAP and are under the control of the clinician.

Table 50.11 Independent Risk Factors for Ventilator-Associated Pneumonia in Multivariate Analysis of Data from Published Studies

Host Factors	Intervention Factors
Serum albumin, <2.2 g/dL	Histamine H_2 receptor blockers ± antacids
Age, ≥60 years	Paralytic agents, continuous intravenous sedation
Acute respiratory distress syndrome (ARDS)	Receipt of >4 units of blood
Chronic obstructive pulmonary disease or other chronic pulmonary diseases	Intracranial pressure monitoring
Coma or impaired consciousness	Mechanical ventilation in excess of 48 hours
Burns, trauma	Positive end-expiratory pressure
Organ failure	Frequent ventilator circuit changes
Advanced severity of illness	Reintubation
Large-volume gastric aspiration	Nasogastric tube
Gastric colonization and high gastric pH	Supine head position
Upper respiratory tract colonization	Transport out of the intensive care unit
Sinusitis	Prior antibiotic therapy

Modified from Chastre J, Fagon JY: Ventilator-associated pneumonia. Am J Respir Crit Care Med 2002;165:867-903.

TREATMENT

Treatment of VAP is discussed in Chapter 42 (Pneumonia: Considerations for the Critically Ill Patient), under "Therapy."

PREVENTION

With an understanding of pathogenesis and epidemiology in hand, clinicians caring for mechanically ventilated patients can implement preventive strategies that can materially reduce the risk of VAP (Table 50.12). Both the CDC HICPAC and Canadian Critical Care Trials Group offer evidence-based guidelines for the prevention of VAP.[135,440] Their recommendations are very similar, with minor differences. The Canadian guideline focuses exclusively on specific interventions for the prevention of VAP,[440] whereas the HICPAC guideline incorporates additional guidance for the prevention of nosocomial influenza, legionellosis, and invasive filamentous fungal infections in the hospital.[135] Recommendations from both guidelines can be divided into general, nonpharmacologic, and pharmacologic preventive measures (see Table 50.12).[441] The general measures employed to reduce VAP including education, infection control, hand hygiene, and reliable disinfection and sterilization of respiratory care equipment are discussed elsewhere in this chapter.

Nonpharmacologic Preventive Measures

Avoiding prolonged intubation and reintubation—if avoiding intubation altogether is not feasible—offers the greatest promise for reducing an individual patient's risk of

Table 50.12 Recommendations for the Prevention of Ventilator-Associated Pneumonia

Preventive Measure	HICPAC Grade*	CCCTG Recommendation
General Measures		
• Educate all health care workers involved with the care of mechanically ventilated patients on the risks and methods of preventing ventilator-associated pneumonia.	IA	—
• Perform adequate hand hygiene between patient contacts.	IA	—
• Use gloves for handling respiratory secretions or objects contaminated with respiratory secretions.	IB	—
• Conduct surveillance for bacterial pneumonia in ICU patients using NNIS definitions. Include data on causative organisms and their antimicrobial susceptibility patterns. Express data as rates to assist intrahospital comparisons.	IB	—
• Do not routinely perform cultures of patients, equipment, or environment in the absence of an outbreak.	II	—
• Thoroughly clean all devices to be sterilized and disinfected.	IA	—
• Use steam sterilization or wet heat pasteurization for reprocessing of heat-stable semicritical devices and low-temperature sterilization for heat- or moisture-sensitive devices.	IA	—
• Use sterile water for rinsing reusable semicritical devices.	IB	—
• Change ventilator circuits only when they become soiled.	IA	Recommended
• Periodically drain and discard condensate from ventilator circuits.	IB	—
• Clean, disinfect, rinse with sterile water, and dry in-line nebulizers between treatments on the same patient.	IB	—
• When possible, use aerosolized medications in single-use vials.	IB	—
Nonpharmacologic Measures to Reduce Pneumonia		
• Oral (non-nasal) intubation	IB	Recommended
• Remove nasogastric and endotracheal tubes as soon as clinically feasible.	IB	—
• Avoid unnecessary reintubation.	II	—
• When feasible, use noninvasive ventilation to avoid the need for intubation or reintubation.	II	—
• Early tracheostomy	—	No recommendation
• Semirecumbent positioning of the patient	II	Recommended
• Implement a comprehensive oral hygiene program for mechanically ventilated patients.	II	—
• If feasible, use an endotracheal catheter that allows for continuous or frequent subglottic suctioning.	II	Consider
• Humidification with heat and moisture exchanger (HME)	NR	Recommended†
• Closed multiuse catheters for airway secretion suctioning	NR	Recommended
• Kinetic bed therapy	NR	Consider
Pharmacologic Measures to Reduce Pneumonia		
• Immunize all patients at risk for pneumococcal infection.	IA	—
• Immunize all patients at risk for influenza.	IA	—
• Routine use of chlorhexidine oral rinse	NR	—
• Targeted use of chlorhexidine oral rinse in post–cardiac surgery patients	II	—
• Oral decontamination with topical antimicrobial agents	NR	—
• Preferential use of sucralfate for stress bleeding prophylaxis	NR	Not recommended
• Selective digestive decontamination	NR	Not recommended‡
• Acidification of gastric feedings	NR	—
• Systemic antimicrobials to prevent development of pneumonia	NR	Not recommended‡
• Cycling of antibiotic classes to reduce resistance in the ICU	NR	—

CCCTG, Canadian Critical Care Trials Group; CDC, Centers for Disease Control and Prevention; HICPAC, Healthcare Infection Control Practices Advisory Committee; ICU, intensive care unit; NNIS, National Nosocomial Infections Surveillance System.

Modified from Tablan OC, Anderson LJ, Besser R, et al: Guidelines for preventing health-care-associated pneumonia, 2003: Recommendations of CDC and the Healthcare Infection Control Practices Advisory Committee. MMWR Recomm Rep 2004;53(RR-3):1-36; and Dodek P, Keenan S, Cook D, et al: Evidence-based clinical practice guideline for the prevention of ventilator-associated pneumonia. Ann Intern Med 2004;141:305-313.

*Taken from CDC/HICPAC system of weighting recommendations based on scientific evidence. IA, strongly recommended for implementation and supported by well-designed experimental, clinical, or epidemiologic studies. IB, strongly recommended for implementation and supported by some experimental, clinical, or epidemiologic studies and a strong theoretical rationale. IC, required by state or federal regulations, rules, or standards. II, suggested for implementation and supported by suggestive clinical or epidemiologic trials or a theoretic rationale. Unresolved issue, an unresolved issue for which evidence is insufficient or no consensus regarding efficacy exists. NR, no recommendation for or against at this time.

†Recommended in patients without hemoptysis or high minute ventilation. Exchanger should be replaced weekly.

‡Topical or systemic antimicrobial agents alone are not recommended. Insufficient evidence on antibiotic resistance and cost-effectiveness exists to recommend combination topical and systemic therapy.

developing VAP.[431] The use of noninvasive ventilation in order to avoid endotracheal intubation has been shown to be successful in reducing rates of nosocomial pneumonia in a number of studies[442,443] and may abrogate the need for reintubation in selected patients who prematurely extubate themselves.[135] The implementation of weaning protocols has also been shown to significantly reduce the duration of mechanical ventilation,[444,445] health care costs,[444,445] and institutional rates of VAP.[446,447] Early tracheostomy—within 1 week of intubation—has been advocated as a method for reducing the risk of VAP in patients likely to require prolonged mechanical ventilation. However, randomized trials, admittedly of limited power, have not found significant benefit with this approach[448] and early tracheostomy is not currently recommended by most authorities.[135,440]

As noted earlier, supine positioning of the mechanically ventilated patient's head has been shown to increase the risk of gastroesophageal-pharyngeal aspiration.[437] A simple solution to this threat is to elevate the head of the patient's bed 35 to 45 degrees. Drakulovic and colleagues[449] found that patients whose torso and head were kept elevated at 45 degrees had much lower rates of microbiologically confirmed pneumonia compared with patients cared for in a 0-degree supine position (5% versus 23%, p = 0.018).[449] In reality, maintaining elevation of the head in excess of 45 degrees on a consistent basis is actually quite difficult and uncommonly achieved in practice. A recent randomized study that sought to maintain head elevation above 45 degrees for 85% of the study period found that head elevation in the intervention arm only averaged 28.1 degrees.[450] Perhaps as a result of failure to successfully achieve adequate elevation, no reductions in the rate of VAP were seen.

Although data on the effect that comprehensive oral care has on risk of infection are limited,[451] maintaining adequate dental hygiene is considered an important component of VAP prevention.[135] Binkley and colleagues[452] found that although a majority of nurses caring for patients undergoing mechanical ventilation appreciated the importance of dental hygiene, the methods used to provide this varied considerably. Until more data are available on specific dental hygienic practices, it is recommended that mechanically ventilated patients have their teeth brushed daily, undergo oral cleansing every 2 to 4 hours, undergo routine suctioning to reduce accumulation of fluids in the oropharynx, and have a mouth moisturizer applied to their lips to prevent cracking.[453] The periodic instillation of a topical oral antiseptic solution is an additional promising intervention[453] and is discussed under pharmacologic preventive measures later.

The use of a modified endotracheal tube that has a separate ventral drainage tube for continuous or intermittent suctioning of subglottic secretions has been evaluated in a number of studies.[454,455] Subglottic suctioning reduced the rate of VAP significantly in all but one of these studies.[455] However, in this latter study, the time to onset of VAP was delayed significantly (5.9 days versus 2.9 days, p = 0.006),[455] and recent evidence-based guidelines have recommended the use of endotracheal tubes that allow for suctioning of subglottic secretions.[135,440] Nevertheless, the use of an endotracheal tube that allows for subglottic suctioning did not reduce the duration of mechanical ventilation or rate of ICU mortality in the studies done, which, coupled with the increased cost of the tube and propensity of the suction lumen to occlude, has limited wider adoption of this technology in practice.[456]

The evidence that heat and moisture exchangers (HMEs) are associated with a reduced risk of VAP is mixed. Only one of six published trials found a statistically significant reduction in VAP with use of HMEs (RR 0.41, 95% CI 0.20 to 0.86, p = 0.02).[457] However, pooling data from a recent systematic review[458] and a subsequently published randomized trial[459] shows that HMEs reduce the risk of VAP by 38% (RR 0.62, 95% CI 0.43 to 0.89, p = 0.012). The use of HMEs has been recommended by authors of a systematic review[460] and is currently recommended by the Canadian Critical Care Trials Group.[440] However, HICPAC made no recommendation for the use of HMEs because five of six published trials failed to demonstrate a statistically significant reduction in the rate of VAP.[135] Heat exchange moisturizers become readily occluded in patients with airway hemorrhage and can increase airway resistance. As a result, they should not be used in patients with hemoptysis or those requiring a high-minute ventilation.[440] Finally, the membranes of HMEs can become colonized with bacteria and should be replaced weekly, according to current guidelines.[440]

The availability of in-line multiuse suction catheters abrogates the need to open and manipulate the endotracheal circuit, theoretically reducing the risk of exogenous contamination.[461] Despite their theoretical benefit, prospective studies have not consistently showed that in-line suction catheters are associated with a reduced risk of VAP.[462-464] Although in-line suction catheters do not appear to increase the risk of VAP, they are more time efficient for nursing personnel and respiratory therapists, and are more cost effective than open suction catheters.[440] Kollef and colleagues[465] found that rates of VAP were identical in patients randomized to as-needed changes of their inline suction catheter versus those who had their catheter changed every 24 hours (14.7% vs. 14.8%). As a result, there is no compelling evidence that in-line suction catheters should be periodically changed, unless clinically indicated.

Pharmacologic Preventive Measures

Antacids and H_2-blockers have been used extensively in the ICU setting to prevent stress ulcer bleeding but have been associated with an increased risk of developing VAP because they lead to bacterial overgrowth of the gastric contents.[56] Sucralfate prevents stress ulcer bleeding without reducing gastric pH but is more difficult to administer and is less effective than acid-reducing agents.[435] The results of clinical trials examining these two competing strategies for preventing gastrointestinal hemorrhage in the ICU have been mixed, with earlier trials favoring the use of sucralfate.[56] However, more recently published trials suggest only a small incremental increased risk of VAP with H_2-blockers,[435,466,467] and most experts feel that this risk is more than offset by their superior capacity to prevent stress ulcer bleeding.[135,440]

Selective digestive decontamination (SDD) is one of the most extensively studied preventive interventions in critical care medicine, yet the role for SDD continues to generate vigorous debate as to its overall benefit.[468,469] A more detailed discussion on the risks and benefits of this intervention is provided later in this chapter. Most U.S. experts believe that SDD has the potential to increase infection caused by multiresistant bacteria, particularly in settings with high rates of endemic antimicrobial resistance.[470,471] Until well-designed multicenter trials are done, proving that SDD does not adversely effect the ICU ecology, it is likely that North American guidelines will continue to discourage its use.[135,440]

The isolated use of parenteral antimicrobials for prevention of VAP has not met with much success,[470] but selective antimicrobial decontamination of the oropharynx, without the use of enteral or systemic agents, reduced the risk of VAP nearly 70% (RR = 0.33, 95% CI 0.16 to 0.67, p = 0.001) in one trial.[411] This study reemphasized the primary role of oropharyngeal colonization in the pathogenesis of VAP but engenders the same concerns as SDD over its potential for promoting antimicrobial resistance. However, it has facilitated the idea that topical decolonization of the oropharynx with *nonantimicrobial* agents might be able to materially reduce the risk of VAP without the potential for emergence of antimicrobial resistance. A meta-analysis of seven randomized trials that enrolled 914 mechanically ventilated patients found that topical chlorhexidine applied to the oropharynx reduced the risk of VAP by nearly 30% (RR = 0.74, 95% CI 0.56 to 0.96, p = 0.02), although there was no significant impact on mortality.[413] The beneficial effects of chlorhexidine appear to be most pronounced in post–cardiac surgery patients,[472,473] prompting HICPAC to recommend its use in this subpopulation.[135]

CATHETER-ASSOCIATED URINARY TRACT INFECTION

INCIDENCE AND IMPACT

Each year, urinary catheters are inserted in more than 5 million patients in acute-care hospitals and extended-care facilities.[474] Catheter-associated urinary tract infection (CAUTI) is one of the most common infections in ICUs, and incidence rates are highest in burn, neurologic, neurosurgical, and trauma ICUs, with intermediate risk in surgical and medical ICUs, and lowest risk in coronary care units (see Table 50.1).[25]

Nosocomial bacteriuria or candiduria develops in up to 25% of patients requiring a urinary catheter for more than 7 days, with a daily risk of 5%.[474] CAUTI is the second most common cause of nosocomial bloodstream infection[475]; some studies have also found increased mortality rates associated with CAUTI.[476] Although most CAUTIs are asymptomatic,[477] rarely extend hospitalization, and add only $500 to $1000 to the direct costs of acute-care hospitalization,[478] asymptomatic infections commonly precipitate unnecessary antimicrobial-drug therapy.[479] CAUTIs comprise perhaps the largest institutional reservoir of nosocomial antibiotic-resistant pathogens, the most important of which are multidrug-resistant Enterobacteriaceae other than *Escherichia coli* such as *Klebsiella, Enterobacter, Proteus,* and *Citrobacter; Pseudomonas aeruginosa;* enterococci and staphylococci; and *Candida* spp.[480]

PATHOGENESIS

Excluding rare hematogenously derived pyelonephritis, caused almost exclusively by *S. aureus,* most microorganisms causing endemic CAUTI derive from the patient's own colonic and perineal flora or from the hands of health care personnel and gain access to the patient's urinary tract during catheter insertion or manipulation of the collection system.[265] Organisms gain access in one of two ways. Extraluminal contamination may occur early, by direct inoculation when the catheter is inserted, or later, by organisms ascending from the perineum by capillary action in the thin mucous film between the external catheter surface and the urethral wall. Intraluminal contamination occurs by reflux of microorganisms gaining access to the catheter lumen from failure of closed drainage or contamination of urine in the collection bag. Recent studies suggest that CAUTIs most frequently stem from microorganisms gaining access to the bladder extraluminally,[481] but both routes are important.

Most infected urinary catheters are covered by a thick biofilm containing the infecting microorganisms embedded in a matrix of host proteins and microbial exoglycocalyx.[482] A biofilm forms on the intraluminal or extraluminal surface of the implanted catheter, or both, usually advancing in a retrograde fashion. The role of the biofilm in the pathogenesis of CAUTI has not been established. However, anti-infective–impregnated and silver-hydrogel catheters, which inhibit adherence of microorganisms to the catheter surface, significantly reduce the risk of CAUTI,[483] particularly infections caused by gram-positive organisms or yeasts, which are most likely to be acquired extraluminally from the periurethral flora. These data suggest that microbial adherence to the catheter surface is important in the pathogenesis of many, but not all, CAUTIs. Infections in which the biofilm does not play a pathogenic role are probably caused by mass transport of intraluminal contaminants into the bladder by retrograde reflux of microbe-laden urine when a catheter or collection system is moved or manipulated.

PREVENTION

Several catheter-care practices are universally recommended to prevent or at least delay the onset of CAUTI[265]: most importantly, avoiding unnecessary catheterizations; considering using a condom catheter in a male or a suprapubic catheter; having trained professionals insert catheters aseptically; removing the catheter as soon as no longer needed; maintaining uncompromising closed drainage; ensuring dependent drainage as much as possible; minimizing manipulations of the system; and separating catheterized patients geographically on the patient care unit.

As noted earlier, technologic innovations to prevent nosocomial infection are most likely to be effective if they are based on a clear understanding of the pathogenesis and epidemiology of the infection. Novel technologies must be designed to block CAUTI by either the extraluminal or intraluminal routes, or both. Medicated catheters, which reduce adherence of microorganisms to the catheter surface, may confer the greatest benefit for preventing CAUTI. Two catheters impregnated with anti-infective solutions have been studied in randomized trials, one impregnated with the urinary antiseptic nitrofurazone[484] and the other with a new broad-spectrum antimicrobial-drug combination, minocycline and rifampin.[485] Both catheters showed a modest reduction in bacterial CAUTIs; however, the studies were small, and the risk of selection of antimicrobial drug–resistant uropathogens was not satisfactorily resolved. Silver compounds have also been studied for coating urinary catheters. A meta-analysis of eight randomized trials comparing silver oxide or silver alloy catheters with standard nonimpregnated catheters found that silver alloy, but not silver oxide, catheters were associated with a reduced risk of CAUTI.[486] Recommendations for the prevention of CAUTI are summarized in Table 50.13.[133]

CONTROL OF ANTIBIOTIC RESISTANCE

During the past 55 years, more than 14 different classes of parenteral antimicrobials and several hundred antimicrobial compounds have been introduced into clinical use. In the 1960s, public health officials confidently declared that the war against infectious diseases was almost over. Unfortunately, it is not clear which side will be victorious. Although the greatest strides in our struggles with infectious diseases have resulted from improvements in hygiene and social conditions, the growing losses of our antibiotic armamentarium as a result of surging bacterial resistance could ultimately be disastrous for ICU patients if the tide is not stemmed.

EVOLUTION OF ANTIBIOTIC RESISTANCE IN INTENSIVE CARE UNITS

Antimicrobial resistance has evolved through several phases. In the 1970s and 1980s, resistance of aerobic gram-negative bacilli was the major concern, and *P. aeruginosa,* with its broad range of intrinsic and acquired resistances, was the quintessential nosocomial pathogen. By the 1990s, the availability of antibiotics from a variety of distinct classes—aminoglycosides, broad-spectrum penicillins (e.g., piperacillin), monobactams (e.g., aztreonam), carbapenems (e.g., imipenem), β-lactam–β-lactamase inhibitors (e.g., piperacillin-tazobactam), trimethoprim-sulfamethoxazole, and fluoroquinolones—promised a respite from concerns about resistance in aerobic gram-negative bacilli. During this period, however, gram-positive cocci gained prominence, and MRSA, β-lactam–resistant coagulase-negative staphylococci, and VRE became the major problem nosocomial pathogens. Antibiotic pressure, deriving first from the widespread use of third-generation cephalosporin antibiotics in hospitals, is often cited as a major factor in the emergence of MRSA. Co-emerging as nosocomial pathogens with MRSA have been methicillin-resistant coagulase-negative staphylococci, which have become the leading cause of IVD-related BSI and prosthesis-related surgical site infections.

In the early 1990s VRE burst onto the hospital and ICU scene in the United States and within a few years became entrenched in most tertiary medical centers (see Fig. 50.2). Heavy use of vancomycin, often as empiric treatment in response to concerns about MRSA, was probably the initial factor driving the emergence of VRE. In most settings, however, exposure to cephalosporins and antimicrobials with antianaerobic activity have emerged as the greatest risk factors for nosocomial colonization or infection by VRE. The mid-1990s witnessed growing problems with resistance in fungi and shifts to non–*Candida albicans* species, representing the effects of heavy empirical use of azoles such as fluconazole in hospitals during this period.

FORCES DRIVING RESISTANCE

To a large extent, the emergence of antimicrobial resistance reflects the combined effects of genetic selection, antibiotic pressures, and the frequency of cross-infection in ICUs.[47] For some resistance mechanisms (e.g., extended-spectrum β-lactamases [ESBLs] that confer resistance to third-generation cephalosporins such as ceftazidime), a shift of a single amino acid in existing resistance genes can lead to new, inactivating enzymes. For other resistant bacteria, such as penicillin-resistant pneumococci, multiple resistance genes must be cobbled together in a specific, exacting sequence, which may take years to evolve, emerge, and spread.

Antibiotic pressures provide the necessary darwinian forces that amplify these genetic changes.[487] Usually, resistance emerges to a specific agent that is used most heavily and, hence, provides the greatest pressure. In some instances, genetic linkage of resistance mechanisms to unrelated classes of antimicrobials results in the capacity of heavy use of one drug class to select for resistance to a different class. For example, use of trimethoprim-sulfamethoxazole has been associated statistically with the emergence of ceftazidime-resistant *E. coli* and *K. pneumoniae* as a result of linkage on a single plasmid of genes that encode production of ESBLs and trimethoprim-sulfamethoxazole resistance. A large proportion of extended-spectrum β-lactamase–producing gram-negative bacilli are also resistant to fluoroquinolones.[488,489]

In epidemiologic and clinical studies of antibiotic resistance, there is always a proportion of patients in whom resistance is found without exposure to the problem antibiotic. These patients usually have other important risk factors, such as increased severity of underlying disease, extremes of age, presence of invasive devices, recent surgery, or proximity to patients who are infected or colonized with antibiotic-resistant bacteria. In these cases the presence of antibiotic-resistant strains is most often the consequence of patient-to-patient spread, usually on the contaminated hands of HCWs; occasionally, spread results from a contaminated common source, such as an inadequately cleaned piece of equipment. Studies of HCW hand hygiene show that rates of handwashing between patient contacts range from 25% to 50%, at best, and are inadequate to control resistance, especially in ICUs, where the staff are extremely busy and less likely to be attentive to hand hygiene.[168]

CONTROLLING ANTIMICROBIAL RESISTANCE IN THE INTENSIVE CARE UNIT

Stemming the tide of antimicrobial resistance requires a multifaceted approach, especially in ICUs, where antibiotic pressures and lapses in hospital hygiene are usually greatest. First, active surveillance for resistant bacteria is essential to

Table 50.13 CDC/HICPAC Guideline Recommendations for Prevention of Catheter-Associated Urinary Tract Infection

Recommendation	Strength*
Appropriate Urinary Catheter Use	
• Insert catheters only for appropriate indications: ◦ Appropriate indications (based primarily on expert consensus) include acute urinary retention or bladder outlet obstruction; measurement of urinary output in critically ill patients; perioperative use for selected surgical procedures—remove as soon as possible; promoting healing of open sacral wounds in incontinent patients; prolonged immobilization from multiple traumatic injuries; and improved comfort for end-of-life care. ◦ Inappropriate indications (based primarily on expert consensus) include substitute for nursing care of the patient with incontinence; obtaining urine for diagnostic tests when patient can void; and prolonged postoperative use without appropriate indications.	IB
• Promptly remove catheter when no longer needed.	IB
• Consider alternatives to use of indwelling urethral catheters in select patients (e.g., external catheters in cooperative male patients without urinary retention or bladder outlet obstruction; intermittent catheterization in spinal cord injury patients or patients with bladder emptying dysfunction).	II
• Further research is needed regarding use of suprapubic catheters as alternative to indwelling urethral catheters.	NR
Urinary Catheter Insertion	
• Perform hand hygiene before and after insertion or manipulation of catheter.	IB
• Only properly trained personnel should insert and maintain catheters.	IB
• Insert catheter using aseptic technique and sterile equipment (sterile gloves, drape, antiseptic or sterile solution for periurethral cleaning).	IB
• Properly secure catheter to prevent movement and urethral traction.	IB
• Use smallest bore catheter possible that allows for good drainage, to minimize bladder neck and urethral trauma.	II
Urinary Catheter Maintenance	
• Maintain a closed drainage system; if break in aseptic technique, disconnection, or leakage occurs, replace catheter and collecting system.	IB
• Maintain unobstructed urine flow (e.g., keep collecting bag below level of bladder at all times; keep catheter and collecting tube free from kinking; empty collecting bag regularly).	IB
• Use standard precautions, including the use of gloves and gown as appropriate, during any manipulation of catheter or collecting system.	IB
• Do not change catheters or drainage bags at routine, fixed intervals.	II
• Do not use systemic antimicrobials to prevent CAUTI.	IB
• Do not clean periurethral area with antiseptics; routine hygiene is appropriate (e.g., cleansing meatal surface during bathing).	IB
• Unless obstruction is anticipated, bladder irrigation is not recommended.	II
• If obstruction occurs, change catheter.	IB
• Irrigation of bladder with antimicrobials and instillation of antiseptic or antimicrobial solutions into drainage bags are not recommended.	II
• Obtain urine samples aseptically.	IB
• If CAUTI rate is not decreasing after implementing a comprehensive strategy to reduce CAUTI rates, consider using antimicrobial/antiseptic-impregnated catheters.	IB
• Further research is needed on use of bacterial interference (i.e., bladder inoculation with a nonpathogenic bacterial strain) to prevent CAUTI.	NR
• Further research is needed regarding spatial separation of patients with catheters to prevent transmission of pathogens colonizing urinary drainage systems.	NR
Other Measures	
• Implement quality improvement strategies to enhance appropriate use of catheters and to reduce the risk of CAUTI.	IB
• Ensure that health care personnel are given periodic training regarding catheter insertion, maintenance, and removal; CAUTI; and alternatives to indwelling catheters.	IB
• Consider surveillance for CAUTI when indicated.	II
• Do not routinely screen catheterized patients for asymptomatic bacteriuria.	II

*IA, strong recommendation supported by high- to moderate-quality evidence suggesting net clinical benefit or harm. IB, strong recommendation supported by low-quality evidence suggesting net clinical benefit or harm or an accepted practice (e.g., aseptic technique) supported by low- to very-low-quality evidence. IC, strong recommendation required by state or federal regulation. II, weak recommendation supported by any-quality evidence suggesting a trade-off between clinical benefit and harm. No recommendation/unresolved issue (NR), unresolved issue for which there is low- to very-low-quality evidence with uncertain tradeoffs between benefit and harm.

CAUTI, catheter-associated urinary tract infection.

Data from Gould CV, Umscheid CA, Agarwal RK, Kuntz G, Pegues DA; Healthcare Infection Control Practices Advisory Committee. Guideline for prevention of catheter-associated urinary tract infections 2009. Infect Control Hosp Epidemiol 2010;31(4):319-26.

provide an understanding of local problems and needs. To support surveillance and treatment, cultures must be obtained from suspected sites of infection before empiric antibiotic therapy is initiated. The benefit of routine surveillance cultures (e.g., periodic cultures of sputum specimens or rectal swabs) for assessing rates of colonization by resistant bacteria in ICUs will depend on how such cultures are used.

Second, when rates of resistance begin to increase, molecular typing, such as by pulsed-field gel electrophoresis, can differentiate spread of a single strain (clonal expansion)—which suggests person-to-person or common source transmission—from spread of multiple strains (polyclonal expansion), which suggests emergence of resistance in individual patients as a result of antibiotic pressures or exogenous introduction of multiple resistant strains. Often, these problems—clonal and polyclonal—coexist.

Third, the importance of hand hygiene must be stressed at all times. Aggressive hand hygiene campaigns, with adherence monitoring and feedback of ward and even individual results, may achieve compliance rates as high as 70%. For some situations (e.g., when there is extensive patient colonization by antibiotic-resistant bacteria), these levels of adherence may not be sufficient to control cross-infection. Response to this problem has been to encourage "universal gloving," in addition to wider use of alcohol-based hand rubs (a "belt-and-suspender" approach) to bridge the gap left by incomplete attention to hand hygiene even in the best of circumstances. Use of universal gloving has been successful in controlling the spread of aminoglycoside-resistant gram-negative bacilli in ICUs and *C. difficile*–related diarrhea.[228,245] Because patients' intact skin and the environment in patient rooms may be a source of resistant bacteria, such as VRE, we recommend that disposable examination gloves be worn for all contact with ICU patients or their environment. Because gloves are not a total barrier, they must be removed and hands disinfected by an alcohol hand rub between patient contacts.

Fourth, antimicrobial stewardship is essential (Table 50.14).[257] The primary goal of antimicrobial stewardship is to optimize clinical outcomes while minimizing unintended consequences of antimicrobial use such as toxicity, emergence of resistance, and *C. difficile*–associated diarrhea. Because antimicrobial use drives antimicrobial resistance, the frequency of inappropriate antimicrobial use can be used as a surrogate marker for antimicrobial resistance. Both antimicrobial stewardship and a comprehensive infection control program are essential to limiting the emergence and transmission of antimicrobial-resistant pathogens. Most studies assessing the utility of antimicrobial stewardship have focused on adults in ICUs, where the burden of antimicrobial resistance is greatest.

A comprehensive evidence-based stewardship program to combat antimicrobial resistance is typically a multifaceted, multidisciplinary program; the size and complexity of the management team and the specific measures applied to optimize prescribing vary on the basis of local antimicrobial use patterns, resistance trends, and available resources. The two core strategies that provide the foundation for a successful antimicrobial stewardship program are (1) prospective audits, with intervention and feedback, and (2) formulary restriction and preauthorization.[257]

Several studies have shown that prospective audits of antimicrobial use with intervention and feedback are an effective means of reducing inappropriate antimicrobial use.[490,491] In a randomized trial conducted at a 600-bed tertiary teaching hospital, inpatients receiving parenteral antimicrobial therapy were randomized to an intervention group that received suggestions for optimal antimicrobial use from an infectious disease physician or to no interventions. Physicians in the intervention group implemented 85% of the suggestions they received, which resulted in 1.6 fewer days of parenteral therapy and $400 savings per patient. Similar results have been noted in trials undertaken in community hospitals.[490] If daily review of antimicrobial use is not feasible, review of antimicrobial usage 3 days a week may still have a significant impact. Effective auditing with intervention and feedback can be undertaken most easily with automated computer surveillance of antimicrobial use, allowing the targeting of specific units where the problems are greatest.

Formulary restriction and preauthorization requirements for specific agents are now common in most hospitals. Antimicrobial restriction is unequivocally the most effective method of controlling antimicrobial use.[492,493] However, it is unclear whether antimicrobial restriction achieves the more important outcome, reducing antimicrobial resistance. Several studies of outbreaks of *C. difficile*–associated diarrhea have shown abrupt cessation of the outbreak following restriction (and greatly reduced use) of one or more key antimicrobials such as clindamycin or third-generation cephalosporins.[492] However, other studies have documented inexorably rising resistance rates in nosocomial pathogens despite a rigorous program of antimicrobial restriction.[494] One explanation for this increase in resistance may be the compensatory increase in usage of broad-spectrum antimicrobials other than the restricted agent, thus counteracting any benefit of restriction. Furthermore, restricting the use of a single drug to reduce antimicrobial resistance may be ineffective because cross-resistance in bacterial species to more than one class of antimicrobials is the rule in nosocomial organisms.

One or both of the core strategies should be adopted and supplemented by close collaboration among a core antimicrobial stewardship team, infection control personnel, health care providers, and hospital administration.

Beyond the two major mechanisms of antimicrobial stewardship mentioned earlier, other elements that should be incorporated into an institutional antimicrobial stewardship program include education of health care providers; however, passive educational efforts such as conference presentations, teaching sessions, and provision of guidelines are only marginally effective in the absence of other active interventions.[495] Clinical practice guidelines are being introduced with increasing frequency; however, the impact of these guidelines on provider behavior and clinical outcomes has been difficult to measure. Guidelines tailored to local antimicrobial resistance patterns and antimicrobial use trends may have more impact than a generic clinical pathway.

Table 50.14 Recommendations for Developing an Institutional Program to Enhance Antimicrobial Stewardship

Recommendation	Level of Evidence*
• Create a multidisciplinary antimicrobial stewardship team, including an infectious disease physician and a clinical pharmacist with infectious disease training.	A-II
• Include, if possible, a clinical microbiologist, an information systems specialist, an infection control professional, and the hospital epidemiologist.	A-III
• Foster collaboration between the antimicrobial stewardship team and the hospital infection control committee.	A-III
• Create a climate of support and collaboration between the antimicrobial stewardship team and the hospital administration and medical staff leadership.	A-III
• Develop infrastructure to measure antimicrobial use, and track use on ongoing basis.	A-II
• Employ a system of prospective audit of antimicrobial use with direct interaction and feedback to the prescriber by an infectious disease physician or a clinical pharmacist with infectious disease training.	A-I
• Use formulary restrictions and preauthorization requirement to reduce antimicrobial use and cost.	A-II
• Provide education to health care providers regarding stewardship strategies.	A-III
• Education must be combined with active interventions to improve antimicrobial prescribing practices.	B-II
• Develop evidence-based multidisciplinary guidelines incorporating local microbiology and resistance patterns to improve antimicrobial utilization.	A-I
• No recommendation can be made regarding antimicrobial cycling as a means of preventing or reducing antimicrobial resistance.	C-II
• Use antimicrobial order forms as a component of antimicrobial stewardship.	B-II
• No recommendation can be made regarding the routine use of combination therapy to prevent emergence of resistance.	C-II
• Streamline or de-escalate antimicrobial therapy on the basis of culture results.	A-II
• Optimize antimicrobial dosing on the basis of individual patient characteristics, causative organisms, site of infection, and pharmacokinetic and pharmacodynamic characteristics of the drug.	A-II
• Use health care information technology such as electronic medical records, computerized physician order entry, and clinical decision support to improve antimicrobial prescribing.	B-II
• Use computer-based surveillance for more efficient targeting of antimicrobial interventions, tracking of resistance patterns, and identification of nosocomial infections and adverse drug reactions.	B-II
• Engage the clinical microbiology laboratory to participate in antimicrobial stewardship by providing patient-specific culture and susceptibility data and by assisting infection control efforts in the surveillance of resistant organisms and in the molecular epidemiologic investigation of outbreaks.	A-III
• Determine the impact of antimicrobial stewardship by measuring process and outcomes.	B-III

*Based on the Infectious Diseases Society of America grading system for ranking recommendations in clinical guidelines. A, good evidence to support a recommendation for use; B, moderate evidence to support a recommendation for use; C, poor evidence to support a recommendation for use; I, evidence from >1 properly randomized, controlled trial; II, evidence from >1 well-designed clinical trial, without randomization, from cohort or case-controlled analytic studies, or from multiple time-series; III, evidence from expert opinion.

Modified from Dellit TH, Owens RC, McGowan JE Jr, et al: Infectious Diseases Society of America and the Society for Healthcare Epidemiology of America guidelines for developing an institutional program to enhance antimicrobial stewardship. Clin Infect Dis 2007;44:159-177.

Interest has been sparked in ICUs by the reborn concept of antibiotic cycling.[496,497] The most recent experiences have evaluated switch therapy[498] for empiric antibiotic use, rather than actual cycling, and have shown beneficial reductions in resistance among gram-negative bacilli[499] and in the prevalence of VRE. Such approaches, as well as true cycling through different antimicrobial classes, may be effective over limited periods in closed environments such as ICUs, by transiently reducing selection pressure and thus resistance to the restricted agent. Yet studies have thus far not shown a consistent long-term benefit with cycling, and mathematical models do not predict that cycling will be an effective measure to reduce antimicrobial resistance.[500]

Antimicrobial order forms reduce antimicrobial usage with automatic stop orders and the requirement for physician justification.[501] Streamlining or de-escalation of therapy based on culture data is an essential component of appropriate antimicrobial use, with studies showing substantial reductions in days of antimicrobial use and cost savings.[502,503]

Computer order entry provides needed information at the moment in a neutral, nonjudgmental, fact-based format; this system is efficient, well accepted, and holds the promise to change prescribing behaviors materially.[504,505]

Effective antimicrobial stewardship programs can be financially self-supporting and improve patient care. Studies have shown reductions in antimicrobial usage from 22% to 36%, with annual savings of $200,000 to $900,000 in larger teaching hospitals and community hospitals. A recent guideline from the Infectious Diseases Society of America and the Society for Healthcare Epidemiology of America provides detailed recommendations for developing institutional programs of antimicrobial stewardship, which are summarized in Table 50.14.[257]

AVANT GARDE INFECTION CONTROL MEASURES

SELECTIVE DIGESTIVE DECONTAMINATION

Intense interest has arisen in Europe and the United States[463-465] over the use of "selective digestive decontamination" (SDD) for the prevention of bacterial pneumonia and other nosocomial infections in mechanically ventilated ICU patients. This novel therapy is based on the premise that the upper respiratory tract flora exists in a continuum with the gastrointestinal flora and that these mucosal microorganisms make up the major reservoir of pathogens causing pneumonia and many other nosocomial infections, especially in mechanically ventilated patients. Most ventilated ICU patients have a nasogastric tube that provides a direct conduit for reflux of microorganisms from the heavily colonized stomach to the oropharynx, from which organisms gain access to the lower respiratory tract.

SDD consists of four components: (1) a broad-spectrum parenteral antibiotic given for approximately 3 days to treat infections incubating at the time of admission to the ICU; (2) topical antimicrobials (usually polymyxin E, tobramycin, and amphotericin B) periodically applied to the oropharynx and instilled into the gut for a variable period, usually for the entire duration of ICU stay, to reduce the mucosal burden of gram-negative bacteria and yeasts while preserving the anaerobic flora; (3) a reemphasized adherence to hand hygiene to prevent nosocomial transmission of bacteria, and in some European centers, empiric barrier isolation; and (4) serial surveillance cultures of the oropharynx and rectum to monitor the efficacy of the treatment.[506,507]

Twelve meta-analyses assessing the efficacy of SDD for reducing infection and mortality rate have been published (Table 50.15).[508-519] All have found a reduction in pneumonia. Some, but not all, have found reduced mortality rate. However, a review showed that the results of the meta-analyses were inversely related to study design,[520] which in the case of SDD may overestimate its efficacy. Most studies and meta-analyses of SDD did not make a distinction between parenteral and topical SDD; the few meta-analyses that undertook subgroup analyses found that topical antibiotics alone reduced infection but not mortality rate.[513] A recently published large clinical trial of SDD and selective oropharyngeal decontamination in 5939 ICU patients showed a large reduction in ICU-acquired bacteremia due to gram-negative bacilli and *S. aureus,* and an estimated reduction in mortality rate of 3.5 percentage points with SDD and 2.9 percentage points with selective oropharyngeal decontamination, providing further evidence of the efficacy of SDD.[521]

However, the greatest deterrent to widespread acceptance of SDD is the fear that it will promote the emergence and spread of antimicrobial-resistant microorganisms. Antibiotic pressure is without question the single most powerful force driving the selection of resistant microorganisms, and any strategy for prevention of infection in the ICU that has the potential to increase infections caused by multiresistant organisms must be approached very cautiously. A number of studies underlie the concern of promoting antimicrobial resistance with SDD. Numerous studies have documented major shifts in the microbial ecology of the ICU with the use of SDD.[522-525] In a study by Lingnau and colleagues,[522] 4.5 years of SDD with ciprofloxacin led to a marked increase in MRSA infection from 17% to 81% and of ciprofloxacin-resistant *S. aureus* from 33% to 80%. The number of infections caused by other multiresistant bacteria such as *Acinetobacter* was also increased by SDD.[522]

A distinction must also be made between the risk to an individual receiving SDD of infection caused by a resistant pathogen and the institutional risk of an increased prevalence of antimicrobial-resistant organisms related to the use of SDD. Although both consequences are undesirable, given the skyrocketing rates of endemic nosocomial MRSA and VRE infections worldwide, any—however small—potential for increased antimicrobial resistance must be taken seriously.[526] In order to better address this issue, well-designed, cluster-randomized trials that employ multilevel modeling and specifically address the effects of SDD on antimicrobial resistance across the entire spectrum of microbial pathogens at the institutional level are necessary. Until such data are available, we believe that continued North American concerns about the effects of SDD on antimicrobial resistance are justified, particularly in institutions where MRSA and VRE are endemic, which encompasses virtually all larger hospitals. Given that other effective measures for the prevention of nosocomial infection exist, we believe that SDD should be restricted to select patients, such as certain trauma patients, or as a potential adjunctive control measure for a nosocomial outbreak caused by multiply resistant organisms.[527]

Randomized trials have identified several novel measures for prevention of VAP such as semirecumbent positioning[449] and subglottic suction endotracheal tubes.[528] We believe that these approaches are ecologically more attractive control measures for ventilated ICU patients than prophylactic topical and systemic antibiotics.

PREEMPTIVE BARRIER ISOLATION

Having fewer patients in a room, improving the facilities for handwashing, and using cohort nursing (i.e., assigning each nurse to designated patients) have reduced the incidence of endemic nosocomial infection in neonatal and pediatric ICUs.[172,529] Complicated forms of protective isolation have reduced the high rates of nosocomial infection in patients with profound granulocytopenia[530] or full-thickness burns.[172,244] Moreover, the routine use of gowns and gloves on a special pediatric unit was associated with a marked decline in the incidence of nosocomial infection with RSV,[81] and the routine use of gloves for all patient contacts was shown to reduce the incidence of nosocomial *C. difficile* infection nearly fivefold in a large veterans hospital.[245]

Unfortunately, the few studies that have prospectively evaluated protective isolation of ICU patients have been performed in newborns and pediatric patients and have yielded conflicting and generally disappointing results[531-534];

Table 50.15 Meta-analyses of Randomized Controlled Trials (RCTs) of Selective Digestive Decontamination

Study	No. of RCTs Included	Description	Pneumonia Point Estimate OR or RR (95% CI)	Mortality Point Estimate OR or RR (95% CI)
Vandenbroucke-Grauls, 1991[508]	6	Medical and surgical patients	0.12 (0.08-0.19)	0.70 (0.45-1.09)
SDD Trialists Collaborative Group, 1993[509]	22	Medical and surgical patients	0.37 (0.31-0.43)	0.90 (0.79-1.04)
Kollef, 1994[510]	16	Medical and surgical patients	0.28 (0.21-0.38)	0.90 (0.74-1.1)
Heyland et al, 1994[511]	25	Medical and surgical patients	0.46 (0.39-0.56)	0.87 (0.79-0.97)
Hurley, 1995[512]	26	Medical and surgical patients	0.35 (0.30-0.42)	0.86 (0.74-0.99)
D'Amico et al, 1998[513]	33	Medical and surgical patients	0.35 (0.29-0.41)	0.88 (0.78-0.98)
Nathens et al, 1999[514]	21	Medical and surgical patients	Medical: 0.45 (0.33-0.62) Surgical: 0.19 (0.15-0.26)	Medical: 0.91 (0.71-1.18) Surgical: 0.70 (0.52-0.93)
Safdar et al, 2004[515]	4	Liver transplant patients	0.88 (0.73-1.09)*	0.82 (0.22-2.45)
Liberati et al, 2004[516]	36	Medical and surgical patients	0.35 (0.29-0.41)	0.78 (0.68-0.89)
Silvestri et al, 2005[517]	42	Medical and surgical patients	0.30 (0.17-0.53)†	NR
Silvestri et al, 2007[518]	51	Medical and surgical patients	0.73 (0.59-0.90)‡	0.80 (0.69-0.94)
Liberati et al, 2009[519]	36	Medical and surgical patients	0.28 (0.20-0.38)	0.75 (0.65-0.87)

*Overall infection.
†Fungal infections.
‡Bloodstream infection.
OR, odds ratio; RR, relative risk.
Studies cited in table (column 1) may be found in the complete list of references for this chapter provided online.

however, most of these studies had major weaknesses in design.[247] More recently, several studies have shown that preemptive use of barrier precautions can effectively reduce the spread of multiresistant organisms such as MRSA or VRE in epidemic[535,536] and endemic settings (Table 50.16).[81,245,532,537-545] If colonization by nosocomial organisms could be prevented or at least delayed until invasive devices are removed, the incidence of infection might be significantly reduced.

One major prospective trial that assessed the efficacy of simple protective isolation—which we prefer to call *preemptive barrier precautions*—to reduce the incidence of nosocomial infection during pediatric intensive care studied 70 high-risk children over 30 months who were not immunosuppressed but who required prolonged mechanical ventilatory support and exposure to invasive devices in a pediatric ICU and were randomized to receive standard care without any special precautions or preemptive barrier isolation, with the use of disposable nonwoven polypropylene gowns and nonsterile latex gloves for all patient contacts.[537] Risk factors predisposing patients to infection were comparable in the two groups. Nosocomial colonization occurred later among isolated patients (median 12 vs. 7 days) and was associated with subsequent infection in 2 patients, as compared with 12 patients given standard care. Among children who were isolated, the interval before the first infection was significantly longer (median, 20 vs. 8 days), the daily infection rate was twofold lower (86 vs. 44 infections per 1000 ICU days), and there were 50% fewer days with fever. The benefit of isolation was most notable after 7 days of ICU care. Isolation was well tolerated by patients and their families. Unannounced monitoring showed that children in each group were touched and handled indiscernibly by hospital personnel and families.

The study concluded that the use of disposable high-barrier gowns and gloves for the care of select high-risk children who require prolonged ICU care can substantially reduce the incidence of nosocomial infection, is well tolerated, and does not compromise the delivery of care. Simple forms of protective isolation as a general control measure would also seem preferable to attempts to suppress nosocomial colonization with SDD. Further studies are necessary to determine the cost effectiveness of prophylactic barrier precautions in the ICU and especially the efficacy of protective isolation in adult surgical ICUs, where the incidence of nosocomial infection is as high as 35%. Studies should also determine the relative importance of wearing a gown, as compared with wearing gloves alone.

Patients with prolonged severe granulocytopenia or those who are receiving high dosages of corticosteroids, usually as part of immunosuppressive regimens to prevent transplant rejection, are at risk for invasive pulmonary infection caused by *Aspergillus* species, *Zygomycetes*, and other filamentous airborne fungi, which is associated with high mortality rate.[40-42,546] The risk of invasive infection appears to be directly related to the counts of airborne fungi, and numerous outbreaks have been linked to building construction or failure of air-control systems. Studies have shown that the isolation of vulnerable patients in positive-pressure rooms with spore-free HEPA-filtered air greatly reduces the risk of invasive infection.[40,42] HEPA-filtered ICU rooms should be available for the care of patients who have received bone marrow or solid organ transplants and who require intensive care, especially in the early post-transplant period or during the treatment of rejection, when dosages of immunosuppressive drugs are high.

Preemptive use of barrier isolation precautions (gowns and gloves) and providing dedicated patient care items

Table 50.16 Studies of Preemptive Barrier Isolation to Contain Spread of Multiresistant Organisms

Organism/Infection Requiring Use of Preemptive Barrier Isolation Precautions for All High-Risk Patients	Control of Epidemic Spread		Control of Endemic Infections			
			Before-After and Nonrandomized Trials		Randomized Trials	
	No. of Outbreaks	No. Totally Controlled	Study	RR (95% CI)	Study	RR (95% CI)
Methicillin-resistant *Staphylococcus aureus*	2[535]	2 (100%)[535]	Safdar[542]	0.36 (0.13-0.98)*	None	
Vancomycin-resistant enterococci	2[535,536]	2 (100%)[535,536]	Montecalvo[544]	0.22 (0.05-0.92)*	None	
			Slaughter[541]	2.66 (1.00-6.77)†		
			Morris[545]	1.18 (NR)†		
			Srinivasan[543]	0.47 (NR)*		
			All studies	0.22-2.66		
Resistant gram-negative bacilli	None		McManus[622]	0.38 (0.31-0.46)*	None	
Clostridium difficile	None		Johnson[245]	0.19 (NR)*	None	
Other						
Necrotizing enterocolitis			Agbayani[532]	0.13 (0.02-0.84)*		
Respiratory syncytial virus			Leclair[81]	0.34 (0.17-0.60)*		
All nosocomial infections			Slaughter[541]	1.51 (0.74-3.12)†	Slota[538]	0.48 (NR)*
					Klein[537]	0.19 (0.05-0.70)*
					Koss[540]	1.86 (1.10-3.16)*

*$p < 0.05$.
†$p > 0.05$.
NR, not reported; RR, relative risk.
Studies cited (by main author) in table may be found in the complete list of references for this chapter provided online.

such as stethoscopes and sphygmomanometers in all high-risk patients from the time of admission is a simple and effective strategy to prevent HCWs from acquiring hand contamination by multiresistant organisms when having contact with patients with unrecognized colonization or infection and to block transmission to other as yet uncolonized patients.

GOALS FOR THE FUTURE

Clearly, nosocomial infection is one of the most important causes of iatrogenic morbidity and death in patients who require prolonged life-support care in an ICU. Much has been learned over the past 3 decades about the relative risks and especially the pathogenesis and epidemiology of these infections, information that has provided the scientific underpinnings for preventive strategies that have proved effective. However, there is an urgent need for better research to prevent nosocomial infection in ICU patients (Box 50.4),[604] particularly with respect to strategies to prevent colonization by multiresistant microorganisms, and to prevent infection even if colonization has already occurred.[28]

Most of our understanding of the epidemiology of nosocomial infection, especially in ICUs, is based on studies of epidemics. Well-designed studies are necessary to better define the epidemiology of *endemic* nosocomial infections, especially those caused by resistant staphylococci, enterococci and gram-negative bacilli, and yeasts. The importance of hand carriage of pathogens by hospital personnel, the role of airborne transmission in the ICU, and the relevance of contamination of the inanimate hospital environment by resistant pathogens all need to be better delineated, as well as the factors influencing nosocomial colonization and superinfection by resistant bacteria and yeasts.

In addition, larger and more sophisticated studies, using multivariate techniques of statistical analysis to define risk factors for the major forms of nosocomial infection in the ICU, are necessary to guide allocation of infection control resources and to target future research efforts.

Considering that the period of greatly increased susceptibility to infection of ICU patients is limited—until the invasive devices have been removed—a major commitment must be made to devise and evaluate strategies for blocking transmission of organisms between patients and preventing, or at least delaying, nosocomial colonization.

One of the oldest yet most important infection control measures—hand hygiene—is still done almost indifferently by HCWs in most hospitals including within ICUs. Innovative approaches are necessary to improve the frequency *and the quality* of handwashing after patient contacts likely to result in acquisition of nosocomial organisms. Exactly how should hands be washed for maximal benefit and with what agents? The question can be posed: Could very frequent handwashing, which approaches 40 times per 8-hour shift in neonatal ICUs, increase the potential for transmission of microorganisms, such as methicillin-resistant coagulase-negative staphylococci? Should the frequency of handwashing, as well as the agents used, be critically reexamined?

Box 50.4 Directions for Future Research in Nosocomial Infection Control

Studies to better define the epidemiology of endemic nosocomial infections:

- Especially those caused by resistant staphylococci, gram-negative bacilli, and *Candida*
- The relevance of hand carriage of pathogens by hospital personnel
- The role of airborne transmission
- The relative importance of contamination of the inanimate hospital environment, especially with methicillin-resistant *S. aureus, C. difficile,* and other resistant organisms
- The biologic factors influencing colonization by nosocomial organisms
- The factors governing superinfection by resistant bacteria and *Candida*
- Better understanding of risk factors predisposing to infection, especially in the ICU, to guide allocation of resources in infection control and focus research efforts

Innovative strategies to prevent nosocomial colonization and interrupt cross-infection, especially in ICUs:

- New approaches to improving compliance with and improving the effectiveness of handwashing between patients
- Various types of barrier precautions (forms of protective isolation)
- The true efficacy and cost-benefit ratio of selective digestive decontamination, with careful assessment of the ecologic effects of long-term use
- Dedicated device care teams
- Large, randomized clinical trials of the various cutaneous antiseptics available, with infection, rather than colonization, as the index of comparison, for handwashing by personnel, site disinfection with invasive devices, patient bathing, and decolonization

Research on devices:

- Innovative designs to implicitly reduce contamination
- Colonization-resistant polymers, possibly incorporating antimicrobials onto the surface or into the polymer itself
- Better techniques of use to enhance safety
- Cost-effective "needleless" systems to protect health care personnel
- Improved laboratory tests to identify infection more accurately and rapidly, especially tracheobronchitis and pneumonia, to reduce unnecessary antibiotic therapy yet permit early therapy to avert progression to life-threatening sepsis
- Measures to restrict and improve the use of antibiotics, especially in ICUs
- Expanded, more effective approaches to education in infection control for health care personnel, especially physicians, with respect to handwashing, use of isolation, invasive devices, and use of antibiotics

Modified from Maki DG: Risk factors for nosocomial infection in intensive care. "Devices vs. nature" and goals for the next decade. Arch Intern Med 1989;149:30-35.
ICU, intensive care unit.

Beyond a certain frequency, more may not necessarily be better. Should handwashing machines, which substantially augment degerming,[605,606] be adopted widely? Could regular application of chlorhexidine-containing evaporative lotions, used without water, replace some of the conventional handwashing or at least compensate for the suboptimal handwashing currently practiced?[225,607,608] Large clinical trials, ideally in multiple centers, are necessary to ascertain the efficacy or lack of efficacy of innovative approaches to hand degerming in reducing infections in high-risk patients, particularly in nurseries and ICUs.

Whereas SDD with topical nonabsorbable antibiotics has shown promise for the prevention of nosocomial respiratory infection in ICU patients, as noted, the potential effect on the microbial ecology of the ICU must be viewed with caution, and the cost-benefit and long-term effects of SDD need better clarification. The uses of simple barrier precautions to prevent colonization and infection have shown promise and warrant further study, especially in ICUs.

Studies have shown that the use of dedicated intravenous therapy teams, consisting of trained nurses or technicians to ensure a high level of aseptic technique during catheter insertion and in follow-up care of the catheter, has been associated with greatly reduced rates of catheter-related infection and appears to be cost effective.[327,328,609] The use of teams of trained ICU personnel to insert all urethral catheters and provide follow-up care for these catheters, all intravascular devices, and percutaneous tubes in the ICU deserves study.

Remarkably, there have been few comparative clinical trials of the various chemical antiseptics available for disinfecting skin before inserting intravascular devices or assisting in surgery or studies of antiseptic handwashing agents. Large, randomized clinical trials, ideally in multiple centers, are necessary in which infection, rather than cutaneous colonization or positive cultures, is used as the index of comparison.

Considerable evidence indicates that the material used in construction of an implanted device plays an important role in the pathogenesis of device-related infection, namely, whether the material provides an attractive surface for adherence by pathogenic microorganisms such as coagulase-negative staphylococci. Studies are necessary to delineate fully the molecular mechanisms of microbial adherence to prosthetic surfaces to develop new materials intrinsically resistant to colonization for use with implantable devices and to design devices that intrinsically deny microbial access.

Increased use of diagnostic tests has greatly increased awareness of infectious diseases. Improved laboratory techniques to identify infection more accurately and rapidly, especially methods to reliably distinguish colonization of the lower respiratory tract from early infection that merits antimicrobial therapy, could greatly reduce unnecessary antimicrobial therapy yet detect infections earlier, before they progress to sepsis with multiple-organ failure.

Antimicrobials are not used optimally in most ICUs, and there is much overuse in hospitals, particularly of extended-spectrum penicillins and cephalosporins, carbapenems, vancomycin, and fluoroquinolones. Antibiotic pressure has had a powerful effect on the hospital microbial ecology and, as noted previously, on the profile of nosocomial infection, especially in ICUs. We must and can do better.

Last, but certainly not least, many physicians remain remarkably oblivious to the most basic precepts of infection control, and nurses are in general far better informed and are a more effective force for ensuring compliance with infection control practices. More effective ways to communicate essential information on nosocomial infection control to hospital personnel, especially with regard to handwashing, aseptic use of devices, and antibiotic therapy, and to apply it more consistently in all hospitals, would have vast immediate benefits.

KEY POINTS

- Patients in modern-day ICUs experience rates of nosocomial infection three to five times higher than non-ICU hospitalized patients. Rates of primary bacteremia and nosocomial pneumonia are up to 10 times higher.
- Patients who are severely immunocompromised or who are critically ill and have high severity of illness scores have a substantially increased risk of nosocomial infection. However, most nosocomial infections in the ICU appear causally to be most directly related to lifesaving technology, particularly invasive devices such as endotracheal tubes and mechanical ventilatory support, urethral and intravascular catheters, and intraventricular catheters, which facilitate colonization by nosocomial organisms and greatly increase vulnerability to infection.
- The major reservoir of bacterial nosocomial pathogens, and possibly *Candida* as well, in the ICU is the colonized or infected patient. Most infections begin with nosocomial colonization by organisms acquired from the hands of noncolonized HCWs. Increasing evidence suggests that antibiotic-resistant organisms, particularly MRSA, resistant enterococci, and *C. difficile,* may also be acquired from the inanimate environment immediately surrounding the patient. *Mycobacterium tuberculosis, Legionella, Aspergillus,* influenza A virus, varicella-zoster virus, measles, mumps, and the highly virulent SARS human coronavirus are transmitted by the airborne route.
- ICUs are uniquely conducive to the epidemic spread of nosocomial organisms of all types, especially antibiotic-resistant bacteria and even *Candida;* more than half of all hospital epidemics occur in ICUs.
- An active, visible institutional infection control program can prevent up to one third of nosocomial infections. Surveillance of infection, whether total or focused, and education of all personnel are the most essential components of the program.
- Use of a chlorhexidine-containing agent for handwashing between patients will reduce endemic nosocomial infections in the ICU by at least 30%. The regular use of waterless alcohol-containing hand rubs or gels may

KEY POINTS (Continued)

provide comparable benefit in prevention of cross-infection.

- Stringent attention to isolation precautions, especially use of disposable gloves and a gown for contacts with patients known to be infected or colonized by resistant organisms, is mandatory to minimize cross-infection and prevent outbreaks. Misuse of gloves as part of universal precautions may, paradoxically, increase the risk of nosocomial infection.
- Modern-day ICUs must have adequate numbers of special negative-pressure isolation rooms for the care of patients with suspected or proven pulmonary tuberculosis and other airborne infections, such as varicella-zoster virus.
- Patients who have undergone recent bone marrow transplants or who have received intensive chemotherapy and are experiencing prolonged severe granulocytopenia should receive ICU care in special HEPA-filtered positive-pressure isolation rooms to protect them from devastating deep *Aspergillus* and other filamentous fungal infection.
- Meticulous attention to aseptic technique and the use of *maximal* barrier precautions—long-sleeved sterile surgical gown, mask and head cover, as well as sterile gloves—during the insertion of central venous catheters; the use of 2% chlorhexidine solutions for cutaneous antisepsis; avoiding insertion into the femoral veins; and prompt removal of catheters as soon as they are no longer necessary can reduce the incidence of catheter-related bloodstream infection at least threefold.
- Studies suggest that the prophylactic use of simple barrier precautions, vis-à-vis protective isolation, may provide protection against all types of ICU-acquired infections. Protective isolation is more appealing ecologically than the use of SDD.
- Measures to avert needle sticks and other sharps injuries are the most important aspect of universal precautions; these measures are necessary to protect the HCWs from HIV and other bloodborne viruses.
- A crisis of antibiotic resistance exists in ICUs. The progressive increase in antibiotic resistance of nosocomial staphylococci (methicillin), gram-negative bacilli (aminoglycosides and expanded-spectrum β-lactams), and enterococci (vancomycin or ampicillin), and the sixfold increase in *Candida* infections during the past 2 decades indicates that it is of highest priority to reduce antimicrobial pressure within ICUs.
- Novel technology holds the greatest promise for prevention of nosocomial infection in general, particularly the development of medical devices that are intrinsically resistant to infection.
- Identifying more effective ways to communicate knowledge of infection control to hospital personnel, especially with regard to handwashing, aseptic use of devices, and antibiotic therapy, and to apply it consistently in all hospitals would have vast immediate benefits.

SELECTED REFERENCES

34. O'Grady NP, Barie PS, Bartlett JG, et al: Guidelines for evaluation of new fever in critically ill adult patients: 2008 update from the American College of Critical Care Medicine and the Infectious Diseases Society of America. Crit Care Med 2008;36:1330-1349.
132. O'Grady NP, Alexander M, Burns LA, et al: Healthcare Infection Control Practices Advisory Committee (HICPAC). Guidelines for the prevention of intravascular catheter-related infections. Clin Infect Dis 2011;52(9):e162-193.
133. Gould CV, Umscheid CA, Agarwal RK, et al: Healthcare Infection Control Practices Advisory Committee. Guideline for prevention of catheter-associated urinary tract infections 2009. Infect Control Hosp Epidemiol 2010;31(4):319-326.
134. Hooton TM, Bradley SF, Cardenas DD, et al: Infectious Diseases Society of America. Diagnosis, prevention, and treatment of catheter-associated urinary tract infection in adults: 2009 International Clinical Practice Guidelines from the Infectious Diseases Society of America. Clin Infect Dis 2010;50(5):625-663.
174. Boyce JM, Pittet D, Healthcare Infection Control Practices Advisory Committee: Society for Healthcare Epidemiology of America. Association for Professionals in Infection Control. Infectious Diseases Society of America. Hand Hygiene Task Force Guideline for Hand Hygiene in Health-Care Settings: Recommendations of the Healthcare Infection Control Practices Advisory Committee and the HICPAC/SHEA/APIC/IDSA Hand Hygiene Task Force. Infect Control Hosp Epidemiol 2002;23(12 Suppl):S3-40.
177. Siegel JD, Rhinehart E, Jackson M, Chiarello L, Health Care Infection Control Practices Advisory Committee: 2007 Guideline for Isolation Precautions: Preventing Transmission of Infectious Agents in Health Care Settings. Am J Infect Control 2007;35(10 Suppl 2):S65-164.
184. Centers for Disease Control and Prevention: Guidelines for preventing health-care-associated pneumonia, 2003. Recommendations of the CDC and the Healthcare Infection Control Practices Advisory Committee. MMWR Morb Mortal Wkly Rep 2004;53: RR-3.
257. Dellit TH, Owens RC, McGowan JE Jr, et al: Infectious Diseases Society of America and the Society for Healthcare Epidemiology of America guidelines for developing an institutional program to enhance antimicrobial stewardship. Clin Infect Dis 2007;44:159-177.
263. Mangram AJ, Horan TC, Pearson ML, et al: Guideline for Prevention of Surgical Site Infection, 1999. Centers for Disease Control and Prevention (CDC) Hospital Infection Control Practices Advisory Committee. Am J Infect Control 1999;27:97-132.
275. Mermel LA, Allon M, Bouza E, et al: Clinical practice guidelines for the diagnosis and management of intravascular catheter-related infection: 2009 Update by the Infectious Diseases Society of America. Clin Infect Dis 2009;49(1):1-45.
389. Guidelines for the management of adults with hospital-acquired, ventilator-associated, and healthcare-associated pneumonia. Am J Respir Crit Care Med 2005;171:388-416.

The complete list of references can be found at www.expertconsult.com.

51 Principles Governing Antimicrobial Therapy in the Intensive Care Unit

Hollis O'Neal | Christopher B. Thomas | George Karam

CHAPTER OUTLINE

In the critical care setting, the selection of optimal antibiotic therapy often entails a two-stage process: empiric therapy, followed by directed therapy once the pathogen and type of infection are clearly identified. Figure 51.1 incorporates this progression in antibiotic therapy and summarizes some principles that contribute to the goal of preserving the antibiotic armamentarium while attempting to achieve optimal clinical efficacy—the components of antibiotic stewardship. A challenge for the critical care physician is to recognize that antibiotic therapy for critically ill patients has potential ramifications for other patients in that unit over the following weeks. If antibiotic-resistant organisms or organisms with certain virulence factors are selected by a pattern of antibiotic use, those pathogens can become part of the ecology of intensive care units (ICUs) and can then be transmitted to other patients. See Figure 51.2 for clinical examples of the principles of empiric therapy. In a joint 2007 guideline paper for the development of an institutional program to enhance antimicrobial stewardship, the Infectious Diseases Society of America (IDSA) and the Society for Healthcare Epidemiology of America (SHEA) wrote on the importance of education as an essential element in any program designed to influence prescribing behavior.[1] This chapter focuses on the elements of antibiotic stewardship that play a clinically relevant role in the use of antibiotics prescribed to patients in ICUs. Knowledge of these variables is essential in clinical practice and can serve as the basis for the insights necessary for an enhanced level of antibiotic prescribing.

ADEQUACY OF INITIAL EMPIRIC ANTIBIOTIC THERAPY

For many years clinicians felt that antibiotic therapy could be adjusted on day 2 or 3 into a clinical course, once either bacterial susceptibility was known or the clinical course of the patient had been defined, with no negative aspects of such changes. Beginning in the 1990s, several reports challenging this tenet were published regarding such infectious disease processes as sepsis and ventilator-associated pneumonia (VAP).[2-8] In these reports investigators used the term *inadequate* to describe situations in which the organism causing an infection was not covered with antibiotic therapy as indicated by in vitro susceptibility. The published studies exhibited variability in sample size, inconclusiveness regarding whether isolated organisms were pathogens or colonizers, and lack of consistent identification of confounders that may contribute to mortality rates. On the basis of such variables, it is not possible to definitively prove that such inadequate therapy increased mortality rates. Nevertheless, the consensus of multiple studies concerned with adequate versus inadequate initial therapy in the critically ill led to the interpretation that initial inadequate therapy contributed to mortality rates.[9]

Shortly after the reports emphasizing the importance of initial, adequate therapy, a growing awareness of other important variables that influenced clinical outcomes in ICU patients began to emerge. In a 2005 joint guideline

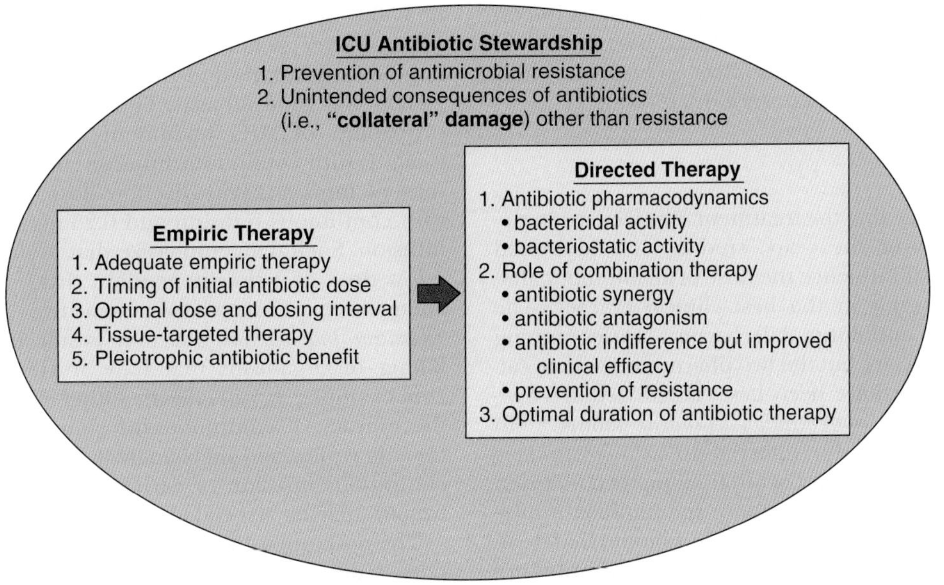

Figure 51.1 Principles governing antibiotic therapy in the intensive care unit. This concept map lists principles that influence antibiotic prescription for an individual patient, first in empiric and then in directed therapy. Antibiotic selection at all times occurs within the context of the entire intensive care unit, raising principles relevant to antibiotic stewardship that may conflict or compete with those influencing individual antibiotic prescription.

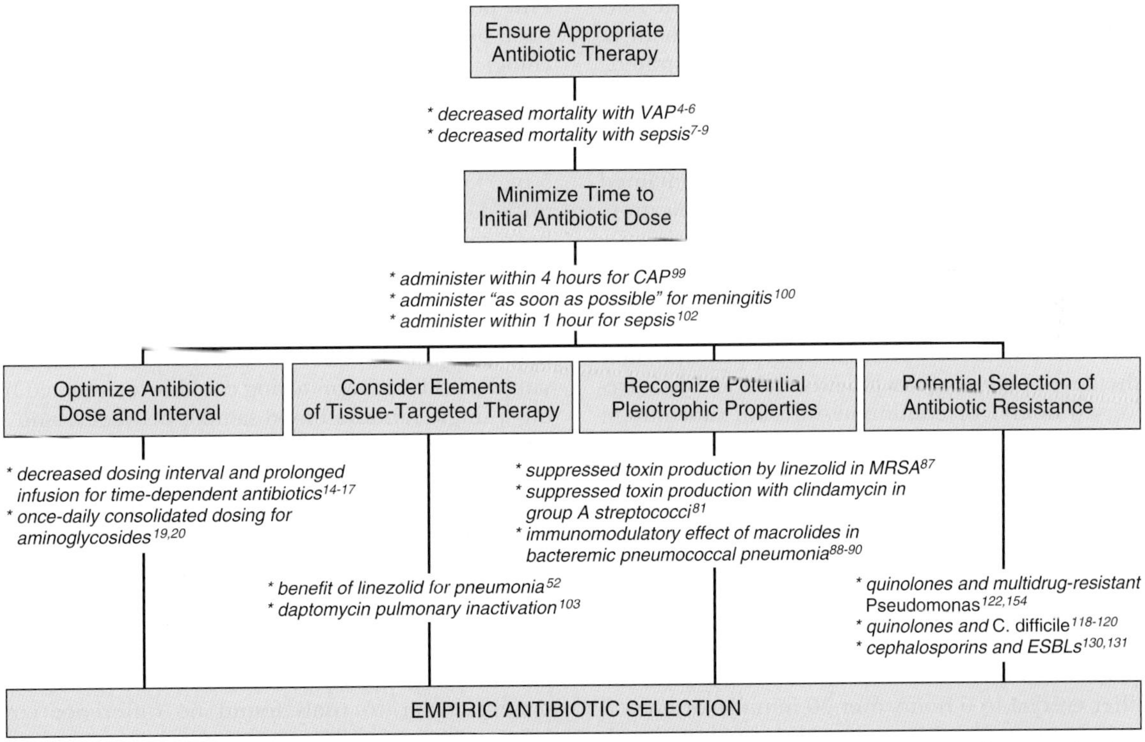

Figure 51.2 Selection of empiric antibiotic therapy in the intensive care unit. This algorithm incorporates specific examples from the text to illustrate how empiric antibiotic-prescribing principles can sequentially or concurrently influence the ultimate selection of an appropriate empiric agent.

for management of patients with hospital-acquired pneumonia (HAP), VAP, and health care–associated pneumonia (HCAP), the American Thoracic Society (ATS) and the IDSA modified definitions for the terms used in the selection of antibiotic therapy.[10] *Inappropriate* replaced the term *inadequate;* furthermore, *adequate* was adopted to refer to therapy that included not only the correct antibiotic based on the susceptibility of the organism but also optimal dose, correct route of administration, and use, if necessary, of combination therapy.[10]

A review of the literature suggests that other variables also play important roles in the determination of optimal clinical outcomes in patients in the ICU, including timing of antibiotic administration and certain pharmacologic properties of the agents selected. Awareness of such factors is important in the development of the knowledge base regarding adequate antibiotic therapy and its effect on both morbidity and mortality rates. These factors are discussed next.

OPTIMAL DOSE

As the literature regarding the treatment of infections in the ICU has evolved over the years, studies have identified several elements that influence the dose of an antibiotic that is most likely to result in the best clinical efficacy. The manner in which antibiotics kill bacteria varies among different classes of drugs, but the two pharmacodynamic categories of killing that have been best categorized are *time-dependent* killing and *concentration-dependent* killing.[11] In time-dependent killing, also referred to as *concentration-independent* killing, maximum bacterial killing occurs when the drug concentration remains above the minimal inhibitory concentration (MIC). Examples of antibiotics that demonstrate time-dependent killing include β-lactam antibiotics (i.e., penicillins, cephalosporins, carbapenems, and monobactams) and vancomycin. Conversely, in concentration-dependent killing, maximum bacterial killing occurs when the peak drug concentration is approximately 10 times the MIC. Examples of agents with concentration-dependent killing are fluoroquinolones and aminoglycosides. The relevance of such antibiotic properties in the management of patients with serious infections has been well demonstrated.

The pharmacologic properties of vancomycin have been nicely summarized, emphasizing the fact that vancomycin exhibits time-dependent killing.[12] Accordingly, the length of time that concentrations of vancomycin are maintained above the pathogen's MIC is critical to bacterial eradication, with a key variable in the treatment of pneumonia being the percentage of time that drug levels in the alveolar space exceed the MIC. As drug levels decline, organisms have the potential to regrow, increasing the chance of clinical failure. The clinical relevance of this pharmacologic principle may support the development of the practice habit of more frequent (every 6 hours) or continuous-infusion vancomycin dosing for infections like pneumonia in which vancomycin penetration to the target site may not be optimal.

Because a goal with time-dependent antibiotics is to maintain levels above the MIC of the organism for as long as possible during the dosing cycle, research has explored extended-infusion dosing of several time-dependent agents, including β-lactam antibiotics and vancomycin. In a study of 194 patients with infection caused by *Pseudomonas aeruginosa*, piperacillin-tazobactam was administered intravenously either every 4 to 6 hours over 30 minutes or every 8 hours over 4 hours.[13] The 14-day mortality rate was significantly lower among patients who received extended-infusion therapy than among patients who received intermittent-infusion therapy (12.2% versus 31.6%, respectively; $P = 0.04$). In another study designed to assess blood levels of antibiotic based on both dose and pattern of administration, meropenem was administered to two study groups, each with eight healthy volunteers.[14] One group received 500 mg as an intravenous infusion over 30 minutes three times a day or a 250-mg loading dose followed by a 1500-mg continuous infusion over 24 hours; the second group received 1000 mg as an intravenous infusion over 30 minutes three times a day or a 500-mg loading dose followed by a 3000-mg continuous infusion over 24 hours. Investigators performed pharmacokinetic calculations and used Monte Carlo simulations for 10,000 simulated subjects. The results of the analyses of the probability of MIC attainment with the high dose were 4 mg/L with continuous infusion and 0.5 mg/L with intermittent infusion. With the low dose, results were 2 mg/L with continuous infusion and 0.25 mg/L with intermittent infusion. Such data emphasize that intermittent infusion of a low dose of a time-dependent drug may result in MICs adequate to treat relatively sensitive organisms such as *Klebsiella pneumoniae* but may result in less-than-optimal killing of organisms that have intrinsically higher MICs (for example, *P. aeruginosa*). Other reports have explored the efficacy of continuous-infusion vancomycin.[15,16] A systematic review and meta-analysis suggests that extended or continuous infusion of carbapenems or piperacillin/tazobactam may be associated with lower mortality.[17]

The postantibiotic effect (PAE), in which microbial killing persists despite loss of detectable serum levels, complements the concentration-dependent killing of gram-negative bacilli exhibited by aminoglycosides, and these two properties may serve as the basis for once-daily aminoglycoside therapy.[18] It has been suggested that giving the same total dose in larger concentration less often will result in better killing, longer PAE period, and reduced aminoglycoside toxicity that has been associated with elevated trough levels. Such pharmacologic and clinical data were the foundation for the move toward once-daily aminoglycoside dosing.

In such a dosing schedule, the single doses of gentamicin or tobramycin that have been used once daily have included 5 mg/kg and 7 mg/kg of body weight. The experience with once-daily therapy using 7 mg/kg in 2184 adult patients has been reported.[19] Excluded from such therapy were patients with ascites, burns involving greater than 20% total body surface area, pregnancy, end-stage renal disease requiring dialysis, and enterococcal endocarditis. The review stated that it was unnecessary to draw standard peak and trough samples and that monitoring could be completed by obtaining a single random blood sample between 6 and 14 hours after the start of an aminoglycoside infusion. The treating clinician could subsequently adjust the dosing interval in accordance with a provided nomogram. Several important observations were made in this large group of patients: (1) Despite the prolonged drug-free period, bacterial regrowth was not clinically evident; (2) no increase in either ototoxicity or nephrotoxicity was found; and (3) efficacy was promoted in a cost-effective manner.[19] A meta-analysis evaluating the safety and efficacy of once-daily aminoglycosides in 1200 patients from 16 trials found no difference concerning efficacy and safety between single-dose and multiple-dose regimens.[20]

To achieve optimal clinical benefits while minimizing the unintended consequences of selecting resistant bacteria, clinicians must simultaneously consider multiple variables when using concentration-dependent drugs in the treatment of serious infections. In a study of lower respiratory tract infections caused by *P. aeruginosa*, ciprofloxacin was administered intravenously as a dose of 200 to 300 mg every 12 hours.[21] Resistance emerged at a rate greater than 70% during therapy. This was similar to the 75% rate predicted by a pharmacodynamic study.[22] By contrast, a randomized comparison of imipenem and ciprofloxacin for treatment of nosocomial pneumonia used a ciprofloxacin regimen of 400 mg given intravenously every 8 hours and noted emergence of resistance during therapy in 33% of cases in which *Pseudomonas* was the causative pathogen.[23] This rate was similar to the 38% predicted by the pharmacodynamic study previously cited.[22] These data emphasize the importance of considering not only the dosing interval but also the dose of antibiotic administered when using concentration-dependent antibiotics to treat infections in the critically ill.

In addition to dosing interval and initial dose, antibiotic clearance plays an integral role in adequacy of antibiotic therapy. Although it is routinely accepted that reductions in antibiotic dosing are appropriate in advancing acute kidney injury,[24] clinicians may fail to escalate drug administration in the increasingly reported clinical phenomenon of augmented renal clearance (ARC).[25] ARC is defined as the enhanced renal elimination of circulating solutes due to an increased creatinine clearance (CrCl > 130 mL/minute/1.73 m^2). Prevalence of ARC is higher in burn,[26] major trauma,[27] traumatic brain injury,[28] and febrile neutropenic[29] ICU patients; however, it is difficult to traditionally recognize as derived estimates of glomerular filtration, such as the modification of diet in renal disease (MDRD) equation and Cockcroft-Gault (CG) formula are less accurate than direct measurement.[30] In 48 ICU patients with measured CrCl, Udy and colleagues demonstrated that CrCl values 130 mL/minute/1.73 m^2 or greater were associated with initial trough concentrations of β-lactams less than MIC in 82% ($P < 0.001$). Moreover, CrCl remained a significant predictor of subtherapeutic concentrations after multivariate analysis.[31] ARC has importance in vancomycin dosing as well. Baptista and associates performed a prospective, single-center, observational cohort study of 93 consecutive septic patients in the ICU treated with vancomycin by continuous infusion after a weight-based loading dose. Investigators compared patients with and without ARC. A statistically significant correlation between subtherapeutic vancomycin serum concentration and ARC was observed in the first 3 days of treatment.[32]

An interaction between renal clearance and hypoalbuminemia also plays a prominent role in pharmacokinetics. In fact, Ulldemolins and colleagues demonstrated that in critically ill patients with hypoalbuminemia, unbound flucloxacillin concentrations fell below concentrations necessary for treatment of methicillin-susceptible *Staphylococcus aureus* (MSSA) 4 hours after standard bolus infusions.[33] The combination of increased volume of distribution due to hypoalbuminemia combined with ARC presents a daily situation in which lower achieved antibacterial exposures could result in subtherapeutic dosing, particularly for time-dependent antibiotics.[34] Because accurate and timely drug exposure is necessary for optimal clinical benefit,[3] ARC and associated factors like hypoalbuminemia must be identified to prevent subtherapeutic pharmacologic treatment.

PENETRATION AT THE SITE OF INFECTION: TISSUE-TARGETED THERAPY

The importance of antibiotic pharmacokinetic properties has recently received heightened attention for the treatment of pneumonia caused by multidrug-resistant gram-positive cocci. Indeed, pulmonary pharmacokinetics underlie the findings that the use of linezolid for pneumonia caused by methicillin-resistant *S. aureus* (MRSA), when compared with vancomycin in traditional regimens, results in improved clinical outcomes.[35-38] Understanding the relevance of pharmacokinetic properties will help the critical care physician navigate through the recent published literature for these infections.

Pulmonary pharmacokinetics specifically address the tissue penetration and distribution of antibiotics within the lung.[39] Early studies investigating antibiotic penetration in pulmonary infections occurring in the ICU were related to aminoglycosides and fluoroquinolones. Although aminoglycoside levels in the interstitium of the lung are acceptable, levels in pulmonary secretions reach a mean of only about 20% of the concomitant serum level.[40] By contrast, the concentrations of quinolones in lung tissue significantly exceed the concomitant serum concentrations, and levels in bronchial secretions also have been reported to exceed those in serum.[41] Despite the fact that quinolones have better penetration into the lung and less potential for nephrotoxicity than aminoglycosides, available data show a trend toward improved survival in patients with VAP treated with an aminoglycoside-containing, but not with a quinolone-containing, combination.[42] A concern with fluoroquinolones in combination therapy directed against gram-negative organisms is the selection of resistance, particularly in organisms such as *P. aeruginosa,* in which the resultant resistance may be to multiple classes of antibiotics.[43] Because of the coexistent potential for clinical efficacy and nephrotoxicity with aminoglycosides, some investigators have suggested, on the basis of clinical trials, discontinuation of the aminoglycoside after 5 days if the patient is improving.[44]

Existing pharmacokinetic evidence reveals the extremely poor lung tissue penetration of vancomycin. Cruciani and associates investigated vancomycin pharmacokinetics in 30 human lung tissue sections after administration of a 1-g dose over 1 hour.[45] A comparison of serum-to-tissue concentration over the dosing interval was used to generate a graph allowing determination of a concentration ratio. Overall, the serum-to-lung tissue concentration ratio was determined to be 21%. Not surprisingly, investigation has confirmed even poorer penetration into epithelial lining fluid.[46] These data raise concern that the traditional dosing regimens of vancomycin (1 g given intravenously every 12 hours) and low target serum trough concentrations (5 to 10 μg/mL) will generate lung tissue concentrations below the MIC for *S. aureus.* The issues surrounding suboptimal vancomycin dosing are reflected in the 2005 published ATS/IDSA guidelines for treatment for adults with HAP, VAP, and HCAP, in which it was noted that retrospective pharmacokinetic modeling suggested that the vancomycin failures may be related to inadequate dosing. Because of these concerns the authors recommend that trough levels for vancomycin should be 15 to 20 μg/mL.[10] This recommendation of intensified vancomycin dosing is supported in a joint vancomycin clinical guideline for treating all complicated infectious caused by MRSA.[47]

In contrast with the poor pulmonary pharmacokinetic properties of vancomycin, several studies of linezolid confirm excellent lung penetration in healthy volunteer subjects and with in vitro modeling.[48-50] Boselli and coworkers investigated the steady-state plasma pharmacokinetic variables and epithelial lining fluid concentrations of linezolid administered to critically ill patients with VAP.[51] Epithelial lining fluid concentrations of linezolid approximated 100% of corresponding plasma values, with drug concentrations that exceeded the susceptibility breakpoint (4 mg/mL) for *S. aureus* throughout the greater part of the dosing interval. The principle of antibiotic pharmacokinetics has supported the conclusion that linezolid is superior to vancomycin in traditional dosing regimens for MRSA pneumonia based on retrospective analysis of the two multinational, double-blind, randomized studies published to date.[38] A subsequent randomized, controlled clinical trial of linezolid versus vancomycin in the treatment of nosocomial pneumonia favored linezolid; furthermore, a subgroup analysis of this investigation did not suggest a benefit in those patients with vancomycin troughs of 15 mg/L or more on day 3.[52]

In light of the difficulty in achieving adequate drug levels in pulmonary tissue, many clinicians consider the use of topical, aerosolized antibiotics to deliver drug directly to the site of infection. The agents most commonly employed in this manner are tobramycin and colistin.[53] Most of our experience with, and evidence supporting, nebulized tobramycin originates from small studies and meta-analyses assessing the utility of these agents in the management of chronic respiratory disease such as cystic fibrosis, not in the treatment of acute infection.[54] Although the risk of toxicity appears lower with the administration of nebulized tobramycin, certain populations, such as those with renal insufficiency, may be at risk.[55] Because of the increasing prevalence of multidrug-resistant gram-negative organisms such as *Acinetobacter baumannii* and *P. aeruginosa*, clinicians have employed colistimethate via intravenous infusion[56] or aerosolization[57,58] as therapy for VAP and HAP. Intravenous colistimethate appears to be safe (with a risk of nephrotoxicity similar to that for intravenous aminoglycosides) and effective, though there are few randomized, controlled trials from which to draw firm conclusions; furthermore, the optimal dosing strategy is unclear.[59] Although the aerosolized route of colistimethate administration appears to be safe,[60] its efficacy has not been established.

ROLE OF COMBINATION THERAPY

SYNERGY

One of the most frequently cited justifications for combination therapy is for the achievement of synergy, in which antimicrobial combinations are more effective than single agents. The best-recognized example of synergistic antimicrobial therapy is in treatment of enterococcal endocarditis, in which treatment with penicillin or ampicillin alone has been associated with a high rate of relapse when compared with therapy with penicillin or ampicillin in combination with streptomycin or gentamicin.[61,62] Discussions of combination therapy have raised the question of whether the use of multiple drugs in the treatment of an infection may result in improved clinical outcomes. For example, in the treatment of bacteremia with *S. aureus*, some investigators have used a semisynthetic penicillinase-resistant penicillin (e.g., nafcillin or oxacillin) in combination with a brief course (3 to 5 days) of an aminoglycoside, based on data showing more rapid clearing of bacteremia.[63] Data from this trial did not show a decrease in mortality rates in the study population of nonaddicts with primarily left-sided endocarditis caused by *S. aureus* when compared with those patients who received nafcillin alone. For *P. aeruginosa* the mechanism of synergy between antipseudomonal penicillins and aminoglycosides is similar to that of enterococci.[64] Despite this microbiologic observation, the presence or absence of synergy seemed less important in a different trial assessing outcomes in patients with *P. aeruginosa* bacteremia; rather, this investigation explored combination therapy given in an attempt to prevent the emergence of resistance.[65]

In contrast with the beneficial effect of synergy, a combination regimen may result in the detrimental effect of antagonism. The classic example of such an effect was with the treatment of pneumococcal meningitis in the 1950s, in which the fatality rate among patients who received penicillin alone was 21%, in contrast with 79% among those who received both penicillin (a bactericidal agent) plus chlortetracycline (a bacteriostatic agent).[66]

The clinical importance of antagonism has increased in the era of community-associated methicillin-resistant *S. aureus* (CA-MRSA). Published evidence supports the fact that MRSA is an independent predictor of mortality rate, ICU length of stay, and overall cost of care.[67-70] Because a limited number of therapeutic options exist for the treatment of severe, invasive MRSA infections, effort has been made to identify the in vitro activity of antibiotic combinations that may have clinical applicability. Although the intent of using antibiotic combinations is to achieve additive or synergistic effects, the use of combinations may have the unintended effect of antagonism.

A study using 10 different strains of *S. aureus* found an overall pattern of antibiotic indifference (no combination effect) in combinations of linezolid with fusidic acid, rifampin, or gentamicin. On the other hand, the combination of linezolid with ciprofloxacin or vancomycin resulted in slight antagonism and reduced bactericidal effect when linezolid was combined with ciprofloxacin and vancomycin against the same strains of staphylococci.[71] A subsequent study using the checkerboard broth microdilution method tested linezolid in combination with 28 different antimicrobial agents—including vancomycin and several fluoroquinolones—and demonstrated no antagonistic effect.[72] Sahuquillo and colleagues reproduced the effect of antibiotic indifference with vancomycin, but they noted antagonism with levofloxacin in two of the five *S. aureus* isolates tested.[73]

Another investigation used the rabbit model of aortic valve endocarditis to evaluate 5-day treatment regimens of linezolid alone, vancomycin alone, and linezolid in combination with vancomycin in 40 rabbits infected with an MRSA strain.[74] Those treated with vancomycin alone demonstrated greater mean reductions in valvular vegetation bacterial counts than those in the other treatment groups ($P = 0.05$). Vancomycin also sterilized aortic valve vegetations in three of eight rabbits; by contrast, none of the rabbits treated with linezolid had sterile aortic valve vegetations. A noteworthy finding in this study was that the treatment regimen of linezolid plus vancomycin lowered the peak linezolid levels in serum to below those obtained with regimens with linezolid alone. Even though in vitro synergy testing revealed additive or indifferent activity between the two drugs, the rabbit model revealed in vivo antagonism. A potential explanation offered by the investigators for the observed antagonism between vancomycin and linezolid was the effect of combining a bacteriostatic (linezolid) with a bactericidal drug (vancomycin). The observed reduction in peak linezolid levels in serum with the combination of the two drugs suggests a role for additional mechanisms in the interaction between the two antibiotics. Unfortunately, the clinical significance of these findings is not yet known.

In the absence of definitive data on optimal management of *S. aureus* infections in seriously ill patients, a pattern has emerged in some health care systems to prescribe combination therapy for this pathogen. The overall assessment of the data is that antibiotic indifference appears to best characterize the drug interaction profile of linezolid with vancomycin. Because some data, albeit unsubstantiated in controlled clinical trials, seem to cast doubt on the advisability of the combination of linezolid with vancomycin[71] and the fluoroquinolones,[73] it is important for the intensivist to be aware of the potential consequences of doing so. In short, the role of combination therapy in the treatment of serious MRSA infection, except in a few specific instances, is unclear.[75]

ENHANCED EFFICACY AGAINST A PATHOGEN

A common question in clinical medicine is whether combination therapy will result in increased efficacy against a pathogen via a mechanism other than synergy. In an attempt to find a more definitive answer to this question, a meta-analysis of 64 trials with 7586 patients comparing β-lactam monotherapy versus β-lactam plus an aminoglycoside in immunocompetent patients with sepsis was conducted.[76] This report did not identify a statistically significant advantage of combination therapy among the 1835 patients with gram-negative infections for whom the data were analyzed. In contrast with the results in the previously cited study,[65] no improved survival was observed for the 426 patients who had infection caused by *P. aeruginosa*. An additional finding was that the rates of development of resistance did not differ in the two treatment groups. Nephrotoxicity, however, developed significantly more often in those patients who received combination therapy.

PREVENTION OF THE EMERGENCE OF RESISTANCE

Clinicians frequently use combination therapy for *P. aeruginosa* in an attempt to prevent the emergence of resistance. Despite the importance of this subject, no definitive data are available to prove that combination therapy will prevent the emergence of *Pseudomonas* resistance;[77] however, results of clinical trials[23] and concern about this possibility based on limited data have been the basis for such use of combination therapy. A meta-analysis of eight randomized controlled clinical trials compared β-lactam monotherapy and β-lactam plus aminoglycoside combination therapy to assess if combination therapy may decrease the risk of the emergence of resistance.[78] Among initially antimicrobial-susceptible isolates in this analysis, combination therapy did not impact the development of antimicrobial resistance. Furthermore, in the meta-analysis of 64 trials comparing β-lactam monotherapy and β-lactam plus aminoglycoside combination therapy in immunocompetent patients with sepsis, there was no difference in the rate of development of resistance.[76]

INCREASED OPPORTUNITY FOR ACHIEVING APPROPRIATE THERAPY

Even though issues of synergy and reduction in the emergence of resistance frequently are invoked in discussions of combination therapy, the relevant data do not prove consistent benefits. In patients in the intensive care setting, an important advantage of combination therapy is that it provides the clinician with broader antibacterial coverage for potentially multidrug-resistant microorganisms.[79] Additionally, because inappropriate initial therapy may result in increased mortality rate, a combination of antibiotics has the potential benefit of providing coverage against a pathogen that may not be the most likely on a statistical basis but is a reasonable consideration in life-threatening clinical settings confronting the critical care physician. The use of antibiotic combinations for empiric therapy increases the probability that at least one of the agents will have activity against the causative organism.

IMMUNOMODULATING EFFECT OF ANTIBIOTICS

Although most classification schemes group antibiotics according to their chemical structure and spectrum of coverage, certain antibiotics may possess additional properties that have important clinical implications. The interaction of antibiotics with host immune response, bacterial population kinetics, and bacterial gene expression for exotoxin production are examples of the pleiotropic, or "off target," properties of antibiotics. For the critical care physician, this is especially relevant in the treatment of life-threatening infection caused by gram-positive cocci and may be the basis for combination therapy in the treatment of infections caused by such pathogens.

Streptococcal toxic shock syndrome is a clinical infection in which bacteria produce exotoxins that act as host superantigens, precipitating shock, multiple organ failure, and death. Although *Streptococcus pyogenes* demonstrates exquisite in vitro sensitivity to penicillin, experimental studies of infection by this pathogen have demonstrated reduced efficacy against organisms in the stationary phase of bacterial growth. This phenomenon has been termed the Eagle effect, whereby high organism population density and slow organism division make treatment with an antibiotic dependent on cell wall synthesis ineffective.[80] Some cite the Eagle effect as a justification for use of the bacteriostatic antibiotic clindamycin in the treatment of toxic shock syndrome. In addition, clindamycin is an antibiotic that inhibits bacterial protein synthesis, and this pharmacodynamic property is independent of the stage of bacterial growth.[81] Clindamycin inhibits bacterial exotoxin production, facilitates phagocytosis of *S. pyogenes* by inhibiting M protein synthesis, and suppresses the production of penicillin-binding proteins (PBPs). Furthermore, evidence exists that demonstrates clindamycin has immunomodulatory effects, suppressing monocyte synthesis of tumor necrosis factor-α (TNF-α).[82,83] All of these pleiotropic qualities have resulted in the recommendation for clindamycin use in necrotizing skin or soft tissue infections and toxic shock syndrome caused by *S. pyogenes*.[81]

The dramatic increase in the worldwide incidence of highly virulent, community-acquired infection with CA-MRSA has resulted in increasing reports of necrotizing skin and soft tissue infections as well as necrotizing pneumonia confronting the critical care physician.[84-86] CA-MRSA virulence has been attributed to expression of several virulence factors: α-hemolysins (AH), toxic shock syndrome toxin-1 (TSST-1), staphylococcal enterotoxin B, and Panton-Valentine leukocidin (PVL). The association of staphylococcal virulence with the current CA-MRSA epidemic prompted Stevens and colleagues to investigate the impact of antibiotics on the expression of virulence-associated exotoxin genes.[87] These investigators were able to demonstrate markedly suppressed in vitro production of staphylococcal toxin genes by clindamycin and linezolid such that no PVL production was noted up to 12 hours after antibiotic administration. Of interest, subinhibitory concentrations of the cell wall–active agent nafcillin were found to increase toxin production. These findings led the investigators to conclude that the inhibition of protein synthesis is an important consideration in the selection of antimicrobial agents for treatment of serious infections caused by toxin-producing gram-positive cocci.[87]

A growing body of evidence exists to support the benefit of macrolide therapy for bacteremic pneumonia caused by *Streptococcus pneumoniae*.[88-96] Although multiple explanations have been proposed, efficacy appears to extend beyond the drug's spectrum of antimicrobial activity. The macrolide class of antibiotics exerts a broad range of immunomodulatory effects, including suppression of harmful interleukin host responses and inhibition of neutrophil oxidant burst and degranulation.[88-90] These pleiotropic effects have received an increasing focus of attention and further illustrate how immune modulation influences recommendations for therapy in the intensive care setting.

TIMING

The impact of the timing of antibiotic therapy has been addressed in several ways with regard to patients in the ICU. In an analysis based on 107 consecutive patients receiving mechanical ventilation and antibiotic treatment for VAP, Iregui and colleagues noted that 30.8% (33 of 107) received antibiotic treatment that was delayed for 24 hours or more after initially meeting diagnostic criteria for VAP; these patients were classified as having initially delayed appropriate antibiotic therapy (IDAAT).[97] Two major variables were identified in these patients with IDAAT: (1) a delay in writing an antibiotic order (in 75.8% of the cases); and (2) the presence of a bacterial species resistant to the initially prescribed antibiotic regimen (in 18.2%). The investigators found that hospital mortality rate was 69.7% for the patients with IDAAT, in contrast with only 28.4% for the patients without IDAAT ($P < 0.01$). An earlier study noted that, in patients with VAP, modification of the antibiotic regimen to cover pathogens based on the susceptibility report did not eliminate the increased mortality rate associated with inadequate empiric therapy.[5] Acknowledgment of this finding was the basis for the statement that secondary modifications of an initially failing antibiotic regimen do not substantially improve the outcome for critically ill patients.[98] These results challenge the clinician to promptly order antibiotics that cover the involved pathogens even before culture results are available.

The importance of antibiotic timing in patients with community-acquired pneumonia was assessed in a retrospective cohort study of pneumonia in 18,209 Medicare patients.[99] In this trial, conducted in a random sample of inpatients 65 years of age or older with community-acquired pneumonia who had not received antibiotics as outpatients, the influence on clinical outcome was assessed for use of antibiotics prescribed according to standard guidelines published at the time of the analysis and not identification of pathogens isolated from the patients. Of the patients who received antibiotics within 4 hours of hospital arrival, 83.2% were prescribed a guideline-recommended regimen, in contrast with 71.8% of the patients who received antibiotics after 4 hours of arrival. The results of this analysis found an association between the administration of antibiotics within 4 hours of hospital arrival and a decrease in mortality rate and length of stay. The investigators postulated that antibiotics may interrupt or minimize the effects of the acute lung injury process that occurs as part of the systemic inflammatory response in patients with bacterial pneumonia.

The IDSA practice guidelines for management of adult patients with meningitis note the lack of prospective clinical data on the relationship of the timing of antimicrobial administration of antimicrobial agents to clinical outcome in patients with bacterial meningitis.[100] Data from a retrospective cohort study of 269 adult patients with community-acquired bacterial meningitis provide some insights into the timing of antibiotic therapy in the absence of definitive recommendations.[101] Using these and other data, the IDSA acknowledged that evidence for definitive recommendations is inadequate and concluded that a reasonable assumption is to administer treatment for bacterial meningitis before the infection advances to a high level of clinical severity.[100] Referring to meningitis as a "neurologic emergency," the guideline recommended that appropriate therapy for meningitis be initiated as soon as possible after the diagnosis is considered to be likely.[100] In support of the importance of prompt timing, this document also noted the potential in certain patients for administration of antibiotics before hospital admission if the patient initially presents outside the hospital.

For the critical care clinician, sepsis is a clinical entity in which adequate antibiotic therapy has been associated with improved clinical outcomes.[2,3,7,8,79] In recognition of the importance of prompt therapy in influencing clinical outcomes in patients with sepsis, the 2008 Surviving Sepsis Campaign guidelines offered a specific recommendation regarding the timing of antimicrobial therapy for the septic patient: "Intravenous antibiotic therapy should be started as early as possible and within the first hour of recognition of septic shock and severe sepsis without septic shock.

Appropriate cultures should be obtained before initiating antibiotic therapy but should not prevent prompt administration of antimicrobial therapy."[102]

SPECIAL PHARMACOLOGIC PROPERTIES

As the focus of antibiotic research has expanded beyond the characterization of in vitro properties for a particular agent, the importance of antibiotic performance at the in vivo target tissue level is becoming increasingly recognized. It was with the 2003 introduction of a novel antibiotic, daptomycin, for treatment of infections caused by resistant gram-positive cocci that the relevance of "organ-specific deactivation" initially was described.[103] Daptomycin is an intravenous cyclic lipopeptide with rapid, concentration-dependent killing and bactericidal activity against a broad spectrum of gram-positive cocci.[104-106] It demonstrates a unique mechanism of action, with calcium-dependent insertion into the phospholipid bacterial cell membrane. This results in cell depolarization via potassium efflux, causing disruption of DNA, RNA, and protein synthesis.[107]

As a result of two multicenter, randomized controlled trials comparing it with penicillinase-resistant penicillin or vancomycin,[108] daptomycin, at a daily dose of 4 mg/kg (for patients with CrCl greater than 30 mL/minute), received U.S. Food and Drug Administration (FDA) approval for the treatment of complicated skin and soft tissue infections. A subsequent randomized, open-label trial investigated use of daptomycin in *S. aureus* bacteremia and endocarditis.[109] This trial prompted FDA approval of daptomycin for treatment of *S. aureus* bacteremia, including right-sided endocarditis, at a daily intravenous dose of 6 mg/kg.

Phase 3 clinical trials also were conducted for the treatment of community-acquired pneumonia in hospitalized patients. Despite daptomycin's potent in vitro bactericidal activity against *S. pneumoniae*, clinical outcomes were disappointing and inferior to those with the comparator, ceftriaxone. Although daptomycin is known to exhibit poor penetration into epithelial lining fluid, the reason for treatment failure was not fully elucidated until Silverman and colleagues described a unique organ-specific inactivation process.[103] Daptomycin's inactivation was linked to its mechanism of bactericidal action: calcium-dependent membrane lipid binding.[103,107,110,111] Using a mouse model, investigators demonstrated drug sequestration and inactivation by binding to phospholipid vesicles that are found in pulmonary surfactant.[103] For this reason daptomycin is not considered an appropriate therapeutic agent for treatment of pneumonia, largely because of the presence of surfactant at the target tissue. This phenomenon appears to be unique to daptomycin[103] but raises the question of unrecognized organ-specific inactivation for other classes of antibiotics and other target organs.

Recent antibiotic developments have introduced the possibility of managing life-threatening infections with antimicrobial agents administered at a prolonged dosing interval. A long drug half-life ($T_{1/2}$) is conducive to completion of treatment courses in the outpatient setting and maximizes patient compliance. In the context of critical care, exploiting an antibiotic's $T_{1/2}$ historically has been used in settings such as hemodialysis with end-stage renal disease. Less frequent antibiotic dosing diminishes the burden of intravenous access and increases the possibility of treatment outside an intensive care environment.

UNINTENDED CONSEQUENCES OF ANTIBIOTIC THERAPY

Traditional teaching about antibiotics focused on three classic parameters: efficacy, safety, and cost-effectiveness. With respect to safety, the major considerations were allergic reactions and adverse effects. Within the pandemic of antibiotic resistance, an important new safety issue should be added: unintended consequences of antibiotic therapy. An insightful report termed such unintended consequences the "collateral damage" of antibiotics.[112] In this report, *collateral damage* referred to the ecologic adverse effect of selecting drug-resistant organisms and the unwanted development of colonization or infection with multidrug-resistant organisms. Some important new considerations recently described in the literature, however, may influence initial antibiotic selection for serious infections in the ICU.

The increasing prevalence of MRSA infections in patients in the critical care setting has required an ongoing evaluation of factors that propagate and sustain such a pattern of resistance. The role of inadequate handwashing in the spread of nosocomial MRSA in hospitals has been well known for many years.[113] As rates of MRSA have increased in infections such as HAP,[114] increased emphasis has been placed on other variables that contribute to the role that MRSA now plays as the etiologic agent of HAP and VAP. In recognition of the infectious disease concept that colonization is an antecedent event to infection, attention has been directed to factors that may increase colonization by MRSA. Bisognano and colleagues provided preliminary evidence by evaluating the occurrence and frequency of increased adhesion in clinical isolates of fluoroquinolone-resistant MRSA and MSSA. This increased adhesion was mediated by fluoroquinolone-induced increases in fibronectin-binding proteins (FnBPs).[115] Although this report does not prove that suboptimal levels of fluoroquinolones contribute in a clinically significant way to increased production of FnBPs and higher levels of bacterial attachment, the data do challenge the clinician to consider unintended antibiotic consequences as an explanation for increasing rates of infection with MRSA.

In addition to infection with MRSA, a problem that has gained increasing attention in recent years has been infection by strains of *Clostridium difficile* with markedly increased levels of toxin production.[116] A postulated cause for this increase in toxin production is the phenomenon of hypermutation. Spontaneous mutations that lead to bacterial resistance occur with a frequency that generally is in the range from 10^{-6} to 10^{-8}. Hypermutation has been used to refer to a situation in which the mutation rate exceeds that recognized for spontaneous mutations.[117] Certain factors may lead to genetic damage in bacteria with a resultant increase in the potential for a mutation that can lead to resistance, and antibiotics that have an effect on DNA have been shown with in vitro experiments to potentially contribute to this predisposition to resistance.[117]

The data regarding the role of antibiotics in causing DNA damage that leads to increased resistance via hypermutation become relevant when one considers potential mechanisms for the increasing toxin production in *C. difficile* that has led to such problems as toxic megacolon, bowel perforation, and death. In an attempt to better understand outbreaks of clinical disease caused by toxin-producing strains of *C. difficile*, the genetics of epidemic strains were studied.[118,119] In these studies, an 18-base-pair deletion in the *tcd*C gene, which normally downregulates production of toxins A and B, was noted. An additional finding was the presence of binary toxin genes. These factors were thought to contribute to the hyperproduction of toxin expressed in clinical outbreaks. The epidemiologic analysis of these outbreaks identified fluoroquinolone therapy as a risk factor in recent *C. difficile* outbreaks.[118-120] These observations challenge the critical care clinician to again consider the potential of unintended antibiotic consequences in the selection of empiric antibiotic therapy in seriously ill patients.

In addition to *C. difficile*, the effect of antibiotics on toxin production has been studied in gram-positive organisms. In a study investigating the effects that cell wall–active antibiotics and protein synthesis inhibitors have on transcription and translation of genes for PVL, AH, and TSST-1, Miller and associates demonstrated that subinhibitory concentrations of nafcillin induced and prolonged messenger RNA (mRNA) expression for PVL, AH, and TSST-1.[86] A clinical interpretation of these data suggested by the investigators is that inadvertent use of β-lactam antibiotics to treat MRSA infections may contribute to worse outcomes.

Even though such processes as DNA damage leading to hypermutation and increases in virulence factors are important considerations in discussions about unintended consequences, the most mature knowledge base related to the collateral damage of antibiotics is the risk of these agents to contribute to the expression of bacterial resistance.

CLINICIAN RESPONSES TO MULTIDRUG RESISTANCE

In the studies addressing increased mortality rates associated with inadequate initial antimicrobial therapy for serious infections,[2-7] unanticipated bacterial resistance was a frequent reason for not initially selecting a drug to which the organism was susceptible. An important insight is provided in the study by Trouillet and colleagues, who evaluated the risk factors for resistance in patients with VAP.[121] The conclusions of that study were that use of antibiotics within the past 15 days and mechanical ventilation of at least 7 days' duration were the most important factors. When these two parameters were used in subcategories to evaluate the predisposition for selecting resistant organisms, antibiotic use was a more influential factor than was mechanical ventilation. This fact highlights the dual role that antibiotics play in the ICU: (1) treatment of infection and (2) potential selection of the resistant organisms that lead to the next episode of infection. The challenge for the clinician is to achieve the appropriate degree of balance between these two opposing effects.

Integral to effective antibiotic stewardship in the ICU is an understanding of those factors that lead to the expression of antibiotic resistance. A basic understanding of the mechanisms of resistance and the organisms that express them can lead to more effective empiric therapy and a more efficient de-escalation process.

MECHANISMS OF ACTION AND OF RESISTANCE

On the most fundamental level, an antibiotic must bind to a target site before the pharmacologic property that kills the organism can be invoked. As examples, β-lactams bind to PBPs to prevent synthesis of the bacterial cell wall, and fluroquinolones bind to DNA gyrase to prevent replication of the genetic elements required for bacterial replication. For an antibiotic to reach its target site, there must be penetration through the outermost part of the bacterial cell wall. Impermeability of those sites precludes the drug from getting to its target site. Once an antibiotic enters the outermost portion of the bacterial cell wall but before it binds to its target site, there are two potential mechanisms by which the drug can be precluded from having its effect: one is enzymatic destruction of the antibiotic; the other is extrusion of the drug from the bacteria via pumps referred to as efflux pumps. Because of the importance of enzymatic destruction and of efflux that leads to the drug resistance encountered in the critical care setting, these two mechanisms of action will be discussed in some detail. However, it is important to consider the importance of target-site binding and of impaired penetration because both of these mechanisms of resistance have practical implications for the clinician.

BINDING TO A TARGET SITE

Although there are multiple sites to which antibiotics might bind and thereby exert their mechanism of action, the one that is probably the most relevant in clinical practice is the binding of β-lactam antibiotics to PBPs. PBPs are best considered as enzymes on the innermost part of the bacterial cell wall that play a role in the synthesis of that structure. When bacteria have alteration in their PBPs such that antibiotics can no longer bind to that site, then those organisms have a mechanism by which they demonstrate resistance to that antibiotic. In clinical medicine, the two most important examples of resistance mediated via altered PBPs are methicillin resistance in *S. aureus* and penicillin resistance in *S. pneumoniae*. The significance of this for the clinician is probably best represented by a relatively common practice. Assume that a patient has an infection presumed to be caused by *S. pneumoniae* that is unresponsive to penicillin. An uninformed practice pattern is the addition of a β-lactamase inhibitor like clavulanic acid to a drug like amoxicillin as the next agent used in an attempt to treat that infection. Because the resistance in penicillin-resistant *S. pneumoniae* is not via β-lactamase production but rather via altered PBPs, the β-lactamase inhibitor adds nothing to the regimen. In contrast, a higher dose of penicillin might overcome the problem of decreased binding of the antibiotic to the PBPs, with the resultant effect of improved efficacy.

PENETRATION THROUGH THE BACTERIAL CELL WALL

For an antibiotic to reach its target binding site, it must penetrate the bacterial cell wall. One route that can be used by certain antibiotics is through trimers of proteins referred to as porins, which are located in the bacterial cell wall.

Originally intended as a point of access for nutrients into the bacteria and excretory products out of the bacteria, porin channels have been used as the route of entry for certain antibiotics, most notably, the carbapenems. When an organism becomes deficient in these porins, then carbapenems are not able to enter the bacteria, which ultimately leads to a lack of binding to PBPs and resultant clinical resistance. The most important example of resistance mediated by porin channel closure is the resistance of *P. aeruginosa* to carbapenems. For the clinician in the ICU, it is important to know that *P. aeruginosa* possesses three mechanisms of resistance regulated by genetic operons on the chromosome: (1) AmpC β-lactamases; (2) efflux pumps; and (3) outer membrane porin alterations.[122,123] Because the clinician will not have information at the time of empiric therapy regarding which, if any, of these mechanisms might be in play in the *P. aeruginosa* being targeted, regimens for infections like hospital-acquired pneumonia often target more than one of these mechanisms of pseudomonal resistance.[10]

Table 51.1 Characteristics of Type 1 β-Lactamase–Expressing Organisms

Common β-Lactamase–Expressing Organisms*	Susceptible Substrate	Stable Antibiotics
Serratia	Penicillins	Aminoglycosides
P. aeruginosa	β-Lactamase inhibitors	Carbapenems
Indole-positive *Proteus*	First-, second-, and third-generation cephalosporins	Fluoroquinolones
Citrobacter	Monobactam	Fourth-generation cephalosporins†
Enterobacter		

*"SPICE" (or "SPACE") Bugs: If *Acinetobacter* is substituted for indole-positive *Proteus*, then the mnemonic SPACE applies.
†Not as predictably stable as the other three classes.

ENZYMATIC DEGRADATION

Enzymatic degradation of antibiotics is one of the most widespread and variable mechanisms of antibiotic resistance available to microorganisms. Furthermore, although resistance in gram-negative bacilli may occur by any of the aforementioned mechanisms, one that provides a foundation for understanding the interaction between antibiotic use and antibiotic resistance is β-lactamase. These enzymes have the ability to cleave, and thereby render ineffective, the four-membered β-lactam ring that is common to all the β-lactam antibiotics (i.e., penicillins, cephalosporins, carbapenems, and monobactams) as well as the β-lactamase inhibitors (i.e., clavulanic acid, sulbactam, and tazobactam). Because researchers have identified countless β-lactamase enzymes, clinicians must employ a clinically relevant classification system to categorize them into practical groups. The most widely used classification system of β-lactamase enzymes places them into four distinct functional classes (i.e., Ambler classes A, B, C, and D). This system can be further simplified to consider three types of β-lactamases with relevance to clinical medicine: (1) AmpC *β-lactamase* (which is a class C β-lactamase also referred to as a type 1 enzyme), (2) extended-spectrum β-lactamase**s** (ESBLs), and (3) carbapenemases.

Type 1 β-lactamase

Type 1 β-lactamases (AmpCs) are chromosomally mediated, with the product of the *ampC* gene (hence the term AmpC β-lactamases) being the archetype. See Table 51.1 for organisms commonly felt to produce type 1 β-lactamase, their substrate, and antibiotics felt to be stable in the presence of the enzyme. According to data from the Centers for Disease Control and Prevention's National Nosocomial Infections Surveillance (NNIS) system, these organisms account for 10% to 33% of nosocomial infections involving blood, surgical site, urine, and lung.[124] Even though these pathogens do not always produce type 1 enzymes, this potential does exist and must be taken into consideration if initial antibiotic therapy is to be appropriate. Because type 1 β-lactamases have an affinity for cephalosporins (and have therefore been referred to by some authors as cephalosporinases), third-generation cephalosporins are not predictably stable in the presence of type 1 enzymes.[125] Also lacking stability are the β-lactamase inhibitors, of which tazobactam is the most likely to resist destruction by these enzymes.

Exposure to specific antibiotics may influence a microorganism's ability to produce type 1 β-lactamases. In a classic paper from the infectious diseases literature, two mechanisms have been described by which this occurs: (1) induction and (2) the selection of spontaneous mutant strains (previously referred to as stable de-repression).[126] Sanders and Sanders[126] explored the property of induction when they performed an investigation in which they incubated an organism with the potential to produce type 1 β-lactamases overnight in the presence of antibiotic. After this incubation, they performed an assay for type 1 β-lactamase. If they subsequently detected the enzyme, they described the process as induction. Strong inducing antibiotics identified in this report were cefoxitin, imipenem, and clavulanic acid. Of note, upon removal of the inducing antibiotic, the β-lactamase production ceased before the next dose of drug was due to be given. The investigators thus described induction as a reversible in vitro phenomenon.[126]

In the years since the description of induction as an in vitro phenomenon, no definitive evidence has been accumulated demonstrating that induction in gram-negative organisms leads to clinically significant resistance in patients; however, the *ampC* gene product can lead to alarming resistance patterns through another mechanism.

What has been proved to occur in patients is the selection of spontaneous mutant strains of bacteria.[126] As stated earlier, organisms that possess the *ampC* gene typically possess complex regulatory mechanisms that prevent overexpression of the gene; however, a certain number of bacteria within clinical isolates (often in the 10^{-6} to 10^{-7} range) will have spontaneous mutation(s) that allows them to overproduce type 1 β-lactamase.[126] When certain broad-spectrum antibiotics are given, the sensitive nonmutated organisms are killed; however, the genetic mutant strains proliferate and become the predominant organisms. Once this occurs, the clinical isolate will now exhibit resistance to a broad range of β-lactam antibiotics. Most notable of the antibiotics that have been described in the literature to select these "stably de-repressed" mutants are the third-generation cephalosporins.[127,128]

A clinically relevant lesson can be learned from the story of how type 1 β-lactamases lead to the expression of resistance. In the overwhelming majority of instances with gram-negative organisms, antibiotics do not cause induction of resistance, but rather certain antibiotics efficiently kill susceptible organisms while leaving resistant mutants to proliferate, thereby selecting the resistant microbes to flourish. This process of selection, not induction, is the basis for most of the resistance that is encountered in the clinical setting; thus, when clinicians suspect infection with organisms capable of producing type 1 β-lactamase, they should avoid certain antibiotics (i.e., antibiotics that provide good substrate for the product enzyme) that efficiently select these mutants.

Extended-Spectrum β-Lactamases

An increasingly common problem facing clinicians and clinical microbiologists is the presence of ESBLs, which are broad-spectrum β-lactamase enzymes produced by such pathogens as *Klebsiella, Escherichia coli, Enterobacter,* and *Proteus.* First described in the 1980s, these enzymes may occur on the basis of a change of only one amino acid in the β-lactamases normally produced by these pathogens.[129] Despite the minimal structural change, the enzymes have the capacity to inactivate many broad-spectrum β-lactam drugs. Of note, use of any of several classes of antibiotics, notably third-generation cephalosporins and fluoroquinolones, has been identified as a risk factor for selecting ESBLs.[130,131]

The resistance that occurs in such ESBL producers is of importance for the clinician in initial antibiotic selection in two regards. First, with β-lactam antibiotic therapy, even antibiotics that generally are stable in the presence of β-lactamases may not have predictable activity. Inferior outcomes associated with extended-spectrum cephalosporins such as cefepime and with β-lactam/β-lactamase inhibitor combinations, such as piperacillin-tazobactam, have been described;[132] one proposed mechanism is inoculum effect, with diminished susceptibility as the size of the inoculum is increased from 10^5 to 10^7 organisms.[132,133] An alternative explanation for the lack of activity by certain β-lactam antibiotics has been proposed by Craig and Bhavnani.[134] As the number of bacterial colony-forming units (CFUs) increases from 5×10^5 to 5×10^7, approximately 100 times more β-lactamase is released from bacteria lysed after antibiotic exposure. Variations in antibiotic efficacy may rest on the increased release of enzyme in infections with larger inoculums of organisms (e.g., pneumonia and intra-abdominal abscess). Thus, in vitro susceptibility may not predict in vivo outcome for treatment of infectious diseases.

Unlike the type 1 β-lactamase, the ESBL is not chromosomal; rather, it is carried on a large plasmid, which may contain genetic material encoding the machinery that conveys resistance to many classes of antibiotics. For example, the resistance genes for aminoglycosides may be located on the same plasmid as those encoding an ESBL. As a result, gentamicin and tobramycin resistance often occurs in ESBL producers.[133] With fluoroquinolones, multiple mechanisms may contribute to quinolone resistance in ESBL producers. Topoisomerase mutations (i.e., target modification) may be associated with decreased binding. The *qnr* gene codes for a protein that wraps around DNA gyrase, thereby preventing quinolones from attaching to target binding sites.[135,136] In addition, ESBL-producing organisms may possess efflux pumps, and because fluoroquinolones are subject to extrusion from bacteria by means of these pumps, efflux is a potential mechanism of quinolone resistance in ESBL producers.[137]

During the early years of infection with ESBL-producing organisms, infections occurred almost exclusively in either hospitalized patients or in those who had been exposed to antibiotics. In the early 2000s, ESBL infections that occurred in the community setting in patients who had never been hospitalized and who had not been previously exposed to antibiotic were reported.[138] Risk factors for ESBL infections included rates in the 35% range of infections caused by ESBL-producing organisms in patients who had no previous health care contact.[139] With the awareness of community ESBL infections came the identification of large increases within relatively short periods of time of specific types of ESBLs (e.g., the enzyme CTX-M, which refers to a cefotaximase that was initially identified in Munich, Germany) occurring predominately in urinary tract isolates of *E. coli* in community settings.[140] Perhaps the best explanation for why infection with ESBL-producing pathogens might originate in the community setting in patients without the risk factors for either selective antibiotic pressure or person-to-person spread of the organism was suggested in the review by Jacoby and Munoz-Price.[133] Genes for CTX-M–type enzymes are found on the chromosome of *Kluyvera,* a genus of rarely pathogenic commensal organisms found in the gastrointestinal tract. The postulation was that pathogenic organisms such as *E. coli* producing CTX-M–type enzymes appear to have emerged by plasmid acquisition of β-lactamase genes from commensal organisms with which they have close proximity in an environmental reservoir (e.g., the gastrointestinal tract). It is awareness of such a trend for community-acquired resistant pathogens that may influence the initial empiric therapy of patients with either a gastrointestinal or urinary tract source of infection who present ill enough to require ICU admission.

Although infection with ESBL-producing organisms has been associated with significant clinical consequences, no definitive recommendations exist for how to optimally treat such infections, and no antibiotic presently on the market has an FDA-approved indication for treating infections caused by ESBL-producing pathogens. In the absence of such data but with the important ramifications of such infections, recommendations must be extracted from the medical literature. The reviews by Jacoby and Munoz-Price[133] and by Paterson and Bonomo[129] have listed carbapenems as a drug of choice for infections caused by ESBL-producing pathogens. Influencing this recommendation are the facts that (1) ESBL-producing pathogens are often resistant to fluoroquinolones and aminoglycosides because resistance mechanisms for these classes of antibiotics are often carried on the same large plasmid containing the genetic elements for ESBL production and (2) carbapenems (although β-lactam agents) are paradoxically stable in the presence of ESBLs.

It is important for the clinician to consider whether one carbapenem might be more favorable than another for the treatment of infections caused by ESBL-producing organisms. In the era of antimicrobial stewardship, a principle of importance in such considerations is whether the collateral damage of antibiotics that may result in selecting resistant strains of *P. aeruginosa* can be prevented. Although not a universally accepted tenet, the concept of pseudomonal sparing is of potential importance. The clinical approach to carbapenems that is useful in such a consideration is to divide this class of antibiotics into those agents with activity against *P. aeruginosa* (i.e., imipenem, meropenem, doripenem) versus the carbapenems without significant activity against *P. aeruginosa* (i.e., ertapenem). Incorporating the data from Sanders and Sanders,[126] selection of strains of resistant *P. aeruginosa* occurs when a spontaneous mutant with the genetics for drug resistance is allowed to grow because sensitive nonmutant strains of the organism have been killed by antibiotic therapy. Although numerous references regarding antibiotic selective pressure leading to drug-resistant *P. aeruginosa* have been published, two publications are representative of how a process might be favored by pseudomonal-active antibiotics.

In a 2-year case-control study of 2613 patients admitted to three ICUs in a large teaching hospital in Paris, France, prolonged receipt of antibiotics with specific antipseudomonal activity, most notably ciprofloxacin, was associated with the emergence of multidrug-resistant *P. aeruginosa*.[141] The authors concluded that if treatment with an antibiotic active against gram-negative bacteria is needed, agents with little antipseudomonal activity should be preferred over those with specific antipseudomonal activity to limit the emergence of multidrug-resistant *P. aeruginosa*. Using data from 779 isolates of carbapenem-resistant *P. aeruginosa*, Carmeli and colleagues showed by univariate analysis that the risk factors for isolation of carbapenem-resistant *P. aeruginosa* were the administration of group 2 carbapenems (imipenem, meropenem) ($P < 0.0001$), aminoglycosides ($P = 0.034$), or penicillins ($P = 0.05$).[142] The group 1 carbapenem ertapenem was not associated with imipenem-resistant *P. aeruginosa* ($P = 0.2$).

Since the introduction of ertapenem onto the market, there have been theoretical concerns that use of this nonpseudomonal carbapenem might select for strains of carbapenem-resistant *P. aeruginosa*. Ecology studies conducted over the first 9 years that ertapenem was on the market specifically addressed this concern, and those studies have been published in a review article on the topic.[143] Results from the 10 clinical studies evaluating the effect of ertapenem use on the susceptibility of *Pseudomonas* to carbapenems uniformly showed that ertapenem use did not result in decreased *Pseudomonas* susceptibility to the antipseudomonal carbapenems.

With the increasing prevalence of ESBL infections, including those in the community setting that might be severe enough to require ICU admission, an unanswered question is whether noncarbapenem therapy might be appropriate for some patients. This question was addressed in a post-hoc analysis from Spain of patients from six published prospective cohorts who had bloodstream infections due to ESBL-producing strains of *E. coli*.[144] Most of these patients had the urinary tract as the site of origin of the bloodstream infection. These results suggested that amoxicillin/clavulanic acid and piperacillin/tazobactam might be suitable alternatives to carbapenems for treating patients with bloodstream infections due to ESBL-producing *E. coli* if the isolate was susceptible in vitro to these agents. Unanswered by the review is the optimal management of ESBL-producing *E. coli* bloodstream infections originating outside the urinary tract and of infections caused by pathogens other than *E. coli* that produce ESBLs.

Of the mechanisms of resistance encountered in clinical practice, the story of ESBLs is illustrative of two insightful philosophical points in antibiotics prescribing. First, the community pattern of ESBL resistance in patients without classic risk factors for any form of bacterial resistance challenges the clinician to consider such a mechanism in any patient who presents with severe infection of the gastrointestinal or genitourinary tract. Such clinical situations highlight the importance of stratification of antibiotic therapy based on severity of illness, especially given the data about inappropriate antibiotics as a risk factor for increased mortality rate in serious infections. Second, the increasingly faced dilemma of broad patterns of resistance in *P. aeruginosa* in an era with a paucity of new antibiotic drug development challenges the clinician to judiciously use antibiotics in an attempt to preserve the antibiotics presently available. The concept of pseudomonal-sparing is therefore reasonable to incorporate when possible into antibiotic selection.

Carbapenemases

Carbapenemase is the name used for those β-lactamases that have the ability to inactivate carbapenems, which at the present time is the broadest class of antimicrobial agents available to the ICU physician. To understand carbapenemases in a clinically applicable manner requires a fundamental set of facts. The numerous types of β-lactamases that exist today can be subdivided based on the foundation of their chemical structure: those that have a serine base; and those that have a metallobase. Within that subdivision, one can then approach the four Ambler classes of β-lactamases: classes A, B, C, and D. Class B β-lactamases have a metallobase, and the initial carbapenemases described clinically were class B metalloenzymes. An example from clinical practice of a class B metalloenzyme is the New Delhi metallo-β-lactamase (NDM) found in certain Enterobacteriaceae. After the identification of metallo-β-lactamases, microbiologists began identifying serine-based β-lactamases that were in Ambler group A (which is the same class in which the majority of ESBLs are found). These enzymes were produced by *K. pneumoniae* and were subsequently referred to as KPCs (*K. pneumoniae* carbapenemases). Although there are also class D serine-based carbapenemases such as the OXA-type enzymes produced by organisms like *Acinetobacter* species, the class A and class B carbapenemases are the ones that are most important today in clinical practice.

The name *carbapenemase* has the potential to be misleading. In an insightful discussion of carbapenemases written at the time when these enzymes were just beginning to be commonly recognized as causes of clinical infections, it was acknowledged that KPC carbapenemases in actuality hydrolyze β-lactams of all classes, with the most efficient hydrolysis observed for nitrocefin, cephalothin, cephaloridine, benzylpenicillin, ampicillin, and piperacillin.[145] That review went on to state that the carbapenems imipenem and meropenem, as well as the β-lactam antibiotics cefotaxime and aztreonam, were hydrolyzed with one tenth the efficiency of the penicillins and early cephalosporins. The microbiologically important message was that the KPC family of carbapenemases has a broad hydrolysis spectrum that includes most β-lactam antibiotics. It is with such a basic science foundation that one can begin to approach the role of antibiotics in selecting organisms that produce carbapenemases.

There has been an inclination by some clinicians to assume based on the name *carbapenemase* that carbapenem antibiotics are the most likely to select such a pattern of resistance. Although a definitive answer for such a question cannot be found from prospective clinical trials, multiple reports in the literature support the conclusion that several classes of antibiotics have been linked to subsequent infection with carbapenemase-producing bacteria. As a basic piece of information, one can assume that patients become colonized with such resistant pathogens and that any broad-spectrum antibiotic has the ability to kill the normal flora and thereby allow the resistant strains to grow and to cause clinical disease. In the absence of identifying a specific class of antibiotics responsible for selecting carbapenemase-producing bacteria, there has been a focus in the medical literature to identify other variables that contribute to the problem. Two representative papers provide an important insight related to the association between prior antimicrobial therapy and the subsequent identification of carbapenemase-producing bacteria. In a 4-year case-control study (n = 102), the only covariate independently associated with carbapenem-resistant Enterobacteriaceae in all multivariate analyses was the cumulative number of prior antibiotic exposures.[146] A 26-month double case-control study (n = 96 ESBL-CRKP and 55 ESBL-CSKP) from Greece identified both prior cumulative exposure to antibiotics and increasing duration of prior treatment as risk factors.[147] Shown in this study to be associated with the isolation of carbapenemases was therapy with β-lactam/β-lactamase inhibitor or with the combination of fluoroquinolone and carbapenem. These data are consistent with previous reports that no particular class of antibiotic is the predominant predisposing factor for selection of carbapenemase production. Knowledge of this information by the ICU physician is important because it (1) debunks the myth that carbapenemases are selected only by one class of antibiotics (and, therefore, that restriction of only one class of antibiotics can manage such a problem) and (2) supports the intensity and duration of antibiotic therapy as the most important variables in creating the milieu in which carbapenemase-producing bacteria are selected.

Therapy for infections caused by carbapenemase-producing bacteria has been extremely challenging, and at the present time there are neither definitive nor predictable recommendations that guarantee clinical success. In the absence of such data, the clinician is challenged to make clinically relevant deductions from the published literature. The findings from 15 studies and reports in treating infections caused by KPCs showed success rates of 75% with aminoglycosides, 73% with polymyxin combinations, 71% with tigecycline, 40% with carbapenems, and 14% with polymyxin monotherapy.[148] At the time of writing of this chapter, the antimicrobial agents accepted as having the most potential activity based on in vitro susceptibility are tigecycline, polymyxins, and aztreonam.[149] There are evolving data suggesting a potential role for carbapenems as a therapeutic option if (1) the MIC of the infecting organism is 4 mg/L or less and (2) the carbapenem is given in combination with another active agent.[150]

The examples of carbapenem resistance (whether on the basis of carbapenemase or other mechanism of resistance) in *Pseudomonas, Acinetobacter, Stenotrophomonas*, and *Klebsiella* underscore an important concept in antimicrobial therapy for the critical care clinician, for whom such patterns of resistance are becoming increasingly prevalent in the ICU. When multidrug resistance occurs, it cannot be predictably assumed that such resistance is on the basis of exposure to the broadest class of antibiotic to which the organism is resistant. To accept such a flawed assessment could result in limited use of that class of antibiotic, which could then shift to increased use of the actual class of antibiotic that led to the pattern of resistance. The other clinically relevant observation in many of the recently described outbreaks is that inadequate infection control contributed to the spread of resistant strains that had been selected by antibiotics.[132,151,152]

EFFLUX PUMPS

Efflux pumps are three-component systems, contained within the bacterial cell wall, that allow bacteria to eliminate antibiotics that have entered. Initially described in 1980 as a mechanism of resistance in tetracyclines, efflux was recognized in 1988 as a contributor to fluoroquinolone resistance.[153] In recent years, the contribution of efflux to clinical resistance has broadened, with important implications for treatment of serious infections. The composition of this system has been nicely detailed.[154,155] The pump itself (also referred to as the transporter) lies in the cytoplasmic membrane and is designated MexB, MexD, or MexF. It is attached via a linker lipoprotein (MexA, MexC, or MexE) in the periplasm to the third component, the exit portal (OprM, OprJ, or OprN), which lies in the outer membrane. These three components of the efflux pump normally are under repressor gene control and therefore are not clinically active.

P. aeruginosa has several efflux systems, with MexAB-OprM and MexEF-OprN having particular clinical significance: The MexAB-OprM system contributes to both intrinsic and acquired resistance; and the MexEF-OprN system contributes only to acquired resistance.[156] The MexAB-OprM system is expressed constitutively in cells grown in standard laboratory media, where it contributes to intrinsic resistance to a number of antimicrobials, including fluoroquinolones, tetracyclines, piperacillin, cefepime, aztreonam, and certain carbapenems.[123] Of the β-lactams, only carbapenems appear to be poor substrates for MexAB-OprM; however, different carbapenems vary with regard to their susceptibility to efflux. Meropenem and doripenem are subject to efflux, and expression of the MexAB-OprM efflux system has been correlated with resistance to meropenem.[157] By contrast, imipenem is not subject to efflux.[156] It has been suggested that this may be due to the need for efflux systems with MexAB-OprM to access their substrates within the cytoplasmic membrane. Meropenem is much more amphiphilic than imipenem, which may explain why imipenem does not act as a substrate for MexAB-OprM whereas meropenem does.[157] Such a microbiologic property may explain why a gram-negative isolate may be susceptible to imipenem but resistant to meropenem.

The ability of fluoroquinolones to select certain *nfxc* (*mexT*) mutants has been discussed.[122,154] In addition to resistance to fluoroquinolones, these mutants may have decreased susceptibility and even clinical resistance to carbapenems (e.g., imipenem, meropenem) that occurs on the basis of either closure of porin channels in the outer membrane of the bacterial cell wall (with resultant impermeability) or upregulation of an efflux pump (which allows the bacteria to eliminate drug that has penetrated the organism's cell wall). Such newly recognized information may help explain patterns of increasing carbapenem resistance in health care institutions in which carbapenem use has not recently increased.

THE CLINICAL RELEVANCE FOR UNDERSTANDING ANTIBIOTIC RESISTANCE

An understanding of this concept takes on significance with the increasingly common problem in ICUs of the development of resistance to multiple antibiotics. Referred to as multidrug-resistant organisms, these pathogens may be the cause of clinical failure of antibiotic treatment if an inappropriate therapeutic regimen is used. A common mistake in clinical practice is to assume that the major predisposition to a pattern of resistance is the overuse of the broadest category of antibiotic to which a pathogen is resistant. Several examples are important in the understanding of this concept.

A classic example of multidrug resistance in gram-negative organisms is the resistance in *P. aeruginosa*. As previously noted, multiple resistance mechanisms regulated by genetic operons on the chromosomes of *P. aeruginosa* have been described, including efflux pumps, AmpC β-lactamases, and outer membrane porin closure.[122,158] For infections such as HAP and VAP, in which *P. aeruginosa* is a pathogen targeted with empiric therapy and for which fluoroquinolones are offered as an option in the initial regimen,[10,15,159] data on the risk of fluoroquinolones leading to multidrug resistance via efflux mechanisms become especially noteworthy. Additionally, because of the ability of certain organisms such as *P. aeruginosa* to express multiple mechanisms of resistance, many experts recommend avoiding the use of traditional antipseudomonal agents (i.e., a pseudomonal-sparing regimen) when treating infections in which *Pseudomonas* is not a suspected pathogen, as the use of overuse these agents may result in the development of multidrug resistance in *Pseudomonas* isolates.[141]

The experience with carbapenem-resistant *A. baumannii* in Brooklyn, New York, provides an important insight into the problem of selection of resistance by one class of antibiotic to an entirely different class. In a study to evaluate the endemicity of *A. baumannii*, all unique patient isolates of this pathogen were collected from 15 Brooklyn hospitals over a 3-month period.[152] Antibiotic susceptibilities, ribotyping, and the relationship between antibiotic use and resistance rates were determined. Among the 224 carbapenem-resistant strains of *A. baumannii*, ribotyping demonstrated that one strain accounted for two thirds of the isolates and was present in all of the 15 participating hospitals. The strongest predisposition to selection for this pathogen was cephalosporin use. Known *A. baumannii* resistance mechanisms include chromosomally associated β-lactamases and porin protein mutations,[160] so it can be assumed that this represents selection of carbapenem-resistant mutant strains by the cephalosporins.

A retrospective analysis of critically ill trauma patients with late-onset gram-negative pneumonia showed that the antibiotic most associated with pneumonia due to *Stenotrophomonas maltophilia* was cefepime.[161] These data on cephalosporins as a risk factor for *S. maltophilia* infection are similar to those in an earlier report that identified use of ceftazidime and imipenem as associated with similar rates of *S. maltophilia* acquisition in hospitalized patients.[162] The suggestion by these reports is that broad-spectrum agents, more so than one specific agent, may kill sensitive bacteria and allow pathogens such as *Stenotrophomonas* to become clinically expressed.

DE-ESCALATION

The concept of de-escalation therapy incorporates the dual goals of (1) initially attempting to decrease mortality rate by selecting the appropriate antibiotic for empiric therapy but (2) decreasing the time that a patient is exposed to the broad-spectrum therapy that might be necessary to get initial therapy administered correctly.

DECREASING BROADNESS OR NUMBER OF AGENTS

Classically, there have been three ways that de-escalation can occur. The most intuitively understood is changing from a broad-spectrum agent to a narrower spectrum agent based on culture and sensitivity data. As is well known to those who practice in the intensive care setting, culture data are often negative in the sickest patients, and the option of de-escalating based on culture data is often not available. The de-escalating process becomes less clear when diagnostic studies do not yield an obvious pathogen. Perhaps an appropriate manner of employing the information gained by a negative culture is to allow the nonrecovery of certain organisms to influence the alteration of an existing regimen. HAP, including VAP, provides a clinically applicable example of this concept. In an attempt to minimize mortality rates, patients with HAP typically receive as empiric therapy a three-drug regimen that includes coverage against MRSA and *P. aeruginosa*. Guidelines of the ATS/IDSA for HAP have suggested that clinically improving patients not on antibiotics when cultures are obtained may have therapy against MRSA and *P. aeruginosa* stopped if sputum cultures are negative for these pathogens.[10]

A third technique for de-escalating is to shorten the duration of therapy.

DURATION OF THERAPY

Because antibiotics may be a risk factor for resistance,[121] it is important in the process of antibiotic stewardship to identify opportunities to minimize exposure to these therapeutic agents. One possibility is by decreasing the duration of therapy to the shortest duration necessary to achieve an optimal clinical outcome.[163] Often the decisions regarding traditional durations of therapy find their basis not in controlled trials or prospective studies, but rather in expert opinion. Although certain infections, such as *S. aureus* bacteremia, require well-defined and often prolonged durations of intravenous therapy,[164,165] trials in VAP have challenged some of the classic tenets and have resulted in recommendations for shorter durations of therapy when compared to the traditional regimens.

Dennesen and coworkers[166] evaluated the response to antimicrobial therapy administered according to ATS guidelines in 27 patients diagnosed with VAP in a study that initially used a bronchoalveolar lavage (BAL) along with clinical parameters to confirm the diagnosis of VAP but subsequently used semiquantitative tracheal aspirates for microbiologic surveillance. All patients in this study received appropriate antibiotic therapy. After initiation of antibiotic therapy, T_{max} (maximal temperature over a 24-hour period), PaO_2/FIO_2 (ratio used to quantify impairment of oxygen gas exchange in the lung), white blood cell count, and semiquantitative cultures of endotracheal aspirate were monitored. Resolution of clinical parameters occurred primarily within the first 6 days of therapy. Using cultures of endotracheal aspirates, the investigators found that colonization with *P. aeruginosa* persisted throughout the duration of treatment, whereas colonization with *S. aureus, H. influenzae,* and *S. pneumoniae* resolved shortly after initiation of therapy. Acquired colonization, predominantly with resistant pathogens such as *P. aeruginosa* or members of Enterobacteriaceae, usually occurred in week 2 and frequently preceded a recurrent episode of lung infection. On the basis of these data, it was suggested that 7 days may be an appropriate duration of therapy for patients with VAP.

Ibrahim and colleagues[167] evaluated a clinical guideline for the treatment of VAP using 7 days of therapy. A total of 102 patients were prospectively evaluated, 50 before institution of the guidelines and 52 after institution. In addition to more frequent choice of adequate initial antibiotic treatment after implementation of the clinical guideline, patients also had shorter antibiotic courses when treated under the guideline. No mortality rate difference was noted between the two groups. As was the case with the study by Dennesen and coworkers,[166] a second episode of VAP was more likely to occur in the patients receiving the longer, traditional duration of therapy.

Chastre and associates[168] conducted a prospective, multicenter, randomized, double-blind study of 401 patients with VAP confirmed by quantitative cultures obtained by bronchoscopic protected specimen brush (PSB) or BAL, or both. Only patients who had received initial appropriate antibiotic therapy were included. Therapy was divided into two categories: short course, which was given for 8 days in 197 patients, versus long course, which was given for 15 days in 204 patients. Clinical efficacy was similar between the short-course and long-course groups. Because slightly more patients with nonfermenting gram-negative bacilli (e.g., *P. aeruginosa* and *A. baumannii*) assigned to the 8-day regimen had pulmonary infection recurrences, the investigators were unable to demonstrate the noninferiority of the 8-day regimen for infection by such pathogens compared with the 15-day course of therapy. Multiresistant pathogens more frequently caused recurrences in patients who received the 15-day regimen. Even though the findings from this study do not definitively prove that therapy for HAP or VAP can be limited to 7 days, they lend support to the findings by Dennesen[166] and Ibrahim[167] and their colleagues.

MINIMIZING CLINICAL RESISTANCE

In the absence of a significant pipeline of antibiotics for treating multidrug-resistant organisms, it is important for the clinician to use antibiotics judiciously so that currently available agents are active for as long as possible. Several approaches toward achieving this goal have been described.

For many years, the standard approach to antibiotic prescribing occurred in a homogeneous manner in which a single antibiotic or limited numbers of antibiotics were used as the "workhorse" agents in empiric therapy.[169] Such an approach to antibiotic prescribing often was associated with restricted formularies, the thought being that limiting broad-spectrum agents might prevent the emergence of resistance. Unfortunately, this approach did not take into consideration the possibility that the inadequate therapy in seriously ill patients might not be reversible when the initial antibiotics were changed to the correct agents once susceptibilities were known. In addition, it was during this era of restricted formularies that the proliferation of bacterial resistance began to occur. Because an inherent risk with homogeneous antibiotic use is the selective pressure that when applied can lead to resistance, other approaches must be considered.

Heterogeneous antibiotic use, in which antibiotic selection is based not on hospital mandates but rather on issues related both to the patient and the pathogens involved in the infectious process, may decrease selective pressure.[169] Heterogeneity can be achieved in any of several ways. A strategy by which multiple or all classes of antibiotics are available for use (i.e., antibiotic heterogeneity) has been suggested as part of a broader effort aimed at curtailing antibiotic resistance within ICUs. As a potential alternative to cycling, a mathematical model was developed to compare antibiotic cycling with *mixing,* in which antibiotic variation is random as opposed to the regulation that occurs with a process like antibiotic cycling.[170] The premise for such a comparison is that mixing imposes greater fluctuation in selective conditions, thereby yielding greater heterogeneity than occurs with cycling. In this study, the results were underlaid by a simple ecologic explanation that led to the conclusion that cycling is unlikely to be effective and may even hinder resistance control and that mixing may yield more favorable results in terms of preserving antibiotic susceptibility.

In contrast with homogeneous antibiotic use, which was developed to control resistance, heterogeneous use is aimed at managing resistance.[169] Because resistance at some level

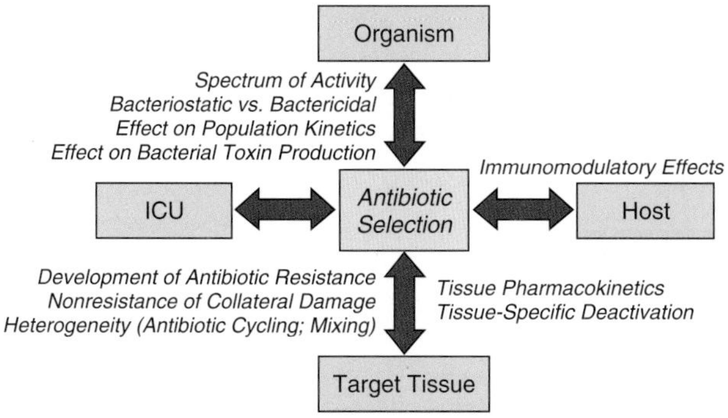

Figure 51.3 The interplay of antibiotic selection with principles relevant to host, organism, intensive care unit, and target tissue. Adequate antibiotic therapy is dictated by more than matching spectrum of antibiotic activity with a pathogen's in vitro susceptibility.

is an inevitable part of medical practice, the latter approach seems more insightful.

CONCLUSIONS

At a time when bacterial resistance is becoming more prevalent but during which antibiotic development is relatively stagnant, the critical care clinician is faced with the somewhat daunting challenge of achieving clinical efficacy without compromising the antibiotic armamentarium that exists at present. For this to be accomplished, the interplay of several important concepts will drive the decision process. As depicted in Figure 51.3, these considerations include the organism, the host, and the targeted tissue, as well as specific issues related to the ICU itself.

Armed with the knowledge of these variables, health care providers now have the foundation for achieving the first goal of antibiotic stewardship—education. Nevertheless, in the recently developed guideline for antibiotic stewardship, it was acknowledged that education alone, without incorporation of active intervention, is only marginally effective in changing antimicrobial prescribing practices and has not demonstrated a sustained effect. An understanding of the principles governing antimicrobial selection in the ICU should better position critical care clinicians for practicing the art of antibiotic prescribing in a manner that both achieves efficacy for optimal outcome and preserves the integrity of the antibiotics available for this task.

KEY POINTS

- Initial appropriate antibiotic therapy (defined as matching antibiotic to pathogen susceptibility), with early dose administration, reduces mortality rate in the treatment of serious infections.
- Adequate antibiotic therapy extends beyond appropriate therapy and includes dose optimization, ensuring target tissue penetration, and consideration of combination therapy.
- Empiric and directed antibiotic regimens for the individual patient also are influenced by factors that the critical care physician must recognize: time- versus concentration-dependent killing; synergy versus

KEY POINTS (Continued)

antagonism; immunomodulatory antibiotic properties; inhibition of bacterial protein synthesis; and organ-specific deactivation.

- In selecting antibiotics for serious infections, the clinician should consider not only the individual therapeutic efficacy but also the potential for unintended antibiotic consequences, such as selection of resistant microorganisms.
- Because antibiotic therapy is a risk factor for selecting resistant microorganisms, antibiotics should not be broader in coverage, or given longer, than necessary. Initial broad and aggressive antibiotic therapy should, therefore, be rapidly de-escalated as soon as is clinically possible.
- It is important to recognize that resistance to a class of antibiotics may be selected by therapy with an entirely different class of drugs.
- With the increasing prevalence of community-acquired mechanisms of resistance such as ESBL production, it is important to stratify initial therapeutic options based on severity of illness.
- Knowledge of the mechanisms by which antibiotic-resistant bacteria are selected may lead to more judicious patterns of antibiotic use that may help to manage the evolving patterns of resistance that are occurring globally.

SELECTED REFERENCES

1. Dellit TH, Owens RC, McGowan JE, et al: Infectious Diseases Society of America and the Society for Healthcare Epidemiology of America guidelines for developing an institutional program to enhance antimicrobial stewardship. Clin Infect Dis 2007; 44(2):159-177.
8. Kumar A, Ellis P, Arabi Y, et al: Initiation of inappropriate antimicrobial therapy results in a fivefold reduction of survival in human septic shock. Chest 2009;136(5):1237-1248.
11. Ebert SC, Craig WA: Pharmacodynamic properties of antibiotics: Application to drug monitoring and dosage regimen design. Infect Control Hosp Epidemiol 1990;11(6):319-326.
25. Udy AA, Roberts JA, Boots RJ, et al: Augmented renal clearance: Implications for antibacterial dosing in the critically ill. Clin Pharmacokinet 2010;49(1):1-16.
52. Wunderink RG, Niederman MS, Kollef MH, et al: Linezolid in methicillin-resistant *Staphylococcus aureus* nosocomial pneumonia: A randomized, controlled study. Clin Infect Dis 2012; 54(5):621-629.
98. Höffken G, Niederman MS: Nosocomial pneumonia: The importance of a de-escalating strategy for antibiotic treatment of pneumonia in the ICU. Chest 2002;122(6):2183-2196.
112. Paterson DL: "Collateral damage" from cephalosporin or quinolone antibiotic therapy. Clin Infect Dis 2004;38(Suppl 4):S341-S345.
133. Jacoby GA, Munoz-Price LS: The new beta-lactamases. N Engl J Med 2005;352(4):380-391.
143. Nicolau DP, Carmeli Y, Crank CW, et al: Carbapenem stewardship: Does ertapenem affect *Pseudomonas* susceptibility to other carbapenems? A review of the evidence. Int J Antimicrob Agents 2012;39(1):11-15.
163. Hayashi Y, Paterson DL: Strategies for reduction in duration of antibiotic use in hospitalized patients. Clin Infect Dis 2011; 52(10):1232-1240.

The complete list of references can be found at www.expertconsult.com.

52 Antifungal and Antiviral Therapy

Luis Ostrosky-Zeichner | John H. Rex

CHAPTER OUTLINE

Over the past 2 decades, fungal and viral diseases have become progressively more important to the critical care specialist. Increasing populations of immunocompromised hosts with serious fungal and viral infections often require critical care, and patients hospitalized in critical care units are also susceptible to these infections. Effective management of these conditions requires not only use of the appropriate anti-infective agents but in-depth knowledge of their pharmacodynamic/pharmacokinetic properties, as well as awareness of their physiologic effects, toxicities, and drug interactions. Recent years have also brought important antifungal and antiviral drug developments, giving the clinician an ever-increasing arsenal of therapeutic choices.

SYSTEMIC ANTIFUNGAL AGENTS

This chapter will focus on systemic antifungal therapy as it is relevant to the critical care setting. Topical therapy of candidiasis and therapy of other systemic fungal infections will be omitted or only briefly reviewed. The interested reader is referred to the Infectious Diseases Society of America (IDSA) guidelines on the topic.[1]

POLYENES

Polyenes act by binding to ergosterol in the fungal cytoplasmic membrane, causing ionic leakage and osmotic instability.[2] Additionally, they cause oxidation of the cytoplasmic membrane.[2] Polyenes are fungicidal in most settings and the most prominent members of the family are amphotericin B and nystatin. Both drugs have important toxic effects that often limit their use in patients with organ/system failure. Newer formulations of the drugs have been developed to reduce this limitation.

AMPHOTERICIN B AND ITS LIPID FORMULATIONS

Amphotericin B is produced by *Streptomyces nodosus* and is one of the oldest and most widely used antifungal agents. There is much experience with its use in mycoses and hosts, and it is usually the comparison standard for new therapies.[3] Because of significant acute and chronic toxicities, there is an extensive anecdotal literature describing ways to ameliorate these toxicities, as well as limitations of all these strategies.[4] The advent of lipid-based formulations of amphotericin B has enhanced our ability to limit toxicities and provide adequate courses of therapy.[5]

Amphotericin B has in vitro and in vivo activity against most isolates of *Candida* spp., *Cryptococcus neoformans*, *Histoplasma capsulatum*, *Blastomyces dermatitidis*, *Mucorales*, *Coccidioides immitis*, *Paracoccidioides brasiliensis*, *Aspergillus* spp., *Fusarium* spp., and *Sporothrix schenckii*.[6] The activity of amphotericin B is so broad that it is almost easier to think of this in terms of the few species that are consistently less susceptible or actually resistant to amphotericin B: *Aspergillus terreus*,[7] *Trichosporon* spp.,[8] and *Pseudallescheria boydii* (*Scedosporium prolificans*).[9] One species of *Candida*, *C. lusitaniae*, readily becomes resistant to the polyenes.[10] Resistance among isolates of *Candida* is otherwise rare.[11,12]

Amphotericin B is hydrophobic and is combined with deoxycholate to permit intravenous (IV) administration in an aqueous solvent. Once in the bloodstream, it dissociates and binds to plasma proteins and lipoproteins. It is stored in the liver and other organs and slowly eliminated. Drug metabolism is complex and not affected by renal or liver failure.[3] Hemodialysis and peritoneal dialysis do not remove the drug. Measuring drug levels is possible[13] but not of obvious clinical relevance. Cerebrospinal fluid (CSF) penetration is poor. Although amphotericin B is primarily used in IV infusion, it can also be used topically for localized gastrointestinal (GI) or urinary infections or instilled directly to treat central nervous system (CNS) infections.

The most common toxicity is the systemic reaction associated with IV infusion, thought to be caused by release of inflammatory mediators from monocytes and macrophages and producing fever, hypotension, and on occasion severe dyspnea. Two forms of renal toxicity are seen. First, a very acute form of renal dysfunction appears to be related to amphotericin B–induced renal arteriolar constriction.[14] Second, cumulative dose-dependent tubular damage is almost invariably seen if significant doses are given. The tubular injury is characterized by potassium/magnesium wasting and azotemia. It is generally reversible when the drug is stopped, but it is also particularly aggravated if the patient is volume depleted or given other nephrotoxic drugs. The renal injury also reduces erythropoietin production[15] and thus causes a mild anemia during chronic therapy (the hematocrit will typically fall to about 30%). Finally, amphotericin B may precipitate cardiac arrhythmias, especially if the patient is already hypokalemic and hypomagnesemic.[16-19] The deoxycholate formulation of amphotericin B is given intravenously at 0.5 to 1.0 mg/kg/day, but it can also be administered every other day by doubling the dose. To avoid producing a precipitate, it must be diluted in an electrolyte-free solution at no more than 0.1 mg/mL. It should be administered over no less than 1 hour and most authorities prefer a 2- to 3-hour infusion.[20] Because the occasional patient reacts violently to the drug, an initial test dose of 1 mg of the drug may be given prior to infusing the entire first dose. Premedication with acetaminophen, diphenhydramine, and steroids may be used if the patient develops reactions to the infusion. Volume loading appears to reduce nephrotoxicity, and many authorities give (if possible) 500 to 1000 mL normal saline just prior to each dose of amphotericin B. Administration via a central line is advisable because amphotericin B given peripherally often produces phlebitis.

Treatment goals have been traditionally and arbitrarily cumulative (such as a total of 1 or 2 g), but a time-based approached is increasingly used for some diseases (e.g., for candidemia, in which 2 weeks of therapy at 0.6-0.7 mg/kg after the last positive blood culture has been shown to produce a late relapse rate of about 1%).[21] Although the importance of therapy in the typical patient is unclear,[22,23] candiduria is sometimes treated with amphotericin B bladder washes. A typical dose is 50 mg of amphotericin B diluted in 1000 mL of water and irrigated over 24 hours. A small number of intracranial fungal infections benefit from intrathecal dosing at 0.1 to 0.5 mg three times per week, but expert advice should be sought if this therapy is considered.

There are three lipid-based formulations of the drug: amphotericin B colloidal dispersion (ABCD, marketed as Amphotec and Amphocil), amphotericin B lipid complex (ABLC, marketed as Abelcet), and liposomal amphotericin (L-AmB, marketed as AmBisome). The names of these compounds are often confusing. Only one of the drugs (L-AmB) is a true liposome. However, it is not uncommon for physicians to refer to therapy with these compounds in general as therapy with "liposomal amphotericin B." The preferred terminology is "lipid-associated formulation of amphotericin B" (LFAB).[5] When speaking of specific compounds, we find that use of the names ABCD, ABLC, and AmBisome minimizes confusion.

All three LFABs have comparable efficacy among themselves and when compared to regular amphotericin B, but significantly less nephrotoxicity.[5,24] They are also thought to be concentrated and distributed in the reticuloendothelial system, theoretically achieving higher tissue dose delivery and concentration. The lipid carrier does, however, dramatically change the pharmacology and delivery of these compounds, and higher doses than are typical for amphotericin B are both safe and necessary for optimal activity: The licensed dosages are 5 mg/kg/day (ABLC), 3 to 6 mg/kg/day (ABCD), and 3 to 5 mg/kg/day (AmBisome). The optimal dosage of these compounds is unclear and the agents appear generally equipotent. Dosages of approximately 3 mg/kg/day would appear suitable for treatment of most serious *Candida* infections. Doses of at least 5 mg/kg/day are used for mold infections, with some authors recommending even higher doses.[25-27] However, a recent study showed no advantage to using 10 mg/kg/day over 3 mg/kg/day for invasive aspergillosis and other invasive mold infections.[28]

All three LFABs appear active against the same range of fungal infections that can be treated with amphotericin B. The compounds do differ in their relative toxicities.[24] ABCD appears to have significant administration-related toxicity and is not often used. AmBisome and ABLC are both well tolerated, but AmBisome has been associated with somewhat less nephrotoxicity in some patient settings.[29] Some patients will tolerate one formulation better than another.[30,31]

Because of the cost of the LFABs, there has been great interest in the concept of making a pseudo-LFAB by suspending amphotericin B deoxycholate in commercially available lipid emulsions.[32-34] This practice does not, however, consistently reduce toxicity.[35] This may be due to preparation-dependent precipitation of the amphotericin B noted by some[36,37] but not all[38] authors. Most authorities have concluded that further work with this approach should be undertaken as part of a controlled clinical trial that addresses these issues.[39] A recent meta-analysis on the use of these formulations has been published, but because of heterogeneity, the results are inconclusive.[40]

The cost of the LFABs is significant, but the counterbalancing reduction in nephrotoxicity is also valuable and should be considered when choosing an LFAB versus a conventional amphotericin B.[41] A recent study of the impact of nephrotoxicity of amphotericin B deoxycholate in patients with invasive aspergillosis suggested that this patient population suffered significant morbidity due to the amphotericin B itself.[42] Use of amphotericin B deoxycholate produces significant nephrotoxicity in about 30% of patients, increasing hospital length of stay and hospitalization costs by nearly $30,000.[43,44] Nevertheless, the context of amphotericin B–induced toxicity should also be considered. A rise of the creatinine to 3 mg/dL in an otherwise well patient who is being treated with amphotericin B for (say) osteoarticular sporotrichosis may be clinically imperceptible owing to the fact that the patient has no other acute medical problems. On the other hand, a rise in creatinine from 1 mg/dL to 2 mg/dL may be disastrous in a surgical patient who is also suffering from nosocomial pneumonia and cardiac insufficiency. No firm guidelines in this area have yet to emerge. We currently believe that an LFAB is appropriate for patients who have failed amphotericin B deoxycholate (FDA [Food and Drug Administration] indication), or who are intolerant of amphotericin B deoxycholate (FDA indication), or who are highly likely to be intolerant (no FDA indication). We define intolerance broadly: a creatinine clearance (CrCl) less than 50% of the normal for the patient's age or a fall in CrCl with therapy. Predicting intolerance is difficult, but such factors as concomitant use of highly nephrotoxic agents (e.g., an aminoglycoside) or underlying primary/intrinsic renal disease (e.g., diabetes mellitus) associated renal dysfunction should be considered.

FLUCYTOSINE

Flucytosine (5-FC) is the fluorine analog of cytosine.[45] It was originally synthesized as an antineoplastic agent, but poor antitumor activity and discovery of its antifungal properties led to its further development as an antifungal agent. It acts by deamination to 5-fluorouracil and then conversion to a noncompetitive inhibitor of thymidylate synthase that interferes with fungal DNA and RNA synthesis. It has been demonstrated effective in cryptococcosis, candidiasis, and chromomycosis, being the drug of choice for the latter infection. Drug resistance in vivo develops quickly, so the standard practice is to combine it with another agent.[46,47] 5-FC is water soluble and has high bioavailability. Protein binding is negligible and approximately 90% is excreted in urine. CSF penetration is good, and both hemodialysis and peritoneal dialysis remove it. It is teratogenic in rats and therefore contraindicated during pregnancy. Adverse effects include rash, diarrhea, and hepatic dysfunction. High blood levels (>100 μg/mL) are associated with profound leukopenia and thrombocytopenia.[48] This has prompted the recommendation of monitoring drug levels, renal/liver function, and blood counts in patients receiving 5-FC. Dosage of 150 mg/kg/day divided in four doses has usually been suggested, but recent in vivo[49] and human experience[50] suggests that dosage of 100 mg/kg/day (again, divided into four doses) may be as effective and better tolerated. Renal failure requires dosage adjustment to half the dose if CrCl is 25 to 50 mL/minute and a quarter dose if it falls below 25 mL/minute. Patients on hemodialysis should be given the latter dose after dialysis. Combination with amphotericin requires constant monitoring of toxicity parameters and dose adjustment. The target blood level is approximately 50 μg/mL. Most experts would discontinue use of this agent if blood counts start dropping, regardless of the blood levels.

THE AZOLE ANTIFUNGAL AGENTS

The introduction of this class of drugs was a major advance in antifungal therapy, because they offer both IV and oral formulations for the treatment of systemic mycosis. Their widespread use has also prompted the emergence of resistance. Azoles act by blocking the activity of lanosterol demethylase, a cytochrome enzyme in both fungal and mammalian cells. Fungal cell membrane synthesis of ergosterol is inhibited and other sterol intermediates are substituted in the membrane, resulting in a nonviable cell. This effect is much slower than that of amphotericin, so these drugs are generally regarded as fungistatic. Because these drugs reduce production of the ergosterol to which polyenes must bind to produce their effect, there is a potential for the azoles and polyenes to appear antagonistic. However, these effects are drug-, organism-, and model-dependent and a range of effects may be seen. This area is complex and has recently been reviewed.[51,52] At present, use of such combinations should be avoided outside a clinical trial. All of the azoles have the ability to interfere with mammalian sterol synthesis. This was most notable with ketoconazole, which can produce gynecomastia and adrenal insufficiency.[53,54] Subsequent azoles have been selected for lack of such effects. All of the azoles can, however, produce hepatic dysfunction. The most common pattern is that of increased transminases. However, any form of dysfunction may be seen. This can be life-threatening if not recognized. The hepatic dysfunction is reversible upon discontinuation of the offending azole.

Another concern with azoles is drug interactions. This becomes particularly important in the critical care setting in which many drugs are being used concomitantly. Table 52.1 summarizes the most important drug interactions that have been reported. The critical interactions generally have to do with drugs cleared by the liver. Some agents (e.g., rifampin and phenobarbital) induce the enzymes that clear the azoles. In other cases, the azole interferes with clearance of another agent (e.g., the azoles predictably increase blood levels of cyclosporine). It is not possible to list all of the known interactions. Consultation with a pharmacy specialist is suggested when using azoles in the setting of polypharmacy, particularly in the critical care setting and when caring for patients with multiple comorbid conditions.

Table 52.1 Selected Azole-Drug Interactions*

Azole Drug	Alters Levels of:	Levels Altered by:	Azole Drug	Alters Levels of:	Levels Altered by:
Fluconazole	Cisapride	Rifampin	Voriconazole	Sirolimus	Rifampin
	Cyclosporine			Rifabutin	Efavirenz
	Diazepam			Efavirenz	Rifabutin
	Glipizide			Ritonavir	Ritonavir
	Glyburide			Terfenadine	Carbamazepine
	Midazolam			Astemizole	Phenytoin
	Phenytoin			Cisapride	
	Rifabutin			Pimozide	
	Sulfonylureas			Quinidine	
	Tacrolimus			Cyclosporine	
	Terfenadine			Methadone	
	Warfarins and coumarins			Tacrolimus	
				Phenytoin	
Itraconazole	Astemizole	Carbamazepine		Warfarin	
	Cisapride	Didanosine (DDI)		Omeprazole	
	Cyclosporine	Histamine H_2 blockers	Posaconazole	Sirolimus	Efavirenz
	Diazepam			Tacrolimus	Rifabutin
	Digoxin	Phenobarbital		Cyclosporine	Phenytoin
	Dihydropyridines	Phenytoin		Pimozide	Cimetidine
	Lovastatin	Proton pump inhibitors		Quinidine	Esomeprazole
	Methylprednisolone			Simvastatin	Metoclopramide
	Midazolam	Rifabutin		Ergot alkaloids	
	Phenytoin	Rifampin		Midazolam	
	Quinidine	Sucralfate		Ritonavir	
	Ritonavir			Atazanavir	
	Sulfonylureas			Vinca alkaloids	
	Terfenadine			Calcium channel blockers	
	Vinca alkaloids			Digoxin	
	Warfarins and coumarins			Glipizide	

*Generally, azoles tend to increase the levels of other drugs, whereas other drugs tend to decrease the level of the azole. This list is not meant to be comprehensive, and the practitioner should review the full prescribing information. Consultation with a pharmacy specialist is recommended when azoles are going to be used in complex polypharmacy situations.

FLUCONAZOLE

Fluconazole is one of the newer triazoles that has in vitro and in vivo activity mainly against yeast, such as *Candida* spp. and *Cryptococcus neoformans.* It also has efficacy against *Coccidioides immitis, Histoplasma capsulatum,* and *Blastomyces dermatitidis.* Unfortunately resistance (mediated by increased production of target enzymes, efflux pumps, and mutations in target enzyme) has become a problem, particularly in *Candida albicans* (mutation to resistance is seen), *C. glabrata* (has intrinsically lower susceptibility and may become highly resistant), and *C. krusei* (intrinsically highly resistant).[55,56] Nevertheless, fluconazole is still very active against most strains causing invasive candidiasis, and higher doses can be used for those organisms that are in the "susceptible-dose dependent" range. Fluconazole is water soluble and is available in oral and IV presentations that produce similar blood levels. Bioavailability is excellent and it is well absorbed regardless of the gastric contents. It has a long half-life and can be administered in a single daily dose. It exhibits little binding to serum proteins and is widely distributed in all body fluids. CSF penetration is particularly high, making it particularly useful in the treatment of CNS infections such as cryptococcosis and coccidioidomycosis. Fluconazole is excreted by the kidneys and dosing should be adjusted in proportion to the CrCl. The most common adverse effects are nausea and vomiting. Skin rash is infrequent but can be severe. Hepatitis has also been reported. The usual dose is 400 to 800 mg (or 6-8 mg/kg) per day by mouth or IV, but doses as high as 2 g/day have been tolerated.[57]

ITRACONAZOLE

Itraconazole is a triazole antifungal agent with a wider spectrum than fluconazole. It has in vitro and in vivo activity against *Candida* spp., *Aspergillus* spp., *Histoplasma* spp., *Blastomyces dermatitidis, Sporothrix schenckii, Trichophyton* spp., *Cryptococcus neoformans, Coccidioides immitis,* and *Paracoccidioides brasiliensis.*[58,59] The resistance issues observed for fluconazole are also an issue with itraconazole.[56] Itraconazole was initially available only in a capsule form that has unpredictable bioavailability. Absorption of the capsule formulation is optimized by ingestion with food.[60] Two new formulations have recently been introduced. First, there is a solution in cyclodextrin for oral administration that significantly enhances bioavailability and is now preferred over the capsule for producing maximal blood levels.[61] Second, an IV formulation (again, in a cyclodextrin carrier) has recently become available. The IV formulation is valuable in that it quickly and reliably produces significant blood levels.[62-64] Itraconazole is highly protein bound and has a prolonged half-life. CSF penetration is negligible, so it is not generally used for CNS infections. Itraconazole is metabolized by the liver and dosing does not need to be modified in renal failure. However, the cyclodextrin carrier used in the IV formulation *is* cleared by the kidneys and its behavior in patients with renal dysfunction is not known. Thus, this formulation of itraconazole should not be used in patients with a CrCl less than 25 mL/hour.

Adverse effects are mainly GI, with nausea, vomiting, and abdominal pain occurring in up to 10% of patients. Hepatitis is uncommon but liver enzyme monitoring is recommended. Because itraconazole, and its major metabolite hydroxyitraconazole, are inhibitors of CYP3A4, drug interactions are a major issue and the most common ones are summarized in Table 52.1.

The usual oral dosage is 100 to 400 mg/day and the oral solution formulation is now preferred. Giving the daily oral dose as two divided doses appears to maximize blood levels. IV dosing is 200 mg twice a day for 2 days and then 200 mg IV every day for a maximum of 14 days. Efficacy is related to plasma concentration, and serum levels can be obtained from national reference laboratories. Such testing is warranted if oral itraconazole is being used to treat a serious fungal infection. Although minimal efficacious blood levels have not been defined, the point of testing is to ensure that at least some level is being obtained. Levels of at least 250 ng/mL are desirable.

VORICONAZOLE

Voriconazole is one of the newest triazoles to arrive into the market. It is licensed for the treatment of invasive candidiasis and invasive aspergillosis, as well as for the treatment of *Fusarium* and *Scedosporium* infections. It is considered as the treatment of choice for invasive aspergillosis.[65] Voriconazole was not inferior to amphotericin B followed by fluconazole in a large clinical trial, but it is unknown if it has any advantages over fluconazole or the echinocandins for treating infections by fluconazole-resistant *C. glabrata.*[66,67] Although it has activity against the endemic mycoses, data are limited at this point, so it is not recommended for routine use in these infections at this time.[68,69]

A relevant gap in its activity is the class of Zygomycetes (such as *Mucor* spp., *Absidia* spp., and *Rhizopus* spp.). Although there have been multiple reports of breakthrough Zygomycetes infections in patients receiving voriconazole prophylaxis or treatment, a causal relationship has not been established.[70,71] Nevertheless, clinicians should be aware that this drug does not have activity against these organisms, and thus it should not be used for empirical therapy of mold infections if Zygomycetes are in the differential diagnosis.

Voriconazole is available in oral (tablets and suspension) and IV formulations, with 96% bioavailability. Usual dosing is 4 to 6 mg/kg IV every 12 hours or 200 to 300 mg orally every 12 hours. Voriconazole has nonlinear pharmacokinetics; thus, increasing the dose will not necessarily increase blood levels. Routine blood level measurement to document absorption is now recommended, although blood levels associated with specific efficacy and safety margins have not been established. Voriconazole is metabolized by the human hepatic cytochrome P-450 enzymes, CYP2C19, CYP2C9, and CYP3A4, and has extensive drug interactions with many drugs commonly used in the critical care setting. Consultation with a pharmacy specialist is recommended for patients on multiple drugs. Like itraconazole, the IV formulation is prepared in a cyclodextrin-based formulation, and thus it is not recommended for use in patients with CrCl less than 50 mL/minute. In such patients the oral formulation may be safely used. Adverse events include self-limited visual disturbances and hallucinations, infrequent reports of hepatic insufficiency, and as with the other azoles, rare reports of arrhythmias and QT prolongation. Monitoring of liver enzymes is recommended during voriconazole therapy.[72-74]

POSACONAZOLE

Posaconazole is the newest triazole in the market and although licensed primarily for prophylaxis of fungal infections in high-risk patients,[75] it does have promising activity against mold infections, in particular infections by the Zygomycetes and *Fusarium.*[76] It has also shown excellent in vitro and in vivo activity against *Candida* spp. with demonstrated efficacy in esophageal disease. It is available only in an oral formulation.[77,78]

ECHINOCANDINS

The echinocandin antifungal agents represent an entirely new class of antifungal drugs. There are three echinocandins on the market at this time: caspofungin, micafungin, and anidulafungin. These agents are cyclic lipohexapeptides that act via inhibition of glucan synthesis.[79] Preclinical studies have shown efficacy against all species of *Candida* without any evidence for cross-resistance with polyenes or azoles, *Aspergillus* spp., and selected other fungi.[80,81] Although the target enzyme is present in most fungi, the echinocandins are not active against *C. neoformans* and molds other than *Aspergillus.* The echinocandins appear to be rapidly fungicidal for *Candida* spp., but their activity against *Aspergillus* may be better described as fungistatic.[82] Nonetheless, they are quite active in animal models of both candidiasis and aspergillosis.[83,84] These drugs have a long half-life, permitting once-daily dosing, and are excreted in the liver. They do not interfere with the cytochrome system and they are not known to be nephrotoxic, having otherwise remarkable safety profiles. At this time, differences between the three drugs appear to be subtle, requiring further study.

CASPOFUNGIN

Caspofungin was the first echinocandin in the market. It has excellent in vitro and in vivo activity against *Aspergillus* and *Candida* spp. It has demonstrated efficacy for the treatment of invasive candidiasis, treatment of invasive aspergillosis, and empirical therapy of fungal infections in the setting of febrile neutropenia.[85-87] The usual dosing includes loading with 70 mg IV, followed by 50 mg IV every 24 hours. The safety profile is good with mild elevation of liver enzymes. Patients with hepatic insufficiency (Child-Pugh class B or C) require dosage adjustment to 35 mg/kg IV every 24 hours.[68,88,89] Drug interactions are infrequent, but it is recommended to monitor cyclosporine levels in patients receiving caspofungin.[90] A recent clinical trial showed that higher doses of caspofungin (100 mg/day) are well tolerated but do not necessarily translate into additional clinical benefits.[91]

MICAFUNGIN

Micafungin is approved by the by the FDA for the treatment of esophageal candidiasis, prophylaxis of *Candida* infections in stem cell transplant patients, and treatment of candidemia. Although micafungin has excellent in vitro and in vivo activity against *Aspergillus* and *Candida* spp., clinical data on invasive aspergillosis are limited.[92,93] Micafungin has demonstrated efficacy both for the treatment of invasive candidiasis and as a prophylactic agent for fungal infections in allogeneic stem cell transplant recipients.[94-96] The prophylactic dose is 50 mg IV every 24 hours, and the therapeutic dose for invasive candidiasis is 100 mg IV every 24 hours. As with the other echinocandins, the most frequent adverse event is mild elevation of liver enzymes. No dosage adjustment is required in the setting of renal insufficiency or moderate hepatic insufficiency. Mild drug interactions have been reported with concomitant use of sirolimus and nifedipine.

ANIDULAFUNGIN

As with the other echinocandins, anidulafungin has excellent in vitro and in vivo activity against *Aspergillus* and *Candida* spp.[97] It is currently indicated for the treatment of invasive candidiasis, having demonstrated noninferiority, and perhaps superiority, in a clinical trial versus fluconazole.[98] The usual dosing includes a loading dose of 200 mg IV, followed by 100 mg IV every 24 hours. Anidulafungin does not require dosage adjustment for patients with renal or hepatic failure and no significant drug interactions are reported.[97,99,100]

SPECIFIC INDICATIONS AND USES FOR ANTIFUNGAL THERAPY

Although the precise diagnosis of a fungal infection may be laborious, time-consuming, and delayed, therapy should never be withheld in a critically ill patient with suspected or confirmed fungal infection. Empirical therapy will often be started with amphotericin B or one of its lipid preparations and then tailored according to the final identification of the organism. This section presents generally accepted treatment recommendations for the most commonly encountered fungal infections in the critical care setting. Infections by less common fungi may be particularly severe and rapidly progressive and require consultation with an infectious diseases specialist for appropriate treatment. Table 52.2 summarizes the most often encountered fungal diseases in the critical care setting with their generally accepted treatment options. Figure 52.1 presents our approach for the critically ill patient with fungemia.

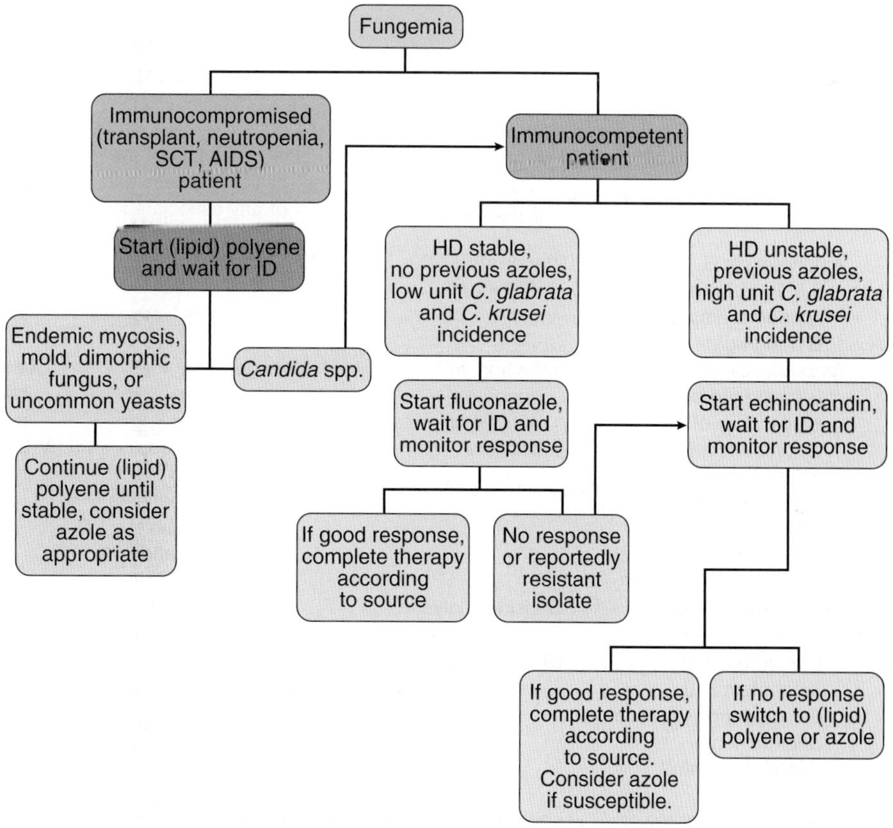

Figure 52.1 Treating the critically ill patient with fungemia. HD, hemodynamically; ID, identification to species level; SCT, stem cell transplant. (Modified from Ostrosky-Zeichner L, Pappas PG: Invasive candidiasis in the intensive care unit. Crit Care Med 2006;34:857-863.)

Table 52.2 Summary of Therapeutic Choices for Fungal Diseases Most Commonly Encountered in the Critical Care Setting

Fungal Disease	Therapy of Choice	Alternative Therapy	Duration of Treatment	Comments
Candidiasis				
Oral candidiasis	Nystatin 200,000-U lozenges qid or 500,000-U suspension swish and swallow qid	Fluconazole 200 mg single dose or 100 mg/day PO	3-5 days	
Mucosal nonoral candidiasis	Topical azole	Fluconazole 200 mg first dose, then 100 mg/day	7-14 days	
Candidemia and most forms of disseminated candidiasis	Amphotericin B 0.5-0.6 mg/kg/d or lipid preparation of amphotericin B 3 mg/kg/d; fluconazole 400 mg qd; voriconazole 4-6 mg/kg/q12h; caspofungin 50 mg/d; anidulafungin 100 mg/d; *or* micafungin 100 mg/d		14 days after bloodstream clearance for uncomplicated candidemia; until resolution of sites of infection if disseminated	Line removal recommended Assess for dissemination A candin or lipid amphotericin B usually preferred for initial therapy if patient is unstable or infected with a non-*albicans* species Loading doses recommended for caspofungin and anidulafungin
Urinary candidiasis	Fluconazole 200 mg first day, then 100 mg/day *or* amphotericin B 0.3 mg/kg IV single dose	Amphotericin B bladder washes, 50 mg/1000 mL H_2O in continuous irrigation for 2 days	7-14 days	Asymptomatic funguria does not require treatment but may be a sign of dissemination in compromised hosts Urinary catheter removal is very useful
Peritonitis	As for disseminated candidiasis			Removal of dialysis catheter is helpful Surgical débridement if abscess present
Aspergillosis	Voriconazole 4-6 mg/kg/q12h	Lipid preparation of amphotericin B 3 mg/kg/d	Until resolution of the clinical process and of any associated immunosuppression	May require surgical treatment
Histoplasmosis	Amphotericin B 0.5-1 mg/kg/d or liposomal amphotericin B 5 mg/kg/d	Itraconazole 200-400 mg/d	3-12 months	Lifelong suppression needed in HIV-infected patients
Cryptococcosis (in HIV-infected patients)	Amphotericin B 0.5-0.7 mg/kg/d or lipid preparation of amphotericin B 3-5 mg/kg/d + 5-FC induction 25 mg/kg/q6h, fluconazole 400 mg/d maintenance	Induction with fluconazole 400 mg/d in stable patients	Managed very differently in HIV-infected (lifelong therapy needed) and uninfected patients (cure is possible) Expert consultation advised	Consider frequent LP to relieve intracranial pressure V-P shunts may be necessary
Zygomycosis	Amphotericin B 0.8-1.5 mg/kg/d or lipid preparation of amphotericin B 3-5 mg/kg/d + surgical débridement + metabolic control	Consider polyene + caspofungin Limited experience with posaconazole		Surgical débridement is critical

5-FC, 5-flucytosine; HIV, human immunodeficiency virus; LP, lumbar puncture; V-P, ventriculoperitoneal.

CANDIDA INFECTIONS

Although *C. albicans* remains the most common pathogen in oropharyngeal and cutaneous candidiasis, non-*albicans* species of *Candida* are increasingly frequent causes of invasive candidiasis.[101] Guidelines and reviews for therapy of candidiasis in the intensive care setting have recently been published.[102-105] These guidelines are extensive and will not be repeated in detail. Rather, the text will focus on several clinical situations in which candidal infections are particularly challenging for the critical care specialist.

CANDIDEMIA AND DISSEMINATED CANDIDIASIS

The diagnosis of disseminated candidiasis is always a challenge.[106] There is no single tool that conclusively makes this diagnosis. Isolation of *Candida* from the bloodstream is simply the most obvious form of disseminated candidiasis, but clinical experience makes it obvious that disseminated candidiasis can occur in the absence of detectable fungemia.

Candidemia may be treated initially with either fluconazole, voriconazole, amphotericin B (or its lipid preparations), or an echinocandin. In the critically ill and unstable patient, an echinocandin or amphotericin B lipid preparations is preferred because of the broader spectrum of activity and more rapid onset of action.[104,107] Owing to their greater safety, echinocandins are increasingly viewed as the initial agents of choice, and in fact, both the anidulafungin study and recent patient level meta-analysis of the candidemia clinical trials suggest that initial therapy with echinocandins may be superior to initial therapy with azoles.[98,108]

The susceptibility of *Candida* to the currently available antifungal agents can generally be predicted if the species of the infecting isolate is known.[10,12,101,109-117] Bloodstream isolates of *C. albicans*, *C. tropicalis*, and *C. parapsilosis* are generally susceptible to fluconazole and amphotericin B. Isolates of *C. glabrata* and *C. krusei* will often (if not always, as is the case with *C. krusei*) be resistant to fluconazole. Isolates of *C. lusitaniae* may be resistant to amphotericin B. Antifungal susceptibility testing is becoming increasingly important as a guide in the treatment of these infections.[118] In particular, detection of fluconazole resistance is very valuable, as it provides support for continued use of echinocandins or polyenes.

Although all *Candida* spp. are generally considered to be susceptible to echinocandins, *C. parapsilosis* has higher minimum inhibitory concentrations (MICs) than the other *Candida* spp. This, however, has not translated into reduced activity in clinical trials.[85,119] Once the organism is speciated, or if the prevalence of more resistant species is low, therapy may be switched to fluconazole. Fluconazole has demonstrated to be as effective in clearing candidemia as amphotericin B in immunocompetent hosts. Duration of treatment is 14 days following the last positive culture,[21] and if a central line is present, removal is highly recommended. If evidence of disseminated candidiasis is found, therapy should be prolonged to at least 4 weeks to ensure proper organ clearance.

THE INTRAVENOUS CATHETER IN CANDIDEMIC PATIENTS

Although long an area of contention, current data strongly suggest that candidemia is often related to (if not primarily propagated by) a central venous catheter. Central venous catheters in particular have been found to be both a risk factor for developing candidemia[120-123] and associated with persistent fungemia.[121] Removal of the catheter has been associated with shorter duration of subsequent candidemia[124] and improved patient outcome.[125,126] Unique to the species of *Candida*, candidemia with *C. parapsilosis* is almost always due to a catheter.[127,128] The situation may be different for neutropenic patients, particularly those who have permanent, lower-risk catheters such as Hickman catheters. Such catheters may of course become infected, but these patients may also have candidemia due to entry of the organisms from the gut into the bloodstream. This concept is supported by demonstrations that *Candida* can enter the bloodstream from the gut,[129] by the relative lack of effect of catheter removal in a large cohort of cancer patients,[128] and by the frequent demonstration of gut wall invasion in patients who die with disseminated candidiasis.[130,131] Unfortunately, there is no convincing way to tell if a given catheter is involved. Differential quantitative blood cultures through the line and from a peripheral site have been suggested to be one approach to resolving this problem,[132] but this technique remains controversial.[133] On a practical basis, serious consideration to line removal should be given if fungemia persists for more than a few days. A recent patient level meta-analysis of the major candidemia clinical trials has confirmed a mortality rate reduction and microbiologic cure benefit for this approach.[108]

MUCOSAL INFECTIONS AND COLONIZATION

Although there are many risk factors for development of disseminated candidiasis, colonization at one or more nonsterile sites represents an unusually strong risk factor.[134] As discussed earlier, local oral and mucosal candidiasis should thus be considered as a predictor of possible invasive disease in the critically ill or immunocompromised host.[135,136] Esophageal candidiasis does require systemic treatment. Fluconazole is generally preferred here, although amphotericin B and the candins can also be used.

CANDIDURIA

Treatment of asymptomatic candiduria produces only temporary clearing of the urine and is probably not indicated.[22,23] However, candiduria should probably be treated in symptomatic patients, immunocompromised patients, low-birth-weight infants, renal transplant patients, and patients who will undergo urologic manipulation or surgery.[102] If treatment is indicated, systemic therapy with amphotericin or fluconazole is preferred, and amphotericin bladder washes should be reserved for patients with renal insufficiency and low renal clearance. Removal of the urinary catheter is by itself a useful intervention and should always be considered.

OTHER FORMS OF INVASIVE CANDIDIASIS

There are many other possible forms of invasive candidiasis: meningitis, endocarditis, and osteomyelitis, just to name a few. This area has recently been reviewed,[103] and for most forms of this disease there are very few specific studies on therapy. The largest body of data will always be anecdotal reports of use of amphotericin B, and for essentially every form there are at least a few reports of successful therapy with fluconazole. In general, amphotericin B is preferred when the infection is most acute, when data on the nature of the infection are still being generated in the laboratory, or when the patient has previously received azole therapy. Fluconazole provides a good way to step down to an oral agent to complete therapy of infections due to susceptible isolates. Data for the echinocandins are starting to accumulate for these chronic infections.[137] Removal of foreign body and standard surgical drainage are often key as well. An excellent example of the need to remove foreign bodies is found in treatment of dialysis catheter-related peritoneal candidiasis in which catheter removal is important. Surgical drainage is of course important in candidal peritonitis related to gut injury and fecal spillage.

CRYPTOCOCCOSIS

Treatment of cryptococcosis has recently been reviewed.[138,139] Cryptococcal meningitis in non–human immunodeficiency virus (HIV)-infected adults continues to be seen sporadically. The majority of the published experience as to treatment is with amphotericin B given for 4 to 6 weeks.[140,141] Because this therapy is curative in approximately two thirds of patients, this approach is warranted. Expert consultation is also appropriate for this relatively uncommon infection.[142,143]

On the other hand, cryptococcal meningitis in the HIV-infected patient is a well-established and common problem. Meningeal cryptococcosis in this setting should be treated with a 2-week course of IV amphotericin B or its lipid preparations,[139,144,145] followed by life-long suppression with fluconazole.[146,147] Current trends favor also using 5-FC unless there is a contraindication.[50] Although itraconazole does not penetrate the CSF, anecdotal evidence has shown that it may be useful in treating CNS disease, although it is apparently less potent as a long-term therapy.[148]

For all forms of cryptococcal meningitis, intracranial hypertension should be aggressively treated with repeated lumbar puctures or a CSF shunt.[149,150] The addition of steroids and other immune modulating agents to antifungal therapy has shown promising results in animal models,[151] and clinical trials are being conducted. The immune reconstitution syndrome plays a major role in cryptococcal-related morbidity in HIV patients and the current recommendation is to delay antiretroviral therapy for a few weeks after treatment for cryptococcosis is started.[139]

ASPERGILLOSIS

Treatment of aspergillosis has been extensively reviewed.[152-154] Invasive aspergillosis should be considered in any severely immunocompromised patient with an unexplained pulmonary or sinonasal process. Biopsy is normally required for definitive diagnosis, although a new generation of galactomannan-based serodiagnostic tests may prove useful as adjuncts to diagnosis.[155,156] Although amphotericin B has classically been the initial treatment of choice for invasive aspergillosis, the current treatment of choice is voriconazole[65,74] or a lipid preparation of amphotericin B. Aggressive surgical management is necessary and curative in some cases.[106,157] Itraconazole has historically been an option for the treatment of aspergillosis in patients who are intolerant or refractory to amphotericin B, but newer and more effective azoles are now available.[158] Overall, the outlook for invasive aspergillosis is critically dependent on recovery of immune function. Without this, the prognosis is usually dismal. Of note, recent studies have documented an increase in incidence of invasive aspergillosis in nonhematology, nontransplant patients seen in the intensive care unit (ICU), such as chronic obstructive pulmonary disease and autoimmune diseases.[159,160] This trend should be monitored, and the critical care specialist should be suspicious when cultures of *Aspergillus* from a bronchoalveolar lavage or diagnostic markers such as galactomannan are positive.[161]

HISTOPLASMOSIS

The initial treatment of choice for severe acute histoplasmosis is an amphotericin B preparation.[162-164] Noncritical cases may be treated with itraconazole 200 to 400 mg/day. Fluconazole is only moderately effective and should not be used as primary therapy.[165] Successful treatment results in a decrease of serum and urine *Histoplasma* antigen.[166] Duration of therapy is a function of disease form and underlying immune status. HIV-infected patients with disseminated disease should be treated as acute histoplasmosis and maintained on life-long suppression with itraconazole. Liposomal amphotericin B has shown excellent efficacy in this setting.[167] Non-HIV-infected patients may require from 3 to 12 months of therapy, and expert consultation is generally advised.

MUCORMYCOSIS

The treatment of choice for mucormycosis (infections typically caused by *Mucor* spp., *Rhizopus* spp., and *Absidia* spp.) is aggressive surgical débridement and prompt start of high-dose amphotericin B or a lipid preparation.[168] Follow-up therapy with itraconazole may be warranted, and expert consultation is advised. Posaconazole has shown efficacy in this setting.[78] More recently, and despite the lack of in vitro activity of echinocandins against these agents, investigators have shown in vitro synergy and excellent clinical outcomes with the combination of amphotericin B and caspofungin.[169] Correction of metabolic abnormalities (acidosis, iron overload, and hyperglycemia) should also be pursued aggressively.

OTHER FUNGAL INFECTIONS

Other fungal infections, such as blastomycosis, fusariosis, and infection by *Trichosporon* spp., *Coccidioides immitis, Malassezia furfur,* and *Penicillium* spp. may be occasionally encountered in the critical care setting, particularly when caring for immunocompromised hosts. Although amphotericin B is probably the best empirical drug for any characterized suspected fungal infection, it is not very effective against some of these pathogens. Guidelines for treating some of these infections have been published.[1] Expert consultation should be promptly obtained.

AREAS OF CONTROVERSY IN ANTIFUNGAL THERAPY

EMPIRICAL ANTIFUNGAL THERAPY FOR THE FEBRILE ICU PATIENT

Fever in the ICU patient is a complex problem that requires prompt evaluation for many possible sources, including infection, atelectasis, pulmonary embolism, drug fever, thermoregulatory dysfunction, and many more.[170] Infection by *Candida* should be suspected when the patient has risk factors such as immunocompromise, broad-spectrum antibiotic therapy, parenteral nutrition, steroids, surgery (especially if the gut wall is transected), urinary catheters, and burns.[171,172]

Unfortunately, making a diagnosis of invasive candidiasis is difficult. In the most straightforward scenario, the patient is febrile and has positive blood cultures for *Candida.* On other occasions, biopsy or aspiration is used to make a clear-cut diagnosis of a localized abscess due to *Candida.* These situations are, however, the exception. Far more common is the scenario of a persistently febrile ICU patient with a combination of the previously mentioned risk factors. In this setting, we place great importance on the presence of positive cultures from nonsterile sites such as wounds, sputum, or stool. The key concept is that presence of *Candida* at any of these sites significantly increases the likelihood of developing invasive disease.[134,173] Positive cultures from the urine are also considered in this context (even though that is normally a sterile site). Candiduria in the afebrile patient is generally a clinical non-event that does not require therapy,[22,23] but candiduria in the febrile ICU patient at the very least represents colonization and increased risk of invasive disease and at the worse represents actual upper urinary tract infection. A similar logic applies to *Candida* in the sputum. Pneumonia due to *Candida* occurs but is generally clinically inapparent.[174] The presence of *Candida* in the sputum more often means that the gut, and thus the patient, is colonized. This, in turn, is a risk factor as discussed previously.

Research has shown conclusively that delays to appropriate antifungal therapy in ICU patients with invasive candidiasis are associated with increased mortality rates.[175] The latest version of the IDSA guidelines recommend empirical antifungal therapy in critically ill patients who are deemed to be at high risk for the infection based on a variety of recently available scoring systems and risk assessment strategies.[105,176-180] On the other hand, there is a negative multicenter study that failed to show a benefit to fluconazole in this setting.[181]

ANTIFUNGAL PROPHYLAXIS IN THE ICU

Prevention is always preferred to therapy, and this is certainly true for invasive candidiasis. Although prevention of mucosal disease can be achieved with almost any regimen, prevention of invasive disease has consistently required systemic therapy. Both fluconazole and amphotericin B are effective in the right setting. The key is to select patient populations with a meaningful chance of contracting invasive candidiasis. The value of prophylaxis has been shown convincingly for bone marrow transplantation patients[182,183] and selected liver transplant patients.[184-187] Studies of patients receiving standard chemotherapy for leukemia have shown a trend favoring prophylaxis,[188,189] but the lower rates of disease in the control group lower the statistical power of the studies. To further confuse matters, even a group that sounds homogeneous (e.g., allogeneic bone marrow transplant recipients) really is not—different forms of chemotherapy and degrees of graft-versus-host disease produce different levels of risk. This point was driven home in an editorial emphasizing the range of variation within the category of "neutropenic patient."[190]

In practical terms, three major studies have demonstrated benefits to prophylaxis of invasive candidiasis in the ICU.[191-193] No study or meta-analysis has shown benefits in terms of mortality rates, however.[194-197] These studies have the limitation of being single center studies and having limited numbers of patients. Most experts would agree with the fact that routine use of antifungal prophylaxis should be reserved for units with a high incidence of invasive candidiasis or for carefully selected patients at the highest risk.[103,105]

DURATION OF THERAPY AND ACCUMULATED DOSING

Optimum dose and duration of therapy have not been clearly defined in most fungal infections. Most of the recommended doses and guidelines presented in this chapter have been developed empirically or from extrapolation from other infections or animal models. Response and duration of treatment should be evaluated primarily on a clinical basis when feasible. Surrogate markers such as cell wall antigens or antibody assays, as well as imaging when appropriate, have also shown to be useful in infections such as cryptococcosis, histoplasmosis, and aspergillosis.

MEASUREMENT OF DRUG LEVELS

Drug level monitoring is theoretically justified to assure efficacy and avoid toxicity. However, drug level monitoring during antifungal therapy is relatively new and should not be carried out routinely because there is a lack of information on its clinical correlation and meaning. Situations in which drug level monitoring has proved to be useful are itraconazole levels to verify adequate absorption when using the oral forms of this compound, 5-FC levels to watch for possible myelotoxicity, and voriconazole/posaconazole levels to document absorption of the drugs when given orally.[198,199]

SUSCEPTIBILITY TESTING

The Clinical Laboratory Standards Institute has published a guideline for standardized antifungal susceptibility testing that has been widely adopted[200] and subsequently revised. This methodology is recommended for testing *Candida* and *Cryptococcus* spp. and breakpoints have been developed.[201] Antifungal susceptibility testing is now widely available and should be considered when treating serious *Candida* infections, when treatment failure occurs, or when toxicity or side effects limit the use of a particular drug. It should also be remembered that pharmacology, safety, published experience, and drug interactions must be considered along with susceptibility when selecting a therapy.[102,105] Mold susceptibility has also been standardized but is not routinely recommended.

ANTIVIRAL AGENTS

Antiviral chemotherapy has made great advances since the 1980s. Before then a diagnosis of a life-threatening viral infection meant mostly supportive therapy and patience. Although still limited, today we have a host of treatment options for herpetic infections; upper and lower respiratory illness by influenza, cytomegalovirus (CMV), and respiratory syncytial virus (RSV); and some relatively exotic systemic diseases. Therapy for HIV, hepatitis B, and hepatitis C infection has also made gigantic leaps, but it is usually not undertaken in the critical care setting and is thus beyond the scope of this chapter. Table 52.3 summarizes the currently available non-HIV specific antiviral drugs and their general spectrum.

ACYCLOVIR, FAMCICLOVIR, AND VALACYCLOVIR

Acyclovir is a nucleoside analog of guanine that has in vitro and in vivo activity against several viruses in the herpesvirus family, particularly against herpes simplex virus type 1 (HSV-1), HSV-2, varicella-zoster virus (VZV), and Epstein-Barr virus (EBV). High concentrations also inhibit CMV. It inhibits DNA polymerase causing DNA chain termination.[202-204] Acyclovir is the treatment of choice for severe herpetic infections in immunocompetent and immunocompromised hosts. Resistance due to viral thymidine kinase mutations or, less often, DNA polymerase mutations may emerge in patients with severe immunocompromise such as transplant recipients and advanced HIV infection during treatment of HSV and VZV infections.[205-207] Acyclovir has also been used for CMV prophylaxis in transplant patients.[208,209] Acyclovir is available in oral, IV, and topical forms. Bioavailability of the oral form is poor (15-21%), requiring high dosage/frequent doses. Protein binding is less than 20%. CSF penetration is low, but acyclovir is active for CNS infections. The topical form is virtually unabsorbed. The half-life is short and the drug is cleared by the kidneys, so dosage adjustment in renal failure and hemodyalisis is required. Supplementation is not needed in peritoneal dialysis. Side effects are uncommon.[210] The main concern with acyclovir therapy is the crystallization of the drug in the renal tubules, leading to renal failure. Aggressive hydration and monitoring of renal function are recommended during IV acyclovir therapy. Oral acyclovir may cause nausea and vomiting. The usual oral dose is 200 to 800 mg every 4 hours. The IV dosing range for severe infections is 8 to 12 mg/kg IV every 8 hours. Proven encephalitis is treated with 10 to 12 mg/kg every 8 hours for 14 to 21 days. Doses of up to 20 mg/kg may be more effective in premature infants.[211]

Famciclovir, the prodrug of penciclovir (a guanosine analog),[212,213] is a well-absorbed oral agent that has shown excellent activity against first-episode or recurrent genital herpes and HSV/VZV infection in both HIV and immunocompetent hosts.[214-216] A dose of 500 mg orally three times a day was shown to be as effective as acyclovir for treatment of herpes zoster.[217]

Valacyclovir, an analog of acyclovir that has a similar profile of side effects, is now available in oral formulations with the advantage of longer dosing intervals. It appears comparable to acyclovir for treatment of mucocutaneous HSV infections, but more effective in herpes zoster. It is also effective orally for prophylaxis of CMV in renal transplant patients.[218] The dosing range is 500 to 1000 mg orally two to three times a day.[219-221] Although absorption is excellent, there is little data to support treating invasive disease, such as CNS disease, with this drug.

GANCICLOVIR AND VALGANCICLOVIR

Ganciclovir is another nucleoside analog of guanine but has a slightly wider antiviral spectrum than acyclovir. It is highly active against CMV, as well as HSV-1, HSV-2, and EBV. Like acyclovir it acts by interference with DNA polymerase, but it is not an obligate chain terminator. Resistance to ganciclovir by CMV and HSV is increasingly reported. HSV isolates that are thymidine kinase–deficient and thus resistant

Table 52.3 Spectrum of Antiviral Agents

Susceptible Virus	Acyclovir/ Valacyclovir/ Famciclovir	Ganciclovir/ Valganciclovir	Foscarnet	Cidofovir	Amantadine/ Rimantadine	Ribavirin	Oseltamivir/ Zanamivir
HSV-1	++*	++	++	++	0	0	0
HSV-2	++*	++	++	++	0	0	0
VZV	++*	++	++	++	0	0	0
CMV	±*	++*	++	++	0	0	0
EBV	+	++	++	++	0	0	0
Influenza A	0	0	0	0	++*	+	++*
Influenza B	0	0	0	0	0	+	++*

CMV, cytomegalovirus; EBV, Epstein-Barr virus; HSV, herpes simplex virus; VZV, varicella-zoster virus.
0, no known activity; ±, active under specific circumstances; +, active; ++, very active.
*Resistant strains reported.

to acyclovir will also be resistant to ganciclovir.[207,222] It is mainly indicated in prophylaxis, treatment, and suppression of CMV syndromes in immunocompromised patients.[208,223-227] Ganciclovir is available in oral, intraocular, and IV forms, the first two being useful only in chronic suppression of CMV disease. Once it reaches the bloodstream it has body-wide distribution, low protein binding, and low CNS penetration. Excretion is renal and dosage adjustment is required in renal failure. Ganciclovir is removed by hemodialysis, and therefore it should be administered after dialysis. Side effects of IV ganciclovir include severe neutropenia (40%), thrombocytopenia (20%), phlebitis, rash, increased liver enzymes, and azotemia. The nephrotoxicity is potentiated by concomitant use of nephrotoxic agents and acyclovir. Ganciclovir should not be used in pregnant women because it is known to be teratogenic. The usual dose in acute infection is 5 mg/kg every 12 hours. Maintenance therapy at 5 mg/kg IV every day should be continued as long as the patient is immunocompromised. Discontinuation of therapy in acquired immunodeficiency syndrome (AIDS) patients appears feasible following immune reconstitution.[208,223,228,229] An intraocular delivery system is also available as an adjunct to the treatment of CMV retinitis.

Valganciclovir is an L-valyl ester of ganciclovir that has significantly increased bioavailability over previous oral formulations of ganciclovir, resulting in levels previously unattainable with the traditional formulations. It allows for prophylaxis and treatment of CMV infections with an oral alternative. The usual dose for prophylaxis is 900 mg orally every 24 hours, and for treatment the recommended induction dose is 900 mg orally every 12 hours, followed by a maintenance dose of 900 mg orally every 24 hours. This drug requires adjustment for patients with renal impairment.[230,231]

CIDOFOVIR

Cidofovir is a nucleotide analog with activity against most herpesviruses. Its activation is not virus-enzyme dependent, so it has activity against most acyclovir-resistant HSV and ganciclovir-resistant CMV. Resistant strains have also been reported, and synergy with ganciclovir and foscarnet has been reported. Oral bioavailability is very low. It is 6% protein bound and is excreted by the kidneys.[232,233] Its side effects include neutropenia and nephrotoxicity, which can manifest as proteinuria, azotemia, and a Fanconi-like renal syndrome. It has been shown to be teratogenic and mutagenic and is contraindicated in pregnancy. It is currently licensed for CMV retinitis in HIV infection but has also shown activity against acyclovir-resistant HSV.[234,235] The usual dose is 5 mg/kg every week for 2 weeks, then 5 mg/kg every other week.

FOSCARNET

Foscarnet is a pyrophosphate analog that has antiviral activity against the herpesviruses, HIV, and hepatitis B virus. Its mechanism of action is interference with DNA polymerase or reverse transcriptase to block effective viral replication. Viral isolates that are resistant to ganciclovir or acyclovir are often susceptible to foscarnet, but primary resistance to foscarnet has also been described, particularly in HIV-infected patients.[205,206,236-238] The main therapeutic indication of foscarnet is ganciclovir-resistant CMV disease. Foscarnet is only available in IV formulations and it has body-wide distribution. Protein binding is 15% and it has good CSF penetration. The drug is excreted almost intact by the kidneys and requires very careful dosage adjustment in renal failure. Foscarnet is removed by hemodialysis but should be avoided in patients with severe renal dysfunction. Its main side effect is nephrotoxicity, which occurs in most patients but is reversible when therapy is stopped.[239] Dosage adjustment should be made by following the CrCl closely. Hypocalcemia and hypercalcemia as well as phosphate abnormalities are common, so monitoring of electrolytes is also recommended. The usual dose is 60 mg/kg every 8 hours for CMV infections and 40 mg/kg every 8 hours for treating acyclovir-resistant HSV infections.

AMANTADINE AND RIMANTADINE

Amantadine is a tricyclic amine inhibitor of influenza A virus. Its mechanism of action involves inhibition of the transmembrane domain of the viral M2 protein, thus preventing viral uncoating during early stages of replication. It has activity against influenza A but no clinical activity against influenza B.[240-243] Resistant strains can be developed in vitro and are also seen in household and nursing home contacts exposed to persons treated for acute influenza. It is indicated in influenza A prophylaxis and treatment and also for management of Parkinson's disease and drug-induced extrapyramidal reactions. It is well absorbed orally and has body-wide distribution. It is 67% bound to plasma proteins and excreted unchanged in the urine by glomerular filtration and tubular secretion. The usual adult dosage for both prophylaxis and treatment is 100 mg twice a day. The dosage must be reduced in elderly patients and patients with renal insufficiency. In individuals who are 65 or older, the dose should be reduced to 100 mg every day. The dose for a CrCl less than 10 mL/minute is 200 mg per week. The most common adverse events are related to the CNS and correlate directly with high levels. Patients may present with confusion, seizures, hallucinations, and coma. Amantadine also causes GI upset.

Rimantadine is another tryciclic amine with similar properties, spectrum, and indications as amantadine.[244,245] The main difference lies in its extensive metabolism by the liver and its minimal renal clearance, but it also requires dosage adjustment in advanced liver and kidney insufficiency (CrCl < 10 mL/minute) as well as in the elderly. Its major advantage is less frequent CNS toxicity. Dosage is 100 mg twice a day.

RIBAVIRIN

Ribavirin is a triazole nucleoside analog that has broad-spectrum antiviral activity. It is effective in vitro against RSV, influenza A and B, HSV, HIV, hepatitis C virus, and viruses causing hemorrhagic fevers.[215,246-248] Its currently approved clinical indications are treatment of pediatric patients with severe RSV infection, and in combination with injected interferon alfa and ribavirin capsules, it is approved for treatment of chronic hepatitis C.[249,250] The IV form has been shown to reduce mortality rate in Korean/Asian hemorrhagic fever with renal syndrome.[251] Its mechanism of action is not fully understood and intrinsic resistance has not been reported. It is available in oral, aerosolized, and IV formulations. It has high bioavailability through the oral or aerosolized forms and it is metabolized by the liver. Toxicity in the aerosolized formulation consists primarily of severe bronchospasm and cardiac rhythm abnormalities. The IV formulation also causes hemolytic anemia. Use in ventilated patients requires experienced personnel because environmental leaking and diffusion are common.[252] Recommended dosage is 1.1 g/day of ribavirin administered by continuous aerozolization for 12 to 18 hours/day for 3 to 7 days. It should not be combined with other aerosolized medications. Induction of bronchospasm is common, and scheduled use of a bronchodilator may be required during ribarvirin therapy.

OSELTAMIVIR

Oseltamivir is a sialic acid neuraminidase inhibitor that has recently become available for the treatment of both influenza A and B.[253-255] Its mechanism of action is inhibition of the viral neuraminidase, causing in turn inhibition of virus release from infected cells and spread in the respiratory tract. Drug resistance has already been reported in vitro in strains with mutations that cause changes in the viral neuraminidase or hemagglutinin. In clinical studies of adults, only 1% to 2% of posttreatment strains showed evidence of mutations with decreased neuraminidase susceptibility. Recent reports have mentioned infrequent resistance in avian influenza and H1N1 strains [256-258] Cross-resistance between oseltamivir and zanamivir, the other member of the class, has also been observed in vitro. It is indicated for the prevention and early treatment of uncomplicated acute influenza A and B.[259] Major clinical trials have demonstrated that oseltamivir reduces the duration, severity, and rate of complications requiring antibiotic use.[255] Its role in complicated cases such as those seen in the critical care setting is unclear at this time, although the 2009 H1N1 epidemic contributed a wealth of data related to its use in critically ill patients.[260,261] Oseltamivir is available in an oral form, which has greater than 75% bioavailability. The drug is converted to oseltamivir carboxylate that is eliminated unchanged in the urine. Less than 20% of the dose is eliminated in feces. Dose adjustment is recommended for renal failure and geriatric patients when CrCl is less than 30 mL/minute.[262] The recommended dose in such settings is 75 mg orally every 24 hours for 5 days. Clinically relevant drug interactions have not been identified. Side effects, which include nausea, vomiting, and abdominal pain, are usually mild. The recommended dosage is 75 mg orally twice daily for 5 days and it is recommended that treatment is begun within 2 days of symptom onset. New formulations of IV oseltamivir are being developed.[263]

ZANAMIVIR

Zanamivir is another sialic acid analog neuraminidase inhibitor that was recently approved for the treatment of both influenza A and B.[253,264] Much like oseltamivir, its mechanism of action is by neuraminidase inhibition with subsequent inhibition of viral release and spread. Resistant strains have also been identified in vitro, and a resistant strain was also recovered from an immunocompromised patient with influenza B after 2 weeks of nebulized treatment.[265,266] It is indicated in acute cases of influenza with early onset of treatment.[254,267-269] Trials on patients with more severe disease are ongoing.[270,271] Experience is also building with its use in prophylaxis.[240,272,273] Zanamivir is available in a powder form for oral inhalation. A new IV formulation is also under development.[274] Approximately 4% to 17% of the dose is absorbed and less than 10% of the drug is protein bound. It is excreted unchanged in the urine and unabsorbed drug is cleared in the feces. No dosage adjustment in renal or hepatic failure is recommended at this time, but experience is limited. Zanamivir does not have significant drug interactions.[275,276] Bronchospasm may be precipitated particularly in patients with underlying lung disease.[277] The recommended dose is 10 mg (two inhalations) twice a day for 5 days.

SPECIFIC INDICATIONS AND USES FOR ANTIVIRAL THERAPY

HERPES SIMPLEX AND VARICELLA-ZOSTER

Acyclovir, famciclovir, and valacyclovir are the drugs of choice in the treatment of virtually all severe herpetic infections.[203,204, 215, 278-285] The greater oral bioavailability of famciclovir and valacyclovir makes these agents very attractive, especially for treatment of VZV. Although primary HSV-1 and -2 infections can be treated orally, immunocompromised patients or severely ill patients will require IV therapy. A high index of suspicion for dissemination should be maintained in immunocompromised patients—mild, localized, or atypical disease may progress to fulminant disease. Duration of therapy in this setting is usually 7 to 14 days.

Herpetic encephalitis has had a substantial decrease in morbidity and mortality rates since acyclovir was introduced. Being one of the few forms of viral encephalitis for which there is a treatment, empirical use of the drug is justified when viral disease is suspected and until it is ruled out. HSV polymerase chain reaction (PCR) of CSF is a very sensitive and specific test for the diagnosis of this disease. The usual dose is 10 to 12 mg/kg every 8 hours for 14 to 21 days. Visceral infections, including esophagitis, hepatitis, pneumonia, and disseminated disease, are frequent in immunocompromised patients and should be treated with 5 to 10 mg/kg every 8 hours for 14 to 21 days. HSV may also cause aseptic meningitis without encephalitis in setting of primary or recurrent genital HSV infection. Unlike the focal necrotizing disease seen with HSV encephalitis, this form of the disease is a mild self-limited aseptic meningitis with a good prognosis.

Finally, acyclovir-resistant HSV infections, which are an increasing problem in the immunocompromised population,[206,207, 286,287] can be treated with foscarnet or cidofovir.

Primary VZV infection (chickenpox) should be treated in all adults, especially in the immunocompromised.[278,281,285,288,289] Reactivation (shingles) should be treated because treatment has been shown to decrease duration and intensity of symptoms.[290,291] Mild cases may be treated with oral famciclovir or valacyclovir. Severe cases (disseminated, immunocompromised patients with involvement of more than one dermatome, or ophthalmic involvement) should be treated with IV acyclovir. It is important to remember that these patients are contagious and should be suitably isolated using airborne precautions. As with HSV, resistant strains may be treated with foscarnet.[292,293]

CYTOMEGALOVIRUS INFECTION

CMV infections require treatment in immunocompromised patients. Populations at increased risk of the disease are HIV-infected patients and transplant recipients. In HIV patients, both retinal and visceral involvement are initially treated with IV ganciclovir at 5 mg/kg every 12 hours for 2 weeks.[208,223,224] Valganciclovir is a suitable oral formulation for the treatment of this infection. Various maintenance options are increasingly available (including ganciclovir ocular implants) but are beyond the scope of this chapter. Resistant cases may be treated with foscarnet 60 mg/kg every 8 hours for 2 weeks [229,236] or cidofovir. Clinical and laboratory monitoring while on either of these drugs is essential to avoid therapy-related complications. Refractory cases may be treated with cidofovir.

In the transplant patient, the combination of ganciclovir and IV immunoglobulin is now the treatment of choice for CMV pneumonia.[223,294-296] High doses of acyclovir are useful as prophylaxis of CMV in the transplant patient but not in the HIV setting. Ganciclovir-resistant strains should be treated with foscarnet.

INFLUENZA

Clear benefit in the treatment of influenza is consistently seen only when patients are treated early in the course of the disease.[253,297-300] Therapeutic options (which can also be used prophylactically) include amantadine/rimantadine, oseltamivir, and zanamivir.[301-306] In patients who present later in the course of the disease, the benefits of therapy are unstudied. Prevention of complications has not been clearly demonstrated. Further trials are required to demonstrate whether one class of drugs is superior to the other and whether they have a role in the critically ill patient. Rapid diagnosis of influenza is now available through different techniques that detect viral components in upper respiratory tract samples. These techniques are useful in detecting and treating infected hospitalized patients early and in regional surveillance of influenza. However, a negative test does not completely rule out influenza, and empirical therapy of ambulatory patients with a clinical syndrome strongly suggesting influenza is probably appropriate.

Avian and pandemic influenza have received much attention from the scientific community and the media in the past 2 years. Considerable efforts are being carried out for surveillance, prompt detection, and containment of these diseases.[307-310] Critical care specialists should have increased awareness and involve infection control and public health authorities in patients with particularly severe forms of influenza with the appropriate epidemiologic background. Suspected and confirmed cases should be placed on airborne precautions. As mentioned earlier, although there are scarce reports of neuraminidase inhibitor resistance in some avian influenza strains, these viruses appear to be generally susceptible to oseltamivir and zanamivir.[256,257]

The 2009 H1N1 epidemic virtually changed how we manage influenza in critically ill patients. During this epidemic oseltamvir and zanamivir were frequently used late in the disease and at high doses, also in the setting of extracorporeal membrane oxygenation (ECMO), with variable results.[261, 270, 311-313] At this point the true value of these agents is still unknown, although most experts agree that at the very least they may decrease viral shedding and transmission.

An important consideration is vaccination and postexposure prophylaxis in health care personnel working in acute and chronic care facilities. Appropriate vaccination and influenza control measures in both health care personnel and patients has proved to be effective in decreasing disease and even mortality rates in patients.[314-316]

OTHER VIRAL INFECTIONS

Other potentially treatable viral infections that may be encountered in the critical care setting include parvovirus, for which treatment with IV immunoglobulin has shown some beneficial effects;[317-319] enterovirus, for which a new drug called pleconaril showed only marginal benefits in the setting of meningitis;[320,321] and hemorrhagic fevers and hantavirus, for which ribavirin may be considered despite lack of definitive proof of efficacy.[248] Dengue and yellow fever can be particularly severe and are most effectively managed with aggressive supportive care.

KEY POINTS

- Amphotericin B and its lipid preparations are the treatment of choice for all critically ill patients with an undiagnosed fungal infection. Once diagnosis is made, other therapeutic options may be considered.
- Fluconazole has excellent antifungal activity, mainly against yeasts, but resistance is possible and clinically relevant.
- The echinocandins are a class of antifungal agents with activity against *Candida* and *Aspergillus* with proven efficacy and remarkable safety profiles. They are now considered the treatment of choice for candidemia in critically ill patients.
- Combinations of antifungal agents should be approached carefully, being clearly beneficial only in selected entities such as CNS disease and endocarditis.
- Empirical antifungal use and antifungal prophylaxis in the ICU setting remain controversial and should be reserved for carefully selected units and patients.
- Uncommon and serious mycoses require expert consultation.
- Acyclovir and its analogs are the drugs of choice for treatment of HSV and VZV infections. The new oral formulations (famciclovir and valacyclovir) have

Continued on following page

KEY POINTS (Continued)

greater bioavailability and are preferred in ambulatory patients.

- Ganciclovir is the drug of choice for treatment of CMV infection in immunocompromised hosts. Immunoglobulin therapy is added to this in transplant patients with pneumonia.
- Critical care specialists should have a high index of suspicion for avian and pandemic influenza. Suspected or confirmed cases should be placed on airborne precautions and treated with neuraminidase inhibitors.
- Resistance is an increasing problem in both antifungal and antiviral therapy.

SELECTED REFERENCES

42. Wingard JR, Kubilis P, Lee L, et al: Clinical significance of nephrotoxicity in patients treated with amphotericin B for suspected or proven aspergillosis. Clin Infect Dis 1999;29(6):1402-1407.
65. Herbrecht R, Denning DW, Patterson TF, et al: Voriconazole versus amphotericin B for primary therapy of invasive aspergillosis. N Engl J Med 2002;347(6):408-415.
72. Boucher HW, Groll AH, Chiou CC, Walsh TJ: Newer systemic antifungal agents: Pharmacokinetics, safety and efficacy. Drugs 2004;64(18):1997-2020.
85. Mora-Duarte J, Betts R, Rotstein C, et al: Comparison of caspofungin and amphotericin B for invasive candidiasis. N Engl J Med 2002;347(25):2020-2029.
98. Reboli AC, Rotstein C, Pappas PG, et al: Anidulafungin versus fluconazole for invasive candidiasis. N Engl J Med 2007;356(24):2472-2482.
105. Pappas PG, Kauffman CA, Andes D, et al: Clinical practice guidelines for the management of candidiasis: 2009 update by the Infectious Diseases Society of America. Clin Infect Dis 2009;48(5):503-535.
139. Perfect JR, Dismukes WE, Dromer F, et al: Clinical practice guidelines for the management of cryptococcal disease: 2010 update by the Infectious Diseases Society of America. Clin Infect Dis 2010;50(3):291-322.
154. Walsh TJ, Anaissie EJ, Denning DW, et al: Treatment of aspergillosis: Clinical practice guidelines of the Infectious Diseases Society of America. Clin Infect Dis 2008;46(3):327-360.
181. Schuster MG, Edwards JE Jr, Sobel JD, et al: Empirical fluconazole versus placebo for intensive care unit patients: A randomized trial. Ann Intern Med 2008;149(2):83-90.
261. Rodriguez A, Diaz E, Martin-Loeches I, et al: Impact of early oseltamivir treatment on outcome in critically ill patients with 2009 pandemic influenza A. J Antimicrob Chemother 2011;66(5):1140-1149.

The complete list of references can be found at www.expertconsult.com.

53

Critically Ill Immunosuppressed Host

Henry Masur

CHAPTER OUTLINE

Patients often become immunosuppressed due to congenital or acquired disease. Additional patients become immunosuppressed because of the therapies that are being used to manage an expanding number of serious underlying conditions. Immunosuppressed patients present special management issues because (1) opportunistic infections often require special diagnostic tests; (2) opportunistic infections can be fulminant but can present without the usual expected signs and symptoms; and (3) patients are often receiving multiple unfamiliar drugs, which can have complex interactions that can lead to reduced drug efficacy or increased toxicity for the drugs related to the immunosuppressive illness or for drugs used for the management of critical care complications.

This chapter emphasizes the important ways in which immunosuppressed patients differ from immunologically normal individuals in terms of infectious complications. The noninfectious complications of immunosuppression are reviewed in Chapter 80.

DEFINITION

Patients who are at increased risk for infectious complications because of a deficiency in any of their host defense mechanisms are referred to as *compromised* hosts. Almost all patients in the intensive care unit (ICU) are compromised because devices, such as intravascular catheters, compromise their physical barriers of defense. Patients are termed *immunocompromised* or *immunosuppressed* if their defect specifically involves immune response (i.e., their innate immunity or their acquired immunity). Patients who have defects in inflammatory response, such as neutropenia or congenital leukocyte abnormalities, are also considered immunosuppressed in most reviews.

HOST DEFENSE MECHANISMS

The microbial complications that any patient develops in the ICU are determined by general, nonspecific barriers; innate immunity; acquired specific immunity; and environmental exposures. Nonspecific barriers include anatomic barriers such as intact skin and mucous membranes; chemical barriers, such as gastric acidity or urine pH; and flushing mechanisms, such as urinary flow or mucociliary transport in the lungs. Organisms that breach these barriers encounter nonspecific and innate host factors termed the *acute phase response*. Acute phase responses trigger a cascade of acquired specific immune responses including mononuclear phagocytes and antibodies, which also trigger a cascade of effector molecules and nonspecific inflammatory responses.[1]

Infections result from normal flora that colonize mucosal or cutaneous surfaces or from abnormal flora that are introduced by surface-to-surface contact, inhalation, ingestion, trauma, or medical procedures. Table 53.1 lists organisms that cause disease when specific anatomic defenses are disrupted in individuals with normal microbial flora. Patients with abnormal flora will develop disease that reflects unique, disease-specific characteristics of the host, the abnormal environment, and modifying factors such as drugs. Infections that result from common defects in the inflammatory or immunologic systems are detailed in Table 53.2.

Immunosuppressed patients are complicated because they generally have multiple factors that change the causes and manifestations of their infectious complications. Patients with hematologic malignancies, for instance, may be predisposed to infection because their leukemia or lymphoma has eliminated functional cells from their bone marrow. In addition, however, ablative chemotherapy may

Table 53.1 Normal Flora That Can Cause Disease When Anatomic Barriers Are Disrupted

Compromised Host Defense: Anatomic Disruption	Bacteria	Fungi
Oral cavity, esophagus	α-Hemolytic streptococci, oral anaerobes	*Candida* species
Lower gastrointestinal tract	Enterococci	*Candida* species
	Enteric organisms	
	Anaerobes	
Skin	Gram-positive bacilli	*Candida* species
	Staphylococci, streptococci	*Aspergillus*
	Corynebacterium, Bacillus species	
	Mycobacterium fortuitum, Mycobacterium chelonei	
Urinary tract	Enterococci	*Candida* species
	Enteric organisms	

Table 53.2 Infections Associated with Common Defects in Inflammatory or Immunologic Response

Host Defect	Examples of Associated Diseases/Therapies	Common Etiologic Agents of Infection
Inflammatory Response		
Neutropenia	Hematologic malignancies, cytotoxic chemotherapy, aplastic anemia	Gram-negative bacilli, *Staphylococcus aureus, Candida* species, *Aspergillus* species
Complement System		
C3	Congenital liver disease Systemic lupus erythematosus	*S. aureus, Staphylococcus pneumoniae, Pseudomonas* species, *Proteus* species
Alternate pathway	Sickle cell disease	*S. pneumoniae, Salmonella*
Immune Response		
T lymphocyte deficiency/ dysfunction	Thymic aplasia, thymic hypoplasia, Hodgkin disease, sarcoid	*Listeria monocytogenes, Mycobacterium* species, *Candida* species, *Aspergillus* species, *Cryptococcus neoformans,* herpes simplex, herpes zoster
	Human immunodeficiency virus infection	*Pneumocystis jiroveci,* cytomegalovirus, herpes simplex virus, *Mycobacterium avium* complex, *C. neoformans, Candida* species
	Mucocutaneous candidiasis	*Candida* species
B-cell deficiency/ dysfunction	Splenectomy, chronic lymphocytic leukemia, hypogammaglobulinemia, chronic lymphocytic leukemia, multiple myeloma, dysgammaglobulinemia	*S. pneumoniae,* other streptococci, *Haemophilus influenzae, Neisseria meningitidis, Babesia* species, *Capnocytophaga, Giardia lamblia, P. jiroveci,* enteroviruses
	Selective IgA deficiency	*G. lamblia,* viral hepatitis, *S. pneumoniae, H. influenzae*
Mixed T- and B-cell deficiency/dysfunction	Common variable hypogammaglobulinemia	*P. jiroveci,* cytomegalovirus, *S. pneumoniae, H. influenzae,* varicella virus, other bacteria

IgA, immunoglobulin A.

have eroded their mucosal surfaces and may have also altered their cellular immune responses or their neutrophil function.

Because of these host defense defects, organisms may cause local tissue destruction due to primary infection or reactivation and may gain access to the capillaries and lymphatics with unusual facility. Microbes that usually do not cause disease, such as BK virus, *Cytomegalovirus* (CMV), *Aspergillus*, and *Mucor*, can cause devastating organ damage or systemic inflammatory syndromes.

Recognition of which host defense mechanisms are disrupted enables the clinician to focus diagnostic, therapeutic, and prophylactic management and optimize patient outcome. For instance, if a patient presents with severe hypoxemia and diffuse pulmonary infiltrates, a health care provider who recognizes a prior splenectomy as the major predisposition to infection would focus the diagnostic evaluation and the empiric therapy on *Streptococcus pneumoniae* and *Haemophilus influenzae*.[2,3] By contrast, if the patient's major predisposition to infection was human immunodeficiency virus (HIV) infection with a $CD4^+$ T lymphocyte count below 50 cells/μL, the health care provider would focus on *Pneumocystis jiroveci* and *S. pneumoniae*.[4,5] However, additional history is also necessary: if the

Table 53.3 Modification of Standard Empiric Therapy in Patients with Neutropenia

Clinical Event	Possible Modifications of Standard Empiric Therapy
Breakthrough bacteremia	For gram-positive isolate (e.g., *Staphylococcus aureus*): Add vancomycin or daptomycin or linezolid until susceptibility pattern of isolate is known. For gram-negative isolate: Add two new agents likely to have activity until susceptibility pattern of pathogen is known.
Cellulitis or catheter-associated infection	Add vancomycin or daptomycin.
Severe necrotizing mucositis or gingivitis	Add specific antianaerobic agent (e.g., metronidazole, meropenem, imipenem, piperacillin-tazobactam) plus agent with activity against streptococci; consider acyclovir.
Ulcerative mucositis or gingivitis	Add acyclovir and anaerobic coverage.
Esophagitis	Add fluconazole or caspofungin; consider adding acyclovir.
Pneumonitis, diffuse or interstitial	Add trimethoprim-sulfamethoxazole and azithromycin or levofloxacin or moxifloxacin (plus broad-spectrum antibiotics if the patient is granulocytopenic).
Perianal tenderness	Include anaerobic agents such as metronidazole, imipenem, meropenem, or piperacillin-tazobactam.
Abdominal involvement	Add antianaerobic agent (e.g., metronidazole, meropenem, imipenem, piperacillin-tazobactam).

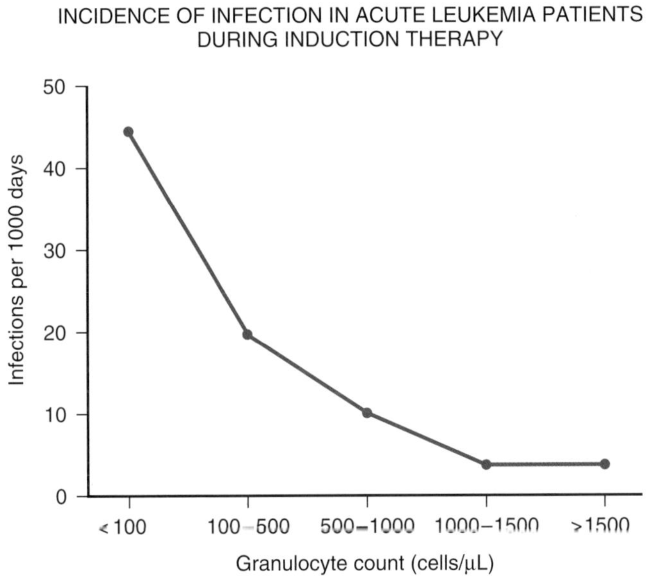

Figure 53.1 Incidence of infection in acute leukemia patients during induction therapy. (From Bodey GP, Buckley M, Sathe YS, Freireich EJ: Quantitative relationships between circulating leukocytes and infection in patients with acute leukemia. Ann Intern Med 1966;64(2):328-340.)

pneumonia occurs during an influenza outbreak, after exposure to a water aerosol (*Legionella*), or after a seizure (aspiration), the likely cause is plausibly linked to the precipitating event.

Immune competence should ideally be measurable by objective laboratory parameters. In fact, the risk for opportunistic infection in patients with HIV infection can be assessed by clinical laboratories with a high degree of accuracy by measuring the number of circulating $CD4^+$ T lymphocytes. The susceptibility of cancer patients to opportunistic bacterial and *Candida* infections can be assessed by measuring the number of circulating neutrophils (Fig. 53.1), and treatment algorithms have been established for managing fever in such patients (Figs. 53.2 to 53.4) and Table 53.3).[6] The predisposition of patients with certain congenital immunodeficiencies can be assessed by measuring serum immunoglobulin levels.[7] Unfortunately, however, for a large number of immunodeficiencies, such as those associated with antilymphocyte monoclonal antibodies or corticosteroids, no objective laboratory measures have been validated as predicting the risk of infection. Moreover, each parameter must be validated for each specific disease entity: for instance, although $CD4^+$ T-cell counts are excellent predictors of opportunistic infection predisposition for patients with HIV/AIDS (acquired immunodeficiency syndrome) (Fig. 53.5), they are not clinically useful for other immunosuppressive disorders.

Clinical series that document the frequency, the timing, and the causative organisms associated with infectious complications are extremely valuable for managing specific populations of immunosuppressed patients. Timelines that depict the time periods of vulnerability following stem cell transplantation (Figs. 53.6 and 53.7) and solid organ transplants (Fig. 53.8) are very useful for clinicians in terms of guiding diagnostic evaluations and for guiding empiric therapy. However, a specific microbial diagnosis should be established for each syndrome that presents in an immunosuppressed patient because the range of possible pathogens is quite broad, and the timelines and laboratory parameters cannot take into account all of the individual patient variables that influence the infectious complications that develop. Although it is useful to narrow the list of likely pathogens by analyzing risk factors, identifying the true causative agents allows therapy to be focused, avoiding unnecessary toxicity and allowing specific therapy to be optimized for efficacy and safety.

GENERAL APPROACH TO MANAGEMENT

With regard to infectious complications, effective management of immunosuppressed patients requires an understanding of several basic tenets of care.

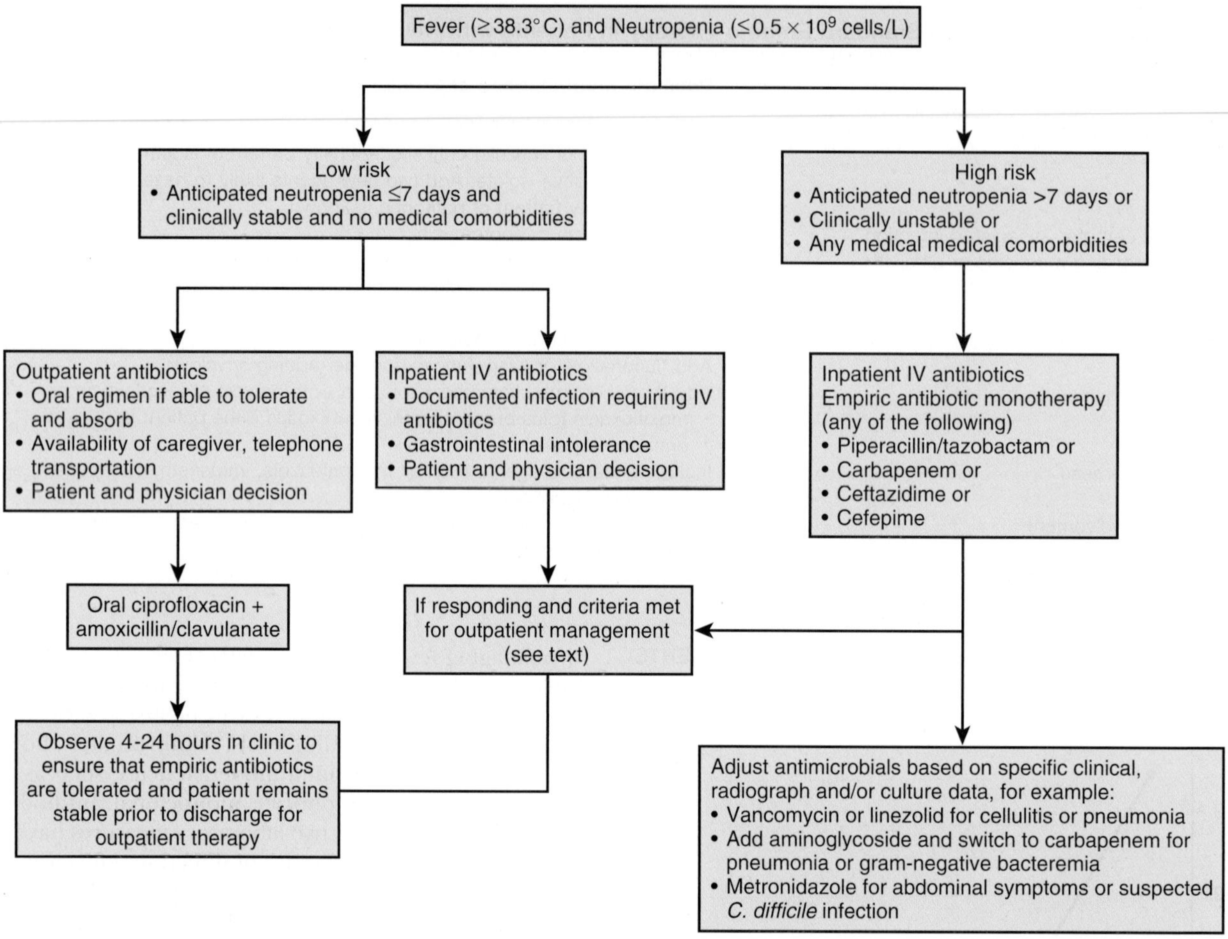

Figure 53.2 Initial management of fever and neutropenia. (From Freifeld AG, Bow EJ, Sepkowitz KA, et al: Clinical practice guideline for the use of antimicrobial agents in neutropenic patients with cancer: 2010 update by the Infectious Diseases Society of America. Clin Infect Dis 2011;52(4):e56-e93, used by permission of Oxford University Press.)

1. Life-threatening complications often present with subtle symptoms and signs that can easily be overlooked.

   Because immunocompromised patients may lack inflammatory and immunologic mediators, the clinical manifestations of infections are often less prominent and less impressive than in immunocompetent patients with similar complications. Thus, clinicians must recognize that even subtle changes in temperature, skin color, tenderness, catheter site appearance, chest radiograph, or abdominal examination may warrant an aggressive diagnostic evaluation and early institution of broad-spectrum empiric therapy.
2. Fever is not invariably present when patients are infected.

   Fever and infection are often seen as equivalent. However, most clinicians recognize that in any patient population there are many noninfectious causes of fever. Conversely, many patients with infection do not have fever: some infected patients may in fact be hypothermic. Corticosteroids and blunted neutropenia are often implicated in the suppression of fever. When dealing with immunosuppressed patients, clinicians need to keep these concepts in mind so that patients do not get unnecessary antibiotics when there is a likely noninfectious cause of the fever. Similarly, afebrile patients with syndromes that could be infectious need consideration for prompt antimicrobial therapy even if there is no measurable temperature elevation.

   For immunosuppressed patients, it is invariably preferable to assume that fever is due to infection and to treat empirically until the situation is fully evaluated. Although many cases of fever and neutropenia may well be noninfectious, the consequences of late treatment are so dire that prompt and broad-spectrum initiation of antimicrobial therapy should almost always be the default management approach.
3. Patients are predisposed to deteriorate precipitously.

   Although all ICU patients demand prompt attention and vigorous diagnostic and therapeutic management, many types of immunosuppression can be associated with especially precipitous clinical deterioration despite their innocuous presentation. Thus, infected patients who are neutropenic or who have undergone splenectomy, for example, are especially likely to have a fulminant course.
4. Diagnostic evaluation needs to be prompt and definitive.

   As indicated earlier, patients with life-threatening infection may present with subtle symptoms and signs that progress rapidly to become florid: these early

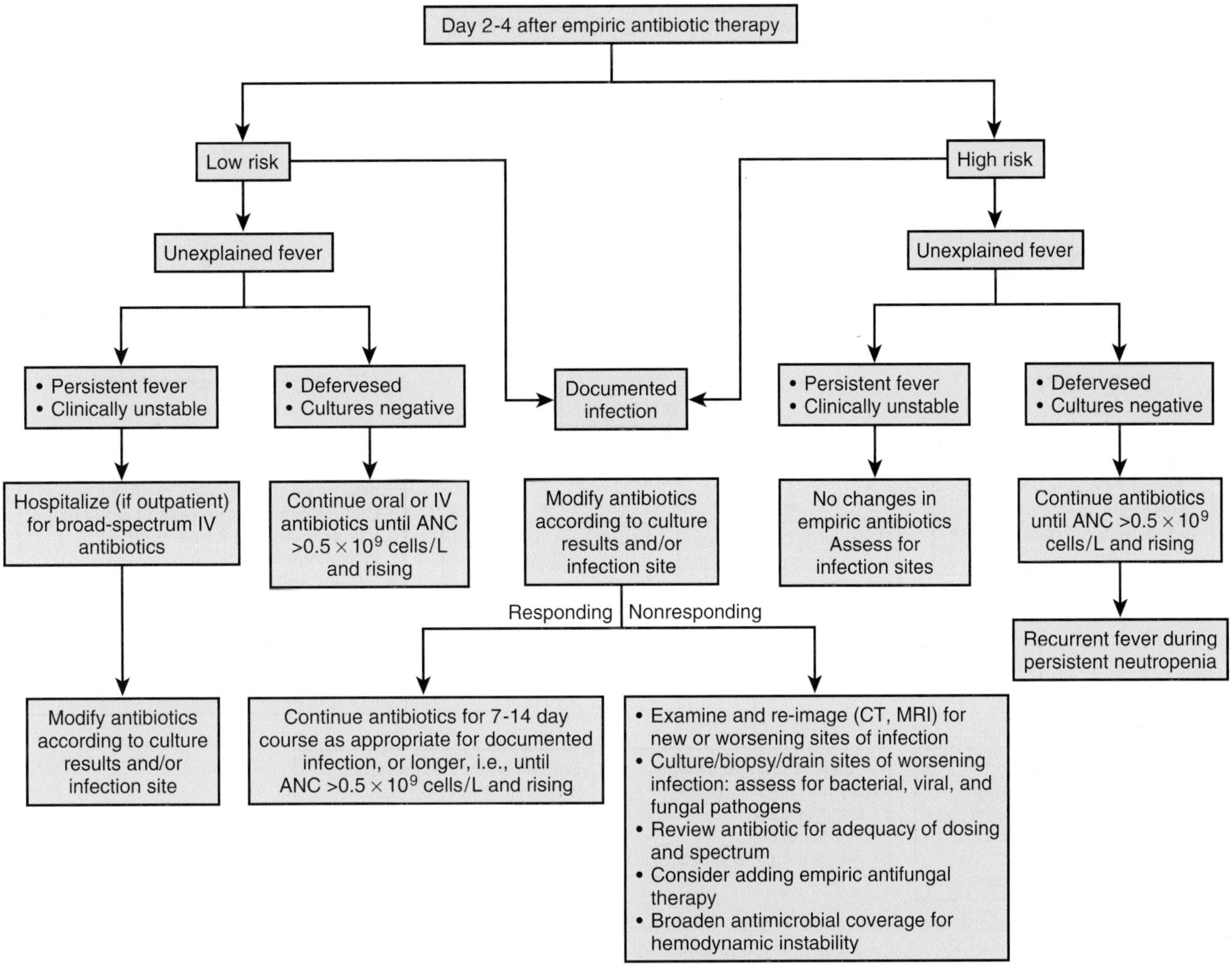

Figure 53.3 Reassessment after 2 to 4 days of empiric antibiotic therapy. ANC, absolute neutrophil count; CT, computed tomography; IV, intravenous; MRI, magnetic resonance imaging. (From Freifeld AG, Bow EJ, Sepkowitz KA, et al: Clinical practice guideline for the use of antimicrobial agents in neutropenic patients with cancer: 2010 update by the Infectious Diseases Society of America. Clin Infect Dis 2011;52(4):e56-e93, used by permission of Oxford University Press.)

manifestations merit aggressive attempts to define the anatomy of the lesion and the causative microbial pathogen. Because the spectrum of potential pathogens in such patients usually includes a wide array of microorganisms (e.g., viruses, fungi, protozoa, and bacteria), clinicians must be certain that appropriate specimens are obtained and the appropriate microbiologic and histologic tests are ordered to identify common, as well as uncommon or unusual, pathogens. This choice requires knowledge of the patient's underlying immunosuppressive disorder. Invasive diagnostic techniques such as bronchoalveolar lavage or tissue biopsies should be performed with less hesitancy than in immunologically normal patients. Patients often have enhanced risk factors for invasive procedures, such as thrombocytopenia, coagulation factor deficiencies, or compromised organ function. However, the benefit of definitive diagnosis often outweighs these risks when the procedures are performed by experienced operators. It is also important to recognize that timing is important: delay in scheduling diagnostic procedures may result in the patient being too hypoxic for bronchoscopy, too unstable for computed tomography (CT) scan or magnetic resonance imaging (MRI), or too coagulopathic for a lumbar puncture or needle aspirate of a fluid collection.

5. Infections may be community acquired, nosocomial, or latent, emphasizing the need for a thorough history of the patient's prior infections and exposures in order to assure the proper diagnostic tests and the optimal empiric therapeutic regimens.
6. Not all infections are related to the underlying disease or immunosuppression.

Immunosuppressed patients may be admitted to the ICU with an infection related to their immunosuppression. However, they may also develop infections that occur in normal hosts. Thus, aspiration pneumonia, catheter-related infections, influenza, mycoplasma infection, syphilis, or malaria may occur in relation to activities of daily living, substance abuse, travel, or community exposures.

7. Empiric therapy should be started promptly.

Time to appropriate antibiotics is an important correlate of successful outcome in any patient outcome,

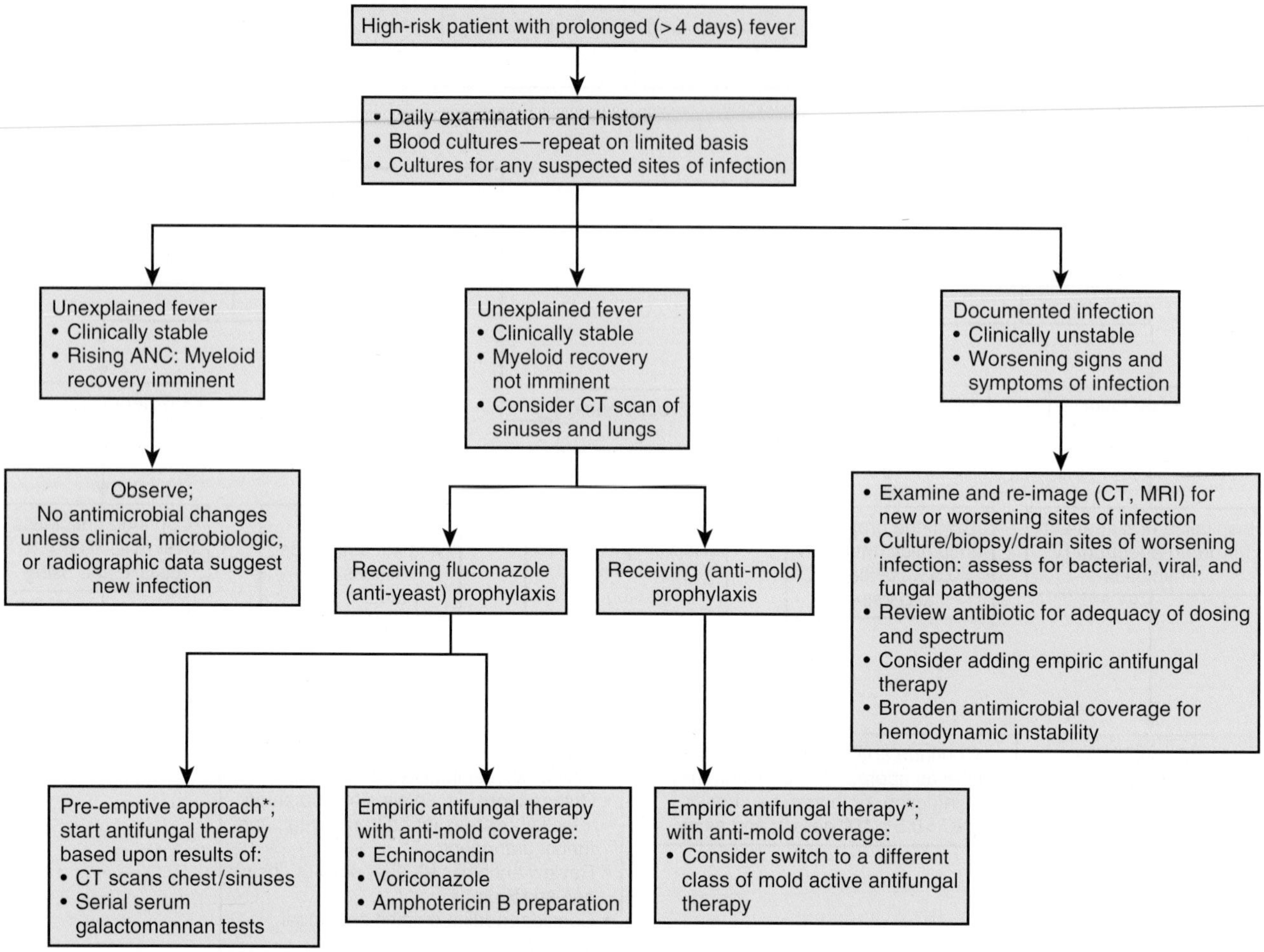
High-risk patient with prolonged (>4 days) fever
• Daily examination and history
• Blood cultures—repeat on limited basis
• Cultures for any suspected sites of infection
Unexplained fever
• Clinically stable
• Rising ANC: Myeloid recovery imminent
Unexplained fever
• Clinically stable
• Myeloid recovery not imminent
• Consider CT scan of sinuses and lungs
Documented infection
• Clinically unstable
• Worsening signs and symptoms of infection
Observe;
No antimicrobial changes unless clinical, microbiologic, or radiographic data suggest new infection
Receiving fluconazole (anti-yeast) prophylaxis
Receiving (anti-mold) prophylaxis
• Examine and re-image (CT, MRI) for new or worsening sites of infection
• Culture/biopsy/drain sites of worsening infection: assess for bacterial, viral, and fungal pathogens
• Review antibiotic for adequacy of dosing and spectrum
• Consider adding empiric antifungal therapy
• Broaden antimicrobial coverage for hemodynamic instability
Pre-emptive approach*; start antifungal therapy based upon results of:
• CT scans chest/sinuses
• Serial serum galactomannan tests
Empiric antifungal therapy with anti-mold coverage:
• Echinocandin
• Voriconazole
• Amphotericin B preparation
Empiric antifungal therapy*; with anti-mold coverage:
• Consider switch to a different class of mold active antifungal therapy

Figure 53.4 High-risk patient with fever after 4 days of empiric antibiotics. *C. difficile, Clostridium difficile*; IV, intravenous. (From Freifeld AG, Bow EJ, Sepkowitz KA, et al: Clinical practice guideline for the use of antimicrobial agents in neutropenic patients with cancer: 2010 update by the Infectious Diseases Society of America, Clin Infect Dis 2011;52(4):e56-e93, used by permission of Oxford University Press.)

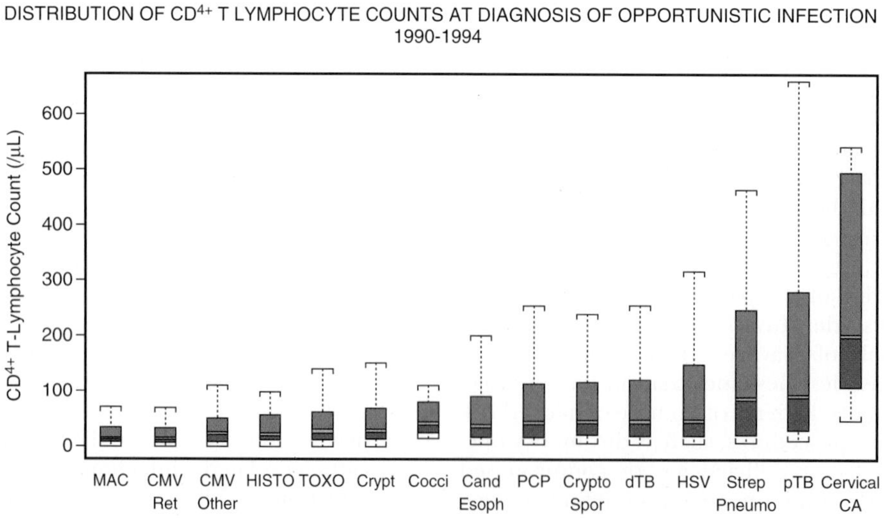

Figure 53.5 CD4+ cell count range for common manifestations of acquired immunodeficiency syndrome. Cand Esoph, *Candida* esophagitis; cervical CA, cervical cancer; CMV Other, other cytomegalovirus diseases; CMV Ret, cytomegalovirus retinitis; Cocci, coccidioidomycosis; Crypt, cryptococcosis; Crypto Spor, cryptosporidiosis; dTB, disseminated tuberculosis; HISTO, histoplasmosis; HSV, herpes simplex virus; MAC, *Mycobacterium avium* complex; PCP, *Pneumocystis jiroveci* pneumonia; pTB, pulmonary tuberculosis; Strep Pneumo, *Streptococcus* pneumonia; TOXO, toxoplasmosis.

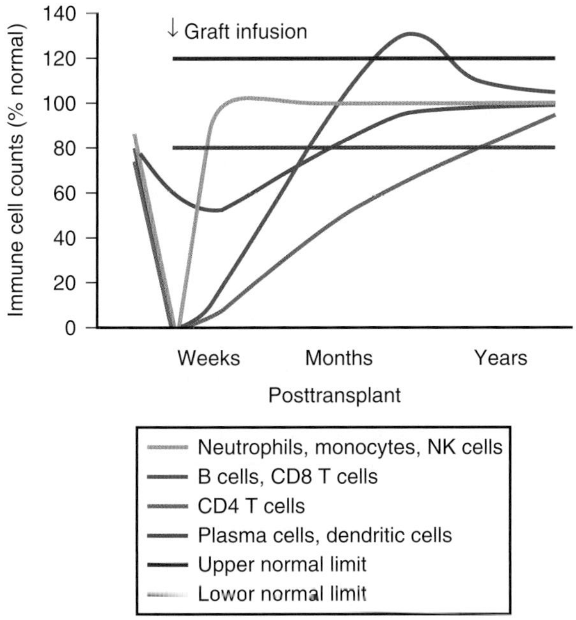

Figure 53.6 Approximate immune cell counts (expressed as percentage of normal counts) peri- and post-MA HCT. Nadirs are higher and occur later after NMA than MA transplantation, as recipient cells persist after NMA transplant for several weeks to months (in the presence of GVHD) or longer (in the absence of GVHD). The orange line represents the innate immune cells (e.g., neutrophils, monocytes, and NK cells), the recovery of which is influenced by the graft type (fastest with filgrastim-mobilized blood stem cells, intermediate with marrow, and slowest with UCB). The green line represents the recovery of $CD8^+$ T cells and B cells, the counts of which may transiently become supranormal. B cell recovery is influenced by graft type (fastest after CB transplant), and is delayed by GVHD and its treatment. The blue line represents the recovery of relatively radiotherapy/chemotherapy-resistant cells such as plasma cells, tissue dendritic cells (e.g., Langerhans cells) and, perhaps, tissue macrophages/microglia. The nadir of these cells may be lower in patients with aGVHD because of graft-versus-host plasma cell/Langerhans cell effect. The red line represents $CD4^+$ T cells, the recovery of which is influenced primarily by T cell content of the graft and patient age (faster in children than adults). aGVHD, acute graft-versus-host disease; GVHD, graft-versus-host disease; HCT, hematopoietic cell transplantation; MA, myeloablative; NK, natural killer; NMA, nonmyeloablative; UBC, umbilical cord blood. (From Storek J: Immunological reconstitution after hematopoietic cell transplantation—its relation to the contents of the graft. Expert Opin Biol Ther (Informa) 2008;8:583-597. Reproduced with permission of Informa Healthcare [Storek J: Immunological reconstitution after hematopoietic cell transplantation—its relation to the contents of the graft. Expert Opin Biol Ther (Informa) 2008;8:583-597], and Elsevier [Tomblyn M, Chiller T, Einsele H, et al: Guidelines for preventing infectious complications among hematopoietic cell transplantation recipients: A global perspective. Biol Blood Marrow Transplant 2009;15:1143-1238.])

but time is especially important in these patients, who are prone to deteriorate rapidly. Thus, the clinician must assure that the drugs are received by the patient and that there are no delaying factors related to pharmacy preparation, team communication, vascular access, or other factors.

Intensivists are more and more aware of the importance for all patients of "time to antibiotics," that is, the importance of starting antibiotics sooner rather than later, and including a drug that is active against the pathogen that is ultimately shown to be the causative organism.[8,9]

8. Empiric therapy should be broad spectrum.

   Antimicrobial stewardship is an important principle for preserving antibiotic efficacy on a population basis and for reducing unnecessary drug toxicities. However, given the breadth of pathogens that can cause the disease, and the often precipitous and sometimes irreversible clinical decline in this patient population, empiric regimens should be rational but very broad spectrum, with rapid narrowing of the regimen as further diagnostic information becomes available.

9. Antibiotic therapy should be narrowed when the causative organism is known, and monotherapy is usually adequate.

   The development of potent β-lactam and quinolone drugs in the 1980s and 1990s provided single agents that appear to be as effective as combination therapy for the treatment of gram-negative bacillary infections.[10-15]

   For aerobic gram-positive cocci, drugs such as oxacillin, vancomycin, and daptomycin appear to be as active as any combination regimen, except for endocarditis and infections involving prosthetic devices. Similarly, for most fungal and viral diseases, no combination therapy is documented to be more potent than the appropriate single-drug therapy.

   Exceptions may occur when pathogens are not highly susceptible to any available agent. However, both the microbial environment and the patient usually benefit from narrowing of the antibiotic regimen so that unnecessary toxicity and unneeded microbial resistance are not facilitated.

10. Foreign bodies and infectious foci should be assessed promptly for drainage or removal.

    When immunosuppressed patients are infected or septic, prompt consideration should be given to replacing all intravascular catheters and to assessing the patient for drainable foci of infection. Antimicrobial therapy may not be effective until such foci are drained or removed. Because some intravascular lines are not easy to replace or drainage procedures in some complicated patients may entail considerable potential morbidity, such decisions require considerable judgment.

11. Consideration should be given to reducing the level of immunosuppression.

    There is no proven survival benefit to interventions meant to augment or improve the immune or inflammatory response such as granulocyte colony-stimulating factor, neutrophil transfusions, or cytokines. It is plausible to reduce immunosuppression by reducing the dose of corticosteroid or other immunosuppressive agent if that is clinically feasible. Some institutions administer granulocyte infusions or colony-stimulating factors for patients with established infections. There is no documentation that such interventions improve survival, and deleterious effects, especially from granulocyte transfusions, can be life-threatening.[16,17]

12. The effectiveness and safety of antimicrobial therapy should be monitored regularly.

    ICU patients characteristically require attentive monitoring to assure the adequacy and safety of therapy. Immunocompromised patients often have multiple

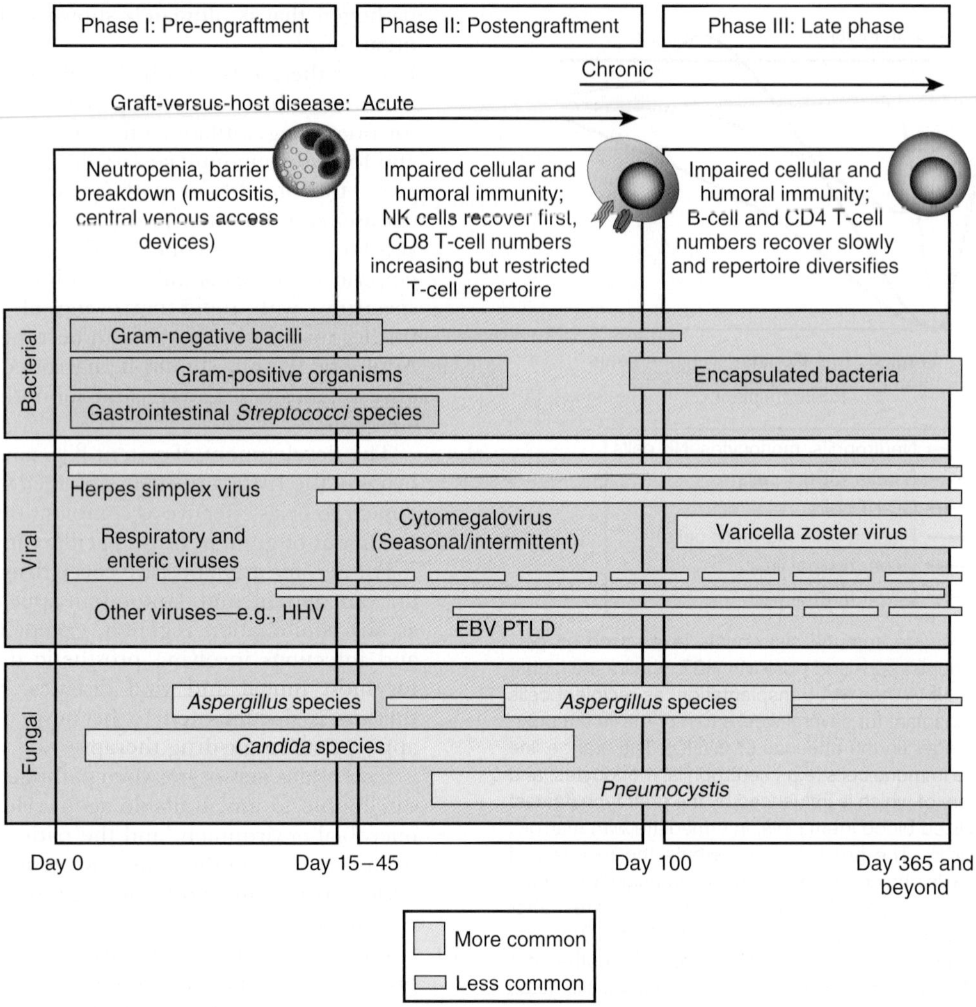

Figure 53.7 Phases of opportunistic infections among allogeneic HCT recipients. EBV, Epstein-Barr virus; HCT, hematopoietic cell transplantation; HHV6, human herpes virus 6; PTLD, posttransplant lymphoproliferative disease. (From Tomblyn M, Chiller T, Einsele H, et al: Guidelines for preventing infectious complications among hematopoietic cell transplantation recipients: A global perspective. Biol Blood Marrow Transplant 2009;15:1143-1238.)

prior and concurrent insults to their renal and hepatic function, and they often receive multiple drugs that can produce drug-drug interactions. Further, their volume of distributions may change dramatically from day to day. Thus, monitoring the pharmacokinetics and assessing potential toxicities are especially important in these patient populations. Moreover, because response to therapy may be less robust than in immunocompetent patients, serial antigen titers or polymerase chain reaction (PCR) titers, as well as serial imaging studies, can be important to assure the adequacy of the management plan. Therapy must often be continued longer than in immunologically normal patients while awaiting return of immunologic or inflammatory host response, or awaiting a sluggish therapeutic response in the face of ongoing immunosuppression.

13. Noninfectious syndromes can masquerade as infections and can be life-threatening.

Clinicians dealing with specific populations must be familiar with the noninfectious syndromes that occur, such as graft-versus-host disease, immune reconstitution syndrome, bronchiolitis obliterans, cardiomyopathy/pulmonary edema, and veno-occlusive disease of the liver. Failure to recognize these entities deprives patients of appropriate therapy, and exposes them to the toxicities and expense of unnecessary antimicrobial therapy.

MANAGEMENT OF SPECIFIC PATIENT POPULATIONS

CANCER PATIENTS WITH NEUTROPENIA

GENERAL PRINCIPLES

Cytotoxic therapy–induced neutropenia is a major predisposition to infection.[6] Neutrophil counts below 1000 cells/μL (the total absolute number of polymorphonuclear neutrophils plus bands) increase susceptibility to infection in a linear fashion (i.e., the lower the neutrophil count, the greater the degree of susceptibility)[18] (see Fig. 53.1). Although most research studies use 500 cells/μL as an arbitrary definition of neutropenia, intensivists must recognize that susceptibility increases as the neutrophil count declines below 500 to 1000 cells/μL. A patient with a neutrophil

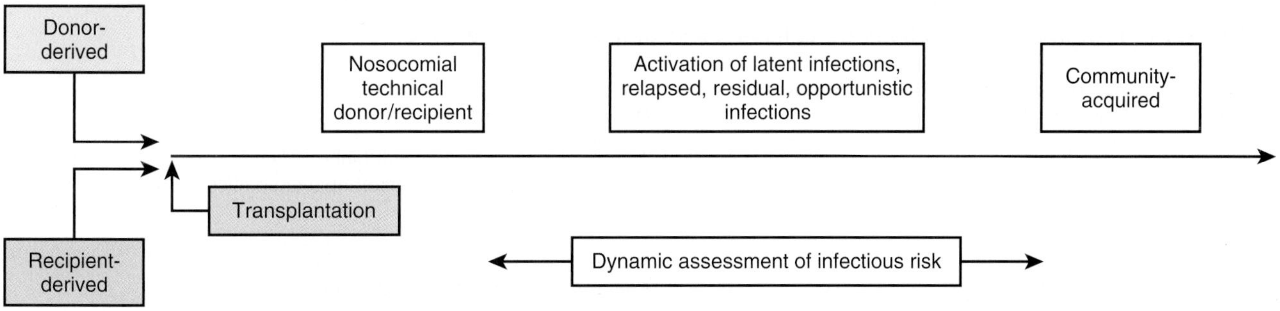

Common infections in solid organ transplantation recipients

Antimicrobial-resistant species: • MRSA • VRE • Candida species (non-albicans) Aspiration Line infection Wound infection Anastamotic leaks/ischemia Clostridium difficile colitis Donor-derived (uncommon): HSV, LCMV, rabies, West Nile Recipient-derived (colonization): Aspergillus, Pseudomonas	With PCP and antiviral (CMV, HBV) prophylaxis: • BK polyomavirus nephropathy • Clostridium difficile colitis • Hepatitis C virus • Adenovirus, influenza • *Cryptococcus neoformans* • *M. tuberculosis* Anastamotic complications Without prophylaxis add: Pneumocystis Herpes viruses (HSZ, VZV, CMV, EBV) Hepatitis B virus *Listeria, Nocardia, Toxoplasma, Stronglyoides, Leishmania, Trypanosoma cruzi*	Community-acquired pneumonia, urinary tract infection: *Aspergillus*, atypical molds, *Mucor* species, *Nocardia*, *Rhodococcus* species Late viral: • CMV (colitis/retinitis) • Hepatitis (HBV, HCV) • HSV encephalitis • Community-acquired (SARS, West Nile) • JC polyomarvirus (PML), skin cancer, lymphoma (PTLD)

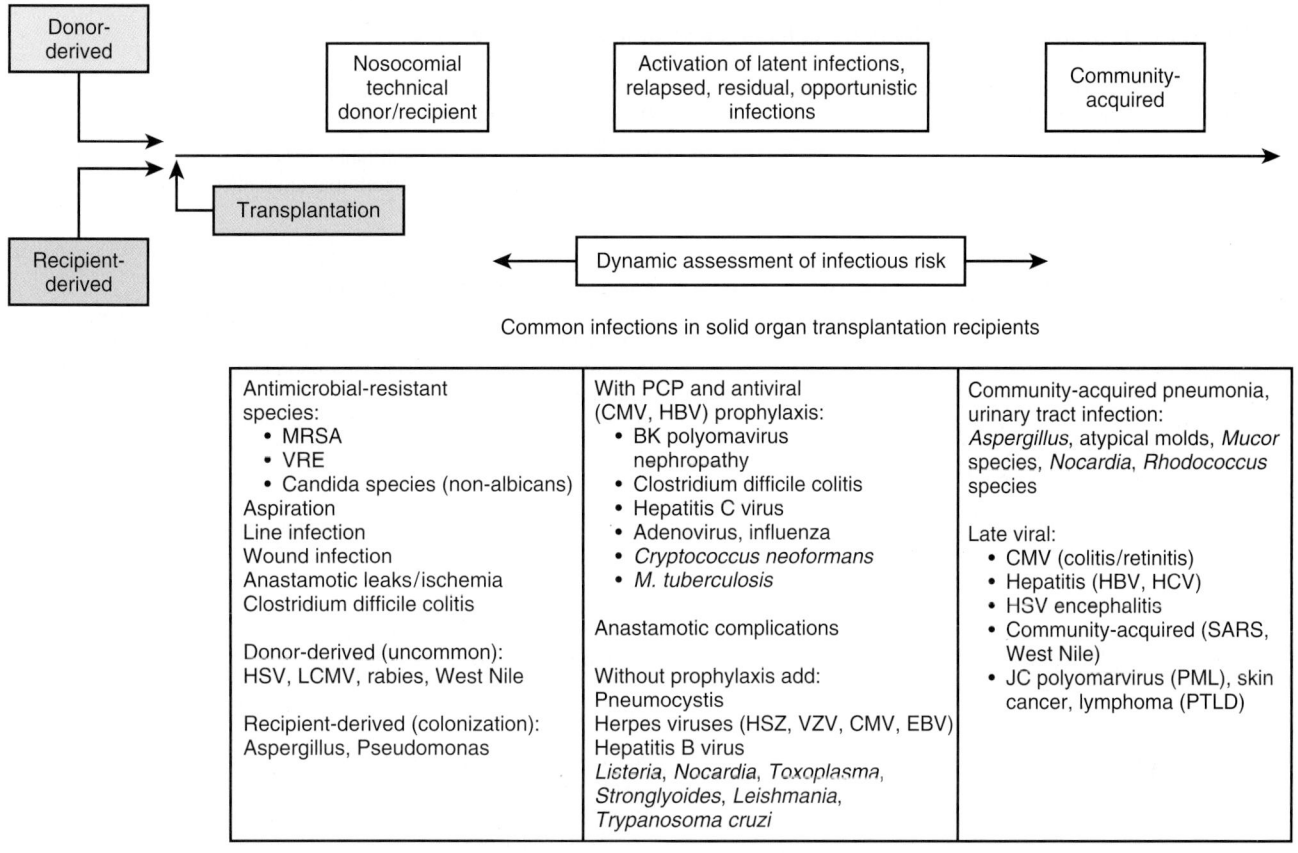

Figure 53.8 Usual sequence of infection after solid organ transplantation. (From Fishman JA: Infection in the solid organ transplant recipient. In Basow DS (ed): UpToDate. Waltham, MA, UpToDate, 2012.)

count of 100 cells/µL is much more vulnerable to infection than a patient with 500 or 1000 cells/µL, and a patient with zero neutrophils is at much higher risk for fulminant infection than a patient with 50 or 100 cells/µL. The trajectory of the neutrophil count is also important: a patient with a neutrophil count of 1500 cells/µL whose counts are dropping precipitously should best be treated like a patient with absolute neutropenia. Similarly, a patient with 500 neutrophils/µL whose counts are rising quickly is not nearly as vulnerable to a poor outcome as a patient with a count of 500 neutrophils/µL that is stable.

Patients with neutropenia are generally divided into high-risk and low-risk patients based on their likelihood of developing severe infectious complications. Markers for high risk include neutropenia for more than 7 days' duration and neutrophil count less than 100 cells/µL, as well as obvious signs of a life-threatening process such as hypotension, obtundation, pneumonia, or severe abdominal pain. As Figures 53.2 to 53.4 outline, this risk assessment is used in designating empiric regimens.

Thus, although the absolute neutrophil count is an essential factor to follow, the duration of neutropenia, the functional capability of neutrophils, the integrity of physical barriers such as the skin and gastrointestinal mucosa, the patient's microbiologic environment (endogenous and exogenous flora), and the status of other immune mechanisms also contribute to the infectious syndromes that will develop.

In the 1960s and 1970s, aerobic gram-negative bacilli such as *Escherichia coli, Klebsiella pneumoniae,* and *Pseudomonas aeruginosa* predominated as pathogens in neutropenic patients. In the 1990s the spectrum of causative pathogens in neutropenic patients shifted from a predominance of gram-negative bacilli to a majority of gram-positive cocci including streptococci, staphylococci (including oxacillin-resistant *Staphylococcus aureus*), and enterococci (including vancomycin-resistant *enterococci*).[10,12-15,19-21] *Candida* species have also become more frequent as pathogens, especially as patients are on broad-spectrum antibacterials and have long-term venous access devices in place.

More recently, highly resistant gram-negative bacilli have become major threats for nosocomial transmission. Clinicians must consider the possibility that a patient may be colonized and then infected with a *Stenotrophomonas*, a *Burkholderia*, or a carbapenemase-producing gram-negative Enterobacteriaceae such as a *Klebsiella*, an *Enterobacter*, or an *E. coli* that has developed mechanisms that evade currently marketed drugs.[22-26]

The management of febrile, neutropenic fever is reviewed in a guideline that is widely used to direct care in North America.[6] Figures 53.2 to 53.4 summarize important aspects of management. Table 53.3 also provides a summary of useful management information. Table 53.4 outlines common prevention strategies that will modify the spectrum of causative pathogens. Box 53.1 summarizes the organisms that most often cause disease in neutropenic patients.

Table 53.4 Prevention of Infectious Complications in Compromised Patients

Method/Agent to Prevent Acquisition of, Suppress, or Eliminate Microbial Flora	Description/Example
Isolation	Total protective isolation with high-efficiency particulate air filters and absorbable or nonabsorbable antibiotics for bone marrow transplant recipient
Prophylactic antibacterial drugs	
Ciprofloxacin	Reduce bacterial infections in neutropenic patients
Trimethoprim-sulfamethoxazole	Suppress flora in patients with chronic bronchitis
Penicillin	Reduce frequency of streptococcal infections after splenectomy or in rheumatic valvular disease or graft-versus-host disease
Clarithromycin	Prevention of *Mycobacterium avium* complex infection in patients with advanced HIV disease
Isoniazid	Prevention of tuberculosis in PPD-positive individuals
Nonabsorbable broad-spectrum agents (i.e., aminoglycoside, plus bacitracin)	Gut decontamination for neutropenic patients
Prophylactic antiviral drugs	
Oral acyclovir or valganciclovir, or IV ganciclovir	Reduce frequency of CMV disease after transplantation
Rimantadine, oseltamivir	Prevent influenza
Prophylactic antifungal drugs	
Fluconazole	Prevent recurrent candidiasis
Liposomal amphotericin B or voriconazole or caspofungin	Prevent *Candida* or mold infections
Trimethoprim-sulfamethoxazole	Prevent *Pneumocystis* pneumonia
Prophylactic antiprotozoal/anthelmintic drugs	
Albendazole or ivermectin	Prevent disseminated strongyloidiasis in high-risk patients
Augmentation of host defenses	
Immunization	Pneumococcal and *Haemophilus* vaccine for patients before splenectomy
Immune serum globulin	Augment levels in deficient patients (e.g., common variable immunodeficiency)
Fresh frozen plasma	Augment complement levels in deficient patients
Neutrophil transfusions	Augment inflammatory response in neutropenic patients or patients with chronic functional neutrophil disorders
Lymphocyte or other mononuclear cell transfusions	Experimental therapies for tumors, various immunodeficiencies
Bone marrow or stem cell transplantion	Reconstitute patients with congenital immunodeficiencies or certain acquired cytopenias
Bone marrow human stem cell stimulation	G-CSF or GM-CSF to increase neutrophil or mononuclear cell quantity and function
Gene therapy	Replace genes to allow normal function

AIDS, acquired immunodeficiency syndrome; CMV, cytomegalovirus; G-CSF, granulocyte colony-stimulating factor; GM-CSF, granulocyte-monocyte colony-stimulating factor; HIV, human immunodeficiency virus; PPD, purified protein derivative.

Patients with neutropenia are generally suspected of being infected if the clinical syndrome is consistent with infection, or if the temperature is at least 38.3° C on one occasion or 38.1° C on two separate occasions. An elevated temperature alone should trigger the institution of broad-spectrum antimicrobials in almost all situations. Given this emphasis of using temperature as an indicator for starting antimicrobial therapy, using a validated technique to measure temperature is important. Although pulmonary artery or urinary catheter thermistors appear to provide the most accurate measurement, most experienced ICUs use tympanic membrane thermistors. Rectal probes are avoided in order to reduce the induction of perirectal infections in neutropenic patients, and to reduce the potential for fecal pathogen transmission. As noted earlier, although fever is almost always a reason to start antimicrobial therapy in this patient population, the absence of fever should not be the grounds for avoiding antimicrobials if a patient has other symptoms or signs suggesting infection. The threshold for starting antimicrobials should be very low, i.e., if there is a suspicion of infection, a broad-spectrum regimen should be started.

As noted earlier, the initial regimen should not be parsimonious in terms of spectrum. Because this population of patients is susceptible to a wide variety of bacterial and fungal pathogens, a very wide broad-spectrum regimen should be used. There are many potential regimens, each of which must be tailored to the local experience with the patient population and the hospital, specific patient factors such as evidence of prior colonization or recent antimicrobial therapy, and clinical manifestations suggesting infection. Popular regimens would include (1) meropenem or cefepime or piperacillin-tazobactam for broad-spectrum antibacterial activity plus (2) vancomycin or daptomycin for staphylococcal infections[27,28] plus (3) ciprofloxacin or moxifloxacin or aztreonam for broader gram-negative bacillus coverage. Many experienced clinicians would add an echinocandin for anti-*Candida* activity given the frequency of

Box 53.1 Common Bacterial Pathogens in Neutropenic Patients

Common Gram-Positive Pathogens

Coagulase-negative staphylococci
Staphylococcus aureus, including methicillin-resistant strains
Enterococcus species, including vancomycin-resistant strains
Viridans group streptococci
Streptococcus pneumonia
Streptococcus pyogenes

Common Gram-Negative Pathogens

Escherichia coli
Klebsiella species
Enterobacter species
Pseudomonas aeruginosa
Citrobacter species
Acinetobacter species
Stenotrophomonas maltophilia

From Freifeld AG, Bow EJ, Sepkowitz KA, et al: Clinical practice guideline for the use of antimicrobial agents in neutropenic patients with cancer: 2010 update by the Infectious Diseases Society of America. Clin Infect Dis 2011;52:e56-e93, used by permission of Oxford University Press.

Box 53.2 Indications for Addition of Antibiotics Active against Gram-Positive Organisms to Empiric Regimen for Fever and Neutropenia

Hemodynamic instability or other evidence of severe sepsis
Pneumonia documented radiographically
Positive blood culture for gram-positive bacteria, before final identification and availability of susceptibility testing results
Clinical evidence suggestive of serious catheter-related infection (e.g., chills or rigors with infusion through catheter, cellulitis around the catheter entry/exit site)
Skin or soft tissue infection at any site
Colonization with methicillin-resistant *Staphylococcus aureus*, vancomycin-resistant enterococci, or penicillin-resistant *Streptococcus pneumoniae*
Severe mucositis, if fluoroquinolone prophylaxis has been given and ceftazidime is used for empiric therapy

From Freifeld AG, Bow EJ, Sepkowitz KA, et al: Clinical practice guideline for the use of antimicrobial agents in neutropenic patients with cancer: 2010 update by the Infectious Diseases Society of America. Clin Infect Dis 2011;52:e56-e93, used by permission of Oxford University Press.

intravascular catheter-associated infections due to *Candida* species.[29-33] Intensivists need to work closely with their infectious disease consultants, microbiology laboratories, and referring teams to develop regimens that are optimal for their hospital environment, for the patient population involved, and for the specific, unique patient who is being managed.

Empiric antiviral therapy is not usually initiated unless there is a specific reason to suspect a viral process. Antiviral agents would generally be added only if a specific viral process such as CMV colitis or disseminated herpes simplex were suspected.

For the duration of neutropenia (when the neutropenia is expected to be time-limited), broad-spectrum therapy must be continued. When a specific causative organism is identified, antimicrobial therapy should be optimized for that organism. However, unlike other immunologically normal patients, the broad-spectrum "background" (i.e., meropenem or piperacillin-tazobactam or cefepime or ceftazidime) must be continued until the neutropenia resolves, on the assumption that a patient who develops one infection is likely to develop or manifest another infectious process while the neutropenia persists.

Coverage for methicillin-resistant *Staphylococcus aureus* (MRSA) does not necessarily need to be continued if no MRSA is identified. There are environmental advantages to reducing vancomycin exposure.

As noted previously, there is no documented reason, even in this population, to use combination therapy to treat a specific pathogen in most situations, although combination therapy is needed for the empiric approach for the duration of neutropenia (Box 53.2). In rare situations, if the causative organism is not susceptible to agents with well-documented efficacy, combination therapy may be an appropriate strategy out of desperation. As an example, for treating enteric carbapenemase-producing organisms, a combination of tigecycline plus colistin plus an aminoglycoside might be desirable given the high minimum inhibitory concentrations for all antibiotics for these organisms and the dreadful clinical results with any therapeutic intervention.[34-38]

For patients with fever and neutropenia, the cause of the fever is historically documented in only 50% to 60% of patients. The duration of therapy once empiric antimicrobials are started depends on the evolution of the neutrophil count, the patient's clinical status, and the results of diagnostic tests. If the patient defervesces and looks clinically well, however, the broad-spectrum regimen should not be stopped until the neutrophil count is above 500 to 750 cells/µL, preferably on two occasions, and the patient has received at least 10 to 14 days of therapy.

If a neutropenic patient is started on antibacterial therapy without fungal therapy, and defervescence has not occurred by days 3 to 5, an antifungal agent should be added (Figs. 53.3 and 53.4). The choice of antifungal agent depends on the patient population and the patient's specific history. In the current era many patients have been receiving short- or long-term prophylaxis with fluconazole, voriconazole, or posaconazole. Although in general clinicians could add fluconazole, an echinocandin (e.g., caspofungin or micafungin or anidulofungin) or liposomal amphotericin B can also be used. An echinocandin is often a preferred choice if the patient has been on long-term azole prophylaxis and if a mold infection is not suspected.[39-42]

As patients receive chemoprophylaxis with quinolones or azoles during periods of intense neutropenia or immunosuppression, breakthrough pathogens are more and more likely to be resistant to the prophylactic agents.[40,42] Thus empiric regimens must be chosen with keen attention to the drugs that patients have received in the recent past, as well as pathogens they have previously been colonized or infected with.

DIAGNOSTIC APPROACH

Patients with fever and neutropenia require aggressive diagnostic efforts to identify the cause of fever so that the appropriate antimicrobial agent is used and appropriate procedures (e.g., surgical drainage, removal of a foreign body such as a catheter) can be performed. All febrile neutropenic patients should at a minimum have two blood cultures drawn, with one drawn peripherally and one drawn through the lumen of the indwelling catheter that has either been in the longest or is most suspicious for being infected. Other sites should be cultured as clinically indicated.

Regular physical examination is necessary to identify sites that merit more focused investigation. With impaired inflammatory response, findings on examination may be subtle. Knowledge of the specific immunologic defect is important so that when cultures of blood, sputum, urine, or other appropriate body fluids or body sites are performed, special microbiologic approaches can be used to detect viruses, fungi, helminths, protozoa, and bacteria as indicated by the clinical situation. Imaging studies are also important because intra-abdominal, intrathoracic, intracerebral, and musculoskeletal processes can be clinically subtle and may not be associated with identifiable organisms in the bloodstream. A growing array of antigen detection systems and molecular and high-performance chromatographic tests are being investigated to facilitate diagnosis.

Some of these approaches, despite their promising initial reports, are not yet clinically practical because of their level of sensitivity, specificity, or the cost or expertise required to perform them adequately. For instance, the PCR test for *Pneumocystis* is so sensitive that there is no clear separation of patients who are colonized with *Pneumocystis* (and whose pulmonary dysfunction is due to another process), and the serum β-glucan antigen detection system is so nonspecific that some clinicians are not confidant that the test provides useful information.[43-45] Similarly, the PCR test for respiratory syncytial virus (RSV) or influenza or parainfluenza is so sensitive that immunosuppressed patients may shed small quantities of virus for many weeks after acute infection, confusing the diagnosis of the new pulmonary processes that occur after the acute viral infection is over, and at a time when another process is causing fever or pulmonary manifestations. Thus, these new tests must be interpreted with caution.

EMPIRIC AND SPECIFIC ANTIMICROBIAL THERAPY

Outside the ICU, stable patients with fever and neutropenia, and no obvious source of infection, are treated with a broad-spectrum regimen, as mentioned previously, that covers all likely pathogens. Recommended regimens for the "backbone" agent include a carbapenem with antipseudomonas activity (e.g., meropenem or imipenem), a β-lactam β-lactamase combination with antipseudomonas activity (e.g., piperacillin-tazobactam), and a broad-spectrum cephalosporin with antipseudomonas activity (e.g., cefepime or ceftazidime). Although vancomycin is not necessarily indicated for empiric therapy of fever and neutropenia, in the ICU an antistaphylococcal drug (e.g., vancomycin or daptomycin) is usually added if the patient has a long-term intravascular catheter in place and may be appropriate empirically in every patient who merits ICU admission until the causative pathogen is known. Because patients with fever and neutropenia have almost always had extensive exposure to hospital-acquired pathogens and to antimicrobials, clinicians must adjust the empiric regimens to fit the patient's situation. Adding colistin plus tigecycline empirically might be appropriate for someone hospitalized during an outbreak of highly resistant *Acinetobacter* or *Klebsiella.*

Patients in the ICU are by definition either unstable hemodynamically or medically fragile due to concurrent disease. In such situations, many clinicians would expand antibacterial coverage with a second broad-spectrum drug (e.g., a quinolone such as ciprofloxacin), aztreonam, or an aminoglycoside (e.g., gentamicin or tobramycin).[20,46-51]

A substantial number of febrile, neutropenic patients fail to improve in terms of fever or other manifestations. Once febrile and neutropenic patients are started on empiric therapy, if no causative process or organism is detected, one of the first three scenarios listed here is likely to be encountered. Figures 53.2 to 53.4 list some of the therapeutic options for such patients.

1. The patient defervesces and remains stable but the source remains unknown. In this case the empiric regimen is usually continued for a minimum of 7 to 10 days, and must be continued until the neutrophil count is over 500 to 1000 cells/μL unless no end is likely with the neutropenia.
2. The patient remains febrile and stable but the source remains unknown. Failure to improve may result from poor immune response, a need for drainage or necessity to remove foreign bodies, the use of drugs without activity against the causative organism, or a noninfectious process including drug allergy (i.e., fever resulting from a drug such as phenytoin or an antimicrobial agent). The potential causative processes need to be aggressively reassessed on a regular basis by physical examination, history, cultures, and imaging techniques. Most centers add antifungal therapy empirically at day 4 to day 7 of therapy if patients remain febrile.[6,40,52] Fluconazole, liposomal amphotericin B, caspofungin, or voriconazole may be used: In some situations fluconazole would be less attractive either because the patient has received fluconazole prophylaxis or because molds are suspected.[41] The toxicity profile of amphotericin B, even in its liposomal form, has led many clinicians to prefer voriconazole or one of the echinocandins (i.e., caspofungin, micafungin, or anidulafungin).[32,53-56]
3. The patient deteriorates clinically but the source remains unknown. In this case continued evaluation for infectious and noninfectious sources of the infection should be pursued, and further empiric changes to the antimicrobial regimen should be considered.
4. The source of the infection is identified. The drug and the duration of therapy depend on the causative syndrome and microorganism. Table 53.3 lists some common scenarios. Rarely should the therapy be discontinued while the patient is neutropenic. Rarely is combination therapy necessary unless the causative organisms are multiple (suspected or confirmed) or (as described earlier)

the causative organism is not highly susceptible to available antimicrobial agents.[12-16,18-21,49]

A common problem in febrile, neutropenic patients is managing indwelling intravascular lines.[57,58] In general, these lines may be left in place initially if examination of the site reveals no indication of infection and the patient is hemodynamically stable. Blood cultures should be drawn through the catheter. Although some experts advocate drawing a culture through each port of each catheter, obtaining this many blood cultures is often not feasible because of time, cost, and volume of blood. If a patient is hemodynamically unstable and fails to respond promptly to fluid administration, it is prudent to remove the line in case an infected catheter is the source of the sepsis. Failure to remove the foreign body in this situation probably increases the likelihood of an unfavorable outcome. Should blood cultures become positive and should the suspicion be high that the catheter is the source, antibacterial therapy may be successful in some settings (e.g., if the pathogen is a bacterium that is relatively sensitive to antibacterial therapy), thus avoiding the need to remove the catheter. Situations suggesting that catheter removal is necessary include hemodynamic instability despite aggressive fluid resuscitation, tunnel infection, or infections resulting from fungi or relatively antibiotic-resistant bacteria such as *P. aeruginosa*.

Granulocyte transfusions have not been proved in randomized trials to improve survival in clinical settings probably because of the inability to administer a large number of cells with adequate frequency.[16,17] However, many clinicians are convinced that matched white blood cell transfusions are helpful in managing life-threatening infections when patients are neutropenic and will use them when such cells are available. The manipulation of immune response with cytokines, cytokine inhibitors, or immunoglobulins is the subject of considerable investigation: Such interventions may reduce the duration of fever or the incidence of infections when used empirically, but in no setting have they been clearly shown to improve survival when administered after an infection has been documented. Algorithms for managing fever in neutropenic patients are provided in Figures 53.2 to 53.4. Table 53.3 suggests modifications of standard empiric regimens in certain common clinical scenarios.

PREVENTION OF INFECTION

Given the experience with frequent and severe infectious complications in cancer patients with neutropenia, it has been logical to attempt to prevent infection. Most microorganisms causing disease in this patient population arise from endogenous gastrointestinal, cutaneous, or respiratory flora. Total protected environments probably reduce frequency of infection, but this approach is expensive and inconvenient. Trying to prove a consistent beneficial impact on survival has been difficult, and thus such isolation is rarely used anymore. Some experts are enthusiastic about placing patients in positive-pressure rooms so that pathogens do not enter via particles and droplets from outside the room. This type of isolation has not clearly improved outcome, however, and is not a standard of care.[59,60] In Europe, there is more enthusiasm for such an approach than in the United States. Controversies over interpretation of data and concern that such antibiotic pressure will encourage the development of drug-resistant bacteria and fungi have diminished widespread acceptance in the United States.

Systemic antibacterial prophylaxis and systemic antifungal prophylaxis have been shown in some studies to reduce the number of infections, but their lack of effect on patient survival, their cost, and their impact on the emergence of resistance have made many clinicians reluctant to use them. Anti-*Pneumocystis* prophylaxis is, in contrast, highly effective in susceptible populations. Prophylaxis for CMV is rarely used unless the patient has received a solid organ or human stem cell transplant. Table 53.4 summarizes general strategies of infection prevention in immunosuppressed patients including patients with neutropenia.

PATIENTS WITH HIV/AIDS

Opportunistic infections continue to occur in three groups of HIV-infected patients: (1) those who are unaware of their HIV status until they develop an opportunistic infection or tumor such as *Pneumocystis* pneumonia or *Toxoplasma* encephalitis or Kaposi sarcoma; (2) those who are unable or unwilling to receive appropriate therapy; and (3) those who fail antiretroviral therapy and opportunistic infection prophylaxis.[4,61-65] In the United States, only about 20% to 40% of patients with HIV infection have a viral load under 50 copies/μL; thus, the majority of patients are not aware of their infection, not linked to care, or not able to adhere to an effective regimen.[66] It is notable that half of all HIV-infected patients are located in 12 large cities: in those areas, patients frequently come to emergency rooms and ICUs with opportunistic infections that are preventable with earlier antiretroviral therapy plus anti-infective chemoprophylaxis if these patients were successfully engaged in care.[67]

Patients with HIV infection who are well controlled by antiretroviral drugs do not develop the classic complications of immunosuppression because their immunosuppression is subtle once their viral load is less than 50 copies/μL and their CD4 cell count rises, especially if it is greater than 200 cells/μL. Patients with CD4 counts greater than 200 cells/μL and viral loads less than 50 copies/μL may be seen in ICUs because of medical or surgical issues unrelated to their HIV infection. Such patients may also develop accelerated "processes of aging," which include accelerated coronary artery disease, stroke, renal disease, or hepatic disease, but these processes appear to be related to enhanced chronic inflammation and not to immunosuppression.[68-70]

SPECTRUM OF CLINICAL MANIFESTATIONS

Patients with HIV infection develop clinical disease as a result of three basic processes: (1) opportunistic infections and tumors that are enabled by HIV-induced immunosuppression; (2) the direct effect of HIV on specific organs (e.g., cardiomyopathy, enteropathy, dementia); or (3) immunologically mediated processes (e.g., glomerulonephritis, thrombocytopenia).

MANAGEMENT OF ANTIRETROVIRAL DRUGS

For any HIV-infected patient in the ICU, clinicians must be cognizant of the need for careful management of antiretroviral drugs.[71] If patients are not receiving antiretroviral drugs at the time of ICU admission, the ICU is not a desirable setting for initiating them: patient commitment to long-term adherence is difficult to assess when patients are critically ill, and drug toxicities and interactions will be hard to assess.[72,73] There is virtually no indication to start antiretroviral therapy acutely in the ICU following the diagnosis of an acute opportunistic infection with the rare exception of rapidly progressive forms of untreatable diseases such as JC virus encephalitis or cryptosporidiosis.

If patients enter the ICU already receiving antiretroviral therapy, an expert in HIV management should be consulted about the benefits of continuing the drugs rather than interrupting them. There is ample evidence that even brief interruption of antiretroviral drugs can have deleterious effects in terms of long-term loss of CD4 cells and in terms of the occurrence of opportunistic infections. However, administration of antiretroviral drugs in the ICU is challenging. Almost all commonly used antiretroviral drugs are available only in oral formulations, and thus absorption is often uncertain in critically ill patients. Subtherapeutic concentrations of antiretroviral drugs can select for drug resistance mutations, producing virus that is irrevocably nonsusceptible to the suboptimally dosed drug, sometimes with cross-class resistance. Many antiretroviral drugs affect cytochrome P-450 hepatic enzymes, resulting in altered pharmacokinetics for many non-AIDS-related drugs, which may substantially alter the efficacy or safety of the non-AIDS drug. Similarly, non-AIDS-related drugs can alter antiretroviral drug kinetics, resulting in drug serum levels that are above or below therapeutic targets, leading to viral resistance or drug toxicity. Stopping antiretroviral drugs may be the least harmful option. However, given the different half-lives of various antiretroviral agents, such discontinuation should be done in consultation with an HIV-experienced clinician.

Clinicians should refer to the Guidelines for Prevention and Treatment of Opportunistic Infections in HIV-Infected Adults and Adolescents and the Guidelines for Antiretrovial Therapy in Adults and Adolescents for more detailed discussion on when to initiate antiretroviral therapy in the setting of a specific opportunistic infection.[74]

DIAGNOSIS OF OPPORTUNISTIC INFECTIONS

The $CD4^+$ T lymphocyte cell number continues to be a useful marker for predicting the occurrence of opportunistic infections in patients with HIV infection.[5] This relationship of $CD4^+$ T lymphocyte count to the occurrence of opportunistic infection continues to be as valid in the era of antiretroviral therapy as it was before the licensing of the first antiretroviral agent, zidovudine, in 1987.[75] Figure 53.5 demonstrates the typical relationship of $CD4^+$ T lymphocyte counts to the occurrence of opportunistic infections. Knowledge of this relationship permits the focusing of diagnostic, therapeutic, and prophylactic management.

For instance, if a patient with HIV infection and a $CD4^+$ T lymphocyte count of 700 cells/μL presents with diffuse pulmonary infiltrates, the diagnostic evaluation and empiric antimicrobial regimen should focus on common, nonopportunistic pathogens such as *Mycoplasma, Legionella,* and *Chlamydia* organisms, as well as common community-acquired viruses such as influenza plus opportunistic infections that occur at high $CD4^+$ T lymphocyte counts, such as *Mycobacterium tuberculosis* or *S. pneumoniae.* In contrast, if the same patient had a $CD4^+$ T lymphocyte count fewer than 50 cells/μL, the evaluation and empiric regimen would focus on pneumocystosis, pneumococcal pneumonia, and tuberculosis, although the previously mentioned processes that occur at high $CD4^+$ T lymphocyte counts can also occur at lower $CD4^+$ T lymphocyte counts.

Keeping in mind that $CD4^+$ T lymphocyte counts are useful predictors of susceptibility to infection is important, but they are not perfect. Occasionally, patients will develop opportunistic infections at "uncharacteristically" high $CD4^+$ T lymphocyte counts. For instance, 5% to 10% of cases of pneumocystosis occur at $CD4^+$ T lymphocyte counts greater than 200 cells/μL.[76] Clinical parameters can provide additional clues; for example, oral *candidiasis,* a previous opportunistic infection, a prior episode of pneumonia, or high viral load are independent risk factors for the occurrence of *Pneumocystis jiroveci* pneumonia (PCP), and logically for other infections as well.

A frequent question is whether an HIV-infected patient's prior $CD4^+$ T lymphocyte count nadir affects the likelihood of an opportunistic infection occurring if antiretroviral therapy has stimulated a $CD4^+$ T lymphocyte count rise. Specifically, if a patient has a $CD4^+$ T lymphocyte count of 400 cells/μL while receiving antiretroviral therapy and that patient's $CD4^+$ T lymphocyte count was 50 cells/μL before antiretroviral therapy, is that patient at greater risk for developing an opportunistic infection than another patient whose current $CD4^+$ T lymphocyte count is 400 cells/μL but whose nadir before antiretroviral therapy was 250 cells/μL? The data suggest that these two patients have comparable risk (i.e., the current $CD4^+$ T lymphocyte count is the most important predictor of risk and the earlier nadir has only minor influence on opportunistic infection susceptibility).

Like other immunosuppressed individuals, patients with HIV infection and low $CD4^+$ T lymphocyte counts require a prompt attempt to define the specific cause of their clinical syndrome. Like patients with neutropenia, fevers of unknown origin are not common. However, patients often present with specific syndromes such as pneumonia, meningitis, focal neurologic abnormalities, chorioretinitis, or diarrhea. Patients can deteriorate quickly, and the range of causative organisms is broad. Thus, as with patients with neutropenia, HIV-infected individuals need specific microbiologic and pathologic tests to determine the specific cause of their syndrome so that the appropriate therapy can be initiated, and so that unnecessary drugs can be eliminated.

In evaluating the differential diagnosis of infectious syndromes in patients with HIV (and in every other patient population as well), geography is an important part of the history. Tuberculosis is always a concern because of the extraordinary susceptibility of HIV-infected patients for developing active disease once they have been exposed.[77-79] It is notable, however, that although HIV and tuberculosis overlap in many patients in much of the developing world, in the United States only 10% of cases of tuberculosis occur in HIV-infected patients.[80] In many urban settings in the United States, each pulmonary evaluation should include smears and cultures for *M. tuberculosis,* both to diagnose the appropriate cause of the pulmonary dysfunction and to assist in determining which respiratory precautions are appropriate. However, in the United States where only about 11,000 cases of new tuberculosis occur per year, and where 50% of cases occur in immigrants, the likelihood of tuberculosis in a U.S. native with no known exposure is quite low, in contrast to a recent immigrant from a highly endemic area.[80]

In some areas of the country, such as the Ohio River Valley including Indianapolis, histoplasmosis is as common as pneumocystosis in causing diffuse pulmonary infiltrates. In the southwestern United States, coccidioidomycosis must be recognized as a cause of pulmonary infiltrates. The clinical presentations of tuberculosis, histoplasmosis, coccidioidomycosis, cryptococcosis, and toxoplasmosis can be clinically indistinguishable from PCP. Thus for HIV-infected patients with pulmonary infiltrates in an ICU, prolonged empiric therapy is discouraged in favor of vigorous efforts to establish a specific diagnosis.

CLINICAL SYNDROMES

HIV-infected patients are admitted to ICUs for major syndromes such as respiratory insufficiency, cerebral dysfunction, septic shock, hepatic or renal failure, and drug toxicities. However, patients with HIV infection also come to ICUs for routine procedures and routine postoperative care. In those situations their management ordinarily requires no extraordinary measures, with two exceptions, in addition to careful consideration of how to manage antiretroviral drugs.

First, as noted earlier, intensivists must consult with HIV specialists about management of antiretroviral drugs. The imprudent continuation of these drugs or the imprudent discontinuation of these drugs can have lifelong consequences for the patient that can be substantially avoided with proper consultation.

Second, drug interactions involving drugs used during procedures and certain antiretroviral drugs can have important clinical consequences. Many of the protease inhibitors and the non-nucleoside reverse transcriptase inhibitors that are now the backbone of antiretroviral therapy can inhibit or enhance the metabolism of drugs that depend on the cytochrome P-450 system. Thus, the half-lives of certain analgesics, sedatives, and hypnotics can be prolonged in HIV-infected patients who are taking ritonavir, for example. This pharmacokinetic effect is also relevant for a host of other therapeutic agents used in the ICU and may affect their efficacy or safety. Clinicians need to be familiar with these interactions when selecting new therapies for procedures or for clinical entities. Given how complicated these interactions are, consultation with a specialist, e.g., a pharmacologist or infectious disease specialist, is appropriate for any HIV patient admitted to the ICU when antiretroviral drugs are involved.

The therapies for specific opportunistic pathogens are summarized in Table 53.5.

RESPIRATORY INSUFFICIENCY

Patients with HIV infection can develop severe pulmonary dysfunction because of common community-acquired pathogens such as *S. pneumonia, Legionella, Mycoplasma,* and *Chlamydia;* adenovirus; influenza; or respiratory syncytial virus, as well as other opportunistic viruses and fungi. Thus the diagnostic evaluation needs to be comprehensive, emphasizing direct smears of sputum or bronchoalveolar lavage. It is important to recognize that the clinical presentations produced by many causative agents can be similar. For instance, histoplasmosis, tuberculosis, and nonspecific interstitial pneumonitis can present identically to PCP.[76,77,81,82] Thus although empiric diagnosis and empiric therapy may be reasonable as initial approaches to some patients with HIV infection and mild pneumonitis, such an approach is usually not appropriate for patients in an ICU.

Evaluation of induced sputum is the first step in the diagnostic approach to PCP. Sensitivity can be as high as 80% to 95% at many hospitals (at some institutions the yield is considerably lower).[83] Specificity should be 100% in an experienced laboratory. Other pathogens, including mycobacteria, fungi, and routine bacteria, can be identified in sputum as well. For intubated patients, respiratory secretions obtained by deep intratracheal suctioning are also likely to be useful, although they have not been as carefully studied as induced sputum. Should the diagnosis not be established by evaluation of sputum or intratracheal secretions, bronchoscopy should be performed. Bronchoalveolar lavage should diagnose almost 100% of cases of PCP, even if patients have already received 7 to 10 days of empiric therapy at the time of the diagnostic procedure.[76] A diagnosis of PCP is established by visualizing one or more clusters of organisms. Some laboratories are now using PCR to diagnose PCP, but this test is not standardized and is likely to be highly sensitive but not highly specific for identifying *Pneumocystis* as the cause of the pulmonary dysfunction.[44,84]

Diagnostic criteria for other opportunistic infections are reviewed in Chapters 12 and 42. CMV merits special mention. CMV pneumonia almost never occurs in patients with HIV infection, as opposed to patients with solid organ or stem cell transplants. CMV should be considered the cause only if other causative processes have been ruled out, and there is convincing histologic or cytologic evidence. Culture of sputum or bronchoalveolar lavage for CMV does not provide useful information; in particular, patients with $CD4^+$ T lymphocyte counts below 100 cells/μL will predictably have CMV present in their secretion independent of whether or not pulmonary disease is present.[85] A diagnosis of CMV pneumonia in this patient population is suggested by cytologic test and confirmed by the presence of multiple inclusion bodies in lung tissue obtained by transbronchial or open lung biopsy.

Similarly, *Mycobacterium avium* complex (MAC) and herpes simplex virus (HSV) can often be found in respiratory secretions of patients with HIV/AIDS by culture or by nucleic acid amplification tests, but these organisms almost never cause pneumonia in patients with HIV infection. In other patient populations they can clearly cause pneumonia, but the dearth of CMV, MAC, and HSV pneumonia in this patient population emphasizes the point that it is important to know from published literature what the clinical likelihood is for different microbial processes.

Fungal pneumonias other than PCP are generally diagnosed by direct microscopy or culture of respiratory secretions (sputum or bronchoalveolar lavage). *Candida* organisms almost never cause pneumonia in patients with HIV infection. The frequency of *Cryptococcus, Histoplasma,*

Text continued on p. 929

Table 53.5 Treatment of AIDS-Associated Opportunistic Infections

Opportunistic Infection	Preferred Therapy	Alternative Therapy	Other Comments
Pneumocystis pneumonia (PCP)	Patients who develop PCP despite TMP-SMX prophylaxis can usually be treated with standard doses of TMP-SMX Duration of PCP treatment: 21 days *For Moderate to Severe PCP:* TMP-SMX: (TMP 15-20 mg and SMX 75-100 mg/kg/day) IV given q6h or q8h may switch to PO after clinical improvement *For Mild to Moderate PCP:* TMP-SMX: (TMP 15-20 mg and SMX 75-100 mg/kg/day), given PO in 3 divided doses, *or* TMP-SMX: (160 mg/800 mg or DS) 2 tablets PO tid *Secondary Prophylaxis, after completion of PCP treatment:* TMP-SMX DS: 1 tablet PO daily *or* TMP-SMX (80 mg/400 mg or SS): 1 tablet PO daily	*For Moderate to Severe PCP:* Pentamidine 4 mg/kg IV daily infused over ≥60 minutes; can reduce dose to 3 mg/kg IV daily because of toxicities, *or* Primaquine 30 mg (base) PO daily + (clindamycin 600 mg q6h IV or 900 mg IV q8h) or (clindamycin 300 mg PO q6h or 450 mg PO q8h) *For Mild to Moderate PCP:* Dapsone 100 mg PO daily + TMP 5 mg/kg PO tid, *or* Primaquine 30 mg (base) PO daily + (clindamycin 300 mg PO q6h or 450 mg PO q8h), *or* Atovaquone 750 mg PO bid with food *Secondary Prophylaxis, after completion of PCP treatment:* TMP-SMX DS: 1 tablet PO tiw, *or* Dapsone 100 mg PO daily, *or* Dapsone 50 mg PO daily + (pyrimethamine 50 mg + leucovorin 25 mg) PO weekly, *or* (Dapsone 200 mg + pyrimethamine 75 mg + leucovorin 25 mg) PO weekly, *or* Aerosolized pentamidine 300 mg monthly via Respirgard II nebulizer, *or* Atovaquone 1500 mg PO daily, *or* (Atovaquone 1500 mg + pyrimethamine 25 mg + leucovorin 10 mg) PO daily	*Indications for Adjunctive Corticosteroids* PaO_2 <70 mm Hg at room air, *or* Alveolar-arterial O_2 gradient >35 mm Hg *Prednisone Doses (beginning as early as possible and within 72 hours of pcp therapy):* Days 1-5: 40 mg PO bid Days 6-10: 40 mg PO daily Days 11-21: 20 mg PO daily IV methylprednisolone can be administered as 75% of prednisone dose. Benefit of corticosteroid if started after 72 hours of treatment is unknown, but some clinicians will use it for moderate-to-severe PCP. Whenever possible, patients should be tested for G6PD before use of dapsone or primaquine. Alternative therapy should be used in patients found to have G6PD deficiency. Patients who are receiving pyrimethamine/sulfadiazine for treatment or suppression of toxoplasmosis do not require additional PCP prophylaxis. If TMP-SMX is discontinued because of a mild adverse reaction, re-institution should be considered after the reaction resolves. The dose can be increased gradually (desensitization), reduced, or the frequency modified. TMP-SMX should be permanently discontinued in patients with possible or definite Stevens-Johnson syndrome or toxic epidermal necrosis.

Toxoplasma gondii encephalitis	*Treatment of Acute Infection:* Pyrimethamine 200 mg PO 1 time, followed by weight-based therapy: If <60 kg, pyrimethamine 50 mg PO once daily + sulfadiazine 1000 mg PO q6h – leucovorin 10-25 mg PO once daily If ≥60 kg, pyrimethamine 75 mg PO once daily + sulfadiazine 1500 mg PO q6h – leucovorin 10-25 mg PO once daily Leucovorin dose can be increased to 50 mg daily or bid *Duration for Acute Therapy:* At least 6 weeks; longer duration if clinical or radiologic disease is extensive or response is incomplete at 6 weeks *Chronic Maintenance Therapy:* Pyrimethamine 25-50 mg PO daily + sulfadiazine 2000-4000 mg PO daily (in 2-4 divided doses) + leucovorin 10-25 mg PO daily (AI)	*Treatment of Acute Infection:* Pyrimethamine (leucovorin)* + clindamycin 600 mg IV or PO q6h *or* TMP-SMX (TMP 5 mg/kg and SMX 25 mg/kg) IV or PO bid, *or* Atovaquone 1500 mg PO bid with food + pyrimethamine (leucovorin), *or* Atovaquone 1500 mg PO BID with food + sulfadiazine 1000-1500 mg PO q6h (weight-based dosing, as in preferred therapy) *or* Atovaquone 1500 mg PO bid with food, *or* Pyrimethamine (leucovorin)* + azithromycin 900-1200 mg PO daily *Chronic Maintenance Therapy:* Clindamycin 600 mg PO q8h + (pyrimethamine 25-50 mg + leucovorin 10-25 mg) PO daily or TMP-SMX DS 1 tablet bid, *or* Atovaquone 750-1500 mg PO bid + (pyrimethamine 25 mg + leucovorin 10 mg) PO daily, *or* Atovaquone 750-1500 mg PO bid + sulfadiazine 2000-4000 mg PO daily (in 2-4 divided doses), *or* Atovaquone 750-1500 mg PO bid with food *Pyrimethamine and leucovorin doses are the same as for preferred therapy.	Adjunctive corticosteroids (e.g., dexamethasone) should only be administered when clinically indicated to treat mass effect associated with focal lesions or associated edema; discontinue as soon as clinically feasible. Anticonvulsants should be administered to patients with a history of seizures and continued through acute treatment, but should not be used as seizure prophylaxis. If clindamycin is used in place of sulfadiazine, additional therapy must be added to prevent PCP.

Continued on following page

Table 53.5 Treatment of AIDS-Associated Opportunistic Infections (Continued)

Opportunistic Infection	Preferred Therapy	Alternative Therapy	Other Comments
Mycobacterium tuberculosis disease (TB)	After collecting specimen for culture and molecular diagnostic tests, empiric TB treatment should be started in individuals with clinical and radiographic presentation suggestive of TB. Refer to Table 53.3 for dosing recommendations. *Initial Phase (2 months, given daily, 5-7 times/week by DOT):* INH + [RIF or RFB] + PZA + EMB *Continuation Phase:* INH + (RIF or RFB) daily (5-7 times/week) or tiw *Total Duration of Therapy (for drug-susceptible TB):* Pulmonary TB: 6 months Pulmonary TB and culture-positive after 2 months of TB treatment: 9 months Extrapulmonary TB w/CNS infection: 9-12 months; Extrapulmonary TB w/bone or joint involvement: 6 to 9 months; Extrapulmonary TB in other sites: 6 months Total duration of therapy should be based on number of doses received, not on calendar time	*Treatment for Drug-Resistant TB* *Resistant to INH:* (RIF or RFB) + EMB + PZA + (moxifloxacin or levofloxacin) for 2 months; followed by (RIF or RFB) + EMB + (moxifloxacin or levofloxacin) for 7 months *Resistant to Rifamycins ± Other Drugs:* Regimen and duration of treatment should be individualized based on resistance pattern, clinical and microbiologic responses, and in close consultation with experienced specialists	Adjunctive corticosteroid improves survival for TB meningitis and pericarditis. See text for drug, dose, and duration recommendations. RIF *is not recommended* for patients receiving HIV PI because of its induction of PI metabolism. RFB is a less potent CYP3A4 inducer than RIF and is preferred in patients receiving PIs. Once weekly rifapentine can result in development of rifamycin resistance in HIV-infected patients and *is not recommended*. Therapeutic drug monitoring should be considered in patients receiving rifamycin and interacting ART. Paradoxical IRIS that is not severe can be treated with NSAIDs without a change in TB or HIV therapy. For severe IRIS reaction, consider prednisone and taper over 4 weeks based on clinical symptoms. For example: *If receiving RIF:* prednisone 1.5 mg/kg/day for 2 weeks, then 0.75 mg/kg/day for 2 weeks *If receiving RFB:* prednisone 1.0 mg/kg/day for 2 weeks, then 0.5 mg/kg/day for 2 weeks A more gradual tapering schedule over a few months may be necessary for some patients.
Disseminated *Mycobacterium avium* complex (MAC) disease	*At Least 2 Drugs as Initial Therapy with:* Clarithromycin 500 mg PO bid + ethambutol 15 mg/kg PO daily, *or* Azithromycin 500-600 mg + ethambutol 15 mg/kg PO daily if drug interaction or intolerance precludes the use of clarithromycin *Duration:* At least 12 months of therapy, can discontinue if no signs and symptoms of MAC disease and sustained (>6 months) CD4 count >100 cells/μL in response to ART	Addition of a third or fourth drug should be considered for patients with advanced immunosuppression (CD4 counts <50 cells/μL), high mycobacterial loads (>2 log CFU/mL of blood), or in the absence of effective ART. *Third or Fourth Drug Options May Include:* RFB 300 mg PO daily (dosage adjustment may be necessary based on drug interactions), Amikacin 10-15 mg/kg IV daily, *or* Streptomycin 1 g IV or IM daily, *or* Moxifloxacin 400 mg PO daily or levofloxacin 500 mg PO daily	Testing of susceptibility to clarithromycin and azithromycin is recommended. NSAIDs can be used for patients who experience moderate to severe symptoms attributed to IRIS. If IRIS symptoms persist, short-term (4-8 weeks) systemic corticosteroids (equivalent to 20-40 mg prednisone) can be used.

Bacterial respiratory diseases *(with focus on pneumonia)*	Empiric antibiotic therapy should be initiated promptly for patients presenting with clinical and radiographic evidence consistent with bacterial pneumonia. The recommendations listed are suggested empiric therapy. The regimen should be modified as needed once microbiologic results are available. *Empiric Outpatient Therapy:* A PO β-lactam + a PO macrolide (azithromycin or clarithromycin) *Preferred β-lactams*: high-dose amoxicillin or amoxicillin/clavulanate *Alternative β-lactams*: cefpodoxime or cefuroxime, *or* *For penicillin-allergic patients:* Levofloxacin 750 mg PO once daily, or moxifloxacin 400 mg PO once daily *Duration:* 7-10 days (a minimum of 5 days). Patients should be afebrile for 48-72 hours and clinically stable before stopping antibiotics. *Empiric Therapy for Non-ICU Hospitalized Patients:* An IV β-lactam + a macrolide (azithromycin or clarithromycin) *Preferred β-lactams:* ceftriaxone, cefotaxime, or ampicillin-sulbactam *For penicillin-allergic patients:* Levofloxacin, 750 mg IV once daily, *or* moxifloxacin, 400 mg IV once daily *Empiric Therapy for ICU Patients:* An IV β-lactam + IV azithromycin , *or* An IV β-lactam + (levofloxacin 750 mg IV once daily or moxifloxacin 400 mg IV once daily) *Preferred β-lactams*: ceftriaxone, cefotaxime, or ampicillin-sulbactam *Empiric Therapy for Patients at Risk of* Pseudomonas *Pneumonia:* An IV antipneumococcal, antipseudomonal β-lactam + ciprofloxacin 400 mg IV q8-12h or levofloxacin 750 mg IV once daily *Preferred β-lactams*: piperacillin-tazobactam, cefepime, imipenem, or meropenem *Empiric Therapy for Patients at Risk for Methicillin-Resistant* Staphylococcus aureus *Pneumonia:* Add vancomycin IV or linezolid (IV or PO) to the baseline regimen Addition of clindamycin to vancomycin (but not to linezolid) can be considered for severe necrotizing pneumonia to minimize bacterial toxin production	*Empiric Outpatient Therapy:* A PO β-lactam + PO doxycycline *Preferred β-lactams*: high-dose amoxicillin or amoxicillin/clavulanate *Alternative β-lactams*: cefpodoxime or cefuroxime *Empiric Therapy for Non-ICU Hospitalized Patients:* An IV β-lactam + doxycycline *Empiric Therapy for ICU Patients:* *For penicillin-allergic patients:* Aztreonam IV + (levofloxacin 750 mg IV once daily or moxifloxacin 400 mg IV once daily) *Empiric Therapy for Patients at Risk of Pseudomonas Pneumonia:* An IV antipneumococcal, antipseudomonal β-lactam + an aminoglycoside + azithromycin, *or* Above β-lactam + an aminoglycoside + (levofloxacin 750 mg IV once daily or moxifloxacin 400 mg IV once daily), *or* *For penicillin-allergic patients*: Replace the β-lactam with aztreonam	Fluoroquinolones should be used with caution in patients in whom TB is suspected but is not being treated. Empiric therapy with a macrolide alone is not routinely recommended, because of increasing pneumococcal resistance. Patients receiving a macrolide for MAC prophylaxis should not receive macrolide monotherapy for empiric treatment of bacterial pneumonia. For patients begun on IV antibiotic therapy, switching to PO should be considered when they are clinically improved and able to tolerate oral medications. Chemoprophylaxis can be considered for patients with frequent recurrences of serious bacterial pneumonia. Clinicians should be cautious about using antibiotics to prevent recurrences because of the potential for developing drug resistance and drug toxicities.

Continued on following page

Table 53.5 Treatment of AIDS-Associated Opportunistic Infections (Continued)

Opportunistic Infection	Preferred Therapy	Alternative Therapy	Other Comments
Bacterial enteric infections *Empiric therapy pending definitive diagnosis*	Diagnostic fecal specimens should be obtained before initiation of empiric antibiotic therapy. Empiric antibiotic therapy is indicated for patients with advanced HIV (CD4 count <200 cells/μL or concomitant AIDS-defining illnesses), with clinically severe diarrhea (>6 stools/day) and/or accompanying fever or chills. *Empiric Therapy:* Ciprofloxacin 500-750 mg PO (or 400 mg IV) q12h Therapy should be adjusted based on the results of diagnostic workup. For patients with chronic diarrhea (>14 days) without severe clinical signs, empiric antibiotics therapy is not necessary; can withhold treatment until a diagnosis is made.	*Empiric Therapy:* Ceftriaxone 1 g IV q24h, *or* Cefotaxime 1 g IV q8h	Hospitalization with IV antibiotics should be considered in patients with marked nausea, vomiting, diarrhea, electrolyte abnormalities, acidosis, and blood pressure instability. Oral or IV rehydration if indicated. Antimotility agents should be avoided if there is concern about inflammatory diarrhea, including *Clostridium difficile*–associated diarrhea. If no clinical response after 5-7 days, consider follow-up stool culture with antibiotic susceptibility testing or alternative diagnostic tests (e.g., toxin assays, molecular testing), alternative diagnosis, or antibiotic resistance.
Salmonellosis	All HIV-infected patients with salmonellosis should be treated because of high risk of bacteremia. Ciprofloxacin 500-750 mg PO (or 400 mg IV) q12h, if susceptible *Duration of Therapy:* *For gastroenteritis without bacteremia:* If CD4 count ≥200 cells/μL: 7-14 days If CD4 count <200 cells/μL: 2-6 weeks *For gastroenteritis with bacteremia:* If CD4 count ≥200/μL: 14 days; longer duration if bacteremia persists or if the infection is complicated (e.g., if metastatic foci of infection are present) If CD4 count <200 cells/μL: 2-6 weeks *Secondary Prophylaxis Should Be Considered for:* Patients with recurrent *Salmonella* gastroenteritis ± bacteremia, *or* Patients with CD4 <200 cells/μL with severe diarrhea	Levofloxacin 750 mg (PO or IV) q24h, *or* Moxifloxacin 400 mg (PO or IV) q24h, *or* TMP, 160 mg-SMX 800 mg (PO or IV) q12h, *or* Ceftriaxone 1 g IV q24h, *or* Cefotaxime 1 g IV q8h	Oral or IV rehydration if indicated. Antimotility agents should be avoided. The role of long-term secondary prophylaxis in patients with recurrent *Salmonella* bacteremia is not well established. Must weigh benefit against risks of long-term antibiotic exposure Effective ART may reduce the frequency, severity, and recurrence of *Salmonella* infections.

Mucocutaneous candidiasis	*For Oropharyngeal Candidiasis; Initial Episodes (for 7-14 days):* *Oral therapy* Fluconazole 100 mg PO daily, *or* *Topical therapy* Clotrimazole troches, 10 mg PO 5 times daily, *or* Miconazole mucoadhesive buccal 50-mg tablet—apply to mucosal surface over the canine fossa once daily (do not swallow, chew, or crush) *For Esophageal Candidiasis (for 14-21 days):* Fluconazole 100 mg (up to 400 mg) PO or IV daily, *or* Itraconazole oral solution 200 mg PO daily *For Uncomplicated Vulvovaginal Candidiasis:* Oral fluconazole 150 mg for 1 dose, *or* Topical azoles (clotrimazole, butoconazole, miconazole, tioconazole, or terconazole) for 3-7 days *For Severe or Recurrent Vulvovaginal Candidiasis:* Fluconazole 100-200 mg PO daily for ≥7 days, *or* Topical antifungal ≥7 days	*For Oropharyngeal Candidiasis; Initial Episodes (for 7-14 days):* *Oral therapy* Itraconazole oral solution 200 mg PO daily, *or* Posaconazole oral solution 400 mg PO bid for 1 day, then 400 mg daily *Topical therapy* Nystatin suspension 4-6 mL qid or 1-2 flavored pastilles 4-5 times daily *For Esophageal Candidiasis (for 14-21 days):* Voriconazole 200 mg PO or IV bid, *or* Posaconazole 400 mg PO bid, *or* Anidulafungin 100 mg IV 1 time, then 50 mg IV daily, *or* Caspofungin 50 mg IV daily, *or* Micafungin 150 mg IV daily, *or* Amphotericin B deoxycholate 0.6 mg/kg IV daily, *or* Lipid formulation of amphotericin B 3-4 mg/kg IV daily *For Uncomplicated Vulvovaginal Candidiasis:* Itraconazole oral solution 200 mg PO daily for 3-7 days	Chronic or prolonged use of azoles may promote development of resistance. Higher relapse rate for esophageal candidiasis seen with echinocandins than with fluconazole use. Suppressive therapy usually not recommended unless patients have frequent or severe recurrences. *If Decision Is to Use Suppressive Therapy:* *Oropharyngeal candidiasis:* Fluconazole 100 mg PO daily or tiw Itraconazole oral solution 200 mg PO daily *Esophageal candidiasis:* Fluconazole 100-200 mg PO daily Posaconazole 400 mg PO bid *Vulvovaginal candidiasis:* Fluconazole 150 mg PO once weekly

Continued on following page

Table 53.5 Treatment of AIDS-Associated Opportunistic Infections (Continued)

Opportunistic Infection	Preferred Therapy	Alternative Therapy	Other Comments
Cryptococcosis	*Cryptococcal Meningitis* *Induction Therapy (for at least 2 weeks, followed by consolidation therapy):* Liposomal amphotericin B 3-4 mg/kg IV daily + flucytosine 25 mg/kg PO qid (Note: Flucytosine dose should be adjusted in patients with renal dysfunction.) *Consolidation Therapy (for at least 8 weeks followed by maintenance therapy):* Fluconazole 400 mg PO (or IV) daily *Maintenance therapy:* Fluconazole 200 mg PO daily for at least 12 months *For Non-CNS, Extrapulmonary Cryptococcosis and Diffuse Pulmonary Disease:* Treatment same as for cryptococcal meningitis *Non-CNS Cryptococcosis with Mild to Moderate Symptoms and Focal Pulmonary Infiltrates:* Fluconazole, 400 mg PO daily for 12 months	*Cryptococcal Meningitis* *Induction Therapy (for at least 2 weeks, followed by consolidation therapy):* Amphotericin B deoxycholate 0.7 mg/kg IV daily + flucytosine 25 mg/kg PO qid, *or* Amphotericin B lipid complex 5 mg/kg IV daily + flucytosine 25 mg/kg PO qid, *or* Liposomal amphotericin B 3-4 mg/kg IV daily + fluconazole 800 mg PO or IV daily, *or* Amphotericin B deoxycholate 0.7 mg/kg IV daily + fluconazole 800 mg PO or IV daily, *or* Fluconazole 400-800 mg PO or IV daily + flucytosine 25 mg/kg PO qid, *or* Fluconazole 1200 mg PO or IV daily *Consolidation Therapy (for at least 8 weeks followed by maintenance therapy):* Itraconazole 200 mg PO bid for 8 weeks—less effective than fluconazole *Maintenance therapy:* No alternative therapy recommendation	Addition of flucytosine to amphotericin B has been associated with more rapid sterilization of CSF and decreased risk for subsequent relapse. Patients receiving flucytosine should have either blood levels monitored (peak level 2 hours after dose should be 30-80 µg/mL) or close monitoring of blood counts for development of cytopenia. Dosage should be adjusted in patients with renal insufficiency. Opening pressure should always be measured when an LP is performed Repeated LPs or CSF shunting are essential to effectively manage increased intracranial pressure. Corticosteroids and mannitol are ineffective in reducing ICP and are *not* recommended. Some specialists recommend a brief course of corticosteroid for management of severe IRIS symptoms.

Histoplasmosis	*Moderately Severe to Severe Disseminated Disease Induction Therapy (for at least 2 weeks or until clinically improved):* Liposomal amphotericin B 3 mg/kg IV daily *Maintenance Therapy* Itraconazole 200 mg PO tid for 3 days, then 200 mg PO bid *Less Severe Disseminated Disease* *Induction and Maintenance Therapy:* Itraconazole 200 mg PO tid for 3 days, then 200 mg PO bid *Duration of Therapy:* At least 12 months *Meningitis* *Induction Therapy (4-6 weeks):* Liposomal amphotericin B 5 mg/kg/day *Maintenance Therapy:* Itraconazole 200 mg PO bid to tid for ≥1 year and until resolution of abnormal CSF findings *Long-Term Suppression Therapy:* *For patients with severe disseminated or CNS infection after completion of at least 12 months of therapy; and those who relapse despite appropriate therapy* Itraconazole 200 mg PO daily	*Moderately Severe to Severe Disseminated Disease Induction Therapy (for at least 2 weeks or until clinically improved):* Amphotericin B lipid complex 3 mg/kg IV daily, *or* Amphotericin B cholesteryl sulfate complete 3 mg/kg IV daily *Alternatives to Itraconazole for Maintenance Therapy or Treatment of Less Severe Disease:* Voriconazole 400 mg PO bid for 1 day, then 200 mg bid, *or* Posaconazole 400 mg PO bid Fluconazole 800 mg PO daily *Meningitis:* No alternative therapy recommendation *Long-Term Suppression Therapy:* Fluconazole 400 mg PO daily	Itraconazole, posaconazole, and voriconazole may have significant interactions with certain ARV agents. These interactions are complex and can be bidirectional. Therapeutic drug monitoring and dosage adjustment may be necessary to ensure triazole antifungal and ARV efficacy and reduce concentration-related toxicities. Random serum concentration of itraconazole + hydroitraconazole should be >1 μg/mL. Clinical experience with voriconazole or posaconazole in the treatment of histoplasmosis is limited. Acute pulmonary histoplasmosis in HIV-infected patients with CD4 counts >300 cells/μL should be managed as nonimmunocompromised host.

Continued on following page

Table 53.5 Treatment of AIDS-Associated Opportunistic Infections (Continued)

Opportunistic Infection	Preferred Therapy	Alternative Therapy	Other Comments
Coccidioidomycosis	*Clinically Mild Infections (e.g., focal pneumonia):* Fluconazole 400 mg PO daily *or* Itraconazole 200 mg PO bid *Severe, Nonmeningeal Infection (diffuse pulmonary infection or severely ill patients with extrathoracic, disseminated disease):* Amphotericin B deoxycholate 0.7-1.0 mg/kg IV daily Lipid formulation amphotericin B 4-6 mg/kg IV daily Duration of therapy: continue until clinical improvement, then switch to an azole *Meningeal Infections:* Fluconazole 400-800 mg IV or PO daily *Chronic Suppressive Therapy:* Fluconazole 400 mg PO daily, *or* Itraconazole 200 mg PO bid	*Mild Infections (focal pneumonia) for patients who failed to respond to fluconazole or itraconazole:* Posaconazole 200 mg PO bid, *or* Voriconazole 200 mg PO bid *Severe, Nonmeningeal Infection (diffuse pulmonary infection or severely ill patients with extrathoracic, disseminated disease):* Some specialists will add a triazole (fluconazole or itraconazole, with itraconazole preferred for bone disease) 400 mg per day to amphotericin B therapy and continue triazole once amphotericin B is stopped *Meningeal Infections:* Itraconazole 200 mg PO tid for 3 days, then 200 mg PO bid, *or* Posaconazole 200 mg PO bid, *or* Voriconazole 200-400 mg PO bid, *or* Intrathecal amphotericin B deoxycholate, when triazole antifungals are ineffective *Chronic suppressive therapy:* Posaconazole 200 mg PO bid, *or* Voriconazole 200 mg PO bid	Some patients with meningitis may develop hydrocephalus and require CSF shunting. Therapy should be continued indefinitely in patients with diffuse pulmonary or disseminated diseases because relapse can occur in 25-33% of HIV-negative patients. It can also occur in HIV-infected patients with CD4 counts >250 cells/μL Therapy should be lifelong in patients with meningeal infections because relapse occurs in 80% of HIV-infected patients after discontinuation of triazole therapy. Itraconazole, posaconazole, and voriconazole may have significant interactions with certain ARV agents. These interactions are complex and can be bidirectional. Therapeutic drug monitoring and dosage adjustment may be necessary to ensure triazole antifungal and antiretroviral efficacy and reduce concentration-related toxicities. Intrathecal amphotericin B should only be given in consultation with a specialist and administered by an individual with experience with the technique.
Aspergillosis, invasive	*Preferred Therapy:* Voriconazole 6 mg/kg IV q12h for 1 day, then 4 mg/kg IV q12h, followed by voriconazole 200 mg PO q12h after clinical improvement *Duration of Therapy:* Until CD4 cell count >200 cells/μL and the infection appears to be resolved	*Alternative Therapy:* Lipid formulation of amphotericin B 5 mg/kg IV daily, *or* Amphotericin B deoxycholate 1 mg/kg IV daily, *or* Caspofungin 70 mg IV 1 time, then 50 mg IV daily, *or* Micafungin 100-150 mg IV daily, *or* Anidulafungin 200 mg IV 1 time, then 100 mg IV daily, *or* Posaconazole 200 mg PO qid, then, after condition improved, 400 mg PO bid	Potential for significant pharmacokinetic interactions between certain ARV agents and voriconazole; they should be used cautiously in these situations. Consider therapeutic drug monitoring and dosage adjustment if necessary.

Cytomegalovirus (CMV) disease	*CMV Retinitis Induction Therapy for Immediate Sight-Threatening Lesions (adjacent to the optic nerve or fovea)* *Consult ophthalmologist; ganciclovir implant no longer available:* Ganciclovir 5 mg/kg IV q12h for 14-21 days followed by Valganciclovir 900 mg PO bid *For Small Peripheral Lesions:* Valganciclovir 900 mg PO bid for 14-21 days One dose of intravitreal ganciclovir can be administered immediately after diagnosis until steady state plasma ganciclovir concentration is achieved with oral valganciclovir *Chronic Maintenance (secondary prophylaxis):* Valganciclovir 900 mg PO daily (for small peripheral lesion). *CMV Esophagitis or Colitis:* Ganciclovir 5 mg/kg IV q12h; may switch to valganciclovir 900 mg PO q12h once patient can tolerate oral therapy Duration: 21-42 days or until symptoms have resolved Maintenance therapy is usually not necessary, but should be considered after relapses. *Well-Documented, Histologically Confirmed CMV Pneumonia:* Experience for treating CMV pneumonitis in HIV patients is limited. Use of IV ganciclovir or IV foscarnet is reasonable (doses same as for CMV retinitis) The optimal duration of therapy and the role of oral valganciclovir have not been established. *CMV Neurologic Disease* Note: Treatment should be initiated promptly. Ganciclovir 5 mg/kg IV q12h + (foscarnet 90 mg/kg IV q12h or 60 mg/kg IV q8h) to stabilize disease and maximize response, continue until symptomatic improvement and resolution of neurologic symptoms The optimal duration of therapy and the role of oral valganciclovir have not been established.	*CMV Retinitis Induction Therapy:* Ganciclovir 5 mg/kg IV q12h for 14-21 days, *or* Foscarnet 90 mg/kg IV q12h or 60 mg q8h for 14-21 days, *or* Cidofovir 5 mg/kg/week IV for 2 weeks; saline hydration before and after therapy and probenecid, 2 g PO 3 hours before dose, followed by 1 g PO 2 hours and 8 hours after the dose (total of 4 g). (Note: This regimen should be avoided in patients with sulfa allergy because of cross-hypersensitivity with probenecid.) *Chronic Maintenance (secondary prophylaxis):* Ganciclovir 5 mg/kg IV 5-7 times weekly, *or* Foscarnet 90-120 mg/kg IV once daily, *or* Cidofovir 5 mg/kg IV every other week with saline hydration and probenecid as above *CMV Esophagitis or Colitis:* Foscarnet 90 mg/kg IV q12h or 60 mg/kg q8h for patients with treatment-limiting toxicities to ganciclovir or with ganciclovir resistance, *or* Valganciclovir 900 mg PO q12h in milder disease and if able to tolerate PO therapy, *or* For mild cases, if ART can be initiated without delay, consider withholding CMV therapy. Duration: 21-42 days or until symptoms have resolved	The choice of therapy for CMV retinitis should be individualized, based on location and severity of the lesions, level of immunosuppression, and other factors (e.g., concomitant medications and ability to adhere to treatment). The choice of chronic maintenance therapy (route of administration and drug choices) should be made in consultation with an ophthalmologist. Considerations should include the anatomic location of the retinal lesion, vision in the contralateral eye, the patients' immunologic and virologic status and response to ART. Patients with CMV retinitis who discontinue maintenance therapy should undergo regular eye examinations—optimally every 3 months—for early detection of relapse IRU, and then annually after immune reconstitution . IRU may develop in the setting of immune reconstitution. *Treatment of IRU* Periocular corticosteroid or short courses of systemic steroid. Initial therapy in patients with CMV retinitis, esophagitis, colitis, and pneumonitis should include initiation or optimization of ART.

Continued on following page

Table 53.5 Treatment of AIDS-Associated Opportunistic Infections (Continued)

Opportunistic Infection	Preferred Therapy	Alternative Therapy	Other Comments
Herpes simplex virus (HSV) disease	*Orolabial Lesions (for 5-10 days):* Valacyclovir 1 g PO bid *or* Famciclovir 500 mg PO bid *or* Acyclovir 400 mg PO tid *Initial or Recurrent Genital HSV (for 5-14 days):* Valacyclovir 1 g PO bid, *or* Famciclovir 500 mg PO bid, *or* Acyclovir 400 mg PO tid *Severe Mucocutaneous HSV:* Initial therapy acyclovir 5 mg/kg IV q8h After lesions begin to regress, change to PO therapy as above. Continue until lesions are completely healed. *Chronic Suppressive Therapy for patients with severe recurrences of genital herpes or patients who want to minimize frequency of recurrences:* Valacyclovir 500 mg PO bid Famciclovir 500 mg PO bid Acyclovir 400 mg PO bid Continue indefinitely regardless of CD4 cell count.	*For Acyclovir-Resistant HSV* *Preferred Therapy:* Foscarnet 80-120 mg/kg/day IV in 2-3 divided doses until clinical response *Alternative Therapy* IV cidofovir (dosage as in CMV retinitis), *or* Topical trifluridine, *or* Topical cidofovir, *or* Topical imiquimod *Duration of Therapy:* 21-28 days or longer	Patients with HSV infections can be treated with episodic therapy when symptomatic lesions occur, or with daily suppressive therapy to prevent recurrences. Topical formulations of trifluridine and cidofovir are not commercially available. Extemporaneous compounding of topical products can be prepared using trifluridine ophthalmic solution and the IV formulation of cidofovir.

Varicella-zoster virus (VZV) disease	*Primary Varicella Infection (Chickenpox):* *Uncomplicated Cases (for 5-7 days):* Valacyclovir 1 g PO tid *or* Famciclovir 500 mg PO tid *Severe or Complicated Cases:* Acyclovir 10-15 mg/kg IV q8h for 7-10 days May switch to oral valacyclovir, famciclovir, or acyclovir after defervescence if no evidence of visceral involvement *Herpes Zoster (Shingles) Acute Localized Dermatomal:* For 7-10 days; consider longer duration if lesions are slow to resolve Valacyclovir 1 g PO tid *or* Famciclovir 500 mg tid *Extensive Cutaneous Lesion or Visceral Involvement:* Acyclovir 10-15 mg/kg IV q8h until clinical improvement is evident May switch to PO therapy (valacyclovir, famciclovir, or acyclovir) after clinical improvement (i.e., when no new vesicle formation or improvement of signs and symptoms of visceral VZV), to complete a 10-14 day course *Progressive Outer Retinal Necrosis (PORN):* Ganciclovir 5 mg/kg + foscarnet 90 mg/kg IV q12h + ganciclovir 2 mg/0.05 mL ± foscarnet 1.2 mg/0.05 mL intravitreal injection biw *or* Initiate or optimize ART *Acute Retinal Necrosis (ARN):* Acyclovir 10 mg/kg IV q8h for 10-14 days, followed by valacyclovir 1 g PO tid for 6 weeks	*Primary Varicella Infection (Chickenpox)* *Uncomplicated Cases (for 5-7 days):* Acyclovir 800 mg PO 5 times/day *Herpes Zoster (Shingles)* *Acute Localized Dermatomal:* For 7-10 days; consider longer duration if lesions are slow to resolve Acyclovir 800 mg PO 5 times/day	In managing VZV retinitis: Consultation with an ophthalmologist experienced in management of VZV retinitis is strongly recommended. Duration of therapy for VZV retinitis is not well defined, and should be determined based on clinical, virologic, immunologic, and ophthalmologic responses. Optimization of ART is recommended for serious and difficult-to-treat VZV infections (e.g., retinitis, encephalitis).

Continued on following page

Table 53.5 Treatment of AIDS-Associated Opportunistic Infections (Continued)

Opportunistic Infection	Preferred Therapy	Alternative Therapy	Other Comments
Progressive multifocal leukoencephalopathy (PML) (JC virus infections)	There is no specific antiviral therapy for JC virus infection. The main treatment approach is to reverse the immunosuppression caused by HIV. Initiate ART immediately in ART-naïve patients Optimize ART in patients who develop PML in phase of HIV viremia on ART	None.	Corticosteroids may be used for PML-IRIS characterized by contrast enhancement, edema or mass effect, and with clinical deterioration.

ACTG, AIDS Clinical Trials Group; ART, antiretroviral therapy; ARV, antiretroviral; ATV/r, ritonavir-boosted atazanavir; bid, twice a day; biw, twice weekly; BOC, boceprevir; CD4, CD4 T lymphocyte cell; CDC, The Centers for Disease Control and Prevention; CFU, colony-forming unit; CNS, central nervous system; CSF, cerebrospinal fluid; CYP3A4, cytochrome P-450 3A4; ddI, didanosine; DOT, directly observed therapy; DS, double strength; EFV, efavirenz; EMB, ethambutol; G6PD, glucose-6-phosphate dehydrogenase; GI, gastrointestinal; ICP, intracranial pressure; ICU, intensive care unit; IM, intramuscular; IND, investigational new drug; INH, isoniazid; IRIS, immune reconstitution inflammatory syndrome; IV, intravenous; LP, lumbar puncture; mm Hg, millimeters of mercury; NNRTI, non-nucleoside reverse transcriptase inhibitor; NRTI, nucleoside reverse transcriptase inhibitor; NSAID, nonsteroidal anti-inflammatory drugs; PegIFN, pegylated interferon; PI, protease inhibitor; PO, oral; PORN, progressive outer retinal necrosis; PZA, pyrazinamide; qAM, every morning; qid, four times a day; q(n)h, every "n" hours; qPM, every evening; RBV, ribavirin; RFB, rifabutin; RIF, rifampin; SQ, subcutaneous; SS, single strength; tid, three times daily, tiw, three times weekly; TVR, telaprevir; TMP-SMX, trimethoprim-sulfamethoxazole; ZDV, zidovudine.

Quality of Evidence for the Recommendation:

I: One or more randomized trials with clinical outcomes and/or validated laboratory endpoints

II: One or more well-designed, nonrandomized trials or observational cohort studies with long-term clinical outcomes

III: Expert opinion

Blastomyces, and *Coccidioides* as causes of pneumonia depends on the geographic exposure of the patient. Among these mycoses, antigen detection techniques can be useful for finding *Cryptococcus* and *Histoplasma* organisms.

Therapy of opportunistic infections is summarized in Table 53.5.[74] While awaiting a specific diagnosis, it is reasonable to initiate empiric therapy in patients ill enough to merit admission to an ICU. For patients with a CD4+ T lymphocyte count greater than 250 to 300 cells/μL, levofloxacin or moxifloxacin and ceftriaxone or azithromycin and ampicillin-sulbactam would be reasonable choices. For patients with CD4+ T lymphocyte counts below 200 to 250 cells/μL, levofloxacin or moxifloxacin plus trimethoprim-sulfamethoxazole or pentamidine plus levofloxacin or moxifloxacin would be potential regimens.

If PCP is documented, trimethoprim-sulfamethoxazole is always the drug of choice in patients who can tolerate it. Table 53.5 lists alternatives for sulfa-intolerant individuals. Regardless of which specific anti-*Pneumocystis* regimen is used, corticosteroid therapy is indicated for any patient who presents with an oxygen pressure (Po_2) below 70 mm Hg or an alveolar-arterial gradient higher than 30 mm Hg.[86-88] Patients with an initial Po_2 lower than 70 mm Hg are the subgroup with substantial mortality risk for whom corticosteroids have been shown to provide a survival benefit. Corticosteroids also provide more rapid resolution of pulmonary manifestations in patients who present with better pulmonary function, but survival in this population is so high that clinical trials have not been able to show survival benefit and thus corticosteroids are not conventionally recommended for patients who present with a room air Po_2 greater than 70 mm Hg. Some experts are concerned that corticosteroid use will be associated with reactivation of latent infections such as CMV or tuberculosis. However, reactivation of life-threatening infections has not been associated with this corticosteroid regimen.

How should a patient with AIDS-associated PCP be managed if there is no improvement, or if there is deterioration, after 5 to 10 days of therapy? The median time to improvement in clinical variables is 4 to 8 days; therefore, changes in therapy are probably not warranted before 5 to 10 days. At that point the accuracy of the diagnosis should be reassessed: Consideration should be given to repeat bronchoscopy with bronchoalveolar lavage or, perhaps, transbronchial biopsy to determine if CMV, fungi, mycobacteria, or a nosocomial bacterial process is present. Noninfectious processes such as congestive heart failure or tumor (e.g., Kaposi sarcoma) must also be considered. If pneumocystosis is the only causative process that can be identified, corticosteroids should be added to the regimen if they have not been already. Whether switching from one anti-*Pneumocystis* agent to another or whether adding a second agent is helpful has not been determined by clinical trials. Some human pneumocystosis isolates carry resistance mutations to sulfonamides, but such testing is available only in a few research centers, and the clinical significance of these mutations is unknown. Most experts add parenteral pentamidine to trimethoprim-sulfamethoxazole. Parenteral clindamycin-primaquine could be used as salvage regimens as well. Patients who have not improved after 14 to 21 days of therapy with specific chemotherapy plus corticosteroids have an exceedingly poor prognosis.

Should patients with AIDS-related PCP be intubated and provided with mechanical ventilation? The mortality rate for such patient populations was 70% to 80% in several series in the early 1980s.[89,90] Since that era, supportive care has improved, and treatment modalities for concurrent infectious and noninfectious processes have become more effective. Patient selection for ventilatory support is probably also improving. Patients who have multiple active opportunistic infections, substantial weight loss, and no response to 14 days of therapy have a worse prognosis than previously ambulatory patients who develop respiratory failure during the first few days of therapy. Thus decisions about ICU support for patients with HIV infection and respiratory failure need to be individualized on the basis of a realistic assessment of prognosis, the availability of resources, and the preference of the individual patient.

As indicated earlier, the ICU is not an ideal setting for initiating antiretroviral therapy. It should be noted, however, that for PCP, early initiation of antiretroviral therapy is generally associated with increased survival and thus therapy generally should not be delayed.[73] However, the studies that have been done had very few patients with life-threatening manifestations of their acute opportunistic infection. Thus, for patients ill enough to be in the ICU, the initiation of antiretroviral therapy might be associated with an immune reconstitution syndrome that could make respiratory support difficult or impossible. Moreover, patients in the ICU may not be able to absorb oral antiretroviral therapy, or might have complicated drug interactions with other necessary drugs. Thus, decisions to start antiretroviral therapy in the ICU require considerable thought and do not lend themselves to simple algorithms.

CENTRAL NERVOUS SYSTEM DYSFUNCTION

Meningitis

In HIV-infected patients with CD4+ counts greater than 200 cells/μL, the causes of meningitis do not differ markedly from those in the normal population: *S. pneumonia* and *Neisseria meningitidis* are the most common causes. For patients with CD4+ counts lower than 100 cells/μL, *Cryptococcus neoformans* is common.[91]

A diagnosis of cryptococcal meningitis is typically established by lumbar puncture: essentially 100% of patients with HIV-related cryptococcal meningitis should have a positive cerebrospinal fluid (CSF) cryptococcal antigen and CSF culture. Most patients will have an elevated CSF protein, low glucose, and elevated mononuclear cell count. Most will also have a positive serum cryptococcal antigen.

The therapy of choice for cryptococcal meningitis is liposomal amphotericin B for at least 2 weeks, plus flucytosine. Fluconazole should not be used for initial therapy, although it can be used after the initial 2 weeks if patients have a good clinical response.[92]

Some patients with cryptococcal meningitis have symptomatic elevations of CSF pressure. Such patients should have therapeutic lumbar punctures to remove enough CSF to reduce the pressure to 20 to 25 cm H_2O. Multiple lumbar punctures may be needed. If after multiple lumbar punctures the patient still have symptomatic elevation of CSF pressure greater than 20 to 25 cm H_2O, the insertion of a ventricular shunt should be considered, although there are no specific guidelines regarding when to place such a shunt. Corticosteroids should not generally be used to treat elevated intracranial pressure in this situation.[93-95]

FOCAL CENTRAL NERVOUS SYSTEM LESIONS

Patients with HIV infection and CD4 counts less than 100 cells/μL may present with focal motor lesions, altered mental status, or seizures. Although the differential diagnosis is extensive, the major considerations are toxoplasmosis and lymphoma.[96,97]

Central nervous system (CNS) toxoplasmosis may present as one or multiple lesions that represent reactivation of latent disease. Lesions are characteristically enhancing in a ringlike pattern and typically occur in the basal ganglia, but many different radiologic presentations have been documented.

All patients with CNS toxoplasmosis are IgG seropositive for toxoplasmosis using sensitive assays. However, some laboratories use less sensitive assays and thus some patients may appear to be seronegative. If lumbar puncture can be performed, a PCR for toxoplasmosis is positive in about 50% of cases, although there is no standardization of these *Toxoplasma* PCRs, making results variable from laboratory to laboratory.[98] The standard practice for HIV-infected patients with CD4 counts less than 200 cells/μL is to undergo an empiric trial of oral sulfadiazine plus pyrimethamine plus leucovorin. Most patients who have toxoplasmosis will show clinical and radiologic improvement within 2 weeks. If such improvement has not been documented, and the diagnosis is in doubt, a needle biopsy of the intracranial lesion should be considered.[99-101]

CNS lymphoma can present identically to CNS lymphoma. A negative serum IgG for toxoplasmosis, and a negative CSF toxoplasma PCR should suggest lymphoma.[102] Most patients with CNS lymphoma will have a positive CSF PCR for EBV (Epstein-Barr virus), although this test is neither 100% sensitive nor 100% specific for lymphoma. Patients who are CSF EBV PCR negative or in whom the diagnosis is uncertain may require a brain biopsy to document the lymphoma.

Therapy for lymphoma is one of several chemotherapeutic regimens. Patients continue to have a poor prognosis, but benefit from immune reconstitution with antiretroviral therapy.

FOCAL WHITE MATTER LESIONS

In patients with HIV, JC virus encephalitis (also known as progressive multifocal encephalopathy) causes focal white matter lesions that are associated with progressive motor, sensory, and neurocognitive dysfunction.[103] A small fraction of patients can present with rapidly progressive cognitive decline.

The CT scan or MRI images of JC virus encephalitis are characteristic of this disease. Diagnosis is usually confirmed by CSF PCR for JC virus. There is no specific therapy. Patients may stabilize or improve if antiretroviral therapy results in immune reconstitution.[104]

DIFFUSE ENCEPHALOPATHY

Patients with HIV infection can develop significant cognitive dysfunction due to nonfocal entities including HIV encephalopathy and CMV encephalitis. HIV encephalitis characteristically progresses slowly and has ventricular enlargement and cerebral atrophy on brain imaging. The CSF is unremarkable, and there is no diagnostic CSF test.

CMV encephalitis, in contrast, is rapid in progression and has a neutrophilic pleocytosis in the CSF and a positive CSF PCR for CMV.[105,106] Imaging shows either periventricular enhancement or focal nodules. Therapy is typically not successful in reversing the cerebral dysfunction. Either ganciclovir, foscarnet, or a combination of both drugs can be used in addition to the institution of antiretroviral therapy.

DIARRHEA

Patients with HIV infection and CD4 counts below 100 cells/μL can develop severe diarrhea due to a wide range of opportunistic pathogens including CMV, cryptosporidiosis, or enteric bacteria such as *Salmonella*, *Shigella*, or *Campylobacter*. Diarrhea in HIV-infected patients can be so severe that patients can have life-threatening malabsorption, electrolyte abnormalities, and bowel perforations. Patients need a thorough stool evaluation for common pathogens such as *Clostridium difficile*, which is the most common cause of diarrhea in this patient population, even though it is not an opportunistic pathogen. If stool cultures are negative, testing samples for ova and parasites might be indicated if there is a history compatible with exposure.

For patients with negative evaluation of multiple stool samples, a sigmoidoscopy with biopsy is indicated to assess the presence of CMV. CMV colitis occurs exclusively in patients with $CD4^+$ T lymphocyte counts lower than 100 cells/μL. CMV colitis is best diagnosed by biopsy: there is no reliable correlation with serum CMV PCR or with stool culture or PCR for CMV. The therapy of choice for CMV colitis is intravenous ganciclovir. Intravenous foscarnet is also effective but is more toxic. Oral valganciclovir is not indicated for patients with severe diarrhea but can be used as maintenance therapy once the CMV colitis is controlled. The most effective remedy for CMV colitis is immune reconstitution with antiretroviral therapy. As soon as absorption seems likely, antiretroviral therapy should be initiated.

HYPOTENSION

Patients with HIV infection develop hypotension resulting from the same types of disorders as with non-HIV-infected individuals—sepsis from a primary infection or a wound or device (especially an intravascular access device), fluid depletion from vomiting or diarrhea, and hemorrhage from a gastrointestinal lesion are examples of common causes. The evaluation of hypotension in a patient with HIV infection must take into account factors particular to this patient population: HIV-infected patients are susceptible to opportunistic infections; they undergo many procedures that can be associated with infectious complications; and they receive an array of drugs, some of which have cardiovascular effects. Thus, evaluating hypotension in this patient population requires a comprehensive and thorough approach. A differential diagnosis of the major causes is shown in Table 53.6. Adrenal function always deserves special attention

Table 53.6 Causes of Hypotension in Patients with HIV Infection

Process	Examples of Causes
Distributive Shock	
Septic shock	
Bacterial	Pneumococcal or *Haemophilus* pneumonia
	Vascular access infection
	Surgical wound
Viral	CMV infection, disseminated VZV infection
Fungal	*Histoplasma, Coccidioides, Cryptococcus* organisms
	Vascular access–related candidemia
	Pneumocystis jiroveci pneumonia
Adrenal insufficiency	Tuberculosis, fungal disease, CMV infection, HIV infection
Oligemic shock	
Dehydration	Bacterial diarrhea
	C. difficile diarrhea
Gastrointestinal hemorrhage	CMV colitis
	Gastrointestinal lymphoma
Cardiogenic Shock	
Cardiomyopathy	HIV infection
Endocarditis	Bacterial pathogens related to intravenous drug abuse
Extracardiac Obstruction	
Pericardial tamponade	Lymphoma, Kaposi sarcoma, primary effusion lymphoma
	Fungal infection, tuberculosis
Pericardial constriction	Tuberculosis, fungal infection
Massive pulmonary embolus	Inactivity, inanition

CMV, cytomegalovirus; HIV, human immunodeficiency virus; VZV, varicella-zoster virus.

because several viral processes, fungal and mycobacterial diseases, HIV, and drugs can suppress the adrenal axis and either cause hypotension or exacerbate it.

PREVENTION OF OPPORTUNISTIC INFECTION

Intensivists usually focus on the management of acute processes, but if attention is not provided to opportunistic infection prevention, patients hospitalized for one process may develop a second life-threatening process given the high incidence of opportunistic infections.

Patients with HIV infection typically receive several antimicrobial agents to reduce the likelihood they will acquire opportunistic infections. *Primary prophylaxis* is the term used to indicate strategies that reduce the likelihood of an initial episode of a disease process. *Secondary prophylaxis* is the term used to indicate strategies that prevent recurrences or relapses. *Chronic suppressive therapy* is identical to secondary prophylaxis: This refers to regimens that are continued after the initial therapeutic course to prevent relapses.

All patients with HIV infection and $CD4^+$ T lymphocyte counts below 200 cells/μL typically receive anti-*Pneumocystis* prophylaxis. Trimethoprim-sulfamethoxazole is the regimen of choice. Patients who actually take this drug have very few breakthroughs of PCP and receive considerable protection against toxoplasmosis and certain routine bacterial infections. Alternative regimens include monthly dapsone, weekly dapsone-pyrimethamine, or daily aerosol pentamidine. Prophylaxis against *M. avium* complex is recommended for patients with $CD4^+$ T lymphocyte counts under 100 cells/μL; clarithromycin and azithromycin are currently the drugs of choice.[74]

Some clinicians also use fluconazole or acyclovir prophylaxis to reduce the frequency of fungal and viral processes, respectively, although this is not recommended because of issues of cost, pill burden, and the emergence of resistant pathogens. Isoniazid prophylaxis is important for any patient with a tuberculin skin test that shows more than 5 mm of induration or a history of substantial recent exposure.

HIV TRANSMISSION IN THE INTENSIVE CARE UNIT

Transmission of HIV is an issue that requires attention in the ICU.[107-109] No evidence exists that HIV-infected health care professionals can infect patients, regardless of what procedure they perform, with the exception of two unusual and unexplained events. Intensivists should realize that although there are no federal policies defining how HIV-infected practitioners should be credentialed and monitored, many hospitals have policies and procedures. Some are modeled after guidelines from the Society of Healthcare Epidemiology.[108,110]

HIV patients pose a risk to health care professionals.[107-110] This risk can be substantially reduced by staff education, by strict monitoring for compliance with universal precautions, and by having proper equipment. Almost all HIV transmission has occurred in an occupational setting as a result of injuries involving sharp instruments (e.g., needles, scalpels). The risk of such injuries is about one case of HIV transmission per 250 injuries, but the likelihood of transmission in an individual accident depends on the amount of viremia at the time of the accident (late-stage patients generally have more circulating virus than do early-stage patients) and the nature of the accident. Most authorities recommend immediate prophylaxis if a significant injury occurs involving an HIV-infected patient. Considerable debate exists over the optimal choice of drugs and the optimal duration of therapy, but it is clear that initiating therapy within a period of hours rather than days is best. Many authorities now advocate an antiretroviral regimen for any situation when the patient and health care provider determine that therapy is appropriate, and continue that for 4 to 6 weeks. If providers have questions about appropriate medical treatment for occupational exposures, 24-hour assistance is available from the Clinicians' Post Exposure Prophylaxis Hotline (PEPline) at 1-888-448-4911 (http://www.nccc.ucsf.edu).[111]

Since surveillance of injuries began, 57 documented cases of occupational transmission of HIV infection have occurred, and 138 possible cases have been documented. More cases involve nurses or phlebotomists than physicians.

No transmission in the operating suite has been documented. There have been no documented cases of transmission for over a decade.

HUMAN STEM CELL, BONE MARROW, AND SOLID ORGAN TRANSPLANT RECIPIENTS

Solid organ transplant recipients and human stem cell recipients have much in common in terms of life-threatening complications that bring them to the ICU. Each of these populations is immunosuppressed and susceptible to opportunistic infections. Each of these populations receives immunosuppressive drugs that have direct toxicities and that may cause clinically important drug interactions with other medications.

Although these patient groups have much in common, they also have many profound differences. Their degrees of immunosuppression are very different: kidney transplant recipients, for example, do not have the same magnitude of risk for opportunistic infection as liver transplant recipients or human stem cell transplant recipients. The time period of severe immunosuppression differs with each patient group. Last, the specific organ being transplanted has an obvious major impact on the complications likely to be encountered: a transplanted liver must be dealt with much differently than a transplanted lung or transplanted stem cells in terms of the infectious and noninfectious complications that are likely to occur.

The field of transplantation is also evolving rapidly. The supportive care in ICUs has evolved over the past decade. Similarly, the immunosuppressive regimens and the prophylactic and therapeutic regimens employed to prevent and treat complications have changed dramatically, rendering some older timelines and guidelines less relevant in the current era.

Timelines are useful to provide clinicians with a general understanding of when infectious and noninfectious complications occur after a transplant procedure. Figure 53.6 demonstrates the typical return of cells and cell function after a stem cell transplant. Figures 53.7 and 53.8 demonstrate timelines typical for stem cell and solid organ transplant infections. However, the occurrence of complications will vary depending on the details of transplant management that may be unique to an institution or a specific protocol, so that these figures should not be considered as inviolable.

The following general principles are useful to keep in mind when approaching transplant recipients, in addition to the principles listed at the beginning of the chapter:

- The risk of infection is related to the "net state of immunosuppression," which is related to the function of the patient's pretransplant immune status, conditioning regimens, antirejection chemotherapy, as well as severity of illness and nutritional status. Net immunosuppression cannot be measured easily: it involves the number and function of neutrophils, T lymphocytes, and B lymphocytes. Although neutrophil number is a highly reliable surrogate for susceptibility to bacterial diseases, measures of cellular immune function, which are relevant to many viral and fungal pathogens, are not reliable surrogates in terms of sensitivity or specificity for predicting disease. Thus, susceptibility to viral and fungal pathogens is more difficult to predict.
- The risk of noninfectious complications is dependent on the organ transplanted and the immunosuppressive regimen used.
- Distinguishing infectious from noninfectious complications can be challenging, emphasizing the need for a broad consideration of causes of fever, hypotension, or organ-related syndromes, and the institution of prompt diagnostic tests that focus on both infectious and noninfectious causes.
- With solid organ transplants or stem cell transplants, the donor is a source of infection if the donor had an unrecognized transmissible infection at the time of organ donation, or if the donor had a latent infection that was transmitted with the donated organ.
- With solid organ transplants, complications of the surgical procedure must be considered when postoperative complications occur.
- Organ transplant recipients characteristically have extensive contact with health care environments and may have been receiving antimicrobial prophylaxis: these factors influence the spectrum of likely causative organisms.
- Diagnostic studies for infections rely more and more on molecular testing, although tissue biopsy and cultures of blood and suspicious body fluids and anatomic areas remain important. Tissue biopsies can be especially useful for differentiating infectious and noninfectious causes.
- Drug levels and microbial markers of infection must be carefully monitored to enhance the likelihood of effective therapy and minimize the likelihood of drug-related toxicities.

DIAGNOSTIC APPROACH

The management of organ transplant recipients focuses on algorithmic monitoring of neutrophil and lymphocyte number, organ function, drug levels, prophylactic drugs, and microbiologic parameters. Most patients will be managed by standard practice protocols that routinely order tests at intervals appropriate for the time period after transplant and for the patient's clinical status.

Programs often have specific targets for drug levels for immunosuppressive drugs. Given the drug interactions that occur in the ICU due to polypharmacy, and other factors altering pharmacokinetics, drugs levels must be monitored closely.

INFECTIOUS COMPLICATIONS OF TRANSPLANTATION

Cytomegalovirus

CMV is one of the most prominent pathogens for solid organ and stem cell transplant recipients. In urban areas of the United States, 60% to 70% of the population is seropositive for CMV, and thus either or both donor and recipient may have latent CMV infection at the time of the transplant procedure. In these populations, transplants from CMV-positive donors to CMV-negative recipients carry particular risk for reactivation of CMV disease in the organ recipient. In addition, any CMV-positive recipient is at risk for CMV disease during the period of immunosuppression.

CMV seronegative patients may acquire primary CMV infection from a CMV-infected organ. Acquisition from CMV-infected blood or blood products is becoming less and less likely since blood products have been screened or filtered.

Laboratory monitoring of patients for evidence of CMV disease using a DNA amplification assay is an important feature in efforts to reduce morbidity and mortality rates resulting from CMV. (CMV antigen detection in buffy coat smears is used less and less commonly and cannot be used in neutropenic patients.) Intensivists need to understand how to interpret these assays in terms of starting empiric, preemptive, or definitive therapy even though the assays are not standardized nor have they been studied in many adequately powered trials.

A seroconversion of a serum PCR test for CMV is usually an indication to treat CMV preemptively or therapeutically in most organ transplant recipients. Some programs make distinctions between low and high positive values based on copy number, and some require more than one consecutive low copy positive to be considered an indication for therapy: each institution has its own approach based on its own experience or the experience of a group with a convincing record for successful outcome.

Serial monitoring of CMV PCR or buffy coat antigen permits the use of preemptive therapy, that is, the use of CMV therapy at a time when there is laboratory evidence of infection but no clinical evidence of disease.

CMV disease in these populations may occur with serologic evidence of CMV infection (i.e., colitis or pneumonitis may occur when the serum CMV PCR is negative). Thus, treatment should be started either preemptively or when there is histologic or cytologic evidence of disease.

CMV disease can cause substantial morbidity and mortality risks including fever, hypotension, pneumonitis, hepatitis, glomerulitis, enteritis, and allograft injury. The availability of ganciclovir, foscarnet, and cidofovir has enabled these conditions to be treated successfully in many instances, although all three of these drugs are associated with substantial toxicity. Ganciclovir is the drug which has been studied most extensively. However, its toxicity on bone marrow, and especially on neutrophil counts, makes this an undesirable drug for many stem cell transplant programs.

Whether immune globulin (either immune globulin or specific hyperimmune globulin) adds anything to the potency of therapeutic regimens is not clear, although some programs administer these products when they are available.

Pneumocystis Pneumonia

PCP has been reported in recipients of most types of organ transplants. Most organ transplant programs use PCP prophylaxis during the period of perceived susceptibility, although there can be underappreciation of the duration of true risk, leading to premature discontinuation of prophylaxis.[30,112] Trimethoprim-sulfamethoxazole is usually the prophylactic agent of choice because it is more effective than other agents, is well tolerated, and reduces the frequency of urinary tract infections and other potential complications (e.g., disease resulting from *Nocardia, S. pneumoniae,* and *Haemophilus* organisms). However, trimethoprim-sulfamethoxazole is moderately immunosuppressive, and thus some human stem cell transplant programs prefer aerosolized pentamidine or oral atovaquone for prophylaxis.

As noted for other patient populations, diagnosis of PCP is usually based on demonstration of organisms by immunofluorescence in sputum or bronchoalveolar lavage. There is no reliable serologic test for PCP. Lung biopsy is rarely necessary to document PCP given the sensitivity of bronchoalveolar lavage and immunofluorescent staining at most medical centers.

The therapy of choice is trimethoprim-sulfamethoxazole, even if the patient was on trimethoprim-sulfamethoxazole prophylaxis at the time that acute disease developed. Intravenous pentamidine or oral primaquine combined with intravenous clindamycin are alternative therapies. It is logical to use corticosteroids for patients with moderate or severe PCP, as adjunct therapy, but the literature supporting this recommendation is not nearly as robust as the literature supporting the use of corticosteroids for HIV-associated PCP.

Fungal Infections

The spectrum of causative fungal organisms is changing because of changes in antifungal prophylactic regimens.[113,114] With the use of fluconazole prophylaxis, *Candida albicans* infections became less common and molds, especially *Aspergillus,* became more important pathogens, as did fluconazole-resistant *Candida.* Some programs are now using voriconazole prophylaxis, which has resulted in the development of disease due to voriconazole-resistant molds such as *Mucor* and certain non-*albicans Candida.* Thus, clinicians must know which antifungal prophylaxis has been used in order to anticipate which complications will occur.

Candida infections have traditionally been a major threat to transplant recipients. Mucosal candidiasis is a common complication. Esophageal candidiasis can lead to bloodstream infections as can *Candida* invasion of ulcerated bowel or perhaps intact bowel in neutropenic patients. Hepatosplenic candidiasis can be a cause of prolonged fever and systemic sepsis which is difficult to diagnose without CT or MRI of the liver and spleen and biopsy of suspicious lesions. Catheter-related *Candida* sepsis has also been a well-documented complication of transplantation.

Diagnosis of *Candida* requires culture of blood or the affected organ or a tissue biopsy. Serologic assays based on β-glucan detection are popular. However, these tests are not highly sensitive or specific, and there is considerable variability in assay performance from specimen to specimen and laboratory to laboratory.

The widespread use of azole prophylaxis has reduced the frequency of *Candida albicans* disease. Azole-resistant *Candida,* such as *Candida krusei* or *Candida glabrata,* are replacing *C. albicans* as pathogens.

The therapy of choice for *Candida* disease depends on the species of *Candida* recovered and its drug susceptibility. Echinocandins are active against almost all *Candida* species, as is amphotericin B. Azoles are not ideal initial choices in the ICU because of the risk to the patient if the causative *Candida* is azole sensitive. Most laboratories will perform azole susceptibility testing for *C. albicans,* and perhaps for other species.

Mold infections are becoming increasingly prominent causes of posttransplant morbidity because of the high degree of immunosuppression that many patients are exposed to, and because of the use of azole antifungal prophylaxis, which prevents most *Candida* infections but is not active against all molds such as certain species of *Aspergillus, Mucor,* and *Fusarium.*

Mold infections are best documented by tissue biopsy, although such biopsies are not always feasible due to the anatomic location of the suspicious lesion, the severity of patient illness, or the presence of a severe coagulopathy. Serologic tests are not yet highly sensitive and specific. Although some clinicians are enthusiastic about using the galactomannan test in the bronchoalveolar lavage or blood, this test is not optimally sensitive for molds, especially when used on serum.[115-118] Many clinicians are less enthusiastic about the serum β-glucan test, which was popular as a test for fungal disease, but which is increasingly seen as insensitive, nonspecific, and subject to laboratory variation.[63,119-123]

Respiratory Viruses Including Respiratory Syncytial Virus

Diffuse pulmonary infiltrates in any patient population may be caused by respiratory viruses. It is especially important to identify the presence of respiratory viruses because they are transmissible to other patients, hospital staff, and families. Most respiratory viruses are not true opportunistic pathogens, and thus, there is little evidence that they occur more frequently or cause more severe disease in transplant recipients than in immunocompetent patients. Transplant recipients may shed influenza, RSV, adenovirus, or coronavirus, for example, for longer periods of time following acute infection than immunocompetent patients, but their pulmonary disease is not necessarily more severe or more prolonged.

RSV is one respiratory virus that is opportunistic, however, in stem cell transplant recipients. Although RSV can, like other community-acquired viruses, cause disease in any patient population, it is especially lethal in those with stem cell transplants. Thus, RSV must be specifically sought in this patient population, as well as their visitors and health care providers, so that it does not spread to highly susceptible patients. RSV is best diagnosed by nasopharyngeal washes and molecular testing or by molecular testing of bronchoalveolar lavage.[124-126]

Many clinicians treat RSV pneumonia in transplant recipients with aerosolized ribavirin, monoclonal antibody against RSV, or both, but the efficacy of these regimens is controversial.[127,128]

NONINFECTIOUS COMPLICATIONS IN HUMAN STEM CELL TRANSPLANT RECIPIENTS

Graft-Versus-Host Disease

For human stem cell transplant recipients, the effects of the graft-attacking host cells rather than just the tumor can cause clinically significant disease that may be mild, severe, or even life-threatening. Typical manifestations are rash ("skin graft-versus-host disease") and diarrhea ("gut graft-versus-host disease"). These manifestations are difficult to distinguish from other causes of rash or diarrhea without tissue biopsy. It is important to make a specific diagnosis, however, because the treatment of graft-versus-host disease is to increase immunosuppression. If the diarrhea is caused by an infectious agent such as CMV, or the rash is due to disseminated herpes simplex, the appropriate treatment would be the opposite (i.e., reduction in immunosuppression in conjunction with specific therapy against the pathogen).

Immune Reconstitution Syndrome

For human stem cell transplant recipients, stem cell engraftment and return of neutrophils may be accompanied by inflammatory syndromes that can mimic infectious diseases. This syndrome is usually defined by a return of circulating neutrophil count in conjunction with exacerbation of inflammation at a new or preexistent site of infection or inflammation. There is no specific diagnostic test for this syndrome: it is a diagnosis of exclusion, and infectious causes must be carefully sought.

Toxicities of Immunosuppressive Drugs

Diagnosis and therapy of opportunistic infections and nosocomial infections should follow the guidelines given in Chapters 51 to 53 and 55. In choosing therapies, attention must be focused on the toxicities of antimicrobial agents and how they influence the outcome of the transplanted organ. In addition, drug interactions are important, especially with cyclosporine. Drugs that alter hepatic metabolism, such as rifampin, rifabutin, and fluconazole, can have substantial influence on cyclosporine levels and thus need to be used with careful pharmacologic attention. Finally, clinicians must recognize that new immunosuppressive regimens and changing prophylactic regimens are changing the spectrum of infectious complications. As mentioned earlier, fungal infections are increasingly likely to be caused by species other than *C. albicans:* non-*albicans Candida, Fusarium,* and *Rhizopus* are recognized with increasing frequency. Similarly, prophylaxis with valganciclovir is reducing CMV disease and pushing disease that does occur later and later in relation to the transplant procedure. Viruses such as HHV-6 and BK virus are causing disease. Thus, clinicians need to look for a changing spectrum of pathogens, as well as changing manifestations if the morbidity and death caused by infection are to be managed optimally.

KEY POINTS

- Knowledge of a patient's specific defects in immunologic and inflammatory response helps predict which opportunistic pathogens are most likely to occur.
- ICUs are increasingly successful in enabling immunosuppressed patients to survive acute crises, especially if the defect in immunologic or inflammatory function is reversible over time or by replacement therapy.

KEY POINTS (Continued)

- For neutropenic patients, gram-positive cocci have become more frequent than gram-negative bacilli as causes of life-threatening illness.
- Resistance to antimicrobial agents is becoming a major problem including bacteria (e.g., carbapenase-producing Enterobacteriaceae, MRSA, vancomycin-resistant enterococci, and penicillin-resistant pneumococci) and fungi (e.g., fluconazole-resistant *Candida* organisms) as well as PCP, and viruses (e.g., acyclovir-resistant herpes simplex and ganciclovir-resistant CMV).
- In neutropenic patients, broad-spectrum empiric therapy should be considered when treating any febrile process, with reduction in antimicrobial drugs once the severity of the illness and the causative process are better defined.
- A substantial fraction of HIV-infected patients with PCP-related respiratory failure can survive mechanical support and be discharged from the hospital.
- Adjunctive corticosteroid therapy is indicated for respiratory failure related to PCP.
- Organ transplant recipients develop opportunistic infections at relatively predictable points depending on the type of transplantation and the specific immunosuppressive regimen used.

SELECTED REFERENCES

3. Di Sabatino A, Carsetti R, Corazza GR: Post-splenectomy and hyposplenic states. Lancet 2011;378(9785):86-97.
4. Kaplan JE, Benson C, Holmes KH, et al: Guidelines for prevention and treatment of opportunistic infections in HIV-infected adults and adolescents: Recommendations from CDC, the National Institutes of Health, and the HIV Medicine Association of the Infectious Diseases Society of America. MMWR Recomm Rep 2009;58(RR-4):1-207; quiz CE201-204.
6. Freifeld AG, Bow EJ, Sepkowitz KA, et al: Clinical practice guideline for the use of antimicrobial agents in neutropenic patients with cancer: 2010 update by the Infectious Diseases Society of America. Clin Infect Dis 2011;52(4):e56-93.
8. Kumar A, Roberts D, Wood KE, et al: Duration of hypotension before initiation of effective antimicrobial therapy is the critical determinant of survival in human septic shock. Crit Care Med 2006;34(6):1589-1596.
39. Center for International Blood and Marrow Transplant Research (CIBMTR), National Marrow Donor Program (NMDP), European Blood and Marrow Transplant Group (EBMT), et al: Guidelines for preventing infectious complications among hematopoietic cell transplant recipients: A global perspective. Bone Marrow Transplant 2009;44(8):453-558.
58. O'Grady NP, Alexander M, Burns LA, et al: Guidelines for the prevention of intravascular catheter-related infections. Am J Infect Control 2011;39(4 Suppl 1):S1-34.
61. Crothers K, Huang L, Goulet JL, et al: HIV infection and risk for incident pulmonary diseases in the combination antiretroviral therapy era. Am J Respir Crit Care Med 2011;183(3):388-395.
71. Panel on Antiretroviral Guidelines for Adults and Adolescents: Guidelines for the use of antiretroviral agents in HIV-1-infected adults and adolescents. Washington, DC, Department of Health and Human Services, 2012; available at http://www.aidsinfo.nih.gov/contentfiles/lvguidelines/adultandadolescentgl.pdf. Accessed on August 28, 2012.
73. Zolopa A, Andersen J, Powderly W, et al: Early antiretroviral therapy reduces AIDS progression/death in individuals with acute opportunistic infections: A multicenter randomized strategy trial. PLoS One 2009;4(5):e5575.
80. Gordin FM, Masur H: Current approaches to tuberculosis in the United States. JAMA 2012;308(3):283-289.

The complete list of references can be found at www.expertconsult.com.

54 Specific Infections with Critical Care Implications

Henry S. Fraimow | Annette C. Reboli

CHAPTER OUTLINE

Infections and their complications, including severe sepsis and septic shock, are major indications for admission to critical care units worldwide. An enormous variety of infections can result in critical illness, and review of all of these syndromes is beyond the scope of this chapter. The diseases discussed here include the most common infectious syndromes likely to be encountered by critical care specialists, as well as less common infections of particular epidemiologic importance or those conditions in which critical care management is an essential component of management. The topics of community-acquired pneumonia, urinary tract infections, and nosocomial infections including device-associated infections are addressed specifically in other chapters.

OVERWHELMING INFECTIONS OF THE CENTRAL NERVOUS SYSTEM

Most patients with serious central nervous system (CNS) infections will require either admission to an intensive care unit (ICU) or the participation of a critical care specialist in their management. This is because of the severity of these infections at the time of presentation, the need for rapid initiation of diagnostic and therapeutic interventions to optimize outcomes, and the potential for rapid progression with development of fulminant and devastating complications. The major acute CNS infectious syndromes include bacterial meningitis, encephalitis, brain abscess, and spinal epidural abscess, although other primary and secondary infectious syndromes can present catastrophically, such as nonbacterial infectious meningitis, suppurative intracranial thrombophlebitis, and mycotic aneurysms. The presentations of all of these infectious syndromes may overlap, and they may also mimic the presentations of noninfectious CNS catastrophes such as stroke or hemorrhage.

ACUTE BACTERIAL MENINGITIS

EPIDEMIOLOGY, PATHOGENESIS, RISK FACTORS, AND CLINICAL PRESENTATION

The annual incidence of bacterial meningitis in individuals older than 16 years of age in developed countries has been steadily decreasing and was estimated at less than 2 cases per 100,000 in the United States in 2006-2007.[1-3] In recent studies from the United States and the Netherlands, the predominant organisms in microbiologically confirmed cases of bacterial meningitis in adolescents and adults were *Streptococcus pneumoniae* (45-60%), *Neisseria meningitidis* (15-30%), *Haemophilus influenzae* (7%), and *Listeria monocytogenes* (5%),[2-4] with no pathogen identified in approximately 10% of cases.[1,2] *Streptococcus agalactiae* (group B β-hemolytic streptococcus) has also recently emerged as an important cause of meningitis in adults, causing over 5% of cases of microbiologically defined episodes in the United States from 1998 to 2007. In some studies, rates of culture-negative cases were as high as 25%.[5] Important recent changes in microbiologic causes of bacterial meningitis reflect the impact of current vaccination strategies. These changes include the marked reduction in cases of of *H. influenzae* meningitis in both children and adults, and the introduction of the conjugated pediatric pneumococcal vaccine that has resulted in decreased rates of invasive childhood pneumococcal disease in children and adults.[3,6] A new meningococcal vaccine, which has the potential to diminish the rates of meningococcal disease in high-risk populations, has also been approved for use in adolescents and high-risk adult populations.[7] Another important trend is the increase in prevalence of nosocomial meningitis.[4] The microbiology of nosocomial meningitis differs from that of community-acquired cases, including higher rates of staphylococcal infection and infection due to a variety of aerobic gram-negative organisms.

The major route of acquisition of bacterial meningitis follows colonization of the nasopharynx with subsequent hematogenous spread and invasion of cerebrospinal fluid (CSF). Less frequently, infection occurs from hematogenous dissemination from distant sites or from other localized intracranial focal infections including sinusitis, mastoiditis, or otitis, or it is secondary to trauma or neurosurgery. In addition to trauma and contiguous focal infectious processes facilitating invasion of the CSF by bacteria, there is a wide variety of immunologic deficits that result in impaired clearance of encapsulated organisms. These include organism-specific deficits such as terminal complement deficiencies predisposing to meningococcal disease, as well as more general deficits such as immunoglobulin deficiencies, splenectomy, alcoholism, cirrhosis, diabetes mellitus, and human immunodeficiency virus (HIV) infection.[2,4] Patients with defects leading to impaired cell-mediated immunity including advanced age and general debility, as well as hematologic malignancies, chemotherapy, and use of tumor necrosis factor (TNF)-β inhibitors, are predisposed to *Listeria* infection.[8]

The presenting symptoms of bacterial meningitis include fever, headache, stiff neck, and altered sensorium. In the recent large series of 696 cases from the Netherlands, 95% had at least two of these four symptoms, although only 44% had all of the classic triad of headache, fever, and stiff neck.[2] Other important presenting symptoms in this cohort included nausea in 74%, focal neurologic deficits in one third of cases, and Glasgow Coma Score of less than 8 in 14% of cases.[2] Rash, especially a petechial or purpural rash that may be an important clue for the diagnosis of meningococcal meningitis, was seen in 26%.[2] Presenting symptoms alone without CSF findings or microbiologic data cannot adequately distinguish between bacterial meningitis and viral or other aseptic meningitis. However, certain features are more suggestive of bacterial rather than viral origin including winter versus summer onset, rapid progression of disease, presentation in shock, and presence of another focal site of bacterial infection such as sinusitis, otitis, or pneumonia. In addition to viruses, other nonbacterial infections including cryptococcosis, tuberculous meningitis, rickettsial diseases, Lyme disease, and syphilis are in the differential diagnoses of acute bacterial meningitis.

DIAGNOSTIC STRATEGIES AND EARLY MANAGEMENT OF SUSPECTED BACTERIAL MENINGITIS

The early management of suspected bacterial meningitis requires careful coordination and appropriate sequencing of the procedures necessary for establishing the diagnosis (lumbar puncture and imaging studies) and the interventions necessary for optimal treatment (antibiotics and dexamethasone). Rapid initiation of therapy leads to improved outcomes but may decrease specific microbiologic yield on CSF analysis.[1,5] Similarly, although lumbar puncture can usually be performed safely without any imaging studies, computed tomography (CT) scan may be required to minimize the risk of this procedure, leading to potential delays in institution of antimicrobial therapy.[9] Recent reviews and published practice guidelines have tried to place these competing urgencies in perspective, using data culled from multiple recent prospective studies and randomized trials.[1,5] One algorithm for early management of bacterial meningitis is shown in Figure 54.1.

The primary tenet of these algorithms is that the initiation of treatment assumes highest priority and thus any delay in performing a lumbar puncture because of the need for imaging or because of other patient-specific contraindications should not delay the administration of antibiotic therapy. Brain herniation is a feared but rare complication of lumbar puncture when performed for diagnosis of suspected meningitis in patients with elevated intracranial pressure.[10] One recent study of a cohort of 301 patients with

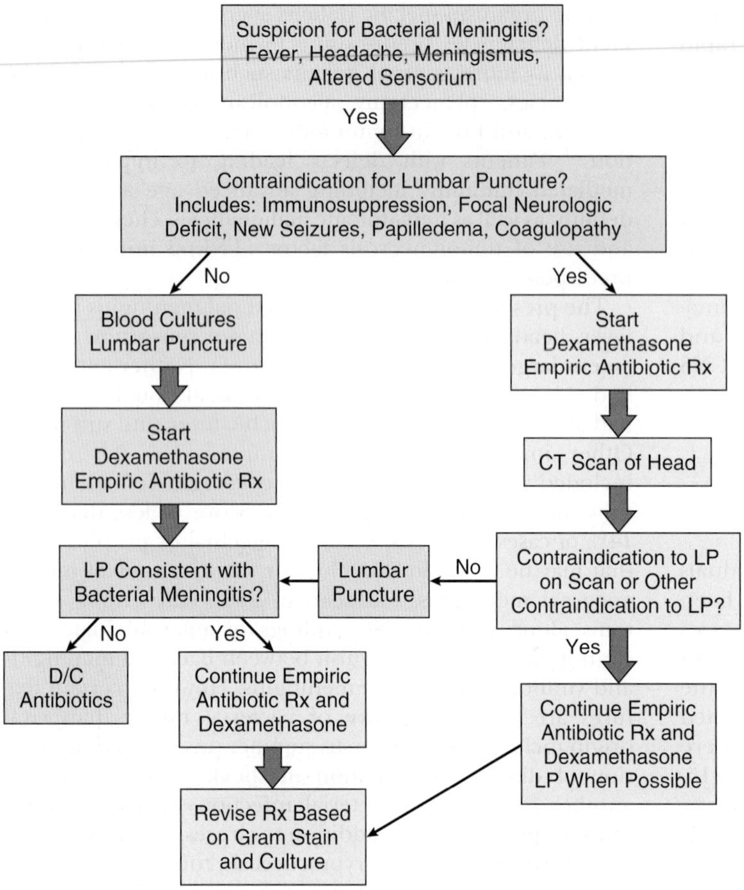

Figure 54.1 Algorithm for early management of suspected bacterial meningitis including determining when to suspect the diagnosis, when imaging should be performed prior to lumbar puncture, and when to initiate or discontinue empiric antibacterial therapy and adjuvant steroids. (Modified with permission from van de Beek D, de Gans J, Tunkel AR, et al: Community-acquired bacterial meningitis in adults. N Engl J Med 2006;354:44-53; and Tunkel AR, Hartman BJ, Kaplan SL, et al: Practice guidelines for the management of bacterial meningitis. Clin Infect Dis 2004;39:1267-1284.)

suspected bacterial meningitis described the relative safety of lumbar puncture without CT scanning in patients without specific clinical contraindications.[9] Proposed criteria for performing imaging prior to lumbar puncture include new-onset seizures, prior CNS disease, immunocompromised state, papilledema, focal neurologic deficits, or moderate to severe impairment of consciousness.[5] Only approximately 45% of patients with bacterial meningitis will have criteria for neuroimaging prior to lumbar puncture, although it remains standard practice in many hospitals for all patients with suspected meningitis to undergo imaging first.[1,5] The main purpose of early imaging is to find evidence of brain shift and both noncontrast CT and magnetic resonance imaging (MRI) can be used for this purpose. Considerations for the optimal imaging modality may be different when imaging tests are done to manage subsequent complications of meningitis or to better define space-occupying lesions. Other specific contraindications to lumbar puncture include coagulopathies and presence of local processeses overlying the lumbar puncture site such as stasis ulcers, burns, or cellulitis.

The diagnosis of bacterial meningitis relies heavily on analysis of CSF parameters including opening pressure, cell count, protein, glucose, and Gram stain and culture. Typically, patients with bacterial meningitis have elevated opening pressures of 200 to 500 mm H_2O, including 40% with opening pressure greater than 400 mm in one recent cohort.[2,5] White blood cell (WBC) counts may range from 100 to 10,000 cells/mm^3, most commonly in the 1000 to 5000 range; very low CSF WBC counts are associated with a worse prognosis.[4,5] Usually there is a polymorphonuclear (PMN) cell predominance of 80% or greater, although up to 10% will have a lymphocytic predominance, particularly early on. CSF-to-serum glucose ratios are less than 0.4, and CSF protein levels are nearly always increased.[5] In a study comparing cohorts of patients with bacterial and viral meningitis, CSF glucose ratios of less than 0.31, total WBC counts of greater than 2000, and total PMN cell counts of greater than 1180 have been predictive of bacterial rather than viral meningitis.[11] Other studies have suggested that protein values of greater than 0.5 g/L and WBC counts greater than 100 are also independently predictive of bacterial meningitis.[12] Gram stains are positive in 60% to 90% of cases of bacterial meningitis, and results on Gram stain are reported to be 97% specific as to cause.[5] Yield of Gram stain is higher on specimens concentrated by Cytospin centrifuge. Highest diagnostic yield from Gram staining is for *S. pneumoniae* meningitis; Gram stains in *Listeria* meningitis are positive in only one third of cases because of the lower inoculum of bacteria in the CSF. Clinicians should also be aware that preliminary "stat" Gram stains done during off-hours are more likely to be misinterpreted; thus, stains should always be reviewed by trained clinical microbiologists before modifying therapy based on a Gram stain report. In untreated patients, cultures will ultimately be positive in up to 90% of cases. Initiation of antibiotic therapy prior to lumbar puncture will not significantly alter cell count, protein, glucose, and even Gram stain results but will decrease CSF culture yield by up to 20%.[5,12] Blood cultures should be performed in all patients with suspected bacterial meningitis prior to initiation of antibiotics, even if the lumbar puncture is delayed.

Additional CSF and blood tests have been used to confirm a diagnosis of bacterial meningitis or help distinguish bacterial from viral disease. Latex agglutination tests for bacterial antigens, although initially reported to have good sensitivity and specificity for diagnosis of specific bacterial meningitis pathogens, have more recently been shown to contribute little to the management of most patients with suspected meningitis.[12] Polymerase chain reaction (PCR) of CSF for bacterial deoxyribonucleic acid (DNA) may be useful to confirm an etiologic diagnosis in culture-negative cases, especially those with prior antibiotic therapy, but is not routinely available in most hospitals. Elevated serum C-reactive protein (CRP) levels (>20 mg/L) and elevated serum procalcitonin (>0.5 ng/mL) are not specific for bacterial meningitis but had high predictive value in distinguishing between cohorts of children with bacterial and viral meningitis.[12] The level of soluble triggering receptor on myeloid cells in CSF has also been reported to distinguish between bacterial and viral meningitis.[12] Additional CSF studies may be useful for diagnosis of other specific infections such as CSF cryptococcal antigen and Venereal Disease Research Laboratory (VDRL) slide test.

Initial antibiotic therapy for suspected bacterial meningitis is most commonly initiated in the absence of culture and even Gram stain data. Initial empiric therapy must include agents active against the most likely pathogens based on the patient's age and underlying illnesses and modified for other specific risk factors such as nosocomial acquisition (Table 54.1). Treatment regimens must take into account local rates of antimicrobial resistance, particularly rates of high-level resistance to penicillin and third-generation cephalosporins in *S. pneumoniae.* Standard regimens include vancomycin administered at doses targeted to achieve adequate CSF levels (serum troughs of 15 to 20 μg/mL) and a third-generation cephalosporin, either ceftriaxone or cefotaxime. In areas with increased rates of resistance to third-generation cephalosporins, rifampin may be added. When there is risk for *Listeria* infection based on age greater than 50 or on other specific risk factors such as alcoholism or altered immunity, high-dose ampicillin is included in the treatment regimen. For patients with nosocomial or postprocedure-related infections, cefotaxime or ceftriaxone may be changed to an agent with improved activity against nosocomial gram-negative organisms including *Pseudomonas aeruginosa.* Initial empiric therapy is modified on the basis of identification and susceptibility data of isolated pathogens. Standard recommended treatment durations are 7 days for meningococcal disease and *H. influenzae,* 10 to 14 days for S. *pneumoniae,* and 21 or more days for *Listeria.*[1,5]

Studies in high-income countries have demonstrated the benefits of adjuvant dexamethasone in decreasing mortality rates and neurologic sequelae in patients with bacterial meningitis, and adjuvant steroids are now part of meningitis practice guidelines in the United States and Europe.[5,13,14] In one large, randomized, placebo-controlled trial of 301 adults with suspected bacterial meningitis and cloudy CSF, adjuvant dexamethasone decreased mortality rates from 15% to 7% and decreased unfavorable outcomes from 25% to 15%.[13] Benefits of corticosteroids were most evident in those with pneumococcal infection and those with a moderately impaired level of consciousness; patients with meningococcal disease had generally better outcomes with or without corticosteroids. More recent

Table 54.1 Treatment of Bacterial Meningitis in Adults*

Patient Group	Most Likely Pathogens	Empiric Antibiotic Therapy	Comments
Age 15-50 yr No risk factors†	*Streptococcus pneumoniae, Neisseria meningitidis*	Vancomycin + third-generation cephalosporin‡	Adjuvant dexamethasone§
Age 15-50 yr plus risk factors†	*S. pneumoniae, N. meningitidis, Listeria monocytogenes, Haemophilus influenzae*	Vancomycin + third-generation cephalosporin‡ + ampicillin	Adjuvant dexamethasone§
Age >50 yr ± risk factors	*S. pneumoniae, N. meningitidis, L. monocytogenes*, aerobic gram-negative rods	Vancomycin + third-generation cephalosporin‡ + ampicillin	Adjuvant dexamethasone§
Trauma, postneurosurgical, or other nosocomial infection	*Staphylococcus aureus*, coagulase-negative staphylococci, aerobic gram-negative rods	Vancomycin + *Pseudomonas*-active agent‖	Consider intrathecal therapy¶

*Patients older than 15 years of age.

†Risk factors: altered immunity including human immunodeficiency virus (HIV) infection and alcoholism.

‡Third-generation cephalosporin: ceftriaxone or cefotaxime; for highly penicillin-allergic patients an alternative would be aztreonam or a fluoroquinolone.

§Evidence for benefit of adjuvant dexamethasone is limited. Consider addition of rifampin in settings with high rates of cephalosporin resistance.

‖ Includes cefepime or ceftazidime; alternatives include aztreonam, meropenem, and ciprofloxacin.

¶For multiresistant organisms or catheter-related infections. Most recent experience is with aminoglycosides or polymyxins.

Modified with permission from van de Beek D, de Gans J, Tunkel AR, et al: Community-acquired bacterial meningitis in adults. N Engl J Med 2006;354:44-53; and Tunkel AR, Hartman BJ, Kaplan SL, et al: Practice guidelines for the management of bacterial meningitis. Clin Infect Dis 2004;39:1267-1284.

trials from resource-limited settings including Malawi and Vietnam have failed to confirm the benefits of adjuvant steroids, even in those with documented pneumococcal infection, calling into question the generalizability of use of steroids in all settings.[12,14] A recent meta-analysis was unable to clearly demonstrate benefits or harm with use of adjuvant corticosteroids.[14] If steroids are to be used, the standard regimen based on published and animal studies is 10 mg of dexamethasone every 6 hours for 4 days and initiated prior to or concurrent with the first dose of antibiotics.[1,5] Any benefit of steroids initiated after onset of antibiotic therapy is unknown. Patients with suspected or confirmed meningococcal meningitis should be placed in isolation to prevent nosocomial transmission via respiratory droplets for the first 24 hours of therapy. Meningococcal prophylaxis is indicated for household and other close contacts of meningococcal cases including first responders. Conversely, patients with Gram stains and clinical presentations consistent with non-meningococcal disease should also be quickly identified, to eliminate unnecessary use of meningococcal prophylaxis.

COMPLICATIONS, ICU MONITORING, AND PROGNOSIS

Patients with bacterial meningitis often require ICU monitoring either for complications evident at the time of presentation or for observation for complications that may subsequently develop during their course. Criteria for admission to an ICU have been proposed (Table 54.2)[1] and include sepsis and septic shock, respiratory compromise or pulmonary infiltrates, those with high risk of brain herniation, moderately impaired and deteriorating level of consciousness, new or evolving neurologic deficits, and presence of seizures. Some authorities feel that all patients with bacterial meningitis may benefit from intensive monitoring early on for presence of new neurologic signs or subtle seizures and for effective control of agitation.[15] Patients with generally good outcomes can be defined early in their course on the basis of age, Glasgow Coma Score, APACHE II score, absence of focal neurologic abnormalities, and favorable laboratory features, but these stratification schemes will still fail to identify some patients with more complicated courses.[2,16]

Major complications that occur during the course of bacterial meningitis have been summarized by van de Beek and colleagues[1,2,12] and include deteriorating level of consciousness, which may be caused by development of meningoencephalitis (15% to 20% of cases), seizures (15% to 23%), brain edema (6% to 10%), and hydrocephalus (3% to 8%). Mannitol, hyperventilation, repeated lumbar punctures, prophylactic lumbar drainage, prophylactic ventriculostomy, and other modalities have all been proposed for management of increasing intracranial pressure. Increased pressure is associated with worse prognosis, but no single approach for treatment has been confirmed to be effective in all cases.[1,17] Patients with severely increased pressure with impending herniation may require ventriculostomy with continuous CSF pressure monitoring. All patients should be monitored for seizures including nonfocal seizures that may only manifest as worsening level of consciousness, but routine use of prophylactic antiepileptic medication is not currently recommended.[1,5] Focal neurologic deficits early in the course of meningitis are most often caused by cerebrovascular complications or arteritis secondary to inflammation or less commonly to venous infarcts. The most common late neurologic complication is hearing loss, described in up to 20% of patients overall and in up to 34% of those with pneumococcal meningitis.[1,2] The incidence of hearing loss may be decreased in dexamethasone-treated patients.[13] Subdural empyema, brain abscess, and hemorrhage are all rare but potentially catastrophic complications of bacterial meningitis.

Table 54.2 Indications for Intensive Care Unit (ICU) Monitoring and Management for Bacterial Meningitis

Indication	ICU Management
Sepsis and shock	Hemodynamic support and monitoring, early goal-directed therapy
Pulmonary infiltrates or respiratory compromise	Airway management, monitoring of oxygenation, non-invasive or invasive ventilatory support
Glasgow Coma Scale score <10	Monitoring of examination; monitor for development of increased ICP, hydrocephalus, and seizures
Deteriorating level of consciousness	Monitoring of examination; monitor for development of increased ICP, hydrocephalus, and seizures
New or evolving neurologic deficits	Monitoring of examination; monitor for development of increased ICP, hydrocephalus, and seizures
Evidence of increased ICP	Consider intracranial pressure monitoring; osmotic diuretics
Acute hydrocephalus	Repeated lumbar puncture, lumbar drain, or ventriculostomy
Seizures	Continuous EEG monitoring, antiepileptic agents
Severe agitation	Careful sedation
Hyperglycemia	Maintain normoglycemic state with insulin therapy
Hyperpyrexia	Cooling modalities for fever >40° C

EEG, electroencephalogram; ICP, intracranial pressure.
Modified with permission from van de Beek D, de Gans J, Tunkel AR, et al: Community-acquired bacterial meningitis in adults. N Engl J Med 2006;354:44-53.

Repeat lumbar punctures are no longer routinely performed in patients with bacterial meningitis who are improving but are indicated in patients with worsening or suboptimal clinical response at 48 hours.[5] Repeat CSF analysis is also indicated in patients with more resistant organisms such as highly cephalosporin-resistant *S. pneumoniae*, especially when treated with dexamethasone, because steroids may decrease antibiotic penetration into the CSF and delay sterilization.[18] Repeat imaging by MRI or enhanced CT scan should be performed in patients with clinical deterioration or persistent decreased level of consciousness to assess for the complications listed earlier.

Overall mortality rates for bacterial meningitis are reported to be approximately 20% but vary by organism, and an additional 14% will have moderate or major neurologic sequelae.[1] Prognosis for meningococcal meningitis is better than for pneumococcal infection. Late neuropsychiatric cognitive effects are seen in up to 10% of cases of bacterial meningitis.

ENCEPHALITIS

The other major CNS infectious syndrome besides bacterial meningitis that may present with fever, headache, altered sensorium, and meningeal signs is acute encephalitis, which is most commonly viral. Although there is significant overlap between clinical presentations of patients with bacterial meningitis and viral encephalitis, the presentation of viral encephalitis is dominated by evidence of parenchymal brain dysfunction including moderate to severely impaired sensorium, delirium, psychosis, focal neurologic findings, and seizures.[19,20] The presence of meningismus is more variable, but most patients will have some evidence of meningeal enhancement on imaging and inflammatory cells in CSF.

A large number of viruses can cause encephalitis, but management strategies focus on the most common causes and those most likely to respond to specific interventions, particularly encephalitis caused by herpes simplex virus (HSV).[19-22] Other important causes with worldwide distribution include other herpesviruses including varicella-zoster virus; Epstein-Barr virus; and cytomegalovirus (CMV), especially in immunocompromised patients.[19,20,21] Influenza virus, mumps, measles, and enteroviruses such as enterovirus 71 are also important causes of acute viral encephalitis worldwide. Acute HIV infection can also occasionally present as a potentially treatable cause of fulminant meningoencephalitis.[21] Acute presentations of progressive multifocal leukoencephaly caused by JC virus are also increasingly reported in HIV infected and other immunocompromised patients.[23] In addition to those viruses seen worldwide, there are a variety of vector-borne viruses with regional and seasonal distributions.[19,21] Important pathogens include eastern, western, and Venezuelan equine encephalitides; Japanese B encephalitis; St. Louis encephalitis; La Crosse encephalitis; and Nipah encephalomyelitis. Recently, West Nile encephalitis emerged as a major pathogen in the United States. West Nile first appeared in New York City in 1999, but cases are now distributed throughout the country, demonstrating the potentially unpredictable and dramatic spread of emerging vector-borne pathogens.[24,25] Rabies, although extremely rare in developed countries, also needs to be considered in the differential diagnosis of fulminant encephalitis, both for its epidemiologic implications and because of recent reports of survival for patients with this previously universally fatal infection with aggressive ICU management protocols.[26] In addition to viral infections, many atypical bacteria, fungi, and protozoal organisms can present as acute meningoencephalitis.[19] Particularly important to consider early in the differential diagnosis are infections that may respond to specific antimicrobial therapy including rickettsial diseases such as Rocky Mountain spotted fever (RMSF) and meningoencephalitis from spirochetal infections including neurosyphilis and Lyme disease.[27,28] Important clues to these diseases include epidemiologic history and associated clinical features such as rash. Data from the California Encephalitis Project, in which cases of suspected infectious encephalitis underwent an aggressive evaluation for a variety of infectious agents, suggest that the cause of at least 50% to 60% of cases of presumed infectious encephalitis remains undefined, and in 10% a noninfectious diagnosis was ultimately established.[29]

Herpes simplex encephalitis is the most common sporadic cause of serious viral meningoencephalitis, causing 3% to 10% of cases of infectious encephalitis in adults and with an estimated frequency of about 1000 to 2000 cases per year in the United States.[21,22,29] Ninety percent of cases are caused by HSV type 1, usually occurring in adults as reactivation disease and not primary infection; HSV type 2 commonly causes aseptic meningitis but much less commonly presents as fulminant encephalitis.[22,30] Herpes encephalitis is an acute necrotizing process, typically causing hemorrhagic necrosis with particular predilection for the frontotemporal lobes and cingulated gyrus. Mortality rates are up to 70% in untreated cases, with 95% of those surviving having serious neurologic sequelae.[21,22] Cases of herpes encephalitis beyond the neonatal period occur throughout life, but the highest case rates occur in younger individuals (younger than 20 years old) and in adults older than age 50 (half of cases). Presentation may include a prodromal viral syndrome in 50% of cases, followed by a generally rapid onset of headache, confusion, and altered level of consciousness. Meningismus, focal neurologic findings, and seizures are also common.[20-22] In one series of patients with encephalitis, of which 37% were caused by HSV, focal CNS disease was much more likely than diffuse CNS disease to be caused by HSV.[31] The approach to cases of suspected herpes encephalitis, as well as other viral or unknown encephalitides, includes early initiation of antiviral therapy and concurrent rapid clinical evaluation that includes imaging, CSF studies, and electroencephalogram (EEG) to establish a diagnosis.[19,20,22] MRI is considered the imaging modality of choice. MRI is positive in more than 90% of cases, often showing changes of edema and necrosis in the medial temporal lobes, insular cortex, and cingulate gyrus as soon as 2 to 3 days into the illness.[32] EEGs will be abnormal in nearly all cases, but early findings may be nonspecific and the characteristic periodic lateralizing epileptiform discharges may not be seen until later in the course.[22] CSF findings include low- to moderate-grade lymphocytic pleocytosis in 85% and elevated protein in 80%; elevated red blood cell count and mildly decreased glucose are common but not universal, and cell counts may be completely normal in 8%.[22,30] Likelihood of HSV encephalitis is extremely low with CSF WBC count of fewer than 5 cells/mm^3 and protein levels of less than 50 mg/dL.[33] The International Herpes Management Forum has issued guidelines for confirmation of the diagnosis and for treatment.[22] PCR of CSF for HSV DNA has replaced brain biopsy as the diagnostic method of choice for HSV encephalitis. Based on data from two trials comparing PCR with the gold standard of brain biopsy, sensitivity of PCR was 98% and specificity was 94% for diagnosing HSV encephalitis; the negative predictive value of PCR on CSF obtained more than 72 hours into the course of illness was close to 100% for excluding HSV.[22,34,35] PCR has also expanded understanding of the range of clinical presentations of HSV encephalitis including recognition of less severe cases.[31] Viral culture has low sensitivity in older children and adults and is not recommended, and CSF and serum antibody studies have little role in the diagnosis.[19,22] Treatment should be initiated on the basis of clinical suspicion pending PCR results using high-dose intravenous (IV) acyclovir at doses of 10 mg/kg every 8 hours and continued for 14 to 21 days, or until PCR results are available or an alternative diagnosis is established. Extrapolating from results in neonates, a positive CSF PCR for HSV at the end of treatment may be an indication to prolong therapy, especially if clinical response has been suboptimal.[19]

WEST NILE VIRUS ENCEPHALITIS

In the 12 years since it first appeared in the Western hemisphere, West Nile virus (WNV) has become a major infectious cause of invasive neurologic disease throughout the United States, with more than 1000 cases from 40 states reported in 2010.[24,36] WNV is a mosquito-borne arbovirus affecting birds, mammals, and humans. Of human cases, 80% are asymptomatic and most of the remainder have West Nile fever, but 1% will develop neuroinvasive disease manifesting as meningitis, encephalitis, or a polio-like flaccid paralysis syndrome.[24,25] Risk of encephalitis increases with age or with immunosuppression, particularly organ transplantation, and manifestations can range from mild disorientation to coma and death.[24] Parkinson-like tremors are also commonly reported. The flaccid paralysis syndrome, caused by viral infection of anterior horn cells, may have abrupt onset and patients may require prolonged ventilatory support. The fatality rate is 9% for WNV neuroinvasive syndromes, and survivors may have prolonged symptoms. In some patients, flaccid paralysis has not resolved after 1 to 2 years.[24] CSF findings of WNV are similar to those of other viral infections with lymphocytic pleocytosis predominating. Neuroimaging may be normal, but some scans may demonstrate abnormal signal in the basal ganglia, thalamus, and other deep brain structures or abnormal signal in anterior horn cells of the spinal cord.[25,37] Diagnosis is confirmed by the finding of WNV-specific IgM antibodies in CSF and serum or by nucleic acid–based PCR of CSF, serum, or other fluids.[19,24] Treatment is primarily supportive; multiple interventions including ribavirin, interferon (INF)-α, immunoglobulin, and other agents have been reported in individual cases and case series, but there are currently no good outcome data to support the use of any specific therapy.

BRAIN ABSCESS

Brain abscesses are focal infections of brain parenchyma, occurring from direct spread from local, contiguous infection (ear, sinuses, mastoid, bacterial meningitis); from hematogenous spread of infecting organisms from distant sites; or by direct inoculation from trauma or surgery.[38,39] Modern imaging modalities have improved the initial management and follow-up care of patients with brain abscess, but it is less certain that this has significantly affected overall outcome. Presenting symptoms may be indistinguishable from those of other CNS infections, with fever, headache, and focal neurologic findings predominating.[38-40] Seizures and decreased level of consciousness are also seen. Sepsis was noted in 18% of cases in one recent series.[41] Duration of symptoms prior to presentation is typically much longer than that of bacterial meningitis or viral encephalitis. Microbiology reflects the source of the original infection and most commonly includes streptococci, staphylococci, oral anaerobes, and enteric gram-negative organisms, but multiple other bacterial, fungal, tuberculous, and atypical organisms can also be found.[38-40] In areas of high HIV prevalence, opportunistic brain infections, especially toxoplasmosis, have become more prevalent than typical pyogenic abscesses, and knowledge of HIV status is crucial to initial management of suspected infectious mass lesions.[42]

The diagnosis of brain abscess is suggested by the clinical presentation and imaging findings by either CT or MRI showing enhancing parenchymal lesions, usually with surrounding inflammatory changes.[38,39] Radiographic appearance may be indistinguishable from a malignant lesion. Management of suspected abscess includes either stereotactic aspiration or surgical drainage to both establish a microbiologic diagnosis and for primary treatment of the abscess. Smaller lesions (<1 cm) can be treated with antibiotics alone, but larger lesions will require either aspiration or open drainage.[38,39] Recent studies have confirmed earlier findings that aspiration may result in lower mortality rates and less residual neurologic deficit than surgical resection.[43] Duration of treatment is until resolution of the abscess on serial imaging studies. Unlike bacterial brain abscesses, toxoplasmosis lesions in patients with AIDS are usually multiple and may respond to empiric toxoplasmosis therapy without need for further invasive diagnostic procedures.[42]

SPINAL EPIDURAL ABSCESS

Spinal epidural infections most commonly arise by contiguous spread of infection into the spinal canal as a complication of vertebral infections or, less commonly, as a complication of epidural procedures such as epidural injections or epidural catheterization.[44-46] Vertebral infections result from hematogenous infection of vertebral bodies or disk space or by direct introduction of organisms from surgery or trauma. In addition to affecting the vertebral bodies and intervertebral disk spaces, vertebral osteomyelitis may expand into surrounding paravertebral soft tissues and spinal canal and even rarely into the medullary spinal cord. Paravertebral and epidural infections can rapidly progress, resulting in severe neurologic symptoms from compression of nerve roots or the spinal cord, or by infarction of the spinal cord from inflammation and vasculitis of vertebral arteries.[45,47] Thus an aggressive diagnostic and therapeutic approach is necessary to prevent catastrophic consequences such as irreversible paraplegia and death.

The incidence of spinal epidural infection from large retrospective reviews is reported as approximately 0.2 to 2 cases per 10,000 hospital admissions, but the frequency of this diagnosis may be increasing, perhaps because of improvements in radiographic diagnosis and increasing prevalence of risk factors.[45] Incidence in adults increases with age older than 30 years; important predisposing factors include diabetes, injection drug use, alcoholism, immunosuppression, underlying spinal disorders, trauma, invasive procedures, and extraspinal sites of infection that cause significant bacteremia.[45,46] Infections can occur at any level of the spinal cord, although most series report predominance of lumbar involvement. Approximately two thirds of infections are caused by *Staphylococcus aureus* including methicillin-resistant *S. aureus* (MRSA) with a variety of other gram-positive organisms (coagulase-negative staphylococci, viridans streptococci, β-hemolytic streptococci), as well as gram-negative organisms all reported in lesser numbers.[41-46] Granulomatous infections including tuberculosis and brucellosis remain major causes of vertebral and epidural infection in many areas of the world.[47] Approximately 10% of episodes are culture-negative.[45]

Presenting symptoms are extremely nonspecific and include back pain in more than 95% of cases and fever in two thirds of cases.[44,45] Thirty percent of cases will present with evidence of early neurologic deficits such as muscle weakness, incontinence, or sensory deficits, and up to one third will have evidence of some paralysis on examination.[44-46] Associated laboratory features include leukocytosis in two thirds of cases and elevated erythrocyte sedimentation rate (ESR) in nearly all cases. The most sensitive imaging modality is MRI with gadolinium, with reported sensitivity of greater than 95%, but most infections were also visualized on CT and unenhanced MRI.[44,45] Standard therapy previously included emergent surgical drainage of the abscess and systemic antibiotic therapy. However, over the past 2 decades there has been an emerging literature on more conservative medical management employing percutaneous aspiration and antibiotics without open surgical drainage.[44-46] These reports have suggested that outcomes are similar or better (i.e., less neurologic sequelae) compared to surgery.[44] No trials have directly compared treatment modalities, and retrospective analyses have not identified risk factors for worse outcomes with medical therapy alone. Indications for surgery include neurologic progression on treatment or lack of clinical response, thus those managed without surgery require careful monitoring.[44,45] Surgery may also be the preferred treatment for those with more severe neurologic deficits on initial presentation, though these patients have worse outcomes overall regardless of treatment modality.[44,45]

FULMINANT ENDOVASCULAR INFECTIONS

Infectious endocarditis and other endovascular infections are common causes of bacteremia and sepsis syndromes, and these patients are frequently admitted to critical care units for management of sepsis and other complications. Often, the diagnosis of endovascular infection is unsuspected, and initiation of appropriate treatment is delayed. Even relatively stable patients with bacterial endocarditis, especially those with left-sided endocarditis, require careful monitoring and management of potential major complications including heart failure and other cardiac events and septic emboli. The role of early surgical intervention has become increasingly appreciated in the management of complicated bacterial endocarditis, especially *S. aureus* endocarditis.

ACUTE INFECTIVE ENDOCARDITIS

Several large case series published since 2005 have addressed changes in the epidemiology of bacterial endocarditis over the past 2 decades.[48,49] The annual incidence of endocarditis of 5 to 7 cases per 100,000 has not changed significantly over time.[48] However, the International Collaboration on Endocarditis Prospective Cohort Study, a multicenter study of 1779 cases from 39 medical centers in 16 countries, has illustrated the recent changes in microbiology and clinical presentation of bacterial endocarditis.[49] In this cohort, as well as other recent cohorts, *S. aureus* rather than viridans streptococci were the predominant pathogens and increasing numbers of cases were considered either nosocomially acquired or health care associated.[49] *S. aureus* endocarditis is associated with a significantly higher mortality rate, higher rate of stroke and other systemic embolization, and higher rate of sustained bacteremia than endocarditis caused by other organisms.[49-51] The increased antibiotic resistance in organisms causing endocarditis, especially the increasing rates of MRSA, are reflected in the recent guidelines for diagnosis, treatment, and management of complications of endocarditis from the American Heart Association.[50] Other important recent epidemiologic trends are the decreased importance of congenital valvular and rheumatic disease as predispositions, the increasing age of cases, and the increased role of hemodialysis and indwelling cardiac devices such as pacemakers and implantable defibrillators as risk factors.[49-52]

Infectious endocarditis must be considered in the differential diagnosis of a broad range of clinical syndromes. Fever is the single most common presenting symptom, often accompanied by other constitutional symptoms of anorexia, weight loss, and fatigue. Onset may be acute or subacute with tendency toward more acute presentations with *S. aureus* infections. Signs and symptoms may be consequences of direct cardiac effects of infection including new or changing heart murmur, worsening congestive heart failure and valvular dysfunction, or onset of heart block from myocardial abscesses.[50] The clinical presentation may also be dominated by systemic manifestations of emboli or immune complex disease including such findings as skin lesions, splenomegaly, glomerulonephritis, cerebrovascular events, and other acute vascular embolic events. Patients with acute, fulminant endocarditis, particularly *S. aureus* endocarditis, may present with concurrent cardiogenic and septic shock.

Clinical criteria have been developed and prospectively evaluated for the diagnosis of infective endocarditis.[53,54] The most current version of these, the Modified Duke Criteria for Diagnosis of Infective Endocarditis (Box 54.1), relies primarily on blood culture data and echocardiographic findings as the two major clinical criteria for diagnosis; additional minor clinical criteria (fever, underlying predisposition, embolic phenomena, immunologic phenomena) can also be used as supporting evidence for determining confirmed or suspected cases.[54] Patients with endocarditis have sustained bacteremia; in the absence of prior antibiotic therapy the yield of at least one positive blood culture after three sets are drawn is greater than 90%, and typically multiple cultures are positive. Thus two to three separate sets of blood culture should always be obtained in suspected endocarditis prior to initiation of therapy. Culture-negative cases may be attributed to prior antimicrobial therapy or to infection caused by fastidious or difficult-to-cultivate organisms.[50] Follow-up blood cultures are critical to document sterilization of blood and should be repeated frequently until

Box 54.1 Definition of Infective Endocarditis (IE) According to the Modified Duke Criteria

Definite IE

Pathologic Criteria

Microorganisms demonstrated by culture or histologic examination of a vegetation, a vegetation that has embolized, or an intracardiac abscess specimen; OR

Pathologic lesions (as earlier) confirmed by histologic examination as showing active endocarditis

Clinical Criteria

2 *major* criteria OR
1 *major* and 3 *minor* criteria OR
5 *minor* criteria

Possible IE

1 *major* and 1 *minor* criteria OR
3 *minor* criteria

Rejected Diagnosis

Firm alternative diagnosis explaining evidence of IE; OR
Resolution of IE syndrome with antibiotic therapy for <4 days; OR
No evidence of IE at surgery or autopsy after antibiotic therapy <4 days; OR
Does not meet at least minimal criteria for possible IE

Definition of Terms Used in the Foregoing Criteria

Major Criteria

Blood culture or other supportive microbiologic data for IE
- Typical organisms consistent with IE (viridans streptococci, *Streptococcus bovis*, HACEK group,* *S. aureus*, community-acquired enterococci) from two separate blood cultures in absence of a primary focus
- Microorganisms consistent with IE from persistently positive blood cultures: at least 2 positive cultures drawn >12 hours apart; or all of 3 or a majority of ≥4 separate cultures drawn over at least 1 hour
- Single positive blood culture or positive results on serologic testing for *Coxiella burnetii*

Evidence of endocardial involvement
- Echocardiogram positive for IE defined as follows: oscillating intracardiac mass on valve or supporting structures, in the path of regurgitant jets, or on implanted material in the absence of an alternative anatomic explanation; or abscess; or new partial dehiscence of prosthetic valve or new valvular regurgitation (worsening or changing or preexisting murmur not sufficient)

Minor Criteria

Predisposition: predisposing heart condition or injection drug use (IDU)
Fever: temperature >38° C
Vascular phenomena: major arterial emboli, septic pulmonary infarcts, mycotic aneurysm, intracranial hemorrhage, conjunctival hemorrhages, and Janeway's lesions
Immunologic phenomena: glomerulonephritis, Osler's nodes, Roth's spots, and rheumatoid factor
Microbiologic evidence: positive blood culture but does not meet a major criterion as noted earlier or serologic evidence of active infection with organism consistent with IE (excludes single positive culture for coagulase-negative staphylococci)

*HACEK: *Haemophilus*, *Actinobacillus*, *Cardiobacterium*, *Eikenella*, *Kingella*.
Modified from Li JS, Sexton DJ, Mick N, et al: Proposed modifications to the Duke Criteria for the Diagnosis of Infective Endocarditis. Clin Infect Dis 2000;30:633-638.

negative. Echocardiography should be performed on all patients with suspected endocarditis.[50,52] When possible, transesophageal echocardiography (TEE) is the preferred modality in adults. Sensitivity of TEE is reported to be as high as 95% for native valve infection compared with 60% to 75% for transthoracic echocardiography (TTE) and is significantly better than TTE for diagnosis of prosthetic valve infection and for detection of complications such as perivalvular abscess that may affect management.[50] In children and uncomplicated adult cases, in which TTE is diagnostic, TEE may not be necessary. If initial studies are negative, TEE should be repeated in 7 to 10 days if clinical suspicion remains high.[50]

Embolic complications may occur at any time during the course of infective endocarditis with overall incidence of 20% to 50%; risk decreases but still remains significant after initiation of antimicrobial therapy, especially with larger vegetations, and remains high for up to 2 to 3 weeks.[50,55,56] Risks for embolization include specific organisms, especially *S. aureus*, *Candida*, HACEK* organisms, and *Abiotrophia*; increased vegetation size (>10 mm) and mobility as determined by echocardiography; mitral versus aortic valve involvement; and anterior versus posterior location on the mitral valve.[50] More than half of clinically manifesting emboli involve the CNS, most commonly in the middle cerebral artery distribution.[50,55] In addition to emboli, other risks for a fatal outcome include congestive heart failure, abnormal mental status, comorbid conditions, higher APACHE score, and *S. aureus* infection.[49-51] Congestive heart failure appears to have the highest association with death.[49-51] Medical therapy (versus surgical therapy) was also associated with higher 6-month mortality rates in recent studies.[51,52]

The decision to perform emergent or urgent valvular surgery on patients with active endocarditis remains complex. Indications for surgery can be broadly classified into those related to management of heart failure, management of uncontrolled infection, and management of embolization, and decisions are also impacted by patient status and available surgical expertise. Traditional indications for surgery include refractory congestive heart failure; persistent infection despite optimal antimicrobial therapy; fungal or other difficult-to-treat organisms; one or more emboli during the first weeks of antimicrobial therapy; and valvular

*HACEK is an acronym formed from the names of bacteria involved: *Haemophilus*, *Actinobacillus*, *Cardiobacterium*, *Eikenella*, and *Kingella* spp.

Table 54.3 Possible Indications for Emergent or Urgent Surgical Intervention for Acute Infective Endocarditis

Indication	Details/Comments
Clinical Indications	
Refractory congestive heart failure	Most common single indication for surgery
Severe valvular decompensation	Usually acute mitral or aortic insufficiency but also valve obstruction. Less commonly, severe tricuspid regurgitation
Emboli and recurrent emboli	Especially with 1 or more events occurring during first 1 to 2 weeks of antimicrobial therapy
Persistent infection/sepsis	Persistent positive blood cultures after 7 days of optimal antibiotic treatment and no other source
Difficult-to-eradicate organisms	Fungal endocarditis, highly resistant bacteria; staphylococcal or gram-negative prosthetic valve endocarditis (controversial)
Extension of infection into myocardium	Evidence of new heart block, echocardiographic findings as listed below
Echocardiographic Indications	
Evidence of valve decompensation	Dehiscence, rupture, perforation, fistula, perivalvular abscess
Vegetation characteristics	>10 mm in size, especially on anterior mitral valve and emboli; increase in size despite treatment; >15 mm in size on aortic, mitral, or prosthetic valve; >20 mm in size on tricuspid valve
Other Possible Indications	
Complicated prosthetic valve infection	As defined by TEE findings; high failure rate for medical therapy alone
?Any left-sided *Staphylococcus aureus* infection	Early surgical management may be associated with lower mortality

TEE, transesophageal echocardiography.
Modified from Baddour LM, Wilson WR, Bayer AS, et al: Infective endocarditis: Diagnosis, antimicrobial therapy, and management of complications, a statement for healthcare professionals from the Committee on Rheumatic Fever, Endocarditis, and Kawasaki Disease, Council on Cardiovascular Disease in the Young, and the Councils on Clinical Cardiology, Stroke, and Cardiovascular Surgery and Anesthesia, American Heart Association. Circulation 2005;111:e394-e433; and Thuny F, Grisoli D, Collart F, et al: Management of infective endocarditis: Challenges and perspectives. Lancet 2012;379 (9819): 965-975.

complications of dehiscence, perforation, fistula, and large perivalvular abscesses (Table 54.3).[50] Vegetation size and location are also emerging as possible independent indications for surgery.[50] The risk of infecting a new prosthetic valve during surgery for active endocarditis is only 2% to 3%; thus active infection is not a contraindication to surgery that is indicated for complications associated with high mortality rate.[50] Reviews of recent studies have confirmed the decreased mortality rates of cohorts of patients who were managed with early surgical intervention, especially those with left-sided *S. aureus* endocarditis, though there are no randomized controlled trials completed that address this.[50,52] The optimal surgical procedure and the role of more conservative procedures such as vegetation resection remain incompletely defined, though resection of vegetations is frequently done in isolated, refractory right-sided endocarditis. The majority of patients who survive an episode of left-sided endocarditis who are not operated on initially will ultimately require valve replacement within the next 15 years.[50]

Anticoagulation in patients with active endocarditis can present difficult management dilemmas. Anticoagulation has been considered to be relatively contraindicated in active endocarditis because of the risk of hemorrhagic CNS events.[50,57] However, data from a recent case cohort study suggest that risk of warfarin therapy in acute left-sided native valve endocarditis has been overestimated.[57] In patients already on anticoagulation for mechanical valves or other specific indications, warfarin should be switched to heparin therapy during the initial phase of therapy, especially in cases in which surgical intervention is being considered. Anticoagulation should be discontinued if possible after acute CNS embolic events. Neurologic events, most commonly embolic events but also mycotic aneurysms, are the second leading cause of death in acute endocarditis after heart failure. Decisions on timing of surgery and management of anticoagulation perioperatively and postoperatively in patients with CNS events are particularly challenging.

Optimal antibiotic therapy for patients with infective endocarditis is outlined in the American Heart Association guidelines, though there are more recent specific recommendations for treatment of MRSA valvular infections.[50,58] Individual treatment regimens including choice of antibiotic, need for combination therapy, and duration of therapy are based on the organism, susceptibility data, location of infected valve, and whether the infection is complicated or uncomplicated. Left-sided *S. aureus* endocarditis is generally treated for 6 weeks with a parenteral β-lactam or vancomycin. Addition of gentamicin for native valve disease is no longer recommended due to risk of nephrotoxicity.[59] MRSA infections require treatment with vancomycin or daptomycin. Uncomplicated right-sided endocarditis in injection drug users may have a more benign course, and there is evidence for use of shorter courses of therapy and even for use of oral therapy in selected patients. Treatment of viridans streptococcal endocarditis is 4 weeks of a β-lactam or vancomycin, and gentamicin is added for disease caused by relatively penicillin-resistant strains. Selected patients with uncomplicated viridans streptococcal infections have been treated with 2 weeks of combination therapy. β-Lactam therapy for susceptible isolates is always preferred to vancomycin in nonallergic patients. Enterococcal endocarditis is usually treated for 4 to 6 weeks with synergistic combinations of a penicillin or vancomycin and an aminoglycoside, but regimens need to be modified on the basis of strain resistance patterns in view of increasing rates of penicillin, vancomycin, and high-level aminoglycoside resistance. Prosthetic valve infections require longer treatment courses and use of combination therapy, and failure rates of medical therapy for prosthetic valve disease are high.[50]

DEVICE-RELATED ENDOVASCULAR INFECTIONS

Endovascular infections other than valvular infections have become increasingly common as causes of bacteremia and sepsis. This is related to the increased use of indwelling devices including vascular catheters for chemotherapy and other long-term parenteral therapies, use of accesses for hemodialysis, and the expanding indications for implantable cardiac devices for patients with congestive heart failure and arrhythmias. Infection is the most common serious complication of peripherally inserted central venous catheters (PICCs), tunneled catheters, and totally implanted intravascular devices.[60] Patients presenting with sepsis and focal findings related to the catheter such as tunnel infection, port abscess, or cellulitis; those with associated venous thrombosis; and those with concurrent endocarditis or osteomyelitis require removal of the catheter.[60] Management is more difficult in patients with sepsis or bacteremia without local signs of infection when removal of the catheter is not a trivial procedure. Diagnosis of the catheter as the source of a bacteremia can sometimes be made with use of paired central and peripheral blood cultures. Positive central and negative peripheral cultures or central cultures that are positive significantly earlier than peripheral cultures implicate the catheter as the source.[60] The majority of infected permanent catheters require removal; selected uncomplicated catheter infections in nonseptic patients whose bloodstream has sterilized on antibiotics can be treated with catheter retention and antibiotic therapy, especially infections caused by coagulase-negative staphylococci and other less virulent organisms.[60] Algorithms for the management of suspected and confirmed line infections in patients with long-term access devices are shown in Figure 54.2A. Antibiotic lock therapy is a strategy in which antibiotic solutions are used to fill the catheter lumen to maintain high antibiotic concentrations in the catheter and catheter hub and yield higher rates of catheter salvage than parenteral antibiotics alone.[60] Hemodialysis catheter infections pose particular management challenges because of the high prevalence of infection in these patients as well as the need to preserve dialysis access. An algorithm for management of tunneled hemodialysis catheters is shown in Figure 54.2B. Hemodialysis has emerged as a major risk factor for endocarditis in recent studies. Catheter salvage strategies and guidewire exchange strategies are employed more frequently in hemodialysis catheter–associated infections than in other populations.[60,61]

Indications for placement of implantable cardioverter-defibrillator devices (ICDs) in patients with cardiac disease have recently been expanded, resulting in increased number of ICDs and increased prevalence of pacemaker and ICD infections.[62,63] Rates of pacemaker and ICD infections have increased out of proportion to increased rates of ultilization of these devices, and in population-based studies infection rates range from 1 to 3 infections per 1000 device years.[62] Infections include site and generator pocket infections and infections of the leads. Lead infections, which account for probably half of all infections, may be complicated by sepsis and septic shock, suppurative thrombophlebitis, and endocarditis and almost always require explantation of the device.[62] Diagnosis is typically made by blood cultures and TEE, which may show vegetations on the leads or associated endocarditis. The most common organisms are coagulase-negative staphylococci and *S. aureus* in 80% of cases. Most infected leads can now be removed through percutaneous extraction procedures rather than open surgical explantation, but the expertise and technology for this are not available at all hospitals. Devices should not be replaced until bacteremia has completely resolved.

PRIMARY BACTEREMIAS

In 10% to 30% of patients presenting from the community with bacteremia and sepsis, the primary source of the bacteremia remains unknown, even after careful clinical and radiographic evaluation.[64,65] This includes patients with infections manifesting with a primary bacteremia, as well as those with probable secondary bacteremia from an occult focus. Bacteremia of unknown cause is associated with higher mortality rate.[64] Primary bacteremias are more common with certain microorganisms and with specific host predispositions. These syndromes, if unrecognized, have particularly high morbidity and mortality rates. Patients with impairment in immunoglobulin production or function and impaired or absent splenic function are predisposed to infections with encapsulated organisms such as S. *pneumoniae, N. meningitidis, H. influenzae,* and group B streptococcus.[66] Patients with advanced liver disease and cirrhosis are predisposed to these, as well as a variety of other spontaneous bacteremias.[67] Patients with cell-mediated immune defects may present with other unusual bacteremias such as *Listeria* and *Salmonella* sepsis. Severe neutropenia greatly increases the risk of spontaneous bacteremia and sepsis from endogenous gastrointestinal flora, and the management of fever in neutropenic patients includes empiric initiation of broad-spectrum antibacterial therapy.[68] Several important specific bacteremia syndromes are described as follows.

MENINGOCOCCEMIA AND MENINGOCOCCAL SEPSIS

Invasive meningococcal disease can present as either bacterial meningitis or as the syndrome of meningococcemia with meningococcal sepsis without meningitis.[7] The

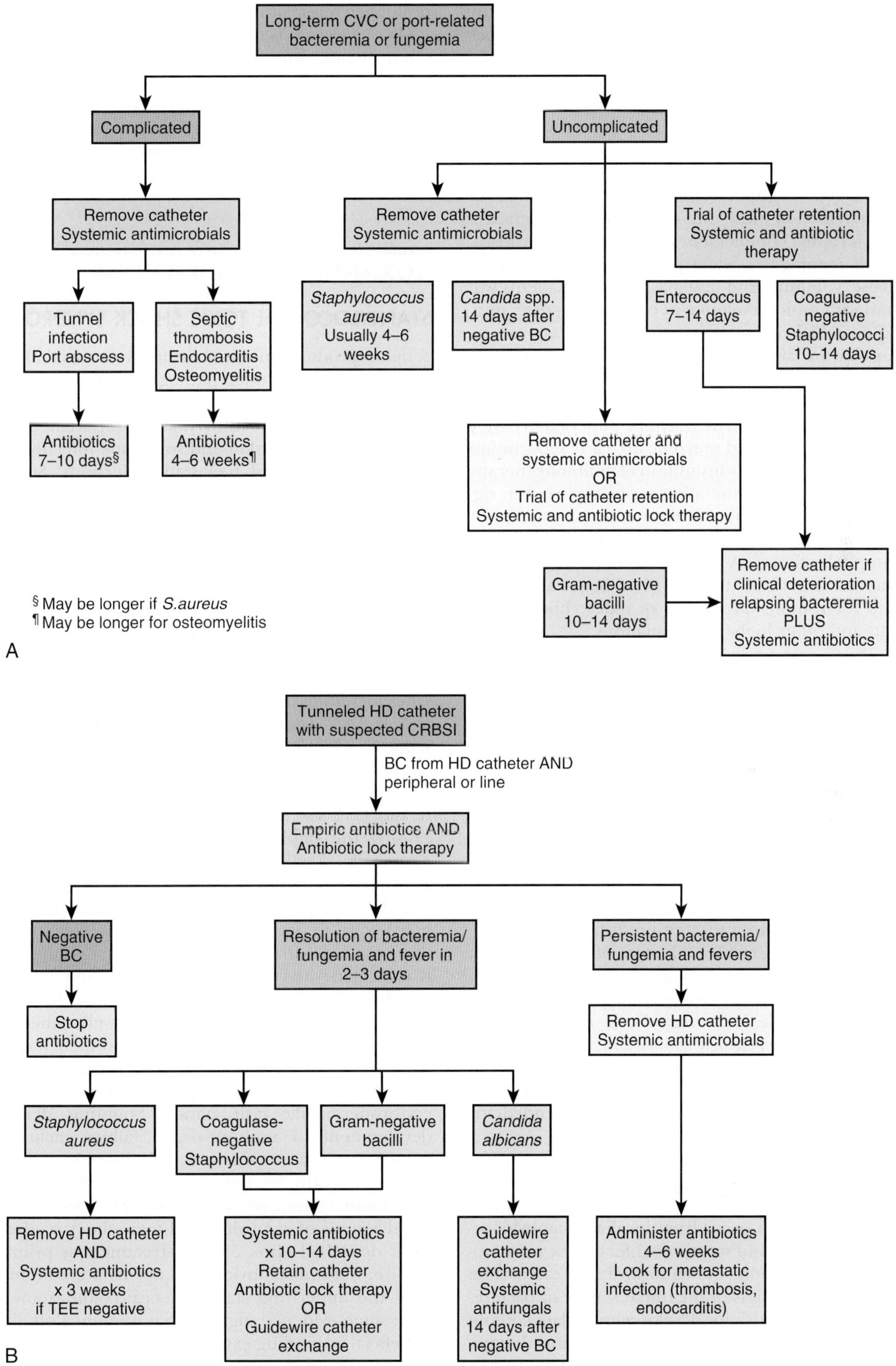

Figure 54.2 Algorithms for management of catheter-related bloodstream infection (CRSBI) in bacteremic patients with long-term central venous catheter or ports (**A**) and for suspected CRSBI in patients with tunneled hemodialysis catheters (**B**) including indications for removal versus attempt at salvage of infected indwelling long-term catheters. BC, blood culture; TEE, transesophageal echocardiography. (Data from Mermel LA, Allon M, Bouzon E, et al: Clinical practice guidelines for the diagnosis and management of intravascular catheter-related infection: 2009 update by the Infectious Diseases Society of America. Clin Infect Dis 2009;49(1):1-45.)

proportion of primary meningococcemia cases and severity of disease manifestations depend in part on the serotypes present in the community but are also heavily influenced by host genetic makeup. The annual incidence of meningococcal disease in the United States is approximately 1 case per 100,000, with mortality rate of 10% to 14% and significant residual morbidity in up to 20%.[7] Besides young children, adolescents and young adults ages 11 to 19 are at increased risk for meningococcal disease, but risk persists throughout life and is increased in those with certain immune deficiencies such as terminal complement deficiency and cirrhosis.[7] Patients with meningococcemia present with fever, headache, malaise, vomiting, and myalgias.[69,70] Most patients will also present with rapid development of a characteristic nonblanching petechial or purpuric rash, but the rash can be maculopapular or absent. Early symptoms that may be important clues to the diagnosis are leg pains and cold hands and feet.[69] If untreated, disease may progress rapidly within 24 hours to fulminant purpura and hemorrhagic shock. The keys to improved outcome are early recognition and aggressive therapy. Early institution of antibiotic therapy with a penicillin or third-generation cephalosporin can significantly improve outcomes. PCR of blood is useful for diagnosis, especially in patients who received antibiotics prior to hospitalization.[7,69] A tetravalent conjugated polysaccharide vaccine is available in the United States and is recommended for routine vaccination of older children and adolescents and other high-risk populations.[7]

PRIMARY PNEUMOCOCCAL BACTEREMIA

Pneumococcal bacteremia is most commonly a consequence of pneumococcal pneumonia, but 5% to 10% of episodes occur without an identified underlying focus.[71] Severe episodes may present with fulminant sepsis and purpura fulminans clinically indistinguishable from meningococcal sepsis. Important risk factors for pneumococcal sepsis include asplenia and hyposplenism, HIV infection, sickle cell disease, alcoholism, malignancy, and other immunocompromised states, although this syndrome can occur in otherwise healthy adults and children without predisposing risks.[72] *S. pneumoniae* causes 50% to 90% of cases of the fulminant sepsis syndrome that occurs in postsplenectomy or functionally asplenic patients.[67] Other causes of the postsplenectomy sepsis syndrome include *N. meningitidis; H. influenzae;* and, less commonly, *Capnocytophaga canimorsus, Escherichia coli, Salmonella,* and the vector-borne parasitic infections malaria and babesiosis. Immunization with pneumococcal, meningococcal, and *H. influenzae* vaccines is recommended for those at risk for postsplenectomy sepsis.[66]

STAPHYLOCOCCUS AUREUS BACTEREMIA

S. aureus bacteremia can occur from localized staphylococcal disease such as skin and soft tissue infection or pneumonia, endovascular infection, and endocarditis. It can also be of occult origin. Regardless of the initial source of bacteremia, there is significant risk for development of late complications including endocarditis, bone and joint disease, infections of prosthetic devices, or other metastatic foci in up to one third of cases.[58,73] Features associated with complicated *S. aureus* bacteremia include prolonged bacteremia, prolonged fever, and embolic lesions. Longer-course therapy (at least 4 weeks) is recommended for patients with complicated disease, whereas 2 weeks of treatment may be adequate for selected patients with uncomplicated bacteremia when endocarditis has been excluded.[74] TEE is recommended to exclude endocarditis in patients with otherwise clinically uncomplicated *S. aureus* bacteremia when short-course therapy is being considered.[73,74]

TOXIN-MEDIATED INFECTIONS

STAPHYLOCOCCAL TOXIC SHOCK SYNDROME

S. aureus produces multiple virulence factors that contribute to its success as a human pathogen. These virulence factors potentiate local adherence, tissue invasion, and avoidance of host defenses, all features that are important in the pathogenesis of localized skin and soft tissue infection, pneumonia, bacteremia, and metastatic infections. Staphylococci also produce a variety of exotoxins that are released into the systemic circulation to act at distant sites.[75] Some of these exotoxins are directly pathogenic to specific cells, such as exfoliatoxin B, which causes staphylococcal scalded skin syndrome. Other exotoxins function as potent superantigens, antigens that bypass the intermediate T-cell antigen processing steps by binding directly to Vβ domains on T-cell receptors. This causes direct activation of multiple T-cell classes resulting in unopposed release of large amounts of cytokines including interleukin (IL) 2, IL-4, IL-6, IFN-γ, TNF-α, and IL-1β.[75] The resulting "cytokine storm" can lead to septic shock, multiorgan failure, and death.

The most well-studied staphylococcal superantigens are the pyrogenic antigens TSST-1 and TSST-2 and enterotoxins B and C. TSST-1 and TSST-2 are the primary exotoxins causing the staphylococcal toxic shock syndrome.[75] First described in 1979 as a unique syndrome primarily associated with menstruating women using super absorbent brands of tampons, staphylococcal toxic shock syndrome is now known to occur potentially from infection or colonization at any site with an exotoxin-producing strain.[76,77] Disease is associated with conditions leading to exotoxin production in a host who lacks preexisting antibodies to TSST-1. The overall incidence of this syndrome, as well as the proportion of cases associated with menstruating women, has decreased since 1980.[76] Toxic shock syndrome is characterized by the acute onset of fever, hypotension, myalgia, scarlatiniform or erythroderma-like rash, nausea, vomiting, diarrhea, and development of multiple-organ failure including renal failure, elevated liver enzymes, and disseminated intravascular coagulopathy.[76,77] Typically the rash will evolve and cause late desquamation of hands and feet. Specific criteria for the diagnosis of staphylococcal toxic shock syndrome have been described (Box 54.2).[76] Treatment is primarily supportive, but antistaphylococcal agents are administered to treat the underlying staphylococcal colonization or infection; some evidence suggests that immunoglobulin may be beneficial by binding exotoxin and attenuating the cytokine response. Staphylococcal strains producing the staphylococcal enterotoxins B and C have been implicated in some nonmenstrual-associated cases.[75]

Box 54.2 Criteria for Diagnosis of Staphylococcal and Streptococcal Toxic Shock Syndromes

Staphylococcal Toxic Shock—CDC Criteria

1. Fever >38.9° C or >102° F
2. Rash (diffuse macular erythroderma)
3. Desquamation 1-2 weeks after onset, particularly of the palms and soles
4. Hypotension: systolic blood pressure <90 mm Hg for adults or orthostatic hypotension
5. Multisystem involvement with 3 or more of the following:
   Gastrointestinal: vomiting or diarrhea at onset of illness
   Muscular: severe myalgia or CK levels at least 2× upper limit of normal
   Mucous membrane: vaginal, oropharyngeal, or conjunctival hyperemia
   Renal: BUN or serum creatinine at least 2× upper limit of normal or >5 leukocytes per high-power field without UTI
   Hepatic: total bilirubin, AST, or ALT at least 2× upper limit of normal
   Hematologic: platelets ≤100,000/mL
   CNS: disoriented or alterations in level of consciousness without focal neurologic signs when fever and hypotension are absent
6. Negative results on tests, if obtained
   Blood, throat, or cerebrospinal fluid cultures (blood may be positive for *S. aureus*)
   Rise in body titer to Rocky Mountain spotted fever, leptospirosis, or measles antigen

Case Classification

Probable: 5 of the 6 clinical findings above
Confirmed: All 6 clinical findings including desquamation

Streptococcal Toxic Shock Syndrome

A. Isolation of group A streptococci
   1. From a sterile body site
   2. From a nonsterile body site
B. Clinical signs of severity
   1. Hypotension
   2. Clinical and laboratory abnormalities (2 or more):
      Renal impairment
      Coagulopathy
      Liver abnormalities
      Acute respiratory distress syndrome
      Extensive tissue necrosis (i.e., necrotizing fasciitis)
      Erythematous rash

Case Classification

Definite: A1 plus B (1 + 2)
Probable: A2 plus B (1 + 2)

ALT, alanine aminotransferase; AST, aspartate aminotransferase; BUN, blood urea nitrogen; CDC, Centers for Disease Control and Prevention; CNS, central nervous system; CK, creatine kinase; UTI, urinary tract infection.

Modified from Haijeh RA, Reingold A, Weil A, et al: Toxic shock syndrome in the United States: Surveillance update, 1979-1996. Emerg Infect Dis 1999;5:807-810; and Stevens DI: Streptococcal toxic-shock syndrome: Spectrum of disease, pathogenesis, and new concepts in treatment. Emerg Infect Dis 1995;1:69-78.

STREPTOCOCCAL TOXIC SHOCK SYNDROME

Group A β-hemolytic streptococci are also capable of producing a toxic shock–like syndrome analogous to staphylococcal toxic shock syndrome.[78,79] Most often this is seen in the setting of severe bacteremic streptococcal soft tissue infection or with streptococcal necrotizing fasciitis. In one large survey of invasive streptococcal infections in Ontario, 13% were complicated by toxic shock syndrome, and the mortality rate of these infections was 81%.[79] The pathogenesis of this syndrome is attributed to streptococcal pyrotoxins functioning as superantigens but may also involve binding of streptococcal M protein-fibrinogen complexes to PMN cells causing PMN activation and endothelial damage. Clinical criteria for the diagnosis of streptococcal toxic shock syndrome have been defined (see Box 54.2).[78] In addition to use of antibiotics that decrease toxin production in vitro, such as clindamycin and linezolid, IV immunoglobulin (IVIG) has been used for treatment though clinical evidence for benefit of IVIG is limited.[80] Other streptococcal species have also been reported to produce a toxic shock–like illness including viridans streptococci; groups B, C, and G β-hemolytic streptococci; and *Streptococcus suis.*

CLOSTRIDIAL TOXIC SHOCK SYNDROME

A rare, generally fatal syndrome of toxic shock has been reported following medical abortion with oral mifepristone and vaginal misoprostol.[81] This syndrome has also been seen complicating endometritis after live births and is due to *Clostridium sordellii.* Clinical findings include tachycardia, hypotension, edema, hemoconcentration, and profound leukocytosis, and generally the absence of fever. Optimal management of this syndrome remains poorly defined.

TETANUS

Tetanus is a syndrome of increased muscle rigidity and convulsive spasms caused by a toxin produced by the environmental spore-forming anaerobic bacterium *Clostridium tetani.*[82] Since the introduction of routine immunization, tetanus has become increasingly rare, with the number of U.S. cases decreasing from 560 cases in 1947 to only 233 cases from 2001 to 2008 with case fatality rate of 13%.[82] Clinical disease is caused by contamination of wounds, most commonly traumatic wounds, with bacterial spores. Spores then germinate and produce toxins including tetanospasmin, a highly potent neurotoxin that inhibits neurotransmitter release, resulting in blockage of inhibitor impulses and unopposed muscle contractions. Cases predominate in the summer or wet season, and disease is now most commonly seen in older adults because of either missed primary immunization or waning effects of childhood immunization.[82] The most common syndrome is that of generalized tetanus with descending symptoms of trismus (lockjaw), difficulty swallowing, muscle rigidity, and spasms. Symptoms may persist for several weeks, and complete recovery may take months. Complications include laryngospasm, fractures, hypertension, nosocomial infections, and death. Treatment is primarily supportive, although metronidazole or penicillin may be given to treat potentially infected or colonized wounds. Patients require admission to an ICU for control of rigidity and spasms with benzodiazepines or neuromuscular blocking agents and for ventilator support. Human tetanus immunoglobulin may be administered, but this only binds free toxin, so there may be little benefit by the time of clinical presentation. Routine childhood and adult immunization with tetanus toxoid remains the primary strategy for preventing this rare but often fatal condition. Guidelines for use of immunoglobulin and vaccination in management of potentially infected wounds have been published.[82]

BOTULISM

Clostridium botulinum is an anaerobic spore-forming bacterium that produces botulinum toxin, a family of closely related but immunologically distinct polypeptide toxins that are among the most potent neurologically acting poisons known.[83] Other, less common clostridial species can also produce botulinum toxin. Botulinum toxin binds irreversibly to synaptic complexes, affecting ganglionic synapses, presympathetic synapses, and neuromuscular junctions. Clinical syndromes include those caused by ingestion of preformed toxin such as food botulism and those resulting from acquisition of the organism and production of toxin in vivo such as infant botulism in very young children and wound botulism from contaminated wounds, most commonly seen in injection drug users. Patients present initially with cranial nerve dysfunction and evolve to descending paralysis without sensory or cognitive effects. Diagnosis is made on clinical grounds; testing of food products or human samples in the United States is performed by the Centers for Disease Prevention and Control (CDC). Treatment is primarily supportive, but equine type-specific antitoxin is available through the CDC.[83] Antitoxin is only effective in binding free toxin if given in the first 72 hours. Because of its potency, environmental stability, and potential for aerosolization, botulinum toxin is considered a potential agent of bioterrorism.[83]

DIPHTHERIA

Diphtheria is caused by toxigenic strains of the bacterial species *Corynebacterium diphtheriae*. This disease has become extremely rare in the United States secondary to universal vaccination with diphtheria toxoid vaccine, with an average of one confirmed case per year.[84] Patients with respiratory diphtheria present with sore throat; low-grade fever; occasional neck swelling; and the characteristic grayish adherent membrane covering the tonsils, throat, or nose.[84] Complications include myocarditis, polyneuritis, and airway obstruction, with mortality rates of 5% to 10%. Outbreaks of diphtheria continue to occur in many parts of the world.

SERIOUS SKIN AND SKIN STRUCTURE INFECTIONS

Serious skin and soft tissue infections are characterized by rapidly progressive inflammation and necrosis of skin, subcutaneous fat, and fascia. Occasionally, muscle is also involved. Several terms have been used to describe these infections: *necrotizing fasciitis; synergistic necrotizing cellulitis; progressive bacterial synergistic gangrene; anaerobic cellulitis*; and, when muscle is involved with clostridial infection, *clostridial myonecrosis (gas gangrene)*.[85] Differentiating among these entities is difficult and somewhat artificial. A variety of features of some of the most important necrotizing skin and soft tissue infections are shown in Table 54.4. Microbiologically, these infections may be caused by a single pathogen such as group A β-hemolytic streptococcus; however, they are more frequently polymicrobial in nature. Risk factors for these infections include diabetes, old age, peripheral vascular disease, malignancy, alcoholism, renal failure, and immunosuppressive therapy. Infection may follow traumatic injuries that become contaminated by soil. The primary traumatic event may be relatively minor. Initial signs and symptoms may be similar to a severe cellulitis. Early findings include fever, tachycardia, moderate to severe pain, and swelling and induration of the skin.[86] Late findings include severe pain or even anesthesia, skin necrosis, hemorrhagic bullae, crepitus, drainage, and signs of systemic inflammatory response syndrome or severe sepsis including multiorgan failure.[86] Laboratory tests usually demonstrate leukocytosis and metabolic acidosis. Plain radiographs may reveal gas in the soft tissues. CT or MRI is useful in delineating extent of disease or the presence of soft tissue gas. Diagnostic evaluation should also include blood cultures, Gram staining of tissue exudates, and aerobic and anaerobic cultures obtained at surgery or from a needle aspiration. Incision and exploration or biopsy can even be done at the bedside to obtain material for Gram stain, culture, and histologic evaluation.

Once a necrotizing soft tissue infection has been identified, prompt therapy is important. Early aggressive surgical débridement is essential.[87] Because most cases of necrotizing skin infection are polymicrobial, empiric antibiotic coverage should be sufficiently broad spectrum to cover gram-positive cocci, gram-negative bacilli, and anaerobes. A reasonable empirical regimen might consist of a β-lactam/β-lactamase inhibitor or a carbapenem combined with vancomycin or another agent effective against MRSA. Antibiotic therapy can subsequently be adjusted on the basis of results of cultures and sensitivities.[88] In cases of group A β-hemolytic streptococcal infection, penicillin plus clindamycin is the therapy of choice. Clindamycin is effective in turning off toxin production. Linezolid also has similar activity.[89] IVIG may be a useful adjuvant therapy for streptococcal toxic shock.[80,90]

NECROTIZING FASCIITIS

Necrotizing fasciitis is an uncommon, severe infection that causes necrosis of the subcutaneous tissue and fascia with sparing of the underlying muscle. Two predominant types, based on microbiology, are described. In type I, at least one anaerobic species is isolated along with one or more facultative anaerobes and members of the Enterobacteriaceae.[85,91] This form of necrotizing fasciitis most commonly affects the extremities but may involve the abdominal wall, postoperative wounds, perianal area, and groin. It occurs following trauma or a variety of surgical procedures, perirectal abscess, decubitus ulcer, or perforation of the intestines. Patients at increased risk include those with diabetes mellitus, alcoholism, and injection drug use. The involved area is initially

Table 54.4 Differentiating Features of Necrotizing Skin and Soft Tissue Infections

Feature	Progressive Bacterial Synergistic Gangrene	Nonclostridial Anaerobic Cellulitis	Clostridial Myonecrosis (Gas Gangrene)	Necrotizing Fasciitis Type 1	Necrotizing Fasciitis Type 2
Risk factors	Surgery, ileostomy, colostomy, chronic ulceration	Diabetes mellitus	Trauma, surgery	Diabetes mellitus, surgery, perineal infection	Trauma, surgery, none
Microbiology	Microaerophilic streptococci plus *Staphylococcus aureus*	Non–spore-forming anaerobes ± coliforms, streptococci, *S. aureus*	*Clostridium* spp.	Polymicrobial (Enterobacteriaceae plus anaerobes)	Group A streptococci
Course	Slow	Slow or rapid	Very rapid	Rapid	Very rapid
Pain	+++	++/+++	++++	+++/++++	++++
Gas formation	–	++++	++	++	–
Appearance	Central necrotic ulcer, erythematous periphery	Erythematous skin necrosis	Bullae, necrosis	Bullae, skin	Bullae, necrotic skin and tissue
Drainage	Purulent if present	Purulent	Serosanguineous	"Dishwater," seropurulent	Serous if present
Depth of involvement	Skin, soft tissue	Skin, soft tissue	Muscle	Fascia	Fascia
Systemic toxicity	±	+++/++++	++++	+++/++++	++++

–, absent; ±, occasionally present; +, minimal; ++, mild; +++, moderate; ++++, marked or severe.

erythematous and painful, but over several days skin changes include color changes, formation of bullae, and cutaneous gangrene. The involved area becomes anesthetic secondary to thrombosis of small blood vessels and destruction of superficial nerves. Anesthesia may develop before the appearance of skin necrosis and is an important clue to the presence of necrotizing fasciitis rather than simple cellulitis.[86] Subcutaneous gas is often present, and systemic toxicity is common.[91] When the lesion is probed at the bedside or in the operating room, there is no resistance along tissue planes. In type II (also known as hemolytic streptococcal gangrene), group A streptococci are generally isolated alone or in combination with *S. aureus*.[92] These strains usually produce pyrogenic exotoxin A. Periodically, group C or group G streptococci are causative organisms. Infection usually develops at a site of trauma but may occur in the absence of an obvious portal of entry.[91] The involved area is extremely painful, erythematous, and edematous. Infection spreads widely in deep fascial planes with relative sparing of the overlying skin and therefore may not be recognized. This form of necrotizing fasciitis is present in approximately 50% of cases of streptococcal toxic shock syndrome.[92] Over several days, the skin becomes dusky and bullae develop. Bullae then rupture and evolve into an area covered by necrotic eschar, often resembling a third-degree burn. Streptococci can usually be cultured from fluid of the early bullae and frequently from blood. Complications include metastatic abscess formation, and the mortality rate from this infection is high.

Fournier's gangrene is a form of necrotizing fasciitis that involves the male perineum, usually the scrotum, but can involve the penis, the perineum, or the abdominal wall. It is caused by anaerobic streptococci along with other bacteria such as *E. coli*; *S. aureus*; β-hemolytic streptococci; *Proteus* species; a variety of anaerobes; and, on occasion, *Pseudomonas* species.[93] The first symptoms are commonly scrotal swelling and pain followed by progressive necrosis of scrotal skin and subcutaneous tissues.[93] The patient may appear toxic. Initially the patient may be erroneously diagnosed with an acute abdomen unless the genitalia are examined. Gangrene of the perineum and sometimes the penis may develop. Urgent and aggressive surgery is necessary along with broad-spectrum antibiotics.

CLOSTRIDIAL MYONECROSIS (GAS GANGRENE)

Gas gangrene is a life-threatening infection of skeletal muscle caused by *Clostridium* species. It should be suspected when the Gram stain of drainage reveals gram-positive bacilli in a patient who is critically ill. Penicillin G is the drug of choice with or without clindamycin. Aggressive surgical exploration and débridement is the mainstay of therapy. The role of hyperbaric oxygen therapy in the treatment of clostridial myonecrosis or in the treatment of necrotizing fasciitis remains controversial. If used, it must be used as an adjunct to surgery.[94]

VIBRIO INFECTIONS

Various *Vibrio* species including *Vibrio vulnificus* have caused mild to severe cellulitis in patients who sustained lacerations or puncture wounds when in contact with saltwater in the southeastern United States and the Gulf of Mexico. Septicemia with secondary necrotizing soft tissue infection may occur after ingestion of raw or undercooked shellfish in immunocompromised hosts, especially those with cirrhosis.[95] An increased incidence of *Vibrio* infections has been described as a result of flooding after natural disasters. Doxycycline, third-generation cephalosporins, and fluoroquinolones are effective therapies, along with aggressive surgical débridement of necrotic tissue.

COMMUNITY-ACQUIRED MRSA

During the past decade, community-associated MRSA (CA-MRSA) infections among persons without health care–associated risk factors have emerged in several geographic areas and have become endemic in some areas.[96] Many of these strains carry the staphylococcal cassette chromosome mec type IV element and the gene encoding Panton-Valentine leukocidin, a toxin that promotes tissue destruction.[97,98] Although most CA-MRSA infections are mild skin and soft tissue infections, severe, life-threatening cases of necrotizing fasciitis, myonecrosis, necrotizing pneumonia, and sepsis have occurred.[97,98] For patients with invasive infections caused by CA-MRSA, vancomycin and linezolid are appropriate therapeutic options.[99] CA-MRSA strains are often susceptible to clindamycin, doxycycline, and trimethoprim/sulfamethoxazole.

SERIOUS GASTROINTESTINAL AND INTRA-ABDOMINAL INFECTIONS

BACTEREMIA ASSOCIATED WITH DIARRHEAL ILLNESS

Of the enteric pathogens, *Salmonella* species are most likely to cause bacteremia and serious infection. Enteric fever is usually caused by *Salmonella enterica* serotype typhi and rarely by *Salmonella paratyphi, Salmonella choleraesuis, Yersinia enterocolitica,* or *Campylobacter fetus.*[100] Features of classic typhoidal fever caused by *S. enterica* include sustained fever, bacteremia, headache, and abdominal pain. Physical findings include "rose spots," which are 2- to 4-mm discrete, irregular, blanching pink macules that are often seen on the anterior chest; hepatosplenomegaly; and relative bradycardia. Multiorgan system dysfunction can occur as a consequence of metastatic infection or immune complex deposition.[101] Intestinal bleeding or perforation may occur as a result of hyperplasia of the lymphoid tissue in the terminal ileum. Diarrhea is seen in less than 50% of cases and only early in the illness. Constipation is a frequent later complaint. The following specimens should be sent for culture: stool, blood, or bone marrow. Serologic findings may provide supportive evidence or may be useful in epidemiologic evaluation.

Therapeutic options include third-generation cephalosporins, fluoroquinolones, and trimethoprim/sulfamethoxazole. Antimicrobial resistance has been reported. Treatment for uncomplicated cases is 12 to 14 days; 30 days of therapy may be necessary for metastatic foci. Metastatic foci are relatively common in the setting of bacteremia. Infection may involve gallbladder, spleen, bone, joints, and the meninges. There is a propensity to infect preexisting intravascular lesions such as atherosclerotic plaques and aneurysms. Sickle cell anemia and the presence of an orthopedic prosthesis are risk factors for osteomyelitis.[101] Meningitis tends to occur in young children.[101]

PERITONITIS

Peritonitis is a localized or general inflammation of the peritoneal cavity that is generally caused by bacteria or fungi but may be caused by a variety of noninfectious agents such as gastric contents, talc, or bile salts. Infective peritonitis has been classified as primary, secondary, or tertiary. Peritonitis is primary when it is not related directly to other intra-abdominal processes.[102] This classification includes spontaneous bacterial peritonitis (SBP), which occurs in patients with underlying ascites from cirrhosis or nephrotic syndrome, and tuberculous peritonitis. Secondary peritonitis most often arises from an enteric source or pelvic focus and includes peritonitis following an acute perforation of the gastrointestinal tract, intestinal necrosis, postoperative peritonitis that may be secondary to an anastomotic leak, and posttraumatic peritonitis following blunt or penetrating abdominal trauma. Intestinal ischemia and frank necrotic bowel may be caused by a variety of processes including malignancies, vascular insufficiency, volvulus, or intussusception.[102] Rupture of an abscess in the pancreas, liver, or spleen or, rarely, rupture of a distended gallbladder can also cause peritonitis. Localized lower abdominal peritonitis can also result from gynecologic infections such as salpingitis and endometritis. Tertiary peritonitis is described as occurring when clinical and systemic signs of peritonitis persist or recur after treatment for secondary peritonitis. A distinct form of device-associated peritonitis is seen in patients undergoing peritoneal dialysis.

Bacterial peritonitis is typically caused by flora of the large intestine including aerobes, with *E. coli* being the most frequent, and anaerobes, of which *Bacteroides fragilis* is the predominant isolate.[103] Common symptoms include localized or generalized abdominal pain, nausea, and vomiting. Treatment with corticosteroids may mask typical signs and symptoms, delaying the diagnosis. Signs may include abdominal rigidity, distention, fever, and an overall toxic appearance. A rigid abdomen may be seen in the early stages of an acute peritonitis, although it may be absent in a peritonitis that progresses more slowly, such as that caused by tuberculosis, or when sterile bile, pancreatic fluid, or urine leaks into the peritoneal cavity. As intraperitoneal fluid accumulates, abdominal distention and an ileus occur. The WBC count is usually elevated. Bacteremia may occur, and the sepsis syndrome may develop as peritonitis evolves. Aspiration of peritoneal fluid is an essential part of the evaluation for peritonitis. Laparoscopy or laparotomy may be necessary. Studies performed on peritoneal fluid should include a cell count with differential blood cell count, amylase, Gram stain and aerobic and anaerobic culture, acid-fast smear and culture, and fungal smear and culture.

The primary cause of secondary peritonitis should be sought and eliminated if possible. Liver function tests and a serum amylase level may define a source in the liver, gallbladder, or pancreas. A plain film of the abdomen or a chest radiograph may reveal free air under the diaphragm in the case of a ruptured viscus. A CT scan of the abdomen may reveal an underlying intra-abdominal abscess or other focal process. Antibiotic therapy to cover gram-negative bacillary organisms and anaerobes should be initiated. Options for empiric therapy include combinations such as a third- or fourth-generation cephalosporin or a fluoroquinolone with metronidazole or monotherapy with a β-lactam/β-lactamase inhibitor combination, a carbapenem, or a glycylcycline such as tigecycline.[104-107] The optimal duration of therapy is not well defined, although nonbacteremic patients are generally treated for 7 to 10 days.[103] Regimens as short as 2 days of treatment may be adequate in uncomplicated situations with adequate surgical source control and in those with penetrating trauma. Bacteremic patients are generally treated for a total of 14 days using a combination of IV followed by oral therapy.

SBP is caused by the translocation of enteric organisms to regional lymph nodes, which produce bacteremia and ultimately seeding of ascitic fluid.[108] Periodically a urinary tract infection may be the source of bacteremia. SBP occurs most commonly in adults with cirrhosis, nephrotic syndrome, or systemic lupus erythematosus.[108,109] Coliforms are the most common pathogens in adults, accounting for 70% of infections, with *E. coli* being the most common isolate followed by *Klebsiella* species. Gram-positive cocci may be seen in up to 20% of cases and anaerobes in less than 5%. Generally SBP is monomicrobial in contrast to the polymicrobial nature of most other forms of peritonitis. Findings of SBP may be subtle, so a high index of suspicion is necessary. Ascites is almost always present.[108] Fever and abdominal pain are seen in the majority of patients. New onset or worsening of hepatic encephalopathy may be seen. Some patients may have abdominal tenderness or rebound tenderness, but these findings are less frequent than in other forms of peritonitis. The most useful diagnostic test is a paracentesis.[108-110] SBP is defined by an ascitic segmented neutrophil count of at least 250 cells/mm^3 with or without a positive fluid culture and no obvious intra-abdominal source of infection.[109,110] The pH of ascitic fluid is low in SBP, whereas that of sterile ascitic fluid is the same as in serum.[110] Despite the low sensitivity (≈33%), Gram staining of ascitic fluid should be performed. Patients with other infections of the abdomen, such as tuberculous peritonitis, secondary bacterial peritonitis caused by perforation, or peritonitis caused by noninfectious processes including pancreatitis or malignancy, also may show elevated neutrophil counts. Presence of a single organism generally supports the diagnosis of SBP, although there is a variant of SBP caused by traumatic entry into the bowel during paracentesis that may be polymicrobial, and conversely, gram-negative bacillary organisms may occur as sole pathogens in secondary peritonitis. If mixed gram-positive and gram-negative bacteria are seen, an intestinal perforation is the more likely source.[110] Peritoneal fluid should be cultured aerobically and anaerobically. Blood cultures should also be performed and are positive in up to 75% of patients with SBP.[109] Other than for symptom relief, a repeat paracentesis is necessary only when the patient fails to have a clinical response or when an unusual organism is isolated. Treatment is usually continued for a total of 7 to 10 days, although some experts have suggested that a 5- to 7-day course of IV therapy may be adequate.[109,111,112] Most studies show a high mortality rate of 30% to 40% for this syndrome, and after an initial episode of SBP, the probability of recurrence within 1 year is 70%.[108,111]

INTRA-ABDOMINAL ABSCESS

Considering the presence of a potential intra-abdominal abscess in febrile patients without any obvious cause of fever is important, especially if there is a predisposing condition such as diverticulitis, inflammatory bowel disease, or a history of recent abdominal surgery or abdominal trauma. Intra-abdominal abscess formation may complicate either primary or secondary peritonitis. The processes that typically predispose to intra-abdominal abscess formation are the same as those that cause secondary peritonitis and include perforation, complicated acute cholecystitis, suppurative cholangitis, acute appendicitis, diverticulitis, intestinal malignancy, surgical procedures, blunt or penetrating trauma, or intestinal ischemia from a mesenteric vascular occlusion, an intestinal obstruction, or a volvulus. Most commonly, abscesses are postoperative complications of trauma or of gastrointestinal or biliary surgery.[113] Abscesses can be found anywhere within the abdomen including the retroperitoneal space. Generally their location is in proximity with the original site of contamination, but they may develop at distant sites.[114] One example of distal infection is subphrenic abscess, which may be a consequence of a perforated appendix. Symptoms of intra-abdominal abscess may include fever, chills, anorexia, weight loss, and abdominal pain. Unexplained fever may be the only sign of an occult intra-abdominal abscess. An abdominal CT scan is the imaging modality of choice for diagnosis of abdominal abscess. Drainage is essential to establish the diagnosis, obtain microbiology to target antimicrobial therapy, and achieve therapeutic success. This may be accomplished by the insertion of percutaneous catheters, or by laparoscopic or operative drainage.[113,114] Large abscesses cannot be eradicated by antibiotic therapy alone. Criteria for considering percutaneous drainage include the presence of a well-defined fluid collection and a safe percutaneous route of access.[115] Drains should remain in place until drainage volume is minimal, usually less than 10 mL in a 24-hour period.

A repeat CT scan should be performed to demonstrate complete collapse of the abscess cavity.[113] Indications for operative surgical drainage rather than percutaneous drainage include the following situations: (1) Percutaneous drainage cannot be performed safely; (2) percutaneous drainage fails; (3) there are multiple interloop abscesses; (4) there is a coagulopathy; or (5) there is infected pancreatic necrosis. Antibiotic therapy is indicated to treat inflammation in the surrounding tissue and to prevent metastatic infection and sepsis from bacteremia. Antibiotic coverage should be directed at abdominal flora including aerobic and anaerobic organisms even if anaerobes are not isolated.[103,112,113] Mortality rate with undrained pancreatic, hepatic, or retroperitoneal abscesses is reported to be 45% to 100%.[114] An approach to the management of intra-abdominal abscesses is outlined in Figure 54.3.

BILIARY TRACT INFECTIONS

Infections of the biliary tract, including the gallbladder and the common bile duct, are usually associated with obstruction to the flow of bile. The biliary tract of healthy individuals is sterile. In acute cholecystitis, infection of the

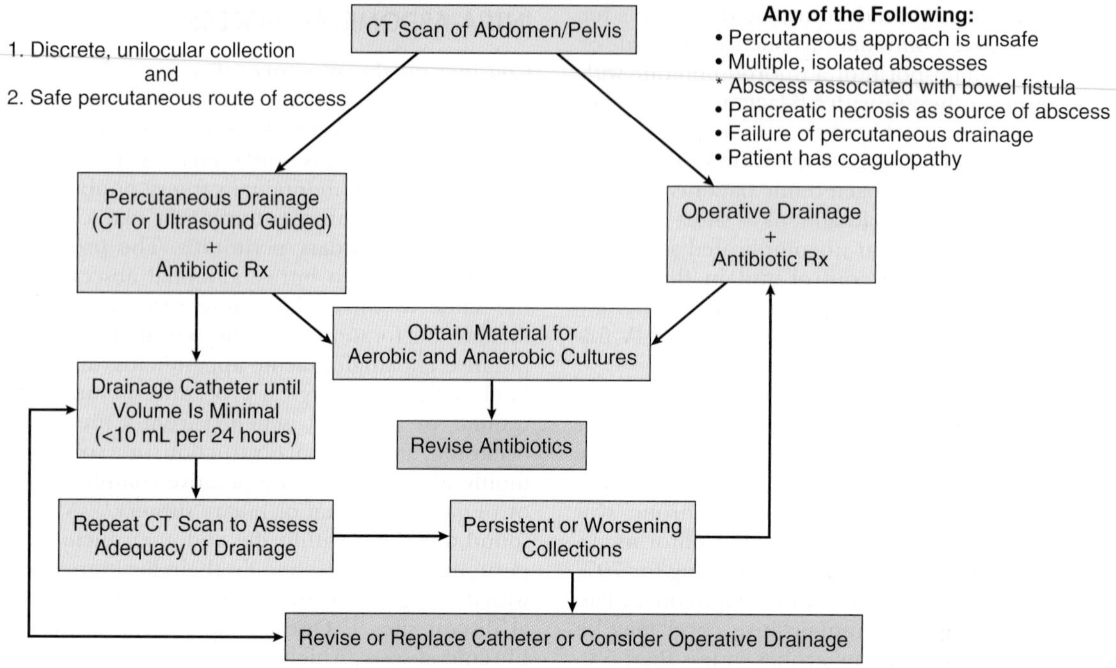

Figure 54.3 Approach to management of intra-abdominal abscesses including indications for consideration of percutaneous versus operative drainage.

gallbladder is most commonly caused by microorganisms that are generally part of the normal intestinal flora.[116] Most biliary infections are polymicrobial, and anaerobes are more frequently isolated in the elderly and in those with common bile duct manipulation or prior biliary procedures. The source of bacteria is presumed to be the duodenum.[116] Many antibiotics achieve good levels in the bile in the absence of obstruction; however, when obstruction of the hepatic ducts or the common bile duct is present, the levels of such antibiotics are often subtherapeutic. Antibiotic therapy is adjunctive to decompression/drainage, which can be accomplished surgically, percutaneously, or endoscopically via endoscopic retrograde cholangiopancreatography (ERCP). Antibiotics prevent the development of bacteremia, progression of infection, and development of liver abscesses. Cultures of blood and bile should be obtained. Empiric antibiotic therapy should generally be directed at gram-negative bacteria. In patients who are critically ill, the elderly, and those with prior common bile duct and complex biliary procedures, antianaerobic and antienterococcal therapy should also be instituted.

Acute acalculous cholecystitis is an acute inflammation of the gallbladder that occurs in the absence of gallstones. Individuals at risk include debilitated, hospitalized patients such as those who have had major surgical procedures, prolonged intensive care stays, hyperalimentation, or predisposing conditions that result in bile stasis, cholecystoparesis, or gallbladder ischemia.[116] The symptoms and findings are similar to those of calculous cholecystitis and include fever, right upper quadrant abdominal pain, nausea, vomiting, leukocytosis, and elevated liver function tests with an obstructive pattern. Diagnostic imaging modalities include ultrasonography, CT scanning, and hepatoiminodiacetic acid (HIDA) scanning. If an open or laparoscopic cholecystectomy cannot be accomplished because of the patient's underlying condition, then urgent percutaneous cholecystostomy should be performed. In addition, broad-spectrum antibiotics should be instituted.

Acute cholangitis is a serious infection with high morbidity and mortality rates. The most common cause of acute cholangitis is obstruction and subsequent infection associated with stones in the common bile duct, which have usually migrated from the gallbladder. Other causes of biliary tract infection include malignant obstruction of the bile duct secondary to pancreatic cancer, cholangiocarcinoma, cancer of the papilla of Vater, or portahepatic metastases. Periodically biliary strictures, pancreatitis, and infection with the intestinal nematode *Ascaris lumbricoides* can cause obstruction. Bacteria enter the bile duct from the gastrointestinal tract through the bloodstream or lymphatics.[117] The most common presenting symptoms are fever, abdominal pain, and jaundice, also known as *Charcot's triad*. Septic shock may occur if treatment is delayed. Blood cultures should be obtained, and ultrasound or CT scanning should be performed. Broad-spectrum antibiotics should be initiated, and biliary decompression accomplished either endoscopically with an endoscopic sphincterotomy, via a percutaneous transhepatic biliary drainage procedure, or by surgical decompression. Endoscopic or percutaneous procedures may be the initial treatment of choice in patients who are seriously ill and at high risk for complications. Elective surgery, which generally includes cholecystectomy and bile duct exploration, can be deferred to a later date when the patient has stabilized.

PANCREATIC INFECTIONS

Although acute pancreatitis is usually a sterile inflammatory process, infectious complications may occur. In addition, a variety of viral infections (rubella; coxsackievirus type B;

mumps; Epstein-Barr virus; CMV; and hepatitis A, B, and C); *Mycoplasma pneumoniae*; and parasites such as *A. lumbricoides* have been implicated as causes of pancreatitis.[118] Some patients may develop sterile or infected pancreatic or peripancreatic necrosis, infected pancreatic pseudocysts, or abscess formation as complications of acute pancreatitis.[118] Sterile necrosis of either the parenchyma or the duct system usually occurs very early in the clinical course of severe pancreatitis. Risk for infection increases as necrosis becomes more extensive. Of patients with acute pancreatitis, only approximately 5% develop pancreatic infections; however, the highest mortality rate from pancreatitis occurs in these patients.[118] The incidence of infection increases over the first few weeks and peaks during the third and fourth weeks. Patients with extensive necrosis, those who are very ill, and those with early infection have the highest mortality rates.[118] CT scan with high-dose contrast agent is the most useful modality for predicting who is at risk for the development of infection. Between 40% and 70% of those with more than 30% necrosis seen on CT scan will ultimately become infected.[118] If gas bubbles are seen in the region of the pancreas, it should be presumed that infection is present. Clinically, it is extremely difficult to determine whether patients with necrotizing pancreatitis have superimposed infection because sterile pancreatic necrosis may cause leukocytosis and fever even in the absence of infection, and approximately 50% of infected patients may not show early clinical signs of infection. CT-guided fine-needle aspiration of necrotic pancreatic tissue for Gram stain and aerobic and anaerobic culture is a useful procedure to determine the presence of infection.[118] The microbiologic picture resembles that of the intestinal flora. *E. coli* is most frequently isolated, followed by *Klebsiella pneumoniae, Enterococcus* species, *Pseudomonas* species, and *S. aureus.*[102] Fifteen percent of organisms isolated are intestinal anaerobes. Treatment of pancreatic infection usually involves débridement of infected tissue or drainage of infected pseudocysts or abscesses combined with antimicrobial therapy based on cultures of the infected site. Surgical management often requires multiple staged procedures. Antibiotics that penetrate into pancreatic tissue include the carbapenems, especially imipenem, fluoroquinolones, piperacillin, advanced generation cephalosporins, and metronidazole.[103]

CLOSTRIDIUM DIFFICILE COLITIS

Manifestations of *Clostridium difficile* infection may range from asymptomatic carriage to a fulminant, relapsing, or life-threatening colitis.[119,120] Antibiotics or chemotherapeutic agents have been associated with alteration of normal bowel flora and growth of *C. difficile.*[119,120] Diarrhea may develop while a patient is receiving antibiotics or several weeks after completion of a course of antibiotics. Only strains that produce toxins are capable of causing diarrhea or colitis.[119,120] Common symptoms include fever, which may be either low grade or high, crampy abdominal pain, and diarrhea, which is watery, profuse, and foul smelling. Approximately 50% of patients will have leukocytes in smears of the stool.[119,120] Leukocytosis is common. The diagnosis is established by assaying the stool for *C. difficile* toxin. Complications of severe disease include electrolyte derangements, dehydration, toxic megacolon, and colonic perforation. Some patients may have little or no diarrhea but present with toxic megacolon, colonic perforation, peritonitis, or even septic shock without other localizing symptoms. An epidemic strain of *C. difficile,* NAP1/027, has enhanced toxin production and causes outbreaks of illness characterized by increased severity, poorer response to antibiotic therapy, and frequent relapse.[121] Oral metronidazole remains first-line treatment for mild to moderate disease; empiric therapy with oral metronidazole should be started while testing for *C. difficile* toxin is being performed. If patients do not have a favorable response within 3 to 5 days, they should be switched to oral vancomycin. Oral vancomycin should be administered to those with severe infection or unresponsiveness to or intolerance of metronidazole. For patients who are unable to tolerate oral medication, IV metronidazole, vancomycin retention enemas, or vancomycin instillation through a colonic catheter should be administered. Surgery is indicated for complications such as severe toxic megacolon and colonic perforation. A variety of surgical procedures including diverting ileostomy, cecostomy, colostomy, and subtotal colectomy have been performed to manage toxic megacolon. Subtotal colectomy is considered the procedure of choice for the management of fulminant toxic megacolon.

LIFE-THREATENING INFECTIONS OF THE HEAD AND NECK

LUDWIG'S ANGINA, LATERAL PHARYNGEAL SPACE INFECTIONS, AND PERITONSILLAR ABSCESS

Infections arising from the flora of the mouth and posterior pharynx can involve the fascial planes of the neck and have the potential to progress rapidly and cause serious life-threatening illness.[122,123] In general, these infections are polymicrobial and the microbiology reflects the normal flora of the mouth. These infections spread rapidly through contiguous fascial spaces and it is essential that they be diagnosed and treated expeditiously to prevent serious sequelae such as airway obstruction, hematogenous infection, and mediastinitis. Potentially life-threatening infections of the head and neck may involve three cervical spaces. Fascial planes both separate and connect these areas. The spaces and infectious manifestations are as follows, and representative images are shown in Figure 54.4:

1. The submandibular space may be affected by infection involving the flora of the mouth and tongue. A bilateral cellulitis of the soft tissue, known as *Ludwig's angina,* is the most important type of infection in the submandibular space. Manifestations of this infection include enlargement of the tongue and submandibular swelling. An odontogenic focus is the origin of infection of 70% to 90% of cases.[123,124]
2. The lateral pharyngeal space consists of an anterior and a posterior compartment divided by the styloid process. The anterior compartment is composed of musculature, and the posterior compartment has nerves and blood vessels. Infection in the anterior compartment causes soft tissue swelling that results in unilateral trismus caused by

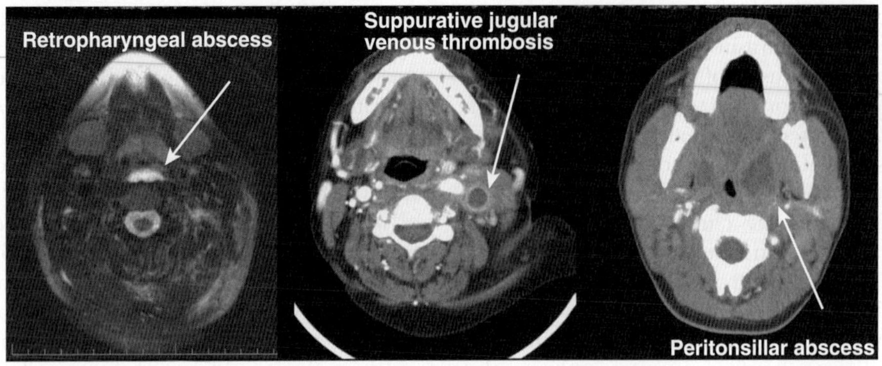

Figure 54.4 Magnetic resonance imaging and computed tomography images showing a variety of life-threatening head and neck infections including retropharyngeal abscess (**A**), suppurative jugular venous thrombosis (**B**), and peritonsillar abscess (**C**). (Images provided by Dr. Joshua Brody, Department of Radiology, the Cooper Health System, Camden, NJ.)

irritation of the internal pterygoid muscle, induration and swelling along the angle of the jaw, bulging of the palatine tonsil into the posterior pharynx, and systemic toxicity. Patients may present with unilateral neck or jaw pain along with ear pain and dysphagia. Pain may worsen when the head is turned because of compression of infected tissue. Dental infection, upper respiratory infection, pharyngitis, and otitis media with mastoiditis may all cause lateral pharyngeal space infection.[125] The carotid sheath is within the posterior compartment and contains the internal carotid artery, the internal jugular vein, the vagus nerve, cranial nerves IX through XII, and lymph nodes. When infection occurs in this space, patients most commonly present with signs of sepsis without localizing signs at the neck. Generally signs and symptoms are related to complications from involvement of the neurovascular structures. The most common complication is suppurative jugular venous thrombosis. Bacteremia and septic emboli may be seen. The carotid artery may also rupture. The carotid sheath is dense and not easily penetrated, so generally arterial erosion is usually a complication of infections of longer duration (1 to 2 weeks). Intermittent bleeding from the mouth or nose may precede rupture.[124] Cranial nerve palsies or Horner's syndrome may occur.

3. The retropharyngeal space contains an area that extends from the base of the skull to the diaphragm and hence is a portal for neck infections to extend into the chest. Infections of the retropharyngeal space or prevertebral space may spread as a result of extension through this area. Retropharyngeal space abscesses are relatively uncommon and are most often seen in young children. These abscesses usually result from odontogenic infection, penetrating trauma, or peritonsillar abscess. Peritonsillar abscess, also known as "quinsy," is an unusual complication of acute tonsillitis seen predominantly in adolescents and young adults. Patients usually present with fever, pharyngitis, odynophagia, dysphagia, trismus, drooling, and a muffled voice that has been described as "hot potato" in quality. On examination there is usually swelling of the anterior tonsillar pillars and soft palate. The most common symptoms of retropharyngeal space infection in adults are fever, dysphagia, pharyngeal pain, dyspnea, noisy breathing, and stiff neck. A lateral radiograph of the neck may reveal prevertebral soft tissue swelling. Any deep neck infection has the potential to spread to the mediastinum via the retropharyngeal space.

Other potential complications of infection of the oral cavity are aspiration pneumonia and lung abscess. Because most of these infections originate from an odontogenic focus, the microbiology reflects polymicrobial oral flora and generally includes *Bacteroides* species, aerobic streptococci, microaerophilic streptococci, peptostreptococci, fusobacteria, *Veillonella* species, and *Actinomyces* species. On occasion, enteric gram-negative bacilli, *P. aeruginosa,* or *S. aureus* may play a role.[125]

Deep neck infections are medical and surgical emergencies. Complications include hematogenous dissemination with sepsis syndrome, airway obstruction, necrotizing pneumonia or empyema, osteomyelitis of the mandible or maxilla, mediastinitis, or intracranial extension and cavernous sinus thrombosis. A contrast CT scan or MRI of the neck is important to help define the anatomy including the vascular structures and to indicate potential need for drainage. Consultation should be obtained from an otolaryngologist. When patients have dyspnea, stridor, or an inability to handle secretions, an artificial airway should be established. Airway obstruction is most likely to occur in infections of the submandibular space. Surgically obtained specimens should be cultured aerobically and anaerobically. For patients with peritonsillar abscess, high-dose IV penicillin is the therapy of choice. Other treatment options include clindamycin or ampicillin-sulbactam. Patients with peritonsillar abscess should undergo incision and drainage to prevent spontaneous rupture, aspiration pneumonia, airway obstruction, or dissection of infection into the lateral retropharyngeal space. Surgical drainage is especially important for infections involving the retropharyngeal and lateral pharyngeal space. Approximately half of cases of Ludwig's angina in the submandibular space can be cured without surgical intervention.[124]

LEMIERRE SYNDROME

Lemierre syndrome (postanginal sepsis) is a fulminant infectious syndrome caused by acute oropharyngeal infection that is complicated by secondary septic thrombophlebitis of the internal jugular vein. It is usually seen in healthy adolescents or young adults. *Fusobacterium* species are most commonly implicated. Complications include septicemia, pneumonia, empyema, meningitis, brain abscess, and vocal cord paralysis. This infection may complicate a routine case of infectious mononucleosis.[126] Therapy usually consists of surgical drainage of the focus and broad-spectrum IV antibiotic therapy.

EPIGLOTTITIS

Acute infectious epiglottitis is an inflammatory process of the epiglottis, supraglottis, and surrounding soft tissues.[127] Since the near disappearance of invasive *H. influenzae* infections in children following universal immunization, acute epiglottitis has become primarily a disease of adults, with an annual incidence of 1 case per 100,000 and peak incidence from ages 40 to 50. Patients present with severe pharyngitis; pain on swallowing; fever; and, less commonly, shortness of breath, hoarseness, and muffled voice. Findings on examination include marked anterior neck tenderness, lymphadenopathy, drooling, and respiratory distress.[127,128] The standard of diagnosis for suspected epiglottitis in adults is visualization of the epiglottis with indirect laryngoscopy.[127] Radiography has low sensitivity and specificity. Treatment includes maintenance of an airway; depending on severity and rapidity of onset of symptoms, this may include emergent tracheostomy, elective intubation, or only close observation in an ICU for the mildest cases.[127] Antibiotics active against the most commonly implicated pathogens, *H. influenzae* and β-hemolytic streptococci, are administered, and corticosteroids are generally recommended.[127,128] Disease may be more aggressive in HIV-infected or other immunocompromised individuals.

MEDIASTINITIS

Acute mediastinitis is an infection of mediastinal structures that can develop from direct extension of pharyngeal and neck infections (descending necrotizing mediastinitis), from esophageal trauma or rupture, or as a complication of cardiothoracic surgical procedures.[129] Descending necrotizing mediastinitis and mediastinitis from esophageal procedures have both become uncommon, and most cases are seen as complications of cardiothoracic surgery procedures or from trauma.[129,130] Symptoms of mediastinitis may initially be mild, but as disease progresses, patients will develop chest pain; dysphagia; and respiratory distress, as well as fever, tachycardia, crepitus, and localized swelling. Sepsis is common. Patients with postcardiothoracic mediastinitis will generally have evidence of local or deep sternal wound infection. Leukocytosis is typical. Plain films may show mediastinal widening; mediastinal air-fluid levels; and subcutaneous, mediastinal, or pericardial air. CT is more sensitive than plain radiographs for diagnosis; contrast esophagography with water-soluble contrast is the optimal study for esophageal perforation.[129]

Treatment of infection related to descending neck infection or esophageal perforation requires broad-spectrum antibiotics directed at oropharyngeal flora including streptococci, oral anaerobes, and gram-negative bacilli in addition to surgical intervention.[129] Mediastinitis following cardiothoracic surgery is most commonly caused by staphylococci, but a large variety of other gram-positive and gram-negative organisms have been implicated. Treatment requires surgical drainage and débridement along with antibiotic therapy.[130]

SERIOUS VECTOR-BORNE INFECTIONS

ROCKY MOUNTAIN SPOTTED FEVER

Tick-borne rickettsial diseases cause severe illness and death in otherwise healthy individuals. Although the various rickettsial diseases may have distinct epidemiologic and etiologic differences, they are clinically similar.[131] RMSF is caused by *Rickettsia rickettsii*, which is a gram-negative, obligate, intracellular bacterium. Infection is transmitted to humans by a variety of ticks but most frequently by the dog tick, *Dermacentor variabilis*. The incidence is greatest in the southeastern and south central United States. The vast majority of cases occur from April to September. Reported risks for infection include living in wooded areas and exposure to dogs. *R. rickettsii* infects endothelial cells, resulting in vasculitis, which leads to the characteristic rash and involvement of the lungs, brain, and other organs.[131-134] Following an incubation period of 3 to 12 days, patients frequently present with fever, rash, and evidence or history of a tick bite, although 30% to 40% of patients do not recall a tick bite.[131] Other symptoms include chills; myalgias; nausea; vomiting; abdominal pain that may be severe enough to mimic an acute abdomen; diarrhea; headache; photophobia; mental status changes; conjunctival injection; and, periodically, cough or arrhythmias secondary to myocarditis. The rash is classically an erythematous macular rash that appears initially on the ankles/soles and wrists/palms and spreads centripetally to the arms, legs, trunk, neck, and face.[132-134] The lesions evolve to become petechial. The rash typically appears after 2 to 6 days of illness. Although rash is the hallmark of this illness, up to 20% of patients are "spotless" or have an atypical rash at presentation.[135] The most characteristic laboratory abnormality is thrombocytopenia. The WBC count is usually normal but more than two thirds of cases have increased band forms. The creatine phosphokinase level may be elevated, as may transaminases and bilirubin.[131] The chest radiograph may reveal infiltrates consistent with pneumonitis or acute respiratory distress syndrome (ARDS). RMSF is frequently a severe illness. Serious complications, in addition to ARDS, include renal failure, disseminated intravascular coagulopathy (DIC), hemophagocytic syndrome, meningoencephalitis, and gangrene.[131]

Rickettsial infections may be difficult to diagnose. The best way to establish the diagnosis of RMSF in patients with a rash is by obtaining a skin biopsy for immunohistochemical or direct immunofluorescent staining. This test has a sensitivity of 70% and specificity of 100%.[132] PCR can also be performed on tissue specimens.[131] However, both immunohistochemical staining and RMFS PCR may not be readily available in many institutions. Serologic testing by indirect immunofluorescence or enzyme-linked immunosorbent assay (ELISA) may also be performed. Empiric treatment with doxycycline should be instituted for suspected RMSF before laboratory confirmation of a diagnosis. Distinguishing RMSF from meningococcemia is especially important. Gastrointestinal symptoms, a pulse-temperature disparity, periorbital edema, edema of the extremities, conjunctival injection, hepatosplenomegaly, and elevated serum transaminases are more likely in RMSF. If there is any doubt as to which infection is present, treatment for both should be instituted empirically.

EHRLICHIOSES AND ANAPLASMOSIS

Illnesses that cause fever and rash are listed in Box 54.3. Other serious rickettsial diseases include ehrlichioses and anaplasmosis, caused by *Ehrlichia chaffeensis*, *E. ewingii,* and *Anaplasma phagocytophilium*, respectively.[131] They have a similar presentation, but rash is much less commonly seen than in RMSF. These infections are transmitted by ticks and are distributed across the United States and Europe. All are intracellular pathogens that infect leukocytes. Common laboratory abnormalities include leukopenia, relative lymphopenia, presence of atypical lymphocytes, eosinopenia, and thrombocytopenia.[136] Anemia and renal involvement are rare. PCR of serum is now the rapid diagnostic test of choice. Blood smear microscopy might reveal the presence of morulae in infected leukocytes, which is highly suggestive of anaplasmosis or, less commonly, ehrlichiosis.[131] Serologic results can also be diagnostic. Complications include ARDS, bleeding, rhabdomyolysis, and myocarditis.[136]

MALARIA

Malaria is a protozoan infection transmitted by female anopheline mosquitoes. The severity of malaria infection depends on a variety of factors including host immunity and age and the species of malaria. Of the four main human pathogens, *Plasmodium falciparum* causes the most serious infection. Chloroquine-resistant *P. falciparum* has spread through many parts of the world. The incubation period of *P. falciparum* is approximately 12 days. It parasitizes all ages of red blood cells and causes the highest degree of parasitemia of any of the species.[137] *P. falciparum* has worldwide distribution and causes a severe illness frequently termed *blackwater fever*. Common symptoms and signs include fever, chills, headache, myalgia, arthralgia, and hepatosplenomegaly. Other symptoms include jaundice, vomiting, diarrhea, and nonproductive cough.[137] Severe malaria is a multisystem illness with a mortality rate of up to 25% in the nonimmune, untreated patient.[137] Defining criteria for severe malaria include (1) severe normocytic anemia, (2) renal failure, (3) pulmonary edema, (4) hypoglycemia, (5) shock, (6) DIC, (7) metabolic acidosis, and (8) cerebral involvement with coma or generalized seizures. Other signs or symptoms frequently present in severe disease include altered mental status, prostration, jaundice, and high-grade fever.[137,138] Additional laboratory features include thrombocytopenia, elevated transaminases, hyperbilirubinemia, evidence of coagulopathy, elevated blood urea nitrogen (BUN) and creatinine levels, and macroscopic hemoglobinuria. Levels of parasitemia are often high. Patients may develop pulmonary edema, or pulmonary edema may occur after successful treatment of parasitemia. ARDS or secondary infection with bacterial pneumonia may also occur.

The differential diagnosis is broad and includes bacterial sepsis, meningitis, rickettsial infections, pneumonia, viral hemorrhagic fever, leptospirosis, severe influenza, meningococcemia, typhoid fever, and viral hepatitis. The diagnostic test of choice is the thick/thin peripheral Giemsa-stained blood smear, which confirms the diagnosis. Rapid diagnostic tests are becoming increasingly useful. However, patients from an endemic area may occasionally present with another serious illness that may be erroneously attributed to malaria because of incidental parasitemia. Treatment for severe malaria regardless of species consists of IV quinine (not available in the United States) or IV quinidine combined with IV doxycycline or IV clindamycin.[139,140] When using quinidine, continuous cardiac monitoring should be performed. IV artesunate is available as an investigational new drug through the CDC for those with severe malaria who are unable to obtain IV quinidine or who are intolerant to it, have a contraindication, or have failed therapy. IV therapy should be continued until the parasite density is less than 1% and oral therapy can be tolerated. Adjunctive therapy for severe malaria may include exchange transfusion, although this is controversial.[139] In addition, broad-spectrum antibiotics for bacterial sepsis and pneumonia should be given if there is concern for secondary bacterial infection.

Box 54.3 Differential Diagnosis of Fever with Maculopapular or Petechial Rash

- Rocky Mountain spotted fever
- Meningococcal disease
- Enteroviral infection (echovirus and coxsackievirus)
- Human herpesvirus 6 infection (roseola)
- Human parvovirus B19 infection (fifth disease)
- Epstein-Barr virus infection
- Disseminated gonococcal infection
- Murine typhus
- Ehrlichioses
- Group A streptococcal pharyngitis
- *Mycoplasma pneumoniae* Infection
- Leptospirosis
- Secondary syphilis
- Kawasaki disease
- Thrombotic thrombocytopenic purpura (TTP)
- Drug reactions
- Immune complex–mediated illness
- Toxic shock syndrome
- Erythema multiforme
- Stevens-Johnson syndrome

DENGUE

Hemorrhagic fever is caused by a variety of viruses, and the hallmark is bleeding. Generally dengue has a geographic endemicity, being seen predominantly in Africa, South America, and Asia. Dengue is transmitted by mosquitoes and has no other reservoir except humans. It is now endemic in at least 112 countries worldwide including many parts of the Caribbean, Mexico, Puerto Rico, and Central America and has recently reemerged in the United States in the Florida Keys and along the Mexican border.[141-144] In many areas the mosquito vector is *Aedes aegypti*. This mosquito species has adapted to man-made conditions, and therefore urban transmission is frequent. The virus has four serotypes, each with a number of genotypes.[143] Dengue is generally divided into four clinical syndromes: a mild influenza-like illness; classic dengue (characterized by fever, retro-orbital headache, severe bone pain and myalgia, maculopapular rash, and nausea and vomiting); dengue hemorrhagic fever (DHF); and dengue shock syndrome (DSS).[141] DHF or DSS may manifest after a few days of typical dengue symptoms, and classically symptoms start as the temperature normalizes.[144] Those with DHF have bleeding, petechiae, ascites, pleural effusion, and sometimes encephalopathy. Laboratory features include hemoconcentration, leukopenia, elevated transaminases, and thrombocytopenia.[144] The differential diagnosis includes many of the infectious entities also in the differential diagnosis of malaria. Noninfectious illnesses in the differential diagnosis include hemolytic uremic syndrome and thrombotic thrombocytopenic purpura. Diagnosis is established serologically, and treatment is supportive.[143]

SEVERE VIRAL INFECTIONS

HANTAVIRUS PULMONARY SYNDROME

Acute infections caused by species of hantavirus are transmitted to humans from rodents and are characterized by nephritis and hemorrhage or by a syndrome of acute noncardiogenic pulmonary edema.[145] Four hantaviruses are associated with hantavirus pulmonary syndrome (HPS). This syndrome was first recognized in the southwestern United States. Rodents, especially deer mice, are the host. Transmission to humans occurs by inhalation of aerosols of rodent urine or feces. Initial symptoms of HPS resemble those of influenza and consist of fever, myalgia, headache, and gastrointestinal symptoms. Two to 15 days later, acute noncardiogenic pulmonary edema and shock develop.[146-148] Laboratory findings at this stage include leukocytosis, hemoconcentration, and thrombocytopenia. Chest radiographic findings include increased vascular markings consistent with pulmonary edema, bilateral infiltrates, and pleural effusions.[149] Treatment is supportive and consists of ventilator support and treatment of shock. This syndrome has a high mortality rate of 50% to 70%, but those who survive improve rapidly after 5 to 7 days and often have complete recovery within 2 to 3 weeks.

INFLUENZA

Influenza results from infection with influenza A or B virus. Infection occurs in yearly epidemics, typically during the winter in temperate climates, with occasional worldwide epidemics referred to as *pandemics*, which occur when there is antigenic shift (a major antigenic change resulting in a new subtype of influenza A).[150] These viruses are spread from person to person primarily through coughing and sneezing.[151] Onset of symptoms is abrupt and occurs after an incubation period of a day or two.[152] Symptoms include fever, chills, headache, myalgia, sore throat, and malaise.[153] Respiratory symptoms, especially a dry cough, are usually present. As systemic signs and symptoms decrease, respiratory complaints become more prominent. Of these, cough is the most frequent and may persist 1 to 2 weeks after fever resolves. Leukocytosis is common early in the illness, and mild leukopenia may be observed later. Most cases are not associated with any significant complications, but when complications do occur, pulmonary complications are the most frequent. Two types of pulmonary complications are recognized: primary influenza viral pneumonia and secondary bacterial pneumonia.[154] Primary influenza viral pneumonia occurs mainly in individuals with cardiovascular disease or in pregnant women. Rapid progression of fever, cough, dyspnea, and hypoxemia usually occurs. Chest radiographs reveal bilateral findings consistent with pulmonary edema. Patients may develop ARDS. Culture of the sputum fails to reveal significant bacteria, whereas molecular diagnostic tests and viral cultures will demonstrate influenza virus. Severe influenza viral pneumonia requires intensive monitoring and support. Mortality rate is high.

Secondary bacterial pneumonia is more common than primary viral pneumonia. It occurs most often in the elderly or those with preexisting pulmonary disease. Following a classic influenza syndrome and a period of improvement of a few days, there is recrudescence of fever and cough accompanied by sputum production and consolidation on chest radiograph. Gram stain and culture of sputum most often demonstrate *S. pneumoniae*, *H. influenzae*, or *S. aureus*. Other rare complications of influenza include Reye syndrome, which is an often fatal CNS and hepatic complication, myositis, transverse myelitis, myocarditis, and pericarditis.[155] Influenza virus is readily isolated from nasal or throat specimens, sputum, or tracheal secretions in the first 2 or 3 days of illness. The neuraminidase inhibitors, inhaled zanamivir and oral oseltamivir, are active against influenza A and B viruses and are effective in treating acute influenza if started early in the illness.[150] Secondary bacterial pneumonia should be treated with antibiotics. A pandemic with H1N1 occurred in 2009 and public health readiness continues for the next pandemic.[156] Respiratory syncytial virus is emerging as an important cause of serious illness in the elderly and high-risk adults with clinical manifestations, length of hospital stay, use of ICU, and mortality rates similar to influenza.[157]

POTENTIAL AGENTS OF BIOTERRORISM

Potential agents of bioterrorism include rare infections that may occur sporadically in specific epidemiologic settings, such as anthrax, as well as diseases considered eradicated, such as smallpox. Features of these illnesses are their potential to cause illness and death, the potential for large-scale dissemination, their ability to cause public disruption, and the requirement for specific public health interventions in the setting of an outbreak. Illness is generally severe, and infected patients are likely to require admission to critical care units. Recognition of these syndromes by clinicians is crucial to triggering the appropriate medical, public health, and governmental response.

ANTHRAX

Bacillus anthracis, the causative agent of anthrax, is an aerobic, gram-positive, sporulating bacillus. When human infection occurs, spores germinate in blood and tissue. Human infection can be of three types: (1) cutaneous, (2) inhalational, and (3) gastrointestinal.[158] Cutaneous is the most common and characteristically appears as a painless papule that evolves to a vesicular stage and then to a depressed black eschar surrounded by a ring of vesicles. Untreated, it carries a mortality rate of approximately 20%.[158]

The inhalational form is the form most likely to be encountered in the critical care setting. After an incubation period of generally 1 to 7 days but potentially up to 60 days, patients present with fever, malaise, dry cough, and an influenza-like illness. Progression to severe respiratory distress and septic shock occurs. The hallmark of this infection is a hemorrhagic mediastinitis.[158,159] Mortality rate has been as high as 85%. In virtually all cases, chest radiographs are abnormal and show either a widened mediastinum or pleural effusions. CT scan is particularly sensitive in detecting mediastinal changes.[160] Blood cultures are positive in 70% of cases. Clinical suspicion should be raised by the sudden appearance of multiple cases of severe influenza-like illness with a fulminant course and high mortality rates. The diagnosis is generally established by culturing the organism from blood, CSF, pleural fluid, or vesicular fluid; by PCR; or by biopsy. Therapy is initially empiric and consists of the combination of ciprofloxacin or doxycycline plus clindamycin and rifampin.[158,159]

SMALLPOX

Smallpox is caused by the variola virus. This serious infection is highly contagious and fatal in about 30% of cases. Two major clinical forms exist, with the most common being variola major. This is a severe form with extensive rash and high fever. After an incubation period of 12 to 14 days, patients develop high fever, malaise, headache, myalgias, and vomiting. The rash appears initially as small intraoral spots and within 24 hours develops on the face, then spreads to the legs, feet, arms, and hands.[161] The rash appears as papules, which are filled with a thick, opaque fluid and have a depressed center. They evolve into pustules, which are raised, round, and firm to the touch. The differential diagnosis includes varicella. Treatment is supportive. The antiviral agent cidofovir may have activity.[162]

PLAGUE

The causative agent of plague is *Yersinia pestis,* an aerobic gram-negative bacillus. The three clinical forms are (1) bubonic, (2) pneumonic, and (3) septicemic.[163,164] Pneumonic plague is transmitted person to person through inhalation of contaminated aerosols and is highly contagious. After an incubation period of 2 to 3 days, patients develop fever, chills, headache, hemoptysis, dyspnea, stridor, cyanosis, respiratory failure, circulatory collapse, and bleeding.[163,164] Diagnosis is based on clinical suspicion and confirmed by culture. Treatment is with streptomycin and doxycycline.[163,164]

TULAREMIA

Tularemia is caused by *Franciscella tularensis,* which is a gram-negative coccobacillus. Types of infection include ulceroglandular, typhoidal, and pneumonic. If there were to be an intentional release of this agent, infection would likely occur via the aerosol route.[165,166] Symptoms include cough, substernal pain, abdominal pain, prostration, fever, chills, and headache. Diagnosis is established by culture onto special media or by serologic testing. Treatment is with streptomycin.

VIRAL HEMORRHAGIC FEVERS

Viral hemorrhagic fevers are caused by several different families of viruses. Symptoms generally include fever, myalgia, hemorrhage, shock, coma, seizures, and possibly renal failure. The diagnosis is established by viral isolation or serologically. Treatment involves supportive care. The antiviral agent ribavirin may have a role in treatment.[167]

KEY POINTS

- Of patients with bacterial meningitis, 95% will have at least two of the following symptoms: fever, headache, stiff neck, and altered sensorium.
- Morbidity and mortality rates of bacterial meningitis are decreased with prompt administration of antibiotics.
- When dexamethasone is administered as adjunctive therapy for bacterial meningitis, it should be given prior to or concurrent with initial antibiotic doses.
- The standard for diagnosis of herpes encephalitis is PCR of CSF, and treatment for suspected herpes encephalitis should be continued until PCR results are back.
- *S. aureus* has become the most common cause of bacterial endocarditis, and *S. aureus* endocarditis is associated with a high risk of complications and high mortality rates.
- Major indications for surgery in acute endocarditis include congestive heart failure, persistent bacteremia and sepsis, ongoing emboli on appropriate antibiotic therapy, and local valvular complications such as dehiscence and perivalvular abscess.
- Staphylococcal and streptococcal toxic shock syndromes are mediated by systemic effects of bacterial exotoxins that trigger massive release of cytokines.
- Necrotizing fasciitis, although uncommon, is a severe infection that causes necrosis of subcutaneous tissue and fascia and requires prompt identification and therapy to minimize morbidity and mortality rates.
- CA-MRSA is an emerging pathogen that can cause life-threatening illness including necrotizing skin infections, pneumonia, and sepsis.

KEY POINTS (Continued)

- Empiric antibiotic therapy for bacterial peritonitis should be directed at gram-negative bacillary organisms and anaerobes.
- The presence of an intra-abdominal abscess should be entertained in febrile patients without any obvious cause of fever or in the seriously ill patient who is on corticosteroid therapy.
- An epidemic strain of *C. difficile* has enhanced toxin production and causes increased severity of illness, poorer response to therapy, and frequent relapse.
- Serious infections of the head and neck are polymicrobial and most frequently have an odontogenic source.
- Serious complications of influenza include primary influenza viral pneumonia, bacterial pneumonia, Reye syndrome, and myocarditis/pericarditis.

SELECTED REFERENCES

1. van de Beek D, de Gans J, Tunkel AR, et al: Community-acquired bacterial meningitis in adults. N Engl J Med 2006;354:44-53.
22. Tyler KL: Herpes simplex virus infections of the central nervous system: Encephalitis and meningitis, including Mollaret's. Herpes 2004;11(Suppl 2):57A-64A.
45. Reishaus E, Waldbaur H, Seeling W: Spinal epidural abscess: A meta-analysis of 915 cases. Neurosurg Rev 2000;232:175 202.
50. Baddour LM, Wilson WR, Bayer AS, et al: Infective endocarditis: Diagnosis, antimicrobial therapy, and management of complications, a statement for healthcare professionals from the Committee on Rheumatic Fever, Endocarditis, and Kawasaki Disease, Council on Cardiovascular Disease in the Young, and the Councils on Clinical Cardiology, Stroke, and Cardiovascular Surgery and Anesthesia, American Heart Association. Circulation 2005;111: e394-e433.
58. Liu C, Bayer A, Cosgrove SE et al: Clinical practice guidelines by the Infectious Diseases Society of America for the treatment of methicillin-resistant *Staphylococcus aureus* infections in adults and children. Clin Infect Dis 2011;52(3):e18-e55.
60. Mermel LA, Allon M, Bouzon E, et al: Clinical practice guidelines for the diagnosis and management of intravascular catheter-related infection: 2009 update by the Infectious Diseases Society of America. Clin Infect Dis 2009;49(1):1-45.
85. Ustin JS, Malangoni MA: Necrotizing soft tissue infections. Crit Care Med 2011;39(9):2156-2162.
95. Chiang SR, Chuang YC: *Vibrio vulnificus* infection: Clinical manifestations, pathogenesis, and antimicrobial therapy. J Microbiol Immunol Infect 2003;36(2):81-88.
98. Kollef MH, Micek ST: Methicillin-resistant *Staphylococcus aureus*: A new community-acquired pathogen? Curr Opin Infect Dis 2006;19:161-168.
103. Solomkin JS, Mazuski JE, Bradley JS, et al: Diagnosis and management of complicated intra-abdominal infection in adults and children: Guidelines by the Surgical Infection Society and the Infectious Diseases Society of America. Clin Infect Dis 2010;50(2):133-164.
119. Bobo LD, Dubberke ER, Kollef M: *Clostridium difficile* in the ICU: The struggle continues. Chest 2011;140(6):1643-1653.
122. Reynolds SC, Chow AW: Life-threatening infections of the peripharyngeal and deep fascial spaces of the head and neck. Infect Dis Clin North Am 2007;21(2):557-576.
133. Walker DH, Paddock CD, Dumler JS: Emerging and re-emerging tick-transmitted rickettseial and ehrlichial infections. Med Clin North Am 2008;92(6):1345-1361.
140. Sarkar PK, Ahluwalia G, Vijayan VK, et al: Critical care aspects of malaria. J Intensive Care Med 2010;25(2):93-103.
145. Stollenwerk N, Harper RW, Sandrock CE: Bench-to-bedside review: Rare and common viral infections in the intensive care unit—linking pathophysiology to clinical presentation. Crit Care 2008;12(4):219.

The complete list of references can be found at www.expertconsult.com.

PART 5

RENAL DISEASE AND METABOLIC DISORDERS IN THE CRITICALLY ILL

Acute Kidney Injury

55

Paul M. Palevsky

CHAPTER OUTLINE

DEFINITION

The primary function of the kidneys is the excretion of metabolic waste products and the maintenance of the composition of body fluids through regulation of water, electrolyte, and acid-base excretion. Acute kidney injury (AKI) describes a sudden decrease in glomerular filtration rate (GFR), resulting in the retention of metabolic waste products and dysregulation of fluid, electrolyte, and acid-base homeostasis.[1-3] AKI, however, does not represent a discrete disease. Rather, AKI is a heterogeneous spectrum that includes hemodynamic perturbations that disrupt normal renal perfusion and decrease GFR without causing overt parenchymal injury; partial or complete obstruction to urine flow; and acute parenchymal injury resulting in glomerular, interstitial, tubular, or vascular dysfunction. Although all forms of AKI can occur in those who are critically ill, the most common causes in this population include hemodynamically mediated prerenal dysfunction and *acute tubular necrosis* (ATN) arising as a result of ischemia-reperfusion injury, nephrotoxin exposure, or sepsis.

The term *acute kidney injury* has largely replaced the older terminology of *acute renal failure* (ARF).[3-6] Implicit in this older terminology was a focus on the most severe presentations of acute kidney dysfunction, generally characterized by overt organ failure. The term *AKI* attempts to broaden the focus to include less severe episodes that, although not resulting in overt organ failure, are associated with increased risks of morbidity and mortality, particularly in the critically ill. However, the use of the term *injury* may incorrectly connote the presence of parenchymal organ damage, which may be absent in a number of forms of AKI, particularly in hemodynamically mediated prerenal states and acute obstructive uropathy. In this chapter, the term AKI will be used to describe the entire spectrum of the syndrome, and the term ARF will be restricted to severe organ failure requiring renal replacement therapy. Often, the terms ATN and AKI have been used interchangeably; although ATN is the most common form of intrinsic AKI, particularly in critically ill patients, the terms are not synonymous, because ATN represents only one of the multiple forms of AKI.

The cardinal manifestation of AKI is the retention of metabolic waste products, most notably creatinine and urea.[1,2] Decreased urine output may also be a manifestation of AKI; however, the urine output in AKI can be highly variable, ranging from virtual anuria (<100 mL/day) to

Additional online-only material indicated by icon.

polyuria (>3 L/day).[1] In addition, transient oliguria (urine volume <400 mL/day) may occur in the absence of decreased kidney function in patients with intravascular volume depletion as the physiologic response to volume depletion due to an increase in tubular salt in water reabsorption.[7] In contrast, persistent oliguria despite adequate volume resuscitation is virtually always a manifestation of AKI.[7] Although the presence of oliguria complicates management, increasing the risk of volume overload, hyperkalemia, and other electrolyte disturbances, and is associated with a greater mortality risk, therapeutic interventions to augment urine output have not been shown to improve outcomes.

A wide array of operational definitions have been used to define AKI based primarily on relative or absolute changes in serum creatinine concentration.[14] The first attempt at developing a consensus definition was undertaken by the Acute Dialysis Quality Initiative in 2002[15]; the resultant RIFLE criteria consisted of three strata ("Risk," "Injury," and "Failure") based on the magnitude of increase in serum creatinine and the duration of oliguria as well as two outcome stages ("Loss" of kidney function and "End-Stage" kidney disease) (Table 55.1). In the RIFLE criteria, the "Risk," "Injury," and "Failure" strata were defined based on an increase in serum creatinine developing over 7 days of 50%, 100%, or 200%, respectively, relative to baseline or oliguria, defined as a urine output of less than 0.5 mL/kg/hour for more than 6 hours ("Risk") or 12 hours ("Injury") or a urine output of less than 0.3 mL/kg/hour for more than 24 hours or anuria for more than 12 hours ("Failure"). These three strata were proposed as providing increasing specificity, although decreasing sensitivity, for the diagnosis of AKI. The outcome criteria were defined based on continued need for renal replacement therapy for more than 4 weeks ("Loss") or more than 3 months ("Failure"). The RIFLE criteria were subsequently modified by the Acute Kidney Injury Network (AKIN) with the addition of an absolute increase in serum creatinine of more than 0.3 mg/dL to the definition of AKI, a decrease in the time frame for the increase in serum creatinine from 7 days to no more than 48 hours, and by dropping the two outcome criteria.[4,5] More recently, the Kidney Disease Improving Global Outcomes (KDIGO) Clinical Practice Guideline for Acute Kidney Injury harmonized the RIFLE and AKIN definitions, maintaining the three stages, but specifying that the 0.3-mg/dL increase in serum creatinine was to have developed over no more than 48 hours but that the greater than 50% increase could occur over up to 7 days (see Table 55.1).[3]

The development of a standardized operational definition and staging system has introduced a degree of uniformity to clinical trials of AKI; however, their utility in the bedside care of patients remains uncertain. The definitions have increased recognition of less severe episodes of AKI, but data are lacking to demonstrate that use of these criteria can meaningfully guide patient care. Several important shortcomings to these definitions and staging criteria must also be recognized. First, as previously discussed, there is poor correlation between change in serum creatinine and actual GFR in the non–steady-state conditions that are present in AKI. Thus, there may be discordance between the level of GFR and the AKI staging. For example, within

Table 55.1 RIFLE, AKIN, and KDIGO Definitions and Staging of Acute Kidney Injury

	Serum Creatinine Criteria			
	RIFLE	AKIN	KDIGO	**Urine Output Criteria**
Definition	Increase in serum creatinine of >50% developing over <7 days	Increase in serum creatinine of 0.3 mg/dL or >50% developing over <48 hours	Increase in serum creatinine of 0.3 mg/dL developing over 48 hours or >50% developing over 7 days	Urine output of <0.5 mg/kg/hour for >6 hours
Staging				
RIFLE–Risk AKIN/KDIGO Stage 1	Increase in serum creatinine of >50%	Increase in serum creatinine of 0.3 mg/dL or >50%	Increase in serum creatinine of 0.3 mg/dL or >50%	Urine output of <0.5 mg/kg/hour for >6 hours
RIFLE–Injury AKIN/KDIGO Stage 2	Increase in serum creatinine of >100%	Increase in serum creatinine of >100%	Increase in serum creatinine of >100%	Urine output of <0.5 mg/kg/hour for >12 hours
RIFLE–Failure AKIN/KDIGO Stage 3	Increase in serum creatinine of >200%	Increase in serum creatinine of >100%	Increase in serum creatinine of >100%	Urine output of <0.3 mg/kg/hour for >12 hours or anuria for >12 hours
RIFLE–Loss	Need for renal replacement therapy for >4 weeks			
RIFLE–End Stage	Need for renal replacement therapy for >3 months			

AKIN, Acute Kidney Injury Network; KDIGO, Kidney Disease Improving Global Outcomes; RIFLE, Risk, Injury, Failure, Loss, End-Stage.

the first 24 hours following an acute ischemic insult the GFR may be essentially zero, but there will have been insufficient time for the serum creatinine to rise beyond the 50% threshold for stage 1 disease; by the time the serum creatinine has increased to a level to fulfill the criteria for stage 3 AKI, the GFR may already be improving. Second, the definition of AKI using the serum creatinine criteria requires a valid referent baseline serum creatinine measurement, which is often unavailable. Third, the reliance of the staging systems on relative changes in serum creatinine makes the staging system highly dependent on baseline kidney function. Because the maximal daily rise in serum creatinine is dependent upon relative muscle mass and not on kidney function, the time to progress from stage 1 to stage 2 or from stage 2 to stage 3 will be longer for a patient with a baseline serum creatinine of 1.4 mg/dL than for a similar patient with a baseline serum creatinine of 0.7 mg/dL. Fourth, concordance between the serum creatinine and urine output criteria has not been established and urine output may be highly dependent upon other factors, including intravascular volume resuscitation and diuretic administration. Fifth, the staging system is focused entirely on the magnitude of the peak excursion in serum creatinine and not on duration of AKI, which may be an independent predictor of outcomes. Sixth, although studies validating these criteria have demonstrated that the AKI stage correlates with increasing mortality risk, it is not clear that mortality risk is the appropriate measure of disease severity. Finally, these classification systems treat AKI as a single disease rather than as a widely heterogeneous syndrome and do not take into consideration the underlying cause of AKI. Despite these shortcomings, the use of these standardized definitions and staging systems has enhanced comparisons across epidemiologic studies and facilitated the design of clinical trials.

EPIDEMIOLOGY

Estimates of the incidence of AKI are highly dependent on both the precise definition employed and the characteristics of the patient population studied. Many of the epidemiologic studies that have been published either preceded the development of the standardized definitions just described[16-24] or have utilized administrative data that do not correlate with these definitions.[25-28] In addition, there are important differences in the distribution of the different types of AKI among patients who develop AKI prior to hospitalization, on general medical-surgical wards, or in the intensive care unit. As a result, published estimates of the incidence of AKI in hospitalized patients have ranged from as high as 44%, using a 0.3-mg/dL change in serum creatinine as the definition to less than 1% when the definition was based on an increase is serum creatinine of more than 2 mg/L, with most estimates of the incidence of AKI ranging from 3% to 7% of the overall hospital population and 10% to 35% of critically ill patients, and 5% to 6% of the ICU (intensive care unit) population having AKI severe enough to require renal replacement therapy.[16-24]

The incidence of AKI has increased substantially over the past several decades. In an analysis of data from the National Hospital Discharge Survey in the United States conducted by the Centers for Disease Control and Prevention, the incidence of AKI among hospitalized patients increased from 18 per 100,000 population in 1980 to 365 per 100,000 population in 2005 with similar trends present in analyses of data from the U.S. National Inpatient Sample and a 5% sample of hospitalized Medicare beneficiaries.[28] These data need to be interpreted with some caution; however, administrative coding for AKI is incomplete, capturing only 20% to 30% of all episodes, and trends over time may be subject to bias from changes in administrative coding practices.[29] However, similar trends were observed in an analysis of administrative and clinical data from Kaiser Permanente of Northern California, an integrated health care delivery system.[30] Using laboratory creatinine data to confirm the diagnosis of AKI, the incidence of AKI not requiring renal replacement therapy increased from 323 to 522 cases per 100,000 person-years between 1996 and 2003; over the same time period, the incidence of AKI requiring renal replacement therapy increased from 19.5 to 29.5 cases per 100,000 person-years. Epidemiologic studies have consistently found that AKI is more prevalent in men and in African Americans and increases in incidence with increasing age.[25,26] Increasing risk of AKI is also associated with severity of baseline chronic kidney disease (CKD). In the aforementioned study from Kaiser Permanente of Northern California, the risk of developing AKI requiring dialysis was approximately double in patients with a baseline estimated GFR between 45 and 60 mL/minute/1.73 m^2 as compared to patients with an estimated GFR greater than 60 mL/minute/1.73 m^2, with the risk increasing to more than 40-fold among patients with a premorbid estimated GFR less than 15 mL/minute/1.73 m^2.[31] Other identified independent risk factors for the development of AKI include diabetes mellitus, hypertension, and the presence of proteinuria.[31,32]

Although AKI is common in critically ill patients, robust epidemiologic data are lacking as the majority of published studies represent the experience at single centers or limited numbers of ICUs.[19-23,33,34] In addition to varying criteria used to define AKI, the incidence of AKI is also highly dependent upon the characteristics of the ICU population. As shown in Figure 55.1, the incidence of AKI is lower in the cardiac care unit and in patients after coronary artery bypass grafting, being 5% to 10%,[35,36] as compared to patients with severe trauma,[37] burns,[38] and following liver and allogeneic bone marrow transplant, in whom AKI occurs in 20% to 40%.[39] The patterns of AKI in the ICU differ from those seen in the general hospital population (Table 55.2). Patients with ICU-associated AKI are younger, are more likely to be male, are more likely to have acute tubular necrosis as compared to prerenal AKI or obstructive disease, are more likely to have AKI in association with multisystem organ failure as opposed to isolated AKI, are more likely to require renal replacement therapy, and have markedly higher mortality rates.[19] Sepsis is the most common predisposing condition for the development of AKI in critically ill patients, contributing to the development of AKI in as many as half of all cases.[19,21,22,24] Other conditions associated with the development of AKI in ICU patients include major surgery, cardiogenic shock, hypovolemia, medication-associated toxicity, and advanced liver disease (Table 55.3).[19,21,22,24] Two distinct patterns of ICU-associated AKI have been described: early-onset AKI is present on ICU admission or within the first 48 hours of ICU stay, and

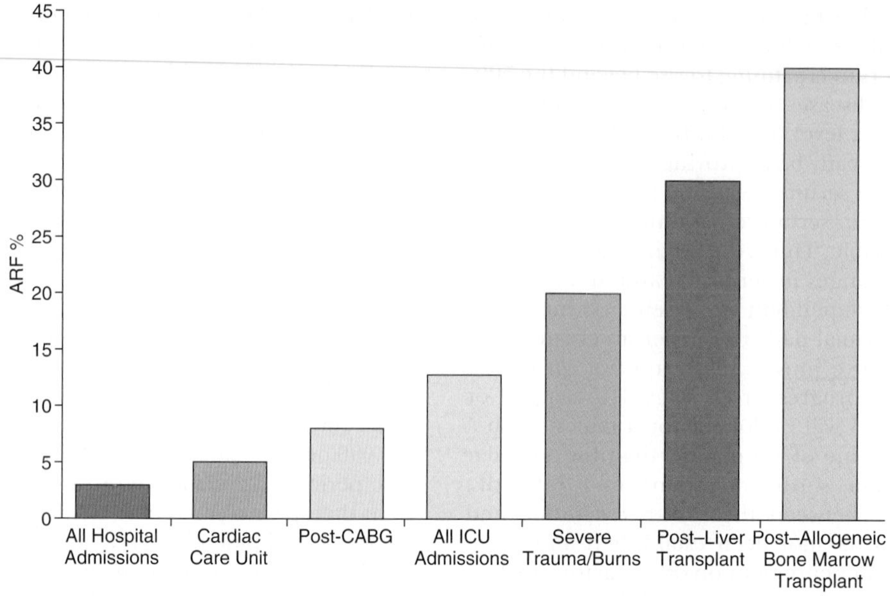

Figure 55.1 Frequency of acute renal failure in selected hospital settings.

Table 55.2 Comparison of Intensive Care Unit (ICU)– and General Hospital Ward–Associated Acute Kidney Injury

Feature	ICU	Non-ICU
Number of patients	253	495
Gender (% male)	72.7	61.4
Age (years)	56.4 ± 16.4	62.6 ± 18.8
Cause (%)		
Prerenal	17.8	28.1
Postrenal	0.8	14.7
Acute tubular necrosis	75.9	37.6
Other	3.2	16.5
Acute-on-chronic	7.9	15.2
Multiple organ dysfunction	89	31
Renal replacement therapy (%)	70.8	18.4
Mortality rate (%)		
Overall	71.5	31.5
By diagnosis:		
Prerenal	78.6	37.1
Acute tubular necrosis	42.2	29.5
Acute-on-chronic	75.0	24.0

From Liano F, Junco E, Pascual J, et al. The spectrum of acute renal failure in the intensive care unit compared with that seen in other settings. Kidney Int 1998;53(Suppl 66):S16-S24.

Table 55.3 Factors Associated with Acute Kidney Injury in the Intensive Care Unit Setting

Factor	Frequency (%)
Multiorgan failure	30-75
Sepsis	30-50
Drugs/medications	20-40
Postoperative state	15-35
Cardiogenic shock	15-30
Hypovolemia	15-30
Liver failure	5-10

late-onset AKI develops after more than 48 hours of ICU care.[23] Delayed-onset AKI is more likely to be due to postischemic or sepsis-associated AKI and is associated with higher mortality rates.

PATHOGENESIS

AKI can be divided into three broad etiologic categories: prerenal AKI, intrinsic AKI, and postrenal (obstructive AKI). Prerenal states (Box 55.1) are characterized by effective hypoperfusion of the kidneys leading to a decrease in GFR in the absence of overt parenchymal damage to the kidneys. Postrenal or obstructive AKI is characterized by acute obstruction of the urinary tract, including ureters or bladder outlet (Box 55.2). In intrinsic AKI, acute injury to the renal parenchyma underlies the development of kidney dysfunction, as is seen in acute tubular necrosis (ATN), acute interstitial nephritis (AIN), and acute glomerulonephritis (AGN) (Box 55.3). Categorizing the forms of AKI in this fashion is useful for didactic purposes and is helpful in guiding the initial assessment of the patient with AKI, but substantial overlap may exist among these categories, particularly between prerenal and intrinsic causes of AKI. For example, renal hypoperfusion may cause a spectrum of renal dysfunction ranging from mild prerenal azotemia to overt ATN, depending upon its severity and duration. Even in patients with classic clinical presentations of volume depletion–associated prerenal AKI sensitive clinical markers of tubular injury may be elevated.[40] Thus, precise categorization of the cause of AKI into one of these categories may not be possible, and overlap and transition among categories may occur.

Box 55.1 Mechanisms and Causes of Prerenal Acute Kidney Injury

Extracellular Fluid Volume Loss

Hemorrhage
Gastrointestinal losses (vomiting, nasogastric drainage, diarrhea, enterocutaneous fistula)
Renal losses (diuretics, osmotic diuresis, diabetes insipidus)
Cutaneous losses (burns, heat stroke)

Extracellular Fluid Sequestration

Gastrointestinal (pancreatitis, peritonitis, ileus)
Muscle crush injury
Capillary leak syndrome (allergic, interleukin therapy, sepsis)

Decreased Cardiac Output

Congestive heart failure
Cardiogenic shock
Pericardial disease
Sepsis

Systemic Vasodilation

Sepsis
Cirrhosis
Anaphylaxis
Medications

Altered Intrarenal Hemodynamics

Sepsis
Hepatorenal syndrome
Hypercalcemia
Medications—catecholamines, vasopressin, nonsteroidal anti-inflammatory drugs, angiotensin-converting enzyme inhibitors, angiotensin receptor blockers, direct renin inhibitors
Iodinated radiocontrast media

Increased Renal Venous Pressure

Abdominal compartment syndrome
Congestive heart failure

Box 55.2 Causes of Postrenal (Obstructive) Acute Kidney Injury

Upper Urinary Tract Obstruction

Intrinsic Obstruction

Nephrolithiasis
Blood clot
Papillary necrosis
Urothelial malignancy
Fungus ball
Stricture

Extrinsic Obstruction

Pelvic or retroperitoneal adenopathy
Pelvic or retroperitoneal tumors
Retroperitoneal hematoma
Retroperitoneal fibrosis
Endometriosis
Granulomatous disease
Surgical ligation

Lower Urinary Tract Obstruction

Benign prostatic hypertrophy
Prostate cancer
Bladder cancer
Bladder stones
Neurogenic bladder
Fungus ball
Urethral valves
Urethral stricture

PRERENAL ACUTE KIDNEY INJURY

Prerenal azotemia caused by extracellular fluid volume loss or volume sequestration, reduced cardiac output, systemic vasodilation, intrarenal vasoconstriction, or increased renal venous pressure is the most common cause of AKI (see Box 55.1), contributing to the development 30% to 60% of all cases.[17-19,24] The primary pathogenesis of prerenal azotemia is a decrease in effective glomerular perfusion. This form of AKI, if treated early, is usually readily reversible; however, if left untreated, renal ischemia with resultant ATN may result.

In classic forms of prerenal azotemia, reduced renal perfusion pressure and afferent arteriolar constriction combine to lower glomerular capillary hydrostatic pressure and the formation of glomerular ultrafiltrate.[1,41,42] Prerenal azotemia develops when the capacity of the usual physiologic responses to hypovolemia is exceeded and GFR falls. In response to hypovolemia there is a decrease in mean arterial pressure, triggering baroreceptors that ultimately lead to activation of the sympathetic nervous system, activation of the renin-angiotensin-aldosterone system (RAAS), and secretion of the antidiuretic hormone vasopressin. Activation of the renal sympathetic nerves constricts the afferent (preglomerular) arterioles and stimulates release of renin from the juxtaglomerular apparatus. Renin secretion is also directly stimulated in response to hypovolemia by changes in intrarenal hemodynamics. Secretion of renin activates a cascade in which angiotensinogen is cleaved to form angiotensin I, which is then cleaved by angiotensin-converting enzyme released by local endothelium to form angiotensin II. Angiotensin II stimulates both afferent and efferent (postglomerular) arteriolar vasoconstriction; however, the effect on the afferent vessel is opposed by vasodilatory prostaglandins, kallikrein, kinins, and nitric oxide.[43,44] The net effect is to maintain the tone of the afferent arteriole while constricting the efferent vessel, returning intraglomerular pressure and glomerular ultrafiltration toward normal. In addition, angiotensin II stimulates proximal tubular sodium reabsorption and, through its action as an aldosterone secretagogue, increases plasma aldosterone levels and stimulates distal tubular sodium reabsorption. Increased vasopressin levels stimulate water and urea reabsorption in the collecting duct. The net effect of modest hypovolemia is maintenance of the GFR at near normal levels accompanied by production of concentrated urine with low sodium content and a decrease in the fractional excretion of urea. When effective volume depletion exceeds the normal physiologic compensatory mechanisms, the GFR falls and overt prerenal AKI ensues.

Multiple medications can exacerbate the development of prerenal AKI. The prerenal form of AKI complicating

Box 55.3 Causes of Intrinsic Acute Kidney Injury

Acute Tubular Necrosis

Ischemia/hypoperfusion
- Hypovolemia
- Hypotension
- Hemorrhage shock
- Cardiogenic shock
- Post–cardiac surgery
- Post–cardiac arrest
- Prolonged prerenal state

Nephrotoxic
- *Endogenous toxins:*
- Myoglobin (rhabdomyolysis)
- Hemoglobin (intravascular hemolysis)
- *Exogenous toxins:*
- Aminoglycosides
- Amphotericin B
- Vancomycin
- Cisplatin
- Ifosfamide
- Foscarnet
- Tenofovir
- Iodinated radiocontrast media
- Acetaminophen
- Intravenous immune globulin
- Sepsis

Acute Interstitial Nephritis

Drug-induced
- Penicillins
- Cephalosporins
- Sulfonamides
- Quinolones
- Vancomycin
- Rifampin
- Proton pump inhibitors
- Phenytoin
- Allopurinol
- Nonsteroidal anti-inflammatory drugs

Infections—viral, bacterial, mycobacterial, fungal
Malignancy

Acute Glomerulonephritis

Postinfectious glomerulonephritis
Rapidly progressive glomerulonephritis
Anti–glomerular basement membrane (anti-GBM) disease
Anti–neutrophil cytoplasmic antibody (ANCA) disease
Systemic lupus erythematosus
Systemic vasculitis

Acute Vascular Disease

Large vessel disease
- Renal artery thrombosis
- Renal artery embolism
- Renal artery dissection
- Renal vein thrombosis

Renal microvasculature
- Atheroembolic disease
- Malignant hypertension
- Scleroderma renal crisis
- Toxemia of pregnancy
- Hemolytic-uremic syndrome
- Thrombotic thrombocytopenic purpura

Intratubular Obstruction

Crystalline nephropathy
- Tumor lysis syndrome/acute urate nephropathy
- Ethylene glycol poisoning/acute oxalate nephropathy
- Acyclovir
- Methotrexate
- Indinavir
- Triamterene
- Sulfadiazine

Myeloma cast nephropathy

diuretic use is caused by extracellular volume depletion. With nonsteroidal anti-inflammatory drugs (NSAIDs), including both nonselective and cyclooxygenase 2 (COX-2)–selective agents, the inhibition of cyclooxygenase leads to depletion of renal vasodilatory prostaglandins that normally counteract the afferent arteriolar constricting effect of angiotensin II and increased renal adrenergic tone.[45-47] In situations in which vasoconstrictor mechanisms are activated, such as volume depletion, heart failure, sepsis, cirrhosis, and nephrotic syndrome, and in patients with chronic kidney disease, the use of NSAIDs may result in severe afferent vasoconstriction, severely reducing glomerular capillary filtration pressure and causing AKI. If promptly discontinued, NSAID-induced AKI can be reversible; however, if NSAIDs continue to be administered ATN may ensue.

Angiotensin-converting enzyme inhibitors (ACEIs), angiotensin receptor blockers (ARBs), and direct renin inhibitors act by inhibiting the RAAS. Inhibition of angiotensin II production by direct renin inhibitors and ACEIs or blockade of its action by ARBs prevents angiotensin II–mediated constriction of the efferent arteriole and diminishes glomerular capillary filtration pressure. Although this effect is desirable in preventing hyperfiltration injury in patients with CKD, the use of these agents may contribute to the development of AKI in the setting of renal hypoperfusion, when maintenance of glomerular filtration is dependent upon activation of renin and angiotensin II.[48] This is particularly likely to happen when therapy is initiated or escalated and volume depletion or hypotension supervenes in patients with renal artery stenosis, CKD, heart failure, or liver disease. The prerenal azotemia that may develop in these settings is usually reversible if the offending agent is promptly discontinued; however, these agents have also been associated with an increased risk of ATN.[49]

Although the majority of forms of prerenal AKI are mediated by decreased renal perfusion, altered intrarenal hemodynamics may result in decreased GFR despite increased organ perfusion. Early in sepsis, renal perfusion may be increased; however, GFR may fall as the result of decreased efferent arteriolar tone, resulting in decreased glomerular capillary filtration pressure.[50]

Increases in renal venous pressure may also contribute to the development of prerenal AKI. As renal venous pressure increases, renal perfusion pressure falls; in addition, renal parenchymal pressure increases as venous pressure rises, narrowing the pressure gradient driving glomerular filtration.[51,52] Two settings in which renal venous congestion results in a prerenal state are the abdominal compartment syndrome and heart failure. Abdominal compartment syndrome (ACS) typically develops in critically ill patients, most commonly in the setting of trauma with abdominal hemorrhage, abdominal surgery, massive fluid resuscitation, liver transplantation, and gastrointestinal conditions including peritonitis and pancreatitis. ACS is defined by an intra-abdominal pressure of 20 mm Hg or higher associated with dysfunction of one or more organ systems.[53] However, intra-abdominal pressures lower than 20 mm Hg may be associated with ACS, while values higher than this threshold do not universally lead to the ACS.[54-57] Oliguria, which can lead to anuria, often develops and, as is true for other forms of AKI associated with impaired renal perfusion, urine sodium concentration is commonly reduced. Renal venous congestion associated with modest increases in intra-abdominal pressure has also been shown to contribute to the acute renal dysfunction accompanying acute decompensated heart failure.[58,59]

POSTRENAL ACUTE KIDNEY INJURY

AKI resulting from obstruction usually accounts for fewer than 5% of ICU-associated AKI.[19] Urinary tract obstruction may occur at any level of the renal collecting system, beginning at the renal pelvis and ending at the urethra (see Box 55.2). Obstruction above the level of the bladder is referred to as upper tract obstruction and may result from either intrinsic (intraluminal) or extrinsic disease. The development of AKI from upper tract obstruction requires the presence of bilateral obstruction or unilateral obstruction in the setting of a single functioning kidney or dysfunction of the contralateral kidney. Common causes for upper tract obstruction include luminal obstruction from ureteric calculi, blood clots, urothelial tumors, sloughed renal papillae or ureteral strictures, and external compression from retroperitoneal and pelvic tumors, adenopathy, hematomas, or retroperitoneal fibrosis. More commonly, obstruction occurs at the level of the bladder neck or urethra, as may occur with benign prostatic hypertrophy or prostate cancer, bladder tumors, and bladder stones. Neurogenic bladder dysfunction associated with diabetes mellitus, autonomic neuropathy, and spinal cord disease may also contribute to the development of obstructive disease. Treatment with narcotics and agents with anticholinergic action may exacerbate subclinical voiding dysfunction and precipitate acute urinary retention in the setting of acute illness.

Patients with obstructive disease may present with anuria if obstruction is complete, with normal or even increased urine volume in the setting of partial obstruction, or with fluctuating urine output with periods of anuria alternating with rapid passage of urine as the pressure in the collecting system rises and overcomes the obstructing disease. In the acute phase of obstruction, intratubular pressure rises, resulting in a reduction in glomerular filtration pressure. As the obstruction persists, renal blood flow diminishes, intratubular pressures fall toward normal, but GFR remains severely depressed. Relief of the obstruction with placement of a bladder catheter for lower tract obstruction or ureteral stents or percutaneous nephrostomy tubes for upper tract obstruction usually results in prompt return of GFR if the duration of obstruction has not been excessive.[60]

INTRINSIC ACUTE KIDNEY INJURY

The causes of intrinsic AKI can be categorized based on the anatomic compartments of the kidney that are involved (see Box 55.3). Using this approach, intrinsic AKI is commonly divided into tubular, interstitial, glomerular, and vascular processes. In addition, in a variety of settings the primary pathophysiology consists of intratubular deposition of crystals or protein. These latter syndromes could be considered as a subset of acute tubular disease, but given the striking difference in pathogenesis, these disorders will be discussed separately in this chapter. It is also important to recognize that although this approach provides a construct for understanding the multitude of causes of intrinsic AKI, there are substantial overlaps among categories. Thus, small vessel vasculitides with predominant glomerular involvement could be classified either with acute glomerulonephritis or as a renal vascular disorder. Similarly, interstitial inflammation may play a substantial role in the pathogenesis of ATN, blurring the distinction with acute interstitial nephritis (AIN).

ACUTE TUBULAR NECROSIS

The most common intrinsic cause of AKI is ATN, accounting for 85% to 90% of intrinsic ICU-associated AKI.[19,24] The causes of ATN can be broken down into three major categories: ischemia-reperfusion injury, nephrotoxins, and sepsis (see Box 55.3). There is, however, significant overlap between septic and ischemic ATN; many, although not all, cases of sepsis-associated ATN develop in the setting of septic shock, and sepsis-associated ATN has frequently been classified as a subcategory of ischemic ATN.[61] Data suggest, however, that sepsis-associated ATN has unique features and may develop in the absence of overt renal ischemia and should be considered as a separate etiologic category.[62-64] Nephrotoxic ATN can result from toxicity from the endogenous heme pigments myoglobin and hemoglobin or may be caused by exogenous toxins, most commonly medications such as aminoglycosides, amphotericin B, and cisplatin. In many patients, multiple etiologic factors are present and the ATN must be characterized as multifactorial.

A description of the pathophysiologic mechanisms thought to underlie ischemic, septic, and nephrotoxic causes of ATN are provided in the online supplement at www.expertconsult.com.

ACUTE INTERSTITIAL NEPHRITIS

AIN constitutes approximately 5% to 10% of intrinsic AKI in the ICU setting and is defined by the presence of lymphocytic infiltration of the kidney (see Box 55.3). AIN is most commonly related to medication use but may also be associated with a wide variety of infections, autoimmune disorders, and malignancy.[88] The most common offending medications include penicillin, cephalosporin, sulfonamide, and quinolone antibiotics; proton pump inhibitors; phenytoin; allopurinol; and NSAIDs. The classic presentation of medication-associated AIN includes fever, rash, and eosinophilia; however, this complete triad is present in fewer than one third of patients and is unusual in NSAID-associated AIN. Characteristic urinary findings include hematuria and pyuria and white blood cell casts in the absence of infection. Eosinophiluria may also be present but is neither a sensitive nor a specific finding. Although the diagnosis may be made based on clinical setting, history of medication use, and urinary findings, definitive diagnosis usually requires kidney biopsy.

ACUTE GLOMERULONEPHRITIS

Acute glomerular disease is an uncommon cause of AKI in the ICU. These forms can include postinfectious glomerulonephritis, rapidly progressive glomerulonephritis, systemic lupus erythematosus, and a broad range of systemic vasculitides with renal involvement. The characteristic finding in acute glomerular disease is the presence of dysmorphic red blood cells and red blood cell casts on urinalysis. Although serologic tests may help guide the diagnosis, definitive diagnosis usually requires kidney biopsy. Prompt diagnosis of acute glomerular disease is critical for guiding therapy with time to initiation of treatment being a critical factor in the response to therapy.

Several causes of acute glomerular disease deserve special mention because they often present as pulmonary-renal syndromes with acute glomerular disease and pulmonary hemorrhage. These causes include anti–glomerular basement membrane (anti-GBM) disease, antineutrophil cytoplasmic antibody (ANCA)–associated vasculitis (granulomatosis with polyangiitis or microscopic polyarteritis), and systemic lupus erythematosus.

ACUTE VASCULAR SYNDROMES

Acute vascular syndromes are divided into large vessel (renal artery and renal vein) and small vessel disease. Large vessel diseases include thrombosis, thromboembolism and dissection of the renal arteries, and renal vein thrombosis.[89,90] Acute arterial or venous occlusion may present with renal infarction. With unilateral or subtotal disease, the presentation usually consists of pain and hematuria. Lactate dehydrogenase levels will be elevated and the diagnosis made by contrast-enhanced computed tomography (CT) or nuclear scintigraphy. As with obstructive disease, AKI is the presenting manifestation only when there is bilateral involvement or unilateral disease with an absent or nonfunctional contralateral kidney.

Multiple conditions can affect the renal microvasculature and present with AKI, including the systemic vasculitides (discussed earlier) that present with primarily glomerular involvement. Other diseases with predominant renal microvascular involvement leading to AKI include malignant hypertension, scleroderma renal crisis, toxemia of pregnancy, and the microangiopathic hemolytic diseases, hemolytic-uremic syndrome, and thrombotic thrombocytopenic purpura. Atheroembolic disease represents another important disease of the renal microvasculature that may present as acute or subacute kidney disease.[91,92] Atheroembolic disease is characterized by the systemic showering of atheromatous debris to the distal branches of the arterial tree. Although atheroembolism may occur spontaneously, it develops most commonly after cardiac or aortic angiography or surgery, or in association with systemic anticoagulation or thrombolytic therapy. Involvement is generally systemic with common manifestations including cutaneous livedo reticularis and digital ischemia and gastrointestinal, hepatic, and nervous system involvement. Because the kidneys receive approximately 20% of the cardiac output, renal involvement is common, ranging from renal infarction to AKI to a subacute and stuttering decline in kidney function.

INTRATUBULAR OBSTRUCTION

AKI may also occur as the result of crystalline or proteinaceous obstruction of the renal tubules. In acute tumor lysis syndrome, AKI often results from intratubular deposition of uric acid.[93,94] Following ethylene glycol ingestion and in certain inborn errors of metabolism, the major mechanism for development of AKI is intratubular deposition of calcium oxalate. A number of medications have also been associated with acute crystalline nephropathy, including acyclovir, methotrexate, indinavir, triamterene, and sulfadiazine.[95,96] In multiple myeloma, tubular obstruction by monoclonal light chains (Bence-Jones protein) is the cause of acute myeloma kidney disease.[97,98]

CLINICAL MANIFESTATIONS

The manifestations of AKI may range from asymptomatic laboratory abnormalities associated with early or mild disease to a constellation of symptoms including oliguria, volume overload, and overt uremic manifestations accompanied by acidosis and electrolyte derangements. A fundamental difficulty in the diagnosis of AKI is the absence of reliable bedside methods to reliably measure GFR and rapidly detect changes in kidney function. Most commonly AKI is recognized based on increases in the concentration of urea or creatinine in the blood or as the result of sustained decreases in urine output.

RETENTION OF FILTRATION MARKERS

Urea and creatinine are primarily excreted by glomerular filtration. A sudden decrease in GFR will result in rising concentrations of these solutes in the blood. However, the relationship between the GFR and their concentration is nonlinear and may be affected by a variety of other factors.

UREA

Urea is the major end product of nitrogen metabolism. Blood urea concentration, commonly assayed as blood urea nitrogen (BUN), is dependent upon the balance between hepatic synthesis and renal excretion. Increased urea generation resulting in elevations in the BUN in the absence of a marked decrease in GFR may result from high dietary protein intake, amino acid loading during parenteral nutrition, and the endogenous protein load from gastrointestinal hemorrhage as well as in hypercatabolic states associated with fever, sepsis, and glucocorticoid administration or inhibition of protein synthesis as may be seen with tetracycline antibiotics. Hypercatabolic states may also result in increases in BUN during AKI that exceed the increase of 10 to 20 mg/dL/day that usually is typically associated with absence of glomerular filtration.[99] Normally, filtered urea is partially reabsorbed along the length of the nephron, with increased reabsorption in states of low urine flow. In volume depletion, severe heart failure, and obstructive uropathy, increased tubular reabsorption of urea often results in increases in the BUN that are disproportionate to the fall in GFR. This variability in the synthesis of urea and the non-GFR-related factors that influence its urinary excretion render the BUN a less reliable marker of GFR than the serum creatinine concentration. However, the level of BUN generally correlates with symptoms of renal failure, with uremic manifestations usually absent until the BUN is greater than 100 mg/dL.

CREATININE

Creatinine is derived from the nonenzymatic hydrolysis of creatine, which is usually released at a constant rate from skeletal muscle and is excreted primarily by filtration at the glomerulus. In patients with normal kidney function, less than 10% of creatinine excretion occurs by tubular secretion, although this percentage increases in CKD. There is essentially no tubular reabsorption of creatinine. This relationship allows creatinine to serve as a reliable endogenous marker of glomerular filtration when the creatinine concentration is in steady state. Because much of the interindividual variability in creatinine production can be accounted for based on demographic and clinical variables including age, gender, race, and weight, it is possible to reliably estimate creatinine clearance or GFR from the serum creatinine concentration.[8-10,12] The confidence intervals around these estimates are wide, however, and these estimates should not be interpreted as precise measures of kidney function. In the absence of glomerular filtration, serum creatinine typically increases by 1 to 2 mg/dL/day.[100] This increase is influenced by numerous factors including the magnitude of decrement in GFR, the rate of creatinine production, and changes in the volume of distribution.[100] For example, creatinine production may be reduced in sepsis,[101] and increased in the setting of skeletal muscle injury (rhabdomyolysis). Aggressive volume resuscitation may also mask any increase in serum creatinine through dilution.[102] Thus, although a sudden increase in serum creatinine concentration is the most common parameter triggering recognition of AKI, the use of estimating equations for GFR are not reliable in critically ill patients with AKI. There are several other factors that may also impair the reliability of serum creatinine as a marker of kidney function in critical illness. Some medications, most notably trimethoprim and cimetidine, block tubular secretion of creatinine, leading to an increase in serum creatinine concentration in the absence of decreased kidney function.[103] This effect is generally minimal in patients with normal kidney function, but the increase in serum creatinine may exceed 30% in patients with underlying CKD. Reported creatinine concentrations may also be increased as a result of chemical interference with some assay methods by ketone bodies or by medications, such as cefoxitin.[103] One final drawback to the use of creatinine as a marker of kidney function in patients with AKI is the inverse relationship between serum creatinine concentrations and GFR. Thus, significant reductions in GFR may occur prior to the serum creatinine concentration being recognized as increasing.

CYSTATIN C

Given the drawbacks to urea and creatinine as markers of kidney function, other readily available markers of GFR have been sought. The use of exogenous filtration markers such as inulin, iothalamate, or iohexol is cumbersome and not practical for the recognition of abrupt changes in kidney function. Cystatin C has been proposed as a more sensitive endogenous marker of GFR, including in ICU patients.[104-106] Cystatin C is a cysteine protease inhibitor that is released into the bloodstream at a constant rate from all nucleated cells. It is readily filtered at the glomerulus and reabsorbed and catabolized by renal proximal tubular epithelial cells such that virtually no cystatin C appears in the urine. The interindividual variability in cystatin C production appears to be less than that for creatinine. Thus, in steady-state situations cystatin C may be a more reliable marker of GFR.[107] In addition, the serum half-life of cystatin C is shorter than that of creatinine, making it a more sensitive marker for acute changes in GFR.[104-106] However, cystatin C assays are not currently readily available in the acute setting, and the optimal place for cystatin C in the detection of AKI in at-risk critically ill patients remains to be determined.

MARKERS OF TUBULAR INJURY

A number of markers of tubular injury have been proposed as novel diagnostic tests for the early diagnosis of AKI. These markers include kidney injury molecule-1 (KIM-1),[108,109] neutrophil gelatinase-associated lipocalin (NGAL),[110-116] interleukin 18 (IL-18),[114-118] liver fatty acid binding protein (L-FABP)[40,119] and α- and π-glutathione-*S*-transferase (GST),[120,121] among others. Even though these markers have shown promise, their role in the clinical care of patients at risk for AKI remains uncertain.

OLIGOANURIA

Decreased urine output represents a second major reason for recognition of AKI. Sustained oliguria, which is usually defined as a urine output of less than 400 to 500 mL/day, or a sustained urine output of less than 20 mL/hour, in the absence of overt volume depletion almost always indicates the presence of AKI.[7] Although oliguria is often considered to be a cardinal feature of AKI, most cases of AKI in the critically ill are nonoliguric.[122] Thus, although sustained oliguria should suggest prompt the evaluation for AKI, the presence of a well-maintained urine output should not be construed to represent the presence of adequate kidney function. Anuria (the absence of urine output) always demands prompt attention. True anuria is most often caused by complete urinary obstruction but may also be seen with vascular catastrophes with bilateral renal infarction and less commonly with severe rapidly progressive glomerulonephritis. Rarely, severe ATN may result in a short period of complete anuria.

DETECTION OF BIOCHEMICAL OR CLINICAL COMPLICATIONS

An additional way in which AKI may come to the attention of the clinician is by the detection of one of the biochemical or clinical consequences of the loss of kidney function. Thus, occasionally, the development of fluid overload, mental status changes, hyperkalemia, metabolic acidosis, hypocalcemia, hyperphosphatemia, hyperuricemia, or anemia may be the initially recognized manifestation of AKI.

DIAGNOSTIC APPROACH

GENERAL ASPECTS

The first step in evaluating the patient with AKI is to determine whether it is primarily prerenal or postrenal in origin or is due to intrinsic renal disease. Although this division is useful for conceptualizing and categorizing the causes of AKI, it is important to recognize that many patients may not fall neatly into a single category. For example, prerenal azotemia and ischemic ATN fall on a continuum; a process that may start out as pure prerenal azotemia may evolve over time into ischemic ATN. This blurring between these broad categories is further evidenced by the fact that markers of tubular epithelial cell injury are elevated in patients with classic presentations of prerenal azotemia.[40] Moreover, most cases of AKI encountered in ICU patients have more than a single cause,* with the single most common condition predisposing to AKI in the critically ill patient being sepsis and with the majority of patients having AKI in the setting of multiple organ failure.[24,61,125] The evaluation of the patient should begin with a careful review of the history and physical examination with particular attention to hemodynamic status, episodes of hypotension and infection, and the record of medication administration. Assessment of voiding function and postvoiding residual bladder volume should be performed to exclude bladder outlet obstruction. This step should then be followed by microscopic examination of the urine and evaluation of urine electrolytes. Renal imaging may be necessary to evaluate for upper tract obstruction or to evaluate for patency of the renal vasculature. In a minority of patients, a renal biopsy will be required for definitive diagnosis.

HISTORY, PHYSICAL EXAMINATION, AND RECORD REVIEW

The initial step in attempting to identify the cause of AKI should be a thorough history, physical examination, and review of the medical record. The overall clinical setting, recent events in the patient's illness, use of medications, and possible toxic exposures should be noted, with particular attention to events during the 1- to 2-day interval prior to the onset of AKI. A history of vomiting, blood loss, diarrhea, diuretic use, burns, or symptoms compatible with decompensation of heart failure or of liver disease suggests potential prerenal azotemia. A history of prostatism with intermittency, hesitancy, or decrease in the force of the urinary stream; history of urologic, gynecologic, or other pelvic or retroperitoneal malignancy; flank or suprapubic pain; or hematuria or pyuria may suggest obstructive (postrenal) disease. The history of a systemic disorder, fever, rash, vascular disease, or musculoskeletal complaints is compatible with a renovascular, glomerular, or interstitial disorder. Review of the medical record should focus on indices of volume status including intake and output records, serial weights, and serial measurements of blood pressure to help assess for risk factors for intravascular volume depletion and prerenal azotemia. Delineation of the pattern of urine output is often helpful. Finally, a careful review of medication records to assess for exposure to potential nephrotoxins is critical.[46,79]

The physical examination should focus on assessing for evidence of intravascular volume depletion, such as orthostatic changes in pulse and blood pressure, dry mucous membranes, decreased skin turgor, longitudinal tongue furrows, and absence of sweat in the axilla and inguinal regions.[126] A fall in systolic blood pressure of more than 20 mm Hg and in diastolic blood pressure of more than 10 mm Hg accompanied by an increase in heart rate of more than 30 beats per minute is suggestive of intravascular volume depletion. However, these findings are neither sensitive nor specific. Orthostatic changes in blood pressure may be absent in some patients despite significant intravascular volume depletion and may be observed in the absence of volume depletion in patients with autonomic dysfunction and in the elderly. Examination for neck vein distention, pulmonary rales, ventricular gallops, and pedal edema may indicate the presence of heart failure. Occasionally, a chest radiograph, cardiac function testing (i.e., an echocardiogram or nuclear gated blood pool scan), or assessment of plasma brain natriuretic peptide (BNP) or *N*-terminal pro-BNP (NT-proBNP) levels may assist in the diagnosis of heart failure. Accurate assessment of extracellular fluid volume status and cardiac function may be difficult on clinical grounds, particularly in immobilized, mechanically ventilated ICU patients, and invasive monitoring of central venous pressure, or less commonly, pulmonary artery and pulmonary capillary occlusion pressure, and assessment of cardiac output may be helpful. Assessment for ascites and abdominal distention may assist in the diagnosis of AKI associated with liver disease or the abdominal compartment syndrome. Abdominal palpation to detect flank, suprapubic or central abdominal masses may be helpful in assessing the presence of obstructive uropathy or for an abdominal aortic aneurysm with possible renovascular compromise. A bladder scan or placement of a bladder catheter to assess postvoid bladder volume in patients who do not have an indwelling bladder catheter should be performed to help exclude bladder outlet obstruction as a cause of obstructive uropathy. A rectal and pelvic examination may also be helpful in assessing for possible causes of obstructive uropathy. Careful examination of the skin may detect rashes compatible with a drug-induced eruption, which may suggest drug-induced acute interstitial nephritis; palpable purpura, suggesting a microangiopathic hemolytic anemia such as hemolytic-uremic syndrome or thrombotic thrombocytopenic purpura or a systemic vasculitis, such as

*See references 18, 19, 21, 22, 24, 123, and 124.

cryoglobulinemia; and *livedo reticularis* or digital ischemia, suggesting atheroembolic disease.

URINALYSIS AND URINE INDICES

Assessment of urine composition and examination of the urine sediment can assist in determining the cause of AKI (Table 55.4). The electrolyte composition of the urine may be helpful in differentiating between prerenal azotemia and ATN.[127-130] In prerenal azotemia, renal tubular function is intact and the tubules avidly reabsorb sodium in an effort to restore extracellular fluid volume and renal perfusion to normal. Thus, in prerenal azotemia, urine sodium concentrations are usually less than 20 mmol/L and the fractional excretion of sodium [calculated as $(U_{Na}/P_{Na}) \div (U_{Cr}/P_{Cr})$, where U_{Na} is the urine sodium concentration, P_{Na} is the plasma or serum sodium concentration, U_{Cr} is the urine creatinine concentration, and P_{Cr} is the plasma or serum creatinine concentration] is less than 1%. In contrast, in ATN, the damaged renal tubular cells fail to reabsorb sodium normally, perhaps because of loss of cellular polarity, with a resultant urine sodium concentration greater than 40 mmol/L and a fractional excretion of sodium above 2%. It needs to be recognized, however, that these urinary electrolyte findings are not absolute. Thus, increased fractional excretion of sodium may occur in prerenal states when diuretics have been administered, in patients with underlying CKD who may take several days after the onset of volume depletion to maximize sodium conservation, in the presence of glycosuria or other osmotic diuresis, or in the presence of bicarbonaturia. A fractional excretion of sodium of less than 1% may be present in multiple settings other than prerenal azotemia, including in the absence of any kidney disease and in many forms of glomerulonephritis, in microangiopathic hemolytic anemia, and in some forms of ATN, including radiocontrast-associated AKI, myoglobinuric ATN, early sepsis-associated ATN, and nonoliguric ATN.[131,132] The fractional excretion of urea [calculated as $(U_{urea}/P_{urea}) \div (U_{Cr}/P_{Cr})$, where U_{urea} is the urine urea nitrogen concentration, P_{urea} is the blood urea nitrogen concentration, U_{Cr} is the urine creatinine concentration, and P_{Cr} is the plasma or serum creatinine concentration] has been proposed as an alternative index of tubular function for the diagnosis of prerenal azotemia in patients who have received diuretic therapy.[133-136] The normal fractional excretion of urea is greater than 60%; in reversible prerenal states, values typically fall to less than 35%. Urinary chemical indices are not of value in establishing the diagnosis of obstructive uropathy.

Urine microscopy is also often very helpful in determining the cause of AKI.[137-141] A normal urine sediment suggests the presence of either a prerenal or postrenal cause of AKI, although obstructive uropathy may be associated with hematuria, pyuria, or crystalluria. In the presence of proteinuria a urinary sediment containing abundant cells or casts suggests an intrinsic cause of AKI. Specifically, the presence of many renal tubular epithelial cells, epithelial cell casts, or pigmented (muddy brown) granular casts suggests the diagnosis of ATN and has been associated with increased risk for greater severity of disease.[141,142] The presence of white blood cells and white blood cell casts suggests AIN. Although eosinophiluria may be seen in association with interstitial nephritis, it is also associated with atheroembolic disease and with urinary tract infections, and the specificity and sensitivity of this finding are limited.[143] The presence of dysmorphic red blood cells (which are best seen using phase contrast microscopy) and red blood cell casts suggests the presence of an acute glomerulonephritis or vasculitis

Table 55.4 Urinalysis Findings in Acute Kidney Injury (AKI)

Etiologic Disorder	Urine Chemistry	Urine Sediment
Prerenal	U_{Na} <20 mmol/L FE_{Na} <1% FE_{urea} <35%	Normal or nearly normal (hyaline casts and rare granular casts)
Acute tubular necrosis	U_{Na} >40 mmol/L FE_{Na} >2% FE_{urea} >60%	Renal tubular epithelial cells, epithelial cell casts, coarse pigmented (muddy brown) casts
Acute interstitial nephritis	Variable; U_{Na} may be >40 mmol/L, FE_{Na} may be >2%	Red blood cells, white blood cells, white blood cell casts, eosinophils
Acute glomerulonephritis	Variable; U_{Na} may be <20 mmol/L, FE_{Na} may be <1%	Red blood cells (dysmorphic), red blood cell casts
Acute vascular disease	Variable; U_{Na} may be <20 mmol/L, FE_{Na} may be <1%	Red blood cells, red blood cell casts in HUS/TTP, eosinophils in atheroembolic disease
Crystal-associated AKI	Variable	Crystalluria Uric acid crystals in tumor lysis syndrome Calcium oxalate crystals in ethylene glycol ingestion Drug crystals (acyclovir, methotrexate, indinavir, triamterene, sulfadiazine)
Obstructive	Variable; early U_{Na} may be <20 mmol/L, FE_{Na} may be <1%; late U_{Na} may be >40 mmol/L, FE_{Na} may be >2%	Normal or red blood cells, white blood cells and crystals

FE_{Na}, fractional excretion of sodium; FE_{urea}, fractional excretion of urea; HUS, hemolytic-uremic syndrome; TTP, thrombotic thrombocytopenic purpura; U_{Na}, urine sodium concentration.

involving the kidney. A urine dipstick test that is positive for red blood cells in the absence of red blood cells on microscopy suggests the presence of either hemoglobinuria or myoglobinuria. Heavy crystalluria suggests the presence of crystalline intratubular obstruction with uric acid crystals suggestive of tumor lysis syndrome, oxalate crystals suggestive of ethylene glycol ingestion, and drug crystals associated with drug-induced nephropathy. The presence of heavy proteinuria with negative or only trace protein by dipstick and only minimal albuminuria suggests the presence of light chains in the urine and a diagnosis of acute myeloma kidney.

RADIOLOGIC IMAGING

Imaging of the kidneys and bladder is required for the diagnosis of obstructive kidney disease.[144,145] The usual initial test is a renal ultrasound. Rarely, the presence of extensive retroperitoneal disease may give a false-negative ultrasonographic result (so-called nondilated obstructive uropathy).[146] Non-contrast-enhanced computed tomography (CT) or magnetic resonance imaging (MRI) may be helpful in this setting to delineate the presence or absence of retroperitoneal disease. Non-contrast-enhanced CT scanning is also the initial diagnostic test of choice for the evaluation of obstruction from nephrolithiasis. Intravenous radiocontrast administration should be avoided in patients with AKI due to the risk of worsening kidney function from superimposed contrast nephropathy. Similarly, the use of gadolinium-containing contrast agents is contraindicated in AKI due to the risk of inducing nephrogenic systemic fibrosis.[147,148] Cystoscopic retrograde or percutaneous antegrade pyelography is occasionally necessary both diagnostically and for the treatment of obstructive disease. Imaging studies may also be helpful for the diagnosis of renovascular disease, renal vein thrombosis, and renal infarction.

OTHER LABORATORY TESTING

A careful review of other standard laboratory tests may be helpful in identifying the cause of AKI. A markedly elevated creatinine phosphokinase (CPK) suggests the diagnosis of rhabdomyolysis. A disproportionately elevated serum potassium, phosphate, and uric acid accompanied by elevated lactate dehydrogenase (LDH) suggests diffuse tissue destruction, as occurs in AKI complicating both rhabdomyolysis and the tumor lysis syndrome. An elevated LDH may also be seen in patients with renal infarction.[89] Findings on the hemogram and peripheral blood smear may also be informative. The presence of anemia and rouleaux formation, particularly if accompanied by an increase in serum globulins and hypercalcemia may suggest the presence of multiple myeloma. Eosinophilia is associated with allergic interstitial nephritis, atheroembolic disease and polyarteritis nodosa. Thrombocytopenia and microangiopathic hemolytic anemia may be seen in vasculitis; hemolytic-uremic syndrome; thrombotic thrombocytopenic purpura; disseminated intravascular coagulation, which is often seen in association with sepsis; scleroderma renal crisis; and malignant hypertension. If a glomerulonephritis or vasculitis is suspected, specific serologic testing may be indicated, including serum complement levels, antinuclear antibody (ANA), anti-double-stranded DNA, antineutrophilic cytoplasmic antibodies (ANCA), anti–glomerular basement membrane (anti-GBM) antibodies, hepatitis B and C virus, rheumatoid factor, and serum cryoglobulins.

NOVEL BIOMARKERS

A number of novel biomarkers, including kidney injury molecule-1 (KIM-1),[108,109] neutrophil gelatinase-associated lipocalin (NGAL),[110-116] interleukin 18 (IL-18),[114-118] liver fatty acid binding protein (L-FABP),[40,119] and α- and π-glutathione-*S*-transferase (GST),[120,121] have been proposed both as a means for early diagnosis of AKI and as a means for differentiating between prerenal and intrinsic causes of AKI. For example, elevations in NGAL have been shown to predict progression of AKI and ultimate need for renal replacement therapy.[149] However, these biomarkers may also be increased in prerenal disease.[40] At present, the optimal role of these biomarkers in the evaluation of patients with AKI remains uncertain.

RENAL BIOPSY

Renal biopsy is usually reserved for patients in whom prerenal and obstructive causes of AKI have been excluded and the cause of intrinsic AKI remains unclear.[150,151] Kidney biopsy is particularly useful for the diagnosis of acute glomerulonephritis, vasculitis, and interstitial nephritis, in which definitive diagnosis is required to guide specific therapy with corticosteroids or immunosuppresion. The precise indications for a kidney biopsy in the critically ill patient with AKI are not established. Factors such as the lack of clinical or laboratory clues to the cause of the AKI and the presence of features atypical for ATN (such as heavy proteinuria, dysmorphic red blood cells, and red blood cell casts on urinalysis, or the presence of an unexplained pulmonary-renal syndrome) are reasonable indications for proceeding with a biopsy. The primary risk of kidney biopsy is postbiopsy hemorrhage, with increased risk seen in patients with poorly controlled hypertension, coagulopathy, thrombocytopenia, or uremic platelet dysfunction. Experience has demonstrated, however, that kidney biopsy can be safely performed even in ICU patients undergoing mechanical ventilation.[152]

PREVENTION

As previously described, the major risk factors predisposing to the development of AKI in the ICU setting are decreased renal perfusion, nephrotoxicity from medications and contrast media, and septic shock. Thus, efforts to prevent AKI should be directed at maintaining renal perfusion and avoiding hypotension, selecting and dosing medications to minimize the risk of nephrotoxicity, and preventing nosocomial infections.

MAINTENANCE OF RENAL PERFUSION

Intravascular volume expansion for the maintenance of renal perfusion in high-risk patients is one of the simplest interventions for the prevention of AKI. Volume administration has been shown to decrease the risk of AKI in a variety of clinical settings including myoglobinuric and hemoglobinuric AKI,[153-155] radiocontrast nephropathy,[156,157] and aminoglycoside- and amphotericin-associated nephrotoxicity.[158,159] Fluid administration has also been shown to decrease the risk of intratubular obstruction from crystal deposition in the tumor lysis syndrome[160] and in the drug-induced crystalline nephropathies.[95,96] The role of volume administration for the prevention of AKI in sepsis is more challenging.[61,161] Septic shock is associated with relative vasodilation and increased vascular permeability leading to sequestration of extracellular fluid volume and renal hypoperfusion. In addition, although sepsis is a hyperdynamic state with increased cardiac output, relative myocardial depression is common. The use of goal-directed fluid resuscitation in early sepsis has been advocated, and data suggest a modest reduction in the incidence of AKI.[162,163] However, fluid resuscitation in this setting is not without risk. Although fluid challenges can result in stabilization and improvement in renal function, persistent fluid challenges should be avoided if either no improvement in kidney function or worsening oxygenation from pulmonary vascular congestion occurs. The selection of fluid has also been subject to considerable scrutiny. The use of synthetic colloids as compared to saline is thought to provide greater expansion of the intravascular space. Recent studies, however have suggested that hydroxyethyl starch is associated with an increased risk of AKI and mortality in critically ill patients, and in particular, in patients with severe sepsis.[164-167]

The role of renal vasodilators, including dopamine and fenoldopam, to maintain renal perfusion has also been advocated in the past. Multiple studies have demonstrated, however, that this strategy does not reduce the risk of AKI.[168-177] Thus the use of these agents cannot be advocated for the prevention of AKI.

AVOIDANCE OF NEPHROTOXICITY

Many of the medications used for the treatment of critically ill patients carry a risk for nephrotoxicity, with pharmacologic agent–associated nephrotoxicity accounting for approximately one quarter of ICU-associated AKI.[19,46,79,178] Common nephrotoxins include radiocontrast agents, ACEIs, ARBs, direct renin inhibitors, NSAIDs, and aminoglycosides. Other nephrotoxins that are less frequently encountered or are used in highly selective populations include amphotericin B, pentamidine, vancomycin, colistin, cisplatin, and high doses of methotrexate and acyclovir, intravenous immunoglobulin (IVIG), and nucleoside inhibitors.

Several general principles are involved in avoiding drug-induced nephrotoxicity: (1) recognizing the nephrotoxic potential of selected pharmacologic agents; (2) knowing which patient populations are at high risk; (3) weighing the risk-benefit ratio for use of a potential nephrotoxin in each patient; (4) considering the use of alternative non-nephrotoxic agents; (5) using the smallest effective dose of each potential nephrotoxin for the briefest interval possible; (6) monitoring blood levels of nephrotoxic agents, when available; (7) frequently monitoring kidney function; and (8) having a surveillance system for early detection of drug-related nephrotoxicity (Box 55.4).

Box 55.4 Strategies to Minimize Risk of Nephrotoxic Acute Kidney Injury

- Recognize agents with nephrotoxic potential.
- Recognize high-risk patients.
- Avoid nephrotoxic agents if possible.
- If nephrotoxic agent must be used, use the smallest dose necessary.
- Use the least nephrotoxic formulation.
- Monitor drug levels if available.
- Monitor kidney function.
- Maintain volume-expanded state.
- Avoid concomitant administration of other nephrotoxic agents.
- Use automatic stop orders to force periodic reevaluation of need for nephrotoxin.

Risk factors for aminoglycoside nephrotoxicity include the use of high doses, prolonged duration of therapy, decreased renal perfusion, associated liver disease, concomitant nephrotoxin administration, and possibly, advanced age.[80,81,83] In patients in whom aminoglycoside therapy is considered, clear goals for the use of the agent and plans for duration of therapy need to be formulated to ensure that treatment duration is no longer than absolutely necessary. Euvolemia and adequate renal perfusion should be maintained, concomitant nephrotoxins should be avoided, dosage should be adjusted based on measurement of plasma levels, and kidney function should be monitored on an ongoing basis. The observation that antimicrobial efficacy of aminoglycosides persists even after the drug levels in the blood have fallen below the minimal bactericidal concentration (postantibiotic killing) has led to the development of once-daily dosing regimens that provide higher peak levels but with less frequent dosing.[81,179-181] These regimens have been shown to result in rates of bacteriologic cure comparable with standard dosing regimens but are associated with lower rates of AKI.

Vancomycin is an antibiotic that has been associated with an increasing incidence of AKI as a result of both increased utilization and the targeting of higher drug levels.[182,183] Although many cases of putative vancomycin nephrotoxicity merely represent elevated drug levels due to decreased renal clearance, the use of higher doses has been associated with an increase in nephrotoxicity. Adjustment of dosing in response to close monitoring of blood levels, especially in patients with fluctuating kidney function, should minimize the risk of drug-induced AKI. Nephrotoxicity of drugs may be reduced through changes in formulation. For example, the use of lipid emulsions of amphotericin B is associated with reduced risk of amphotericin-induced AKI.[184]

NSAIDs often induce AKI by causing renal vasoconstriction, especially in settings where the renal circulation is dependent on angiotensin.[45,185] Less frequently, NSAIDs cause an interstitial nephritis, often accompanied by glomerular involvement with heavy proteinuria. Patients at risk for the development of NSAID-induced AKI include individuals with volume depletion, shock, hypotension, cardiac or liver disease, advanced age, and underlying CKD. Any patient with one or more of these risk factors should be carefully monitored for changes in kidney function associated with NSAID therapy. The same patient population at risk for NSAID-induced AKI is also at greatest risk for an abrupt decrease in kidney function following initiation or adjustment in the dose of ACEIs, ARBs, or direct renin inhibitors.[48] In addition, patients with bilateral renal artery stenosis or unilateral renal artery stenosis with a nonfunctional or absent contralateral kidney are also at increased risk for AKI with inhibition of the renin-angiotensin-aldosterone system.

PREVENTION OF CONTRAST-INDUCED ACUTE KIDNEY INJURY

Beyond the preceding general interventions, prevention of AKI requires that the insult to the kidney be timed in such a fashion that preventive strategies can be implemented prospectively. Contrast-induced AKI (CI-AKI) following the administration of iodinated radiocontrast media represents one of these few situations. Cardiac surgery represents another such setting; however, other than minimizing time on cardiopulmonary bypass and avoiding intraoperative and postoperative decreases in renal perfusion, there are no proven strategies for the prevention of cardiac surgery–associated AKI.

Risk factors for CI-AKI are well defined, with the single most important risk factor being preexisting CKD. In patients with normal kidney function, the risk of CI-AKI is much lower than 1% but increases in a graded fashion with severity of CKD.[186,187] Other risk factors include increasing age, diabetes mellitus, congestive heart failure, volume depletion, and concomitant NSAID use.[85] Utilization of alternative imaging modalities is the most effective means of preventing CI-AKI; however, when that is not possible strategies should be implemented to minimize the risk of nephrotoxicity. The primary intervention for prevention of CI-AKI is administration of isotonic intravenous fluids prior to and following the administration of contrast medium,[157,188] although the optimal composition and rate of fluid administration are not known. Studies comparing the relative benefits of isotonic saline and isotonic sodium bicarbonate have yielded conflicting results.[189-192] In hospitalized patients the administration of either isotonic saline or isotonic sodium bicarbonate at a rate of 1 mL/kg/hour for 12 hours prior to and 12 hours following the procedure is recommended[3]; however, alternative regimens involving more rapid fluid administration for a shorter duration may be equally efficacious.

Multiple pharmacologic agents have been evaluated, but most of them are not beneficial for preventing CI-AKI, including mannitol, furosemide, dopamine, fenoldopam, and calcium channel blockers.[176,193-197] Trials of other agents, including natriuretic peptides, aminophylline and theophylline, statins, and ascorbic acid have yielded conflicting results.[198-207] *N*-acetylcysteine (NAC), an antioxidant with vasodilatory properties, has been evaluated for the prevention of CI-AKI in multiple clinical trials. The rationale for the use of NAC relates to its capacity to scavenge reactive oxygen species, reduce the depletion of glutathione, and stimulate the production of vasodilatory mediators including nitric oxide.[208,209] These clinical trials of both oral and intravenous NAC have yielded contradictory findings.[210-218] Although it is uncertain whether NAC is beneficial in preventing CI-AKI, in its oral form it is both safe and inexpensive. For this reason, some, but not all, practice guidelines have recommended its use, with the important caveat that it should not be employed in lieu of intravenous fluids for the prevention of CI-AKI.[3,219]

Renal replacement therapies for the prevention of CI-AKI are ineffective, and the use of "prophylactic" hemodialysis has been associated with harm.[220-222] Although hemofiltration has been suggested to decrease the postprocedural increase in serum creatinine, the interpretation of these studies is confounded by the lowering of serum creatinine by the intervention.[223,224] Given the risks associated with intravenous line placement along with a lack of clear benefit, the use of dialysis or hemofiltration to prevent CI-AKI is not recommended.[225]

MANAGEMENT OF ESTABLISHED ACUTE KIDNEY INJURY

There is no specific management for the vast majority of patients with established AKI. Patients with prerenal azotemia should have intravascular volume deficits corrected and cardiac function optimized. Patients with hepatorenal syndrome may respond to vasoconstrictor therapy to reverse the splanchnic and peripheral vasodilation that underlies the development of the syndrome.[226,227] Abdominal compartment syndrome is treated with abdominal decompression.[53,54] Obstructive (postrenal) kidney disease is treated by mechanical relief of obstruction. The primary management of acute interstitial nephritis is discontinuation of the inciting agent; in patients with persistent AKI there may be a role for treatment with glucocorticoids. The treatment of AKI developing as a result of acute glomerulonephritis or renal involvement by vasculitis is dependent upon the precise cause and may include glucocorticoids and immunomodulatory therapy. Once AKI has developed and treatable or reversible causes have been excluded, the general therapeutic approach outlined in Box 55.5 is followed. Optimization of extracellular fluid volume status, cardiac index,

Box 55.5 General Therapeutic Approach to Established Acute Kidney Injury

- Correct prerenal factors and maintain euvolemic state.
- Attempt to establish a urine output if the patient remains oliguric despite correction of prerenal factors and exclusion of obstructive uropathy.
- Monitor for clinical and biochemical complications.
- Carefully monitor all drug therapy, dose-reducing medications for reduced glomerular filtration rate (GFR).
- Provide adequate nutrition.
- Reduce risk for infection.
- Use renal replacement therapy when indicated.

and maintenance of perfusion and oxygenation of vital organs are considered first.

MANAGEMENT OF VOLUME STATUS

Once volume status and cardiac output have been optimized, if the patient remains oliguric the use of a short trial of diuretics to establish urine output can be considered. Although nonoliguric forms of ATN are associated with significantly lower risk of morbidity and mortality than oliguric forms, the primary rationale for a trial of diuretic therapy is to facilitate volume management.[122] There is no evidence that conversion of ATN from an oliguric to a nonoliguric form alters risk of morbidity and mortality,[228,229] and if a diuretic response is not seen after one or two doses, diuretic agents should be discontinued. The utility of diuretic therapy is supported by a *post hoc* analysis of data from 306 patients from the Acute Respiratory Distress Syndrome Network's Fluid and Catheter Treatment Trial (FACTT) who developed AKI.[230] Positive fluid balance after development of AKI was associated with increased mortality rate; higher doses of furosemide had a protective effect on mortality rate, although this effect was attenuated after adjustment for fluid balance. Thus, the benefit of diuretics was thought to be mediated by fluid balance. No threshold dose of furosemide was observed above which the mortality rate increased.

In contrast to the use of diuretics, the use of renal vasodilators, including dopamine, fenoldopam, and atrial natriuretic peptide (ANP), has not been shown to be beneficial in AKI. Low-dose dopamine increases renal blood flow and to a lesser extent GFR in experimental animals and in healthy human volunteers and inhibits sodium reabsorption in the proximal tubule. However, in prospective clinical trials, low-dose dopamine has not been demonstrated to prevent or alter the course of ischemic or nephrotoxic ATN.[168-175] In a meta-analysis, the use of low-dose dopamine was associated with a transient increase in urine output on day 1 but had no impact on the development or progression of AKI, need for renal replacement therapy, or mortality rate.[174] Thus, the use of low-dose dopamine in the treatment of AKI is not justified.[231,232] Fenoldopam is a selective dopamine (DA1) receptor agonist.[233] In a randomized controlled trial of ICU patients with early ATN, fenoldopam failed to reduce mortality rate or the need for renal replacement therapy.[177] Similarly, anaritide, a synthetic analog of ANP, failed to show clinically significant improvement in dialysis-free survival rate or overall mortality rate in patients with ATN.[234] Although there was an improvement in dialysis-free survival rate in the subset of patients who were oliguric, this benefit was not confirmed in a subsequent study.[235]

PREVENTING, MONITORING, AND TREATING COMPLICATIONS

AKI is associated with the development of numerous electrolyte and acid-base disturbances, including most commonly hyperkalemia, hyponatremia, hyperphosphatemia, hypo- and (less commonly) hypercalcemia, hypermagnesemia, hyperuricemia, and metabolic acidosis. In addition, AKI is associated with anemia, bleeding diatheses, increased risk of infections, and dysfunction of other organ systems, including cardiovascular dysfunction, respiratory failure, gastrointestinal complications, and neurologic disturbances.

A detailed discussion of these complications can be found in the online supplement at www.expertconsult.com.

MEDICATION DOSING CONSIDERATIONS

Most pharmacologic agents are eliminated, at least in part, by the kidneys. Thus, use of standard doses and dosing intervals of many pharmacologic agents in patients with AKI can lead to accumulation of active drug or metabolites, with subsequent drug-induced morbidity and death. To avoid medication-induced toxicity in AKI, scrutiny of the medication list is essential. All medications not essential for care should be eliminated. A thorough understanding of the pathways of drug metabolism and elimination and the potential side effects of each drug used is mandatory. Excellent, up-to-date resources of this information are readily available.[265] Careful monitoring of clinical and biochemical parameters and drug levels is indicated, especially for agents with narrow therapeutic indices that are eliminated by the kidneys. In addition, further dosage adjustments may be required when renal replacement therapy is provided, especially for antibiotics to ensure that adequate therapeutic levels are achieved.

NUTRITIONAL CONSIDERATIONS

Nutritional support for patients with AKI must be considered in the overall context of associated comorbid conditions and other aspects of the management of critically ill patients.[266-269] The optimal nutritional support in critically ill patients with AKI is often influenced more by the nature of underlying illness and the type and frequency of renal replacement therapy rather than the AKI per se. The presence of oliguria and of high protein catabolic rates becomes an important consideration in the nutritional management of patients with severe ICU-associated AKI.[266-269] When possible, nutrition should be provided via the enteral route, as even small amounts of luminal nutrition help maintain intestinal integrity and decrease the risk of bacterial translocation. However, enteral nutrition is often insufficient to meet patient requirements and parenteral nutrition is often necessary. Caloric intake should generally be 25 to 30 kcal/kg/day and even in hypercatabolic patients, energy intake should not exceed 35 kcal/kg/day.[270] In noncatabolic patients, a protein intake of 1 to 1.3 g/kg/day is generally sufficient to achieve positive nitrogen balance. In hypercatabolic patients and patients receiving continuous renal replacement therapy, protein catabolic rates may reach 1.5 to 1.7 g/kg/day and higher protein intakes are ineffective in achieving positive nitrogen balance.[271] Current recommendations are that catabolic patients with AKI should receive 1.2 to 1.5 g/kg of protein and amino acids on a daily basis, even after adjusting for amino acid losses that occur during renal replacement therapy.[269,272] Careful attention must be paid to fluid volume and electrolyte content of nutritional formulations so as to minimize the risk of exacerbating volume overload or causing serious mineral and electrolyte disturbances.

RENAL REPLACEMENT THERAPY

In patients with severe AKI, renal replacement therapy (RRT) is the cornerstone of supportive management. The goal of renal replacement therapy is to permit the removal of fluids and solutes that accumulate in renal failure, thereby restoring the composition and volume of the extracellular fluids and preventing the complications of uremia. A detailed technical guide to the performance of RRT is beyond the scope of this chapter; the following discussion will provide an overview of RRT with a focus on the key management issues of selection of modality, timing of initiation of therapy, and appropriate intensity of therapy.

MODALITIES OF RENAL REPLACEMENT THERAPY

The available modalities of RRT include conventional intermittent hemodialysis (IHD); the various forms of continuous renal replacement therapy (CRRT) including continuous hemodialysis, continuous hemofiltration, and continuous hemodiafiltration; the hybrid modalities of prolonged intermittent renal replacement therapy (PIRRT; also known as extended duration dialysis[273-275] [EDD] or sustained low-efficiency dialysis [SLED])[276,277]; and peritoneal dialysis.[278,279]

In IHD and PIRRT, vascular access is generally achieved using large-bore double lumen venous catheters in the internal jugular, subclavian, or femoral veins. Because of concern of causing subclavian stenoses that might impair future angioaccess for chronic dialysis in patients who do not recover kidney function, internal jugular and femoral catheters are generally preferred over subclavian catheters.[3] CRRT was initially described using an arteriovenous extracorporeal circuit with inflow through a large-bore arterial catheter and return through a venous catheter. Although these arteriovenous modalities allowed for technical simplicity, they have been largely replaced by pumped venovenous extracorporeal circuits that allow for blood flow rates that are higher and are independent of mean arterial pressure and avoid the complications of prolonged arterial cannulation.[273-275]

Solute removal during RRT may occur by diffusion down a concentration gradient from the blood, across a semipermeable membrane, into dialysate or by convective transport of solute across the membrane during ultrafiltration. Fluid removal occurs by ultrafiltration, driven by either a hydrostatic or osmotic pressure gradient across the semipermeable dialysis or filtration membrane. In conventional IHD, the patient's blood passes through a semipermeable hemodialyzer countercurrent to the flow of dialysate on the opposite side of the dialysis membrane. The dialysis solution has a composition that approximates the normal electrolyte composition of extracellular fluids. Solutes that accumulate in kidney failure diffuse across the dialysis membrane from blood into dialysate. Fluid removal is achieved by applying a negative pressure across the membrane to permit the desired ultrafiltration rate. Treatment duration and frequency are variable, dictated by the patient's metabolic and volume status.

The CRRTs utilize either diffusive hemodialysis, convective hemofiltration, or a combination of diffusion and convection in continuous hemofiltration. As in intermittent hemodialysis, in continuous hemodialysis blood and dialysate flow in opposite directions on the two sides of the dialysis membrane; solute removal occurs by diffusion down a concentration gradient and ultrafiltration is driven by hydrostatic forces. The ultrafiltration during continuous hemodialysis is set at the level necessary to achieve the desired daily fluid removal. In addition to the duration of therapy, the major difference between intermittent and continuous hemodialysis is the dialysate flow rate. In intermittent hemodialysis, dialysate flow rates (typically 500 to 800 mL/minute) are equal to or greater than blood flow rates, allowing rapid solute clearance. In continuous hemodialysis, the dialysate flow rate (typically 15 to 50 mL/minute) is slow compared to that of the blood, permitting virtual equilibration of low-molecular-weight solutes such as urea between the blood and dialysate. Thus, solute clearance for low-molecular-weight solutes approximates the dialysate flow rate. Although the instantaneous clearance rate during continuous hemodialysis is much lower than during conventional IHD, the daily or weekly clearance is greater due to the longer duration of therapy.

In continuous hemofiltration, a high ultrafiltration rate is generated, and physiologic replacement fluid is administered at a rate equal to the difference between the high ultrafiltration rate and the desired rate of fluid removal. No dialysate is used, solute removal occurs exclusively by convection, and clearance is approximately equal to the ultrafiltration rate. Because the ability of solutes to diffuse across a dialysis membrane is inversely related to their molecular weight, while convective transport is limited primarily by the pore size of the membrane, hemofiltration provides more efficient clearance of higher molecular weight (>500-1500 KDa) solutes. Although it has been proposed that augmented removal of higher molecular weight solutes with hemofiltration as compared to hemodialysis would be of clinical benefit, particularly in patients with sepsis-associated AKI, this has not been borne out in clinical practice. In continuous hemodiafiltration, the dialysate flow of continuous hemodialysis is added to the convective ultrafiltration of continuous hemofiltration. Because of their prolonged duration, the net ultrafiltration rate (the difference between the ultrafiltration rate and infusion of replacement fluid) required to attain the same daily fluid removal is lower with CRRT than with IHD. As a result, CRRT is generally considered to cause less hemodynamic stress than conventional IHD.

Prolonged intermittent renal replacement therapy is a modification of conventional IHD, utilizing lower blood and dialysate flow rates while prolonging the treatment duration to 8 to 16 hours as compared to the usual 3- to 5-hour IHD treatment.[276,277] As with the continuous therapies, by prolonging the treatment duration and decreasing the rate of net ultrafiltration, the hemodynamic stress on the patient is minimized.

In peritoneal dialysis, dialysate with a high sugar concentration is instilled into the peritoneal membrane. Solute transport occurs by diffusion across the peritoneal membrane down the concentration gradient from blood to dialysate. The high osmolality resulting from the sugar in the dialysate provides an osmotic gradient for ultrafiltration. Because this is also a continuous therapy it has the same general benefit with regard to hemodynamic stability as CRRT, but the regulation of ultrafiltration is less precise. In addition, the use of glucose as the predominant sugar to generate the osmotic gradient predisposes to the development of hyperglycemia. In addition, the ability to perform peritoneal dialysis may be limited by recent abdominal surgery or intra-abdominal disease.

There has been considerable debate regarding which modality is most appropriate for use in critically ill patients with AKI. Current data suggest that no individual modality of RRT provides either better patient survival or recovery of kidney function.[3,280] Comparing outcomes between modalities in observational studies is complicated by the fact that patients treated with continuous or extended duration therapy are more likely to have greater severity of illness and be hemodynamically unstable. Not unexpectedly, observational studies have generally found higher unadjusted mortality rates when comparing CRRT to conventional IHD.[281-287] Randomized controlled trials have generally found no survival benefit when comparing continuous and intermittent therapies.[288-293] For example, in the Hemodiafe study, the largest of the randomized controlled trials comparing IHD and CRRT, which enrolled 360 patients who were well matched with regard to severity of illness across 21 ICUs in France, there was no difference in either survival or recovery of kidney function.[292] Recent systematic reviews and meta-analyses have confirmed the absence of differences in mortality rate or recovery of kidney function across modalities[294-296] but have suggested that continuous therapy is more effective at attaining negative fluid balance[263] but is more expensive.[295] Based on these data, the Kidney Disease Improving Global Outcomes (KDIGO) Clinical Practice Guidelines for Acute Kidney Injury has recommended that continuous and intermittent modalities of RRT be used as complementary therapies, although with the suggestion that CRRT be used preferentially for hemodynamically unstable patients.[297] In patients with acute brain injury or increased intracranial pressure, CRRT is associated with better preservation of cerebral perfusion than IHD and is the more appropriate modality of RRT.[298-302]

Only limited comparisons between PIRRT and the other modalities of therapy are available and have demonstrated similar hemodynamic stability and metabolic control[303-305] and comparable clinical outcomes.[306] Peritoneal dialysis (PD) has long been used as a dialytic therapy in AKI, although its use has declined as the use of CRRT has increased. There are only a limited number of studies that have compared outcomes with PD to outcomes with other modalities of renal support in AKI.[307-310] Although one study demonstrated poorer survival with PD than with continuous hemofiltration,[307] others have demonstrated biochemical and patient outcomes with high-volume peritoneal dialysis that are comparable to those seen with intermittent hemodialysis.[308-310]

In the absence of data suggesting better survival or recovery of kidney function with any one modality of RRT, these modalities should be considered to be complementary.[3] In general, the slower continuous (CRRT) and prolonged intermittent (PIRRT) modalities may be more optimal therapies for patients who are hemodynamically unstable. The choice of modality, however, should also reflect the local availability and expertise of the practitioners prescribing RRT and the nursing staff delivering the therapy.

Box 55.6 Indications for Initiation of Renal Replacement Therapy in Acute Kidney Injury

Conventional Indications

- Volume overload unresponsive to diuretic therapy
- Electrolyte and acid-base disturbances refractory to medical management
  - Hyperkalemia
  - Metabolic acidosis
  - Severe hypernatremia
  - Severe hyperphosphatemia
- Overt uremic symptoms
  - Encephalopathy
  - Pericarditis

Relative Indications

- Progressive azotemia
- Persistent oliguria

TIMING OF INITIATION OF RENAL REPLACEMENT THERAPY

Standard indications for initiation of renal replacement therapy include volume overload unresponsive to diuretic therapy; electrolyte and acid-base disturbances refractory to medical management, particularly severe hyperkalemia and metabolic acidosis; and overt uremia, characterized pericarditis or encephalopathy (Box 55.6). Common practice, however, is to initiate RRT preemptively, well before the development of these advanced complications, in patients with severe AKI in whom imminent recovery of kidney function is unlikely. Uncertainty in predicting if and when kidney function will recover creates a clinical conundrum: the earlier the initiation of therapy, the greater the probability of dialyzing patients who, if managed conservatively, might have recovered kidney function and survived without needing RRT.

The clinical data guiding current practice regarding the optimal timing of initiation of RRT is weak, derived primarily from retrospective and observational cohort studies and small, underpowered prospective trials. Several observational studies published in the 1960s and early 1970s concluded that mortality rates were higher when dialysis was initiated late, when the BUN was above 160 to 200 mg/dL, as compared to earlier initiation, when the BUN was approximately 90 to 150 mg/dL.[311-313] Two subsequent small prospective studies compared more intensive and earlier initiation of therapy to more "conventional" management.[314,315] In the first, a study of 18 patients with posttraumatic AKI, 5 of 8 patients (64%) assigned to the more intensive regimen which maintained the predialysis BUN below 70 mg/dL and serum creatinine below 5 mg/dL survived, as compared to 2 of 10 patients (20%) assigned to the less intensive strategy in which dialysis was not performed until the BUN approached 150 mg/dL, the creatinine reached 10 mg/dL, or other indications for dialysis were present ($p = 0.14$).[314] In the subsequent study, 34 patients with severe AKI were assigned to either an intensive regimen, designed to maintain the predialysis BUN less than 60 mg/dL and serum creatinine less than 5 mg/dL or to a delayed and less intensive regimen, in which the BUN was allowed to reach 100 mg/dL and the serum creatinine 9 mg/dL when their serum creatinine reached 8 mg/dL.[315] Initiation of dialysis was 2 days earlier in the more intensive regimen. The mortality rate was slightly higher (59% vs. 47%) with the earlier and more intensive strategy; however, this difference did not reach statistical significance. On the basis of these data, the conventional approach to management of RRT in AKI has been to initiate therapy prophylactically, in the absence of specific metabolic indications or symptoms, when the BUN rises to approximately 80 to 100 mg/dL.

A number of more recent retrospective and observational studies have suggested that even earlier initiation of RRT may be associated with better survival.[316-328] For example, in a retrospective analysis of timing of initiation of CRRT in 100 consecutive patients with posttraumatic AKI, 39% of patients who were started on CRRT when their BUN was less than 60 mg/dL survived as compared to 20% of patients in whom CRRT was not begun until their BUN was more than 60 mg/dL.[316] Only one small randomized trial has attempted to rigorously evaluate the timing of initiation of therapy. In this study of 106 critically ill patients with AKI randomized to early high-volume, early low-volume, and late low-volume continuous venovenous hemodiafiltration (CVVHDF), there was no difference in survival between early and late initiation of therapy.[329] A recent systematic review and meta-analysis of studies comparing early and late initiation of renal support published between 1985 and 2010, which included 15 unique studies, found an odds ratio for 28-day mortality rate of 0.45 associated with early initiation of renal support but noted that the methodologic quality of the included studies was low.[330] However, there is an important methodologic flaw underlying the majority of studies that have evaluated the timing of RRT. In restricting their analyses to patients who actually received RRT, either "early" or "late," these studies excluded the large number of patients who did not receive "early" RRT and either recovered kidney function and survived or died prior to reaching the criteria for "late" initiation of RRT.

The issue of severity of volume overload as an indication for initiation of renal support has garnered considerable attention and deserves special mention. The severity of volume overload at initiation of RRT is a strong predictor of fatality.[263,331-333] For example, in a cohort of pediatric patients, there was an increase in mortality rate from 29% in patients whose fluid gain was less than 10% of premorbid body weight at the time of initiation of CRRT as opposed to 66% in patients with 20% or greater fluid overload at initiation of therapy and an adjusted odds ratio of death of 8.5 associated with 20% or greater fluid overload.[333] Similarly, in a cohort of 396 critically ill adult patients, the presence of greater than 10% fluid overload at initiation of RRT was associated with an odds ratio of death of 2.1.[263] Although these data provide a strong caution regarding overly aggressive volume administration in patients with AKI, the hypothesis that earlier initiation of renal support to prevent or reverse volume overload still needs to be tested in prospective clinical trials.

INTENSITY OF RENAL SUPPORT IN ACUTE KIDNEY INJURY

Assessment of the dose of both IHD and PIRRT is dependent on both the intensity of therapy delivered with each individual treatment, usually quantified in terms of urea reduction ratio or the fractional clearance of urea (Kt/V_{urea}), and the frequency with which the treatments are provided. For the continuous therapies, dose is usually expressed in terms of the total effluent flow (dialysate plus ultrafiltrate) normalized to body weight. Several small clinical trials suggested that an augmented dose of RRT, either as intermittent hemodialysis or CRRT, improves survival.[334-336] These results were not consistent, however, across all studies[329,337] and were not confirmed in two large multicenter randomized controlled trials.[125,338] The Veterans Administration/National Institutes of Health (VA/NIH) Acute Renal Failure Trial Network (ATN) study randomized 1124 critically ill patients to lower- or higher-intensity RRT using a strategy that allowed patients to shift between modalities as hemodynamic status changed over time.[125] In the intensive arm, continuous venovenous hemodiafiltration (CVVHDF) was provided with a total effluent flow of 35 mL/kg/hour and conventional and prolonged intermittent hemodialysis were provided six times per week (daily, except Sunday); in the less intensive arm, the dose of CVVHDF was 20 mL/kg/hour and conventional and prolonged intermittent hemodialysis was provided three times per week (every other day, except Sunday). In the more intensive arm, 60-day all-cause mortality rate was 54% as compared to 52% in the less intensive arm. The Randomized Evaluation of Normal Versus Augmented Level (RENAL) Replacement Therapy study randomized 1508 patients in 35 ICUs in Australia and New Zealand to two doses of CVVHDF (25 or 40 mL/kg/hour) during their ICU stay. The survival rate to 90 days was 55.3% in both treatment arms.

The results of these two studies do not support the concept that more intensive renal support results in improved outcomes. It is recommended that intermittent hemodialysis be provided to deliver a total weekly therapy equivalent to that used in the ATN study (a target Kt/V_{urea} of 1.2-1.4 per treatment delivered three times per week).[3] More frequent IHD may be necessary, however, for fluid management in extremely hypercatabolic patients and for control of severe hyperkalemia. For patients treated with CRRT, the recommended delivered dose of therapy is an effluent flow rate of 20 to 25 mL/kg/hour.[3] Achieving this target dose may require the prescription of a slightly higher dose (25 to 30 mL/kg/hour) and careful attention to minimization of interruptions of therapy.

PROGNOSIS AND OUTCOMES

The mortality rate associated with AKI is high, although there is significant variation based on underlying cause, with much higher mortality rates associated with intrinsic forms of AKI than with prerenal or postrenal disease. In intrinsic AKI short-term mortality rates are approximately 50% and have changed little over the past 3 decades.* It is speculated

*See references 17, 21, 22, 24, 334, 339-350.

that this lack of improvement despite significant advances in supportive care most likely reflects a decrease in the proportion of patients presenting with isolated AKI, and a corresponding increase in the percentage of patients with AKI accompanied by multiple-organ dysfunction.[22,24,351,352] In patients with sepsis-associated AKI, mortality rates are as high as 60% to 90%.[17,61,341,351]

Multiple factors are associated with mortality risk in AKI and include male gender, advanced age, oliguria (<400 mL/day), a rise in the serum creatinine value of greater than 3 mg/dL, and coexistent sepsis or nonrenal organ failure. In general, these factors reflect severity of renal injury and overall severity of illness. However, even less severe AKI is associated with an increase in mortality risk. In a study of patients undergoing cardiothoracic surgery, increases in serum creatinine less than 0.6 mg/dL were independently associated with a nearly twofold increase in the 30-day mortality rate.[353] Similarly, small increments in serum creatinine following radiocontrast agent administration, even if transient, are associated with increased rates of short- and long-term mortality.[187,253,354,355] It remains unclear, however, whether such transient increases in serum creatinine actually mediate the adverse long-term outcomes or merely represent a biochemical marker of risk.[356]

In addition to the very high short-term mortality rate associated with AKI, there is also an increased risk of longer-term morbidity and mortality. It was previously believed that if a patient with AKI survived the acute episode the prognosis was good, with approximately 90% of patients having complete recovery of kidney function, 5% remaining dialysis dependent, and an additional 5% developing progressive deterioration in kidney function after initially recovering function. More recent data suggested a less optimistic prognosis. In recent clinical trials of RRT in AKI, rates of recovery have been highly variable.[125,338,357] In the RENAL study, fewer than 10% of patients remained dialysis dependent as compared to 25% of surviving patients in the ATN study and 40% of patients in the Hanover Dialysis Outcomes study. The reason for this variability in recovery of kidney function across studies is unclear and may reflect differences in patterns of care or may reflect differences in the study population.

Approximately half of patients who recover renal function can be demonstrated to have subclinical kidney disease including modest decrements in GFR, defects in tubular function and urinary concentration, and tubulointerstitial scarring on kidney biopsy.[358-361] More importantly, patients who recover from AKI are at increased risk of progressive CKD and are at increased risk for the development of end-stage renal disease (ESRD).[31,362-365] For example, in a 5% representative sample of elderly Medicare beneficiaries AKI in the absence of underlying CKD was independently associated with a 13-fold hazard for the development of ESRD within 2 years while AKI that developed in the setting of preexistent CKD was associated with a greater than 41-fold hazard for the development of ESRD.[362] Similarly, in a population-based cohort study using data from Ontario, Canada, 3769 patients who developed AKI that required temporary dialysis had a more than threefold increased risk for the development of ESRD over 3 years as compared to 13,598 matched control subjects who were hospitalized but did not develop AKI.[363] In a similar analysis using data from 562,799 patients hospitalized in the Kaiser-Permanente of Northern California health system, AKI requiring transient dialysis was associated with a twofold increased risk of death over 6 years of follow-up and a 28-fold increased risk of developing progressive CKD.[31] Mild AKI has also been associated with an increased risk of AKI. For example, increases in serum creatinine of as little as 0.3 to 0.5 mg/dL following an acute MI were independently associated with a greater than twofold increased hazard for ESRD and an approximately 25% increased hazard for long-term mortality.[364]

AKI is associated with prolongation of the length of hospitalization and substantial health resource utilization.[284,345,366-368] In 1999, the cost of treating an episode of AKI was estimated to be $50,000 per Quality Adjusted Life Year (QALY).[369] In a more recent analysis, quality adjusted survival was poor among 153 ICU survivors who had recovered from AKI as compared to an age- and gender-matched community population.[370] Although quality adjusted survival in this cohort was poor (15 quality adjusted years per 100 patient-years in the first year following discharge), the survivors' self-perceived health satisfaction was not significantly different from that of the general population.[370] Similar poor health-related quality of life was also observed in a follow-up of 415 subjects who participated in the ATN study and survived at least 60 days, with 27% of respondents' health status corresponding to levels considered by the general population to be equivalent to or worse than death.[371]

KEY POINTS

- Acute kidney injury is a common complication in critically ill patients and is accompanied by high rates of morbidity and mortality.
- The diagnosis of acute kidney injury is based on increases in the serum creatinine concentration or persistent oliguria despite adequate volume resuscitation.
- Multiple different pathogenic mechanisms can result in the development of acute kidney injury, including functional, hemodynamically mediated (prerenal) acute kidney injury, urinary tract obstruction (postrenal) acute kidney injury, and intrinsic acute kidney injury.
- Acute tubular necrosis, developing as the result of ischemia-reperfusion injury, nephrotoxic exposure, or sepsis, is the most common form of intrinsic acute kidney injury.
- The primary clinical manifestations of acute kidney injury include retention of nitrogenous waste products and disordered volume, electrolyte, and acid-base homeostasis.
- The initial assessment and management of the patient with acute kidney injury should focus on the identification and treatment of reversible etiologies including volume depletion, organ hypoperfusion, and urinary tract obstruction.

Continued on following page

KEY POINTS (Continued)

- Efforts to prevent AKI should be directed at maintaining renal perfusion and avoiding hypotension, selecting and dosing medications to minimize the risk of nephrotoxicity, and preventing nosocomial infections.
- Treatment of acute kidney injury is supportive, including optimizing volume status, treating electrolyte and acid-base disturbances, providing adequate nutrition, and dose adjusting renally excreted medications to prevent drug toxicity.
- In patients with severe AKI, renal replacement therapy should be employed to maintain volume status, correct electrolyte and acid-base disturbances, and remove the metabolic waste products responsible for the development of uremia.
- The majority of patients surviving an episode of acute kidney injury will recover kidney function; however, survivors are at increased risk for the development of chronic kidney disease and need for long-term dialysis.

SUGGESTED REFERENCES

3. KDIGO Clinical Practice Guideline for Acute Kidney Injury. Kidney Int Suppl 2012;2:1-138.
15. Bellomo R, Ronco C, Kellum JA, et al: Acute renal failure—Definition, outcome measures, animal models, fluid therapy and information technology needs: The Second International Consensus Conference of the Acute Dialysis Quality Initiative (ADQI) Group. Crit Care 2004;8:R204-212.
28. Hospitalization discharge diagnoses for kidney disease—United States, 1980-2005. MMWR Morb Mortal Wkly Rep 2008;57:309-312.
32. Grams ME, Astor BC, Bash LD, et al: Albuminuria and estimated glomerular filtration rate independently associate with acute kidney injury. J Am Soc Nephrol 2010;21:1757-1764.
120. Koyner JL, Vaidya VS, Bennett MR, et al: Urinary biomarkers in the clinical prognosis and early detection of acute kidney injury. Clin J Am Soc Nephrol 2010;5:2154-2165.
125. Palevsky PM, Zhang JH, O'Connor TZ, et al: Intensity of renal support in critically ill patients with acute kidney injury. N Engl J Med 2008;359:7-20.
265. Brier ME, Aronoff GR: Drug Prescribing in Renal Failure, 5th ed. Philadelphia, American College of Physicians, 2007.
338. Bellomo R, Cass A, Cole L, et al: Intensity of continuous renal-replacement therapy in critically ill patients. N Engl J Med 2009;361:1627-1638.
362. Ishani A, Xue JL, Himmelfarb J, et al: Acute kidney injury increases risk of ESRD among elderly. J Am Soc Nephrol 2009;20:223-228.
363. Wald R, Quinn RR, Luo J, et al: Chronic dialysis and death among survivors of acute kidney injury requiring dialysis. JAMA 2009;302:1179-1185.

The complete list of references can be found at www.expertconsult.com.

Chronic Kidney Disease

56

Christopher B. McFadden

CHAPTER OUTLINE

INTRODUCTION

Chronic kidney disease (CKD) is a common diagnosis in adult medicine.[1-6] In order to properly identify patients at risk for adverse outcomes and disease progression, extensive work has focused on early and appropriate classification over the last 10 years. In particular, the National Kidney Foundation (NKF) proposed a classification system for CKD in 2002 using estimated glomerular filtration rate (eGFR) as a method to categorize patients.[7,8] Table 56.1 describes current NKF guidelines of CKD. In regard to critical care, CKD patients have higher mortality rate following critical illnesses.[9] Understanding this population's physiology and underlying disease state may aid caregivers in attempting to improve this outcome.

This chapter will aim to define CKD and discuss the physiology of CKD in terms of blood pressure (BP), electrolytes, bone structure, and anemia. An emphasis will be given to the intensive care unit (ICU) management of these problems. When available, evidence-based guidelines will be reviewed and discussed. Unfortunately, the ICU management of CKD patients often is not guided by evidence-based therapy. As a result, guidelines developed from other populations will be reviewed with appropriate scrutiny.

DEFINITION AND ETIOLOGY

As previously stated, currently CKD is staged in a five-tier system based on eGFR (see Table 56.1). The diagnosis relies on abnormal kidney function or urinalysis findings for 3 months or more. The serum creatinine as well as age, sex, gender, and race is used to generate an eGFR from a quadratic equation derived from the Modification of Diet in Renal Disease Study.[7] Most CKD patients do not progress to end-stage renal disease (ESRD), however, because of the very high cardiovascular and noncardiovascular mortality rate associated with this at-risk population.[10-13] Proposals exist to more clearly define elderly subjects with CKD stage 3 disease at risk for disease progression, though this practice has not become standard.[14-16]

Causes for CKD are broad and often multifactorial. Frequently, however, diabetes mellitus and hypertension play a major role. Hypertension may lead to kidney damage in the form of nephrosclerosis or chronic renal ischemia due to atherosclerotic vascular disease. An important recent development is the recognition that the higher prevalence of nondiabetic kidney disease in the African-American population may be due to genetic risk conferred by inherited variants in the apolipoprotein L1 gene (*APOL1*).[17] Additional causes include immune-mediated glomerular diseases such as systemic lupus erythematosus, IgA nephropathy, membranous nephropathy, and other often preexisting glomerulonephritides. Glomerulonephritis may be active as evidenced by hematuria and proteinuria or may have occurred in the patient's past, leading to abnormal kidney function but a relatively bland urinalysis. Alternatively, primary tubulointerstitial diseases could exist owing to reflux nephropathy, sarcoidosis, chronic infections, allergic reactions, or side effects from medications such as cyclophosphamide (Cytoxan) and lithium. In general, the diagnosis of CKD should warrant a higher index of suspicion for concurrent, and potentially undiagnosed, cardiovascular disease (CVD).

The CKD population is at risk for deterioration in kidney function during a hospitalization stay, particularly if a critical illness is present. Potential causative factors for this are listed in Box 56.1. Importantly, acute tubular necrosis may occur without obvious hypotension, and patients with reduced kidney function are more at risk for this complication.[18]

DIAGNOSIS

Intrinsic to the eGFR formula, as well as other estimates of renal function from the serum creatinine, is the

Table 56.1 Chronic Kidney Disease Stages

Stage	eGFR (mL/min/ 1.73 m²)	Urinalysis Findings
1	≥90	Hematuria, proteinuria, or imaging abnormalities at >3 months
2	60-89	Hematuria, proteinuria, or imaging abnormalities at >3 months
3	30-59	↑ or normal
4	15-29	↑ or normal
5	0-14	↑ or normal

eGFR, estimated glomerular filtration rate.

Box 56.1 Factors Leading to Deterioration in Renal Function During Hospitalization in Patients with Chronic Kidney Disease

Volume depletion: prerenal, including "normotensive" sepsis, renal vasoconstriction due to medications or hypercalcemia
Obstruction
Renal vascular disease: atherosclerotic with volume depletion, thrombotic, or embolic disease
Upper urinary tract infection: bilateral or unilateral with single kidney including a kidney transplant
Nephrotoxic medications: allergic inflammation, tubular injury
Glomerular disease: IgA or postinfectious related to infection

IgA, immunoglobulin A.

Box 56.2 Factors That May Alter Serum Creatinine (Cr) Level

Endogenous

Reduced muscle mass: ↓
Hyperbilirubinemia: ↓

Exogenous

Medications inhibiting tubular secretion (trimethoprim, cimetidine): ↑

Medications Interfering with Laboratory Assays*

Flucytosine and cefoxitin: ↑
Catecholamines: ↓

*Varies by assay type used.

presumption that a patient's serum creatinine is stable. This finding may not be the case in ICU patients; as a result, imprecision should be expected in kidney function estimation in ICU patients.[19] Serum creatinine is now recognized to potentially underestimate the level of renal function in a large population of patients, particularly those with low weight, small muscle mass, and liver disease.[20] Additionally, both endogenous and exogenous factors can influence the measurement of serum creatinine.[21-24] Box 56.2 describes situations in which serum creatinine measurements may not adequately reflect kidney function. Importantly, some vasoactive substances can impart a negative interference on creatinine values if the creatinine sample is obtained from a central line used for vasopressors.[25] Nonetheless, creatinine variation has improved since values have been standardized to reference values.[26,27]

In general, current guidelines recognize the importance of stage 3 through 5 kidney disease for prognostication in outpatient and inpatient outcomes. Proteinuria is now associated with increased cardiovascular risk at all glomerular filtration rates (GFRs), including normal GFRs.[28] Even mild kidney dysfunction, defined typically as a serum creatinine level over 1.5 mg/dL or GFR below 60 mL/minute, is associated with worse outcomes after coronary artery bypass graft (CABG), cardiac valvular, and general surgery.[29-33]

Concern exists about the accuracy of the Modification of Diet in Renal Disease (MDRD) equation at higher GFRs. For example, the newer creatinine-based CKD-EPI formula equation leads to a lower prevalence rate of CKD stage 3 than the MDRD equation, as more patients have an eGFR above 60 mL/minute.[34-36] Measurement of serum cystatin C levels, a protein produced by all nucleated cells and freely filtered by the glomerulus, may provide more accurate estimates of kidney function than creatinine-based equations, particularly when kidney function is close to normal.[37] Cystatin C may also provide prognostic information about future cardiovascular events.[12] In fact, cystatin C has been proposed as a marker of "preclinical" kidney disease based on worse cardiovascular outcomes in elderly subjects with higher cystatin C levels.[38] Despite a growing body of literature, use of cystatin C is not routine in clinical practice.

When serum creatinine is stable and the eGFR formula is felt to inaccurately measure kidney function, creatinine clearance can be measured by using a 24-hour urine collection through the following formula:

$$\text{Creatinine clearance (dL/24 hours)} = (\text{Urine creatinine (mg/dL)} \times (\text{volume of urine (dL)}))/\text{Plasma creatinine (mg/dL)}$$

In this equation, units will need to be converted from dL/24 hours to mL/minute by a conversion factor of 0.0694.

If this measure is pursued, clinicians are counseled to pay close attention to units as well as the expectation that men excrete 1500 to 2500 mg/day of creatinine and women excrete 1000 to 1500 mg/day of creatinine.[39] If a lower amount of urinary creatinine is obtained, the possibility of an undercollection should be considered. It is also worthwhile to note that historically, drug dosing has been determined by creatinine clearance and not eGFR.

In summary, estimating kidney function in ICU patients may be challenging because of the absence of steady-state conditions and irregularities in body size and fluid compartments. Critical care providers need to understand the strengths and weaknesses of measuring kidney function in these patients.

PHYSIOLOGY

HYPERTENSION

Over 80% of CKD patients with eGFR less than 60 mL/minute have hypertension.[5] This has several important impacts on the management of ICU patients. First, long-standing hypertension, if uncontrolled, leads to adaptations in autoregulation. Autoregulation refers to the ability of blood vessels to constrict and dilate in the presence of hypertension and hypotension, respectively. Consequently, patients become acclimated to BPs near their "typical" BP and may not tolerate lower BPs despite these apparent lower values appearing in the normal range. A consequence of this may be hypoperfusion to the kidneys as well as the brain, heart, intestine, and other critical organs at BP levels that appear normal. If a history of poorly controlled hypertension is obtained, an astute clinician should aim to keep BP close to the level the patient being treated is used to. This very much requires individualized attention and thorough history taking.

Second, CKD leads to sodium retention.[40,41] The most notable ICU impact this will have is the potential for volume retention and the need for diuretics to manage hypertension in the CKD population.[42-44] Several mechanisms lead to the development of hypertension in the CKD population. They include upregulation of the renin-angiotensin system, increased sympathetic nervous system activity, and impairment of endothelial-dependent arterial smooth muscle relaxation.[45-51] Owing to the preceding mechanisms, CKD patients may develop more edema and volume overload with equivalent amounts of intravenous (IV) fluids. One worthwhile consideration, however, is that sodium retention associated with CKD may be counterbalanced by sodium loss from excessively high BP levels. This phenomenon, known as pressure natriuresis, may explain the rapid drops observed in BP in hypertension emergencies once excess sympathetic activity is controlled.

ELECTROLYTE DISORDERS

SODIUM

Sodium homeostasis in patients with CKD is abnormal. With increased loss of sodium in the urine, but declining numbers of functioning nephrons, sodium balance is maintained.[52] Though CKD patients are sodium "avid" and tend toward states of volume overload, they are less able to increase sodium retention in times of need and subsequently are also at risk for volume depletion. In comparison, subjects with normal renal function can quickly increase sodium absorption and avoid volume-depleted states.[53] Tubulointerstitial disease and obstructive uropathy may be particularly at risk for episodes of volume depletion due to their recognized inability to increase sodium reabsorption in times of volume depletion.[54]

Patients with CKD thus are a group at risk for both volume depletion as well as volume overload. ICU illnesses may confound this because of irregularities in physical examination findings in this population. Specifically, elevated BP and edema in the CKD population are frequently present but do not represent states of intravascular volume overload. In summary, close attention to assessment of volume status and need for supplemental fluids or diuresis is warranted in the CKD population.

When volume overload is present, iatrogenic sources may be playing a role. Potential sources of sodium include maintenance IV fluids (including bicarbonate), antibiotics, and nutritional sources including total parenteral nutrition (TPN). Tracking fluid intake and output ("Is and Os") does not clearly differentiate between the electrolyte makeup of the various sources. Consequently, volume overload may develop insidiously. When volume overload develops, the standard approach involves minimizing sodium-containing sources and initiating a diuretic regimen. Diuretics range from the more gentle thiazide diuretics, which are ineffective with a GFR below 30 mL/minute, to more potent loop diuretics. In general, if significant volume removal is desired, a diuretic regimen twice a day (every 12 hours) should be prescribed to avoid excess sodium reabsorption in the period after the major diuretic effect.[55] Chronic administration of diuretics, prior to ICU admission, may lead to adaptive processes necessitating higher diuretic doses, combination therapy, or alternative approaches to volume overload states.[56-59] Torsemide is the loop diuretic that may be closest to lasting 24 hours.[60] Doses of loop diuretics need to be increased as renal function declines. Significant variability in loop diuretic kinetics exist; if a dose does not yield an increase in urine output within 2 hours, consideration should be given to increasing the dose. Alternatively, continuous infusion of loop diuretics may provide a better diuresis with less toxicity.[61,62] Typically infusion rates of furosemide are 10 to 40 mg/hour. When a loop diuretic drip is ordered, a bolus should be given prior to initiating therapy to avoid a significant delay in efficacy.

Diuretic failure is common in the CKD population. Potential explanations in an ICU population include acute kidney injury, inadequate dosing, and distal tubular hypertrophy due to chronic diuretic use. When high-dose loop diuretics do not achieve adequate diuresis, the addition of metolazone may improve urine output. Historically, metolazone is given 30 minutes prior to the loop diuretics, though it may be efficacious if given at other times as well. Finally, isolated ultrafiltration or potentially dialysis may be required for volume removal. Significant attention has been given to the importance of elevated intra-abdominal pressures leading to a reduction in renal function and, potentially, ability to respond to diuretics.[63-68]

WATER

Water concentration and dilution are abnormal in CKD patients. Normal patients can dilute and concentrate urine within a range of 40 to 1400 mOsm/kg.[69] CKD leads to a narrower range of urine osmolality. Specifically, patients with advanced CKD have a urine osmolality much closer to 300 mOsm/kg; the ability to adjust urine osmolality declines as urine function worsens.[70] Consequently, patients with CKD are prone both to hypernatremia and hyponatremia. Loop diuretics may further worsen the kidney's ability to concentrate and dilute urine.[71]

The approach to hypernatremia and hyponatremia is similar to that in other patients. In hypernatremia cases, concurrent illnesses often lead to patients being unable to obtain water for themselves; a high urine output due to hyperglycemia or a high urea concentration may worsen this. Elevated urea, as with high serum glucose levels, functions as an osmolar agent in the tubular lumen and creates a state of relative antidiuretic hormone (ADH) resistance with the potential for substantial free water loss.[72]

Hypernatremia can lead to significant agitation and should be treated aggressively with increased water either intravenously, in the form of hypotonic IV fluids, or enterally. When severe, an estimation of free water deficit is appropriate. Unexplained polyuria with a low urine osmolality, hypernatremia, and CKD in an ICU patient with unclear history should warrant an investigation for previous lithium use.[73]

Hyponatremia reflects irregularities in water excretion in the vast majority of cases. CKD patients are less able to excrete water owing to the inability to lower urine osmolality.[74] Sources of water include IV fluids, medications mixed in dextrose, and enteral sources. Patients often are not aware or not forthcoming in the amount of water they drink, though this is less an issue in ICU patients. The approach for most CKD patients is similar to that in other cases of hyponatremia, which involve looking for and reducing causes of increased water intake. Importantly, sodium abnormalities in the CKD patient, both with and without congestive heart failure, are associated with a higher mortality rate.[75]

POTASSIUM

Potassium (K^+) regulation is an essential function of the kidneys in normal states. CKD patients routinely maintain serum K^+ in the normal range despite losing up to 90% of renal function.[76,77] Mechanisms underlying the maintenance of normal serum K^+ in advanced CKD include increased K^+ excretion per functioning nephron, increased gastrointestinal (GI) elimination of K^+, and increased uptake of K^+ by cells.[78] Diabetes mellitus, however, may exacerbate the development of hyperkalemia due to the presence of a distal tubular acidosis (type 4) from aldosterone resistance. Hypokalemia may also be present due to current diuretic use or renovascular hypertension.[79] Its presence is associated with a higher risk of death and future ESRD needs in the CKD population.[80]

ICU patients with CKD represent a population prone to irregularities in K^+ homeostasis, in particular, hyperkalemia.[81,82] Potential causes of hyperkalemia include insulin deficiency, hypoaldosteronism, and a loss of normal intestinal function, which plays a role in increased potassium excretion in CKD patients. Decreased blood flow to muscle and intestines in times of critical illness may impede potassium cellular uptake and excretion, respectively. Tissue ischemia from trauma, hypoxia, or tumor lysis is associated with an elevation in K^+ which may occur quickly.[83] One additional clinical consideration is that CKD patients who are fasting may develop surprising levels of hyperkalemia without any apparent cause due to low levels of insulin.[84] Glucose-containing IV fluids may avoid this.

The evaluation of hyperkalemia in CKD patients begins with assessing the cause. Typically, this includes close scrutiny of medications, IV fluids, and types of nutritional support. Frequently, ICU patients receive nutrition very different from what the body is used to and cannot manage a higher load of K^+, especially in states of relative tissue perfusion. Importantly, many CKD patients are on diuretics as part of their routine outpatient medications; simply stopping these medications may lead to states of hyperkalemia. Hyperosmolality leads to a K^+ shift out of cells caused by solvent drag; in its most common presentation, hyperglycemia, this can be reversed quickly with the use of insulin. Metabolic acidosis may be associated with hyperkalemia though organic acidosis states appear to cause less hyperkalemia than nonorganic acid–induced states.[85]

Medications are an important and growing cause of hyperkalemia. Congestive heart failure and proteinuric renal disease remain as two indications for possible dual renin-angiotensin-aldosterone blockade; hyperkalemia has been observed more frequently since the publication of the RALES trial.[86] Box 56.3 lists some common causes of hyperkalemia in the CKD population and the associated mechanisms.[87] The presence of hyperkalemia should warrant close attention to affected patients as its presence is associated with increased mortality rate.[88]

Box 56.3 Causes of Hyperkalemia, with Associated Mechanisms, in Patients with Chronic Kidney Disease in the Intensive Care Unit (ICU) Setting

Medications

Trimethoprim—↓ renal K^+ excretion[135,136]
NSAIDs, ACE inhibitors, ARBs—↓ renal K^+ excretion
Heparin—↓ aldosterone synthesis[137]
Beta blockers, nonselective—↓ cellular K^+ uptake[138]
Triamterene, spironolactone, amiloride—↓ renal K^+ excretion
Digoxin overdose—↓ cellular K^+ uptake[139]
Succinylcholine use with trauma/critical illness—↑ K^+ release from cells[140]
Pencillin G—↑ K^+ load[141,142]

Clinical Conditions

Renal tubular acidosis (associated with diabetes)—↓ renal K^+ excretion
Thrombocytosis—K^+ release *after* phlebotomy[143]
Insulin deficiency—↓ cellular K^+ uptake
Cell death (tumor lysis, rhabdomyolysis)—↑ K^+ load

ACE, angiotensin-converting enzyme; ARB, angiotensin receptor blockers; NSAIDs, nonsteroidal anti-inflammatory drugs.
Superscript numbers indicate references provided online.

METABOLIC ACIDOSIS

The kidneys and lungs regulate acid excretion by the body. Kidney excretion of acid occurs through two mechanisms: as protons bound to anions such as phosphate and through ammoniagenesis. As kidney function declines below a GFR of 30 mL/minute, the excess excretion of protons by each remaining functional nephron is no longer able to keep serum bicarbonate in the normal range. As a result, bicarbonate levels in CKD patients frequently range in the 18 to 22 mmol/L range due to a modest increase in the serum anion gap.[89] A recent trial showed sodium bicarbonate, supplemented orally, could delay kidney disease progression (Fig. 56.1).[90]

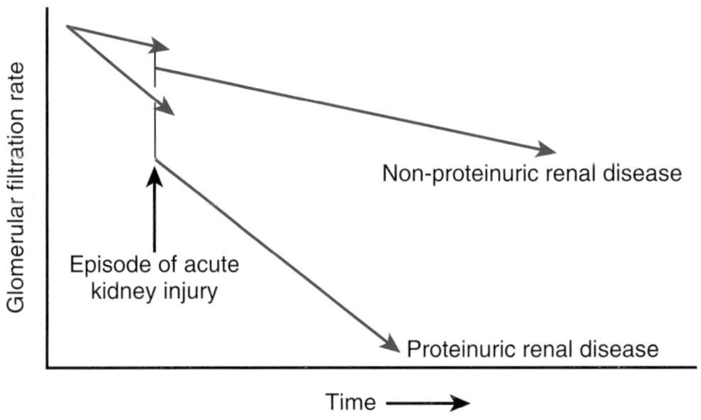

Figure 56.1 Rate of decline in renal function over time showing higher rate of decline in patients with proteinuric renal disease *and* potential for episodes of acute kidney injury to hasten kidney disease progression.

In ICU CKD patients, serum bicarbonate and anion gaps are often further worsened by concurrent conditions including lactic acidosis, ketoacidosis, or dilution due to aggressive volume resuscitation. The latter case, dilutional acidosis, will present with a worsening serum bicarbonate in the days following admission to the ICU and institution of IV fluids; the anion gap should not change significantly. In general, an anion gap over 20 should warrant a workup for other causes of increased acid generation. Medications may also worsen acidosis in the CKD population owing to disturbances in ammonia production as well as excess acid production in the form of lactic acid, keto acids, and pyroglutamic acids.[91,92]

MINERAL BONE DISORDER

Substantial information has developed in the last several years about the mechanisms leading to abnormal calcium and bone metabolism in patients with CKD. Historically, this disorder was named "renal osteodystrophy." The current preferred term is CKD mineral bone disorder.[93] The main developments reflects the growing importance of FGF-23 on phosphate and parathyroid regulation and the relaxation of guidelines for strict parathyroid hormone (PTH) control at least in the ESRD population.[94]

FGF-23 is a phosphaturic protein produced by bone. Phosphaturia occurs as a result of decreased expression of NaPi-2a cotransporters in renal proximal tubular cells.[95] In addition, FGF-23 leads to a reduction in 1,25(OH)2D production by the kidney.[96] Its concentration increases earlier in the course of CKD than PTH. These adaptations initially keep calcium and phosphorus levels well maintained despite progressively increased serum FGF-23 and PTH levels.

From an ICU patient perspective, hypocalcemia will routinely be encountered owing to the preceding developments. Hypocalcemia, in the absence of other causes, suggests renal disease is chronic. Serum phosphorus levels may similarly be elevated as GFR declines. Dietary phosphorus restriction and phosphorus binders are the primary treatments for this. There are limited prospective data evaluating the best management of CKD mineral bone disorder, and therapy is for the most part dictated by nonrandomized studies and consensus guidelines. Elevations of FGF-23 are associated with a higher risk of mortality across multiple levels of kidney function.[97] Important issues for anyone caring for CKD patients with abnormalities of calcium bone deposition in the ICU include the following:

- Avoidance of phosphorus-containing GI stimulants because of risk of systemic absorption and acute kidney injury
- Recognition that hypocalcemia may be chronic: typically, patients become adapted to this with a normal ionized calcium due to concurrent metabolic acidosis. Rapidly raising pH may lower serum calcium levels acutely and predispose patients to arrhythmias.[98]
- Consideration for other causes of hypocalcemia and hyperphosphatemia, in particular, cell death from rhabdomyolysis and tumor lysis syndrome

ANEMIA AND HEMATOLOGIC DISEASE

Erythropoietin is produced by the kidney and stimulates hematopoiesis in the bone marrow. CKD is associated with a reduction in erythropoietin levels and consequent anemia. As CKD progresses toward ESRD, anemia becomes more severe.[99] As a general rule, most ESRD patients receive supplemental erythropoietin to increase their hemoglobin (Hb) level and avoid transfusions.

Two large trials published in 2006 significantly altered the management of anemia of CKD.[100,101] The CHOIR and CREATE trials both showed, in a well-designed format, that randomization to a normal Hb did not improve outcomes and increased some adverse events. As a result, goal Hb levels have dropped closer to 10.0 g/dL in general practice and the use of these medications has fallen substantially. These trials reinforced earlier data that showed that aiming for a normal Hb, achieved through supplemental erythropoietin, in the CKD population was dangerous.[102] Similar results were noted with darbapoietin alpha.[103] These studies clearly show adverse events from supraphysiologic Hbs in CKD patients. The impact of relative reductions in Hb in critically ill CKD patients is not well studied.

In CKD with critical illnesses the problems of anemia are often magnified. How the anemia of CKD impacts hospital course is not well understood. The current preference of minimizing transfusions and keeping Hbs in a lower range, based on trials for the most part on non-CKD patients, has led to a reduction in Hb in CKD patients as well.[104-106] It is important to consider that CKD patients may not be able to recover Hb after acute illness because of reduced erythropoietin production.

Acute drops in Hb in ICU CKD patients should be managed similar to those in non-CKD patients. Chronic anemia should not be presumed to be due to CKD, and routine evaluations should still occur, including stool studies and iron status assessment. CKD patients, when blood urea nitrogen (BUN) levels increase above 100 mg/dL, are more prone to bleeding because of irregularities in platelet functional activity.[107-109] Dialysis may reduce the risk of bleeding due to azotemia and "uremic platelets," though variable data on this point exist.[110-112] Additionally, desmopressin will stimulate von Willebrand factor release acutely though tachyphylaxis develops after the first dose.[113,114] Finally, conjugated estrogens may provide a sustained reduction in bleeding complications in CKD patients who have recurrent

GI bleeding.[115] Low-molecular-weight heparin clearance is reduced in patients with low GFRs. Appropriate dose reductions should occur; currently, no guidelines exist for dosing these medications with a GFR below 15 mL/minute, and their use in these settings should be avoided.

END-STAGE RENAL DISEASE

Patients with ESRD make up a large and growing percentage of the CKD population. In the United States, 90% of this population receives renal replacement therapy (RRT) in the form of in-center hemodialysis at the time of dialysis initiation.[5] Efforts are under way to move more of this care to the patient's home in the form of home hemodialysis or peritoneal dialysis.

ESRD patients have a higher mortality rate when admitted to ICUs.[116,117] Indications for admission may be dialysis specific such as access complications or volume overload or may be due to other comorbid illnesses. Most commonly, indications include cardiovascular causes including acute coronary syndromes and strokes, other infectious causes, and GI hemorrhages. Commonly used ICU prognostic scoring systems such as Apache II and III, Simplified Acute Physiology Score (SAPS) II, and Sequential Organ Failure provide reasonable prognostication of patients with ESRD.[118]

Attention to a dialysis patient's access for ESRD is essential in the care of any ICU ESRD patient. Arteriovenous fistulas (AVFs) and arteriovenous grafts (AVGs) may potentially occlude during hypotension.[119] Loss of dialysis access due to complications from hypotension or potential iatrogenic causes such as restraints could pose a severe hardship for the patient upon recovery from the current illness.[120-122] A relatively recently recognized issue is the need to avoid brachial and subclavian access whenever possible in patient who may currently or imminently need an AVF or AVG. The reason is the frequent development of venous stenosis or thrombosis, which could hamper future access maturation; studies show a high prevalence of thrombosis, over 30%, following peripherally inserted central catheter (PICC) line placement.[123] Tunneled intrajugular catheters are an appropriate option in this population.[124] Subclavian lines, even temporarily, pose similar complication risks. Currently, the Kidney Disease Outcomes Quality Initiative (KDOQI), sponsored by the National Kidney Foundation, recommends not placing PICC lines in patients with CKD.[125]

Common causes of infection in the ESRD population are cellulitis, pneumonia, bacteremia, and pycocystitis.[126] In the absence of a clear cause of infections, a high index of suspicion for access infection should be maintained for ESRD patients presenting with unexplained sepsis if a tunneled dialysis catheter is being used. Generally, catheters do not show signs of infection. Initially, antibiotic therapy should broadly cover gram-positive and gram-negative organisms as these are the most common organisms associated with infection.[127] Vancomycin and gentamicin, prescribed with a loading dose to achieve therapeutic targets based on local sensitivity data, are standard regimens. Considering the prevalence of methicillin-resistant *Staphylococcus aureus* (MRSA), a cephalosporin-only regimen may significantly delay effective therapy.[128] An important consideration is the peritoneal dialysis patient who still makes urine. If feasible, these patients should not receive aminoglycoside therapy in order to maintain their important residual renal function. Instead, a third-generation cephalosporin should be used. Whenever possible, old culture results should be used to guide initial treatment as antibiotic resistance is commonplace. When a tunnel infection is suspected in a hemodialysis patient, as evidenced by an erythematous track around the course of the catheter or purulent drainage from the tunnel itself, catheter removal should urgently occur. When an AVG is infected, urgent removal or resection should also occur. Old, occluded AVGs may represent a source for chronic indolent infections and inflammation.[129]

Ideal fluid management in ESRD patients with sepsis requires close monitoring and repeat assessments. Limited data exist to guide the clinician, and in states of classic sepsis, appropriate volume resuscitation should occur. Nonetheless, thoughtful consideration as to when to moderate fluid repletion in the septic, intubated ESRD patient may improve subsequent ventilator weaning.

KIDNEY TRANSPLANT PATIENTS

Data from the 2008 USRDS survey show that patients with a functioning kidney transplant make up 30% of all ESRD patients.[5] Infectious and cardiovascular complications are the most frequent complications requiring admission to an ICU.

The risk of infection in a kidney transplant patient is complex and related to a number of factors including the health of the allograft, specific donor and recipient factors (CMV status, for example), adequate prophylaxis, up-to-date and effective vaccination, and the level of immunosuppression.[130] In the early post-transplant period, generally defined as 1 month or less, typical postoperative complications, including *Clostridium difficile*–associated colitis, are most common. In months 1 to 6 following transplantation, opportunistic infections and viral infections are the predominant source of infection due to the residual effects of induction immunosuppression. After 6 months, typical community-acquired organisms remain the primary source of infection. Infection with cytomegalovirus is an important cause of morbidity in the transplant population and may be present outside the first 6 months. Specific guidelines exist regarding prophylaxis, screening, and treatment for CMV infection in the solid organ transplant patient.[131]

DRUG DOSING

Drug dosing in CKD patients requires close attention to current levels of kidney function and an understanding of the risks and benefits of the medication prescribed. Two points are worthy of specific attention. First, drug dosing has historically been defined by creatinine clearance and not eGFR.[132,133] The second is that CKD patients, particularly with advanced disease, are a population that is understudied in terms of medication dosing.[134] Antibiotic dosing in the critically ill patient is an area in which the toxicity of overdosage needs to be balanced against the possibility of

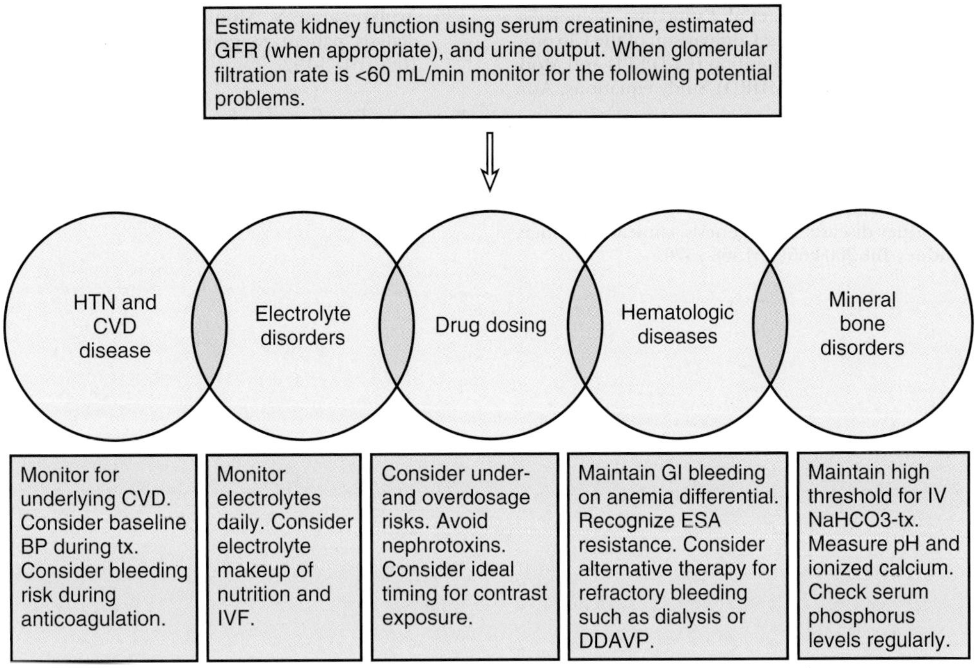

Figure 56.2 Select management principles for patients with chronic kidney disease.

subtherapeutic dosing. Recognizing that serum creatinine may not reflect true GFR is an important part of this process.

SUMMARY

The prevalence of CKD and ESRD in the ICU has increased and this population is prone to poor outcomes. Ideal care of this population includes the recognition that serum creatinine may not reflect GFR, patients are prone to volume overload and volume depletion, and abnormalities in Hb, pH, calcium, and phosphorus may reflect normal and not abnormal physiology. Drug dosing needs to be tailored to individuals, and risks of underdosage as well as overdosage must be considered. See Figure 56-2 for a summary of management principles for CKD.

KEY POINTS

- CKD patients frequently die of CVD; a low index of suspicion for occult CVD should guide caregivers.
- Serum creatinine frequently does not accurately reflect current level of kidney function in the ICU patient.
- CKD is associated with sodium retention and a higher prevalence of hypertension. Acute BP control should take into account baseline BP control to avoid tissue underperfusion.
- Electrolyte disorders, in particular hyperkalemia, in the ICU CKD population, are frequent.
- Acute treatment of chronic metabolic acidosis may lead to iatrogenic falls in serum calcium.

KEY POINTS (Continued)

- Brachial and subclavian access is relatively contraindicated in the advanced CKD and ESRD population owing to their future impact on maturing vascular access for dialysis.
- Drug dosing in CKD patients is poorly studied. Clinicians should be cautious of under- and overdosage issues.

SELECTED REFERENCES

1. Coresh J, Astor BC, Greene T, et al: Prevalence of chronic kidney disease and decreased kidney function in the adult US population: Third National Health and Nutrition Examination Survey. Am J Kidney Dis 2003;41(1):1-12.
7. Levey AS, Coresh J, Balk E, et al: National Kidney Foundation practice guidelines for chronic kidney disease: Evaluation, classification, and stratification. Ann Intern Med 2003;139(2): 137-147.
10. Go AS, Chertow GM, Fan D, et al: Chronic kidney disease and the risks of death, cardiovascular events, and hospitalization. N Engl J Med 2004;351(13):1296-1305.
16. Abutaleb N: Why we should sub-divide CKD stage 3 into early (3a) and late (3b) components. Nephrol Dial Transplant 2007; 22(9):2728-2729.
17. Freedman BI, Kopp JB, Langefeld CD, et al: The apolipoprotein L1 (APOL1) gene and nondiabetic nephropathy in African Americans. J Am Soc Nephrol 2010;21(9):1422-1426.
21. Srisawasdi P, Chaichanajarernkul U, Teerakanjana N, et al: Exogenous interferences with Jaffe creatinine assays: Addition of sodium dodecyl sulfate to reagent eliminates bilirubin and total protein interference with Jaffe methods. J Clin Lab Anal 2010;24(3):123-133.
26. Panteghini M: Enzymatic assays for creatinine: Time for action. Clin Chem Lab Med 2008;46(4):567-572.

34. Korhonen PE, Kivela SL, Aarnio PT, et al: Estimating glomerular filtration rate in hypertensive subjects: Comparison of the Chronic Kidney Disease Epidemiology Collaboration (CKD-EPI) and Modification of Diet in Renal Disease (MDRD) Study equations. Ann Med 2012;44(5):487-493.
41. Rodriguez-Iturbe B, Johnson RJ: The role of renal microvascular disease and interstitial inflammation in salt-sensitive hypertension. Hypertens Res 2010;33(10):975-980.
51. Neumann J, Ligtenberg G, Koomans HA, et al: Sympathetic hyperactivity in chronic kidney disease: Pathogenesis, clinical relevance, and treatment. Kidney Int 2004;65(5):1568-1576.
126. Arulkumaran N, Montero RM, Singer M: Management of the dialysis patient in general intensive care. Br J Anaesth 2012;108(2):183-192.

The complete list of references can be found at www.expertconsult.com.

Acid-Base, Electrolyte, and Metabolic Abnormalities

57

Jason A. Kline | Lawrence S. Weisberg

CHAPTER OUTLINE

Acid-base, electrolyte, and metabolic disturbances are common in the intensive care unit (ICU). Indeed, critically ill patients often suffer from compound acid-base and electrolyte disorders. Successful evaluation and management of such patients requires recognition of common patterns (e.g., hypokalemia and metabolic alkalosis), and an ability to discern one disorder from another. This chapter is intended to provide intensivists with the tools they need for diagnosis and treatment of the acid-base, electrolyte, and metabolic disorders encountered in the care of critically ill patients. By reviewing the elements of normal physiology in these areas, and presenting a general diagnostic scheme for each condition, we hope to provide readers with a foundation for approaching not only common, but novel and complex disorders.

ACID-BASE HOMEOSTASIS

Normal acid-base balance depends on the cooperation of at least two vital organ systems: the lungs and the kidneys. The gastrointestinal (GI) tract also is involved in many acid-base disturbances. Multiorgan system involvement, therefore, provides the backdrop for the acid-base disorders commonly seen in critically ill patients.

NORMAL ACID-BASE PHYSIOLOGY

Normal biochemical and physiologic function requires that the extracellular pH be maintained within a very narrow range. Although the "normal" range of pH in clinical laboratories is 7.35 to 7.45 pH units, the actual pH in vivo varies considerably less.[1] This tight control is maintained by a complex homeostatic mechanism involving buffers and the elimination of volatile acid by respiration.

The principal extracellular buffer system is the carbonic acid/bicarbonate pair. The equilibrium relationships of the components of this system are illustrated as follows:[1]

$$H_2O + CO_2 \leftrightarrow H_2CO_3 \leftrightarrow H^+ + HCO_3^-$$

From these relationships, the Henderson-Hasselbalch equation is derived:

$$pH = pK + \log_{10} \frac{HCO_3^-}{\alpha_{CO2} \cdot PCO_2}$$

In this equation, α_{CO2} is the solubility coefficient of CO_2 (0.03), and pK is the equilibrium constant for this buffer pair (6.1). Rearrangement yields the Henderson equation:

$$H^+ = 24 \cdot \frac{PCO_2}{HCO_3^-}$$

It is apparent from this equation that disturbances in the proton concentration of the extracellular fluid (ECF) (and blood) may be due to perturbation in the numerator, the denominator, or both. Disturbances that affect the P_{CO_2} primarily are called *respiratory* disturbances, and those that affect the HCO_3^- primarily are called *metabolic*.

Acid-base homeostasis depends on compensation for a primary disturbance. Compensation for a respiratory disturbance is metabolic, and compensation for a metabolic disturbance is respiratory. Furthermore, it is clear from the previous equations that in order to mitigate the change in proton concentration or pH, the direction of the compensation must be the same as the direction of the primary disturbance. Thus, consumption of bicarbonate will be accompanied by hyperventilation and a consequent reduction in P_{CO_2}. A simple acid-base disturbance is considered to consist of the primary disturbance *and* its normal compensation. A complex acid-base disturbance consists of more than one primary disturbance. In order to detect complex acid-base disturbances, one must be familiar with both the direction and magnitude of normal compensation (shown in Table 57.1).[2] More than one metabolic disturbance may coexist (e.g., metabolic acidosis and metabolic alkalosis), but only one respiratory disturbance is possible at a time.

In the present section, we will discuss disorders that affect the metabolic component of acid-base homeostasis: metabolic acidosis and metabolic alkalosis. Respiratory disturbances affecting acid-base balance will be discussed elsewhere (Chapters 37 and 40).

METABOLIC ACIDOSIS

DEFINITION AND CLASSIFICATION

A metabolic acidosis is a process that, if unopposed, would cause *acidemia* (a high hydrogen ion concentration, or low pH, of the blood) by reducing the extracellular bicarbonate concentration. The extracellular bicarbonate concentration may be reduced by either addition of acid and consequent consumption of bicarbonate, or by primary loss of bicarbonate.

An adult eating a normal diet generates 16,000 to 20,000 mmol of acid a day.[3] Almost all of that acid is in the form of carbonic acid, resulting from CO_2 and water generation in the metabolism of carbohydrates and fats. Individuals with normal ventilatory capacity eliminate this prodigious acid load through the lungs, thus the term *volatile acid*. The remainder of the daily acid load, about 1 mmol/kg body weight per day, derives from metabolism of phosphate- and sulfate-rich protein (yielding phosphoric and sulfuric acid). These nonvolatile or *fixed acids* are buffered, primarily by extracellular bicarbonate under normal circumstances. The kidneys are responsible for regenerating the consumed bicarbonate by secreting hydrogen ions (protons) in the distal nephron. These secreted protons must be buffered in the tubule lumen in order to allow elimination of the daily fixed acid load within the physiologic constraint of the minimum urinary pH. The urinary buffers are composed of the filtered sodium salts of the phosphoric acid and ammonia, which is synthesized in the proximal tubule and acidified in the collecting duct to form ammonium (NH_4^+). Under conditions of acid loading, the normal kidney reabsorbs all the filtered bicarbonate in the proximal tubule. Urinary net acid excretion therefore comprises phosphoric acid (so-called titratable acidity, because it is quantified by titrating the urine with alkali to pH 7.40) and ammonium, less any excreted bicarbonate.[4]

Many factors modify the kidney's capacity to regulate acid-base balance. For example, renal ammoniagenesis is stimulated by acidemia, and inhibited by alkalemia, and thus participates in a homeostatic feedback loop.[1] Hyperkalemia inhibits and hypokalemia stimulates renal ammoniagenesis. Hypokalemia further stimulates acid secretion by activating the Na^+-H^+ exchanger in the proximal tubule and the H^+/K^+-ATPase in the collecting duct. Finally, aldosterone stimulates both proton and K^+ secretion in the collecting duct. For these reasons, hypokalemia tends to perpetuate a metabolic alkalosis, and hyperkalemia a metabolic acidosis.[1]

Metabolic acidosis can be caused by excessive production of fixed acid, decreased renal secretion of fixed acid, or loss of bicarbonate, either through the kidney or through the intestine.[4] The net effect of any of these processes is a reduction in the blood bicarbonate concentration. The plasma *anion gap* helps to distinguish among the various causes of metabolic acidosis. Of course, because of charge neutrality, the sum of the concentration of all cations in the plasma is equal to the sum of all the anions. By convention, however, the anion gap is defined as the difference between the plasma sodium concentration and the sum of the bicarbonate and chloride concentrations. It represents the concentration of anions that are normally unmeasured by a basic metabolic chemistry panel.[5] The anion gap normally is about 8 mmol/L, but it varies widely according to the methods employed by the clinical chemistry laboratory.[6] The anion gap is composed mainly of albumin, along with phosphates, sulfates, and organic anions.

Table 57.1 Expected Compensation for Simple Acid-Base Disorders

Disorder	Primary Disturbance	Compensation	Magnitude	Time to Completion
Metabolic acidosis	↓ $[HCO_3^-]$	↓ P_{CO_2}	1.5 • $[HCO_3^-]$ + 8	12-24 hours
Metabolic alkalosis	↑ $[HCO_3^-]$	↑ P_{CO_2}	0.9 • $[HCO_3^-]$ + 9	12-24 hours
Respiratory acidosis, acute	↑ P_{CO_2}	↑ $[HCO_3^-]$	1 mmol/L/10 mm Hg	<6 hours
Respiratory acidosis, chronic	↑ P_{CO_2}	↑ $[HCO_3^-]$	3.5 mmol/L/10 mm Hg	>5 days
Respiratory alkalosis, acute	↓ P_{CO_2}	↓ $[HCO_3^-]$	2 mmol/L/10 mm Hg	<6 hours
Respiratory alkalosis, chronic	↓ P_{CO_2}	↓ $[HCO_3^-]$	5 mmol/L/10 mm Hg	>7 days

There are two important pitfalls in the interpretation of the anion gap. First, because the anion gap is proportional to the plasma albumin concentration, hypoalbuminemia (common in critically ill patients) will lower the "baseline" anion gap (by approximately 2.5 mmol/L for each g/dL decline in the albumin concentration).[7] Thus, profound hypoalbuminemia may falsely lower the anion gap, and thus mask a high anion gap acidosis. Second, alkalemia increases the anion gap by causing lactate generation and by titrating plasma buffers, most notably albumin.[8] (Thus, in respiratory alkalosis, the bicarbonate concentration will be low in compensation, and the anion gap may be elevated, giving a false impression of a high anion gap metabolic acidosis by inspection of the electrolytes alone.)

If bicarbonate is lost (e.g., through diarrhea), or hydrochloric acid is gained (e.g., renal tubular acidosis or administration of unbuffered amino acid solutions[9]), the bicarbonate concentration falls with a commensurate increase in the plasma chloride concentration; thus the anion gap is unchanged. If, on the other hand, bicarbonate is lost in buffering an organic acid such as lactic acid or a ketoacid, the decrement in the bicarbonate concentration is more or less matched by an increase in the anion gap. These processes are illustrated in Figure 57.1.

Box 57.1 lists the causes of hyperchloremic metabolic acidosis. Two diagnoses are of particular interest in the critical care arena. First is the posthypocapnic metabolic acidosis, in which bicarbonate falls in compensation for a chronic respiratory alkalosis. When "normal" ventilation is restored, the pH falls until bicarbonate can be retained, giving the appearance of a hyperchloremic metabolic acidosis. This emphasizes the importance of observation over time in the analysis of acid-base status. The second entity of interest is a so-called dilutional hyperchloremic acidosis. This is seen in patients who are rapidly resuscitated with large volumes of isotonic saline solution. The acidosis traditionally has been attributed to dilution of blood bicarbonate. Analysis based on physical-chemistry principles may better explain the phenomenon (see later).[10]

The differential diagnosis of high anion gap metabolic acidosis is limited (Box 57.2). The most common cause in critically ill patients is a lactic acidosis. The causes of lactic acidosis are numerous. As shown in Box 57.3, they are divided into type A (imbalance between tissue oxygen demand and supply) and type B (impaired oxygen utilization).[5] Diabetic ketoacidosis (DKA) (Chapter 58) and intoxications (Chapter 68) are discussed elsewhere. Two causes of high anion gap acidosis recently added to the differential diagnosis, and of particular relevance to intensivists, are *pyroglutamic acidosis* and intoxication with *propylene glycol*.

Pyroglutamic acid is a metabolic intermediate in the γ-glutamyl cycle, one product of which is glutathione. Pyroglutamic acidosis may be congenital (caused by one of several enzyme deficiencies) or acquired.[8] The acquired syndrome may be caused by acetaminophen (which depletes glutathione, leading to uninhibited pyroglutamic acid synthesis), β-lactam antibiotics, or glycine deficiency. The

Box 57.1 Causes of Hyperchloremic Metabolic Acidosis

Extrarenal Loss of Base

Diarrhea
Pancreatic fistula
Ureteral diversion

Extrarenal Gain of Acid

Ammonium chloride
Hydrochloric acid
Sodium chloride

Renal Loss of Base

Type II renal tubular acidosis
Posthypocapnic state
Excretion of organic anions (bicarbonate precursors)
Toluene inhalation (glue sniffing)
Diabetic ketoacidosis

Renal Acid Excretory Defect

Type IV renal tubular acidosis
- Chronic kidney disease
- Hypoaldosteronism
- Urinary tract obstruction

Type I renal tubular acidosis
- Sickle cell nephropathy
- Lupus nephritis
- Renal transplant

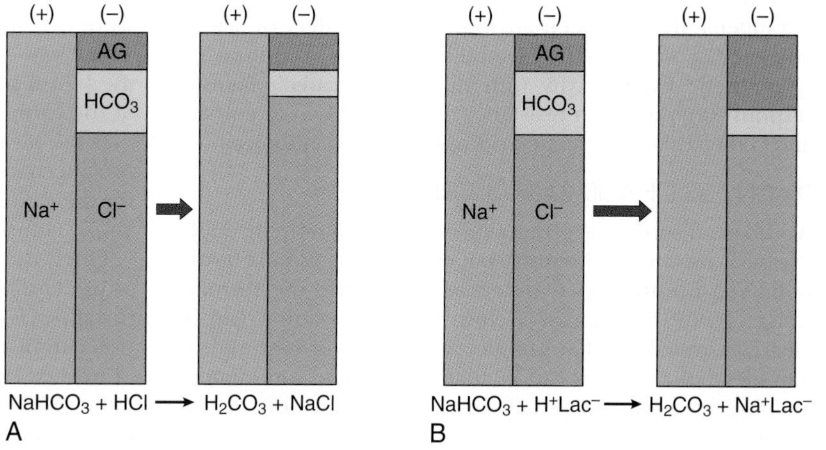

Figure 57.1 The generation of hyperchloremic and anion gap (AG) acidoses. Blocks represent the ionic composition of the plasma, cations (+) to the left and anions (−) to the right. In each of the panels (A and B), the bar to the left represents the basal or normal state. The AG is shown in red. **A,** The change in the ionic composition of the plasma when hydrochloric acid is added. The chloride concentration increases as bicarbonate is consumed. **B,** The effect of addition of an organic acid such as lactic acid, in which case the bicarbonate is consumed and the AG increases proportionately. Cl, chloride; H_2CO_3, carbonic acid; Na, sodium; $NaHCO_3$, sodium bicarbonate.

Box 57.2 Causes of High Anion Gap Metabolic Acidosis

Ketoacidoses
- Diabetic
- Alcoholic
- Starvation

Intoxications
- Methanol
- Ethylene glycol
- Propylene glycol
- Salicylate

Pyroglutamic acidosis
- Congenital
- Acquired

Lactic acidosis (see Box 57-3)

Uremic acidosis

acidosis may be profound and the anion gap greater than 30 mmol/L.[11] Definitive diagnosis is made by urinary screen for organic acids. In practice, however, circumstantial evidence suggests the acquired syndrome and the diagnosis is supported by a favorable response to appropriate intervention.

Propylene glycol is a solvent for medications, many of which are commonly infused intravenously in critically ill patients, such as lorazepam, nitroglycerin, etomidate, and phenytoin. Propylene glycol is metabolized by alcohol dehydrogenase to lactic acid. High anion gap acidosis has been associated with high- and even low-dose infusions, particularly of lorazepam.[7,12] Thus, development of a high anion gap acidosis in a critically ill patient should prompt a search for a source of propylene glycol, because withdrawal of the agent will promptly alleviate the acidosis.

CONSEQUENCES OF ACIDEMIA

It has been generally accepted that severe acidemia (pH < 7.20) is associated with a variety of deleterious effects. Of particular concern are the cardiovascular effects, including pressure-resistant arterial vasodilation, venoconstriction, diminished myocardial contractility, and impaired hepatic and renal perfusion.[13] (Some controversy exists as to which of these effects are directly caused by acidemia.[4]) A predisposition to malignant arrhythmias has been reported in vitro and in animal models. Finally, numerous metabolic derangements have been attributed to the effect of acidemia on key enzymes in metabolic pathways, resulting in sympathetic hyperactivity with diminished catecholamine responsiveness; insulin resistance and suppressed glycolysis; and reduced hepatic lactic acid uptake and metabolism.[14]

DIAGNOSIS OF ACID-BASE DISORDERS

Acid-base disorders are revealed most commonly through the basic metabolic chemistry panel, when the plasma bicarbonate concentration is noted to be outside the normal range. If the bicarbonate is low, and if the anion gap is clearly elevated on that sample, a diagnosis of high anion gap metabolic acidosis can be made with some confidence, keeping in mind the pitfalls in the interpretation of the anion gap mentioned earlier.[7]

Box 57.3 Causes of Lactic Acidosis

Type A (Tissue Oxygen Supply: Demand Mismatch)

Decreased tissue oxygen delivery
- Shock
- Hypoxemia
- Severe anemia
- Carbon monoxide poisoning

Increased tissue oxygen demand
- Grand mal seizure
- Extreme exercise

Type B (Impaired Tissue Oxygen Utilization)

Sepsis/systemic inflammatory response syndrome

Diabetes mellitus

Malignancy

Thiamine deficiency

Inborn errors of metabolism

Human immunodeficiency virus infection

Malaria

Drugs/toxins
- Ethanol
- Metformin
- Zidovudine
- Didanosine
- Stavudine
- Lamivudine
- Zalcitabine
- Salicylate
- Propofol
- Niacin
- Isoniazid
- Nitroprusside
- Cyanide
- Catecholamines
- Cocaine
- Acetaminophen
- Streptozotocin
- Sorbitol/fructose
- Carboplatin
- Entecavir
- Linezolid

Liver failure

Alkalemia

D-Lactic Acidosis

If the bicarbonate is low and the anion gap normal, two possibilities exist: either a hyperchloremic metabolic acidosis or a respiratory alkalosis with metabolic compensation. These two entities can be distinguished by examination of the blood pH and blood gases, a low pH being diagnostic of the former.

If the bicarbonate concentration is high, again there are two alternative diagnoses, requiring blood pH measurement for their differentiation: either a metabolic alkalosis or metabolic compensation for a respiratory acidosis.

Once the primary disturbance has been identified, the astute clinician, recognizing the possibility of a mixed disturbance, is obligated to ask, "Is that all there is?" This question can be answered only by an understanding of the rules of normal compensation for simple acid-base disorders (see Table 57.1).[2] Knowing at least the expected direction of compensation will allow the clinician to diagnose the most obvious mixed disturbances. For example, if the pH is low, the bicarbonate is low, and the P_{CO_2} is above 40 mm Hg, there is clearly a mixed metabolic and respiratory acidosis. Similarly, if the pH is high, the bicarbonate is high, and the P_{CO_2} is below 40 mm Hg, the diagnosis is a mixed respiratory and metabolic alkalosis. More subtle mixed disorders can be diagnosed only by understanding not only the expected direction, but the expected magnitude of compensation. This will allow one to conclude, for example, whether the hyperventilation in a patient with metabolic acidosis is appropriate (expected compensation), inadequate (a separate respiratory acidosis), or excessive (a separate respiratory alkalosis).

The preceding method permits the diagnosis of simple and dual acid-base disorders. Triple acid-base disorders can be diagnosed only by comparing the change in the anion gap with the change in the plasma bicarbonate concentration. Most simply conceived, the fall in the bicarbonate should equal the rise in the anion gap (see Fig. 57.1). If the rise in the anion gap exceeds the fall in the bicarbonate, a metabolic alkalosis is said to be present in addition to the high anion gap acidosis. Conversely, if the fall in the bicarbonate exceeds the rise in the anion gap, mixed hyperchloremic and high anion gap acidoses are said to coexist. Although this analysis is useful in the case of large discrepancies, in more subtle cases it is confounded by theoretical and practical considerations.[5,15]

The classical approach to acid-base disorders described earlier has been challenged recently by proponents of a physical-chemistry approach described originally by Stewart.[16] According to this method, the pH of the blood depends on the ionization of water by the difference in the concentration of so-called strong ions (the strong ion difference, or SID). The SID offers a quantitative approach to measuring the degree of acidosis in hyperchloremic metabolic acidosis. Although there is evidence that this approach may offer prognostic capabilities in patients with severe sepsis and septic shock with hyperchloremic metabolic acidosis, the complexity of the equations for calculating the SID may make this method cumbersome in clinical settings.[17] The main utility of this construct in the critical care setting seems to be its explanation of a hyperchloremic metabolic acidosis in patients who receive large volumes of isotonic saline.

TREATMENT OF METABOLIC ACIDOSIS

Treatment of metabolic acidosis is aimed at reversing the adverse consequences of acidemia. Treatment of hyperchloremic metabolic acidosis is straightforward. In cases of acute metabolic acidosis, treatment depends on successful therapy of the underlying cause (e.g., diarrhea) and correction of the bicarbonate deficit, usually in the form of sodium bicarbonate. One can estimate the bicarbonate deficit as follows:

$$HCO_3^- \text{ deficit} = \left([HCO_3^-]_{\text{final}} - [HCO_3^-]_{\text{initial}}\right) \times (\text{volume of distribution of } HCO_3^-)$$

The difficulty in accurately estimating this value arises from two factors: First, the apparent volume of distribution of bicarbonate varies more than twofold—from 50% of body weight to 100% of body weight—and is inversely proportional to the initial bicarbonate concentration.[18] Second, there are often many simultaneous processes in a critically ill patient that tend to ameliorate or exacerbate the metabolic acidosis, such as vomiting, shock, and liver failure. In order to avoid overshoot alkalemia, it is prudent to estimate the volume of distribution to be 50% of the body weight[14] and to target an increase in the bicarbonate concentration of no more than 8 mmol/L over 12 to 24 hours.

Sodium bicarbonate generally is considered to be the alkalinizing agent of choice for severe acidemia. Alternative alkalinizing agents such as citrate, acetate, and lactate, which under normal circumstances are oxidized in the liver to bicarbonate, should not be used to treat acidemia in patients with suspected or confirmed hepatic impairment or circulatory compromise. The sodium bicarbonate should be administered as a continuous infusion, the concentration of which should be guided by the patient's serum sodium concentration. Bolus injection of undiluted ampules of sodium bicarbonate (1000 mmol/L) should be used with great restraint and only in patients with the most severe acidemia because of the risk of hyperosmolality. Large volumes of any bicarbonate solution can lead to volume overload, a reduction in the ionized calcium concentration (see "Hypocalcemia"), and increased generation of CO_2. This last effect will tend to cause a respiratory acidosis in patients with ventilatory insufficiency. Plasma electrolytes and blood gases must be monitored frequently to guide adjustments in the composition of the solution and its rate of infusion.

Tris(hydroxymethyl)aminomethane, or THAM, is an amino alcohol that buffers without generating CO_2. It has the advantage, therefore, of avoiding a superimposed respiratory acidosis. It has been used successfully in animals and humans with various metabolic acidoses.[13,19] It is eliminated by the kidney, and thus should be used with caution in the setting of renal insufficiency. Risks include hyperkalemia, hypoglycemia, and hepatic necrosis (in neonates).[7]

The treatment of choice for lactic acidosis is reversal of the underlying cause of the acidosis (see Box 57.3). Pending resolution of the underlying disorder, however, the intensivist is often confronted with an unstable patient who is profoundly acidemic. Treatment at this stage is controversial.[5,13] The debate has focused on the potentially deleterious effects of bicarbonate administration in lactic acidosis.[20] In addition to the effects mentioned earlier, bicarbonate in animal models of lactic acidosis has been associated with increased lactate generation, reduction in intracellular pH, increased venous P_{CO_2}, and reduction in cardiac output. (This last effect correlates well with the reduction in ionized calcium concentration.[13]) Studies in humans likewise show no improvement in cardiac output, morbidity rate, or mortality rate with bicarbonate.[13] Continuous venovenous hemodialysis (e.g., CVVHD) may be a promising tool for treating lactic acidosis, because it provides large amounts of bicarbonate without the risks of volume overload or hypocalcemia. There are several reported cases of successful treatment of metformin-associated lactic acidosis using continuous hemodialysis.[21,22] Because of its superior short-term clearance compared with continuous renal replacement therapy, however, conventional hemodialysis remains the preferred treatment for metformin intoxication.[23] Treatment of DKA and the acidoses associated with other intoxications are discussed in Chapters 58 and 68, respectively.

METABOLIC ALKALOSIS

DEFINITION AND CLASSIFICATION

Metabolic alkalosis is a process leading to accumulation of extracellular bicarbonate that, if unopposed, will result in an increase in the plasma pH (alkalemia). It can be caused either by a gain of bicarbonate or a loss of fixed acid from the ECF. The causes of metabolic alkalosis have been described.[24] In its pure form, it is accompanied by hypoventilation (CO_2 retention).[2]

From a pathophysiologic perspective, metabolic alkalosis is divided into those factors that generate the alkalosis and those factors that maintain or perpetuate it.[24,25] Metabolic alkalosis is generated by addition of bicarbonate to the blood. This can occur either by loss of acid from the body or by addition of exogenous alkali. Loss of acid may be from the stomach (e.g., vomiting or nasogastric suction) or kidney. Renal acid loss is enhanced by a high rate of sodium delivery to the distal nephron, high circulating mineralocorticoid levels, potassium depletion, and high rates of ammoniagenesis.

Because of the kidney's prodigious ability to excrete bicarbonate, however, addition of bicarbonate to the blood is not sufficient to cause a sustained metabolic alkalosis. Some mechanism(s) to maintain the alkalosis must prevail. The most common mechanism contributing to the maintenance of metabolic alkalosis is volume depletion, either absolute or relative (e.g., congestive heart failure), which (1) reduces glomerular filtration, (2) enhances tubular bicarbonate reabsorption, and (3) causes secondary hyperaldosteronism, further enhancing urinary acidification. Another common perpetuating factor is potassium depletion, which stimulates proton secretion at several sites along the nephron.[24-26]

Patients with metabolic alkalosis and signs of volume expansion—especially hypertension—usually have excess mineralocorticoid as the explanation for the metabolic alkalosis. Aldosterone and glucocorticoids (other than dexamethasone) stimulate renal loss of acid and potassium, and thereby generate and maintain the alkalosis.

Most cases of clinically significant metabolic alkalosis are maintained by loss of chloride or potassium. Although total body sodium (and hence, volume) derangements are not directly responsible for the generation and maintenance of the metabolic alkalosis, potassium and chloride depletion are commonly seen in settings of volume depletion or excess. Therefore, from a clinical standpoint, it is useful to approach the patient with metabolic alkalosis centering on the history and physical examination, with special attention to the ECF volume status, followed by sequential analysis of blood chemistries.[26] Causes of metabolic alkalosis are shown in Box 57.4. One entity unique to critically ill patients is posthypercapnic metabolic alkalosis. This syndrome is caused by abrupt treatment (usually with tracheal intubation and mechanical ventilation) of a chronic respiratory acidosis. The renal bicarbonate retention that compensated for the chronic respiratory acidosis persists (because of volume depletion) after restoration of a normal P_{CO_2}, resulting in the high pH and high plasma bicarbonate characteristic of metabolic alkalosis. The key to the diagnosis is the history and sequential analysis of blood chemistries.[24]

Box 57.4 Causes of Metabolic Alkalosis

Intravascular Volume Depletion, Absolute or "Effective"

- Gastrointestinal acid loss
  - Vomiting or nasogastric suction
  - Villous adenoma
  - Chloride diarrhea
- Renal acid loss
  - Diuretics (loop, thiazide)
  - Bartter syndrome
  - Gitelman syndrome
  - Magnesium depletion
  - Posthypercapnic state
  - Congestive heart failure
  - Hepatic cirrhosis/ascites

Intravascular Volume Expansion

- High renin, high aldosterone
  - Renal artery stenosis
  - Accelerated hypertension
  - Renin-secreting tumor
- Low renin, high aldosterone
  - Primary aldosteronism
- Low renin, low aldosterone
  - Cushing syndrome or disease
  - Exogenous mineralocorticoid
  - Apparent mineralocorticoid excess syndrome
  - Liddle syndrome
- Renal insufficiency
  - Exogenous alkali load
  - Milk-alkali syndrome

Adapted from Palmer BF, Alpern RJ: Metabolic alkalosis. J Am Soc Nephrol 1997;8(9):1462-1469.

CLINICAL CONSEQUENCES

Alkalemia in critically ill patients is associated with increased mortality rate.[27] Patients with combined metabolic and respiratory alkalosis have a higher mortality rate than those with respiratory alkalosis alone, and mortality rate in alkalemia is roughly proportional to the pH.[27] Although no causal relationship between alkalemia and mortality rate has been established, the pathophysiology of alkalemia is far from benign.[25]

First, metabolic alkalosis suppresses ventilation, causing CO_2 retention and relative hypoxemia.[28] Second, alkalemia acutely increases hemoglobin's oxygen affinity (Bohr effect). Third, respiratory alkalosis causes vasoconstriction, particularly in the cerebral circulation.[25] All these processes tend to decrease tissue oxygen delivery.[29] (Note that chronic alkalemia inhibits 2,3-diphosphoglycerate synthesis, allowing normalization of the oxyhemoglobin desaturation curve, mitigating tissue hypoxia to some extent.) These alterations in tissue oxygen delivery could be responsible at least in part for some of the clinical manifestations of metabolic alkalosis.

Because alkalemia causes a decrease in ionized calcium concentration (see discussion under "Calcium Homeostasis"), many of the neuromuscular manifestations of metabolic alkalosis overlap with those of hypocalcemia, including paresthesias, tetany, and a predisposition to seizures.[1] The acutely diminished tissue oxygen delivery to the brain may contribute to initial confusion and obtundation seen with metabolic alkalosis.

Metabolic alkalosis often is accompanied by hypokalemia and hypomagnesemia. Thus, there is an association between alkalosis and arrythmias,[24] but an independent effect of the alkalosis on cardiac arrythmogenesis has not been established.

Increases in blood lactate concentration may occur in patients with metabolic alkalosis due to upregulation of phosphofructokinase and thus glycolysis, and because of tissue hypoxia (see earlier).[8] With severe metabolic alkalosis (arterial pH above 7.55), the tissue hypoxia may be so marked that compensatory hypoventilation will be overridden by hypoxic drive, resulting in a normal to low arterial P_{CO_2} and elevated blood lactate levels (so-called "lactic alkalosis").[30]

TREATMENT

Treatment of metabolic alkalosis entails correcting the factor(s) responsible for its maintenance and, if possible, correcting the factor that generated the alkalosis. Once the underlying diagnosis is clear (see Box 57.4), therapy is usually straightforward. If the metabolic alkalosis is maintained by chloride depletion and ECF volume contraction, the intravascular volume should be restored to normal, usually with intravenous isotonic saline.[24,25] Potassium should be given, as KCl, to replace any deficits (see "Disorders of Potassium Homeostasis"), because potassium depletion perpetuates the metabolic alkalosis. If nasogastric suction cannot be stopped, acid loss can be reduced by the use of H_2 blockers and proton pump inhibitors.

Treating patients with metabolic alkalosis in the setting of volume overload and diminished effective circulating volume (e.g., congestive heart failure, hepatic cirrhosis) is more challenging, because saline infusion is contraindicated. Unless hyperkalemia is present, chloride should be replenished with KCl supplementation. In rare cases of concurent hyperkalemia, acetazolamide (a carbonic anydrase inhibitor) may be of benefit as it produces a bicarbonate diuresis. Acetazolamide should be avoided in patients with hypokalemia, because the alkaline diuresis will cause renal potassium wasting.[24] Another potential complication of acetazolamide administration, particularly in patients with impending ventilatory failure, is worsening of hypercapnia owing to inhibition of red blood cell carbonic anhydrase and impaired CO_2 transport.[25] Hydrochloric acid infusion, as a 0.1 to 0.25 N solution, has been used with success in patients with severe metabolic alkalosis ($pH > 7.55$ and systemic instability such as encephalopathy or cardiac arrhythmia[24]) refractory to conventional measures.[25,31] Correction of the metabolic disturbances has been reported with infusion of 0.25 N HCl at 100 mL/hour over about 12 hours.[31] Extreme care must be taken to ensure that the infusion catheter is properly positioned within the vena cava, because the solution is highly caustic. Plasma chemistries must be monitored frequently in order to avoid overcorrection. If renal function is severely impaired or medical therapy is not possible, hemodialysis against a low-bicarbonate bath may be used.[24]

In states of primary mineralocorticoid excess, an aldosterone antagonist such as spironolactone should be used until the underlying abnormality can be corrected. Other potassium-sparing diuretics, such as amiloride and triamterene, are useful as well and are essential in managing the rare patient with Liddle syndrome.

POTASSIUM HOMEOSTASIS

NORMAL POTASSIUM PHYSIOLOGY

Disorders of potassium (K) homeostasis are common in hospitalized patients and may be associated with severe adverse clinical outcomes, including death.[32,33] Prevention and proper treatment of hyper- and hypokalemia depend on an understanding of the underlying physiology.

The total body potassium content of a 70-kg adult is about 3500 mmol, of which only 2% (about 70 mmol) is extracellular.[34] This uneven distribution reflects the large potassium concentration gradient between the intracellular (Ki ≈140 mmol/L) and the extracellular (Ke ≈ 4.5 mmol/L) space, a gradient that is maintained by the intrinsic ion permeabilities of cell membranes and by Na^+/K^+-ATPase, the sodium-potassium pump.[35] The Ke : Ki ratio largely determines the resting membrane potential of cells and thus is crucial for proper function of excitable tissues (muscle and nerve).[35] Small absolute changes in Ke will perturb the ratio significantly. Therefore, disturbances of Ke (measured as changes in plasma potassium concentration, or P_K) may have serious, even fatal, consequences mainly in the form of excitable tissue dysfunction.

It is not surprising, therefore, that the extracellular potassium concentration is tightly regulated. In fact, two separate and cooperative systems participate in potassium homeostasis. One system regulates *external potassium balance*: the total body parity of potassium elimination with potassium intake. The other system regulates *internal potassium balance*: the distribution of potassium between the intracellular and extracellular fluid compartments. This latter system provides a short-term defense against changes in the plasma potassium concentration (P_K) that might otherwise result from total body potassium losses or gains.

REGULATION OF INTERNAL POTASSIUM BALANCE

Internal potassium balance serves to protect against changes in Ke; potassium tends to move out of cells during potassium depletion and into cells following potassium intake. This process tends to prevent drastic alterations of Ke : Ki.[36,37] The factors that influence internal potassium balance include hormones, acid-base status, plasma tonicity, exercise, and cell integrity (Box 57.5).

The direction and magnitude of an *acid-base*-related change in P_K depend on the nature and the duration of the disturbance. The most consistent and pronounced relationship between changes in pH and P_K occurs in acute mineral (hyperchloremic) acidosis, where there is a strong inverse relationship between these two variables.[38-40] Interestingly, *hypo*kalemia is seen with prolonged mineral acidosis in patients with normal renal function and reflects increased renal potassium excretion.[39] Unlike mineral acidoses, however, even severe acute organic (high anion gap)

Box 57.5 Factors Affecting Internal Potassium Balance

Factors Causing Cellular Potassium Influx

Insulin
β_2-Adrenergic receptor agonist
(Metabolic alkalosis)*

Factors Causing Cellular Potassium Efflux

Cell ischemia/lysis
Exercise
Plasma hypertonicity
α-Adrenergic receptor agonist
(Metabolic acidosis)*

*Factors shown in paretheses have a minor or variable effect. See text.

acidoses are not usually associated with hyperkalemia.[41-44] Indeed, organic acidoses, such as lactic acidosis, actually tend to cause cellular potassium uptake.[41] Nonetheless, factors coincident with the acidosis may alter P_K. For example, mesenteric ischemia may result in both lactic acidosis (from anaerobic metabolism) and hyperkalemia. Even the hyperkalemia so commonly seen in patients with DKA does not result from the acidemia; rather, it appears to be a consequence of the characteristic insulin deficiency and hyperglycemia (see discussion of hypertonicity in the next paragraph).[44] Respiratory disturbances typically alter P_K less than metabolic disturbances. Alkaloses, respiratory or metabolic, have less effect on P_K than their corresponding acidoses.[38] Bicarbonate administration, which was once thought to reduce the P_K by stimulating cellular potassium uptake,[45] is now known to have very little if any immediate effect on internal potassium balance,[46,47] except perhaps in patients with preexisting severe metabolic acidosis.[41] It is clear, however, that longstanding alkalemia causes urinary potassium losses that may over time result in profound potassium depletion.[48]

Hypertonicity, as seen with hypertonic fluid administration[49] or diabetic hyperglycemic states,[50] leads to hyperkalemia, probably as a result of potassium efflux from cells by way of solvent drag. Fatal hyperkalemia has been attributed to this phenomenon in diabetic patients with end-stage renal disease (ESRD).[51]

Exercise causes a transient shift of potassium out of cells. Clinically significant hyperkalemia may result from exercise[52,53] (and clinically misleading local venous hyperkalemia results from fist clenching during phlebotomy[54]).

REGULATION OF EXTERNAL POTASSIUM BALANCE

In contrast to the prodigious capacity of the kidney to excrete potassium,[55] renal potassium conservation is imperfect and explains why significant potassium depletion and hypokalemia may result from dietary potassium deficiency alone.[56]

Normally, 90% to 95% of dietary potassium is eliminated through the kidney, and only about 5% to 10% through the intestine. It is the kidney that is almost entirely responsible for matching potassium output to potassium intake in order to maintain total body potassium constant.[57] The majority of potassium excreted by the kidney derives from potassium secretion in the distal nephron (connecting tubule and collecting duct).[57] Virtually all regulation of potassium excretion takes place at this site in the nephron, under the influence of two principal factors: the rate of flow and sodium delivery through that part of the nephron, and the effect of aldosterone.[57] Potassium secretion is directly proportional to flow rate and sodium delivery through the distal nephron, explaining in part why diuretic use often is accompanied by hypokalemia.

Metabolic acidosis with acidemia results in inhibition of renal potassium secretion.[41] In contrast, metabolic alkalosis and bicarbonate delivery to the distal nephron stimulate kaliuresis by increasing the electrochemical "driving force" for potassium secretion.[57] Other anions that are poorly reabsorbed in the distal nephron (e.g., synthetic penicillins) have a similar effect to stimulate potassium secretion.[58]

It is well established that aldosterone participates in a homeostatic feedback loop with P_K such that increases in P_K stimulate adrenal aldosterone production, which in turn reduces P_K primarily by stimulating renal potassium excretion.[57] Hypokalemia is a prominent feature of primary aldosteronism (Conn syndrome) because the high circulating aldosterone levels are accompanied by volume expansion and thus a high rate of sodium delivery to the distal nephron. When circulating aldosterone levels are high due to volume depletion (secondary aldosteronism), the increase in distal potassium secretion is offset by a decrease in distal nephron flow, thus mitigating renal potassium loss. Indeed, it is only when patients with secondary hyperaldosteronism (e.g., in congestive heart failure or hepatic cirrhosis) are treated with diuretic drugs that distal nephron flow is increased and hypokalemia may ensue.

Magnesium deficiency is associated with renal potassium wasting and may result in severe potassium depletion.[59] Because magnesium, like calcium, acts to stabilize excitable membranes, the deleterious effects of hypokalemia on the myocardium are magnified by concurrent hypomagnesemia (see "Clinical Manifestations" later).[60]

The effect of dexamethasone (a pure glucocorticoid) to enhance renal potassium excretion appears to result entirely from hemodynamic changes that cause an increase in glomerular filtration rate and distal flow rate. All other glucocorticoids tend to further stimulate potassium secretion in proportion to their mineralocorticoid activity.[57]

DISORDERS OF POTASSIUM HOMEOSTASIS

Disorders of potassium homeostasis may be conveniently divided according to the duration of the disturbance: acute (<48 hours' duration) or chronic. Such a distinction is particularly applicable to the medical intensive care setting where blood chemistries are sampled frequently and a patient's condition and therapy may change radically over a short time. In addition, the approach to treatment varies according to the acuity of the disturbance. The treatment of acute disturbances is largely independent of their cause, whereas the rational treatment of chronic disturbances depends on understanding their pathogenesis.

Box 57.6 Causes of Acute Hyperkalemia

Excessive Potassium Intake
- Oral
- Intravenous
- Blood transfusion
- Cardioplegic solutions

Transcellular Potassium Shift
- With acute renal failure
  - Rhabdomyolysis
  - Tumor lysis syndrome
- Tissue infarction
  - Mesenteric
  - Limb
- Hypertonicity
  - Hyperglycemia
- Metabolic acidosis
- Drug-induced
  - Digitalis intoxication
  - Succinylcholine
- Hyperkalemic periodic paralysis
- Pseudohyperkalemia
  - Thrombocytosis
  - Leukocytosis
  - In vitro hemolysis
  - Fist clenching with phlebotomy

ACUTE HYPERKALEMIA (BOX 57.6)

Excessive Potassium Intake

Given an acute potassium load, a normal individual will excrete about 50% in the urine and transport about 90% of the remainder into cells over 4 to 6 hours.[61] It is possible to overwhelm this adaptive mechanism such that if too much potassium is taken in too quickly, significant hyperkalemia will result. Such events are almost always iatrogenic (i.e., overly aggressive potassium replacement therapy).[62] One's ability to tolerate a potassium load declines with disordered internal balance (see later) and impaired renal potassium excretory capacity.[63] In such circumstances, an otherwise tolerable increase in potassium intake may cause clinically significant hyperkalemia: Doses of oral potassium supplements as small as 30 to 45 mmol have resulted in severe hyperkalemia in patients with impaired external or internal potassium homeostasis.[64]

KCl, used as a supplement, is the drug most commonly implicated in acute hyperkalemia.[63,65] Banked blood represents a trivial potassium load under most circumstances, because a unit of fresh banked blood, either whole or packed cells, contains only about 7 mmol of potassium.[66] (The potassium concentration in banked blood does increase substantially as the blood ages, however.[67]) Thus, severe hyperkalemia would result only from massive transfusion of compatible blood.[67,68] Infants[69] or patients with renal insufficiency may develop hyperkalemia from an otherwise tolerable transfusion.

Patients undergoing open heart surgery are exposed to cardioplegic solutions containing KCl typically at about 16 mmol/L,[70] which may lead to clinically significant hyperkalemia in the postoperative period, especially in patients with diabetes mellitus with or without renal failure.[71]

Abnormal Potassium Distribution

Acute hyperkalemia may result from sudden redistribution of intracellular potassium to the extracellular space. If only 2% of intracellular potassium were to leak unopposed from cells, P_K would immediately double. Fortunately, such dramatic circumstances are rarely encountered. Nevertheless, smaller degrees of potassium redistribution commonly result in clinically significant hyperkalemia.

Among the most impressive syndromes associated with acute hyperkalemia are those involving *rapid cell lysis*. The *tumor lysis syndrome* results from treatment of chemosensitive bulky tumors with release of intracellular contents, including potassium, into the ECF.[72] Extreme hyperkalemia even causing sudden death[73] has featured prominently in some series of patients. Most of such patients were in renal failure from acute uric acid nephropathy, thus impairing their ability to excrete the potassium load.[73] *Rhabdomyolysis*, either traumatic or nontraumatic, may result in sudden massive influx of potassium to the extracellular space.[74] Hyperkalemia is present in about 40% of patients upon presentation with rhabdomyolysis[75] and is more common among patients whose course is complicated by oliguric acute renal failure.[76] Rhabdomyolysis is commonly associated with the use of alcohol[75] and cocaine.[77] Extreme hyperkalemia in this latter context has been reported.[78] Statin drugs are frequently associated with rhabdomyolysis,[79] rarely causing extreme hyperkalemia.[80] Other circumstances that may result in redistributive hyperkalemia include severe extensive burns, hemolytic transfusion reactions, and mesenteric ischemia or infarction.

Pharmacologic Agents

Two drugs may rarely cause acute hyperkalemia by redistribution: digitalis glycosides and succinylcholine. Massive digitalis overdose has been associated with extreme hyperkalemia.[81,82] Succinylcholine depolarizes the motor end plate and in normal individuals causes a trivial amount of potassium leak from muscle, resulting in an increase in P_K by about 0.5 mmol/L.[83] In patients with neuromuscular disorders, muscle damage, or prolonged immobilization, however, muscle depolarization may be more widespread, causing severe hyperkalemia.[84] Prolonged use of nondepolarizing neuromuscular blockers in critically ill patients may predispose to succinylcholine-induced hyperkalemia.[85]

Hyperkalemic Periodic Paralysis

This rare syndrome of episodic hyperkalemia and paralysis is caused by a mutation of the skeletal muscle sodium channel, inherited in an autosomal dominant pattern.[86] Attacks may be precipitated by exercise, fasting, exposure to cold, and potassium administration, and prevented by frequent carbohydrate snacks. Attacks are usually brief and treatment consists of carbohydrate ingestion. Severe attacks may require intravenous glucose infusions.[87]

Acute Renal Failure

Hyperkalemia accompanies acute renal failure in 30% to 50% of cases. It is seen most commonly in oliguric renal failure. Contributing factors include tissue destruction (e.g., tumor lysis syndrome, rhabdomyolysis) and increased catabolism.[88]

Pseudohyperkalemia

Pseudohyperkalemia refers to a measured potassium level that is higher than that circulating in the patient's blood. It has a number of possible causes. First, it may be caused by efflux of potassium out of blood cells in the test tube after phlebotomy. This may be seen in a *serum* specimen in cases of thrombocytosis[89] or leukocytosis,[90] when the clot causes cell lysis in vitro. These days, many clinical laboratories measure electrolytes in plasma (unclotted) specimens. Even under these conditions, extreme leukocytosis may cause pseudohyperkalemia if the specimen is chilled for a long time before the plasma is separated, leading to passive potassium leak from cells.[91] Hemolysis during specimen collection will falsely raise P_K *or* plasma potassium concentration by liberating intraerythrocyte potassium. Second, if the patient's arm is exercised by fist clenching with a tourniquet in place before the specimen is drawn, the sampled blood potassium concentration will rise significantly as a result of local muscle release of intracellular potassium.[54]

ACUTE HYPOKALEMIA

Hypokalemia that develops over hours is virtually always the result of redistribution of potassium from the extracellular to the intracellular space. The causes of acute hypokalemia are summarized in Box 57.7. Selected causes are discussed as follows.

Treatment of Diabetic Ketoacidosis

It is well recognized that patients presenting in DKA are always severely depleted in total body potassium as a result of glucose-driven osmotic diuresis, poor nutrition, and vomiting during the development of DKA.[44] Paradoxically, most patients in DKA have a normal P_K upon admission.[92] Insulin deficiency and hyperglycemia appear to account for the preservation of a normal P_K despite severe total body potassium depletion.[44] Once therapy for DKA is instituted, however, P_K typically plummets as potassium is rapidly taken up by cells. Potassium replacement at rates up to 120 mmol per hour have been reported, with total potassium supplementation of 600 to 800 mmol within the first 24 hours of treatment.[93] Hypokalemia in this setting may lead to respiratory arrest.[94]

Box 57.7 Causes of Acute Hypokalemia

- Treatment of diabetic ketoacidosis
- Refeeding syndrome
- Rapid cell production
  - Vitamin B_{12} treatment of pernicious anemia
  - GM-CSF treatment of leukopenia
- Pharmacologic agents
  - β_2-Adrenergic receptor agonists
  - Epinephrine
  - Soluble barium salts
- Hypokalemic periodic paralysis
  - Familial
  - Sporadic
  - Thyrotoxic
- Pseudohypokalemia

GM-CSF, granulocyte-macrophage colony-stimulating factor.

Refeeding

A situation analogous to DKA arises during aggressive refeeding after prolonged starvation or with aggressive "hyperalimentation" of chronically ill patients. The glucose-stimulated hyperinsulinemia and tissue anabolism shift potassium into cells, rapidly depleting extracellular potassium.[95] Death in the setting of refeeding has been reported and may be partly due to rapid cellular uptake of other ions (e.g., phosphorus, magnesium).[96]

Pharmacologic Agents

Specific *β_2-adrenergic receptor agonists* (e.g., albuterol) may cause electrophysiologically significant hypokalemia, especially when given to patients who are potassium depleted from the use of diuretic drugs.[97] *Epinephrine*, given intravenously in a dose about 5% of that recommended for cardiac resuscitation, causes a fall in P_K by about 1 mmol/L.[98] Such a dose achieves plasma levels of epinephrine comparable to those seen after acute myocardial infarction and may explain the transient hypokalemia following resuscitation from cardiac arrest even without the use of exogenous epinephrine (postresuscitation hypokalemia).[99,100] A rare cause of severe hypokalemia is poisoning with *soluble barium salts* such as chloride, carbonate, hydroxide, and sulfide. Soluble barium salts are used in pesticides and some depilatories, which may be ingested accidentally or intentionally.[101] Thiopentone, a barbiturate used to induce coma for refractory intracranial hypertension, is associated with redistributive hypokalemia in the majority of treated patients within 12 hours of initiating therapy.[102]

Hypokalemic Periodic Paralysis

Three forms of this rare syndrome have been described: familial, sporadic, and thyrotoxic.[103,104] All have in common attacks of muscle weakness accompanied by acute hypokalemia caused by cellular potassium uptake. Death may occur due to ventilatory failure or cardiac dysrhythmias. The *familial* variety—resulting from a skeletal muscle calcium channelopathy[86]—is inherited in an autosomal dominant pattern, with onset of clinical manifestations typically in the second decade of life. Attacks may occur after carbohydrate or salt ingestion or exercise. Administration of potassium orally or intavenously will abort an acute attack but is ineffective in preventing attacks.[103] The *sporadic* variety of hypokalemic periodic paralysis is identical to the familial form except for the absence of a hereditary pattern. *Thyrotoxic* periodic paralysis was first described in Asians but is now recognized to be nearly ubiquitous.[104] The usual onset of symptoms is in the third decade. Severe hypophosphatemia may accompany the hypokalemia.[105] Treatment of the disorder is the same as treatment of hyperthyroidism.

Pseudohypokalemia

Severe leukocytosis may cause spuriously low plasma potassium concentrations if blood cells are left in contact with the plasma for a long time at room temperature or higher. This phenomenon results from ongoing cell metabolism in vitro with glucose and potassium uptake.[59] Unexpected hypokalemia and hypoglycemia in the setting of leukocytosis should alert the clinician to this phenomenon.

CHRONIC HYPERKALEMIA

Renal Failure

Patients with chronic kidney disease tend to maintain a normal P_K until renal function declines to about 10% of normal.[106] Aldosterone and insulin both appear to play a role in the extrarenal potassium adaptation in chronic kidney disease.[107] This explains why patients with chronic kidney disease who are mineralocorticoid or insulin deficient have a particular predisposition to hyperkalemia.[108]

Mineralocorticoid Deficiency

Mineralocorticoid deficiency may result from global adrenal insufficiency (*Addison's disease*) or from selective defects in the renin-angiotensin-aldosterone axis (see Chapter 59). Hyperkalemia in the setting of unexplained hypotension should immediately raise one's suspicion for adrenal insufficiency. A common setting for isolated mineralocorticoid deficiency is the syndrome of *hyporeninemic hypoaldosteronism.*[108] This syndrome is most often seen in elderly patients with diabetes mellitus and moderate renal insufficiency. Hyperkalemia is a universal finding. An associated hyperchloremic metabolic acidosis (type IV renal tubular acidosis) is characteristic.[108] In addition to diabetes mellitus, two other systemic diseases are associated with this syndrome: the acquired immunodeficiency syndrome[109,110] and systemic lupus erythematosus.[111]

Aldosterone deficiency may be induced by a variety of pharmacologic agents acting at different sites in the renin-angiotensin-aldosterone axis. *β-Adrenergic receptor blockers* and, to a greater extent, *cyclooxygenase inhibitors* (COX-1 and COX-2) predispose patients to hyperkalemia by suppressing renin release.[112] As a general rule, COX inhibitors should be avoided in patients with renal insufficiency or who are otherwise prone to hyperkalemia either because of diabetes or the use of other implicated drugs. *Converting enzyme inhibitors* and *angiotensin receptor blockers* decrease aldosterone biosynthesis. These drugs are reported to be implicated in 10% to 38% of hyperkalemia in hospitalized patients.[113] Volume depletion and hypotension increase the risk of hyperkalemia with all these agents.

High- and low-dose *heparin* therapy decreases circulating aldosterone levels by selectively inhibiting aldosterone biosynthesis.[114] Hyperkalemia is seen with the use of low-molecular-weight heparins as well, particularly in patients with diabetes mellitus.[115]

Renal Potassium Secretory Defect

An isolated defect in renal potassium secretion (often with a renal tubular acidosis) is associated with *sickle cell disease* or trait,[116] *systemic lupus erythematosus,*[111] and after *renal transplantation.*[117] In this last circumstance, the hyperkalemia is exacerbated by the use of *cyclosporine* and *tacrolimus* for immunosuppresion.[118,119] A syndrome of hyperkalemic (type IV) distal renal tubular acidosis is seen in patients with *urinary tract obstruction.*[120]

The so-called *potassium-sparing diuretics* (spironolactone, eplerenone, amiloride, and triamterene) impair renal potassium excretion by blocking sodium reabsorption in the distal nephron. Two antibiotics, *pentamidine*[121] and *trimethoprim,*[122,123] cause hyperkalemia, occasionally severe, by blocking sodium reabsorption in the distal nephron.

CHRONIC HYPOKALEMIA

Chronic hypokalemia is virtually always the result of altered external balance: insufficient potassium intake, excessive potassium losses, or a combination of the two. Losses most often are either GI or renal.

Inadequate Potassium Intake

Because renal potassium conservation is not perfect, severe dietary potassium restriction will cause hypokalemia in 3 to 7 days in normal humans.[56] In one series of hypokalemic hospitalized patients, inadequate potassium supplementation during intravenous therapy contributed to the development of severe hypokalemia in 45% of cases and was the sole cause in 6%.[124] Other disorders associated with nutritional hypokalemia include anorexia nervosa, alcoholism, and malignancy.

Excessive Potassium Losses

Hypokalemia may develop as a result of both upper and lower GI fluid losses, but the pathogenesis is quite different in the two situations. With *diarrhea,* the potassium is lost from the gut.[125] *Gastric fluid losses* (e.g., vomiting or gastric suction) are associated with hypokalemia. Paradoxically, however, most of the potassium losses are renal, not gastric. Gastric fluid potassium concentration is only 5 to 10 mmol/L. Thus, only massive gastric fluid losses would, alone, significantly deplete total body potassium stores. The gastric fluid losses, however, stimulate renal potassium secretion in several ways. First, by generating a metabolic alkalosis and increasing bicarbonate delivery to the distal nephron, potassium secretion is stimulated. The metabolic alkalosis also leads to cellular proton loss and potassium uptake that, in renal epithelial cells, enhances potassium secretion. Finally, the volume contraction that usually accompanies GI fluid losses causes secondary aldosteronism, which further augments urinary potassium losses. Thus, in this situation, urinary potassium concentration is typically high while urinary chloride concentration is low due to volume contraction. (Urinary sodium losses may be high because of natriuresis obligated by the bicarbonaturia.)

All *diuretics* work by inhibiting sodium and chloride reabsorption by the nephron. Those drugs that act proximal to the potassium secretory site in the nephron promote a kaliuresis by increasing delivery of fluid distally and causing secondary aldosteronism. Thus, hypokalemia frequently accompanies the use of the two most common classes of diuretics: thiazides and loop diuretics.[126] Carbonic anhydrase inhibitors exert an additional kaliuretic effect by shunting bicarbonate-rich, chloride-poor fluid to the distal nephron.[127] Combining two potassium-wasting diuretics for added diuretic effect (e.g., furosemide plus metolazone) can result in severe hypokalemia. In such cases, P_K has been found to fall below 3.5 mmol/L in over 80% of patients and below 3.0 mmol/L in more than half.[126]

Various antibiotic agents may cause renal potassium wasting and thereby hypokalemia; 90% of patients receiving *amphotericin B* require potassium supplementation.[128] *Penicillin* antibiotics, particularly polyanionic derivatives such as carbenicillin and ticarcillin, have been associated with hypokalemia.[129]

Mineralocorticoids predispose to hypokalemia by stimulating renal potassium excretion. Mineralocorticoid excess may be *primary*[130] (Conn syndrome) or *secondary* to diminished real or "effective" circulating volume. All glucocorticoid drugs except dexamethasone possess some mineralocorticoid activity. Therefore, prolonged administration of these agents can cause severe hypokalemia. In edematous patients with secondary aldosteronism (e.g., congestive heart failure, hepatic cirrhosis) hypokalemia commonly ensues only when diuretic therapy enhances distal nephron flow rate.

Magnesium deficiency is associated with renal potassium wasting and may result in severe potassium depletion (see later). Because magnesium, like calcium, acts to stabilize excitable membranes, the deleterious effects of hypokalemia on the myocardium are magnified by concurrent hypomagnesemia.[131] The intensive care setting is fraught with potential causes of hypomagnesemia (see discussion under "Magnesium Homeostasis").

Hypercalcemia causes a salt and water diuresis and is therefore commonly associated with renal hypokalemia (see "Calcium Homeostasis").[132] In one series, one third of hypercalcemic patients were hypokalemic with no other predisposing factors; the prevalence was 52% in patients with hypercalcemia of malignancy. P_K was inversely proportional to the plasma calcium concentration.[133]

Several inborn tubular transport abnormalities are associated with chronic hypokalemia (and metabolic alkalosis). *Bartter* and *Gitelman* syndromes are associated with volume contraction and normal blood pressure, and *Liddle* syndrome with hypertension.[134]

CLINICAL MANIFESTATIONS OF POTASSIUM IMBALANCE

Alterations in P_K have a variety of adverse clinical consequences, the expression of which may be magnified in the critically ill patient. The most serious of these manifestations are those involving excitable tissues.

CLINICAL MANIFESTATIONS OF HYPERKALEMIA

Cardiac Effects

Hyperkalemia depolarizes the cell membrane, slows ventricular conduction, and decreases the duration of the action potential. These changes produce the classic electrocardiogram (ECG) manifestations of hyperkalemia including (in order of their usual appearance) peaked T waves, prolongation of the PR interval, widening of the QRS complex, loss of the P wave, "sine wave" configuration or ventricular fibrillation, and asystole.[135,136] These ECG changes may be modified by a multitude of factors such as ECF, pH, calcium concentration, sodium concentration, and the rate of rise of P_K.[135]

ECG changes may not accompany changes in P_K. If present, these ECG changes certainly suggest hyperkalemia. However, in the absence of the classic ECG changes, the clinician should not be lulled into a false sense of security when evaluating a hyperkalemic patient. Normal ECGs occur despite extreme hyperkalemia,[137] and the first cardiac manifestation of hyperkalemia may be ventricular fibrillation.[138] Consequently, P_K greater than 6.5 mmol/L, even with a normal ECG, should be treated as an emergency (see "Treatment of Potassium Imbalance").

Neuromuscular Effects

Hyperkalemia may result in paresthesias and weakness progressing to a flaccid paralysis, which typically spares the diaphragm. Reflexes are depressed or absent. Cranial nerves are rarely involved and sensory changes are minimal.[139]

Metabolic Effects

Hyperkalemia decreases renal ammoniagenesis, which by itself may produce a mild hyperchloremic metabolic acidosis[140] and will limit the kidney's ability to excrete an acid load and thus prevent correction of a metabolic acidosis.[141]

CLINICAL MANIFESTATIONS OF HYPOKALEMIA

Although less immediately life threatening than hyperkalemia, hypokalemia has many detrimental effects in critically ill patients. Along with cardiac and neuromuscular manifestations are many more subtle effects.

Cardiac Effects

Hypokalemia hyperpolarizes the cell membrane and prolongs the cardiac action potential.[142] These changes are associated with the following ECG manifestations: ST-segment depression, a decrease in T-wave amplitude, and an increase in U-wave amplitude.[135,136] However, because all of these changes are nonspecific, the ECG is an even less reliable index of hypokalemia than it is of hyperkalemia.

Hypokalemia may be associated with an increased incidence of arrhythmias and conduction defects. It is well established that potassium depletion increases the cardiac toxicity of digitalis glycosides.[143] However, controversy exists as to whether hypokalemia per se induces ventricular arrhythmias in patients not taking digitalis. There is an increase in benign ventricular ectopy in hypokalemic patients without acute myocardial ischemia.[144] The clinical importance of this observation is unclear. In individuals hospitalized with acute myocardial infarction, however, a correlation between hypokalemia and ventricular tachycardia and fibrillation was observed.[145] Because potassium repletion did not reduce the occurrence of these arrhythmias, it is unlikely that hypokalemia was the sole arrhythmogenic factor.[145] A recent study of patients presenting with acute myocardial infarction showed a U-shaped relationship between mean in-hospital P_K and mortality rate, such that P_K less than 3.5 mmol/L or greater than 4.5 mmol/L were each associated with higher in-hospital mortality rates. The lowest mortality rate was seen in patients with P_K 3.5 to 4.0 mmol/L, implying that potassium supplementation to achieve higher concentrations was not justifiable.[146]

Neuromuscular Effects

Modest hypokalemia generally presents as weakness, myalgias, muscle fatigue, and "restless" legs. With more severe hypokalemia (less than 2 mmol/L), paralysis may supervene. This usually involves the extremities but may progress to include the trunk and muscles of ventilation. As with hyperkalemia, cranial nerves typically are spared and sensory function usually remains intact.[59] It is important to note that these manifestations may be masked by concomitant hypocalcemia and may only appear when calcium is replenished. Conversely, in patients with hypokalemia and hypocalcemia, tetany may develop only after potassium replacement.[59] Smooth muscle dysfunction (ileus, gastroparesis) is more commonly seen with hypokalemia than with hyperkalemia.

In addition to the effects of potassium depletion on the electrical properties of the neuromuscular system, profound hypokalemia may result in muscle injury and frank rhabdomyolysis, even in bed-bound patients.[147]

Miscellaneous Effects

Hypokalemia and potassium depletion are associated with glucose intolerance,[148] increased protein catabolism, polydipsia and polyuria,[59] and metabolic alkalosis.[149]

EVALUATION OF DISORDERS OF POTASSIUM HOMEOSTASIS

The diagnostic approach to disorders of potassium homeostasis may be focused by dividing them according to their duration: acute (or of unknown duration) versus chronic.

EVALUATION OF ACUTE HYPERKALEMIA

When P_K rises abruptly or if P_K is high (greater than 6.5 mmol/L) on initial presentation of the patient, the first step is to obtain an ECG to look for electrophysiologic evidence of hyperkalemia. In the presence of such signs, treatment for hyperkalemia should begin urgently (see "Treatment of Potassium Imbalance"). At the same time, an unclotted blood sample should be obtained, using meticulous phlebotomy technique, for another set of electrolytes, glucose, blood urea nitrogen (BUN) and creatinine, and complete blood count (CBC). Urine should be tested for heme pigments to exclude acute rhabdomyolysis or hemolysis. The patient's list of medications and diet should be reviewed promptly, looking for exogenous sources of potassium and drugs that may impair potassium tolerance (see Box 57.6).

EVALUATION OF CHRONIC HYPERKALEMIA

Figure 57.2 outlines an approach to the patient with hyperkalemia lasting for days. Failure to stimulate cortisol release with a cosyntropin stimulation test (see Chapter 59) supports a diagnosis of Addison's disease. Absent that diagnosis, the patient is likely to have either selective aldosterone deficiency or tubular unresponsiveness to aldosterone. Assessment of the renin-angiotensin-aldosterone axis is most simply done by measuring plasma renin activity (PRA) and aldosterone levels in the basal and diuretic/posture-stimulated state.[108] Tubular unresponsiveness to aldosterone is assessed by measuring the potassium secretory effect of 9a-fludrocortisone (9a-F, Florinef). One index of the driving force for potassium secretion that may be useful in this regard is the transtubular potassium gradient (TTKG), calculated as follows:

$$TTKG = \frac{U_K}{P_K} \times \frac{P_{osm}}{U_{osm}}$$

where P_{osm} and U_{osm} are plasma and urine osmolalities, respectively.[150] A spot urine potassium : creatinine ratio may be used instead of the TTKG.

EVALUATION OF ACUTE HYPOKALEMIA

Hypokalemia accompanied by serious cardiac or neuromuscular manifestations is an emergency. Likewise, urgent therapy is indicated for profound hypokalemia (P_K less than 2.0 mmol/L) even in the absence of clinical complications. In addition, moderate hypokalemia (P_K less than 3.0 mmol/L) in patients taking digitalis,[143] and perhaps with acute myocardial ischemia,[145] should be treated urgently because of the risk of ventricular arrhythmias. In all these situations, it is imperative that the blood specimen be

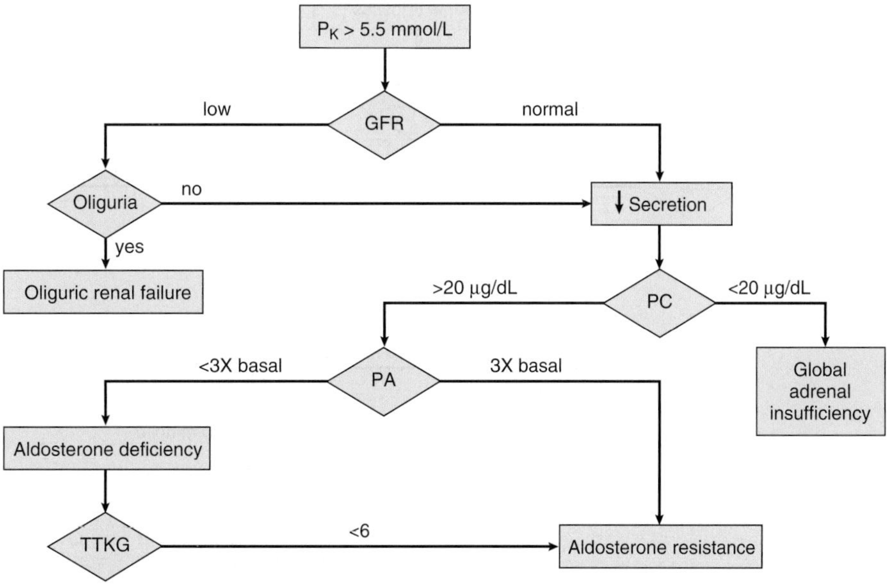

Figure 57.2 Diagnostic evaluation of chronic hyperkalemia. GFR, glomerular filtration rate; PA, stimulated plasma aldosterone (see text); PC, stimulated plasma cortisol (see Chapter 59); TTKG, transtubular potassium gradient (see text).

obtained and handled properly, especially in patients with leukocytosis, because rapid administration of potassium to a patient with pseudohypokalemia may cause severe hyperkalemia.

The remainder of the evaluation of acute hypokalemia derives mainly from the patient's history, with an emphasis on treatments causing cellular potassium uptake (e.g., insulin, β-adrenergic agonists) or a rapid increase in tissue anabolism, and a history of periodic paralysis. Patients who are hypokalemic upon presentation should be evaluated as though their hypokalemia were acute.

EVALUATION OF CHRONIC HYPOKALEMIA

Once acute hypokalemia and transient potassium redistribution have been excluded, one should next determine whether the kidney is responding appropriately to the potassium deficit or whether it is contributing to the problem. This is best done by measuring the 24-hour urinary excretion of potassium during potassium repletion (Fig. 57.3). Potassium excretion less than 20 mmol per day suggests appropriate renal potassium conservation and points to extrarenal (lower GI or skin) potassium losses, recovery from diuretic-induced hypokalemia, or chronically potassium-deficient diet. Excretion of greater than 20 mmol per day is evidence of inadequate renal potassium conservation indicating a renal cause of the hypokalemia. Renal potassium losses associated with normal systemic blood pressure are most commonly seen with the use of thiazide or loop diuretics and are accompanied by a metabolic alkalosis. Other causes of hypokalemia with metabolic alkalosis in a normotensive patient include gastric fluid loss and Bartter and Gitelman syndromes. These are separable most often by history, but if not, the urinary chloride measurement will be helpful, being low with gastric fluid losses. Renal hypokalemia may accompany a renal tubular acidosis, in which case the plasma bicarbonate will be low.

Mineralocorticoid excess may be the cause if the renal potassium loss is associated with systemic hypertension, and the renin-aldosterone axis should be studied with basal and saline-suppressed blood hormone measurements. High PRA and aldosterone levels suggest renal artery stenosis, malignant hypertension, or rarely a renin-secreting tumor. Low PRA and high aldosterone levels indicate primary aldosteronism. When both PRA and aldosterone levels are low, one should suspect the syndrome of apparent mineralocorticoid excess, Cushing syndrome, or rarely Liddle syndrome. Note that Cushing syndrome due to ectopic adrenocorticotropic hormone (ACTH) secretion often is not accompanied by typical cushingoid features.[151]

TREATMENT OF POTASSIUM IMBALANCE

In general, the initial treatment of acute severe potassium imbalance is independent of the cause of the disturbance, whereas the rational therapy for chronic hyper- or hypokalemia depends on an understanding of its pathogenesis.

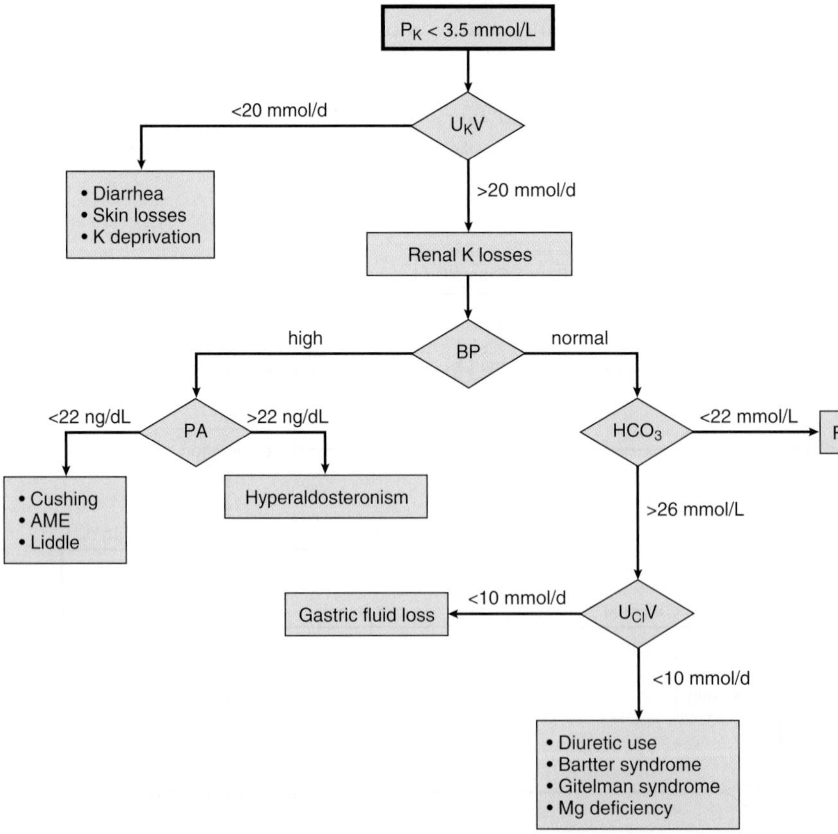

Figure 57.3 Diagnostic evaluation of chronic hypokalemia. AME, syndrome of apparent mineralocorticoid excess; BP, blood pressure; PA, stimulated plasma aldosterone (see text); RTA, renal tubular acidosis; $U_{Cl}V$, urinary chloride excretion; U_KV, urinary potassium excretion.

TREATMENT OF ACUTE HYPERKALEMIA

In considering when hyperkalemia constitutes an emergency, two points should be kept in mind. First, the electrophysiologic effects of hyperkalemia are directly proportional to both the absolute P_K and its rate of rise.[135] Second, although the ECG manifestations of hyperkalemia are generally progressive and proportional to the P_K, ventricular fibrillation may be the first ECG disturbance of hyperkalemia;[138] conversely, a normal ECG may be seen with extreme hyperkalemia.[137] Thus, it is apparent that neither the ECG nor the P_K alone is an adequate index of the urgency of hyperkalemia, and that the clinical context must be considered when assessing a hyperkalemic patient. Because most patients manifest hyperkalemic ECG changes at P_K greater than 6.7 mmol/L,[136] hyperkalemia should be treated emergently for (1) P_K greater than 6.5 mmol/L and (2) ECG manifestations of hyperkalemia regardless of the P_K.[152]

Therapy of acute or severe hyperkalemia is directed at preventing or ameliorating its untoward electrophysiologic effects on the myocardium. The goals of therapy, in chronologic order, are as follows (Table 57.2):

1. Antagonize the effect of potassium on excitable cell membranes.
2. Redistribute extracellular potassium into cells.
3. Enhance elimination of potassium from the body.

Membrane Antagonism

Calcium. Calcium directly antagonizes the myocardial effects of hyperkalemia without lowering P_K.[153] During treatment with calcium, the ECG should be monitored continuously. The dose may be repeated in 5 minutes if there is no improvement in the ECG, or if the ECG deteriorates after an initial improvement.[152] There are several case reports of sudden death in patients given intravenous calcium while also receiving digitalis glycosides.[154] Although these observations do not provide clear guidance, it may be wise to administer intravenous calcium with caution to patients known or strongly suspected of having toxic levels of digitalis glycosides.

Hypertonic Saline. Intravenous hypertonic sodium chloride has been shown to reverse the ECG changes of hyperkalemia in patients with concurrent hyponatremia.[155] Whether hypertonic saline is effective in the treatment of eunatremic patients has not been established. Moreover, the extracellular volume load imposed by hypertonic saline argues against its use.

Redistribution of Potassium into Cells

Insulin. Insulin reliably lowers P_K in a dose-dependent manner. An intravenous dose of 10 units of regular insulin given as a bolus along with an intravenous bolus of dextrose (25-40 g as a 50% solution) to adult patients lowers the P_K by about 1 mmol/L.[156,157] After the initial bolus, a dextrose infusion should be started, because a single bolus of 25 g of dextrose has been shown to be inadequate to prevent hypoglycemia at 60 minutes.[156] There seems to be no advantage of a continuous insulin infusion over a bolus injection.[40] Insulin should be used without dextrose in hyperglycemic patients; indeed, the cause of the hyperkalemia in those patients may be the hyperglycemia itself.[50]

Albuterol. P_K has been shown to decline by 0.6 mmol/L after inhalation of 10 mg of albuterol, and by about 1.0 mmol/L after 20 mg in patients with ESRD.[158] The effect of insulin is additive with that of albuterol, with the

Table 57.2 Emergency Treatment of Hyperkalemia

Agent/Intervention	Dose	Onset	Duration	Complications
Membrane Stabilization				
Calcium gluconate (10%)	10 mL IV over 10 min	Immediate	30-60 min	Hypercalcemia
Hypertonic (3%) sodium chloride	50 mL IV push	Immediate	Unknown	Volume overload Hypertonicity
Redistribution				
Insulin (short-acting)	10 units IV push, with 25-40 g dextrose (50% sol'n)	20 min	4-6 h	Hypoglycemia
Albuterol	20 mg in 4 mL normal saline solution, nebulized over 10 min	30 min	2 h	Tachycardia Inconsistent response
Elimination				
Loop diuretics				
Furosemide	40-80 mg IV	15 min	2-3 h	Volume depletion
Bumetanide	2-4 mg IV			
Sodium bicarbonate	150 mmol/L IV at variable rate	Hours	Duration of infusion	Metabolic alkalosis Volume overload
Sodium polystyrene sulfonate (SPS) (Kayexalate, Kionex)	15-30 g in 15-30 mL 70% sorbitol PO	>2 h	4-6 h	Variable effect Intestinal necrosis
Hemodialysis		Immediate	3 h	Arrhythmias

combination reported to result in a decline in P_K by about 1.2 mmol/L at 60 minutes.[156] Even among patients not taking beta blockers, as many as 40% appear to be resistant to the hypokalemic effect of albuterol.[156,158] For that reason, albuterol should never be used alone for the treatment of urgent hyperkalemia.

Bicarbonate. The putative benefits of a bolus injection of sodium bicarbonate in the emergency treatment of hyperkalemia pervaded the literature until the past decade. Ironically, this dogma was based on studies using a prolonged (4-6 hours) infusion of bicarbonate.[45] It has now been clearly demonstrated that short-term bicarbonate infusion does not reduce P_K in patients with dialysis-dependent kidney failure, implying that it does not cause potassium shift into cells.[46,47,159]

Elimination of Potassium from the Body

Enhanced Renal Elimination. Hyperkalemia occurs most often in patients with renal insufficiency. However, renal potassium excretion may be enhanced even in patients with moderate renal failure by increasing distal nephron flow. This may be accomplished with *saline* or *sodium bicarbonate infusions* and may be enhanced further by the use of *loop diuretics.* Diuretic-induced volume contraction must be avoided because this will lead to decreased distal nephron flow and reduced potassium excretion.[152]

Exchange Resin. Sodium polystyrene sulfonate (SPS, Kayexalate, Kionex) is a cation exchange resin that exhanges sodium for secreted potassium in the colon. Each gram of resin binds approximately 0.65 mmol of potassium in vivo, although the effect is highly variable and unpredictable.[40] The resin causes constipation and hence almost always is given with a cathartic. It is more effective when given orally than by retention enema.[40]

There are two concerns with the use of SPS for the treatment of urgent hyperkalemia. The first is its slow effect. When given orally, the onset of action is at least 2 hours and the maximum effect may not be seen for 6 hours or more. One recent study in hemodialysis patients failed to show any effect on P_K after an oral dose of SPS.[160] The second concern with SPS is its possible toxicity. There are numerous case reports of patients who developed intestinal necrosis after exposure to SPS in sorbitol as an enema[161-163] and orally.[164] A retrospective study estimated the incidence of colonic necrosis to be 1.8% among postoperative patients.[164] For these reasons, some authorities consider the use of SPS to be unjustifiable.[165]

Dialysis. *Hemodialysis* is the dialytic method of choice for removal of potassium from the body. P_K falls by over 1 mmol/L in the first 60 minutes of hemodialysis and a total of 2 mmol/L by 180 minutes, after which it reaches a plateau.[40] Rebound always occurs after dialysis, with 35% of the reduction abolished after an hour and nearly 70% after 6 hours.[40] There is controversy as to whether dialysis for severe hyperkalemia precipitates serious ventricular arrhythmias. Because of the possibility, patients dialyzed for severe hyperkalemia should have continuous ECG monitoring.[40] The rate of potassium removal with *peritoneal dialysis* is much slower than with hemodialysis.[40]

TREATMENT OF CHRONIC HYPERKALEMIA

As established previously, chronic hyperkalemia always implies deficient renal potassium excretion. It follows that the therapy of chronic hyperkalemia is primarily directed toward stimulating renal potassium excretion while limiting potassium intake. For all adults with chronic hyperkalemia, daily potassium intake should be restricted to 60 mmol. All drugs known to impair either internal or external potassium balance should be eliminated if possible. Finally, all patients with chronic hyperkalemia should be evaluated for occult urinary tract obstruction.

Further therapy of the persistently hyperkalemic patient should be guided by the diagnostic evaluation outlined in Figure 57.2. In cases of mineralocorticoid unresponsiveness or when mineralocorticoid treatment is complicated by fluid overload, a *thiazide* or *loop diuretic* can be added to the regimen. This will restore normal volume status and enhance renal tubular potassium secretion in many mineralocorticoid-resistant patients. It is crucial to avoid diuretic-induced volume depletion, however, because this will exacerbate the renal potassium secretory defect.

Patients who fail to respond to the previously mentioned measures with an increase in TTKG or urine potassium : creatinine ratio and a decrease in P_K may be given sodium bicarbonate, which will stimulate renal potassium secretion. This is especially appropriate for patients whose chronic hyperkalemia is accompanied by a renal tubular acidosis (type IV RTA). The usual dose is 1 to 2 mmol bicarbonate per kg body weight per day in three or four divided doses.[152]

TREATMENT OF ACUTE HYPOKALEMIA

A low P_K almost always indicates a large total body potassium deficit. In fact, P_K decreases by approximately 0.3 mmol/L for each decrement of 100 mmol total body potassium.[166] But if potassium is replenished too quickly, the homeostatic mechanisms that defend P_K will be overwhelmed and P_K will rise abruptly. The rate of rise of P_K with potassium administration can be greatly altered by factors that affect internal potassium balance. For example, during treatment of DKA with insulin, cellular uptake of potassium may be massive, obligating enormous replacement doses of potassium. Conversely, insulin deficiency markedly impairs tolerance to a potassium load.[61]

See "Evaluation of Acute Hypokalemia" for definitions of urgent hypokalemia. Limited information exists on which to base a rational prescription of KCl in an emergency.[61,167,168]

Based on the available literature, we can estimate that nondiabetic patients with normal renal function should respond well to a 1- to 2-hour infusion of KCl at 0.6 mmol/kg/hour given intravenously in saline. In patients with renal failure of any degree, the infusion rate should be halved (0.3 mmol/kg/hour). Patients with diabetes mellitus not being treated for DKA or hyperglycemia should receive no more than 0.2 mmol/kg/hour, or about 0.1 mmol/kg/hour in the setting of renal failure. For severe hypokalemia, the ECG should be monitored continuously and the infusion stopped immediately if signs of hyperkalemia develop. The maximum increase in P_K is seen at the end of the infusion, and about 50% of the increase is lost over the next 2 to 3 hours when a new steady state is achieved. Thus, P_K

should be measured at the end of the infusion. If the patient is still dangerously hypokalemic at this point, additional potassium may be given. If at the end of the infusion P_K is in an acceptable range, the measurement should be repeated 2 to 3 hours later when disposal of potassium load is complete in order to determine the need for further treatment.[152]

Hypokalemia in the setting of aggressive "refeeding," and especially in the treatment of severe DKA, should be treated initially as described earlier. Frequent monitoring of P_K with rapid laboratory turnaround time is critical for proper management.

Hypokalemia that is not life threatening is best treated with oral potassium replacement. It is important to recognize that GI absorption of an oral dose of KCl elixir is essentially complete. Dangerous hyperkalemia can occur in entirely normal individuals following KCl ingestion.[169] The maximum increase in P_K is seen 1.5 to 2 hours after an oral potassium load. Thus, a sensible oral dose of KCl in moderate hypokalemia should probably not exceed the hourly intravenous doses proposed earlier. There is no reason to give a simultaneous oral and intravenous potassium dose; serious hyperkalemia may ensue.

TREATMENT OF CHRONIC HYPOKALEMIA

The treatment of chronic hypokalemia depends entirely on identifying and, if possible, remediating the cause (see Fig. 57.3). When the cause of the excessive potassium loss cannot be treated specifically, maintenance potassium supplementation is needed.

WATER HOMEOSTASIS

Hyponatremia and hypernatremia reflect disorders of water homeostasis. They are common disorders in critically ill patients and are associated with increased morbidity and mortality rates.[170,171]

PHYSIOLOGY OF WATER HOMEOSTASIS

Normal plasma sodium concentration varies very little, even less than the "normal" range of clinical laboratories (135-145 mmol/L). This tight regulation depends on the following elements: (1) pituitary secretion of arginine vasopressin (AVP; also known as antidiuretic hormone, or ADH) that varies over a wide range in response to physiologic stimuli; (2) kidneys that are capable of responding to circulating vasopressin by varying the urine concentration; (3) intact thirst; and (4) access to water.

Tonicity or *effective osmolality* describes the capacity of particles in solution to effect water movement across a semipermeable membrane such as the cell membrane. The normal response to water ingestion (of sufficient magnitude to lower the plasma osmolality even slightly) is the excretion of maximally dilute urine (urine osmolality <100 mOsm/kg). The underlying physiologic sequence is as follows: The plasma *hypotonicity* is sensed by the cells making up the hypothalamic osmostat. These hypothalamic nuclei then proportionately reduce their synthesis of AVP, also known as ADH, leading to diminished AVP release into the circulation by the posterior pituitary. The lower circulating AVP concentration, in turn, results in the insertion of proportionately fewer water channels into the collecting duct of the kidney. This, in turn, creates a more water-impermeable conduit, preventing water reabsorption and allowing excretion of the dilute urine elaborated by the more proximal segments of the nephron.[172]

Conversely, plasma hypertonicity leads to higher circulating AVP concentration and proportionately higher water permeability of the collecting duct, and the excretion of a concentrated urine.[172]

Figure 57.4 shows the relationship between plasma osmolality, plasma AVP concentration, and urine osmolality. The normal "set point" is a plasma osmolality of about 285 mOsm/kg. Notice that the minimum urine osmolality is about 50 mOsm/kg, and the maximum is about 1200 mOsm/kg.[173]

When plasma osmolality rises beyond 290 to 295 mOsm/kg, the *thirst* center of the hypothalamus is stimulated. At that point, neurologically intact individuals with access to water will drink until the plasma osmolality returns to normal.[173]

NONOSMOTIC VASOPRESSIN RELEASE

It is important to recognize that plasma osmolality is not the only determinant of AVP synthesis and release. Low arterial blood pressure and low effective arterial volume powerfully stimulate AVP release.[173] This baroreceptor-mediated AVP release is teleologic, because water retention is an important component in the defense against hypovolemia. So primal is this circulatory defense that the baroreceptor stimulation predominates over any osmolal effect on AVP release.[173] Thus, a volume-contracted or hypotensive individual will have high circulating AVP levels even if his plasma osmolality is low. In addition, circulating AVP levels rise with pain, stress, nausea, hypoxia, hypercapnia, and a variety of medications, most notably epinephrine and high doses of narcotic analgesics.[173]

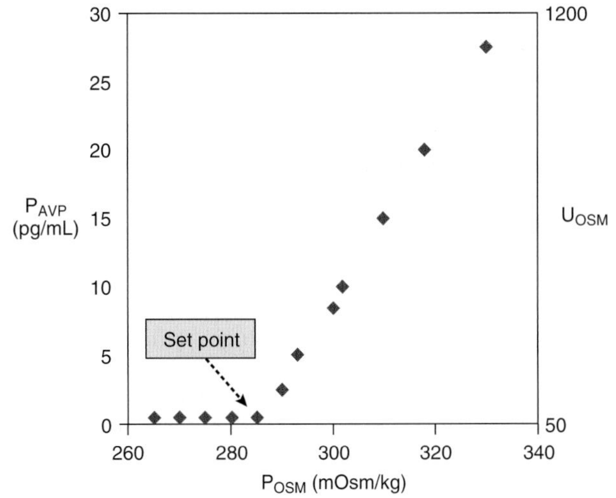

Figure 57.4 Typical example of the relationship between plasma osmolality (P_{osm}), plasma vasopressin concentration (P_{AVP}), and urine osmolality (U_{osm}). P_{AVP} and U_{osm} vary around the *set point* to maintain P_{osm} within the range of normal.

HYPONATREMIA

EPIDEMIOLOGY AND CLINICAL MANIFESTATIONS

Hyponatremia (plasma sodium concentration < 135 mmol/L) is one of the most common electrolyte disorders, found in approximately 3% of hospitalized patients and as many as 30% of patients in ICUs.[170]

The clinical manifestations of hyponatremia are largely attributed to intracellular volume expansion (cellular edema), which occurs only when hyponatremia is associated with hypotonicity. Intracellular volume expansion is of greatest consequence in the brain, where it is translated into increased intracranial pressure because of the rigid calvarium.[174]

PATHOPHYSIOLOGY

The pathophysiology of hypotonic hyponatremia has important implications for its management. Most cells—especially brain cells—have adaptive mechanisms for mitigating tonicity-related volume changes.[174] Cell volume peaks 1 to 2 hours after the onset of acute hypotonicity. Thereafter, solute and water are lost from cells, and cell volume returns toward normal. After several days of sustained hypotonicity, cell volume is restored nearly to normal.[174]

The morbidity and mortality risks associated with hypotonic hyponatremia are influenced by several factors, including the magnitude and rate of development of the hyponatremia, the patient's age and gender, and the nature and severity of any underlying diseases.[174] The very young and very old, women, and alcoholics appear to be at particular risk.[175] Cell-volume adaptation to hypotonicity may be deficient in premenopausal women, who suffer more frequent and more severe neurologic consequences than men with equivalent degrees of hypotonicity.[176]

Neurologic symptoms usually do not occur until the plasma sodium concentration falls below 125 mmol/L, at which point the patient may complain of anorexia, nausea, and malaise. Between 120 and 110 mmol/L, headache, lethargy, confusion, agitation, and obtundation may be seen. More severe symptoms (seizures, coma) may occur with levels below 110 mmol/L.[177] Focal neurologic findings are unusual but do occur, and transtentorial cerebral herniation has been described in severe cases, especially in young women following surgery.[176] In that setting, hypoxemia is common and often is associated with noncardiogenic pulmonary edema.[178] Hypoxia appears to exacerbate the cerebral damage in hyponatremia.[179]

Although symptoms generally resolve with correction of the hypotonicity, permanent neurologic deficits may occur, particularly in acute severe hypotonicity, when the brain's volume-regulatory defenses may be overwhelmed.[176] Profound hypotonicity that develops in less than 24 hours may be associated with residual neurologic deficits and has a 50% mortality rate in some populations.[176] In contrast, when hypotonicity develops more gradually, symptoms are both less common and less severe. Indeed, patients with chronic hyponatremia, even in the range of 115 to 120 mmol/L, may be completely asymptomatic.[174]

DIFFERENTIAL DIAGNOSIS

Hyponatremia may coexist with a normal, high, or low plasma osmolality. Thus, the diagnostic algorithm for hyponatremia (see Fig. 57.2) begins with an assessment of the plasma osmolality (P_{osm}). This may be estimated by the following formula:

$$\text{estimated } P_{osm} = (2 \times P_{Na}) + \frac{P_{gluc}}{18} + \frac{BUN}{2.8}$$

where P_{gluc} is the plasma glucose concentration and BUN is blood urea nitrogen concentration, both in mg/dL. If there is a suspicion that an unmeasured, osmotically effective solute may be implicated (e.g., mannitol or glycerol), the P_{osm} should be measured directly.

Isotonic hyponatremia (also known as *factitious hyponatremia* or *pseudohyponatremia*) is a laboratory artifact seen with analytic techniques that measure the mass of sodium per unit volume of plasma sampled.[180] It is seen in the presence of marked hypertriglyceridemia or paraproteinemia, when the measurement method involves a predilution step. Direct potentiometry (which uses an ion-selective electrode in undiluted plasma) avoids this problem.[180]

Hypertonic hyponatremia results from the presence in ECF of abnormal amounts of osmotically effective solutes other than sodium (e.g., glucose, mannitol, or glycerol). The osmotic pressure exerted by the nonsodium solute leads to redistribution of water from the intracellular to the ECF compartment, resulting in cellular dehydration and hyponatremia. The hyponatremia is real (not *pseudo*-), but it is accompanied by *hyper*tonicity and a *decrease* in cellular volume.

Hypotonic hyponatremia is almost always caused by an inability of the kidney to excrete sufficient electrolyte-free water to match water intake. This may occur either because the normal diluting capacity of the kidney is overwhelmed by excessive water intake or because the diluting capacity of the kidney is impaired. These alternatives usually can be distinguished by measuring the urine osmolality. A urine osmolality less than 100 mOsm/kg in a patient with hypotonic hyponatremia points to excessive water intake as the cause (Fig. 57.5). It is a prodigious feat for an individual eating a normal diet to overwhelm the normal diluting capacity of the kidney. Estimates are that one can ingest (and excrete) about 20 L of water a day without affecting the plasma osmolality appreciably.[173] Thus, patients who develop hyponatremia from so-called *psychogenic* or *primary polydipsia*—usually patients with obsessive-compulsive disorder or psychosis—typically have concurrent urinary diluting defects, either in association with the underlying mental illness or perhaps as a side effect of psychotropic or anticonvulsant medications.[181]

Not all patients with hypotonic hyponatremia and a dilute urine have primary polydipsia. The patient may be ingesting a diet so deficient in protein and salt that he excretes very little solute in the urine. In that situation (called *beer potomania* for obvious reasons,[182] although the syndrome has been seen in other patients with very low daily solute intake[183]) the low daily solute excretion limits the total amount of water that can be eliminated even with a maximally dilute urine (i.e., maximum urine volume = solute excretion ÷ minimum U_{osm}). This might reduce the maximum water excretion to only 3 to 4 L/day, a quantity easily exceeded by an enthusiastic beer drinker.

A urine osmolality above 100 mOsm/kg in the face of hypotonic hyponatremia signifies impaired urinary diluting

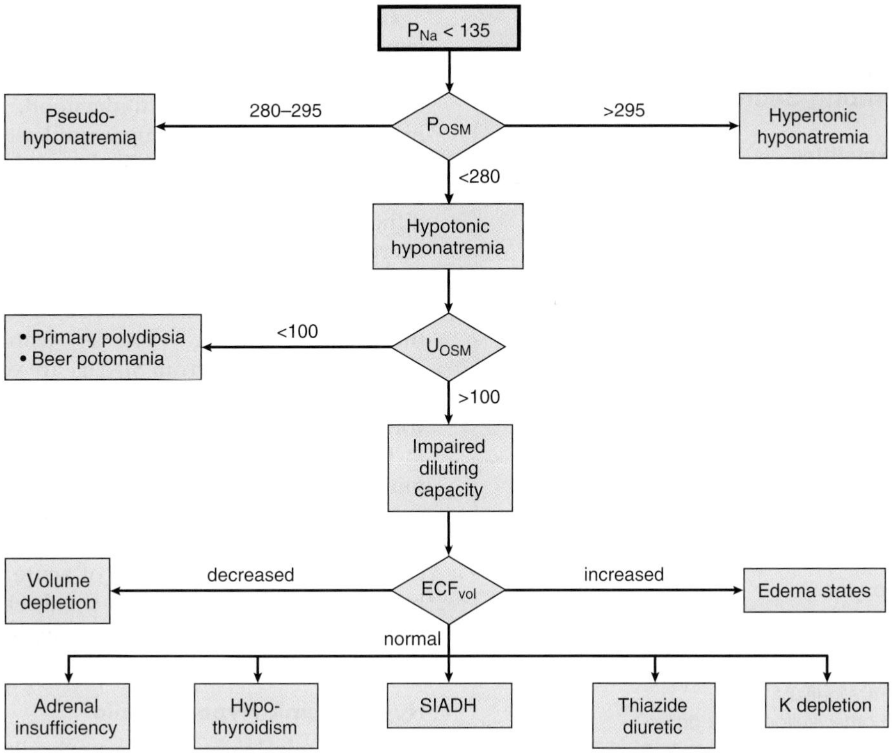

Figure 57.5 Diagnostic evaluation of hyponatremia. ECF_{vol}, extracellular fluid volume status; P_{Na}, plasma sodium concentration; P_{osm}, plasma osmolality (mOsm/kg); SIADH, syndrome of inappropriate antidiuretic hormone secretion; U_{osm}, urine osmolality (mOsm/kg).

capacity. The concentrated urine usually reflects a high circulating AVP level. Because circulating AVP is affected by systemic hemodynamics as well as osmolality, assessment of the patient's ECF volume status and hemodynamics is crucial at this juncture. Hypotonic hyponatremia may be associated with normal, decreased, or increased extracellular volume.

Euvolemic Hyponatremia

Patients with pure water excess appear clinically euvolemic because excess water distributes throughout the total body water space; only one third of total body water is extracellular (and only one twelfth is intravascular). The only evidence of the slight intravascular volume expansion is low BUN and plasma uric acid concentration.[184] The paradigm of euvolemic hyponatremia with a concentrated urine is the syndrome of inappropriate antidiuretic hormone secretion (SIADH). It is characterized by elevated circulating AVP (ADH) levels that are inappropriate to vasopressin's two physiologic stimuli (i.e., osmotic or hemodynamic).[185] Hypotonic hyponatremia in patients with SIADH develops to the extent that water ingestion exceeds water eliminated by insensible, GI, and renal routes. Because the normal response to extracellular hypotonicity is the elaboration of maximally dilute urine (urine osmolality < 100 mOsm/kg), the urine need only be inappropriately concentrated (i.e., >100 mOsm/kg) to be compatible with a diagnosis of SIADH.

Because hypothyroidism[186] and glucocorticoid insufficiency[187] may impair urinary dilution, patients in whom a diagnosis of SIADH is entertained should undergo appropriate tests of thyroid and adrenocortical function. (see Chapter 59.)

Once a diagnosis of SIADH is made, its cause must be established, because the cause may have important implications in its own right and may be easily remediable. Box 57.8 lists important causes of SIADH. They fall into five major categories: intracranial abnormalities, intrathoracic abnormalities, tumors, drugs, and idiopathic. An important variant of SIADH is the *reset osmostat syndrome*,[188] in which vasopressin levels are regulated normally by tonicity but around a lower "set point" than normal. This syndrome is seen most often in patients who are severely debilitated (e.g., malnutrition, metastatic cancer, advanced tuberculosis) and may account for up to one third of cases of SIADH. The diagnosis of reset osmostat syndrome has important therapeutic implications, as will be discussed later.

Hypovolemic Hyponatremia

The urinary diluting impairment in hypovolemia is mediated both by decreased delivery of fluid to the diluting segments of the nephron and by hemodynamically stimulated vasopressin release. Thus, the volume-contracted patient cannot excrete electrolyte-free water normally, and even in the face of modest water ingestion readily may become hyponatremic.

The cause of the volume contraction usually is obvious (e.g., hemorrhage, vomiting, diarrhea, diuretics). When it is not, the urine sodium concentration can be helpful in distinguishing between renal and extrarenal solute losses. Renal losses (e.g., as a result of diuretic medications) are usually reflected by sodium wasting, and extrarenal losses

Box 57.8 Causes of Syndrome of Inappropriate Antidiuretic Hormone Secretion

Intracranial Abnormalities

Infection
Stroke
Hemorrhage
Tumor

Intrathoracic Abnormalities

Malignancy
Pulmonary abscess
Pneumonia
Pleural effusion
Pneumothorax
Chest wall deformity

Drugs

Antidiuretic drugs (vasopressin, 1-deamino-8-D-arginine vasopressin [DDAVP], oxytocin)
Narcotic analgesics
Antidepressant medications
Amiodarone
Major antipsychotic medications
Chlorpropamide and other sulfonylurea drugs
Carbamazepine
Cyclophosphamide
Methotrexate
Interferon-α
Vinca alkaloids
Platinum compounds
Melphalan
Isofosfamide
MDMA (Ecstasy)

Extracranial Tumors

Small cell lung carcinoma
Pancreatic cancer
Others

HIV/AIDS

Hereditary

Gain-of-function mutation of vasopressin-2 receptor

Miscellaneous

Guillain-Barré syndrome
Nausea
Stress
Pain
Acute psychosis
Legionella infection

Idiopathic

AIDS, acquired immunodeficiency syndrome; HIV, human immunodeficiency virus.

are usually accompanied by sodium conservation (urine sodium concentration < 10 mM). Exceptions occur in the recovery phase after diuretic therapy and in metabolic alkalosis due to vomiting. In the latter situation, the urine chloride concentration tends to be very low and is the best indicator of extracellular volume depletion.[189,190]

Cerebral salt wasting may be responsible for hypovolemic hyponatremia in patients with intracranial pathology (e.g., tumors, hemorrhage). The pathogenesis of the urinary salt wasting is incompletely understood. The mechanism of hyponatremia in this setting is similar to that of other hypovolemic states. As a hyponatremic syndrome in patients with central nervous system disease, cerebral salt wasting is often difficult to distinguish from SIADH because urinary sodium excretion tends to be high. Particularly confusing in patients with cerebral salt wasting is the finding of *hypo*uricemia, which is thought to reflect impaired solute reabsorption in the proximal tubule.[191] The key features that distinguish cerebral salt wasting from SIADH are volume depletion and urinary sodium excretion inappropriate to the patient's volume status.[191]

The hyponatremia associated with *diuretic treatment* is multifactorial in origin. Insofar as diuretics produce overt volume depletion, they can cause hyponatremia by the mechanisms discussed previously. Thiazides have been associated with the development of acute severe, symptomatic hyponatremia, particularly in small, elderly women, in the absence of overt signs of volume depletion.[192] The cause of this often precipitous syndrome remains uncertain.[193]

Hypervolemic Hyponatremia

Hypervolemic hyponatremia generally is seen in patients who cannot excrete sodium normally because they have either severe renal failure or one of the pathologic edema-forming states (e.g., congestive heart failure, hepatic cirrhosis, nephrotic syndrome). Patients with advanced chronic kidney disease are predisposed to hyponatremia.[194] Acute oliguric renal failure or end-stage (dialysis-dependent) renal failure will be accompanied by hyponatremia to the extent that water intake exceeds insensible and GI water elimination (see Chapter 55).

Hyponatremia is seen in over 20% of patients presenting with decompensated congestive heart failure and over 30% of patients admitted to hospital with complications of hepatic cirrhosis.[195] The hormonal milieu of such patients is typical of intravascular volume depletion, even though the absolute intravascular volume typically is increased. Thus, these disorders are said to be characterized by *reduced effective circulating volume.*[196] Because of the perceived intravascular volume depletion, renal diluting ability is compromised for reasons similar to those in hypovolemic hyponatremia.

Hyponatremia in Endurance-Sports Athletes

The incidence of hyponatremia, with serum sodium less than 135 mmol/L, is approximately 15% in marathon and triathalon athletes; 0.6% of runners develop severe hyponatremia with serum sodium levels less than 120 mEq/L.[195] The three major risk factors associated with hyponatremia in this setting includes body mass index (BMI) less than 20, racing time more than 4 hours, and weight gain related to excessive fluid intake during the race. Fluid overload is the most important factor in the development of hyponatremia for runners.[195]

MANAGEMENT AND COMPLICATIONS

Hyponatremia per se requires treatment only when it is associated with hypotonicity. Hypertonic hyponatremia responds to the treatment of the underlying disorder, most commonly a hyperosmolar hyperglycemic state (see Chapter 58).

The therapy of hypotonic hyponatremia must be tailored to (1) the patient's signs and symptoms, and (2) the duration of the disorder.[175] Severe hyponatremia (plasma sodium concentration < 115 mmol/L) can be life threatening, especially if it develops rapidly.[177,197] The therapy of symptomatic hyponatremia, irrespective of cause, is directed at raising ECF tonicity to shift water out of the intracellular space, thereby ameliorating cerebral edema. The rate of correction, however, must be carefully regulated. Overly rapid correction, particularly in patients with chronic hyponatremia, in whom cell volume adaptations may be complete, can produce *osmotic demyelination syndrome.*[198,199] Osmotic demyelination syndrome is associated with a variety of sometimes irreversible neurologic deficits (e.g., dysarthria, dysphagia, behavioral disturbances, ataxia, quadriplegia, coma), which typically develop 3 to 10 days after treatment.[200] Additional risk factors for osmotic demyelination include hypokalemia, malnutrition, alcoholism, advanced age, female gender, and the postoperative state, particularly after orthotopic liver transplantation.[201-203]

For patients with chronic hyponatremia (>48 hours duration) or hyponatremia of unknown duration, the plasma sodium concentration should be raised by a maximum of 0.5 mmol/L/hour, 8 to 10 mmol/L in the first 24 hours[199] and 20 mmol/L over the first 48 hours. Care should be taken to avoid *over*correcting the plasma sodium concentration.[187,200] In grave situations (plasma sodium concentration < 105 mmol/L or in the presence of seizure or coma), initial therapy can be more aggressive (targeting a change in the plasma sodium concentration of 1 to 2 mmol/L/hour for the first few hours), but the recommended daily target should not be exceeded.[187,200]

Correction of severe symptomatic hypotonic hyponatremia, regardless of cause, should be accomplished with hypertonic (3%) saline (sodium concentration 513 mmol/L). The volume of 3% saline required can be estimated by the following formula:

$$\text{volume of 3\% saline (L/24 hours)} = \text{target change } P_{Na} \text{ (mmol/L/24 hours)} \times \text{TBW (L)} \div 513$$

For example, in a 70-kg man with a plasma sodium concentration of 105 mmol/L and total body water (TBW) of 42 L (60% of body weight), the amount of sodium needed to raise the plasma sodium concentration by 10 mmol/L is 10 × 42, or 420 mmol. Therefore, 420 ÷ 513 or 0.82 L of 3% saline would be required in the first 24 hours, or 34 mL/hour. It is important to recognize that the calculation provides only a very rough guideline. The plasma sodium concentration must be monitored frequently during treatment to adjust the rate of correction. If the rate of correction begins to exceed the target rate, the hypertonic saline infusion should be stopped; rarely, it may be necessary to administer water (enterally or intravenously) or even desmopressin[204] in order to prevent overly rapid correction or overcorrection. Rapid extracellular volume expansion with hypertonic saline may precipitate pulmonary edema, particularly in patients with underlying heart disease. Thus, patients receiving 3% saline should be assessed frequently for evidence of volume overload. One may administer a loop diuretic if necessary, recognizing that this will enhance electrolyte-free water clearance and accelerate the correction. Rarely, administration of isotonic (normal) saline to patients with SIADH paradoxically may *lower* the plasma sodium concentration if the urine osmolality remains high—a process that has been called *desalination.*[205]

The treatment of chronic asymptomatic hypotonicity should be directed at correcting the pathophysiologic mechanisms involved in generating the hypotonic state. Because euvolemic hyponatremia represents pure water excess, treatment depends on restricting water intake to less than the daily water output. Patients with SIADH excrete little or no electrolyte-free water in the urine. Therefore, if water intake is limited to less than the amount of insensible water losses (approximately 10 mL/kg/day), the plasma sodium concentration will slowly rise. Patients with the reset osmostat variant of SIADH characteristically do not develop progressive hypotonicity, and therapy is rarely required.

If the cause of SIADH cannot be corrected and if water restriction is poorly tolerated or ineffective, a specific vasopressin (V_2) receptor antagonist (VRA) can be used.[206] Conivaptan (parenteral) and tolvaptan (oral) were the first VRAs to be approved by the U.S. Food and Drug Administration for clinical use. These agents have changed the management of patients with SIADH.[207] Tolvaptan reliably increases P_{Na} concentration, but hyponatremia recurs within 1 week after the medication is discontinued.[208] For patients admitted with hyponatremia related to decompensated congestive heart failure, tolvaptan along with diuretic therapy improves most signs and symptoms of heart failure within 1 week,[209] although no effect on 24-month mortality rate or heart failure morbidity has been demonstrated.[210] Before the introduction of VRAs, demeclocycline (a tetracycline antibiotic that increases electrolyte-free water excretion by inhibiting vasopressin-mediated water reabsorption in the collecting duct) was commonly used to treat patients with SIADH. Demeclocycline is contraindicated in patients with renal disease, hepatic cirrhosis, or congestive heart failure because drug related renal insufficiency has been described in these situations.[206] Neither VRAs nor demeclocycline are indicated for the treatment of acute, severe hyponatremia.

Therapy of hypovolemic hyponatremia should be directed at restoring intravascular volume with intravenous isotonic saline while identifying and correcting the cause of the excessive solute loss. Volume repletion readily elicits a water diuresis by increasing the delivery of fluid to the renal diluting segments and suppressing vasopressin release. As with all categories of hypotonic hyponatremia, the rate of correction must be carefully controlled.

The treatment of diuretic-induced hyponatremia is straightforward: Withdrawing the offending drug, liberalizing salt intake, and replenishing body potassium stores usually correct the disorder. Severe symptomatic hyponatremia in this setting should be treated with hypertonic saline as detailed earlier. Patients must be watched carefully after correction of the hyponatremia because relapse may occur for up to a week.[193]

Resolution of the hyponatremia associated with any of the pathologic edematous disorders ultimately depends on effective treatment of the underlying disease. Regardless of the specific therapy of the underlying disorder, the mainstay

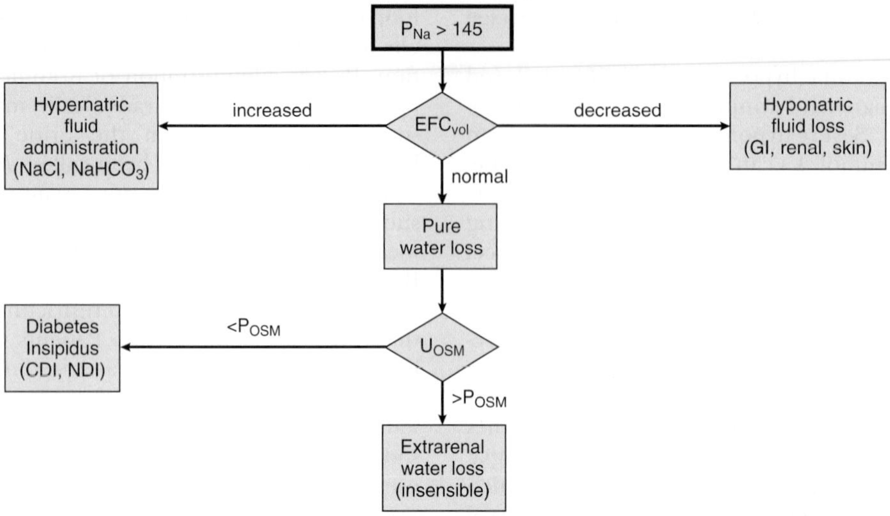

Figure 57.6 Diagnostic evaluation of hypernatremia. See Figure 57.3 legend for abbreviations. CDI, central diabetes insipidus; GI, gastrointestinal; NDI, nephrogenic diabetes insipidus.

of therapy for the hyponatremic edematous patient remains salt and water restriction. Diuretics are often a double-edged sword in the hyponatremic edematous patient: They may be needed to treat pulmonary vascular congestion, peripheral edema, and ascites but if used to excess can produce further decrements in effective arterial blood volume and exacerbate water retention. Strategies directed at increasing effective arterial blood volume (e.g., afterload reduction with angiotensin-converting enzyme inhibitors[211,212]) have had some success in increasing electrolyte-free water excretion and ameliorating hyponatremia in patients with congestive heart failure. VRAs are likely to facilitate treatment of hypervolemic hyponatremia (see earlier).[207]

HYPERNATREMIA

EPIDEMIOLOGY AND CLINICAL MANIFESTATIONS

Hypernatremia is common in critically ill patients, being present on admission in about 9% of patients and developing during the course of the ICU stay in another 6%.[213] It is associated with a significantly higher mortality rate than is seen in patients without hypernatremia.[213]

Sustained hypernatremia develops in patients whose water output exceeds their input. Water ingestion can defend against the development of hypernatremia even when water losses are prodigious. For that reason, hypernatremia upon presentation to the hospital occurs most commonly in patients who are incapacitated: those who have impaired thirst sensation, who cannot access water, or who cannot express their need for water (e.g., infants and patients with neurologic impairments). Similar predispositions prevail among critically ill patients. Thus, the development of hypernatremia in hospitalized patients is considered to be iatrogenic, reflecting an incomplete understanding of the factors that lead to hypernatremia.[213] The increased mortality rate seen in patients with hypernatremia probably is due to their underlying vulnerabilities rather than an effect of the hypernatremia itself.[214]

The clinical manifestations of hypernatremia are proportional to the magnitude and rate of rise of the plasma sodium concentration and are attributable to intracellular volume contraction. To counteract cellular volume contraction, cells begin to adapt within minutes by allowing the influx of electrolytes, thus mitigating cell shrinkage. When hypernatremia lasts more than a few hours, brain cells generate new *organic osmolytes.* This leads to further water movement back into brain cells, restoring cell volume nearly to normal after about 3 days.[215] Thus, chronic progressive hypernatremia is associated with fewer and milder symptoms than acute severe hypernatremia. Most often, patients with longstanding hypernatremia present with weakness, lethargy, and confusion. Seizure and coma may supervene. Acute severe hypernatremia in infants and small children is associated with intracranial bleeding,[216] presumably caused by brain shrinkage and traction on the penetrating vessels. There is some controversy, however, as to whether the hypernatremia in that situation is the cause or the effect of the intracranial hemorrhage.[217]

DIFFERENTIAL DIAGNOSIS

The plasma sodium concentration reflects the ratio of body sodium content to total body water. Thus, hypernatremia (plasma sodium concentration > 145 mmol/L) can result from loss of pure water alone, loss of *hyponatric** fluid, or a gain of sodium or *hypernatric* fluid. It is important to distinguish among these paths to hypernatremia because they have diagnostic and therapeutic implications (Fig. 57.6).

Euvolemic Hypernatremia

Hypernatremic patients who appear euvolemic most likely have pure water loss as an explanation for their hypernatremia. This is because the water is lost from all body compartments proportionately; only one twelfth of the water loss is intravascular. For example, a 60-kg woman with a 3 L pure

**Hyponatric* and *hypernatric* are used here to refer to a fluid with a sodium concentration less than (or greater than) that of plasma.

water loss would experience an intravascular loss of only 250 mL (clinically imperceptible) but would develop a plasma sodium concentration of 155 mmol/L.* Pure water can be lost either through the skin and respiratory tract (so-called *insensible* losses) or in urine.

Insensible losses amount to about 10 mL/kg/day under normal environmental conditions in an afebrile individual with a normal respiratory rate. A hot environment, fever, or rapid respiratory rate may double that rate.[173] Note that a patient on a mechanical ventilator using humidified gas will lose no water through the respiratory tract.

The loss of large amounts of dilute, electrolyte-free water in the urine is typical of *diabetes insipidus* (DI). DI may be central (CDI) or nephrogenic (NDI) depending on whether the defect is in vasopressin release from the posterior pituitary or in renal response to circulating vasopressin, respectively. The causes of DI are shown in Box 57.9. Most cases of CDI, especially those following trauma or intracranial surgery, are self-limited, lasting 3 to 5 days. Of special interest to intensivists is a classic triphasic syndrome that may be seen following severe head trauma:

1. Initially, there is abrupt cessation of vasopressin release from the posterior pituitary, accompanied by polyuria.
2. About a week later, an antidiuretic phase ensues, characterized by urinary concentration and water retention with a tendency toward hyponatremia, lasting 5 to 6 days. This appears to result from the release of stored vasopressin from the degenerating hypothalamic neurons.
3. Persistent CDI recurs when the vasopressin stores are depleted.[218]

Regardless of the cause, patients with DI of either type usually have a plasma sodium concentration within the normal range because their water ingestion matches their urinary water output. They develop hypernatremia only with water deprivation due to mental or physical incapacity or neglect. An awareness of the causes of DI, a careful history, and familiarity with the differential diagnosis of polyuria will prevent hypernatremia in these circumstances.

Hypovolemic Hypernatremia

The loss of salt and water, with the water loss greater than the sodium loss, will lead to hypernatremia and volume depletion, manifested by orthostatic or persistent hypotension and tachycardia and evidence of organ underperfusion (e.g., acute renal failure, lactic acidosis). For example, if the 60-kg woman whose plasma sodium concentration rose to 155 mmol/L (see earlier) had lost the equivalent of half-isotonic saline instead of pure water, her intravascular volume would have contracted by 750 mL, enough to cause at least orthostatic hypotension and tachycardia.

A common cause of hypovolemic hypernatremia is the loss of GI fluids.[219] Most GI fluids have an electrolyte concentration below that of plasma: The concentration of sodium plus potassium in stool is roughly constant at 110 to 120 mmol/L over a wide range of stool volume.[125] Gastric fluid has an even lower electrolyte concentration: about 40 to 50 mmol/L total cation concentration.[220] Diuresis, either osmotic (glucose-, mannitol-, or urea-induced) or medication-induced, causes the loss of urine with an electrolyte concentration less than that of plasma, leading to volume contraction and hypernatremia. The loss of sweat, which contains some sodium, can cause hypovolemic hypernatremia in individuals who exercise vigorously in a hot environment. If the cause of the fluid loss is not apparent from the history or the physical examination, a urinary chloride concentration less than 10 mmol/L in the face of hypovolemic hypernatremia suggests that the electrolyte loss is extrarenal (cutaneous or GI).

*The expected change in the serum sodium concentration is calculated as follows: [initial total body water volume] × [serum sodium concentration initial] ÷ [final total body water volume]; 30 L × 140 mmol/L ÷ 27 L = 155 mmol/L.

Box 57.9 Causes of Diabetes Insipidus

Central Diabetes Insipidus

- Posthypophysectomy
- Posttraumatic
- Granulomatous diseases
  - Histiocytosis
  - Sarcoidosis
- Infections
  - Meningitis
  - Encephalitis
- Inflammatory/autoimmune hypophysitis
- Vascular
  - Hypoxia
  - Thrombotic or embolic stroke
  - Hemorrhagic stroke
- Neoplastic
  - Craniopharyngioma
  - Pituitary adenoma
  - Lymphoma
  - Meningioma
- Drugs or toxins
  - Ethanol
  - Snake venom
- Congenital/hereditary

Nephrogenic Diabetes Insipidus

- Drug-induced
  - Lithium
  - Demeclocycline
  - Cisplatin
  - Ethanol
- Hypokalemia
- Hypercalcemia
- Vascular
  - Sickle cell anemia
- Infiltrating lesions
  - Sarcoidosis
  - Multiple myeloma
  - Amyloidosis
  - Sjögren syndrome
- Congenital
  - Autosomal recessive: aquaporin-2 water channel gene mutations
  - X-linked recessive: arginine vasopressin (AVP) V_2 receptor gene mutations

Hypervolemic Hypernatremia

Hypervolemic hypernatremia is relatively uncommon. It results most often from the administration of hypertonic sodium salts to patients without free access to water.[219] Patients show signs of extracellular volume expansion (e.g., hypertension, edema, congestive heart failure, and pulmonary edema). In infants, this syndrome has been caused by erroneous preparation of dietary formula using salt instead of sugar; in adult outpatients, it may be caused by ingestion of a concentrated salt solution, usually for its emetic effect.[221] The risk of death is substantial and seems to be proportional to the plasma sodium concentration.[221]

In hospitalized adults, hypervolemic hypernatremia it is most often iatrogenic, caused by intravenous administration of undiluted sodium bicarbonate (formulated at 1 mEq/mL or 1000 mmol/L) or sodium chloride (3% [513 mmol/L] or 23.5% [4019 mmol/L]). Not all hypervolemic hypernatremia results from the administration of hypertonic fluids. It may be seen in a volume-expanded patient who then loses hypotonic fluid.[222]

TREATMENT

The initial treatment of the hypernatremic patient depends on his or her volume status. For patients with pure water losses (euvolemic), therapy has two goals: (1) reduction or replacement of ongoing water losses, and (2) replacement of the existing water deficit.

If the water losses are urinary (see Fig. 57.6) and due to CDI, ADH should be administered. Several formulations are available (Table 57.3). In the acute (postsurgical or posttraumatic) setting, L-arginine vasopressin may be used either subcutaneously or intravenously, although the latter route may be associated with hypertension and coronary spasm and should therefore be used with extreme caution.[223] The advantage of vasopressin in this setting is its short half-life, which allows the physician to repeatedly assess the need for continued hormone replacement, especially when the disorder may be self-limited. Desmopressin (DDAVP) is a synthetic analog of vasopressin that has no vasoconstrictor properties, thus avoiding the risks of hypertension and myocardial ischemia. The treatment of the urinary water losses associated with NDI are best treated with thiazide diuretics with or without COX inhibitors. Because most of these agents are orally administered, treatment of NDI in the critically ill patient often consists of urinary water replacement until he or she is able to take medications by mouth.

The current body water deficit can be estimated by the following formula:

$$\text{Water deficit (liters)} = \text{TBW } (1 - [140 \div \text{current } P_{Na}])$$

where TBW is total body water in liters (estimated as about 0.5 × lean body weight [kg] in women and 0.6 × lean body weight in men). For example, a 60-kg woman presenting with a plasma sodium concentration of 160 mmol/L is estimated to have a total body water deficit of 30 (1 – 0.875), or 3.75 L. This formula provides only a rough estimate of the water deficit.

The rate of water replacement should be proportional to the rapidity with which the hypernatremia developed.[215] Thus, if the hypernatremia had developed over only a few hours (such as in postsurgical or posttraumatic DI), it can be corrected just as quickly. On the other hand, hypernatremia of more than a day's duration, or of unknown duration, must be correctly slowly in order to avoid cerebral edema. In general, one should aim to correct half the water deficit in the first 24 hours and the remainder over the next 24 to 48 hours.

Water is best administered enterally, as tap water. If that route is unavailable, 5% dextrose in water (D_5W) may be used, with the understanding that the capacity to metabolize glucose is limited to about 15 g/hour in a critically ill adult.[224] Thus, even in nondiabetic patients, the administration of more than 300 mL/hour of D_5W is likely to result in hyperglycemia, which may be relatively resistant to insulin administration. Hyperglycemia will exacerbate urinary water losses by causing an osmotic diuresis. Half-normal (0.45%) saline may be a good alternative, as long as one recognizes that only half the administered volume is electrolyte-free water and that the sodium load may cause unwanted volume expansion.

Regardless of the degree of hypernatremia, normal (.9%) saline should be given intravenously to patients who present with obvious volume depletion, manifested by hypotension, tachycardia, and evidence of impaired tissue perfusion. This is consistent with the first principles of emergency and critical care, prioritizing the adequacy of the circulation. Only

Table 57.3 Pharmacologic Treatment of Central Diabetes Insipidus

Agent	Total Daily Dose	Frequency of Administration	Time to Onset (h)	Duration of Action (h)	Comments
Arginine vasopressin, 20 units/mL	5-10 units subcutaneous	q2-4h	1-2	2-6	Intravenous route may cause vasoconstriction and coronary spasm
Desmopressin acetate (DDAVP)					
10 µg/0.1 mL intranasal	10-40 µg intranasal	Daily or bid	1-2	8-12	
4 µg/mL injection	2-4 µg IV or subcutaneous	Daily or bid	1-2	8-12	

Adapted from Singer I, Oster JR, Fishman LM: The management of diabetes insipidus in adults. Arch Intern Med 1997;157(12):1293-1301.

after the extracellular volume deficits have been largely corrected may the physician direct his or her attention to the total body water deficit (see earlier).

Patients with hypervolemic hypernatremia need reduction in their extracellular and intravascular volume before their water deficit can be corrected. Failure to do so will exacerbate the volume overload. For patients with adequate renal function, this may be accomplished with the use of diuretic drugs. Loop diuretics tend to cause the excretion of an isotonic urine. Replacement of that urine volume with pure water will allow correction of the hypervolemia and the hypernatremia simultaneously.

Because of the imprecision of the estimation formulas and the failure of the foregoing analysis to take account of other fluids and electrolytes both administered and lost, it is crucial that the plasma electrolytes be monitored frequently during the correction of hypernatremia, especially in view of the dire consequences of overly rapid correction.

CALCIUM HOMEOSTASIS

Calcium (Ca) is required for bone mineralization, muscle contraction, nerve conduction, and blood coagulation. It is required for cell division, hormone secretion, phagocytosis, chemotaxis, and activation of numerous intracellular second messengers.[225] Calcium is also responsible for activation of calcium-dependent phospholipases and proteases, generation of free radicals, release of cytokines, and inhibition of adenosine triphosphate (ATP) production in the face of ischemic injury. Thus calcium plays a central role in physiologic as well as pathologic conditions.[226]

NORMAL CALCIUM PHYSIOLOGY

Calcium is the most abundant cation in the body. The total body calcium content of an average adult is approximately 1 kg, 99% of which is found in bones and teeth, with only 1% in plasma and soft tissues.[227] Calcium homeostasis is achieved with the cooperation of several organs, including the skeleton, the gut, and the kidney, under the influence of several hormones, mainly vitamin D, parathyroid hormone (PTH), and calcitonin.

CALCIUM INTAKE AND ABSORPTION

The typical daily dietary intake of calcium for an average adult in North America is 800 to 1000 mg. The main dietary source of calcium is milk and other dairy products; it is also available in the form of fortified food and calcium-containing supplements. Approximately 20% of dietary calcium is absorbed by intestine. Intestinal absorptive capacity increases with calcium deprivation and under certain physiologic conditions such as growth spurt in children, pregnancy, and lactation.[228] Intestinal absorption occurs via both passive paracellular and active transcellular pathways. Vitamin D increases the active transport of calcium across the intestinal membranes.[227]

RENAL HANDLING OF CALCIUM

The filtered load of calcium (the product of glomerular filtration rate and the plasma concentration of ultrafilterable calcium) is about 10 g/day. Calcium balance is maintained when the kidneys excrete about 200 mg/day (the intestinal absorptive load). Thus, the fractional excretion of calcium is only about 2%.[227,228] Of the 98% of filtered calcium reabsorbed along the nephron, 60% is reabsorbed in the proximal tubule. Approximately 15% of the filtered calcium is reabsorbed in the thick ascending limb of loop of Henle (TAL). The reabsorption of calcium in TAL is mostly passive and proportional to the lumen-positive voltage generated by the furosemide-inhibitable Na-K-Cl cotransporter (NKCC2) channel and potassium recycling via renal outer medullary potassium (ROMK) channels. There is also some active transcellular transport, which is under the influence of PTH and calcitonin.[227,228] In the distal tubule, approximately 10% to 15% of filtered calcium is reabsorbed via active transcellular pathways. The apical membranes of distal convoluted tubules (DCT) and connecting tubules (CNT) contain highly selective epithelial calcium channels (TRPV-5)[227,228] that facilitate calcium entry into the cells. PTH increases the density and open probability of TRPV-5 channels.[229]

Volume expansion, hypercalcemia, acute and chronic acidosis, and loop diuretics reduce the renal calcium reabsorption and result in hypercalciuria. Conversely, hypocalcemia, alkalosis, PTH, calcitriol, and thiazide diuretics enhance renal calcium reabsorption and cause hypocalciuria.

REGULATION OF PLASMA CALCIUM

Normal plasma calcium concentration is 8.8 to 10.4 mg/dL. In plasma, calcium exists in two forms: protein-bound and *ultrafilterable* (permeant across the glomerular filtration barrier). Approximately 40% of plasma calcium is bound to plasma proteins (predominantly albumin), cannot cross the biologic membranes, and is thus physiologically inert. The ultrafilterable portion of plasma calcium makes up the remaining 60% of plasma calcium and consists of calcium complexed with various anions like citrate, phosphate, and lactate (about 10%) and free, ionized calcium (Ca^{2+})—the biologically active form—accounting for about 50% of plasma levels.[230]

Plasma Ca^{2+} concentration is tightly regulated. Several factors play an important role in maintaining plasma Ca^{2+} concentration within a narrow range (about 4.4-5.2 mg/dL or 1.1-1.3 mmol/L). The principal regulators are PTH, vitamin D_3, and Ca^{2+} itself.

Ca^{2+} acts as a ligand for calcium-sensing receptors (CaSR) present on the chief cells of the parathyroid glands. A rise in plasma Ca^{2+} concentration results in activation of CaSR, which in turn inhibits PTH secretion. Conversely, a fall in Ca^{2+} concentration inhibits CaSR, increasing PTH secretion. PTH mobilizes the calcium from bone stores, stimulates renal calcium reabsorption, and increases the conversion of $25(OH)D_3$ to $1,25(OH)_2D_3$, the most active form of vitamin D_3. Activated vitamin D_3 increases intestinal calcium absorption. All these systems work in concert to keep the Ca^{2+} levels within physiologic levels.[225]

PLASMA CALCIUM MEASUREMENT

Ca^{2+} is the physiologically important moiety, yet total calcium is most often measured in clinical laboratories. Under normal circumstances, there is a fairly constant relationship between total and ionized calcium (see earlier), but in critically ill patients, this relationship may be disturbed such that total calcium no longer provides a reliable index of the physiologically important calcium concentration. The two major factors affecting the ratio of ionized to total calcium are acid-base status and plasma protein concentration.

Acidemia causes displacement of calcium ions from albumin by protons and results in a relative increase in Ca^{2+}. Conversely, alkalemia increases calcium binding to albumin, causing a relative fall in Ca^{2+} levels while total plasma calcium concentration remains unchanged.[225,227]

Changes in the concentration of plasma protein, especially albumin, result in alterations in total calcium concentration: Hypoalbuminemia, common in critically ill patients, causes a reduction in total calcium concentration; hyperalbuminemia (e.g., in states of severe volume contraction) tends to cause an increase in total plasma Ca. Numerous formulas have been proposed to adjust the total calcium concentration for changes in plasma albumin concentration.[231] The most commonly used formula is based on the observation that each gram of albumin binds about 0.8 mg calcium at physiologic pH:

$$Ca_{corrected} = Ca_{observed} + (0.8 \cdot [4.0 - albumin])$$

Unfortunately, the corrected calcium correlates very poorly with Ca^{2+} in various critically ill populations, typically with a very low sensitivity for diagnosis of true hypocalcemia.[231-233]

The reasons for this discrepancy are manifold, including concurrent acid-base disorders, high circulating concentrations of free fatty acids,[234] and infusions of heparin, citrate, and bicarbonate.[233] Therefore, in critically ill patients, direct measurement of Ca^{2+} is recommended for assessing physiologic calcium concentration.

HYPOCALCEMIA

EPIDEMIOLOGY

Hypocalcemia is extremely common in critically ill patients. The prevalence of ionized hypocalcemia is reported to be 60% to 85% among medical, surgical, and trauma ICU patients.[235-238] Risk factors for the development of hypocalcemia in critically ill patients include advanced age, sepsis, acute renal failure, multiple blood transfusion, malnutrition, magnesium deficiency, severe shock, and colloid volume resuscitation.[238,239] Mortality rate is higher in hypocalcemic patients[236,240,241] but does not appear to be independently associated with hypocalcemia.[237,238]

CAUSES OF HYPOCALCEMIA

Causes of hypocalcemia are shown in Box 57.10. Hypocalcemia may be caused by disorders involving the hormonal regulators of calcium homeostasis, PTH, and vitamin D; redistribution of calcium; drugs; and miscellaneous influences. We will discuss causes of particular relevance to the critical care setting.

Box 57.10 Causes of Hypocalcemia

Hypoparathyroidism

- Acquired
  - Parathyroidectomy
  - Infiltrative or malignant disease
- Congenital
- Idiopathic

Vitamin D Deficiency

- Malnutrition
- Malabsorption
- Liver disease
- Kidney disease

Redistribution

- Tissue sequestration
  - Acute pancreatitis
  - Rhabdomyolysis
- Complexation
  - Alkali
  - Citrated blood-product transfusions
  - Citrate anticoagulation in continuous renal replacement therapy
  - Plasmapheresis
  - Bicarbonate infusion for metabolic acidosis
  - Phosphate
  - Tumor lysis syndrome
  - Fleet enemas and phosphate-containing laxatives
  - Rhabdomyolysis
- Ethylenediamine tetra-acetic acid (EDTA)

Drugs

- Cisplatin
- Bisphosphonates
- Plicamycin

Miscellaneous

- Sepsis/systemic inflammatory response syndrome
- Hypomagnesemia
- Acute renal failure

Hypoparathyroidism

Parathyriodectomy, for hyperparathyroidism or "incidentally" with thyroidectomy, may cause postoperative hypocalcemia. Risk factors for developing hypocalcemia include subtotal parathyroidectomy and simultaneous thyroidectomy. Profound, long-lasting hypocalcemia may develop as part of the "hungry bone" syndrome, in which calcium is sequestered into the rapidly remineralizing bone.[242] Hypomagnesemia may contribute to the hypocalcemia (see discussion under "Magnesium Homeostasis").

Vitamin D Deficiency

Vitamin D deficiency is common in elderly, institutionalized patients due to poor dietary intake and inadequate sunlight exposure. Diseases involving liver and small intestine may result in poor absorption of vitamin D. For conversion to its most active form, vitamin D requires hydroxylation in liver and kidney. Frequently, critically ill patients suffer from liver and kidney dysfunction, which results in impaired vitamin D synthesis and predisposes to hypocalcemia.[226] Vitamin D deficiency (level <20 ng/dL) upon admission to a medical ICU has been associated with increased mortality rate.[243] Whether vitamin D supplementation to critically ill patients will reduce mortality rate remains to be determined.

Redistribution

Citrate is useful as a preservative and anticoagulant for blood components precisely because it chelates calcium and thereby inhibits the coagulation cascade. The calcium citrate complex is then metabolized in liver, where citrate is converted into bicarbonate, and ionized calcium is released into the circulation. Massive blood transfusion may result in ionized hypocalcemia due to chelation of calcium by citrate. However, hypocalcemia is transient in patients with normal liver function and ionized calcium levels return to normal levels within 15 minutes of transfusion.[244] Citrate also may be used for anticoagulation of the dialysis circuit for continuous renal replacement therapy (CVVHD and variants). Under those conditions, calcium typically is infused through a central venous line to prevent hypocalcemia. Inadequate calcium replacement or concomitant liver failure may result in clinically significant hypocalcemia. In the latter case, with citrate accumulation, the total calcium may be misleadingly normal, but the Ca^{2+} is low.[245,246] Hypocalcemia is frequently reported with plasmapheresis where citrate is used for anticoagulation.[247] Sodium *bicarbonate* to treat metabolic acidosis may cause hypocalcemia from calcium binding to albumin and formation of carbonate complexes. Similarly, abrupt alkalinization from hemodialysis against a bicarbonate bath may precipitate symptomatic hypocalcemia.

Phosphate binds with calcium to form insoluble calcium phosphate complexes. Under normal physiologic conditions, calcium and phosphorus levels are tightly regulated, preventing significant complexation. Any condition that causes acute increase in phosphate levels, however, can cause complexation and resultant ionized hypocalcemia. Examples include endogenous phosphorus overload as in the tumor lysis syndrome[72] and exogenous phosphorus overload from laxatives and cathartics.[248-251] Patients with impaired renal function are at particular risk.[249] (See discussion under "Phosphorus Homeostasis.")

Hypocalcemia in *rhabdomyolysis* is multifactorial and involves calcium deposition in injured muscles, formation of calcium-phosphate complex due to hyperphosphatemia, and acute renal failure causing decreased synthesis of vitamin D.[252]

Ionized hypocalcemia is reported in up to 85% of patients suffering from acute severe *pancreatitis*.[253] The cause of hypocalcemia in this setting us unclear. Calcium has been shown to accumulate in pancreas, liver, and skeletal muscle in an animal model of acute pancreatitis.[254] Low[255] and high[256,257] levels of PTH have been reported. Experimental elevation in free fatty acids, both circulating[258] (as might be seen in the hypertriglyceridemia of acute pancreatitis) and intraperitoneal,[259] have been associated with the hypocalcemia of acute pancreatitis. Finally, high circulating endotoxin levels may have a role.[253]

Drugs

Bisphosphonates are used for the treatment of osteoporosis and hypercalcemia. They act by impairing osteoclast function and reducing osteoclast numbers. Bisphosphonate-induced hypocalcemia has been reported in patients with renal failure, hypoparathyroidism, or vitamin D deficiency.[260] Other drugs such as colchicine, plicamycin (formerly mithramycin), and calcitonin also decrease bone release of calcium.[227]

Sepsis/Systemic Inflammatory Response Syndrome

Hypocalcemia is common in patients suffering from sepsis or systemic inflammatory response syndrome.[236,240] The cause probably is multifactorial.[261] Among the proposed mechanisms are calcium sequestration,[262,263] an effect of inflammatory cytokines,[264] calcitonin precursors,[264,265] hypomagnesemia[266] with inappropriate hypoparathyroidism,[261] and probable PTH resistance.[264,267] Vitamin D deficiency, from malnutrition and inability to hydroxylate vitamin D due to coexisting liver and kidney dysfunction, also has been implicated.[261] The hypocalcemia may serve to protect vulnerable cells from the deleterious effects of calcium during sepsis. Indeed, calcium administration in this setting may be detrimental.[261]

CLINICAL MANIFESTATIONS

Hypocalcemia affects predominantly the neuromuscular and cardiovascular systems. Neuromuscular manifestations include paraesthesias (perioral and acral), hyperactive reflexes, tetany (carpopedal spasm and other muscle spasm), and seizures.[227] Laryngospasm and bronchospasm may supervene, leading to respiratory arrest.[225] Tetany may be provoked by tapping over the facial nerve and noting ipsilateral facial muscle twitching (Chvostek sign) and transiently occluding the brachial artery with a tourniquet and noting carpal spasm (Trousseau sign), although neither of these signs is specific for hypocalcemia. Prolonged hypocalcemia lasting more than 36 hours has been associated with the development of critical illness polyneuropathy and myopathy.[268] Psychiatric manifestations include anxiety, irritability, confusion, and psychosis.[225]

Cardiovascular findings include a prolonged QT interval and, in severe hypocalcemia, bradycardia, hypotension refractory to fluids and pressors, heart block, heart failure, and cardiac arrest.[226]

Symptoms and signs of hypocalcemia depend on the degree of depression of ionized calcium levels and the rate of decline.[227] Mild hypocalcemia (ionized calcium > 3.2 mg/dL) usually is well tolerated.

DIAGNOSIS

When hypocalcemia is suspected in a critically ill patient, the diagnosis should be established by direct measurement of ionized calcium levels (see "Plasma Calcium Measurement"). If ionized hypocalcemia is confirmed, plasma magnesium and phosphorus should be measured. Further diagnostic evaluation derives from the differential diagnosis (see Box 57.10). Without PTH levels and vitamin D levels, the diagnosis of hypocalcemia remains obscure in the majority of critically ill patients.[236]

TREATMENT

Therapy of hypocalcemia depends on its severity. Hypocalcemia (ionized Ca < 3.2 mg/dL) accompanied by serious cardiovascular or neuromuscular signs should be treated urgently. Calcium gluconate (10% in 10 mL containing 90 mg elemental calcium) can be given over 5 to 10 minutes, followed by calcium gluconate infusion (500-1000 mg in 500 mL 5% dextrose) over 6 hours.[227] Calcium chloride (10% in 10 mL containing 272 mg elemental calcium) contains more calcium and can rapidly increase plasma calcium levels, however, it is more irritating to the veins and must be given by a central venous catheter. Patients with renal failure, hyperphosphatemia, and serious hypocalcemia may require dialysis.

Patients receiving intravenous calcium should have frequent measurement of the ionized calcium. They should be monitored for side effects of calcium administration including hypertension, skin flushing, nausea, vomiting, and chest pain.

Intravenous calcium should be reserved for patients who have severe hypocalcemia or who are incapable of taking calcium orally. Administration of intravenous calcium can cause complexing with phosphorus and ectopic calcification.

Critically ill patients with mild hypocalcemia (iCa > 3.2 mg/dL) tend to have few if any manifestations. Patients with longstanding or chronic hypocalcemia (e.g., due to vitamin D deficiency or hypoparathyroidism) should receive oral calcium supplementation. Calcium is available as carbonate, citrate, phosphate, and lactate salt. Calcium requirement varies between 1 and 4 g elemental calcium daily and must be given in divided doses. Vitamin D can be added with calcium to enhance intestinal absorption.

Several points in the management of hypocalcemia should be borne in mind. First, in cases of concomitant mild hypocalcemia with hyperphosphatemia (e.g., renal failure), the hyperphosphatemia should be corrected using phosphate binders because that alone will often lead to correction of the hypocalcemia. Second, magnesium deficits should be corrected because that may restore normal calcium physiology even without calcium supplementation (see discussion under "Magnesium Homeostasis"). Finally, concurrent severe metabolic acidosis should await correction of the hypocalcemia, because correction of the acidosis will be likely to worsen the ionized hypocalcemia and precipitate tetany.

HYPERCALCEMIA

Hypercalcemia has been reported in 15% to 30% of critically ill patients, [267,269] and thus appears to be less common than hypocalcemia. It is more common in patients with higher severity of illness and in those with concurrent renal failure.[267,269]

CAUSES OF HYPERCALCEMIA

Box 57.11 lists causes of hypercalcemia. About 90% of hypercalcemia in ambulatory and non-ICU patients is caused by only two entities: primary hyperparathyroidism and malignancy.[225] The spectrum is a bit broader in critically ill patients.

Box 57.11 Causes of Hypercalcemia

- Primary hyperparathyroidism
- Malignancy
  - Parathyroid hormone related peptide (PTHrP)
  - Ectopic parathyroid hormone
  - Vitamin D mediated
  - Lytic bone lesions
- Vitamin D
  - Exogenous
  - Endogenous
- Hyperthyroidism
- Adrenal insufficiency
- Rhabdomyolysis, recovery
- Immobilization
- Drugs
  - Thiazide
  - Lithium
  - Vitamin D/calcium supplements
  - Vitamin A

Primary Hyperparathyroidism

Primary hyperparathyroidism is the most common cause of hypercalcemia, accounting for more than 50% of cases in ambulatory patients. Specific causes include benign adenoma (80-90%), hyperplasia (10-20%), and carcinoma (1%). Biochemical abnormalities include elevated circulating intact PTH, hypercalcemia, and hypophosphatemia.[225]

Malignancies

Hypercalcemia is rarely the presenting sign of a malignancy; most malignancies are advanced at the time hypercalcemia develops. About 40% of hypercalcemia in hospitalized patients has been associated with cancer.[270] Almost 80% of malignancy-related hypercalcemia is secondary to the secretion of *parathyroid hormone-related peptide* (PTHrP) by the malignant cells.[270] PTHrP is not detected by clinical laboratory assays for PTH. Numerous types of malignancies are associated with PTHrP-mediated hypercalcemia including breast,[271] renal cell, and ovarian carcinomas[225] and hematologic malignancies.[272]

Increased production of 1,25-$(OH)_2D_3$ by malignant cells is one of the causes of hypercalcemia in patients with lymphomas.[273,274] Finally, osteolytic bone lesions from advanced cancers such as breast, lung, and multiple myeloma frequently result in hypercalcemia.[225]

Rhabdomyolysis

Rhabdomyolysis associated with acute renal failure commonly produces hypocalcemia during the initial phase (see "Hypocalcemia"). Approximately 30% of patients, mostly young men, develop hypercalcemia during resolution of the acute renal failure.[275] Release from injured muscles of previously sequestered calcium appears to be the basis for the hypercalcemia.[275,276] PTH is appropriately suppressed according to most[277,278] but not all[279] studies. Vitamin D levels may be elevated[277,279] or suppressed;[252,278] its contribution to the syndrome is unclear. Whatever the underlying mechanism, the hypercalcemia is usually mild and self-limited.[275]

Immobilization

Immobilization is associated with hypercalcemia due to increased bone resorption. Risk factors include duration of bed rest, spinal cord injury, multiple skeletal fractures, and underlying disorders leading to increased bone resorption (e.g., Paget disease, malignancy).[280,281] Although hypercalcemia is usually modest and completely reversible with activity, calcitonin and bisphosphonates can be used with success if treatment is required.[280]

Medications

A small percentage (5-10%) of patients treated with *lithium* develop hypercalcemia due to lithium-induced hyperparathyroidism.[225] Hyperparathyroidism may or may not be reversible on discontinuation of therapy. *Thiazide diuretics* increase tubular reabsorption of calcium and are well known to cause modest hypercalcemia, which reverts back to normal upon discontinuation of therapy. More severe hypercalcemia should prompt an evaluation for occult hyperparathyroidism. *Vitamin A* may increase osteoclast-mediated bone resorption and cause hypercalcemia.

Milk-Alkali Syndrome

This syndrome comprises hypercalcemia (often extreme), metabolic alkalosis, and acute renal failure. It is seen in patients who ingest large quantities of alkaline calcium salts (e.g., calcium carbonate), often with vitamin D preparations.[282] Because of the increasing use of these medications to prevent or treat osteoporosis, the incidence of this syndrome, once considered rare, appears to be increasing.[283]

CLINICAL MANIFESTATIONS

Clinical manifestations of hypercalcemia depend on the rate of increase and absolute level of plasma calcium. The most serious manifestations are *neurologic* and *cardiovascular*. Patients may experience muscle weakness, fatigue, depression, and altered mental status. At extremely high levels, stupor and coma may ensue.[225,230] Prolonged hypercalcemia lasting longer than 36 hours has been associated with the development of critical illness polyneuropathy and myopathy.[268] Hypercalcemia causes an increased rate of cardiac repolarization and results in shortened QT interval. Conduction disturbances and malignant arrhythmias have been reported with hypercalcemia.[284,285]

Hypercalcemia may lead to acute renal failure from volume depletion and renal vasoconstriction and polyuria and polydipsia due to NDI.[225,230] GI symptoms include anorexia, nausea, vomiting, and constipation. Peptic ulcer disease and acute pancreatitis are exceedingly rare, especially in the acute setting.[225]

DIAGNOSIS

The diagnosis of hypercalcemia often is apparent from the history, with an understanding of the differential diagnosis (see Box 57.11). In cases of sustained or unexplained hypercalcemia, assays for intact PTH and vitamin D metabolites are of great value. An assay for PTHrP rarely is necessary in the evaluation of hypercalcemia in a critically ill patient, because in most patients with hypercalcemia of malignancy, the cancer is advanced and the diagnosis will be obvious when the PTH and vitamin D levels are shown to be suppressed.

TREATMENT

The treatment strategy for hypercalcemia depends on the severity of the disturbance and on its underlying cause. Identification of the probable cause of the hypercalcemia is important both for the immediate and long-term management.

Mild hypercalcemia (total Ca $\leq$ 12 mg/dL or 3 mmol/L) is usually caused by primary hyperparathyroidism, thiazide diuretics, calcium and vitamin D supplements, lithium, and immobilization. Treatment should begin with withdrawal of the offending agent (if possible). Volume deficits should be replaced orally if possible. Early mobilization should be encouraged. Loop diuretics should be avoided in patients with mild asymptomatic hypercalcemia as they may exacerbate the volume depletion, leading to increased renal calcium reabsorption.

The immediate treatment of moderate hypercalcemia (total Ca > 12 mg/dL or 3 mmol/L, and $\leq$ 14 mg/dL or 3.5 mmol/L) includes the measures discussed earlier, as well as intravenous volume expansion with isotonic saline. A loop diuretic will enhance renal excretion of calcium, but care must be taken to avoid volume depletion.

Severe hypercalcemia (total Ca >14 mg/dL or 3.5 mmol/L), even in the absence of signs and symptoms, should be treated as an emergency. Strategies for treatment include (1) enhanced calcium elimination; (2) reduced bone resorption; (3) decreased gut absorption of Ca; and (4) identification and treatment of the underlying cause.

Enhanced Calcium Elimination

Forced diuresis is the mainstay of treatment. *Volume expansion* with normal saline should be instituted immediately at a rate of 200 to 300 mL/hour. The net fluid balance in adults should be positive approximately 2 L in 24 hours. Caution must be taken to avoid symptomatic volume overload in patients with impaired myocardial performance and/or renal insufficiency.

Once the volume deficit is adequately replaced, *loop diuretics* should be added to enhance renal calcium excretion. A dose of loop diuretic that at least doubles the rate of urine output can be given as often as every 8 hours.

For patients with congestive heart failure unresponsive to diuretics, or with advanced kidney failure, *dialysis* should be considered. Hemodialysis against a solution containing 2.0 mEq/L calcium is very effective in decreasing plasma calcium levels. Lower calcium baths are likely to cause hypotension[286] and precipitate tetany.

Reduced Bone Resorption

Several agents are available for the management of hypercalcemia. *Bisphosphonates* inhibit the osteoclast functions and number and inhibit bone turnover. They are well tolerated, although nephrotoxicity may develop if administered too quickly.[230] Pamidronate (60-90 mg intravenously) reduces the plasma calcium in 48 to 72 hours and the effect may last for a month.[230] Zoledronic acid may be even more efficacious.[287] With the advent of bisphosphonates, two older agents have fallen into disfavor: *Calcitonin* has rapid onset of action but tachyphylaxis occurs within 48 to 72 hours. *Plicamycin* (formerly mithramycin) has unacceptable liver, renal, and bone marrow toxicity.

Decreased Gut Calcium Absorption

If endogenous vitamin D overproduction is implicated in the hypercalcemia (e.g., lymphoma, sarcoidosis), corticosteroids will lower the plasma calcium, at least partly by decreasing gut calcium absorption.

MAGNESIUM HOMEOSTASIS

Disorders of magnesium balance may be the most commonly seen electrolyte abnormalities in the ICU. Hypomagnesemia, the more common disorder, is seen in 12% of hospitalized patients and up to 65% of critically ill patients.[288-290] Because of magnesium's involvement in a host of critical physiologic functions,[291] its derangement can be expected to result in a variety of manifestations.

NORMAL MAGNESIUM PHYSIOLOGY

The normal adult total body magnesium content is approximately 24 g or 2000 mEq, 50% to 60% of which is found in bones and 40% to 50% in the intracellular compartment, mainly in the muscles and soft tissues. Only about 1% of total body magnesium is in the extracellular space, the normal concentration range being 1.8 to 2.3 mg/dL (1.5-1.9 mEq/L or about 0.7-1.0 mmol/L).[228] In plasma, 20% to 30% of magnesium is bound to protein, mainly albumin, with the rest (70-80%) in a form that is filterable across the glomerulus.[228] Magnesium is taken up slowly into cells, under no known hormonal control.

Magnesium is a major constituent of chlorophyll, and therefore green vegetables are a good dietary source. Also, magnesium is found in grains, cereals, meat, and seafood.[228,292] The normal adult diet contains about 300 mg of magnesium.[293] Under normal circumstances, about one third of that is absorbed in the small bowel; there is some obligatory secretion in that segment as well, along with some minor reabsorption downstream in the colon.[288] This results in net absorption of about 100 mg/day. (Magnesium absorption is highly dependent on dietary magnesium content, however, and can increase to up to 70-80% of dietary intake under conditions of magnesium deprivation.[228]) Unlike calcium absorption, magnesium absorption from the intestine does not seem to depend significantly on vitamin D.[228,294] The small intestinal secretion of magnesium normally amounts to a loss of only about 20 mg a day. With acute or chronic diarrhea, however, GI losses can be substantial.[228]

The filtered load of magnesium (the product of the glomerular filtration rate and the plasma concentration of ultrafilterable magnesium) is about 2500 mg/day. In order to maintain external magnesium balance, the renal excretion of magnesium must equal the intestinal absorption, or about 100 mg/day. Thus, the fractional excretion of magnesium ($Mg_{excreted} \div Mg_{filtered}$) is about 4% under normal conditions.[228] With magnesium depletion, the fractional excretion of magnesium can fall to less than 1%, and with magnesium loading, it can rise to match the excess in the filtered load.[228] This modulation in magnesium excretion is largely due to changes in plasma magnesium concentration.

The major site of renal magnesium reabsorption (60-70% of the filtered load) is the TAL. This tubular segment is responsible for most of the modulation in magnesium excretion. Magnesium reabsorption here is largely passive and depends on a lumen-positive voltage generated by the (diuretic-inhibitable) NKCC2 channel and potassium recycling via the ROMK channels.[228] This explains why loop diuretics increase urinary magnesium excretion and tend to cause hypomagnesemia. Other factors that inhibit magnesium reabsorption in the TAL include volume expansion, hypercalcemia, hypophosphatemia, and to a lesser extent metabolic acidosis. Conversely, volume depletion, hypocalcemia, and metabolic alkalosis increase magnesium reabsorption. About 10% of filtered magnesium is reabsorbed in the distal convoluted tubule. Reabsorption at this site is stimulated by potassium-sparing diuretics like amiloride.[288]

Magnesium plays a vital role in cellular physiology. It catalyzes over 300 enzymatic reactions and is an integral part of all ATP-dependent reactions.[291] It is involved in synthesis of proteins, energy-rich compounds, and electron and proton transporters; DNA and RNA transcription; translation of mRNA; and regulation of mitochondrial function.[291,295] There is evidence that magnesium helps regulate intracellular calcium concentration, especially in vascular smooth muscle, and thereby affects vascular tone.[295] In vitro studies suggest a role for magnesium in inflammation and immunity, though clinical confirmation is lacking.[295]

ASSESSMENT OF BODY MAGNESIUM STATUS

Because extracellular magnesium accounts for only about 1% of total body magnesium, plasma magnesium is a poor reflection of body magnesium status. Nonetheless, magnesium status is most commonly assessed by measuring plasma magnesium levels. Like calcium, magnesium circulates in the plasma in bound and free (ionized) forms, the latter being the metabolically active form. Determination of Mg^{2+} is clinically impractical, and there is no reliable correlation with serum albumin concentration. Moreover, the relationship between low Mg^{2+} concentration and increased morbidity and mortality rate in critically ill patients has yet to be clearly established.[296-298] Thus, the available literature does not support the superiority of the measurement of Mg^{2+} over the cheaper and widely available total serum magnesium levels.

The magnesium loading test has been proposed as a more sensitive measure of total body magnesium stores than the plasma magnesium concentration. In theory, magnesium-depleted individuals will translocate more of the administered magnesium load into cells and excrete a lower proportion in the urine over 24 hours.[266,288,295] Because the test requires a 24-hour urine collection, and must be limited to patients who have normal renal function and who are not on medications that affect magnesium excretion (see later), the test is impractical.

HYPOMAGNESEMIA

EPIDEMIOLOGY

Patients with malnutrition, chronic alcoholism, or congestive heart failure on loop diuretics; patients in the postoperative period (especially after open heart surgery); and patients with cancer are at higher risk than general ICU population.[288-290,299]

CAUSES

The causes of hypomagnesemia can be divided into four main categories: (1) insufficient intake, (2) renal loss, (3) extrarenal loss, and (4) redistribution (Box 57.12).

The renal causes can be distinguished from the others by measuring 24-hour urinary magnesium excretion or, more practically, the fractional excretion of magnesium (FE_{Mg}), calculated as follows:[288]

$$FE_{Mg} = \frac{U_{Mg} \times P_{Cr}}{(0.7 \times P_{Mg}) \times U_{Cr}} \times 100$$

where U_{Mg} and P_{Mg} are the urine and plasma concentrations of Mg, respectively, and U_{Cr} and P_{Cr} are the urine and plasma concentrations of creatinine, respectively. (P_{Mg} is multiplied by 0.7, which represents the ultrafilterable fraction of magnesium.) A 24-hour urinary magnesium excretion of more than about 25 mg, or FE_{Mg} greater than 2%, is consistent with renal hypomagnesemia.[225,288] Most hypomagnesemia in critically ill patients is multifactorial.

Box 57.12 Causes of Hypomagnesemia

Deficient Intake

- Magnesium-deficient parenteral nutrition
- Protein-calorie malnutrition
- Alcoholism

Renal Loss

- Drug induced
  - Loop diuretics
  - Thiazide diuretics
  - Aminoglycosides
  - Amphotericin B
  - Cisplatin
  - Cetuximab
  - Foscarnet
  - Pentamidine
- Volume expansion
- Osmotic diuresis (e.g., hyperglycemia)
- Alcohol
- Hypercalcemia
- Tubular dysfunction
  - Recovery from acute tubular necrosis
  - Bartter syndrome
  - Gitelman syndrome

Gastrointestinal

- Small intestine resection
- Inflammatory bowel disease
- Jejunoileal bypass surgery
- Diarrhea
- Steatorrhea
- Malabsorption syndromes
- Proton pump inhibitors

Redistribution

- Acute pancreatitis
- "Hungry bone" syndrome

Deficient Intake

The prevalence of hypomagnesemia is chronic alcoholics is approximately 20% to 30%. Hypomagnesemia in alcoholics is multifactorial and results from decreased dietary intake, increased renal loss, and acute pancreatitis.[288] Parenteral nutrition is an important cause of hypomagnesemia in the ICU. Patients receiving parenteral nutrition have a higher daily magnesium requirement for unknown reasons.[225]

Gastrointestinal Losses

Diarrheal fluid contains high concentration of magnesium, up to 16 mg/dL,[225,295] and hypomagnesemia is a common finding in patients suffering from acute or chronic diarrhea from any cause. Because intestinal absorption of magnesium occurs primarily in jejunum and ileum, conditions such as celiac disease, inflammatory bowel disease, extensive small bowel resection, and jejunoileal bypass surgery for obesity are frequently associated with intestinal magnesium wasting.[288]

Renal Losses

Medications are perhaps the most important cause of renal magnesium wasting in critically ill patients. Loop diuretics are commonly used at high doses. Aminoglycosides may cause asymptomatic hypomagnesemia 3 to 4 days after initiation of therapy; typically it resolves after cessation of therapy.[225,300] Almost all patients who receive cisplatin develop renal magnesium wasting and hypomagnesemia, which may persist for months after discontinuation of therapy.[301] Most of the patients who receive intravenous pentamidine therapy develop renal magnesium wasting and hypomagnesemia that may last for 1 to 2 months after cessation of the therapy.[225] The renal magnesium wasting associated with chronic alcohol use may take up to a month to resolve with abstinence.[288]

Redistribution

Hypomagnesemia is reported in up to 20% of patients with acute pancreatitis.[200,205] The proposed mechanism is saponification of necrotic fat with magnesium and calcium. The mechanism of hypomagnesemia with the "hungry bone" syndrome (following parathyroidectomy for hyperparathyroidism) is rapid bone uptake of magnesium during remineralization.

CLINICAL MANIFESTATIONS

Hypomagnesemia in critically ill patients has been associated with a twofold increase in mortality rate, even after adjustment for severity of illness.[302] (The observation that magnesium supplementation has not been shown to improve outcome[288] suggests that hypomagnesemia may be a marker for pejorative conditions not captured by severity of illness scores.)

The signs and symptoms of hypomagnesemia are cardiovascular, neuromuscular, and metabolic, and are shown in Box 57.13.[225,288,291,295] There is little evidence that hypomagnesemia is associated with arrhythmias in otherwise healthy individuals. In the setting of acute myocardial ischemia, however, even mild hypomagnesemia has been associated with increased frequency of ventricular arrythmias.[288] Results of recent large clinical trials, however, have shown no benefit to magnesium supplementation in this setting in the absence

Box 57.13 Clinical Manifestations of Hypomagnesemia

Cardiovascular
Ventricular arrhythmias
- Torsades de pointes
- Ventricular fibrillation; premature ventricular contractions
- Increased digitalis toxicity

Conduction disturbances
- Prolonged QT interval
- Prolonged QRS duration
- ST-segment depression
- Peaked T wave

Neuromuscular
Muscle weakness
Tetany
Horizontal and vertical nystagmus
Choreoathetoid movements
Seizures

Metabolic
Hypokalemia, refractory
Hypocalcemia, refractory

of overt hypomagnesemia.[295] Torsades de pointes is a malignant ventricular arrhythmia associated with magnesium deficiency or drugs that prolong the QT interval. Magnesium is the treatment of choice. Magnesium supplementation after cardiopulmonary bypass may reduce the frequency of ventricular ectopy.

The hypocalcemia associated with hypomagnesemia is caused by both hypoparathyroidism and bone resistance to PTH. The hypokalemia is caused by renal potassium wasting and will not resolve until the hypomagnesemia is corrected.[303,304]

TREATMENT

In patients who have malignant cardiac arrhythmias (ventricular fibrillation or torsades de pointes) or seizure attributed to hypomagnesemia, intravenous magnesium (2 g of magnesium sulfate over minutes) must be given immediately (see Chapter 31 for details).

Less urgent cases, but those in which signs and symptoms are present, may be treated with magnesium sulfate 6 g intravenously in the first 24 hours followed by 3 to 4 g daily for the next 2 to 6 days.[225,288,295] Because translocation of magnesium into cells is a slow process, and because urinary excretion is proportional to the plasma magnesium level, more rapid infusion rates are associated with urinary magnesium wasting that defeats the purpose of the therapy. Effective intravenous infusions should be given over 8 to 12 hours.[288] For patients with impaired renal function, the dose should be reduced by 50% to 75% and serum magnesium levels should be monitored frequently. Patients should be monitored closely for symptoms and signs of hypermagnesemia (see later).

Patients with refractory hypokalemia in the setting of hypomagnesemia, who are receiving high doses of potassium, must be monitored closely for the development of hyperkalemia once the magnesium is being replenished.

Box 57.14 Causes of Hypermagnesemia

Patients with Renal Insufficiency
Magnesium-containing antacids (e.g., magnesium aluminum hydroxide)
Magnesium-containing laxatives or enemas (e.g., magnesium citrate)

Patients with Normal Renal Function
Treatment of preeclampsia or eclampsia
Treatment of hypomagnesemia

Miscellaneous
Hypothyroidism
Hyperparathyroidism
Addison's disease
Lithium treatment

For mild asymptomatic hypomagnesemia, patients who can tolerate oral medication should receive oral magnesium salts (e.g., magnesium chloride, 500 mg slow release tablets, 10-12 per day in divided doses). High doses of oral magnesium salts may cause diarrhea.

HYPERMAGNESEMIA

CAUSES

Hypermagnesemia is much less common than hypomagnesemia. Patients with normal renal function have prodigious capacity to excrete excess magnesium through the kidneys.[225] Thus, hypermagnesemia is seen only in patients with compromised renal function receiving enteral or parenteral Mg or in patients with normal renal function receiving massive exogenous magnesium (e.g., treatment for preeclampsia and eclampsia).[225] The causes of hypermagnesemia are shown in Box 57.14.

CLINICAL MANIFESTATIONS

The clinical manifestations of hypermagnesemia (Box 57.15) are largely due to the effects on the heart, nerve, and smooth muscle. Initial manifestations, with plasma concentrations of 4 to 6 mg/dL, include nausea and vomiting, hypotension, and flushing. More severe effects, including death,[305] are seen with levels exceeding 6 mg/dL.

TREATMENT

Treatment of hypermagnesemia depends on severity of symptoms and the patient's renal function. Patients with adequate renal function and mild asymptomatic hypermagnesemia require no treatment except to remove all sources of exogenous magnesium. The half-time of elimination of magnesium is about 28 hours.[225] Magnesium excretion may be enhanced by saline infusion and the use of loop diuretics.[225] (Care must be taken to prevent hypokalemia and metabolic alkalosis.) Patients with symptomatic hypermagnesemia, especially with cardiovascular manifestations, require urgent treatment. The recommended therapy is calcium gluconate 1 g intravenously over 5 minutes.

Patients with acute or chronic renal failure and symptomatic hypermagnesemia will require dialysis to remove excess

Box 57.15 Clinical Manifestations of Hypermagnesemia

Cardiovascular
- Hypotension
- Facial flushing
- Bradycardia
- Sinoatrial or atrioventricular heart block
- Asystole

Gastrointestinal
- Nausea and vomiting
- Ileus

Neuromuscular
- Hyporeflexia
- Flaccid skeletal muscle paralysis
- Respiratory muscle weakness and paralysis
- Lethargy
- Coma

Urinary retention

magnesium. Hemodialysis removes magnesium efficiently, yielding a 30% to 50% reduction in predialysis serum magnesium levels after a 3- to 4-hour treatment.[225]

PHOSPHORUS HOMEOSTASIS

Phosphorus has an essential role in normal physiology. It is necessary for skeletal integrity; energy economy (formation of high-energy phosphate bonds); nucleic acid, lipid, and protein structure; cell signaling; and buffering.[228] It is not surprising, therefore, that disorders of phosphorus homeostasis have diverse manifestations.[306-308] Hypophosphatemia is considerably more common in hospitalized and critically ill patients than hyperphosphatemia.

NORMAL PHOSPHORUS HOMEOSTASIS

Total body phosphorus amounts to about 700 g in an adult. About 85% resides in the skeleton, about 15% in soft tissues, and only about 1% in blood.[227] Circulating phosphorus is mostly in the form of inorganic phosphates. The normal plasma concentration of phosphorus is 2.5 to 4.5 mg/dL, also expressed as a phosphate concentration of 0.9 to 1.45 mmol/L. (Phosphate concentration should not be expressed in mEq/L because the average valence of plasma phosphates—a mixture of HPO_4^{2-} and $H_2PO_4^-$—changes with pH.[309]) Of that circulating phosphorus, about 75% is free and ultrafilterable; 25% being protein bound.[228]

A normal adult diet includes about 1000 mg of phosphorus per day. Stool contains about 300 mg, so the net absorption (mostly in the small intestine under the influence of vitamin D) is about 70%. The dietary and secreted phosphorus may be bound into insoluble, nonabsorbable salts by cations such as Al^{3+}, Ca^{2+}, and Mg^{2+}. Thus, the kidney is responsible for excreting about 700 mg phosphorus per day. Almost all phosphorus reabsorption takes place in the proximal tubule. The most important regulators of renal phosphorus excretion are PTH, fibroblast growth factor (FGF)-23, and dietary phosphorus content. PTH increases phosphorus excretion.[227] FGF-23, a phosphotonin released by osteocytes and osteoblasts in bone, increases urinary phosphorus excretion.[310] Renal excretion of phosphorus is proportional to the dietary intake. Other factors that increase renal phosphorus excretion include extracellular volume expansion, acute hypercalcemia, diuretics, and glucocorticoids.[227,228] Acid-base disorders have a variable effect on phosphorus reabsorption depending on their direction and duration,[227,228] with one exception: Respiratory alkalosis causes a marked decrease in renal phosphorus excretion by causing redistributive hypophosphatemia[307] (see later).

Phosphorus homeostasis depends on PTH, FGF-23, and vitamin D. PTH and FGF-23 cause phosphaturia by decreasing renal proximal tubule reabsorption. Active vitamin D inhibits PTH release. Vitamin D activation (1-α-hydroxylation) in the kidney is inhibited by FGF-23 and hyperphosphatemia. This, in turn, reduces intestinal phosphorus absorption and allows increased PTH secretion, causing phosphaturia and returning plasma phosphorus toward normal. Hypophosphatemia reverses this physiology, allowing increased gut absorption and reduced renal excretion of phosphorus.

HYPOPHOSPHATEMIA

Hypophosphatemia is common in critically ill patients. It has been reported in 29% of adult surgical patients (and 45% of patients with one or more risk factors for hypophosphatemia) and—liberally defined—in 76% of pediatric ICU patients.[311] Patients with malnutrition, uncontrolled diabetes mellitus, sepsis, and chronic alcoholism are at high risk for hypophosphatemia.[312] It is associated with a marked increase in mortality rate in patients with sepsis,[313] and serum phosphorus concentration is inversely correlated with APACHE II after liver resection.[314] In these situations, the serum phosphorus concentration probably is a marker of severity of illness. If severe, however, hypophosphatemia itself may cause serious complications.

CAUSES OF HYPOPHOSPHATEMIA

The causes of hypophosphatemia classically are divided into three general categories: (1) redistribution from the extracellular to the intracellular space, (2) increased renal excretion, and (3) decreased intestinal absorption (Box 57.16). It is important to recognize that many factors have several different effects on phosphorus homeostasis.

Redistribution

Respiratory alkalosis causes intracellular phosphate shift (by stimulating glycolysis) and can cause severe symptomatic hypophosphatemia. Respiratory alkalosis is commonly encountered in ICU patients because of sepsis or liver failure and is seen in patients requiring mechanical ventilation; in the latter case, the degree of hypophosphatemia is proportional to the pH.[225,315] *Sepsis* is commonly associated with hypophosphatemia, probably due to hyperventilation and respiratory alkalosis. Rapid *refeeding* of patients with malnutrition may result in significant hypophosphatemia due to insulin-mediated intracellular phosphate shift. In one study of ICU patients, refeeding hypophosphatemia developed in 34% of patients after 48 hours of starvation and was predicted by the prealbumin concentration. Profound hypophosphatemia (<1 mmol/dL) occurred in 10%

Box 57.16 Cause of Hypophosphatemia

Redistribution

Acute respiratory alkalosis
Refeeding syndrome
Treatment of diabetic ketoacidosis
"Hungry bone" syndrome—postparathyroidectomy
Leukemia

Increased Renal Excretion

Hyperparathyroidism
Vitamin D deficiency or resistance
Volume expansion
Postobstructive diuresis
Recovery from acute tubular necrosis
Fanconi syndrome
Postrenal transplantation
Drugs
- Acetazolamide
- Corticosteroids

Inherited disorders
Tumor-induced osteomalacia

Decreased Intestinal Absorption

Malnutrition
Phosphate-binding medications
Chronic diarrhea
Chronic alcoholism

Box 57.17 Clinical Manifestations of Hypophosphatemia

Skeletal muscle
- Weakness
- Rhabdomyolysis

Decreased cardiac output
Hematologic
- Erythrocytes
- Decreased 2,3-DPG (2,3-diphosphoglycerate)
- Decreased tissue oxygen delivery
- Spherocytosis
- Hemolysis
- Impaired leukocyte function
- Impaired platelet function

Neurologic
- Anorexia
- Irritability
- Confusion
- Paresthesias
- Ataxia
- Seizure
- Coma

Skeletal
- Bone pain
- Pseudofractures
- Osteomalacia

Insulin resistance

of patients.[316] Patients with anorexia nervosa, uncontrolled diabetes mellitus, chronic malnutrition, and chronic alcoholism are at a particularly high risk of developing refeeding syndrome. *Leukemia* in the leukemic phase[317] and with rapid leukocyte reconstitution after bone marrow transplant[318] has been reported to cause severe redistributive hypophosphatemia.

DKA is associated with phosphorus efflux from cells and increased urinary phosphate excretion, resulting in severe total body phosphorus depletion (often with a deceptively normal presenting serum phosphorus concentration).[307] Initiation of insulin therapy in such patients results in intracellular phosphate shift and can result in profound, symptomatic hypophosphatemia.[307]

Increased Renal Excretion

Any cause of *primary hyperparathyroidism* will cause phosphaturia and tend to cause hypophosphatemia. Hyperparathyroidism due to hypocalcemia or *vitamin D deficiency* or *resistance* is similarly associated with hypophosphatemia. The exception is the secondary hyperparathyroidism of chronic kidney disease, in which hyperphosphatemia due to decreased renal phosphorus elimination is characteristic. Vitamin D deficiency or resistance also causes hypophosphatemia from decreased intestinal phosphate absorption. Extracellular volume expansion increases the filtered phosphorus load and dilutes the luminal concentration of phosphorus, resulting in phosphaturia. *Ethanol* and *glycosuria* both decrease proximal tubule phosphate reabsorption.[225,307] All *diuretic drugs*, but particularly those with proximal tubular effects such as acetazolamide and, to a lesser degree, thiazides, cause phosphaturia.

Decreased Intestinal Absorption

Salts of Al^{3+} and Ca^{2+}, formulated for oral administration as antacids or as phosphate-binding medications, can cause malabsorptive hypophosphatemia. Chronic diarrhea and steatorrhea may cause reduced intestinal phosphate absorption directly and by way of vitamin D deficiency and cause hypophosphatemia.

The hypophosphatemia commonly associated with *chronic alcohol ingestion* is multifactorial. Dietary phosphorus deficiency, malabsorption, antacid ingestion, hypocalcemia, secondary hyperparathyroidism, hypomagnesemia, and an ethanol-induced renal tubular defect all have been implicated.[307]

CLINICAL MANIFESTATIONS

Important clinical manifestations of hypophosphatemia are shown in Box 57.17. Most patients are asymptomatic until plasma phosphorus falls below 1.5 mg/dL or about 0.5 mmol/L. The most severe manifestations, such as hemolysis, spontaneous rhabdomyolysis, seizure, or coma, are not commonly seen with phosphorus above 1 mg/dL (0.3 mmol/L). Acute clinical manifestations are thought to be largely due to altered cellular energy economy.[225,227,306,307]

TREATMENT

The therapy of hypophosphatemia starts with its prevention. In critically ill patients, this depends on recognition and correction of the factors that lead to hypophosphatemia. The astute clinician will be able to anticipate the development of hypophosphatemia (in refeeding, for example), monitor the patient appropriately, and supplement phosphorus accordingly. Patients on total parenteral nutrition should receive adequate phosphorus for their level of renal function (see Chapter 82).[309]

The exact method of phosphorus supplementation in hypophosphatemia depends on the severity of the disturbance and the patient's underlying condition. In mild to moderate hypophosphatemia (>1.5 mg/dL or about 0.5 mmol/L) oral replacement is usually sufficient. Skim milk is an excellent source of phosphorus and provides 900 mg/L of inorganic phosphate. In patients who cannot tolerate milk, oral sodium phosphate, formulated to provide 250 mg of phosphate in each tablet, can be used. Alternatively, Fleet Phospho-soda can be give to provide 60 mmol of phosphorus per day, divided into three doses of 5 mL each.[227] Supplementation should continue for several days in order to replenish phosphorus deficits adequately. Administration of sufficient doses of oral phosphorus preparations very commonly causes diarrhea, limiting its usefulness.

Patients with severe hyperphosphatemia (<1.5 mg/dL), or those for whom the enteral route is not an option, require intravenous phosphorus repletion. In such patients, the recommended dose is 2.5 to 5.0 mg (0.08-0.16 mmol) per kg body weight over 6 hours, doses at the higher end of the range being reserved for profound, symptomatic hypophosphatemia.[227,309] A recent study used a more aggressive, weight-based protocol in critically ill patients and found it to be safe and effective.[319] Clinicians should recognize that the administered intravenous phosphorus can complex with circulating calcium, leading to a decrease in Ca^{2+} (with attendant hypotension and tetany) and metastatic calcification. The use of potassium salts of phosphate for repletion of phosphorus deficits has been associated with dangerous hyperkalemia. For that reason, potassium deficits and phosphorus deficits should be treated separately.[309]

HYPERPHOSPHATEMIA

Hyperphosphatemia (plasma phosphorus > 5.0 mg/dL or a phosphate concentration > 1.6 mmol/L) most often is associated with renal dysfunction. Massive influx of phosphorus into the extracellular space, however, either from endogenous sources or exogenous, can overwhelm normal renal excretory mechanisms and lead to severe hyperphosphatemia.

CAUSES OF HYPERPHOSPHATEMIA

Hyperphosphatemia may be caused by (1) redistribution of phosphorus from the intracellular to the extracellular space, (2) increased phosphorus intake, and (3) decreased renal excretion of phosphorus (Box 57.18). It is important to recognize that most hyperphosphatemia is multifactorial.

Box 57.18 Causes of Hyperphosphatemia

- Redistribution
  - Tumor lysis syndrome
  - Rhabdomyolysis
  - Pancreatitis
  - Respiratory acidosis
  - Lactic acidosis
  - Diabetic ketoacidosis
- Increased intake
  - Phosphate-containing enemas and laxatives
  - Intravenous phosphate
  - Hypervitaminosis D
- Decreased renal excretion
  - Acute renal failure
  - Chronic kidney disease
  - Hypoparathyroidism
- Pseudohyperphosphatemia

Redistribution

Hyperphosphatemia is a common complication of the *tumor lysis syndrome.*[72] Similarly, rhabdomyolysis often is associated with hyperphosphatemia, especially when it is complicated by acute renal failure.[74,320] Less commonly recognized causes of redistributive hyperphosphatemia include acute and chronic respiratory acidosis, acute pancreatitis,[321] DKA,[322] and lactic acidosis.[323]

Increased Intake

Exogenous administration of phosphorus is unlikely to cause hyperphosphatemia unless renal function is compromised. Several cases have been reported of potentially life-threatening hyperphosphatemia and hypocalcemia after the use of phosphate-containing laxatives and enemas, especially in children and elderly.* Overly aggressive parenteral phosphorus supplementation can cause hyperphosphatemia. Hypervitaminosis D causes increased intestinal uptake of phosphorus and a decrease in PTH, both of which predispose to hyperphosphatemia.

Decreased Renal Excretion

Acute renal failure is associated with elevated phosphate levels due to inability of kidneys to excrete phosphate load. This is particularly pronounced in patients in whom acute renal failure is caused by the tumor lysis syndrome or rhabdomyolysis. Advanced chronic kidney disease (GFR < 25 mL/minute) commonly is associated with hyperphosphatemia. Such patients are particularly susceptible to developing severe and life-threatening hyperphosphatemia if they are exposed to acute increase in serum phosphate levels. Hypoparathyroidism of any cause is associated with impaired renal phosphorus excretion.

Pseudohyperphosphatemia

Spurious increases in the measured plasma phosphorus concentration are reported to be caused by contamination of the blood sample with phosphate-buffered saline as a diluent for heparin[326] or during sample processing by the laboratory.[327] Even microliter volumes of the contaminant can cause significant elevations in the measured phosphorus.[326] Paraproteinemia can also cause pseudophyperphosphatemia.

CLINICAL MANIFESTATIONS OF HYPERPHOSPHATEMIA

Phosphate complexes with circulating calcium, reducing the concentration of Ca^{2+}. Thus, most of the clinical

*248, 250, 251, 324, 325.

consequences of hyperphosphatemia are the same as those of hypocalcemia (see earlier). In addition, ectopic deposition of calcium phosphate salts can occur, especially when the calcium-phosphorus product exceeds 70 mg/dL.[227] Such ectopic calcification in the heart can cause conduction and rhythm disturbances.[328]

Because phosphate is an "unmeasured ion," hyperphosphatemia causes increases in the anion gap. Extreme hyperphosphatemia can cause shocking elevations in the anion gap. One case of hyperphosphatemia from Phospho-soda intoxication (serum phosphorus 62.5 mg/dL) was associated with an anion gap of 51 mmol/L.[329] In order to estimate the contribution of phosphorus to the anion gap, one must know not only the plasma concentration of phosphorus but the pH, because the valence of phosphate varies with pH, from 1.8 mEq/mmol at pH 7.4 to 1.6 mEq/L at pH 7.0.[309] Because extreme hyperphosphatemia can be caused by lactic or ketoacidosis (see earlier), an elevated anion gap in the setting of hyperphosphatemia should never be attributed to the hyperphosphatemia itself without further investigation.

TREATMENT OF HYPERPHOSPHATEMIA

Treatment of hyperphosphatemia consists of reducing the phosphate intake and enhancing the removal of excess phosphate. If the patient is taking oral diet, dietary phosphate should be restricted to less than 800 mg/day. Oral phosphate binders can be added with meals to decrease intestinal phosphate absorption.

Patients with normal renal function can be treated with saline diuresis to increase renal phosphate excretion. Acetazolamide can be added to enhance phosphaturia, taking care to avoid a metabolic acidosis. Patients with severe hyperphosphatemia with coexisting renal failure may require renal replacement therapy in the form of intermittent or continuous hemodialysis.

KEY POINTS

- Acid-base disorders often provide a window into underlying pathology. Optimal diagnosis of acid-base disorders requires familiarity with the rules of normal compensation and the pitfalls characteristic of critical illness.
- Acute hyperkalemia may result from exogenous potassium administration or redistribution from cells. Acute hypokalemia always is caused by redistribution.
- Patients, particularly women, are predisposed to catastrophic hyponatremia if hypotonic fluids are administered in the postoperative period.
- The treatment of acute symptomatic hyponatremia is largely independent of its cause, whereas the treatment of chronic hyponatremia depends critically on the underlying pathophysiology.

KEY POINTS (Continued)

- Hypernatremia in hospitalized patients should be considered iatrogenic, reflecting insufficient recognition of the causes of water loss and inadequate water replacement in vulnerable patients.
- Plasma calcium concentration, corrected for the plasma albumin concentration, correlates poorly with Ca^{2+} in critically ill patients. If possible, Ca^{2+} should be directly measured when considering disorders of calcium homeostasis.
- The clinical manifestations of many metabolic disorders have common features (e.g., hypocalcemia, hypomagnesemia, hyperphosphatemia, metabolic alkalosis) relating to their overlapping pathophysiology.

SELECTED REFERENCES

7. Gauthier PM, Szerlip HM: Metabolic acidosis in the intensive care unit. Crit Care Clin 2002;18(2):289-308, vi.
20. Rachoin JS, Weisberg LS, McFadden CB: Treatment of lactic acidosis: Appropriate confusion. J Hosp Med 2010;5(4):E1-E7.
26. Gennari FJ: Pathophysiology of metabolic alkalosis: A new classification based on the centrality of stimulated collecting duct ion transport. Am J Kidney Dis 2011;58(4):626-636.
36. Sterns RH, Cox M, Feig PU, Singer I: Internal potassium balance and the control of the plasma potassium concentration. Medicine (Baltimore) 1981;60(5):339-354.
41. Aronson PS, Giebisch G: Effects of pH on potassium: New explanations for old observations. J Am Soc Nephrol 2011; 22(11):1981-1989.
59. Weiner ID, Wingo CS: Hypokalemia—Consequences, causes, and correction. J Am Soc Nephrol 1997;8(7):1179-1188.
113. Palmer BF: Managing hyperkalemia caused by inhibitors of the renin-angiotensin-aldosterone system. N Engl J Med 2004; 351(6):585-592.
139. Weiner ID, Wingo CS: Hyperkalemia: A potential silent killer. J Am Soc Nephrol 1998;9(8):1535-1543.
159. Weisberg LS: Management of severe hyperkalemia. Crit Care Med 2008;36(12):3246-3251.
185. Verbalis JG: Disorders of body water homeostasis. Best Pract Res Clin Endocrinol Metab 2003;17(4):471-503.
189. Kamel KS, Ethier JH, Richardson RM, et al: Urine electrolytes and osmolality: When and how to use them. Am J Nephrol 1990; 10(2):89-102.
196. Schrier RW, Gurevich AK, Cadnapaphornchai MA: Pathogenesis and management of sodium and water retention in cardiac failure and cirrhosis. Semin Nephrol 2001;21(2):157-172.
213. Palevsky PM, Bhagrath R, Greenberg A: Hypernatremia in hospitalized patients. Ann Intern Med 1996;124(2):197-203.
238. Zivin JR, Gooley T, Zager RA, Ryan MJ: Hypocalcemia: A pervasive metabolic abnormality in the critically ill. Am J Kidney Dis 2001;37(4):689-698.
288. Agus ZS: Hypomagnesemia. J Am Soc Nephrol 1999;10(7): 1616-1622.
295. Tong GM, Rude RK: Magnesium deficiency in critical illness. J Intensive Care Med 2005;20(1):3-17.
310. Juppner H: Phosphate and FGF-23. Kidney Int Suppl 2011;(121):S24-S27.

The complete list of references can be found at www.expertconsult.com.

58

Acute Diabetic Emergencies, Glycemic Control, and Hypoglycemia

Marc Laufgraben | Steven T. Kaufman

CHAPTER OUTLINE

DIABETES MELLITUS: EPIDEMIOLOGY AND CLASSIFICATION

Diabetes mellitus (DM) is the fourth to fifth most common cause of death in developed countries and is one of the most common noncommunicable diseases globally.[1] DM affects nearly 27 million individuals in the United States and 366 million adults aged 20 to 79 years worldwide.[2] Nearly half of those with diabetes are undiagnosed.[2] The worldwide incidence of DM is expected to reach 552 million by 2030 with the prevalence of diabetes increasing in every country.[2] Diabetes is the leading cause of kidney failure, nontraumatic lower limb amputations, and new cases of blindness among adults in the United States, and is a major cause of heart disease and stroke.[3]

Diabetes is generally classified as follows:

1. *Type 1 diabetes*—autoimmune β-cell destruction resulting in an absolute insulin deficiency
2. *Type 2 diabetes*—progressive defects resulting in increased insulin resistance and a relative insulin deficiency
3. *Gestational diabetes*—diabetes appearing during pregnancy
4. *Diabetes due to other causes*—such as genetic defects in β-cell function, genetic defects in insulin action, diseases of the exocrine pancreas (such as cystic fibrosis, pancreatitis, or pancreatectomy), and drug- or chemical-induced diabetes[4]

Type 2 diabetes accounts for 90% to 95% of DM in the United States.[3] The epidemic of type 2 DM has been attributed to the increasing rates of obesity.

In patients with diabetes, absolute or relative insulin deficiency leads to hyperglycemia from decreased glucose utilization in peripheral tissues (especially skeletal muscle) and increased hepatic glucose output from glycogenolysis and gluconeogenesis.[5] Proteolysis and lipolysis are also increased, providing the amino acids and free fatty acids that are the substrate for gluconeogenesis and alternative fuel sources such as ketones. The various actions of insulin are shown in Box 58.1.[6]

DIABETIC KETOACIDOSIS AND THE HYPERGLYCEMIC HYPEROSMOLAR STATE

Diabetic ketoacidosis (DKA) and hyperglycemic hyperosmolar state (HHS) are both part of an overlapping process of decompensated hyperglycemia.[7] A significant imbalance between insulin and its counterregulatory hormones

Table 58.1 Diagnostic Criteria for Diabetic Ketoacidosis (DKA) and Hyperglycemic Hyperosmolar Syndrome (HHS)

	DKA			
Criterion	**Mild**	**Moderate**	**Severe**	**HHS**
Plasma glucose (mg/dL)	>250	>250	>250	>600
Arterial pH	7.25-7.3	7-7.24	<7	>7.3
Serum bicarbonate (mEq/L)	15-18	10-<15	<10	>15
Urine ketones*	Positive	Positive	Positive	Small
Serum ketones*	Positive	Positive	Positive	Small
Effective serum osmolality (mOsm/kg)†	Variable	Variable	Variable	>300
Anion gap	>10	>12	>12	Variable
Alteration in sensorium or mental obtundation	Alert	Alert/drowsy	Stupor/coma	Stupor/coma

*Nitroprusside reaction method.
†Calculation: 2 [measured Na^+] + [glucose]/18.
Copyright ©2004 American Diabetes Association. Modified from Kitabchi AE, Umpierrez GE, Murphy MB, et al: Hyperglycemic crises in diabetes. Diabetes Care 2004:27:S94-S102, used with permission from the American Diabetes Association.

Box 58.1 Actions of Insulin on Target Organs

Adipose Tissue

Increased glucose entry
Increased fatty acid synthesis
Increased glycerol phosphate synthesis
Increased triglyceride deposition
Activation of lipoprotein lipase
Inhibition of hormone-sensitive lipase

Liver

Decreased ketogenesis
Increased protein synthesis
Increased lipid synthesis
Decreased glucose output via increased glycogen synthesis and decreased gluconeogenesis

Muscle

Increased glucose entry
Increased glycogen synthesis
Increased amino acid uptake
Increased protein synthesis in ribosomes
Decreased protein catabolism
Decreased release of gluconeogenic amino acids
Increased ketone uptake
Increased K^+ uptake

General

Increased cell growth

From Barrett KE, Barman SM, Boitano S, Brooks H: Endocrine functions of the pancreas and regulation of carbohydrate metabolism. In Barrett KE, Barman SM, Boitano S, Brooks H (eds): Ganong's Review of Medical Physiology, 23rd ed. New York, McGraw-Hill, 2010, Chap. 21.

(especially glucagon) leads to DKA, a severe metabolic state of hyperglycemia and acidemia from abnormal metabolism of fats, lipids, and carbohydrates.[8] DKA is common complication of type 1 DM and is also seen, albeit less frequently, in type 2 DM. The combined findings of serum glucose greater than 250 mg/dL, a pH less than 7.30 with an elevated anion gap, and elevated serum ketones are consistent with DKA.

HHS is a state of hyperglycemia associated with osmotic diuresis and dehydration. HHS is defined by glucose levels greater than 600 mg/dL, an elevated serum osmolality, a lack of significant acidemia or ketosis, and typically a change in mental status. HHS has replaced the term "hyperglycemic, hyperosmolar nonketotic coma" because patients may present with a mild elevation in urine or serum ketones and may have a variety of mental status changes other than coma. A careful evaluation of history, physical examination, and laboratory values helps differentiate DKA from HHS (Table 58.1) and assists in distinguishing DKA and HHS from other conditions with overlapping clinical presentation.[9]

EPIDEMIOLOGY

DKA has high morbidity rates, mortality rates, and financial costs despite numerous advances in the treatment of DM. The incidence of DKA in the United States is estimated at 5.9 to 12.9 cases per 100,000 people.[10,11] The 120,000 patients admitted to the hospital for DKA each year[12] account for approximately $1.4 billion in hospital reimbursement.[13] DKA carries a mortality rate of 1% to 5%.[9,14] Though the highest mortality rate is in the elderly and in patients with comorbid conditions, DKA remains the leading cause of death in diabetic patients below the age of 24.[15]

Although most patients will have a history of diabetes, 27% to 37% of patients with DKA carry no prior diagnosis.[16,17] This is especially true in young children.[18] Although the development of DKA is classically associated with type 1 DM, some patients lack the classic clinical presentation, autoimmune markers, or diminished β-cell reserve of type 1 diabetes.[19-21] This subgroup, known as "ketosis-prone type 2 diabetes," represents patients with type 2 DM who present with DKA and often are African American or Latino, male, middle-aged, and overweight or obese; have a family history of diabetes; and have newly diagnosed diabetes.[22,23] Patients with ketosis-prone type 2 DM account for 1 in 5 cases of

DKA.[22] Patients with "classic" type 2 diabetes may also develop DKA in situations of extreme stress.

HHS occurs far less commonly than DKA, with an estimated prevalence of 1 in 1000,[24] though the increasing incidence of type 2 DM is expected to increase the prevalence of HHS. HHS typically occurs in patients with type 2 DM and 30% to 40% cases of HHS may be the initial finding leading to diagnosis of type 2 DM.[25,26] The mortality rate in HHS tends to be higher than in DKA, with the patient's comorbid conditions and severity of presentation significantly affecting risk of death.[27]

PATHOPHYSIOLOGY

The pathophysiology of DKA is driven by insulin deficiency and a rise in the counterregulatory hormones, particularly glucagon, but also epinephrine, cortisol, and growth hormone (Fig. 58.1).[28,29] Insulin deficiency results in decreased glucose uptake by peripheral tissues, resulting in elevated serum glucose levels, and hyperglycemia worsens when an increase in glucagon (and an imbalanced insulin/glucagon ratio) results in unrestrained hepatic glycogenolysis and gluconeogenesis.[9,24,28] Osmotic diuresis results in total body loss of water and electrolytes, causing intravascular volume depletion. Cellular dehydration occurs as water and electrolytes move from the intracellular to extracellular space. With volume depletion, impaired renal function limits the clearance of glucose and worsens the hyperglycemia.[9,24] In an insulin-deficient state proteolysis and lipolysis drive accelerated gluconeogenesis as amino acids and free fatty acids are shunted to the liver.[30] At the same time, oxidation of free fatty acids results in the production of the keto acids acetoacetate and β-hydroxybutyrate.[9,24] These weak acids react with bicarbonate and diminish the body's bicarbonate stores. The development of metabolic acidosis in DKA results when the increase in acid production exceeds the body's buffering capacity.[31]

HHS is also caused by a relative insulin deficiency and a rise in counterregulatory hormones. Decreased peripheral glucose uptake and increased glycogenolysis and gluconeogenesis result in hyperglycemia followed by osmotic diuresis with volume depletion and dehydration. However, the amount of insulin is sufficient to limit the oxidation of free fatty acids,[9] and significant keto acid production does not

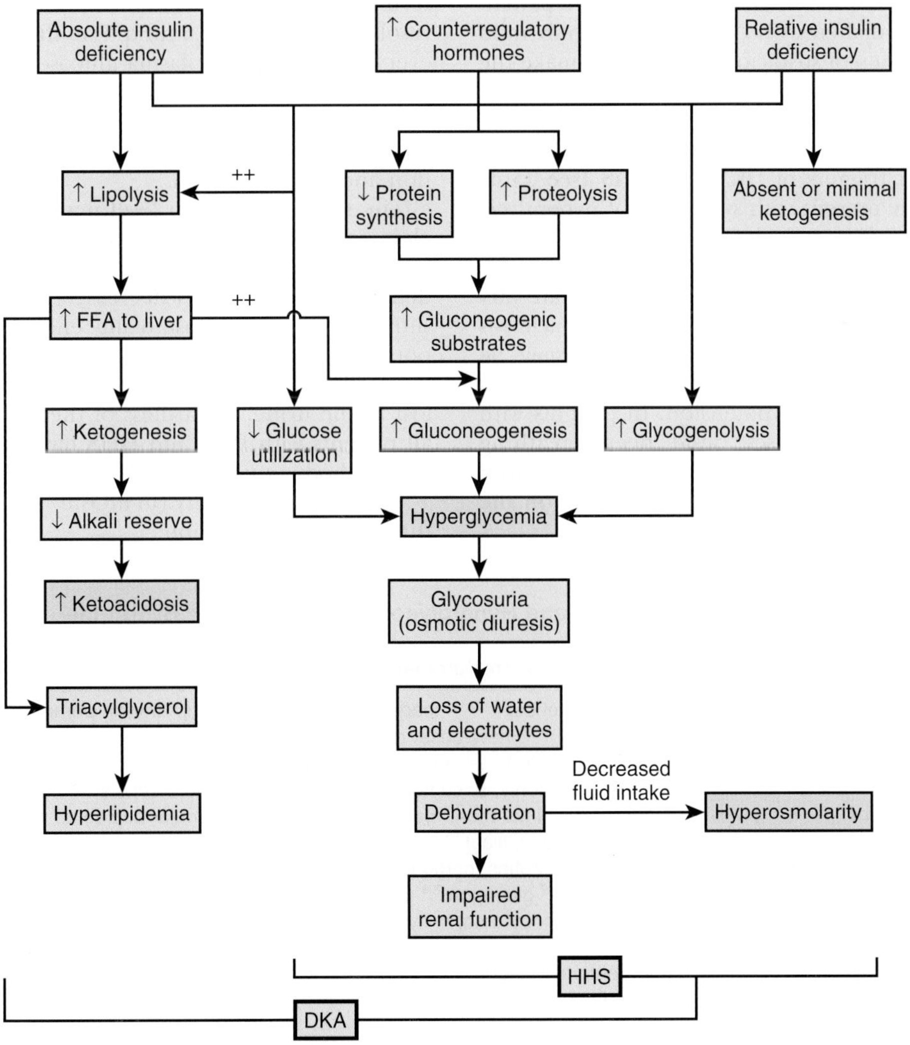

Figure 58.1 Pathogenesis of diabetic ketoacidosis (DKA) and hyperglycemic hyperosmolar state (HHS): stress, infection, or insufficient insulin. FFA, free fatty acid. (From Kitabchi AE, Umpierrez GE, Miles JM, Fisher JN: Hyperglycemic crises in adult patients with diabetes. Diabetes Care 2009;32(7):1335-1343.)

occur. In the absence of ketoacidosis, the process of dehydration is allowed to continue for longer than in DKA, and patients present with significant hyperosmolarity.

PRECIPITATING FACTORS

The precipitating factors for the development of DKA and HHS are listed in the Table 58.2. Omission of antidiabetic medications is an important factor in the development of DKA and HHS. Omission of insulin may result in DKA in a patient with type 1 diabetes in a matter of hours. In contrast, the development of HHS (or DKA) in a patient with type 2 diabetes occurs over days to weeks in a patient omitting insulin or oral agents. In addition to the factors listed in the table, impaired thirst or lack of access to water, particularly in the elderly, will contribute to the development of HHS.[32] Eating disorders may account for up to 20% of cases of recurrent DKA.[9]

PRESENTATION

The presentation of DKA and HHS varies with the severity of the metabolic derangement and any intercurrent illnesses or comorbid conditions. DKA can occur in a patient without a history of diabetes who presents with only mild symptoms; a high index of suspicion is needed to make the diagnosis in this setting, particularly in children under the age of 6. A detailed evaluation should reveal precipitating factors, especially infection and medication nonadherence, which are common triggers of DKA and HHS (see Table 58.2).[24] Patients may present with symptoms of hyperglycemia (polyuria, polyphagia, polydipsia, or blurred vision) or with nonspecific symptoms of fatigue, abdominal pain, nausea, vomiting, and headache. Mental status can vary from somnolence to lethargy and even coma as the acidosis or hyperosmolarity worsens. Volume depletion may be manifested by tachycardia, poor skin turgor, dry mucous membranes, and orthostatic hypotension. In patients with DKA, metabolic acidosis causes rapid deep breathing (known as Kussmaul respiration), and acetone (derived from acetoacetate) can be sensed as a fruity smell on the patient's breath.

DIAGNOSIS

The diagnosis of DKA is based on a serum glucose level greater than 250 mg/dL, presence of ketones, arterial pH less than 7.3, and a CO_2 concentration less than 18 mmol/L.[5,9] The anion gap will be elevated, reflecting the presence of the unmeasured keto acids. The laboratory findings and changes in mental status help the clinician gauge the severity of DKA and distinguish DKA from HHS. Although arterial blood had previously been the standard for determining pH, current evidence supports the use of venous pH as a less expensive, more accessible alternative.[33,34] Exceptions to the typical presentation include pregnant patients or those with poor oral intake who may have a serum glucose value below 250 mg/dL, or even in the normal range.[35,36] In patients with severe vomiting, the bicarbonate value may be normal or elevated.

The serum sodium may be normal, low, or elevated depending on the degree of dehydration and hyperglycemia. Patients with hyperglycemia have dilutional hyponatremia from a shift in fluids from the intracellular to extracellular compartment. The serum sodium may be "corrected" for hyperglycemia (i.e., adjusted to estimate the serum sodium concentration once the hyperglycemia has resolved) by adding 1.6 mEq/L to the measured sodium for every 100 mg/dL of plasma glucose above 100 mg/dL. As the measured serum sodium will underestimate the "corrected" sodium level in patients, measured serum sodium in the "normal" range may represent significant dehydration and hypernatremia.

The serum potassium level may also be normal, low, or elevated depending on factors such as the degree of acidosis or osmotic diuresis and the duration of the process. Insulin deficiency and acidosis decrease cellular uptake of potassium, although hyperosmolality enhances cellular efflux of potassium.[37] Large amounts of potassium shift from the intracellular space to the extracellular space and are then lost in the urine. Regardless of the serum potassium level, all patients with DKA and HHS have substantial depletion of total body potassium.[9,37,38]

The serum osmolality (in mOsm/kg) can be estimated by the following calculation:

Table 58.2 Causes of Diabetic Ketoacidosis and Hyperglycemic Hyperosmolar Syndrome

Etiologic Factor/Condition	Diagnoses with Comments
Inadequate insulin	Nonadherence,[25,193,194] inadequate insulin regimen,[34] insulin pump failure or omission of insulin,[195,196] new-onset diabetes[197]
Infections	Any moderate to severe infectious process[29,198] Most commonly, pneumonia, urinary tract infection, sepsis[9]
Acute medical conditions	Myocardial infarction,[9] pancreatitis,[41] cerebrovascular accident,[9] arterial thrombosis (mesenteric, iliac)[199]
Interference with glucose metabolism or insulin secretion[32]	Thiazide diuretics, corticosteroids,[200] second-generation (atypical) antipsychotics,[201] FK506,[202] glucagon,[203] sympathomimetic agents (albuterol, terbutaline, dobutamine)[204]
Endocrine disturbance	Pheochromocytoma,[205] hyperthyroidism,[206] acromegaly,[207] hemochromatosis[208]
Substance abuse	Cocaine[209]
Nutritional factors	Parenteral nutrition[210]
Immune modulation	Interferon[211]

Superscript numbers refer to references provided online for this chapter.

$$2[\text{measured Na}^+] + [\text{glucose (mg/dL)}/18] + [\text{BUN (mg/dL)}/2.8]$$

Serum osmolarity is generally normal or mildly elevated in DKA but is often profoundly elevated in patients with HHS.

Semiquantitative nitroprusside assays for urine and serum ketones are commonly employed but test only for acetone and acetoacetate, not β-hydroxybutyrate. This can be problematic, although β-hydroxybutyrate is the predominant keto acid, accounting for 75% of the keto acid load in DKA.[39] In addition, nitroprusside assays may remain positive long after resolution of the metabolic acidosis, so serial measurements may be misleading and are not recommended. Quantitative assays for β-hydroxybutyrate are available and may be useful for diagnosis, especially if the nitroprusside test is negative. A small pilot study found that a serum level above 3.5 mmol/L has 100% specificity for DKA.[40] Unlike the nitroprusside assay, the β-hydroxybutyrate test can also be used to monitor the management of DKA because appropriate treatment will be accompanied by a progressive fall in β-hydroxybutyrate levels.

The diagnostic criteria that distinguish HHS from DKA include higher plasma glucose (>600 mg/dL), a lack of acidosis ($pH > 7.3$, $CO_2 > 18$ mEq/L), more profound dehydration (serum osmolality > 320 mOsm/kg), and a change in mental status.[9] Patients with HHS often have low levels of ketones (β-hydroxybutyrate between 0.3 and 3.0 mmol/L) compared with DKA patients, whose β-hydroxybutyrate levels will be greater than 3.0 mmol/L.

Initial laboratory studies should include electrolytes, phosphorus, blood urea nitrogen (BUN), creatinine, urinalysis, complete blood count with differential, and electrocardiogram (see Table 58.2). Further evaluation should be undertaken based on the patient's presentation. A variety of laboratory abnormalities are frequently seen in DKA. Amylase, from both salivary and pancreatic sources, may be increased in up to 90% of patients with DKA. Lipase, normally a sensitive marker for pancreatitis, may also be elevated in DKA. However, the clinician should be aware that 10% to 15% of DKA patients do have concomitant pancreatitis.[41,42] Leukocytosis of 10,000 to 15,000 white blood cells/mm^3 is common, but levels greater than 25,000 cells/mm^3 or the presence of greater than 10% band neutrophils should increase the clinical suspicion for an active infection. Elevated hemoglobin due to the volume depletion may be present. High liver function studies occur commonly, especially in patients with fatty liver,[43] and mild increases in creatine kinase and troponin may occur in the absence of myocardial damage.[44]

Intercurrent illnesses contribute to the morbidity and mortality rates in a hyperglycemic emergency, and every patient with DKA or HHS should undergo a thorough assessment with a focus on infectious and cardiovascular causes.[34] Appropriate management should be started immediately and continue concurrent to the treatment of the DKA and HHS.

Additional causes of acidosis or ketosis should be considered in the differential diagnosis including starvation ketosis; alcoholic ketoacidosis; lactic acidosis; intoxication from methanol, salicylate, or ethylene glycol; chronic renal failure; and rhabdomyolysis.[34]

MANAGEMENT

The treatment of HHS and DKA in adults and children follows similar principles of intravenous (IV) fluid, insulin, and electrolyte management. Children require more attention to weight-based regimens for fluid management in order to avoid cerebral edema.[45] The details of the management of HHS and DKA in patients older than 20 years are detailed in Figure 58.2.

FLUID REPLACEMENT

Although hyperglycemia drives the cascade of osmotic diuresis, volume depletion, and renal insufficiency, the process is reversed with appropriate fluid replacement.[46] In both DKA and HHS, normal saline solution should be started at 15 to 20 mL/kg body weight per hour initially (maximum of 1 L/hour), with hourly assessments of fluid status and urine output.[46] The infusion rate can be lowered to 250 to 500 mL/hour once the blood pressure stabilizes.

Once the sodium corrects to the eunatremic or hypernatremic level the fluids should be changed to one half normal saline solutions. Fluid rates are titrated based on the response to treatment and volume status. Patients with congestive heart failure (CHF), an acute myocardial infarction (MI), evidence of volume overload, or anuria warrant less aggressive fluid replacement and close monitoring of volume status. To avoid hypoglycemia, dextrose should be added to the IV fluids once the glucose drops below 250 mg/dL. Addition of dextrose to the IV fluid allows for the continued infusion of insulin that is necessary for the correction of ketoacidosis in DKA.

INSULIN

An initial bolus of regular insulin is typically given at 0.1 to 0.15 units/kg body weight followed by an IV insulin infusion at 0.1 unit/hour, though there is little evidence to support the need for an initial bolus.[47,48] Higher dose insulin regimens are not beneficial.[49,50] In patients receiving IV insulin, point of care testing should be performed every 1 to 2 hours and may be changed to every 2 hours once the patient is stable. Although subcutaneous (SC) and intramuscular (IM) insulin protocols can treat DKA or HHS, the initial response to glucose lowering is slower, and SC or IM regimens are generally reserved for emergent situations (i.e., a DKA patient with severe hyperkalemia and electrocardiographic [ECG] changes) in which IV access has been delayed.[49,51]

With the initial correction of volume depletion, particularly in HHS, the glucose level may fall precipitously. Thereafter, glucose levels should make a steady decline of 50 to 75 mg/dL each hour.[34] There is no advantage to a more rapid improvement in the glucose level. The rate of insulin infusion may be adjusted to allow the glucose to trend downward at an appropriate rate. Once the glucose level decreases to less than 250 mg/dL, dextrose is added to the IV fluid to allow for the continued insulin infusion necessary to resolve the acidosis, because the fall in glucose will precede normalization of the acid-base status.[9] By this point, the insulin infusion rate will usually have been adjusted to 0.02 to 0.05 unit/hour.

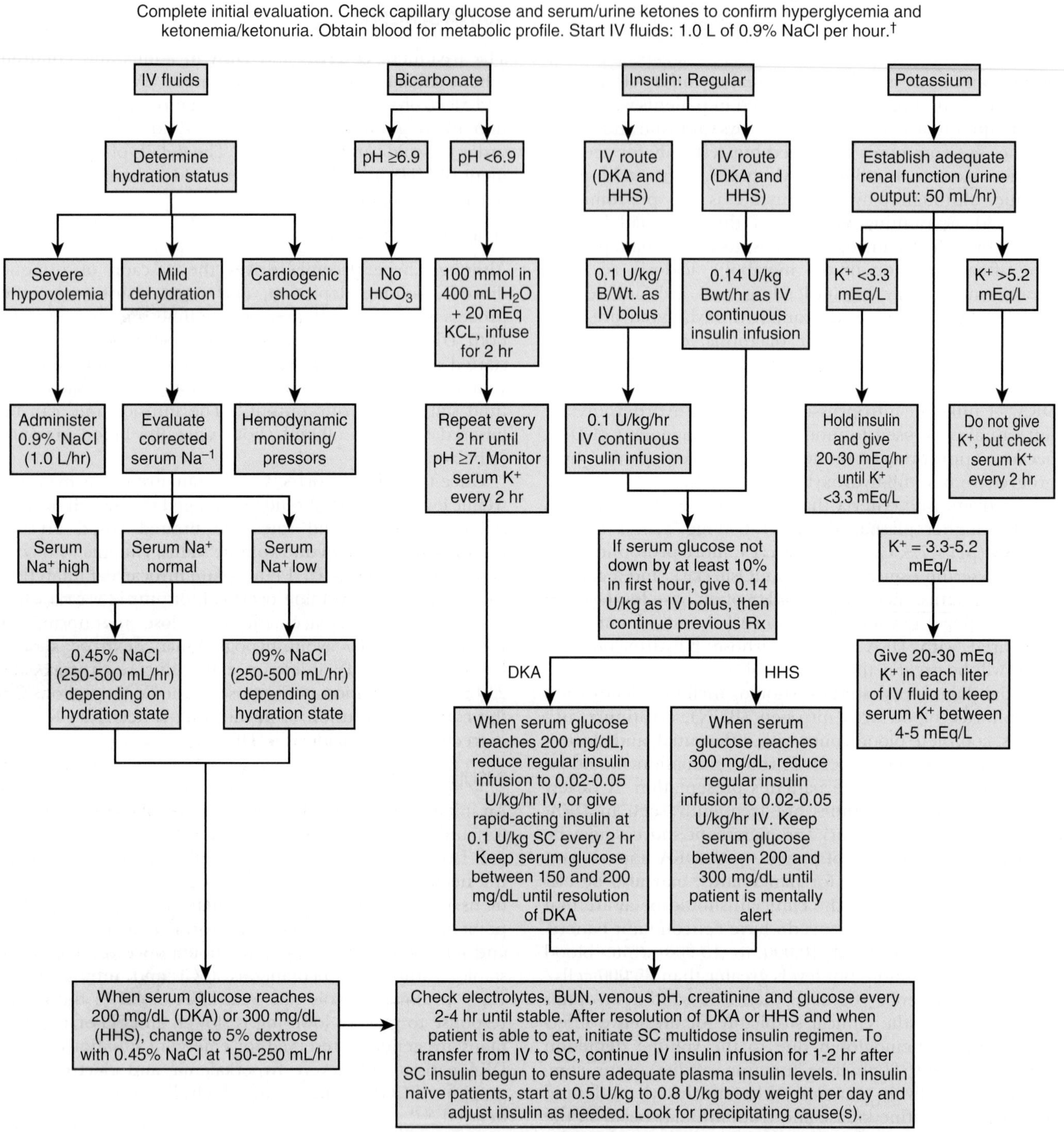

Figure 58.2 Protocol for the management of adult patients with diabetic ketoacidosis (DKA) or hyperglycemic hyperosmolar state (HHS). DKA diagnostic criteria: blood glucose 250 mg/dL, arterial pH 7.3, bicarbonate 15 mEq/L, and moderate ketonuria or ketonemia. HHS diagnostic criteria: serum glucose greater than 600 mg/dL, arterial pH greater than 7.3, serum bicarbonate greater than 15 mEq/L, and minimal ketonuria and ketonemia. †15 to 20 mL/kg/hour; ‡serum Na should be corrected for hyperglycemia (for each 100 mg/dL glucose, add 1.6 mEq to sodium value for corrected serum value). Bwt, body weight; IV, intravenous; SC, subcutaneous. (From Kitabchi AE, Umpierrez GE, Miles JM, Fisher JN: Hyperglycemic crises in adult patients with diabetes. Diabetes Care 2009;32(7):1335-1343.)

The insulin infusion should be continued until resolution of the hyperglycemic crisis. In DKA, resolution of ketoacidosis is indicated by a normalization of the anion gap or a drop in the β-hydroxybutyrate level to less than 3 mmol/L.[52] In HHS, resolution is indicated by correction of the fluid and electrolyte abnormalities. Once the acute abnormalities have resolved and the glucose level has improved to less than 200 mg/dL, the patient can be transitioned to scheduled SC insulin. Patients should be placed on a physiologic insulin regimen, which includes a basal insulin (NPH, glargine, or detemir) and a mealtime, or "nutritional," insulin (regular, lispro, aspart, or glulisine). NPH and regular insulin are associated with higher rates of hypoglycemia.[53] The use of corrective ("sliding scale") insulin as the sole SC insulin strategy is never appropriate in a patient recovering from DKA. Most protocols call for 80% to 100% of the calculated daily insulin requirements to be started based on a stable insulin infusion.[54-57] The insulin doses are divided into 50% basal and 50% nutritional insulin.

Older age, higher IV insulin requirements, and greater blood glucose variation decrease the chance of a successful transition.[56] Other potential pitfalls include discontinuing the IV insulin without initiating physiologic insulin, and over- or underestimating the 24-hour insulin requirements based on fluctuating insulin infusion rates. Despite pressures in a busy intensive care unit (ICU) to transition patients off IV insulin, the SC insulin needs to be calculated based on the relatively stable IV insulin requirements over 4 to 6 hours prior to the transition.[57] IV insulin should not be discontinued until at least 2 hours after the start of basal insulin. A protocol for the successful transition from IV to SC insulin is listed in Box 58.2.[58]

POTASSIUM

Patients with DKA or HHS may initially present with hyperkalemia or hypokalemia, each with significant potential cardiac consequences. Tall peaked T waves in the precordial leads are the first ECG sign of hyperkalemia as the potassium increases above 5.5 mmol/L. As potassium levels increase to greater than 6.5 mmol/L, additional ECG changes emerge: prolonged PR interval, decreased amplitude of P waves, and a widening of the QRS complex. As the potassium increases to greater than 8.0 mmol/L more ominous changes occur, including loss of P waves; intraventricular, fascicular, and bundle branch blocks; and widening of the QRS complex, ultimately resulting in asystole.[59] Conversely, hypokalemia also increases the risk of cardiac arrhythmia. ECG changes in hypokalemia include broad flat T waves, ST-segment depression, and QT interval prolongation.[60] Additionally, hypokalemia decreases myocardial contractility.[60]

Treatment with volume expansion and insulin will lower serum potassium levels as potassium shifts from the extracellular to intracellular space. Electrolytes should be monitored every 2 to 4 hours in the early stages of DKA.[9,32] For a potassium concentration greater than 5 mmol/L, serum K^+ testing should be repeated every 1 to 2 hours. Potassium replacement should be started once the potassium decreases into the normal range and the patient is producing urine. Once serum potassium is below 5 mmol/L, patients should receive KCl 5 mEq/hour via the IV fluid, and the rate can be increased to 10 mEq/hour if the serum K^+ is below

Box 58.2 Important Steps in Transition from Insulin Infusion to Subcutaneous (SC) Insulin

Step 1: Is the patient stable enough for transition?
Hypotension, active sepsis, use of pressors, and intubation are contraindications to transition because these factors are recognized to be associated with unreliable subcutaneous insulin absorption, with continued need for the most flexible dosing due to frequently changing insulin requirements.

Step 2: Does the patient need to switch to scheduled SC insulin?

Yes:	*No:*
Type 1 DM all patients	Type 2 DM in patients with a recent mean infusion rate <0.5 unit/hour
Type 2 DM in patients on home insulin regimen	Stress hyperglycemia or previously unrecognized DM if infusion rate <1 unit/hour or if HbA_{1c} is near normal
Type 2 DM in patients with a recent mean infusion rate ≥0.5 unit/hour	

Step 3: If transition is needed, calculate a total daily dose (TDD) of insulin. The TDD is an estimate of the 24-hour insulin requirement when the patient is receiving full nutrition.

- Determine mean insulin infusion rate from last 6-8 hours.
- Calculate 24-hour insulin dose based on this rate, and reduce the 24-hour dose by 20%.
  - Multiply hourly insulin infusion rate by 20 (80% of 24) to arrive at a safety-adjusted 24-hour insulin dose.
- Determine if this total is the TDD or basal dose based on current nutrition.
  - If the infusion was providing both the basal and nutritional needs of the patient (i.e., continuous tube feeds), this will be the TDD.

  OR
  - If the infusion was not covering significant nutrition, this *could* be the basal insulin dose.

Step 4: Construct a basal/bolus regimen tailored to the patient's nutritional situation, building safeguards for any changes in nutritional intake and uncertainties about reliability of intake. Several options are again available.

- *Basal*: glargine, detemir, or NPH
  1. Dose is 40-50% of TDD.

  OR

  2. Adjusted 24-hour intravenous requirement can be given as all basal.
- *Nutritional*: The remainder of TDD is scheduled nutritional insulin in divided doses. In general, these doses need to be adjusted down for <100% nutritional intake, and the orders should allow for administering nutritional insulin just AFTER observed meal to allow an assessment of intake. Several options are available for estimating the initial doses:
  1. Use 50% of the TDD as nutritional coverage, and divide this amount by 3 to determine the scheduled meal dose. Hold if patient does not eat more than 50% of each meal.
  2. Use a more conservative start of 0.1-0.2 × basal dose for each meal.
  3. Use carbohydrate counting to cover nutritional intake.

Step 5: Be sure to give SC insulin BEFORE the infusion stops.

- Basal glargine and detemir ideally are given at least 2 hours before infusion is discontinued.
- Shorter lead times (30 minutes) are possible if rapid-acting insulin is given with basal insulin.

DM, diabetes mellitus; HbA_{1c}, hemoglobin A_{1c} (glycosylated hemoglobin).
Modified from O'Malley CW, Emanuele, M, Halasyamani L, Amin AN. Bridge over troubled waters: safe and effective transitions of the inpatient with hyperglycemia. J Hops Med 2008, 3(S5):S55-65.

4 mmol/L. Lower doses should be used if the patient has evidence of impaired renal function.

BICARBONATE

The metabolic acidosis of DKA impairs myocardial contractility, affects oxyhemoglobin dissociation and tissue oxygen delivery, inhibits intracellular enzymes, alters cellular metabolism, and may result in vital organ dysfunction.[61] Correction of acidosis focuses on the correction of insulin deficiency and volume depletion, as well as any other underlying conditions that may be contributing to the acidosis. Although the administration of bicarbonate would appear to be a reasonable consideration, multiple trials of bicarbonate replacement in DKA patients have demonstrated no benefit.[61,62] Furthermore, the use of IV bicarbonate may result in complications.[34,40] Bicarbonate therapy has been associated with hypokalemia, intracellular acidosis, and tissue hypoxia.[47] On the other hand, a potential benefit for bicarbonate therapy in those individuals with severe acidemia ($pH < 6.9$)[62,63] has been suggested, though the literature is limited. In patients with pH less than 6.9, the use of sodium bicarbonate (100 mmol sodium bicarbonate in 400 mL sterile water with 20 mEq KCl, administered at a rate of 200 mL/hour for 2 hours, and then repeating every 2 hours) may be considered until the pH is greater than 6.9.[9]

PHOSPHATE

Phosphate levels initially may be normal to elevated, but usually decline with treatment.[64] There is no evidence to support the routine use of phosphate replacement in patients with DKA.[65,66] Nevertheless, severe hypophosphatemia may impair oxygen delivery and cause muscle fatigue, and selective replacement is suggested in patients with phosphate levels less than 1.0 mg/dL, anemia, respiratory failure, or CHF.[9,67] Correcting the phosphorus level improves tissue oxygenation and restores the body's buffering capacity. Phosphate is generally replaced as a potassium salt.[68] To avoid complications, particularly hypocalcemia, phosphorus replacement should be limited to 40 to 50 mmol of potassium phosphate at approximately 3 to 4 mmol/hour. The potassium being provided in other IV fluids may need to be adjusted to account for the potassium infused as part of the phosphorus replacement.[68]

HYPERCHLOREMIC ACIDOSIS

The development of hyperchloremic acidosis occurs in DKA because the ability to completely regenerate bicarbonate is hampered by the urinary loss of keto acids, which normally act as substrate for the re-formation of bicarbonate. To maintain the appropriate balance of cations and anions, chloride ions from the infused saline will partially compensate for the lack of bicarbonate. As the ketoacidosis resolves, a hyperchloremic acidosis (with a normal anion gap) may ensue. This benign process resolves gradually in the hours to days after the saline infusion is reduced or stopped.[68]

COMPLICATIONS OF THE MANAGEMENT OF HYPERGLYCEMIC EMERGENCIES

Management of hyperglycemic emergencies is associated with several complications, the most common being iatrogenic hypoglycemia from aggressive insulin dosing. Frequent monitoring of glucose (every 1-2 hours) and down-titration of insulin doses as the glucose approaches normal are appropriate strategies to prevent hypoglycemia. The addition of dextrose-containing IV fluid is suggested when the glucose level drops below 250 mg/dL to allow for the continued insulin infusion necessary to restore the acid-base balance.

Cerebral edema is the one of the most feared complications of hyperglycemic crisis. Classically, cerebral edema has been reported in children with DKA. It occurs in 0.5% to 1% of all DKA cases[69,70] and carries a mortality rate of 20%. Survivors are at risk for residual neurologic problems.[45] Although cerebral edema is occasionally seen in adults with HHS, it is rare in adults with DKA and children with HHS.[71] Children who present with (1) low partial pressures of arterial carbon dioxide and (2) high serum urea nitrogen concentrations and (3) are treated with bicarbonate are at increased risk for cerebral edema. The exact cause of cerebral edema remains unknown. It does not appear to be associated with the initial level of hyperosmolarity or more rapid correction of the hyperosmolarity.[72,73] Cerebral ischemia, and not changes in osmolality, may be the causal factor in patients who develop cerebral edema.[73] Nevertheless, care should be taken to avoid rapid changes in glucose and osmolarity, especially in younger patients. The clinician should also be aware of the signs of cerebral edema, which include headache, persistent vomiting, hypertension, bradycardia, and neurologic changes.

Attention to the diagnosis and management of any infections or cardiovascular events is imperative. Other complications of the management of DKA and HHS include hypokalemia, hypophosphatemia, acute renal failure, and shock. Appropriate management of hyperglycemic emergencies with close attention to fluid and electrolyte balance minimizes these complications. Less common problems can include rhabdomyolysis,[74] thrombosis and stroke,[75] pneumomediastinum,[76] and memory loss with decreased cognitive function in children.[77]

PREVENTION

Despite improvements in insulin treatment and glucose monitoring[78] the incidence of DKA is increasing.[3] Prevention is paramount. Health care providers should recognize signs of DM in all age groups. Patients with DM and their caregivers should be familiar with sick day recommendations (Box 58.3), and patients with type 1 DM should check urine ketones by dipstick if the glucose is greater than 240 mg/dL.[79] Home measurement of serum ketones with a commercial glucometer may allow earlier detection of DKA and decreased hospital visits,[80] though most meters lack this capability.

Nonadherence to medical regimens is often cited as the cause of recurrent DKA, and in fact, 5% of patients account for more than 25% of all cases of DKA.[81] Health care providers need to recognize disparities in the health care system that limit access to appropriate DM care or otherwise contribute to nonadherence with insulin or other antidiabetic medications. Diabetes education enhances patient knowledge of appropriate monitoring and prevention of DKA,[82] and diabetes educators are an excellent resource to help

Box 58.3 Sick Day Management Protocol for Diabetic Patients[212,213]

Examples of "Sick Day" Scenarios

- Feeling sick or presence of fever for 2 days or longer without getting better
- Vomiting or diarrhea for more than 6 hours

Management

General Measures

- Check blood sugar levels at least every 4 hours, but when values are changing quickly, check more often.
- Check urine or blood ketones.
- Modify usual insulin regimen according to a plan developed by the diabetes physician or team.
- Maintain adequate food and fluid intake. If your appetite is poor, aim for consumption of 50 g of carbohydrate every 3-4 hours. If you are nauseous, high-carbohydrate liquids, such as regular (not diet) soft drinks or juice, or frozen juice bars, sherbet, pudding, creamed soups, or fruit-flavored yogurt usually are tolerated. Broth also is a good alternative.

Taking Medications When You Are Sick

- If you are eating: Continue taking your pills for diabetes or your insulin. Your blood sugar may continue to rise because of your illness.
- If you are nauseous or vomiting or otherwise cannot take your medicines:
  - Continue to take your long-acting insulin (Lantus, Levemir, NPH).
  - Call your doctor and discuss whether you need to adjust your short- or rapid-acting insulin dose (regular, lispro [Humalog], aspart [Novolog], glulisine [Apidra]) or your other diabetes medicines.

Examples of When to Call Physician or Diabetes Team

- If glucose levels are higher than 240 mg/dL despite taking extra insulin according to a sick day plan
- If you take diabetes pills and blood sugar is still above 240 mg/dL before meals and remains there for more than 24 hours
- If symptoms/signs develop that might signal DKA or dehydration, such as dizziness, trouble breathing, fruity breath, or dry and cracked lips or tongue

DKA, diabetic ketoacidosis.

assess a patient's barriers to optimal care including financial, social, and cultural issues.[82]

GLYCEMIC CONTROL IN THE INTENSIVE CARE UNIT

EPIDEMIOLOGY AND SIGNIFICANCE OF HYPERGLYCEMIA

Hyperglycemia is a common occurrence in hospitalized patients and is associated with increased morbidity and mortality rates,[83-85] including higher rates of surgical infections after cardiothoracic surgery,[86,87] increased mortality rates after MI,[88-90] and poor outcome in critically ill patients.[91,92] Forty percent of patients in the ICU and 80% of those undergoing cardiac surgery have elevated glucose levels.[93] Of hyperglycemic patients in the hospital, two thirds have a history of diabetes, although the remainder have no prior history.[85] This latter group includes patients with previously unrecognized diabetes as well as those with "stress hyperglycemia" (patients who are normoglycemic on follow-up testing). Only 15% of patients with new-onset hyperglycemia have confirmed diabetes 1 year after the hospital admission.[94] Hyperglycemic patients with no prior history of diabetes have a worse prognosis than patients with preexisting diabetes, including greater mortality rates after MI[83] and a significantly increased 30-day and 1-year mortality rate.[95] This is particularly true of patients with stress hyperglycemia, a condition of acutely elevated glucose related to illness-related increases in counterregulatory hormones seen (Fig. 58.3)[93] in patients with otherwise normal glucose metabolism. Stress hyperglycemia is consistently associated with increased adjusted mortality rates for patients with unstable angina, acute MI, CHF, arrhythmia, ischemic and hemorrhagic stroke, gastrointestinal bleeding, acute renal failure, pneumonia, pulmonary embolism, and sepsis.[96]

Glucose variability, measured as the standard deviation of glucose excursions around the mean, adds to the metabolic burden.[97] Glycemic variability may be a better predictor of morbidity and mortality rates than the level of hyperglycemia in patients with preexisting diabetes.[98-100] In a retrospective analysis, the odds ratio for ICU death is significantly greater in patients with higher hourly change in glucose.[101] Glycemic variability may be a better predictor of morbidity and mortality rates than the level of hyperglycemia in patients with preexisting diabetes.[98-100]

SYNOPSIS OF TRIALS OF GLYCEMIC CONTROL

The benefits of improved glucose control were initially suggested by several retrospective or nonrandomized trials in patients with acute MI,[102] with stroke,[84] after coronary artery bypass surgery,[87] and in the ICU.[103] A landmark single-center prospective study in surgical ICU patients was published in 2001, in which intensive insulin therapy (IIT) was reported to decrease ICU and in-hospital mortality rates, as well as significant comorbid conditions such as bloodstream infections, acute renal failure requiring dialysis or hemofiltration, the median number of red blood cell transfusions, critical-illness polyneuropathy, and prolonged mechanical ventilation. The number of patients who received red-cell transfusions did not differ significantly between the two groups. However, the median number of transfusions in the intensive-treatment group was only half that in the conventional-treatment group. This difference was not due to more liberal use of transfusions in the conventional-treatment group, as indicated by the lower hemoglobin and hematocrit values in that group.[104] Based on this study, many ICUs initiated IV insulin protocols designed to achieve glucose levels in the 70- to 110-mg/dL range. Soon, however, enthusiasm over the benefits of normoglycemia from IIT in the critically ill patient were tempered by (1) an inability to extend the initial results across multiple centers,[105,106] (2) concern over the risk of hypoglycemia,[105,106] (3) questions

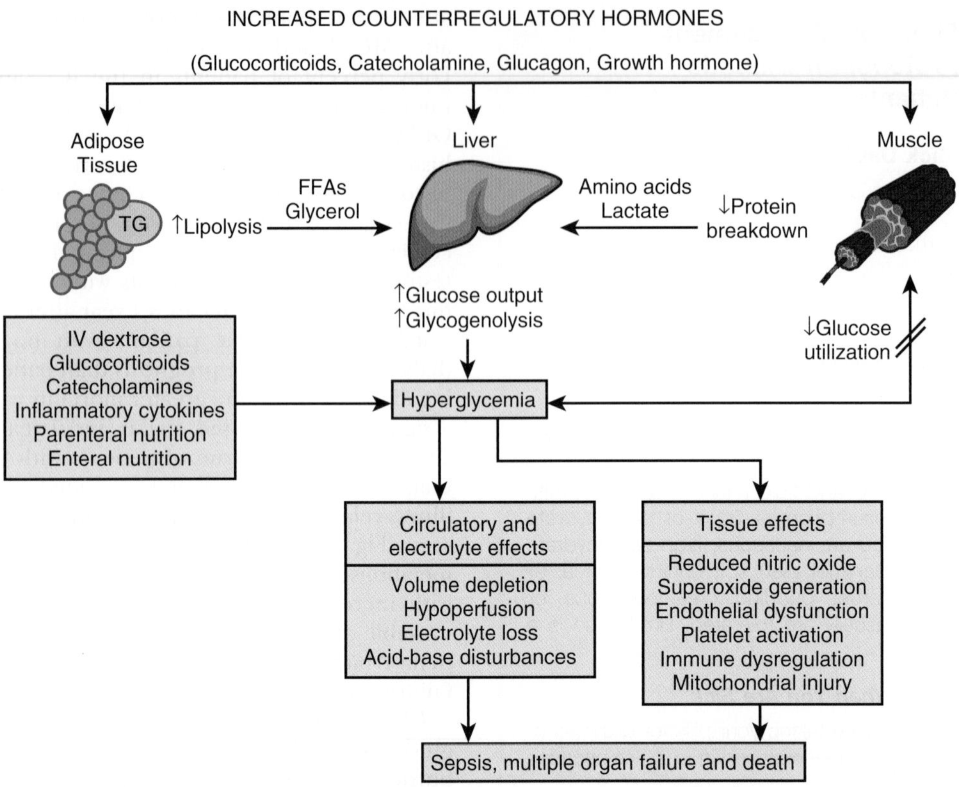

Figure 58.3 Pathogenesis of stress hyperglycemia. Stress hyperglycemia results from increased hepatic glucose production and impaired glucose utilization in peripheral tissues. Excess counterregulatory hormones (glucagon, cortisol, catecholamines, and growth hormone) increase lipolysis and protein breakdown (proteolysis), and impair glucose utilization by peripheral tissues. Hyperglycemia causes osmotic diuresis that leads to hypovolemia, decreased glomerular filtration rate, and worsening hyperglycemia. At the cellular level increased blood glucose levels result in mitochondrial injury by generating reactive oxygen species and endothelial dysfunction by inhibiting nitric oxide production. Hyperglycemia increases levels of proinflammatory cytokines such as tumor necrosis factor-α (TNF-α), and interleukin 6 (IL-6), leading to immune system dysfunction, and increases plasminogen activator inhibitor-1 and fibrinogen, causing platelet aggregation and hypercoagulable state. These changes can eventually lead to increased risk of infection, impaired wound healing, multiple organ failure, prolonged hospital stay, and death. (From Farrokhi F, Smiley D, Umpierrez GE: Glycemic control in non-diabetic critically ill patients. Best Pract Res Clin Endocrinol Metab 2011;25:813-824.)

over the role of early nutrition,[104] and (4) a less pronounced improvement for patients with preexisting diabetes.[107] Additionally, nonrandomized and observational studies suggested a J-shaped curve for mortality rate related to glycemic control in the ICU with increasing mortality rate for glucose levels less than 90 mg/dL and greater than 120 mg/dL.[96,103,108-110] In the NICE-SUGAR (Normoglycemia in Intensive Care Evaluation—Survival Using Glucose Algorithm Regulation) study,[111] a randomized controlled, multicenter trial, in which ICU patients were randomized to intensive glycemic control or conventional glucose control, no mortality rate benefit was seen with IIT. In a meta-analysis of studies evaluating the impact of intensive glycemic control, including the results from NICE-SUGAR, the relative risk of death was not significantly different with IIT compared with conventional therapy, but the risk of severe hypoglycemia was significantly greater.[112] Figure 58.4 summarizes key studies on the impact of intensive glycemic control.

The foremost obstacle to the use of IIT is hypoglycemia. Patients managed with IIT for tight glycemic control have significantly greater rates and duration of hypoglycemia.[112,113] Hypoglycemia from insulin therapy increases mortality risks in critically ill patients,[105,114-118] which may mitigate any benefits of tight glucose control.[104] As expected, use of glucose control algorithms modified for a higher glucose target range significantly reduces the risk of severe hypoglycemia.[119,120]

INTRAVENOUS INSULIN PROTOCOLS

A standardized insulin protocol should be used to maintain goal glucose levels and reduce hypoglycemic episodes. Current practice requires the clinician to consider the multiple factors affecting glucose control, such as changes in nutrition, medication or medical acuity, and proactively respond to avoid large fluctuations in glucose levels. An effective IV insulin protocol allows for titration of IV insulin in the setting of changing glucose levels. Multiple published insulin protocols are available,[54,57,121-126] though any protocol will need to be adapted and adjusted to fit the needs of the local environment. A multidisciplinary team consisting of intensivists, endocrinologists, nurses, and pharmacologists should be involved in the development, implementation, and continued evaluation of IV insulin protocols.

TECHNICAL ISSUES IN MEASURING GLUCOSE

Accurate measurement of glucose in the ICU is essential to maintain glycemic control and limit the risk of severe hypoglycemia. The use of IIT magnified the importance of

Title	N	Setting	Blood plasma sups (mEq/L (mmol))		Blood glucose achieved [mg/dl 9mmol/l)[b]		Primary outcome	End point rate (%)		ARR (%)[c]	RRR (%)[c]	Odds ratio (95% CI)
			Intensive	Conventional	Intensive	Conventional		Intensive	Conventional			
DIGAMI (ref. 33),1995	620	CCU (AMI)	126-196 (7-10.9)	Usual care	173 (9.6)	211 (11.7)	1-year mortality	18.6	26.1	7.5	29[d]	NR
Van den Berghe et al. (ref. 5), 2001	1,548	SICU	80-110 (4.4-6.1)	180-200 (10-11)	103 (5.7)	153 (8.5)	ICU mortality	4.6	8.0	3.4	42	0.58 (0.38-0.78)[d]
DIGAMI 2 (ref. 34), 2005	1253	CCU (AMI)	126-180 (7-10) (groups 1 and 2)	Usual care (group 3)	164 (9.1)	180 (10)	2-year mortality	Group 1, 23.4; group 2, 21.2	Group 3, 17.9	—[e]	—[e]	NR
Van den Berghe et al. (ref. 16), 2006	1200	MICU	80-110 (4.4-6.1)	180-200 (10-11)	111 (6.2)	153 (8.5)	Hospital mortality	37.3	40.0	2.7	7.0	0.94 (0.84-1.06)[e]
HI-5 (ref. 35), 2006	240	CCU (Ami) (GIK)	72-180 (4-10)	Usual care <288	149 (8.3)	162 (9)	6-month mortality	7.9	6.1	−1.8[e]	−30[e]	NR
GuControl (ref. 27), 2007[f]	1101	ICU	80-110 (4.4-6.1)	140–180 (7.8-10)	118 (6.5)	144 (8)	ICU mortality	16.7	15.2	−1.5	−10	1.10 (0.84-1.44)[e]
Gandhi et al. (ref. 36), 2007	399	Operating room	80-110 (4.4-6.1)	<200 (<11)	114 (6.3)	157 (8.7)	Composite[g]	44	46	2	4.3	1.0 (0.8-1.2)[e]
VISEP (ref. 13), 2008	537[h]	ICU	80-110 (4.4-6.1)	180-200 (10-11)	112 (6.2)	151 (8.4)	28-day mortality	24.7	26.0	1.3	5.0	0.89 (0.58-1.38)[e,i]
De La Rosa et al. (ref. 28), 2008[f]	504	SICU MICU	80-110 (4.4-6.1)	180-200 (10-11)	117 (6.5)	148 (8.2)	28-day mortality	36.6	32.4	−4.2[e]	−13[e]	NR
NICE-SUGAR (ref. 14) 2009	6104	ICU	81-108 (4.5-6)	≤180 (≤10)	115 (6.4)	145 (8.0)	3-month mortality	27.5	24.9	−2.6	−10.6	1.14 (1.02-1.28)[d]

[a]ARR, absolute risk reduction; CCU, coronary care unit; GIK, glucose-insulin-potassium; MICU, medical ICU; NR, not reported; RRR, relative risk reduction; SICU, surgical ICU. [b]Mean morning blood glucose concentrations (except for GluControl, which reported mean overall blood glucose concentrations). [c]Intensive group versus conventional group. [d]$P < 0.05$. [e]Not significant ($P < 0.05$). [f]Presented as abstract only. [g]Composite of death, sternal infection, prolonged ventilation, cardiac arrhythmias, stroke, and renal failure at 30 days. [h]Only patients with sepsis. [i]Personal communication, Dr. Frank Brunkhorst.

Figure 58.4 Summary data of selected randomized controlled trials of intensive insulin therapy in critically ill patients (>200 randomized patients). ARR, absolute risk reduction; CCU, coronary care unit; GIK, glucose-insulin-potassium; MICU, medical ICU; NR, not reported; RRR, relative risk reduction; SICU, surgical ICU. (From Moghissi ES, Korytkowski MT, DiNardo M, et al: American Association of Clinical Endocrinologists and American Diabetes Association consensus statement on inpatient glycemic control. Diabetes Care 2009;32(6):1119-1131; Endocr Pract 2009;15(4):353-369.)

accurate point of care (POC) glucose monitoring. In the ICU measurements of glucose are affected by the clinical status of the patient, by certain medications, and by the type of blood sample.[127] Anemia may falsely elevate POC glucose levels, which can mask hypoglycemia.[128-130] This deserves attention given the high prevalence of anemia routinely encountered in ICUs.[131] The accuracy of POC testing is also affected by several other common conditions (e.g., acidosis, hypothermia, and hypotension) and medications (dopamine, mannitol, acetaminophen, and pressor use).[132-135] The rates of intrapatient variability in glucose measurements are lowest from arterial samples. Variability increases in venous sampling with the greatest variability in capillary blood. Arterial blood analysis correlates better with central laboratory glucose values than capillary blood measurements. During hypoglycemia, the discrepancy is exaggerated. POC capillary and whole blood samples from patients with poor peripheral perfusion overestimate the laboratory glucose level by 20% in a significant proportion of samples.[136] The difference between capillary and arterial blood glucose measurements has led most insulin protocols for ICUs to recommend the use of arterial blood measurements when available.[136]

Subcutaneous electrochemical sensors can measure glucose levels in the interstitial fluid and report an average glucose level every 1 to 10 minutes, although a lag time of 8 to 18 minutes exists between blood glucose and interstitial glucose equilibration.[137] Determining trends in glucose, the devices may provide earlier detection of hypoglycemia and hyperglycemia. Several small studies found excellent accuracy for continuous glucose monitoring (CGM) in the ICU as compared to POC testing.[137-140] However, there is currently insufficient evidence to support the general use of CGM in the ICU.[141]

CURRENT GUIDELINES FOR GLYCEMIC CONTROL

The current guidelines for glycemic control in the ICU have transitioned from declarations for tight glycemic control (based on observational and retrospective data and a single-site randomized controlled study) to more moderated goals taking into account the increased mortality rate associated with hypoglycemia and the limited benefit from tight glycemic control seen in other trials.[105,106,142,143]

The 2009 American Academy of Clinical Endocrinologists and American Diabetes Association Consensus Statement on Inpatient Glycemic Control[122] recommends insulin therapy for persistent hyperglycemia at a threshold no greater than 180 mg/dL, with a target range for glucose levels in the ICU of 140 to 180 mg/dL. The guideline recommends treatment with IV insulin using an established protocol associated with low rates of hypoglycemia and frequent glucose monitoring.

The 2012 Surviving Sepsis Guidelines (2012)[144] recommend:

- Initiating an IV insulin protocol in ICU patients with severe sepsis who have two consecutive blood glucose levels greater than 180 mg/dL
- Targeting a blood glucose level less than 180 mg/dL
- Providing a glucose calorie source to all patients on IV insulin
- Monitoring glucose levels every 1 to 2 hours until infusion rates are stable, then every 4 hours
- Interpreting POC capillary blood glucose testing with caution, keeping in mind that this may overestimate arterial blood glucose or plasma glucose

THE EFFECT OF PARENTERAL NUTRITION, ENTERAL NUTRITION, AND GLUCOCORTICOIDS ON GLYCEMIC CONTROL

Changes in nutrition and glucocorticoid dosing occur commonly, often quickly, in the intensively ill patient. Even when changes in enteral or parenteral nutrition are planned, or the patient is on a prescribed steroid taper, insulin adjustments need to be considered proactively to minimize glycemic variability.

Enteral feeding preparations have high concentrations of carbohydrates, and are associated with an increase in glucose concentration.[145,146] Similarly, the majority of patients with type 2 DM who are not on insulin prior to ICU admission require insulin to maintain glycemic control once parenteral nutrition is initiated.[147] It is advisable to begin an IV or SC insulin regimen at the onset of total parenteral nutrition/peripheral parenteral nutrition (TPN/PPN) use,[122] or alternatively, regular insulin can be added to parenteral nutrition. When nutrition is held or discontinued, the insulin dosing will usually need to be reduced, or dextrose-containing IV fluid started, to reduce the risk of hypoglycemia.

Glucocorticoid-induced hyperglycemia is common in the critically ill patient. Glucocorticoids decrease insulin sensitivity, impair glucose disposal, and increase hepatic insulin resistance.[148] All patients should have regularly scheduled glucose monitoring for the first 48 hours after steroids are initiated. Subcutaneous insulin therapy may be started for glucocorticoid-induced hyperglycemia with an initial total daily dose (TDD) of 0.3 to 0.5 unit per kg body weight. IV insulin infusion is appropriate for moderate to severe hyperglycemia.[149] In patients started on insulin for glucocorticoid-induced hyperglycemia, the insulin dose will need to be titrated for changes in steroid dose.

SUBCUTANEOUS INSULIN USE IN THE HOSPITALIZED PATIENT

Insulin is the therapy of choice for glucose control in the ICU. Oral agents and noninsulin injectable agents should be discontinued on admission. The multiple contraindications and the inability to make rapid adjustments for changes in clinical or nutritional status make noninsulin therapy poorly suited for the care of the critically ill patient. The onset, peak, and duration of action of the currently available insulin preparations are listed in (Table 58.3). Insulin can be categorized based on the physiologic profile: basal insulin is either long or intermediate duration; short- or rapid-acting insulin is used for prandial control and for the correction of hyperglycemia. The lack of a defined peak and prolonged action profile make glargine (Lantus) and detemir (Levemir) advantageous for use as a basal insulin. Glargine is typically dosed once daily and detemir one to two times daily. NPH has an intermediate duration of action

Table 58.3 Onset, Peak, and Duration of Action of Currently Available Insulin Preparations

Insulin Preparation	Onset of Action	Peak Action	Duration of Action
Lispro	5-15 min	30-90 min	3-5 hr
Aspart	5-15 min	30-90 min	3-5 hr
Glulisine	5-15 min	30-90 min	3-5 hr
Regular	30-60 min	2-3 hr	5-8 hr
NPH	2-4 hr	4-10 hr	12-20 hr
Detemir	2-4 hr	Relatively peakless	Up to 24 hr
Glargine	2-4 hr	Relatively peakless	20-24 hr

with peak effect at 6 to 8 hours after dosing and is usually dosed twice daily.

With a variety of insulin regimens available, the practitioner has several options available to manage hospitalized patients with diabetes or stress hyperglycemia. Patients who are not eating or who are receiving continuous nutrition (enteral or parenteral) should have a basal insulin in place. The basal insulin is given SC, or in the case of parenteral nutrition, regular insulin may be added to the PPN or TPN at an initial dose of 1 unit for each 15 g of dextrose.[150] In a patient on continuous nutrition or NPO (nothing by mouth), glargine is dosed daily, detemir every 12 to 24 hours, or NPH every 8 to 12 hours. No research is available to support the use of one basal insulin over another in the hospitalized patient. The potential risk of NPH is the peak effect, although the longer duration of glargine and detemir may result in longer periods of hypoglycemia. Glucose monitoring should be performed every 4 to 8 hours, depending on the stability of the patient.

In patients tolerating scheduled meals, a prandial insulin should be added. Lispro, aspart, and glulisine each have a more physiologic profile with a quicker onset of action, time to peak, and shorter duration of action than regular insulin. The use of a rapid-acting insulin analog is associated with better glycemic control compared to regular insulin.[151] In patients who are eating, glucose monitoring is usually performed before the meal and at bedtime.

The lack of flexibility with premixed insulin (Humulin 70/30, Novolin 70/30, Novolog 70/30, and Humalog 75/25) makes their use less suitable for the hospital. Each of the premixed insulin preparations contains 70% to 75% NPH for intermediate-acting insulin and 25% to 30% of regular insulin or a rapid-acting insulin analog (lispro or aspart). Though not an optimal practice, if the practitioner wishes to continue a successful home regimen of premixed insulin in a hospitalized patient, the component doses of NPH and lispro, aspart, or regular insulin can be given separately.

In the hospitalized patient, there are several methods for determining insulin dosing for a basal-bolus regimen:

1. A weight-based protocol[152] can be utilized, typically starting at 0.3 to 0.6 unit/kg body weight depending on the patient's weight and risk factors for insulin sensitivity (body mass index [BMI] < 25, hepatic insufficiency, renal insufficiency) or insulin resistance (morbid obesity, sepsis, glucocorticoids). A weight-based regimen is helpful in initiating an SC insulin regimen in a patient with new-onset hyperglycemia or a patient who is on a noninsulin antidiabetic regimen with or without basal insulin. Fifty percent of the dose is given as basal insulin, and the remaining 50% is divided into three mealtime boluses.
2. The patient's home insulin basal-bolus dose can be restarted if the patient has good outpatient glucose control, based on a recent hemoglobin A_{1c} (HbA_{1c}) or a reliable history. The results of an HbA_{1c} obtained in the past 3 months will give insight into the efficacy of the patient's outpatient medical regimen, and may also help to determine if a patient without a history of diabetes has unrecognized DM versus stress hyperglycemia.
3. A premixed insulin regimen can be changed to basal-bolus by adding the TDD of insulin and then giving 50% as basal insulin and 50% as nutritional (mealtime) insulin.
4. An insulin regimen can be determined based on the IV insulin infusion requirements.

The use of correctional (sliding) scale insulin as sole therapy cannot be promoted for the patient with hyperglycemia. Reliance on sliding scale insulin is associated with worse glycemic control in hospitalized patients.[153,154] In particular, patients with type 1 DM always require physiologic insulin dosing including a basal insulin to prevent the development of DKA. Correctional insulin doses may be used as an adjunct to a physiologic insulin regimen. Doses of correctional insulin should be aligned to the TDD of prescribed insulin; thus, a patient requiring 100 units of insulin a day will require more correctional dose insulin than a patient whose TDD is 30 units. The clinician can calculate the expected change in glucose for 1 unit of regular or rapid-acting insulin analog using the "Rule of 1500" formula: 1500/TDD = expected decrease in glucose (in mg/dL) for 1 unit of correctional dose insulin. For insulin-sensitive patients (e.g., type 1 DM, BMI < 25 kg/m^2, end-stage renal disease [ESRD], or hepatic failure), 1800 rather than 1500 is used for the numerator.

HYPOGLYCEMIA

As noted in the previous section, hypoglycemia is the main deterrent to good glycemic control[155] and is associated with higher rates of morbidity and mortality in the ICU.[105,120,156,157] Under normal circumstances the fasting glucose is 70 to 90 mg/dL.[158] Although only 1.5% of patients without DM or who are pre-DM will have clinically significant hypoglycemia,[114] the critically ill patient is at enhanced risk of hypoglycemia due to underlying illness as well as the use of medications that can lower glucose.

PHYSIOLOGIC RESPONSE TO HYPOGLYCEMIA

The physiologic response to hypoglycemia is mediated through neural and humoral pathways and that involves both a reduction in insulin and activation of the

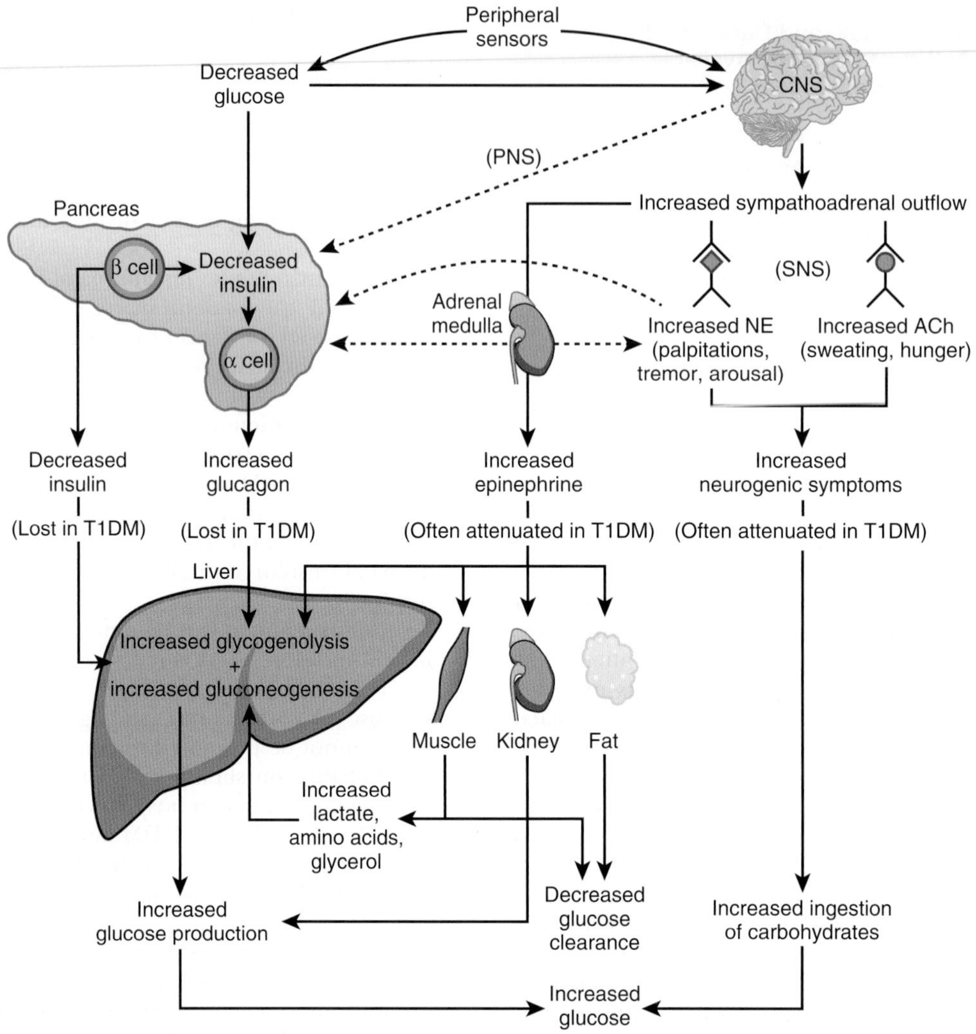

Figure 58.5 Physiologic and behavioral defenses against hypoglycemia in humans. α-cell, pancreatic islet alpha cells; ACh, acetylcholine; β-cell, pancreatic islet beta cells; NE, norepinephrine; PNS, parasympathetic nervous system; SNS, sympathetic nervous system; T1DM, type 1 diabetes. (From Cryer PE: Mechanisms of sympathoadrenal failure and hypoglycemia in diabetes. J Clin Invest 2006;116:1470-1473, used with permission of the American Society of Clinical Investigation.)

counterregulatory response[159] (Fig. 58.5). The first humoral response to a decreasing glucose is inhibition of insulin secretion when the glucose level drops to less than 80 mg/dL.[159,160] The drop in insulin level causes decreased peripheral glucose utilization, as well as increased glucose production through glycogenolysis and gluconeogenesis.[161] Glucagon, epinephrine, and growth hormone secretion increases as glucose levels fall below 70 mg/dL.[159,160] Cortisol release increases as the glucose drops below 60 mg/dL. Of the counterregulatory hormones, glucagon plays the key role in the minute-to-minute prevention of hypoglycemia.[162] If glucagon secretion is diminished (e.g., in longstanding autoimmune diabetes), epinephrine release becomes critical for the reversal of hypoglycemia. Under normal circumstances, cortisol and growth hormone are not essential in the prevention of hypoglycemia but are necessary in the absence of glucagon.[159] The stepwise response to hypoglycemia and the redundancy in the counterregulatory hormones suggest the physiologic importance placed on the prevention of hypoglycemia.[159]

Table 58.4 Clinical Symptoms of Hypoglycemia

Sympathoadrenal	Neuroglycopenic
Tremor	Tiredness or drowsiness
Palpitations	Difficulty thinking
Diaphoresis	Confusion
Nervousness	Blurred vision
Anxiety or apprehension	Slurred speech
Hunger	Dizziness, weakness
Pallor	Abnormal or belligerent behavior
	Seizure
	Coma or death

SYMPTOMS

The symptoms of hypoglycemia can be thought of as either sympathoadrenal or neuroglycopenic (Table 58.4). The sympathoadrenal symptoms are mediated through both β- and α-adrenergic and cholinergic pathways, and begin as the glucose decreases to less than 60 mg/dL.[163] These symptoms include cholinergic-mediated complaints of diaphoresis and hunger and adrenergic-related symptoms of tremulousness, palpitations, and anxiety.[163]

Neuroglycopenic symptoms represent the effects of low glucose on the brain. Although the brain is responsible for 50% of the body's glucose use under physiologic conditions,[164,165] it can neither generate glucose nor store glycogen. Thus, the brain requires a constant source of glucose.[164,165] The onset of neuroglycopenic symptoms represents a drop in glucose below the critical level of glucose transport across the blood-brain barrier to meet the brain's metabolic demands.[166] Initial neuroglycopenic symptoms include the sensation of warmth, difficulty concentrating, weakness, fatigue, dizziness, difficulty speaking, and blurred vision.[163] As glucose falls, these effects may progress to confusion, behavioral change, lethargy, seizure, and coma. The severity of symptoms may be altered by the degree of hypoglycemia, the rate of fall in glucose levels, and the blunting of the hypoglycemic response from either medication or habituation from recurrent hypoglycemia.[165,167]

HYPOGLYCEMIA IN PATIENTS WITH DIABETES OR WHO RECEIVE INSULIN

Although insulin is necessary to manage hyperglycemia in hospitalized patients, it is also the major risk factor for hypoglycemia. Additional risks for hypoglycemia are seen in (1) patients with comorbid conditions such sepsis, organ failure, or malnutrition; (2) patients receiving medications such as beta blockers that mask the neurogenic symptoms of hypoglycemia; or (3) patients who do not have the capacity to respond to a hypoglycemic episode (e.g., sedated patients).

In patients with diabetes, hypoglycemia occurs with decreased or interrupted carbohydrate consumption, increased glucose utilization from elevated energy expenditure, or an increase in insulin to a degree that overwhelms the glucose counterregulatory system. The source of insulin may be exogenous, from an insulin injection or infusion, or endogenous, caused by an insulin secretagogue drug such as a sulfonylurea or a glinide. A detailed description of the onset, peak, and duration of the various types of insulin is given in the earlier section "Glycemic Control in the Intensive Care Unit." Sulfonylurea drugs such as chlorpropamide, tolbutamide, and glyburide, which have extended half-lives and are renally metabolized, predispose to prolonged hypoglycemia, particularly in patients with renal insufficiency.[168] Newer agents such as glipizide and glimepiride have dual hepatic and renal metabolism, which decreases the risk of prolonged hypoglycemia. The shorter duration of action of the glinides (repaglinide and nateglinide) reduce the risk of prolonged hypoglycemia. Diabetes medication affecting insulin resistance or carbohydrate consumption (i.e., metformin, thiazolidinediones, α-glucosidase inhibitors [AGIs], dipeptidyl peptidase IV inhibitors, amylin or incretin mimetics, bile acid sequestrants, or bromocriptine) do not typically cause clinically significant hypoglycemia unless taken in combination with insulin or an insulin secretagogue.

HYPOGLYCEMIC UNAWARENESS (HYPOGLYCEMIA-ASSOCIATED AUTONOMIC FAILURE)

Recurrent episodes of hypoglycemia,[169] particularly those that occur with sleep[170,171] or exercise,[172,173] blunt the normal response to hypoglycemia. This condition, known as hypoglycemia-associated autonomic failure (HAAF), reflects decreased adrenomedullary and sympathetic neural responses, and results in defective counterregulation and diminished symptoms of hypoglycemia, called hypoglycemic unawareness. The risk of severe hypoglycemia is markedly increased in patients with HAAF.[174] Furthermore, the response to glucagon and epinephrine may already be blunted in the critically ill patient,[158,175] further increasing the hypoglycemic risk.

Over time, patients with type 1 diabetes develop diminished α-cell production of glucagon, leaving these patients at even higher risk of hypoglycemia. The inability of patients with type 1 DM to appropriately regulate insulin and glucagon secretion is associated with a 25 times greater risk of iatrogenic hypoglycemia. The absence of both β-cell (insulin) and α-cell (glucagon)[176] function also occurs following pancreatectomy and results in significant glycemic instability.[176]

MANAGEMENT OF HYPOGLYCEMIA IN PATIENTS WITH DIABETES

A hypoglycemic patient with a history of diabetes should be evaluated for the frequency and severity of the hypoglycemic episodes, timing and dose of insulin or insulin secretagogues, missed or lower carbohydrate meals, increased physical activity, or new-onset hepatic or renal dysfunction. The risk of severe hypoglycemia increases with intensive glucose control.[177] Although an HbA_{1c} less than 7% can indicate excellent glucose control, it may also suggest an enhanced risk of hypoglycemia, particularly in the elderly.

Published protocols on the management of hypoglycemia are available.[57,178,179] Patients who can eat should receive 15 to 20 g of carbohydrates with recheck of the glucose level in 15 to 20 minutes.[180] If the glucose remains less than 70 mg/dL,[178] the protocol should be repeated. A snack or small meal should follow once the hypoglycemic episode has resolved. Overtreatment with unmeasured carbohydrates such as fruit juice (with or without added sugar) increases the likelihood of rebound hyperglycemia and glycemic variability. Measured amounts of dextrose with glucose gel packets or glucose tablets offer more accurate dosing of carbohydrates. In the patient with IV access who is NPO or is unable to consume oral carbohydrates (including patients with impaired level of consciousness due to hypoglycemia), low glucose levels can be managed with 25 g of 50% dextrose (1 amp).[159] The use of glucagon should be limited to those patients with neuroglycopenic symptoms who have no IV access. The glycemic response to IV dextrose or glucagon may lead to moderate hyperglycemia.

It is important to be aware that in some instances (e.g., the use of long-acting insulin, or insulin secretagogues with long half-lives), there is increased risk that hypoglycemia will recur after initial treatment. The clinician needs to evaluate each episode of hypoglycemia for the underlying causes and adjust either the insulin dose, nutrition, or both.

Table 58.5 Risk Factors for Hypoglycemia in the Hospitalized Patient[118,214]

Risk Factor	Prevention
Initiation of insulin	Individualized insulin dosing
Inappropriate timing of mealtime insulin	Mealtime insulin boluses up to 15 minutes before or 15 minutes after meal
Overuse or overdosing of correctional doses of insulin	Individualized insulin dosing based on total daily insulin requirements
Change in nutrition	Standardized orders to adjust insulin or add intravenous fluids with dextrose
Reduction in corticosteroid dose	Adjust insulin doses as steroid dose tapered

Superscript numbers refer to references provided online.

Table 58.6 Causes of Hypoglycemia in Adults

Ill or Medicated Individual	Seemingly Well Individual
1. Drugs Insulin or insulin secretagogue Alcohol Others 2. Critical illnesses Hepatic, renal, or cardiac failure Sepsis (including malaria) Inanition 3. Hormone deficiency Cortisol Glucagon and epinephrine (in insulin-deficient diabetes mellitus) 4. Non–islet cell tumor	1. Endogenous hyperinsulinism Insulinoma Functional cell disorders (nesidioblastosis) Noninsulinoma pancreatogenous hypoglycemia Post–gastric bypass hypoglycemia Insulin autoimmune hypoglycemia Antibody to insulin Antibody to insulin receptor Insulin secretagogue Other 2. Accidental or malicious administration of antidiabetic agents

From Cryer PE, Axelrod L, Grossman AB, et al: Evaluation and management of adult hypoglycemic disorders: An Endocrine Society Clinical Practice Guideline. J Clin Endocrinol Metab 2009;94(3):709-728.

Other caveats exist in the management of hypoglycemia. First, glucagon induces glycogenolysis and thus is not effective in patients who are glycogen-depleted such as those with alcohol abuse. Second, although mild or moderate cases of hypoglycemia related to insulin secretagogues respond well to treatment with oral carbohydrates or dextrose, the recommended treatment of sulfonylurea overdose is octreotide 100 µg,[181] which decreases the insulin secretion. Third, AGIs block the digestion of disaccharides, and therefore, treatment of hypoglycemia with disaccharides such as sucrose (cane sugar) or lactose (in milk) will be ineffective in patients taking AGIs. Oral glucose (dextrose), a monosaccharide, should be used.

PREVENTION

Forethought is required to prevent hypoglycemia in the ICU, but the prevention of hypoglycemia can be forgotten in the midst of multiple competing interests. Intensivists need to remain attentive to the increased risk for hypoglycemia as the patient's illness status, nutritional status, and medications change[182] (Table 58.5). Particular attention should be given to the titration of insulin doses when steroids or epinephrine are being tapered.

A dependence on correctional dose insulin ("sliding scales") rather than scheduled basal-bolus insulin regimens has become endemic in many hospitals. This practice is to be strongly discouraged. The reliance on correctional insulin as the sole glycemic management strategy is associated with poor glycemic control and increased hypoglycemia, although a physiologic, basal-bolus insulin regimen improves glycemic control.[57]

HYPOGLYCEMIA IN PATIENTS WITHOUT DIABETES

Because of the tiered physiologic mechanisms to protect against low blood glucose, hypoglycemia is unusual in nondiabetic patients. Only 1.5% of hypoglycemic episodes occur in patients without diabetes or who are not receiving insulin,[167] and most conditions or medications will not cause hypoglycemia unless multiple factors occur simultaneously.[167] The acute management of hypoglycemia is similar in diabetic and nondiabetic individuals, but nondiabetic patients presenting with hypoglycemia require a careful diagnostic evaluation.

DIAGNOSIS

All patients considered to have hypoglycemia should meet the criteria for "Whipple's triad": symptoms consistent with hypoglycemia, a low glucose level at the time of the symptoms, and prompt resolution of the symptoms with correction of hypoglycemia. The differential diagnosis of hypoglycemia can be broadly divided into those causes most commonly seen in otherwise healthy patients versus those seen in patients with underlying illness (Table 58.6). Essentially any critical illness can cause hypoglycemia, though this should remain a diagnosis of exclusion after consideration of any other potential causes.

A large number of medications have been reported to cause hypoglycemia (Table 58.7). Other than insulin and insulin secretagogues, most of these agents cause hypoglycemia only in rare instances.

Ethanol inhibits gluconeogenesis[167] by depleting hepatic nicotinamide adenine dinucleotide (NAD), impairs the counterregulatory actions of cortisol and growth hormone, and delays the response to glucagon and epinephrine. At particular risk of alcohol-induced hypoglycemia are alcoholic patients who are simultaneously malnourished and therefore glycogen-depleted as well.

In general adults with deficiencies of cortisol, with or without growth hormone deficiency, are not at increased

Table 58.7 Examples of Medications Implicated as Causative Agents for Hypoglycemia

Suspected Mechanism	Agent(s)
Accidental or malicious administration of antidiabetic agents	Insulins, sulfonylureas, glinides
Increased insulin or decreased clearance	Quinine, pentamidine, isoniazid, lithium, haloperidol, chloroquine, indomethacin[214]
Decreased hepatic glucose output	Alcohol, unripe akee fruit
Autoimmune	Isoniazid, interferon-α, hydralazine, procainamide, sulfhydryl-containing drugs
Interactions with sulfonylureas	Phenylbutazone, colchicine, paracetamol
Beta cell toxicity	Pentaminide
Unknown mechanism	Sulfonamide, salicylates, warfarin, octreotide

risk of hypoglycemia unless another condition such as pregnancy or alcohol intoxication is present. Patients with primary adrenal insufficiency who are on appropriate steroid replacement do not have an increased risk of hypoglycemia. The management of hypoglycemia related to adrenal crisis should include carbohydrates and stress dose steroids.

Given the liver's crucial role in glucose homeostasis, it is not surprising that patients with hepatic insufficiency, particularly acute liver disease, are susceptible to hypoglycemia. The kidneys are responsible for limited gluconeogenesis under normal conditions, though alterations in fasting glucose levels are not recognized until end-stage renal disease.[183] Most renal patients with significant hypoglycemia are cachectic, and therefore lack the fat or muscle stores for gluconeogenesis.

In sepsis, an increased risk of hypoglycemia results from increased glucose utilization followed by decreased glucose production[184] and decreased responsiveness to changes in insulin and glucagon.[159,185] Cachexia is a rare cause of hypoglycemia,[159,186] but has been reported in patients with severe muscle wasting or fat depletion who are therefore unable to generate glucose via gluconeogenesis. Malnourished patients are more likely to develop hypoglycemia in the setting of another disorder with increased risk of low blood sugar, such as renal insufficiency or alcohol abuse.

Insulinomas are rare (less than 1 in 250,000 patient-years) β-cell tumors that produce insulin. The tumors do not have an age or ethnic predominance, but do occur slightly more frequently in women.[187] Patients present with recurrent hypoglycemia associated with neuroglycopenic symptoms. Increasingly, hypoglycemia has been reported in patients following gastric bypass with a roux-en-Y procedure. Typically, the episodes occur postprandially. The precise mechanism of this phenomenon is an area of active investigation.

<u>Suggested protocol for a prolonged diagnostic fast</u>

- Date the onset of the fast as the time of the last food intake.
- Discontinue all nonessential medications.
- Allow the patient to drink calorie-free beverages. Ensure that the patient is active during waking hours.
- Collect samples for plasma glucose, insulin, C-peptide, proinsulin, and beta-hydroxybutyrate every 6 h until the plasma glucose concentration is less than 60 mg/dL; at that point the frequency of sampling should be increased to every 1 to 2 h.
- Samples for plasma insulin, C-peptide, and proinsulin should be sent for analysis only in those samples in which the plasma glucose concentration is less than 60 mg/dL.
- End the fast when the plasma glucose concentration is less than 45 mg/dL and the patient has symptoms and/or signs of hypoglycemia (or if 72 h have elapsed without symptoms).
- The decision to end the fast before 72 h should not be based on a low plasma glucose concentration alone, in the absence of symptoms or signs, because some healthy individuals, especially women and children, have low glucose levels during prolonged fasting.
- Alternatively, the fast can be ended when the plasma glucose concentration is less than 55 mg/dL without symptoms or signs if Whipple's triad was documented unequivocally on a prior occasion.
- A low plasma glucose concentration is a necessary, albeit not in itself sufficient, finding for the diagnosis of hypoglycemia. Therefore, the decision to end the fast should be based on laboratory-measured plasma glucose concentrations, not those estimated with a point-of care.

Figure 58.6 Suggested protocol for a prolonged diagnostic fast. (From Cryer PE, Axelrod L, Grossman AB, et al: Evaluation and management of adult hypoglycemic disorders: An Endocrine Society Clinical Practice Guideline. J Clin Endocrinol Metab 2009;94(3):709-728.)

APPROACH TO THE NONDIABETIC PATIENT WITH HYPOGLYCEMIA

Patients in the ICU often have multiple reasons to become hypoglycemic. A standardized approach to the evaluation of hypoglycemia reduces the risk of unnecessary testing. A thorough history, physical examination, and review of laboratory results often give clues to the cause of the hypoglycemia.[188] When a cause is evident, appropriate steps should be taken both to correct the offending problem and to increase nutritional support while the problem is being addressed. Once the acute hypoglycemic episode is treated, the appropriate steps should be taken to avoid recurrent hypoglycemia.

In a patient who satisfies Whipple's triad but lacks an obvious cause for hypoglycemia, levels of glucose, cortisol, insulin, C-peptide, proinsulin, and β-hydroxybutyrate, as well as a urine screen for sulfonylurea, should be measured during an episode of spontaneous hypoglycemia.[188-190] Some patients may need to have hypoglycemia provoked by a prolonged (up to 72 hours) fast.[188,190,191] A protocol for a prolonged fast[188,192] is listed in Figure 58.6,[188] though this is not recommended in critically ill patients and should be deferred until the patient is stable. Response of glucose to IV injection of 1.0 mg glucagon may be useful in certain cases, and measurement of insulin antibodies is useful in cases in which antibody-induced hypoglycemia is suspected. An interpretation of laboratory values in hypoglycemia is presented in Table 58.8.[188]

In a patient with documented endogenous hyperinsulinemic hypoglycemia with negative testing for oral

Table 58.8 Patterns of Clinical and Serum Chemistry Findings after Fasting or a Mixed Meal

Symptoms/ Signs	Glucose (mg/dL)	Insulin (μU/mL)	C-peptide (nmol/L)	Proinsulin (pmol/L)	β-Hydroxy-butyrate (mmol/L)	Glucose Increase after Glucagon (mg/dL)	Circulating Oral Hypoglycemic Agent	Antibody to Insulin	Diagnostic Interpretation
No	<55	<3	<.2	<5	>2.7	<25	No	No	Normal
Yes	<55	≫3	<.2	<5	≤2.7	>25	No	Neg (Pos)	Exogenous insulin
Yes	<55	≥3	≥.2	≥5	≤2.7	>25	No	Neg	Insulinoma, post–gastric bypass hypoglycemia
Yes	<55	≥3	≥.2	≥5	≤2.7	>25	Yes	Neg	Oral hypoglycemic agent
Yes	<55	≥3	≫.2	≫5	≤2.7	>25	No	Pos	Insulin autoimmune
Yes	<55	<3	<.2	<5	≤2.7	>25	No	Neg	IGF mediated
Yes	<55	<3	<.2	<5	>2.7	<25	No	Neg	Not insulin (or IGF)-mediated

IGF, insulin-like growth factor.

hypoglycemic agents and insulin antibodies, an insulinoma is sought by imaging with computed tomography, magnetic resonance imaging, or transabdominal ultrasound. Invasive imaging with endoscopic ultrasound also be performed in cases in which noninvasive imaging is unrevealing.

KEY POINTS

- Despite advances in the management of critical illness, DKA and HHS remain life-threatening emergencies.
- DKA and HHS are often precipitated by interruption of insulin treatment or an illness such as infection, but may also be the initial presentation of diabetes.
- Use of IV insulin allows for the frequent dose adjustment necessary for the successful management of hyperglycemic emergencies.
- Attention to potassium replacement is a cornerstone of the management of hyperglycemic emergencies.
- The ultimate goal of DKA management is to correct the acidosis, and the ultimate goal of HHS management is to correct the hyperosmolarity.
- Goal glucose levels for the critically ill patient are 140 to 180 mg/dL, with attention also given to avoidance of hypoglycemia.
- An HbA_{1c} on admission distinguishes between stress hyperglycemia and previously unrecognized DM, and helps guide therapy at the time of discharge.
- A physiologic insulin regimen, not oral hypoglycemic agents, is the appropriate strategy for glucose control in the hospitalized patient.
- Supplemental insulin doses ("sliding scale") can be given for unanticipated hyperglycemia, but should never be the sole therapy for hospitalized patients with diabetes.

KEY POINTS (Continued)

- Recurrent hypoglycemia blunts the normal counterregulatory response in patients with type 1 DM and predisposes to severe hypoglycemia.

SELECTED REFERENCES

9. Kitabchi AE, Umpierrez GE, Miles JM, Fisher JN: Hyperglycemic crises in adult patients with diabetes. Diabetes Care 2009;32(7):1335-1343.
26. Trence DL, Hirsch IB: Hyperglycemic crises in diabetes mellitus type 2. Endocrinol Metab Clin North Am 2001;30(4):817-831.
32. Nyenwe EA, Kitabchi AE: Evidence-based management of hyperglycemic emergencies in diabetes mellitus. Diabetes Res Clin Pract 2011;94(3):340-351.
47. Kitabchi AE, Umpierrez GE, Fisher JN, et al: Thirty years of personal experience in hyperglycemic crises: Diabetic ketoacidosis and hyperglycemic hyperosmolar state. J Clin Endocrinol Metab 2008;93:1541-1552.
93. Farrokhi F, Smiley D, Umpierrez GE: Glycemic control in non-diabetic critically ill patients. Best Pract Res Clin Endocrinol Metab 2011;25:813-824.
112. Griesdale DE, de Souza RJ, van Dam RM, et al: Intensive insulin therapy and mortality among critically ill patients: A meta-analysis including NICE-SUGAR study data. Can Med Assoc J 2009;180(8):821-827. Epub 2009 Mar 24.
121. Moghissi ES: Insulin strategies for managing inpatient and outpatient hyperglycemia and diabetes. Mt Sinai J Med 2008;75:558-566.
188. Cryer PE, Axelrod L, Grossman AB, et al: Evaluation and management of adult hypoglycemic disorders: An Endocrine Society Clinical Practice Guideline. J Clin Endocrinol Metab 2009;94(3):709-728.
190. Service F: Diagnostic approach to adults with hypoglycemic disorders. Endocrinol Metab Clin 1999;28(3):519-532.
192. Service F: Classification of hypoglycemic disorders. Endocrinol Metab Clin North Am 1999;28(3):501-517.

The complete list of references can be found at www.expertconsult.com.

59

Adrenal Insufficiency in the Critically Ill Patient

Rekha Lakshmanan | Robert W. Taylor

CHAPTER OUTLINE

Adrenal diseases are infrequent primary admitting diagnoses to the intensive care unit (ICU). However, patients with unrecognized or previously diagnosed disease of the hypothalamic-pituitary-adrenal (HPA) axis may demonstrate severe decompensation in the setting of other critical illness.

Adrenal insufficiency (AI) is by far the most common adrenal disorder seen in the ICU and is the focus of this chapter. It occurs more frequently in critically ill patients than in general hospitalized patients and represents a true emergency that requires rapid diagnosis and treatment. If missed, the condition can be fatal. In addition, because critical illness is often the precipitant of overt AI, the intensivist may have the first and only chance to make the diagnosis.[1]

Primary AI results from a subtotal or complete destruction of the adrenal cortex (>90%) and results in cortisol, aldosterone, and androgen deficiency. Multiple causes of primary AI include autoimmune destruction (Addison's disease), polyendocrine deficiency syndrome, infections (e.g., tuberculosis, fungus), vascular compromise, primary or metastatic cancer, amyloidosis, and surgical removal of the adrenal glands.

Secondary AI is much more common than primary AI and can be traced to a lack of adrenocorticotropic hormone (ACTH). Without ACTH to stimulate the adrenal glands, production of cortisol falls but aldosterone secretion remains intact. The most common cause of secondary AI is the inadvertent abrupt withdrawal of therapeutic exogenous corticosteroids. Another cause of secondary AI is the surgical removal of benign or noncancerous, ACTH-producing tumors of the pituitary gland (Cushing syndrome). In this case the source of ACTH is suddenly removed, and replacement hormones must be taken until normal ACTH and cortisol production resumes.

Less commonly, secondary AI occurs when the pituitary gland reduces or ceases production of ACTH. This can occur for a variety of reasons including tumors or infections of the area, loss of blood flow to the pituitary, radiation for the treatment of pituitary tumors, total or subtotal removal of the hypothalamus, and surgical removal of the pituitary gland.

The term relative adrenal insufficiency has been replaced in recent literature by critical illness–related corticosteroid insufficiency (CIRCI),[2,3] which in simple terms is inadequate corticosteroid activity for the severity of the illness of a patient. Similar to type II diabetes (relative insulin deficiency), CIRCI is thought to arise because of corticosteroid tissue resistance and inadequate circulating levels of free cortisol.

Patients at risk of AI vary from young athletes on steroids to persons taking adrenal extracts for "adrenal fatigue syndrome." Also at risk are those receiving chronic topical glucocorticoids for dermatologic disorders. Patients who are on glucocorticoids and inhibitors (such as itraconazole, diltiazem) of CYP3A4 are at risk as well.[4] For all these reasons the intensivist must understand clinical problems associated with the HPA axis and the use of glucocorticoid hormones.

INCIDENCE AND PREVALENCE

The actual incidence of acute AI is unknown. The incidence of HPA axis failure varies depending on the criteria used to make the diagnosis and the patient population studied. The overall incidence of AI in critically ill patients is estimated to be as high as 60% in patients with severe sepsis and septic shock.[5] At least 90% of both adrenal glands must be destroyed before clinical and biochemical manifestations of AI occur. Tissue hypoxia, a relatively common disorder in critically ill patients, has little effect on the synthesis of cortisol. Secondary AI may be more common than primary AI. The clinical presentation of secondary AI is relatively nonspecific and often resembles other conditions common in the ICU. Hence it is not uncommon to attribute the clinical features resulting from acute AI to commonly seen medical conditions in the ICU.[6]

PATHOPHYSIOLOGY

To understand the pathogenesis of adrenal diseases one must understand the physiology of the adrenal glands and the causes that result in the disruption of the physiologic process.

The adrenal glands are pyramid-shaped, each weighing about 5 to 10 g, and located just superior to their respective kidneys. The left adrenal gland is usually slightly more cephalad than the right. Each adrenal gland is composed of an inner medulla and outer cortex. These layers are embryologically, anatomically, and physiologically distinct. The adrenal cortex is responsible for the secretion of multiple steroid hormones. The adrenal medulla is responsible for the secretion of catecholamines.

The adrenal cortex is composed of three zones: the outer zona glomerulosa, inner zona fasciculata, and zona reticularis. The zona glomerulosa secretes the mineralocorticoid aldosterone in response to angiotensin, ACTH, and a high circulating potassium concentration. The zona fasciculata and zona reticularis secrete glucocorticoids and adrenal androgens.

The principal mineralocorticoid is aldosterone, which is regulated not only by ACTH but also by serum sodium and potassium levels and by the renin-angiotensin system.[7,8] Mineralocorticoids exert their primary effect on distal renal tubule cells, resulting in renal sodium retention at the expense of potassium loss in the urine. A third major class of adrenal steroids is the sex hormones: dehydroepiandrosterone (DHEA), DHEA-sulfate, and androstenedione. Like the glucocorticoids, ACTH primarily regulates these steroid hormones. They function mainly as precursors for the primary circulating androgen, testosterone, and also may undergo separate conversion to estrogen hormones. In critically ill patients, glucocorticoids are the steroid hormones of greatest concern and therefore remain the focus of the remainder of this discussion.

GLUCOCORTICOID SYNTHESIS

Glucocorticoid synthesis is regulated by (1) a negative feedback mechanism involving cortisol and adrenal steroids, (2) a diurnal rhythm, and (3) stress. The hypothalamus and the pituitary gland closely regulate adrenal hormone production. Corticotropin-releasing hormone (CRH) is produced in the hypothalamus and acts on specialized cells in the pituitary, stimulating production of ACTH, which serves, in turn, to stimulate adrenal cortical cells to produce numerous steroid hormones, including cortisol. Adrenal hormones have a negative influence at the level of the hypothalamus and the pituitary, inhibiting CRH and ACTH release. The adrenal gland in turn ceases its secretory activity until the cortisol concentration returns to normal. When serum cortisol levels are below normal, secretion of CRH and ACTH increases, stimulating the adrenal glands to produce cortisol until its level normalizes. Therefore, abnormalities in circulating serum levels of adrenal steroid hormone can be caused by either adrenal or hypothalamic pituitary disease. Because ACTH possesses α-melanocyte-stimulating hormone activity, excessive production of ACTH is associated with hyperpigmentation.

Cortisol is normally secreted in a diurnal pattern. The circulating cortisol level is increased in the morning hours, at approximately 8 AM. Serum cortisol concentrations decrease throughout the remainder of the day.[9] Similarly, the serum cortisol response to ACTH stimulation also varies in a circadian rhythm. Afternoon responsiveness is much greater because of the decreased circadian level of cortisol at that time. In addition, cortisol is secreted in a series of pulses rather than in a continuous fashion. These factors contribute to make interpretation of a random cortisol level and the ACTH-stimulated value difficult.

"Stress" (exemplified by sepsis, major surgery, or trauma) also affects glucocorticoid synthesis.[10-12] The *stress response* is characterized by continuous ACTH secretion despite a high serum cortisol concentration. Stress overrides all other regulatory mechanisms of cortisol secretion by the adrenal cortex and increases cortisol secretion irrespective of the time of day or the current serum cortisol concentration. The mechanism by which the HPA axis is regulated during stress is not clearly understood. Periventricular neurons in the hypothalamus respond to stress by increasing the levels of CRH messenger ribonucleic acid (mRNA).[13,14] It has been shown that production of the cytokines interleukin 1 (IL-1), interleukin 6 (IL-6), and tumor necrosis factor-α (TNF-α) also plays an important role in the regulation of the HPA axis.[15-19] The cortisol secretion that occurs because of the activation of the HPA axis causes an inhibitory effect not only on the secretion of CRH and ACTH but also on the liberation of interleukins.[20] Thus, there is a functional loop between immune activation and regulation of the HPA axis during stress.

The stress response is biphasic, consisting of an early phase in which both ACTH and cortisol are elevated and a late phase in which the serum cortisol level is elevated but the serum ACTH level is paradoxically low.[8] This is explained by the fact that endothelin and atrial natriuretic peptide are both elevated in severe illnesses. Endothelin increases cortisol production by the adrenals, whereas the atrial natriuretic peptide inhibits ACTH production by acting at the hypothalamic-pituitary level. Vasopressin and angiotensin II can increase ACTH secretion during stress conditions, such as sepsis and septic shock

Acute respiratory failure causes a 50% to 100% rise in serum cortisol concentration. A twofold to sixfold rise occurs with septic shock and following surgical procedures and trauma. The rise in serum cortisol correlates positively with severity of illness[6] and negatively with survival.[7]

The normal daily output of cortisol by the adrenal glands is 20 to 30 mg. The normal adrenal gland secretes about 10 to 12 times the normal daily output of cortisol when under maximal physiologic stress. Hence approximately 200 to 300 mg of hydrocortisone or its equivalent is considered a daily "stress dose" of glucocorticoid.

GLUCOCORTICOID ACTIONS

After uptake of free hormone from the circulation, the effects of cortisol and aldosterone are mediated by binding to intracellular receptors termed the glucocorticoid receptor and the mineralocorticoid receptor.

CARDIOVASCULAR EFFECTS

Glucocorticoids help to maintain vascular tone and cardiac contractility. The presence of glucocorticoids is important to the physiologic effects of catecholamines on vascular smooth muscle. Glucocorticoids affect blood pressure by different mechanisms including direct action of glucocorticoids on the vasculature, permissive effects of the glucocorticoids on the vasopressor action of catecholamines, and glucocorticoid-induced decrease in the levels of prostaglandin E_2 and kallikrein (vasodilators). Angiotensinogen synthesis is increased by glucocorticoids.[21] Glucocorticoids increase the synthesis of β-adrenergic receptors, reverse β_2-adrenergic receptor dysfunction, and increase the coupling of the receptor with the second messenger system.[22]

Two hemodynamic states have been described during acute AI:

1. Low cardiac output, high systemic vascular resistance shock is caused by both decreased myocardial contractility and decreased preload.
2. High cardiac output, low systemic vascular resistance shock mimics septic shock.[23] It appears that patients with AI present initially with a combination of cardiogenic shock and hypovolemic shock. Intravascular volume expansion with intravenous fluids results in an increase in cardiac output and a lowering of systemic vascular resistance. The hemodynamic profile that one sees depends on the timing of pulmonary artery catheter placement during the course of treatment in an individual patient. Thus, the hypotension of AI can mimic cardiogenic, hypovolemic, or septic shock (depending on when the hemodynamic assessment was made) and may be poorly responsive or unresponsive to treatment with fluids and vasopressors in the absence of glucocorticoid therapy.

METABOLIC EFFECTS

Glucocorticoid hormones have profound influence on carbohydrate metabolism. A major action is on gluconeogenesis. Glucocorticoids increase hepatic glycogen and glucose by inducing the synthesis of hepatic enzymes and increasing the availability of gluconeogenic substrates. This is because of glucocorticoid-induced proteolytic activity on peripheral tissues, which causes mobilization of glycogenic amino acid precursors from peripheral supporting structures such as bone, skin, muscle, and connective tissue because of protein breakdown and inhibition of protein synthesis. Glucocorticoids decrease the peripheral uptake and utilization of glucose. They have a permissive effect on other hormones such as glucagon and catecholamines, thus serving to increase the circulating glucose concentration, which in turn increases insulin secretion.

Glucocorticoids also affect fat and protein metabolism. They increase lipolysis both directly and indirectly by action on other hormones. Glucocorticoids regulate fatty acid mobilization by enhancing activation of cellular lipase by lipid-mobilizing hormones (e.g., catecholamines, pituitary peptides). They elevate free fatty acid levels in the plasma and enhance any tendency to ketosis. Glucocorticoids stimulate peripheral protein metabolism, using the amino acid products as gluconeogenic precursors. Glucocorticoids inhibit RNA synthesis in most body tissues, but in the liver they stimulate RNA synthesis.

RENAL EFFECTS

Glucocorticoids bind to the mineralocorticoid receptors in renal tubules and increase sodium reabsorption and excretion of potassium and hydrogen ions. Glucocorticoids increase the glomerular filtration rate, proximal tubular epithelial sodium transport, and free water clearance.[21] Glucocorticoids also increase free water excretion by inhibiting the release of antidiuretic hormone (ADH).

IMMUNOLOGIC EFFECTS

Glucocorticoids suppress immunologic responses, and this is the basis for their use in the treatment of autoimmune and inflammatory disorders. In the peripheral blood, they redistribute lymphocytes from the intravascular compartment to the lymphoid pool in the spleen, lymph nodes, and bone marrow. They therefore decrease lymphocyte counts, but neutrophil counts increase after glucocorticoid administration. Eosinophil counts fall, due to eosinophil apoptosis. The immunologic actions of glucocorticoids are mediated through T and B lymphocytes. Glucocorticoids inhibit immunoglobulin synthesis and cytokine production from lymphocytes. Glucocorticoids also inhibit monocyte differentiation into macrophages and plasminogen activators.[21]

Glucocorticoids mediate anti-inflammatory effects by stabilizing lysosomal membranes. They also decrease the release of inflammatory mediators such as histamine, cytokines, and prostaglandins.

The immunologic actions of glucocorticoids are only significant in circumstances in which they are present in supraphysiologic amounts such as markedly increased endogenous production or exogenous administration.

GASTROINTESTINAL EFFECTS

It has been postulated that CRH inhibits the release of motilin, a duodenal hormone that is responsible for the initiation of peristaltic contractions, which begin in the stomach and propagate distally. Glucocorticoids decrease

CRH production and thus inhibit gastric and intestinal motility. This could explain the vomiting, constipation, and abdominal pain seen in cortisol deficiency. Glucocorticoids can also increase risk of peptic ulcer disease and pancreatitis.

CALCIUM METABOLISM

Glucocorticoids lower serum calcium levels by several mechanisms. They inhibit calcium absorption from the gut, decrease renal calcium reabsorption (which results in hypercalciuria), and promote shift of calcium from the extracellular compartment to the intracellular compartment. Glucocorticoids inhibit osteoblast function and cause osteoporosis, which occurs in approximately 50% of patients who require long-term glucocorticoids.[24] Avascular necrosis is a dreaded complication.[21] It mainly affects the femoral head and causes pain and collapse of the bone, often necessitating hip replacement. This effect is not necessarily dose dependent.

OTHER EFFECTS

Glucocorticoids have many other effects, including the ability to produce significant mood changes and even psychosis in some patients. Glucocorticoids have an association with cataract formation and increased intraocular pressure both by increasing aqueous humor production and decreasing drainage. They also affect the production and action of a number of other hormones including insulin, thyroid hormones, and gonadal hormones.

Aldosterone secretion is regulated mainly by the renin-angiotensin system. The most potent modulator of this system is renal perfusion. Hyperkalemia inhibits production of renin but increases the synthesis of aldosterone. Aldosterone increases sodium reabsorption in the collecting tubules and at the same time causes potassium and hydrogen ion excretion. This is mediated by the Na^+/K^+ pump in the presence of the enzyme Na^+/K^+-ATPase and results in sodium and water retention and an increase in intravascular volume.[21]

Hyperkalemia, hyponatremia, non–anion gap metabolic acidosis, hemoconcentration, and hypovolemia provide important clinical clues to the diagnosis of primary AI. Because ACTH is not a potent regulator of aldosterone secretion, secondary AI is usually not associated with hyperkalemia. Hyponatremia and hypovolemia may be present in secondary AI but not to the degree found in primary AI. The renin-angiotensin system is activated during AI and serves as a defense mechanism to improve the low intravascular volume and the altered vasomotor tone that results from aldosterone and cortisol deficiency.[25,26]

Box 59.1 Causes of Primary Adrenal Insufficiency

- Autoimmune (idiopathic) 80% (most common cause)
- Infections
  - Tuberculosis (second most common cause)
  - *Pneumococcus* infection
  - Histoplasmosis
  - Coccidioidomycosis
  - Blastomycosis
  - *Meningococcus* infection
  - Cryptococcosis
  - Candidiasis
  - *Torulopsis* infection
  - Cytomegalovirus infection
- Acquired immunodeficiency syndrome
- Neoplasia
  - Metastatic carcinoma
  - Lymphoma
- Infiltrative diseases
  - Amyloidosis
  - Sarcoidosis
  - Hemochromatosis
- Adrenal hemorrhage
- Sepsis
- Anticoagulants
- Coagulopathy
- Trauma
- Prior surgery
- Difficult pregnancy
- Vasculitis
- Postadrenal venography
- Medications
  - Ketoconazole
  - Phenytoin
  - Phenobarbital
  - Rifampin
  - Etomidate
  - Fluorouracil
  - Metyrapone
- Miscellaneous
  - Irradiation
  - Bilateral adrenalectomy
- Congenital conditions

ETIOLOGY AND PATHOGENESIS

Causes of primary AI have been previously discussed and are shown in Box 59.1.

AUTOIMMUNE DISEASE

Autoimmune disease (Addison's disease) is currently the most common cause of primary AI and accounts for approximately 80% of cases. For many years tuberculosis was the most common cause. AI may occur as isolated disease or as part of a polyglandular autoimmune syndrome associated with thyroiditis, diabetes mellitus (Schmidt's syndrome), hypogonadism, vitiligo, and pernicious anemia.[27-29] Autoimmune AI is more common in women than men and usually occurs in the third to fifth decades of life. The mean duration of symptoms before diagnosis is approximately 3 years. In this disorder high levels of circulating autoantibodies attack the cytoplasm of adrenal cortical cells and inhibit synthesis of glucocorticoids.[27,28]

INFECTIOUS DISEASE

TUBERCULOSIS

The second most common cause of primary AI is adrenal gland destruction by *Mycobacterium tuberculosis.* This infection currently accounts for less than 20% of cases.[30] This usually occurs in the presence of tuberculosis elsewhere in the body, especially with involvement of the lungs, genitourinary system, and gastrointestinal system. AI is usually manifest years after the initial presentation of tuberculosis.[31] The mean duration of symptoms of AI prior to diagnosis is 6 to 9 months. AI secondary to tuberculosis occurs with equal frequency in men and women. In contrast to autoimmune adrenalitis, tuberculosis-induced adrenal disease is not associated with other endocrine diseases. In addition, with tuberculosis the adrenal glands are enlarged and may be calcified. In contrast, the adrenal glands in autoimmune adrenalitis are usually atrophied and noncalcified.

FUNGAL DISEASE

Fungal disease can also cause primary AI. *Histoplasma capsulatum* is the most common organism. As seen in tuberculosis, fungal infection is usually disseminated and involves organs other than the adrenal glands. Adrenal involvement may be seen during the active phase or may develop years later after the disease has become "inactive." Sarosi and colleagues[32] reported that more than 50% of patients with disseminated histoplasmosis had AI, and AI was the most common cause of death.

ACQUIRED IMMUNODEFICIENCY SYNDROME

Patients with acquired immunodeficiency syndrome (AIDS) are at risk of developing AI by several different mechanisms. Fungal infections are more common in this patient population, and disseminated disease may involve the adrenal glands. Similarly, mycobacterial infection, cytomegalovirus infection, and Kaposi sarcoma may cause involvement of the adrenals in up to 50% of patients.[3] In addition, sepsis and spontaneous adrenal hemorrhage are also seen in this group of patients. Because patients with human immunodeficiency virus (HIV) infection now survive longer, an increased incidence of AI is likely.

NEOPLASIA

Neoplastic metastasis to the adrenal glands has been found on autopsy in 27% to 40% of patients who die of malignancy.[33-36] Yet metastatic carcinoma accounts for less than 1% of cases of primary AI.[33] This finding is explained by the tremendous functional reserve possessed by the adrenal glands. More than 90% of the adrenal gland must be destroyed before hypofunction occurs. Many patients with metastasis to the adrenals do not develop hormonal deficiency.[37] The most common neoplasms to involve the adrenals are lung cancer, breast cancer, melanoma, and lymphoma.[35] AI usually occurs in the setting of widespread metastatic disease and is rarely the initial manifestation of malignancy.

MEDICATIONS

Certain medications can cause AI. Of particular interest to the intensivist are ketoconazole, phenytoin, phenobarbital, rifampin, and etomidate. Ketoconazole decreases glucocorticoid production and is also a glucocorticoid receptor antagonist. Etomidate decreases glucocorticoid production. Phenytoin, rifampin, and barbiturates increase the catabolism of glucocorticoids. These medications can precipitate acute AI by decreasing glucocorticoid production or function in a patient who has compromised adrenal reserve.

ADRENAL HEMORRHAGE

Adrenal hemorrhage is an important but uncommon cause of AI in the ICU. The association of adrenal hemorrhage with fulminant sepsis was first described with *Neisseria meningitidis* (Waterhouse-Friderichsen syndrome). Infections with *Streptococcus pneumoniae, Pseudomonas* species, and *Haemophilus influenzae* type b can also cause this syndrome.

Besides the infectious causes, other conditions may predispose to adrenal hemorrhage, including severe illness (particularly cardiac disease), coagulopathy, anticoagulant therapy, thromboembolism, burns, and trauma.[38] Under these circumstances the typical signs and symptoms of AI are often mistaken for those of other common conditions. Typical settings include the patient who is in the first or second postoperative week or a patient who has been started recently on anticoagulation therapy. Common findings include abdominal, back, flank, or chest pain; nausea; vomiting; fever; altered mental status; orthostatic hypotension; and a sudden drop in hematocrit. The hemodynamic crisis associated with adrenal hemorrhage occurs 1 to 3 days after the initial hemorrhage.

ETIOLOGY OF SECONDARY ADRENAL INSUFFICIENCY

Causes of secondary AI have been discussed previously and are shown in Box 59.2. Secondary AI occurs because of a decrease in ACTH caused by either hypothalamic-pituitary disease or suppression of the HPA axis as a result of glucocorticoid therapy. The most common cause today is discontinuation of corticosteroid therapy. Chronic glucocorticoid therapy leads to HPA axis suppression with resulting secondary AI if glucocorticoids are abruptly discontinued. With the exception of AI because of discontinuation of chronic glucocorticoid therapy, secondary adrenocortical insufficiency is much less common than primary AI. Isolated ACTH deficiency is rare, and ACTH is the last pituitary hormone to be impaired by enlarging sellar and suprasellar tumors.

Most patients admitted to the ICU with secondary AI have recently received steroid therapy or have taken steroids within the year prior to admission. No clear evidence indicates that detailing the duration or dose of steroid therapy predisposes patients to adrenal suppression. Doses of 25 mg of prednisone twice a day for 2 days, 12.5 mg per day for 6 months, or 5 mg per day for 5 years have all been shown to cause adrenal suppression. On the other hand, studies have shown that prednisone in doses less than 40 mg per day given every morning for 5 to 7 days did not cause adrenal suppression.[39]

As a practical guideline, all patients who have taken 40 mg of prednisone per day or its equivalent for a period greater than 2 or 3 weeks should be considered to be adrenal insufficient until proved otherwise. If glucocorticoids have been given to a patient for more than 1 to 2 weeks, they should be tapered off to allow time for the adrenal glands to recover function. AI can occur in response to stress as long as 1 year after steroids are discontinued.[40] All of these patients should be evaluated for adrenal function and

Box 59.2 Causes of Secondary Adrenal Insufficiency (AI)

Glucocorticoid therapy (most common cause of secondary AI)
Neoplastic
- Pituitary adenoma
- Meningioma
- Craniopharyngioma
- Metastatic carcinoma
  - Breast
  - Lung
  - Gastrointestinal
  - Lymphoma
  - Leukemia

Vascular
- Pituitary apoplexy
- Sheehan's syndrome
- Sickle cell disease
- Intracranial aneurysm
- Cavernous sinus thrombosis
- Vasculitis
- Eclampsia

Infection
- Tuberculosis
- Fungal infection
- Malaria
- Actinomycosis
- Viral infection

Autoimmune disorders
Infiltrative disorders
- Sarcoidosis
- Hemochromatosis

Irradiation
Head trauma and pituitary surgery
Isolated adrenocorticotropic hormone deficiency

Box 59.3 Common Symptoms and Signs of Adrenal Insufficiency

Symptoms
- Weakness
- Fatigue
- Anorexia
- Gastrointestinal symptoms (nausea, vomiting, abdominal pain, diarrhea, constipation, and weight loss)
- Orthostatic symptoms
- Myalgias
- Arthralgias

Signs
- Weight loss
- Orthostatic hypotension
- Hyperpigmentation
- Vitiligo
- Confusion/psychosis

Box 59.4 Common Laboratory Findings in Adrenal Insufficiency

- Hyponatremia
- Hyperkalemia
- Acidosis
- Prerenal azotemia
- Hypoglycemia
- Lymphocytosis
- Eosinophilia

should be treated with stress doses of steroids during the interim period.

CLINICAL FEATURES

Common symptoms and signs of AI are shown in Box 59.3. The symptoms, signs, and general laboratory data seen in AI are nonspecific. However, when taken together they form a pattern of findings that should suggest the possibility of AI. Patients with acute AI share many characteristics with patients who have chronic AI, but the symptoms are usually more severe in the acute setting. Virtually all patients complain of weakness, fatigue, and loss of appetite. They also complain of nausea and diarrhea with occasional vomiting and abdominal pain. Infrequently, patients note myalgias, arthralgias, and dizziness caused by orthostatic hypotension. Weight loss can occur. The classic presentation of acute AI is a patient with unexplained hemodynamic instability who is unresponsive to intravascular volume resuscitation and use of vasopressors. Patients with primary AI may have hyperpigmentation of the tongue, buccal mucosa, palmar creases, and scar tissue. This is caused by increased production of ACTH from the pituitary. Hyperpigmentation is notably absent in secondary AI. If the underlying problem is autoimmune adrenalitis, the patient may have vitiligo, pernicious anemia, or one of the other associated endocrinopathies.

DIAGNOSIS

The diagnosis of AI demands a high index of suspicion. The classic symptoms, signs, and laboratory findings of AI are not commonly seen. The consequences of missing the diagnosis can be lethal, but if the diagnosis is made the condition can usually be treated easily. If the diagnosis of AI is being considered, the patient's history should be carefully reviewed for use of steroids (especially in the past year), exposure to tuberculosis, use of anticoagulant therapy, presence of sepsis, or history of cancer that may have metastasized to the adrenals. Patients on high doses of steroids can develop AI when subjected to stress.

LABORATORY FINDINGS

Laboratory evaluation of patients with suspected AI is essential. In a patient with acute worsening of a chronic hypoadrenal state, the common laboratory findings shown in Box 59.4 are more likely to be present and are likely to be more pronounced. Electrolyte abnormalities depend on the type of deficiency: a combined glucocorticoid and mineralocorticoid deficiency (typically seen in primary AI) or an isolated glucocorticoid deficiency (characteristic of secondary AI).

Patients who have a combined deficiency may show hyponatremia, hyperkalemia, decreased serum bicarbonate, and increased blood urea nitrogen (BUN). This is primarily caused by the mineralocorticoid deficiency, which leads to renal sodium loss, potassium retention, and dehydration with acidosis and prerenal azotemia. Patients with secondary adrenocortical deficiency usually have milder electrolyte abnormalities. Their normal adrenal glands are able to produce sufficient amounts of mineralocorticoid even in the absence of ACTH stimulation. They usually have mild hyponatremia with normal potassium levels, and they show little evidence of dehydration. Patients with AI may also have hypoglycemia. This occurs as a result of increased utilization of glucose and decreased gluconeogenesis in the face of glucocorticoid deficiency.

DIAGNOSTIC TESTS

When there is a high suspicion of AI, hormonal testing is necessary to confirm the diagnosis. The laboratory evaluations most commonly used to detect AI in critically ill patients are the random serum cortisol level and the rapid ACTH stimulation test.

SERUM CORTISOL LEVEL

The biochemical diagnosis of AI is controversial. It is based on the demonstration of decreased cortisol production. Most clinical laboratories routinely measure total rather than free cortisol levels. Experts have recently suggested that measurement of free cortisol levels makes more physiologic sense, but studies have not helped establish diagnostic thresholds for free cortisol levels.[41] In addition, variability of cortisol assays can confound the diagnosis of AI.[42]

Given the controversy in diagnosis, the following recommendations are made. A randomly measured serum cortisol level that exceeds 44 μg/dL makes the diagnosis of adrenocortical deficiency unlikely.[5] Serum cortisol levels increase significantly in patients with normal adrenal function who are in shock and critically ill. The finding of a random serum cortisol level of less than 10 μg/dL in this setting is highly suggestive of compromised adrenal function and should prompt treatment or a confirmatory ACTH stimulation test.[5]

One must be careful in the interpretation of random serum cortisol levels in patients treated with several commonly used drugs in the ICU. Propofol produces a temporary reduction in serum cortisol levels. However, it does not seem to inhibit adrenal responsiveness to ACTH. Etomidate, on the other hand, is associated with a reduced serum cortisol concentration despite ACTH stimulation.[43]

RAPID ACTH STIMULATION TEST

The ACTH stimulation test measures the response of the adrenal gland to stimulation by exogenous ACTH. This test can be performed at any time of the day because the normal diurnal variation of cortisol is lost in the setting of critical illness. A blood sample is drawn, and a baseline serum cortisol level is measured. Cosyntropin (synthetic ACTH) 250 μg is then administered intravenously. Repeat samples are drawn at 60 minutes. Although controversial, some studies have shown that a low dose of ACTH (1 to 5 μg) produces a similar response as the 250 μg dose, especially in patients with AI that is recent or new onset.[44,45]

An increase in serum cortisol of less than 9 μg/dL following 250 μg of cosyntropin is highly suggestive of AI regardless of the baseline cortisol level. An increase in serum cortisol of greater than 17 μg/dL or total cortisol level of 44 μg/dL or greater suggests adrenal competence. When the baseline cortisol level is between 10 and 44 μg/dL, and the cortisol increment after cosyntropin stimulation is between 9 and 17 μg/dL, metyrapone testing is needed to assess adrenal function.[5]

The rapid ACTH stimulation test is a relatively simple test for evaluating AI.[46] It does not, however, differentiate between primary and secondary AI. To differentiate between primary and secondary AI, a basal plasma ACTH determination is made. A serum cortisol measurement is then made following a continuous 48-hour infusion of ACTH. An increased basal ACTH (>250 pg/mL) or a serum cortisol level (<20 μg/dL) after 48 hours of ACTH stimulation is compatible with primary AI. On the other hand, a decreased basal ACTH and a high cortisol level after ACTH administration suggest secondary AI.

CRITICAL ILLNESS–RELATED CORTICOSTEROID INSUFFICIENCY

The term critical illness–related corticosteroid insufficiency (CIRCI) describes HPA axis dysfunction in critical illness, which is defined as a cellular corticosteroid activity that is inadequate for the severity of the patient's illness. The use of the term relative adrenal insufficiency is no longer recommended by some authors.

Despite no conclusive evidence of benefit, in the 1950s, 1960s, and into the 1970s cortisol at low doses over days was often used in patients with severe manifestations of sepsis to counter the AI that was assumed to be present. This was based on autopsy studies that revealed adrenal necrosis in patients dying with severe infection. The subsequent recognition of the systemic effects of inflammation in sepsis and the discovery that the majority of patients in septic shock had normal or increased cortisol levels led to a paradigm shift in treating septic shock with massive doses of steroids given for a short period of time. This practice was based on animal studies showing that large doses of steroids given prior to boluses of endotoxin or gram-negative bacteria prevented death.[42] Clinical trials testing the utility of several large doses of steroids in patients with septic shock failed to show benefit.[47,48]

One study in patients with septic shock demonstrated that regardless of baseline cortisol level, the inability to raise the cortisol level following ACTH stimulation by at least 10 μg/dL signified poor prognosis.[49] Of this poor prognostic group, the higher the baseline cortisol level with failure to produce a 10 μg/dL increase, the worse the prognosis.

MANAGEMENT

Once the diagnosis of AI is made, a search for the cause should be initiated as the patient is being stabilized. To rule out tuberculosis, a purified protein derivative (PPD) skin test must be placed and a chest radiograph performed. An abnormal prothrombin time, partial thromboplastin time, or platelet count may point to an unsuspected coagulopathy suggesting the possibility of adrenal hemorrhage. Antiadrenal antibodies are found in about 70% of patients with autoimmune adrenal disease and in less than 0.1% of normal subjects.[50] Computed tomography scanning of the abdomen is useful in determining the size and presence of calcification of the adrenal glands. Adrenal calcification can be seen in 53% of cases of tuberculosis.[51]

Management of AI can be best accomplished by identifying the degree of acuteness and severity of the patient's illness at the time of presentation.[52]

PREEXISTING ADRENAL INSUFFICIENCY

Patients who are known to have AI or who have received glucocorticoid therapy in the past year should receive stress doses of corticosteroids during critical illnesses and during surgical procedures. Hydrocortisone 100 mg IV bolus is administered followed by 100 mg as an intravenous infusion every 6 to 8 hours. Isotonic saline is administered intravenously in volumes sufficient to support blood pressure. Five percent dextrose in isotonic saline may be used in the hypoglycemic patient. Once the acute insult has resolved, the hydrocortisone should be tapered to a maintenance dose. The replacement dose is usually 5 mg of prednisone or 30 mg of hydrocortisone each day.

Patients with known AI scheduled for operation should continue the existing steroid dose prior to surgery. The morning of the operation hydrocortisone 100 mg is given intravenously. During the operation a 100-mg hydrocortisone infusion is given. Following surgery 100 mg of hydrocortisone is administered intravenously every 8 hours during the first postoperative day. The dose is then tapered back to the baseline steroid dose over the next 3 to 4 days.

Adequate instruction is important in this group of patients. Patients with AI should be advised to wear a medical alert bracelet. These patients should be provided with a parenteral form of glucocorticoid and taught to self-administer the drug in case of emergency. They should be taught about the clinical situations in which increased amounts of glucocorticoids are required.

HEMODYNAMICALLY STABLE PATIENT

A patient who is suspected of having AI and who is hemodynamically stable should be managed in the following manner. A serum cortisol level and a rapid ACTH stimulation test should be performed prior to initiation of stress doses of corticosteroids. Hypovolemia should be treated with isotonic saline. If the diagnosis of AI is confirmed, hydrocortisone 100 mg should be administered as an intravenous infusion every 6 to 8 hours.

HEMODYNAMICALLY UNSTABLE PATIENT

Acute AI is a life-threatening emergency and requires immediate and aggressive therapy to ensure prompt recovery. A patient who is suspected of having AI and who is hemodynamically unstable should be managed in the following manner. Immediate glucocorticoid therapy and intravenous administration of isotonic fluids are warranted. Blood should be obtained for baseline serum cortisol concentration, electrolytes, glucose, BUN, and creatinine.

The dose of hydrocortisone is 100 mg IV bolus followed by 100 mg IV every 6 hours. After the patient has stabilized, the hydrocortisone is tapered at 10 to 15 mg per day until a maintenance dose of 30 mg per day is achieved.

Vigorous intravascular volume expansion with saline-containing solutions is recommended. Volume resuscitation is usually initiated with 0.9% normal saline. Dextrose 5% in saline is added to prevent hypoglycemia. The patient's fluid, electrolyte, and glucose status should be carefully monitored during resuscitation. In general, patients with acute AI have a deficit that is approximately 20% of their extracellular space. The rapidity of infusion depends on the patient's hemodynamic status and the presence or absence of underlying cardiovascular disease. A pulmonary artery catheter may be helpful in monitoring hemodynamic status and guiding fluid therapy. Vasopressors may be necessary in the initial stages to maintain an adequate blood pressure to ensure tissue perfusion. In general, if the hypotension is caused by AI, improvement in blood pressure should be seen within 6 hours of corticosteroid therapy.

Mineralocorticoid administration is usually not required initially during acute AI, because the large doses of hydrocortisone provide adequate mineralocorticoid activity. Once the acute event has resolved and the hydrocortisone is tapered to less than 100 mg per day, mineralocorticoids should be started. Fludrocortisone is recommended at a dose of 0.05 to 0.20 mg per day. Excess mineralocorticoids can cause congestive heart failure, hypokalemia, and metabolic alkalosis.

In patients with concurrent hypothyroidism, glucocorticoid replacement should begin prior to thyroid hormone replacement. Administration of thyroid hormone increases the metabolism of glucocorticoids. Thus treatment with thyroid hormone before glucocorticoid therapy might worsen the hypoadrenal state and precipitate AI.

Reversal of the underlying cause of adrenal dysfunction is an important aspect of treatment. The precipitation of acute adrenal failure is provoked by another acute process and thus the causes of both primary and secondary AI should be sought. Prophylactic use of antibiotics is not beneficial, but specific infections should be treated aggressively with appropriate antibiotic therapy.

SEVERE SEPSIS AND SEPTIC SHOCK

Six randomized clinical trials suggest that replacement of moderate-dose hydrocortisone (200-300 mg/day) decreases the need for vasopressor support in patients with septic shock.[2,53] Among them, the two larger trials were better powered to detect a survival difference but had differing results. These differences were attributed in part to varying demographics and other factors. In the Corticus study, hydrocortisone did not decrease mortality rate in both responders and nonresponders to ACTH, but the patients who received hydrocortisone had more rapid resolution of shock, which has been seen in other studies as well. These results were different from the Annane study, in which the nonresponders to ACTH had both reduction in mortality

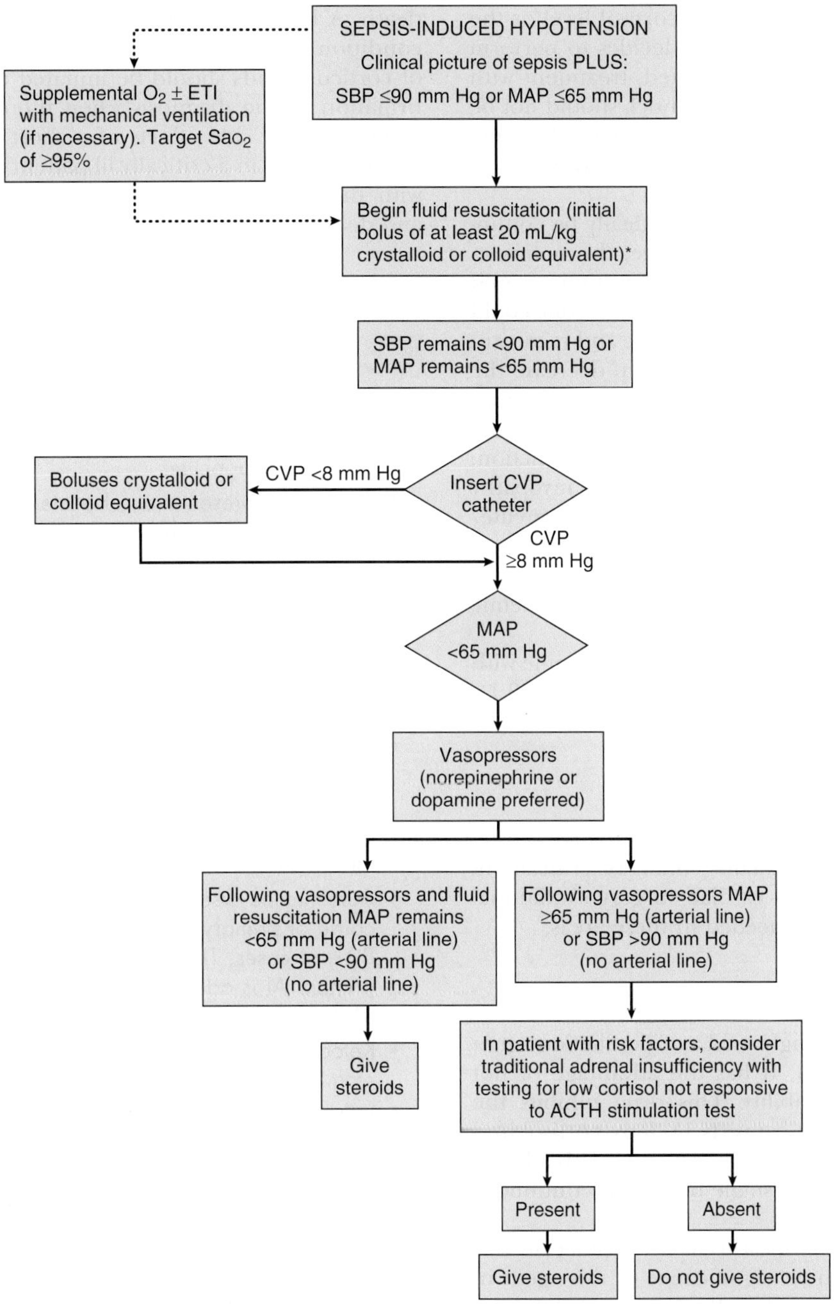

* In circumstances where MAP is judged to be critically low, vasopressors may be started at any point in this algorithm.

Figure 59.1 Algorithm for management of severe sepsis/septic shock. CVP, central venous pressure; ETI, endotracheal intubation; MAP, mean arterial pressure; SBP, systolic blood pressure.

rate and reversal of shock. The differences were attributed in part to the fact that in the Annane study, the patients enrolled were sicker, patients had higher SAPS II scores, and time to enrollment differed (8 hours versus 72 hours in the Corticus study). The Corticus study was published some years after the Annane study; it is possible that variations in the supportive care of the critically ill with advances in the care of the septic patient in the last few years could have made it difficult to show a mortality rate difference in Corticus. More patients in the Corticus study had a surgical source of sepsis, and thus source control may have played a bigger role in improving outcomes. In addition, fludrocortisones was not administered in the Corticus study. The duration of steroid therapy was different in the two studies, and this could have caused the differing results. In addition, Corticus had a higher rate of superinfection. Compounding all these issues is the difficulty surrounding the accurate diagnosis of AI.[53,54] However, in a recent study, the addition of enteral fludrocortisone did not result in a significant improvement in hospital mortality rates.[55]

In the trials mentioned here, there was resolution of shock in both responders and nonresponders to ACTH stimulation. The decision to treat patients with septic shock with hydrocortisone should, therefore, probably not be based on the results of a random total cortisol level or the response to cosyntropin. If a clinician decides to perform an ACTH test, until the test is performed, treatment with dexamethasone in patients with septic shock should not be done because of the possibility that a single dose of a long-acting corticosteroid may cause prolonged suppression of the hypothalamic-pituitary axis.[2]

Once initiated, hydrocortisone should ideally be continued for about 7 days. At the present time, the optimum duration of therapy is not clear, but data from studies would suggest that abrupt discontinuation of hydrocortisone could precipitate a rebound inflammatory response and recurrent shock. The ideal dose of steroid should help decrease the proinflammatory responses and at the same time minimize adverse effects, such as interference with wound healing, and decrease any negative impact on immune function. From studies, it appears that adverse effects of myopathy and superinfections are more common with doses greater than 200 to 300 mg/day of hydrocortisone. Hydrocortisone can be administered as a bolus dose or as a continuous infusion. Continuous infusions tend to cause less glycemic fluctuations.

To date, no studies document an improved outcome with corticosteroid use in the absence of septic shock (Fig. 59.1).

ADDITIONAL INDICATIONS FOR CORTICOSTEROIDS

Observational studies suggest that stress doses of corticosteroids may have a role in the management of critically ill patients with liver failure and cardiac surgery. Additional large randomized studies are needed in these areas.[3]

ETOMIDATE

Etomidate is a drug increasingly used as an induction agent for endotracheal intubation. It has the advantage of not causing hemodynamic instability. This drug inhibits the 11β-hydroxylase enzyme that converts 11-deoxycortisol into cortisol in the adrenal gland, and can cause AI. This adverse event has been described with single bolus and continuous infusions.

Additional randomized clinical trials are needed in this area to determine the clinical significance of this agent in causing AI septic shock and the effect on mortality rate, given that the incidence of AI in septic patients can be as high as 60%.[43]

SUMMARY

Management of acute AI involves prompt diagnosis and immediate treatment to prevent cardiovascular collapse and death. A high index of suspicion is necessary because the condition can be lethal if missed. Therapy with stress doses of corticosteroids should be initiated even before the confirmation of the diagnosis when there is a high index of suspicion. The side effects of a short course of high-dose corticosteroids in a critically ill patient are minor compared with the possible consequence of cardiovascular collapse and death.

KEY POINTS

- AI is a true emergency and requires rapid diagnosis.
- Common symptoms of AI include weakness, fatigue, and loss of appetite.
- The classic presentation of acute AI is a patient with unexplained hemodynamic instability who is unresponsive to intravascular volume resuscitation and use of vasopressors. AI can mimic cardiogenic, hypovolemic, or septic shock.
- Secondary AI is more common than primary AI. The most common cause of secondary AI is discontinuation of corticosteroid therapy.
- Patients who have taken 40 mg of prednisone per day or its equivalent for a period longer than 2 or 3 weeks during the past year should be considered to be adrenal insufficient until proved otherwise.
- Autoimmune disease is currently the most common cause of primary AI and accounts for approximately 80% of cases. The second most common cause of primary AI is adrenal gland destruction by *Mycobacterium tuberculosis*.
- Ketoconazole, phenytoin, phenobarbital, rifampin, and etomidate can cause AI.
- When there is a high suspicion of AI, hormonal testing is necessary to confirm the diagnosis.
- Therapy with stress doses of corticosteroids should be initiated even before the confirmation of the diagnosis when there is a high index of suspicion. The side effects of a short course of high-dose corticosteroids in a critically ill patient are minor compared with the possible consequence of cardiovascular collapse and death.

The complete list of references can be found at www.expertconsult.com.

Thyroid Disorders

60

Susan S. Braithwaite

CHAPTER OUTLINE

This chapter addresses nonthyroidal illness syndrome and critical illnesses or complications during critical illness that are manifestations of thyroid disease.

THYROID PHYSIOLOGY

Thyroid hormone exerts profound multisystemic actions. A patient developing clinically apparent thyroid dysfunction may experience some symptoms soon after onset, but a change of thyroid hormone availability is slow to exhibit its full effect. On the other hand, patients with established hyperthyroidism or hypothyroidism may destabilize quickly in response to intercurrent illness or medical and surgical interventions.

CELLULAR EFFECTS OF THYROID HORMONE

Thyroid hormone action is initiated by the binding of nuclear hormone receptors activated by 3,5,3′-triiodothyronine (T_3) to nuclear thyroid hormone response elements, in which the hormone-receptor complex acts as a transcription factor.[1] In addition, T_3 exerts rapid nontranscriptional extranuclear effects that are especially important in cardiovascular physiology.[2] Transporters necessary for cellular uptake of thyroid hormone recently have been recognized.[3] Thyroxine (T_4) acts as a prohormone for T_3 and itself is only weakly interactive with thyroid hormone receptors. The compound 3,3′,5′-triiodothyronine(reverse T_3) is almost devoid of metabolic activity (Fig. 60.1).

PERIPHERAL AND INTRATHYROIDAL CONVERSIONS OF T_4 AND T_3

Normally about 80% of circulating T_3 and probably greater than 90% of circulating reverse T_3 are derived from circulating T_4. Peripheral production of T_3 is modulated by the availability of T_4, by peripheral cellular uptake of T_4, and by the activities of the enzymes identified as iodothyronine selenodeiodinase 1 (D1), selenodeiodinase 2 (D2), and selenodeiodinase 3 (D3). The enzymes affecting peripheral levels of circulating thyroid hormone and tissue levels of T_3 either convert T_4 to T_3, also removing reverse T_3 by deiodination (the D1 and D2 enzymes), or deiodinate and thus inactivate T_3 (the D3 enzyme) and convert T_4 to reverse T_3 (the D3 enzyme)[4,5] (see Fig. 60.1).

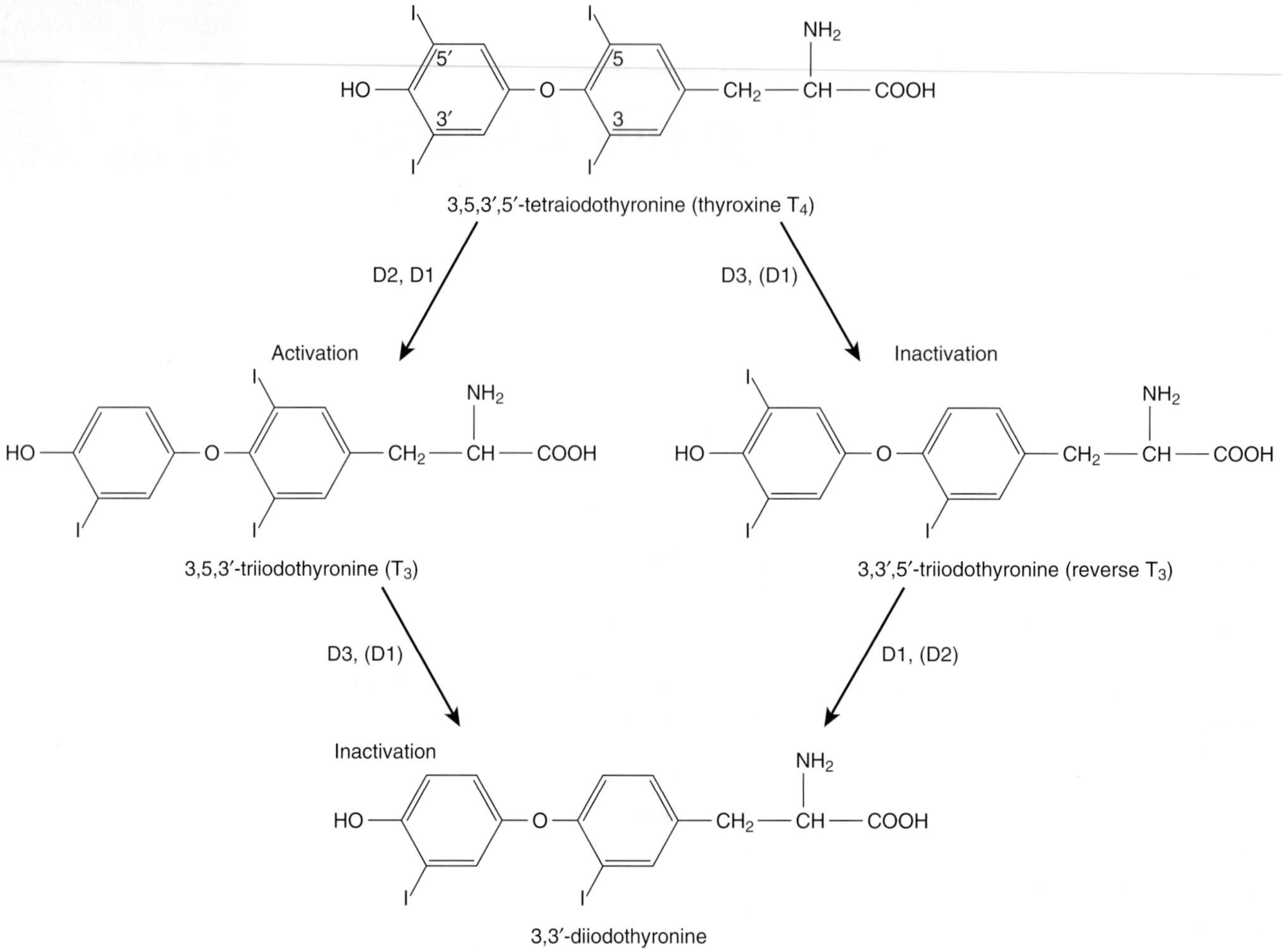

Figure 60.1 Enyzmatic conversion of iodothyronines by iodothyronine selenodeiodinase 1 (D1), iodothyronine selenodeiodinase 2 (D2), and iodothyronine selenodeiodinase 3 (D3). T_3 is the metabolically active hormone (3,5,3′-triiodothyronine). Reverse T_3 is metabolically inactive (3,3′,5′-triiodothyronine). T_4 is converted to T_3 by the activating action of the D1 and D2 enzymes. Reverse T_3 is deiodinated by the D1 and D2 enzymes. T_3 is deiodinated and inactivated principally by the D3 enzyme. (Adapted with permission from Figure 1 of Bianco AC, Salvatore D, Gereben B, et al: Biochemistry, cellular and molecular biology, and physiological roles of the iodothyronine selenodeiodinases. Endocr Rev 2002;23:38-89.)

HORMONE TRANSPORT

Circulating T_4 is carried about 49% to 64% by thyroxine-binding globulin (TBG), 12% to 13% by transthyretin, and 7% to 9% by albumin. T_3 is carried 80% by TBG, 9% by transthyretin, and 11% by albumin.[6] A small fraction is transported by lipoproteins. About 0.03% of circulating T_4 and 0.3% of T_3 is free or unbound. TBG is produced by the liver, and transthyretin by the liver and choroid plexus. The approximate half-lives of circulating transport proteins are transthyretin, 2 days; TBG, 5 days; and albumin, 15 days.[6] Recent research suggests that TBG allows targeted delivery of T_4 to tissues, for example, at sites of inflammation.[7] The unbound fraction of circulating hormone gains access to peripheral tissues and pituitary, determines metabolic status, and participates in feedback inhibition of the pituitary.

Unbound circulating hormone remains in a dynamic equilibrium with hormone provided by thyroid output, carried on transport proteins, or taken up or released by peripheral tissues. The half-life of circulating hormone is about 1 week for T_4 and 1 day for T_3. Deiodination occurs in many tissues, and the partially metabolized moieties are excreted in bile. Some enterohepatic recirculation occurs.

THYROID FUNCTION

Thyroid function is regulated by cyclic adenosine monophosphate (cAMP)-dependent events initiated by binding of thyroid-stimulating hormone (thyrotropin; TSH) to the thyroid follicular cell membrane TSH receptor. TSH stimulation leads to consumption of colloid and the release of thyroglobulin (TG), T_4, T_3, and reverse T_3. Activation of the TSH receptor promotes conversion of T_4 to T_3 within the thyroid and proportionately increased secretion of T_3 by the thyroid. Thyroidal autoregulation is influenced by the availability of iodine.

PITUITARY AND HYPOTHALAMIC FUNCTION

Pituitary TSH and hypothalamic thyrotropin-releasing hormone (TRH) are ultimately necessary for regulation of adequate thyroid hormonogenesis and thyroid hormone secretion. On the principle of feedback inhibition and in the absence of central disease, an inverse relationship between circulating levels of TSH and free T_4 is expected. The D2 enzyme in hypothalamic tanycytes in animal models is thought to be responsible for conversion of T_4 to T_3, allowing for local regulation by hypothalamic tissue levels of T_3, dependent upon not only circulating hormone levels but also local deiodinase activity.

DIAGNOSTIC APPROACH TO THYROID DISEASE

HISTORY, PHYSICAL EXAMINATION, AND RECORD REVIEW

In critical illness, ambiguity of thyroid function tests is commonplace. The obstacles to laboratory assessment augment the importance of record review, history, and physical examination. When overt thyroid dysfunction is present, the history and physical examination usually yield multisystemic positive findings.[8]

CASE FINDING BY SCREENING

Ambulatory patients who should be screened and periodically monitored for thyroid dysfunction include those with a history of previous thyroid surgery or radioactive iodine therapy; those with deterioration of cardiac function or weight loss; and those receiving lithium, amiodarone, α-interferon, interleukin 2 therapy, tyrosine kinase inhibitors, and other medications affecting thyroid function.

In a meta-analysis of earlier studies, the frequency of thyroid disease ascertainable by screening hospitalized patients was similar to that among outpatients, about 1% to 2%.[9] In the hospital the relatively low case-finding rate and the confounding effect of nonthyroidal illness have been viewed as impediments to general screening of unselected patients, except possibly among elderly women.[10,11] However, one study in which TSH and free T_4 index were performed on sera drawn at the time of admission from 364 consecutive patients suggested that the rate of nonthyroidal illness syndrome (7.4%) was exceeded by the combined rates of unsuspected thyroidal failure (5.8%), subclinical hypothyroidism (6%), and hyperthyroidism (2%).[12] Among critical care patients, the case-finding rate for thyroid disease during screening is not known with confidence. Clinical suspicion of thyroid disease based on patient symptoms or findings should, of course, result in testing.

ASSAYS AND IMAGING

Among critically ill patients, the TSH assay taken alone may yield misleading results, and the utility of most commercial methods for determining free thyroid hormone levels is limited.[13-17] Thyroid function test results may change on a daily basis. The best course of action is not to screen with a single test but to order a potentially useful battery of tests from the outset.

SIMULTANEITY OF SAMPLING OF TROPHIC AND TARGET HORMONE

In normal health, the trophic hormone TSH and the circulating target gland thyroid hormones exhibit the characteristics of regulation by feedback inhibition. Thyroidal autonomy or primary thyroidal failure can be diagnosed if unambiguous reciprocal changes of TSH and target gland hormone are seen, each into the clearly abnormal range. In order to interpret the relationship between trophic and target hormones, it is essential that measurements of TSH and thyroid hormones, and any assessments of hormone binding, should be performed on samples of blood that were obtained simultaneously.

THYROID-STIMULATING HORMONE

Reasons for misleading TSH results, some of which apply to critically ill patients, include nonequilibrium conditions in which thyroid status has recently fluctuated, acute psychiatric illness, nonthyroidal illness syndrome, central causes of hyperthyroidism or hypothyroidism, and the effects of medication.[18-20] The distribution of TSH results in nonthyroidal illness syndrome may overlap with the range seen in thyrotoxicosis. Conversely, in mild cases of subclinical thyrotoxicosis, for example, in nodular thyroid disease at the earliest stages of autonomy, TSH suppression may be minimal. The indication for measuring TSH is to support a diagnosis of primary hypothyroidism or hyperthyroidism.

ESTIMATES OF FREE THYROXINE

Although with some exceptions most free T_4 assays perform well in the ambulatory setting, in critically ill patients some commercial assays for free T_4 yield low results that cannot be verified by an equilibrium dialysis method.[14,17] The indication for ordering a free T_4 rather than total T_4 assay is to assess thyroid function in the presence of suspected abnormalities of thyroid hormone transport or to clarify the significance of an abnormal total T_4 result in a patient whose clinical condition appears euthyroid. A normal result of a free T_4 determination together with a normal TSH is reassuring.

FREE T_4 BY EQUILIBRIUM DIALYSIS OR ULTRAFILTRATION

High levels of free T_4 may occur in the early stages of sepsis (see discussion under "Nonthyroidal Illness Syndrome"). By most assay methods, high estimates of free T_4 also may occur in the presence of acute elevations of free fatty acids or drugs including furosemide, heparin, or enoxaparin that directly or indirectly cause inhibition of T_4 binding to transport proteins, such that there actually is an in vitro elevation of free T_4 (see later discussion under "Medication Effects"). When elevation of free T_4 is caused by such effects, not only standard commercial assays but also free T_4 assays by equilibrium dialysis or ultrafiltration are likely to report an elevation of free T_4.

A free T_4 assay by equilibrium dialysis or ultrafiltration may help resolve the meaning of a low estimation of free T_4 determined by other commercial methods. In critical care medicine the principal indication for ordering a free T_4

assay by equilibrium dialysis or ultrafiltration is the concern that other free T_4 methods might yield false low results.

TOTAL THYROXINE

In order to avoid risk of misinterpretation of free T_4 elevations, the total T_4 should be one of the front-line tests among patients treated with furosemide in high dosage, heparin, or enoxaparin. If the TSH and total T_4 both are normal, then the patient is probably euthyroid.

When the patient condition predicts that free T_4 methods may yield spurious low results, or when a free T_4 assay has yielded a low result in a patient having low or normal TSH, a confirming test to discount central hypothyroidism is desirable. The institutional turnaround time for a total T_4 assay may be faster than for the gold standard test, a free T_4 assay by equilibrium dialysis or ultrafiltration. The total T_4 may be measured, together with an estimate of binding by transport proteins.

The indication for ordering a total T_4 assay is to discount hyperthyroidism in the presence of misleading free T_4 elevations in euthyroid patients, to provide reassurance when considered together with an estimate of thyroid hormone binding that central hypothyroidism may be absent, or to demonstrate the presence and quantitate the severity of hypothyroidism or hyperthyroidism.[13]

T_3 UPTAKE OR THYROXINE-BINDING GLOBULIN AND CALCULATED FREE T_4 INDEX

The T_3 uptake, together with a determination of total T_4, is used in index methods to provide information about hormone transport and to help estimate free T_4. In critically ill patients with hypothyroxinemia, the free T_4 index frequently is misleading. Nevertheless, when hypothyroxinemia by a free hormone estimate is present but its interpretation is uncertain, for example, when the TSH is normal or low, it is advantageous to review a second independent assay such as the T_3 resin uptake or a direct measurement of TBG to see whether qualitatively the result is consistent with reduced T_4 binding sites on circulating transport proteins. Elevation of T_3 uptake accompanied by low total T_4 suggests reduced hormone binding to transport proteins, consistent with nonthyroidal illness syndrome. Nonelevated T_3 uptake or low T_3 resin uptake accompanied by hypothyroxinemia in the face of nonthyroidal illness suggests the possibility of hypothyroidism (Table 60.1).

Table 60.1 Use of Total T_4 and T_3 Uptake to Calculate Free Thyroxine Index (FTI)

	Total T_4	T_3 Uptake	Physiology Reflected by Test Results
Normal	Normal	Normal	Normal
Increased binding sites	↑	↓	Normal
Reduced binding sites	↓	↑	Normal
Hyperthyroid	↑	↑	↑
Hypothyroid	↓	↓	↓

T_3, triiodothyronine; T_4, thyroxine.

The index methods generally are inferior to the membrane dialysis or ultrafiltration methods of determining free T_4, but the rapid turnaround time of the index method is advantageous. The combination of low T_4 with normal or low TSH may raise consideration of central hypothyroidism. The indication for an index method for free T_4 in this setting is to use the resin uptake or TBG measurement to provide qualitative evidence for a competing explanation for low T_4, namely, that T_4 carriage by transport proteins may be reduced.

THYROXINE-BINDING GLOBULIN

The transport protein TBG can be directly measured, and the result can be used together with a determination of total T_4 as one method of calculating a free T_4 index. TBG levels are increased in hepatitis, hepatoma, and human immunodeficiency virus (HIV) infection. The indication for ordering a TBG or T_3 resin uptake for calculation of a free T_4 index is to provide qualitative information about the significance of a low total T_4 in a setting in which the commercial free T_4 assay is judged to be unreliable. The TBG may used, together with the total T_4, to help discount suspicion of central hypothyroidism.

TOTAL T_3

Like T_4, the total T_3 is affected by alterations of binding to hormone transport proteins. Measurement of T_3 should not be employed to evaluate the possibility of hypothyroidism or to evaluate the significance of a low T_4. Under intense TSH stimulation, the failing thyroid preferentially secretes T_3 rather than T_4, so that patients with T_4 reduction due to primary hypothyroidism still may maintain normal T_3 levels. The main indication for measuring total T_3 is suspicion of T_3 toxicosis or hyperthyroidism in patients lacking hyperthyroxinemia. If the TSH is suppressed to less than 0.1 μIU/mL but T_4 is normal, measurement of T_3 is necessary. T_3 also is measured to evaluate for amiodarone-induced thyrotoxicosis.

FREE T_3

Free T_3 sometimes is found to be normal among patients with nonthyroidal illness syndrome having low total T_3, helping offset suspicion of secondary hypothyroidism due to organic pituitary or hypothalamic disease. Methodologic limitations in critically ill patients may result in variability of findings between assay systems. Chopra and colleagues reported that by direct equilibrium dialysis radioimmunoassay in nonthyroidal illness syndrome serum free T_3 concentration was normal in approximately 83% of patients with low total T_3.[21-23] The indication for ordering the free T_3 test is to confirm or exclude T_3 toxicosis in patients suspected of having thyroid transport abnormalities, such that reliance upon total T_3 might be inappropriate. Free T_3 also may help identify amiodarone-induced thyrotoxicosis.

REVERSE T_3

If T_3 and T_4 are low, and if hypothyroidism is present, then the reverse T_3 may be low. In contrast, in nonthyroidal illness syndrome, even though the T_3 and T_4 may be low, the concentration of reverse T_3 potentially is high, but not invariably so. Slow laboratory turnaround and frequency of normal reverse T_3 results in nonthyroidal illness syndrome limit the usefulness of reverse T_3 measurement. The indication for ordering reverse T_3 is to differentiate intrinsic hypothyroidism from nonthyroidal illness syndrome.

SERUM ALBUMIN

In some circumstances, opposite changes of albumin and TBG are seen, for example, in hepatitis. However, when low T_4 levels are present, a finding of concomitant hypoalbuminemia usually permits the caregiver tentatively to attribute the low T_4 results to reduction of circulating transport proteins, including TBG.

ANTITHYROID PEROXIDASE AND ANTITHYROGLOBULIN ANTIBODIES

In sufficient titer, positive antibodies strongly suggest autoimmune thyroid disease. In the critical care setting the principal indication for antithyroid antibody determination is to evaluate the significance of a modest TSH elevation.

THYROID-STIMULATING HORMONE RECEPTOR ANTIBODIES

A sensitive assay for TSH receptor antibodies may suggest the classification of hyperthyroidism as Graves' disease.

RADIOIODINE UPTAKE AND THYROID SCAN

The radioactive iodine uptake is a number, expressed as a percentage of uptake counted 24 hours after administration of a small dose of radioactive iodine, and the scan provides an image. The radioactive iodine uptake test helps differentiate low-uptake forms of hyperthyroidism (amiodarone- or iodine-induced thyrotoxicosis, thyroiditis, factitious hyperthyroidism, and others) from high-uptake forms of hyperthyroidism (Graves' disease, toxic adenoma, and toxic multinodular goiter). These tests often are postponed until 4 to 6 weeks after the last use of an iodinated contrast medium. The utility of the radioactive iodine uptake and thyroid scan is to identify the cause of hyperthyroidism to help decide between therapeutic alternatives.

ULTRASONOGRAPHY AND COMPUTED TOMOGRAPHY

Examination of the thoracic inlet in cases of large compressive goiters is best accomplished with computed tomography (CT). The indication for thyroid ultrasonography is to obtain information about the size, texture, vascularity, and nodularity of the thyroid and to evaluate other structures in the neck.

"BEST PANEL" FOR CRITICALLY ILL PATIENTS

For confirmation of a suspected diagnosis of thyroid dysfunction, a panel rather than a single test is recommended at the outset. The TSH should not be used as monoscreening in the hospital (Fig. 60.2). The initial "best panel" is whichever has the faster turnaround time or weekend availability, or both, at the laboratory used by the institution. The initial panel should include either a calculated free T_4 index (utilizing T_3 uptake or TBG together with total T_4) or a free T_4 estimate by any other method having rapid turnaround time, together with total T_4 and TSH. These initial panels will yield unambiguous results in most cases of critical illness that are caused or complicated by preexisting clinically

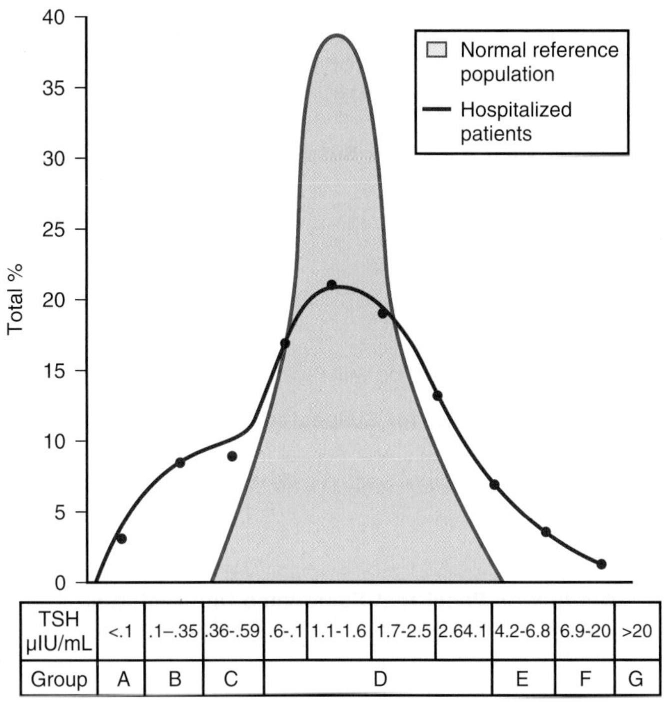

Figure 60.2 Frequency of observation of values of serum thyroid-stimulating hormone (TSH) in each of seven ranges among normal ambulatory patients (*solid line*) and in the hospital setting (*dashed line*). The observed frequency distribution spans a broader range of TSH values during hospitalization, partly because TSH suppression occurs during illness or consequent to administration of medications, and partly because TSH overshoot occurs during recovery. (Adapted with permission from Spencer C, Eigen A, Shen D, et al: Specificity of sensitive assays of thyrotropin (TSH) used to screen for thyroid disease in hospitalized patients. Clin Chem 1987;33(8):1391-1396.)

significant primary hypothyroidism or hyperthyroidism. Furthermore, the findings of normal TSH and normal or elevated free T_4 with normal total T_4 suggest euthyroidism. The isolated finding of free T_4 elevation may result from sepsis or the effects of furosemide, heparin or enoxaparin.

If clinical examination suggests hyperthyroidism and marked suppression of TSH is present, but if hyperthyroxinemia cannot be demonstrated, then the next step is to draw simultaneously TSH and total and free T_3.

If the free T_4 and TSH considered as a hormone pair appear discordant (both values high or both values low), and if the explanation or management is not straightforward, a consultation should be obtained. However, in the setting of nonthyroidal illness, if low T_4, low free T_4 estimate, and normal or low TSH are demonstrated during screening, to discount suspicion of secondary hypothyroidism it is sometimes helpful to order TSH, free T_4 by equilibrium dialysis, and morning cortisol (Box 60.1).

MEDICATION EFFECTS

When unexpected thyroid function test results are reported, a medication review should be conducted. Drugs may alter the results of thyroid function tests either in vivo or in vitro without affecting thyroid function. Additionally, drugs not designed to treat hypothyroidism or hyperthyroidism may

Box 60.1 "Best Panel" and Follow-up Studies for Critically Ill Patients

Initial "Best Panel" for Suspected Thyroid Disease

TSH
Total T_4
T_3 uptake or TBG
Calculated free T_4 index

or

TSH
Total T_4
Free T_4 by any method with rapid turnaround

Confirming Panel for Suspected Hyperthyroidism

(Reserved for patients with normal free T_4 and suppressed TSH or for amiodarone-treated patients)

TSH
Total T_3
Free T_3

Confirming Panel that Sometimes Differentiates Suspected Nonthyroidal Illness Syndrome from Central Hypothyroidism

TSH
Free T_4 by equilibrium dialysis or by ultrafiltration
AM cortisol

T_3, triiodothyronine; T_4, thyroxine; TBG, thyroxine-binding globulin; TSH, thyroid-stimulating hormone.

Table 60.2 Thyroid Function Test Abnormalities Induced by Medication in Euthyroid Patients

Abnormality	Etiologic Agent(s)*
Low TSH	Glucocorticoids Dopamine and congeners Octreotide
High T_4, high free T_4, low T_3	Amiodarone
High free T_4	Heparin and enoxaparin Salicylates and congeners Furosemide
High total T_4	Estrogen Oral contraceptives Tamoxifen Raloxifene 5-Fluorouracil
Low T_4	Salicylates and congeners Glucocorticoids
Low total T_4 and sometimes low free T_4	Phenytoin Carbamazepine
Other Thyroid Dysfunction	
Hypothyroidism or hyperthyroidism	Amiodarone Interferon-α Lithium Iodides Radiographic contrast agents
High TSH signifying hypothyroidism	Tyrosine kinase inhibitors

T_3, triiodothyronine; T_4, thyroxine; TSH, thyroid-stimulating hormone.
*Commonly implicated agents. This list is not exhaustive.

alter thyroid function.[15-17] Periodic monitoring before and during long-term use should occur during use of a drug that is recognized to be a potential cause of thyroid dysfunction. Medication effects are summarized in Table 60.2.

Suppression of TSH is seen during use of dopaminergic drugs, glucocorticoids, and octreotide. High total T_4 can result from elevation of transport proteins, as seen during pregnancy or during treatment with estrogen, oral contraceptives, tamoxifen, raloxifene, 5-fluorouracil, and other medications, or resulting from hereditary or acquired disorders affecting hormone transport protein concentration, such as hepatitis. If the only abnormality is increased concentration of carrier proteins, then total T_4 will be high, but TSH will be normal and in an appropriate assay system the free T_4 will be normal.

Lowering of total T_4 may result from reduction of thyroid hormone transport protein concentration, as may be seen during treatment with glucocorticoids. Lowering of total T_4 may occur during use of drugs that cause displacement of thyroid hormone from binding proteins, as seen during treatment with salicylates and congeners, phenytoin, and carbamazepine. If the only abnormality is reduced concentration of carrier proteins, then TSH will be normal and in an appropriate assay system the free T_4 often will be normal. However, during use of drugs that may cause acute displacement of thyroid hormone from transport proteins, misleading elevations of free T_4 or free T_3 may occur. These drugs notably include furosemide and heparin, given subcutaneously or even given at the low doses used to flush intravenous lines, or enoxaparin. The lipoprotein lipase activity of heparin causes release of free fatty acids, which in turn reduce thyroid hormone binding to transport proteins, resulting in elevation of free T_4.

Selective lowering of T_3 levels without reduction of T_4 levels may result from inhibition of peripheral conversion of T_4 to T_3, as may occur during use of glucocorticoids, beta blockers, iodinated cholecystographic contrast agents, and amiodarone.

TSH elevation signifying hypothyroidism or TSH suppression signifying hyperthyroidism may result, or patients may remain euthyroid during treatment with any of the following: interferon-α,[24,25] lithium,[26,27] iodinated contrast agents,[28] iodine,[29] and amiodarone.[30-35] During use of iodine-containing medications, hyperthyroidism of the Jod-Basedow type due to the iodine content of the drug may fail to self-resolve. However, when the mechanism of hyperthyroidism is destructive thyroiditis, as may be seen during some cases of interferon-α-induced hyperthyroidism and type 2 amiodarone-induced thyrotoxicosis, a possible sequence is hyperthyroidism followed by hypothyroidism.[31,32] The prevalence of amiodarone-induced hypothyroidism has been variably reported, but it may be seen in up to 22% of treated patients from iodine-sufficient regions,[35] and its occurrence may be increased in the presence of positive antithyroid antibodies.[30,33] The combined findings of elevation of total and free T_4 together with reduction of T_3 occur in euthyroid persons receiving amiodarone; these findings taken alone, when seen together with a normal TSH, do not indicate thyroid dysfunction

Box 60.2 Possible Outcomes of Amiodarone Therapy

Euthyroidism
Normal TSH
High T_4 and free T_4
Low T_3

Hypothyroidism
High TSH
Normal or low T_4 and free T_4

Hyperthyroidism
Low TSH
High T_3 and free T_3

T_3, triiodothyronine; T_4, thyroxine; TSH, thyroid-stimulating hormone.

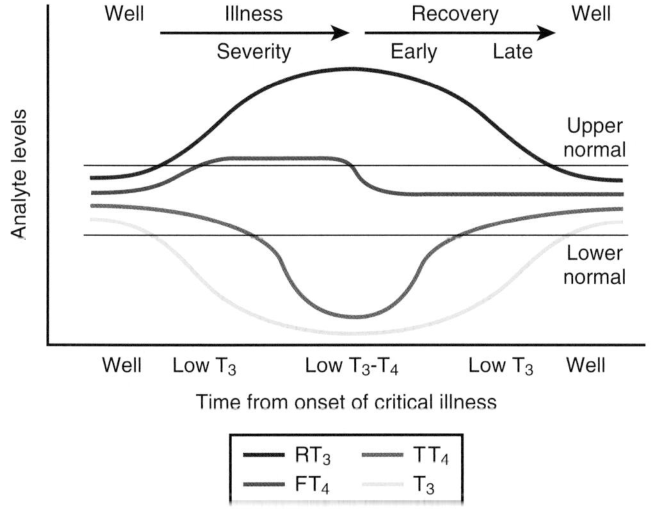

Figure 60.3 Nonthyroidal illness syndrome. The time course of concentration of circulating iodothyronine levels are shown qualitatively during evolution of nonthyroidal illness syndrome. A characteristic sequence involves first the development of a low total T_3, initially with normal T_4 or sometimes with high free T_4. Characteristically, as T_3 falls, reverse T_3 (RT_3) rises. With duration of illness, as thyroid hormone transport protein concentrations decline, concentrations of total T_3 and total T_4 (TT_4) both are affected, and total T_4 levels fall. Later, during the greatest severity of the illness, there may be low thyroid-stimulating hormone (TSH) and low free T_4, a predictor of higher mortality risk. During recovery, TSH overshoots the normal range (not shown) as T_4 rises. Finally, after recovery, tests become normal. (Adapted with permission from Figure 1[56]: In turn, Chopra had reproduced this from Nicoloff et al.)

(Box 60.2). High TSH signifying hypothyroidism may be caused by tyrosine kinase inhibitors including sunitinib, imatinib, motesanib, and sorafenib.[36-41]

NONTHYROIDAL ILLNESS SYNDROME

Nonthyroidal illness syndrome is usually recognized as a constellation of laboratory findings of uncertain clinical significance, discovered on thyroid function testing among patients having acute medical or surgical illness, the more pronounced abnormalities being associated with worse prognosis, and characterized by resolution after recovery from illness (Fig. 60.3). Although the severity of illness often makes clinical assessment difficult, patients usually appear clinically euthyroid. Laboratory findings of nonthyroidal illness syndrome may occur with psychiatric illness, starvation, congestive heart failure, acute and chronic renal failure, acquired immunodeficiency syndrome (AIDS), postoperative status, trauma, and in general with critical illness.[19,42-62]

High free T_4 without elevation of total T_4, seen in the early stages of nonthyroidal illness, may be associated with use of certain drugs or with sepsis. Otherwise, during development of nonthyroidal illness syndrome, reduction of circulating T_3 is one of the earliest and most consistently observed findings, possibly seen in over 70% of patients, depending upon the duration and severity of the illness.[42,43] The decline of T_3 often is accompanied by a rise of reverse T_3. Patients with chronic renal failure who have low T_3 do not invariably have high reverse T_3 levels,[44,45] and patients with HIV may have low reverse T_3.[52]

The additional finding of a low T_4 together with low T_3, a combination not usually seen at the onset, suggests nonthyroidal illness syndrome of greater severity and duration. Some cases of low total T_4 during the subacute stage of nonthyroidal illness are caused by transport protein deficiency alone, not necessarily accompanied by decline of free T_4, whereas others may result from TSH suppression. Not all patients experience progression to the stage of TSH suppression. If the free T_4, as evaluated by equilibrium dialysis, is low at the same time that TSH is low, biochemical differentiation between nonthyroidal illness syndrome and central hypothyroidism due to pituitary or hypothalamic disease is often not possible. In fact, nonthyroidal illness syndrome may be a cause of functional central hypothyroidism.

During recovery from nonthyroidal illness the TSH often is mildly elevated above the normal ambulatory reference range, and the free T_4 is normal. The differential diagnosis includes subclinical primary hypothyroidism. After recovery from nonthyroidal illness syndrome, thyroid function tests are normal. There are of course exceptions to the described sequence. Not all of the findings are seen in every case.

INCIDENCE

Among hospitalized patients, intrinsic thyroid disease is less common than nonthyroidal illness syndrome.[9,11,47] The prevalence of nonthyroidal illness syndrome among patients with psychiatric disease has been reported to be about 10%, often manifesting as elevated TSH or elevated T_4.[19,55] Abnormalities of thyroid function tests interpreted as euthyroid sick syndrome were found in 51.5% of elderly patients undergoing emergency surgery.[57] Hypothyroxinemia without TSH elevation was reported in 22% of critically ill patients in one study.[46] In another study of intensive care unit patients, depending upon the duration of illness and patient outcome, the findings of low total T_3 approached 70% to 80%, and about half of patients had low total T_4.[59]

PATHOGENESIS OF THE LABORATORY FINDINGS

The laboratory findings of nonthyroidal illness have been recognized for years, but the understanding of the pathogenesis of the findings has undergone rapid evolution in recent years, accompanied by controversy on the relative importance of each of several mechanisms in producing the observed features.

In order to understand the mechanisms for observed alterations of iodothyronine molecules (T_4, T_3, and reverse T_3) during nonthyroidal illness, under conditions of health and illness with and without specific interventions, there would need to be comparative human data on each of the following: tissue-specific functions of thyroid hormone; actual tissue levels of T_4 and T_3; cellular uptake of thyroid hormones; activity of each of the deiodinase enzymes in each tissue of interest, including hypothalamus and pituitary, thyroid, liver, muscle, and other tissues; tissue-specific direct and indirect mechanisms of regulation of each deiodinase enzyme, including enzyme-regulating effects of iodothyronines, cytokines, and drugs; contribution of each tissue and each of the three deiodinase enzymes to circulating levels of T_3; the role of transport proteins in targeted delivery of thyroid hormone in health if any and in illness; and any adaptative or maladaptative effects of the alterations of iodothyronine availability seen in illness. Much of our present knowledge derives from experimental animal models and is complicated by possible ambiguity of experimental assay results for deiodinase enzyme activity and by the necessarily inferential nature of human data.[5,7,63-96]

Alterations of T_3 and reverse T_3 usually precede reductions of T_4. Peripherally, there is reduced production of T_3 by 5′-deiodination of T_4, reduced removal of reverse T_3 by 5′-deiodination, and increased removal of T_3 by deiodination (see Fig. 60.1). The reduction in circulating T_3 is believed to result from a combination of mechanisms, including changes of cellular uptake of T_4, reduced activity of deiodinase enzymes that normally catalyze peripheral conversion of T_4 to T_3, inactivation of T_3 by deiodination resulting from activity of the D3 enzyme, and possibly decline of hypothalamic TRH resulting from an enzymatically mediated increase of T_3 production in the tanycytes.[5] The role of cytokines in mediating some of these changes has been explored.[71,76-79,81,84] Because T_3 may amplify its own production at the tissue level by activating the D2 enzyme, a decline of central TSH drive to the thyroid indirectly could reduce peripheral production of T_3. With acknowledgment that the finding of free T_3 abnormalities may be method-dependent, studies suggest that in some but not all patients having low total T_3, the results of free T_3 assays may be normal.[21-23]

Elevations of free T_4 sometimes occur in nonthyroidal illness, often accompanied by low or low normal total T_4, and without TSH suppression. The isolated finding of free T_4 elevation in vivo at least in some instances may represent artifact, such as could be introduced by nonselective beta blockers, furosemide, or free fatty acids (see previously, under "Assays and Imaging"). Mechanisms leading to high free T_4 in the early stages of sepsis have been controversial. Circulating inhibitors of binding of T_4 to transport proteins may be present such as nonesterified fatty acids.[65,67-69,72] Additionally, cleavage by elastases or consumption of the TBG molecule by serine proteases may occur at sites of inflammation, possibly leading to release of free T_4 to the circulation and permitting targeted delivery of T_4 at sites of inflammation.[82,83,85]

Patients with both low T_4 and low T_3 generally have disease of greater severity and longer duration. Early studies of hormone kinetics in the setting of low T_4 were consistent with reduced binding to vascular sites.[64,66] A low serum albumin level often, but not always, permits the caregiver to predict that TBG will be low. Hypoalbuminemia is highly associated with nonthyroidal illness syndrome.[57,60] Reduced concentration of transport proteins is a prevalent finding among cases of nonthyroidal illness presenting with low T_4 and low T_3.[49] Inhibitors of hormone binding to transport proteins also may result in low total concentrations of circulating thyroid hormone.

With use of an assay having low risk of artifact, most patients including those with low total T_4 have normal free T_4. However, low free T_4 also may be demonstrated among other patients with nonthyroidal illness syndrome. The question of the true levels of circulating free T_4 remains unresolved, dogged by issues of assay artifact and heterogeneity within the patient population.

The more severely ill patients with nonthyroidal illness syndrome, usually those having low T_4 levels, as well as low T_3, may have low circulating levels of TSH.[51,80,81,87,88] Central production of TRH and TSH may be reduced by inflammatory mediators. In a human autopsy study, reduced TRH gene expression was demonstrated among patients with an antemortem finding of low T_3.[80] In animal studies, it has been suggested that central conversion of T_4 to the active hormone T_3 in hypothalamic tanycytes under the action of the D2 enzyme, by producing local hyperthyroidism under conditions of illness, may act as a negative feedback signal that reduces hypothalamic release of TRH and pituitary release of TSH.[5,88,92,94,96] Therefore, in prolonged or severe nonthyroidal illness syndrome, a central mechanism may contribute to the findings of low T_4 and low T_3.

Investigationally, after TNF-α administration, as during recovery following nonthyroidal illness, there may be temporary overshoot of TSH into the mildly elevated range, accompanied by rising T_4.[51,81]

Presently it is unknown whether nonthyroidal illness syndrome is adaptive or maladaptive. In starvation, low T_3 syndrome may promote protein sparing.[97] Human trials have not been conducted with a sufficient number of randomized, critically ill human subjects to resolve the question of whether thyroid hormone therapy is beneficial. In a nonrandomized study of patients with sepsis, T_3 was used to reduce dopamine dependence.[98] Treatment with T_3 for human burn injury showed no benefit.[99] In a small study of critically ill patients with low T_3 and low T_4, therapy with T_4 did not correct the low T_3 or improve the prognosis,[100] and T_4 for nonthyroidal illness may increase mortality rate among acute renal failure patients.[101]

NONTHYROIDAL ILLNESS SYNDROME AMONG CARDIAC PATIENTS

Low T_3 or low T_3 and T_4 levels are observed in the setting of advanced heart failure, after revascularization, and after myocardial infarction, providing a rationale for therapeutic trials of treatment with thyroid hormone among cardiac patients.[102-121] Among patients with severely impaired left ventricular performance, the use of intravenous T_3 as an alternative to standard therapy (such as dopamine) and the compatibility or usefulness of T_3 in combination with other inotropic and vasodilating regimens requires further research. Correction of any reversible ischemia should first be achieved. Use of intravenous T_3 shows promise as an inotrope and vasodilator.[104,111] In the setting of advanced heart failure, coronary bypass or valve surgery, correction of congenital heart lesions, or in the treatment of transplantation donors and recipients, the benefits that have been attributed to intravenous T_3 therapy include improvement of cardiac index with reduction of systemic vascular resistance,[104,111] a reduction in postoperative episodes of atrial fibrillation,[107] reduction in estimated mortality rate among high-risk patients,[109] a reduced requirement for inotropic support and mechanical devices,[112,113] a lower incidence of postoperative myocardial ischemia,[113] improved cardiac allograft function,[102] and improved neuroendocrine profile with improved ventricular performance.[121] Whether the apparently beneficial cardiac effects of T_3 administration are pharmacologic effects or at least partially the effects of physiologic replacement of a true hormone deficiency are unclear. Overall, the use of T_3 for cardiac indications has not gained widespread acceptance.

APPROACH TO MANAGEMENT AND THERAPEUTIC ALTERNATIVES

It is unknown whether the spontaneously developing alterations of tissue exposure to thyroid hormone during nonthyroidal illness are advantageous or disadvantageous to the patient. Although there is interest in evaluating T_3 therapy for nonthyroidal illness syndrome, it is expected that differences in outcome resulting from such treatment will be small and difficult to demonstrate.[62,122-125] Proposed approaches have not been adequately studied for safety or efficacy in critically ill patients having nonthyroidal illness syndrome. A special niche may exist for the use of T_3 in the treatment of cardiac patients who require hemodynamic support. As a precaution, it is noted that high levels of T_3 have been identified as a risk factor for coronary events.[126] Although future research may bring about changes in the standard of care, at the present time for nonthyroidal illness syndrome most experts recommend observation without thyroid hormone treatment, with reevaluation of thyroid function tests after recovery. The philosophy of nontreatment would imply that there is no obligation to order thyroid tests unless thyroid disease is suspected.

Treatment for possible hypopituitarism is offered when caregivers believe the clinical evaluation and results of thyroid tests do not permit exclusion of intrinsic disease of the thyroid, pituitary, or hypothalamus. If the patient is euthyroid and free of reversible myocardial ischemia and if adequacy of cortisol production is assured by measurement or by concomitant administration, then treatment with thyroid hormone will probably do no harm.

IMPLICATION FOR PROGNOSIS

Normal T_3 is a favorable prognostic indicator, whereas the biochemical findings of low T_3 or other findings of nonthyroidal illness syndrome predict worse outcomes of critical illness in general.[46,110,118,127-140]

HYPOTHYROIDISM AND MYXEDEMA COMA

HYPOTHYROIDISM

Common causes of hypothyroidism include autoimmune destruction (Hashimoto's thyroiditis) or previous surgery or radioiodine ablation therapy for hyperthyroidism, as well as medication-induced causes. Patients with antithyroid antibodies may be at special risk of iodine- or amiodarone-induced hypothyroidism. The manifestations of hypothyroidism are dependent not only on the severity of hormone deficiency by laboratory testing but also the duration of hypothyroidism.

INCIDENCE

In contrast to the high frequency of finding the laboratory manifestations of nonthyroidal illness syndrome in the intensive care unit, among outpatients the prevalence of spontaneous hypothyroidism is relatively low, found in 1% to 2% in iodine-replete communities, and more commonly found in women than in men.[141-143] An age-related increase of incidence of hypothyroidism exists, and the prevalence is higher in women. The appearance of overt hypothyroidism is predicted by prior isolated TSH elevation and positive antithyroid antibodies. Hypothyroidism can be induced by iodine, amiodarone, lithium, or tyrosine kinase inhibitors.

PATHOPHYSIOLOGY

Patients with severe hypothyroidism have reduced calorigenesis and oxygen consumption. Many metabolic processes proceed at a markedly reduced rate. Glycosaminoglycan metabolism is impeded, resulting in widespread tissue deposition of hyaluronan (hyaluronic acid). A contributory factor in the production of generalized edema is transcapillary albumin escape.[144] Slowing of the metabolism of lipoproteins results in secondary hyperlipidemia. Hypercholesterolemia is common. Hypometabolism affects conversion of carotene to vitamin A and the rate of removal of vitamin K.

Reduced ventilatory responses to hypoxia and hypercapnia appear to have a dominantly central mechanism, and there may be upper airway obstruction.[145-150] The effusions of myxedema contain high concentrations of protein and cholesterol. Pericardial effusion is more characteristic than pericardial tamponade.[151-154] Vasoconstriction with or without hypertension exists. The mechanisms of resistance to catecholamine effects are complex and controversial. There is reduced responsiveness to adrenergic stimuli but actual elevation of circulating norepinephrine concentration.[155-157] Myocardial contractility, oxygen consumption, ejection time, diastolic ventricular compliance, stroke volume, heart rate, and cardiac index are reduced and systemic vascular resistance is increased.[115,119,120] The left ventricular end-diastolic pressure is not necessarily elevated in myxedema and the cardiac index may increase in response to exercise.[158-161] Nevetheless, when TSH is higher than 10 μIU/mL, there is an increased risk for congestive heart failure even at the stage of subclinical hypothyroidism.[162-164] An increased occurrence of coronary artery disease also may exist.[165-170] Hypomotility of the bowels is common. There may be coexistent iron losses as a result of menorrhagia or gastrointestinal bleeding. Malabsorption of vitamin B_{12} and folic acid may occur. A reduction in atrial natriuretic factor production may occur,[171] as well as a reduction of the glomerular filtration rate. The kidney cannot excrete a water load effectively, but antidiuretic hormone deficiency cannot be consistently implicated when hyponatremia and defective intrarenal mechanisms are suspected.[172-174] Calcium loading can result in hypercalcemia. Hyperuricemia commonly results from underexcretion of uric acid. Pituitary overproduction of prolactin but retarded responsiveness of the pituitary-adrenal axis to appropriate challenges may occur in myxedema.

CLINICAL MANIFESTATIONS

An adult patient with longstanding hypothyroidism will have multisystemic findings. Constitutional symptoms include cold intolerance, fatigue, constipation, and weight gain, the latter not invariably observed and usually modest. Dry, brittle hair may be noted. Sleep apnea may occur. Women may have galactorrhea or menorrhagia. Myopathic and arthritic complaints can lead to misdiagnosis of a primary rheumatic disorder. Patients may have carpal tunnel syndrome. A history of somnolence, dementia, syncope, or seizures may exist.

Hypertension may be attributable to myxedema. The thyroid is often atrophic but may be goitrous. The following characteristics often permit clinical diagnosis: a deep, husky quality of the voice; slow mode of speech; involuntary blepharoptosis; torpid expression; facial bloating; eyelid and infraorbital edema; sallowness, facial pallor; hearing loss; bradycardia, distant muffled heart tones; cool, dry, coarse skin; nonpitting edema of the supraclavicular fossae, hands, legs, and feet[144]; bruising; and the delayed relaxation of deep tendon reflexes. The patient may present with adynamic ileus.

Despite the reduction of glomerular filtration rate, the serum creatinine and blood urea nitrogen (BUN) are normal. Macrocytic anemia may be present with or without vitamin B_{12} deficiency, and iron deficiency is common. The erythrocyte sedimentation rate is modestly elevated. Elevation of muscle enzymes is seen in advanced cases. Unless a creatine kinase (CK) is measured, abnormal aspartate aminotransferase (AST) and alanine aminotransferase (ALT) levels of muscle origin may be misinterpreted as representative of liver dysfunction. An electrocardiogram (ECG) may show sinus bradycardia, first-degree atrioventricular (AV) block, low voltage QRS complexes, and nonspecific T-wave changes.

DIAGNOSTIC APPROACH

The TSH level of patients with untreated primary hypothyroidism can be lowered into the normal range by critical illness, but only rarely.[175] Sometimes the severity of TSH elevation is blunted by the myxedema itself, with extreme hypothyroxinemia accompanied by TSH levels that are elevated but may be less than 20 μIU/mL. In most cases of advanced hypothyroidism the TSH will be above the normal reference range and the T_4 and free T_4 will be low. Therefore, in general, during nonthyroidal illness the laboratory diagnosis of coexistent primary hypothyroidism is straightforward (see Fig. 60.2).

Milder cases of hypothyroidism potentially can be confused with the recovery phase of nonthyroidal illness syndrome, when transitory TSH elevation commonly occurs. The patient should be examined for goiter. The finding of subnormal free T_4, positive antithyroid peroxidase antibodies, or TSH above 20 μIU/mL sometimes signifies intrinsic thyroid disease.[18,51] Outpatient reassessment should occur.

In critically ill patients the diagnosis of secondary hypothyroidism is not straightforward. When a low free T_4 level by equilibrium dialysis and low TSH level are present, the question arises of whether the findings signify central hypothyroidism for any reason other than nonthyroidal illness syndrome. The most pressing immediate need would be to recognize and treat cortisol deficiency or pituitary mass effect. History of prior reproductive dysfunction, examination of cranial nerve function and mental status, and measurements of cortisol and other pituitary and target gland hormones, including follicle-stimulating hormone (FSH) and luteinizing hormone (LH) among postmenopausal women, may suggest preexisting pituitary dysfunction with or without tumor or the new occurrence of pituitary apoplexy or may help provide evidence of intactness of pituitary function. However, some critically ill patients lacking intrinsic hypothalamic or pituitary disease may have features of "eugonadal sick" syndrome as well as nonthyroidal illness syndrome. Measurement of cortisol or free cortisol may be of special value.[54] The diagnosis of pituitary tumor or apoplexy is confirmed by pituitary magnetic resonance imaging (MRI) or CT scanning.

APPROACH TO MANAGEMENT

Replacement therapy for hypothyroidism can be provided as levothyroxine (thyroxine, T_4) or liothyronine (triiodothyronine, T_3), each of which is available for oral or intravenous administration, but T_4 is the preferred hormone for the treatment of ambulatory patients and most hospitalized patients.[176-191] Normally, production of T_3 from T_4 occurs rapidly. Because of the prolonged half-life of T_4, after each daily dose or after short-term interruption of chronic T_4 therapy there are stable blood levels of T_4 and T_3.[178,179] An ambulatory hypothyroid patient, when treated with T_4 in dosage sufficient to maintain euthyroidism (normal TSH), often has normal T_3 but blood levels of T_4 slightly above the mean for a euthyroid patient.[183] A patient whose T_4 dose requirement was established before hospitalization generally should be maintained on the same dose, if it can be given orally. The oral absorption of T_4 is impeded by intestinal disease or concomitant administration of iron, sucralfate, cholestyramine, colestipol, calcium, and other drugs.[185] Enteric administration of T_4 should be separated from these drugs by at least 2 to 4 hours.

When T_4 therapy is given for overt hypothyroidism, whole body oxygen consumption and myocardial work load increase. If coronary artery disease is present, the myocardial demand for increased oxygen consumption may not be met. The risks of angina, arrhythmia, or myocardial infarction indicate the need that introduction of thyroid hormone treatment of older patients should be cautious and gradual, using starting doses less than full replacement, making incremental small doses until full replacement is achieved by biochemical parameters, with assessment of tolerance before each adjustment, and with willingness to aim for less than full replacement in case of poor tolerance. Despite the need for a cautious approach in patients who may have heart disease, the long-range goal is to reduce risk for dyslipidemia, heart failure, and coronary atherosclerosis.[192-198] Even younger patients sometimes may experience discomfort if replacement is introduced too quickly, experiencing myopathic symptoms that may worsen at first but eventually will resolve if treatment continues, or, rarely, cardiac symptoms.[198] In case of intolerance during initiation, the risk for abandonment of treatment may be reduced if a temporary T_4 dose reduction is made, with intent to work back more gradually toward full replacement. An uncommon outcome during initiation of treatment in children is increased pseudotumor cerebri.

To initiate therapy for overt hypothyroidism, patients with abrupt development of hypothyroidism or young patients may be started on full replacement doses of T_4. To reduce the risk of discomfort during initiation, young patients with longstanding severe untreated hypothyroidism may be started at a dose of levothyroxine 0.05 mg/day. Older patients or those with coronary artery disease should start with levothyroxine 0.025 mg/day. Increments of levothyroxine 0.0125 to 0.025 mg for older patients are made at about 3-week intervals until it is estimated that the patient is close to full replacement, and then the free T_4 and TSH levels are rechecked. After a dosage adjustment of T_4 therapy, 6 weeks is necessary before biochemical reevaluation will reflect a steady-state condition. After upward titration of the dose, the average adult requirement for hypothyroidism is about 0.112 mg/day levothyroxine orally. For elderly patients the dose is lower than for younger patients,[180,183] and for subclinical or early hypothyroidism, the dose of levothyroxine necessary to normalize the TSH may be as low as 0.05 to 0.075 mg/day.

It may be stated anecdotally that atrial arrhythmias are no contraindication to providing replacement therapy for hypothyroidism.[195] Development of hypothyroidism during lithium or amiodarone therapy does not require drug discontinuation but may require thyroid hormone replacement.

Subclinical hypothyroidism refers to persistent TSH elevation with normal free T_4 and absence of characteristic symptoms of hypothyroidism. Mild or subclinical hypothyroidism is not likely to present short-term risks to a critically ill patient. However, evidence suggests increased long-term morbidity, including heart failure, from untreated subclinical hypothyroidism.[162,164] Therefore, follow-up in the ambulatory setting is appropriate to determine whether TSH elevation is persistent.

The hypothyroidism associated with medication use may remit if the initiating agent is later withdrawn, so that determination of a treatment plan for hypothyroidism in part depends upon the drug and in part depends upon the severity of symptoms and duration of intended treatment with the drug held responsible for the development of hypothyroidism (Fig. 60.4).

Continuation of Established Thyroid Hormone Therapy During NPO Status

For prolonged NPO (nil per os, nothing by mouth) status or during continuous administration of substances that may impair absorption of levothyroxine or for other indications, intravenous levothyroxine may be provided daily to substitute for enteral administration, in reduced amount compared to the ambulatory daily dose, with subsequent monitoring.* The fractional gastrointestinal absorption of a tablet of levothyroxine has been reported to be about 81%, considerably higher than the earlier estimate of 48%.[183] However, concomitant administration of other substances, including calcium carbonate, may diminish absorption.[186] Intestinal malabsorption and, anecdotally, development of severe right-sided heart failure may result in unusually high dose requirements for oral levothyroxine therapy. More than half of patients receiving enteral levothyroxine may develop subclinical or overt hypothyroidism after 2 to 3 weeks if a previously established levothyroxine dose is maintained concomitantly with continuous enteral feedings.[189] Owing to the long half-life of levothyroxine and delayed tissue response to dosage adjustments, manifestations of myxedema evolve only slowly after interruption of therapy, so that interruption of levothyroxine during short-term NPO status generally is inconsequential. The American Association of Clinical Endocrinologists and the American Thyroid Association (AACE-ATA) guideline recommends that "Patients resuming L-thyroxine therapy after interruption (less than 6 weeks) and without an intercurrent cardiac event or marked weight loss may resume their previously employed full replacement doses."[191] For patients whose oral intake will be curtailed for a prolonged interval, the usual enteral dose of levothyroxine should be reduced by 20% to 40% to arrive at a dose for intravenous therapy.[176,183,188]

Precautions in the Care of the Hypothyroid Patient and Sensitivity to Pharmacologic Agents

The patient who has not yet been rendered euthyroid by therapy is at risk of water intoxication by overly vigorous intravenous fluid administration. There is risk of oversedation and central nervous system (CNS) suppression from sedative and analgesic drugs, which are metabolized and excreted abnormally slowly in the presence of hypothyroidism. The slow metabolism of drugs contributes to the marked propensity of hypothyroid patients to experience the effects of overdosage, especially with respect to digoxin, narcotics, sedatives, and analgesics. These drugs and digitalis should be given with caution, in reduced dosage. Perhaps because of reduced clearance of vitamin K, however, there is resistance to warfarin. Warfarin sensitivity may increase during treatment.

Preparation of the Patient with Untreated Hypothyroidism for Emergency Surgery or Coronary Revascularization

Subclinical hypothyroidism has not been shown to increase operative risk.[200] For patients with overt hypothyroidism, there is increased risk of perioperative complications such as sensitivity to analgesics and anesthesia, prolonged ventilator dependence, hypotension, water intoxication, and iatrogenic myxedema coma. Elective surgery should be deferred until euthyroidism is attained. For emergency surgery, younger patients without coronary disease should be prepared as if they already had myxedema coma, using a

*See References 176, 183, 185-187, 189, 190, 199.

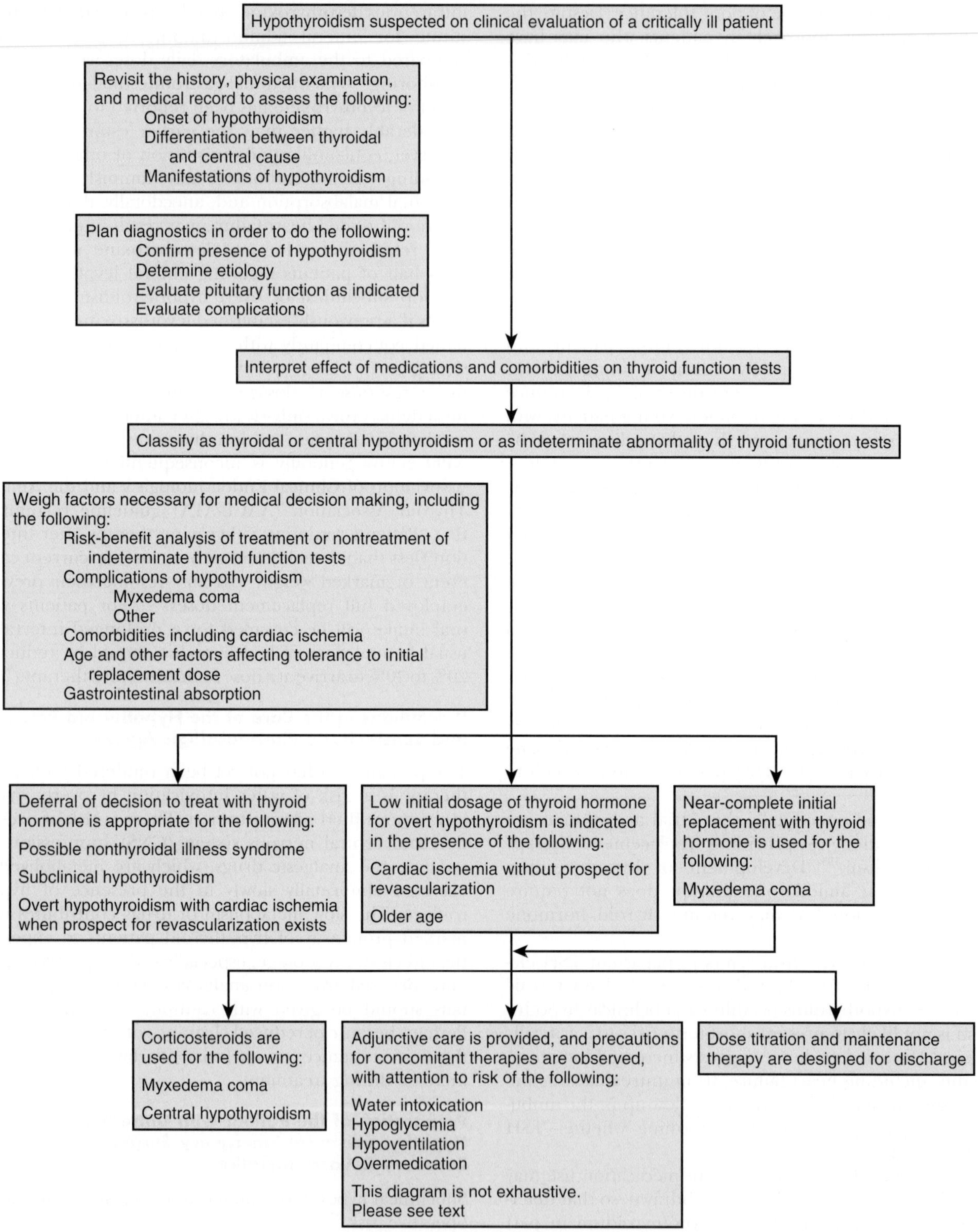

Figure 60.4 Approach to management for hypothyroidism.

preoperative intravenous bolus of levothyroxine, depending on age and transport protein status, as described later (see "Myxedema Coma"), and providing hydrocortisone coverage, with other precautions as described earlier (see "Precautions in the Care of the Hypothyroid Patient"). The risk of undiagnosed coronary insufficiency has to be considered in determining the preoperative levothyroxine replacement regimen of older patients. Emergency surgery should be deferred for 24 to 48 hours after initiation of thyroid hormone treatment if possible.[188,201,202]

Patients who are candidates for correction of reversible myocardial ischemia generally should undergo revascularization before one attempts to treat their hypothyroidism. The risks of immediate thyroid hormone replacement before noncardiac surgery should be weighed against the probably acceptable risks of successful operation without levothyroxine pretreatment.[188,194,203-212]

A protocol for patients with correctable coronary artery disease, or for others having surgery despite incompletely corrected hypothyroidism, might be to use light preoperative analgesia and sedation, avoid water intoxication, administer glucose as small volumes of concentrated dextrose solutions, be prepared to support ventilation for prolonged intervals postoperatively, provide hydrocortisone 100 mg starting immediately preoperatively and every 8 hours on the first postoperative day, taper and discontinue hydrocortisone over 5 to 7 days, and for those not yet treated, to initiate intravenous levothyroxine 0.05 mg daily in the immediate postoperative period.

PROGNOSIS

New onset of angina, myocardial infarction, or sudden death may occur within days or weeks after initiation of treatment for hypothyroidism.[192,193] Secondary hyperlipidemia and most clinical manifestations of juvenile hypothyroidism and adult myxedema are reversible after therapy, although some features, such as anemia, may require months for correction.

MYXEDEMA COMA

HISTORY AND INCIDENCE

Our present-day knowledge of myxedema coma derives from isolated case reports and small retrospective series.[213-234] Historically, the low doses of thyroid hormone normally used to initiate treatment of uncomplicated hypothyroidism, when administered enterally for myxedema coma, failed to prevent fatalities. The mortality rate was probably higher than 80%. In 1964 it was demonstrated that intravenous replacement with 500 μg levothyroxine, a dose calculated to nearly replete body stores of T_4, improved the rate of survival.[218] Liothyronine (triiodothyronine, T_3) for intravenous injection later became commercially available.

PATHOGENESIS

Myxedema coma arising in the community can generally be divided into episodes that arise spontaneously and those that arise in connection with a precipitating illness or event. Those arising spontaneously tend to occur during the colder months of the year. Precipitating factors may include congestive heart failure, pneumonia or other infection, bleeding, administration of hypotonic fluids, sedative and analgesic drugs, or anesthesia and surgery. The particular risk of hypoventilation probably is increased by the presence of heart failure, obesity, pleural or other restrictive disease, chronic obstructive lung disease, neuromuscular disease, or exposure to drugs that reduce respiratory drive.[146,147]

CLINICAL MANIFESTATIONS AND DIAGNOSIS

Myxedema coma presents with a constellation of findings including physical evidence of advanced hypothyroidism, stupor, bradycardia, hypotension, hypothermia, alveolar hypoventilation, obstipation, or ileus, and sometimes water intoxication or hypoglycemia.[224] Patients are often elderly. The condition if untreated progresses to fatal hypotension.

In the cases of myxedema coma arising spontaneously in the community, stupor progresses over several days, and families report that the number of hours spent sleeping has gradually increased to include most of a 24-hour period. Seizures have been reported.[221] In history taking it is important to ask whether the patient with suspected myxedema coma formerly was diagnosed with hypothyroidism or formerly was treated with radioactive iodine or surgery for overactive thyroid. On physical examination overt manifestations of myxedema are apparent. The patient often can be aroused and will make monosyllabic responses to questioning before lapsing back into stupor. Breathing is stertorous. Some patients with an infectious process may not have a fever. The most ominous sign of impending myxedema coma for a hypothyroid patient under inpatient observation is progressive hypothermia.

In contrast to patients with nonthyroidal illness syndrome, the laboratory evaluation will demonstrate low free T_4 and high TSH in the majority of true cases of myxedema coma. Myxedema coma resulting from pituitary failure is uncommon.[227]

APPROACH TO MANAGEMENT

Before initiating therapy for myxedema coma, the caregiver should question whether the hypothyroid patient is experiencing a self-limited consequence of a definable precipitating event. Stupor may be induced by sedatives and analgesics, especially opiates, and may resolve without rapid thyroid hormone replacement. Hyponatremia may be induced by intravenous fluid therapy. Short-term ventilator dependency may result from surgery. Yet each of these complications by itself does not require rapid replacement of thyroid hormone therapy unless conservative management fails.

A blood sample should be withdrawn for determination of TSH, free T_4, and serum cortisol levels before treatment is initiated. In the presence of progressive hypothermia and with a clinical picture of advanced myxedema, therapy should be initiated before the return of the results of thyroid function tests. If the TSH level is not elevated, the diagnosis of myxedema coma must be questioned. The needed initial dose of levothyroxine is unlikely to cause adverse effects, should the laboratory studies unexpectedly suggest euthyroidism or nonthyroidal illness syndrome.

The patient should be treated in an intensive care unit. Complications during treatment of myxedema coma include gastrointestinal bleeding and intracranial hemorrhage, which may result from coagulopathy resulting from myxedema itself. Pressors are generally ineffective in combating hypotension and may precipitate arrhythmia. Efforts at rewarming the patient may precipitate shock as a result of vasodilation in an individual whose cardiac output cannot match the demand. Treatment should include fluid restriction, avoidance of hypotonic fluids, administration of glucose as concentrated solutions if required, avoidance of pressors, and use of ordinary blankets for rewarming. Respiration should be supported as needed to treat alveolar hypoventilation.

The author would advise restricting use of a 400- to 500-μg levothyroxine intravenous bolus to those patients whose myxedema coma arose in the community without obvious precipitating cause and who are known to have normal serum albumin and absence of cardiac risk factors. If the patient is hypoalbuminemic or the serum albumin is unknown, or if the patient has cardiac risk factors, an initial 200- to 300-μg levothyroxine intravenous bolus should be used for myxedema coma, and, if coexistent precipitating illness is present, combination therapy with liothyronine (triiodothyronine, T_3) could be considered. If an albumin level is subsequently reported normal and if the patient demonstrates no arrhythmia or manifestations of cardiac ischemia, 100 μg of levothyroxine can be added every several hours to bring the cumulative dose up to 500 μg in the first 24 hours. Such replacement provides protection against relapsing hormonal deficiency in a way that short-acting T_3 monotherapy cannot. The oral route is unsatisfactory for initial therapy because of the likelihood of ileus or delayed absorption. After intravenous treatment, T_4 can be withheld for several days until the patient is able to take medication orally, or 50 μg of levothyroxine daily can be administered intravenously beginning on the second day. Hydrocortisone 100 mg every 8 hours is given during the first 24 hours. Glucocorticoids are tapered and discontinued before discharge. There should be a low threshold for evaluation for the presence of coronary artery disease.

THERAPEUTIC ALTERNATIVES

There is not sufficient evidence to strongly advocate for or against therapy with liothyronine (triiodothyronine, T_3). Arguments in favor of intravenous levothyroxine as monotherapy include its long history of successful use, its ability to prevent relapsing of hypothyroidism, avoidance of supranormal levels of T_3, and the observation that in the absence of intercurrent illness T_3 levels become normal within 24 hours.

Theoretical controversy continues to exist on whether to include intravenous liothyronine in the initial treatment plan. Some authorities recommend using both hormones at the outset, especially if coexistent illnesses are present that might impede conversion of T_4 to T_3.[227,234] Additional arguments in favor of including liothyronine relate to the delayed conversion of T_4 that is seen in hypometabolic patients and the more rapid effect on tissues when T_3 therapy is used.[181] In combination therapy, the recommended intravenous doses are approximately 10 μg of liothyronine initially and 10 μg of liothyronine every 8 to 12 hours on the first day, combined with an initial loading dose of about 200 to 250 μg levothyroxine. This treatment is followed by approximately 100 μg of levothyroxine daily intravenously on the second day and 50 μcg levothyroxine daily thereafter. On the other hand, it has been speculated that some cases of fatality were caused by relatively high T_3 levels attained early in therapy.[225] Conventional treatment with levothyroxine alone has not been shown to be inferior and is generally effective.

PROGNOSIS

Patient findings associated with fatality have included old age, cerebrovascular bleeding, or myocardial infarction during treatment[213,225,226,229] or suspected coronary events after recovery.[218] In a series of 11 cases the level of consciousness, Glasgow score, and APACHE II score were predictive of death.[232] Treatment factors associated with fatality may include overly gradual oral regimen of replacement of thyroid hormone, high replacement doses of thyroid hormone [liothyronine (triiodothyronine, T_3) doses = 75 μg/day, levothyroxine doses = 500 μg/day], or high measured levels of T_3 during treatment.[213,225,229] Within 6 to 36 hours most patients treated with T_4 in sufficient dosage experience a rise of temperature and blood pressure; improvement of mentation; and through peripheral conversion of T_4, correction of low T_3 levels.

HYPERTHYROIDISM, THYROID STORM, THYROCARDIAC CRISIS, AND CORONARY ARTERY SPASM

HYPERTHYROIDISM

In the United States, with reference to the uptake of radioactive iodine during diagnostic testing, the common causes of high-uptake hyperthyroidism are Graves' disease, toxic multinodular goiter, and toxic adenoma. Low-uptake causes of endogenous hyperthyroidism are recognized, having a self-limited course, and medications may cause hyperthyroidism.

PREVALENCE AND INCIDENCE

The age-related incidence of hyperthyroidism depends on the cause of hyperthyroidism.[141-143,235,236] The prevalence of overt hyperthyroidism is between 0.5% and 2% in women, and is 10 times more common in women than in men in iodine replete areas, with an annual incidence rate of 0.4 per 1000 women and 0.1 per 1000 men.[141,143] In Sweden the overall incidences of Graves' disease, toxic multinodular goiter, and toxic adenoma were 17.7, 5.4, and 2.7 per 100,000 persons per year, respectively, but the peak age-specific incidence of toxic multinodular goiter and toxic adenoma occurred in the 80-plus age group: 31.5 per 100,000 persons per year.[235] In the ambulatory setting among adult patients, the overall prevalence of subclinical hyperthyroidism (isolated TSH suppression) is 0.5% to 6.3%, with variability dependent on population under study, inclusion or exclusion of patients with thyroid disease, and definition of threshold TSH for inclusion.[141-143]

PATHOGENESIS

In the hyperthyroidism of Graves' disease, the TSH receptor/G protein/adenylyl cyclase complex is activated by abnormal thyroid-stimulating immunoglobulins with affinity for the TSH receptor. The associated phenomena of orbitopathy and dermopathy also are thought to result from autoimmune processes. In some cases of hyperthyroidism resulting from toxic adenoma, a G protein mutation is demonstrable that results in activation of the membrane adenylyl cyclase associated with the TSH receptor complex. Plummer's disease (toxic multinodular goiter) is most commonly seen in older patients and represents a late outcome in the natural history of euthyroid multinodular goiter. Because of TSH suppression, in toxic multinodular goiter the internodular thyroidal tissue is metabolically inactive in accumulating iodine.

In susceptible individuals, especially those from iodine-deficient regions of the world or with preexisting nodular thyroid disease, hyperthyroidism can be produced by iodine (Jod-Basedow phenomenon). Hyperthyroidism can be produced by glandular destruction, as in thyroiditis, characterized by having low radioactive iodine uptake. Common causes of low-uptake hyperthyroidism include silent thyroiditis, postpartum thyroiditis, subacute thyroiditis, and exogenous thyroid hormone. Substances implicated in drug-induced forms of destructive thyroiditis causing hyperthyroidism include amiodarone, lithium, interferon-α, interleukin 2, iodine, and iodinated contrast agents.[236] Two different mechanisms of hyperthyroidism are possible during amiodarone therapy: iodine-induced thyrotoxicosis and drug-induced thyroiditis.

In general, intense activation of the TSH receptor complex results in an increased ratio of T_3 to T_4 resulting from direct thyroidal T_3 secretion. The augmentation of thyroidal T_3 release of hyperthyroid patients may result in part from enhancement of the thyroidal type 2 deiodinase activity.[237] The altered ratio of T_3 to T_4 is not observed in destructive hyperthyroidism.[238]

Hyperthyroidism is characterized by hypermetabolism and increased thermogenesis. There is enhanced target organ response to sympathoadrenal stimuli. Multisystemic changes of organ physiology occur. Of special interest to the intensivist is the pathophysiology of the cardiac manifestations, discussed in the section on "Thyrocardiac Crisis and Coronary Spasm."

CLINICAL MANIFESTATIONS

Intubation and central lines may prevent adequate palpation of the thyroid. If thyroidal bruit is detected on auscultation of the upper poles of the lateral lobes of the thyroid in a hyperthyroid patient, the classification of the cause of hyperthyroidism as Graves' disease essentially is assured. The eyes, nails, and skin should be examined for evidence of orbitopathy, onycholysis, fine skin quality (smooth elbows), or dermopathy ("pretibial myxedema"). The remainder of the physical examination is likely to yield findings that are suggestive of hyperthyroidism but nonspecific, such as hyperhidrosis, atrial arrhythmia, hyperdynamic heart, precordial lift, systolic ejection murmur, S_3 gallop, restlessness, hyperkinesia, agitation, or briskness of Achilles reflexes. In severe cases, adrenal reserve may be insufficient.[239] A different spectrum of symptoms and signs has been reported in the elderly, who may appear apathetic or depressed, and among whom the average number of thyrotoxic symptoms may be as low as two, with dominance of weight loss, proximal myopathy, tremor, and cardiac manifestations such as heart failure, sinus tachycardia, or atrial fibrillation.[240-243]

DIAGNOSTIC APPROACH

Laboratory Diagnosis

The laboratory findings will include TSH below 0.1 μIU/mL and usually elevation of total and free T_4. If the T_4 level is normal and TSH is below 0.1 μIU/mL, elevated T_3 will identify T_3 toxicosis. Diagnosis of amiodarone-induced thyrotoxicosis requires demonstration of low TSH, and a T_3 level higher than the low levels typical of the euthyroid amiodarone-treated patient.

T_4 Hyperthyroidism

The finding of high T_4 without high T_3, although atypical of hyperthyroidism, sometimes occurs after surgery, during exposure to substances that block conversion of T_4 to T_3, among the elderly or the critically ill, or sporadically. During the acute illness, differentiation between euthyroid hyperthyroxinemia and hyperthyroidism may be difficult.[244-248]

Subclinical Hyperthyroidism

Stable TSH suppression outside the critical care setting, sustained over several months, in the absence of drug effects or pituitary or hypothalamic disease, and without concomitant iodothyronine elevations, suggests subclinical hyperthyroidism. Patients with toxic nodular goiters in the early years of their disease may have TSH suppressions that are only marginal, and yet the diagnosis of subclinical hyperthyroidism can be suspected by thyroid palpation and confirmed by finding autonomous nodularity on thyroid scanning.

Determining the Cause

Classification of hyperthyroidism according to radioiodine uptake provides information about the expected course of the thyrotoxicosis and appropriateness of treatment alternatives. The so-called high-uptake forms of hyperthyroidism (Graves' disease, toxic adenoma, toxic multinodular goiter, and TSH-secreting pituitary adenoma) are appropriately treated with thionamide drugs. The low-uptake forms caused by destructive thyroiditis or iodine are treated primarily by beta blockers and possibly corticosteroids, depending upon cause and severity, and are self-limited in duration. In high-uptake forms of hyperthyroidism, a 24-hour radioiodine uptake evaluation sometimes yields intermediate range or normal results, suggesting mild disease or an unrecognized source of exogenous iodide. In toxic adenoma and toxic multinodular goiter, even though these disorders are classified as high-uptake forms of hyperthyroidism, a normal or high normal uptake is common (see discussion under "Diagnostic Approach to Thyroid Disease"). In the critical care setting, radioiodine uptake and scanning tests may be impracticable. Ultrasonography may define the vascularity of the gland and the presence or absence of nodularity. A thyroidal bruit, endocrine orbitopathy, or high levels of antibodies to the TSH receptor may suggest that Graves' disease is the probable cause of hyperthyroidism.

APPROACH TO MANAGEMENT

If endogenous hyperthyroidism was recognized before hospitalization, and if biochemical euthyroidism had been maintained until the time of admission by use of a stable dosage of antithyroid medication, the established dose probably should be maintained during the critical illness.

For those having subclinical hyperthyroidism, the 2011 Hyperthyroidism Management Guidelines of the American Thyroid Association and the American Association of Clinical Endocrinologists suggest that persistent findings of TSH at 0.1 μIU/mL or below over 3 to 6 months should lead to determination of cause, with a decision for treatment or observation determined by patient characteristics.[162,164,236]

For those critically ill patients having overt hyperthyroidism classifiable as a probable high-uptake form, generally treatment should consist of antithyroid medication (Fig. 60.5). Management of most aspects of overt hyperthyroidism are addressed in the guideline, including many of the issues important to critical care medicine.[236] The drugs used in treatment of hyperthyroidism include the

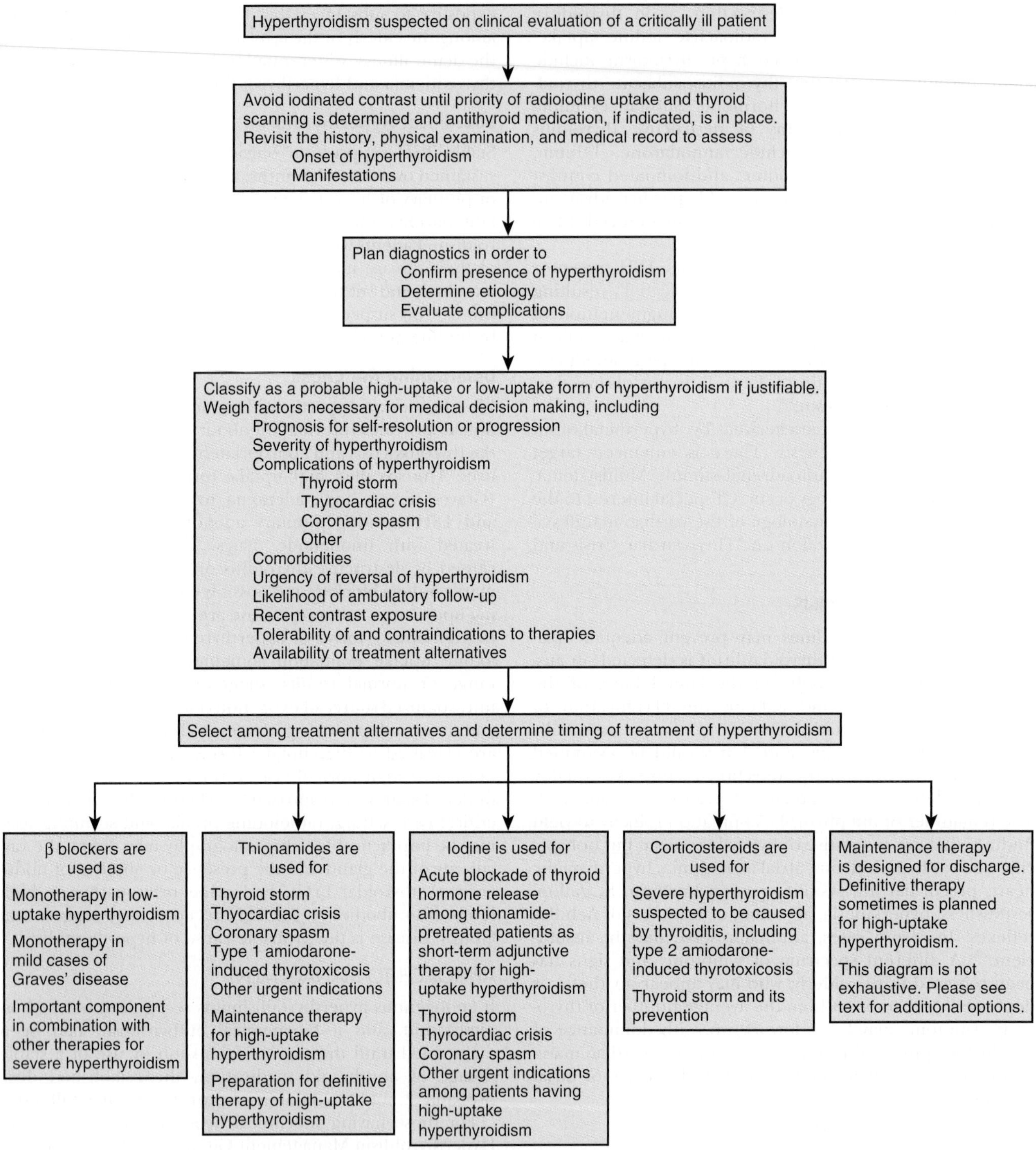

Figure 60.5 Approach to management for hyperthyroidism.

thionamides propylthiouracil and the longer-acting drug methimazole.[249-259] Thionamides inhibit the coupling of moieties on TG and organification of iodide, thus preventing storage and synthesis of thyroid hormone. By inhibiting 5′-monodeiodination of T_4 by the D1 enzyme, propylthiouracil reduces peripheral conversion of T_4 to T_3.[249,260] To initiate therapy it is common practice to start with a relatively higher dose than will be required for maintenance and to choose a dosage on the basis of the apparent clinical severity of hyperthyroidism and size of the thyroid gland. Methimazole can cause a reversible cholestatic picture of hepatic injury. Propylthiouracil, however, can cause irreversible hepatic necrosis resulting in fatality.[256] Both drugs can cause neutropenia or agranulocytosis.[261] A rare adverse effect of propylthiouracil is antineutrophil cytoplasmic antibody–positive vasculitis. Methimazole taken in the first trimester of pregnancy has been associated with aplasia cutis and choanal atresia of the neonate. When thionamide drug therapy is chosen, except for hyperthyroidism during the first trimester of pregnancy, for thyroid storm, or for patients having a history of a minor reaction to methimazole, because of the difference in severity of potential hepatotoxicity, the preferred drug for virtually every patient is methimazole rather than propylthiouracil.[236] For uncomplicated hyperthyroidism the initial daily dosage might be propylthiouracil 50 to 150 mg every 8 hours or methimazole 10 mg twice daily. After control is achieved, methimazole usually is converted to once-daily therapy and, after gradual dose reduction, sometimes is given in doses as little as 5 mg daily. Once control is achieved, methimazole may be given as a single daily dose. Propylthiouracil may be reduced to as little as 50 mg two or three times daily but must be administered in a divided dosage to prevent escape.

During hyperthyroidism beta-blocker therapy is the preferred method of controlling tachycardia and peripheral manifestations of sensitivity to catecholamines. Among the beta blockers, there is the greatest experience with propranolol. The metabolism of propranolol is enhanced, and blood levels are highly variable in hyperthyroidism. Most patients requiring enteral propranolol for hyperthyroidism should begin with 10 to 40 mg every 6 hours. Other beta blockers have been used, and some advocate cardioselective agents.[262-278] Definitive treatment of hyperthyroidism consists of radioactive iodine or surgery. Use of radioiodine therapy is inappropriate for low-uptake hyperthyroidism.

Conservative management of low-uptake causes of hyperthyroidism consists of observation or beta blockers. In cases of amiodarone-induced thyrotoxicosis, in order to define a treatment strategy that might include corticosteroids, an effort should be made to classify the hyperthyroidism as type 1 or type 2 amiodarone-induced thyrotoxicosis.

Classification and Management of Amiodarone-Induced Thyrotoxicosis

Hyperthyroidism may occur in up to 6% of amiodarone-treated patients in iodine-sufficient regions, and in up to 9.6% or more of treated patients in iodine-deficient regions.[30,236] A regimen recommended for detection of thyroid dysfunction during amiodarone therapy is to check before and at 1 and 3 months following initiation, and then at 3- to 6-month intervals thereafter.[236] Amiodarone-induced thyrotoxicosis may be recognized by characteristic clinical and laboratory findings, including tachycardia, weight loss, proximal muscle weakness, low TSH, and high or high normal T_3 and free T_3.[279-292] Classification as type 1 or type 2 amiodarone-induced thyrotoxicosis is based on the mechanism of the hyperthyroidism. Type 1 amiodarone-induced thyrotoxicosis is a Jod-Basedow type of hyperthyroidism consequent to the high iodine content of amiodarone, likely to be associated with preexisting nodular goiter or, less commonly, Graves' disease. On color flow Doppler examination, the gland may appear hypervascular. Despite the iodine exposure from amiodarone, the radioiodine uptake, though relatively low, may be measurable, and technetium MIBI (methoxyisobutylisonitrile) scanning may show areas of uptake. Type 2 amiodarone-induced thyrotoxicosis, now by far the more common type, results from a drug-related destructive thyroiditis, often occurring in a patient having no prior history of known thyroid disease and not having thyroidal enlargement, sometimes recognized by markedly diminished vascularity on color flow Doppler examination.[284,289] Radioiodine uptake is negligible or absent. When the differentiation can be made, type 1 and type 2 amiodarone-induced thyrotoxicosis are addressed by different management strategies.[291] In type 1 amiodarone-induced thyrotoxicosis, thionamide therapy is used. Because there is unlikely to be a full response during continuation of amiodarone, the usual recommendation is to interrupt amiodarone for type 1 amiodarone-induced thyrotoxicosis. Once the iodine stores from the previous treatment have dissipated, radioactive iodine may be administered to ablate the thyroid in preparation for reinstitution of amiodarone, especially if hyperthyroidism still is demonstrable. Sometimes surgery is the best option available for the treatment of resistant cases of type 1 amiodarone-induced thyrotoxicosis.[279] Postoperatively amiodarone may be reinstituted.

For type 2 amiodarone-induced hyperthyroidism, the course of the hyperthyroidism may be transitory, with subsequent development of hypothyroidism among some patients.[31,32] Glucocorticoids promote resolution of type 2 amiodarone-induced thyrotoxicosis.[280,290] During glucocorticoid therapy it is not necessary to interrupt amiodarone.[288,292] A typical starting dose is 30 mg prednisone daily.[292] Because there may be mixed types or indeterminate presentations in which the classification of the amiodarone-induced thyrotoxicosis may be uncertain, in actual practice thionamides and glucocorticoids both may be used during initiation of treatment. In this country, perchlorate, another option, is not available.

Precautions in the Care of the Hyperthyroid Patient

Thyrotoxic patients display enhanced susceptibility to sympathetic stimuli and adrenergic drugs. They may be volume depleted and may not tolerate excessive diuresis. Before administering contrast material, the physician should consider whether the radioactive iodine uptake or thyroid scanning tests can be deferred. Administration of a thionamide should precede use of iodinated substances.

Preparation of the Thyrotoxic Patient for Emergency Nonthyroidal Surgery

Elective surgery should be deferred until euthyroidism is attained. In deciding whether to operate, the risk of perioperative fatality due to hyperthyroidism has to be weighed against the strength of the medical indications for immediate surgery. Before emergency surgery, the risk of thyroid storm obligates the caregiver to prepare the patient with antithyroid treatment.[293-295] For newly diagnosed patients with endogenous hyperthyroidism requiring rapid preparation for emergency surgery, preoperatively propylthiouracil 200 mg every 4 hours or methimazole 20 mg every 4 hours has been recommended.[294] At least 2 hours after the first dose of propylthiouracil, the patient should receive iodide. Ipodate or iopanoic acid (as described later in the section on treatment of thyroid storm) are potentially useful but unavailable in many countries. In the absence of contraindications, propranolol orally in a dosage up to 20 to 40 mg four times per day or more should be started. The regimen should be continued in the immediate postoperative period by use of a nasogastric tube if necessary. By the time of discharge methimazole would be the preferred thionamide, and the dose should be tapered. Glucocorticoids also may have a role in preoperative preparation, initially 100 mg hydrocortisone every 8 hours.

ALTERNATIVES FOR TREATMENT

For patients who cannot take oral medications, antithyroid drugs can be prepared for rectal administration.[251,252] Patients with a history of minor skin reactions to one thionamide may be treated with the other. Patients with a history of hepatocellular jaundice during propylthiouracil therapy may be treated with methimazole.[254,257] Lithium has been used for the control of hyperthyroidism in patients unable to use propylthiouracil or methimazole, starting at a dose of 300 mg twice per day.[254,296-299] The ability of the radiographic contrast agents iopanoic acid and ipodate to inhibit thyroid hormone release, peripheral conversion of T_4, and possibly nuclear binding of T_3 has been exploited in certain hyperthyroid states including cases of destructive hyperthyroidism and in thionamide intolerance.[300-305] The use of radiographic contrast agents usually should be adjunctive to thionamides and beta-blocker therapy. Instances of escape after prolonged use of iodinated substances have been reported.[302] Therefore, if a radiographic contrast agent is used as an antithyroid medication without antecedent and concomitant thionamide medication, some patients will require thyroidectomy as soon as reasonable control has been obtained.[295] Recommended daily doses are ipodate 500 to 1000 mg orally or iopanoic acid 500 mg twice daily. These iodinated oral cholecystographic agents have not been clinically available in the United States recently.

For patients with contraindications to the use of beta blockers, older regimens included guanethidine[306] or reserpine,[307] which are seldom used at present. For control of heart rate in patients with reversible airway disease, diltiazem is an alternative to beta blockers.[308,309] Iodine has been used to reduce vascularity of the thyroid and inhibit thyroid function. Brief treatment with iodine may hasten clinical recovery by acutely blocking release of thyroid hormone (see section "Thyroid Storm and Thyrocardiac Crisis"). Thionamide administration must precede use of iodine, and must be continued during treatment. Accidental gastrointestinal injuries have been reported.[310-312]

PROGNOSIS

After a treatment course with thionamides administered for as long as 18 to 24 months, a variably reported percentage of patients with Graves' disease (probably <50%) will be in remission. Some will develop hypothyroidism as a result of Hashimoto's disease. With toxic adenoma, remission of hyperthyroidism is uncommon. With toxic multinodular goiter, hyperthyroidism is persistent. Low-uptake forms of hyperthyroidism are self-limited conditions, and hyperthyroidism usually resolves within 6 months. If there is an offending drug, the mechanism of hyperthyroidism and the importance of the drug to patient well-being have to be weighed in deciding whether discontinuation should be advised. Storage of amiodarone in adipose tissue may prolong the episode of thyroid dysfunction. The hyperthyroidism of destructive thyroiditis, as may be seen with lithium therapy or type 2 amiodarone-induced hyperthyroidism, may self-resolve with the passage of time, or the thyrotoxicosis may be followed by a more prolonged period of hypothyroidism.

Socioeconomic factors coupled with a lapse in care may account for some of the long-term morbidity and mortality risks associated with hyperthyroidism.[313] Some cardiovascular abnormalities may persist after treatment of hyperthyroidism. Some but not all epidemiologic studies suggest that an increased overall mortality risk is associated with a history of hyperthyroidism, even after radioiodine treatment.[314-322]

THYROID STORM

Thyroid storm is a potentially lethal complication of hyperthyroidism, managed in the critical care setting.[231,236,323-327] In a hyperthyroid patient the diagnosis of this emergency is based on the clinical presentation.*

HISTORY AND INCIDENCE

In the present day, thyroid storm is seen after the development of intercurrent illness or infection, operative intervention for nonthyroidal illness, or infrequently after exposure to medications that exacerbate either the severity of hyperthyroidism or patient sensitivity to thyroid hormone excess. Initially this entity was recognized as a complication of thyroidectomy for hyperthyroidism that had been performed in unprepared patients.[328] In an early series, two thirds of the patients died[329]; postmortem examinations were not illuminating. After it was recognized that patients should be rendered euthyroid before thyroidectomy, the incidence of storm after thyroidectomy declined, and the literature began to focus on nonsurgical precipitating factors.[331,332] As early as 1960, after the use of reserpine and glucocorticoids was added to therapy with antithyroid medication and iodide, it was reported that the mortality rate from thyroid storm had been reduced from 60% or 70% nearly to 25%.[332] In 1966 the importance of initiating thionamide therapy before iodide administration was emphasized.[334] By employing guanethidine as reported in 1969[306] or reserpine therapy reported in 1970,[307] the mortality rate of thyroid storm in small series was as low as 7% and 0%, respectively. By the mid-1970s the use of propranolol had largely replaced earlier methods of attaining sympathetic blockade.[262,264,266,337]

Thyroid storm is a relatively infrequent reason for admission to critical care units. Even before the existence of modern antithyroid therapy, the estimated incidence of thyroid storm among patients hospitalized for hyperthyroidism was only 7%.[332]

PATHOGENESIS

Graves' hyperthyroidism is the most common thyroid disorder identified with thyroid storm, but storm has also been associated with toxic multinodular goiter, amiodarone-induced hyperthyroidism,[282] and rarely exogenous thyroid hormone overdosage.[330,345,347,363] Precipitating factors precede the development of thyroid storm in the

*See References 239, 247, 262, 278, 297, 306, 307, 328-375.

majority of cases. Identifiable events accompanying thyroid storm may include infection,[335] surgery,[328,329,335,372] administration of radioactive iodine,[331,341,357] recent exposure to iodine or iodinated contrast dye, or withdrawal of inorganic iodide,[329,354] trauma,[48,361,368] parturition,[333] diabetic ketoacidosis,[358,366] status epilepticus and stroke,[351] pulmonary embolism,[332] pseudoephedrine administration,[346] other precipitating events, discontinuation of antithyroid medication,[331] or a lapse in care.[340] In the absence of thionamide therapy, administration of iodine-containing compounds floods the gland with iodine, but inhibition of hormone release by iodine may be incomplete or temporary, and thyroid storm may occur during continued administration of iodine.[329] Recently instituted or incompletely effective thionamide therapy does not necessarily protect against storm induced by radiation thyroiditis.[344] Reliance on lithium[297] or propranolol[265] as monotherapy for preoperative preparation may be responsible for thyroid storm.

In thyroid storm the T_3 and total T_4 levels are not different from levels in uncomplicated cases of hyperthyroidism, but the dialyzable fraction of T_4 (the percentage that is free) is higher.[338,339] This finding has been taken to support the idea that the medical illness may cause acute unbinding of thyroid hormone from transport proteins. Relative adrenal insufficiency may be present.

CLINICAL MANIFESTATIONS AND DIAGNOSIS

The definition of thyroid storm has come to include a constellation of fever greater than 100° F, tachycardia out of proportion to fever, and exaggerated manifestations of thyrotoxicosis affecting at least two other of the following systems: cardiac, gastrointestinal, or neurologic.[332] A clinical scoring system for identifying thyroid storm has been endorsed in which identification of a precipitating factor is one diagnostic criterion.[236,324] The system also identifies a range of scores that is used to classify a patient's presentation as impending thyroid storm. Cardiac findings may include marked tachycardia out of proportion to fever, atrial arrhythmia, heart failure, shock, ventricular tachycardia, and ventricular fibrillation.[352,364,360,371] Gastrointestinal symptoms include hyperdefecation, diarrhea, vomiting, abdominal pain, acute abdomen,[349,350,370] and jaundice or liver failure.[353,355,356,375] Hepatic failure usually is a result of right-sided heart failure. Rhabdomyolysis may occur.[342] Neurologic features include tremulousness, agitation, hyperkinesia, muscle weakness, delirium or psychosis, apathy, prostration, seizures, or obtundation. Brisk contraction and relaxation time often are observed when deep tendon reflexes are elicited. Fever is the hallmark of the condition, sometimes as high as 106° F. As a practical matter, even if another underlying cause of fever is identified, any febrile patient (temperature >100° F) who has known hyperthyroidism with marked tachycardia or exaggerated manifestations of hyperthyroidism is best treated as having impending thyroid storm.

No specific laboratory finding defines the presence of thyroid storm, but rather, thyroid storm is defined by the characteristic clinical picture, which will be accompanied by laboratory findings of TSH suppression and generally free T_4 elevation. Measurement of T_3 is not necessary unless free T_4 levels are normal.[336] Rarely, in the presence of coexisting illness, the T_4 may be elevated but total T_3 may be normal.[247]

APPROACH TO MANAGEMENT

Although thionamides block the synthesis of thyroid hormone, this effect will not benefit the patient until several weeks later, when thyroid glandular stores of preformed hormone have been discharged. To block hormone release acutely, iodide is administered. Thionamide pretreatment with a loading dose is essential to induce a biosynthetic blockade that will prevent flooding of the gland with iodide, with the attendant future risk of exacerbation of hyperthyroidism. Glucocorticoid therapy is employed to correct potential relative adrenal insufficiency.[239] Beta blockers combat cardiac sensitivity to catecholamines and reduce central and peripheral neurologic manifestations of hyperthyroidism. Propylthiouracil, glucocorticoids, and propranolol block conversion of T_4 to T_3.

Treatment of thyroid storm requires thionamide, beta blocker, and glucocorticoid doses higher than usually required for ordinary care. There is no comparative evidence that would support specific titration rules or a preference among differing dose ranges that have been recommended for thionamides and beta blockers.[231,236,323-326,337] Nevertheless, although incomplete response to beta blockers could require upward dose titration, caution should be exercised in the initial dosing, and tolerance to the initial dose should be demonstrated.

A reasonable starting regimen is an initial propylthiouracil loading dose of 600 mg, and thereafter a continued dose of 200 mg every 4 hours, or 1200 mg daily in divided dosage, given orally or by nasogastric tube. The literature suggests that the initial propylthiouracil loading dose may be as high as 1000 mg, with a continued dose of 250 mg every 4 hours, or 1500 mg daily. Propylthiouracil inhibits peripheral conversion of T_4 to T_3 and therefore is favored over methimazole in thyroid storm. Alternatively, methimazole 60 to 80 mg per day in divided dosage may be used.[324,325,337] These doses are reduced as the patient begins to respond. Beginning 1 to 2 hours after the loading dose of propylthiouracil or methimazole, saturated solution of potassium iodide, 5 drops every 6 hours, is given, or Lugol's solution, 30 drops daily in divided dosage three to four times a day. Hydrocortisone is administered in a dose of 100 mg every 8 hours. Beta-blocker therapy is considered to be one of the mainstays of therapy, useful for control of tachyarrhythmias and other manifestations of the characteristic increased sensitivity to catecholamines. Although the literature on beta-blocker therapy during thyroid storm acknowledges use of or requirement for extremely high doses in some cases, nevertheless adverse effects including hypotension or cardiorespiratory arrest also may be seen in conjunction with beta-blocker therapy.[277,278] For patients having evidence of heart failure or hypotension or developing these findings during treatment, beta blockers must be given during hemodynamic monitoring with great caution, and alternative methods of controlling heart rate and rhythm should be considered. Despite evidence that extremely high doses may be required by some patients, a starting oral dose of propranolol as low as 20 to 40 mg every 6 hours has been recommended.[325] The propranolol dose requirement may be as high 480 mg daily, given as 60 to 80 mg propranolol every 4 hours, or 80 to 120 mg every 6 hours.[231,323,326] With monitoring of blood pressure and rhythm, while awaiting the effects of orally administered propranolol, 0.5 to 1 mg propranolol intravenously may be cautiously provided; the dose may be increased to 2 to 3 mg over 15 minutes if tolerated.[324] Digoxin is used for atrial fibrillation. The underlying cause of thyroid storm must be identified and treated, cultures made, and in general empiric antibiotics may be considered until infection is excluded. Because salicylates may promote unbinding of thyroid hormone from transport proteins, for control of fever, acetaminophen is preferred, and cooling blankets may be required. Hemodynamic monitoring should be provided as appropriate. Fluid and electrolyte replacement are necessary, and administration of vitamins is prudent.

Often, propylthiouracil is tapered by the time of discharge to 300 to 600 mg daily in divided dosage, or methimazole to a dose of 30 to 60 mg, with intent for further outpatient dose reduction. The glucocorticoids are tapered and discontinued, and the iodide dose is reduced to 2 drops three times per day. The iodide therapy is discontinued within 2 weeks. In consideration of the desirability of future radioactive iodine therapy, it is important to anticipate potential financial, philosophic, or emotional barriers to follow-up care and definitive therapy.

THERAPEUTIC ALTERNATIVES

For thyroid storm propylthiouracil normally is administered enterally, but the rectal route for administration has been described.[253,259] Lithium is not a substitute for thionamide therapy unless unacceptable intolerance to thionamide therapy has been demonstrated. The initial dose of lithium in this setting is 300 mg every 6 hours.[325] The route of administration of iodide may be sublingual or rectal by retention enemas.[253,350] Ipodate therapy 500 mg once or twice daily and iopanoic acid are effective, but these agents presently have become unavailable in many countries.[305] For patients at risk of cardiac decompensation, the rapid-acting drug esmolol may replace propranolol as initial intravenous therapy, used while awaiting the effects of orally administered cautious doses of propranolol.[275] Adjuncts to therapy, reserved for resistant cases, include peritoneal dialysis, plasma exchange, or plasmapheresis.* Thyroidectomy also has been used successfully for iodine-induced storm and failure of medical management.[354,359,362]

PROGNOSIS

Clinical markers suggesting a poor prognosis include delay in therapy, coma, jaundice, and shock. Normalization of temperature, drop of heart rate, and improved mental status are favorable signs. With treatment as described earlier, a sharp reduction of circulating thyroid hormone concentration is observable by the second hospital day, but it may be several days before adequate stabilization of clinical manifestations is seen.[325]

THYROCARDIAC CRISIS AND CORONARY ARTERY SPASM

In most cases of overt hyperthyroidism and in thyroid storm, cardiac manifestations are one component of a multisystem presentation. Chest discomfort is not an uncommon complaint among patients with hyperthyroidism, even among the young, and usually has benign significance. Characteristic anginal symptoms are uncommon. Sometimes, however, cardiac manifestations dominate the clinical presentation, especially in the elderly or in patients whose cardiac events emerge suddenly.* Whereas the full evolution of most manifestations of hyperthyroidism emerge over an extended period, the sudden onset of thyrocardiac effects may complicate any form of thyrotoxicosis, even fleeting or recent-onset thyrotoxicosis, such as that resulting from subacute thyroiditis or overdosage of thyroid hormone, and may occur among young patients. In the absence of other criteria permitting a diagnosis of thyroid storm, thyrocardiac symptoms may present with a medical crisis.

PREVALENCE AND INCIDENCE OF THYROCARDIAC DISEASE

Thyrocardiac crises without storm are relatively more common than thyroid storm.[376-379] Preexisting heart disease and age older than 60 are risk factors for manifestations of thyrocardiac disease.[377,379,380] Among 462 patients with hyperthyroidism who had no associated organic heart disease and who were referred for radioactive iodine, a 1958 study reported the prevalence to be atrial fibrillation 10%, congestive heart failure with atrial fibrillation 5%, and congestive heart failure with sinus rhythm 0.6%.[377] In a study of unselected hyperthyroid patients, the prevalence was atrial fibrillation 9% and congestive heart failure 6%.[379] In the Framingham Heart Study, for persons with TSH levels 0.1 μIU/mL or less compared with persons with normal TSH, the relative risk of atrial fibrillation was 3.1 (95% confidence interval, 1.7 to 5.5). Among patients with TSH suppression of less severity (i.e., >0.1 μIU/mL), the risk for atrial fibrillation was comparable with the risk among people with normal TSH.[381] After emergency presentation with atrial fibrillation, screening for hyperthyroidism may be justified by the possibility of detecting unrecognized cases of hyperthyroidism.[382,385] No body of literature exists on predictors of myocardial infarction, ventricular arrhythmia, or sudden death. The occurrence of coronary ischemic events during hyperthyroidism had been considered to be surprisingly low. In an early series of unselected hyperthyroid patients, 2 of 200 died as a result of myocardial infarction.[379] In one study, high levels of T_3 on admission were associated with the presence of a coronary event and also predicted subsequent coronary events over a 3-year follow-up period.[126] Isolated case reports document the occurrence of sudden death or coronary spasm even among young patients.

PATHOPHYSIOLOGY

Structural and regulatory proteins in the heart are encoded by genes regulated by T_3.[115] Despite the low levels of circulating catecholamines, the physiology of a hyperthyroid patient resembles a hyperadrenergic state.[386] Sinus tachycardia is the most common arrhythmia in uncomplicated hyperthyroidism. On examination there are characteristically tachycardia at rest, widened pulse pressure, and systolic hypertension. The patient with hyperthyroid heart disease has a high left ventricular ejection fraction at rest, high

*See References 343, 344, 365, 367, 373, 374.

*See References 115, 119, 120, 126, 376-385.

cardiac output, subnormal response to exercise, and sometimes rate-related heart failure.[376] Physiologic abnormalities include decreased systemic vascular resistance; increased blood volume; increased work load; increased contractility; shortening of systolic contraction and diastolic relaxation times; and reduction of contractile reserve. Hyperthyroidism reduces serum cholesterol.

CLINICAL MANIFESTATIONS

Thyrocardiac crises are potentially seen without the complete picture of thyroid storm—in particular, without fever. Thyrocardiac crises otherwise can be divided into several major problems, including atrial arrhythmias and thromboembolism*; heart failure and manifestations of cardiomyopathy[376,380,399-410]; the rare complications of conduction disturbance,[411] ventricular arrhythmia,[412] and sudden death[413-415]; and coronary artery spasm. Coronary artery spasm is increasingly recognized as a potentially reversible complication of uncontrolled hyperthyroidism, sometimes seen in young women, infrequently complicated by myocardial infarction.[416-428]

APPROACH TO MANAGEMENT

If a thyrocardiac crisis is present, β-blockade is part of the therapy unless contraindications are present. In treating atrial fibrillation digoxin is used, and for congestive heart failure digoxin and furosemide are used. If some degree of systolic cardiac dysfunction may be present, β-blockade may result in hypotension and should be instituted with careful monitoring. For patients with tachycardia-related congestive heart failure, the use of beta blockers in doses equivalent to 20 mg propranolol every 6 hours may be well tolerated, and the dose may be titrated up to 40 or 80 mg every 6 hours. However, in low-output heart failure or heart disease of other causes complicated by hyperthyroidism, administration of beta blockers must be approached with caution if these agents are used at all.[380] Diltiazem also must be used with caution because it may have negative inotropic effects. Thionamides should be given in relatively high dosage, such as such as 20 mg methimazole daily every 8 hours. Two hours after the first dose of methimazole, SSKI (potassium iodide oral solution) 5 drops every 6 hours may be started. Iodide is tapered to 2 drops three times per day before discharge and is discontinued after 7 to 14 days. Patients in atrial fibrillation resulting from hyperthyroidism generally should receive anticoagulation therapy according to the same criteria as other patients. For thyrocardiac crises, treatment with glucocorticoids is seldom indicated. A reduction of methimazole dose usually is indicated once the initial response is assured.

After medical stabilization, definitive therapy with radioactive iodine usually is offered to patients who have experienced thyrocardiac symptoms.[378] Radiation thyroiditis or interruption of antithyroid medication to permit radioiodine administration can cause patient destabilization. Pretreatment with thionamide medication usually should be offered for about 2 months in the absence of contraindications. For patients in atrial fibrillation, the frequency of spontaneous conversion to sinus rhythm is greater if relatively large ablative doses of radioactive iodine are used, sufficient to bring about prompt development of hypothyroidism.[391] Thionamide therapy must be withheld temporarily to permit radioiodine treatment, but if antithyroid medication is reinstituted after radioiodine treatment, any recurrence of hyperthyroidism is usually corrected within 4 to 6 weeks.

Patients who do not spontaneously convert to sinus rhythm generally should be rendered euthyroid before elective cardioversion is attempted; otherwise, there is a greater risk of relapse of atrial fibrillation after cardioversion. It has been suggested that because no spontaneous conversions occurred more than 16 weeks after attainment of euthyroidism, the ideal timing for elective cardioversion is at that time.[390,396] Hyperthyroid patients are more sensitive to warfarin than others. The immediate risks of anticoagulation sometimes must be weighed against the desirability of postponing elective cardioversion. The guidelines of the Seventh ACCP Conference on Antithrombotic and Thrombolytic Therapy recommended that because the incidence of thromboembolic events in patients with thyrotoxic atrial fibrillation appeared similar to other causes of atrial fibrillation, antithrombotic therapies should be chosen based on the presence of validated stroke risk factors.[398]

In cases of anginal pain and coronary vasospasm, aggressive medical treatment of vasospasm and hyperthyroidism is indicated.

PROGNOSIS

Even in young adult patients, atrial fibrillation may be complicated by thromboembolism resulting in fatal or disabling cerebrovascular accidents.[387,388,395]

About 37% to 61% of patients may experience spontaneous conversion of atrial fibrillation after attainment of euthyroidism, mostly within 6 weeks.[377,390] Absence of congestive heart failure is a favorable prognostic predictor of spontaneous conversion. Other patients may be successfully cardioverted. The absence of other heart disease, short duration of atrial fibrillation, and younger age predict successful conversion and maintenance of sinus rhythm.

As a result of treatment of hyperthyroidism, a patient with heart failure caused by thyrotoxic heart disease experiences improved ability to augment cardiac output during exercise.[399] With treatment of thyrotoxicosis alone, about 41% of patients with congestive heart failure and thyrotoxicosis who receive radioactive iodine experience relief of heart failure.[377] For the rare patient having hyperthyroidism and anginal chest pain caused by coronary artery spasm, isolated published case reports emphasize reversibility of anginal symptoms after successful treatment of hyperthyroidism.

Lipid status should be reevaluated after correction of hyperthyroidism.

KEY POINTS

- In unstable patients, sampling of TSH, thyroid hormone concentrations, and any assessments of hormone binding should occur simultaneously.
- Low TSH is attributable to dopamine or glucocorticoid therapy in some critically ill patients.

*See References 308, 381, 382, 385, 387-398.

Continued on following page

KEY POINTS (Continued)

- High free T_4 is attributable to furosemide, heparin, or sepsis in some critically ill patients.
- Thyroid function test abnormalities that resolve after recovery are common in critical illness (nonthyroidal illness syndrome).
- Low T_3 is the earliest finding of nonthyroidal illness syndrome, resulting from impaired peripheral activation of T_4 (impaired peripheral conversion of T_4 to T_3) and enhanced deactivation of T_3 (deactivating conversion of T_3 to T_2).
- Low transport protein concentrations, low total T_4, and low TSH are seen in more longstanding or severe cases of nonthyroidal illness syndrome.
- Biochemical differentiation between nonthyroidal illness syndrome and intrinsic hypofunction of the pituitary or hypothalamus may be impossible until after recovery.
- Because it is unknown whether the changes of nonthyroidal illness syndrome are detrimental to the patient, the present-day standard of care does not require thyroid hormone treatment.
- T_3 has inotropic and vasodilatory effects.
- The rise of total T_4 and T_3 into the normal range that occurs during recovery from severe nonthyroidal illness syndrome may be accompanied by TSH elevation above the normal ambulatory range.
- Findings of low T_4, low free T_4, and high TSH generally signify hypothyroidism.
- Findings of high T_4, high free T_4, and low TSH generally signify hyperthyroidism.
- Among patients treated for established hypothyroidism, brief interruption of levothyroxine therapy confers negligible medical risk. Concomitantly administered substances may interfere with enteral absorption of levothyroxine. Conversion to intravenous administration of levothyroxine in the treatment of established hypothyroidism requires a dosage reduction.
- The patient having untreated hypothyroidism is at risk for hypoventilation, congestive heart failure, water intoxication, relative adrenal insufficiency, sensitivity to sedatives and analgesics, hypometabolism of administered medications, and resistance to warfarin.
- If replacement with levothyroxine is introduced too quickly, the patient having untreated hypothyroidism with coexistent heart disease is at risk for arrhythmia, exacerbated heart failure, or myocardial infarction.
- In the treatment of myxedema coma, the benefits of rapid replacement with levothyroxine outweigh the risks. Outcomes depend on additional supportive measures.
- Myxedema coma, thyroid storm, and thyrocardiac crisis are diagnosed by clinical evidence of the emergency condition and biochemical verification of thyroid status and are often appropriately treated in a critical care unit.

KEY POINTS (Continued)

- Clinical and biochemical control of hyperthyroidism should be attained before elective surgery.
- Coronary vasospasm may occur during hyperthyroidism and remit with control of hyperthyroidism.

SELECTED REFERENCES

5. Gereben B, Zavacki AM, Ribich S, et al: Cellular and molecular basis of deiodinase-regulated thyroid hormone signaling. Endocr Rev 2008;29(7):898-938.
13. Stockigt JR: Free thyroid hormone measurement. A critical appraisal. Endocrinol Metab Clin North Am 2001;30(2):265-289.
16. Dufour DR: Laboratory tests of thyroid function: Uses and limitations. Endocrinol Metab Clin North Am 2007;36(3):579-594.
18. Spencer C, Eigen A, Shen D, et al: Specificity of sensitive assays of thyrotropin (TSH) used to screen for thyroid disease in hospitalized patients. Clin Chem 1987;33(8):1391-1396.
43. Bermudez F, Surks MI, Oppenheimer JH: High incidence of decreased serum triiodothyronine concentration in patients with nonthyroidal disease. J Clin Endocrinol Metab 1975;41(1):27-40.
56. Chopra IJ: Nonthyroidal illness syndrome or euthyroid sick syndrome? Endocr Pract 1996;2(1):45-52.
83. Jirasakuldech B, Schussler GC, Yap MG, et al: A characteristic serpin cleavage product of thyroxine-binding globulin appears in sepsis sera. J Clin Endocrinol Metab 2000;85(11):3996-3999.
96. Warner MH, Beckett GJ: Mechanisms behind the non-thyroidal illness syndrome: An update. J Endocrinol 2010;205(1):1-13.
120. Klein I, Danzi S: Thyroid disease and the heart. Circulation 2007;116(15):1725-1735.
177. Ridgway EC, McCammon JA, Benotti J, Maloof F: Acute metabolic responses in myxedema to large doses of intravenous l-thyroxine. Ann Intern Med 1972;77(4):549-555.
191. Garber JR, Cobin RH, Gharib H, et al: Clinical Practice Guidelines for Hypothyroidism in Adults: Co-sponsored by American Association of Clinical Endocrinologists and the American Thyroid Association. Endocr Pract 2012;Sept 11:1-207. [Epub ahead of print.]
234. Wartofsky L: Myxedema coma. In Braverman LE, Cooper DS (eds): Werner and Ingbar's The Thyroid: A Fundamental and Clinical Text, 10th ed. Philadelphia, Lippincott Williams & Wilkins, 2012, pp 600-605.
236. Bahn RS, Burch HB, Cooper DS, et al: Hyperthyroidism and other causes of thyrotoxicosis: Management guidelines of the American Thyroid Association and American Association of Clinical Endocrinologists. Endocr Practice 2011;17(3):456-520.
257. Cooper DS: Antithyroid drugs. N Engl J Med 2005;352(9):905-917.
291. Bogazzi F, Bartalena L, Martino E: Approach to the patient with amiodarone-induced thyrotoxicosis. J Clin Endocrinol Metab 2010;95(6):2529-2535.
292. Eskes SA, Endert E, Fliers E, et al: Treatment of amiodarone-induced thyrotoxicosis type 2: A randomized clinical trial. J Clin Endocrinol Metab 2012;97(2):499-506.
326. Nayak B, Burman K: Thyrotoxicosis and thyroid storm. Endocrinol Metab Clin North Am 2006;35(4):663-686.
393. Sawin CT, Geller A, Wolf PA, et al: Low serum thyrotropin concentrations as a risk factor for atrial fibrillation in older persons. N Engl J Med 1994;331(19):1249-1252.
416. Resnekov L, Falicov RE: Thyrotoxicosis and lactate-producing angina pectoris with normal coronary arteries. Br Heart J 1977;39(10):1051-1057.

The complete list of references can be found at www.expertconsult.com.

PART 6

NEUROLOGIC DISEASE IN THE CRITICALLY ILL

Coma

61

Axel Rosengart | Sea Mi Park | Karen Berger | Igor Ougorets

CHAPTER OUTLINE

CONCEPT AND TERMINOLOGY OF IMPAIRED CONSCIOUSNESS

Alteration of consciousness is a frequent admission diagnosis to critical care services. Most patients require immediate and often extensive diagnostic workup as both time to diagnosis and treatment initiation are decisive factors for brain recovery. To the public, the portrayal of coma is overly optimistic as 89% of "comatose" patients in a meta-analysis of 64 characters in American soap dramas regained consciousness and around 92% "survived" coma.[1] In contrast, medical experience does not compare as favorably, as only about 50% of patients survive in an unselected coma population.[2-4] Therefore, defining coma in a succinct and operational manner will provide a deeper understanding of the depth of brain injury and avoid miscommunications and unrealistic prognostications.

Consciousness can be viewed as the patient's responses to internal and external stimulation and his or her awareness of self and the environment. These two basic components of consciousness, arousal and awareness, are clinically used to classify the state of consciousness, but, strictly speaking, the qualitative examination of arousal should be separated from the quantitative assessment of the patient's self- and environmental awareness and cognitive function. These interdependent components are regulated by different neuroanatomic domains within the central nervous system. Arousal and ensuing wakefulness are tightly dependent on the network function of the ascending reticular activating system (ARAS), namely, the midbrain reticular formation, mesencephalic nucleus and tegmentum, thalamic intralaminar (centromedian) nucleus, and dorsal hypothalamus. These build a network of brainstem and diencephalic centers with a strong connection to the cerebral cortices. Self-awareness and the spectrum of cognitive interactions with the environment are the purview of the hemispheres. Simplistically, the hemispheres are structured into three functional systems: units that receive, process, and store sensory information; units that generate and regulate motor activity; and units responsible for programming, regulating, and verifying actions. These three functional systems operate as an intercortical network; relate, as a whole, to the experience of awareness; and allow cognitive performance. The partition of arousal network and intercortical (cognitive) network implies that the level of self-awareness and cognitive performance cannot be examined in a patient with lack of arousal. In other words, in a person with a quantitatively reduced state of consciousness, the qualitative assessment of the content of consciousness is not possible. Practically speaking, the assessment of content (i.e., testing a patient's cognitive abilities and thinking) should be done after the best level of arousal has been achieved. A fully aroused person can express completely normal or deficient awareness and cognitive performance. Conversely, failure of arousal renders it impossible to test awareness and cognition.

When evaluating a patient's mental status, the state of consciousness should be viewed as a continuum ranging from the patient who has full alertness and cognitive lucidity to the deeply comatose patient; it is not an all-or-nothing phenomenon.[5] An all-or-nothing approach limits the interpretation of remaining brain function and, hence, diagnostic certainty. Furthermore, the duration and time development of coma are helpful diagnostic features and should complement the quantitative and qualitative assessment of consciousness. Standard classification systems categorize consciousness based on systematic testing of arousal, awareness, and content. Table 61.1 classifies various abnormalities of consciousness, and the following section delineates clinically important syndromes.

In the *awake* state, the examination allows the clinician to test a person for the degree of self-awareness and intactness of cognitive function. Drowsiness, sleepiness, and *lethargy* resemble reduced spontaneous physical and mental activities in a person who cannot sustain wakefulness without repeated external stimulation. They are somewhat comparable to the experience of lighter sleep, though drowsy patients almost always have reduced attention and concentration and some degree of associated mild confusion. Although sleep and pathologic states of consciousness share common features—for instance, the sleeping person is unaware of his or her resembling unconsciousness—quick reversal to full consciousness is a classic feature of sleep.

A *stuporous patient* (from Latin *stupure*, meaning "insensible") requires repeated, stronger stimuli to show some arousal, and these patients may or may not open their eyes. Full arousal and alertness are not achieved and with continuing external stimulation, restlessness and stereotypic motor responses are observed, but without the appropriate cognitive interactions. A deep stuporous state closer to coma is differentiated by European clinicians and is referred to as *sopor* (from Latin *sopor*, meaning "deep sleep").

Coma (from Greek κῶμα, or "deep sleep") is a continuous state of unresponsiveness identified by an inability to arouse to vigorous (noxious) external or internal stimuli. The degree of coma can differ; lighter stages (sometimes denoted as semicoma) can be identified by brief moaning to strong stimulation and associated observed changes in autonomic function; whereas the deepest coma examination shows an absence of any response, including brainstem reflex responses (i.e., lack of oculo- and pupillomotoric responses). Some cyclic autonomic activity such as the sleep-wake cycle and changes in motor tone may coexist. A detailed discussion of coma is provided in the classic textbook by Plum and Posner.[6]

The *vegetative state* is characterized by the complete absence of behavioral evidence for self- or environmental awareness. This state can follow coma and identifies a state in which brainstem and diencephalic (thalamic) activity is present to a degree that clinical signs of spontaneous or stimulus-induced arousal and sleep-wake cycles are observed. Patients often show blink responses to light; intermittent eye movements (sometimes erroneously interpreted as following objects or looking at family members); stimulus-sensitive automatisms such as swallowing, bruxism, and moaning; or primitive motor responses. If this state lasts longer than 30 days, it is referred to as persistent vegetative state (PVS) and is used as a descriptive clinical syndrome rather than a disease-specific entity. The most common causes include cardiac arrest, head trauma, severe brain infections, and various causes of thalamic injury. Vegetative states can also be seen in the terminal phase of degenerative illnesses such as Alzheimer's disease. Ambiguous terms for PVS such as *apallic syndrome* and *neocortical death* should be avoided.[2,7]

Minimal conscious state can be diagnosed in patients displaying some but often inconsistent behavioral evidence of awareness of the environment, but they cannot communicate their content and are unable to follow instructions reliably.[8] It describes a large group of patients who are different from vegetative patients in that they demonstrate some signs of awareness of themselves and their surroundings, albeit inconsistently.

As mentioned earlier, the time progression and persistence of the impairment can be used to further classify abnormalities of consciousness. *Delirium* is classified as a mental disorder because it involves a fluctuating level of consciousness and pervasive impairment in mental, behavioral, and emotional functioning. It is commonly acute in onset and short in duration and is frequently correlated to a specific etiology such as medications, anesthesia, or sleep deprivation. The criteria for delirium listed in the fourth edition of the *Diagnostic and Statistical Manual of Mental Disorders* (DSM-IV) include a disturbance of consciousness with reduced the ability to sustain or shift attention and focus. In our experience, attention and concentration deficits are always present in delirious patients and accompanied by a variable degree of cognitive dysfunction unattributed to preexisting dementia. The dysfunctions of this acute syndrome include memory deficits, disorientation, disturbance of language and situational perception, and disorganized behavior. Other delirium markers are its acute onset and tendency to fluctuate along a spectrum of hyperactive (i.e., agitation, restlessness, emotional labiality), hypoactive (withdrawal, flat affect, apathy, decreased responsiveness), or mixed presentations. Concurrent or sequential appearance of features of both hyper- and hypoactive states is not unusual. The history, physical examination, and ancillary test results frequently indicate that the disturbance is caused by an underlying medical or situational condition.

Dementia is a chronic condition in which content of consciousness is affected initially, but in advanced stages reduced levels of arousal are seen. Dementia is generally progressive and affects memory and at least two other cognitive domains such as language, executive function, planning motor tasks, and recognition. Dementing illnesses include a variety of intrinsic degenerative diseases of the cerebral hemispheres, but they also result from many other causes such as traumatic brain injury and hydrocephalus. The underlying etiology can be reversible (i.e., after correction of a vitamin deficiency) or irreversible (Lewy body dementia). Additionally, disease progression can be highly variable, lasting weeks to years, often with fluctuating severity, or be static after the initial impact injury. Anxiety, depression, and agitation may alternate and greatly complicate the disease course. The anatomically affected neurologic structures are commonly a result of bihemispheric cortical dysfunction; however, subcortical structures (i.e., vascular dementia from multifocal small vessel disease) can also represent the predominant pathology.

Akinetic mutism is a silent, alert-appearing immobility of a patient with injury to the hypothalamus or basal forebrain. It manifests as apparent depressed levels of consciousness in a patient with well-formed sleep-wake cycles and with little or no evidence of awareness or spontaneous motor activity. Various etiologies can present or lead to an akinetic mute state, and it is imperative to have a rigorous neurologic examination and careful review of neuroimaging and electroencephalography (EEG). The term *locked-in syndrome* was introduced by Plum and Posner to describe the

Table 61.1 Classifications and Descriptions of Abnormalities of Consciousness

Terminology	Consciousness (Arousal, Awareness)		Content and Cognitive Function	Involuntary Response			Voluntary Response	Main and Essential Dysfunctional Structure or System
	Arousal (Level of Responsiveness to External Stimuli)	Awareness (Awareness of Self and Environment)		Brainstem Reflexes	Autonomic Reflexes	Auditory/Visual Response		
Physiologic sleep	Normal with various degree of stimuli	Normal with various degree of stimuli	Preserved	Preserved	Preserved	Preserved	Preserved with various degree of stimuli	Normal
Dementia (subacute or chronic)	Normal to abnormal depending on disease progression	Normal to abnormal depending on disease progression	Variable impaired	Preserved	Preserved	Preserved	Preserved until the damage is too extensive and severe	Cerebral cortex
Akinetic mutism or abulia (subacute or chronic)	Normal or depressed level, but hard to assess due to very slow response	Normal or depressed level, but hard to assess due to very slow response	Normal or depressed level, but hard to assess due to very slow response	Preserved	Preserved	Preserved	Impaired or very slow response or almost quadriplegic	Hypothalamic or basal forebrain injury
Drowsiness or hypersomnia (subacute or chronic)	Variable, with light stimuli	Variable with light stimuli	Preserved	Preserved	Preserved	Preserved	Preserved with light stimuli	Normal to variable lesion with damage in RAS
Lethargy	Variable with light stimuli	Variable with light stimuli	Preserved	Preserved	Preserved	Preserved	Preserved with light stimuli	Normal to variable lesion with damage in RAS
Confusion or delirium (acute)	Variable with light stimuli	Variable with light stimuli	Variable impaired	Preserved	Preserved	Preserved	Preserved with light stimuli	Normal to variable lesion with damage in RAS
Stupor (acute)	Variable with strong stimuli	Variable with strong stimuli	Inaccessible	Variable impaired	Variable impaired	Preserved	Variable impaired	Normal to variable lesion with damage in RAS
Minimal conscious state (subacute or chronic)	Impaired, but shows subtle signs of arousal	Impaired, but shows subtle signs of awareness	Inaccessible	Variable impaired	Variable impaired, sleep-wake cycle preserved	Localize sound location/ inconsistent command following/ sustained visual fixation/sustained visual pursuit	Localize noxious stimuli/reaches for object/ voluntary scratching	Normal to variable lesion with damage in RAS
Vegetative state (subacute or chronic)	Impaired, but shows subtle signs of arousal	Absence with strong stimuli	Inaccessible	Variable impaired	Variable impaired, sleep-wake cycle preserved	Variable impaired, startle/brief orienting to sound/variable impaired/brief visual fixation	Occasional aimless movement	Cerebral cortex, thalamocortical disconnections or RAS
Coma (acute)	Absence with strong stimuli	Absence with strong stimuli	Inaccessible	Absence	Impaired, postural/motor reflex preserved	Absence	Absence	Diffuse brain damage or RAS
Brain death (subacute or chronic)	Absence with strong stimuli	Absence with strong stimuli	Inaccessible	Absence	Impaired, postural/motor reflex preserved	Absence	Absence	Diffuse brain damage or RAS

RAS, reticular activating system.

quadriplegia and anarthria resulting from the disruption of corticospinal and corticobulbar pathways, respectively. The extent of the deficits in patients with locked-in syndromes can vary, but these patients are aware of the environment and can hear and understand what is discussed around them. They may retain some ability of oculomotor (i.e., ability to open eyes) or other residual cranial nerve function. These patients are also anarthric or severely dysarthric with varying degrees of motor deficits ranging from complete quadriplegia to quadriparesis. As consciousness is preserved, communication is possible using vertical or lateral eye movements or blinking of the eyelid to signal yes/no responses. The majority of cases are caused by basilar artery occlusion leading to brainstem infarction in the ventral pons, yet numerous other etiologies have been described. *Abulia* (from the Greek meaning "lack of will") is an apathetic state in which the patient is awake, has normal sleep-wake cycle, and is very slow to respond to stimuli. Mental function is usually normal when tested with sufficient stimulation. It is secondary to bilateral frontal lobe disease and in severe instances may mimic or progress to akinetic mutism.

NEUROANATOMY, NEUROTRANSMITTER, AND PATHOLOGY

Consciousness, which consists of three main parts, largely depends on the integrity of brain structure for arousal (Fig. 61.1). The ascending reticular activating system (ARAS) is the lowest order arousal system, consisting of a set of brainstem nuclei located within the brainstem and interconnected by neuronal circuits. The ARAS relays arousal signals to the more rostral thalami, which, in turn, act as hemispheric gatekeepers of arousal and regulate consciousness and sleep-wake transitions. In turn, thalamic activated cerebral cortices allow cognitive processing, which then determines the overall content of consciousness.[6] Structural damage to or metabolic-chemical derangements of any or all of these elements will affect consciousness. Important components of the ARAS[9-11] include the midbrain reticular formation, mesencephalic nuclei (dorsal raphe nucleus, pedunculopontine tegmental nucleus, locus coeruleus), and ventral tegmental areas. Those areas have rich connections to thalamic intralaminar nuclei and further frontally reaching projections to the tuberomammillary nucleus, lateral hypothalamus, and basal forebrain.

The ascending arousal system of the brainstem contains different neurotransmitter systems. Main cholinergic projections include the ascending mesopontine tegmental and basal forebrain pathways projecting to the thalami and to virtually all subcortical and cortical structures. These projections usually function as synaptic facilitators but at times can act as depressors of transmission.[12] Glutamate is the main transmitter influencing the firing patterns of tegmental cholinergic neurons.[13] The adrenergic component of the ARAS is closely associated with the noradrenergic neurons of the midbrain locus coeruleus. It runs in parallel with cholinergic projections rostrally to the cortical areas but also descends caudally within the spinal cord.[14] Hypocretin/orexin neurons within the hypothalamus activate both adrenergic and cholinergic pathways and coordinate activity of the entire ARAS system, enhancing complementary and synergistic control of arousal and locomotion.[15] Histamine-releasing cells from the hypothalamus and tuberomammillary neurons are active during the qualitative activation needed for cognition and EEG activation, but they remain silent during sleep.[16-18]

The main inhibitor of the arousal system is γ-aminobutyric acid (GABA), without which normal sleep does not occur. The GABAergic circuitry is located in the midbrain and pons, but its activity is regulated and sustained by forebrain structures.[19] It is thought that the GABAergic system's main function is to contain and channel the spread of arousal, both spontaneously and in response to a stimulus. GABAergic processes are responsible for the occurrence of paradoxical sleep (deep sleep characterized by a brain wave pattern similar to that of wakefulness, rapid eye movements, and heavier breathing but without motor responses). The name "waking neurons" has been given to the serotonergic dorsal raphe nucleus in the midbrain,[20] which receives convergent excitatory input from the noradrenaline, histamine, and hypocretin/orexin arousal systems[21,22] as the main activator of the ARAS. Cortical signals that pass through the

AROUSAL STRUCTURE AND MAIN NEUROTRANSMITTER

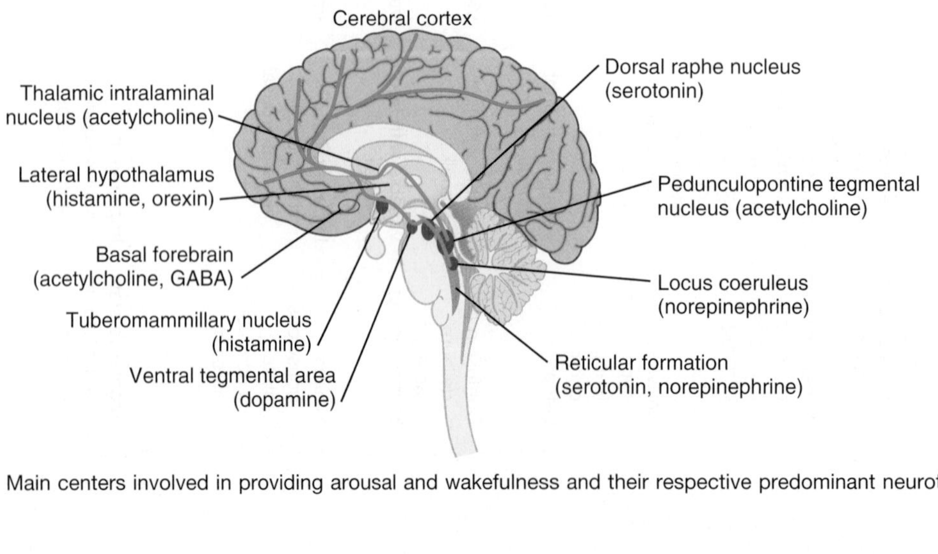

Figure 61.1 Main centers involved in providing arousal and wakefulness and their respective predominant neurotransmitters.

striatum (caudate and putamen) are refined by the action of dopamine. Dopaminergic neurons are tonically active and stimulate or inhibit cortical neurons depending on various environmental influences (pain, hunger, etc.).[23,24] It is thought that many sensory signals that reach conscious awareness pass through this basal ganglia loop with dopamine as the modulating neurotransmitter. Koch and colleagues suggested that coalitions of neurons compete to dominate conscious thoughts and activities at any given time point and, hence, dopaminergic innervation may facilitate the transient domination of conscious awareness by certain sets of neuron coalitions.[25] Therefore, it seems that arousal is an event with a defined time distribution, which is tightly orchestrated by a few key neurotransmitters. As we know, there is no singular "arousal neurotransmitter."[10,26]

PATHOLOGY SEEN IN PATIENTS WITH IMPAIRED CONSCIOUSNESS

There are four major pathologies that can cause severe, acute, and global reductions of consciousness.[6,27] (1) One of these pathologies is the presence of diffuse, global, or extensive multifocal bilateral dysfunction of the cerebral cortex. In this injury mechanism, the cortical gray matter is diffusely impaired and so are cortical-subcortical excitatory feedback loops. The clinical examination will reveal disinhibited autonomic brainstem reflexes, which have also been described as "reticular shock." (2) Another is injury to the paramedian gray matter from the level of the nucleus parabrachialis of the pons (tegmentum) and reaching to the midbrain pretectal areas and ventral posterior hypothalamus. An injury of this type damages the ascending arousal system and normal cortical activation. The affected structures are predominantly the paramedian gray matter, extending rostrally from the level of the nucleus parabrachialis of the pons (tegmentum) and reaching rostrally as far as the adjacent pretectal area and ventral posterior hypothalamus. (3) The widespread disconnection of the cortex from subcortical activating mechanisms acts pathophysiologically to produce effects similar to both of the previously mentioned conditions. (4) Finally, cortical and subcortical arousal mechanisms can be affected by a variety of diffuse disorders and to various degrees—for example, metabolic encephalopathy in a patient with acute liver failure.

APPROACH TO COMA

The initial approach to stupor and coma is based on the principle that all alterations in arousal are acute, life-threatening emergencies. Urgent steps are required to prevent or minimize permanent brain damage from reversible causes. Patient evaluation and treatment must occur simultaneously. Serial examinations with accurate documentation are necessary to determine a change in the patient's status. Accordingly, management decisions (therapeutic and diagnostic) must be made. The clinical approach to an unconscious patient entails the following steps: (1) emergency treatment; (2) history (from relatives, friends, and emergency medical personnel); (3) general physical examination; (4) neurologic profile, the key to categorizing the nature of coma; and (5) specific management.

EMERGENCY MANAGEMENT

Initial assessment must focus on vital signs to determine appropriate resuscitation measures; diagnostic processes can occur later. Urgent and sometimes empiric therapy must be given to avoid additional brain insults.

OXYGENATION AND INTUBATION

Oxygenation must be ensured by establishing an airway for ventilation of the lungs. The threshold for intubation should be low in a comatose patient, even if respiratory function is sufficient for proper ventilation and oxygenation. The level of consciousness may deteriorate, and breathing may decompensate suddenly and unexpectedly. An open airway must be ensured and protected from aspiration of vomitus and blood. If severe neck injury is a possibility or has not been excluded, intubation should be performed by the most skilled practitioner without extension of the patient's neck. Mask-bag-assisted ventilation should continue during the examination if necessary. Signs of arousal include dilated, reactive pupils, copious tears, diaphoresis, tachycardia, and systemic hypertension.

A brief neurologic examination is mandatory before any sedative or paralytic required for intubation is administered. The key points of a rapid neurologic examination are the following:[28]

- Assessment of level of arousal and level of consciousness (i.e., coma, stupor, lethargy)
- Pupillary size and response to light
- Abnormalities of eye movements (i.e., disconjugate eyes; unilateral gaze paralysis; lack of voluntary movements)
- Grimacing and motor responses to noxious stimulation
- Abnormal plantar response (Babinski's sign)

The preferred route of emergency intubation is orotracheal, which can be performed rapidly, safely, and reliably with inline stabilization of the neck in patients with suspected cervical spine injury. Intubation causes intense reflexive cardiovascular stimulation that may lead to a deleterious elevation of intracranial pressure (ICP). Therefore, the patient should be adequately sedated. Etomidate is the preferred sedative in patients with suspected ICP elevation as it reliably facilitates induction in less than 1 minute with a duration of action of 4 to 6 minutes. Propofol is another anesthetic agent that does not increase ICP; however, its hypotensive effects, which can ultimately decrease cerebral perfusion pressure, often limit its use. Both medications result in a dose-dependent decrease of cerebral metabolic rate that reduces cerebral blood flow and ICP. Ketamine has a fast onset, but it may elevate ICP and should generally be avoided. Midazolam can alter the patient's mental status and may prohibit a postintubation examination.

RESPIRATION/PEEP

The effect of positive end expiratory pressure (PEEP) on ICP is only partly predictable for a number of reasons. Lung and pleural pressures are transmitted to the cerebrospinal fluid (CSF) column through intravertebral spaces and the vertebral venous plexus, and to the jugular venous system through the superior vena cava. The effect of PEEP on ICP depends on both intracranial and pulmonary compliance and changes over time. ICP responses are not limited to PEEP but also relate to mean airway pressure, which can be elevated by many factors other than PEEP, including peak airway pressure and inspiratory time. Furthermore, the position of the patient's head and upper body can significantly affect ICP. A nasogastric tube should be placed to facilitate gastric lavage, decompression, and to reduce the risks for aspiration.

CIRCULATION

Circulation must be maintained at a level always ensuring adequate cerebral perfusion pressure. In any patient with suspected brain injury, resuscitation fluids include isotonic solutions such as normal saline or lactated Ringer's solution. An initial systemic mean arterial pressure (MAP) of approximately 100 mm Hg is adequate and safe for most patients (unless intracranial bleeding is suspected). Because cerebral perfusion pressure (CPP) equals the difference between MAP and ICP, CPP-matching ICP therapy targets a CPP from 60 to 70 mm Hg in most instances. Invasive ICP monitoring is mandatory if ICP elevations are suspected. While obtaining venous access, blood samples should be collected for anticipated tests. Hypotension may be treated by replacing blood and volume losses and vasoactive agents may be utilized (if volume and cardiac status is adequate) to maintain target MAP and systolic blood pressures. Hypertension should be aggressively managed with intravenous antihypertensive agents that do not elevate ICP by their vasodilatory effects. Thus labetalol and nicardipine are generally preferred and commonly used for managing uncontrolled hypertension. In most cases, including patients with intracranial hemorrhage, systolic and diastolic blood pressures of less than 160 mm Hg and 90 mm Hg, respectively, are tolerated and maintained. Urine output should be at least 0.5 mL/kg/hour and accurate measurement requires bladder catheterization.

GLUCOSE AND THIAMINE

Hypoglycemia is a frequent cause of altered consciousness and also leads to secondary brain injury if uncorrected. Glucose (25 g as a 50% dextrose solution) should be administered intravenously and immediately after blood is drawn for baseline values, as the benefits of empiric glucose in preventing possible hypoglycemic brain damage outweigh the risk of hyperglycemia. Thiamine (100 mg) may be given with the glucose infusion to prevent precipitation of Wernicke's encephalopathy as seen in malnourished, thiamine-depleted patients receiving glucose infusions. In rare circumstances, an established thiamine deficiency can cause coma.

SEIZURES

Repeated generalized seizures such as impact seizures invariably lead to secondary brain injury and should be treated aggressively with an intravenous benzodiazepine. Lorazepam, in 4-mg doses administered at 2 mg/min, has become the preferred agent due to its longer duration of action; however diazepam and midazolam are effective alternatives. Subsequent seizure control is maintained with an intravenous antiepileptic. Although there is no proven drug of choice, first-line agents generally include phenytoin (15 to 20 mg/kg intravenous (IV) bolus at a maximum rate of 50 mg/min), fosphenytoin (15- to 20-mg PE/kg IV bolus at a maximum rate of 150 mg/min), or valproic acid (20- to 40-mg/kg IV bolus). Fosphenytoin is often selected due to its faster rate of administration and lower risk of hypotension (as it is not formulated with propylene glycol). Drug levels for these agents should be drawn following the loading dose and maintenance dosing should be initiated. Corrected total target levels for phenytoin (and fosphenytoin) are 15 to 20 mcg/mL; free levels can be drawn in patients who are critically ill or have low protein stores with a target of 1.5 to 2 mcg/mL. Valproic acid target levels are 50-100 mcg/mL. Seizure breakthrough requires immediate administration of benzodiazepines and loading of a second anticonvulsant. Continuous video EEG monitoring is frequently employed to detect nonconvulsive seizures.

SEDATION AND PARALYSIS

Sedation is often required to facilitate comfort with respiratory support, to counteract agitation, or to treat elevated ICP. Short-acting medications given as continuous infusions such as propofol or dexmedetomidine are preferred. However, deeper sedation, especially in patients with seizures, may require a midazolam infusion. Because of the accumulation of its active metabolite in patients with renal dysfunction, extended durations of midazolam should be avoided or interrupted if possible. Sedation should be titrated to a predefined goal using a validated sedation scale. The Richmond Agitation Sedation Scale (RASS) is commonly used and a goal range of 0 (alert and calm) to −2 (light sedation, briefly awakens with eye contact to voice) is appropriate for most patients. Hourly interruption of sedation is needed to obtain serial neurologic examinations, except in paralyzed patients or those in whom awakening leads to deterioration of ICP. Additional analgesia (i.e., intravenous intermittent morphine [2 to 4 mg every 3 to 4 hours] or a fentanyl infusion) is often needed in postoperative patients or patients with traumatic injuries. Patients with critically high ICP should be paralyzed as part of the treatment regimen for increased intracranial hypertension, but only after initiation of both a sedative and analgesic.

REVERSAL OF DRUG OVERDOSE

Drug overdose is the largest single cause (30%) of coma in the emergency department. Most drug overdoses are treated by supportive measures alone. Certain antagonists, however, specifically reverse the effects of coma-producing drugs. Intravenous naloxone (0.4 to 2 mg) is used as "test" antidote for opiate-induced coma, and it acts as a μ-receptor antagonist. Caution is needed as the reversal of narcotic effect may precipitate acute withdrawal in an opiate addict. In suspected opiate coma, the minimum naloxone dose (not completely reversal) should be given to establish the diagnosis by pupillary dilation and to reverse depressed breathing and consciousness. Due to its short half-life, patients who respond to naloxone reversal may require additional doses or a continuous infusion to avoid rebound sedation and respiratory depression. Intravenous flumazenil antagonizes benzodiazepine-induced coma and can be administered in 0.2-mg doses every minute for a maximum of 1 mg. In patients who initially respond to flumazenil reversal but experience recurrent sedation, flumazenil 1 mg may be redosed every 20 minutes with a max of 3 mg/hour.[29]

Careful consideration should be given prior to administration of flumazenil as patients may experience benzodiazepine-withdrawal seizures. Thus, whereas naloxone is commonly used with minimal serious adverse effects, the use of flumazenil should be restricted to select, low-risk cases. The sedative effects of drugs with anticholinergic properties, particularly tricyclic antidepressants, can be reversed with 1 to 2 mg physostigmine intravenously (duration of action about 45 to 60 minutes). Pretreatment with 0.5 mg atropine will reduce the risk for symptomatic bradycardia. Of note, only full awakening is characteristic of an anticholinergic drug overdose because physostigmine has nonspecific arousal properties.

BODY TEMPERATURE

Hyperthermia is detrimental in brain injury as it increases brain metabolic demands and facilitates secondary brain injury.[30] Elevated temperature greater than 104° F (40° C) requires immediate, lifesaving cooling measures, even before the underlying cause is determined and treated. In 2002, two research groups independently published that lowering the body temperature to 33° C for 12 or 24 hours in comatose survivors of cardiac arrest resulted in nearly doubling the number of patients being discharged home or to rehabilitation. Generally speaking, no patient with acute brain injury should be allowed to be hyperthermic, and modern technology provides a variety types of noninvasive and invasive cooling equipment suitable to maintain any target core temperature desired. Core temperatures of less than 93° F (34° C) on admission should be slowly elevated to above 35° C to reduce the risks of unwanted side effects from uncontrolled, persistent hypothermia.

HISTORY

Once the patient's condition and vital signs have been stabilized, clues to the cause of coma should be sought by interviewing relatives, friends, bystanders, or medical personnel who may have observed the patient before or during the decline in consciousness. The history should address witnessed events, evolution of coma, recent medical and surgical histories, and medication/drug intake.

PHYSICAL EXAMINATION

A systematic, detailed examination is necessary when approaching a comatose patient (Box 61.1, Table 61.2). Important findings include evidence of trauma, acute or chronic medical illnesses, ingestion of drugs (needle marks, alcohol breath), and the presence of nuchal rigidity.

As outlined earlier, an in-depth physical and neurologic examination followed by serial neurologic evaluations (i.e., hourly) is the most important, indispensable, and readily available method of assessing a comatose patient.[31] However, in coma patients the examination remains limited in detecting changes in brain function. Nevertheless, the astute clinician will carefully evaluate for changes in findings (i.e., the appearance of new asymmetry in examination or focal deficits, progressive loss of brainstem reflexes, or loss of reflex motor responses). Finding progression of impairment is of immense clinical value as it indicates a new or worsening "intracranial emergency" demanding immediate clarification and stabilization. Skilled neurologic examination is challenging and provides a limited surveillance window of brain tissue at risk. Intracranial monitoring and, if needed, repeated head imaging have become the standard of care in neurocritical care units.

The differential diagnosis of a comatose patient is supported by the patient's risk factor profile, activity at symptom onset, and disease progression. Acute, devastating headaches with nausea and vomiting quickly followed by impaired consciousness in a hypertensive patient with a history of smoking should be rapidly worked up for subarachnoid or intracerebral hemorrhage. Deterioration of consciousness hours after head injury necessitates immediate exclusion of newly emerging, delayed intracranial hematoma with intracranial pressure crisis. In contrast, the slow progression of a focal neurologic deficit evolving to generalized depressed consciousness in an elderly individual directs toward an intracranial metastasis with secondary seizures. Increased intracranial pressure is a common denominator of many acute and subacute central nervous system (CNS) injuries. Typical manifestations include headaches from the dural stretch of trigeminal (V) sensory fibers; intractable nausea and recurrent vomiting often associated with visual disturbances; some neurologic deficits on detailed examination; and, in later stages, reduction in level of alertness.

When performing the neurologic examination, monitoring vital signs can be utilized as part of the autonomic nervous system evaluation. For example, appearance of systolic hypertension, vagal bradycardia, and respiratory irregularity is known as Cushing's triad and indicates increased ICP. In addition, changes in the pattern of respiration in a spontaneously breathing patient can help localize the level

Box 61.1 Neurologic Profile: A Modified Glasgow Coma Scale

Verbal Response
- Oriented speech
- Confused conversation
- Inappropriate speech
- Incomprehensible speech
- No speech

Eye Opening
- Spontaneous
- Response to verbal stimuli
- Response to noxious stimuli
- None

Motor Response
- Obeys
- Localizes
- Withdraws (flexion)
- Abnormal flexion
- None

Pupillary Reaction
- Present
- Absent

Spontaneous Eye Movement
- Orienting
- Roving conjugate
- Roving disconjugate
- Miscellaneous abnormal movements
- None

Oculocephalic Response
- Normal (unpredictable)
- Full
- Minimal
- None

Oculovestibular Response
- Normal (nystagmus)
- Tonic conjugate
- Minimal or disconjugate
- None

Deep Tendon Reflexes
- Normal
- Increased
- Absent

Table 61.2 Correlation Between Levels of Brain Function and Clinical Signs

Structure	Function	Clinical Sign
Cerebral cortex	Conscious behavior	Speech (including any sounds)
		Purposeful movement
		Spontaneous
		To command
		To pain
Brainstem activating and sensory pathways (reticular activating system)	Sleep-wake cycle	Eye opening
		Spontaneous
		To command
		To path
Brainstem motor pathways	Reflex limb movements	Flexor posturing (decorticate)
		Extensor posturing (decerebrate)
Midbrain CN III	Innervation of ciliary muscle and certain extraocular muscles	Pupillary reactivity
Pontomesencephalic MLF	Connects pontine gaze center with CN III nucleus	Internuclear ophthalmoplegia
Upper pons		
CN V	Facial and corneal	Corneal reflex-sensory
CN VIII	Facial muscle innervation	Corneal reflex-motor response
		Blink
		Grimace
Lower pons		
CN VIII (vestibular portion) connects by brainstem pathways with CN III, IV, VI	Reflex eye movements	Doll's eyes
		Caloric responses
Pontomedullary junction pressure	Spontaneous breathing	Breathing and blood pressure do not require mechanical or chemical support
	Maintained blood pressure	
Spinal cord	Primitive protective responses	Deep tendon reflexes
		Babinski response

CN, cranial, nerve; MLF, medial longitudinal fasciculus.

of injury. Abnormalities of respiration can range from apnea to hyperpnea with undulating crescendo-decrescendo patterns as well as complete irregularity of breathing with erratic pauses that finally terminate in complete apnea. This "autonomic survey" and observing for spontaneous patient movements are followed by the assessment of a patient's level of arousal. The reduction in response to external stimulations provides the basis for commonly used classification schemes such as the Glasgow Coma Scale (GCS). If the patient's level of alertness permits, then orientation, attention and concentration span and intactness of cognitive functions are examined next. This is followed by a detailed assessment of cranial nerve, motor, and peripheral reflex status. Optic nerve head edema (papilledema) is an important and, if present, a reliable manifestation of raised ICP. Additional findings of increased ICP on fundoscopy include venous engorgement, loss of venous pulsation, optic disk hemorrhage with increased disk diameter, and blurring of its margins. Compression of the third nerve is a result of a variety of intracranial processes, including uncal herniation and aneurysms of the posterior communicating artery. It is identified by pupillary dilatation, ptosis, and various degrees of ophthalmoparesis except for abduction and intorsion-depression. A sixth nerve palsy, typically a nonlocalizing sign, is identified by abduction deficit and is seen in patients with elevated ICP or hydrocephalus and stretching of the nerve but is also present in patients with intrinsic brainstem injury (i.e., strokes). Patients with acute intracranial mass lesions and increased ICP commonly develop herniation syndromes—that is, shifting of brain tissue from areas with higher regional ICP toward areas with normal ICP. If the mass lesion is predominantly located within one hemisphere, the main force vector will shift the brain primarily laterally across the midline and toward the opposite hemisphere as it impresses on the upper brainstem and thalamic structures during lateral displacement. More centrally located mass lesions (i.e., acute, obstructive hydrocephalus or global brain swelling as seen in fulminant encephalitis or hepatic encephalopathy) will to the contrary lead primarily to downward herniation with the main force vector impressing upon the brainstem. Different herniation syndromes have different clinical presentations and therapeutic approaches. When intracranial hypertension remains uncontrolled and escalates uniformly central, downward herniation occurs involving increasingly more brainstem structures in a rostrocaudal fashion. The terminal event is complete brainstem destruction resulting invariably in brain death. During this course, progressive loss of brainstem reflexes can be determined on examination and at this stage, the patient is deeply comatose. Injury to the fifth cranial nerve nucleus within the pons results in loss of the corneal reflex. A vestibulocochlear nerve nucleus compromise results in loss of the oculocephalic reflex and manifests as "doll's eyes" or the inability to maintain eye position as the head moves. Medullary injury with damage to the ninth and tenth nerves results in loss of lower cranial nerve reflexes including the absence of gag and cough reflexes.

Ipsilateral hemiparesis indicates the possibility of uncal herniation causing compression of the contralateral cerebral peduncle as temporal lobe tissue herniates into the space between the tentorium and brainstem. For example, a left-sided subdural hematoma causing temporal herniation pushes the opposite cerebral peduncle and its motor fibers against the right tentorial edge (right-sided Kernohan's notch) leading to a hemiparesis on the same side as the hemispheric lesion. Posturing is involuntary flexion or extension of the arms or legs spontaneously or elicited by stimulation, and it is included in the Glasgow Coma Scale as a measure of the severity of brain injury. Three types of posturing can be observed depending on the level of brain injury: decorticate (flexor), decerebrate (extensor), and opisthotonos (body arching along the craniospinal axis) posturing. Injury involving the brainstem above or below the red nucleus in the midbrain leads to decorticate and decerebrate posturing, respectively. Of note, flexion or extension can be witnessed either unilaterally or bilaterally, is sometimes seen only intermittently, and can involve one or all extremities. Decorticate posturing commonly indicates damage of the cerebral hemispheres, the internal capsule, and the thalamus, possibly also involving the uppermost brainstem. Decerebrate posturing is involuntary extension of both upper (elbow) and lower extremities indicating brainstem damage below the midbrain. Progression from decorticate to decerebrate posturing is indicative of progressive transtentorial herniation. Opisthotonic posturing is an infrequently encountered sign seen with severe brainstem injury or extrapyramidal lesions involving the axial muscles. Importantly, increasing downward pressure leads to dysfunction first at the level of the diencephalon (i.e., thalami), next affecting the upper and middle sections of the brainstem (midbrain and pons), and ultimately impeding medullary function leading to deep coma without any reflexes or motor responses (flaccidity). Once complete rostrocaudal herniation has occurred, the patient is brain dead.

ASSESSMENT OF COMA: GENERAL ASPECTS

Correctly characterizing disorders of consciousness continues to pose interesting clinical questions and diagnostic challenges with important ethical consequences (Box 61.2). Not only may an individual patient acutely fluctuate in his or her examination findings, but recovery may take place over prolonged time periods, necessitating constant reassessments. To address this uncertainty, standardized neurobehavioral assessments have become the best tool for categorizing coma and its transitional stages. Predicting long-term outcome has significantly improved when utilizing standardized assessments. Generally speaking, clinical and electrophysiologic markers of coma and its transitional states remain unsatisfactory. The reader is reminded that larger observational studies identified a high rate of misdiagnoses (>40%),[32] especially in patients in vegetative state, when assessment is made on clinical grounds only.

Box 61.2 Characteristics of Categories in Coma

Supratentorial Mass Lesion Affecting the Diencephalon/Brainstem

Initial focal cerebral dysfunction
Dysfunction progresses rostral to caudal
Signs reflect dysfunction at one level
Signs often asymmetric

Infratentorial Structural Lesion

Symptoms of brainstem dysfunction or sudden onset coma
Brainstem signs precede/accompany coma
Cranial nerve and oculovestibular dysfunction
Early onset of abnormal respiratory patterns

Metabolic-Toxic Coma

Confusion/stupor precede motor signs
Motor signs usually symmetric
Pupil responses generally preserved
Myoclonus, asterixis, tremulousness, and generalized seizures common
Acid-based imbalance common with compensatory ventilatory changes

Psychogenic Coma

Eyelids squeezed shut
Pupils reactive or dilated, unreactive (cycloplegics)
Oculocephalic reflex unpredictable; nystagmus on caloric tests
Motor tone normal or inconsistent
No pathologic reflexes
Awake-pattern EEG

EEG, electroencephalogram.

STANDARDIZED NEUROBEHAVIORAL ASSESSMENT

The behavioral diagnosis of the level of consciousness in severely brain-damaged patients remains challenging. To improve differential diagnostic evaluations, evidence-based recommendations endorse neurobehavioral characteristics using standardized tools.[33] The Coma Recovery Scale-Revised (CRS-R) has excellent content validity and is a solid tool addressing all established differential diagnostic criteria. To differentiate vegetative, minimally conscious state (MCS) or emerging MCS, several other tools have demonstrated good validity, including the Sensory Modality Assessment Technique (SMART), Sensory Stimulation Assessment Measure (SSAM), Wessex Head Injury Matrix (WHIM), and Stimulation Profile (WNSSP). The FOUR and CRS-R tools showed substantial evidence of good interpreter reliability. Our recommendations are to use the Coma Recovery Scale-Revised (CRS-R)[32] as a valid and reliable tool in most situations for differential diagnostic assessments. With reservations, the SMART, WNSSP, SSAM, WHIM, and DOCS can be used. The lack of evidence with respect to content validity, standardization, and reliability make the FOUR, INNS, Glasgow Coma Scale, Swedish Reaction Level Scale-1985, Loewenstein Communication Scale, and CLOCS undesirable.

NEUROIMAGING

Novel neuroimaging modalities have not only provided additional insight into residual brain function in patients with disorders of consciousness but have also raised ethical discussions concerning the clinical management of these patients. Neuroimaging studies have provided considerable evidence for the existence of major functional differences in patients with vegetative state (VS) and minimally conscious state (MCS).[34-37] For example, positron emission tomography (PET) and functional MRI (fMRI) studies delineated more extended cerebral processing in response to various external stimuli of modalities in patients with MCS.[35,36,38] Resting state fMRI studies identified that MCS patients have preservations of functional connectivity to higher-order associative cortices, such as default networks.[37,39] Complementary to these results, brain tissue integrity, as assessed by diffusion weighted imaging and gray matter volumetry, is more preserved in MCS as compared to VS.[34,40] These findings correlate to the relative improved long-term prognosis in MCS.[41]

Currently, MR imaging is the procedure of choice for structural and functional imaging of the brain. Further experience with MR tractography (DTI), estimating the extent of brain connectivity, and MR spectroscopy, evaluating regional neuronal chemistry, will enhance outcome predictions in patients with severe brain injury. In addition, passive, active-response, and resting-state functional MRI paradigms are currently being validated to help in differentiating impaired states of consciousness. The combination of clinical examination and standardized coma assessment with structural and functional imaging currently seems to provide the best estimates for long-term outcome.

CONVENTIONAL MAGNETIC RESONANCE IMAGING (MRI)

Commonly available morphologic MRI acquisitions include non-contrast-enhanced sagittal T1, axial diffusion, axial fluid attenuated inversion recovery (FLAIR), axial T2, coronal T2* (or gradient echo [GRE]) sequences as well as 3D T1-weighted volume acquisitions.

FLAIR and T2-SE sequences are commonly used to delineate, measure, and monitor the extent and impact of acute brain injury. Common pathologies seen include brain edema, contusions, intracerebral, dural or subarachnoid blood, herniation syndromes, and hydrocephalus. T2* (also called GRE) and susceptibility-weighted imaging (SWI) are helpful for delineating blood product and detecting hemorrhagic diffuse axonal injuries (DAI). In traumatic Brain Injury (TBI) patients, the total number of lesions detected on FLAIR and T2* has been shown to inversely correlate with admission GCS score.[42,43] Three-dimensional rendering allows evaluating and quantifying brain atrophy after injury.[44] Conventional MRI is useful in TBI patients. Lesions in the pons, midbrain, and basal ganglia, especially when bilateral, correlate with poor outcome. However, the contrary may not be true as MRI may fail to explain why some vegetative state or marked cognitively impaired patients have minimal or no lesions. Further advanced imaging studies would be especially helpful for those patients (discussed later). Diffusion tensor imaging (DTI) can be viewed as an extension of diffusion-weighted imaging (DWI) where diffusion restricted water molecule movement (i.e., water trapped in ischemic cells or, in DTI, confined to axonal spaces) is preferentially visualized. As with most conventional MRI techniques, obtaining results with DTI is independent of the coma or sedation status of a patient.[45] Serial changes in white matter DTI metrics can be used as surrogate markers to evaluate treatment responses even when clinical scores cannot be obtained.[46] Whole brain white matter and regional DTI measures have become sensitive markers of TBI impact correlating with acute and discharge injury severity, especially when adjusted for age, gender, and admission GCS score.[47,48]

PROTON MAGNETIC RESONANCE SPECTROSCOPY (MRS)

MRS reveals noninvasively regional, metabolic information of targeted brain regions correlating with the functional neuronal state of the examined sample region. To assess brain function, comprehensive MRS protocols looking for changes in axial chemical shift imaging at the level of the cortical white matter,[49,50] splenium,[51] basal ganglia (thalamus),[52] insular cortex, and pons[42] have been used. Using this approach, it is possible to detect posttraumatic neurochemical damage and neuronal dysfunction in brain areas where conventional MR imaging techniques show no abnormalities.[53] In a TBI case-control study, the *N*-acetylaspartate (NAA)/creatinine (Cr) ratio correlated as a good neuronal marker with the overall recovery (and therefore lack as reliable index of unfavorable outcome after TBI), whereas less consistency was found using the choline (Cho)/Cr[54] or NAA/Cho ratios.[55] Moreover, early posttraumatic spectroscopic assessment of axonal damage is clinically relevant for prognostication, and significant increases in brain lactate levels seem to be a dependable index of injury severity and outcome in TBI.[56]

POSITRON EMISSION TOMOGRAPHY (PET)

18-fluorodeoxyglucose (FDG)-PET delineates glucose utilization deficiencies and, hence, it provides insights to neuronal energy metabolism correlating to regional, functional performance. For example, in acute vegetative state, overall glucose utilization was significantly reduced to 50% to 70% in comparison with age-matched, healthy controls.[57] As expected, patients with locked-in syndrome (i.e., pontine lesions) showed normal cortical metabolism. TBI patients with diffuse axonal injury had neuronal hyperglycolysis and metabolic depression.[58] 1C-Flumazenil (FMZ)-PET measures the density of benzodiazepine receptors (BZRs) providing an estimate of neuronal integrity.[15] O-H_2O PET imaging delineates activation-induced changes in regional cerebral blood flow in response to passive external (auditory, somatosensory or visual) stimulation. The combination of preserved activation of primary cortices (i.e., visual) but lack of co-activation of secondary processing areas provides evidence that "higher-order" associative cortical networks are disconnected from the primary sensory cortex.[38,59-63] Thalamocortical disconnections have also been reported using this technique.[64]

FUNCTIONAL MRI (fMRI)

Functional MR imaging provides activity measures of brain regions at rest and after both passive (internal, though-induced) and active (external, command-induced) stimulation.[65] Such acquisitions can obtain estimates of average metabolic activity in relatively short time periods (i.e., 10 minutes) compared to PET (~30 minutes).[66] fMRI has been shown to be a good predictor of outcome in patients with impaired consciousness.[67-72] The previously discussed PET evidence of preserved but isolated (disconnected) cortical activation areas in a patients in vegetative state was corroborated by fMRI.[39,73-76]

ELECTROPHYSIOLOGY

EEG

Although a single electroencephalography (EEG) study can be a helpful diagnostic tool (i.e., to identify seizures), diagnostic certainty improves with continuous or serial EEG monitoring. Reactivity that is the increase in brain wave frequencies with patient stimulation has been used to assess thalamocortical function. For example, a patient with renal or hepatic dysfunction may have slowed background rhythms with triphasic waves and preserved or absence reactivity. Cerebral hypoxia, drug intoxications, and sedative medications as well as other CNS depressants produce abnormal EEG patterns including burst suppression, alpha coma, and spindle coma. Focal EEG slowing with or without evidence of abnormal excitability (i.e., focal spikes) can be found in comatose patients with structural lesions, either focal cortical, focal deep-seated diencephalic or mesencephalic reticular formation, or diffuse bihemispheric. Furthermore, EEG is the primary diagnostic tool to identify patients with impaired consciousness due to nonconvulsive seizures or status epilepticus.

Interpreting EEG can be challenging for anyone not trained in neurophysiology. However, despite the numerous etiologies leading to coma, EEG in coma patients is dominated by a few stereotypic patterns generally providing good indicators of the depth of the coma. Separating three common themes of interpretations will aid the nonexpert in utilizing EEG for diagnosis and prognosis in patients with disorders of consciousness. EEG findings can be categorized into responsiveness (reactivity to acoustic, painful, and photic stimuli), brain wave frequency abnormalities (focal or global), and specific EEG patterns (i.e., seizure discharges). Keeping this categorization in mind, commonly encountered EEG findings will be discussed next.

In patients with *alpha coma* the underlying brain wave activity is predominantly in the (normal) alpha range, from 8 to 12 Hz. In contrast to the normal EEG in a healthy, awake person, the EEG pattern found in comatose patients lacks alpha reactivity, implying a significant disturbance of thalamocortical pathways. In 36 patients in alpha coma,[77] one third showed anterior predominance and two thirds (66%) showed uniform distribution of alpha activity. Three major brain-injury categories have been observed in alpha coma:[78,79] status postcardiorespiratory arrest (anoxic encephalopathy), toxic encephalopathies, and de-efferentiated (locked-in) state (i.e., pontine hemorrhage).

Theta coma and *alpha-theta coma* patients show slower brain wave activities in the theta 4- to 7-Hz range (theta coma), which in some is superseded by a predominance of alpha activity (alpha-theta coma).[80] In many coma patients, the alpha and theta activities will change after about 5 days to a more permanent pattern at which time the EEG may be uniformly slow and depressed. EEG reactivity may emerge in subsequent studies as a relatively favorable sign; however, resolution into a burst-suppression pattern without reactivity signifies unfavorable outcome after anoxic encephalopathy.[80]

Beta coma consists of fast activities in the 12- to 16-Hz range, usually with frontal predominance. Interspersed alpha, theta, delta, and spindle (sleep)-like activities can be found. The most frequent cause for beta coma is sedative-hypnotic overdose from substances such as benzodiazepines and barbiturates.[81]

Intermittent rhythmic delta activity (IRDA) consists of low amplitude, slow 2- to 3-Hz sinusoidal waves. Those waves can appear intermittently during the early stages of impairment of consciousness and soon after loss of alpha rhythm.[78] This nonspecific pattern can be seen in many metabolic and toxic encephalopathies, hemispheric lesions, acute brain injuries, and other conditions affecting cortical and subcortical structures diffusely. The prognosis of IRDA depends on the underlying etiology.

Continuous high-voltage delta activity consists of arrhythmic, high-amplitude, polymorphic 1- to 2-Hz delta activity. This pattern is seen in later stages of coma and may evolve out of theta coma. This contrasts with the slow, nonreactive theta and delta coma EEG of low amplitude (<20 μV) and without reactivity.

Spindle coma consists of an EEG pattern predominated by 11- to 14-Hz spindle discharges, which are generally symmetric and synchronous, appearing as sleeplike oscillations on a background rhythm dominated by theta and delta activities. It resembles the EEG of a sleeping person and additional findings include anterior, low-voltage rhythmic bursts, K complexes, vertex waves, and delta slowing. However, in these patients, wakefulness is not regained after stimulation and depth of consciousness does not fluctuate in spindle coma. These patterns indicate dysfunction at the brainstem level. Traumatic brain injury, anoxic encephalopathy, infectious encephalitis, drug-induced and metabolic encephalopathy, as well as postictal states can lead to this EEG finding.[82-84] The prognosis of spindle coma is uncertain, as both positive[85-87] and negative outcomes[84] have been reported.

Periodic lateralized epileptiform discharges (PLEDs) occur asymmetrically (lateralized) and are episodic in nature. Morphologically, variations include sharp waves, spikes, slow waves, or a combination of these followed by a slow wave with a periodicity ranging from 0.3 to several seconds.[88] PLEDs are nonspecific and can be seen in a wide variety of brain injuries such as after cortical ischemia and with brain tumors. They are also associated with recent seizures, alcohol withdrawal, and toxic-metabolic encephalopathy among many others.[89] In contrast, generalized periodic epileptiform discharges (GPEDs) are seen bilaterally and typically occur at a frequency of <1 Hz. Subclassifications define the interval between discharges and include periodic short-interval diffuse discharges (PSIDDs), periodic long-interval diffuse discharges (PLIDDs), and suppression burst patterns.[90] GPEDs are seen after global brain injury—for example, after hypoxic or hepatic encephalopathy, drug intoxication, but also with various degenerative disorders.[90]

Bilateral independent periodic lateralized epileptiform discharges (BIPLEDs) are slow (<1 Hz), bilateral independent epileptiform activity[91] seen in coma due to bihemispheric lesions. For example, after anoxic encephalopathy and infections, they are associated with a poorer prognosis[91] and about two times higher overall mortality than patients with PLEDS.[91,92]

The *burst-suppression* pattern identifies an EEG demonstrating generalized, synchronous bursting of slow but mixed-frequency waves of high-voltage alternating periodically interspersing within longer periods of isoelectric (flat) EEG. It identifies abnormal cortical excitability,[93] and with deepening coma, the isoelectric periods become longer. Main etiologies include anoxic encephalopathy, severe intoxication, or sedative/anesthesia-induced coma states. The overall prognosis is determined by the underlying etiology.[94]

Triphasic waves are distinct, blunt delta waves (~2 to 3 Hz) consisting of a high-voltage positive wave preceded and followed by lower amplitude negative waves. This nonspecific EEG can be seen in various brain injuries, among them serotoninergic syndrome, Creutzfeldt-Jacob disease, lithium and baclofen toxicity, hepatic and renal insufficiency, and neuroleptic malignant syndrome.[95]

Studies have identified that different EEG patterns seen in patients with hypoxic (postarrest) encephalopathy include suppression, burst suppression, alpha and theta coma, complete generalized suppression (<10 μV), and generalized periodic complexes in combination with burst suppression. Unfortunately, common to all of them is the poor correlation to long-term outcome.[94]

EVENT-RELATED POTENTIALS (ERPs)

These EEG potentials are identifiable after signal-averaging EEG-derived potentials evoked by a specific sensory, cognitive, or motor stimulus. Under normal circumstances, the brain generates event-related, neuronal (electrical) responses to stimulation. This neuronal activation can be detected by surface EEG; however, it requires specific mathematical processing of the EEG signal to identify brain oscillations that are time and phase locked to particular events (stimuli). Detection of such event-related potentials in patients with impaired consciousness has been interpreted as the brain's ability to process stimulus information and for cortical movement preparation. Advantages of this approach include detected signals that have an excellent time-stimulus correlation within the millisecond range helpful to relate a particular stimulus to certain cortical processing. The method is low cost and noninvasive, and it can be used to monitor the brain function. Fast processors have allowed the development of brain-computer interfaces based on event-related signal responses that assist communication with brain-injured patients. Several ERP paradigms have been developed allowing identification of specific response signals. The N1-P2 complex has been identified in visual ERPs and its presence interpreted as a negative correlation to repressiveness.[96] The P300 (or P3) is an average, positive potential with a latency of about 300 milliseconds. It is generated when a patient mentally reacts to a defined cognitive stimulus and is related to positive outcomes in coma.[97] Cognitive responses to command have been verified in patients with complete locked-in syndrome after basilar artery thrombosis.[98]

EVOKED POTENTIALS

Brainstem auditory evoked responses (BAER) are a series of seven potentials recorded at specific time intervals at the skull after defined auditory stimulation employing headphones. Based on the redundancy and interconnections of the auditory pathways, BAER are robust and can be obtained in many patients with depressed level of consciousness, including patients under anesthesia or deep sedation. This implies that the absence of BAER, or its lemniscal complexes III-IV reflecting the integrity of upper brainstem, uniformly infers a poorer prognosis in coma (i.e., 3 to 6 days after head injury).[99] In addition, BAER have been employed as a "brainstem monitoring" tool to identify progressive downward brain herniation. Frequently, in clinical settings, BAER monitoring is combined with somatosensory evoked potential (SEP) and EEG monitoring. Somatosensory evoked potentials (SSEP) are a series of peaks recorded over the neck and scalp in response to electrical stimulation of a peripheral nerve, usually the median nerve. The N13 wave is a negative peak at 13 milliseconds reflecting activity at the cervical cord, whereas the N20 is a negative peak at 20 milliseconds reflecting the earliest cortical activity. Longer latency responses are also seen at 25, 35, 45, 70, and 95 milliseconds, reflecting higher cortical processing. Multimodality evoked potentials (MEP) combine simultaneous brainstem auditory, somatosensory, and visual evoked potential monitoring[100] in order to enhance the predictive value of evoked potential monitoring—for example, in TBI patients[101] or during induced barbiturate coma where examinations cannot be obtained.[102]

CEREBRAL BLOOD FLOW MONITORING

Transcranial Doppler (TCD) records the velocity and pulsatility of cerebral blood flow, allowing hemodynamic analysis, despite the use of sedatives or moderate hypothermia. TCD has been utilized for serial examinations in comatose patients after initial recovery from cardiac arrest in order to detect and treat early cerebral hemodynamic changes. If a patient has an appropriate temporal ultrasound window, TCD can determine cerebral perfusion arrest and, hence, can be used as an ancillary study to determine brain death.[103] Further, velocity and pulsatility indices correlate as a noninvasive measure with ICP elevations and also identify the delayed presence of a hyperemic flow pattern—that is, high velocities with low pulsatility as seen in patients with intracranial hypertension from hyperemia.[104]

XENON-ENHANCED CT SCANNING

Xenon CT utilizes the diffusion of xenon into the CNS to determine cerebral blood flow (CBF)[105] in order to assess perfusion deficits after a traumatic brain injury.[105] Using hyperventilation, xenon CT can be used to estimate cerebral vasoreactivity, a marker correlating with outcome in comatose TBI patients.[106]

GENERAL TREATMENT APPROACH

The immediate goals in a comatose patient are stabilization of vital signs, rapid diagnosis, immediate treatment to reverse the primary injury (i.e., recanalization of cerebral blood flow), and minimization of further nervous system damage from secondary injury (i.e., brain swelling). These general goals are greatly facilitated by a team approach of medical and nursing staff with expertise in acute brain injuries. Successive care steps in managing coma of unknown etiology include (1) immediate exclusion of most harmful brain injuries (i.e., intracranial bleeding from an unsecured aneurysm), (2) sequentially ruling out alternative diagnoses, (3) determining the precise injury type leading to coma, (4) stabilization and reversal of primary brain injury, and (5) intensive brain monitoring (serial examinations, imaging, ICP, etc.) with watchful anticipation and early treatment of secondary injuries. It is of utmost importance to remember that the "time is brain" concept holds true for each of these care steps. Acute coma should be viewed as a "brain arrest" and approached with similar urgency and diligence as cardiac arrest.

If known, initial coma evaluation must take the injury mechanism into account. For example, in trauma victims, empiric cervical spine stabilization and early detection of an unstable c-spine injury by reconstructed cervical CT will be needed (i.e., before evaluating oculocephalic responses). Endotracheal intubation is frequently required due to the risk of aspiration and the need to maintain an open upper airway in an unconscious patient. Prehospital endotracheal intubation was associated with a significant decrease in mortality from 36% to 26% in patients with blunt injury and a GCS ≤ 8, especially those with severe head injury by anatomic criteria.[107] Furthermore, mechanical ventilation is required to avoid oxygen desaturations (of the brain) or to induce therapeutic hypocapnia to acutely lower uncontrolled ICP. Early tracheotomy is often indicated in moderate to severe brain injuries. For example, a GCS of ≤4 on day 3 of injury or a Simplified Acute Physiology Score (SAPS)[108] of >15 on day 4 can indicate tracheotomy with 84% positive predictive value.[109] There are many benefits of early tracheotomy including increased patient comfort and subsequent reduction in sedatives and analgesics and ease of oral and pulmonary care, and its association with shorter duration of mechanical ventilation and ICU length of stay.[110] At our institution we commonly perform bedside tracheotomy, which is a safe bedside procedure that circumvents the need to transport patients with brain injury and reduces overall costs.[111]

Any correctable coma etiology such as abnormal glucose and electrolyte levels, hypotension, hypoxemia, or abnormal core temperatures should be managed immediately. Intravenous access is immediately established for the administration of resuscitation fluids, administration of contrast, and therapeutic care. Infusion of hypotonic solutions should be avoided to prevent deterioration of intracranial swelling, and there is a definite role for immediate ICP monitoring (i.e., using an external ventricular drain, which also allows the release of CSF) in any acute brain injury with the potential for ICP. The management of raised ICP is discussed in Chapter 16.

TRAUMATIC AND NONTRAUMATIC COMA

Coma is a descriptive term based on examination findings and can result from a range of heterogeneous etiologies that are classically grouped into traumatic versus nontraumatic coma. As outlined earlier, other stages of impaired consciousness, including vegetative state, typically follow nonremitting acute coma. Usually after 1 month of coma, the term *persistent vegetative state* is used for both nontraumatic and traumatic etiologies; however, some authors prefer the term *permanent vegetative state* 3 months after nontraumatic and 1 year after traumatic injury. Notably, these terms do not imply irreversibility and do not exclude the potential for further recovery.[112]

Dividing coma into traumatic and nontraumatic etiologies is useful as each group is predominated by different demographics and disease prognosis. Often patients with traumatic brain injury achieve greater functional and cognitive improvements than patients suffering from acquired cerebrovascular or anoxic injury. In a longitudinal, prospective study of 192 traumatic, 104 cerebrovascular, and 33 anoxic brain injury patients, male gender was prevalent in all etiologies. Patients with traumatic brain injury were younger and had shorter admission/rehabilitation intervals, greater functional and cognitive outcomes, and a higher frequency of returning home. In contrast, patients with anoxic brain injury achieved the lowest grade of functional and cognitive recovery.

COMA AFTER SEVERE TRAUMATIC BRAIN INJURY

Therapeutic interventions following severe traumatic brain injury (TBI; GCS ≤ 8) should focus on blocking the primary injury process and preventing or reducing secondary brain injury. Primary injury in severe TBI includes hematoma formation, diffuse axonal injury after high-velocity injury (i.e., vehicle collisions, falls from great height), and ischemic brain injury due to traumatic vascular lesions (i.e., arterial dissection in the neck). Immediate arrest of ongoing primary injury (i.e., by acute recanalization of a dissected arterial occlusion or reversing anticoagulation during ongoing intracerebral bleeding) should be attempted whenever possible. Unfortunately, little can be done to treat or reverse the primary injury in TBI. Secondary brain injuries after TBI are common and include increased brain swelling leading to ICP elevations, brain tissue shifts (herniation) and critical reduction in cerebral perfusion pressure, formation of new hematoma, prolonged seizures, hypoxia, neurogenic/hypovolemic hypotension, uncontrolled hyperventilation, hypoglycemia, thromboembolism from venous thrombosis, and so on. Therefore, early TBI management strategies should focus on prevention and early recognition of such complications and a combination of intracranial (i.e., ICP, brain temperature, brain oxygen tension and perfusion) and systemic monitoring as well as repeated neuroimaging is indicated in the patients.

Noncontrast CT is the most common imaging evaluation tool in TBI patients. A cervical spine CT with reconstructed views and head and neck CT angiogram (CTA) are often added during initial evaluation, if injury to the neck and arteries, respectively, is suspected. Bone and brain windows should be reviewed separately and in experienced hands. Head imaging has a good sensitivity for the presence of pathologic air, skull fractures, hemorrhagic lesions, abnormalities of the brain parenchyma (i.e., shift), and obstruction of CSF spaces (hydrocephalus). Injury to the neuroanatomic structures of consciousness or the presence of additional etiologies for coma (i.e., alcohol) should be considered when disparities between CT findings and examination exist. In this setting, appropriate additional screening and further imaging diagnostics (i.e., MRI) must be initiated.[113] Compared to CT, MRI has a higher sensitivity to detect diffuse axonal injury (DAI); however, this advantage has not translated into improved clinical outcomes as there is currently no treatment for this condition. However, both the detection of DAI and delineating injury of major motor (i.e., corticospinal) tracts on diffusion tensor imaging (DTI) can be utilized together with the clinical course to prognosticate TBI.[114] MR spectroscopy (MRS) provides additional "chemical" information, especially of the white matter injury process.[115]

The presence and severity of secondary brain injury should constantly be assessed and managed throughout the acute phase of TBI. Its time course can be variable but is somewhat predictable: for example, ranging from hours (i.e., development of new hematoma) to 1 to 3 days for brain edema development to several days as seen in late brain ischemia from vasospasm due to traumatic subarachnoid blood. There is only limited evidence to support the use of ICP monitoring. ICP monitoring has evolved as an essential tool and also one of the earliest monitoring tools in clinical practice; thus many believe clinical trials cannot ethically be justified. Current TBI management guidelines recommend its use in severe TBI. Of note, head imaging cannot predict ICP. Furthermore, treating for elevated ICP (other than empirically in the emergency setting) and not monitoring ICP can be deleterious and result in a poor outcome.[116] In addition to ICP, other brain monitoring techniques utilized in modern TBI management include jugular venous and transcranial oxygen saturations ($SjvO_2$; NIRS), brain tissue oxygen tension (btO_2), brain tissue metabolism (microdialysis) and temperature, direct brain perfusion, transcranial Doppler sonography, and electrophysiologic studies such as EEG and evoked potentials. A discussion of these techniques is beyond the scope of this chapter and the reader is referred to recent reviews.

The management of severe TBI includes emergent decompressive craniectomy in controlling intractable ICP, especially if deterioration is associated with hematoma evacuation and there is some evidence that there will be positive outcomes in surviving patients.[117-128] Although timing of decompressive craniectomy remains controversial, early referral seems most intuitive. The Brain Trauma Foundation's Guidelines for Management of Severe Traumatic Brain Injury regard craniectomy as an option after TBI to manage patients with intracerebral hemorrhage (ICH) and the resultant increased ICP refractory to medical management.[116] Intravenous mannitol and hypertonic saline solutions are a main building block in the management of increased ICP.[129-141] The superiority of one over the other is uncertain, and both approaches are routinely used in the management of severe TBI.[142] Therapeutic hypothermia is postulated to exert neuroprotective effects by several mechanisms, including reducing cerebral metabolic rate/requirement, modulating apoptosis or programmed cell death, reducing intracellular calcium/toxic excitatory neurotransmitters/inflammation, and preserving protein synthesis.[116,143-151] However, the reported impact on neurologic outcome in severe TBI remains inconsistent and a meta-analysis of randomized controlled trials suggests its lack of benefit in severe TBI.[143,144] We utilize hypothermia as last resort therapy and commonly, together with pentobarbital therapy and ICP-matching, CPP elevation to protect the brain from otherwise intractable ICP elevations. Until well-designed, randomized controlled trials are available, its use must be weighed against potential side effects such as an increased incidence in pneumonia and coagulation abnormalities, among others.[143,151]

The initial GCS seems to be a reasonable marker to predict mortality from severe TBI. To further improve prediction, models include a combination of clinical data, imaging results, GCS score, and patient demographics.[152] In a large, traumatic coma databank study,[153] patients with severe injury (GCS 3 to 8) had approximately 36% mortality. In 170 patients, the GCS 5 hours postinjury was compared to the Glasgow Outcome Scale (GOS) at 1 month and positive recovery was seen in 99% of mild TBI (GCS 13 to 15), 71% of moderate TBI(GCS 9 to 12), and in only 35% of severe TBI. In contrast, only 2% to 3% of patients with mild TBI (GCS 13 to 15) died. Generally speaking, clinical outcome after TBI is more variable than in nontraumatic coma (i.e., after hypoxia).[154] Furthermore, outcome predictions for patients with intermediate GCS scores identify that a midline shift of less than 4.1 mm on initial CT scanning had a significantly higher favorable outcome rate compared with patients with a larger shift.[155]

Biomarkers after traumatic brain injury (TBI), such as cellular glial fibrillary acidic protein (GFAP) and S100B released with astrocyte injury, may offer diagnostic and prognostic tools in addition to clinical indices. In 79 patients with TBI (GSC $\leq$ 12), identified intracranial mass lesion, pupillary reactivity, GFAP, and S100B were the strongest predictors of death and unfavorable outcome, with S100B as the strongest single predictor of unfavorable outcome with 100% discrimination.[156] Somatosensory evoked potentials in 58 TBI patients unconscious for >30 days were compared with outcome at 12 months[157] and showed an excellent prediction for outcome (persistent coma or MCS, 92% and 86%, respectively) at 12 months when combined with age, sex, and GCS.[157] Furthermore, among electrophysiologic testing, SEP and BAEP are more sensitive than EEG (i.e., 45% to 60% sensitive versus 35%) and if EEG and SEP show opposing results, generally speaking, prognosis is linked to the better test result.[158] The results of multimodality evoked potentials can be used as a reliable prognostic indicator (91% accuracy) in TBI patients.[101]

The International Mission for Prognosis and Analysis of Clinical Trials in TBI (IMPACT) is a prognostic model predicting 6-month functional outcome (Glasgow Outcome Scale [GOS]) and mortality in 587 patients with severe TBI (mean age 38 $\pm$ 17 years). At the 6th month, the median GOS was 3 (IQR 3) and 6-month mortality 41%, and age, motor score, pupillary reactivity, head CT findings, secondary insults, and laboratory values displayed good prediction ability for unfavorable outcome and mortality.[159] In another study of 428 isolated, older adult TBI cases, the in-hospital death rate was 28%, and increasing age, decreasing GCS, and injury type were significant independent predictors of in-hospital mortality. At the 6-month follow-up, age < 75 years and with systolic blood pressure (BP) on arrival at hospital of 131 to 150 mm Hg had higher likelihood of living independently at follow-up. No patients with a GCS <

9 had a favorable 6-month outcome, and most of them died, with the survival rate for brainstem injury at 21%.[160]

COMA AFTER CARDIAC ARREST

Cardiac arrest affects more than 300,000 people each year in the United States alone and anoxic-ischemic encephalopathy is among the leading causes of mortality and morbidity. Since the publication of two pivotal trials in 2002 utilizing systemic cooling, the outcome for patients in coma after out-of-hospital ventricular fibrillation arrest has significantly improved. Simultaneously, prognostication after arrest in patients has become more complicated as the literature is lacking new prospective outcome studies integrating the advantages of hypothermia treatment.

The retrospective landmark study by Levy and colleagues,[161] which reviewed postcardiac arrest outcome of 210 patients studied in the mid-1970s, is still commonly applied for prognostication. However, several inherent epidemiologic shortcomings of this study exist in addition to the fact that postcardiac arrest management has obviously advanced. The American Academy of Neurology published guidelines in 2006[162] based on an in-depth review of the available literature; however, most studies included were performed without the use of hypothermia. The guideline defines poor outcome either as coma or death at 1 month or severe disability at 6 months. Further, the absence of brainstem reflexes or absence of extensor motor responses at 72 hours was shown to be highly specific (or have a false positive rate near zero) and so were absence of somatosensory evoked responses (SSEPs) and a high level of neuron-specific enolase (NSE).

Hypothermia has multiple actions not only within the CNS but also systemically. Among them are depression of neuronal activity, amelioration of intracellular postischemic reactions mitigating secondary cell injury, cardiac arrhythmias, hypocoagulability, decrease in immune defense, and reduction in drug metabolism and clearance. Notably, the latter can lead to misinterpretation of the prolonged effects of sedatives and paralytics. Therefore, interpretation of the neurologic examination and prognostication in patients undergoing hypothermia or rewarming is complex and challenging. Generally speaking and without the use of hypothermia, absence of brainstem reflexes implies that the cortex is severely affected as the brainstem neurons are more resistant to hypoxia-ischemia. Absence of pupillary reflexes at 72 hours predicts poor outcome with high specificity; however, the opposite, the presence of reflexive pupils, only predicts good outcome in about 21%. Studies performed after the introduction of hypothermia[163-165] delineate predictive findings for absent papillary responses but delineate that the corneal reflex seems to be more vulnerable to prolonged sedative and hypothermic effects. With respect to motor responses, studies performed prior to hypothermia identify a high predictive value for poor outcome for the absence of motor responses at 72 hours, a clinical finding that outperformed even SSEP prediction.[166] On the contrary, studies suggest that the lack of motor responses does not invariably predict poor outcome in patients treated with hypothermia (i.e., positive predictive values 92% and negative predictive value 85%) and exceptions have been reported.[163-165,167]

Electroencephalography (EEG) is used in postcardiac arrest patients to determine outcome but also to differentiate myoclonus from shivering and detect seizures. Generalized EEG suppression, burst suppression with or without epileptiform activity, and a flat background with intermittent generalized periodic complexes are indicators of poorer prognosis. The opposite is true for finding reactivity and variability of the EEG pattern in patients treated with or without cooling. Larger prospective studies are currently lacking; however, some reports identify some hypothermia-treated patients with postanoxic status epilepticus who can achieve good outcome,[168] especially when the status evolves from a continuous EEG pattern and not from burst suppression.[169] As seizures and status epilepticus are seen in up to 65% of patients with less severe cortical damage, continuous EEG is indicated to guide management and prognostication in many postarrest patients.

According to current practice parameters from 2006, the absence of the N20 (primary cortical somatosensory) wave on SSEPs in the first 3 days after cardiac arrest identifies a high likelihood for poor outcome. In contrast, only about 41% of patients with present N20 wave will recover. Prognosticating based on SSEP findings in patients treated with hypothermia has only been reported in a few smaller studies with uncertain overall results[170,171]; however, SSEP likely remains useful as evoked potentials are relatively resistant to metabolic and temperature derangements. Also, the NSE is a frequently used and validated biochemical marker used for prognostication. Levels >33 mcg/L at 72 hours or earlier were found to have zero false predictive rate in patients treated without hypothermia. However, hypothermia decreases NSE levels. Some studies have shown that a similar cutoff also holds true for the hypothermia-treated patient population,[172-174] whereas others found unacceptable false-positive rates for the cutoff value 33 mcg/L.[175,176] With respect to imaging, certain MRI findings such as severe cortical abnormalities on diffusion-weighted imaging have been shown to correlate to poor outcome,[177] but imaging studies often report on smaller patient numbers and are performed unblinded, reducing their value for prediction. Some studies identify that most patients who regained consciousness had normal cortical structures, some of them despite involvement of the deep gray nuclei.[178,179]

Myoclonic status epilepticus are generalized, multifocal, repetitive muscle jerks involving some or all parts of the body. They are frequently seen within 24 hours after arrest, and EEG often shows burst suppression or bursts of generalized spikes. Whether myoclonic discharges actually represent seizures remains controversial, and as patients may have severe cortical damage and clinical myoclonus at the same time, it is postulated that myoclonus status epilepticus is subcortical in origin. In contrast, postanoxic status epilepticus is cortical in origin (but some overlap to myoclonic status may exist), whereas the posthypoxic myoclonus (Lance-Adams syndrome) is generally seen after primary respiratory failure. It is triggered by startle, often subsides over time, and the patient may be aware and distressed by it. Myoclonic status epilepticus has been associated with poor prognosis and remains poor even in the setting of hypothermia.[163,165]

Given these results it seems prudent to forecast the postarrest patient treated with hypothermia 72 hours after the event. Examination should take place at least 12 hours after termination of all sedatives and later if concomitant renal and liver damage are confounding factors. Prognostic variables associated with but not invariably predictive of poor outcomes are (1) absences of brainstem reflexes, (2) absence of motor responses or extensor posturing, (3) EEG abnormalities including generalized suppressions or periodic complexes on suppressed background and a burst suppression pattern with generalized epileptiform activity, (4) myoclonic status epilepticus, (5) MRI with widespread cortical injury on DWI or CT with loss of gray-white matter differentiation and sulcal effacement, (6) high NSE levels, and (7) absence of N20 on SSEP.

ETHICAL CONSIDERATIONS

A surrogate decision maker is a person who directs care when the patient is unable to provide consent. Legally and ethically, surrogate decisions should follow the expressed wishes of the patient. In the absence of known prior wishes, surrogates should utilize the best standard with respect to what the patient would do when confronted by the circumstance. A surrogate designated by the patient has precedence over other potential decision makers and is delineated by an advanced directive, also called a health care proxy, health care agent, or durable power of attorney for health care. In contrast, a living will expresses patient preferences but does not authorize a surrogate decision maker or spokesperson. If there is no designated surrogate, family members and close friends are selected in order of their relationship to the patient; the highest priority is given to the spouse, then parents, then children, then siblings followed by other relatives and finally friends. In a comatose patient, surrogates or family members may authorize a do no resuscitate (DNR) order or request limitations of care (i.e., no hemodialysis). Approximately two thirds of DNR orders are put into place by surrogate decision makers.[180]

It is important to strive for the best possible diagnostic and prognostic correctness when discussing a DNR order or withdrawal of care. Understandably, relatives and surrogates place a great deal of decision making on the significance of conscious experience and the level of expected patient interactions with the environment (recovery). Therefore, the diagnostic accuracy of a patient's present level of consciousness is requested from the treating physician as well as the best estimate of improvement of consciousness.[181] Identifying medical futility in a patient with markedly impaired consciousness allows the surrogate and physician to withdraw life-supporting therapy. However, surrogate decision making may change if a patient is in a minimal conscious state, as this disorder implies different prognostication, especially in TBI patients.[182] Further, it is important for physicians to reiterate to the family that coma progression into the vegetative state is not considered an improvement. This progression is seen in most coma patients and sleep-wake cycles, roving eye movements, startle, and other witnessed phenomena are merely reflexive and do not indicate consciousness or awareness. Of note, "persistence" is a diagnosis given to a patient who remains in a vegetative state for greater than 1 month. This state is considered permanent when it persists for 3 months after anoxic brain injury and 12 months after TBI.[2] Greater prognostic uncertainties exist for patients in a state of minimal consciousness, as these patients have consistent evidence of consciousness, awareness, and, in some, the ability to communicate. Because these patients have an unpredictable recovery, it is necessary to continue standardized assessment and therapy.

Physicians and care teams should utilize the latest medical evidence when discussing the probability of recovery from impaired consciousness with the family and surrogate decision maker. Further, it should be delineated that prognostication is inherently difficult. Outcome studies include a broader patient spectrum with a range of brain injury mechanisms. Furthermore, recovery is a dynamic and fluctuating process with marked individual variations. Such discussions require a delicate balance of perspectives on the need for clinical decision making and the inevitable fact of remaining medical uncertainties. Discussions with families and surrogates should include a thorough investigation about what the patient would have decided facing the inevitable scenario of permanent impaired (cognitive and physical) existence. This includes the importance of respecting a surrogate's decision that ongoing life support would have been unacceptable with the patient's wishes.

KEY POINTS

- Coma is a state of pathologic unresponsiveness from which the patient cannot be aroused. The eyes are closed, and only reflex responses or no responses at all can be elicited from the patient when applying vigorous stimulation.
- The cause of coma is diverse and follows neuronal injury, reversible or irreversible, to both cerebral hemispheres or to the reticular activating system in the diencephalon and brainstem.
- A supratentorial mass legion located within one hemisphere can induce a lateral herniation syndrome with lateral torsion of the midbrain plus uncal herniation. In contrast a mass lesion located within the brain midline (i.e., acute hydrocephalus) primarily lead to downward herniation with rostocaudal compression of the brainstem.
- An acute mass lesion below the tentorium (i.e., a cerebellar hemorrhage) early on compresses the brainstem, leading to cranial nerve deficits, obstructed CSF outflow resulting in hydrocephalus, and, if large enough, herniation of brain tissue upward through the tentorium and downward through the foramen magnum. On examination these patients may present with a complete lack of all cranial nerve and motor function, yet hemispheric function may be preserved.
- Initial attention must focus on the restoration of respiratory, hemodynamic, and metabolic homeostasis in parallel with a search to identify the cause and acuity of the coma state. Generally, a comatose patient's recovery depends on appropriate treatment of the underlying disorder but also very much on

KEY POINTS (Continued)

monitoring and stabilizing brain function (ICP, perfusion, etc.).

- Status epilepticus is characterized by either clinically detectable (convulsive) or EEG-identified (nonconvulsive) seizure activity. Both require immediate and aggressive treatment to avoid permanent brain damage.
- Alteration in cognitive function (especially attention and concentration deficit) is the earliest manifestation of metabolic encephalopathy. Some disease processes may provide specific diagnostic clues.
- The neurologic examination consists of an assessment of the level of arousal determined by eye opening, verbal responses, and reflex or purposeful movements in response to noxious stimulation of the face, arms, and legs. Neuro-ophthalmologic function is evaluated by spontaneous eye movements, pupillary size and response to light, oculocephalic responses (doll's eyes), and oculovestibular (ice water caloric) responses. Autonomic function is assessed by the respiratory pattern and observing the monitored vital sign changes before and during examination.

SELECTED REFERENCES

2. Medical aspects of the persistent vegetative state (2). The Multi-Society Task Force on PVS. N Engl J Med 1994;330:1572-1579.
3. Hamel MB, Goldman L, Teno J, et al: Identification of comatose patients at high risk for death or severe disability. JAMA 1995;273:1842-1848.
7. Medical aspects of the persistent vegetative state (1). The Multi-Society Task Force on PVS. N Engl J Med 1994;330:1499-1508.
28. Goldberg S: The Four Minute Neurologic Exam. Miami, FL, Medmaster, 1992.
41. Luaute J, Maucort-Boulch D, Tell L, et al: Long-term outcomes of chronic minimally conscious and vegetative states. Neurology 2010;75:246-252.
56. Marino S, Zei E, Battaglini M, et al: Acute metabolic brain changes following traumatic brain injury and their relevance to clinical severity and outcome. J Neurol Neurosurg Psychiatry 2007;78: 501-507.
168. Rossetti AO, Logroscino G, Liaudet L, et al: Status epilepticus: An independent outcome predictor after cerebral anoxia. Neurology 2007;69:255-260.
175. Fugate JE, Wijdicks EF, Mandrekar J, et al: Predictors of neurologic outcome in hypothermia after cardiac arrest. Ann Neurol 2010;68:907-914.
181. Giacino JT, Kalmar K: Diagnostic and prognostic guidelines for the vegetative and minimally conscious states. Neuropsychol Rehabil 2005;15:166-174.
182. Lammi MH, Smith VH, Tate RL, Taylor CM: The minimally conscious state and recovery potential: A follow-up study 2 to 5 years after traumatic brain injury. Arch Phys Med Rehabil 2005;86: 746-754.

The complete list of references can be found at www.expertconsult.com.

62 Neurologic Criteria for Death in Adults

Fred Rincon

CHAPTER OUTLINE

The clinical examination in brain death is the most unequivocal in neurology. Most of the time, establishing the diagnosis of brain death on clinical grounds is not a difficult task, as long as providers follow established protocols and guidelines for the interpretation of findings during clinical examination.[1,2] However, there may be confusion based on the variability of the interpretation of current guidelines,[3,4] hurdles to clinical examination in specific patient populations such as trauma victims, laws from specific jurisdictions, and the changing face of outcomes after severe brain injury in an era of advancements in critical care and resuscitative medicine. In this chapter we will review current procedures and recommendations for the evaluation of comatose patients presumed brain dead, the concept of brain death substantiated by anatomic and physiologic bases, important concepts for the determination of brain death in the setting of novel interventions such as hypothermia and extracorporeal circulation, and how to avoid pitfalls during the evaluation of patients presumed brain dead.

HISTORICAL PERSPECTIVE AND DEFINITIONS

The concept of brain death is modern to medicine but the definition of death has historically been associated with physiologic cessation of cardiopulmonary function. With advancements in mechanical ventilation, life support, and resuscitation medicine, a new state in which a patient's cardiopulmonary functions could be sustained in the absence of neurologic function emerged. In 1959, Mollaret and Goulon described 23 patients with irreversible coma, whose clinical syndrome was characterized by the absence of brainstem function, spontaneous respiratory function, and cardiovascular collapse that ensued without the use of vasopressors, in what became the birth of the concept of brain death.[5] In 1963, Harvard neurologists proposed that a patient be certified as dead in the setting of coma, absence of brainstem reflexes, apnea for 30 minutes, and an isoelectric electroencephalogram (EEG) tracing in all leads for more than 30 minutes,[6] despite the presence of cardiac function. The first guideline (the Harvard criteria) for deciding brain death was established in 1968.[7] This concept has been accepted worldwide, although its fundamental meaning is not exactly globally uniform yet. Some countries, such as the United States, accept the concept of brain death as "whole brain death," which is defined as irreversible loss of all cortical and brainstem function. The Medical Royal Colleges of the United Kingdom established the definition of brain death on a "lower brain" concept of brainstem death.[8] In the opinion of the Royal Medical College, permanent unconsciousness secondary to neuronal death of brainstem structures such as the reticular activating system (RAS) is irreversible.[8]

In 1981, a Presidential Commission in the United States was formed to address the issue of death by neurologic criteria.[9] The President's Commission established the foundations of the criteria currently used in the United States for the diagnosis of brain death: the cause of brain death should be known and irreversible and no improvement in neurologic condition should occur during a period of observation; the period of observation was left at the discretion of the physician, but periods of 6 to 12 hours were recommended depending on the availability of confirmatory testing such as EEG or cerebral perfusion scans.[9] Though the President's Commission suggested periods of observation of 24 hours for cases of ischemia-anoxia,[9] more recent clinical experience in the era of therapeutic hypothermia and published guidelines suggest a period of observation of up to 72 hours in patients with hypoxic-ischemic coma.[10] The President's Commission guidelines for the determination of brain death culminated in a proposal for a legal definition that led to the Uniform Determination of Death Act (UDDA) in 1981. Under the law, the determination of death must be made with accepted medical standards and can be established only if an individual "has sustained either: 1) irreversible cessation of circulatory and respiratory functions, or 2) irreversible cessation of all functions of the entire brain, including the brain stem."

In 1995, the American Academy of Neurology (AAN) published the practice parameter to delineate the medical standards for the determination of brain death.[11] The guideline emphasized the three clinical findings necessary to confirm irreversible cessation of all brain functions including the brainstem: (1) known cause and presence of coma, (2) absence of brainstem reflexes, and (3) apnea.[11] Despite this publication, there is considerable practice variation in the adherence to the AAN guidelines for the determination of brain death, particularly in areas related to definitions of acceptable core temperature, number of required examinations, ancillary testing to be used,[3] and deficiencies in documentation.[3] In response to this phenomenon, the AAN published an evidence-based update of the 1995 Practice Parameter[12] to answer the main questions related to practice variability in the determination of brain death.[3,13]

In the United States, most state laws have adopted the UDDA, and some have added their own amendments. All states and the District of Columbia have statutes for determining brain death based on the UDDA, but certain statutes differ in minor points such as the requirement that determination of brain death should be done by two different physicians, the use of confirmatory testing, and the notification of next of kin before the declaration of brain death. To this end, it is important for the practitioner to understand local hospital policies for the declaration of brain death that should abide by the laws of their respective jurisdictions. Additional information about specific status in jurisdictions of the United States can be downloaded from http://www.braindeath.org.

DETERMINATION OF BRAIN DEATH

The most common causes of brain death in the adult population are traumatic brain injury (TBI), aneurysmal subarachnoid hemorrhage (SAH), hypoxic-ischemic injury, and fulminant hepatic failure.[14] It is estimated that the diagnosis of brain death is made at least 25 to 30 times a year in large referral centers, but this number may be lower in nonacademic centers.[14] The determination of brain death is based on the UDDA and supported by the AAN Practice Parameter.[11,12] The diagnosis is based on the establishment of three main criteria: (1) known cause and presence of coma, (2) absence of brainstem reflexes, and (3) apnea. Therefore, the clinical diagnosis, when considering accepted guidelines, is the most unequivocal in neurology.

In general, most jurisdictions require that the determination of brain death be made by a licensed physician, which in most of the cases should be an attending physician who has experience in the assessment of comatose patients and the legal requirements applicable to the jurisdiction of practice. Some centers require the testing to be performed by two different physicians, and some centers require one of these physicians to be a neurologist, neurosurgeon, or critical care specialist. In the United States, 42% of top neuroscience centers required the brain death examination to be documented by a neurologist or neurosurgeon and only 35% required that an attending neurologist or neurosurgeon be involved; of the 42% centers, residents could document the examination in up to 65% of the centers.[3] In those circumstances in which the patient is a potential organ donor, the clinical team may not be directly involved with the discussions of organ procurement, as a conflict of interest may be apparent.

CLINICAL EVALUATION OF COMA AND PREREQUISITES

Practitioners should first determine the cause of coma by history, physical examination, neuroimaging, and laboratory testing. Exclusion of central nervous system (CNS) depressants should be attempted by careful history taking, drug screen testing, and calculation of drug clearance using the rule of five times the drugs half-life (assuming a normal hepatic and renal function) or drug plasma levels below therapeutic ranges.[12] In the setting of abnormal hepatic or renal function, or after use of therapeutic hypothermia, caution should be taken before entertaining the diagnosis of brain death based on changes in drug metabolism inherent to these clinical settings, and to avoid catastrophic and embarrassing misdiagnoses.[15] In these circumstances, more than recommended times for observation are suggested or the use of confirmatory testing may be sought. The legal limit for ethanol is a blood alcohol content of 0.08%, which is a practical threshold below which an examination to determine brain death could reasonably proceed.[12] In those patients exposed to pentobarbital for the management of intracranial hypertension, an accepted level in which a clinical examination can proceed without chance of confounding is 10 μg/mL.[12] There should be no temporal administration of neuromuscular blockers and this can be assessed definitely by the presence of train-of-four twitches with maximal ulnar stimulation. Acid-base status and electrolyte levels must not be severely deviated from the norm, but the presence of signs and symptoms of *diabetes insipidus* does not preclude the diagnosis of brain death; however, treatment with fluids and vasopressors such as vasopressin will target both sodium and blood pressure requirements to allow for adequate neurologic assessment. With more cardiac arrest survivors being exposed to therapeutic hypothermia, practitioners should now achieve a normal core temperature, defined as near-normal temperature or core temperature higher than 36° C, before attempting to determine brain death. Patients should have normal blood pressure, defined as systolic blood pressure (SBP) equal to or higher than 100 mm Hg, as the neurologic examination is usually reliable at this level of blood pressure.

A temporal cause of severe brain injury must be established. Irreversibility from neurologic injury is recognized by the extent of the injury, the devastation in neurologic findings, and the lack of improvement. Neuroimaging is useful in establishing an acute neurologic catastrophe that

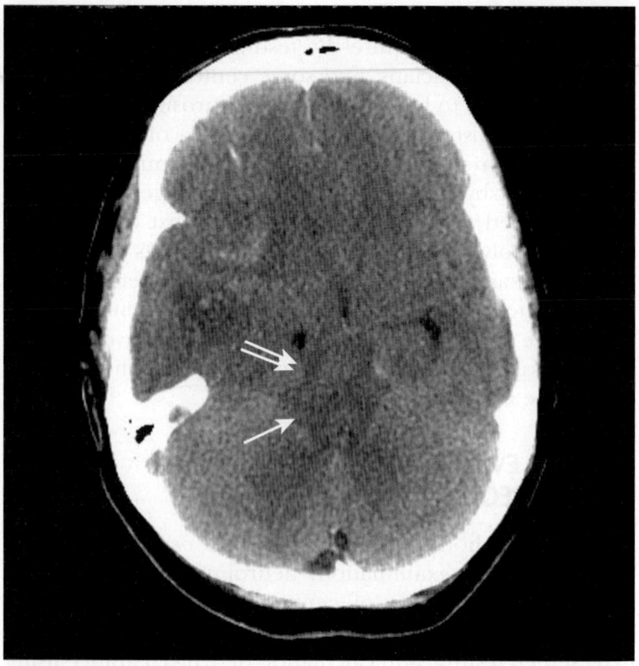

Figure 62.1 Computed tomography scan of a young patient with traumatic brain injury showing right frontal contusion, mild subarachnoid hemorrhage, and severe cerebral edema. The patient has suffered bilateral transtentorial uncal herniations (*double arrow*, for right-sided uncus); note that the horn of the right lateral ventricle has been pushed toward the midline. The perimesencephalic cisterns are effaced (*single arrow*). There is slight hypodensity in the midbrain suggesting edema or ischemia.

is compatible with the clinical diagnosis. In most cases, a computed tomography (CT) scan will reveal specific findings such as diffuse cerebral edema, mass lesions with severe shift of midline structures, and herniation (Fig. 62.1).

Coma is established by the lack of all evidence of responsiveness. That is, eye opening or eye movement to noxious stimuli must be absent. The motor responses to noxious stimuli should not be flexor or extensor but spinally mediated. The clinical differentiation of motor responses may require experience and specific training in neurology or neurosurgery. When flexor posturing of the upper extremities and extension of the lower extremities (decorticate) or extensor posturing of both the upper and lower extremities (decerebrate) is observed, the diagnosis of brain death cannot be entertained and an additional period of observation is recommended (Fig. 62.2). The basis of these responses is related to the patency of the rubrospinal and vestibulospinal tracts, and lower segments of the medulla that connect with the spinal cord.[16] Brain death patients typically exhibit spinal cord–mediated motor responses characterized by "en bloc" flexor responses of the lower extremities with flexion of the hip, flexion of the knee, and dorsiflexion of the ankle and toes (the so-called triple flexion response or Babinski en bloc spinal cord sign) (see Fig. 62.2). More complex movements that have been referred to as brain death–associated reflexes (Lazarus sign, spinal man, spinal reflexes, or spinal automatisms) have been described in patients who otherwise meet all other brain death criteria.[17] When in doubt, the neurologic examination of a comatose patient becomes equivocal, and in these circumstances, additional observation or a confirmatory test may be warranted.

ABSENCE OF BRAINSTEM REFLEXES

All segments of the brainstem should be tested in the clinical examination. The highest segments are examined by documentation of the pupillary response to bright light in both eyes (cranial nerves II and III). The usual presentation is dilated fixed pupils, which may be asymmetrical. Constricted pupils may mean drug intoxication or lesions at the level of the pons causing de-efferentation from sympathetic fibers and unopposed activation of parasympathetic centers located in the rostral area of the midbrain (Edinger-Westphal nucleus). Absence of ocular movements using oculocephalic and oculovestibular reflex testing can be achieved after assuring integrity of the cervical spine (cranial nerves III, IV, VI, and VIII [vestibular part]). The oculocephalic reflex is tested by briskly rotating the head side to side and vertically. Vertical oculocephalic movements are important for the determination of brain death as injuries in the lateral portions of the pons may manifest with bilateral palsies of horizontal eye movements but would spare the vertical eye movements. The oculovestibular or cold-caloric reflex is tested by irrigating each ear with 50 mL of iced water and observing the response for up to 1 minute. The absence of corneal reflexes (cranial nerves VII, V, and others) is demonstrated by touching the cornea with a cotton swab or gauze. Painful noxious stimulation in the cranium, trunk, or limbs should not produce any facial movement or grimacing (cranial nerve VII). Absence of pharyngeal (cranial nerve IX) or gag reflex (cranial nerve IX) is demonstrated by stimulating the back of the mouth or oropharynx with a suction device or tongue blade. The tracheal reflex (cranial nerve X) is tested by examining the cough response to tracheal stimulation provided by suctioning. Additional cranial nerve reflexes such as the "jaw jerk" (cranial nerve V) may be assessed for completeness and to follow established guidelines.[11] Any unanticipated movements of any segment of the face, trunk, or limbs during brainstem examination implies intact brainstem efferent connections and precludes the diagnosis of brain death. In trauma victims with facial trauma in whom adequate examination of brainstem patency cannot be substantiated, the use of confirmatory testing may be warranted.

Deviations from accepted guidelines during clinical examination of comatose patients presumed brain dead may be associated with false-positive results, so a thorough examination of all segments of the brainstem is required. Areas of particular deviation from the AAN Practice Parameter for the determination of brain death include failure of testing for pain above the foramen magnum, the oculocephalic reflex, the jaw-jerk reflex, and establishing the absence of spontaneous respirations[3] (Fig. 62.3).

APNEA

Complete absence of breathing drive must exist to confirm the diagnosis of brain death. The absence of respiratory drive is tested with a CO_2 challenge, which requires all of the following: (1) normotension, (2) normothermia, (3)

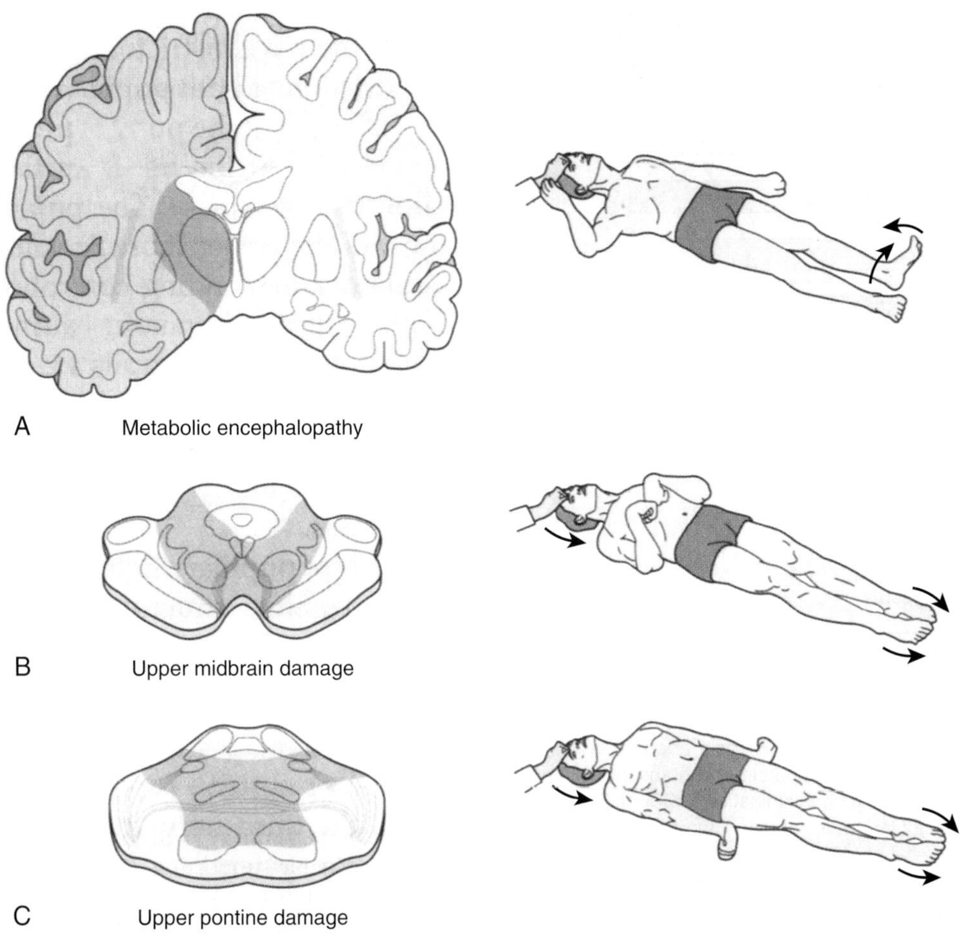

Figure 62.2 The motor response to painful stimulation during the examination of comatose patients. **A,** Localization with right upper extremity and dorsiflexion of ankle and toe. **B,** Flexor posturing of the upper extremities and extension of the lower extremities (decorticate rigidity). **C,** Extensor posturing of both the upper and lower extremities (decerebrate rigidity). Note that the response of the lower extremities is always extensor in both flexor and extensor posturing. (From Saper CB: Brain stem modulation of sensation, movement, and consciousness. In Kandel ER, Schwartz JH, Jessell TM (eds): Principles of Neural Science. New York, McGraw-Hill, 2000, pp 889-909. Used with permission from McGraw-Hill.)

euvolemia, (4) eucapnia ($Pa{CO_2}$ 35-45 mm Hg), (5) absence of hypoxia, and (6) no prior evidence of CO_2 retention (chronic obstructive pulmonary disease [COPD], severe obesity, or sleep apnea syndrome).[12] The test is started by preoxygenating the patient with 1.0 $F{IO_2}$ for 10 minutes to achieve a $Pa{O_2}$ of more than 200 mm Hg using a respiratory rate of 10 per minute to achieve eucapnia. If the patient remains hemodynamically stable and with oxygen saturation more than 95%, the patient is disconnected from the ventilator and oxygenation is preserved by placing a catheter through the endotracheal tube and close to the level of the carina delivering O_2 at 1.0 $F{IO_2}$ with a flow of 6 L/minute. During the following 8 to 10 minutes, the practitioner should look carefully for respiratory movements (abdominal or chest excursions and may include a brief gasp).[12] The test should be aborted if oxygen saturation drifts lower than 85% for more than 30 seconds. If this is the case, the test can be repeated later using a T-piece, continuous positive airway pressure (CPAP) with 10 cm H_2O, and O_2 with 1.0 $F{IO_2}$ with a flow of 12 L/minute.[12,18] The test is considered positive if respiratory movements are absent and the $Pa{CO_2}$ is higher than 60 mm Hg or 20 mm Hg change from baseline supporting the diagnosis of brain death.[12]

Pitfalls in the diagnosis of brain death may be related to circumstances involving interference with the appropriate clinical diagnosis of brain death such as patients with (1) facial trauma (inability to appropriately examine cranial nerve responses or to elicit sensory/motor responses from stimulation above the level of the foramen magnum), (2) preexisting pupillary abnormalities, (3) toxic levels of anesthetics, sedatives, tricyclic antidepressants, anticholinergics, antiepileptics, or neuromuscular blocking agents, and (4) severe chronic respiratory acidosis (COPD, severe obesity, or sleep apnea syndrome). In these circumstances, a confirmatory test may be warranted.

CONFIRMATORY TESTING

The role of confirmatory testing in brain death differs among jurisdictions.[19] In the United States and the United Kingdom, they are discretionary.[11,12,20] According to the AAN guidelines, confirmatory tests are required only when specific components of the clinical examination cannot be reliably assessed.[11,12] In some European countries such as Italy, France, and the Netherlands, among others, these tests

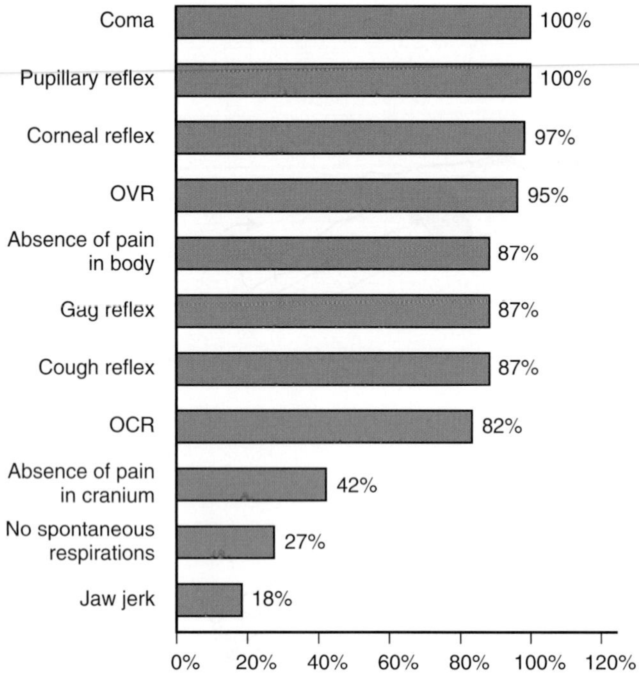

Figure 62.3 Variability during clinical examination of brain dead patients in top neuroscience centers of the United States. Poor compliance occurred mainly during testing of pain above the foramen magnum and the jaw jerk, as well as documenting absence of spontaneous respirations in brain death examination. OCR, oculocephalic reflex; OVR, oculovestibular reflex. (From Greer DM, Varelas PN, Haque S, Wijdicks EF: Variability of brain death determination guidelines in leading US neurologic institutions. Neurology 2008;70:284-289. Used with permission from Lippincott Williams & Wilkins.)

Table 62.1 Historical Time Frame for Confirmatory Tests Used in Determination of Brain Death

Year	Reported Study*	Test
1959	Löfstedt and von Reis[39]	Cerebral angiogram
1959	Fischgold and Mathis[40]	EEG
1969	Goodman et al[41]	Nuclear brain scan
1974	Yoneda et al[42]	TCD
1976	Starr[43]	BAEP
1978	Rappaport et al[45]	CT angiogram
1978	Rangel[46]	CT angiogram
1981	Goldie et al[44]	SSEP
1992	Jones and Barnes[47]	MRI

*Studies cited in complete list of references for this chapter provided online.

BAEP, brainstem auditory evoked potential; CT, computed tomography; EEG, electroencephalography; MRI, magnetic resonance imaging; SSEP, somatosensory evoked potential; TCD, transcranial Doppler.

Adapted from Wijdicks EF: The case against confirmatory tests for determining brain death in adults. Neurology 2010;75:77-83; used with permission from Lippincott Williams & Wilkins.

are mandatory,[19,20] however, there is still significant variability in the approach to determining brain death in the world.[19]

A specialist in the neurosciences and any other skilled physician should be able to determine brain death using clinical criteria alone, so the main purpose of confirmatory testing besides being a diagnostic safeguard is to support the diagnosis of brain death in the setting of failure to complete a thorough neurologic examination or an apnea test. The important thing about confirmatory testing is that these tests should never replace the clinical examination and should never be ordered before attempts to complete a thorough neurologic examination.[21]

ORIGINS OF CONFIRMATORY TESTING IN BRAIN DEATH

In the earlier years of refining the clinical picture of brain death, there was a desire to demonstrate absence of brain function with information different from clinical data. In the 1950s Jouvet[22] in France and C. Miller Fisher[23] in the United States began to use electrocerebral science to study a group of patients who would have poor neurologic outcomes. Although these studies provided the basis for defining brain death by the Ad Hoc Committee of the Harvard Medical School[7] a year later, Beecher, who served as the chairman of the committee, mentioned in an editorial that EEG was "not essential to a diagnosis of reversible coma, but provides valuable supporting data"[24] and this statement was later endorsed by the American Neurological Association.[25] Additional confirmatory tests, which can be divided into those that test for electrical function and those that test for blood flow, have been introduced and are aimed at confirming cerebral death (Table 62.1). Electrophysiologic tests include EEG, brainstem auditory evoked potentials (BAERs), and somatosensory evoked potentials (SSEPs); blood flow tests include four-vessel cerebral angiography, transcranial Doppler (TCD), CT angiogram, magnetic resonance (MR) angiogram, and nuclear brain scan (Fig. 62.4). More recent ancillary tests used for the determination of brain death include the bispectral index scale monitor[26] (BIS, mathematical algorithm of EEG), jugular bulb venous oxygen saturation ($Sjvo_2$),[27] and brain tissue oxygenation ($Pbto_2$).[28]

ACCURACY OF CONFIRMATORY TESTS

Practitioners must be careful at the time of interpreting the results of confirmatory tests and be knowledgeable of the technology being used, as there are disparities in the accuracy of confirmatory tests that could lead to potential pitfalls in the determination of brain death (Box 62.1). Based on the absence of gold standards from a physiologic and pathologic perspective,[29] the results of confirmatory testing may confound the practitioner in two ways: tests can be labeled as false positives or false negatives when they are compared against each other. False positives occur when the test suggests brain death and the patient does not meet clinical criteria. False negatives are more common (Table 62.2), and they occur when the patient is clinically brain dead but the test shows otherwise,[21] which may be more common with EEG.[30]

Table 62.2 False-Negative Rates with Confirmatory Tests Used in Determination of Brain Death

Reported Study*	No. of Patients	Test†	False-Negative Rate
Petty et al, 1990[48]	23	TCD	10% (2 patients)
Flowers and Patel, 1997[49]	219	Nuclear brain scan	3% (6 patients)
Munari et al, 2005[50]	20	Nuclear brain scan	5% (1 patient)
De Freitas and Andre, 2006[51]	270	TCD	17% (47 patients)
Quesnel et al, 2007[52]	21	CTA	50% (10 patients)
Combes et al, 2007[53]	30	CTA	23% (13 patients)
Escudero et al, 2009[54]	27	CTA	7% (2 patients)

*Studies cited in complete list of references for this chapter provided online.
†All tests evaluated by comparison with clinical confirmation of brain death.
CTA, computed tomographic angiogram; TCD, transcranial Doppler.
Adapted from Wijdicks EF: The case against confirmatory tests for determining brain death in adults. Neurology 2010;75:77-83; used with permission from Lippincott Williams & Wilkins.

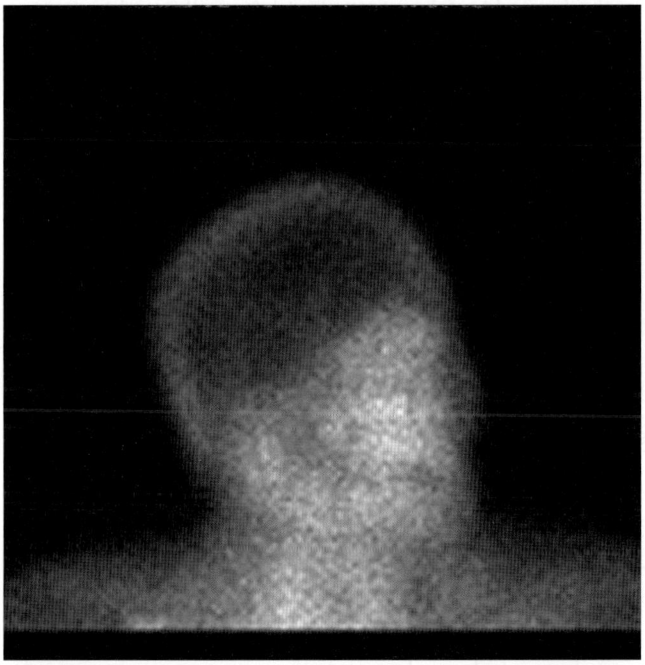

Figure 62.4 Nuclear brain scan of a brain dead patient showing no cerebral blood flow. (Used with permission from the Society of Critical Care Medicine.)

Box 62.1 Potential Pitfalls with Confirmatory Tests Used in Determination of Brain Death

Cerebral angiogram
- Image variability with injection of arch or selective arteries
- Image variability with injection and/or push technique
- No guideline for interpretation, operator-dependent

TCD
- Technically difficult and skill-dependent
- Normal findings in anoxic-ischemic injury

EEG
- Artifacts in intensive care settings
- Information from mostly cortex

SSEP
- Absent in comatose patients without brain death

CT angiogram
- Interpretation difficulties
- Retained blood flow reported in 205 cases
- Possibility to miss flow states because of rapid acquisition of images
- Delayed flow in low flow states (e.g., shock, heart failure)

Nuclear brain scan
- Areas of perfusion in thalamus in patients with anoxic injury or skull defect

CT, computed tomography; EEG, electroencephalogram; SSEP, somatosensory evoked potential; TCD, transcranial Doppler.
Adapted from Wijdicks EF: The case against confirmatory tests for determining brain death in adults. Neurology 2010;75:77-83; used with permission from Lippincott Williams & Wilkins.

RECOMMENDATIONS FOR CONFIRMATORY TESTING

Current evidence-based guidelines from the AAN recommend the use of only one confirmatory test for the determination of brain death in those cases in which an additional period of observation, or an apnea test, or clinical examination is not feasible to fully establish the clinical criteria of brain death.[12] In a large study of brain death determination at the Mayo Clinic, the apnea test was aborted in 3% of patients and in 7% of patients the apnea test was not performed as it was not deemed to be safe, a situation that occurred more frequently in patients with polytrauma or with chest trauma.[31] In practice, practitioners should anticipate that 1 in 10 patients with devastating neurologic injury will be unable to have an apnea test, and declaration of brain death may not be possible on clinical grounds. Families should be informed about the unlikely event of meaningful recovery and in these circumstances, if the patient is a candidate for organ donation, donation after circulatory determination of death (DCDD) may be considered; most hospitals have protocols for donation under DCDD,[21] and this approach could potentially increase the supply of deceased donor organs.[32]

SPECIAL CIRCUMSTANCES

DETERMINATION OF BRAIN DEATH AFTER CARDIAC ARREST IN THE ERA OF THERAPEUTIC HYPOTHERMIA

About 450,000 Americans have cardiac arrest annually.[33] The face of prognostication after cardiac arrest has changed in recent years based on clinical trials suggesting a robust effect of therapeutic hypothermia on clinical outcomes.[34] In 2006, the AAN published an algorithm to facilitate prognostic determination in patients who are resuscitated within 24 hours after cardiac arrest[10] (Fig. 62.5). The algorithm may require modification as more information accrues on the effects of hypothermia and with validation of other tests for poor and favorable outcomes[35] but the most important feature of the new clinical practice parameter was the recommendation to practitioners to wait at least 24 hours before entertaining the diagnosis of brain death. Despite the practice parameter a recent study shows that prognostication after cardiac arrest occurs on the basis of insufficient clinical data, which may lead to early withdrawals on the basis of self-fulfilling prophecies of doom.[36]

EXTRACORPOREAL MEMBRANE OXYGENATION

Extracorporeal membrane oxygenation (ECMO) is increasingly used as a means of extracirculatory support to patients in severe, reversible cardiac or respiratory failure. Patients presumed to have brain death may have earlier withdrawal of ECMO support,[37] which would limit the possibility of organ donation in patients who would otherwise be declared brain dead. In these circumstances, confirmatory testing may be warranted. A protocol of apnea testing involving the addition of CO_2 to the oxygenator to a target of 60 mm Hg or more than 20 mm Hg from the baseline normal CO_2 value may be used in lieu of the conventional protocol for apnea testing, but this protocol requires future validation.[38]

CONCLUSIONS

In the United States, current legislation allows physicians to determine death on the basis of neurologic criteria. The diagnosis of brain death on clinical grounds is not a difficult task, as long as providers follow established protocols and guidelines for the interpretation of findings during the

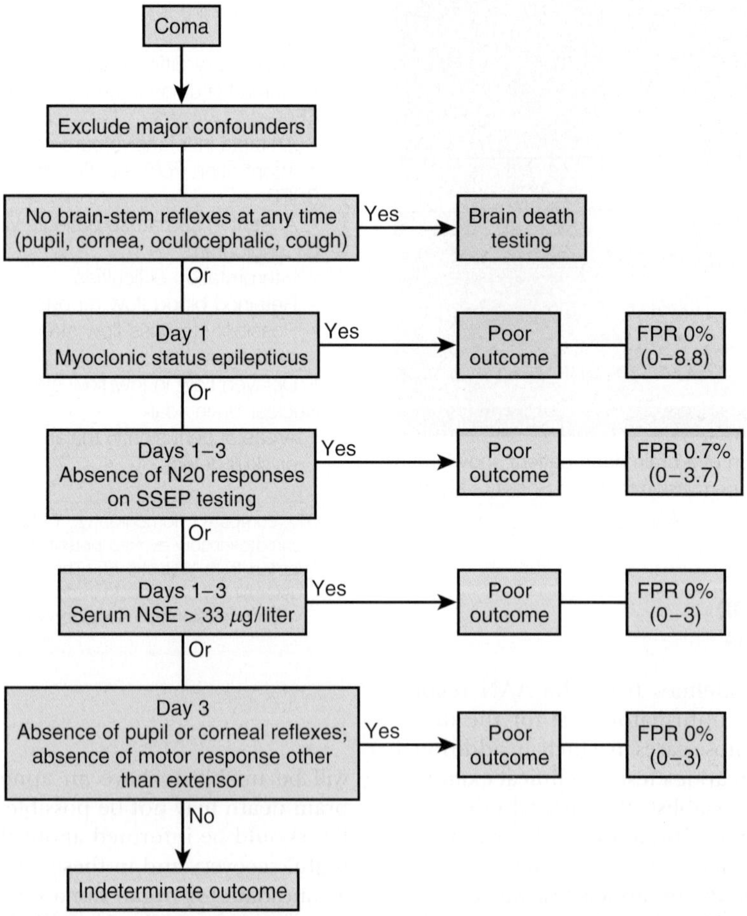

Figure 62.5 Decision algorithm for use in outcome prediction for comatose survivors of cardiac arrest. (From Wijdicks EF, Hijdra A, Young GB, et al: Practice parameter: Prediction of outcome in comatose survivors after cardiopulmonary resuscitation (an evidence-based review): Report of the Quality Standards Subcommittee of the American Academy of Neurology. Neurology 2006;67:203-210. Used with permission from Lippincott Williams & Wilkins.)

clinical examination. The establishment of a known cause and presence of coma, the absence of brainstem reflexes, and apnea supports the diagnosis of brain death. Most jurisdictions require that the determination of brain death be made by a licensed physician, which in most of the cases should be an attending physician who has experience in the assessment of comatose patients and the legal requirements applicable to the jurisdiction of practice. When in doubt, an additional period of observation or a confirmatory test should be done to support in the determination of brain death.

KEY POINTS

- The clinical examination of brain dead patients is the most unequivocal in neurology.
- The determination of brain death in a comatose patient with catastrophic neurologic injury requires several consecutive steps supported by well-established guidelines.
- When the clinical diagnosis is in doubt or interferences to obtain a thorough clinical examination are present, a confirmatory test may be used to determine brain death in adults.
- Confirmatory testing should not be used in lieu of clinical examination, and when indicated, only one confirmatory test should be performed.
- A period of observation of up to 24 hours after cardiac arrest in patients exposed to therapeutic hypothermia may be required before fully entertaining the determination of brain death.

SELECTED REFERENCES

2. Flowers WM Jr, Patel BR: Accuracy of clinical evaluation in the determination of brain death. South Med J 2000;93:203-206.
3. Greer DM, Varelas PN, Haque S, Wijdicks EF: Variability of brain death determination guidelines in leading US neurologic institutions. Neurology 2008;70:284-289.
10. Wijdicks EF, Hijdra A, Young GB, et al: Practice parameter: Prediction of outcome in comatose survivors after cardiopulmonary resuscitation (an evidence-based review): Report of the Quality Standards Subcommittee of the American Academy of Neurology. Neurology 2006;67:203-210.
11. The Quality Standards Subcommittee of the American Academy of Neurology: Practice parameters for determining brain death in adults (summary statement). Neurology 1995;45:1012-1014.
12. Wijdicks EF, Varelas PN, Gronseth GS, Greer DM: Evidence-based guideline update: Determining brain death in adults: Report of the Quality Standards Subcommittee of the American Academy of Neurology. Neurology 2010;74:1911-1918.
14. Wijdicks EF: The diagnosis of brain death. N Engl J Med 2001; 344:1215-1221.
21. Wijdicks EF: The case against confirmatory tests for determining brain death in adults. Neurology 2010;75:77-83.
29. Wijdicks EF, Pfeifer EA: Neuropathology of brain death in the modern transplant era. Neurology 2008;70:1234-1237.
35. Young GB: Clinical practice. Neurologic prognosis after cardiac arrest. N Engl J Med 2009;361:605-611.
36. Perman SM, Kirkpatrick JN, Reitsma AM, et al: Timing of neuroprognostication in postcardiac arrest therapeutic hypothermia. Crit Care Med 2012;40:719-724.

The complete list of references can be found at www.expertconsult.com.

63 Stroke

Thomas R. Mirsen

CHAPTER OUTLINE

HISTORICAL BACKGROUND

Stroke has a major impact in the United States, with an estimated yearly incidence of 731,100 new and recurrent strokes[1] from 1993-1994. In 1997, 821,760 stroke admissions occurred in this country.[2] Stroke constitutes the third leading cause of death and is a major cause of disability.[3] Although stroke is a lesser cause of disability than heart disease,[4] the population of stroke survivors continues to increase, in part because of a fall in mortality rate.[5] Historically, stroke was not emphasized in the critical care setting because of the limited scope of interventions in the past. In the early 1990s, neurologic diseases, including but not limited to stroke, accounted for a mere 6% to 7% of admissions to critical care units.[6] Now there is acute treatment for stroke, namely, the use of tissue plasminogen activator (tPA) for ischemic stroke within 3 hours of symptom onset,[7] as well as intra-arterial (IA) thrombolysis for as long as 6 hours following stroke onset.[8] A clot removal device (mechanical embolus removal in cerebral ischemia, or MERCI)[9] has been approved, and newer, likely more effective, devices[10] may become available shortly. Thrombolytic agents designed to work within a 9-hour time window, in conjunction with sophisticated imaging, have being studied, although they have not yet been shown to be useful.[11] The great danger with the use of these agents is the risk of intracerebral hemorrhage (ICH). Frequent monitoring, as often as every 15 minutes following administration of a thrombolytic, is standard for patients so treated, and observation in a critical care unit is required.

Consequently, critical care physicians need to learn about this condition, which has become a regular part of their professional lives, particularly in centers that devote themselves to the care of stroke patients. In one critical care unit with which the author is familiar, ischemic stroke accounts for 3% of the primary admissions and hemorrhagic stroke for 5.4%.[12]

OVERVIEW

This chapter reviews the general diagnosis and treatment of ischemic stroke. It describes the following:

- The specific interventions available
- Their rationale and utility
- New developments in the area
- The reasons for critical care consultation

Stroke is traditionally defined as a focal neurologic deficit of presumed vascular onset, lasting 24 hours or longer, as opposed to transient ischemic attack (TIA), which is an episode shorter than 24 hours in duration.[13] Many TIAs actually last for less than 60 minutes.[14]

Stroke symptoms, including retinal TIA *(amaurosis fugax),* arise either from the territory fed by the internal carotid artery or from the vertebrobasilar system. The carotid, through its major branches, the anterior cerebral arteries (ACAs) and middle cerebral arteries (MCAs), provides blood to the major portion of the cerebral hemispheres. The vertebrobasilar system, in contrast, perfuses the brainstem and cerebellum, as well as the inferior and medial aspects of the occipital and temporal lobes, and the thalamus.

Carotid symptoms, as listed in Box 63.1, primarily consist of hemisensory loss, hemiparesis, and retinal ischemia (monocular blindness). Left hemispheric ischemia, generally in the perisylvian area, may result in varying degrees of aphasia.[15] Involvement of the sensory association areas within the right parietal lobe can produce the phenomenon of neglect.[16] In neglect, a stimulus is felt when it is alone but not in the presence of a competing stimulus. For example, a touch on the left hand or an object in the left visual field may be perceived when alone, but not when another stimulus is simultaneously presented, generally on the right side (double simultaneous stimulation). In that instance the

Box 63.1 Stroke Symptoms

Carotid Distribution

1. Hemiparesis
2. Hemisensory loss
3. Aphasia
4. Retinal ischemia
5. Neglect
6. Homonymous hemianopia

Vertebrobasilar Distribution

1. Motor dysfunction—crossed or bilateral
2. Sensory loss—crossed or bilateral
3. Gait ataxia
4. Homonymous hemianopia
5. Diplopia, dysphagia, dysarthria, vertigo, hiccups—none of these alone qualify as stroke/transient ischemia attack symptoms
6. Combinations of the above

Symptoms Not Considered Vascular in Origin

1. Syncope or presyncope
2. Dizziness, "wooziness," giddiness
3. Impaired vision associated with alteration of consciousness
4. Any of the following in isolation: amnesia, confusion, vertigo, diplopia, dysphagia, dysarthria
5. Tonic or clonic motor activity
6. March of sensory or motor deficits
7. Focal symptoms in association with migraine
8. Bowel or bladder incontinence

Modified from Hachinski V, Norris JW: The Acute Stroke. Philadelphia, FA Davis, 1985.

right-sided stimulus alone is perceived. In extreme circumstances, affected individuals may not recognize the left side of the body as being theirs (*anosognosia*), as described memorably by Oliver Sacks in *The Man Who Mistook His Wife for a Hat.*[17]

Box 63.1 lists symptoms resulting from ischemia in the vertebrobasilar territory, which includes the cerebellum, brainstem, and the medial aspect of the occipital lobe, as well as the thalamus and the inferomedial portions of the temporal lobe. As a result, vertebrobasilar ischemia can produce cranial nerve dysfunction, nystagmus, cerebellar dysmetria, ataxia, and long tract signs such as sensory loss or motor impairment. These may involve one or both sides of the body. Memory disorders and visual field deficits also occur. In extreme circumstances, when the basilar artery becomes occluded, coma or quadriparesis may develop, although the presentation may vary, as described by Kubik and Adams[18] in 1946. As a result of coma or quadriparesis, mechanical ventilation may be required, and the prognosis in such patients is grim. In one study,[19] 22 of 25 patients died, and the other 3 lingered in the "locked-in syndrome."[20] This frightening manifestation of basilar occlusion, secondary to pontine infarction, leaves patients chronically limited to eye blinking as their sole means of communication.

Differentiating between carotid and vertebrobasilar symptoms is important. There exists intervention to repair carotid stenosis, which is most effective following stroke

Box 63.2 Common Seizure Symptoms

Incontinence
Tongue-biting
Tonic movements
Clonic movements
Jacksonian march (sensory, motor, or both)
Automatisms (grimacing, chewing)

or TIA in the distribution of the affected vessel. Failure to recognize symptoms as originating from the vertebrobasilar territory may lead to unwarranted intervention for carotid narrowing.

Likewise, one must not label complaints that are not cerebrovascular in nature as stroke (see Box 63.1). Syncope, wooziness, and the like usually reflect systemic hypotension as opposed to focal ischemia. The still widespread practice of studying carotid vessels—most often through ultrasound—following the development of syncope should be abandoned because syncope does not result from ischemic stroke.

In Box 63.1, item 4 under "Symptoms Not Considered Vascular in Origin" draws attention to the fact that certain symptoms may represent stroke when associated with other symptoms but not in isolation. Vertigo, for instance, can result from disease of the semicircular canals. If other complaints or findings referable to the posterior fossa of the brain (brainstem and cerebellum) coexist, such as those listed in Box 63.1 under "Vertebrobasilar Distribution," the symptoms may indeed localize there. Similarly, amnesia alone may follow a seizure or result from transient global amnesia as opposed to stroke, and so on.

The items listed in Box 63.2 reflect the presence of seizures. Seizure onset may be unwitnessed, and in the hospital only postictal deficits, such as aphasia or hemiparesis, may be observed. The appearance of any number of positive phenomena will draw attention to the correct diagnosis. These phenomena contrast with the abolition of normal function that happens with stroke and instead represent abnormal activity resulting from uncontrolled electrical discharges. Occasionally, however, limb shaking may represent carotid ischemia, usually as the result of hemodynamic compromise in the territory of the ipsilateral carotid artery.[21] Dreifuss[22] gives a comprehensive classification of epilepsy types and symptoms.

Migraine can also be associated with focal neurologic complaints. Commonest among these are visual complaints including scotomas, whether scintillating or not. The most dramatic manifestation is hemiplegic migraine, which raises the fear of ICH at first presentation. Aphasia and paresthesia are also described. Silberstein and colleagues[23] have reviewed the manifestations of migraine.

Box 63.3 lists those entities that most frequently mimic stroke. Hypoglycemia may produce focal neurologic deficits. Occasionally a mass lesion such as tumor or subdural hematoma may present with fluctuating deficits or be revealed by seizure activity that may be confused with stroke. In the case of subdural hematoma in the elderly, the inciting trauma may have been minor or forgotten. Headache may be prominent, mild, or even absent. Mass lesions and hemorrhage are frequently marked by confusion, decreased

Box 63.3 Stroke Mimics

Intracerebral hemorrhage
Seizure
Migraine
Hypoglycemia
Tumor

level of consciousness, or headache, but if the lesion is small, these symptoms may not appear. Consequently, blood sugar measurements and computed tomography (CT) scans (without contrast) are obligatory in all instances of suspected stroke. Within the first 6 hours of the event, CT may well be negative, even in instances of major infarction such as that involving the entire MCA watershed. Thus CT finds its greatest utility not in confirming the clinical diagnosis but in excluding the presence of small hemorrhages. Neurologists have relied on clinical findings to diagnose stroke, especially in the hyperacute phase (0 to 6 hours), when CT is least helpful.

ADVANCES IN RADIOLOGY

With the advent of diffusion-weighted imaging (DWI), magnetic resonance imaging (MRI) scans (Fig. 63.1) can now be used to detect acute cerebral ischemia within the initial 6-hour period following symptom onset.[24] This allows the clinician to confirm or exclude the presence of stroke in doubtful cases. Most commonly, such circumstances involve the possibility of a new lesion in a previously injured area of the brain. For example, in the case of a new seizure originating from the hemisphere affected by a prior stroke, DWI can show whether the new event is seizure alone or caused by a new stroke. By the same token, if a newly delirious or febrile patient should manifest worsening of a preexisting neurologic deficit, DWI will clarify whether the worsening stems from the intercurrent injury or from a coincident new stroke. DWI can also reveal silent areas of cerebral ischemia, which sometimes appear simultaneously with the area of injury that presents symptomatically as stroke. The coincident development of ischemia in different vascular territories may indicate the presence of an unusual mechanism of infarction, such as vasculitis, hypercoagulable state, or cardiac source of emboli. MRI has been proved to be just as effective as CT in detecting ICH,[25] thus potentially removing an extra step (the initial head CT) from the stroke evaluation. Unfortunately, MRI is less immediately available than CT, requires more time and cooperation from the patient, and may not be feasible in the face of claustrophobia or of ferromagnetic implants/fragments within the body.

Both CT and MRI technology can delineate the cerebral vasculature in detail, starting from the aortic arch and extending to the vicinity of the circle of Willis. Computed tomographic angiography (CTA) has been shown to be reliable in studying the intracranial vasculature[26] and the extracranial segment of the carotid artery (Fig. 63.2).[27] Magnetic resonance angiography (MRA) is superior to ultrasound in detecting carotid artery stenosis in the neck[28] and is effective

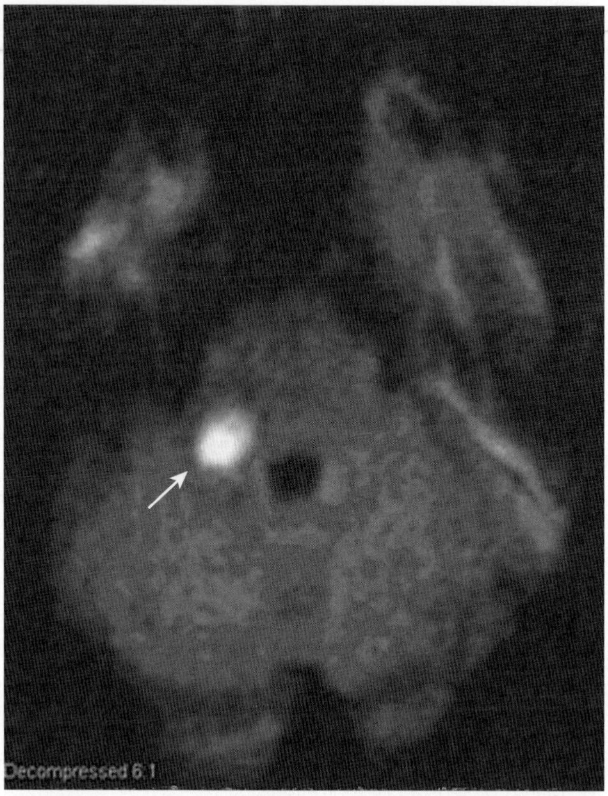

Figure 63.1 Cerebral infarction as shown by diffusion-weighted imaging *(arrow)* on magnetic resonance imaging. Hyperdensity in the right middle cerebellar peduncle is demonstrated.

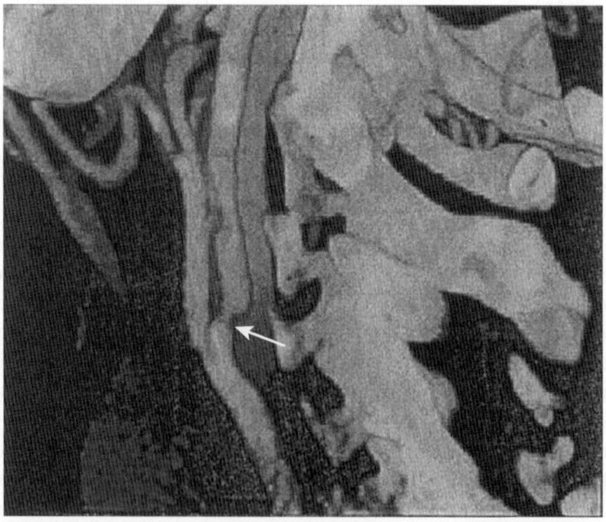

Figure 63.2 Computed tomography angiogram of the extracranial carotid artery. An area of stenosis *(arrow)* is shown in the internal carotid artery.

as well intracranially[29] (Figs. 63.3 and 63.4), although its specificity and sensitivity in both instances are likely to improve. CTA has its own limitations, namely, the difficulty in performing the study in patients with contrast dye allergies. Because of these new techniques, the performance of conventional cerebral angiography is limited to specific indications, as outlined in Box 63.4.

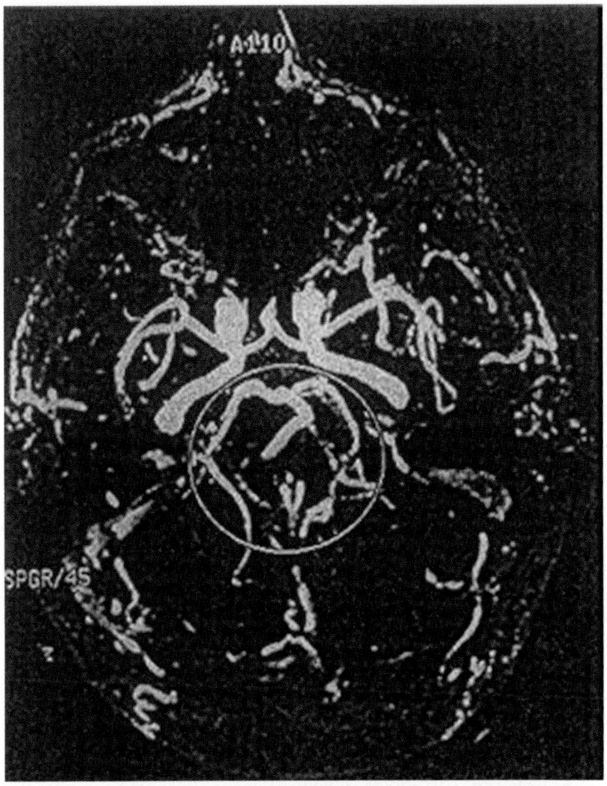

Figure 63.3 Magnetic resonance angiogram demonstrating circle of Willis *(highlighted)* and its vertebrobasilar component *(circle)*.

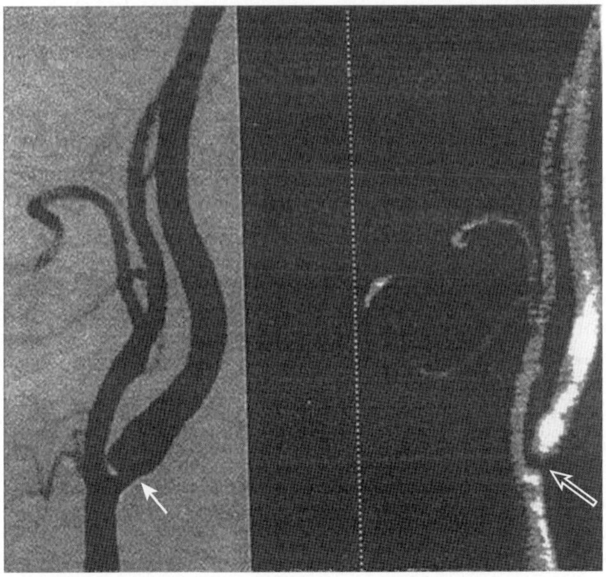

Figure 63.4 Shown are magnetic resonance angiography *(left)* and computed tomographic angiography *(right)* of the extracranial carotid artery in a patient with internal carotid artery stenosis *(arrows)* located above the common carotid bifurcation.

Box 63.4 Indications for Conventional Cerebral Angiography

- To ascertain the precise degree of arterial stenosis, most often of the extracranial carotid artery, in doubtful cases
- To detect and map intracranial aneurysms and arteriovenous malformations
- To determine patterns of collateral flow in the brain
- To diagnose vasculitis
- To detect intraluminal thrombus
- To enable intra-arterial thrombolysis or mechanical clot extraction
- For the performance of carotid angiography and stenting

Box 63.5 Thrombolysis Inclusion Criteria at 0-3 Hours

Acute ischemic stroke with clearly defined time of onset
Neurologic deficit measurable using the NIH Stroke Scale
CT scan of the brain without evidence of intracerebral hemorrhage
Age 18 years or older

CT, computed tomography; NIH, National Institutes of Health.

THROMBOLYSIS IN STROKE

The era of thrombolysis in acute stroke began with the publication of the NINDS (National Institute of Neurological Disorders and Stroke) tPA trial in 1995.[7] This groundbreaking study was the first to demonstrate a beneficial effect of tPA when given to patients presenting within 3 hours of the onset of the event. Depending on the criteria used to determine favorable outcome at 3 months, roughly an additional 11% to 13% of subjects receiving tPA recovered with little or no disability. If one uses the National Institutes of Health stroke scale (NIHSS) (Table 63.1) score, a reliable measure[30] to measure disability, the improvement was from 20% with minimal or no disability with placebo to 31% with tPA. This was counterbalanced by an increase in the rate of ICH, from 0.6% in the placebo group to 6.4% in the tPA cohort. Half the subjects in the placebo group who suffered ICH died, whereas the mortality rate from ICH in the tPA cohort was 2.9% (less than half). Hemorrhage following tPA use occupies the same area of the brain affected by the initial thrombosis in most but not all cases.[31]

Strict inclusion (Box 63.5) and exclusion (Box 63.6) criteria are applied to attempt to minimize the risk of ICH. The safety and efficacy of thrombolysis have not been analyzed in children. The time of onset of symptoms is taken to be the last time that the patient was seen to be normal. For example, an individual who went to sleep at 10 PM and awoke at 6 AM, immediately hemiplegic, will not qualify for tPA therapy. One who awoke at 4 AM, went back to sleep, and awoke again at 6 AM with stroke symptoms may be treated with tPA, but only up to 7 AM. A person who awoke at 6 AM, was briefly normal, and developed stroke symptoms at 6:05 AM may be treated until 9:05 AM.

The blood glucose must be determined before initiating tPA therapy to avoid misdiagnosing hypoglycemia as stroke (see Box 63.3). A CT scan of the head is essential to look for a mass, most often an ICH or subdural hematoma. The CT must also be scrutinized for the presence of early ischemic changes, such as sulcal effacement, hypolucency within the brain, or loss of definition between structures within the

Table 63.1 National Institutes of Health (NIH) Stroke Scale

Component	Description	No. of Points
1a. Level of consciousness (LOC)	Alert	0
	Drowsy	1
	Stuporous	2
	Coma	3
1b. LOC questions	Answers both correctly	0
	Answers one correctly	1
	Incorrect	2
1c. LOC commands	Obeys both correctly	0
	Obeys one correctly	1
	Incorrect	2
2. Best gaze	Normal	0
	Partial gaze palsy	1
	Forced deviation	2
3. Visual field	No visual loss	0
	Partial hemianopia	1
	Complete hemianopia	2
	Bilateral hemianopia	3
4. Facial palsy	Normal	0
	Minor	1
	Partial	2
	Complete	3
5. Motor arm	No drift	0
	Drift	1
	Some effort against gravity	2
	No effort against gravity	3
	Plegia	4
6. Motor leg	No drift	0
	Drift	1
	Some effort against gravity	2
	No effort against gravity	3
	Plegia	4
7. Limb ataxia	Absent	0
	Present in upper or lower	1
	Present in both	2
8. Sensory	Normal	0
	Partial loss	1
	Dense loss	2
9. Best language	No aphasia	0
	Mild to moderate aphasia	1
	Severe aphasia	2
	Mute	3
10. Dysarthria	Normal articulation	0
	Mild to moderate dysarthria	1
	Near unintelligible or worse	2
11. Extinction and inattention	No neglect	0
	Partial neglect	1
	Complete neglect	2

brain, or for the presence of a hyperdense MCA, suggestive of thrombosis.[32] Whether ischemic changes on CT predict a heightened risk of hemorrhagic transformation is controversial.[31,33] However, CT findings appear more commonly among subjects with scans performed relatively late in the course of their stroke.[33] Hence their appearance should prompt reevaluation of the time of onset of the stroke. Prior ICH, recent stroke, and hypertension at presentation are believed to increase the risk of sustaining ICH. Avoiding systemic bleeding, which may result in hypotension and worsening of the neurologic deficit, is also important. Extremes of blood glucose or the presence of a coincident seizure make the neurologic deficit seem worse than it is, rendering calculation of a risk-benefit ratio more difficult.

Box 63.6 Thrombolysis Exclusion Criteria at 0-3 Hours

Stroke or serious head injury within the past 3 months
Major surgery within the previous 14 days
Prior history of intracerebral hemorrhage
Systolic blood pressure >185 mm Hg or diastolic blood pressure >110 mm Hg
Rapid neurologic improvement or minor deficit
Symptoms suggestive of subarachnoid hemorrhage
Gastrointestinal or genitourinary hemorrhage within the previous 21 days
Evidence of significant bleeding or fracture on examination
Arterial puncture at a noncompressible site within the previous 7 days
Seizure with postictal residual neurologic deficits
Anticoagulation or heparin use within 48 hours before treatment and elevated PTT
Prothrombin time greater than 15 seconds or INR greater than 1.7
Platelet count less than 100,000/μL
Blood glucose less than 50 mg/dL or greater than 400 mg/dL
Recent use of low-molecular-weight heparin
Large myocardial infarction in the past 3 months
CT scan of the brain with hypodensity involving less than one third of the cerebral hemisphere

Caution should be exercised in treating:

- Patients with major deficits
- Patients who have undergone lumbar puncture or organ biopsy within the preceding 7 days
- Patients with hyperglycemia (>400 mg/dL)

CT, computed tomography; INR, international normalized ratio; PTT, partial thromboplastin time.

Two blood tests must be checked before embarking on thrombolysis: a blood sugar, as mentioned earlier, and a platelet count. If the patient is on anticoagulant therapy, the prothrombin time/international normalized ratio or partial thromboplastin time must be available before deciding whether to proceed with treatment. If a patient is not known to be receiving anticoagulants at baseline, but the coagulation profile proves abnormal, the infusion must be stopped if thrombolysis is still ongoing at the time that the abnormal value returns. If a patient is receiving low-molecular-weight heparin, there is no rapid way of determining the degree of anticoagulation, and intervention must be withheld. Testing for the activity of factor Xa antagonists is not yet standardized, although a normal thrombin time may suggest that thrombolysis is safe.[34]

If the blood pressure is elevated (>180 mm Hg systolic or 110 mm Hg diastolic), a modest dosage of labetalol, 5 to 10 mg IV (intravenous), may be given and repeated if necessary, up to a maximum dosage of 40 mg. Nitropaste is a less exact alternative but has the advantage that it can be removed. A nicardipine drip may be employed as well, which constitutes a change from prior guidelines. If the blood pressure subsequently rebounds to an undesirable range, tPA should not be given. If the pressure should rise above 180 mm Hg systolic or 105 mm Hg diastolic subsequent to starting the tPA infusion, it is paramount to bring it down using IV infusions of antihypertensive agents (Table 63.2).[35] In this context, it is worth emphasizing that blood pressure should be treated acutely only when there exists a specific indication for doing so, as defined in the table.

tPA should not be given in the presence of a deficit mild enough that reasonable recovery may be expected within 3 months. However, there is not a clear cutoff based on the NIHSS to identify those patients whose deficits are too mild to warrant intervention. The choice falls to the treating physician. For instance, a partial hemisensory loss, facial palsy, or mild dysarthria would not normally warrant treatment with tPA when appearing in isolation. A hemianopia in a bedridden elderly subject residing in a nursing facility may not be considered deserving of thrombolysis by some physicians. However, an active middle-aged person presenting with an isolated hemianopia would probably be treated more aggressively by most doctors. The most difficult choices exist in the setting of mild motor or speech deficits. Such deficits may recover well, but a percentage of subjects will worsen while in the hospital and then no longer be candidates for rescue using thrombolysis. Unfortunately, we

Table 63.2 Approach to Elevated Blood Pressure in Acute Ischemic Stroke

Blood Pressure Level (mm Hg)	Treatment
A. Not Eligible for Thrombolytic Therapy	
Systolic <220 mm Hg OR diastolic <120 mm Hg	Observe unless other end-organ involvement (e.g., aortic dissection, acute myocardial infarction, pulmonary edema, hypertensive encephalopathy) Treat other symptoms of stroke (e.g., headache, pain, agitation, nausea, vomiting) Treat other acute complications of stroke including hypoxia, increased intracranial pressure, seizures, and hypoglycemia
Systolic >220 mm Hg OR diastolic 121-140 mm Hg	Labetalol 10-20 mg IV over 1-2 min May repeat or double every 10 min (maximum dose 300 mg) OR Nicardipine 5 mg/hr IV infusion as initial dose; titrate to desired effect by increasing 2.5 mg/hr every 5 min to maximum of 15 mg/hr Aim for a 10-15% reduction in blood pressure
Diastolic >140 mm Hg	Nitroprusside 0.5 µg/kg/min IV infusion as initial dose with continuous blood pressure monitoring Aim for a 10-15% reduction in blood pressure
B. Eligible for Thrombolytic Therapy	
Pretreatment	
Systolic >185 mm Hg OR diastolic >110 mm Hg	Labetalol 10 to 20 mg IV over 1 to 2 min, may repeat _1; OR Nitropaste 1 to 2 inches OR Nicardipine infusion, 5 mg/hr, titrate up by 2.5 mg/hr at 5- to 15-min intervals, maximum dose 15 mg/hr; when desired blood pressure attained, reduce to 3 mg/hr If blood pressure does not decline and remains >185/110 mm Hg, do not administer rtPA
During/after Treatment	
1. Monitor blood pressure	Check blood pressure every 15 min for 2 hr, then every 30 min for 6 hr, and finally every hour for 16 hr
2. Diastolic >140 mm Hg	Sodium nitroprusside 0.5 µg/kg/min IV infusion as initial dose and titrate to desired blood pressure
3. Systolic >230 mm Hg OR diastolic 121-140 mm Hg	Labetalol 10 µg IV over 1-2 min May repeat or double labetalol every 10 min to maximum dose of 300 mg; or give initial labetalol dose, then start labetalol drip at 2-8 mg/min OR Nicardipine 5 mg/hr IV infusion as initial dose and titrate to desired effect by increasing 2.5 mg/hr every 5 min to maximum of 15 mg/hr; if blood pressure is not controlled by labetalol, consider sodium nitroprusside
4. Systolic 180-230 mm Hg OR diastolic 105-120 mm Hg	Labetalol 10 mg IV over 1-2 min May repeat or double labetalol every 10-20 min to maximum dose of 300 mg; or give initial labetalol dose, then start labetalol drip at 2-8 mg/min

rtPA, recombinant tissue plasminogen activator.

From Adams HP, del Zoppo G, Alberts MJ, et al: Guidelines for the early management of adults with ischemic stroke. Stroke 2007;38:1655-1711.

presently lack a tool to predict which subjects will worsen during their acute hospital stay.

Subjects who have been on antiplatelet agents such as aspirin before their event may receive tPA, but no anticoagulants or antiplatelet agents should be given for the 24 hours following the start of tPA therapy. Arterial punctures, nasogastric tubes, and catheterization should be avoided unless they are essential to care, in order to minimize the risk of bleeding.

Hypotension may develop, raising the concern of systemic hemorrhage. Of course, hypotension may have a variety of other causes. The most feared event following tPA use is the development of ICH. The presenting signs and symptoms appear in Box 63.7. Most are self-explanatory. Hypertension is a compensatory response to increased intracranial pressure (ICP), to maintain cerebral perfusion, and bradycardia occurs secondary to it.

The steps to be taken with suspected ICH appear in Box 63.8. It is relatively uncommon for neurosurgeons to intervene on hemorrhages in the setting of tPA because of the risk of further bleeding into the surgical bed. Systemic hemorrhage is handled in a similar fashion, but transfusion may also be necessary. Platelets should be administered if the count is significantly decreased (<50,000 cells/μL).

The benefit of tPA is greatest in the instances of the smallest vascular occlusions (lacunar, as opposed to cortical, infarcts). Older subjects with particularly severe strokes are most likely to have a poor outcome, but even in this group tPA remains beneficial overall.[36] The sooner tPA is administered, the higher the likelihood of successful recovery, as shown by a meta-analysis[37] of thrombolysis trials. A residual benefit of tPA exists, as far out as 6 hours from the ictus. Two studies[38,39] that specifically examined treatment beyond 3 hours failed to show a benefit of administration of tPA within a 5- or 6-hour time frame. More recently, however, the ECASS-III (European Cooperative Acute Stroke Study III) trial[40] established the utility of tPA administration in the 3.0- to 4.5-hour period following stroke onset. The inclusion and exclusion criteria are more restrictive than those for treatment within 3.0 hours (Boxes 63.9 and 63.10). Initially, there was some concern about the administration of tPA within the 3.0- to 4.5-hour window to subjects with a history both of prior stroke and of diabetes. A statistical analysis[41] based on datasets from large registries suggests that neither factor predisposes to poor outcome in reality. No doubt there exists a subgroup of subjects presenting beyond 4.5 hours that remains amenable to treatment, but this group cannot yet be identified.

Box 63.7 Signs and Symptoms of Intracerebral Hemorrhage

New neurologic deficits
Worsening of existing neurologic deficits
Headache
Nausea, vomiting
Decreased level of consciousness, coma
Marked hypertension
Bradycardia

Box 63.8 Management of Suspected Intracerebral Hemorrhage after Use of Tissue Plasminogen Activator (tPA)

Discontinue the tPA infusion if it remains in progress.
Obtain CT scan of the head (noncontrast) STAT.
Order PT, PTT, platelet count, fibrinogen level STAT.
Type and crossmatch blood.
Arrange for neurosurgery consultation.
Administer fresh frozen plasma or cryoprecipitate (4 to 8 units).

CT, computed tomography; PT, prothrombin time; PTT, partial thromboplastin time.

Box 63.9 Thrombolysis Inclusion Criteria at 3.0-4.5 Hours

Age 18 to 80 years
Onset of stroke symptoms 3.0 to 4.5 hours before initiation of study drug
Stroke symptoms present for at least 30 minutes with no significant improvement before treatment

Box 63.10 Thrombolysis Exclusion Criteria at 3.0-4.5 Hours

Intracranial hemorrhage
Time of symptom onset unknown
Symptoms rapidly subsiding or only minor before start of infusion
Severe stroke as assessed clinically (e.g., NIHSS score >25) or by appropriate imaging techniques*
Seizure at onset of stroke
Stroke or serious head trauma within previous 3 months
Administration of heparin within 48 hours preceding onset of stroke, with an activated partial thromboplastin time at presentation exceeding the upper limit of the normal range
Platelet count of less than 100,000/μL
Systolic pressure greater than 185 mm Hg or diastolic pressure greater than 110 mm Hg, or aggressive treatment (intravenous medication) necessary to reduce blood pressure to these limits
Blood glucose less than 50 mg/dL or greater than 400 mg/dL
Symptoms suggestive of subarachnoid hemorrhage, even if CT scan was normal in appearance
Oral anticoagulant treatment
Major surgery or severe trauma within previous 3 months
Other major disorders associated with an increased risk of bleeding

*A severe stroke as assessed by imaging was defined as a stroke involving more than one third of the middle cerebral artery territory. On the NIHSS, total scores range from 0 to 42, with higher values reflecting more severe cerebral infarcts.
CT, computed tomography; NIHSS, National Institutes of Health Stroke Scale.

Various authors have identified different predictors of ICH following treatment with tPA. Levy and colleagues[42] identified the dosage of tPA given, the age of the subjects, and diastolic hypertension as pertinent factors. Larrue and colleagues[31] also found age to heighten the risk of development of ICH, but not the degree of hypertension or the time to treatment. It has become clear that tPA can be given safely in the community[43] and that complication rates of tPA use can be lowered to a satisfactory level by careful adherence to the exclusion criteria.[44]

IA thrombolysis can be used to treat acute ischemic stroke beyond the 3-hour time window for IV tPA. Basilar thrombosis has been treated as late as 24 hours after the onset of symptoms using this approach.[45] Other subjects with occlusion of the proximal (M1 or M2) segments of the MCA have been successfully treated between 3 and 6 hours following stroke onset. The utility of this approach rests on the PROACT II (Prolyse in Acute Cerebral Thromboembolism II) trial,[8] a study using a novel agent, prourokinase (pro-UK). In contrast to the IV tPA trial, aspirin was allowed in the first 24 hours following stroke onset and heparin was used acutely following pro-UK to prevent vascular occlusion. To enter the study, the upper age limit was 85 years and the minimum NIHSS score was 11.

The trial showed a 40% rate of favorable neurologic outcome at 3 months following IA thrombolysis, as opposed to 25% in the control group. The rate of ICH with clinical deterioration at 24 hours following study entry was 10% in the pro-UK group, as opposed to 2% in the placebo group. Although pro-UK itself has not been approved for use in this country, IA tPA is used for subjects who cannot be treated within 3 hours with IV tPA, and, despite the absence of studies, as rescue therapy following IV tPA use. The inclusion and exclusion criteria are similar to those for IV tPA. The availability of mechanical clot extraction, as summarized later, means that subjects who do not qualify for IA tPA may still receive treatment, again in the absence of definitive trials. Apparent predictors of hemorrhagic transformation of cerebral infarct in patients subjected to IA thrombolysis appear in Box 63.11.[46] In another study,[47] 36 subjects underwent IA thrombolysis for stroke within 2 weeks of major surgery (mean time from surgery to treatment of 21.5 hours). Nine of the subjects (25%) died, but only three died of hemorrhagic complications, suggesting that IA thrombolysis may be considered following major surgery when IV thrombolysis is contraindicated. The smaller dosage of thrombolytic (0.2 mg/kg vs. 0.9 mg/kg) used may render the IA approach safe in this setting. IA thrombolysis is also used when cardiac catheterization is complicated by stroke, in large part because of immediate access to the vascular tree. This approach, although reasonable, has not been studied systematically.[48]

Box 63.11 Predictors of Hemorrhagic Transformation of Cerebral Infarction after Intra-arterial tPA

- Higher NIHSS score
- Longer time to arterial recanalization
- Hyperglycemia
- Lower platelet count

NIHSS, National Institutes of Health Stroke Scale; tPA, tissue plasminogen activator.

The use of a 0.6-mg/kg systemic bolus of IV tPA acutely, followed by IA thrombolysis if shown necessary by immediate angiography, was examined by the IMS (Interventional Management of Stroke) II trial.[49] A microcatheter was employed, when feasible, to allow for ultrasound-assisted clot lysis in addition to local instillation of tPA. There were trends toward higher incidence of ICH, but better clinical outcomes overall, when compared to the original NINDS tPA trial. The IMS III trial,[50] a randomized comparison of IV tPA against IV/IA therapy, the latter enhanced by mechanical clot extraction, has begun.

Neurointerventionalists attempt to heighten the effectiveness of local thrombolytics by using catheters to mechanically disrupt clots. Such an approach is difficult to assess in a standardized fashion. There exist data on the MERCI device, designed to extract clot via the endovascular approach without thrombolysis. Initially, this approach was tested in subjects ineligible for tPA,[9] but it has also been tested subsequently in subjects previously treated with IV tPA.[51] Even though a trend toward increased ICH emerged, vessel recanalization rates were relatively high, approaching 70% in patients also treated with IA tPA. This intervention was used, when needed, to dissolve clot resistant to device intervention or to treat inaccessible distal thrombus. A newer and possibly more effective device, Solitaire,[10] may shortly be available.

Such devices have been compared to each other, but not to placebo. Available data consist of series of patients treated with a device compared with historical control subjects. The data focus on the rate of recanalization of the occluded vessel and only secondarily on clinical outcome. The limitations of such an analysis are discussed in detail elsewhere.[52] Mechanical clot extraction will find a role in the acute treatment of ischemic stroke, which remains to be defined.

Radiologic imaging has been proposed as a tool to determine when individual subjects may be suitable for IA intervention, regardless of time from stroke onset. Specific patients may, by virtue of good collateral flow, possess a significant area of ischemic but viable brain that may be salvaged by endovascular treatment, even if beyond standard time windows. This algorithm may apply particularly to "wake-up" strokes. Computed perfusion tomography (CT perfusion) can be used to estimate the size of the ischemic area but not infarcted area at presentation,[53] and diffusion-weighted/perfusion-weighted MRI may identify those patients who will benefit from intervention.[54] However, these tools need validation and standardization in large studies in order to attain clinical efficacy.

SYMPTOMATIC CAROTID DISEASE/STENTING

Carotid endarterectomy (CEA) dramatically reduces stroke risk in patients with cerebral or retinal ischemia who prove to harbor a significant carotid stenosis ipsilateral to the affected cerebral hemisphere. Two separate randomized controlled trials[55,56] have shown similar results. In NASCET (North American Symptomatic Carotid Endarterectomy Trial),[56] the risk of stroke fell from 26% over 2 years in the nonsurgical group to 9% over 2 years in the surgical group, with a surgical morbidity and mortality rate of 5.6%. The patients had stenosis of 70% or greater. A more modest benefit was seen in men with stenoses between 50% and 69%; namely, they showed a reduction in stroke risk from 22.2% over 5 years without surgery to 14.9% over 5 years with surgery. This is an absolute reduction of the stroke rate of 7.3% over 5 years, as opposed to an absolute reduction of 17% over 2 years in the group with stenosis greater than 70%. Superior surgical skill is necessary in order to lower the surgical morbidity and mortality rates to a point that the procedure remains beneficial in this cohort.

In order for endarterectomy to be beneficial, there must be a reasonable expectation of survival without other major disability over a 5-year period. Thus subjects with moderately advanced dementia, hepatic failure, or renal failure are generally not considered suitable candidates.

Other considerations help determine which patients carry an increased risk of poor outcome acutely from endarterectomy. As far back as 1975, Sundt and colleagues[57] recognized that poor or unstable neurologic status, as well as cerebral ischemia within 24 hours of surgery, identified a group at high surgical risk. These authors also related high risk to the following: congestive heart failure, recent cardiac ischemia, marked hypertension, emphysema, age older than 70, and severe obesity. The presence of a contralateral carotid occlusion places subjects at extremely high risk of stroke if left untreated but also carries a high morbidity and mortality risk acutely.[58]

The likelihood of stroke in patients with carotid stenosis rises steadily with increasing severity of stenosis greater than 70%[56] and then decreases again as the stenosis reaches 94% to 99%. However, surgery remains beneficial in this range.[59] In addition, hemispheric symptoms predict roughly twice the danger of stroke as do isolated retinal symptoms.[60] The presence of ulceration in conjunction with stenosis, as detected angiographically, increases the risk of stroke. This effect is most marked when associated with the highest degrees of stenosis and becomes progressively more modest as the degree of stenosis decreases toward 70%.[61]

A meta-analysis[62] has shown that men benefit more from carotid surgery than women. In contrast to Sundt and colleagues'[57] prior findings, there is greater benefit of the procedure in persons older than 75 years. The most important finding to emerge from this report, however, is the dramatic benefit when endarterectomy is performed within 2 weeks of the sentinel event, which diminishes rapidly if surgery is delayed. The previously established surgical practice, to wait for 4 to 6 weeks following stroke or TIA before proceeding with surgery, has become untenable. When severe disability exists, endarterectomy may be reasonably delayed in order to see if sufficient recovery occurs to warrant intervention. However, carotid revascularization, whether by means of endarterectomy or, as discussed later, carotid angioplasty and stenting (CAS), should be undertaken acutely in the absence of major neurologic disability.

Protected CAS has been compared with CEA in a controlled, randomized trial.[63] Study participants were 18 years old or older and had either a greater than 50% symptomatic stenosis or a greater than 80% asymptomatic stenosis. They were at high risk, as defined by at least one of the factors listed in Box 63.12.

Box 63.12 High-Risk Criteria for Entry into the SAPPHIRE Trial

- Clinically significant heart disease: congestive heart failure, abnormal stress test, or need for open heart surgery
- Severe pulmonary disease
- Contralateral carotid artery occlusion
- Contralateral laryngeal nerve palsy
- Previous radical neck surgery
- Previous radiation therapy to the neck
- Carotid restenosis after endarterectomy
- Age older than 80 years

SAPPHIRE, Stenting and Angioplasty with Protection in Patients at High Risk for Endarterectomy.

SAPPHIRE (Stenting and Angioplasty with Protection in Patients at High Risk for Endarterectomy) trial showed a trend favoring CAS for the incidence of death and major ipsilateral stroke, both in the year following intervention. These gains fell short of statistical significance, perhaps because the study was terminated prematurely. The CAS group benefited significantly as far as reduction of hospital length of stay (by 1 day) and reduction in the incidence of laryngeal nerve palsy. Lastly, there was a significant decline in the rate of myocardial infarction (MI) at 1 month following intervention in the CAS group when compared with endarterectomy, caused primarily by a fall in the incidence of non-Q-wave MI. Some of this benefit may reflect the use of clopidogrel in addition to aspirin for 2 to 4 weeks following treatment in the CAS group, whereas the endarterectomy subjects received only aspirin. In summary, the study showed that CAS was not inferior to endarterectomy and perhaps was superior in certain respects. The durability of these results is not known because of limited follow-up. A more important question involves the necessity of intervention. The authors do not systematically distinguish between symptomatic and asymptomatic subjects in their report. Is the benefit of stenting more evident in the symptomatic group? Do the patients with significant systemic illness (cardiac or pulmonary disease) survive long enough to warrant the initial risk of any intervention? There is no control group treated with medical therapy alone for comparison.

In conclusion, SAPPHIRE establishes CAS as a practical alternative to endarterectomy in a somewhat heterogeneous high-risk population. It is intuitively attractive because it is less invasive. The clinician must still decide who will benefit from the procedure on an individual basis. CAS will find an important role in the management of subjects with symptomatic carotid stenosis who are awaiting coronary artery bypass surgery. The requisite use of clopidogrel following stenting will mandate a delay of 6 weeks before proceeding with surgery.

Subsequently published studies, SPACE (Stent-Protected Angioplasty versus Carotid Endarterectomy)[64] and EVA-3S (Endarterectomy Versus Angioplasty in Patients with

Symptomatic Severe Carotid Stenosis),[65] have been used to cast doubt on the efficacy of CAS in a population of patients with significant symptomatic stenosis, free of such elevated risk. SPACE shows a trend, not reaching statistical significance, toward more stroke and death acutely with CAS than with CEA. Over subsequent 2-year follow-up, the stroke and death risk is the same in either group. However, there appears to be more restenosis in the CAS group, and it is clear that CEA is superior in patients older than 68 years of age. SPACE has flaws. The severity of stenosis was assessed by carotid ultrasound alone, without further validation. Distal protection devices were employed in only a quarter of the CAS patients. Although the authors state that the incidence of periprocedural stroke was not affected by the use of such devices, it is not clear how the decision was taken to use them.

EVA-3S shows that the complication rate of CAS is much higher (9.6%) than the complication rate of CEA (3.6%), without a consequent improvement in natural history over 4-year follow-up. These results may be peculiar to this trial, in which the surgical complication rate was much lower than the CAS complication rate. In this study, CEA seems to be preferable for those older than 70, for men, and for those with stroke either previously or at presentation.

The most recently published trials, CAVATAS (Carotid And Vertebral Artery Transluminal Angioplasty Study)[66] and CREST (Carotid Revascularization Endarterectomy versus Stenting Trial),[67] are more definitive. They include both symptomatic and asymptomatic subjects. CAVATAS is an earlier study using a mix of angioplasty and stenting. It shows that endovascular treatment carries a higher risk of small perioperative stroke, although it does protect from cranial nerve injury. Overall, there is no substantive difference between the two treatments. There may be a higher risk of stroke, among both older patients and those patients suffering from cardiac disease, and there may be a higher risk of restenosis with angioplasty. CREST, the largest and most recent trial, reveals an increased risk of stroke acutely with stenting, although endarterectomy acutely is associated with an increased risk of heart attack—this latter risk, however, is not associated with increasing mortality risk. Over 2.5 years of follow-up, there is no significant difference in outcome between the two treatments. Endarterectomy appears to be superior, again, in older patients over 70. Recovery from nonfatal MI is less problematic than recovery from stroke, and the increased stroke risk in the CAS group is early in the patients' course. The results of this study argue against adoption of CAS as an alternative to CEA, particularly as it does not appear to confer a survival benefit, as hoped, to older subjects.

A comment on intracranial angioplasty and stenting is also in order. The realization that warfarin is not superior[68] to high-dose aspirin for stroke prevention in the setting of symptomatic intracranial arterial stenosis led to the performance of the SAMMPRIS (Stenting and Aggressive Medical Management for Preventing Recurrent Stroke in Intracranial Stenosis) trial.[69] This was a randomized comparison of intracranial angioplasty and stenting versus intensive medical therapy, including the use of aspirin in conjunction with clopidogrel, for symptomatic intracranial stenosis. The study was stopped prematurely because of a very high risk of periprocedural stroke following intervention, and a very low risk of stroke in the medically treated group. Consequently, it is difficult to support the routine performance of intracranial angioplasty and stenting on symptomatic vessels, but combined therapy with aspirin and clopidogrel may be considered.

ANTICOAGULATION IN STROKE

Anticoagulants occupy an important but limited place in stroke therapy. The acute use of heparin in unselected stroke patients was studied some years ago but not justified.[70] More recently, the treatment with warfarin of subjects presenting with symptomatic intracranial stenosis has proved no better than therapy with high-dose (1300 mg daily) aspirin. This use of warfarin produced increased morbidity, in part because of an increased risk of major hemorrhage, primarily gastrointestinal (GI).[68] When warfarin is given to unselected stroke patients in a population including a slight majority of subjects with lacunar stroke, it confers no advantage relative to aspirin.[71] Warfarin does not reduce the incidence of stroke among subjects with a decreased ejection fraction (<35%) when compared to aspirin.[72]

Warfarin clearly prevents stroke among subjects suffering from nonrheumatic atrial fibrillation, even if they have never had a stroke or TIA.[73] The risk of stroke falls by 64%, a robust and consistent effect that aspirin cannot equal. The CHADS2[74] score (Box 63.13) is used commonly to assess the risk of stroke; the higher the score, the higher the risk. Individuals younger than 65 years of age with atrial fibrillation who have no significant vascular risk factors are at low risk and do not need anticoagulation. Such individuals are rare in clinical practice. The risk of systemic hemorrhage and of ICH with warfarin use in this setting is low. A combination of clopidogrel and low-dose aspirin[75] is inferior to warfarin in stroke prevention among patients with atrial fibrillation. The bleeding risk is actually lower with warfarin than with the antiplatelet combination. However, combination therapy with aspirin and clopidogrel is superior to aspirin alone among patients thought unsuitable for anticoagulant use,[76] although the combination does raise the risk of major hemorrhage somewhat.

Individuals with atrial fibrillation who sustain a minor stroke or TIA have a high stroke risk (12% per year), which

Box 63.13 Components of the CHADS2 Score

Congestive heart failure	1 point
Hypertension (consistently >140/90 mm Hg or on therapy)	1 point
Age older than 75 years	1 point
Diabetes mellitus	1 point
Prior **s**troke or TIA	2 points

CHADS2, Congestive heart failure, Hypertension, Age >75, Diabetes mellitus, and prior Stroke or transient ischemic attack; TIA, transient ischemic attack.

falls to 4% per year upon treatment with warfarin. A 2.8% yearly risk of all bleeding complications with warfarin exists, as opposed to 0.7% with placebo. Aspirin is nearly as safe as placebo, but it reduces the stroke risk only modestly.[77] It remains uncertain when in the course of stroke to initiate anticoagulant therapy. A randomized trial[78] has compared a form of low-molecular-weight heparin (dalteparin) to 160 mg of aspirin in patients with stroke and atrial fibrillation. Treatment began within 30 hours of stroke onset, and the risk of recurrent stroke at 14 days was determined. This proved to be 8%. Dalteparin was equivalent to aspirin. This study was not powered to demonstrate a more modest beneficial effect of dalteparin, which may or may not be present. Nevertheless, this study urges caution on those who would treat completed stroke acutely with anticoagulants. The exclusion criteria for the study serve as a guideline as to when not to treat with anticoagulants. Patients with severe strokes and those with marked elevation of blood pressure were not entered. Acute anticoagulation in the face of stroke should be withheld if there is a sizable infarct as measured by the NIHSS (perhaps a score of ≥12) or on CT (>⅓ of MCA territory), which could progress to herniation and death as a result of hemorrhage into the infarct bed. The 185/110 mm Hg cutoff measurement used in the NINDS tPA trial may give some idea of the range of hypertension that would cause one to withhold acute treatment with anticoagulants.

In contrast, one should move quickly to anticoagulation following a TIA occurring in conjunction with atrial fibrillation or any other recognized indication for anticoagulation. Minor strokes that begin with potentially devastating deficits but go on to resolve substantially should receive anticoagulation if its use is indicated. These recommendations seem appropriate in view of the high risk of stroke recurrence in atrial fibrillation, as cited previously.[77]

Other indications for anticoagulation appear in Box 63.14. Some, such as the presence of rheumatic heart disease with atrial fibrillation, prosthetic heart valve, or deep venous thrombosis (DVT), are long established. Anticoagulation carries more urgency when a DVT coexists with a communication across the atrial septum, such as patent foramen ovale (PFO), because there is risk of both recurrent stroke and pulmonary embolism.

The utility of warfarin is limited by the need for regular blood work, and by difficulty in regulating its dosage. Factor II and factor Xa inhibitors have recently been studied for stroke prevention in the setting of atrial fibrillation. Dabigatran (Pradaxa) and rivaroxaban (Xarelto) are marketed in the United States. Another, apixaban, reduces the risk of stroke[79]—when compared to aspirin—in patients deemed unsuitable for warfarin use, without an increase in major or intracranial hemorrhage. When compared directly to warfarin, apixaban reduces the risk not only of stroke but also of both intracranial hemorrhage and of serious hemorrhage.[80] Rivaroxaban[81] appears equivalent to warfarin in stroke prevention, and it is less likely to produce intracranial hemorrhage but carries a higher risk of major GI hemorrhage. Dabigatran, at the dosage of 150 mg daily,[82] is associated with a smaller stroke risk and, like rivaroxaban, a lesser risk of intracranial hemorrhage but a higher risk of major GI hemorrhage, when compared to warfarin.

Box 63.14 Indications for Anticoagulation in Stroke

- Atrial fibrillation, with or without rheumatic heart disease
- Prosthetic heart valve
- Deep venous thrombosis, with or without the potential for paradoxical embolus
- Hypercoagulable state
- Venous sinus thrombosis
- Arterial dissection

The main concern with these agents is the lack of means to reverse their effect in the setting of hemorrhage. One patient taking dabigatran has died[83] from relatively minor head trauma leading to progressive intracranial hemorrhage. It may be possible to reverse the effects of rivaroxaban, but not dabigatran, through the use of prothrombin complex concentrate,[84] although dabigatran may be cleared through dialysis.[85] Fortunately, these agents have short half-lives and are cleared rapidly.[86] Nevertheless, care is enjoined in their use, both in the setting of renal insufficiency, and in conjunction with aspirin.[87] Hemorrhage in patients using factor II and factor Xa antagonists will remain troublesome until means to reverse the anticoagulation produced by these agents are developed, together with the capability to monitor the process in real time. For now, fear of this complication will limit the use of these agents.

Venous sinus thrombosis is an uncommon condition that manifests with headache and papilledema, as well as focal symptoms, and often leads to ICH.[88] Diagnosis is by magnetic resonance venography.[89] Treatment is with heparin acutely, even in the presence of ICH.[90] More recent reports have established the safety of low-molecular-weight heparin followed by 3 months of warfarin therapy for this condition, although only a trend toward favorable outcome emerged.[91] Retrograde thrombolysis through the venous system with tPA in conjunction with IV heparin is effective in more serious cases.[92]

Spontaneous dissection of the carotid and vertebral arteries is the subject of a review by Schievink.[93] This is a significant cause of stroke in younger individuals. Carotid dissection often presents with neck pain, radiating to the head, and with components of Horner's syndrome (ptosis, miosis, and anhidrosis). Vertebral dissection presents with pain in the neck or back of the head initially. Either may proceed to cerebral infarction or to retinal infarction in the case of carotid dissection. MRA diagnoses carotid dissection quite accurately, and vertebral dissection less so.[94] Anticoagulation is commonly employed but has not been subjected to a rigorous trial. The presence of dissection does not appear to contraindicate the performance of thrombolysis by whatever route.[95]

Box 63.15 lists the hypercoagulable states.[96] Most of these lead mainly to the development of venous thrombosis, although antiphospholipid antibodies and the lupus anticoagulant may produce both venous and arterial thrombosis. The duration of anticoagulation rests on the judgment of the treating physician. Three to 6 months of therapy is commonly undertaken if the episode of thrombosis is isolated.

Box 63.15 Causes of Hypercoagulable States

Protein C deficiency
Protein S deficiency
Antithrombin III deficiency
Factor V Leiden
Prothrombin gene mutation
Antiphosphilipid antibodies
Lupus anticoagulant

ANTIPLATELET AGENTS IN STROKE

Secondary stroke prevention continues to depend on aspirin, as it has for many years. A meta-analysis carried out in 1994[97] showed that antiplatelet therapy, primarily with aspirin, reduces the risk of stroke, MI, and vascular death in aggregate by 25%. This analysis did not discriminate among those subjects treated primarily for heart disease and those treated for cerebral ischemia. A similar analysis[98] focusing only on the latter found a lesser benefit of aspirin, on the order of 13%. The optimal dosage of aspirin remains unknown. One study[99] failed to show a difference in outcome when comparing dosages of 30 mg and 283 mg. Another[100] revealed no difference in efficacy between 300 mg and 1200 mg of aspirin a day. In both reports, the lesser dosage led to fewer significant bleeding episodes.

The limited effect of aspirin on stroke recurrence, coupled with the seeming failure of increases in dosage to further reduce stroke risk, led to a search for other antiplatelet agents. Ticlopidine enjoyed brief popularity but was found to produce agranulocytosis (<1500 neutrophils/μL) in 2.4% of subjects, which was severe (<450/μL) in 0.8%.[101] Thrombotic thrombocytopenic purpura, fatal in 4 of 13 cases, also occurred.[102] Both the need for regular blood monitoring and the risk of a severe and potentially fatal complication led to the virtual abandonment of this agent.

Another thienopyridine, clopidogrel, was studied in the CAPRIE (Clopidogrel versus Aspirin in Patients at Risk of Ischemic Events) trial.[103] It exhibited minimal benefit compared with aspirin in preventing vascular events both in patients presenting with stroke and in those manifesting with MI. Nevertheless, it was approved for use primarily on the strength of its ability to reduce the development of vascular events in subjects presenting with peripheral arterial disease. It has won wide support and has subsequently proved quite useful, administered together with aspirin, in the treatment of unstable angina[104] and acute MI[105,106] and following stent placement in the coronary vessels.[107]

Physicians have used clopidogrel in conjunction with aspirin for stroke prevention in the expectation that the combination would prove superior to clopidogrel in isolation. However, a comparison between the use of 75 mg of aspirin together with 75 mg of clopidogrel and the use of clopidogrel alone revealed no benefit of combination therapy, just a heightened risk of GI hemorrhage.[108] Another study[109] failed to show a benefit of combination therapy when compared with the use of aspirin alone in preventing stroke, MI, or vascular death. In addition, the risk of "moderate" hemorrhage was increased in the group receiving combination therapy. Patients, in order to enter this study, had to have either established vascular disease or, in a minority, multiple vascular risk factors. The study as published does not assess the risks or benefits of combination therapy relative to aspirin in subjects randomized for stroke alone. Nevertheless, the results do not support the chronic use of combination therapy in the prevention of acute vascular syndromes and death of vascular origin. Perhaps combination therapy may be useful in the setting of acute cerebral ischemia, as it is for acute coronary syndromes with ST-segment elevation.[105,106] Certainly the use of aspirin is recognized as beneficial in acute stroke when instituted within 48 hours,[110] and one may imagine, on the basis of the cardiac data, that clopidogrel may also benefit stroke acutely. A study is ongoing[111] to address this possibility, but results will not be available soon.

An alternative to the use of aspirin or clopidogrel is the combination of low-dose aspirin in conjunction with extended-release dipyridamole (ASA + ER/DP). The initial aspirin and dipyridamole study, ESPS (European Stroke Prevention Study),[112] showed a striking benefit of the combination of 990 mg of aspirin and 75 mg of dipyridamole daily in reducing stroke by 38%. This result raised the question of whether the high aspirin dosage or the addition of dipyridamole was responsible for the dramatic improvement in outcome. A second trial, ESPS-2,[113] revealed a similar benefit using a regimen of 50 mg of aspirin and 400 mg of ER/DP per day. The effect of the two agents was additive. However, there was no improvement in mortality rate or in the rate of MI in any of the treatment groups (ASA, ER/DP, or ASA + ER/DP) when compared with placebo in ESPS-2. This contrasts with the results of ESPS, in which combination therapy did reduce both the rate of vascular death and, in the intention-to-treat analysis, that of MI. Thus both the active regimen used in ESPS and the combination therapy used in ESPS-2 significantly reduced the rate of recurrent stroke. However, only in ESPS, which used a much higher aspirin dosage, was there a reduction in the rate of MI and vascular death.

As already noted, previous studies[99,100] have not revealed significant differences in outcome on the basis of the aspirin dosage used but the numbers enrolled in these trials are relatively modest and differences cannot be definitively excluded.

A recent large randomized trial with roughly 20,000 patients (PRoFESS [Prevention Regimen for Effectively avoiding Second Strokes]) compared ASA + ER/DP to clopidogrel in the prevention of stroke, MI, and death among patients presenting with stroke.[114] The two treatments proved equivalent overall, but the rate of ICH was increased in the ASA + ER/DP group. Because ASA + ER/DP needs to be taken twice daily, has more side effects (headache, primarily), and has no cost advantage, the study has not led to its widespread use.

In conclusion, the area of antiplatelet therapy for stroke has evolved. Clopidogrel remains the drug of choice under certain restricted circumstances (Box 63.16). Clinicians often change therapy from one antiplatelet agent to another following the development of a cerebral ischemic event, but one must expect a significant failure rate with any of these agents. Whether such a strategy is beneficial is unclear. Aspirin will remain the agent of choice for most patients,

Box 63.16 Indications for the Use of Clopidogrel after Cerebral Ischemia

Recent acute coronary syndromes
Recent stent placement
Absolute aspirin intolerance including aspirin allergy
Coexistent symptomatic peripheral arterial disease

particularly when one considers the cost of the alternatives. Combination therapy with aspirin and dipyridamole may find a niche in individuals with cerebrovascular disease who are at risk for the development of GI hemorrhage.

PATENT FORAMEN OVALE

PFO is a recently recognized cause of cardiac embolization to the brain. PFO is detected by two-dimensional echocardiography with injection of agitated saline or by transesophageal study. In one report it appeared in 18% of young control subjects and in 40% of subjects with cryptogenic stroke. PFO was more common as well in younger as opposed to older patients with cryptogenic stroke (stroke of unknown origin following standard evaluation).[115] The combination of PFO with atrial septal aneurysm in stroke patients younger than the age of 55 is associated with a high (15.2% over 4 years) risk of recurrent stroke.[116] Others[117] have found a large diameter (>4 mm) of the PFO to predict increased risk of stroke recurrence. PFO can be treated with warfarin, aspirin, surgical closure, and now endovascular closure. No data suggest conclusively that one treatment surpasses the others,[118] as confirmed by the recently published CLOSURE I trial.[119] In this study, PFO closure did not lead to fewer strokes than did medical therapy. Neither the size of the interatrial shunt nor the presence of an associated atrial septal aneurysm influenced the results. Moreover, PFO closure, aside from procedural complications, was related to a significantly increased risk of atrial fibrillation. At this time, closure of a PFO may be indicated in the absence of another explanation for multifocal infarction.

MASSIVE HEMISPHERIC CEREBRAL INFARCT

Infarction of the entire MCA territory leads to the development of the "malignant MCA" syndrome.[120] This major injury leads to death in 78% of cases in the first week after the ictus, as the result of cerebral edema leading to transtentorial herniation, and the survivors are quite disabled. Brain swelling peaks at 3 to 5 days following stroke onset.

The presence of early CT changes, namely, hypodensity of more than 50% of the MCA territory, indicates a poor prognosis.[121] In the absence of appropriate intervention, midline displacement of the pineal gland greater than 4 mm predicts death reliably. Large volume of infarction (Fig. 63.5) and displacement of the septum pellucidum also indicate a poor outcome.[122] At initial presentation, aphasia or neglect may be present, depending on the hemisphere affected. Characteristically, the patients display hemiplegia and a dense hemisensory loss, although the leg may be relatively spared. Quite often, there is a forced eye deviation and hemianopia may coexist. Mortality rate is higher in older individuals with this syndrome,[123] but transtentorial herniation is a more significant cause of death among younger subjects with ischemic stroke.[124] Presumably younger individuals have less cerebral atrophy and less room within the cranial vault to accommodate brain swelling.

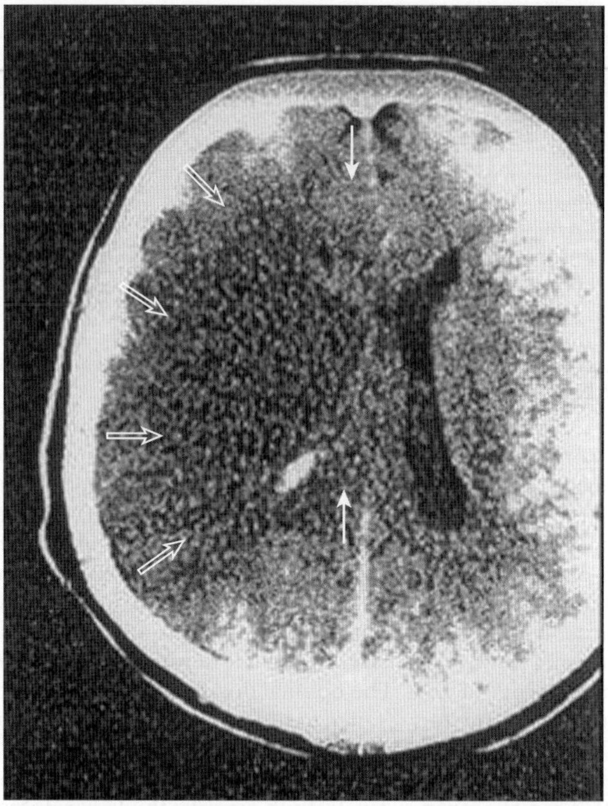

Figure 63.5 Massive middle cerebral artery (MCA) infarct. Hypolucency of the entire right MCA territory *(open arrows)* and compression of the right lateral ventricle *(white arrows)* are demonstrated.

Treatment of this syndrome has so far proved disappointing, as reviewed by different authors.[125-127] The review by Wijdicks[127] is particularly comprehensive. Standard therapies include hyperventilation and the administration of IV mannitol. Mannitol is a dehydrating agent, an osmotic diuretic, which aims at reducing cerebral volume and thus ICP. It is given initially at a dosage of 1 g/kg, followed by recurrent dosing four times daily with 0.25 to 0.5 g/kg. The goal of therapy is a serum osmolality of 315 to 320 mOsm/L. Mechanical ventilation with hyperventilation produces hypocarbia, which leads to cerebral vasoconstriction, reduced cerebral blood volume, and decreased ICP. The target range for $Paco_2$ is not well defined. Steiner and colleagues[126] state that lowering Pco_2 from "35 to 29 mm Hg lowers ICP by 25% to 30% in most subjects." The benefit of these interventions in clinical practice appears to be short-lived. Because hyperventilation is associated with decreased blood flow, it should be viewed as a temporizing measure only.

More promising therapies include hypothermia and decompressive hemicraniectomy. Hypothermia in one pilot trial[128] lowered ICP temporarily when instituted within 14 hours of onset of major MCA stroke. Hypothermia has also been employed[129] shortly after thrombolysis. The use of a device placed in the inferior vena cava lowers body temperature much more quickly than surface cooling,[130] although there is a concern regarding the development of DVT. Hypothermia to 33° C for 24 hours, following tPA administration within 6 hours of stroke onset, is safe, apart from an increased risk of pneumonia.[131] A larger randomized trial of hypothermia following thrombolysis, ICTuS2/3 (Intravascular Cooling in the Treatment of Stroke 2/3 Trial),[132] is under way.

Decompressive hemicraniectomy with durotomy in early studies appeared beneficial when compared with medical treatment,[133] particularly when intervention occurred before the appearance of signs of incipient herniation.[134] However, the surgically treated patients in these two reports differed significantly from the control patients. The surgical patients were younger, and subjects with large left hemispheric infarcts producing global aphasia were not considered for surgery. Some, if not all, of the benefit in the surgically treated group may be explained by this imbalance between the control and treated groups. More recently, three randomized trials have been carried out,[135-137] and a preplanned pooled analysis[138] of their results published. Two of these studies were terminated prematurely,[135,136] all the studies revealed reductions in mortality rate, but benefits in functional outcome were lesser and not consistently significant. The pooled analysis, looking at the benefit of hemicraniectomy in patients younger than 60 years of age treated within 48 hours, showed significant benefits both in mortality rate and in functional outcome, such that hemicraniectomy has been adopted into general practice. A further study, DESTINY II,[139] will examine the efficacy of this intervention among subjects older than 60.

Surgical intervention also exists for cerebellar infarction, which, when large, may expand and place pressure on the brainstem.[140] Both ventriculostomy to relieve hydrocephalus acutely and decompressive craniotomy are employed. The main determinant of survival and recovery is the absence of coma on presentation. Surgery is the accepted treatment, but the exact timing of intervention remains uncertain.[141]

CRITICAL CARE CONSULTATION

Critical care consultation for stroke patients is indicated for a number of reasons (Box 63.17).

Box 63.17 Indications for Critical Care Consultation

Intubation and mechanical ventilation
Administration of continuous infusions of antihypertensive agents
Administration of pressor agents
Monitoring not feasible in other settings
Intraventricular drainage
Induction and maintenance of hypothermia

SUMMARY

In conclusion, stroke therapy is advancing significantly. Thrombolysis and endovascular therapy have developed over the past 20 years. Advances in radiology have improved imaging of strokes and of blood vessels and may come to play a role in patient selection for acute intervention. Endarterectomy has become established in the treatment of carotid disease and angioplasty and stenting for the treatment of high-risk cases. New anticoagulants have appeared, although they are not free of risk. No longer is aspirin the only antiplatelet agent available. Decompressive surgery can save lives that would otherwise be lost. Hypothermia may soon join these other therapies in the physician's armamentarium. Much of this activity has taken place in the critical care unit. One may hope that the next 20 years will bring further revelations. As our means for intervention increase, so will the role of critical care in reducing death and disability from stroke.

KEY POINTS

- Determine time of onset of all new strokes.
- Consider IV thrombolysis with tPA if within 3 hours of onset.
- Consider IA thrombolysis for basilar thrombosis or if within 6 hours of stroke onset.
- Consider rescue therapy with mechanical clot extraction or IA thrombolysis.
- Observe published guidelines for blood pressure control.
- Use MRI and MRA or CT and CTA to visualize the brain and its vasculature.
- Proceed promptly to carotid endarterectomy or carotid angioplasty and stenting.
- Apply anticoagulants when indicated.
- Use antiplatelet agents according to specific indications.
- Treat malignant MCA infarction with craniectomy.
- Consider surgical intervention for large cerebellar infarcts.

SELECTED REFERENCES

7. The National Institute of Neurological Disorders and Stroke t-PA Stroke Study Group: Tissue plasminogen activator for acute ischemic stroke. N Engl J Med 1995;333;1581-1587.
10. Saver JL, Jahan R, Levy E, et al: Primary Results of the SOLITAIRE with the Intention for Thrombectomy (SWIFT) Multicenter, Randomized Clinical Trial. Abstract presented at the International Stroke Conference, New Orleans, LA, Feb. 3, 2012.
19. Wijdicks EFM, Scott JP: Outcome in patients with acute basilar artery occlusion requiring mechanical ventilation. Stroke 1996; 27:1301-1303.
24. Tong DC, Yenari MA, Albers GW, et al: Correlation of perfusion- and diffusion-weighted MRI with NIHSS score in acute (<6.5 hour) ischemic stroke. Neurology 1999;50:864-869.

25. Fiebach JB, Schellinger PD, Gass A, et al, for the Kompetenznetzwerk Schlaganfall B5: Stroke magnetic resonance imaging is accurate in hyperacute intracerebral hemorrhage: A multicenter study on the validity of stroke imaging. Stroke 2004;35:502-506.
40. Hacke W, Kaste M, Bluhmki E, et al: Thrombolysis with alteplase 3 to 4.5 hours after aute ischemic stroke. N Engl J Med 2008;359:1317-1329.
67. Brott TG, Hobson RW, Howard G, et al: Stenting verus endarterectomy for treatment of carotid-artery stenosis. New Engl J Med 2010:363:11-23.
69. Chimowitz MI, Lynn MJ, Derdeyn CP, et al: Stenting versus aggressive medical therapy for intracranial arterial stenosis. N Engl J Med 2011;365:993-1003.
114. Sacco RL, Diener H-C, Yusuf S, et al: Aspirin and extended-release dipyridamole versus clopidogrel for recurrent stroke. N Engl J Med 2008;359:1238-1251.
118. Messe SR, Silverman IE, Kizer JR, et al: Practice parameter: Recurrent stroke with patent foramen ovale and atrial septal aneurysm. Report of the Quality Standards Subcommittee of the American Academy of Neurology. Neurology 2004;62:1042-1050.

The complete list of references can be found at www.expertconsult.com.

64

Muscular Paralysis: Myasthenia Gravis and Guillaine-Barré Syndrome

Manoj K. Mittal | Eelco F. M. Wijdicks

CHAPTER OUTLINE

Acute neuromuscular disorders may be suspected in patients with acute hypercapnic respiratory failure. They usually present with acute, subacute, or chronic dyspnea, tachypnea, and tachycardia. They may also have associated oropharyngeal weakness manifested by nasal voice, poor cough, and problems in handling secretions. Neuromuscular respiratory failure is associated with the use of accessory muscles of respiration and paradoxical breathing. Neuromuscular weakness–induced acute respiratory failure seen in the intensive care unit (ICU) involves patients with Guillain-Barré syndrome (GBS) or an exacerbation of previously diagnosed myasthenia gravis (MG). The management of patients with these disorders is different from that of patients with primary or secondary pulmonary disease and requires challenging decisions on all aspects of care.

This chapter provides a concise overview of pathophysiology, diagnosis, and optimal management of acute neuromuscular respiratory failure as a result of GBS and MG.

CLINICAL PRESENTATION

MYASTHENIA GRAVIS

MG is an autoimmune disease of defective neurotransmission leading to fatigable muscle weakness. The incidence is 0.5 to 5 cases per 100,000. Its pathogenesis can be summarized briefly as an antibody reaction at the antigen epitopes of the acetylcholine receptor (AChR), eventually leading to destruction and simplification of the junctional fold and widening synaptic cleft.[1] Onset may be at any age but tends to be earlier in women (mean age 28 years) than in men (mean age 42 years). MG results in either transient or persistent focal or generalized fatigability or weakness. In more than half of the cases, the initial symptoms involve the eyes, presenting as ptosis, diplopia, or ophthalmoparesis.

Myasthenic crisis is arbitrarily defined as MG complicated by respiratory failure requiring mechanical ventilation or delayed extubation for more than 24 hours in an already intubated myasthenic patient. It is seen in 10% to 60% of MG patients typically within the first 12 months of disease onset.[2,3] The need for ventilatory assistance usually follows onset of weakness of diaphragmatic or accessory respiratory muscles, but mechanical ventilation also may become necessary because of airway collapse from oropharyngeal muscle weakness, stridor from vocal cord weakness, or the inability to clear secretions.[4] One third of the patients may have recurrent myasthenic crises.[5]

Common precipitating causes include viral or bacterial infection in 48% (pneumonia, respiratory infection, or sepsis), aspiration in 10%, reduction of pyridostigmine in 19%, and initiation of steroids in 7% patients.[6,7] Changes in medication may relate to the recent addition of corticosteroid, dose reduction, or high-dose acetylcholinesterase inhibitors. Other precipitating factors may be physical trauma, surgical procedures (particularly thyroidectomy), pregnancy, emotional stress, or exposure to drugs with neuromuscular blocking action such as aminoglycosides. No precipitating factor can be identified for myasthenic crisis in 30% patients.[6,7]

Myasthenic crisis requires urgent evaluation and treatment. The mortality rate for myasthenic crisis has declined from a nearly always fatal outcome in the 1920s to 4.5% in the new millennium with the discovery and application of acetylcholinesterase compounds, mechanical ventilation, immunosuppressive agents, and more recently, plasma exchange and intravenous immunoglobulin (IVIG).[8] Timely diagnosis and appropriate treatment with IVIG or plasma exchange for patients with bulbar and respiratory muscle weakness have helped to reduce the mortality rate and total hospital stay from myasthenic crisis, but care of a patient with MG may be prolonged and complicated. Median hospital stay after a myasthenic crisis is 4 to 6 weeks.

GUILLAIN-BARRÉ SYNDROME

GBS is an acute, monophasic, inflammatory, demyelinating polyneuropathy, also known as acute inflammatory demyelinating polyneuropathy (AIDP). Its incidence is 1 to 2 cases per 100,000 people and remains fairly constant across the continents. GBS commonly is precipitated by an infection, but the immunopathogenesis has remained elusive since its original description in 1916. *Campylobacter jejuni,* cytomegalovirus, and Epstein-Barr virus predominate as preceding infection pathogens.[9] Symptoms and signs usually progress within 1 to 2 weeks.

The diagnosis of GBS often is straightforward. Severe back pain and limb paresthesias, starting in the ankles and wrists with a "tight band" feeling, are typical presenting signs. The paresthesias gradually scatter over the limbs and move proximally. Although paresthesias are often the presenting symptoms, sensory modalities remain normal to mildly impaired. Weakness begins in the more proximal muscles, causing difficulty with climbing stairs and getting out of a chair, and is notable 1 or 2 days after the onset of paresthesias. Symmetrical weak muscles are accompanied by depressed or absent deep tendon reflexes. Mostly legs are more involved than arms, creating the impression of an ascending paralysis. Facial and oropharyngeal muscles are affected in 50% of the cases, and weakness of these muscle groups may be the initial manifestation. Patients may also have staccato speech (ability to speak only short sentences) and small tidal volume with increased respiratory rate. Respiratory failure, if it occurs, commonly appears within 1 week after the onset of paresthesias.[10] Dysautonomia occurs in up to 70% of the cases, manifesting as arrhythmias, tachycardia, diaphoresis, labile blood pressures, urinary retention, or ileus.

Cerebrospinal fluid (CSF) analysis typically shows high protein content with a normal white blood cell count (the classic albuminocytologic dissociation). More than 10 white blood cells may be seen although this number is unusual but is more common in associated disorders such as Lyme disease, sarcoidosis, and AIDS.[11] Electrophysiologic studies are more useful for diagnosis and less useful for prognostication. The typical finding involves demyelination seen as conduction block or increased conduction velocities. Specific tests for proximal nerve involvement seen early in the disease course include recording of F waves and nerve signal abnormalities like dispersion or dropout in signal. Prolonged F wave may be the only finding early on. Needle electromyography may be normal in the first 2 weeks. Recovery often starts after the second week. Progression over 8 weeks more likely suggests the diagnosis to chronic inflammatory demyelinating polyneuropathy (CIDP).

ACUTE NEUROMUSCULAR RESPIRATORY FAILURE

PATHOPHYSIOLOGY

During respiration, lungs can expand and recoil in two ways: by downward and upward movement of the diaphragm to lengthen and shorten the chest cavity, and by elevation and depression of the ribs to increase and decrease the anteroposterior diameter of the chest (Fig. 64.1). Normal quiet breathing is largely accomplished by contraction of the diaphragm.

In neuromuscular respiratory failure, ventilatory function is compromised through two mechanisms: (1) respiratory muscle weakness or fatigue (involving the diaphragm and the intercostal muscles), and (2) oropharyngeal weakness, which leads to obstruction of the upper airway and inability to clear secretions. The neuromuscular respiratory failure follows the following pattern: failure of diaphragm and

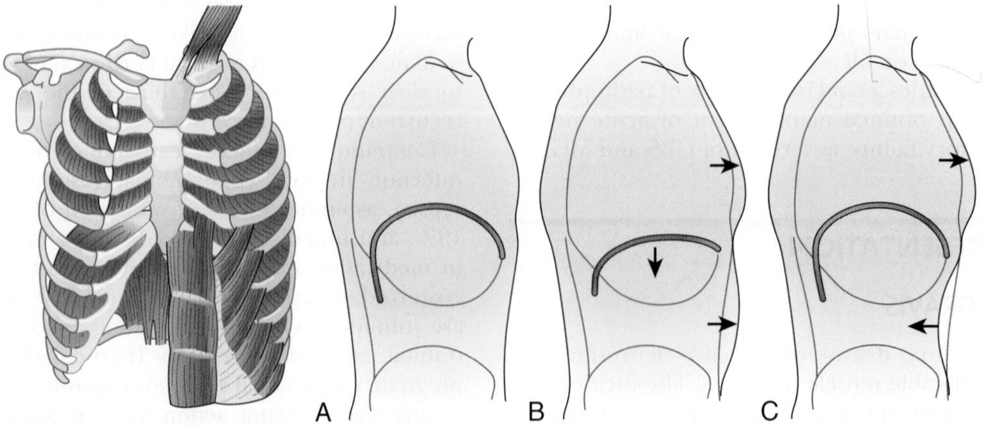

Figure 64.1 Normal mechanism of breathing and paradoxical breathing in neuromuscular respiratory failure. Normal position of diaphragm (**A**). Normal mechanism: during inspiration, a downward movement of the diaphragm pushes the abdominal contents down and out as the rib margins are lifted and moved out, causing both the chest and abdomen to rise (**B**). Paradoxical breathing: with diaphragmatic weakness or paralysis, the diaphragm moves up rather than down during inspiration, and the abdomen moves in, contracting during chest rise (**C**).

intercostal muscles followed by use of accessory muscles resulting in hypoventilation and atelectasis, further leading to shunting and hypoxia. Respiratory muscle weakness leads to shallow low tidal volume breathing and poor gas exchange leading to tachypnea and later hypercapnia. Oropharyngeal muscle weakness leads to aspiration pneumonitis and could further worsens the hypoxia. Clinically, the patient will pause frequently during speech and breathlessness improves in an upright position (Fig. 64.2).

Pulmonary studies typically reveal a pure ventilatory defect with otherwise normal pulmonary parenchyma. The ventilatory defect may worsen with the development of atelectasis. Neuromuscular weakness of the respiratory muscles is characterized by the inability to generate or maintain normal respiratory pressures. The degree of involvement of the inspiratory and the expiratory muscles is variable, and the clinical manifestations reflect the compromise of both muscle groups. Ventilation remains intact until diaphragm involvement becomes significant.

The first indication of diaphragmatic weakness is alveolar hypoventilation and impaired CO_2 exchange. These changes are followed by an increase in respiratory rate as a compensatory mechanism to attempt to maintain minute ventilation. Later, accessory muscles of ventilation are recruited in response to increased ventilatory demand. Paradoxical breathing, also known as thoracoabdominal asynchrony, occurs with severe respiratory weakness. Normally, the abdomen and chest expand and contract in a synchronized fashion. During inspiration, a downward movement of the diaphragm pushes the abdominal contents down and out as the rib margins are lifted and moved out, causing both chest and abdomen to rise. With diaphragmatic weakness or paralysis, the diaphragm moves up rather than down during inspiration, and the abdomen moves in, contracting during chest rise. This is known as "paradoxical breathing" and can be visualized with fluoroscopy (see Fig. 64.1). The ventilatory drive response to an increase in CO_2 in patients with GBS and MG has been studied and was found to be unlikely to contribute to hypoventilation during ventilatory failure.[12] Ventilatory drive increases during acute hypoventilation, and the ventilatory drive response to CO_2 remains intact, even when the minute ventilation response to CO_2 is poor.

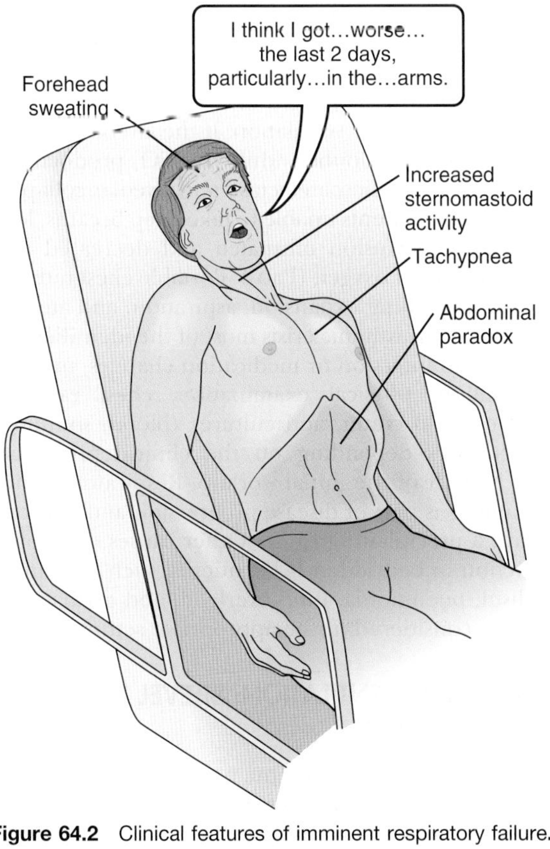

Figure 64.2 Clinical features of imminent respiratory failure.

Although the upper airway muscles do not contribute directly to chest expansion or collapse, they are essential for keeping the airways open during respiration. They play an important role in preventing collapse of the pharynx during inspiration and preventing aspiration during swallowing. With the exception of laryngeal muscles, oropharyngeal muscles have a higher proportion of fast fibers. Their weakness can be seen early on in MG and later in GBS (Fig. 64.3). Slow fibers have a higher fatigue resistance than fast fibers due to their highly oxidative metabolism. The diaphragm has an equal proportion of slow and fast muscle fibers, which in association with small fiber size, high aerobic oxidative enzyme activity, and large number of capillaries make it resistant to fatigue.[13]

CLINICAL EVALUATION

The first step in evaluation of neuromuscular respiratory failure is assessment of clinical features along with bedside pulmonary function tests.

Clinical predictors of worsening neuromuscular respiratory failure in both GBS and MG patients include difficulty handling secretions, restlessness, use of accessory muscles of respiration, rapidly progressing neuromuscular failure, and increasing oxygen requirements. Aspiration or major atelectasis on chest radiograph, evidence of respiratory infection, and failure to improve on bilevel positive airway pressure (BiPAP) are other indicators for worsening neuromuscular respiratory failure.

Frequent (at least four times daily) assessment of pulmonary function should be instituted using bedside spirometry. Although bedside spirometry is often done for respiratory evaluation in both MG and GBS, it is less reliable for MG as patients' results often vary depending on their activity level prior to the testing. Patients should be coached for spirometry as they may have difficulty making an adequate seal around the mouthpiece of the spirometer. Poor effort and leak around the mouthpiece may lead to lower vital capacity (VC), maximal inspiratory pressure (PImax), and maximal expiratory pressure (PEmax) than expected based on arterial blood gas (ABG) and chest x-ray studies. VC, the volume of exhaled air after maximal inspiration, is 60 to 70 mL/kg in normal persons, and is determined primarily by the size of the thorax and lungs. In neuromuscular respiratory failure, reduction of VC to 30 mL/kg is associated with weak cough, accumulation of oropharyngeal secretions, atelectasis, and hypoxemia. Another measure of respiratory muscle strength is the ability to generate negative pressure with inspiratory effort. In normal persons, respiratory muscles cause pleural and alveolar pressures to change by approximately 3 cm H_2O during the breathing cycle. Maximal

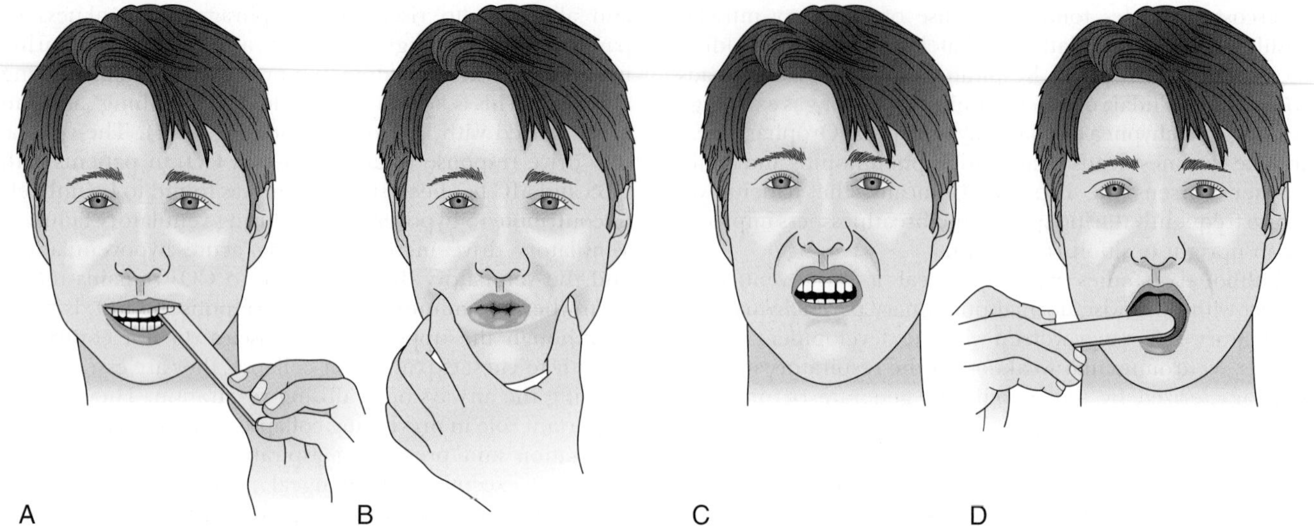

Figure 64.3 Clinical examination of pertinent features in myasthenia gravis. **A,** Biting on tongue depressor to assess masseter weakness. **B,** Puffing out cheeks and resisting pressure from examiner's fingers. **C,** Ptosis and typical snarl of bifacial weakness. **D,** Pushing away tongue depressor with tongue.

Box 64.1 Pathophysiologic Changes with Neuromuscular Failure

- Normal respiratory function is present with VC of 65 mL/kg.
- Poor cough is evident with accumulation of secretions and with VC of 30 mL/kg.
- With VC of 20 mL/kg, the sigh mechanism is impaired, and atelectasis and hypoxia develop.
- Sigh is lost with VC of 15 mL/kg, and atelectasis and shunting appear.
- Hypoventilation starts with VC of 10 mL/kg.
- Hypercapnia develops with VC between 5 and 10 mL/kg.

VC, vital capacity.

pressure generation can be determined by blocking the upper airway and recording mouth pressure changes during inspiratory effort. PImax measures the strength of the diaphragm and other muscles of inspiration and reflects the ability to maintain normal lung expansion and avoid atelectasis. A maximal PImax is −114 cm H_2O in young men and −67 cm H_2O in young women (normal, exceeding −70 cm H_2O). PEmax measures strength of the muscles of expiration and correlates with strength of cough and ability to clear secretions from the airway[12] (Box 64.1). PEmax averages 160 cm H_2O in young men and 95 cm H_2O in young women (normal, greater than 100 cm H_2O). This means that the respiratory muscles are capable of generating more than 30 times the amount of force necessary for tidal breathing.[14] Worsening bedside spirometry can identify MG and GBS patients requiring invasive or noninvasive mechanical ventilation (NMV). An easy way to remember bedside pulmonary indicators of respiratory failure in GBS is the so-called 20/30/40 rule, with VC less than 20 mL/kg, a PImax less negative than −30 cm H_2O, and a PEmax less than 40 cm H_2O.

A simple bedside test, asking patients to count to 20 without the need of an additional respiration, may identify early neuromuscular respiratory weakness.

Bedside ABG may be helpful for to look for hypercapnia and hypoxia. It is important to recognize that in patients with neuromuscular respiratory failure and imminent respiratory arrest, ABG analysis results often remain relatively normal until severe respiratory muscle weakness or total failure develops. ABG analysis performed early after development of a rapid, shallow breathing pattern may show a decreased arterial partial pressure of carbon dioxide (Pa_{CO_2}). This change is followed by progressive inspiratory muscle weakness, leading to hypoventilation and hypercapnia. The P_{CO_2} in alveolar gas or arterial blood is inversely related to the alveolar ventilation. If the alveolar ventilation is halved, the P_{CO_2} doubles while the CO_2 production rate remains constant. Microatelectasis and alveolar collapse also can develop in patients unable to take deep breaths, leading to ventilation-perfusion mismatch and decreased arterial partial pressure of oxygen (Pa_{O_2}). Portable chest radiograph may show poor lung expansion, aspiration, and atelectasis.

Because in myasthenic crisis most of the identified causes are related to infection or medication changes, medication reconciliation, physical examination, chest radiograph, complete blood count, and cultures (blood, sputum, and other cultures depending on the clinical presentation) should be part of the initial workup. Respiratory failure in GBS patients is part of disease progression and may or may not have a precipitating cause. Other causes of respiratory dysfunction in bedridden ICU patients, such as pulmonary embolism, pneumonia, fluid overload, and cardiac failure, should be considered in the appropriate setting.

NONINVASIVE VENTILATION: BILEVEL POSITIVE AIRWAY PRESSURE

Traditionally, patients with acute neuromuscular respiratory failure are ventilated by invasive mechanical ventilation. Prolonged endotracheal intubation, however, is associated with discomfort and ventilator-associated complications.[7] In both MG and GBS, mortality and morbidity rates are strongly tied to the duration of invasive mechanical ventilation. NMV is being used increasingly to manage acute deterioration in patients with neuromuscular failure.[15] Downsides of NMV are, in patients with associated bulbar weakness, upper airway collapse with increased airway resistance, and lack of airway protection from secretions.

Noninvasive mechanical ventilation using BiPAP ventilation (inspiration and expiration pressure application) in acute respiratory failure caused by MG was shown to be effective in a group of patients with MG from the Mayo Clinic.[15] The mean duration of BiPAP was 4.3 days. NMV averted endotracheal intubation in 14 cases of severe MG exacerbation, even in the presence of bulbar weakness. In this study, the presence of hypercapnia (Pa_{CO_2} greater than 45 mm Hg) at onset predicted NMV failure and subsequent intubation. Lower PEmax on arrival was associated with longer ventilator duration.[15] In contrast with the findings with MG, data on use of NMV in GBS is scarce. One study warned against its use because improvement following initiation of NMV did not prevent emergency intubation in patients with GBS.[16]

MECHANICAL VENTILATION: ENDOTRACHEAL INTUBATION

MYASTHENIA GRAVIS

Although several parameters traditionally have been suggested for intubation in MG patients (VC less than 15 mL/kg, PImax less than −30), the fluctuating nature of the disease and frequently associated facial muscle weakness give these parameters limited positive predictive power.[17,18] PImax worsening of 30% or more may predict patients at higher risk of requiring mechanical or noninvasive ventilation.[18] Ventilatory support is unlikely to be needed when VC is more than 20 mL/kg.

Assessment of respiratory function in MG patients should use a range of criteria including symptoms of breathlessness, paradoxical abdominal wall motion, bulbar nerve palsy, and ABG analysis to look for the presence of hypercapnia or hypoxia. As discussed earlier, patients with Pa_{CO_2} greater than 45 mm Hg usually are unresponsive to noninvasive ventilation and should be managed with endotracheal intubation. However, hypercapnia alone is not always a mandatory indication for mechanical ventilation, and this decision should take into consideration the patient's ease of respiration, level of consciousness, and stability of Pa_{CO_2}.[18] MG patients who are positive for anti-MuSK (muscle-specific kinase) antibodies are at a greater risk for the development of respiratory compromise and bulbar symptoms and should be watched more closely.[19-21]

Invasive mechanical ventilation in patients with MG can be avoided in a majority of cases with early implementation of rapid immunomodulatory treatments and noninvasive ventilation.[15] Mechanical ventilation has been associated with atelectasis and cardiac, infectious, and veno-occlusive complications.[8] MG patients requiring mechanical ventilation have high mortality rates of 4% to 17%, with common causes of death identified as acute respiratory distress syndrome, disseminated intravascular coagulation, cardiac failure, and multiorgan failure.[6] Duration of mechanical ventilation usually ranges from 1 to 4 weeks. Age more than 50 years, preintubation serum bicarbonate level of 30 mmol/L or more, and peak VC less than 25 mL/kg in the first week after intubation were noted to be the three independent predictors of prolonged intubation.[7] Major medical complications secondary to myasthenic crisis are related to days on mechanical ventilation. Fever is the most common complication (occurring in 70% of patients), followed by pneumonia (in 50%) and atelectasis (in 40%). Half of those who survive an MG crisis are functionally dependent at discharge, more commonly with intubation period more than 2 weeks.[7]

GUILLAIN-BARRÉ SYNDROME

Mechanical ventilation is required in 20% to 30% of patients with GBS.[22,23] A majority of complications in GBS occur during this stage. The decision of when to intubate GBS patients with respiratory failure has been discretionary. It requires a clinical choice between premature intubation with possible secondary risk of tracheal and pulmonary injury or watchful observation, which could lead to the need for emergency intubation. GBS patients requiring emergency intubation had prolonged mechanical ventilation and anoxic brain injury if associated with respiratory arrest.[24]

Several clinical factors have been proposed to predict when to intervene. Predictive factors for intubation include rapid progression, dysautonomia, bilateral facial palsy, and oropharyngeal weakness.[25] Serial measurements on pulmonary function testing are essential in anticipating the need for mechanical ventilation. As previously mentioned, the 20/30/40 rule may help to predict the need for mechanical ventilation.[5] Profound abnormalities of phrenic nerve conduction time and findings on diaphragmatic electromyography may predict the need for mechanical ventilation.[26]

Duration of mechanical ventilation in patients with GBS ranges from 18 to 49 days.[27-29] Inspiratory pressures and ABG tests immediately preceding intubation do not predict the need for prolonged ventilation.[23,29] IVIG and plasma exchange have been shown to reduce the duration of ventilation in randomized trials.[30] Prolonged intubation (14 days) was found to be associated with increased morbidity and mortality rates, mainly due to increased risk of ventilator-associated pneumonia and longer duration of mechanical ventilation.[31] Mechanical ventilation–related respiratory complications such as pneumonia and tracheobronchitis occur in more than half of GBS patients. An increase in ICU stay also increased the number of systemic infections.[10] Complications are less common if the ICU stay is less than 3 weeks. Independent ambulation can be seen in up to 80% of patients who survive from the acute phase of GBS.[10] Patients may take 2 months to 10 years for independent ambulation.[32] ICU complications, prolonged mechanical ventilation, and early axonal abnormalities are associated with slower recovery.[7] Advanced age and delay in transfer to ICU are independent factors predictive of poor outcome.[33]

Aggressive respiratory therapy, including frequent suctioning and use of ventilatory strategies aiming at minimizing atelectasis, should be emphasized. If no improvement is noted, aggressive respiratory management should include tracheostomy to allow more efficient bronchial clearing and reduction in the work of breathing imposed by the endotracheal tube. Tracheostomy and its timing are debated topics. The need for tracheostomy is more likely in the elderly and in the presence of preexisting pulmonary disease.[23] A majority of patients with GBS-associated neuromuscular failure and mechanical ventilation undergo tracheostomy (up to 89%).[31] Tracheostomy should be postponed until the third week in patients who show some clinical improvement. This provides a period of assessment during which neuromuscular respiratory function may improve in response to treatment, and up to 50% of these patients (those showing improvement) could be spared from tracheostomy by waiting until the third week.

Percutaneous tracheostomy may allow transfer of unstable patients to the operating room, thereby decreasing the incidence of wound infection, reducing cost, and providing better cosmetic results. Tracheostomy-related complications include short-term complications such as bleeding from the tracheostomy site, early cuff leak, wound infection, wound breakdown, and self-decannulation; long-term complications include minor voice change.[34] Percutaneous tracheostomy decreases the incidence of complications such as tracheal obstruction and pneumothorax, which are seen more often in open tracheostomy.[35] With the current neurocritical care availability for GBS patients, the mortality rate has decreased to less than 5%.[32,33]

EXTUBATION TRIALS

Weaning from mechanical ventilation should be guided by improvement in strength and normalization of values on serial pulmonary function tests. Diaphragmatic weakness may reverse before extremity weakness; thus, the timing of weaning should not be gauged solely by recovery of extremity muscle strength.

The weaning process in patients with MG often is challenging because of the fluctuating nature of the disease. Reintubation is not uncommon. In a review of 26 episodes of myasthenic crisis, the reintubation rate was 27%. In selected patients, noninvasive ventilation can be used for bridging during the weaning process to prevent reintubation.[36] Older age, pneumonia, and atelectasis are major risk factors for poor outcome.[37] Weaning trials may begin when VC exceeds 15 mL/kg, Pɪmax exceeds −30 cm H_2O, and oxygenation is adequate on inspired oxygen concentrations (FIO_2) of 40% or less. It is important to reintroduce cholinesterase inhibitors before extubation trials are initiated. Weaning methods may vary. Patients can be switched to continuous positive airway pressure (CPAP) with pressure support ventilation (PSV) and the level decreased 1 to 3 cm H_2O each day. A decrease in tidal volume and an increase in respiratory and heart rates are indicators of fatigue. Once the patient demonstrates good endurance at low pressure support (5 cm H_2O), usually for more than 2 hours, extubation can be accomplished. After extubation, incentive spirometry is helpful to reduce the risk of atelectasis and reintubation.[38]

In GBS, weaning from mechanical ventilation should be undertaken as early as possible because of the number of significant complications related to prolonged intubation.[39] After intubation, however, respiratory function parameters often continue to fall. Reducing intermittent mandatory ventilation rate or reducing pressure support level can be used as weaning approaches, at the discretion of the treating physician. However, one should anticipate weeks on the ventilator. The weaning process can be initiated once VC reaches 25 mL/kg and spontaneous tidal volumes of 10 to 12 mL/kg are attained. Pɪmax exceeding −50 cm H_2O and VC improvement by 4 mL/kg from preintubation to preextubation are associated with successful extubation.[40] Extubation often is delayed if dysautonomia is still present. Electrophysiologic testing can be helpful while deciding for extubation. Established risk factors for poor outcome in GBS are electrophysiologic evidence of axonal degeneration, preceding diarrheal illness, and rapid disease progression.[29]

MANAGEMENT

MYASTHENIA GRAVIS

Treatment of MG is geared toward identifying the typical causes of crisis (Fig. 64.4). Common causes of myasthenic crisis as mentioned earlier include infection, aspiration, surgery (especially thymectomy), and changes in medication. A careful review of medications, including over-the-counter preparations, is needed. Postoperative complications may be reduced in MG patients with baseline minimal bulbar or respiratory muscle weakness by preoperative plasma exchange or IVIG.[2]

The issue of cholinergic crisis is controversial. Cholinergic crisis is believed to occur as a result of overtreatment with acetylcholinesterase inhibitors. It may manifest with copious respiratory secretions and fasciculations from nicotinic toxicity. Historically, when the treatment of MG was limited to use of acetylcholinesterase inhibitors, overdose could lead to MG crisis, but this entity is now infrequently encountered, and its importance may have been overstated.[41] In a retrospective review of 73 episodes of myasthenic crisis, no instances of cholinergic crisis were identified.[7] In another review of 27 patients, only one patient had cholinergic crisis.[6] To avoid any confusion during the acute management of myasthenic crisis, it is recommended to discontinue acetylcholinesterase inhibitors during invasive mechanical ventilation. During NMV, this decision should be made on a case-by-case basis, depending on the patient's response to acetylcholinesterase inhibitors.

The mainstay of immunotherapy for the short-term treatment of myasthenic crisis is plasma exchange. Plasma exchange directly removes AChR antibodies from the circulation, and clinical improvement roughly correlates with the degree of elimination as reflected in AChR antibody levels. Although widely used and considered effective, plasmapheresis for MG crisis has not been compared with sham exchange in a controlled trial. A total of 5 to 7 exchanges typically are done over 2 weeks, and 2 to 4 L of plasma is removed with each exchange. One randomized controlled trial did not show any difference in efficacy when plasma exchange was done daily versus every other day.[42] Improvement usually is noted within days and can be quite dramatic, although some patients may not show evidence of response until weeks after therapy. The effects of plasma exchange may last up to 3 months. Major complications of plasma

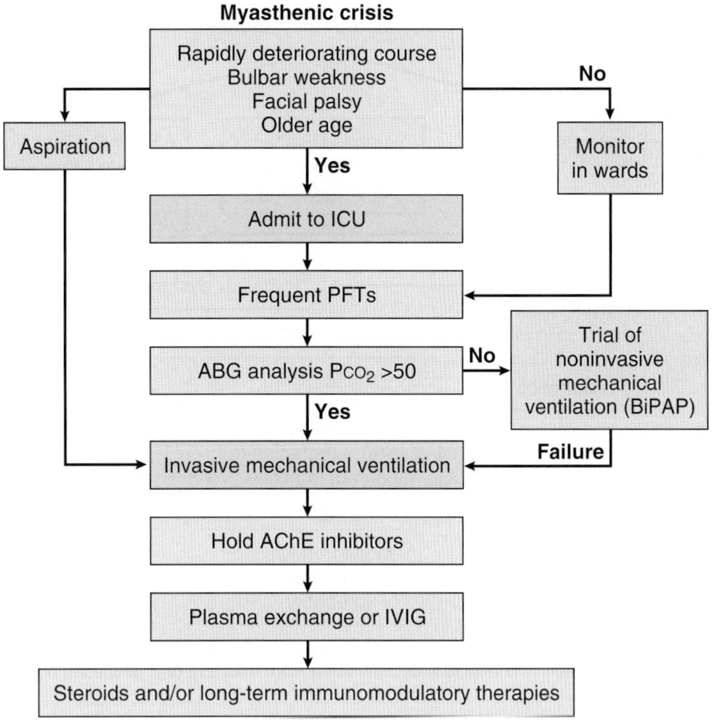

Figure 64.4 Clinical flowchart for the management of myasthenic crisis. ABG, arterial blood gas; AChE, acetyl cholinesterase; BiPAP, bilevel positive airway pressure; ICU, intensive care unit; IVIG, intravenous immunoglobulin; PFTs, pulmonary function tests.

exchange are problems with vascular access (including infection, local thrombosis, and vascular perforation), hypotension, transient electrolyte disturbances, and heparin-induced thrombocytopenia.

IVIG is also used in the management of MG but much less in myasthenic crisis. Its mechanism of action in MG is less certain, but it is believed to work by introduction of anti-idiotype antibodies and reduced AChR antibody production achieved through negative feedback. IVIG when compared to placebo clearly showed benefit for MG patients in a randomized controlled trial.[43] It often is employed in a dose of 0.4 g/kg of body weight given over 5 days (total dose of 2 g/kg), although a recent randomized clinical trial found no significant superiority of 2 g/kg over 1 g/kg of IVIG in MG exacerbation.[44] IVIG is better tolerated as compared to a plasma exchange. Side effects related to IVIG treatment are often mild and include headache, chills, fever, and nausea. These manifestations are related to the rate of infusion. Major side effects, independent of infusion rate, are acute renal failure, thrombotic events, and anaphylaxis.

A recent randomized controlled trial comparing IVIG and plasma exchange found both therapies to be equally efficacious in MG patients, but it did not include severely affected MG patients or patients in myasthenic crisis.[45] Trials comparing plasma exchange and IVIG found more rapid onset of improvement in clinical measures of MG, as well as earlier time to extubation, with early (in the first 2 weeks) institution of plasmapheresis, but did not find any significant difference on long-term follow-up evaluation.[46,47] One study found plasma exchange also to be effective in patients in whom IVIG has failed.[48] Plasma exchange is generally preferred as first-line therapy in MG crisis. High-dose corticosteroids can transiently worsen the neuromuscular weakness associated with MG during early stages of treatment in up to 50% of patients. For this reason, during myasthenic crisis, it is recommended to start steroids only after initiation of plasma exchange or IVIG treatments and then to continue until a remission occurs.[17]

Complete thymectomy is indicated in cases of thymoma-associated MG. Thymectomy is controversial in patients without thymoma. In a 17-year follow-up study of 110 MG patients, post-thymectomy myasthenic crisis episodes were fewer, were less severe, required less ventilatory support, and had reduced ICU stay when compared to a nonsurgical group.[49] Desflurane plus remifentanil was found to be a better anesthetic combination than propofol plus remifentanil in MG patients undergoing video-assisted thoracoscopic-extended thymectomy due to its reversible muscle relaxation effect and faster recovery with no increase in side effects.[50] Empiric thymectomy in the elderly is likely to be less effective because of atrophy of the thymus.

Post-thymectomy myasthenic crisis is not uncommon and can be seen in up to 30% of patients. Most of these patients (65%) present within the first 6 months.[51] Alternate day oral corticosteroids reduce immediate postoperative myasthenic crisis to 5% based on a retrospective series.[52] Plasma exchange and IVIG can also be useful to prevent deterioration preoperatively in patients undergoing thymectomy or other surgery. Preoperative plasma exchange was found to reduce the incidence of postoperative myasthenic crisis and improve long-term outcome.[53] In a retrospective study, predictors of postoperative myasthenic crisis were preoperative oropharyngeal weakness, preoperative serum anti-AChR antibody level greater than 100 nmol/L, and intraoperative blood loss greater than 1 L.[54] Previous history of myasthenic crisis and presence of thymoma are other significant predictors for post-thymectomy myasthenic crisis.[55] Delaying

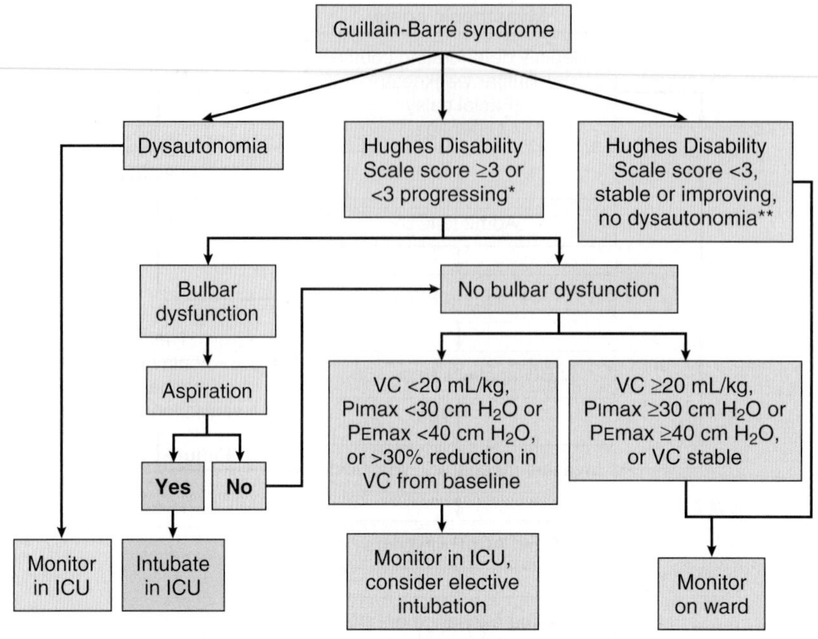

Figure 64.5 Flowchart based on clinical and respiratory factors in the management of Guillain-Barré syndrome. ICU, intensive care unit; PEmax, maximum expiratory pressure; PImax, maximum inspiratory pressure; VC, vital capacity.

thymectomy until immunosuppressive treatment has been initiated and bulbar symptoms are resolved may be beneficial in avoiding postoperative myasthenic crisis. Postoperative myasthenic crisis leads to prolonged mechanical ventilation and need for tracheostomy. Improvement after thymectomy may not be seen for months or even years.

GUILLAIN-BARRÉ SYNDROME

The management of patients with GBS can be challenging because of its unpredictable course, potential for rapid deterioration, and high chances for respiratory failure (Fig. 64.5). Any patient with worsening weakness on initial evaluation or presentation will need admission and observation in an ICU. However, only 1 in 3 patients will deteriorate significantly enough to mandate further or prolonged ICU monitoring and possibly intubation.

Main modalities of acute treatment are plasma exchange or IVIG, both of which are recommended for nonambulatory patients with GBS who present within 4 weeks of disease onset. Large multicenter trials have established the effectiveness of plasma exchange in GBS.[56,57] Earlier clinical improvement, reduced need for mechanical ventilation, and faster recovery have been shown with plasma exchange. A systematic review of six randomized trials in 2002 found that plasma exchange was superior to supportive care.[58] Plasma exchange was most effective when started within 7 days of symptom onset; however, an improvement in outcome was still observed if treatment was instituted up to 30 days after onset of symptoms in the North American study. Two plasma exchanges are superior to none in mild GBS, and four exchanges are superior to two in moderately severe GBS. However, six exchanges were not superior to four in severe GBS requiring mechanical ventilation.[59]

No randomized trials have been conducted to compare IVIG with placebo for the treatment of GBS, but IVIG was shown to be as effective as plasma exchange for the treatment of GBS by a Cochrane systematic review of five trials.[60] Analysis found no significant difference between plasma exchange and IVIG in disability scores at 4 weeks; however, treatment effect was faster with plasma exchange as compared to IVIG.[46] Combining IVIG with plasma exchange also has been tried and was found not to have additional benefit.[61] Corticosteroids alone have no significant benefit in GBS. Intravenous methylprednisolone in combination with IVIG may hasten recovery but does not significantly affect the long-term outcome or neuropathic pain from GBS.[62,63] One third of the patients felt completely cured at 12 months, changed their job due to GBS, and did not function at home as well as before in a self-administered questionnaire containing questions on their physical status at homecoming and at 12 months.[64]

KEY POINTS

- Clinical examination and pulmonary function tests form the basis of assessment in patients with neuromuscular respiratory failure.
- VC less than 20 mL/kg, PImax less than −30 cm H_2O, and PEmax less than 40 cm H_2O usually will indicate the need for mechanical ventilation in patients with GBS (20/30/40 rule).
- In myasthenic crisis, pulmonary function tests have a limited positive predictive value. Respiratory support

KEY POINTS (Continued)

is unlikely to be needed when VC is more than 20 mL/kg.

- NMV is the first-line treatment in respiratory failure secondary to MG when P_{CO_2} level is less than 45 mm Hg and definitive therapy is rapidly initiated. This can prevent intubation up to 60% of the time.
- NMV is not beneficial in respiratory failure secondary to GBS and can even be detrimental by masking further respiratory decline.
- Timing for tracheostomy in GBS is unclear, but waiting for 2 to 3 weeks in patients showing improvement may prevent the need for tracheostomy in up to 50% of cases.
- Both IVIG and plasma exchange probably are equal in efficacy for the treatment of GBS.
- In treatment of ventilatory failure secondary to MG, plasma exchange is superior to use of IVIG. Plasma exchange or IVIG must be followed by long-term immunosuppression.

SELECTED REFERENCES

5. Lawn ND, Fletcher DD, Henderson RD, et al: Anticipating Mechanical Ventilation in Guillain-Barre Syndrome. Arch Neurol 2001;58: 893-898.
16. Wijdicks EF, Roy TK: BiPAP in early guillain-barre syndrome may fail. Can J Neurol Sci 2006;33:105-106.
36. Rabinstein A, Wijdicks EFM: BiPAP in acute respiratory failure due to myasthenic crisis may prevent intubation. Neurology 2002;59: 1647-1649.
37. Rabinstein A, Mueller-Kronast N: Risk of extubation failure in patients with myasthenic crisis. Neurocritical Care 2005;3: 213-215.
42. Trikha I, Singh S, Goyal V, et al: Comparative efficacy of low dose, daily versus alternate day plasma exchange in severe myasthenia gravis. Journal of Neurology 2007;254:989-995.
45. Barth D, Nabavi Nouri M, Ng E, et al: Comparison of IVIg and PLEX in patients with myasthenia gravis. Neurology 2011;76: 2017-2023.
58. Raphael JC, Chevret S, Hughes RA, et al: Plasma exchange for Guillain-Barre syndrome. Cochrane Database Syst Rev 2002: CD001798.
60. Hughes RA, Swan AV, van Doorn PA: Intravenous immunoglobulin for Guillain-Barre syndrome. Cochrane Database Syst Rev 2010: CD002063.
62. van Koningsveld R, Schmitz PIM, van der Meché FGA, et al: Effect of methylprednisolone when added to standard treatment with intravenous immunoglobulin for Guillain-Barré syndrome: randomised trial. The Lancet 2004;363:192-196.
64. Bernsen RAJAM, De Jager AEJ, Van Der Meché FGA, et al: How Guillain–Barré patients experience their functioning after 1 year. Acta Neurologica Scandinavica 2005;112:51-56.

The complete list of references can be found at www.expertconsult.com.

65 Seizures in the Critically Ill

Thomas P. Bleck

CHAPTER OUTLINE

Seizures complicate the course of about 3% of adult patients admitted to intensive care units (ICUs) for non-neurologic conditions[1] and occur more frequently in specialized neuroscience ICUs.[2] The medical and economic impact of seizures in these patients confers a significance on these events out of proportion to their incidence. Seizures are often the first indication of a central nervous system (CNS) complication in these patients, making their rapid etiologic diagnosis mandatory. Furthermore, because epilepsy is a common disorder (affecting about 2% of the general population), patients with preexisting seizure disorders will occasionally require ICU admission for intercurrent conditions. The intensivist usually manages the initial treatment of these patients, so he or she must be familiar with the indications and risks of the potential therapies as they affect the already critically ill patient. In addition, the patient who develops status epilepticus (SE), whether already in the ICU or not, will often require the care of a critical care specialist in addition to a neurologist.

HISTORY

Although seizures have been recognized at least since Hippocratic times, their relatively high rate of occurrence in critically ill patients has only recently been recognized. Seizures as a side effect of critical care treatments (e.g., as a complication of lidocaine infusion for ventricular arrhythmias) are also a recent phenomenon.

The first recorded description of SE is by Gavasetti in 1586.[3,4] Sir Thomas Willis described the complications of untreated SE in 1667:

> *… as to what further belongs to the prognostication of the Disease, if it end not about the time of ripe age, neither can be driven away by the use of medicines, there happens yet a diverse event in several sick Patients, for it either ends immediately in Death, or is changed into some other Disease, to wit, the Palsie, stupidite, or melancholly, for the most part incurable. As to the former, whenas the fits are often repeated, and every time grow more cruell, the animal functions are quickly debilitated; and from thence, by the taint, by degrees brought on by the Spirits, and the Nerves serving the Praecordia, the vital function is by little and little enervated, till at length, the whole body languishing, and the pulse is loosned, and at length ceasing, at last the vital flame is extinguished.*[5]

Attempts at treating SE in the nineteenth century included bromide,[6] morphine,[7] and ice applications. Barbiturates were introduced in 1912, followed by the identification and use of phenytoin in 1937; these were the first rational treatments for SE.[8] Paraldehyde gained brief prominence in the next decades.[9] The most recent major improvement is the use of benzodiazepines, pioneered by the French in the 1960s.[10]

EPIDEMIOLOGY

Few data are available concerning the epidemiology of seizures in ICU patients. A 10-year retrospective study of all ICU patients at the Mayo Clinic reported approximately 7 patients with seizures per 1000 ICU admissions.[11] In a 2-year prospective study of a medical ICU, we acquired approximately 35 patients with seizures per 1000 admissions.[1] These

Table 65.1 Etiology of Status Epilepticus at San Francisco General Hospital

	Distribution (%)			
	1970-1980 (*N* = 98)		1980-1989 (*N* = 152)	
Etiologic Factor/Disorder	Prior Seizures	No Prior Seizures	Prior Seizures	No Prior Seizures
Ethanol-related	11	4	25	12
Anticonvulsant noncompliance	27	0	41	0
Drug toxicity	0	10	5	10
Refractory epilepsy		(Not used)	8	0
CNS infection*	0	4	2	10
Trauma	1	2	2	6
Tumor	0	4	2	7
Metabolic*	3	5	2	4
Stroke*	4	11	2	5
Anoxia*	0	4	0	6
Other	11	5	3	5

CNS, central nervous system.
*Conditions most likely to result in admission to intensive care unit (ICU).

analyses are not strictly comparable, because the patient populations and methods of detection differed. The incidence of seizures is probably higher in pediatric ICUs than in medical ICUs.[12-14]

Certain ICU patients appear to be at increased risk for seizures, but the degree of that increased risk has not been quantified. Patients with renal failure or with an altered blood-brain barrier who receive imipenem-cilastatin are an obvious example, but other patients receiving this antibiotic (or γ-aminobutyric acid [GABA] antagonists such as penicillin) occasionally seize. Cefepime has emerged as a cause of nonconvulsive seizures and SE, especially in patients with renal insufficiency.[15] Transplant patients, especially those receiving cyclosporine, appear to have an increased risk for convulsions. Patients who rapidly become hypo-osmolar from any cause are also at risk. Nonketotic hyperglycemia patients have a high likelihood of partial seizures; this is a rare instance of a metabolic disorder producing focal neurologic syndromes.[16] Less commonly, diabetic ketoacidosis may also produce partial seizures.[17]

The epidemiology of SE is somewhat better understood. Estimates of the incidence of generalized convulsive SE in the United States range from 50,000 cases/year[18] to 250,000 cases/year.[19] Some portion of this discrepancy may be due to differences in definitions. The larger estimate comes from the only population-based data available and may be more accurate. Similarly large variations occur in mortality rate estimates, from 1% to 2% in the former study to 22% in the latter. This disagreement stems, at least in part, from a conceptual discordance: the smaller number attempts to determine mortality rate that the authors directly attribute to SE, while the larger figure reflects the overall mortality rate for SE patients, in whom death was frequently a consequence of the cause of the underlying disease rather than SE itself. In the latter study, for example, anoxia was the cause of SE in adults with the highest mortality rate. In many of the reports surveyed in the earlier review, these patients were not included.

A number of important risk factors have emerged from the Richmond study. When SE lasted longer than 1 hour, the mortality rate was 32%; when it lasted less than 1 hour, the mortality rate was only 2.7%. SE caused by anoxia was associated with a mortality rate of about 70% in adults, but the corresponding rate in children was less than 10%. After the age of 12 months, the mortality rate of SE rose with increasing age. In their study, the commonest cause of SE in adults was stroke, followed thereafter by withdrawal from anticonvulsant drug therapy; cryptogenic (or idiopathic) SE; and SE related to ethanol withdrawal, anoxia, and metabolic disorders. Systemic infection was the most commonly diagnosed cause of SE in children; this was followed by congenital abnormalities, anoxia, metabolic disorders, anticonvulsant drug withdrawal, CNS infections, and trauma. Although brain tumors seldom caused SE in children, such patients experienced a nearly 50% mortality rate.

Towne and colleagues demonstrated that 8% of an unselected series of comatose medical ICU patients had unsuspected nonconvulsive status epilepticus (NCSE).[20] In septic ICU patients, Oddo and colleagues showed that about 30% have periodic epileptiform activity or NCSE when recorded for 24 hours or longer.[21]

Hospital-based series of SE patients are usually subject to considerable selection bias regarding cause. The data in Table 65.1, based upon 20 years of experience in San Francisco, are of great interest because almost all patients with SE in the city of San Francisco who began to seize outside the hospital are included.[22-24]

Between 6% and 12% of epilepsy patients present with SE,[25] and about 20% of seizure patients will experience an episode of SE within 5 years of their first seizure.[11]

NOSOLOGY AND SEMIOLOGY

Numerous systems have evolved for the classification of seizures; the most frequently used today is that of the

Box 65.1 International Classification of Epileptic Seizures

I. Partial seizures (seizures beginning locally)
  A. Simple partial seizures (consciousness not impaired) (SPS)
    1. With motor symptoms
    2. With somatosensory or special sensory symptoms
    3. With autonomic symptoms
    4. With psychic symptoms
  B. Complex partial seizures (with impairment of consciousness) (CPS)
    1. Beginning as SPS and progressing to impairment of consciousness
      a. Without automatisms
      b. With automatisms
    2. With impairment of consciousness at onset
      a. With no other features
      b. With features of SPS
      c. With automatisms
  C. Partial seizures (simple or complex), secondarily generalized
II. Primary generalized seizures (bilaterally symmetric, without localized onset)
  A. Absence seizures
    1. True absence ("petit mal")
    2. Atypical absence
  B. Myoclonic seizures
  C. Clonic seizures
  D. Tonic seizures
  E. Tonic-clonic seizures ("grand mal") (generalized tonic-clonic [GTC])
  F. Atonic seizures
III. Unclassified seizures

From Commission on Classification and Terminology of the International League Against Epilepsy: Proposal for revised clinical and electroencephalographic classification of epileptic seizures. Epilepsia 1981;22:489-501.

International League Against Epilepsy[26] (Box 65.1). This schema allows classification based primarily on clinical criteria, without inferences about cause. Although a more recent proposal for terminology has been published, it is not yet widely accepted.[27] It is important because of its predictive value for cause, prognosis, and treatment decisions in ICU patients. *Simple partial* seizures arise focally in the cerebral cortex, without taking over either the limbic system or subcortical nuclei. The patient remains aware of the environment during the ictus, and except for the seizure itself appears unchanged. Bilateral limbic system dysfunction results in a *complex partial* seizure; the patient's awareness and ability to interact with the environment are diminished (but not always completely abolished). *Automatisms* are movements that the patient seems to make without being aware of them; typical automatisms include swallowing, masticatory movements, and fumbling with nearby items. *Secondary generalization* implies invasion of either the other hemisphere (with loss of consciousness) or, more commonly, subcortical structures, with the development of a generalized convulsion.

Primary generalized seizures seem to arise from the entire cerebral cortex and the diencephalon at the same time; there are no visible focal phenomena. Consciousness is lost from the start of the seizure. True *absence* seizures are usually confined to childhood; they consist of the abrupt onset of a blank stare usually lasting 5 to 15 seconds, without lateralizing phenomena, from which the patient abruptly returns to normal. Atypical absence is usually seen in children who have the Lennox-Gastaut syndrome. *Myoclonic* seizures begin with brief, bilaterally synchronous jerks without an initial change in consciousness, followed by a generalized convulsion. They occur in several of the genetic epilepsies, but in the ICU are more commonly the consequences of anoxia or metabolic disturbances.[28] *Clonic* seizures involve repetitive movements; they may be generalized (synchronous movements of all extremities and both sides of the face) or partial (e.g., one side of the face and the arm of the same side). *Tonic* seizures are episodes of tonic extension of the arms, legs, and trunk; they must be distinguished from decerebrate rigidity and from tetanic spasms.[29] *Tonic-clonic* seizures begin with tonic extension, followed by a brief phase of rapid vibration of the extremities, evolving into bilaterally synchronous clonus, and concluding with a postictal phase in which incontinence is common and brief apnea is occasionally noted. They may be primarily generalized or, more commonly, occur as the manifestation of spread of a partial seizure. Only those seizures that are known to involve progression through the tonic and clonic stages should be called tonic-clonic.

When seizures occur in ICU patients, clinical judgment is required to apply this system. Patients whose consciousness is already altered by drugs, hypotension, sepsis, or intracranial disease may be difficult to diagnose regarding the "simple" or "complex" nature of their partial seizures.

SE is classified by a somewhat similar system, with alterations to match the observable clinical phenomena (Box 65.2).[30] Again, the ability to use clinical observation without inferences about cause is important. *Generalized convulsive SE* (GCSE) is the type most commonly encountered in ICUs, and poses the greatest risk to the patient. GCSE may be either primarily generalized, as in the intoxicated patient, or may represent secondary generalization, as in the patient with a brain abscess who develops GCSE. *Tonic* SE is usually seen in children or adolescents with a history of severe CNS dysfunction. *Nonconvulsive* SE (NCSE) in the ICU is most commonly the consequence of partially treated GCSE. Some authors use this as a general term for any SE involving altered consciousness without convulsive movements. Although conceptually useful, this blurs the distinctions among absence SE, partially treated GCSE, and *complex partial* SE (CPSE), which have different causes and treatments. *Epilepsia partialis continua* (EPC) is a special form of partial SE in which a small area of the body makes repetitive movements, sometimes for months or years following a CNS insult.

PATHOGENESIS

Clinical SE has a large variety of causes. The relative frequencies of causes depend upon the definition of SE employed (e.g., if repetitive, stereotyped myoclonic activity after a cardiorespiratory arrest is considered SE, then the frequency of such arrests as a cause of SE will rise).

The reported "causes" of SE can be separated, if imperfectly, into predispositions and precipitants. *Predispositions*

Box 65.2 Clinical Classification of Status Epilepticus (SE)

I. Generalized seizures
  A. Generalized convulsive SE (GCSE)
    1. Primary generalized SE
      a. Tonic-clonic SE
      b. Myoclonic SE
      c. Clonic-tonic-clonic SE
    2. Secondarily generalized SE
      a. Partial seizure with secondary generalization
      b. Tonic SE
  B. Nonconvulsive SE (NCSE)
    1. Absence SE (petit mal status)
    2. Atypical absence SE (e.g., in Lennox-Gastaut syndrome)
    3. Atonic SE
    4. NCSE as a sequel of partially treated GCSE
II. Partial SE
  A. Simple partial SE
    1. Typical
    2. Epilepsia partialis continua (EPC)
  B. Complex partial SE (CPSE)
III. Neonatal SE

Adapted from Ettinger AB, Shinnar S: New-onset seizures in an elderly hospitalized population. Neurology 1993;43:489.

are relatively fixed conditions that increase the likelihood of SE, such as a brain tumor, in the presence of a precipitant. *Precipitants*, in contrast, are transient conditions that can produce SE in most, if not all, people but will tend to affect those with predispositions at lesser degrees of severity (e.g., barbiturate withdrawal).

For experimental purposes, the nosologic division of SE into partial (focal) or generalized based on the type of seizure produced works well, as does the recognition of convulsive and nonconvulsive seizure types. One must recognize that these are models of *acute SE*; they are not chronic conditions that occasionally produce SE, as are many of the afflictions of patients. Nevertheless, they have substantial explanatory power for understanding the neuronal and systemic processes of SE, for studying its consequences, and for predicting responses to therapy.

PATHOPHYSIOLOGY

The causes and effects of SE at the cellular, brain, and systemic levels are interrelated, but their individual analysis is useful for understanding them and their therapeutic implications. One must first understand the consequences of a single seizure and then contrast this information with the effects of prolonged or frequent seizures merging into SE. Longer durations of SE produce more profound alterations with an increasing likelihood of permanence, and of becoming refractory to treatment. Figure 65.1 illustrates the variety of processes involved in a single seizure and in the transition to SE.[31]

The ionic events of a seizure follow the opening of ion channels coupled to excitatory amino acid (EAA) receptors. Although the endogenous ligands of these channels are glutamate and aspartate, the channels are named for synthetic compounds that potently activate them. From the standpoint of the intensivist concerned with SE, three channels are particularly important because their activation may raise intracellular free calcium to toxic concentrations. The first channels primarily conduct sodium ions (the AMPA [amino-3-hydroxy-5-methyl-4-isoxazolepropionic acid] channels). The second are the *N*-methyl-D-aspartate (NMDA) channels, which admit sodium and calcium when the cell has been depolarized (which relieves the resting blockade of the ionophore by magnesium). The third, the metabotropic or ACPD (aminocyclopentane-trans-1,3-dicarboxylic acid) channels, mobilize calcium from intracellular stores via coupling to G-protein-linked second messengers.

These EAA systems are normally crucial for learning and memory. Many drugs that block these systems, such as ketamine, are too toxic to use as chronic anticonvulsants. However, the deleterious consequences of SE, and the brief period during which they would be needed, suggest that similar agents may prove to have a role in the management of SE. Counterregulatory ionic events are also triggered by the epileptiform discharge; the most important is activation of inhibitory interneurons, which feed back to the bursting cells via $GABA_A$ synapses.

The cellular consequences of the excessive EAA channel activation include (1) accumulation of toxic concentrations of free intracellular calcium; (2) activation of autolytic enzyme systems; (3) production of oxygen-derived free radicals; (4) generation of nitric oxide, which both enhances subsequent excitation and serves as a toxin; (5) phosphorylation of several enzyme and receptor systems, making seizures likely; and (6) increasing intracellular osmolality, thereby producing neuronal swelling. If adenosine triphosphate (ATP) production should fail (because the substrate becomes inadequate or is diverted into EAA-related events), membrane ion exchange systems stop functioning, and the neuron swells further. These events are responsible for the neuronal damage associated with SE.

Many other important biophysical and biochemical alterations occur during and after SE. The intense neuronal activity activates immediate-early genes and produces heat shock proteins, providing strong indications of the deleterious effects of SE and insight into the mechanisms by which neurons protect themselves.[32] Wasterlain's group summarized the many mechanisms through which SE damages the nervous system.[33]

Absence SE is an exception among these conditions. It appears to consist of rhythmically increased inhibition and does not produce clinical sequelae or neuropathologic abnormalities.

The mechanisms that terminate seizure activity are uncertain. Given the relative rarity of SE in a population in which at least 1 in 50 patients has had a seizure, one must infer that these mechanisms are generally effective. The leading candidates for seizure terminating systems are inhibitory mechanisms, primarily GABAergic neuronal aggregates. This hypothesis receives strong support from the clinical observation that human SE frequently follows withdrawal from GABA agonists (e.g., benzodiazepines).

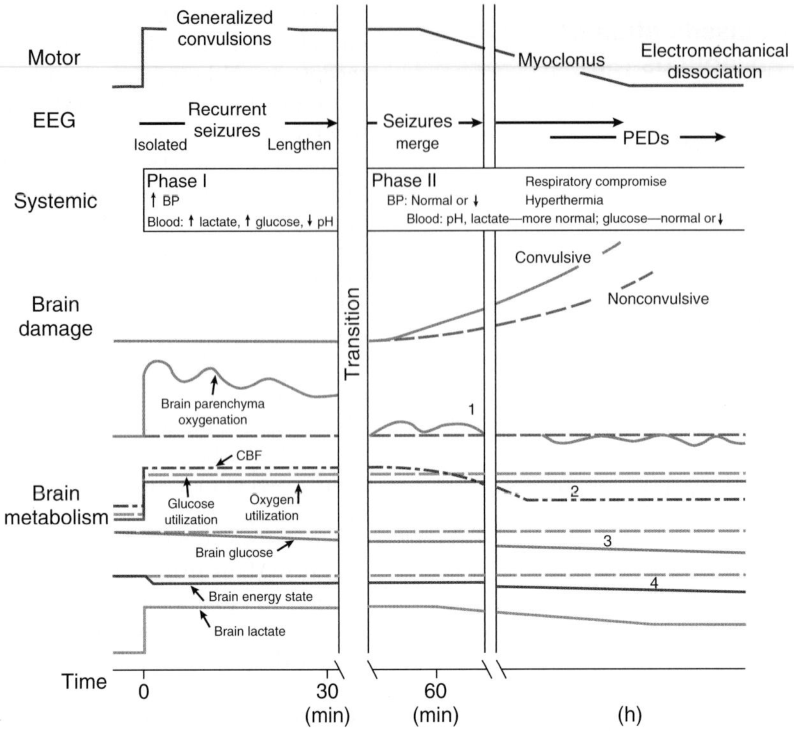

Figure 65.1 Pathophysiology of status epilepticus (SE). Summary of pathophysiologic events during experimental SE. Note that the abscissa is discontinuous. Numerals in figure indicate the following events: *1*, loss of cortical responsiveness to changes in oxygen tension; *2*, a fall in cerebral blood flow; *3*, depletion of brain glucose; and *4*, a decline in the total brain energy state. (Adapted from Lothman EW, Bertram EH: Epileptogenic effects of status epilepticus. Epilepsia 1993;34[Suppl 1]:S59-S70.)

Table 65.2 Electrographic-Clinical Correlations in Generalized Convulsive Status Epilepticus

Stage	Typical Clinical Manifestations*	Electroencephalographic Features
1	Tonic-clonic convulsions; hypertension and hyperglycemia common	Discrete seizures with interictal slowing
2	Low- or medium-amplitude clonic activity, with rare convulsions	Waxing and waning of ictal discharges
3	Slight, but frequent, clonic activity, often confined to the eyes, face, or hands	Continuous ictal discharges
4	Rare episodes of slight clonic activity; hypotension and hypoglycemia become manifest	Continuous ictal discharges punctuated by flat periods
5	Coma without other manifestations of seizure activity	Periodic epileptiform discharges on a flat background

*The clinical manifestations may vary considerably, depending on the underlying neuropathophysiologic process (and its anatomy), systemic diseases, and medications. In particular, stages of the electrographic progression may be sufficiently brief to be overlooked. Partially treating status epilepticus may dissociate the clinical and electrographic features.

The electrical phenomena of SE at the whole brain level, as seen in the scalp electroencephalogram (EEG), reflect the seizure type that initiates SE (Fig. 65.2). Thus, absence SE begins with a generalized 3-Hz wave-and-spike EEG pattern. During the course of SE, there will usually be some slowing of this rhythm, but the wave-and-spike characteristic persists. In contrast, GCSE goes through the sequence of EEG changes outlined in Table 65.2. The initial high-frequency discharge becomes progressively less well formed over minutes; this pattern implies that neuronal activity is less synchronous. Whether this indicates that inhibitory systems are attempting to terminate SE, a progressive decay in the ability of synaptic mechanisms to maintain synchrony, or global deterioration in neuronal function remains to be determined.

The repetitive firing that characterizes SE alters the extracellular microenvironment. The most important change is probably the elevation of the extracellular potassium concentration. Although extruding potassium is an effective strategy to maintain normal electronegativity, the excessive amounts of potassium ejected during SE overcome the ability of astrocytes to buffer it. Patients with cerebral edema, glial scarring, or alien tissue lesions have extracellular space abnormalities that impair the potassium buffering ability of glial cells. Raising extracellular potassium is a potent epileptogenic stimulus.

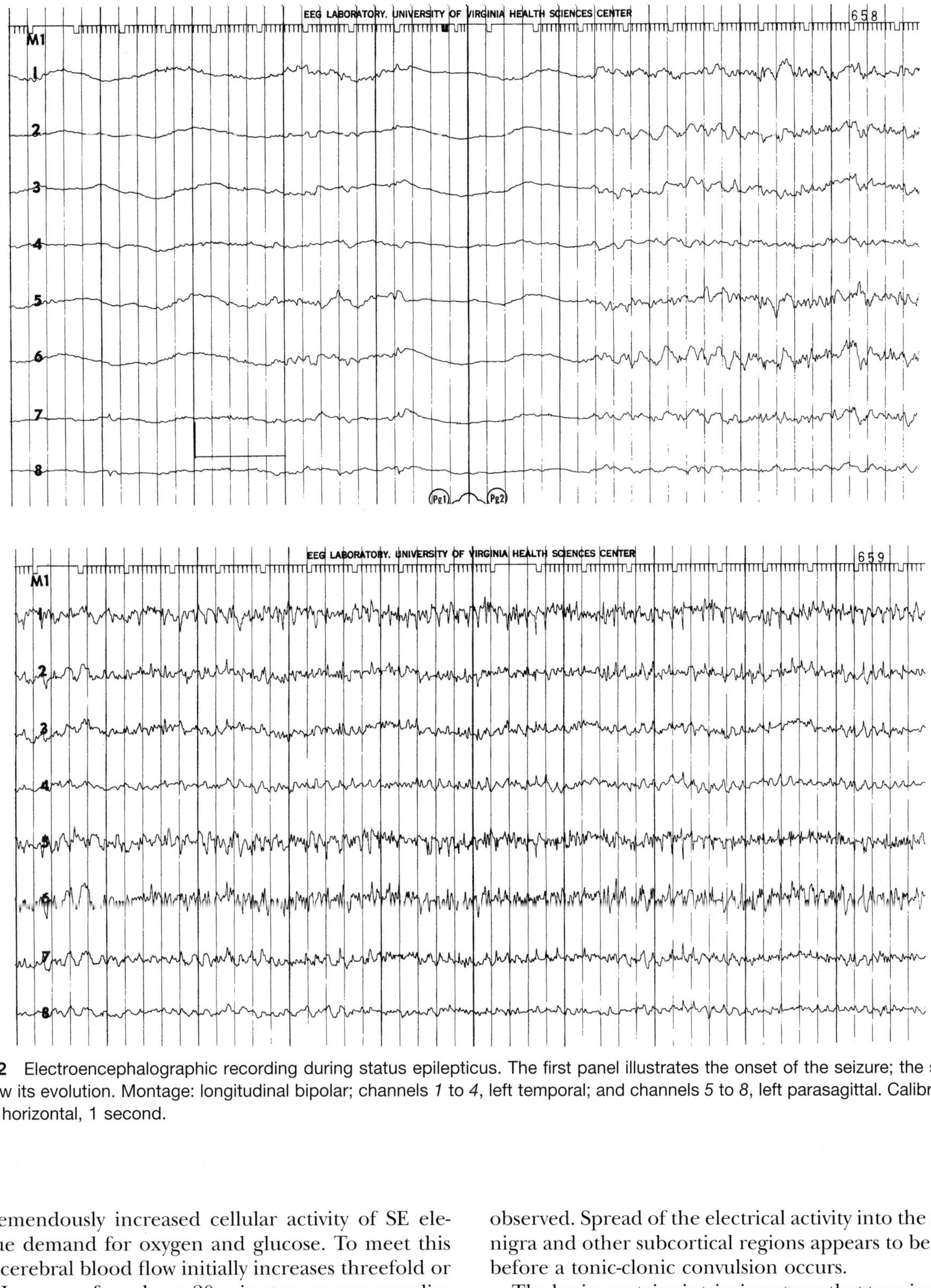

Figure 65.2 Electroencephalographic recording during status epilepticus. The first panel illustrates the onset of the seizure; the subsequent panels show its evolution. Montage: longitudinal bipolar; channels *1* to *4*, left temporal; and channels *5* to *8*, left parasagittal. Calibration: vertical, 50 μv; horizontal, 1 second.

The tremendously increased cellular activity of SE elevates tissue demand for oxygen and glucose. To meet this demand, cerebral blood flow initially increases threefold or greater. However, after about 20 minutes, energy supplies become exhausted. This accentuates the demand for local catabolism in order to support ion pumps (in a vain attempt to restore the internal milieu during the flood of sodium and calcium). Many researchers believe that this is the major cause of epileptic brain damage in GCSE. Other forms of SE may not be subject to such severe hypercatabolism, but still pose a risk.

When partial seizures generalize, subcortical structures begin to play an active role in the clinical phenomena observed. Spread of the electrical activity into the substantia nigra and other subcortical regions appears to be necessary before a tonic-clonic convulsion occurs.

The brain contains intrinsic systems that terminate seizure activity; both local GABAergic interneurons and inhibitory thalamic neurons are involved. Whether these systems have evolved, at least in part, for protection against seizures, or whether this effect is an epiphenomenon of some other physiologic function, is unresolved.

SE can produce cerebral edema, which follows ictal damage to the blood-brain barrier.

Prolonged SE produces chronic neuropathologic changes. Prior to the 1970s, these changes were often attributed

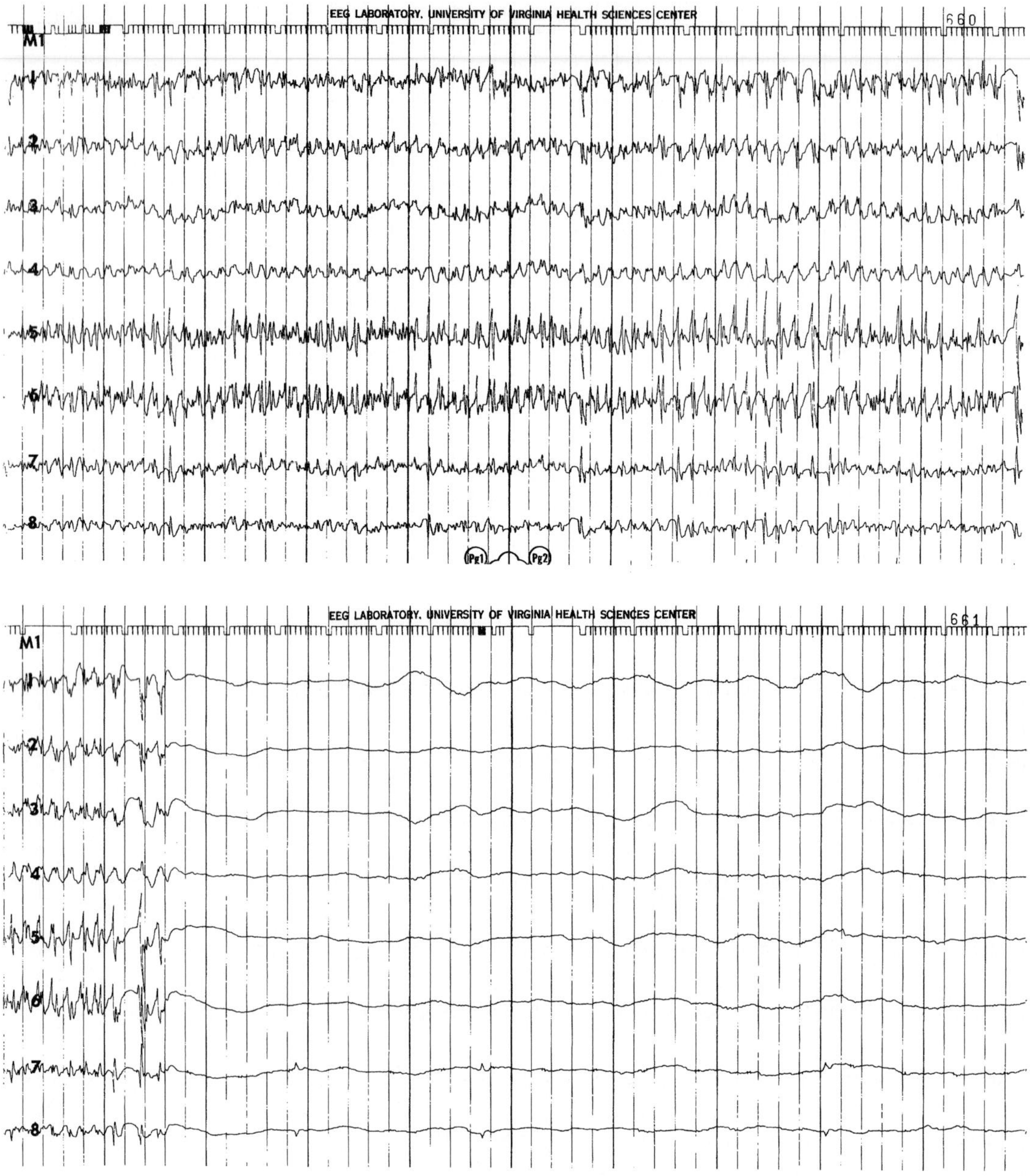

Figure 65.2, cont'd

to the systemic effects of SE (e.g., hypoxia and hyperthermia). However, SE itself produces these changes even in patients who are paralyzed, ventilated, and maintained at normal temperature and blood pressure. The hippocampus, which is one of the most important areas for memory function, contains the most susceptible neurons, but the cerebral cortex is also vulnerable. These regions express high densities of EAA receptors, and may be relatively deficient in systems for handling unusual elevations of free intracellular calcium. Cells that contain nitric oxide synthase seem relatively protected.

In addition to damaging the CNS, GCSE produces serious, often life-threatening, systemic effects.[34] Pressures in the systemic arterial system (under sympathetic control) and in the pulmonary arterial system (raised via efferents from pontine and medullary centers) are dramatically elevated from the moment of seizure onset. Epinephrine and cortisol release prompts further elevations of systemic arterial pressure, and also produces hyperglycemia. Increased muscular work raises the circulating lactate concentration. Respiration becomes ineffective; both airway obstruction and diaphragmatic contraction impede air movement. The consequent hypoxia further elevates lactate levels. Ventilatory failure impairs CO_2 excretion while CO_2 production increases markedly, adding a respiratory component to the acidosis. In GCSE, the arterial blood pH frequently falls below 7.0. The muscular work accelerates heat production; when coupled with decreased dermal blood flow (produced by sympathetic stimulation), GCSE can quickly raise the core temperature to 40° C or higher.

If GCSE is not completely controlled within the first 20 minutes, motor activity begins to diminish in intensity, and ventilation usually improves. Therefore, even without treatment, the metabolic acidosis improves. Core temperature may continue to climb, however, probably reflecting hypothalamic dysfunction. The initial hyperglycemia diminishes; after an hour or more, hepatic gluconeogenesis may fail, and hypoglycemia develops.

GCSE patients frequently suffer secondary complications as well. Aspiration of oral or gastric contents commonly produces chemical pneumonitis, with bacterial pneumonia often following. Rhabdomyolysis is common, and is occasionally followed by acute renal failure. Compression fractures, joint dislocations, and tendon avulsions are other common sequelae of GCSE.

CLINICAL MANIFESTATIONS

RECOGNITION OF SEIZURES

Because of the close observation patients receive in the critical care setting, most seizures are witnessed. The partial onset of a secondarily generalized convulsion, a finding of important diagnostic significance, is more likely to be seen and properly described in the ICU than on regular hospital floors or in the community. Three problems occur in ICU seizure recognition: (1) complex partial seizures in patients with already impaired awareness, (2) seizures in patients receiving neuromuscular junction blockade, and (3) the misinterpretation of movement disorders and psychiatric disturbances as seizures. (In any ICU patient who develops abnormal movements or unexplained changes in awareness, thiamine deficiency should be excluded immediately by giving thiamine.)

ICU patients often have altered awareness in the absence of seizures, reflecting their underlying condition, complications of those conditions (such as septic encephalopathy[35]), and drugs that depress alertness (intentionally or not). Although clonic motor activity in these patients remains visible, it may be difficult to tell whether a subsequent further decline in alertness reflects a seizure or some other process. In this situation, an EEG is required to make the diagnosis of a complex partial seizure. Although the detailed interpretation of EEGs is beyond the scope of this chapter, the intensivist can easily learn to recognize basic seizure types and other important EEG abnormalities in critically ill patients.[36]

Patients receiving neuromuscular junction blocking agents will not manifest any of the usual signs of seizures. Because most such patients receive concomitant sedation with GABA agonists (e.g., benzodiazepines), the likelihood of seizures is small. The autonomic signs of seizures (hypertension, tachycardia, pupillary dilation) are not readily distinguished from the effects of pain or the patient's response to inadequate sedation. Thus, any patient who manifests these findings and who has a potential reason for seizures (e.g., intracranial disease) should have an EEG to exclude this possibility.

Many sorts of abnormal movements occur in patients with severe metabolic disturbances or anoxic brain damage. Some of them can be distinguished from seizures by observation; such movements are frequently evoked or exacerbated by sensory stimuli and can sometimes be suppressed by changing the patient's posture. However, Hirsch and colleagues have demonstrated that seizures in ICU patients may be induced by external stimuli[37]; if any doubt about the nature of such movements persists, an EEG should be performed.

During therapeutic cooling for patients in a coma after cardiac arrest, seizures may be difficult to detect clinically, especially when neuromuscular junction blockade is used.[38] EEG monitoring should be performed.[39]

MANIFESTATIONS OF STATUS EPILEPTICUS

The neurologic manifestations of SE depend on the type of SE and, for the partial forms, the area of cortex from which the abnormality arises. Box 65.2 summarizes the types of SE encountered in clinical practice. This section will focus on the varieties of SE seen most frequently among ICU patients.

Primary GCSE usually begins as tonic extension of the trunk and extremities, without any preceding focal ictal activity. If the patient was awake before onset, no aura is reported, and consciousness is immediately lost. After several seconds of tonic extension, the extremities begin to vibrate; this phase gives way to clonic (rhythmic) extension of the extremities, with flexion occurring during each brief relaxation. Usually, this clonic phase will wane in intensity over 1 to 3 minutes. The patient developing SE may then repeat the cycle of tonic activity followed by clonic movements, or may continue to have intermittent bursts of clonic activity without recovery between. Less commonly encountered forms of GCSE are *myoclonic SE,* in which bursts of brief myoclonic jerks increase in intensity until a convulsion occurs, and *clonic-tonic-clonic SE,* in which a period of clonic activity precedes the first tonic contraction. Myoclonic SE is particularly common in patients with anoxic encephalopathy or metabolic disturbances, particularly renal failure.

Secondarily generalized SE in the ICU begins with a partial (focal) seizure, which progresses to a tonic-clonic convulsion. Even under the watchful eye of the ICU staff, the initial focal clinical activity may be overlooked. Because this type of seizure is very strong evidence of a structural brain lesion, care should be taken to elicit evidence of any lateralized movement. *Tonic SE* is almost always confined to patients (usually children) with serious preexisting cerebral disorders. Its importance in critical care practice follows from the observation that benzodiazepines may *precipitate* tonic SE; paradoxically, these agents are also used to treat it.

There are several forms of generalized *NCSE.* Of greatest importance to intensivists is NCSE as a sequel of inadequately treated GCSE. In this circumstance, a patient with GCSE is treated with one or more anticonvulsants, often in inadequate doses, after which visible convulsive activity stops. However, the patient does not awaken (or otherwise return to baseline), and SE is actually continuing. As a rule, patients are expected to begin to awaken within 15 to 20 minutes after the successful termination of SE; many will regain consciousness much faster. Those who have not begun to awaken after 20 minutes should be assumed to have entered NCSE. This form of SE is sometimes termed *subtle SE,* and careful observation will often reveal low-amplitude clonic activity in some part of the body (most commonly, the face or the hands). Most investigators view NCSE as an extremely dangerous problem, because the neuronally destructive effects of SE continue unabated, often for several hours. *This condition requires emergent treatment under EEG monitoring* to prevent further cortical damage. There are no clinical criteria, which indicate when therapy has finally become effective.

The usual form of *partial SE* in the ICU follows a stroke or is seen in patients with rapidly expanding cerebral masses (e.g., abscesses). Although clonic motor activity is the most easily recognized form, the seizure will take on the functional characteristics of the adjacent functional tissue. Thus, somatosensory or special sensory manifestations may occur; the ICU patient who is already neurologically impaired may not be able to report these symptoms. Aphasic SE may occur if the seizure begins in a language area; this must be distinguished from a stroke. Physical examination usually reveals at least some mild lateralizing findings.

EPC is a special type of partial SE in which repetitive movements are confined to a small portion of the body (typically the thumb), and may last for months or years. This type of SE is most commonly associated with nonketotic hyperosmolar hyperglycemia and does not respond to conventional anticonvulsant treatment.

CPSE presents with a state of diminished awareness, although frank loss of consciousness is rarely noted. The patient may exhibit automatisms, but commonly the diagnosis comes as a surprise when an EEG is obtained.

DIAGNOSTIC APPROACH

THE INTENSIVE CARE UNIT PATIENT WITH NEW-ONSET SEIZURES

When a patient already in an ICU has a seizure, the staff has a natural tendency to try in some way to stop the ictus. This may, unfortunately, lead to both diagnostic obscuration and iatrogenic complications. Beyond trying to protect the patient from harm, very little can be done with sufficient rapidity to influence the course of the seizure. In particular, padded tongue blades (or similar items) should not be placed in the mouth, because they are more likely to obstruct the airway than to preserve it. Similarly, most patients have stopped seizing before any medication, even administered into a preexisting intravenous line, can reach the brain in an effective concentration. A common scenario is the administration of intravenous diazepam (DZ), which begins to take effect after the seizure is over; the patient is now both postictal and pharmacologically sedated and becomes apneic.

The most important "intervention" during a single seizure is careful observation. This is the best time to collect evidence of a partial onset, which implies structural brain disease. The postictal examination is similarly valuable; language, motor, sensory, or reflex abnormalities after an apparently generalized convulsion should also be viewed as evidence of focal disease.

In addition to the standard historical information to be requested from patients and family members after a seizure, the ICU patient has several special predispositions that must be investigated. Medications are an important cause of ICU seizures, especially in patients with diminished renal or hepatic function, or with damage to the blood-brain barrier. Imipenem-cilastatin is a common cause of seizures in this setting, but other antibiotics may also be offenders. The neurotoxic desmethyl metabolite of meperidine accumulates in renal failure; it also may produce seizures in patients with normal renal function. A complete list of potentially epileptogenic drugs is beyond the scope of this chapter; the medications of any patient who seizes should be reviewed with this possibility in mind.

Drug withdrawal is another common problem. Although ethanol withdrawal is the most common offender, discontinuing any hypnosedative agent (e.g., barbiturates, benzodiazepines, other sedatives) may prompt convulsions 24 to 96 hours later. This may be a particular problem in the ICU, where such agents may be withheld from patients because the staff is afraid that the drug's effects will obscure the neurologic examination.

The physical examination should be conducted with special emphasis on the points mentioned earlier for the postictal examination. In addition, evidence of cardiovascular disease (as a source for cerebral emboli) and systemic infection should be sought. Careful examination of the skin and fundi are sometimes revealing. The presence of papilledema is obviously important, but its absence does exclude increased intracranial pressure.

In addition to routine biochemical studies, screening for drugs of abuse should be performed on patients with unexplained seizures. Cocaine has emerged as a prominent cause of seizures in many urban hospitals.[40] One area of controversy involves the importance of divalent cation disturbances in adult seizures. Hypocalcemia is rarely a cause of seizures beyond the neonatal period, and its discovery should not be the end of the diagnostic workup. Hyperparathyroidism has been linked anecdotally to seizures, with the inference that parathormone is neurotoxic. Similarly, hypomagnesemia has an unwarranted reputation as a cause of seizures, especially in the malnourished alcoholic patient.

In our prospective study of neurologic complications in medical ICU patients, 38 of 61 patients (62%) with seizures had a vascular, infectious, or neoplastic explanation for their fits.[1] Computed tomography (CT) or magnetic resonance imaging (MRI) should be performed on all ICU patients with new seizures, with a few exceptions. Hypoglycemia and nonketotic hyperosmolar hyperglycemia will commonly produce seizures (even partial seizures), and such patients might be treated for their metabolic disturbance and observed if there is no other indication of neurologic disease. With currently available technology, there are almost no patients who cannot be transported to undergo CT scanning. Although MRI is preferable diagnostically in most situations, the magnetic field precludes infusion pumps and other metallic devices (nonferromagnetic ventilators are available). The decision whether to administer contrast agent for a CT or MRI scan depends on the clinical setting and on the appearance of the plain scan.

The EEG is a vital diagnostic tool for the seizure patient. Partial seizures usually have EEG abnormalities, which begin in, and may remain confined to, the area of cortex producing the seizures. Primary generalized seizures, in contrast, appear to start over the entire cortex at once. Areas of postictal slowing or depressed amplitude provide clues to the focal cause of the seizures, and interictal epileptiform activity helps to classify the type of seizure and guide the patient's subsequent treatment. In patients who do not begin to awaken soon after seizures have apparently been controlled, an emergent EEG is necessary to exclude NCSE.

The need for a lumbar puncture (LP) depends on the clinical situation. In view of the common causes of seizures in the critical care setting, those who need cerebrospinal fluid (CSF) analysis will usually require a CT scan before the LP. If a CNS infection is suspected in such patients, empiric antibiotic treatment should be strongly considered while these studies are being performed, rather than waiting for the scan to be performed and CSF results to be obtained.

THE PATIENT PRESENTING WITH OR DEVELOPING STATUS EPILEPTICUS

In contrast to the ICU patient with a single or a few seizures, the SE patient will require concomitant diagnostic and therapeutic efforts. The first issue is to make a diagnosis of SE. Because most seizures stop within 5 to 7 minutes,[41] it is reasonable to begin treatment after 5 minutes of continuous seizure activity or after the second or third seizure occurring without recovery between the spells. The available treatments are discussed later.

SE has a limited differential diagnosis. GCSE might rarely be confused with decerebrate posturing, but the evolutionary nature of the former and the stimulus sensitivity of the latter make their clinical distinction straightforward. Generalized tetanus patients are awake during their spasms, and almost always flex their arms rather than extending them.[20] The distinction of seizures from movement disorders and psychiatric conditions is discussed earlier.

EEG monitoring is frequently useful in SE,[42] but treatment should not be delayed to obtain it when the diagnosis is apparent. A variety of EEG findings may be present, depending on the type of SE and its duration (see Table 65.2) The most typical pattern early in SE is that of rhythmic, high-frequency (>12 Hz) activity that increases in amplitude and decreases in frequency, finally terminating abruptly and leaving postictal low-amplitude slowing in its wake. CPSE patients often lack such organized discharges, but may instead have waxing and waning rhythmic activity in one or several head regions. Such a pattern requires a high index of suspicion in order to correctly diagnose CPSE; a diagnostic trial of an intravenous benzodiazepine is often necessary. Patients who develop refractory SE or experience seizures during neuromuscular blockade will require continuous EEG monitoring. The technology to perform such monitoring outside specialized epilepsy centers is only now becoming available.

MANAGEMENT APPROACH

THE INTENSIVE CARE UNIT PATIENT WITH NEW-ONSET SEIZURES

Deciding whether to administer anticonvulsants to an ICU patient who experiences a single seizure or a few seizures requires a provisional etiologic diagnosis, an estimate of the likelihood of seizure recurrence, and an understanding of the utility and limitations of available anticonvulsants. For example, the patient who seizes during ethanol withdrawal will probably not benefit from chronic anticonvulsant treatment, and the administration of phenytoin (PHT) will not prevent more withdrawal convulsions during the same episode. Such a patient may need prophylaxis against delirium tremens with benzodiazepines, but the seizures themselves seldom require treatment. The patient who seizes during barbiturate or benzodiazepine withdrawal, in contrast, should usually receive short-term treatment (usually with lorazepam [LRZ]) to prevent the development of SE. Seizures due to drug intoxications or metabolic disturbances should similarly be treated for a brief period, but do not indicate chronic anticonvulsant therapy.

The ICU patient with CNS disease who has even a single seizure should usually be started on a chronic anticonvulsant regimen, with the decision to continue medication reviewed prior to hospital discharge. It is now apparent that initiating anticonvulsant therapy after the first *unprovoked* (e.g., not drug- or withdrawal-related) seizure helps delay the onset of subsequent seizures, but does not change their eventual incidence.[43] Starting treatment after the first seizure in a critically ill patient who has a condition predictive of seizure recurrence may be even more important if the patient's problems include coagulopathies, myocardial ischemia, or other conditions that would be seriously complicated by a convulsion.

The Neurocritical Care Society recently published extensive guidelines for the treatment of SE,[44] which should be consulted for detailed information about the drugs discussed briefly here.

In the ICU setting, PHT (20 mg/kg loading dose, no faster than 50 mg/minute, followed by an initial maintenance dose of 5 mg/kg/day) is often chosen to prevent subsequent seizures because of its relative ease of administration. Slowing the infusion rate to less than 25 mg/minute can usually prevent hypotension and cardiac arrhythmias that may complicate its rapid intravenous administration. Because of the possible precipitation of third-degree atrioventricular (AV) block, an external cardiac pacemaker should be available when patients with conduction abnormalities receive intravenous PHT. Patients who are not actively seizing can be loaded enterally over 6 to 12 hours. Although fosphenytoin is safer than PHT, if it extravasates, this agent does not have less cardiovascular toxicity. Fosphenytoin can also be used for intramuscular loading; PHT (pH 12) should not be administered intramuscularly because it produces myonecrosis.

The total PHT serum concentration should be kept in the "therapeutic" range of 10 to 20 μg/mL while the patient is in the ICU, unless further seizures occur; the level may then be increased until signs of toxicity occur. If the patient is unable to express these signs (e.g., ataxia) because of his or her underlying condition or its treatment, failure to prevent seizures at a concentration of 25 μg/mL is usually an indication to add phenobarbital (PB) (see later). Although the usual goal of chronic anticonvulsant treatment is to administer the smallest dose of a tolerated single agent that completely controls seizures, such an approach is often impossible in the critical care environment. When the patient is more stable, an attempt to decrease minor side effects or to convert to monotherapy may then be made.

PHT is normally about 90% protein bound. Patients with renal dysfunction will have lower total PHT levels for a given dose because the drug is displaced from its binding sites, but the "free" (unbound) level is not affected. Thus, in renal failure patients, and perhaps in others who are receiving highly protein bound drugs (which will compete for PHT binding sites), it may be advantageous to measure free PHT levels. Because only the free fraction is significantly metabolized, the dose need not be altered with changing renal function. Calculations of the unbound concentration based on the serum albumin concentration are unreliable. The half-life for PHT clearance in patients with normal liver function varies from about 20 hours for the intravenous form and the oral solution to over 24 hours for the extended-release oral capsules. Hence, a new steady-state serum concentration will take 4 to 6 days to establish. The drug need not be given more often than every 12 hours; the dosage interval for the enteral forms depends on the preparation but may be even longer. Hepatic dysfunction will mandate a decrease in the maintenance dose; if the serum albumin is very low, the loading dose can be reduced as well.

Hypersensitivity to PHT is the major adverse effect of concern to the intensivist. This allergy may be manifested solely as fever, but more commonly includes a rash and eosinophilia. Febrile reactions appear to be more common with intravenous than with enteral loading. The Stevens-Johnson syndrome occurs rarely. The diagnosis and management of adverse reactions to PHT and other anticonvulsants have been reviewed.[45] PHT is associated with a number of long-term adverse effects in patients with subarachnoid or intracerebral hemorrhage.[46]

PB (10-20 mg/kg loading dose, followed by an initial maintenance dose of 1.5 mg/kg/day) remains useful as an anticonvulsant for patients who cannot tolerate PHT, or who have breakthrough seizures after *adequate* PHT loading. The target level for PB in ICU patients should be 20 to 40 μg/mL. Either hepatic or renal dysfunction may affect PB metabolism. The half-life for PB clearance is about 96 hours. Thus, maintenance doses of this agent need be given only once a day, and a steady-state level will take about 3 weeks to be established. Sedation is the major adverse effect; allergy is rare.

Carbamazepine, one of the most useful chronic anticonvulsants, is seldom introduced to critically ill patients because its insolubility has precluded a parenteral formulation. Oral loading with carbamazepine in conscious patients may produce coma lasting several days. It should be recalled as a cause of hyponatremia in patients receiving it chronically.

Valproate should be avoided in settings in which liver disease or hyperammonemia may be problems but is otherwise a useful drug available both orally and intravenously. A loading dose of 30 mg/kg is reasonable.

The place of the newer anticonvulsants in critical care is not well established. Levetiracetam has gained substantial popularity because of its limited drug interactions; it is predominantly excreted by the kidney, so the dose must be adjusted in renal insufficiency. The usual dose for seizure prevention is between 500 and 1500 mg/day, although doses up to 6 g/day have been employed. The role of serum concentrations for assessment of efficacy or toxicity is not yet established. Lacosamide is also available intravenously and is started at a dose of 200 mg twice daily.

STATUS EPILEPTICUS

The patient in GCSE has an obvious medical emergency; unfortunately, the NCSE and CPSE patients also require emergent treatment but are less straightforward to recognize. In a patient with any of these three conditions, the clinician must move quickly to stop seizures in order to prevent further brain destruction.[47] A suggested management protocol for these conditions is presented in Box 65.3, and Figure 65.3 shows a management algorithm for SE. Patients with simple partial SE or EPC appear to be at substantially less risk of developing widespread cerebral damage and also appear less likely to respond to the aggressive approach outlined in Box 65.3. In this group, correction of underlying problems, if possible (such as nonketotic hyperosmolar hyperglycemia), is most important. Of the available anticonvulsants, PB seems most likely to be efficacious. These patients are often loaded with PHT in the hope that this agent will prevent secondary generalization, but the actual value of this practice is unknown.

Some frequent errors in the use of medications to terminate SE include (1) use of inadequate doses of potentially effective agents and, conversely, (2) continued administration of drugs that are ineffective in the patient being treated. The first point most frequently applies to PHT; the proverbial "gram of Dilantin" is not adequate for patients weighing more than 50 kg.

SPECIFIC AGENTS

Benzodiazepines

LRZ is emerging as the agent of first choice for terminating SE. A study in the Veterans Affairs medical system compared LRZ, DZ followed by PHT, PHT alone, and PB as first-line agents and demonstrated that LRZ is the definitive agent of first choice.[48] The advantages of LRZ over PHT include (1) its longer duration of action against SE (4-14 hours as opposed to 20 minutes) and (2) a higher initial response rate.[49] One study concluded that children receiving PHT for SE were far more likely to require intubation for ventilatory failure than comparable children receiving LRZ[50]; the same was true for all ages in the San Francisco Prehospital Status Study.[51] PHT and LRZ remain the only agents in this class with FDA indications for SE. In Europe, midazolam (MDZ) or clonazepam is often used initially. MDZ is exceptionally useful for refractory SE, but it is hampered by tachyphylaxis,[52] which occurs because the $GABA_A$ receptors bearing benzodiazepine-sensitive subunits are removed from the neuronal cell membrane and replaced with receptors bearing benzodiazepine-insensitive ones.[53] Respiratory depression is the major adverse effect of all agents in this class when administered intravenously.

Data from the Veterans Affairs cooperative trial indicate that the use of other conventional agents after failure of the first one is very unlikely to terminate SE.[49]

Box 65.3 Suggested Therapeutic Sequence for Terminating Status Epilepticus (SE)

I. Establish airway.
Often the most rapid way to accomplish this is to rapidly terminate SE. If endotracheal intubation under neuromuscular junction blockade is necessary, use a nondepolarizing agent such as rapacuronium (1.5 mg/kg) or vecuronium (0.1 mg/kg). If increased intracranial pressure is a concern, premedicate with lidocaine (1 mg/kg) or thiopental (4-5 mg/kg). If these agents are used, the patient should be considered still to be in SE until neuromuscular transmission is reestablished, or until an EEG demonstrates that SE is no longer present.

II. Determine blood pressure.
If the patient is hypotensive, begin volume replacement and/or vasoactive agents as clinically indicated. Patients with GCSE who present with hypotension will usually require admission to a critical care unit. (Hypertension should not be treated until SE is controlled, because terminating SE will usually substantially correct it, and many of the agents used to terminate SE can produce hypotension).

III. Unless the patient is known to be normo- or hyperglycemic, administer dextrose (1 mg/kg) and thiamine (1 mg/kg).

IV. Terminate SE.
We recommend the following pharmacologic protocol (see text for discussion of these and alternative agents). Be cognizant of the potential of these drugs to eliminate the visible convulsive movements of GCSE while leaving the patient in nonconvulsive SE. Patients who do not begin to respond to external stimuli 15 minutes after the apparent termination of GCSE should be considered at risk for nonconvulsive SE and undergo emergency EEG monitoring.

A. Administer LRZ 0.1 mg/kg at 0.04 mg/kg/min.
This drug should be diluted in an equal volume of the solution being used for intravenous infusion, because it is quite viscous. Most adult patients who will respond have done so by a total dose of 8 mg. The latency of effect is debated, but lack of response after 5 minutes should be considered a failure.

B. Give MDZ if SE persists.
Administer MDZ 0.2 mg/kg as a bolus, followed by an infusion of 0.1-2.0 mg/kg/hr to achieve seizure control (as determined by EEG monitoring). We routinely intubate patients at this stage if this has not already been accomplished. Patients reaching this stage should be treated in a critical care unit.

C. Give propofol if MDZ is not effective.
Should the patient's SE not be controlled with MDZ, administer propofol at a dose of 50-250 µg/kg/min. Prolonged infusions of propofol have hemodynamic consequences similar to those with pentobarbital. Alternative agents include valproate, ketamine, and levetiracetam.

D. Give pentobarbital if propofol is not effective.
If propofol fails, use pentobarbital 12 mg/kg at 0.2-0.4 mg/kg/min as tolerated, followed by an infusion of 0.25-2.0 mg/kg/hr as determined by EEG monitoring (with a goal of burst suppression). Most patients will require systemic and pulmonary arterial catheterization, with fluid and vasoactive therapy as indicated to maintain blood pressure. Other complications of this treatment are discussed in the text.

V. Prevent recurrence of SE.
The choice of drugs depends greatly on the contributing/causative disorder and the patient's medical and social situation. In general, patients who have not previously received anticonvulsants whose SE is easily controlled often respond well to chronic treatment with PHT or carbamazepine. By contrast, others (e.g., patients with acute encephalitis) will require two or three anticonvulsants at "toxic" levels (e.g., PB in doses greater than 100 µg/mL) to be weaned from MDZ or pentobarbital, and may still have occasional seizures.

VI. Treat complications.

A. Rhabdomyolysis
Rhabdomyolysis should be treated with a vigorous saline diuresis to prevent acute renal failure, urinary alkalinization may be a useful adjunct. If definitive treatment of GCSE takes longer than expected because of hypotension or arrhythmias, neuromuscular junction blockade under EEG monitoring might be considered.

B. Hyperthermia
Hyperthermia usually remits rapidly after termination of SE. External cooling usually suffices if the core temperature remains elevated. In rare instances, cool peritoneal lavage or extracorporeal blood cooling may be required. High-dose pentobarbital generally produces poikilothermia.

C. Cerebral edema
The treatment of cerebral edema secondary to SE has not been well studied. When substantial edema is present, SE and cerebral edema are likely to be manifestations of the same underlying condition. Hyperventilation and mannitol may be valuable if edema is life-threatening. Edema due to SE is vasogenic, so steroids may be useful as well.

EEG, electroencephalogram; GCSE, generalized convulsive status epilepticus; LRZ, lorazepam; MDZ, midazolam; PB, phenobarbital; PHT, phenytoin.

Hydantoins

PHT is an effective anti-SE agent but cannot be delivered rapidly enough to be used as a first-line agent. Its major advantage is a very long duration of action once an adequate dose has been administered (the 20-mg/kg loading dose reliably produces a total serum concentration above 20 µg/mL for 24 hours). Concerns about its intravenous administration were discussed earlier. If the patient is no longer in SE during PHT administration, a slower rate should be employed.

PHT is highly insoluble, and it must be dissolved in sodium hydroxide and propylene glycol at a pH greater than 11 to remain in solution. Therefore, extravasation can produce severe necrosis. The drug can also cause thrombophlebitis, which may result in the "purple glove syndrome."[54]

Fosphenytoin is a PHT prodrug, which is converted to PHT by phosphatases with a half-life of about 7 minutes. It is prescribed in "PHT equivalents," so the loading dose remains 20 mg/kg. The maximal recommended rate of infusion is 150 mg/minute, but it should be started more slowly and increased to this rate if tolerated. Because it is water-soluble, extravasation does not pose the problem of skin and soft tissue necrosis.

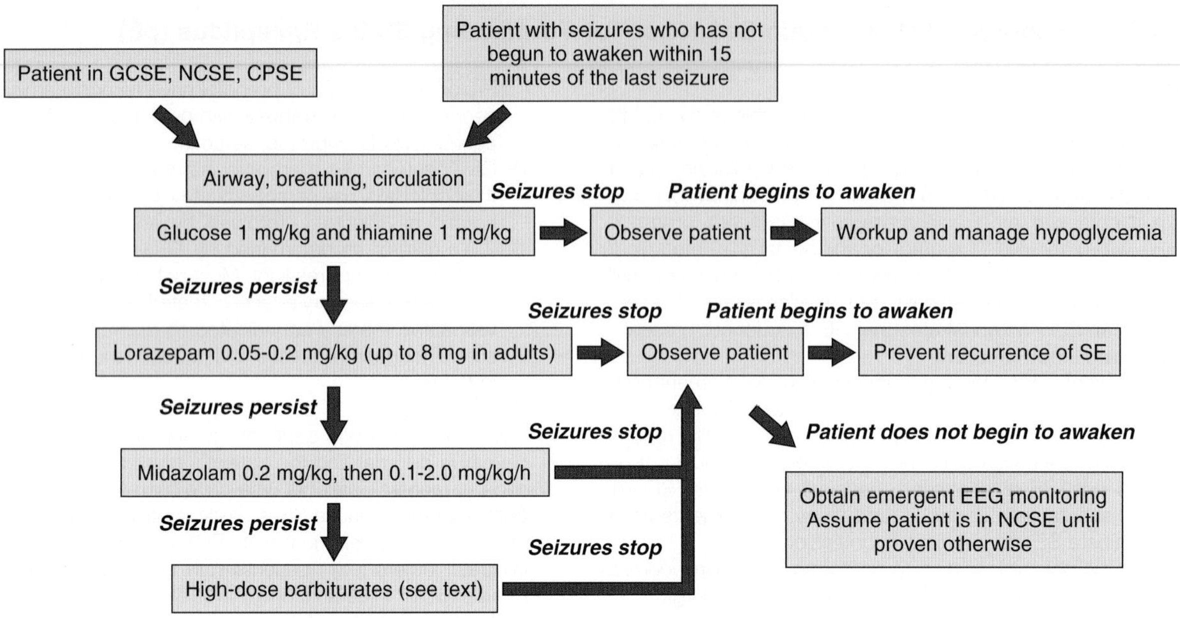

Figure 65.3 Management algorithm for status epilepticus.

Hydantoins should not be used in absence SE, as they may worsen the condition.

Barbiturates

PB has long been one of the major anti-SE agents. Some advocate it as a first-line drug,[55] but it is rarely used in this role. It has classically been a third-line agent for control of SE, after a benzodiazepine and PHT. Its utility in SE is diminished by the length of time required to obtain a therapeutic effect in patients who have already failed with a benzodiazepine and PHT. It remains an important agent in patients with simple partial SE, and in preparing patients to be withdrawn from high-dose pentobarbital.

Pentobarbital and thiopental are commonly reserved for the control of refractory SE, although thiopental is not currently available in the United States. Although these agents will be effective if used in large enough doses, side effects often limit their use[56] or may even be fatal.[57] They are important when other rapidly available modalities have failed (see Box 65.3).

Valproate

Intravenous valproate, given in a dose of 20 to 30 mg/kg, has gained popularity for the treatment of SE because it does not produce respiratory depression or marked sedation. It has been successful in case series[58,59] but has not been directly compared to the other available agents. Hypotension may occur with large doses.[60] This drug should be avoided if the patient has an inborn error of metabolism affecting the liver, as it may precipitate fulminant hepatic failure.[61] Valproate has a number of drug interactions that limit its utility in the ICU.[62]

Isoflurane and Desflurane

The inhalational anesthetics isoflurane and desflurane are effective in controlling refractory SE, but the difficulties involved in delivering the gases (such as the requirement for an anesthesia machine) and the need for a gas scavenging system have essentially confined their use to the operating suite or the recovery area.[63] Advances in delivery systems may make its use in the ICU more reasonable, but long-term use is potentially hepatotoxic.

Propofol

Propofol has been reported effective in refractory SE in doses up to 250 μg/kg/minute[64] but has not been directly compared with other drugs. It theoretically offers a lower risk of respiratory depression and more rapid recovery of consciousness after the agent is stopped. We use it in SE patients who have failed or become resistant to MDZ.[65] One should observe for evidence of the propofol infusion syndrome and stop the drug should a metabolic acidosis or evidence of muscle injury develop.

Ketamine

Although only anecdotes and small case series are available, ketamine appears to be a useful agent for the termination of refractory SE.[66] Its NMDA blocking effect distinguishes it from the other agents discussed here, and it carries theoretical advantages in terms of brain protection.[67] Its intrinsic sympathomimetic effect makes it a useful choice in hypotensive patients, and it does not markedly impair ventilation. The appropriate dose in SE has not been established; we use a loading dose of 1 to 5 mg/kg, with an infusion rate of 10 to 50 μg/kg/minute.

Levetiracetam

Levetiracetam is now available for intravenous use, but its role in SE remains to be determined. The effective dose in adults is reported to be between 1 and 6 g/day.[68] Oral administration may be useful for maintenance.[69]

Lacosamide

Lacosamide, which is available for both intravenous and oral use, is typically started at 200 mg twice daily and may be increased to 400 mg twice daily if needed.[70]

The management of "super-refractory" SE has long been an area of contention. These patients may require general anesthesia for a month or longer, while the stimulus for epileptogenicity comes under control or remits. Some of these patients are now recognized to have an autoimmune or paraneoplastic cause for their condition, which requires immunologic therapy.[71] Although these patients sometimes seem hopeless, it is important to remember that 35% will return to their premorbid level of function.[72]

CONTROVERSIAL MANAGEMENT ISSUES

Controversy remains regarding the long-term neurologic consequences of two clinical conditions: periodic lateralized epileptiform discharges (PLEDs) and EPC. PLEDs are an EEG phenomenon usually seen in the setting of large acute strokes or rapidly expanding mass lesions (e.g., tumors or abscesses). Less commonly, acute metabolic or toxic disorders will "reactivate" PLEDs in the vicinity of an old lesion. The EEG activity signifies the repetitive, synchronous firing of large numbers of neurons near the lesion; there is occasionally contralateral myoclonic jerking of the hand or face. Expert opinion is divided regarding the possibly epileptic nature of these phenomena. Patients who have clinical seizures (i.e., other than the myoclonic jerks) should receive anticonvulsants. The myoclonic movements associated with PLEDs are difficult to suppress without resorting to high-dose barbiturates or benzodiazepines. The data available do not suggest that suppressing the electrical phenomenon improves outcome.

EPC is usually diagnosed in a patient who has an isolated repetitive movement (usually of the hand or face), often following an infectious or vascular insult, or in the setting of nonketotic hyperglycemia.[73] The movement may persist for months or years. Most patients receive anticonvulsants to prevent spread of the discharge, but these agents seldom affect EPC itself. Attempts at treatment with high-dose barbiturates result in short-term suppression of the movement, but it usually returns as the drug levels decline.

Another area of contention concerns the periodic epileptiform discharges occasionally seen after respiratory or cardiac arrests. Because experimental studies show that neurons in anoxic animals exhibit epileptiform behavior, some have raised the possibility that these discharges are a form of SE and should therefore be treated. Although this possibility has not been systematically studied in humans, the lack even of anecdotes of neurologic improvement with anticonvulsant treatment suggests that currently available anticonvulsant drugs do not improve patient outcome in this condition. If it is associated with myoclonus that the family finds disconcerting, suppression of the movements with neuromuscular junction blockers may be useful. High-dose barbiturates or benzodiazepines will also stop the movements, but they obscure the neurologic examination and complicate the possible diagnosis of brain death. These drugs do not improve prognosis in postanoxic patients.

PROGNOSIS

Wijdicks and Sharbrough reported that 34% of patients experiencing a seizure in any ICU at the Mayo Clinic died during that hospitalization.[11] In our prospective study of neurologic complications in medical ICU patients,[10] having even one seizure while in the unit for a non-neurologic reason doubled the patient's in-hospital mortality rate. This effect on prognosis appeared to be due to the effect of the cause of the ictus, rather than the seizure itself.

Three major factors determine the outcome of SE: the type of SE, its cause, and its duration. In general, GCSE carries the worst prognosis for neurologic recovery as a consequence of SE itself; myoclonic SE following an anoxic episode carries a very poor prognosis for survival. CPSE produces some risk of limbic system damage, usually manifested by memory dysfunction. Simple partial SE may produce neuronal damage, but this is difficult to discern from the effect of the lesion that commonly produces this form of SE. At the far end of the spectrum, absence SE does not seem to carry a risk of neurologic deterioration.

Most studies of SE outcome have concentrated on mortality rates in GCSE. Hauser[18] summarized the data available in 1990, showing mortality rates for SE to vary from 1% to 53%. The few studies that attempted to distinguish the mortality rate due to SE from that of the underlying disease attributed rates of 1% to 7% to SE and 2% to 25% to its cause. The Virginia Commonwealth University population-based studies have analyzed the mortality risks for various aspects of GCSE.[12] SE lasting longer than 1 hour was associated with a 10-fold increase in mortality rate when compared to SE lasting less than 1 hour. Other causes associated with marked increases in mortality rate were anoxia, intracranial hemorrhages, tumors, infections, and trauma.

Very few findings are available regarding the functional status of GCSE survivors, and none reliably allows a distinction between the effects of SE and its causes. A review of intellectual impairment as an outcome of SE concluded intellectual abilities probably did decline as a consequence of SE.[74] Survivors of SE frequently have memory and behavioral disorders out of proportion to any structural damage produced by the cause of their seizures. This observation is supported by a wealth of experimental data and argues strongly for the rapid and effective control of SE. The prognosis of CPSE is less certain, but case reports of severe memory deficits following prolonged CPSE have appeared.[75]

The effect of the treatment of SE on the risk of subsequent epilepsy is uncertain. Experimental studies suggest that SE does lower the threshold for subsequent seizures.[76]

KEY POINTS

- Seizures lasting longer than 1 hour markedly increase mortality risk compared to seizures lasting less than 1 hour.
- Primary generalized seizures arise from the entire cerebral cortex without evidence of focal point.
- In addition to damaging the CNS, GCSE produces serious, often life-threatening, systemic effects that include cardiovascular, respiratory, and muscular systems.

Continued on following page

KEY POINTS (Continued)

- Hypersensitivity to PHT is the major adverse effect of concern to the intensivist. This allergy may be manifested solely as fever but more commonly includes a rash and eosinophilia. Rarely Stevens-Johnson syndrome occurs.
- The patient who seizes during ethanol withdrawal will probably not benefit from chronic anticonvulsant treatment, and the administration of PHT will not prevent more withdrawal convulsions during the same episode.
- Errors in the use of medications to terminate SE include (1) use of inadequate doses of potentially effective agents and, conversely, (2) continued administration of drugs that are ineffective in the patient being treated.
- Myoclonic SE following an anoxic episode carries a very poor prognosis for survival.

SELECTED REFERENCES

2. Varelas PN, Mirski M: Treatment of seizures in the neurologic intensive care unit. Curr Treat Options Neurol 2007;9:136-145.
11. Wijdicks EFM, Sharbrough FW: New-onset seizures in critically ill patients. Neurology 1993;43:1042-1044.
21. Oddo M, Carrera E, Claassen J, et al: Continuous electroencephalography in the medical intensive care unit. Crit Care Med 2009;37:2051-2056.
38. Geocadin RG, Koenig MA, Stevens RD, Peberdy MA: Intensive care for brain injury after cardiac arrest: Therapeutic hypothermia and related neuroprotective strategies. Crit Care Clin 2006;22:619-636.
44. Brophy G, Bell R, Claassen J, et al: Guidelines for the evaluation and management of status epilepticus. Neurocrit Care 2012;17(1):3-23.
48. Treiman DM, Meyers PD, Walton NY, et al: A comparison of four treatments for generalized convulsive status epilepticus. Veterans Affairs Status Epilepticus Cooperative Study Group. N Engl J Med 1998;339:792-798.
57. Bleck TP: High-dose pentobarbital treatment of refractory status epilepticus: A meta-analysis of published studies. Epilepsia 1992;33:5.
58. Venkataraman V, Wheless JW: Safety of rapid intravenous infusion of valproate loading doses in epilepsy patients. Epilepsy Res 1999;35:147-153.
64. Stecker MM, Kramer TH, Raps EC, et al: Treatment of refractory status epilepticus with propofol: Clinical and pharmacokinetic findings. Epilepsia 1998;39:18-26.
66. Sheth RD, Gidal BE: Refractory status epilepticus: Response to ketamine. Neurology 1998;51:1765-1766.

The complete list of references can be found at www.expertconsult.com.

66

Head Injury

Alan R. Turtz | H. Warren Goldman

CHAPTER OUTLINE

INTRODUCTION

In the context of critical care medicine, the management of severe head injuries remains the Achilles' heel of neurosurgery, as borne out by our own observations over three decades of practice at academic centers. Although revolutionary advances now allow imaging of the brain and spinal cord with greatly improved speed and anatomic detail, translation of this resource into better outcomes has been disappointing. The search for a neuroprotective agent that can consistently prevent the deadly cascade of events that leads to irreparable brain damage remains for future investigators as of this writing.

Key to optimizing clinical outcomes has been the recognition that the time from injury to surgery must be as short as possible to minimize the secondary manifestations of serious brain trauma. Other valuable lessons from clinical experience reported in the literature are that glucocorticoids have no significant therapeutic benefit in managing severe head injuries and that hyperventilation, very effective in reducing high intracranial pressure (ICP), must be used judiciously; otherwise, it may become more harmful than helpful.

It also has been demonstrated that the management of serious brain trauma requires specialty teams consisting of experienced neurosurgeons, traumatologists, and intensivists (specifically, neurointensivists) working together in a dedicated unit equipped and staffed to optimally care for these patients. In the absence of such facilities, outcomes suffer.[1-3]

Finally, the introduction of a simple-to-use and highly predictable neurologic status scoring system, the Glasgow Coma Scale (GCS), has enabled meaningful multidisciplinary communication from the accident scene through intensive care and beyond, resulting in efficient and timely triage and treatment of these patients in tenuous conditions.

INCIDENCE

The Centers for Disease Control and Prevention report the number of patients sustaining a traumatic brain injury (TBI) to be at least 1.7 million per year in the United States. Approximately 80% of patients are released from the emergency department, 275,000 are admitted, and 52,000 die. Nearly a third of all traumatic deaths in the U.S. involve a head injury. The ages most likely to sustain a TBI are children up to 4 years old and adults over 64, with adults greater than 74 years old having the highest rates of hospitalization and death associated with head injury.[4] Teenagers and young adults continue to be at high risk for sustaining TBI, but the range has decreased over the past 20 years from between 15 and 24 to between 15 and 19[4,5]. The incidence of head injury has been shown to be inversely proportional to economic status,[6] and has remained up to three times more common in males in every age group over the past several decades.[4,7,8] In the United States, falls are the most common cause of TBI and are responsible for half of the head-injured children up to 14 years of age and 60% of the adults over the age of 64.[4] Although the frequency of head injury related to motor vehicle crashes has decreased over the years to a little less than 20%, these crashes are the second leading cause of head injury in all age groups and result in the largest percentage of TBI-related deaths.[4,9] The incidence of TBI worldwide is difficult to quantify but is estimated to be at least 10 million people a year, with traffic accidents accounting for more than half, and falls being the second leading cause;[10] this is the opposite distribution seen in the United States[4]. Violence is estimated to cause about 10% of head injuries throughout the world,[10] as well as in the U.S.[4], but there is significant variability in the specific mechanisms. For example, between 1997 and 2007 in the U.S., firearms were related to just over a third of all lethal TBIs, compared to a single hospital in South Africa that reported its experience with more than 300 stab wounds to the brain.[11]

DIAGNOSTIC APPROACH

The presenting neurologic condition of patients with head injuries is the primary factor in determining the initial management and prognosis. When a detailed history is unavailable, it is important to keep in mind that loss of consciousness may have preceded and in fact caused the traumatic event, such as aneurysmal subarachnoid hemorrhage (SAH), hypoglycemia, intoxication, or syncope. Level of consciousness is one of the most important neurologic considerations in managing a head-injured patient. Neurosurgical patients generally have an alteration in level of consciousness from either brainstem or bilateral cerebral hemispheric involvement. This may be secondary to poor perfusion due to high ICP or brainstem compression, both of which require neurosurgical intervention. Therefore, an accurate tool to measure level of consciousness is essential. Many clinical assessment tools are available for use in the critical care setting.[12-24]

GLASGOW COMA SCALE

Ideally, using the GCS, a nurse, medical student, paramedic, physician assistant, intensivist, trauma surgeon, emergency medicine physician, neurologist, and neurosurgeon all should obtain the same score when assessing a patient. The GCS system is not perfect, but it has proved itself to be, overall, a practical, straightforward grading system that can be used by health professionals in various fields and at different levels to produce reliable results.[25-30] The GCS has become the most widely used assessment tool and is considered the gold standard for the evaluation of patients with head injuries.[12]

The GCS is a measure of level of consciousness and does not take into account focal deficits. It is based on eye opening (1-4), verbal response (1-5), and motor response (1-6) (Table 66.1). A patient with a normal level of consciousness should have the highest possible score of 15. The lowest score possible is 3, not 0 as might be expected. An intubated patient technically gets a 1 for verbal response and is assigned 1T (for Tube) for the verbal score. It is important to identify the score for each observed variable tested. For example, a typical score for an intubated patient with decorticate posturing probably would be E1 + V1T + M3 = 5T (where E denotes eye opening, V is verbal response, and M is motor response). It also is important to realize the shortcoming of this system in evaluating patients with dementia or aphasia. A point to keep in mind is that the GCS attempts to put a numeric value on level of consciousness, with 15 being representative of normal. If a demented patient from a nursing home presents with a normal level of consciousness after a fall but doesn't know what day it is, the GCS would be calculated as E4 + V4 + M6 = 14. A GCS score of 14 describes a patient with an abnormal level of consciousness but fails to accurately communicate this particular patient's condition. Likewise, clinicians must use caution when applying the GCS to patients with aphasia. Conversely, patients with profound focal deficits and a normal level of consciousness should have a GCS score of 15. Another problematic case is that of a quadriplegic patient with a normal level of consciousness who is able to blink the eyes or stick out the tongue upon command, thereby giving a top score of 6 on the motor assessment.

Table 66.1 Glasgow Coma Scale

Component	Score
Eye Opening	
Spontaneously	4
To voice	3
To pain	2
No response	1
Verbal	
Oriented	5
Disoriented	4
Inappropriate	3
Incomprehensible sounds	2
No response	1
Motor	
Following commands	6
Localizing to pain	5
Withdrawing to pain	4
Abnormal flexion	3
Abnormal extension	2
No response	1

The GCS has been used to predict outcome.[31] The motor score itself has predictive value as well.[32] The GCS score should be calculated after hemodynamic and pulmonary resuscitation and without sedatives or muscle relaxants.[33]

Aggressive implementation of early sedation and intubation in severely head-injured patients compromises the ability to determine an accurate GCS score.[34]

COMPUTED TOMOGRAPHY CLASSIFICATION: MARSHALL CLASSIFICATION

A useful classification of brain injuries by findings on computed tomography (CT) has been devised by Marshall and colleagues. This CT classification, presented in Table 66.2, can serve as a guide in describing scans and has strong predictive power.[34,35]

Table 66.2 Marshall Computed Tomography Classification

Category	Definition
Diffuse injury I (no visible pathology)	No visible intracranial pathology seen on computed tomography scan
Diffuse injury II	Cisterns are present with midline shift of 0-5 mm or lesion densities present no high- or mixed-density lesion > 25 cm^3 may include bone fragments and foreign bodies
Diffuse injury III (swelling)	Cisterns compressed or absent with midline shift of 0-5 mm; no high- or mixed-density lesion > 25 cm^3
Diffuse injury IV (shift)	Midline shift > 5 mm; no high or mixed-density lesion > 25 cm^3
Evacuated mass lesion	Any lesion surgically evacuated
Nonevacuated mass lesion	High- or mixed-density lesion > 25 cm^3; not surgically evacuated

From Marshall LF, Marshall SB, Klauber MR, et al: A new classification of head injury based on computerized tomography. J Neurosurg 1991;75:S14-S20.

Maas and associates have proposed a scoring system with better predictive power (Table 66.3), with a sum total adjusted to be consistent with the GCS.[34] Table 66.4 presents a mortality prediction chart based on this classification.

This scoring system is best used as one piece of data in the overall clinical assessment in considering a patient's prognosis.[36]

PREDICTION OF OUTCOMES

Severe brain injury outcomes can be accurately predicted using four variables: age, GCS score on admission (especially motor score), CT characteristics, and presence of ischemic and hemodynamic secondary insults. Using these four predictors, numerous investigators have used statistical modeling techniques to predict up to 80% or more of outcomes.[37]

Head injuries generally are classified as mild (GCS score of 13 to 15), moderate (GCS score of 9 to 12), or severe,[3-8] although the evidence may be sufficient to include a GCS score of 13 in the moderate category.[38]

CT scanning is the diagnostic imaging study of choice in trauma. Plain x-ray films of the skull are rarely indicated as a screening study for head-injured patients. Outcomes with the strategy of obtaining CT scans in all head-injured patients are superior to those with other management strategies. The incidence of missed surgical lesions in mildly head-injured patients by CT scanning is 0.028%.[39-42]

PRIMARY HEAD INJURY

Primary head injury can be defined as the damage that occurs at the moment of impact and can take the form of skull fractures, surface contusions and lacerations, diffuse axonal injury, or diffuse vascular injury.[42] Some authors include the contusions and hematomas that form as a direct and immediate effect of the impact as part of the primary injury as well.[43] These hemorrhages may manifest with significant mass effect requiring surgical intervention.

Emergent neurosurgical intervention is designed to prevent permanent damage to the central nervous system (CNS) in general and to the reticular activating system in particular. Located in the brainstem, the reticular activating system is what allows a meaningful, awake condition; if it is destroyed, the patient will be vegetative. The surgical management of head-injured patients typically is driven by the presence of pathologic masses (hematomas) in anatomic spaces. These spaces are best described by reviewing the anatomic layers.

In virtually all cases of head injury seen in clinical practice, the pathogenic mechanism is an impact. The first

Table 66.3 Prognostic Score Chart for Probability of Mortality in Patients with Severe or Moderate Traumatic Brain Injury by Computed Tomography Characteristics

Predictor	Score
Basal Cisterns	
Normal	0
Compressed	1
Absent	2
Midline Shift	
No shift or shift < 5 mm	0
Shift > 5 mm	1
Epidural Mass Lesion	
Present	0
Absent	1
Intraventricular Blood or tSAH	
Absent	0
Present	1
Sum Score*	+1

*The sum score can be used to obtain the predicted probability of mortality (see Table 66.4). The authors chose to add plus 1 to make the grading numerically consistent with the grading of the motor score of the GCS and with the Marshall CT classification. tSAH, traumatic subarachnoid hemorrhage.

Table 66.4 Computed Tomography Classification by Prediction Score

Score	Mortality Rate (%)
1	0
2	6.8
3	16.0
4	26.0
5	53.0
6	61.0

layer involved is the scalp, the layers of which are best remembered by the pneumonic SCALP: S for skin, C for connective tissue, A for galea aponeurosis, L for the loose connective tissue layer, and P for periosteum. The scalp is the thickest skin in the body and absorbs some of the energy delivered to the head during impact. The scalp has a rich blood supply with relatively large blood vessels situated in the space where the connective tissue meets the galea. A large laceration has the potential for heavy blood loss and needs to be managed with local, direct pressure until surgical repair can be accomplished. Care must be taken in applying pressure if there is an underlying depressed skull fracture or, especially, a skull defect as is seen in missile injuries. It should be noted that an unattended, serious scalp laceration does have the potential for blood loss to the point of hemodynamic instability, but this is the only exception to the rule that an adult cannot lose enough blood from any intracranial hemorrhage to cause hypovolemic shock and hemodynamic instability. Blood clots within the scalp usually are limited to the loose connective tissue layer and are referred to as subgaleal hematomas, which may be a feature of massive injuries or a sign of coagulopathy but rarely require treatment other than direct pressure if active bleeding is suspected. A cephalohematoma is a blood clot that expands in the potential space between the periosteum and the skull; this lesion is limited to neonates.

SKULL FRACTURES

The next layer involved in trauma is the skull, composed of outer and inner tables with the intervening vascular diploic space. Skull fractures are best considered as involving the cranial vault or the skull base. Cranial vault fractures are further divided into linear or depressed and open or closed. In general, closed, linear fractures of the cranial vault do not require any specific treatment.

Basilar skull fractures typically are linear and involve the anterior cranial base and the petrous part of the temporal bone. These fractures have the potential for an associated dural laceration adjacent to potentially contaminated paranasal sinuses, or the external ear canal if the tympanic membrane is disrupted. This allows the potential for a cerebrospinal fluid (CSF) fistula to develop, as well as meningitis. Clinical signs of a fracture of the petrous portion of the temporal bone include hemotympanum with or without tympanic membrane disruption, hearing loss, CSF otorrhea, and Battle sign. The cranial nerves that course through the temporal bone include the facial, acoustic, and vestibular nerves; therefore, associated vestibular dysfunction or facial weakness may be noted (Fig. 66.1). Anterior cranial base fractures may be associated with "raccoon eyes," anosmia, and CSF rhinorrhea. It is important to remember that when a fracture of the floor of the anterior cranial base is suspected, a nasogastric tube should not be inserted, because of the risk of intracranial penetration (Fig. 66.2).

The use of prophylactic antibiotics in basilar skull fractures has been debated but generally is not recommended. When CSF leak does occur, the break in the tissue usually will heal with conservative treatment over the course of a week, unless the defect is very large or a bony spicule is identified. Keeping the patient's head elevated and possibly using external CSF diversion after a few days are reasonable nonoperative methods; however, if the leak persists, surgical repair is indicated.[44]

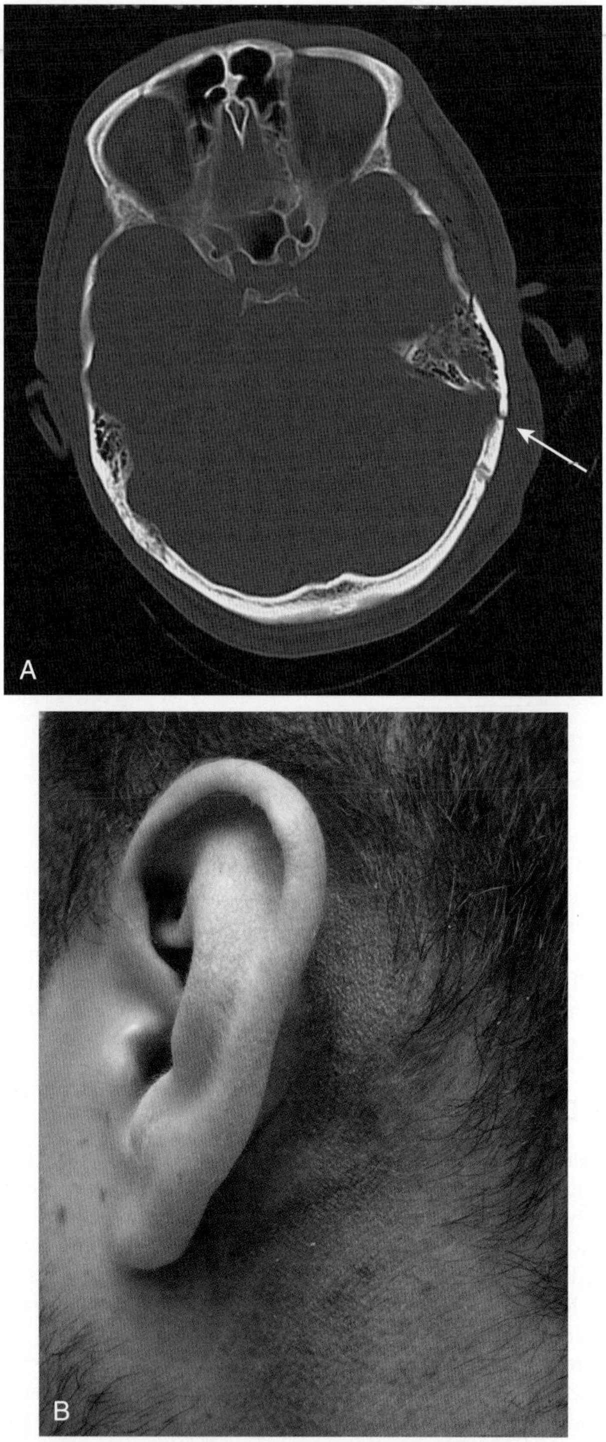

Figure 66.1 **A,** Axial computed tomography image demonstrating skull base fracture (*arrow*) through the petrous portion of the temporal bone. **B,** Battle sign.

Most depressed skull fractures occur in men younger than 30 years of age.[45] Despite very little literature to support any particular management strategy, closed depressed skull fractures generally are operated on if the extent of depression is greater than the full thickness of the adjacent skull, with the theoretical benefits of improved cosmetic result, a

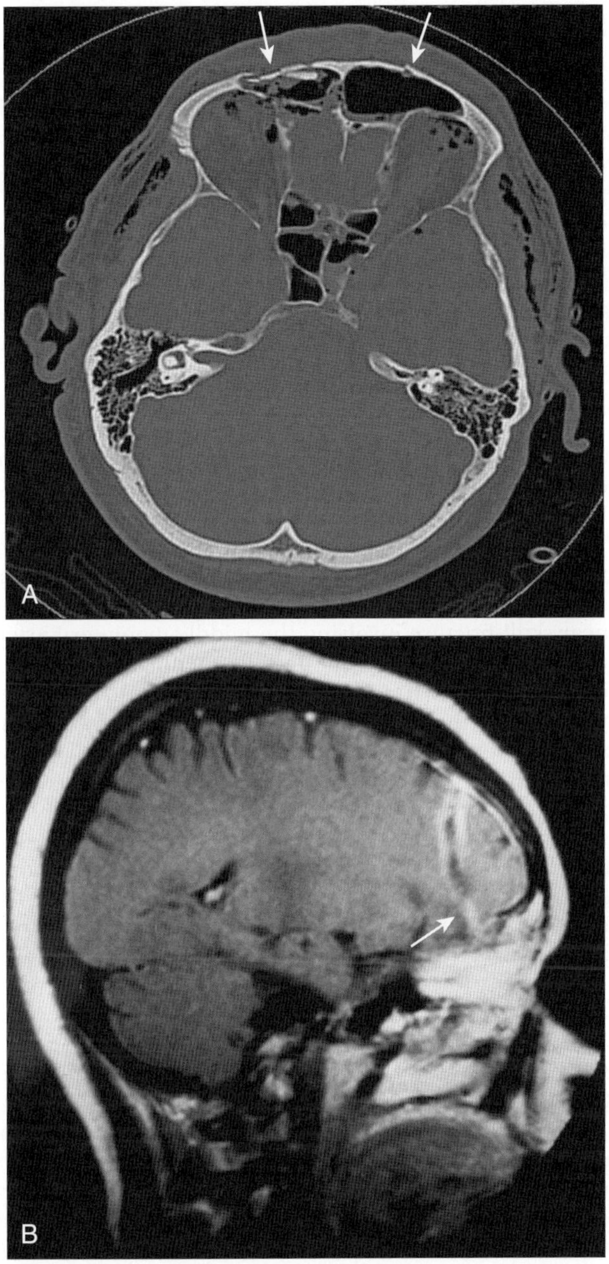

Figure 66.2 **A,** Preoperative axial computed tomography image demonstrates multiple anterior cranial base fractures involving the cribriform plate and posterior wall of the frontal sinus *(arrows)* in a 50-year-old man who fell off a ladder onto his face. The patient sustained minimal brain injury from the impact because the facial and anterior frontal sinuses absorbed much of the energy, cushioning the brain during impact, much like an air bag. **B,** Image from a preoperative sagittal T1 MRI study without contrast demonstrates the tract of a nasogastric tube through the frontal lobe in a 42-year-old woman with an anterior cranial base defect *(arrow)*.

decrease in late-onset posttraumatic epilepsy, and a reduction in the incidence of persistent neurologic deficit.[46] Most depressed skull fractures, however, are open[45] (Fig. 66.3), meaning that a scalp laceration with galeal disruption overlying the fracture is present.

Open depressed skull fractures may be associated with significant morbidity and mortality.[45,47] Infection rates are

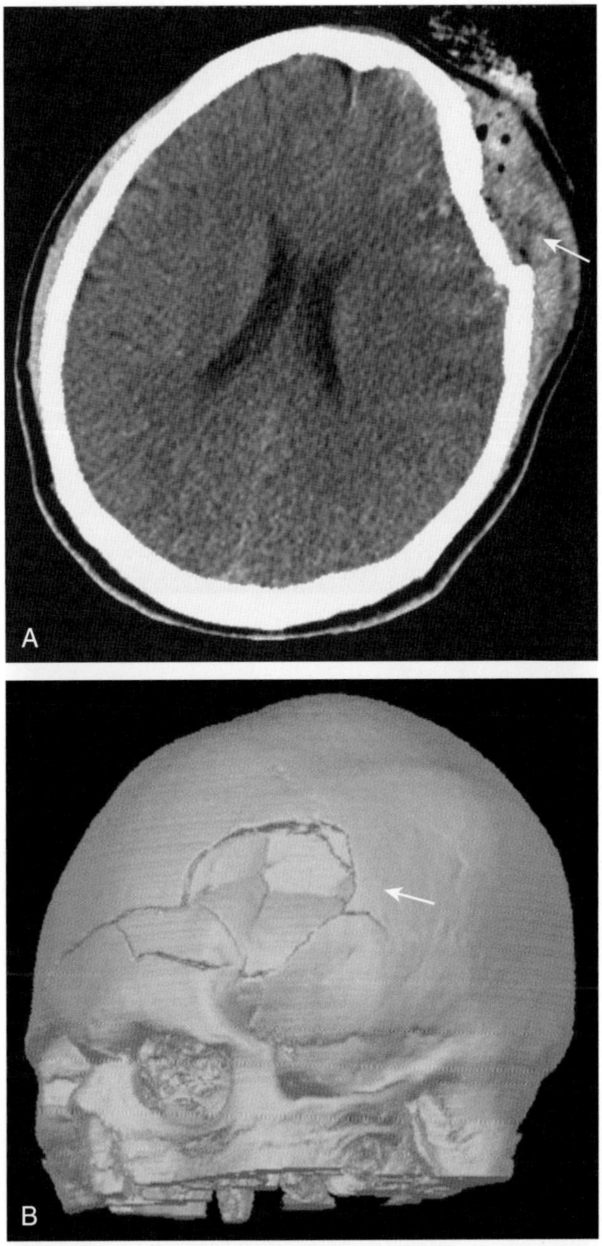

Figure 66.3 Depressed skull fracture. **A,** Brain window *(arrow)*. **B,** Computed tomography three-dimensional reconstruction also demonstrates the depressed skull fracture *(arrow)*.

reported to be between 1.9% and 10.6%,[46-50] with neurologic morbidity and mortality rates of approximately 11% each[46] and an incidence of late epilepsy up to 15%.[51]

By convention, open depressed cranial vault fractures are treated surgically, with debridement and elevation, primarily to attempt to decrease the incidence of infection. Open depressed cranial fractures may be treated nonoperatively if clinical and radiographic examination reveals no evidence of dural penetration, significant intracranial hematoma, depression greater than 1 cm, frontal sinus involvement, gross cosmetic deformity, wound infection, pneumocephalus, or gross wound contamination.[46]

A special type of depressed fracture is fracture of the frontal sinus. Depression of the fracture may require surgery

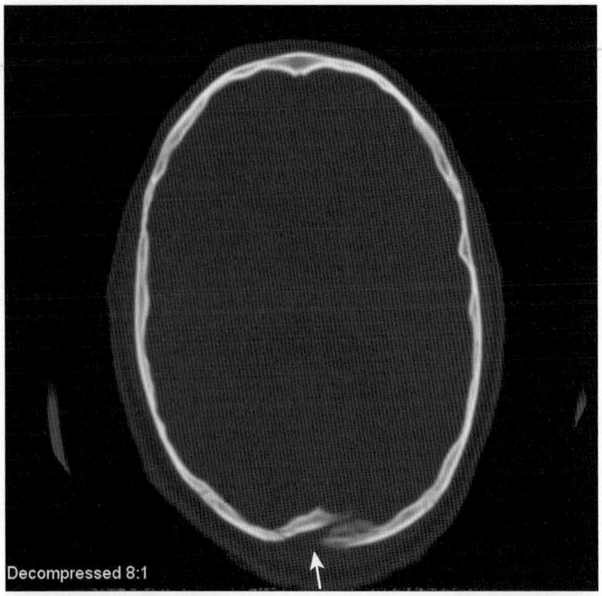

A

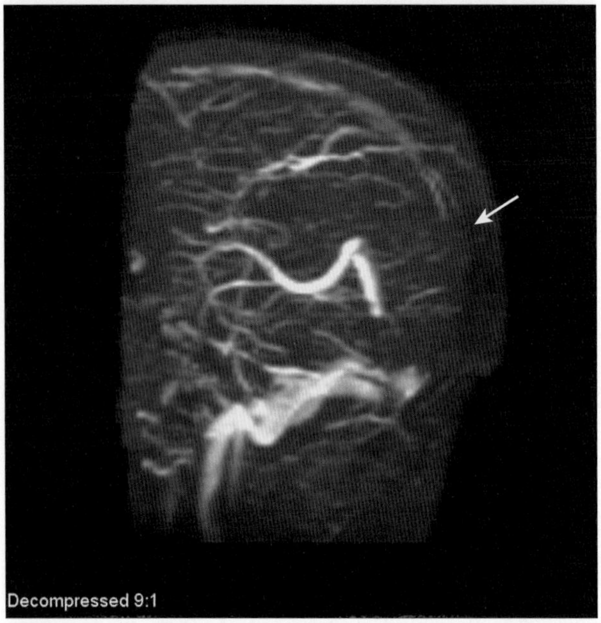

B

Figure 66.4 Depressed skull fracture requiring urgent decompressive surgery. The patient was a 32-year-old man hit on the back of the head by a metal beam at a construction site who presented with a deteriorating level of consciousness. **A,** Axial computed tomography scan demonstrates an open depressed skull fracture *(arrow)* at the level of the superior sagittal sinus (SSS) that extended down to the confluence of the transverse and SSS. **B,** Sagittal magnetic resonance venogram demonstrates occlusion of venous outflow *(arrow)* at the level of the fracture, which necessitated emergency surgical decompression and repair of the SSS.

to prevent CNS infection and CSF leak (Fig. 66.4). Another special type of depressed fracture involves a major dural venous sinus (see Fig. 66.4). Under these circumstances, the risks associated with surgery are increased, and elevation of the fracture fragment generally is reserved for significant compromise of venous drainage.[44]

EPIDURAL HEMATOMA

The next anatomic layer after the skull is the dura, which is the periosteum of the inner table of the skull and, as such, is tightly adherent to the bone. The potential space between the inner table of the skull and the dura is the *epidural space.* Epidural hematomas (EDHs) form in this potential space between the skull and the dura. The most common mechanism for the development of an EDH is a motor vehicle crash (in 53% of the cases), followed by falls (in 30%) and assault (in 8%).[52-60] Typically, bleeding results from damage to the middle meningeal artery, but an EDH also can occur from injury to the middle meningeal vein, diploic veins, or the venous sinuses.[60]

EDHs generally occur in the temporal and temporoparietal regions (Fig. 66.5).[52,57,61-64] A useful way to describe the development of an EDH is to follow the events that take place when a patient presents with an initial lucid interval following brief loss of consciousness after head trauma. A lucid interval occurs when a patient initially is rendered unconscious from a concussive head injury that causes a linear skull fracture involving the middle meningeal artery or one of its branches. The middle meningeal artery is a dural vessel that runs half in the dura and half through the groove in the inner table of the skull. When a fracture extends across the bony groove of the artery, it will tear and bleed. Because the dura is tightly adherent to the inner table of the skull, significant force is needed to push the dura off the inner table. An arterial hemorrhage generally has enough pressure to strip the dura off the bone, converting the potential epidural space into a mass. The bony attachment of the dura becomes progressively stronger with age; therefore, the dura of a younger patient requires less force to push it off the bone than would be required in an older patient. Not surprisingly, the mean age of patients with EDH is between 20 and 30 years of age,[53-55,63-70] and EDHs are unusual in patients older than 50.[60]

The growing epidural mass commonly compresses the anterior temporal lobe, which usually will not cause a major detectable neurologic deficit early in the course in the emergency department. During this so-called lucid component of the lucid interval, the patient regains consciousness from the concussive injury while the EDH is expanding and compressing the relatively silent anterior temporal lobe. The medial part of the temporal lobe, the uncas, lies just lateral to the brainstem at the level of the third cranial nerve (oculomotor nerve), which runs alongside the tentorial edge. When the EDH enlarges to the point at which it pushes the uncas of the temporal lobe over the tentorial edge, rapid development of a third nerve palsy, along with brainstem compression, is possible—which, at this level, will cause a contralateral hemiparesis from direct compression of the cerebral peduncle and a decrease in level of consciousness from the effect on the reticular activating system. The classic signs at this point are coma with a dilated pupil ipsilateral to the EDH and a contralateral hemiparesis. Occasionally, instead of directly compressing the ipsilateral cerebral peduncle, the herniating uncas can shift the brainstem into the contralateral tentorial edge, a relatively sharp rigid structure. This can damage the brainstem on the side opposite the EDH and cause a hemiparesis ipsilateral to the

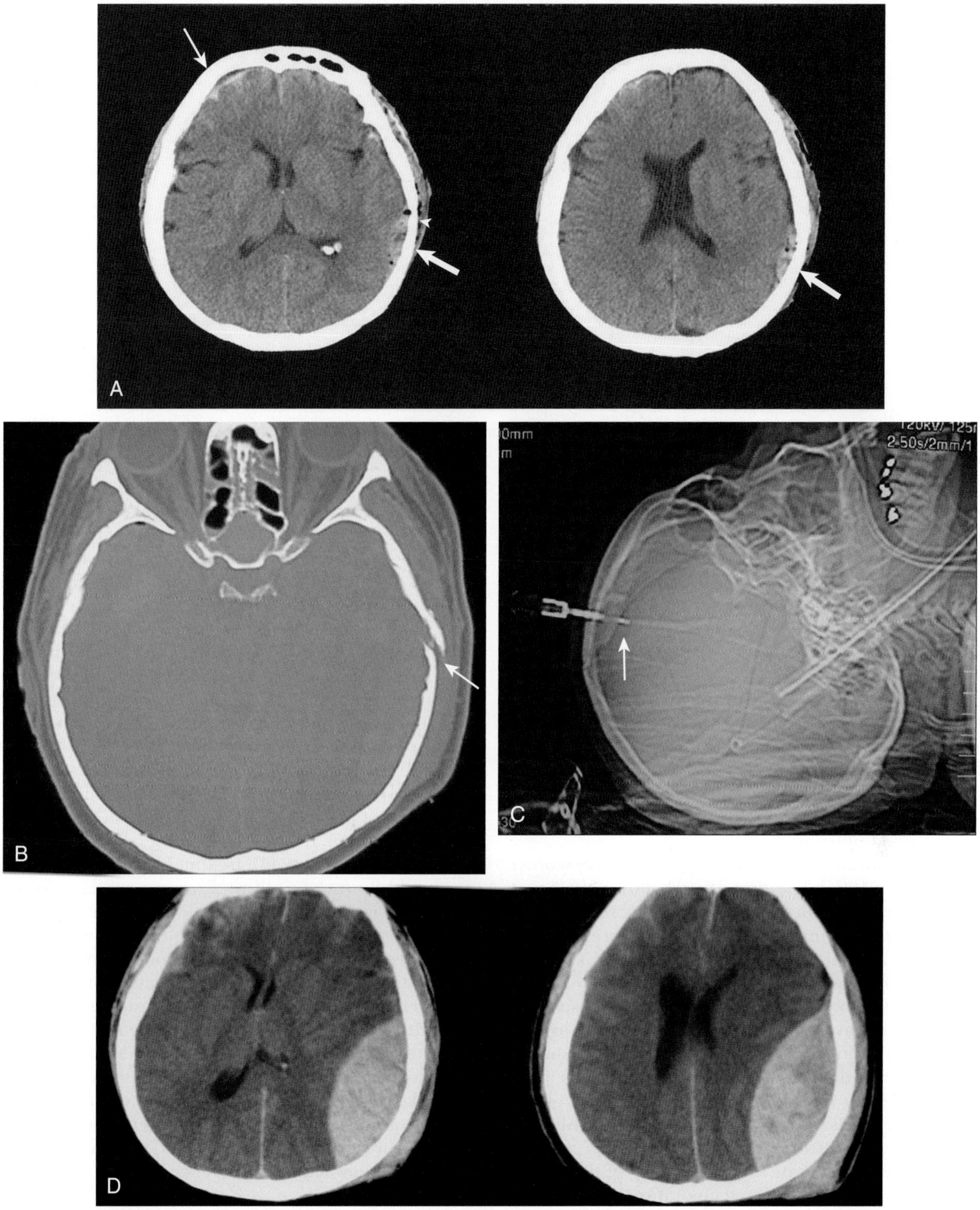

Figure 66.5 The patient was a 58-year-old female pedestrian who was hit by a car and unconscious at the accident scene. She was combative on presentation, pharmacologically paralyzed, and intubated in the trauma bay. **A,** Computed tomography (CT) image shows a small left temporal epidural hematoma without significant mass effect *(large arrow)*. Note the right frontal traumatic subarachnoid hemorrhage *(small, thin arrow)* and the small amount of air *(arrowhead)* from the associated open, linear fracture *(arrow)*, seen in **B.** There is no significant mass effect, and an intracranial pressure monitor *(arrow)* was placed, seen in **C.** Intracranial pressure (ICP) steadily increased shortly after placement, and immediate follow-up CT scans, shown in **D,** reveal marked expansion of the epidural hematoma with mass effect and shift requiring emergency craniotomy.

Continued on following page

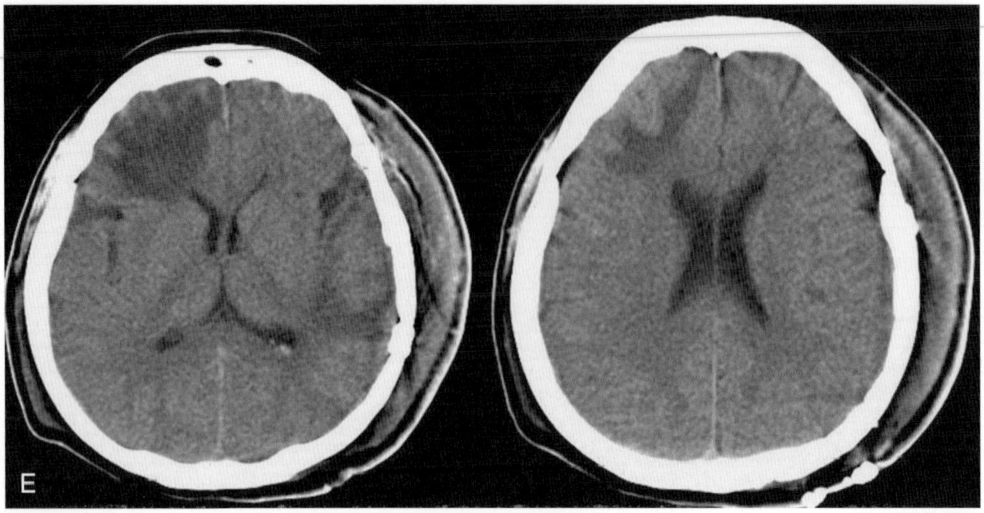

Figure 66.5, cont'd E, Postoperative CT scans reveal adequate decompression of surgical clot, with subsequent development of edema on the right side of the brain.

side of the hematoma. This is known as Kernohan's notch phenomenon.

Taking a general view, the patient goes from unconscious at the time of impact from a concussive injury, to awake, to unconscious again secondary to brainstem compression—hence the term *lucid interval.* The lucid interval is observed in close to half of the patients undergoing surgery for EDH.*

Pupillary abnormalities occur in approximately 20% to 30% of patients with surgical EDH.[52,54,59,60,67] Cranial fractures are present in between 70% and 95% of the cases.[54,60,68,70,74,75] Associated intracranial lesions are found in 30% to 50% of adults with surgical EDHs,[†] and subdural or parenchymal lesions in association with EDH lower the chance of a good outcome.[60]

The overall mortality rate (for all ages and GCS scores) is approximately 10%.[‡] The time lapse between the onset of pupillary abnormalities and surgery determines outcome,[61,66,80] but the single most important predictor of outcome in patients operated on for EDH is the GCS score on admission and before surgery.[52,53,55,61,81-83]

Not all EDHs, however, require surgery. No prospective randomized trials have been conducted to compare surgical treatment with nonoperative management, nor should there be. Available data describe nonsurgical management in selected cases. In one study, approximately 10% of the total number of EDHs were treated nonoperatively. All were conscious with a GCS score greater than 11 and a midline shift on CT scan of less than 10 mm. Not one of these nonoperative hematomas was in the temporal region.[84]

Another study reported findings in a group of 57 selected patients treated nonoperatively with an initial GCS score of 10 or higher, with maximum hematoma thickness less than 13 mm, with five clots located in the temporal region, but only one patient had a midline shift on CT.[53]

An interesting approach for dealing with thin, acute EDHs in an early stage has been reported in a small, isolated series of patients using endovascular techniques to occlude the middle meningeal artery.[85] Surgical decision making for an acute EDH is based on GCS score, pupillary findings, comorbid conditions, CT findings, age, and, in delayed decisions, ICP. Guidelines for the surgical management of acute EDH published in 2006 recommend surgical evacuation of an EDH less than 30 mL in volume. Smaller hematomas in patients with a GCS score greater than 8 and without focal deficits, clot thickness less than 15 mm, and less than 5 mm of midline shift may be considered for nonoperative management. Close neurologic monitoring and serial CT scanning are essential. Of importance, a temporal location for an EDH is associated with failure of nonoperative management and should lower the threshold for surgery.[60]

Because time between neurologic deterioration and surgery is critical, the question of whether a patient with an acute EDH should receive treatment at the nearest hospital or should be transferred to a trauma center is important. The issue is whether or not a non-neurosurgeon should operate on a patient deteriorating from an acute EDH as a true emergency. One suboptimally controlled study reported worse outcomes in a small group of patients who underwent emergency operations by non-neurosurgeons and attributed this mainly to the technical inadequacy of the operation.[59,60] Other studies have documented worse outcomes in patients transferred from outlying hospitals for surgery.[52,73] The take-home message is that EDHs are extra-axial hemorrhages located adjacent to the brainstem that can represent a true neurosurgical emergency, and that rapid, competent decompression makes a difference.

SUBDURAL HEMATOMA

Proceeding deep to the skull, the next space is the subdural space. Unlike the potential epidural space, the subdural space is a real space. It is a compartment that follows the contour of the brain, which is how it appears on a CT scan (Fig. 66.6). Anatomically, bridging veins course through the subdural space from the cerebral hemispheres to the superior sagittal sinus. As the brain accelerates within the skull after impact, these veins can stretch and tear.[86]

The source of bleeding also can be from a cortical artery[87,88] or vein. These hematomas typically form over the

*See references 52, 55, 60, 65, 69, 71-73.
†See references 52, 54, 55, 57-60, 63-67, 73, 76, 77.
‡See references 54, 55, 64, 65, 68, 72, 73, 78, 79.

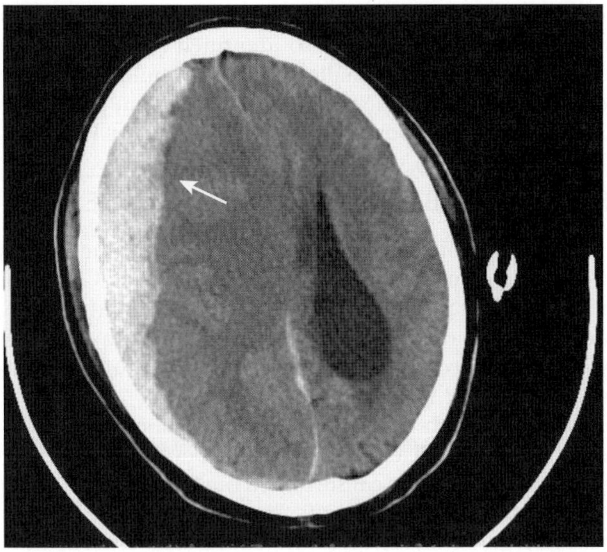

Figure 66.6 Axial computed tomography scan demonstrating a typical acute subdural hematoma *(arrow)*. Note that the hematoma expands the subdural space and follows the contour of the brain as it generates severe extra-axial mass effect and shift.

surface or between the cerebral hemispheres, along the tentorium, or between the temporal lobe and base of the skull.

An acute subdural hematoma (SDH), as defined by Bullock and colleagues, appears within 14 days of injury,[60] although some authors consider an SDH to be subacute when signs and symptoms develop between 3 and 20 days after trauma.[89]

Acute SDHs consist of clotted blood, which is fibrous and often adherent to adjacent tissue. The blood remains clotted for several days. After this time, the clot gradually and progressively lyses, resulting in a mixture of clot and fluid. After several weeks, the clot is liquefied and becomes a chronic SDH. Chronic SDHs may manifest weeks or months after what may have been mild or insignificant trauma. Chronic SDHs occur more often in elderly patients and individuals who have more intracranial space because of cortical atrophy. A membrane often surrounds these hematomas, and the collection of fluid may slowly grow in size because of repeated small bleeds or accumulation of fluid transudate from the membrane.[86]

The incidence of acute SDHs is approximately 20% in severe traumatic brain injury,[60,90-93] and the mean age is between 31 and 47 years, with most of the patients being men.[60,94-97] The mechanism of injury differs between age groups, with patients older than 65 more commonly presenting after a fall, and younger patients being involved more often in a motor vehicle crash,[60,98-100] which, among comatose patients with acute SDH, is the most common mechanism of injury.[60,91,93,101]

Between 37% and 80% of patients with acute SDH present with a GCS score of 8 or lower,[60,65,71,94,97,102] and the overall mortality rate is between 40% and 60%.* Mortality rates among comatose patients requiring surgery are somewhat higher, with reported rates between 57% and 68%.† Acute

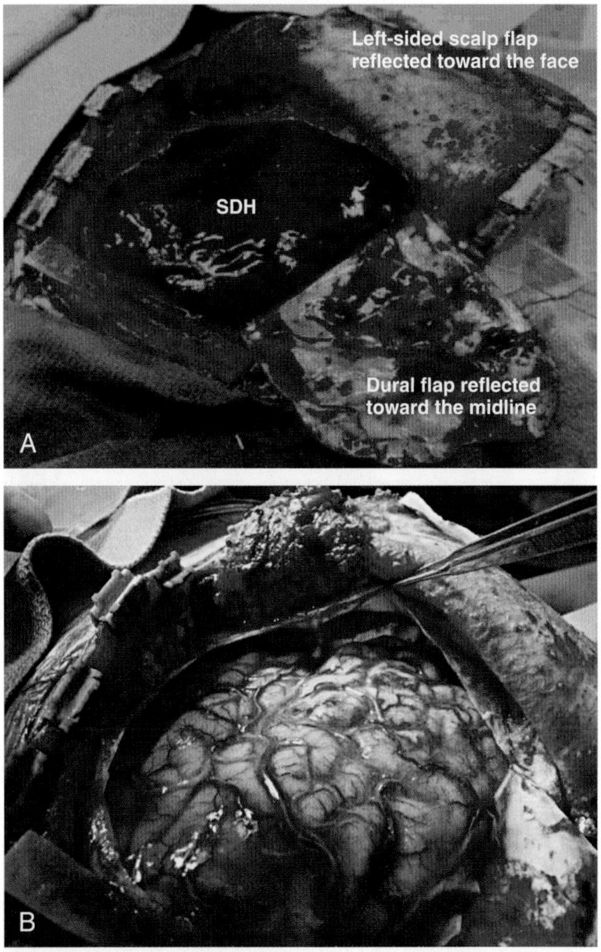

Figure 66.7 **A,** Intraoperative view of a solid subdural hematoma (SDH) on the surface of the brain. **B,** Decompressed brain with demonstration of evacuated subdural space.

subdural hematomas frequently are associated with other brain injuries,[97,102] which is one of the reasons why the mortality rate is relatively high.

A simple acute SDH is a subdural, extra-axial hematoma without any other associated brain injury (Fig. 66.7). A complex SDH is associated with parenchymal injury (Fig. 66.8).[107,108] Fewer than half of acute SDHs requiring surgery are isolated, simple lesions.[60,97,102]

One useful method to identify the presence of associated injury is to measure the thickness of the subdural clot relative to the amount of brain shift on the CT scan. If the amount of shift is directly proportional to the thickness of the extra-axial clot, the injury is likely to be simple and only the brain compressed. However, if the amount of shift is more than expected as indicated by the size of the hematoma, then additional parenchymal brain injury probably is present under the clot, causing additive mass effect. Not surprisingly, the mortality for complex injuries is higher than that for simple SDHs.[107,108]

In addition to the obvious compressive effects that an SDH generates, the available evidence points to a direct toxic effect of the blood itself on the underlying cortex, thereby compounding the problem.[109,110]

Age is an important factor in acute SDHs. There is a significant increase in poor outcome among patients older than 60 years of age with severe head injury in

*See references 60, 66, 92, 95, 96, 103-106.
†See references 60, 76, 81, 91, 92, 101, 106.

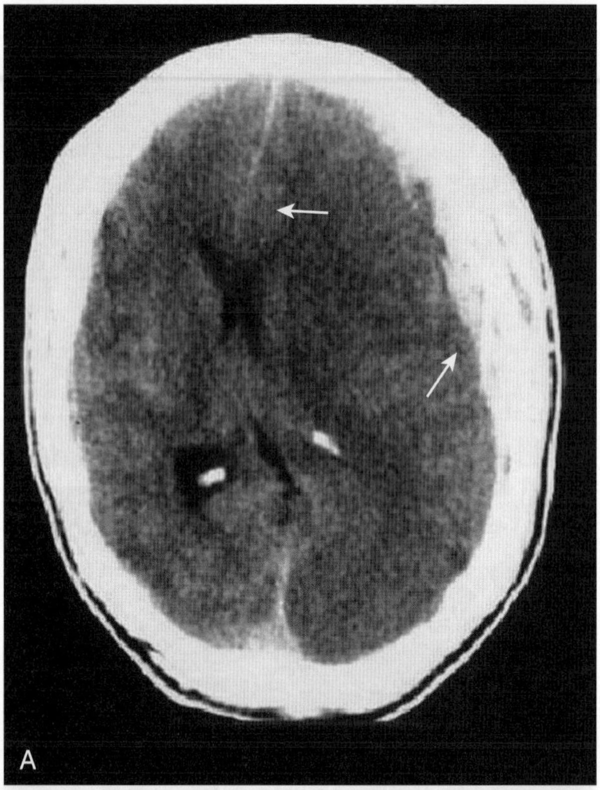

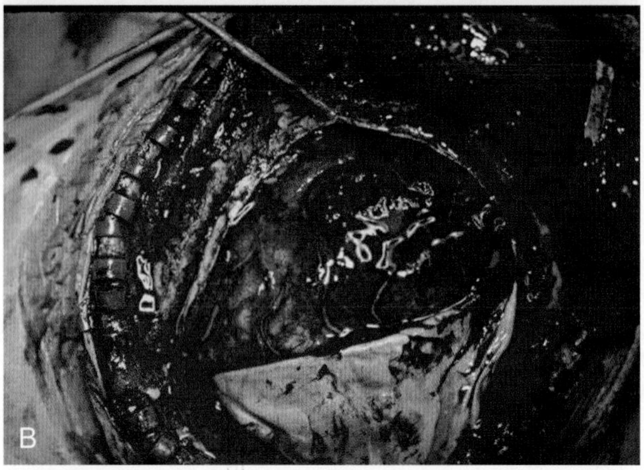

Figure 66.8 **A,** Computed tomography scan of acute, complex left-sided subdural hematoma (SDH) *(lower arrow)* with mass effect *(upper arrow)* out of proportion to the size of the clot, indicating more than just the effect of an extra-axial compressive mass—that is, intrinsic, parenchymal brain injury with edema. **B,** Intraoperative photograph of decompressed brain reveals hemorrhagic, inflamed, and edematous brain swelling out through the cranial defect. Compare with the intraoperative photograph of the simple SDH in Figure 66.7.

general.[93,98-101,111,112] Older patients with an acute SDH and a low GCS score do especially poorly.[98-101,111,112]

The decision for immediate surgery is dependent on GCS score, age, pupillary examination, comorbidities, CT findings, and salvageability with respect to the patient's level of injury. In addition to all of these factors, decision making for delayed surgery is dependent on clinical course and ICP.[60]

On the basis of a contemporary search of the literature, Bullock and colleagues found that CT parameters of a midline shift greater than 5 mm and a clot thickness greater than 10 mm were independent factors requiring surgery in salvageable patients. They also identified a select group of comatose patients with smaller SDHs who could be managed nonoperatively if the patients remained neurologically stable with normal pupils and ICP of 20 mm or less.[60]

TRAUMATIC SUBARACHNOID HEMORRHAGE

The subarachnoid space is a CSF-filled compartment within which are the major cerebral blood vessels. The CSF within the subarachnoid space fills the basal cisterns and interdigitates into the cortical sulci. Traumatic SAH can be caused by bleeding of cortical arteries, veins, or brain surface cerebral contusions.[113]

In contrast with hemorrhages in other locations, SAH is not a discrete surgical clot that requires evacuation. Trauma is the most common cause of SAH; a ruptured aneurysm is the most common cause of a spontaneous SAH. Aneurysmal SAH generally involves the suprasellar cistern, where the circle of Willis lies. Traumatic SAH can be found as small-volume hemorrhages in the sylvian fissures and especially in the interpeduncular cistern. Traumatic SAH also commonly involves the cerebral convexity and can fill cortical sulci, which can sometimes mimic sulcal effacement[114] (Fig. 66.9A).

Occasionally, the distribution of the hemorrhage may be hard to differentiate from an aneurysmal hemorrhage. Under this circumstance, a vascular study should be obtained (Fig. 66.9B). Cerebral vasospasm following aneurysmal SAH is a common, well-described problem with an unclear pathogenesis. Increasing evidence suggests that SAH from trauma also may cause clinically significant cerebral vasospasm, which may be responsible for ischemia and infarction.[115,116]

Clearly the incidence of clinically relevant cerebral vasospasm is less than what is seen in aneurysmal SAH; however, posttraumatic SAH may cause ischemia during the acute as well as the delayed phase.[115,117]

In severe nonpenetrating head injury, the degree of SAH can be predictive of outcome,[118,119] and although traumatic SAH can be an isolated finding, it is commonly associated with other intracranial injuries.[120]

Traumatic SAH can be a marker of severe primary injury and the amount of blood can also be an independent predictor of the development and progression of intraparenchymal contusions[113] (Fig. 66.9C).

INTRAPARENCHYMAL CONTUSIONS AND HEMATOMAS

Traumatic parenchymal mass lesions are common and are reported in 13% to 35% of severe traumatic brain injury.[121-127] Contusions consist of heterogeneous areas of necrosis, pulping, infarction, hemorrhage, and edema.[89,128,129] Hemorrhagic contusions are mixtures of blood and edematous cerebral parenchyma that also have a heterogeneous appearance on CT.[89] Contusions commonly occur in the frontal and temporal lobes both at the poles and on the inferior surfaces as a result of contact with the rough, bony skull base[130] (Fig. 66.10A).

Contusions typically involve the crests of the gyri but in more severe injury may extend into the substance of the

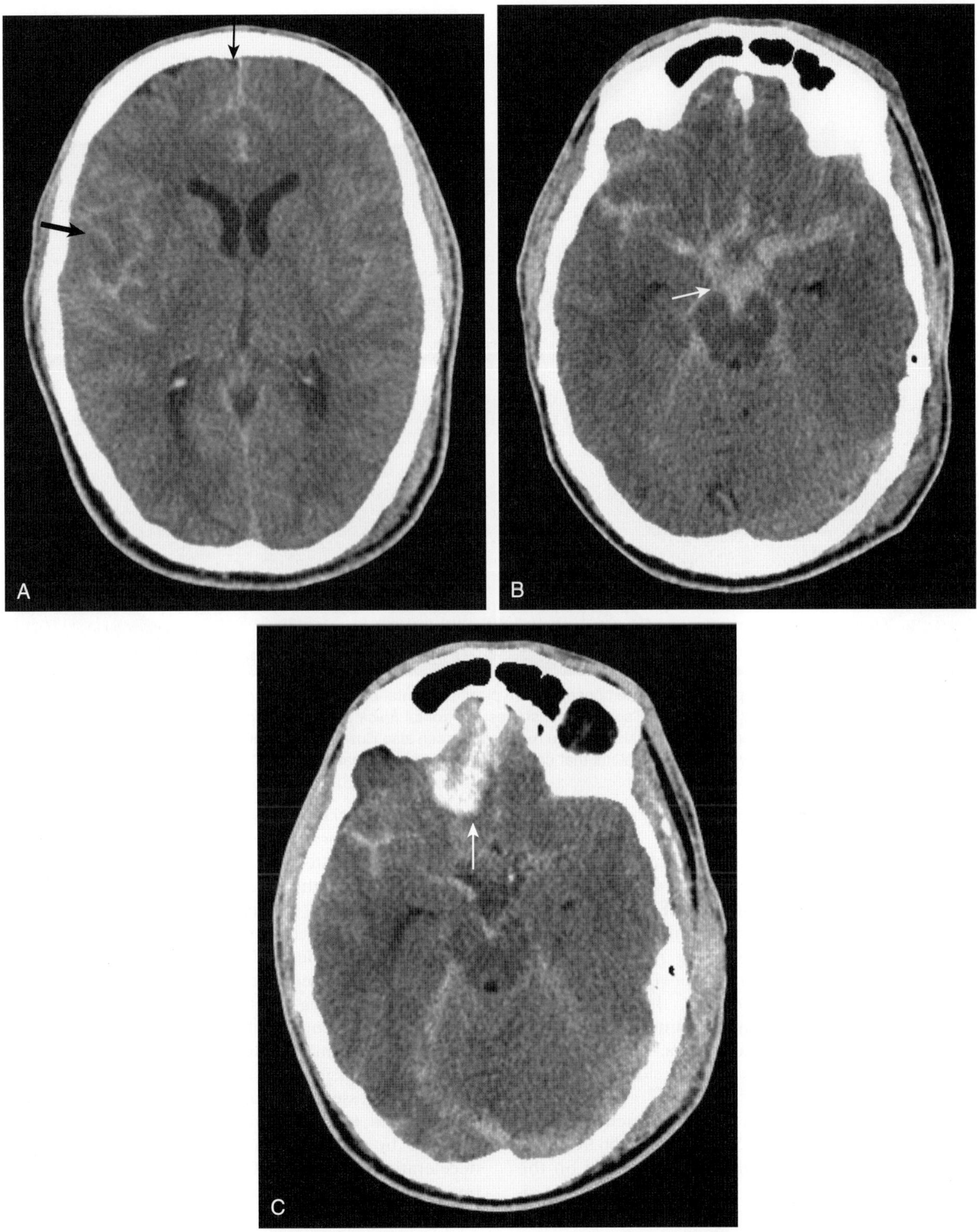

Figure 66.9 The patient was a 25-year-old man who sustained a brain injury in a motorcycle accident. **A,** Computed tomography (CT) scan immediately after the accident demonstrates traumatic subarachnoid hemorrhage (SAH) in cortical sulci *(thick arrow)* and anterior interhemispheric fissure *(thin arrow)*. **B,** CT scan at the level of the circle of Willis reveals a distribution of subarachnoid blood *(arrow)* throughout the suprasellar cistern, a pattern similar to that seen with a ruptured aneurysm. Findings on an immediate cerebral angiogram to rule out an aneurysm were normal. **C,** Follow-up CT scan obtained 8.5 hours later demonstrates an intraparenchymal contusion *(arrow)* that was not seen on the initial study, with rapid clearing of the traumatic SAH in the suprasellar cistern.

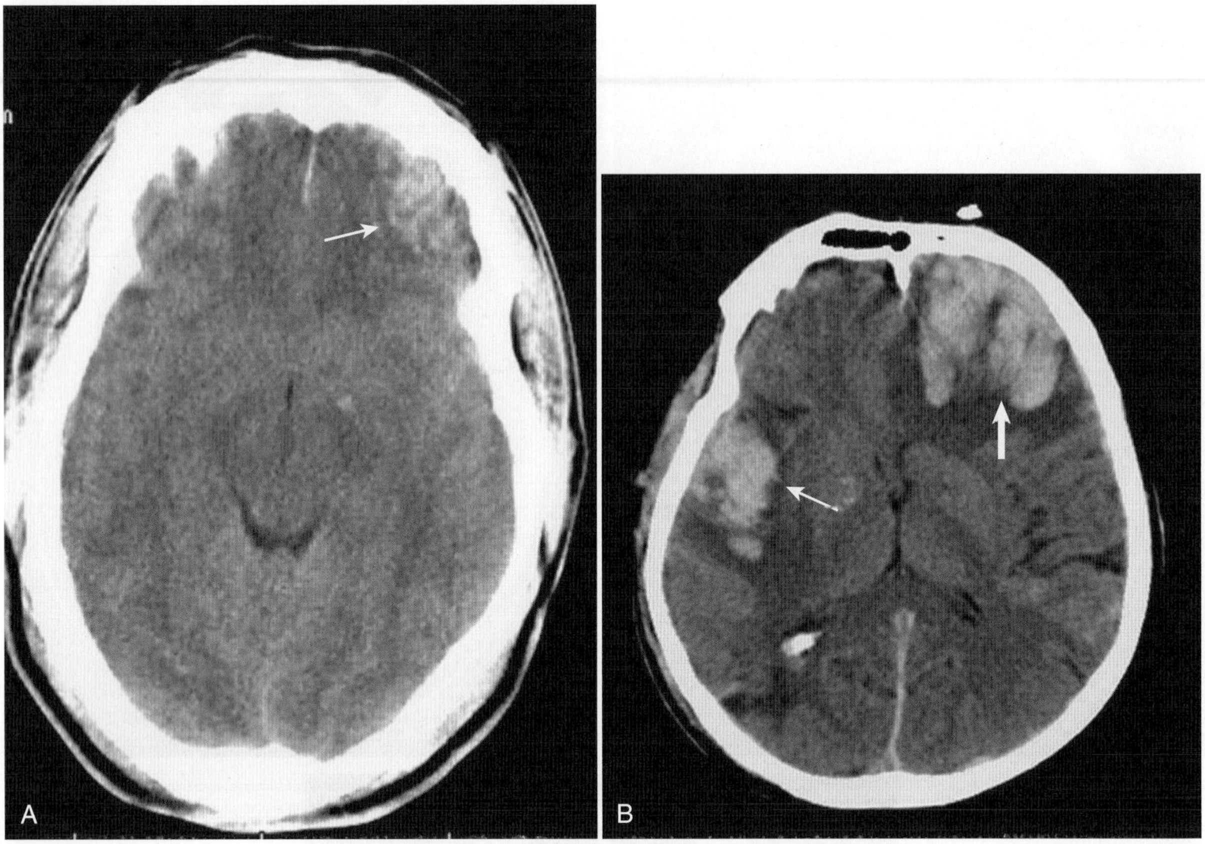

Figure 66.10 **A,** Computed tomography (CT) scan demonstrates a typical left frontal basal contusion *(arrow)* where the brain interfaces with the rough base of the anterior cranial fossa. **B,** CT scan demonstrates left frontal *(thick arrow)* and right temporal hemorrhagic *(thin arrow)* contusions. The floor of the middle (temporal) fossa also is quite rough. This scan also illustrates the continuum from contusion to hematoma. Note the large, homogeneous areas within the contusions that could be classified as hematomas.

white matter. If the pia-arachnoid is torn, contusions are classified as cortical lacerations.[130-132]

Contusions represent one end of a spectrum of injury on which hematomas, which are well-defined, homogeneous collections of blood, are the other end (Fig. 66.10B). The amount of energy delivered may have only been enough to cause failure of small vessels, resulting in contusions. If more energy is delivered, failure of larger vessels may occur, resulting in hematomas. Alternatively, the hemorrhagic component of a contusion may continue to bleed and coalesce into a more discrete hematoma. In general, the most common traumatic parenchymal lesions are contusions,[89] and they tend to evolve.[122,126,127,133,134]

Risk factors for the progression of intraparenchymal hemorrhage include the presence of SAH (see Fig. 66.9C), and subdural hematoma, as well as the size of the clot on the initial CT scan. Enlargement of contusions occurs approximately 40% of the time, which justifies early follow-up CT scanning.[135] In addition to the problem of progressive enlargement of existing contusions is a phenomenon of delayed appearance of traumatic intracerebral contusions (DITCH). DITCH is defined as a new contusion identified on a CT scan in an area of brain that was normal on the admission CT scan. These delayed hemorrhages are reported to occur in up to 7% of patients with severe head injuries.[90]

Contusions can be subdivided into two groups. *Coup* contusions occur in the brain tissue under the impact site and usually are associated with an acceleration injury. *Contrecoup* contusions are located away from the point of impact and usually are associated with a deceleration injury.[130,131,136-138]

Understanding the biomechanics of how a contrecoup contusion develops is useful. In general, biologic tissues tolerate strain better if they are deformed slowly rather than quickly. For example, a 150-mL hematoma with accumulation of blood over minutes is likely to be lethal, whereas a 150-mL slow-growing meningioma may have no appreciable effect on the patient's level of consciousness. In trauma, the cause of tissue damage may be any of three types of induced strains: compression, tension, and shear. The skull, brain, and blood vessels will tolerate compression better than tension, and tension better than shear. These strains are induced by contact or inertia (relative to acceleration-deceleration), or both. Contact injuries are a result of impact, which may cause inward deformation of the skull with local effects, and of shock waves, which can produce remote effects. As a consequence of contact the head is set in motion, which leads to inertial injury. Inertial injuries may cause damage by differential acceleration of the skull and brain. In addition, acceleration-deceleration can independently produce strains in the brain itself. The two clinically relevant types of acceleration are translational (when the brain moves in a straight line) and angular. Most injuries are a combination of both.[139]

These effects are best illustrated by a case example of a 37-year-old man who falls from a height onto the back of his

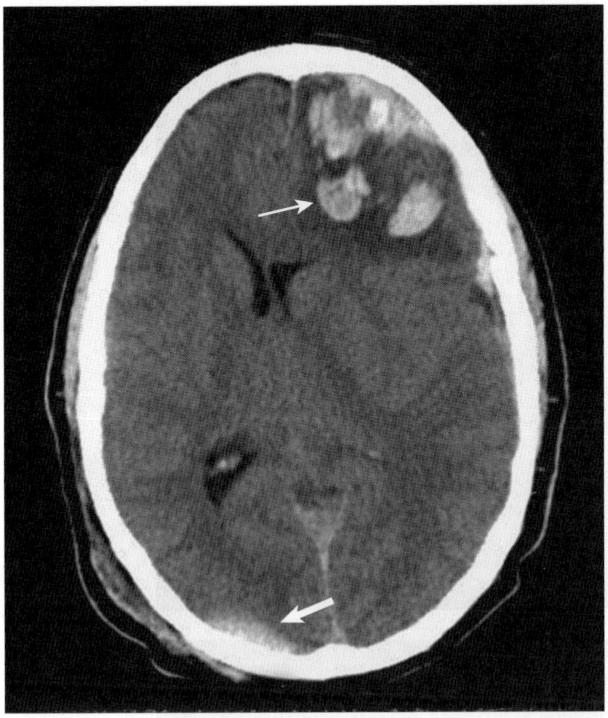

Figure 66.11 Computed tomography scan demonstrates a relatively small right occipital hemorrhage *(thick arrow)* underlying the point of impact as confirmed by the overlying soft tissue swelling of the scalp and a large, left frontal hemorrhagic contrecoup contusion *(thin arrow)*.

head and presents with a deteriorating level of consciousness. His CT scan (Fig. 66.11) reveals soft tissue swelling at the point of impact in the right occipital region with a small underlying hemorrhage, as well as a large, hemorrhagic contusion in the left frontal lobe. The mechanism involved is primarily translational (linear) deceleration. The skull stops suddenly as it hits the ground, but the brain continues to move toward the impact site, where compression is induced (Fig. 66.12).

As the brain is moving toward the inner table of the skull at the impact site, it also is moving away from the skull on the opposite side, creating regions of low pressure and tensile strains. Contributing to the extensive tissue damage in the left frontal lobe also may be movement of the brain across the rough surface of the anterior cranial base.[89,139]

The same amount of energy is delivered to the brain in nearly a straight line, with the compressive injury at the point of impact resulting in much less damage than the contrecoup injury caused by tension. In view of the dramatic differential susceptibilities of the brain and blood vessels to compressive and tensile strains induced in trauma, it is understandable that diffuse injuries can be caused by seemingly less violent trauma when the head undergoes an injury with a large component of angular acceleration-deceleration. This is the motion that can induce shearing strains, which the tissues tolerate poorly (see "Diffuse Axonal Injury" later on).

Surgical decision making is more straightforward for epidural and subdural types of hematomas, in which the extra-axial mass causing compression is simply on the surface of the brain. Contusions and hematomas, however, are intra-axial masses intimately associated with surrounding regions of brain that may be salvageable. It is one thing to surgically evacuate an extra-axial hematoma *compressing* the dominant frontal lobe, and quite another to operate on a large contusion *within* the dominant frontal lobe.

In 2006, guidelines were published after a thorough review of the relevant but scientifically weak literature. The reviewers reported that patients with parenchymal mass lesions and signs of progressive neurologic deterioration referable to the lesion, medically refractory intracranial hypertension, or signs of mass effect on CT scan should be treated operatively. Patients with GCS scores of 6 to 8 with frontal or temporal contusions greater than 20 cc in volume with midline shift of at least 5 mm or cisternal compression on CT scan and patients with any lesion greater than 50 cc in volume should receive operative treatment. Patients with parenchymal mass lesions who do not show evidence of neurologic compromise, whose ICP is controlled, and who demonstrate no significant signs of mass effect on CT scan may be managed nonoperatively with intensive monitoring and serial imaging. For patients with refractory intracranial hypertension and diffuse parenchymal injury with clinical and radiographic evidence for impending transtentorial herniation, the guidelines also recommended, as treatment options, subtemporal decompression, temporal lobectomy, or hemispheric decompressive craniectomy (Fig. 66.13). With regard to timing of surgery, the literature supports a bifrontal decompressive craniectomy within 48 hours of injury as a treatment option for patients with diffuse, medically refractory posttraumatic cerebral edema and resultant intracranial hypertension.[127]

HYPOTHALAMIC-PITUITARY INJURY

Injury to the pituitary and hypothalamus can complicate head injury. A prolonged loss of consciousness often is reported in patients with such injuries. Up to 80% of cases are associated with a fracture through the skull base. Injuries include (in decreasing order of frequency) pericapsular hemorrhage, hypothalamic infarction, posterior pituitary hemorrhage, anterior pituitary infarction, and rupture of the infundibulum.[140-142] Clinically measurable decreases in pituitary hormone production are not seen until at least 75% of the gland is destroyed. Complete loss of production requires destruction of at least 90% of the gland.

Derangements in pituitary function can result in decreased production of any of the pituitary hormones. Of particular clinical significance is impairment of adrenocorticotropic hormone release that can result in secondary adrenal insufficiency (Addison's disease). Physiologic stressors such as trauma, surgery, or infection can result in addisonian crisis, with potentially life-threatening results. Diabetes insipidus has been reported in a significant number of severe head injuries, with a high percentage of cases remaining permanent.[143] Injuries to the pituitary often are not suspected in the acute period, and the diagnosis of hypopituitarism is therefore often delayed (Fig. 66.14).

DIFFUSE AXONAL INJURY

The term *diffuse axonal injury* (DAI) describes brain damage in a group of patients who become immediately

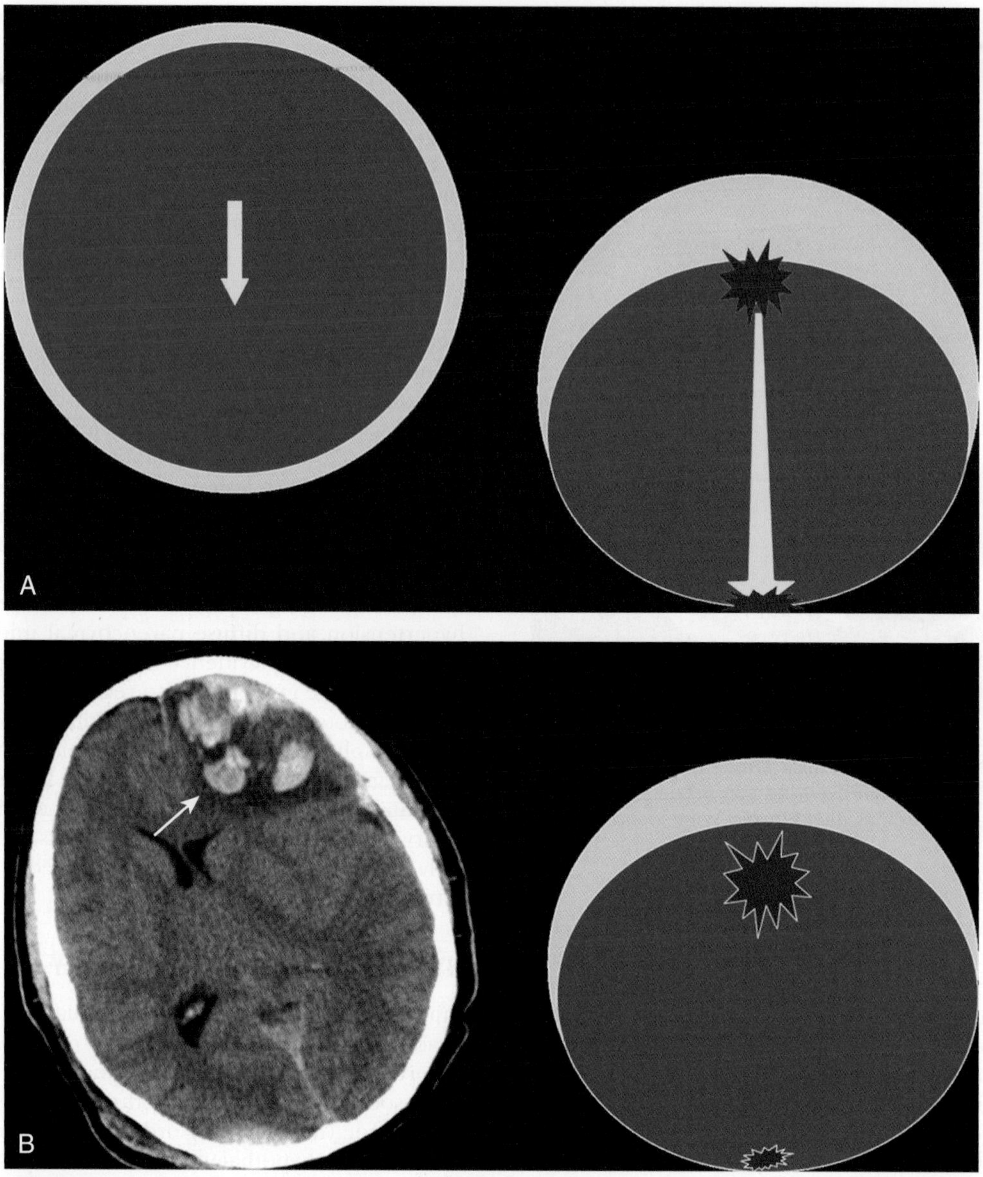

Figure 66.12 **A,** Schematic representing the head falling in a straight line. Rapid deceleration of the skull occurs as the brain continues to move toward the impact site. The energy is applied in a linear trajectory, resulting in a compressive strain generated at the impact site and a tensile strain at the opposite point *(right diagram)*. The same energy delivered to the brain results in more damage by tension than compression. **B,** A comparison of this schematic with that for a similar mechanism of injury would demonstrate why a contrecoup contusion (*arrow* on computed tomography scan, *left*) generally is more severe than the injury sustained as a result of compression at the point of impact.

unconscious or go into coma at the time of the head trauma.[81] Depending on the severity of the injury, patients may have mild, moderate, or severe DAI. A large number of patients with severe head injury will have DAI. Because of the gradient acceleration difference of certain brain areas during primary impact, shearing forces at the gray-white junction, corpus callosum, or brainstem may occur.[131,144] The result of these forces will be diffuse tearing of axons and small blood vessels. These lesions initially may be hemorrhagic, but as they become chronic, shrinking, softening, and scarring ensue, often with cyst formation.[42,145] The lesions usually are microscopic but can be large and macroscopic. Although small, focal, petechial hemorrhages may be visualized, the initial CT scan often is normal.[146] Most of the clinical and experimental studies support that the diffuse injury occurs at the time of initial impact and is not the result of other adverse factors, such as decreased brain oxygenation, increased ICP, or brain swelling,[145,147] although these factors tend to accentuate the amount of damage.

The term *gliding contusions* originally was introduced by Lindenberg and Freytag[148] to describe hemorrhagic lesions in parasagittal white matter; this brain injury concept has been reanalyzed.[149] Gliding contusions frequently are found in association with DAI and acute subdural hematomas. Two mechanisms have been considered in relation to the formation of these contusions. First, during angular acceleration, more movement and displacement of the cortical gray matter occur than of the deep white matter; accordingly, most of the tissue injury occurs at the gray-white junction because shearing strains predominate. The

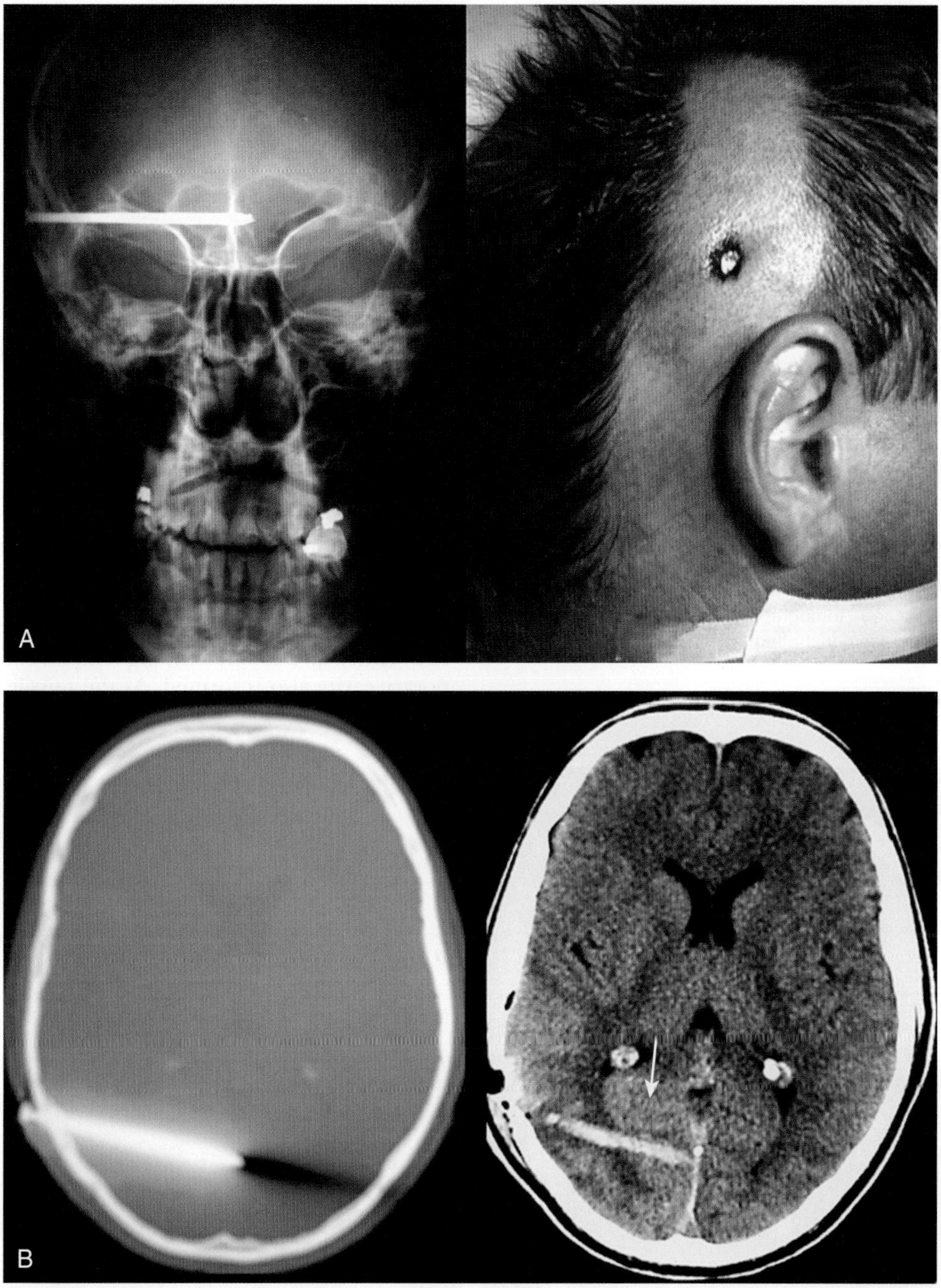

Figure 66.13 A 32-year-old man presented awake and alert after accidental discharge of a nail gun to the head while working at a construction site. **A,** *Left*, An anteroposterior radiograph of the skull demonstrates the nail. *Right*, On this intraoperative photograph, the head of the nail can be seen indenting the surface of the scalp. **B,** Preoperative bone-windowed computed tomography (CT) scan *(left)* and immediate postoperative brain-windowed CT scan *(right)* demonstrate the blood-stained tract after removal.

second mechanism involves excessive displacement of the bridging veins during brain acceleration. Patients with severe DAI who survive may be profoundly disabled, but some patients with mild or moderate DAI may recover with mild or no disability.[81] The importance of recognizing DAI in the initial evaluation cannot be overstressed; this will affect the management and outcome. Clinically, these patients will have impaired consciousness secondary to bicortical damage, possibly in association with unremarkable imaging findings and normal ICP.

PENETRATING BRAIN INJURY

It is estimated that between 6000 to 7000 people die each year in the United States from gunshot wounds to the brain.[130-139,150-152]

CLASSIFICATION

Low-velocity penetrating brain injuries include wounds from nail guns, arrows, and knives and some types of gunshot wounds (Fig. 66.15). Gunshot wounds are divided into

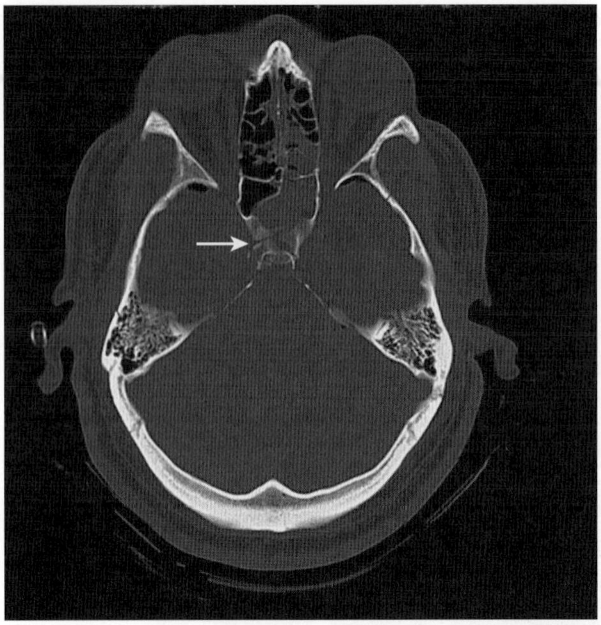

Figure 66.14 Computed tomography scan through the skull base in bone window demonstrating fractures through the sella turcica *(arrow).*

low-velocity injuries, such as from civilian handguns and shrapnel, and high-velocity injuries, from rifles and military weapons[152] (see Table 66.1).

An Israeli report described an intermediate type of injury from spherical bolts whereby the ball bearings used by suicide bombers, having unique ballistics, may cause a type of "stab wound" injury to the brain.[152]

BALLISTICS

The biomechanics of penetrating brain injury (PBI) are important and require an understanding of the dynamics of projectiles—that is, ballistics. Ballistics can be divided into three phases. The first phase, internal ballistics, deals with the source of the projectile and its intrinsic dynamics (e.g., rifle, bomb). External ballistics, the second phase, focuses on the flight of the projectile itself and the deviation of its longitudinal axis relative to the line of flight, referred to as yaw motion. Collision of the projectile with any object during this external phase will change the speed, angle, and yaw. The third phase is referred to as terminal ballistics, which is the physical interaction between the projectile and the body.[152]

As the projectile directly crushes tissue, it forms a permanent cavity, and as surrounding tissue is compressed, a temporary cavity also is formed. As the missile breaks through

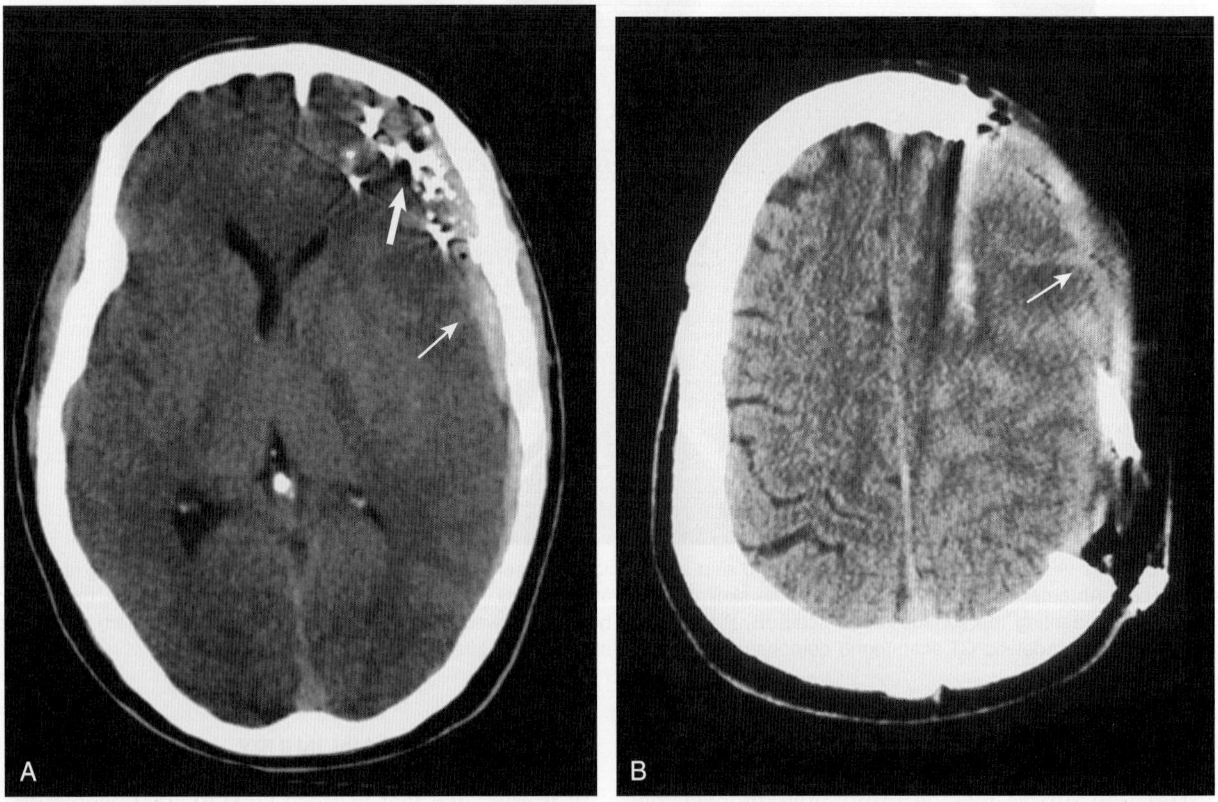

Figure 66.15 The patient was a 27-year-old man with a self-inflicted gunshot wound to the head who presented with a deteriorating level of consciousness. The patient put the muzzle of a handgun to the right medial orbital roof. The bullet traversed the frontal sinus and traveled through the left frontal lobe. **A,** Computed tomography (CT) scan demonstrates bullet fragments *(thick arrow)* and an associated left frontotemporal acute subdural hematoma *(thin arrow),* requiring surgical evacuation and hemicraniectomy for anticipated swelling. **B,** Postoperative CT scan demonstrates edematous hemisphere herniating out through the cranial defect *(arrow)*. There was damage to the anterior cranial base with contamination secondary to involvement of the frontal sinus. Surgical repair of the skull base was delayed because of the anticipated cerebral edema, and the patient was placed on antibiotics. When the cerebral swelling resolved, there was no evidence of cerebrospinal fluid (CSF) rhinorrhea or infection. The patient never required the delayed repair of the anterior cranial base anticipated. He made an excellent neurologic recovery and returned to work as a professional recruiter several months after replacement of his cranial bone flap.

the skull, secondary projectiles of bone fragments may be generated, causing independent, secondary permanent and temporary cavities.[152-156]

Terminal ballistics are influenced by many factors, such as size, shape, and stability of the penetrating object; however, most authors (but not all) believe that entrance velocity is the most important factor in determining the degree of tissue damage.[152,153,155,157-159] Experimental evidence has demonstrated an immediate increase in ICP with a pressure wave transmitted throughout the cranial cavity, which probably accounts for the transient respiratory arrest observed in PBI.[152,160] High-velocity injuries (velocity greater than 320 meters per second) cause shock waves that emanate from the front of the missile. These shock waves can reflect off the inside of the skull and summate, producing significant pressure gradients with remote effects.

INITIAL RESUSCITATION

Initial resuscitation in the trauma bay should be in accordance with current recommendations for head-injured patients in general. During this initial resuscitation, it is important to recognize that hypotension in PBI either is a terminal event or is related to other injuries. Once resuscitation has been accomplished, a CT scan is essential. Although skull films seldom add to the information obtained from a CT scan,[152] our group has found plain films to be very helpful in PBI, particularly in industrial accidents, in which the shape of the penetrating object may be unknown.

SURGICAL MANAGEMENT

Most of what is known about the surgical management of PBI comes from the battlefield, beginning with World War I, when Harvey Cushing, the father of American neurosurgery, described his technique of en bloc craniectomy under aseptic conditions; thorough debridement of scalp, bone, brain, metal, and bone fragments; and watertight closure of the scalp. Using this management strategy a century ago, in the absence of antibiotics, Cushing reported a significant drop in postoperative mortality from 55% to 28%.[161,162]

Mortality decreased even further in World War II, primarily because neurosurgical personnel were present in forward military hospitals and antibiotics were introduced. The operative approach, however, was largely the same: that of radical debridement. Treatment consisted of four tiers: emergent life-saving maneuvers through hemostasis and cerebral decompression; prevention of infection through extensive debridement; preservation of nervous tissue through prevention of meningocerebral scars; and restoration of anatomic structures through accurate closure of the dura and scalp. Although untested against other management strategies, this approach became the standard of treatment for PBI by default. Indeed, in the U.S. military, thorough debridement of intracranial bone and metal fragments was official military policy through the Vietnam War.[162]

The overall mortality rate from PBI sustained during relatively modern wartime conditions ranges from 8% to 43% and generally is considered to be in the 20% range.[162-171] The mortality rate from military gunshot wounds has been reported to be 2.5 to 4 times more than from shrapnel.[162-165,170] Of interest, mortality rates from wartime PBIs in the U.S. military from World War II through the Vietnam War did not change significantly,[172] which is consistent with the relatively unchanged management strategy of complete removal of intracranial bone or metal fragments, using repeated surgery as necessary.[173]

Aggressive debridement was intended to reduce complications such as infection, epilepsy, and cerebral edema. However, studies reveal that additional surgery to remove retained fragments results in significant morbidity and mortality.[170,174,175]

The use of broad-spectrum antibiotics in recent wars has resulted in data suggesting that retained bone fragments are not independently associated with an increased risk of infection. Therefore, aggressive debridement is no longer supported.[162,176] The use of broad-spectrum antibiotics in PBI has now become universal.[152]

Multiple studies have looked at post-PBI epilepsy and reported an incidence of 22% to 53%.[167,177,178] Several studies suggest that it is not necessary to remove all bone fragments in order to decrease the chance of developing epilepsy, but the value of removing metal fragments in this regard remains unclear.[162,167,169,177,178] In military PBI, it appears that vigorous debridement is associated with increased morbidity and mortality and is not necessary to prevent infection, has no obvious efficacy in preventing epilepsy, and does not appear to improve survival.[162]

A CSF leak resulting from a PBI is the variable most highly correlated with intracranial infection.* One study found that most CSF leaks appeared within 2 weeks of the injury and less than half of them closed spontaneously. The incidence of infection was approximately 10 times higher in the group with CSF fistulas than in the group without leaks, and the mortality was greater as well.[181] Because CSF leaks are the primary predictor of the development of intracranial infection,[167,169,171] it is important to fix or prevent a CSF leak; therefore, a watertight closure of the scalp entry wound is necessary.[181]

To accomplish this objective, various surgical interventions are available. Small entrance wounds without underlying surgical pathology may be cleaned up and closed in the emergency department.[182] Complex entry wounds or those with underlying surgical pathology will require more extensive surgical manipulation, which may include extending the incision to allow vigorous superficial debridement; complete excision of devitalized tissues including muscle, fascia, and periosteum; extension and debridement of the bony entry or exit site by craniectomy; and similarly generous debridement of the dural opening with watertight closure, using grafting as necessary.†

PREDICTIVE FACTORS

Increased mortality in penetrating head injury is associated with increasing age, suicide attempts, hypotension, coagulopathy (particularly with lower GCS scores), respiratory distress, low GCS score, bilateral fixed and dilated pupils, high ICP, and cisternal effacement on CT scan. Mortality also is increased with traumatic injuries in which a missile tract perforates the skull (through-and-through injury) or with injuries that involve both hemispheres, multiple lobes, or the ventricular system.[162]

In civilian gunshot wounds to the head, a specific vector analysis from Los Angeles County demonstrated a region of

---

*See references 162, 166, 167, 170, 179-182.
†See references 161, 168, 170, 172, 183, 184.

involvement that resulted in 100% fatality and is designated as the zona fatalis. This region comprises the midbody of the ventricle, the body of the corpus callosum, and the cingulum.[184]

No effect has been demonstrated for weapon caliber on outcome, independent of total kinetic energy, and no relation between midline shift and outcome has been established.[162]

SPECIAL PROBLEMS

Special problems that may be encountered with PBI include those associated with craniofacial entrance wounds: an increased incidence of hematoma formation, direct vascular injury, extensive contamination due to paranasal sinus involvement (see Fig. 66.15), and CSF fistulas.[152]

Other special problems include dural venous sinus involvement, tangential wounds, and traumatic aneurysms, with 0.4% to 0.7% of all intracranial aneurysms being caused by penetrating trauma.[185]

In PBI, mechanical loading of the cerebral vasculature, by either the contact forces of the projectile or the shearing forces of a pulsating temporary cavity, may cause partial or complete transection of an arterial wall. Such damage can result in SAH or formation of intracerebral and intraventricular hematomas.[162,186,187]

Damage to the arterial wall also may cause the development of a traumatic intracranial aneurysm (TICA). TICAs are primarily false aneurysms, which could heal or change in size over time, but they are especially vulnerable to rupture and can lead to delayed traumatic intracerebral hematoma or SAH or both.[185,188-190]

Patients with an increased risk of vascular injury include cases in which the trajectory passes through or near the sylvian fissure, supraclinoid carotid, cavernous sinus, or a major venous sinus. The development of substantial and otherwise unexplained SAH or delayed hematoma also should prompt consideration of a vascular injury.[162]

Cerebral angiography (CTA or conventional) remains the usual technique to detect intracranial aneurysms.[187,189,191] Because a majority of traumatic intracranial aneurysms are not true aneurysms, excluding the aneurysm by clipping may not be possible and may require trapping between clips on the parent vessel.[162]

COURSE IN THE INTENSIVE CARE UNIT

Not surprisingly, intracranial hypertension is common after PBI.[181,192-194] Early ICP monitoring should be considered when the ICU clinician is unable to assess the patient's neurologic status accurately; if the need to evacuate a mass lesion is unclear; or if CT scanning suggests elevated ICP.[162] Another practical use for ICP monitoring is ongoing assessment of a patient with a depressed level of consciousness to look for an early sign of progressive intracranial pathology, which may require repeated imaging and surgical decompression.[181,192,194]

Cerebral autoregulation may be defective after PBI[181,192,194]; cerebral edema can appear extremely rapidly, contributing to medically refractory intracranial hypertension. Systemic hypertension may exacerbate intracranial hypertension after PBI.[162]

Treatment is not necessarily futile, and some patients with intracranial hypertension can be managed successfully and survive with acceptable morbidity.[181,192,194,195] However, the literature does not clearly relate successful treatment of intracranial hypertension after PBI to an improved outcome. Not enough good data are available to guide management strategies for intracranial hypertension after PBI. It cannot be assumed that the intracranial pathology is the same as in nonpenetrating traumatic brain injury. Because of the paucity of data, however, treatment generally follows the methods for nonpenetrating traumatic brain injury as outlined in Guidelines for the Management of Severe Traumatic Brain Injury.[162,196]

Harrington and Apostolides have proposed a treatment algorithm for patients with gunshot wounds to the head. Patients who have lesions causing mass effect and a postresuscitation GCS score of 7 or greater undergo surgery, and patients with a GCS score of 3 or 4 with bilaterally fixed pupils after resuscitation receive no treatment beyond wound closure. In patients with GCS scores of 5 or 6, treatment should be individualized, depending on pupillary findings and other conditions.[197]

SECONDARY HEAD INJURY

BASIC CONCEPTS

Management of primary head injury generally entails the surgical management of head-injured patients and typically is driven by the presence of pathologic masses (hematomas) in anatomic spaces. Management of secondary head injury usually involves the nonsurgical management of these patients and deals with the pathologic derangement of physiologic processes.

The three functional volumetric compartments in the head are blood, brain, and CSF. The volumes of these three functional compartments are approximately 1200 mL for brain, 150 mL for CSF, and roughly 150 mL for the variable blood compartment. The total volume of the intracranial compartment is relatively fixed and relatively incompressible. Therefore, if volume is added to one of these three compartments, a compensatory loss of volume from another compartment will occur; otherwise, ICP will rise. To illustrate this point, a pressure-volume curve for the intracranial compartment is shown in Figure 66.16. Initially, as volume is added to the system, no significant change in pressure occurs. With cerebral edema, for example, as the brain compartment increases in volume, venous capacitance vessels collapse, which moves blood volume out of the system; therefore, overall net volume does not change and ICP remains stable. As the brain continues to swell and increase in volume, the ventricles become smaller as CSF moves out of the system, again keeping overall net volume and ICP relatively stable. At some point the system loses this buffering capacity, and as more injury-related volume accumulates, ICP starts to rise. The rise in ICP is gradual, progressive, and nonlinear. As the system continues to get stressed with additional volume, it progressively loses compliance and, in effect, gets stiffer. The result is that increasingly smaller volumes introduced into the system result in higher changes in ICP. Using MRI methods to study cerebral edema, Marmarou and colleagues noted a rise in ICP when edema was only 1% higher than the normal water content

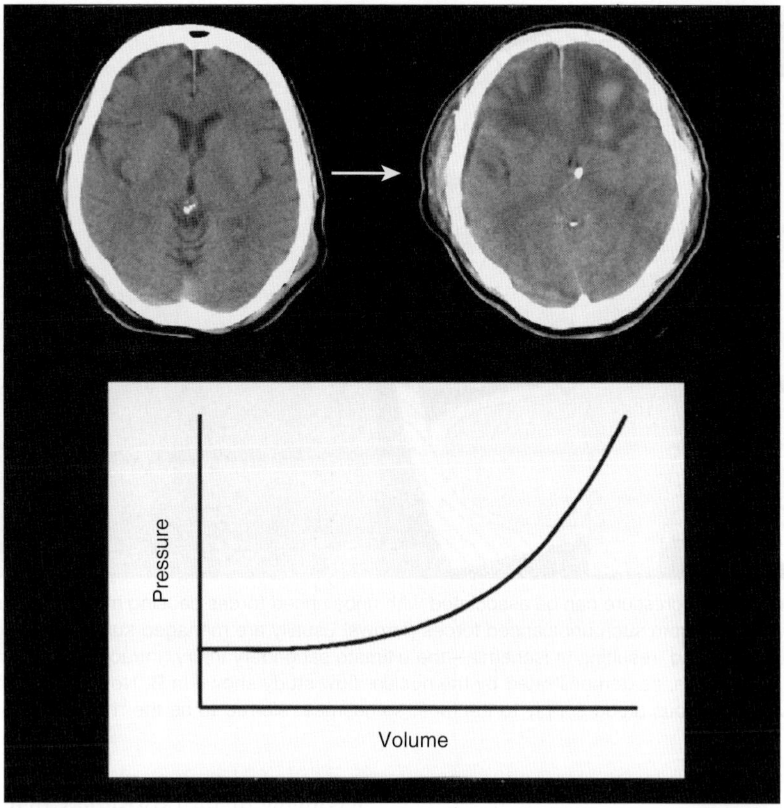

Figure 66.16 Pressure-volume curve of the intracranial compartment using cerebral edema as an example (see text). The computed tomography (CT) scan above the graph on the *left* is an image of a normal brain. The CT scan on the *right* demonstrates severe cerebral edema in a trauma patient with obliteration of most of the subarachnoid space, reducing cerebrospinal fluid (CSF) volume to make room for the swelling brain. Initially, as CSF moves out of the system, overall net volume does not change significantly. This part of the process is represented by the flat part of the curve toward the *left* and reflects the buffering capacity of the brain to respond to gradual increases in volume.

of brain tissue. These investigators also showed that when water content increased in a contused hemisphere, ICP increased exponentially. These findings demonstrate the importance of small changes in intracranial volume, particularly when the buffering capacity of the system has been exhausted.[198]

Increased ICP may be associated with mass effect secondary to unbalanced forces, causing direct, mechanical compressive damage to involved structures. This condition generally necessitates surgical decompression in the operating room. Increased ICP also may result in inadequate perfusion. This condition generally requires medical management in the ICU (Fig. 66.17).

The heart delivers blood at a given mean arterial blood pressure (MABP), the systemic perfusion pressure, to the base of the skull. The blood pressure then has to overcome whatever pressure is inside the head for blood flow to get in, and whatever is left over will be the pressure that perfuses the brain—that is, cerebral perfusion pressure (CPP). Simple in concept and calculation, CPP is defined as the mean arterial blood pressure minus ICP (CPP = MABP – ICP). It is the physiologic variable that defines the pressure gradient driving cerebral blood flow (CBF) and metabolic delivery and is therefore closely related to ischemia.[199,200]

Technically, the MABP should be measured as the mean carotid pressure with the arterial line transducer zeroed at the level of the foramen of Monro (as opposed to the right atrium),[201] but this approach is not common in clinical practice. Normal values generally are considered to be 60 to 80 mm Hg for CPP and approximately 10 mm Hg or less for ICP.

The ultimate cause of secondary injury is typically ischemic, and the fundamental goal in dealing with severe traumatic brain injury is to ensure adequate CBF relative to the metabolic demand of the brain. It is, however, impractical to continuously measure CBF at the bedside. Fortunately, CBF is dependent on CPP—which can easily and continuously be measured at bedside. Therefore, a fundamental management strategy for treating a head-injured patient is to maintain adequate CPP by lowering ICP, accomplished by reducing intracranial volume.

Surgical methods for reducing intracranial volume include evacuating an intracranial hematoma, removing part of the frontal or temporal lobe, and placing a ventriculostomy to drain CSF. Other methods for reducing intracranial volume are applicable in the ICU setting, where management strategies are directed at treating volume in the blood and brain compartments.

CEREBRAL BLOOD VOLUME

In discussing cerebral blood volume, it is useful to divide this topic into the arterial and venous compartments.

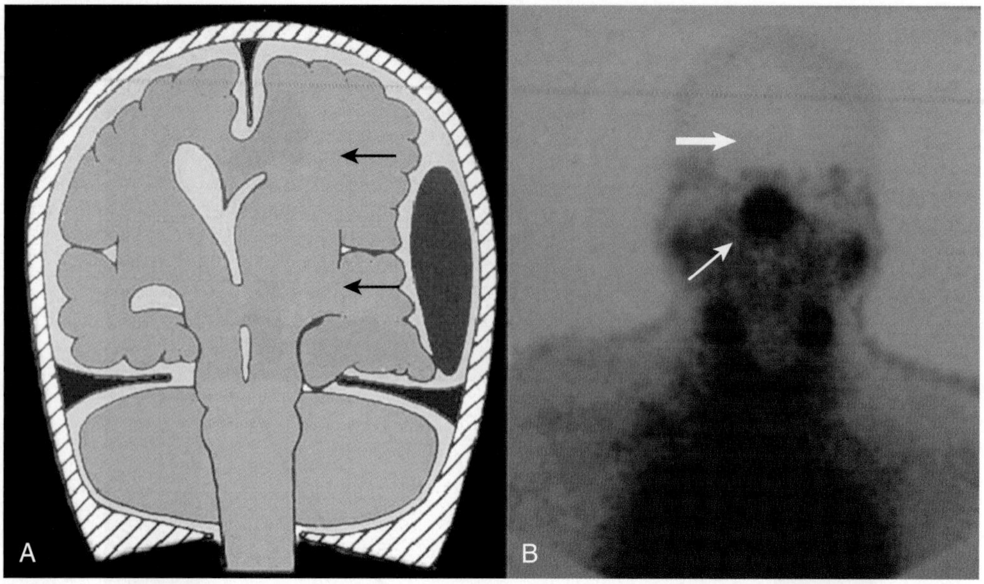

Figure 66.17 **A,** Increased intracranial pressure can be associated with unbalanced forces causing mass effect, shift, and possibly herniation. The resultant pathostructural changes from such unbalanced forces *(arrows)* usually are managed surgically. With increased intracranial pressure, cerebral perfusion may be impaired, resulting in ischemia—the ultimate secondary injury. Intractable intracranial hypertension and inadequate perfusion can lead to brain death, as demonstrated by the nuclear flow study shown in **B.** Note the absence of flow to the brain *(thick arrow),* compared with the overly generous blood supply to the face, sometimes referred to as the "hot nose sign" *(thin arrow).*

ARTERIAL BLOOD COMPARTMENT

Blood Pressure

Systemic blood pressure has a direct effect on arterial cerebral blood volume. Normally, CBF will remain relatively constant over a wide range of perfusion pressures as cerebrovascular resistance (CVR) automatically adjusts. The autoregulation curve (Fig. 66.18) demonstrates the relationship among CBF, perfusion pressure, and cerebrovascular resistance. As MABP goes up, CVR increases in order to maintain a stable CBF.

The CVR increases by vasoconstriction, which reduces the volume of blood in the brain. Conversely, as MAPB drops, CVR goes down by means of vasodilation, which increases the volume of blood in the brain. This is a very powerful system; a cerebral arteriole has the ability to change its diameter by up to 200%. It also is quite fast, responding to sudden changes in pressure within 3 to 5 seconds.

Most people have had the experience of suddenly jumping out of bed after having been recumbent for several hours and then feeling the "lights going out" as the cerebral vasculature rapidly dilates in response to the sudden drop in perfusion pressure and CBF; after several seconds, the lights come back on as cerebrovascular status is restored, as reflected by flattening of the autoregulation curve.

A normal MABP for a young, healthy adult is approximately between 70 and 90 mm Hg, and a normal ICP generally is considered to be approximately 10 mm Hg or less, which is consistent with a normal range of CPP values between 60 and 80 mm Hg. Although the normal ranges are at the low end of the autoregulation curve, there is the ability to autoregulate between perfusion pressures ranging from 50 to 150 mm Hg. It is clear from the autoregulation curve that CBF becomes a direct, linear function of MABP when outside the ability of the cerebrovascular bed to maximally dilate (MABP less than 50 mm Hg) or constrict (MABP greater than 150 mm Hg).

The normal range of 50 to 150 mm Hg is not rigidly fixed, and individual variations are common. A hypotensive patient with an MABP of 20 mm Hg clearly is in shock, but what about a 21-year-old athlete who has just had surgery for a ruptured appendix with an MABP of 45 mm Hg? Clearly a clinical assessment is necessary in borderline situations, and one of the most important indicators of shock is a change in mental status. In this example, if the athlete demonstrates a change in mental status, he is likely to be off his autoregulation curve and in shock.

At the other end of the spectrum is systemic hypertension. Is a 74-year-old patient with longstanding hypertension who presents with an MABP exceeding 150 mm Hg by a few points having a hypertensive crisis? Again, a change in mental status may be the indicator that autoregulatory capacity has been exceeded, and the patient may be diagnosed with hypertensive encephalopathy.

CVR often is increased by trauma. At the beginning of the autoregulation curve, CBF is zero at a perfusion pressure greater than zero. A measurable pressure in the vessel exists, yet no blood flow occurs, indicating vascular collapse (see Fig. 66.18). The cerebrovasculature in its resting state is collapsed; it takes a certain amount of energy (pressure) to open the vessels. These vessels each have critical opening and closing pressures. After a head injury, free radicals can be released, which tend to make biologic tissues less compliant. This in turn may make it more difficult for the vessels to stay open—that is, more pressure is required to keep the vessels from closing, which could shift the autoregulation curve to the right (see Fig. 66.18).[202-205] This is the theoretical basis for the studies that led to the earlier recommendations to keep the minimum CPP in head-injured patients above normal values—that is, at 70 mm Hg or greater.[206]

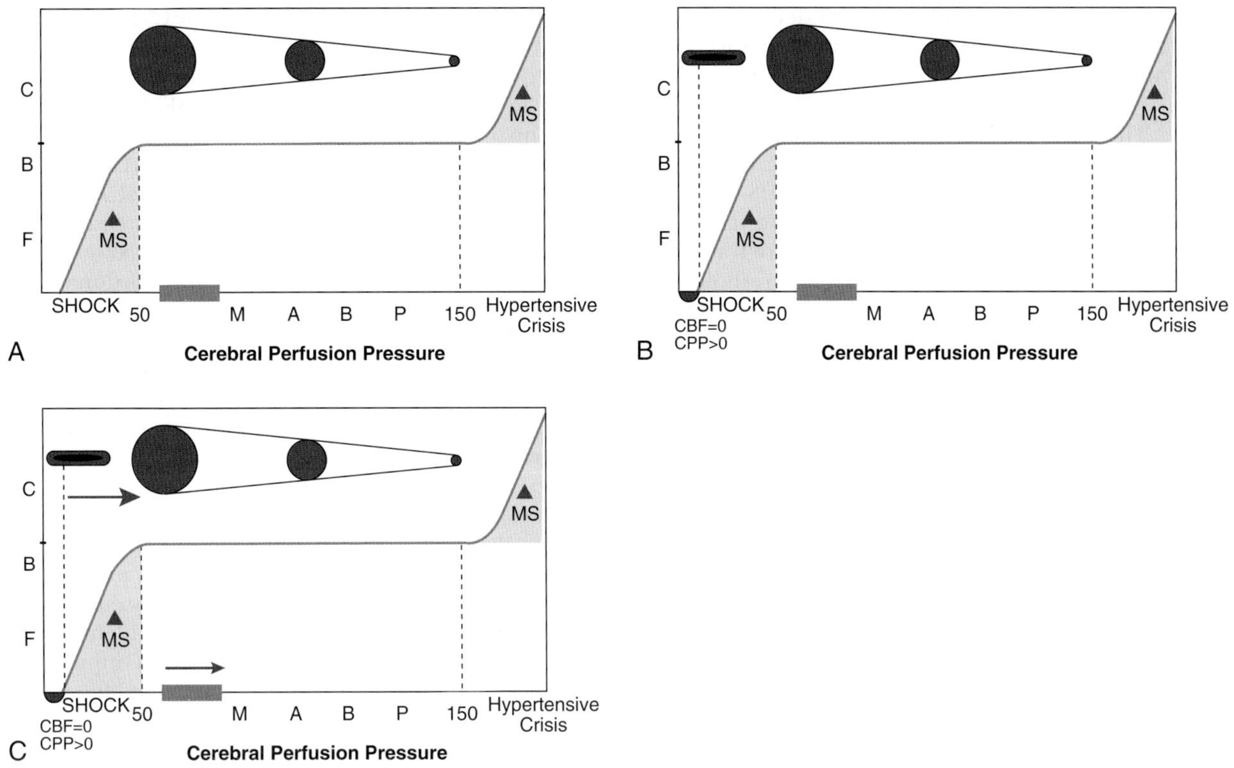

Figure 66.18 A, The autoregulation curve demonstrates how the brain maintains a relatively constant CBF over a wide range of perfusion pressures by changing the caliber (resistance) of the cerebral vasculature, which necessarily leads to changes in intracranial volume. Under normal circumstances, when ICP is negligible, the MABP is equivalent to cPP; however, when ICP is elevated, it is the CPP that is "read" by the brain. CPP will drive CBF, causing changes in cerebrovascular resistance, unless overridden by other superimposed processes such as hyperventilation, which may be pathologic or intentionally altered for a therapeutic effect. Although we have the ability to autoregulate over a wide range of perfusion pressures, the normal range is at the lower end of the curve *(horizontal green bar)*. **B,** The normal resting state of the cerebrovasculature is collapsed. These vessels have critical opening and closing pressures that are slightly different from each other. With the vessel open, it typically will collapse at a slightly lower pressure than is required to open it from a collapsed state. **C,** After a significant injury, the potential exists to increase the critical closing pressure, which could shift the autoregulation curve to the right. CBF, cerebral blood flow; CPP, cerebral perfusion pressure; MABP, mean arterial blood pressure; MS, mental status.

Cerebral Perfusion Pressure

A low perfusion pressure jeopardizes ischemic regions of the brain. Increasing intravascular hydrostatic pressure by increasing CPP can help improve cerebral perfusion. Although CPP can be manipulated and enhancement of CPP may help to avoid both global and regional ischemia, the level at which CPP is best maintained is not entirely clear,[206] and considerable interest has been directed toward attempts to determine the optimum CPP for a head-injured patient. Some studies suggest that increasing CPP to greater than 70 mm Hg leads to improved outcomes.[207]

A combination of studies of traumatic brain injury in which CPP was actively maintained at approximately 70 mm Hg in patients with a GCS score less than 8 reported a mean mortality rate of 21%, which was substantially less than the 40% mortality rate reported for similar patients in the Traumatic Coma Data Bank (TCDB). Good recovery and moderate disability rates were 54% in the patients whose CPP values were maintained in the 70 mm Hg range, compared with the 37% reported in the TCDB. However, it could not be concluded that the improved outcomes in these studies were a result of CPP management because none of the reported studies was a randomized, prospective trial of this treatment[200,205,208-212]; and in some, another treatment was actually the focus of the study.[208,209]

In a prospective study of 21 patients with severe traumatic brain injury in whom brain tissue PO_2 ($BtiO_2$) was monitored, ischemic episodes during the first week after injury were associated with unfavorable neurologic outcomes. Elevation of the CPP improved $BtiO_2$, but raising CPP above 68 mm Hg did not cause a further increase in $BtiO_2$. In the investigators' analysis, a CPP greater than 60 mm Hg emerged as the most important factor determining a sufficient $Btio_2$.[200,213]

Another prospective, controlled trial of 189 adult patients with a motor GCS score of 5 or lower within 12 hours of head injury randomized patients to an "ICP-targeted protocol" in which CPP was kept above 50 mm Hg or to a "CBF-targeted protocol" in which CPP was kept above 70 mm Hg. The investigators in this study found no significant difference in outcome. In this trial, the mean CPP for patients managed in the CBF-targeted protocol was 76 mm Hg and for those in the ICP-targeted protocol, 72 mm Hg. These differences were small but statistically significant.[214]

Contant and associates used data from this trial to examine risk factors for acute respiratory distress syndrome (ARDS) and consequences of its development. The risk of ARDS was five times greater among patients in the CBF-targeted group than in those in the ICP-targeted group and was associated with a more frequent use of epinephrine and a higher dose of dopamine.[199,215] Patients in whom ARDS developed were two and a half times more likely to develop refractory intracranial hypertension[215] and almost three times more likely to be in a vegetative state or dead at 6 months after injury.[215,216] These outcomes may be a direct consequence of ARDS, and the related therapeutic limitations of treating raised ICP and low CPP in the presence of ARDS.[199]

Analysis of data from a study investigating the value of a neuroprotective agent in 427 patients with severe traumatic brain injury revealed that the critical CPP threshold was 60 mm Hg. Although CPPs that were persistently less than 60 mm Hg were associated with a significant decline in outcomes, no effect on neurologic outcomes was observed for patients who had CPPs that were higher, and specifically no difference was observed among those who averaged 60 mm Hg and those at 70 mm Hg or higher.[199,217]

In 1995 and 2000, the Brain Trauma Foundation in cooperation with the American Association of Neurological Surgeons and the Joint Section for Trauma and Critical Care published guidelines for the management of severe head injury. From the data available, based on the theoretical need to increase the minimum CPP because of a change in critical closing pressures (see Fig. 66.18), the guidelines recommended maintaining a minimum CPP of 70 mm Hg or greater—10 mm Hg above the accepted norm. In 2003, this group updated the recommendation for CPP management and published a guideline that CPP should be maintained at a minimum of 60 mm Hg. In the absence of cerebral ischemia, aggressive attempts to maintain CPP above 70 mm Hg with fluids and pressors should be avoided because of the risk of ARDS.[199] In 2007, the recommendations were again modified with a level 3 recommendation to target CPP values within the range of 50 to 70 mm Hg.[200] Clearly, guidelines change as new data become available and the reader is strongly advised to check for the most up-to-date recommendations.

CARBON DIOXIDE

Carbon dioxide is a powerful regulator of cerebrovascular resistance. At any given physiologic perfusion pressure, $Paco_2$ can act rapidly and severely to affect CBF in a linear fashion by vasodilating or vasoconstricting the cerebrovascular bed. For every mm Hg change in $Paco_2$, a 3% change in CBF can occur.[218]

Allowing the $Paco_2$ to rise to levels between 60 and 80 mm Hg can result in a doubling of CBF, through vasodilation with a concomitant increase in cerebral blood volume (CBV). Conversely, aggressive hyperventilation of a patient down to a $Paco_2$ of 20 mm Hg or less can result in CBFs being cut in half, along with a reduction in CBV. Hyperventilation was a mainstay in the therapeutic management strategy of treating head-injured patients because it had such immediate and measurable effects on ICP. Lowering $Paco_2$ causes rapid vasoconstriction, resulting in reduced CBV, which translates to reduced intracranial volume, which lowers ICP and increases CPP. However, hyperventilation reduces ICP by taking blood *away* from the brain, when the goal is to prevent ischemia. As seen on the autoregulation curve, the cerebrovasculature is fine-tuned to the existing perfusion pressure, providing a normal level of CBF. Aggressive hyperventilation can override the normal effect of MABP and cause a marked increase in CVR to the point at which a very high perfusion pressure would be needed to match the degree of severe vasoconstriction induced in order to maintain a normal level of CBF. This is the mechanism involved when a normal person hyperventilates, vasoconstricts, and becomes lightheaded as CBF falls. It is important to recognize that this individual has a normal MABP, ICP, and CBF before the $Paco_2$ decreases.

Despite the fact that hyperventilation lowers ICP, the degree of vasoconstriction can be disproportionate relative to the enhancement in CPP. For example, at an MABP of 80 mm Hg with an ICP of 30 mm Hg and a CPP of 50 mm Hg, aggressive hyperventilation could reduce ICP to 15 by reducing intracranial volume, thereby improving CPP to 65. But aggressive hyperventilation can cause severe vasoconstriction. At maximal vasoconstriction, the cerebrovascular bed would need an MABP of 150 mm Hg with a normal ICP in order to maintain a normal CBF.

The data on CBF in severely head-injured patients indicate that phases of CBF change over time after traumatic brain injury, with hypoperfusion occurring in the first 24 hours.[218] Multiple studies have identified brain ischemia in up to 35% of serious head injuries within the first 12 hours.[200,218-224] It appears that this reduction happens almost immediately. Mean CBF values measured less than 4 hours after head injury in adults were 32 mL/100 g/minute in survivors and 20 mL per 100 g per minute in nonsurvivors (normal CBF is 55 mL/100 g/minute).[224] Low cerebral blood flow, to ischemic levels (less than 18 mL/100 g/minute), was observed in 31% of patients with severe head injury measured an average of 3 hours after trauma.[200,225]

Because of the consistent data regarding reduced CBF early after trauma, attempts at further reductions using hyperventilation have come under close scrutiny. Some evidence suggests that hyperventilation carries a particular risk of causing cerebral hypoxia when $Paco_2$ is 30 mm Hg or less, or within the first 24 hours[226,227] because of a further reduction of an already low CBF.[225] It has become clear that hyperventilation decreases $BtiO_2$ because of decreased CBF in most patients, which negates the perceived benefit of improving intracranial and cerebral perfusion pressures.[213,226,227-232]

On the basis of principles reflecting a high degree of clinical certainty, the Brain Trauma Foundation (BTF) in 1995 and 2000 recommended that in the absence of increased ICP, chronic prolonged hyperventilation therapy (Pco_2 of 25 mm Hg or less) should be avoided after severe traumatic brain injury.[233]

On the basis of principles reflecting a moderate degree of clinical certainty, this group recommended that the use of prophylactic hyperventilation (Pco_2 less than 35 mm Hg) therapy during the first 24 hours after severe traumatic brain injury should be avoided because it can compromise cerebral perfusion during a time when CBF is reduced. On the basis of principles for which there is unclear clinical certainty, the group recommended that hyperventilation therapy may be necessary for brief periods during acute neurologic deterioration, or for longer periods in the presence of intracranial hypertension refractory to sedation, paralysis, CSF drainage, and osmotic diuretics.[234]

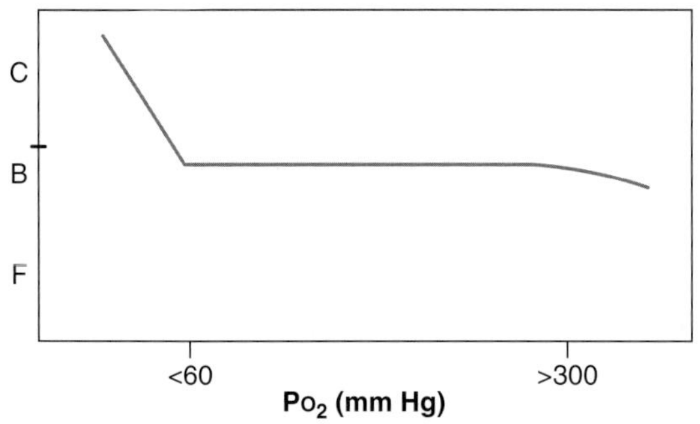

Figure 66.19 Graph demonstrating the relationship of cerebral blood flow (CBF) to oxygen (Po_2). Within a physiologic range, oxygen is of no use as a therapeutic tool. The cerebral vasculature will vasodilate under hypoxic conditions, so hypoxia must be avoided.

OXYGEN

Within a normal physiologic range, oxygen causes little or no change in CBF (Fig. 66.19). Beyond a PaO_2 of approximately 300 mm Hg, CBF can begin to wane. Oxygenation does become very important at PaO_2 levels considered to be hypoxic. Below a PaO_2 of 60 mm Hg in most head-injured patients, the cerebrovasculature can vasodilate rapidly, causing an increase in CBV with poorly oxygenated blood, with an attendant increase in intracranial volume and pressure.

With careful clinical monitoring, our group has observed ICP spikes as a result of acute oxygen desaturation before a change in the pulse oximeter reading. With a moderate degree of clinical certainty, the BTF has recommended that hypoxia, defined as apnea or cyanosis in the field or a PaO_2 less than 60 mm Hg, must be scrupulously avoided or corrected immediately. Therefore, in contrast with $Paco_2$, manipulation of PaO_2 is not a useful tool for medical management of a head-injured patient, and hypoxia must be avoided.[200]

In view of the powerful effects of hypoxia and hypercarbia, it is no surprise that early intubation in significant head injury is important.

METABOLISM

Under normal circumstances, the cerebral metabolic rate of oxygen ($CMRO_2$) is directly related to CBF; this is referred to as a coupled relationship. As metabolic demand increases, the cerebrovasculature will vasodilate to supply an appropriate increase in CBF; and, conversely as $CMRo_2$ decreases, the cerebrovasculature will vasoconstrict to maintain a coupled relationship between supply and demand. As demand exceeds supply and the ability of the brain to extract more oxygen wanes, ischemia develops. Therefore, whatever increases the $CMRO_2$ will cause an appropriate vasodilatory response in the brain with its attendant increase in CBV and, potentially, ICP, with a resultant decrease in CPP. Clearly, if the primary event is an increase in demand and the end result is a reduction in supply, the gap between supply and demand increases, and with it the potential for ischemia. Under physiologic conditions whereby the $CMRO_2$ is coupled to CBF, various clinical states will demonstrate an appropriate balance of the two. For example, a comatose patient will have low $CMRO_2$, and a patient having a generalized seizure will have a high $CMRO_2$.

The metabolic state of the brain is sensitive to changes in temperature; lower temperatures lower $CMRO_2$, and vice versa. Recognition of this relationship has led to interest in using hypothermia as a therapeutic tool in severe head injury, both as a way to lower ICP and as a neuroprotective strategy by reducing demand in the face of limited supply. Although hypothermia can be a useful adjunct to standard treatments for controlling elevated ICP it is difficult to find good data to prove a benefit in outcome. Clifton and associates found that ICP was lower in patients managed with hypothermia, but no improvement in outcome was observed, and the complication rate was higher than in a normothermic group. These investigators concluded that lowering body temperature to 33° C within 8 hours after injury was not effective in improving outcomes in patients with brain injuries.[235] A Cochrane review of therapeutic hypothermia for head injury looked at 14 trials with more than 1000 participants and found no evidence that hypothermia is beneficial in the treatment of head injury, and that it increased the risk of pneumonia nearly twofold.[236] A different meta-analysis using clinical trials of moderate or poor quality, identified preliminary findings suggesting a greater decrease in mortality risk when target temperatures are maintained for more than 48 hours, as well as an association with better outcomes.[237,238]

Although it is not clear that routine use of prophylactic hypothermia is helpful, hyperthermia is believed to be harmful to a severely head-injured patient.[239] As the temperature rises, so does the $CMRO_2$, with a concomitant increase in CBV. If the patient has lost enough compliance then small changes in intracranial volume can result in big changes in ICP (see Fig. 66.16), and CPP can fall.

A frequent scenario is development of a fever in a trauma patient with a high ICP and poor compliance who is barely meeting metabolic needs. Metabolic requirements increase as CBV and ICP increase and CPP decreases, widening the gap between supply and demand, resulting in ischemia.

Another consideration in the management of $CMRO_2$ is drug effect. Pentobarbital is the gold standard drug for reducing cerebral metabolism and can be used in cases of refractory intracranial hypertension to induce a barbiturate coma. A condition of burst suppression is achieved, meaning that the continuous EEG recording demonstrates periods of an isoelectric tracing (straight line) interrupted by bursts of cortical electrical activity. This therapy results in vasoconstriction appropriate for the degree of reduction in metabolism, with an attendant decrease in ICP. This has the theoretical advantage of improving supply to a brain with reduced metabolic demands. However, despite the evidence for cerebral protection in experimental models, little clinical evidence is available to suggest that barbiturates improve outcome after severe head injuries in humans. Other drugs that reduce the $CMRO_2$ and CBF are other barbiturates such as thiopental, as well as the substituted phenol propofol, the hypnotic agent etomidate, and the water-soluble short-acting benzodiazepine midazolam.[239]

VISCOSITY

When autoregulation is intact, lowering viscosity of the blood improves flow dynamics and results in an appropriate increase in CVR to maintain a constant, normal CBF.[240-244]

This vasoconstriction reduces intracranial volume. From a rheologic standpoint, there is an advantage to lowering viscosity by hemodilution, but this is at the expense of oxygen-carrying capacity. Reducing the hematocrit from 45% to 30% can theoretically double CBF, yet oxygen-carrying capacity would be reduced by only a third. By generalizing experimental and clinical data involving ischemia and hematocrit, it is reasonable to consider an optimum hematocrit of approximately 30% to 35%.[245]

A common mechanism for lowering viscosity in traumatic head injury is the use of mannitol, which causes an immediate influx of extravascular water, leading to hemodilution. The vasoconstriction resulting from this reduction in viscosity allows the same CBF and oxygen delivery to be maintained by means of smaller vessels and with a lower intracranial volume (see later section, "Hyperosmolar Therapy"). In addition, mannitol will dehydrate the red blood cells themselves by about 15%, which further improves blood flow dynamics.[245]

VENOUS BLOOD COMPARTMENT

In general, vascular organization of most organ systems is anatomically similar—for example, the renal artery travels with the renal vein. The brain, however, has two entirely different anatomic systems for arterial supply and venous drainage. The paired carotid and vertebral arteries provide the arterial supply to the brain but have no corresponding venous counterparts. Blood leaves the brain through cortical and deep draining veins that empty into the superior sagittal, transverse, and sigmoid sinuses. These dural sinuses are open, semirigid structures that empty into bilateral jugular veins, which communicate directly with the right heart through the superior vena cava. There are no valves in this entire venous system. This means that right heart pressures are in direct continuity with the superior sagittal sinus within the intracranial compartment. When measured with the subject lying supine, ICP cannot be lower than central venous pressure. Of more importance, right heart pressures will be directly transmitted to the intracranial compartment, a relevant dynamic involved with a Valsalva maneuver.

During a Valsalva maneuver, intrathoracic pressure elevates and venous return to the right heart goes down. Decreased venous return means decreased venous outflow from the brain. This results in a rapid, instantaneous increase in CBV as the arterial side continues to supply the brain with blood that is not getting physiologic draining. A Valsalva maneuver also will decrease cardiac output along with a decrease in venous return, but it is a disproportionate change. A common neurosurgical practice is to have the anesthesiologist induce a controlled Valsalva maneuver toward the end of a brain operation during the final stages of hemostasis, just before beginning the closure. Intrathoracic pressure is elevated to approximately 30 mm Hg for 10 seconds as the surgeon looks for any areas of bleeding while the brain immediately physically and visibly swells as it engorges with blood. An intrathoracic pressure of 30 mm Hg will overcome a normal CVP and essentially interrupt venous outflow from the brain. The concomitant decrease in cardiac output with a pressure of 30 mm Hg will have much less of an effect than on the venous side; therefore, a relatively large volume of arterial blood will continue to fill the brain. Even a normal brain with normal compliance will immediately "feel" the effect of decreased venous outflow because it happens faster than the buffering capacity of the brain can handle (see Fig. 66.16). In fact, one mechanism the brain will use to buffer increases in volume is to collapse venous capacitance vessels, which, in the case of decreased venous outflow from the brain, becomes part of the problem, not the solution.

Other common ways in which venous outflow from the brain can be compromised is with anything that interferes with jugular venous drainage such as a tight-fitting rigid cervical collar or thrombosis from an internal jugular line. It is not uncommon to have dominant venous outflow on one side and, following head rotation to that side, increased resistance to venous outflow. Obviously, gravity also will have a role, with head elevation enhancing venous outflow from the brain. We generally keep our patients with the head elevated at 30 degrees, with neck straight and free of lines, with a good-fitting cervical collar that is not too tight.

BRAIN COMPARTMENT

Another functional volumetric compartment is the brain itself. One of the consequences of traumatic brain injury is an acute increase in total brain water.[246]

The volume of the brain parenchyma can be affected by therapeutic dehydration induced with the use of osmotic agents. These agents can be used to treat cerebral edema in an effort to remove a pathologic accumulation of fluid. Dehydration also can be used to manipulate the volume status of an otherwise normal but threatened brain compartment in order to emergently manage an increase in ICP as a temporizing measure before surgery, such as with extra-axial hematoma or hydrocephalus. The agents most commonly used to effect these changes are mannitol and hypertonic saline.

CEREBRAL EDEMA

By definition, brain edema is an abnormal accumulation of fluid within the brain parenchyma that produces a volumetric enlargement of the brain tissue.[198] The three types of cerebral edema are vasogenic, neurotoxic, and cytotoxic. Vasogenic edema occurs when the blood-brain barrier opens, resulting in movement of vascular fluid into the extracellular spaces of the brain.[247] Neurotoxic edema involves astrocytic and dendritic swelling secondary to the neurotoxic effects of excitatory amino acids, particularly glutamate, seen with reperfusion.[198] Cytotoxic edema results from retention of water within swollen cells, most commonly found in stroke, in which interruption of energy supply leads to pump failure and an intracellular increase in sodium and water.[198]

It is ischemia, associated with energy failure at the level of mitochondria, that contributes to cytotoxic brain edema and intracranial hypertension.[246-254] Earlier studies led to the general acceptance that traumatic brain swelling was primarily a result of vascular engorgement, which caused increased ICP.[255-259] Although opinions differ, more recent work has demonstrated that cerebral edema may be primarily responsible for brain swelling, not vascular engorgement.[251,260] Marmarou and colleagues have used sophisticated MRI techniques to demonstrate that traumatic brain edema is predominantly a cellular phenomenon in both focal and diffuse brain injury.[198]

Although cellular edema predominates, it is likely that edema formation in head injury is complicated, with time-dependent contributions of both vasogenic and cytotoxic mechanisms. Experimental evidence points to transient compromise of the blood-brain barrier occurring immediately after injury, with resultant vasogenic edema. Studies indicate early closure of the blood-brain barrier, after which cytotoxic, cellular edema predominates.[198,261-263]

HYPEROSMOLAR THERAPY

Mannitol

Mannitol, an inert six-carbon alcohol of the corresponding sugar mannose, causes cellular dehydration by increasing serum osmolarity. The use of mannitol in head-injured patients to lower ICP is based on two mechanisms of action of this drug: It establishes an osmotic gradient across the blood-brain barrier to reduce water content,[264,265] and it causes cerebral vasoconstriction through rheologic effects that decrease blood viscosity and enhance CBF and MABP (see earlier section, "Viscosity").[245,266,267] This vascular mechanism of action has a strong, independent effect, such that CBF can be enhanced even when ICP is not substantially reduced.[268,269]

With head-injured patients, mannitol is used in two clinical scenarios. The first is that of a comatose trauma patient with a surgical clot, when mannitol is given on the way to the operating room to buy time until emergent decompression is accomplished. Generally, higher doses of up to 1.2 to 1.4 g per kg can be given in this scenario.[270,271]

The second clinical scenario is one of cerebral edema, when mannitol is given to control ICP. Unlike with its use for emergency surgical clots, there is no consensus on the optimal dosing regimen of mannitol in the ICU to manage ICP. Doses ranging from 0.25 g per kg to 1.0 g per kg may be effective. Mannitol can be given in response to high ICP, or it can be used prophylactically regardless of ICP, using serum osmolarity as an end point of treatment,[272] although some evidence indicates that it is most effective when used in the presence of high ICP or low perfusion pressure.[267,273]

Regardless of how mannitol is used, because of its osmotic diuresis, replacement of urinary water and electrolyte losses is critical, to avoid hypovolemia and hypotension. Mannitol typically is given as a bolus at a rate not to exceed 0.1 g per kg per minute in order to avoid hypotension.[272] Caution should be exercised in patients with a propensity toward congestive heart failure, because the early effects of bolus administration cause intravascular volume expansion.[272]

Mannitol can extravasate into the interstitium of the brain, with breakdown of the blood-brain barrier, which may be a cause of cerebral edema. This is thought to be less of an issue with bolus dosing as opposed to continuous infusion.[274] Because of this particular concern with mannitol toxicity, many clinicians prefer to use the smallest doses of mannitol necessary, and to administer it only for proven intracranial hypertension.[275]

Another concern is renal failure, which is a rare complication of mannitol therapy. It is generally believed that the kidneys are at risk above a serum osmolarity of 320 mOsm per L[276,277]; however, kidney damage may in fact be due to high serum concentrations of mannitol itself, as opposed to high serum osmolarity. It is suggested that keeping the osmolar gap (measured serum osmolarity minus calculated serum osmolarity) below 55 mOsm per kg of H_2O may be better than using serum osmolarity alone to direct mannitol therapy.[272,277]

To summarize, mannitol therapy in the ICU is effective given as boluses for elevated ICP while keeping the patient normovolemic and hyperosmolar with an osmolar gap less than 55 mOsm per kg.

Furosemide, a loop diuretic, has some effectiveness for removing extracellular fluid from the brain. Although it does not work as fast as mannitol, furosemide commonly is used in conjunction with that agent because of a synergistic effect on ICP.[278]

HYPERTONIC SALINE

In many ICUs, hypertonic saline is being used with increasing frequency for the treatment of raised ICP in patients with traumatic brain injury.[279] It is known that patients with hypotension after severe traumatic brain injury have twice the mortality rate of normotensive patients[280]; therefore, aggressive resuscitation with intravenous fluids is recommended in the guidelines for the management of patients with severe traumatic brain injury.[281] However, the real concern for the development of cerebral edema is reason enough to limit the amount of free water available to the injured brain during this early period. The use of hypertonic saline, both to increase mean arterial pressure and to decrease ICP, is a logical and promising approach to limit secondary injury and improve neurologic outcome.

The rapid infusion of a small volume of hypertonic solution originally was designed for the prehospital treatment of hemorrhagic shock,[282-285] and a trial found a trend toward a reduction of ICP in a double-blind, randomized, controlled trial of prehospital fluid resuscitation using hypertonic saline in comatose and hypotensive head-injured patients (although no improvement in outcome was demonstrated).[286]

The rapid infusion of small volumes of hypertonic solution leads to an osmotic gradient that mobilizes parenchymal fluid into the vascular compartment,[287,288] resulting in hemodilution, endothelial shrinkage, and improved blood flow in the microcirculation,[289,290] as well as improved cardiac output.[282,283,291] Hypertonic saline has been shown to reduce brain bulk and ICP[292-295] and to be effective in lowering ICP both in bolus form and as a maintenance fluid.[296-298]

It is widely believed that the mechanism of action of both hypertonic saline and mannitol in reducing ICP is their hyperosmolar properties, although additional mechanisms are likely to be in play. Some authors have found hypertonic saline to be more effective than mannitol in selected patients.[299,300]

Concerns about central pontine myelinolysis and acute renal failure appear to be unfounded on the basis of clinical experience; however, a rebound effect may occur in some patients.[301] A trial also reported no episodes of acute anemia or hypokalemia associated with 23.4% saline administration, nor were there any episodes of convulsions, congestive heart failure, or coagulopathy after the administration of hypertonic saline.[299]

In the United States, 3% sodium chloride is readily available. An initial dose of 1.5 to 3.0 mL per kg with a target for a serum sodium concentration of approximately 155 mEq per L is reasonable,[295] although 23.4% saline has been shown to be safe and effective in the treatment of intracranial hypertension.[299] As with hyperosmolar therapy for mannitol, it is important to maintain a normovolemic state at all times during treatment.

CEREBROSPINAL FLUID COMPARTMENT

CSF is produced mostly by the choroid plexus located in the ventricles. CSF flows from the lateral ventricles (first two ventricles) through the foramina of Monro into the third ventricle, and from there the fluid moves through the aqueduct of Sylvius to the fourth ventricle. From the fourth ventricle, CSF moves out of the ventricular system through the foramen of Magendie in the midline and the foramina of Luschka laterally. CSF then enters the subarachnoid space of the brain and spinal cord and circulates around the surface of the cerebellum and brainstem as it comes up through the tentorial hiatus, thus forming the basal cisterns. The clear and colorless fluid migrates over the cerebral hemispheres toward the midline, where, through a semiactive process, it is transported from the subarachnoid space into the superior sagittal sinus.

CSF is made at a continuous rate of approximately 0.3 mL per minute. With a total volume of approximately 150 mL (roughly 10% of intracranial volume), the entire CSF volume is replaced three times a day. A little less than one third of the total volume is in the ventricular system.

In severe head injury, CSF can be displaced out of the intracranial compartment as pressure differences between the superior sagittal sinus and the intracranial compartment increase (see Fig. 66.16). The spinal CSF compartment also is an important physiologic sink, and this contribution of CSF flow to ICP is another justification for nursing traumatic brain-injured patients with the head elevated.[300]

A standard way of managing the CSF compartment in the trauma patient is by draining CSF through an indwelling ventricular catheter (ventriculostomy). This has proved to be a relatively safe and effective tool in lowering intracranial volume and pressure, although ventricles in younger trauma patients commonly are smaller and harder to access and have less CSF to drain. Ventricular drainage is discussed further in Chapter 17.

SPECIFIC TREATMENT CONSIDERATIONS

CRANIECTOMY

Craniectomy is an alternative to the medical and direct surgical methods for reducing intracranial volume. This is a surgical strategy for managing a dangerous increase in intracranial volume by expanding the size of the intracranial compartment. The necessary expansion is accomplished by removing a large portion of the skull and opening the dura (see Fig. 66.13).

Intractable intracranial hypertension despite maximal medical therapy is associated with a high risk of morbidity and death.[301-303] In one multicenter trial, an 86% mortality rate was found among patients whose condition failed to respond to an induced pentobarbital coma[304]—the last line of defense in medical management. Similarly, a significant relationship has been recognized between an ICP higher than 25 mm Hg and a poor outcome.[305]

Because of these ominous facts, craniectomy to increase the space available for the swollen brain has been used to lower ICP, although early outcome studies of hemicraniectomy yielded poor results.[306-308] More contemporary experiences, however, have achieved better results. In 2006, Aarabi and colleagues reviewed 10 reports published since 1988, with a total of 323 patients treated with decompressive craniectomy for posttraumatic brain swelling and intractable intracranial hypertension, and calculated a collective mortality rate of 22.3%, with good outcomes in 48.3%, with the rest of the patients (29.4%) remaining severely disabled or vegetative. These results compared favorably with six previous reports in which the mortality rates ranged from 42% to 100% when ICP greater than 20 mm Hg remained refractory to medical management. Reported complications included subgaleal collections, which resolved over the course of weeks to months; delayed wound healing; bone flap resorption and infections; increased swelling and hemorrhagic contusions; and parenchymal lucencies, possibly due to ischemia.*

In addition to the demonstrated improvement in outcome, contrast-enhanced ultrasonography has been used to assess cerebral perfusion after decompressive craniectomy and found an average fivefold improvement in microvascular blood flow.[319] A technical point worth emphasizing is that a decompressive craniectomy must be sufficiently large in order to be helpful.[320]

MANAGEMENT OF INTRACRANIAL HYPERTENSION

Acute, severe traumatic brain injury is a dynamic process with the potential for dangerous changes that can evolve over hours to days; therefore, all patients need to be observed closely. Ideally, ongoing assessment by neurologic examination should be at least hourly. In most patients with a GCS score of 8 or less, however, airway protection mechanisms will be impaired, necessitating intubation and, therefore, sedation, which makes an accurate neurologic assessment problematic. An ICP measuring device usually is needed at this point to adequately monitor the patient, in lieu of a reliable examination (see Chapter 16 on ICP monitoring).

The medical management of intracranial hypertension in the ICU generally occurs after surgical decompression of hematomas causing unbalanced forces, or in patients without a surgical lesion. This management strategy generally is divided into tiers of therapy. The first tier is sedation, analgesia, and intubation without hyperventilation, keeping the head elevated and the neck straight and uncompressed. The routine use of paralytics may increase the risk of pulmonary complications; therefore, muscle relaxants should be used for ICP control when sedation is inadequate.[321] If

*See references 10, 217, 287, 301, 305, 309-318.

ICP exceeds 20 mm Hg[322] despite these maneuvers, moving to the next level of care is indicated, which includes CSF drainage if a ventriculostomy is being used, mannitol, or hypertonic saline. Beyond the first 24 hours, mild hyperventilation to keep P_{CO_2} in the mid-30s can be used. Throughout the clinical course it also is necessary to maintain an adequate CPP of at least 60 mm Hg by ensuring normovolemia and a safe MABP. If ICP is refractory to these treatments, the next step is use of decompressive hemicraniectomies or barbiturate coma (or both). Historically, surgical decompression has been reserved as a radical, end-of-the-line treatment after the patient has failed to respond to burst suppression barbiturate coma; however, craniectomy is moving up in the treatment algorithm of most centers (Fig. 66.20).

When ICP goes up, it is important to understand why and then try to correct the underlying problem if possible. In any given head-injured patient in whom the brain has lost its buffering capacity, with resultant poor compliance, small increases in intracranial volume can cause a significant rise in pressure. When ICP rises, CPP goes down. This usually will result in a decrease in CVR and vasodilation, with its attendant increase in cerebral blood volume and increase in intracranial volume. This of course leads to a further increase in ICP, and the cycle perpetuates itself. This is the mechanism of a plateau wave.[245]

In managing these patients, it is critical to try to determine the source of the problem. Perhaps the patient became hypovolemic and the blood pressure dropped, or a ventilator change caused hypercarbia or hypoxia. Maybe the patient is inadequately sedated or having an unrecognized seizure while pharmacologically paralyzed. The problem may be as simple as a high fever or a rigid cervical collar compressing the jugular veins. Whatever is driving this process must be corrected to break this dangerous plateau wave.

If the cause cannot be determined, a new CT scan may need to be taken, and therapeutic maneuvers should be employed to help turn things around, such as increasing sedation, further head elevation, ventricular drainage, administration of mannitol or hypertonic saline, pressors when needed, and brief periods of gentle hyperventilation.

ANTICOAGULATION

It is intuitive that severe coagulopathy is associated with increased mortality after head injury.[323-331] Penetrating or blunt brain injury can be associated with the massive release of thromboplastin from neuronal tissue, thereby initiating the coagulation process, which evolves to an exaggerated fibrinolytic response and disseminated intra-vascular coagulopathy (DIC).[324] This brain injury–induced coagulopathy may lead to significant secondary injury and delay the invasive monitoring necessary for the aggressive management of intracranial hypertension.[332] The criteria for the diagnosis of DIC include abnormal clotting studies, thrombocytopenia, low fibrinogen, and, in some cases, elevation in levels of products of fibrinolysis (D-dimer or fibrin degradation products).[327] The DIC caused by head trauma is relatively common and frequently is detected by a prolonged prothrombin time and elevated international normalized ratio (INR). Its presence may be an indication for more intense clinical observation and follow-up CT scanning. An important component of DIC is coagulation; however, in the setting of active bleeding, anticoagulation is not indicated. The therapeutic focus is on hemostasis and replacement of diluted or consumed blood elements and components.[328-329]

Typical treatment of coagulopathy consists of fresh frozen plasma (FFP) administration; however, use of FFP can be problematic. This product takes time to administer, so that a relatively large volume of fluid may be given to a head-injured patient when it is important to avoid hypervolemia. Other concerns are the possibility of blood-borne disease transmission and, as reported in a rare case, transfusion-related acute lung injury. Another important issue is the variable effect FFP can have on brain injury–induced coagulopathy, such that it ultimately may fail to correct the coagulopathy.

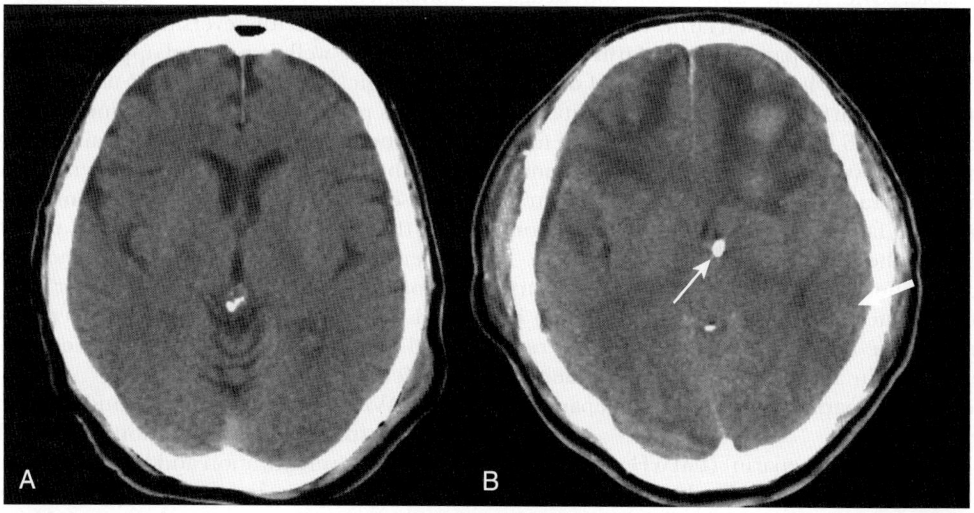

Figure 66.20 **A,** Computed tomography (CT) image of a normal brain. **B,** CT scan of the brain of a patient with severe traumatic brain injury and medically intractable intracranial hypertension. Between the poorly controlled cerebral edema and the indwelling ventriculostomy, almost no cerebrospinal fluid can be identified on the scan, which shows complete obliteration of cortical sulci *(thick arrow)* and basal cisterns *(thin arrow)*. Given the absence of shift, bilateral hemicraniectomies were required.

Preliminary data indicate that recombinant activated factor VII (rFVIIa) provides a rapid and successful correction of coagulopathy in head-injured patients.[326] Originally developed for the treatment of hemophiliacs, rFVIIa also may be helpful in reversing the effects of anticoagulants and antiplatelet drugs.[326,330-340] It is a vitamin K–dependent glycoprotein, similar to the human plasma-derived factor VIIa, which appears to promote hemostasis by activating the extrinsic pathway of the coagulation cascade.[341] Its mechanism of action is not fully understood but includes interaction with platelets or tissue factor to augment thrombin generation and platelet activation.[330,332,334,335] Factor VIIa seems to be the bottleneck, the critical factor most depleted when patients are profoundly anticoagulated.[342] The use of rFVIIa to correct a coagulopathy before neurosurgical intervention was reported in 1998 in a hemophiliac patient with an EDH requiring craniotomy for evacuation.[343] Although not specifically evaluated for use in DIC, rFVIIa has been administered to neurosurgical patients in whom DIC was likely to be present.[329,338] Recombinant FVIIa has been used in the absence of hemophilia for neurosurgical emergencies such as EDH and SDH, SAH and intracerebral hemorrhage, tumor resection, and during placement of ICP monitors.[333,336,338,340] A retrospective study found improved outcomes, without complications, when rFVIIa was used for coagulopathic patients requiring urgent neurosurgical intervention.[344] The incidence of thrombosis after rFVIIa is low, but thrombosis is an extremely important potential complication[334,338,339,345,346] and of particular concern in DIC.[328] Precise dosing for conditions other than hemophilia has not been confirmed[332]; the Food and Drug Administration (FDA) has approved rFVIIa only for use in hemophilia; other uses are considered off-label.

In addition to the coagulopathy induced by a brain injury, neurosurgeons and intensivists often are faced with managing patients with traumatic intracranial hemorrhage who are pharmacologically anticoagulated. The use of these drugs is expected to increase as the population ages.[329] These patients must have normal coagulation rapidly restored to prevent further bleeding and to make surgical intervention possible. One of the more common drugs encountered in clinical practice is warfarin; a typical scenario is one in which an elderly patient on warfarin sodium (Coumadin) falls and hits her head. It takes about 4 days to normalize coagulation if warfarin is stopped. With vitamin K, full reversal begins 4 to 6 hours after administration and takes about 24 hours to lower the INR. FFP contains vitamin K–dependent factors, is rapidly effective, and is given intravenously. Recombinant factor VIIa also can be used to normalize coagulation in these patients.[329,336,347,348]

In hospitalized patients on heparin, reversal occurs approximately 60 minutes after an intravenous infusion is stopped. If it needs to be reversed faster, protamine is recommended. Desmopressin also has been recommended to reverse the effects of heparin. Subcutaneous heparin is usually not reversed.[329]

With low-molecular-weight heparin (LMWH), a partial thromboplastin time (PTT) is variably altered and not a reliable measure of its effect. Reversal of LMWH effect with protamine is variable in humans.[329]

A common situation is the presentation of a head-injured patient on an antiplatelet agent such as aspirin or other nonsteroidal anti-inflammatory drug (NSAID). Acetylsalicylic acid (ASA) inhibits platelet aggregation for the life of the affected platelet, which is approximately 10 days. This occurs even at the lowest dose of 81 mg per day. A period of 5 to 6 days typically is needed after stopping aspirin to replace approximately half of the circulating platelets (10% per 24 hours). The effect of ASA on platelets is complete and irreversible. If treatment is necessary, platelet transfusion is given to provide unaffected platelets as long as no ASA remains in the circulation. Desmopressin (DDAVP) may secondarily improve platelet adhesion to endothelial defects and is therefore also recommended to overcome aspirin-induced platelet dysfunction. Other NSAIDs have various anticoagulant effects. If significant NSAID use has occurred before a neurosurgical emergency, the same interventional strategy may apply. Data confirming efficacy in counteracting an anticoagulant effect, however, are not available.[329]

Other antiplatelet agents include adenosine diphosphate (ADP) and glycoprotein receptor-blocking agents. Clopidogrel and ticlopidine irreversibly alter platelet aggregation[349-352] through a mechanism that is additive to the antiplatelet effects of aspirin. The platelets are permanently affected; once the drug is stopped, recovery of normal platelet function requires about a week until new platelets are produced. Rapid correction requires platelet transfusion, and DDAVP also may have a beneficial, short-term effect.[329]

Abciximab, eptifibatide, and tirofiban are highly effective in generating 80% to 95% reversible inhibition in platelet aggregation.[349,350,352-355] Stopping the medication allows return of normal platelet function in approximately 48 hours for abciximab and in 4 to 8 hours for the others. Platelet transfusion increases the proportion of unaffected platelets and is the primary intervention.[329]

Fibrinolytic and thrombolytic agents disrupt formed clots.[355-357] These drugs have a prolonged half-life and frequently are used in combination with heparin or other agents to ensure continued therapeutic anticoagulation. Because circulating fibrinogen is decreased during thrombolysis, cryoprecipitate, a source of concentrated fibrinogen, is the basis for reversing treatment.[329] Although these agents have well-recognized applications for cardiac[358] and neurologic[359,360] problems, their use generally is not seen in patients presenting with head injury.

Hypothermia also is known to cause and worsen coagulation abnormalities,[332,361] the treatment for which is rewarming. Certain medical conditions also may affect coagulation, and therefore may be important as underlying factors in patients with a head injury. DDAVP increases the release of factor VIII and von Willebrand factor and is used to treat mild hemophilia A, von Willebrand disease, and chronic renal and liver disease, as well as acquired and congenital platelet disorders.[361,362-365]

DDAVP has a significant antidiuretic effect and will increase free water reabsorption in the kidney, potentially leading to overhydration and hyponatremia. This may cause serious problems in a severely head-injured patient with cerebral edema, poor compliance, and high ICP.

Unintended, iatrogenic worsening of coagulopathy may result with use of hetastarch solutions, which may be administered to increase intravascular volume. These solutions may lower von Willebrand factor levels and alter platelet function. Low-molecular-weight hetastarch preparations are available that may cause less severe changes; however, if the patient requires correction of a coagulation abnormality, these solutions should be avoided if possible.[365-368]

NUTRITIONAL SUPPORT

Replacement of 140% of resting metabolic expenditure in nonparalyzed patients and 100% resting metabolic expenditure in paralyzed patients using enteral or parenteral formulas containing at least 15% of calories as protein by the seventh day after injury is recommended.[3,369]

ROLE OF STEROID THERAPY

On the basis of class 1 evidence originating from a prospective randomized trial comparing dexamethasone and placebo in 300 head-injured patients, dexamethasone was found to be ineffective in improving outcome or reducing ICP in patients with severe brain injury.[3,312] Methylprednisolone, when given in high doses to moderate and severe head-injured patients, is associated with increased mortality.[370] Therefore, the use of steroids is not recommended in their management.

CONCLUSIONS

The management of traumatic brain injury will remain for the foreseeable future a major medical and surgical challenge. Despite concentrated basic research directed at elucidating the metabolic factors that mediate the transition from primary to secondary tissue damage, nothing has been found that might have clinical efficacy. As the percentage of the population older than 70 years of age continues to rise, ICU physicians will face an ethical dilemma when dealing with brain hemorrhages in this age group. Subdural hematoma in an 86-year-old with mild dementia on warfarin sodium (Coumadin) for atrial fibrillation is becoming one of the most common presentations in an active trauma center. At present, intensivists are left with the application of best protocol-driven critical care management, supported by a high index of suspicion for surgically correctable lesions, the judicious use of decompressive hemicraniectomy, and a societal commitment to protective and preventive programs.

KEY POINTS

- The management of severe head injuries remains a major challenge to neurosurgeons.
- The time from injury to surgery must be as short as possible to minimize the secondary manifestations of serious brain trauma.
- Hyperventilation, although very effective in reducing high intracranial pressure (ICP), must be used judiciously; otherwise, it may become more harmful than helpful. Glucocorticoids have no significant therapeutic benefit in managing severe head injuries.
- A simple-to-use and highly predictable neurologic status scoring system, the GCS, has enabled meaningful multidisciplinary communication from the accident scene through intensive care and beyond, resulting in efficient and timely triage and treatment of these patients.
- Mannitol is used in head-injured patients to lower ICP. This drug exerts its beneficial effect through two mechanisms of action: It establishes an osmotic gradient across the blood-brain barrier to reduce water content, and it causes cerebral vasoconstriction through blood flow dynamic effects that decrease blood viscosity and enhance cerebral blood flow and mean arterial blood pressure.
- The use of hypertonic saline to increase mean arterial pressure and decrease ICP is a logical and promising approach to limit secondary injury and improve neurologic outcome.
- Craniectomy can be used to increase the space available for the swollen brain, thereby lowering ICP.

SELECTED REFERENCES

1. Varelas PN, Eastwood D, Yun HJ, et al: Impact of a neurointensivist on outcomes in patients with head trauma treated in a neurosciences intensive care unit. J Neurosurg 2006;104:713-719.
3. Bullock R, Chestnut R, Clifton G, et al: Guidelines for the management of severe traumatic brain injury. A joint initiative of The Brain Trauma Foundation, The American Association of Neurological Surgeons, Congress of Neurological Surgeons, Joint Section on Neurotrauma and Critical Care. 2001.
135. Chang EF, Meeker M, Holland MC: Acute traumatic intraparenchymal hemorrhage: Risk factors for progression in the early post-injury period. Neurosurgery 2006;58:647-656.
200. Brain Trauma Foundation: Guidelines for the management of severe traumatic brain injury, 3rd edition. Chap. 9, Cerebral perfusion thresholds. Journal of Neurotrauma 2007;24(1)S-59-S-64.
228. Kiening KL, Sarrafzadeh AS, Stover JF, Unterberg AW: Should I monitor brain tissue Po_2? In Valadka AB, Andrews BT (eds): Neurotrauma. New York, Thieme Medical Publishers, 2005, pp 62-67.
248. Aarabi B, Hesdorffer D, Ahn E, et al: Outcome following decompressive cranietomy for malignant swelling due to severe head injury. J Neurosurg 2006;104:469-479.
252. Marmarou A, Fatouros PP, Barzo P, et al: Contribution of edema and cerebral blood volume to traumatic brain swelling in head injured patients. J Neurosurg 2000;93:183-193.
300. Ware ML, Nemani VM, Meeker M, et al: Effects of 23.4% sodium chloride solution in reducing intracranial pressure in patients with traumatic brain injury: A preliminary study. Neurosurgery 2005;57:727-736.
330. Powner DJ, Hartwell EA, Hoots WK: Counteracting the effects of anticoagulants and antiplatelet agents during neurosurgical emergencies. Neurosurg 2005;57:823-831.
370. Roberts I, Yates D, Sandercock P, et al: Effect of intravenous corticosteroids on death within 14 days in 10,008 adults with clinically significant head injury (MRC CRASH trial): Randomized placebo controlled trial. Lancet 2004;364:1321-1328.

The complete list of references can be found at www.expertconsult.com.

PART 7

PHYSICAL AND TOXIC INJURY IN THE CRITICALLY ILL

67

Critical Care Management of the Severely Burned Patient

Jeffrey R. Saffle

CHAPTER OUTLINE

INTRODUCTION

Patients suffering major burn injuries present unique challenges in both the types and magnitude of management problems. Fluid resuscitation, pulmonary dysfunction, metabolic stress, and infections complicating burns may surpass similar problems in other intensive care unit (ICU) populations, and treatment is further complicated by abnormal drug pharmacology, severe pain, and psychosocial stress, all superimposed on the need for multiple major surgical procedures and prolonged rehabilitation.

This chapter will review the critical care management of burned adults. It will be apparent that in many areas existing literature is neither comprehensive nor rigorously "evidence-based."[1] In providing a rationale for treatment, therefore, it is often necessary to extrapolate from studies in other disorders, particularly trauma. This may or may not be valid, particularly in such "burn-specific" areas as fluid resuscitation, inhalation injury, and nutritional support. These issues will be discussed as they arise, but readers will need to interpret this information for themselves.

INCIDENCE AND SURVIVAL FROM BURN INJURY

The incidence of burn injury has declined in the United States throughout recent decades. From the 1960s to the early 1990s, reported burns decreased from 10.2 to approximately 4.2 injuries per 1000 Americans annually, or about 1.25 million injuries[2]; hospitalizations decreased from over 90,000 to approximately 52,000/year; and deaths decreased at least 40%, from 9000/year to 5500/year. These trends are likely to continue.

Simultaneously, survival from burns has improved dramatically. During World War II, burns of 40% total body surface area (TBSA) produced a 50% mortality rate; today a similar mortality rate is seen with burns of over 80% TBSA.[3] Survival rate is lower—though still improved—for the elderly, and even higher for children and young adults.[4] These accomplishments are due to cumulative advances in fluid resuscitation, critical care, nutrition, surgery, and skin substitutes. However, it has been the organization of specialized burn centers around a consolidated team of experts that has made this success possible.[5]

Burn survival has been repeatedly shown to correlate with three major factors: patient age, burn size, and the presence of inhalation injury. Pulmonary damage from smoke inhalation is itself a serious injury, and can as much as double the mortality rate from cutaneous burns alone.[3,5] Ryan and colleagues found that burn size 40% TBSA or greater, age 60 years or older, and inhalation injury contributed to the mortality rate in a stepwise manner; patients with all three had a mortality rate of 90% (Table 67.1).[6]

This experience has two important implications for current and future burn treatment. First, mortality risk for many patients is now so low that almost no injury is too large to preclude survival. The decision to intentionally withhold treatment is now rare and is based on predicted quality of life rather than predicted fatality itself. Second, it has necessitated unprecedented research and interest on the rehabilitation of patients who increasingly survive catastrophic injuries. Functional outcomes of burn treatment, including quality of life and return to work, are now the most relevant measures of successful care for all patients.[7,8]

However, the decline in burns has had other unintended consequences, which create challenges to the provision of effective burn care in many areas. As burns have decreased, so has the number of burn centers in the United States. There are now over 25% fewer burn centers than in 1970[9]; only 60 facilities in the United States are currently verified by the American Burn Association (ABA) and American College of Surgeons (ACS).[10] This reduced number limits access to specialized burn care for many Americans. For the same reason, the experience of most physicians with even basic burn care has been dramatically reduced; many U.S. doctors—even surgeons—receive little or no burn training. As a result, important errors in initial burn assessment are made commonly by primary care providers,[11-13] leading to significant under- or (mostly) overtriage, care that is sometimes inadequate, and further stress on the few remaining centers, which now must cover larger referral areas.[14,15]

PATHOPHYSIOLOGY OF BURNS

Although the term *burn* strictly denotes injury caused by heat from flames and scalding liquids, other agents including chemicals, electric current, ionizing radiation, and friction produce nearly identical coagulative necrosis of tissues. The magnitude of such injury depends on the intensity of the source (temperature, voltage, pH, etc.) and the duration of contact, and the clinical severity of a burn is a function of the depth and extent of injury; these factors determine what skin structures are destroyed, the magnitude of response, and the ability of the wound to heal. Accurate assessment of burn wounds is essential in determining appropriate treatment and in predicting outcome.

The outermost *epidermis* of the skin is a thin layer of metabolically active cells that provides a specialized barrier to moisture, bacteria, and chemicals. Burns limited to the epidermis display redness and mild pain without blisters. The underlying *dermis* is much thicker, containing large amounts of structural proteins, which provide strength and flexibility to the skin. Burns extending into the dermis (second-degree, or partial-thickness burns) can vary greatly in appearance and severity. Superficial dermal burns are red, painful, and moist, with prominent fluid-filled blisters, but coagulative necrosis of deeper injuries effectively seals off the skin surface, producing a dry wound. Hair follicles and sweat glands lined with epidermis penetrate through the dermis and serve as a source of epidermal regeneration as partial-thickness injuries heal. Full-thickness or third-degree burns destroy the entire dermis. Such injuries may be a variety of colors, but are invariably dry and relatively insensate. The coagulated dermis is constricted and rigid; as fluid accumulates beneath it, tissue pressure can increase to a dangerous degree, causing vascular compromise and compartmental compression (see later).

Cutaneous injury generates intense inflammation with protean systemic manifestations that persist even after wound coverage is attained. Immediately following injury,

Table 67.1 Risk Factors for Death from Burn Injuries*

No. of Risk Factors	Age >60 yr	Burns ≥40% TBSA	Inhalation Injury	No. of Patients	No. of Deaths	Mortality (%)
0	No	No	No	1314	3	0.2
1	No	No	Yes	112	5	4
1	No	Yes	No	31	1	3
1	Yes	No	No	75	4	5
2	No	Yes	Yes	79	21	27
2	Yes	No	Yes	30	12	39
2	Yes	Yes	No	1	0	0
3	Yes	Yes	Yes	22	21	95
TOTALS				1665	67	4.0

*This table indicates the three risk factors universally accepted to affect burn patient mortality rate, their prevalence, and relative contribution to mortality rate. These data are similar to those from many modern burn centers. Note that overall mortality rate is only 4% and that most patients are relatively young and have limited burn wounds, placing them at little risk of dying.

TBSA, total body surface area.

Adapted with permission from Ryan CM, Schoenfeld DA, Thorpe WP, et al: Objective estimates of the probability of death from burn injuries. N Engl J Med 1998;338(6):362-366.

release of inflammatory mediators causes widespread loss of capillary integrity and depletion of intravascular volume, as well as depressed myocardial contractility, increased peripheral vascular resistance, and systemic hypoperfusion. This shock state can be rapidly lethal, but with adequate support, hemodynamic stability is restored within 24 to 48 hours and is thereafter characterized by increased cardiac output and decreased vascular resistance. This process is fueled by a cascade of local and systemic inflammatory mediators and includes sustained release of epinephrine, cortisol, and glucagon, which generate hypermetabolism, autocannibalism of body protein stores, and glucose intolerance, which persist well into rehabilitation (see "Metabolic Support and Gastrointestinal Management," later).

An even more obvious consequence of burn injury is the burn wound itself. Burned skin quickly accumulates a coating of tenacious *eschar* comprising dried serum and necrotic dermis. Minor burn injuries can often be allowed to heal spontaneously as eschar sloughs and new epidermis emerges from deep appendages to cover the wounds. But the eschar of deep or extensive injuries is extremely susceptible to infection, which has historically been a frequent cause of death. Prompt removal of eschar and coverage with intact skin is essential to control sepsis, ameliorate inflammation, reduce scarring, and optimize functional long-term outcomes. This is a major goal of early burn treatment.

ACUTE CARE OF THE BURNED PATIENT

Acute burn treatment can be divided into four phases, which are outlined in Figure 67.1. *Initial assessment* is the process of stabilizing the acutely injured patient, treating

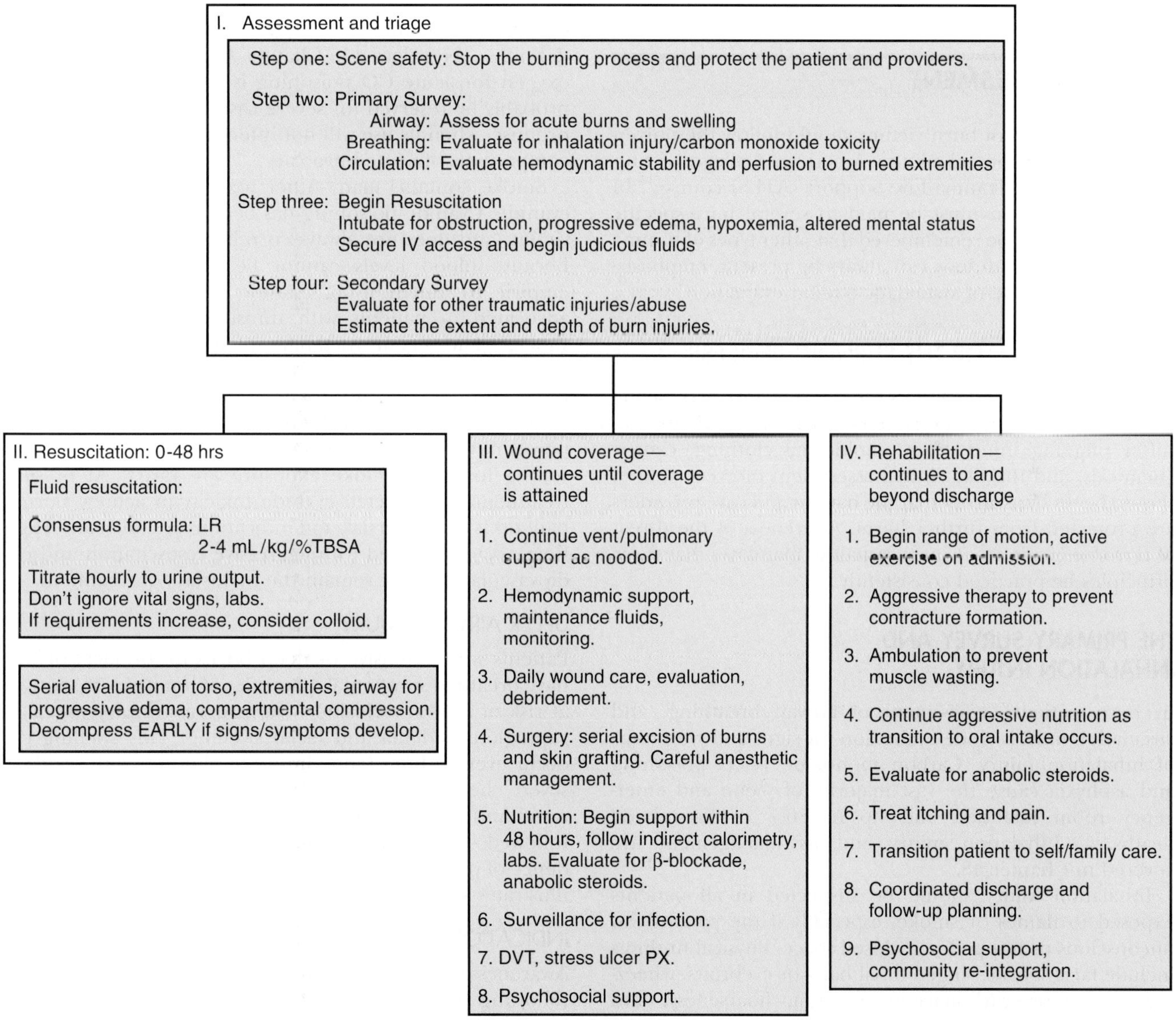
I. Assessment and triage
Step one: Scene safety: Stop the burning process and protect the patient and providers.
Step two: Primary Survey:
Airway: Assess for acute burns and swelling
Breathing: Evaluate for inhalation injury/carbon monoxide toxicity
Circulation: Evaluate hemodynamic stability and perfusion to burned extremities
Step three: Begin Resuscitation
Intubate for obstruction, progressive edema, hypoxemia, altered mental status
Secure IV access and begin judicious fluids
Step four: Secondary Survey
Evaluate for other traumatic injuries/abuse
Estimate the extent and depth of burn injuries.
II. Resuscitation: 0-48 hrs
Fluid resuscitation:
Consensus formula: LR
2-4 mL/kg/%TBSA
Titrate hourly to urine output.
Don't ignore vital signs, labs.
If requirements increase, consider colloid.
Serial evaluation of torso, extremities, airway for progressive edema, compartmental compression.
Decompress EARLY if signs/symptoms develop.
III. Wound coverage—continues until coverage is attained
1. Continue vent/pulmonary support as needed.
2. Hemodynamic support, maintenance fluids, monitoring.
3. Daily wound care, evaluation, debridement.
4. Surgery: serial excision of burns and skin grafting. Careful anesthetic management.
5. Nutrition: Begin support within 48 hours, follow indirect calorimetry, labs. Evaluate for β-blockade, anabolic steroids.
6. Surveillance for infection.
7. DVT, stress ulcer PX.
8. Psychosocial support.
IV. Rehabilitation—continues to and beyond discharge
1. Begin range of motion, active exercise on admission.
2. Aggressive therapy to prevent contracture formation.
3. Ambulation to prevent muscle wasting.
4. Continue aggressive nutrition as transition to oral intake occurs.
5. Evaluate for anabolic steroids.
6. Treat itching and pain.
7. Transition patient to self/family care.
8. Coordinated discharge and follow-up planning.
9. Psychosocial support, community re-integration.

Figure 67.1 Schematic representation of acute burn treatment. Initial assessment and triage should follow the principles of advanced trauma life support, but particular attention must be paid to burn-specific conditions, including protection from additional injury and the presence of inhalation injury, acute edema formation, and major fluid requirements. Following this immediate care, ongoing burn treatment consists of acute fluid resuscitation, wound coverage, and rehabilitation. These phases are shown in overlapping boxes to indicate that, even though the importance of each varies as burn care proceeds, they are often performed simultaneously, and consideration of the importance of each should be borne in mind throughout the course of treatment. See text for additional details.

immediate life-threatening injuries, and preparing for inpatient care. The first 48 hours following injury constitute *acute resuscitation,* focused on initial assessment, airway support, and fluid replacement. The *wound coverage* phase then ensues, in which the major goal of treatment is surgical excision and closure of burn wounds. Ventilator management, metabolic support, control of infection and pain, physical therapy, and other supportive measures are essential adjuncts during this period. The goals of the final *rehabilitation* phase include scar control, optimizing function, and return to independent living. This period can last for months and continue long past discharge. Obviously these phases overlap: discoveries made during initial assessment may require prolonged management; many units begin surgical excision even before resuscitation is completed, and several aspects of rehabilitation—physical therapy, psychosocial support, nutrition, etc.—should start essentially at the time of injury.

INITIAL ASSESSMENT

Initial assessment of burn victims should follow the universally accepted protocol of the American College of Surgeons' Advanced Trauma Life Support (ATLS) course.[16] In doing so, attention must be paid to several burn-specific issues, but it must be remembered that other types of trauma or preexisting conditions can always be present, emphasizing the importance of systematic patient evaluation.

SCENE SAFETY: STOP THE BURNING PROCESS

Though many burned patients receive appropriate on-scene care from first responders, remember that patients can suffer ongoing injury from smoldering clothing, caustic chemicals, and the like. Initial assessment of every patient should begin by assuring that the patient and care providers are protected from further harm. Awareness of the threat of terrorist incidents or mass casualties mandates that these principles be practiced consistently.

THE PRIMARY SURVEY AND INHALATION INJURY

In burn patients, assessment of airway, breathing, and circulation must include evaluation for signs and symptoms of inhalation injury. Carbon monoxide (CO) poisoning and asphyxia cause the vast majority of scene and emergency room fatalities, and up to 80% of fire-related deaths.[17,18] Inhalation injury and its management are covered in Chapter 48.

Inhalation injury should be suspected in all patients exposed to flames or smoke, especially if the patient was unconscious or trapped in a closed space. Physical findings include facial burns, singed nasal hairs or eyebrows, wheezing or stridor, carbonaceous sputum, hoarseness, and anxiety. These findings should alert the examiner to the possible need for airway support.[19]

Inhalation injury is classically considered to consist of three distinct entities: CO poisoning, upper airway injury, and lower airway injury (the "true" inhalation injury). Although patients can frequently present with a combination of all three problems, this classification is worthwhile because of the different pathologic processes and time courses with which these injuries present.

CARBON MONOXIDE POISONING

CO is a product of incomplete combustion, and its highest concentrations occur in indoor fires, where its effects may be amplified by flame-induced oxygen depletion.[20] CO displaces oxygen binding, producing systemic hypoxia despite normal oxygen tension. The most common symptoms are mental status changes, varying from headache to coma, which can present without burn injuries or respiratory distress and be overlooked easily. Classic "cherry red cyanosis" appearance is absent in many victims or can be obscured by soot or burns. Importantly, pulse oximetry is inaccurate in the presence of CO. Direct measurement of carboxyhemoglobin concentration should be performed but should never delay treatment. Patients are at greatest risk on presentation, and immediate application of oxygen is often definitive. As reviewed in Chapter 48, the use of hyperbaric oxygen for acute CO poisoning is controversial; it should probably be reserved for severe cases with neurologic compromise, when its use will not interfere with other essential components of acute burn care.

Smoke contains many other toxic chemicals, including cyanide. Cyanide poisoning has been documented in burn victims and does not always correlate with CO exposure.[21] Because blood levels cannot be obtained immediately, empiric treatment using cyanide antidote kits has been advocated in patients with unusually severe acidosis or shock.[22] The recent availability of hydroxocobalamin as a cyanide antidote, which has few side effects, has led to both renewed interest in the treatment of cyanide toxicity and aggressive marketing of the drug. However, a recent review points out that confirmed cases of significant cyanide poisoning following smoke exposure are rare.[23] At present, treatment of suspected cyanide toxicity in acutely burned patients is controversial, and indications are unclear.[24] High-flow oxygen coupled with aggressive resuscitation and cardiovascular support remain the mainstays of treatment.

UPPER AIRWAY INJURY

Patients with extensive or deep burns to the face, or who have breathed substantial quantities of hot gases or soot, are at risk of airway occlusion from progressive pharyngeal or supraglottic edema and facial swelling. This swelling can occur even without flame injury in children with scalds or severe chemical burns. Edema formation can be extremely rapid and progress for at least 24 hours. Patients must be followed serially, and intubated early and electively if evidence of progressive airway compromise occurs. Figure 67.2 illustrates such a case.

INDICATIONS FOR INTUBATION

Awareness of the potential for acute airway compromise following burn injury has led to a liberal attitude toward intubation that is probably appropriate. "When in doubt, intubate" expresses many physicians' attitude toward this problem. However, this dictum has sometimes led to indiscriminate and unnecessary intubation of patients with even minor facial burns.[25] The presence of inhalation injury does not mandate intubation, and airway compromise can be

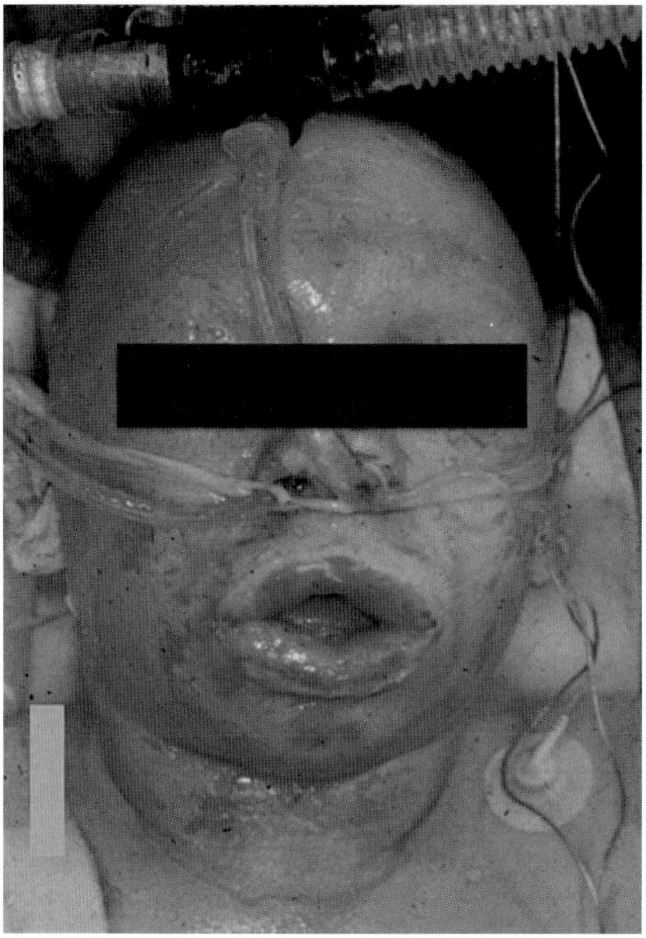

Figure 67.2 This young man was burned playing with matches and gasoline, sustaining burns to 60% total body surface area, including his entire face. On presentation, he was alert and breathing comfortably. Arterial blood gases (including carboxyhemoglobin) and chest x-ray findings were normal. Based on the extent and location of his injuries, elective nasotracheal intubation was performed. Six hours later, the patient displays massive facial edema. Eyes are swollen shut, and oral excursion is severely restricted. If he lost his endotracheal tube at this point, his airway could not be maintained. Note that the tube is tied around his head securely, not taped in position. He will need to remain intubated for at least 3 to 5 days until most of this edema resolves.

life-threatening even in the absence of inhalation injury. Indications for intubation, as in all trauma patients, are based on symptoms found on initial assessment, including altered mental status, refractory hypoxemia, and signs of impending airway obstruction including wheezing, stridor, dyspnea, and progressive facial swelling. Emergency tracheostomy or cricothyroidotomy, which should rarely be needed if intubation is performed in a timely manner, can be an extremely challenging procedure in the setting of massive head and neck swelling.

PULMONARY ("TRUE") INHALATION INJURY

Exposure of the bronchi and small airways to toxic smoke causes chemical injury to the epithelium, which can progress to mucosal sloughing, mucous plugging, bronchiectasis, hypoxemia, and pneumonia. Clinical signs of this problem may be absent for up to 72 hours after exposure,

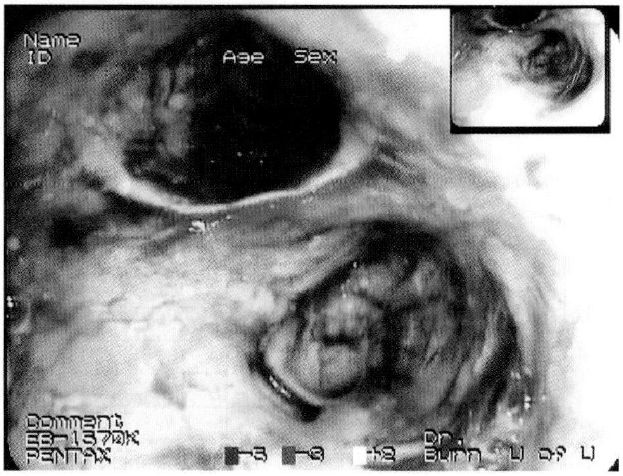

Figure 67.3 Bronchoscopic appearance of the carina of a man who was dragged unconscious from a burning house. Carbonaceous deposits are apparent in his trachea, and more extensively in the mainstem bronchi. This finding is diagnostic of inhalation injury.

and initial chest radiographs are usually normal.[26] Patients with immediate respiratory distress, stridor, or hypoxemia are much more likely to have upper airway injury. Even in the absence of symptoms, patients suspected of having inhalation injury require hospital admission and close observation. Fiberoptic bronchoscopy demonstrating carbonaceous debris, erythema, or mucosal sloughing is highly sensitive for diagnosis of inhalation injury and can facilitate immediate intubation if injury is confirmed[27] (Fig. 67.3). Inhalation injury is discussed further in Chapter 48.

BEGIN RESUSCITATION

Following quick initial assessment, intravenous resuscitation and other support should be initiated.

THE SECONDARY SURVEY

As resuscitation is beginning, a thorough head-to-toe examination is performed. Burn victims frequently suffer other trauma, which can be obscured by overlying burns (see later). Much of the subsequent care of the burn patient is based on assessment of the extent and depth of injury, including fluid resuscitation, nutritional requirements, surgery, and in extreme cases, the decision to provide aggressive treatment. For these reasons, the burn wound should be washed and thoroughly debrided and then documented as accurately as possible, preferably by an experienced clinician. Rough estimates of burn size are often made using the "rule of nines"; more accurate detailed documentation can be done using the Lund and Browder chart (Fig. 67.4). Computerized programs are also becoming popular, such as the Sage diagram (www.sagediagram.com). In evaluating smaller injuries, another useful rule is that the area of the patient's palm (with fingers) equals about 1% of his/her TBSA.

BURNS AND MULTIPLE TRAUMA

The many mishaps that cause burns often cause other trauma as well. These situations can include explosions

BURN ESTIMATE AND DIAGRAM
AGE VERSUS AREA

Area	Birth 1 yr	1–4 yr	5–9 yr	10–14 yr	15 yr	Adult	2 degrees	3 degrees	Total	Donor Areas
Head	19	17	13	11	9	7				
Neck	2	2	2	2	2	2				
Ant. Trunk	13	13	13	13	13	13				
Post. Trunk	13	13	13	13	13	13				
R. Buttock	2½	2½	2½	2½	2½	2½				
L. Buttock	2½	2½	2½	2½	2½	2½				
Genitalia	1	1	1	1	1	1				
R. U. Arm	4	4	4	4	4	4				
L. U. Arm	4	4	4	4	4	4				
R. L. Arm	3	3	3	3	3	3				
L. L. Arm	3	3	3	3	3	3				
R. Hand	2½	2½	2½	2½	2½	2½				
L. Hand	2½	2½	2½	2½	2½	2½				
R. Thigh	5½	6½	8	8½	9	9½				
L. Thigh	5½	6½	8	8½	9	9½				
R. Leg	5	5	5½	6	6½	7				
L. Leg	5	5	5½	6	6½	7				
R. Foot	3½	3½	3½	3½	3½	3½				
L. Foot	3½	3½	3½	3½	3½	3½				
						TOTAL				

Cause of Burn ______________________

Date of Burn ____________

Time of Burn ____________

Age ____________

Sex ____________

Weight ____________

BURN DIAGRAM

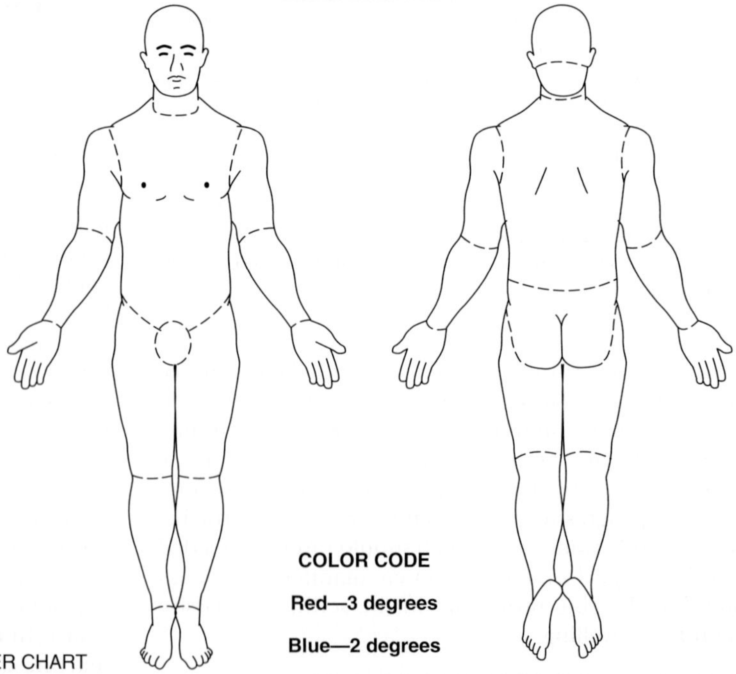

COLOR CODE

Red—3 degrees

Blue—2 degrees

LUND AND BROWDER CHART

Figure 67.4 The Lund and Browder chart is in widespread use in burn centers for diagramming and calculating burn extent and depth. The chart divides the body into small areas and gives the relative percent total body surface area for each area for different age groups. With a little practice, physicians can estimate burns quite accurately. To do so, evaluate wounds after they have been washed and debrided. Inspect each area carefully and attempt to distinguish between partial- and full-thickness burn wounds. Total burn size is calculated by adding individual body areas.

(blasts, falls, projectile wounds), electrocutions (tetany-induced fractures, falls), fires in motor vehicle or airplane crashes, and escaping fires (lacerations, falls). Combined burn/trauma injuries are particularly likely following assault or child abuse and should increase suspicion for such causes.[28]

The combined mortality rates for burns and trauma appear to be at least additive compared to either injury alone.[29,30] Thorough evaluation of all potential injuries according to ATLS guidelines is imperative and can be challenging in burn patients: the discoloration, pain, and swelling of burn wounds, for example, can conceal underlying fractures[31]; and burns of the torso or acute inhalation injury can obscure a pneumothorax or other injuries. For this reason, it is important not to focus too heavily on burn injuries in performing the secondary survey.

In addition, care should be provided by a multispecialty team with expertise in managing all injuries. Treatment of many traumatic injuries takes priority over definitive burn care and mandates immediate operation. Because fresh burn wounds are initially—and briefly—free of bacteria, laparotomy, craniotomy, repair of lacerations, and operative fixation of fractures should be performed immediately, and no later than 12 to 24 hours after burn.[32,33] This approach will minimize risk of infections, permit early mobilization, and facilitate access to burn wounds for dressings and surgery. These interventions can be performed safely provided essential components of burn care—including airway support, temperature control, and aggressive fluid resuscitation—are instituted immediately and continued through surgery. Close coordination between the burn center and trauma center will optimize outcome for these patients.

THE RESUSCITATION PHASE

BURN SHOCK

Following initial evaluation, the primary focus of early burn treatment is fluid resuscitation. The goals of resuscitation are to support organ function while avoiding complications of over- or underadministration of fluid.[34] This task can be challenging given the huge fluid shifts and cardiovascular effects of acute burns. Development of effective protocols for resuscitation represents one of the major advancements in burn care in this century.

The magnitude of fluid shifts following a major burn can exceed those of any other injury. At the cellular level, burn injury immediately impairs membrane adenosine triphosphatase (ATPase) activity and reduces transmembrane potential,[35,36] resulting in increased intracellular sodium and extracellular potassium concentrations, cellular swelling, and acidosis. Fluid resuscitation only partially corrects these abnormalities, which may require several days to resolve completely as local inflammation subsides.

These events present clinically as a profound inflammatory response, causing increased capillary permeability and massive tissue edema at the expense of intravascular volume. Immediate release of histamine and serotonin increase local perfusion, initiate capillary leakage, and potentiate vasoconstriction caused by massive catecholamine secretion.[36-38] Tumor necrosis factor (TNF)-α produces myocardial depression and activates a number of other vasoactive mediators.[39] Prostaglandins, leukotrienes, oxygen radicals, products of platelet activation and coagulation, and a cascade of cytokines also contribute to these abnormalities.[40,41] Alterations in local blood flow increase arteriolar tone and pressure and dilate postcapillary venules, causing local capillary perfusion to become less selective and increased, favoring extensive edema formation.

The forces that control transcapillary fluid flux are summarized in Starling's equation[42]; their alterations in burn injury have been reviewed by Demling[43] (Table 67.2). The greatest edema formation occurs almost immediately within the wound, caused by near-total permeability to even very large (35 nm) molecules,[44] and permitting protein-rich plasma to pour into the interstitium.[45] Maximum protein extravasation occurs within the first hour of injury, and both its duration and magnitude are proportional to burn size.[46,47]

Even after local capillary integrity normalizes within 8 to 12 hours, edema formation continues in unburned as well as burned tissues.[48] Depletion of intravascular proteins, further diluted by crystalloid resuscitation,[49] eliminates the oncotic pressure gradient (see $\pi p - \pi i$ in Table 67.2), which maintains intravascular volume. Hypoproteinemia alone can mimic burn edema, and infusions of colloid can almost completely prevent edema in unburned tissues.[50,51] Progressive edema also alters the configuration of interstitial collagen and hyaluronic acid, which are normally densely coiled to limit fluid influx.[52] Burn injury disrupts this "safety valve" configuration, increasing compliance, producing osmotically active molecular fragments, and generating negative ("sucking") interstitial pressure[53] and extremely rapid fluid sequestion.[48] Though this gradient is neutralized within a few hours, compliance continues to increase as interstitial gel is hydrated, allowing liters of fluid to accumulate with little change in hydrostatic pressure[54] and permitting edema to persist for weeks following injury.

Cardiac output falls within minutes of injury, reaching 50% to 60% of normal within an hour, although systemic vascular resistance (SVR) increases dramatically. Both changes occur far faster than the depletion of intravascular volume[45,55] and regardless of fluid resuscitation. Release of catecholamines and other vasoactive mediators clearly increases SVR, but the decrease in cardiac output is harder to explain. Researchers have long postulated the existence of a "myocardial depressant factor,"[56] though no such substance has been isolated. It seems more likely that cardiac output is impaired by the combination of increased SVR, volume depletion, and actions of TNF-α, endotoxin, and other chemicals. One clinically important side effect of capillary permeability is hemoconcentration—a marked rise in hematocrit as plasma is sieved out of the bloodstream into the interstitium—which increases blood viscosity and further impairs cardiac output.

Cardiac output begins to recover within a few hours of injury and requires 12 to 24 hours to normalize, even with vigorous resuscitation. SVR follows an opposite course, peaking quickly and then declining to near-normal within 24 to 48 hours (Fig. 67.5). Following these initial changes a chronic hyperdynamic circulation is maintained, with cardiac output persisting well above normal, and marked

Table 67.2 Starling Forces and Capillary Permeability*

Starling's formula: $Q = Kf\,(Pcap - Pi) + \sigma\,(\pi p - \pi i)$

Symbol	Definition	Alteration in Burn Injury
Q	Net rate of fluid passage across the capillary membrane	Increased dramatically as a result of changes in all component forces
Kf	Filtration coefficient; consists of two components:	
	The surface area of the capillary system	Increased as a result of increased local blood flow, perfusing more capillaries
	Compliance of the interstitium	Increased owing to alterations in molecular configuration (see text)
Pcap	Capillary hydrostatic pressure	Increased as a result of arterial vasoconstriction
Pi	Interstitial hydrostatic pressure	Decreased secondary to changes in molecular configuration of the interstitium (see text)
σ	Reflection coefficient—describes the permeability of the capillary to macromolecules	Greatly increased permeability to even large molecules; in burned skin, this value approximates 0.3
	Ordinarily this is quite limited; a coefficient of 1.0 indicates that no protein can pass across the membrane; a coefficient of zero implies total permeability. For normal skin, this value is approximately 0.9.	This effect appears largely limited to burned tissues; generation of edema formation in nonburned tissues depends more on changes in colloid oncotic pressure and interstitial compliance.
πp	Plasma colloid oncotic pressure	Progressively reduced
	Each gram of albumin generates approximately 4 mm Hg of oncotic pressure; normal πp is 20 mm Hg.	Most direct leakage of albumin is into burned tissues, but as this occurs, πp is reduced systemically. This is further diluted by crystalloid resuscitation
πi	Interstitial colloid oncotic pressure	Reduced slightly, but this effect is limited owing to changes in interstitial compliance
Pcap – Pi	The difference in hydrostatic pressure across the capillary membrane	Increased owing to increased hydrostatic pressure; little or no increase in interstitial pressure
	The greater the gradient, the more rapid the flow of fluid. Normal gradient is 10-12 mm Hg.	
$\pi p - \pi i$	The difference in oncotic pressure across the capillary membrane	Reduced owing to dilution of plasma proteins; little change in interstitial pressure

*See discussion in Demling RH: The burn edema process: Current concepts. J Burn Care Rehabil 2005;26:207-227.
Adapted with permission from Ryan CM, Schoenfeld DA, Thorpe WP, et al: Objective estimates of the probability of death from burn injuries. N Engl J Med 1998;338:362-366.

vasodilation and decreased SVR often persisting even after wound coverage is attained.

FLUID RESUSCITATION OF BURN PATIENTS

Before World War II, patients with even moderate burns usually died within a few days because of progressive shock and renal failure. In 1942, surgeons Oliver Cope and Francis Moore designed the first formal resuscitation regimen to treat victims of the Cocoanut Grove nightclub fire, with substantial improvements in survival.[36] With continued refinements, today almost all patients can be resuscitated successfully, and renal failure complicating burn injury is rare. A host of formulas have been developed, almost all based on body weight and burn size, and utilizing various combinations of crystalloid and colloid solutions. The archetype and most widely used of such regimens is the Parkland formula, designed by Baxter.[35] He demonstrated that a volume of lactated Ringer's (LR) solution equal to 4 mL per kilogram body weight for each percent TBSA burned (4 mL/kg/%TBSA), given in the first 24 hours after injury, would maintain urine output of 50 to 70 mL/hour, replete blood volume, and restore cellular transmembrane potential and cardiac output in most patients. Half this calculated volume is given in the first 8 hours after burn, the remainder over the next 16 hours. The intravenous rate is adjusted hourly to maintain urine output and is decreased gradually until a "maintenance" rate is reached at approximately 24 hours.

Maintenance requirements for burn patients are also increased due to ongoing evaporative and metabolic losses, and continued fluid support is essential even after resuscitation is complete. A popular formula to estimate these requirements is that developed by Warden:[57]

24-hour maintenance fluid requirements
= Evaporative water losses + normal insensible losses

In this equation,

Evaporative water losses = (35 + %TBSA burn) × m^2 × 24 hours
Normal insensible losses = (1500 × m^2) per 24 hours
m^2 = body surface area in square meters

This experience forms the basis of modern burn resuscitation. But despite widespread acceptance of the principles of fluid replacement, disagreement persists over almost every aspect of practical management, and the practice of

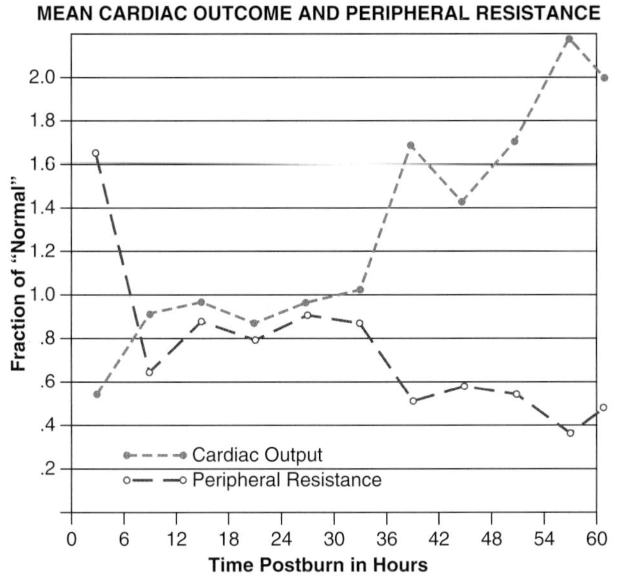

Figure 67.5 This classic graph shows characteristic postburn changes in cardiac output and peripheral vascular resistance in a group of seven patients (mean burn size 64.5% total body surface area [TBSA]) resuscitated with the Brooke formula (lactated Ringer's [LR] solution, 1.5 mL/kg/%TBSA, albumin, 0.5 mL/kg/%TBSA, plus 2000 mL dextrose/water in the first 24 hours). Cardiac output falls acutely, before blood volume has changed appreciably, then rebounds gradually, with return to normal by 24 to 36 hours, and thereafter remaining above normal. Peripheral vascular resistance shows an opposite effect. (From Pruitt BA Jr, Mason AD Jr, Moncrief JA: Hemodynamic changes in the early postburn patient: The influence of fluid administration and of a vasodilator (hydralazine). J Trauma 1971;11:36-46.)

resuscitation varies significantly among units. One example exists in defining the end points of resuscitation. Successful resuscitation requires meticulous monitoring and adjustment of resuscitation based on patient response. Traditional resuscitation relies almost exclusively on hourly urine output for this purpose, so the amount of fluid required for resuscitation depends partly on the urine output targeted. Baxter used an output of 50 to 70 mL/hour; several other formulas that accept outputs of 0.5 mL/kg/hour (1.0 mL/kg/hour in children) call for LR infusion rates between 2 and 3 mL/kg/%TBSA, and are also in widespread use.[34,36]

THE PHENOMENON OF "FLUID CREEP"

Clinicians have long accepted the consensus that patients should receive as little fluid as possible to maintain organ perfusion.[58] But several patient groups routinely require more resuscitation fluid than predicted by the Parkland formula, including patients with inhalation injury,[59] those with multiple trauma and electrical burns, patients in whom resuscitation is substantially delayed,[4] and patients with alcohol or drug abuse.[60] Inexperienced clinicians often make substantial errors in estimating burn size, which can result in significant under- or overestimation of fluid requirements.[11] Careful monitoring of resuscitation and individualized fluid therapy can often obviate these problems.

But in recent years a widespread tendency for patients to receive increasing quantities of resuscitation fluid has been observed, a phenomenon dubbed "fluid creep" by Pruitt.[61] Cancio and associates found that 63% of their recent patients required a mean of 6.1 ± 0.22 mL/kg/%TBSA for resuscitation despite very modest urine output.[62] Others have documented such increased fluid requirements in up to 100% of patients.[63-65] The potential complications of fluid creep are far from benign, including extremity and abdominal compartment syndromes, worsening pulmonary dysfunction, and more frequent and prolonged endotracheal intubation. Figure 67.6 illustrates the actual resuscitation of a child who required an excessive amount of crystalloid to achieve successful resuscitation and maintain adequate urine output.

This departure from tradition is probably due to several influences. First, the successful resuscitation of patients with massive burns appears to routinely require increased fluid volumes.[62] In Baxter's initial report of 277 patients, 89% of those with burns 60% TBSA or greater died.[45] However, modern survival is much better and owes some of its success to persisting with aggressive fluid resuscitation beyond the confines of the Parkland formula.

Second, it appears that fluid creep perpetuates itself. Overly zealous initial fluid administration—often performed in the field—increases serum protein depletion, generating a vicious circle of reduced oncotic pressure and enhanced edema, which in turn increases crystalloid requirements. This mechanism also helps explain the occurrence of resuscitation failure, in which fluid requirements actually escalate despite adequate—or excessive—crystalloid administration.[66] The use of colloid-containing fluids can arrest this cycle and restore oncotic pressure but adds to overall fluid requirements as well.

Fluid creep has probably also been encouraged by resuscitation trends in other ICU populations. Traditional burn resuscitation formulas permit significant deficits in vascular volume and cardiac output to persist until the end of 24 hours.[45] The routine observation of hematocrits as high as 70% during resuscitation is consistent with this concept. Both lactic acid (LA) and base deficit (BD) remain elevated throughout traditional resuscitation,[67] which also fails to reflect changes in cardiac output and oxygen delivery (VO_2).[68] In contrast, resuscitation in other shock states has been increasingly directed at normalizing LA and BD, and optimizing cardiac output, VO_2, and pulmonary wedge pressure.[69,70] As this concept gained acceptance in critical care, burn clinicians have become more inclined to monitor these parameters and to respond to abnormalities by increasing fluid support.

However, this approach may not be valid in burns. Although it is accepted that patients' ability to achieve optimal values of cardiac output and VO_2 correlates strongly with outcome, it is less clear whether exaggerated fluid infusion, invasive monitoring, and inotropic support can change nonresponders into responders and thus improve survival.[71] Optimizing VO_2 and improved survival in one group of patients with severe burns,[72] but both Kaups and colleagues[64] and Choi and coworkers[65] were unable to determine if resuscitation aimed at normalizing elevated BD was effective or beneficial. In other studies of goal-directed therapy in burns, attaining target values of cardiac output, VO_2, or wedge pressure routinely required more fluid—as much as four times Parkland calculations—without obvious improvement in survival,[73,74] and potential increase in edema-related

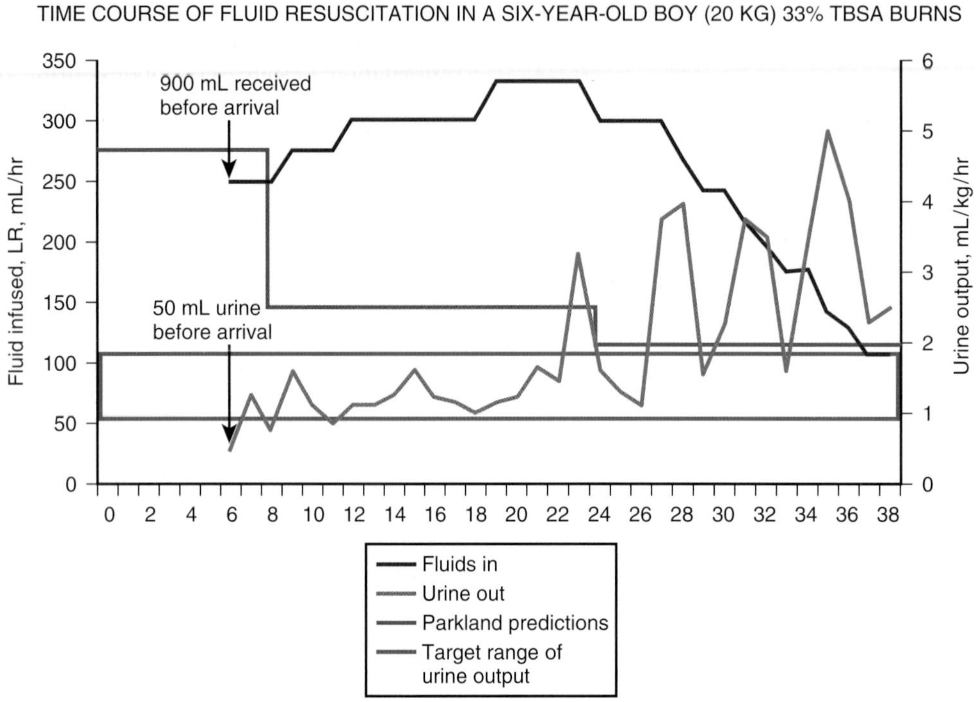

Figure 67.6 Time course of fluid resuscitation for a 6-year-old boy (20 kg) with 33% total body surface area (TBSA) scald burns. He arrived at the burn center 6 hours after injury, having received 900 mL of lactated Ringer's (LR) solution prior to arrival. Fluid resuscitation was started according to the Parkland formula *(heavy dashed line);* nurses were instructed to maintain urine output between 0.9 and 1.8 mL/kg/hour *(dotted line).* Initial resuscitation was close to Parkland guidelines, but beginning at about 10 hours after burn, fluid requirements increased progressively until about 22 hours, when urine output finally began to rise, and fluids were tapered in a stepwise manner according to protocol. The patient reached his calculated maintenance fluid rate of 106 mL/hour at hour 36. Total resuscitation received was 11.38 mL/kg/%TBSA. He had no difficulties with compartment syndromes or respiratory distress. This case illustrates the occurrence of "fluid creep" that has been experienced frequently in modern burn care.

complications, which appear directly related to the fluid volume administered.[75,76]

It is clear that the optimal method of monitoring and delivering burn resuscitation has yet to be determined. Although fluid creep is widespread, most burn centers still base fluid administration primarily on urine output. Invasive hemodynamic monitoring does not appear beneficial for routine use, though it may be helpful in guiding therapy in individuals who are clearly failing to respond to traditional resuscitation, including elderly patients or those with massive injuries, cardiac disease, associated multiple trauma, or severe pulmonary dysfunction.

HYPERTONIC RESUSCITATION

Crystalloid solutions remain the mainstay of all resuscitation regimens as they are inexpensive, well tolerated, readily available, and easily mobilized and excreted. The effective component of crystalloid is sodium,[77] which has led to the use of hypertonic saline solutions to satisfy capillary and cellular leakage while minimizing fluid volume and edema.[78,79] Solutions containing as much sodium as 300 mEq/L result in delivery of almost identical quantities of sodium as LR solution with substantially less volume.[80] Hypertonic saline resuscitation has been advocated for children[81] and the elderly,[82] who tolerate under- and overresuscitation poorly, as well as for patients with head injuries,[83] and for field and combat resuscitation when the weight of available solutions must be minimized.[84,85]

Hypertonic saline resuscitation carries the risk of significant hypernatremia, hyperchloremia, acidosis, and hyperosmolarity, and requires careful monitoring. In addition, savings in initial fluid requirements may be balanced by increased free water retention later.[86] Hypertonic saline has been associated with increased mortality risk in at least one study, possibly related to increased renal failure.[86] However, it is still used selectively in some burn centers[79,87] and remains an option in acute burn management.

CRYSTALLOID VERSUS COLLOID

Because of the indiscriminate nature of early postburn capillary leakage, colloids are not superior to crystalloids in initial burn resuscitation.[55] For this and other reasons, colloid use in resuscitation of all types has been condemned.[88] However, capillary integrity is largely restored by the end of 24 hours after injury, and colloids given at this time can effectively restore oncotic pressure, expand plasma volume, and reduce secondary edema in unburned tissue,[35,51] including possible prevention of abdominal compartment syndrome.[89]

Colloids used in burn resuscitation have included albumin, plasma protein fraction (Plasmanate), fresh frozen plasma, and the synthetic colloids dextran and hetastarch. Routine albumin administration is a component of the traditional Evans and Brooke formulas[36,55] and was originally used at the end of Parkland resuscitation.[35] In a widely quoted randomized trial, Goodwin and associates found that albumin-based resuscitation required less total fluid than solution alone but was associated with a sustained increase in extravascular lung water.[90] Critics have also pointed out that routine albumin supplementation has no apparent benefits.[91] Nonetheless, albumin remains a popular colloid; its current use varies among burn centers from routine administration within 8 to 12 hours of injury,[50,57] to selective use as "rescue" in problem resuscitations, to near-total interdiction. Fresh frozen plasma has also been used successfully[92]; its colloid effect probably explains much of the efficacy of plasma exchange therapy in complex burn resuscitations.[93] Both low-molecular-weight dextran and hetastarch have been used in burn resuscitation and appear as effective as albumin in maintaining oncotic pressure and limiting edema in unburned tissues.[51,94,95] They offer advantages of long shelf life, availability, freedom from disease transmission, and lower cost. However, hetastarch has been associated with rare anaphylaxis and dose-dependent coagulopathy and bleeding, which limits is use in large volumes.[96]

Colloid is probably unnecessary for resuscitation of most patients with uncomplicated injuries. With increasing burn size, the benefits of colloid administration, restricted to use after the first 8 to 12 hours after burn, may be significant in reducing total fluid requirements and edema-related complications. Many centers now utilize LR solution for the first hours after injury, followed by hypertonic saline, colloid, or both to reduce edema as resuscitation is completed.[57] The patient illustrated in Figure 67.6 would be a very appropriate candidate for this form of "rescue" therapy, which would likely have reduced his ongoing fluid requirements. This area of resuscitation is extremely controversial and will benefit from randomized multicenter trials.

PHARMACOLOGIC MANIPULATION OF RESUSCITATION

Improved understanding of the pathophysiology of burn shock has led investigators to attempt to reduce its severity by blocking some of its specific chemical mediators. These efforts have included use of vasodilators such as hydralazine, histamine blockade using cimetidine, the serotonin antagonist ketanserin, and anti-inflammatory drugs such as hydrocortisone and ibuprofen.[43,55,97-99] Large doses of the antioxidant vitamin C has been shown to decrease fluid requirements in clinical burn resuscitation.[100] Many of these efforts have shown modest benefits, though none has found its way into widespread clinical use. The possibility of developing an effective "cocktail" to ameliorate the effects of burn shock holds promise for the future.

PRACTICING EFFECTIVE RESUSCITATION

A bewildering array of regimens (and opinions) are in current use for burn resuscitation. In attempting to practice resuscitation effectively, the clinician must decide on a protocol that is uniform and easy to apply by nurses, yet flexible enough to permit individualized therapy and provide appropriate "escapes" for patients who are unstable.

An example of the protocol used at the University of Utah is included in Figure 67.7. The protocol is based on the Parkland formula, but contains an option for the use of LR/albumin to arrest escalating fluid requirements. It requires nurses to adjust infusions based on hourly urine output, but mandates that physicians be contacted if worrisome parameters develop. We have found this protocol effective in resuscitating the vast majority of patients without frequent input from physicians. Similar protocols are in use in a number of burn centers.

COMPLICATIONS OF EDEMA

Although the quantity of edema in both burned and unburned tissue is affected by fluid resuscitation, it is also true that substantial swelling occurs regardless of the resuscitation used. Swelling within the face, eyes, extremities, and torso can have catastrophic consequences if untreated, and it is essential to remember that edema is progressive for 24 hours following burn injury; an area that is soft and pliable on admission may become tensely swollen within hours or overnight. Clinicians must be aware of the potential for these complications, follow serial examinations, and treat them as they develop.

FACIAL SWELLING

Full-thickness facial burns can swell massively and produce complete airway obstruction within an hour or 2 of injury, as illustrated in Figure 67.2. As discussed under initial assessment, endotracheal intubation is essential in this setting and should be performed early and electively.

Continued facial swelling may preclude safe extubation for several days following injury, and inadvertent extubation in this period can be disastrous. Tubes must be secured carefully; patients may require sedation or paralysis to ensure this. As edema begins to resolve within 48 to 72 hours, extubation should not be attempted until patients can open their eyes and breathe spontaneously and an air leak can be demonstrated with the cuff deflated. Early tracheostomy may provide a more comfortable and secure airway for patients with large injuries.

OCULAR SWELLING

Elevated intraocular pressures (IOPs) have been documented in burn patients and appear to correlate with resuscitation volume. No data exist on the consequences of this phenomenon, but the risk of optic nerve ischemia and permanent visual loss may exist. Lateral canthotomy has been recommended for patients with persistently high IOPs.[101,102] Measurement of IOP during acute burn resuscitation may be warranted in patients with severe facial injuries and eyelid edema.

EXTREMITY COMPARTMENT SYNDROMES

Burns probably constitute the most common cause of extremity compartment syndromes. The pathophysiology is identical to that which accompanies fractures, crush injuries, and so on with the notable exception that in burn patients the constricting layer is the burn eschar, not the underlying fascia, so that incision through the burn wound—"escharotomy"—is required to relieve compression.

Failure to diagnose circulatory embarrassment of a burned extremity can lead to progressive ischemia, myonecrosis, and amputation. Because this can develop insidiously in burned extremities that are soft on presentation, a high index of suspicion and performance of serial examinations are essential. Compartmental compression is most likely

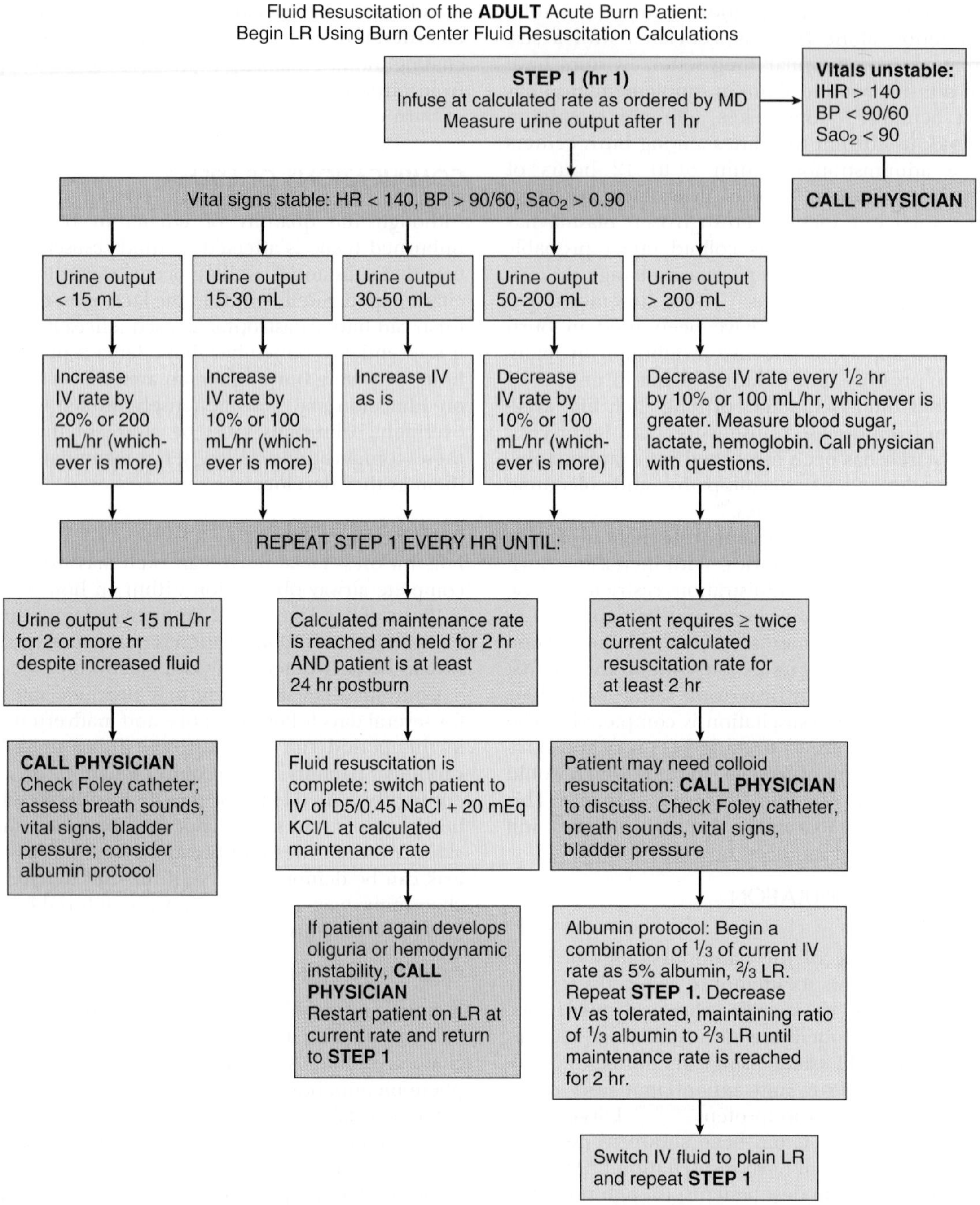

Figure 67.7 Burn fluid resuscitation protocol used at the University of Utah. Physicians order an initial infusion rate of lactated Ringer's solution based on Parkland calculations, and indicate the target maintenance rate. Nursing staff measures hourly urine output, and increases or decreases fluids based on this response. If patients develop unexpected changes in vital signs, or fail to respond appropriately, physicians are contacted. An option for the use of colloid-containing resuscitation is included for patients whose requirements fail to decline. This regimen permits close titration of fluids without requiring hourly physician input.

following full-thickness, circumferential extremity burns but can develop in the absence of these findings, even in unburned extremities in patients who require excessive resuscitation volumes, particularly children.

Swollen extremities should be initially treated with elevation and avoidance of constricting dressings. Classic findings of pain, paralysis, pallor, paresthesia, pulselessness (the "five Ps") may be difficult beneath burn injuries or in intubated patients, and may not develop until irreversible ischemia has occurred. Similarly, limb-threatening compression can exist despite persistent palpable or Doppler pulses.[103] For these reasons, some authorities perform escharotomies based on a general impression of extremity swelling, or even prophylactically. Alternatively, many clinicians monitor intramuscular pressure to determine the need for decompression. This procedure is easily done by inserting a large-bore (18-gauge) needle attached to a pressure transducer through the eschar into the underlying muscle.

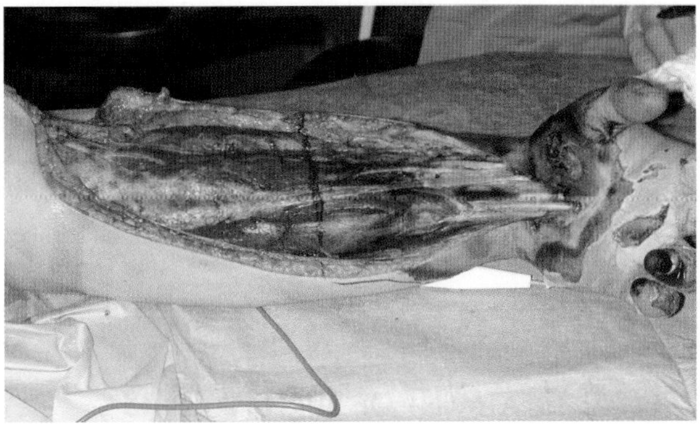

Figure 67.8 Massively swollen forearm following high-voltage electrocution injury. Simple escharotomy of the distal forearm and hand failed to decompress the extremity, so extensive fasciotomy was performed to above the elbow. The skin edges are widely separated by edema. Proximal forearm muscles are viable, but tissues distal to the drawn line—the line of anticipated amputation—are clearly necrotic. The wrist and fingers are "frozen" in flexion caused by contraction of damaged muscles.

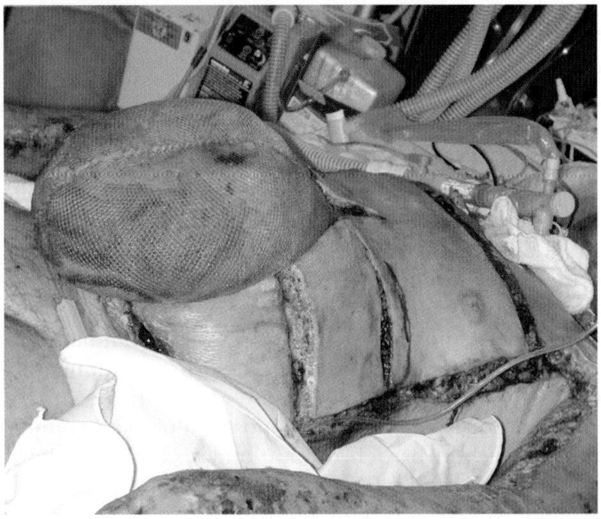

Figure 67.9 Complications of edema in an elderly man with 70% total body surface area burns. Facial edema is massive; tracheostomy has been performed to provide secure, long-term airway support. Escharotomies on upper extremities and multiple torso escharotomies have resulted in increased swelling and separation of wound edges. Despite these measures, abdominal compartment syndrome necessitated bedside laparotomy and placement of a synthetic mesh "silo" to contain eviscerated abdominal contents. As edema resolved over several days, viscera were gradually returned to the abdomen and the silo was trimmed, until closure of the fascia was possible. The other escharotomy wounds were covered with skin grafts.

Pressures that exceed 30 cm H_2O in the relaxed extremity indicate compromised capillary perfusion and mandate decompression.[104] Measurements should be repeated following escharotomy; pressures that remain elevated indicate the need to deepen or extend incisions or to proceed with fasciotomy. This may be particularly likely in patients with very deep burns, associated trauma, or electrical injury (Fig. 67.8).

Escharotomies can often be done at the bedside using electrocautery and appropriate analgesia. Longitudinal incisions should run the length of the burn wound, be placed medially and laterally on the supinated limb to avoid major nerves and vessels, and facilitate resurfacing with skin grafts. Incisions must penetrate through the burn until the wound edges "pop open," and pressure is clearly relieved. Incisions in burned hands should extend at least to the metacarpophalangeal joints; performance of individual digit escharotomies has some support[105] but is often omitted. As an alternative, the use of enzymatic debriding agents to provide chemical escharotomy is popular in some centers.[106]

TORSO COMPARTMENT SYNDROMES

Recent awareness of massive abdominal swelling as a cause of cardiorespiratory compromise has led to protocols for monitoring intra-abdominal pressure and performing decompressive laparotomy in many ICU populations. In burn patients, occurrence of abdominal compartment syndrome has accompanied reports of fluid creep, as discussed earlier,[75] though it can clearly develop in the absence of excessive resuscitation. Patients with major (≥25% TBSA) burns and extensive torso injuries or who require large resuscitation volumes (≥500 mL/hour[76]) should have routine monitoring of bladder pressures.[76,107] The finding of intra-abdominal hypertension in the absence of clinical symptoms should prompt other measures to reduce abdominal pressure.[108] There is evidence that both hypertonic saline and colloid-based resuscitation can prevent the development of abdominal compartment syndrome[79,89]; removal of peritoneal fluid with dialysis catheters has also been effective.[109] Unfortunately, many patients with abdominal compartment syndrome present with diffuse retroperitoneal swelling rather than free peritoneal fluid; diagnostic ultrasound can make this decision and guide catheter placement if free fluid is seen.

Like other edema-related complications, abdominal hypertension can develop insidiously and then present precipitously with oliguria and critical hypotension and respiratory embarrassment. In patients with deep burns of the chest or abdomen, performance of torso escharotomy—sometimes repeatedly—will often improve ventilation and obviate laparotomy. Patients in whom other measures fail or symptoms progress rapidly should undergo immediate decompressive laparotomy, at the bedside if necessary. Delayed decompression may worsen shock and even lead to intestinal necrosis, although prompt decompression will both improve survival and reduce ongoing resuscitation requirements.[110] Containment of the exposed viscera by mesh or plastic silos may be needed following laparotomy, as widely used "vac-pack" dressings[111] may be impossible to secure over burn eschar. As edema resolves, every effort should be made to reduce abdominal contents and obtain fascial closure through repeated wound revisions. Figure 67.9 illustrates a patient in whom numerous complications of edema—massive facial swelling, extremity compartment syndromes, and abdominal compartment syndrome—have occurred simultaneously. Although the mortality rate of abdominal compartment syndrome in burn patients is high,[112] this likely reflects the severity of the underlying burn more than this complication itself.

ACUTE RENAL FAILURE

The development of effective protocols for fluid resuscitation has greatly reduced the incidence of acute renal failure (ARF) during initial burn treatment. ARF may still develop if resuscitation is delayed or inadequate,[113] particularly in patients with high-voltage electrical injuries or extremely deep burns, in whom pigment-induced nephropathy from myoglobin/hemoglobin is possible. Patients with visibly red or black urine should have resuscitation increased to produce urine outputs of 50 to 100 mL/hour. A one-time initial dose of an osmotic diuretic such as mannitol to stimulate urine production, and alkalinization of the urine by adding bicarbonate to intravenous fluids, is also widely practiced.[114,115]

ARF in burn patients is now most often a late complication of infection or dehydration and continues to have a high mortality rate.[116] Clearly its prevention is the best management strategy through meticulous fluid management and infection control. When ARF develops, patients should be treated with dialysis according to standard indications. Continuous renal replacement therapy can be particularly effective in managing patients who tolerate intermittent dialysis poorly.[117] Nutritional support should not be reduced in this setting; rather, patients should continue to receive the calories and protein they require and undergo dialysis as needed.

ELECTROLYTE ABNORMALITIES

Although almost any disturbance of electrolytes can occur during the course of an acute burn, several characteristic patterns are seen. Most frequent are disturbances in serum sodium concentration. Massive resuscitation with LR solution (sodium content 130 mEq/L) results in the infusion of a large sodium load. Following resuscitation, urine output will be less reflective of intravascular volume, and serum sodium concentration will reflect free water balance. The formula given previously for maintenance fluids following resuscitation provides only a rough estimate of individual requirements, which can also be affected by fever, ventilator support, hyperglycemia, and other abnormalities. Progressive hyponatremia should prompt a reduction in total free water intake, although hypernatremia should be treated with increased free water. Dehydration can develop insidiously despite adequate daily urine output.

Hypokalemia may occur immediately after burn related to epinephrine release from injury,[118] although hyperkalemia can result from cellular injury and acidosis. Both are usually short-lived and rarely require treatment. Thereafter, potassium levels often drop below normal, and patients may require substantial supplementation. Elevated aldosterone secretion following burn injury contributes to chronic hypokalemia and alkalosis.[119] Magnesium levels also commonly drop, and supplementation of both potassium and magnesium is required as part of the "refeeding" effect of aggressive nutritional support.

Hypophosphatemia is also extremely common from multiple causes including catecholamine secretion, metabolic alkalosis, impaired renal phosphate absorption, and increased excretion during postresuscitation diuresis.[120] Phosphate levels typically reach a nadir 2 to 5 days after injury, and afterward rebound slowly. Significant hypophosphatemia can lead to cardiac dysfunction, reduced red blood cell survival, and neurologic abnormalities, particularly during refeeding. Substantial phosphate supplementation may be needed throughout the wound coverage phase of burn treatment. Routine monitoring and replacement of all electrolytes should be performed at least until patients no longer require intravenous fluids.

THE WOUND COVERAGE PHASE

SURGICAL TREATMENT OF BURN PATIENTS

Although effective fluid resuscitation has reduced the acute mortality risk of burned patients, aggressive surgery has produced the greatest advancement in overall survival from burns. Early excision of wounds and coverage with skin or skin substitutes work to remove burn eschar as a major source of infection, shorten the period of severe hypermetabolism, relieve pain, improve function, and permit earlier mobilization and preservation of muscle mass.

Burn eschar left in place eventually separates from underlying tissue through the action of leukocyte enzymes. Bacterial infection facilitates this process, and burn eschar is an ideal medium for bacterial growth. In the era before routine excision, many patients died from sepsis while awaiting eschar separation while experiencing unremitting pain and prolonged muscle wasting. Surgical excision of burns was first practiced in the early twentieth century but produced high mortality rates from blood loss and anesthesia. Beginning in the 1970s, improved support has permitted aggressive excision of major burns with increased survival and decreased length of stay.[121,122-124] Early excision is now considered a standard of care. A detailed discussion of these techniques is beyond the scope of this chapter. However, intensivists must be aware of the principles of surgical treatment and be able to support patients pre- and postoperatively.[125]

INDICATIONS AND TIMING OF SURGERY

The larger the burn injury, the more acute the need for early excision. Patients with small (<10-15% TBSA) burns can be followed for up to 14 days to evaluate healing, but when burn size exceeds 25% to 30% TBSA, a widely accepted goal is removal of essentially all of the burn wound within 7 days of injury. Muller and Herndon excise the entire wound in a single procedure even while fluid resuscitation is ongoing,[126] but most units practice a staged approach, removing 15% to 20% TBSA at each operation.

En bloc excision of skin and subcutaneous tissue to vascularized fascia is rapid and relatively bloodless and creates a reliable bed for skin grafting. It is often practiced in the elderly and for particularly deep burns. However, fascial excisions are disfiguring and cause substantial problems with joint stiffness and pain. Far more common today is "tangential excision," in which thin slices of tissue are removed until a viable bed of dermis or subcutaneous fat is reached. This requires more skill and time and produces more blood loss, but long-term results are unquestionably superior.

Unless covered, excised wounds will desiccate and develop a new layer of necrotic tissue—in essence, a second eschar—with attendant metabolic stress, pain, and infection. The ultimate goal of excision is autografting—coverage with the patient's own skin. Burns excised within 7 to 10 days of injury are usually quite clean, and are often autografted immediately, providing prompt wound closure and facilitating early mobility. If donor sites are limited, autografts can be meshed to expand and cover more area. Excised wounds can be covered with antibiotic-soaked dressings to maintain tissue viability and combat infection for a few days. In recent years, a variety of skin substitutes have been utilized when donors are not available or if burns appear infected or poorly vascularized. The most widely used material is cadaver allograft skin obtained from tissue banks. Like autograft, allograft permits vascular ingrowth and take—sometimes for weeks—though this tissue is always eventually rejected. Allograft placement reduces bacterial colonization and pain, retards wound contraction, creates a clean, vascular bed, and can serve as a test for subsequent autografting. Cultured epithelial autografts (cultured skin) can be used to cover extensive areas but are expensive, fragile, and prone to loss from infection. They are best used over a scaffolding of intact or allograft dermis, and meticulous wound care is essential for success. A variety of synthetic and processed skin are also available, including synthetic dermis (Integra), acellular dermal matrix (Alloderm), amniotic membrane, collagen-bound polymer membranes (Biobrane, Transcyte), and others. Products still in development combine synthetic dermis with cultured epidermis, providing the potential for future one-step complete skin replacement.[127] All of these products require experience and skill to utilize successfully.

HEMODYNAMIC SUPPORT

In acutely burned patients blood pressure is sustained by elevated catecholamine levels, though blood volume may remain below normal and hematocrit artificially high. With induction of anesthesia, adrenergic blockade and vasodilation can produce sudden hypotension as these hidden hypovolemia and anemia are revealed. In addition, surgical excision of old or infected burn wounds may stimulate bacteremia and potentiate hemodynamic instability.[128] The surgical team should prepare for these contingencies by continuing liberal fluid infusions during surgery and anticipating blood loss. Major burn excisions produce significant bleeding, which is often underestimated by surgeons. The blood loss from excision of 1% of the body surface area of an adult has been estimated at approximately 100 mL.[129] Use of tourniquets for excision, performance of staged excisions, and use of subdermal clysis of epinephrine-containing solutions—the Pitkin procedure—can all help reduce intraoperative bleeding.[130]

TEMPERATURE CONTROL

Burn patients often display mild to moderate fever secondary to hypermetabolism and also have accelerated evaporative heat loss. In the operating room, exposure and suppression of metabolism increase the risk of hypothermia, which can be very hard to correct. Temperature should be monitored carefully, patient warming devices should always be used in the operating room, and the room itself should be kept warm. Limiting operations to 2 to 3 hours is also helpful in avoiding hypothermia.

BURN PHARMACOLOGY AND ANESTHESIA

Depolarizing muscle relaxants (succinylcholine) should not be used in patients with acute injuries,[131] but burn patients are also relatively resistant to nondepolarizing agents and frequently require increased dosage. Induction agents that produce vasodilation, such as propofol, may potentiate hypotension, and should be used with caution. Ketamine maintains hemodynamic stability, and can be used effectively in surgery or for bedside procedures and dressing changes.[132] Pharmacokinetics and dynamics of many other drugs are also significantly altered in burn patients.[133] Increased volume of distribution, decreased albumin binding, and increased renal blood flow necessitate monitoring and individualized dosing of many drugs.[134]

PAIN CONTROL

Pain management is notoriously difficult in burn patients, who often require remarkable quantities of narcotics and sedatives throughout their hospital course. Although altered pharmacology undoubtedly plays a role in this process, extreme levels of sustained pain are typical, and tachyphylaxis often develops during long-term administration of opioids. Patient-controlled analgesia (PCA) can be effective, but use may be limited by impaired consciousness and hand function.[135] Nonopioid analgesics such as ibuprofen and toradol can be useful adjuncts in patients with cutaneous injuries. Finally, behavior modifications such as relaxation therapy, hypnosis, and virtual reality can be extremely helpful in overcoming the anxiety of dressing changes and physical therapy. Careful assessment of pain and anxiety and individualized dosing regimens are essential for successful management of burn patients.[136]

PULMONARY MANAGEMENT

A variety of pulmonary problems occur frequently in burn patients and can require simultaneous treatment. Initial airway compromise, discussed previously, can be isolated and self-limited, but frequently contributes to pulmonary infection and inflammation. Acute respiratory distress syndrome (ARDS) can occur in the absence of inhalation injury, or components of both disorders can coexist and complement each other. Pulmonary edema or large pleural effusions can complicate fluid resuscitation. Aspiration, narcotic-induced respiratory depression, atelectasis and immobilization from bed rest, associated chest trauma, pulmonary thromboembolism, barotrauma, and pneumothorax/hemothorax following central line placement are all encountered in the management of major burns.

Chapter 48 provides a detailed discussion of the pathophysiology and treatment of the pulmonary complications of burn injury. Recent evidence suggests that inadequate fluid resuscitation may actually accentuate pulmonary damage[137]; burn patients with inhalation injuries require increased resuscitation volumes[59] and should be resuscitated at least as aggressively as other burn patients. Pulmonary artery catheterization may be helpful in patients with severe lung injuries who require high ventilator pressures. Although colloid-based resuscitation may be associated with persistently increased extravascular lung water,[90] this does not appear to be the case with crystalloid, even in patients who require substantially more fluid than Parkland requirements.[74]

A number of reports have focused on techniques to improve oxygenation in burn patients with severe acute lung injury, including extracorporeal membrane oxygenation,[138] inhaled nitric oxide,[139] and novel ventilator strategies such as high-frequency volume diffusive,[140] oscillation,[141] or percussive ventilation.[142] However, these modalities are limited in their availability and usefulness, and clear-cut indications for each have not been developed. The use of permissive hypercapnia may be beneficial,[143] though other protective lung strategies have not been evaluated in burns. The vast majority of burn patients can be managed effectively with conventional ventilation techniques, and death purely from hypoxia is rare.

Multiple organ failure is the most common cause of death in burn patients,[144,145] very frequently triggered by ongoing pulmonary infection, which can be severe and persistent.[146] This pneumonia is usually ventilator associated; intubation facilitates contamination of the lower airways already primed for infection by the mucosal sloughing, mucous plugging, and atelectasis caused by inhalation injury. Frequent cultures and aggressive antibiotic use are necessary for successful treatment. The use of ventilator bundles, including frequent suctioning and chest physiotherapy, elevation of the head of the bed, closed suction techniques, postpyloric feeding, and frequent oral care, may also be helpful.[147] The use of heparin and acetylcysteine aerosols—sometimes combined with bronchodilators—to liquefy and mobilize casts and debris has shown some promise in pediatric patients.[148] Improved mobilization of secretions may also be the mechanism by which percussive or oscillatory ventilation is beneficial.[142] Fiberoptic bronchoscopy and bronchoalveolar lavage can be used both for diagnosis of pneumonia and as a therapeutic maneuver to clear tenacious plugs and improve ventilation.[19] Based on limited evidence, neither corticosteroids nor prophylactic antibiotics appear to be helpful in treating respiratory failure or preventing pneumonia.[149] The performance of tracheostomy in patients who fail initial attempts at extubation may or may not reduce infections[150] but unquestionably provides a more comfortable and secure airway for long-term ventilator support.

CARDIOVASCULAR COMPLICATIONS AND CARE

As mentioned previously, the immediate response to burn injury consists of reduced cardiac output and increased peripheral resistance, followed by gradual return of both values to near-normal at the end of resuscitation, after which markedly elevated cardiac output and reduced peripheral resistance persists through wound coverage and into rehabilitation (see Fig. 67.5). This response is so characteristic that invasive hemodynamic monitoring is rarely needed during resuscitation.

Catecholamine stimulation of cardiac function often results in hypertension, which can be difficult to manage, as well as sustained tachycardia and tachyarrhythmias. Beta blockade is useful in treating these problems, and may be indicated for routine administration as well. Beta blockers are tolerated well in this situation, and may even contribute to improved outcomes.[151]

Hypotension can also occur in burn patients during acute care. Obligatory postresuscitation diuresis coupled with increased evaporative and metabolic fluid losses favors development of occult volume depletion. Progressive hypernatremia or azotemia and sustained tachycardia provide clues to this diagnosis, which may require aggressive fluid support. Persistent hypotension should lead to a search for sepsis. Invasive monitoring may be helpful in this setting as well; however, the classic hemodynamic picture of sepsis—increased cardiac output and reduced peripheral resistance—is also the characteristic postburn response, so that such monitoring will likely be more useful in guiding therapy than in diagnosis.

ADRENAL INSUFFICIENCY

Recent studies have demonstrated a surprisingly high frequency of absolute or relative adrenal insufficiency in critical care patients, including burns, which may increase mortality risk from shock and sepsis.[152,153] However, the quoted incidence of this problem has varied greatly, depending on the diagnostic criteria used and the populations studied.[154-157] No systematic evaluation of adrenal insufficiency has been conducted in burn patients. The incidence of this complication remains unknown,[158] but may be more common than previously suspected, and should be considered in burn patients with refractory hypotension.

INFECTION CONTROL

BURN WOUND INFECTIONS

Historically overwhelming burn wound sepsis was a major cause of death in patients who survived resuscitation. Over the past 50 years, the use of systemic and topical antibiotics coupled with surgical excision and skin grafting has dramatically decreased this problem. However, infection in burn wounds remains an important source of morbidity and mortality risks. As with other infections, the development of increasingly effective antibiotics has been matched by rapid adaptation of microbial pathogens. The initial use of antibiotics in World War II controlled *Streptococcus* and *Staphylococcus* infections, but these were supplanted by gram-negative organisms, particularly *Pseudomonas.* In the 1960s and 1970s, development of silver nitrate solution, mafenide acetate (Sulfamylon) and silver sulfadiazine (Silvadene, Thermazene) were effective in combating these infections, but microflora continued to evolve. Today, burn wound infections are increasingly caused by multiply resistant gram-negative organisms, *Acinetobacter,* methicillin-resistant *Staphylococcus, Candida,* and fungi.[159] Individual patients may display a similar progression of wound colonization as therapy and antibiotic administration continue.

Established principles of infection control remain a critical component of burn care. Essentially every open wound should be treated with topical agents until healed. The time-tested agents sulfadiazene and mafenide remain effective against a wide range of bacteria, and still constitute the first line for acute burn treatment despite some limitations. Silver sulfadiazine has been associated with neutropenia, though this is usually a transient phenomenon in the early postburn period (see later). Mafenide is a carbonic anhydrase inhibitor that can generate significant metabolic acidosis if used on large areas and has also been linked to the emergence of fungal infections.[160] A number of newer topical agents are now available, including silver-containing dressings (Acticoat, Acquacel-Ag), cerium-silver nitrate, mupirocin (Bactroban), chlorhexidine, betadine, and others. The choice of agent and technique should be adjusted based on culture results and wound appearance, and can often be reduced as wounds heal. Silver-containing agents and topical antifungals such as nystatin are effective against yeast and mold infections, and antibiotic solutions including mafenide and silver nitrate are widely used to soak fresh skin grafts and some skin substitutes. The so-called melting graft syndrome has been attributed to chronic infection with *Staphylococcus* species[161]; topical mupirocin may be particularly effective in this setting.

In addition to topical antibiotics, meticulous wound cleansing and debridement should be performed at least daily and wounds inspected carefully. Findings suggestive of invasive infection include green or black discoloration, purulent exudate, extending erythema or tissue necrosis, conversion of superficial-appearing burns to deep wounds, development of satellite lesions (ecthyma gangrenosum), and loss of vascularized skin grafts. Any of these findings should prompt careful culturing of wounds, escalating or changing topical and systemic antibiotics, and possibly surgery.

Surface cultures of burn wounds will identify dominant organisms, but cannot distinguish between invasive infection and colonization. Burn wound biopsies can be obtained for quantitative culture; bacterial counts of 10^5 per gram of tissue or more has been used as a criterion for invasive burn wound sepsis. However, false-positive results are frequent; wounds may be heavily colonized without bacterial invasion, and biopsies must be obtained in exactly the right place.[162] Histologic demonstration of organisms penetrating into viable tissue and capillaries remains a valid diagnostic finding.[159] However, many centers lack an experienced pathologist to read these samples accurately, so routine biopsies are now used infrequently. Daily examination of wounds and clinical suspicion remain the most important tools for prompt diagnosis of burn wound infection. Once detected, burn wound sepsis is best treated by aggressive, total wound excision, broad-spectrum systemic coverage, and topical antibiotic soaks in preparation for allograft or autograft placement. Burn wound sepsis is an extremely serious complication and should involve every member of the burn team.

OTHER INFECTIONS

Modern methods of infection prevention and control have contributed to decreased rates of many types of infections in burn patients. With the decline in burn wound infections, pneumonia has emerged as the most common infection in burn patients. Central venous catheter infections—particularly from *Candida*—also remain a constant threat[163] and can contribute to bacterial endocarditis, particularly if lines are allowed to reach the atrium or ventricle.[164] Neither routine catheter changes nor rewires have been shown to decrease infectious risks.[165] The current use of peripherally inserted central catheters (PICC lines) may or may not reduce the risks of catheter-related infection,[166] but regardless of the line or site used, adherence to accepted principles of catheter placement and care[167] and prompt removal of catheters when possible should be practiced. Improved wound management, nutrition, and hygiene have all but eliminated such historically important infections as suppurative thrombophlebitis, chondritis of the ear, and suppurative parotitis as clinical problems.

Diagnosis of infection can be difficult in burn patients. Fever, leukocytosis, and tachycardia are all normal consequences of acute burn injury, and standard criteria for the diagnosis of systemic inflammatory response syndrome (SIRS) and sepsis are difficult to interpret.[168] Low-grade fever may be sustained during acute treatment, but any increase in temperature above 38.5° C, especially when accompanied by increases in white blood cells (WBCs) or heart rate, should prompt an evaluation for infection, including appropriate cultures. The once-common policy of obtaining routine surveillance cultures of blood, urine, or wounds has been shown to have relatively low yield and a high incidence of false-positive results.[169] Some units use swab cultures to detect colonization and to track dominant flora for epidemiologic reasons. The value of measuring specific biomarkers to detect infection, including C-reactive protein and procalcitonin, has been inconsistent and remains controversial.[170,171]

Systemic prophylactic antibiotics have not been shown to reduce burn wound or other infections and should not be used.[172,173] As in all ICU patients, antibiotic use should be guided by the clinical situation and culture results. As noted previously, burn patients often exhibit abnormal drug kinetics and require increased antibiotic dosing and careful monitoring of antibiotic efficacy. The clinical pharmacist is an essential member of the burn team for this and other reasons. The isolation of burn patients through universal precautions and the separation of infected patients by cohort nursing should be practiced as routine components of infection control. The practice of selective digestive decontamination in burn patients is controversial; although some centers report benefits,[174] and some no effect,[175] from this time-consuming technique, it is not routinely practiced in U.S. burn centers.

METABOLIC SUPPORT AND GASTROINTESTINAL MANAGEMENT

THE HYPERMETABOLISM OF BURN INJURY

Burns induce the greatest hypermetabolic response of any injury. This response typically follows the ebb and flow pattern described over 70 years ago,[176] in which initial (24-72 hours) reduced energy expenditure is followed by increasing metabolism, which peaks 10 to 14 days after injury and then tapers slowly as wound healing progresses. The degree of hypermetabolism correlates with burn size but appears to level off with burns of 40% to 50% TBSA, above which no further increase is seen.[177] This response is sustained by the secretion of catecholamines, cortisol, and glucagon that persists until after wounds are closed. Together these hormones accelerate catabolism through breakdown of skeletal muscle, reduced uptake of fats, and opposition to the effects of insulin.[178,179] The result is obligatory muscle wasting to support gluconeogenesis; lipids have very little protein-sparing effect, and even exogenous glucose is limited in its ability to prevent protein wasting.[180]

In the 1970s burn patients frequently demonstrated prolonged calorie and protein consumption that exceeded twice normal and caused fatal inanition within a few weeks of injury.[181-184] Modern burn treatment—aggressive excision and wound coverage, control of sepsis and pain, mechanical ventilation, and improved environmental control—have all helped reduce both the duration and magnitude of this response.[177,185,186] Nonetheless, significant hypermetabolism persists well after burn wounds are closed, and careful nutritional support is a requirement for the successful care of burn patients.[187]

ROUTE AND TIMING OF NUTRITIONAL SUPPORT

The superiority of enteral nutrition is widely accepted,[188] and may be especially true for burn patients. Enteral nutrition nourishes bowel mucosa, preserves blood supply, reduces permeability, and improves associated immune function.[189-191] In trauma and ICU patients, early and aggressive enteral nutrition appears to decrease infectious complications, but total parenteral nutrition (TPN) has been associated with an increased mortality rate in burn patients,[192,193] and it also promotes development of fatty liver.[194] It may even be preferable to withhold nutrition entirely for limited periods, rather than use TPN.

Enteral feeding should begin as quickly as practical following injury, especially if patients will not be able to eat within 5 to 7 days. In contrast to early studies,[195] immediate enteral feedings have not been consistently shown to reduce hypermetabolism,[196] but do decrease calorie deficit and improve nitrogen balance.[197,198] Feedings can be started within a few hours of injury, and continued even through surgical procedures.[199] The routine use of promotility agents has not been studied in burn patients[200]; it is also unclear whether small intestinal feedings are superior to gastric feedings; both can have complications, and both require careful monitoring.

ENERGY REQUIREMENTS

Dozens of regimens have been used to estimate the caloric needs of burn patients, including the famous Curreri formula.[201] However, static formulas cannot accommodate the major fluctuations that occur over time and between individuals of different ages and burn sizes.[202] In addition, because modern burn treatment has reduced hypermetabolism, older formulas overestimate requirements significantly.[203] Current recommended caloric intake for adults with major burns is 120% to 150% of Harris-Benedict estimates of basal needs.[204] Many centers also use indirect calorimetry to measure energy expenditure and to detect significant under- or overfeeding.[205] Regardless, support should still be increased during periods of peak energy expenditure to avoid underfeeding, and reduced later to avoid overfeeding.

Whatever regimen is chosen, the practical difficulties of delivering nutritional support are substantial.[206,207] Interruptions in feedings, fluctuations in energy consumption caused by fever and activity, and delivery of empty calories in glucose solutions all frustrate attempts to tailor individual nutrition exactly, which may explain why the superiority of indirect calorimetry-based nutrition has not been proved.[202] Involvement of the team—including a dietician—in implementing, assessing, and adjusting feedings is probably more important than adherence to predetermined estimations.[208]

ENTERAL FORMULAS

Chapter 82 provides details on the composition of many commercially available enteral formulas which can be used in burn patients. Specific components of effective enteral formulas include the following:

Carbohydrates and Glucose Control

The catabolism of burn injury makes carbohydrates the preferred energy source, but also worsens hyperglycemia. Recent studies have demonstrated the value of meticulous glucose control in ICU populations in reducing organ failure, length of stay, and inflammation.[209,210] These benefits are likely seen in burn patients as well,[211] but hormonally mediated resistance to insulin—the so-called diabetes of injury—makes attaining control a major challenge. Many burn units use hyperglycemia protocols, which require frequent (or continuous) dosing of insulin and careful monitoring. Oral hypoglycemics appear helpful in this effort[212]; in addition, giving limited calories as fat helps reduce the glucose burden required by these patients.

Fat

A certain (small) quantity of dietary fat is an essential nutrient. Lipolysis is suppressed in burn patients, as is the ability to utilize exogenous fat as an energy source. Fat intake should be restricted to less than 30% of total nonprotein calories, or about 1 g/kg/day[213] or less[214,215]; withholding fat entirely from TPN for substantial periods may be beneficial.[188,216] In addition, products high in ω-3 free fatty acids (FFAs) and correspondingly low in ω-6 FFAs may improve glucose control and reduce infections.[217,218] Most clinical experience has been obtained with the use of immune-enhancing diets (IEDs) (see later) in which the effects of individual components have been difficult to assess.

Protein

Accelerated proteolysis is often the most important characteristic of burn-induced hypermetabolism. A major goal of nutrition is to reduce or replace protein losses, which can exceed ½ lb of lean body mass per day. Providing adequate calories alone will not reduce muscle breakdown,[219] so increased protein must be provided as well. Protein requirements increase with burn size[220,221]; appropriate provision of dietary protein has resulted in reduced infections and a lower mortality rate in patients with major injuries.[222] Current recommendations are 1.5 to 2.0 g of protein/kg/day (up to 3.0 g/kg/day in children),[205,208,223] which corresponds to a nonprotein calorie/nitrogen ratio of 100:1 or less. Nitrogen balance should be monitored regularly.

Specific Amino Acids

The amino acids arginine (Arg) and glutamine (Glu) play enhanced roles in critical illness. Both are depleted rapidly in burn patients, and are considered conditionally essential.[219,224] Glutamine is important in energy transport, as a precursor of glutathione[225] and as a nutrient for enterocytes, helping to preserve bowel integrity and limit permeability.[226-228] In burn patients provision of up to 25 g Glu/day, given parenterally[229] or enterally,[230] has been associated with improved visceral protein levels and reduced infectious mortality rate and length of stay. Glutamine supplementation has been recommended[188] but is not routinely practiced. Glutamine is almost totally absent from TPN formulas, which may explain some of the benefits of enteral nutrition in burn patients.

Arginine enhances natural killer cell function and nitric oxide (NO) synthesis, promoting inflammation and resistance to infection.[231,232] Specific studies of arginine supplementation have not been performed in burn patients, but arginine has been incorporated into complex immune-enhancing diets (IEDs) containing ω-3 FFAs, arginine, glutamine, and RNA, among other components.[233] These diets have shown benefits in some surgical populations,[234] but deleterious or no effects in patients with sepsis or pneumonia,[235] and their widespread use has been questioned.[188] Few data are available on IEDs in burn patients,[236] but the mixed results in other groups suggest that components should be studied separately before incorporating them into cocktails with even more unpredictable effects. Most burn centers simply use high-protein diets rather than these specialized and expensive formulas.

Other Nutrients

A number of micronutrients—including vitamins A, C, and D, iron, zinc, and others—are important in wound healing and may be depleted following burn injury,[237] and some supplementation has been recommended.[238] Many centers simply administer multivitamins, which is probably adequate.[178,239] Commercial enteral formulas also contain far more than the recommended daily dietary allowances of many vitamins and trace elements.

MONITORING NUTRITIONAL SUPPORT

Because burn injury alters many parameters of nutritional status, monitoring nutrition can be as difficult as providing it. For example, substantial weight gain invariably accompanies fluid resuscitation,[240] although overfeeding can increase body fat even as protein stores are depleted.[241,242] As a result, patients have often lost more lean body mass than is reflected by weight alone.[243] Nitrogen balance studies can be useful, but sedation and bed rest make attaining positive nitrogen balance difficult,[244] emphasizing the need to continue physical therapy even during acute care. Serum protein markers are often distorted; levels of albumin,[245] prealbumin, and transferrin[205,246] fall quickly following injury, and recover only very slowly even with appropriate nutrition. Perhaps the best marker of nutritional adequacy in burn patients is their overall status, including vital signs, wound healing, and functional improvement. Body weight, nitrogen balance, and protein markers may be most useful in tracking trends in individuals.[247]

MODULATION OF HYPERMETABOLISM

Burn-related hormonal changes complicate the provision of nutritional support, but also provide mechanisms by which hypermetabolism can be manipulated. Recent studies have shown promising results, and suggest that manipulation of the metabolic response to injury may become routine in the future. A variety of approaches have been utilized, including beta blockade with propranolol, low-dose insulin infusions, use of counterregulatory hormones such as insulin-like growth factor-1 (IGF-1), or anabolic agents such as testosterone and oxandrolone.[248] The use of propranolol appears to be a safe, low-cost way to ameliorate both the cardiovascular response and hypermetabolic muscle wasting that occur during acute burn care.[249] Administration of the synthetic oral androgen oxandrolone has been shown to reduce muscle breakdown, speed rehabilitation, and lead to decreased length of stay in hospitalized patients.[250,251] Although none of these therapies is now routine, they are becoming more widespread. Recommendations for their routine use will need to await larger controlled trials to demonstrate efficacy.

GASTROINTESTINAL COMPLICATIONS IN BURN PATIENTS

Although the incidence of most gastrointestinal (GI) complications has decreased dramatically with improved resuscitation and control of infection, a number of problems are frequent or serious enough to deserve discussion.

Acute Cholecystitis

Cholecystitis—usually acalculous—can have a number of causes, including gallbladder ischemia from shock and dehydration,[252] biliary stasis from narcotics and TPN, bile pigment loads from hemolysis and transfusion, and bacterial seeding from sepsis. With more effective control of these factors, acute cholecystitis is now rare; a recent review documented just 20 cases among 10,762 acutely burned patients (0.18%), with progressive declines in recent years.[253] Fever, leukocytosis, feeding intolerance, and abdominal pain are characteristic findings, though they may be difficult to sort out in acutely ill patients. Ultrasound and computed tomography (CT) scanning are preferred for confirmation of diagnosis; biliary scintigraphy can have a high false-positive rate. Treatment has traditionally consisted of prompt cholecystectomy, though placement of cholecystostomy tubes under ultrasound guidance can provide definitive treatment in many patients.[254] With prompt diagnosis, the mortality rate from this complication should be low.

Hepatic Enzyme Elevation

Immediately following burn injury, hemolysis and ileus can contribute to a cholestatic picture, which should resolve within a few days. Some degree of chronic fatty infiltration of the liver may be inevitable in patients with major burns, and mild enzyme elevations are often seen, which is exacerbated by overfeeding and the use of TPN.[194] Severe hepatic steatosis may be both a cause and consequence of sepsis, and correlates with increased mortality rate.

Pancreatitis

Pancreatitis can also result from systemic hypoperfusion and secondary sepsis. In contrast to cholecystitis, the incidence of pancreatitis may be increasing as more severely injured patients now survive burn shock. Ryan and colleagues documented hyperamylasemia in 40% of patients with large burns, with an associated increased mortality rate and length of stay,[255] although pancreatic pseudocysts and abscesses were quite rare. Pancreatic enzymes should be measured in patients with feeding intolerance, abdominal pain, or nausea; in many cases, transient bowel rest and fluid support will be effective treatment. Use of TPN should be avoided unless pancreatitis is unusually severe and prolonged.

Gastrointestinal Bleeding

Although the time-honored eponym Curling's ulcer has sometimes been considered a unique entity, burn patients develop the stress ulcerations typical among acutely ill patients. Mucosal erosions and atrophy can occur within 72 hours of injury and progress to large (often multiple) ulcerations of the prepyloric area or duodenum. Their primary cause is thought to be gastric mucosal hypoperfusion from shock or sepsis; the role of *Helicobacter pylori* infection is unclear.[256,257] Modern treatment strategies including aggressive fluid resuscitation, suppression or neutralization of gastric acid, and early enteral feeding have resulted in a dramatic decline in the incidence of this complication from as high as 86% in early postmortem studies[258] to less than 2% today. Bleeding is more frequent with large injuries and in patients with coagulopathy, prolonged mechanical ventilation, and sepsis. Aggressive evaluation of any observed GI bleeding should be undertaken. Most patients can be controlled with endoscopic maneuvers and continuous proton pump inhibitors. Surgery for acute upper GI bleeding is now rarely required.[259]

Ileus and Intestinal Necrosis

Ileus occurs routinely following acute burns, and oral intake should be withheld at least until resuscitation is completed. Impaired intestinal motility can be aggravated by narcotics, infection, and ventilatory support. Severe colonic ileus—Ogilvie's syndrome—can occur in this setting,[260] and overly aggressive enteral feeding can rarely lead to bowel distention, ischemia, necrosis, perforation, and death.[261,262] For this reason, feedings should be monitored carefully, and held if obstipation, distention, or pain becomes significant. CT scanning can confirm bowel dilatation or free air, in which case immediate laparotomy is mandatory.

Diarrhea

Diarrhea is extremely common with enteral feedings, and can be a major problem in management. The cause is often multifactorial,[263] including high osmotic loads, overfeeding, enteral medications, and infections including *Cytomegalovirus* and *Clostridium difficile*.[264] Treatment options include enteral opiates such as Imodium or paregoric or the use of fiber-containing products. However, fiber can clog small-diameter tubes and has been blamed for intestinal distention and necrosis,[265] and slowing intestinal transit can potentiate infectious diarrhea. Often simply holding feedings for a few hours will suffice; diarrhea unresponsive to simple measures should prompt a search for infectious causes, inside or outside the bowel.[266]

HEMATOLOGIC CONSIDERATIONS

RED BLOOD CELLS

Hemoconcentration, which accompanies burn shock, can result in hematocrits of 70% or higher. This will theoretically produce sludging and increased vascular resistance, though clinical problems with thrombosis are rare. As resuscitation proceeds hematocrits fall progressively, and are usually below normal by the end of 48 hours. Thereafter, anemia often persists or worsens until wound coverage is obtained. Several mechanisms contribute to this finding.[267] First, burn injury destroys red blood cells directly; significant hemolysis can occur within minutes of injury and produce hemoglobinuria or jaundice. Burn-induced alterations in red blood cell metabolism result in spherocytosis, increased membrane fragility, and shortened red blood cell survival. Erythropoietic response is blunted, apparently at the stem cell level,[268] and erythropoietin supplementation is not helpful.[269] Acute hemorrhage from surgery, and more gradual blood loss from wound debridements add to these effects.

The issue of appropriate transfusion trigger is controversial in burn patients. No systematic trial of transfusion thresholds has been performed, and no standard is universally accepted,[270] though limited evidence supports the practice of conservative transfusion in burn patients as in other ICU populations. In a multicenter review, Palmieri and coworkers found that transfusions correlated with both mortality risk and infectious episodes in major burns,[271] which underscores that transfusions should be based on physiologic assessment and not given routinely.

WHITE BLOOD CELLS

Immediately after burn, leukocytosis and WBC demargination are nonspecific components of the stress response. As with red blood cells, WBC numbers decline following resuscitation, reaching a nadir that is often well below normal on postburn days 2 to 5. In the past, this has been attributed to the use of silver sulfadiazine, but this decline appears to occur regardless of whether this topical agent is used and resolves spontaneously. Thereafter, WBC levels reflect systemic infection and stress. Leukocytosis is common with acute infections, but neutropenia is a far more ominous finding in severe sepsis and may suggest bone marrow failure. Granulopoiesis is accelerated following injury, and is mediated at least partially by catecholamines. Treatment with colony-stimulating factors has not been routinely practiced.

PLATELETS

Platelets and coagulation factors are also consumed in the early postburn period; platelet counts below 100,000/μL and coagulopathy are common for the first few days, and supplementation may be needed if major excisions are anticipated. Subsequently, both rebound to supranormal levels. During wound coverage, patients may demonstrate platelet counts in excess of 1,000,000/μL, and fibrinogen levels may exceed twice normal. These are reactive abnormalities and do not require treatment.[272] Platelet counts are a sensitive indicator of infection; a falling platelet count occurring after the first few days should suggest sepsis, and is associated with a poor prognosis.[273]

THROMBOEMBOLISM

Systemic inflammation, a hypercoagulable state, and frequent immobilization might all suggest that thromboembolic complications are common in burn patients. In fact, reported incidences of clinically apparent deep venous thrombosis (DVT) and pulmonary embolism (PE) are low.[274] However, prospective evaluation of burn patients suggests an incidence of DVT/PE similar to that of other moderate- to high-risk populations.[275] At present, no consensus exists on the issue of DVT prophylaxis in burn patients. Some centers use it routinely, but many centers provide it for high-risk patients, including the obese and patients with large burns, lower extremity burns, or femoral venous lines.

THE REHABILITATION PHASE

Although the focus of this chapter is the acute care of burn patients, it must be remembered that rehabilitation begins at the time of injury. The physical therapist is an essential member of the acute burn team, and therapy should begin before resuscitation is completed. Physical therapy, mobilization, and prevention of skin breakdown and muscle wasting can have profound effects on the overall success of acute burn care. Immobility and inactivity result in rapid depletion of muscle mass and function; other complications include demineralization of bone and pathologic fractures,[276] myositis ossificans, and extensive contracture formation. Therapeutic exercise regimens, beginning during acute care and continuing beyond hospital discharge, can result in improved function and well-being, and increased chances of return to independent living.[277]

KEY POINTS

- Carbon monoxide poisoning and asphyxia are the most immediate causes of death in burn patients exposed to smoke. High-flow oxygen should be administered to all patients immediately.
- Acute airway obstruction can occur at any time during the first 24 hours of injury, even in the absence of smoke inhalation. Early and elective endotracheal intubation should be performed in patients who develop wheezing, stridor, dyspnea, or significant facial swelling.
- Following initial assessment, fluid resuscitation is the primary goal of initial burn treatment. Fluid resuscitation should be instituted using a formula based on body weight and burn size, such as the Parkland formula, and adjusted to maintain urine output of 0.5 to 1.0 mL/hour.
- During the first 8 to 12 hours after burn, crystalloid solutions such as lactated Ringer's solution should be the sole fluids used for burn resuscitation. After that time, the addition of colloid-containing solutions may be helpful in limiting edema in unburned tissues.
- Invasive hemodynamic monitoring with Swan-Ganz catheters and inotropic fluid support should be reserved for problem patients who are not responding to standard fluid resuscitation.
- Edema in both burned and unburned tissue is progressive throughout fluid resuscitation and may progress rapidly. Intubation should be performed if facial swelling is severe or increasing.

KEY POINTS (Continued)

- Extremities with full-thickness or circumferential burns should be monitored with measurements of intramuscular pressure, and escharotomies performed if pressures exceed 30 cm H_2O. Fasciotomies should be performed if pressures fail to improve with escharotomy.
- Torso compartment syndromes can present with sudden and life-threatening hypotension, oliguria, and respiratory distress. Bladder pressures should be measured in patients with extensive torso injuries. Torso escharotomies should be performed initially, but decompressive laparotomy may be required in patients with progressive compromise.
- Multiple trauma in burn patients can be managed using standard approaches, as long as fluid resuscitation is continued.
- Surgical excision and skin grafting of burn wounds require specialized attention to fluid support, blood loss, temperature control, and drug pharmacology.
- Pain control is difficult in burn patients, who often require increased quantities of narcotics. Routine pain assessment and individualized dosing are necessary for successful pain control.
- Acute lung injury is the most common organ failure in burn patients, and pneumonia is the most common infection. Meticulous pulmonary toilet, ventilator support, and antibiotic treatment guided by culture results are all important components of care.
- Burn wound infections remain common in burn patients. Careful wound cleansing, debridement, and examination should be performed daily. Burn wound biopsies can be used to confirm diagnosis and direct therapy, but clinical evaluation remains the most important method for diagnosing these infections.
- Suspected or confirmed burn wound sepsis requires immediate excision of the wound, along with topical and systemic antibiotics.
- Aggressive nutritional support of burn patients is an essential component of care. Enteral nutrition should be started immediately after injury, and consist of a high-calorie, high-protein diet that is relatively low in fat. Commercially available tube feedings also contain sufficient vitamins and trace elements for effective support. Use of immune-enhancing diets is controversial.
- GI complications of burn injury can include acalculous cholecystitis, pancreatitis, ileus, and ischemic necrosis of the bowel.
- Prophylaxis against deep venous thrombosis is not routinely practiced in burn patients, but is probably indicated for patients with a prior history of thromboembolism, patients with extensive lower extremity injuries, and those who are obese.
- Rehabilitation is an essential component of burn treatment and begins with initial care.

SELECTED REFERENCES

1. Saffle JR (ed): Practice guidelines for burn care. J Burn Care Rehabil 2001;22:S1-69.
11. Saffle JR, Edelman L, Morris SE: Regional air transport of burn patients: A case for telemedicine? J Trauma 2004;57:57-64.
15. Klein MB, Kramer CB, Nelson J, et al: Geographic access to burn center hospitals. JAMA 2009;302:1774-1781.
19. Fitzpatrick J, Cioffi W: Diagnosis and treatment of inhalation injury. In Herndon D (ed): Total Burn Care. Philadelphia, WB Saunders, 2002, pp 232-241.
33. Purdue GF, Hunt JL: Multiple trauma and the burn patient. Am J Surg 1989;158:536-539.
73. Barton RG, Saffle JR, Morris SE, et al: Resuscitation of thermally injured patients with oxygen transport criteria as goals of therapy. J Burn Care Rehabil 1997;18:1-9.
148. Saffle JR, Morris SE, Edelman L: Early tracheostomy does not improve outcome in burn patients. J Burn Care Rehabil 2002; 23:431-438.
186. Heyland DK, Dhaliwal R, Drover JW, et al: Canadian clinical practice guidelines for nutrition support in mechanically ventilated, critically ill adult patients. J Parenter Enteral Nutr 2003;27: 355-373.
190. Herndon D, Stein M, Rutan T, et al: Failure of TPN supplementation to improve liver function, immunity, and mortality in thermally injured patients. J Trauma 1987;27:195-204.
227. Wischmeyer PE, Lynch J, Liedel J, et al: Glutamine administration reduces gram-negative bacteremia in severely burned patients: A prospective, randomized, double-blind trial versus isonitrogenous control. Crit Care Med 2001;29:2075-2080.

The complete list of references can be found at www.expertconsult.com.

Poisonings

68

Janice L. Zimmerman

CHAPTER OUTLINE

Poisonings may result from intentional or unintentional ingestion, inhalation, or skin contact. Toxic complications can also result from therapeutic use of medications. Although mortality rate from toxin exposures is low, patients requiring hospitalization are often cared for in the intensive care unit (ICU). Limited evidence-based information on management of poisonings is available because the variety of drugs and doses that patients are exposed to limit the ability to conduct clinical trials of specific interventions. In addition, animal and human volunteer studies fail to fully replicate the clinical situations that are commonly encountered. Therapeutic recommendations are based on extrapolation of data from animal models, human volunteer studies, case reports, pharmacokinetic information, known pathophysiology, consensus opinion, and a limited number of clinical trials. Toxicologists and local poison control centers are valuable sources of additional information for the clinician.

The approach to the poisoned patient requires an organized evaluation and management plan that often requires the input of emergency physicians, primary care physicians, intensive care clinicians, and clinical pharmacists. The basic steps include initial resuscitation and stabilization, diagnosis, gastrointestinal (GI) decontamination and toxin elimination, institution of specific antidotes or interventions, and supportive care. This chapter addresses these components of management in regard to poisonings most likely to be encountered in ICU patients. Although discussed separately, these steps are usually initiated concurrently in a severely ill patient.

RESUSCITATION AND STABILIZATION

The initial management of seriously ill poisoned patients requires assessment of airway patency, breathing difficulties, circulatory problems, and the level of consciousness. These issues, along with immediate resuscitation interventions, are usually addressed in the emergency department but may be continued in the ICU (Box 68.1).

DIAGNOSIS

HISTORY

A complete history should be obtained regarding the involved substance or substances including the route of exposure, quantity used, time of exposure, form of medication (regular or sustained-release), and chronicity of use to determine the significance of the presenting symptoms. Specifically, the clinician should inquire about the patient's baseline mental and health status and the medical, occupational, and social history. A detailed medication history should include information about over-the-counter, prescription, illicit, and nutritional or herbal medications. Intentional ingestions often involve multiple coingestants or alcohol, or both. Additional or corroborating information should be obtained from family, friends, paramedics, or witnesses, if available. All available containers found at the site should be brought in with the patient.

Box 68.1 Approach to Resuscitation and Stabilization of the Poisoned Patient

Assess airway and breathing:
- Supplemental oxygen for patients with low oxyhemoglobin saturation; F_{IO_2} 1.0 for carbon monoxide or cyanide exposure
- Intubation and mechanical ventilation for airway protection or with obstruction, hypoventilation, or hypoxemia

Assess hemodynamic status:
- Isotonic fluids initially for hypotension; vasopressor if condition is refractory to fluids
- Treat significant arrhythmias

Assess mental status:[1]

Consider the following for altered mental status:
- 50% glucose (25-50 g IV)
- Thiamine (100 mg IV)
- Naloxone (0.4-2 mg IV or IM initially)
- Flumazenil (not routinely recommended)*

*See section on benzodiazepines for further information.

Table 68.1 Drug Effects on Vital Signs

Increased	Decreased
Blood Pressure	
Amphetamines	Antihypertensive agents
Anticholinergics	Cyanide
Cocaine	Cyclic antidepressants
Ephedrine	Ethanol, other alcohols
Phencyclidine	Iron
Sympathomimetic agents	Opioids
	Organophosphates/carbamates
	Sedative-hypnotics
Heart Rate	
Amphetamines	Beta blockers
Anticholinergics	Calcium channel blockers
Antihistamines	Clonidine
Caffeine	Digitalis glycosides
Carbon monoxide	Gamma hydroxybutyrate
Cocaine	Lithium
Cyanide	Opioids
Cyclic antidepressants	Organophosphates/carbamates
Ephedrine	Physostigmine
Ethanol	Sedative-hypnotics
Phencyclidine	
Theophylline	
Respiratory Rate	
Alcohols	Ethanol, other alcohols
Amphetamines	Gamma hydroxybutyrate
Anticholinergics	Opioids
Carbon monoxide	Organophosphates
Hydrocarbons	Sedative-hypnotics
Salicylates	
Theophylline	
Temperature	
Amphetamines	Beta blockers
Anticholinergics	Carbon monoxide
Cocaine	Ethanol
Cyclic antidepressants	Gamma hydroxybutyrate
Lithium	Hypoglycemic agents
Phencyclidine	Opioids
Salicylates	Sedative-hypnotics
Theophylline	

PHYSICAL EXAMINATION

The initial physical examination should focus on vital signs and neurologic findings that may provide physiologic clues to the toxicologic cause. Many toxic substances affect the autonomic nervous system, which is responsible for changes in vital signs mediated by the sympathetic and parasympathetic pathways. Attention to these initial and subsequent clinical signs is of paramount importance in identifying patterns or changes suggesting a particular drug or category of drugs (Table 68.1). Changes in the clinical examination after a therapeutic intervention or the administration of an antidote should be noted. Continued monitoring and reevaluation are necessary because drug effects may not be present on initial evaluation.

Altered mental status is common in a toxicologic emergency. A detailed assessment of neurologic status should be made to determine if there is any alteration in level (stupor/coma or agitation) or content of consciousness (confusion/delirium).[1] The evaluation should include an assessment of pupillary reactivity, ocular movements, and motor responses. Ruling out structural versus toxic or metabolic reasons for the altered state is important. Drug-induced seizures are often difficult to treat and may respond only to specific antidotal therapy. In general, benzodiazepines are more effective in terminating drug-induced seizures than other agents.

Pupils should be assessed for size and reactivity, and ocular movements should be evaluated for the presence of sustained nystagmus. Agents associated with miosis include organophosphates/carbamates (mydriasis also seen), other cholinergic agents, opioids, acetone, clonidine, phencyclidine, phenothiazines, and nicotine. Both anticholinergics and sympathomimetics may cause mydriasis; the pupils are reactive to light with cocaine but unreactive in diphenhydramine overdose. Opioid withdrawal may also result in dilated pupils. The assessment may be difficult in the setting of multiple coingestants, whereby the response may be blocked or partially manifested. Horizontal nystagmus is commonly seen with alcohols, lithium, carbamazepine, solvents, and primidone. Phenytoin, sedative-hypnotics, and phencyclidine may cause a combination of vertical, horizontal, or rotatory nystagmus.

The clinical examination should also include evaluation of bowel sounds (decreased/hyperactive), skin (wet/dry), and mucosa (secretions).

TOXIDROMES

A complex of signs and symptoms may be identified by physical examination and grouped into a toxic syndrome, or "toxidrome." In many cases, recognition of this toxic pattern is more important than identifying a specific offending agent. Identifying a toxidrome enables the clinician to

Table 68.2 Toxidromes

Drug Group	Vital Signs: BP	HR	RR	T	Additional Manifestations: Mental Status	Pupil Size	Peristalsis	Diaphoresis	Other
Sympathomimetic (adrenergic) agents	±	↑	↑	↑	Altered, agitation	↑	↑	↑	Flushing, potential for seizures
Anticholinergic agents	±	↑	±	↑	Altered, hallucinations	↑	↓	↓	Dry mucous membranes, thirst, flushing, urinary retention
Cholinergic (muscarinic, nicotinic) agents	±	±	—	—	Altered	±	↑	↑	Salivation, lacrimation, urination, emesis, bronchorrhea, fasciculations
Opioids	↓	↓	↓	↓	Altered, sedation	↓	↓	↓	Hyporeflexia
Sedative-hypnotics or ethanol	↓	↓	↓	↓	Altered, sedation	±	↓	↓	Hyporeflexia

BP, blood pressure; HR, heart rate; RR, respiratory rate; T, temperature; ↑, increase; ↓, decrease; ±, variable; —, change unlikely.
Adapted from Nelson NS, Lewin NA, Howland MA, et al: Initial evaluation of the patient: Vital signs and toxic syndromes. In Nelson NS, Lewin NA, Howland MA, et al (eds): Goldfrank's Toxicologic Emergencies, 9th ed. New York, McGraw-Hill Medical, 2011, p 33.

initiate the assessment, derive a differential diagnosis, and formulate a treatment plan. The most typical toxidromes are listed in Table 68.2.[2] Importantly, the clinician should note that patients may not present with a classic toxidrome due to variable manifestations of toxins and overlapping features that exist between toxidromes.

LABORATORY TESTS

A laboratory test for a patient exposed to toxic agents should be helpful in diagnosis or monitoring.[3] Select laboratory examinations may be used when appropriate to determine the three gaps of toxicology—the anion gap, the osmolar gap, and the oxygen saturation gap. An arterial blood gas (ABG) analysis will identify hypoxemia or hypoventilation, as well as acid-base abnormalities. Agents associated with a gap in oxygen saturation (>5% difference between measured and calculated saturation) include carbon monoxide (CO) and methemoglobin inducers. In these exposures, a pulse oximeter inaccurately reflects the oxygen saturation of tissues and co-oximetry is necessary to identify abnormal hemoglobins. Determination of electrolytes with blood urea nitrogen (BUN) and creatinine will detect renal abnormalities and allow calculation of the anion gap. Some common drugs associated with an anion gap acidosis are listed in Box 68.2. Hypoperfusion must also be considered as a cause of metabolic acidosis. An osmolar gap (>10 mOsm/L) may be caused by any small particle (toxin) that increases the measured osmolarity as measured by freezing point depression. Such agents include ethanol, ethylene glycol, glycerol, isopropyl alcohol, mannitol, methanol, propylene glycol, and sorbitol. An electrocardiogram (ECG) should be obtained when potential cardiac toxicity exists.

A qualitative urine drug screen is a combination of tests that serves to identify common drugs encountered in overdoses. However, a "tox screen" is usually unnecessary because the results rarely alter management, many toxins are not detectable, and positive results do not assess severity of exposure. Quantitative determination of drug/toxin concentrations in blood is indicated by history and clinical examination to diagnose the intensity of toxicity, monitor the treatment or course of a patient, or define indications for specific interventions. Serum concentration measurements may be required as criteria for therapy or to assess the effectiveness of therapy. Because of the ubiquity of acetaminophen in over-the-counter and prescription preparations and the potential for significant morbidity and even death, a level should be obtained in any suspected polydrug ingestion.

Box 68.2 Selected Agents Associated with Anion Gap Acidosis

Acetaminophen
Carbon monoxide
Cyanide
Ethylene glycol
Iron
Isoniazid
Metformin
Methanol
Propofol
Propylene glycol
Salicylates
Toluene
Valproic acid

GASTROINTESTINAL DECONTAMINATION

GI decontamination techniques in the poisoned patient with an oral ingestion have included gastric emptying procedures (ipecac-induced emesis, gastric lavage), adsorption of drugs (activated charcoal), and increasing transit through the GI tract (cathartics, whole bowel irrigation [WBI]). Use of these interventions has decreased due to uncertain evidence of benefit and recognition of adverse effects of the techniques.[4] The consideration of a GI decontamination technique depends on the toxicity of the substance ingested, potential for deterioration in respiratory and mental status, severity of symptoms, dose, time since ingestion, presence of spontaneous emesis, and contraindications of the procedure.

Ipecac, which contains emetic alkaloids, stimulates gastric mucosal sensory receptors and the chemoreceptor trigger zone in the brain to produce vomiting. The amount of ingested drug removed by ipecac-induced emesis is highly variable, and no benefit of ipecac has been confirmed even when administered less than 60 minutes after ingestion. Currently, ipecac is not used in the management of adult poisoning victims.[5] Complications that have been associated with ipecac administration include aspiration pneumonitis, esophageal rupture, Mallory-Weiss tear, pneumomediastinum, and protracted vomiting that can delay administration of activated charcoal.

Gastric lavage with a large bore (36- to 40-French) orogastric tube is a technique used to empty the stomach of orally ingested substances that can be associated with significant complications. After insertion of the tube, lavage is accomplished with sequential 250 mL aliquots of normal saline or water until no pill fragments are retrieved. Intubation for airway protection is required before the procedure in patients with a depressed level of consciousness or potential for sedation. No clear benefit of gastric lavage has been demonstrated, even when instituted in obtunded patients presenting within 1 hour of ingestion.[6] Gastric lavage should not be employed routinely in the management of poisoned patients.[7] In rare circumstances, gastric lavage may be considered with ingestion of a life-threatening amount of toxin when the procedure can be instituted within 60 minutes of ingestion or a significant amount of toxin is still likely to be present in the stomach. The clinician must consider contraindications and the potential risks before performing gastric lavage in an overdose patient. Serious complications include aspiration pneumonitis, esophageal perforation, and cardiovascular instability. Gastric lavage is contraindicated with ingestions of substances such as acid, alkali, or hydrocarbons when the risk of aspiration is increased. Patients with a risk of GI perforation or severe bleeding diathesis or who are combative should also not be subjected to gastric lavage.

Single-dose activated charcoal is one of the more frequently used interventions for GI decontamination. Activated charcoal potentially adsorbs the toxin in the GI tract and minimizes systemic absorption. The optimum dose of activated charcoal has not been established, but the usual dose for adults is 25 to 100 g (1 g/kg). Activated charcoal is not effective in adsorbing iron, lithium, cyanide, strong acids and bases, alcohols, and some hydrocarbons. Some clinical studies examining the use of activated charcoal versus no intervention found no improvement in outcomes.[8,9] Volunteer studies suggest that the greatest benefit of administering activated charcoal may be within 1 hour of ingestion.[10] Use of activated charcoal may be considered when a potentially toxic amount of a substance adsorbed by charcoal has been ingested within 1 hour.[11,12] Later administration may be appropriate if clinical factors suggest the ingested substance has not yet been completely absorbed. Activated charcoal is contraindicated in patients with a depressed level of consciousness unless intubated, when administration increases the risk of aspiration, or the patient is known or suspected to have a GI perforation. Few complications are associated with the appropriate use of single-dose activated charcoal. Emesis has been reported but may be related to sorbitol administered with charcoal or the ingested toxin.

Cathartics have been administered in poisoning ingestions based on the hypothesis that absorption and overall bioavailability of the agent are decreased by reducing contact time in the GI tract. Sorbitol (70% solution with activated charcoal) is the most commonly used cathartic, but magnesium citrate and magnesium sulfate have also been used. No clinical studies have demonstrated beneficial effects of cathartics in poisoned patients. A cathartic alone has no role in the management of poisonings, and even the routine use of a cathartic in combination with activated charcoal cannot be recommended.[13] If a cathartic is used, only a single dose should be administered. A cathartic should not be administered in patients with ileus, GI obstruction or perforation, recent GI surgery, or hemodynamic instability. Complications of cathartics include nausea, vomiting, and abdominal cramping. Multiple doses of magnesium-containing cathartics may result in significant dehydration and electrolyte abnormalities.

WBI has been proposed as a technique to prevent absorption of ingested poisons by rapidly expelling the bowel contents. WBI involves the enteral administration (usually by nasogastric tube) of large volumes (1 to 2 L/hour in adults) of polyethylene glycol electrolyte lavage solution; this is continued until the rectal effluent is clear or elimination of the toxin has been confirmed. During the procedure, the head of the bed should be elevated to 45 degrees to decrease the likelihood of vomiting and aspiration. No clinical trials have assessed the impact of WBI on patient outcomes. Currently, there are no established indications for WBI, but it may be considered for potentially toxic ingestions of sustained-release or enteric-coated drugs, iron, and illicit drug packets.[14] WBI is contraindicated in the presence of ileus, GI obstruction or perforation, GI bleeding, hemodynamic instability, or intractable vomiting. In the patient with decreased level of consciousness or respiratory depression, the airway must be protected before instituting WBI.

ENHANCED ELIMINATION

Multiple-dose activated charcoal (MDAC) therapy involves the repeat oral administration of activated charcoal to prevent absorption of drug that persists in the GI tract and to enhance elimination of drugs already absorbed into the body by functioning as an adsorbent "sink" at several sites in the gut.[15] First, it can interrupt enterohepatic circulation of drugs or metabolites that are actively secreted into bile. Second, it can adsorb drugs or metabolites that enter the gut by active secretion or passive diffusion and prevent reabsorption. Finally, it may prevent desorption of drugs, particularly acidic substances that bind two to three times less avidly to activated charcoal in the alkalotic milieu of the intestinal lumen than in the acidic environment of the stomach. Drugs with a prolonged elimination half-life after overdose and small volume of distribution are more likely to have elimination enhanced significantly by MDAC.

One suggested regimen for administering MDAC is to follow the initial dose of activated charcoal with 0.5 to 1 g/kg every 4 hours. Alternatively, it is possible to administer charcoal as an aqueous solution by continuous infusion via a nasogastric tube at a rate of 0.25 to 0.5 g/kg/hour (not <12.5 g/hour). Additionally, the smaller doses (and volumes) administered more frequently may reduce the likelihood of vomiting. It may still be necessary to give an antiemetic intravenously to ensure effective administration. The dosing schedule will be dictated by clinical parameters such as patient cooperation, level of consciousness, the presence of ileus and vomiting, laboratory parameters, plasma concentrations of drug, and clinical improvement. Patients receiving MDAC should be monitored carefully for the development of constipation or obstruction and for the prevention of aspiration.

There is no convincing evidence that MDAC reduces morbidity and mortality rates in poisoned patients.[16] However, MDAC may be considered if the patient has ingested a life-threatening amount of carbamazepine, dapsone, phenobarbital, quinine, or theophylline and may obviate the need for invasive extracorporeal techniques. Insufficient evidence exists to support routine use of MDAC in ingestions of other substances.

Forced diuresis involves the intravenous (IV) administration of large volumes of isotonic fluids and diuretics to enhance renal excretion of drug or metabolite. This method is of limited clinical benefit and should not be used because of the potential for fluid overload and acid-base disturbances.

Urinary alkalinization is beneficial in increasing renal clearance of weak acids such as salicylates and phenobarbital. These weak acids are ionized at alkaline urine pH, trapped in the renal tubules, and not reabsorbed. Alkalinization can be initiated by adding 88 to 132 mEq sodium bicarbonate to 1 L of 5% dextrose in water (D_5W). Urine pH should be tested every hour, and the rate of the bicarbonate infusion should be titrated to achieve a urine pH of 7.5 to 8.5. Alkalinization may be difficult to achieve if metabolic acidosis is present. Hypokalemia is a common complication and requires correction to facilitate urinary alkalinization. Increasing the urine pH with carbonic anhydrase inhibitors such as acetazolamide is not recommended because metabolic acidosis will worsen. Urine alkalinization can be considered in patients with significant salicylate ingestions who do not require hemodialysis. Phenobarbital poisonings are more effectively treated with MDAC.[17]

Hemodialysis is useful to increase the clearance of certain drugs and metabolites, as well as to correct metabolic acidosis induced by some substances. The concentration gradient of the unbound toxin provides the driving force for clearance. The following criteria should be applied to a drug to determine the potential for enhanced elimination by hemodialysis: low volume of distribution (<1 L/kg), single-compartment kinetics, low endogenous clearance (<4 mL/minute/kg), molecular weight less than 500 daltons, water solubility, and low plasma protein binding. Drugs for which hemodialysis should be considered in the presence of a significant intoxication include methanol, ethylene glycol, salicylates, lithium, valproic acid, boric acid, and thallium. The usual complications of hemodialysis may occur, particularly in unstable patients. Hemoperfusion is a form of extracorporeal toxin removal, whereby whole blood is passed through an adsorbent-containing (charcoal) cartridge. In general, if a compound is well adsorbed by activated charcoal, then charcoal hemoperfusion clearance may exceed that of hemodialysis. In contrast to hemodialysis, substances with a high degree of plasma protein binding can be removed. However, advancements in hemodialysis and the limited availability of hemoperfusion cartridges have resulted in decreased utilization of hemoperfusion. Charcoal hemoperfusion is effective for elimination of carbamazepine, phenobarbital, phenytoin, and theophylline. Lithium and other heavy metals are not well removed by hemoperfusion. Charcoal hemoperfusion is generally performed for 4 to 6 hours at flow rates of 250 to 400 mL/minute. The risks of hemoperfusion are similar to those of hemodialysis. Additionally, hypoglycemia, hypocalcemia, and hypothermia may occur.

Continuous renal replacement therapies have been used less frequently for drug removal in the treatment of poisoning.[18] Clearance rates achieved with these techniques are considerably lower than those achieved with hemodialysis. Such therapy may be instituted after hemodialysis or hemoperfusion to further remove the drug after it slowly redistributes from tissue to blood. This is a potential option for agents such as lithium or procainamide. Continuous renal replacement techniques may be advantageous in hemodynamically unstable patients who cannot tolerate conventional hemodialysis or hemoperfusion. Despite many case reports demonstrating significant drug clearance, there are no data demonstrating that these techniques affect outcome.

SPECIFIC POISONINGS

ALCOHOLS

ETHYLENE GLYCOL AND METHANOL

Methanol and ethylene glycol are toxic alcohols that have similar properties in overdose. Toxicity can occur through ingestion, inhalation, or dermal absorption. Cardiopulmonary and central nervous system (CNS) symptoms are common, and both agents can produce an anion gap metabolic acidosis and an osmolar gap. However, absence of an osmolar gap or anion gap does not exclude a toxic ingestion. The osmolar gap may be normal if all alcohol is metabolized to acid metabolites, and an anion gap may be normal if metabolism of alcohol has not yet produced acid metabolites (e.g., concomitant ethanol ingestion or early presentation). If toxic alcohol ingestion is suspected, regardless of whether the patient is symptomatic, blood should be immediately sent for serum methanol, ethylene glycol, and ethanol levels, and definitive treatment initiated based on the clinical history and acid-base status. Significant toxicity is associated with methanol and ethylene glycol levels greater than 50 mg/dL. The severity of pH, serum bicarbonate, and anion gap abnormalities appears to be directly correlated with the likelihood of survival.

Ethylene glycol is found in antifreeze and deicing solutions. Ethylene glycol causes acidemia as a result of metabolism by alcohol dehydrogenase to glycolic and oxalic acid.

Oxalate crystals in the urine may be detected with a Wood's lamp or on microscopic examination, but they may not be present in the majority of exposed patients. Three classic phases of ethylene glycol toxicity have been described: neurologic, cardiopulmonary, and renal. During the first 0.5 to 12 hours after ingestion, ethylene glycol produces transient inebriation without the usual odor of ethanol, along with GI symptoms (nausea, vomiting). After toxic metabolites form (4 to 12 hours after ingestion), a metabolic acidosis develops along with CNS depression. The CNS symptoms may progress to coma associated with hypotonia, hyporeflexia, and occasionally seizures, meningismus, and cerebral edema. In the second stage (12 to 24 hours after ingestion), tachycardia and hypertension often occur along with progression of metabolic acidosis. Hypoxia may result from aspiration, heart failure, or acute respiratory distress syndrome. Death is most common in this stage. In the third stage (24 to 72 hours after ingestion), oliguria, flank pain, acute tubular necrosis, and renal failure develop.

Methanol is found in windshield washer fluid, solvents, and bootleg whiskey. It is metabolized by alcohol dehydrogenase to formaldehyde, which is then metabolized by aldehyde dehydrogenase to formic acid. Uncoupling of the mitochondrial oxidative metabolism produces lactic acid. The metabolic derangements are caused by lactic and formic acid; the latter is responsible for ocular disturbances. When methanol is ingested, peak levels occur within 30 to 60 minutes but there is often a latent period of about 24 hours (range 1 to 72 hours) before the development of toxic symptoms or metabolic acidosis. GI (abdominal pain, nausea, vomiting), CNS (dizziness, headache, seizures, coma), and ocular toxicities (blurred vision, photophobia, retinal edema, disc hyperemia, blindness) are seen.

Practice guidelines are available for the treatment of ethylene glycol and methanol intoxication.[19,20] If the patient has symptoms and is significantly acidemic, sodium bicarbonate may be administered as a temporizing measure to enhance formate and oxalate elimination by ion trapping. Fluid overload and hyperosmolarity may become significant problems as a result of bicarbonate administration. Hydration is helpful because ethylene glycol is well excreted by the kidney as long as renal function is maintained. The definitive treatment of intoxication with methanol or ethylene glycol is inhibition of the alcohol's metabolism and hemodialysis to remove the alcohol and toxic metabolites and to correct metabolic abnormalities. Hemodialysis should be considered for the following conditions: deteriorating vital signs despite intensive supportive care, significant metabolic acidosis (pH < 7.25 to 7.3), blood level of methanol or ethylene glycol higher than 25 mg/dL, or any evidence of renal failure or electrolyte imbalances unresponsive to conventional therapy.[19,20]

Antidotal treatment of significant poisoning involves inhibition of alcohol dehydrogenase to prevent metabolism of the alcohols to toxic metabolites with ethanol or fomepizole. Ethanol (IV or oral) allows preferential metabolism of ethanol over methanol and ethylene glycol. Ethanol should be administered to maintain a blood level of 100 to 150 mg/dL. A loading dose should be followed by a maintenance infusion according to the established dosing requirements for nondrinkers, drinkers, and during hemodialysis (Table 68.3).[21] Problems encountered during

Table 68.3 Intravenous Administration of 10% Ethanol

	Amount (mL) Infused over 1 Hour, as Tolerated, by Body Weight			
Dosing	30 kg	50 kg	70 kg	100 kg
Loading Dose*				
Loading dose of 0.8 g/kg of 10% ethanol†	240	400	560	800
Maintenance Dose‡	**Infusion Rate (mL/hr) by Body Weight**			
	30 kg	50 kg	70 kg	100 kg
Normal Maintenance Range§				
80 mg/kg/hr	24	40	56	80
110 mg/kg/hr	33	55	77	110
130 mg/kg/hr	39	65	91	130
Maintenance Dose for Chronic Alcoholic				
150 mg/kg/hr	45	75	105	150
Dose Required during Hemodialysis				
250 mg/kg/hr	75	125	175	250
300 mg/kg/hr	90	150	210	300
350 mg/kg/hr	105	175	245	350

*A 10% vol/vol concentration yields approximately 100 mg/mL.
†For a 5% concentration, multiply the amount by 2.
‡Infusion to be started immediately after the loading dose. Concentrations above 10% are not recommended for intravenous administration. The dose schedule is based on the premise that the patient initially has a zero ethanol level. The aim of therapy is to maintain a serum ethanol level of 100 to 150 mg/dL, but constant monitoring of the ethanol level is required because of wide variations in endogenous metabolic capacity. Ethanol will be removed by hemodialysis.
§Rounded to the nearest milliliter.
Adapted from Howland MA: Antidotes in depth: Ethanol. In Nelson NS, Lewin NA, Howland MA, et al (eds): Goldfrank's Toxicologic Emergencies, 9th ed. New York, McGraw-Hill Medical, 2011, p 1419.

ethanol administration include CNS depression, hypoglycemia, dehydration, and fluctuating serum concentrations. A second IV line using 0.9% sodium chloride may be necessary to avoid development of hyponatremia because of the large free water content and significant hypertonicity (1713 mOsm/L) of 10% ethanol solution. Advance notice should be given to the pharmacy to allow sufficient time to locate enough ethanol for administering and preparing the solution. If IV ethanol is not available, oral ethanol can be used.

Fomepizole, a competitive inhibitor of alcohol dehydrogenase, is approved for use in ethylene glycol and methanol overdose.[22] It is easier to administer than ethanol, does not cause sedation, and is associated with fewer severe and serious adverse events.[23] Fomepizole administration should be considered instead of ethanol if the patient develops altered consciousness, seizures, or a significant metabolic acidosis. Although fomepizole appears to be equally effective, there are no data to demonstrate its comparative efficacy or cost-effectiveness. Administration of ethanol or fomepizole should continue after dialysis until the serum ethylene glycol or methanol concentration is undetectable or less than 20 mg/dL or acidosis is resolved and the patient is asymptomatic. In the absence of renal dysfunction and a significant metabolic acidosis, the use of fomepizole potentially could obviate the need for hemodialysis, even though the serum ethylene glycol or methanol concentration exceeds 50 mg/dL.[24] If patients with high serum concentrations of ethylene glycol are not treated with hemodialysis, then their acid-base balance should be monitored closely and hemodialysis instituted if a metabolic acidosis develops.[19]

Additional therapeutic measures for ethylene glycol ingestions may include thiamine 100 mg IV and pyridoxine 50 mg every 6 hours until the ethylene glycol level is zero and no acidosis persists. If the patient becomes hypocalcemic as a result of precipitation of calcium oxalate crystals, calcium should be replaced. In methanol overdose, it may be reasonable to also administer IV folate (folinic or folic acids) at 50 to 75 mg IV every 4 hours for at least 24 hours to provide the cofactor for enhancing formic acid elimination.

ISOPROPYL ALCOHOL

Isopropyl alcohol may also be ingested, particularly by chronic alcoholics with no access to ethanol. It is found in rubbing alcohol and some hand sanitizers in high concentrations. Oral absorption occurs rapidly (within 0.5 hour), and it undergoes metabolism to acetone, carbon dioxide, and water. Symptoms may include severe abdominal pain, GI bleeding, nausea, and vomiting. Isopropyl alcohol is two to three times more potent than ethanol as a CNS depressant, and acetone is comparable with ethanol. Patients frequently present with headache, lethargy, ataxia, or coma. Respiratory depression occurs secondary to the CNS depression. Laboratory findings include an osmolar gap without a metabolic acidosis. Patients may, however, have a fruity odor on their breath from acetone, and ketonemia and ketonuria may also be present. Treatment is supportive with fluid administration for significant dehydration. Hemodialysis should be considered when isopropyl alcohol levels exceed 400 to 500 mg/dL, evidence of hypoperfusion exists, coma is present, or a failure to respond to supportive therapy is noted.

PROPYLENE GLYCOL

Propylene glycol is another alcohol that can cause toxicity in critically ill patients receiving high doses of IV medications containing the alcohol as a solvent. Medications that contain propylene glycol include lorazepam, diazepam, phenobarbital, pentobarbital, nitroglycerin, phenytoin, esmolol, etomidate, and sulfamethoxazole/trimethoprim. Propylene glycol toxicity is more commonly observed with lorazepam because of the use of high doses in some patients, the frequency of use for sedation in ICUs, and the high concentration of propylene glycol—approximately 830 mg/mL.[25] Common manifestations of propylene glycol accumulation are anion gap metabolic acidosis and increased osmolar gap.[26] Additional toxicities include renal dysfunction, hemolysis, cardiac arrhythmias, seizures, and CNS depression or agitation. Clinical studies suggest that an elevated osmolar gap correlates with propylene glycol accumulation. Accumulation can occur when doses of lorazepam exceed 0.1 mg/kg/hour and when renal or hepatic insufficiency is present. Although toxicity is more common after long periods of lorazepam infusion (>3 days), toxicity has occurred with short-term, high-dose use. The treatment of choice is to stop the lorazepam infusion and sedate with an agent that does not contain propylene glycol. Hemodialysis removes propylene glycol but is usually not required unless severe renal dysfunction develops.

ANALGESICS

ACETAMINOPHEN

Acetaminophen (*N*-acetyl-*p*-aminophenol [APAP]) is present in a large number of prescription and over-the-counter medications and is frequently a coingestant with other drugs. In addition, unintentional overdoses result from patients unknowingly ingesting multiple products containing acetaminophen (particularly acetaminophen-narcotic combinations). Because APAP overdose may result in significant hepatotoxicity and even death that is preventable, it is important to recognize and initiate appropriate therapy. With higher doses of APAP, a greater proportion is hepatically metabolized by the cytochrome P-450 system of mixed function oxidases (CYP450) to the toxic metabolite, *N*-acetyl-*p*-benzoquinoneimine (NAPQI), which can result in cell injury and death. Hepatic glutathione facilitates detoxification and elimination of NAPQI with therapeutic doses of APAP, but glutathione supply is overwhelmed in APAP overdoses. The clinical course of APAP toxicity has been divided into stages on the basis of the development of hepatotoxicity (Table 68.4).[27]

If possible, an estimate of the quantity and dosage form of APAP ingested and the time of ingestion should be obtained. In adults, hepatic toxicity can occur after ingestion of more than 7.5 to 10 g during 8 hours or less but has been reported with exposures of 4 g. The maximum daily dose of acetaminophen has been reduced to 3 g because of concerns for toxicity.[28] The risk of toxicity may be increased in patients with low glutathione stores (malnutrition, fasting state, chronic alcoholism) or induction of CYP450 enzymes (chronic alcoholism, phenytoin or carbamazepine use). For patients with a recent single, acute ingestion, an acetaminophen level should be obtained at least 4 hours after ingestion. Liver enzymes only need to be evaluated if the APAP

Table 68.4 Stages of Acetaminophen Toxicity

Stage	Time Course (after Ingestion)	Characteristics
I	0-24 hours	Asymptomatic or nausea, vomiting; normal LFTs
II	24-72 hours (latent stage)	Right upper quadrant pain; abnormal LFTs and PT; renal dysfunction possible
III	72-96 hours (hepatic stage)	Encephalopathy, jaundice, bleeding, renal dysfunction; maximal hepatic injury, synthetic dysfunction
IV	4 days-2 weeks (recovery stage)	Recovery of liver function

LFT, liver function tests; PT, prothrombin time.

level indicates potential toxicity or the clinical examination suggests hepatic injury. If the time of ingestion is unknown, an APAP level should be obtained on admission. An APAP level and liver function tests should be determined in patients presenting late, patients with multiple ingestions over time, or chronic ingesters of APAP.

Activated charcoal does adsorb acetaminophen, and it is reasonable to administer charcoal up to 2 hours after ingestion. Acetaminophen is absorbed rapidly from the GI tract, so later use of charcoal is not warranted unless gastric emptying is likely to be delayed. Administration of activated charcoal will not interfere with subsequent administration of oral *N*-acetylcysteine (NAC) therapy.

NAC is the antidote for APAP poisoning, but the optimal route and duration of treatment are still debated.[29] NAC limits toxicity by combining with NAPQI and by serving as a precursor of glutathione, which inactivates NAPQI. For patients with a single, acute ingestion of APAP, the serum acetaminophen level assessed at least 4 hours after ingestion is compared with the Rumack-Matthew nomogram. Treatment with NAC is initiated in the United States if the value falls above the lower possible hepatotoxicity line. Only the initial APAP level is used in making the decision to initiate or continue NAC treatment. Subsequent levels are unnecessary unless extended-release preparations are ingested (see following). The Rumack-Matthew nomogram is not useful for patients with multiple ingestions of APAP over time, chronic ingesters, or those ingesting extended-release forms (see following discussion). If acetaminophen levels are not available, NAC treatment should be initiated if more than 150 mg/kg or 10 g acetaminophen is ingested. For extended-release APAP, a second level 4 hours after an initial nontoxic level should be evaluated to assess for delayed absorption. If the second value is above the lower line on the Rumack-Matthew nomogram, NAC is initiated.

NAC is most effective in preventing toxicity if administered within 8 hours of ingestion. NAC therapy can be initiated pending results of the acetaminophen level if the patient is presenting late or APAP level results will be delayed. The oral regimen for NAC includes a loading dose of 140 mg/kg followed by 17 oral maintenance doses of 70 mg/kg administered 4 hours apart (72-hour regimen). Due to the odor of the oral form, a nasogastric tube may need to be placed for administration, and antiemetic therapy may be necessary to control vomiting that occurs in up to 50% of patients. If the patient vomits the loading dose or any maintenance dose within 1 hour of administration, the dose should be repeated. IV NAC is administered as a loading dose of 150 mg/kg over 60 minutes followed by 50 mg/kg infused over 4 hours and then 100 mg/kg infused over 16 hours (21-hour regimen). Anaphylactoid reactions may occur in 14% to 18% of patients with IV NAC. Oral and IV regimens of administering NAC are similar in efficacy.[30] However, the oral regimen may be more appropriate in patients who present later after ingestion (>18 hours) and when large amounts of APAP are ingested due to the higher dose of administered NAC.[31,32] If the patient has a serum APAP level in the potentially toxic range, the aspartate aminotransferase (AST) or alanine aminotransferase (ALT) level should be evaluated daily. If abnormal, additional tests such as bilirubin, prothrombin time, creatinine, BUN, blood glucose, and electrolytes should also be obtained. In patients with elevated liver enzymes, NAC may be continued beyond the full course of therapy until transaminases are decreasing.

Chronic ingesters of APAP or patients with multiple ingestions over time are problematic when determining the need to administer NAC. Presentation beyond 24 hours after ingestion makes the APAP level essentially useless, and there are no established guidelines for administration of NAC in these circumstances. A marker of toxicity that may be useful is the evaluation of AST and ALT. If enzymes are elevated at the time of presentation (>50 IU/L) or the APAP level is greater than 10 μg/mL (>10 μmol/L), a course of NAC should be strongly considered.[33] A course of NAC should also be administered to patients with hepatic failure caused by APAP.

Patients with evidence of toxicity from APAP should be monitored for signs and symptoms of hepatic failure. This includes evaluating mental status and frequently assessing blood glucose. In cases in which fulminant hepatic failure develops, appropriate consultation with a hepatologist should be obtained. Transplant may be an option in severe cases.

OPIOIDS

Illicit and prescription opioids can result in a toxidrome characterized by depressed level of consciousness, respiratory depression, and miosis. However, manifestations may be variable depending on the drug used and presence of other drugs or alcohol. Miosis is not seen with meperidine, propoxyphene, and tramadol toxicity. Additional clinical findings may include hypotension, pulmonary edema, bronchospasm (heroin), ileus, nausea, vomiting, and pruritus. Seizures may be a manifestation of toxicity with meperidine, propoxyphene, and tramadol. Methadone use is associated with QT interval prolongation and ventricular arrhythmias.

Prescription opioids obtained from physicians or illicitly now account for almost 40% of all poisoning deaths in the

United States and affect all age groups.[34] The agents most commonly involved in deaths include methadone, oxycodone, and hydrocodone.[35] Toxicity depends on the potency of the agent, dose ingested, tolerance of the individual, and concomitant use of other drugs. These prescription opioids have overshadowed deaths due to heroin. Heroin is rapidly absorbed by all routes of administration including IV, intranasal, intramuscular, subcutaneous, and inhalation, but most fatal overdoses occur with IV administration. IV fentanyl (sometimes extracted from analgesic patches) is also associated with fatalities. Diagnosis of an opioid overdose is made by characteristic clinical findings, exposure history, qualitative urine toxicology assay, and response to naloxone. Qualitative urine assays may not detect all opioid derivatives (e.g., fentanyl).

The immediate priorities in a patient with opioid toxicity are support of ventilation, correction of hypotension, and reversal of the toxic effects with an opioid antagonist. If reversal of respiratory depression cannot be accomplished quickly, intubation may be necessary. Isotonic fluids should be administered for hypotension. Naloxone, a potent competitive opioid antagonist, is the antidote for opioid toxicity. It can be administered intravenously, intramuscularly, subcutaneously, by sublingual injection, or through an endotracheal tube. The initial dose of naloxone in a suspected opioid overdose is 0.04 to 2 mg; the lower dose should be considered in patients suspected of chronic addiction to avoid precipitating acute withdrawal symptoms. The goal of therapy is to restore adequate spontaneous respirations rather than complete arousal. Doses of naloxone up to 10 to 20 mg may be required to reverse the effects of synthetic opioids such as pentazocine, methadone, and fentanyl. The effects of naloxone last approximately 60 to 90 minutes, necessitating continued observation of the patient for resedation. Patients may require continuous infusion of naloxone to maintain adequate respirations, particularly with long-acting opioids. The dose for infusion is typically one half to two thirds of the initial amount of naloxone that reversed the respiratory depression administered on an hourly basis. Adjustments of the dose should be made to achieve clinical end points and avoid withdrawal symptoms. Nalmefene, a long-acting opioid antagonist, has also been used to treat opioid overdoses, but prolonged withdrawal symptoms may be a concern.[36] Potential acetaminophen toxicity should be considered in patients ingesting opioids formulated with acetaminophen. Patients should also be observed for potential complications of opioid overdose including aspiration pneumonitis and noncardiogenic pulmonary edema. Noncardiogenic pulmonary edema is usually self-limited (24 to 36 hours) and managed with supportive care that may include intubation and mechanical ventilation.[37] Other complications that may be related to injection drug use include wound botulism, endocarditis, rhabdomyolysis, and compartment syndrome.

SALICYLATES

Salicylates should be considered as a potential toxin if a metabolic acidosis with an anion gap of unknown cause is present. The uncoupling of mitochondrial oxidative phosphorylation by salicylates results in metabolic acidosis and hyperthermia, and the stimulation of medullary respiratory centers results in tachypnea and respiratory alkalosis. Initial symptoms of toxicity include tinnitus and nausea or vomiting. Systemic acidosis promotes penetration of salicylate into the CNS, resulting in a depressed level of consciousness, coma, and seizures. Coagulopathy, transient hepatotoxicity, and hypoglycemia may also develop. Noncardiogenic pulmonary edema occurs more frequently in chronic salicylate toxicity than in acute overdose. The organ dysfunction and acid-base findings of salicylate intoxication can mimic sepsis and mislead clinicians.

Activated charcoal can be used for GI decontamination. Salicylates in large ingestions or enteric-coated forms can result in gastric concretions providing a depot for continued absorption; multiple doses of activated charcoal can be considered in this situation or when levels continue to rise despite other therapy.[16,38] A salicylate ingestion is considered toxic if symptoms are present, if more than 150 mg/kg has been ingested, or if levels are higher than 35 mg/dL at 6 hours after ingestion. The Done nomogram was developed in pediatric ingestions and does not provide good clinical correlation with toxicity in adults. Acute intoxication with salicylate levels in excess of 35 mg/dL at 6 hours after ingestion should be treated with sodium bicarbonate to alkalinize the urine to a pH 7 to 8, which increases the renal clearance of salicylate metabolites through ion trapping.[17] Hypokalemia will develop with correction of metabolic acidosis and must be corrected for urine alkalinization to be achieved. Alkalemia shifts the gradient of movement of salicylate from brain and tissues to blood.

Fluid status must be closely monitored, along with coagulation parameters, complete blood count, ABGs, electrolytes, and urine pH. Hemodialysis may be required for levels greater than 100 mg/dL in an acute ingestion, seizures, persistent alteration in mental status, refractory acidosis, persistent electrolyte abnormalities despite adequate therapy, or fluid overload resulting from sodium bicarbonate therapy. Additional indications for hemodialysis may include congestive heart failure (relative), noncardiogenic pulmonary edema, hepatotoxicity with coagulopathy, or renal insufficiency

CARBON MONOXIDE

Carbon monoxide (CO) poisoning may be accidental or intentional and continues to be a significant cause of morbidity in the United States. Sources of CO include motor vehicle exhaust fumes, gasoline-powered generators, poorly functioning heating systems, and inhaled smoke. CO binds to hemoglobin with an affinity 200 to 250 times greater than oxygen. Toxicities result from impaired release of oxygen at the tissue level, causing cellular hypoxia and possibly direct CO-mediated damage at the cellular level. The clinical manifestations of CO poisoning are nonspecific and may suggest other illnesses unless exposure is known or suspected. Headache, nausea, and vomiting are common. Cellular hypoxia may also result in confusion, angina, arrhythmias, syncope, and seizures. Tachycardia and tachypnea are frequently present as compensatory mechanisms for hypoxia. Classic findings of cherry red lips, cyanosis, and retinal hemorrhages occur rarely. Symptoms can range from mild to severe, and carboxyhemoglobin levels do not necessarily correlate with symptom severity. After recovery from acute CO exposure, delayed neuropsychiatric sequelae may occur.

Diagnosis requires a high level of suspicion. Carboxyhemoglobin levels can be measured in venous or arterial blood and must be interpreted carefully. Carboxyhemoglobin levels may be as high as 10% in smokers and are higher in urban compared with rural areas. An elevated level of carboxyhemoglobin may often be diagnostic, but a normal level does not rule out the diagnosis. The carboxyhemoglobin level may have decreased because of removal of the patient from the exposure and intervention with oxygen before hospital arrival.

Management of CO poisoning includes a detailed evaluation of neurologic and cardiorespiratory status. Acid-base status should be determined and an ECG examined for evidence of ischemia or arrhythmia. Oxygen is the antidote and shortens the half-life of carboxyhemoglobin by competing for binding with hemoglobin. High-concentration oxygen should be instituted as soon as possible and continued until the carboxyhemoglobin level has decreased to normal. Pulse oximetry overestimates arterial oxygenation because carboxyhemoglobin is misinterpreted as oxyhemoglobin. Analysis of arterial blood by co-oximetry is required for an accurate assessment of oxygen content. Intubation may be necessary in patients exposed to CO from fire. Hyperbaric oxygen therapy shortens the half-life of carboxyhemoglobin to 15 to 30 minutes compared with 40 to 80 minutes when patients breathe 100% oxygen. However, controversy exists over the specific indications for instituting hyperbaric oxygen therapy in CO poisoning.[39-41] Coma has been used as an indication for hyperbaric oxygen therapy; other suggested indications include a period of unconsciousness, neurologic findings other than headache, carboxyhemoglobin level greater than 40%, pregnancy with carboxyhemoglobin level greater than 15%, cardiac ischemia or arrhythmia, history of ischemic heart disease with carboxyhemoglobin level greater than 20%, and symptoms that do not resolve with normobaric oxygen after 4 to 6 hours. Hyperbaric oxygen treatment may decrease postexposure cognitive deficits.[42]

CARDIOVASCULAR DRUGS

Cardiovascular drugs are in the top five categories of substances involved in adult overdose exposures and a leading cause of fatalities from overdose.[4] Although a large number of cardiovascular drugs are available, the most clinically relevant agents are beta blockers, calcium channel blockers, and digoxin. Note that the clinical manifestations and management of beta-blocker and calcium channel blocker toxicity are very similar.[43]

BETA BLOCKERS

β-Adrenergic blockers differ in their lipid solubility, oral availability, first-pass effect, protein binding, metabolism, β-1 selectivity, membrane stabilization, and intrinsic sympathomimetic activity. Clinical findings with beta-blocker toxicity include bradycardia, atrioventricular (AV) conduction abnormalities (QRS prolongation, first-degree AV block), and hypotension. The hypotension is primarily due to the negative inotropic effects of these agents. With the exception of sotalol, ventricular fibrillation and other arrhythmias are not usually seen. The more lipophilic β-adrenergic antagonists such as propranolol, metoprolol, acebutolol, and timolol can cause delirium, coma, and seizures. Hypoglycemia is rare in adults. Toxicity generally occurs within 6 hours of ingestion of immediate-release preparations. Ingestion of sotalol or extended-release preparations may result in delayed toxicity, and these patients should be observed for 24 hours or longer if absorption is delayed. Propranolol is associated with the highest mortality rate, which may reflect its greater toxicity attributable to membrane-stabilizing effects.[44] Bradyarrhythmias and asystole usually precede death.

GI decontamination with gastric lavage may be considered if there is a large ingestion of propranolol or other more toxic agent and the patient presents within the first hour, even if symptoms are absent. Because of the risk of vagal stimulation, pretreatment with atropine may be indicated. Orogastric lavage may also be a consideration in patients with significant symptoms if the drug is suspected to still be present in the stomach. Activated charcoal is another option for GI decontamination in patients who present early after ingestion. WBI may be considered in ingestions of sustained-release preparations. Extracorporeal removal is ineffective for lipid-soluble beta blockers because of the large volume of distribution. Hemodialysis may be rarely considered for atenolol, a water-soluble beta blocker.

The primary goal of treatment is to reverse hypotension rather than to increase heart rate. Increases in heart rate do not always result in improvements in blood pressure. Although atropine is frequently administered for bradycardia, it is usually ineffective for beta-blocker and calcium channel blocker toxicity. Isotonic fluids can be administered for hypotension, but caution is warranted due to the negative inotropic effects of beta blockers on myocardial function. Pharmacologic interventions that have been used in beta-blocker overdoses include glucagon, calcium, catecholamines, insulin euglycemia therapy, and phosphodiesterase inhibitors.[43] IV lipid emulsion has recently been reported to be effective in refractory cases. Although clinical trials are lacking, glucagon is considered to be the appropriate initial intervention and is administered as 2 to 5 mg IV followed by a dose of 10 mg if necessary. If there is a positive clinical response, a continuous infusion (usually 2 to 10 mg/hour) is necessary owing to the short duration of action of glucagon. Glucagon is a chronotropic and inotropic agent that stimulates cyclic adenosine monophosphate (cAMP) by bypassing adrenergic receptors.[45] Adverse effects of glucagon include nausea, vomiting, hyperglycemia, and hypocalcemia.

Calcium salts should be considered as the next intervention for reversing hypotension that does not respond to glucagon if digoxin ingestion has been excluded.[43,46] Calcium chloride 10% (1 g by slow IV push) may be administered initially, and up to 3 g is recommended. Calcium chloride is preferred over calcium gluconate because it contains three times the amount of elemental calcium. It is best administered through a central venous catheter to avoid the possibility of skin necrosis from extravasation. If access is limited, 10% calcium gluconate can be administered but an increased dose is required.

High-dose regular insulin infusions and glucose administration to maintain euglycemia have been shown to be effective in beta-blocker and calcium channel blocker toxicity.[46,47] The beneficial effect may be caused in part by the metabolic effects of decreasing cardiac uptake of free fatty acids and increasing carbohydrate use. Reported insulin doses have been variable, but a reasonable initial dose is 0.5 units/hour with titration based on clinical response. It is also reasonable to administer a bolus insulin dose prior to initiation of the infusion. A glucose infusion should be initiated at the same time and a glucose bolus may also be needed. Careful monitoring of glucose and potassium is required.

Catecholamine infusions are frequently administered in beta-blocker toxicity concomitantly with other interventions. No agent is known to be more effective than others and response to various agents is often inconsistent in these clinical situations. Very large doses may be required because the β-adrenergic receptors are blocked; as a result, tachyarrhythmias can occur. The combination of dobutamine and norepinephrine may allow for titration of desired effects against cardiac output and blood pressure. Alternatively, phenylephrine may be used in conjunction with dobutamine. Epinephrine has been shown to be more effective than isoproterenol.[48] Infusion of any vasoactive agent should be started at usual doses and rapidly escalated to achieve a clinical response, but it should be stopped if there is a further fall in blood pressure or no beneficial effect.

Phosphodiesterase inhibitors such as milrinone and enoximone have been reported to be effective in some cases of human ingestions.[43,46] These agents may be useful in patients who fail other pharmacologic interventions, although experience is limited and they may cause further hypotension through peripheral vasodilation. Invasive hemodynamic monitoring may be needed in some patients.

Recent reports suggest that a bolus administration of 20% lipid emulsion (100 mL) may be beneficial in beta-blocker and calcium channel blocker cardiovascular toxicity refractory to other interventions. An additional infusion of 0.25 mL/kg/minute has been used in some cases. The exact mechanism of effect is unknown, but it has been proposed that lipids serve as a "sink" for the toxin that reduces free drug levels and limits distribution to tissues. Another possibility is that the fatty acids of lipids improve inotropy by increasing intracellular calcium concentrations.[49]

Ventricular pacing (transthoracic or transvenous) may be considered, but electrical capture is often unsuccessful. Even when pacing increases the heart rate, blood pressure often fails to improve. Intra-aortic balloon pump and cardiopulmonary bypass are potential options to maintain circulation until drug is metabolized in the unstable patient unresponsive to other interventions.

CALCIUM CHANNEL BLOCKERS

Calcium channel blockers selectively inhibit calcium movement in cardiac or vascular smooth muscle membranes during the slow inward phase of excitation-contraction. These agents have varying degrees of negative inotropic effect (verapamil), vasodilatory effect (nifedipine, diltiazem), depression of rate of discharge of the sinus node (verapamil, diltiazem), and slowed conduction through the AV node (verapamil, diltiazem). All are well absorbed with clinically significant protein binding (80%) and a large volume of distribution. All undergo extensive hepatic metabolism, many through the cytochrome P-450 system, and have varying degrees of active metabolites.

Signs and symptoms of toxicity occur within 6 hours for immediate release formulations but are delayed 6 to 18 hours for sustained-release preparations.[50] Gastric concretions often form, acting as a further reservoir for sustained absorption. Nausea, vomiting, and hypotension are usually accompanied by bradycardia with verapamil and diltiazem or reflex tachycardia with nifedipine. Conduction abnormalities associated with verapamil and diltiazem may include first-degree block, Wenckebach block, junctional rhythm, third-degree AV block, and AV dissociation. Hypoperfusion secondary to decreased cardiac output may lead to tissue ischemia and metabolic acidosis. The patient may present with CNS symptoms such as lethargy, confusion, and coma. Hyperglycemia can result from a decrease in insulin secretion and insulin resistance and may be a marker of severe exposure.

Activated charcoal is the preferred method of GI decontamination in recent ingestions. Because of the hepatic metabolism of calcium channel blockers, the parent and active metabolites exhibit enterohepatic circulation. However, once absorbed, calcium channel blockers decrease cardiac output and may lead to mesenteric ischemia and diminished bowel motility, which is a relative contraindication to MDAC. WBI may be considered for removing sustained-release preparations.

As with beta blockers, initial treatment of calcium channel blocker overdose should be aimed at treating hypotension and significant conduction defects. Interventions include the same pharmacologic interventions as for beta blockers with a change in order of administration. Calcium salts should be administered initially in toxicity due to calcium channel blockers.[44,46] Repeat boluses of calcium may be needed every 10 minutes. If blood pressure improves with calcium, an infusion is usually needed owing to the transient effect of bolus doses of calcium. Doses up to 0.4 mL/kg/hour of 10% calcium chloride may be needed. Ionized calcium concentrations can be monitored, but high serum concentrations may be necessary for beneficial effects. Glucagon has also been reported to be beneficial in toxicity due to calcium channel blockers and it should be considered as a second intervention if there is no response to calcium.[45] Glucagon is dosed as in beta-blocker overdoses. A continuous infusion of glucagon can be titrated to maintain blood pressure, cardiac output, and sinus rhythm. Insulin-glucose infusions have also been evaluated as an adjunctive treatment in severe cases and should be considered if calcium and glucagon are ineffective.[47] As with beta-blocker overdose, large doses of catecholamines may be required. Administration of lipid emulsion can be considered in refractory cases.[49] Transthoracic or transvenous pacing may be considered but are often ineffective. Refractory hypotension may require intra-aortic balloon pump or cardiopulmonary bypass.

DIGOXIN

Cardiac glycosides inhibit active transport of Na^+ and K^+ across cell membranes by reversibly binding to a specific site on the Na^+/K^+-ATPase. The alterations in cardiac rate and rhythm occurring in digitalis toxicity can produce almost every type of arrhythmia. Toxicity results from the complex influence of digitalis on the electrophysiologic properties of the heart, as well as the cumulative result of the direct, vagotonic, and antiadrenergic actions of digitalis. Toxicity should be suspected if there is evidence of increased automaticity (ectopic rhythms) or depressed conduction (prolonged PR interval, AV node blockade, decreased QT interval). Early in acute intoxication, depression of sinoatrial (SA) or AV node function may be reversed by atropine, but atropine subsequently does not reverse the direct and vagomimetic actions of the drug. Noncardiac manifestations of acute digitalis intoxication include anorexia, confusion, nausea or vomiting, and increased K^+ concentrations.

GI decontamination in digoxin overdose consists of activated charcoal, if the timing is appropriate. Late administration of activated charcoal or MDAC may be considered due to enterohepatic metabolism of the drug.[16] Steroid-binding resins such as cholestyramine and colestipol have also been used to prevent further absorption from the GI tract and reduce serum half-life in the same manner as charcoal. Forced diuresis, hemoperfusion, and hemodialysis are not effective in hastening the elimination of digoxin because of the large volume of distribution (4 to 10 L/kg). Only 1% of total body stores of digoxin is present in the serum; of that, 25% is protein bound.

The treatment for life-threatening digitalis toxicity is administration of digoxin-specific antibody fragments.[51] Administration of digoxin-specific antibody fragments results in a sharp decrease in free digoxin levels, an increase in total serum digoxin, an increase in renal excretion of digoxin bound to Fab, and a decrease of serum potassium toward normal. The time to response is approximately 30 minutes (range 20 to 90 minutes). Indications for administration of digoxin-specific antibody fragments include severe ventricular arrhythmias, progressive bradyarrhythmias unresponsive to atropine, potassium concentration greater than 5 mEq/L in the setting of suspected digoxin toxicity, rapidly progressive cardiac or GI symptoms, an increasing potassium concentration, serum digoxin concentration greater than 15 ng/mL at any time or more than 10 ng/mL at steady state, ingestion of more than 10 mg of digoxin in a previously healthy adult, and to establish the diagnosis. In the event that digoxin-specific fragments are not immediately available, phenytoin (50 mg/minute up to 1000 mg) or lidocaine may be administered until control of the arrhythmia is achieved. Atropine may work for severe supraventricular bradyarrhythmias or varying degrees of AV block if administered early. Beta blockers may be used for supraventricular and ventricular tachycardias. Magnesium sulfate may be an effective temporizing measure for the treatment of ventricular arrhythmias in the absence of digoxin-specific antibodies, even in the presence of hypermagnesemia. All class Ia antiarrhythmic drugs are contraindicated. Isoproterenol should be avoided because there is an increased risk of ventricular ectopy in the presence of toxic digoxin levels. Transthoracic or transvenous pacing has limited value in this setting.[52]

Hypokalemia, hyperkalemia, and hypomagnesemia can exacerbate digitalis cardiotoxicity and should be aggressively corrected. When hyperkalemia exists with toxic digoxin levels and ECG evidence of potassium toxicity, the serum potassium should be treated with conventional interventions if digoxin-specific Fab fragments are not immediately available. Calcium chloride, in the presence of digitalis toxicity, can theoretically be disastrous because intracellular hypercalcemia already exists. Intractable ventricular fibrillation or tachycardia may result.

After digoxin-specific antibodies have been administered, serum digoxin levels are no longer reliable because they represent free and bound digoxin. The digoxin-specific antibodies are effective even in anephric patients. In renal insufficiency, the Fab half-life is prolonged 10-fold with no change in volume of distribution. Fab concentrations remain detectable for 2 to 3 weeks. Although there is no dissociation of the complex in renal insufficiency, free digoxin levels rebound (redistribution from tissue sites) and Fab fragments leave the vascular space over 7 to 14 days.[53] During this time symptoms may recur and a second dose may be necessary.

CYANIDE

Inhalation or ingestion of cyanide is rare but can produce severe poisoning rapidly leading to death. A history of potential cyanide exposure is extremely important in suggesting the diagnosis because rapid cyanide assays are not available and clinical manifestations are nonspecific.[54] Cyanide exposure may occur from incomplete combustion of products containing carbon and nitrogen in fires and from industrial processes such as electroplating, metal refining, photography, fumigation, and gold or silver extraction. Cyanogenic substances are also found in a variety of plants, although severe toxicity is rare. Iatrogenic cyanide intoxication may occur during nitroprusside administration with high doses or in the presence of hepatic dysfunction.

Cyanide is a nonspecific inhibitor of enzymes; inhibition of mitochondrial cytochrome oxidase results in anaerobic metabolism with decreased adenosine triphosphate (ATP) production, lactic acidosis, and decreased oxygen utilization. Clinical characteristics of acute cyanide poisoning are rapid deterioration, loss of consciousness, anion gap metabolic acidosis, and cardiopulmonary failure. CNS signs and symptoms include headache, anxiety, agitation, confusion, seizures, and coma. Cardiovascular responses manifest as initial bradycardia and hypertension, followed by hypotension with reflex tachycardia that can progress to terminal bradycardia and hypotension. Ventricular arrhythmias and myocardial ischemia also occur. Pulmonary findings include cardiogenic and noncardiogenic pulmonary edema. GI symptoms of abdominal pain, nausea, and vomiting are less common. A bitter almond odor from vomitus or gastric contents is described in cyanide poisonings but may not be present and is often not detectable by health care personnel.

Early diagnosis, rapid administration of antidote, and aggressive supportive care are necessary to stabilize patients with severe cyanide poisoning. A cyanide level may be requested for confirmation, but results will not be available to guide immediate care. Intubation and mechanical ventilation are usually required. Fluids, inotropes, and vasopressors may be indicated for hypotension. If the poison was ingested, gastric lavage may be indicated but should not delay the administration of antidote. As soon as cyanide poisoning is suspected, a cyanide antidote kit or equivalent should be used. The kit contains amyl nitrite ampules, 3% sodium nitrite, and 25% sodium thiosulfate. Amyl nitrite is used as the first agent when lack of IV access delays the administration of sodium nitrite. It is an immediate source of nitrite that oxidizes hemoglobin to methemoglobin, which has a higher affinity for cyanide than cytochrome oxidase. Cyanmethemoglobin is formed, which eventually dissociates, but at such a rate that cyanide can be metabolized by hepatic rhodanese. The ampules are crushed in a gauze sponge and initially intermittently inhaled. This is followed by IV administration of 300 mg of sodium nitrite (10 mL 3% solution) as soon as possible. The optimum methemoglobin level that should be achieved is unknown, but clinical responses have occurred with levels of 3.6% to 9.2%. The second component of the antidote package is 25% sodium thiosulfate (12.5 g for adults), which provides sulfur for conversion of cyanide to thiocyanate by hepatic rhodanese. Thiocyanate is then excreted by the kidneys.

Hydroxocobalamin, a vitamin B_{12} precursor administered at an initial dose of 5 g, is commonly used in Europe for acute cyanide poisoning and has been available in the United States since 2006.[55] It displaces cyanide from the cytochrome oxidase and forms cyanocobalamin, which is then excreted in the urine or metabolized by hepatic rhodanese. A second dose of 5 g can be administered for severe poisoning or lack of clinical response. Thiosulfate is administered with hydroxocobalamin. Hyperbaric oxygen has also been proposed for treating cyanide toxicity, but data supporting efficacy are not available.

DIETARY AND NUTRITIONAL AGENTS

Dietary and nutritional products are categorized as supplements and can be marketed without testing for safety or efficacy. Although some herbs and supplements may have inherent toxicity, poisoning may result from product misuse, contamination of the product, or through interaction with other medications.[56-58] Patients and their families should always be questioned regarding use of nutritional supplements, herbal preparations, energy drinks, or natural remedies when considering possible toxin exposure as a cause of clinical abnormalities. Adverse effects resulting from these products should be reported to the U.S. Food and Drug Administration. Table 68.5 contains a partial list of toxicities that may result in or complicate critical illness.

Herbal teas may contain aconitine or digoxin-like substances.[59] Management is usually supportive. A digoxin level should be obtained in any patient demonstrating symptoms consistent with digoxin toxicity. The level may not correlate with clinical findings because numerous cardiac glycosides will not cross-react in the digoxin immunoassay. With significant toxicity, digoxin-specific antibodies should be administered.

Products containing ephedrine and ephedrine-free products are often used for weight loss. These products can result in manifestations similar to a sympathomimetic syndrome with cardiovascular and cerebrovascular complications.[60-62] Similarly, caffeinated energy drinks can precipitate atrial and ventricular arrhythmias.[63]

Toxicity from ingestion of herbal preparations and nutritional supplements may result from product contaminants.

Table 68.5 Toxicities of Selected Dietary and Nutritional Agents

Agent	Toxic Effect(s)
Herbal teas	
Aconitine	Bradycardia, ventricular tachycardia and fibrillation, hypersalivation, GI disturbances, muscle weakness
Cardiac glycosides (digoxin-like factors)	Arrhythmias, GI disturbances, visual disturbances
Energy drinks (caffeine, xanthine alkaloids)	Arrhythmias, cardiac arrest
Weight loss products	
Ephedrine (ma huang)	Sympathomimetic syndrome, intracranial hemorrhage, seizures, arrhythmias, myocardial infarction, stroke, hepatic failure, rhabdomyolysis, death
Ephedrine-free supplements (bitter orange, synephrine, octopamine)	Myocardial ischemia, syncope, stroke, ischemic colitis
Ginkgo biloba	Bleeding (cerebral or extracerebral)
Ginseng	Hypoglycemia, potential bleeding
Garlic	Bleeding
Kava kava	Hepatic failure, potentiation of anesthetics

GI, gastrointestinal.

Products may contain heavy metals, unlisted drugs, or other ingredients.[64] The California Department of Health Services, Food and Drug Branch, screened 260 Asian patent medicine products and found 32% contained undeclared pharmaceuticals or heavy metals.[65] Unusual symptoms or toxidromes in patients ingesting such products may require the assistance of the local health department or toxicologist to identify a possible toxin. Additional information about specific agents can be found at www.herbmed.org or www.mskcc.org/aboutherbs.

METHEMOGLOBIN INDUCERS

Methemoglobin results from the oxidation of ferrous iron in hemoglobin to ferric iron. Methemoglobin is not able to bind oxygen and high concentrations lead to a functional anemia which results in cellular hypoxia by limiting oxygen delivery. The most common inducers of methemoglobin in the health care setting are topical spray anesthetics (benzocaine, tetracaine, butyl aminobenzoate) and dapsone. Procedures utilizing topical anesthetics that are associated with the development of methemoglobinemia are transesophageal echocardiography, GI endoscopy, intubation, and bronchoscopy.[66,67] Predisposing factors include sepsis, anemia, and hospitalization. Dapsone may cause prolonged methemoglobinemia in patients with acquired immunodeficiency syndrome (AIDS) because of its long half-life.

Clinical manifestations are related to the impaired oxygen delivery, and the severity varies with the concentration. Cyanosis is apparent when methemoglobin concentrations are 10% or greater due to the deep color of methemoglobin. Concentrations of 20% to 50% may cause headache, dyspnea, dizziness, and fatigue and concentrations greater than 50% can result in metabolic acidosis, arrhythmias, tachypnea, seizures, lethargy, and depressed level of consciousness. Diagnosis requires measurement of methemoglobin concentrations in arterial or venous blood gas assays by co-oximetry. Pulse oximetry is not usually accurate for determining the presence or concentration of methemoglobin depending on the specific characteristics of the monitor. A helpful clue is the observance of a saturation gap between the measured oxyhemoglobin saturation by pulse oximeter and the calculated oxyhemoglobin saturation provided by ABG assay. In the presence of methemoglobin, the calculated concentration will be higher than the measured saturation by pulse oximeter. Co-oximetry is required to identify the abnormal hemoglobin.

Methylene blue is the antidote for methemoglobinemia and should be administered when there are significant symptoms indicating impaired oxygen delivery.[68] In addition, individuals with lower methemoglobin concentrations may also warrant treatment if further oxidant stress may increase the concentrations. High-flow oxygen should be administered. The usual dose of methylene blue is 1 to 2 mg/kg IV over 5 minutes. Clinical improvement in symptoms and cyanosis is usually evident within a few minutes. A second dose can be administered if cyanosis does not resolve within 1 hour. Although there is concern for methylene blue causing hemolysis in patients with glucose-6-phosphate dehydrogenase (G-6-PD) deficiency, this information will not usually be known at the time of treatment and methylene blue should not be withheld in symptomatic patients.

Table 68.6 Signs and Symptoms of Cholinesterase Poisoning

Muscarinic Effects	Nicotinic Effects	CNS Effects
Salivation	Muscle fasciculations, cramping, weakness	Restlessness
Lacrimation	Diaphragmatic fatigue	Headache
Urination	Respiratory failure	Tremor
Diarrhea	Areflexia	Drowsiness
Nausea, vomiting	Paralysis	Confusion, delirium
Bronchorrhea	Tachycardia	Slurred speech
Bronchoconstriction	Mydriasis	Ataxia
Miosis		Seizures
Bradycardia		Psychosis
		Respiratory depression

CNS, central nervous system.

ORGANOPHOSPHATE AND CARBAMATE AGENTS

Organophosphates and carbamates are cholinesterase inhibitors and are usually a component of insecticides. However, nerve agents used in chemical warfare such as sarin and VX are also organophosphate compounds. Cholinesterase inhibitors exert toxicity by blocking the activity of acetylcholinesterase resulting in acetylcholine accumulation at cholinergic receptors. When organophosphates or carbamates bind to acetylcholinesterase, they form a conjugate that is infinitely more stable than the acetylcholine-acetylcholinesterase conjugate. The carbamate-acetylcholinesterase bond spontaneously hydrolyzes in minutes to hours so that acetylcholinesterase is eventually regenerated (reversible binding). Carbamates do penetrate the CNS based on clinical symptoms and autopsy studies.[69] Most carbamate poisonings spontaneously resolve within 24 to 48 hours and do not have significant morbidity or mortality risk. Phosphorylated or phosphonylated enzymes, however, degrade over days to weeks, making acetylcholinesterase essentially inactive (irreversible binding). For the physiologic enzyme activity to return, new enzyme must be generated or antidote given. After the acetylcholinesterase is phosphorylated over 24 to 48 hours, "aging" occurs, and the enzyme can no longer spontaneously hydrolyze and is permanently inactivated.[70]

Organophosphates may be absorbed by virtually any route including transdermal, transconjunctival, inhalation, across the GI or genitourinary mucosa, and through direct injection. Onset of systemic symptoms may occur in 5 minutes with inhalation, and most patients will develop symptoms within 12 hours of ingestion, unless exposure to fat-soluble organophosphates (e.g., fenthion, clorfenthion) has occurred or if significant metabolic activation must occur (e.g., parathion, malathion). Signs and symptoms of cholinesterase poisoning are listed in Table 68.6. Pulmonary toxicity from bronchorrhea, bronchospasm, and respiratory depression is the primary concern.[71]

Early intubation is usually indicated with significant toxicity, and succinylcholine should be avoided because of prolonged paralysis. Initially, atropine 2 to 4 mg is given IV and repeated every 5 minutes. If there are no CNS symptoms, glycopyrrolate may be substituted. The end point of atropinization is clearing of secretions. Tachycardia is not a contraindication to atropine use because it may represent hypoxia and autonomic stimulation. The tachycardia may resolve with improved oxygenation. In massive exposures, hundreds of milligrams of atropine may be required over days or weeks. A continuous infusion of atropine should be initiated at 0.05 mg/kg/hour and titrated to effect. After the patient is adequately stabilized, atropine must be carefully and slowly withdrawn because secretions will likely return if the drug is still bound to acetylcholinesterase or leaches from fat stores.

Atropine does not reverse nicotinic effects, and patients with significant respiratory muscle weakness require the use of pralidoxime. Pralidoxime is a nucleophilic oxime that regenerates acetylcholinesterase at muscarinic, nicotinic, and CNS sites. It may also prevent continued toxicity by scavenging the remaining organophosphate molecules. Treatment with pralidoxime may be most effective when started early. It may have benefit beyond the 48-hour aging limit, although the mechanisms have not been clearly elucidated. It should be continued as long as atropine is continued. The evidence for benefit of any oxime in pesticide poisoning is limited.[72] Pralidoxime is usually administered as a loading dose (1 to 2 g in normal saline 500 mL administered over 30 minutes) and then as a continuous infusion at 200 to 500 mg/hour to maintain serum levels higher than 4 μg/L.[73] Other dosing regimens have also been proposed.[71] Pralidoxime may also be protective against the development of the intermediate syndrome and other long-term neurologic sequelae. Pralidoxime therapy is usually not needed if the toxin is known to be a carbamate.

In addition to acute toxicity, organophosphates may cause persistent effects, which may manifest while the patient is in the ICU and last several weeks to months. These include organophosphate-induced delayed neurotoxicity and delayed polyneuropathy that occur 1 to 3 weeks after exposure.[74] Recovery may occur gradually or not at all. The third complication is intermediate syndrome.[75] The syndrome develops 24 to 96 hours after resolution of an acute, severe cholinergic crisis, and patients develop acute respiratory paralysis, weakness in the bulbar musculature, nuchal weakness, proximal limb weakness, and depressed reflexes. Electromyography studies show decremental conduction with repetitive nerve stimulation and suggest both presynaptic and postsynaptic nerve impairment. Recovery takes 2 to 4 times longer than the development.

PSYCHOTROPIC DRUGS

CYCLIC ANTIDEPRESSANTS

Deaths caused by overdose with cyclic antidepressants are declining because of the increasing use of alternative antidepressants.[4] The principal toxicities of cyclic antidepressants result from central and peripheral anticholinergic activity, α-adrenergic antagonism, and inhibition of norepinephrine reuptake. They also exert a membrane-depressant local anesthetic effect on the myocardium by blocking rapid sodium influx during phase 0 of the action potential. Primary toxicities include depressed level of consciousness, wide-complex arrhythmias, seizures, and hypotension. Acidosis, hypoxia, and seizures may increase the risk of wide-complex arrhythmias. Anticholinergic effects include mydriasis, fever, dry skin, delirium, agitation, tachycardia, ileus, and urinary retention. Life-threatening events usually occur within 6 hours of ingestion, most often in the first 2 hours.[76] Several electrocardiographic criteria have been proposed to predict complications: QRS duration greater than 0.1 second correlates with risk of seizures, QRS duration greater than 0.16 second correlates with increased risk of arrhythmias, and the presence of an R wave in lead aVR greater than 3 mm predicts seizures and arrhythmias.[77,78] However, the performance of these criteria in predicting complications including death is relatively poor.[79]

If poisoning with a cyclic antidepressant is suspected, electrocardiographic monitoring should be instituted and IV access obtained. Intubation may be needed in patients with CNS depression who are unable to protect their airway. If wide-complex arrhythmias (or ECG changes described previously), hypotension, or seizures are present, stabilization requires immediate alkalinization of the blood and sodium loading with sodium bicarbonate.[80] Sodium bicarbonate should be administered in 50 to 100 mEq (1 to 2 mEq/kg) boluses to alkalinize the blood pH to 7.5 to 7.55. Clinical end points are normalization (narrowing) of the QRS complex, reestablishment of an adequate blood pressure, and termination of seizure activity. Alkalinization appears to decrease the free drug by increasing protein binding and shifting the concentration gradient away from tissues back into the main compartment. Sodium loading may have a greater benefit by overcoming the blockade of the myocardial sodium channels. The bolus doses of sodium bicarbonate should be immediately followed with a continuous infusion, which can be prepared by adding 150 mEq $NaHCO_3$ (sodium bicarbonate) to 1 L of D_5W. This should be titrated to the desired blood pH, QRS interval, and blood pressure. The infusion may be discontinued after 4 to 6 hours if the width of the QRS complex remains less than 100 ms without the administration of sodium bicarbonate. Hyperventilation to achieve blood alkalinization may be less effective but useful in patients who cannot tolerate the sodium and volume load or in those who develop pulmonary edema from treatment with sodium bicarbonate.[80,81] Hyperventilation without the administration of sodium bicarbonate may also be considered for patients with cerebral edema, head trauma, or poorly controlled congestive heart failure. Hypertonic saline has been effective in treating cardiac toxicity refractory to initial blood alkalinization.[82,83]

If torsades de pointes is associated with QT prolongation, magnesium sulfate 1 to 2 g IV over 2 to 5 minutes should be administered.[80] Hypotension refractory to volume expansion is best treated with a direct-acting catecholamine such as norepinephrine or phenylephrine in the setting of depleted norepinephrine stores.[84] An inotropic agent such as dobutamine can be added if hypotension is the result of depressed myocardial contractility and decreased cardiac output. If hypotension remains refractory to fluids and vasopressors, the use of an intra-aortic balloon pump may be considered as a temporizing measure. Recently, IV lipid emulsion has been reported to successfully treat hemodynamic instability associated with cyclic antidepressant toxicity.[49,85]

After the patient with a known or suspected cyclic antidepressant overdose has been stabilized and the airway protected, activated charcoal is indicated. Gastric lavage should only be performed if the patient is seriously ill and the ingestion occurred within 1 hour of presentation. A second dose of activated charcoal may be given in several hours if it seems plausible that the drug still remains in the GI tract in the case of a massive ingestion or hypotension. MDAC to enhance elimination is not warranted given the extremely large volume of distribution (10 to 50 L/kg) and the low-protein binding of cyclic antidepressants.[16] Forced diuresis, hemodialysis, and hemoperfusion are ineffective. Physostigmine should also be avoided because of the potential anticholinergic toxicity of seizures and asystole.

If the patient has had altered mental status, seizures, or cardiac arrhythmia, the patient should remain in the ICU for 12 hours after all supportive therapeutic interventions have been discontinued. If the patient remains asymptomatic with a normal ECG during this phase of observation, the patient may then be transferred for additional care.

LITHIUM

Although lithium is used to treat bipolar affective disorder and other psychiatric disorders, its narrow therapeutic index predisposes to toxicity.[86] After oral ingestion, lithium is absorbed within 1 to 2 hours, reaching peak blood levels in 2 to 4 hours with regular preparations or in 4 to 12 hours with sustained-release preparations. Lithium does not bind to plasma proteins and is excreted almost entirely by the kidneys. Toxicity may occur with acute, acute on chronic, or chronic ingestions. Drugs that increase lithium reabsorption (angiotensin-converting enzyme [ACE] inhibitors, thiazides, nonsteroidal anti-inflammatory drugs), sodium restriction, volume depletion, and intrinsic renal dysfunction increase the risk of toxicity. Lithium levels do not necessarily correlate with toxic symptoms. With an acute ingestion, the patient may be asymptomatic with a lithium level of 6 to 8 mmol/L. In chronic lithium ingestion, a high total-body lithium burden results in more immediate toxicity at lower serum levels.

The clinical presentation of patients with lithium toxicity varies with the type of ingestion. In an acute ingestion, nausea, vomiting, and diarrhea occur early with CNS symptoms developing later because of a delay in tissue distribution. In chronic ingestions, neurologic abnormalities are usually the major presenting manifestations. Patients with acute on chronic ingestions may manifest GI and neurologic symptoms. Neurologic abnormalities include tremor, hyperreflexia, agitation, fasciculations, clonus, and altered mental status. Confusion may be followed by lethargy, coma, and seizures. The tremor, hyperreflexia, and clonus usually precede altered mental status. Lithium can impair urine-concentrating ability in acute ingestions and cause nephrogenic diabetes insipidus and renal dysfunction in chronic ingestions that result in volume depletion. Although myocardial dysfunction and rhythm abnormalities have been reported in lithium toxicity, they occur infrequently. Lithium toxicity may produce flattened or inverted T waves and U waves on ECG.

Lithium toxicity is confirmed by assessment of the serum lithium level. A lithium level should be assessed immediately and 2 hours later to evaluate for increasing levels. Levels higher than 2.5 mmol/L in a chronic ingestion or higher than 4 mmol/L in an acute ingestion are potentially life-threatening. Renal function and volume status should also be assessed.

Management decisions in treating lithium toxicity may depend on the type of ingestion (acute versus chronic) and the product ingested (regular versus sustained-release). Lithium is not adsorbed by activated charcoal, but charcoal may be administered if other drugs are ingested or suspected. A forced diuresis is not effective in enhancing lithium excretion, but isotonic saline should be administered to replete and maintain intravascular volume and promote adequate urine output.[87] Diuretics can worsen lithium toxicity and should be avoided. WBI has been proposed for GI decontamination with acute or acute on chronic ingestions, ingestion of sustained-release products, or when serial lithium levels are rising. Despite lack of proven clinical benefit, this approach may be considered with appropriate precautions. Hemodialysis is effective in removing lithium, but controversy exists on the indications for treatment and duration of therapy. Proposed indications that have not been validated include renal dysfunction, severe neurologic dysfunction, inability to tolerate fluid replacement, lithium level higher than 4 mmol/L in an acute overdose, and lithium level higher than 2.5 mmol/L in chronic toxicity. The lithium level, duration of exposure, and severity of clinical symptoms should be balanced against risks of the procedure before initiating hemodialysis. Hemodialysis clears lithium only from the plasma, and a rebound increase can develop from drug redistribution. A lithium level should be assessed immediately after hemodialysis and 6 to 8 hours later. Repeat dialysis can be considered if the lithium level increases or neurologic toxicity persists at that time. Although a lithium level of 1 mmol/L is often recommended as the end point for hemodialysis, no systematic investigations have established the ideal end point for optimal outcome. Because of redistribution of lithium, improvement of neurologic toxicity lags behind the decrease in plasma level. Prolonged monitoring of lithium levels may be necessary, especially when sustained-release preparations are ingested. Continuous venovenous hemodiafiltration has also been used to remove lithium and may be associated with less rebound.[88] This technique results in a slower lithium clearance compared with hemodialysis and is not recommended if hemodialysis is available and can be tolerated. Sodium polystyrene sulfonate resin has been proposed to bind and remove lithium, but it is not currently recommended and may result in hypokalemia, hypernatremia, and fluid overload. Aminophylline and low-dose dopamine infusions have also been proposed to enhance lithium excretion, but no evidence of clinical efficacy exists and they should not be used.[87]

SELECTIVE SEROTONIN REUPTAKE INHIBITORS

Selective serotonin reuptake inhibitors (SSRIs) and related antidepressants are frequently prescribed for depression and other disorders. They have decreased lethality and fewer adverse cardiovascular effects compared with cyclic antidepressants.[89] Most fatalities involving SSRIs involve coingestion of other substances. Manifestations of an acute SSRI overdose may include nausea, vomiting, dizziness, blurred vision, and rarely CNS depression. Seizures and a wide QRS occur rarely but may be more likely with citalopram and bupropion, a unicyclic antidepressant. A syndrome characteristic of SSRIs is the serotonin syndrome, which may occur after a single dose, high dose, overdose, or when combined with other serotonergic agents.[90] The pathophysiology is related to excessive stimulation of central and peripheral serotonergic receptors. Clinical manifestations include altered mental status ranging from agitation to coma; autonomic dysfunction including diaphoresis, tachycardia, hyperthermia, unstable blood pressure, and diarrhea; and neuromuscular abnormalities that may range from tremors to myoclonus and rigidity.[91] Severe cases may be complicated by rhabdomyolysis, renal failure, disseminated intravascular coagulation, or acute respiratory distress syndrome.

Management of an acute overdose of SSRIs is largely supportive. Gastric lavage is not warranted because of the low toxicity of these compounds, but use of activated charcoal may be considered. An ECG should be obtained to assess for the rare occurrence of a wide QRS complex or other electrocardiographic abnormality. Although clinical experience is limited, there are reports of sodium bicarbonate administration resulting in narrowing of the QRS complex. The treatment of serotonin syndrome is primarily supportive therapy after discontinuing the precipitating agents. Intubation and mechanical ventilation may be necessary for patients with significant alteration of mental status. Benzodiazepines are useful for control of agitation and external cooling for sustained hyperthermia. Rarely, neuromuscular blockers may be necessary for control of muscle rigidity or tremor. The syndrome usually resolves in 24 to 72 hours. Treatment of patients with serotonin antagonists has been proposed, but experience is limited to case reports. Cyproheptadine in varying dose regimens (12 to 32 mg/24 hour) has been most commonly recommended as a treatment option. Currently there is no role for the use of bromocriptine or dantrolene.[91]

SEDATIVES

BENZODIAZEPINES

Although ingestions are relatively common, fatalities from benzodiazepines alone are uncommon. Benzodiazepine overdose results in a typical sedative-hypnotic toxidrome characterized by depressed level of consciousness, respiratory depression, hyporeflexia, and potentially hypotension and bradycardia. The clinical manifestations may be exacerbated by concomitant ingestion of other agents with sedating properties, such as ethanol, opioids, or antidepressants. Alprazolam is commonly seen in overdoses due to wide availability and may result in greater toxicity than other benzodiazepines.[92] Flunitrazepam is a benzodiazepine not approved for use in the United States that has been associated with sexual assault. Diagnosis of benzodiazepine ingestion is primarily based on the history and clinical manifestations. Many benzodiazepines can be detected in qualitative urine toxicology assays, but a negative test does not rule out ingestion. If warranted, gas chromatography/mass spectrometry can be requested for definitive detection.

Managing benzodiazepine ingestions should be guided by the clinical presentation of the patient. The airway is assessed and stabilized if necessary. Activated charcoal is the primary method of GI decontamination for recent ingestions. Supportive care with intubation and mechanical ventilation may be necessary for patients with significant toxicity. Hypotension usually responds to volume infusion.

Flumazenil is a competitive benzodiazepine receptor antagonist that will reverse the sedative effects of benzodiazepines. It may be a helpful diagnostic tool in evaluating an overdose patient but should not be routinely used as a substitute for adequate airway protection.[93] A dose greater than 1 mg is seldom necessary in overdose victims. The short half-life of flumazenil (0.7 to 1.3 hours) makes resedation likely because of the longer half-life of benzodiazepines. Continuous monitoring must be instituted if flumazenil is used to arouse the patient. Flumazenil use has been associated with seizures in patients with chronic benzodiazepine use and when cyclic antidepressants are present.[93] It is best to avoid flumazenil in those situations and in patients with a seizure disorder or when a drug capable of causing seizures has been ingested. Slow titration of flumazenil (0.1 mg/minute) and limiting the total dose to 1 mg may minimize the risk of seizures. If seizures occur with flumazenil, benzodiazepines (often in higher doses) may be effective.

GAMMA HYDROXYBUTYRATE

Gamma hydroxybutyrate (GHB), a naturally occurring substance found in the brain and peripheral tissues, is banned in the United States except for the treatment for narcolepsy. It is one of several agents characterized as a "date rape" drug and has been promoted to build muscle, improve performance, produce euphoria, induce fat loss, and enhance sleep. Several deaths have been attributed to GHB and related agents.[94] The drug is usually available as a colorless, odorless liquid with a mild, salty taste that is easy to mask in drinks. GHB is rapidly absorbed from the stomach (usually within 10 to 15 minutes) and readily crosses the blood-brain barrier. It is metabolized to carbon dioxide and water without active metabolites. Stimulatory effects occur from resulting increased dopamine levels in the brain and sedative effects by potentiation of endogenous opioids. The manifestations of GHB toxicity are dose related and include agitation, coma, seizures, respiratory depression, and vomiting.[95] Other effects include amnesia, tremors, myoclonus, hypotonia, hypothermia, decreased cardiac output, and bradycardia. Coma and respiratory depression may be potentiated by the concomitant use of ethanol. GHB is not routinely detected by urine toxicology assays but can be detected in plasma or urine by gas chromatographic and mass spectrophotometric techniques. Diagnosis is usually determined by the clinical course and history of exposure elicited after the patient recovers. Gamma butyrolactone (GBL), also known as 2(3H)-furanone dihydro, and 1,4-butanediol (BD), also called tetramethylene glycol, have been abused with the same adverse effects as GHB including death. Both agents are metabolized in the body to GHB.[94]

No antidote for GHB, GBL, or BD exists. The primary management for ingestion of these drugs is supportive care with particular attention to airway protection and ventilation. In some cases, intubation and mechanical ventilation are required. Gastric lavage and activated charcoal are not indicated because of the small amounts involved and the rapid absorption. Naloxone and flumazenil are of no benefit. Patients with mild intoxication may be observed in the emergency department and released after symptoms resolve. A rapid recovery of consciousness from an obtunded condition is frequently observed. In patients requiring intubation and mechanical ventilation, symptoms can be expected to resolve within 2 to 96 hours unless complications such as aspiration or anoxic injury have occurred. The concomitant use of alcohol may prolong the CNS depression. Although physostigmine has been used to awaken patients with GHB intoxication, its use is not recommended.[96]

A withdrawal syndrome has been described in patients who frequently ingest high doses of GHB (every 1 to 3 hours).[97] Mild symptoms such as anxiety, insomnia, nausea, vomiting, and tremors begin within 6 hours of the last dose and may progress to severe delirium with autonomic instability (usually mild) requiring hospitalization and sedation. The duration of symptoms requiring treatment may be as long as 2 weeks. Benzodiazepines are the initial choice for management, and high doses may be required. Propofol and barbiturates have also been used successfully.

PROPOFOL

Propofol is a sedative-hypnotic used for general anesthesia, procedural sedation, more prolonged sedation in critically ill patients, and treatment of status epilepticus. It has also been implicated in abuse, accidental overdose, suicide, and even murder.[98] The critical care clinician should be aware of a potentially fatal toxicity associated with more prolonged infusions of propofol known as propofol-related infusion syndrome (PRIS).[99] The syndrome is usually associated with doses of propofol greater than 4 mg/kg/hour for longer than 48 hours' duration. However, metabolic acidosis has been reported within 1 to 4 hours after the initiation of propofol infusion. Predisposing factors that have been associated with PRIS include young age, CNS or respiratory illness, vasopressor use, glucocorticoid use, greater severity of illness, sepsis, and impaired oxygen delivery. Mortality rates of 18% to 80% have been reported.[99] Clinical features of the syndrome can include refractory bradycardia progressing to asystole, other arrhythmias, myocardial failure, lactic acidosis, rhabdomyolysis, renal failure, and hypertriglyceridemia.[100] The pathophysiology is hypothesized to be related to mitochondrial utilization of free fatty acids and genetic predisposition.

Propofol infusions should be limited to less than 4 mg/kg/hour and no longer than 48 hours of infusion when possible. Prompt recognition of early signs of PRIS (elevated serum lactate, elevated creatine kinase, hypertriglyceridemia) is essential for successful intervention. Another clinical clue to possible PRIS is the unexplained need for increasing doses of pressor or inotropic agents. Management includes discontinuation of propofol and the use of alternative sedative agents. The most effective treatment for severe PRIS is cardiorespiratory support and hemodialysis or hemofiltration to decrease blood levels of metabolic acids and lipids.[100]

STIMULANTS

AMPHETAMINES/METHAMPHETAMINES

Amphetamines, methamphetamines, and related agents cause central and peripheral release of catecholamines, which result in a sympathomimetic/adrenergic toxidrome characterized by tachycardia, hyperthermia, diaphoresis, agitation, hypertension, and mydriasis. Hallucinations (visual and tactile) and acute psychoses are frequently observed. The clinical manifestations associated with abuse of these agents may last up to 24 hours due to the longer duration of pharmacologic effects. The acute adverse consequences are similar to those seen with cocaine abuse (see following) and include myocardial ischemia and arrhythmias, pulmonary hypertension, seizures, intracranial hemorrhage, stroke, hepatotoxicity, rhabdomyolysis, necrotizing vasculitis, and death.[101] Chronic use of these drugs may result in dilated cardiomyopathy.[102] Poor oral hygiene and severe dental caries ("meth mouth") can be clues to chronic methamphetamine use.[103]

Methamphetamine hydrochloride in a crystalline form called "ice," "crank," or "crystal" is one of the most popular drugs in this class. It has high purity and can be orally ingested, smoked, insufflated nasally, or injected intravenously. An amphetamine-like drug (3-4-methylenedioxymethamphetamine) is a designer drug commonly known as Ecstasy, XTC, or MDMA that acts as a stimulant and hallucinogen.[104] It results in serotonin release in the brain with inhibition of serotonin reuptake and has been reported to produce serotonin syndrome. Complications are usually a result of the drug effects and excessive physical activity. Complications include hyperthermia, hyponatremia (excessive water intake or syndrome of inappropriate antidiuretic hormone secretion), rhabdomyolysis, renal failure, cardiac collapse, cerebral infarction/hemorrhage, and multiple organ failure. MDMA and other amphetamines will usually be detected on qualitative toxicology assays of urine but false positives and negatives occur.

Management of amphetamine intoxication is primarily supportive. Gastric lavage is not recommended because absorption after oral ingestion is usually complete when patients present. Activated charcoal may be considered if a recent oral ingestion is known to have occurred. Further interventions are dependent on patient complaints and clinical findings. A careful assessment for complications should be made including measurement of core temperature, obtaining an ECG, and evaluating laboratory data for evidence of renal dysfunction and rhabdomyolysis. IV hydration for possible rhabdomyolysis is warranted in individuals with known exertional activities pending creatine phosphokinase (CPK) results. Benzodiazepines, often in high doses, are used to control agitation. Haloperidol should be reserved for patients who do not have an adequate response to benzodiazepines. Seizures are best treated with benzodiazepines.

COCAINE

Cocaine abuse is a global problem that results in significant medical complications.[105] Cocaine hydrochloride is water soluble and can be injected intravenously, ingested, or snorted intranasally. Crack or rock cocaine is the alkaloid form primarily abused by inhalation. The onset, peak, and duration of physiologic effects of cocaine vary with the route of use, form of cocaine used, and concomitant use of other drugs.[105] Both forms of cocaine are absorbed from all mucosal surfaces and undergo hydrolysis by plasma and liver cholinesterases. The major metabolites, benzoylecgonine and ecgonine methyl ester, are excreted in the urine and can be detected by qualitative urine assays. The metabolites of cocaine may be detectable in urine for 24 to 36 hours after use, but prolonged detection can occur in frequent users of high doses.

Cocaine inhibits the presynaptic reuptake of biogenic amines such as norepinephrine, dopamine, and serotonin throughout the body including the CNS. Characteristic clinical findings of a sympathomimetic syndrome include tachycardia, mydriasis, hypertension, hyperthermia, diaphoresis, euphoria, and agitation. The sympathetic stimulation also results in multiple potential complications (Box 68.3). Complications such as myocardial ischemia or cerebral infarction may occur several days after the last use of cocaine. Complications of transporting cocaine in body cavities may include rupture of packets with drug absorption and bowel obstruction.

No specific antidote exists for cocaine. Treatment is primarily aimed at detecting complications, intervening as

Box 68.3 Complications Associated with Cocaine Use

Cardiovascular

Myocardial ischemia, infarction
Arrhythmias
Aortic dissection, rupture
Hypertension
Atherosclerosis
Cardiomyopathy
Vasculitis

Central Nervous System

Seizures
Cerebral infarction
Transient ischemic attack
Intracranial hemorrhage (intraparenchymal, intraventricular, subarachnoid)
Cerebral vasculitis
Cognitive dysfunction

Pulmonary

Bronchospasm
Barotrauma
Noncardiogenic edema
Pulmonary hypertension

Renal

Renal infarction
Renal failure
Scleroderma renal crisis

Gastrointestinal

Mesenteric ischemia, infarction
Gastrointestinal tract perforations

Metabolic

Hyperthermia
Rhabdomyolysis
Weight loss
Multiple organ failure

Other

Deep venous thrombosis
Skin ischemia
Dystonic reactions

indicated, and preventing further injury. Benzodiazepines should be used liberally for control of agitation. Haloperidol is reserved for overt psychosis because of its potential for lowering the seizure threshold.

No large clinical trials have evaluated therapeutic strategies for myocardial ischemia resulting from cocaine use. Aspirin should be administered if the risk of intracranial hemorrhage is low because a significant number of patients have thrombotic occlusion as the cause of ischemia. Benzodiazepines and nitroglycerin are first-line agents for relief of chest pain, but small clinical studies have yielded conflicting results on the benefit of combining the agents.[106] α-Adrenergic blockers such as phentolamine and calcium channel blockers have been recommended as second-line treatment for unrelieved pain but are rarely necessary.[106] Beta blockers were often considered to be contraindicated in the management of potential ischemia related to cocaine because of the potential for unopposed α-adrenergic-mediated vasoconstriction leading to elevated blood pressures. However, beta-blocker use was not found to be detrimental in two retrospective studies of patients with recent cocaine use and may be beneficial in some patients.[107,108] It may be appropriate to avoid administration of beta blockers in patients manifesting acute sympathomimetic findings. In addition, routine use of IV beta blockers is no longer recommended for acute coronary syndromes. Reperfusion interventions, primarily percutaneous coronary interventions, should be considered for patients with myocardial infarction.[106] Ventricular arrhythmias are not common and may be related to cocaine blockade of myocardial sodium channels leading to QRS and QT interval prolongation. Wide complex arrhythmias may respond to treatment with sodium bicarbonate.[109] Class IA antiarrhythmic drugs such as procainamide should be avoided. Treatment of life-threatening arrhythmias should otherwise follow advanced life support guidelines.

Cerebral complications should be managed by standard interventions specific for the injury. Seizures are best managed with benzodiazepines. The reported incidence of underlying vascular malformations in intracranial hemorrhage has been variable, but if present these problems may require specific intervention. Severe hyperthermia is managed the same as heat stroke with either conductive or evaporative cooling.[110] When there is suspicion of rhabdomyolysis, IV hydration should be instituted immediately pending assessment of renal function and CPK levels. Asymptomatic transporters of cocaine packets should be managed conservatively with activated charcoal, possible WBI, and supportive care. Surgery is reserved for patients exhibiting manifestations of cocaine poisoning or GI perforation or obstruction.[111] Contamination of cocaine with other drugs or fillers can result in toxicities that are not directly related to the effects of cocaine. Levamisole, an anthelminthic agent used in veterinary medicine, has been found in cocaine supplies and linked to the development of agranulocytosis.[112] Agranulocytosis resolves when drug use is discontinued. Retiform purpura and skin necrosis secondary to thrombotic vasculopathy have also been linked to cocaine contaminated with levamisole.[113,114] The potential for suicidal intent should be recognized in cocaine abusers, and psychiatric consultation may be appropriate after stabilization.

MEPHEDRONE/METHYLENEDIOXYPYROVALERONE (BATH SALTS)

Mephedrone and 3.4-methylenedioxpyrovalerone (MDPV) are synthetic stimulants marketed in products sold as bath salts to avoid regulation. MDPV inhibits reuptake of dopamine and norepinephrine, and mephedrone may act as a monoamine reuptake inhibitor.[115] Street names include Ivory Wave, Bliss, White Lightning, Vanilla Sky, Hurricane Charlie, White Knight, and others. The products have been ingested, snorted, smoked, and injected and are often used in combination with alcohol or other drugs. These agents are not detected by qualitative toxicology screens.

Clinical manifestations are similar to those of other stimulant drugs and include agitation, tachycardia, hyperthermia, hypertension, mydriasis, chest pain, palpitations, seizures, hallucinations, delusions, and paranoia.[115,116] Symptoms may be prolonged for more than 24 hours after use of mephedrone despite a short expected half-life.[116] Management includes IV benzodiazepines for significant agitation and psychotic symptoms. Symptoms may recur as sedation wears off, requiring repeat dosing. A thorough clinical evaluation is required to identify other complications such as rhabdomyolysis, myocardial ischemia, and organ dysfunction. Seizures are best treated with IV benzodiazepines.

VALPROIC ACID

Use of valproic acid (VPA) for seizure disorders, psychiatric disorders, migraine prophylaxis, and neuropathic pain has resulted in increased toxicity reported with therapeutic doses and overdoses. The most common manifestation of toxicity in overdoses is CNS depression with higher drug levels associated with an increased incidence of coma and respiratory depression requiring intubation.[117] Cerebral edema may occur 48 to 72 hours after overdoses and may be related to hyperammonemia that usually occurs in the absence of hepatotoxicity. The increase in ammonia is not well understood but may be related to carnitine deficiency, renal abnormalities, or defects in the urea cycle.[117] Large VPA ingestions can result in refractory hypotension. Pancreatitis has been associated with chronic ingestion and acute overdose. Metabolic abnormalities of VPA toxicity include hypernatremia, hyperammonemia, anion gap metabolic acidosis, hypocalcemia, and acute renal failure. Hepatotoxicity is rare with VPA overdoses, but mild, asymptomatic abnormalities may occur with chronic use.

Initial and serial VPA levels should be obtained because of delayed peak serum levels in overdose. Patients may be comatose with normal serum VPA concentrations caused by unmeasured metabolites. An ammonia level should be obtained in patients with altered level of consciousness. Activated charcoal should be administered if the patient presents early after ingestion. MDAC may be beneficial because of a potential enterohepatic recirculation of drug, but routine use is not currently recommended. Although VPA is highly protein bound, protein binding is saturated at high serum concentrations resulting in more free drug being available for removal by extracorporeal techniques. Hemoperfusion, combined hemodialysis-hemoperfusion, or high flux hemodialysis may be considered in patients with severe or persistent hemodynamic instability, coma, or metabolic acidosis.[118] No antidote exists for VPA toxicity, but L-carnitine administration has been proposed for patients with VPA toxicity and hyperammonemia. Chronic VPA therapy has been associated with carnitine deficiency and case reports suggest that L-carnitine administration is safe.[119] However, there is no evidence that L-carnitine alters clinical outcome and more rigorous study is needed. Dosing of L-carnitine in reports has been variable but a suggested regimen is 100 mg/kg IV bolus or infusion over 15 to 30 minutes, followed by 50 mg/kg (maximum 3 g/dose) every 8 hours until the ammonia level is decreasing and the patient clinically improves.[119]

KEY POINTS

- Evaluating and managing the poisoned patient involves resuscitation and stabilization, diagnosis, GI decontamination and toxin elimination, institution of specific antidotes or interventions, and supportive care.
- In the poisoned patient with altered mental status, hypertonic dextrose, thiamine, and naloxone should be considered for administration.
- Patterns of signs and symptoms identified by physical examination may often suggest a toxidrome that is associated with classes of toxins.
- Single-dose activated charcoal is most effective when administered within 1 hour of toxin ingestion; later administration may be appropriate if clinical factors suggest the toxin has not yet been completely absorbed.
- Recognition of potential acetaminophen toxicity is essential for appropriate treatment and prevention of morbidity.
- Findings of bradycardia and hypotension should suggest possible ingestion of a beta blocker or calcium channel blocker.
- Dietary and nutritional supplements can result in significant cardiac and cerebrovascular toxicities.
- Cyclic antidepressant toxicity with increased QRS duration or wide complex tachyarrhythmia requires immediate alkalinization of the blood with sodium bicarbonate or hyperventilation.
- The initial treatment for patients presenting with a clinical syndrome suggesting a stimulant toxin (cocaine, amphetamines, bath salts) is IV benzodiazepines for control of agitation.
- Be aware of potential toxicities that can develop in ICU patients exposed to propylene glycol–containing medications, topical anesthetics, and propofol.

SELECTED REFERENCES

2. Nelson NS, Lewin NA, Howland MA, et al: Initial evaluation of the patient: Vital signs and toxic syndromes. In Nelson NS, Lewin NA, Howland MA, et al (eds): Goldfrank's Toxicologic Emergencies, 9th ed. New York, McGraw-Hill Medical, 2011, p 33.
25. Wilson KC, Reardon C, Theodore AC, Farber HW: Propylene glycol toxicity: A severe iatrogenic illness in ICU patients receiving IV benzodiazepines. Chest 2005;128(3):1674.
30. Brok J, Buckley N, Gluud C: Interventions for paracetamol (acetaminophen) overdose. Cochrane Database Syst Rev 2006;(2):CD003328.
46. Kerns W: Management of β-adrenergic blocker and calcium channel antagonist toxicity. Emerg Med Clin North Am 2007;25:309.
49. Cave G, Harvey M: Intravenous lipid emulsion as antidote beyond local anesthetic toxicity: A systematic review. Acad Emerg Med 2009;16:815.

80. Bradberry SM, Thanacoody HKR, Watt BE, et al: Management of the cardiovascular complications of tricyclic antidepressant poisoning: Role of sodium bicarbonate. Toxicol Rev 2005;24:195.
91. Boyer EW, Shannon M: The serotonin syndrome. N Engl J Med 2005;352:1112.
105. Goldstein Ram, DesLauriers C, Burda AM: Cocaine: History, social implications, and toxicity—A review. Dis Mon 2009;55:6.
106. McCord J, Jneid H, Hollander JE, et al: Management of cocaine-associated chest pain and myocardial infarction. A statement from the American Heart Association Acute Cardiac Care Committee of the Council on Clinical Cardiology. Circulation 2008;117:1897.
118. Licari E, Calzavacca P, Warrillow SJ, Bellomo R: Life-threatening sodium valproate overdose: A comparison of two approaches to treatment. Crit Care Med 2009;37:3161.

The complete list of references can be found at www.expertconsult.com.

69 Hypothermia, Hyperthermia, and Rhabdomyolysis

Zoulficar Kobeissi | Christopher B. McFadden

CHAPTER OUTLINE

HYPOTHERMIA

Cold exposure has been recognized as a cause of death since ancient times. In the year 492 BC, the Persians were sailing to launch their attack against the Greeks when they encountered bad weather and lost about 300 ships and 20,000 soldiers. Herodotus wrote, "… some were dashed by the rocks, and some of them did not know how to swim and perished for that cause, others again by reason of *cold*."

In order to recognize hypothermia, it must be possible to measure a temperature. The first thermometer for clinical use was invented in 1612. It was a foot long and required 20 minutes to register a temperature. The invention of the mercury thermometer by Fahrenheit in 1714 made the tool more practical. However, it was not until the late nineteenth century that the thermometer became a clinical tool. This use was established after the invention of a small thermometer that only required 5 minutes to obtain a temperature (1866) and after Carl Wunderlich's publication (1868), which presented data on nearly 25,000 patients and analyzed temperature variation in 32 diseases. In the early 1900s, temperature was routinely measured and physiologic experiments started to appear. By the 1930s to 1940s, therapeutic hypothermia for malignancy and anesthesia was investigated. By the middle of the twentieth century, accidental hypothermia was established as a disease entity.[1]

This section discusses the epidemiology, definition, pathophysiology, clinical diagnosis, clinical manifestations, and management of hypothermia.

EPIDEMIOLOGY

Accidental hypothermia continues to be a public health problem. The Centers for Disease Control and Prevention (CDC) reports that between 1979 and 2002, a total of 16,555 deaths in the United States (average of 689 per year, range 417-1021) were attributed to excessive natural cold.[2]

Approximately 50% of all hypothermia-related deaths occur in persons older than 65. The age-adjusted mortality rate is three times higher for men than it is for women. In blacks and other races, the mortality rate is higher than that of whites.[2,3] Blacks have decreased heat production and lower rectal temperatures in response to cold exposure.[4] Other populations at risk include the elderly, people with preexisting chronic medical conditions, and people suffering from alcoholism and drug intoxication.[2,3,5] Emerging populations include wilderness enthusiasts and winter sport participants.[6]

Despite advances in medical care, hypothermia remains a challenge to health care providers, with in-hospital mortality rate reaching 40%,[7] and an overall mortality rate ranging from 17% to 80%.[8] The prompt recognition and appropriate management play a key role in improving outcomes.

DEFINITION

Hypothermia is defined as a core body temperature lower than 35° C (<95° F). It has been further classified by severity according to the degree by which the core temperature has decreased from baseline into mild, moderate, and severe. Mild hypothermia is defined by a core body temperature of 32° to 35° C (90-95° F). Moderate hypothermia reflects a core body temperature of 28° to 32° C (82-90° F). Severe hypothermia is a core body temperature of less than 28° C (less than 82° F). Some reports refer to severe hypothermia below 30° C. In trauma patients, hypothermia carries a poorer prognosis. In this case, the definition is even more conservative, with severe hypothermia starting below 32° C. This subclassification has important implications regarding the anticipated physiologic changes and subsequently the use of appropriate therapeutic modalities.[9,10]

HEAT REGULATION

Body temperature is regulated through a balance between heat production and heat dissipation.[11] Heat production occurs mostly from the metabolic activity of energy-consuming processes within the viscera, namely, the heart, liver, and brain. Heat production in these organs is estimated to be between 40 and 60 kcal/m^2/hour. Normally heat production is increased by food intake and muscle activity. Different stresses such as fever, infection, and cold exposure also increase heat production.

Heat loss occurs through different forms. Radiation cooling (infrared emissions) accounts for approximately 60% of heat loss. It occurs primarily from the head and unisolated parts of the body. Conduction (direct transfer of heat to an adjacent cooler object) and convection (direct transfer of heat to convective air currents) account for around 10% to 15% of heat loss. Evaporation from the skin and respiratory tract accounts for 25% to 30%. Conduction is an important mechanism in immersion accidents because thermal conduction of water is 30 times that of air. Convection is important in windy conditions by removing the warm isolating layer of air around the body.[6,10,11]

Upon cold exposure, the hypothalamus initiates mechanisms for heat conservation and heat production. Heat conservation is achieved by peripheral vasoconstriction, reducing heat conduction to the skin, and behavioral responses such as wearing more clothes and seeking a warmer environment. Heat production is achieved through stimulation of muscular activity via shivering, which can increase the basal metabolic rate by two to five times. A nonshivering thermogenesis occurs via increased levels of catecholamines and thyroxine.[12]

This coordinated physiologic response occurs typically for temperatures between 32° and 35° C. It only lasts for few hours, after which muscle fatigue and glycogen depletion ensue. As the core temperature drops below 32° C (90° F), shivering thermogenesis abates, and nonshivering thermogenesis slows down. By temperatures below 20° to 24° C, the different mechanisms of heat production completely fail.[13]

CLINICAL PRESENTATION

ETIOLOGIC FACTORS (FIG. 69.1)

Factors that predispose to hypothermia are related to impaired thermoregulation, increased heat loss, and decreased heat production. A combination of these factors is often noted in a hypothermic patient.

1. *Impaired thermoregulation* is of critical importance in the elderly, mentally ill, and patients with chronic medical conditions such as Parkinson's disease, stroke, multiple sclerosis, and diabetes mellitus. Such populations are often on multiple medications including anxiolytics, antidepressants, phenothiazines, barbiturates, opioids, antipsychotics, oral antihyperglycemics, beta blockers, and alpha blockers. These drugs can cause further impairment in thermoregulation.[14] In addition, the elderly and chronically ill may suffer from maladaptive behavior (decreased mobility, and inability to communicate effectively), which increases the chance of remaining in an environment with prolonged cold exposure.[14]
2. *Increased heat loss* can be environmental or nonenvironmental.
   a. Hypothermia commonly occurs during winter weather and in cold climates. People with inadequate insulation and continued cold exposure are especially at risk.
   b. Patients with dermatologic dysfunction such as burns, psoriasis, and exfoliative dermatitis can have increased heat loss.
   c. Large amounts of unheated intravenous fluid resuscitation, whether crystalloids or blood, coupled with unheated humidified oxygen, predispose hospital and trauma patients to greater heat loss.
   d. Conditions that cause vasodilation should be highlighted in this category and include alcohol, anesthesia, and toxins released in disease entities such as sepsis.
3. *Decreased heat production* is noted in some specific types of disorders:
   a. Endocrine dysfunction such as hypopituitarism, hypothyroidism, hypoadrenalism, and hypoglycemia.
   b. Malnutrition and starvation, which cause decreased insulative subcutaneous fat and are often associated with hypoglycemia.
   c. Conditions that alter the level of consciousness, causing decreased shivering mechanism. Drugs such as phenothiazines and tricyclic antidepressants as well as alcohol can induce impairment of shivering.[6]

DIAGNOSIS

Diagnosis should be performed using a thermometer probe capable of measuring temperatures as low as 25° C (77° F). This instrument could be a rectal, esophageal, or bladder probe. It should be noted that standard clinical thermometers do not register below 34.4° C (94.4° F).[15] Combined

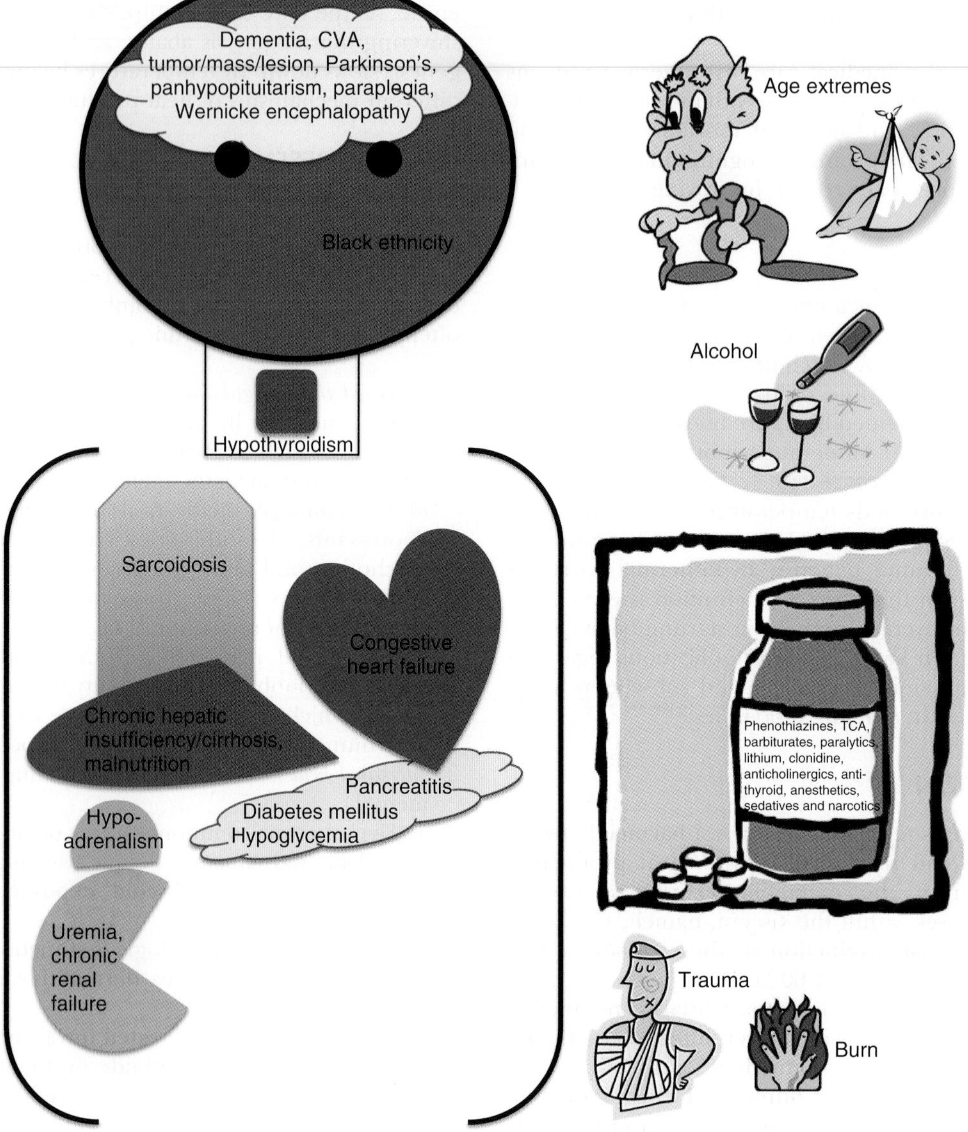

Figure 69.1 Diseases and factors associated with hypothermia.

methods for temperature monitoring may allow better detection of further changes.

END-ORGAN MANIFESTATIONS (FIG. 69.2)

Although hypothermia is divided into three stages, it is important to note that the physiologic changes follow a continuum. The initial mechanisms mimic intense sympathetic stimulation, which fades as body temperature drops. Almost every organ in the body is affected by hypothermia.[16]

Cerebral Effects

Hypothermia is associated with progressive decrease in neuronal metabolism between 35° C and 25° C. This protective effect of hypothermia allows better tolerance to periods of cardiocirculatory collapse in contrast with the normothermic state.[6,17,18] Neurologic symptoms starts with mild hypothermia. Between 34° and 35° C, loss of fine motor skills, lack of coordination, dysarthria, and amnesia take place. Ataxia and apathy are noted around 33° C.[19] Below 32° C, progressive decrease in level of consciousness and pupillary dilation develops. Cerebrovascular autoregulation is lost below 25° C. Deep tendon reflexes diminish and flaccid muscular tone takes place below 27° C. By 23° C, corneal and oculocephalic reflexes are absent. The electroencephalogram (EEG) pattern flattens at 19° to 20° C. The lowest temperature reported for an adult survival with hypothermia is 13.7° C.[6,15,20] Therefore, one has to be very careful in assessing brain death when a patient remains hypothermic.[8]

Cardiovascular Effects

The initial response (34-36° C) includes increased heart rate, blood pressure, and carbon dioxide secondary to elevated catecholamine production and peripheral vasoconstriction.[6] This is associated with marked increase in oxygen consumption. A core temperature decrease of as little as

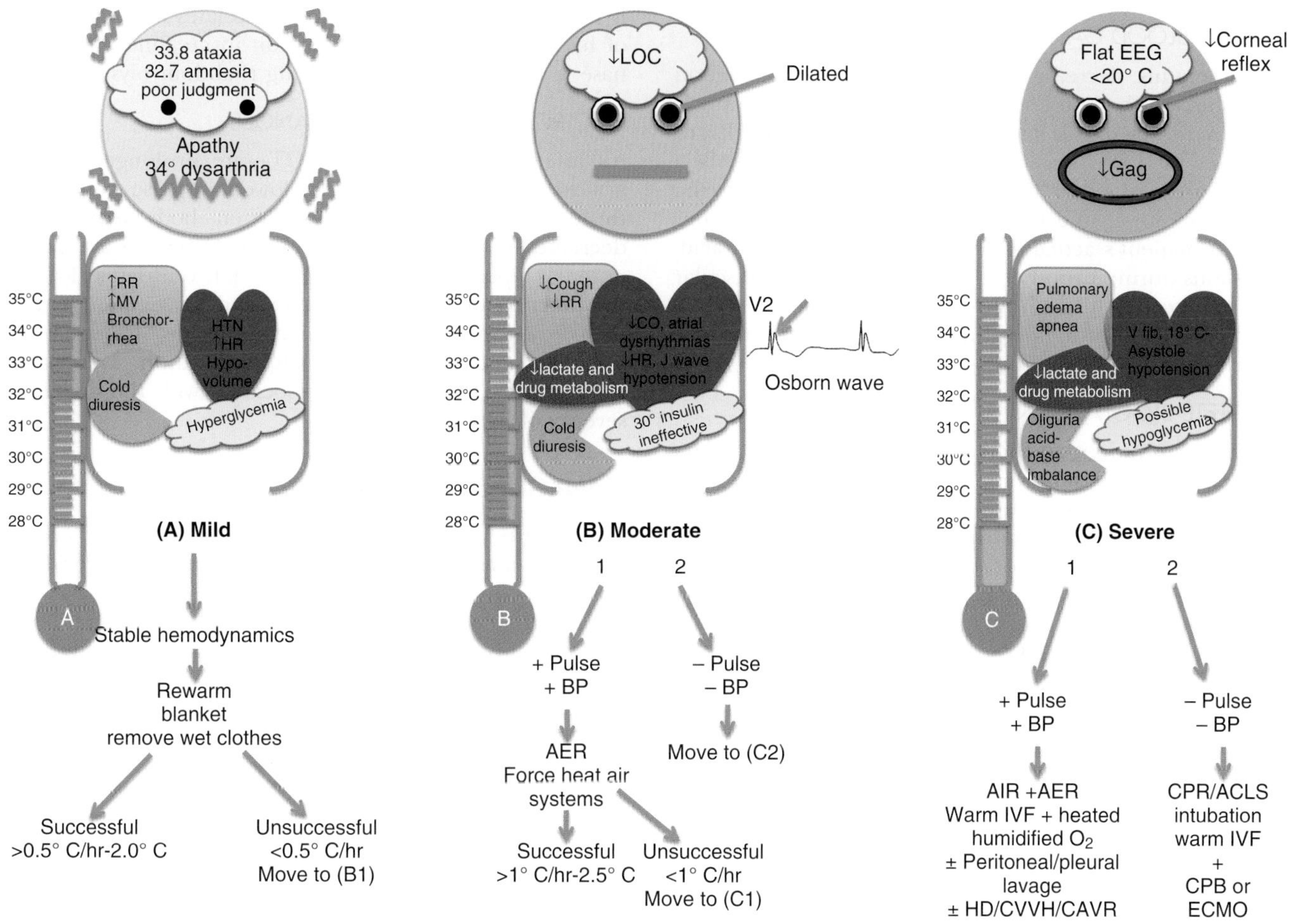

Figure 69.2 Hypothermia: clinical presentation and treatment approach.

0.3° C is associated with a 7% increase in oxygen consumption. The increase in oxygen requirement results in anaerobic metabolism, acidosis, and significant cardiopulmonary stress, further worsening the abnormal physiology of hypothermia.[16] Below 34° C, progressive bradycardia and decrease in cardiac output and blood pressure take place. Below 28° C, 50% of patients show bradycardia with a 50% decrease in heart rate. Bradycardia is chiefly related to progressive decreased spontaneous depolarization of pacemaker cells. The conduction system is also affected, with prolongation initially noted in the PR interval, then QRS complex, then QT intervals.[21] Atropine is ineffective. The myocardium becomes irritable. As temperature falls lower than 32° C, atrial fibrillation is common, usually preceding ventricular fibrillation that may occur spontaneously when temperature falls below 28° C (82° F). Asystole usually occurs at temperatures less than 25° C.[22]

Respiratory Changes

Early in hypothermia (34-36° C) the respiratory drive is stimulated. The minute ventilation increases in response to increased oxygen consumption and CO_2 production. Below 33° C, respiratory depression takes place. Minute ventilation decreases. Depressed cough reflex and ciliary action coupled with increased production of mucus (bronchorrhea) increase the risk of atelectasis and aspiration. Noncardiogenic pulmonary edema has also been reported.[23,24]

Renal Changes

The initial response to hypothermia includes increased renal blood flow secondary to an increase in blood pressure and cardiac output, inducing diuresis. As hypothermia progresses below 32° C and cardiac output declines, renal blood flow and glomerular filtration rate decrease. This response sets the stage for acute renal failure but without affecting urinary output secondary to impaired renal tubular sodium reabsorption, a condition that maintains ongoing diuresis (cold diuresis). This response explains why hypothermia patients may present with profound intravascular volume depletion.[6,16,25]

Gastrointestinal Changes

Ileus, bowel wall edema, depressed hepatic detoxification, punctate gastric erosions, and rarely hemorrhagic pancreatitis are among the gastrointestinal manifestations of hypothermia.[16]

LABORATORY EVALUATION

Laboratory evaluations should be obtained to assess metabolic status and organ dysfunction. The following are common laboratory findings during hypothermia. They usually change with rewarming and require frequent monitoring.

ARTERIAL BLOOD GASES

As temperature decreases, the oxyhemoglobin dissociation curve shifts to the left. For every 1° C drop in temperature, pH increases by 0.015, Pao_2 decreases by 7.2%, and $Paco_2$ decreases by 4.4%. Because all arterial blood gas (ABG) samples are warmed to 37° C (98.6° F) when measured, the pH appears lower and the Pao_2 and $Paco_2$ appear higher than the patient's actual values. Most knowledge on acid-base status during hypothermia comes from cardiovascular surgery reports. Although most literature does not recommend correction of temperature to guide therapy, the use of corrected values should be strictly individualized.[26-28]

COMPLETE BLOOD COUNT

Hemoconcentration, an increase in hematocrit secondary to a decrease in plasma volume, is common (2% for each 1° C decrease in temperature). An initial low hemoglobin suggests acute hemorrhage or preexisting anemia. White blood cells (WBCs) may decrease; therefore, any history suggestive of infection should prompt treatment with antibiotics in high-risk groups such as the elderly, neonates, and the immunocompromised.[29]

COAGULATION FACTORS

Hypothermia induces inhibition of coagulation factors. It also induces thrombocytopenia secondary to bone marrow suppression and splenic and hepatic sequestration, as well as reduction in platelet adhesions and aggregation. Prolonged bleeding time and clotting times are common. Coagulation tests in the laboratory are performed under 37° C. If normal, they may not negate the presence of underlying hypothermia-induced coagulopathy. The key treatment in this condition is rewarming, not supplementation of coagulation factors.[30,31] Rewarming, however, increases the clotting response. Clinicians should use caution during this process, as patients are more susceptible to negative cardiovascular events.[4]

BLOOD UREA NITROGEN/CREATININE/ ELECTROLYTES

As mentioned earlier, acute renal failure with intravascular volume depletion and decreased renal perfusion is encountered. This is usually associated with higher levels of blood urea nitrogen (BUN) and creatinine (Cr) secondary to decreased clearance. Recurrent evaluation of electrolytes is essential during rewarming because no consistent pattern is present. Either hypo- or hyperkalemia may complicate the course of hypothermia and should be corrected promptly. Hypothermia masks the usual electrocardiogram (ECG) changes seen in normal hyperkalemia.[6,8,16]

BLOOD GLUCOSE

Hyperglycemia is initially noted as hypothermia inhibits insulin release and insulin uptake by membrane receptors at temperatures less than 30° C. It is further exacerbated by increased catecholamines. Insulin at these temperatures is ineffective. Exogenous insulin should be avoided, as it may cause rebound hypoglycemia during rewarming.[32]

OTHER LABORATORY ABNORMALITIES

Hyperamylasemia is common and may be related to a preexisting pancreatitis or pancreatitis induced by hypothermia. Hyperamylasemia correlates with the severity of hypothermia. Variable elevation in creatine phosphokinase levels may reflect underlying rhabdomyolysis.

ELECTROCARDIOGRAPHY CHANGES

All intervals—PR, QRS, and QT—are prolonged secondary to hypothermia-induced slowed impulse conduction through potassium channels. When body temperature decreases below 33° C (91.4° F), the J (Osborn) wave may be noted as a positive deflection in the left ventricular leads at the junction of the QRS complex and ST segment in 25% to 30% of patients. The presence of this wave is not pathognomonic and has no prognostic implication. The magnitude of the Osborn wave is associated with the degree of severity of hypothermia.[12,21]

MANAGEMENT (SEE FIG. 69.2)

The severity of hypothermia, clinical findings, and comorbid conditions of the patient are important factors for determining the aggressiveness of resuscitation techniques. Once hypothermia is confirmed, assessment and treatment of the critically ill patient should take place simultaneously. Some patients with hypothermia and cardiac arrest achieved an almost complete recovery despite prolonged resuscitation with a temperature as low as 13.7° C. Patients with moderate or severe hypothermia should be resuscitated until adequate rewarming is achieved before declaring efforts as unsuccessful.[33-35]

INITIAL STABILIZATION

Removal of wet clothing and moving the patient to a warm environment for protection against continued heat loss are essential. Rough movements of the patient's body during physical assessment should be avoided as it could precipitate serious cardiac arrhythmias. Continuous monitoring of cardiac status and core temperature should be established without delay. Similar to any emergency situation, airway, breathing, and circulation should be evaluated promptly in the hypothermic patient.

AIRWAY/BREATHING SUPPORT

Chest rigidity and decreased diaphragmatic movement impede adequate ventilation. Oxygenation may be insufficient secondary to underlying aspiration or pulmonary edema. Supplemental oxygen should be provided to alert patients with intact airway reflexes pending full assessment of oxygenation status. Hypothermic patients with apnea, deteriorating mental status, or loss of protective reflexes should undergo endotracheal intubation. The oropharyngeal route is preferred. Jaw maneuvering could be difficult in this category of patients secondary to muscle rigidity. Neuromuscular blocking agents do not have a role as they are ineffective at temperatures below 30° C. Intubation with a smaller endotracheal tube may be attempted. Intubation is unlikely to induce dysrhythmias in hypothermic patients.[8]

CARDIOCIRCULATORY SUPPORT

Volume Resuscitation

Most patients with moderate to severe hypothermia suffer from volume depletion. Continuous warmed intravenous fluids (40-42° C) should be administered. Peripheral large-gauge catheters are the preferred route of administration. The femoral vein is the preferred site if a central line is anticipated. Volume status should be monitored continuously during rewarming, as peripheral vasodilation and hypotension are likely to occur.[36]

Cardiac Resuscitation

Patients with moderate to severe hypothermia should undergo a thorough evaluation, looking for signs of cardiac output or peripheral blood flow. Echocardiography and Doppler ultrasound can be utilized for this purpose. Cardiopulmonary resuscitation should be performed immediately if no pulse or a nonperfusing rhythm (ventricular fibrillation or asystole) is established.[37-39]

Defibrillation. The hypothermic heart may be unresponsive to cardioactive drugs, attempted electric pacing, and defibrillation. Most arrhythmias other than ventricular fibrillation tend to convert spontaneously with rewarming. Sinus bradycardia does not require pacing or pharmacologic intervention. Ventricular fibrillation or tachycardia without a pulse requires initial defibrillation with maximum energy. If unsuccessful, rewarming is initiated. Defibrillation is reattempted after every 1° to 2° C increase in core temperature or when temperature rises above 30° to 32° C.[37-39]

Cardioactive Drugs. The antiarrhythmic and vasoactive drug efficacy in moderate to severe hypothermia is not well determined. It is mainly based on animal studies. Epinephrine and vasopressin may increase coronary perfusion but not survival. According to the American Heart Association 2010 guidelines, it may be reasonable to consider administration of a vasopressor during cardiac arrest according to the standard ACLS (advanced cardiac life support) algorithm concurrent with rewarming strategies. Isolated use of antiarrhythmics does not appear to be beneficial. In general, these drugs are withheld until rewarming achieves a temperature above 30° C, and then the lowest effective dose should be administered. Caution should be exercised not to administer these drugs repeatedly, as toxic accumulation can occur secondary to decreased metabolism. As normothermia is approached (above 35° C), standard drug protocols are used.[37-39]

ADDITIONAL SUPPORT

A nasogastric or orogastric tube should be placed in patients with moderate to severe hypothermia to relieve gastric distention. This tube also might help reduce vomiting and aspiration secondary to gastric dysmotility. A urinary catheter is also essential to monitor urine output and assess volume resuscitation efforts. Intra-arterial catheters for pressure monitoring should be used selectively. A Doppler ultrasound device may be necessary. Pulse oximetry is unlikely to be accurate given the poor perfusion to the extremities.

REWARMING METHODS

There are several methods of rewarming. Selection depends on the severity of hypothermia and the clinical condition of the patient. Controlled clinical studies and interventional studies are limited, and evidence-based protocols are lacking. Absence of a developed protocol led to the use of a wide variety of treatment strategies, depending on the expertise and previous exposure of the clinical teams and hospital resources.[40]

Passive External Rewarming

Passive external rewarming is the method of choice for hemodynamically stable patients with mild hypothermia (above 32° C), adequate physiologic reserve, and intact mechanism of shivering. Treatment includes placement of patients in a warm environment, removal of wet clothing, and application of insulating materials, such as blankets, to prevent heat loss. This method is expected to raise core temperature by 0.5° to 2.0° C per hour.[6] If unsuccessful, active rewarming is initiated.

Active Rewarming

Active External Rewarming. Active external rewarming (AER) is applied to patients with a core temperature between 86° and 92° F (30-34° C) without potential compromise of airway or hemodynamic status. It involves one or a combination of techniques, including warming blankets, heating pads, radiant energy, and forced heated air systems. Few complications (such as thermal injuries in the form of skin burns) have been reported using these methods. "After drop" is a phenomenon that was reported as a complication of AER. When the extremities and the trunk are warmed simultaneously, cold acidemic blood returns to the central circulation from the periphery secondary to vasodilation, causing a paradoxical decrease in core temperature. This drop worsens acidemia, precipitating hypotension and arrhythmias that can be fatal. Therefore, it is advised to apply rewarming strategies to the trunk before the extremities.[41,42]

Estimated rates of rewarming using this method ranges from 0.8° C with heating blankets up to 2.5° C per hour with the forced air rewarming systems. This forced air system is the most widely used by clinicians because it is easy and effective.[41,42]

Active Internal Rewarming. Active internal rewarming (AIR) is used for patients with moderate to severe hypothermia (under 86° F or 30° C) with adequate hemodynamics, in conjunction with AER.[43] Methods include administration of warmed intravenous fluids (40-42° C) and warmed humidified air (40-45° C) through a mask or endotracheal tube. Intravenous fluids alone are not adequate but prevent further heat loss. It is estimated that an average 1 L crystalloid (40-42° C) for a 70-kg person will increase the temperature by 0.3°. Rewarming by heated oxygen by endotracheal tube is more effective than a facemask. A total rate of 1° to 2.5° C per hour is anticipated by this method.[15,43,44] Gastric bladder and colonic irrigation are of limited value secondary to their small surface area.

Peritoneal and Pleural Lavage

If rewarming is inadequate, more aggressive methods include peritoneal and pleural lavage. In pleural irrigation, two large-bore (36F or greater) thoracotomy tubes are used. One tube is placed at the midclavicular line and is connected to saline at 42° C (107.2° F). The other tube is placed at the posterior axillary line and is connected to a chest tube drainage.[45]

Peritoneal lavage and dialysis are achieved by placement of a peritoneal catheter (8F) into the peritoneum and infusing 10 to 20 mL/kg of warmed 42° C isotonic fluid. The fluid is kept in the peritoneal cavity before it is removed.[15]

Extracorporeal Methods of Rewarming

This approach is the most effective method in raising core body temperature.

Hemodialysis. Hemodialysis is appropriate for patients with severe hypothermia and accompanying hyperkalemia and renal failure. The benefit is that hemodialysis is widely available and practical. It is portable and efficient. The rewarming rate ranges between 2° and 4° C per hour, but it requires the absence of circulatory collapse.[46]

Continuous Arteriovenous Rewarming. Continuous arteriovenous rewarming (CAVR) has the ability to maintain circulation, correct hypoxia, and replenish intravascular volume without the need for systemic anticoagulation. The rate of rewarming ranges between 3° and 4° C per hour and requires a systolic blood pressure of at least 60 mm Hg to be performed.

Continuous Venovenous Hemofiltration. Continuous venovenous hemofiltration (CVVH) has also been reported to achieve successful rewarming. It is widely available, can be performed with lower blood pressure, but provides slow rewarming rates (1-3° C per hour). It does not provide full circulatory support, and volume resuscitation is necessary when cardiac output is inadequate. Chest compressions and ventilation must be continued until the return of spontaneous circulation. However, it may prove to be an alternative to CAVR when limited by profound hypotension.

Cardiopulmonary Bypass. Cardiopulmonary bypass (CPB) is the standard of care for patients with severe hypothermia, apnea, and cardiac arrest or hemodynamic instability. It provides rapid rewarming rates (8-12° C per hour) while maintaining oxygenation, circulation, and rapid correction of metabolic derangements. However, the need for CPB in hypothermic trauma patients may be limited secondary to the need for systemic anticoagulation. In addition, the expert teams required for CPB make the implementation somewhat challenging.[6,15,38] Portable CPB systems are available.

Extracorporeal Membrane Oxygenation. There is a growing body of evidence that extracorporeal membrane oxygenation (ECMO) could be more preferable to CPB. It has the same rate of rewarming (8-12° C per hour).[38] In patients undergoing rewarming, ECMO may reduce the risk of multiorgan failure secondary to reperfusion. It can be continued for several days and needs less anticoagulation.

Endovascular Temperature Control Device. Endovascular temperature control device has been reported in recent years as another tool for rewarming in patients with severe hypothermia. It is generally placed in the emergency department in cool comatose survivors of cardiac arrest. It can also be used to warm patients with accidental hypothermia. Because the same device is used in both sets of patients, the operation of the equipment is familiar to both the emergency department and ICU staff. The only procedure required to place this device is a central venous catheter, which is less invasive than CPB or pleural lavage.

PROGNOSIS

Different reports on the outcome of moderate to severe hypothermic patients have been variable. Multiple confounding factors exist that make it difficult to predict survival. Older age, lower core body temperature, indoor exposure, submersion, trauma, toxin ingestion, prehospital hemodynamic status, BUN and potassium levels, the need for intubation, and presence or absence of asphyxiation are significant predictors of outcome. For patients undergoing CPB for hypothermia and hemodynamic instability, favorable factors for survival are associated with younger age, higher arterial pH, lower Pa_{CO_2}, lower serum potassium levels, and the absence of asphyxia and suffocation.[18] Many patients die even after achieving adequate rewarming secondary to multiorgan failure. Knowing its detrimental outcome, an important approach should pursue prevention. In general, hypothermia is a preventable condition. Public health education and preparedness should be directed toward populations at risk.

HYPERTHERMIA

HISTORY AND INCIDENCE

Innumerable military campaigns throughout history were lost as a result of heat illness, long before the enemy ever raised a weapon. In modern times, the Israeli Six-Day War during the late 1960s provides the best example of the ravages of heat illness. The Israeli army had forced water consumption policies, by the clock, including strict disciplinary measures for evidence of heat injury due to negligence. By contrast, the Egyptian army did not have well-enforced policies. In the end, the Israeli army's heat injury statistics were negligible, but more than 50% of the Egyptian soldiers in the same locale suffered from heat illnesses that rendered them unable to effectively perform their expected tasks.

Heatstroke and hyperthermia have been identified as the environmental diseases least frequently monitored by epidemiology systems in the United States. Serious heat illness has received considerable recent attention owing to catastrophic heat waves in the United States and Europe, the deaths of high-profile athletes, and military deployments. The exact incidence of heatstroke in the United States is unknown. The CDC reported that between the years 1987 and 1988, 1092 death certificates listed excessive heat as either a primary or a secondary cause.[47] It is suspected that a number of other heat-related severe illnesses and deaths occur each year that are attributed to other causes. Guidelines from the National Association of Medical Examiners suggest that in cases in which the measured antemortem body temperature at the time of collapse was 105° F (40.6° C) or higher, the cause of death should be certified as heatstroke or hyperthermia. Deaths also may be certified as heatstroke or hyperthermia with lower body temperatures when cooling has been attempted before arrival at the hospital or when the clinical history includes mental status changes and elevated liver and muscle enzymes.[48]

PATHOGENESIS

Heatstroke is a complex syndrome of end-organ dysfunction initiated by hyperthermia that occurs when heat accumulation in the body overwhelms heat-dissipating mechanisms. The diagnosis of heatstroke should be considered in patients with core body temperatures greater than 41° C, or in patients with a core temperature of 40.6° C and concomitant mental status changes. Because anhidrosis is a late finding and sweating may be observed in severely hyperthermic patients, diaphoresis should not be considered a discriminatory finding. Heatstroke traditionally is subdivided into exertional and nonexertional causes. Box 69.1 outlines examples of diseases and conditions within each of these categories. To understand the pathogenesis of heatstroke, the systemic and cellular responses to heat stress must be appreciated. These responses include thermoregulation (with acclimatization), an acute-phase response, and a response that involves the production of heat shock proteins.

THERMOREGULATION

At basal metabolic levels, less than 100 kcal of metabolic heat is generated per hour. However, when physical activity increases, heat production may rise as high as 900 kcal/hour. This level of heat production is capable of raising the core body temperature by 1° C every 5 to 8 minutes. Heat is dissipated via evaporation, conduction or radiation, and convectional losses. Cutaneous vasodilation results in heat loss through all of these physical mechanisms except evaporation. Unfortunately, when the ambient temperature exceeds body temperature, only evaporative losses associated with perspiration actually dissipate heat. Perspiration can produce a maximum rate of heat loss of approximately 400 to 650 kcal/hour in acclimatized persons. When heat production exceeds this threshold, body temperature quickly begins to rise.

Box 69.1 Conditions and Diseases Associated with Heatstroke

Exertional Causes

Environmental: high ambient temperatures/humidity
Physiologic: lack of physical conditioning, inadequate acclimatization, or overexertion

Nonexertional Causes

Environmental: high ambient temperatures/humidity, lack of air conditioning, lack of shrubbery/trees around dwelling, height of home above ground level
Physiologic: age older than 65 years, alcoholism, congestive heart failure, renal failure, diabetes mellitus, chronic obstructive pulmonary disease, dementia, schizophrenia, cystic fibrosis, thyrotoxicosis, hypokalemia, dehydration
Drugs: alcohol, antidopaminergics, anticholinergics, amphetamines, beta blockers, butyrophenones, cocaine, diuretics, hallucinogens, tricyclic antidepressants

ACCLIMATIZATION

Acclimatization is a physiologic term that collectively describes various adaptive responses to repeated heat stress. Many of these responses are directed at conserving plasma volume. They include decreased total sweat sodium concentration and nonreflexively increased aldosterone secretion. In addition, acclimatized people tend to drink greater volumes of water and have measurable increases in extracellular fluid volume beyond that of nonacclimatized persons. Ultimately, maximum cardiac output and stroke volume increase, while maximum heart rate and O_2 consumption decrease (improved efficiency per unit of metabolic work expended).[49] Similarly, the net amount of heat generated per unit of work expended also decreases.

ACUTE-PHASE RESPONSE

The acute-phase response, involving endothelial cells, leukocytes, and epithelial cells, protects body tissues from heat-induced tissue injury. A variety of immunomodulatory and inflammatory cytokines are released in response to increased endogenous or environmental heat, including interleukin 6 (IL-6), tumor necrosis factor-α (TNF-α), IL-10, IL-12, and interferon.

HEAT SHOCK RESPONSE

Cells respond to heat by production of inducible heat shock proteins that help induce a state of tolerance to heat stress. These proteins function as molecular chaperones that bind to partially folded or misfolded proteins and thereby prevent their irreversible denaturation. Heat shock proteins also may help regulate the baroreceptor reflex response during heat stress, abating hypotension and bradycardia.

PREDISPOSING FACTORS

The epidemiology of heatstroke parallels that of hypothermia—nonexertional heatstroke is seen in elderly, alcoholic, or otherwise debilitated patients in urban areas. By contrast, exertional heatstroke develops in otherwise healthy people who overexert themselves in exceedingly hot or humid conditions. Like hypothermia, heatstroke most often develops in patients with impaired thermoregulation. Antidopaminergic drugs, alcohol, and primary central nervous system (CNS) disorders are common denominators in many patients.[49] A number of environmental and socioeconomic conditions have been associated in recent years with heatstroke.[50,51] A lack of air conditioning and a lack of trees or shrubbery around homes are commonly observed in patients presenting with heatstroke. People who are apartment bound, particularly those on higher floors, also appear to be at higher risk during summer heat waves. Finally, elderly patients not only have diminished temperature perception but also do not produce the same volume of sweat, placing them at higher risk for the development of heatstroke.

Many drugs, "recreational" and prescription, are associated with an increased risk of hyperthermia and deserve further emphasis. Cocaine causes generalized sympathetic activation and loss of response to environmental cues. It is rapidly becoming a leading cause of heatstroke in many urban emergency departments. Beta blockers, on the other hand, have been implicated in heatstroke through a drug-mediated direct decrease in sweat gland production. Diuretics decrease baseline circulating plasma volume, leading to decreased sweat production. Hypokalemia decreases sweat gland output as well, and barbiturates can even cause sweat gland necrosis. When a heat wave arrives in an urban area, any one or several of the foregoing factors combined can lead to outbreaks of heat injury.

PRESENTATION AND CLINICAL MANIFESTATIONS

Nonexertional heatstroke may manifest insidiously.[52] An urban setting and the recognized presence of a heat wave may be the best available diagnostic clues. Some form of CNS dysfunction is nearly universal in patients with nonexertional heatstroke. The spectrum of dysfunction ranges from increased irritability and confusion to stupor and coma. Hyperpyrexia often is the most specific physical finding. In many cases, the presentation of an elderly patient with an altered mental status, irritability, and a high fever suggests sepsis. However, epidemiologic associations, concurrent debilitating disease, and the impact of medications that limit thermoregulation should be considered before limiting therapy to empiric antibiotics and antipyretic medications.

Exertional heatstroke typically occurs more suddenly and with a more self-evident clinical history.[53] Severe dehydration, anhidrosis, and extreme hyperpyrexia are common in external heatstroke. Affected persons appear hyperdynamic, with tachycardia, increased cardiac output, and peripheral arterial vasodilation. CNS dysfunction is somewhat less common in this patient subset. Initially, thermoregulation is intact in patients with exertional hyperthermia. At high core body temperatures, however, metabolic activity overwhelms normal heat dissipation mechanisms, and clear-cut disruption of normal thermoregulation may then appear. Hyperthermia is further accelerated by the loss of effective sweating for evaporative heat dissipation. Myocardial dysfunction with depression of left ventricular ejection fraction also has been described after heatstroke, which resolves with treatment.[54]

In addition to alterations of consciousness, hallucinations, focal neurologic deficits, various cranial nerve abnormalities, and opisthotonos are well described. Seizures occur in greater than half of these patients and may be related strictly to core body temperature or to concomitant disorders of free water-electrolyte balance. Decerebrate posturing also is rarely observed in some patients without other known mechanisms of acute brain injury. Many patients may suffer residual defects such as dementia, personality changes, focal deficits, cerebellar changes, or pyramidal findings. Nevertheless, many patients also proceed to complete recovery, suggesting that early findings should not deter acute management.[51]

DIAGNOSTIC APPROACH

In addition to CNS dysfunction, rhabdomyolysis is a frequent feature of exertional hyperthermia. Manifestations sometimes include tender, edematous muscles and "cola-colored" urine, but the condition more commonly is defined by elevation in total creatine kinase (CK), serum aldolase, uric acid, or serum potassium (alone or in combination). Hyperkalemia in this situation may be life-threatening.

Acute renal failure occurs in up to one third of patients with heatstroke.[55] It is considerably more common in patients in whom rhabdomyolysis is a feature (i.e., with myoglobinuria or urate nephropathy). However, direct heat injury and renal hypoperfusion also may contribute. Acute tubular necrosis in heatstroke typically manifests with oliguria, non-nephrotic range proteinuria, and abundant granular cast formation.

Evidence of hepatocellular injury is present to some degree in essentially all patients with heatstroke and is attributed principally to a direct toxic effect of hyperthermia on hepatocytes.[56] Elevation of serum transaminases is a cardinal feature of this toxicity and often is observed within 30 minutes of syndrome onset. So prevalent is this finding that the absence of transaminitis should cast serious doubt on the diagnosis of heatstroke. Histologic changes including centrilobular necrosis have been observed within 24 hours of heat injury and evolve over the ensuing days. Transaminase and lactate dehydrogenase levels typically peak on the third or fourth hospital day, and depending upon the extent of injury, these changes may be accompanied by increased alkaline phosphatase levels, hyperbilirubinemia, and a prolonged prothrombin time. Overall, fulminant hepatic necrosis is rare; however, hepatic insufficiency contributes to late morbidity and death in patients who survive the initial resuscitation.[57] Prolongation of coagulation times also may be due to disseminated intravascular coagulation (DIC). Although DIC also is rare, it is a marker of poor prognosis when present. Clinical manifestations of DIC range from isolated laboratory abnormalities to generalized bleeding. In patients with heatstroke, DIC may exacerbate hepatic injury and is associated with the development of acute respiratory distress syndrome (ARDS). In fact, the codevelopment of DIC and ARDS in patients with heatstroke is predictive of a high mortality rate (>75%). Qualitative coagulation function (including platelet function) also may be impaired by heat injury. The clinical effects of these impairments are variable.

A range of electrolyte abnormalities related to renal failure and dehydration in heatstroke victims has been well described and includes hyponatremia, hypocalcemia, hypokalemia (hyperkalemia in patients with acute tubular necrosis or rhabdomyolysis), hypophosphatemia, and hypomagnesemia. Of these, hyponatremia and free water excess may produce severe neurologic effects including central pontine myelinolysis (CPM). CPM has been reported in patients with heatstroke who receive aggressive prehospital resuscitation with hypotonic solutions. Serum osmolality should be carefully monitored during volume resuscitation, and intravenous solutions should be modified accordingly. Severe lactic acidosis is especially common in patients with exertional heat injury.[58] Finally, arterial blood gas results are influenced by temperature in a fashion opposite that described with hypothermia (Box 69.2).

APPROACH TO MANAGEMENT

Duration of extreme hyperpyrexia is the single most important determinant of morbidity and fatality in all patients with heatstroke (both exertional and nonexertional). Therefore, expeditious cooling should be initiated

Box 69.2 Temperature Correction Factors for Arterial Blood Gas (ABG) Specimens*

ABG Component Correction Factor

pH + 0.015 (37 − T_c)
PaO_2 − 0.072 (37 − T_c) × PaO_2
$PaCO_2$ − 0.044 (37 − T_c) × $PaCO_2$

Example

A patient presents with a core temperature of 32° C with the following ABG values: pH = 7.12, $PaCO_2$ = 52 mm Hg, and PaO_2 = 52 mm Hg. Corrections for temperature are as follows:

pH = 7.12 + [0.015 (37 − 32)] = 7.195
PaO_2 = 52 − [0.072 (37 − 32) × 52] = 33.28 mm Hg
$PaCO_2$ = 52 − [0.044 (37 − 32) × 52] = 40.56 mm Hg

These corrections also may be used for hyperthermia.

*ABG values not corrected for temperature in significantly hypothermic patients yield falsely low pH and falsely elevated $PaCO_2$ and PaO_2 values.
T_c, core temperature.

simultaneously with other basic and advanced life support modalities. Indeed, a review of outcome data for heatstroke victims during the Chicago heat wave of 1995 suggested that computed tomography imaging of the brain contributed little to patient management and simply delayed efforts to rapidly cool the patient.[59] General supportive measures and specific measures for cooling the patient are discussed next.

SUPPORTIVE MEASURES

Intravascular volume restoration must be individualized. In general, patients with exertional hypothermia are severely hypovolemic. Hemodynamic monitoring has demonstrated that patients may manifest two distinct responses to heatstroke: (1) a hyperdynamic response with an elevated cardiac index (CI) and depressed systemic vascular resistance (SVR) and (2) a hypodynamic response with depressed CI and elevated SVR.[55] Although the hypodynamic response may be more common in older patients with preexisting medical problems and classic heatstroke, severe hyperthermia can lead to myocardial dysfunction even in young, healthy adults without preexisting cardiac disease. Overzealous volume resuscitation in this setting can produce significant pulmonary congestion. The rapid restoration of an adequate perfusion pressure without pressor support is a reasonable goal, and if this is achieved, further volume resuscitation should proceed at a more measured pace. Pulmonary artery catheterization is recommended early in the clinical course for patients with unclear cardiovascular physiology. Finally, isoproterenol traditionally has been considered the inotrope of choice for patients with severely depressed myocardial performance. Its lack of α-activity ensures that heat dissipation is not impeded. Dobutamine may be a more rational choice, however, because it has considerably fewer myocardial irritant and arrhythmogenic properties.

Seizures are treated according to standard guidelines. Benzodiazepines are used for acute, ongoing convulsive activity. Dilantin is useful for added control or prophylaxis; however, hypotension with rapid intravenous infusion should be anticipated. Barbiturates also are effective antiseizure drugs but should be reserved as second-line therapeutic agents because of their theoretical impediment to sweat formation and heat dissipation.

Acute renal failure should be approached aggressively in patients with rhabdomyolysis. Intravascular volume repletion should be promptly accomplished, with continued infusion of volume to produce forced diuresis. Mannitol or loop diuretics may be of value to maintain appropriate urine output. Hyperkalemia management may be challenging. The clinician should not hesitate to administer glucose, insulin, and calcium in patients with ECG changes. Subsequent sodium polystyrene sulfonate (Kayexalate) dosing may also be required.

COOLING MEASURES

Effective heat dissipation depends on the rapid transfer of heat from the core to the skin and from the skin to the external environment. In persons with hyperthermia, transfer of heat from the core to the skin is facilitated by active cutaneous vasodilation. Therapeutic cooling techniques are therefore aimed at accelerating the transfer of heat from the skin to the environment without compromising the flow of blood to the skin, which can be accomplished by increasing the temperature gradient between the skin and the environment (for cooling by conduction) or by increasing the gradient of water vapor pressure between the skin and the environment (for cooling by evaporation), as well as by increasing the velocity of air adjacent to the skin (for cooling by convection).

Core body temperature should be rapidly cooled to a goal of 38° to 39° C. The most effective approaches to lowering the core temperature are immersion and evaporative methods. Of these, efficacy data related to ice-water immersion modalities historically have been better defined, with observed cooling rates of up to 0.13° C per minute. Similar efficacy has been noted with cool-water immersion as well, which should be less uncomfortable for both patient and staff members. Unfortunately, water immersion is not practical for many critically ill patients. Monitoring and treatment for arrhythmias, seizures, and other sequelae are problematic while the patient is immersed in a tub.

Evaporative techniques are quite effective and allow the ICU patient to be placed on a bed or other supportive surface and treated accordingly. The patient is repeatedly wetted with tepid water (not alcohol) or sprayed with water mist while warm air from a fan is blown across the body surface. Evaporative cooling by this method has shown a faster cooling rate in a canine model that is as effective as aggressive peritoneal lavage cooling, reaching rates as high as 0.32° C per minute.[60] An aggressive approach to cooling the heatstroke victim, whatever the approach, is most important. Other adjuncts to cooling include rectal, intraperitoneal, and gastric lavage with iced saline. These techniques are effective at rapidly lowering core temperature but are cumbersome and generally unnecessary and may lead to unwanted iatrogenesis.

Efforts to cool a patient should be discontinued when the core temperature falls to 38° to 39° C. At that point, a continued fall by 1° or 2° C is expected. Dantrolene sodium has been used in some patients but was found to be ineffective in a double-blinded randomized study.[61,62] Chlorpromazine may be useful in patients in whom shivering develops during active cooling efforts; however, if neuroleptic malignant syndrome (NMS) is in the differential diagnosis (and it often is), meperidine may be a better option than an antidopaminergic agent in patients with normal renal function.

SPECIFIC HYPERTHERMIC SYNDROMES

Malignant hyperthermia (MH) and NMS deserve special emphasis because of their potentially catastrophic impact on critically ill patients, particularly when they are not promptly recognized. MH is associated with use of certain anesthetic agents and can lead to profound skeletal muscle contraction and the subsequent development of life-threatening hyperthermia and other complications. NMS is caused by a variety of antipsychotic drugs and also leads to sustained muscular contraction and hyperthermia.

MALIGNANT HYPERTHERMIA

MH develops in approximately 1 of 15,000 patients who undergo surgical procedures requiring general anesthesia. The vast majority of cases are associated with either halothane or succinylcholine use; however, a variety of other drugs also have been implicated. Box 69.3 outlines these agents by type. Unlike in heatstroke, endogenous heat production is solely responsible for the observed hyperpyrexia. MH constitutes a true medical emergency because of the rapid tempo at which severe sequelae evolve. Better recognition of this syndrome and modern treatment techniques, however, have reduced mortality rates from 70% to approximately 10% in recent years.

Box 69.3 Anesthetics Associated with the Development of Malignant Hyperthermia and Neuroleptic Malignant Syndrome

Malignant Hyperthermia

Volatile Anesthetics

Cyclopropane, diethyl ether, enflurane, ethylene, halothane, isoflurane, methoxyflurane, sevoflurane

Muscle Relaxants

Succinylcholine, decamethonium

Neuroleptic Malignant Syndrome

Phenothiazines

Fluphenazine, chlorpromazine, levomepromazine, thioridazine, trimeprazine, trifluoroperazine, prochlorperazine

Butyrophenones

Haloperidol, bromoperidol, droperidol

Dibenzoxepine

Loxapine

Dopamine-Depleting Drugs

Alpha-methyltyrosine, tetrabenzamine

Dopaminergic Agent Withdrawal

Levodopa-carbidopa, amantadine

PATHOGENESIS

MH results from a rapid, sustained increase in myoplasmic Ca^{2+} levels in response to halogenated anesthetics and depolarizing neuromuscular blocking agents. Susceptibility to MH results from mutations in calcium channel proteins that mediate excitation-contraction coupling, with the ryanodine receptor calcium release channel (RyR1) representing the major locus. The mode of inheritance appears to be autosomal dominant, with variable penetrance. The phenomenon occurs in persons who have a mutation in the ryanodine type 1 receptor, resulting in a defective protein in the skeletal muscle sarcoplasmic reticulum membrane.[63] The uncontrolled rise in the myoplasmic Ca^{2+} concentration disables the troponin inhibition of actin and myosin, resulting in uncontrolled muscle tetany. This surge in muscle metabolic activity causes thermogenesis to increase exponentially and is rapidly followed by total body rigidity and extreme hyperpyrexia.

Numerous familial myopathies (such as Evans myopathy, King-Denborough syndrome, and central core disease) have been associated with the reaction.[64,65] Curiously, this genetic predisposition does not translate into the predictable development of MH. That is, an initial challenge with an anesthetic drug that leads to MH does not consistently predict whether or not MH will occur with future exposures to the same drug. Measured contraction in caffeine or halothane preparations of muscle biopsy specimens is the most reliable predictor of risk for MH.

PRESENTATION

MH is characterized by the triad of (1) severe hyperthermia, (2) muscle rigidity, and (3) metabolic acidosis. MH usually is an acute and rapidly progressive process; however, many reports suggest that the syndrome may vary considerably in severity and rate of progression. In the anesthesia setting, capnography may provide the earliest clue of impending MH, as end-tidal CO_2 rises in response to the increased metabolic rate. Clinical harbingers of impending MH include masseter muscle rigidity or trismus and tachycardia, which is reported to occur in greater than 95% of patients.[64] Cyanosis, increased blood pressure, and increased respiratory rate all may be observed with the onset of the reaction as the hypermetabolic response is triggered.

Muscle rigidity may explosively progress from localized masseter contraction to diffuse rigidity of skeletal muscle groups. When uninterrupted, this process will lead to progressive, severe hyperthermia. Extreme hyperpyrexia is considered a late finding in MH. Mortality risk has been related to peak core body temperature, reflecting both MH severity and delayed recognition. With progressing rigidity, a mixed metabolic and respiratory acidosis may occur, along with a variety of other electrolyte abnormalities, including hyperkalemia, hypercalcemia, and hypermagnesemia. Severe chest wall rigidity may even prevent adequate mechanical ventilation, leading to life-threatening hypoxemia and hypoventilation. Rhabdomyolysis is reflected in elevated CK levels, usually greater than 1500 U/L and often greater than 10,000 U/L. Myoglobinuria may produce acute tubular necrosis with oliguric renal failure and severe DIC. High fever may result in myocardial dysfunction, pulmonary edema, and cerebral edema.

DIAGNOSIS

Susceptibility to MH can be identified unequivocally only by an in vitro muscle test. Fascicles of muscle obtained from the thigh by biopsy are exposed to halothane and separately to increasing concentrations of caffeine in vitro. The muscle contractures are increased in persons who are susceptible to MH. This test is now widely used to identify susceptibility to MH in patients who have had a reaction to inhaled halogenated anesthetics or suxamethonium that is suggestive of MH. If the test results in the propositus are positive, testing can be offered to first-degree relatives for genetic counseling. Patients whose biopsied muscle demonstrates a contracture to 3% halothane of 0.5 g or more and a contracture to 2 mmol/L caffeine of 0.2 g or more are considered to be susceptible to MH.[66] An in vitro contracture test is the gold standard for diagnosing susceptibility to MH. Two different protocols are used. European laboratories use the protocol devised by Ellis in Leeds with incremental doses of halothane up to 2% and incremental doses of caffeine. In the United States, a single dose of 3% halothane and incremental doses of caffeine are used. The two protocols give essentially the same results.[67]

TREATMENT

By far, the most important measure for MH is the immediate cessation of any suspected triggering agents. If anesthesia must be maintained, nontriggering agents should be used. Agents considered safe in MH include barbiturates, narcotics, benzodiazepines, and propofol, to name only a few. Nondepolarizing neuromuscular blockers such as vecuronium or atracurium, although also considered safe in these patients, will do nothing to abort the MH reaction because the primary disease resides within the skeletal muscle cell itself—beyond the neuromuscular junction.

In addition to discontinuing offending agents, sodium dantrolene should be administered. Sodium dantrolene initially was tested as an antimicrobial; however, dantrolene was found to produce muscle weakness by blocking the Ca^{2+} efflux from the sarcoplasmic reticulum. The agent is capable of reversing the MH reaction by lowering myoplasmic Ca^{2+} concentrations. The onset of action usually is within 2 to 3 minutes, with initial responses including muscle relaxation, decreasing heart rate, and decreasing core body temperature. Muscle weakness may follow drug administration, but this should never limit proper therapy. After the initial response, dantrolene may be dosed orally for 24 to 48 hours. Late recurrences of MH have been reported if inadequate dantrolene dosing occurs. Intravenous preparations of dantrolene contain significant amounts of mannitol, which may produce a subsequent osmotic diuresis. Although this reaction may be desirable in patients with rhabdomyolysis, volume and electrolyte management should take this effect into account.

Systemic cooling may be best achieved in these complex patients with evaporative techniques, cooling blankets, cold saline infusion, or ice packs. Because of its similar actions on myoplasmic Ca^{2+} concentration, procainamide was the drug of choice for this syndrome before the advent of dantrolene therapy. Cardiac dysrhythmias not responding to electrolyte correction may be safely treated with procainamide or lidocaine. Numerous reports suggest that intravenous calcium may be safely infused for toxic hyperkalemia. Diltiazem and verapamil may interact with dantrolene to produce hyperkalemia; therefore, these agents should be avoided. Although the effects of MH on cardiac muscle remain unclear, some authors advocate that cardiac glycosides also should be avoided because they increase intracellular Ca^{2+} concentration.

NEUROLEPTIC MALIGNANT SYNDROME

NMS is an idiosyncratic reaction to neuroleptic drugs and other antidopaminergic agents. A number of drugs that are known to be associated with NMS are listed in Box 69.3. NMS is characterized by muscle rigidity and altered mental status, followed by autonomic instability and hyperthermia. However, temperature elevations generally are less extreme than in MH and are not as life-threatening.

NMS is reported to occur in up to 2% to 3% of all patients receiving neuroleptic medications. The reaction typically develops within a few days of initiating therapy and almost always appears within the first 30 days. Curiously, NMS also occurs rarely in some patients after many years on a stable dosing regimen. Of importance, NMS also can occur in response to the withdrawal of central dopaminergic agonists such as bromocriptine or levodopa-carbidopa.

PATHOPHYSIOLOGY

Some investigators suspect that the genetic predisposition to MH also defines patients at risk for NMS, but most work has failed to demonstrate a relationship between NMS and altered sarcolemmal membrane calcium permeability. Unlike in MH, patients with NMS appear to have both increased heat production and impaired central thermoregulation, compromising heat dissipation. In these patients, a decrease in central dopaminergic tone also results in extrapyramidal signs of skeletal muscle rigidity and tremor and may account for alterations in mental status due to effects in the mesolimbic system and mesocortical pathways.[68] Finally, even though altered central thermoregulation may contribute to hyperthermia in NMS, rapid resolution of fever after administration of neuromuscular relaxing agents or dantrolene suggests that hyperthermia is due primarily to increased heat generation by skeletal muscle rigidity.

PRESENTATION

NMS should be considered when fever, muscular rigidity, catatonia, or dystonia occur in the setting of neuroleptic drug administration. Recent reviews have suggested the following criteria for the diagnosis of NMS: treatment with neuroleptics within 7 days; hyperthermia with core temperatures greater than 38° C; muscle rigidity; exclusion of other systemic or drug-related illness; and any five of the following: altered mental status, tachycardia, hypertension or hypotension, tachypnea or hypoxia, diaphoresis or sialorrhea, tremor, incontinence, CK elevation or myoglobinuria, leukocytosis, or metabolic acidosis.[68,69]

Altered mental status commonly precedes the onset of other symptoms and may manifest as confusion or agitation. More severe cases may progress to obtundation or coma, or may manifest as a mute catatonia that is difficult to differentiate from lethal catatonia. Muscle rigidity typically involves the neck, shoulders, and limbs but may compromise ventilation if chest wall involvement is severe. Other neuromuscular findings are diverse and may include dysarthria, dyskinesias, ataxia, or tremors.

Autonomic findings typically include diaphoresis, hypertension, and tachycardia. However, hypotension may develop in some patients. Fever is a late finding and usually occurs in the range of 38° to 42° C. When fever exceeds 42° C, it may cause end-organ damage like that seen in other hyperthermia syndromes.

Rhabdomyolysis occurs often, though it usually is of a milder caliber than that observed in MH or exertional heatstroke. Elevations in serum transaminases, BUN, and serum Cr often are seen, as well as a leukocytosis.

TREATMENT

When NMS is suspected, the offending drug should be discontinued immediately and supportive measures initiated. Volume resuscitation, physical measures for cooling, and monitoring of cardiopulmonary and renal parameters should be instituted immediately. Pharmacologic options for the treatment of NMS are more numerous than for other hyperthermia syndromes, because they may be directed toward restoring central dopaminergic tone or reducing peripheral rigidity until the neuroleptic effects subside.

Dopamine agonists such as bromocriptine, amantadine, and levodopa-carbidopa have been successfully employed in NMS.[68,70] These agents act to directly increase central dopaminergic tone, thereby antagonizing the various effects of neuroleptic dopamine blockade. Regimens include bromocriptine or amantidine for up to 10 days before tapering, If a levodopa-carbidopa combination is used, it should be dosed four times a day owing to its shorter half-life. Some authors advocate avoiding central dopamine agonists if the diagnosis is unclear or if psychosis remains in the differential diagnosis, to avoid acutely exacerbating the psychotic state or contributing to a lethal catatonia.

Sodium dantrolene has been successfully used in numerous small series. The muscle relaxation that occurs helps to reduce temperature and decrease the sequelae of prolonged rigidity. Neuromuscular blockers also are effective at decreasing skeletal muscle tone, and in patients with high fever and autonomic instability, these agents offer a rapid means of establishing therapeutic effects. Combinations of central dopamine agonists and peripheral-acting agents have not as yet demonstrated a significant advantage over either treatment alone. Electroconvulsive therapy (ECT) has been used in a number of reports, but its advantages over supportive care alone have not been adequately assessed.[70] Furthermore, the need for anesthesia presents an additional hazard that may complicate management in these patients.

Airway-protective reflexes should be vigilantly assessed because dystonia and impaired bulbar functions increase the risk of gastric aspiration in patients with NMS. Morbidity and mortality risks in these cases often arise from pulmonary complications such as aspiration, pneumonia, ARDS, or pulmonary embolism. Cardiac complications such as arrhythmias or myocardial infarction in more fulminant cases also contribute to fatality in these patients. As in all of the hyperthermia syndromes, worsening rhabdomyolysis and acute renal failure have been identified as signs of poor prognosis.

RHABDOMYOLYSIS

Rhabdomyolysis is a pathologic state in which the necrosis of muscle cells, through trauma, toxins, medications, or other causes, leads to an excess of intracellular solutes in the extracellular compartments. Target organ damage can range from minimal to severe depending on the degree of necrosis; the main consequences are metabolic abnormalities and acute kidney injury (AKI). Our understanding of the pathophysiology of rhabdomyolysis has evolved with an emphasis on early diagnosis and treatment, often in the setting of major catastrophes. The first report in the English literature, describing four cases of crush injury in Britain during World War II, was recently republished.[71]

EPIDEMIOLOGY

The incidence of rhabdomyolysis is dependent on the population undergoing analysis and the diagnostic criteria being used. It is recognized as a major cause of fatality following severe musculoskeletal injury from trauma.[72] Following the 1999 Marmara earthquake in northwestern Turkey, 8.9% of hospitalized patients required renal replacement therapy for crush-related injuries.[73] Recently, a particular focus has been the ability of the HMG-CoA reductase (3-hydroxy-3-methyl-glutaryl-CoA reductase) inhibitor class of medications to cause rhabdomyolysis. Though likely a class phenomenon and rare overall, the incidence of rhabdomyolysis is not equivalent for all medications and is increased with the addition of other specific agents, in particular gemfibrozil, other fibrates, or cyclosporine.[74,75] Additional causes of rhabdomyolysis are listed in Box 69.4.[76-81] A recent review noted exogenous toxins, both prescribed and illicit, to be responsible for nearly 50% of cases.[82]

Two additional scenarios that have received significant attention include "propofol infusion syndrome" and the potential for patients with sickle cell trait (SCT) to develop rhabdomyolysis. Both of these situations occur in younger patients. Propofol is rarely associated with a syndrome of metabolic acidosis and rhabdomyolysis. Risk factors include high-dose infusions over a prolonged period and a young age.[83-86] SCT with subsequent rhabdomyolysis due to exertional sickling is now recognized as a cause for sudden deaths in young patients during strenuous workouts, in particular, football.[87-93]

Box 69.4 Causes of Rhabdomyolysis*

Trauma/crush injuries
Prolonged immobilization
Electrical injury
Excessive muscular activity
- Excessive exertion especially in sickle cell trait patients
- Malignant hyperthermia
- Neuroleptic malignant syndrome

Infections
- Bacterial infections, in particular, those involving organisms causing pneumonia, muscle inflammation (pyomyositis), or sepsis
- Viral infections including those due to human immunodeficiency virus, influenza virus, coxsackievirus, and Epstein-Barr virus

Medications†
- HMG-CoA reductase inhibitors
- Gemfibrozil
- Paraphenylenediamine (hair dye)
- Phenothiazines
- Theophylline

Toxins
- Cocaine
- Carbon monoxide
- Amphetamines including *N*-benzylpiperazine (BZP)-based medications
- Alcohol
- *Tricholoma equestre* (wild mushrooms)
- Hemlock
- Animal venoms

Metabolic myopathies[123]
- Carnitine palmitoyl transferase deficiency
- Mitochondrial respiratory chain deficiencies
- McArdle disease
- Phosphofructokinase deficiency

*In addition to the causes listed here, risk factors include excessive heat, hyponatremia, hypophosphatemia, and hypokalemia.[124-127]
†Additional medications have been associated with rhabdomyolysis.[76,128]
*Studies cited in this table may be found in the complete list of references for this chapter provided online.
HMG-CoA, 3-hydroxy-3-methyl-glutaryl-coenzyme A.

The epidemiology of rhabdomyolysis is limited by a lack of uniformity regarding the critical value in CK elevation needed to make the diagnosis. Threshold values above which rhabdomyolysis may occur vary and have ranged from 1000 to 10,000 U/L, though 5000 to 10,000 U/L are most common.[94] From an intensivist's perspective, CK elevations less than 5000 U/L should not be associated with myoglobin-induced renal failure unless clear additive causes such as volume depletion, sepsis, or radiocontrast are also present.

PATHOPHYSIOLOGY

The primary event in rhabdomyolysis is muscle cell necrosis resulting in the accumulation of sodium and calcium intracellularly; disruption of the cell membrane and excessive requirements for adenosine triphosphate accelerate this insult.[95,96] As muscle cells undergo necrosis, intracellular substances are released and include potassium, uric acid, phosphorus, lactic acid, and myoglobin. Under normal circumstances, haptoglobin binds any free myoglobin, thus prohibiting filtration across the glomerulus. As the haptoglobin binding is overwhelmed, free myoglobin is filtered and injures renal tubular cells. This process involves free radical toxicity. Additional causes include volume depletion, renal vasoconstriction, and tubular obstruction.[76,97] Myoglobin and urinary tubular-protein casts are more prone to precipitation at a lower pH in experimental models. As a result, inducing an alkaline diuresis has been a traditional part of therapy for cases of rhabdomyolysis.[98]

Research has suggested that it is the reperfusion of ischemic muscle as much as the ischemia itself that produces a high burden of oxygen-derived free radicals with subsequent cellular lipid membrane injury.[99] As renal function worsens, particularly when accompanied by intravascular volume depletion and renal failure, patients cannot excrete the high load of metabolites associated with muscle death, especially potassium.

Myoglobin release occurs across a spectrum of physical injuries from moderate exercise to lethal crush injuries. Myoglobinemia was noted in 39% of a cohort of Marine recruits, illustrating the frequency of mild muscle cell necrosis with strenuous exercise.[100] Obviously, not all such injuries lead to AKI. Beyond the actual amount of muscle necrosis, the development of AKI is most dependent on the degree of volume depletion present during the initial insult and the rapidity with which it is restored. Many of the syndromes that lead to the development of rhabdomyolysis, such as very strenuous exercise, crush injuries, or intoxications, are accompanied by volume depletion.

CLINICAL PRESENTATION

Patients with rhabdomyolysis present with a variety of symptoms. Often there is a history of injury, weakness, or muscle pain. Dark red or brown urine may or may not be present, depending on the amount of muscle necrosis and delay from injury. Frequently, the history is limited because of altered sensorium; clues include unexplained acidosis, hyperkalemia, hyperuricemia, hypocalcemia, elevations in CK not consistent with myocardial infarction, and unexplained renal failure. Recurrent presentations warrant an evaluation for a metabolic myopathy.[101] Screening for rhabdomyolysis, through serial CK measurements, may be worthwhile in high-risk obese patients (body mass index over 56 kg/m^2) undergoing gastric bypass surgery.[102]

In most instances, serum CK will increase during the initial 48 hours of hospitalization. In a retrospective review of patients admitted to an ICU with rhabdomyolysis, defined as a CK greater than 10,000 U/L, significantly higher CK levels were associated with renal failure.[103] In the group with renal failure, the mean CK levels were 47,194 and 55,366 U/L at admission and peak, respectively; in the group without renal failure, the same levels were 17,531 and 28,643 U/L.

Although myoglobin is the most important protein in terms of nephrotoxicity, serum CK is routinely used in clinical practice as a marker of disease severity. This inconsistency is due to the widespread availability of the CK assay. Myoglobin clearance is not dependent on the kidneys and thus levels peak before CK levels.[104] Consequently, the CK levels being monitored for disease activity may not correlate with the timing of the renal injury. AKI due to peak CK levels less than 5000 U/L should not be attributed to rhabdomyolysis unless the diagnosis was made substantially after the peak period of muscle cell necrosis; in this scenario, the CK levels will have decreased from a previously undocumented level.

The change of serum Cr in nonrhabdomyolysis oliguric AKI is usually not more than 1 mg/dL/24 hours. In rhabdomyolysis, Cr enters the intravascular compartment at a higher rate due to cell lysis, yielding an unusually rapid rise in serum Cr. In an early report, Grossman and associates noted a rise in Cr frequently greater than 2.5 mg/dL/day.[105] Speculation exists that this change in Cr may, in part, be due to the larger than average size in patients affected with rhabdomyolysis.[106] These same authors noted the impressive rate of renal recovery from rhabdomyolysis-induced AKI seen in the majority of patients; this high rate of recovery is now well recognized.

SPECIFIC TREATMENT REQUIREMENTS

The most important intervention to limit renal complications of crush-related injuries is early and aggressive volume resuscitation. Delays in initiation of intravenous fluid are associated with a higher frequency of patients requiring renal replacement therapy.[107] The damaged muscle cells provide a large reservoir for fluid sequestration; as a result large volumes of intravenous fluids have to be given and, ideally, should be instituted as early as possible, even on-site before victims of crush injuries are freed.[78,108] A debate exists in the medical literature regarding the ideal type of volume resuscitation. As previously mentioned, alkaline diuresis has been shown in animal models to decrease the formation of myoglobin casts and subsequent AKI.[98] Similarly, mannitol is an agent favored for its proposed ability to scavenge free radicals and to reduce tissue swelling due to osmotically induced fluid removal from damaged muscle.[109,110] These treatments have not been validated in well-designed, prospective trials. Retrospective studies suggest no benefit with the addition of mannitol or alkaline diuresis over normal saline alone.[111] In addition, there are potential risks to volume expansion with bicarbonate-based solutions or mannitol. They include the increased risk of calcium-phosphate complex formation and hypocalcemia from an increase in pH and the development of a hyperosmolar state when renal failure limits mannitol excretion. Finally, mannitol may *increase* the risk of renal failure in certain populations.[112] Risk factors for mannitol-induced AKI include kidney dysfunction, high-dose mannitol therapy, and use of cyclosporin A. In summary, volume expansion irrespective of the type of agent is the most important treatment modality. The focus on adequate diuresis is appropriate but presumes myoglobin-induced renal damage is ongoing. Intensivists often encounter patients whose myoglobin load is falling and whose renal insult has already occurred. Though the Cr may continue to rise, the onset of oliguria suggests limited benefit from further aggressive volume resuscitation, presuming adequate intravascular volume has been restored. In fact, given the good prognosis of AKI, overzealous volume resuscitation risks pulmonary compromise.

Historically, extremely aggressive volume resuscitation was pursued with an initial goal diuresis of up to 12 L/day, presuming intact renal function. Less aggressive volume resuscitation may be equally protective though data are lacking. The focus on diuresis downplays the importance of establishing and maintaining adequate intravascular volume. Central venous pressure or other means to monitor intravascular pressure may be more useful to determine adequate resuscitation. It is also likely that the rapidity with which volume status is restored, irrespective of the type or quantity of diuresis, is the key determininant. Unfortunately, these guidelines are poorly studied in a prospective format.

In the setting of AKI requiring renal replacement therapy, the ideal modality is the one most easily accessible, assuming hemodynamic stability. Options include hemodialysis, peritoneal dialysis, and continuous modalities. Though continuous renal replacement modalities provide the best theoretical protection from ongoing metabolic and volume complications, its superiority has not been verified in rigorous trials. In cases associated with large-scale injuries such as earthquakes, the remaining infrastructure often dictates which dialytic modality can and should be provided.[72,113] Historically, peritoneal dialysis has not been considered adequate in its ability to remove the large solute load present with rhabdomyolysis.[114] Nonetheless, if it is the only available modality its potential role in managing rhabdomyolysis may be improved with more frequent exchanges. It should be noted that no traditional renal replacement method has the capability of removing myoglobin because of its size. However, considering the rapid extrarenal clearance of myoglobin it is unclear if therapy focused on myoglobin clearance will provide any superiority over current care. A novel approach recently evaluated the use of super high-flux (SHF) membranes to clear myoglobin during continous venovenous hemofiltration.[115,116] The authors demonstrated a fivefold increase in myoglobin removal but did acknowledge the potential for the removal of albumin, clotting factors, and protein-bound medications.

Hypocalcemia is common in rhabdomyolysis and may provide challenging management choices. Calcium entry into necrotic muscle cells often causes profound hypocalcemia. Calcium supplementation should be reserved for those patients with symptomatic hypocalcemia as hypercalcemia is a frequent finding during disease recovery.[117] In addition, rapid increases in serum pH through the administration of intravenous bicarbonate may worsen hypocalcemia. Rasburicase has been reported to reduce hyperuricemia in young patients with rhabdomyolysis.[118]

Additional issues include close monitoring for limb ischemia due to compartment syndromes induced by muscle damage and subsequent fluid sequestration. Intracompartmental pressure monitoring may predict the need for intervention though research has suggested additional factors, most importantly hypotension and the difference between mean arterial pressure and intracompartmental pressures, influence whether compartment syndrome develops.[119] The history, logic, and disappointing results of early and aggressive fasciotomy have recently been described.[120] Mannitol is postulated to "decompress" intracompartmental edema in acute muscle compartment syndromes. Animal data support an acute reduction in intracompartmental pressures[121]; long-term tissue protection and human outcomes have not been validated. High-dose corticosteroids have been proposed as a treatment option for refractory cases of rhabdomyolysis but prospective studies are lacking.[122]

In summary, rhabdomyolysis is a frequent, treatable disorder. Extensive metabolic research has yielded a number of clues about the cause of AKI during rhabdomyolysis. Therapy should emphasize aggressive and early volume resuscitation. Renal replacement therapy may be necessary to assist in managing the metabolic complications of patients; patients have a good prognosis for recovery of rhabdomyolysis-induced AKI.

KEY POINTS

- Populations at risk for hypothermia include the elderly, people with preexisting chronic medical conditions, and people suffering from alcoholism and drug intoxication. Emerging populations include wilderness enthusiasts and winter sport participants.
- All intervals—PR, QRS, and QT—are prolonged secondary to hypothermia-induced slowed impulse conduction through potassium channels.
- Patients with moderate or severe hypothermia should be resuscitated until adequate rewarming is achieved before declaring efforts as unsuccessful.
- The diagnosis of heatstroke should be considered in patients with core body temperatures greater than 41°C.
- Severe dehydration, anhidrosis, and extreme hyperpyrexia are common in external heatstroke.
- Myocardial dysfunction with depression of left ventricular ejection fraction also has been described after heatstroke that resolves with treatment.
- Acute renal failure occurs in up to one third of patients with heatstroke.
- Intravascular volume restoration must be individualized. In general, patients with exertional hypothermia are severely hypovolemic.
- The most effective approaches to lowering the core temperature are immersion and evaporative methods.
- By far, the most important measure for MH is the immediate cessation of any suspected triggering agents.
- NMS is characterized by muscle rigidity and altered mental status, followed by autonomic instability and hyperthermia.
- Dopamine agonists such as bromocriptine, amantadine, and levodopa-carbidopa have been successfully employed in treating NMS.
- Rhabdomyolysis is unlikely to occur with a creatine kinase level below 5000 U/L unless volume depletion or another kidney insult is present.

KEY POINTS (Continued)

- Aggressive volume resuscitation is more important than the type of volume replacement given to reduce the risk of myoglobin-induced AKI in cases of rhabdomyolysis.
- Alkaline-based volume resuscitation may worsen hypocalcemia.
- Rhabdomyolysis-associated AKI, including cases requiring renal replacement therapy, has a good prognosis.

SELECTED REFERENCES

12. McCulough L, Arora S: Diagnosis and treatment of hypothermia. Am Fam Physician 2004;70(12):2325-2332.
46. Sultan N, Theakston KD, Butler R, Suri RS: Treatment of severe accidental hypothermia with intermittent hemodialysis. Can J Emerg Med 2009;11(2):174-177.
49. Kilbourne EM, Choi, K, Jones TS, et al: Risk factors for heat stroke. A case control study. JAMA 1982;247:3332.
74. Ballantyne CM, Corsini A, Davidson MH, et al: Risk for myopathy with statin therapy in high-risk patients [see comment]. Arch Internal Med 2003;163(5):553-564.
76. Huerta-Alardin AL, Varon J, Marik PE: Bench-to-bedside review: Rhabdomyolysis—An overview for clinicians. Crit Care 2005; 9(2):158-169.
77. Bosch X, Poch E, Grau JM: Rhabdomyolysis and acute kidney injury. N Engl J Med 2009;361(1):62-72.
83. Amrein S, Amrein K, Amegah-Sakotnik A, et al: Propofol infusion syndrome—A critical incident report highlighting the danger of reexposure. J Neurosurg Anesthesiol 2011;23(3):265-266.
87. Eichner ER: Sickle cell considerations in athletes. Clin Sports Med 2011;30(3):537-549.
94. Allison RC, Bedsole DL: The other medical causes of rhabdomyolysis. Am J Med Sci 2003;326(2):79-88.
98. Zager RA: Studies of mechanisms and protective maneuvers in myoglobinuric acute renal injury. Lab Invest 1989;60(5): 619-629.
101. Lofberg M, Jankala H, Paetau A, et al: Metabolic causes of recurrent rhabdomyolysis. Acta Neurol Scand 1998;98(4):268-275.
104. Lappalainen H, Tiula E, Uotila L, Manttari M: Elimination kinetics of myoglobin and creatine kinase in rhabdomyolysis: Implications for follow-up. Crit Care Med 2002;30(10):2212-2215.
105. Grossman RA, Hamilton RW, Morse BM, et al: Nontraumatic rhabdomyolysis and acute renal failure. N Engl J Med 1974;291(16):807-811.
107. Gunal AI, Celiker H, Dogukan A, et al: Early and vigorous fluid resuscitation prevents acute renal failure in the crush victims of catastrophic earthquakes. J Am Soc Nephrol 2004;15(7): 1862-1867.
111. Brown CV, Rhee P, Chan L, et al: Preventing renal failure in patients with rhabdomyolysis: Do bicarbonate and mannitol make a difference? J Trauma 2004;56(6):1191-1196.
112. Visweswaran P, Massin EK, Dubose TD Jr: Mannitol-induced acute renal failure. J Am Soc Nephrol 1997;8(6):1028-1033.
113. Sever MS, Erek E, Vanholder R, et al, Marmara Earthquake Study G: Treatment modalities and outcome of the renal victims of the Marmara earthquake. Nephron 2002;92(1):64-71.
128. Mor A, Wortmann RL, Mitnick HJ, Pillinger MH: Drugs causing muscle disease. Rheum Dis Clin North Am 2011;37(2):219-231.

The complete list of references can be found at www.expertconsult.com.

PART 8

ADMINISTRATIVE, ETHICAL, AND PSYCHOLOGICAL ISSUES IN THE CARE OF THE CRITICALLY ILL

70

Intensive Care Unit Administration and Performance Improvement

Sean Townsend | Christa Schorr | Carolyn Bekes

CHAPTER OUTLINE

The delivery of critical care services continues to represent a disproportionate share of health care expenditures relative to the proportion of patients who use these services. The federal Medicare program has become the largest provider of health care insurance in the United States and in 2002 accounted for nearly 30% of annual payments to hospitals.[1] An analysis of Medicare admissions in 2000 determined that cases involving a stay in an intensive care unit (ICU) cost nearly three times as much as those limited to the general care wards. Nevertheless, only 83% of the cost of the care of ICU patients was reimbursed, compared with 105% for patients cared for on the general care floors.[2] Over the subsequent 5 years, critical care costs reportedly increased another 44%.[3]

Against this challenging background, ICU administrators must plan for expected needs, improve on the efficiency and quality of care, and adequately staff their organizations. Additional challenges include coping with a pending reduction in the size of the critical care workforce concomitant with an increase in the proportion of patients utilizing these resources. Administrators must respond to pressures from external organizations to meet higher standards of care delivery. These tasks are not insurmountable. The ICU leadership in cooperation with administration is uniquely positioned to respond to these problems. In the ICU, the relatively small number of ICU beds, a compartmentalized physical plant, and the large degree of control that leaders can exert over the environment make it a fertile ground for change.

Accordingly, the principal consideration for ICU administrators becomes a question of what type of structure and leadership their ICU will need to accomplish its mission. Typically, ICUs have been structured along the lines of tertiary, large community, and small community hospitals. These hospitals have different aims and goals and differing capacities to respond to acuity in the care of patients. Likewise, most ICUs have a designated ICU director with roles and responsibilities commensurate with those goals. Standards of care for typical arrangements have been described in the literature.[4] An essential function of ICU administration is to determine and specifically articulate the ICU's compliance with these standards.

Once an ICU's structure and leadership are well established, administrators may turn their attention to addressing the challenges presented by economic, market, and technologic forces. Increasingly, well-run ICUs have striven to promote an ICU culture that aims for efficiency while continuously improving the quality of care provided to patients. Performance improvement seeks to integrate best scientific practice into the care of critically ill patients. Regardless of the type of structure and leadership selected for a particular ICU, a focus on quality improvement can optimize function and build efficiencies to care for critically ill patients. Methodologies such as Six Sigma may be useful.

THE PRESENT-DAY CRITICAL CARE LANDSCAPE

Establishing an agenda for administrators and leaders of ICUs starts with a critical analysis of their current position in critical care delivery. This section describes the ongoing evolution of the critical care landscape in regard to patterns of use, costs, and current configurations.

Surveys of critical care delivery in the United States date back to the early 1990s.[5,6] Reports of the supply and demand of adult critical care were most recently completed in 2000 through a joint effort on behalf of the American Thoracic Society (ATS), the American College of Chest Physicians (ACCP), and the Society of Critical Care Medicine (SCCM).[7] Estimates on current and future requirements for adult critical care and pulmonary medicine physicians in the United States were reported by the Committee on Manpower for the Pulmonary and Critical Care Societies (COMPACCS). Angus and coworkers, on behalf of the COMPACCS group, extended their inquiry in 2006 to profile the organization and distribution of ICU patients and services in the United States.[8]

The initial COMPACCS study concluded that in 1997, intensivists provided care to 36.8% of all ICU patients and that intensivist level care was more common in regions with high managed care penetration. The 2006 update estimated that there were 5980 ICUs in the United States, caring for approximately 55,000 patients per day. Sixty-five percent of ICUs were combined medical-surgical ICUs; 71% were located in nonteaching community hospitals; and 62% of all ICUs were located in hospitals with fewer than 300 beds. Another important finding was the projected shortfall of critical care physicians of 22% by 2020 and 35% by 2030.

In response to the COMPACCS study report, an analysis was requested by the U.S. Senate. In 2006 a report to Congress from the U.S. Department of Health and Human Services' Health Services and Resource Administration (HSRA) updated the findings in COMPACCS, reiterating their projections with respect to the critical care workforce.[9] The HSRA workforce analysis indicated that the growth and aging of the population alone will increase demand for adult intensivist services by at least 38% between 2000 and 2020. Similarly, critical care nursing availability remains woefully inadequate to meet the demand. Proactive recruitment and retention strategies are paramount to maintain high-quality nursing care (Box 70.1).

Box 70.1 Reasons for Nursing Turnover and Retention Strategies

Why Nurses Leave

- Increased market demand
- Heavy workload/inadequate staffing
- Better pay elsewhere
- More flexible scheduling elsewhere
- Better career/developmental opportunities elsewhere
- More desirable work culture elsewhere
- Better benefits elsewhere
- Inadequate managerial skills
- Physician relationships
- Better employer reputation elsewhere

Retention Strategies

- Enhancing supplemental pay plans
- Increasing base pay
- Retention bonuses
- Variable pay/incentives
- Flexible scheduling/shifts
- Addressing staffing needs using rotations/float pools
- Staffing support using unlicensed personnel
- New clinical advancement programs
- Enhanced continuing education
- Regular staff input/surveys
- New processes to assist in delivery of care
- Changing patient care delivery model
- Increasing staff understanding of organizational mission, goals, and initiatives
- Management training/skill building
- Enhancing collaboration with support departments
- Physician relations programs
- New work environment/culture initiatives

From Medical Economics 2000;77:33.

Adapted, displayed, and reprinted with permission from Joint Commission on Accreditation of Healthcare Organization. (2002, August) Health care at the crossroads: Strategies for addressing the evolving nursing crisis, is a copyrighted publication of Advanstar Communication Inc.

The shortfall in supply of intensivists may drive administrators to consider an alternative critical care delivery team model, which may include nonintensivist physicians and physician extenders. Consideration to hopitalists partnering with intensivists as an option to fill the gap in intensivist supply is being addressed by two task forces, first in a publication of the 2004 Framing Options for Critical Care in the United States (FOCCUS) report and second in 2007 Prioritizing the Organization and Management of Intensive Care Services in the United States (PrOMIS) Conference Report.[10,11] Reports from these task forces made three recommendations in an attempt to address the situation: to include (1) uniform protocols for intensive care treatment, (2) a process for certification of physicians providing critical care services with a competency assurance process, and (3) health service research with a focus on outcomes of ICU patients cared for by hospitalists.[12] In another model, use of physician extenders may include physician assistants (PAs) and nurse practitioners (NPs). Limited research exists examining the use of NPs and PAs in the critical care setting with the majority focused on their impact on patient care management. Despite the small sample sizes and limited studies, NPs and PAs have demonstrated enhanced patient flow, improved clinical and financial outcomes for mechanically ventilated patients, reduction in ICU and hospital length of stay, and improved management in the heart failure patient population.[13] Because the lack of intensivist staffing is unlikely to change significantly over the next few years, alternative models may be on the horizon.

Regardless of the expected reductions in available staffing, calls for increased access to intensivists continue with a goal of increasing intensivist coverage in-house around the clock. Despite the challenge by one recent study,[14] multiple studies have demonstrated mortality rate and cost-savings benefits to critically ill patients receiving care by intensivists. Young and Birkmeyer estimated that in the context of 360,000 deaths occurring each year in ICUs, 54,000 lives may be saved annually with intensivist staffing.[15] Similarly, Pronovost and colleagues have estimated that more than $5 billion could be saved annually.[16] A report generated for the Agency for Healthcare Research and Quality (AHRQ) notes that these benefits alone underestimate the potential improvement in the quality of care in terms of fewer complications, avoiding inappropriate utilization, decreased patient suffering, and better end-of-life care.[17]

The Leapfrog Group, a consortium of companies that purchase health care for their employees, convened in an effort to leverage their purchasing power to improve the quality of care. This powerful group has focused on improving four key areas central to patient safety and to cost containment in health care: (1) the use of computerized physician order entry, (2) the oversight of critical care physicians in the care of ICU patients, (3) the use of evidence-based hospital referral systems, and (4) Leapfrog safe practice scores.[18] The influence of this group on both payers and health systems alike has contributed to the increasing demand for intensivists to care for critically ill patients. Unfortunately, the 2006 update to the COMPACCS study suggests that this need has gone essentially unmet. Loosely defining Leapfrog-compliant intensivist coverage for 80% of critically ill patients and the presence of 24-hour in-house physician coverage, Angus and colleagues found that only one in four ICUs had 80% intensivist coverage and that half had no intensivist coverage. Very few hospitals provided in-house physician coverage during off hours: 20% during weekend days, 12% during weekday nights, and 10% during weekend nights. Overall, only 4% of adult ICUs in the United States appeared to meet even a liberal interpretation of Leapfrog standards.[8]

Box 70.2 Examples of Best Practices for Coordinating Care in the Intensive Care Unit (ICU)

Within the ICU

- Specific guidelines and protocols for medical and nursing care
- Physician credentialing for selected procedures (e.g., intubation, invasive monitoring)
- Updated protocols for limiting life-supporting therapy
- Physician rounds made early, facilitating communications and planning by nurses
- Orientation, written guidelines, and close supervision for residents
- Rounds and conferences with pharmacist, dietitian, radiologist
- Emphasis on decentralized services (satellite pharmacy, laboratory, and radiograph viewing) or close to ICU
- Guidelines for nursing change of shift report

Between the ICU and Other Areas

- New nurses oriented to emergency, recovery, step-down units
- Standardized nursing reports for patients transferred from ICU; interunit conferences for long-term, complex cases
- Floor care for hopelessly ill or chronically ventilated patients with a do-not-resuscitate order and other treatment limits
- Direct phone line from visiting area to unit clerk
- Administrative and support services with emphasis on importance of satisfying "internal" customers

From Zimmerman JE, Shortell SM, Rousseau DM, et al: Improving intensive care: Observations based on organizational case studies in nine intensive care units: A prospective, multicenter study. Crit Care Med 1993;21:1443.

IDEALIZED DESIGN FOR CRITICAL CARE PRACTICE

In the face of an emerging demand-driven crisis in critical care, the task of effective ICU administration will only become a more difficult challenge. Nevertheless, efforts must be made to adapt care delivery patterns to the emerging demand crisis. Failure to develop new patterns of critical care delivery will ensure inadequate care for thousands of patients for years to come. In the absence of renewed planning, failure probably will evolve slowly, first affecting vulnerable populations, such as the uninsured and those located in rural areas. As time passes, a larger and larger proportion of Americans will receive less than the ideal standard of care.

A key first step is to halt further deterioration in present practice through effective coordination and communication to mitigate further erosion in practice standards (Boxes 70.2 and 70.3). Strategies to refine critical care delivery and meet predicted needs are present in the literature. Retaining tactics that have proved effective in trauma care are essential in building on current designs to streamline access to critical care. Hospital systems will need to collaborate on the care of critically ill patients in order to distribute critical care equitably as a resource, a social commodity. Finally, a realignment of values among health care leaders to build and reinforce a culture of efficiency, safety, and continuous improvement may stave off mediocrity.

RATIONAL MODEL FOR CRITICAL CARE DELIVERY

Delivery of critical care should attempt to balance the needs of the community with access to the highest quality critical care services within that area. The American College of Surgeons (ACS) set the precedent for national practice standards for specific sets of critically ill patients when trauma centers were organized. When patients sustain injury with possible trauma, their care is initiated at appropriate trauma centers, depending on readiness and capacity to deliver care. Each designated level of classification (levels I to IV) has associated standards designated by the ACS. The structure has redefined the care of trauma patients and has been associated with improved outcomes and decreased mortality rates.[19,20]

Advancement in critical care delivery is feasible using a similar approach. The American College of Critical Care Medicine (ACCM) of the SCCM has developed a system to segregate hospitals into specific categories based on readiness and capacity to deliver critical care services (Box 70.4). These guidelines were first published in 1999 and revised in 2003.[4] Appropriate application of these guidelines provides a gateway in developing collaborative relationships and to ensure a streamlined approach to critical care delivery.

Although the ACCM guidelines set the stage for ideal function of hospitals within each classification, a substantial

Box 70.3 Examples of Best Communication Practices

- Bulletin boards used to highlight important messages
- Communication books for facilitating information transfer
- Regular, consistent staff meetings with a set agenda and staff input
- Brief, group change-of-shift report followed by individual bedside reports
- Nurse manager available to staff through regular visits on all shifts
- Working paging systems; immediate response 24 hours a day, 7 days a week
- Charting systems that are user friendly, clear, and readily available
- Daily rounds promoting high levels of interaction between nurses and physicians
- Multidisciplinary forums for information sharing
- Social workers used to facilitate communication with patients' families
- Open visiting hours for family members
- Rotating shifts for orienting new nurses
- Standard evaluation form for registry/agency nurses

From Zimmerman JE, Shortell SM, Rousseau DM, et al: Improving intensive care: Observations based on organizational case studies in nine intensive care units: A prospective, multicenter study. Crit Care Med 1993;21:1443.

Box 70.4 Levels of Critical Care

Level I critical care: Level I critical care centers have intensive care units (ICUs) that provide comprehensive care for a wide range of disorders requiring intensive care.[4] They require the continuous availability of sophisticated equipment, specialized nurses, and physicians with critical care training. Support services including pharmacy services, respiratory therapy, nutritional services, pastoral care, and social services are comprehensive. Although most of these centers fulfill an academic mission in a teaching hospital setting, some may be community-hospital based.

Level II critical care: Level II critical care centers have the capability to provide comprehensive critical care but may not have resources to care for specific patient populations (e.g., cardiothoracic surgery, neurosurgery, trauma). Although these centers may be able to deliver high-quality care to most critically ill patients, transfer agreements must be established in advance for patients with specific problems. The ICUs in level II centers may or may not have an academic mission.

Level III critical care: Hospitals that have level III capabilities have the ability to provide initial stabilization of critically ill patients, but they are limited in the ability to provide comprehensive critical care. These hospitals require written policies addressing the transfer of critically ill patients to critical care centers that are capable of providing the comprehensive critical care required (level I or level II). These facilities may continue to admit and care for a limited number of ICU patients for whom care is routine and consistent with hospital and community resources.

Adapted from Haupt MT, Bekes CE, Brilli RJ, et al: Guidelines on critical care services and personnel: Recommendations based on a system of categorization of three levels of care. Crit Care Med 2003;3:267-268.

performance gap between compliance with the guidelines and actual practice remains. Administrators should define their mission, thereby determining the range of services that their hospital seeks to effectively offer patients. Instrumental aspects to consider include the population the hospital serves, services provided by neighboring hospitals, and subspecialties of the staff physicians. Other factors that may be informative in redesign include a list of common diagnoses and acuity level in patients who are routinely treated.[4]

Even hospitals that appear to have well-integrated strategies can benefit from review of current operating procedures. As part of the overall strategy for evolution of hospitals into this operating model, it is reasonable to expect a large number of hospitals to be in transition at any given time. Resistance to regionalization at the local level can be anticipated. Local hospital administrators will not want to forgo revenue, community physicians will not want to "lose" patients to the referral hospital, and communities may resist loss of local services.

The specific standards that define level I and level II care are summarized in Box 70.5. Many hospitals will not be able to maintain these standards, and overlap with level II or level III critical care facilities may be considerable. Level II hospitals capable of providing comprehensive care for most diagnoses should attempt to emulate the level I guidelines for most conditions. For instance, a level II institution may not have the resources for optimal treatment of severe burns, but that facility may provide excellent surgical, cardiac, and posttransplantation medical care. Such a facility should aim to meet level I standards for conditions other than severe burns.

For level II or III institutions, a critical requirement of the guidelines is to establish agreements for transfer of patients for higher levels of care. It should be a usual practice in such facilities to stabilize patients with the intention to invoke established agreements to transfer to collaborating facilities.[21] Although completing transfers may be routine for ICU staff, the requirement for agreements established in advance with collaborating institutions to accept transfers may be novel. In order to develop the efficiencies that will be necessary in the emerging critical care environment, these types of prenegotiated arrangements will be necessary to ensure access to needed care.

The requirement to transfer also implies a burden of review on level II and level III centers to understand the treatment options available at more advanced centers with respect to a wide array of diagnoses. Although many administrators may assume that their clinicians maintain a full understanding of treatment options outside their facility, this assumption may be faulty. It is therefore appropriate with respect to specific diagnoses to develop codified procedures that demarcate established points in care suitable for transfer. These procedures may be incorporated as part of the envisioned interhospital agreement to coordinate transfers. Bed availability in the tertiary hospital may require alternative solutions in times of high occupancy.

Box 70.5 Intensive Care Unit (ICU) Leadership

A. A physician Unit Director is required. In general, the director should meet the guidelines for the definition of an intensivist as published by the Society of Critical Care Medicine. Specific requirements for the Unit Director include:
  1. Training, interest, and time availability to give clinical, administrative, and educational direction to the ICU
  2. Board certification in critical care medicine
  3. Time and commitment to maintain active and regular involvement in the care of patients in the unit
  4. Expertise necessary to oversee the administrative aspects of unit management, including formation of policies and procedures, enforcement of unit policies, and the education of unit staff
  5. The ability to ensure the quality, safety, and appropriateness of care in the ICU
  6. Availability (of either the Director or a similarly qualified surrogate) to the unit 24 hours a day, 7 days a week for both clinical and administrative matters
  7. Active involvement in local or national critical care societies
  8. Hospital privileges to perform relevant invasive procedures
  9. Active involvement as an advisor and participant in the organization of the care of the critically ill patient in the community as a whole
  10. Participation in the education of unit staff, other physicians, house staff, and medical staff as indicated
  11. Participation in scholarly activity (case reports, clinical and basic research)
  12. Active participation in the review of the appropriate utilization of ICU resources in the hospital

B. A Nurse Manager is appointed to provide precise lines of authority, responsibility, and accountability for the delivery of high-quality patient care. Specific requirements for the Nurse Manager include:
  1. An RN with a BSN or preferably an MSN degree
  2. Certification in critical care or equivalent graduate education
  3. At least 2 years of experience working in a critical care unit
  4. Previous management experience, including experience with health information systems, quality improvement, risk management activities, and health care economies
  5. Preparation to participate in the on-site education of critical care unit nursing staff and physicians-in-training
  6. Ability to foster a cooperative atmosphere with regard to the training of nurses, physicians, respiratory therapists, and other personnel involved in the care of critical care unit patients
  7. Regular participation in ongoing continuing nursing education
  8. Ability to participate in, and foster cooperation for, scholarly activity in the ICU (e.g., presentations, clinical research)
  9. Knowledge about current advances in the field of critical care nursing
  10. Participation in strategic planning and redesign efforts

From Haupt M, Bekes CE, Bayly RW, et al: Critical care services and personnel: Recommendations based on a system of categorization into two levels of care. American College of Critical Care Medicine of the Society of Critical Care Medicine. Crit Care Med 1999;27:422.

Committing the national critical care infrastructure to reorganization in line with the ACCM guidelines will not shield critical care providers and their patients from evolving demographic and market forces. However, by advancing institutions' understanding of their own critical care infrastructure, needs, and capacity, and by establishing agreements for transfer between hospitals, the initiative will facilitate the movement toward regionalization of care. A study commissioned by the SCCM in 1994 suggested that regionalization of critical care services probably is beneficial to patients, in part by promoting access to larger academic institutions and resources, increasing subspecialty availability, and providing expertise in the care of the critically ill.[22]

In trauma systems, studies suggest that considerable efficiencies have been obtained with regionalization. Both mortality rates and hospital lengths of stay have decreased.[19,23] Transition to level I ACS status has incurred increased costs at some centers, whereas other centers indicate that certification reduced costs.[24,25] Beyond the financial impact of regionalization, the transition to a regional trauma system has promoted interhospital cooperation and promoted more effective resource utilization.[26,27]

FINANCIAL MODELING OF CRITICAL CARE

The need for a transition to more rational structures in the provision of critical care services implies that hospitals will require an accurate accounting of costs and revenues as changes are made. Additionally, ICU quality improvement programs rely on an accurate understanding of costs to measure benefit (or harm) from programs intended to improve the quality of care. Several financial models exist to assess costs in the ICU.[28,29] A given hospital's cost accounting system may determine whether the ICU is viewed as generating a profit or a loss. Traditional methods have focused on the ICU as a cost center but not as a venue that may be revenue generating.[30] Even in cases in which an ICU may always represent a net loss of revenue for an institution, understanding the revenue streams can permit optimization and diminish losses.

STATE OF CRITICAL CARE REIMBURSEMENT

The federal Healthcare Financing Administration, which formerly administered Medicare and Medicaid, was renamed in 2001 the Centers for Medicaid and Medicare Services (CMS). Data from CMS's Medicare Provider Analysis and Review (MEDPAR) database remain the single best public source to support understanding of the financial horizon for hospital administrators. Contributing 30% of annual payments to hospitals in 2002, Medicare is the single largest payer in the U.S. health care system.[1]

Using the MEDPAR database, Cooper and Linde-Zwirble analyzed all hospital admissions during 2000 to determine the incidence, cost, and payment for ICU services.[2] Their findings suggested that more than one fifth of all Medicare cases had an ICU stay with a cost to hospitals of nearly three times as much as floor patients—$14,135 versus $5571. However, ICU cases were paid at a rate only twice that of floor cases—$11,704 versus $5835. This means that only 83% of costs were paid for ICU patients, compared with 105% for floor patients, generating an annual $5.8 billion loss to hospitals when ICU care is required.

Halpern and Pastores describe recent patterns of critical care medicine (CCM) use and costs in the United States from 2000 to 2005. The study analyzed data from the Hospital Cost Report Information System. Results indicate the number of acute care hospitals decreased by 20.6%, hospital beds decreased by 4.2%, yet CCM beds increased by 6.5%. Fifty-two percent to 56% of insurance coverage is attributed to Medicare and Medicaid for both CCM and hospital days. Data show that the critical care payer mix is evolving with an increase in Medicaid recipients using CCM services. The results show the percentage of CCM days by Medicare decreased by 3.8% compared to an increase of 15.5% by Medicaid. From 2000 to 2005 the CCM cost per day rose 44.2% (from $2698 to $3518). With an increase in uninsured and underinsured, development of a plan to understand the impact of the Medicaid population should be considered during strategic planning.[3]

FOCUS ON EXPENDITURES AND REVENUES

In view of the dramatic overall losses that hospitals sustain relative to expenditures on critical care patient services, a natural instinct among ICU administrators is to cut costs by reducing services. Hospital costs are best analyzed as either fixed or variable costs and as either direct or indirect expenditures. Fixed costs represent expenditures related to buildings, equipment, and certain labor costs; variable costs include items dependent on the volume of hospital operations, such as pharmaceutical expenditures and patient care supplies.

Reducing services is a flawed method to contain costs, however, because the fixed costs (and some variable costs) associated with the provision of critical care remain high and the differential savings achieved by limiting access to these services is small. Typically, direct patient care costs can be accounted to individual patients whose care generated those costs, and indirect patient care costs are averaged across all patients admitted to critical care. The indirect costs are not reduced when access to available services is limited. Reliable savings stem from elimination of services, rather than limiting access to or frequency of utilization of services.[31]

Moreover, the availability of sufficient services to care for the population at large remains essential. In line with the need to develop a more rational distribution of critical care delivery as outlined earlier, eliminating unnecessary services due to duplication in the community is appropriate. Once unnecessary or underutilized services have been eliminated, the next most appropriate steps to maximize ICU efficiency involve turning attention away from cost-cutting measures and toward revenue-enhancing strategies.

The development of cost-cutting methods may be further understood in evaluating the various regions of the United States in overall spending differences. Data from the Dartmouth Atlas Project in five U.S. hospital regions from 1992 to 2006 found annual Medicare spending growth rates range from 2.3% to 5% per capita.[32] Understanding this wide range in expenditures in areas with similar technologic and health care access may influence regions/hospitals with higher spending to develop more efficient and effective services.

CRITICAL CARE AS A PRODUCT LINE

Organizing a business plan for the critical care division, Bekes and colleagues[30] isolated the major sources of critical care patients and their relative profit or loss for the division. Analysis via the customary cost accounting methods employed by the hospital demonstrated hospital-to-hospital transfers appeared to produce a majority of the revenue. Focusing on this source of revenue as a unique "product line" enabled these clinician-investigators to promote these services more widely in the surrounding community.

Viable "products" may vary from institution to institution. Factors that may influence whether a particular service offered by the ICU is profitable or not include the availability of critical care resources in the community, the presence or absence of a stable network of hospitals for referrals, and the organizing structure of the institution (academic versus community, tertiary care versus otherwise, and so on). Presuming that the gap in reimbursement for critical care services noted in the Medicare data reflects patterns from other payers, many institutions may not be able to demonstrate a profit from their ICU regardless of identifiable sources of revenue. Nevertheless, in order to stave off losses of even greater magnitude, efforts to identify sources of revenue within critical care units will be essential as the health care market evolves.

CRITICAL CARE QUALITY IMPROVEMENT

Several market forces, as described earlier, in combination with clinicians' drive to provide the best possible care for ICU patients in a safe environment, have created a standard in critical care delivery: quality improvement. Although quality improvement in health care may not seem novel to practitioners involved in the day-to-day delivery of critical care, the field, much like critical care as a specialty, is relatively new. Many organizations and participants have begun to outline the scope of the field, but at present the boundaries of critical care quality improvement are defined only by a consensus of the involved parties. Critical care quality improvement initiatives are less than reified, however, and they are increasingly becoming the lens through which many intensivists view their daily work in the ICU.

BACKGROUND

In 1999, the Institute of Medicine (IOM) of the National Academies published a landmark report, *To Err Is Human: Building a Safer Health System.* The National Academies bring together committees of experts in all areas of scientific and technologic endeavor to address critical national issues and give advice to the federal government and the public. The

IOM report was widely hailed as groundbreaking in view of its documentation of the ways in which the health care system harms patients. Some of the findings about the American health care system included the following: (1) tremendous gaps exist between medical knowledge and practice; (2) adverse events harm patients far too often; (3) too many people do not get the care they need; and (4) the system propagates waste by permitting fragmentation of care and utilization inefficiencies.[33] In *To Err Is Human*, the IOM also estimated that despite incurring costs that are 40% greater than those for the next most expensive nation in terms of health care, 44,000 to 98,000 Americans die each year as a result of errors in their health care.

In 2003, in an exhaustive review of nearly 7000 patient charts across all regions of the United States, McGlynn and colleagues reported that the average defect rate, defined as the percent of cases in which care consistent with 439 indicators of quality was not delivered, approached 45% nationally.[34] Stated otherwise, patients receive the care indicated slightly more than one half of the time. These investigators concluded that the deficits identified in adherence to recommended processes for basic care posed a continuing immediate danger to the health of the American public.

DONABEDIAN FRAMEWORK

Building on work begun by Donabedian, the IOM published *Crossing the Quality Chasm: A New Health System for the 21st Century* in 2001. The report outlined fundamental changes that must be made in order to improve health care in the United States. Donabedian had described three components of quality care—structure, process, and outcome—each of which must be addressed to effectively control and manage quality in health care settings.[35] He proposed that each overarching concept of control should be monitored using specific tools (Table 70.1). The IOM report also refined Donabedian's seven attributes of high-quality health care, proposing instead six primary aims: safety, effectiveness, patient-centeredness, timeliness, efficiency, and equity.[36]

QUALITY IMPROVEMENT LANDSCAPE

Based on formidable critiques of the quality of the U.S. health care system, a variety of organizations either willingly have taken up the challenge to improve health care or, through legislation, have been empowered to improve the delivery of health care in the United States. All of these efforts have led to creation of agencies or activities with relevance to the ICU.

Table 70.1 Relations Between Quality Areas and Management Tools with Their Relative Importance

	Management Tools		
Quality Area	Standards	Guidelines	Indicators
Structures	+++	+	+
Processes	++	+++	++
Results/outcomes	+	++	+++

Reproduced from Frutiger A, Moreno R, Carlet J, et al for the Working Group on Quality Improvement of the European Society of Intensive Care Medicine: A clinician's guide to the use of quality terminology. Intensive Care Med 1998;24:860-863.

AGENCY FOR HEALTHCARE RESEARCH AND QUALITY

Funding for health services research is achieved primarily through grant applications to the AHRQ. Lucian Leape and Donald Berwick report that the Center for Quality Improvement and Safety, a division of AHRQ, has emerged as a leader in education, training, convening agenda setting workshops, disseminating information, developing measures, and facilitating the setting of standards.[37] AHRQ supports and funds efforts to evaluate best practices, medical errors, and development of patient safety indicators. The agency also has articulated an agenda that promotes the advancement of evidence-based best practices.

In 2001, Congress appropriated $50 million in annual funding for general patient safety research through AHRQ. Within 3 years these funds were assigned to an information technology focus. Leape and Berwick, key health care quality opinion leaders, lamented that this initial funding and subsequent reversal both legitimized health services research and at the same time starved these new researchers of the ability to undertake additional efforts.[37] Although investigator-initiated research funding has declined, the previous work of sentinel studies has changed the face of health care. AHRQ's funding in 2009 was allocated to compare alternative treatments for health conditions, reduce threats to patient safety, and advance health information technology.[38]

NATIONAL QUALITY FORUM

The National Quality Forum (NQF) has maintained close alignment with the platform advanced by the AHRQ. The NQF is a private, not-for-profit membership organization created to develop and implement a national strategy for health care quality measurement and reporting. The group seeks to improve American health care through endorsement of consensus-based national standards for the measurement and public reporting of health care performance data. Working with a broad base of health care interests including governmental agencies, insurers, and various medical associations, the NQF has prevailed upon hospitals to report compliance rates with their measures. In 2002 the NQF published a list of 30 evidence-based best practices ready for implementation. This list of practices was expanded in 2005.

THE JOINT COMMISSION

The Joint Commission (JC), formerly the Joint Commission on Accreditation of Healthcare Organizations (JCAHO), evaluates and accredits nearly 15,000 health care organizations and programs in the United States. The Commission, commonly misunderstood to be a governmental agency, is an independent not-for-profit organization. This body seeks to continuously improve the safety and quality of care provided to the public through the provision of health care accreditation and support for services that foster performance improvement in health care organizations.[39]

In 2003, after NQF's publication of evidence-based safe practices, the JC required hospitals to implement 11 of these practices.[40] The JC also has taken a special interest in developing a set of ICU core measures that are at present part of its library of supplemental measures.[41] Reserve measures, unlike the core measures previously proposed by the JC to satisfy its ORYX* performance measurement requirements for accreditation, are available for hospitals that are seeking a set of voluntary measures to monitor ICU care.

The ICU JC reserve measures included six measures:

ICU 1: Ventilator-associated pneumonia (VAP) prevention—patient positioning
ICU 2: Stress ulcer disease (SUD) prophylaxis
ICU 3: Deep vein thrombosis (DVT) prophylaxis
ICU 4: Central line–associated bloodstream infection (CLABSI) rate
ICU 5: ICU length of stay, risk-adjusted
ICU 6: Hospital mortality rate for ICU patients, risk-adjusted[42]

Reporting of the JCAHO ICU core measures was stopped July 1, 2005, after a decision was taken to align the measure set with those under development at CMS and a new entity, the Surgical Care Improvement Project (SCIP). SCIP is a collaboration among CMS, the Centers for Disease Control and Prevention (CDC), and more than 20 surgical organizations. Under this arrangement, JCAHO has agreed to refocus the ICU reserve measures to apply primarily to surgical care. Ultimately, once these standards are evaluated and approved through the NQF consensus process, they will satisfy ORYX performance measurement standards.[43]

ALIGNMENT OF EFFORTS

The alignment of forces interested in promoting evidence-based standards of care has led to efforts to establish a single set of applicable measures for hospitals. Although NQF appears to remain the ultimate clearinghouse for the endorsement of national standardized measures, the Hospital Quality Alliance (HQA) has been instrumental in decreasing fragmentation in the development of national measures for quality of care. The HQA is a public-private collaboration including the CMS, the American Hospital Association, the Federation of American Hospitals, and the Association of American Medical Colleges. The HQA is supported by the AHRQ, NQF, JCAHO, American Medical Association, American Nurses Association, National Association of Children's Hospitals and Related Institutions, Consumer-Purchaser Disclosure Project, AFL-CIO (American Federation of Labor and Congress of Industrial Organizations), AARP, and U.S. Chamber of Commerce.[44]

THE LEAPFROG GROUP: PURCHASERS AND PAYERS

The Leapfrog Group is a coalition of more than 160 large private employers and public purchasers that joined in 2000 to obtain leverage in health care purchasing decisions for employees. The group aims to "leapfrog" over key barriers as goals of their purchasing directives in order to overcome the poor value in the health care marketplace.[45]

Leapfrog relies on a survey of hospital quality and safety to inform its leadership about adherence to Leapfrog standards nationally. Completion of the survey is voluntary; however, it is required for certification of Leapfrog compliance.

THE INSTITUTE FOR HEALTHCARE IMPROVEMENT

The Institute for Healthcare Improvement (IHI) is a not-for-profit organization with the self-declared aim of leading the improvement of health care throughout the world. Founded in 1991, the IHI has as its mission the acceleration of change in health care by cultivating promising concepts for improving patient care and turning those ideas into action. The IHI has championed the use of collaborative methods to produce improvement in health care.

The IHI launched the 100,000 Lives Campaign in 2004 to reduce mortality rate in hospitals throughout the United States. Accomplishments in the campaign prompted the 5 Million Live Campaign over a 2-year period, 2006 to 2008. The aim of the campaign was to reduce morbidity and mortality rates by taking steps to reduce harm and death. More than 2000 facilities committed to pursue 12 interventions to reduce infection, surgical complication, medication errors, and other areas of unreliable care. One of the interventions included recruiting hospital boards to support the process for improvement in care.

Campaign results include 65 hospitals reporting close to a year or more without a VAP and 35 hospitals close to a year or more without a CLASBI. Success across states includes a reported 42% reduction in CLASBI and a 70% reduction in pressure ulcers in 150 organizations across New Jersey.[46]

SPONSORED STATEWIDE AND INTEGRATED HEALTH SYSTEM COLLABORATIVES

As a national quality agenda has become better articulated, several critical care quality improvement projects have emerged at the state level. In Michigan, for instance, the Michigan Health and Hospital Association's (MHA) Keystone Center for Patient Safety & Quality was created in March 2003. In collaboration with patient safety experts at Johns Hopkins University, MHA launched Keystone: ICU, which enjoys the participation of at least 120 ICUs and 70 hospitals. Johns Hopkins University and MHA estimate that the Keystone: ICU project saved 1574 lives, more than 84,000 ICU days, and greater than $175 million.[47,48] This initiative has been expanded to other states such as New Jersey and Rhode Island. Group purchasing organizations such as Veterans Health Administration (VHA) and Premier, Inc. have launched similar national initiatives in critical care quality improvement available to their membership.

PAY FOR PERFORMANCE AND QUALITY REPORTING

Agencies dedicated to critical care quality improvement have had a significant interest in linking quality of care to pay-for-performance. The concept is not a new one as private and public insurers, health care purchasing organizations, and quality improvement thought leaders have

---

*ORYX is the name of the Joint Commission's initiative to integrate performance measures into the accreditation process. It is not an acronym but was chosen because it was viewed as a unique catchword taken from the name of a graceful, swiftly moving animal.

pressed for the establishment of pay-for-performance plans to drive the market toward meeting evidence-based standards.[49,50] Although guidelines were established to ensure the fairness of pay-for-performance plans, most recognize the inevitable increase in such initiatives.[51,52]

Pay for performance has been variously described. One iteration refers to direct payments to physicians from hospitals, or less commonly from insurers, as a reward for high-quality performance. For example, the most recent general practitioner contract in the United Kingdom includes 146 performance measures across seven areas of practice. This contract rewards performance in accordance with the measures with financial incentives.[53] First-year results were recently reported: physicians exceeded projections of their performance and achieved a mean of 91% compliance with clinical guidelines. This resulted in payments estimated at $700 million more than expected.[54] Despite the seeming success of this program, there is no means to detect whether physicians' compliance efforts also may have detracted from quality in unmeasured patterns of care.[55]

Although pay for performance can contribute to improvements in quality of care it may present ethical concerns, whereby clinicians may become focused on scores and the need to meet the quality measure and potentially lose sight of the whole patient.[56] Consideration of plans toward minimizing potential harm through quality measures and public reporting may likely contribute to the transition from quality to payment. Maximizing the CCM team efforts in proactive quality improvement initiatives may be the most effective approach to capitalize on making overall care better.[57]

SPECIFIC QUALITY IMPROVEMENT INTERVENTIONS IN CRITICAL CARE

Several intervention-specific quality improvement initiatives in critical care have emerged in the past decade. Many organizations have committed resources to implement such initiatives based in part on high-profile campaigns to improve care and new regulatory or accreditation standards. Some of the strategies for ICU quality improvement benefit from standardized measures available through the NQF and others; however, as practitioners take notice of the growing imperative to change the way critical care is delivered, many cutting-edge initiatives are moving forward without a consensus on which quality indicators should be applied. Often, specific interventions are coupled to strategies that advance more general goals such as developing a culture of safety in the ICU to prevent harm.

SHEWART MODEL FOR PROCESS IMPROVEMENT

Critical care quality improvement initiatives typically have been executed in the setting of collaborative efforts as initially championed by the IHI and adapted by other groups. The precise mechanisms of implementation for these initiatives vary, but most sponsored quality improvement initiatives encourage the use of small-scale experiments to test new ideas. The principle calls for organizations to make the process of scientific prediction a part of routine work and was first advanced in 1931 by Walter Shewart, a pioneer in industrial quality control. Shewart advocated the use of iterative "plan-do-check-act" (PDCA) cycles to systematically test new ideas, evaluate their results, and, if successful, implement them.[58] More recently, the IHI has advocated a similar structure known as the Model for Improvement[59] (Fig. 70.1).

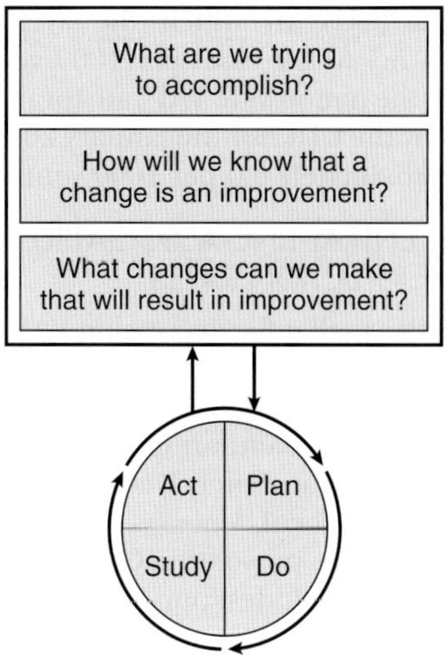

Figure 70.1 Institute for Healthcare Improvement model for quality improvement. (From Langley GL, Nolan KM, Nolan TW, et al: The Improvement Guide: A Practical Approach to Enhancing Organization Performance. San Francisco, Jossey-Bass, 1996.)

DECREASING VENTILATOR-ASSOCIATED PNEUMONIA RATES

Reducing mortality risk due to VAP requires an organized process that guarantees the early recognition of pneumonia along with the uniform and consistent application of the best evidence-based practices. Despite variability in clinical definitions to establish valid criteria to diagnose VAP, institutions have devoted considerable effort to combating VAP rates. The most recent evidence suggests the selection of diagnostic criteria may be irrelevant to outcomes. The CDC, however, has offered a clinical definition of VAP that has been widely adopted by the quality organizations cited earlier.[60]

The prototypical collaborative effort to decrease VAP rates has been use of the "ventilator bundle" promulgated by the IHI. The IHI ventilator initiative was initially launched to describe a pattern of best practices for ventilated patients, not to decrease VAP rates. A careful review of the literature on the care of ventilated patients produced four well-evidenced recommendations: elevation of head of the bed to 30 degrees, provision of a daily awakening or "sedation vacation," application of DVT prophylaxis, and provision of peptic ulcer disease prophylaxis. Although not components of IHI's ventilator bundle, several other practices with varying supporting evidence have become commonly applied as well, including the use of oral care techniques and subglottic suctioning.

Between July 2002 and January 2004, multidisciplinary improvement teams from 61 health care organizations participated in an IHI collaborative that included use of the ventilator bundle. Thirty-five of these teams consistently collected data on ventilator bundle element adherence and VAP rates. An average 44.5% reduction in the incidence of VAP was observed in these groups.[61] Sixteen units were medical-surgical ICUs, in which the average VAP rate decreased from 5.5 to 2.7 cases per 1000 ventilator days.[61] By comparison, the nationwide VAP rate for medical-surgical ICUs reported by the CDC for the January 2002 to June 2003 period was approximately 6.0 per 1000 ventilator days.[62]

DECREASING CENTRAL LINE–ASSOCIATED BLOODSTREAM INFECTION RATES

In an effort similar to that for decreasing VAP rates, decreasing CLABSIs has been a national priority in critical care quality improvement. The CDC has produced a standard measure that defines prevention of these infections as part of the National Healthcare Safety Network's (NHSN) patient safety component protocol.[60]

A typical approach to preventing CLABSIs has been advocated by the IHI and includes four elements of care: proper hand hygiene, use of chlorhexidine for skin antisepsis, routine application of maximal barrier precautions, and optimal site selection. In 2004, Berenholtz and colleagues reported that in using a similar strategy, the rate of CLABSIs fell from 11.3 to 0 per 1000 catheter days.[63] These results were estimated to have prevented 43 catheter-related bloodstream infections, 559 additional days in the ICU, and 8 deaths.[63] Cost savings were estimated to be $1,824,447.[63]

DEPLOYING RAPID RESPONSE TEAMS

The rapid response team (RRT)—sometimes referred to in the literature as a medical emergency team (MET)—is a team of nurses and other health care professionals (respiratory therapists, pharmacists, emergency department personnel, and others) who bring critical care expertise to the bedside. The teams may or may not include physicians. The essential concept is intervening to prevent harm when nursing staff is urgently concerned about a patient's well-being. The key goal is to act before "failure to rescue" occurs and a patient has suffered a cardiac or respiratory arrest.[64]

The evidence supporting RRT adoption is mixed. Nevertheless, many hospitals have detected the need to have such a team to respond to urgent patient issues when physicians or housestaff may not be readily available. Several facilities that have implemented RRTs have reported a reduction in cardiac arrests and deaths, as well as a reduction in ICU and hospital bed days among survivors of cardiac arrest.[65-67] Despite these findings, a single comprehensive negative trial has been published on the effects of MET/RRTs. Eleven hospitals functioned as usual, and 12 introduced a MET system. The investigators concluded that although the introduction of the MET system led to an increase in calls to the team, it did not substantially affect the incidence of cardiac arrest, unplanned ICU admissions, or unexpected death.[68]

RESUSCITATION AND TREATMENT FOR SEVERE SEPSIS OR SEPTIC SHOCK

Unique among projects to improve the quality of care for critically ill patients, the Surviving Sepsis Campaign (SSC) was formed in 2003 with the joint cooperation of the SCCM, the European Society of Intensive Care Medicine (ESICM), and the International Sepsis Forum (ISF). Evidence-based guidelines for the treatment of severe sepsis and septic shock were published in 2004 with an updated version published in 2008 and a second revision scheduled for publication in early 2012.[69,70] Partnering with the IHI, the SSC transformed into a global performance improvement program to extend the campaign guidelines to the bedside.[71] The campaign included the development of sepsis bundles, educational material, recruitment of sites and local physician and nurse champions, launch meetings, and a secure database for data collection and outcome measures. Campaign results from 15,022 subjects at 165 international sites report a significant increase in bundle compliance and unadjusted mortality rate decrease from 37% to 30.8% over a 2-year period.[72]

ESTABLISHING MULTIDISCIPLINARY ROUNDS

Multidisciplinary rounds enable all members of the team caring for critically ill patients to come together formally and offer their expertise as cases in the ICU are reviewed. Multidisciplinary rounds have been established in critical care units with various structures, either nurse-led or physician-led, meeting daily or regularly during the week.

Experience with applying multidisciplinary rounds suggests that although initial meetings may be wide-ranging and unstructured, they can become a vital adjunct to patient care. Specifically, they provide an opportunity for disciplines to share their knowledge of patient care needs and focus the entire care team on common goals. Surveys of institutional perceptions of the state of safety in ICUs have led to the establishment of multidisciplinary rounds.[73] These rounds are a mainstay of the effort to change the culture of ICUs from compartmentalized care based upon a single discipline's knowledge to a more holistic approach integrating the talents of the many services caring for critically ill patients.[74]

ASSESSING DAILY PATIENT GOALS

Daily goals assessment allows all parties involved in the care of patients to formally keep track of plans established on either patient care rounds or multidisciplinary rounds and to verify their completion. This typically has been achieved in critical care units by using a daily goals worksheet completed by the rounding team.

One such tool was evaluated by Johns Hopkins University, the VHA, and the IHI in a prospective study. The tool was designed to facilitate explicit communication in the ICU, allow for independent redundancy to monitor key practices, empower nursing to carry out clear plans, increase nurse morale, and avoid duplicate work. The worksheets aimed to reduce ICU length of stay and mortality rate while increasing the care team's understanding of the daily goals for patients in the ICU. In addition, the worksheets were used to document specific items that must be accomplished for patients to leave the ICU; to identify the greatest safety risk to a particular ICU patient; to institute a reminder system that identifies key processes for patients on ventilators; to document the scheduled laboratory tests for a patient; to compile information about the age, number, and sites of catheters; and to organize daily work flow to include communication with the family.

All patients admitted to a 16-bed surgical oncology ICU were eligible for inclusion. The outcome variables assessed were ICU length of stay and percent of ICU residents and nurses who understood the goals of care for patients in the ICU. Baseline measurements were compared with measurements of understanding after implementation of a daily goals form. At baseline, less than 10% of residents and nurses understood the goals of care for the day. After implementing the daily goals form, greater than 95% of nurses and residents understood the goals of care for the day. After implementation of the ICU Daily Goals Worksheet, ICU length of stay decreased from a mean of 2.2 days to 1.1 days.[75]

PRACTICE MANAGEMENT-CLINICIAN-FAMILY COMMUNICATION

Protocols, guidelines, and toolkits have improved process and outcomes in numerous areas of critical care. Application of these techniques to advance communication with family members of the critically ill are interdependent upon a partnership between clinicians and family members, which is frequently not a recognized goal.[76] Discussions with family members geared toward establishing treatment goals are important in promoting patient-family–centered care.

Clinician-family meetings are intended to share information related to the patient condition and prognosis and for the family to discuss care preference, family concerns, and goals of treatment.[77] Early effective communication with patients and family members is imperative in shared decision making as they are an integral part of the care in the critically ill.

The American College of Critical Care Medicine Task Force 2004 to 2005 recognized the need for clinicians to develop a care plan and partner with patients and family members to improve outcomes.[78] Family members often act as surrogate decision makers for the critically ill, which has been reportedly linked to anxiety, depression, and fatality. Methods to decrease stress include clinicians adapting to the family preference in decision making using a stepwise approach progressing toward improved decision making for the critically ill patient.[76,79]

Clinician-family conferences should be conducted within 72 hours of ICU admission. Preconferences have been suggested to improve the family experience with future conferences. Increased family satisfaction has been reported when clinicians spend more time listening than talking. Clinical-family communication has been summarized in a mnemonic and used as a framework for communication (Box 70.6). As part of an in interventional study reported by Lautrette and associates, application of the VALUE conference approach resulted in significant reduction in family symptoms of anxiety, depression, and posttraumatic stress disorder 90 days after the patient's death.[80] Use of printed information, staff champions, and consulting services are necessary resources to facilitate intensive communication.[81] Documentation of the pertinent conference details and treatment goals are essential to assist future clinician-clinician and clinician-family communication throughout the patient's ICU and hospital stay.

Box 70.6 Value: A Five-Step Approach to Improving Communication in Intensive Care Unit with Families of Deceased Patients

V	Value and appreciate statements by family members.
A	Acknowledge family emotions.
L	Listen to the family.
U	Understand who the patient was as a person.
E	Elicit questions from the family.

From Lautrette A, Darmon M, Megarbane B, et al. A communication strategy and brochure for relatives of patients dying in the ICU. N Engl J Med 22007;356:469-478.

OPEN VERSUS CLOSED INTENSIVE CARE UNITS: INTENSIVIST-LED MODEL

A prime example of a structural change (as in the Donabedian model described earlier) that may lead to improvement in the quality of care includes the establishment of an intensivist-led ICU service in medical ICUs. Although in other ICUs, such as neurosurgical units or pediatric units, it is commonly expected that the attending physician is an intensivist trained in that specialty, this has not been the rule in medical ICUs. Typically, mixed medical-surgical ICUs in the United States are "open" in that any physician on staff may admit patients to the ICU and write orders for care of that patient. A recent well-developed literature suggests that "closed" ICUs in which only medical intensivists care for medical patients may be associated with decreased morbidity and mortality rates and length of stay.[82] Reorganizing ICU physician services in one organization by implementing an intensivist infrastructure has resulted in a 14% absolute risk reduction in mortality.[83]

Despite these findings, a number of barriers exist to adopting a "closed" model of care. These include excess inpatient bed capacity; reimbursement strategies that provide an incentive for nonintensivists to stay involved in ICU care; internal political barriers among the medical staff that hamper closure; and the growth of the hospitalist movement and an associated unwillingness to relinquish control of patients when admitted to the ICU. Some intensivists have adopted a "consultative" model, rather than providing 24-hour patient coverage.[84]

CULTURE TRANSFORMATION AND ORGANIZATIONAL LEARNING

The ultimate goal of clinical quality improvement work of any sort remains that of creating a culture of enduring change that can absorb new initiatives and sustain gains earned in prior improvement efforts. Underscoring the long-term strategy of ICU culture change in describing improvement initiatives cannot be overestimated. If insufficient attention is paid to the context in which improvement efforts are set into motion, an environment unfamiliar with testing changes and hostile to deviations from routine will frustrate the project itself. To this end, as clinical initiatives are advanced, concern must be maintained for executing projects so as to encourage collaboration and cooperation among the persons who work in the ICU. Typically, these strategies involve crafting of change teams, devising and testing protocols to incorporate the concerns of the frontline users of the protocols, and adapting to local cultural needs and traditions while bringing in new ideas. In the course of this work, colleagues cease contemplating their work as discrete projects that can be finalized. Instead, they learn to constantly revise protocols and strategies in response to feedback from the front-line users. If these ideals are maintained in the rollout of key initiatives and structural changes, often a change in mindset from an organization of independent actors to one in which collaborative efforts promote organizational learning can take hold. Unfortunately, to make these cultural transformations gracefully, no scientific procedure is available that can guide the way. The talents of committed and patient people are essential.

KEY POINTS

- Critical care represents a disproportionate share of health care expenditures relative to the proportion of patients who access these services.
- Demand for critical care physician and nursing care will exceed supply in the next 20 years, prompting novel critical care team models.
- Administrative solutions to an emerging critical care crisis are possible and rely on efficiencies that may be obtained in care delivery.
- Market forces and clinicians' drive to provide the best possible care for ICU patients have created a new standard in critical care delivery: quality improvement.
- Multiple interventions have been identified to reduce mortality risk in critical care patients but require consistent performance.
- Optimizing clinician-patient-family communication includes a family meeting within 72 hours using a stepwise approach toward achievement of patient-family–centered goals.

SELECTED REFERENCES

3. Halpern N, Pastores SM: Critical care medicine in the United States 2000-2005: An analysis of bed numbers, occupancy rates, payer mix, and costs. Crit Care Med 2010;38:65-71.
8. Angus DC, Shorr AF, White A, et al: on behalf of the Committee on Manpower for Pulmonary and Critical Care Societies (COMPACCS): Critical care delivery in the United States: Distribution of services and compliance with Leapfrog recommendations. Crit Care Med 2006;34:1016-1024.
11. Barnato A, Kahn JM, Rubenfeld GD, et al: Prioritizing the organization and management of intensive care services in the United States: The PrOMIS conference. Crit Care Med 2007;35: 1103-1111.
21. Guidelines Committee of the American College of Critical Care Medicine, Society of Critical Care Medicine and American Association of Critical-Care Nurses Transfer Guidelines Task Force: Guidelines for the transfer of critically ill patients. Crit Care Med 1993;21:931-937.
30. Bekes CE, Dellinger RP, Brooks D, et al: Critical care medicine as a distinct product line with substantial financial profitability: The role of business planning. Crit Care Med 2004;32:1207-1214.
32. Fisher ES, Bynum JP, Skinner JS: Slowing the growth of health care costs—Lessons from regional variation. N Engl J Med 2012;360: 849-852.
48. Robeznieks A: ICU effort saved lives, money: Organizers. More than 70 hospitals took part in the Keystone: ICU program. Mod Health Care 2005;35:16.
57. Kahn JM: Linking payment to quality-opportunities and challenges for critical care. Am J Respir Crit Care Med 2011;184:491-502.
72. Levy MM, Dellinger RP, Townsend SR, et al: The Surviving Sepsis Campaign: Results of an international guideline-based performance improvement program targeting severe sepsis. Crit Care Med 2010;38(2):367-374.
78. Davidson JE, Powers K, Kedayat KM, et al: Clinical practice guidelines for support of the family in the patient-centered intensive care unit: American College of Critical Care Medicine Task Force 2004-2005. Crit Care Med 2007;35:605-622.

The complete list of references can be found at www.expertconsult.com.

71

Ethical Considerations in Managing Critically Ill Patients

Marion Danis | Emily Bellavance | Henry Silverman

CHAPTER OUTLINE

Critical illnesses and the interventions necessary to address them pose many ethical dilemmas for clinicians. Therefore, it is not surprising that critical care physicians encounter ethical dilemmas more often than do general internists.[1] The most frequent predicaments relate to end-of-life care, including decisions about termination of medical treatment, respect for patient autonomy, and conflicts among various parties involved in patient care. Less frequent quandaries stem from concerns about equitable use of resources, truth telling, religious and cultural differences, and professional conduct. On rare occasions, critical care providers must be prepared to address the extraordinary demands related to disasters because the skills and resources at their command offer key components of a well-organized disaster response.

The first section of this chapter focuses on ethical considerations in the everyday operation of the intensive care unit (ICU). The second section discusses the difficult ethical issues involved in decisions at the end of life. The third section discusses ethical questions involved in research in the ICU. Clinical practice and clinical research are fundamentally distinct enterprises, with different aims and different ethical requirements. In research, the interests of the patient are not the sole priority; but at the same time, the human subjects of ICU research must be protected. The chapter concludes with brief consideration of the ethics of disaster response.

THE DOCTOR-PATIENT RELATIONSHIP

Critical illness stresses the relationship between patients and hospital staff members caring for them. Patients with life-threatening illness often are frightened and feel isolated. Physicians and nurses often must make crucial decisions quickly and despite uncertainty about the consequences of various options. In addition, key decisions frequently must be made while patients are cognitively impaired or unable to communicate. Thus, a combination of the disease process and medical interventions often deprives patients of the power to control their lives.

As a rule, clinicians should follow the same ethical guidance in critical care situations as in less stressful contexts:[2] They should treat patients with respect. They should deal honestly with patients and should not reveal confidences entrusted to them, unless the well-being of others is threatened. They should act in good faith, keep promises and commitments, and try faithfully to meet fiduciary responsibilities to patients.

At the same time, ICU staff must balance competing moral obligations that may limit or override obligations to fidelity to one particular patient, such as the needs of other patients who are currently under their care or may need their care in the future. Various models of decision making have been proposed—ranging from an *informative* model, in which patients make the decisions quite independently after the clinician has offered sufficient information, to a more *paternalistic* model, in which clinicians make decisions based on their judgment of what is in the best interest of the patient.[3] A commonly accepted model today is a *deliberative* model, in which the clinician gives the patient information about his or her condition and the medical options, along with their advantages and disadvantages, and the patient explains his or her values and preferences, and together they reach a treatment decision. This model must be adapted to the extreme circumstance of critical illness.[4,5] Leaders in the field of critical care medicine have endorsed a model of decision making, shared decision making, that recognizes that patients and their surrogates will vary in their desire to participate in decision making, but generally all will feel most comfortable with decisions if they have been given sufficient information to be able to understand and trust the decision process.[6-9]

Clinicians in the ICU should assess each patient's cognitive ability, provide information, and involve the patient or the patient's family in decisions about his or her treatment to the extent feasible.

Most physicians do not follow the same model with every patient or in every encounter. Regardless of the model adopted, clinicians should heed the elements of good ethical practice when making their decisions (Box 71.1). ICU clinicians also should be attentive to the many facets of patients' lives that influence their views and preferences. For example, patients' families play a large role in shaping their experiences and beliefs and in supporting them, particularly when they are sick. Ethicists in North America initially took an approach to patient autonomy that ignored the family, but more recent thought has recognized the importance of the family's supportive role.[10,11]

Clinicians also should be sensitive to the needs of the family when a patient is sick.[12] Among these, according to a survey of family members in ICU waiting rooms, are the need to talk about negative feelings such as guilt and anger; to talk about the possibility of the patient's death; to be told what to expect before they go into the ICU for the first time; to visit at any time; to talk to the same nurse every day; to receive explanations that are understandable; to feel that there is hope; to have good food available in the hospital; to be assured that it is all right to leave the hospital for a while; and to feel accepted by the staff.[13]

Members of the ICU staff also should take note of the religious affiliation and cultural identity of their patients. However, they should not stereotype patients and presume to know what patients want based on their affiliation, but rather should be ready to inquire about each patient's views and should be respectful of diverse beliefs[14,15] (Box 71.2).

Box 71.1 Elements of Good Ethical Practice in Medical Decisions in the Intensive Care Unit

- Careful assessment of the patient's condition
- Evaluation of the risks and benefits of therapeutic options
- Clear communication with the patient or proxy to inform about options and identify plan of care
- Identification and respect for a competent patient's or proxy's preferences
- Plan of care based on clinical assessment and mutually identified goals
- Toleration of uncertainty when making decisions
- Toleration of disagreement between parties
- Ongoing dialogue to resolve difficult situations

COMMUNICATION WITH PATIENTS

From an ethical standpoint, communication is an important component of respect for patients; it is an indispensable ingredient for learning about patients' needs, values, and preferences. Many factors undermine communication with patients and with families in the ICU: insufficient time for staff members and patients to get to know one another and develop a trusting relationship, discomfort or fear of talking about illness and death, focus on the patient's physiologic function, and lack of a conducive setting for communication. However, taking time to talk to patients and families on a daily basis is a crucial element of respectful care.

Often, the ICU clinician must convey bad news. Recommendations for breaking bad news include the following[16]:

- Use a location that is comfortable, quiet, and private.
- Set aside adequate time for discussion.
- Check what the patient or family already knows.
- Give some warning that there will be unfortunate news.
- Let the patient's desire for information guide the discussion.
- Elicit and address the patient's reactions and concerns.
- Foster an appropriate level of hope.
- Be honest, caring, and empathic.

Communication with ventilated patients is particularly difficult. Clinicians should make every effort to use techniques designed to overcome communication barriers with ventilated patients.[17]

DECISION MAKING FOR COGNITIVELY IMPAIRED PATIENTS

Because many patients are, or may become, cognitively impaired, clinicians should frequently and repeatedly assess patients' capacity to understand their situation and make decisions. Judging the capacity of patients to make decisions can be difficult.[18,19] Table 71.1 shows recommendations for assessing the relevant criteria: the ability to communicate a

Box 71.2 Guiding Questions for Attending to Diverse Perspectives of Critically Ill Patients

Language

- What language do the patient and family prefer to use to discuss illness and disease? How openly do they wish to discuss diagnosis, prognosis, and death itself?

Religion

- What is their religious background and how avid is their religious affiliation?
- What do the patient and family think about the sanctity of life, and how do they conceive of death?
- Do they believe in miracles? Do they believe in an afterlife? Do they believe the body should be handled in a certain way after death?

Social, Political, and Historical Context

- Do any of the following factors affect the attitudes of the patient and family: the patient's status in the family, country of origin, or experiences such as poverty, refugee status, past discrimination, or lack of access to care?

Beliefs About Illness

- What do the patient and family believe are the causal agents in illness, and how do these relate to the dying process?

Decision-Making Style

- Who makes decisions about matters of importance in the family?
- Are the patient and family fatalistic about the course of events, or do they wish to take active control of events?

Social Support and Resources

- What resources, including community and religious leaders, family members, and language translators, are available to aid in the complex effort of interpreting cultural dimensions of a patient's illness?

Adapted from Koenig B, Gates-Williams J: Understanding cultural differences in caring for dying patients. West J Med 1995;163: 244-249.

choice, to understand the relevant information, to appreciate the situation and its consequences, and to reason about treatment options. When patients are capable of decision making, they should be involved to the extent that they desire. Patients who have not prepared advance directives should be asked if they would like to prepare such a directive and should be asked to designate someone to hold durable power of attorney for them.

When such a conversation is not possible and no advance directive exists, clinicians should be aware that most states have laws that determine who has legal decision-making status for persons who have not assigned durable powers of attorney. When no family member or other surrogate is available to make decisions on behalf of a decisionally incapacitated patient who needs emergency treatment, the physician in charge should carefully document the pressing necessity for treatment even without consent.

COLLABORATIVE CARE

Care in the ICU is provided by a multidisciplinary team; good collaboration among its members is essential. Paying attention to the perspectives of all team members and respecting their skills and clinical judgment are ethically important and are associated with improved clinical outcomes.[20] Collaboration is valuable not only for individual patients' care but also to achieve optimal function of the unit as a whole.[21]

AVOIDING CONFLICTS IN THE INTENSIVE CARE UNIT

Because of the high stakes and emotional tension surrounding the care of critically ill patients, conflicts often arise among patients, family members, and staff. Strategies for avoiding conflict are worth pursuing because it often is difficult to resolve conflicts once they have arisen.

Conflict avoidance tactics should include the following: giving frequent information to families about patients' status, including realistic assessment of outcomes; acknowledging uncertainty regarding predictions, so that forecasts that do not come to pass are not an undue source of disappointment; coordinating the provision of information among ICU staff members, so that the patient and family receive consistent information about the patient's status and plans for care; and eliciting patient and family concerns.

JUSTICE-RELATED ISSUES

Because critical care is expensive and limited in supply, clinicians should deliver critical care services in a manner that distributes the benefits fairly. Much of the ethics literature has focused attention on making decisions that will allocate critical care resources justly. The issue is one of distributive justice; it arises most frequently when clinicians decide whether to admit or discharge patients from the ICU, and when they face triage decisions during periods in which resources are limited. Less obvious instances obtain whenever a clinician considers whether to use a marginally beneficial intervention.

Several dominant, contending theories of distributive justice provide plausible underpinnings for making such decisions. *Utilitarian* theory is based on the tenet that one should act in a manner that promotes the greatest happiness for the greatest number of people. An act is morally right if it brings about a greater amount of good than any other possible act under the circumstances. Such an assessment is *consequentialist* in that it is based on expected outcome. *Egalitarianism* is another prominent contender. This view holds that all humans are equal and should be treated equally in similar circumstances. *Social contract* theory holds that a just arrangement can be identified by asking rational persons to consider what scheme they would agree to if they had no idea whether or when it might be applied to themselves.

The ethical theory most commonly applied to decisions about admission, discharge, and triage is a utilitarian one. In other words, those patients who are expected to gain the most benefit from intensive care are considered the ones

Table 71.1 Legally Relevant Criteria for Decision-Making Capacity and Approaches to Assessment of the Patient

Criterion	Patient's Task	Physician's Assessment Approach	Questions for Clinical Assessment*	Comments
Communicate a choice	Clearly indicate preferred treatment option	Encourage patient to paraphrase disclosed information regarding medical condition and treatment	*Have you decided whether to follow your doctor's (or my) recommendations for treatment?* *Can you tell me what that decision is?* If no decision, *What is making it hard for you to decide?*	Frequent reversals of choice due to psychiatric or neurologic conditions may indicate lack of capacity.
Understand the relevant information	Grasp fundamental meaning of information communicated by physician	Encourage patient to paraphrase disclosed information regarding medical condition and treatment	*Please tell me in your own words what your doctor (or I) told you about:* • *the problem with your health now* • *the recommended treatment* • *the possible benefits and risks (or discomforts) of the treatment* • *any alternative treatments and their risks and benefits* • *the risks and benefits of no treatment*	Information to be understood includes nature of patient's condition, nature and purpose of proposed treatment, possible benefits and risks of that treatment, and alternative approaches (including no treatment) and their benefits and risks.
Appreciate the situation and its consequences	Acknowledge medical condition and likely consequences of treatment options	Ask patient to describe views of medical condition, proposed treatment, and likely outcomes	*What do you believe is wrong with your health now?* *Do you believe that that you need some kind of treatment?* *What is the treatment likely to do for you?* *What makes you believe it will have that effect?* *What do you believe will happen if you are not treated?* *Why do you think your doctor has (or I have) recommended this treatment?*	Courts have recognized that patients who do not acknowledge their illnesses (often referred to as "lack of insight") cannot make valid decisions about treatment. Delusions or pathologic levels of distortion or denial are the most common causes of impairment.
Reason about treatment options	Engage in rational process of manipulating the relevant information	Ask patient to compare treatment options and consequences and to offer reasons for selection of option	*How did you decide to accept or reject the recommended treatment?* *What makes* (chosen option) *better than* (rejected option)?	This criterion focuses on the process by which a decision is reached, not the outcome of the patient's choice, because patients have the right to make "unreasonable" choices.

*Responses need not be verbal.

From Appelbaum PS: Assessment of patients' competence to consent to treatment. N Engl J Med 2007;357:1834-1840.

who should receive it. Accordingly, patients who are so severely ill that they are likely to die despite intervention and patients who are so minimally sick that intensive care will not add to the likelihood of their survival should not be admitted to ICU. Patients whose conditions are chronic and devastating, such as those in a permanent vegetative state, often are included among patients who should not receive intensive care for any acute life-threatening events, because their underlying illnesses are not amenable to improvement.

Of interest, Baker and Strosberg have argued that the assumption that triage is based on a utilitarian theory of justice is not correct.[22] They point out that triage was developed by Larrey, surgeon general of Napoleon's army, as a strategy for systematically handling the wounded so that those who had to be attended to first got care without regard to rank, in keeping with the French Revolutionary commitment to liberty, equality, and fraternity. Baker and Strosberg suggest that an egalitarian form of triage is advantageous because the public is likely to voluntarily comply with it. Persons with normal "rational self-interest" would agree with it because it improves everyone's chances of survival. The chances of survival of the fatally wounded and the slightly wounded would not be significantly altered by deferred treatment. This optimal arrangement thus also is compatible with a social contract theory of justice.[23]

Although triage strategies have relied on the probability of survival, some authors have argued that this is too crude an outcome measure to guide triage. Engelhardt and Rie have suggested that critical decisions to admit, continue care, or discharge patients should be based on a more complete formula that includes probability of successful outcome, quality of life, predicted length of life remaining, and cost of therapy.[24]

ADMISSION CRITERIA

The Task Force on Guidelines of the Society of Critical Care Medicine (SCCM) and the American College of Critical Care Medicine (ACCM) have published recommendations for ICU admission and discharge.[25,26] Each ICU should create a specific policy that explicitly articulates admission and discharge criteria and defines the services that it provides to the population served. Compliance with the policy should be monitored, and the policy should be revised as needed. Any decision to deny a patient admission should be made by clinicians who are familiar with expert opinion and relevant literature and should use established guidelines. Standardized criteria and guidelines facilitate fair rationing because they enhance the likelihood that patients will be treated similarly.

DISCHARGE CRITERIA

Discharge decisions should be guided by an assessment that less care is necessary and should take patient safety into account. Decisions to transfer a patient from the ICU to other hospital facilities should always be accompanied by good communication with the receiving team to avoid oversights and errors in care.[27] Straightforward indications would include, at one extreme, improvement in medical condition that obviates the need for further intensive therapy or, at the other extreme, a decision to end intensive care because of impending death. The ethically challenging aspect of discharge criteria involves the question of discharge when a patient's probability of survival is expected to be only minimally improved by remaining in the ICU, but the probability is not zero.

TRIAGE

Triage decisions should be made explicitly and without bias. Ethnicity, race, gender, social status, sexual preference, and financial status should not be considered.[26] Factors that are appropriate to consider include probability of survival; likely functional outcome; age; chronic underlying conditions; marginal benefit to be gained; and preferences expressed by the patient or surrogate.[28] When the ICU is full, patients already in the ICU should not necessarily be given priority if someone else stands to benefit more from the care.[29] Like many ethically difficult decisions, triage decisions can be made more manageable by thinking proactively, every day, about the disposition of patients. For example, ICU physicians should regularly review the status of all patients in the unit to assess their degree of readiness for discharge in case the need for new admissions arises.[27] Application of this kind of strategy should involve cooperation with other patient care units in the hospital to arrange smooth transfer.

Even when policies are in place for fair triage through an admission approval process by a designated individual, attempts to circumvent admission rules by seeking permission from ICU clinicians or administrators who are on duty in the ICU are fairly common.[30] Therefore, policies should be designed to anticipate—and resist—such backdoor efforts.

In addition to decisions about admission, discharge, and triage, ICU physicians frequently must deal with the question of whether to offer or withhold treatments from patients with ultimately fatal injuries or illnesses. The ethical reasoning behind decisions to ration possibly beneficial interventions should be clear in the clinician's mind[31]; this issue is discussed more fully later in the section on termination of medical care.

Because expected benefit is a crucial factor in decision making, it is important for critical care physicians to understand the limits of prognostic guidelines for patients with life-threatening illnesses.[32] Physicians should recognize the degree of uncertainty that surrounds mortality estimates. Although it is useful to consider a patient's expected outcome, and to use this prognosis to guide decisions, a false sense of certainty can lead to mistakes. Furthermore, communicating prognostic information with a false sense of certainty can lead to misunderstanding and subsequent distrust on the part of families. Prognostic scoring systems can serve as a useful baseline on which to build treatment recommendations, but firm thresholds should not be set. For a patient with a very uncertain prognosis, trying different treatments for short periods can avoid extended inappropriate treatments without denying care that has a minute chance of working. Medical decision making requires more than functional assessment and prediction. Scoring systems can provide an unbiased measure to help inform physicians' decisions, but such measures should not be adopted as absolute guides.[32]

DISPARITY IN USE AND OUTCOME OF INTENSIVE CARE

Critical care clinicians should be aware that a number of studies show a pattern of disparity in use of intensive care that is the result of forces outside the ICU itself. Patients of lower socioeconomic status have higher mortality rates.[33] Patients who lack health insurance are less likely to be admitted to hospitals; once hospitalized, however, they are more likely to be admitted to the ICU and more likely to die in the hospital.[34] Patients with private attending physicians are likely to stay longer in the ICU. Intensive care providers should try to prevent inequitable use of resources in the delivery of critical care services.

ETHICS CONSULTATION IN THE INTENSIVE CARE UNIT

In view of the many ethical dilemmas that arise in the ICU, proactive ethics consultation can be useful for reducing conflicts over treatment and for planning wise use of resources, as supported by good evidence.[35]

THE ETHICS OF END-OF-LIFE CARE

The contemporary practice of critical care medicine includes consideration of the ethical issues surrounding end-of-life care including the definition of death, the ethical justification and legal precedent for withdrawing and withholding treatment, the concept of futility in administering treatments, and ethical issues in transitioning a patient to palliative care.

DEFINING DEATH

Given the emphasis on life and death decisions in intensive care, it is prudent for the critical care practitioners to be aware of the many philosophical questions surrounding the definition of death.[36] In any consideration of the definition of death, it is useful to recognize that death is more of a process than an instantaneous event and that the boundary between life and death is not perfectly sharp. The specification of any standard will require some arbitrary line drawing that has ethical implications.[36]

Historically, death has been defined both legally and medically as the moment at which cardiac and respiratory function has irreversibly stopped. This definition of death has been termed the cardiopulmonary standard of death. The concept of using neurologic criteria to establish death did not emerge until the 1960s with the advent of mechanical ventilation, which allowed for circulation of oxygenated blood in the absence of brainstem function and called into question whether the cardiopulmonary criteria for determining death were sufficient for all patients. Advances in cadaveric organ transplantation also stimulated the question of whether separate neurologic criteria should be determined for death, which would allow the procurement of viable organs from patients meeting a separate set of neurologic criteria.

In 1968, the Ad Hoc Committee of the Harvard Medical School to Examine the Definition of Brain Death determined that severely brain injured patients meeting certain diagnostic criteria could be declared dead prior to the cessation of cardiopulmonary function.[37] The use of neurologic criteria to determine death was subsequently accepted by some states in the United States. However, confusion remained with regard to what constituted "brain death"; specifically whether total brain nonfunction or brainstem nonfunction sufficiently fulfilled neurologic criteria for death. In response to the variability in state statutes regarding brain death, the President's Commission for the Study of Ethical Problems in Medicine published a uniform statute for determining brain death, called the Uniform Determination of Death Act (UDDA). According to the UDDA, "an individual who has sustained either 1) irreversible cessation of circulatory and respiratory function or 2) irreversible cessation of all functions of the entire brain, including the brainstem is dead. A determination of death must be made in accordance with accepted medical standards."[38]

The ethical justification for using neurologic criteria to determine death relies on the presumption that in brain death, the body of the patient is no longer "a somatically integrated whole" and that in the absence of whole brain function, maintaining circulation, even with cardiorespiratory support, will stop imminently within a defined period of time.[39]

Recently the use of brain death criteria has been questioned in the medical and bioethical community. Opponents of using brain death criteria cite the uncertainty in determining physiologic death by neurologic parameters. There is evidence that even in the setting of whole brain death many homeostatic functions can persist, including maintenance of body temperature, wound healing, the gestation of a fetus in a pregnant patient, and sexual maturation and growth in pediatric patients who fulfill the neurologic criteria for death.[40] In addition, cardiopulmonary death does not always occur in a timely fashion after brain death and in rare cases may take weeks or years to occur after brain death has been declared.[41] Notably, arguments against neurologic standards of death do not preclude the ethical permissibility of withdrawing supportive care when the criteria of brain death have been met, but question whether these criteria alone constitute the death of the patient.

In response to concerns regarding brain death as a legitimate determinant of human death, the President's Council on Bioethics revisited the philosophical and clinical dilemmas surrounding this issue in 2008.[39] The council's ultimate conclusions were to support neurologic criteria of brain death with an alternative argument regarding defining death as the inability of the organism to function as "a somatically integrated whole." Rather, "total brain failure" constitutes death as the patient, "is no longer able to carry out the fundamental work of a living organism. Such a patient has lost—and lost irreversibly—a fundamental openness to the surrounding environment as well as the capacity and drive to act on this environment on his or her own behalf . . . a living organism engages in self-sustaining, need-driven activities critical to and constitutive of its commerce with the surrounding world. These activities are authentic signs of active ongoing life. When these signs are absent, and these activities have ceased, then a judgment that the organism as a whole has died can be made with confidence."

Currently all 50 states and the District of Columbia have adopted the UDDA definition of brain death by statute or judicial decision. Two states, New Jersey and New York, have specific laws or regulations to address religious objections to neurologically based declarations of death.[42] Similarly, over 90 countries use neurologic criteria to determine death in addition to traditional cardiopulmonary criteria.[43] The cultural variability in accepting neurologic criteria to determine brain death is exemplified in the organ transplant laws in China and Japan. In 2003, the Chinese Ministry of Public Health drafted a proposal to outline neurologic criteria that would define death in the absence of cardiopulmonary arrest. However, legislation approving the use of brain death criteria was not endorsed, lacking support from the public and health care professionals.[43] Prior to 2010, Japan's Organ Transplant Law only recognized brain death when the patient had given prior written consent to be an organ donor and the family did not object to the donation. This law has since been revised to allow a determination of death based on neurologic criteria for the purposes of organ donation with family consent so long as the donor did not previously refuse organ donation. However, the revision still does not address whether neurologic criteria for death are sufficient in the absence of an anticipated organ donation.[44]

WITHHOLDING AND WITHDRAWING LIFE-SUSTAINING TREATMENT

The first suggestion that physicians should withhold medical interventions from terminally ill patients probably dates to Hippocrates's injunction to "refuse to treat those [patients] who are overmastered by their disease, realizing that in such cases medicine is powerless."[45] In 1835, Jacob Bigelow urged members of the Massachusetts Medical Society to withhold "therapies"—such as cathartics and emetics—from hopelessly ill patients.[46] In 1848, John Warren, the surgeon who performed the first operation with ether anesthesia, urged that ether should be used "in mitigating the agonies of death."[47] In 1958, Pope Pius XII, in response to questions about resuscitating patients and maintaining comatose patients on respirators, stated that physicians had no obligation to use such "extraordinary" means to forestall death.[48] The concept that the mere extension of life is not always in the best interest of the patient is perhaps even more apparent in current times, when advances in medical technology have led to the seemingly indefinite prolongation of the lives of the critically and terminally ill.[49]

Many physicians find withdrawing life-sustaining treatment more difficult than withholding treatment. However, from a bioethical perspective, there is little distinction between withholding and withdrawing life-sustaining treatments.[50] Competent patients have the right to refuse medical care and can use whatever criteria they deem acceptable; it is their values that guide the choice.[51] Every medical intervention, including artificial nutrition and hydration, may be terminated under some conditions.

The right to refuse medical interventions, including life-sustaining treatment, is supported by legal precedent (Table 71.2). Court decisions have sanctioned the withholding or withdrawal of respirators, chemotherapy, blood transfusions, hemodialysis, and major surgical operations. In its 1990 *Cruzan* decision, the U.S. Supreme Court recognized that competent patients have a constitutional right to refuse medical care.[52]

Competent patients need not be terminally ill to exercise the right to refuse interventions; they have the right regardless of health status. Moreover, the right applies both to withholding proposed treatments and to discontinuing initiated treatments. This does not, however, imply that patients have a correlative right to demand treatment.[53,54]

In theory, the right of patients to refuse medical therapy can be limited by state interests in the preservation of life, prevention of suicide, protection of third parties such as children, and preservation of the integrity of the medical profession.[54] In practice, these interests almost never override the rights of competent patients or of incapacitated patients who have left explicit advance directives.

ADVANCE CARE DIRECTIVES AND DURABLE POWERS OF ATTORNEY

Most patients at the end of life will have lost decision-making ability due to medical or cognitive incapacity. Advance care directives or appointed surrogate decision makers with instructions regarding the patient's wishes serve as a critical resource in preserving patient autonomy in end-of-life care.

There are two types of advance care planning documents: living wills and proxy statements. *Living wills* or instructional directives are advisory documents specifying the patient's preferences to specific care decisions. State-specific forms that people can fill in to draw up advance directives are available on the Internet.[55] Some advance directives, such as the Medical Directive, enumerate different scenarios and interventions for the patient to choose from.[56] Among these, some are for general use and others are designed for use by patients with a specific disease, such as cancer.[57] Less specific directives can be general statements of not wanting life-sustaining interventions or forms that describe the values that should guide specific terminal care decisions. Of importance, a person does not have to use a state-specific form because "a living will or health care power of attorney that does not strictly follow the statutory [state] form is also valid in most states" and the U.S. Supreme Court has ruled that a person has a constitutional right to refuse medical treatments.[58] Practitioners should be aware that living wills may have some legal limitations. For instance, in 25 states, a living will is not valid if a woman is pregnant; specific state statutes should be reviewed in caring for a pregnant patient.

The health care *proxy statement*, sometimes called a durable power of attorney for health care, specifies a person selected by the patient to make decisions. A combined directive includes both instructions and the designation of a proxy; the directive should clearly indicate whether the specified patient preferences or the proxy's choice should take precedence if they conflict.[56]

Many states permit clear and explicit verbal statements to be legally binding even if not written down.[58] However, such statements must be very explicit. In the *Wendland* case, a

Table 71.2 Major Legal Cases Regarding the Withholding or Withdrawing of Medical Interventions

Case and Citation	Year	State	Facts	Decision
In re Quinlan, 70 N.J. 10	1976	NJ	A 21-year-old woman in a persistent vegetative state was dependent on a respirator, artificial nutrition, and hydration.	The right to privacy includes a right to refuse medical care and extends to incompetent patients. Patient's guardian can withdraw her respirator. No need for judicial review in most cases.
Superintendent of Belchertown v. Saikewicz, 373 Mass. 728	1977	MA	A 67-year-old retarded man with a mental age of 2 years 8 months who had always lived in a state institution developed acute myelomonocytic leukemia. Did he have to receive chemotherapy?	All persons, including incompetent persons, have the right to refuse medical treatment. Using substituted judgment, the court determined that the patient would not want chemotherapy.
In re Eichner (Brother Fox), 52 N.Y.2d 262	1981	NY	An 83-year-old priest was in a persistent vegetative state after a cardiac arrest. Before the event, he had publicly stated that he would not want to be respirator-dependent if he were vegetative.	Patients have the right to determine the course of their own medical care. Patient's wishes were known, even if not expressed in writing. Respirator should be withdrawn.
In re Conroy, 98 N.J. 321	1985	NJ	An 84-year-old bedridden, totally impaired woman with organic brain syndrome was being fed by a nasogastric tube. Her nephew requested removal of the tube.	Nasogastric tube feedings are medical interventions that can be withdrawn.
Brophy v. New England Sinai Hospital, 398 Mass. 417	1986	MA	A 49-year-old man in a persistent vegetative state after a ruptured aneurysm was maintained by gastric tube feedings. He had no written living will but had explicitly stated that he would never want to live on life support systems.	Common law and the constitutional right of privacy give a person the right to refuse medical treatment. The patient's wishes are clearly known from explicit conversations. The gastric tube can be withdrawn.
Bouvia v. Superior Court, 225 Cal. Rptr. 297	1986	CA	A 29-year-old mentally competent woman with cerebral palsy that left her almost completely immobile and totally unable to care for herself requested that a nasogastric tube to supplement her inadequate oral intake be withdrawn.	The patient has the "right to refuse any medical treatment even that which may save or prolong her life."
In re Jobes, 108 N.J. 394	1987	NJ	A 32-year-old woman in a permanent vegetative state was receiving J-tube feedings. Her husband and parents request withdrawal of the feedings. She left no clear written or verbal indication of her wishes.	Incompetent patients have the right to refuse medical care even if they have left no clear indication of their wishes. Using substituted judgment the family can exercise her right to withdraw the J-tube feedings.
Cruzan v. Director of Missouri Department of Health, 110 S. Ct. 2841	1990	U.S.	A 33-year-old woman in a persistent vegetative state was maintained by gastric tube nutrition and hydration. Her parents requested that these tube feedings be terminated.	Voting 8 to 1, the Supreme Court ruled that patients have a constitutional right to refuse medical care and that this applies to artificial nutrition and hydration. If there was no clear and convincing written or oral statement of the patient's wishes, states could regulate how families exercise the right.
In re Helga Wanglie, Fourth Judicial District PX-91–283, Minnesota (Hennepin County)	1991	MN	An 85-year-old woman in a persistent vegetative state was maintained on a respirator. After months, physicians suggested withdrawal of life-sustaining treatment because the patient was receiving no benefit. The family refused withdrawal.	The husband should represent the patient's interests, and his refusal to discontinue the respirator is binding.

Table 71.2 Major Legal Cases Regarding the Withholding or Withdrawing of Medical Interventions (Continued)

Case and Citation	Year	State	Facts	Decision
Wendland v. Wendland, 110 Cal. Rptr. 2d 412	2001	CA	A 42-year-old conscious man with severe cognitive impairments, hemiparesis, and limited communication who was not terminally ill required a feeding tube. The feeding tube fell out and needed to be replaced. After authorizing replacement of the feeding tube three times, wife refused replacement.	Patients have a right to refuse all medical treatments including life-sustaining treatments. This right can be exercised for mentally incompetent patients through advance care directives. For patients who are terminally ill, in a persistent vegetative state, or comatose who have not completed an advance care directive, proxies who have not been formally appointed can terminate interventions. However, for mentally incompetent but conscious patients, "clear and convincing" evidence of the patient's wishes is needed before life-sustaining treatment can be stopped.
In re guardianship of Schiavo, No. 90–20–8GD-003, 2000 WL 34546715 (Fla. Cir. Ct. Feb. 11, 2000)	2005	FL	In February 1990, Terri Schiavo collapsed in her apartment. She was resuscitated but left in a persistent vegetative state not requiring a respirator but receiving artificial nutrition and hydration. Many attempts were made to rehabilitate her, including thalamic stimulation. In May 1998, her husband filed a motion to remove the nasogastric tube. This engendered conflict between her husband and her parents. Her parents claimed she would not want feedings ended and that her husband should not be the guardian. In 2000, a judge heard the case about her medical condition and wishes, and who should be her guardian. The judge ruled she was in a persistent vegetative state, her husband could make decisions for her, and she made oral declarations indicating she would not want to be kept alive in a persistent vegetative state. In 2003, Florida legislature passed "Terri's Law" to give the governor power to intervene. Over 7 years, 14 appeals and 5 suits in Federal District Court led to removal and reinsertion of the feeding tube three times. In March 2005, the feeding tube was removed and Terri Schiavo died.	Terri Schiavo's husband is the rightful guardian, there is oral evidence of patient's wishes, and based on her wishes, her husband has the authority to make the decision to remove the feeding tube. Terri's Law violates the Florida constitution.

42-year-old man suffered permanent brain damage and hemiparesis in a car accident.[59] The California Supreme Court ruled that when the patient is conscious and there is no advance care directive, there must be "clear and convincing" evidence of the patient's view in order to permit withdrawal of a feeding tube.[59] "Clear and convincing" evidence requires prior comments to refer to the specific intervention in the specific circumstances of the patient, not a similar health state.

In 1984, California passed the first law recognizing the appointment of a designated proxy for health care decisions; by 2007, all 50 states and the District of Columbia had enacted statutes recognizing the durable power of attorney for health care decisions. There are some limitations. For instance, although most states permit proxies to terminate life-sustaining treatments, Alaska prohibits such decisions by proxies. In other states, orally appointed proxies are limited to a particular hospitalization or episode of illness.

Nevertheless, it appears that any properly filled-out, formal advance care document or durable power of attorney designation, whether or not it conforms to a state's specific document, is protected by the U.S. Constitution and must be honored.[52]

Although advance directives can be helpful in guiding clinicians and family members, many patients have not prepared them. Despite polling data showing that approximately 80% of Americans endorse the use of advance directives, and passage in 1990 of the federal Patient Self-Determination Act (PSDA), which requires hospitals and other health care facilities to inform patients about their right to complete an advance care directive, less than 30% of the adult population in the United States has a formally prepared advance directive.[60] The use of advance care directives may be more prevalent in older adults. Silveira and colleagues used data from the Health and Retirement Study to survey the proxies of patients 60 years and older who had died between 2000 and 2006 and found that approximately 47% of these patients had advance directives.[61]

However, even when advance care directives have been prepared, they frequently are not in the patient's medical record, and the patient's physician may not be aware of the existence or content of the document.[62,63] In addition, recent studies suggest that most advance directives are either proxy forms or standard living wills, and that few have any specific directions from the patient.[64] Finally, studies confirm that proxies and family members tend to be poorly informed about patients' wishes regarding end-of-life care and therefore are unlikely to make decisions as the patient would.[65,66] Even if specific treatment courses are outlined, these directives may be outdated as preferences change with time or the patient's medical condition evolves. Ideally, advance directives should be revisited with the patient over time with family members or a physician with whom the patient has a long-term relationship.

For mentally incapacitated patients who appointed a surrogate decision maker but did not give specific indications of their wishes, or who never completed an advance care directive, four guiding decision criteria have been proposed: (1) futility of treatment, (2) the ordinary versus extraordinary care distinction, (3) substituted judgment, and (4) best interests.

FUTILE TREATMENTS

In the late 1980s and early 1990s, some argued that physicians could ethically terminate futile treatments.[67] However, citing medial futility as an ethical and legal justification for the withdrawal of life-sustaining treatments is not a clear-cut endeavor and has been criticized as inadvisable.[68,69] The term *futility* carries both quantitative and qualitative meanings. There is little, if any, agreement among health care professionals as to what numeric threshold of probability should be considered an indication of futility. Medical futility also has a qualitative aspect that implies that the objective of the proposed treatment is not worthwhile.[42] The qualitative definition of futility can be especially problematic when patients or their surrogate decision makers disagree with physicians about what constitutes a worthwhile outcome. In addition, a declaration by clinicians that a treatment is futile can marginalize patients and surrogates by effectively revoking their participation in treatment decisions. Thus, the ambiguities in defining medical futility and the potential for alienation of patients and family members have led some bioethicists to propose that the term futility be replaced by the terms "medically inappropriate" or "surgically inappropriate" to more accurately describe an assessment that reflects a professional opinion rather than a summation of value.[70]

Nonetheless, some states including Texas, Virginia, Maryland, and California have enacted so-called medical futility laws.[71] These laws protect physicians from liability if they terminate life-sustaining treatments against family wishes. In Texas, if the medical team and the hospital ethics committee believe that interventions should be terminated, but the patient's family disagrees, the hospital is supposed to seek another institution willing to provide treatment.[71] If, after 10 days, this fails, then the hospital and the physician may unilaterally withdraw treatments determined to be futile; however, the family may appeal to a state court. Early data suggest that the law increases futility consultations with the ethics committee, and that most families concur with withdrawal decision.[71]

Some hospitals have enacted "unilateral DNR" (do not resuscitate) policies to allow clinicians to provide a DNR order in cases in which consensus cannot be reached with families and there is medical opinion that resuscitation would not affect a patient's outcome. Because the ethical justification for unilateral DNR relies on the medical assessment that resuscitation efforts will not achieve the desired outcome (i.e., resuscitation is futile) the unilateral DNR remains a controversial policy. If a unilateral DNR is being considered by a physician, a second opinion by another physician and a hospital ethics committee consultation should be considered.[42]

"Partial codes" and "slow codes" describe resuscitation efforts that are selective or foreshortened in the setting in which the medical team believes resuscitation efforts to be inappropriate and the patient's family or proxy will not agree to a recommended DNR order. Slow codes have been historically almost universally repudiated in the bioethics community. The American College of Physicians Ethics Manual cautions against slow codes as "deceptive, half-hearted resuscitation efforts."[72] Ultimately slow and partial codes threaten the ethical principles of autonomy and beneficence. By neither attempting a full resuscitation nor invoking a unilateral DNR, the patient's or surrogate's decision is disregarded while administering a nonbeneficial treatment. However, more recently Lantos and Meadow have defended the practice of partial and slow codes when communication has been exhausted and intractable disagreements about cardiopulmonary resuscitation (CPR) persist.[73-75] Supporters of the slow or partial code cite the symbolic value of CPR and delineate specific circumstances in which such a limited code would be ethically permissible such as when resuscitation will almost certainly be ineffective, the surrogate decision makers understand that death is inevitable, and the surrogates "cannot bring themselves to agree to a do-not-resuscitate order."[73] When compared to enforcing a unilateral DNR on a surrogate or family member, such a compromise may be a more compassionate option for those responsible for making a decision on DNR status. However, arguments supporting limited resuscitation are almost always focused exclusively on the welfare of the surrogates, rather than the patient under the physician's care. Therefore, slow and partial codes should not be considered an acceptable practice in the care of critically ill patients.

ORDINARY/EXTRAORDINARY CARE

Following Pope Pius XII's and Roman Catholic teachings, some ethicists advocate a distinction between ordinary and extraordinary care: Ordinary care is considered to be mandatory, whereas extraordinary care may be withheld or withdrawn.[48] One commentator for the Catholic Hospital Association explained this distinction as follows:

> *Ordinary* means of preserving life are all medicines, treatments, and operations, which offer a reasonable hope of benefit for the patient and which can be obtained and used without excessive expense, pain, or inconvenience. . . . *Extraordinary* means of preserving life mean all medicines, treatments, and operations, which cannot be obtained without excessive expense, pain, or other inconvenience, or which, if used, would not offer reasonable hope of benefit.[76]

Many ethicists and courts have concluded that this distinction is too vague and has "too many conflicting meanings" to be helpful in guiding surrogate decision makers and physicians.[53,54,77,78] As one lawyer noted, ordinary and extraordinary are "extremely fact-sensitive, relative terms. . . . What is ordinary for one patient under particular circumstances may be extraordinary for the same patient under different circumstances, or for a different patient under the same circumstances."[78] Thus, the ordinary versus extraordinary distinction should not be used to justify decisions about stopping treatment.[54]

SUBSTITUTED JUDGMENT

The standard of substituted judgment is based on preserving the patient's right of self-determination in the absence of decisional capacity. Many courts advocate use of the substituted judgment criterion. Substituted judgment holds that the surrogate decision maker should try to imagine what the patient would do if the patient were competent.[77] That is, the surrogate should try to "ascertain the incompetent person's actual interests and preferences" and to make the decision that "would be made by the incompetent person, if that person were competent."[79]

An emphasis on substituted judgment when counseling patients' surrogates in end-of-life care can sometimes help alleviate feelings of overwhelming responsibility and guilt if the decision is to proceed with withdrawal or withholding life-sustaining treatments. Similarly, in scenarios in which family members of the patient disagree on end-of-life decisions, focusing the conversation on what the patient would have wanted can, at times, help to resolve controversies.

In the absence of specific guidance from the patient, substituted judgment involves surmising what a patient would want, rather than a guaranteed fulfillment of the patient's wishes.[54,80] Of note, patients who were surveyed varied regarding the extent to which they want families to strictly adhere to their personal wishes in making end-of-life decisions on their behalf.[81]

BEST INTERESTS

The best-interests criterion holds that treatment decisions should be made based on balancing benefits and risks and should select those treatments in which the benefits maximally outweigh the burdens of treatment.[53,54] When the patient's wishes are truly unknown or cannot be inferred, the best-interests standard should take precedent.

For the best-interests standard to work, there must be some "objective, societally shared criteria" about what constitutes benefits and burdens.[82] However, as is made clear by many court cases involving conflict between family members, or between family members and the medical team, no objective way of determining benefits and burdens, and how they should be balanced, has been recognized. One court suggested that burdens should be determined solely by levels of pain.[53] However, many people consider a permanent vegetative state to be a serious burden that they want to avoid, even if they do not feel pain. In the absence of an objective best-interests standard, families largely decide what constitutes a benefit or burden from their estimation of a patient's personal values.

As a matter of practice, physicians rely on family members to make decisions that they feel are best and only object if these decisions seem to demand treatments that the physician considers nonbeneficial. Without a perfect solution to the problems raised by proxy decision making, this approach may be the most reasonable one in difficult circumstances.

ETHICAL ISSUES IN TRANSITIONING PATIENTS TO PALLIATIVE CARE

Critical care clinicians have a particularly challenging responsibility when taking care of patients whose chances of survival are uncertain. Under such circumstances, clinicians need to understand how to use prediction tools such as the Acute Physiology and Chronic Health Evaluation (APACHE) tool or the Simplified Acute Physiology Score (SAPS) system, or SAPS II, to estimate the likelihood of survival. Awareness of the limited predictive ability of these tools is important for the ICU physician, who at the same time will use them to trigger decisions and interventions as part of a systematic approach to improving care.[83]

Although prognosis is uncertain, clinicians are advised to attend to the dual goals of prolonging life and palliating symptoms. As a patient's prognosis becomes increasingly worse, consideration needs to be given to withholding or withdrawing life-sustaining treatments. Useful guidelines for withdrawing life support are shown in Box 71.3.

Because decisions to limit life support should be shared with patients or their families, clinicians should be familiar with the important components of discussing these decisions. These components are summarized in Box 71.4.

Critically ill patients require relief of symptoms regardless of their prognosis. Once a patient is thought to be dying, the focus of care increasingly shifts away from combined efforts to prolong life and palliate symptoms to more exclusive focus on palliative care. Critical care clinicians should aim to deliver high-quality palliative care (Box 71.5).

When the decision is made to withdraw treatment and focus on comfort care, necessary palliative interventions to

Box 71.3 Guiding Principles of Withdrawing Life Support

1. The goal of withdrawing life-sustaining treatment is to remove treatments that are no longer desired or do not provide comfort to the patient.
2. The withholding of life-sustaining treatments is morally and legally equivalent to their withdrawal.
3. Actions with the sole goal of hastening death are morally and legally problematic.
4. Any treatment can be withheld or withdrawn.
5. Withdrawal of life-sustaining treatment is a medical procedure.
6. *Corollary to principles 1 and 2*: When circumstances justify withholding a life-sustaining treatment, consideration should be given to withdrawing current life-sustaining treatment.

From Rubenfeld GD, Gordon SW: Principles and practice of withdrawing life-sustaining treatments in the ICU. In Curtis JR, Rubenfeld GD (eds): Managing Death in the Intensive Care Unit. New York, Oxford University Press, 2001.

Box 71.4 Components of a Discussion about End-of-Life Care in the Intensive Care Unit

Making Preparations before a Discussion about End-of-Life Care

Review previous knowledge about the patient and family.
Review previous knowledge about the patient's attitudes and reactions.
Review your knowledge of the disease—prognosis, treatment options.
Review your own personal feelings, attitudes, biases, and grief reactions.
Plan the location and setting: a quiet, private place.
Have advance discussion with the family about who will be present.

Holding a Discussion about End-of-Life Care in the Intensive Care Unit

Introduce everyone present.
If appropriate, set the tone in a nonthreatening way: "This is a discussion I have with all my patients."
Find out what the patient and family understand.
Find out how much the patient and family want to know.
Be aware that some patients do not want to discuss end-of-life care.
Discuss prognosis frankly in a way that is meaningful to the patient.
Do not discourage all hope.
Avoid temptation to give too much medical detail.
Make it clear that withholding life-sustaining treatment is not withholding caring.
Use repetition to show that you understand what the patient or family member is saying.
Acknowledge strong emotions and use reflection to encourage patients or families to talk about their emotions.
Tolerate silence.

Finishing a Discussion of End-of-Life Care in the Intensive Care Unit

Achieve common understanding of the disease and treatment issues.
Make a recommendation about treatment.
Ask if there are any questions.
Ensure that a basic follow-up plan is in place, and make sure the patient or appropriate family member knows how to reach you for questions.

Modified from Curtis JR, Patrick DL: How to discuss dying and death in the ICU. In Curtis JR, Rubenfeld GD (eds): Managing Death in the Intensive Care Unit. New York, Oxford University Press, 2001.

relieve pain, alleviate air hunger, or assuage anxiety may cause the unintended effect of hastening death. The doctrine of double effect provides the ethical justification for providing care that may have harmful effects. This principle relies on the distinction between an intended versus a foreseen but unintended effect of treatment[50]. There are a number of critics of this doctrine[84]; some opponents of the doctrine of double effect deny that the distinction between intended and merely foreseen consequences has moral significance. Regardless of whether one relies on this doctrine, most clinicians and medical ethicists endorse the view that if the goals of care have shifted to alleviating symptoms of pain and discomfort, administering interventions to achieve these goals is ethically and legally permissible even if doing so results in hastening the patient's death.

PALLIATIVE SEDATION

Palliative sedation is a controversial practice in part due to the lack of a consistent definition. Administering sedatives to a dying patient in a titrated fashion for the purposes of specific symptom relief is an accepted practice in palliative care. However, the term palliative sedation has also been used to describe the practice of providing continuous sedation to the dying patient for the purposes of maintaining a sustained level of unconsciousness. In 2008, the American Medical Association (AMA) condoned the use of palliative sedation to unconsciousness to relieve intractable clinical symptoms unresponsive to "aggressive symptom-specific treatments." A palliative care team should be consulted to ensure that all other treatment options have been exhausted. Informed consent must be obtained from the patient or the patient's surrogate. Obtaining consent should include a thorough discussion addressing the degree and length of sedation with respect to achieving an intermittent or constant level of unconsciousness. The AMA Code of Ethics does not condone the use of palliative sedation to unconsciousness for the purposes of relieving existential suffering such as feelings of death anxiety, social isolation, or loss of control, citing that these symptoms are more appropriately and effectively addressed by alternative measures.[85] Other professional organizations including the American Academy of Hospice and Palliative Medicine (AAHPM) and the National Hospice and Palliative Care Organization (NHPCO) have released similar policy statements and recommendations and additionally recommend an interdisciplinary approach involving palliative care expertise.[86,87] The NHPCO recognized the controversy surrounding palliative

Box 71.5 Quality Measures for Palliative and End-of-Life Care

Patient and Family-Centered Decision Making
Assessment of the patient's decisional capacity
Documentation of a surrogate decision maker within 24 hours
Documentation of the presence and, if present, contents of advance directive
Documentation of the goals of care
Communication within team and with the patient and the family
Documentation of timely physician communication with the family
Documentation of timely interdisciplinary clinician-family conference

Continuity of Care
Transition of key information with transfer of the patient out of the intensive care unit (ICU)
Policy of continuity of nursing service
Emotional and practical support for patient and family
Open visitation policy for family members
Documentation that psychosocial support has been offered

Symptom Management and Comfort Care
Documentation of pain assessment and management
Documentation of respiratory distress assessment and management
Protocol for analgesia and sedation in terminal withdrawal or mechanical ventilation
Appropriate medications available during withdrawal of mechanical ventilation

Spiritual Support for Patients and Family
Documentation that spiritual support was offered
Emotional and organizational support for clinicians
Opportunity to review experience of caring for dying patients by ICU clinicians

From Mularski RA, Curtis JR, Billings JA, et al: Proposed quality measures for palliative care in the critically ill: A consensus from the Robert Wood Johnson Foundation Critical Care Workgroup. Crit Care Med 2006;34:S404-S411.

sedation to unconsciousness for relief of existential suffering and the panel was unable to reach an agreement on recommendations regarding this practice.[86]

EUTHANASIA AND PHYSICIAN-ASSISTED SUICIDE

Administering treatments to hasten death as a way to relieve pain and discomfort falls into the realm of euthanasia and physician-assisted suicide. The term *euthanasia* requires clarification. So-called passive euthanasia is the withdrawal or withholding of life-sustaining medical interventions and is widely accepted as both ethical and legal. "Indirect euthanasia"—such as increasing narcotic dosage to ease a patient's pain, even if this has the consequence of hastening the patient's death—also is a misnomer; it generally has been deemed both ethical and legal for more than 100 years.[88] Almost all commentators agree that involuntary and nonvoluntary active euthanasia are unethical because they end the life of a patient without consent. Consequently, the focus of debate is on physician-assisted suicide and voluntary, active euthanasia. To avoid confusion, use of the term *euthanasia* should be restricted to voluntary, active euthanasia.

Proponents typically cite four reasons to justify physician-assisted suicide or euthanasia.[88,89] First, they claim that euthanasia ensures patients' autonomy. How a person dies is essential to that person's values. Therefore, to respect patients' autonomy, it is mandatory to respect their wishes regarding the manner and timing of their death, through euthanasia and physician-assisted suicide.[90,91] Second, for some patients, dying causes pain and suffering. A main purpose of euthanasia or physician-assisted suicide is a comfortable, quick death. Hence, euthanasia or physician-assisted suicide furthers beneficence, which is one of the major principles of medical ethics.[90,91] Third, euthanasia and physician-assisted suicide are morally equivalent to terminating life-sustaining treatments. The goal is the same: a peaceful, painless death. Furthermore, there is no difference between an act of omission and an act of commission.[91] Finally, the potential adverse consequences of legalization are speculative.

Opponents of euthanasia and physician-assisted suicide offer four parallel but opposite arguments. First, autonomy does not justify euthanasia or physician-assisted suicide.[92-94] Autonomy does not mean a person should be permitted to do anything he or she wishes. Both Kant[94a] and Mill[94b] thought that a person's autonomy could be limited to prevent voluntary dueling or slavery. Similarly, one could argue that because euthanasia and physician-assisted suicide are aimed at ending autonomy, they can be limited without infringing autonomy. Second, many terminally ill patients receive inadequate treatment for pain, fatigue, and depression. With proper treatment, few people would experience pain and suffering of a level sufficient to justify euthanasia or physician-assisted suicide. Third, acts of omission and acts of commission are not equivalent. The ethical validity of an act does not depend solely on its final result but also stems from the intention of the person performing it. When physicians stop a medical intervention, they are stopping unwanted bodily intrusion, not trying to end a person's life; euthanasia and physician-assisted suicide do aim to end a person's life.[38,92-94] Finally, permitting euthanasia and physician-assisted suicide would have a variety of well-documented adverse consequences. These effects include disruption of the doctor-patient relationship, intrusion of the courts, and possibly extension of euthanasia to children, mentally incapacitated patients, and others.[94]

Although the U.S. Supreme Court has upheld the right of patients to reject medical treatment, the Court ruled unanimously in 1997 that there is no constitutional right to euthanasia or physician-assisted suicide.[95] Of importance, the U.S. Supreme Court did permit individual states to legalize these interventions. Oregon and Washington state have enacted legislation permitting physician-assisted suicide.[96,97] The Supreme Court of the state of Montana has ruled that prohibition of physician-assisted suicide is against the state's constitution.[98]

The Netherlands and Belgium have legalized both euthanasia and physician-assisted suicide. Their legislation included the following safeguards: The patient must have unbearable pain and suffering that cannot be medically relieved; the patient must be competent and must repeatedly request to have his or her life ended; and the physician must consult a second physician.[99] In 2008, Luxembourg legalized euthanasia for patients with a "grave and incurable" condition. The physician must first consult a colleague and the patient must have repeatedly asked for the intervention.[100]

For a brief period the Northern Territory of Australia had legalized euthanasia, but this was rescinded by the national legislature.[101] In Switzerland assisted suicide is legal and the assistance need not be provided by a physician.[102]

After receiving a request for euthanasia or physician-assisted suicide, health care providers should carefully clarify the request with empathetic, open-ended questions to help elucidate the underlying cause. Health care providers must reassure the patient of their continued care and commitment. The patient should be educated about alternative, less controversial options, such as symptom management and withdrawal of any unwanted treatments. Physicians also should discuss the realities of euthanasia and physician-assisted suicide, because the patient may have misconceptions about their effectiveness and the legal implications of the choice.

In addition, the physician should reevaluate the patient's condition—not just for physical and psychological symptoms but also for lack of social support and spiritual fulfillment and need for care, which are strongly associated with interest in euthanasia and physician-assisted suicide. The physician should reassess whether additional interventions are required, including psychiatric evaluation, palliative care consultations, availability of skilled or unskilled home health care, and pastoral services. Obviously, the patient and family should be reassured that the physician will not abandon them and will provide care and attend to the patient's symptoms and needs.

RESEARCH IN CRITICALLY ILL PATIENTS

Research involving critically ill patients in the ICU presents special ethical challenges. Chief among these challenges is the recognition of the distinction between clinical care and research. Although clinical medicine aims at providing optimal medical care for individual patients, clinical research lies outside the context of the doctor-patient relationship. It is designed to answer a scientific question, with the aim of promoting the medical good of future patients. Research abuses occur when interest in advancing science is allowed to outweigh concern for protection of human research participants. Adherence to ethical principles for research serves to minimize the possibility of such abuses and enhances the public trust in the research endeavor.

HISTORY AND FUNDAMENTALS OF HUMAN RESEARCH ETHICS

Among the first documented experiments with human subjects were vaccination trials in the 1700s. In these early trials, many physicians used themselves or their family members as test subjects. Even these early practices were not without some formulations of research ethics. In 1865, the French physiologist Claude Bernard wrote that the first principle of medical morality "consists in never performing on man an experiment which might be harmful to him to any extent, even though the result might be highly advantageous to science."[103] Louis Pasteur is reported to have "agonized" over performing a previously untried intervention in humans, even though he was confident of the results obtained through animal trials. He finally did so only when he was convinced that the death of the first test subject "appeared inevitable."[104]

The rise of the experimental method in medicine in the late nineteenth century led to an acceleration of the progress of medicine. Clinical trials became large-scale endeavors, but many trials targeted vulnerable groups of persons who could not protect their own interests, such as orphans, the mentally ill, and prisoners. During this era, no formal codes of research ethics existed to guide scientists in their experiments.

In the twentieth century, the medical experiments conducted by German physicians on concentration camp prisoners during World War II ushered in a new era of research ethics. After the war, 23 Nazi doctors and scientists were put on trial at Nuremberg for the torture and murder of concentration camp inmates who were used as research subjects. Most were convicted and sentenced to death or prison terms ranging from 10 years to life.[105]

The Nuremberg judges were convinced that the Hippocratic Oath alone could not serve as an adequate foundation for ethical research. Accordingly, their principles for research, which became known as the Nuremberg Code, were meant to protect subject welfare as well as basic human rights.[106,107] They formed the basis of the research ethics codes that are used internationally today.

The Nuremberg Code's first principle was stated as a basic human right: "The voluntary consent of the human subject is absolutely essential." Another basic right of research subjects was the right to withdraw from an experiment at any time. The other eight principles aimed to protect the welfare of human subjects by insisting, for example, that only qualified scientists conduct the research, that physical and mental suffering are avoided, and that risks are balanced against the importance of the scientific problem to be solved.

In the United States, the fundamental ethical guidelines for medical research were set out in 1974 by the National Commission for the Protection of Human Subjects in Biomedical and Behavioral Research, which was established by Congress after a series of ethical scandals in the 1960s and 1970s. In its *Belmont Report*, the Commission outlined three basic ethical principles for the conduct of medical research: *respect for persons; beneficence*; and *justice*[108] (Table 71.3).

Respect for Persons. Respect for persons requires that people should be treated as autonomous agents and that those with diminished capacity, such as children or the mentally ill, are entitled to special protection. To respect autonomy is to give weight to a person's considered opinions and choices. To show lack of respect for autonomy is to repudiate a person's considered judgments, to deny the person the freedom to act on those considered judgments, or to withhold information necessary to make a considered judgment, when there are no compelling reasons to do so. Respect for persons is manifested in the informed consent *process, in which potential subjects are provided with information about the experiment and then are allowed to decide whether to participate.*

Beneficence/Nonmaleficence. Treating people in an ethical manner means not only respecting their decisions but also making

Table 71.3 Principles and Derived Requirements for Ethical Research

Respect for Persons	**Beneficence; Nonmaleficence**	**Justice**
Persons should be treated as autonomous agents Persons with diminished autonomy need protection	Minimize possible harms Maximize societal and potential individual benefits	Fairness in distribution of risks and potential benefits of research to all groups Fairness in selection of subjects
Informed Consent	**Social Value**	**Fair Subject Selection**
Disclosure of information Understanding of information Voluntariness of decisions Surrogate consent for vulnerable persons	Research will lead to knowledge that will improve societal health	Vulnerable subjects are not targeted for enrollment because of their compromised position Aims of research dictate subject selection When possible, less burdened groups of persons should bear the risks of research
	Scientific Validity	
	Research will produce reliable and valid data Selected subjects are likely to be recipients of future benefits	
	Favorable Risk-Benefit Ratio	
	Risks are identified Risks are minimized Benefits are maximized Risks are reasonable when compared to potential benefits to subject and society	
	Independent Review	
	Persons free from controlling influences review research to enhance implementation of ethical requirements and enhance subject protection	

efforts to secure their well-being. Such treatment falls under the principle of beneficence, which obliges physician-researchers to (1) do no harm and (2) maximize possible benefits and minimize possible harms. Beneficence requires that investigators and members of institutional review boards (IRBs) analyze the risks and benefits to the subjects, making sure that anticipated risks are proportional to the potential benefits. Risk should be minimized as much as possible.

Justice. Justice requires that the benefits and burdens of research be distributed equitably. Subjects should not be chosen simply because they are available and easy to manipulate. In addition, subjects who are likely to benefit from a study should not be excluded. Finally, whenever research supported by public funds leads to the development of therapeutic devices and procedures, these should be available not only to the wealthy but to all society; and such research should not unduly involve groups who are unlikely to benefit from the research.

The U.S. federal regulations and most international regulations governing research with human beings are largely based on these principles.

PUTTING PRINCIPLES INTO PRACTICE: APPLICATIONS

Although ethics codes and regulations exist to ensure the ethical conduct of research, what is needed is a systematic and coherent framework for evaluating the ethics of human subject research that incorporates all relevant ethical considerations. Stemming from the principles of research ethics, several *requirements* have been proposed to ensure the ethical conduct of research set out in the Belmont Report (see Table 71.3).

SCIENTIFIC VALIDITY

Clinical trials must be designed to answer valuable scientific questions with the necessary methodologic rigor to validly claim any scientific conclusions. The large number of therapeutic interventions required in the care of the critically ill creates special challenges in the conduct of clinical trials in the ICU.

The ideal clinical trial establishes whether therapeutic interventions work and determines the overall benefits and risks of each alternative. This is achieved by limiting the effects of chance, bias, and confounding. The need for scientific rigor also must be balanced against other requirements of clinical trials, such as protection of subjects' rights and welfare as well as minimizing the cost and the number of subjects necessary for enrollment to achieve significant results.[109]

An important ethical construct in clinical trials is that of clinical *equipoise*.[110] This concept refers to the existence of an "honest, professional disagreement among expert clinicians" concerning the relative benefits and harms of the interventions being tested.[110] The presence of clinical equipoise serves two important goals.[111] It assures a physician that random selection of the intervention that a research participant will receive is ethically permissible, as neither of the interventions in the study groups dominates the other in terms of perceived safety and efficacy. Accordingly, the welfare of research subjects is not knowingly sacrificed for the interests of future patients. The other goal ensures that the results of the research will disturb clinical equipoise and hence yield reliable, generalizable information regarding the standard of care. The randomized controlled trial (RCT) is a formal method of resolving uncertainty about scientific knowledge, although well-conducted observational cohort and case-control studies also can provide valuable information to disturb equipoise and might lead to better human subject protections.[112,113] Several research methods have raised specific ethical issues in critical care research and deserve special mention. Some examples follow.

Placebo Controls

Clinical research involving placebo controls in circumstances in which an established therapeutic alternative is not available is not ethically problematic. In this situation, an experimental intervention (e.g., a new drug) is compared with a placebo and both may be superimposed on the current standard of care for the enrolled research participants. Placebo controls have been used in trials of critical care treatments for a wide range of conditions, including asthma and pulmonary hypertension.[114,115]

In contrast, the use of a placebo control group, when a proven effective treatment exists for the medical condition, does raise ethical issues. Critics of placebo-controlled trials contend that when effective treatments exist, placing patients in a placebo group is not only unethical but also unwise. They argue that no scientific or clinical value derives from determining whether an investigational drug is better than an inert placebo; instead, they say, an experimental treatment should be compared with a standard treatment, to demonstrate which is better.[116,117]

Advocates of placebo-controlled studies argue that such studies are not only ethical but indeed necessary under many circumstances.[118-120] For example, an experimental therapy may have fewer side effects or may be more effective for particular subgroups of patients, but these effects might not be recognized in active-control trials. Moreover, demonstrating that a new treatment is equivalent to an existing treatment may not prove that the new treatment is effective; both treatments could be ineffective. And comparing an experimental treatment with an existing treatment would require many more patients in each arm of the study than are necessary for a placebo-controlled trial.

To be sure, a placebo-controlled trial would be unethical when life-saving—or at least life-prolonging—treatment is available, and if patients assigned to receive placebo would be substantially more likely to suffer serious harm than those assigned to receive the investigational agent. Such trials involving diseases that are less serious, however, may be ethically appropriate if compelling methodologic reasons exist to conduct a placebo-controlled trial, and if the known harm associated with forgoing standard of care treatment in the placebo group would be mild to moderate in degree and reversible.

Choice of Control in Clinical Trials Comparing a New Intervention with the Current Standard of Care

If a new intervention is going to be compared to contemporary standard practice the control must be representative of current practices both to permit a useful comparison and to protect the welfare of research participants, as the inclusion of such a control group allows a trial to be stopped early if the tested intervention has a mortality rate or survival rate that is significantly higher than standard practices.[121]

The difficulty in control group selection is made more manifest when current practices of critical care practitioners are variable. Accordingly, the choice of control group may involve a set protocol that is designated as the standard of care, and there are constraints on all treatment in both the experimental and standard-of-care control groups. Such constraints serve to improve the signal-to-noise ratio and increase the likelihood of finding difference between the tested interventions.[122] However, the cost of using such control groups that enhance scientific validity is reduced generalizability and a potential to increase the risk of harm to enrolled research subjects.[109,122,123]

In recognition of this concern, several critical care trials have used so-called "usual care" control groups whereby the control group represents the broad range of current practices and care is individualized for each patient. Several important critical care studies,[124-128] including those involving mechanical ventilation,[129-131] have proved to be extremely informative.[132] Surveys and observational studies of clinicians' practice patterns would help ensure that such control groups reflect usual care. An international trial evaluating two target ranges for glycemic control in ICU patients took such an approach.[133]

INFORMED CONSENT

Informed consent is the ethical prerequisite for all clinical trials involving human beings. The informed consent process respects subjects' autonomy and ensures that they are not to be used merely as a means to another's end.[134] It also provides research subjects a mechanism to protect themselves.[135,136] Practices regarding obtaining informed consent from critically ill patients differ among researchers; for example, there is a difference in the extent to which participants consent personally rather than having a surrogate do so.[137]

Valid informed consent consists of three major elements: disclosure of information, subject competence to make a decision, and voluntariness of the decision.[138]

Disclosure of Information

The basic elements of information that should be communicated to potential subjects and their surrogates include a full description of any reasonably foreseeable risks or discomforts a subject may experience, and full disclosure of other procedures or courses of treatment that are available[139,140] (Box 71.6). Some of these elements are absent in many informed consent forms, including those used in critical care clinical trials.[141,142] Recommendations for writing informed consent forms for critical care studies have been published.[143]

Decision-Making Capacity

In order to give valid informed consent to research, potential research participants must be able to understand the information given to them, to understand or appreciate their situation and its consequences, to be able to rationally consider information in light of their underlying values, and to be able to commit to a decision.

Critical care investigators face a difficult task of recruiting research subjects who may have diminished capacity to give valid informed consent. Patients with acute illnesses often have limitations in their decision-making capabilities due to a number of factors, including the presence of delirium, their underlying illness, or the use of sedatives and

Box 71.6 Required Basic Elements of Informed Consent for Research in Critically Ill Patients

Element 1: Description of Research

a. Purpose of the research
b. A statement that the study involves research
c. Expected duration of the subject's participation
d. Description of the procedures to be followed and identification of any procedures that are experimental

Element 2: Risk

Description of any reasonably foreseeable risks or discomforts to the subject

Element 3: Benefits

Description of benefits that might reasonably be expected from the research:
a. To the subject
b. To others

Element 4: Alternatives

Disclosure of alternative procedures or courses of treatment, if any, that might be advantageous to the subject

Element 5: Confidentiality

Assurance of confidentiality

Element 6: Risk Management

For research involving more than minimal risk, if research injury occurs:
a. An explanation as to whether any compensation is available
b. An explanation as to whether any medical treatments are available

Element 7: Contact Information

a. An explanation of whom to contact for answers to questions about the research
b. An explanation of whom to contact for questions about the research subjects' rights
c. An explanation of whom to contact in the event of a research-related injury

Element 8: Voluntariness

a. Voluntariness of participation
b. Assurance that subject may discontinue participation without penalty or loss of benefits to which the subject is otherwise entitled

analgesics.[144-146] Understanding is less complete in severely ill patients than in healthier patients.[147] Research participants enrolled in clinical trials often have limited understanding of the research to which they have consented.[148,149] Many potential participants may not understand certain concepts of randomization, the notion of a placebo design, research risks, and the distinction between research and clinical care. Understanding is less complete in severely ill patients than in healthier patients.[147] Investigators should make special efforts to ensure that potential research participants understand these general concepts and their implications for the specific study participants may be consenting to.

Investigators also should keep in mind that written descriptions of the research may not be effective in conveying information—particularly if the written material is so long and technical that potential research participants do not read it fully. Information given verbally can enhance understanding by giving research participants the opportunity to engage in a dialogue with the investigator. The opportunity for such a dialogue for patients receiving ventilatory support is difficult, and hence, the feasibility of enrolling such individuals with their own informed consent might be ethically problematic. One approach to such potential research participants who have some degree of decisional capacity is to obtain their assent in conjunction with proxy consent.[137]

Regarding the distinction between research and clinical care, patients and families have a strong tendency to inaccurately attribute therapeutic intent to the research.[150] Physician-investigators should explicitly refute such a "therapeutic misconception" and should dispel any notion that a clinical trial is designed to or will provide patients with direct benefits, or that the research substitutes for clinical care.[108,151]

Finally, the research community often assumes that research participants derive benefits solely from participating in a research study—even if they are receiving inert placebo—because of the extra monitoring and superior care associated with academic "centers of excellence." Such an "inclusion benefit," however, has not been proved.[152,153]

Voluntariness

Valid informed consent requires that patients' decisions to enroll in clinical trials are free from coercion—including a fear, justified or not, that they may be harmed in some way if they do not enroll in the clinical trial.[108] The institutional setting of the research may be a source of subtle or covert coercion. Critically ill patients often lack decisional capacity. Patients may feel they have little choice but to participate in research when "their doctor" asks them to do so—particularly if their treating physician occupies the dual role of clinician-investigator. Accordingly, someone other than the treating physician should obtain informed consent from patients.[154,155]

Another factor that may affect voluntariness is the presence of undue influence, which occurs when offers to induce enrollment, such as financial payments or free medical care, are of such magnitude that they influence subjects' decisions.[156]

PROXY CONSENT

Ethically acceptable research may proceed with critically ill patients who are—or are at risk of becoming—decisionally impaired, if the investigators receive appropriate proxy consent.[157,158] U.S. and European standards require proxy or surrogate decision makers to be legally authorized to provide such consent. In the United States, the legal representative for the patient is determined by the applicable state laws.

If possible, surrogate decision makers should follow the "substituted judgment" standard: They should make a good-faith judgment of what the subjects would have decided if capable of making a decision themselves. As discussed earlier, however, surrogates often do not know patients' previous preferences.[159,160] Therefore, they also should consider what would be in the best interests of the patient.

Investigators should appreciate that family members of critically ill patients have high levels of anxiety and psychological distress that might impair their ability to give adequate informed consent for research participation for incapacitated patients.[161,162]

If research participants who were entered into a trial through proxy consent regain decisional capacity during the trial, investigators should obtain their informed consent for continuing their participation.[163] Such retrospective consent should be sought even when the research procedures have been completed, because research participants have a right to know that they have participated in a trial and that further data may be collected. Whether participants should be given the right to withdraw the data obtained from them when they were unconscious is an unsettled issue. This is a sound proposal, ethically speaking, but from a methodologic standpoint it is arguable because it could ruin the comparability of study groups.

WAIVER OF INFORMED CONSENT

In some circumstances, the informed consent requirement can be waived—but only when an IRB finds that all of the following conditions are met:[139]

- The research involves no more than minimal risk to the research participants.
- The waiver or alteration of informed consent requirements will not adversely affect the rights and welfare of the research participants.
- The research could not practicably be carried out without the waiver or alteration.
- Whenever appropriate, the participants will be provided with additional pertinent information after participation.

Under U.S. regulations, research may be characterized as minimal risk if "the probability and magnitude of harms or discomforts anticipated in the research are not greater in and of themselves than those ordinarily encountered in daily life or during the performance of routine physical or psychological examinations or tests."[164] In other words, the types of minimal risks that are considered socially acceptable, such as in driving to work or crossing a street, or those encountered in routine physical or psychological evaluations, are acceptable in research.

An IRB can grant a waiver of informed consent for research assessing interventions in medical conditions that frequently occur in emergency situations such as cardiac arrest, stroke, shock, severe arrhythmias, and life-threatening traumatic injury. Patients with these conditions cannot give consent, and the narrow time window in which treatment must be given often does not afford sufficient time to obtain consent from a legal representative. A trial assessing the safety and efficacy of an infusion of low-dose steroid in severe septic shock provides a good example.[165]

Various countries and regions have differing regulations governing such research. In 1996, the U.S. government specified several mechanisms under which research involving incapacitated research participants in emergency situations can be allowed without informed consent of a legally authorized representative.[166] But these procedures have been criticized as unnecessarily complicated and burdensome.[167-169]

A European Directive regarding clinical research involving drugs contains no provisions for waiver of informed consent for research in emergencies. Some European countries, however, provide for possible waivers in their own regulations.[170]

Australia's National Statement on Ethical Conduct in Research Involving Humans allows an ethics committee to approve research without prior consent provided that (1) inclusion in the research is not contrary to the interest of the patient; (2) the research is intended to be therapeutic, and the research intervention poses no more risk than that inherent in the patient's condition and alternative methods of treatment; (3) the research is based on valid scientific hypotheses that support a reasonable possibility of benefit over standard care; and (4) as soon as reasonably possible, the patient or the patient's relatives or legal representatives, or both, will be informed of the patient's inclusion in the research and of the option to withdraw from the research without any reduction in quality of care.[171]

Regulations in Canada stipulate that research in the emergency setting may proceed under the following conditions: if a serious threat to the prospective subject requires immediate intervention,[172] if no standard efficacious care exists or the research offers a real possibility of direct benefit to the subject in comparison with standard care, or if the risk of harm is not greater than that involved in standard efficacious care or is clearly justified by direct benefit to the subject.

ANALYSIS OF RISKS AND BENEFITS

The U.S. federal regulations require that risks to research participants are reasonable in relation to anticipated benefits, if any, to the research participants, and the importance of the knowledge that may reasonably be expected to result. This assessment of the potential risks involves three steps.[157] First, the risks and discomforts of the trial must be identified; these factors include not only the physical risks but also psychological, economic, and social risks, including those that might emanate from breaches of confidentiality. Second, the risks must be minimized by changing the study design if possible—for example, excluding research participants who are at substantially higher risk, replacing invasive procedures with less risky procedures, or providing enhanced safety monitoring, for example, additional blood studies to monitor for safety. Finally, the risks must be reasonable when weighed against potential benefits to the research participants and to society. In weighing risks and benefits, some ethicists have found it useful to use a component analysis, which distinguishes between procedures with potential for benefiting research participants and procedures that merely answer a scientific question, without offering a potential direct benefit to research participants.[158,173]

Within a component analysis, a study should be acceptable only if the risk of each component of the research—that is, each procedure the researchers will carry out—is justified separately by the corresponding potential benefit. Hence, a procedure that has no potential to benefit the subject but is designed solely to answer a research question is justified only if the risks of that procedure are reasonable in relation to its potential to generate scientific knowledge—a so-called risk-knowledge calculus. Procedures that may directly benefit the research participant are justified only if the risks are reasonable in relation to the potential benefit and the potential scientific knowledge meets an additional standard of equipoise: There must be genuine uncertainty about whether the balance of risks and potential benefits of the experimental intervention are superior to those of accepted practice.

A component analysis is intended to avoid what has been termed the "fallacy of the package deal" in which the potential benefits of one intervention are considered to justify the risks of a another intervention in the study.[174]

Justifying risks by the separate components of the study does not imply that there is no upper limit to acceptable risk.[175] However, what the risk threshold should be is debatable. When investigational procedures do not offer a prospect of direct benefit to the patient, commentators have argued that the risk should be capped at the level of minimal risk.[176,177] This position reflects the concern that vulnerable subjects should not be put at undue risk for the sake of society and that such research is exploitative. However, advocating such a risk ceiling would seriously impair important research. Instead of restricting such research, a desirable alternative might be to institute a safeguard for this risk level, such as the "necessity requirement." Such a safeguard would provide that decisionally impaired research participants can be enrolled in research only when their participation is scientifically necessary—for example, when the desired information cannot be obtained by enrolling adults who can consent. To provide supplemental protection, some guidelines reinforce the necessity requirement with a "subject condition" requirement, under which the research must involve a condition from which the subject suffers.

CORE SAFEGUARDS FOR VULNERABLE SUBJECTS

The U.S. federal regulations state that when some or all of the research participants are likely to be vulnerable because of intrinsic factors, such as lack of capacity to make decisions, or because of situations that threaten voluntary choice, such as coercive settings or undue inducements, additional safeguards must be included in the study to protect the rights and welfare of these individuals.

Although the U.S. regulations are silent regarding specific safeguards to provide additional protections to adults unable to provide consent, other guidelines have proposed examples of specific safeguards.[178] These safeguards include (1) assessment of potential research participants' decision-making capacity; (2) respect for potential participants' assent and dissent; (3) "necessity" requirement to ensure that research cannot be performed without enrolling incapacitated adults; (4) "subject-condition" requirement, whereby the research involves a condition from which the subject suffers; (5) an independent participation monitor to monitor participants' involvement as they progress through the study protocol; and (6) an independent and (7) sufficient evidence of subjects' prior preferences and interests.

Additional protections for vulnerable people and groups should be based on the level of risk of the procedures that will be involved.[172,175,179] For example, for research involving potential direct benefits that pose more than minimal risk, additional protections for vulnerable subjects could include designating independent monitors to witness the informed consent process or to determine when it might be appropriate to withdraw the subject from the study.[177,180]

MONITORING FOR SAFETY OF RESEARCH PARTICIPANTS

The welfare of participants in clinical trials is overseen not just by IRBs and research ethics committees, which approve protocols before a trial can begin, but also by data and safety monitoring boards (DSMBs), which monitor data from ongoing trials, particularly large, multicenter trials.[181] The role of DSMBs is to collect data that otherwise might not be aggregated until much later in a trial and to watch for unexpected adverse results that might necessitate halting the trial—or unexpected beneficial results that might justify making the experimental therapy more widely available.

Investigators should be vigilant in observing and reporting adverse events to their research ethics committees and other regulatory agencies. Although interpretation of individual adverse events may be problematic for IRBs, these ethics committees do need to conduct effective continuing reviews. DSMBs should review individual reported adverse events, as well as aggregate data on mortality rates or other outcome trends. By using preplanned statistical analyses, DSMBs can determine when trials should be stopped early to avoid continued exposure of participants to inferior treatments.

RESEARCH IN THE INTERNATIONAL CONTEXT

In September 2011, the U.S. Presidential Commission for the Study of Bioethical Issues published a review of U.S. Public Health Service-led studies in Guatemala involving the intentional exposure and infection of vulnerable populations that occurred between 1946 and 1948 during the study of penicillin to prevent and treat infection. The Commission concluded that "the experiments involved gross ethical violations."[182]

The Commission reviewed domestic and international contemporary human subjects protection rules and standards to ensure that federally funded scientific studies are conducted ethically.[183] This review was relevant as an increasing number of federally sponsored and pharmaceutical sponsored research is being performed in the developing world. Furthermore, commentators have recommended collaborations with colleagues in the developing world to address global disparities in critical illness and to care for those who become critically ill due to the consequences of natural disasters, acts of war, pandemics, and bioterrorism. Investigators and sponsors of such research need to ensure that it is not exploitative of the indigenous populations and is culturally sensitive.

COLLECTION AND STORAGE OF TISSUE SAMPLES FOR FUTURE UNSPECIFIED RESEARCH, PARTICULARLY GENETIC RESEARCH

Recent advances in genetics, molecular biology, and biomedical technologies have increased the scientific value of research on stored biologic samples and have spurred the development of genetic databases and biobanks. The collection, storage, and use of biologic samples in future research from acutely ill patients raise unique logistical and ethical challenges,[184] particularly regarding confidentiality, accuracy of substituted judgments, ownership, and the commercialization of stored biologic samples. There has also been a lack of consensus regarding the type and quality of informed consent needed to collect and store samples for future, unspecified research.[185] Finally, as research has become increasingly globalized, ethical issues also arise from collaborative international research in which samples are collected in developing countries and then exported for analysis to developed countries.[186]

RESPONSE TO DISASTER

Critical care practitioners may be called upon to participate in responding to natural and human-made disasters. As such they should be familiar with crisis standards of care developed by the Institute of Medicine (IOM)[187] and recommendations from the European Society of Intensive Care Medicine regarding benchmarks for management of critical illness when disasters occur. They are obliged to be well prepared with regard to key functions and assets including triage, infrastructure, essential equipment, sufficient personnel, protection of staff and patients, medical procedures, hospital policy, coordination and collaboration with interface units, registration and reporting, administrative policies, and education.[188] The IOM committee has argued that when crisis standards of care prevail, as when ordinary standards are in effect, health care practitioners must adhere to ethical norms. Conditions of overwhelming scarcity limit autonomous choices for both patients and practitioners regarding the allocation of scarce health care resources but do not permit actions that violate ethical norms. It has recognized that ethical considerations are one of the key elements of crisis standards of care protocols and that the most relevant ethical considerations are fairness, duty to care, duty to steward resources, transparency, consistency, proportionality, and accountability.[189]

KEY POINTS

- The goals of the ICU team are to resolve life-threatening illness, to prolong life, and to relieve suffering.
- ICU providers should understand concepts of biomedical ethics including beneficence, nonmaleficence, autonomy, justice, truth telling, and confidentiality.
- When a diagnostic or therapeutic option is not medically indicated, a physician should not make it available.
- Given the likelihood that critically ill patients may be unable to participate in life-sustaining treatment decisions, clinicians should make efforts to promote advance care planning—use of advance directives—and should anticipate the need for limited treatment orders in advance of life-threatening events.
- Competent patients have the legal right to refuse medical treatments, even if physicians believe that such treatments are indicated. Patients do not, however, have a correlative right to demand treatment.
- Withholding or withdrawing life-sustaining treatment—with the informed consent of the patient or surrogate decision maker, or in compliance with advance directives—is both valid and quite common. However, state laws regulating the authority of surrogate decision makers vary.
- Active euthanasia—for example, administering a fatal overdose of a narcotic with the express purpose of ending life—and physician-assisted suicide are illegal in most states but are the subject of intense ethical debate.
- Research lies outside the context of the doctor-patient relationship. In medical practice, physicians' primary obligation is to protect the best interests of their patients. Researchers have dual interests of advancing medical science and protecting the rights and welfare of human subjects. Physicians engaged in clinical research should make certain that their patients understand the difference.
- Heightened awareness of the principles and requirements that govern such research would enhance the ability of the research community to conduct such research ethically and to maintain the public trust in the research endeavor.
- Critical care practitioners should be prepared to coordinate care with other providers during disasters and should act ethically within the guidelines of crisis standards of care.

SELECTED REFERENCES

12. Davidson JE, Powers K, Hedayat KM, et al: Clinical practice guidelines for support of the family in the patient-centered intensive care unit: American College of Critical Care Task Force 2004-2005. Crit Care Med 2007;5:2-18.
18. Appelbaum PS: Assessment of patients' competence to consent to treatment. N Engl J Med 2007;357:1834-1840.
31. Truog RD, Brock DW, Cook DJ, et al: Rationing in the intensive care unit. Crit Care Med 2006;34:958-963; quiz 971.
39. Snead OC: President's Council on Bioethics. Controversies in the determination of death. Washington, DC, President's Council on Bioethics, 2008. Available at http://bioethics.georgetown.edu/pcbe/reports/death/chapter1.html. Accessed April 18, 2012.
50 Beauchamp TL, Childress JF: Principles of Biomedical Ethics, 6th ed. New York, Oxford University Press, 2009.
62. Teno J, Lynn J, Wenger N, et al: Advance directives for seriously ill hospitalized patients: Effectiveness with the patient self-determination act and the SUPPORT intervention. SUPPORT Investigators. Study to Understand Prognoses and Preferences for Outcomes and Risks of Treatment. J Am Geriatr Soc 1997;45:500-507.
85. American Medical Association Code of Ethics. Available at http://www.acponline.org/running_practice/ethics/manual/manual6th.htm. Accessed April 15, 2012.
108. National Commission for the Protection of Human Subjects of Biomedical and Behavioral Research: The Belmont Report: Ethical Principles and Guidelines for the Protection of Human Subjects of Research. Washington, DC, U.S. Government Printing Office, 1979.
137. Silverman H: Protecting vulnerable research subjects in critical care trials: Enhancing the informed consent process and recommendations for safeguards. Ann Intensive Care 2011;1:8.
151. Miller FG, Rosenstein DL: The therapeutic orientation to clinical trials. N Engl J Med 2003;348:1383-1386.
157. Emanuel EJ, Wendler D, Grady C: What makes clinical research ethical? JAMA 2000;283:2701-2711.

The complete list of references can be found at www.expertconsult.com.

72

Delirium, Sleep, and Mental Health Disturbances in Critical Illness

Dustin M. Hipp | E. Wesley Ely

CHAPTER OUTLINE

OVERVIEW

An admission to the intensive care unit (ICU) is recognized by both the lay public and medical professionals to be a life-threatening event in most circumstances that is immediately made more distressing and sinister by the onset of delirium and severe sleep derangements during the ICU stay. Upon survival, however, these worries are often replaced over the ensuing months and years by mental health disturbances that can be crippling to survivors. We are now aware of the sometimes life-changing ramifications of brain and behavioral disorders that ICU survivors suffer. In the past 15 or so years, data have been published that clearly illustrate a spectrum of acquired or exacerbated "neck-up" disorders that often dismantle the lives of these patients and seriously delay their recovery. Most notable among these disorders is a potentially life-altering "dementia-like" brain injury that occurs in 60% to 80% of ICU survivors that is most often characterized by memory deficits and executive dysfunction. These problems have real-world implications because they diminish patients' ability to work, drive, shop, monitor finances, and remember the names of their friends, relatives, and coworkers. These extremely troublesome neuropsychological deficits are compounded by mood disorders such as major depression and posttraumatic stress disorder (PTSD). These two diagnoses (depression and PTSD) are underdiagnosed despite their occurrence in 20% to 30% and 10% to 20% of ICU survivors, respectively. As a profession, we are just beginning to address the risk factors for these newly acquired diseases.

Having acknowledged the preceding realities of the states of survival of critical illness, it is also true that advances in clinical medicine have resulted in dramatic improvements in survival in a host of medical conditions, such as acute respiratory distress syndrome (ARDS) and sepsis. In general, 1- to 3-month mortality rates for both of these common ICU admission diagnoses in most cohorts is now in the 20% to 35% range, whereas in the 1990s these mortality rates were in the 40% to 60% range. As a result of the increased confidence in survival, both the lay public and health care professionals are now increasingly focused on preservation of cognitive abilities, prevention of functional decline, and the quality of life among patients who survive critical illness.[1-5] The potential of being left cognitively impaired is a major determinant of patients' treatment preferences at the end of life, with 9 of every 10 patients preferring death to severe cognitive impairment.[6] In support of this reality, in a report from the international "Surviving Intensive Care" 2002 Roundtable Conference held in Brussels,[7] the need for future investigations in neurocognitive abnormalities among survivors of intensive care received the strongest recommendation from the international panel of experts. Physicians and health care providers in ICUs are accustomed to recognizing multiple organ dysfunction syndrome (MODS),[8-11] with therapy focused on the causes and treatment of respiratory, cardiovascular, renal, and hepatic dysfunction. There are increasing data on the syndrome of brain dysfunction during and following the ICU. This chapter focuses on the cognitive and mental health disturbances of critical illness, with emphasis on delirium and sleep disturbances during critical illness, as well as a brief discussion of PTSD, long-term cognitive impairment (LTCI), and depression after critical illness.

ACUTE BRAIN DYSFUNCTION OR DELIRIUM

DEFINITION

Delirium is defined by American Psychiatric Association's *Diagnostic and Statistical Manual of Mental Disorders*, 4th revised edition (DSM-IV),[12] as a disturbance of consciousness with the cornerstone component of inattention[13] being the pivotal feature of the diagnosis. This alarmingly common form of brain dysfunction often develops acutely (hours to days) in critically ill patients and fluctuates over time. Many different terms have been used to describe this spectrum of cognitive impairment in critically ill patients, including ICU psychosis, ICU syndrome, acute confusional state, septic encephalopathy, and acute brain failure.[14-16] The current consensus of many authorities is to use the unifying term *delirium* and subcategorize according to the level of alertness (hyperactive, hypoactive, or mixed).[17] We will take this approach in this chapter.

PREVALENCE AND SUBTYPES

Although the prevalence of delirium in medical ICU cohort studies has been reported to be between 20% and 80%,[18-20] more general ranges are practical depending on the severity of illness and the delirium detection instrument used, such as 40% to 60% in nonventilated and 60% to 80% in ventilated ICU patients.[21] Unfortunately, because delirium is usually "quietly" manifested by negative symptoms, it remains unrecognized by the clinician in a majority of the patients experiencing this complication,[22,23] and it may be incorrectly attributed to dementia, depression, or just an "expected" occurrence in the critically ill, elderly patient.[22] Peterson and associates[24] reported on delirium subtypes from a cohort of ventilated and nonventilated ICU patients in whom delirium was monitored. They found the rates of these subtypes in the ICU to be 1.6% for hyperactive, 43.5% for hypoactive, and 54.1% for mixed.[25]

Hyperactive delirium, which is rare in the pure form and associated with a better overall prognosis,[26] is characterized by agitation, restlessness, attempting to remove catheters or tubes, hitting, biting, and emotional lability.[17,27] This subtype was in the past referred to by the misnomer "ICU psychosis." Hypoactive delirium, on the other hand, is very common and in many circumstances actually more deleterious for the patient in the long run.[26] Unfortunately, it remains unrecognized in 66% to 84% of patients, whether being treated in the ICU, hospital ward, or emergency department.[23,28-30] This delirium subtype is characterized by withdrawal, flat affect, apathy, lethargy, and decreased responsiveness.[26,31,32] Some authorities continue to refer to the hypoactive delirium as "encephalopathy" and the hyperactive subtype as "delirium or ICU psychosis." Because of the fluctuating nature of delirium, patients may present with a mixed clinical picture or may sequentially experience both of these subtypes. Many critical care providers would have the incorrect impression that hyperactive delirium is far more common, perhaps because affected patients attract attention because of their immediate threat to self and others. Unless routine monitoring for delirium is implemented as part of an overall ICU bundle such as the ABCDEs (spontaneous Awakening trials, spontaneous Breathing trials, Coordination of care and Choice of sedative, Delirium monitoring and management, and Early mobility),[33,34] the majority of delirium episodes, especially the "quiet" (hypoactive) form, will be missed.

PROGNOSTIC SIGNIFICANCE

In non-ICU populations, the development of delirium in the hospital is associated with an in-hospital mortality rate of 25% to 33%, prolonged hospital stay, and three times greater likelihood of discharge to a nursing home.[35-37] In a three-site study of non-ICU medical patients, delirium was found to be an independent predictor of the combined outcome of death or nursing home placement.[38] McCusker and colleagues[39] found a 2.11 adjusted hazard ratio for dying in association with the development of delirium. This mortality rate increase has now been shown to be independent of dementia status.[40] Furthermore, three prospective studies have found that delirium was associated with a higher risk for dementia during the 2 to 3 years after hospitalization in non-ICU patient populations.[41-43]

Among medical ICU patients, delirium has been shown to be a strong predictor of longer duration of mechanical ventilation, longer length of ICU stay, higher costs, prolonged neuropsychological dysfunction, and even death.[44-47] The development of delirium was associated with a threefold increase in risk of death after data were controlled for preexisting comorbid conditions, severity of illness, coma, and the use of sedative and analgesic medications.[44] Three separate cohort studies have shown that the duration of delirium (in a dose-dependent sort of relationship) is an independent predictor of increased subsequent death, with the most commonly cited finding being that every day a patient spends in ICU delirium portends a 10% higher risk of death even after adjusting for relevant covariates such as severity of illness, age, psychoactive medication use, and coma.[44,48,49] In addition, it is now shown that the duration of delirium is an independent predictor of LTCI in general medical and surgical ICU patients who in the past were not suspected of having long-term dementia-like abnormalities.[50]

PATHOPHYSIOLOGY

The mechanisms of delirium remain a very promising area of neuroscientific study and likely relate to those factors leading to LTCI, which are as follows:

NEUROTRANSMITTERS

From a neuroscience perspective, delirium is thought to be related to imbalances in the synthesis, release, and inactivation of neurotransmitters modulating the control of cognitive function, behavior, and mood.[26,32] Three of the neurotransmitter systems involved in the pathophysiology of delirium are dopamine, γ-aminobutyric acid (GABA), and acetylcholine.[15,51,52] Whereas dopamine increases excitability of neurons, GABA and acetylcholine decrease neuronal excitability.[15] An imbalance in one or more of these neurotransmitters results in neuronal instability and unpredictable neurotransmission. In general, an excess of dopamine and depletion of acetylcholine are two major physiologic problems believed to be central to delirium.[53] Other neurotransmitter systems thought to be involved in the development of delirium are serotonin imbalance, endorphin hyperfunction, and increased central noradrenergic activity.[26,51]

INFLAMMATORY MEDIATORS

Other factors thought to be mechanistically deliriogenic in ICU patients are inflammatory abnormalities induced by endotoxins and cytokines.[54-57] The inflammatory mediators produced in sepsis, such as tumor necrosis factor-α (TNF-α), interleukin 1, and other cytokines and chemokines, initiate a cascade that leads to endothelial damage, thrombin formation, and microvascular compromise.[58] Animal models show that these inflammatory mediators cross the blood-brain barrier,[59] increase vascular permeability in the brain,[60] and result in electroencephalography (EEG) changes consistent with those seen in septic patients with delirium.[61,62] Release of inflammatory mediators may occur from (1) decreased cerebral blood flow, a result of the formation of microaggregates of fibrin, platelets, neutrophils, and erythrocytes in the cerebral microvasculature, (2) cerebral vasoconstriction occurring in response to (α_1-adrenergic receptor activity[63]; or (3) interference with neurotransmitter synthesis and neurotransmission.[64]

IMPAIRED OXIDATIVE METABOLISM

One hypothesis attempts to explain acute delirium as a behavioral manifestation of a "widespread reduction of cerebral oxidative metabolism resulting in an imbalance of neurotransmission."[65] On the basis of a series of investigations in which they evaluated delirious patients using EEG, Engel and Romano[66] postulated that delirium is a state of "cerebral insufficiency," that is, a global failure of cerebral oxidative metabolism. Their work showed that delirium is associated with diffuse slowing on EEG, a finding believed to represent a reduction in brain metabolism.

CHOLINERGIC DEFICIENCY

Blass and colleagues[67] offered a possible link between the state of cerebral insufficiency proposed by Engel and Romano[66] and the hypothesis of cholinergic blockade by suggesting that impaired oxidative metabolism in the brain results in a cholinergic deficiency. The finding that hypoxia impairs acetylcholine synthesis supports this hypothesis.[68] This reduction in cholinergic function leads to an increase in the level of glutamate, dopamine, and norepinephrine in the brain. Additionally, serotonin and GABA levels are reduced; all of these changes contribute to delirium.

LARGE NEUTRAL AMINO ACID IN DELIRIUM

Changes in the plasma levels of various amino acid precursors of cerebral neurotransmitters may affect their function, thus contributing to the development of delirium.[69] The amino acid entry into the brain is regulated by a sodium-independent large neutral amino acid transporter type 1 (LAT1).[70] The essential amino acid tryptophan, which is the precursor for serotonin, competes with several large neutral amino acids (LNAAs), such as tyrosine, phenylalanine, valine, leucine, and isoleucine, for transport across the blood-brain barrier via the LAT1 transporter.[70] This competition determines its uptake into the brain.[70] Recently, alterations in plasma tryptophan and tyrosine levels were identified as independent risk factors for the transition to clinical delirium.[71] Increased activation of the kynurenine pathway, which is involved in the metabolism of tryptophan and the formation of neurotoxins, has also been linked to fewer days alive and without acute brain dysfunction in critically ill patients.[72] Another amino acid that may play an important role in the pathogenesis of delirium is phenylalanine.[65] Like tryptophan, phenylalanine competes with the other LNAAs (tyrosine, tryptophan, valine, leucine, and isoleucine) for transport across the blood-brain barrier. An increase in the cerebral uptake of tyrosine and phenylalanine compared with the other LNAAs leads to greater availability of precursors for both dopamine and norepinephrine, two neurotransmitters that have been implicated in the pathogenesis of delirium.[65]

INFLAMMATION

It is important to realize that although delirium may occur as a result of perturbations in other organ systems, the brain responds to systemic infections and injury with an inflammatory response of its own that also involves cytokine production, cell infiltration, and tissue damage.[73,74] Reports indicate that local inflammation in the brain and subsequent activation of these central nervous system immune responses are accompanied by manifestations of systemic inflammation,[52,75,76] including production of large amounts of peripherally produced TNF-α, interleukin 10, and interferon-γ.[73,77-79] Thus, it is postulated that the brain can become an engine of inflammation, driving the development, resolution, or both, of MODS. Van Gool and associates propose that this self-propelling inflammation, in the context of microglial activation, could help explain the association between delirium and LTCI.[80] Surprisingly, van Gool points out that animal models have shown activated microglia can remain primed for months following injury, allowing ample time for ongoing injury long beyond the period of an ICU stay. This factors into hypothesis generation when designing neuroimaging studies in ICU survivors and will serve as fascinating topics for future study.

RISK FACTORS FOR DELIRIUM

Although non-ICU cohort studies have identified numerous risk factors for the development of delirium,[37] only a few studies have examined these factors in the ICU population. Baseline risk factors that predispose patients to a greater degree of vulnerability for delirium include Alzheimer's disease, chronic illness, advanced age, and depression.[15,81,82] Dubois and coworkers[83] found that preexisting hypertension and smoking (presumably because of relative hypoperfusion and nicotine withdrawal, respectively) were significantly associated with the development of ICU delirium. Another investigation reported that preexisting dementia was a significant risk factor for the development of delirium in the post-ICU period.[19] A new area of investigation is genetic predisposition to delirium, as the apolipoprotein E4 polymorphism was found to predict delirium that lasted nearly twice as long as patients without the polymorphism.[84] Further studies have continued to suggest this association.[85]

Precipitating and iatrogenic risk factors represent areas of potential modification and, thus, intervention for delirium prevention and treatment. Precipitating factors are hypoxia, metabolic disturbances, electrolyte imbalances, withdrawal syndromes, acute infection (systemic and intracranial), seizures, dehydration, hyperthermia, sleep deprivation, head trauma, vascular disorders, and intracranial space-occupying lesions.[15,81,82]

In practical terms, the risk factors for delirium can be divided into the following categories: (1) host factors, (2) the acute illness itself, and (3) iatrogenic or environmental factors (Box 72.1). Although delirium may be a function of patients' specific underlying illness, it may also be due to medical management issues and thus may have preventable causes. Of these risk factors, sedative and analgesic medications and sleep deprivation appear to be the leading iatrogenic and hence possibly preventable risk factors for delirium. There are conflicting data on the association of anticholinergics, corticosteroids, histamine H_2 antagonists, and anticonvulsants with the development of delirium in ICU patients.[22,86-88]

SEDATIVES AND ANALGESIC AGENTS CONTRIBUTING TO DELIRIUM

Sedative and analgesic medications are routinely administered to patients undergoing mechanical ventilation, in accordance with widely recognized clinical practice guidelines by the Society of Critical Care Medicine (SCCM),[89] in order to reduce pain and anxiety. Investigations have shown that continuous intravenous sedation is associated with prolonged mechanical ventilation and greater morbidity.[90] Similarly, associations between psychoactive medications and worsening cognitive outcomes have been reported in postoperative patients. Marcantonio and colleagues,[91] studying postoperative patients in whom delirium developed, found an association between use of benzodiazepines and meperidine and the occurrence of delirium. Dubois and coworkers[83] have shown that opiates (morphine and meperidine) administered either intravenously or via an epidural catheter may be associated with the development of delirium in medical/surgical ICU patients. Studies such as these have generated concern about whether such drugs were actually responsible for the development of delirium or were given as a result of delirium.

Our group has studied this temporal relationship between the administration of sedatives and analgesics and delirium.[92] To do so, one must make repeated cognitive assessments and must be able to assess the risk factors a patient is exposed to in between these assessments in order to study which of these factors is associated with a transition or a change in cognitive status to or from normal, delirium, or coma. In our study, lorazepam was found to be an independent risk factor for daily transition to delirium, and fentanyl, morphine, and propofol were associated with higher but not statistically significant odds ratios for such transition (Fig. 72.1).[92] Increasing age and APACHE II (Acute Physiology and Chronic Health Evaluation II) scores were also independent predictors of transitioning to delirium (Figs. 72.2 and 72.3).[92] Similar associations between another benzodiazepine, midazolam, and transition to delirium have been found in another study conducted in our trauma and surgical ICU patients.[21]

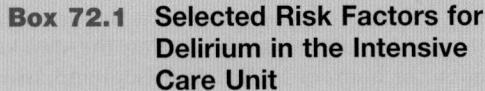

Box 72.1 Selected Risk Factors for Delirium in the Intensive Care Unit

Patient Factors

Age
Baseline comorbid conditions
Baseline cognitive impairment
Genetic predisposition (?)
Acute illness
Sepsis
Hypoxemia*
Global severity of illness score
Metabolic disturbances

Iatrogenic or Environmental Factors

Metabolic disturbances*
Anticholinergic medications*
Sedative and analgesic medications*
Sleep disturbances*

*Potentially modifiable factor.

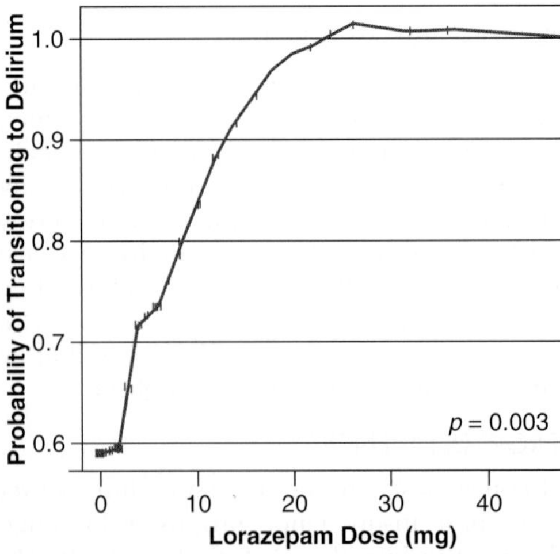

Figure 72.1 Lorazepam dose versus probability of transitioning to delirium. The probability of transitioning to delirium increased with the dose of lorazepam administered in the previous 24 hours. This incremental risk was large at low doses and plateaued at around 20 mg/day. (From Pandharipande P, Shintani A, Truman P, et al: Lorazepam is an independent risk factor for transitioning to delirium in intensive care unit patients. Anesthesiology 2006;104:21-26. Used with permission from Lippincott Williams & Wilkins.)

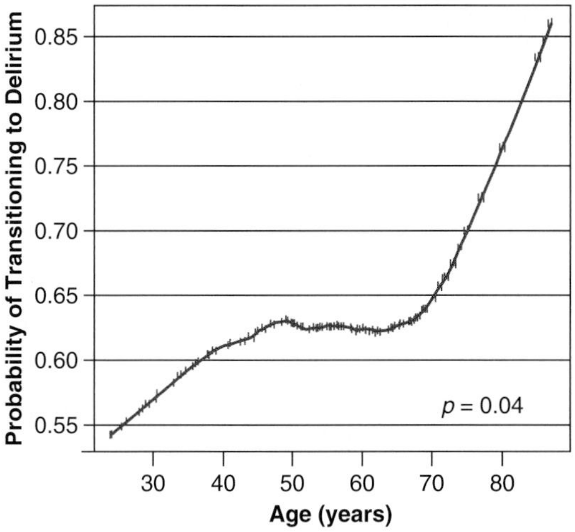

Figure 72.2 Age versus the probability of transitioning to delirium. The most notable finding related to age was that probability of transitioning to delirium increased dramatically for each year of life after 65 years. (From Pandharipande P, Shintani A, Truman P, et al: Lorazepam is an independent risk factor for transitioning to delirium in intensive care unit patients. Anesthesiology 2006;104:21-26. Used with permission from Lippincott Williams & Wilkins.)

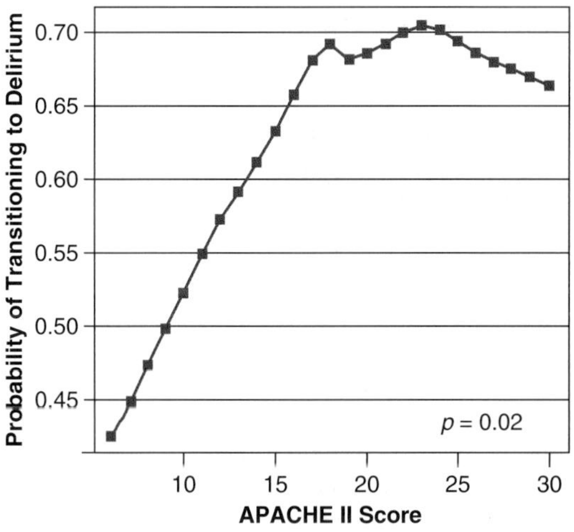

Figure 72.3 Severity of illness versus the probability of transitioning to delirium. The probability of transitioning to delirium increased dramatically for each additional point in APACHE II (Acute Physiology and Chronic Health Evaluation II) severity of illness score until it reached a plateau score of 18. (From Pandharipande P, Shintani A, Truman P, et al: Lorazepam is an independent risk factor for transitioning to delirium in intensive care unit patients. Anesthesiology 2006;104:21-26. Used with permission from Lippincott Williams & Wilkins.)

At this time it is not clear whether this association between benzodiazepines, and possibly opioids, and delirium is related to the pharmacokinetic properties of the agents or the pharmacodynamics of the drug. Benzodiazepines and propofol have high affinity for the GABA receptor in the central nervous system.[93] This GABA-mimetic effect can alter levels of numerous neurotransmitters believed to be deliriogenic.[64,94] Novel sedative agents that are GABA receptor-sparing (such as the α_2-agonists) may help reduce some of the cognitive dysfunction seen in ICU patients. It is important to note that the data for opioids and delirium are not as consistent as those for the benzodiazepines. Although meperidine has been associated with delirium in most of the published studies, evidence for both fentanyl and morphine has been less convincing.[83,91,95] Morrison and colleagues[95] conducted a prospective observational trial in patients who had undergone hip surgery and found that patients whose pain was well controlled with morphine were less likely to demonstrate delirium than those who received other opioids. These investigations point to the importance of the judicious use of psychoactive medications, with a focus on adequate analgesia.[96] One hopes that ongoing randomized controlled trials will pave the way to the development of sedation and analgesic guidelines for the prevention or reduction of the occurrence of delirium due to the administration of these psychoactive drugs.

DIAGNOSIS

The development of tools such as the Intensive Care Delirium Screening Checklist (ICDSC)[18] and the Confusion Assessment Method for the ICU (CAM-ICU)[20] have allowed for the rapid diagnosis of delirium in patients by nonpsychiatric physicians and other health care personnel even while such patients are mechanically ventilated. The SCCM has proposed guidelines for more routine and more diligent monitoring of delirium using reliable and validated scales.[89]

Diagnosis of delirium is a two-step process. Level of arousal is first measured with the use of a standardized sedation scale, like the Richmond Agitation-Sedation Scale (RASS) (Fig. 72.4).[97,98] This is a 10-point scale with scores ranging from +4 to –5, score of 0 denoting a calm and alert patient. Positive RASS scores denote positive or aggressive symptomatology ranging from +1 (mild restlessness) to +4 (dangerous agitation). The negative RASS scores differentiate between response to verbal commands (scores –1 to –3) and physical stimulus (scores –4 and –5). If the patient's RASS score is –4 or –5 or not arousable by verbal commands, no further evaluation for delirium is performed, because the patient is comatose and is unable to be assessed for delirium. For patients who are arousable (RASS scores of –3 and higher), delirium can be assessed with the ICDSC[18] or by the CAM-ICU.[20] The ICDSC assesses eight features of delirium: altered level of consciousness, inattention, disorientation, hallucinations, psychomotor agitation/retardation, inappropriate mood/speech, sleep/wake cycle disturbance, and symptom fluctuation. The sensitivity and specificity of this tool are 99% and 64%, respectively.[18] The CAM-ICU, which can be performed in about 60 to 90 seconds,[99] comprises four features that assess the following: acute change or fluctuation of mental status (feature 1), inattention (feature 2), disorganized thinking (feature 3), and an altered level of consciousness (feature 4).

To be diagnosed as delirious, a patient must have a RASS score of –3 or higher, with an acute change or fluctuation in mental status (feature 1), accompanied by inattention (feature 2) and either disorganized thinking (feature 3) or an altered level of consciousness (feature 4). A complete description of the CAM-ICU as well as training materials, including translations and clinical vignettes, can be found at our website (www.icudelirium.org).

Recently, a meta-analysis evaluated the accuracy of the CAM-ICU and the ICDSC for the diagnosis of ICU delirium.[100] This investigation included nine studies evaluating

Linking Sedation and Delirium Monitoring:
A Two-Step Approach to Assess Consciousness

Step One: Sedation Assessment
The Richmond Agitation and Sedation Scale: The RASS

Score	Term	Description	
+4	Combative	Overly combative, violent, immediate danger to staff	
+3	Very agitated	Pulls or removes tube(s) or catheter(s); aggressive	
+2	Agitated	Frequent non-purposeful movement, fights ventilator	
+1	Restless	Anxious but movements not aggressive vigorous	
0	Alert and calm		
−1	Drowsy	Not fully alert, but has sustained awakening (eye-opening/eye contact) to *voice* **(≥10 seconds)**	Verbal Stimulation
−2	Light sedation	Briefly awakens with eye contact to *voice* **(<10 seconds)**	
−3	Moderate sedation	Movement or eye opening to *voice* **(but no eye contact)**	
−4	Deep sedation	No response to voice, but movement or eye opening to *physical* stimulation	Physical Stimulation
−5	Unarousable	No response to *voice or physical* stimulation	

If RASS is −4 or −5, then **Stop** and **Reassess** patient at later time.
If RASS is above −4 (−3 through +4), then **Proceed to Step Two.**

Step Two: Delirium Assessment

Feature 1: Acute onset of mental status changes or a fluctuating course

And

Feature 2: Inattention

And

Feature 3: Disorganized thinking OR **Feature 4:** Altered level of consciousness

= DELIRIUM

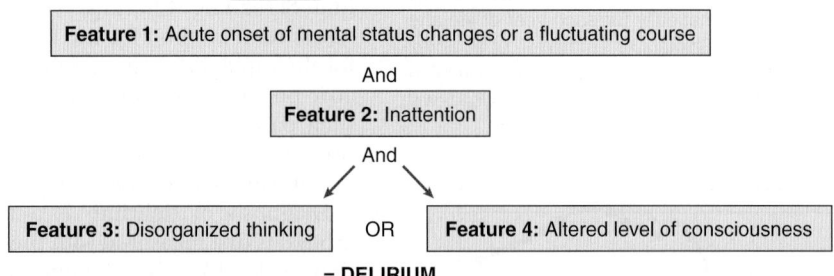

Figure 72.4 Richmond Agitation-Sedation Scale (RASS) and the Confusion Assessment Method for the ICU (CAM-ICU). This sedation scale and delirium instrument can be used together as a two-step approach to assess consciousness and diagnose delirium. Patients are considered to have delirium if they have RASS scores of −3 and higher and are assessed by CAM-ICU as "positive" by having both features 1 and 2 and either feature 3 or feature 4. (Data from references 19, 85, 86, and 148 [available online].)

the CAM-ICU (N = 969 total patients) and four studies evaluating the ICDSC (N= 361). The authors calculated the pooled sensitivity of the CAM-ICU to be 80% (95% confidence interval [CI]: 77.1-82.6%) and specificity of 95.9% (95% CI: 94.8-96.8%). The pooled sensitivity and specificity of the ICDSC were 74% (95% CI: 65.3-81.5%) and 81.9% (95% CI: 76.7-86.4%). They concluded that both delirium scales can be used as a screening tool, and that the CAM-ICU was an excellent diagnostic tool and the ICDSC had moderate sensitivity and good specificity.[100]

PREVENTION AND MANAGEMENT

PRIMARY PREVENTION AND NONPHARMACOLOGIC APPROACHES

In a trial of 852 general medical patients older than 70 years,[101] implementation of strategies for primary prevention of delirium resulted in a 40% reduction in the odds for development of delirium (15% in control subjects vs. 9.9% in the intervention patients). The protocol focused on optimization of risk factors via the following methods: repeated reorientation of the patient by trained volunteers and nurses, provision of cognitively stimulating activities for the patient three times per day, a nonpharmacologic sleep protocol to enhance normalization of sleep/wake cycles, early mobilization activities and range-of-motion exercises, timely removal of catheters and physical restraints, institution of the use of eyeglasses and magnifying lenses, use of hearing aids and earwax disimpaction, and early correction of dehydration.[101] Unfortunately, this intervention did not show sustained benefit during the 6 months of follow-up.[102] Later studies of delirium were unable to reproduce this success in reducing the incidence of delirium.[103,104]

Milisen and associates[105] and Lundstrom and coworkers,[106] who studied the implementation of multifactorial and multidisciplinary educational strategies, reported decreases in the duration and severity of delirium in patients cared for by staff who had received delirium-specific education.[105,106] Milisen and associates[105] measured the impact on delirium of implementing a nurse-led intervention program that involved delirium education for the nursing staff, systematic cognitive screening, availability of consultative services from a delirium resource nurse, and scheduled pain protocol on delirium. These researchers reported that although the program had no effect on the incidence of delirium, the duration and severity of delirium were significantly lower.[105] Lundstrom and coworkers[106] reported that in patients on a ward where the staff participated in specific educational activities focused on delirium and where the bedside nursing care was reorganized to provide more continuity of patient-centered care, duration of delirium and hospital stay were shorter and mortality rate was lower than in control patients. Cole and colleagues[104] found no difference in delirium rates between patients cared for by an intervention nurse and patients who received standard care. All of these nonpharmacologic "protocolization of care" studies focused on non-ICU patient populations. Clearly such investigations must be designed and conducted in the ICU (rather than simply extrapolated from non-ICU studies).

Although primary prevention of delirium is preferred, some delirium is inevitable in the ICU. In patients exhibiting delirium, the basic tenets of patient management, such as restoration of sleep/wake cycles, timely removal of catheters, early mobilization, minimization of unnecessary noise/stimuli, and frequent reorientation, should be applied liberally. Additionally, it should be emphasized that although sedative and analgesic agents have a very important role in patient comfort, health care professionals must also strive to achieve the right balance of administering these drugs through greater focus on reducing unnecessary or overzealous use. Instituting daily interruption of sedatives and analgesics, protocolizing their delivery, and instituting target-based sedation have all been shown to improve patient outcomes, although the studies reporting these results have not specifically looked at delirium rate or duration.[107-109] Studies have also shown a benefit for pain control using morphine in the prevention of delirium, because pain itself can be a risk factor for the development of delirium. Family involvement can also be very helpful in reorienting and soothing some delirious patients. It is important to teach family members about the fluctuating course of delirium as well as how they can detect it. Preventive and management strategies for delirium in the ICU represent an important area for future investigation.

PHARMACOLOGIC THERAPY

Medications should be used for delirium only after adequate attention has been given to correction of modifiable contributing factors (e.g., sleep disturbance, restraints), as discussed previously. It is important to remember that delirium could be a manifestation of an acute, life-threatening problem that requires immediate attention (such as hypoxia, hypercarbia, hypoglycemia, metabolic derangement, or shock). After such concerns have been addressed, pharmacologic management should be considered. It should be recognized that although agents used to treat delirium are intended to improve cognition, they all have psychoactive effects that may further cloud the sensorium and promote a longer overall duration of cognitive impairment. Therefore, until we have outcomes data that confirm beneficial effects of treatment, these drugs should be used judiciously in the smallest possible dose and for the shortest time necessary, a practice infrequently adhered to in most ICUs. Indeed, some cases prove refractory to all "cocktail" approaches to sedation and delirium therapy, and in these cases, a trial of complete cessation of all psychoactive drugs should be considered. Some reports have described the utility of dexmedetomidine (an α_2-agonist) as an adjunct to assist with weaning patients from all psychoactive medications.[110] Preliminary results from a prospective, randomized, yet unblinded trial in postoperative patients who had undergone cardiac surgery showed that sedation with dexmedetomidine at sternal closure was associated with an 8% incidence of postoperative delirium compared with 50% for either propofol or benzodiazepines.[111]

Benzodiazepines, which are used most commonly in the ICU for sedation, are not recommended for the management of delirium because of the likelihood of oversedation, exacerbation of confusion, and respiratory suppression. However, they remain the drugs of choice for the treatment of delirium tremens (and other withdrawal syndromes) and seizures. The amnestic qualities of benzodiazepines make these agents especially useful when noxious or unpleasant procedures are required. It is likely, however, that residual accumulation of these drugs may lead to prolonged delirium long after they have been discontinued. In certain populations, particularly elderly patients with underlying dementia, benzodiazepines may increase confusion and agitation. In such cases, one may try to take advantage of the sedative effects of haloperidol in lieu of continuing the benzodiazepine therapy.

Currently, no drugs are approved by the U.S. Food and Drug Administration (FDA) for the treatment of delirium. The SCCM guidelines[89] recommend haloperidol as the drug of choice, with the acknowledgment that this recommendation is based on sparse outcome data from nonrandomized case series and anecdotal reports (i.e., level C data). Nevertheless, haloperidol is a "typical" butyrophenone antipsychotic, which is the most widely used neuroleptic agent for delirium.[112] It does not suppress the respiratory drive and works as a dopamine receptor antagonist by blocking the δ_2-opioid receptor, resulting in treatment of positive symptoms (hallucinations, unstructured thought patterns, etc.) and producing a variable sedative effect. There are data to suggest that haloperidol may have some anti-inflammatory properties,[113,114] though this is theoretical in terms of a helpful pharmacologic effect on disease (such as septic delirium) at this point and requires further study.

In the non-ICU setting, the recommended starting dose of haloperidol is 0.5 to 1.0 mg orally or parenterally, with repeated doses every 20 to 30 minutes until the desired effect is achieved. In the ICU, a recommended starting dose would be 2 to 5 mg every 6 to 12 hours (intravenous, intramuscular, or oral), with maximal effective doses usually in the neighborhood of 20 mg/day. This dose range will usually be adequate to achieve the "theoretically optimal" 60% δ_2-receptor blockage[115] while avoiding complete δ_2-receptor saturation associated with the adverse effects cited later. Because of the urgency of the situation in many ICU patients—due to the potential for inadvertent removal of central lines, endotracheal tubes, or even aortic balloon pumps—much higher doses of haloperidol or a sedative are often used. Unfortunately, there are few data from formal pharmacologic investigations to guide dosage recommendations in the ICU. Once calm, the patient can usually be managed with much lower maintenance doses of haloperidol.

Neither haloperidol nor similar agents (i.e., droperidol and chlorpromazine) have been extensively studied for ICU use.[89] Newer "atypical" antipsychotic agents (e.g., risperidone, ziprasidone, quetiapine, and olanzapine) may also prove helpful for delirium.[116] The rationale behind use of the atypical antipsychotics rather than haloperidol (especially in hypoactive/mixed subtypes of delirium) is theoretical and centers on the fact that they affect not only dopamine but also other potentially key neurotransmitters such as serotonin, acetylcholine, and norepinephrine.[116-119] The use of haloperidol has been reported to have a mortality benefit in a retrospective analysis of critically ill, mechanically ventilated patients.[114] Kalisvaart and associates[120] showed that low-dose haloperidol prophylaxis reduced the duration and severity of delirium in elderly patients recovering from hip surgery, even though the actual prevalence of delirium was not reduced. A more recent study by Wang and coworkers[121] also studied prophylactic haloperidol administration after cardiac surgery and actually did find a lower incidence of postoperative delirium associated with haloperidol, though this study was of a low severity of illness cohort and may not apply to truly critically ill patients with septic shock and ARDS. Skrobik and colleagues[116] reported that olanzapine and haloperidol were equally efficacious in treating ICU delirium in both medical and surgical patients but that olanzapine had fewer side effects (again findings from a moderately ill group that must be confirmed and tested against placebo).

Adequately powered prospective, randomized placebo-controlled trials of antipsychotics are not available to date and must be performed to provide clinicians with evidence-based guidelines for preventing and treating delirium. Although there are prospective studies that begin to examine the safety and efficacy of antipsychotics such as amisulpride,[122] quetiapine,[122-124] and risperidone,[125,126] these are generally small and quite heterogeneous in design population studied, dosing regimens, and the use of delirium assessment tools. A National Institutes of Health (NIH)-sponsored large prospective randomized placebo-controlled trial called MIND-USA is currently under way to investigate further the utility, risk, and benefit of both haloperidol and the atypical antipsychotic ziprasidone. The pilot study, called the MIND (Minimizing the Incidence of Delirium) trial,[127] established feasibility in a population of mechanically ventilated medical and surgical ICU patients and laid the groundwork for future research.

Kato and coworkers[128] reported a case study that suggests that genotyping may affect the choice of antipsychotic drugs. They showed that a patient with the CYP2D6 genotype had persistent delirium and demonstrated severe extrapyramidal symptoms when treated with risperidone. When quetiapine (metabolized by CYP3A4) was used instead, the patient's delirium cleared within 2 days without side effects. This case report is not proof of a positive effect of antipsychotics; yet it is interesting and suggests that pharmacogenetics may play an important role in medication choices in the near future.

Adverse effects of typical and atypical antipsychotics include hypotension, acute dystonias, extrapyramidal effects, laryngeal spasm, malignant hyperthermia, glucose and lipid dysregulation, and anticholinergic effects such as dry mouth, constipation, and urinary retention. Perhaps the most immediately life-threatening adverse effect of antipsychotics is torsades de pointes, and these agents should not be given to patients with prolonged QT intervals unless absolutely necessary. Patents who receive substantial quantities of typical or atypical antipsychotics or coadministered arrhythmogenic drugs should be monitored closely with electrocardiography. In early 2005, the FDA issued an alert that atypical antipsychotic medications are associated with a mortality risk among elderly patients. This warning was supported by a meta-analysis of a large volume of data from outpatient treatment of patients with dementia who were experiencing psychotic symptoms that resulted in their receiving antipsychotic medications.[129] Similar associations with higher stroke risk and fatality have been reported by other investigators.[130,131] Subsequently, other studies have suggested that this higher risk of death in non-ICU elderly patients treated with antipsychotics may not be limited to the atypical antipsychotic agents; Schneider and colleagues[130] found that the conventional antipsychotic haloperidol had an even higher mortality risk.

Along with haloperidol and the atypical antipsychotics for the treatment of acute brain dysfunction, a growing body of literature suggests a role for sedatives such as the α_2-agonist dexmedetomidine in the pharmacologic management of delirium. The MENDS (Maximizing Efficacy of Targeted Sedation and Reducing Neurological Dysfunction) trial[132] compared dexmedetomidine to lorazepam for targeted sedation greater than 24 hours in 106 mechanically ventilated patients. Sedation with dexmedetomidine resulted in more days alive without coma or delirium and lower prevalence of coma compared to sedation with lorazepam. Subgroup analysis also demonstrated that sedation with dexmedetomidine reduced the daily risk of delirium, particularly in patients with sepsis.[133] The SEDCOM (Safety and Efficacy of Dexmedetomidine Compared with Midazolam) trial[134] compared dexmedetomidine to midazolam, another commonly used benzodiazepine in the ICU. This large prospective trial showed significantly lower prevalence of delirium in patients receiving dexmedetomidine compared to midazolam, an effect observed within 1 day of initiating sedation and sustained throughout the week of study drug administration.[134] In 2012, the MIDEX and PRODEX trials compared midazolam to dexmedetomidine (MIDEX) and propofol (preferred usual care) to dexmedetomidine (PRODEX) in mechanically ventilated patients requiring long-term sedation. These large trials, which together enrolled nearly 1000 patients, showed that dexmedetomidine was not inferior to midazolam or propofol for targeted light to moderate sedation and was found to be associated with improved communication between the patients and others involved in their care. Dexmedetomidine also reduced time to extubation and was associated with fewer neurocognitive disorders (including delirium) than propofol.[135] In each trial, the reproducible significant adverse effect associated with dexmedetomidine was bradycardia, which typically resolved without event and infrequently required adjunctive treatment beyond discontinuation of the drug.[135]

Other agents such as the cholinesterase inhibitors have proved unsuccessful in the management of ICU delirium. Given the hypothesis that delirium was associated with excess dopamine and a central cholinergic deficiency, it was logical to test the cholinesterase inhibitors such as rivastigmine, used in treating dementia, for the management of ICU delirium. However, in 2010, a large placebo-controlled trial evaluating rivastigmine as an adjunct to usual care with haloperidol was halted early due to increased mortality risk and longer duration of delirium in patients receiving rivastigmine.[136] Other agents such as ondansetron[137] and melatonin[138] are being considered for the treatment of ICU delirium but thus far have little support in the literature.

Protocols and evidence-based strategies for prevention and treatment of delirium will no doubt emerge as more evidence becomes available from ongoing randomized clinical trials of both nonpharmacologic and pharmacologic strategies. To assist readers in developing a delirium management algorithm in their respective clinical arenas, we have provided an empiric protocol largely based on the current SCCM clinical practice guidelines (Fig. 72.5). At this time, we have few data as to which antipsychotic medications are most suitable for delirium. The nonpharmacologic interventions recommended in this protocol have shown beneficial results in non-ICU patients, but the extrapolation to ICU populations is speculative. Nevertheless, such data emphasize the need for more research in this area and underscore the importance of exercising caution in the treatment of delirium. We wish to emphasize that protocols such as the ABCDEs of critical care[33,34] must be updated regularly with new data and also individualized at each medical center to form an integrated approach to delirium monitoring, sedation targeting, and delirium management in critically ill ICU patients.

By way of summary regarding delirium management, the main thrust of our approach as health care professionals must begin with treatment of the underlying disease processes that are leading to brain dysfunction, then drug removal, and then modification of the environmental factors (hearing and vision aids, removal of restraints and early mobility, and sleep hygiene), which can be summarized via the mnemonic Dr. DRE (Diseases, Drug Removal, Environment). These are nicely summarized and operationalized in the evidence-based ABCDEs of ICU care, which stands for spontaneous Awakening trials, spontaneous Breathing trials, Coordination of care and Choice of sedative, Delirium monitoring and management, and Early mobility.[33,34] Only after these issues are addressed is it appropriate to add another medication such as an antipsychotic into the mix of the individual pharmacopeia for any patient.

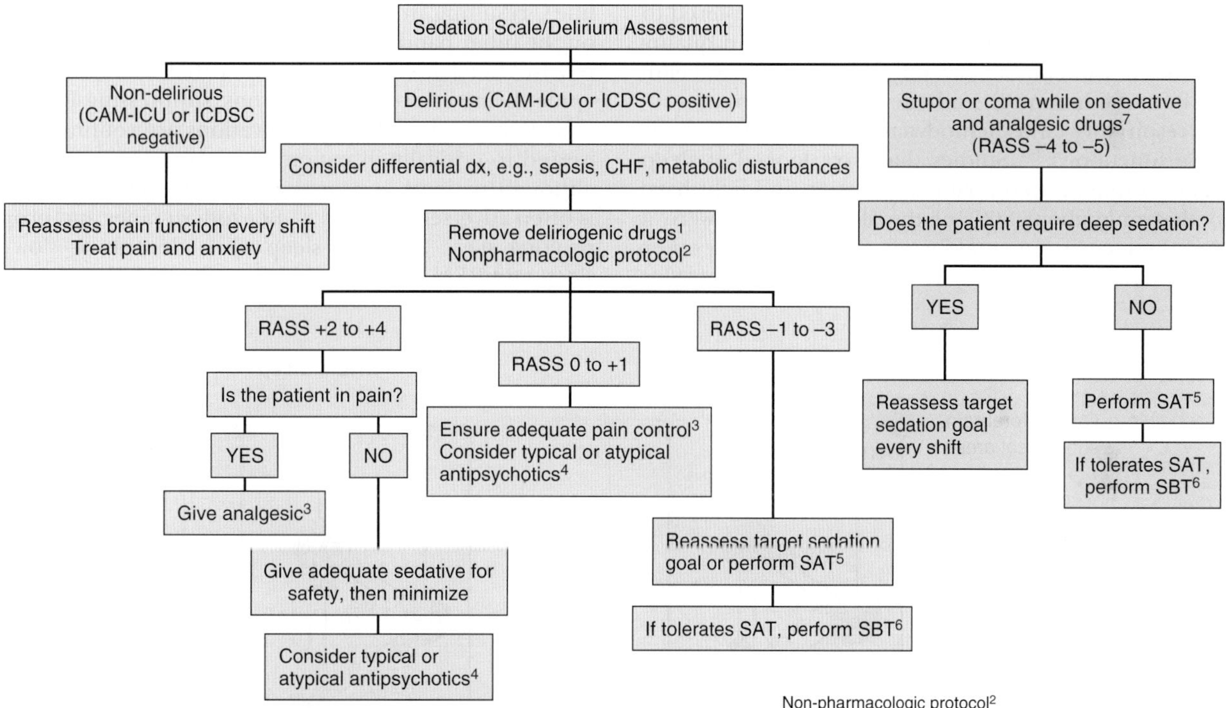

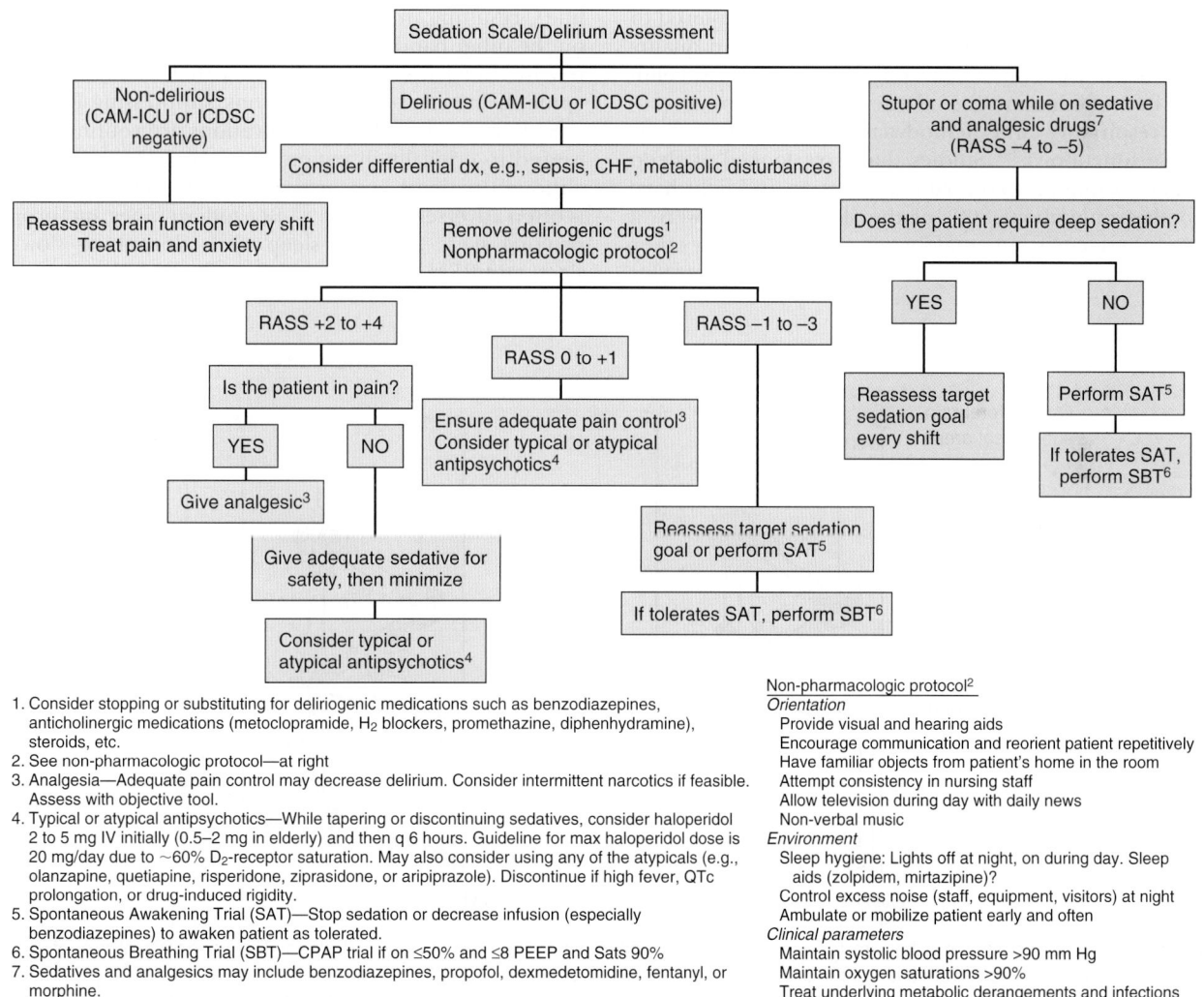

1. Consider stopping or substituting for deliriogenic medications such as benzodiazepines, anticholinergic medications (metoclopramide, H_2 blockers, promethazine, diphenhydramine), steroids, etc.
2. See non-pharmacologic protocol—at right
3. Analgesia—Adequate pain control may decrease delirium. Consider intermittent narcotics if feasible. Assess with objective tool.
4. Typical or atypical antipsychotics—While tapering or discontinuing sedatives, consider haloperidol 2 to 5 mg IV initially (0.5–2 mg in elderly) and then q 6 hours. Guideline for max haloperidol dose is 20 mg/day due to ~60% D_2-receptor saturation. May also consider using any of the atypicals (e.g., olanzapine, quetiapine, risperidone, ziprasidone, or aripiprazole). Discontinue if high fever, QTc prolongation, or drug-induced rigidity.
5. Spontaneous Awakening Trial (SAT)—Stop sedation or decrease infusion (especially benzodiazepines) to awaken patient as tolerated.
6. Spontaneous Breathing Trial (SBT)—CPAP trial if on ≤50% and ≤8 PEEP and Sats 90%
7. Sedatives and analgesics may include benzodiazepines, propofol, dexmedetomidine, fentanyl, or morphine.

Non-pharmacologic protocol[2]

Orientation
- Provide visual and hearing aids
- Encourage communication and reorient patient repetitively
- Have familiar objects from patient's home in the room
- Attempt consistency in nursing staff
- Allow television during day with daily news
- Non-verbal music

Environment
- Sleep hygiene: Lights off at night, on during day. Sleep aids (zolpidem, mirtazipine)?
- Control excess noise (staff, equipment, visitors) at night
- Ambulate or mobilize patient early and often

Clinical parameters
- Maintain systolic blood pressure >90 mm Hg
- Maintain oxygen saturations >90%
- Treat underlying metabolic derangements and infections

Figure 72.5 Delirium protocol. This empiric protocol, which is based largely on the current Society of Critical Care Medicine's clinical practice guidelines, is the algorithm we use to treat delirium in our intensive care units (ICUs). We wish to emphasize that such protocols need to be updated regularly with new data and also individualized at each medical center. Specific recommendations about the choice of antipsychotics to treat delirium have not been described, because limited data are available regarding the appropriate drug to use in ICU patients. The nonpharmacologic interventions recommended in this protocol have been shown to have beneficial results in non-ICU patients, but the extrapolation to ICU populations is speculative. CAM-ICU, Confusion Assessment Method for the ICU; ICDSC, Intensive Care Delirium Screening Checklist; RASS, Richmond Agitation-Sedation Scale; Sats, saturations.

SLEEP DISRUPTION IN THE CRITICALLY ILL

The sleep cycle is divided into rapid eye movement (REM) sleep and non-REM (NREM) sleep.[139] NREM sleep is further divided into four stages according to an increasing depth of sleep.[111] A normal sleep cycle lasts approximately 90 minutes, cycling continuously between REM and NREM sleep. Stages 3 and 4 of the NREM sleep represent slow-wave or more restful sleep.[139]

Critically ill patients have severe sleep deprivation with disruption of sleep architecture. The average amount of sleep in the ICU has been measured to be about 2 hours out of 24 hours, with less than 6% of it spent in REM sleep. In a study by Cooper and associates,[140] the majority of the patients had abnormal sleep patterns. The causes of sleep deprivation in the ICU have been extensively reported. They consist of excessive noise and lighting, patient care activities such as procedures and baths, metabolic consequences of critical illness, mechanical ventilation, and the sedative and analgesic medications that are administered to these patients.[141] This disturbance in duration and quality of sleep has detrimental effects on protein synthesis, cellular and humoral immunity, and energy expenditure, resulting in respiratory and hemodynamic effects as well as cognitive function.[141,142] Studies that have looked at sleep disturbances due to noise, patient activities, and light have found that only about 30% of the sleep arousals were a result of these environmental factors, suggesting that other patient factors or management issues play an important role.[143] Of these, it is interesting that the psychoactive medications are common risk factors for both delirium and sleep disturbances, whereas sleep deprivation can itself lead to delirium.

NEUROTRANSMISSION IN SLEEP

The ventrolateral preoptic (VLPO) nucleus in the anterior hypothalamus is the major area of the brain that controls sleep induction and maintenance.[144] Its major neurotransmitter is GABA, and during the awake state, the GABA release from the VLPO nucleus is inhibited by norepinephrine (NE) from the locus coeruleus.[144] With the inhibition of GABA, neurotransmitters such as orexin, serotonin, histamine, and acetylcholine are released, resulting in a state of wakefulness (Fig. 72.6). During NREM sleep, norepinephrine release diminishes, thus removing the inhibitory effect on release of GABA from the VLPO nucleus. The firing of GABA neurons inhibits the neurotransmitters of wakefulness (orexin, serotonin, histamine, and acetylcholine), resulting in NREM sleep (see Fig. 72.6). REM sleep, on the other hand, is facilitated by neurons in the pons that release acetylcholine. Studies show that serotonin and norepinephrine inhibit these neurons, suppressing REM sleep.

Sedative and analgesic medications are routinely administered to critically ill patients to promote sleep. However, although patients appear sedated, their sleep architecture is often adversely affected.[139] Benzodiazepines and propofol prolong stage 2 NREM sleep while decreasing slow-wave sleep and REM sleep. Opioids, on the other hand, increase

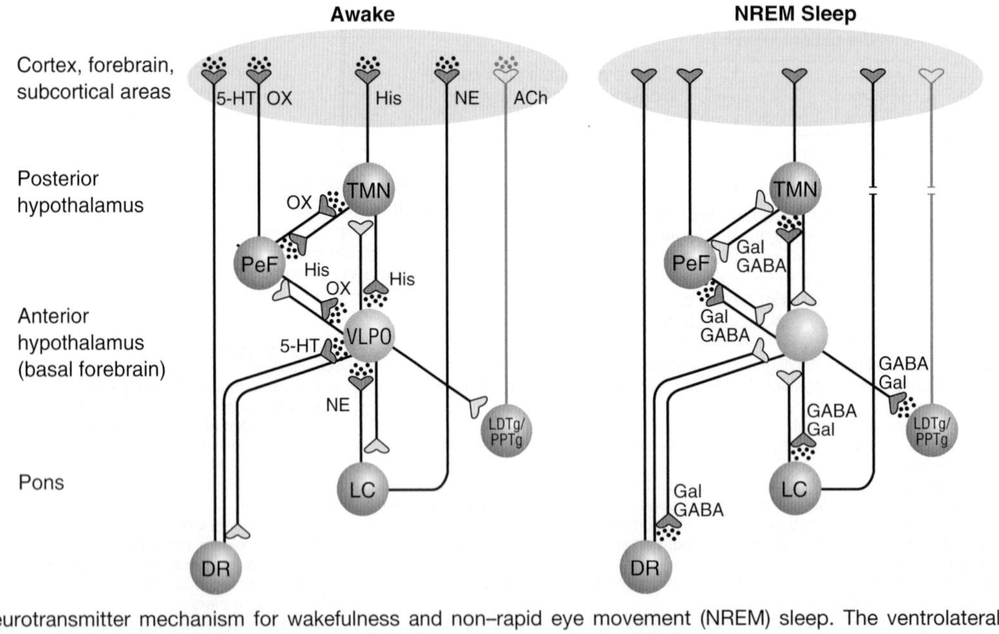

Figure 72.6 Neurotransmitter mechanism for wakefulness and non–rapid eye movement (NREM) sleep. The ventrolateral preoptic (VLPO) nucleus in the anterior hypothalamus is the major area of the brain that controls sleep induction and maintenance. Its major neurotransmitter is γ-aminobutyric acid (GABA), and during the awake state, GABA release from the VLPO nucleus is inhibited by norepinephrine (NE) from the locus coeruleus (LC). With the inhibition of GABA, neurotransmitters such as orexin (OX), serotonin (5-HT), histamine (His), and acetylcholine (ACh) are released, resulting in a state of wakefulness. During NREM sleep, there is a hierarchical sequence of changes in which inhibition of the LC disinhibits the VLPO nucleus to release GABA and galanin (Gal) at the projections that terminate at the tuberomamillary nucleus (TMN). These inhibitory neurotransmitters inhibit firing of the TMN projections to the cortical and subcortical regions. LDTg, laterodorsal tegmental nucleus; PPTg, pedunculopontine tegmental nucleus. (From Analgesics: Receptor ligands: Alpha 2 adrenergic receptor agonists. In Evers AS, Maze M: Anesthetic Pharmacology: Physiologic Principles and Clinical Practice. St. Louis, Churchill Livingstone, 2004. Used with permission from Dr. Mervyn Maze and Elsevier, Inc.)

stage 1 NREM sleep while decreasing slow-wave and REM sleep. It is hypothesized that one of the reasons that dexmedetomidine allows for less time in acute brain dysfunction (delirium) is that its effect in the locus coeruleus (rather than the VLPO nucleus, which is the site of action of benzodiazepines and propofol) leads to a more normal pattern of sleep. This effect has not been convincingly shown beyond animal models to date. Numerous other medications routinely administered to critically ill patients affect sleep architecture. These include antiarrhythmic agents, inotropes and vasopressors, antibiotics, antidepressants, steroids, anticonvulsants, and bronchodilators.[139] The effects of some of these compounds on sleep patterns are summarized in Table 72.1.

Although they lack anxiolytic properties, ω_1-receptor agonists such as zolpidem may preserve REM as well as slow-wave sleep.[145] Similarly, mirtazapine, a noradrenergic and specific serotonergic antidepressant, has been studied in healthy volunteers and has been shown to improve sleep efficiency, reducing the number and duration of awakenings.[146] The slow-wave sleep time was also increased, whereas stage 1 sleep time was reduced significantly. This agent had no significant effect on REM sleep variables.[147] An investigation of the use of dexmedetomidine (an α_2-agonist) in rats shows that it mimics and increases NREM sleep[144] but decreases REM sleep. By acting on the locus coeruleus, dexmedetomidine inhibits the release of norepinephrine, thus causing GABA output from the VLPO nucleus and inhibition of the neurotransmitters of wakefulness to produce a NREM sleep pattern. In contrast, benzodiazepines and propofol exert their sedative action on the VLPO nucleus to increase GABA and decrease the neurotransmitters such as orexin, histamine, and serotonin but without affecting norepinephrine release from the locus coeruleus. Further clinical trials are required to ascertain the role of these medications in improving the quality and quantity of sleep in critically ill patients and to see whether such improvement may better the cognitive outcomes in ICU patients.

POSTTRAUMATIC STRESS DISORDER

DEFINITION AND DIAGNOSTIC CRITERIA

The DSM-IV[12] defines PTSD as a potentially debilitating psychiatric condition that develops as the result of exposure to a traumatic occurrence, in which the person experienced, witnessed, or was confronted with an event or events that involved actual or threatened death or serious injury, or a threat to the physical integrity of self or others and that generates intense feelings of fear, helplessness, or horror in the person exposed to the trauma. This condition is characterized by a constellation of symptoms in the following three domains:

- Symptoms of reexperiencing (e.g., intrusive thoughts and upsetting recollections of the trauma, recurrent dreams or nightmares, and flashbacks)
- Symptoms of avoidance and emotional numbing (e.g., efforts to avoid conversations, places, and thoughts associated with the trauma; detachment from others; and a restricted range of affect)

Table 72.1 Drugs Commonly Used in the Intensive Care Unit and Their Effects on Sleep Patterns

Drug Class/Individual Drug	Sleep Disorder Induced/Reported	Possible Mechanism
Benzodiazepines	↓ REM, ↓ SWS	γ-Aminobutyric acid type A (GABA[A]) receptor stimulation
Opioids	↓ REM, ↓ SWS	μ-Opioid receptor stimulation
Clonidine	↓ REM	α_2-Adrenergic receptor stimulation
Nonsteroidal anti-inflammatory drugs	↓ TST, ↓ SE	Prostaglandin synthesis inhibition
Norepinephrine/epinephrine	Insomnia, ↓ REM, ↓ SWS	α_1-Adrenergic receptor stimulation
Dopamine	Insomnia, ↓ REM, ↓ SWS	δ_2-Opioid receptor stimulation/α_1-adrenergic receptor stimulation
β-Blockers	Insomnia, ↓ REM, nightmares	Central nervous system β-blockade by lipophilic agents
Amiodarone	Nightmares	Unknown mechanism
Corticosteroids	Insomnia, ↓ REM, ↓ SWS	Reduced melatonin secretion
Aminophylline	Insomnia, ↓ REM, ↓ SWS, ↓ TST, ↓ SE	Adenosine receptor antagonism
Quinolones	Insomnia	GABA(A) receptor inhibition
Tricyclic antidepressants	↓ REM	Antimuscarinic activity and α_1-adrenergic receptor stimulation
Selective serotonin reuptake inhibitors	↓ REM, ↓ TST, ↓ SE	Increased serotonergic activity
Phenytoin	↑ Sleep fragmentation	Inhibition of neuronal calcium influx
Phenobarbital	↓ REM	Increased GABA(A) activity
Carbamazepine	↓ REM	Adenosine receptor stimulation and/or serotonergic activity

REM, rapid eye movement (sleep); SE, sleep efficiency; SWS, slow-wave sleep; TST, total sleep time.

Reproduced with permission from Bourne RS, Mills GH: Sleep disruption in critically ill patients—Pharmacological considerations. Anaesthesia 2004;59:374-384.

- Symptoms of increased arousal (e.g., sleep disruption, hypervigilance, and exaggerated startle response)

These symptoms must meet two criteria to be diagnosed as PTSD, as follows:

1. Symptoms must cause significant impairment in social, occupational, or other important functional domains.
2. Symptoms must be present for at least 1 month after exposure to the traumatic event or events.

PREVALENCE OF ICU-RELATED POSTTRAUMATIC STRESS DISORDER

The prevalence rates reported in studies on PTSD after critical illness vary widely (5% to >50%) and differ according to whether the specific outcome in question is a diagnosis of PTSD or merely the presence of PTSD symptoms. In the eight investigations that focused on the identification of subjects with PTSD (as opposed to those with PTSD symptoms), prevalence rates ranged from 9.7% to approximately 40%.[147] The prevalence of PTSD differed depending on the time of assessment, with higher rates identified in closer proximity to the time of hospital discharge. In investigations that included serial evaluations, patients generally demonstrated a decrease in symptoms over time. For example, Kapfhammer and colleagues[148] reported that 43.5% of study subjects had PTSD at discharge (although according to the DSM-IV, PTSD cannot be diagnosed until 4 weeks after exposure to the "traumatic stressor"), whereas 23.9% suffered from PTSD an average of 8 years later. Prevalence rates tend to be higher among some specific ICU populations, such as patients with sepsis or ARDS (25% to 40% at follow-up), in comparison with general medical ICU cohorts.[148]

RISK FACTORS FOR POSTTRAUMATIC STRESS DISORDER

A number of subject characteristics appear to raise the risk of PTSD symptoms or an actual diagnosis of PTSD, although consensus among the studies reviewed is limited. Reported risk factors include delusional memories of the ICU, a greater number of traumatic memories of the ICU, longer ICU length of stay or duration of mechanical ventilation or both, younger age, prior mental health history, female gender, and higher levels of sedation and neuromuscular blockade.[149] No studies have investigated the association between delirium and PTSD.

CONCEPTUAL EXPLANATIONS FOR POSTTRAUMATIC STRESS DISORDER AFTER CRITICAL ILLNESS

Although the stresses associated with ICU hospitalization may differ from events typically described as "traumatic experiences," there are a variety of conceptual explanations for the development of PTSD following critical illness. They include (1) profound feelings of helplessness associated with the experience of critical illness, (2) high rates of preexisting psychiatric morbidity that may characterize ICU patients,[150] (3) cognitive impairment, including decreased working memory, which may limit individual abilities to suppress intrusive thoughts,[150] and (4) multiple traumatic episodes associated with anxiety, panic, or pain that occur during ICU hospitalization, such as intubations, extubations, nightmares, and respiratory distress.[151,152]

The frequency of anxiety-provoking episodes during ICU hospitalization might partly explain the association between higher levels of sedation and increased PTSD symptoms, in that anxious patients may receive more sedatives. Brewin and Holmes[153] suggest that immobilization with incomplete sedation promotes a dissociative experience that may be a PTSD risk factor.

A significant percentage of patients treated in the ICU have chronic medical illnesses,[154,155] which may increase anxiety or susceptibility to anxiety reactions. The presence of such stressors may have a cumulative effect on an individual's coping resources, leading to a greater vulnerability to PTSD. This concept is bolstered by evidence from numerous studies as well as the theoretical work of Turner and Lloyd,[156] which supports the notion that healthy coping responses are impeded by the "accumulated burden of adversity" associated with illness or disease.[157-159] Although the contribution of cumulative illness to the development of PTSD has not been assessed in ICU populations, investigations support an association between accumulated medical burden and higher risk of PTSD. For example, accident victims (without chronic medical illnesses) who are admitted to the trauma ICU have a lower prevalence of PTSD than their medical ICU counterparts (with multiple chronic diseases).[160] Alternatively, patients with chronic cardiovascular disease who have undergone cardiac surgery have relatively high rates of PTSD, which correlate positively with preoperative disease severity.[151]

The relationship between cognitive function and PTSD is a subject of ongoing debate, particularly as it relates to the role of memory in mediating the development of PTSD.[161] The importance of specific, explicit memories (memories pertaining to facts and events, which are accessible to consciousness)[162,163] in the generation and maintenance of PTSD is difficult to estimate because they are the basis for nightmares, flashbacks, and intrusive thoughts and contribute to symptoms of avoidance and reexperiencing. Although a detailed treatment of these issues is beyond the scope of this chapter, we briefly discuss several key findings from the literature as they relate to ICU populations.

The preponderance of evidence suggests that the absence of episodic memory for a traumatic event is protective against the development of PTSD, because a majority of studies have shown that the risk of PTSD is markedly lower in individuals unable to recall a traumatic event than in those with explicit memory of it.[164-168] The literature is not unanimous and is narrow in scope, with virtually all relevant studies having been conducted on victims of motor vehicle accidents or other traumas with concomitant traumatic brain injury.[169] Theories of information processing suggest that traumatic memories can be encoded implicitly during periods of impaired consciousness and may provide the basis for the generation of PTSD symptoms even if patients are not consciously aware of the memories.[170-173] Additionally, during periods of impaired consciousness, the encoding of emotional experiences such as panic and severe pain appears to be sufficient for the generation of PTSD symptoms.[174]

Many ICU patients report little if any conscious awareness of their critical illness, although as Jones and associates[175] have reported, delusional memories, often with violent and paranoid themes, are pervasive among such patients. Distorted and fragmentary memories may be vestiges of the nightmares, hallucinations, or delusions induced by critical illness, a variety of medications, or other causes and may be particularly likely to occur during delirium, which is ubiquitous in critically ill, mechanically ventilated patients.[16,176] Sedative medications may constitute one factor that mediates the development of delusional memories.[177] Delusional memories may exist in the absence of factual memories, which provide markers of reality and may serve to orient the patient. For example, daily sedative interruption has been found to be associated with fewer symptoms of PTSD,[178] suggesting that even limited factual memories from brief awakening may reduce PTSD. In addition, delusional memories tend to be stable over time and are significantly more persistent than factual memories.[179] Delusional memories may be more refractory to the normal cognitive processes of habituation and reappraisal because they are not well integrated into the long-term memory. Although research is limited, the presence of delusional memories of the ICU is associated with higher levels of anxiety and PTSD.[180,181]

LONG-TERM COGNITIVE IMPAIRMENT AFTER CRITICAL ILLNESS

Medical and surgical management of critical illnesses can, and frequently does, result in de novo neurocognitive impairments. Approximately one third or more of ICU survivors have LTCI.[182] It is difficult to make comparisons among studies owing to differences in definitions of neurocognitive sequelae, administered neuropsychological tests, time to follow-up, patient population, study design (prospective vs. retrospective), and inclusion of a control group. Nevertheless, current data suggest that neurocognitive impairments are extremely common in survivors of critical illness.

Currently, 10 cohort studies totaling approximately 455 patients have assessed LTCI after critical illness.[182-192] The populations of the patient cohorts include patients with ARDS, acute lung injury, and respiratory failure in the ICU[182,183,187,189-192] as well as two studies in general ICU patients.[184,188] The time to neurocognitive assessments was variable, with the majority occurring during the first year after hospital discharge. Three studies assessed patients more than 1 year later. A prospective longitudinal study monitored patients at hospital discharge and then at 1 and 2 years after hospital discharge,[193] and two retrospective studies assessed the patients at approximately 6 years after hospital discharge.[187,191]

The evidence from the 10 cohorts suggests that 25% to 78% of ICU survivors experience neurocognitive impairments.[182-192] Among specific populations, such as patients with ARDS, the prevalence of LTCI is even greater; it may be as high as 78% at hospital discharge, 46% at 1 year,[183] and 25% at 6 years.[191] Hopkins and colleagues[183] assessed ARDS patients' premorbid estimated intelligence quotient (IQ) and found it was significantly higher than the patients' measured IQ at hospital discharge. However, the patients' measured IQ improved to their premorbid level by 1-year follow-up, with no additional improvement at 2 years. The finding that patients recovered over time with regard to intelligence does not necessarily suggest a comparable recovery in all cognitive domains, because data from traumatic and anoxic brain injury literature suggest that some neurocognitive abilities are more likely to improve than others.[194]

A 2004 study found that neurocognitive impairments occur in 70% of ARDS patients at hospital discharge, 45% at 1 year, and 47% at 2 years.[193] The neurocognitive test scores of the ARDS survivors with neurocognitive sequelae (≈50% of survivors) fell below the sixth percentile of the normal distribution of cognitive function. These ARDS survivors had marked difficulty with tasks that require executive function, memory, attention, or quick mental processing. The neurocognitive impairments in critically patients are similar to those reported in medical ICU survivors[182] after carbon monoxide poisoning[195] and several years after elective coronary artery bypass graft surgery.[196]

In addition to ARDS survivors, neurocognitive impairments have been reported in the general population of critically ill patients. Jackson and colleagues,[182] evaluating 34 medical ICU survivors at 6 months, found that 33% had LTCI (using a very conservative definition of impairment as two test scores 2 standard deviations below the mean or three test scores 1.5 standard deviations below the mean). The neurocognitive impairments were similar to those reported in ARDS survivors; they included mental processing speed, memory, language, and visuospatial abilities. Additional support for cognitive impairment in the general critically ill population comes from a prospective cohort of 32 critically ill patients who underwent long-term mechanical ventilation (>5 days). The patients were evaluated at hospital discharge and 6 months later.[185] Of the patients who received long-term mechanical ventilation, 91% at hospital discharge and 41% at 6 months had impairments in attention, memory, mental processing speed, and executive function.[185]

Girard and colleagues showed that the duration of delirium was an independent predictor of LTCI at 1-year follow-up even after adjusting for relevant covariates.[50] It is hoped that other ongoing investigations will provide information about the risk factors for the development of LTCI and help guide interventions for prevention of the rather debilitating sequelae of critical illness that affect a person's quality of life.

DEPRESSION

Many ICU survivors experience significant affective symptoms, such as depression and anxiety.[197] The prevalence and severity of affective disorders, including symptoms of depression and anxiety in ICU survivors, range from less than 10% to 58%.[147,182,183,190,198] Depression has been reported to occur in up to 30% of ICU survivors,[182] and it is estimated that 47% have clinically significant anxiety.[197] Indeed, the high rates of depression among ICU survivors may be related to the cognitive impairment they experience, although this issue has not been evaluated in ICU cohorts. Affective disorders such as depression, PTSD, and anxiety may adversely affect test performance, especially if severe.[199,200] Moderate to severe depression may result in decreased effort and low motivation, which may in turn lower neuropsychological test scores in cognitive domains such as psychomotor speed and attention.[201,202] Moderate to severe anxiety, however, may lead to increased distractibility and blocked thoughts or words.[203,204] In some cases, severe depression may mimic symptoms of cognitive impairment, although there are important differences between these conditions. In general, individuals with depression retain the ability to learn and do not forget as rapidly, do not display significant decrements in language, are inconsistent with regard to orientation to time and date, and are typically more self-aware than their cognitively impaired counterparts.[205-207]

A variety of instruments are available for use in the assessment of affective function. Tools such as the Geriatric Depression Scale-Short Form (GDS-SF),[208] the Beck Depression Inventory (BDI),[209] the Center for Epidemiologic Studies Depression Scale (CES-D),[210] and the Hospital Anxiety-Depression Scale (HADS)[211] assess depression. Anxiety can be assessed with the HADS[211] or the Beck Anxiety Inventory (BAI).[212] Discussion of these tools is beyond the scope of this chapter.

CONCLUDING THOUGHTS

How might we incorporate these issues into our life as a health care professional? It is important as you see patients being newly admitted to the ICU with diseases such as severe sepsis or an exacerbation of COPD to remind yourself that during subsequent days under your care, these patients will acquire new "neck-up" and "neck-down" (brain plus neuromuscular) diseases. It is imperative that these two new elements of disease burden become a major focus of medical attention during and following these patients' ICU stays. It is also important to recognize that these two categories of disability are inextricably linked. As we work to identify methods of intervention to prevent and treat these disabilities, it may be helpful to focus on modifiable aspects of care such as reducing total exposure to psychoactive medications, reducing duration of delirium, mitigating sleep deficits and derangements, and minimizing periods of immobilization.

KEY POINTS

- Delirium is a disturbance of consciousness heralded by the cardinal manifestation of inattention, accompanied by a change in cognition or perceptual disturbance that develops over a short time and has a fluctuating course.
- The prevalence of delirium in medical and surgical ICU studies has been reported to be 60% to 80% in cohorts restricted to those receiving mechanical ventilation and around 40% to 60% in ICU cohorts of nonventilated patients.

KEY POINTS (Continued)

- Delirium is an independent predictor of longer duration of mechanical ventilation, longer ICU stays, higher costs, and a threefold higher risk of dying within 6 months or an increase of 10% risk of death per day of delirium.
- The development of tools such as the ICDSC and the CAM-ICU have allowed for the rapid diagnosis of delirium in patients by nonpsychiatric physicians and health care personnel even during mechanical ventilation.
- Sedative and analgesic medications and sleep disturbances in the ICU may be modifiable risk factors of delirium.
- The main thrust of delirium management must begin with treatment of the underlying disease processes that are leading to brain dysfunction, then drug removal (not addition), and then modification of the environmental factors (hearing and vision aids, removal of restraints and early mobility, and sleep hygiene). Summarize these via the mnemonic Dr. DRE. These are nicely summarized and operationalized in the evidence-based ABCDEs of ICU care.
- Only after these issues are addressed is it appropriate to add another medication such as an antipsychotic into the mix of the individual pharmacopeia for any patient. Which medication to add (e.g., antipsychotic) is a point of ongoing investigation.
- Critically ill patients often have severe sleep deprivation with disruption of sleep architecture that is made worse by most sedative medications.
- The average amount of sleep in ICU patients has been measured to be about 2 hours in a 24-hour period, less than 6% of which is REM sleep often because of REM suppression from medications such as benzodiazepines and propofol.
- PTSD is a potentially debilitating psychiatric condition, which develops in 5% to 50% of ICU survivors as the result of exposure to a traumatic occurrence that generates intense feelings of fear, helplessness, or horror.
- Medical and surgical management of critical illnesses is associated with long-term neurocognitive impairments in approximately two thirds of ICU survivors. This form of cognitive impairment mimics dementia in many patients as they suffer from moderate to severe deficits in memory, executive dysfunction, and other domains with profound ecologic validity.
- Between one third and two thirds of ICU survivors experience significant affective symptoms, such as depression and anxiety, which serve as another ongoing aspect of suffering that all too often remains undiagnosed and therefore unaddressed by the medical teams caring for ICU survivors.

SELECTED REFERENCES

20. Ely EW, Inouye SK, Bernard GR, et al: Delirium in mechanically ventilated patients: Validity and reliability of the confusion assessment method for the intensive care unit (CAM-ICU). JAMA 2001;286:2703-2710.
33. Vasilevskis EE, Ely EW, Speroff T, et al: Reducing iatrogenic risks: ICU-acquired delirium and weakness—Crossing the quality chasm. Chest 2010;138(5):1224-1233.
44. Ely EW, Shintani A, Truman B, et al: Delirium as a predictor of mortality in mechanically ventilated patients in the intensive care unit. JAMA 2004;291:1753-1762.
50. Girard TD, Jackson JC, Pandharipande PP, et al: Delirium as a predictor of long-term cognitive impairment in survivors of critical illness. Crit Care Med 2010;38:1513-1520.
92. Pandharipande P, Shintani A, Truman P, et al: Lorazepam is an independent risk factor for transitioning to delirium in intensive care unit patients. Anesthesiology 2006;104:21-26.
98. Ely EW, Truman B, Shintani A, et al: Monitoring sedation status over time in ICU patients: Reliability and validity of the Richmond Agitation-Sedation Scale (RASS). JAMA 2003;289:2983-2991.
109. Kress JP, Pohlman AS, O'Connor MF, Hall JB: Daily interruption of sedative infusions in critically ill patients undergoing mechanical ventilation. N Engl J Med 2000;342:1471-1477.
132. Pandharipande PP, Pun BT, Herr DL, et al: Effect of sedation with dexmedetomidine vs lorazepam on acute brain dysfunction in mechanically ventilated patients: The MENDS randomized controlled trial. JAMA 2007;298(22):2644-2653.
134. Riker RR, Shehabi Y, Bokesch PM, et al: Dexmedetomidine vs midazolam for sedation of critically ill patients: A randomized trial. JAMA 2009;301(5):489-499.
183. Hopkins RO, Weaver LK, Pope D, et al: Neuropsychological sequelae and impaired health status in survivors of severe acute respiratory distress syndrome. Am J Respir Crit Care Med 1999;160:50-56.

The complete list of references can be found at www.expertconsult.com.

73 Severity of Illness Scoring Systems

Rui Moreno

When you can measure a phenomenon about which you are talking and express it in numbers, you know something about it. But, when you can not express it in numbers, your knowledge is vague and unsatisfactory. It may be the beginning of knowledge, but you progressed very little toward the state of science.

LORD KELVIN (1824-1907)

CHAPTER OUTLINE

The goal of intensive care is to provide the highest quality of treatment in order to achieve the best outcomes for critically ill patients. Although intensive care medicine has developed rapidly over the years, there exists, still, little scientific evidence as to what treatments and practices are really effective in the real world. Moreover, intensive care now faces major economic challenges, which increase the need to provide evidence not only on the effectiveness but also on the efficiency of practices. Intensive care is, however, a complex process, which is carried out on very heterogeneous populations and is influenced by several variables, including cultural background and different structure and organization of the health care systems. It is, therefore, extremely difficult to reduce the quality of intensive care to something measurable, to quantify it and then to compare it among different institutions. Also, in recent years, patient safety as a necessary dimension in the evaluation of quality of the care provided has become mandatory, leading to major changes in the way benchmarking should be evaluated and reported.[1]

Although quality encompasses a variety of dimensions, the main interest to date is focused on effectiveness and efficiency: It is clear that other issues are less relevant if the care being provided is either ineffective or harmful. Therefore, the priority must be to evaluate effectiveness. The instruments available to measure effectiveness in intensive care derive from the science of outcome research. The starting point for this science was the high degree of variability in medical processes, which was found during the first part of the twentieth century, when epidemiologic research was developing. The variation in medical practices led to the search for the "optimal" therapy for each syndrome or disease through the repeated performance of randomized controlled trials (RCTs). However, the undertaking of RCTs in intensive care is fraught with ethical and other difficulties. For this reason, observational studies to evaluate the effects of intensive care treatment are still frequently employed and sometimes more informative than prior RCTs.[2] Outcome research provides the methods necessary to compare different patients or groups of patients, especially different institutions. Risk adjustment (also called case-mix adjustment) is the method of choice to standardize the severity of illness of the individual or groups of patients. The purpose of risk adjustment is to take into account all of the characteristics of patients known to affect their outcome, in order to understand the differences due to the treatment received and the conditions (timing, setting, standardization) in which that treatment has been delivered.

Conceptually, the quantification of individual patients should be made by the use of severity scores, and the evaluation of groups of patients is done by summing up the probabilities of death given by the model for each individual patient and its comparison with actual fatality.

This chapter intends to describe the different methods and systems that are available for the purpose of accessing and comparing severity of illness and outcome in critically ill patients. Starting with a brief historical outline of the development of scoring systems over time, the reader should then become familiar with the way such systems have been designed and constructed. In succession, the chapter will describe available systems with their applications and limitations. Finally, the text will focus on the potential applications of these systems at both the patient level and the intensive care unit (ICU) level.

HISTORICAL PERSPECTIVE

Scoring systems have been broadly used in medicine for several decades. In 1953 Virginia Apgar[3] published a very simple scoring tool, the first general severity score designed to be applicable to a general population of newborn children. It was composed of five variables, easily evaluated at the patient's bedside, that reflect cardiopulmonary and central nervous system function. Its simplicity and accuracy have never been improved on, and any child born in a hospital today receives an Apgar score at 1 and 5 minutes after birth. Nearly 50 years ago Dr. Apgar commented on the state of research in neonatal resuscitation: "Seldom have there been such imaginative ideas, such enthusiasms and dislikes, and such unscientific observations and study about one clinical picture." She suggested that part of the solution to this problem would be a "simple, clear classification or grading of newborn infants which can be used as the basis for discussion and comparison of the results of obstetric practices, types of maternal pain relief and the effects of resuscitation." Thirty years later, physicians working in ICUs found themselves using the same tools and applying them in the same way.

Efforts to improve risk assessment during the 1960s and 1970s were directed at improving our ability to quickly select those patients most likely to benefit from promising new treatments. For example, Child and Turcotte[4] created a score to measure the severity of liver disease and estimate mortality risk for patients undergoing shunting. In 1967, Kilipp and Kimball classified the severity of acute myocardial infarction by the presence and severity of signs of congestive heart failure.[5] In 1974 Teasdale and Jennett introduced the Glasgow Coma Scale (GCS) for reproducibly evaluating the severity of coma.[6] The usefulness of the GCS score has been confirmed by the consistent relationship between poor outcome and a reduced score among patients with a variety of diseases. The GCS score is reliable and easy to perform, but problems with the timing of evaluation, the use of sedation, inter- and intraobserver variability, and its use in prognostication have caused strong controversies.[7] Nevertheless, the GCS remains the most widely used neurologic measure for risk assessment.

The 1980s brought an explosive increase in the use of new technology and therapies in critical care. The rapidity of change and the large and growing investment in these high-cost services prompted demands for better evidence for the indications and benefit of critical care. For this reason several researchers developed systems to evaluate and compare the severity of illness and outcome of critically ill patients. The first of these systems was the Acute Physiology And Chronic Health Evaluation (APACHE) system, published by Knaus and associates in 1981,[8] followed soon after by Le Gall and colleagues with the Simplified Acute Physiology Score (SAPS).[9] The APACHE system was latter updated to APACHE II,[10] and a new system, the Mortality Probability Model (MPM), joined the group.[11] By the beginning of the 1990s different systems were available to describe and classify ICU populations, to compare severity of illness, and to predict mortality risk in their patients. These systems performed well, but there were concerns about errors in prediction caused by differences in patient selection and lead-time bias. There were also concerns about the size and representativeness of the databases used to develop the three systems and about poor calibration within patient subgroups and across geographic locations. These concerns, in part, led to the development of their subsequent versions such as APACHE III,[12] the SAPS II,[13] and the MPM II,[14] all published between 1991 and 1993.

During the mid-1990s, the need to quantify not only mortality but also morbidity risks in specific groups of patients became evident and led to the development of the so-called organ dysfunction scores, such as the Multiple Organ Dysfunction Score (MODS),[15] the Logistic Organ Dysfunction System (LODS) score,[16] and the Sequential Organ Failure Assessment (SOFA) score.[17]

SEVERITY OF ILLNESS ASSESSMENT AND OUTCOME PREDICTION

The evaluation of severity of illness in the critically ill patient is made through the use of severity scores and outcome prediction models. This distinction is crucial to understanding the differences, limitations of use, and aims of each one.

- Severity scores are instruments that aim at stratifying patients based on their severity, assigning to each patient an increasing score as the severity of the illness increases.
- Outcome prediction models, apart from their ability to stratify patients according to their severity, aim at predicting a certain outcome (usually the vital status at hospital discharge) based on a given set of prognostic variables and a certain modeling equation.

The development of this kind of system, applicable to heterogeneous groups of critically ill patients, started in the 1980s (Table 73.1). The first general severity of illness score applicable to most critically ill patients was the APACHE score.[8] Developed in the George Washington University Medical Center in 1981 by William Knaus and coworkers, the APACHE system was created to evaluate, in an accurate and reproducible form, the severity of disease in this population.[18-20] Two years later, Jean-Roger Le Gall and coworkers published a simplified version of this model, the SAPS.[21] This model soon became very popular in Europe, especially in France. Another simplification of the original

Table 73.1 General Severity Scores and Outcome Prediction Models

Characteristic	APACHE	SAPS	APACHE II	MPM*	APACHE III	SAPS II	MPM II†	SAPS 3	APACHE IV	MPM_0 III
Year	1981	1984	1985	1988	1991	1993	1993	2005	2006	2007
No. of countries	1	1	1	1	1	12	12	35	1	1
No. of ICUs	2	8	13	1	40	137	140	303	104	135
No. of patients	705	679	5815	2783	17,440	12,997	19,124	16,784	110,558	124,855
Selection of variables and their weights	Panel of experts	Panel of experts	Panel of experts	Multiple logistic regression	Multiple logistic regression	Multiple logistic regression	Multiple logistic regression	Multiple logistic regression	Multiple logistic regression	Multiple logistic regression
Variables										
Age	No	Yes	Yes	Yes	Yes	Yes	Yes	Yes	Yes	Yes
Origin	No	No	No	No	Yes	No	No	Yes	Yes	No
Surgical status	No	No	Yes	Yes	Yes	Yes	Yes	Yes	Yes	Yes
Chronic health status	Yes	No	Yes	Yes	Yes	Yes	Yes	Yes	Yes	Yes
Physiology	Yes	Yes	Yes	Yes	Yes	Yes	Yes	Yes	Yes	Yes
Acute diagnosis	No	No	Yes	No	Yes	No	Yes	Yes	Yes	Yes
No. of variables	34	14	17	11	26	17	15‡	20	142	16 (+1)
Score	Yes	Yes	Yes	No	Yes	Yes	No	Yes	Yes	No
Mortality prediction	No	No	Yes	Yes	Yes	Yes	Yes	Yes	Yes	Yes

*These models are based on previous versions, developed by the same investigators (Lemeshow et al[11,181]; see online list of references for this chapter).
†The numbers presented are those for the admission component of the model (MPM II0). MPM II24 was developed using data for 15,925 patients from the same ICUs.
‡MPM II24 uses only 13 variables.
APACHE, Acute Physiology and Chronic Health Evaluation; ICUs, intensive care units; MPM, Mortality Probability Model; SAPS, Simplified Acute Physiology Score.

APACHE system, the APACHE II, was published in 1985 by the same authors of the original model.[10] This system introduced the prediction of mortality risk, providing a major reason for ICU admission from a list comprising 50 operative and nonoperative diagnoses. The MPM,[22] developed by Stanley Lemeshow, provided additional contributions for the prediction of prognosis, using logistic regression techniques. Further developments in this field include the third version of the APACHE system (APACHE III)[12] and the second versions of the SAPS (SAPS II)[13] and MPM (MPM II).[14] All of them use multiple logistic regression to select and weight the variables and are able to compute the probability of hospital mortality risk for groups of critically ill patients. It has been demonstrated that they perform better than their old counterparts,[23,24] and they represented the state of the art in this field by the end of the last century.

Since the early 1990s, owing to the progressive lack of calibration of these models, the performance of these instruments began to slowly deteriorate with the passage of time. Differences in the baseline characteristics of the admitted patients, in the circumstances of the ICU admission, and in the availability of general and specific therapeutic measures introduced an increasing gap between actual mortality rate and predicted mortality risk.[25] Overall, in the last years of the century, there was an increase in the mean age of the admitted patients, a larger number of chronically sick patients and immunosuppressed patients, and an increase in the number of ICU admissions due to sepsis.[26,27] Although most of the models kept an acceptable discrimination, their calibration (or prognostic accuracy) deteriorated to such a point that major changes were needed.

An inappropriate use of these instruments outside their sampling space was responsible also for some misapplication of the instruments, especially for risk adjustment in clinical trials.[28-30]

In the early 2000s, several attempts were made to improve the old models. However, a new generation of general outcome prediction models was built that included models such as the MPM III developed in the IMPACT database in the United States,[31] new models based on computerized analysis by hierarchical regression developed by some of the authors of the APACHE systems,[32] the APACHE IV,[33] and the SAPS 3 admission model, developed by hierarchical regression in a worldwide database.[34,35] Models based on other statistical techniques such as artificial neural networks and genetic algorithms have been proposed but, besides academic use, they never became used widely.[36,37] These approaches have been revised more than once,[38] and will be summarized later.

RECALIBRATING AND EXPANDING EXISTING MODELS

All the existing general outcome prediction models used logistic regression equations to estimate the probabilities of a given outcome in a patient with a certain set of predictive variables. Consequently, the first approach to improve the calibration of a model when the original model is not able to adequately describe the population is to customize the model.[39] Several methods and suggestions have been proposed for this exercise,[40] based usually on one of two strategies:

- First-level customization, or the customization of the logit, developing a new equation relaying the score to the probability, such as one proposed by Le Gall or Apolone.[41,42]
- Second-level customization, or the customization of the coefficients of the variables in the model as described for the MPM II_0 model,[39] which can be made either by keeping unchanged the relative weight of the variables in the model or eventually by changing also these weights (this latter technique involves the limit of second-level customization: from this point forward, so the researcher is developing a new model and not customizing an existing one). Usually the researcher customizing an existing model assumes that the relative weight of the variables in the model is constant.

Both of these methods have been used in the past with a partial success in increasing the prognostic ability of the models.[39,43] However, both fail when the problem of the score is on discrimination or in its poor performance in subgroups of patients (poor uniformity of fit).[44] This fact can be justified by the lack of additional variables, more predictive in this specific context. The addition of new variables to an existing model has been done before[45,46] and can be an appropriate approach in some cases. It can lead to very complex models, needs the collection of special data, and is also more expensive and time-consuming. The best tradeoff between the burden of data collection and accuracy should be tailored case by case. It should be noted that the aim of first-level customization, which is nothing more than a mathematical translation of the original logit in order to get a different probability of mortality risk, is to improve the calibration of a model and not to improve discrimination. It should therefore not be considered when the improvement of this parameter is considered important.

A third level of customization can be imagined, through the introduction in the model of new prognostic variables and the recomputation of the weights and coefficients for all variables, but—as mentioned before this technique crosses the borders of customizing a model versus building a new predictive model. In past years, all these approaches have been tried.[47-49]

BUILDING NEW MODELS

Three general outcome prediction models have been developed and finally published: the SAPS 3 admission model in 2005, the APACHE IV in 2006, and the MPM III in 2007.[50]

THE SAPS 3 ADMISSION MODEL

Developed by Rui Moreno, Philipp Metnitz, Eduardo Almeida, and Jean-Roger Le Gall on behalf of the SAPS 3 Outcomes Research Group, the SAPS 3 model was published in 2005.[34,35] The study used a total of 19,577 patients consecutively admitted to 307 ICUs all over the world from 14 October to 15 December 2002. This high-quality multinational database was built to reflect the heterogeneity of current ICU case mix and typology all over the world, trying not to focus only on Western Europe and the United States. Consequently, the SAPS 3 database better reflects important differences in patients' and health care systems' baseline characteristics that are known to affect outcome. These include, for example, different genetic makeups, different styles of living, and a heterogeneous distribution of major diseases within different regions, as well as issues such as access to the health care system in general and to intensive care in particular, or differences in availability and use of major diagnostic and therapeutic measures within the ICUs. Although the integration of ICUs outside Europe and the United States surely increased its representativeness, it must be acknowledged that the extent to which the SAPS 3 database reflects case mix on ICUs worldwide cannot be determined yet.

Based on data collected at ICU admission (±1 hour), the authors developed regression coefficients by using multilevel logistic regression to estimate the probability of hospital death. The final model, which comprises 20 variables, exhibited good discrimination without major differences across patient typologies; calibration was also satisfactory. Customized equations for major areas of the world were computed and demonstrate a good overall goodness of fit. It is interesting that the determinant of hospital mortality probability changed remarkably from the early 1990s,[12] with chronic health status and circumstances of ICU admission now being responsible for almost three fourths of the prognostic power of the model.

To allow all interested parties to see the calculation of SAPS 3, completely free of charge, extensive electronic supplementary material (http://dx.doi.org/10.1007/s00134-005-2762-6 and http://dx.doi.org/10.1007/s00134-005-2763-5, both accessed 30/06/2013) was published together with the study reports, including the complete and detailed description of all variables as well as additional information about SAPS 3 performance. Moreover, the SORG provides at the project website (www.saps3.org) several additional resources: First, a Microsoft Excel sheet is available and can be used to calculate a SAPS 3 "on the fly." Second, a small Microsoft Access database allows for the calculation, storage, and export of SAPS 3 data elements.

However, as all outcome prediction models, SAPS 3 is slowly losing calibration, as recently demonstrated by several groups.[51-55] It seems to keep a good level of reliability and discrimination, but a recalibration process, which can be relatively easy to perform, must be done in the following years.

THE APACHE IV MODEL

In early 2006, Jack E. Zimmerman, one of the original authors of the original APACHE models, published in collaboration with colleagues from Cerner Corporation (Vienna, VA) the APACHE IV model.[33] The study was based on a database of 110,558 consecutive admissions during 2002 and 2003 to 104 ICUs in 45 U.S. hospitals participating in the APACHE III database. The APACHE IV model uses the worst values during the first 24 hours in the ICU and a multivariate logistic regression procedure to estimate the probability of hospital death.

Predictor variables were similar to those in APACHE III, but new variables were added and different statistical modeling has been used. The accuracy of APACHE IV predictions was analyzed in the overall database and in major patient subgroups. APACHE IV had good discrimination and calibration. For 90% of 116 ICU admission diagnoses, the ratio of observed to predicted mortality was not significantly different from 1.0. Predictions were compared with the APACHE III versions developed 7 and 14 years previously: there was little change in discrimination, but aggregate mortality risk was systematically overestimated as model age increased. When examined across disease, predictive accuracy was maintained for some diagnoses but for others seemed to reflect changes in practice or therapy. A predictive model for risk-adjusted ICU length of stay was also published by the same group.[56] More information about the model and the possibility to compute the probability of death for individual patients is available at the website of Cerner Corporation (www.criticaloutcomes.cerner.com).

THE MPM_0 III MODEL

The MPM_0 III was published by Tom Higgins and associates in 2007.[50] It was developed using data from ICUs in the United States participating in the project IMPACT but there is almost no published data to evaluate its behavior outside the development cohort. As for the previous MPM models, the MPM_0 III does not allow the computation of a score but estimates directly the probability of death in the hospital.

DEVELOPING PREDICTIVE MODELS

SELECTING THE TARGET POPULATION

Although named "general," most of the existing models are not applicable to all ICU patients. Patients with burns, admitted with coronary ischemia (or to rule out myocardial infarction), who were young (less than 16 or 18 years of age), in the postoperative phase of cardiac surgery, or with a very short length of ICU stay were explicitly excluded from the development of the majority of systems. This limitation is especially important when we evaluate specialized ICUs, with a particular case mix, but can also be important in general ICUs. In many cases, the application of exclusion criteria can imply the analysis of just a small proportion of the admitted patients, resulting in significant errors.

OUTCOME SELECTION

Outcome selection identifies the end point of interest, and at a minimum, the selected outcome should be as follows:

- A relatively common event
- Easily defined, recognized, and measured
- Clinically relevant
- Independent of therapeutic decisions

Fatality meets all the preceding criteria; however, there are confounding factors to be considered when using death as an outcome. The location of the patient at the time of death can considerably reduce hospital mortality rates. For example, in a study of 116,340 ICU patients, a significant decline in the ratio of observed and predicted death was attributed to a decrease in hospital mortality rate as a result of earlier discharge of patients with a high severity of illness to skilled nursing facilities.[57] In the APACHE III study, a significant regional difference in mortality rate was entirely secondary to variations in hospital length of stay.[58] Improvements in therapy, such as the use of thrombolysis in myocardial infarction or steroids in *Pneumocystis* pneumonia and the acquired immunodeficiency syndrome[59] can dramatically reduce hospital mortality rate. Increases in the use of advance directives, do-not-resuscitate orders, and limitation or withdrawal of therapy all increase hospital mortality rates.

Variations in any of the previous factors will lead to differences between observed and predicted deaths that have little to do with case mix or effectiveness of therapy. Predictive instruments directed at long-term mortality predictions provide accurate prognostic estimates within the first month of hospital discharge, but their accuracy falls off considerably thereafter, because other factors, such as HIV infection or malignancy, dominate the long-term survival pattern.[45] Owing to these caveats, fatality is the most useful outcome for designing general severity of illness scores and predictive instruments.

Other outcome measures represent important issues in improving ICU care. These issues include the following:

- Morbidity and complication rates
- Organ dysfunction
- Resource use
- Duration of mechanical ventilation, use of pulmonary artery catheters
- Quality of life after ICU/hospital discharge
- Length of stay in the ICU

Case-mix adjustment is indispensable for studying morbidity, resource utilization, and length of stay. Although these outcomes are difficult to define and are sensitive to local conditions, they are related to the cost of care and have therefore been useful in measuring and comparing ICU efficiency.

All current outcome prediction models aim at predicting vital status at hospital discharge. It is thus incorrect to use them to predict other outcomes, such as the vital status at ICU discharge. This approach will result in a gross underestimation of mortality rates.[60]

DATA COLLECTION

The next step in the development of a general outcome prediction model is the evaluation, selection, and registration of the predictive variables. At this stage major attention should be given to the variable definitions as well as to the time frames for data collection.[61-63] Very frequently models have been applied incorrectly, the most common errors being related to the following:

- The definitions of the variables
- The time frames for the evaluation and registration of the data
- The frequency of measurement and registration of the variables
- The applied exclusion criteria
- Data handling before analysis

It should be noted that all existing models have been calibrated for nonautomated (i.e., manual) data collection. The use of electronic patient data management systems (with high sampling rates) has been demonstrated to have a significant impact on the results:[64,65] the higher the sampling rate, the more outliers will be found and thus scores will be higher. The evaluation of intra- and interobserver reliability should always be described and reported, together with the frequency of missing values.

SELECTION OF VARIABLES

The number of variables used in severity and prognostic systems is influenced by the data collection burden, statistical considerations, measurement reliability, and frequency. Variable selection reflects a balance between adding variables with a diminishing impact on outcome and limiting variables to the strongest predictors to ease data collection and minimize processing errors. Variables should have these characteristics:

- Readily available and clinically relevant
- Plausible relationship to outcome and easily defined and measured
- Independent of treatment processes
- Verifiable by checks of data accuracy

Initial selection of variables can be either deductive (subjective), using terms that are known or suspected to influence outcome, or inductive (objective) using any deviation from homeostasis or normal health status. The deductive approach employs a group of experts, who supply a consensus regarding the measurements and events most strongly associated with the outcome. This approach is faster and requires less computational work; APACHE I and SAPS I both started this way. A purely inductive strategy, used by MPM, begins with the database, and tests candidate variables with a plausible relationship to outcome. In the SAPS 3 model several complementary methods have been used, such as logistic regression on mutually exclusive categories built using smoothed curves based on LOWESS (locally weighted scatterplot smoothing),[66] and multiple additive regression trees (MART).[67]

As a practical matter, neither technique is used exclusively; all systems now use a combination of these techniques. Variables that have been used in severity and prognostic systems include the following:

- Age
- Chronic disease status or comorbid conditions
- Circumstances of ICU admission
- Physiologic measures
- Reasons for ICU admission and admitting diagnoses
- Cardiopulmonary resuscitation (CPR), mechanical ventilation prior to ICU admission
- Location and length of stay before admission
- Emergency surgery and operative status

Predictor variables should be easily defined and reliably measured to ensure uniform data collection and minimize scoring variations. For statistical purposes, variables are considered dichotomous (e.g., surgery or not), categoric (e.g., disease classification or patient location before admission), or continuous (blood pressure or heart rate). With very large sample sizes, some continuous variables may be rendered dichotomous or categorical if it is discovered that there are strong and biologically sound threshold values beyond which their numerical value has no additional significance.

Weights for ICU admission diagnosis or reason for ICU admission (e.g., asthma vs. acute respiratory distress syndrome) significantly augment prognostic accuracy because a similar extent of physiologic derangement reflects substantial variations in mortality risk for different diseases. Interestingly, the circumstance of ICU admission such as the planned or unplanned character of the admission has been demonstrated to be very important. Systems that include weights for admitting diagnosis must have sufficient numbers of patients in each disease category to perform statistical analyses. Predictive instruments that ignore admitting diagnosis reduce the data collection burden, but perform poorly in ICUs with a case mix that differs significantly from the development database.

Location and length of stay before ICU admission account, at least partly, for lead-time bias, which has an important impact on outcome. For example, a patient treated for 2 days and then admitted to the ICU is at greater risk of death than a patient with the same diagnosis and severity of illness admitted from the emergency department.

The accuracy of any scoring system depends on the quality of the database from which it was developed. Even with well-defined variables, significant interobserver variability is reported.[68,69]

In calculating the scores, several practical issues should be discussed.[70,71] First, exactly which value for any parameter should be considered? It is true that for many of the more simple variables, several measurements will be taken during any 24-hour period. Should the lowest, highest, or an average be taken as the representative value of that day? There is a general consensus that, for the purposes of the score, the worst value in any 24-hour period should be considered. Second, what about missing values? Should the last known value repeatedly be considered as representative until a new value is obtained, or should the mean value between two successive values be taken? Both options make assumptions that may influence the reliability of the score. The first option assumes that we have no knowledge of the evolution of values with time and the second assumes that changes are usually fairly predictable and regular. However, we prefer this second option because values may be missing for several days and repeating the last known value may involve considerable errors in calculation. In addition, changes in most of the variables measured (platelet count, bilirubin, urea) are, in fact, usually fairly regular, moving up or down in a systematic manner.

VALIDATION OF THE MODEL

All predictive models developed for outcome prediction need, of course, to be validated, that is, to demonstrate their ability to predict the outcome under evaluation. Three aspects should be evaluated in this context: the first aspect is the calibration, or the degree of correspondence between the predictions of the model and observed results. The second is discrimination, or the capability of the model to distinguish observations with a positive outcome from those with a negative outcome. The third is the uniformity of fit of the model, which is related to the performance over various subgroups of patients.

The evaluation of the calibration and discrimination has been named *goodness of fit*. The evaluation of the performance of the model in major subgroups has been named *uniformity of fit*.

GOODNESS OF FIT

The evaluation of the goodness of fit comprises the evaluation of calibration and discrimination in the analyzed population. Calibration evaluates the degree of correspondence between the estimated probabilities of fatality and the actual fatality in the analyzed sample. Several methods are usually proposed: observed/estimated (O/E) mortality ratios, Flora's Z score,[72] Hosmer-Lemeshow goodness of fit tests,[73-75] and Cox calibration regression and calibration curves.

O/E mortality ratios are computed by dividing the observed fatality (in other words, the number of deaths) by the predicted fatality (in other words, the sum of the probabilities of death of all patients in the sample). In a perfectly calibrated model this value should be 1.

Hosmer-Lemeshow goodness of fit tests are two chi-square statistics proposed for the formal evaluation of the calibration of predictive models.[73-75] In the $\hat{H}$ test, patients are classified into 10 groups according to their probabilities of death. Then, a chi-square statistic is used to compare the observed number of deaths and the predicted number of survivors with the observed number of deaths and the observed number of survivors in each of the groups. The formula is (Equation 1):

$$\hat{C}_g = \hat{H}_g = \sum_{l=1}^{g} \frac{(o_1 - e_1)^2}{e_1(1-\bar{\pi}_1)}$$

with g being the number of groups (usually 10), o the number of events observed in group l, e the number of events expected in the same group, and $\bar{\pi}_1$ the mean estimated probability, always in group l. The resulting statistic is then compared with a chi-square table with 8 degrees of freedom (model development) or 10 degrees of freedom (model validation), in order to know if the observed differences can be explained exclusively by random fluctuation. The Hosmer-Lemeshow $\hat{C}$ test is similar, with the 10 groups containing an equal number of patients. Hosmer and Lemeshow demonstrated that the grouping method used on the $\hat{C}$ statistics behaves better when most of the probabilities are low.[73]

These tests are nowadays considered to be mandatory for the evaluation of calibration,[76] although they are subject to criticism.[77,78] It should be stressed that the analyzed sample must be large enough to have the power to detect the lack of agreement between predicted and observed mortality rates.[40]

The Hosmer-Lemeshow tests are very sensitive to the size of the sample. When the sample is small, the test is usually underpowered to detect poor fit; when the sample size is very large, even minor, insignificant differences between the predicted and the observed fatality will result in a significant chi-square; for this reason, more and more investigators, especially those dealing with large databases, prefer to use the Cox calibration regression, in which the relation between the expected and the observed probabilities is assessed by logistic regression with hospital death being the dependent variable and the natural logarithm of the odds of the probabilities given by the model being the independent variable. If the intercept is 0 and the slope of the model 1, then the calibration is perfect.[49]

This is the one of the best methods to provide the user with a quantitative measure of calibration, but it does not indicate fully the deviations between observed and predicted mortality rates, in particular in the direction, extent, and risk classes affected by these deviations. This last information is more or less provided by the traditional calibration plot, which, however, is not a real curve (single points are theoretically independent from each other), is not a formal statistical method, and consequently does not provide the uncertainty of the estimate. Another weak point of the most commonly used calibration assessment methods (i.e., the Hosmer–Lemeshow statistics combined with the traditional calibration plot) is that they average the risk of patients in each decile, thus not using the entire information carried by each patient. These shortcomings were recently addressed by a new statistical approach, the GiViTI calibration belt,[53] recently used by Poole and colleagues in the comparison of the calibration of SAPS II and 3.[53] However, it is also not perfect, because most of the time there is a left (low-risk) deviation of the distribution of risks and the test becomes less helpful and informative. Calibration curves are also used to describe the calibration of a predictive model. These types of graphics compare observed and predicted mortality risks. They can be misleading, because the number of patients usually decreases from left to right (when we move from low probabilities to high probabilities), and as a consequence, even small differences in high-severity groups appear visually more important than small differences in low-probability groups. It should be stressed that calibration curves are not a formal statistical test.

Discrimination evaluates the capability of the model to distinguish between patients who die from patients who survive. This evaluation can be made using a nonparametric test such as Harrell's C index, using the order of magnitude of the error.[79] This index measures the probability of, for any two patients chosen randomly, the one with the greater probability to have the outcome of interest (to be dead). It has been shown that this index is directly related with the area under the receiver operating characteristic (ROC) curve and that it can be obtained as the parameter of the Mann-Whitney-Wilcox statistic.[80] Additional computations can be used to compute the confidence interval of this measure.[81]

The concept of the area under the ROC curve is derived from psychophysical tests. In an ROC curve, a series of two by two contingency tables are built, varying from the smallest to the largest score value. For each table the rate of true-positive (or sensitivity) and the false-positive rate (or 1 minus the specificity) are calculated. The final plot of all possible pairs of rates of true-positives versus false-positives gives then the visual representation of the ROC curve.

The interpretation of the area under the ROC curve is easy: a virtual model with a perfect discrimination would have an area of 1.0, a model with a discrimination no better than chance has an area of 0.5. Discriminative abilities are said to be satisfactory when the ROC curve is greater than 0.70. General outcome prediction models usually have areas greater than 0.80. Several methods have been described to compare the areas under two (or more) ROC curves,[82-84] but they can be misleading if the shape of the curves is different.[85]

Other measures have been utilized, based on classification tables, with describing sensitivity, specificity, positive and negative predictive values, and the correct classification rates. However because these calculations must use a fixed cutoff (usually 10%, 50%, or 90%), their value is limited.

The relative importance of calibration and discrimination depends on the intended use of the model. Some authors advise that for group comparison calibration is especially important[86] and that for decisions involving individual patients both parameters are important.[87]

UNIFORMITY OF FIT

The evaluation of calibration and discrimination in the analyzed sample is nowadays current practice. More complex is the identification of subgroups of patients when the behavior of the model is nonoptimal. These subgroups can be viewed as influential observations in model building and their contribution for the global error of the model can be vary large.[88]

The most important subgroups are related to the case-mix characteristics that can be eventually related to the outcome of interest:

- The intrahospital location before ICU admission
- The surgical status
- The degree of physiologic reserve (age, comorbid conditions)
- The acute diagnosis (including the presence, site, and extension of infection at ICU admission)

Although some authors such as Rowan and Goldhill in the United Kingdom[89,90] and Apolone and Sicignano in Italy[42,91] have suggested that the behavior of a model can depend to a significant extent on the case mix of the sample, no consensus exists about the subpopulations that should mandatorily be analyzed.[44]

UPDATING SEVERITY SCORES

Changes in the characteristics of the populations, changes in the therapy of major diseases, and the introduction of new diagnostic methods all imply modifications that result in necessary updates. Moreover, the use of a model outside its development population can eventually imply its modification and adaptation.

USING A SEVERITY OF ILLNESS SCORE

CALCULATING A SEVERITY OF ILLNESS SCORE

Using the original score sheets (or a computer software, well developed and validated), a score is assigned to each variable, depending on its deviation from normal values. The arithmetic sum of these variable scores (the sum score) represents the severity score for that patient, which is then used in the equation to predict hospital death. As described earlier, this approach was not chosen by any of the MPM systems, in which the variables are directly used to compute a probability of death in the hospital by a logistic regression equation.

TRANSFORMING THE SCORE INTO A PROBABILITY OF DEATH

The transformation of the severity score into a probability of death in the hospital uses a logistic regression equation. The dependent variable (hospital mortality) y is related to the set of independent (predictive) variables by the equation:

$$y = b_0 + b_1x_1 + b_2x_2 \ldots b_kx_k$$

with b_0 being the intercept of the model, x_1 to x_k the predictive variables and b_1 to b_k the estimated regression coefficients. The probability of death is then given by:

$$\text{Probability of death} = \frac{e^{\text{logit}}}{1 + e^{\text{logit}}}$$

with the logit being y as described before. The logistic transformation included in this equation allows the S-shaped relationship between the two variables to become linear (on the logit scale). In the extremes of the score (very low or very high values) changes in the probability of death are small; for intermediate values, even small changes in the score are associated with very large changes in the probability of death. This ensures that outliers do not influence the prediction too much.

APPLICATION OF A SEVERITY OF ILLNESS SCORE: EVALUATION OF PATIENTS

All existing models aim at predicting an outcome (vital status at hospital discharge) based on a given set of variables: they estimate the outcome of a patient with a certain clinical condition (defined by the registered variables), treated in a hypothetical reference ICU. Several issues, however, need to be taken into account in order to apply one of the previously described models in another population:

- Patient selection
- Evaluation and registration of the predictive variables
- Evaluation and registration of the outcome
- Computation of the severity score
- Transformation of the score in a probability of death

After validation, the utility and applicability of a model must be evaluated. Literature is full of models developed in large populations that failed, when applied within other contexts.[42,43,89,92-96] Thus, this question can only be answered by validating the model in its final population. The potential applications of a model—and consequently its utility—are different for individual patients and for groups.[97]

EVALUATING INDIVIDUAL PATIENTS

Some evidence exists that suggests that statistical methods behave better than clinicians in predicting outcome,[98-105] or that they can help clinicians in the decision-making process.[106-108] This opinion is, however, controversial,[109-111] especially for decisions to withdraw or to withhold therapy.[112] Moreover, the application of different models to the same patient results frequently in very different predictions.[113] Thus, application of these models to individual patients for decision making is not recommended.[114]

It should not be forgotten that such statistical models are of a probabilistic nature. A well-calibrated model, applied to an individual patient may, for example, predict a hospital mortality rate of 46% for this individual; this, however, just means that for a group of 100 patients with a similar severity of illness, 46 patients are predicted to die; it makes no statement if the individual patient is included in the 46% who will eventually die or in the 54% who will eventually survive.

If should be noted that severity scores have been proposed for applications as diverse as to determine the use of total parenteral nutrition[115] or the identification of futility in intensive care medicine.[116] Some authors demonstrated that knowledge of predictive information will not have an adverse effect on the quality of care, helping at the same time to decrease the consumption of resources and to increase the availability of beds.[117]

One field in which the scientific community agrees consensually is the stratification of patients for inclusion into clinical trials and for the comparison of the balance of randomization to different groups.[118]

EVALUATING GROUPS OF PATIENTS

At a group level, general outcome prediction models have been proposed for two objectives: distribution of resources and performance evaluation. Several studies were published describing methods used to identify and to characterize patients with a low risk of death.[119-123] This type of patient, who requires only basic monitoring and general care, could eventually be transferred to other areas of the hospital.[108,124] One could, however, also argue that these patients have a low mortality risk only because they have been monitored and cared for in an ICU.[125] Also, the use of current instruments is not recommended as a triage instrument in the emergency department,[126] and also the use of early physiologic indicators outside the ICU is being questioned.[127]

Moreover, patient costs in the ICU depend on the amount of required (and utilized) nursing workload use. Patient characteristics (diagnosis, degree of physiologic dysfunction) are thus not the only determinants: costs depend also on the practices and policies in a given ICU. To focus our attention on the effective use of nursing workload[128] or the dynamic evolution of the patient[129,130] seems thus a more promising strategy than those approaches based exclusively on the condition of the patients during the first hours in the ICU or in the O/E length of stay in the ICU.[58,131,132]

On the other hand, general outcome prediction models have been proposed to identify patients who require more resources.[133] Unfortunately, these patients only rarely can be identified at ICU admission, because their degree of physiologic dysfunction during the first 24 hours in the ICU tends usually to be moderate, although very variable.[134-136] And even if some day these patients might be well identified, the question of what to do with this information remains.

Another important area in which these type of models have been used is evaluation of ICU performance. Several investigators proposed the use of standardized mortality ratios (SMR) for performance evaluation, assuming that current models can take into account the main determinants of mortality risk.[137] The SMR is computed by dividing the observed mortality rate by the averaged predicted mortality rate (the sum of the individual probabilities of death of all the patients in the sample). Additional computations can be made to estimate the confidence interval of this ratio.[138]

The interpretation of the SMR is easy: a ratio lower than 1 implies a performance better than the reference population and a ratio greater than 1 indicates a performance worse than the reference population. This methodology has been used for international comparison of ICUs,* comparison of hospitals,† ICU evaluation,[143-146] management evaluation,[142,147,148] and the influence of organization and management factors on the performance of the ICU.[149]

Before applying this methodology, six questions should always be answered:

1. Can we evaluate and register all the data needed for the computation of the models?
2. Can the models be used in the large majority of our patients?
3. Are existent models able to control for the main patient characteristics related to mortality?
4. Has the reference population been well chosen and are the models well calibrated to this population?
5. Is the sample size large enough to draw meaningful differences?
6. Is vital status at ICU discharge the main performance indicator?

Each of these assumptions has been questioned in past years and there is no definitive answer at this time. However, most investigators believe that performance is multidimensional and consequently that it should be evaluated in several dimensions.[25,150] The problem of sample size seems especially important with respect to the risk of a type II error (in other words, to say that there are no differences when they exist).

Moreover, the comparison between observed and predicted might make more sense if done separately in low-, intermediate-, and high-risk patients, because the performance of an ICU can change according to the severity of the admitted patients. This approach was advocated in the past based on theoretical concerns,[151-153] but was used only in a small number of studies.[149,154] Multilevel modeling with varying slopes can be an answer for the developers of such models.[25,155]

ORGAN DYSFUNCTION/FAILURE SCORING SYSTEMS

Organ failure scores are designed to describe organ dysfunction/failure more than to predict survival. In the development of organ function scores, three important principles need to be remembered.[17] First, organ failure is not a simple all-or-nothing phenomenon; rather, a spectrum or continuum of organ dysfunction exists from very mild altered function to total organ failure. Second, organ failure is not a static process and the degree of dysfunction may vary with time during the course of disease so that scores need to be calculated repeatedly. Third, the variables chosen to evaluate each organ need to be objective, simple, and available but reliable, routinely measured in every institution, specific to the organ in question, and independent of patient variables, so that the score can be easily calculated for any patient in any ICU. Interobserver variability in scoring can be a problem with more complex systems[63,156] and the use of simple, unequivocal variables can avoid this potential problem. Ideally, scores should be independent of therapeutic variables, as stressed by Marshall and coworkers,[15] but in fact, this is virtually impossible to achieve as all factors are more or less treatment dependent. For example, the Pao_2/Fio_2 ratio is dependent on ventilatory conditions and positive end-expiratory pressure (PEEP), platelet count may be influenced by platelet transfusions, urea levels are affected by hemofiltration, and so on.

The process of organ function description is relatively new and there is no general agreement on which organs to assess and which parameters to use. Many different scoring systems have been developed for assessing organ dysfunction,[15-17,157-165] differing in the organ systems included in the score, the definitions used for organ dysfunction, and the grading scale used.[71,166] The majority of scores include six key organ systems—cardiovascular, respiratory, hematologic, central nervous, renal, and hepatic—with other systems, such as the gastrointestinal system, less commonly included. Early scoring systems assessed organ failure as either present or absent, but this approach is very dependent on where the limits for organ function are set, and newer scores consider organ failure as a spectrum of dysfunction. Most scores have been developed in the general ICU population, but some were aimed specifically at the septic patient.[17,158,159,163,164] Three of the more recently developed systems will be discussed later, the main difference between them being in their definition of cardiovascular system dysfunction (Table 73.2).

MULTIPLE ORGAN DYSFUNCTION SCORE

This scoring system was developed by a literature review of clinical studies of multiple organ failure from 1969 to 1993.[15] Optimal descriptors of organ dysfunction were thus identified and validated against a clinical database. Six organ systems were chosen, and a score of 0 to 4 allotted for each organ according to function (0 being normal function through 4 for most severe dysfunction) with a maximum score of 24. The worst score for each organ system in each 24-hour period is taken for calculation of the aggregate score. A high initial Multiple Organ Dysfunction Score (MODS) correlated with ICU mortality risk and the delta MODS (calculated as the MODS over the whole ICU stay less the admission MODS) was even more predictive of outcome.[15] In a study of 368 critically ill patients the MODS was found to better describe outcome groups than the APACHE II or the organ failure score, although the predicted risk of mortality was similar for all scoring systems.[167] The MODS has been used to assess organ dysfunction in clinical studies of various groups of critically ill patients, including those with severe sepsis.[168-171]

*See references 19, 69, 89, 93, 139, 140.
†See references 18, 58, 94, 95, 131, 137, 141, 142.

Table 73.2 Organ Dysfunction/Failure Scoring Systems

Organ System	MODS*	SOFA†	LOD‡
Respiratory	Pao_2/Fio_2 ratio	Pao_2/Fio_2 ratio Mechanical ventilation	Pao_2/Fio_2 ratio Mechanical ventilation
Cardiovascular	Pressure-adjusted HR	MAP Use of vasoactive agents	SAPS HR
Renal	Creatinine	Creatinine Urinary output	Creatinine Urinary output Urea
Hematologic	Platelets	Platelets	Platelets WBCs
Neurologic	GCS	GCS	GCS
Hepatic	Bilirubin	Bilirubin	Bilirubin Prothrombin time

*Data from Marshall JC, Cook DA, Christou NV, et al: Multiple organ dysfunction score: A reliable descriptor of a complex clinical outcome. Crit Care Med 1995;23:1638-1652.

†Data from Vincent J-L, Moreno R, Takala J, et al: The SOFA (Sepsis-related Organ Failure Assessment) score to describe organ dysfunction/failure. Intensive Care Med 1996;22:707-710.

‡Data from Le Gall JR, Klar J, Lemeshow S, et al, The ICU Scoring Group: The logistic organ dysfunction system. A new way to assess organ dysfunction in the intensive care unit. JAMA 1996;276:802-810.

GCS, Glasgow Coma Scale; HR, heart rate; LOD, Logistic Organ Dysfunction; MAP, mean arterial pressure; MODS, Multiple Organ Dysfunction Score; SAPS, Simplified Acute Physiology Score; SOFA, Sequential Organ Failure Assessment; WBC, white blood cells.

SEQUENTIAL ORGAN FAILURE ASSESSMENT SCORE

The sequential organ failure assessment (SOFA) score was developed in 1994 during a consensus conference organized by the European Society of Intensive Care and Emergency Medicine in an attempt to provide a means of quantitatively and objectively describing the degree of organ failure over time in individual, and groups of, septic patients.[17] Initially termed the *sepsis-related organ failure assessment score,* the score was then renamed the *sequential organ failure assessment* because it was realized that it could be applied equally to nonseptic patients. In devising the score, the participants of the conference decided to limit to six the number of systems studied: respiratory, coagulation, hepatic, cardiovascular, central nervous system, renal. A score of 0 is given for normal function through 4 for most abnormal, and the worst values on each day are recorded. Individual organ function can thus be assessed and monitored over time, and an overall global score can also be calculated. A high total SOFA score (SOFA max) and a high delta SOFA (the total maximum SOFA minus the admission total SOFA) have been shown to be related to a worse outcome,[129,172] and the total score has been shown to increase over time in nonsurvivors compared to survivors.[172] The SOFA score has been used for organ failure assessment in several clinical trials, including one in septic shock patients.[173-176]

LOGISTIC ORGAN DYSFUNCTION SYSTEM SCORE

This score was developed in 1996 using multiple logistic regression applied to selected variables from a large database of ICU patients.[16] To calculate the score, each organ system receives points according to the worst value for any variable for that system on that day. If no organ dysfunction is present, the score is 0, rising to a maximum of 5. As the relative severity of organ dysfunction differs between organ systems, the Logistic Organ Dysfunction System (LODS) score allows for the maximum of 5 points to be awarded only to the neurologic, renal, and cardiovascular systems. For maximum dysfunction of the pulmonary and coagulation systems, a maximum of 3 points can be given for the most severe levels of dysfunction; and for the liver, the most severe dysfunction receives only 1 point. Thus, the total maximum score is 22. The LODS score is designed to be used as a once-only measure of organ dysfunction in the first 24 hours of ICU admission, rather than as a repeated assessment measure. The LODS system is quite complex and seldom used; nevertheless, it has been used to assess organ dysfunction in clinical studies.[177]

COMPARISON OF THE DESCRIBED SYSTEMS

The main difference among the three described models is the method chosen for the evaluation of the cardiovascular dysfunction: SOFA uses blood pressure and the level of adrenergic support, MODS uses a composed variable (heart rate × ratio of central venous pressure) and mean arterial pressure (heart rate × central venous pressure/mean arterial pressure), and LOD score uses the heart rate and the systolic blood pressure. There are now a few comparisons among them, not describing clinically significant differences.

Mixed models, integrating organ failure assessment scores, and general severity scores have been published,[162,178] but they never gained widespread acceptance.

SCORING SYSTEMS FOR SPECIFIC CLINICAL CONDITIONS

Several scoring systems have been developed to be applied on a subsample of patients with specific clinical conditions, such as for cardiac surgery, severe sepsis and septic shock, trauma, and acute renal failure. These systems, given their specificity and limited applicability, will not be covered here, but the reader should realize that they can be extremely helpful when dealing with patients with trauma or in the postoperative stage of cardiac surgery.

DIRECTIONS FOR FURTHER RESEARCH

In the last year a new generation of general outcome prediction models has been developed. More complex than their old counterparts, relying heavily in computerized data registry and analysis (although the SAPS 3 model can be still computed by hand), incorporating more extensively the reasons and circumstances responsible or associated with ICU admission, these instruments must now be evaluated outside their development populations.

The choice between them remains largely subjective and depends on the reference database that the user wants to use: the U.S. centers participating in the APACHE III database or a more heterogeneous sample of ICUs across all major regions of the globe. The absence of any fee regarding the SAPS 3 model and the existence of equations specific for each region of the world should be weighted with the paid participation in a continuous database program, providing a more professional support and analysis of the data.

No matter the model chosen, users should keep in mind that the accuracy of these models is dynamic and should be periodically retested, and that when accuracy deteriorates these models must be revised and updated. Also, it is important to remember that these instruments have been developed to be used in populations of patients with critical illness and not in individual patients; consequently, their use in individual patients should always be complementary and not alternative to the use of clinical evaluation, because statistical predictive methods are prone to error, especially in the individual patient.[179,180]

KEY POINTS

- Scoring systems have been broadly used in medicine for several decades, both for clinical research and for the evaluation of ICU effectiveness.
- The evaluation of severity of illness in the critically ill patient is made through the use of severity scores and (general) prognostic models. Severity scores are instruments that aim at stratifying patients based on their severity, assigning to each patient an increasing score as the severity of illness increases. General prognostic models, apart from their ability to stratify patients according to their severity, aim at predicting a certain outcome based on a given set of prognostic variables and a certain modeling equation.
- Several different systems are available to describe and classify ICU populations, to compare severity of illness, and to predict mortality risk in their patients. These systems perform well globally, but there are still

KEY POINTS (Continued)

concerns about errors in prediction caused by differences in patient selection, lead-time bias, sample size, representativeness of the databases used to develop the systems, and poor calibration within patient subgroups and across geographic locations.[182]

- The most widely used general outcome prognostic systems for adults are the APACHE II, III, and IV; the SAPS II and 3; and the MPM II and III.
- At the patient level, severity scores and prognostic models have been used for purposes as diverse as determining the use of total parenteral nutrition, the identification of futility in intensive care medicine, the use of new therapies in sepsis, the stratification of patients for inclusion into clinical trials, and the analysis of the balance of randomization in different groups during clinical trials. At the group level, general outcome prediction models have been proposed for the allocation of resources and performance evaluation, through the use of the observed to expected mortality ratio or SMR.
- Organ failure scores are designed to describe in a repetitive way the presence and degree of organ dysfunction/failure in critically ill patients. Most of them evaluate six key organ systems (cardiovascular, respiratory, hematologic, central nervous, renal, and hepatic), with other systems, such as the gastrointestinal system, less commonly included. All of them use a combination of physiologic and therapeutic variables to access organ dysfunction/failure.
- Disease-specific scoring systems have been developed to be applied on more specific populations with specific clinical conditions, such as cardiac surgery or trauma. Models specifically developed to be used in neonates or children are also available.
- The choice between existing systems remains largely subjective and depends on the reference database that the user wants to use: the U.S. centers participating in the APACHE II or IV database or a more heterogeneous sample of ICUs across all major regions of the globe (as in SAPS 3). Complexity, cost, and the existence of equations specific for each region of the world should be weighted as well as the participation in a continuous database program, providing a more professional support and analysis of the data. No matter the model chosen, accuracy should be periodically retested and revised and updated as it deteriorates. The models should be complementary, and they should not be used as an alternative to clinical evaluation.

SELECTED REFERENCES

10. Knaus WA, Draper EA, Wagner DP, Zimmerman JE: APACHE II: A severity of disease classification system. Crit Care Med 1985; 13:818-829.

12. Knaus WA, Wagner DP, Draper EA, et al: The APACHE III prognostic system. Risk prediction of hospital mortality for critically ill hospitalized adults. Chest 1991;100:1619-1636.

13. Le Gall JR, Lemeshow S, Saulnier F: A new simplified acute physiology score (SAPS II) based on a European/North American multicenter study. JAMA 1993;270:2957-2963.
17. Vincent J-L, Moreno R, Takala J, et al: The SOFA (Sepsis-related Organ Failure Assessment) score to describe organ dysfunction/failure. Intensive Care Med 1996;22:707-710.
25. Moreno R, Matos R: The "new" scores: What problems have been fixed, and what remain. Curr Opin Crit Care 2000;6:158-165.
34. Metnitz PG, Moreno RP, Almeida E, et al, SAPS 3 Investigators: SAPS 3. From evaluation of the patient to evaluation of the intensive care unit. Part 1: Objectives, methods and cohort description. Intensive Care Med 2005;31:1336-1344.
35. Moreno RP, Metnitz PG, Almeida E, et al, SAPS 3 Investigators: SAPS 3. From evaluation of the patient to evaluation of the intensive care unit. Part 2: Development of a prognostic model for hospital mortality at ICU admission. Intensive Care Medicine 2005;31:1345-1355.
49. Harrison DA, Brady AR, Parry GJ, et al: Recalibration of risk prediction models in a large multicenter cohort of admissions to adult, general critical care units in the United Kingdom. Crit Care Med 2006;34:1378-1388.
56. Zimmerman JE, Kramer AA, McNair DS, et al: Intensive care unit length of stay: Benchmarking based on Acute Physiology and Chronic Health Evaluation (APACHE) IV. Crit Care Med 2006;34:2517-2529.
86. Schuster DP: Predicting outcome after ICU admission. The art and science of assessing risk. Chest 1992;102:1861-1870.
129. Moreno R, Vincent J-L, Matos R, et al, on behalf of the working group on "sepsis-related problems" of the European Society of Intensive Care Medicine: The use of maximum SOFA score to quantify organ dysfunction/failure in intensive care. Results of a prospective, multicentre study. Intensive Care Med 1999;25: 686-696.
172. Vincent J-L, de Mendonça A, Cantraine F, et al, on behalf of the working group on "sepsis-related problems" of the European Society of Intensive Care Medicine: Use of the SOFA score to assess the incidence of organ dysfunction/failure in intensive care units: Results of a multicentric, prospective study. Crit Care Med 1998;26:1793-1800.

The complete list of references can be found at www.expertconsult.com.

74

Education and Training in Intensive Care Medicine

Nandan Gautam | Julian Bion

CHAPTER OUTLINE

Training programs in intensive care medicine (ICM) vary worldwide in content, assessment, and duration, influenced heavily by domestic traditions and training structures. Even countries and health care communities that have much in common may differ significantly in curriculum content, delivery, assessment, accreditation, and requirements for continuing professional development, particularly when ICM exists as multiple subspecialities. In many countries the resources available to support training and education are inadequate, aggravated in the European context by legislation that requires workplace-based education to be delivered within the 48-hour weekly limit on working hours.

These challenges have acted as a stimulus to develop web-based methods of knowledge dissemination, workplace-based approaches to reflective learning, and e-portfolios for documentation of learning outcomes. Since 2003 there have been a number of successful initiatives to harmonize the outcomes of training through common competencies and the development of international standards for programs of training in ICM. Further work is needed to develop techniques of training and reliable methods of assessment, particularly in the domain of human factors and behavioral skills, framed by the ethos of life long learning as a device for improving the care that we offer to our patients and families.

TRAINING ASPIRATIONS FOR INTENSIVE CARE MEDICINE

The purpose of any medical education program should be to integrate knowledge, skills, attitudes, and behaviors within a sound ethical and professional framework that encourages reflective life long learning, with the aim of producing competent and caring practitioners who possess both team-working and leadership capacities. Achieving this objective requires a firm focus on the needs of patients and confident and effective structures and processes for training and education. The American College of Critical Care Medicine states,[1] "*Critical care medicine trainees and faculty must acquire and maintain the skills necessary to provide state-of-the art clinical care to critically ill patients, to improve patient outcomes, optimize intensive care unit utilization, and continue to advance the theory and practice of critical care medicine. This should be accomplished in an environment dedicated to compassionate and ethical care.*" To this statement one could add: *using the knowledge and resources of a multiprofessional team and involvement of patients and caregivers.*

THE TRAINING ENVIRONMENT

Training and service are necessary companions. In the last 20 years, health systems worldwide have seen that patients' expectations of safe and reliable health care are not always satisfied.[2,3] It is reasonable for patients to expect that their care should be delivered by fully trained specialists and not by less experienced individuals or those in training grades. However, this expectation is made difficult to satisfy by cost pressures, rationing, increased throughput, staffing limitations, and reduced hours of work for trainees.[4,5] These challenges are a particular problem for acute and emergency care, including critical care,[6] but it is in precisely these areas that some of the most innovative solutions can be found.

Physician assistants or extended-role nurse practitioners are now active in many roles. In ICM, the United Kingdom has developed a program for advanced critical care practitioners[7] derived from the physicians' Competency-Based Training in Intensive Care Medicine (CoBaTrICE) program. Critical care and outreach, medical emergency teams,[8] and the United Kingdom's hospital at night and 24/7 teams[9] all involve senior nurses with diagnostic and management training. In the United States, growth of the hospitalist movement into a new specialty demonstrates how the clinical demands of acutely ill patients can have an impact on training and education.[10] The National Organization of Nurse Practitioner Faculties has developed a national program of competencies that includes diagnostic algorithms and treatment based on protocols,[11] and many of the competencies are centered around management of acutely ill or physiologically unstable patients. Acutely ill patients are thus necessarily cared for by multiple teams involving physicians, nurses, and allied health care professionals. Such teams have rapidly changing membership, and colleagues often do not know each other well. Accurate and comprehensive clinical handoffs/handovers need to be standardized in order to ensure continuity of care. This care needs to be supplemented by objective processes that pick up measures of physiologic deterioration, escalate concerns in a timely and appropriate manner, and can call upon the best person at the right time, every time. Training to acquire these complex skills in the acute and emergency care environment must be embedded in undergraduate curricula for all health care professionals.[12,13]

CURRENT TRAINING IN INTENSIVE CARE MEDICINE

The emergence of critical care medicine from the poliomyelitis epidemics of the 1950s was underpinned by developments in cardiorespiratory pathophysiology and organ system support led by anesthesiology and respiratory medicine. The safety record of anesthesiology combined with better technology and drugs has enabled increasingly complex surgery and has extended the role of the anesthetist into postoperative intensive care. Respiratory physicians also have a traditional association with critical care, particularly in the United States, where they remain the most numerous specialists within critical care medicine. Principles of ICM are a mandatory component of many specialty training programs worldwide, but the extent to which this training is recognized as specialist ICM training varies. Specialists from other primary disciplines such as surgery and internal and emergency medicine (and pediatrics) participate in critical care, but with varying degrees of access to, or inclusion of, competencies in ICM.

In a survey of 41 countries carried out by the CoBaTrICE Collaboration[14] under the aegis of the European Society for Intensive Care Medicine (ESICM), 54 different ICM training programs were identified (37 within the European region) that ranged in duration from 3 months to 6 years (most frequently 2 years). Entry criteria were significantly different between some countries with regard to the structure and format of the training program. Nursing surveys demonstrate similar diversity in their training programs. The CoBaTrICE survey was updated for European Region countries in 2009,[15] and demonstrated that although progress had been made on convergence in speciality status and shared competencies there were still significant deficiencies in standards for assessment, quality assurance, and infrastructure support for training. Currently 10 European Region countries use the harmonized CoBaTrICE competencies.

Most countries observe one or more of the following models of ICM training: primary specialty (critical care training directly after medical school), subspecialty (critical care training as an exclusive component of a primary discipline), or supraspecialty training (a common critical care training shared by multiple primary specialties).

In *primary specialty* training, ICM is regarded as a fully independent specialty with a separate training program accessed directly from the undergraduate level or from a common stem at internship or residency. This training may be undertaken in addition to a complementary primary specialty, commonly anesthesiology or internal medicine.

Subspecialty refers to ICM training within a parent specialty and exclusive to it. In the majority of such systems, ICM training can be accessed only through anesthesiology. Other disciplines, such as internal medicine and surgery, may offer their own subspecialty training in ICM. These separate routes may be related to each other but are administered differently and often have different components. Certification will reflect the base specialty but often documents subspecialty status also.

Supraspecialty training is the most common model. Here, a primary specialty is chosen and intensive care training is grafted onto it, either in a modular or in a single-block format. Certification in ICM requires certification in the primary specialty also. It allows a number of specialties to access common ICM training. In practice, however, the specialties remain predominantly anesthesiology, internal medicine (adult and pediatric), and respiratory medicine. ICM is now a primary speciality in Spain, the United Kingdom, Switzerland, Australia, and New Zealand; all except Spain also offer dual certification in ICM and another primary speciality.

Outside the CoBaTrICE program and those countries that have adopted it, few national programs define the outcomes of training explicitly in terms of the competencies expected of a specialist in ICM. There is tacit acknowledgment that the terms "attending," "consultant," and "specialist" may have administrative and logistic equivalence within individual countries and that a "good" specialist in one country is likely to be as well equipped with knowledge and skills as a good specialist in another, but there is little evidence to prove this, whereas there is solid evidence that standards of assessment and quality assurance vary widely between countries and even between different speciality programs within countries.[15]

Specialist status in all these schemes is obtained through some combination of time spent in the program, competency-based assessments, case reports, submission of diploma theses, oral (viva voce) examination, and clinical examination. There does not as yet exist an enforced recertification process specifically for ICM in any country, nor is there an agreed-upon standard for benchmarking intensive care units or training programs against international peers, though such standards are now being developed.[16] For example, the United Kingdom has now established a multicollegiate Faculty of Intensive Care Medicine responsible for the new primary specialist training program in ICM, and for standards of revalidation and peer review.[17,18]

COMPETENCY-BASED TRAINING

Competencies are a method for describing the knowledge, skills, attitudes, and behavior expected of specialists in terms of what they are able to do. Several national regulatory bodies for physicians have started to modify their training programs from syllabus-based, examination-driven systems to programs based on competencies assessed in the workplace, particularly the United Kingdom, Canada (using the CanMEDS framework[19]), and the United States. The challenge for trainers and trainees is to develop robust methods for workplace-based assessment and to create the necessary flexibility within training programs to allow time-based training to be replaced by programs in which trainees acquire competencies at different rates. This has been made more difficult by limitations on working hours.[4,5] The resultant friction between service and training has led to poor use of assessment tools and an increasing belief that excellence in some has been sacrificed for a basic level of competence in many.[20]

The CoBaTrICE Collaboration was formed in 2003 to harmonize standards of training in ICM internationally, first by defining outcomes of specialist ICM training and then by developing guidance and standards for assessment of competence and program infrastructure and quality assurance.[21,22] The underlying principle of this initiative was the concept that an ICM specialist trained in one country should have the same core skills and abilities as one trained in another, thereby ensuring a common standard of clinical competence. This follows the European Union ethos of free movement of professionals and mutual recognition of medical qualifications between member states.[23] Competency-based training makes convergence possible by defining the outcomes of specialist training—a common "end product"—rather than enforcing rigid structures and processes of training. A minimum standard of knowledge, skills, attitudes, and behavior is defined a priori and applied to existing structures and processes of training; acquisition and assessment of competence occur during training in the workplace.

DEFINING CORE COMPETENCIES

The CoBaTrICE project has used consensus techniques—an extensive international consultation process using a modified online Delphi involving more than 500 clinicians in more than 50 countries, an eight-country postal survey of patients and relatives, and an expert nominal group—to define the core competencies required of a specialist in ICM.[21,24] These competencies have been linked to a comprehensive syllabus, relevant educational resources, and guidance for the standardized assessment of competence in the workplace via a dedicated website.[22] Since its launch in September 2006, 10 national training programs have adopted CoBaTrICE, and others have made use of the materials. In 2008, the second phase of the project developed international standards for national training programs in ICM,[16] and further refined the methods of assessment of competence. The implementation and long-term evaluation of the CoBaTrICE program will be necessary to assess its impact on an individual's competence and harmonization of ICM training. In the United States, a multisociety initiative has used a similar methodology to the CoBaTrICE program to create common competencies.[25]

EVOLVING PROFESSIONAL ROLES: IMPLICATIONS FOR TRAINING

The CoBaTrICE Delphi demonstrated the importance that intensive care clinicians attach not only to the acquisition of procedural technical skills but equally to aspects of professionalism—communication skills, attitudes and behavior, governance, team working, and judgment.[24] The intensivist is akin to an "acute general practitioner," a family doctor with enhanced role in acute medicine, physiology, diagnostics, palliative care, research, ethics, and with added technical ability. Most importantly they are the team leaders and orchestrators (and providers) of care, and their competencies must therefore include these team-management, integration-of-care skills. Competency-based training makes this possible by explicitly identifying which skills are shared in common and which are peculiar to specific disciplines. Thus, although weaning from ventilation,[26] instigation of renal replacement, nutritional support, prophylaxis for venous thromboembolism, and chest pain management pathways,[27] among others, can be nurse led and protocol driven, the intensivist provides a strategic, integrating, and continuity role as much as a technical one. Opportunities for collaboration between critical care physicians and hospitalists can also be clarified in this manner. In this model, hierarchies become flatter, practitioners become more patient focused, and the intensivist's leadership skills must include the capacity for collaborative decision making while continuing to assume final responsibility for patient care. As nonphysician roles increase and extend, it is essential that their schemes for training be coordinated and better integrated with those for physicians, ideally starting at undergraduate level.[28]

PRACTICAL IMPLICATIONS OF COMPETENCY-BASED TRAINING

Concerns about competency-based training include the perception that competencies describe a "craftsman" rather than a "professional" and that "being a good doctor" is too complex to be defined by lists of skills or activities.[29-31] This may be an artificial distinction, because both may aspire to excellence through constant practice and reflection. The professional has the privilege of self-regulation based on defined standards of practice, which emphasizes the importance of revalidation and recertification. The minimum standard for revalidation should include the competencies of a specialist, plus evidence of excellence, which may include the domains of research, teaching, professional development, role modeling, and high-quality patient care demonstrated through processes or outcomes. A minimum safe standard is where professional training starts, not where it ends.

The *duration of training* is determined by the acquisition of competencies, not by a fixed and arbitrary period in training, although training programs will of course need to continue to set a minimum time. The practical implication is that some trainees may not meet the expected targets and will require remedial training or more focused attention. The key to this is adequate supervision by "trained trainers" supported by all senior staff. Monitoring progress is essential to avoid discovering problems too late for effective remediation, such as at the end of training, or after specialist accreditation through adverse events or clinical complaints. The cost implications of having senior faculty with time to mentor, assess, and develop their trainees is considerable. In larger programs, it becomes even more important to bridge the distance between trainer and trainee, because shift working and arduous schedules disrupt opportunities for apprentice-based relationships.

Documentation is a crucial component of training because it provides the evidence on which the trainee makes the case for being accepted as competent or, indeed, excellent. Portfolios are the responsibility of the trainee but require review by the trainer designated as mentor or supervisor for that trainee. It seems likely that most training programs will move from traditional paper-based methods to e-portfolios as technology evolves. This change brings with it both advantages and disadvantages (Box 74.1). A particular advantage of Internet-based technologies is the ability to link competencies and syllabi to the rapidly expanding repository of web-based educational resources.[32] They may also make it easier to deliver educational interventions in the workplace during clinical work rather than limiting provision of education to office hours.[33]

Maintenance of competence has become an increasingly regulated activity for specialists, incorporating the distinct but related processes of accredited continuing medical education (CME) or continuing professional development (CPD), appraisal, revalidation, and recertification or maintenance of certification. Standards for recertification vary widely.[34] Several countries now have mandated processes, including Australia, New Zealand, Canada, the United States, and from 2013 the United Kingdom. Maintenance of certification in the United States is based on demonstrating competence in six domains,[35] and in the United Kingdom in four domains.[36] The process for revalidation for intensive care specialists in the United Kingdom has recently been defined.[37]

Access to educational materials is another important consideration. Service pressures and budgetary constraints mean that education will need to be delivered locally, supplemented by distance-learning programs combined with self-assessment. To work well, education needs to be integrated with the clinical and training environment, be available in a timely manner, and be placed in context—for example, during a ward round or immediately after seeing a patient with a particular condition. Computers and clinical decision support systems can provide this, but careful collaborative development by information technology experts, clinicians, and educators is required. Linking educational resources to competencies is a necessary step in building and maintaining competency-based systems of training. It is now more common for trainees to look to smartphone applications to access knowledge and procedural guidance than traditional texts. This is both a useful and problematic innovation. The Internet allows both peer-reviewed and entirely unedited repositories of knowledge to be created, many of which are excellent, some less so.

Box 74.1 E-Portfolios: Analysis of Utility

Strengths

- Facilitates remote communication between trainee and trainer
- Integrates with whole career: life long learning and revalidation
- Easy to update
- Secure central database
- Links to Internet, e-resources
- Portable: smartphone/phone/laptop
- Facilitates audit, monitoring, identifying gaps in knowledge

Weaknesses

- Data security
- Loss of passwords/access/firewalls
- Overemphasis on detail and "box ticking"
- Electronic communication not as good as face to face
- Expensive technical support and maintenance

Opportunities

- International integration
- Facilitates pedagogic research
- Update reminders/diary
- Link to educational resources
- Documentation of course attendance and skills acquisition

Threats

- Data loss, confidentiality
- Cheating
- Internet access speeds diminished with large volume of users

ASSESSMENT

Workplace-based assessment of competence (Box 74.2)[38-46] is not generally problematic for the majority of trainees, but the potential complexity of assessment becomes apparent when there is a trainee in difficulty or when an adverse assessment results in litigation or revelations of serial malpractice later in life. Why was the problem not detected earlier? Whose responsibility is it to undertake assessment? How should it be performed? How often should assessments be made? How reliable and repeatable are the methods used, and how does one deal with disagreement between different trainers?

For any program of training, a system of evaluation must exist to test the validity of the teaching method, the content,

Box 74.2 Workplace-Based Assessment Methods

Direct Observation

- Direct observation of skills (e.g., DOPS, OSATS)[50,51]
  Direct observation of a physician performing diagnostic and interventional procedures during normal ("routine") clinical practice—used to assess the doctor-patient interaction and the process as a whole, not just the procedure itself
- Clinical evaluation exercise (CEX)[52,53]
  A "snapshot" observation of a normal (i.e., routine) clinical encounter
- Audiovisual records
  Assessment of real-time video-recorded consultations using a structured rating scale
- Multisource feedback (MSF)[49]
  Patients' or colleagues' views of the physician's professional attitudes and behavior in day-to-day practice are collected on a structured rating form; completed forms are returned to a central point and summarized. Feedback is then provided during a meeting between the doctor and the reviewer. MSF also is termed 360-degree assessment, peer assessment, or team assessment of behavior

Case Reviews and Analysis

- Case-based discussion or chart-stimulated recall
  Use of an actual written record to focus structured discussion about a case
- Structured case histories
  A written report summarizing a case that has been encountered and, with reference to the relevant literature, reflecting on the management of that case

DOPS, directly observed procedural skills; OSATS, objective structured assessment of technical skills.
Superscript numbers refer to specific references provided online for this chapter.

and its application. If the curriculum is to have an assessment component, it too requires regular evaluation to ensure that it remains valid, that is, repeatable and consistent between observers. The ultimate test is whether the curriculum and method of testing lead to improvements in health care. Miller's hierarchy of learning[47] suggests that whereas undergraduate training is more focused on the acquisition of knowledge, postgraduate training places increasing importance on performance, and assessment strategies must therefore focus at the "action" level or on "what one does." Assessments need to take into account the trainees' abilities and previous experience, the complexity of the tasks that they perform, and the context. In a variation of the Miller pyramid, the route to becoming a true specialist might be a training ladder, with step 1 (the novice) representing the acquisition of knowledge; step 2 (the trainee) the period of training, which will vary in duration and intensity, depending on needs; step 3 (the competent new specialist) indicating independence; and step 4 (the expert) with experience and further training beyond basic competencies. The steps are not truly rigid because in reality, skills and knowledge are learned together and experiences and practice occur at all stages in training. This schema is equally applicable to all disciplines.

Definitions of competencies serve to guide the assessment process. Descriptions of what physicians should be able to do create a benchmark against which judgments can be made of clinical performance ("docs," rather than "can do"). A range of methods and tools may be used to assess training, but assessment of physicians' performance at work is still in its infancy.[48] Assessment must go beyond technical skills to include aspects of professionalism, attitudes, and behavior: communication skills, familiarity with current knowledge, shared decision making, respect for autonomy, and compassion. Techniques for the assessment of holistic professionalism include "360-degree assessment," also called multisource feedback.[49,50] This technique involves actively seeking the opinion of others on the team, both one's peers and junior colleagues and, where appropriate, patients and relatives, about one's performance.

During training these assessments should be formative—that is, they should contribute to learning and not be a final pass/fail judgment. This traditional "apprentice-master" model requires frequent observation during routine clinical work by an experienced trainer and works well for the majority of trainees. However, the model may need to be supplemented by formal methods involving more objective assessment of performance. The assessments should be documented in the trainee's portfolio and combined with annual appraisal. A more novel technique is based on video recording of team behaviors during ward rounds.[51]

Institutions need to allow protected time for trainers to be trained in formal assessment techniques and time to carry them out within employment contracts. It is important that all members of the team contribute to teaching and to training assessments; it cannot be the sole responsibility of one individual.

DELIVERING TRAINING AND ASSESSMENT IN THE WORKPLACE: ROLE OF SIMULATION

Simulators in health care are not a new concept. The Romans had birthing phantoms made from various leathers and bone to teach midwifery. Indeed early vivisectionists would have claimed operations on animals improved performance of the surgeon when dealing with patients. Simulated clinical environments and patient or equipment simulators have long seemed a highly effective solution to the problems of providing effective individual and team training. Modern medical simulators come in various guises, from simple anatomic models, to part task trainers, to complex virtual reality systems (Table 74.1). However, the most important part of a simulator is not the technology, but the faculty who write the scenario and, more importantly, debrief the students after simulation. Simulated cases lend themselves well to acute care settings. Here, a number of discrete interventions carried out on a single "patient" by various members of the team can be evaluated, subsequently can be viewed in private or during group discussion, and can be of assistance in understanding team working. Rare critical events associated with high rates of mortality or morbidity will not be encountered with

Table 74.1 Categories of Simulators Used in Medicine

Simulator Type	Description	Example	Uses	Relative Cost
Diagrams and static models	Basic anatomic representations	Circulatory system	Largely illustrative	Low
Part task trainers	Anatomically correct models that have simple moving parts demonstrating one or more processes	Airway manikin with inflatable bladders representing lungs	Clinical skills and procedural training to look at individual tasks	Low
Computer simulation software	Computer- or web-based programs that can recreate physiologic processes and the responses to interventions	ACLS Sim*	Rehearsal of treatment algorithms and practice in applying knowledge	Low
Complex task trainers	Anatomically correct models with a number of elements that can be manipulated and respond to manipulation to produce physiologically credible effects	Resusci-Annie† ALS training manikins with inflatable lungs, rhythm generators for electrocardiographic analysis	More complex scenario–based training when multiple interventions are required	Medium
Intermediate-fidelity manikins	Anatomically correct human manikins that demonstrate automated and instructor-driven responses to a range of interventions	Instructor-driven manikins: Laerdal Sim Man‡	Complex multiuser scenario–based training and assessment	Medium to high
High-fidelity manikins	Anatomically correct human manikins equipped with response algorithms that can mimic the physiologic responses of numerous patient types to a range of interventions and environmental changes	Instructor- and algorithm-driven manikins: Meti-Human Patient Simulator (Meti-HPS)§	Complex multiuser scenario–based training and assessment	High
Virtual (VR) reality trainers	Simple VR trainers are available that largely resemble complex task trainers Experimental systems will ultimately be able to recreate any clinical situation in any environment.	Training and assessing complex tasks Full-blown recreations of events True telemedicine		Very high

*ACLS Sim is a computer screen–based Advanced Cardiac Life Support training program that tests applied knowledge of resuscitation treatment algorithms. Further information is available at www.acls.net/sim.htm.

†Resusci-Annie is an ALS trainer manikin made by Laerdal Medical AS, Stavanger, Norway. Further information is available at www.laerdal.com.

‡Sim Man is the universal patient simulator made by Laerdal Medical AS, Stavanger, Norway. Further information is available at www.laerdal.com.

§Meti-HPS is the human patient simulator made by Medical Education Technologies, Inc., Sarasota, FL. Further information is available at www.meti.com.

ALCS, advanced cardiac life support; ALS, advanced life support.

From Gautam N: Uses of Human Patient Simulators for Critical Care Training [thesis for diploma in intensive care medicine]. London, Intercollegiate Board for Training in Intensive Care Medicine (IBTICM), 2004.

sufficient frequency in normal clinical practice for all clinicians to gain proficiency in their avoidance and management, but they can easily be incorporated in simulations. This ability to re create complex and infrequent but highly significant clinical scenarios improves the consistency and repeatability of assessment.

Critical incident training has been carried out in industry for many years, most notably in aviation. High-fidelity aircraft simulators have been in routine use by flight and cabin crews for many years. Human patient simulators (HPS) offer physiologically accurate responses, haptic feedback, integration with patient records, and high-quality closed capture video recording. Such intermediate and high-fidelity manikins are freely and widely available. However, there remains little standardization in the way they are used for training or assessment. Also, the considerable setup fees are dwarfed by the faculty costs in using these systems to their best. Often, then, items bought with the best intention are not used as part of any integrated training scheme and exist as novelty.

A number of studies have demonstrated that knowledge acquisition is faster when using simulations to support traditional learning methods. This context-specific learning also allows better retention of knowledge but only up to a point. Skills acquisition is also faster if first taught on simulators, but those taught on more conventional lines soon catch up, and after a period of similar clinical practice, differences in performance are negligible.

Areas in which simulators are frequently used are the advanced life support courses, the Fundamentals of Critical Care Support course developed by the Society of Critical Care Medicine (SCCM),[52] and the European Society of Intensive Care Medicine's PACT (Patient-centered Acute Care Training) program.[53]

The pressures to deliver service rather than training, the reduction in trainees' working hours, and the need for quality assurance in training have led to more effective teaching methods and credible assessment tools. Simulation assessment is efficient, repeatable, and reliable; and the scenarios can be well integrated with the clinical environment to allow short and focused training opportunities linked to debriefing.

SUMMARY

Critical care medicine provides important training opportunities for all clinicians and is an ideal environment in which to gain proficiency in technical skills, team working, ethics, and professionalism. Training in ICM should start at the undergraduate level to maximize these opportunities. A universal set of core competencies can be expanded according to local requirements and be used to foster shared team-based skills in acute care across different disciplines. Health care systems need to invest in education in the workplace, with access to information integrated with clinical work, support for trainers, and the development of workplace-based methods for assessment. Portfolios should become reflective life long learning documents for specialists, as much as for trainees. Pedagogic research is needed to evaluate education programs as quality improvement implementation devices for translating research knowledge into better patient care.

KEY POINTS

- Critical care training is heterogeneous in access, process, and certification.
- There appears to be growing consensus on the core knowledge and skills needed to practice intensive care.
- Internationally recognized competency-based training should ensure a minimum knowledge and skill base for specialists and allow meaningful comparisons.
- Continuous workplace assessments and appraisals will be needed for revalidation.
- Service delivery pressures will require greater use of specialist nonphysician grades to operate within protocol-driven frameworks. Competency-based training will allow integration of their training with that of physicians.
- Simulators and simulated environments will increasingly be used for team training and to adequately prepare staff to deal with uncommon situations.
- The reduced length of training will lead to better trained but less experienced individuals entering the specialist workforce. This emphasizes the need for continuing medical education integrated with clinical practice and formal "protected" training sessions conducted by experienced clinical educators.
- There are significant resource implications associated with life long training and assessment schemes with mutual recognition across international borders.

SELECTED REFERENCES

1. Dorman T, Angood PB, Angus DC, et al: Guidelines for critical care medicine training and continuing medical education. Crit Care Med 2004;32(1):263-272.
7. The national education and competence framework for advanced critical care practitioners. London, Department of Health, 2008. Available at http://www.dh.gov.uk/en/Publicationsandstatistics/Publications/PublicationsPolicyAndGuidance/DH_084011. Accessed June 2012.
14. Barrett H, Bion JF, on behalf of the CoBaTrICE Collaboration: An international survey of training in adult intensive care medicine. Intensive Care Med 2005;31:552-561.
16. The CoBaTrICE Collaboration: International standards for programmes of training in intensive care medicine in Europe. Special article. Intensive Care Med 2011;37:385-393.
17. Faculty of Intensive Care Medicine. Available at http://www.ficm.ac.uk/
20. Tooke J: Aspiring to excellence: Final report of the independent inquiry into modernising medical careers. London, MMC Inquiry, 2008. Available at www.mmcinquiry.org.uk.
25. Buckley JD, Addrizzo-Harris DJ, Clay AS, et al: Multisociety task force recommendations of competencies in pulmonary and critical care medicine. Am J Respir Crit Care Med 2009;180(4):290-295.
30. Leung W: Competency based medical training: Review. BMJ 2002;325:693-695.
31. Gonczi A: Review of international trends and developments in competency based education and training. In Argulles A, Gonczi A (eds): Competency Based Education and Training: A World Perspective. Balderas, Mexico, Noriega Editores, 2000.
49. Evans R, Elwyn G, Edwards A: Review of instruments for peer assessment of physicians. BMJ 2004;328:1240.

The complete list of references can be found at www.expertconsult.com.

PART 9

OTHER CRITICAL CARE DISORDERS AND ISSUES IN THE CRITICALLY ILL

75

Diagnosis and Management of Liver Failure in the Adult

Nick Murphy

CHAPTER OUTLINE

Liver failure is most often encountered as result of decompensation of chronic liver disease but can also occur de novo in patients with previously normal livers. These patients are often described as having fulminant or acute liver failure depending on the definition used.

Liver failure is characterized by a constellation of physical signs and symptoms including jaundice, coagulopathy, and encephalopathy. Not all of these need be present for a diagnosis to be made, but as the syndrome progresses they are usually present to varying degrees. Liver failure progresses to multiple organ failure and ultimately death in a large proportion of patients, and supportive care plus removal of the primary cause is the mainstay of treatment. In a small group liver transplantation may be indicated. Liver support systems are being actively investigated and may, in the future, have the ability to bridge a patient to recovery or transplantation.

DECOMPENSATION OF CHRONIC LIVER DISEASE

"Decompensation" in cirrhosis of the liver is a term used to describe the onset of visible signs of portal hypertension such as the development of ascites and variceal bleeding. These signs and symptoms can also be described as "symptomatic" cirrhosis, with the onset of liver failure in symptomatic cirrhosis described as "decompensation." One often leads to the other, but for the purposes of this chapter decompensation will refer to the onset of liver failure.

The pathologic basis of acute decompensation in chronic liver disease or acute on chronic liver failure (AoCLF) is incompletely understood but is thought to be precipitated by systemic inflammation, and if looked for hard enough, some signs or symptoms of infection will be seen in most patients.[1,2] Patients with well-compensated cirrhosis often decompensate following a defined event. The precipitants can be split into two types: (1) those due to direct liver insult, such as ischemia, a toxic insult such as alcohol, or a superimposed viral infection and (2) those in which the liver is affected as a bystander in a systemic inflammatory process, such as following an episode of sepsis or a gastrointestinal bleed. This can be contrasted to the progressive liver failure of end-stage cirrhosis. Both present with similar clinical pictures but in AoCLF there remains the possibility of improvement and reversibility, and if these patients do recover they end up back on the previous mortality trajectory.[1,2]

Differentiating between the two is difficult but the presence of a precipitating factor and history can be useful. In patients with end-stage liver cirrhosis there is often a history of gradual deterioration in biochemical parameters, clinical status, and other organ function whereas in AoCLF there is often an acute deterioration. Organ support in the former setting is of dubious utility as it is almost always futile (Fig. 75.1).

One group has proposed a working definition for AoCLF as "acute deterioration in liver function over a period of 2-4 weeks, usually associated with a precipitating event, leading to severe deterioration in clinical status, with jaundice and hepatic encephalopathy and or hepatorenal syndrome (HRS), with a high SOFA/APACHE II score."[1]

Additional online-only material indicated by icon.

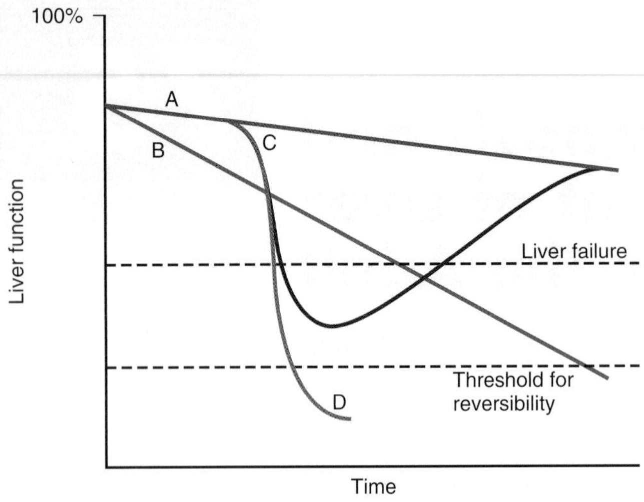

Figure 75.1 Graphs A and B represent the trajectory of liver function in cirrhosis. B is indicative of a patient with progressive end-stage disease. A has a more shallow trajectory until there is a precipitating event, at which time either graphs C or D can be followed. C recovers with intervention back to the previous trajectory, but D does not.

AoCLF often occurs with multiple organ dysfunction. This may be because of the underlying precipitating event such as pneumonia or bacterial peritonitis or as a result of the severe deterioration in liver function. Often it is difficult to distinguish which came first. Renal failure is the most common organ failure associated with AoCLF and it is the severity of organ dysfunction that dictates the outcome.[3]

PRECIPITATING FACTORS OF ACUTE ON CHRONIC LIVER FAILURE

ALCOHOLIC HEPATITIS

Alcoholic hepatitis is a common manifestation of alcohol abuse. Between 20% and 30% of heavy drinkers will present with it at some time. The clinical picture is variable from a relatively mild syndrome associated with loss of appetite, nausea, and vomiting with right upper quadrant pain to severe life-threatening liver decompensation, but the most obvious sign is the sudden onset of jaundice, and this can be the first indication of liver disease in a heavy drinker. Overall, following first presentation, 35% to 50% of patients will die within the first month of diagnosis.[4] It usually presents following a bout of heavy drinking and often occurs on a background of cirrhosis. Patients frequently deteriorate after stopping alcohol. This may be due to the immunosuppressive effects of alcohol. In patients without cirrhosis abstinence and nutritional support can lead to a marked improvement in liver function over time.

Features suggestive of malnutrition such as muscle wasting and vitamin deficiency are seen commonly. In severe decompensation other intercurrent illnesses such as pneumonia or urinary tract infection or a gastrointestinal bleed are often present. Systemic inflammation may be the precipitant of decompensation in these patients.[5]

PORTAL HYPERTENSIVE BLEEDING

Portal hypertension is a significant complication of chronic liver disease leading to the formation of portosystemic collateral vessels. Of these vessels, the most significant clinically are those that occur in the wall of the stomach and esophagus. In patients with portal hypertension as a result of cirrhosis the development of gastrointestinal varices occurs in approximately 60% at the time of diagnosis.[11] The incidence of the first acute bleed in an unselected patient is relatively low at about 5% per year but it can be catastrophic when it occurs.[12] The mortality rate associated with the event has fallen over the past 20 years from approximately 30% to 50% to about 20% and control of the initial bleeding episode is achieved in about 90% of patients.[13] Half of all fatalities occur in the first 5 days following an acute bleed and about half of them are due to uncontrolled bleeding and the rest are due to multiple organ failure. This pattern remains the same when mortality rate in the first 6 weeks following the first bleed is examined.[13]

The use of antibiotic prophylaxis has been shown to reduce the incidence of infection in this group of patients and to improve short-term mortality rate.[20,21] It has been proposed that infection is the precipitant to an acute increase in portal pressure that may trigger bleeding.[22]

BACTERIAL PERITONITIS

Patients with chronic liver disease are at increased risk of infection. The immunosuppression associated with chronic liver disease is incompletely understood but relates to a range of factors including an impaired innate and adaptive immune response.[23,24]

In cirrhotic patients with ascites, decompensation to liver failure is often precipitated by infection. Bacterial peritonitis is a common and severe complication. It can be completely asymptomatic but can present with a range of symptoms and signs including local signs of peritonitis, abdominal pain, diarrhea, and signs of systemic inflammation such as fever, rigors, raised white blood cell count, hypotension, and tachycardia.[25]

Bacterial peritonitis is often spontaneous, without any obvious source, although it can be secondary to other intra-abdominal disease. It is generally caused by aerobic gram-negative bacteria, although gram-positive bacteria including methicillin-resistant *Staphylococcus aureus* (MRSA) should be suspected if there is treatment failure, especially if the patient has been taking prophylactic antibiotics.[26] In any patient with ascites and decompensation of liver disease, spontaneous bacterial peritonitis (SBP) should be suspected. Diagnosis is demonstrated by sampling of the ascitic fluid. An absolute leukocyte count in ascitic fluid of greater than 250/μL is diagnostic. Antibiotics should be started as soon as SBP is suspected, following blood culture and a diagnostic ascitic tap. Empiric broad-spectrum antibiotic coverage for gram-negative and MRSA organisms (depending on local prevalence) should be started until cultures are available.

Renal failure is a significant complication of SBP in patients with cirrhosis and is discussed later. The use of human albumin solution (HAS) in SBP has been shown to reduce the incidence of progression to renal failure and should be considered in this setting.[25]

SUPPORTIVE MANAGEMENT IN CRITICAL CARE

The presentation of AoCLD will depend on the precipitating event or events but the clinical picture and pattern of organ failure will on the whole look very similar. Hyperbilirubinemia and the resulting jaundice are almost universal, as are other biochemical manifestations of poor liver function. Plasma protein production is deranged, leading to a prolongation of prothrombin time and hypoalbuminemia. Thrombocytopenia due to hypersplenism and sepsis is also characteristic. The effects on the coagulation system are complex, however, as there is a concurrent reduction in the production of endogenous anticoagulant proteins in the liver resulting a relative rebalancing. Infection leads to consumption of factors and platelets and so the use of thromboelastography is recommended in bleeding patients. Lower levels of factors can result in difficulties maintaining coagulation during times of stress, particularly during infections, and evidence of a heparin-like effect has been shown.[27] It is also interesting to note that the incidence of thromboembolism is not lower in patients with cirrhosis even in the setting of a prolonged international normalization ratio (INR), suggesting that standard measures of coagulation are unreliable.[28]

The pattern of circulatory changes associated with cirrhosis is distinctive. Hypotension and an increase in cardiac output are typical, resulting in a hyperdynamic circulation. Peripheral vasodilatation, however, is not distributed evenly and occurs mainly in the splanchnic circulation as a result of sinusoidal portal hypertension. Splanchnic vasodilatation results in effective arterial underfilling with the resulting activation of compensatory mechanisms.[29] During decompensation circulatory changes become more pronounced with an increase in portal pressure; systemic vasodilatation worsens and blood pressure drops further and becomes less responsive to vasopressor support. Recent work shows that cardiac output may fall in those who develop hepatorenal failure, as do cardiac filling pressures and pulmonary artery pressure. These changes point toward some form of cardiac depressant factor associated with decompensation.[29] There is a reduction in intrarenal blood flow, due to the activation of compensatory mechanisms designed to maintain arterial volume, such as the renin-angiotensin system and sympathetic nervous system. This results in a further reduction in glomerular filtration rate (GFR) and urine output. Cardiac function may be further compromised by liver failure–associated cardiomyopathy, which is manifested by a low or normal cardiac output in the setting of reduced afterload.[30] There may also be a relative hypovolemia in the setting of a normal or raised central venous pressure because of raised intra-abdominal pressure due to ascites. Echocardiography is very helpful in the delineation of any cardiac dysfunction and can help assess pulmonary artery pressure to assess if the patient has portopulmonary hypertension.[31] A pulmonary artery (PA) catheter should be used if there is any doubt.

Acute kidney injury (AKI) is the most common form of organ dysfunction seen in patients with AoCLF and has significant attributable mortality risk.[32] There are four main causes: those associated with bacterial infection are the most common, followed by hypovolemia and parenchymal disease, with hepatorenal failure the least common.[3] However, hepatorenal failure has a particularly poor outcome. The diagnosis of AKI in the setting of liver disease is problematic, as conventional measures of renal function are less indicative of renal function.

Hepatorenal syndrome is a severe and progressive reduction in renal function in patients with severe liver disease and presents in two clinical patterns, type 1 and type 2. Hepatorenal syndrome represents the renovascular response to the profound circulatory changes associated with cirrhosis. Type 2 HRS is characterized by a less severe and more gradual reduction in renal function associated with diuretic-resistant ascites and hyponatremia. It is usually seen in association with end-stage cirrhosis. Type 1 HRS is characterized by the rapid decline in renal function defined as a 100% increase in serum creatinine to a level greater than 221 mmol/L or a 50% reduction in 24-hour creatinine clearance to a level less than 20 mL/minute in less than 2 weeks.[33] Initially HRS is potentially reversible as the kidneys are functionally normal; however, the longer the circulatory changes last without reestablishing the GFR, the less likely are the kidneys to recover, and the distinction between HRS and acute tubular necrosis becomes less clear. In most patients there is a precipitating event, while in others it occurs in close proximity to an event such as the resolution of SBP. The diagnosis is made by the exclusion of other causes and is based on criteria developed by the International Ascites Club.[33]

AKI in the setting of AoCLF is managed along conventional lines. Hypovolemia is corrected and diuretics are stopped. Potentially nephrotoxic drugs are stopped, and the underlying precipitating event is managed.

Until recently there was no effective treatment for patients with HRS other than liver transplantation, but over the past 15 years observational and interventional studies have shown that countering the compensatory circulatory changes that promote intrarenal vasoconstriction with use of systemic and selective vasoconstrictors plus plasma volume expansion with albumin can lead to significant improvement in renal function.[34] The aim of therapy is to focus vasoconstriction on the dilated splanchnic vessels, resulting in a redistribution of the blood volume back into the systemic arterial circulation. Over time this results in suppression of the compensatory mechanisms; a reduction in plasma renin activity, sympathetic activity, and circulating catecholamines; and an associated increase in GFR, sodium excretion, and urine output.[35] Many different vasoconstrictors have been tried in this setting. The drug most commonly studied is terlipressin and it is often given with 20% human albumin solution (HAS). This approach has been subjected to a randomized controlled clinical trial in which the addition of albumin was associated with an improvement in outcome.[36] Evidence suggests that vasoconstrictor therapy, with or without plasma volume expansion, results in an improvement in renal function in about a third of patients with type I HRS. The best predictors of response to therapy is the baseline serum creatinine, and those who do respond have a significant rise in their arterial pressure.[34,37]

Hepatic encephalopathy (HE) is almost universal during decompensation of chronic liver disease and is characterized by loss of normal day/night differentiation, confusion, somnolence, asterixis, hyperreflexia, and progression to coma. It is reversible in the event of recovery of liver function or removal of the precipitating event. The etiology of hepatic encephalopathy is incompletely understood but relates to the inability of the failing liver to clear circulating toxins, most notably ammonia. There are other important factors including minor degrees of cerebral edema and systemic inflammation. Interaction of these components leads to the profound levels of encephalopathy seen in AoCLF.

Ammonia production in the gut is important in the pathogenesis. Ammonia is usually cleared from the portal circulation in the liver. The mainstays of treatment are colonic cleansing with enemas and enteral disaccharides such as lactulose. Both of these procedures have been shown to improve encephalopathy grades. The restriction of protein, once fashionable in patients with liver disease, is contraindicated. The majority of these patients are malnourished and adequate enteral nutrition is essential.[38]

Patients with AoCLD and high grades of HE will require intubation and ventilation, if not because of hypoxia, then to allow airway protection. Airway protection is most frequently needed in patients with bleeding esophageal or gastric varices requiring endoscopic therapy for large volume hematemesis in the presence of HE and a difficult or prolonged endoscopic procedure. Patients with AoCLD are usually exquisitely sensitive to sedative and anesthetic agents. Even small doses of benzodiazepines can cause prolonged coma. Care should be exercised in their use and shorter-acting agents such as propofol are preferred.

Large volume paracentesis should be considered in any patient with tense ascites. There is evidence that large volume paracentesis improves lung mechanics and oxygenation in nonventilated patients but data in ventilated patients are lacking.[39-41] Hepatic hydrothorax is a persistent pleural effusion, almost always associated with ascites, usually on the right side of the chest. It can be massive in size, containing many liters of fluid, and is thought to be due to communication from the peritoneum. Management can be difficult. Direct drainage with thoracocentesis is usually inadvisable as the fluid accumulation is persistent, leading to continued need for chest tube placement, which carries the risk of infection. Management should be directed at the ascites and includes diuretics, salt restriction, and paracentesis. TIPS can be used to control both ascites and hydrothorax but is associated with worsening encephalopathy grade in some patients.[42]

Adrenal dysfunction in patients with critical illness has been documented extensively, particularly in patients with septic shock.[43] Studies have suggested an improvement in outcome with steroid use but subsequent investigations have been less clear. Currently recommendations suggest steroid treatment should not be based on adrenal stimulation and should be reserved for those with vasopressor-resistant septic shock or early acute respiratory distress syndrome (ARDS) within 14 days of onset.[43] Patients with liver failure have been shown to have a high incidence of adrenal suppression as well, although it is not clear if this has a different etiology to other critically ill patients. Patients with adrenal suppression have worse hepatic and renal function, more organ failure, and a higher intensive care unit (ICU) and hospital mortality rate.[44] There remains, however, a lack of consensus regarding definitions of adrenal dysfunction and appropriate testing in patients with liver disease and in which patients require treatment.[45] However, in patients with cirrhosis and septic shock admitted to the ICU with adrenal insufficiency as defined by a suboptimal response to ACTH stimulation, replacement of hydrocortisone (50 mg every 6 hours) results in a higher incidence of shock resolution and hospital survival when compared to historical control subjects.[46]

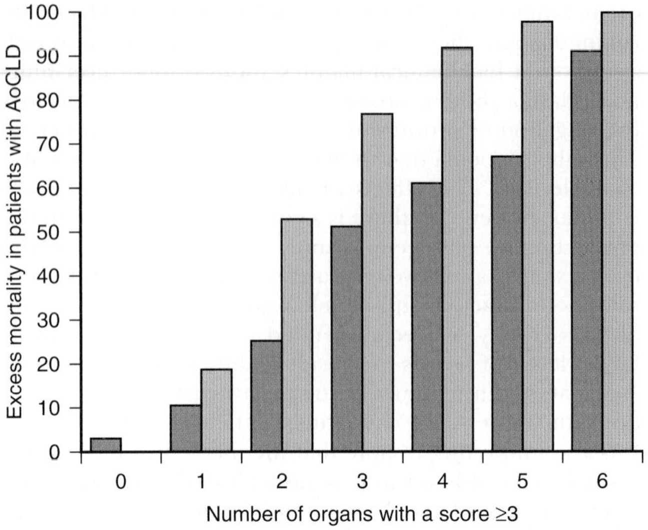

Figure 75.2 This graph shows the relative mortality rates associated with the number of failing organs as defined by a SOFA (sequential organ failure) score of greater than 3. In patients with cirrhosis (*yellow bars*) there is an excess mortality rate at each position. Blue bars, unselected group.

OUTCOME AND DATA ON ICU USE IN DECOMPENSATED CIRRHOSIS

Despite ICU care, the outcome in patients with decompensated cirrhosis is poor. In one study overall cumulative mortality rates were 36% in the critical care unit, 46% in the hospital, and 56% at 6-month follow-up.[47]

In patients who require organ support within the critical care environment a number of observations can be made. Derangement of acute physiology at admission is a predictor of outcome, as it is for unselected patients admitted to the ICU.[48] In addition, the number of organs requiring support also is predictive of outcome, as it is in unselected patients.[47,49] If you compare the number of organs failing (defined as an organ-specific SOFA score greater than 3) there is an excess mortality rate associated with cirrhosis when compared to an unselected group (Fig. 75.2).[50] Patients with cirrhosis and three organ systems requiring support have a mortality rate in excess of 90% in some studies.[49] Severity of liver disease at admission has a significant bearing on outcome irrespective of indication for admission to the ICU.[49,51]

ACUTE (FULMINANT) LIVER FAILURE

Acute liver failure (ALF) is a syndrome manifested by the rapid cessation of normal function in individuals with previously normal livers. The rate of decline in function dictates the manner in which the syndrome manifests and influences the outcome. The cause is the main influence on the rate of progression and the likelihood of spontaneous recovery.[52]

The pathologic basis of the massive hepatic necrosis was described in detail by Lucké and Mallory following the Second World War in 1946.[53] The presence of the American army in East Asia and Africa resulted in exposure to both epidemic and serum hepatitis, and data regarding the clinical course of the syndrome and its pathologic features were collated via the army medical services.

In 1970 Trey and Davidson introduced the term *fulminant hepatic failure* (FHF) to encompass the current clinicopathologic understanding of the syndrome.[54] This definition was an attempt to encapsulate the clinical course and to differentiate it from decompensation of chronic liver disease. They described a syndrome of rapidly progressing liver failure (within 8 weeks) in which the defining point was the onset of hepatic encephalopathy following the onset of symptoms in someone without previous liver disease. They make the point that the syndrome is potentially reversible in some patients. This definition is still used today; however, it has become clear that this definition is too narrow and that subgroups exist. This point is important as these subgroups predict the likely prognosis and potential for survival without a liver transplant.[52]

The rate of progression from the onset of jaundice or other initial symptoms (such as fatigue or acute viral illness) to development of encephalopathy is used to define subgroups. This in part relates to the cause of liver failure and to the way the pathologic expression of the pattern of organ failure presents. For example, patients with significant acetaminophen-induced hepatotoxicity will generally present with liver failure within 7 days of ingestion, unless ingestion was staggered over a period of time when the timing of liver insult is difficult to define. Patients often present with cardiovascular collapse and renal failure before they become encephalopathic. In contrast, patients presenting with seronegative hepatitis (unknown cause) can have a very variable presentation, some with a prolonged illness over a period of months, resulting in a patient who is deeply jaundiced with evidence of portal hypertension, such as ascites, at the onset of encephalopathy, and others with a relatively short presentation period. These two extreme ends of the syndrome split the group into hyperacute and subacute, with ALF in the middle. Interestingly, it is the hyperacute group that has the best chance for spontaneous recovery, although this group has the highest risk of cerebral edema. The subacute group has the worse prognosis with medical management alone.[52]

ALF is rare, with about 1 to 6 cases per 1 million of the population in the developed world.[55] The incidence in the rest of the world is less clear because of the paucity of data (Box 75.1).

Box 75.1 Hyperacute, Acute, and Subacute Liver Failure

Hyperacute liver failure

- Jaundice to encephalopathy within 7 days—usually secondary to paracetamol hepatotoxicity

Acute liver failure

- Jaundice to encephalopathy in 8 to 28 days

Subacute liver failure

- Jaundice to encephalopathy in 29 days to 6 months

ETIOLOGY

Worldwide, and in the developing world in particular, approximately 95% to 100% of patients presenting with ALF will have viral hepatitis.[56] Within the United Kingdom and as recently reported in the United States, paracetamol (acetaminophen) hepatotoxicity is the leading cause of ALF. This is followed by liver failure of unknown cause or seronegative hepatitis.[57,58]

The pattern of ALF within the United Kingdom and United States has been changing over the past 30 years.[57,58] Up until the late 1990s, the rate of hospital admission due to paracetamol ingestion had risen year by year. In the United Kingdom paracetamol overdose (POD) is usually due to deliberate self-harm. In contrast, the U.S. data suggest that over half of all patients with ALF due to POD were due to therapeutic misadventure. Some doubts have been expressed regarding this interpretation as misadventure in some cases that appear to be occult suicide attempts.[58,59]

In 1998 legislation was introduced in the United Kingdom to restrict the over-the-counter sale of paracetamol to 16 tablets from most retail outlets and 32 from pharmacies in the form of blister packs. Interpretation of the effects of the legislation have proved to be complex, in a large part because there were no prospective audits initiated at the time to study it. Early interpretation suggested that admissions to hospital, severe liver toxicity, and transplantation for POD fell.[60] The picture is more complex, though. Death rates have fallen; however, much of this reduction can be related to the withdrawal of co-proxamol during the mid-2000s. Co-proxamol, a combination of paracetamol and dextropropoxyphene (a mild opioid), was a prescription-only medication associated with a high degree of fatality if taken in overdose, most of this out of hospital and attributed to the effects of dextropropoxyphene on respiratory depression.[61] Admission to hospital because of POD has continued to rise year by year but the number of pills taken on average has fallen and so the case fatality rate is lower. The numbers of patients being referred to transplant centers is also lower than before the legislation, but the number of patients transplanted has remained about the same, indicating the small number of determined overdoses and misadventure cases has remained relatively stable.

In the United Kingdom and the United States, the incidence of acute hepatitis A virus (HAV) and hepatitis B virus (HBV) infection has fallen dramatically since the 1980s[57,58] (Figs. 75.3 and 75.4).

Less than 1% of acute hepatitis A or B progress to ALF. In the United States and United Kingdom, as a proportion of the total, the number of admissions with ALF due to viral hepatitis has fallen steadily and is currently responsible for less than 5% of all admissions in the United Kingdom and 11% in the United States.[57,58]

Indeterminate hepatitis (non-A to E hepatitis, seronegative ALF, non-A/non-B hepatitis) is often presumed to be viral in origin and is the most common presentation excluding POD in the United Kingdom and United States along with viral hepatitis in the developing world. It is a diagnosis of exclusion and, as diagnostic capabilities improve, is falling in incidence in some centers.[57]

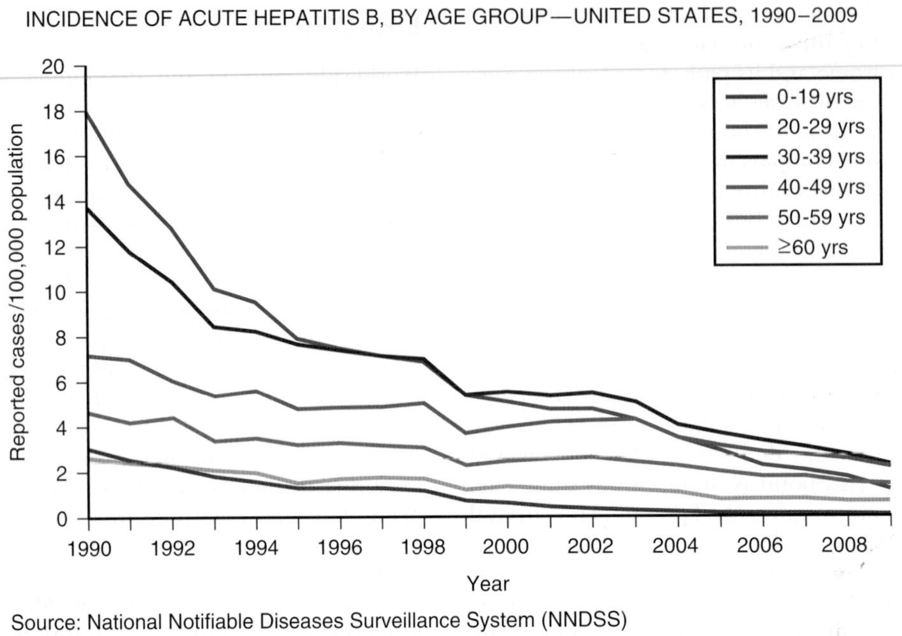

Figure 75.3 The incidence of acute hepatitis B in the United States by age group 1990-2009. The incidence has fallen in all age groups over this time. (From National Notifiable Diseases Surveillance System).

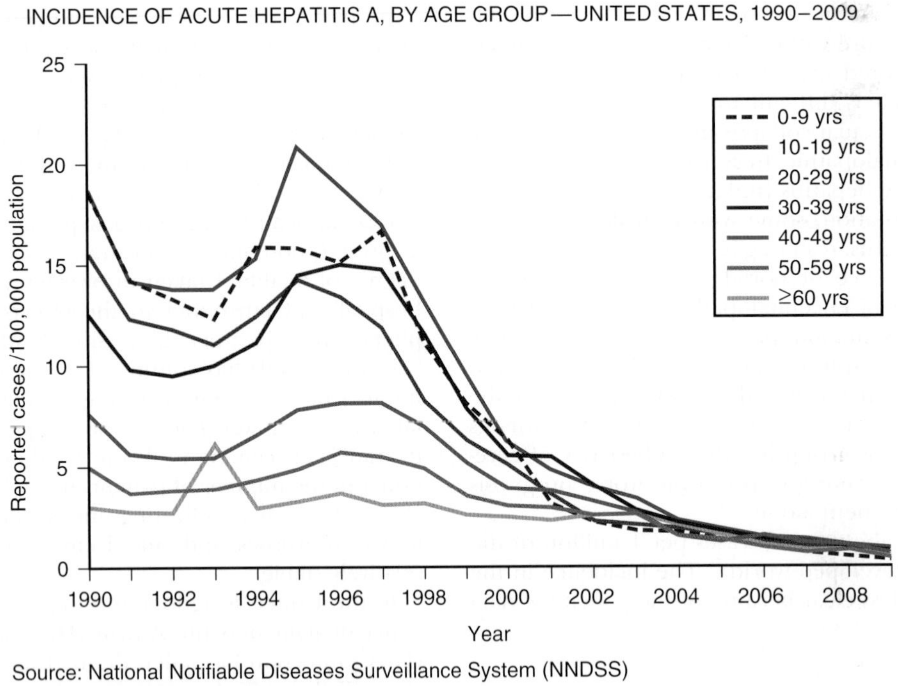

Figure 75.4 The incidence of acute hepatitis A in the United States by age group, 1990-2009. The incidence has fallen in all age groups in recent years. (From National Notifiable Diseases Surveillance System).

ACETAMINOPHEN (PARACETAMOL)

Acetaminophen-induced liver failure is the cause of the vast majority of hyperacute liver failure. Acetaminophen poisoning is a common cause of presentation to acute and emergency departments in the United Kingdom and United States; however, the case progression to ALF following paracetamol ingestion is rare at just 0.6% of all presentations in the United Kingdom.[62]

It was in the mid-1960s that the main mechanisms of paracetamol-induced liver injury were elucidated. The scheme outline by various groups revealed the production of electrophilic quinone imine (*N*-acetyl-*p*-benzoquinone imine, NAPQI), which covalently binds to hepatic proteins, was central to the resultant centrilobular necrosis seen following poisoning. The two major pathways for metabolism are the glucuronidation and sulfation of the phenolic group, with the metabolites produced excreted in the urine. In therapeutic doses approximately 80% of the drug is metabolized via these two pathways and 5% to 10% is excreted unchanged in the urine. The remainder is metabolized via the hepatic mixed function oxidase, cytochrome P-450, to produce NAPQI.

Following poisoning the half-life of acetaminophen is greatly prolonged because of the saturation of glucuronidation and sulfate conjugation. As a result, there is an increase in the quantity of NAPQI produced. NAPQI is extremely reactive in biologic systems and has a short half-life. Following poisoning, reaction of NAPQI occurs within the centrilobular portions of the liver and leads to necrosis in experimental models. It reacts with cellular constituents in a covalent and noncovalent manner. The exact mechanisms by which NAPQI induces cell death are incompletely understood but include the deactivation of critical cellular proteins, the induction of reactive oxygen species, and the activation of Kupffer cells.[63] The loss of regulatory protein function results in abnormal calcium homeostasis and resultant energy failure within the cell and mitochondria.[63] Other events such as noncovalent interaction with intracellular signaling and lipid peroxidation also contribute to the toxicity of this molecule. Following this primary toxic phase there is a secondary or extrinsic phase. This extrinsic phase is equated with the recruitment of immune cells to the liver. The liver is one of the major immune organs of the body. Up to 35% of the liver is made up of nonparenchymal cells, including endothelium, Kupffer cells, and resident lymphocytes. These cells, together with macrophages within the liver, perform a major role in immune regulation and in the filtering of antigens from the gut contents via the portal circulation. They are also implicated in the pathologic processes that occur following liver insult. Massive activation of immune cells in response to the intrinsic cellular damage induces the release of cytokines and chemokines both locally and into the systemic circulation.[64,65]

The pathophysiologic consequences of severe liver injury result from a combination of factors, including the release of cytokines and other inflammatory molecules resulting from the necrosis of hepatocytes and activation of local and systemic immune cells, and from the loss of metabolic activity related to a critical reduction in liver cell mass. The relative contribution of these factors is not completely clear but is debated and has led to attempts at therapy including temporizing hepatectomy and nonbiologic liver assist devices.

The minimum dose that can induce hepatic damage appears to be about 125 mg/kg. This represents 15500-mg tablets in a 60-kg individual, although hepatic necrosis has been recorded at much lower doses, especially if associated with hepatic enzyme induction. Doses above 250 mg/kg (30500-mg tablets in a 60-kg individual) will often produce damage, and doses in excess of 350 mg/kg invariably produce significant damage.[66]

The symptoms over the first 24 hours following a significant intake of paracetamol, irrespective of amount ingested, are usually nausea and vomiting. During the following 4 to 5 days, if liver failure ensues, there is a gradual worsening of the patient's general condition. Those with significant overdose should be admitted to the hospital and monitored closely.

The antidote for acetaminophen poisoning is *N*-acetylcysteine (NAC). It provides complete protection against hepatotoxicity if given within 12 hours of nonstaggered ingestion.[67] Within 12 hours, if the time from ingestion is known with certainty and a plasma acetaminophen level is obtained, reference can be made to the nomogram to see if the potential for hepatotoxicity is present. The nomograms are unreliable if the time from ingestion is uncertain or if there was staggered ingestion over a period of time, as often occurs with therapeutic misadventure or repeated overdose. The use of alcohol often accompanies ingestion, making timing unreliable. Situations that alter normal cytochrome P-450 function such as drug induction, (chronic ethanol use, phenytoin, and isoniazid) again render the information unreliable.[68] The use of the nomogram as the only basis for the decision to withhold NAC therapy is to be discouraged because of the uncertainty associated with this timing and the catastrophic potential if NAC is erroneously withheld (Fig. 75.5).

The main effect of NAC is to increase hepatic glutathione production. This promotes the conjugation of NAPQI and its subsequent excretion. In addition, NAC may act as an antioxidant within and outside the liver. It is most effective if given within the first 8 hours following overdose but is still effective following this, although less so. There is some evidence that NAC is effective when administered to the patient up to 72 hours following poisoning, although the mechanism of action is unclear and probably relates to antioxidant effects rather than to any effect on acetaminophen metabolism.[69] The role of NAC in established ALF from any cause is more controversial despite widespread use, but recent data have lent support to its use certainly at lower coma grades. However, the mechanism of action is unclear.[70,71]

VIRAL HEPATITIS

Both epidemic and serum hepatitis were recognized well before the viral form was discovered. In the seminal work of Lucké and Mallory in 1946, they describe 196 patients who died of ALF following both epidemic hepatitis and serum hepatitis, related to the administration of blood products during World War II.[53]

ALF following acute viral hepatitis is uncommon, with a reported incidence of 0.2% to 1% depending on the underlying cause.[72] Liver failure following viral hepatitis tends to run an acute or hyperacute course with the onset of encephalopathy occurring within days or weeks of the first symptoms.[73]

Hepatitis A is now rare in the United States and Western Europe but is still a common form of acute enterally transmitted hepatitis in the underdeveloped world where it is mainly a mild and self-limiting illness of children.[73,74] Infection with hepatitis A carries the lowest risk of conversion to acute hepatic failure of all the hepatotropic viruses. In the West the incidence of ALF following hepatitis A appears to be higher than in the endemic areas. It occurs more commonly in adults and is more severe. Persistent infection with hepatitis A has also been reported[75] and even recurring following liver transplantation.[76] Diagnosis is made on the basis of IgM antibodies at the time of hospitalization although false-negative results can occur.[77]

Hepatitis B may lead to ALF is several settings. It occurs most commonly following acute infection but can occur following an acute increase in viral replication following immunosuppressive therapy such as cancer chemotherapy or steroids as well as with coinfection with other viral agents such as delta virus. The host immune response is thought to be responsible for the severity of reaction to the virus,

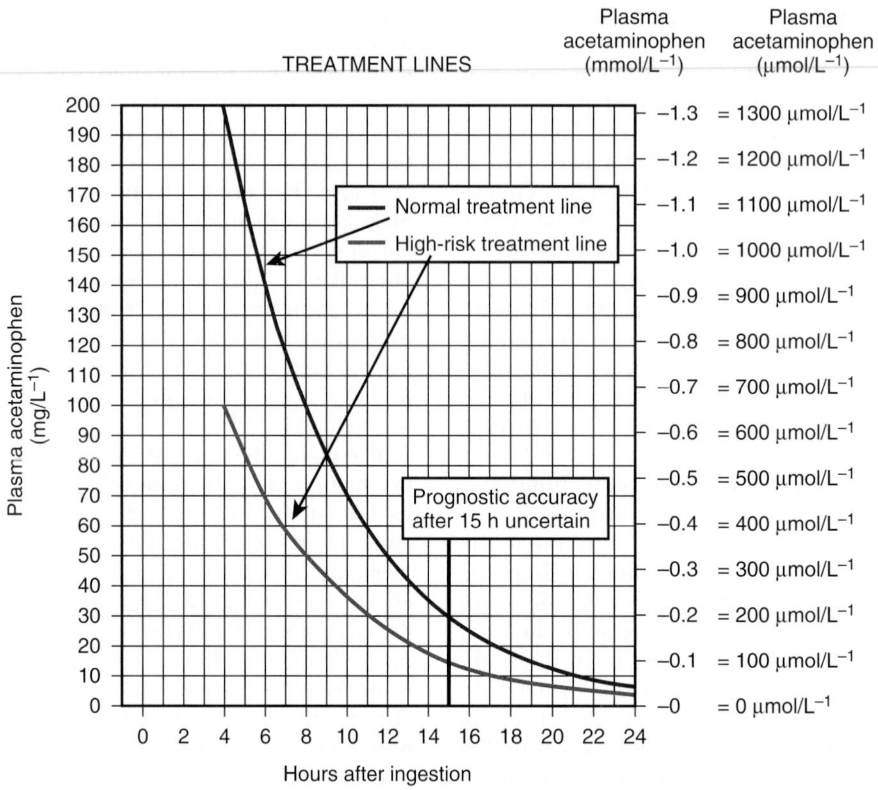

Figure 75.5 Normal treatment line and high-risk treatment line for the initiation of *N*-acetylcysteine treatment based on serum acetaminophen levels and hours following ingestion. The high-risk line has been adopted as the standard and only treatment line in the UK. This is to avoid confusion and to reduce the risk of under-treatment in patients with chronically induced hepatic enzymes, such as those receiving anti-epileptic medication, chronic ethanol abusers, or smokers. If there is any doubt about the number of hours since ingestion, or if there is any suggestion of a staggered overdose or chronic over-ingestion, NAC should be administered. (Drug Safety Update September 2012, vol 6, issue 2: A1.)

subsequent clearance, and the induction of ALF. This can be seen following the withdrawal of immunosuppressive therapy when there is a very active immune response to the increased viral load. In acute infection surface antigen (HBsAg) is often negative but IgM antibodies to the viral core (HBcAb) will usually be positive. Mutations to the precore stop codon or the core promotor region of the viral genome may be associated with a higher incidence of ALF.[78] These particular genes code for HBeAg, and lack of this antigen is associated with a more profound immune response. There have been reports of a very high incidence of ALF associated with outbreaks of acute hepatitis B in the setting of intravenous drug use and chronic hepatitis C infection.[79] Lamivudine antiviral therapy for acute HBV-induced hepatitis has been tried, but because of the lack of controlled trials, it is difficult to know if it or other drugs like it help.[80]

Hepatitis C, as a cause of ALF, is rare in northern Europe and the United States but has been described.[81] There is a wide spectrum of clinical presentation associated with acute infection with the more florid presentation associated with a more rapid clearance rate, suggesting that the magnitude of the initial immune response is important.[82] Liver failure associated with acute infection appears to be more common in India and the Far East.[83] Acute infection may contribute to decompensation in patients with preexisting liver disease, and hepatitis C seropositivity may predispose to liver failure when coinfection with another hepatotropic virus is present.[83]

Hepatitis E is likely the most common cause of ALF worldwide and certainly for the Indian subcontinent.[83] In the Far East acute HBV infection is the most common cause of ALF due to the high levels of endemicity.[84]

The existence of hepatitis E was inferred before serologic evidence was available by a process of exclusion. It was long assumed that most if not all epidemic enteric hepatitis was due to the A virus. When serologic markers for hepatitis A became available in the early 1980s it was apparent that the majority of waterborne epidemic hepatitis were due to other agents, producing a syndrome similar clinically to hepatitis A.[85] Hepatitis E does not produce a chronic infection and in the vast majority is a self-limiting infection that occurs most commonly in young adults, in contrast to hepatitis A, which is primarily an infection of children. The incidence of hepatitis E associated with ALF is low, with a case-related mortality rate reported at about 0.5% to 4% in the general population but with a much higher mortality rate in pregnancy, as high as 20% in the third trimester. Pregnancy itself appears to be a risk factor for ALF, with a quarter of all infected female patients reported as pregnant in one series. However, this may not be particular to hepatitis E but rather due to the high incidence of epidemic hepatitis E in a relatively immunosuppressed state and pregnant patients do not have a worse prognosis compared to nonpregnant patients with ALF due to hepatitis E.[83,86]

Five genotypes have been described with 1 to 4 infecting humans and genotype 5 infecting only birds. Genotype 1 is the most common in Asia, with genotype 2 more common in Africa and South America. Genotype 3 can infect both human and animals, whereas genotype 1 and 2 have been described only in humans.[87] In the West, travel to endemic areas is a risk factor, but sporadic cases are now being seen more commonly in the developed world. Some of these cases have been associated with contact with animals.[87]

Seronegative hepatitis is the second most common cause of ALF worldwide in most published series. In northern Europe and the United States it comes in behind paracetamol toxicity, and in the developing world it is second to acute viral hepatitis (Figs. 75.6 and 75.7).

Seronegative hepatitis can be conveniently thought of as a single entity. In reality it is probably an amalgam of various causes that have defied definition or characterization, including acute presentations of autoimmune hepatitis, idiosyncratic drug reactions, and viruses.[88,89] Seronegative hepatitis has a variable clinical presentation including a slow insidious onset of general malaise, jaundice, and ascites followed by progressive signs and symptoms of liver failure. At presentation the patient may be deeply jaundiced and may already have ascites and splenomegaly. It can also present with a hyperacute picture. The pattern of signs, symptoms, and organ failure is dictated by the rate of progression. In subacute seronegative hepatitis, the presenting clinical picture can be similar to that of decompensated chronic liver disease, causing occasional diagnostic difficulty. A liver biopsy is sometimes needed to differentiate between the two.

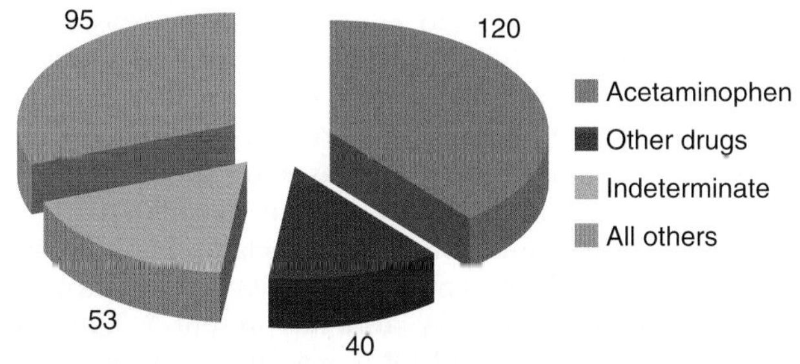

Figure 75.6 Etiology of acute liver failure in the United States 1998-2001 based on 17 centers. (From Ostapowicz G, Fontana RJ, Schiodt FV, et al: Results of a prospective study of acute liver failure at 17 tertiary care centers in the United States. Ann Intern Med 2002;137:947-954.)

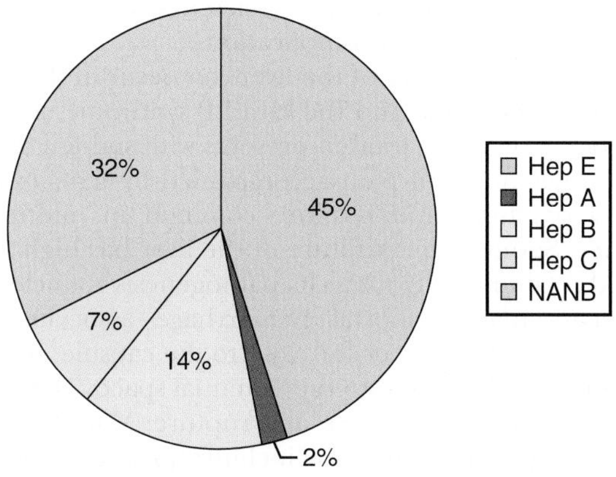

Figure 75.7 Causes of acute liver failure in an Indian center 1989-1996. (From Khuroo MS, Kamili S: Aetiology and prognostic factors in acute liver failure in India. J Viral Hepat 2003;10(3):224-231.)

ACUTE PRESENTATION OF AUTOIMMUNE HEPATITIS

Autoimmune hepatitis can occur at any time of life from childhood until old age. It is more common in women with a male/female ratio of 1:3. Presentation can be asymptomatic, discovered following routine laboratory testing, or more commonly, the infection may present with jaundice and general malaise. In rare cases autoimmune hepatitis can present as ALF.[90] Unfortunately there are no serologic tests with sufficient sensitivity or specificity to make the diagnosis certain. Patterns of markers in the right clinical setting and in the absence of other causes may be useful.[91] The diagnosis of autoimmune hepatitis in the setting of ALF is difficult and a degree of uncertainty often lasts. Classically there is a combination of elevated immunoglobulin levels, autoantibodies, and confirmatory histologic evidence of hepatitis in the absence of active viral markers. Elevation of autoantibodies is often seen in patients with ALF due to other causes such as drug-induced liver disease.[90] Liver failure should be assessed in the same way as for other causes, and once signs of encephalopathy become apparent, standard prognostic criteria apply. The role of steroids is unproved but should be considered in patients prior to the onset of encephalopathy. Once the patient is listed for transplantation steroid use is controversial because of increased risk of infection.

DRUG-INDUCED LIVER DISEASE

The liver is a major site for drug metabolism in the body. Metabolism of xenobiotics (a chemical which is found in an organism but which is not normally produced or expected to be present in it) takes place in a series of specialized enzyme reactions that increase the water solubility of lipophilic molecules by the incorporation of polar groups. Drug metabolism often involves a number of processes. Intermediates produced during the process are sometimes more toxic than the parent drug and can cause liver damage by a number of mechanisms.

Drug-induced liver disease may be due to a known dose-dependent toxicity, as with paracetamol. Alternatively, unpredictable, rare, idiosyncratic reactions can occur with any drug with a frequency of about 1 in 1000 to 1 in 100,000 patient prescriptions.[68] Drug-induced liver failure can mimic all forms of acute and chronic liver disease. However, the predominant clinical presentation consists of either acute hepatitis or cholestatic liver disease. The former has a reported mortality rate of 10% irrespective of the drug.

The patterns of injury associated with these idiosyncratic reactions relate to the mechanism of damage and the cells involved.[92] Many patterns have been described but it is massive hepatic necrosis that most often presents as ALF. Liver failure associated with severe cholestasis and veno-occlusive disease is also seen.[92]

Liver injury usually is seen within 6 months following the initiation of therapy. Even if the diagnosis of drug-induced liver failure is considered, a search for other possible causes should be performed. Although any drug is capable of inducing liver injury, more common causes include herbal remedies and recreationally used drugs such as "ecstasy" and cocaine. If suspected, a comprehensive history with a timetable of drug initiation should be constructed. Management includes stopping the offending drug and supportive

Table 75.1 Idiosyncratic Drug Reactions and Effects on Cells

Type of Reaction	Effect on Cells	Examples of Drugs
Hepatocellular	Direct effect or production by enzyme-drug adduct leads to cell dysfunction, membrane dysfunction, cytotoxic T-cell response	Isoniazid, trazodone, diclofenac, nefazodone, venlafaxine, lovastatin
Cholestasis	Injury to canalicular membrane and transporters	Chlorpromazine, estrogen, erythromycin and its derivatives
Immunoallergic	Enzyme-drug adducts on cell surface induce IgE response	Halothane, phenytoin, sulfamethoxazole
Granulomatous	Macrophages, lymphocytes infiltrate hepatic lobule	Diltiazem, sulfa drugs, quinidine
Microvesicular fat	Altered mitochondrial respiration, beta-oxidation leads to lactic acidosis and triglyceride accumulation	Didanosine, tetracycline, acetylsalicylic acid, valproic acid
Steatohepatitis	Multifactorial	Amiodarone, tamoxifen
Autoimmune	Cytotoxic lymphocyte response directed at hepatocyte membrane components	Nitrofurantoin, methyldopa, lovastatin, minocycline
Fibrosis	Activation of stellate cells	Methotrexate, excess vitamin A
Vascular collapse	Causes ischemic or hypoxic injury	Nicotinic acid, cocaine, methylenedioxymethamphetamine
Oncogenesis	Encourages tumor formation	Oral contraceptives, androgens
Mixed	Cytoplasmic and canalicular injury, direct damage to bile ducts	Amoxicillin-clavulanate, carbamazepine, herbs, cyclosporine, methimazole, troglitazone

IgE, immunoglobulin E.
From Lee WM: Drug-induced hepatotoxicity. N Engl J Med 2003;349(5):474-485.

care. Transplantation should be considered once liver failure occurs as the outcome from drug-induced liver failure, other than that induced by paracetamol, can be poor.[93] Presentation profiles for various drugs causing ALF are shown in Table 75.1.[68]

PREGNANCY-INDUCED LIVER DISEASE

In general, pregnancy-associated liver failure has the best prognosis when compared to all other causes of ALF, and prompt recovery can be expected with delivery of the fetus in most cases, if recognized early enough. Pregnancy-associated liver failure can present in several ways including the syndromes of preeclampsia and the HELLP syndrome (hemolysis, elevated liver function tests, and low platelets), liver rupture, and acute fatty liver of pregnancy.[94] Any cause of ALF can occur during pregnancy, and in particular viral hepatitis can be particularly fulminant in its course. This is especially true for hepatitis E and herpes simplex virus infection.

Although originally thought to be a variant of preeclampsia there is evidence that HELLP syndrome may be a separate entity and in fact more related to acute fatty liver of pregnancy.[95] Both HELLP and preeclampsia appear to be related to an endothelial injury, possibly immunologically initiated with activation of the coagulation and complement cascades and an imbalance of prostaglandin and thromboxane resulting in increased vascular tone, microangiopathic hemolytic anemia, and vascular thrombosis.[96] About 2% to 12% of severe preeclampsia is complicated by HELLP.[94] HELLP is thought to occur in approximately 1 in every 1000 live deliveries and patients usually present in the third trimester with nonspecific signs often seen in preeclampsia such as weight gain due to edema and hypertension. In addition, right upper quadrant pain accompanied by nausea and vomiting is commonly seen. Laboratory abnormalities include hyperbilirubinemia due to liver dysfunction and evidence of hemolysis. Transaminases are modestly raised and the platelet count is usually less than 100,000/μL. Liver biopsy, while commonly normal in preeclampsia, shows specific changes of periportal necrosis and fibrin microthrombi. Microvascular steatosis may also be present.[96] The liver failure associated with HELLP is manifest as a prolonged prothrombin time and ascites. Renal failure is common. Maternal mortality rate is low but fetal mortality rate has been reported to be between 20% and 60%, although some reports suggest this is lower at 7% and associated with twin pregnancies.[96-98] The treatment of choice is delivery of the baby. Conservative therapy is associated with an increase in both maternal and fetal complications.

Spontaneous rupture of the liver can occur in the setting of both preeclampsia and the HELLP syndrome, although it can occur de novo. It often presents with sudden onset of right upper quadrant pain accompanied by signs of hypovolemia or shock and is more common in multiparous women.[96] Spontaneous rupture of the liver has high maternal and fetal mortality rates. Its pathogenesis is unclear but it appears that periportal hemorrhage associated with HELLP syndrome may occur close to the capsule, resulting in lifting and bleeding into the potential space. These areas of the capsule then coalesce and rupture. Management of this devastating complication includes prompt delivery of the fetus, local surgical control with packs, and aggressive management of the accompanying coagulopathy. Embolization of any feeding vessels in the liver may be of utility if such skills are available. Hepatectomy followed by liver transplantation can be lifesaving and has been performed.

Acute fatty liver of pregnancy (AFLP) occurs during the third trimester of pregnancy and should be considered in any patient exhibiting signs of liver dysfunction. It is uncommon with an incidence of approximately 1 in 6659 live births.[99] If left untreated, maternal and fetal mortality rates are high. The treatment of choice is delivery and prompt recovery can then be expected. There is usually a prodromal illness over a couple of weeks with nonspecific symptoms progressing to jaundice and encephalopathy. Symptoms and signs of preeclampsia or HELLP syndrome are seen in a third of cases and there is some evidence of a common origin due to a fetal fatty acid metabolism disorder.[95] Diagnosis is critical and it should be differentiated from viral hepatitis or hepatic failure due to other causes. Liver biopsy can aid in the diagnosis and can be performed via the jugular route if coagulopathy precludes the conventional approach. Characteristic zone 3 microvesicular steatosis is seen. Delivery is the best treatment if diagnosed early. Characteristic features include normoblasts on blood smears and high serum urate. Bleeding can be a major problem during operative delivery. On occasion transplantation may be the only viable option. Triggers for transplantation in pregnancy-induced liver failure are not well defined and the Kings College Criteria perform poorly. Arterial lactate in the setting of encephalopathy appears to be the best predictor.[98]

WILSON'S DISEASE

Wilson's disease is a rare autosomal recessive disorder resulting from copper toxicity with primarily brain and liver manifestation. It usually presents in the second or third decade of life, although it can present from early childhood until late middle age.[100] The disease can present with predominantly liver or neurologic symptoms. Neurologic symptoms relate to the distribution of copper to the basal ganglia and result in movement disorders. Patients presenting with liver disease may presents with an active hepatitis, established cirrhosis, or ALF. Other signs such as Kayser-Fleischer rings are associated but not pathognomonic for Wilson's disease. These greenish brown rings in the cornea result from the deposition of copper.

ALF due to Wilson's disease can present at any age but more commonly presents in the early 20s. High urinary copper excretion is possibly the most predictable laboratory finding, although the patient may be anuric on presentation. A low serum ceruloplasmin is an additional indicator but again is unreliable in ALF. A high serum bilirubin in combination with modest elevations of transaminases and alkaline phosphatase is often seen, as is intravascular hemolysis, contributing to the raised bilirubin level. Patients with severe liver failure due to Wilson's disease have an almost 100% mortality rate without liver transplantation, which should be considered as soon as the diagnosis is made.[100] There is debate as to whether liver failure secondary to Wilson's disease is truly ALF, as cirrhosis is invariably present on liver biopsy at the time of presentation. Nevertheless, many patients present acutely and the presentation is often catastrophic. In this sense the timing of the onset and the lack of previous symptoms place fulminant Wilson's disease in the ALF group. In an uncontrolled series the administration of D-penicillamine before the onset of encephalopathy was associated with survival.[101]

NEOPLASTIC INFILTRATION

Poorly differentiated solid tumors such as breast and lung and hematologic malignancies can sometimes present with a syndrome of liver failure. There is often diagnostic delay and difficulty.

The syndrome can be considered as part of the hypoxic hepatitis group as zone 3 necrosis is often seen. The metabolic demand of the neoplastic cells and congestion within the liver sinusoids results in infarction of hepatocytes. Hepatosplenomegaly and a raised alkaline phosphatase are often present. Other stigmata including palpable lymphadenopathy and marrow or peripheral blood film changes may be present. Imaging may be diagnostic, especially with massive hepatomegaly, but biopsy may be required.[102]

BUDD-CHIARI SYNDROME

ALF secondary to Budd-Chiari syndrome is usually fatal without transplantation. The syndrome is defined as outflow obstruction to the hepatic veins and the underlying pathogenesis is thrombosis in the majority but tumor invasion or vascular membrane obstruction may be the cause. This is a rare disorder that occurs predominantly in young adults and affects more women than men. Overall, the 5-year survival rate varies from 50% to 80% in different series.[103] The vast majority of patients with the syndrome have at least one predisposing clotting abnormality, either congenital or acquired, such as a malignancy, myeloproliferative disorders, protein C or S deficiency, polycythemia rubra vera, lupus anticoagulant, antithrombin III deficiency, antiphospholipid syndrome, etc.[104] The fulminant form of the syndrome in which the patient develops encephalopathy within 8 weeks of the onset of symptoms is rare, and it is much more common for Budd-Chiari syndrome to present in a subacute form over a 3- or 4-month period, characterized by ascites, abdominal pain and hepatomegaly, jaundice, coagulopathy, and raised AST and alkaline phosphatase. Others present with signs of portal hypertension, including refractory ascites and variceal bleeding, and relatively intact hepatocellular function. The diagnosis is made with the combination of clinical presentation and imaging, including Doppler ultrasound studies of the hepatic vessels, plus or minus liver histologic examination, usually via the jugular route because of coagulopathy. Management of the syndrome depends on the manner in which it presents and the underlying cause. Medical management of the syndrome involves the use of anticoagulants and diuretics in an attempt to control ascites. Thrombolysis can be attempted in selected patients with recent onset disease.[105] In patients in whom there is progression to signs and symptoms of liver cell failure some sort of portosystemic shunting procedure may reduce symptoms and prevent progression of the disease, allowing time for collateral vessels to develop. Transjugular intrahepatic portosystemic shunt (TIPSS) is most often attempted unless there is evidence of a hypertrophied caudate lobe and inferior vena cava compression, making mesoatrial shunting a better option. In patients with signs of liver failure care must be used when considering a TIPSS procedure, as this can precipitate decompensation and rapid progression to ALF.[106] Liver transplantation is ultimately the only option in many patients in which there is a failure of medical and shunt therapy as well as in the fulminant presentation of the syndrome.[107] Anticoagulation is usually necessary in the immediate postoperative period.

VENO-OCCLUSIVE DISEASE OF THE LIVER

Veno-occlusive disease (VOD) of the liver is a nonthrombotic obstruction of the sinusoids, which may extend to the central veins, in the absence of thrombosis or other underlying disorder of the hepatic veins.[108] As a result of a toxic challenge there is acute damage to the endothelial cells, followed by their detachment and their embolization in the central area of the lobule, where they cause a postsinusoidal outflow block.[108] The most common cause is myeloablative chemotherapy induction regimens in preparation for bone marrow transplantation (BMT), being seen in up to 54% in some older series.[109] Other toxins are known to cause it and it was first described in children following the ingestion of herbal teas in South Africa and it represents a nonspecific response to certain noxious stimuli. Particular induction regimens such as high-dose cyclophosphamide and total body irradiation are implicated in the pathogenesis. The more aggressive induction regimens appear to result in a higher incidence of VOD. Recent reduction in incidence may be due to a reduction in the use of myeloablative regimens and better monitoring of plasma drug concentrations.[110] The symptoms of VOD usually occur within 2 weeks of BMT. The development of jaundice, hepatomegaly, abdominal pain, and encephalopathy in the setting of recent BMT strongly suggests the diagnosis. Severe cases are characterized by evidence of hepatocellular necrosis and a high AST concentration. In 25% of cases, which are characterized as severe, the syndrome is progressive, leading to ALF.[111] Treatment options in these patients are limited as the outcome is poor with medical management or liver transplantation, although there is hope that newer therapies such as defibrotide (a deoxyribonucleic acid derivative anticoagulant with multiple modes of action), if initiated early before the onset of multiple organ failure, may improve the outlook. In addition, the prophylactic use has been tried in several noncontrolled reports.[108]

HYPOXIC (ISCHEMIC) HEPATITIS

"Shock liver," "ischemic hepatitis," or more recently hypoxic hepatitis is the most common cause of significant rise in serum aminotransferase (S-AT) seen in hospitalized patients (Fig. 75.8).

There is often an underlying chronic reduction in oxygen delivery to the liver due to comorbid disease states such as congestive cardiac failure or chronic respiratory failure. There is then a subsequent sudden acute drop in oxygen delivery due to a decrease in cardiac output or further hypoxia.

Diagnostically, there are three conditions that should be met: the appropriate clinical setting of circulatory, cardiac, or respiratory failure with a massive rise in S-AT and the exclusion of other causes of massive hepatic necrosis such as viral or drug-induced liver failure.[102]

In patients with chronic congestive heart failure (CCHF), liver congestion is common. This is usually manifest as mild abnormalities of liver function tests, a prolonged prothrombin time, and mild ascites in some. Hepatic congestion is usually clinically unapparent unless jaundice is present, which can occur following multiple bouts of CCHF. Chronic congestion can lead to fibrosis and ultimately cirrhosis in some patients. Acute rises in serum transaminase and prolongation in prothrombin time, representing acute hepatic necrosis, most commonly develop in patients with CCHF when there is a sudden drop in cardiac output due to an event such as an arrhythmia or myocardial infarction. It is relatively uncommon for the liver to become involved during shock states because of the huge redundancy in blood supply and the ability of the portal system to compensate for any reduction in hepatic arterial flow. If, however, portal flow is already compromised due to passive congestion, then an acute drop in hepatic blood flow can result in ischemia. It is uncommon for hypoxic hepatitis to occur without a recognizable precipitant, but it can occur due to a silent myocardial infarction or arrhythmia, for example. It can occur before the diagnosis of CCHF has been made or be the primary diagnostic event in a younger patient with a cardiomyopathy. Clinically, severe ischemic hepatitis becomes apparent between 24 and 48 hours following an event and is manifest as huge rises in S-AT (up to 10-20 times normal). There is prolongation of the prothrombin time, encephalopathy, hypoglycemia, jaundice, and renal failure. The syndrome is usually self-limiting once the hemodynamic disturbance has receded, and there is a rapid fall in serum transaminases (usually 50% in the first 72 hours).[112] Occasionally, progressive liver cellular failure leads rapidly to death. Management should be aimed at investigating and supporting the underlying cause.

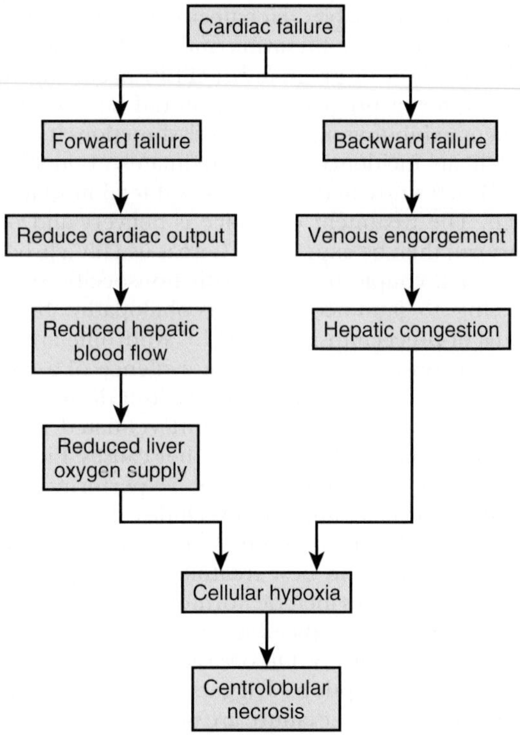

Figure 75.8 The most common cause of hypoxic hepatitis results from a combination of liver congestion due to chronic cardiac failure and an acute drop in cardiac output causing liver ischemia.

HEAT STROKE

Liver failure in the setting of heat stroke can be considered to be part of the hypoxic hepatitis group of causes. The argument for its inclusion here is the zone 3 necrosis seen in the liver following autopsy in patients who survive long enough for a reperfusion injury to occur.[102] The pathophysiology is complex but is probably related to dehydration and cardiovascular collapse plus increased oxygen demand and acute cardiac failure.[102] Exertional heat stroke may occur in new recruits to the army or police force engaging in physical initiation programs. It can also occur in unacclimatized athletes in hot conditions or with drug overdoses such as cocaine and hyperpyrexia syndrome such as those induced by MDMA (methylenedioxy-*N*-methylamphetamine). It is a potentially devastating syndrome that can lead to multiple organ failure and death. It ranges from mild involvement to ALF and is seen to develop during the first few days following the event. Management is supportive and the majority improves over a period of days to weeks. Liver transplantation has been used in severe cases but the outcome is poor owing to coincident organ failure.[113]

MUSHROOM POISONING

There are many types of poisonous fungi in the world that are responsible for a variety of disorders that can be classified according to the type of poisoning and the timing of onset.[114] There are a number of fungi associated with the induction of liver failure following ingestion. Of these, the most common and most deadly are of the genus *Amanita*. *Amanita* associated hepatotoxicity follows a triphasic response after ingestion. The first is a self-limiting, nonspecific gastrointestinal upset that occurs within the first 6 to 24 hours. Nausea and vomiting, abdominal cramps, and diarrhea are often seen and it can mimic food poisoning. This is followed by a period of recovery and a few days later by progressive liver failure.

Management is essentially supportive, although many specific therapies have been tried in the treatment of *Amanita* toxicity such as high-dose penicillin, silibinin, cimetidine, and NAC, but none has been shown to improve outcome. Liver transplantation should be considered for patients with severe liver failure and standard criteria apply.[114]

CLINICAL COURSE

HISTORY AND PHYSICAL EXAMINATION

The presentation and clinical course of ALF depends on its cause and the rate of progression of the syndrome. This varies widely from admission via an emergency department following a paracetamol overdose or acute viral hepatitis versus admission from a hepatology outpatient department in a patient with progressive jaundice and ascites. Owing to its relative rarity the diagnosis can often be missed during initial contact and this delay may detrimentally influence the outcome.

The history will initially focus on the rate of progression of the illness and any clues to the cause. The first symptoms are often the onset of jaundice (typically noticed by a relative). Any history of foreign travel or high-risk behavioral activity (intravenous drug use or unprotected sex) associated with the contraction of viral hepatitis should be investigated. A thorough drug history should be taken for prescribed and recreational drug use for the preceding 6 to 10 weeks. Drug therapy or recreational use that can induce or inhibit hepatic enzymes should be noted. If the patient is unable to provide this information, the relatives and the patient's primary care physician should be contacted for help.

The history may be self-evident in the case of paracetamol hepatotoxicity, especially if the patient is self-presenting following deliberate self-harm. However, therapeutic misadventure, which is a relatively common cause of hepatotoxicity, especially in the United States, may not be obvious unless considered by the physician.[115] Any patient presenting with coma should have a drug screen (including paracetamol).

Subacute liver failure has, by definition, a more insidious onset. Jaundice is often preceded by nonspecific symptoms of fatigue and general malaise. Abnormal liver enzymes will often be revealed during the initial workup. Subsequent investigations will include viral, iron, copper and genetic studies and, in addition, attempt to rule out decompensation of chronic liver disease as a cause the current symptoms and signs. Liver biopsy may be considered in subacute liver failure (Fig. 75.9).

INITIAL RESUSCITATION AND EMERGENCY CARE

Patients presenting with acute or hyperacute liver failure tend to follow a similar course irrespective of cause. Initial therapy and emergency care will be dictated by the condition of the patient at presentation. Liver failure is a multisystem disease and can progress very rapidly to multiple organ failure.

Patients presenting with rapidly progressive hepatic encephalopathy via the emergency care system will often be intubated and ventilated at the time of or shortly after admission. The emergency physicians will often perform a head computed tomography (CT) scan because of diagnostic uncertainty.

The symptoms and signs of hepatic encephalopathy in ALF are subjectively different from those seen in decompensated chronic liver disease or in patients with stable chronic encephalopathy. Agitation and aggressive behavior are more common in ALF. This may be based on an increased turnover of the excitatory neurotransmitter glutamate in ALF associated with an acute increase in cerebral ammonia uptake.[116]

The West Haven criteria, designed to assess coma grade in patients with cirrhosis, are often applied to patients with ALF and are useful because of familiarity.[117] However, once the patient becomes unconscious at grade IV encephalopathy, the scale does not provide any further information and is too crude to provide a clinically useful description of the level of consciousness. The Glasgow Coma Scale score, while not assessed specifically in this setting, is useful in relating clinical information to others.[118] Encephalopathy grade can progress very quickly, especially with hyperacute presentation. Intubation and sedation are recommended once grade III encephalopathy is achieved because of the attendant risks to airway and possibilities of raised intracranial pressure, discussed later. Figure 75.10 describes encephalopathy grade and Glasgow Coma Scale score.

Early contact with a regional liver center should be made in any patient with signs of acute severe liver dysfunction as

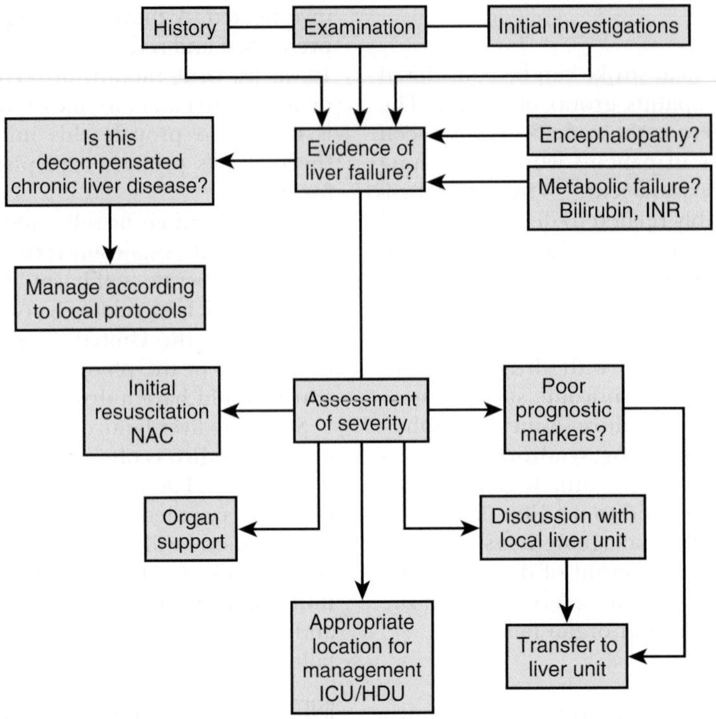

Figure 75.9 Initial management of a patient presenting with liver failure. HDU, high dependency unit; ICU, intensive care unit; INR, international normalized ratio; NAC, *N*-acetylcysteine.

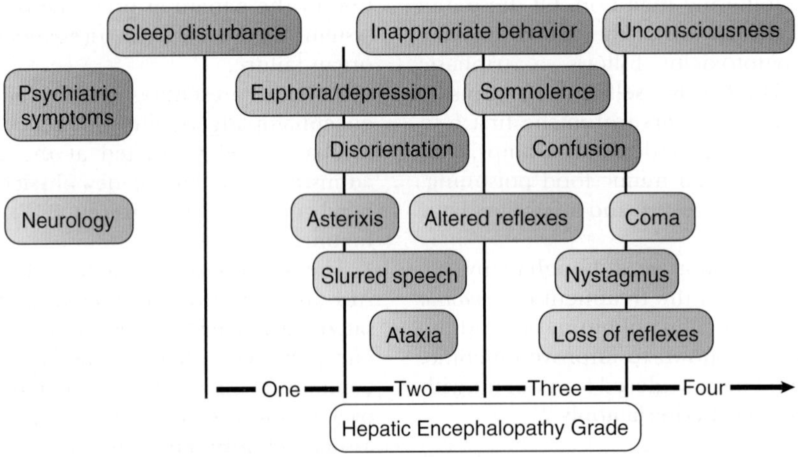

Figure 75.10 Hepatic encephalopathy grade in acute liver failure.

serial blood results and clinical signs can be relayed to the center over the phone. POD patients can often be managed over the phone but plans for transfer can be made well in advance, if necessary. As liver failure progresses over the next several days, a number of organ systems may become affected.

Following the safe and appropriate management of airway and breathing, focus can be directed to the correction of any circulatory dysfunction. Patients with ALF can progress rapidly to circulatory shock. The circulatory changes associated with ALF are predictable, usually associated with systemic vasodilatation and relative hypovolemia. This can be profound and require significant volume resuscitation. It is easy to underestimate the amount of fluid required in the early stages of ALF and the use of prognostic markers is unreliable before adequate circulatory function is restored. Monitoring at this stage should include a central venous catheter and direct arterial access for both blood pressure monitoring and for repeated blood tests. Care must be given to serum electrolytes because they often become deranged during this initial period. In particular, hyponatremia and hypophosphatemia are common.[119-121] This may be due to excess quantities of hypotonic fluid administration. A typical flowsheet of investigations of a patient presenting with paracetamol poisoning from a referring hospital is shown in Box 75.2.

Regardless of cause, patients with significant liver damage or signs of secondary organ dysfunction should be managed within the ICU. The speed at which patients deteriorate can be very rapid and it is not uncommon for hepatic

Box 75.2 Acetaminophen Overdose Case Example: Laboratory Data

A 20-year-old woman, an intravenous drug user, took a 250-tablet overdose (500 mg of acetaminophen) the day before presentation at the hospital emergency department. She received *N*-acetylcysteine alanine transaminase 25 hours after the ingestion. The patient was then transferred and listed for transplantation.

Dates	7/10/2003	8/10/2003 AM	8/10/2003 PM	9/10/2003 AM
INR No	2.08	3.17	3.79	6.2
Bilirubin = mmol/L	12	37		35
AST/ALT = U/L	273/223	8535/4254		15,734/10,060
Alk Phos = U/L				100
Alb = g/L	52	45		30
Glucose = mmol/L	4.1		7.5	5.2
Urea = mmol/L		5.5		3.0
Creatinine = μmol/L		86	83	128
pH		7.38	7.41	7.39
Lactate = mmol/L			5.4	

Alk Phos, alkaline phosphatase; AST/ALT, aspartate transaminase/alanine transaminase; INR, international normalized ratio.

Table 75.2 Initial Investigation and Common Findings

Laboratory Test	Finding(s)
Complete blood count	Platelets often low
Urea and electrolytes	Serum sodium often low, especially in paracetamol hepatotoxicity
	Urea often low because of reduced production
	Serum creatinine is useful prognostic marker
Liver enzymes	Serum AST/ALT variable, very high in paracetamol toxicity
	Bilirubin is prognostic marker in nonparacetamol liver failure
	Also can be high in Wilson's disease from hemolysis
Phosphate	Often low, especially in paracetamol toxicity
	High level indicative of poor prognosis; suggests lack of regeneration
Magnesium	Often low
Prothrombin time, international normalized ratio (INR)	Very sensitive indicator of liver function
	Has prognostic significance in all forms of acute liver failure
	May improve with vitamin K in deficiency states
Viral serology for all known hepatotropic viruses	
Urinary copper, plasma ceruloplasmin if Wilson's disease is suspected	Ceruloplasmin level often very low but can be normal
	Urine copper usually high
Arterial ammonia	Has some prognostic value and may be an indicator of cerebral edema in patients at risk
Arterial whole blood lactate	Very sensitive marker for liver function, particularly in paracetamol toxicity
	High level indicative of poor prognosis
Serum glucose	Hypoglycemia common
β-Human chorionic gonadotropin in women	Unwanted pregnancy can be a precipitant of deliberate self-harm

AST/ALT, aspartate transaminase/alanine transaminase.

encephalopathy to progress from grade 0 to grade IV over several hours.

For prognostic reasons it is important not to avoid correcting any biochemical coagulopathy at this stage if possible. Despite quite significant prolongation of prothrombin time, bleeding from line sites is uncommon in the initial stages of ALF. In fact, there is evidence that the patients are prothrombotic in vivo.[122]

INVESTIGATION IN A PATIENT WITH SUSPECTED ACUTE LIVER FAILURE

Initial investigations provide a baseline from which important diagnostic and prognostic information is taken. Serial blood test measurements should be performed as severity and prognosis are assessed over time from initial presentation (Table 75.2). Depending on the manner and speed of presentation, a complete blood count, clotting tests, liver function tests, arterial blood gas measurements, and ammonia levels should be performed twice daily, if not more often, in the early stages to assess progression of the illness. A liver ultrasound scan to assess liver size and blood supply should be performed.

TRANSFER CRITERIA GUIDE

ALF is a sporadic syndrome with a case incidence of about 2000 per year in the United States.[123] Management is complex and liver transplantation is the only effective therapy in severe cases. Transfer to a unit with experience in the management of these patients, preferably one with a liver transplant program, will provide optimal care. It is often difficult to decide when or whether to transfer a patient with acute liver dysfunction, and this decision will vary according to cause and presentation. The best described clinical course is that following severe paracetamol poisoning after a deliberate overdose.[52] Staggered overdose and therapeutic misadventure are less predictable in their clinical course but often have a poor outcome and can be considered a poor prognostic risk factor.[124]

The following criteria for transfer are based on expert opinion and have not been subjected to rigorous study and err on the side of caution[72] (Fig. 75.11):

- In patients with a subacute presentation it is better to transfer patients before they have progressed to grade II encephalopathy because of the additional complications associated with transferring ventilated patients.
- Patients with acute or hyperacute liver failure showing signs of early encephalopathy should be intubated and ventilated prior to transfer. This can occasionally result in disagreement between referring hospitals and receiving liver units on how the transfer should be managed. There are many anecdotal stories from liver units around the world describing patients who become unmanageable during transfer in planes, helicopters, and road ambulances resulting in injury to patients and staff.
- Heroic transfers are almost always inappropriate. Patients should not be considered for transfer if they are on rapidly accelerating inotropic support, have severe hypoxemia, or already have fixed dilated pupils. There is little point a patient dying in an ambulance.

MANAGEMENT

SUPPORTIVE CARE

Airway and Ventilation

Patients with ALF who reach grade II or III encephalopathy require intubation and ventilation to provide safe management in the setting of increasing agitation, protection of the airway from stomach contents, or transfer from peripheral hospitals. In patients with severe liver failure it can be expected that encephalopathy grade will progress, and so waiting until some predefined stage before intubation often delays adequate resuscitation and monitoring.

Controlled ventilation to a normal $Paco_2$ is recommended at this stage. The use of hyperventilation is not indicated without further monitoring.[125,126]

Circulation

The circulatory changes associated with ALF can be profound.[127] The pathologic basis for this are incompletely understood, but similar in many ways to changes observed in patients with a systemic inflammatory response due to sepsis or trauma. The pattern observed depends on the cause and the rate of onset of the syndrome. In hyperacute liver failure due to paracetamol overdose, patients can develop fulminant peripheral cardiovascular collapse that can be an early mode of death.[128] Others with a more subacute onset can develop peripheral vascular changes similar to those with decompensated chronic liver disease and hepatorenal failure.

Fluid resuscitation should be commenced as soon as possible after presentation and should be directed by invasive monitoring. The type of fluid used for resuscitation has not been subjected to controlled trials in this setting but large volumes of hypotonic fluids should be avoided as this

Referral to specialist unit after paracetamol ingestion. Any of these criteria should prompt referral.

Day 2	Day 3	Day 4
Arterial pH < 7.30	Arterial pH < 7.30	INR > 6 or PT > 100 s
INR > 3.0 or PT > 50 s	INR > 3.0 or PT > 50 s	Progressive rise in PT to any level
Oliguria	Oliguria	Oliguria
Creatinine > 300 μmol/L	Creatinine > 300 μmol/L	Creatinine > 300 μmol/L
Hypoglycemia	Encephalopathy	Encephalopathy
	Severe thrombocytopenia	Severe thrombocytopenia

INR, international normalized ratio; PT, prothrombin time.

Referral to specialist unit in non-paracetamol ingestion etiologies. The presence of any of these criteria should prompt referral.

Hyperacute	Acute	Subacute
Encephalopathy	Encephalopathy	Encephalopathy
Hypoglycemia	Hypoglycemia	Hypoglycemia (less common)
Prothrombin time > 20 s	Prothrombin time > 20 s	Prothrombin time > 20 s
INR > 2.0	INR > 2.0	INR > 1.5
Renal failure	Renal failure	Renal failure
Hyperpyrexia		Serum sodium < 130 μmol/L
		Shrinking liver volume

INR, international normalized ratio.

Figure 75.11 Transfer criteria to a specialist unit. INR, international normalized ratio; PT, prothrombin time. (From O'Grady JG: Acute liver failure. Postgrad Med J 2005;81(953):148-154.)

may contribute to cerebral swelling seen in this group, and it has been shown that hypertonic saline infusion reduces the incidence of intracranial hypertension in patients with ALF.[119]

If following adequate fluid resuscitation mean arterial pressure remains less than 65 mm Hg, a vasopressor should be commenced. Norepinephrine is the vasopressor of choice as it induces vasoconstriction without the induction of lactate production as often seen with the use of epinephrine, although epinephrine has been used in this setting successfully.

Vasopressin and its longer acting analog terlipressin have been used as vasopressors in septic and cardiogenic shock.[129,130] Terlipressin results in profound systemic vasoconstriction and, if used inappropriately, has the potential to reduce cardiac output and hence oxygen delivery. It has been shown to increase intracranial hypertension in ALF due to an increase in cerebral blood volume because of the breakdown in cerebrovascular autoregulation.[131] However, the data are mixed and a more recent study suggests that terlipressin may be a useful adjunct to norepinephrine in ALF.[132] Because of this uncertainty, monitoring of ICP should be considered if it is used.

The majority of patients presenting with ALF are young adults, and as a result, comorbid cardiac dysfunction is usually absent. Cardiac depression has been reported in association with POD.[128] On occasion cardiac disease can present as ALF in the case of ischemic hepatitis.

Relative adrenal insufficiency has been shown to occur in patients with septic shock and in patients with decompensated chronic liver disease and ALF.[44,133-135] The use of stress doses of corticosteroids in ALF has been shown to reduce norepinephrine requirements in patients with ALF.[136] The effect on outcome is uncertain, though.

Renal Support

Renal failure is common in ALF with a reported incidence of up to 70%.[137] Paracetamol causes direct renal tubular dysfunction, possibly by affecting membrane protein function and occasionally renal failure is the predominant organ affected.[138,139] As a result, renal failure can be expected in this setting. Although it is most commonly associated with POD, the incidence in other causes, such as Wilson's disease due to the direct toxic effects of copper, is also high but it is less prominent in ALF due to viral hepatitis or seronegative hepatitis.

There remains debate regarding the cause, pathology, and definition of renal dysfunction in critical illness despite a huge amount of effort.[140] The term *acute tubular necrosis* is inadequate in the setting of critical illness when it fails to describe the full spectrum of renal dysfunction. This is even truer in the setting of ALF. In addition, the use of *hepatorenal syndrome* in ALF is also inappropriate because this term does not adequately describe the often rapid clinical deterioration. This is not to say that altered systemic and renal hemodynamics do not contribute to the pathophysiology of renal failure as they do in critical illness in general. In the subacute presentation of this syndrome early renal dysfunction can be similar in presentation to that seen in end-stage chronic liver disease with sodium and water retention in the absence of intrinsic renal damage.[141]

Management of renal failure is essentially the same as in ALF and other forms of multiple organ failure and consists of maintenance of intravascular volume, cardiac output, and mean arterial pressure.[123,142]

Extracorporeal renal support is necessary in most patients with ALF at some time. Continuous venovenous hemofiltration (CVVH) is the most efficient and safest method for renal support and should be started early.[143] Indications for the early use of renal support are not just limited to oliguria. CVVH has been shown to improve hemodynamic stability in patients with critical illness and has been used as salvage therapy in patients on high-dose vasopressor.[144] High-volume hemofiltration (4000 mL/hour ultrafiltrate exchange) has been studied in ALF and has been shown to reduce serum lactate, base deficit, and norepinephrine requirements when compared to historical control subjects.[145] Evidence for survival benefit for high-dose renal replacement therapy in critical illness is lacking, however, and recent high-quality studies suggest that there is a ceiling of dose, above which there is no additional survival benefit.[146,147]

Patients with liver failure do not tolerate the lactate load associated with lactate-buffered replacement fluid during CVVH. In fact, the rapid infusion of lactate can induce a systemic acidosis in this setting.[148] Also, the infusion of large quantities of lactate-containing fluid reduces the utility of serum lactate as one of the most important prognostic indicators.[149] As a consequence, the use of bicarbonate hemofiltration is recommended.[150]

CVVH can often be performed successfully without anticoagulation in ALF. If required, a loading dose of 2000 units of heparin and thereafter 500 to 1000 units an hour, depending on the activated clotting time, can be used if needed to allow CVVH. If bleeding is a problem or there is severe thrombocytopenia, epoprostenol should be instituted (2.5-5 ng/kg/minute) either alone or in association with low-dose heparin (100 units/hour). Blood flow rates of 200 mL/minute and above will help with filter life.

INTRACRANIAL HYPERTENSION

Etiology

The hallmark of liver failure is the development of hepatic encephalopathy, which with severe liver failure progresses to deep coma. In addition to the progressive coma, early reports of patients with signs of raised ICP were noted in the literature.[151] What is less clear is whether they possess a common cause. Certainly patients with subacute liver failure can develop a deep coma without signs of cerebral edema, but patients with signs of intracranial hypertension (ICH) always develop high-grade encephalopathy prior to this.

Cerebral edema was noted and commented on in the seminal clinicopathologic review of servicemen presenting with fulminant epidemic hepatitis during the East Asian campaign of the Second World War.[53] However, the recognition that cerebral edema was a distinct clinical entity and cause of death associated with ALF did not become clear until much later.[151,152]

The recognition that brain swelling is an important component of ALF is now well established. Management strategies place the risk of ICH at the forefront of care, and prophylactic therapy, monitoring, and treatment are widely debated in the literature.[153,154] The incidence of cerebral edema in ALF is not completely clear and is dependent on the cause of liver failure, the severity, and the rate of onset. It is important to distinguish between ICH and cerebral edema. The former requires the measurement of pressure within the cranial vault and results in brain ischemia and signs of tentorial herniation. The latter is difficult to define clinically and depends on how hard you look. CT and postmortem studies have suggested an incidence of between 50% and 80% of those with high-grade encephalopathy.[151,155] The pathologic changes of cerebral edema and ICH in ALF are not completely understood, but in recent years progress has been made in understanding the processes involved.[156]

An increase in cerebral blood flow may induce ICH by a number of mechanisms and induce further cerebral swelling. This could occur due to an increased flux of potentially toxic metabolites such as ammonia or by an increase in cerebral water content because of an increase in cerebrovascular hydrostatic pressure. The blood-brain barrier has been considered to remain intact in ALF but recent evidence suggests that there is some impairment, although the degree to which this contributes to cerebral swelling is still being debated.[161,167]

Cerebrovascular autoregulation is lost in ALF.[165,168] The cause is unknown but a gradual cerebral vasoparesis concurs with clinical observation. Autoregulation can be restored by hyperventilation and mild hypothermia but not by the use of indomethacin.[169] It has been suggested that the increase in astrocyte glutamine plays a role in this gradual vasoparalysis and loss of autoregulation by the induction of local nitric oxide or carbon monoxide.[156] It is relatively common to find a patient with a high ICP and jugular venous oxygen saturation above 80%. This suggests a state of luxury perfusion (unregulated blood supply in excess of demand) in which an increase in cerebral blood volume in an already swollen brain accounts for the associated increase in ICP.[170]

Management

In the management of ICH in ALF it is important to target those at risk. The development of ICH sets the management of ALF apart from other forms of critical illness and it remains a leading cause of death despite advances in the understanding of the etiology ALF and management of ALF patients.[172,173] Monitoring the pressure within the cranial vault is difficult and invasive. Despite investigation, a reliable noninvasive method for the evaluation of cerebral blood flow, cerebral oxygenation, and ICP remains elusive.[174]

There are important points that need to be considered when managing a patient with ALF and possible raised ICP:

- Prediction of patients at risk of ICH
- How to monitor the brain
- Prophylactic management
- Treatment of established ICH

Predicting Intracranial Hypertension

In ALF the development of cerebral edema is seen in patients with the shortest time between the development of jaundice and the onset of encephalopathy.[52] A fulminating presentation, lack of time for cerebral adaptation, and systemic burden of a necrotic liver appear to be the likely reasons. Patients with paracetamol toxicity make up the largest number in this group. Other causes can fall into the hyperacute group including patients with ALF due to hepatotrophic viruses, particularly HBV. In contrast, patients with subacute liver failure have a smaller risk.

It has been suggested that the incidence of ICH following paracetamol toxicity has fallen since the mid-1980s.[175] However, it still represents a significant complication in this setting. Recent work from King's College Hospital in London suggests an incidence of 20% to 30% in all patients with ALF. Data from our own unit suggest that ICH is implicated in the death of 25% of all patients with ALF and 35% of those following paracetamol-induced toxicity.[172,173]

Young age has consistently been found to be a risk factor.[151,173] Arterial ammonia concentration has been shown to correlate with death and cerebral herniation.[158,159,173,176] Recent commentary suggests that arterial ammonia should be measured serially in all patients with ALF and that ICP monitoring be instituted if the concentration is greater than or equal to 150 μmol/L.[170]

Serum sodium is often low in patients with ALF. In a consecutive group of patients with ALF from POD admitted to King's Hospital liver intensive care unit, 65% were hyponatremic on arrival (Will Bernal, personal communication). Hyponatremia is associated with a poor outcome in ALF,[177] and data have shown an inverse relationship between ICP and serum sodium in patients with ALF[178]) (Box 75.3).

The severity of the inflammatory response and organ failure are positively associated with the risk of developing ICH. Systemic inflammation may exacerbate ICH in a brain primed by ALF.[173]

Monitoring the Brain

There are a number of monitoring devices and methods that can be undertaken to screen for raised ICP or cerebral ischemia or both. Some of these devices are more invasive than others and the possible risks and benefits need to be understood.

Computed tomography is a standard investigation in any patient with suspected intracranial disease. Cerebral edema can be recognized in CT scans of patients with ALF and the severity correlates crudely to encephalopathy grade, but the correlation between imaging and severity of ICP measurement is poor.[155,179] As little additional information is gained, very careful consideration should be undertaken before transporting this very sick group of patients to the CT scanner. Occasionally there are diagnostic difficulties or a

Box 75.3 Risk Factors for Brain Swelling in Acute Liver Failure

Are there risk factors for ICH?

- Less than 40 years of age
- Very low or high JV O_2 sat
- Significant organ dysfunction requiring support
- Severe hyponatremia <130 mmol/L
- Arterial ammonia >150 μmol/L
- Pupillary abnormalities or seizures
- High temperature, tachycardia, hypotension, signs of infection

suspected complication of ICP bolt insertion and CT scanning might be considered.

Functional brain imaging, using single positron emission tomography (SPECT), has been used to investigate the distribution of cerebral blood flow in ALF and magnetic resonance imaging (MRI) scanning has been used to investigate the distribution of intracerebral water, but neither has found a place in clinical practice.[126,180,181]

In patients with suspected ICH the direct monitoring of cerebral oxygenation and blood flow are appealing but current methods have technical and clinical limitations. Tissue Po_2 and interstitial metabolites, using intraparenchymal probes, have been investigated in traumatic brain injury and to a limited extent in ALF.[116,182] They have the advantage in traumatic injury of providing localized information around the area of injury. The use of cerebral microdialysis (sampling of the cerebral interstitial fluid using a microcoaxial catheter with a semipermeable membrane) remains a research tool in ALF at the present time.

Methods used for the estimation of global cerebral oxygenation include the sampling of jugular venous (JV) blood for oxygen saturation, and products of metabolism such as lactate. A JV saturation of less than 55% suggests an ischemic brain. This can be due to a reduction in blood flow in excess of demand because of brain swelling or cerebral vasoconstriction due to hypocarbia, if the patient is being hyperventilated. An increase in demand due to seizure activity can also manifest as a reduction in JV saturation.[183] High jugular saturation (>80%) may represent a hyperemic brain, and steps can be taken to reduce cerebral blood volume if ICP is raised. Very high JV saturation is often seen as a terminal event and may represent a complete loss of oxygen extraction by the brain (Fig. 75.12).

Near infrared spectroscopy is a noninvasive technique used to assess the oxygen content of various organs. It can be used to determine cerebral oxygenation and changes in cerebral perfusion in ALF and warrants further investigation.

Noninvasive measurement of cerebral blood flow using transcranial Doppler (TCD) has been investigated in ALF. In one study it was found to be predictive of changes in cerebral blood flow induced by hyperventilation.[184] More recent investigation has shown changes in TCD waveform as ICP increases, but it is not clear how reproducible these results are.[185]

The recognition that ICP is raised in a significant proportion of patients with ALF and that this is implicated in significant rates of morbidity and mortality has led to the use of direct measurement of ICP with various forms of monitoring.[151,186] These techniques, although fully supported internationally in traumatic brain injury, are controversial in the field of ALF and there remains a dichotomy of opinion in most countries, with some units using them and others not.[153,154,187,188]

Controversy revolves around the lack of evidence of improved outcome with the monitoring of ICP and the risk of intracranial bleeding complicating insertion. The reported risk of bleeding, from survey data, is between 10% and 20% overall, the majority of which is not clinically significant. Mortality rate has been reported at between 1% and 3% (Alistair Lee, Edinburgh, UK, personal communication).[186,188] The risk of bleeding following placement is higher than that seen following traumatic brain injury. There is uncontrolled evidence that activated factor VII can reduce this risk.[189]

It has not been possible to prove that ICP monitoring improves survival in ALF, as a randomized controlled clinical trial has not been performed to evaluate it. However, it is generally accepted that medical intervention can reduce ICP and prevent cerebral ischemia and brain herniation in patients with ALF.[170] Published data suggest that having an ICP monitor increases the intervention rate compared to

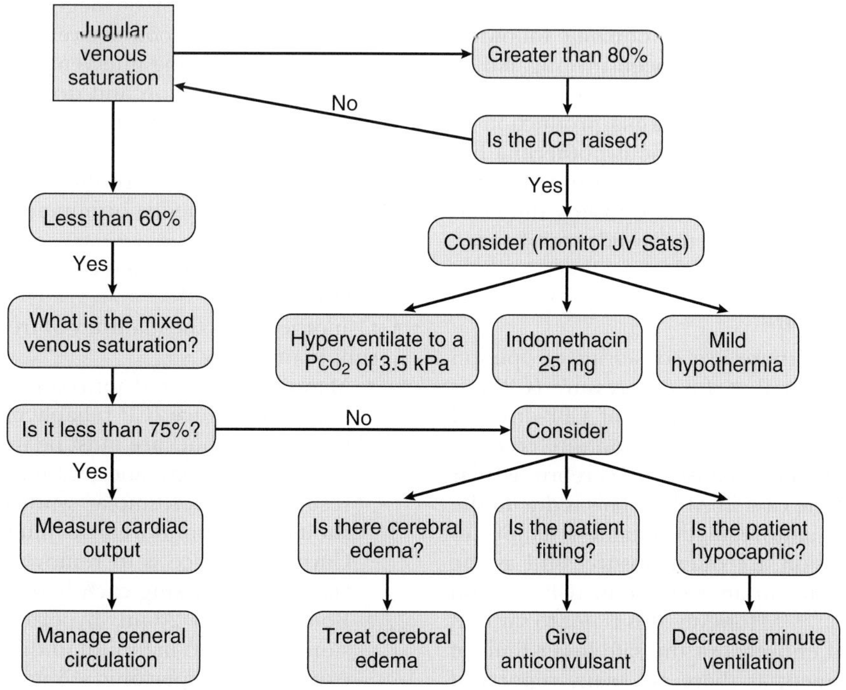

Figure 75.12 Monitoring cerebral oxygenation with jugular bulb sampling. ICP, intracranial pressure; JV, jugular venous; Sats, saturation.

patients without and increases the length of survival in the critical care unit, if not overall survival.[190] The majority of patients with ALF die of multiple organ failure due to sepsis. Intervention to reduce ICP may just prevent early cerebral death.

Although the risks of monitoring are documented, the risks of not monitoring are less clear. Without monitoring ICP there is a tendency toward therapeutic paralysis because of uncertainty and a tendency to manage all patients as if they had raised ICP. The reassurance of a normal ICP enables a reduction in sedation and paralysis. It enables tracheal suctioning and other nursing care without the uncertainty of worsening an unknown ICP. With ICP monitoring modest increases in ICP can be treated early before clinical signs suggest impending brain herniation. Monitoring ICP enables the calculation of cerebral perfusion pressure and, together with the monitoring of jugular oxygen saturation, allows a more complete picture of cerebral perfusion and oxygenation. The use of ICP monitoring has been advocated in the setting of liver transplantation for ALF and, of course, enables continued clinical research into the management of cerebral edema.

Prophylactic Measures

In patients at high risk of cerebral edema a number of prophylactic interventions have been shown to reduce the incidence of ICH.

Serum sodium is often low in patients with ALF. In a consecutive group of patients with ALF from POD admitted to King's Hospital liver intensive care unit, 65% were hyponatremic on arrival (Will Bernal, personal communication). Hyponatremia is associated with a poor outcome in ALF.[177] Based on retrospective data showing an inverse relationship between ICP and serum sodium in patients with ALF, moderate hypernatremia was investigated as a possible prophylactic intervention.[119,178] Maintaining serum sodium between 145 and 155 mmol/L using hypertonic saline was found to reduce ICP from baseline and reduce the incidence of surges in ICP.[119] Hypothermia improves outcome following out-of-hospital cardiac arrest and has been investigated in patients with traumatic brain injury. Early reports suggest hypothermia can reduce ICP and ammonia production in patients with ALF. However, prophylactic hypothermia has not been shown to reduce the incidence or improve outcome in this setting.[191] Simple measures such as raising the head of the bed to a 30-degree angle and the avoidance of excessive stimulation are also prudent.

Cerebral Perfusion Pressure

In traumatic brain injury there is a consensus of opinion supporting the use of cerebral perfusion pressure (CPP) as a treatment goal.[187] In ALF the concept of CPP-directed therapy is less useful. To assume a correlation with cerebral blood flow there has to be a consistent cerebrovascular resistance, which is not the case in ALF.[170] This is due to the loss of cerebrovascular autoregulation, and attempts to increase cerebral perfusion are often unsuccessful as the use of a vasopressor results in an increase in ICP as brain blood volume increases.[131,192] However, this is not to say that CPP should be ignored entirely but the safe lower limit of CPP has yet to be defined, as there are many reports of patients surviving with normal cerebral function despite a low CCP.[193] The normal lower limit of cerebral autoregulation is reached at a mean arterial blood pressure of about 50 mm Hg, below which flow becomes pressure dependent. In patients with absent autoregulation, such as in ALF, CCP should probably be maintained above 40 mm Hg (the normal lower limit of autoregulation with an ICP of 10 mm Hg or less), but no data exist to back this statement up. Maintenance of CPP in ALF is best achieved by decreasing ICP and aiming for a mean arterial pressure with fluid and a vasopressor that does not increase ICP above 25 mm Hg. Attempting to improve cerebral oxygen balance is also attractive in this setting. This may be attempted with intravenous indomethacin (has been shown to improve CPP without compromising cerebral oxygenation), hypothermia, increased sedation, and hyperventilation.[169,194-196] Monitoring cerebral oxygenation is very useful during such a maneuver.

General Management of Patients with Raised Intracranial Pressure

In patients at risk of or with suspected cerebral edema, prophylactic measures should be instituted. The decision to insert an ICP bolt or not will have to be made by the clinical team. If inserted, there is the potential to manage ICP.

ICP is normally less than 15 mm Hg in an adult. The definition of ICH is not precise and will vary among patients. Available data are derived from patients with traumatic brain injury (TBI) where observational studies suggest that intervention to reduce pressure should be instituted between 20 and 25 mm Hg, although pupillary abnormalities and brain herniation can occur at lower pressures.[187] There have not been any studies investigating treatment threshold in ALF and so similar thresholds to traumatic brain injury are used.

The management of ICH is usually escalated along standard algorithms (Figs. 75.13 and 75.14). Elevate the patient to an angle of 30 degrees and avoid tight straps around the neck to encourage venous drainage. ICP tends to increase during nursing intervention. If the ICP rises following nursing intervention and does not resolve after several minutes it implies poor intracranial compliance. Treatment is usually instituted for a sustained rise in ICP (more than 10 minutes over the treatment threshold) or clinical signs suggesting cerebral ischemia or impending herniation.

- Sedation should be increased. Propofol is probably the agent of choice.[194]
- Osmotherapy is the mainstay of treatment following these simple measures.
  - Mannitol as a rapid infusion (0.5-1.0 g/kg) has been shown to reduce ICP reliably in ALF.[197] The dose can be repeated but care must be used in renal failure due to accumulation, and multiple administrations can result in a hyperosmolar syndrome. Plasma osmolality should be monitored if multiple doses are used. Current practice is to remove 500 mL of ultrafiltrate via CVVH following each bolus dose of mannitol.
  - Bolus doses of 20 mL hypertonic saline (30%) has a similar effect to mannitol in this setting in the author's experience. Hypertonic saline has a higher reflectance coefficient at the blood-brain barrier compared to

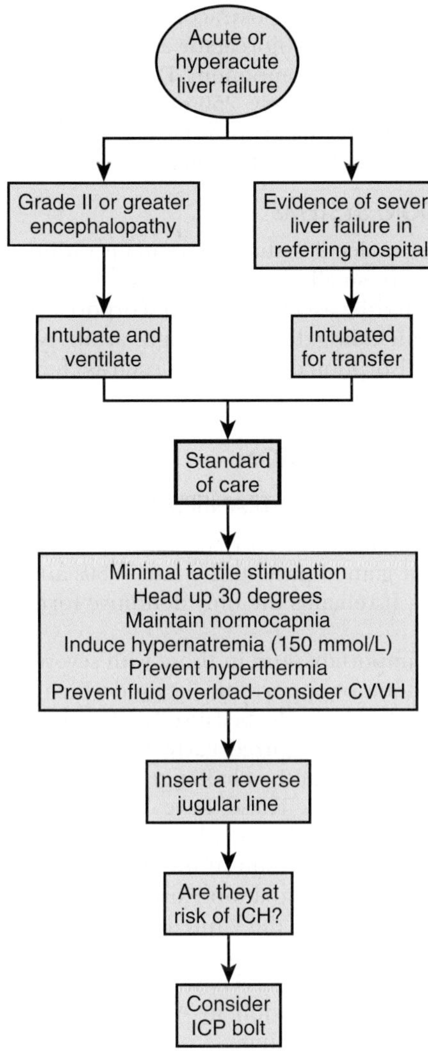

Figure 75.13 Initial management of patient with high-grade encephalopathy. CVVH, continuous venovenous hemofiltration; ICH, intracranial hypertension; ICP, intracranial pressure.

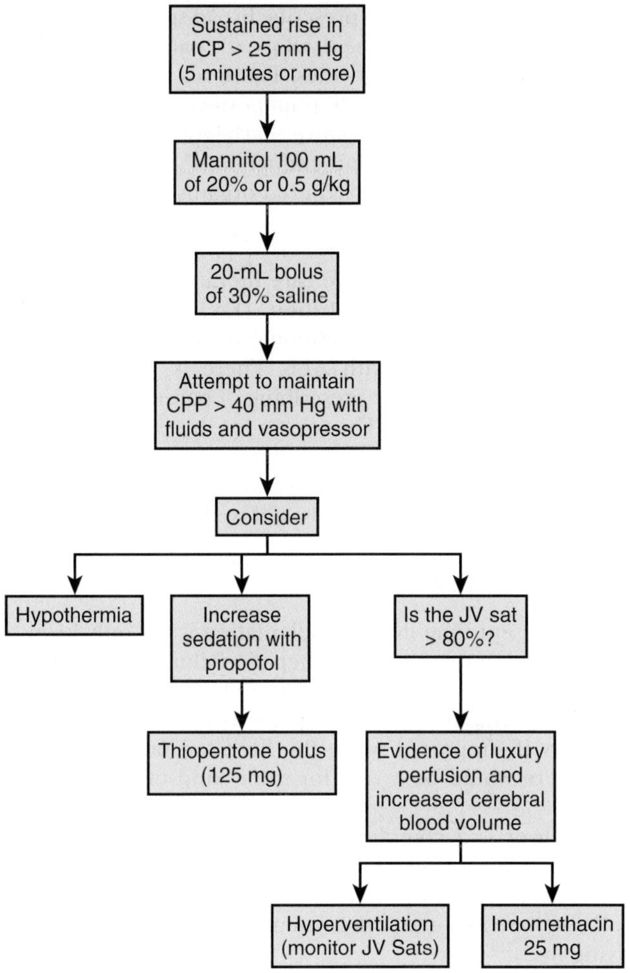

Figure 75.14 Management of a sustained rise in intracranial pressure. CPP, cerebral perfusion pressure; ICP, intracranial pressure; JV, jugular venous; Sats, saturation.

mannitol and there appears to be less tachyphylaxis to multiple administration.[119]

In patients with a raised ICP and cerebral hyperemia, suggested by a JV oxygen saturation of 80% or greater (luxury perfusion), short-term hyperventilation will induce cerebral vasoconstriction and reduce blood volume. This maneuver has been shown not to impair cerebral oxygenation but close monitoring of cerebral oxygenation should be employed if it is attempted.[195] Short-term hyperventilation has not been shown to improve outcome in ALF but does prolong survival in the ICU.[198] Hyperventilation may be lifesaving and may buy time for definitive treatment (transplantation). Indomethacin induces cerebral vasoconstriction and reduces ICP in patients with both traumatic brain injury and ALF without impairing cerebral oxygenation, although confirmatory studies are needed.[169]

Seizures

Ammonia toxicity and cerebral edema are associated with seizure activity and it has been recognized that subclinical seizures occur more commonly than previously thought.[183] The use of mechanical ventilation facilitated by sedatives and muscular paralysis can mask clinical signs. Seizures adversely affect cerebral oxygen consumption and may contribute to cerebral edema and are a cause of low jugular oxygen saturation. It has been suggested that prophylactic phenytoin be used in all patients with ALF and high-grade encephalopathy. Others have questioned this approach because of the significant side effects and apparent lack of effect on outcome.[199] If confirmed, seizure activity should be managed along standard management guidelines.

INFECTION AND IMMUNOSUPPRESSION

Patients with ALF have multiple immune defects and are susceptible to infections.[200] Infection is a common cause of progression and complication in ALF.[201] Antibiotic prophylaxis has been shown to reduce the incidence of infection and enable transplantation to proceed but has not been shown to improve survival. Selective decontamination of the digestive tract has not been shown to be superior to intravenous antibiotics alone.[200,202] More recent work has shown how the microbiologic flora of a liver unit has changed over the past 20 years—for example, bacteremia appearing later in the ICU stay and being predominantly gram-negative in nature.[203]

It is current practice to prescribe broad-spectrum antibacterial and antifungal medication to patients with ALF depending on local sensitivities. There is a general trend to the timing of infection with gram-positive infections occurring earlier than gram-negative. Early gram-negative infections tend to be less resistant "endogenous" bacteria followed later by resistant hospital-acquired organisms.[204,205]

NUTRITION

Within the general intensive care literature there is a consensus toward enteral nutrition (EN) as the route of choice.[206] There are few additional data on which to base decisions in patients with ALF. There is, however, wide regional variation in the prescribing of parenteral nutrition (PN) compared to EN. The reason for this is unclear as EN is associated with a reduction in infectious complications.[206] However, it is clear that some centers prefer PN.[207] Nutritional requirements in ALF are not well understood.

ARTIFICIAL LIVER SUPPORT

At the present time liver transplantation is the only form of definitive therapy for severe hepatic failure. However, the scarcity of organs and potential for delay in transplantation, together with a proportion of patients who will make a full recovery if supported while the liver regenerates, suggest that there would be a role for some kind of liver support system.

The liver is a complex organ, and to be an ideal liver replacement, any system has to support a wide range of biosynthetic and metabolic functions. Any working system will also have to counter the systemic burden of the necrotic, dying liver.[216]

Artificial liver support can be split into two main approaches. In the first there is an attempt to simulate or replace all or most of the functions of the liver. These systems include hepatocytes either from human or animal sources. Another view of liver failure suggests that toxins either excreted by the dying liver or not metabolized because of an acute reduction in function are responsible for the majority of the signs and symptoms. In this view extracorporeal blood purification with dialysis or adsorption techniques are employed and serum proteins not produced are replaced with plasma (Box 75.4).

BIOLOGIC SYSTEMS

Biologic systems consist of a bioreactor within which the cellular biomass is contained, and a mechanism of containing and separating the biomass from the circulation of the patient. They require an extracorporeal system to deliver blood or plasma to the bioreactor and may also contain an adsorption or dialysis component. Data from liver resection suggest that approximately 250 mL of liver by volume is required to prevent death from liver failure. This typically represents 20% to 30% of liver mass.[217]

Box 75.4 Functions of the Liver

- Excretion of bilirubin, cholesterol, hormones, and drugs
- Metabolism of fats, proteins, and carbohydrates
- Enzyme activation
- Storage of glycogen, vitamins, and minerals and regulation of glucose levels
- Synthesis of plasma proteins such as albumin, clotting factors, and bile production
- Blood detoxification and purification
- Immune regulation

NONBIOLOGIC SYSTEMS

Many of the molecules that accumulate within the blood during ALF are small or middle-sized.[216] These molecules can be targeted by a variety of extracorporeal purification techniques, including dialysis through various types of membranes and adsorption onto carriers such as charcoal, resins, or albumin.

LIVER TRANSPLANTATION

WHEN AND WHOM TO TRANSPLANT

Liver transplantation for ALF was used sporadically during the 1980s but gained pace in the late 1980s and now has a huge impact. It remains the only definitive form of therapy for some.

Timing is important, and in those with severe liver injury there is a window of opportunity beyond which transplantation often becomes futile because of deteriorating organ function.[228] It was recognized early in the history of transplantation for ALF that the challenge was to develop robust prognostic indicators. These have to be sensitive, early enough to provide maximum advantage to the patient, and specific enough not to result in unnecessary transplants.

A "super-urgent" designation exists in the national transplant sharing scheme in the United Kingdom with a similar "category 1A" designation in the United States (see http://www.unos.org/ for details). These categories recognize the role of early transplantation in ALF and the detrimental effect of delay in this setting.

In the United Kingdom, the super-urgent designation (Box 75.5) is closely linked to the prognostic score developed in King's College Hospital in the late 1980s using retrospective multivariate analysis with prospective validation.[229] The prognostic criteria have been subsequently validated in other centers and shown to be robust.[230] Other criteria have been developed.[231]

The criteria are not perfect. First, despite their good specificity (i.e., if the patient meets criteria the patient is likely to die), the sensitivity and negative predictive value are not as good, and there is a substantial proportion of patients who will die without ever reaching transplant criteria. In addition, awaiting positive criteria can lead to delay in listing and worsening of organ failure that often then preclude listing. This contributes to the fact that published rates of transplantation in those who reach criteria are only 50% following POD.[232] Clinical practice has changed since this designation was first defined. For example, it is rare to see a patient following POD with a pH below 7.3 or a creatinine above 300 mmol/L because of improved resuscitation and early renal support at the referring hospital. Because of these factors, ongoing efforts to establish markers that increase sensitivity and occur even earlier in the course of the syndrome, while maintaining good specificity and not reducing the positive predictive value to unacceptable levels leading to unnecessary transplants, continue.

Box 75.5 Prognostic Indicators for Liver Transplantation

Category 1: Paracetamol: pH <7.25 more than 24 hours after overdose and after fluid resuscitation
Category 2: Paracetamol: coexisting prothrombin time >100 seconds or INR >6.5, serum creatinine >300 μmol/L or anuria, grade 3-4 encephalopathy
Category 3: Paracetamol: serum lactate >3.5 mmol/L on admission or >3.0 mmol/L more than 24 hours after overdose and after fluid resuscitation
Category 4: Paracetamol: two of three criteria from category 2 with clinical evidence of deterioration (e.g., increased ICP, FiO_2 >50%, increasing inotrope requirements) in the absence of clinical sepsis
Category 5: Etiology: hepatitis A, hepatitis B, idiosyncratic drug reaction, seronegative hepatitis; prothrombin time >100 seconds or INR >6.5 and any grade of encephalopathy
Category 6: Etiology: hepatitis A, hepatitis B, idiosyncratic drug reaction, seronegative hepatitis; any grade of encephalopathy and any three from the following: unfavorable etiology (idiosyncratic drug reaction, seronegative hepatitis), age >40 years, jaundice to encephalopathy time >7 days, serum bilirubin >300 μmol/L, prothrombin time >50 seconds or INR >3.5
Category 7: Etiology: acute presentation of Wilson's disease, acute presentation of Budd-Chiari syndrome; combination of coagulopathy and any degree of encephalopathy
Category 8: Hepatic artery thrombosis within 14 days of liver transplantation
Category 9: Early graft dysfunction with at least two of the following: AST >10,000, INR >3.0, serum lactate >3 mmol/L, absence of bile production

AST, aspartate transaminase; ICP, intracranial pressure; INR, international normalized ratio.

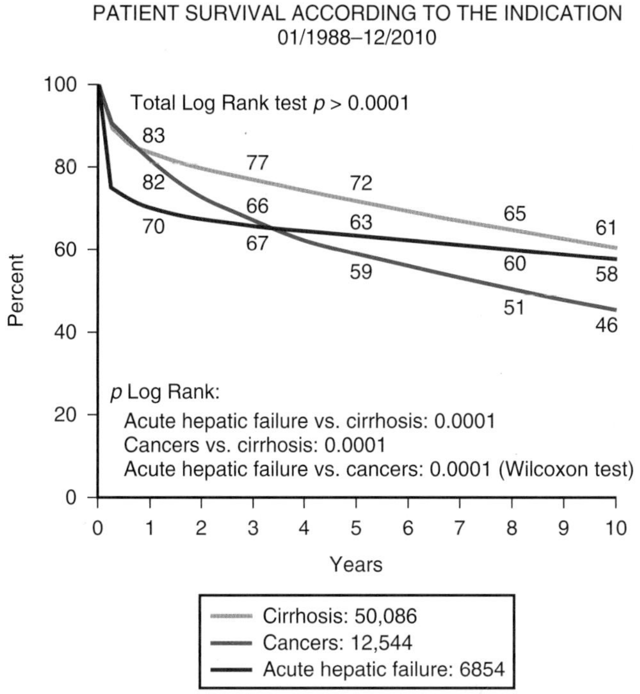

Figure 75.15 Patient survival according to the first indication for liver transplant. (From European Liver and Intestine Transplant Association, accessed at http:www.eltr.org.)

Serum phosphate levels are higher in nonsurvivors following both POD and in other causes of ALF.[120,233] However, there appears to be an unacceptable overlap and others have suggested that the use of serum phosphate does not provide any additional benefit to existing markers.[121,234,235] Other factors investigated include α-fetoprotein levels and nuclear magnetic resonance (NMR) analysis of peripheral blood.[120,236] Acute physiologic scoring as a basis for prediction has also been utilized.[237]

The liver plays a central role in lactate metabolism. In fact, in patients with severe liver necrosis the liver changes from being a consumer of lactate to being a net producer.[209] Arterial blood lactate levels have been shown to improve the sensitivity and maintain the specificity if added to the original King's College Hospital criteria and are achieved earlier in the course of the syndrome.[149] However, the additional advantage of lactate over the original criteria has been questioned by some.[238]

On the practical issue of actually managing patients with fulminant hepatic failure some room for clinical interpretation has been included in the super-urgent listing rules. For example, there is a group of patients who do not achieve King's College Hospital criteria but subsequently die, usually of cerebral edema or multiple organ failure secondary to sepsis.[172,175] These patients often have worse acute physiologic scores compared to survivors.[232,237] As a result the U.K. super-urgent criteria allow an assessment of deteriorating acute physiology based on cardiovascular, respiratory, or cerebral disease. Similarly, the UNOS 1A criteria allow for patients "not expected to survive a further 7 days."

OUTCOME FROM TRANSPLANTATION

In Europe the 1-year survival rate following transplantation for ALF is worse than that seen in chronic liver disease. The excess mortality rate is seen in the first month or so after transplantation. This represents the severity of organ dysfunction seen prior to transplantation in ALF. Following this initial period, the curve flattens and the survival rate is actually better than that of patients with chronic liver disease (Fig. 75.15). This probably represents a younger age group and less disease recurrence. There is a huge degree of heterogeneity in ALF, and those transplanted with seronegative hepatitis display a better survival profile than patients transplanted for other causes, although they exhibit a similar early mortality rate while in the ICU.[89]

A tremendous amount of research effort has been put into the search for prognostic criteria on which to base the decision to transplant patients with ALF; however, much less information is available about the prediction of fatality following transplantation. This is important, as decisions to withdraw from the waiting list based on severity are difficult.

There appear to be both recipient and donor factors that help predict the outcome from transplantation in ALF.[89,232,239] In theory, the severity of illness and organ dysfunction prior to transplantation should predict outcome. However, because unstable patients tend to be either not listed or withdrawn from the waiting list, there is inherent bias in retrospective analysis. Age of the recipient is a significant factor, certainly for seronegative ALF, but also in POD, in which age is often used to exclude listing.[232] In non-paracetamol ALF, serum creatinine at the time of transplantation is a predictor of 2-month survival. Following POD, time from ingestion to transplantation has been shown to be a good predictor of 2-month survival; all patients transplanted later than 6 days from ingestion died. APACHE III score at transplantation and the severity of metabolic acidosis are also predictive.[239]

Donor factors found to be important are the use of reduced size grafts in paracetamol-induced ALF and evidence of early graft dysfunction as defined by a high AST or INR in the early postoperative period. In addition a high donor body mass index (BMI) is a risk factor for death in seronegative hepatitis.[89,232]

In 2012 a review of the European liver transplant database for patients transplanted following ALF was done in which 4903 patients were evaluated. The 1-, 5-, and 10-year patient and graft survival rates were 74%, 68%, and 63%, respectively. Death and graft loss were independently associated with male recipients, recipients older than 50 years, incompatible ABO matching, donors older than 60 years, and reduced size graft. Recipients over 50 receiving a graft >60 years old had a 57% 1-year mortality rate or graft loss.[240]

The conclusions from this review suggest that older recipients with severe preoperative organ dysfunction are less able to tolerate poor early graft function, often seen with marginal grafts. Therefore, in order to achieve the best graft and patient survival there should be matching of the organ to the recipient, but this is difficult because of time constraints.

AUXILIARY TRANSPLANTATION

Auxiliary partial liver transplantation has many theoretical advantages compared to standard orthotopic transplantation in ALF. It can be performed orthotopically (i.e., in the same place as the original liver) or heterotopically (e.g., in the left iliac fossa). These days it is always performed as a partial orthotopic transplant with a native left lobe in situ in adults and a right lobe in children using an adult left lobe graft, depending on size.

It provides the potential to support the patient during the acute phase of liver failure, enabling regeneration of the native liver. This is attractive because in a number of patients immunosuppressive drugs can be withdrawn, allowing the graft to atrophy or be removed, and eliminating the risks associated with lifelong immunosuppression. Data on this procedure have been accumulating since the mid-1990s. Initial reports suggested that the procedure was associated with a high incidence of technical problems, primary dysfunction, and retransplantation. Later reports, however, suggest that many of these issues are resolving with greater experience in patient and graft selection. The best outcome has been seen in patients aged younger than 40 years with either acute viral hepatitis or paracetamol hepatotoxicity in which 1-year graft and patient survival are similar to those for standard transplantation for ALF. Withdrawal of immunosuppression can be achieved in 30% to 70% of patients transplanted.[241-243]

LIVING RELATED LOBE DONATION

In many countries the only chance of transplantation for ALF is in a living related donation of a liver lobe. This is most often performed in children when an adult left lobe can be used. In adults, a right lobe is usually required, increasing the risk to the donor. With the worldwide shortage of donor organs, living related transplantation for ALF is widely accepted in many countries but not all. There are significant issues related to living related transplantation in ALF including a donor mortality rate of 1% and major morbidity rate of 40% to 60%. There are also ethical implications of adequately preparing the donor, medically and psychologically, in a time of acute crisis.[244]

KEY POINTS

- Liver failure can occur with a background of cirrhosis, when it is often termed *acute on chronic liver failure* (AoCLF), or it can occur de novo in a previously healthy individual due to a toxic, immunologic, hypoxic, or infective cause, when it is termed *acute liver failure* (ALF) or fulminant liver failure.
- Liver failure, defined by the onset of hepatic encephalopathy and progressive failure in hepatic metabolic activity, progresses to multiple organ failure and ultimately death in a large proportion of patients, and supportive care is the mainstay of therapy.
- AoCLF is seen much more commonly than ALF. It is most often seen in the setting of advanced, decompensated cirrhosis with portal hypertension. It is usually precipitated by some intercurrent event such as sepsis or an upper gastrointestinal bleed. Therapy is aimed at the treatment of sepsis and aggressive management of the circulation.
- Worldwide, particularly in the developing world, approximately 95% to 100% of patients presenting with ALF will have viral hepatitis.
- Acetaminophen poisoning is the most common cause of ALF in northern Europe and the United States. It can be treated successfully in the majority of patients with NAC, if given within the first 12 hours following nonstaggered ingestion.
- The presentation and clinical course of ALF depends on its cause and the rate of progression of the syndrome.
- Liver failure following viral hepatitis is rare and tends to run an acute or hyperacute course, with the onset of encephalopathy occurring within days or weeks of the first symptoms.
- The West Haven criteria, designed to assess coma grade in patients with cirrhosis, are often applied to patients with ALF and are useful because of their familiarity.
- Intracranial hypertension secondary to cerebral edema often complicates severe hyperacute liver failure and remains a leading cause of death.
- Management of ALF is complex, and liver transplantation is the only effective therapy in severe cases.

SELECTED REFERENCES

2. Katoonizadeh A, Laleman W, Verslype C, et al: Early features of acute-on-chronic alcoholic liver failure: A prospective cohort study. Gut 2010;59(11):1561-1569.
25. European Association for the Study of the Liver: EASL clinical practice guidelines on the management of ascites, spontaneous bacterial peritonitis, and hepatorenal syndrome in cirrhosis. J Hepatol 2010;53(3):397-417.
30. Olson JC, Kamath PS: Acute-on-chronic liver failure: Concept, natural history, and prognosis. Curr Opin Crit Care 2011; 17(2):165-169.
73. Schiodt FV, Davern TJ, Shakil AO, et al: Viral hepatitis-related acute liver failure. Am J Gastroenterol 2003;98(2):448-453.
97. Hamid SS, Jafri SM, Khan H, et al: Fulminant hepatic failure in pregnant women: Acute fatty liver or acute viral hepatitis? J Hepatol 1996;25(1):20-27.
127. Ellis A, Wendon J: Circulatory, respiratory, cerebral, and renal derangements in acute liver failure: Pathophysiology and management. Semin Liver Dis 1996;16(4):379-388.
170. Toftengi F, Larsen FS: Management of patients with fulminant hepatic failure and brain edema. Metab Brain Dis 2004; 19(3-4):207-214.
186. Blei AT, Olafsson S, Webster S, Levy R: Complications of intracranial pressure monitoring in fulminant hepatic failure. Lancet 1993;341(8838):157-158.
200. Rolando N, Philpott-Howard J, Williams R: Bacterial and fungal infection in acute liver failure. Semin Liver Dis 1996;16(4): 389-402.
230. Anand AC, Nightingale P, Neuberger JM: Early indicators of prognosis in fulminant hepatic failure: An assessment of the King's criteria. J Hepatol 1997;26(1):62-68.

The complete list of references can be found at www.expertconsult.com.

76 Gastrointestinal Bleeding

Louis Chaptini | Steven Peikin

CHAPTER OUTLINE

Gastrointestinal (GI) bleeding encompasses a wide range of diagnoses with multiple types of lesions and bleeding that can occur virtually anywhere in the GI tract. Acute GI bleeding is often an emergency that can be alarming to both the patient and physician. Management and the outcome of GI bleeding depend on both the severity of the bleeding and any comorbid conditions present at the time of the bleeding. Acute GI bleeding often requires close monitoring and management in an intensive care unit (ICU). Management of such bleeding relies on a team approach that involves the expertise of an intensivist, gastroenterologist (endoscopist), radiologist, and surgeon.

More than 300,000 annual hospitalizations in the United States are attributed to GI bleeding.[1] Upper GI bleeding accounts for most of these hospitalizations, with an incidence rate of 100 cases per 100,000,[1] whereas the incidence of lower GI bleeding is estimated at 20 to 27 cases per 100,000.[2,3] Mortality rates vary depending on the source of the bleeding. Most nonvariceal upper GI bleeding studies document mortality rates approximating 10%.[4,5] These rates have not changed over the past 2 decades despite the evolution of acid suppression therapy, which is probably explained by an aging population with increased comorbid diseases. Mortality rates for lower GI bleeding are usually in the range of 5%.[6,7]

CLINICAL PRESENTATION

INITIAL EVALUATION AND RESUSCITATION

The clinical findings in a patient with GI bleeding are crucial in determining the site, cause, and rate of bleeding. The first step in clinical evaluation is to assess the severity of the bleeding. This is done primarily by measuring hemodynamic parameters in an attempt to quantify the amount of blood volume lost (Table 76.1).[8] Because bleeding can represent a dynamic ongoing situation, continuous monitoring of hemodynamics is necessary to guide resuscitation efforts and provide key prognostic information. In patients with GI bleeding, two large-bore intravenous catheters should be placed immediately on arrival to restore euvolemia.

The hematocrit at initial evaluation may not reflect the severity of the bleeding because very recent loss of both plasma and red blood cells leads to a percentage of red blood cells in the remaining blood (which defines the hematocrit) that is close to the same value. The hematocrit drops when hemodilution occurs as extravascular fluid enters the vascular space to restore volume, a process that may take up to 72 hours (Fig. 76.1).[9]

The rapidity of blood and colloid infusion depends in part on the patient's cardiovascular condition. Placement of a central venous pressure catheter can help one base decisions on more objective findings. Several recent studies found that transfusion was associated with higher risk for nosocomial infection, multiorgan dysfunction, acute respiratory distress syndrome, and death.[10] Current transfusion trends are to administer blood to patients with hemoglobin less than 7 mg/dL and to avoid transfusion when it's above 10 mg/dL. However, the threshold for blood transfusion should take into consideration the patient's underlying condition, hemodynamic status, and markers of tissue hypoxemia.[11] In patients with conditions associated with defects in platelet or coagulation factors, these substances should be replaced. Patients requiring massive transfusion of packed

Table 76.1 Hemodynamics, Vital Signs, and Blood Loss

Hemodynamics and Vital Signs	% Blood Loss (Fraction of Intravascular Volume)	Bleeding Type
Shock (resting hypotension)	20-25	Massive
Postural (orthostatic tachycardia or hypotension)	10-20	Moderate
Normal	<10	Minor

From Rockey DC: Gastrointestinal bleeding. Gastroenterol Clin North Am 2005;34:581-588.

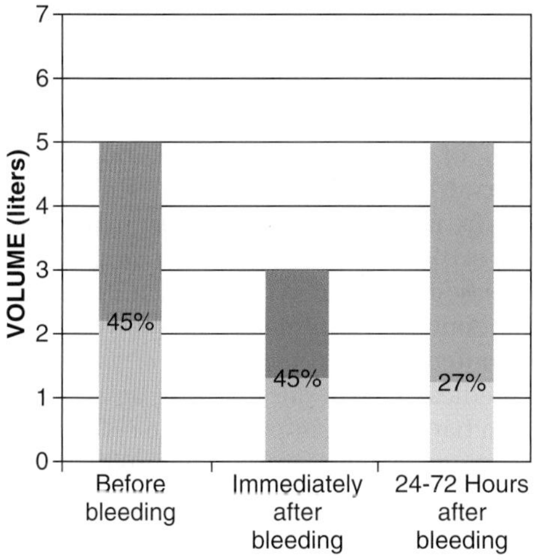

Figure 76.1 Plasma volumes *(solid bars)*, red blood cell volumes *(pale bars)*, and hematocrit values (%) before bleeding and after blood loss of 2 L. A baseline hematocrit level of 45% is assumed. (From Rockey DC: Gastrointestinal bleeding. In Feldman M, Friedman LS, Sleisenger MH [eds]: Sleisenger and Fordtran's Gastrointestinal and Liver Disease, 7th ed. Philadelphia, WB Saunders, 2002, pp 221-248.)

red blood cells require fresh frozen plasma and platelets. Hypocalcemia can develop in these patients because of the large amount of citrate received with massive transfusion, and thus calcium replacement should be considered, especially in individuals with end-stage liver disease and heart failure, in whom citrate metabolism may be impaired.[12] The initial evaluation of patients with nonvariceal upper GI bleeding should include risk stratification of patients into low- and high-risk categories for rebleeding and death based on clinical, laboratory, and when available, endoscopic criteria.[10] This allows appropriate intervention and minimizes morbidity and mortality risks. The most extensively validated scores for risk stratification are the Blatchford and Rockall scores[13,14] (Tables 76.2 and 76.3). Similarly, risk stratification in lower GI bleeding helps in guiding the management of these patients. Hemodynamic instability, ongoing hematochezia, and comorbid illnesses have been consistently associated with poor outcome in lower GI bleeding.[15]

Table 76.2 Blatchford Score for Gastrointestinal Bleeding*

Admission Parameter	Score Value
Urea (mg/dL)	
≥6.5 to <8.0	2
≥8 to <10	3
≥10 to <25	4
≥25	6
Hemoglobin (g/dL)	
Men	
≥12 to <13	1
≥10 to <12	3
<10	6
Women	
≥10 to <12	1
<10	6
Systolic blood pressure (mm Hg)	
100 to 109	1
90 to 99	3
<90	3
Other parameters	
Pulse >100	1
Melena at presentation	1
Syncope	2
Hepatic disease	2
Cardiac failure	2

*The score is calculated by adding the points from each variable. A score of zero is associated with a low risk of the need for endoscopic intervention

From Blatchford O, Murray WR, Blatchford M: A risk score to predict need for treatment for upper-gastrointestinal haemorrhage. Lancet 2000;356:1318-1321.

Box 76.1 Historical Features in the Assessment of Gastrointestinal Bleeding

- Age
- Previous bleeding
- Previous gastrointestinal disease
- Previous surgery
- Underlying medical disorder (especially liver disease)
- Nonsteroidal anti-inflammatory drugs
- Abdominal pain
- Change in bowel habits
- Weight loss or anorexia
- History of oropharyngeal disease

From Rockey DC: Gastrointestinal bleeding. Gastroenterol Clin North Am 2005;34:581-588.

HISTORY AND CLINICAL FINDINGS

After hemodynamic stabilization is achieved, a careful history and clinical examination are imperative to make a preliminary assessment of the location and cause of the bleeding. Important historical features in the evaluation of GI bleeding are shown in Box 76.1.[8]

Hematemesis typically points to an upper source of bleeding, proximal to the ligament of Treitz. In rare cases,

Table 76.3 Rockall Scoring System for Risk of Rebleeding and Death in Acute Gastrointestinal Bleeding*

	Points			
Variable	0	1	2	3
Age (years)	<60	60 to 79	>80	
Shock	No shock (systolic BP >100 mm Hg, pulse <100)	Tachycardia (systolic BP >100 mm Hg, pulse >100)	Hypotension (systolic BP <100 mm Hg, pulse >100)	
Comorbidity	Nil major		Cardiac failure, ischemic heart disease, any major comorbid condition	Renal failure, liver failure, disseminated malignancy
Diagnosis	Mallory-Weiss tear, no lesion, and no SRH	All other diagnoses	Malignancy of upper GI tract	
Major SRH	None or dark spot		Blood in upper GI tract, adherent clot, visible or spurting vessel	

BP, blood pressure; GI, gastrointestinal; SRH, stigma(ta) of recent hemorrhage.
*The score is calculated by adding the points from each variable. A score of 2 or less is associated with a low risk of further bleeding or death.
From Rockall TA, Logan RF, Delvin HB, et al: Risk assessment after acute upper gastrointestinal haemorrhage. Gut 1996;38:316-321.

hematemesis can be a sign of swallowed blood from oral, pharyngeal, or nasal bleeding. Melena is defined as black tarry stool with a glistering sheen and results from degradation of blood in the GI tract. At least 50 mL of blood in the upper GI tract is required to cause melena, although volumes up to 100 mL may be clinically silent.[16] Melena usually indicates upper GI bleeding, but its source may be the small bowel and sometimes even the proximal part of the colon when the volume of blood is too small to cause hematochezia. Coffee-ground emesis is typically a sign of recent, but currently inactive upper GI bleeding, and its appearance is caused by the acid's effect on blood in the lumen. Hematochezia is generally associated with colonic bleeding but can also be caused by more proximal bleeding. Proximal bleeding in association with hematochezia is usually more hemodynamically significant.

Other symptoms at initial evaluation can help in narrowing the differential diagnosis. Abdominal pain before or at the time of the bleeding episode can be a sign of underlying peptic ulcer disease (PUD), mesenteric or colonic ischemia, perforation, or even intestinal infarction. Multiple episodes of vomiting and retching preceding the bleeding episode should alert one to the presence of a Mallory-Weiss tear.

A previous history of bleeding from PUD, esophageal or gastric varices, diverticulosis, or vascular ectasia puts these diagnoses high on the differential diagnosis list. A history of abdominal vascular surgery adds aortoenteric fistula to this list. In patients with known liver disease, the possibility of bleeding from conditions associated with portal hypertension, such as esophageal or gastric varices and portal gastropathy, should be raised. One should also look for risk factors for chronic liver disease, such as a history of chronic alcohol abuse and chronic hepatitis.

GI bleeding in elderly patients is usually caused by conditions less commonly encountered in younger patients (i.e., diverticulosis, vascular ectasia, ischemic colitis), whereas in younger patients, bleeding from sources such as varices, ulcer disease, and esophagitis is more common.

Ingestion of aspirin and other nonsteroidal anti-inflammatory drugs (NSAIDs) increases the risk of bleeding from PUD. In patients taking anticoagulant medications, bleeding most often results from underlying GI disease such as ulcer disease or vascular ectasia, even in the setting of a supratherapeutic international normalized ratio, and should not be attributed to the anticoagulation itself.

Other medical conditions present at the time of the bleeding can have a large impact on the resuscitation efforts and subsequent management. Bleeding patients with a history of coronary artery disease are at increased risk for myocardial infarction, and restoration of volume and oxygenation should be an immediate goal. Patients with pulmonary disease may need airway intubation before sedation when endoscopy is being contemplated.

Physical examination should look for evidence of chronic liver disease such as spider angiomas, gynecomastia, splenomegaly, and ascites. The presence of these signs suggests the possibility of portal hypertension. Telangiectases of the skin or mucous membranes and lips raise the possibility of hereditary hemorrhagic telangiectasia (Osler-Weber-Rendu disease). Acanthosis nigricans can be a sign of GI malignancy (especially gastric cancer). The presence of purpura suggests vascular diseases such as Schönlein-Henoch purpura or polyarteritis nodosa. Tenderness with or without peritoneal signs on abdominal examination may indicate PUD, ischemia, or perforation. The abdominal examination should include percussion and palpation to look for organomegaly and masses. Bedside examination of the character of the stool is a necessary measure that provides critical information about the source and severity of the bleeding episode. Bright red blood per rectum, maroon-colored stools, and melena suggest active bleeding, whereas brown stools indicate less aggressive bleeding.

The use of a nasogastric tube in patients presenting with GI bleeding is a common practice but at the same time controversial. The presumed benefits of nasogastric lavage include confirmation of an upper GI source of bleeding, better visualization during endoscopy, and prediction of high-risk lesions such as an oozing or spurting lesion and nonbleeding visible vessel. A bloody aspirate suggests, with some degree of certainty, an upper source of bleeding because false-positive results are rare and generally related to nasogastric trauma.[17] In one study looking at patients presenting with suspected upper GI bleeding, 45% of cases with a bloody aspirate were associated with a high-risk lesion on endoscopy versus 15% when the aspirate was clear or bilious.[18] Identifying patients with high-risk lesions is important because those patients have the worst outcome and early endoscopic therapy may have the most benefit. However, the positive and negative predictive values of a bloody aspirate for high-risk lesions are only 45% and 85%, respectively, which makes basing the decision of an early endoscopy on the information obtained by the nasogastric lavage controversial. In a recent retrospective study looking at the impact of performance of nasogastric lavage, this practice was associated with earlier time to endoscopy but had no effect on mortality rate, length of hospital stay, surgery, or transfusion requirements.[19] In our opinion, if an upper endoscopy is planned in the next 12 to 24 hours after presentation of a patient with suspected upper GI bleeding, nasogastric lavage should be avoided owing to lack of proven benefit and major discomfort and pain inflicted to the patient. In the setting of hematochezia with hemodynamic instability, extremely brisk upper GI bleeding should be suspected, and a positive nasogastric aspirate can confirm this suspicion.

DIAGNOSTIC TESTS

The initial laboratory evaluation in patients with GI bleeding should include a complete blood count, liver enzymes, prothrombin time, blood urea nitrogen (BUN), and creatinine. As mentioned earlier, the first hematocrit level may be falsely reassuring, so management decisions should rely on other parameters such as hemodynamics and the nature of the bleeding. A high white blood cell count should alert one to the presence of ischemia or infarction. Thrombocytopenia can be a sign of portal hypertension, and a critically low platelet count, as well as a high prothrombin time, should be addressed immediately by transfusion of platelets and fresh frozen plasma. An elevation in the BUN level out of proportion to creatinine is compatible with upper GI bleeding but may also be seen with intravascular volume depletion from any source of bleeding. In one study, this ratio was significantly higher in patients with upper GI bleeding than in those with lower GI bleeding (22.5 ± 11.5 vs. 15.9 ± 8.2; $p = 0.001$); however, the degree of overlap shows the poor discriminatory value of this ratio.[20] In another study, a ratio greater than 36 had a specificity of 27% and a sensitivity of 90% for upper GI bleeding.[21]

After initial resuscitation and stabilization, a diagnostic plan should be initiated. Several diagnostic tools are available, including endoscopy, radionuclide imaging, and angiography. These tests are aimed at detecting the location, source, and activity of bleeding. Other tests may be necessary in specific clinical situations, such as computed tomography (CT) scanning when abdominal pain is a prominent complaint to rule out ischemia, infarction, and perforation. Endoscopy and to some extent angiography have the advantage of allowing both diagnosis and therapy.

THERAPEUTIC OPTIONS

In addition to controlling the current episode of bleeding, treatment is also aimed at preventing recurrent bleeding. The available forms of therapy are pharmacologic, endoscopic, angiographic, and surgical. They are often complementary and require a multidisciplinary team approach. Use of these different modalities varies with the specific cause and source of bleeding.

Advances in potent acid suppression with the advent of proton pump inhibitors (PPIs) and the progress made in endoscopic technology have revolutionized the management of GI bleeding. Effective acid suppression has an established role in decreasing bleeding recurrence. Different endoscopic treatment modalities can be used alone or in combination during endoscopy and have been shown to decrease bleeding recurrence. Such modalities include injection, cautery, and mechanical therapy.

Detailed approaches to the diagnostic and therapeutic options will be highlighted in specific sections of this chapter.

UPPER GASTROINTESTINAL BLEEDING

DIFFERENTIAL DIAGNOSIS

NONVARICEAL BLEEDING

Nonvariceal upper GI bleeding remains a significant cause of death and morbidity despite recent advances in pharmacologic and endoscopic therapy. The cause of nonvariceal bleeding encompasses a large array of diagnoses involving multiple organs above the ligament of Treitz and at times outside the GI tract. The causes and frequency of nonvariceal bleeding are listed in Table 76.4.[22]

Peptic Ulcer Disease

PUD traditionally refers to gastric and duodenal ulcers, gastritis, and duodenitis. A number of population-based and

Table 76.4 Causes of Nonvariceal Upper Gastrointestinal Bleeding

Diagnosis	Incidence (%)
Peptic ulcer	30-50
Mallory-Weiss tear	15-20
Erosive gastritis or duodenitis	10-15
Esophagitis	5-10
Malignancy	1-2
Angiodysplasia or vascular malformations	5
Other	5

From Ferguson CB, Mitchell RM: Nonvariceal upper gastrointestinal bleeding: Standard and new treatment. Gastroenterol Clin North Am 2005;34:607-621.

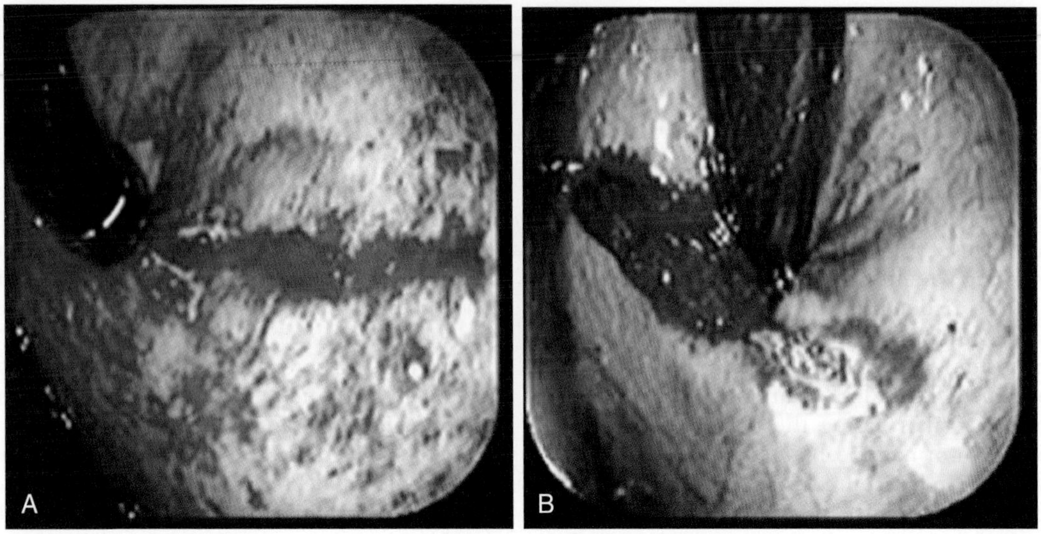

Figure 76.2 **A,** Mallory-Weiss tear in the cardia of the stomach. Active bleeding is seen. **B,** The same tear seen in A after injection with epinephrine and coagulation. The bleeding is controlled. (From Schmulewitz N, O'Connor JB: Esophageal disease caused by medication, radiation and internal trauma. In DiMarino AJ, Benjamin S [eds]: Gastrointestinal Disease: An Endoscopic Approach, 2nd ed. Thorofare, NJ, Slack, 2002, pp 245-262.)

prospective studies rank PUD as the most common source of acute upper GI bleeding, with PUD representing up to 50% of all such cases.[23] However, recent analysis from the Clinical Outcomes Research Initiative (CORI) database reported that the most common endoscopic finding in persons with acute upper GI bleeding was "mucosal abnormality" (40%), and gastric or duodenal ulcers were found in 20.6%.[24] Eradication of *Helicobacter pylori* and extensive use of PPIs are probably responsible for this observed decline in the frequency of PUD.

The most important factors predisposing to ulcer disease include acid, *H. pylori* infection, and NSAIDs; however, the role of some of these risk factors in inducing ulcer bleeding remains unclear. Indirect evidence regarding the role of acid in ulcer bleeding comes from data showing that acid suppression by PPIs in patients with active or recent bleeding reduces the risk for rebleeding.[25] Evidence of the association between NSAIDs and ulcer bleeding is strong and comes from both placebo-controlled and case-control studies.[26,27]

The pathogenesis of bleeding from an ulcer involves aneurysmal dilation with an intense arteritis associated with a marked inflammatory response.[28] When eroding into large vessels, ulcers can cause catastrophic bleeding. This most commonly occurs in the posterior portion of the duodenal bulb, where ulcers can erode directly into the pancreaticoduodenal artery.

Other Sources of Nonvariceal Upper Gastrointestinal Bleeding

Mallory-Weiss tears (MWTs) are mucosal and occasionally submucosal lacerations caused by sudden increases in pressure within the cardia and lower esophagus produced by retching. MWTs are responsible for 5% to 15% of upper GI bleeding.[23] The majority of upper GI bleeding caused by MWTs stops spontaneously and does not require any blood transfusion or endoscopic treatment. However, some cases are severe enough to require endoscopic hemostasis and occasionally angiography with embolization or even surgery. A history of retching on arrival at the emergency department is not always present.[29] Endoscopically, tears are usually 1.5 to 2 cm in length and occur at the gastroesophageal junction or, most commonly, in the proximal part of the stomach (Fig. 76.2).

Angiodysplasia, also referred to as arteriovenous malformation or vascular ectasia, is another source of upper GI bleeding and accounts for approximately 5% to 10% of cases.[23] It occurs in inherited syndromes such as hereditary hemorrhagic telangiectasia (Osler-Weber-Rendu syndrome) and blue rubber bleb nevus syndrome, but most cases are acquired.[30] The association of angiodysplasia with medical conditions such as renal failure, aortic stenosis, connective tissue disease (scleroderma), and von Willebrand disease has been recognized, but the evidence for these associations is limited.[23,31]

Dieulafoy's lesion is an underrecognized cause of upper GI bleeding and is described as a visible vessel protruding from a small mucosal defect without any underlying ulcer.[23] It has also been called "caliber-persistent artery" in submucosal tissue. Bleeding from Dieulafoy's lesion represents less than 5% of cases of upper GI bleeding.[32,33] The lesion is generally located on the lesser curvature within 6 cm of the gastroesophageal junction and can be difficult to detect because of its small size and normal surrounding mucosa (Fig. 76.3).[31]

Benign and malignant neoplasms are responsible for less than 5% of upper GI bleeding.[34] Bleeding can be the initial symptom of tumors originating from the esophagus, stomach, or small intestine. These neoplasms can be primary malignancies, such as adenocarcinoma of the esophagus, stomach, or duodenum; squamous cell carcinoma of the esophagus; and gastric or duodenal lymphomas.

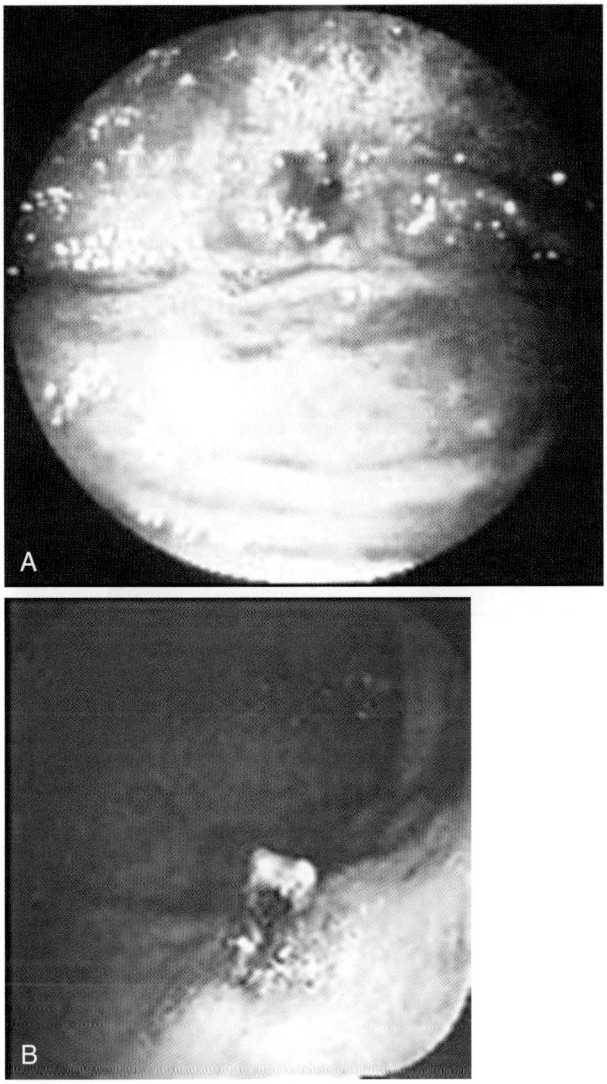

Figure 76.3 **A** and **B,** Endoscopic appearance of Dieulafoy's lesion in the proximal part of the stomach. (From Bashir RM, Al-Kawas FH: Vascular lesions of the stomach. In DiMarino AJ, Benjamin S [eds]: Gastrointestinal Disease: An Endoscopic Approach, 2nd ed. Thorofare, NJ, Slack, 2002, pp 535-550.)

Gastrointestinal stromal cell tumors (GISTs), carcinoid tumors, and lipomas are examples of benign tumors that can cause upper GI bleeding.[23]

Upper GI bleeding from an aortoenteric fistula is very rare but should be considered in the appropriate clinical setting (such as a patient with a history of aortic aneurysm repair). Fistulas are generally located in the third portion of the duodenum. Patients will frequently have a small hemorrhage first, known as a "herald bleed," that occurs before a major hemorrhage.[35]

Another rare cause of upper GI bleeding is hemobilia. It can occur after liver biopsy or hepatobiliary tree instrumentation (such as with endoscopic retrograde cholangiopancreatography [ERCP]) or from biliary tumors.

Hemosuccus pancreaticus is an uncommon cause of upper GI bleeding that occurs secondary to pseudoaneurysm formation and rupture into the pancreatic duct as a complication of a pancreatic pseudocyst in patients with chronic pancreatitis.[36]

BLEEDING SECONDARY TO PORTAL HYPERTENSION

Portal hypertension is defined by a hepatic venous pressure gradient (HVPG) greater than 5 mm Hg. HVPG represents the difference between portal vein pressure and free hepatic vein pressure. Portal hypertension is most commonly related to cirrhosis but can be secondary to a variety of other conditions. It has been classified as prehepatic, hepatic, and posthepatic, depending on the location of the obstruction to flow. Examples of noncirrhotic portal hypertension include portal vein thrombosis, Budd-Chiari syndrome, and constrictive pericarditis. In the presence of portal hypertension, the development of portosystemic collateral venous drainage results in the formation of varices. Varices develop most commonly in the distal portion of the esophagus and the stomach. Ectopic varices can be seen in the duodenum, jejunum, or colon; at the level of stomas (ileostomy and colostomy); and in the anorectal region.

Most portal hypertensive bleeding results from ruptured esophageal varices, but clinically significant bleeding can also be secondary to gastric varices, portal gastropathy, and ectopic varices.

Esophageal Varices

The incidence of varices among all cirrhotic patients is around 50%. However, if monitored long enough, varices eventually develop in most cirrhotics.[37] Variceal hemorrhage occurs in a third of cirrhotic patients with varices. Although portal hypertension is defined by an HVPG greater than 5 mm Hg, Garcia-Tsao and colleagues showed that varices do not develop and hence do not bleed as long as the HVPG is less than 12 mm Hg.[38] However, once this threshold is reached, there is poor correlation between the pressure gradient and the risk for bleeding. Other risk factors associated with variceal bleeding include the degree of liver disease (provided by Child's classification), variceal location and size (higher risk near the gastroesophageal junction and with large varices), and the presence of particular endoscopic signs (red wale markings suggestive of dilated longitudinal venules, cherry-red spots, and hematocystic spots consisting of small red dots or a reddish blister-like formation on the variceal surface and the white or purple nipple sign on a varix) (Fig. 76.4).[37,39]

Gastric Varices

Sarin and colleagues classified gastric varices into two groups: (1) isolated gastric varices (IGVs) and (2) gastroesophageal varices (GEVs) that are continuous with esophageal varices and extending to the cardia (GEV 1) or to the fundus (GEV 2).[40] The authors found that GEV 1 was the most common type of gastric varix but IGV was the type that bleeds the most. Although the incidence of bleeding from gastric varices is in the range of 10% to 36%, it is usually massive and associated with high mortality rates.[41]

DIAGNOSTIC EVALUATION

ENDOSCOPIC EXAMINATION

After the initial evaluation, resuscitation, and stabilization of a patient with upper GI bleeding, effort is directed at localization and treatment of the hemorrhage. Endoscopy has become the preferred diagnostic and therapeutic

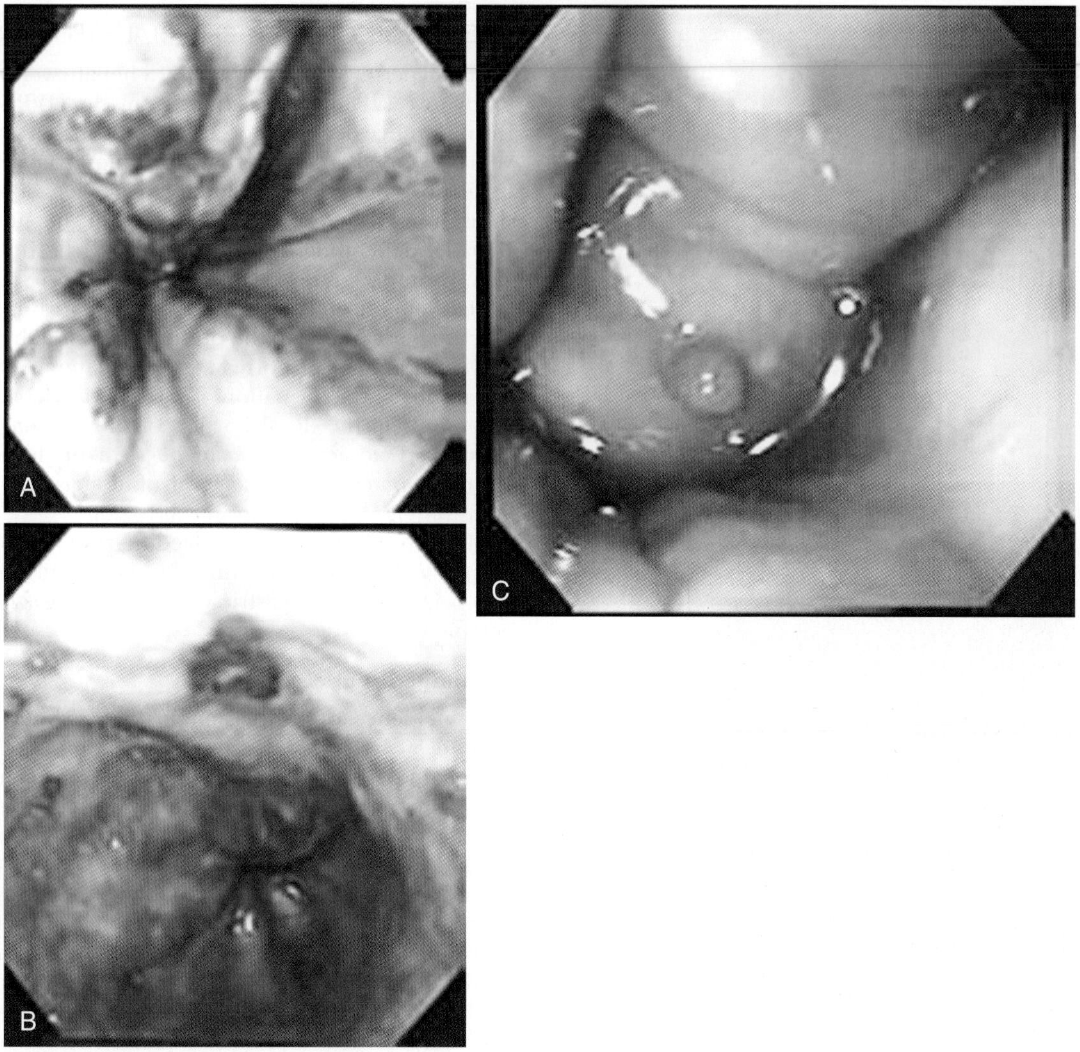

Figure 76.4 A to C, Esophageal varices with red color and white nipple signs. (From Sheikh RA, Prindiville TP, Trudeau W: Gastrointestinal bleeding in portal hypertension. In DiMarino AJ, Benjamin S [eds]: Gastrointestinal Disease: An Endoscopic Approach, 2nd ed. Thorofare, NJ, Slack, 2002, pp 605-644.)

modality for upper GI bleeding because of its accuracy and low complication rate. With its use, a specific diagnosis can be achieved in 95% of patients. The use of promotility agents such as metoclopramide and intravenous erythromycin (250 mg by intravenous bolus or 3 mg/kg over a 30-minute period) before the endoscopic examination can significantly improve mucosal visibility by promoting gastric motility and emptying of gastric contents.[42-44] An analysis of data from erythromycin trials showed that pre-endoscopic erythromycin was cost effective.[45]

The optimal timing of endoscopy remains a balance between clinical need and resources and is still subject to controversy.[22] Recent guidelines recommend the performance of upper endoscopy within 24 hours in patients with suspected nonvariceal upper GI bleeding.[11] Endoscopy has to be delayed or deferred in selected high-risk patients such as patients with bowel perforation or acute coronary syndrome. In a meta-analysis looking at timing of endoscopy, no significant reduction in rebleeding, surgery, or mortality rate was found with urgent endoscopy (1 to 12 hours) compared with later endoscopy (more than 12 hours).[11] In a subset of patients with bloody gastric lavage, length of hospital stay and blood tranfusion requirements were significantly lower in the urgent endoscopy group (within 12 hours).[46]

One major role of endoscopy is to identify stigmata of recent hemorrhage known to correlate well with an increased risk for rebleeding and thus a need for endoscopic therapy. Rates of rebleeding with these specific endoscopic findings are summarized in Table 76.5.[47]

NONENDOSCOPIC ASSESSMENT

When endoscopy is not able to be performed or has not yielded a definitive diagnosis, angiography and radionuclide imaging may be useful alternatives. Such endoscopic failures are most often related to anatomic situations (i.e., strictures or surgical alterations) preventing full endoscopy. Esophagography and upper GI series are no longer used as part of the diagnostic evaluation of patients with upper GI bleeding.

Table 76.5 Stigmata of Ulcer Hemorrhage and Risk for Recurrent Bleeding without Endoscopic Therapy

Endoscopic Finding	Risk for Recurrent Bleeding without Therapy
Active arterial (spurting) bleeding	Approaches 100%
Nonbleeding visible vessel ("pigmented protuberance")	Up to 50%
Nonbleeding adherent clot	30-35%
Ulcer oozing (without other stigmata)	10-27%
Flat spots	<8%
Clean-based ulcers	<3%

From ASGE Standards of Practice Committee: ASGE guideline: The role of endoscopy in acute nonvariceal upper GI-hemorrhage. Gastrointest Endosc 1999;49:145-152; and from ASGE Standards of Practice Committee: ASGE guideline: The role of endoscopy in acute nonvariceal upper GI-hemorrhage. Gastrointest Endosc 1999;49:145-152.

THERAPEUTIC ALTERNATIVES

NONVARICEAL BLEEDING

Pharmacotherapy

Acid suppression has been shown to play a role in the inactivation of pepsin, optimization of platelet function, and inhibition of fibrinolysis. Subsequently, clot stabilization and ulcer healing may be more effective and rapid within a less acidic environment. This constitutes the rationale for acid suppressive therapy in patients with bleeding peptic ulcers.

Treatment with PPI before the performance of upper endoscopy has been shown to down-stage the endoscopic lesion and decrease the need for endoscopic intervention.[11] However, a meta-analysis including studies assessing oral, intravenous, and high-dose PPI failed to show significant differences in rates of mortality, rebleeding, or surgery between, the pre-endoscopic PPI therapy and control groups.[48]

Once endoscopy is performed, the role of PPI therapy becomes more obvious. In patients found to have high-risk lesions treated endoscopically, an intravenous bolus followed by continuous-infusion PPI therapy is indicated.[11] The use of a continuous infusion is supported by data showing that maintenance of intragastric pH at greater than 6 after endoscopic hemostasis is associated with the lowest rebleeding rates and that this goal can be achieved only by bolus administration of a PPI followed by a constant infusion.[49] Strong data from several studies showed significant benefit in rebleeding, surgery, and mortality rates with high-dose intravenous PPI therapy after endoscopic treatment.[50] Other reports suggest similar benefits from low-dose intravenous and high-dose oral PPI therapy but these remain to be confirmed in larger studies.

Other agents with different mechanisms of action have been studied in patients with upper GI bleeding. A reduction in splanchnic blood flow with somatostatin and its analogs (such as octreotide) is an attractive measure in patients with upper GI bleeding and has been the subject of several trials, with conflicting results.[51-53] To date, the available data are not convincingly in favor of using these agents in patients with nonvariceal upper GI bleeding, even though some authors find them useful in patients who are bleeding uncontrollably while awaiting endoscopy or surgery or in whom surgery is contraindicated.[51]

Endoscopic Therapy

Endoscopic therapy for nonvariceal upper GI bleeding in patients with high-risk lesions has been shown to reduce the rate of rebleeding, need for surgery, and mortality rate.[54] It is indicated in patients with active bleeding, spurting arterial vessels, and nonbleeding visible vessels in an underlying ulcer.[47] When a clot is found in an ulcer bed, targeted irrigation in an attempt at dislodgement with treatment of the underlying lesion is indicated. If the clot remains adherent after irrigation, endoscopic therapy (injection followed by snaring of the clot) may be considered but intensive PPI therapy alone may be sufficient.[11] Different forms of endoscopic therapy include injection technique, thermal technique, and mechanical technique. In many cases a combination of these modalities is used to treat a single bleeding lesion or one at high risk of bleeding.

Injection therapy results in hemostasis, probably from a combination of vascular tamponade and pharmacologic effect of the injected agent. Agents used for injection include normal saline solution, epinephrine, and sclerosants such as ethanol, ethanolamine, and polidocanol. In addition to the local tamponade effect of normal saline solution and epinephrine, the latter has a vasoconstricting effect. Sclerosant agents work by causing direct tissue injury and thrombosis.[47] Another class of agents used during injection therapy includes thrombin, fibrin, and cyanoacrylate glue. These agents create a primary tissue seal at the bleeding site. Epinephrine at a concentration of 1:10,000 or 1:20,000 is the most commonly used agent, sometimes in conjunction with other agents or techniques.

Thermal therapy consists of the delivery of heat to the mucosa, which results in edema, coagulation of tissue proteins, and contraction of arteries. When heat is delivered through a contact probe, an additional effect is achieved by mechanical compression of the target artery before delivery of the heat.

Thermal energy can be delivered through noncontact techniques such as the neodymium:yttrium-aluminum-garnet (Nd:YAG) and argon lasers and argon plasma coagulation (APC). The laser technique has been abandoned because of its high cost and the high risk of complications associated with its use. In APC, the argon gas forms a plasma and acts as an electrical conductor of the current, thereby resulting in coagulation of superficial tissues. Despite comparable results with the heater probe technique when used for ulcer bleeding,[55] APC is used primarily for the treatment of superficial lesions such as vascular abnormalities.[47]

Contact thermal techniques refer to the delivery of heat through direct contact of the mucosa with heater probes or electrocautery probes (monopolar and bipolar probes). The heater probe is an aluminum cylinder that delivers a programmed amount of energy (heat) through its end or sides to the tissue. The catheter tip can also be used to apply firm pressure on the bleeding point or the visible vessel.

Electrocautery probes use an electrical current that passes from the electrode tip through the patient's body to a grounding plate (monopolar) or flows between two or more electrodes at the probe tip (bipolar or multipolar). The advantage of the bipolar (multipolar) probe is that the concentration of current at the level of the tip results in less depth of tissue injury and lower potential for perforation.

Mechanical therapy refers to the use of a device that causes physical tamponade of a bleeding site. Such devices include metallic clips, sewing devices, rubber band ligation, and endoloops. Metallic clips are the most studied of these devices and have shown variable success, probably because of the difficulty encountered with their placement. Some authors have suggested the use of clips in combination with other endoscopic treatments.[51]

The choice of endoscopic therapy depends on the stigmata of ulcer hemorrhage and the experience of the endoscopist. Monotherapy with epinephrine injection has been shown to be more effective than medical therapy in patients with high-risk lesions. However, it is inferior to other monotherapies (thermal or mechanical) or to combination therapy that uses two or more methods.[11] Epinephrine plus a second method significantly reduces rates of rebleeding, surgery, and mortality when compared to epinephrine alone.[56]

Angiographic Therapy

Angiography can be useful as a potential diagnostic and therapeutic modality in specific cases of upper GI bleeding when endoscopy cannot be performed or fails to reveal the bleeding site and when endoscopic hemostasis is unsuccessful. It is also considered in patients who are poor surgical candidates.

Angiographic or "transcatheter" intervention in cases of upper GI bleeding involves two techniques: infusion of vasoconstricting medication and mechanical occlusion (embolization) of the arterial supply responsible for the hemorrhage. Vasopressin infusion induces vasoconstriction and results in cessation of bleeding in 70% to 80% of cases initially, but rebleeding occurs in up to 20%. Complications can range from problems related to arterial access to pulmonary edema and myocardial depression.[57] Vasopressin infusion has lost favor with the advent of embolization. Transcatheter embolization has become the mainstay for the radiographic treatment of nonvariceal upper GI bleeding and comes second after endoscopic therapy in most centers.[58] The embolic material used can be temporary (such as a gelatin sponge and autologous clot) or permanent (such as coils). Clinical success with embolization ranges from 52% to 91%. Potential complications of embolization include ischemia and perforation.[58]

Surgical Therapy

When endoscopic hemostasis fails to control the bleeding or when hemorrhage recurs after successful control of bleeding, surgical intervention provides an alternative therapeutic option. The main goal of surgery is control of active bleeding and prevention of exsanguination, with a secondary aim to prevent recurrent ulceration. The choice of operation depends on the location of the bleeding lesion and the surgeon's expertise. Truncal vagotomy with antrectomy and vagotomy with pyloroplasty are examples of operations performed in cases of nonvariceal upper GI bleeding. Total gastrectomy is rarely indicated. Because recurrent ulcers can be prevented by avoiding NSAIDs, eliminating *H. pylori* if present, or administering prophylactic PPI therapy, most ulcer operations for acute bleeding focus on oversewing the ulcer rather than performing the more definitive surgeries just listed.

VARICEAL BLEEDING

Pharmacotherapy

Pharmacologic agents used in the treatment of acute variceal bleeding are aimed at reducing portal pressure by either decreasing portal blood flow or reducing intrahepatic resistance. Infusion of vasoactive agents constitutes an adjunct to endoscopic therapy and often precedes endoscopy when suspicion of variceal bleeding is high.

Vasopressin, terlipressin, somatostatin, and somatostatin analogs (octreotide and lanreotide) all induce constriction of the splanchnic vasculature and result in a decrease in portal blood flow. Vasopressin causes systemic vasoconstriction, as well as splanchnic vasoconstriction, and can lead to adverse effects such as myocardial ischemia and infarction and cerebrovascular accidents.[59] These dangerous side effects led to the combination of vasopressin with other agents and the search for analogs with a better safety profile.

In one study, the combination of vasopressin with nitroglycerin resulted in a reduction in side effects and improved efficacy over vasopressin alone.[59] Nitroglycerin, a potent venous dilator, decreases the hemodynamic side effects of vasopressin and at the same time reduces intrahepatic resistance, thereby resulting in a further reduction in portal pressure.

Terlipressin is a synthetic analog of vasopressin with a longer duration of action and fewer side effects than vasopressin. Unlike other vasoactive agents, terlipressin has been shown to reduce mortality rate when compared with placebo.[60] At present, terlipressin is not available in the United States.

Somatostatin is a naturally occurring peptide that induces splanchnic vasoconstriction without affecting the systemic circulation and thus results in a decrease in portal pressure. When compared with vasopressin, somatostatin was equivalent in bleeding control but had significantly fewer side effects.[61] Further data suggested that somatostatin has the greatest effect when used in conjunction with endoscopic therapy.[62,63] Octreotide, a somatostatin analog, is approved for use in variceal bleeding in the United States. Meta-analyses looking at the efficacy of octreotide led to controversial results.[61,64] One meta-analysis of trials of somatostatin analogs in general showed a negligible effect.[65] However, octreotide appears to be useful as an adjunct to endoscopic therapy.[66,67] At present, because of its excellent safety profile and easy availability, octreotide (50-μg bolus followed by a 50-μg/hour continuous infusion for 3 to 5 days) is almost always used in conjunction with endoscopic therapy.

The use of prophylactic antibiotics in patients with variceal bleeding has been shown to decrease the mortality rate in several randomized controlled trials.[62] The rationale behind antibiotic prophylaxis derives from the fact that bacterial infection is present in up to 20% of patients with cirrhosis who are admitted with variceal bleeding and that infection develops in as many as 50% of patients while hospitalized.[68] The mortality rate is significantly higher in infected cirrhotic patients than in noninfected cirrhotics.[69,70] Furthermore, infected cirrhotic patients have a higher rate of variceal rebleeding.[71] This is probably due to the presence of cytokines and endotoxins that induce hematologic abnormalities such as platelet dysfunction and activation of the coagulation and fibrinolytic systems.[62] A recently updated meta-analysis showed that antibiotic prophylaxis significantly reduced the all-cause mortality rate, bacterial infection mortality rate, rebleeding events, and length of hospital stay.[72] Prophylaxis benefits were observed regardless of the type of antibiotic used. Nonabsorbable antibiotics, quinolones, and more recently cephalosporins have all been used with good success. Recent concerns have been raised about bacterial resistance and potential decreased benefit with quinolones in some geographic areas.[72]

The use of recombinant factor VIIa in cirrhotic patients with upper GI bleeding has been attractive because cirrhotic patients will often have deficiencies in coagulation factors and factor VII in particular. In a randomized controlled trial investigating the use of this factor, Bosch and coworkers[73] demonstrated benefit in the rate of rebleeding only in the subgroup of patients with advanced cirrhosis (Child-Pugh grades B and C). A 2010 retrospective study (Flower and colleagues) showed no benefits in mortality rate reduction when recombinant factor VII was used in patients with upper GI bleeding.[74] Further studies are needed before the routine use of this expensive therapy can be recommended.

Endoscopic Therapy

Endoscopic sclerotherapy and endoscopic band ligation are the mainstays of therapy for acute variceal bleeding. These procedures are successful in achieving hemostasis in 80% to 90% of patients.[62]

Sclerotherapy consists of intravariceal or paravariceal injection of a sclerosant agent such as sodium tetradecyl sulfate or ethanolamine. These agents provoke a severe inflammatory reaction within or around the varix that leads to variceal thrombosis and obliteration. Despite its high effectiveness in controlling bleeding, the complication rate with sclerotherapy can be as high as 40%.[75] Complications range from local effects, such as deep ulcers causing rebleeding, odynophagia, and in some cases perforation to bacteremia and systemic complications such as pleural and pericardial effusion. Esophageal stricture is the most common long-term side effect of sclerotherapy. Once the acute bleeding is controlled, repeated sessions of sclerotherapy are required to eradicate the varices and prevent rebleeding.

Endoscopic band ligation consists of the placement of a ligating device on the tip of the endoscope, and elastic rings are placed over the targeted varix (Fig. 76.5). With the availability of multiband ligating devices, 5 to 10 bands can be deployed in one session. Band ligation has a lower rate of complication (including the rebleeding rate in some but not all studies[76]) than sclerotherapy does, but it can be difficult to perform during acute bleeding.[62] Superficial mucosal ulceration occurs when the elastic ring and underlying tissue slough off. Transient chest discomfort and dysphagia are common after band ligation. Band ligation also has the advantage of achieving eradication of varices with fewer endoscopic sessions than are typically needed for sclerotherapy.[76]

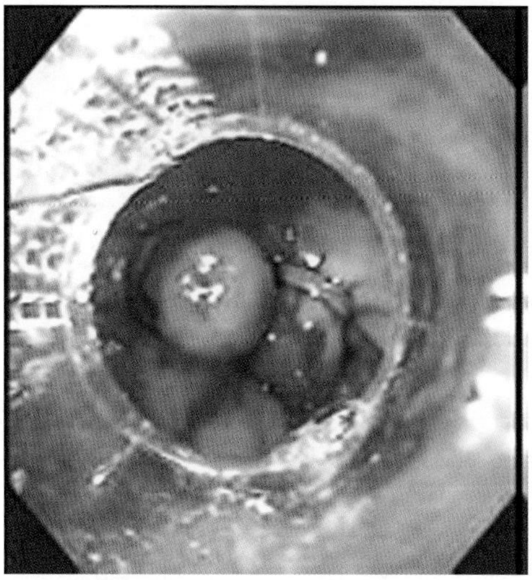

Figure 76.5 Esophageal varices immediately after band ligation. (From Bashir RM, Al Kawas FH: Vascular lesions of the stomach. In DiMarino AJ, Benjamin S [eds]: Gastrointestinal Disease: An Endoscopic Approach, 2nd ed. Thorofare, NJ, Slack, 2002, pp 245-262.)

A meta-analysis of 10 randomized clinical trials showed an almost significant benefit of endoscopic band ligation over sclerotherapy in the initial control of bleeding.[77] A practice guideline by the American Association for the Study of Liver Diseases recommends the use of endoscopic band ligation as the preferred form of endoscopic therapy and the use of sclerotherapy when band ligation is not technically feasible.[67]

Balloon Tamponade

The use of balloon tamponade in the control of active variceal bleeding comes as a last resort when other forms of therapy are not available or fail to achieve hemostasis. Three balloons have been used for this purpose: the Minnesota tube, the Sengstaken-Blakemore tube, and the Linton-Nachlas tube. Control of bleeding with these tubes depends on patient selection, the concomitant use of other therapies, and the experience of the staff using them. With the advent of other therapies and the increasing experience of endoscopists in sclerotherapy and endoscopic banding, experience in the use of tamponade balloons decreased substantially. A major concern with the use of these tubes is the high risk of rebleeding after deflation of the balloon, in addition to the risk of esophageal rupture. Balloon tamponade should be used only as a temporary means of stabilization and as a bridge to a more definitive form of therapy. Figure 76.6 illustrates the steps used to control bleeding with a balloon. The use of a fully covered self-expandable metallic stent has shown some promise in control of variceal bleeding.[78]

Transjugular Intrahepatic Portosystemic Shunt

The transjugular intrahepatic portosystemic shunt (TIPS) procedure involves the creation of a low-resistance channel between the portal vein and the hepatic vein through which blood is shunted from the portal to the systemic circulation.

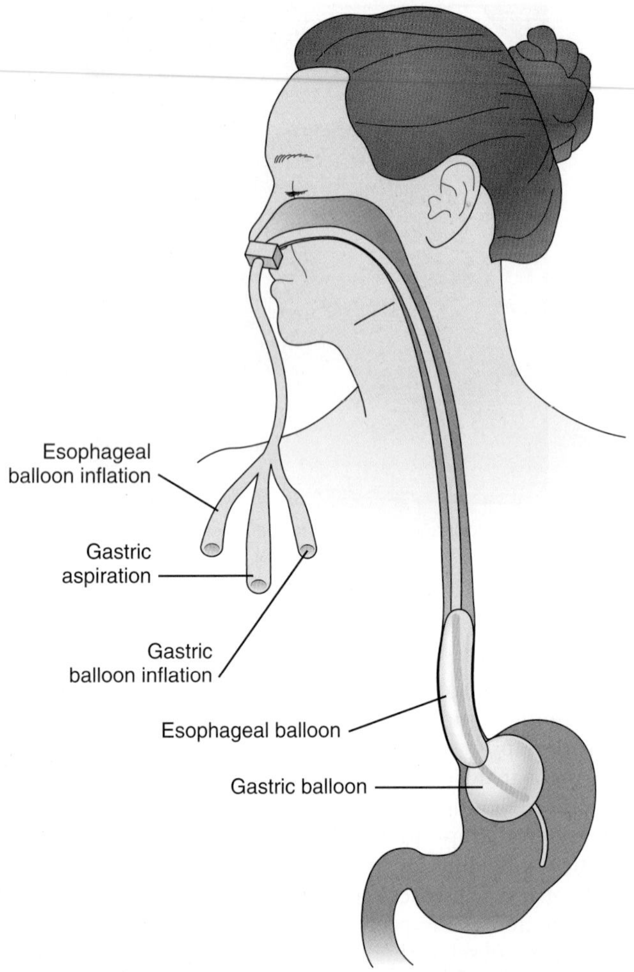

Figure 76.6 Sengstaken-Blakemore tube. The tube is passed to at least the 50-cm mark. The gastric balloon is then inflated with the full recommended volume of air (usually 450-500 mL). Portable chest radiograph should be obtained to check for proper placement. The tube is pulled back gently until resistance is felt against the diaphragm. If bleeding persists from the aspiration port, the esophageal balloon is inflated to the lowest pressure needed to stop bleeding (usually 30-45 mm Hg).

Via an angiographic technique, an expandable metal stent is deployed across this channel and results in a significant decrease in portal pressure. This technique allows the creation of a portosystemic shunt without requiring general anesthesia and major surgery. TIPS is indicated in situations in which acute variceal bleeding is refractory to endoscopic and pharmacologic therapy. It has been shown to control bleeding in more than 90% of patients, with a rebleeding rate of less than 20%.[79,80] In 2010 data (Garcia-Tsao and colleagues) showed that early TIPS (within 24 to 48 hours of admission) was associated with significant decrease in mortality rate in high-risk patients (with HVPG >20 mm Hg or with Child-Pugh class C disease).[81] However, the mortality rate after the TIPS procedure in the setting of acute uncontrollable variceal bleeding is between 30% and 40%.[62] A major complication associated with this procedure is the development of encephalopathy in 10% to 20% of patients. Stenosis and complete occlusion of the shunt occur in 5% to 15% of the cases, requiring revision.

Surgical Therapy

Surgical creation of portosystemic shunts has been used for decompression of the portal system to treat and prevent variceal bleeding. The various forms of surgical shunts include portacaval shunts, distal splenorenal shunts, and partial shunts. Revascularization of the esophagus is another surgical option for the treatment of variceal bleeding. Interest in surgery has declined over the years because of the advent of the less invasive endoscopic and TIPS procedures. At present, surgery is considered only when medical and endoscopic therapy fails to control bleeding and TIPS is not available.[62]

STRESS-RELATED MUCOSAL DISEASE

The term *stress-related mucosal disease* (SRMD) covers a spectrum of conditions ranging from superficial mucosal damage to focal deep mucosal damage (stress ulcers). The terms *stress ulcer, stress gastritis, stress erosions,* and *stress lesions* are used interchangeably in the literature. SRMD is defined as mucosal abnormalities of the upper GI tract that occur with extreme physiologic stress, typically in the ICU.

The incidence of endoscopically documented gastric lesions in patients in the ICU ranges from 74% to 100%.[82] The lesions are typically, but not exclusively, located in the fundus and body of the stomach. However, most of these lesions are of little significance because healing occurs rapidly. Clinically evident bleeding, defined as blood in a nasogastric aspirate, hematemesis, and melena, occurs in 5% to 25% of patients in the ICU. Clinically important bleeding, however, is defined as overt bleeding associated with one of the following within 24 hours of the onset of the bleeding: a drop in systolic blood pressure of greater than 20 mm Hg, an increase in the pulse rate of more than 20 beats per minute and a 10-mm Hg drop in systolic blood pressure, or a decrease in hemoglobin of greater than 2 g/dL requiring blood transfusion and failure of hemoglobin to increase by the number of units transfused minus 2 g/dL.[83] Clinically important bleeding affects only 3% to 6% of critically ill patients.[84]

The pathogenesis of SRMD involves a disruption in the balance between aggressive and protective factors that leads to gastric mucosal damage. Adequate microcirculation in the upper GI tract is the most important defense mechanism against luminal aggressors such as acid and enzyme secretion, as well as infection. The role of the microcirculation is to provide nutrients and eliminate toxic oxygen-derived free radicals. In the presence of severe physiologic stress, disruption of intramucosal blood flow leads to a number of events, including the formation of toxic oxygen-derived radicals, a decrease in the synthesis of cytoprotective prostaglandins and mucus production, and a reduction in bicarbonate secretion resulting in an increase in intramural acidity (Fig. 76.7).[82,84] These events create a favorable setting for mucosal injury and ulceration.[85,86] Subsequent reperfusion also plays a major role in the development of lesions.[86]

Identification of critically ill patients at risk for significant bleeding from SRMD has been the subject of several studies. A landmark study by Cook and associates[83] demonstrated a

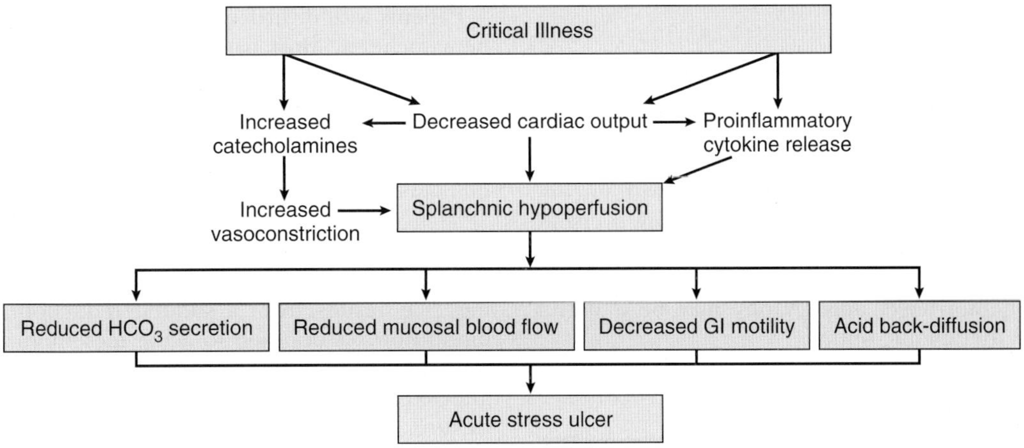

Figure 76.7 Pathophysiology of stress ulcers. (From Mutlu GM, Mutlu EA, Factor P: GI complications in patients receiving mechanical ventilation. Chest 2001;119:1222-1241.)

significant increase in the risk for bleeding from SRMD in patients requiring mechanical ventilation for more than 48 hours and in those with coagulopathy (defined as thrombocytopenia [platelet count <50,000/mL^3], an international normalized ratio above 1.5, or a partial thromboplastin time more than 2.0 times the control value). Other risk factors such as shock, sepsis, renal failure, liver failure, and glucocorticoids were identified, but the association with bleeding was not statistically significant. Risk factors associated with the presence of SRMD (not necessarily bleeding) include recent major surgery, major trauma, severe burns (Curling's ulcers), head trauma or coma (Cushing's ulcers), and multiple organ failure.[87-89] Further understanding of the risk factors associated with bleeding from SRMD will help in directing prophylactic therapy to patients who will benefit most from this therapy.[90]

The reported mortality rates in critically ill patients with bleeding from SRMD ranges from 46% to 77%.[83,91,92] These high rates are most likely due to the underlying disease and not directly related to GI bleeding. However, they reveal the importance of significant bleeding as a sign of the degree of severity of the primary illness.

PROPHYLAXIS

As mentioned earlier, the risk for bleeding from SRMD is significantly increased in patients undergoing prolonged mechanical ventilation and in those with coagulopathy. Such patients should benefit from the different forms of prophylaxis available.

The role of enteral nutrition in prophylaxis for SRMD is controversial.[93,94] The rationale behind the use of enteral nutrition derives from its ability to improve blood flow to the stomach and sustain mucosal immunity and integrity.[95] However, experimental data in hemodynamically compromised animals showed an increase in tissue hypoxia when enteral nutrition was administered.[96] Furthermore, in one study the degree of acid suppression was reduced in patients receiving H_2 receptor antagonists (H_2RAs) or PPIs with concomitant enteral feeding.[97]

When compared with placebo, antacids have been shown to decrease bleeding in patients with SRMD.[98] However, antacids require frequent dosing and monitoring of pH and are not practical to use, especially with the advent of other effective agents for prophylaxis.

Sucralfate works by coating the gastric mucosa and forming a thin protective layer between the mucosa and the gastric acid in the lumen without affecting acid secretion and intragastric pH. The use of sucralfate for the prevention of bleeding in patients with SRMD gained interest because of theoretical concern about gram-negative bacterial overgrowth when the pH of the stomach is increased by the use of H_2RAs or PPIs, which can potentially lead to nosocomial pneumonia. Conflicting results were reported regarding this issue, but a large trial by Cook and colleagues in which ranitidine and sucralfate were compared showed no significant difference in the development of nosocomial pneumonia.[99] In this same trial, the incidence of clinically important bleeding was significantly lower with ranitidine. Other studies demonstrated comparable efficacy between sucralfate and antacids and H_2RAs in terms of prevention of SRMD.[100,101] One drawback to the use of sucralfate is that it may decrease the absorption of other concomitantly administered oral drugs.

Intravenous H_2RAs are the most widely used pharmacologic agents for the prophylaxis of bleeding in patients with SRMD. A meta-analysis of studies looking at the role of H_2RAs in SRMD demonstrated a decrease in the incidence of clinically important bleeding.[98] Furthermore, H_2RAs were more effective than antacids in preventing bleeding.[98,102] Despite better control of gastric pH with continuous infusion of H_2RAs, bolus infusion has been shown to be as effective in preventing bleeding.[98,103] One major concern is the development of tolerance to H_2RAs when administered for a prolonged period.

In recent years PPIs have gained wider use in the prevention of bleeding from SRMD because of their ease of dosing, effective and predictable acid suppression, lack of need for regular gastric pH monitoring, and lack of tolerance as encountered with H_2RAs.[95] A recent meta-analysis compared the efficacy of PPIs versus H_2RAs in the prophylaxis of stress-related mucosal bleeding in critically ill patients at risk of bleeding. It demonstrated that PPI prophylaxis significantly decreased rates of clinically significant bleeding compared with H_2RAs without affecting the development of nosocomial pneumonia or mortality rates.[104]

TREATMENT

Endoscopy is the principal diagnostic and therapeutic procedure used in patients with bleeding from SRMD. The same endoscopic techniques used for hemostasis in peptic ulcer bleeding are used in SRMD when an actively bleeding lesion is found. Surgery is reserved for patients with uncontrolled hemorrhage and usually involves vagotomy, oversewing of bleeding sites, and in rare cases, subtotal or total gastrectomy.[95] In poor surgical candidates with severe uncontrolled hemorrhage, angiography may be a useful diagnostic and therapeutic option.

LOWER GASTROINTESTINAL BLEEDING

DIFFERENTIAL DIAGNOSIS

Lower GI bleeding is defined as bleeding that originates from a source distal to the ligament of Treitz. It is caused by a diverse range of bleeding sources and can range from trivial to life-threatening bleeding. It can also be acute, arbitrarily defined as less than 3 days' duration and possibly resulting in hemodynamic compromise, or chronic, extending over a period of several days or longer and usually less severe in terms of the amount of blood loss.[105] Sources of lower GI bleeding and their incidence from several large studies are listed in Table 76.6.[106-113]

DIVERTICULAR BLEEDING

Diverticular bleeding, the most common source of lower GI bleeding, accounts for up to 40% of cases.[105] Diverticular disease is more common in the elderly. It affects up to two thirds of people older than 80 years. Only 3% to 15% of patients with diverticulosis experience diverticular bleeding.[105]

Patients with diverticular bleeding typically have painless hematochezia. Most patients will stop bleeding spontaneously, but the bleeding can recur in 10% to 40% of cases.[114]

The bleeding is thought to occur after repetitive trauma to the vasa recta (nutrient arteries) that stretch over the diverticular dome.[115] NSAIDs have been associated with increased risk for diverticular bleeding.[116]

ISCHEMIC COLITIS AND OTHER FORMS OF COLITIS

Ischemic colitis accounts for up to 19% of lower GI bleeding.[105] It results from a sudden reduction in mesenteric blood flow. As opposed to acute mesenteric ischemia, this reduction is transient and reversible. The typical regions affected are the "watershed" areas of the colon: the splenic flexure, the rectosigmoid junction, and the right colon. Ischemia is precipitated by any event that compromises colonic blood flow. Clinically, patients have a sudden onset of abdominal pain, followed by hematochezia within 24 hours. Endoscopically, ischemia is suspected in the presence of bluish hemorrhagic nodules from submucosal bleeding, cyanotic or necrotic mucosa with hemorrhagic ulcerations, or segmental distribution with an abrupt transition between injured and normal mucosa (Fig. 76.8).[105] Most cases of ischemic colitis resolve spontaneously with supportive treatment. Rare cases require surgery (if peritoneal signs are present) or develop chronic ischemic colitis with stricture formation. Ischemic colitis is a common cause of lower GI bleeding in patients in the ICU because of the frequent hemodynamic instability in this setting.[117]

Infectious colitis, radiation colitis, and inflammatory bowel diseases can also result in bloody diarrhea, but the bleeding is rarely severe.

ANGIODYSPLASIA

Estimates of angiodysplasia as a source of lower GI bleeding vary widely and reach 37% in some reports.[108] Current data suggest that acute bleeding caused by angiodysplasia is less

Table 76.6 Sources of Lower Gastrointestinal Bleeding

	No. of Affected Patients (%)							
Study	Diverticulosis	Angiodysplasia	Cancer/ Polyp	Colitis/ Ulcers*	Anorectal†	Others‡	Unknown	Totals
Jensen and Machicado[107]	13 (20)	24 (37)	9 (14)	7 (11)	3 (5)	3 (5)	5 (8)	64
Longstreth[108]	91 (41)	6 (3)	20 (9)	35 (16)	10 (5)	31 (14)	26 (12)	219
Farrands and Taylor[109]	30 (29)	6 (6)	38 (36)	20 (19)	5 (5)	5 (5)	1 (1)	105
Bramley et al.[110]	60 (24)	17 (7)	25 (10)	52 (21)	22 (9)	11 (4)	64 (25)	251
Colacchio et al.[111]	98 (55)	13 (7)	14 (8)	11 (6)	5 (3)	5 (3)	32 (18)	178
Richter et al.[112]	51 (48)	13 (12)	12 (11)	6 (6)	3 (3)	7 (6)	15 (14)	107
Rossini et al.[113]	60 (15)	16 (4)	122 (30)	92 (22)	0 (0)	47 (11)	72 (18)	409
Totals	403 (33)	95 (8)	240 (19)	223 (18)	48 (4)	109 (8)	215 (16)	1333

*Includes inflammatory bowel disease, infectious colitis, ischemic colitis, radiation colitis, vasculitis, and inflammation of unknown origin.
†Includes hemorrhoids, anal fissure, and idiopathic rectal ulcers.
‡Includes postpolypectomy bleeding, aortocolonic fistula, trauma from fecal impaction, and anastomotic bleeding.
Studies cited in this table may be found in the complete list of references for this chapter provided online.
From Zuckerman GR, Prakash C: Acute lower intestinal bleeding. Part II: Etiology, therapy, and outcomes. Gastrointest Endosc 1999;49:228-238.

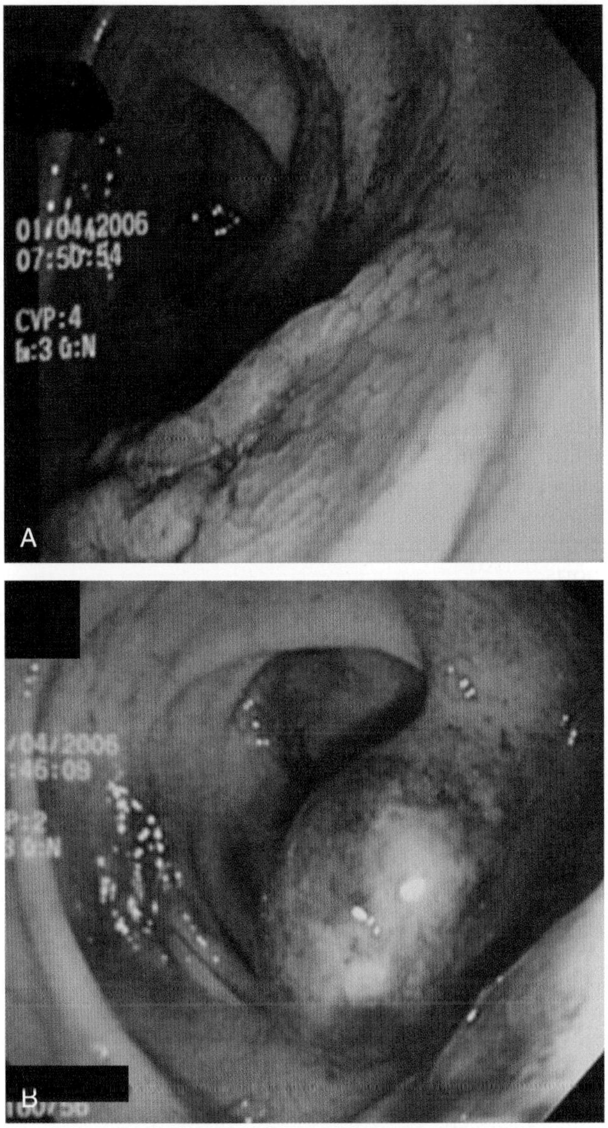

Figure 76.8 A and **B,** Ischemic colitis.

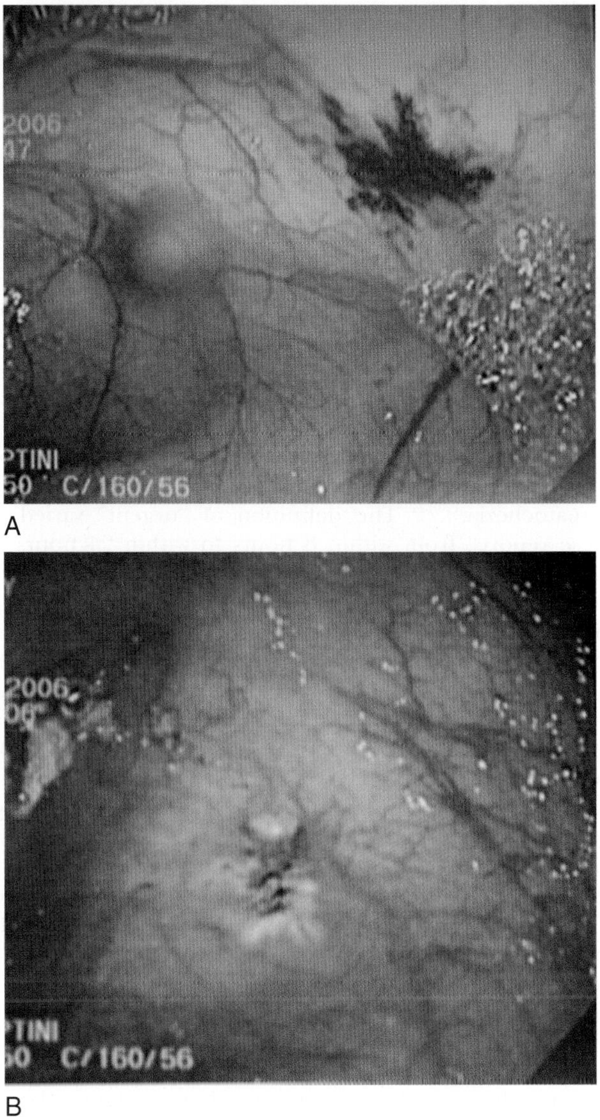

Figure 76.9 A, Angiodysplasia in the cecum. **B,** Same lesion after thermal therapy (electrocauterization).

frequent than previously thought, with most cases demonstrating iron deficiency anemia and occult blood loss.[115] These lesions are seen predominantly in the elderly. They appear endoscopically as red, flat lesions with ectatic blood vessels radiating from a central feeding vessel, usually in the right colon (Fig. 76.9). Overt bleeding from angiodysplasia is usually brisk and painless and cannot be distinguished from diverticular bleeding. Endoscopic treatment is highly effective and safe and prevents bleeding episodes from recurring.

OTHER SOURCES OF LOWER GASTROINTESTINAL BLEEDING

Acute significant bleeding from colonic neoplasia and polyps is uncommon despite reports in which it accounts for up to 36% of cases.[112] Cancer and polyps are thought to bleed from erosions on the surface.

Postpolypectomy bleeding occurs in 1% to 6% of patients undergoing colonoscopic polypectomy.[115] Bleeding can be immediate or delayed up to 3 weeks after the procedure. Risk factors for postpolypectomy bleeding include large size, sessile morphologic appearance, and right colonic location.[118]

Anorectal sources of lower GI bleeding include hemorrhoids, anorectal fissures, stercoral ulcers, and proctitis. Hemorrhoids can cause significant bleeding and may sometimes require endoscopic or surgical intervention. Bleeding from rectal ulcers is common in elderly bedridden patients and in critically ill patients.[106]

Small bowel sources of lower GI bleeding include angiodysplasia (most frequent), lymphoma, small bowel ulcers, and Crohn's disease.[115] Small bowel lesions are typically more difficult to identify and require more diagnostic procedures.[119]

DIAGNOSTIC EVALUATION

COLONOSCOPY

After initial evaluation, stabilization, and exclusion of an upper GI source, management shifts to localization of the lower GI bleeding site. Colonoscopy is an attractive choice in this setting because it offers the best opportunity for early diagnosis and subsequent management. In the past, colonoscopy used to be performed in an expectant manner, after cessation of bleeding and colonic preparation. Concern about poor visibility, the potential for complications, and the adverse effects of bowel preparation in the setting of bleeding is behind the reluctance in performing "urgent" colonoscopy. Over the past decade, early colonoscopy has gained interest in the management of lower GI bleeding. Several reports have shown that early (or urgent) colonoscopy is safe and has high diagnostic yield in patients with hematochezia.[120-124] The definition of "urgent" varied in these reports, from within 8 hours to within 24 hours of initial evaluation. This approach was also associated with shorter hospital stay.[125] Bowel preparation is generally recommended before urgent colonoscopy to improve visibility and prevent complications related to poor visibility. Polyethylene glycol lavage solution by mouth or through a nasogastric tube is commonly used in these cases. It can be administered at a rate of approximately 1 L every 30 to 45 minutes.[105] Some authors have proposed the use of colonoscopy without bowel preparation and have shown high diagnostic yield with this approach.[126] Despite the fact that urgent colonoscopy improves the diagnostic yield and leads to more frequent endoscopic therapy, there is still controversy regarding its impact on important outcomes such as mortality rate, rebleeding, and the need for surgery.[122,124] Jensen and colleagues[122] showed that urgent colonoscopy with endoscopic treatment in a group of patients with active diverticular bleeding (versus a historical group that did not receive endoscopic treatment) may prevent recurrent bleeding and the need for surgery. Another randomized trial compared urgent colonoscopy with a standard care algorithm in which radionuclide scanning, followed, if positive, by angiography, was used in patients with suspected active bleeding versus expectant colonoscopy in those without active bleeding. This trial showed that a definite source of bleeding was found more often in urgent colonoscopy patients. However, no difference in mortality rate, surgery, and rebleeding was found in the two groups.[124] A more recent trial looking at the benefit of urgent versus elective colonoscopy (<12 hours vs. 36 to 60 hours from presentation) showed no evidence of improving clinical outcomes such as rebleeding, transfusion requirements, and hospital length of stay. A major limitation of this trial was that the study was terminated before reaching the prespecified sample size.[127] In conclusion, the optimal timing of colonoscopy in patients with lower GI bleeding has not been determined and it is unknown if early performance of colonoscopy affects major outcomes such as rebleeding and mortality rate.[15]

RADIONUCLIDE SCANNING

The use of radionuclide scanning (also known as a technetium-labeled red blood cell scan) in patients with lower GI bleeding is highly controversial. It has been used for several decades as a method for localization of the bleeding source.[115] A main advantage of radionuclide scanning is its sensitivity for bleeding at a rate as low as 0.05 to 0.1 mL/minute, in addition to its noninvasive nature.[115] It also can be repeated in cases of intermittent bleeding. On the other hand, this diagnostic modality lacks therapeutic capability, has variable accuracy, and may delay other diagnostic and therapeutic procedures. A review of data from several studies of radionuclide scanning for lower GI bleeding in which radionuclide scintigraphy findings were confirmed by a different test found the accuracy of a positive test to be 66%.[15] Localization improves when scans are positive within 2 hours of injection. A common practice in the setting of ongoing lower GI bleeding is to perform radionuclide scanning as a screening test before angiography and in some cases as a guide to surgery. The problem with this approach is the inconsistent and widely variable accuracy and the high rate of false-positive results in different reports.[115,128,129]

ANGIOGRAPHY

Angiography is less sensitive than radionuclide scanning in the detection of active bleeding. It can detect bleeding at a rate of 0.5 to 1.0 mL/minute. In addition to its role in accurate localization of bleeding lesions, angiography offers therapeutic possibilities. As with radionuclide scanning, the ability of angiography to detect the bleeding source varies widely among studies, from 20% to 70%.[115] This variation is due to several factors, including patient selection (higher diagnostic yield in patients with positive radionuclide scanning), the severity and intermittent nature of the bleeding, procedural delay, and venous or small vessel bleeding.[115] In one study, a systolic blood pressure of less than 90 mm Hg and a requirement of at least 5 units of blood within a 24-hour period have been shown to predict a positive angiography (85% when both criteria were present).[130] Angiography is usually performed in patients with ongoing lower GI bleeding with or without a positive radionuclide scan. This sequence in management was the standard approach to ongoing bleeding up until recently, when colonoscopy started gaining interest in the setting of acute bleeding (as opposed to expectant elective colonoscopy). When angiographic therapy fails or is not available after localization of the bleeding, the findings are used to guide surgical resection. Angiography can cause serious complications such as contrast reactions, arterial thrombosis and dissection, and catheter site infection and bleeding. Thus, it should be used in carefully selected patients.

COMPUTED TOMOGRAPHY

CT gained interest in the setting of GI bleeding after the recent introduction of multidetector row CT. It enables the accurate acquisition of arterial images, which can show contrast extravasation in areas of active bleeding.[15] It can detect bleeding rates as low as 0.3 to 0.5 mL/minute. The yield for lower GI bleeding ranges from 25% to 95% and is highest in severe ongoing bleeding. The advantages of CT are its wide availability and the added diagnostic yield of cross-sectional imaging, but exposure to radiation and contrast and, like radionuclide scanning, the inability to deliver therapy constitute some of the disadvantages of this technique.[15]

THERAPEUTIC ALTERNATIVES

ENDOSCOPIC THERAPY

Data on the effectiveness of endoscopic therapy for lesions causing lower GI bleeding are limited. However, the experience from published series suggests that this form of therapy is likely to be beneficial. Methods of endoscopic hemostasis are similar to those used for upper GI bleeding and include injection therapy, thermal therapy (APC and heater and electrocautery probes), and mechanical therapy (hemoclips).[131] Several studies showed that clipping is very effective modality for diverticular bleeding with a low rate of early rebleeding.[15]

ANGIOGRAPHIC THERAPY

When angiography identifies the bleeding site in cases of lower GI bleeding, hemostasis can be achieved by the intra-arterial infusion of vasopressin or superselective embolization. Infusion of vasopressin can control bleeding in up to 91% of cases,[131] but complications develop in 10% to 20% and include arrhythmia, pulmonary edema, and ischemia.[131] Furthermore, rebleeding occurs in as many as 50% of cases.[131] In early studies, transcatheter embolization carried a high risk for bowel infarction, but current superselective techniques using smaller catheters with various agents (gelatin sponge, microcoils, and polyvinyl alcohol particles) appear to be more effective and safer than the old techniques. Review of several studies using superselective techniques showed that immediate hemostasis was achieved in 96% of cases and rebleeding within 30 days occurred in 22%.[15] Since the advent of these new techniques, embolization has become the preferred modality when angiographic therapy is contemplated.

SURGICAL THERAPY

Surgery is indicated in cases of recurrent bleeding (especially diverticular) and massive ongoing bleeding with high transfusion requirements (generally more than 6 units of packed red blood cells in a 24-hour period).[105] Accurate localization of the site of bleeding preoperatively is crucial so that segmental rather than subtotal colectomy can be performed. Unfortunately, the accuracy of radionuclide scanning in localization of the bleeding is variable, and hence it should not be used as a guide for surgery. Colonoscopy and angiography may be used as a guide for surgery in cases in which bleeding is initially identified and possibly treated through these modalities and then recurs and requires surgery.

OBSCURE GASTROINTESTINAL BLEEDING

Obscure GI bleeding is bleeding that persists or recurs without an obvious source identified on upper and lower endoscopy. Obscure bleeding can be occult (positive fecal occult blood testing without frank recognizable blood loss) or overt (clinically evident). Obscure bleeding can be very challenging to the physician and, in cases of overt massive bleeding, life-threatening to the patient. The initial approach to the problem is the same as with upper and lower GI bleeding and includes resuscitation and stabilization, followed by a search for the source.

DIFFERENTIAL DIAGNOSIS

Missed lesions on upper and lower endoscopy should be considered first in the workup of obscure bleeding. Causes difficult to identify on routine endoscopy include hemosuccus pancreaticus, hemobilia, aortoenteric fistula, Dieulafoy's ulcer, and extraesophageal varices. Small bowel lesions are another source of obscure bleeding and include tumors (lymphomas, carcinoids, adenocarcinomas), vascular ectasia, NSAID-induced ulcers, Meckel's diverticulum, and other less common causes.[132]

DIAGNOSTIC EVALUATION

Repeat upper and lower endoscopy is usually warranted at least once after the index endoscopy, with the uncommon and subtle lesions just listed kept in mind. When the patient has active ongoing bleeding, radionuclide scanning and angiography should be considered. In young patients, Meckel's diverticulum scan may be helpful. If all these tests are negative, the focus should shift to evaluation of the small bowel. Radiographic, endoscopic, and surgical modalities are used for this purpose.

Small bowel follow-through (SBFT) and enteroclysis (which is a modified form of SBFT) should be performed only when Crohn's disease or malignancy is suspected. These modalities have lost favor with the advent of capsule endoscopy and device-assisted enteroscopy (except in cases in which there may be narrowing of the small bowel). Small bowel push enteroscopy can be very helpful in identifying and, in some cases, treating lesions in the small bowel that are responsible for obscure bleeding. Unfortunately, it can examine only 50 to 150 cm of small bowel.[133] Device-assisted enteroscopy (double and single balloon enteroscopy and spiral enteroscopy) has comparable diagnostic yield to capsule endoscopy but has the advantage of performing therapeutic interventions and obtaining biopsies.[134]

Capsule endoscopy gained large interest in evaluation of the small bowel because of its ability to examine the entire small bowel and its noninvasive nature. It consists of swallowing a pill-sized camera with sufficient battery life to image the entire small bowel. Studies have supported the role of capsule endoscopy in the evaluation of obscure GI bleeding with an overall diagnostic yield of 55% to 70%.[132] The diagnostic yield is even higher when it is administered to patients with ongoing bleeding (87% to 92%).[135,136] In our opinion, efforts should be made to perform capsule endoscopy in patients with obscure overt bleeding while still in the hospital instead of waiting until discharge (which is the current standard practice in most centers). In patients who can tolerate an invasive procedure, device-assisted enteroscopy can be used when available and has the advantage of therapeutic ability. However, this procedure only achieves total enteroscopy in 29% of patients. Other limitations include limited availability, time, and sedation requirements. The procedure's risk of complications is low (less than 1%).[134]

Exploratory laparotomy is generally the last option in the evaluation of obscure GI bleeding. When combined with intraoperative enteroscopy, the diagnostic yield reaches 50% to 100%.[132]

CONCLUSION

In summary, acute GI bleeding is a life-threatening emergency that requires a quick response and a coordinated team approach. Acute management is the same regardless of the source of bleeding (Fig. 76.10) and should be orchestrated by a critical care team. The prime direction in resuscitation should be restoration of euvolemia. Once a source is suspected, specific management and therapeutic options are considered and may require communication with gastroenterologists, surgeons, and interventional radiologists. Prevention of bleeding from SRMD is indicated in a specific population of critically ill patients. Endoscopy plays a major role in the diagnosis and management of acute GI bleeding. Endoscopic therapy with standard and innovative techniques has been shown to have a major impact on the prognosis of bleeding patients.

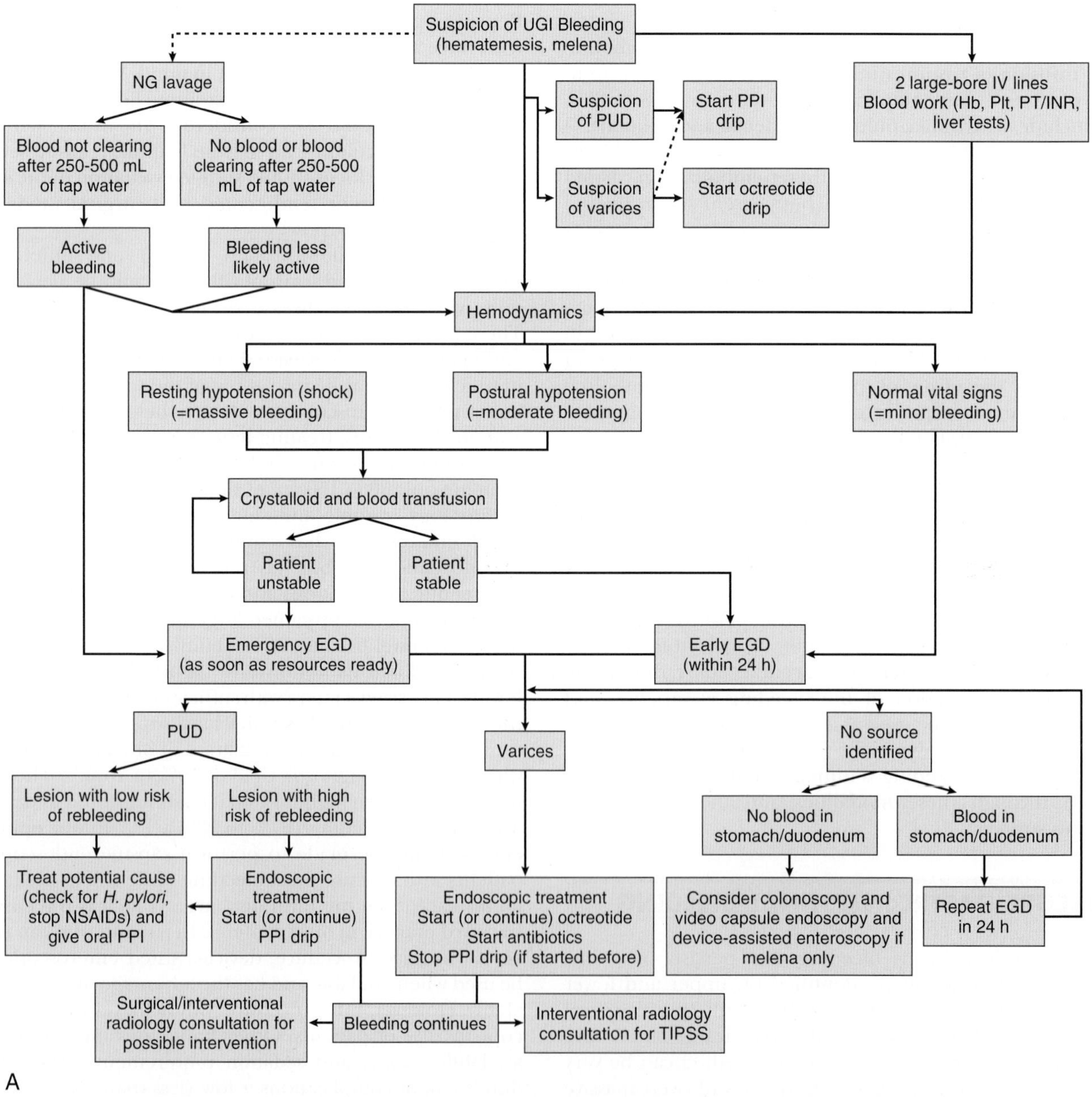

Figure 76.10 A, Approach to managing upper gastrointestinal bleeding in critical care patients.

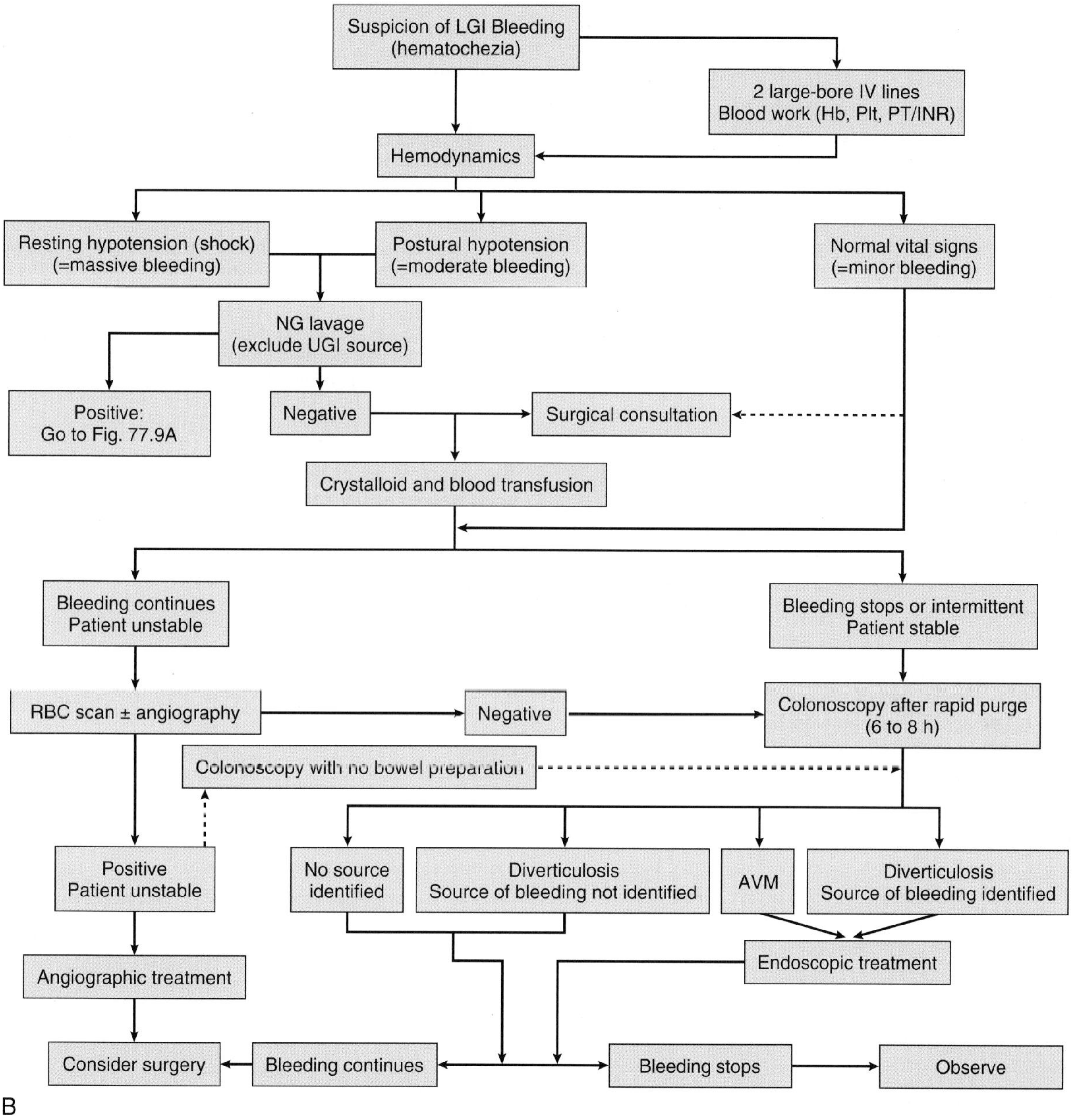

Figure 76.10, cont'd B, Approach to managing lower gastrointestinal bleeding in critical care patients. AVM, arteriovenous malformation; EGD, esophagogastroduodenoscopy; Hb, hemoglobin; INR, international normalized ratio; LGI, lower gastrointestinal; NG, nasogastric; NSAIDs, nonsteroidal anti-inflammatory drugs; Plt, platelets; PPI, proton pump inhibitor; PT, prothrombin time; PUD, peptic ulcer disease; RBC, red blood cell; TIPSS, transjugular intrahepatic portosystemic stent shunt; UGI, upper gastrointestinal.

KEY POINTS

- The history gives important clues regarding the cause of the acute GI bleeding and helps direct initial management.
- Management of GI bleeding relies on a team approach involving an intensivist, endoscopist, radiologist, and surgeon.
- The prime direction of evaluation and resuscitation in a bleeding patient should be restoration of euvolemia.
- SRMD is a common source of upper GI bleeding in physiologically stressed patients, and prophylaxis with acid suppressants should be given to patients with coagulopathy and those undergoing prolonged mechanical ventilation.
- PPIs in drip form should be given to patients with upper GI bleeding after endoscopic treatment of lesions with a high risk of rebleeding.
- Antibiotic therapy decreases the mortality rate in patients with variceal bleeding. It should be given empirically along with vasoactive agents (octreotide).
- Several forms of endoscopic therapy are effective for nonvariceal bleeding, including injection, thermal, and mechanical therapy.
- Endoscopic band ligation is the most commonly used and preferred technique for the treatment of bleeding varices.
- Early colonoscopy has become an attractive choice in lower GI bleeding because of its diagnostic and therapeutic abilities.
- Videocapsule endoscopy has an important role in the evaluation of patients with obscure overt GI bleeding, and efforts should aim at performing it in hospitalized patients. Device-assisted enteroscopy has the benefit, when available, of therapeutic ability and should be performed in the appropriate setting.

SELECTED REFERENCES

11. Barkun AN, Bardou M, Kuipers EJ: International consensus recommendations on the management of patients with nonvariceal upper gastrointestinal bleeding. Ann Intern Med 2010;152:101-113.
13. Blatchford O, Murray WR, Blatchford M: A risk score to predict need for treatment for upper-gastrointestinal haemorrhage. Lancet 2000;356:1318-1321.
14. Rockall TA, Logan RF, Delvin HB, et al: Risk assessment after acute upper gastrointestinal haemorrhage. Gut 1996;38:316-321.
19. Huang ES, Karsan S, Kanwal F, et al: Impact of nasogastric lavage on outcomes in acute GI bleeding. Gastrointest Endosc 2011;74:971-980.
22. Ferguson CB, Mitchell RM: Nonvariceal upper gastrointestinal bleeding: Standard and new treatment. Gastroenterol Clin North Am 2005;34:607-621.
47. ASGE Standards of Practice Committee: ASGE guideline: The role of endoscopy in acute nonvariceal upper-GI hemorrhage. Gastrointest Endosc 2004;60:497-504.
50. Laine L, McQuaid KR: Endoscopic therapy for bleeding ulcers: An evidence-based approach based on meta-analyses of randomized controlled trials. Clin Gastroenterol Hepatol 2009;7:33-47.
62. Zaman A, Chalasani N: Bleeding caused by portal hypertension. Gastroenterol Clin North Am 2005;34:623-642.
67. Garcia-Tsao G, Sanyal AJ, Norman GD, Carey W: Prevention and management of gastroesophageal varices and variceal hemorrhage in cirrhosis. Hepatology 2007;46:922-938.
81. Garcia-Tsao G, Bosch J: Management of varices and variceal hemorrhage in cirrhosis. N Engl J Med 2010;362(9):823-832.

The complete list of references can be found at www.expertconsult.com.

77 Acute Pancreatitis

John C. Marshall

CHAPTER OUTLINE

INTRODUCTION

Acute pancreatitis is a complex disease with a highly variable clinical course. It is responsible for more than 200,000 hospital admissions each year in the United States,[1] and it has an annual incidence of 10 to 80 cases in 100,000 in the developed world.[2-5] Incidence rates have been increasing.[6] For reasons that are unknown, there is seasonal variation in rates of the disease, the incidence being maximal in the spring and fall.[7] The crude mortality rate for patients who are hospitalized with acute pancreatitis is less than 2%,[8] and the majority of patients with acute pancreatitis experience a benign and self-limited disease, resulting in a hospital stay of only several days and no significant lasting sequelae. In a small percentage of patients, however, acute pancreatitis is sufficiently severe to lead to admission to an intensive care or high dependency unit, and a complicated clinical course with a mortality risk that may exceed 20%.[1,9] These latter patients can present the intensivist with formidable challenges during the course of their illness, but if they recover, as most do, they can return to their premorbid state of health with no significant diminution in quality of life.

The prognosis for patients with severe acute pancreatitis has improved considerably since Ranson proposed his widely used severity criteria. In the mid-1970s, the mortality for patients with severe pancreatitis approached 100%[10]; today the risk is less than one quarter of that figure.[11,12] This improved outcome can be ascribed in part to general improvements in the care of critically ill patients and, more important, to fundamental changes in the approach to the medical and surgical care of the patient with acute pancreatitis that, in turn, reflect an evolving understanding of the pathophysiology of the disease.

DEFINITIONS AND TERMINOLOGY

Pancreatitis is an acute inflammatory disorder that arises as a consequence of the activation of pancreatic digestive enzymes within the parenchyma of the gland and the surrounding tissues of the peritoneal cavity and retroperitoneum. Its evolution and complications are variable and give rise to terminology that is both confusing and imprecise. The most widely used classification system is that known as the Atlanta classification from 1992[13] (Table 77.1). Its reproducibility, however, is poor,[14] and it is easier to conceptualize the disease as a spectrum of overlapping abnormalities resulting from the leakage of activated pancreatic enzymes, the host response to local tissue injury, and the superimposed complication of infection of what is initially a sterile process (Fig. 77.1).

In the mildest form of the disease, leakage of activated enzymes is minimal, and the most prominent manifestation is pancreatic edema secondary to a local inflammatory process. In more severe cases, pancreatic ductal disruption results in leakage of pancreatic enzymes into adjacent tissues. If the leakage occurs anteriorly into the peritoneal cavity, fluid collections will be evident. The local peritoneal inflammatory response triggers coagulation and fibrin deposition, walling the collection off and creating a pseudocyst, so called because it is a fluid collection that lacks an

Table 77.1 The Atlanta Classification System for Acute Pancreatitis

Term	Definition
Acute pancreatitis	Acute inflammation of the pancreas with variable involvement of peripancreatic and remote tissues
Mild acute pancreatitis	Edema of pancreas; benign clinical course with minimal organ dysfunction and full recovery
Severe acute pancreatitis	Evidence of pancreatic necrosis; complications of infection, pseudocyst; clinical course characterized by organ failure
Acute fluid collection	Pancreatic or peripancreatic fluid, evident early in course of disease, and lacking wall
Pancreatic pseudocyst	Contained collection of pancreatic juice within a capsule of fibrous tissue and arising following an episode of acute pancreatitis
Pancreatic necrosis	Diffuse or focal loss of viability of pancreatic parenchyma or peripancreatic fat, evident as nonenhancing tissue on a contrast-enhanced CT scan
Pancreatic abscess	Localized collection of pus within pancreas or peripancreatic region and containing little or no necrotic material

Adapted from Bradley EL: A clinically based classification system for acute pancreatitis. Arch Surg 1993;128:586-590.

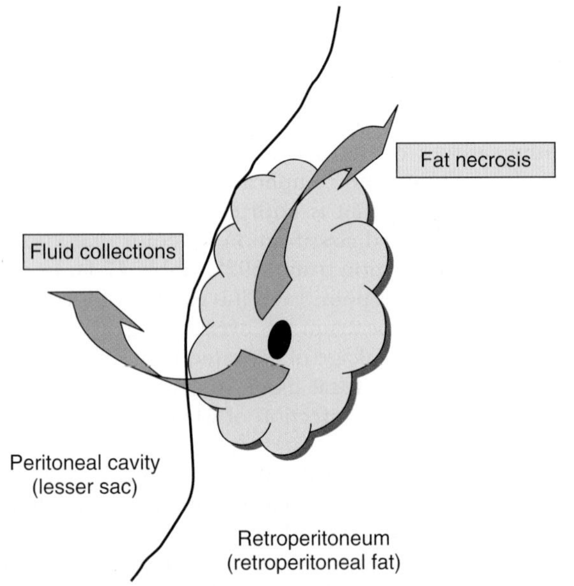

Figure 77.1 Disruption of the pancreatic ductal system results in leakage of activated digestive enzymes into the peripancreatic tissues. When the predominant direction is anteriorly into the lesser sac, the result is one or more fluid collections that either resolve or coalesce to form a pseudocyst. Leakage posteriorly into the fatty tissues of the retroperitoneum results in fat necrosis.

epithelial lining. Drainage of the pancreatic ascites through the diaphragm can create a pleural effusion; typically this is seen on the left. Marked elevation of the amylase level in the pleural fluid establishes the collection as pancreatic juice, rather than as a reaction to an inflammatory process on the abdominal side of the diaphragm. Alternatively, if leakage is into the fatty tissues of the retroperitoneum, necrosis predominates, although small loculated fluid collections are often present. Often in patients with severe acute pancreatitis, computerized tomography shows evidence of both intraperitoneal and retroperitoneal involvement. The older term, *hemorrhagic pancreatitis,* describes the sequelae of extension of retroperitoneal necrosis into blood vessels of the retroperitoneum. Extraperitoneal tracking of the resulting hematoma gives rise to Grey-Turner's sign when the ecchymosis is evident in the flanks and Cullen's sign when it tracks anteriorly through the falciform ligament to present at the umbilicus.[15]

Both necrotic tissue and fluid collections can become secondarily infected with bacteria and fungi from the gastrointestinal tract, the former giving rise to infected pancreatic or peripancreatic necrosis and the latter to an infected pseudocyst or pancreatic abscess—the latter terms being largely interchangeable.

PATHOGENESIS

Acute pancreatitis arises in the pancreas through the leakage of activated pancreatic enzymes into pancreatic and peripancreatic tissues. The characteristic clinical syndrome, however, reflects the activation of a massive systemic inflammatory response to that local tissue injury, mediated through the activation of the inflammasome—a multiprotein intracellular complex that leads to the activation of the key inflammatory cytokine, interleukin-1.[16]

Beyond its role as an endocrine organ, the pancreas plays a fundamental role in the digestion of foodstuffs through the production of enzymes that degrade the major constituents of ingested food: protein (proteases), fat (lipases), starch (amylase), and nucleic acids (nucleases). Pancreatic enzymes are synthesized by the acinar cells lining the pancreatic ductal system and released from the cell as inactive zymogens.[17] They pass via the pancreatic duct into the lumen of the duodenum, where they are activated by mucosal enzymes such as enterokinase, and so become capable of degrading their target substrates. Under normal circumstances, activation is vigorously inhibited within the pancreas itself through sequestration of newly synthesized enzymes within zymogen granules, and further through the local action of a specific inhibitor of trypsin activation called SPINK.[18] The importance of normal mechanisms that inhibit trypsin activation is underlined by the observation that genetic mutations in the SPINK gene associated with reduced activity have been implicated in the pathogenesis of hereditary pancreatitis.[19]

Acute pancreatitis arises through the activation of pancreatic enzymes within the pancreas itself, possibly through the activity of lysosomal hydrolases in the acinar cell and initiating autodigestion of the pancreas and surrounding tissues.[20,21] Activation of trypsinogen to trypsin appears to be a critical event during the early pathogenesis of the acute process,[22,23] and an increase in intracellular calcium concentrations may contribute to activation of trypsinogen.[24] Trypsinogen can also be activated by lysosomal cathepsin B within the acinar cell.[25] Pancreatic acinar cells can die by either necrosis or apoptosis. Necrotic death is characterized by cell lysis, with the leakage of intracellular constituents into the surrounding microenvironment and the activation of an acute inflammatory response. Neutrophil recruitment in response to the local tissue injury has been implicated in the amplification of cellular damage in acute pancreatitis.[26-28] Apoptotic death, in contrast, is noninflammatory. Cells are degraded into membrane-bound vesicles that are taken up by fixed tissue macrophages. Phagocytosis of an apoptotic cell not only prevents the local activation of inflammation but triggers transcriptional programs in the phagocytosing cell that are anti-inflammatory and reparative in nature, with up-regulation of counter-inflammatory cytokines such as interleukin-10 (IL-10).[29] The local cellular injury in acute pancreatitis can also be conceptualized as an imbalance between necrotic and apoptotic cell death. Activation of caspases—the intracellular enzymes that mediate apoptosis—attenuate the severity of pancreatitis,[30] whereas severe pancreatitis is associated with reduced levels of IL-10.[31]

Activated pancreatic enzymes injure not only cells of the pancreas but also those of surrounding tissues. Fat cells appear to be particularly vulnerable, and the disease tends to be more severe in the obese because of the greater amount of peripancreatic fat necrosis.[32] However, the degradative effects of pancreatic enzymes, and the secondary tissue injury resulting from the host response, can injure other structures in the vicinity of the pancreas, in particular, the transverse colon, and major vessels such as the splenic artery and vein.[33] Pancreatitis rapidly evolves from an inflammatory disease of the pancreas to a chemical burn of the retroperitoneum.

The pathogenesis of the clinical syndrome is further complicated by the presence of the gastrointestinal tract immediately adjacent to the pancreas (Fig. 77.2). The head of the pancreas lies within the curve of the duodenum, immediately behind the stomach and above the transverse colon.

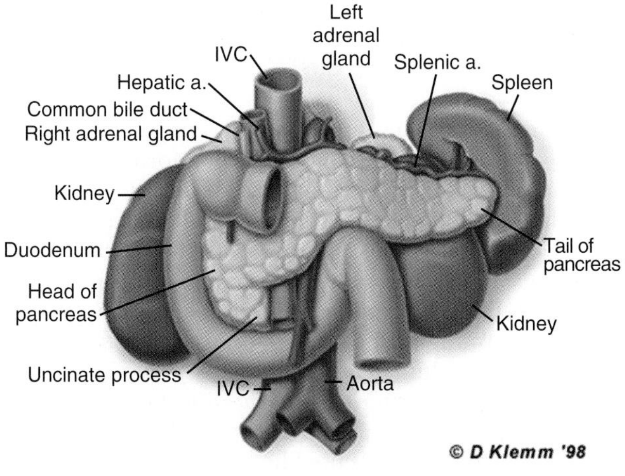

Figure 77.2 The pancreas is a retroperitoneal organ, lying posterior to the stomach, within the curve of the duodenum. It lies in immediate proximity to a number of large blood vessels including the splenic artery and vein, the superior mesenteric artery and vein, and the portal vein.

Damage to terminal feeding vessels in the colonic fat caused by activated pancreatic enzymes can result in focal perforation of the colon, with leakage of colonic bacteria into the peritoneal cavity.[34] Although the stomach and duodenum are only lightly colonized in health, the local ileus induced by the acute pancreatic inflammation promotes proximal gut overgrowth with enteric bacteria.[35] In addition, changes in gut mucosal barrier function arising from local inflammation and the absence of enteral nutrients promote the translocation of luminal bacteria and of bacterial products such as endotoxin into the injured or necrotic peripancreatic tissues.[36]

Ultimately in the more severe cases, the clinical syndrome evolves as a result of a systemically activated inflammatory response, with the same changes in microvascular blood flow, endothelial permeability, and inflammatory mediator release that characterize bacterial sepsis.[37]

ETIOLOGY AND RISK FACTORS

Acute pancreatitis has many causes, although 80% of cases in the developed world result from either alcohol or gallstones (Table 77.2). The mechanism of alcohol-induced pancreatitis is unclear. The acinar cell of the pancreas is capable of metabolizing alcohol and also appears to be the primary target of alcohol-mediated pancreatic injury.[38] In vitro studies show that alcohol reduces the sensitivity of isolated acini to zymogen activation by cholecystokinin.[39] Gallstone pancreatitis appears to be a consequence of a transient acute increase in pancreatic ductal pressures associated with passage of a small gallstone through the sphincter of Oddi in patients with a common channel for the bile

Table 77.2 Causes of Acute Pancreatitis

Congenital	
Anatomic abnormalities: Pancreas divisum, choledochocele, periampullary diverticulum	
Familial pancreatitis	
Cystic fibrosis	
Hereditary angioedema	
Acquired	
Toxic:	Alcohol, scorpion venom
Obstructive:	Gallstones, duodenojejunal intussusception
Metabolic:	Hypercalcemia, hypertriglyceridemia
Trauma:	Blunt/penetrating
	Induced by endoscopic retrograde cholangiopancreatography (ERCP)
	Operative
Drugs:	Thiazides, corticosteroids
Ischemia:	Low flow state
Infectious:	Mumps, HIV, cytomegalovirus (CMV), other viral infections, *Salmonella*, ascariasis, tuberculosis, brucellosis, leptospirosis
Autoimmune disease:	Systemic lupus erythematosus
Idiopathic	

and pancreatic ducts.[40] True obstruction of the duct is uncommon, and approximately 90% of patients will be found to have gallstones in the stool, implicating the passage of the stone, rather than an obstructing mechanism, in the etiology of the resulting pancreatic inflammation. The list of drugs implicated in the etiology of acute pancreatitis is long[41]; some of the more prominent associations are shown in Table 77.2.

Genetic factors have been associated with the development of acute pancreatitis. A polymorphism in the secretory trypsin inhibitor (SPINK1) gene is associated with an increased risk for acute pancreatitis,[42] as are mutations in the cystic fibrosis transmembrane conductance regulator (CFTR) gene,[43] and PRSS1.[44] Polymorphisms in the genes for tumor necrosis factor α (TNFα) and heat shock protein 70 have also been linked to an increased risk for acute pancreatitis,[45] although the association is less clear.

CLINICAL PRESENTATION AND DIAGNOSIS

Acute pancreatitis typically presents as severe acute epigastric pain that radiates to the back, a reflection of the retroperitoneal position of the pancreas. Nausea and vomiting are common associated symptoms. From the perspective of the intensivist, the predominant manifestations of severe acute pancreatitis are those that reflect hemodynamic instability secondary to an activated systemic inflammatory response. These can evolve with alarming rapidity, and the severity of the process is frequently not appreciated until it is quite advanced.

The causes of shock in the patient with acute pancreatitis are multifactorial. Initially, the acute inflammatory process in the retroperitoneum elicits local inflammation, with an outpouring of fluid into the relatively confined space of the retroperitoneum or into the peritoneal cavity itself. Intra-abdominal inflammation evokes secondary ileus within the gastrointestinal tract, and fluid is sequestered here, increasing the relative intravascular volume deficit. Nausea, vomiting, and a reluctance to take fluids by mouth further exacerbate this fluid deficit. As the process evolves, a systemic inflammatory response to the local abdominal process results in diffuse vasodilatation and capillary leak syndrome. In aggregate, the effective loss of intravascular volume can be enormous, and so the initial resuscitation may require large volumes of intravenous fluid. Acute hypocalcemia may also contribute to the clinical picture of cardiovascular compromise. Indeed the classical prognostic criteria articulated by Ranson (Table 77.3) emphasize the importance of acute inflammation (white cell count), and the secondary hemodynamic (fluid sequestration, base excess, blood urea nitrogen [BUN], and hematocrit) and metabolic (glucose, calcium) sequelae in determining the ultimate prognosis.

The diagnosis of pancreatitis is usually straightforward, based on the combination of clinical manifestations and characteristic biochemical findings of elevations in the circulating levels of amylase and lipase, the latter being somewhat more accurate diagnostically.[46] The diagnosis can be confirmed, and the severity of the disease evaluated by computerized tomography (Fig. 77.3), using the grading system developed by Balthazar[47] (Table 77.4).

Table 77.3 Ranson's Criteria in Acute Pancreatitis

On Admission	Over First 48 Hours
Age > 55 years	Po_2 < 60 mm Hg
White cell count > 16,000/μL	Estimated fluid sequestration > 6 L
Blood sugar > 11.1 mmol/L (200 mg/dL)	Calcium < 2 mm/L (8 mg/dL)
LDH > 350 IU/L	Hematocrit fall < 10%
AST > 250 IU/L	BUN rise > 1.8 mmol/L (5 mg/dL)
	Base excess > −4 mEq/L

LDH, Lactate dehydrogenase; AST, aspartate aminotransferase; BUN, blood urea nitrogen.
From Ranson JH, Rifkind KM, Roses DF, et al: Prognostic signs and the role of operative management in acute pancreatitis. Surg Gynecol Obstet 1974;139:69-81.

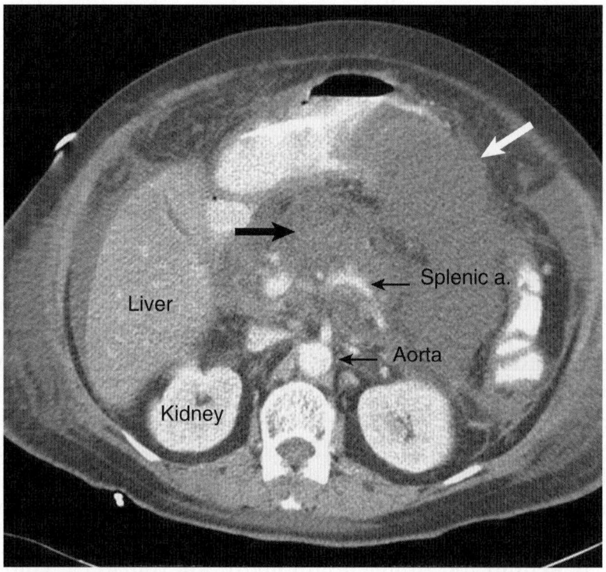

Figure 77.3 CT findings in severe acute pancreatitis (Balthazar grade E). Note the combination of pancreatic necrosis *(black arrow)* and fluid and debris *(white arrow)* and the intimate relationship of the inflamed pancreas to the splenic artery.

An initial assessment of the severity of the disease is useful primarily for deciding the optimal venue for the early management of the patient, as at least some of the delayed morbidity of acute pancreatitis can be reduced through aggressive initial resuscitation and support. Various approaches have been used to quantify disease severity. Ranson identified 11 variables—5 at initial presentation and 6 over the ensuing 48 hours—that correlated in a graded fashion with the ultimate risk of mortality (see Table 77.3). The Glasgow-Imrie criteria are a modification of Ranson's scale and represent an alternate model of severity scoring. In head-to-head studies, Acute Physiology, Age, and Chronic Health Evaluation (APACHE) II—a generic severity of illness scale—performs at least as well as the Ranson or Glasgow-Imrie criteria in predicting hospital survival.[48] Moreover, even simpler scales appear to provide comparable prognostic information.[23,49] Various biochemical measures,

Table 77.4 Balthazar Grading of CT Findings in Acute Pancreatitis

Grade	Findings
Grade A	Normal pancreas
Grade B	Pancreatic enlargement
Grade C	Pancreatic or peripancreatic inflammation
Grade D	Single peripancreatic fluid collection
Grade E	2 or more pancreatic collections and/or retroperitoneal air

From Balthazar EJ: CT diagnosis and staging of acute pancreatitis. Radiol Clin North Am 1989;27:19-37.

including C-reactive protein, procalcitonin, interleukin-6, and trypsinogen activation peptide (TAP), are purported to differentiate mild and severe pancreatitis early during the clinical evolution of the disease[50-52]; their clinical utility is unclear. Persistence of clinical manifestations of systemic inflammation beyond 48 hours is also associated with subsequent organ dysfunction and a higher mortality.[53] Precision in prognostication is far less important than early recognition of the patient for whom close monitoring and aggressive resuscitation can alter the clinical course, and a low threshold for management in a more controlled and monitored setting is an important factor in reducing the complications of pancreatitis.[54]

EARLY MANAGEMENT OF THE CRITICALLY ILL PATIENT WITH ACUTE PANCREATITIS

INITIAL RESUSCITATION

Intravascular fluid deficits early in the course of pancreatitis can be substantial. Early aggressive fluid resuscitation is the cornerstone of initial successful management.[55] Volume status should be monitored with a urinary catheter and central venous catheter, and although studies in the specific setting of pancreatitis have not been performed, there is every reason to believe that the principles of goal-directed resuscitation should be followed.[56] There are no data to support a preference for colloids or crystalloids during resuscitation; the key, however, is to administer sufficient volumes rapidly enough to restore an adequate circulating volume.[57] Typically this comprises many liters of fluid, and not infrequently, the sickest patients will receive more than 10 to 15 L of fluid resuscitation over the first 24 hours. Such aggressive resuscitation is best carried out within the well-monitored environment of the intensive care unit (ICU).

Although aggressive fluid resuscitation can minimize later complications such as pancreatic necrosis and acute renal failure, in the patient with increased vascular permeability it carries a high risk of complications related to interstitial edema. Frequently patients will require endotracheal intubation and mechanical ventilation. Development of the abdominal compartment syndrome is a relatively common and underdiagnosed complication of resuscitated acute pancreatitis.[58] Intra-abdominal pressure can be measured by transducing a urinary catheter in the bladder. Normal pressures approximate the central venous pressure, whereas pressures greater than 20 cm H_2O indicate intra-abdominal hypertension, and pressures greater than 30 cm H_2O indicate a compartment syndrome and carry an increased risk of ischemic injury because of impairment of visceral venous drainage. In severe cases, management requires abdominal decompression by laparotomy. The need for laparotomy in the patient with acute pancreatitis may be avoided by the use of continuous venovenous hemofiltration[59] or decompressive anterior abdominal fasciotomy.[60]

Box 77.1 Common Microbial Isolates in Pancreatic and Peripancreatic Infections

Organism

Gram-Negative Aerobes

E. coli
Klebsiella
Pseudomonas
Proteus
Enterobacter

Gram-Positive Aerobes

Enterococcus
Staphylococcus aureus
Staphylococcus epidermidis

Anerobes

Bacteroides

Fungi

Candida

INFECTION PROPHYLAXIS

Infection is a common complication of acute necrotizing pancreatitis, and its development is associated with an increased risk of morbidity and mortality.[61] For the patient with severe acute pancreatitis, these infections may arise within the injured or necrotic peripancreatic tissues or at distant sites as nosocomial infection in a critically ill patient.

The characteristic microbial flora of peripancreatic infection includes organisms normally resident within the gastrointestinal tract[62] and organisms that characteristically colonize the proximal gastrointestinal tract of the critically ill patient[35] (Box 77.1). Anaerobes may be present but are uncommon, whereas organisms such as *Candida, Enterococci*, and coagulase-negative *Staphylococci* are encountered with increasing frequency.[63,64] This infecting flora reflects the role of the gastrointestinal tract as the reservoir of organisms inducing superinfection during acute pancreatitis.[65]

Infection of necrotic tissue in the retroperitoneum can arise by one of several routes. Bacteremic spread from a distant site, retrograde passage up the pancreatic duct, and direct extension through a defect in the adjacent gastrointestinal tract are all plausible mechanisms. However, the most significant mechanism of infection appears to be as a consequence of the translocation of viable microorganisms across an anatomically gastrointestinal (GI) tract, from either the colon or the small intestine. Bacterial translocation is readily demonstrable in animal models of acute pancreatitis,[66,67] and indirect evidence suggests that the phenomenon contributes to infectious complications in human pancreatitis.[68] Patients with severe pancreatitis, for example, have higher rates of proximal gut colonization with the same enteric organisms that produce infection,[69] and intestinal colonization invariably precedes the development of invasive infection.[70] Moreover, suppression of pathologic gut colonization reduces the risk of infection.[71]

Host-microbial interactions within the GI tract are complex,[72,73] and the changes that occur in pancreatitis are much more than a state of generalized leakiness. Colectomy, for example, increases rates of small bowel microbial colonization and bacterial translocation.[74] Moreover, the anaerobic flora of the gut provides a barrier to intestinal mucosal colonization with pathogenic aerobes and inhibits bacterial translocation.[75] Thus, anaerobes are uncommonly found in pancreatic infections, and the isolation of an anaerobic organism from an area of infected pancreatic necrosis is highly suggestive of a physical breach of the gastrointestinal tract.

Infection of pancreatic necrosis is a relatively late event, occurring maximally during the second or third week after the onset of the acute disease.[76] However, circulating bacterial DNA[77] or endotoxin from gram-negative bacteria[78] can be detected early during the course of the disease.

The role of antibiotic prophylaxis, however, is controversial. An early meta-analysis of randomized controlled trials of prophylactic antibiotics for patients with acute pancreatitis concluded that prophylaxis can improve survival without significantly altering rates of pancreatic infection.[79] A consensus conference of critical care organizations, however, has recommended that routine antibiotic prophylaxis should not be used in the absence of more compelling evidence from randomized controlled trials,[54] and more recent compilations of data from clinical trials fail to show clear evidence of benefit for antibiotic prophylaxis.[80] A push for conservatism is driven by three principal factors: the low methodological quality of trials supporting antibiotic prophylaxis, concern regarding the adverse ecologic consequences of prolonged broad-spectrum antibiotic administration, and the increasing use of an alternate prophylactic strategy, enteral feeding.[81] One of the most influential studies of prophylactic antibiotics in pancreatitis, for example, reported a significant survival improvement associated with antibiotic prophylaxis in a cohort of 60 patients[82]; in that study, however, antibiotic use had no impact on rates of pancreatic infection, and fully three quarters of patients in the control arm received antibiotics early in the course of their disease. The prevention of pathologic gut colonization through the use of selective digestive tract decontamination has been shown to reduce rates of pancreatic infectious complications[71] and to reduce mortality associated with gram-negative infections.[83] Whether antifungal prophylaxis is efficacious is also controversial.[84,85]

NUTRITIONAL SUPPORT

In contrast to the persistent controversy regarding the utility of antibiotic prophylaxis in severe acute pancreatitis, it is now generally accepted that patients do better and, in particular, experience less infectious and inflammatory morbidity if they are fed enterally rather than parenterally. Enteral feeding is associated with maintained epithelial barrier function as well as reduced rates of translocation of endotoxin and viable bacteria in experimental animals.[86,87] A meta-analysis of eight trials recruiting 348 patients found a lower rate of infectious complications (relative risk [RR] 0.39; 95% confidence interval [CI] 0.23 to 0.65), a reduced need for operative intervention (RR 0.44; 95% CI 0.29 to 0.67), a reduced risk of organ failure (RR 0.55; 95% CI 0.37 to 0.81), and a reduced risk of death (RR 0.50; 95% CI 0.28 to 0.91).[88]

Current guidelines recommend the early institution of enteral feeds in patients with severe acute pancreatitis, supplemented, as needed, with parenteral support to meet full nutritional requirements.[54,89,90] Although the presence of gastric ileus in acute pancreatitis has resulted in a preference for the nasojejunal rather than the nasogastric route of feeding, there is no evidence of the inferiority of nasogastric feeding in more recent clinical trials.[91,92] Similarly, there is no compelling evidence at present to favor any particular nutritional formulation.

ADJUVANT THERAPY

Despite a substantial body of literature suggesting a benefit for a variety of different adjuvant treatments in preclinical models, there is no evidence for any specific therapy in human disease. A systematic review of the use of cimetidine found no evidence that suppression of gastric acid secretion improved outcome, but rather a trend to a higher risk of complications.[93] Pooled data from small studies have suggested that somatostatin or octreotide can improve survival for patients with severe acute pancreatitis,[94] but data from larger, more robust trials are lacking. Protease inhibitors have also been suggested to reduce mortality in moderate to severe pancreatitis.[95]

Platelet-activating factor (PAF) is a potent pro-inflammatory lipid mediator that has been implicated in the local and remote manifestations of acute pancreatitis.[96] Inhibition of PAF with either a receptor antagonist[97] or through the administration of recombinant PAF acetylhydrolase—the enzyme responsible for degrading PAF[98]—results in attenuation of injury in animal models. Unfortunately, despite early promise in phase II clinical trials,[99,100] a phase III trial failed to show any benefit for adjuvant treatment with the PAF receptor antagonist, lexipafant, in 290 patients with severe acute pancreatitis.[101]

Other strategies such as inhibition of TNF or blockade of interleukin-1 have shown promise in preclinical models but have not been evaluated in human disease.[102]

ENDOSCOPIC RETROGRADE CHOLANGIOPANCREATOGRAPHY (ERCP) IN ACUTE GALLSTONE PANCREATITIS

Gallstone pancreatitis is caused by a gallstone that has migrated from the gallbladder into the common bile duct producing transient obstruction of the pancreatic duct. This pathogenetic mechanism raises the possibility that measures to relieve the obstruction at the level of the sphincter of

Oddi might reduce the severity of the disease. This possibility has been evaluated in at least four clinical trials, the pooled data from which suggest benefit for patients with severe pancreatitis in reducing subsequent complications.[103] It is unclear whether the benefit extends to all patients or simply to the subset of patients with persistent common bile duct obstruction and concomitant cholangitis.[104,105]

MANAGEMENT OF THE LATE COMPLICATIONS OF SEVERE ACUTE PANCREATITIS

It is apparent from the foregoing that the early management of the patient with severe acute pancreatitis is focused primarily on adequate resuscitation and organ support. Early lethal postresuscitation complications are uncommon[106] and include intestinal ischemia (typically secondary to a low flow state or mesenteric venous thrombosis following delayed resuscitation)[107] and bleeding secondary to erosion into a major vessel. In the absence of these catastrophic and fortunately rare complications, the subsequent management of the critically ill patient with acute pancreatitis involves optimal intensive care,[108] close monitoring, and patience.

PANCREATIC PSEUDOCYSTS

Serial evaluation by computerized tomography shows that the diffuse fluid collections evident in early pancreatitis coalesce to form discrete cystlike collections contained within an organized capsule of fibrin and termed a *pseudocyst.* Typically these arise in the lesser sac, between the pancreas and the posterior wall of the stomach (Fig. 77.4). Management is expectant in the absence of complications,[109] and rarely is intervention required in the ICU setting. The most common symptom precipitating drainage is persistent pain or symptoms of gastric obstruction. Other important complications include infection and hemorrhage into the cyst.

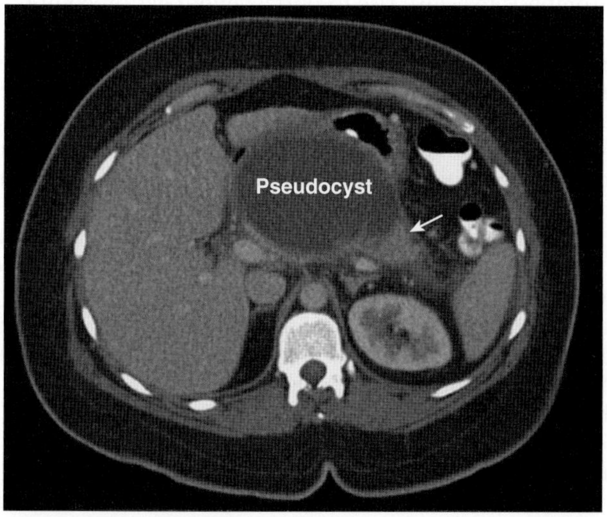

Figure 77.4 A maturing pancreatic pseudocyst, evident as a well-circumscribed fluid collection in the lesser sac, compressing the residual pancreas *(white arrow).*

The classic approach to the management of a pancreatic pseudocyst involved waiting until the fibrous capsule of the cyst had matured, then draining the cyst into the back wall of the stomach. Open surgical pseudocyst gastrostomy has largely given way to less invasive approaches, creating a cyst gastrostomy by radiologic image guided,[110] endoscopic,[111] or laparoscopic approaches.[112] A pseudocyst forms because of injury to the main pancreatic duct, or one of its branches, and persists because of obstruction to the flow of pancreatic juice through the duct. If that obstruction persists, then external drainage will result in a persistent pancreaticocutaneous fistula. Thus, regardless of how it is accomplished, drainage into the stomach avoids this complication by replacing the external fistula with an internal fistula that is without clinical importance. Open operation may be required for massive hemorrhage; angiographic embolization of the bleeding vessel is another alternative.[113]

INFECTED NECROSIS AND PANCREATIC ABSCESS

One of the more significant advances in the management of severe pancreatitis has been the adoption of a policy of surgical conservatism in managing patients with suspected pancreatic or peripancreatic infection. Case series demonstrate improved survival rates when surgery is delayed,[114-118] and a single randomized trial showed that delaying surgical intervention for at least 2 weeks in patients with necrotizing pancreatitis improves clinical outcomes.[119] This improved outcome can be attributed to a reduced frequency of major bleeding complications associated with the debridement of necrotic, infected retroperitoneal tissue.

Just as serial evaluation reveals localization of pancreatic fluid collections, serial study of areas of pancreatic necrosis shows that they too coalesce with time, becoming more circumscribed and, importantly, developing a wall of granulation tissue between the areas of necrosis and viable surrounding tissues. It is this clear demarcation between viable and nonviable tissue that renders operative intervention safe and obviates the need for repeat operation or open-abdomen approaches. Typically, the process of demarcation takes 3 to 4 weeks or longer to occur; thus, surgical intervention, if contemplated, should be deferred. A strategy of surgical conservatism in the face of a patient with clinical manifestations of sepsis and ongoing organ dysfunction may appear counterintuitive, but it is both well tolerated and safer than the alternative.[120]

There is general consensus that the indication for operative intervention in a patient with severe pancreatitis is infected necrosis; sterile necrosis should be managed conservatively.[115,121,122] The diagnosis of infection of pancreatic necrosis can be challenging to establish, for clinical manifestations of systemic inflammation are common in the acutely ill patient with pancreatitis, even in the absence of infection, as are nosocomial infections in sites other than the necrotic retroperitoneal tissues. A diagnosis of infection may be suggested by new elevations in levels of procalcitonin[123,124] or by computed tomography (CT) findings of air in the necrotic tissues (Fig. 77.5). However, definitive diagnosis of infection is best established by CT-guided fine-needle aspiration of the peripancreatic necrotic tissues.[125]

Documentation of infection on a fine-needle aspirate is not an absolute indication for operative intervention.

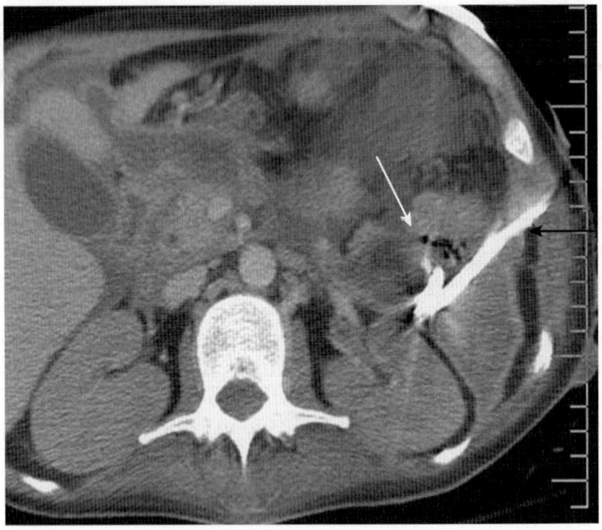

Figure 77.5 Infected pancreatic necrosis *(white arrow);* the fluid component of the collection was decompressed with a percutaneously placed drain *(black arrow),* allowing delayed laparoscopic debridement.

Antibiotics should be administered as guided by the results of culture and sensitivity and then source control options evaluated. Early in the course of the disease, before the demarcation of necrotic and viable tissues, percutaneous drainage of the fluid component of the collection can temporize until operative intervention is safer (see Fig. 77.5). Percutaneous drainage alone may be curative,[126,127] and there is even evolving literature indicating that some patients with infected pancreatic necrosis can be successfully managed nonoperatively.[128,129]

The surgical management of infected pancreatic necrosis entails the debridement of the necrotic retroperitoneal tissues and drainage of the resulting cavity. Approaches span the surgical spectrum from minimal access techniques[130-132] to open abdomen approaches.[133,134] Improved clinical outcomes have also been seen with the use of less invasive, staged procedures. van Santvoort and colleagues reported a randomized controlled trial of a staged approach to pancreatic necrosectomy, consisting of initial percutaneous drainage of the liquid elements of a pancreatic infection, followed by a minimally invasive necrosectomy, using the drain tract as a route of access.[12] The minimally invasive approach resulted in significantly lower rates of major complications and new-onset organ dysfunction, as well as lower rates of delayed complications including diabetes and incisional hernia. This same group has also reported lower rates of new organ dysfunction and pancreatic fistula when patients were managed by transgastric endoscopic necrosectomy when compared with open necrosectomy.[135]

In general, the optimal approach is the one that entails the least anatomic and physiologic upset to the patient. An open laparotomy can be performed using either a midline or bilateral subcostal incision. With the aid of a recent CT scan to guide the dissection, the infected retroperitoneal necrosis is approached either through the gastrocolic omentum and the lesser sac or through the inferior aspect of the transverse mesocolon. Dissection is performed largely blindly and bluntly, evacuating necrotic retroperitoneal fat and pus. Soft drains are left in the resulting cavity to provide egress for pancreatic juice, and the abdomen can usually be closed primarily. If there is evidence of significant involvement of the mesocolon or preoperative cultures yield anaerobic organisms, a proximal diverting ileostomy may be added to minimize contamination from the adjacent colon. If the patient is likely to require prolonged ICU care, an operative feeding jejunostomy can facilitate nutritional support.

Laparoscopic techniques have the added advantage of permitting direct visualization of the abscess cavity,[132,136,137] but they may be challenging if there is extensive or multiloculated areas of necrosis. Infected necrosis can also be approached via the flank, using a nephroscope or laparoscope to aid in visualization of the abscess contents.[138] Further insights into the role of minimally invasive approaches should emerge from several ongoing clinical trials.[112,139] The role for open abdomen approaches in the management of infected pancreatic necrosis is diminishing as surgical practice shifts to delayed intervention with more minimally invasive techniques.[140]

Peritoneal lavage with the objective of evacuating activated pancreatic enzymes enjoyed a period of popularity[141] but is now used less frequently. Some authors recommend continuous postoperative lavage following pancreatic necrosectomy,[140] though the benefits of this approach are unproven.

VASCULAR COMPLICATIONS OF NECROTIZING PANCREATITIS

The vascular complications of acute pancreatitis include both thrombosis and hemorrhage.[142,143] Thrombosis of the splenic, superior mesenteric, and portal veins develops as a consequence of the pro-thrombotic effects of the adjacent inflamed pancreas and reduced flow prior to full resuscitation. Less commonly, more distant vessels such as the inferior vena cava or renal veins may thrombose. Venous thrombosis may give rise to portal venous gas on computed tomography; in the absence of clinical findings dictating a need for emergent intervention, both the venous thrombosis and the associated CT findings can be managed conservatively.[144] Treatment consists of anticoagulation; intestinal infarction secondary to venous thrombosis in patients with acute pancreatitis carries a prohibitive mortality, even with surgery.

Erosion of the retroperitoneal inflammatory process into a major artery can produce bleeding into either the peritoneal cavity or the gut lumen, in which case it presents as a gastrointestinal hemorrhage. Commonly involved vessels include the splenic artery, the gastroduodenal artery, and the pancreaticoduodenal arcade.[145] Operative exposure is challenging in the face of acute retroperitoneal inflammation, and whenever feasible, bleeding is best managed by angiographic embolization.[113]

An algorithm summarizing the key elements in the management of the patient with severe acute pancreatitis is provided in Figure 77.6.

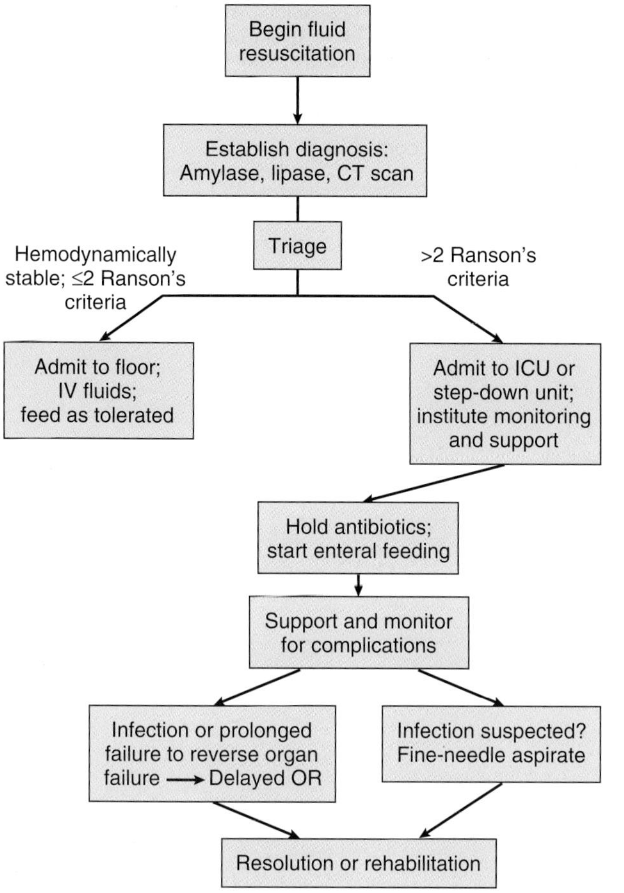

Figure 77.6 Approach to the patient with acute pancreatitis. CT, computed tomography; ICU, intensive care unit; IV, intravenous; OR, operation.

LONG-TERM OUTCOME AND QUALITY OF LIFE

Acute necrotizing pancreatitis can be an enormously challenging process to treat. The ICU and hospital stay is often prolonged, and in addition to operative procedures undertaken during the acute episode, there is often a need for later intervention to close a stoma, repair an incisional hernia, or excise the gallbladder. Yet there is ample evidence that patients who survive their acute illness return to a health-related quality of life that is no different from age-matched controls.[146-149] Abnormalities of both endocrine and exocrine function are commonly evident at follow-up,[150] and approximately one third of survivors of severe necrotizing pancreatitis develop diabetes.[151]

CONCLUSIONS

Necrotizing pancreatitis is a challenging but enormously satisfying disease to manage. Current management approaches are supportive, with treatment directed at correcting complications of the disease process. Adjunctive treatment strategies that target the pathologic host inflammatory response are not yet available but should emerge. Although the outcome is heavily dependent on disease severity, with early and aggressive resuscitation, optimal supportive care in an intensive care unit, and judicious and delayed intervention to manage infected necrosis, the overwhelming majority of patients survive and are rehabilitated to an excellent quality of life.

KEY POINTS

- The initial presentation of severe acute pancreatitis can be subtle; early objective quantification of disease severity is important to guide resuscitation and informing decisions regarding patient disposition.
- Aggressive fluid resuscitation is the cornerstone of successful management. Large volumes of intravenous fluids must often be given, and the development of acute respiratory failure with a need for endotracheal intubation and admission to an intensive care unit is neither uncommon nor undesirable.
- The role of prophylactic antibiotics is controversial; in the absence of more compelling evidence of efficacy, their use is discouraged.
- Nutritional support should be instituted early, and by the enteral route, reserving parenteral nutrition for patients who cannot meet their caloric needs by the enteral route.
- There is, at present, no established role for other adjuvant treatments, and support postresuscitation is entirely supportive.
- Serial CT scans can document the severity of the disease and monitor its progression; CT-guided fine-needle aspiration is the diagnostic technique of choice to identify infected necrosis.
- The management of infected necrosis consists of culture-guided systemic antibiotics and delayed surgical intervention. There is an increasing role for minimally invasive techniques of pancreatic debridement and even for nonoperative management of infected necrosis.
- Despite the complexity and morbidity of the acute episode, the long-term health-related quality of life for survivors of acute necrotizing pancreatitis is excellent.

SELECTED REFERENCES

1. Whitcomb DC: Clinical practice: Acute pancreatitis. N Engl J Med 2006;354:2142-2150.
12. van Santvoort HC, Besselink MG, Bakker OJ, et al: A step-up approach or open necrosectomy for necrotizing pancreatitis. N Engl J Med 2010;362:1491-1502.
47. Balthazar EJ: Acute pancreatitis: Assessment of severity with clinical and CT evaluation. Radiology 2002;223:603-613.
54. Nathens AB, Curtis JR, Beale RJ, et al: Management of the critically ill patient with severe acute pancreatitis. Crit Care Med 2004;32:2524-2536.
61. Isenmann R, Rau B, Beger HG: Bacterial infection and extent of necrosis are determinants of organ failure in patients with acute necrotizing pancreatitis. Br J Surg 2007;86:1020-1024.

80. Villatoro E, Mulla M, Larvin M: Antibiotic therapy for prophylaxis against infection of pancreatic necrosis in acute pancreatitis. Cochrane Database Syst Rev 2010:CD002941.
88. Al-Omran M, Albalawi ZH, Tashkandi MF, Al-Ansary LA: Enteral versus parenteral nutrition for acute pancreatitis. Cochrane Database Syst Rev 2010;CD002837.
119. Mier J, Leon EL, Castillo A, et al: Early versus late necrosectomy in severe necrotizing pancreatitis. Am J Surg 1997;173:71-75.
125. Rau B, Pralle U, Mayer JM, Beger HG: Role of ultrasonographically guided fine-needle aspiration cytology in the diagnosis of infected pancreatic necrosis. Br J Surg 1998;85:179-184.
147. Halonen KI, Pettila V, Leppaniemi AK, et al: Long-term health-related quality of life in survivors of severe acute pancreatitis. Intensive Care Med 2003;29:782-786.

The complete list of references can be found at www.expertconsult.com.

78

Hemorrhagic and Thrombotic Disorders

Neil A. Lachant

CHAPTER OUTLINE

APPROACH TO A CRITICALLY ILL PATIENT WITH HEMORRHAGE OR THROMBOSIS

In the patient with acute hemorrhage or thrombosis, the history taker must be a detective interviewing the patient, family members, and outside health care providers. Useful information includes a personal or family history of a known bleeding disorder; bleeding after previous trauma, surgery, or dental procedures; a personal history of recent bleeding, bruising, or menorrhagia; and a history of liver or kidney disease, malabsorption, or recent chemotherapy. Perhaps the most challenging is obtaining a medication history, particularly as it may relate to covert heparin exposure. The use of anticoagulants, antiplatelet agents, aspirin, and nonsteroidal anti-inflammatory drugs (NSAIDs) should be determined. Recently started or intermittently used medications (e.g., quinine) that may cause thrombocytopenia should be elicited. In a hypercoagulable patient, a personal or family history of a known thrombophilic defect, thrombosis, recurrent miscarriage, or stillbirth may be useful.

The physical examination can be used to assess active problems, although physical signs of hemorrhage or thrombosis can be subtle. As examples, petechiae or purpura may develop only in dependent areas in a bedridden patient. The digits and skin should be carefully examined for signs of ischemia or necrosis.

LABORATORY TESTS OF COAGULATION

Although not reflective of the current model of coagulation, the integrity of coagulation is routinely tested by a limited set of in vitro assays (Fig. 78.1). The prothrombin time (PT) reflects the cascade of reactions traditionally called the extrinsic pathway, whereas the activated partial thromboplastin time (aPTT) reflects the intrinsic pathway. They intersect in the common pathway. The thrombin time (TT) measures the rate of conversion of fibrinogen to insoluble fibrin polymer after thrombin is added to plasma. A prolonged TT may be due to an inhibitor of thrombin (e.g., heparin, direct thrombin inhibitor [DTI]), hypofibrinogenemia or dysfibrinogenemia, fibrin degradation products (FDPs), and rarely paraproteins. The only specific coagulation factor that is routinely measured is fibrinogen. These four tests can usually localize abnormalities in the coagulation cascade.

Once a coagulopathy has been identified, the next step is to determine whether it is due to a factor deficiency or a circulating inhibitor. In the inhibitor or mixing study, the

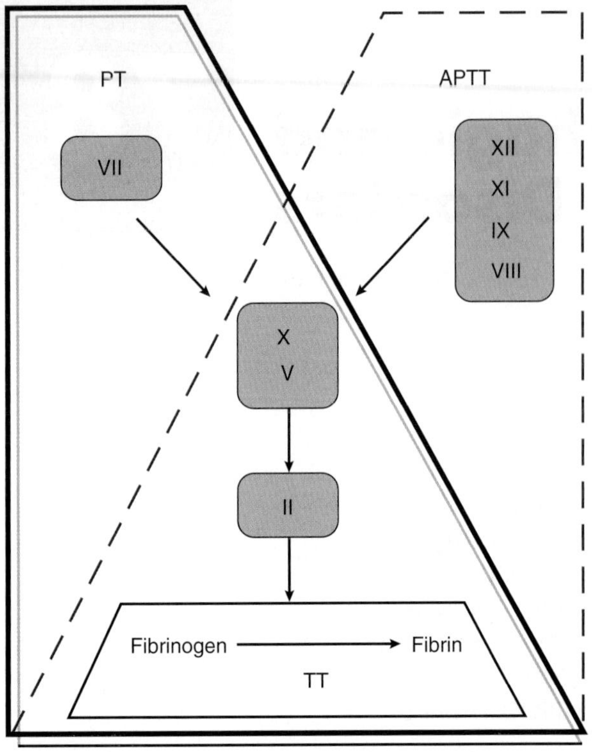

Figure 78.1 Coagulation factors evaluated in routine coagulation assays. aPTT, activated partial thromboplastin time; PT, prothrombin time; TT, thrombin time.

Box 78.1 Common Causes of Thrombocytopenia in Critically Ill Patients

Decreased Production

Drugs (e.g., thiazides, linezolid)
Ethanol
Liver disease
Right-sided heart failure

Increased Destruction/Consumption

Bacteremia/sepsis
Drugs
Disseminated intravascular coagulation
Massive bleeding/transfusions
Pulmonary artery catheter
Intra-aortic balloon pump
Ventricular assist device
Idiopathic thrombocytopenic purpura
Burns
Post-transfusion purpura
Thrombotic thrombocytopenic purpura
Antiphospholipid syndrome

Splenic Sequestration

Portal hypertension
Hypothermia

patient's plasma is mixed with an equal volume of normal pooled plasma. Normalization of the PT or aPTT in such a "mixing study" reflects a deficiency of one or more coagulation factors. It also implies that administration of fresh frozen plasma (FFP) should correct the coagulopathy. A further diagnosis requires specific factor assays. If there is partial or no correction in the mixing study, an inhibitor is suspected—most often contaminating heparin or a lupus anticoagulant.

The template bleeding time (BT) assesses in vivo platelet function in patients with a normal platelet count. It is used as a screen for disorders of platelet function. The concept of using the BT to predict surgical bleeding is archaic.

DISORDERS OF PLATELETS

THROMBOCYTOPENIA

MECHANISMS AND GENERAL MANAGEMENT

Thrombocytopenia is common in the intensive care unit (ICU). It has been estimated that 23% to 41% of patients in the ICU have a platelet count less than 100,000/μL, and 10% to 17% have a count less than 5000/μL.[1] Common causes of thrombocytopenia in the ICU are shown in Box 78.1. In complex, acutely ill patients, many of these mechanisms may operate simultaneously. Severe sepsis is the most common cause of thrombocytopenia in the ICU.[2]

Frequently, thrombocytopenia must be managed without a specific diagnosis. Medications should be reviewed for potential offending agents.[3,4] Inhibitors of platelet function should be avoided with platelet counts below 50,000/μL. If there is bleeding or if invasive procedures are anticipated, platelet transfusions should be given, unless contraindicated, to elevate the platelet count above 50,000/μL. In life-threatening situations, the goal should be a platelet count higher than 100,000/μL. In nonbleeding patients, maintenance of a platelet count above 10,000/μL (20,000/μL with fever or infection) with prophylactic transfusions is usually adequate.[5]

PSEUDOTHROMBOCYTOPENIA

Pseudothrombocytopenia is a laboratory artifact.[6] The platelet count is factitiously lowered because of the presence of naturally occurring antibodies that cause platelet agglutination in the presence of ethylenediaminetetraacetic acid (EDTA) at room temperature. The diagnosis is suspected by finding platelet clumps on the peripheral blood smear. Repeating the platelet count with a different anticoagulant such as citrate will generally produce a normal platelet count.

DRUG-INDUCED THROMBOCYTOPENIA

A limited number of drugs have evidence-based data to support a causal role in the development of thrombocytopenia.[3,4,7,8] Medications commonly used in the ICU can cause thrombocytopenia (Box 78.2). Drug-induced thrombocytopenia most commonly occurs 7 to 21 days after exposure to the offending agent. Clinical manifestations can range from an asymptomatic decrease in platelets to life-threatening bleeding. The diagnosis is established by (1) finding a temporal relationship between starting the drug

Box 78.2 Drugs Commonly Causing Thrombocytopenia in the Intensive Care Unit

Abciximab
Carbamazepine
Cephalosporins
Clopidogrel
Digoxin
Eptifibatide
Heparins
Hydrochlorothiazide
Linezolid
Quinidine
Quinine
Ranitidine
Tirofiban
Trimethoprim/sulfamethoxazole
Vancomycin

and the fall in the platelet count, (2) having no alternative diagnosis, and (3) having the platelet count recover after removal of the putative offending agent. Unfortunately, this is usually difficult to establish in the typical ICU patient. Treatment is based on removing the putative offending agent and initiating a drug of another class if possible. Though often used, steroids in general have not been shown to hasten the rate of platelet recovery. In severe thrombocytopenia with bleeding such as seen with quinine, intravenous immunoglobulin (IVIG) (1 g/kg/day for 2 days) and platelet transfusion are beneficial.

GLYCOPROTEIN IIB/IIIA INHIBITORS

All platelet glycoprotein (GP) IIb/IIIa inhibitors have been associated with severe thrombocytopenia that can occur within hours of exposure (up to 2 weeks with abciximab).[7] Heparin induced thrombocytopenia (HIT) is the main differential diagnosis. Bleeding is very uncommon with HIT because of the strong prothrombotic state. Conversely, with GP IIb/IIIa inhibitor-associated thrombocytopenia, bleeding or hematoma formation may occur, especially at the site of the sheath. A platelet count less than 20,000/µL and clinical bleeding are indications for platelet transfusion. The use of IVIG and corticosteroids is not evidence based.

IMMUNE THROMBOCYTOPENIC PURPURA

Immune thrombocytopenic purpura results from the destruction of IgG-coated platelets in the reticuloendothelial system, primarily the spleen. There is no compensatory increase in thrombopoiesis. Anemia, if present, may be autoimmune (Evans syndrome) or due to bleeding and iron deficiency. Immune thrombocytopenia may be primary (idiopathic [ITP]) or secondary. The differential diagnosis includes pseudothrombocytopenia; immune thrombocytopenia secondary to systemic lupus, human immunodeficiency virus (HIV) infection, or hepatitis C; and drug-induced thrombocytopenia.

Guidelines for the diagnosis and management of ITP have been developed.[9,10] Indications for therapy in ITP are platelet count less than 20,000 to 30,000/µL or clinical bleeding. Corticosteroids (prednisone, 1 mg/kg/day, or pulse dexamethasone, 40 mg/day for 4 days monthly) are the usual initial therapy for ITP.[9,10] Individuals with ITP in the ICU usually have severe or life-threatening bleeding. Several modalities of therapy should be used in concert to raise the platelet count in urgent situations (methylprednisolone, 1 g/day for 3 days, and IVIG, 1 g/kg/day for 2 days). Although platelets may be destroyed quickly, platelet transfusions should still be used as initial therapy. The response to platelet transfusion may improve after IVIG is given. Anti-Rh(D) IgG (WinRho), 50 to 75 µg/kg, has also been used.[11] Because the dose of anti-Rh(D) must be reduced in face of anemia, its use may be problematic in a patient with severe bleeding. Anti-Rh(D) IgG is ineffective in Rh-negative patients and after splenectomy. ε-Aminocaproic acid (4-5 g IV followed by either 2-4 g IV every 4 hours or 0.5-1.0 g/hour continuous IV infusion [maximum 24 g/24 hours]) may be useful for mucosal bleeding and severe menorrhagia.

POST-TRANSFUSION PURPURA

Post-transfusion purpura (PTP) is a rare condition characterized by acute, severe immune-mediated thrombocytopenia. PTP occurs in human platelet antigen-1 (HPA-1) negative individuals who receive HPA-1 positive platelets (most commonly as a contaminant in packed red blood cells [RBCs]). These individuals have previously been sensitized to HPA-1 through transfusion or pregnancy. Usually 7 to 10 days after reexposure to HPA-1, an anamnestic response occurs, resulting in a precipitous fall in the platelet count. Petechiae and bleeding are common. IVIG and plasma exchange are effective.[12]

ACQUIRED PLATELET DYSFUNCTION

MEDICATION-INDUCED ABNORMALITIES

Aspirin irreversibly acetylates cyclooxygenase (COX), inhibiting platelet function for the life of the platelet (7 to 10 days). The aspirin effect can be overcome with platelet transfusion or the infusion of desmopressin (DDAVP). The effect of NSAIDs is reversible and disappears as the drug is cleared, usually within 24 to 48 hours for ibuprofen. The risk of bleeding from NSAIDs is lowest with ibuprofen and greatest with ketorolac. The thienopyridine clopidogrel tightly binds the platelet ADP P2Y12 receptor. Clopidogrel should be withheld for 5 to 7 days before elective surgery or invasive procedures.[13] In an emergency, platelet transfusion can be tried, but platelet function may not be fully restored because of circulating active clopidogrel metabolites, which have a half-life of 8 hours and bind to the transfused platelets. Prasugrel is a new thienopyridine whose active metabolites have a 4-hour half-life. COX-2 inhibitors don't affect platelet function.

RENAL FAILURE

The hemorrhagic diathesis of renal failure is the result of metabolic derangements related to uremic toxins.[14] Bleeding may worsen when the hematocrit falls below 30% due to a rheologic phenomenon in which rapidly flowing RBCs gravitate to the center of the streaming blood and force the platelets toward the vessel wall. Uremic bleeding is uncommon in the modern era of dialysis.[15] For clinical bleeding, intravenous DDAVP (0.3 µg/kg given over 30 minutes) is often therapeutic.[14] If the hematocrit is less than 30%, the patient should be transfused with packed RBCs.[14,15] An alternative to DDAVP is cryoprecipitate (10 bags every 12 to 24 hours).[14] Intravenous conjugated estrogen, 0.6 mg/kg/day for 5 days, is also effective.[14] An unexpected "coagulopathy" (prolonged aPTT and TT) may develop as a result of delayed clearance of heparin after dialysis. If available, an anti–factor Xa assay will show the presence of heparin.

THROMBOCYTOSIS

Although not as common as thrombocytopenia, reactive thrombocytosis (splenectomy, surgery, or bleeding) may be seen in the ICU. Reactive thrombocytosis does not have an increased risk of thrombosis. Antiplatelet therapy is not needed even for platelet counts higher than 1,000,000/µL.

COMPLEX THROMBOHEMORRHAGIC DISORDERS

HEPARIN-INDUCED THROMBOCYTOPENIA

Although commonly looked for, HIT is an uncommon cause of thrombocytopenia in the ICU.[2,16] HIT is a paradoxical condition in which modest thrombocytopenia may be associated with devastating heparin-induced thrombocytopenia thrombosis (HITT). Thus, the entire health care team needs to be vigilant for the development of HIT in any patient receiving heparin. HIT has been associated with all types of heparin (unfractionated [UFH] and low-molecular-weight [LMWH]), at any dose, and by any route, including flushes and heparin-coated catheters.[1,17] The incidence of HIT has been estimated to be less than 1% of patients in the ICU.[2,16,18] HIT occurs in three time intervals. Classic HIT occurs 5 to 15 days after the initiation of heparin. Rapid-onset HIT develops hours to 1 to 2 days after heparin is started in individuals who have preformed circulating antibodies from a previous exposure to heparin, usually in the last 2 months. Classic and rapid-onset HIT may be manifested as thrombocytopenia with or without thrombosis [HIT(T)]. Delayed-onset HIT occurs an average of 12 days after the discontinuation of heparin and is manifested as isolated thrombosis. The thrombocytopenia of HIT is usually modest with an average platelet count of 50,000 to 60,000/µL.[19] Severe thrombocytopenia (<10,000/µL) should suggest an alternative diagnosis. HIT may be associated with a normal platelet count if there is a baseline thrombocytosis (e.g., postoperatively). HIT may be manifested as isolated thrombocytopenia or thrombocytopenia with potentially devastating thrombosis. Venous complications include deep venous thrombosis (DVT), pulmonary embolism (PE), cerebral sinus thrombosis, infarctive adrenal hemorrhage, and skin necrosis at the heparin injection site. Arterial complications include iliofemoral artery thrombosis, digital ischemia, myocardial infarction, stroke, and mesenteric artery thrombosis.

HIT is an immune-mediated process in which the heparin–platelet factor 4 complex becomes immunogenic. Antibodies are formed that activate platelets, causing the release of thrombogenic microparticles.[16,19] The antibodies can also activate monocytes and endothelial cells.

Box 78.3 Clinical Situations to Suspect Heparin-Induced Thrombocytopenia

Current Use of Heparin or Heparin Exposure within 40 Days and at Least One of the Following:

- Platelets <100,000/µL
- Platelets <50% of baseline or <50% of the maximum level if reactive thrombocytosis is present
- Platelets less than baseline 5 days after open heart surgery
- New arterial or venous thrombotic event
- Inflammation or necrosis at heparin injection sites
- Acute allergic or anaphylactic reaction to a heparin bolus

Recent Admission to a Hospital, Nursing, or Rehabilitation Facility Plus

- A new venous thromboembolic event
- A new arterial ischemic event

The diagnosis of HIT is clinicopathologic. HIT should be thought of in appropriate clinical situations (Box 78.3). The "4T" score has been used to predict the likelihood (pretest probability) of HIT (Table 78.1).[16,20] The HEP score, devised by an expert consensus panel, has recently been validated.[21] Although the decision to initiate therapy should be based on the clinical likelihood of HIT, laboratory testing should be used for the retrospective confirmation of the pretest likelihood of HIT. The complexities of HIT antibody testing are reviewed elsewhere.[16,22] In general, a strongly positive HIT enzyme-linked immunosorbent assay (ELISA) and strongly positive serotonin release assay (SRA) with a high pretest probability confirm the diagnosis of HIT, whereas a negative ELISA and SRA make the diagnosis of HIT unlikely with a low pretest probability. In other situations, clinical judgment prevails in establishing or excluding a diagnosis of HIT, especially because ELISA and SRA testing from commercial labs has not been validated in clinical studies.[1,16,22]

Once the diagnosis of HIT is thought to be likely, all heparin should be discontinued. Heparin-coated pulmonary artery catheters should be replaced with noncoated catheters. Catheters for dialysis or apheresis should be locked with 4% citrate or tissue plasminogen activator. The patient's chart and bedside should be labeled *heparin allergy*. Platelet transfusions should be avoided except for life-threatening bleeding, given the anecdotal observations of acute thrombosis occurring after platelet transfusion. A patient with life- or limb-threatening arterial thrombosis should be evaluated for surgical intervention. Anticoagulation with a DTI (Table 78.2) should be initiated in all patients unless contraindicated. LMWH is contraindicated in HIT caused by UFH. Conversion to warfarin can be considered after a minimum of 5 days of DTI therapy if the platelet count has returned to normal (suggesting that the process has cooled off and the patient is no longer hyperprothrombotic) and no future invasive procedures are planned. Simply discontinuing heparin therapy and not starting a DTI is inappropriate because occult thrombosis may have already developed.[23] Starting or continuing warfarin monotherapy is also contraindicated because of the risk

Table 78.1 Determining Pretest Probability of Heparin-Induced Thrombocytopenia (HIT): The "4 Ts"

Points	Thrombocytopenia	Timing of Onset of Thrombocytopenia (or Other Serious Sequelae)*	Thrombosis or Other Sequelae	OTher Causes of Thrombocytopenia
2	>50% decrease and nadir >20,000/µL	Day 5-10 or <1 day with recent heparin (past 30 days)	Proven new thrombosis, skin necrosis, or acute systemic reaction to heparin bolus	None evident
1	30-50% decrease or nadir of 10,000-19,000/µL	>Day 10 or timing unclear or <1 day with recent heparin (past 31-100 days)	Progressive or recurrent thrombosis, erythematous skin lesions, suspected thrombosis (not proved)	Possible
0	<30% decrease or nadir of <10,000/µL	<Day 4 (no recent heparin)	None	Definite

Pretest probability score: 0-3 points = low (<5%), 4-5 points = intermediate (physician judgment), 6-8 points = high (>80%).
*First day of heparin exposure = day 0.
Adapted from Lo GK, Juhl D, Warkentin TE, et al: Evaluation of pretest clinical score (4 T's) for the diagnosis of heparin-induced thrombocytopenia in two clinical settings. J Thromb Haemost 2006:4:759.

Table 78.2 Parenteral Anticoagulant Doses

Anticoagulant	Dosage: Prophylactic	Therapeutic: Initial	Therapeutic: Maintenance	Therapeutic: Optimal Level
Unfractionated heparin	5000 U SC q8h	80 U/kg by IV bolus	18 U/kg/h by continuous IV infusion	aPTT range corresponding to 0.3-0.7 U/mL
Enoxaparin	40 mg SC qd	1 mg/kg SC q12h	Continue at initial dose	0.5-1.0 U/mL obtained 3.5-4.0 h after the dose
Fondaparinux	2.5 mg SC qd	*<50 kg*: 5 mg SC qd *50-100 kg*: 7.5 mg SC qd *>100 kg*: 10 mg SC qd	Continue at initial dose	None
Argatroban	None	No bolus	2 µg/kg/min CI	aPTT 1.5-3.0 × patient's baseline
Liver disease			0.5 µg/kg/min CI	
ICU (i.e., open heart surgery, CHF)*	None	No bolus	0.5 µg/kg/min CI	aPTT 1.5-3.0 × patient's baseline
Lepirudin (Ccr ≥60 mL/min)	25 mg SC q12h	No bolus	0.15 mg/kg/h CI	aPTT 1.5-2.5 × midnormal
*ICU**				
No life-threatening thrombosis	25 mg SC q12h	No bolus	0.05-0.10 mg/kg/h CI	aPTT 1.5-2.5 × midnormal
Life-threatening thrombosis	None	0.2 mg/kg	0.05-0.10 mg/kg/h CI	APTT 1.5-2.5 × midnormal
Bivalirudin	None	No bolus	0.15 mg/kg/h	aPTT 1.5-2.5 × patient's baseline (or midnormal) aPTT

aPTT, activated partial thromboplastin time; Ccr, creatinine clearance; CHF, congestive heart failure; CI, continuous infusion; ICU, intensive care unit; qd, once daily; SC, subcutaneously.
*Suggested dose modification in ICU patients.
Data from Selleng K, Warkentin TE, Greinacher A. Heparin-induced thrombocytopenia in intensive care patients. Crit Care Med 2007;35:1165-1176.

of venous limb gangrene.[24] If warfarin has been given at the time HIT is diagnosed, vitamin K should be given to replenish proteins C and S. If invasive procedures are needed (e.g., tracheostomy, pacemaker), it is best to delay them, if medically safe, until the platelet count is normal to minimize the risk of developing thrombosis during the time that DTI therapy is withheld. Inferior vena cava (IVC) filters should be avoided because of the risk of vena cava thrombosis. Patients with active HIT may need percutaneous coronary intervention (PCI). Argatroban has been approved by the Food and Drug Administration (FDA) for use during PCI in patients with HIT.[25] Though not FDA approved, bivalirudin has been used safely in this situation.[26] In a patient who has active HIT or persistent HIT antibodies and who needs open heart surgery, medical management is recommended until the antibody becomes negative. If urgent surgery is needed, bivalirudin is most commonly used.[27] For the patient with a past history of HIT who needs open heart surgery and is currently HIT antibody negative, heparin can be used during bypass and a DTI started as soon as it is surgically safe postoperatively.[28]

THROMBOTIC THROMBOCYTOPENIC PURPURA

Thrombotic thrombocytopenic purpura (TTP) is a relatively rare disorder whose hallmarks are thrombocytopenia, microangiopathic hemolytic anemia (MAHA), and neurologic dysfunction. The diagnosis of TTP should be considered in any patient with unexplained thrombocytopenia and MAHA.[29] TTP is the clinical manifestation of a heterogeneous group of underlying disorders driven by different pathophysiologic processes. Although most cases of TTP are idiopathic, TTP may be associated with exposure to drugs (e.g., ticlopidine, clopidogrel, quinine, mitomycin C, gemcitabine, cyclosporine), pregnancy, HIV infection, and bone marrow transplantation.[30] The morphologic hallmark of TTP is hyaline thrombi in precapillary arterioles composed primarily of platelets. Classic TTP is due to an immune-mediated deficiency of the metalloproteinase ADAMTS13, which cleaves ultralarge multimers of von Willebrand factor (vWF) into smaller forms that are less platelet reactive.[31] Deficiency of this enzyme allows ultralarge forms of vWF that are normally sequestered in the endothelium to bind platelets and form microthrombi in the circulation. Conversely, ADAMTS13 activity is normal in TTP associated with bone marrow transplantation and the hemolytic-uremic syndrome.[30,31] Organ dysfunction is due to microvascular thrombosis. Commonly involved organs are the brain, kidneys, heart, and pancreas. It is critical to establish the diagnosis quickly because TTP can be rapidly fatal if not properly treated.

The core laboratory features of TTP are those of MAHA (more than two schistocytes per oil immersion field on a peripheral smear, increased lactate dehydrogenase, and very low haptoglobin). The differential diagnosis includes disseminated intravascular coagulation (DIC), severe vasculitis, eclampsia, HELLP (hemolysis, elevated liver enzymes, and low platelet count) syndrome, malignant hypertension, sepsis, and malignancy.

Once the diagnosis of TTP is thought to be likely, therapy should be initiated quickly because of the proclivity of the disease to progress rapidly. All patients should initially be treated in the ICU. Platelet transfusions should be avoided except for life-threatening bleeding because of anecdotal reports of acute decompensation after platelet transfusions. A large-bore catheter will need to be placed, even in the face of severe thrombocytopenia, because the mainstay and only evidence-based component of therapy for TTP is plasma exchange.[32,32a] Most commonly, 1.5 plasma volumes are exchanged daily with FFP. A clue that TTP is the correct diagnosis is the color of the plasma removed from the first plasmapheresis. A red or brown color suggests free hemoglobin from intravascular hemolysis. If plasma exchange cannot be initiated in a timely manner, infusion of 30 mL/kg of FFP daily can be a temporizing maneuver.[32] Corticosteroids (e.g., prednisone, 1 mg/kg/day) are commonly used as well.[32a] The use of antiplatelet agents, which may increase the risk of bleeding, and vincristine is controversial.[33] In patients who do not respond to initial therapy, rituximab is an attractive second-line therapy.[30,34]

HEMOLYTIC-UREMIC SYNDROME

Hemolytic-uremic syndrome (HUS), the triad of thrombocytopenia, MAHA, and acute kidney injury, is most commonly due to infection with Shiga toxin–producing *Escherichia coli* in children.[35] Adult atypical HUS (aHUS) is not Shiga toxin associated. It may be idiopathic or associated with calcineurin inhibitors (cyclosporin, tacrolimus), pregnancy, and HIV. aHUS is associated with low C3 and is a complement deposition disease. Mutations in complement factor H (CFH) are found in a minority of cases. Although not as efficacious as when used for TTP, plasma exchange is used for aHUS. The anti-C5 antibody eculizumab (Soliris) has been FDA approved for the treatment of aHUS.[36] Plasma exchange should be initiated while waiting to obtain eculizumab. Supplemental eculizumab dosing is required after each plasma exchange.[37] Patients need to receive quadravalent meningococcal vaccine before starting eculizumab.

DISSEMINATED INTRAVASCULAR COAGULATION

DIC is always a manifestation of a severe underlying pathologic process (Box 78.4). The final common pathway is the

Box 78.4 Common Causes of Disseminated Intravascular Coagulation

Acute

Infection
- Bacteria
- Fungus
- Virus
- *Rickettsia*

Complications of pregnancy
- Abruptio placentae
- Amniotic fluid embolism

Tissue trauma
Tissue hypoperfusion
Acute hemolytic transfusion reaction

Chronic

Neoplasia
- Adenocarcinoma

Liver disease
Retained dead fetus

Localized

Aortic aneurysm
Cavernous hemangioma

generation of thrombin, which produces microthrombi that can lead to organ dysfunction.[38] In the process, natural anticoagulants are consumed and fibrinolysis is activated. Circulating FDPs, along with the consumption of platelets and coagulation factors, lead to a bleeding diathesis. The balance between these competing processes results in the clinical manifestations in any particular individual.

The clinical manifestations of DIC are protean. Microvascular thromboses produce ischemia in many tissues, including the brain (delirium, coma), skin (digital gangrene, purpura fulminans), kidney, lungs (acute respiratory distress syndrome), gastrointestinal tract (mucosal ulceration), and blood (MAHA). The bleeding associated with DIC is due to the combination of depletion of coagulation factors, thrombocytopenia, inhibitory effects of FDPs on coagulation and platelet function, and tissue necrosis with ulceration. Common manifestations are intracerebral hemorrhage, global oozing at lines and venipuncture sites, hematuria, epistaxis, and gingival and gastrointestinal bleeding.

There are no strict, evidence-based laboratory criteria for the diagnosis of DIC.[38] The diagnosis is based on identifying an underlying predisposition, the clinical features, and laboratory testing. The most common laboratory features of DIC are thrombocytopenia, elevated FDP or D-dimers, and decreased fibrinogen. The PT and aPTT may or may not be prolonged, depending on the sensitivity of the assay, degree of baseline elevation of coagulation factors as acute-phase reactants, the rate of consumption of coagulation factors, and the amount of FDPs released. An absolute decrease in fibrinogen is very suggestive of DIC. However, fibrinogen activity in the normal range may still be consistent with DIC because fibrinogen is an acute-phase reactant and its level may be inappropriately low for the underlying physiologic state.[39] Serial measurement of fibrinogen is often useful. Schistocytes are seen in half the cases. Although the natural anticoagulants antithrombin (AT) (previously called AT-III) and proteins C and S are decreased, and thrombin-antithrombin complexes are increased, their levels usually cannot be measured in real time and are of limited clinical value.

The International Society of Thrombosis and Haemostasis (ISTH) has developed a scoring system for the identification of overt DIC using four commonly available tests (platelets, prothrombin time, FDPs such as D-dimer or soluble fibrin monomer, and fibrinogen) (Table 78.3), which has been prospectively validated.[40,41] It is important to remember that all the laboratory abnormalities seen in DIC can be caused by other disease processes. Vitamin K deficiency,[42] a heparin-contaminated blood sample, or a lupus anticoagulant can cause a coagulopathy, whereas elevations in FDPs can be seen with metastatic cancer or can be found after surgery or trauma. Other microangiopathies cause thrombocytopenia and RBC fragmentation. Liver failure can produce a constellation of laboratory abnormalities indistinguishable from those observed in DIC.[43]

The most important principle in the management of DIC is to treat the underlying cause. If the driving process cannot be controlled, the DIC will progress unabated. Hypothermia and acidosis should be corrected because they interfere with the function of coagulation factors.

Table 78.3 Original ISTH Scoring System for Overt Disseminated Intravascular Coagulation (DIC) and the Modified ISTH Scoring System for Overt DIC in Severe Sepsis

Test	Score
Platelet count (per μL)	
≥100,000	0
50,000-99,999	1
<50,000	2
D-dimer (μg/mL)	
≤0.39 (upper limit of normal)	0
0.40-4.0	2
>4.0	3
Prothrombin time prolongation (s)	
≤3	0
>3 but <6	1
≥6	2
Fibrinogen (mg/dL)	
>100	0
<100	1

Original ISTH score: (platelets + D-dimer + PT + fibrinogen) ≥ 5 signifies overt DIC.

Modified ISTH score: (platelets + D-dimer + PT) ≥ 5 signifies overt DIC in severe sepsis.

ISTH, International Society of Thrombosis and Haemostasis; PT, prothrombin time.

Adapted from Taylor FB, Toh CH, Hoots WK, et al: Towards definition, clinical and laboratory criteria, and a scoring system for disseminated intravascular coagulation. Thromb Haemost 2001;86:1327; and Dhainaut J-F, Yan SB, Joyce DE, et al: Treatment effects of drotrecogin alfa (activated) in patients with severe sepsis with or without overt disseminated intravascular coagulation. J Thromb Haemost 2003;2:1924.

If the diagnosis is suspected only because of laboratory abnormalities, management should be conservative. Alternative, potentially correctable processes should be kept in mind, such as vitamin K deficiency and drug-induced thrombocytopenia.

If clinically significant bleeding becomes apparent, a patient with overt DIC should receive blood component therapy (cryoprecipitate if fibrinogen is less than 100 mg/dL, FFP, and platelets). A realistic goal is to keep the fibrinogen level 100 to 150 mg/dL, the aPTT close to normal, and the platelet count greater than 50,000/μL. Heparin is not routinely used for the treatment of DIC. Heparin may be helpful for ischemic manifestations (e.g., digital ischemia, purpura fulminans). A continuous infusion at a rate of 7 U/kg/hour is a reasonable starting dose.

Other treatment modalities have been tried in DIC. The use of AT concentrates showed no significant decrease in mortality rate.[44] Activated protein C (drotrecogin alfa) used for the treatment of sepsis has been withdrawn from the U.S. market. Because of the intense fibrinolytic activity in DIC, antifibrinolytic agents (ε-aminocaproic acid and tranexamic acid) have been tried in an attempt to reduce bleeding. In general, failure rates have been quite high, and serious thromboses have occurred because the lysis of diffuse microthrombi was suppressed.

DISORDERS OF HEMOSTASIS

It has been estimated that 16% of ICU patients have bleeding caused by a coagulation defect and another 66% have abnormal coagulation test results.

ARTIFACTS

A common cause of an unexplained prolongation of the aPTT is unsuspected heparin in the line from which the blood was drawn. A diagnostic clue is a prolonged TT with a normal fibrinogen. A heparin level (anti–factor Xa assay) will confirm the diagnosis. Although venous access is often an issue in the ICU, blood for coagulation studies should be drawn by venipuncture if possible.

COAGULATION FACTOR ABNORMALITIES

ACQUIRED DEFICIENCIES OF PROCOAGULANTS

Vitamin K Deficiency

Vitamin K is essential for the post-translational modification (γ-carboxylation) of factors II, VII, IX, and X and proteins C and S. The daily requirement of vitamin K is 50 µg. Normal daily intake of vitamin K is 200 µg from the diet and 200 µg from intestinal flora. Thus, vitamin K deficiency occurs commonly in the ICU in the patient who is not being fed and who is receiving antibiotics that alter the gut flora. Vitamin K stores last approximately 1 week.

Because factor VII has the shortest half-life (approximately 4 hours), early vitamin K deficiency is manifested by an isolated prolongation of the PT. As factors II, IX, and X become depleted, the aPTT will become prolonged. Vitamin K deficiency is common in critically ill patients and may result in serious bleeding.[42] Treatment of vitamin K deficiency depends on the clinical situation. In a nonbleeding patient, vitamin K should be given enterally if the gut is working. Subcutaneous vitamin K should be avoided if the gut is working because of its erratic absorption, especially in face of impaired tissue perfusion and because anaphylactic reactions have been reported with subcutaneous vitamin K.[45] In a bleeding patient, FFP will correct the coagulopathy most quickly. In critically ill patients with an urgent need for vitamin K replacement, phytonadione may be administered intravenously if the benefits are thought to outweigh the risk of anaphylaxis. Vitamin K should be given no faster than 1 mg/minute with cardiorespiratory monitoring because anaphylactic reactions can occur even at this slow infusion rate.[45] One milligram of vitamin K twice a week can prevent vitamin K deficiency.

Liver Disease

The perturbation of hemostasis in liver disease is complex. All hemostatic factors except for vWF and plasminogen activator inhibitor-1 are synthesized in the liver. Loss of the ability to synthesize factor VII is disproportionately greater in patients with liver disease than in those receiving warfarin. Thus, the bleeding risk of a prolonged international normalized ratio (INR) from liver disease is not as great as the same INR with warfarin therapy.[46] As outlined later, changes in factor VIII/vWF, and decreased synthesis of natural anticoagulants and fibrinolytic proteins, may help keep the patient with liver disease in hemostatic balance,[43] making the autoanticoagulation of liver disease promulgated among house staff a myth.

Although hepatic dysfunction is most commonly associated with bleeding, the risk of thrombosis has been underappreciated.[43] Synthesis of hemostatic proteins becomes impaired when the albumin falls below 2.5 g/dL. Similar to vitamin K deficiency, the earliest abnormality is a reduction in factor VII. In more severe liver disease, the other coagulation factors become deficient. Factor V and fibrinogen do not usually decrease significantly until the liver failure is severe. In contrast, the activities of factor VIII and vWF are normal or elevated. AT, proteins C and S, and plasminogen are decreased. Hepatic clearance of activated procoagulants and FDP is reduced. Thrombocytopenia may develop due to decreased thrombopoietin production or splenic sequestration. Advanced liver disease may also be complicated by vitamin K deficiency from malnutrition and decreased vitamin K absorption due to cholestasis.

A variety of approaches have been used to treat the coagulopathy of liver disease. If the patient is not bleeding, a trial of vitamin K can be given for 3 days to see if the coagulopathy corrects. Because all patients with liver disease have some degree of biliary obstruction and fat malabsorption, the subcutaneous route is preferred over oral administration. Although the risk of anaphylaxis with intravenous vitamin K is low, it is not generally recommended empirically in a patient with liver disease because of the low likelihood that vitamin K will completely correct the coagulopathy.[45] If bleeding is a problem, FFP should be administered. Because the relationship between the levels of coagulation factors and the PT/PTT is nonlinear, the greater the prolongation of the PT and PTT, the greater the chance of correction with FFP. However, it is difficult to normalize the PT.[47] On average, a unit of FFP increases all coagulation factors by 6% to 7%. A typical patient with the coagulopathy of liver disease may have approximately 10% to 15% of the normal level of coagulation factors. If a factor level of 50% of normal is needed for hemostasis, 6 units of FFP would be expected to correct the bleeding diathesis. The PT and PTT may still be prolonged, however, depending upon the sensitivities of PT and PTT assays. The PT (and aPTT) should be checked immediately after the FFP is administered. Given the short half-life of factor VII, waiting until the next morning's routine blood draw will produce a prolongation of at least the PT and give the impression that the coagulopathy is uncorrectable.

Massive Transfusion

Massive volume replacement (>1 blood volume in less than 24 hours) may not give the liver sufficient time to replace coagulation factors. In a hemodynamically stable patient, coagulation studies should be followed serially and FFP infused when a coagulopathy develops. Conversely, exsanguinating patients should be managed with balanced transfusion of RBC:FFP:platelets in a ratio of 1:1:1 (either 1 unit of single donor or 6 units or random donor platelets).[48]

ACQUIRED CIRCULATING INHIBITORS

FACTOR VIII INHIBITORS

The clinical manifestations of factor VIII inhibitors can range from an unexplained prolongation of the aPTT to severe bleeding. The aPTT is markedly prolonged with a normal BT, PT, TT, and fibrinogen. The mixing study does not correct. Further evaluation includes factor VIII, IX, XI, and XII activities and a lupus anticoagulant panel; hematomas should not be drained except in severe circumstances (e.g., compartment syndrome) because of the risk for bleeding, even with replacement therapy. Treatment options depend on the severity of the inhibitor. A low-titer inhibitor (<5 Bethesda units [BU]) may be treated with factor VIII infusion (200 U/kg every 8 to 12 hours). For a high-titer antibody (>5 BU), the treatment options are recombinant human factor VIIa (rH-VIIa; NovoSeven) and virally inactivated concentrates containing activated coagulation factors (FEIBA [factor eight inhibitor bypass activity]). The dose of rH-VIIa is 90 μg/kg, which can be repeated every 2 hours until the bleeding stops. rH-VIIa carries a risk of thrombotic and ischemic events even in individuals with severe coagulopathy.[49] Coagulation studies are not used to adjust the dose. The PT always falls below the lower end of normal. The FEIBA dose is 50 to 100 U/kg, which is repeated every 6 to 12 hours (maximum daily dose 200 U/kg/day due to thrombotic risk). A total of 500 units of heparin can be added to each bag to prevent infusion phlebitis. The clinical response to FEIBA is monitored.

FACTOR V INHIBITOR

Topical thrombin (a.k.a. fibrin glue) is ubiquitously used in the operating room. Bovine thrombin is contaminated with factor V. Approximately 7 to 10 days after the use of fibrin glue, the PT and aPTT may prolong as a result of the development of antibodies against bovine factor V and rarely factor II. Bleeding is uncommon because platelet factor V is protected from the antibody.

INHERITED DEFICIENCIES OF PROCOAGULANTS

Management of critically ill patients with inherited coagulopathies requires specialized expertise. A hematologist or coagulationist should be consulted. Laboratory measurement of coagulation factor activity should be available on site.

VON WILLEBRAND DISEASE

von Willebrand disease (vWD) is the most common inherited coagulopathy. Synthesized in the vascular endothelium and megakaryocytes, vWF is the ligand that binds to the platelet GP Ib/IX/V complex and promotes platelet adhesion in vivo. vWF is a complex multimeric protein, with the largest molecular weight forms having the greatest platelet-binding capacity. Factor VIII procoagulant, which is synthesized by the liver, circulates bound to vWF.

vWD is inherited in an autosomal dominant manner with partial penetrance. The clinical features, diagnosis, and subclassification of vWD are reviewed elsewhere.[50]

Patients with vWD in the ICU most commonly have had major surgery, closed head trauma, major trauma, or life-threatening hemorrhage. The goal of therapy is to increase vWF activity and factor VIII activity to 100% of normal and to maintain them above 50%. Two virally inactivated factor VIII concentrates available in the United States (Humate-P and Alphanate) are rich enough in vWF to be of clinical use for treating vWD. The other brands of factor VIII concentrate do not contain enough vWF to be of clinical value. rH-VIII, used in hemophilia A, is of no benefit in vWD. The dose is 40 to 50 U/kg of vWF followed by 20 to 25 U/kg every 12 hours. Peak and trough levels of factor VIII (and vWF activity if available) should be obtained to help guide therapy. Doses should be rounded to the size of the nearest vial, if possible, so that these expensive factors are not wasted. In an emergency situation in a smaller facility that does not stock hemostatic factors on site, cryoprecipitate can be used at a dose of two bags per 5 kg followed by one bag per 5 kg every 12 hours until the patient can be transferred to a referral center. In mild cases of type I vWD, DDAVP may be adequate for promoting hemostasis. Repeat doses may be given every 12 hours, although tachyphylaxis will likely develop due to exhaustion of vWF stores in the Weibel-Palade bodies of the endothelium. Patients should be monitored for hyponatremia, especially if large volumes of fluid are given.

FACTOR VIII DEFICIENCY

Factor VIII deficiency (hemophilia A) is an X-linked recessive disorder that occurs in approximately 1 in 10,000 white males. Bleeding characteristically occurs in the joints, soft tissues, and gastrointestinal tract. Although the platelet count should be normal, individuals with hemophilia A complicated by hepatitis C or HIV infection (primarily from exposure to contaminated blood products prior to the era of viral inactivation) may have a concomitant immune thrombocytopenia.

For major surgery, closed-head trauma, major trauma, or life-threatening hemorrhage, the factor VIII level should be raised to 100% and then maintained continuously above 50% for the first 5 to 7 days and above 40% for an additional 5 to 7 days. rH-VIII is the treatment of choice because it has no risk of viral infection. One unit of factor VIII per kilogram should raise the plasma factor VIII activity by 2%. Thus, the initial dose is 50 U/kg followed by 25 U/kg every 8 hours. Peak and trough factor VIII levels should be obtained after the first dose and at least daily. In an emergency situation if rH-VIII is not available, virally inactivated factor VIII would be the treatment of choice. The dosing schema is similar to that of rH-VIII. In an emergency situation in a smaller facility that does not stock hemostatic factors on site, cryoprecipitate can be given every 8 hours until the patient can be transferred. Similar to vWD, DDAVP can be given for mild or moderate factor VIII deficiency in known DDAVP responders. As the hemophilia population ages, coronary artery disease (CAD) is becoming an increasing problem. Individuals with hemophilia A should be supported through indicated cardiac procedures and surgery.[51]

FACTOR IX DEFICIENCY

Except for the rate of spontaneous mutations, the clinical picture of factor IX deficiency (hemophilia B) is indistinguishable from that of hemophilia A. The laboratory features are similar except factor IX activity is decreased and factor VIII activity is normal. The treatment of choice is rH-IX. Because of differences in the volume of distribution in comparison to rH-VIII, the initial loading dose of rH-IX is 100 U/kg followed by half the dose every 12 hours. At least 30% of individuals require a higher dose. Thus, it is not unreasonable to start with a dose of 125 to 150 U/kg, especially in a patient whom you do not want to underdose. Peak and trough levels should be monitored. If rH-IX is not available in an emergency situation, virally inactivated prothrombin complex concentrate (PCC) can be used. The initial dose is factor IX 100 U/kg followed by 50 U/kg every 12 hours. DDAVP and cryoprecipitate are not effective.

FACTOR XI DEFICIENCY

Factor XI deficiency is an autosomal recessive disorder most commonly seen in Ashkenazi Jews. The bleeding history is variable, ranging from menorrhagia to bleeding with delivery or surgery. Therapy depends on the clinical situation.[52] For severe deficiency, FFP (10 to 20 mL/kg followed by 3 to 6 mL/kg every 6 hours) is used. The goal is factor XI activity greater than 40% to 45%. Individuals with factor XI deficiency may be seen in the ICU because factor XI deficiency is not protective against coronary artery disease. These individuals may require emergency cardiac catheterization and coronary intervention.[53] Clopidogrel has been given safely after coronary stenting.[54]

VENOUS THROMBOEMBOLISM

Venous thromboembolism (VTE) is common in critically ill patients. Twenty-nine percent of medical ICU patients have been found to have asymptomatic lower extremity DVT, although 5.8% and 4.2% have symptomatic DVT and PE, respectively.[55] Most patients admitted to the ICU have multiple risk factors including recent surgery, trauma, sepsis, malignancy, immobilization, stroke, advanced age, heart or respiratory failure, previous VTE, and indwelling catheters.[55-57]

DEEP VENOUS THROMBOSIS PROPHYLAXIS

All patients admitted to the ICU should be evaluated for their risk for DVT. The perceived risk of thrombosis and bleeding needs to be assessed in each ICU patient.[55] In medical patients, options are LMWH and UFH.[55] In medical patients with a high bleeding risk, mechanical prophylaxis (graded compression stockings and intermittent pneumatic compression devices) is recommended.[55] Beyond the size limitations of this chapter, specific recommendations for DVT prophylaxis are available for trauma, abdominal/pelvic, thoracic, cardiac, and neurologic surgery.[58]

THERAPY FOR VENOUS THROMBOEMBOLISM

In the noncritical care setting, VTE is routinely treated with at least 5 days of UFH, LMWH, or fondaparinux (see Table 78.2), followed by warfarin.[59] In the ICU, intravenous UFH is the safest mode of anticoagulation give its rapid reversabilty for procedures or bleeding. LMWH has the disadvantages of a longer half-life and being only partially reversed with protamine. As discussed in the section on anticoagulation, fondaparinux should not be used routinely in the ICU. ICU patients should not be transitioned to warfarin given their risk of bleeding and frequent need for invasive procedures. Warfarin is hard to regulate due to frequent drug interactions (especially with antibiotics) and erratic oral intake. Warfarin may stick to feeding tubes.[60] Warfarin is absorbed in the upper small bowel and may not be absorbed if given via J-tube.[61]

INFERIOR VENA CAVA FILTER

Approximately 80% of PE occur as a result of the lower extremity DVT. IVC filter placement is indicated in two situations: (1) acute DVT and a contraindication to anticoagulation (e.g., recent intracranial hemorrhage or stroke, recent neurologic or ophthalmologic surgery, active gastrointestinal hemorrhage, cerebral metastasis with a high risk of bleeding [e.g., melanoma, renal cell, seminoma][62]), and (2) recurrent PE despite therapeutic anticoagulation. Filters may have some benefit in face of PE causing hypotension.[59] IVC filters are not indicated for PE without DVT. IVC filters do not eliminate all risk of PE and do not decrease mortality rates.[59] There is an approximate 10% risk of thrombosis at the filter insertion site.[59]

CATASTROPHIC ANTIPHOSPHOLIPID SYNDROME

Catastrophic antiphospholipid syndrome is an uncommon disorder manifested as multiple organ dysfunction secondary to microvascular thrombi. The diagnosis should be considered in patients with an acute onset of more than three of the following: respiratory failure, stroke or other neurologic impairment, abnormal liver function, renal impairment, skin infarction, and thrombocytopenia. Laboratory testing should show evidence of antiphospholipid antibodies. Though not evidence based, empiric therapy has centered around the combined use of high-dose corticosteroids, anticoagulation, and plasma exchange or IVIG.

ANTICOAGULANTS

A variety of parenteral and oral anticoagulants acting through different mechanisms are commercially available with many more in development. Commonly used dosing schema are shown in Table 78.2.

HEPARIN, HEPARIN DERIVATIVES, AND HEPARINOID

HEPARIN

Heparin is a glycosaminoglycan that anticoagulates blood by augmenting the activity of AT.[63] Complexes of heparin and AT inhibit thrombin, factor Xa, and other procoagulant proteases. The first five sugars of heparin bind to AT. The additional sugars determine the protein binding properties and pharmacokinetics of UFH and LMWH.[63]

UNFRACTIONATED HEPARIN

Binding of heparin to AT varies markedly between individuals, making monitoring a requirement. The anti–factor IIa property of heparin is measured by the aPTT. Because the anti-IIa and anti-Xa properties of UFH are equal, UFH is usually monitored by the aPTT.

The goal of therapeutic heparin is to maintain the aPTT in a range that corresponds to a heparin level of 0.3 to 0.7 U/mL.[63] Given the marked variability in aPTT response to heparin because of differences in reagents and laboratory equipment, this range needs to be determined in each laboratory. Because some hospitals do not have a heparin protocol, an adaptation of the Raschke nomogram is shown in Table 78.4.[63,64] An aPTT ratio of 1.5 to 2.5 times the control value correlates very poorly with the anti-Xa heparin assay and should not be used. The dose of heparin is weight based. No adjustments are needed for obesity, hepatic dysfunction, or renal impairment. The hemoglobin and platelet count should be monitored daily as surveillance for occult bleeding and HIT. Overanticoagulation with heparin can usually be managed by simply interrupting the infusion. With serious bleeding, heparin can be reversed immediately with intravenous protamine sulfate.[63] One milligram of protamine will neutralize 100 units of heparin. If bleeding occurs during the constant infusion, the amount of heparin given during the previous 2 hours should be used for the calculation. Thus, a patient bleeding after a 5000-unit heparin bolus will need 50 mg of protamine, whereas a patient receiving a 1250 U/hour infusion will need only 25 mg of protamine. Protamine should be given slowly over 1 to 3 minutes to minimize the risk for hypotension and bradycardia. The risk for anaphylaxis is increased in those who have received protamine zinc insulin or who have had a vasectomy.

LOW-MOLECULAR-WEIGHT HEPARIN

The properties of LMWH vary significantly from those of UFH.[63] The anti-Xa:anti-IIa ratio of LMWH is approximately 4:1. Thus, LMWH does not significantly affect the aPTT. There is little protein binding, allowing for predictable renal excretion. The properties of the available LMWHs (enoxaparin, dalteparin, tinzaparin) are different. Their kinetics and dosing are not interchangeable.[63] In a normal-sized adult (50 to 150 kg) with normal renal function, monitoring is not necessary. If monitoring is necessary (weight outside the usual range, impaired renal function, pregnancy), anti-Xa activity is measured 3.5 to 4.0 hours after an enoxaparin dose. The therapeutic range for enoxaparin (1 mg/kg every 12 hours) is 0.5 to 1.0 U/mL. LMWH is only 60% reversible by protamine.[63] If bleeding occurs within 8 hours of a LMWH injection, 1 mg of protamine per 100 anti-Xa units should be given. Because of the kinetics of LMWH, a second protamine dose of 0.5 mg per 100 anti-Xa units should be given if the bleeding persists.[63]

Table 78.4 Heparin Dosing Nomogram

Anti–Factor Xa (U/mL)	aPTT
Initial dose	80 U/kg bolus, then 18 U/kg/hour
<0.15	80 U/kg bolus, increase by 4 U/kg/hour
0.15-0.29	40 U/kg bolus, increase by 2 U/kg/hour
0.30-0.70	No change
0.71-0.85	Decrease infusion by 2 U/kg/hour
>0.85	Hold 1 hour, decrease infusion by 3 U/kg/hour

aPTT, activated partial thromboplastin time.
Adapted from Raschke RA, Reilly BM, Guidry JR, et al: The weight based heparin dosing nomogram compared with a "standard care" nomogram: A randomized controlled trial. Ann Intern Med 1993;119:874.

PENTASACCHARIDE

Fondaparinux (Arixtra) is a synthetic analog of the first five sugars of heparin. Due to its small size, it is a pure factor Xa antagonist. Fondaparinux is approved for treatment of DVT and PE and for DVT prophylaxis in orthopedic and abdominal surgery. Although not FDA approved, fondaparinux has been used off-label for the prophylaxis and treatment of HIT(T).[16] As a result of its 18- to 21-hour half-life, its use in the ICU is limited because it is not rapidly cleared in a patient population that needs frequent procedures, that has a high risk of bleeding, and often has renal impairment (contraindicated with creatine clearance [Ccr] < 30 mL/minute). It does not prolong the PT, aPTT, or TT. It can be measured in the anti-Xa assay calibrated for fondaparinux. It is not reversed by protamine. Bleeding due to pentasaccharide should be supported by transfusion. rH-VIIa can be tried.

HEPARINOID

Danaparoid is a mixture of sulfated glycosaminoglycans, distinct from heparin, that produces an anticoagulant effect primarily by enhancing the activity of AT. Danaparoid is primarily used in the setting of HIT. Dosing schema are available for most clinical situations.[65] If monitoring is necessary, such as during renal failure, anti-Xa activity must be determined. Though no longer available in the United States, danaparoid is available in Canada and Europe.

DIRECT THROMBIN INHIBITORS

As the name implies, DTIs directly bind to and inhibit the function of thrombin. Because of their expense, parenteral DTIs are generally reserved for the treatment of patients with HIT(T) or true heparin allergy. Although none of them have an antidote, rH-VIIa has anecdotally been used off-label to stop life-threatening bleeding. Oral DTIs have recently become available.

Argatroban is an arginine analog with a 40-minute half-life. It is metabolized in the liver, and its half-life increases to around 140 minutes with hepatic dysfunction. Because of its short half-life, an initial bolus is not needed. Although argatroban is monitored by the aPTT, it has a significant effect on the PT.[66] Argatroban monotherapy will approximately double the INR and can markedly prolong the INR with warfarin cotherapy. As long as the aPTT is therapeutic, this exaggerated increase in INR does not increase the bleeding risk.

Hirudin is a family of recombinant proteins originally extracted from the salivary glands of leeches.[67] Lepirudin is used subcutaneously or intravenously. The half-life of intravenous lepirudin is 80 to 180 minutes but extends to days with severe renal failure. Although lepirudin can be removed by hemofiltration, the filters are not approved for use in the United States.[68] It should not be used in those with sulfite sensitivity. Approximately 40% of individuals exposed to lepirudin will develop antilepirudin antibodies, which will impair drug excretion and which may cause anaphylaxis on reexposure. Lepirudin is no longer produced for the European Union.

Bivalirudin is a reversible synthetic analog of hirudin. Bivalirudine has the advantage of a 25-minute half-life. Although it is cleared primarily by intravascular proteolysis, the dose must be reduced with renal dysfunction. Although not FDA approved, bivalirudin is used off-label in many centers for systemic anticoagulation for HIT(T).[69] It is also used off-label for bypass surgery in individuals with HIT.[27]

Dabigatran (Pradaxa) is the first FDA approved oral DTI. It is approved for prevention of stroke and systemic embolization with nonvalvular atrial fibrillation.[70] It should be used with extreme caution in the elderly, especially because of the risk of bleeding due to overestimation of the Ccr and risk of trauma in the infirm. The dose is 150 mg twice a day (if Ccr > 30 mL/minute). Although not FDA approved, dabigatran has shown efficacy for the treatment of VTE.[71] It binds free and clot bound thrombin, and is primarily cleared via the kidneys with a half-life of 12 to 17 hours.[72] Drugs that are metabolized via P-glycoprotein may alter metabolism of dabigatran, which is a prodrug. There is no standardized laboratory test to measure the dabigatran level. Thus, in a patient who is having bleeding or thrombotic events while taking dabigatran, there is no test to tell whether the event may be related to over- or underanticoagulation. Given its sensitivity, a normal TT suggests that there is no dabigatran present. How long dabigatran should be discontinued before procedures depends upon the renal function and the bleeding risk of the procedure.[72] Dabigatran has no antidote. In the bleeding patient, in addition to supportive care and transfusion, the use of activated charcoal (if within 2 hours of ingestion), FEIBA, rH-VIIA, and dialysis have been suggested. Although antifibrinolytics have been shown to decrease bleeding after trauma,[73] they should be used with trepidation with FEIBA and rH-VIIa because of the risk of thrombosis.

ORAL FACTOR XA INHIBITORS[74]

Oral factor Xa inhibitors are undergoing clinical trials for a variety of indications. Because there are no evidence-based data regarding the reversal of oral factor Xa inhibitors in the bleeding patient, they should be used with caution in the ICU.

APIXIBAN

Apixiban (Eliquis), 5 mg twice a day, has been shown to be superior to warfarin for stroke prevention in atrial fibrillation and is under FDA review.[75] Its elimination is fecal and renal with an 8- to 15-hour half-life. Platelet GP and strong CYP3A4 inhibitors significantly increase its plasma concentration.

RIVAROXABAN

Rivaroxaban (Xarelto), 20 mg daily, is FDA approved for the prevention of stroke and systemic embolization with nonvalvular atrial fibrillation, and doses of 10 mg daily have been approved for the prevention of VTE with knee and hip replacement surgery.[76] Although not FDA approved, it has been shown to be efficacious for the treatment of DVT and PE.[77] It has a 5- to 9-hour half-life (9-13 hours in the elderly) and is metabolized primarily via the cytochrome system. Combined platelet GP and strong CYP3A4 inhibitors may significantly increase the plasma concentration of rivaroxaban. It should be avoided in face of significant hepatic dysfunction, and dose reduction is required for a Ccr less than 50 mL/minute. It should be discontinued at least 24 hours before surgery. Rivaroxaban activity can be measured by the anti-Xa assay used to monitor heparins. Unfortunately, at the time of this writing, standards to calibrate the assay are not available in the United States. Prolongation of the INR by rivaroxaban has been reversed with the use of PCC in healthy volunteers.[78] There are no data on the efficacy of PCC in bleeding patients. Rivaroxaban is not dialyzable.

Box 78.5 Reversal of Warfarin

International Normalized Ratio (INR) < 4.5, No Bleeding

- Lower dose or
- Omit dose and restart at a lower dose

INR > 4.5 but <10.0, No Significant Bleeding

- Omit 1 or 2 doses and restart at a lower dose, or
- For rapid reversal (e.g., surgery), vitamin K, 3 to 5 mg orally
  INR should decrease in 24 hours
  Give another 1 to 2 mg if the goal is not reached

INR > 10.0, No Significant Bleeding

- Hold warfarin and
- Give vitamin K, 5 to 10 mg orally
  The INR should be significantly reduced in 24 to 48 hours
  Give additional vitamin K orally if needed
  Resume warfarin when the INR is therapeutic

Any INR, Major Bleeding

- Hold warfarin
- Vitamin K, 5-10 mg by slow intravenous infusion
- Repeat vitamin K every 12 hours as needed
- If urgent correction needed (in order of preference)
  Quadravalent prothrombin complex concentrate
  Fresh frozen plasma
  Recombinant human factor VIIa

Adapted from Hirsch J, Raschke R: Heparin and low molecular weight heparin: The seventh ACCP conference on antithrombotic and thrombolytic therapy. Chest 2004;126:188S; Ageno W, Gallus AS, Wittkowsky A, et al: Oral anticoagulant therapy: Antithombotic therapy and prevention of thrombosis, 9th ed. ACCP evidence-based clinical practice guidelines. Chest 2012;141;e44S-e88S.

WARFARIN

The vitamin K antagonist warfarin decreases the activities of factors II, VII, IX, and X and proteins C and S. Although prolongation of the PT is often seen within the first 24 to 48 hours after initiation of warfarin due to the decrease in factor VII, 4 to 5 days are required for factors II and X to drop to antithrombotic levels.

The response to warfarin is variable and is affected by many factors common in the ICU, such as poor nutrition (vitamin K deficiency), liver dysfunction, and coadministration of medications that affect warfarin pharmacokinetics. It is not uncommon for patients to become overanticoagulated with warfarin. An approach to warfarin reversal is shown in Box 78.5.[79,80]

KEY POINTS

- Hemorrhagic and thrombotic complications in a critically ill patient can usually be anticipated and avoided by careful history taking and physical examination. Routine laboratory tests (platelet count, PT, aPTT, TT, fibrinogen) are helpful in evaluating hemorrhagic disorders but not thrombotic disorders.
- Vitamin K deficiency is a relatively common coagulopathy in critically ill patients, and it is easily treated if recognized.
- von Willebrand disease, the most common inherited coagulopathy, varies highly in clinical severity. Humate-P and Alphanate are the only "factor VIII" concentrates that are therapeutic.
- The bleeding diathesis of uremia can improve with several different treatments, including dialysis, DDAVP, intravenous administration of estrogens, and cryoprecipitate.
- Idiopathic thrombocytopenic purpura (ITP) in adults is usually chronic. If life threatening, several modalities are available for urgent elevation of the platelet count.
- Disseminated intravascular coagulation (DIC) is always a secondary disease process. Treatment must be focused on the underlying cause. If bleeding occurs, blood components should be given. Heparin is generally reserved for clinically evident thrombosis.
- Thrombotic thrombocytopenic purpura (TTP) is a clinical diagnosis associated with multiple inciting events. It is often fatal unless recognized early and treated with plasma exchange.

KEY POINTS (Continued)

- Heparin-induced thrombocytopenia with thrombosis may be life threatening. It should be looked for in any patient with thrombocytopenia who has been exposed to heparin. It can be managed with DTIs.
- Deep venous thrombosis is common in critically ill patients. Prophylactic treatment should be considered for every patient in the ICU. Intravenous UFH is often the safest treatment of established DVT in the critical care setting.
- Novel oral direct thrombin and factor Xa inhibitors are being used with increasing frequency. They have no antidotes for bleeding and there are no evidence-based protocols for their reversal.

SELECTED REFERENCES

2. Greinacher A, Selleng K: Thrombocytopenia in the intensive care unit patient. Hematol Am Soc Hematol Educ Program 2010; 2010:135-143.
10. Neunert C, Lim W, Crowther M, et al: The American Society of Hematology 2011 evidence-based practice guideline for immune thrombocytopenia. Blood 2011;117:4190-4207.
16. Linkins L-A, Dans AL, Moores LK, et al: Treatment and prevention of heparin-induced thrombocytopenia: Antithombotic therapy and prevention of thrombosis, 9th ed. ACCP evidence-based clinical practice guidelines. Chest 2012;141:e495S-e530S.
20. Lo GK, Juhl D, Warkentin TE, et al: Evaluation of pretest clinical score (4 T's) for the diagnosis of heparin-induced thrombocytopenia in two clinical settings. J Thromb Haemost 2006;4:759-765.
29. George JN: Thrombotic thrombocytopenic purpura. N Engl J Med 2006;354:1927-1935.
43. Lisman T, Porte RJ: Rebalanced hemostasis in patients with liver disease: Evidence and clinical consequences. Blood 2010,116. 878-885.
47. Abdel-Wahab OL, Healey B, Dzik WH: Effect of fresh-frozen plasma transfusion on prothrombin time and bleeding in patients with mild coagulation abnormalities. Transfusion 2006;46:1279-1285.
55. Kahn SR, Lim W, Dunn AS, et al: Prevention of VTE in nonsurgical patients: Antithombotic therapy and prevention of thrombosis, 9th ed. ACCP evidence-based clinical practice guidelines. Chest 2012;141:e195S-e226S.
63. Garcia DA, Baglin TP, Weitz JI, et al: Parenteral anticoagulants: Antithombotic therapy and prevention of thrombosis, 9th ed. ACCP evidence-based clinical practice guidelines. Chest 2012; 141:e24S-e43S.
73. CRASH-2 Trial Collaborators: Effects of tranexamic acid on death, vascular occlusive events, and blood transfusion in trauma patients with significant haemorrhage (CRASH-2): A randomized, placebo-controlled trial. Lancet 2010;376:23-32.

The complete list of references can be found at www.expertconsult.com.

79 Use of Blood Components in the Intensive Care Unit

Michael C. Shen | Janice L. Zimmerman

CHAPTER OUTLINE

Transfusion of blood components is a frequent intervention in hospitalized patients, particularly in critically ill patients. An estimated 22,628,000 units of red blood cells (RBCs), platelets, plasma, and cryoprecipitate were transfused in 2008 in the United States.[1] RBC transfusion is often utilized to optimize oxygen-carrying capacity and tissue perfusion that may be due to blood loss, inadequate marrow function, and RBC destruction. Additionally, hemostatic disorders may necessitate the administration of other blood components such as plasma, platelet concentrates, or cryoprecipitate.

Blood components should be considered therapeutic agents with potential benefits as well as adverse effects. Unlike pharmaceutical agents, however, blood components have fewer objective indications for use and no therapeutic index relating dose to safety. Although infectious risks of blood component transfusion have diminished, recognition of risks such as immunomodulation and transfusion-related acute lung injury (TRALI) has increased. Programs of patient blood management are proposed to determine appropriate evidence-based use of blood components and to minimize use of blood products.[2] Although more quality evidence has become available to guide clinical decisions in transfusion, many questions remain to be explored through clinical trials, particularly in critically ill patients.

BLOOD COMPONENTS AND INDICATIONS FOR TRANSFUSION

Blood component therapy is used to optimize management of the blood supply. The basic principle of blood component therapy is to use the specific blood product that meets the patient's need. Up to four components (RBCs, plasma, platelets, cryoprecipitate) can be derived from a single whole blood (WB) donation and then distributed to several recipients with differing physiologic needs. Component therapy thus meets the clinical requirements of increased safety, efficacy, and conservation of limited resources. As the variety of available blood product components increases, however, the complexity of transfusion medicine also increases. A WB donation is typically separated into RBCs, a platelet concentrate, and fresh frozen plasma (FFP). The plasma may be further processed into cryoprecipitate and

Table 79.1 Characteristics of Blood Components

Blood Component	Content	Volume (mL)	Plasma (mL)	Shelf Life
Red Cell Products				
Whole blood	RBCs (hct 40-45%), WBCs, plasma, platelets (nonviable)	500-515	~300	21-35 days at 1-6° C (depending on anticoagulant) 24 h if unrefrigerated
Packed RBCs	RBCs (hct 60-80%), WBCs, plasma, platelets (nonviable)	250-300	~25-50 mL	21-42 days at 1-6° C (depending on anticoagulant)
Leukocyte-reduced RBCs (filtered)	RBCs (hct 90%), minimal plasma	200	Minimal	21-42 days at 1-6° C (depending on anticoagulant)
Washed RBC	RBCs (hct 60%), some WBCs	340	0	24 hours
Frozen RBCs	RBCs (hct 90%, minimal WBC and platelets (nonviable)	170-190	0	10 years at −80° C
Platelets				
	Platelets, some WBCs, some RBCs, plasma			Open, 24 hours at 20-24° C with continuous agitation Closed, 5 days at 20-24° C with continuous agitation
Single donor (apheresis)	≥ 3 × 10^11 platelets/unit	~300 (200-400)	~250	
Random donor	≥ 5.5 × 10^10 platelets/unit	50	50	
Plasma-Derived Products				
Fresh frozen plasma (frozen within 6 to 8 hours of phlebotomy)	Plasma with all coagulation factors and inhibitors, complement, fibrinogen, albumin, globulins	*Whole blood donor:* 200-250 *Apheresis donor:* 400-600	200-250 400-600	1 year at −18° C; 24 hours at 1-6° C once thawed
Plasma frozen within 24 hours (separated from whole blood stored at 4-6° C within 24 hours of collection)	Plasma with all coagulation factors and inhibitors but with lower levels of V and VIII; complement, fibrinogen, albumin, globulins	200-250	200-250	1 year at −18° C; 24 hours at 1-6° C once thawed
Cryoprecipitate-reduced plasma (fresh frozen plasma with cold-induced precipitate removed)	Similar to fresh frozen plasma but deficient in XIII, VIII, fibrinogen, and von Willebrand factor	200-225	200-225	1 year at −18° C; 24 hours at 1-6° C once thawed
Cryoprecipitate	Factor VIII (minimum 80 IU), XIII, fibrinogen (minimum 150 mg), von Willebrand factor, plasma, fibronectin	5-20	5-20	1 year at −18° C; 4-6 hours at room temperature once thawed

RBCs, red blood cells; WBCs, white blood cells; hct, hematocrit.

supernatant (cryopoor) plasma. The characteristics of more commonly transfused blood products are described in Table 79.1.

WHOLE BLOOD AND RED BLOOD CELLS

Unseparated venous donor blood with a preservative solution constitutes a WB unit. It contains all blood components, but after less than 24 hours of refrigerated storage, platelet and leukocyte function is lost. With further storage, levels of the labile coagulation factors V and VIII markedly decrease.[3] The growing need for specialized blood components has resulted in processing the majority of blood donations into components, thus limiting the availability of WB. Only 0.03% of total blood transfusions in the United States in 2008 were WB units.[1]

RBCs, commonly known as *packed red blood cells* (PRBCs), are the blood component most commonly transfused to increase RBC mass. PRBCs are derived from the centrifugation or sedimentation of WB and removal of most of the plasma/anticoagulant solution. PRBCs may be further modified to meet the specific needs of patients or blood bank regulations. Leukocyte-reduced PRBCs are the most commonly transfused modified RBC product. Transfusion of blood components containing leukocytes may lead to nonhemolytic febrile transfusion reactions, a greater propensity for platelet alloimmunization, and transmission of pathogens carried by leukocytes, such as cytomegalovirus (CMV). Leukocyte reduction requires filtration of the blood component by a special filter at the time of blood donation and processing or later at the time of transfusion ("bedside filtration"). Leukocyte-reduced RBC units must contain less than 5.0×10^6 leukocytes. Filtration before storage conveys the benefit of removing white blood cells (WBCs) before they can deteriorate and elaborate cytokines and other unwanted substances during storage.[4] Because of proven and theoretical benefits of leukocyte reduction of blood components (discussed later in the section covering the adverse effects of transfusion), many European countries and Canada require that all PRBCs be leukocyte reduced, a process called *universal leukoreduction* (ULR). Some institutions in the United States have also made that decision, but either method of leukocyte reduction adds significantly to the cost of each transfusion, and the benefits of this measure when applied globally have yet to be quantified.[5] Almost 70% of transfused PRBCs are leukoreduced in the United States.[1]

Washing PRBCs involves recentrifuging in normal saline to remove the plasma/preservative solution from the unit. Washing removes 99% of the plasma proteins and 85% of leukocytes. Washing may take an hour or more, limits subsequent storage time to 24 hours, and causes loss of RBCs (10-20%). Washing is not an effective method of leukoreduction. Washed PRBCs may be indicated for patients with febrile transfusion reactions not prevented by leukoreduction, IgA deficiency with documented antibodies to IgA, and history of a previous anaphylactic reaction to blood transfusion.

PRBCs can also be modified by irradiation to inactivate lymphocytes. Transfusion of irradiated blood is indicated in severely immunocompromised patients at risk of graft-versus-host disease (GVHD), such as transplant recipients, those with aggressively treated malignancies, and those with congenital immunodeficiencies. The transfusion of irradiated PRBCs in the United States is increasing and accounted for 10% of blood transfusions in 2008.[1] Irradiation of RBCs reduces RBC viability and increases release of intracellular potassium.

PRBCs can be frozen in cryoprotective solution and stored for extended periods. Frozen RBCs are generally limited to units of special value, such as those with a rare RBC antigen profile or autologous blood donations that need to be stored for future use. A rare-donor registry of frozen PRBCs exists to assist in providing blood to patients with complex or multiple alloantibodies to RBC antigens. Significant advance planning is necessary to acquire and thaw frozen PRBCs for transfusion, thus limiting their use in acute situations.

RBC components suffer some cell loss during storage. The current technology with preservative solutions attempts to optimize cell quality and quantity by using strict criteria to determine the allowable storage time. Nonetheless, as RBC metabolism decreases progressively, a "storage lesion" results, with accumulation of a variety of undesirable substances and loss of cellular function.[6] During storage, a slow rise in the concentration of potassium, lactate, aspartate aminotransferase, lactate dehydrogenase, ammonia, phosphate, and free hemoglobin and a slow decrease in pH and bicarbonate concentration occur. Cytokines and inflammatory mediators such as interleukin 1, interleukin 6, and tumor necrosis factor also accumulate. The pH of freshly stored blood in citrate solution is 7.16, which declines to approximately 6.73 at the end of the unit's shelf life. As potassium leaks from RBCs during storage, levels as high as 25 mEq/L may result. However, each unit transfused supplies at most 7 mEq of potassium, which is usually well tolerated.

During the storage period there is also a progressive decrease in RBC-associated 2,3-diphosphoglycerate (2,3-DPG) and adenosine triphosphate (ATP).[6] A decrease in 2,3-DPG increases the affinity of hemoglobin for oxygen, which shifts the oxygen dissociation curve to the left and decreases oxygen delivery to tissues. There is little evidence, however, that this transient increase in oxygen affinity has clinical importance. After infusion, 2,3-DPG gradually increases as the transfused RBCs circulate, with 25% recovery in 8 hours and full replacement by 24 hours.[7] Decreased ATP during storage diminishes the viability of RBCs after transfusion and is one of the chief factors limiting storage time. There is no currently available storage or rejuvenation solution that optimizes these cellular constituents.

The majority of blood transfusions are in the form of PRBCs, the component indicated for normovolemic patients or those for whom intravascular volume constraints are necessary. Resuscitation in patients requiring increased oxygen-carrying capacity and volume is effectively achieved with the use of PRBCs and crystalloid or colloid solutions. Each unit of PRBCs is expected to raise the hemoglobin concentration by 1 g/dL and the hematocrit by 3% in stable, nonbleeding, average-sized adults.

INDICATIONS FOR RED BLOOD CELL TRANSFUSION

Despite a long tradition of transfusion of RBCs in critically ill patients, the precise indications for transfusion remain a source of debate, and transfusion practices may vary widely among clinicians, ICUs, institutions, and geographic regions. Multiple observational studies document transfusion rates in ICU patients that vary from 17% to 53%,[8-12] and the rate of transfusion increases with longer ICU length of stay.[8,13] There has been a trend over time for use of a lower transfusion threshold in critically ill patients.[14,15]

RBCs should be transfused only to enhance tissue oxygen delivery, but the underlying physiology of anemia, the complex adaptations to anemia, and the potential advantages and disadvantages to particular groups of patients are not as well understood. Determining when an anemic patient would truly benefit from increased oxygen-carrying capacity remains an imprecise task. In addition, mounting evidence argues that transfusions may result in donor-recipient interactions deleterious to the critically ill patient, including the disruption of compensatory physiology, the immunomodulation caused by the presence of foreign cells, and the introduction of unintended plasma contents.

Compensatory mechanisms for acute and chronic anemia are complex and work in concert to maintain oxygenation within the microcirculation.[16,17] Cardiovascular adjustments leading to increased cardiac output include decreased afterload and increased preload resulting from changes in vascular tone, increased myocardial contractility, and elevated heart rate. Lowered blood viscosity permits improved flow of RBCs within capillaries. Blood flow is redistributed to favor critical organs with higher oxygen extraction such as the heart and brain. Pulmonary mechanisms, though contributing relatively little to short-term oxygenation demands, exert potent effects on related metabolic variables. Finally, the hemoglobin molecule can undergo biochemical and conformational changes to enhance the unloading of oxygen at the capillary level. Increased synthesis of RBC 2,3-DPG in anemia results in a rightward shift of the oxyhemoglobin saturation curve and facilitates the release of oxygen to tissues. A rightward shift of the oxyhemoglobin curve can also occur with a decrease in pH (Bohr effect) but the clinical significance is small.[16] All these mechanisms contribute to an oxygen reserve capacity that exceeds baseline requirements by approximately fourfold. Unfortunately, acute illness and chronic morbidities may limit these compensatory mechanisms in critically ill patients. Animal studies and case reports in patients refusing transfusion indicate that an extremely low hematocrit is tolerated if tissue perfusion is adequate.[17-19]

Indirect measurements of tissue oxygen utilization can be derived if patients are monitored invasively with a pulmonary artery catheter, although use of this monitoring tool has significantly decreased in ICUs. Mixed venous oxygen content and arterial oxygen content can be calculated from measured variables. The oxygen extraction ratio (ER), defined as the ratio of oxygen consumption (Vo_2) to total oxygen delivery (Do_2), can be used as a surrogate to determine adequacy of tissue oxygen delivery in the absence of low cardiac output. ER can be calculated by using venous and arterial partial pressures and oxygen saturation values:

$$ER = (Cao_2 - Cvo_2)/Cao_2$$

where the arterial content of oxygen (Cao_2) equals 1.36 × hemoglobin × Sao_2 + 0.003 × Pao_2. The venous oxygen content (Cvo_2) can be calculated by the same formula, replacing the values with mixed venous oxygen saturation ($S\bar{v}o_2$) and venous partial pressure of oxygen (Pvo_2). Because the contribution of dissolved oxygen in plasma to the oxygen-carrying capacity is negligible, ER can be estimated by: $1 - (S\bar{v}o_2/Sao_2)$. The total body ER at baseline is about 25%. A falling Cvo_2 and an ER increasing to greater than 50% have been proposed as indicators of the need for RBC transfusion, but have never been validated in clinical studies.[20]

Although RBC transfusion can increase oxygen-carrying capacity and thus oxygen delivery, it may not improve tissue oxygen consumption. Multiple case series evaluating the effects of RBC transfusion in critically ill patients have failed to document increased oxygen consumption or improvement in lactate level.[21-25] Hypotheses to explain this discrepancy include an increase in blood viscosity limiting microvascular flow and impaired tissue and cellular oxygen utilization.

In practice, clinicians usually rely on the hemoglobin to determine when oxygen-carrying capacity is potentially compromised, despite the limitations noted earlier. Prior transfusion strategies often targeted a hemoglobin goal of greater than 10 g/dL with support of reports that anemia, defined by various criteria, is associated with increased mortality rate in critically ill patients,[26] mechanically ventilated COPD patients,[27] surgical patients who refuse transfusion,[28] and patients undergoing major noncardiac surgery.[29,30] However, the first large multicenter randomized trial of RBC transfusion strategies in the critically ill showed this liberal transfusion strategy may actually be unnecessary and potentially detrimental.[31] The Transfusion Requirement in Critical Care (TRICC) trial compared a liberal (target hemoglobin, 10 to 12 g/dL) with a restrictive (target hemoglobin, 7 to 9 g/dL) RBC transfusion policy in 838 euvolemic patients with hemoglobin less than 9 g/dL within 72 hours of ICU admission. The primary outcome measure of 30-day all-cause mortality rate was not statistically different between the restrictive strategy and the liberal strategy ($p = 0.11$). A secondary outcome measure of overall hospital mortality rate was significantly lower in the restrictive strategy group ($p = 0.05$). The restrictive strategy was superior for subgroups of patients younger than 55 years and patients with lower (<20) APACHE (Acute Physiology, Age, and Chronic Health Evaluation) II scores. In addition, liberal transfusion was not associated with shorter ICU or hospital stays or less organ failure; longer mechanical ventilation times and cardiac events were more frequent in the liberal strategy group. A separate analysis of 713 patients in the study who received mechanical ventilation did not find any significant differences between treatment groups for the duration of mechanical ventilation or extubation success.[32] Similarly, a subgroup analysis of 357 patients from the TRICC study with cardiovascular disease did not find any differences in mortality rates between the restrictive and liberal strategies.[33]

The results of the TRICC study were replicated in a study of transfusion strategy in critically ill pediatric patients.[34] A liberal transfusion threshold of 9.5 g/dL was compared with a restrictive transfusion threshold of 7.0 g/dL. The primary outcomes of death and new or progressive multiple organ dysfunction as well as adverse events were similar in both treatment groups, but 54% of patients in the restrictive group did not receive transfusion as compared to only 2% in the liberal group ($p < 0.001$). Subsequent prospective randomized trials have validated the use of a restrictive transfusion strategy in other adult patient populations.[35-39] Although a small study of liberal (hemoglobin threshold of 10 g/dL) versus restrictive (hemoglobin threshold of 8 g/dL) transfusion in 120 hip fracture surgery patients raised concern for increased cardiovascular complications and mortality rate with a restrictive strategy,[40] a larger trial in 2016 high-risk patients undergoing surgery for hip fracture found no increase in mortality rate and no difference in functional recovery.[35] The Transfusion Requirements After Cardiac Surgery (TRACS) study compared transfusion thresholds of hematocrit less than 30% with hematocrit less than 24% from the start of surgery through the ICU stay.[36] There was no difference in the composite outcome of 30-day all-cause mortality rate and severe morbidity between the liberal and restrictive strategies, and fewer blood products were administered in the restrictive group. These results are similar to those in an earlier study in coronary artery bypass surgery patients that evaluated liberal and restrictive transfusion strategies in the postoperative period.[41]

The TRACS study and the analysis of patients with cardiovascular disease from the TRICC study suggest that RBC transfusion using a hemoglobin threshold of 7 to 8 g/dL in stable patients at risk for myocardial ischemia is well tolerated. However, these studies do not answer the question of whether patients with acute coronary syndromes (current or recent ischemia) would benefit from a liberal transfusion strategy. Results from retrospective and prospective observational studies of anemia and transfusion in acute coronary syndrome patients have yielded conflicting results.[42-45] A recent prospective, randomized pilot study of 45 patients with acute myocardial infarction (MI) and hematocrit 30% or less compared a transfusion threshold of hematocrit less than 24% with hematocrit less than 30%.[46] The composite safety end point of in-hospital death, new MI, or new or worsening heart failure occurred in 38% of the liberal strategy patients versus 13% in the conservative strategy patients ($p = 0.046$). These results suggest that even in acute MI moderate anemia may not be as harmful as the risks involved with transfusions. Larger studies in the future should help determine whether a restrictive transfusion strategy should be adopted in patients with acute coronary syndromes.

Prior guidelines for transfusion of RBCs did not specifically address critically ill patients and were primarily based on consensus rather than evidence.[47-51] Transfusion was usually recommended if hemoglobin was less than 6 or 7 g/dL and not indicated when hemoglobin was greater than 10 g/dL.[48,52] Guidelines of the American Association of Blood Banks[46] and the Society of Critical Care Medicine/Eastern Association for Surgery of Trauma[53] and a Cochrane review[54] provide an evaluation of clinical evidence and more specific recommendations that are applicable to the critically ill. A summary of the guideline recommendations is presented in Box 79.1. Transfusion of single units of RBCs is recommended except in the setting of acute hemorrhage.[53] Implementation of a restrictive transfusion practice as recommended by the guidelines could decrease patient RBC exposure by an estimated 40%.[46] The threshold for administration of RBCs should also be considered as part of a comprehensive, multidisciplinary patient blood management program to detect and treat anemia, reduce surgical blood loss, and optimize hemostasis.[2]

Box 79.1 Guideline Recommendations for Transfusion of Red Blood Cells

American Association of Blood Banks (2012)

- Adhere to a restrictive strategy in hospitalized, hemodynamically stable patients (*strong recommendation*)
  - Adult ICU patients: consider transfusion when hemoglobin ≤7 g/dL
  - Postoperative surgical patients: consider transfusion when hemoglobin ≤8 g/dL or for symptoms (chest pain, heart failure, orthostatic hypotension, tachycardia unresponsive to fluid resuscitation)
- Adhere to a restrictive strategy in hospitalized, hemodynamically stable patients with preexisting cardiovascular disease (*weak recommendation*)
  - Consider transfusion when hemoglobin ≤8 g/dL or for symptoms
- No recommendation for a specific transfusion strategy in hospitalized, hemodynamically stable patients with acute coronary syndrome

Society of Critical Care Medicine/Eastern Association for Surgery of Trauma (2009)

- Transfusion is indicated for patients with hemorrhagic shock and may be indicated for patients with acute hemorrhage and hemodynamic instability or inadequate oxygen delivery.
- Transfusion when hemoglobin is <7 g/dL (*restrictive strategy*) is as effective as transfusion when hemoglobin is <10 g/dL (*liberal strategy*) in critically ill hemodynamically stable patients.
- Transfusion may be beneficial in patients with acute coronary syndromes with hemoglobin <8 g/dL on hospital admission.

ICU, intensive care unit.

PLATELETS

Platelet components are available as random donor units or single donor apheresis units. Because of the limited storage time and the increasing demand for this component, platelets are often subject to supply shortages. A random donor platelet concentrate is obtained by centrifugation from a unit of WB. This type of platelet concentrate contains up to 50% of the leukocytes from the WB unit. The average transfused dose of random donor platelets has been decreasing over time and is now 5 units in the United States.[1] If bags are entered for pooling before transfusion, the platelets must be administered within 4 hours. A single donor apheresis platelet unit contains the equivalent of 4 to 6 units of random donor platelet concentrates. This type of platelet concentrate is considered to be leukoreduced and no additional filtration is needed. Single-donor platelets offer the benefit of reducing the risk of multiple-donor exposure to the recipient, and may also be the only available alternative for recipients who have been alloimmunized by previous platelet transfusions. Apheresis platelets now account for 87% of all platelets transfused in the United States.[1]

Platelets are stored at room temperature to avoid loss of function from refrigeration and are constantly agitated to maximize gas exchange. Some loss of viability and platelet numbers occurs during storage, but 5-day-old platelets still effect hemostasis. The plasma contained in platelet concentrates is a good source of stable coagulation factors and contains diminished but still potentially beneficial amounts of factors V and VIII. Platelet components may be modified by leukocyte reduction, irradiation, and washing similar to that for RBCs. Transfusion of ABO-compatible platelets is desirable but not essential. When ABO-mismatched platelets are given, removal of some of the incompatible plasma can be carried out prior to transfusion. Single donor apheresis platelets may be matched to an alloimmunized recipient for human leukocyte antigens (HLA) or platelet antigens. There is no contraindication to the use of Rh-positive platelets in Rh-negative patients. However, if Rh-positive random donor platelets are administered to Rh-negative women with childbearing potential, Rh immune globulin should be used prophylactically due to the small risk of Rh alloimmunization from RBCs that may be contained in the platelet concentrate. In similar circumstances, Rh immune globulin is not indicated if single donor apheresis platelets are transfused because they contain few RBCs.

Each unit of random donor platelets is expected to increase the platelet count by 10×10^9/L in a typical 70-kg adult. A 1-hour posttransfusion platelet count should be obtained to determine the adequacy of response. The following equation, which relates platelet number and body size to the posttransfusion increment, can be used to assess the effectiveness of the transfusion:

$$\text{Corrected count increment (CCI)} = \frac{\text{Observed rise in platelet count} \times \text{Body surface area (m}^2\text{)}}{\text{Number of platelet units transfused}}$$

A CCI of 10×10^9/L or higher can be considered a good response, whereas a CCI of 5×10^9/L or lower indicates a poor response to transfusion.[55] The increment in platelet count is higher with single-donor apheresis units, ABO-identical platelets, and platelets stored no longer than 3 days.[56,57] However, there is no advantage of these platelet characteristics on prevention of clinical bleeding.[56]

INDICATIONS FOR PLATELET TRANSFUSION

Although the prevalence of thrombocytopenia in the critically ill varies with the definition used and clinical setting, thrombocytopenia is associated with platelet transfusions and increased mortality rate in ICU patients.[58,59] Guidelines for transfusion of platelets are derived from consensus opinion and experience primarily in patients with chemotherapy-induced thrombocytopenia rather than critically ill patients.[48,60-63] Extrapolation of these guidelines to critically ill patients is problematic because the cause, risks, and consequences of thrombocytopenia may be different. Indications for platelet transfusions include active bleeding due to thrombocytopenia or functional platelet defects (therapeutic transfusion) or prevention of bleeding due to thrombocytopenia (prophylactic transfusion). The majority of platelet transfusions in the ICU are performed for prophylactic indications and often do not result in an increase in platelet count.[64]

Suggested indications for platelet transfusion are summarized in Table 79.2. There is good evidence that medical or surgical patients with active bleeding and platelet counts of 50×10^9/L or above will not benefit from transfusion if thrombocytopenia is the only abnormality. Prophylactic platelet transfusions are administered to prevent spontaneous bleeding or bleeding with invasive procedures. The threshold for platelet transfusion prior to invasive procedures is usually recommended as less than 50×10^9/L, but transfusion decisions should take into account the type of procedure, bleeding risks associated with the procedure, consequences of bleeding, and concomitant factors affecting hemostasis. For critical invasive procedures in which even a small amount of bleeding could lead to loss of vital organ function or death, maintaining the platelet count greater than 50×10^9/L is typically preferred. The presence of factors that diminish platelet function, such as certain drugs, foreign intravascular devices (e.g., intra-aortic balloon pump or membrane oxygenator), infection, or uremia, alter this requirement upward. Patients at risk for small but strategically important hemorrhage, such as neurosurgical patients, may need to be maintained at platelet counts of 80 to 100×10^9/L.

Table 79.2 Indications for Platelet Transfusion

Clinical Situation	Platelet Count: $\times 10^9$/L
Therapeutic	
Active bleeding	<50
Prophylactic	
Spontaneous bleeding risk very high	0-10
Spontaneous bleeding risk high with concomitant coagulation abnormality, anticoagulant therapy, sepsis, fever, concurrent antibiotic use, rapidly decreasing count or planned invasive procedure	11-20
Planned invasive procedure	21-50
Consider with platelet dysfunction (uremia, antiplatelet drugs) and planned invasive procedure when other therapies are ineffective	>50

The most appropriate platelet count for procedures that may be performed in critically ill patients, such as placement of central venous catheters and arterial catheters, thoracentesis, and paracentesis, has not been defined. A retrospective study suggests that central venous catheters can be placed safely when the platelet count is greater than or equal to 20×10^9/L.[65]

Patients undergoing cardiac bypass surgery experience a drop in platelet count and often acquire a transient platelet functional defect from damage associated with the bypass apparatus.[66] Most patients do not experience platelet-associated bleeding, however, and prophylactic transfusion in the absence of bleeding is not warranted. In a patient who continues to bleed postoperatively, more likely causes are a localized, surgically correctable lesion or failure to reverse the effects of heparin. If these conditions are excluded, empiric transfusion of platelets may be justified.

Patients without hemorrhage who have platelet counts of 5×10^9/L or lower are at increased risk for significant spontaneous bleeding, and the majority of guidelines propose prophylactic platelet transfusion to prevent hemorrhage at a threshold of 10×10^9/L or less. The recommendations are based on experience in patients with hematologic malignancies and chemotherapy-induced underproduction of platelets. The prior practice of transfusion to maintain the platelet count above 20×10^9/L derives from data published in 1962, which demonstrated an increase in spontaneous bleeding in leukemic patients at that level.[67] However, critical evaluation of the data reveals that serious hemorrhage was not greatly increased until counts fell to 5×10^9/L or lower and that these patients received aspirin for fever, which might have compromised platelet function and enhanced bleeding.

A prospective study of a more conservative platelet transfusion protocol found that major bleeding episodes occurred on 1.9% of days with counts of less than $10 \times 10^9/L$ and on only 0.07% of days with counts of 10 to $20 \times 10^9/L$.[68] Additional studies have confirmed the safety of using less than or equal to $10 \times 10^9/L$ as a prophylactic platelet transfusion threshold in patients with hematologic malignancies or stem cell transplants.[69-72] The trigger for prophylactic platelet transfusion of less than or equal to $10 \times 10^9/L$, however, applies primarily to a specific population of stable thrombocytopenic patients. Factors such as fever, use of anticoagulant or antiplatelet drugs, and invasive procedures must be considered when generating a treatment plan for individual patients. Patients experiencing rapid drops in platelet count may be at greater risk than those at steady state and thus may benefit from transfusion at higher counts. Prospective studies in critically ill patients have not been reported. Benefits to the patient of more conservative use of platelet transfusion include decreased donor exposure, which lessens the risk of transfusion-transmitted disease; fewer febrile and allergic reactions that may complicate the hospital course; and the potential delay or prevention of alloimmunization to HLA and platelet antigens.[73]

Patients thrombocytopenic by virtue of immunologic destructive processes such as idiopathic thrombocytopenic purpura (ITP) receive little benefit from platelet transfusions because transfused platelets are rapidly removed from the circulation. In the event of life-threatening hemorrhage or an extensive surgical procedure, transfusion may prove beneficial for its short-term effect but may require higher doses of platelets. Transfusion may be accomplished effectively by pretreatment with high-dose immunoglobulin or high-dose anti-D antiserum.[74,75] Platelet transfusion is contraindicated in thrombotic thrombocytopenic purpura (TTP),[76] hemolytic-uremic syndrome, and heparin-induced thrombocytopenia. Cautious administration of platelets may be considered in cases of life-threatening thrombocytopenic bleeding.

The development of refractoriness to platelet transfusions due to alloimmunization is a serious event. Poor response to platelet transfusions due to increased platelet consumption also occurs with splenomegaly, fever, trauma and crush injury, burns, disseminated intravascular coagulation (DIC), concomitant drugs, and transfusion of platelets of substandard quality.[77] These factors should be identified and corrected if possible. Alloimmunization is characterized by the development of anti-HLA or platelet-specific antibodies, with resultant immune platelet destruction. As many as 70% of patients receiving multiple RBC or platelet transfusions become immunized.[73] Leukocyte depletion of transfused components can prevent or delay this phenomenon, but it is important to use leukoreduced components early in the course of transfusion therapy.[73,78] When patients fail to achieve expected increments after platelet transfusion, provision of ABO-specific platelet concentrates that are less than 48 hours old may improve the response. If no improvement is seen, the patient should be screened for HLA antibodies or be HLA typed and provided with HLA-compatible single-donor platelets. Alternatively, platelet crossmatching with the patient's serum can be carried out. There is no advantage to unmatched single-donor platelets in this situation.

PLASMA-DERIVED COMPONENTS

PLASMA

Standard FFP is prepared by centrifugation of WB or single-donor apheresis and is frozen within 8 hours of blood donation. Standard FFP contains all coagulation factors (including the labile factors V and VIII) and inhibitors, approximately 400 mg fibrinogen, complement, albumin, and globulins. By convention, the coagulation factors are present in concentrations of 1 U/mL. Plasma that is separated and frozen from refrigerated WB more than 8 hours but within 24 hours of phlebotomy is referred to as PF24. PF24 differs from standard FFP by having lower levels (approximately 15% to 25% reduction) of factors V and VIII, but the decrease in labile factor levels is not considered to be clinically significant. The processing technique for PF24 allows for clinical utilization of plasma collected at distant sites and increases the plasma supply. Cryoprecipitate-reduced plasma (also called *cryopoor plasma*) refers to FFP with the cold-induced precipitate removed. Cryopoor plasma will thus be deficient in factors VIII and XIII, fibrinogen, and von Willebrand factor. In the United States, FFP accounted for 54% of plasma transfusions and PF24 accounted for 39%.[1] The most common method of thawing FFP requires about 30 to 45 minutes in a 37° C water bath. Crossmatching to the recipient is not performed, but FFP must be ABO compatible. Standard FFP is as likely to transmit hepatitis, HIV, and most other transfusion-related infections as cellular components. The following types of pathogen-reduced plasma products are available in some countries outside the United States: solvent/detergent-treated plasma, methylene blue–treated plasma, psoralen- and ultraviolet light–treated plasma, and riboflavin- and ultraviolet light–treated plasma.[79]

Indications for Fresh Frozen Plasma

FFP is frequently transfused inappropriately in critically ill patients who are not bleeding or in whom the international normalized ratio (INR) is less than 1.5.[80,81] Guidelines for transfusion of FFP have been primarily based on expert opinion rather than clinical evidence (Box 79.2).[60,82,83] A summary of practice recommendations for specific clinical circumstances based on a systematic review is presented in Box 79.3. The review emphasized the lack of high-quality evidence on plasma infusion and the need for well-designed trials to address relevant knowledge gaps.[84]

Box 79.2 Guideline Recommendations for Transfusion of Fresh Frozen Plasma

Acquired deficiency of coagulation factors with abnormal coagulation tests AND
- Active bleeding
- OR
- Planned surgery or invasive procedure

Immediate reversal of warfarin effect with active bleeding or planned procedure
Thrombotic thrombocytopenic purpura
Congenital factor deficiency with no alternative therapy
Rare protein deficiencies (protein C or S)

Box 79.3 Recommendations Regarding Fresh Frozen Plasma (FFP) Transfusion in Specific Conditions*

1. Suggest that FFP be transfused to trauma patients requiring massive transfusion
2. Cannot recommend for or against of FFP transfusion at a plasma-to-RBC ratio of 1:3 or more in trauma patients with massive transfusion.
3. Cannot recommend for or against FFP transfusion in patients undergoing surgery in the absence of massive transfusion.
4. Suggest FFP be transfused in patients with warfarin-related intracranial hemorrhage.
5. Cannot recommend for or against FFP transfusion to reverse warfarin in patients without intracranial hemorrhage.
6. Suggest against FFP transfusion in other groups of patients (in the absence of massive transfusion, surgery, bleeding, or overanticoagulation)

*Based on a systematic review.
RBC, red blood cell.
Adapted from Roback JD, Caldwell S, Carson J, et al: Evidence-based practice guidelines for plasma transfusion. Transfusion 2010;50:1227-1239.

FFP should be administered only to provide coagulation factors or plasma proteins that cannot be obtained from safer sources. FFP is commonly used to treat bleeding patients with acquired deficiency of multiple coagulation factors, as in liver disease, DIC, or dilutional coagulopathy. However, changes in INR after FFP transfusion are usually minimal and not clinically significant when the pretransfusion INR is less than 2.0.[81,85] FFP may be indicated for the provision of protein C or S in patients who are deficient and suffering acute thrombosis. FFP should be administered as boluses as rapidly as feasible so that the resulting factor levels achieve hemostasis. The use of FFP infusions is not helpful. Variable doses of FFP have been recommended including 2 units initially (probably underdosage) up to 10 to 15 mL/kg. However, some studies suggest that doses as high as 30 mL/kg may be needed to achieve adequate factor levels.[86] Due to the short half-life of factor VII, FFP should be infused every 6 to 8 hours if bleeding continues. FFP should not be used for volume expansion or as a nutritional source of protein. Anticoagulation induced by heparin, direct thrombin inhibitors (e.g., dabigatran), or direct factor Xa inhibitors (e.g., rivoraxaban) is not reversed by FFP.

Patients do not usually bleed as a result of coagulation factor deficiency when the INR is less than about 2.0, and even then the results are not always predictable.[87] The partial thromboplastin time (PTT) is also not useful in predicting procedural bleeding risk.[88] Prophylactic administration of FFP does not improve patient outcome in the setting of cardiac surgery unless there is bleeding with an associated documented coagulation abnormality.[89] FFP is often requested prophylactically before an invasive procedure when the patient exhibits mild prolongation in coagulation studies. Most of these procedures may be carried out safely without transfusing FFP.[87,90] A randomized trial of FFP versus no FFP in critically ill nonbleeding patients with INR between 1.5 and 3.0 scheduled to undergo central venous catheter placement, thoracentesis, percutaneous tracheostomy, or drainage of abscess or fluid is under way.[91]

Coagulation factors are normally present in the blood far in excess of the minimum levels required for hemostasis. As little as 10% of the normal plasma concentration of several factors will effect hemostasis. Conversely, FFP treatment of acquired multiple deficiencies, as in hepatic failure, is often ineffective because many patients cannot tolerate the infusion volumes required to achieve hemostatic levels of coagulation factors, even transiently.[92] The plasma half-life of transfused factor VII is only 2 to 6 hours. It may be impossible to administer sufficient FFP every few hours without encountering intravascular volume overload. Finally, in some instances, transfusion of seemingly adequate volumes may still fail to correct the coagulopathy.[93] Careful documentation of both the need for FFP and the adequacy and outcomes of therapy is essential.[94]

Transfusion of FFP is associated with significant adverse effects. It is the most commonly implicated blood product in the development of TRALI. Because of the large volumes that may be transfused, FFP administration is a risk factor for transfusion-associated circulatory overload (TACO). Allergic reactions to FFP are usually mild with the exception of anaphylactic reactions to IgA proteins that can occur when plasma is transfused in IgA-deficient patients.

CRYOPRECIPITATE

A total of 1.1 million units of cryoprecipitate were transfused in 2008 in the United States at a mean average cost of $65.10/unit.[1] Cryoprecipitate is prepared by thawing and centrifuging FFP below 6°C and resuspending the precipitated proteins in a small volume of supernatant plasma. Each unit is a concentrated source of factor VIII (≥80 IU), von Willebrand factor (50% of original plasma content), fibrinogen (≥150 mg), factor XIII (30% of original plasma content), and fibronectin. It is considered to be leukoreduced without additional filtration. Cryoprecipitate offers the advantage of transfusing more specific protein and less total volume than an equivalent dose of FFP. Cryoprecipitate does not require crossmatching, but ABO compatibility with the recipient is preferred.

Indications for Cryoprecipitate Transfusion

In the past, cryoprecipitate was used to treat patients with inherited coagulopathies, such as hemophilia A, von Willebrand disease, and factor XIII deficiency. However, the availability of safer specific factor concentrates makes use of cryoprecipitate unwarranted for these conditions unless factor concentrates are unavailable. In the critical care setting, cryoprecipitate is most commonly used to replenish fibrinogen, especially in bleeding patients with hypofibrinogenemia caused by dilutional or consumptive coagulopathy. Transfusion of cryoprecipitate is usually recommended when fibrinogen levels are less than 100 mg/dL in the setting of bleeding or need for an invasive procedure.[83,95,96] Cryoprecipitate also reportedly improves hemostasis in uremic patients, presumably by reversing the functional platelet defect,[97] but desmopressin[98] or conjugated estrogens exert similar effects and should be used preferentially to avoid potential transfusion-related complications. Similar to other blood components, cryoprecipitate is often transfused inappropriately.[99]

The usual dose of cryoprecipitate to treat hypofibrinogenemia is 10 units to start, then 6 to 10 units every 8 hours or as necessary to keep the fibrinogen level above 100 mg/dL. The fibrinogen response will depend on the patient's plasma volume (varies with gender and weight), initial fibrinogen level, and consumption of fibrinogen. A simple formula to start with dosing is number of units = 0.2 × weight (kg).[100] Each unit of cryoprecipitate carries a risk of disease transmission equivalent to that of 1 unit of blood.

ADVERSE EFFECTS OF BLOOD COMPONENT TRANSFUSION

The decision to transfuse blood components must be made with full awareness of the potential risk to the recipient, as well as the expected benefits. For some patients, the benefit from transfusion of a blood product is so obvious that the associated risks are not significant in comparison to the consequences of withholding transfusion. However, the clinician's knowledge of the incidence and management of the adverse effects to transfusion is vital, not only to ensure the best patient care but also to provide appropriate patient education and true informed consent.

Measurable reactions to transfusion occur in about 20% of patients; more serious adverse responses may be expected in only 1% to 2% of transfusions.[101] The nature of these adverse reactions ranges from those that are common but clinically unimportant to those that may cause significant morbidity or death. The Food and Drug Administration reported 58 transfusion-related or potentially transfusion-related deaths in 2011.[102] From 2007 through 2011, TRALI accounted for 43% of fatalities followed by acute hemolytic reactions in 23%.

Why blood component transfusions may be harmful in critical care patients is not well understood. With the modern techniques in screening, storing, and matching RBCs, the mortality rate directly attributable to transfusions is extremely low; however, retrospective data often link increased numbers of transfusions to increased mortality rates.[8,9,12,103] It is difficult to distinguish whether this trend is a function of anemia as a signal for increased severity of illness versus an actual consequence of the transfusion. Nevertheless, the relationship between transfusions and increased mortality rates is concerning, and a better understanding would help both clinicians and patients understand the risks involved with transfusions, as well as to aid investigators to develop new methods of safer transfusions. Potential mechanisms of recipient harm include risk of infections or multiorgan failure via immunomodulatory effects from the introduction during transfusion of unintended lipid breakdown products, cell-signaling factors, and donor-recipient antigen-antibody interactions.

ACUTE TRANSFUSION REACTIONS

The signs and symptoms of severe, life-threatening transfusion reactions are frequently indistinguishable from those of less significant reactions. However, every transfused patient who experiences a significant change in condition, such as an elevation in temperature, change in pulse or blood pressure, dyspnea, or pain, must be promptly and fully evaluated to identify the cause of the reaction and to institute treatment when necessary. The basic approach to all acute reactions should be to maintain a high index of suspicion for acute hemolytic reactions (with RBC components) by stopping the transfusion immediately, maintaining venous access with intravenous fluids, and informing the blood bank laboratory immediately so that the appropriate transfusion reaction protocol can be instituted and posttransfusion specimens obtained. Early recognition of severe transfusion reactions may be lifesaving.

ACUTE HEMOLYTIC TRANSFUSION REACTION

Acute hemolytic transfusion reactions (AHTRs) are caused by the recipient's existing complement-fixing antibodies attaching to donor RBC antigens with resultant intravascular RBC lysis. Non-ABO incompatibility is now more commonly implicated than ABO incompatibility in these incidents.[102] In addition to hemolysis, complement activation stimulates the release of inflammatory mediators and cytokines and can lead to hypotension and vascular collapse. Activation of the coagulation system may result in DIC and bleeding. Acute renal failure may also occur, presumably on the basis of immune complex interactions. Morbidity and mortality rates are directly related to the quantity of incompatible blood transfused, which is why prompt recognition and cessation of transfusion are imperative. Misidentification of the patient, or clerical error, at any time beginning with acquisition of the donor specimen through release of the unit and initiation of infusion is the major cause of AHTRs.[104] It is preferable to transfuse uncrossmatched group O RBCs than to chance ABO incompatibility caused by improper patient and specimen identification procedures.

The most common clinical sign of an AHTR is sudden onset of fever, with or without chills.[105] Other common signs and symptoms include back or flank pain, anxiety, nausea, light-headedness, dyspnea, and hemodynamic instability. In a comatose or anesthetized patient, these symptoms may not be evident; therefore, signs such as hypotension, hemoglobinuria, and diffuse oozing from puncture sites or incisions may be the only notable features.

Immediate management of suspected AHTRs includes cessation of the transfusion; the remainder of care is supportive. Rapid verification of patient and unit identification must be made, not only to confirm the suspected reaction but also to prevent a second patient from receiving a reciprocally incompatible unit if a clerical error has been made. Steroids, heparin, or other pharmacologic interventions have no role in treatment.

FEBRILE NONHEMOLYTIC TRANSFUSION REACTIONS

Febrile nonhemolytic transfusion reactions (FNHTRs) are the most commonly occurring acute reaction to RBC and platelet transfusions. These reactions can cause significant discomfort and must be investigated because they share manifestations with AHTRs and bacterially contaminated blood. Although a temperature increase of 1° C is often used to define an FNHTR, fever may be absent in patients pretreated with antipyretics. Additional clinical signs include chills or rigors usually beginning 1 to 2 hours after the start of the transfusion but occasionally delayed up to 4 to 6 hours. Associated manifestations may include nausea, vomiting, and dyspnea. FNHTRs occur in approximately 1.0% of transfusion episodes but are more common with platelet transfusions (4-31%).[106,107] The cause of FNHTRs varies with the transfused product, but the release or presence of cytokines and pyrogens results in the clinical manifestations. This reaction to RBC transfusion is usually initiated by the interaction of recipient antibodies to donor leukocytes. Nonhemolytic transfusion reactions (NHTRs) with platelet products are most commonly initiated by leukocyte- or platelet-derived cytokines or other biologic response modifiers.[107] Management of NHTRs includes discontinuation of transfusion and initiation of the appropriate transfusion reaction evaluation. Antipyretics such as acetaminophen may be administered. Antihistamines are neither preventive nor therapeutic. Once acute hemolysis is excluded, transfusion of a new unit may be instituted. If repeated NHTRs become problematic, leukocyte-depleted blood components should be supplied. The implementation of universal leukocyte reduction results in a reduction in the frequency of all fever seen after transfusion by only about 12%.[108] Pretreatment with antipyretics or corticosteroids may also minimize FHTRs.

ANAPHYLAXIS

Anaphylactic reactions to blood transfusions are rare but may be life-threatening. The usual cause is recipient antibody to a component of plasma that the patient lacks, most commonly antibody to IgA in IgA-deficient individuals. However, antibodies to other proteins (anti-haptoglobin) have been demonstrated and activated platelet membranes may also play a role.[109,110] The highest rate of anaphylaxis occurs with platelets followed by FFP and RBCs. Signs and symptoms usually begin within minutes after transfusion is initiated and include severe anxiety, flushing, dizziness, dyspnea, bronchospasm, abdominal pain, vomiting, diarrhea, hypotension, and eventually shock. Fever and hemolysis do not occur. Management includes immediate cessation of transfusion and standard therapy for anaphylaxis. If anti-IgA antibodies are determined to be the cause of this reaction, the patient must receive blood components donated by IgA-deficient individuals or, if unavailable, specially prepared washed RBCs and platelet concentrates. Plasma-derived preparations, such as albumin, and immunoglobulins contain varying amounts of IgA and pose a substantial risk in these patients.

ALLERGIC AND URTICARIAL REACTIONS

Hives and pruritus are relatively common cutaneous adverse effects of transfusion and may occur with transfusion of RBCs, platelets, and FFP.[106] They are a hypersensitivity reaction localized to the skin, and their cause is unknown but may include both donor and recipient characteristics. These reactions consist of localized or generalized urticaria beginning shortly after the start of transfusion without fever or signs or symptoms of anaphylaxis or hemolysis. The transfusion should be temporarily interrupted, and antihistamines administered. If the hives resolve in a short time, the same unit of blood may be cautiously restarted. If repeated urticarial reactions occur, premedication with antihistamines may be effective.

DELAYED HEMOLYTIC TRANSFUSION REACTIONS

Delayed hemolytic transfusion reactions (DHTRs) are an uncommon but probably underrecognized reaction to RBC transfusion that result from the stimulation of a primary or secondary (anamnestic) recipient antibody response to foreign RBC antigens. These antibodies are below the limit of detection at the time of transfusion but increase after transfusion. DHTRs typically occur 3 to 14 days after transfusion but may not be recognized because of the lack of a clear temporal association with transfusion. DHTRs are more likely in patients requiring frequent RBC transfusion.[106] Patients may be asymptomatic or experience fever, chills, and an unexplained decline in hematocrit.[111] Transient elevation in unconjugated bilirubin and lactate dehydrogenase may also occur. The diagnosis is established by a positive direct antiglobulin (Coombs) test resulting from recipient antibody coating donor RBCs. The specificity of the antibody is often against such RBC antigens as the Rh family, Kidd, Duffy, or Kell systems. Hemolysis may not occur, but if it does, it is likely to be extravascular and only rarely causes renal failure or DIC.

Prevention of these reactions is difficult. Alloimmunization to foreign RBC antigens occurs in approximately 1% of transfusions.[101] Detection of delayed antibodies is the purpose for requiring a new blood bank specimen every 72 hours if the patient has recently been transfused. Permanent transfusion records should record the occurrence of delayed antibodies, even though they may not be apparent at a later crossmatch.

TRANSFUSION-ASSOCIATED CIRCULATORY OVERLOAD

TACO is estimated to occur in 1:100 to 1:10,000 transfusions and accounts for 15% of transfusion-related fatalities in the United States between 2007 and 2011.[102] It is more likely to occur with RBC or FFP transfusion due to the higher volumes of these blood components.[110] Aside from the inherent volume of the blood components, the concurrently administered normal saline adds to the volume load. Risk factors for TACO include older age, critical care patients, cardiac and renal dysfunction, chronic anemia, increased volume of blood products, and increased rate of transfusion. Clinical manifestations of TACO include dyspnea, orthopnea, cough, and worsening oxygenation due to hydrostatic pulmonary edema. Management options include slowing the rate of transfusion and administration of diuretics. Careful attention to transfusion requirements and the use of volume reduction maneuvers available to the transfusion service can help minimize volume overload in most instances. TACO may be difficult to distinguish clinically from TRALI but TACO is less likely to be associated with fever and hypotension and more likely to be associated with a significantly elevated brain natriuretic peptide (BNP) and hypertension.

TRANSFUSION-RELATED ACUTE LUNG INJURY

TRALI is now the leading cause of transfusion-related deaths in the United States.[102] An increase in incidence of TRALI is likely related to an increased awareness of the syndrome rather than a true increase in frequency of reactions. The reported incidence of TRALI for all blood component transfusions is less than 0.1%, but in the critical care setting, it is reported to be as high as 8% per transfusion.[112] Products containing plasma (e.g., FFP and platelets) appear to have the highest risk, but the reaction has been seen with all types of blood components. Tranfusion of plasma from female donors also increases the risk of TRALI.[112,113] TRALI is defined as the development of acute lung injury (hypoxia and bilateral infiltrates of noncardiac cause) within 6 hours of transfusion in the absence of another more likely cause.[113,114]

In patients without prior respiratory compromise, TRALI manifests as acute hypoxia with the development of rales and diffuse infiltrates on chest radiograph.[115] Recognition of TRALI may be difficult in critically ill patients who may have other reasons for dyspnea or may already require mechanical ventilation. In addition, TRALI and TACO may be difficult to distinguish. Clinical features that favor TRALI over TACO include the presence of fever and leukopenia. Hemodynamic monitoring may aid in differentiation, but is not required for management.

Unlike other forms of acute respiratory distress syndrome (ARDS), TRALI is usually self-limiting and resolves within 1 to 4 days. However, reactions can be severe, and often may necessitate mechanical ventilation. Treatment consists of supportive care, including the prompt management of hypoxia. If mechanical ventilation is required, lung protective ventilation should be implemented, and daily spontaneous breathing trials should be performed to ensure timely extubation upon resolution. Because the inciting factor is derived from the donor product rather than the patient, additional blood products can still be transfused if necessary with low risk of redevelopment.

Studies have suggested several mechanisms in the development of TRALI. The presence of leukocyte antibodies in the donor blood has been consistently linked to many cases, although other triggers such as lipids and biologic response modifiers (cytokines) have also been implicated.[116,117,113] When exposed to donor antibodies, neutrophils that are already recruited to the pulmonary vascular endothelium release inflammatory products, leading to injury of the endothelial cells and increased vascular permeability. Recipient factors are also involved, as blood products from the same donor do not consistently cause TRALI in different recipients. Critically ill patients may be more susceptible to TRALI owing to increased localization of neutrophils in the pulmonary vasculature.

To reduce the risk of TRALI, blood agencies are evaluating possible interventions to reduce the presence of leukocyte antibodies in the donated products. One strategy is to limit donation by multiparous women, who are at high risk of carrying antibodies.[118] Decreasing the duration of storage of blood products may also be beneficial. The number of fatalities due to plasma has been decreasing in the United States, most likely due to reduced plasma transfusion from female donors.[102]

TRANSFUSION-ASSOCIATED GRAFT-VERSUS-HOST DISEASE

Transfusion-associated GVHD (TA-GVHD) is a rare and usually fatal immunologic complication of blood component transfusion.[106] Immunocompromised patients infused with blood components containing viable donor lymphocytes are at risk for engraftment of the allogeneic lymphocytes and ensuing rejection of recipient (host) tissues. Transfusion recipients who are at highest risk include bone marrow and organ transplant recipients, leukemia and lymphoma patients, and recipients of blood donated by relatives. TA-GVHD has been reported in patients after cardiac surgery who received designated donor blood from relatives; presumably, the HLA antigenic differences between donor and recipient were insufficient to stimulate a recipient immune response but sufficient to elicit a donor immune response.[119] The onset of TA-GVHD is usually within 8 to 30 days after transfusion, and it is manifested as fever and skin rash, followed by diarrhea and evidence of liver dysfunction and bone marrow suppression. TA-GVHD differs from that seen in bone marrow transplantation (BMT) by its involvement of the marrow and far greater mortality risk. Treatment is largely ineffective, and mortality rate exceeds 90%.

Irradiation of blood components at 25 Gy prevents TA-GVHD by eliminating the donor lymphocyte mitogenic response. All cellular blood components should be irradiated before transfusion to high-risk patients. The functions of the cellular components of blood are unaffected, although damage to RBC membranes limits the duration of postirradiation storage of PRBCs to 28 days. Blood donated by a relative for any patient should be irradiated, as should HLA-matched or crossmatched platelet products.

TRANSFUSION-RELATED IMMUNOMODULATION

Transfusion-related immunomodulation (TRIM) may potentially have significant adverse effects that affect patient outcome. Allogeneic RBC transfusion has been shown to suppress the recipient's immune response, an effect first noted with kidney transplantation that resulted in increased survival of the transplanted kidney.[120] However, immunosuppression is generally undesirable in critically ill patients, even though the clinical impact of blood component transfusion is not well defined. As noted in previous sections, immunomodulation likely contributes to AHTRs, NHTRs, anaphylaxis, and TRALI. The major clinical issues regarding TRIM center around the association between blood product transfusion and increased risk of infection and increased and more rapid rates of tumor recurrence in surgical oncology patients. The largest prospective trial of colorectal cancer resection, for example, was negative,[121] but a meta-analysis of existing data suggests that an adverse effect on recurrence does exist.[122] Significant heterogeneity exists in the reported studies and makes definitive conclusions difficult.[123] Most retrospective and prospective trials of postoperative or critical care unit infections suggest an adverse effect of blood component transfusion.[124-126]

The precise mechanism of the immunomodulation induced by transfusion has not yet been delineated, and several mechanisms may be involved.[123] Allogeneic plasma, leukocytes and substances that accumulate in stored blood components may contribute to TRIM. Alterations identified in laboratory and clinical transfusion recipients have included depression of the T-helper/T-suppressor lymphocyte ratio, decreased natural killer cell activity, diminished interleukin 2 generation, formation of anti-idiotype antibodies, impairment of phagocytic cell function, and chronic persistence of donor lymphocytes (microchimerism), suggestive of low level GVHD. Difficulties in analysis of human data arise because patients requiring blood component transfusions have conditions that may induce immune changes. There is some evidence from two large clinical trials to suggest that leukocyte reduction of blood components reduces or eliminates this immunomodulatory effect but other results are conflicting.[127,128] Well-designed prospective trials are needed to more clearly elucidate the impact of any immunomodulatory effects of transfusing blood products.

TRANSFUSION-TRANSMITTED INFECTIOUS DISEASES

Transfusion-associated acquired immunodeficiency syndrome (AIDS) has done more to revolutionize transfusion practice than any other transfusion risk by resulting in more conservative blood use, more stringent donor selection criteria, and improved screening tests. The result is that viral transmission rates are now difficult to measure, and the risk of transfusion-related infectious diseases is lower than ever.[46,129] Bacterial infection has become the most common infectious risk.

MICROBIAL AND ENDOTOXIN CONTAMINATION

Several fatalities are reported yearly from the transfusion of blood components contaminated with viable bacteria, with or without the accumulation of endotoxin.[102,130] Platelet concentrates stored at room temperature are particularly prone to bacterial growth, with a reported incidence of 1.13 in 10,000 components with apheresis units having the highest contamination rate.[131] Organisms isolated from platelets and implicated in fatal transfusion reactions include *Staphylococcus* and *Streptococcus* species and gram-negative bacilli. Fatalities resulting from bacterial contamination of refrigerated RBCs have occurred as well and more often involve cryophilic bacteria. RBC transfusions contaminated by *Yersinia enterocolitica* have been consistently reported for a decade.[132] Transfusion reactions caused by bacterial or endotoxin contamination are fortunately quite rare, but the mortality rate exceeds 60%.

Signs and symptoms of reactions caused by microbial contamination overlap those of hemolytic transfusion reactions and consist primarily of fever and hypotension, along with other signs of endotoxic shock. A Gram stain of the implicated unit can be prepared immediately and, if positive, appropriate antibiotic and supportive therapy instituted. Autologous blood components may also be contaminated at the time of collection; therefore, reactions occurring in patients who are receiving their own blood should be evaluated as fully as though they were receiving allogeneic blood.

HEPATITIS

The success of viral screening measures is most clearly illustrated by the fall in the risk for posttransfusion hepatitis over the past 2 decades. The elimination of paid donors in 1972 and the introduction of nucleic acid tests for hepatitis B virus (HBV) and hepatitis C virus (HCV) have resulted in a steady reduction in the rates of posttransfusion hepatitis. The estimated residual risk for HBV is 1 in 2.8 million to 1 in 3.6 million transfused blood components.[133] Although about 30% to 40% of HBV transmissions will result in acute hepatitis, chronic HBV infection develops in less than 10% of such patients. In contrast, the risk for chronic HCV infection after transfusion is higher, nearly 50%, and the long-term risk for mortality related to cirrhosis or hepatocellular carcinoma is about 15% over more than 20 years after posttransfusion hepatitis secondary to HCV.[134,135] The risk of HCV transmission is even lower than HBV with a residual risk estimate of 8.7 per 10 million transfused blood components.[136] The clinical course of hepatitis A is generally milder, and the lack of a chronic carrier state means that with donor screening for symptoms of the acute illness, the risk of transmission is rare.

RETROVIRUSES

Retroviruses known to be capable of transmission by transfusion are human immunodeficiency virus (HIV-1, HIV-2) and human T-cell leukemia/lymphoma virus (HTLV I and II). Transfusion-associated AIDS was initially reported in late 1982.[137] The first report of an associated viral agent did not appear until late 1983, and in March 1985 the screening enzyme-linked immunosorbent assay (ELISA) to detect antibody to HIV-1 was licensed and immediately incorporated into the blood-screening process. Improved confidential donor screening also decreased the risk of infectious units appearing in the donor pool.[138] The discovery that heat treatment decreased transmission resulted in a reduction in transmission by plasma products, especially to persons with hemophilia. Removal of donor units with seropositivity by ELISA was insufficient to prevent transmission of HIV-1. Subsequent development of an assay for the p24 antigen and nucleic acid testing have lowered the risk of transfusion-associated HIV-1 infection to an estimated 1 in 1,467,000 transfused blood components.[136] Despite donor screening and sensitive assays, an extremely small but finite risk of HIV-1 transmission by screened blood transfusions remains. This risk is largely due to the eclipse period (interval between infection and development of detectable concentrations of HIV RNA in plasma) experienced by newly infected donors. The eclipse period for HIV-1 is estimated to be 9 days.[136]

A second retrovirus, HIV-2, first described in residents of countries in West Africa and subsequently detected in migrants to western Europe, causes an immunodeficiency syndrome similar to that caused by HIV-1. Although very few cases of HIV-2 have been reported in the United States[139] and there have been no reported transfusion-transmitted cases, experience with other retroviruses suggests that screening may prevent the majority of potential transmissions. Therefore, donated blood is now screened for the presence of HIV-2.

The retrovirus HTLV-I is the causative agent of adult T-cell leukemia (ATL) and is strongly implicated in the chronic, progressive neurologic disorder termed *tropical spastic paraparesis* or *HTLV-I-associated myelopathy* (TSP/HAM). HTLV-II has been linked to hairy cell leukemia, but no transfusion-transmitted cases have been reported. The virus exhibits strong serologic cross-reactivity with HTLV-I such that screening assays fail to distinguish between the two viruses. Transfusion-transmitted HTLV-I has been demonstrated.[140] TSP/HAM has developed in a small percentage of infected transfusion recipients, but no transfusion-associated cases of ATL have been seen. Approximately 0.025% of donors in the United States are seropositive for HTLV-I and HTLV-II[141]; further testing reveals the majority of them to be HTLV-II. Donated blood is currently screened for antibodies to HTLV-I and HTLV-II.

CYTOMEGALOVIRUS

CMV is a human herpesvirus that establishes latent infection in the host's tissues, particularly leukocytes, and is transmitted by all cellular blood components.[142] Seropositivity, or the presence of antibody, denotes previous exposure to the virus but does not confer protective immunity. Secondary reinfection or reactivation of latent infection can occur. Antibodies to CMV persist for life and serve as a marker indicating the potential for transmission of live virus.

Immunocompetent recipients of transfused CMV-positive blood experience minimal morbidity and mortality risks. The majority are asymptomatic, whereas a heterophile-negative mononucleosis syndrome may develop in a few. Immunocompromised patients, however, may suffer life-threatening manifestations such as severe interstitial pneumonitis, gastroenteritis, hepatitis, or disseminated disease. Several groups of patients are at particular risk (Box 79.4),[143] and these patients should receive blood incapable of transmitting the virus. Screening of donated blood for CMV is not routine but can be performed quickly if necessary. Because the prevalence of donor seropositivity is quite high, CMV-seronegative blood may not be readily available. Blood that is leukocyte depleted may be as effective as seronegative blood in the prevention of CMV transmission, although a meta-analysis of clinical trials comparing the two methods suggests that CMV-negative blood products might have a slight advantage over leukocyte-depleted products.[144]

PARASITES

Many blood-borne parasites may be transmitted by transfusion, although this is a rare occurrence in the United States because of donor screening questions and the low endemicity of implicated agents. Changing immigration patterns and global travel, however, make transfusion-transmitted parasites an increasing concern.

On a worldwide basis, malaria is the most important transfusion-transmitted infective parasite, although only a few cases are reported in the United States each year.[145] Such infections are manifested by delayed fever, chills, diaphoresis, and hemolysis, often masked by underlying medical conditions. Fatalities have occurred. Babesiosis, a tick-borne disease caused by *Babesia microti,* is endemic in regions of the northeastern United States. Transfusion-transmitted cases have been reported, with asplenic, elderly, or immunocompromised patients being particularly susceptible.[146] Babesiosis was the leading cause of infectious transfusion-related fatality in the United States from 2007 to 2011, and there are no effective methods of donor screening or testing.[102] With increases in the number of Central and South American immigrants to North America, Chagas' disease, transmitted by the protozoan parasite *Trypanosoma cruzi,* has emerged as a potential transfusion-transmissible infection.[147] Other parasitic diseases that have been transmitted by transfusion include toxoplasmosis, leishmaniasis, and Lyme disease.

Box 79.4 Patients for Whom Cytomegalovirus-Safe Blood Components Are Strongly Recommended

Seronegative pregnant women
Seronegative premature infants weighing less than 1200 g
Seronegative allogeneic or autologous bone marrow transplant recipients
Seronegative transplant recipients of seronegative organs

EMERGING INFECTIONS IN TRANSFUSION MEDICINE

Human parvovirus B19 has been recognized as a pathogen capable of transmission by transfusion, with typical clinical findings and the potential for aplastic anemia. Epstein-Barr virus infection with a typical mononucleosis-like illness has been reported after transfusion. West Nile virus can also be transmitted by transfusion. H2N1 influenza, severe acute respiratory syndrome (SARS), and other new viral infections should be capable of transmission by transfusion, although cases have not been reported and the prevalence of asymptomatic disease is unknown. A rising concern is the transmission of prion disease, either Creutzfeldt-Jacob disease or bovine spongiform encephalopathy (BSE). Donor referral criteria were implemented in 1987 for these diseases, and transfusion transmission of BSE has been reported in the United Kingdom.

SPECIAL TRANSFUSION SITUATIONS IN THE CRITICAL CARE SETTING

MASSIVE TRANSFUSION

Massive transfusion is commonly defined as the administration of blood components in excess of one blood volume or greater than or equal to 10 units PRBCs within a 24-hour period, although other definitions have been used in the literature and for resuscitation protocols.[148] Massive transfusion, especially in the range of 20 or more units of blood products, causes complications not generally seen in usual transfusion practice: accumulation of undesirable substances present within stored blood and dilutional depletion of normal blood constituents that are lacking in stored units. Trauma victims, surgical patients undergoing complex or emergent procedures, and patients with vascular or coagulation disorders may require massive transfusion in the critical care setting. The first priority in such patients is to stop the bleeding but transfusion of blood products occurs simultaneously to maintain hemostasis and ensure oxygen-carrying capacity. Survival is determined more by the nature and degree of the patient's injuries or medical conditions than by the transfusions, but the presence of adverse effects of massive transfusion can complicate a patient's course in the ICU.

Transfusion of large quantities of RBCs deficient in functional platelets often results in hemostatic defects and thrombocytopenia. Platelet counts consistently decrease in inverse proportion to the amount of blood administered, with the hemostatically significant level of $50 \times 10^9/L$ reached after 20 units.[149] Functional defects have also been noted.[150] Despite these laboratory changes, severe diffuse bleeding develops in less than 20% of massively transfused patients, and no laboratory studies alone are predictive. Prophylactic platelet transfusions were not shown to be of benefit in older studies.[151] Platelet counts may return to hemostatically effective levels quickly in patients with normal marrow function.

Resuscitation of massively bleeding patients with PRBCs in combination with crystalloids will usually result in hemodilution to about 60% of normal coagulation factor levels after the transfusion of about 10 units; this factor level can usually maintain normal hemostasis. However, if crystalloids are given in excess of PRBCs less plasma protein may remain after 10 units are transfused. Bleeding is unlikely until prothrombin time (PT), INR, and PTT prolongations exceed 1.5 to 1.8 times the midpoint normal range, the equivalent of an INR approaching 2.0.[149] Prophylactic administration of FFP was also not effective in preventing diffuse bleeding in older studies.[152] Based on the earlier studies, previous recommendations suggested that transfusion of blood components in massive bleeding should be based on measured or anticipated results of platelet count and coagulation studies (laboratory driven).

More recently some trauma centers have adopted a protocol approach (formula driven) to replacing platelets and plasma when massive transfusion is required, usually with a set ratio of RBC to platelet and FFP infusions (e.g., 3:1:1 or less).[153,154] Variable ratios have been used and the optimal ratio of blood products is not defined. Although the published experiences from these retrospective, nonrandomized studies are generally positive, confirmation is needed from well-designed prospective randomized studies to avoid bias, particularly survival bias that favors higher plasma to RBC ratios.[155,156] Additional reports have also suggested that early transfusion of FFP may not improve outcomes and may predispose to organ failure.[157,158] Until higher quality evidence can support the use of specific blood product ratios in massive transfusion, it is difficult to support this practice.

Blood preservative solutions contain citrate, which anticoagulates stored blood by binding ionized calcium. WB contains approximately 1.8 g of citrate/citric acid per unit in the plasma fraction. Patients with normal liver function can metabolize the citrate load in 1 unit of WB in 5 minutes, but hepatic impairment may extend removal to 15 minutes or longer. Toxicity may result when citrate is administered in excess of the metabolic capacity, thereby causing a decrease in ionized calcium levels.[159] Although paresthesias, cramps, and myoclonus can result from citrate excess, the principal danger of hypocalcemia is depression of myocardial contractility and potential prolongation of the QT interval. Because the effects of citrate are transient and the use of PRBCs containing little residual citrated plasma is far more common than massive transfusion with WB, routine administration of calcium is not indicated; clinically significant rebound hypercalcemia may result. Calcium infusion should be limited to hypoperfused patients with hepatic or cardiac failure who manifest citrate toxicity. Hypomagnesemia is common in patients with massive transfusion, and it is often associated with hypocalcemia.[160] Citrate binds magnesium as well as calcium and may play a role in the development of hypomagnesemia.[148] Hypomagnesemia does not appear to impact outcomes in massively transfused patients.

Potassium leaks from RBCs during storage, and up to 7 mEq of extracellular potassium may accumulate in each unit. Irradiation of RBCs increases extracellular potassium. However, dangerous levels of potassium rarely develop in adults from transfused blood; the potassium level is more likely to be determined by the patient's acid-base status.[161] Studies of massively transfused patients have demonstrated a wide range of potassium levels, with hypokalemia seen as frequently as hyperkalemia. Because of the complexity of physiologic changes during resuscitation, it is impossible to predict the net effect of massive transfusion on serum potassium levels. Potassium levels need to be monitored closely in patients receiving large amount of PRBCs.

The pH of stored blood drops during storage, from 7.16 at the time of collection to as low as 6.73 after several weeks of storage. The administration of large quantities of acidic blood, together with the metabolic acidosis common in these patients before resuscitation, would lead one to expect worsening acidosis as the outcome of massive transfusion. However, patients are more likely to exhibit metabolic alkalosis at the end of the transfusion episode,[161,162] partly because of improved tissue perfusion and the metabolism of citrate and lactate to bicarbonate. Patients in renal failure may be unable to handle the bicarbonate load and require dialysis. Acidosis persisting after transfusion suggests inadequate tissue perfusion.[159] Empiric administration of bicarbonate to counter the acid load is not warranted and may contribute to the deleterious effects of hypercapnia in patients with impaired ventilation.

RBC components are stored at approximately 4° C and require 30 to 45 minutes to warm to room temperature. Elective transfusions at standard flow rates are tolerated without the need to warm the blood; however, core body temperature, measured by esophageal probe, can fall to 30° C or lower with the administration of large volumes of cold blood over a period of 1 to 2 hours.[163] Adverse effects of hypothermia include a decreased heart rate and myocardial contractility, cardiac arrhythmias, increased affinity of hemoglobin for oxygen resulting in decreased tissue oxygen delivery, DIC, and impaired ability to metabolize the citrate load of stored blood. Both blood warmers and patient warming may be instituted during massive transfusion, and patient core temperature should be monitored during resuscitative efforts.

Whether massive transfusion in and of itself is a cause of ARDS is another source of controversy. There are theoretical reasons why massive transfusion might precipitate ARDS because all cellular transfusions contain damaged or activated WBCs, cell membranes, aggregated platelets, and microthrombi, all of which are capable of lodging in and damaging pulmonary capillaries. Despite this possibility, neither microfiltration of transfusions nor routine leukocyte depletion has shown a significant impact on the incidence of ARDS in massively transfused patients.[164] Certainly, other causes of ARDS exist in patients who undergo massive transfusion, and the possibility of TACO and TRALI should be considered in the evaluation of patients with hypoxia and diffuse pulmonary infiltrates after massive transfusion.

AUTOIMMUNE HEMOLYTIC ANEMIA

Patients with autoimmune hemolytic anemia (AIHA) have an autoantibody, usually of broad specificity, that fixes itself to their RBCs and triggers extravascular immune-mediated destruction. Patients with AIHA have a positive direct antiglobulin test (DAT, commonly known as the Coombs test)[165] and varying degrees of hemolysis, and their autoantibodies cause agglutination of RBCs from all donors during crossmatching. If the hemolysis is brisk, patients may require RBC transfusion to support oxygen needs before medical management is effective. Hence, transfusion is difficult because agglutination during crossmatching interferes with proper definition of compatible units of RBCs and because the transfused RBCs are themselves subject to the same immune hemolysis as the host RBCs. Many blood banks have methods for depletion of autoantibodies from the recipient's plasma and elution of antibodies from RBCs to arrive at a proper crossmatch.[166] Although such crossmatches are time consuming and not generally available on an emergency basis, they can be lifesaving. Criteria for transfusion should remain the same as for other recipients.

NECESSARY TRANSFUSION OF INCOMPATIBLE BLOOD

RBCs are crossmatched for RBC antigens in the ABO and $Rh_0(D)$ group and for other RBC antigens when antibodies are present. However, there are several hundred other RBC antigens in the human family and with repeated transfusion recipients may become alloimmunized to other antigens. Generally, alloimmunization occurs in approximately 1% of transfusions, but the prevalence of alloantibodies is higher in chronically transfused, relatively immunocompetent patients, especially African Americans, whose distribution of RBC antigens has significant variation from the white population. Alloimmunization may present difficulties in crossmatching of blood to the point that compatible blood must be obtained from rare-donor registries, if at all. In some patients the alloantibody is never precisely identified, yet the majority of blood available for transfusion is incompatible. The delay engendered by working with multiple or unidentified antibodies may be unacceptable in some critical care situations in which the need for oxygen-carrying capacity leaves no choice but to transfuse incompatible blood. The behavior of these antibodies in the laboratory may assist in predicting the clinical outcome of the incompatible transfusion.[167] Special procedures such as clearance studies, flow cytometry, and in vivo crossmatching (cautious administration of a small aliquot of blood, with subsequent observation of serum and urine for evidence of hemolysis) are useful if time permits.

Emergency transfusion of type O, Rh-negative uncrossmatched blood is generally reserved for the resuscitation of trauma patients, for whom the delay in crossmatching may be life-threatening. The risks of alloimmunization to non-ABO antigens are generally accepted as low and a recent study found antigen-incompatible RBCs were transfused in 2.6% of patients who required emergency blood release.[168] Even Rh-positive type O RBCs may be used because rates of alloimmunization to $Rh_0(D)$ are low under the circumstances of emergency transfusion.

TRANSFUSION IN PATIENTS WITH DISSEMINATED INTRAVASCULAR COAGULATION

DIC is a common disorder in critically ill patients that may manifest as severe hemorrhage or thrombosis. Therapy is primarily directed at treating the cause and supporting the patient. Supportive therapy includes the transfusion of blood components needed to correct the bleeding diathesis caused by the consumption of platelets and fibrinogen, in addition to PRBCs to restore oxygen-carrying capacity. Platelets and fibrinogen (as cryoprecipitate) are the most common components used to treat the coagulopathy, but their use risks increasing the microvascular thrombosis of DIC. Heparin anticoagulation is controversial and may increase the risk of bleeding, especially if depleted factors are not replenished. No clinical trials support the routine use of heparin, and randomized trials of other components and coagulation inhibitors have uniformly been negative.

HEPATIC FAILURE

Cirrhotic patients or those with fulminant hepatic failure have a variety of hemostatic disorders that complicate transfusion management of a bleeding patient.[169] Hepatic synthesis of coagulation factors may be markedly diminished, thereby necessitating replacement by FFP or cryoprecipitate. Patterns of factor diminution may vary between acute hepatic necrosis and chronic cirrhosis.[170] Associated hemodynamic alterations may make it impossible to administer the volumes required for effective hemostasis, however, and any effect is transient. The use of factor concentrates or antifibrinolytic agents may precipitate thrombosis. Activation of fibrinolysis and decreased clearance of activated factors may produce or mimic chronic DIC, thus further exacerbating the factor deficiencies and impairing coagulation. Abnormal platelet function and thrombocytopenia may contribute to the coagulopathy of liver disease, with concomitant splenomegaly reducing the effectiveness of platelet transfusions. As with DIC, blood product transfusions for coagulopathy of hepatic failure have not demonstrated any long-term benefits, and should be considered only to achieve emergent hemostasis.

ALTERNATIVES TO TRANSFUSION OF BLOOD COMPONENTS

The safest transfusion is one that is not given. Therefore, alternatives to blood component therapy continue to be sought. It may be possible to limit blood component exposure by the appropriate use of pharmacologic agents that promote hemostasis and the administration of recombinant hematopoietic growth factors to stimulate marrow hematopoiesis.

BLOOD SUBSTITUTES

Two types of alternative oxygen carriers are being evaluated for clinical use, but no oxygen-carrying blood substitute is currently approved for use in the United States.[171,172] Perfluorocarbons are hydrophobic molecules with high oxygen-carrying capacity that have to be administered as an emulsion to be soluble in plasma. The perfluorocarbon solutions have failed to demonstrate any utility as intravascular oxygen carriers because of their unfavorable P-50 (oxygen half-saturation pressure) and oxygen off-loading characteristics. The other type of preparation that has been explored in clinical trials is cell-free hemoglobin solutions cross-linked or polymerized by chemical manipulation to prevent rapid clearance from the circulation. Known as hemoglobin-based oxygen carriers (HBOCs), they are intended to provide short-term oxygen-carrying capacity for acutely ill patients and have the advantage of not requiring cross-matching and no risk of infection. Although these proposed products may have a longer shelf-life and are easier to transport, they have many drawbacks. Most have a circulatory half-life of only about 24 hours. The oxygen dissociation curve for these substitutes is also frequently not favorable: either a high FIO_2 is required to "load" these molecules or they are less likely to deliver oxygen efficiently at lower PO_2 levels. Certain preparations of HBOCs are currently in clinical trials. Main concerns for HBOCs have been unfavorable side effects including hypertension, increased cardiovascular mortality risk, and renal dysfunction. Because the hemoglobin source is reclaimed bovine or human RBCs, it is unlikely that patients who do not accept blood components because of their religious beliefs (Jehovah's Witnesses) will accept these types of hemoglobin solutions.

DESMOPRESSIN

The synthetic vasopressin analog, desmopressin (DDAVP), increases plasma factor VIII:c and promotes the release of von Willebrand factor from endothelial stores.[173] DDAVP has provided effective hemostasis in bleeding patients with mild hemophilia A and type I von Willebrand disease and has been used as prophylaxis for patients undergoing surgery. DDAVP reportedly improves platelet function in some patients with qualitative platelet disorders associated with uremia, cirrhosis, and aspirin ingestion. Studies of its efficacy in cardiopulmonary bypass procedures are conflicting, but a subset of these patients may benefit. The chief drawback to its use is tachyphylaxis, which develops in essentially all cases after short-term repeated administration.

ANTIFIBRINOLYTIC AGENTS

The lysine analogs ε-aminocaproic acid and tranexamic acid inhibit fibrinolysis by blocking the binding of plasminogen and plasmin to fibrin. These antifibrinolytic agents may decrease bleeding and thus the need for homologous blood components in patients with hemophilia, thrombocytopenia, and systemic fibrinolysis. A novel and effective use of tranexamic acid involves administration as a mouthwash in preparation for oral surgery in patients with hemophilia or those receiving oral anticoagulant therapy. Tranexamic acid has also been demonstrated to effectively decrease mortality rates in high-risk trauma patients when given at presentation.[174] Use may also be promising in decreasing blood transfusion requirements in high-risk surgical procedures, such as radical prostatectomy.[175] The most serious side effect of these agents when systemically administered is thrombosis; thus, it is important to use them appropriately and monitor the patient carefully during their use.

Aprotinin is a naturally occurring bovine serine protease inhibitor that acts on plasma serine proteases such as plasmin, kallikrein, trypsin, and some coagulation proteins. Aprotinin was previously shown to reduce blood loss in patients undergoing cardiopulmonary bypass surgery by inhibiting fibrinolysis and preventing platelet damage.[176] However, an observational study and a large multicenter randomized trial in cardiovascular surgery patients found that use of aprotinin was associated with an increased mortality rate, and therefore should not be used routinely.[177,178]

VITAMIN K

When time permits, vitamin K is the preferred agent to reverse the coagulopathy induced by warfarin. Normalization of the PT can be seen in as few as 6 to 12 hours. Additionally, selected cirrhotic patients may exhibit improvement in the PT when treated with therapeutic doses of vitamin K. Many patients in critical care units exhibit a prolonged PT, especially if dietary supplements are limited and broad-spectrum antibiotic therapy is given. Vitamin K is a safe and effective agent for reversing this effect. Intravenous administration of vitamin K is associated with a small risk of anaphylaxis, and oral replacement is preferred over subcutaneous administration for more consistent absorption.

HEMATOPOIETIC GROWTH FACTORS

Recombinant erythropoietin (EPO) has dramatically reduced the RBC transfusion requirements of patients with chronic renal failure, in which decreased renal EPO production accounts for the anemia. Studies of EPO efficacy in reducing perioperative RBC transfusion requirements by increasing the yield of predeposited autologous blood or stimulating bone marrow synthesis after surgery have shown benefit in reducing blood transfusion, although preoperative planning and autologous deposits are required.[179] Despite initial promising results, use of EPO in critically ill patients lacked efficacy in decreasing RBC transfusions and increased the risk for thrombotic vascular events.[180] Consideration for EPO administration may be appropriate in select patients who are unable to receive blood transfusions after risks and benefits are addressed.

CELL SALVAGE TECHNOLOGY

Cell salvage equipment has been in clinical use for several decades, and although cell salvage is clearly capable of rescuing otherwise "lost" RBCs, its full impact on transfusions has been poorly documented. Cell salvage generally consists of collection of shed blood from a clean, uncontaminated operating field, followed by removal of the cellular elements and retransfusion into the patient. Cell salvage has been used both intraoperatively and postoperatively, especially in cardiac surgery. Although clinical studies of cell salvage have many methodologic flaws, it does reduce the need for blood transfusion in adult elective cardiac and orthopedic surgery.[181] Risks include bacterial contamination, febrile reactions, triggering of DIC, and coagulopathy as a result of dilution. When combined with acute intraoperative hemodilution, this technology is also potentially cost saving.[182]

LEGAL ISSUES IN TRANSFUSION MEDICINE

Most states regulate blood banking and medical practice, but blood products are regarded as a service, not as a commodity, so standard product liability does not pertain to blood components.[183] However, negligence in the course of preparing, testing, transferring, crossmatching, and administering blood products is still a potential cause for legal action. Every clinician who orders transfusions must be aware that blood components, like drugs, are approved for specific uses and that the indications should be clearly documented in the medical record.

The informed consent of the patient is an important area of potential liability. The Joint Commission has required written patient consent for blood transfusions since 1996. What constitutes adequate informed consent and who is responsible for advising the patient are still debated. Elements of informed consent include an understanding of the need for transfusion, its risks and benefits, and the alternatives, including the risk of not undergoing transfusion, as well as the opportunity to ask questions. Whether the clinician documents informed consent with an individual progress note in the patient record or with a standardized form is generally established as institutional policy. Similarly, institutions vary with respect to policies for consenting adults who are temporarily incompetent, such as sedated patients in the ICU.

A competent adult patient may refuse blood transfusion, and Jehovah's Witnesses commonly do so for religious reasons. Case law is clear in upholding this right of the patient,[184] which extends to care given at such time as the patient may become incompetent (i.e., comatose) after such refusal was expressed before becoming incompetent. Courts will usually order a lifesaving transfusion for minors. Exceptions have been made in the case of some "emancipated minors" who are at the age of reason. Most states have evoked a "special interest" in the welfare of a fetus in ordering transfusions to pregnant women.

The advent of sentinel event reviews and other quality management procedures for patient safety has had an impact on transfusion practice as well. Procedures for patient identification before surgical procedures, including devices such as bar code readers, have also been applied to transfusion practice.

KEY POINTS

- Blood components should be prescribed like therapeutic agents as part of a blood management program.
- RBC transfusion can be considered when the hemoglobin is less than or equal to 7 g/dL for the majority of hemodynamically stable ICU patients. A transfusion threshold of less than 8 g/dL may be appropriate for patients with symptomatic cardiovascular disease and postoperative surgical patients.
- Platelet transfusions are indicated for patients who have active bleeding due to thrombocytopenia or functional platelet defects and for the prevention of bleeding due to thrombocytopenia.
- FFP is indicated for the repletion of coagulation factors in bleeding patients deficient in those factors or to provide specific plasma proteins that cannot be obtained from safer sources.
- Cryoprecipitate is a concentrated source of fibrinogen and selected coagulation factors. Cryoprecipitate may be more helpful than FFP in correcting the hypofibrinogenemia of dilutional or consumptive coagulopathy.
- Adverse reactions to blood components occur in 1% to 2% of transfusion episodes. Adherence to routine protocols for the evaluation of transfusion reactions may save lives.
- Transmission of infectious agents by transfusion has been markedly reduced, and bacterial infection is now the most common infectious complication of transfusion.
- Adverse effects unique to massive transfusion are likely to complicate the management of critically ill or severely injured patients. Component therapy for such patients should remain conservative pending the outcome of prospective studies.
- Informed consent for blood transfusion is a standard of practice. A competent adult has the legal right to refuse blood transfusion.

SELECTED REFERENCES

2. Goodnough LT, Shander A: Patient blood management. Anesthesiology 2012;116:1367-1376.
31. Hebert PC, Wells G, Blajchman MA, et al: A multicenter, randomized, controlled clinical trial of transfusion requirements in critical care. N Engl J Med 1999;340:409-417.
46. Carson JL, Grossman BJ, Kleinman S, et al: Red blood cell transfusion: A clinical practice guideline from the AABB. Ann Intern Med 2012;157:49-58.
53. Napolitano LM, Kurek S, Luchette FA, et al: Clinical practice guideline: Red blood cell transfusion in adult trauma and critical care. Crit Care Med 2009;37:3124-3157.
54. Carson JL, Carless PA, Hebert PC: Transfusion thresholds and other strategies for guiding allogeneic red blood cell transfusion. Cochrane Database Syst Rev 2012;(4):CD002042.

60. College of American Pathologists: Practice parameter for the use of fresh-frozen plasma, cryoprecipitate, and platelets. JAMA 1994;271:777-781.
72. Estcourt L, Stanworth S, Doree C, et al: Prophylactic platelet transfusion for prevention of bleeding in patients with haematological disorders after chemotherapy and stem cell transplantation (Review). Cochrane Database Syst Rev 2012;(5):CD004269.
83. British Committee for Standards in Haematology, Blood Transfusion Task Force: Guidelines for the use of fresh-frozen plasma, cryoprecipitate and cryosupernatant. Br J Haematol 2004;126: 11-28.
84. Roback JD, Caldwell S, Carson J, et al: Evidence-based practice guidelines for plasma transfusion. Transfusion 2010;50:1227-1239.
106. Perrotta PL, Snyder EL: Non-infectious complications of transfusion therapy. Blood Rev 2001;15:69-83.
113. Toy P, Popovsky MA, Abraham E, et al, for the NHLBI Working Group on TRALI: Transfusion-related acute lung injury: Definition and review. Crit Care Med 2005;33:721-726.
154. Phan HH, Wisner DH: Should we increase the ratio of plasma/platelets to red blood cells in massive transfusion: What is the evidence? Vox Sang 2010;98:395-402.

The complete list of references can be found at www.expertconsult.com.

80 Intensive Care of the Cancer Patient

Brendan D. Curti | Dan L. Longo

CHAPTER OUTLINE

The annual estimated incidence of new invasive cancers in the United States in 2012 exceeds 1.6 million, with greater than 570,000 deaths.[1] Long-term remissions and control of advanced cancer are being achieved with targeted therapy, and new immunotherapy agents in many malignancies.[2-6] We are entering an era of "personalized" oncologic care in which treatments are prescribed based on the profile of mutated or overexpressed genes in the tumor specimen. For the treatment of metastatic malignancies, enhanced success has come from the ability to deliver chemotherapy, radiation therapy, immunotherapy, or combination regimens with increased dose intensity. Progress in supportive care and intensive care medicine has allowed oncologists to treat their patients aggressively and support them despite the toxicities inherent in dose-intense treatment modalities. A greater understanding of the mechanisms for these toxicities has also improved care and patient outcomes.

This chapter describes specific oncologic clinical entities and cancer treatment toxicities that require intensive care management. The discussion of these problems is organized according to organ system because cancers are best understood as systemic diseases that can directly or indirectly influence all organ systems. The pathophysiology that gives rise to these clinical circumstances is increasingly understood and is used as the basis for treatment recommendations. Aspects unique to biologic therapies and bone marrow transplantation are treated in separate sections. The ethical aspects of treating cancer patients in the intensive care unit (ICU) are also discussed.

METABOLIC AND ENDOCRINE COMPLICATIONS

Endocrine syndromes associated with malignancies have been described for many years and some clinically significant endocrinopathies are induced by immunotherapy agents, such as ipilimumab, currently used in the treatment of advanced melanoma.[4,7] These problems may manifest as solitary laboratory derangements, such as hypercalcemia or hyperphosphatemia, or can present as clinical syndromes, such as Cushing syndrome in small cell lung cancer. Metabolic disorders can also arise as a consequence of cancer treatment. This is most often seen with chemotherapy for rapidly growing tumors such as leukemias or lymphomas. Abrupt changes in metabolic variables have also been observed after interleukin 2 (IL-2)-based immunotherapy and the rapid in vivo expansion of lymphocytes.[8] The most common of these clinical entities are tumor lysis syndrome (TLS), hypercalcemia, oncogenic osteomalacia, syndrome of inappropriate secretion of antidiuretic hormone (SIADH), adrenal failure, pheochromocytoma, tumor-induced hypoglycemia, and chemotherapy-induced metabolic disturbances.

TUMOR LYSIS SYNDROME

Case reports of metabolic and electrolyte abnormalities after chemotherapy for rapidly growing tumors such as Burkitt's lymphoma and leukemias were first published in the 1950s.[9] Cadman and his colleagues in the 1970s proposed a mechanism that linked these metabolic observations.[10] More recently, TLS has been observed in patients with solid tumors and has been observed in patients receiving immunotherapy, such as IL-2, sunitinib, imatinib, and rituximab.[11-14] TLS after treatment for solid tumors is relatively rare.

TLS is characterized by hyperuricemia, hyperkalemia, hyperphosphatemia, and hypocalcemia.[10] Electrolyte abnormalities can appear as soon as 6 hours after chemotherapy administration and can persist for 5 to 7 days after treatment. The hyperuricemia comes from the massive release of intracellular nucleic acids and their metabolism by xanthine oxidase into uric acid. Urate crystals can form in the renal collecting ducts and result in oliguric and anuric renal failure. Similarly, potassium and phosphate are released from lysing tumor cells, and renal excretion of these intracellular ions is impaired by hyperuricemia. Serum calcium levels drop from ectopic calcium deposition; this becomes more likely as the calcium-phosphorus product increases. Calcium deposition is favored by a calcium-phosphorus product greater than 60 mg^2/dL^2 and becomes severe when the product is more than 75 mg^2/dL^2. The clinical manifestations of TLS depend on which electrolyte derangement predominates. Tetany, confusion, hypotension, dysrhythmias, and sudden death have been reported with TLS. The most effective management approach for this syndrome is to anticipate its occurrence and intervene prospectively. Patients at greatest risk for TLS are those with a diagnosis of a rapidly growing lymphoma or leukemia with high blast counts, and pretreatment levels of lactate dehydrogenase greater than 1500 U/dL and uric acid greater than 10 mg/dL. Pretreatment azotemia is also a poor prognostic sign. Azotemia may be exacerbated by uric acid nephropathy, which is more common with uric acid levels exceeding 20 mg/dL. It is unlikely that TLS will occur in patients at risk who do not develop metabolic changes within 48 hours after receiving chemotherapy. Guidelines for prophylaxis and treatment of TLS are given in Box 80.1. It is important to note that rasburicase poses an oxidative stress and can induce hemolytic anemia in patients with glucose-6-phosphate dehydrogenase (G6PD) deficiency.

Box 80.1 Tumor Lysis Syndrome: Treatment Recommendations

When no metabolic aberration exists:
- Allopurinol 300 mg/day, reduce to 100 mg/day after 3 days of chemotherapy
  OR
- Rasburicase 0.2 mg/kg IV daily × 5 days
- Hydration: 0.45% saline 3000 mL/day
- Initiate chemotherapy within 24-48 hours of admission
- Monitor serum chemistry values every 12-24 hours

When metabolic aberration exists:
- Allopurinol OR rasburicase as above; reduce dose if hyperuricemia controlled or for renal insufficiency
- Hydration with D_5W with 2 ampules/L of $NaCO_3$, add nonthiazide diuretics as needed
- Urinary alkalization to keep urine pH >7.0, may discontinue when serum uric acid level is normal
- Postpone chemotherapy until uric acid decreased and electrolytes stable
- Monitor serum chemistries every 6-8 hours
- Replace calcium with slow intravenous infusion of calcium gluconate (if symptomatic or for ECG changes)
- Treat hyperkalemia and hyperphosphatemia with exchange resins and phosphate binders, respectively

Criteria for hemodialysis in patients unresponsive to the measures listed above:
- Serum potassium >6.0 mEq/L
- Serum uric acid >20 mg/dL
- Serum phosphorus >10 mg/dL
- Fluid overload unresponsive to diuretics

Symptomatic hypercalcemia D_5W, 5% dextrose in water; ECG, electrocardiogram; $NaCO_3$, sodium carbonate.

HYPERCALCEMIA

Hypercalcemia is the most common metabolic abnormality occurring in cancer patients. Approximately 10% to 20% of all cancer patients have hypercalcemia at some point in their course. The clinical symptoms of hypercalcemia are nonspecific and include lethargy, confusion, nausea, and anorexia. Often the clinical symptoms in cancer patients may be subtle because the onset of hypercalcemia is gradual. The mechanism that underlies all cases of cancer-related hypercalcemia is increased calcium resorption from bone due to enhanced osteoclast activity mediated through receptor activator for nuclear factor κB ligand (RANKL).[15] This resorption increase can be due to local action of tumor in bone or to the production of bone-resorbing hormones and cytokines by tumor cells remote from bone. Normally, increased circulating calcium results in decreased parathyroid hormone (PTH) production. When PTH levels decrease, bone resorption and renal tubular reabsorption of calcium decline. Low PTH levels cause a decrease in vitamin D production; thus, gut absorption of calcium is lowered. Although PTH levels are suppressed in cancer patients with hypercalcemia, the destructive action of tumor deposits in bone or the action of tumor-produced hormones on bone maintains high calcium resorption rates. This is accomplished through osteoclast activation and proliferation from factors produced by the tumor, such as interleukin 1 (IL-1), tumor necrosis factor (TNF), prostaglandin E_2, granulocyte-macrophage colony-stimulating factor (GM-CSF), transforming growth factor-α, platelet-derived growth factor, and PTH-related peptides.[16-20] Malignancies that commonly cause hypercalcemia include multiple myeloma, breast carcinoma, epidermoid lung carcinoma, and renal cell carcinoma. Hypercalcemia in lymphoma and leukemia is probably not associated with PTH-related peptide, but rather with the overproduction of activated vitamin D.[20,21]

Cardiac complications and renal dysfunction are the most serious end-organ effects of hypercalcemia. Electrocardiogram (ECG) changes include prolongation of the PR and QRS intervals and shortening of the QT interval. Bradydysrhythmias and bundle branch blocks become more frequent with serum calcium levels greater than 16 mg/dL. These may progress to complete heart block and asystole. Renal dysfunction may also occur because increased serum calcium induces a diuretic effect, which can cause moderate to severe dehydration and prerenal azotemia. This process can result in acute tubular necrosis if untreated.

Management for any symptomatic hypercalcemic patient should begin with intravenous hydration, which may increase renal blood flow and enhance calciuresis.[22] Renal excretion of calcium can be enhanced with furosemide diuresis, although no randomized trials exist to support its use in hypercalcemia. These measures should be viewed as temporizing steps until definitive treatment has been implemented. The bisphosphonates zoledronic acid, pamidronate, alendronate, etidronate, and clodronate have been shown to be highly effective in the long-term treatment of hypercalcemia of malignancy. These agents work by binding to the hydroxyapatite in bone and preventing calcium resorption, although they may also have much more complicated effects on the cell cycle and bone turnover.[23,24] A commonly used bisphosphonate regimen is a single dose of pamidronate (60-90 mg intravenously over 2 to 4 hours) or zoledronic acid (4 mg intravenously over 15 minutes). Doses may be repeated in 3 to 4 days if the calcium does not decline. In addition, therapy directed at controlling the tumor should be implemented. RANKL inhibitors are now available for clinical use (denosumab) that inhibit osteoclast activity induced by malignancy and may be more potent in inhibiting bone resorption compared to bisphosphonates.[25,26] Gallium nitrate can be tried in patients with hypercalcemia unresponsive to bisphosphonates.[27] Calcitonin, glucocorticoids, or mithramycin can also be tried in patients unresponsive to first-line therapies, although these therapies are no longer commonly used owing to potential renal injury. Dialysis may be necessary if renal compromise is severe. Treatment recommendations are summarized in Table 80.1.

Table 80.1 Agents Used for the Management of Hypercalcemia

Drug	Dosage
Pamidronate	90 mg IV over 2 hours
Zoledronic acid	4 mg IV over 15 minutes
Gallium nitrate	200 mg/m^2 by continuous infusion for 5 days
Calcitonin	400 IU SQ every 8 hours
Mithramycin	25 μg/kg IV once or twice per week

IV, intravenously; SQ, subcutaneously.

ONCOGENIC OSTEOMALACIA

Oncogenic osteomalacia is a rare syndrome characterized by severe hypophosphatemia, high serum alkaline phosphatase, aminoaciduria, glycosuria, low levels of 1,25-dihydroxyvitamin D, and normal serum calcium. The syndrome is the result of humoral inhibition of activation of 25-hydroxyvitamin D. Patients present with bone pain and muscle weakness. Hemolysis from hypophosphatemia is a possible sequela of this syndrome. The tumors that give rise to oncogenic osteomalacia are usually vascular mesenchymal tumors, such as hemangiopericytoma. Treatment involves surgical removal of the tumor and phosphate supplementation.

SYNDROME OF INAPPROPRIATE SECRETION OF ANTIDIURETIC HORMONE

SIADH is associated with carcinoid tumors, myeloma, lymphoma, and carcinomas originating in the lung, prostate, esophagus, head and neck, adrenal gland, and pancreas. Cerebral metastasis from any tumor can also give rise to SIADH. Clinical findings are mainly neurologic, often do not correspond precisely to serum sodium levels, and range from mild confusion to coma and seizures. Because the clinical findings are secondary to water intoxication and hyponatremia, treatment involves water restriction (500 mL/day) and control of the primary tumor. More aggressive treatment should be started with 0.9% or 3% saline solution and furosemide diuresis for patients with neurologic deficits from hyponatremia. The rate of intravenous fluid supplementation should be adjusted based on the urinary excretion of sodium and potassium. Correction of severe hyponatremia (sodium less than 125 mEq/L) should take place over 7 to 10 days. Too rapid a correction can lead to serious neurologic sequelae such as central pontine myelinosis. Patients who fail to respond to water restriction can be treated with demeclocycline (600 to 1200 mg daily), which blocks the peripheral action of antidiuretic hormone (ADH). There is also a new class of selective vasopressin V_2-receptor antagonists that compete with native vasopressin, resulting in an increase of free water clearance. Tolvaptan (15-60 mg daily) can be used in patients who do not respond to demeclocycline.

ADRENAL FAILURE

Cancers of the lung, breast, kidney, stomach, and pancreas and melanoma are the tumors that metastasize most often to the adrenal glands. It is estimated that more than 90% of adrenal tissue must be destroyed before clinical manifestations of adrenal insufficiency appear. The clinical signs and symptoms of hypoadrenalism include weakness, gastrointestinal complaints, postural hypotension, dehydration, and electrolyte disturbances. The typical electrolyte profile is hyponatremia, hyperkalemia, and a mild anion gap acidosis.

Adrenal failure has also been observed in patients receiving ipilimumab, an antibody that blocks the effects of an inhibitory protein in T cells known as CTLA-4 (cytotoxic T lymphocyte antigen 4) and is used in the treatment of advanced melanoma.[4] Hypoadrenalism from ipilimumab is usually secondary to panhypopituitarism induced by T-cell–mediated hypophysitis.[28] These patients can present with headache and visual changes from pituitary swelling in addition to the clinical findings of hypoadrenalism as reviewed earlier. Evaluation of these patients should include a contrast-enhanced brain magnetic resonance imaging (MRI), and measurement of serum levels of cortisol, adrenocorticotropic hormone (ACTH), and thyroid-stimulating hormone (TSH).

The diagnosis of hypoadrenalism can be made with a cosyntropin stimulation test. Plasma cortisol levels are obtained before cosyntropin injection (0.25 mg intravenously) and 30 and 60 minutes after injection. A normal response is an increase in plasma cortisol of at least 7.0 mg/dL in 60 minutes. If the cortisol response to cosyntropin stimulation is suboptimal, physiologic doses of glucocorticoids should be administered twice a day (cortisone acetate, 25 mg every morning and 12.5 mg every evening). Mineralocorticoid supplementation is required in some patients (fludrocortisone, 0.05-0.1 mg daily). If the diagnosis of adrenal insufficiency is highly suspected, treatment should begin immediately after completion of the cosyntropin test. For patients in adrenal crisis with circulatory collapse, hydrocortisone should be given at stress doses (100 mg intravenously every 8 hours). This dose of hydrocortisone should also be adequate to supplement mineralocorticoid-deficient patients. Patients receiving glucocorticoids as part of their chemotherapy regimen (usually lymphoma or myeloma patients) or for treatment of brain tumors or metastases, may already have adrenal suppression and require stress-dose glucocorticoid replacement during episodes of neutropenic sepsis or elective surgery.

PHEOCHROMOCYTOMA

Pheochromocytoma is most commonly associated with the multiple endocrine neoplasia syndrome. The clinical features of this tumor are related to episodic catecholamine release and include hypertension, severe headache, cardiac dysrhythmias, pallor, perspiration, and rarely, hypotension. Patients can also present with a multisystem crisis characterized by encephalopathy, hyperpyrexia, and hemodynamic instability.[29] Diagnosis is made by measuring urinary catecholamine metabolites. An elevated vanillylmandelic acid is accurate approximately 90% of the time in making the diagnosis.[30] Patients with borderline catecholamine levels can often be diagnosed with the clonidine suppression test.[31] Localization of pheochromocytomas can be difficult because the tumors can arise anywhere between the base of the brain and the scrotum and can be multicentric. MRI and computed tomography (CT) are helpful in visualizing adrenal abnormalities. Nuclear medicine studies with *m*-[^{111}I]iodobenzylguanidine (MIBG) can be used if the CT scan is negative. MIBG scans are sensitive and specific for detecting ectopic adrenal medullary tissue.[32] Positron emission tomography (PET) imaging and diffusion-weighted MRI can detect sites of disease not apparent on CT or MIBG and can aid in surgical planning.[33-35] Surgical extirpation of the tumor is the only effective treatment. Preoperative control of catechol secretion is necessary and can be attained with long- or short-acting α-adrenergic blockade (phenoxybenzamine 10 mg orally two or three times daily or doxazosin 2-16 mg orally daily). A comparison of preoperative management strategies using long- versus short-acting α-antagonists showed no difference in long-term outcome after surgery, although the incidence of intraoperative hypertension was greater with short-acting medications like doxazosin, terazosin, and prazosin.[36] Tachycardia can be controlled with beta blockers, but these should be started only after phenoxybenzamine. Patients in hypertensive crisis can be managed with α-methyltyrosine or calcium channel blockers such as nifedipine or nicardipine.[37-39]

TUMOR-INDUCED HYPOGLYCEMIA

Functional endocrine tumors can give rise to a variety of clinical syndromes. Most of these problems can be managed outside the ICU; however, tumor-induced hypoglycemia can cause serious consequences including coma, seizures, and focal neurologic deficits. A number of different mechanisms can give rise to hypoglycemia. Autonomous insulin production is most commonly associated with islet cell tumors, whereas production of insulin-like growth factors (IGF-1 or IGF-2) is seen with non–islet cell tumors.[40] Slow-growing mesenchymal tumors such as leiomyosarcoma, mesothelioma, and fibrosarcoma are the most common non–islet cell tumors that cause hypoglycemia.

Treatment should be focused on control of the tumor. Insulinomas are often benign and can be cured by surgical removal. For unresectable malignancies, hypoglycemic episodes can often be reduced with supportive measures such as dietary modification with frequent meals. Insulinomas may respond to diazoxide, an inhibitor of insulin secretion. Glucagon infusions may be beneficial in some patients.[41]

CHEMOTHERAPY-INDUCED METABOLIC DISTURBANCES

A number of chemotherapy drugs can cause potentially severe electrolyte disturbances. Cyclophosphamide is associated with hyponatremia from SIADH. Vinca alkaloids such as vinorelbine and vinblastine also cause SIADH. Cisplatin and carboplatin can cause renal tubular defects resulting in hypokalemia and hypomagnesemia, which can be severe enough to require intravenous replacement. Mithramycin lowers serum calcium by a mechanism that is thought to involve inhibition of the effect of PTH on osteoclasts. Although mithramycin can be used for the treatment of hypercalcemia, it can also cause hypocalcemia in patients with normal serum calcium. Cetuximab, a humanized murine antibody directed against the epidermal growth factor receptor (EGFR) and used to treat colon carcinoma and head and neck cancer is associated with severe and symptomatic hypomagnesemia from inappropriate urinary excretion.[42] Cetuximab may interact with EGFR in the loop of Henle blocking resorption of magnesium and causing secondary hypokalemia and hypocalcemia. Abiraterone, a CYP17 inhibitor of androgen biosynthesis used in men with advanced prostate cancer, also increases adrenal mineralocorticoid synthesis resulting in clinically significant hypokalemia and decreases glucocorticoid synthesis necessitating concurrent administration of prednisone. Everolimus, an oral inhibitor of the mammalian target of rapamycin (mTOR), used in the management of advanced renal cancer and neuroendocrine tumors, can induce severe hyperglycemia requiring insulin.[43,44] The mechanism through which mTOR inhibitors cause hyperglycemia is not fully understood but may involve decreased insulin secretion, direct toxicity to pancreatic β-cells, or impaired suppression of hepatic glucose production.[45]

CARDIAC COMPLICATIONS IN CANCER PATIENTS

Cardiac dysfunction in cancer patients can be secondary to direct mechanical effects of the tumor on the heart, pericardium, or great vessels. Certain chemotherapy drugs, immunotherapy agents, and radiation can also cause treatment-related cardiac problems. Clinical entities that require emergent and chronic management are discussed.

SUPERIOR VENA CAVA SYNDROME

Obstruction of blood flow through the superior vena cava (SVC) can be caused by fibrosis, thrombosis, external compression, or invasion of the vessel by tumor. SVC syndrome can also be caused by thrombus secondary to a central venous access device, which is now a common fixture of oncologic care. Malignancies that involve the mediastinum, such as lung carcinoma and lymphoma, are the most common causes of this syndrome. Facial and upper extremity edema, facial plethora, headache, and tachypnea are the most common clinical presentations. Collateral venous channels may be found on the chest or abdomen. Death from SVC syndrome is rare, but life-threatening respiratory compromise and elevated intracranial pressure can occur. Therapy for SVC syndrome depends on the underlying malignancy; thus, a biopsy is mandatory for optimal management of these patients. If lymphoma or small cell lung carcinoma is the cause of SVC syndrome, initiation of the appropriate chemotherapy regimen can rapidly shrink the mediastinal mass and is the treatment of choice. For tumors not responsive to chemotherapy, radiation therapy given with high initial fractions (3 to 4 Gy/day) can provide symptomatic relief in more than 80% of patients.[46] Thrombolysis has only been studied in catheter-associated SVC syndrome and is effective in this setting.[47] Endovascular stents can restore patency of the SVC in approximately 50% of patients and can result in significant palliation.[48] Improvement is often evident within 72 hours and the patency of occluded endovascular stents can sometimes be restored with angioplasty.

CARDIAC TAMPONADE

Although primary or metastatic tumors of the heart can decrease cardiac output by impairing ventricular outflow, the most frequent causes of cardiac tamponade in cancer patients are metastatic tumors of the breast and lung, and melanoma, lymphomas, and leukemias. Tamponade may occur through either encasement of the heart by tumor or production of a malignant pericardial effusion. The clinical manifestations of tamponade include decreased exercise tolerance, shortness of breath, and cough. Voltage may be decreased on ECG with a pulsus alternans pattern present. Muffled heart tones, a pericardial rub, or an increased paradoxical pulse (i.e., decrease in systolic blood pressure on inspiration exceeds 10 mm Hg) may be present on physical examination. Echocardiography is extremely useful in confirming the diagnosis of tamponade if it is suspected on physical examination. Diastolic collapse of the right atrium or right ventricle on echocardiogram is an indicator of hemodynamic compromise.[49,50] Swan-Ganz catheterization may be helpful to confirm the presence of significant tamponade.

Pericardiocentesis for relief of tamponade is indicated emergently when echocardiographic or clinical evidence of hemodynamic compromise is present. Intravenous infusions of normal saline at high flow rates (100 to 500 mL/hour) may be required to support the patient until a drainage procedure is performed. Although rapid reversal of cardiac filling problems can be accomplished by this procedure, a long-term solution is required. Creation of a pericardial window can prevent the reaccumulation of fluid in more than 90% of patients.[51] Sclerosing agents such as tetracycline and bleomycin have also been used to prevent reaccumulation of pericardial fluid.[52] Sclerosants may be instilled into the pericardial space after adequate drainage has been accomplished and appear to have a success rate comparable to pericardial window procedures. Some centers also perform pericardial windows using video-assisted thoracoscopy, but there have been no prospective randomized studies showing superior clinical outcomes for subxiphoid versus video-assisted thoracoscopy approaches.[53]

TREATMENT-INDUCED CARDIAC DYSFUNCTION

A number of chemotherapy medicines have cardiac toxicities that can be life threatening. Cumulative doses of doxorubicin greater than 450 mg/m^2 are associated with an increased risk for congestive heart failure (CHF). Heart damage from this drug is thought to be from an iron-dependent generation of free radicals, which secondarily cause oxidative damage to lipid membranes and intracellular organelles.[52] This toxicity can present acutely or months after drug administration. It is more prevalent in older patients and those with a history of coronary artery disease, hypertension, tobacco abuse, or chest radiation therapy. Initial management with diuretics, digoxin, and angiotensin blockers is usually of benefit, but heart failure can be progressive. Liposomal encapsulation of doxorubicin or the use of dexrazoxane to prevent oxygen-derived free radical formation, may diminish the cardiac toxicities of this agent.[54-56] Other anthracyclines, such as mitoxantrone and epirubicin, may have a lower incidence of CHF. Furthermore, weekly low-dose boluses or continuous-infusion methods of doxorubicin administration appear to reduce the incidence of clinically significant heart damage. Although anthracycline-induced cardiac damage has generally been considered irreversible, some studies suggest that some improvement in cardiac function may occur with aggressive medical management.[57] Paclitaxel, which is commonly used in ovarian, breast, and lung carcinomas, is associated with bradydysrhythmias.[57,58] Ventricular tachycardia, myocardial infarction, and cardiac ischemia have also been reported. Cyclophosphamide, which is commonly used in breast cancer, lymphoma, and stem cell transplant conditioning regimens, is associated with sporadic instances of CHF, which may be severe and occurs within a few days of cyclophosphamide administration, especially at high doses. Hemorrhagic myocarditis with myonecrosis was seen on autopsy specimens from these patients. These events appear unrelated to cumulative dose or method of administration. CHF from ifosfamide has also been reported.[59] CHF is usually seen approximately 2 weeks after high doses of the drug and appears more frequently in patients with concurrent renal insufficiency. Medical management successfully reverses the heart failure in most patients. CHF is also associated with trastuzumab, an anti-HER2 (human epidermal growth factor receptor 2) antibody used commonly in the management of certain forms of breast carcinoma. The incidence of CHF after trastuzumab in a large randomized trial was between 3% and 4%, and was more common in patients with antecedent cardiac disease, older patients, and those having diminished ejection fraction (EF) after anthracycline-containing chemotherapy.[60] Most patients with trastuzumab-induced cardiac dysfunction have improved symptoms with appropriate medical management for CHF and discontinuation of trastuzumab.

Serial echocardiography studies have been used to assess cardiac toxicities in patients receiving chemotherapy for many years, but subtle alterations in myocardial function can be missed with standard assessment of EF. A decrease in longitudinal strain assessed by Doppler measurements of tissue velocity at baseline and repeated at 3 months after starting anthracyclines or trastuzumab is a more sensitive predictor of cardiac dysfunction than EF[61,62] and may be useful in identifying patients in need of medical management before significant symptoms occur.

Radiation therapy delivered to the chest for the treatment of Hodgkin's disease, lung malignancies, breast cancer, or other neoplasms can result in a number of cardiac toxicities, including radiation pericarditis with tamponade, myocardial fibrosis, and premature coronary artery disease. The toxic effects of radiation therapy are secondary to microvessel fibrosis and may take up to 20 years to appear.[63] After mantle-field radiation therapy, the risk of fatal myocardial infarction is more than three times greater than in age-matched control subjects, although mantle-fields are rarely used currently to treat patients with lymphoma. Nervertheless, it is difficult to treat the mediastinum without also treating the heart.

PULMONARY COMPLICATIONS IN CANCER PATIENTS

Many of the same mechanical issues that influence cardiac dysfunction are also pertinent to pulmonary problems with an underlying neoplasm. Chemotherapy and radiation therapy can also cause lasting and sometimes fatal pulmonary complications. Many of these conditions are difficult to diagnose and can be confused with other clinical entities, such as opportunistic infections. Indeed, pneumonias are the most common pulmonary disorder requiring intensive care. A number of acute and chronic pulmonary presentations are discussed.

LYMPHANGITIC TUMOR INVOLVEMENT

Interstitial lung processes in cancer patients may be due to a variety of infectious insults but can also be caused by direct lymphangitic spread of the tumor. The symptoms of lymphangitic involvement are nonspecific and include dyspnea, nonproductive cough, and hypoxemia. Pulmonary hypertension and cor pulmonale can also be present. The diagnosis can be established by video-assisted thoracoscopic biopsy or transbronchial biopsy. Pulmonary microvascular cytologic specimens obtained with a wedged pulmonary artery catheter may be a less invasive way to make the diagnosis of lymphangitic carcinomatosis.[64] The prognosis of this condition is generally poor, with a life expectancy of 1 to 6 months. Appropriate systemic treatment should be implemented when the site of the primary malignancy is diagnosed.

TREATMENT-INDUCED PULMONARY DYSFUNCTION

A number of chemotherapy agents and radiation therapy can cause pneumonitis leading to chronic pulmonary fibrosis. The chemotherapeutic agents most likely to cause this problem are bleomycin and mitomycin, but other alkylators, nitrosoureas, antimetabolites, gemcitabine, taxanes, and vinca alkaloids can cause pulmonary dysfunction. Inhibitors of the mTOR pathway such as everolimus and temsirolimus used in the treatment of advanced renal cancer can also induce severe pneumonitis.[44,65] Erlotinib, an inhibitor of the phosphorylation of EGFR used in the treatment of advanced lung cancer, can also induce severe and irreversible pneumonitis.[66] The underlying mechanisms for lung injury induced by these agents are not fully understood, but likely involves oxygen-derived free radical toxicity[67] and dysregulation of leukocyte apoptosis regulated by TNF-receptor family members. TRAIL (TNF-related apoptosis-inducing ligand) has shown promise in preclinical models of bleomycin lung injury and may also have antitumor properties.[68] We advocate that cancer patients in need of supplemental oxygen should receive the lowest possible fractional concentration of oxygen that produces a hemoglobin oxygen saturation of greater than 90%. Irreversible lung damage can occur if excessive oxygen is administered to patients receiving bleomycin or radiation therapy. Clinical assessment is crucial to patient management because there are no sensitive or accurate tests to predict the onset or course of bleomycin-induced pulmonary toxicity. The resting diffusion capacity has been used, but is suboptimal to follow patients.[69] Treatment recommendations are based on the recognition of three distinct clinical entities:

1. Patients who have radiographic changes but no symptoms do not require treatment.
2. Glucocorticoids are used for managing pneumonitis induced by chemotherapy, mTOR and EGFR inhibitors, and radiation when fever, cough, shortness of breath, and pulmonary infiltrates are present. The mechanism of glucocorticoid action may involve reducing inflammation and microvessel damage through inhibition of leukotriene synthesis, inducing granulocyte demargination from endothelial cells, and direct toxicity to lymphocytes.
3. There is no effective treatment for patients with chronic pulmonary fibrosis, cor pulmonale, or pulmonary hypertension from chemotherapy or radiation therapy.

DIFFUSE INTERSTITIAL PNEUMONITIS

The differential diagnosis of diffuse pulmonary infiltrates in cancer patients is large. Infectious causes include bacterial, viral, fungal, and protozoal pathogens. Noninfectious causes for diffuse pulmonary infiltrates are neoplasm, autoimmune disease, cardiac failure, leukostasis, pulmonary hemorrhage, and radiation- or chemotherapy-induced pneumonitis. Making a diagnosis on clinical grounds is difficult because the radiographic and physical examination findings are virtually indistinguishable among these diverse causative entities. Performing an open-lung biopsy is often the only way to confirm a diagnosis; however, empiric treatment may result in equally good patient outcomes. A randomized study compared immediate open-lung biopsy followed by therapy directed at the diagnosis versus empiric antibiotics alone without biopsy to treat diffuse pulmonary infiltrates in cancer patients.[70] The antibiotic regimen included trimethoprim-sulfamethoxazole (20 mg/kg/day intravenously) and erythromycin (30 mg/kg/day intravenously, divided into four daily doses). A broad-spectrum antibiotic was added if the patient was neutropenic at the time of diagnosis. There was no significant difference in the outcome for these patients; however, those who received an open lung biopsy had a greater complication rate. Empiric antibiotics are appropriate initial management for diffuse interstitial infiltrates, but patients who do not improve after 4 days of empiric therapy should receive open-lung biopsy.

The decision to place a patient with a cancer diagnosis on ventilator support is often controversial for medical staff and families. It is generally recognized that such patients have a poor prognosis, with a mortality rate approaching 80%. A large multicenter trial prospectively examined prognostic variables for cancer patients requiring ventilatory support.[71] Factors having a statistically significant negative influence on survival were a diagnosis of leukemia, allogeneic stem cell transplantation, progressive cancer, cardiac dysrhythmia, presence of disseminated intravascular coagulation (DIC), and need for vasopressor support. Prior surgery with curative intent was protective and probably relates to a selection bias for patients with physiologic reserve sufficient to tolerate surgery. Although this model is similar to other prognostic models used in the ICU setting, it differs in its emphasis on cancer-specific factors. There also appears to be a positive association between recovery from neutropenia, pneumonia, and acute respiratory distress syndrome (ARDS) requiring mechanical ventilation and an inverse relation to survival in patients with hematologic malignancy.[72] The mortality rate of patients with ARDS during neutropenic recovery was 86.8% versus 51.5% in patients without ARDS in this single institution study. In general, the assessment of the potential reversibility of the organ dysfunction is the critical variable. Most iatrogenic toxicities are reversible, and patients having toxicity from treatment can generally be supported to recovery. Similarly, organ dysfunction from treatable malignancies should be assumed to be reversible. However, when more than three organ systems are failing, the chances of recovery are very small. The decision to place a cancer patient on ventilator support is highly individualized, but such models can assist in counseling families about level-of-care issues.

HEMOPTYSIS

Hemoptysis can be a presenting sign of cancer, especially endobronchial lesions of non–small cell lung cancer. Patients presenting with significant hemoptysis and airway compromise can be palliated with a variety of bronchoscopic techniques including argon or neodymium:yttrium-aluminum-garnet (Nd:YAG) laser, photodynamic therapy, stent placement, endoluminal brachytherapy, or combinations of these techniques.[73] External beam radiation, pulmonary artery embolization, and blood pressure control can also be effective in controlling hemoptysis.

Bevacizumab, a monoclonal antibody against vascular endothelial growth factor, has been used with chemotherapy agents to increase overall response and time-to-progression in lung cancer. Bevacizumab can also cause significant and life-threatening hemoptysis; especially in patients with squamous cell histologic lung cancer.[74] The mechanism of hemoptysis after bevacizumab is collapse of the tumor vasculature resulting in tumor cavitation in proximity to major blood vessels. Because cancer outcomes can be improved with bevacizumab, we endorse an aggressive approach in supporting patients who experience hemoptysis as a result of this or other vascular-targeting agents.

INFECTIOUS COMPLICATIONS IN CANCER PATIENTS

Pancytopenia is perhaps the most common sequela of dose-intense chemotherapy regimens. Fever in the setting of neutropenia in conjunction with bacteremia is a life-threatening complication of many chemotherapy regimens, whether given with adjuvant, palliative, or curative intent. The microbial pathogens that infect neutropenic patients have changed over time. Previously, *Pseudomonas aeruginosa* was one of the most common organisms in this setting, but staphylococci, streptococci, and vancomycin-resistant organisms have become increasingly prevalent.[75] Improved broad-spectrum antibiotics and hematopoietic growth factors have greatly improved the outcome for febrile neutropenic patients,[76,77] many of whom can be managed easily without intensive care interventions. This section focuses on septic shock and the infections that commonly occur as complications of cancer treatment. The infections that arise as a consequence of the severe immune compromise after bone marrow transplant are covered separately.

FEBRILE NEUTROPENIA AND SEPTIC SHOCK

Despite appropriate broad-spectrum antibiotics, approximately 10% of febrile neutropenic patients progress to septic shock. Fluid resuscitation and pressor agents such as phenylephrine, dopamine, dobutamine, and norepinephrine remain standard treatment for the hemodynamic consequences of shock despite advances in understanding the physiology and immunologic sequelae of shock and a growing number of drugs that may influence the pathophysiology of this clinical entity. Treatments aimed at modifying the host reaction to sepsis other than hemodynamic support have not been shown to improve outcomes.

NEUROLOGIC COMPLICATIONS IN CANCER PATIENTS

Brain or spinal cord metastases can often be managed outside the ICU but may require acute intervention if there is evidence of increased intracranial pressure or spinal cord compression. Seizure management in the cancer patient also is discussed.

SPINAL CORD COMPRESSION

The tumors that most often cause spinal cord compression from epidural metastases or bony destruction are carcinomas of the lung, breast, and prostate and multiple myeloma. The level of the spinal cord involvement determines the clinical neurologic deficit. Cervical cord compression can cause quadriplegia or respiratory arrest; thoracic, paraplegia, and lumbar involvement can give rise to loss of bladder and bowel function. If the problem is detected when local or radicular pain is the only symptom, treatment with glucocorticoids, radiation therapy using conventional or conformal techniques, or laminectomy can be highly effective. If the patient presents with a neurologic deficit, such as the inability to walk, the chance of significant improvement is less than 10%.[78] MRI is the diagnostic test of choice for diagnosing epidural metastases. Glucocorticoids should be started emergently for patients who present with myelopathy (dexamethasone 10 mg followed by 4 mg every 6 hours) and imaging obtained as soon as possible. The maximal effect of dexamethasone on alleviating symptoms may not be achieved at total doses of 24 mg/day. If clinical improvement from glucocorticoids is suboptimal, doubling the dose each day up to a maximum of 200 mg/day total dose may improve symptom control until definitive therapy is implemented.[79] The standard of care for cord compression had been glucocorticoids and radiation; however, a randomized trial has shown benefit for decompressive surgery followed by radiation.[80] Eighty-four percent of patients randomized to receive surgery and radiation maintained the ability to walk compared to 57% in the radiation alone group. Better palliation of pain and the duration of ambulation were maintained better in the surgery group. A meta-analysis of 1595 articles describing 2495 patients supports better functional improvement and pain control using surgery with or without postsurgical radiation in the management of malignant spinal cord compression.[81]

BRAIN METASTASES AND HEMORRHAGE

Tumor metastatic to the brain may be a localized problem, amenable to surgical resection with good results.[82] Patients who present with significant peritumoral edema and increased intracranial pressure may suffer brain herniation if acute measures are not taken. Therapy includes high-dose glucocorticoids (dexamethasone 10 mg, followed by 4 mg intravenously every 6 hours), intubation and mechanical hyperventilation to maintain partial pressure of carbon dioxide in arterial blood ($Paco_2$) between 25 and 30 mm Hg, and mannitol diuresis (1.0 to 1.5 g/kg intravenously as a 20% solution). Patients who do not respond may benefit from higher glucocorticoid doses (dexamethasone 25 to 50 mg every 6 hours). After stabilizing the patient with these acute interventions, definitive radiation therapy or surgery can be started. Prophylactic anticonvulsants are often administered; however, this intervention has scant supportive data and should be held in most patients until a seizure has occurred.[83,84] Frontal lobe tumor deposits and brain metastases from melanoma are two situations in which prophylactic antiseizure medication should be considered. Newer radiation techniques such as stereotactic or gamma knife radiosurgery can also be effective in controlling or eradicating brain metastatic disease, although this modality is more appropriate for patients with good functional status and a total volume of metastatic disease less than 12 cm^3.[85]

Dose-intensive therapy for acute leukemia is associated with prolonged thrombocytopenia and the possibility of intracranial hemorrhage. It was previously thought that such events were highly associated with platelet counts less than 20,000 cells/μL[86]; however, the threshold for platelet transfusion used in most medical centers is now 10,000/μL, based on a randomized trial that showed no difference in patient outcome with the more stringent threshold.[87] Other events, such as sepsis and fever, contribute to the likelihood of bleeding with thrombocytopenia. Patients with solid tumors are also less likely than those with leukemia to bleed as a consequence of thrombocytopenia. In cancer patients with suspected intracranial bleeding and thrombocytopenia, the platelet count should be maintained above 50,000 cells/μL. The best strategy to maintain adequate hemostatic function with platelet transfusion support is controversial because platelet kinetics are complex.[88,89] We advocate frequent dosing or continuous infusion of platelets in actively bleeding thrombocytopenic patients who have poor increments in platelet count after transfusion resulting from platelet sensitization. The blood bank should identify human leukocyte antigen (HLA)-matched platelet donors for such patients and maintain an adequate supply of the HLA-matched platelets. Single-donor platelets are often more effective than pooled platelets in this setting.

UNCONTROLLED SEIZURES

In 15% to 30% of patients who develop brain metastases, the initial sign is a generalized seizure.[90] Metabolic disturbances, such as hyponatremia from SIADH, may also cause seizures in cancer patients. Acute control can be obtained with intravenous diazepam (5 mg intravenously every 5 to 10 minutes up to 30 mg). Standard measures to protect the airway, prevent aspiration, and avoid limb injury should also be implemented. After acute control has been attained, phenytoin should be started (15 mg/kg intravenously at a maximum rate of 50 mg/minute, then maintenance doses of 300 mg/day). Phenytoin up-regulates the P-450 system in the liver, which may accelerate the metabolism of certain chemotherapy agents, such as paclitaxel and docetaxel.[91,92] Levetiracetam (1000 mg daily) is also highly effective in the acute and chronic management of seizures induced by brain malignancy.[93] Antiseizure agents that do not influence P-450 cytochromes, like gabapentin, should be used in patients requiring taxane-based chemotherapy. Serum levels of phenytoin and levetiracetam should be monitored.

Seizures, coma, and other neurologic complications can occur with a variety of chemotherapeutic and biologic agents. Most of these toxicities improve with cessation of the causative agent and supportive care. Ifosfamide-induced neurotoxicity has a unique mechanism related to changes in mitochondrial fatty acid oxidation and the accumulation of glutaric acid metabolites.[94] Treatment with methylene blue (200-300 mg orally or intravenously daily), an electron-accepting drug, can reverse and prevent neurologic toxicity during ifosfamide infusion.[95]

GASTROINTESTINAL COMPLICATIONS IN CANCER PATIENTS

Bowel injury is a common cause of morbidity and death in cancer patients. Lymphomatous bowel involvement is relatively common in acquired immunodeficiency syndrome (AIDS)–lymphoma patients[96] and can be a site of metastatic disease in a variety of solid tumors including ovarian cancer, melanoma, and renal cancer. Management of these problems can often be accomplished with meticulous standard care; however, intensive support may be needed for emergent surgical or medical conditions arising from gastrointestinal complications.

TUMOR-INDUCED EMERGENCIES

For most tumor types, obstruction may be related to a localized lesion that is readily amenable to surgical correction. In women with ovarian cancer, the obstruction is often related to loss of peristalsis in long segments of bowel because of diffuse wall invasion by malignancy. Little can be done with surgical intervention in such circumstances. Improvement hinges on the availability of effective chemotherapy. Bowel obstruction or perforation can occur from primary or metastatic tumors. If the patient presents with peritoneal signs of an acute abdomen, then emergent exploratory surgery is indicated.[97] For less clear-cut presentations, abdominal radiographs, CT scans, and endoscopy may be helpful. These patients can be managed initially with bowel rest, nasogastric suction, and anaerobic antibiotic coverage until a diagnosis is made. Somatostatin can provide palliation in some patients, probably by increasing intestinal water resorption.[98]

Biliary obstruction can occur from primary tumors of the pancreas, bile ducts, or gallbladder but more commonly is from tumors metastatic to the porta hepatis, such as breast carcinoma, melanoma, or lymphoma. Ascending cholangitis and sepsis are possible sequelae if bile drainage is not accomplished. A percutaneous or endoscopic approach can be used to decompress the bile ducts emergently. Effective treatment of the primary tumor should be implemented when possible. If the tumor is unlikely to respond to chemotherapy or radiation therapy, palliation with an internal stent or an operative biliary diversion procedure is indicated.

Hemorrhage of an abdominal viscus can occur from chemotherapy or progressing tumor. Identifying the source of the bleeding can be accomplished with endoscopy, CT scan, angiography, or labeled red blood cell studies. Bleeding from ulcers or mucosal irritation from chemotherapy can usually be managed medically or with endoscopic control via heater probe or Nd:YAG laser. If a tumor deposit is the cause, surgical control of the site should be considered. If the patient is not a surgical candidate, an angiographic embolization procedure may provide effective palliation.

CHEMOTHERAPY-INDUCED GASTROINTESTINAL DYSFUNCTION

Typhlitis (ileocecal syndrome) is seen most often in patients with leukemia receiving induction chemotherapy. It presents usually after more than 7 days of neutropenia with watery diarrhea, abdominal distention, and right-sided abdominal tenderness. Bowel rest and antibiotics may be successful in treating this condition, but surgery is required for repeated sepsis, bowel necrosis, or perforation. This syndrome can occur on subsequent cycles of chemotherapy; thus, a colonic diversion procedure may be needed in order to complete chemotherapy.

Colitis can occur in up to 40% of patients who have received ipilimumab of whom 5% experience severe symptoms including high-output diarrhea and intestinal perforation.[4,99] Neutrophilic and lymphocytic infiltrates are evident on biopsy consistent with the idea that ipilimumab elicits autoimmune tissue damage by breaking self-tolerance. Intervention early when symptoms are mild or moderate (e.g., 4-6 stools per day over baseline) is key to avoiding severe or life-threatening colitis. Initial management is to withhold ipilimumab and administer loperamide. If symptoms persist, then a course of glucocorticoids should be started (e.g., prednisone 0.5 mg/kg/day). For patients who have seven or more stools per day, abdominal pain, melena, or hematochezia, then glucocorticoids (e.g., prednisone 1-2 mg/kg/day) should begin promptly with a slow taper when symptoms resolve. Endoscopic evaluation may be helpful. Emergent surgery for perforation is appropriate. TNF inhibitors (e.g., infliximab) can be effective in managing diarrhea from ipilimumab unresponsive to glucocorticoids.[99] Figure 80.1A and B depicts the biopsy findings in ipilimumab colitis and an associated tumor response.

A number of chemotherapy agents can decrease bowel motility resulting in ileus. Examples of such medications are paclitaxel, vincristine, and cytosine arabinoside. Supportive care of the ileus is usually successful, but toxic megacolon can occur and is an indication for surgical management.

A particularly difficult management problem is the severe constipation that can accompany the use of opioid analgesics in patients with advanced cancer. Prophylactic measures are very important, including the use of stool softeners and osmotic laxatives and maintaining patient activity as much as possible. Even with optimal prophylaxis, results are often unsatisfactory. Methylnaltrexone, a μ-opioid receptor antagonist that does not cross the blood-brain barrier, can significantly improve constipation, usually within 4 hours of dosing, without reducing the analgesic effect of narcotics.[100]

A

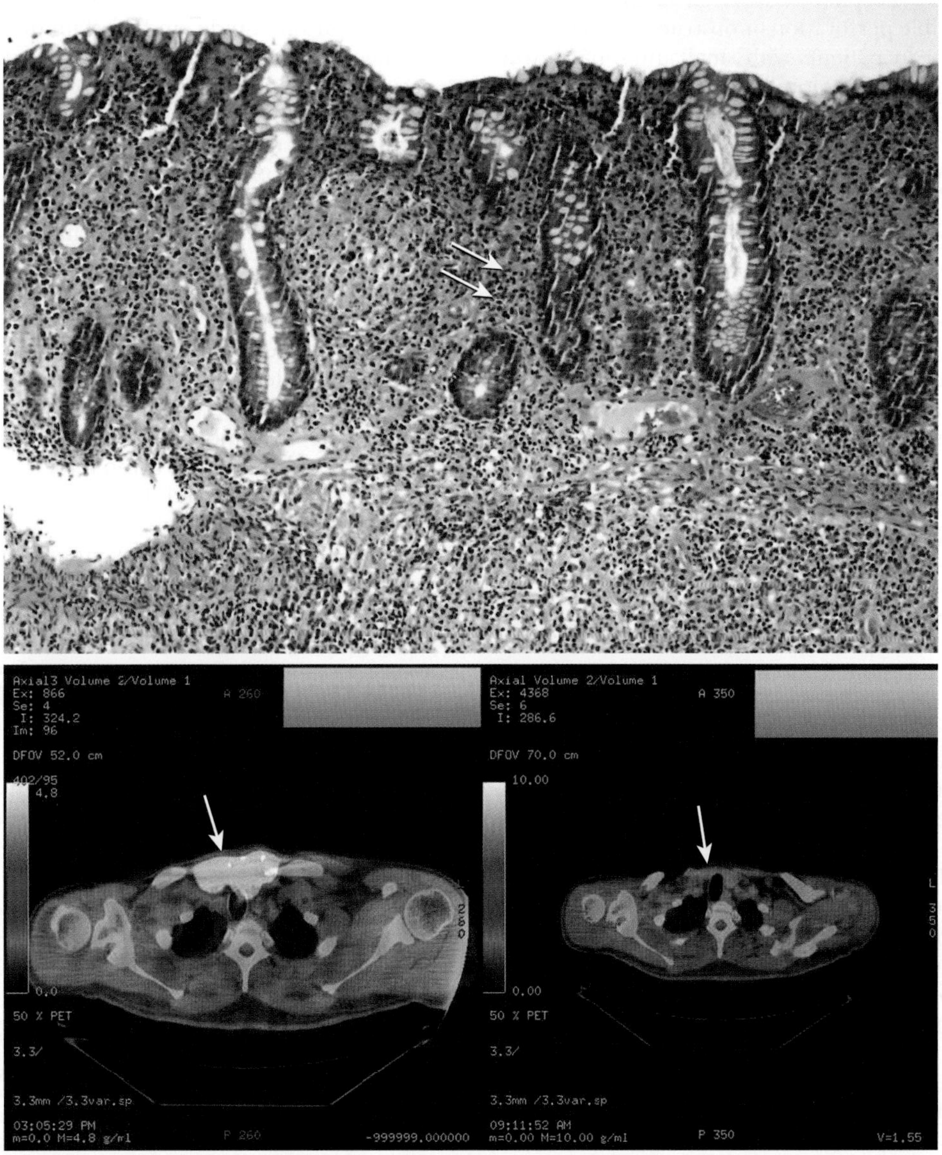

B

Figure 80.1 Ipilimumab enterocolitis and treatment response. **A,** Photomicrograph of a biopsy (hematoxylin and eosin stain, ×100) from the descending colon of a patient with severe diarrhea after ipilimumab immunotherapy. Extensive neutrophilic infiltration of colonic crypts is present *(arrows),* which is a hallmark of ipilimumab enterocolitis. **B,** Before *(left)* and after *(right)* positron emission tomography computed tomography images on the same patient. The large fluorodeoxyglucose (FDG)-avid chest wall melanoma mass *(arrows)* has a standard uptake value (SUV) of 46 that has regressed significantly in size and shows normal FDG uptake (SUV <2) after ipilimumab.

GASTROINTESTINAL LYMPHOMAS

Lymphoma presenting as a gastric or intestinal mass is common in AIDS patients and in patients with B-cell lymphomas arising in mucosal-associated lymphatic tissue (MALT) secondary to *Helicobacter pylori* infection. This situation warrants extreme caution because perforation of an abdominal viscus is a potentially life-threatening complication of potentially curative chemotherapy. Because perforation is a major concern in these patients, initial surgical resection is advocated by some authors.[101,102] Others have noted low rates of abdominal catastrophe in patients treated with chemotherapy and radiation therapy alone.[103] Data from patients with gastric MALT lymphoma treated with antibiotics or radiation therapy suggest that perforation is rare in patients achieving a tumor response.[104] Patients with extensive gastric involvement by lymphoma should start chemotherapy in the hospital with surgical consultation to monitor for possible perforation or obstruction. Perforation is more common in patients with small intestinal involvement with aggressive histologic lymphomas compared to gastric or colon involvement by lymphoma.

GENITOURINARY COMPLICATIONS IN CANCER PATIENTS

Intensive care interventions for genitourinary tract problems may be required for the sequelae of obstruction or primary renal dysfunction. Tumors arising locally, metastatic tumors, and certain chemotherapy drugs can give rise to genitourinary problems. Both tumor-induced and chemotherapy toxicities are discussed.

TUMOR-INDUCED GENITOURINARY DYSFUNCTION

Obstructive uropathy resulting in hydronephrosis can occur at the bladder outlet or anywhere along the path of the ureter. Bladder outlet problems are most commonly caused by local tumor invasion from prostate, bladder, rectosigmoid, cervical, or ovarian neoplasms. Metastatic deposits from gastric, breast, or pancreatic malignancies can also obstruct the bladder outlet. Tumors that arise from retroperitoneal structures or metastasize to the retroperitoneum can cause ureteral obstruction. Examples of tumors that commonly have a retroperitoneal presentation are Hodgkin's and non-Hodgkin's lymphoma, germ cell tumors that metastasize to retroperitoneal lymph nodes, and axial sarcomas. Primary tumors of the ureter can also cause obstruction. If the obstruction and the resulting hydronephrosis are of short duration, percutaneous drainage and decompression are recommended. If there is a concurrent infection, decompression is mandatory and constitutes an oncologic emergency. After a period of 48 to 72 hours, a ureteral stent can be placed using the anterograde or retrograde approach. Furosemide-renal scanning can be used to confirm the presence of kidney function if there is a question about the reversibility of the functional impairment of the obstructed kidney.[105] After stenting, appropriate radiation therapy, chemotherapy, or hormonal treatment should be implemented for control of the malignancy.

Renal function can also be compromised indirectly by malignancies. The nephrotic syndrome is seen in association with several solid tumors, such as colon, gastric, ovarian, and breast carcinomas. Lymphomas, especially those of T-cell origin, and chronic lymphocytic leukemia can also cause nephrotic syndrome and other glomerulopathies. Multiple myeloma and Waldenström's macroglobulinemia can produce amyloid and cryoglobulin deposits in the kidneys, resulting in acute tubular necrosis or interstitial nephritis. Recurrent and chronic pyelonephritis is common in patients with myeloma. Dialysis may be necessary to support the patient until effective antitumor therapy is given.

CHEMOTHERAPY-INDUCED GENITOURINARY COMPLICATIONS

Hemorrhagic cystitis can be caused by acrolein, a metabolite of cyclophosphamide and ifosfamide. This problem can usually be prevented with adequate hydration, bladder irrigation, or the use of thiol-based chemoprotectants, such as mesna. Mesna administration is mandatory for ifosfamide treatment. If the hemorrhagic cystitis is severe and unresponsive to supportive measures and saline bladder irrigation, formalin bladder instillation can be performed under general anesthesia.[106] A 1% formalin solution should be used, but bladder fibrosis and strictures may occur despite this low concentration. Care must be taken to avoid reflux of the formalin up the ureters. Urinary diversion and cystectomy may be required for uncontrolled bleeding.

Methotrexate, an antifolate chemotherapy agent, can precipitate in renal tubules and cause acute tubular necrosis if adequate hydration and urinary alkalinization are not achieved before therapy. If renal toxicity occurs, leucovorin rescue should be started, based on serum levels of methotrexate (Table 80.2 provides details of methotrexate toxicity prevention or reversal). Intravenous fluids containing bicarbonate, furosemide, and mannitol may be helpful in preventing oliguric renal failure.

HEMATOLOGIC COMPLICATIONS IN CANCER PATIENTS

Although clinical prodromes for leukemias may evolve over weeks or months, treatment for these disorders, once

Table 80.2 Leucovorin Rescue for Methotrexate Toxicity

Methotrexate drug levels above 5×10^{-7} at 48 hours after infusion require additional leucovorin rescue as follows:

Drug Level	Leucovorin Dosage
5×10^{-7}	15 mg/m^2 q6h × 8 doses
1×10^{-6}	100 mg/m^2 q6h × 8 doses
2×10^{-6}	200 mg/m^2 q6h × 8 doses

Drug levels should be measured every 24 hours and leucovorin dose adjusted until drug concentration is less than 5×10^{-8}.

diagnosed, is often urgent and requires intensive care support. This support is needed not only to treat a number of well-known disease-related complications, but also to manage chemotherapy toxicities because some of the most dose-intense drug regimens are used against these malignancies.

HYPERLEUKOCYTOSIS

Large numbers of leukemic blasts may be present in acute leukemias or in the late stages of chronic leukemias. When the number of circulating myeloblasts is greater than 100,000 cells/μL, the viscosity of the blood increases because white blood cells are much less deformable than red blood cells. Patients with chronic lymphocytic leukemia can tolerate higher circulating numbers of malignant cells (e.g., 100,000-300,000 cells/μL) without consequence. In acute leukemia, the blasts may invade and weaken the vessel wall, leading to hemorrhage. Hyperleukocytosis chiefly affects the microvasculature in the lungs and the central nervous system. Symptoms can range from mild shortness of breath and blurred vision to pulmonary congestion, hypoxia, intracranial hemorrhage, and TLS (tumor lysis syndrome). Rapid institution of leukapheresis can often decrease leukocyte counts by 20% to 50%.[107] Although the improvement may be transient, chemotherapy treatments for the underlying leukemia can be accomplished with greater safety, and perhaps a lesser degree of TLS.

All-*trans*-retinoic acid (ATRA), used in the treatment of acute promyelocytic leukemia (APL), induces differentiation of leukemic cells.[108] ATRA is associated with a leukocytosis syndrome characterized by fever, dyspnea, and interstitial lung infiltrates on chest radiograph, which can progress to ARDS.[109] ARDS may be secondary to accumulation of differentiated leukemic blasts and their release of cytokines, such as IL-2, in the lung. Leukapheresis is ineffective in this setting; however, the early implementation of glucocorticoids is beneficial (dexamethasone 10-20 mg/day in divided doses).

DISSEMINATED INTRAVASCULAR COAGULATION

DIC can be associated with a variety of solid tumors, including carcinoma of the prostate, lung, breast, and gastrointestinal tract, and melanomas. However, DIC is the hallmark of the clinical presentation for APL. The leukemic blasts in APL manufacture procoagulants, which are released into the circulation, particularly after cytotoxic chemotherapy.[110] The use of ATRA for treating APL has lessened the severity of DIC in this illness, but a new complication has been added (discussed in the previous paragraph). To manage DIC in APL, serial determinations of fibrin split products and fibrinogen levels should be made. Replacement of fibrinogen can be accomplished with cryoprecipitate (1 bag/2 kg of body weight initially, followed by 1 bag/10-15 kg of body weight daily). If DIC worsens after cryoprecipitate, intravenous heparin can be started but should be used cautiously. Antifibrinolytic agents, such as epsilon-aminocaproic acid, should be avoided because they can block the normal dissolution of thrombi and increase organ damage.

The most effective approach to DIC is prevention. Given the reciprocal serious complications associated with using ATRA alone or cytotoxic chemotherapy in the treatment of APL, the DIC and ATRA syndromes are best prevented by using ATRA and combination chemotherapy together so that the mass of cells differentiating in response to ATRA can be reduced to levels by the cytotoxic chemotherapy that do not result in sticking and sludging in the lungs.

BIOLOGIC THERAPY

Advances in molecular biology have made large quantities of cytokines, monoclonal antibodies, and chimeric molecules available for clinical use and testing. Examples of biologically active compounds that have been approved for patient use or are in clinical trials include the interferons (α, β, and γ), interleukins (IL-2, IL-7, IL-15, IL-21), colony-stimulating factors (GM-CSF), monoclonal antibodies (anti-HER2 [trastuzumab, Herceptin], anti-CD20 [rituximab, Rituxan]), T-cell directed antibodies (ipilimumab, anti-PD-1, anti-41BB, anti-OX40), and antibody-radioisotope conjugates (tositumomab [Bexxar]). Intensive basic science and clinical research efforts are ongoing to realize the full potential of these molecules and to understand toxicities, which can be severe and require ICU management. IL-2, which is used to treat metastatic melanoma and renal cancer, is the biologic therapy most likely to induce toxicities requiring ICU management. T-cell–directed antibodies such as ipilimumab are gaining wider use and also have the potential to induce severe toxicity.

INTERLEUKIN 2

IL-2-induced capillary leak is the chief underlying cause for most of its end-organ toxicity. The capillary leak is associated with endothelial relaxation caused by nitric oxide.[111,112] Clinical data also support the notion that nitrate levels are greatly elevated in patients treated with IL-2.[113] In addition, the adhesion of activated lymphocytes to vascular endothelium after IL-2 administration has been shown to cause vascular leak in a rabbit model.[114]

The most common serious manifestation of IL-2–induced capillary leak is hypotension with essentially the same hemodynamic findings of warm shock[115]; thus, effective support for these patients requires the use of parenteral α-adrenergic agonists, such as phenylephrine or dopamine.[116,117] Recommendations for treating cytokine-induced hypotension are given in Table 80.3. Fluid administration, though of transient benefit, often exacerbates the pulmonary capillary leak seen with IL-2. IL-2 infusions can be continued, despite hypotension, with appropriate pressor management. In our clinical experience, phenylephrine doses of up to 500 μg/minute can be tolerated to reverse IL-2–induced hypotension in this selected group of patients who have normal cardiopulmonary function before treatment. IL-2 doses are held until capillary leak has improved sufficiently to warrant a decrease in phenylephrine to less than 100 μg/minute and can be resumed thereafter in the absence of other dose-limiting toxicities.

INTERLEUKIN 2 PULMONARY CAPILLARY LEAK

The clinical manifestations of IL-2 pulmonary toxicity often do not correlate with the severity of radiologic findings.

Table 80.3 Schema for the Treatment of Cytokine-Induced Hypotension

Blood Pressure (BP) (mm Hg)	Treatment
80 < BP < 90 (asymptomatic)	500 mL 0.9% saline bolus followed by intravenous infusion at 150 mL/hr Phenylephrine 50 μg/min IV titrated up to 200 μg/min to maintain systolic BP >90
70 < BP < 80	Maintain or consider increase in phenylephrine dose and add dopamine; titrate to maximum of 20 μg/kg/min to maintain systolic BP >90
BP < 70 or 70 < BP < 80 on maximal phenylephrine dose	Consider: norepinephrine infusion, methylprednisolone
BP unresponsive to above, or cardiac sequelae of hypotension	Hetastarch 250 mg IV bolus q6, methylene blue 1-3 mg/kg IV over 5 min, followed by infusion at same rate if bolus increases BP

Between 70% and 80% of patients receiving IL-2 have some radiographic abnormality, which may consist of pleural effusions, diffuse infiltrates, or focal infiltrates.[118,119]

Because clinically significant pulmonary capillary leak cannot be anticipated by radiographic findings, relatively minor symptoms such as tachypnea need to be carefully evaluated in patients receiving IL-2. Pulse oximetry is sometimes helpful but can be falsely low in patients concurrently receiving phenylephrine for IL-2–induced hypotension; therefore, an arterial blood gas may be required for these patients. Hypoxemia should be treated with oxygen supplementation, which can be delivered initially via nasal cannula, Venturi mask, or positive-pressure airway ventilation. Worsening hypoxemia may sometimes respond to diuresis; however, intubation may be required in some patients. A key to the ventilatory management of IL-2 lung toxicity is to reverse the pulmonary edema through positive end-expiratory pressure and enhancement of renal function. Although high partial pressures of oxygen may be required in the initial treatment of these patients, prolonged oxygen exposure may exacerbate IL-2 toxicity.[116] For this reason, rapid titration of oxygen to maintain arterial partial pressure oxygen greater than or equal to 60 mm Hg is recommended. If diffuse pulmonary infiltrates worsen and an ARDS-like syndrome develops, parenteral glucocorticoids should be administered. The beneficial effect of glucocorticoids may be mediated by the lysis of activated lymphocytes that have been stimulated by IL-2.[120]

INTERLEUKIN 2 RENAL DYSFUNCTION

Hypotension and the systemic capillary leak associated with IL-2 also create renal and liver toxicities. The renal dysfunction typically consists of oliguria and prerenal azotemia with elevated blood urea nitrogen and creatinine.[121,122] Creatinine levels greater than 6.0 mg/dL or 530 μmol/L are often tolerated without modifying IL-2 doses because recovery is rapid after IL-2 treatment is completed without hemodialysis. The associated oliguria mandates meticulous fluid management because pulmonary toxicity may be exacerbated by fluid overload. Furosemide, or other nonthiazide diuretics, can be tried but are infrequently effective and may exacerbate IL-2–related hypotension.

CARDIAC RHYTHM DISTURBANCES AND MYOCARDIAL INFARCTION

IL-2 is associated with a variety of cardiac problems, including nonspecific ST-segment or T-wave changes, dysrhythmias (most commonly supraventricular tachycardia, but ventricular tachycardia can also occur), myocarditis, pericarditis, and myocardial ischemia or infarction. The rhythm disturbances and inflammatory conditions may be secondary to lymphocyte infiltration of the myocardium or pericardium.[123] Cardiac toxicity (with the exception of sinus tachycardia) should be treated initially by holding or discontinuing IL-2 doses. Supraventricular tachycardia may respond to adenosine (12 mg by rapid intravenous bolus) and is our agent of choice when IL-2–induced hypotension is present. If hypotension is present and adenosine is ineffective, intravenous diltiazem at doses between 0.15 and 0.45 mg/kg should be considered (as long as the QRS complex is not prolonged, >0.12 second) because the incidence of hypotension appears to be less than with other calcium channel blockers.[124] Amiodarone is useful in treating atrial fibrillation that occurs in approximately 5% of patients receiving IL-2. After sinus rhythm is reestablished, amiodarone can be continued (200-400 mg orally daily) to prevent or lessen the incidence of atrial fibrillation and IL-2 can generally be continued. Other cardiovascular events should be managed with the same medical and intensive care interventions used for any other acute cardiac patient.

ALLERGIC AND ANAPHYLACTIC REACTIONS TO MONOCLONAL ANTIBODIES

Allergic reactions to monoclonal antibodies occur in 10% to 15% of patients, probably because some agents are chimeric mouse proteins. However, even humanized antibodies can produce shortness of breath, tachycardia, and hypotension, especially with the first infusion. The symptoms may result from complement activation by the antibody and can often be safely managed by slowing or temporarily stopping the antibody infusion. When symptoms abate, the antibody infusion can be resumed at half the initial rate. Mild allergic manifestations, such as urticaria and pruritus, can be managed with oral antihistamines. We advocate a stepwise approach, starting with H_1 blockers (diphenhydramine, 50 mg every 4 hours alternating with hydroxyzine, 50 mg). H_2 blockers (ranitidine 150 mg every 12 hours) may be added if urticaria worsens. Pharyngeal and laryngeal edema can occur, with or without bronchospasm. Clinical manifestations of upper airway edema include drooling, phonation changes, and a sensation of throat pain or tightness. For these more severe presentations, stopping the antibody and a period of observation in the ICU setting is recommended. Parenteral antihistamines should be started, along with inhaled β_1-agonists if bronchospasm is present. Fiberoptic endoscopic examination of the hypopharynx should be performed to determine the extent of the edema. If repeat fiberoptic examination after 4 to 6 hours shows resolution of the edema, resumption of the antibody at the lower dose or reduced flow rate can be considered. If laryngeal edema worsens, intubation may be necessary to protect the airway.

There are rare patients who experience an anaphylactic reaction with circulatory collapse after monoclonal antibody treatment or other immunotherapy. This response is not always predicted by test doses of the antibody. The prognosis for these individuals in our clinical experience is poor, with a mortality rate approaching 100% despite the prompt implementation of intensive care support.

IMMUNE-MEDIATED TOXICITIES FROM T-CELL–DIRECTED THERAPY

A new class of monoclonal antibodies directed at the regulatory pathways of T cells is being developed, and has shown great promise in inducing durable antitumor effects in a variety of solid tumors, myeloma, and leukemia. The four T-cell pathways under investigation are CTLA-4, PD-1, OX40, and 41BB. Thus far, ipilimumab, a monoclonal antibody antagonizing the inhibitory function of CTLA-4, is the only one of these T-cell–targeted antibodies that has been approved by the Food and Drug Administration (FDA) for the treatment of advanced melanoma, but it is likely that more T-cell–directed agents will enter oncologic practice in the future.

The toxicities of ipilimumab have been extensively reviewed[125] and include rash, diarrhea, colitis with perforation, endocrinopathies, hepatocellular injury, fatigue, and pyrexia. The toxicities are presumed due to T-cell activation induced by CTLA-4 blockade by ipilimumab, although the precise mechanism is not well understood. Of these toxicities, immune-mediated colitis has the greatest potential to induce critical illness, as discussed earlier.

SPECIAL CONSIDERATIONS IN BONE MARROW TRANSPLANTATION

High-dose chemotherapy with stem cell support is central to managing many leukemias, myeloma, and lymphoma. It has been used in other illnesses including collagen vascular diseases and aplastic anemia. A number of life-threatening toxicities are unique to this form of dose-intense therapy and require intensive care management. The pathophysiology and treatment recommendations for these entities are discussed later.

ACUTE AND CHRONIC GRAFT-VERSUS-HOST DISEASE

Graft-versus-host (GVH) disease is most commonly seen in the setting of allogeneic transplants but can be observed after syngeneic and autologous transplants. It is well documented that GVH disease can reduce recurrence rates in leukemia[126]; it also lowers overall survival after transplant. The prerequisites for GVH disease are that the graft must include a population of immunologically competent T cells, the graft recipient must be unable to destroy these cells, and tissue antigens must be present in the recipient that are not present in the donor.[127] Studies of the immunobiology of GVH disease suggest that dysregulation of T-cell subsets ($CD4^+$, $CD25^+$, $Foxp3^+$, Treg, and T_H17) are instrumental in the clinical manifestations of GVH disease and represent potential therapeutic targets.[128,129]

The clinical manifestations of GVH include skin rash (maculopapular or diffusely erythematous), liver function abnormalities, and gastrointestinal symptoms including diarrhea, nausea, vomiting, and ileus.[126] These toxicities are graded (I to IV) on a semiquantitative basis. Grade I or II GVH disease has relatively little morbidity, but grade IV GVH disease carries a 100% mortality rate. Treatment of established GVH disease requires suppression of the immune system. The drugs used most commonly to suppress GVH disease are glucocorticoids, cyclosporine, tacrolimus, and methotrexate, which are usually used in combination. Gamma globulin infusions may also be beneficial in the prophylaxis of GVH disease.[130] The mechanism of action of gamma globulin is unknown but may involve binding to Fc receptors, which may prevent T cells from recognizing target tissues.

VENO-OCCLUSIVE DISEASE

Hepatic veno-occlusive disease (VOD) is a clinical syndrome characterized by weight gain (fluid), tender hepatomegaly, and elevations of hepatocellular enzymes and bilirubin. The syndrome is the result of endothelial toxicity from high-dose chemotherapy, and results in a local hypercoagulable state with tissue factor synthesis, down-regulation of thrombomodulin, and release of von Willebrand factor with the resultant formation of blood clots in hepatic veins.[131] The incidence of VOD has diminished with the prophylactic use of heparin.[132] Agents used in the treatment of established VOD include tissue plasminogen activator,[133] antithrombin III,[134] antioxidant therapy,[135] and transjugular intrahepatic portosystemic stent-shunt.[136] Clinical trials using a polydisperse oligonucleotide known as defibrotide[137] are showing activity and defibrotide may be helpful in both the prevention and treatment of VOD. Intensive support is often needed for patients with VOD. Despite aggressive treatment, the mortality rate for severe established VOD approaches 100%.[138] Patients with milder disease may recover with supportive measures. Early recognition and intervention are key factors influencing outcome.

INFECTIOUS COMPLICATIONS OF STEM CELL TRANSPLANTATION

Different facets of immune function return at varying intervals after bone marrow transplant.[139] Integumentary and mucosal barriers are disrupted in the period immediately after myeloablative chemotherapy. For this reason, aerobic bacteria and *Candida* organisms are the most likely pathogens early after transplant. There are decreased neutrophil numbers for the first 2 to 4 weeks after transplant, although the use of colony-stimulating factors shortens the neutrophil recovery period. Until neutrophil numbers increase, herpes simplex virus, *Candida*, *Aspergillus*, and bacterial infections are common. It should be noted that the full chemotactic function of neutrophils does not return for 100 days after transplant. Cellular and humoral immunity defects persist for 1 to 3 months after transplant and may lengthen if GVH disease occurs. Fungal and cytomegalovirus (CMV) infections predominate in this period.[140,141] From 3 months to 1 year after transplant, T cells remain dysfunctional and disordered immunoregulation may occur. Varicella zoster, hepatitis C, *Pneumocystis jiroveci* pneumonia, and pneumococcal pneumonia are the most common infections until T-cell function has recovered. Immune deficits may be moderated by antigen-specific immunity conferred by the transplanted marrow and the use of gamma globulin infusions, which are now routinely given after allogeneic transplant. Antibiotic recommendations in bone marrow transplant are similar to those for other febrile neutropenic cancer patients. Individual recommendations should take into account the frequency of specific microorganisms isolated at a given institution. Trimethoprim-sulfamethoxazole and fluoroquinolone antibiotics (e.g., ciprofloxacin) are routinely used for the prophylaxis of *Pneumocystis* organisms and gram-positive infections, respectively. Invasive fungal infections can be a significant cause of morbidity and death after transplant, but voraconazole prophylaxis or secondary therapy can be effective. CMV responds poorly to single-agent therapy, but the combination of ganciclovir and gamma globulin infusions improves outcome in these patients. Death rates from CMV pneumonitis approached 80% before use of the combination regimen. The use of CMV-negative donors and the elimination of CMV-contaminated leukocytes from platelet and red blood cell transfusions with leukocyte filters have reduced the mortality rate from CMV infection.

There has been ongoing work in using cytotoxic T-lymphocyte (CTL) clones to treat specific opportunistic infections including those from CMV, Epstein-Barr virus (EBV), and adenovirus.[142-144] Augmentation of antiviral activity was conferred with these infusions in most patients.[145] This strategy may prove useful in reducing the number of life-threatening infections in bone marrow transplant, human immunodeficiency virus, and other immunodeficiency states.[142]

CODE STATUS AND INTENSIVE CARE IN CANCER PATIENTS

The high cost of intensive care and the demands placed on these precious resources by all medical and surgical subspecialties mandate that critical care interventions be meted out wisely. Because cost containment has become imperative in medicine practice and health care reform, certain poor prognosis illnesses, including cancer, are perceived by the public and often by medical staff as relative contraindications to cardiopulmonary resuscitation (CPR) or intensive care interventions.[146] Although several studies have shown that CPR in patients with cancer diagnoses has a low success rate (less than 10%),[147,148] the success rate of CPR in noncancer diagnoses is less than 5%.[149] Hospital utilization studies do not support the notion that a disproportionate amount of special care resources are used in terminally ill cancer patients.[150] The central determination in each case should hinge on the answer to a single question: "Is it likely that these abnormalities are reversible?" For nearly all iatrogenic toxicities, the answer is generally yes. For patients with curable tumor types, every effort should be made to support the patient until the long-term prognosis of the underlying tumor can be ascertained. Given that nearly 60% of individuals with a cancer diagnosis are cured of their disease, intensive care interventions are justified.

When viewed in the context of other underlying medical conditions, a cancer diagnosis is neither medically nor ethically a contraindication to intensive care management. The wishes of the individual and the family are central in establishing an appropriate level of care for any patient. In order to better define the level of care desired by individuals with serious or terminal illnesses, the state of Oregon originated a program known as POLST (Physician Orders for Life-Sustaining Treatment), which is now being implemented in at least 15 other states.[151] In cancer patients, the compliance of physicians with documented care preferences is generally greater than 90%, but the timing and extent of this documentation vary.[152] Public awareness of these issues is increasing, and many cancer patients now have such directives, which include living wills, do-not-resuscitate orders, and POLST. These directives can be helpful to the physician and the patient's family, although they sometimes complicate medical management in clinical situations in which reversible conditions exist but for which care might require violating a directive.[153] Patient education and strong support from social work and pastoral and legal services can assist the physician in arriving at the appropriate level of care for each individual.

SUMMARY

Intensive care support can be a critical component of the success of any dose-intense cancer treatment modality. Support of treatment toxicities is justified given the growing improvement in outcome for cancer diagnoses. Understanding of the pathophysiology of a number of clinical entities, such as septic shock and cytokine-induced hypotension, will provide the basis for more rational and effective management of many of these toxicities. However, it is even more important to develop cancer treatments that attack the malignancy and spare the host. This level of therapeutic sophistication is attainable through our increasing knowledge of the molecular basis of malignancy and the physiology of tumors. Even when the goal of therapeutic specificity in oncology is achieved, intensive care will still be salient in the support of patients presenting with the end-organ sequelae of malignancy.

KEY POINTS

- TLS occurs most frequently in rapidly growing lymphomas or leukemias with high myeloblast or lymphoblast counts. The most effective management strategy is to anticipate the occurrence of TLS and initiate allopurinol, hydration, and intensive monitoring before metabolic aberrations occur.

KEY POINTS (Continued)

- Hypercalcemia is the most common metabolic disturbance in cancer patients. Intravenous hydration and bisphosphonates are the initial treatments for hypercalcemia.
- SIADH in cancer patients often presents with neurologic findings. The initial treatment is fluid restriction.
- Treatment of SVC syndrome depends on the underlying histologic diagnosis; therefore, a biopsy is mandatory in previously undiagnosed patients. If SVC is secondary to lymphoma or small cell lung cancer, chemotherapy is the treatment of choice. Radiation with high initial dose fractions can be palliative in more than 80% of patients with malignancies unresponsive to chemotherapy. Endovascular stents can palliate symptoms in a high proportion of patients.
- Central nervous system or spinal metastases can often be managed on an outpatient basis with dexamethasone and radiation treatment. Individual patients may benefit from higher doses of dexamethasone (up to 200 mg/day), and surgery with radiation can achieve significant palliation for some patients.
- DIC is observed in a number of solid tumors and is the hallmark of APL. Serial levels of fibrin split products and fibrinogen will determine the amount of cryoprecipitate needed to replace consumed coagulation proteins. Heparin can be used in patients who do not respond to cryoprecipitate.
- Febrile neutropenia can often be managed outside the ICU with appropriate broad-spectrum antibiotic support. The choice of antibiotics should take into account the microbial pathogens most prevalent in the treating institution.
- Hypotension caused by IL-2 and other cytokines has a pathophysiology similar to that of septic shock, with the induction of nitric oxide and other vasoactive mediators. Phenylephrine is an effective pressor agent for IL-2–induced hypotension. Glucocorticoids may be useful in patients with circulatory collapse or ARDS from IL-2 or other immunotherapy.
- Infections that occur during bone marrow transplant are related to the recovery of different parts of immune function after transplant. Aerobic bacteria and *Candida* infections are most prevalent early, when mucosal barriers are disrupted by myeloablative chemotherapy. Herpes simplex, *Candida*, bacterial, and *Aspergillus* infections are common until neutrophil recovery has occurred. Varicella zoster, hepatitis C, and *Pneumocystis jiroveci* infections are observed up

KEY POINTS (Continued)

to 3 months after transplant until cellular immune function recovers.

- Immune-mediated colitis induced by ipilimumab can be life threatening. Early administration of high-dose glucocorticoids and fluid resuscitation are essential elements of management. Emergent surgery and ICU support may be necessary in some patients.
- A cancer diagnosis is not a contraindication to intensive care management. Dose-intense treatment modalities mandate intensive support and have resulted in improved outcomes for patients with malignancies.

SELECTED REFERENCES

4. Hodi FS, O'Day SJ, McDermott DF, et al: Improved survival with ipilimumab in patients with metastatic melanoma. N Engl J Med 2010;363:711-723.
6. Chapman PB, Hauschild A, Robert C, et al: Improved survival with vemurafenib in melanoma with BRAF V600E mutation. N Engl J Med 2011;364:2507-2516.
26. Stopeck AT, Lipton A, Body JJ, et al: Denosumab compared with zoledronic acid for the treatment of bone metastases in patients with advanced breast cancer: A randomized, double-blind study. J Clin Oncol 2010;28:5132-5139.
36. Weingarten TN, Cata JP, O'Hara JF, et al: Comparison of two preoperative medical management strategies for laparoscopic resection of pheochromocytoma. Urology 2010;76:508 e6-11.
48. Lanciego C, Pangua C, Chacon JI, et al: Endovascular stenting as the first step in the overall management of malignant superior vena cava syndrome. Am J Roentgenol 2009;193:549-558.
53. O'Brien PK, Kucharczuk JC, Marshall MB, et al: Comparative study of subxiphoid versus video-thoracoscopic pericardial "window." Ann Thorac Surg 2005;80:2013-2019.
61. Sawaya H, Sebag IA, Plana JC, et al: Early detection and prediction of cardiotoxicity in chemotherapy-treated patients. Am J Cardiol 2011;107:1375-1380.
72. Rhee CK, Kang JY, Kim YH, et al: Risk factors for acute respiratory distress syndrome during neutropenia recovery in patients with hematologic malignancies. Crit Care 2009;13:R173.
84. Mikkelsen T, Paleologos NA, Robinson PD, et al: The role of prophylactic anticonvulsants in the management of brain metastases: A systematic review and evidence-based clinical practice guideline. J Neurooncol 2010;96:97-102.
99. Beck KE, Blansfield JA, Tran KQ, et al: Enterocolitis in patients with cancer after antibody blockade of cytotoxic T-lymphocyte-associated antigen 4. J Clin Oncol 2006;24:2283-2289.
117. Schwartzentruber DJ: Guidelines for the safe administration of high-dose interleukin-2. J Immunother 2001;24:287-293.
152. Ahluwalia SC, Chuang FL, Antonio AL, et al: Documentation and discussion of preferences for care among patients with advanced cancer. J Oncol Pract 2012;7:361-366.

The complete list of references can be found at www.expertconsult.com.

81 Critical Care Medicine in Pregnancy

Stephen E. Lapinsky

CHAPTER OUTLINE

Management of the critically ill pregnant patient is a situation with which few intensive care physicians gain significant expertise. The usual clinical approach may be altered by the physiologic changes induced by pregnancy, by the relatively uncommon pregnancy-specific conditions, and by perceived limitations on therapy produced by the presence of a fetus (Fig. 81.1).

PHYSIOLOGIC CHANGES IN PREGNANCY

The pregnant woman undergoes a number of physiologic changes affecting various systems relevant to critical care management. From a respiratory perspective, the upper airways develop edema and hyperemia, which may be relevant during endotracheal intubation. Changes in lung volumes occur, with a 10% to 25% decrease in functional residual capacity (FRC), whereas total lung capacity decreases only minimally as the thoracic cage widens to compensate.[1] Forced expiratory volume in 1 second (FEV_1) is not altered by the pregnant state. Lung compliance remains unchanged, but chest wall and total respiratory compliance are reduced.[2]

The rising progesterone level stimulates an increase in ventilation. Tidal volume and minute ventilation increase from the first trimester, reaching 20% to 40% above baseline by term (Table 81.1).[3] A mild respiratory alkalosis is produced with compensatory renal excretion of bicarbonate ($Paco_2$ 28 to 32 mm Hg; HCO_3^- 18 to 21 mEq/L). Oxygen consumption increases because of the demands of the fetus and maternal metabolic processes, reaching levels up to 33% above baseline by term. Arterial Po_2 remains normal throughout pregnancy, but mild hypoxemia caused by an increased alveolar-arterial oxygen tension difference may develop in the supine position, as FRC diminishes near term.

Maternal blood volume and cardiac output increase through pregnancy, reaching a peak at 30% to 50% above baseline levels by about 28 weeks (Fig. 81.2).[4] Hemodynamic measurements by pulmonary artery catheter in the near-term patient demonstrate the increased cardiac output, with a reduced systemic vascular resistance and pulmonary vascular resistance (see Table 81.1).[5] During labor and continuing into the immediate postpartum period, cardiac output is further augmented by the return of 300 to 500 mL of blood to the central circulation.[6]

Oxygen delivery to the fetus is dependent on the maternal arterial oxygen content and the uterine blood flow. Maternal hypotension, alkalosis (e.g., hyperventilation), and endogenous or exogenous catecholamines can vasoconstrict the uterine artery and adversely affect fetal oxygenation.[7] Uterine blood flow is also reduced transiently by

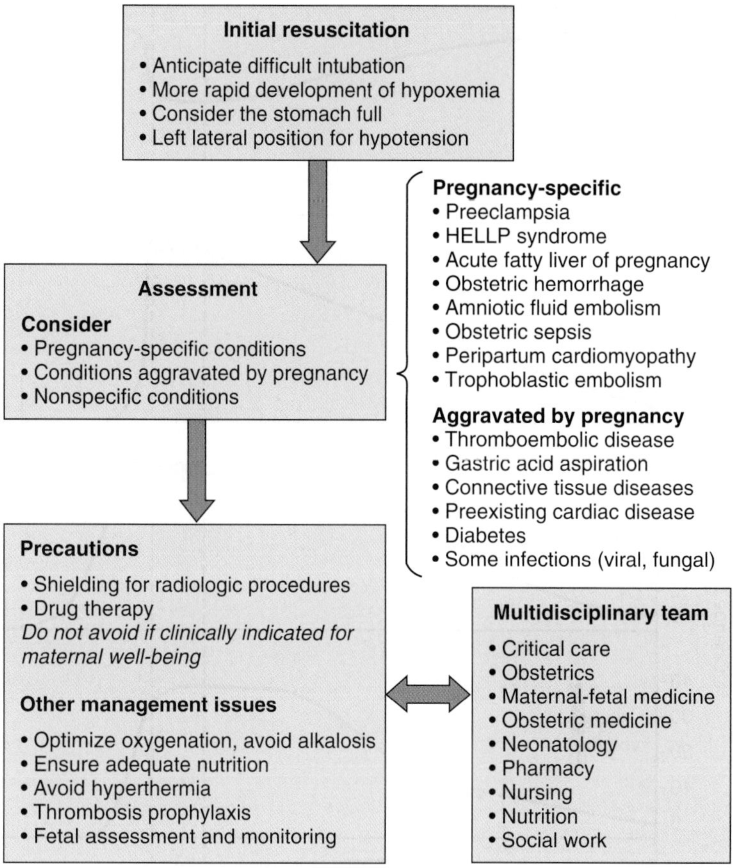

Figure 81.1 Approach to the assessment and management of the critically ill obstetric patient.

Table 81.1 Physiologic Changes in Late Pregnancy

Parameter	Change
Respiratory	
Functional residual capacity	Decreased 10-25%
Minute ventilation	Increased 20-40%
Arterial partial pressure of oxygen	No change
Arterial partial pressure of carbon dioxide	Reduced to 28-32 mm Hg
Serum bicarbonate	Reduced to 18-21 mEq/L
Cardiac	
Heart rate	Increased 10-30%
Pulmonary capillary wedge pressure	No change
Cardiac output	Increased 30-50%
Systemic vascular resistance	Decreased 20-30%
Pulmonary vascular resistance	Decreased 20-30%
Renal	
Glomerular filtration rate	Increased 50%
Creatinine	Decreased (24-68 μmol/L; 0.29-0.77 mg/dL)

uterine contractions. Although umbilical venous blood returning to the fetus has a relatively low oxygen tension, a high oxygen content is maintained by the left shift of the oxygen dissociation curve of fetal hemoglobin.

Glomerular filtration rate increases early in pregnancy, reaching a value 50% above prepregnancy levels in the second trimester, and remains elevated throughout pregnancy (see Fig. 81.2).[8] The normal serum creatinine level is therefore in the range of 0.5 to 0.7 mg/dL (45 to 60 μmol/L). As pregnancy progresses, mild ureteric dilation and mild hydronephrosis may occur as a result of uterine compression and smooth muscle relaxation.

Pregnancy is associated with a reduced lower esophageal sphincter pressure, reaching a nadir at 36 weeks. The position of the stomach is displaced, further decreasing the effectiveness of the gastroesophageal sphincter and reducing gastric emptying. The pregnant woman should therefore always be considered at risk for aspiration of stomach contents, regardless of the time elapsed since her last meal.

The increase in plasma volume is associated with a lesser increase in red blood cell mass causing a physiologic anemia, with a hematocrit of 32% to 34% by the third trimester. A mild leukocytosis occurs with white blood cell count rising further during labor. Platelet counts are usually unchanged, although a condition of benign mild thrombocytopenia may occur.[9] Procoagulant factors rise, contributing to the hypercoagulable state of pregnancy. The erythrocyte sedimentation rate (ESR) rises related to increased levels of plasma globulins.

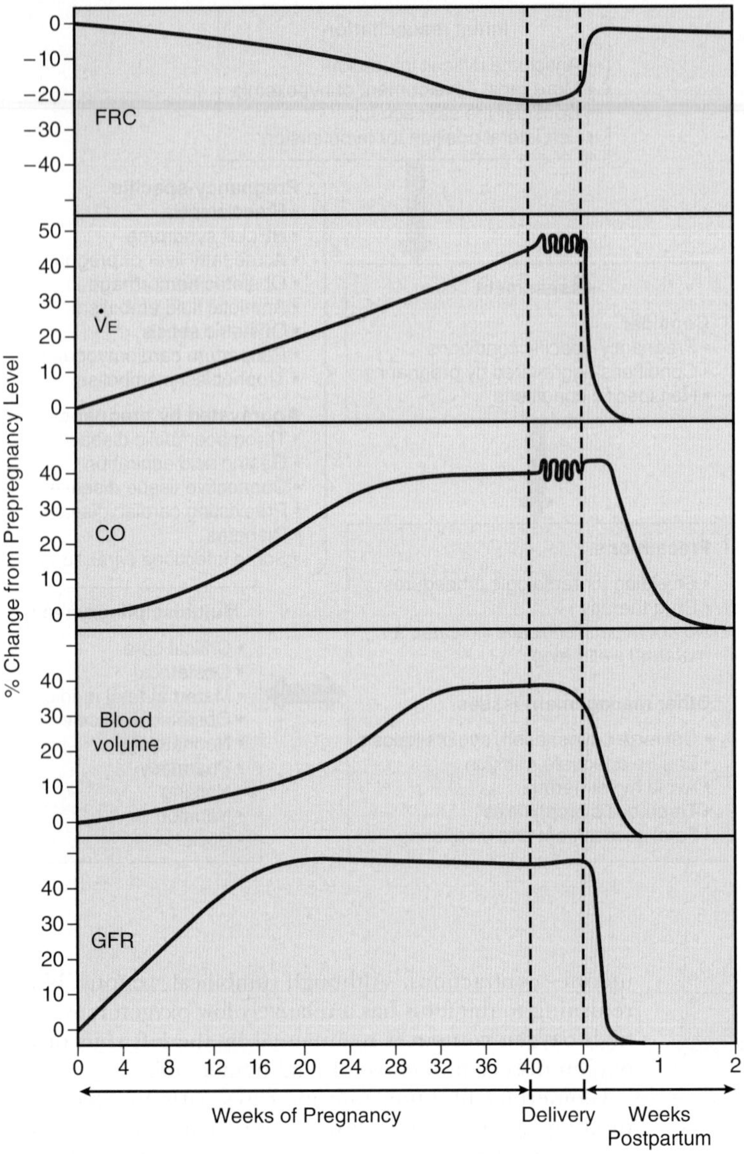

Figure 81.2 Graphic representation of some of the physiologic changes that occur in pregnancy. CO, cardiac output; FRC, functional residual capacity; GFR, glomerular filtration rate; V̇E, minute ventilation. (From Lapinsky SE, Kruczynski K, Slutsky AS: Critical care in the pregnant patient. Am J Respir Crit Care Med 1995;152:427-455.)

CRITICAL CARE MANAGEMENT

GENERAL CARE

POSITIONING

In the supine position the gravid uterus produces mechanical effects on the vena cava and aorta, reducing central venous return. This results in a decrease in cardiac output and hypotension. This "supine hypotensive syndrome" should be considered in hemodynamically unstable patients.[10] Pregnant patients should be positioned on their left side, or at least with the right hip slightly elevated.

NUTRITION

During starvation, maternal body stores are protected at the expense of the fetus and inadequate nutrition may result in intrauterine growth retardation and fetal loss. Growth restriction before 26 weeks' gestation may lead to fetal neurologic impairment. Caloric requirements in pregnancy increase by about 300 kcal/day, and protein intake should be augmented by 20% to 50%. Several nutrients have an increased requirement in pregnancy including iron, folate, and calcium. Total parenteral nutrition (TPN) has been used successfully to provide nutritional support during pregnancy in the patient in whom enteral nutrition is not possible. Blood glucose should be measured frequently in view of the predisposition to hyperglycemia.

THROMBOSIS PROPHYLAXIS

Pregnancy increases the risks of venous thrombosis caused by hypercoagulability and venous stasis. Antithrombotic measures including physical interventions and heparin prophylaxis should be considered.

RADIOLOGIC PROCEDURES AND FETAL RISK

Radiologic investigations are often essential for the assessment and management of the critically ill pregnant patient. Although there are potential risks of exposing the fetus to ionizing radiation, fetal well-being depends on maternal recovery, and appropriate radiologic procedures should not

Table 81.2 Risk of Fetal Radiation Exposure Resulting from Radiologic Studies in the Critically Ill Pregnant Patient

Investigation	Fetal Radiation Exposure (mGy)
Chest radiograph (with abdomen shielded)	0.01
Ventilation-perfusion scan	
Perfusion	0.1-1
Ventilation	0.1-0.4
CT pulmonary angiogram	0.1-4
CT scan of pelvis and abdomen	30-50
Radiation effect on fetus	
Teratogenicity	50-100
Oncogenicity	20-50

CT, computed tomography.

be avoided. Techniques such as shielding the abdomen with lead and using a well-collimated x-ray beam can effectively reduce exposure. With these precautions, estimated fetal radiation exposure can be limited to safe levels for most procedures, although investigations such as abdominal-pelvic computed tomography (CT) will obviously cause significant fetal radiation exposure (Table 81.2).[11]

The adverse effects of fetal exposure to radiation include oncogenicity and teratogenicity. A twofold increased risk of childhood leukemia may result from fetal exposure in the range of 20 to 50 mGy (2 to 5 rads). Most intensive care unit (ICU) procedures can be carried out well below these levels of exposure to the fetus (see Table 81.2). Teratogenicity does not appear to occur at these radiation doses, requiring radiation exposure greater than 50 to 100 mGy (5 to 10 rads). Nonetheless, every effort should be made to minimize uterine exposure, particularly in the first trimester.

DRUG THERAPY IN PREGNANCY

Pharmacotherapy during pregnancy requires consideration of the altered drug clearance, metabolism, and volume of distribution of drugs in pregnancy, and the potential pharmacologic and teratogenic effects on the embryo. A detailed description of drug therapy in pregnancy is beyond the scope of this chapter. Consultation with an obstetrician and pharmacist is essential, and several excellent resources are available.[12,13] Some common ICU drugs are discussed briefly as follows.

CATECHOLAMINES

Catecholamines commonly used in the ICU such as dobutamine, dopamine, norepinephrine, and epinephrine all have the potential to reduce uterine blood flow. Both ephedrine and phenylephrine boluses are used for transient hypotension induced by neuraxial anesthesia. Nonpharmacologic maneuvers such as volume replacement and left lateral positioning are essential to the management of hypotension, and the rapidity of correction of blood pressure may be more important than the specific inotropic agent used. If vasopressor infusion therapy is required to support maternal hemodynamics, this therapy should not be withheld because of concerns for potential adverse effects on the fetus.

SEDATION, ANALGESIA, AND NEUROMUSCULAR BLOCKADE

Little data exist on the preferred drugs for prolonged sedation, analgesia, or neuromuscular blockade in pregnancy. Benzodiazepine use in early pregnancy has been associated with a small risk of congenital malformations, mainly cleft lip and palate. Midazolam crosses the placenta to a lesser degree than diazepam, which can accumulate in the fetus at levels greater than in the mother. Propofol has been used as an induction agent for cesarean section, but a single case report describes the development of non–anion gap acidosis in two pregnant women receiving propofol infusion for neurosurgical procedures.[14] Congenital malformations have not been demonstrated with use of narcotic analgesics such as morphine, meperidine, and fentanyl. The majority of nondepolarizing neuromuscular blocking agents have been shown to cross the placenta including pancuronium, vecuronium, and atracurium, but transfer is unlikely to have clinical effects on the fetus in the short term. Nevertheless, if sedative or paralyzing agents are used in the pregnant woman, this information must be communicated to the neonatologist, who should anticipate the need for ventilatory support for the fetus.

ANTIBIOTICS

Antibiotic regimens similar to those used in the nonpregnant patient are appropriate, with some precautions. Quinolones should probably be avoided because of the potential risk of arthropathy. Tetracyclines produce adverse effects on fetal teeth and bone, and aminoglycosides and sulfonamides should be used with caution.

FETAL OXYGENATION AND MONITORING

Attention to interventions aimed at optimizing fetal oxygenation is important in the management of any critically ill pregnant patient. Depending on gestational age, delivery of the fetus may be the most appropriate intervention. Uteroplacental oxygen delivery can be optimized by increasing oxygen carrying capacity—by blood transfusion, improving maternal cardiac output, and optimizing maternal oxygenation. The simple maneuver of tilting the patient to the left lateral position to increase cardiac output should always be considered.[10]

Continuous electronic monitoring of fetal heart rate (FHR) can be used to identify changes in fetal physiology. Abnormal patterns of FHR have been described with good sensitivity but varying specificity for fetal distress. Fetal tachycardia may occur in the presence of maternal infection or chorioamnionitis, but fetal bradycardia or sinusoidal variation in FHR are more ominous, suggesting fetal hypoxia. Changes in FHR occur in response to uterine activity. Early decelerations coinciding with contractions are benign, but late decelerations beginning beyond the peak in contraction and persisting after the contraction may indicate fetal compromise, particularly if associated with a reduced beat-to-beat variation. Fetal compromise may occur as a result of uteroplacental or fetal pathology but may also indicate maternal illness with reduced uterine oxygen delivery. The fetus may be further assessed by an ultrasound biophysical profile that evaluates factors such as spontaneous movement, breathing action, and amniotic fluid volume. A normal biophysical profile carries a good prognosis.

HEMODYNAMIC MONITORING

In general the indications for use of the pulmonary artery catheter are similar to those in nonobstetric patients, and pregnancy is not a contraindication to invasive hemodynamic monitoring. An awareness of the normal cardiovascular physiologic changes in pregnancy (discussed earlier) is necessary in order to correctly interpret the hemodynamic data obtained.

VENTILATORY SUPPORT

NONINVASIVE VENTILATION

Noninvasive ventilation avoids the adverse effects of endotracheal intubation, such as airway trauma, the increased risk of nosocomial pneumonia, and the complications associated with sedation. This modality is ideally suited to short-term ventilatory support, which is the case in many obstetric complications that reverse rapidly. The major concern with mask ventilation in pregnancy is the risk of aspiration because of the increased intra-abdominal pressure, delayed gastric emptying, and reduced lower esophageal sphincter tone accompanying pregnancy. Noninvasive ventilation should therefore be reserved for the patient who is alert, protecting her airway, and has an expectation of a relatively brief requirement for mechanical ventilatory support.

AIRWAY MANAGEMENT

Failed intubation is more common in the obstetric population than in other anesthetic intubations.[15] The reduced oxygen reserve caused by diminished FRC and increased oxygen consumption produces rapid desaturation in response to apnea or hypoventilation.[16] Preoxygenation with 100% oxygen is beneficial, but respiratory alkalosis must be avoided. In view of the delayed gastric emptying and elevated intra-abdominal pressure, the pregnant patient should always be considered to have a full stomach and appropriate precautions should be taken. Upper airway hyperemia and edema may reduce visualization and necessitate use of a smaller endotracheal tube. The risk of bleeding is increased and nasal intubation should be avoided.

MECHANICAL VENTILATION

The normal $Paco_2$ of about 30 mm Hg in late pregnancy should be considered in the interpretation of arterial blood gases when decisions are made to institute ventilatory support. Data on the prolonged mechanical ventilation of pregnant patients are limited. Hyperventilation should be avoided because this adversely affects uterine blood flow[17] because of the resulting alkalemia as well as the effect of positive-pressure ventilation in reducing cardiac output. The current ventilatory approach of avoiding excessive lung stretch by pressure limitation and permissive hypercapnia has not been assessed in pregnancy. The usual pressure limits (e.g., plateau pressure of 35 cm H_2O) may not be applicable in the near-term patient, in whom chest wall compliance is reduced. Transpulmonary pressures may not be elevated at a plateau pressure of 35 cm H_2O, and higher ventilatory pressures may be acceptable in pregnant patients near term. Although late pregnancy is associated with a mild respiratory alkalosis, maternal hypercapnia up to 60 mm Hg in the presence of adequate oxygenation does not appear to be detrimental to the fetus.[18] Maternal hypercapnia and respiratory acidosis may produce fetal acidosis, but this does not have the same ominous implications as fetal acidosis due to lactic acidosis resulting from fetal hypoxia.[19] However, acidosis produces a right shift of the hemoglobin oxygen dissociation curve, which may negate the beneficial oxygen-carrying characteristics of fetal hemoglobin. If marked respiratory acidosis results from permissive hypercapnia, treatment with bicarbonate may improve maternal and fetal acidemia.

It may be considered that, because of the effects of pregnancy on respiratory physiology, delivery of the pregnant patient will result in improvement in the mother's respiratory status.[20] Limited case series addressing this issue have not found a significant benefit to the mother, and delivery carries a risk of harm.[21,22] Some improvement in oxygenation has been noted, but without improvement in respiratory system compliance or reduction in positive end-expiratory pressure (PEEP) level.[20] Delivery is therefore not indicated purely in the hope of improving "maternal condition." If the fetus is considered viable but is at risk due to severe maternal hypoxia, consultation with a neonatologist may identify a benefit to the fetus in being delivered. Obstetric indications should always determine the mode of delivery.

CARDIOPULMONARY RESUSCITATION

Cardiopulmonary resuscitation requires only minor modifications from standard protocols.[23] Intravenous access should be established above the diaphragm owing to potentially impeded inferior vena caval blood flow. Electrical cardioversion and defibrillation may be performed in pregnancy, but fetal monitoring leads should be removed to prevent electrical arcing. Management in the supine position may cause aortocaval compression, resulting in impaired venous return and inadequate cardiac output. Manual displacement of the uterus to the left should be used, or alternatively a 30-degree left lateral tilt, which may impede cardiac compressions. Appropriate pharmacologic therapy should not be withheld if clinically indicated. Perimortem cesarean section may save the fetus when initial attempts at resuscitation have failed in a woman with a fetus at a viable gestation. Data suggest that infant survival without neurologic sequelae is highest if the postmortem cesarean section is initiated within 4 minutes of cardiac arrest, aiming for delivery within 5 minutes of arrest.

PREGNANCY-SPECIFIC CONDITIONS REQUIRING INTENSIVE CARE UNIT CARE

PREECLAMPSIA

Preeclampsia is a pregnancy-induced condition usually occurring after 20 weeks' gestation, characterized by hypertension and proteinuria.[24] The cause remains unknown but is likely related to a placental abnormality producing a diffuse maternal endothelial effect, which leads to vasospasm and reduced organ perfusion (Fig. 81.3). Preeclampsia and its complications account for 20% to 50% of obstetric admissions to the ICU.[25-27] Less common multisystem diseases should be considered in the differential diagnosis including systemic lupus erythematosus (SLE), thrombotic thrombocytopenic purpura (TTP), and hemolytic-uremic syndrome (HUS) (Table 81.3). Complications of preeclampsia may result in critical illness including pulmonary edema, cerebral edema, renal failure, hypertensive crisis, seizures (eclampsia), and the HELLP (hemolysis, elevated liver enzymes, low platelet count) syndrome (microangiopathic hemolytic anemia, thrombocytopenia, and hepatic involvement).[28]

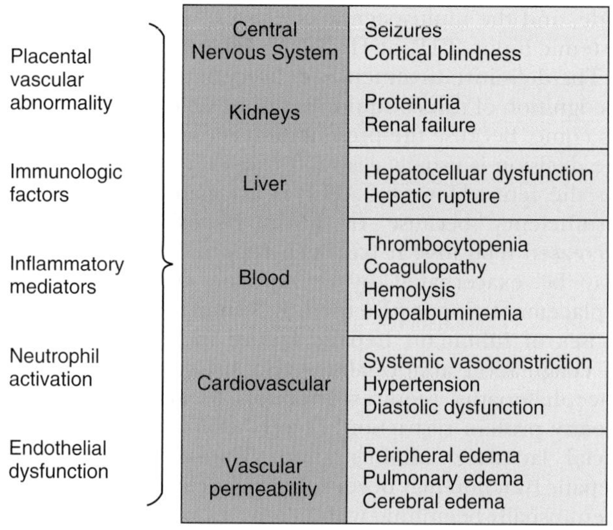

Figure 81.3 Pathophysiology and multiorgan effects of preeclampsia.

The only specific treatment is delivery of the fetus and placenta. Delivery is always in the best interest of the mother, but timing may depend on fetal maturity. The role of antihypertensive therapy is to prevent maternal hypertensive complications, and it does not alter the natural history of the condition or benefit the fetus.[29] Commonly used agents include intravenous hydralazine or labetalol, as well as oral calcium antagonists.[24] Rapid reduction in blood pressure should usually be avoided because of the risk of reducing uteroplacental perfusion. Magnesium sulfate is used for seizure prophylaxis and treatment, giving an initial intravenous bolus (2 to 4 g) followed by an infusion of 1 to 3 g/hour. Toxic magnesium levels may occur (>3.5 mmol/L), particularly in the presence of renal dysfunction, producing respiratory muscle weakness and cardiac conduction defects. Hypocalcemia may be noted during magnesium infusion and should not be corrected routinely because this would negate the therapeutic effects of magnesium. Fluid management in preeclampsia usually requires careful volume expansion, but excessive fluid administration can cause pulmonary or cerebral edema.

HELLP SYNDROME

The HELLP syndrome is a condition associated with preeclampsia, characterized by the development of a microangiopathic hemolytic anemia and a consumptive thrombocytopenia.[28] Reduced hepatic perfusion results in periportal and focal parenchymal necrosis, elevated liver enzymes, and rarely hepatic hemorrhage or rupture. The clinical presentation is often with epigastric or right upper quadrant pain, nausea, vomiting, or evidence of bleeding.

Table 81.3 Differential Diagnosis of Pregnancy-Related Complications

Clinical Finding	Pregnancy-Specific Complications	Nonspecific Complications
1. Hypertension	Preeclampsia	Essential hypertension Secondary hypertension (renal, pheochromocytoma)
2. Thrombocytopenia	Preeclampsia HELLP syndrome Acute fatty liver of pregnancy	TTP ITP Sepsis SLE
3. Abnormal liver enzymes	Preeclampsia HELLP syndrome Acute fatty liver of pregnancy Cholestasis of pregnancy	Viral hepatitis Drug-induced hepatitis Budd-Chiari syndrome
4. Renal dysfunction	Preeclampsia Acute fatty liver of pregnancy Idiopathic postpartum renal failure	Sepsis Hypovolemia/hemorrhage TTP/HUS SLE
5. Pulmonary edema	Preeclampsia Peripartum cardiomyopathy Tocolytic pulmonary edema Amniotic fluid emboli	Valvular heart disease Ischemic heart disease ARDS Aspiration

ARDS, acute respiratory distress syndrome; HELLP, hemolysis, elevated liver enzymes, low platelet count; HUS, hemolytic-uremic syndrome; ITP, idiopathic thrombocytopenic purpura; SLE, systemic lupus erythematosus; TTP, thrombotic thrombocytopenic purpura.

Features of preeclampsia do not occur in all patients, and approximately 30% of patients with HELLP develop the disease only in the postpartum period.

The diagnosis is based on the presence of thrombocytopenia ($<100 \times 10^9$ cells/L), with a moderate elevation of liver enzymes, and microangiopathic hemolytic anemia (increased lactate dehydrogenase, bilirubin, abnormal blood smear). Many patients are found to have a more widespread coagulation defect than just thrombocytopenia. White blood cell count may be elevated, and hypoglycemia is uncommon, in contrast to acute fatty liver of pregnancy (AFLP).

Management includes early delivery if the fetus is viable, blood product support, and management of associated preeclampsia. Dexamethasone initiated prior to delivery has been reported to produce more rapid recovery of thrombocytopenia in some studies but this was not confirmed in the most recent study.[30,31] Delivery may require platelet support, and if cesarean section is necessary, hemorrhage should be anticipated and adequate drains should be inserted. Epidural anesthesia is usually contraindicated in the presence of thrombocytopenia.

The maternal complications of HELLP include hemorrhage, acute respiratory distress syndrome (ARDS), and acute renal failure. An uncommon but catastrophic consequence of the HELLP syndrome is hepatic subcapsular hemorrhage, which occurs in about 2% of patients and can progress to hepatic rupture. Hepatic rupture should be considered in any preeclamptic patient with sudden shock or acute abdominal pain. Management requires aggressive hemodynamic and blood product support, urgent delivery, and invasive control of the hemorrhage with embolization, or laparotomy with packing of the liver. Hemorrhage without rupture may be managed conservatively if the patient remains hemodynamically stable.

Significant overlap exists between HELLP and other multisystem conditions and thrombotic microangiopathies (see Table 81.3). A response to plasmapheresis may be noted in some patients, possibly representing those with TTP or HUS rather than HELLP. Plasmapheresis is recommended for patients with delayed postpartum resolution when severe thrombocytopenia, hemolysis, or organ dysfunction persist more than 72 hours following delivery. The maternal mortality rate for women with HELLP syndrome is reported between 1% and 3% (with isolated reports as high as 25%) and with a significant perinatal mortality rate at 8% to 60%.

ACUTE FATTY LIVER OF PREGNANCY

AFLP is an uncommon condition affecting about 1 in 15,000 pregnancies. Although early reports described acute fulminant hepatic failure with high maternal and fetal mortality rates, the condition is now usually recognized at an earlier stage, allowing early delivery and a significantly improved outcome.[32] Maternal mortality rate has been reported at 0% to 18% with fetal loss of 23% to 60%. The cause of this condition is unknown, but an association with a fetal inborn error of metabolism (L-CHAD [long-chain 3-hydroxyacyl-coenzyme A dehydrogenase] deficiency) has been described.[33] Pathologically, diffuse fatty infiltration of the liver occurs with necrosis and inflammation being mild or absent.

Patients usually present toward the end of the third trimester with a range of onset from as early as 30 weeks' gestation up until the puerperium. Prodromal symptoms of malaise, anorexia, and vomiting may precede the onset of jaundice by 1 to 2 weeks. Abdominal pain may occur, which may be diffuse or localized to the right upper quadrant. Laboratory investigations demonstrate a moderate elevation in transaminase levels (e.g., 300 to 600 units), in contrast with the higher levels occurring in acute hepatitis. The white blood cell count is often elevated and thrombocytopenia and fragmented red blood cells may be demonstrated. Features of hepatic dysfunction such as hypoalbuminemia, hypoglycemia, and coagulopathy occur in more severe cases.

The differential diagnosis of liver disease in pregnancy is wide, and the multisystemic effects of AFLP may resemble systemic lupus, TTP, or HUS (see Table 81.3).

The definitive treatment is delivery of the fetus, and early recognition of this condition is responsible for an improved outcome. Because the presentation is usually close to term, the decision is usually easy and carries little additional risk for the fetus. However, AFLP is associated with placental insufficiency because of fibrin deposition, producing increased fetal loss. It has been reported that this process may be exacerbated by therapeutic coagulation factor replacement. Supportive therapy is similar to that for other causes of fulminant hepatic failure including correction of coagulation abnormalities and hypoglycemia. Hepatic encephalopathy requires attention to airway protection, dietary protein restriction, bowel sterilization, and oral or rectal lactulose administration. Transient worsening of hepatic function may occur following delivery with improvement usually beginning within 2 to 3 days. A small subset of patients continue to deteriorate following delivery, and liver transplantation may be indicated. Complications such as hemorrhage, pancreatitis, renal failure, diabetes insipidus, and infection should be sought and treated.

AMNIOTIC FLUID EMBOLISM

Amniotic fluid embolism is a catastrophic cardiopulmonary complication of pregnancy, carrying a mortality rate of 10% to 86%.[34] It usually occurs in association with labor and delivery but may be precipitated by uterine trauma or manipulations. Amniotic fluid enters the venous circulation and particulate contents or humoral factors produce acute pulmonary hypertension, as well as acute left ventricular dysfunction.[35] The pregnant woman develops sudden onset of dyspnea, hypoxemia, and cardiovascular collapse. The presenting feature may sometimes be seizures related to cerebral hypoxia or acute fetal hypoxia and distress. Many patients with amniotic fluid embolism die within the first hour. No specific diagnostic test is available, and the diagnosis of amniotic fluid embolism is based on a typical clinical picture and exclusion of other conditions such as septic shock, pulmonary thromboembolism, abruptio placentae, tension pneumothorax, or a myocardial ischemic event.

Treatment involves routine resuscitative and supportive measures including mechanical ventilation and inotropic therapy. A role for corticosteroids has been suggested on the basis of the hypothesis that the process may involve an anaphylactoid reaction to amniotic fluid contents.[34]

Survivors of the initial process may develop disseminated intravascular coagulation (DIC) and ARDS. Neurologic damage caused by the initial hypotension and hypoxemia is common.

OBSTETRIC HEMORRHAGE

Uterine blood flow reaches 600 mL/minute near term, subjecting the pregnant patient to the risk of devastating blood loss. Antepartum hemorrhage occurs from disruption of the placenta, such as with placental abruption or a low-lying placenta (placenta previa) as the cervix dilates. Most hemorrhage occurs postpartum because of uterine atony, cervical or vaginal lacerations, or related to antepartum hemorrhage, or associated with coagulopathy. The pregnant woman is physiologically prepared for blood loss and tolerates the loss from a normal vaginal delivery (600 mL) or cesarean section (1000 mL). However, excessive blood loss will result in hypovolemic shock with compromise to fetus and vital organs. The pregnant woman is particularly susceptible to hypoperfusion injury to the kidney. A high incidence of myocardial ischemia has been noted in pregnant women with hemorrhagic shock.

Supportive management of obstetric hemorrhage is similar to that for any cause of hemorrhage and involves rapid volume replacement, supplemental oxygen administration, and red blood cell and blood product support for an associated dilutional coagulopathy. Various pharmacologic agents are utilized to control uterine bleeding. Intramuscular administration of methylergonovine (0.2 mg) may be useful in the presence of uterine atony but is contraindicated in the presence of hypertension.[36] Oxytocin is infused intravenously in a dose greater than that used for augmentation of labor, up to 100 mU/minute (e.g., 40 U in 1000 mL normal saline at 150 mL/hour). This dose may produce an antidiuretic effect and cause hyponatremia. A prostaglandin F_{2a} analog (carboprost tromethamine—Hemabate) given intramuscularly (0.25 mg, repeated every 15 to 90 minutes to maximum 2 mg) or intramyometrially, is effective in controlling hemorrhage.[36,37] Side effects include vomiting, hypertension, bronchoconstriction, and increased intrapulmonary shunt. Obstetricians are increasingly using intrauterine balloon devices to tamponade bleeding.[38] Antibiotic prophylaxis is often given while the balloon is in place and analgesia is essential.

Isolated reports suggest that recombinant factor VIIa may be useful in the management of severe obstetric hemorrhage.[39] If the above-mentioned methods fail to control bleeding, radiologic transcatheter embolization of the internal iliac or uterine artery is usually effective.[40] Surgical exploration with arterial ligation or hysterectomy may become necessary.

PERIPARTUM CARDIOMYOPATHY

Cardiac failure may occur in the absence of preexisting heart disease because of peripartum cardiomyopathy. This idiopathic condition presents in the last month of pregnancy or within 5 months of delivery, with an incidence of approximately 1 in 3500 live births.[41] The clinical presentation is usually after 36 weeks' gestation (in contrast to women with preexisting cardiac disease) and involves the gradual onset of symptoms of heart failure. The diagnosis is made by the demonstration of left ventricular systolic dysfunction and by the exclusion of other causes of cardiomyopathy. During labor and the early postpartum period, tachycardia and increased cardiac output may precipitate acute pulmonary edema.

Treatment is similar to other patients with cardiac failure, although angiotensin-converting enzyme (ACE) inhibitors should be avoided before delivery. Anticoagulation is essential because of the hypercoagulable state of pregnancy and the high incidence of thrombotic complications. A subset of patients may have an inflammatory myocarditis, and immunosuppressive therapy may be considered in those who do not improve after 2 weeks of standard treatment.[41] Although a high mortality rate has been described (10% to 50%), about half of patients recover normal ventricular function.[42]

TOCOLYTIC PULMONARY EDEMA

β-Adrenergic blockers can be used to inhibit uterine contractions in preterm labor, although this is less frequently used because studies have demonstrated a lack of fetal benefit from this practice. A complication of this β-agonist therapy in pregnancy is the development of acute pulmonary edema.[43] Treatment involves discontinuing the β-agonist and supportive treatment including diuresis and oxygen therapy. Failure of the pulmonary edema to resolve within 24 hours should prompt a search for an alternative diagnosis (Table 81.4).

GESTATIONAL TROPHOBLASTIC DISEASE

Pulmonary hypertension and pulmonary edema may occur in the setting of benign hydatidiform mole, as a result of trophoblastic pulmonary embolism. This most commonly occurs during evacuation of the uterus, with a higher incidence of pulmonary complications in the woman later in pregnancy.[44] With supportive treatment resolution occurs within 48 to 72 hours. Molar pregnancy may also be associated with choriocarcinoma, which can produce multiple, discrete, pulmonary metastases.

CONDITIONS NOT SPECIFIC TO PREGNANCY

SEPTIC SHOCK

Changes occur in the immune status in pregnant women, facilitating tolerance to paternally derived fetal antigens. An altered T_H1/T_H2 balance occurs, with the maternal immune response favoring humoral immunity (T_H2 response), and suppressing cell-mediated immunity (T_H1 response), which could be harmful to the fetus.[45] This altered immune response may predispose pregnant women to increased incidence or severity of certain infections, including *Listeria monocytogenes* infection, disseminated herpesvirus infections, varicella, and coccidioidomycosis infections. Human immunodeficiency virus infections should always be considered. Obstetric sepsis in the antepartum period produces chorioamnionitis, but most obstetric sepsis occurs in

Table 81.4 Differential Diagnosis of Acute Respiratory Distress in Pregnancy

Disorder	Distinguishing Features
Pregnancy-Specific	
Amniotic fluid embolism	Cardiorespiratory collapse, seizures, DIC
Pulmonary edema secondary to preeclampsia	Hypertension, proteinuria
ARDS secondary to obstetric sepsis	Evidence of obstetric sepsis, shock
Tocolytic pulmonary edema	Tocolytic administration, rapid improvement
Peripartum cardiomyopathy	Gradual onset, cardiac gallop, cardiomegaly
Trophoblastic embolism	Nodular infiltrate, molar pregnancy
Risk Increased by Pregnancy	
Aspiration pneumonitis	Vomiting, aspiration
Venous thromboembolism	Evidence of DVT, positive $\dot{V}/\dot{Q}$ scan, leg Doppler studies, CT angiogram
Pneumomediastinum	Occurs during delivery, subcutaneous emphysema
Valvular heart disease	Pulmonary edema, cardiac murmur, cardiomegaly
ARDS secondary to sepsis	Evidence of sepsis (e.g., pyelonephritis)
Unrelated to Pregnancy	
Asthma	Features similar to those in nonpregnant patient
Pneumonia	Features similar to those in nonpregnant patient

ARDS, acute respiratory distress syndrome; CT, computed tomography; DIC, disseminated intravascular coagulation; DVT, deep vein thrombosis; $\dot{V}/\dot{Q}$, ventilation-perfusion.

the postpartum period. The most common location of infection is the placental site, causing endometritis, which can spread to become a peritonitis. Episiotomy sites or cesarean section wounds may also become infected. Infections often involve a mixed flora, with microorganisms originating from the vagina (e.g., anaerobes, group B streptococci), intestine (gram-negative organisms, enterococci, anaerobes), sexual transmission (e.g., *Neisseria gonorrhoeae*), or hematogenous spread (e.g., *Listeria*, group A streptococci).[46]

Management of septic shock is similar to that in the nonpregnant patient, with prompt resuscitation with volume expansion. If inotropic therapy is necessary in the antepartum patient, the effects of such drugs on uteroplacental perfusion should be considered. Adequate specimens for culture should be obtained including amniocentesis in the antepartum patient. Ultrasonography may be valuable to identify a source of localized infection and exclude retained products of conception.

Initial empiric antibiotic therapy should provide broad gram-negative, gram-positive, and anaerobic cover. Common regimens use drugs such as ampicillin, gentamicin, and clindamycin; ampicillin/sulbactam; ticarcillin/clavulanate; piperacillin and gentamicin; or carbapenems.[47] Urgent delivery may be required for management of chorioamnionitis with sepsis syndrome.

A poor response to antibiotic therapy may indicate a resistant organism (e.g., *Enterococcus*), a localized abscess, myometrial microabscesses, or septic pelvic thrombophlebitis. Gas in the subcutaneous tissues or uterine wall suggests clostridial gas gangrene. Patients with retained products or devitalized tissue are at significant risk. Toxic shock caused by *Staphylococcus aureus* or *Clostridium sordelli* may occur, often associated with septic abortion. Surgical evacuation of the uterus or laparotomy with débridement or even hysterectomy may be required. Puerperal ovarian vein thrombophlebitis may complicate endometritis, presenting with acute deterioration with fever. The diagnosis can be confirmed with CT or magnetic resonance imaging scanning, and treatment requires anticoagulation and antibiotic therapy. Surgical intervention with venous ligation or excision may be required.

Group A streptococcal necrotizing fasciitis and toxic shock syndrome have been reported to occur unexpectedly following an uncomplicated pregnancy and delivery.[48] Management includes antibiotic therapy with penicillin and clindamycin and early surgical intervention. Intravenous immunoglobulin (2 g/kg) may be beneficial.

ACUTE RESPIRATORY DISTRESS SYNDROME IN PREGNANCY

The pregnant patient is at risk of developing acute lung injury from pregnancy-associated complications and other conditions (see Table 81.4).[49] The pregnant patient appears to be at increased risk of developing pulmonary edema because of the cardiovascular changes, the reduced albumin level occurring in pregnancy, increased capillary leak, and possibly an upregulation of components of the acute inflammatory response.

Management is similar to that in the nonpregnant patient. Adequate maternal oxygenation is essential for fetal well-being, and delivery may benefit both the mother and the fetus.[50] Survival from ARDS is as good as or better than that in the general population, likely because of these patients' young age, lack of comorbid conditions, and the reversibility of many of the predisposing conditions.

PULMONARY THROMBOEMBOLIC DISEASE

Pulmonary thromboembolism is a leading cause of maternal death. Although the risk is significantly increased in pregnant women because of increased coagulation factors, hormonally mediated venous stasis, and local pressure effects, the incidence is relatively low at about 1 per 1000 deliveries. Pulmonary embolism occurs most frequently in the early postpartum period.

Investigation of suspected pulmonary embolism is not different from that in the nonpregnant patient, with duplex ultrasound as the initial investigation. False positives may occur with Doppler alone because of venous obstruction by the gravid uterus. Ventilation-perfusion scanning and CT pulmonary angiography can be performed with low risk of fetal radiation exposure (see Table 81.2).[11]

Warfarin is generally avoided in pregnancy because of the risk of a first trimester embryopathy and central nervous system abnormalities with second- and third-trimester exposure. Heparin does not cross the placenta and can be readily reversed, and low-molecular-weight heparins are safe and effective in pregnancy although less easy to reverse acutely.[51] Thrombolysis has been used successfully in pregnancy but should be limited to life-threatening situations. Transvenous inferior vena caval filters have been used in the pregnant patient, although there is a risk of dislodgement because of venous dilation and pressure effects.

ASTHMA

The hormonal changes of pregnancy can affect asthma variably, with worsening, improvement, or no substantial change occurring. Asthma is a common condition, and acute asthmatic attacks are therefore an important cause of respiratory compromise in pregnancy. In assessment of the patient with a severe acute attack, the reduced $Paco_2$ occurring in late pregnancy should be considered; a normal $Paco_2$ level associated with acidosis may imply respiratory failure. Treatment is similar to the nonpregnant patient, including β-agonists and corticosteroids. Although there is a natural reluctance to prescribe drug therapy in these patients, pregnancy is not an absolute contraindication to systemic corticosteroid therapy.[52] Uncontrolled asthma is more dangerous to the fetus than appropriate drug therapy, and management should highlight the importance of adequate oxygenation.

CARDIAC DISEASE

Overt or occult preexisting heart disease may produce acute cardiac decompensation as the blood volume and cardiac output increase during pregnancy. Women with prior cardiac events, cyanotic disease, or pulmonary hypertension are at particular risk. Patients with mitral and aortic stenosis are at risk of developing hemodynamic deterioration as the physiologic changes peak at about 28 weeks, but mild to moderate regurgitant valvular disease is generally well tolerated.[53] The onset of atrial fibrillation or severe hypertension can precipitate sudden hemodynamic deterioration even in those women with less severe cardiac disease.

Patients with moderate to severe mitral stenosis are likely to experience hemodynamic deterioration during the third trimester or during labor. Treatment is similar to the nonpregnant patient using digoxin and beta blockers to control heart rate and diuretics to reduce left atrial pressure.[54] ACE inhibitors should be avoided. Most patients with mitral stenosis can undergo vaginal delivery with consideration to invasive hemodynamic monitoring during labor and the early postpartum period. Epidural anesthesia is usually better tolerated hemodynamically than general anesthesia during labor and delivery. Electrical cardioversion can be performed safely if indicated.

Severe aortic stenosis is associated with significant risk during pregnancy,[54] with symptoms such as dyspnea, angina, or syncope appearing from late in the second trimester. Percutaneous aortic balloon valvuloplasty can be performed during pregnancy. Spinal and epidural anesthesia during labor may adversely affect hemodynamics because of the vasodilatory effects.

Ischemic heart disease is uncommon in pregnancy but may be missed because of masking of the symptoms, signs, and cardiac enzyme levels by pregnancy. Coronary artery dissection may occur, particularly in the immediate postpartum period. Aortic dissection may occur related to hypertension, aortic coarctation, or Marfan syndrome and is associated with significant maternal and fetal death.[55]

Women with cyanotic congenital heart disease, particularly those with associated pulmonary hypertension, are at significant risk during pregnancy. Because of the inability of the right ventricle to tolerate the increases in cardiac output, primary or secondary pulmonary hypertension is associated with a high mortality rate in pregnancy.[56] New specific treatments are now available, and although clinical trials in pregnancy are lacking, mortality rate appears to be decreasing to some degree.[57] Vasodilators such as prostacyclin (inhaled or intravenous) or inhaled nitric oxide, as well as phosphodiesterase-5 inhibitors such as sildenafil, have been used successfully in pregnancy.[58,59] Endothelin receptor antagonists (e.g., bosentan) are avoided because of potential teratogenicity, and anticoagulation is recommended for most patients. Patients with pulmonary hypertension should be managed in a center with expertise and experience in this area.

TRAUMA

The anatomic and physiologic changes of pregnancy may alter the manifestations and severity of traumatic injury. Uterine injury can produce severe hemorrhage because of the high uterine blood flow and may precipitate placental abruption or rarely uterine rupture. Uterine rupture manifests with maternal shock, abdominal pain, and palpable fetal parts. Penetrating injury to the abdomen predominantly affects the uterus in later pregnancy, but because intra-abdominal viscera are compressed in the upper abdomen, minor injury may result in significant damage.[60] Fractures of the pelvis can produce severe retroperitoneal hemorrhage because of dilation of pelvic veins.

Maternal trauma is associated with a significant increase in fetal loss, due to maternal shock or hypoxia, placental injury, or direct fetal injury.[61] Direct fetal injury resulting from blunt trauma usually involves head injury related to maternal pelvic fracture. Other fetal injuries may occur following blunt or penetrating trauma, sometimes with minimal maternal injury. A high fetal mortality rate occurs in the presence of maternal burns to greater than 30% of the body surface area. Placental abruption is an important cause of fetal demise,[60] and may present with vaginal bleeding, abdominal cramps, uterine tenderness, amniotic fluid leakage, and unexplained fetal distress or maternal hypovolemia. Placental abruption is often complicated by DIC due to release of thromboplastin into the maternal circulation.

Evaluation of the pregnant trauma patient should include a detailed abdominal examination, but physical signs may be affected by changing organ position and the reduced peritoneal sensitivity that occurs in pregnancy.[62] Initial investigations should include blood type including Rh status. Ultrasound is useful for evaluation of the fetus for injury and biophysical profile and to assess intra-abdominal organ damage. Ultrasound-guided paracentesis or diagnostic peritoneal lavage (by open technique, above the uterus) may aid in detecting bowel perforation or intraperitoneal hemorrhage. Transplacental hemorrhage of fetal blood into the maternal circulation may occur and can result in fetal exsanguination and maternal Rh sensitization. Fetomaternal hemorrhage is detected by the Kleihauer-Betke test, which identifies fetal cells in the maternal blood smear, and can estimate the volume of fetal hemorrhage by the percentage of red blood cells of fetal origin. Fetal evaluation includes heart rate assessment by auscultation (possible from 20 weeks) or Doppler probe. Obstetric consultation and continuous fetal cardiotocography are important when the fetus is at a viable gestation.

Care of the severely injured pregnant patient requires a multidisciplinary approach involving the emergency physician, trauma surgeon, obstetrician, intensivist, and neonatologist. Initial resuscitation follows usual principles with efforts directed primarily at stabilizing the mother. Fluid replacement may need to be given more rapidly than in nonpregnant women because of the physiologic increase in plasma volume, and maternal blood pressure and heart rate may not be reliable predictors of the degree of hemorrhage.[62] Left lateral positioning to prevent supine hypotensive syndrome is an important consideration in the hypotensive patient. Rh-negative mothers with abdominal trauma should receive Rh immune globulin even in the presence of a negative Kleihauer-Betke test. Higher doses of Rh immune globulin will be necessary in the presence of significant fetomaternal hemorrhage.

In the unstable mother, management of maternal injuries takes precedence over fetal distress because correction of maternal hemodynamics is beneficial to the fetus. The fetus is extremely vulnerable to hypotension and hypoxemia, and uterine blood flow will be markedly reduced when maternal circulation is compromised. If the mother is stable, cesarean section may be appropriate if the fetus is considered viable, the limits of viability being largely dependent on the level of neonatal care available.

KEY POINTS

- The reduced FRC and increased oxygen consumption in pregnancy result in rapid oxygen desaturation during apnea or intubation.
- Although there is a risk to the fetus from radiologic procedures and drug therapy, necessary investigations and treatment should not be withheld, with appropriate precautions.

KEY POINTS (Continued)

- The various pregnancy-specific conditions should be considered in the differential diagnosis of a critically ill pregnant woman including preeclampsia, HELLP syndrome, acute fatty liver of pregnancy, and amniotic fluid embolism.
- Hypotension may occur in the supine position in late pregnancy because of aortocaval compression—the clinician should position the hypotensive pregnant patient in the left lateral position.
- Management of preeclampsia, the commonest cause of ICU admission, involves delivery of the fetus, seizure prophylaxis with magnesium sulfate, correction of fluid balance, and treatment of hypertension if clinically significant.

SELECTED REFERENCES

1. Elkus R, Popovich J: Respiratory physiology in pregnancy. Clin Chest Med 1992;13:555-565.
10. Kinsella SM, Lohmann G: Supine hypotensive syndrome. Obstet Gynecol 1994;83:774-788.
11. Ratnapalan S, Bentur Y, Koren G: "Doctor, will that x-ray harm my unborn child?" CMAJ 2008;179:1293-1296.
23. Vanden Hoek TL, Morrison LJ, Shuster M, et al: Part 12: Cardiac arrest in special situations: 2010 American Heart Association Guidelines for Cardiopulmonary Resuscitation and Emergency Cardiovascular Care. Circulation 2010;122:S829-S861.
34. Conde-Agudelo A, Romero R: Amniotic fluid embolism: An evidence-based review. Am J Obstet Gynecol 2009;201:445.
38. Georgiou C: Balloon tamponade in the management of postpartum haemorrhage: A review. Br J Gynaecol 2009;116:748.
51. Shannon M, Bates SM, Greer IA, et al: VTE, thrombophilia, antithrombotic therapy, and pregnancy: Antithrombotic therapy and prevention of thrombosis, 9th ed. American College of Chest Physicians Evidence-Based Clinical Practice Guidelines. Chest 2012;141(2 Suppl):e691S-e736S.
57. Bédard E, Dimopoulos K, Gatzoulis MA: Has there been any progress made on pregnancy outcomes among women with pulmonary arterial hypertension? Eur Heart J 2009;30:256-265.

The complete list of references can be found at www.expertconsult.com.

Nutrition Support

82

Richard G. Barton

CHAPTER OUTLINE

MALNUTRITION

Malnutrition is a disorder in body composition in which inadequate macronutrient (protein, carbohydrate, and fat) or micronutrient (vitamins, minerals, and trace elements) intake results in decreased body mass, reduced organ mass, and most important, decreased organ function. Although malnutrition is most frequently associated with a risk for immune dysfunction-related infection, wound healing/fascial dehiscence, and breakdown of surgical anastomoses, it can affect virtually all organ systems when severe. Skeletal muscle wasting, decreased myocardial mass, diastolic cardiac dysfunction and decreased sensitivity to inotropic agents, respiratory insufficiency/need for prolonged mechanical ventilation, renal cortical atrophy, and loss of gastrointestinal absorptive/barrier functions have all been associated with malnutrition.

Malnutrition can occur as a result of combined protein-calorie deficiency (marasmus), predominantly protein deficiency (kwashiorkor), and deficiencies in specific micronutrients, as well as altered metabolism arising from a disease state such as sepsis, burns, or trauma. Critically ill patients may suffer from a combination of these causes. Malnutrition is thought to be present in as many as 25% to 50% of patients on hospital admission and may affect an additional 25% to 30% of patients during their hospital stay. The National Surgical Quality Improvement Program (NSQIP) has shown preoperative serum albumin, a measure of chronic nutritional status, to be an independent predictor of mortality risk in a study of more than 400,000 surgical patients and specifically in patients undergoing colectomy, proctectomy, transurethral resection of bladder tumors, and major lung resection.[1-4] Malnutrition becomes particularly important in critically ill patients, in whom the combination of bed rest and catabolic illnesses such as sepsis, multiple trauma, burns, pancreatitis, and acute respiratory distress syndrome (ARDS) hasten the malnutrition, loss of lean body mass, and organ system dysfunction.

The purpose of this chapter is to contrast starvation and stress metabolism with emphasis on protein, carbohydrate, and fat metabolism; review the basic concepts of nutrition support with regard to energy and substrate requirements; discuss routes of nutrition support; provide an overview of organ-specific nutrition and immunonutrition; briefly summarize nutritional assessment and monitoring; and discuss the complications of nutrition support and their prevention.

STARVATION VERSUS STRESS METABOLISM

Starvation is a clinical situation that develops whenever nutrient supply is inadequate to meet nutrient demand. It is characterized by a specific metabolic adaptive response aimed at preserving lean body mass, as well as by decreased energy expenditure, utilization of alternative fuel sources, and reduced protein wasting. During the initial 12 to 24 hours of starvation, glycogen is the primary oxidative fuel source. Thereafter, gluconeogenesis increases temporarily and glucose synthesized from amino acids becomes the primary fuel source for the production of "obligate" glucose for use by tissues such as the brain and, to some degree, the liver and skeletal muscle. Over time, gluconeogenesis decreases as these organs adapt to ketone bodies as the primary oxidative fuel source, and in the fully adapted starved state, fatty acids, ketones, and glycerol become the primary fuel source in all tissues except the brain and red blood cells. The respiratory quotient (i.e., the ratio of carbon dioxide produced to oxygen consumed) is 0.6 to 0.7 as a result of the use of fat as the primary fuel source. Ultimately, rates of net protein catabolism and ureagenesis are decreased, relative to the fed state, during starvation. From a clinical perspective, it is important to understand that the metabolic response to starvation is reversible with feeding.

Stress metabolism is a generalized response whereby energy and substrate are mobilized to support inflammation, immune function, and tissue repair. It occurs in response to a variety of stimuli such as sepsis, multiple trauma, burns, pancreatitis, bone marrow transplantation, and major surgery. This mobilization of energy and substrate occurs at the expense of lean body mass. It is driven by endocrine hormones such as cortisol, glucagon, and catecholamines, as well as by a multitude of inflammatory mediators. The stress response is often related to some degree of perfusion deficit (shock) and resultant microcirculatory injury. Clinically, the response is characterized by increased energy expenditure and increased oxygen consumption. The stress response is further characterized by hyperglycemia, elevated lactate, and increased urinary nitrogen excretion. The respiratory quotient is often elevated in the range of 0.80 to 0.95 as a result of the use of a mixed oxidative fuel source. Loss of lean body mass occurs more rapidly than with simple starvation because skeletal muscle protein stores become the "fuel" for the stress response. Most important, the malnutrition associated with stress metabolism is less responsive to nutrition support than is starvation metabolism. Reversal of stress-associated malnutrition is dependent not only on the provision of adequate nutrients but also on elimination of the underlying stress response (i.e., control of infection, stabilization of fractures, grafting of burns, or resolution of the inflammatory state). Starvation and stress metabolism are summarized in Table 82.1.

Table 82.1 Starvation Versus Stress Hypermetabolism

Characteristic	Starvation	Hypermetabolism
Energy expenditure	Decreased	Increased
Respiratory quotient	Low (0.7)	High (0.85)
Response to feeding	+++	+
Mediator activation	+	+++
Primary fuels	Fat	Mixed
Gluconeogenesis	+	+++
Proteolysis	+	+++
Protein synthesis	+	++
Ureagenesis/urinary urea nitrogen	+	+++
Ketone formation	++++	+

CARBOHYDRATE METABOLISM IN CRITICAL ILLNESS

Carbohydrate metabolism in critical illness is characterized clinically by hyperglycemia, often described as being due to "insulin resistance" based on increased blood glucose levels in the presence of high circulating levels of insulin. In fact, cellular glucose uptake and oxidation in the critically ill are increased,[5-7] and hyperglycemia is associated with increased glucose production, decreased insulin-mediated glucose uptake, and increased non–insulin-mediated glucose uptake.[5,8]

Glucose production is increased primarily by increased hepatic gluconeogenesis, to a lesser extent by renal gluconeogenesis,[9] and by increased glycogenolysis. Increased glucose production occurs under the influence of glucagon, catecholamines, and cortisol, with glucagon being the most important stimulant of hepatic gluconeogenesis and epinephrine being the primary stimulant of glycogenolysis.[10,11] The hormonal changes observed in critical illness appear to be mediated by cytokines in both the central nervous system and peripheral tissues. Interleukin 1 (IL-1) stimulates the release of adrenocorticotropic hormone, which in turn favors the release of cortisol and glucagon, and tumor necrosis factor (TNF) stimulates increased secretion of glucagon.[12] Gluconeogenic substrates include lactate and alanine, as well as glutamine, glycine, serine, and glycerol. The amino acids used for gluconeogenesis are derived largely from proteolysis in skeletal muscle.

Glucose uptake into cells is regulated by a process of facilitated transport in which a carrier protein promotes the movement of glucose across the cell membrane down its concentration gradient. Three isoforms of this glucose carrier protein (glucose transporter 1 [GLUT-1], GLUT-2, and GLUT-4) are thought to be important in glucose transport.[13] Non–insulin-mediated glucose uptake is dependent on the GLUT-1 isoform, whereas insulin-mediated glucose transport is dependent on the GLUT-4 isoform. During stress, total body glucose uptake is increased, but largely via non–insulin-mediated pathways.[8] Non–insulin-mediated glucose uptake is particularly important in the central nervous system and in tissues rich in macrophages and neutrophils (e.g., lung, liver, intestine, spleen, wound), which use glucose for energy and in the process generate the respiratory burst.[14] Inflammatory cytokines may promote the uptake of glucose by increasing the synthesis, plasma membrane concentration, or activity of the glucose transporter.[15,16] Insulin-mediated glucose transport is suppressed in the liver, heart, and skeletal muscle.[17,18] Hepatic insulin resistance is characterized by elevated circulating levels of insulin-like growth factor-binding protein-1.[17,18] The mechanisms of insulin resistance are incompletely understood, although proinflammatory cytokines may alter insulin receptor signaling.[14,19,20]

The net result of these alterations in carbohydrate metabolism in critical illness is hyperglycemia inasmuch as the liver seems to be unresponsive to high levels of circulating insulin and glucose and continues to synthesize glucose via gluconeogenesis. In other tissues, non–insulin-mediated glucose uptake is enhanced and results in increased glycolytic oxidation to pyruvate and a stoichiometric rise in lactate.[5,6] Although hyperlactatemia is usually thought of as being reflective of anaerobic metabolism, it can be indicative of glycolytic flux and the level of metabolic stress when observed in conjunction with elevated pyruvate.[5]

FAT METABOLISM IN CRITICAL ILLNESS

In both starvation and stress metabolism, fat metabolism is characterized by increased lipolysis and decreased lipogenesis as fat stores are mobilized for energy. In the stressed state there is a marked increase in lipolytic activity in adipose tissue as a result of catecholamine-mediated stimulation of β_2-receptors; cytokines may also participate in this process.[21,22] Fatty acids are released from adipose tissue in quantities that exceed the amount oxidized, and approximately half of these fatty acids are re-esterified in the liver.[23] In this triglyceride–fatty acid cycle, triglycerides and fatty acids are shunted back and forth between the liver and adipose tissue in an apparently futile pathway.[24]

Stress fat metabolism is further characterized by increased oxidation of fatty acids of all chain lengths and decreased plasma levels of medium- and long-chain essential fatty acids relative to the quantities of oleic acid. The latter may reflect preferential oxidation of essential fatty acids, suppressed mobilization because of hyperinsulinemia, or conversion of ω-6 fatty acids to inflammatory mediators.

Hypertriglyceridemia is common in critically ill patients, particularly in the presence of multiple organ dysfunction, and results from the combination of increased hepatic triglyceride production and decreased clearance.[25,26] Hepatic steatosis has classically been attributed to overfeeding because triglycerides are constructed from fatty acids synthesized from excess carbohydrate. This theory has been called into question inasmuch as a substantial proportion of hepatic triglyceride may be synthesized from recycled fatty acids rather than from fatty acids synthesized de novo from carbohydrate.[27] It is possible that fatty infiltration of the liver reflects a cytokine-mediated defect in triglyceride secretion that represents an organ-specific response to critical illness rather than an adverse effect of carbohydrate overfeeding.[28,29] Regardless of the immediate source of the fatty acids used in triglyceride synthesis, experience suggests that clinically apparent fatty infiltration of the liver can be prevented by avoiding overfeeding.

Ketonemia is common in starvation, whereas ketogenesis is decreased in stress metabolism.[30] Acetoacetate continues to be used as an oxidative fuel source, although the reduction of β-hydroxybutyrate to acetoacetate is impaired.[31] With the development of multiple organ dysfunction, there is a progressive decrease in the acetoacetate/β-hydroxybutyrate ratio.[32] This alteration in hepatic redox potential reflects a disturbance in the cellular energy charge that may be associated with hepatic mitochondrial damage by toxic oxygen radicals and other inflammatory mediators.[33]

PROTEIN METABOLISM IN CRITICAL ILLNESS

Protein synthesis is increased in the stressed state relative to that seen in starvation. Protein breakdown is markedly increased in comparison to the synthetic rate, thereby resulting in net protein catabolism and a rapid decrease in lean body mass.[30] There is a net efflux of amino acids from skeletal muscle as protein breakdown via the ubiquitin-proteosome pathway of protein degradation is accelerated by catecholamines, cortisol, and cytokines.[34-37] Amino acid uptake by skeletal muscle is impaired despite excess amino acids circulating in the bloodstream early in the course of stress metabolism; the situation deteriorates further as plasma concentrations of specific amino acids such as leucine begin to fall.[38] Decreased plasma glutamine is known to have deleterious effects on immune function and gastrointestinal barrier function.[39,40] Although it has long been thought that the accelerated protein catabolism associated with critical illness is unresponsive to the provision of amino acids or other fuel sources, the fact that muscle amino acid uptake is in part compromised by decreased plasma levels of specific amino acids suggests the possibility that protein catabolism during stress may be attenuated with the provision of appropriate nutrition support.[41]

Amino acids mobilized from skeletal muscle are redistributed to other areas of the body to support immune function, wound healing, and tissue repair, as well as for the hepatic synthesis of acute-phase proteins, presumably in an attempt to enhance survival. It has recently been demonstrated that endotoxemia induces significant increases in protein synthesis in the liver, spleen, kidney, jejunum, diaphragm, lung, and skin at the expense of skeletal muscle catabolism.[42] Amino acids such as alanine, glutamine, glycine, and serine are used as gluconeogenic substrate, and branched-chain amino acids (leucine, isoleucine, and valine) can be used as an oxidative fuel source, particularly in skeletal muscle. The net result of stress protein metabolism is a rapid decrease in lean body mass that exceeds that associated with bed rest or simple starvation, along with increased ureagenesis, azotemia, and increased urinary nitrogen excretion.

INDICATIONS FOR NUTRITION SUPPORT

Nutrition support should be considered once hemorrhage has been controlled, devitalized tissue débrided, fractures stabilized, and the patient resuscitated from shock. Limited data are available regarding the appropriate timing for the institution of nutrition support, although there are suggestions in the literature that early enteral feeding, within 24 to 72 hours of admission, may help decrease postburn and postinjury hypermetabolism and reduce infectious complications. In general, nutrition support should be initiated in any patient who is malnourished on admission to the intensive care unit (ICU), for any patient who is likely to become malnourished during a long and complicated ICU stay, and for any patient who has not eaten for 5 to 7 days.

GOALS OF NUTRITION SUPPORT

The goals of nutrition support in a critically ill patient are to minimize the effects of starvation to provide appropriate doses of macronutrients and micronutrients, to modulate the metabolic processes of the disease, to minimize complications of nutrition support, and to improve outcomes. More specifically, the goals of nutrition support in the critically ill or injured are to provide sufficient calories to meet the energy requirements of the hypermetabolic state while avoiding the complications associated with overfeeding, provide sufficient protein to attain nitrogen balance or minimize the nitrogen deficit, provide electrolytes to maintain normal levels while taking into account excessive losses or impaired excretion, and provide appropriate vitamins and trace elements with consideration of disease-specific requirements.

NUTRITION SUPPORT IN CRITICAL ILLNESS

CALORIES

In any metabolic state, energy requirements must be met to minimize the use of stored energy reserves and to decrease the loss of lean body mass. In the setting of adapted starvation, the protein-sparing effect of an adequate caloric intake is well recognized; however, in the stressed state, protein catabolism is only partially responsive to caloric intake and continues to a significant degree regardless of caloric intake.[30,41] Overfeeding is of particular concern in a critically ill patient because it can result in excess carbon dioxide production and ventilator dependence,[43] lipogenesis and fatty infiltration of the liver,[44-46] and hyperglycemia with its attendant hyperosmolar and infectious complications.[14,47-49]

The daily caloric requirement depends on total energy expenditure (TEE), which is the sum of basal energy expenditure (BEE), diet-induced thermogenesis (DIT), and activity energy expenditure (AEE). BEE is the caloric expenditure of a person in the recumbent position who has fasted for at least 10 hours. DIT is the energy expended to perform all aspects of food consumption, including eating and hydrolysis and absorption of nutrients, and may account for 15% to 40% of TEE. Resting energy expenditure (REE) is the energy expenditure of a recumbent person who is not fasting and is the sum of BEE and DIT. These relationships can be expressed by the following equations:

$$\text{REE} = \text{BEE} + \text{DIT}$$

$$\text{TEE} = \text{REE} + \text{AEE}$$

Caloric requirement can be estimated by using a number of formulas or can be measured with indirect calorimetry. Most commonly, BEE is estimated with the Harris-Benedict equations, which are based on sex, age, height, and weight and then multiplied by stress and activity factors to estimate caloric requirement. The Harris-Benedict equations are as follows:

For males:

$$\text{BEE} = 66.42 + (13.75 \times \text{Wt [kg]}) + (5.0 \times \text{Ht [cm]}) - (6.77 \times \text{Age [yr]})$$

For females:

$$\text{BEE} = 655.10 + (9.65 \times \text{Wt [kg]}) + 1.85 \times \text{Ht [cm]}) - (4.68 \times \text{Age [yr]})$$

Classically, REE is then estimated by multiplying the calculated BEE by a stress factor ranging from 1.0 in a stable, mechanically ventilated patient to 2.0 in a patient with a 50% total body surface area burn. Stress factors for patients with multiple trauma or sepsis fall somewhere between the two extremes. TEE is estimated by multiplying REE by an activity factor of 1.2 to 1.3 for ambulatory patients. The caloric requirement is decreased to varying degrees (6% to 30%) in mechanically ventilated patients receiving narcotics or sedatives and is reduced by as much as 33% in chemically paralyzed patients.[50] In nonventilated postoperative patients or in patients with decreased lung compliance, energy expenditure related to the work of breathing may increase. Although estimation of energy expenditure is relatively accurate in healthy people, it is much less reliable in critically ill patients because of the heterogeneity of the metabolic response and variations in sedation, work of breathing, and physical activity. Most critically ill patients should receive calories to supply 100% to 120% of calculated BEE. Estimation of energy expenditure in obese patients is particularly difficult. If indirect calorimetry is unavailable, the provision of calories should be based upon body mass index (BMI) and ideal body weight rather than on obesity adjusted body weight.[51]

Indirect calorimetry can be used to measure REE and does not require the addition of estimated stress factors. REE is based on measured oxygen consumption and carbon dioxide production and is calculated according to the Weir equation:

$$\text{REE} = (3.94 \times \dot{V}O_2) + (1.1 \times (\dot{V}CO_2)$$

where VO_2 = oxygen consumption and VCO_2 = carbon dioxide production.

Even when not used routinely, indirect calorimetry can still be helpful in assessing the energy needs of obese patients, to rule out overfeeding in patients with seemingly excessive ventilatory demands, in severely malnourished patients, and in patients with apparently high levels of metabolic stress.

In general, critically ill patients should receive 25 to 30 kcal/kg/day, with sedated mechanically ventilated patients receiving closer to 25 kcal/kg/day. Chemically paralyzed patients generally require 20 kcal/kg/day.[52] In obese patients, hypocaloric feeding may induce some degree of weight loss and improve insulin sensitivity and may decrease ventilator days and length of ICU stay.[52] In patients with a BMI greater than 30, calories should not exceed 60% to 70% of target energy requirements or 11 to 14 kcal/kg actual body weight per day or 22 to 25 kcal/kg ideal body weight per day.[51]

CARBOHYDRATE

Carbohydrate is usually the primary source of calories in human beings. The maximal rate of glucose oxidation is approximately 5 mg/kg/minute, or 7.2 g/kg/day.[53] In stressed patients, part of this maximally tolerated glucose load will be provided by glucose synthesized endogenously from amino acids via gluconeogenesis. In a severely hypermetabolic patient, gluconeogenesis may provide as much as 4 mg/kg/minute of glucose[54] and result in significant hyperglycemia when large exogenous glucose loads are administered. Insulin tends to be ineffective in controlling this hyperglycemia, in part because glucose oxidation may already be maximal, endogenous insulin levels are already high, and insulin-mediated glucose uptake in the liver and

Table 82.2 Nutrition Support in a Hypermetabolic Patient

Nutrient	General Recommendation
Total calories	25-30 kcal/kg/day OR BEE × 1.2-2.0 OR REE by IDC
Glucose	5 g/kg/day OR 20 kcal/kg/day OR 60-70% of calories
Fat	15-40% of calories OR Less than 1 g/kg/day
Amino acids or protein	1.2-2.0 g/kg/day
Trace elements and vitamins	RDA
Electrolytes	Maintain normal levels

BEE, basal energy expenditure; IDC, indirect calorimetry; RDA, recommended dietary allowance; REE, resting energy expenditure.

other tissues is suppressed in a septic and hypermetabolic patient.[17,18] Complications of excess glucose administration include hyperglycemia and its attendant hyperosmolar/infectious complications, excess carbon dioxide production and ventilator dependence, and hepatic steatosis. In general, glucose should initially be provided at a rate of 5 g/kg/day or approximately 20 kcal/kg/day. Carbohydrate should generally constitute 60% to 70% of nonprotein calories in a hypermetabolic patient (Table 82.2).

FAT

In a hypermetabolic patient, fat should constitute 15% to 40% of daily caloric intake, both to prevent essential fatty acid deficiency and to meet caloric needs in the face of a fixed capacity to oxidize glucose. In the starved state, as little as 2% to 5% of calories can be provided as fat, primarily to prevent essential fatty acid deficiency. Substituting lipid calories for carbohydrate calories can reduce carbon dioxide production, although avoiding excess calories in general is probably most important in minimizing carbon dioxide production and ventilator dependence. Complications of excess lipid administration, particularly when given parenterally, include hyperlipemia, immunosuppression, and hypoxemia as a result of both impaired oxygen diffusion and ventilation-perfusion mismatching. In general, a hypermetabolic patient should receive 15% to 40% of calories as fat, not to exceed 1.0 to 1.5 g/kg/day (see Table 82.2).[55]

PROTEIN

Protein needs in a hypermetabolic patient are increased in comparison to those in a patient with simple starvation. Protein catabolism in a stressed patient has long been thought to be unresponsive to protein or amino acid administration or glucose infusion,[56] and attainment of nitrogen balance is thought to depend largely on the support of stress protein synthesis.[41] However, recent evidence suggests that protein catabolism may be attenuated by the provision of appropriate nutrition support.[42] Regardless of the specific mechanisms involved, lean body mass decreases during catabolic illness because of bed rest and inactivity. Amino acids are redistributed from skeletal muscle to support hepatic protein synthesis, the cellular inflammatory response, and gluconeogenesis and are used as oxidative fuel sources. The critically ill or injured patient may require 1.2 to 2.0 g/kg/day to promote nitrogen balance or at least minimize the nitrogen deficit. With the exceptions noted later, the provision of more than 2.0 g/kg/day of protein rarely promotes nitrogen balance and usually results simply in increased urinary nitrogen excretion (see Table 82.2).

To meet the protein requirements of the stressed state and at the same time avoid excess calories and the attendant complications, an injured or septic patient may require nutrition support with a nonprotein calorie-to-nitrogen ratio of 80:1 or 100:1, as compared with a patient with starvation metabolism, who may tolerate a nonprotein calorie-to-nitrogen ratio of 150:1 or higher. The higher protein needs of a patient with catabolic illness can be met with custom-compounded total parenteral nutrition (TPN) or with numerous commercially available enteral formulas specifically designed for such patients (Table 82.3).

In summary, most critically ill patients should receive 1.2 to 2.0 g/kg/day of protein. Obese patients with BMI 30 to 40 should receive at least 2.0 g/kg/day of protein and patients with BMI greater than 40 should receive at least 2.5 g/kg/day in conjunction with hypocaloric feeding.[51] Critically ill patients with renal failure should generally receive 1.25 to 1.75 g/kg/day and those requiring continuous renal replacement therapy (CRRT) may require up to 2.5 g/kg/day.[51]

ELECTROLYTES, VITAMINS, AND TRACE ELEMENTS

Fluid and electrolytes should be provided to maintain adequate urine output and normal serum electrolyte levels. Typical daily electrolyte requirements include sodium 60 to 100 mEq/day, potassium 60 to 100 mEq/day, magnesium 10 to 20 mEq/day, calcium 10 to 15 mEq/day, chloride 80 to 120 mEq/day, and phosphorus 20 to 30 mmol/day.[57] Intravenous amino acid formulations contain acetate, but additional acetate can be added in the setting of metabolic acidosis. Particular attention should be paid to the intracellular electrolytes (potassium, phosphorus, and magnesium), which are required for attainment of nitrogen balance[58] and serum levels of which can fall precipitously when nutrition support is initiated.

The requirements for vitamins and trace elements in critical illness are largely unknown, and in general the recommended dietary allowance (RDA) for both should be provided. Antioxidant vitamins (including vitamins E and ascorbic acid) and trace minerals (including zinc, copper, and particularly selenium) may improve outcome in burns, in trauma, and in critically ill patients requiring mechanical

Table 82.3 Enteral Nutrition Formulas

Type	General Information	Sample Formulas	Concentration (kcal/mL)	Osmolality	Nonprotein Calorie: Nitrogen Ratio	Protein (g/1000 kcal)	Carbohydrate (% kcal)	Fat (% kcal)
Intact Protein								
Standard	Some may be taken by mouth; generally lactose-free, low-residue, and isotonic	Ensure	1.5	525	125:1	41.8	54.3	29
		Osmolite	1.06	300	153:1	35	57	29
		Isosource	1.2	490	149:1	44.2	57	29
		Nutren	1.5	510	131:1	40	45	39
High protein	Similar to above formulas except contain >45 g protein/L	Replete	1.0	300-350	75:1	62.4	45	30
		TraumaCal	1.5	560	91:1	54.7	38	40
		Isosource VHN	1.0	300	77:1	62	50	25
		Promote	1.0	340	75:1	62.5	52	23
Fluid concentrated	Calorically dense (1.5-2.0 kcal/mL), lactose free, moderate-to-high osmolality	Nutren 2.0	2.0	745	131:1	40	39	45
		Deliver 2.0	2.0	640	144:1	37.5	40	45
		TwoCal HN	2.0	690	125.1	41.8	43.2	40.1
Immunity-enhancing	May contain fiber, MCT, fish oil, added vitamins/minerals; 22-25% protein	Immun-Aid	1.0	460	53:1	80	48	20
		Impact	1.0	375	71:1	56	53	25
		Impact with Glutamine	1.3	630	64:1	60	46	30
		Perative	1.3	385	97:1	52.1	54.5	25
Diabetic	33-40% carbohydrate, contains fiber, standard to high protein	DiabetiSource	1.0	360	100:1	50	36	44
		ReSource Diabetic	1.06	300-320	79:1	59.4	36	40
		Glucerna	1.0	355	125:1	41.8	34.3	49
		Glytrol	1.0	380	114:1	45	40	42
Hepatic	High BCAAs, 1.2-1.5 kcal/mL	NutriHep Diet	1.5	690	209:1	26.7	77	12
		Hepatic-Aid II	1.2	560	148:1	36.8	57.3	27.7
Pulmonary	40%-55% fat, lactose free	NutriVent	1.5	330-450	116:1	45	55	55
		NovaSource	1.5	650	102:1	50.1	40	40
		Respalor	1.5	400	102:1	50	40	40
		Oxepa	1.5	493	125:1	41.6	28.1	55.2
		Pulmocare	1.5	475	125:1	41.7	28.2	55.1
Renal	2 kcal/mL, low to standard protein, low to no electrolytes	Renalcal	2.0	600	338:1	17.2	58.1	35
		Suplena	2.0	600	393:1	15	51	43
		Magnacal Renal	2.0	570	180:1	37.5	40	45
		NovaSource	2.0	700-960	140:1	37	40	45
Hydrolyzed Protein								
Immunity-enhancing	Standard to high protein, may have added vitamins/minerals or amino acids	Crucial	1.5	490	67:1	62.7	36	39
		Criticare HN	1.06	650	149:1	35.8	81.5	4.5
		AlitraQ	1.0	575	94:1	52.5	65.7	13.2
GI-compromised	Mix of peptides and amino acids, >40% fat as MCT	Peptamen	1.0	270-380	131:1	40	51	33
		Peptamen VHP	1.0	300-430	75:1	62.5	42	33
		Reabilan	1.0	350	175:1	31.5	52.5	35
		Reabilan HN	1.33	490	117:1	43.8	47.5	35
		SandoSource Peptide	1.0	490	100:1	50	65	15
		Vital HB	1.0	500	125:1	41.7	73.8	9.5
Crystalline amino acids	Powdered form, 8-18% protein, <6% fat	Vivonex T.E.N.	1.0	630	149:1	38	82	3
		Vivonex Plus	1.0	650	115:1	45	76	6

BCAAs, branched-chain amino acids; GI, gastrointestinal; MCT, medium-chain triglyceride.

ventilation[59] and should be provided to all critically ill patients receiving specialized nutrition support.[51] Patients with prolonged diarrhea or large burns or those undergoing dialysis have increased trace element loss and vitamin requirements, and deficiencies can develop if intake is inadequate. Initial limitation of trace elements should be considered in patients with renal failure. Routine supplementation of vitamins is necessary in patients receiving TPN. Typically, one ampule of a standard multivitamin preparation is added to TPN daily. Vitamin K, which is light sensitive, must be added separately in a light-impermeable bag or given by another route once or twice weekly. Excessive doses of vitamin C should be avoided in renal failure because of the accumulation of oxalate. Vitamin A accumulates and should not be supplemented beyond the RDA.[60]

ROUTE AND TIMING OF ADMINISTRATION

Nutrition support can be delivered enterally (via the gastrointestinal tract) or parenterally (via the intravenous route). The preferred route has been the subject of considerable controversy during the past 40 years.

Both routes have advantages and disadvantages, and nitrogen balance can be achieved by either route. TPN does not require an intact or functioning gastrointestinal tract, it is convenient to use, and its use virtually guarantees that the nutrients prescribed will be administered and that these nutrients will appear in the bloodstream. Disadvantages of parenteral nutrition include cost, procedure (central venous catheter)-related complications, an increased likelihood of metabolic complications, including hyperglycemia, and an increased risk of infectious complications. Enteral nutrition is much less expensive, is more physiologic, is associated with fewer metabolic complications such as electrolyte abnormalities and hyperglycemia, and stimulates gut function and preserves mucosal integrity and barrier function better than parenteral nutrition does. Disadvantages of enteral nutrition include the requirement for an intact and functioning gastrointestinal tract, procedure (feeding tube placement)-related complications, pulmonary aspiration, malabsorption, feeding intolerance (pain, vomiting, bloating, diarrhea), and as a result, an inability to deliver the entire nutrient prescription.

The gastrointestinal tract is a major interface between the host and the environment and not only regulates the ingestion and absorption of nutrients but is also responsible for defending the host against noxious microorganisms and toxins.[61] Malnutrition impairs gastrointestinal barrier function,[62] as does the lack of luminal nutrients independent of general nutritional status.[63,64] Enteral nutrition has been shown to promote mucosal growth, improve absorptive capacity, alter digestive enzyme production, improve gut mucosal weight, generate DNA and protein synthesis, and improve the efficiency of nutrient utilization.[65] Enteral nutrition stimulates intestinal contractility; the release of trophic substances such as bile salts, gastrin, and motilin; and the release of secretory IgA.[65a-65d] Enteral nutrition supports commensal bacteria, which in turn degrade bacterial toxins and prevent gut colonization by pathogenic organisms.[65a,65e] Further, enteral nutrition stimulates gut blood flow and supports gut-associated lymphoid tissue (GALT).[65a-65d] Enteral nutrition supports the processing of naïve CD4 helper lymphocytes by exposure to bacterial antigens in the gut. These IgA-producing lymphocytes then migrate to distant organs such as lungs, liver, and kidneys, where they form mucosal-associated lymphoid tissue (MALT) and produce secretory IgA.[65a-65d] T_H2 CD4 helper lymphocytes, the proliferation of which are stimulated by feeding, enter the circulation and have an anti-inflammatory effect.[65a,65f,65g] Enteral nutrients stimulate the proliferation of T_H1 and T_H3 lymphocytes,[65f] which in turn release transforming growth factor–beta (TGF-β), resulting in a further down-regulatory or anti-inflammatory effect.[65a,65f]

Several randomized prospective trials in a variety of critically ill patient populations, including trauma, burns, head injury, major surgery, and acute pancreatitis, have documented the benefits of enteral compared to parenteral nutrition.[66-71] Few studies show a beneficial effect on mortality rate, but most demonstrate reduced infectious morbidity, primarily pneumonia and central line infections. In trauma patients, enteral nutrition has been associated with a reduction in abdominal abscesses.[67] Further, enteral nutrition has been associated with decreased length of hospital stay,[69] and in head injury patients, return of cognitive function.[71] Several meta-analyses comparing enteral to parenteral nutrition have shown significant reductions in infectious complications with the use of enteral nutrition.[72-75]

Parenteral nutrition, although able to maintain overall nutritional status, does not offer the benefits related to gut mucosal integrity and immune function mentioned earlier. Whether this is the primary reason for the increased infection risk associated with parenteral nutrition is less clear. In several of the studies mentioned in previous paragraphs, many of the patients managed with parenteral nutrition received significantly more calories and had a higher incidence of hyperglycemia[73] than did their enterally fed counterparts. In a study in which parenterally fed patients had a higher incidence of sepsis, twice as many patients receiving parenteral nutrition had hyperglycemia as enterally fed patients.[70] More recently, in a large prospective trial comparing tight glucose control with standard glucose control, patients with tight glucose control had significantly lower rates of morbidity, infectious complications, and mortality.[49] Further analysis of these data revealed that when glucose was tightly controlled, there was no difference in infection when patients were nourished parenterally rather than enterally.[77] These data suggest that control of hyperglycemia may be as important as the route of nutrition in minimizing infectious complications.

In summary, because it is less costly and associated with fewer metabolic complications and a lower incidence of infection, the enteral route continues to be the recommended route for nutrition support.[51] That said, in as many as 15% of critically ill patients, enteral nutrition is either contraindicated or not tolerated, and parenteral nutrition remains a viable option, particularly when overfeeding is avoided and hyperglycemia is controlled.[51]

The timing for the initiation of nutrition support in critically ill patients has also been controversial. It has been suggested that enteral nutrition started early (within 24 to 72 hours of admission or the onset of the hypermetabolic insult) is associated with less gut permeability, release of inflammatory cytokines, and reduced systemic endotoxemia.[69] Further, the accumulation of an energy deficit early in the course of an ICU admission has been significantly associated with the occurrence of ARDS, renal failure, pressure ulcers, and the need for surgery[77a] and with longer ICU length of stay and more days of mechanical ventilation.[77,78] In a meta-analysis by Heyland and associates, early enteral nutrition was associated with a trend toward reduced infectious morbidity and mortality rates.[69] A second meta-analysis by Marik and Zaloga demonstrated significant reductions in infectious morbidity and hospital length of stay with early enteral nutrition as compared to delayed feedings.[77] In patients who are hemodynamically stable, it is recommended that enteral nutrition be started within 48 hours of admission.[76]

The early use of TPN to supplement enteral nutrition and thus prevent a caloric deficit has been controversial.[69,71,78] In a recent prospective, randomized, multi-institutional trial 2312 patients were randomized to initiation of parenteral nutrition to supplement insufficient enteral nutrition within 48 hours of ICU admission (early initiation group) and compared to 2328 patients randomized to receive supplementary parenteral nutrition no earlier than 8 days after ICU admission (late initiation group). All patients received early enteral nutrition by protocol and had insulin infused to maintain normoglycemia. The late initiation group was slightly more likely to be discharged alive from the ICU and from the hospital without evidence of decreased functional status. Further, patients in the late initiation group had significantly fewer infections, a significant reduction in the proportion of patients requiring more than 2 days of mechanical ventilation, a significant median reduction of 3 days in the duration of renal replacement therapy, and a mean reduction in health care costs of approximately $1600. These patients were considered to be at nutritional risk but not malnourished on admission based on BMI.[79] These results suggest that early parenteral nutrition, even when used to supplement enteral nutrition, may be harmful and should be avoided unless the patient is chronically malnourished.

TYPES OF NUTRITIONAL FORMULAS

Parenteral nutrition is most commonly administered as a three-in-one solution of dextrose, lipid, and amino acids. TPN order forms typically allow the physician to order "standard" or custom solutions, fluid-restricted solutions, and in some cases, disease-specific solutions such as renal failure or hepatic failure solutions. Electrolytes can usually be added in standard stock concentrations or individually. Vitamins and trace elements are generally added in standard quantities but can be supplemented. H_2 blockers for stress ulcer prophylaxis and regular insulin can also be added.

Enteral formulas are usually premixed with a fixed nonprotein calorie-to-nitrogen ratio, and the needs of a specific patient are generally met by changing the formula. Protein and carbohydrate supplements can be added at the bedside to alter premixed formulas. Enteral formulas can be classified numerous ways, including the form in which protein is provided (e.g., intact protein, hydrolyzed protein [chemically defined or peptide], or crystalline amino acids [elemental]), the quantity of protein contained, the caloric density of the formula, and the disease state for which they were designed. Examples of different formulas are shown in Table 82.3. More detailed information is available elsewhere.[80]

Intact protein solutions contain protein as caseinate or soy isolate–based products that are lactose-free, gluten-free, and low in residue. Such solutions contain 45% to 60% of calories as carbohydrate (oligosaccharides), 20% to 35% of calories as long-chain fats (e.g., linoleic acid), and 15% to 20% of calories as protein. Intact formulas are usually isosmotic and may contain 1 to 2 kcal/mL of solution. Some formulas contain fiber as a means to improve diarrhea or glycemic control. Hydrolyzed formulas provide protein as peptides or amino acids, are generally low in fat, and are designed for patients with gut dysfunction or malabsorption.[81] Elemental solutions contain protein exclusively as amino acids and are intended for similar indications. Controlled studies comparing hydrolyzed or elemental formulas with intact formulas have not demonstrated improved tolerance or outcomes.

High-protein formulas contain more than 45 g protein per 1000 kcal and are designed for patients with increased protein needs, such as patients with catabolic illness.

Calorie-dense formulas are designed for patients in whom fluid restriction is required. They are generally relatively low in protein and not ideal for a stressed patient.

ORGAN-SPECIFIC ENTERAL FORMULAS

Organ-specific formulas are products designed to meet the nutritional requirements of patients with specific organ failures. None has been consistently shown to improve outcomes when compared with conventional formulas.

Pulmonary failure formulas are designed for patients with acute respiratory failure associated with chronic lung disease. They contain at least 50% of calories as fat and thus reduce CO_2 production and decrease the work of breathing relative to high-carbohydrate formulas. Few data suggest a benefit with specific pulmonary formulas, and avoiding overfeeding is more important in reducing ventilatory demand.[82,75]

Hepatic failure formulas were developed for patients with encephalopathy. They contain high concentrations of branched-chain amino acids and reduced concentrations of aromatic amino acids. Although these solutions have been shown to correct the abnormal amino acid profile characteristic of patients with liver failure,[83,84] it is less clear that they actually treat hepatic encephalopathy.[84] Hepatic failure formulas should be reserved for the rare encephalopathic patient who is refractory to lactulose and luminal antibiotics.[51]

Renal failure formulas have reduced concentrations of electrolytes and decreased protein content to minimize nitrogenous waste in patients with renal failure. Patients with acute renal failure frequently have associated catabolic illness and as a result need more protein rather than less. Although these formulas may be useful in patients with electrolyte abnormalities not yet being dialyzed, they are inappropriate for patients with catabolic illness who are undergoing dialysis and particularly CRRT.

IMMUNOMODULATING ENTERAL FORMULAS

Immunomodulating enteral formulas are supplemented with various combinations of specific nutrients, arginine, ω-3 polyunsaturated fatty acids, nucleotides, glutamine, and antioxidants aimed at improving immune function and reducing inflammation in critically ill patients.

Arginine is a nonessential amino acid that has both beneficial and deleterious effects. It is a secretagogue for anabolic hormones, supports T-cell function, detoxifies ammonia, and supports wound healing via metabolism to polyamine and proline.[85,86] An arginine deficiency may develop after trauma or major surgery that is mediated by pathologic release of arginase from granulocytes.[86-88] Arginine deficiency impairs the immune response, which may result in increased infections and in impaired wound healing.[86,87,89] Arginine is a precursor for the synthesis of nitric oxide, which in turn is a modulator of hepatic protein synthesis and vascular tone. This nitric oxide–induced vasodilation may be beneficial in some circumstances but in the setting of severe sepsis and hypotension may aggravate hemodynamic collapse. Further, nitric oxide is metabolized to peroxynitrite,[86,90] which is a potent oxidizing and nitrating agent that may damage mitochondria, increase gut barrier permeability, and promote organ dysfunction.[86,90-95]

Omega-3 *fatty acids* are incorporated into the phospholipid fraction of cell membranes and converted to trienoic prostaglandins and pentaenoic leukotrienes, which are less "inflammatory" than their ω-6 counterparts. Omega-3 fatty acids have been shown to decrease prostaglandin E_2, TNF, and IL-1 production in rat Kupffer cells[96] and alter TNF and IL-1 production in human monocytes.[97] Furthermore, ω-3 fats have been shown to be beneficial in animal models of chronic inflammation and in humans with psoriasis[98] and rheumatoid arthritis.[99]

Glutamine is an important fuel for enterocytes and cells of the immune system. Considered a nonessential amino acid, glutamine may become conditionally essential when skeletal muscle stores and plasma levels become depleted during catabolic illness, thereby resulting in adverse effects on gut barrier and immune function.[100-102] Glutamine has been shown to improve nitrogen balance and decrease bacterial translocation in animals.[103-105] It also promotes the synthesis of glutathione, an important antioxidant. A meta-analysis of 14 randomized trials in which glutamine-supplemented nutrition was compared with standard nutrition demonstrated reduced infectious morbidity and mortality rates with glutamine supplementation, particularly in parenterally nourished surgical patients.[106] Unfortunately, glutamine dipeptide, which is the optimal form for parenteral administration due to stability and the minimal added volume required for infusion, is not currently available in the United States.[86]

Antioxidants such as vitamins A, E, and C; selenium; and *N*-acetylcysteine offer the potential to reduce oxidant injury but have not been studied individually in critically ill patients in terms of clinical outcomes.[107]

Numerous studies comparing immunity-enhancing enteral nutrition with conventional nutrition have produced contradictory results. In a 2001 meta-analysis of 22 studies (2419 patients) in which enteral nutrition supplemented with various combinations of arginine, ω-3 fatty acids, glutamine, and nucleotides was compared with conventional enteral nutrition, the supplemented patients had decreased infectious morbidity but no difference in mortality rates when compared with patients receiving the control diet.[108] The majority of studies demonstrating benefit involved elective surgery patients and not critically ill patients. In the subsequently published and largest (597 patients) randomized trial to date, immunonutrition had no benefit in terms of infectious morbidity, length of hospital stay, number of ventilator days, or mortality rate.[109] In retrospect, it appears that a number of factors may have been responsible for the conflicting results mentioned earlier. First, there was considerable heterogeneity in the patient populations studied (major elective surgery, burns, trauma, sepsis, and ARDS). Second, the immunomodulating enteral formulas studied contained varying combinations of arginine, ω-3 polyunsaturated fatty acids (fish oil), glutamine, and antioxidants. These differences were addressed in a 2008 meta-analysis of 24 studies by Marik and Zaloga in which studies were analyzed by patient type (ICU, burns, and trauma) and by the combination of immunomodulating nutrients in the subject study formula (fish oil, arginine, glutamine, fish oil plus arginine, fish oil plus arginine plus glutamine).[110] All enteral formulas contained antioxidants, primarily selenium, though in varying doses, and could not be studied separately. Overall, the immunomodulating diets had no effect on mortality rate but did demonstrate significant reductions in secondary infections. Mortality rates, infections, and length of stay were significantly reduced only in ICU patients with sepsis, systemic inflammatory response syndrome (SIRS), and ARDS receiving a formula supplemented with fish oil alone.[111-113] Infection and length of stay were reduced in the 13 ICU studies, but this effect disappeared when the three fish oil studies were excluded.[110] It appears that arginine, perhaps due to the preceding mechanisms, counteracts the beneficial effects of fish oil in trauma and ICU patients with sepsis/SIRS.

Currently, the 2009 guidelines for the Provision and Assessment of Nutrition Support Therapy in the Adult Critically Ill Patient, published jointly by the Society of Critical Care Medicine and the American Society for Parenteral and Enteral Nutrition, recommend the use of an immunomodulating enteral formula supplemented with fish oil and antioxidants for patients with acute lung injury/ARDS.[75] Further, these guidelines recommend enteral formulas supplemented with arginine for patients with major surgery, burns, and trauma, but emphasize that such formulas may be harmful in severe sepsis. Finally, the guidelines describe glutamine as possibly beneficial in trauma and burns.[51]

NUTRITIONAL ASSESSMENT AND MONITORING

The history and physical examination remain the mainstay of nutritional assessment, although they are perhaps more useful in the ambulatory setting or in patients with chronic malnutrition.[114] Pertinent historical information includes height and weight, a history of recent weight change, genetic background, recent nutritional intake, and a history of disease that might affect nutrient intake, absorption, or tolerance. The physical examination might, on occasion,

Table 82.4 Selected Vitamin Deficiencies

Vitamin	Function	Signs of Deficiency
Niacin (vitamin B_5)	Component of the coenzymes NAD and NADP, which catalyze oxidation-reduction reactions and play a role in the oxidative catabolism of carbohydrates, proteins, and lipids and the biosynthesis of fatty acids	Pellagra, dermatitis, headaches, loss of memory, dementia, glossitis, diarrhea
Folate (vitamin B_9)	Transfer of single-carbon units; DNA synthesis	Megaloblastic anemia, diarrhea, glossitis
Cyanocobalamin (vitamin B_{12})	Maintains normal folate metabolism; coenzyme in reactions involving isomerizations and reductions; participates in the metabolism of fat, carbohydrate, and protein and in myelin synthesis	Pernicious anemia, glossitis, peripheral neuropathy, spinal cord degeneration
Thiamine	Carbohydrate metabolism coenzyme in oxidative decarboxylation	Paresthesias, impaired memory, nystagmus, congestive heart failure, Wernicke-Korsakoff syndrome
Riboflavin (vitamin B_2)	Electronic transport as flavin nucleotides	Mucositides, dermatitis, cheilosis, vascularization of the cornea, photophobia, decreased vision, lacrimation, impaired wound healing
Pyridoxine (vitamin B_6)	Coenzyme in transformations of amino acids	Neuritis, dermatitis, convulsions
Pantothenic acid	Precursor of coenzyme A (Krebs cycle)	Headache, fatigue, malaise, insomnia, vomiting, abdominal cramps
Biotin	Coenzyme for carboxylation reactions	As with other B vitamins (normally synthesized and absorbed from gut)
Ascorbic acid (vitamin C)	Reducing agent, wound healing, integrity of blood vessels, folate metabolism	Enlargement and keratosis of hair follicles, impaired wound healing, anemia, ecchymosis, lethargy, depression, bleeding
Vitamin A	Normal vision, mucopolysaccharide synthesis, protease release, entry of macrophages and leukocytes into an acute wound, immune stimulation, mucosal integrity	Dermatitis, keratomalacia, xerophthalmia, night blindness
Vitamin D	Calcium and phosphorus homeostasis	Rickets, osteomalacia
Vitamin E	Antioxidant	Hemolysis
Vitamin K	Clotting factors II, VII, IX, X	Bleeding

NAD, nicotinamide-adenine dinucleotide; NADP, nicotinamide-adenine dinucleotide phosphate.

demonstrate abnormal end-organ function that reflects malnutrition, but more commonly it is useful for the assessment of body mass and detection of specific nutrient deficiencies. Signs and symptoms of selected vitamin and mineral deficiencies are presented in Tables 82.4 and 82.5.

Anthropometric measurements such as triceps skinfold thickness (SFT), midarm circumference (MAC), and arm muscle area, which is derived from SFT and MAC, can be used to estimate fat mass and lean body mass.[115] Although serial measurements may be useful in certain patients over long periods, SFT measurements are less reliable in the elderly because of changes in fat distribution and skin compressibility associated with aging[115,116] and are inaccurate in patients with peripheral edema.[117] In general, these measurements are not practical for nutritional monitoring in a recumbent, critically ill patient.[118]

Visceral protein levels have long been used in nutritional assessment and monitoring and can be useful in the appropriate clinical setting. They are affected by a number of variables other than nutritional status, such as hydration state and gastrointestinal and urinary losses, and must therefore be used cautiously in a critically ill patient.

Albumin is contained in a large body pool (4 to 5 g/kg) and has a half-life of 20 days, so it is insensitive to acute changes and responds slowly to nutritional therapy. Serum albumin levels are decreased in nephrotic syndrome, enteropathies, hepatic failure, and dialysis (particularly peritoneal dialysis), as well as in the setting of acute volume expansion. Levels may be increased in the presence of dehydration, hypercortisolemia, and anabolic hormones such as insulin, growth hormone, and estrogen. Although serum albumin levels are useful in predicting surgical mortality rate and monitoring nutritional status over the long term, they are much less useful in monitoring a critically ill patient.[119]

Transferrin is contained in a smaller body pool and has a shorter half-life than albumin does (8 to 10 days), so it is a more sensitive indicator of nutritional status. It is subject to the same influences as mentioned for albumin and, in addition, is affected inversely by serum iron levels.[120]

Retinol-binding protein is a specific carrier involved in vitamin A transport and is linked with thyroxine-binding prealbumin in a constant molar ratio.[121] It has a 12-hour

Table 82.5 Selected Mineral Deficiencies

Trace Element	Function	Signs of Deficiency
Chromium	Glucose tolerance; possible role in maintenance of normal serum lipid levels	Elevated serum lipids, insulin-resistant glucose intolerance
Copper	Metalloenzyme biochemical processes, component of ceruloplasmin, connective tissue metabolism, melanin formation	Anemia, neutropenia, leukopenia, depigmentation of skin
Iron	Constituent of hemoglobin, myoglobin, and the cytochrome enzymes	Microcytic hypochromic anemia, fatigue, faulty digestion, decreased serum iron
Zinc	Essential for the function of many enzymes and a component of lipid, protein, carbohydrate, and nucleic acid metabolism; cell replication and connective tissue synthesis	Dermatitis; impaired wound healing; alopecia; depressed cell-mediated immunity, taste acuity, and dark adaptation; sexual retardation; depressed visceral protein status
Cobalt	Biologic methylation	Pernicious anemia, methylmalonic aciduria
Manganese	Oxidative phosphorylation, fatty acid metabolism, protein and mucopolysaccharide synthesis	Growth retardation, bony abnormalities, central nervous system dysfunction

half-life and is sensitive to synthesis and utilization rates. Levels rise in patients with renal disease[122] and with excess vitamin A administration and are reduced in patients with liver disease, cystic fibrosis, hyperthyroidism, and vitamin A deficiency.

Transthyretin (thyroxine-binding prealbumin) is involved in the transport of thyroid hormone and is a carrier for retinol-binding protein. It has a small body pool and a short half-life (2 to 3 days) and as such may be a sensitive indicator of nutritional status.[123,124] Levels are affected by the same variables that affect albumin and transferrin. Levels are low in patients with hyperthyroidism, cystic fibrosis, chronic illness, and acute stress. Because of its short half-life and ease of measurement, transthyretin is the visceral protein of choice for nutritional assessment and monitoring, although its use in a critically ill patient is controversial. During catabolic illness, hepatic protein synthesis is reprioritized, under the influence of cytokines, with increased synthesis of acute-phase reactant proteins and decreased synthesis of visceral proteins.[125-127] Transthyretin levels fall early in the course of catabolic illness and rise with the subsequent decrease in acute-phase reactant proteins as a result of reversal of the reprioritized hepatic protein synthesis. The association of this response with specific nutrients,[128-131] nitrogen balance,[52,132-135] and outcomes[71,134,136] has been variable. Whether transthyretin levels are reflective of appropriate nutrition support or simply a reflection of the course and severity of the inflammatory response is unclear. An initial transthyretin level lower than 50 mg/L or failure to increase by 40 mg/L per week has been associated with a poor prognosis.[124]

In general, because visceral protein levels are affected by a variety of non-nutritional factors, they are not recommended for the monitoring of nutritional status in critically ill patients.[51]

Nitrogen balance is the nutritional parameter most consistently associated with improved outcomes, and nitrogen balance studies are used routinely in many ICUs to monitor nutrition support. Ideally, positive nitrogen balance is the goal, but minimizing the nitrogen deficit in a critically ill patient is probably more realistic when one considers the fact that proteolysis in the skeletal muscle compartment, which constitutes 70% of body protein stores, is likely to exceed protein synthesis related to the inflammatory response and wound healing, simply because of the size of the compartments involved. Nitrogen balance is calculated as follows:

$$\text{Nitrogen balance (g)} = \text{Nitrogen intake (g)} - \text{Nitrogen output (g)}$$

$$\text{Nitrogen intake (g)} = \text{Protein or amino acid intake (g)}/6.25$$

$$\text{Nitrogen output (g)} = \text{Urinary nitrogen losses (g)} + 2\text{ g (stool and skin losses)}$$

Urinary nitrogen consists of several components, including urea, creatinine, uric acid, ammonia, and amino acids. In health, urea constitutes 90% of urinary nitrogen, whereas in catabolic states, urea may represent as little as 70% of urinary nitrogen. Measurement of total urinary nitrogen (TUN) is complex and not done in most hospitals, whereas urinary urea nitrogen (UUN) is measured routinely. When UUN is used in the calculation of urinary nitrogen excretion, an additional 20% of the UUN is added to account for nonurea nitrogen losses. In the absence of abnormal stool or skin losses, nitrogen output is calculated as

$$\text{Nitrogen output (g)} = \text{TUN (g/24 hours)} + 2\text{ g (stool and skin losses)}$$

or

$$\text{Nitrogen output (g)} = \text{UUN (g/24 hours)} + 20\%\ \text{UUN} + 2\text{ g (stool and skin losses)}$$

Classically, measurement of urinary nitrogen excretion involves a 24-hour urine collection, but recent evidence suggests that a carefully collected 12- or even 6-hour urine collection can be obtained and extrapolated to a 24-hour period.[137] Nitrogen balance is usually calculated weekly.

Numerous techniques for assessment and monitoring of energy balance have been studied, including continuous whole-body calorimetry,[138] the doubly labeled water technique,[138] and nuclear magnetic resonance spectroscopy using ^{31}P,[139] but no method is ideal. Though potentially useful, these methods are either cumbersome, expensive, or impractical for use in critically ill patients.

Indirect calorimetry is used to determine the heat produced by oxidative processes by measuring oxygen consumption and carbon dioxide production, which are then used to calculate REE via the abbreviated Weir equation.[140,141] Indirect calorimetry is widely used at the bedside, convenient, relatively inexpensive, and accurately estimates REE when compared with standard predictive formulas.[142-148] Indirect calorimetry is performed on patients at rest and therefore does not account for energy expenditure during periods of activity. Many clinicians will increase caloric input by 20% to 25% above measured REE to account for physical activity, particularly in patients who are agitated, ambulatory, or involved in intense physical therapy.[149-151]

In addition to the nutrition-specific monitoring techniques mentioned, the usual laboratory values should be monitored for fluid and electrolyte composition, hepatic function, infection, and any coagulopathy that might reflect vitamin K deficiency. In a critically ill patient, serum electrolytes (Na^+, K^+, Cl^-, and HCO_3^-) should be determined daily and as needed. Special attention should be paid to the intracellular electrolytes (K^+, Mg^{2+}, and PO_4^{2-}), which are required for the attainment of nitrogen balance[73] and can fall precipitously when nutrition support, particularly glucose, is initiated. Rapid uptake into cells can result in dangerously low serum levels acutely. Intracellular electrolyte levels should be measured before starting nutrition support, 1 or 2 days after starting support, and at least weekly thereafter. Liver function and coagulation parameters should be evaluated weekly and as needed. Glucose should be measured every 6 hours initially and then as needed; it can be measured as often as every 2 hours when continuous insulin infusions are being used (Fig. 82.1).

COMPLICATIONS OF NUTRITION SUPPORT

Complications of nutrition support include those related to the route of nutrition support and those related to nutrition support in general and are discussed in the following

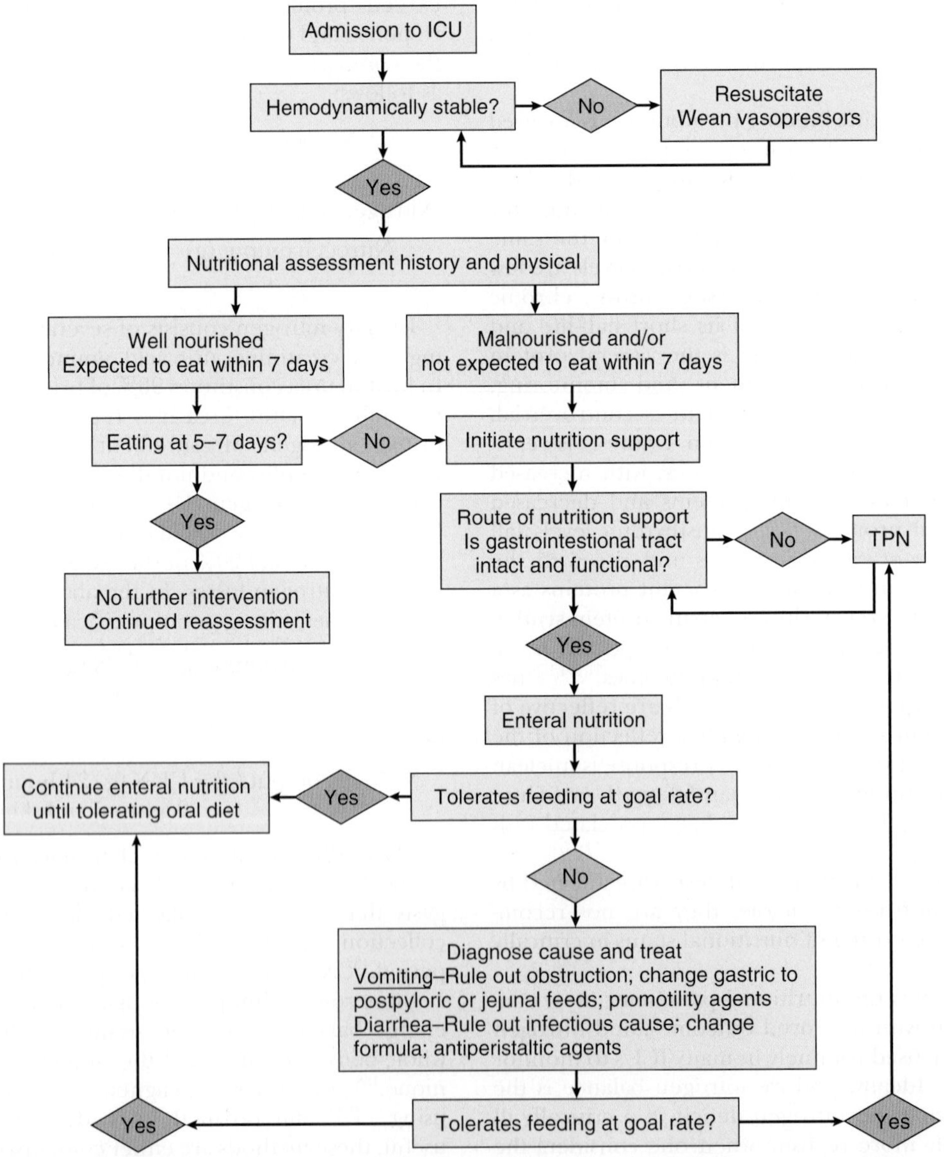

Figure 82.1 Approach to administering nutritional support to a critical care patient. ICU, intensive care unit; TPN, total parenteral nutrition.

paragraphs. Perhaps the most important problem with nutrition support is failure to achieve therapeutic goals. Recommendations for appropriate doses of protein and calories, electrolytes, vitamins, and trace elements are discussed in previous paragraphs.

COMPLICATIONS OF ENTERAL NUTRITION SUPPORT

Complications specific to enteral nutrition support include mechanical or technical complications, gastrointestinal complications, and aspiration pneumonia.

Mechanical and technical complications of enteral nutrition include feeding tube misplacement, gastrointestinal perforation, sinusitis, otitis media, ulceration of the nasal septum, and obstruction of the feeding tube. Proper placement of feeding tubes in the gastrointestinal tract should be confirmed radiographically or with pH testing before feeding is initiated. Auscultatory techniques for confirmation of proper tube placement are unreliable.[152] Nasally placed feeding tubes are a potential cause of sinusitis or otitis media (or both), particularly when stiff, large-bore nasogastric tubes are used as feeding tubes. Soft, small-caliber tubes such as Miller-Frederick or Dobhoff tubes seem to cause sinusitis less frequently. In mechanically ventilated patients, feeding tubes may be placed orally to minimize the incidence of sinusitis.[153] Perforation of the esophagus or other parts of the gastrointestinal tract is a disastrous complication and seems to occur most frequently in the setting of stricture, obstructing tumor, or abnormal anatomy as a result of surgery. In these situations, tube placement under fluoroscopic guidance or endoscopic tube placement should be considered. Dislodgement of the feeding tube is a frequent and frustrating problem and can be disastrous when the tube dislodged is a recent, surgically placed tube such as a gastrostomy or jejunostomy tube. When a surgically placed tube has been present for longer than 1 to 2 weeks, the stomach or intestine should be adherent to the abdominal wall and the tube can usually be replaced through the existing tract, as long as the tube is replaced within a few hours before the tract begins to close. A radiograph with contrast enhancement should be used to verify replacement of the tube in the appropriate location. Dislodgement of a surgically placed tube within a week of placement can result in peritonitis from spillage of enteral formula or gastrointestinal contents into the abdominal cavity. Care should be taken to properly secure all feeding tubes either with sutures and tape or with commercially available fixation systems, and tubes should be protected with appropriate patient restraints and caregiver attention when the patient is being moved. Feeding tube obstruction occurs most frequently when tubes are not routinely flushed or when crushed medications are delivered through the tubes. Tubes should be flushed every 6 hours and after every medication dose. Numerous techniques have been used to clear obstructed tubes, including flushing with cola, pancreatic enzymes, cranberry juice, and streptokinase, although none is universally successful. Clearing a nasoenteric tube with a stylet or wire carries the risk of perforating the gastrointestinal tract and should be avoided unless done under fluoroscopic guidance to ensure that the stylet remains within the tube lumen.

Gastrointestinal complications such as abdominal distention, nausea, vomiting, diarrhea, and constipation occur in approximately 60% of critically ill patients receiving nutrition support.[154] Gastrointestinal motility is often decreased in these patients,[154,155] although gastric stasis and high gastric residual volumes occur more frequently than decreased small intestinal motility does.[155] Potential causes of gastroparesis include increased sympathetic tone, elevated intracranial pressure, opiates, benzodiazepines, dopamine, hyperglycemia, recent abdominal surgery, and pancreatitis. Prokinetic agents such as metoclopramide may restore gastric motility and allow gastric feeding.[156] Postpyloric feeding tube placement will often allow the continuation of enteral nutrition. Advancement of the feeding tube into the proximal jejunum facilitates enteral nutrition in patients with pancreatitis.

Diarrhea occurs in as many as 70% of critically ill patients.[154] Potential causes include antibiotics and other drugs, hyperosmolar formulas, infected solutions, hypoalbuminemia, chronic malnutrition and disuse mucosal atrophy, intolerance to lactose or other nutrients, pancreatic insufficiency, biliary fistula, and short-gut syndrome.

Clostridium difficile overgrowth is perhaps the most serious cause of antibiotic-associated diarrhea, and stool should be assayed for *C. difficile* toxin in every case of persistent diarrhea in the critically ill. *C. difficile* enterocolitis should be treated with appropriate antibiotics. Antibiotics may also cause diarrhea by eliminating the bacteria that ferment dietary fiber into short-chain fatty acids. Short-chain fatty acids are important for maintaining colonic mucosal integrity and enhance water and electrolyte absorption.[157] Enteral formulas should be replaced daily to avoid bacterial contamination of the solution.

A change in formula or more gradual institution of nutrition support can be used to overcome problems caused by nutrient intolerance, disuse atrophy, and short-gut syndrome. Semi-elemental or peptide formulas may reduce diarrhea in patients with mucosal atrophy. H_2 blockers can be used to decrease the contribution of gastric secretions to diarrhea in patients with short-gut syndrome. Drugs with the potential to cause diarrhea should be identified and eliminated if possible. Pancreatic insufficiency should be treated with commercially available pancreatic enzymes. Diarrhea secondary to a biliary fistula may be improved with reinfusion of bile into the intestine distal to the fistula. Once correctable causes of diarrhea have been identified and eliminated, Kaopectate can be given for symptomatic relief. Antiperistaltic agents such as Imodium or opiates should be avoided until infectious causes of diarrhea have been ruled out. Fiber may be used to thicken stool and lessen perineal irritation, but it may be associated with constipation and fecal impaction in critically ill patients. Intractable diarrhea may warrant the discontinuation of enteral nutrition and the initiation of parenteral nutrition.

Aspiration pneumonia is the major infectious complication of enteral nutrition. Bolus feeding carries a higher risk of aspiration than continuous feeding does. Gastric residual volume, which has traditionally been used to assess gastric feeding tolerance, does not appear to correlate with risk for aspiration.[158] Gastric feeding is routinely used in many ICUs, but because a nasogastric tube is one of the leading causes of aspiration, gastric feeding should probably be done with a soft, small-caliber tube designed for feeding. The risk of aspiration associated with gastric feeding may be lower when done via a percutaneous gastrostomy tube,[158] which avoids compromising the function of the gastroesophageal junction and swallowing mechanics. Multiple studies have compared the risk of aspirating gastric versus postpyloric feedings, but the results have been contradictory.[71,150,160] In a recent meta-analysis of seven randomized trials, small bowel feeding was associated with a lower risk of aspiration pneumonia than was gastric feeding.[161] Nursing protocols for the bedside placement of postpyloric feeding tubes have been developed,[162,163] although placement under fluoroscopic guidance is more likely to be successful and is cost-effective.[164] The semirecumbent body position has been shown to significantly reduce aspiration pneumonia as compared with the supine body position.[165]

COMPLICATIONS OF PARENTERAL NUTRITION SUPPORT

The primary complications of parenteral nutrition include mechanical or technical complications and infectious complications. Mechanical and technical complications are related to central venous catheter placement and include pneumothorax, arterial injury, hemothorax, hydrothorax, cardiac arrhythmia, and cardiac perforation with tamponade. The incidence of severe complications with subclavian vein catheterization is 1% to 3%, with an overall complication rate of 5%.[166] The incidence of complications with jugular venous catheterization ranges from 0.1% to 4.2%.[167] Jugular venous catheterization under ultrasound guidance is increasingly being recommended.[168-171] Jugular or subclavian vein thrombosis is a postprocedural complication that is manifested as neck or arm swelling and should be managed by catheter removal and anticoagulation; thrombolytics have also been recommended.[172]

Catheter infection and catheter-associated bloodstream infection are the major infectious complications of parenteral nutrition and occur in 2% to 8% of patients with central venous catheters. The most common infecting organisms are coagulase-negative staphylococci, *Staphylococcus aureus*, and *Candida* species. Infection is more likely when parenteral nutrition is administered through a multilumen catheter than through a single-lumen catheter,[173] although the incidence of infection may be reduced when parenteral nutrition is infused through a dedicated port.[174] Jugular and femoral catheters have higher rates of infection than do subclavian catheters.[175] Dedicated central line care teams and regular dressing change protocols may reduce the incidence of catheter infection.[174] Antibiotic-coated or antibiotic-impregnated catheters are expensive but appear to be effective in reducing catheter-related bloodstream infections.[176] Guidewire exchange is associated with a decreased incidence of technical complications but an increased incidence of catheter infections.[177] Although the possibility of catheter infection increases with time, routine catheter exchange is probably not indicated.[176] Catheters should be replaced, ideally at a fresh site, for obvious site infection, for the evaluation and treatment of fever of unknown origin, and after any positive blood culture. If guidewire exchange is used and the removed catheter proves to be infected, the new catheter often becomes infected during the exchange and should in turn be removed and replaced at a fresh site.

METABOLIC COMPLICATIONS OF NUTRITION SUPPORT

Common metabolic complications of nutrition support include hyperglycemia, hepatobiliary complications, disturbances in water and electrolyte balance, and acid-base abnormalities. Though more common in patients receiving parenteral nutrition, metabolic complications can occur with either form of nutrition support.

Hyperglycemia occurs frequently in critically ill patients receiving nutrition support and is most common in diabetic patients and those with catabolic illness.

Complications related to hyperglycemia include infection, hyperosmolarity, and osmotic diuresis. The first step in the control of blood sugar is avoidance of overfeeding, as discussed previously. Insulin, whether by intermittent dosing or continuous infusion, is the mainstay for maintenance of acceptable blood glucose levels. The appropriate glucose level has been the subject of controversy. In a large, prospective, randomized trial in critically ill surgical patients, tight glucose control (80-120 mg/dL) was associated with significantly decreased mortality rate, infection, neuropathy, and renal failure.[49] In medical ICU patients the same tight glucose control protocol was associated with decreased renal failure, ventilator days, and reduced ICU and hospital length of stay, but not improvements in mortality rate or infection.[178] Subsequently, the NICE-SUGAR trial compared tight glucose control to glucose levels less than 180 mg/dL and demonstrated similar infection and mortality rates and fewer episodes of dangerous hypoglycemia with more liberal glucose control.[179] Currently, most practitioners aim for blood glucose levels below 150 to 180 mg/dL. Symptomatic hypoglycemia has been reported in children after sudden withdrawal of TPN but is rare in adults, and weaning of TPN in adults is not usually necessary.[180]

Hepatobiliary complications of nutrition support include hepatic steatosis (fatty infiltration of the liver) and intrahepatic and extrahepatic cholestasis. Progression to chronic liver disease occurs in premature infants[181] but is rare in adults. Hepatic steatosis may develop after 7 to 21 days of parenteral nutrition and is characterized initially by elevated transaminases. Usually asymptomatic, fatty infiltration can, in severe cases, be accompanied by hepatomegaly and right upper quadrant abdominal pain. Histologically, mild cases are characterized by periportal fat infiltration and severe cases by centrilobular infiltration. Overfeeding, hyperinsulinemia, essential fatty acid deficiency, and carnitine deficiency may predispose to fatty infiltration. Cholestasis occurs later in the course of parenteral nutrition and is characterized by elevations in bilirubin and alkaline phosphatase. Histologically, periportal or pericentral canalicular bile plugging, bile staining of surrounding hepatocytes, and lymphocytic triaditis characterize cholestasis. Cholelithiasis has been linked to long-term TPN use. Gallstone formation is almost certainly related to the lack of enteral feeding and the resultant lack of neural and hormonal stimulation of gallbladder contraction. Other potential but unproven causes of cholestasis include overfeeding, the production of toxic bile acids by intestinal bacteria, hormones, endotoxin, and taurine deficiency.[31,182-185] Management of hepatobiliary complications is aimed at prevention. Overfeeding should be avoided. Cyclical TPN and enteral feeding, even if only partial, may help prevent cholestasis. A trial of oral neomycin and metronidazole may be helpful.[185]

Serum electrolyte levels should be monitored and electrolytes added to or eliminated from TPN as indicated, with consideration of excess losses or abnormal accumulation. Hypernatremia or hyponatremia can be managed by increasing or decreasing free water. Particular attention should be paid to the intracellular electrolytes potassium, magnesium, and phosphorus. In malnourished individuals, these electrolytes rapidly move intracellularly when nutrition support is initiated. In what is termed the refeeding syndrome, serum levels of these intracellular electrolytes fall precipitously, with hypophosphatemia resulting in hemolysis, rhabdomyolysis, and heart failure with hypokalemia and hypomagnesemia leading to cardiac arrhythmias.[186,187] Serum levels of intracellular electrolytes should be corrected before and, in particular, 24 hours after the institution of nutrition support. Abnormally high levels of the intracellular electrolytes are of concern in renal failure and often need to be reduced or eliminated from TPN solutions. Hyperkalemia and hypomagnesemia may lead to weakness and cardiac arrhythmia, and hyperphosphatemia may result in hypotension, hypocalcemia, and metastatic calcification. Hyperphosphatemia is often treated with oral phosphate binders such as calcium carbonate.

Metabolic acidosis related to nutrition support is most commonly due to excess chloride administration and resultant renal bicarbonate losses, but it can also occur as a result of thiamine deficiency with resultant lactic acidosis.[188,189]

KEY POINTS

- Malnutrition is a significant contributor to morbidity and mortality rates in critically ill patients.
- Distinguishing stress metabolism from starvation metabolism is critical to the provision of appropriate nutrition support.
- Critically ill patients may require more energy but are less able to tolerate glucose than starved patients are and require a significant portion of calories as fat.
- Critically ill patients require increased protein to achieve nitrogen balance.
- Enteral nutrition is less costly and more physiologic; is associated with fewer metabolic disturbances; and may be associated with fewer infections than

KEY POINTS (Continued)

parenteral nutrition is and thus remains the preferred route for nutrition support.

- Parenteral nutrition is acceptable when enteral nutrition cannot be used, particularly if blood glucose is tightly controlled.
- Nutrition support should be closely monitored to avoid complications.

SELECTED REFERENCES

49. van den Berghe G, Wouters P, Weekers F, et al: Intensive insulin therapy in the surgical intensive care unit. N Engl J Med 2001;345:1359-1367.
51. McClave SA, Martindale RG, Vanek VW, et al, the A.S.P.E.N: Board of Directors and the American College of Critical Care Medicine: Guidelines for the provision and assessment of nutrition support therapy in the adult critically ill patient. JPEN J Parenter Enteral Nutr 2009;33:277-316.
59 Visser J, Labadarios D, Blaauw R: Micronutrient supplementation for critically ill adults: A systematic review and meta-analysis. Nutrition 2011;27:745-758.
69. Heyland DK, Dhaliwal R, Drover JW, et al, Canadian Critical Care Clinical Practice Guidelines Committee: Canadian clinical practice guidelines for nutrition support in mechanically ventilated, critically ill adult patients. JPEN J Parenter Enteral Nutr 2003;27:355-373.
78. Singer P, Berger MM, van den Berghe G, et al: ESPEN guidelines on parenteral nutrition: Intensive care. Clin Nutr 2009;28: 387-400.
79. Casaer MP, Mesotten D, Hermans G, et al: Early versus late parenteral nutrition in critically ill adults. N Engl J Med 2011;365:506-517.
86. Mizock BA: Immunonutrition and critical illness: An update. Nutrition 2010;26:701-707.
108. Heyland DK, Novak F, Drover JW, et al: Should immunonutrition become routine in critically ill patients? A systematic review of the evidence. JAMA 2001;286:944-953.
110. Marik PE, Zaloga GP: Immunonutrition in critically ill patients: A systematic review and analysis of the literature. Intensive Care Med 2008;34(11):1980-1990.
112. Pontes-Arruda A, Aragao AM, Albuquerque JD: Effects of enteral feeding with eicosapentaenoic acid, gamma-linolenic acid, and antioxidants in mechanically ventilated patients with severe sepsis and septic shock. Crit Care Med 2006;34:2325-2333.
178. van den Berghe G, Wilmer A, Hermans G, et al: Intensive insulin therapy in the medical ICU. N Engl J Med 2006;354:449-461.
179. Finfer S, Chittock DR, Su SY, et al, NICE-SUGAR Study Investigators: Intensive versus conventional glucose control in critically ill patients. N Engl J Med 2009;360(13):1283-1297.

The complete list of references can be found at www.expertconsult.com.

83

Bedside Ultrasonography in the Critical Care Patient

Rebecca L. Ryszkiewicz | Paul E. Marik

CHAPTER OUTLINE

Ultrasonography has become an invaluable tool in the management of critically ill patients. Its safety and portability allow for use at the bedside to provide rapid, detailed information regarding the cardiovascular system and the function and anatomy of certain internal organs. A new generation of portable, battery-powered, inexpensive, hand-carried ultrasound devices has recently become available. The true portability, ease of use, and low cost make these devices ideally suited for use by the intensivist. The safety and utility of bedside ultrasonography performed by adequately trained intensivists has now been well demonstrated. All intensivists should be trained to perform "focused" ultrasound examinations that answer specific questions applicable to the management of critically ill and injured patients. It is important to emphasize that ultrasonography performed by the intensivist is an extension of the patient's evaluation rather than being a discrete imaging procedure. Furthermore, it is performed by the clinician caring for the patient rather than a subspeciality consultant, and it is contemporaneous with the intensivist's evaluation rather than being temporally distinct. This chapter reviews the indications and techniques for extracardiac ultrasonography in the intensive care unit (ICU).

LUNG ULTRASONOGRAPHY

Lung ultrasonography is a valuable tool in the assessment of critically ill patients. The diagnostic accuracy of using ultrasound in the lung to establish the presence of pneumothorax, pleural effusion, lung consolidation, and alveolar-interstitial syndrome has been well established.[1] Lung ultrasonography can be rapidly performed at the bedside and has been shown to significantly aid in the management of critical patients.[2] Lung computed tomography (CT) remains the gold standard for thoracic imaging in the critical care setting, despite its major drawbacks (radiation, cost, transportation), even though portable chest radiography is the most common diagnostic imaging modality.[2-4] Although portable chest radiographs are routinely performed in the ICU, multiple studies have shown limited diagnostic accuracy, with the elimination of routine chest radiographs having no adverse effect on length of stay, readmission, and mortality rates.[5-7] Routine use of bedside lung ultrasound in the ICU has been shown to significantly reduce the number of both chest radiographs and CT scans obtained.[8]

TECHNIQUE AND EQUIPMENT

In normal lung, ultrasound waves are reflected off gas-filled structures, limiting the visualization of lung structures beyond the pleura.[1] The diagnosis of lung disease by ultrasound largely relies on the detection of ultrasound artifacts. To examine the thorax, a high-frequency linear transducer (5-12 MHz) is best used to visualize the relatively superficial pleural line. Lower frequency microconvex and convex transducers (2-5 MHz) can be used to scan the deeper lung parenchyma.[9] Supine positioning is most commonly utilized in the ICU, and lateral decubitus positioning may assist in the visualization of the dorsal aspects of the lower lobes. To

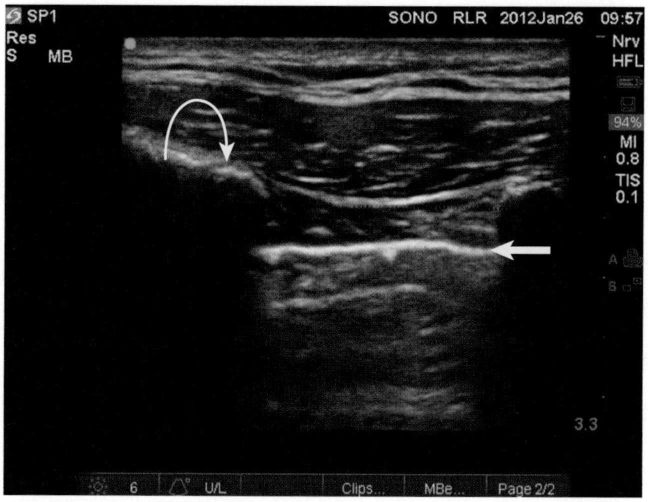

Figure 83.1 The pleural line appears as a hyperechoic horizontal line *(straight arrow)* approximately 0.5 cm deep to the anterior border of the ribs *(curved arrow)*.

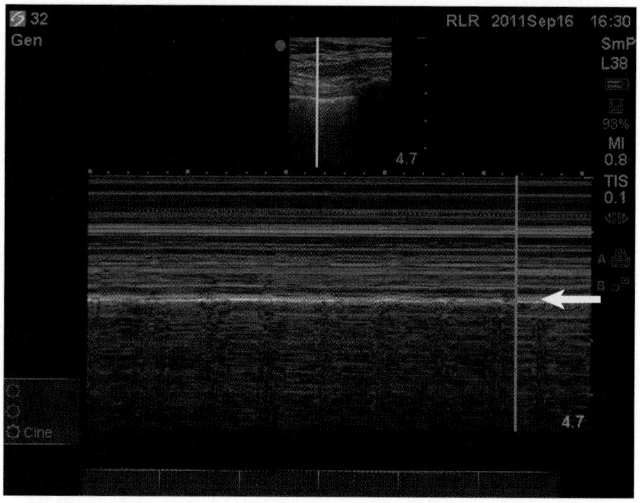

Figure 83.2 M-mode imaging of normal lung tissue, demonstrating the "seashore sign." The linear pattern superior to the pleural line *(arrow)* represents the motionless chest wall, and the granular pattern below the pleural line represents normal lung tissue.

perform lung ultrasonography the transducer should be placed in a longitudinal axis, between two ribs. In this view the pleural interface can be seen as a hyperechoic horizontal line approximately 0.5 cm deep, relative to the anterior border of the ribs[1,10] (Fig. 83.1). This image of the ribs and pleural line is the basic landmark in lung sonography and is often referred to as the *bat sign*.[10,11]

PNEUMOTHORAX

Pneumothorax, defined as a collection of air between the visceral and parietal pleural layers, has a frequency of approximately 6% in the ICU setting.[12] Although screening for pneumothorax with supine anteroposterior (AP) chest radiography is still common in the critical care setting, sensitivities for the diagnosis of pneumothorax average 50%.[13] The sensitivity for diagnosis of pneumothorax by lung ultrasound has been shown to be greater than 95% in multiple large prospective studies.[14] Moreover, lung ultrasound for pneumothorax can be completed in an average of 2 to 3 minutes, significantly faster than obtaining a portable chest radiograph or transport to CT scan.[15] The examination should begin with the transducer placed longitudinally at the midclavicular line at the level of the second to third intercostal space. Sequential movement of the transducer inferior and lateral across multiple rib interspaces will allow for a comprehensive examination of the pleura.[9] This approach should then be repeated on the opposite hemithorax.

Focusing on the pleural line in real time, a sliding type of motion of the visceral and parietal pleura can be observed. This dynamic motion is termed *lung sliding*, and can be seen in normal lung ultrasound (Video 83.1). In the presence of a pneumothorax, air is trapped between the visceral and parietal pleural layers and the dynamic motion of lung sliding will not be detected (Video 83.2). The presence of lung sliding alone has a 100% negative predictive value in the diagnosis of pneumothorax.[16] However, the absence of lung sliding does not rule in the diagnosis of pneumothorax. A number of conditions can result in the absence of lung sliding such as massive atelectasis, acute respiratory distress syndrome (ARDS), pleural adhesions, and severe fibrosis.[9,10] M-mode and power Doppler may be useful when lung sliding is difficult to visualize on real-time B-mode imaging. M-mode analysis of normal lung tissue displays the "seashore sign," a characteristic linear wave pattern representing the motionless chest wall, and below the pleural line a granular pattern represents normal lung motion[17] (Fig. 83.2). M-mode analysis of a pneumothorax demonstrates the "stratosphere sign," a characteristic appearance of exclusively linear lines[10] (Fig. 83.3). Power Doppler will depict motion along the pleural interface, corresponding to normal lung sliding (Fig. 83.4). In the presence of a pneumothorax, no Doppler signal will be detected along the pleural surface. The visualization of the lung point may also be used in the diagnosis of pneumothorax, having a specificity of 100%. The lung point represents the area on the chest wall where normal lung sliding is again appreciated,

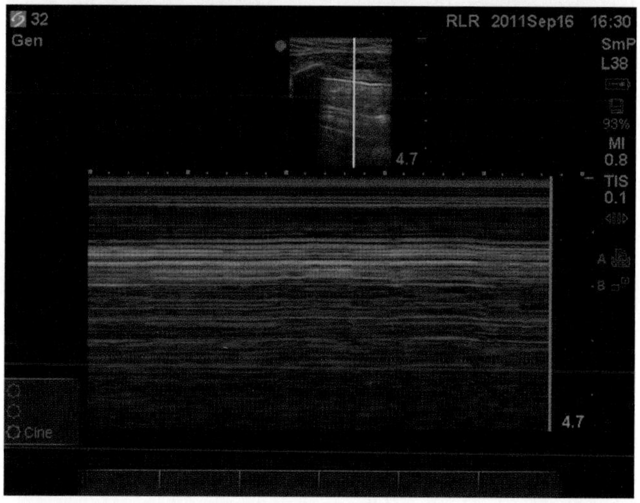

Figure 83.3 M-mode imaging of a pneumothorax, demonstrating the "stratosphere sign." Exclusively horizontal linear lines are displayed.

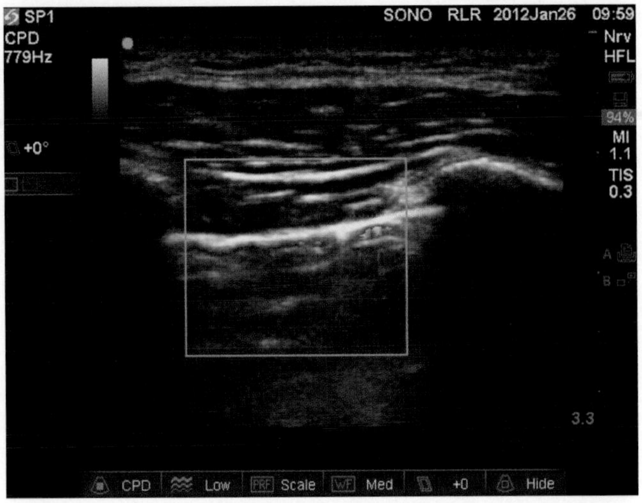

Figure 83.4 Power Doppler of normal lung tissue, which demonstrates the presence of a Doppler signal along the pleural interface.

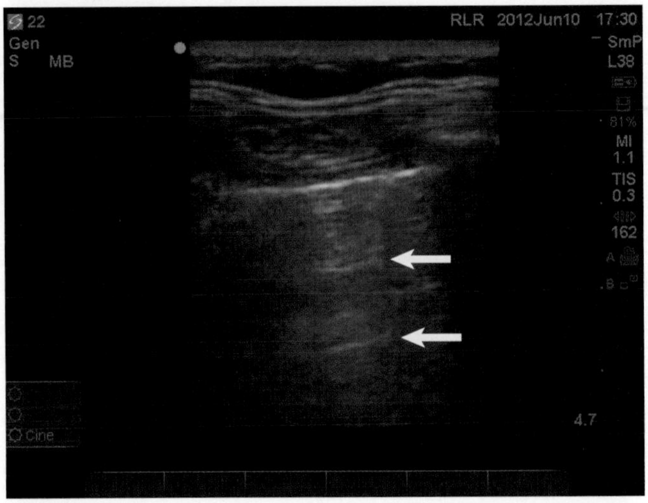

Figure 83.6 A lines, reverberation artifacts, represented as horizontal lines *(arrows)* parallel to the pleural line. A lines are found in a repetitive equidistant pattern below the pleural line.

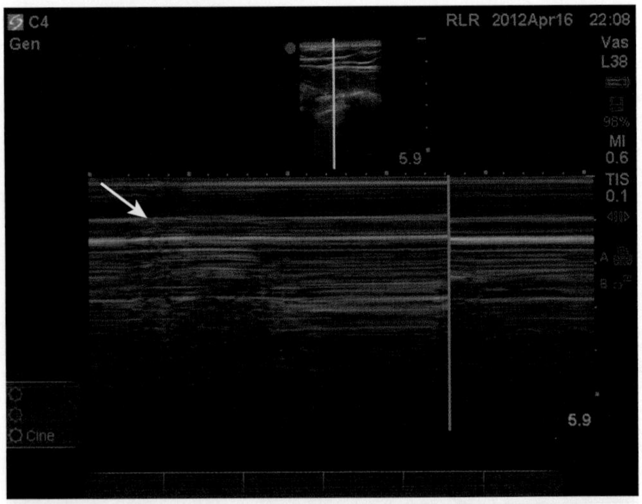

Figure 83.5 M-mode ultrasound imaging of the lung point, correlating with the lateral edge of the pneumothorax.

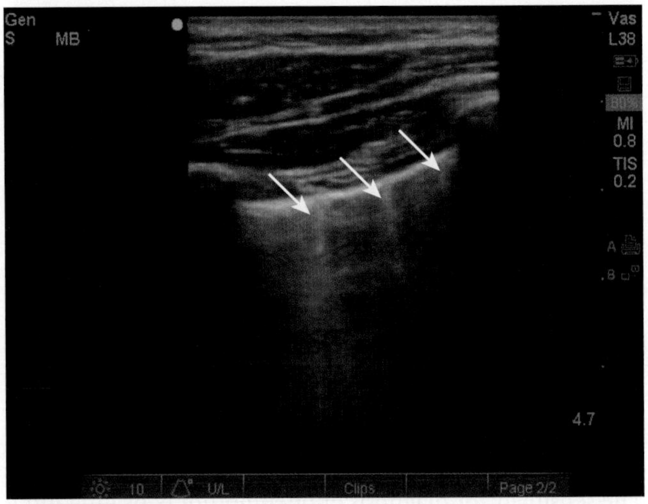

Figure 83.7 B lines, or comet tails, are vertical linear artifacts that extend the entire length of screen.

corresponding to the lateral edge of the pneumothorax (Fig. 83.5). This confirms the absence of visualization of lung sliding was not due to technical errors in lung ultrasound, but rather the presence of pneumothorax.[10]

Two linear artifacts arising from the pleural line are key to the evaluation of pneumothorax by lung ultrasound, A and B lines. A lines are a reverberation artifact of the parietal pleura, represented as horizontal lines in a repetitive pattern (Fig. 83.6). B lines, or comet tails, are described as vertical lines extending the length of the screen, which erase A lines and move with lung sliding[12] (Fig. 83.7). In lung ultrasound, the appreciation of only one B line indicates normal apposition of the parietal and visceral pleura and rules out pneumothorax at that location.[9] Because A lines arise from the parietal pleura, their presence can be appreciated in both normal lung and pneumothorax. The absence of lung sliding with the presence of A lines has a sensitivity of 95% and specificity of 94% in the diagnosis of pneumothorax.[12]

LUNG CONSOLIDATION

Alveolar consolidation, seen in pulmonary edema, bronchopneumonia, lung contusion, and lobar atelectasis, results in the loss of lung aeration replaced by fluid, allowing for ultrasound transmission and imaging.[1] As the ratio of lung tissue to air increases, lung hepatization appears on ultrasound imaging, with the lung parenchyma taking a hepatic tissue-like appearance[3] (Fig. 83.8). Consolidated lung adjacent to the pleura will permit the transmission of ultrasound waves. A prospective clinical study in a medical ICU setting showed that 98% of alveolar consolidations abutted the pleura, allowing for ultrasound assessment. The deep border of alveolar consolidations will typically have an irregular appearance, sometimes referred to as the shred sign, unless the entire lobe is involved.[10] Using CT as the gold standard, ultrasound has a 90% sensitivity and 98% specificity in the diagnosis of alveolar consolidation.[18] Air bronchograms can be visualized within consolidated lung as bright highly

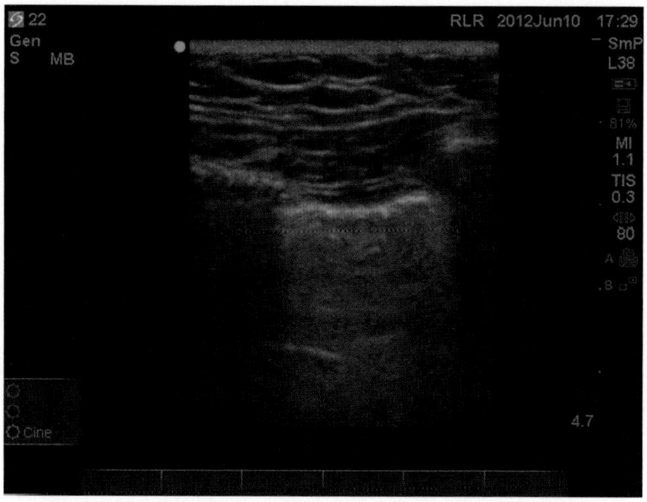

Figure 83.8 Hepatization of lung tissue seen with consolidation.

reflective echogenic lines.[21] Dynamic air bronchograms move centrifugally during inspiration and can typically be seen in pneumonia, as opposed to static air bronchograms of atelectasis.[19]

ALVEOLAR-INTERSTITIAL SYNDROME

Alveolar-interstitial syndrome is a common entity in the ICU, caused acutely by a variety of conditions, including ARDS, acute pulmonary edema, and interstitial pneumonia.[20] Interstitial edema precedes alveolar edema and may be difficult to discern on chest radiograph. Interstitial edema can be visualized on lung ultrasound by demonstrating three or more B lines located between two ribs, defined as lung rockets[21] (Fig. 83.9 and Video 83.3). B lines 7 mm apart correspond to thickened interlobular septa and extravascular lung volume, but B lines 3 mm apart or less correspond to alveolar edema and a ground-glass appearance of the lung.[22] In an acutely dyspneic patient, the detection of lung rockets allows the intensivist to immediately differentiate acute pulmonary edema from chronic obstructive pulmonary disease (COPD). Lung rockets are also unusual in the presence of pulmonary embolism.[10] It is important to remember that B lines may be isolated or confined laterally in the last intercostal space in normal healthy lung.[23]

PLEURAL EFFUSION

The prevalence of pleural effusion is approximately 60% in the ICU setting.[24] Pleural effusion may arise from a variety of conditions, most commonly heart failure, atelectasis, pneumonia, and volume overload. Portable supine chest radiography has poor sensitivity and specificity in the diagnosis of a pleural effusion, but lung ultrasound outperforms both chect radiography and clinical examination. Lung ultrasound can help differentiate pleural effusions from infiltrate or atelectasis, with a sensitivity of 92% and specificity of 93%.[22] Pleural effusions appear as an anechoic area in dependent lung regions (Figs. 83.10 and 83.11). Transudative fluid appears echo-free, and exudative fluid may contain small echogenic debris. In intercostal imaging, pleural effusions will be bordered laterally by rib shadows, superiorly by the parietal pleural line, and inferiorly by the lung line. M-mode analysis demonstrates a decrease in the interpleural distance with inspiration, known as the sinusoid sign[10] (Fig. 83.12). Lung ultrasound can also help estimate volume of pleural fluid. An anteroposterior diameter greater than 5 cm measured at the lung base or fifth intercostal space predicts a pleural effusion fluid volume of greater than 500 mL.[25]

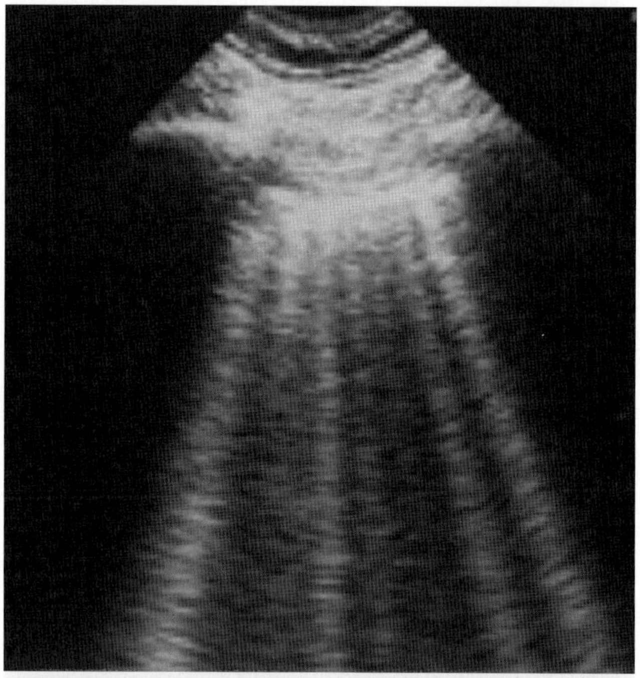

Figure 83.9 Multiple lung rockets visualized as hyperechoic vertical lines extending from the pleural line to the entire length of the image.

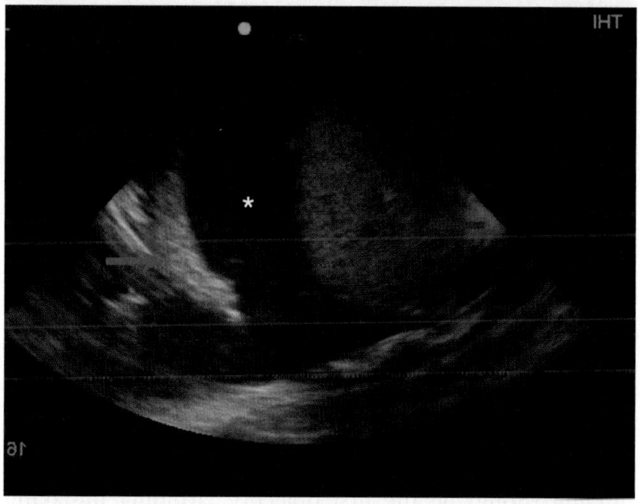

Figure 83.10 A right-sided pleural effusion *(star)* located cranially to the liver *(red arrow)* and seen surrounding lung tissue *(blue arrow)*.

THORACENTESIS

The utilization of ultrasound to determine needle placement in thoracentesis has been shown in multiple studies to

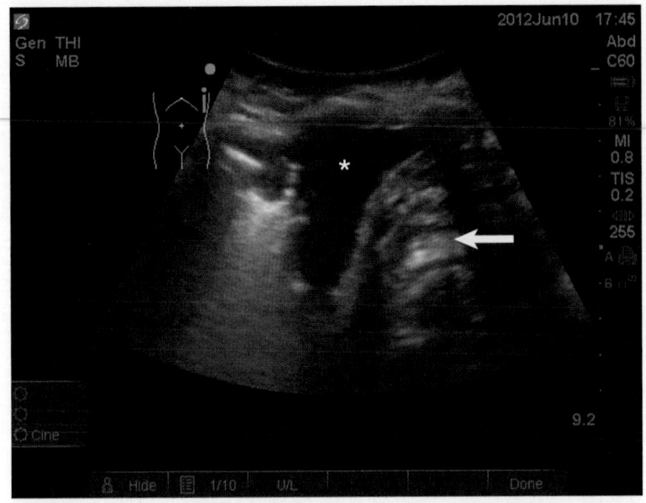

Figure 83.11 Left-sided pleural effusion *(star)*.

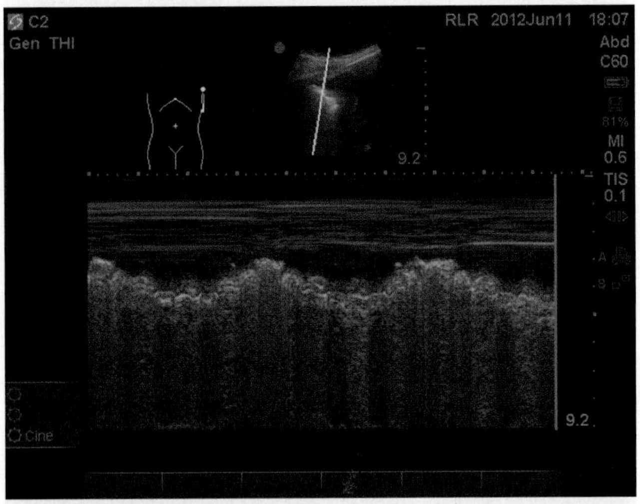

Figure 83.12 M-mode lung imaging demonstrating the sinusoidal sign of pleural effusion.

significantly decrease complication rates, especially that of pneumothorax.[26-28] Localization of fluid above the diaphragm should be the first objective, avoiding mistaking peritoneal for pleural fluid.[28] Once pleural fluid is visualized, the transducer should be moved one interspace above and below to evaluate the extent of the effusion.[29] The chest should be scanned in both the longitudinal and cross-sectional plane and the positions of the heart, diaphragm, and liver/spleen determined. Next, an interpleural measurement (parietal pleura to visceral pleura) of at least 1.5 cm during inspiration should be obtained to allow for safe needle puncture. The potential site of needle puncture should be observed throughout the entire respiratory cycle to evaluate for the appearance of lung, heart, liver, or spleen in the projected needle path.[28] After a safe site has been identified, the skin should be marked and disinfected. It is essential the patient remain in the same position as when the ultrasonography was performed.[30] Real-time guidance is not necessary for needle puncture, but needle insertion should occur within minutes of ultrasound marking.[31]

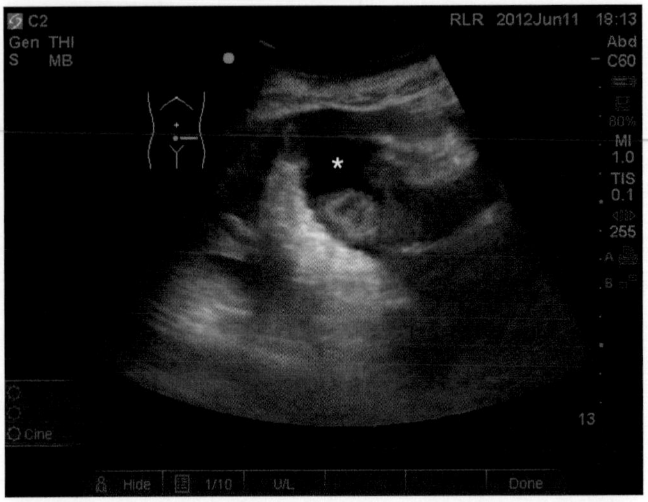

Figure 83.13 Ascites visualized in the left lower quadrant, with loops of bowel demonstrated floating in ascitic fluid *(star)*.

ABDOMINAL ULTRASONOGRAPHY

PARACENTESIS

Paracentesis is a commonly performed procedure in the critical care setting. Bedside ultrasonography prior to every paracentesis improves both the safety and efficacy of this procedure.[32,33] An emergency department study comparing ultrasound-assisted paracentesis versus traditional blind technique showed a 95% success rate with ultrasound guidance versus only 61% with the traditional technique. Moreover, 25% of patients randomized to the ultrasound-assisted technique completely avoided the procedure due to either the absence of ascitic fluid or too little ascitic fluid for aspiration. Two more patients in this group did not receive paracentesis after performance of bedside ultrasound, which revealed a large cystic mass in the left lower quadrant of one patient and a ventral hernia in the other, both of which were mistaken for ascitic fluid and in which performance of paracentesis would have been potentially disastrous.[33]

A low-frequency curved array transducer is preferred. As with the traditional blind technique, the urinary bladder should be decompressed and the patient should be lying supine. Ascites will appear as anechoic fluid within the peritoneal cavity and often loops of bowel will be seen floating within this fluid (Fig. 83.13). Ultrasonographic guidance assists in determining the amount and location of ascitic fluid while mapping the most appropriate point of entry and puncture angle. Measurement of abdominal wall thickness can be performed to determine puncture depth. The location of the urinary bladder, bowel, solid organs, and abdominal wall vasculature may all be visualized for avoidance. Such intra-abdominal structures should be visualized in real time throughout the respiratory cycle to ensure they do not cross into the anticipated needle path. Once an appropriate fluid pocket has been determined, it should be visualized in at least two perpendicular planes to ensure avoidance of critical structures. An estimate of the abdominal wall thickness should be made, as well as the depth of the fluid pocket until critical structures such as bowel or bladder are encountered. Once the site has been mapped and marked, needle puncture may occur. Paracentesis involving small volumes may be better performed with real-time ultrasound guidance, allowing direct visualization of the needle entering the peritoneal space. Most larger volume paracentesis may be performed with mapping of the puncture site and needle with ultrasound guidance, although the actual needle puncture occurs without real-time ultrasound visualization.

THE "FAST" EXAMINATION

The focused assessment with sonography for trauma (FAST) examination has been used by trauma surgeons for decades to identify intra-abdominal fluid.[34] The identification of free fluid—hemoperitoneum or ascites—in the abdomen may also be essential in the critical care setting. Localization of ascitic fluid for paracentesis and hemoperitoneum in the setting of persistent or undifferentiated hypotension may prove beneficial in the ICU.

The FAST examination is based on the principle that in a supine patient, free intraperitoneal fluid will accumulate in the most dependent regions of the peritoneal cavity. The most dependent areas in the male and female are the rectovesical pouch and pouch of Douglas, respectively. Free intraperitoneal fluid in the right upper quadrant will accumulate in Morison's pouch, but fluid in the left upper quadrant will accumulate in the left subphrenic space and splenorenal recess. A prospective study that compared diagnostic peritoneal lavage, CT scanning, and abdominal ultrasound showed an accuracy of 93% for abdominal ultrasound.[35] Moreover, the time required to perform such an examination averages less than 3 minutes.[36]

The FAST examination is performed with either the low-frequency phased array or curvilinear probe. The basic views of the intra-abdominal assessment of the FAST examination include Morison's pouch, left lateral longitudinal, and pelvic views.[34] Starting with Morison's pouch, in the supine patient, the probe is placed in the right midaxillary line at the level of the lower ribs. The right hemidiaphragm, liver, and right kidney should be visualized (Figs. 83.14 and 83.15). Free fluid in Morison's pouch will be appreciated as an anechoic area (Fig. 83.16). Massive hemoperitoneum may be rapidly diagnosed with this single view with a sensitivity of 82% and accuracy of 91%.[37] Next, the left side is evaluated by placing the probe in the posterior axillary line at the level of the lower ribs. The left hemidiaphragm, spleen, and left kidney can all be identified from this view (Fig. 83.17). Free fluid can be appreciated as an anechoic stripe in the subphrenic space and splenorenal recess. Lastly, the pelvic view is obtained by placing the probe in a midline transverse position just above the pubic symphysis. A fluid-filled urinary bladder appears as well-circumscribed anechoic fluid with posterior acoustic enhancement (Fig. 83.18). A longitudinal view can also be obtained by rotating the probe 90 degrees clockwise. In female patients, the uterus may be seen posterior to the urinary bladder and free fluid may be appreciated in the pouch of Douglas. In male patients, the prostate may be seen posterior to the urinary bladder and free fluid may be appreciated in the rectovesical pouch. The FAST examination does have its limitations, with the patient's body habitus greatly affecting the quality

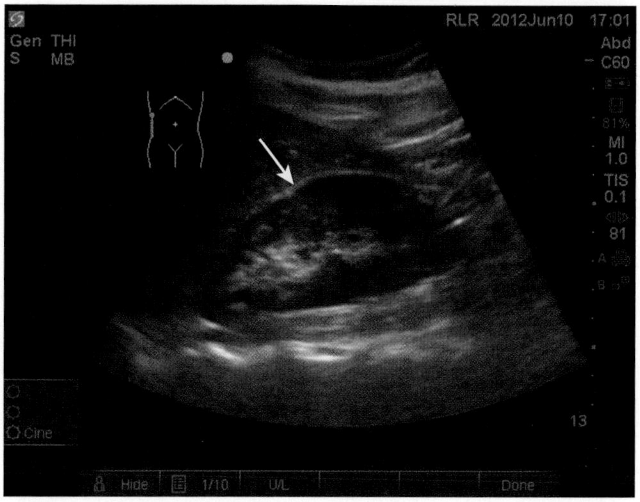

Figure 83.14 FAST (focused assessment with sonography for trauma) imaging of Morison's pouch, demonstrating the interface *(arrow)* between the right kidney and liver.

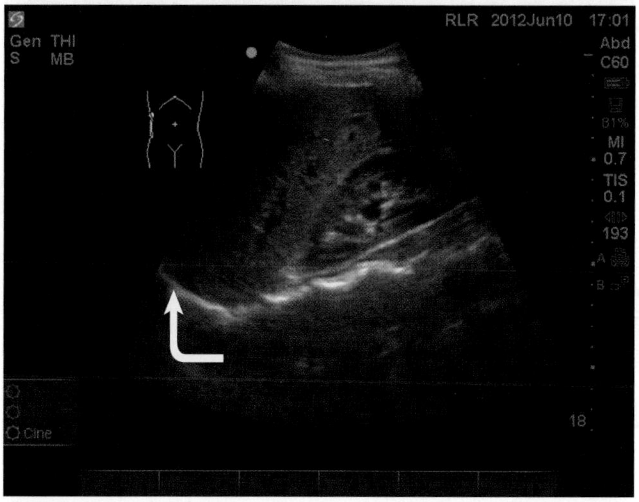

Figure 83.15 Visualization of the right hemidiaphragm *(curved arrow)*, seen as a hyperechoic line located cranial to the liver.

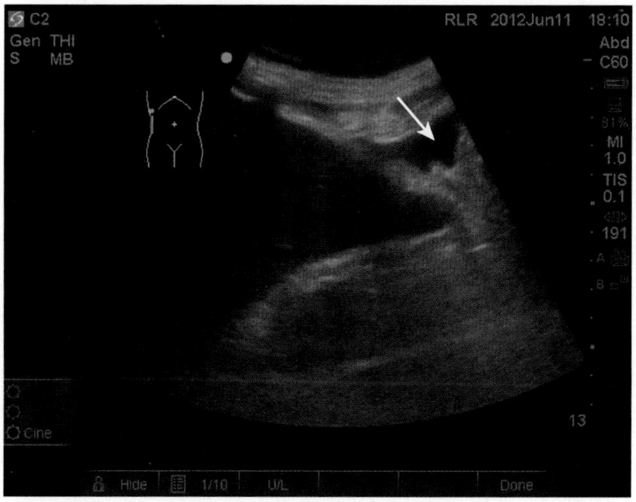

Figure 83.16 Free fluid *(arrow)* visualized near the inferior tip of the liver. The kidney is not visualized in this image.

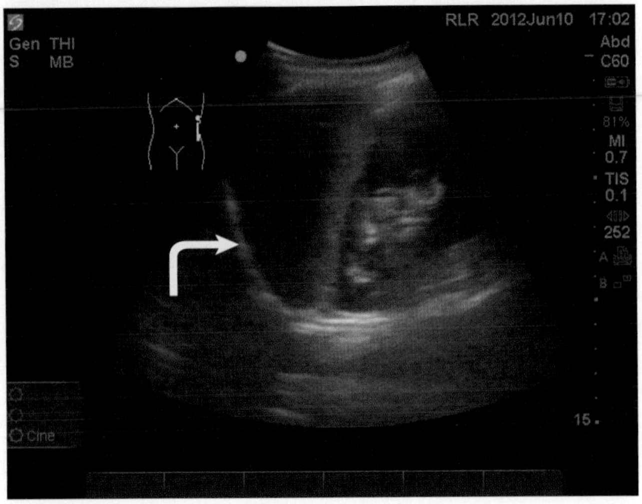

Figure 83.17 FAST (focused assessment with sonography for trauma) imaging of the interface of the spleen and liver, with visualization of the left hemidiaphragm *(curved arrow).*

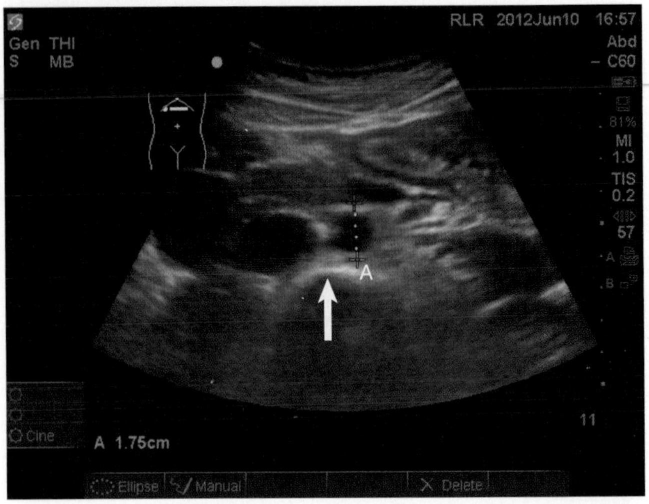

Figure 83.19 Transverse view of the abdominal aorta, which lies anteriorly to the hyperechoic vertebral body *(arrow)* with posterior shadowing. Wall measurements should be obtained measuring the outer to outer wall.

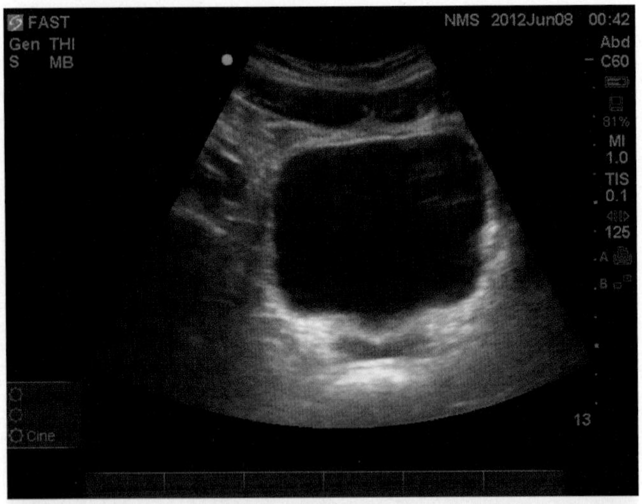

Figure 83.18 A fluid-filled urinary bladder, visualized as a well-circumscribed anechoic structure.

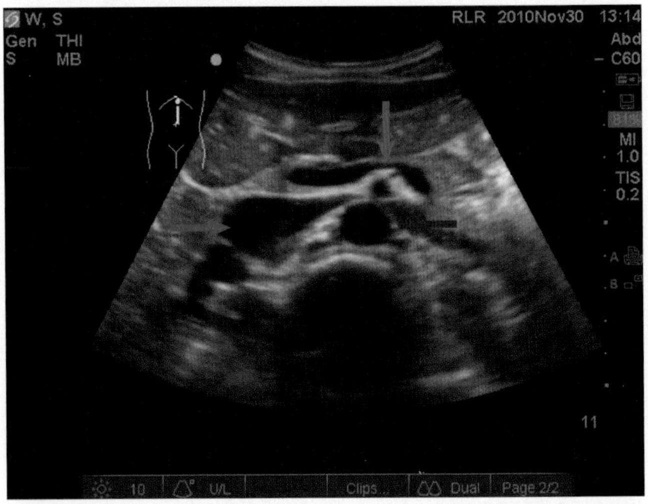

Figure 83.20 A transverse view of the aorta *(red arrow),* with the inferior vena cava visualized to the right *(blue arrow).* The superior mesenteric artery is seen in transverse view anterior to the aorta with the splenic vein coursing horizontally above the superior mesenteric artery *(green arrow).*

of the images obtained. Moreover, ultrasound is capable of identifying free fluid in the abdomen, but it cannot accurately distinguish ascites from hemoperitoneum. Last, ultrasound is not sensitive for the identification of free fluid in the retroperitoneum.

ABDOMINAL AORTA

The abdominal aorta may also be imaged by ultrasonography to diagnose both an abdominal aortic aneurysm (AAA) and dissection. Unexplained hypotension, syncope, dizziness, or cardiac arrest may be caused by a ruptured aneurysm. The prevalence of AAAs is relatively common, ranging from 2% to 5% in adults over the age of 50.[38-42] Bedside ultrasonography in the detection of AAA is highly sensitive, specific, and accurate.[43,44]

The abdominal aorta extends from the level of the diaphragm at approximately the twelfth thoracic vertebra down to its bifurcation into the common iliac arteries around the level of the umbilicus. The aorta can be best visualized with a curvilinear probe, either longitudinal or transverse. Generally the patient will be positioned supine, but if obesity or bowel gas obstructs the images, the patient may be moved into a decubitus position. Starting transverse in the epigastrium with the probe marker to the patient's right, the abdominal aorta is seen lying superiorly and slightly to the left of the patient's spine. The vertebral body appears as a bright hyperechoic structure with posterior shadowing (Fig. 83.19). The most proximal branch seen on ultrasound is the celiac trunk branching off anteriorly, followed by the superior mesenteric artery (SMA) approximately 1 to 2 cm distally (Video 83.4). Continuing caudally, the renal arteries can be appreciated branching off laterally just distal to the SMA. The inferior mesenteric artery and paired gonadal arteries may be difficult to image on bedside ultrasonography. The inferior vena cava (IVC) should also be appreciated coursing to the right of the aorta (Fig. 83.20). Turning

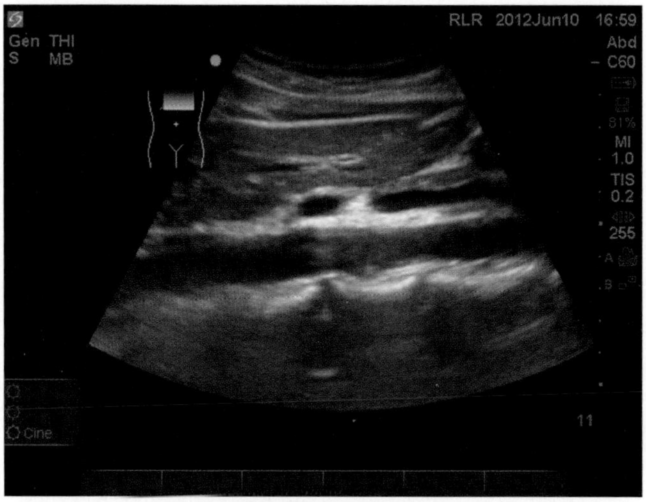

Figure 83.21 A longitudinal view of the abdominal aorta.

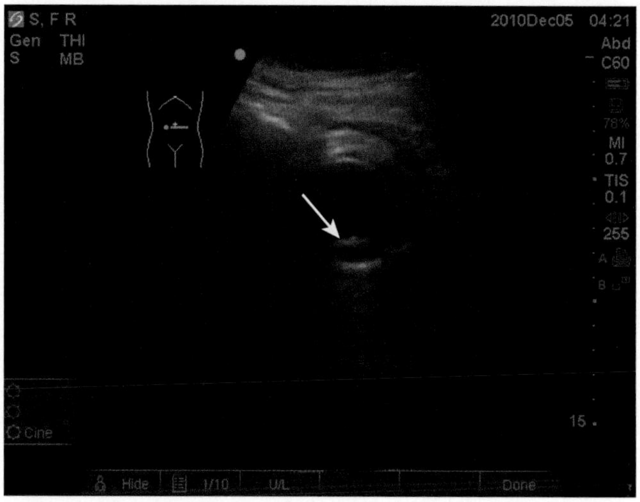

Figure 83.23 An echogenic linear flap, representing an aortic dissection *(arrow),* can be visualized in the abdominal aorta.

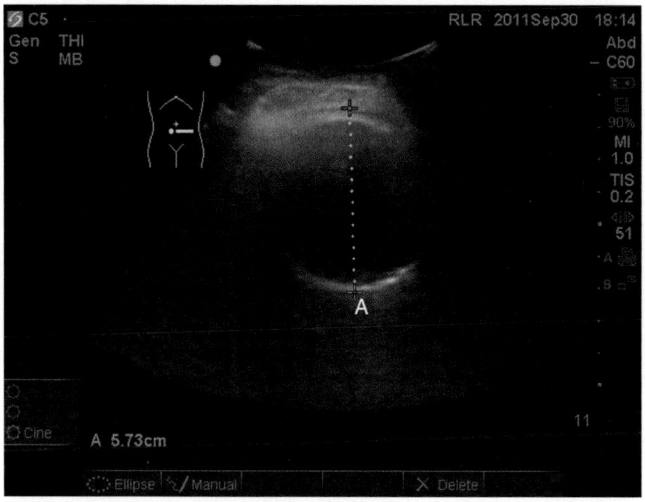

Figure 83.22 Abdominal aortic aneurysm measured in the anteroposterior diameter, outer wall to outer wall.

the probe 90 degrees clockwise allows the aorta to be viewed in the longitudinal plane (Fig. 83.21). Often, the celiac trunk and SMA can be visualized branching from the anterior aspect of the aorta (see Video 83.4). Tilting the probe slightly to the patient's right will place the IVC in view. Care must be taken not to confuse the IVC for the aorta.

Measurements of the abdominal aorta should be taken in the anteroposterior diameter in the transverse orientation. The calipers should be placed on the outer wall to outer wall. Measurements in the longitudinal orientation may lead to underestimation if the image plane is obtained tangentially. Diameters greater than 3 cm are considered to be abnormal (Fig. 83.22). Although the large majority of dissections start in the thoracic aorta, those that extend to the abdominal aorta can be appreciated on abdominal ultrasonography. An echogenic linear flap can be visualized in the abdominal aorta (Fig. 83.23). If appreciated, further imaging modalities should be performed to assess the thoracic aorta.

RENAL ULTRASONOGRAPHY

Acute renal failure is a common diagnosis encountered in those who are critically ill. In the critical care setting, acute renal failure has a mortality rate of 20% to 30%, which increases with each additional organ system involved.[45] Evaluation of acute renal failure begins with determining if the cause is prerenal, postrenal, or intrinsic. Bedside ultrasound can quickly determine if postrenal causes are present, demonstrating a large distended urinary bladder or hydronephrosis.[46-48]

Imaging of the urinary bladder is performed with a curvilinear probe, with the probe marker toward the patient's right in transverse orientation, and with the probe marker toward the patient's head in longitudinal orientation. The probe should be placed just superior to the pubic symphysis. A quick visual assessment of urinary bladder size can be determined. Bladder volume can also be estimated by using the formula width × depth × length × 0.75. A postvoid residual volume greater than 100 mL is consistent with urinary retention.[49] If no ureteral obstruction is present, one can appreciate ureteral flow jets visualized intermittently near the trigone of the urinary bladder. This intermittent flow of urine from the ureter into the urinary bladder is best visualized with the use of color Doppler (Fig. 83.24). If urinary retention is present, the kidneys should next be evaluated for the presence of hydronephrosis. Studies have shown that bedside sonographic evidence of hydronephrosis correlates well with findings on intravenous pyelogram and CT scanning.[37,50] On ultrasound imaging, the kidney parenchyma appears slightly hypoechoic compared to the adjacent liver or spleen. The renal sinus typically appears hyperechoic owing to its high fat content. The collecting system is generally not well visualized with ultrasound unless some degree of hydronephrosis is present.[51]

Ultrasonographically, hydronephrosis is visualized as dilation of the collecting system, which appears dark and anechoic. It can be further classified as mild, moderate, or severe. As the severity worsens, the dilation of the renal pelvis increases, the individual calyces become less distinct,

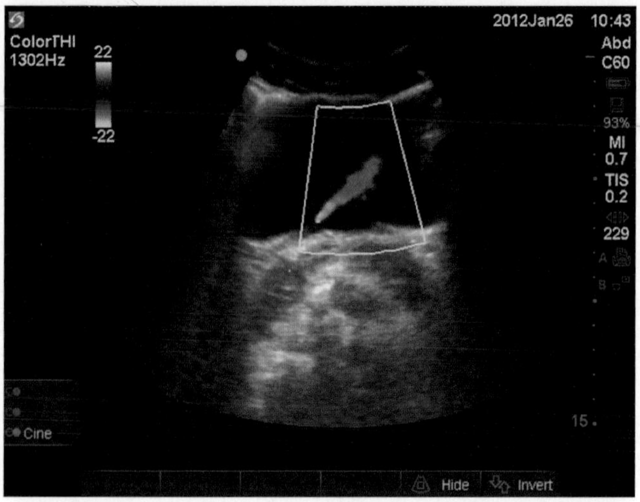

Figure 83.24 A ureteral jet visualized with color Doppler, representing the intermittent flow of urine from the ureter into the urinary bladder. The color box is placed near the urinary trigone when attempting to visualize a ureteral jet.

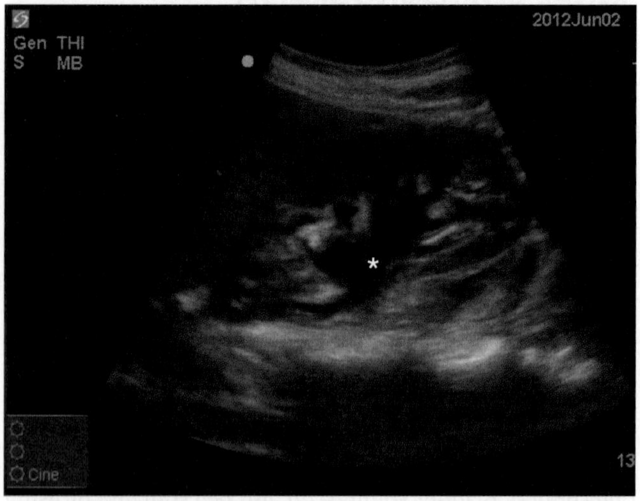

Figure 83.25 Moderate right-sided hydronephrosis, with dilation of the collecting system *(star)*.

and thinning of the renal cortex can be appreciated[52] (Fig. 83.25). Imaging of the right kidney begins with the probe placed in the anterior axillary line, at the subcostal margin. The patient may be lying supine or in the left lateral decubitus position. Once the kidney is identified, slight tilting or sweeping of the probe medially and laterally should be performed to visualize the kidney in its entire longitudinal axis. Turning the probe horizontally to obtain transverse views, sweeping and tilting superiorly and inferiorly, should then be performed. Similarly, when imaging the left kidney, the patient should be placed in either a supine or right lateral decubitus position. The probe should be placed in the posterior axillary line at the subcostal margin and both subcostal and intercostal images may be obtained. Again the probe should be swept or tilted throughout the entire longitudinal axis and then turned 90 degrees to obtain transverse imaging. Normal kidneys measure approximately 9 to 12 cm in length and 4 to 5 cm in width.[53] Typically, small, atrophic, and hyperechoic kidneys are indicative of chronic renal failure. Enlarged kidneys often suggest an acute process, such as infection, renal vein thrombosis, and rejection.[54]

DEEP VENOUS THROMBOSIS ULTRASONOGRAPHY

Venous thromboembolic disease is a common entity encountered in the critical care setting. Despite prophylaxis in the critically ill, the incidence of deep venous thrombosis (DVT) remains around 10% in such populations.[55] Critically ill patients are susceptible to the development of venous thromboembolism from an increased prevalence of risk factors such as immobility, indwelling central venous catheters, cardiac failure, dehydration, and inflammatory states.[55,56] Many studies have shown that an abbreviated physician-performed bedside compression ultrasound scan may be highly accurate in the diagnosis of proximal lower extremity DVT.[57-60] A two-point compression study performed in the emergency department using portable ultrasonography showed a 100% sensitivity and 99% specificity in the diagnosis of proximal lower extremity DVT when compared to lower extremity duplex ultrasonography performed in a radiology department.[58] The efficiency of physician-performed bedside ultrasound is a great advantage in the critical care setting. The average time for completion of bedside DVT ultrasound was 3.5 minutes, compared to 37 minutes, the average time for completion of formal venous ultrasonography.[57] This latter time does not take into account transport of critically ill patients to the radiology department or the possibility that the test may be delayed until an ultrasonography technician is available.

The examination for lower extremity DVT is performed with a high-frequency linear transducer. Images can be obtained with the patient supine, the leg externally rotated, and the knee slightly bent. Veins are best visualized at maximal distention, which is achieved by placing the bed in reverse Trendelenburg positioning at 30 to 45 degrees so that pooling of the venous vasculature occurs, enhancing visualization. The examination begins with visualization of the common femoral vein just beneath the inguinal ligament (Fig. 83.26). In most instances the vein will be easily distinguished from the artery; however, color or pulse wave Doppler may be used to help differentiate the vessels. With color Doppler, arterial flow will appear more pulsatile. In pulse wave Doppler, an arterial waveform will show rapid acceleration and deceleration, and a venous waveform will show continuous flow even during diastole. Once the common femoral vein is identified proximally, downward pressure should be applied to the transducer and the vein should collapse completely (Fig. 83.27). Concern for venous thromboembolism occurs if enough pressure is applied to the transducer to cause deformation of the artery without complete collapse of the vein (Fig. 83.28). The transducer should then be moved approximately 1 cm distally with sequential compression until the common femoral vein is seen branching into the superficial and deep branches. Imaging and compression should continue for 1 to 2 cm beyond this point.

The examination then moves to the popliteal region, where the probe is placed in the popliteal fossa. Identification of the popliteal artery and vein should occur with

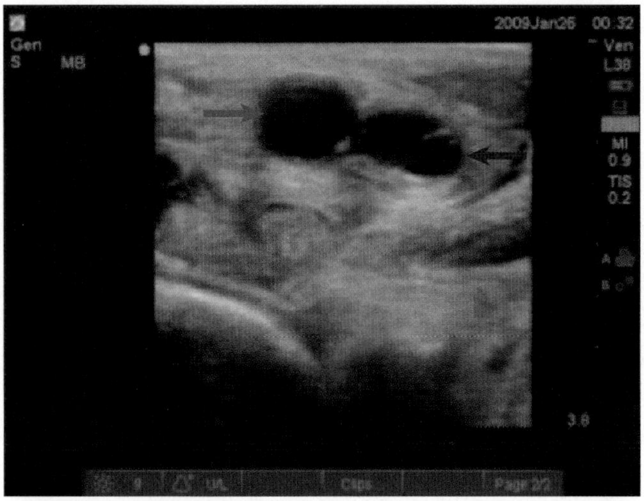

Figure 83.26 Ultrasound examination of the common femoral artery *(blue arrow)* and vein *(red arrow)*.

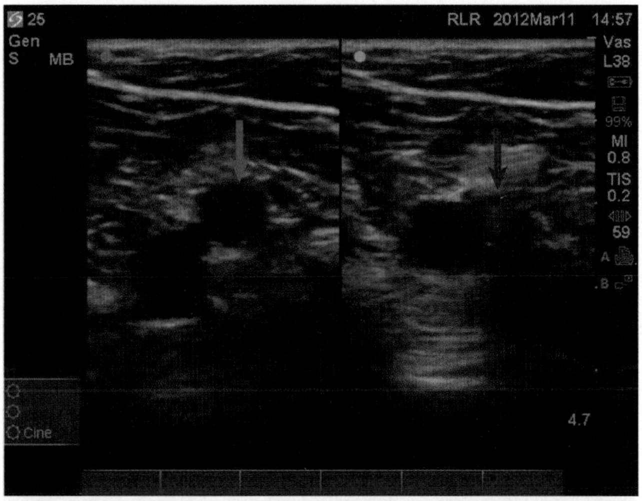

Figure 83.27 The common femoral vein visualized without probe pressure *(blue arrow)*. With gentle pressure placed on the probe, the common femoral vein completely collapses *(red arrow)*.

complete compression of the popliteal vein. Be aware that the popliteal vein may be duplicated and both veins must collapse on examination. Again, sequential compression at approximately 1-cm intervals should occur while moving distally to the trifurcation of the popliteal vein. Proximal DVTs are those located at or above the popliteal vein and imaging of the calf veins is generally not performed in bedside ultrasonography for DVT. While imaging the deep veins of the lower extremity, thrombus may be visualized as echogenic material within the lumen of the vessels under examination. Often this depends both on the age of the thrombus and the quality of the images. Remember, an acute thrombus may not be directly visualized within the lumen because it likely has the same echogenicity as blood.[56] Lastly, upper extremity DVT accounts for approximately 18% of all venous thromboembolic disease.[61] Bedside ultrasonography for the diagnosis of upper extremity DVT is possible but is technically more involved than for lower extremity imaging. The examination will not be discussed further in this chapter.

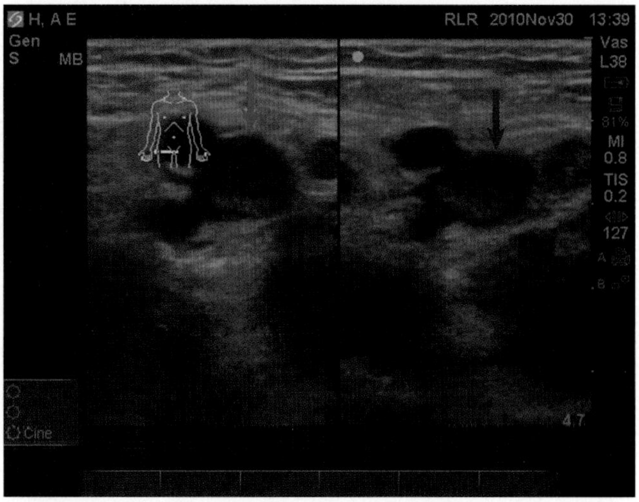

Figure 83.28 The common femoral vein visualized without probe pressure *(blue arrow)*. With the addition of gentle probe pressure, the common femoral vein does not collapse *(red arrow)*. Moreover, echogenic material can be observed inside the lumen of the common femoral vein, representing thrombus.

VASCULAR ACCESS

Central venous catheterization is a common procedure performed in the ICU, with an estimated 5 million central venous lines placed annually in the United States. Central venous access is often essential for volume resuscitation, hemodynamic monitoring, vasopressor therapy, and frequent blood sampling.[62] Traditionally, central venous catheterization was performed with a blind technique, using external anatomic landmarks to assist in vessel location.

Use of Doppler ultrasound for localization of the internal jugular vein in central venous catheterization has been described since 1984.[63] A meta-analysis evaluating both real-time or Doppler assisted ultrasound guidance in central venous cannulation demonstrated that ultrasound guidance significantly decreased catheter placement failure by 64% when compared to standard landmark techniques. Likewise, the use of ultrasound decreased complications during placement by 78% and decreased the need for multiple needle passes by 40%.[62] Common complications of central venous cannulation include carotid artery puncture, neck or mediastinal hematomas, brachial plexus injury, and pneumothorax.[64] Studies evaluating the anatomic variation of the internal jugular vein using two-dimensional ultrasound show that the position of the internal jugular vein was outside the path predicted by external landmark techniques in 5.5% to 12% of cases.[65,66]

Veins and arteries are easily identified with ultrasound. A 7.5- to 10-MHz linear array transducer should be used for vessel imaging. Blood vessels appear black, or anechoic, owing to complete transmission of ultrasound waves. Arteries are pulsatile and difficult to compress with the ultrasound transducer. Veins are nonpulsatile, are easily compressed with the ultrasound transducer, and will distend when the patient performs a Valsalva maneuver or is placed in the Trendelenburg position.[67] The vessel can be viewed in either the longitudinal/long-axis approach or transverse/short-axis approach (Figs. 83.29 to 83.31). The transverse,

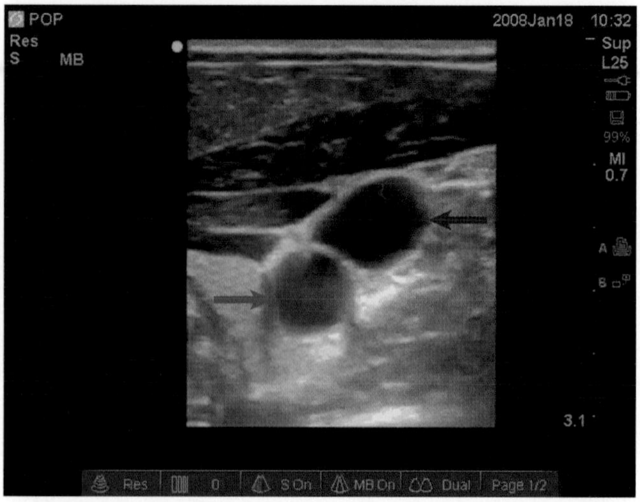

Figure 83.29 Visualization of the internal jugular vein *(red arrow)* slightly lateral to the carotid artery *(blue arrow)*. Notice the carotid is circular, although the internal jugular vein appears slightly flattened.

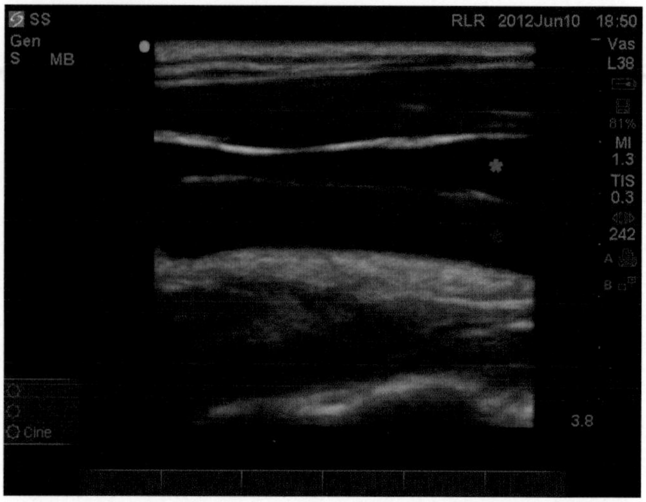

Figure 83.31 Longitudinal imaging of the internal jugular vein *(blue star)* lying anterior to the common carotid artery *(red star)*.

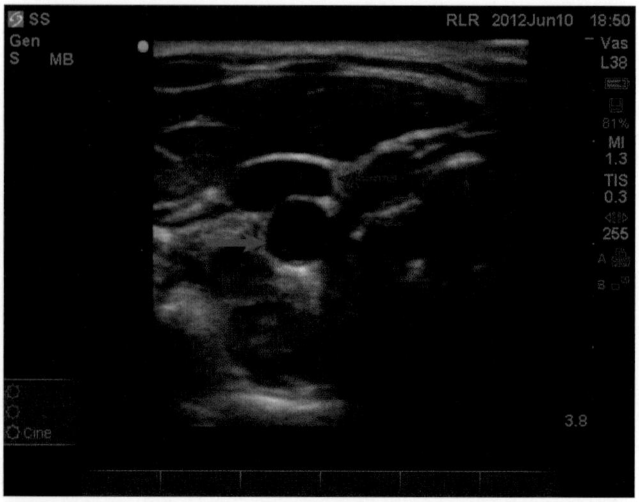

Figure 83.30 Visualization of the internal jugular vein *(red arrow)* lying directly over the common carotid artery *(blue arrow)*.

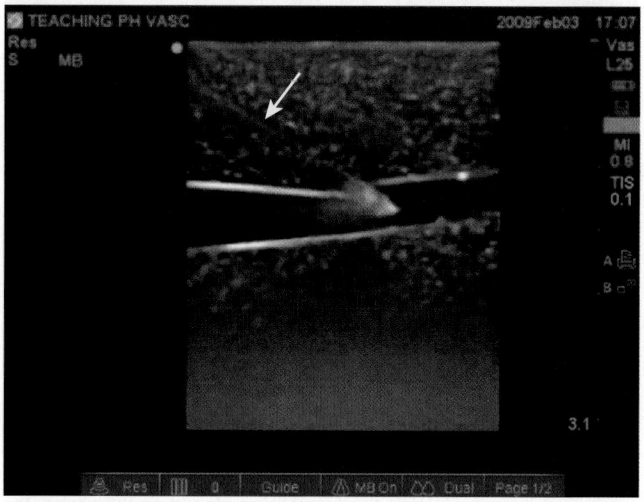

Figure 83.32 Longitudinal vascular orientation, which visualizes the needle *(arrow)* traversing through the superficial soft tissue and puncturing the deeper anterior vessel wall.

short-axis approach has been shown to be easier for novices to learn.[68] In the short-axis view, however, the tip of the needle must remain in axis with the ultrasound beam in order to be visualized.

The dynamic approach uses direct ultrasound guidance to visualize the needle puncturing the vessel in real time (Fig. 83.32). The patient should be prepped in the usual sterile fashion, and the ultrasound transducer should be placed into a sterile transducer cover, and sterile ultrasound gel should be used throughout the procedure. Ultrasound gel must be placed both inside the sterile cover contacting the probe and outside the sterile cover contacting the patient's skin. Holding the transducer in the nondominant hand and the introducer needle in the dominant hand, the operator can visualize the needle tip puncturing the appropriate vessel. The transducer should then be placed down while the guidewire is inserted. Once the guidewire is placed, ultrasound should be used to confirm placement of the wire in the appropriate vessel to avoid inadvertently dilating an artery or soft tissue structures. Needle guidance devices, which attach onto the ultrasound transducer, can be used in the dynamic approach to control needle trajectory.[69] This choice is a technical consideration and is based on operator preference. A static approach may also be used in which the vessel is located using ultrasound guidance to confirm predicted landmark anatomy. The ultrasound transducer is then put down, the patient is prepped in the usual fashion, and the vessel is cannulated without real-time ultrasound imaging. Ultrasound guidance may also be used for arterial or peripheral vein puncture. Arterial puncture of the femoral, axillary, or radial arteries is commonly performed with ultrasound guidance. Similarly, venous access of the deeper cephalic, basilic, and brachial veins can be obtained using ultrasound to assist in visualization.[69]

KEY POINTS

- The true portability, ease of use, and low cost make current ultrasound devices ideally suited for use by the intensivist.
- In the presence of a pneumothorax, air is trapped between the visceral and parietal pleural layers and the dynamic motion of lung sliding will not be detected.
- Consolidated lung adjacent to the pleura will permit the transmission of ultrasound waves.
- In an acutely dyspneic patient, the detection of lung rockets allows the intensivist to immediately differentiate acute pulmonary edema from COPD.
- Lung ultrasound can help differentiate pleural effusions from infiltrate or atelectasis, with a sensitivity of 92% and specificity of 93%.
- With the use of ultrasound during paracentesis the location of the urinary bladder, bowel, solid organs, and abdominal wall vasculature may all be visualized for avoidance.
- The abdominal aorta may be imaged by ultrasonography to diagnose both an AAA and dissection.
- Bedside ultrasound can quickly determine if postrenal causes of acute renal insufficiency are present, demonstrating a large distended urinary bladder or hydronephrosis
- Studies have shown that an abbreviated physician-performed bedside compression ultrasound scan is very accurate in the diagnosis of proximal lower extremity DVT.
- The use of ultrasound has been shown to decrease complications during placement of internal jugular catheters by 78% and decrease the need for multiple needle passes by 40%.

SELECTED REFERENCES

3. Soldati G, Sher S: Bedside lung ultrasound in critical care practice. Minerva Anestesiol 2009;75(9):509-517.
9. Ouellet JF, Ball CG, Panebianco NL, et al: Sonographic diagnosis of pneumothorax. J Emerg Trauma Shock 2011;4(4):504-507.
18. Lichtenstein DA, Lascols N, Mezière G, et al: Ultrasound diagnosis of alveolar consolidation in the critically ill. Intensive Care Med 2004;30(2):276-281.
21. Volpicelli G, Mussa A, Garofalo G, et al: Bedside lung ultrasound in the assessment of alveolar-interstitial syndrome. Am J Emerg Med 2006;24(6):689-696.
25. Roch A, Bojan M, Michelet P, et al: Usefulness of ultrasonography in predicting pleural effusions > 500 mL in patients receiving mechanical ventilation. Chest 2005;127(1):224-232.
30. Beaulieu Y, Marik PE: Bedside ultrasonography in the ICU: Part 2. Chest 2005;128(3):1766-1781.
34. Jehle D, Guarino J, Karamanoukian H: Emergency department ultrasound in the evaluation of blunt abdominal trauma. Am J Emerg Med 1993;11(4):342-346.
43. Tayal VS, Graf CD, Gibbs MA: Prospective study of accuracy and outcome of emergency ultrasound for abdominal aortic aneurysm over two years. Acad Emerg Med 2003;10(8):867-871.
50. Kiely EA, Hartnell GG, Gibson RN, et al: Measurement of bladder volume by real-time ultrasound. Br J Urol 1987;60(1):33-35.
53. Bradnt TD, Neiman HL, Dragowski MJ, et al: Ultrasound assessment of normal renal dimensions. J Ultrasound Med 1982;1(2):49-52.
60. Kory PD, Pellecchia CM, Shiloh AL, et al: Accuracy of ultrasonography performed by critical care physicians for the diagnosis of DVT. Chest 2011;139(3):538-542.
62. Randolph AG, Cook DJ, Gonzales CA, et al: Ultrasound guidance for placement of central venous catheters: A meta-analysis of the literature. Crit Care Med 1996;24(12):2053-2058.
68. Blaivas M, Brannam L, Fernandez E: Short-axis versus long-axis approaches for teaching ultrasound-guided vascular access on a new inanimate model. Acad Emerg Med 2003;10(12):1307-1311.

The complete list of references can be found at www.expertconsult.com.

Index

Page numbers followed by "f" indicate figures, "t" indicate tables, and "b" indicate boxes.

A

J

K

O

P

Q

R

U

V

W